MEDICAL-SURGICAL NURSING
CONCEPTS AND CLINICAL PRACTICE

MEDICAL-SURGICAL NURSING

CONCEPTS AND CLINICAL PRACTICE

EDITED BY

WILMA J. PHIPPS, R.N., Ph.D., F.A.A.N.

Professor and Chairperson of Medical-Surgical Nursing,
Frances Payne Bolton School of Nursing,
Case Western Reserve University;
Director of Medical-Surgical Nursing,
University Hospitals of Cleveland, Cleveland, Ohio

BARBARA C. LONG, R.N., M.S.N.

Associate Professor of Medical-Surgical Nursing,
Frances Payne Bolton School of Nursing,
Case Western Reserve University, Cleveland, Ohio

NANCY FUGATE WOODS, R.N., Ph.D., F.A.A.N.

Professor, Department of Physiological Nursing;
Director, Office for Nursing Research Facilitation,
University of Washington, Seattle, Washington

SECOND EDITION

With 852 illustrations

The C. V. Mosby Company

ST. LOUIS · TORONTO · LONDON 1983

To our colleagues, students, families, and friends
for all their support while this book was in progress

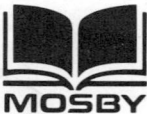

MOSBY

A TRADITION OF PUBLISHING EXCELLENCE

Editors: Thomas Manning, Julie Cardamon

Assistant editor: Bess Arends

Manuscript editors: Mary C. Wright, Millicent Schroeder, Jessica Bender

Book design: Nancy Steinmeyer

Cover design: Diane Beasley

Production: Margaret B. Bridenbaugh, Judith Bamert

Second edition
Copyright © 1983 by The C.V. Mosby Company

Previous edition copyrighted 1979

Printed in the United States of America
The C.V. Mosby Company
11830 Westline Industrial Drive, St. Louis, Missouri 63141

Library of Congress Cataloging in Publication Data

Main entry under title:

Medical-surgical nursing.

   Bibliography: p.
   Includes index.
   1. Nursing. 2. Surgical nursing. I. Phipps,
Wilma J., 1925-   . II. Long, Barbara C.,
1926-   . III. Woods, Nancy Fugate.
[DNLM: 1. Nursing care. WY 150 M4894]
RT41.M49 1983   610.73   82-18886
ISBN 0-8016-3931-X

C/D/D 9 8 7 6 5 4 3   02/A/218

CONTRIBUTORS

Jane E. Anderson, R.N., M.S., Ph.D. Candidate
University of Michigan School of Nursing,
Ann Arbor, Michigan

Sandra Vandam Anderson, R.N., M.S.
Lecturer, College of Nursing,
The University of Arizona,
Tuscon, Arizona

Eleanor E. Bauwens, R.N., Ph.D., F.A.A.N.
Associate Dean and Associate Professor,
College of Nursing,
The University of Arizona,
Tuscon, Arizona

Patricia A. Betrus, R.N., M.N.
Research Instructor,
Psychosocial Nursing,
University of Washington,
Seattle, Washington

Debra C. Broadwell, R.N., M.N., E.T.
Project Director,
Enterostomal Therapy Educational Program,
School of Medicine,
Section of General Surgery,
Emory University,
Atlanta, Georgia

Linda Anne Broseman, R.N., M.S.N.
Formerly Assistant Professor of
Medical-Surgical Nursing,
Frances Payne Bolton School of Nursing,
Case Western Reserve University;
Associate in Nursing,
University Hospitals of Cleveland,
Cleveland, Ohio

Dorothy J. Brundage, R.N., Ph.D., F.A.A.N.
Associate Professor of Nursing,
Duke University School of Nursing,
Durham, North Carolina

Patricia Buergin, R.N., B.S.N.
Senior Clinical Nurse,
University Hospitals of Cleveland,
Cleveland, Ohio

Mary E. Bushong, R.N., M.S.N.
Assistant Professor of Operating and
Recovery Room Nursing,
Frances Payne Bolton School of Nursing,
Case Western Reserve University;
Associate Director of Operating and Recovery Room
Nursing and Director of Ambulatory Surgical Services,
University Hospitals of Cleveland,
Cleveland, Ohio

Virginia L. Cassmeyer, R.N., M.S.N.
Associate Professor of Medical-Surgical Nursing,
School of Nursing, University of Kansas,
Kansas City, Kansas

Lynn Chenoweth, R.N., M.S.N.
Formerly Assistant Professor of
Medical-Surgical Nursing,
Frances Payne Bolton School of Nursing,
Case Western Reserve University,
Cleveland, Ohio

Ella Cinkota, R.N., Ed.M.
Consultant Nurse, Bureau of Maternal
and Child Health,
New York State Department of Health,
Albany, New York

Linda Wagner Craig, R.N., M.S.N.
Psychiatric Nurse Coordinator,
The Mary Imogene Bassett Hospital
(affiliated with Columbia University),
Cooperstown, New York

Ruth F. Craven, R.N., M.N.
Assistant Professor,
Department of Physiological Nursing,
University of Washington,
Seattle, Washington

Barbara J. Daly, R.N., M.S.N., F.A.A.N.
Assistant Clinical Professor of
Medical-Surgical Nursing,
Frances Payne Bolton School of Nursing,
Case Western Reserve University;
Assistant Director of Medical-Surgical Nursing,
University Hospitals of Cleveland,
Cleveland, Ohio

Gretchen Kramer Dery, R.N., M.S.N.
Assistant Professor of Nursing,
Duke University School of Nursing,
Durham, North Carolina

Mariann DiMinno, R.N., M.S.N., Ph.D. Candidate
Committee on Social and Organization Psychology,
University of Chicago,
Chicago, Illinois

Nancy Durham, R.N., M.S.N.
Formerly Assistant Professor of
Medical-Surgical Nursing,
Frances Payne Bolton School of Nursing,
Case Western Reserve University,
Cleveland, Ohio

Elizabeth Cameron Eckstein, R.N., B.S.N.
Infection Control Nurse,
University Hospitals of Cleveland,
Cleveland, Ohio

Fred Farley, R.N., M.S.N.
Clinical Instructor in Medical-Surgical Nursing,
Frances Payne Bolton School of Nursing,
Case Western Reserve University;
Assistant Director, Medical-Surgical Nursing,
University Hospitals of Cleveland,
Cleveland, Ohio

Janet Larson Gelein, R.N., M.S., Ph.D. Candidate
Assistant Professor of Nursing,
University of Rochester,
Rochester, New York

Greer Glazer, R.N., M.S.N.
Instructor in Maternity and Gynecologic Nursing,
Frances Payne Bolton School of Nursing,
Case Western Reserve University;
Associate in Nursing,
University Hospitals of Cleveland,
Cleveland, Ohio

Jean Goeppinger, R.N., Ph.D.
Associate Professor and Director of Primary Nursing
Care in Society Graduate Major,
University of Virginia School of Nursing,
Charlottesville, Virginia

C. Joan Gowin, R.N., M.A., F.A.A.N.
Associate Professor of Nursing,
Frances Payne Bolton School of Nursing,
Case Western Reserve University;
Director of Operating and Recovery Room Nursing,
University Hospitals of Cleveland,
Cleveland, Ohio

Judith L. Greig, R.N., M.S.N.
Instructor in Nursing,
Lakeland Community College,
Mentor, Ohio

Sandra Griffiths, R.N., M.S.N.
Assistant Clinical Instructor of Pediatric Nursing,
Frances Payne Bolton School of Nursing,
Case Western Reserve University;
Nurse Clinician, Pediatric Nursing,
University Hospitals of Cleveland,
Cleveland, Ohio

Donna Williams Hewitt, R.N., M.N.
Assistant Clinical Professor,
Director of Continuing Education,
Duke University School of Nursing,
Durham, North Carolina

Rosemarie Hogan, R.N., M.S.N.
Assistant Professor of Nursing, Kent State University,
Kent, Ohio

Maura A. Hopkins, R.N., M.S.N., C.C.R.N.
Clinical Instructor in Medical-Surgical Nursing,
Frances Payne Bolton School of Nursing,
Case Western Reserve University, Cleveland, Ohio;
Critical Care Clinical Specialist, Veterans
Administration Hospital,
Wade Park, Ohio

Patricia Humphrey, R.N., B.S.N., M.P.H., F.N.P.
Assistant Professor of Nursing,
Duke University School of Nursing,
Durham, North Carolina

Noel Joyce, R.N., M.S.N.
Clinical Instructor in Medical-Surgical Nursing,
Frances Payne Bolton School of Nursing,
Case Western Reserve University;
Administrative Nurse Clinician, University Hospitals
of Cleveland, Cleveland, Ohio

Virginia Burke Karb, R.N., M.S.N.
Assistant Professor of Medical-Surgical Nursing,
University of North Carolina,
Greensboro, North Carolina

Jane Steinman Kaufman, R.N., M.S.
Assistant Professor of Nursing,
Duke University School of Nursing,
Durham, North Carolina

Joan M. Kavanagh, R.N., M.S.N.
Instructor of Medical-Surgical Nursing,
Ursuline College, Cleveland, Ohio

Marjorie Kinney, R.N., M.S.N.
Assistant Professor of Nursing,
Wright State University,
Dayton, Ohio

Mary K. Kirkpatrick, R.N., M.S.N.
Assistant Professor of Nursing,
East Carolina University,
Greenville, North Carolina; Ph.D. Candidate, North
Carolina State University, Raleigh, North Carolina

Marie L. Lobo, R.N., Ph.D.
Assistant Professor,
University of Wisconsin–Milwaukee,
Milwaukee, Wisconsin

Juanita Lee Long, R.N., Ed.D.
Associate Professor of Nursing,
Duke University School of Nursing,
Durham, North Carolina

Paula Lambrecht Miller, R.N., M.S.
Formerly Assistant Clinical Professor of
Medical-Surgical Nursing,
Frances Payne Bolton School of Nursing,
Case Western Reserve University;
Assistant Director of Medical-Surgical Nursing,
University Hospitals of Cleveland,
Cleveland, Ohio

Pamela Holsclaw Mitchell, R.N., M.S., C.N.R.N.,
F.A.A.N.
Professor,
Department of Physiological Nursing,
University of Washington,
Seattle, Washington

Carol J. Mitten, R.N., M.S.N.
Assistant Clinical Professor of
Medical-Surgical Nursing,
Frances Payne Bolton School of Nursing,
Case Western Reserve University;
Assistant Director of Medical-Surgical Nursing,
University Hospitals of Cleveland,
Cleveland, Ohio

Doris M. Molbo, R.N., M.A.
Associate Professor,
Department of Physiological Nursing, and
The American Cancer Society Clinical Professor of
Oncology Nursing,
University of Washington,
Seattle, Washington

Mary Lou Monahan, R.N., M.S.N.
Nurse Clinician, University Hospitals of Cleveland,
Cleveland, Ohio

Janice Neville, D.Sc.
Professor of Nutrition, Case Western Reserve
University,
Cleveland, Ohio

Joan Nivinski, R.N., M.S.N.
Formerly Assistant Clinical Professor of
Pediatric Nursing,
Frances Payne Bolton School of Nursing,
Case Western Reserve University; Nurse Clinician,
Pediatric Nursing, University Hospitals of Cleveland,
Cleveland, Ohio

Alice Norman, R.N., M.S.N.
Assistant Clinical Professor of
Medical-Surgical Nursing,
Frances Payne Bolton School of Nursing,
Case Western Reserve University, Cleveland, Ohio;
Pulmonary Clinical Specialist, Veterans Administration
Hospital, Wade Park, Ohio

Elizabeth Strauss Nosse, R.N., M.S.N.
Formerly Clinical Instructor in
Medical-Surgical Nursing,
Frances Payne Bolton School of Nursing,
Case Western Reserve University;
Administrative Nurse Clinician,
University Hospitals of Cleveland,
Cleveland, Onio

Penny O'Malley, R.N., B.S.N.
Director for Ambulatory Nursing Services,
Cleveland Metropolitan General Hospital,
Cleveland, Ohio

Cheryl Patterson, R.N., M.S.N.
Clinical Instructor in Medical-Surgical Nursing,
Frances Payne Bolton School of Nursing,
Case Western Reserve University;
Administrative Nurse Clinician,
University Hospitals of Cleveland,
Cleveland, Ohio

Debra Power, R.N., M.S.N.
Lecturer,
Department of Physiologic Nursing,
University of Washington,
Seattle, Washington

Antoinette T. Ragucci, R.N., Ph.D.
Associate Professor of Medical-Surgical Nursing,
Frances Payne Bolton School of Nursing,
Case Western Reserve University;
Associate in Nursing,
University Hospitals of Cleveland,
Cleveland, Ohio

Marcia J. Riegger, R.N., B.S.N.
Advanced Clinical Nurse,
University Hospitals of Cleveland,
Cleveland, Ohio

Rebecca Roberts, R.N., M.S.N.
Clinical Instructor in Medical-Surgical Nursing,
Frances Payne Bolton School of Nursing, Case
Western Reserve University; Instructor in
Decentralized Staff Development,
University Hospitals of Cleveland,
Cleveland, Ohio

Elizabeth Schenk, R.N., M.S.N.
Clinical Instructor in Medical-Surgical Nursing,
Frances Payne Bolton School of Nursing,
Case Western Reserve University;
Administrative Nurse Clinician,
University Hospitals of Cleveland,
Cleveland, Ohio

Katherine Schenk, R.N., Ed.D.
Associate Professor Emeritus,
Duke University School of Nursing,
Durham, North Carolina

Barbara Soltis, R.N., M.S.N.
Assistant Professor of Medical-Surgical Nursing,
Frances Payne Bolton School of Nursing,
Case Western Reserve University;
Associate in Nursing, University Hospitals of
Cleveland,
Cleveland, Ohio

Sally Schafer Todd, R.N., M.S.N.
Associate Director of Nursing Education,
Fayetteville Area Health Education Center,
Fayetteville, North Carolina; Clinical Assistant
Professor of Nursing, Duke University School of
Nursing, Durham, North Carolina;
Adjunct Assistant Professor, School of Nursing,
University of North Carolina at Chapel Hill,
Chapel Hill, North Carolina

E. Ronald Wright, Ph.D.
Associate Professor of Microbiology and Administrative
Officer, Instructional Development Programs,
Case Western Reserve University,
Cleveland, Ohio

May Wykle, R.N., Ph.D.
Associate Professor of Psychiatric Nursing,
Frances Payne Bolton School of Nursing,
Case Western Reserve University;
Associate in Nursing, University Hospitals of
Cleveland,
Cleveland, Ohio

Mary A. Wyper, R.N., M.S.N.
Assistant Professor of Medical-Surgical Nursing,
Frances Payne Bolton School of Nursing,
Case Western Reserve University;
Associate in Nursing, University Hospitals of
Cleveland,
Cleveland, Ohio

Deanna Melton Xistris, R.N., M.S.N.
Clinical Specialist in Oncology Nursing,
Hematology-Oncology Associates, Inc.,
Stamford, Connecticut

Karen K. Yoder, R.N., M.N., Ph.D. Student
The University of Michigan School of Nursing,
Ann Arbor, Michigan

PREFACE

The social environments in which nursing is practiced have undergone considerable change in recent years, and as a result the knowledge necessary to practice nursing has grown considerably. Today there are many facets to the nursing role, and nurses practice in more diverse environments than ever before. Central to all of these environments is an encounter between the nurse and the patient or client. In order to enhance the effectiveness of this encounter, the nurse needs information drawn from a wide variety of sources. The purpose of this book is to present information that we believe is relevant to the practice of medical-surgical nursing in the 1980s.

This book is divided into three major parts. In *Part One*, "Perspectives for Nursing Practice," there are two units. *Unit I* examines social, cultural, and environmental perspectives that can be applied to nursing practice, whether it be in the community or in the hospital. In this unit, concepts of health and illness; the systems approach; family, culture, and society; health care delivery systems; epidemiologic approaches to health care; and perspectives for nursing practice are presented. The latter chapter, which is new with this edition, explores some of the conceptual frameworks commonly used in nursing today. All of the concepts presented in Part One can be used to enhance the knowledge base of nurses and are relevant to nursing students and practicing nurses alike.

Unit II looks at those concepts and processes in wide use today. First, the components of the nursing process are presented, with emphasis on the steps of assessment, including data collection and analysis. Key concepts in nurse-client interactions are presented next, followed by an introduction to the problem-oriented system for organizing data. The last chapter in Unit II looks at the issues involved in quality assurance programs and the monitoring of client outcomes. This introduction to client or patient outcomes should prepare the reader to understand the reason for, and the importance of, the outcome criteria presented in the chapters in Part Three of this book.

Throughout the book we have referred to the persons who are recipients of the services of nurses as clients or patients. In our minds the term *client* is most generally accepted as a referrant to persons in nonhospital settings, whereas *patient* is more commonly used to denote those who are in hospitals or other health care institutions. We recognize that some nurses are more comfortable with one term than the other, and for this reason both terms are used in this text.

Part Two, "Stress and Adaptation," consists of two units. Concepts necessary to understanding the processes of stress and adaptation are presented in *Unit III*, "Adaptation." A framework for understanding stress, coping, and adaptation is presented first followed by a new chapter on stress management. Other chapters in the unit are adaptive behavior, maladaptive behavior, adaptation throughout the life cycle, death and dying, neuroendocrine integrating mechanisms, biologic defense mechanisms, and mechanisms for maintaining dynamic equilibrium. The chapters in this unit have been reorganized and expanded to better define and discuss these concepts from behavioral and biologic perspectives. Chapter 18, "Neuroendocrine Integrating Mechanisms," contains the information required to understand the relationships between the parts of the nervous and endocrine systems responsible for the integration of the body functions necessary to the maintenance of a stable internal environment.

Common stressors and their management are discussed in *Unit IV*. These include fluid and electrolyte imbalance, infectious diseases, pain, surgery, neoplasia, sensory overload and sensory deprivation, altered levels of consciousness, altered body image, and chronic illness. Like the chapters in Units I and II, these chapters present basic concepts that are essential to the practice of nursing in the world of today. The chapter on emergencies and disasters that was in this unit in the first edition has been moved to Unit XII, "Environments of Care."

Part Three of this text, "Clinical Interventions for Persons with Medical-Surgical Problems," presents material traditionally found in medical-surgical books. The content is divided into eight units to reflect common problems encountered as pathophysiologic changes occur relative to certain essential body processes. In response to comments from readers the pathophysiology in these chapters has been strengthened by adding new content and by consistent use of the heading "Pathophysiology" so that this content can be readily identified as each problem is presented.

Failures of integrative mechanisms resulting in regulatory problems are presented first, followed by sensorimotor problems, gas transport problems, problems of nutrition, problems of elimination, problems related to sexuality and reproduction, problems related to impaired protective mechanisms, and special environments of care. The units were organized in this manner to allow the content to be presented in a relevant and useful manner. In each of these units a nursing process format is used, with an assessment chapter of the system involved being presented first, followed by an intervention chapter, which discusses various interventions (medical and nursing) commonly used for persons with that impairment. The purpose of the intervention chapter is to present the interventions without going into detail about the pathologic process making the intervention necessary. For example, thoracic surgery is discussed in Chapter 49, "Intervention for the Person with a Respiratory Problem," without discussing pathologic considerations of the lung that make thoracic surgery necessary. Following the intervention chapter is a problems chapter that presents the details of basic pathophysiologic processes which lead to the development of specific disease processes in that body system. Thus cancer of the lung and other pulmonary conditions that may be treated with thoracic surgery are discussed in Chapter 51, "Problems of the Lower Airway."

All chapters have been updated, and many have been revised in response to suggestions from readers. *Unit V*, "Failure of Integrative Mechanisms: Regulatory Problems," contains four chapters: assessment of regulatory mechanisms, intervention for the person with impaired regulatory mechanisms, endocrine dysfunction, and dysfunction of the liver and related structures. In the chapter on endocrine dysfunction the content about the etiology, pathophysiology, and interventions for diabetes has been completely rewritten.

Unit VI, "Sensorimotor Problems," has nine chapters. The first three of these are neurologic assessment, intervention for the person with common neurologic manifestations, and problems of the nervous system. The next three chapters are assessment of the special senses, eye and ear; special sensory problems, eye and ear; and problems of the eye and ear. The last three chapters in this unit are musculoskeletal system assessment, intervention for the person with motor problems, and musculoskeletal problems.

Unit VII, "Gas Transport Problems," has been reorganized so that the content related to the heart and blood vessels is separated from the content on respiratory and airway problems. New to this edition are separate chapters on intervention for the person with a cardiovascular problem and intervention for the person with a respiratory problem. There are nine chapters in the unit, three devoted to the cardiovascular system, a chapter on problems of peripheral circulation, a chapter on problems of the blood and blood-forming tissues, and four chapters on the respiratory system including a separate chapter on the upper airway.

Unit VIII, "Problems of Nutrition," contains five chapters, including assessment of nutritional status and assessment, intervention, and problem chapters related to the upper gastrointestinal tract. In *Unit IX*, "Problems of Elimination," the first three chapters relate to the lower gastrointestinal tract and the last three chapters to the urinary system.

Unit X, "Problems Related to Sexuality and Reproduction," and *Unit XI*, "Problems Related to Impaired Protective Mechanisms," each contain five chapters, presented in the same order as in the first edition.

Unit XII, "Special Environments of Care," contains the chapter on emergencies and disasters mentioned previously as well as three chapters on care of the critically ill patient.

Throughout this revision the emphasis is on assisting the patient or client to improve his or her health by providing appropriate physical care, emotional and social support, and information necessary for self-care. We believe that the patient's or client's significant others, be they family or friends, provide essential support to that person, and therefore we make reference to involving them as appropriate in the care of the individual patient or client.

Many new figures and tables have been added to this edition, and the reference list at the end of each chapter has been divided into contemporary and classic (those published before 1970) references.

It is our hope that this revision will meet the needs of nurses for a reference book that assists them to provide the best possible nursing care to their clients.

Many experts have contributed to this second edition, and we wish to thank each of them. Medical colleagues as well as nursing colleagues have been generous in taking time to review chapters. We also wish to thank all the readers who contributed their thoughtful comments and suggestions about the first edition.

The new illustrations for this edition are the work of Kathleen Jung of Cleveland and Jan Norbisrath of Seattle.

The preparation of the manuscript was done by Beverly Ernst of Seattle and Janet Mitchell and Sondra Patrizi of Cleveland, who deserve special thanks for their help with every aspect of the preparation of the manuscript.

We also wish to thank Mrs. Geraldine Mink, who assisted with the library research for several of the chapters, and Deanna Carroll, M.S.N., who assisted with the last-minute details of this revision.

We are also grateful to Tom Manning, Bess Arends, Fran Mues, and Mary Wright of The C.V. Mosby Company for their assistance and support during the preparation of this second edition.

WILMA J. PHIPPS
BARBARA C. LONG
NANCY FUGATE WOODS

CONTENTS

PART THREE CLINICAL INTERVENTIONS FOR PERSONS WITH MEDICAL-SURGICAL PROBLEMS

PART ONE

PERSPECTIVES
FOR NURSING PRACTICE

SOCIAL, CULTURAL, AND ENVIRONMENTAL PERSPECTIVES

Health and illness, when considered from a clinical perspective, frequently bring to mind definitions rooted in biology. Because they are biologic organisms, people's physical bodies, organs, cells, and even subcellular components are intimately involved with their health statuses; however, the experience of health and illness is inexorably linked to the social, cultural, and physical environments in which they live. This unit explores definitions of *health, illness,* and *disease* from lay as well as professional perspectives. One approach to foster a holistic view of humanity, the *systems perspective,* is considered. The *influence of society and culture on behavior* in times of health and illness is examined. This is followed by exploration of *systems of health care delivery* with an emphasis on models for the delivery of nursing care and a description of an *epidemiologic perspective* for health care, stressing the need for a multicausal approach to understanding health and illness. The unit concludes with an overview of various *perspectives* that may help guide the practice of medical-surgical nursing.

CHAPTER 1

CONCEPTS OF HEALTH AND ILLNESS

GRETCHEN KRAMER DERY

Nicole Peters is 3 months old. She was born with an umbilical hernia. Mr. and Mrs. Peters have been informed by their pediatrician that this is not uncommon. The physician recommends observation as the best approach, since many hernias of this type will resolve without intervention.

Stephen Walters is 7 years old. He was born with no right leg. He walks with crutches and is able to play with the children in his neighborhood. He is not able to be involved in some of the children's more strenuous and highly competitive activities. He attends the neighborhood school and is making satisfactory progress in his studies.

Craig Wellons is a 35-year-old successful insurance salesperson. He is married and has two children. He and his family are financially comfortable and view their life situation as very positive. Unknown to him, atherosclerotic plaques are insidiously forming in his coronary arteries.

Each of the persons described above could be defined as ill or healthy, depending on the perspective of the definer. The purpose of this chapter is to explore concepts of health and illness from the perspective of the patient or client as well as that of the health professional. This chapter begins with a comparison of definitions of health, illness, and disease from lay and medical perspectives. This is followed by an exploration of concepts of health including high-level wellness and a consideration of behavior in health and illness.

Lay and professional perspectives

Lay persons and health professionals alike have notions of health, illness, and disease that guide their behavior.[40] In some instances, the lay and professional definitions vary significantly, which leads to difficulty in communication between the professional who desires to deliver acceptable health care and the lay person who desires to receive health care.[11,49,61]

Health

The medical profession has concentrated on defining the nature of aberrant functioning rather than health. Consequently, "normal" has come to imply the opposite of "abnormal." At one pole is health, which is normal and denoted by the absence of pathologic signs and symptoms. At the opposite pole is disease, which is abnormal and denoted by the presence of pathologic signs and symptoms. Thus some health professionals define health as a negative concept, the absence of disease, the uninteresting opposite of disease.[79]

The nursing profession has leaned toward a definition of health that is broader than the absence of disease, although there is not one universally agreed on definition within the profession. Three models utilized in addition to the nondisease model are the eudaimonistic model, the adaptive model, and the role performance model. The eudaimonistic model defines health as exuberant well-being or self-fulfillment. The adaptive model describes health as the condition of the organism in which it can engage in effective interaction with its physical and social environment. The third model, the role performance model, states that healthy people are those who effectively perform their roles.[71]

As scientific and medical technology increases and greater interventive techniques are forthcoming, potential maneuvers (e.g., genetic modification) to alter health may ultimately force a revolutionary redefinition of the professional concepts of health.[25]

Lay definitions of health reflect both positive and negative aspects. Three orientations to health include:

1. The feeling-state orientation, described as "feeling good"
2. The symptom orientation, characterized by lack of general or specific symptoms of disease
3. The performance orientation, defined as activities that a person who is healthy should be able to perform[84]

Thus the lay view of health is multidimensional.

Disease and illness

The professional orientation defines disease as objective, observable, and quantifiable. Disease involves change in the structure or function of the body or mind of the human organism. A knowledge of anatomy and physiology is essential for studying disease. Objective changes in structure and function are called *signs* of disease. Although the medical profession also looks at subjective information concerning disease, this type of data is often considered as a secondary source for diagnosis. Subjective information about disease is called *symptoms* and includes reports such as perception of pain, anxiety, and nausea. Such perceptions are difficult to quantify and tend to be influenced by a variety of factors, which are not necessarily directly related to the disease process. Thus subjective reports are considered by some professionals to provide less reliable diagnostic information than objective signs. The signs and symptoms of certain diseases tend to recur among geographic, cultural, social, and socioeconomic populations. The frequent recurrence of combinations of signs and symptoms is labeled a clinical *syndrome*. There are, in addition to signs and symptoms, other characteristics of disease, including incidence, onset, course, prognosis, duration, and communicability.[80] *Incidence*, or frequency with which the disease occurs (or more accurately, is diagnosed), results in such labels as "common childhood diseases" and the "common cold" versus such entities as "rare blood dyscrasias." The *onset*, or beginning appearance of signs and symptoms, can be insidious, obvious, gradual, or rapid. The *course* or path, may be smooth, rough, predictable, or unpredictable. The *prognosis*, or ultimate outcome, can be hopeful or guarded or can range from poor to excellent. The *duration*, or length, can be short, long, or permanent. *Acute* and *chronic* are words frequently used to describe duration but have such a diversity of interpretation that there is little universal agreement on their precise meaning. "Chronic" is generally applied to diseases of a long-term nature. *Communicability* refers to the contagious or transmissible quality of a disease. Contrasting examples of communicability are gastric ulcer and venereal disease, the former being noncom-

municable and the latter considered highly communicable.

The terms *disease* and *illness* are commonly used interchangeably by the medical profession, which adds confusion to the attempts to clarify the concepts. It has been noted that the medical definition of disease remains inadequate and essentially conceptually undefined, because there exists a comfortable delusion that everyone knows what it is.[5]

The lay person experiencing a disease regards it from a completely different framework than does the professional treating the disease. Whereas the medical diagnostician considers disease in terms of medical knowledge and objectively evaluates the meaning of signs and symptoms, the lay person generally tends to perceive disease from a subjective, personalized, and *phenomenologic* framework. That is, illness is perceived by the lay person in terms of its meaning to that particular individual.

In a study of lay perceptions of illness, researchers have tried to determine at what point health problems are considered illness by lay persons. The findings suggested that for middle-class Americans being ill meant *having an ailment of recent origin that interfered with one's usual activities*. Interference with usual activities seemed to be the most important criterion lay persons applied to the definition of illness.[81] In another study it was noted that lay persons often perceived disease as *an object or thing that invaded the body*. These individuals regularly referred to a wide spectrum of diseases as objects, that is, invading and foreign "its." They impersonalized both the symptoms and organs involved through the use of depersonalized language.[15]

Illness has been viewed by the lay person at times as a metaphor, especially illness caused by diseases that are overlaid with mystification and wrapped in an aura of inescapable fatality.[72] Persons afflicted with such illnesses provoke dread and social ostracism. Today cancer qualifies as a metaphorical disease, possessing both mythology and mystique. The lay person views cancer as the supreme body insult because the body devours itself through the metastatic process.

Disease can occur in an individual without the person's awareness of illness and without others perceiving illness. On the other hand, a person can feel very ill even though no pathologic processes can be identified.[19]

Concepts of health

Although much of the medical and nursing literature describes disease and illness, increased attention is being devoted to health. Two contemporary concepts of health are Maslow's hierarchy of needs and Dunn's concept of high-level wellness.

Maslow's hierarchy of needs

Maslow[87] describes a hierarchy of needs in which the physiologic needs are considered as most basic, followed by safety, love, esteem, and self-actualization needs. A need that is not satisfied constitutes a motivating factor for an individual.

Needs are generally more unconscious than conscious. Basic needs are not seen as being exclusive determinants of behavior(s), since almost all behaviors have social, cultural, and biologic motivations. Any particular behavioral incident is more likely to be influenced by all the needs in varying degrees than by a single need.

It is necessary to recognize that for most people the needs in the hierarchy exist simultaneously and in differing degrees and that new needs emerge not suddenly but very gradually. At varying times an individual will have different amounts of various needs being met. Lower level needs do not need to be met *completely* before higher level needs can emerge. Maslow suggests that the degree of need satisfaction is positively related to mental health and that, theoretically, total need gratification and ideal health are synonymous.

Physiologic needs

Physiologic needs include hunger, thirst, sleep, and rest. Totally deprived human beings would generally find the physiologic needs to be their major motivating force. All other needs would be pushed into the background or cease to exist for those persons. However, once physiologic needs are satisfied, the higher level needs begin to emerge, and when they are satisfied, new and still higher level needs are manifested.

Safety needs

Safety needs are the second level of needs. For the majority of citizens of developed countries these are not the prime motivators of human behavior. Societies usually succeed in protecting their members from extremes in temperature and from such forms of aggression as assault, murder, and tyranny. In the lower socioeconomic groups of these same societies it is possible that safety needs may not be met and that these safety needs may become the prime motivators of behavior within these segments of the society. In general, however, safety needs are seen as prime motivators only in times of national, natural, or personal crises, for example, war, natural disasters, and illness. When safety needs are satisfied, the need for love and belonging emerges.

Love and belonging needs

Love is associated not only with sexual behavior but also with a desire for affectionate relationships with people in general. Deprivation of love and belonging needs is believed to cause the basic maladjustment seen in the more severe psychopathologies, whereas less severe thwarting of these needs is seen among those who are lonely.

Esteem needs

Esteem needs consist of two subsets. The first includes a desire for strength, achievement, adequacy, mastery, competence, and independence. The second subset is geared toward reputation or prestige entities received from others, as in status dominance, recognition, attention, importance, and appreciation. Thwarting of these needs produces negative feelings, such as inferiority, weakness, and helplessness. Satisfaction of self-esteem needs leads to positive feelings of being useful and necessary in the world.

Self-actualization need

Self-actualization need is the highest need and describes persons continually moving toward achieving their potential. Few persons achieve self-actualization, a need more commonly met during the mature years.

While there is generally a progression in the hierarchy of needs, it is not a rigid scheme of classification. A person who has had basic needs satisfied for a consistent period throughout life demonstrates ability to withstand the thwarting of needs. However, a person's aspiration level may be permanently lowered by consistent deprivation; for example, chronically unemployed persons may be totally satisfied as long as they have enough food, and they may cease to strive for more than that. When a need has been long satisfied and then is deprived, its importance may be undervaluated. For example, many people who have met their physiologic and higher needs throughout life may find the fact that they presently have only one meal a day *not* a potent motivator. Such a situation can frequently be observed among our aged population today.

Dunn's high-level wellness

Dunn describes high-level wellness in relation to the individual, family, community, environment, and society.

Individual high-level wellness is described as integrated functioning oriented toward maximizing individual potential while maintaining balance and purposeful direction in the environment. It includes three components: an upward and forward direction toward higher functional potential; an open-ended future containing challenges to achieve higher potential; and an integrated being, that is, body-mind-spirit participating in the functioning process.[85] Wellness is differentiated from good health. "Good health" is viewed as a relatively passive state of freedom from illness.[4] In fact, in the United States, "normal health" is seen as a sorry state of existence.[28]

Nature of people

Dunn's view of wellness is based on a philosophy of the nature of people that includes the following five aspects. First, each individual functions as a *total personality*. Next, each person possesses enormous *dynamic energy*. Third, each person has and must maintain *peace with inner and outer worlds*. Fourth, each person has a *relationship* between *energy use* and *self-integration*, when self-integration is defined as the interweaving of all the known aspects of life. Finally, each individual possesses an *inner* and an *outer world*. The inner world can be described as each and every body cell composing an organized whole. The outer world refers simply to the individual's environment with all its components. A person must find his or her being and belonging in both worlds. Questions to be explored are: "What and why am I?" and "Where am I going?"

Dunn maintains that humans have the capacity to recognize certain *processes* that help provide them with the answers to the above questions. These processes are being, belonging, becoming, and befitting. In *being*, one can recognize oneself after the neonatal period as something separate and distinct from the remainder of the world. Additionally, if one is a separate part, there must be a whole to which one *belongs*. People grow and develop in all spheres of their being; that is, they are *becoming*. As people grow and become, they individually and selectively make choices; that is, they *befit* themselves for the future.

Cellular commonwealth

From a physiologic standpoint, a person is composed of a cellular commonwealth organized into systems. The optimal functioning of the cellular commonwealth is an essential component of wellness. Each of the body's cells is seen as a unique totality, is made of energy, has an inner and outer world, and is an open system. Protoplasm, the main constituent of cells, has six qualities, which then become qualities of each cell. These qualities or functions are:

1. Irritability: the ability to attract or repel
2. Mobility: the ability to move about, sacrificed by some cells in the name of organization and cooperation
3. Metabolism: the ability to perform chemically
4. Growth and reproduction: the abilities to expand and replicate
5. Adaptability: the ability to be interdependent and to maintain an organized whole

Systems have several functions to perform if the cellular needs are to be met, including keeping ports of entry and exit open, transforming energy and waste, growing, reproducing, and problem solving (including the storage, integration, and use of information).

The overall function served by the commonwealth of cells is maintenance of unity.

Mind

The *mind*, called the emergent mind because of its developing state, is characterized by its potential for problem solving in daily living. The mind's total functioning is not yet fully understood. Problem solving, its chief function, involves eight components: communication, storage, values, imagination, concept of self, integration of self, maturity in wholeness, and purpose.

High-level wellness cannot exist without *communication* and freedom to pick and choose solutions. One of society's greatest crimes against a person is constriction of channels of communication so that the individual cannot problem solve.

Three types of *storage mechanisms* exist for people: memory stored in the nervous system, memory stored in muscles as tension patterns, and chemical memory of cells. Dunn believes that pain and fear can be locked into body tissues and can constitute an ongoing source of increasing tension. Trapped physical pain can raise tension and prevent tissue healing; trapped emotional pain can prolong grieving. For the storage mechanism to function, access to data must be maintained. Blocked accesses must be cleared. Long-standing barriers may require psychotherapy or other therapeutic measures. New blocks caused by recent physical or emotional pain can be diminished or dispersed through discussion and sharing.

Values are essential problem-solving components because they provide a means for selection of options and decision making. The ultimate goal of people can be seen as seeking enhancement of the value attributes or experiences.

Imagination refers to mental synthesis of new ideas from elements experienced separately and appears to be a uniquely human phenomenon. Imagination helps people see alternatives; for example, when problems arise the mind perceives similarity to situations previously encountered, and possible solutions are postulated with freedom of choice. Creative imagination is one part of the problem-solving process whereby people can explore their futures and maximize their potential to reach high-level wellness.

The "self" in the problem-solving process provides the reason for choosing. Although the *self-concept*, or how we see ourselves, tends to be rigid, every "self" is continually changing. If one does not periodically bring the "self" and the self-concept into focus, the "self" idea of oneself may become less and less reality oriented. Self-fulfillment and satisfaction come from what one is, not what one was. Health requires that one be capable of facing the facts about one's self.

Integration of self is the sixth component of problem solving. Integration of body-mind-spirit is more feasible when body and mind are in balance. Rest, sleep, relaxation, and leisure are necessary for body-mind-spirit balance. Mental health, physical health, spiritual health, and social health are possible only when there is balance between the interacting and integrated energy fields of the body-mind-spirit and the environment.

Maturity in wholeness is related to how the body-mind-spirit grows. It is not an end point but varies at different points in the life cycle. The principal expressions of maturity in wholeness lie in the development of conceptual thought, formation of knowledge, self-integration, group integration, and development of purpose. Maturity in wholeness involves understanding of and harmony between the individual and others.

The final component of the problem-solving mechanism is *purpose*. It is in the pursuit of purpose that humans boldly attempt to solve complex problems.

Family, community, and social high-level wellness

To this point high-level wellness has been discussed in relation to the individual. The concept is easily applied to groups. The family is an essential group in our society that fulfills several functions: reproduction, rearing of children, and provision of an emotional setting for the stabilization of the adult personality. Family wellness is reflected in the degree to which the family unit succeeds in providing security for all members; love characterized by caring, responsibility, knowledge of other family members, and shared values; a future with the opportunity to develop to full potential; and integration so that problem solving can be done in unity.

Community wellness does not involve only good sanitation, water supply, living space, lack of crime, or sound businesses but might include concern for beauty and wildlife, an environment conducive to interchange between generations, and decentralization of industry to decrease long commuting hours. *High-level environmental wellness* includes more than absence of air, water, and noise pollution; it assumes people's cooperation with nature.

Social wellness involves a forward direction in *progress*, an open-ended expanding future, and the integration of the society into a total personality. Dunn maintains that societies would benefit from learning to fight *for* things and not against them and that problems must be dealt with on a world basis, for there is no possible unilateral human survival.

Other authors have taken Dunn's concept of high-level wellness and elaborated on it.[8,60,63] The concept of high-level wellness can be applied by health professionals, especially nurses, as they begin to focus attention on the wellness of people rather than focusing exclusively on sickness.[23,39,59] To shift the emphasis in this fashion, wellness needs to be viewed not as a simple category or static entity but as a dynamic process.

An acceptance of the holistic approach outlined in this chapter will not allow the nurse-client relationship to be superficial. It will not be sufficient to know only the name and health care need of the person to be served. A functional relationship will be replaced by one of care and concern for the total person, incorporating full consideration of both inner and outer worlds.[31,32,34]

Behavior in health and illness

Health and illness are usually considered from their clinical perspectives, but it is the social system perspective that has provided practitioners with a wealth of insight into the behavioral aspects of health and illness. Social scientists have examined health and illness in terms of the statuses and roles involved. *Status* refers to the position that could be occupied by members of a society, and *roles* are behaviors of persons who fill a particular status. The individuals of a particular social system share certain common expectations about how people of a specific status should behave in the performance of their roles. These expectations, called *role expectations*, are different for each status. All of these expectations together form the normative framework of a social system. The *norms* outline the expected behaviors for a status. These norms may impose a behavior as obligatory, may prohibit a behavior, or may allow the individual a choice about certain optional behaviors.[42,90] A summary of the social science descriptions of human behavior in health and illness roles follows.

Health behavior

Health behavior is defined as any activity undertaken by persons who believe they are well, for the purpose of preventing or detecting disease or promoting health.

Categories of health behavior

Health behaviors can be classified into three general categories: behaviors geared toward the individual's health, health behavior related to the source and utilization of health care, and individual health behavior in relation to the larger community and health care system as a whole. Each of the three categories describes behaviors geared toward prevention and detection of illness.

The first category, *behaviors geared toward the individual's health,* is admittedly very broad and in need of further research.[10] Preventive behaviors include eating a well-balanced diet, obtaining proper rest, participating in a daily exercise program, and avoiding risk-taking behaviors, such as smoking. Some detection behaviors in this category could include monthly self-examination of the breasts by women, taking one's temperature, weighing oneself regularly, and a host of other activities.

The second category, *health behavior related to the source and utilization of health care,* has received a great deal of study.[86] Preventive behaviors in this category include such activities as receiving immunizations, seeking information about health problems such as warning signals of cancer, or getting fluoride treatment for teeth. Examples of health behaviors directed toward detecting illness in this category include seeking routine screening of vision and hearing, Pap smears, physical examinations, chest x-ray studies, and prenatal and postpartum care.

The third category, *individual health behavior in relation to the larger community and health care system as a whole,* has received comparatively little attention. These behaviors might include individual involvement in health legislation, service as a volunteer in health programs, financial support of health organizations, and voting on health proposals.

Changed health attitudes and resultant changed behaviors could become a major preventive resource. Prevention of chronic disease now depends more on changing life-styles than on modifying the physical world. Health is determined more by what people do to themselves than by what an external infectious agent does to them.

Health belief model

One widely used model for describing health behavior is the health belief model (Fig. 1-1) designed to explain the widespread failure of people to accept low-cost or free health screening and detection measures for asymptomatic disease.

Health behavior, viewed from the perspective of this model, is influenced by several variables. All variables are interpreted from the phenomenologic viewpoint. The major components of the model are individual perceptions about the threat of the disease; modifying factors, including demographic variables and cues to action; and the likelihood of action.

Individual perceptions. The perceived threat of disease results from two factors: perceived susceptibility and perceived seriousness. *Perceived susceptibility* is the extent to which individuals feel threatened with contraction of a disease. The perceived threat, or the

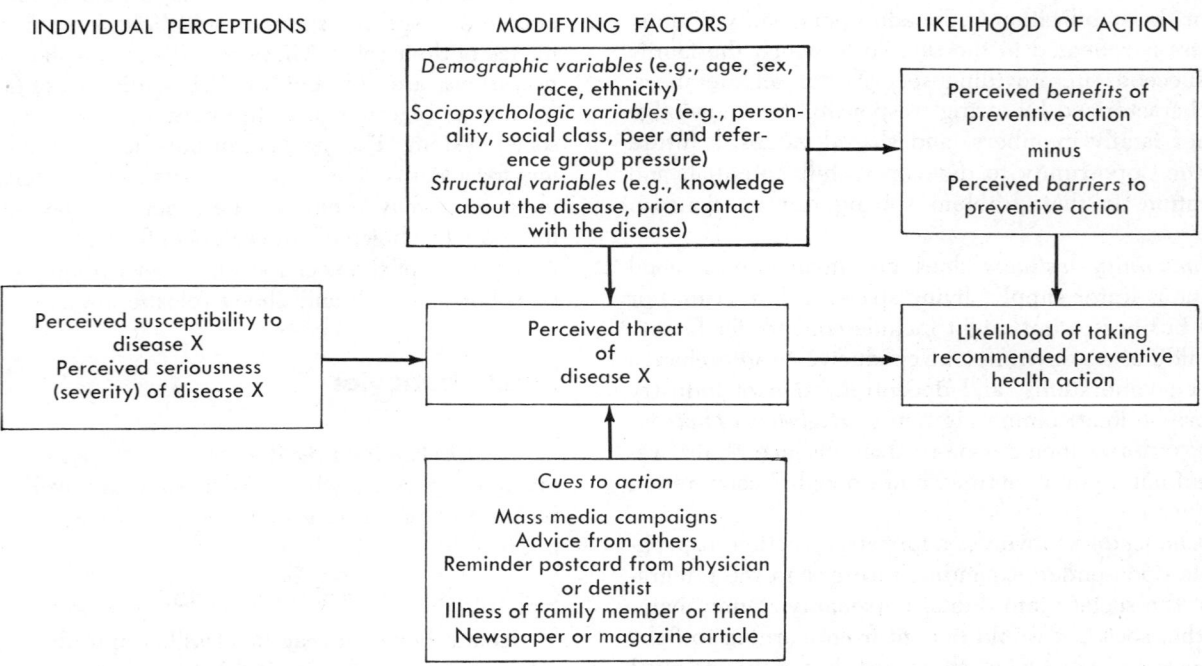

Fig. 1-1. Health belief model. (From Becker, M.H., Drachman, R.H., and Kirscht, J.: Am. J. Public Health **64**:205-216, 1974.)

person's sense of vulnerability, has been demonstrated to be the single best predictor of health utilization behaviors in selected settings.[45] Since this is a phenomenologic or subjective assessment, the individual's perception of risk may be similar to or vary widely from the perception of a health professional. Perceived susceptibility could conceivably range from being very afraid one will contract a certain condition to complete denial of any risk and feelings of invulnerability. Persons who smoke two packages of cigarettes each day may see themselves as highly susceptible to lung cancer or they may deny the risk of contracting the disease.

Perceived *seriousness*, the second factor making up the perceived threat, can be viewed from two perspectives: inherent seriousness and impact on one's lifestyle. A disease such as a brain tumor may be seen as inherently serious inasmuch as the disease process could lead to extensive physical disability or death. The impact of this disease on the person's life-style may also be judged as quite serious inasmuch as it can necessitate drastic adjustments in employment, function, and ability to care for oneself. Perceived seriousness is calculated on the basis of knowledge about a particular condition and constitutes a force leading to action. The actual performance of a particular recommended action is further influenced by two factors: the individual's conviction that performing the health behavior will prevent or modify the disease, and the person's perception of the unpleasantness or cost of performing the health behavior as compared with taking no action. These two factors can be combined in several ways, providing a large range of resultant behaviors.

Modifying factors and likelihood of action. Even though the *perceived threat of the disease* and the *perceived value of the action* are both high, it is possible that the individual involved may elect to engage in no health behavior at all. Cues seem to be necessary to initiate health behavior. These cues are most likely to be external and may take a wide variety of forms, such as a discussion with a friend, a television or newspaper message, or a postcard reminder from the dentist.

People are thought to vary in their susceptibility to cues.[67] In a situation where the perceived value of action and the perceived threat are high, a weak cue may be effective in eliciting health behavior. In another situation where the perceived value of the action and the perceived threat are low, a strong cue would be needed to be effective. The role of cues has been very difficult to determine because of their transient nature.

Other modifying factors include demographic, sociopsychologic, and structural variables. Thus such variables as sex, age, race, ethnic origin, education, occupation, income, and amount of knowledge are considered influential in health behavior.[1,14,63] In general, services for prevention and detection in the United States are used most by the young or middle aged, by those with higher income and greater formal education, and by whites.[66]

Assessment of health belief model

The health belief model is not without problems and limitations. Health services make up only one of many possible arenas for health behaviors, and there is a vast array of health providers other than those trained as professionals. Research demonstrates that only between 6% and 30% of health problems receive medical attention, with the majority of problems being handled by self or home treatment, lay consultation, or consultation with a nonorthodox health practitioner.[22] The health belief model is based on perceived threat of disease, very much in the manner of the medical-clinical model. It does not attempt to provide a mechanism to study causal factors in achieving higher levels of health where perceived threat of a disease entity is not an important variable.

The model is supposedly applied in situations where the behavior is purely voluntary and the individuals are symptom free, yet much of health behavior is a result of social pressure, legal compulsion, and job requirements.[66] It is conceivable that only a small proportion of the population presently takes voluntary health action to detect or prevent disease in the absence of symptoms. But careful study of these people could lead to an understanding of health behavior that would allow health teaching to increase the number of people who would take preventive action. Looking at how people utilize preventive or detection health services does not explain *why* they use such services. Little is known about the stability of health beliefs over time or about the acquisition of health beliefs. There may be different patterns of behavior for beliefs established early in life vs. those established later in life.[7,46,51]

Other research has suggested that health behaviors, no matter how well described and analyzed, might in fact *not* be predictably related to the impetus to seek preventive or diagnostic services.[26] Several items are thought to be significant other than as modifying factors for preventive and promotive health behaviors. Sex, socioeconomic status, and life-style are factors known to influence health behaviors.[33,58] Questions are being asked relative to the interrelationships among preventive and promotive behaviors. Is health behavior unidimensional, that is, are people consistent across health behaviors? Are people who use seat belts the same ones who obtain medical checkups, get preventive dental care, and engage in regular exercise? Or are health behaviors multidimensional, that is, independent and totally unrelated to each other? Or are there differing patterns of behavior; that is, some people are consistent in a variety of health behaviors while other people are inconsistent? Or are some behaviors performed consistently and others inconsistently, that is, preventive vs.

promotive behaviors? There is beginning evidence to support the concept that positive health behaviors are a part of a complex life-style that may reflect the ability to anticipate problems, mobilize to meet them, and cope actively.[44,53] These and other questions about health behaviors are receiving attention through continued research.[55] The cumulative research data presently available does allow the health care professional a beginning framework for identifying known barriers to and supports for preventive and promotive health behaviors.[21]

At-risk role

Research describes four states in which individuals can find themselves while fluctuating between various states of health and illness: healthy, at risk, convalescent, or ill. The term *healthy,* as applied by this study, is reserved for those persons who pursue no dangerous habits such as smoking, who do not engage in certain activities that involve directly some health hazard, and who are not in an age range in which there is a high risk from some designated health threat. Those persons who participate in activities that elevate their risk to a significant degree but who are neither convalescent nor ill are termed *at risk*. Convalescents are those who need treatment or rehabilitation before regaining their full working capacity. *Ill* persons are defined as persons under medical treatment or as individuals who must perform certain activities in addition to receiving medical treatment. Thus those individuals who according to the study are not healthy, convalescent, or ill constitute a group whose health status warrants their behaving in a way that will reduce their risk of illness, that is, assuming the at-risk role.[83]

Phases of the at-risk role

The above study describes four phases of the at-risk role. The first phase involves acquiring information related to a threat through mass media or through participating in screening procedures and applying that data to one's specific situation. The second phase involves validating the credibility of and attitudes toward both the threat and the recommended preventive action in the social milieu, that is, the lay system. The third phase involves pursuing medical validation of the threat and its applicability to the individual. The fourth phase is acceptance of the high-risk status and is accompanied by compliance with behaviors recommended in relation to the threat.[83]

Appraisal of the at-risk role

The tendency of healthy persons to accept the at-risk role is limited by several factors. First, the at-risk role possesses no rights, only responsibilities. The person at risk is expected to maintain the usual healthy-role responsibilities, to change or modify present behavior, and to do this with no right to social recognition for any achievements. Besides these disadvantages, the at-risk role is not time limited. Its appropriate behaviors could be required over a long period. Results of behaviors are not immediately evident, although they may have a positive outcome that is likely to be manifested in the remote future.[65] Further, the at-risk role is *noninstitutionalized,* and the assumption of it depends solely on the individual. That is, the person at risk must take action to reduce the risk status without the benefits of social reinforcement.

Many times the social environment will negatively reinforce the behaviors necessary for the at-risk role by tempting individuals to deviate from those necessary behaviors. Positive reinforcement, if there is any, could come in the form of additional information concerning the health threat.

Two final disadvantages of the at-risk role exist. First, the at-risk role is based on a statistical probability (as opposed to cause and effect) between certain behaviors and the health threat and often relates to diseases for which no cure exists. The role allows for no transfer of responsibility for cure to the medical profession, since the individual can be considered to be responsible for his or her own illness.

The research recommends that three criteria be met before the at-risk role can be implemented and produce viable results in achieving increased levels of wellness in our society. The first involves recognition and acceptance of the at-risk role. The second involves institutionalization of the at-risk role. All medical practitioners, since they are considered to be the legitimizing institution, would need to confirm the at-risk status and reinforce it periodically. The third criterion is the development of norms related to the at-risk role; that is, society would need to begin to regulate the demands and expectations related to this role. This would provide a basis for the social network of the person at risk to exert pressure to conform to those expectations.

Nursing could become involved in implementing the recognition and acceptance of the at-risk role by focusing on the value system of nursing. The validity of the nursing profession could become a significant part of the legitimizing force. Nurse practitioners, community health nurses, and others are presently discovering and validating the existence of the at-risk role in individuals and providing reinforcement to persons who have assumed the at-risk role. The concept of the at-risk role is presently utilized by many nurses teaching in clinics for birth control, hypertension, and obesity. It could easily become an integral part of every nurse's function to assess clients for their at-risk status and to follow through by reinforcing appropriate behaviors.

Illness behavior

Behavior during illness can be considered as a process with distinguishable phases or stages.

Stages of illness

The illness process can be viewed as a five-stage model that facilitates consideration of social, cultural, and psychologic implications of the illness experience. The five stages are symptom experience, assumption of the sick role, medical care contact, dependent patient role, and recovery or rehabilitation. The decisions, behaviors, and outcomes associated with each phase are summarized in Fig. 1-2.[92]

Symptom experience begins as the person makes a *decision* that something is wrong. This decision has three components: physical, cognitive, and emotional. The *physical* aspects include the presence of signs or symptoms, such as nausea, vomiting, or a rash. The *cognitive* aspects include the personal meaning that the signs and symptoms have for the individual. The *emotional* responses to the physical experience and cognitive interpretation constitute the third aspect.

A community survey based on this model demonstrates that pain was the most significant symptom experienced during the first phase, followed by fever and chills and shortness of breath. The initial signs and symptoms were extremely difficult to ignore, were usually severe, were continuous, and could not be alleviated by lay interventions. Most of the individuals, when faced with frightening and serious symptoms, thought immediately of seeking professional health care. This observation supports the premise that the severity of the symptoms determines the rapidity with which the ill individual seeks care from professionals.

Aspects of symptom experience that have meaning to health care professionals include the results of symptom denial, delay in seeking treatment, and possibly the use of illness for social or psychologic purposes as in hypochondriasis. It becomes a problem to establish a suitable balance between denial of symptoms and over-reaction to symptoms (hypochondriasis) at this stage. While chronic illness is insidious in its onset and not immediately productive of serious or incapacitating effects, it is nevertheless a major concern, and it is important that persons thus afflicted be encouraged to seek early health care.

The second stage of illness, the *assumption of the sick role*, involves a decision that one is ill and needs competent care. The ill individual now consults with selected respected lay persons. This serves two purposes. Validation is provided (or not provided) by the friend or relative consulted that the person really is sick. If validation is given, there is a *provisional excuse*

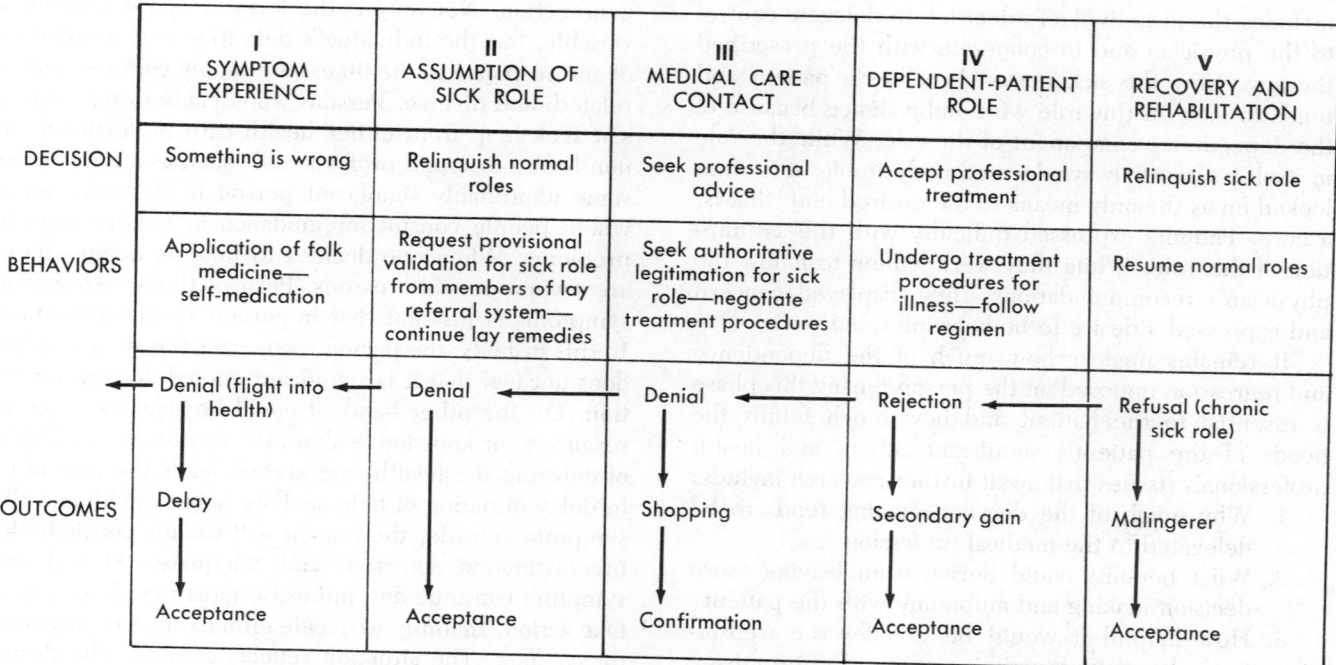

	I SYMPTOM EXPERIENCE	II ASSUMPTION OF SICK ROLE	III MEDICAL CARE CONTACT	IV DEPENDENT-PATIENT ROLE	V RECOVERY AND REHABILITATION
DECISION	Something is wrong	Relinquish normal roles	Seek professional advice	Accept professional treatment	Relinquish sick role
BEHAVIORS	Application of folk medicine—self-medication	Request provisional validation for sick role from members of lay referral system—continue lay remedies	Seek authoritative legitimation for sick role—negotiate treatment procedures	Undergo treatment procedures for illness—follow regimen	Resume normal roles
OUTCOMES	Denial (flight into health) ↓ Delay ↓ Acceptance	Denial ↓ Acceptance	Denial ↓ Shopping ↓ Confirmation	Rejection ↓ Secondary gain ↓ Acceptance	Refusal (chronic sick role) ↓ Malingerer ↓ Acceptance

Fig. 1-2. Stages of illness experience. (From Coe, R.: Sociology of medicine, New York, © 1970, McGraw-Hill Book Co. Used with permission of McGraw-Hill Book Co.)

for nonperformance of usual role obligations. It is provisional because American society requires that a health professional legitimize one's entrance into the sick role.

The ill person seeks *advice* as well as validation. It was found that the majority of people in the survey did discuss their illnesses, usually with one other person, most often their spouse. This discussion occurred before seeking medical help, and almost all discussion took place as soon as the signs and symptoms were noticed.

The majority of the persons consulted by the sick individual also interpreted the signs and symptoms as illness, and most of them recommended seeking professional assistance. Sick persons tended to follow the options suggested by the lay consultant, whether the advice was to seek medical assistance, begin self-treatment, or await further developments. On the whole the discussion process provided a necessary and usually positive impetus toward seeking adequate care.

The *medical care contact stage* involves the decision to seek medical care, that is, to obtain a diagnosis, prognosis, and treatment plan from a medical source. It is here that the person receives authoritative permission to assume the sick role. If such validation is not forthcoming, the sick individual either returns to normal role and status obligations or continues seeking professional opinions until an acceptable diagnosis is found. During this stage most of the individuals in the survey did in fact receive diagnoses, prognoses, and plans of care that they were able to accept.

The fourth stage, the *dependent patient role stage*, includes the ill individual's decision to delegate control to the physician and to cooperate with the prescribed therapy. Now the sick person becomes a patient and tends to look on this role with ambivalence because of the dependency component of the role. While the role in itself is almost always deemed undesirable, it is often looked on as the only means to the desired end, that is, a cure. Patients expressed difficulty with the assumption of this role. While they were willing to follow the physician's recommendations, they displayed concern and expressed a desire to be kept informed.

It remains unclear how much of the dependency and regression imposed on the person during this phase is essential to the patient and how much fulfills the needs of the patient's significant others and health professionals. Issues that await further research include:
1. Why much of the decision making tends to be delegated to the medical profession
2. What benefits could derive from leaving more decision making and autonomy with the patient
3. How helpful it would be to offer the well-informed patient the choice of feasible, promising treatments rather than leave the selection entirely to the professional

The fifth and final stage; *recovery and rehabilitation*, involves the decision to relinquish the sick role. During this phase the individual resumes normal roles and tasks and rejoins the world of the well. In acute limited illness, there are generally no major problems encountered in resuming normal roles. In chronic illness, however, this can be more demanding and the return to normal roles more difficult.

During this phase the majority of persons were being cared for at home and reported satisfaction with their care. It was concluded that most patients are either satisfied with their care or reluctant to complain. Patients who do not successfully accomplish the tasks of this final stage are identified as malingerers.

The major and recurrent concerns of persons during the entire illness experience were variations of questions about chances of full recovery, residual effects of the illness, ability to carry on usual activities, and method of payment for services.

Variations of this model are being developed to further define and analyze illness behavior in specific situations, such as emergency or life-threatening conditions.[2]

Types of illness behavior

Illness behavior can be of various types. The individual can take action for symptom relief, take no action, vacillate, or take counteraction.[80]

Illness behavior involves symptom perception, evaluation, and response. The individual reacts or does not react to such cues or symptoms as pain, discomfort, or malfunction. Not only is the form of illness extremely variable, but the individual's definition and recognition of and response to the illness are highly complex, interrelated, and diverse. Persons who decide to *take action* can seek help from either health care professionals or non-health-oriented professionals, such as a minister or some identifiably significant person in the community whom people consult for guidance in various sorts of problems. When one decides to *take no action*, there are several possible reasons. Perhaps the appearance of symptoms is just not that important to the individual. In this instance the person recognizes the symptom but does not feel that it is significant enough to warrant action. On the other hand, it could be that fear, lack of resources (or knowledge about the resources), or dislike of entering the health care system leads the individual to delay initiation of help-seeking behavior. Should the symptom subside, the person will usually consider the procrastination effective and adequate. Should the symptom continue and intensify, most people will then take action. Inability to decide either way can cause one to *vacillate*. The situation reflects conflict. The desire to take action is present, but some type of cost to the individual remains a significant deterrent. *Taking coun-

teraction is a form of denial. It consists of attempting to demonstrate that no illness exists. This behavior opposes definition and assessment of the symptoms and resists action to alleviate or correct them. This type of response to illness can be labeled *deviant illness behavior,* or "pathological health."[56] The term does not apply, however, to the behaviors demonstrated by persons who, perhaps due to lack of knowledge of the situation, do not realize that the symptoms could be illness related.[80]

The type of illness behavior demonstrated by the individual is probably determined by a number of variables:

1. Visibility and importance of the symptoms
2. Perceived seriousness of the situation
3. Degree of discomfort caused by the symptoms
4. Tolerance threshold of the individual experiencing the symptoms
5. Interpretation of the symptoms
6. Availability and accessibility of treatment resources[88]

Utility of studying illness behavior

Since almost all health care is delivered on the initiative of individuals who choose to seek professional help, the study of illness behavior is very important. If we are to understand how persons select themselves for professional health care, then we must learn more about how they define themselves as ill and decide to take action.[52,57] Attention needs to be focused on the nonusers of health care.

Attempts have been made to define illness behavior by determining the prevalence of signs and symptoms that do *not* receive medical attention but are socially and medically significant and consequential. One hypothesis states that bodily deviations can be potentially contained within social situations, and if contained these deviations will not reach medical attention. There is evidence accumulating that illness or some type of health status deviation is almost an everyday occurrence and will only result in contact with a health professional in highly selected situations.[3]

If too much attention is devoted to examining the characteristics of those who do seek professional care while relatively little attention is turned to those who do not seek care, an unbalanced, or biased, understanding of illness behavior could result. Once the motivating factors influencing both use and nonuse of professional health care are understood, improved educational programs geared toward increasing options for those experiencing illness can be developed. The study of illness behavior can also increase the accuracy of history taking. Response tendencies that are a part of a person's illness behavior pattern, such as denial, adversely influence the diagnostic process. Illness behav-

ior patterns could influence the patient's response to varying treatment modalities; an awareness of these response patterns could improve compliance with therapy regimens.

Sick role

Being sick may result in the person's inability to perform normally expected roles and tasks. Our society has institutionalized a set of expectations and sanctions regarding the behavior of persons unable to perform their usual roles because of illness: the sick role.

Components of the sick role

On assuming the sick role the person is exempted from normal social roles and responsibilities as necessitated by the kind and severity of the illness. Being exempted from normal social roles requires that the illness be legitimized, usually by a physician. The sick person is not considered responsible for an acquired illness; that is, the individual cannot be expected to get well by personal volition. "He can't help it." Being ill is seen as undesirable; the sick person is expected to want to get well and to seek technically competent help.[91]

Three factors produce variations in the sick role: the unique background and experience of the individual, the specific disease process and its severity, and the interactional context in which the person seeks to assume the role. It has been suggested that the demands placed on the individual by roles other than the sick role may cause the greatest variation in assumption of the sick role.[50]

The necessity for legitimizing the illness and seeking competent help confers on the therapeutic agency a method for social control. These agencies are allowed to regulate and define the individual illness process as well as facilitate recovery from the illness state.[91] *Negative control* is exerted through isolating the sick person, both from other sick persons and from the healthy. This accomplishes two goals: the sick cannot reinforce the illness behavior of others, and there does not develop a subculture of sick people; and it decreases the visibility of the sick role and thus decreases the likelihood that healthy people will choose to imitate it.

Society exerts *positive control* by having sick persons place themselves under the control of therapeutic agencies. This places the ill persons in a situation of dependency on health professionals, not on others who are ill.

Assessment of the sick role paradigm

Questions have been raised about the applicability of the sick role paradigm to all types of illnesses.[50] It could be argued that the sick role paradigm is less applicable to the person with a mental illness than to the person with a physical illness, since the mentally ill are seen as more responsible for their illness, mental illness is less acceptable than physical illness as legitimized illness, and those who are mentally ill often maintain the ability to perform their normal social roles.[17,29]

Similar concerns have been raised regarding the applicability of the sick role paradigm to the chronically ill. Health professionals do not encourage the chronically ill to define their states as undesirable but to accept and learn to live with their limitations. The chronically ill often are able to perform some of their social roles and thus are not exempted from total responsibility to society. The maintenance care required by the chronically ill person requires that the individual assume a great deal of responsibility for his or her own condition rather than having the health professional assume such responsibility. The utility of the sick role paradigm has also been questioned for those who are aging, abusing drugs or alcohol, suicidal, or pregnant.[64]

The legitimized sick role requires the seeking of technically competent help, yet most persons do not consult a health professional when ill. Often their illnesses are legitimized by family members or friends. Some individuals simply exempt themselves from their usual roles by going to bed. Individuals with some acute illnesses, such as venereal disease, may desire to get well, seek technically competent help, but continue to perform their usual roles.

Several aspects of the sick role require further research:

1. Whether different groups of people have different expectations of the sick role
2. Which specific role and task exemptions are permissible with which types of illnesses
3. How significant others influence sick role expectations
4. Whether different illnesses elicit different types of sick role behavior
5. Whether people accept responsibility for contracting certain illnesses
6. Whether there are changing behavioral expectations over time while one is experiencing the sick role[37,68]

Deviance, health, and illness

Deviance implies the violation of the norms of a group or society.[42] Persons who are ill might be considered deviant if they are no longer able to meet the expectations associated with their roles.[48]

Deviant behaviors violate norms, nondeviant behaviors do not. Variant behaviors depart from specified norms but are still within a permissible or acceptable range.[76] In this context primary deviance occurs when a person defined as normal commits a deviant act; for example, a non-drug-user experiments once with drugs. Secondary deviance occurs when a person defined as deviant commits a deviant act; for example, a "drug abuser" habitually uses drugs.

Labeling a person as deviant alters the expectations that the person will behave normally and may perpetuate the deviance. Labeling the chronically ill or physically handicapped as deviant results in stereotypic expectations that they will not be able to perform adequately in certain situations. Employers and others may consequently deny the chronically ill or handicapped the opportunity to demonstrate their abilities.

Illness can be differentiated from other forms of deviance, for example, crime and sin. The criminal and the sinner commit their acts volitionally, whereas ill persons lack voluntary control over their health state. The social response to sin and crime is punishment in hopes of eliciting conformity. The social response to the sick person is to use some form of therapy to change the factors that prevent that person from conforming. In all situations there are role changes inasmuch as the sinner, criminal, and ill person are pronounced incapable of accepting full responsibility for their behavior: others must intervene to control their behavior.

Several investigators have criticized the *deviance model* of illness,[5,76] yet others believe that the deviance model has utility for the health field.[82] The deviance model allows labeling of populations as deviant rather than labeling individuals. The labeling of populations, such as smokers, as deviant would then allow health professionals the right and give them the responsibility to change unhealthy situations. This change would be accomplished by social sanctions and pressures and education to change the deviants into conformists. However effective it might be, this approach does little to foster individual autonomy and responsibility for health.[83]

Medicine as an institution is increasingly assuming more responsibility for controlling deviant behaviors.[76, 91] Some behaviors that in previous eras would have been defined as sin or crime and controlled by religious or legal institutions are now being defined as illness and being controlled through medical institutions.

Simultaneously, legal and religious institutions are increasingly adopting medical approaches to control deviance. Churches utilize the mental health model of deviance to provide pastoral counseling similar to psychotherapy. The legal profession often chooses confinement to mental institutions rather than imprisonment, and prisons now frequently define rehabilitation rather than punishment as their goal.

Szasz,[75] a psychiatrist and well-known crusader for the rights of individuals, warns against this medicalization of social deviance. In his view medicine, sociology, psychiatry, and psychology should have nothing to say about whether a person ought to be free to use drugs, commit suicide, engage in homosexual acts, or have delusions. The potential ability to injure or destroy oneself is a basic freedom and there are no grounds for regarding self-injury as a crime to be controlled by police power. Szasz warns of the "therapeutic state," a society in which government, advised by health professionals, increasingly makes individuals' decisions for them. Self-determination is replaced by a powerful medicopsychiatric complex, a subtle and yet real threat to individual liberty. The medicopsychiatric complex has grown in the last decades to a government monopoly that has a strong voice in public policy and legislative decisions. It is armed with federal funds to provide therapy when people get out of line.

Maslow asks for studies of the *positive effects* of deviance, a much neglected area of study. Culture can never be advanced without persons who are not afraid to be different. He asks why these persons are usually seen as pathologic and if deviance can be healthy.[87]

The labeling of behavior as deviant can be confined to those areas that impinge on the rights of others. Certain behaviors that have been labeled deviant are presently being reconsidered. Homosexuality can be used to illustrate this. At one time homosexuality was defined as a psychiatric illness. Now it has been removed from this illness status and is considered one of the variations of normal. Nursing could be a force in preventing the labeling of behaviors as deviant when in fact they are only variant, thus increasing individual freedom and the number of acceptable options available to people.

Summary

Several models of health, disease, and illness have been presented. As health professionals, nurses need to be familiar with such models and the research based on them to enhance the conceptual bases of their practice. If the goal of nursing is to help people move toward improvement of their health status, then the practitioner needs to ascertain the patient's or client's philosophy of health and illness and also the professional's own view of health and illness. The client's concept of health and illness will be an influential modifier of behavior and will be a prime determinant of goals relative to health. How nurses define health and illness will influence the goals they try to set with clients. The nursing interventions selected by individual nurses, and indeed by the nursing profession as a whole, will be determined largely by theoretical beliefs about health and illness. The effective functioning of nurses may be based on their ability to bring their own and their clients' beliefs, theories, and attitudes to the conscious level. At this level the nurse and client can examine, refine, add, or modify knowledge and attitudes of the health and illness process.

REFERENCES AND SELECTED READINGS
Contemporary

1. Alan, D.K., and Boldt, J.: A study of preventive health attitudes and behaviors in a family practice setting, J. Fam. Pract. **11:**77-84, 1980.
2. Alonzo, A.A.: Acute illness behavior: a conceptual exploration and specification, Soc. Sci. Med. **14A:**515-526, 1980.
3. Alonzo, A.A.: Everyday illness: a situational approach to health status deviations, Soc. Sci. Med. **13A:**397-404, 1979.
4. Ardell, D.B.: The nature and implications of high level wellness, or why "normal health" is a rather sorry state of existence, Health Values: Achieving High Level Wellness **3:**17-24, 1979.
5. Armstrong, D.: The structure of medical education, Med. Educ. **11:**244-248, 1977.
6. Becker, M.H.: Research on health behavior (editorial), J. Community Health **3:**97-99, 1977.
7. Becker, M.H., Drachman, R.H., and Kirschit, J.: A new approach to explaining sick-role behavior in low income populations, Am. J. Public Health **64:**205-216, 1974.
8. Bell, J.M.: Stressful life events and coping methods in mental-illness and -wellness behaviors, Nurs. Res. **26:**136-141, 1977.
9. Belloc, N.B.: Relationship of health practices and mortality, Prev. Med. **2:**67-81, 1973.
10. Belloc, N.B., and Breslow, L.: Relationship of physical health status and health practices, Prev. Med. **1:**409-421, 1972.
11. Bibace, R., and Walsh, M.: Development of children's concepts of illness, Pediatrics **66:**912-917, 1980.
12. Breslow, L., and Enstrom, J.E.: Persistence of health habits and their relationship to mortality, Prev. Med. **9:**469-483, 1980.
13. Brown, J., and Raulinson, M.: Relinquishing the sick-role following open heart surgery, J. Health Soc. Behav. **16:**12-27, 1975.
14. Bullough, B.: Poverty, ethnic identity and preventive health care, J. Health Soc. Behav. **13:**347-359, 1972.
15. Cassel, E.J.: Disease as an "it": concepts of disease revealed by patients' presentation of symptoms, Soc. Sci. Med. **10:**143-146, 1976.
16. Chalfant, P., and Kurts, P.: Alcoholics and the sick-role: assessments by social workers, J. Health Soc. Behav. **12:**66-72, 1971.
17. Cheetham, R.W., and Rzadkowolski, A.: Crosscultural psychiatry and the concept of mental illness, S. Afr. Med. J. **58:**320-325, 1975.
18. Coburn, D., and Pope, C.R.: Socioeconomic status and preventive health behavior, J. Health Soc. Behav. **15:**67-78, 1974.
19. Coe, R.: Sociology of medicine, New York, 1970, McGraw-Hill Book Co.
20. Cole, S., and Lejune, R.: Illness and the legitimization of failure, Am. Sociol. Rev. **37:**347-356, 1972.
21. Coulton, C.: Factors related to preventive health behavior: implications for social work intervention, Soc. Work Health Care **3:**297-310, 1978.
22. Demers, R.W., et al.: An explanation of the dimensions of illness behavior, J. Fam. Pract. **11:**1085-1092, 1980.
23. Diekelmann, N.: Wellness: approaches and resources, Nurse Pract. **5:**41-44, 1980.
24. Dolfman, M.: Toward an operational definition of health, J. School Health **43:**206-209, 1974.
25. Dougherty, C.J., and Walker, V.R.: Scientific medicine, tech-

nology, and the concept of health, Ethics Sci. Med. **5**:75-81, 1978.

26. Dowie, J.: The portfolio approach to health behavior, Soc. Sci. Med. **9**:619-631, 1975.

27. Dubos, R.: Man overadapting, Psychology Today **4**:50-53, 1971.

28. Dunn, H.L.: What high level wellness means, Health Values: Achieving High Level Wellness **1**:9-16, 1977.

29. Fabrega, H.: The position of psychiatric illness in biomedical theory: a cultural analysis, J. Med. Philos. **5**:145-168, 1980.

30. Fabrega, H.: Toward a model of illness behavior, Med. Care **11**:470-484, 1973.

31. Fink, D.L.: Holistic health: implications for health planning, Am. J. Health Planning **1**:23-31, 1976.

32. Flynn, P.R.: Holistic health: the art and science of care, Bowie, Md., 1980, Robert J. Brady Co.

33. Fredric, D., and Wolinsky, S.R.: Background attitudinal and behavioral patterns of individuals occupying eight discrete health states, Sociol. Health Illness **3**:31-48, 1981.

34. Fry, P.W.: The scientific method and its impact on holistic health, Sociol. Health Illness **2**:1-7, 1980.

35. Gerson, E.: The social character of illness: deviance of politics? Soc. Sci. Med. **10**:219-224, 1976.

36. Hern, W.M.: The illness parameters of pregnancy, Soc. Sci. Med. **9**:365-372, 1975.

37. Hover, J., and Juelsgaard, N.: The sick role reconceptualized, Nurs. Forum **17**:407-416, 1978.

38. Jago, J.: Hal—old word—new task, Soc. Sci. Med. **9**:1-6, 1975.

39. Jeffers, J.: Wellness: teaching students to assess, Health Values: Achieving High Level Wellness **4**:119-123, 1980.

40. Keller, M.J.: Toward a definition of health, Adv. Nurs. Sci. **4**:43-64, 1980.

41. Kelman, S.: Social organization and the meaning of health, J. Med. Philos. **5**:133-144, 1980.

42. Koltow, M.: Defining health, Med. Hypotheses **6**:1097-1104, 1980.

43. Kurtz, R., and Glacopassi, D.J.: Medical and social work students' perceptions of deviant conditions and sick role incumbency, Soc. Sci. Med. **9**:249-255, 1975.

44. Langlie, J.K.: Interrelationships among preventive health behaviors: a test of competing hypotheses, Public Health Rep. **94**:216-225, 1979.

45. Leavitt, F.: The health belief model and utilization of ambulatory care services, Soc. Sci. Med. **13A**:105-112, 1979.

46. Lewis, C.E., and Lewis, M.A.: Child-initiated health care, J. School Health **49**:144-148, 1980.

47. Lewis, W.R.: Health behavior and quality assurance, Nurs. Clin. North Am. **9**:359-366, 1974.

48. Macleod, A.: Illness as a deviant role: a clue to the rejection of symptoms, Nurs. Times **74**:1400-1401, 1978.

49. Magi, M., and Allander, E.: Toward a theory of perceived and medically defined need, Sociol. Health Illness **3**:49-71, 1981.

50. McKinlay, J.: The sick role: illness and pregnancy, Soc. Sci. Med. **6**:561-572, 1972.

51. Mechanic, D.: The stability of health and illness behavior: results from a sixteen year follow up, Am. J. Public Health **69**:1142-1145, 1979.

52. Mechanic, D.: Effects of psychological distress on perceptions of physical health and use of medical psychiatric facilities, J. Human Stress **4**:26-32, 1978.

53. Mechanic, D., and Cleary, P.: Factors associated with the maintenance of positive health behavior, Prev. Med. **9**:805-814, 1980.

54. Mercer, J.R.: Who is normal? Two perspectives on mild mental retardation. In Jaco, E.G.: Patients, physicians and illness, New York, 1972, The Free Press.

55. Mikhail, B.: The health belief model: a review and critical eval-

uation of the model, research and practice, Adv. Nurs. Sci. **4**:65-82, 1981.

56. Musaph, H.: The right of falling ill: on pathological health behavior, Psychother. Psychosom. **31**:19-23, 1979.

57. Najam, J.M.: Theories of disease causation and the concept of a general susceptibility: a review, Soc. Sci. Med. **14A**:231-237, 1980.

58. Nathanson, C.A.: Sex roles as variables in preventive health behavior, J. Community Health **3**:142-155, 1977.

59. *Oelbaum, C.H.: Hallmarks of adult wellness, Am. J. Nurs. **74**:1623-1625, 1974.

60. Pelletier, K.R.: In search of optimal health, Med. Self-Care, pp. 48-50, Winter 1980.

61. *Peters, B.M.: School-aged children's beliefs about causality of illness: a review of the literature, Matern. Child Nurs. J. **7**:143-154, 1978.

62. Rankin, W.R.: Concepts of illness and care of the ill, Ethics Sci. Med. **6**:239-243, 1979.

63. Reif, A.E.: High level wellness and low level wellness: an overview, Health Values: Achieving High Level Wellness **2**:198-210, 1978.

64. Ries, J.K.: Public acceptance of the disease concept of alcoholism, J. Health Soc. Behav. **18**:338-344, 1977.

65. Robbins, L.C., and Hall, J.H.: Perspective medicine, ed. 2, Indianapolis, 1979, Methodist Hospital of Indiana.

66. Rosenstock, I.: The health belief model and preventive health behavior, Health Educ. Monog. **2**:354-386, 1974.

67. Rosenstock, I.: Historical origins of the health belief model, Health Educ. Monogr. **2**:328-335, 1974.

68. Segall, A.: The sick role concept: understanding illness behavior, J. Health Soc. Behav. **17**:163-170, 1976.

69. Segall, A.: Sociocultural variation in sick role behavioral expectations, Soc. Sci. Med. **10**:47-51, 1976.

70. Shuval, J., and Antonovsky, A.: Illness: a mechanism for coping with failure, Soc. Sci. Med. **7**:259-265, 1973.

71. *Smith, J.A.: The idea of health: a philosophical inquiry, Adv. Nurs. Sci. **3**:43-50, 1981.

72. Sontag, S.: Illness as a metaphor, New York, 1979, Vintage Books.

73. Suchman, E.A.: Accidents and social deviance, J. Health Soc. Behav. **11**:4-15, 1970.

74. Suchman, E.A.: Health attitudes and behavior, Arch. Environ. Health **20**:105-110, 1970.

75. Szasz, T.: Our despotic laws destroy the right to self-control, Psychology Today **8**:19-127, 1974.

76. Twaddle, A.C.: Illness and deviance, Soc. Sci. Med. **7**:751-762, 1973.

77. White, K.L.: Life, death and medicine, San Francisco, 1973, W.H. Freeman & Co., Publishers.

78. Williams, J.S.: Disease as deviance, Soc. Sci. Med. **5**:219-226, 1971.

79. Wilson, R.: The sociology of health: an introduction, New York, 1979, Random House, Inc.

80. Wu, R.: Behavior and illness, Englewood Cliffs, N.J., 1973, Prentice-Hall, Inc.

Classic

81. Apple, D.: How laymen define illness, J. Health Soc. Behav. **1**:219-225, 1960.

82. Baric, L.: Conformity and deviance in health and illness, Int. J. Health Educ. **12**:2-12, 1969.

83. Baric, L.: Recognition of the at-risk role: a means to influence behavior, Int. J. Health Educ. **12**:24-34, 1969.

*References preceded by an asterisk are particularly well suited for student reading.

84. Bauman, B.: Diversities in conceptions of health and physical fitness, J. Health Soc. Behav. **2:**39-46, 1961.

85. Dunn, H.: High-level wellness, Arlington, Va., 1961, R.W. Beatty, Ltd.

86. Kasl, S.V., and Cobb, S.: Health behavior, illness behavior, and sick role behavior, Arch. Environ. Health **12:**246-266, 1966.

87. Maslow, A.H.: Motivation and personality, New York, 1954, Harper & Row, Publishers.

88. Mechanic, D.: Medical sociology: a selective view, New York, 1968, The Free Press.

89. Mechanic, D.: The concept of illness behavior, J. Chronic Dis. **15:**189-194, 1962.

90. Mechanic, D.: Illness behavior and medical diagnosis, J. Health Soc. Behav. **1:**86-94, 1960.

91. Parsons, T.: Definitions of health and illness in the light of American values and social structure. In Jaco, E.G.: Patients, physicians and illness, New York, 1958, The Free Press.

92. Suchman, E.A.: Stages of illness and medical care, J. Health Soc. Behav. **6:**114-128, 1965.

CHAPTER 2

INTRODUCTION TO THE SYSTEMS APPROACH

JANET LARSON GELEIN

Biomedicine is a term applied to medicine in Western nations; it encompasses knowledge, practice, organizations, and social roles.[12] The biomedical model that guides beliefs and actions today in health care has been predominantly influenced by the science of molecular biology. The influence of molecular biology on medicine and the study of disease has resulted in the assumption that disease may be fully accounted for by deviations of measurable biologic variables from the norm. The assumption seems to be that many of the values of key physiologic and chemical variables in humans conform to narrow ranges that are common to the entire species. Deviations from health are viewed in physicalistic terms: the sciences of chemistry and physics are used to explain the phenomena accompanying disease.[12] The limitations of this approach are that it separates the body and the mind and that it neglects the social, psychologic, and behavioral dimensions of illness.

When an individual experiences an alteration in health, that individual's past experiences will determine reactions to the illness and the actions taken in an attempt to regain health. Likewise, society and the culture in which the individual lives will affect perception of and give meaning to the altered states of functioning. "The level of function, the efficiency, and the flexibility of a biologic system are affected by the kind of environment in which the individual lives."[11] Thus cultural, social, and psychologic variables, as well as biologic phenomena, need to be considered in conjunction with alterations in health. The tendency to ignore these variables and to separate the psyche from the soma may be attributable to the lack of models that integrate the various sciences into a unified, holistic perspective of humanity and health.

General systems theory

General systems theory provides a perspective for the consideration of humanity and nature in the context of wholes. It is a model for organizing and examining holistic relationships, an alternative to the reductionistic, physicalistic models that have promoted illness care by specialization around organ systems. The purposes of this chapter are to describe general systems theory and identify fundamental qualities of open systems, to consider the development of a systems approach for nursing, and to explore the application of systems concepts to the developing science of nursing.

Von Bertalanffy, a theoretical biologist, is generally credited with the development of the science of systems. The systems sciences consider a number of different interacting characteristics of nature and examine these characteristics as whole under diverse conditions. The systems sciences grew out of diversity and ever increasing specialization. Scientists from many disciplines, independent of one another, were studying similar problems and exploring similar concepts. However, a common language that would enable investigators from multiple disciplines to communicate with each other was lacking. The development of general systems theory enabled scientists to derive principles that apply to any system, irrespective of the particular properties or elements of the system involved. These principles are valid for systems in general, whatever the nature of their component elements or the relationship of forces between them.

Living systems: basic concepts

A system may broadly be defined as a set of units with relationships among them.[47] These *components*, or units, interact with each other and possess a *boundary*, which is capable of filtering both the kind and rate of flow of inputs that enter the system and outputs that leave the system.[32]

The *state* of a system refers to the value that is given to a set of system variables at a given instant in time. The state of a system changes continuously over time.[43]

One way to evaluate the state of a system is by classifying the system as closed or open. A *closed system* is one that does not exchange matter or energy with its environment. Conventional physics and physical chemistry are limited to the examination of processes in closed systems. The laws of thermodynamics apply only to closed systems. In fact, the second law of thermodynamics states that in a closed system entropy will increase to a maximum and eventually the process will come to a stop at a state of equilibrium.[47] *Entropy*, the energy cost that cannot be recovered from any reaction, accumulates in closed systems. Because matter, energy, or information cannot enter or leave a closed system, the system becomes increasingly disorganized as the amount of stored energy is utilized. In closed systems, entropy is always increasing. As a result order is continuously destroyed.[47]

Living systems are open systems. An *open system* exchanges matter, energy, and information with its environment, has inputs into its boundaries and outputs into the environment, and constantly builds up and breaks down its material components.[47] Although living systems have some characteristics similar to those of closed systems, or systems in equilibrium, we cannot consider living systems as in equilibrium, or closed systems. Even though cells have a certain composition and react to disturbances in ways similar to chemical reactions, there is a fundamental difference between chemical equilibria and metabolizing, living organisms. The organism is *not* a static system for it is not closed to the environment and does not always contain identical components. Rather, it is an open system in a quasi-steady state.

The *steady state* of open systems is maintained by means of a continuous exchange of component matter and energy. Matter is continually entering from the environment and leaving the system to the environment. The openness of a system, then, refers to the ability of the system to exchange matter, energy, or information with its environment.

The steady state of an open system may be defined as a relative state of balance: a dynamic equilibrium. Von Bertalanffy believes that a steady state exists when the composition of the system is relatively constant despite continuous exchange of matter.[47]

Open systems have the capability to import matter as the potential carrier of free energy, or "negative entropy."[47] Negative entropy, or *negentropy*, is the capability of open systems to take in inputs of matter or energy that are higher in complexity of organization than their outputs. Negentropy makes it possible for an open system to restore energy and prevent breakdowns. Living systems adapt through maintaining a steady negentropic state.

Along with the ability to adapt, open systems exhibit a dynamic process called *equifinality*. Whereby closed systems eventually reach thermodynamic equilibrium, open systems may attain a steady state that has a value equifinal or independent of initial conditions. In other words, independent states or goals in open systems may be reached from different initial conditions in different ways at the same time. One example of this concept may be seen in the development of a human being, which may occur from the fertilization of one whole ova or from the fertilization of a divided ovum as with identical twins. Both processes may eventually result in the birth of a normal human infant. Likewise, two infants of different heights and weights may arrive at the same final state, a certain species-specific adult size, despite possible intervening variables disturbing or inhibiting growth in childhood.[47]

Hierarchy of systems

The systems view allows us to understand that humanity is one species with values and intrinsic worth in a hierarchy of nature. Life begins with complex macromolecules, such as genes and viruses, which may be organized and integrated with chemical substances to form cells. Cells may be organized into tissues and organs, which may be further integrated into organisms that are capable of organization into groups, organizations, communities, and societies. This hierarchy of complexity can extend to multinational systems.[23]

When using systems theory it is imperative to identify the level of reference one is using. To avoid confusion the following terms are used in this chapter to identify the level of reference for systems analysis. *System* refers to the identified level on which we are focusing. *Suprasystem* refers to the level above the focal system, and *subsystem* refers to the level below the identified system. All systems tend to function by maintaining steady states, keeping an orderly balance among subsystems within the system, their environments, and suprasystems. There are inputs across the boundary of a system to the subsystems; internal processes that utilize energy, matter, or information; and outputs from the system to suprasystems. Humanity is considered as one system in hierarchical structure of nature that occurs in multiple levels, each level reflecting its own variant of general systems characteristics.

Fundamental qualities of open systems

When defining an open system consideration should be given to three fundamental qualities: structure, process, and function. *Structure* refers to the arrangement of all defined components of a system at a given moment in time. Miller[23] defines the structure of a system as three dimensional, remaining relatively fixed or changing depending on the characteristics of the process of the system at that particular time.

The model of a simple feedback control scheme in Fig. 2-1 illustrates the basic structure of an open system. The *environment* external to an open system consists of all those elements that affect the system and are likewise affected by the system. The *boundary* of a system is permeable and delineates intrasystemic processes from extrasystemic elements. All boundaries of open systems are dynamic in that they function by continually exchanging information, energy, or matter with their environments.[47] The boundary of a system may be viewed as a filter through which inputs and outputs must pass and it functions in a manner that differentiates processes within the system from those outside the boundaries of the system. The boundary controls both the rate and flow of inputs and outputs. The processes within the boundaries of the system (subsystem processes) are mutually attracted or balanced in a way that permits the system to function as a whole. The exchange of energy or the intensity of interaction is greater between elements within the boundary of a system than between those elements outside the boundary.

Process refers to the transformation of energy, information, or matter in a system over time and incorporates the function of a system. *Function* relates to the interaction between component parts.

The exchange of matter, energy, or information between the environment and the identified system occurs through the processes of input, throughput (systems processing), output, and feedback. *Input* to a system occurs when matter, energy, or information is obtained by the system. Once the system absorbs this input, it processes or transforms the information or energy in a way that is useful to its function in a process called *throughput* and then expels or discharges matter, information, and energy in the process of output. *Output* is energy, matter, or information disposed of by the system as a consequence of its function.

Feedback refers to the process of self-regulation in open systems and involves the system's ability to control input and output. Negative feedback reduces deviation and positive feedback amplifies deviation from the steady state. If the system's negative feedback is disrupted, its steady state vanishes, and ultimately its boundary disappears and the system terminates. Feedback mechanisms in open systems allow them to maintain steady states and to adapt.[23]

Adaptation to the environment may be accomplished by means of certain boundary maintenance functions. The boundary can contain undesirable elements in the environment; obtain needed matter, energy, or information (inputs); retain these as necessary; and dispose of unwanted or unnecessary matter (outputs).[34]

It is also suggested that integration and decision making are processes critical to the survival of a system. Integration of the components of a system is essential for the system to function effectively and to persist. The integration of components requires patterns of interaction between the components. Decision making refers to the process by which resources for adaptation and integration are allocated.

Development of a systems approach for nursing

Historical perspective

If we closely examine publications of early nursing leaders we find that some of them seemed to view disease as it more recently was described from a systems perspective. Von Bertalanffy describes disease as a life process that regulates toward normalcy after a disturbance, this regulation toward normalcy being attributable to the equifinality of biologic systems.[47] In 1859 Florence Nightingale expressed similar beliefs about disease. She asserted that all disease was a reparative process and was not necessarily accompanied by suffer-

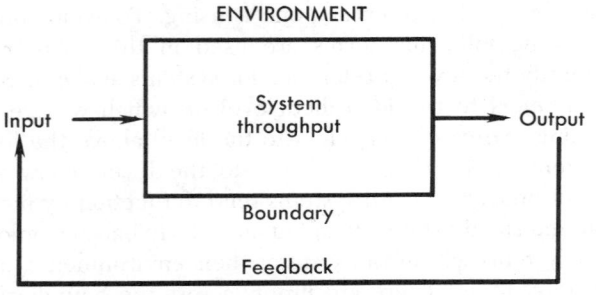

Fig. 2-1. Simple control scheme involves input, throughput, and output. Feedback provides a self-regulating mechanism for the organism.

ing. Nightingale conceived of disease as an effort of nature to repair destructive processes.[44] When disease is viewed as a life process moving toward normalcy, roles of health professionals can be viewed as supplementary to this process.

Von Bertalanffy considers the role of medicine to be an expression of dynamic systems and thus, to the extent possible, maintaining and reestablishing the steady state.[47] Again comparing Von Bertalanffy's ideas about the role of medicine with Florence Nightingale's, we find some similarities. Nightingale considered medicine as doing nothing more than assisting nature—only nature was believed to cure. She suggested that nursing's goal was to assist the patient to attain the optimal condition for nature to act.[44] In 1885, Clara Weeks Shaw, another nursing leader, expressed a view similar to that of Nightingale. She spoke of the role of the nurse as keeping the patient in the state most conducive for natural reparative tendencies.[45] Even though the concepts of systems theory were not refined by Von Bertalanffy until 1968, there are similarities between his statements about disease and medicine and Nightingale's and Shaw's earlier descriptions of disease and the role of nursing.

Rogers[28] would probably be identified as the first nurse to introduce a theoretical basis for nursing that recognized the person as a system whose characteristics are identifiably those of the whole. She proposed a conceptual model for nursing that envisioned the individual as an open system: more than and different from the sum of the parts, continually exchanging matter and energy with the environment.

Since Rogers's writings, several texts have been published in nursing that consider a systems perspective for nursing practice.[5,7,16,26] The reader is encouraged to consult these or other texts for alternative viewpoints on the application of systems theory to nursing practice. The remainder of this chapter *considers one conception* for the application of systems theory to nursing practice. First nursing will be defined and then a systems model for nursing explicated.

Systems definition of nursing

From a systems perspective nursing may be defined as a process that supports, maintains, or helps restore, insofar as possible, the desired steady state of an identified system. As defined earlier, when an identified system is in a steady state, it is in a relative state of balance or in a dynamic state of equilibrium. This relative state of balance, or steady state, does not negate the presence of disease; rather, it assumes a state of wellness. Wellness, on the other hand, assumes integration of social, cultural, psychologic, and biologic functioning in a manner that is oriented to maximize

the potential capabilities of the identified system.[39] The goal of nursing is to promote the maximal health potential of a system and is directed toward supporting, maintaining, or restoring, insofar as possible, a dynamic state of equilibrium: the steady state of an identified system.

Maximal health potential and the steady state of an identified system depend on system variables. For example, if the identified system is an individual, the nurse would assess and define the structure, process, and function of this system. Are there subsystem or suprasystem variables that influence the system's ability to achieve maximal health? If so, what can the nurse and the client design that will support, maintain, or restore a desired steady state? These questions, basic to the process of nursing, are central to a systems perspective for nursing. The following sections of this chapter explain the application of systems concepts.

Applied science of nursing today

Nursing as a developing science draws on many disciplines for knowledge to assist with the assessment of systems and the dynamics associated with health. Fig. 2-2 illustrates the bodies of knowledge useful to nursing and the potential focal systems to which they pertain. Since the biomedical model dominates health care in most Western nations, medicine and nursing are still influenced by the biologic sciences, such as anatomy, physiology, biochemistry, microbiology, and molecular biology. One can see from Fig. 2-2 that the microscopic orientation of the biologic sciences restricts our notions of humanity and health to the subsystem levels of reference. However, if the individual were identified as the focal system (as in Fig. 2-2), organ systems, organs, and cells would be seen as subsystems and the family, community, society, and culture as relevant suprasystems. This approach enables us to examine health from a perspective that includes the relevant suprasystems and illustrates that knowledge of the social sciences is essential for nursing practice.

Subsystem focus

Nurses are familiar with the structure, function, and processes of many organ systems and with the organs, cellular functions, and alterations that frequently occur with disease. For example, systems theory concepts can be readily applied to the cardiovascular system.

The cardiovascular system meets the criteria for a system, since it is a complex of elements in purposeful interaction. The structure of this organ system is composed of the heart, blood vessels, lymphatic vessels and nodes, and the red bone marrow by virtue of its hematopoietic function. The functions of the cardiovascular system are to transport various substances to and

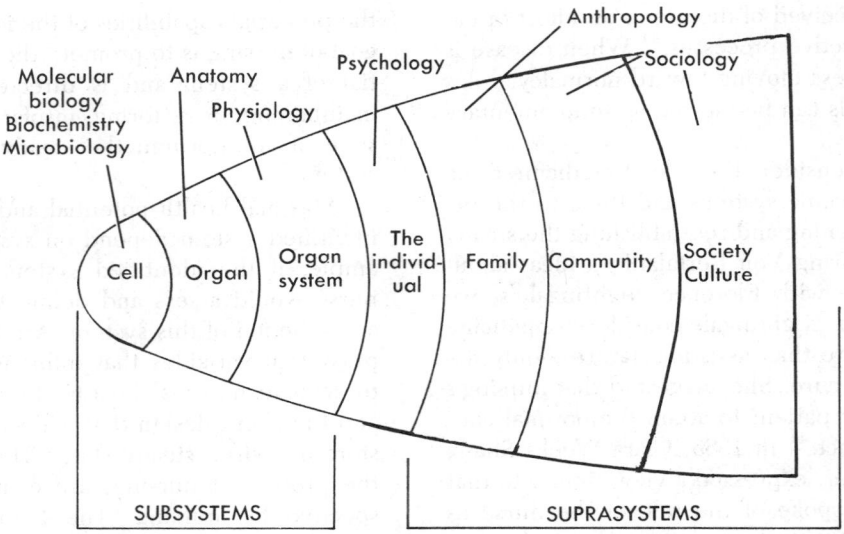

Fig. 2-2. Sciences influencing nursing practice. Molecular biology, biochemistry, microbiology, anatomy, and physiology support our understanding of human subsystems. Knowledge of psychology, anthropology, and sociology contributes to our understanding of humankind as a holistic entity in context of suprasystems.

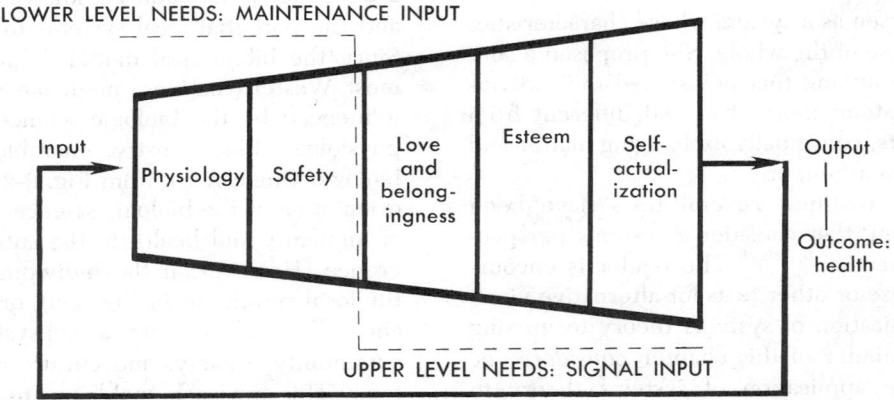

Fig. 2-3. Individual as system: hierarchy of needs. Lower level needs require maintenance input into system, whereas upper level needs require and produce signal input.

from the body cells, to protect the body against invading microorganisms, and to regulate body heat. System processes are accomplished through homeostatic mechanisms related to structures in the organ system: the heart, blood vessels, and blood cells. Starling's law of the heart would be one example of such a process: energy set free at each contraction of the heart is a simple function of the length of the fibers composing its muscular walls.

Individual as a system

The individual as a focal system requires a variety of different inputs from subsystems and suprasystems to maintain a state of health. For example, one conception of humankind and health identifies a hierarchy of needs that the individual as a system is motivated to fulfill. Maslow conceives of full health as individuals actualizing and fulfilling their natural potentialities (see Chapter 1). As shown in Fig. 2-3, the natural potentials of individuals are fulfilled through the satisfaction of five basic needs: physiologic, safety, love and belongingness, self-esteem, and self-actualization needs.[41] The individuals' environment—the suprasystems of family, community, society, and culture—provide a variety of inputs to satisfy the development of these needs. For example, food, fluids, and oxygen nourish cells and promote physiologic functions. A safe environment provides protection, order, and predictability in the world, nurturing survival of the organism. These two needs, physiologic and safety needs, are considered as lower level needs or prerequisites of all living animal systems. Lower level needs require a form of energy that is similar to what Berrien refers to as "maintenance input" in social systems. Maintenance input energizes the system and makes it ready to function.[32] All living systems require some type of maintenance input to survive. However, what distinguishes the human from all other living systems is the motivation to fulfill upper level needs.

The motivation to pursue a range of upper level needs—love and belongingness, self-esteem, and self-actualization—is unique to human beings. Gratification of these needs results in increased happiness, serenity, and richness of inner life. The lack of input to gratify these needs is the most commonly identified core of the low level of health in our society.[41] The form of energy processed from the suprasystem to promote upper level needs may be similar to the input that Berrien has described in social systems as "signal input."[32] *Signal input* is energy-information processed by social systems to produce an output to the suprasystem. This form of energy that satisfies upper level needs, along with the interchange of energy between humans and the environment, advances humanity. Upper level need fulfillment cultivates apperception: self-perceptive consciousness and creativity.

Suprasystem focus: the family

One of the suprasystems of the individual identified in Fig. 2-2 is the family. Like the human subsystems and the individual as a focal system, the family may also be analyzed from a systems perspective. Let us consider one perspective of the family as the focal system and apply some of the concepts of systems theory to this suprasystem of humanity.

Function. The family as a social system performs several essential functions: socialization, selection, recreation, protection, and reproduction.[19] As discussed earlier, the function of a system relates to the interaction between component parts and cannot always be readily distinguished from system processes. One way to describe the function of the family is to consider the family as an open, adaptive, organizationally complex, information-processing system.[20] Families as organiza-

tionally complex systems involve networks of interdependent, causal relations governed by feedback control mechanisms. Like other systems, the family changes as it responds to input from the environment. As an open system the family interchanges matter, energy, and information with the environment and adapts through these frequent processes.

The information processing of family systems involves the relationship between sets, or ensembles, of structured variety. The process of feedback informs parts of the family how to function toward purposeful, goal-seeking activity. What distinguishes family systems from other biologic or mechanical systems is the feedback process, which involves primarily psychic, complex communication processes of information exchange.[35]

Structure. The structure of family systems has been conceptualized in a variety of ways.[4,19,22] To explicate the application of systems concepts, only one systems perspective for the analysis of families will be discussed. Kantor and Lehr[20] describe the family system as one that is composed of three subsystems: the personal subsystem, the family-unit subsystem, and the interpersonal subsystem. These three subsystems interact with each other as well as with systems outside their boundaries.

The *personal subsystem* refers to an individual family member and incorporates self-interests, desires, meanings, and needs of an individual, similar to those discussed earlier. In addition to the characteristics of an individual, or the personal subsystem, members of a family are also part of the family-unit subsystem. *Family-unit subsystem* refers to selected architectural boundaries and social space perimeters that the family uses to establish family territory. Besides the same name and address, families have neighborhoods and associated community elements such as schools, libraries, town centers, and churches. One component of structure related to the family unit is the social space, or the structural enclosure where the family process takes place. The social space perimeter of a family's "territory" is evidenced in the behaviors they signal to others around them. Even though there are no physical walls to block entrance, one is usually aware of the extent to which the family wants others to impinge on their family boundaries. High fences, doorbells, and privately listed telephone numbers all function to limit access to the social space of family subsystems.

Even when others have been admitted to a family unit's space there is no guarantee that they will be allowed to enter the family's *interpersonal* subsystem. The family's interpersonal subsystem involves the interrelationships between individual family members in the realization of three goals: *affect* (intimacy and nurturance), *power* (freedom to decide and acquire money or skills), and *meaning* (philosophical framework for guiding reality).

Process. According to Kantor and Lehr, family members regulate access to power, affect, and meaning through time, space, and energy. Families regulate space through defining safety zones to protect privacy, property, and relationships among family members. Time in families is structured as clock or calendar time, and an understanding of temporal relationships in families is facilitated through examining the family's basic rhythmic patterns. Energy in families is both static and kinetic: kinetic when members expend supplies of energy and static when energy is stored and available for use. The assessment of energy in families provides insight into the balance between supply and demand and the amount of energy available to facilitate the target goals of affect, power, and meaning. The family that has energy to process information and matter to maintain goals so that no one subsystem is consistently denied actualization enables individual family members and the family unit to grow and develop in a healthy way.[20]

Alterations in basic human needs: stress, instability, and disease

Let us return to the individual as the focal system and examine the distinction mentioned earlier between maintenance and signal input, since this often provides insight into the decay and deterioration of social systems. It is postulated that for varied periods of time open systems may be impervious to signal inputs and appear relatively isolated and closed. Human systems, like social systems, begin to deteriorate if they do not interact purposefully with their environments.

To reach full health potential a human system must interact with the environment to satisfy a hierarchy of needs. If individuals are impaired or obstructed in some way from achieving their full potential, their systems become stressed.

Stress is experienced when there is a substantial imbalance between what the environment supports or demands and what the system needs. If matter, energy, or information is lacking or there is an underload of input, the system may experience stress. Likewise, if there is an excess or overload of input, the system must act to correct this excess of matter, energy, or information. Since individual systems have a range of stability within which they function and process inputs of energy, there is a wide range of adaptive potentials. However, there are limits to a system's ability to function and process stress.

One outcome for a system that is stressed is *insta-*

bility. A system that is unstable responds by changing its own state or that of its environment so as to increase its efficiency with respect to its function.[4] Instabilities in an open system do not lead to random behavior; rather, they tend to drive the system to a new dynamic regimen that corresponds to a new state of complexity. When a system is in such a transition, it acquires new possibilities for action.[12] If the system were closed, it would monotonously increase entropy, and the development of maximal disorder would reach a state of equilibrium or rest: death. Open systems, through the exchange of energy with the environment, move through instabilities, fluctuations, transitions, and mutations to new regimens of metabolizing activity for life. Instability promotes order through fluctuation, which mutates toward new dynamic regimens.

The traditional view of disease is that of a deranged condition in an affected organ or organ system, usually precipitated by an agent external to the system. From a systems perspective disease is a life process related to the structure and functions of humanity, due to the equifinality of open systems. Disease is manifested when basic human needs are impeded either through self-selected actions or environmental demands and constraints that obstruct basic need satisfaction. When individuals' basic needs are such that they fail to make rapid enough a perfect adaptive response to the new environments in which they elect to live and function, disease ensues. Dubos cautions that disease cannot be kept at bay through environmental and medical control, since humans cannot control all cosmic forces and because of the human propensity to move on to the unknown.[38] Humans will never live in an environment that is static. Instability is an inevitable outcome as humanity changes and evolves. Disease is one outcome of instability for individuals as they adapt to stress, a transitional state, a time when the system promotes order through fluctuation. In this framework, nursing assists the individual to help restore, insofar as possible, the steady state of the individual's system and provides support during transitions from one dynamic regimen to another dynamic regimen.

Summary

This chapter has considered systems theory as one theory for guiding nursing practice. As the science of nursing evolves, various theories will be defined to explain nursing phenomena. Systems theory as a theory of theories could provide the framework for classifying and defining knowledge as it develops in nursing and assist in relating this knowledge to other disciplines, thus expediting nursing's endeavors to promote the health of the individual as a holistic system.

Education, research, and nursing practice often tend to focus on the subsystem level. The recognition and exploration of psychologic, social, and cultural variables in promoting health will assist nursing exploration of suprasystem variables and encourage options other than the reductionistic, physicalistic, subsystem approach to health care that exists today. Systems theory constructs could guide the understanding of systems and the integration of physical and psychologic principles, since it provides a perspective for considering humanity and nature in the context of wholes.

Basic concepts for living systems were defined, including steady state, negentropy, equifinality, and the distinctions between open and closed systems. The fundamental qualities of an open system—structure, process, and function—were examined, along with boundary and the processes of input, throughput, output, and feedback. System, subsystem, and suprasystem were defined.

A systems perspective for nursing was explicated. Nursing was described as a process that supports, maintains, or helps restore, insofar as possible, the steady state of an identified system. The applied science of nursing was considered as it relates to humanity's subsystems, to an individual system, and to a suprasystem with the family as a focal system. Systems concepts were applied to the subsystem, system, and suprasystems of human beings.

REFERENCES AND SELECTED READINGS
Contemporary

1. Abbey, J.: FANCAP: What is it? In Reihl, J., and Roy, C.: Conceptual models for nursing practice, New York, 1980, Appleton-Century-Crofts.
2. Ackoff, R., and Emory, F.: On purposeful systems, Chicago, 1972, Aldine Publishing Co.
3. Ahad, M.A.: Evolution of nursing science: implications for nursing world wide, Image 13:56-59, 1981.
4. Anderson, R., and Carter, I.: Human behavior in the social environment, Chicago, 1974, Aldine Publishing Co.
5. *Auger, J.: Behavioral systems and nursing, Englewood Cliffs, N.J., 1976, Prentice-Hall, Inc.
6. Broncatello, K.: Auger in action: application of the model, Adv. Nurs. Sci. 2:13-23, 1980.
7. Byrne, M.L., and Thompson, L.: Key concepts for the study and practice of nursing, ed. 2, St. Louis, 1978, The C.V. Mosby Co.
8. *Cassel, J.: Psychiatric epidemiology. In Caplan, G.: An American handbook of psychiatry, New York, 1973, Basic Books, Inc., Publishers.
9. Chinn, P., and Jacobs, M.: A model for theory development in nursing, Adv. Nurs. Sci. 1:1-11, 1978.
10. Clark, J.: A framework for health visiting: a systems approach, Health Visit 53:418-420, 1980. (Parts 1 and 2, 53:487, 1980.)
11. Fabrega, H.: Toward a theory of human disease, J. Nerv. Ment. Dis. 162:229-312, 1976.
12. Fabrega, H.: The need for an ethnomedical science, Science 189:969-975, 1975.
13. Flaskerud, J.H.: Areas of agreement in nursing theory development, Adv. Nurs. Sci. 3:1-7, 1980.
14. Guyton, A.: Textbook of medical physiology, ed. 5, Philadelphia, 1979, W.B. Saunders Co.
15. Jantsch, E.: Design for evolution: self-organization and planning in the life of human systems, New York, 1975, George Braziller, Inc.
16. *Hall, J., and Weaver, B.: A systems approach to community health, Philadelphia, 1977, J.B. Lippincott Co.
17. Hardy, M.: Perspectives on nursing theory, Adv. Nurse. Sci. 1:37-48, 1978.
18. Henry, J., and Stephens, P.: Stress, health, and the social environment, New York, 1977, Springer-Verlag.
19. Horton, T.E.: Conceptual basis for nursing interventions with human systems. In Hall, J., and Weaver, B.: A systems approach to community health, Philadelphia, 1977, J.B. Lippincott Co.
20. Kantor, D., and Lehr, W.: Inside the family, San Francisco, 1975, Jossey-Bass, Inc., Publishers.
21. *Laszlo, E.: The systems view of the world: the natural philosophy of the new developments in the sciences, New York, 1972, George Braziller, Inc.
22. Lewis, J., et al.: No single thread: psychological health in family systems, New York, 1976, Brunner/Mazel, Inc.
23. Miller, J.G.: Living systems, New York, 1978, McGraw-Hill Book Co.
24. Newman, M.: Theory development in nursing, Philadelphia, 1979, F.A. Davis Co.
25. Nordstrom, M.J.: Applying systems theory to a view of the skilled nursing facility: potential barriers to effective rehabilitation measures, A.R.N. J. 4(6):12-16, 1979.
26. Putt, A.: General systems theory applied to nursing, Boston, 1978, Little, Brown & Co.
27. Riehl, J., and Roy, C.: Conceptual models for nursing practice, New York, 1980, Appleton-Century-Crofts.
28. Rogers, M.: The theoretical basis of nursing, Philadelphia, 1970, F.A. Davis Co.
29. Stevens, B.: Nursing theory: analysis, application, and evaluation, Boston, 1979, Little, Brown & Co.
30. Svalastoga, K.: The social system, Copenhagen, 1974, Akademisk Forlag. (Translation.)
31. Watson, J.: Nursing: the philosophy and science of caring, Boston, 1979, Little, Brown & Co.

Classic

32. *Berrien, K.: General and social systems, New Brunswick, N.J., 1968, Rutgers University Press.
33. Boulding, K.: General systems theory, Management Sciences 2:197-208, 1956.
34. Bredemeier, H.C. Cited in Smoyak, S.A.: Toward understanding nursing situations: a transactional paradigm, Nurs. Res. 18:405-411, 1969.
35. Buckley, W.: Sociology and modern systems theory, Englewood Cliffs, N.J., 1967, Prentice-Hall Inc.
36. Dickoff, J., James, P., and Wiedenbach, E.: Theory in practice discipline, Nurs. Res. 17:415-435, 1968.
37. Dubos, R.: Man adapting, New Haven, Conn., 1965, Yale University Press.
38. Dubos, R.: Mirage of health, New York, 1959, Doubleday & Co., Inc.
39. Dunn, H.: High-level wellness, Arlington, Va., 1961, R.W. Beatty, Ltd.
40. Kuhn, T.: The structures of scientific revolutions, Chicago, 1962, The University of Chicago Press.
41. Maslow, A.H.: Motivation and personality, New York, 1954, Harper & Row, Publishers.

*References preceded by an asterisk are particularly well suited for student reading.

42. McKay, R.: Theories, models and systems for nursing, Nurs. Res. **18**:393-400, 1969.
43. *Miller, J.G.: Living systems: basic concepts. In Gray, W., et al.: General systems theory and psychiatry, Boston, 1969, Little, Brown & Co.
44. Nightingale, F.: Notes on nursing: what it is and what it is not, London, 1859 and 1914, Harrison.
45. Shaw, C.W.: A textbook of nursing, ed. 3, New York, 1885 and 1902, D. Appleton and Co.
46. *Vickers, G.: Is adaptability enough? Behav. Sci. **4**:219-234, 1959.
47. *Von Bertalanffy, L.: General systems theory: foundations, development, and applications, New York, 1968, George Braziller, Inc.

CHAPTER 3

SOCIAL AND CULTURAL DIMENSIONS OF HEALTH AND ILLNESS

ANTOINETTE T. RAGUCCI
JEAN GOEPPINGER

Health maintenance, illness, and death are universals of the human condition. Preventive, diagnostic, and curing behaviors have characterized all human groups' responses in coping and adapting to threats to the biologic integrity of the body. The diversity of human responses to events associated with illness, disease,* and death and the adaptive arrangements that must be made by individuals and groups need to be taken into account in nursing interventions. Health and illness behaviors may be viewed as social and cultural phenomena as well as physiologic, pathophysiologic, and psychologic entities.

The purpose of this chapter is to examine the interconnections between acute and chronic disease entities that affect a person's biologic integrity and some social and cultural variables that need to be considered in planning nursing interventions on behalf of patients and clients. Some concepts and findings derived from the specialty areas of medical anthropology and medical and family sociology will be explicated. These include the physical anthropology, or biocultural dimensions, of disease and the social and cultural determinants of health-seeking behavior. To facilitate identification of universal features of human responses to illness as well as responses unique to a group or subculture, a cross-cultural comparative approach is used.

The specialty areas cited above are engaged in the development of a body of knowledge that will advance theoretical as well as applied interests in health and illness care. Medical anthropologists, for the most part, have directed their attention to cultural phenomena associated with illness events and health-seeking behaviors. On the other hand, the medical sociologists' prime focus has been on society and social class variables.[25] Both areas of study use an essentially comparative approach to facilitate the identification of differences and similarities in group responses to health and illness events.

A comparative approach is developing within nursing. One nurse-anthropologist advocates a transcultural nursing approach, which offers a frame of reference that "can offer insight, new relationships, new foci and new dimensions of caring about one's own culture in relation to another."[43] Transcultural health care is defined as an evolving body of knowledge and practices regarding health-illness caring patterns from a comparative perspective of two or more cultures to determine major care features and the health services of cultures.[43]

Psychologic, cultural, and social phenomena are analytically distinct categories. A review of the nursing literature reveals that these dimensions of nursing care are usually subsumed under the headings *psychosocial* or *sociocultural* needs or components. In addition, some medical-surgical nursing literature appears to treat sociocultural or psychosocial considerations of patient care almost as an afterthought. Nursing interventions directed toward ameliorating discomfort and the problems associated with social and cultural variables are usually phrased in general terms of "shoulds" and "oughts." Failure of nurses to distinguish analytically between the physiologic, psychologic, social, and cultural determinants has resulted in many instances of

---

*Distinction is made between *disease* and *illness*. Disease refers to pathologic conditions as defined by contemporary Western biomedical science. Illness is conceptualized as the cultural, social, and psychologic (phenomenologic) construction of a health problem by the patient, family, and associates.[19,21,41]

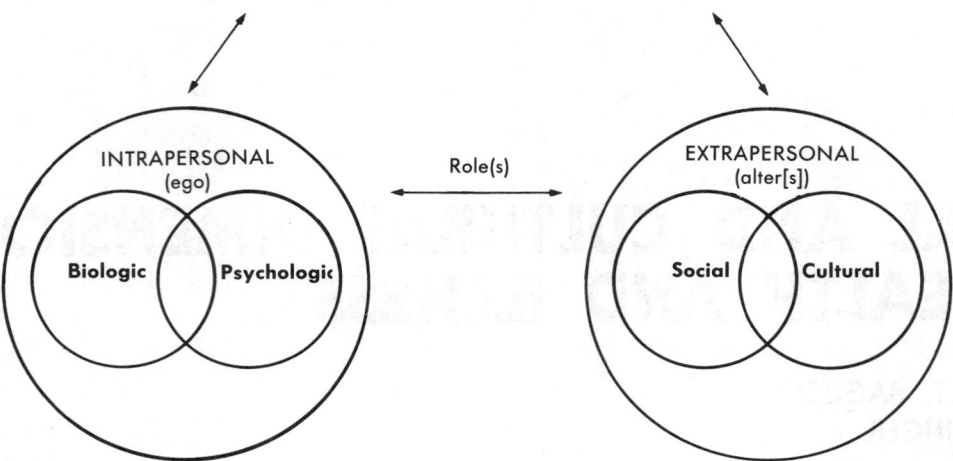

Fig. 3-1. Dimensions of health-seeking behaviors.

Biologic	**Psychologic**	**Social**	**Cultural**
Genotype	Emotional (affective)	Social structure	Value orientations
Phenotype	Basic personality structure	Family and kin networks	Norms
Body systems	Cognitive	Neighborhood	Beliefs: religious, health,
Neurologic	Motivation, etc.	Peer groups	political, etc.
Endocrine		Work groups: factory, office,	Knowledge: arts, sciences,
Cardiopulmonary		hospital, etc.	medical, nursing, etc.
Reproductive, etc.		Institutions: legal, educational,	Customs
		political, health care, etc.	Habits
		Social class	Technology: farm, industrial,
		Status	educational, biomedical, etc.

less attention being paid to the social and cultural components of nursing care.

Fig. 3-1 presents a model delineating the various dimensions of health-seeking behaviors. It can be noted that the extrapersonal factors (social and cultural) affect and in turn are influenced by intrapersonal factors (biologic and psychologic) and environmental factors (ecologic and demographic). The model is intended to convey the analytic distinctiveness of the variables that determine human behaviors.

Social phenomena

Social phenomena are conceptualized as those human actions and interactions that involve two or more persons. Subsumed under the category *social* are the constructs of social structure, social system, and social organization. These constructs are variously defined by sociologists, anthropologists, and other behavioral theorists. In general, *social structure* refers to ongoing, recurring, or patterned relationships. The concept is applied to small groups (e.g., the nuclear family) as well as to large organizations or aggregates (e.g., the community and society).[100] A social structure consists of arrangements of positions or statuses variously created and maintained or a network of relationships among persons.

A *social system* is made up of the interactions of a number of individuals whose relationships to each other are defined and mediated by a system of culturally structured and shared expectations. Thus the analytic unit of the social system is the role (or role sets) that serves to link or relate the individual (ego) to one or more others or alters.[118] A role, which may be interpreted as a unit of society, is differentiated from a status, which defines a person's place or position within a social group or society.[107]

Social roles may be further defined as goal-directed configurations of acts patterned in accordance with cultural value orientations[117] and conforming to the position (status) a person holds in a social group or situation. The behavioral expectations within a role differ across cultures. The underlying assumption of the above definition of social roles is that roles never exist within a vacuum but are considered from the perspective of a social group or context. Roles form social systems that are reciprocally linked by the acts of role partners, such as nurse-patient (dyadic) or nurse-patient-physician (triadic).

Social organization can be defined as the actions of any individual resulting from personal choices and decisions and the actions of others.[96] Social organization is conceptualized as consisting of the working arrangements of a society or processes involved with ordering actions and relationships toward given social goals. Social organization refers to those actions that are directed toward the integration of a society.[96] It is through social organization that the work of a society or cultural group is accomplished. Some categories of social organization are political parties and economic, legal, and health care institutions (hospitals) (Fig. 3-1). The analysis of the hospital as a social system would be concerned with delineating relationships between individuals and groups of individuals according to their social roles, which are culturally defined.

Cultural phenomena

Cultural phenomena include those objects or events that are patterned and arranged into a cultural system whose different parts are interrelated to form values, beliefs, and symbolic systems (Fig. 3-1). The concept of culture is variously defined as the ways of life or designs for living common at any one time to all humankind, the ways of living peculiar to a group or society among whose members there is a greater or lesser degree of interaction, the patterns of behavior peculiar to a group, or special ways of behaving characteristic of a segment of a large and complex society. The classic definition of culture is that of Sir Edward Tylor, who defined culture as "that complex whole which includes knowledge, belief, art, morals, law, custom and any other capabilities and habits acquired by man as a member of society."[129] The notions of holism, continuity, and diversity are implicit in the concept of culture. Kluckhohn and Kelly define culture as a "historically derived system of explicit and implicit designs for living which tend to be shared by all or specifically designated members of a group."[104] Culture is learned behavior transmitted with modifications from generation to generation. Some categories of culture are technology, beliefs, values, and symbols associated with religion, medicine, nursing, politics, and so on.

The concept of *subculture* refers to specific social units or groupings within a society. For example, in America the following may be viewed as subcultures: socioeconomic strata (lower, middle, upper), regional populations (the South, New England), community types (rural or urban), occupational groups, religious groups, and political groups. When considered within the context of American society, a subcultural group may also be defined as one that retains its identity and to a varying degree the customs and language or dialects of the country or region of origin. The term *ethnic* refers to a common and distinctive culture and people whose origins are from the same or related racial, linguistic, and cultural groups.

Ethnicity defines groups on the basis of both common origins and shared symbols and standards of behavior. Within the contemporary American scene, sociologists and anthropologists have identified manifestations of ethnicity termed variously as *old* and *new*, or *behavioral* and *ideologic*.[57,81]

Behavioral ethnicity is based on distinctive values, beliefs, behavioral norms, and language acquired during the process of socialization. These cultural norms serve as the basis for interactions within groups and influence the interaction with members of other ethnic groups and the participation in mainstream social institutions. Behavioral ethnic traits are manifested in the United States primarily by first- and second-generation residents and by ethnic minorities with a history of systematic exclusion from mainstream educational institutions and positions of political power, most notably blacks, Hispanics, and native Americans.[33]

Ideologic ethnicity, on the other hand, is based largely on customs that are neither central to a person's social life nor learned from early socialization. Ideologic ethnics are drawn largely from third- and fourth-generation whites whose behavior in most situations cannot be distinguished from that of other members of the same social class and regional background.[33]

The construct of *health culture* has been developed to refer to "all of the phenomena associated with the maintenance of well-being and problems of sickness with which people cope in traditional ways, in their own social networks."[89] Distinction is also made between popular, lay, or folk health cultures and the orthodox, or "scientific," health culture. Freidson has suggested the use of Redfield's concepts of the "great" and "little" traditions to differentiate modern medical knowledge from that possessed by the lay person.[97] In an era characterized by technologic innovation and complexity and increasing professional specialization, the medical or cultural lag between lay and professional knowledge can be expected to increase rather than decrease. According to Freidson, professional knowledge, then, is the "great tradition" of the contemporary era, and the "little tradition" of medicine refers to the lay person's perceptions and interpretations of modern medical knowledge and practices as well as to traditional or indigenous healing practices.

The social and cultural dimensions of health-seeking behavior (Fig. 3-1) and their link to biologic and environmental variables are discussed next. The psychologic correlates of health-seeking behavior are discussed in Chapter 14.

Biocultural dimension of health and illness

The analysis of direct relationships between culture and specific disease entities provides a fertile field for anthropologic, epidemiologic, and health research. A new field, *biocultural ecology*, has as a major focus the study of human adaptation and homeostasis. The effort is to transcend the fragmentation inherent in the separation of culture, human biology, and ecology or environment.[6]

The study of human populations using this three-way interaction system focuses on specific, localized individuals and populations for whom the environment is taken to represent all relevant variables, external and internal, to the people under study (Fig. 3-1).

Ecologic influences on genetics

Subcultural and ethnic peoples within America, linguistic groups in Africa, and tribal peoples of North and South America and New Guinea provide a number of population groups that are sufficiently distinct to provide the demographic isolates or units required for purposes of study of certain disease entities. For example, the study of the distribution of the sickle cell trait in Africa illustrates the changed ecologic conditions that have led to selective pressures and subsequent evolutionary and genetic changes.[109] Sickle cell polymorphism provides the classic example of cultural and ecologic effects on the genetic and demographic structure of human populations. The introduction of the technologic innovations of iron working and slash-and-burn agriculture changed the tropical rain forest, resulting in stagnant pools of water that served as breeding grounds for mosquitoes carrying the malarial parasite. This ecologic change led to the balanced polymorphism and relatively high frequencies of the allele (alternate gene forms in one chromosome) for hemoglobin S. In the contemporary era, the introduction of another cultural object, DDT, for control of malaria has altered selective processes and resulted in demographic changes whose effects on morbidity, mortality, and perhaps fertility have not yet been fully studied.[6]

The study of many genetic conditions requires consideration of changing social and cultural variables, especially those relating to nutrition or drugs. A well-known case is glucose-6-phosphate dehydrogenase

(G6PD) deficiency. The highest frequency of this sex-linked condition occurs in malarial belts, reaching slightly over 70% in a population of Kurdish Jews on the northern Iraqi border. It is generally assumed that G6PD-deficient individuals possess resistance to malaria in these regions.[6] Over 80 different G6PD variants have been found, many of which are associated with nonspherocytic hemolytic anemia on ingestion of natural foods (e.g., fava beans) or administration of certain antimalarial and antibiotic medications.

Attention to seemingly esoteric cultural practices associated with ritual cannibalism in the Fore tribe in New Guinea provided data instrumental in gaining knowledge about the causative factors that may be operating in some so-called slow-virus diseases. Kuru, a neurologic disease, was originally believed to be of genetic origin. Instead, cannibalism was found to be responsible for the epidemic spread of the disease through the tribes and neighboring groups with whom tribal members intermarried. The incidence of kuru was found to be higher for women and for children of both sexes. Kuru was rare in the men who did not participate in the rituals carried out as marks of respect for the dead. Clinical disease followed 4 to 20 years after eating poorly cooked tissues containing the viral agent.[28,110] Observations in the field combined with epidemiologic and genealogic observations over time and the transmission of kuru to chimpanzees by the oral route did not support the original postulate of genetic origin of the disorder.[28] The Fore tribe provided the natural setting for gaining insight into the probable causes of some neurologic disorders prevalent in Western countries today.

Biocultural dimensions of disease

It has been stated that the word *adaptation* connotes fitness to a particular environment or the possession of traits or attributes that make it possible for individuals to function effectively and to reproduce in this environment.[94] Adaptation, however, may be bought at a high price, and certain peculiarities that are assets in some geographic areas may be handicaps in others. The sickle cell hemoglobin deficit is an example of such a change. Cancer, heart disease, disorders of the cerebral system, and diabetes have all been referred to as diseases of civilization. Many types of *neoplastic disease* have been traced to environmental factors. The incidence of cancer has been shown to vary according to culture and social class.[94] Lung cancer is a common cause of death in the United States, England, Wales, and several other Western countries where cigarette smoking is common. Stomach cancers account for 50% of cancer among men in Iceland and Japan but only 10% in the United States. Liver cancer accounts for one half of all causes of death among the Bantus in Africa and less than 4% in Europe. Breast cancer is eight times more common in Israel than in Japan.[94] Regional variations have been found for skin and lip cancer in the United States and Russia. There are more cases in the south than in the north for both countries.

The etiologic factors in *diabetes* are still poorly understood. Some epidemiologic and genetic evidence suggests that viruses may be involved in causing at least one type of diabetes.[48] Both genetic and environmental factors are believed to play an important role in the high incidence of diabetes in some cultural groups. The high incidence of obesity among some populations is also correlated with the prevalence of diabetes. Changes in the specific components of a cultural group's diet and activity patterns have been identified as leading to an increased expression of diabetes.[70,116] The data accumulating about geographic and cultural differentials in the incidence of diabetes and pathologic complications raise questions relative to the nature of humankind's adaptation to culture change.[116] The increased incidence of diabetes reported for rural migrants to urban centers in Israel,[92] South Africa,[121] and Canada[70] has led some to label diabetes a disease of civilization.[39]

The relationship between increasing urbanization and diabetes morbidity reinforces Neel's hypothesis of diabetes as a "thrifty" genotype.[116] The theory holds that in prehistoric times the prediabetic individual was better equipped to adapt to the environment. The gene or genes responsible for diabetes mellitus permitted gaining extra weight during times of relative plenty and therefore enhanced survival during times of famine. Once these factors no longer existed the diabetic gene once considered functional for survival became a liability.

Studies of the differences in population frequencies of *lactase deficiencies* suggest a genetic as well as an acquired basis.[9] Adults of cultures as diverse as the Thai, Japanese, Andean Indians, and Chinese have inadequate levels of lactase. In the United States the rate for lactase deficiency among adults of predominantly European ancestry is between 10% and 20%. This contrasts with 70% lactase deficiency among adults of African descent.[31] The geographic distribution of the trait supports the hypothesis that primary adult hypolactasia arose after the cultural innovation of the domestication of milk-producing animals and large-scale milk production. McCracken[49] believes that all human populations were originally lactase deficient and that with the development of milk-producing cultures and uninterrupted consumption of milk during the transition years from infancy to childhood, those individuals who could metabolize milk enjoyed a reproductive advantage over those who could not.

Given the high nutritional value placed on milk in the United States and its inclusion in special diets, a reassessment of milk consumption is indicated. Individuals with the enzyme deficiency suffer discomforts such as flatulence, bloating, and diarrhea after ingesting milk; thus, contrary to the popular slogan, some people, especially those of African and Asian origin, do outgrow their need for milk. There is evidence that many lactose-intolerant adults in the milk-drinking culture of the United States simply restrict the amount of milk they drink at any one time to an amount that does not provoke symptoms. In this way they derive some benefits without suffering adverse effects.[32] In addition, cheese, yogurt, sour milk, and other milk products with a lower lactose content may be substituted.

Social and economic influences on disease

The interaction between social class, culture, and illness has been identified in several studies. For example, some social and economic correlates of diabetes mellitus have been identified. Economic deprivation is associated with an increased incidence of diabetes.[16] Diabetes per se may intensify economic deprivation because of the increased cost of carrying out prescribed medical and dietary regimens. In addition, there is an increased probability of work limitations because of sickness, absenteeism, or disability rising out of diabetic complications.[56,115]

Regional and racial differences in the incidence of diabetes have been found. A period of steady increase in diabetic rates for whites was noted in the 1930s. The rates leveled off in the 1940s and have varied little since then. On the other hand, the rates for nonwhites were lower than the rates for whites during most of the century. The pattern began to change in the 1960s. Now the rate for nonwhites is higher, 23 per 100,000 vs. 17 to 18 per 100,000 for whites.[66] Other demographic contrasts relative to the diabetic death rate (age adjusted) are those found to exist in different regions and states within the United States. Alaska has the lowest incidence of deaths, Delaware the highest. Death rates were higher in the eastern and central states and lower in the Rocky Mountain and Pacific states.[66]

The influence of socioeconomic conditions on developmental adaptation has been studied. Poor socioeconomic conditions associated with nutritional limitations represent an environmental stress that is known to influence body size. Using anthropometric* and demographic† measures, researchers studied highland and

Anthropometry is the science and technique of human measurements, specifically of anatomic and physiologic features; *anthropometric* is the adjective form.
†*Demography* is the study of vital and social statistics in their application to ethnology, anthropology, and public health; *demographic* is the adjective form.

lowland migrants living in new settlements (barriados) in a city slum in Peru. They found that parents of small body size (particularly the mother) had significantly greater offspring survivals than parents of large body size. It was hypothesized that women with low growth potential are better adapted to a poor environment than those who grow fast and become tall.[26]

In the American urban setting, the diversity of ethnic and social class groups provides the basis for comparative studies of within-group and between-group similarities and differences. Premigration patterns as well as postmigration histories are available. A study of ethnic differences in the prevalence of anencephaly (cranial neural deficit) and spina bifida (vertebral neural deficit) in Boston revealed the highest rates for children born to mothers who had emigrated from Ireland and lower rates for children of Jewish and Italian origins. There was a marked association with father's occupation, and the rates were twice as high for children born to mothers in ward accommodations as for those born to mothers in private accommodations. The findings suggest cultural determinants as well as the fact that those in the lower socioeconomic group may have had increased exposure to an as yet unidentified environmental factor.[114]

This section provides some data that nurses may find useful for the identification of those groups or populations at risk. Nursing interventions may then be directed toward educational and care activities that will ameliorate or prevent these health care problems.

Social context of health and illness behavior

The articulation of lay and professional knowledge and roles has been studied from the point of view of status differentials in reciprocal, or dyadic, role relationships of patient and physician. This section discusses some functions of family, kin, and community social units in health care systems and social class and cultural variables associated with the "sick role" and the place of the sick in society (see Chapter 1 for definition and discussion of the sick role).

Social class and health and illness

According to social scientists, the utilization of complex medical services calls for a medically sophisticated population with a degree of knowledge and understanding that is lacking in groups with low levels of education.[125,128] The greater the social and cultural distance between participants in a social system, the less likely that they will perceive each other in terms of ideal role types. Therapeutic relations should function at optimum where the professional and the patient are of the same status and hold common values.[128]

A number of sociologic studies have identified some social and psychologic characteristics of the poor that may influence health-seeking behaviors. People in the lower socioeconomic strata are perceived as being less likely than those in the middle class to engage in preventive health behavior and to defer gratification in the interest of long-term goals. The poor tend to have a fatalistic nonachievement orientation with a focus on adjustment or resignation rather than control over natural events or forces. The kin or peer group is preferred to professionals for consultation for solution of common human problems.[105,125] For example, a study of the concepts of health and illness in a Nova Scotian community revealed than when compared with the more affluent members of the society, the lower socioeconomic groups were less informed about illness and health care, were more skeptical of modern medical care, expected a good deal of illness in their lifetime, and had greater difficulty internalizing the sick role.[17]

Studies by nurses of class values as determinants of health-seeking behavior both support and refute the findings relative to class differences in values and health-seeking actions. Based on the findings of a study of maternal activity patterns, it was concluded that a clearer explication of the values of people in the lower class category is needed.[113] In particular, the variations that exist within this class in the ranking or preference for values, the informal social organization, and patterns of communication require further study.[113] The use of preventive health services by low-income women studied by Triplett revealed "ample evidence that there is no magic formula, no convenient stereotype, no generalizations to be made that can relieve the nurse of the responsibility for a careful assessment of each patient."[85] It has also been found that low-income mothers of high-risk infants had values concerning health similar to those of nurses.[8] Nurses, however, perceived the values held by clients as dissimilar, and it was suggested that this misperception by nurses may be a barrier to communication.[8]

Cultural dimension of the sick role

A cross-cultural comparative study of three communities (each with a rural and urban component) in England, Yugoslavia, and the United States tested empirically the notion of cultural relativity in the definition of illness and the assumption of the sick role.[11] It was found that a substantial amount of perceived illness is handled outside the framework of the sick role. A large number of people were validated by the medical profession as ill without the individuals assuming the privileges of the sick role. The study showed that in the English and American communities fewer than one third sought professional advice or reported limitation of usual activities. On the other hand, the proportion reporting limitation of usual work activities in the Yugoslavian community was 59%. In Yugoslavia over half of those who reported limitation of activities failed to seek medical treatment. In a summary of the international cooperative effort to study the cultural dimensions of the sick role, it was concluded that to define people as being ill solely in terms of social adjustment is to disregard a number of people who, using a different set of nonclinical criteria, also define themselves as ill and in some cases as seriously ill.[11]

Gassow and Tracy's study of "impression management" by patients with leprosy describes patients' attempts to alter and control the negative social and emotional responses of others to this stigmatized disease. Impression management refers to efforts people make to create a desired image about themselves and to control the conduct of others by controlling what they say and hear. Patients have developed theories that redefine the disease so that it may be removed from its position as the "idealized maximal horrible illness." Patients function in the role of educators in the attempt to change the public image of the leper. The development of these "educational specialists" has led to a new concept that is descriptive of their function: the career patient status.[99]

The destigmatizing ideology and the concept of a career patient status may be applied to other disease entities. Social organizatins such as the "ostomy clubs" (see p. 1473), the Lost Chord Club for laryngectomees (see p. 1282), and Alcoholics Anonymous are among those groups that use career patients who employ their own theories and concepts to facilitate adaptation as well as to bring about changes in society's attitudes.

Illness referral systems

A concept or construct that may be useful for analysis of people's health and action systems within a community context is that of illness referral systems. An *illness referral system* is conceptualized as a subsystem of the medical system and includes all health actors and their actual or expected behavior in illness situations.[87] Summarizing the definitions of a number of investigators and theorists, Weaver has defined a *medical system* as comprising the "whole complex of a people's beliefs, attitudes, practices and roles associated with concepts of health and disease and with patterns of diagnosis and treatment."[87] The patterns and modes of treatment have meaning only when the totality of social, struc-

tural, and group actions is taken into account.

This construct of an illness referral system is similar to Freidson's conceptualization that a *lay referral system* consists of a "variable lay culture and a network of personal influence along which the patient travels on his way to the physician."[97] Two variants of the lay referral system are identified: an extended and a truncated, or modified, form.[98] The former is found most often among certain indigenous and low socioeconomic cultural groups. The modified version is one in which individuals participate directly with the professional health care giver.

Four distinct phases of the illness referral system as it functioned in a Spanish community have been identified. These phases were used differently by traditional and acculturated Spanish-Americans. The typical traditional Spanish-American family or patient would progress through the following phases: the *self-addressed phase*, or self-perception of a change in health status; the *kinship phase*, in which consultants are members of the patient's own social group; the *community phase*, in which friends, neighbors, and influential community members are sought for help and diagnostic and curing advice; and a *folk specialist phase*, in which culturally recognized practitioners are consulted.[87,98]

This account of the referral system used by Spanish-Americans residing in a southern Rocky Mountain community bears similarity to the system used by residents of immigrant origin, that is, first generation of an Italian-American community in an eastern city.[64] The "home medical specialists" in the Spanish-American subcultural group, who treated minor ailments within the home or neighborhood, functioned in ways that were similar to the "therapeutic women" and "lay medical specialists" in the Italian-American community.[64] The therapeutic women gave traditional or folk prescriptions for the reported emotional or physical ailments of the elderly Italian immigrant women. On the one hand, most of the therapeutic women were immigrants themselves. On the other hand, the lay medical specialists were women of the second generation, or American-born offspring of Italian parents. These women had assumed the functional role of intermediary between the immigrant who lacked language and literary skills in English and the American medical and health care systems. The lay medical specialists were among the first to be consulted by the elderly for help in making a decision about seeking professional medical assistance. In addition, they interpreted prescribed medical and dietary regimens and often were depended on to administer treatments such as eye drops or insulin injections. Their ability to make preliminary or differential diagnoses was enhanced by the intermediary role relationships in which they functioned.

Thus far health and illness actions have been discussed from the perspective of the social context in which these actions take place. Reciprocal role relationships of patient and health care giver, the consequences of environmental and cultural influences on certain disease entities, and the use of alternate health care referral systems have been discussed. Knowledge of family variations in social structural roles and functions provide another dimension for assessing the social and cultural correlates of health-seeking behavior.

Family in health and illness

The family is a basic unit of society. It is probably the single most important social context in which health and illness occur, health-protective activities are performed, illness is identified and resolved, and professional health care is implemented. During the last 2 decades the family has been studied as an independent, dependent, and intervening variable in the illness and treatment of physically and emotionally ill family members.[46] Historically, these studies have considered the family and family health as composites of individual family members and of the health statuses of individual family members, respectively.[90] More recently, however, students in the area have begun to examine the family and family health as something more than composites.[40,52,54] The concept of the effectively functioning family unit has gained prominence.

A focus on the family and its functioning irrespective of whether the family unit or the individual family member is considered the primary client or patient is mandatory for nurses. The site where the nurse practices (hospital, health center, private practice, or home), the thrust of health care offered at the site (primary, secondary, or tertiary), and the nurse's own orientation to practice and expertise determine how the family will be incorporated into health care. The nurse may focus on the individual but recognize that the individual's membership in a family with distinct health values, beliefs, and practices circumscribes the options for nursing care. The nurse may also focus on the family itself. This nurse would ascertain the family's capacities to live, work, and play together and to function as a societal unit and strive to enhance these capacities.

The purpose of this section is to contribute to family-focused nursing by (1) defining the family, (2) sketching useful frames of reference for the nurse working with families and their members, and (3) discussing family competence and its consequences for behavior in health and illness.

Family defined

The American family may be defined by three criteria: kinship, function, and location. The family is generally characterized by (1) any one occurrence or combination of sexual or marital, parental, and sibling rela-

tionships; (2) intensive and inclusive relationships; and (3) cohabitation. Each criterion can be specified more precisely.

In the first criterion, that of *kinship*, the three dyads with biologic or genealogic correlates (sexual or marital, parental, and sibling) imply the existence of three positions or locations for the individual within the family structure: husband-father, wife-mother, and child-sibling. Two conventional forms of family structure are composed of these positions. They are the nuclear or conjugal family and the stem family. The *nuclear family* consists of a man, his wife, and their unmarried or nonadult children. It is based on marital, parental, and sibling dyads and is restricted to a depth of two generations. The *stem family* encompasses three generations: grandparents, parents, and children. Other forms of family structure, such as the single-parent family and the affiliated family, exist, as do countercultural forms such as communes and group marriages and the urban kin networks of impoverished blacks.* Each of these family forms also includes individuals occupying sexual or marital, parental, and sibling positions.

The second criterion defining the family, *intensive and inclusive relationships*, is often contrasted with diffuse and segmented, temporary and expedient relationships. Intensive and inclusive family relationships are notable for their persistence over a substantial period of time and for their concern with basic domestic tasks, for example, the pooling of income, the socialization of the children, the taking of rest or leisure, and the preparation and serving of meals. The criterion also suggests closeness, warmth, and affection as opposed to social distance and compelling moral obligation. The intimate emotional quality of family life results from its chronologic depth and from continuous interaction to ensure that multiple tasks are allocated and completed.

The final criterion, *cohabitation*, may be defined as common or at least proximate residence. Family members usually have one address, sleep under one roof, and eat at the same table.

Frames of reference for family-oriented nursing practice

Since 1960 a number of theories and conceptual frameworks about the family have been developed.[10,37,91] The *developmental, systems,* and *interactional* approaches to family analysis, in particular, have been extensively developed.†

These approaches are salient to family-focused nursing. They suggest that nurses be attentive to such fundamental concepts as stages of family development; family tasks or functions; family structure; and interac-

*References 47, 59, 73, 80, 82.
†References 1, 2, 18, 36, 55, 68.

tion processes within the family and between the family, its kin networks, and its society. Each of these concepts and its relevance to nursing are discussed in turn.

The *stages of family development* are the sequential phases in the family life cycle. The time periods encompass the natural history of most nuclear families, beginning with the simple husband-wife pair, becoming more complex as children are born, stabilizing briefly, becoming less complex after the launching of adult children into jobs and marriage, and eventually dissolving with the deaths of the original conjugal pair. Seven stages are identified in the nuclear family's life cycle: the beginning family, the childbearing family, the family with preschool children, the family with school-aged children, the family with teenagers and young adults, the postparental family, and the aging family.[2]

Family behavior is expected to change predictably as families move from one developmental stage to the next, and a compendium of research efforts testing the utility of this principle has been published.[2] The research indicates that some family behaviors can be predicted by knowing the developmental stage of the family. Other family behaviors are relatively constant, and still others are situational or circumstantial. Prediction is possible because certain family tasks or functions are specific to each stage of the family life cycle. The findings support the proposition that the achievement of a developmental task at one period affects family life at a later period.

Family tasks or *functions* are the activities carried out by the family: the allocation of economic and material resources; the reproduction, recruitment, and release of family members; education and socialization; physical maintenance and protection; and the exchange of affection. The accomplishment of these tasks is imperative for the social life of communities and for the growth of individual family members. At each stage of family development the tasks that have primacy and those that are secondary can be highlighted. Thus, for the aging family in contemporary America, the tasks of ensuring economic survival on a fixed income, of reallocating household responsibilities, and of maintaining or rediscovering intimacy are crucial.

To accomplish these tasks the family develops an *organization* or *structure*. The key elements of the family organization are *positions, roles,* and *norms.* The husband-father, wife-mother, and child-sibling positions are common to the nuclear family. Each position is composed of roles or prescriptions for interpersonal behavior. The husband-father position in the nuclear family often consists of breadwinner, sex partner, companion, teacher, and disciplinarian roles. The role content of a position changes over the family life cycle, as occurs, for instance, with the retirement of the husband-father from active employment. Roles are distinguished from one another by norms (social expectations

for behavior). For example, the normative power structure in the modern family is thought to be egalitarian; an authoritarian role is no longer expected of many husband-fathers. Nurses may properly investigate a family's organization to ascertain if positions are filled and roles developed and played in ways that enhance the functioning of individual family members, the family unit, and the community. Intervention may be required to support or modify a family's organization to better accomplish its tasks.

Interaction processes are another fundamental concept. Interaction between the family and the surrounding society is critical. The family must negotiate for income and services; in turn it must supply society with productive, responsible members. The nurse may be required to mediate between a family and society when the family's and/or the society's activities are inadequate or inappropriate to healthful living.

The family's interaction with noncohabiting kin is also significant. Kin relationships among families range from integrated to isolated. Notwithstanding the current spate of research efforts to prove that the American family is isolated from its kin, relatives do keep in touch, celebrate rituals and ceremonies associated with death, birth, and weddings, and exchange gifts and services.[42,80,96] Nurses may need to intervene to mobilize kin in situations of family crisis, since kin are frequently an essential source of support.[15,42]

Intrafamilial interaction processes are equally important. *Family conflict* is as basic an interaction process as family cohesion. The management of family conflict, not simply the avoidance or resolution of strife and disharmony, has been proposed as essential to healthy family life.[51,78] The nurse might be essential to successful conflict management during transitions from one family development stage to another, the transition to parenthood for example.

Family problem solving, those behaviors selected and implemented by families to accomplish desired tasks, is another intrafamilial interaction process to be considered.[2,50,83] Family problem-solving efforts are perhaps less rational than those of other small work groups or committees and are less problem than solution oriented. The elements in the problem situation are often not open to manipulation and change.[83,88] It is believed that families seldom explicitly define a situation as a problem, seek satisfying solutions, and take action. Rather, they handle the most resistant, unsettling features of the situation in the ways past experience has suggested may be effective. The daily routines and the constant pressure or problematic situations force the family to solve but not to analyze their problems. In addition, many family problems arise either from economic and political events that the family alone is powerless to control or from interpersonal relationships that would require personality changes if solutions were to endure. Families facing the unexpected protracted illness of the breadwinner may, for instance, require nursing assistance to reach workable solutions for problems ranging from the care of the ill individual and role reversal to income maintenance.[14] Families may also benefit from nursing intervention related to the management of problems of everyday life.[74]

The concepts presented above provide some frames of reference for family-focused nursing practice. They suggest broad areas of assessment and intervention that are necessary if the family is to be incorporated into nursing care. The need to develop clinically salient "measures" of these concepts and to examine their relationships to individual, family, and community well-being is obvious. Several recent studies indicate that attempts in this direction have begun.* Tools to assess the health of the family unit have been developed. Tools assessing family health constructs—family structure, family functioning, family competence, and family developmental status—incorporate many, if not all, of the previously discussed concepts. They have been used to examine relationships between the health of the family unit and the health statuses of child and adult family members.†

Competent family in health and illness

One expert has approached the competent family from the perspective of the family's effective functioning as a social unit, "a unit created to allow people to live together and rear children who are themselves physically well and have qualities accepted as desirable by the community concerned."[54] Another expert delineated seven dimensions of family competence: the commitment of family members to family group objectives, communication, pride in the family, self-confidence, judgment, creativity-resourcefulness, and participation.[7] Still another approach was taken by two experienced clinicians whose concept of family functioning included the components of communication, togetherness, closeness, decision making, and child orientation.[62]

All three approaches imply that the family, whether it is a healthy family or a family in trouble, must be treated as a social unit; that effective family functioning or competence may be equated roughly with family health; and that the nature, that is, the health or competence, of the family unit has an impact on individual and societal well-being.

Boardman,[7] for example, studied the relationship between family competence and school absences of children in the second, third, and fourth grades. She found that children with high rates of absenteeism were clustered in families with low competence scores and,

conversely, that children whose families' competence scores were high had few school absences. She also found that three of the components—self-confidence, judgment, and participation in community life—were mainly responsible for the explanatory power of family competence.

Using an abridged version of the same tool, Goeppinger[30] found that as family competence scores increased, the health statuses of her adult respondents improved. Once again the participation component was responsible for much of the power of the family competence tool.

Pratt[63] studied the relationship between family structure and reported illnesses of family members. Families with "energized" or healthy structures were those in which members interacted frequently and extensively with one another, ties to the community were strong, autonomy of individual members was encouraged, family resources supported creative problem solving, and family members coped successfully with the role changes occurring within the family. She found that families with energized structures noted fewer health problems among their members than did families lacking energized structures.

The conclusions of a series of studies carried out by the Rochester Child Health Study Group are consistent with those of Boardman, Goeppinger, and Pratt. The studies examined the relationship between effective family functioning or quality family life and children's responses to chronic illness. Briefly, they revealed that children from families with low family functioning scores adjusted poorly, irrespective of the severity of their diseases. Children with mild, moderately severe, or severe disease adjusted well to their illnesses if their families functioned effectively.[60,62]

The findings of these studies suggest that family health, variously labeled family competence, energized family structure, and effective family functioning, is relevant to elementary school absenteeism, frequency of health problems experienced by family members, adult health status, and children's adjustment to chronic illnesses. They indicate that perhaps the family, as well as the individual child or adult family member, should be the focus of nurses' efforts when individuals are often ill, frequently absent from school or job, or responding inadequately to treatment for chronic illnesses.

The family may also play a part in defining and legitimizing a member's right to assume the sick role and in deciding not only whether a family member will receive care but if it should be provided at home. The process of becoming a patient includes a series of decisions involving family, friends, and health care providers.[5] In general, the role the family may play in the process varies over time and is contingent on the disease condition, its severity and chronicity, the family

---

*References 7, 29, 30, 52, 60-64, 75, 84.
†References 7, 30, 60-64, 75.

members involved, and the degree of familial concern. The mother, for example, may exhibit a great deal of reluctance to accept the sick role. It has been observed that mothers are more likely to seek medical care and advice for their children than for themselves and that they are more willing to define their children than themselves as sick.[111] It is easy to speculate that the mother, the pivotal member of many families, experiences considerable difficulty in fulfilling her obligations when she is ill and thus tends to postpone labeling herself as sick.

The decision as to whether a family member's illness should be treated at home or with the assistance of professional health care providers also tends to be negotiated within the family setting. In one study approximately half of the respondents of low-income urban households consulted a household member about what they should do in the case of a particular symptom.[67] Another study found that the decision to seek professional care for an ill family member generally rested with the wife-mother; half of the respondents would find it fairly difficult to care for a sick member at home for any protracted period of time and would be willing to relinquish the care of the sick to the hospital.[45,46] The ultimate success of the family's involvement in home diagnosis, treatment, and referral to professional sources of care may revolve around restoration of its ability to do the task and preparation to do so. The self-help movement and the parallel disenchantment with the cure rate and iatrogenic effects of "scientific" medicine as reported in the literature may stimulate the family to care for itself more effectively.[37,44]

Some concepts by which the family is linked to the wider society and culture are discussed next. The focus is on the cultural dimensions of health and illness.

Cultural dimensions of health beliefs and practices

Effects of cultural health beliefs and practices

Every culture provides a set of significant questions and potential answers and procedures for arriving at answers to cope with illness events. Effective communication directed toward therapeutic nursing intervention requires that the nurse know something about how the patient and family members perceive and define the illness, its cause, and therapy in general. Assessment of the level of patients' knowledge and understanding of what ails them will permit nurses to identify the medical or cultural lag or discrepancy be-

tween lay and professional knowledge. Nursing care actions may then be directed toward closing the knowledge gap.

The articulation for comparative purposes of folk or lay and modern medicine, that is, the "little tradition" and the "great tradition" has not received much attention by medical-surgical nurses. The reason for this may be a lack of knowledge or the general disregard of many health professionals for folk or laypersons' expressed beliefs and practices. Folk healing actions and beliefs are variously perceived by some health professionals as esoteric, quaint, irrelevant, or scientifically unproved. Yet cultural and individual beliefs about the cause of disease do determine, to a greater or lesser degree, what actions people will take to ameliorate symptoms or prevent illness and whether they will comply with prescribed regimens.

People living in traditional or nontechnologically developed societies have had a long history of medicinal contributions, particularly in pharmacology. It has been estimated that more than 220 medicines have been contributed to the official *U.S. Pharmacopoeia* by indigenous Indian healers of North and South America.[86] Rational therapy employing indigenous botanical drugs was extensive among these Indian groups, and medicinal preparations, such as insulin and penicillin, were anticipated. An effective remedy for scurvy was in use in the New World at a time when the then great tradition of European medicine believed it to be caused by bad air. Among the well-known medicinal preparations contributed by South American Indians are cinchona, coca, curare, and ipecac. The American variety of foxglove was used for its cardiac stimulant qualities hundreds of years before digitalis was discovered in England.[86]

Belief systems do interfere with therapy. For example, in a multidisciplinary study of Quechua Indians living at high altitudes in the Andes, the people gave unexpected resistance to giving blood samples and having blood pressures taken.[4] It was determined that the people believed that blood removal was detrimental because once removed it would not be replaced, and the blood pressure cuff was perceived as extracting blood.

On the other hand, one would expect some resistance to giving blood samples from lay persons whose beliefs about the generation of blood differ from those of conventional modern medicine. One study of southern black migrants in Tucson revealed that people held notions about blood, such as that new blood is constantly being formed, used blood is eliminated through sweat in men and menses in women, and blood loss is weakening.[76] It is reasonable to assume that in any hospital or clinic setting the perception of individuals relative to the common procedure of drawing blood samples will vary according to idiosyncratic or cultural variables.

Assessment of health beliefs

Lay concepts and categories can be arrived at by noting the answers and responses to a number of dimensions expressed as questions about illness episodes.[12]

1. What kind of illness is it (i.e., its name)?
2. How has it been treated (or how will it be treated, or how should it be treated)?
3. What caused the illness?
4. How serious is it?
5. Does the sickness pose a threat to others?
6. How long will the illness last? For example, is it acute or chronic?
7. Was the illness inherited?

These questions originally used for a Malayan population by Colson[12] may be adapted for patients in the American health and medical setting.*

The illness referral system, which defines the social process by which people seek therapy, has been discussed. Cultural responses to the above questions will supply the cognitive categories, the theories about illness causation, prevention, treatment, and prognosis. Cultural categories and criteria for defining illness may be studied by the use of an approach called ethnomedicine. Ethnomedicine is a domain of *ethnoscience,* an approach that seeks to discover and describe the concepts and behavior system of a given culture in accordance with concepts derived from that culture. *Ethnomedicine* is an attempt to elicit the lay person's own definitions of the illness situation without the imposition of a priori categories by health professionals. Clients may not use the same sets of criteria or expectations as members of the health professions for the same illness event. For example, a study of emergency department admissions revealed that lay persons and professionals differed in their definition of what constituted a medical emergency.[20]

Beliefs concerning cause of illness

Beliefs about causation of illness reveal variations across cultural groups. Americans in general attribute illness to physiologic and psychologic causes. People as diverse as the Gadsup of New Guinea[106] and the Azande of Africa[95] stress the social and cultural causes of a number of illnesses. Some ethnic groups, particularly those in the lower socioeconomic class and of rural origin, attribute illness to fate, destiny, or God's will.

Cultural themes pertaining to curing and healing, particularly in regard to nutrition or foods, have been identified. A study of Puerto Rican families in New York revealed that the hot-cold notions associated with the Hippocratic humoral theories continued to find

*See also references 33 and 41.

expression.[33,35] Health, according to the humoral theoretic orientation, was defined as a state of balance among four bodily humors, namely, blood, phlegm, black bile, and bile. An imbalance in these humors results in illness, which causes the body to become excessively dry, cold, hot, wet, or a combination of these qualities. Foods and medicinal herbs are classified as having hot or cold qualities and are prescribed to return the body to its proper balance.

Vestiges of theories directed toward correcting body imbalance form the basis for treatment within a number of ethnic and cultural groups. The New England Yankee, for example, uses apple cider and honey to maintain proper acid-base balance.[103] In a Guatemalan community two concepts, *fresco* (fresh or cool) and *alimento* (highly nutritive substance), were used to accommodate and reinterpret modern health and nutritional beliefs.[13] Fresh or cool substances (carrot juice, tea, chicken, rice) rather than cold were considered the best treatment for "hot" illnesses. Many of the health professionals working with the Guatemalans were not aware of the distinctions people made between highly nutritive substances (alimento) and other foods. The wet-dry polarity forms the basis of the therapeutic beliefs about foods of several eastern and western European groups.[64,122] A balance in the wet and dry foods is believed to be important in maintaining a healthy state. Meals or prescribed diets lacking soups and green leafy vegetables are perceived as "too dry" and detrimental to maintaining the body in its proper state.

The identification by nurses of cultural themes associated with caring and curing behaviors is facilitated within settings such as the hospital, where these behaviors would be more likely to be manifested. Acknowledgement and respectful recognition by nurses of the functional nature of folk or lay persons' beliefs aid in decreasing the social and cultural distance between patient and professional. Beliefs and practices that reinforce or interfere with the physician's and nurse's prescriptions require identification. Nurses may then be able to develop therapeutic plans of care working within the patient's belief system. For example, it was found that Puerto Rican patients receiving diuretics discontinued use of orange juice, a needed source of potassium, when they had a cold because of its "cold" quality.[35] In such cases nurses can suggest alternate potassium-rich foods that do not fall into the "cold" category.

Behaviors associated with pain

The pain experience is a universal component of the human condition, and the phenomena associated with pain have been encountered by all nurses. Health professionals tend to be aware of the psychologic, social, and cultural components of patient pain responses (see Chapter 23 for further discussion of pain). Differences in responses to pain in relation to the variables of ethnicity, religious affiliation, and race have been the subject of several studies.[112,130,131] Zborowski's study was one of the earliest to focus on differentials in cultural responses to pain. The findings of this study are still applied without question by some nurses. However, the study has been critized for its failure to distinguish between pain as a basically physiologic phenomenon and the "pain experience," which has cognitive and emotional components.[130] Social class and generation variables were not adequately controlled in the study, and subsequent studies revealed that immigrant and other groups (e.g., religious and racial) will follow the patterns of the majority group in the society if the subjects are made aware of the ethnic or religious differences.[130] A comprehensive review of research of cultural factors and pain responses concluded that there is a paucity of adequately controlled experimental studies of the pain experience; any attempt to delineate cultural factors in human responses should be made in the wider context of cultural attitudes toward sickness and health; and religious attitudes, insofar as they "influence perception of the physical self," may be an important variable for study.[130]

Pollution behaviors

Beliefs and cultural health practices categorized under the construct *pollution behaviors* are universal components of human behavior. The word *pollution* conveys notions of uncleanness, dirty, untouchable, defilement, taboo, contamination, and disease, especially communicable disease. All cultures have elaborated definitions and rules to ensure a clean or pure state and the means by which those considered unclean or impure may be restored. Most pollution rules spell out prohibitions in relation to food and contact with certain objects or persons. Pollution theories and practices probably have been most fully elaborated for the occupational caste and outcaste systems of India. Food taboos and prohibitions about contact, however, find expression throughout the world.[127] Most nurses are familiar with kosher dietary rules and the food proscriptions of other religious groups, such as the Seventh Day Adventists.

Study of pollution within a cultural context has led to the delineation of some concepts that may be useful for nurses in understanding some of the underlying dynamics of the subtle yet pervasive behaviors associated with pollution.[93] Pollution as a concept has affective and cultural components. All pollution behaviors are perceived as the reaction to any event that is likely to confuse or contradict "cherished classifications" or the usual order of things. Implicit in the pollution concept is the notion of "things out of place" (deviant). Ambiguity and cultural dissonance are other qualities associated with the concept. Cultures have evolved pollution rules (ways of behaving) as an attempt to impose order on existence. Pollution beliefs reinforce the cultural norms and social structure and reduce dissonance.[93]

Rules and rituals that regulate behaviors for the avoidance of pollution vary cross culturally. In some cultures rules about menstrual blood or the menstruating woman have been elaborated. In other cultures the bodies of the dead, certain body excretions, and a wide variety of foods may be avoided or treated in such a way that contact is minimized.

Pollution and pollution behaviors are relevant constructs for nursing. Illness or disease may be viewed as a deviance (deviance from a healthy state), and with illness there is a disruption of the social order (see the discussion of the sick role in Chapter 1.) Some disease entities or physiologic states more than others may be viewed as "dirty" or "things out of place." Leprosy is the classic disease in which affective and cultural behaviors are manifested. Other conditions are colostomy and ureterostomy. Pathologic conditions in which there are increased secretions and incontinence may be viewed as "things out of place." Some persons with diabetes consider it a "dirty" disease because of the need for contact with urine and urine-testing equipment. The fear of defilement or pollution with body secretions and excretions appears to be deeply embedded. Nurses need to be aware of the culturally specific ways in which these beliefs and behaviors are expressed. Nursing care plans may then be developed to assist patients and their families in developing techniques to minimize the distressing features of self-care functions. Nurses have a unique opportunity as they work with clients to systematically collect data about these beliefs and behaviors and share them with other health care providers.

Summary

The social and cultural correlates of health-seeking behavior have been discussed. Social class differences, family organization and practices, and cultural beliefs and values do affect health caring behaviors and actions directed at the prevention, treatment, and amelioration of symptoms of disease. Beliefs about the causation of illness vary according to cultural groups (ethnic or subcultural) and social class. The consideration of similarities and differences within and between groups aids in the identification of health beliefs and actions that are either universal for all people, specific or unique for a group or social class, or idiosyncratic, that is, applicable only to an individual. This comparative frame of reference, which focuses on group variations as well as similarities, will help to decrease the tendency toward stereotyping the behavior of clients. In addition, the cultural or "medical" lag between lay (folk) and professional knowledge and action may be determined. Nursing interventions that acknowledge the discrepancy between these two levels of knowledge may then be planned and instituted.

REFERENCES AND SELECTED READINGS
Contemporary

1. Aldous, J.: Family careers: developmental change in families, New York, 1978, John Wiley & Sons, Inc.
2. Aldous, J.: The developmental approach to family analysis, 2 vols, Minneapolis, 1975, The University of Minnesota Press. (Mimeographed.)
3. Aldous, J., editor: Family problem solving, Hinsdale, Ill., 1971, The Dryden Press.
4. Baker, P.T., and Little, M., editors: Man in the Andes, Stroudsburg, Penn., 1976, Dowden, Hutchinson & Ross, Inc.
5. Becker, M., editor: The health belief model and personal health behavior, Thorofare, N.J., 1974, Charles B. Slack Co.
6. Bennett, K.A., Osborne, R.H., and Miller, R.J.: Biocultural ecology: annual review of anthropology, Palo Alto, Calif., 1975, Annual Reviews Inc.
7. Boardman, V.: School absences, illness and family competence, Ph.D. dissertation, Chapel Hill, N.C., 1972, University of North Carolina.
8. *Brinton, D.M.: Value differences between nurses and low-income families, Nurs. Res. 21:46-52, 1972.
9. Brock, D.J.H.: Inborn errors of metabolism. In Brock, D.J.H., and Mayo, O.: The biochemical genetics of man, New York, 1972, Academic Press, Inc.
10. Burr, W.R., et al., editors: Contemporary theories about the family, Research-based theories (vol. 1) and General theories/theoretical orientations (vol. 2), New York, 1979, The Free Press.
11. *Butler, J.R.: Illness and the sick role: an evaluation in three communities, Br. J. Sociol. 21:241-261, 1970.
12. Colson, A.C.: The prevention of illness in a Malay village: an analysis of concepts and behavior, Overseas Research Center Developing Nations, Monograph series 2, no. 1, Winston-Salem, N.C., 1971, Wake Forest University.
13. Cosminski, S.: Alimento and fresco: nutritional concepts and implications for health care, Hum. Org. 36:203-207, 1977.
14. Craven, R.F., and Sharp, B.H.: The effects of illness on family functions, Nurs. Forum 11:187-193, 1972.
15. *Croog, S.H., Lipson, A., and Levine, S.: Help patterns in severe illness: the roles of kin network, non-family resources and institutions, J. Marriage Fam. 34:32-41, 1972.
16. Davidson, J.K.: Diabetes in socioeconomically deprived neighborhoods. In Diabetes mellitus: diagnosis and treatment, New York, 1971, American Diabetes Association.
17. Davidson, K.R.: Conceptions of illness and health practices in a Nova Scotia community, Can. J. Public Health 61:232-242, 1970.

18. Duvall, E.M.: Family development, ed. 4, Philadelphia, 1971, J.B. Lippincott Co.
19. Eisenberg, L.: Disease and illness: distinction between professional and popular ideas of sickness, Cult. Med. Psychiatry 1:9-23, 1977.
20. *Evaneshko, M., and Bauwens, E.: Cognitive analysis and decision-making. In Leininger, M.: Medical emergencies in health care dimensions, Philadelphia, 1976, F.A. Davis Co.
21. Fabrega, H.: Toward a theory of human disease, J. Nerv. Ment. Dis. 162:299-312, 1976.
22. *Fabrega, H.: The need for an ethnomedical science, Science 189:969-975, 1976.
23. Fabrega, H.: The study of disease in relation to culture, Behav. Sci. 17:183-203, 1972.
24. Firth, R., Hubert, J., and Forge, A.: Families and their relatives, Atlantic Highlands, N.J., 1970, Humanities Press, Inc.
25. Foster, G.: Medical anthropology: some contrasts with medical sociology, Med. Anthropol. Newsl. 6:1-6, 1974.
26. Frisancho, A.R., et al.: Adaptive significance of small body size under poor socio-economic conditions in southern Peru, Am. J. Phys. Anthropol. 39:255-261, 1973.
27. Frisancho, A.R., et al.: Influence of developmental adaptation on lung function at high altitudes, Hum. Biol. 45:583-594, 1973.
28. Gajdusek, D.C.: Unconventional viruses and the origin and disappearance of Kuru, Science 197:943-960, 1977.
29. Geismar, L.L.: Family and community functioning: a manual of measurement for social work practice and policy, Metuchen, N.J., 1971, Scarecrow Press, Inc.
30. Goeppinger, J.: The relationship between familial health and the health status of parents: into the mainstream with health risk reduction, Proceedings of the fifteenth annual meeting of prospective medicine and health hazard appraisal, St. Petersburg, Fla., Oct. 3-6, 1979.
31. Harris, M.: One man's food is another man's whitewash, Nat. Hist. 81:12-13, 1972.
32. Harrison, G.G.: Primary adult lactase deficiency: a problem in anthropologic genetics, Am. Anthrop. 77:812-835, 1975.
33. *Harwood, A., editor: Ethnicity and medical care, Cambridge, Mass., 1981, Harvard University Press.
34. Harwood, A.: Mainland Puerto Ricans. In Harwood, A., editor: Ethnicity and medical care, Cambridge, Mass., 1981, Harvard University Press.
35. Harwood, A.: Hot-cold theory of disease, J.A.M.A. 216:1153-1158, 1971.
36. Heiss, J., editor: Family roles and interaction: an anthology, ed. 2, Chicago, 1976, Rand McNally & Co.
37. Holman, T.B., and Burr, W.R.: Beyond the beyond: the growth of family theories in the 1970's, J. Marriage Fam. 42:729-741, 1980.
38. Illich, I.: Medical nemesis: the expropriation of health, New York, 1976, Pantheon Books, Inc.
39. Judkins, R., and Lieberman, L.: Specialist reports: biomedicine and nutrition, Med. Anthropol. Newsl. 6:14-17, 1974.
40. Kaplan, F.H., and Cassel, J.C., editors: Family and health: an epidemiological approach, Chapel Hill, N.C., 1975, University of North Carolina Press.
41. Kleinman, A., Eisenberg, L., and Good, B.: Culture, illness and care: clinical lessons from anthropologic and cross-cultural research, Ann. Intern. Med. 88:251-258, 1978.
42. Lee, G.R.: Kinship in the seventies: a decade review of research and theory, J. Marriage Fam. 42:923-934, 1980.
43. Leininger, M.: Transcultural health care: issues and conditions, Philadelphia, 1976, F.A. Davis Co.
44. Levin, L.S., Katz, A.H., and Holst, E.: Self care: lay initiatives in health, New York, 1976, Neale Watson Academic Publications, Inc., PRODIST.
45. *Litman, T.J.: The family as a basic unit in health and medical

---

*References preceded by an asterisk are particularly well suited for student reading.

care: a social-behavioral overview, Soc. Sci. Med. **8**:495, 1974.

46. Litman, T.J.: Health care and the family: a three-generation analysis. In Sussman, I.B.: Sourcebook in marriage and the family, ed. 4, Boston, 1974, Houghton Mifflin Co.

47. Macklin, E.D.: Nontraditional family forms: a decade of research, J. Marriage Fam. **42**:905-922, 1980.

48. Maugh, T.H.: Diabetes: model systems indicate virus a cause, Science **188**:436-438, 1975.

49. McCracken, R.D.: Lactase deficiency: an example of dietary evolution, Curr. Anthropol. **12**:479-517, 1971.

50. McCubbin, H.I., et al.: Family stress and coping: a decade review, J. Marriage Fam. **42**:855-871, 1980.

51. McDonald, G.W.: Family power: the assessment of a decade of theory and research, 1970-1979, J. Marriage Fam. **42**:841-854, 1980.

52. McEwen, P.: The social approach to family health, Soc. Sci. Med. **8**:487-493, 1974.

53. Meister, S.B.: Charting a family's developmental status—for intervention and for the record, Matern. Child Nurs. J. **2**:43-48, 1977.

54. Miller, F.J.W.: The epidemiological approach to the family as a unit in health statistics and the measurement of community health, Soc. Sci. Med. **8**:479-482, 1974.

55. Miller, J.R., and Janosik, E.R.: Family-focused care, New York, 1980, McGraw-Hill Book Co.

56. Mills, J.W., Saunders, K., and Martin, F.I.R.: Socioeconomic problems of insulin dependent diabetes, Med. J. Aust. **2**:1040-1044, 1973.

57. Novak, M.: Further reflections on ethnicity, Middletown, Pa., 1977, Jednota Press.

58. Novak, M.: The rise of the unmeltable ethnics, New York, 1972, Macmillan Publishing Co., Inc.

59. Otto, H.A.: Communes: the alternative life style, Sat. Rev., pp. 16-21, April 23, 1971.

60. Pless, I.B., Roghmann, K., and Haggerty, R.J.: Chronic illness, family functioning, and psychological adjustment: a model for the allocation of preventive mental health services, Int. J. Epidemiol. **1**:271-277, 1972.

61. Pless, I.B., and Satterwhite, B.: The families: family functioning and family problems. In Haggerty, R.J., Roghmann, K., and Pless, I.B., editors: Child health in the community, New York, 1975, John Wiley & Sons, Inc.

62. Pless, I.B., and Satterwhite, V.: A measured family function and its application, Soc. Sci. Med. **7**:613-621, 1973.

63. Pratt, L.: Family structure and effective health behavior: the energized family, Boston, 1976, Houghton Mifflin Co.

64. Ragucci, A.T.: Italian Americans. In Harwood, A., editor: Ethnicity and medical care, Cambridge, Mass., 1981, Harvard University Press.

65. Reid, J.M., et al.: Nutrient intake of Pima Indian women: relationship to diabetes mellitus and gallbladder disease, Am. J. Clin. Nutr. **24**:1282-1289, 1971.

66. Report of National Commission on Diabetes, vol. 3, U.S. Department of Health, Education and Welfare, No. (NIH) 76-1019, Washington, D.C., 1975.

67. Richardson, W.: Measuring the urban poor's use of physicians' services in response to illness episodes, Med. Care **18**:132, 1970.

68. Rodgers, R.H.: Family interaction and transaction: the developmental approach, Englewood Cliffs, N.J., 1973, Prentice-Hall, Inc.

69. Salsedo, A.J.: Book reviews, Med. Anthropol. Newsl. **8**:22-23, 1977.

70. Schaefer, O.: The changing health picture in the Canadian North, Can. J. Ophthalmol. **8**:196-204, 1973.

71. Schaefer, O.: When the Eskimo comes to town, Nutr. Today **6**:8-16, 1971.

72. Scott, E.: Family and social network, ed. 2, New York, 1971, The Free Press.

73. Skolnick, A.S., and Skolnick, H.: Family in transition: rethinking marriage, sexuality, child rearing and family organization, ed. 2, Boston, 1979, Little, Brown & Co.

74. Smiley, O.: The family centered approach: a challenge to public health nurses, Can. J. Public Health **63**:424-426, 1972.

75. *Smilkstein, G.: The family in trouble—how to tell, J. Fam. Pract. **2**:19-24, 1975.

76. Snow, L.F.: Folk medical beliefs and their implications for care of patients, Ann. Intern. Med. **81**:82-96, 1974.

77. *Spiegel, J.: Transaction: the interplay between individual, family and society, New York, 1971, Science House Inc.

78. Sprey, J.: Family power and process: toward a conceptual integration. In Cromwell, R., and Olson, D., editors: Power in families, New York, 1975, John Wiley & Sons, Inc.

79. Sprey, J.: Family power structure: a critical comment, J. Marriage Fam. **34**:235-238, 1972.

80. *Stack, C.: All our kin: strategies for survival in a black community, New York, 1974, Harper & Row, Publishers.

81. Stein, H., Hotwood, F., and Hill, R.: The ethnic imperative: examining the new white ethnic movement, University Park, Pa., 1977, State University Press.

82. Sussman, M.B., editor: Nontraditional family forms in the 1970's, Minneapolis, 1972, National Council on Family Relations.

83. Tallman, I.: The family as a small problem solving group, J. Marriage Fam. **32**:94-104, 1970.

84. Tapia, J.A.: The nursing process in family health, Nurs. Outlook **20**:267-270, 1972.

85. Triplett, J.: Characteristics and perceptions of low-income women and use of preventive health services, Nurs. Res. **19**:140-146, 1970.

86. Vogel, V.L.: American Indian medicine, Norman, Okla., 1970, University of Oklahoma Press.

87. Weaver, T.: Use of hypothetical situations in a study of Spanish American illness referral system, Hum. Org. **29**:140-154, 1970.

88. Weick, K.: Group processes, family processes and problem solving. In Aldous, J.: Family problem solving, Hinsdale, Ill., 1971, The Dryden Press.

89. Weidman, H.H., and Egland, J.: A behavioral science perspective in the comparative approach to the delivery of health care, Soc. Sci. Med. **7**:845-860, 1973.

90. World Health Organization Study Group: Statistical indices of family health, World Health Organization Technical Report, Series No. 5871, Geneva, 1976, World Health Organization.

Classic

91. Christenson, H.T., editor: Handbook of marriage and the family. Chicago, 1964, Rand McNally & Co.

92. Cohen, A.M.: Prevalence of diabetes among different ethnic Jewish groups in Israel, Metabolism **10**:50, 1961.

93. Douglas, M.: Pollution. In UNESCO: a dictionary of the behavioral sciences, New York, 1969, The Free Press.

94. Dubos, R.: Man, medicine, and environment, New York, 1968, Mentor Books.

95. Evans-Pritchard, E.E.: Witchcraft, oracles and magic among the Azande, Oxford, England, 1936, Oxford Clarendon Press.

96. Firth, R.: Essays on social organization and values, Atlantic Highlands, N.J., 1969, Humanities Press, Inc.

97. Friedson, E.: Patients' view of medical practice, New York, 1961, Russell Sage Foundation.

98. Freidson, E.: Client control and medical practice, Am. J. Sociol. **65**:374-382, 1960.

99. Gassow, Z., and Tracy, G.S.: Status, ideology and adaptation to stigmatized illness: a study of leprosy, Hum. Org. **27**:316-325, 1968.

100. Gould, J., and Kolb, W.L.: A dictionary of the social sciences, UNESCO, New York, 1969, The Free Press.
101. Goffman, E.: Stigma, Englewood Cliffs, N.J., 1963, Prentice-Hall, Inc.
102. Goffman, E.: The presentation of self in everyday life, New York, 1959, Anchor Books.
103. Jarvis, D.C.: Folk medicine, Greenwich, Conn., 1958, Crest Books.
104. Kluckhohn, C., and Kelly, W.: The concept of culture. In Linton, R.: The science of man in the world crisis, New York, 1945, Columbia University Press.
105. Kluckhohn, F., and Strodtbeck, F.: Variations in value orientations, Evanston, Ill., 1961, Row Peterson & Co.
106. *Leininger, M.: The culture concept and its relevance to nursing, J. Nurs. Educ. **6:**27-37, 1967.
107. Linton, R.: The cultural background of personality, New York, 1945, Appleton-Century-Crofts.
108. Linton, R.: The study of man, New York, 1936, Appleton-Century-Crofts.
109. Livingstone, F.B.: Anthropological implications of sickle cell gene distribution in West Africa, Am. Anthropol. **60:**533-562, 1958.
110. Matthews, J.D., et al.: Kuru and cannibalism, Lancet **2:**449-452, 1968.
111. Mechanic, D.: Influence of mothers on their children's health attitudes and behavior, Pediatrics **33:**4-15, 1964.
112. Meehan, J.P., Stoll, A.M., and Hardy, J.P.: Cutaneous pain threshold in native Alaskan, Indian and Eskimo, J. Appl. Physiol. **6:**397-400, 1954.
113. Milio, N.: Values, social class and community, Nurs. Res. **16:**26-31, 1967.
114. Naggan, L., and MacMalton, B.: Ethnic differences in the prevalence of anencephaly and spina bifida in Boston, Massachusetts, N. Engl. J. Med. **277:**1119-1123, 1967.
115. Nasr, A.N.M., et al.: Absentee experience in a group of employed diabetics, J. Occup. Med. **8:**621-625, 1966.
116. Neel, J.V.: Diabetes mellitus: a "thrifty" genotype rendered detrimental by progress, Am. J. Hum. Genet. **14:**353-362, 1962.
117. Parsons, T.: Definitions of health and illness in the light of American values and social structure. In Jaco, G.E.: Patients, physicians and illness, New York, 1957, The Free Press.
118. Parsons, T., and Shils, E.: Toward a general theory of action, New York, 1962, Torchbooks.
119. Pell, S., and D'Alonzo, C.A.: Sickness and injury experience of employed diabetics, Diabetes **9:**303-310, 1960.
120. Prosnitz, L.R., and Mandell, G.L.: Diabetes mellitus among Navajo and Hopi Indians: the lack of vascular complications, Am. J. Med. Sci. **253:**700-705, 1967.
121. Remoin, D.L.: Ethnic variability in glucose tolerance and insulin secretion, Arch. Intern. Med. **124:**695-700, 1969.
122. Sanders, I.: Balkan village, Lexington, Ky., 1949, University of Kentucky Press.
123. Sarbin, T.R., and Allen, V.L.: Role theory. In Lindsey, G., and Aronson, E.: Handbook of social psychology, ed. 2, Reading, Mass., 1968, Addison-Wesley Publishing Co., Inc.
124. Shostak, A.B.: Blue collar life, New York, 1969, Random House, Inc.
125. Shostak, A.B., and Gomberg, W.: Blue-collar world: studies of the American workers, Englewood Cliffs, N.J., 1964, Prentice-Hall, Inc.
126. *Sigerist, H.: The special position of the sick. In Roemer, M.I.: Henry E. Sigerist on the sociology of medicine, New York, 1960, M.D. Publications.
127. Simoons, F.J.: Eat not this flesh, Madison, Wis., 1967, University of Wisconsin Press.
128. Suchman, E.A.: Social factors in medical deprivation, Am. J. Public Health **55:**1725-1733, 1965.
129. Tylor, E.: Primitive culture, vol. 2, New York, 1974, New York Publ. (English edition.)
130. *Wolff, B.B., and Langley, S.: Cultural factors and the response to pain: a review, Am. Anthropol. **70:**494-501, 1968.
131. Zborowski, M.: Cultural components in response to pain, J. Soc. Issues **8:**16-30, 1952.

CHAPTER 4

SYSTEMS OF HEALTH CARE DELIVERY

KATHERINE SCHENK

Health care in the United States

The system through which health care is obtained by those who need it in the United States is mixed and fragmented. It has been said by some that there is no "health care system" and by others that there are many "systems," which only poorly articulate with each other. The latter is probably more nearly correct. A significant part of the problem is confusion regarding the meaning of *health* and *health care*. To the average citizen health may mean, "I am not ill"; but health care (and, along with that, health insurance) may mean care when *not* healthy, or care needed to bring one back to health. This latter concept traditionally brings to mind the physician and the hospital.

Centers of excellent medical (illness) care are scattered throughout the United States, yet many areas of the country are unserved or underserved by health care personnel and facilities. These centers of excellence are the finest in the world; they are usually in the close environs of universities that have schools of medicine, nursing, and other health sciences. They are also the centers of research in the health sciences. Paradoxically, it is not unusual for many of the underserved to live close to these centers in the urban ghettos as well as in many remote rural areas.

Persons with the means and know-how or those who meet certain specific qualifications (e.g., chronic renal failure) can obtain the finest health and medical care ever known. Other citizens of the United States are more poorly served than citizens in many other modern countries where there is a broad base of at least minimal service for all.

The great diversity of care in the United States is not hard to understand in view of the pluralistic nature of the society—the many national and cultural origins of the citizens, each with varying expectations about health, how it is attained and retained, and the part played by self, family, and others in maintaining health.

In contrast, one might look at Denmark, which has a clear national health policy. It is a comparatively small nation, with a population of about 5 million, compared with 240 million in the United States. It encompasses only about 1/200 of the U.S. land mass. In addition, it has a much more homogeneous population in terms of a common cultural heritage. Many more customs and values are commonly understood and accepted as Danish than is true in the United States. A broadly accepted national approach to dealing with social problems such as housing and unemployment extends to health care. There is a centrally designated institution, the National Board of Health, through which most decisions regarding the national health system are coordinated. This involves all care for citizens, from maintenance and preventive services through surgery and acute care. It involves health personnel from the highly skilled specialists through all preventive and supportive levels to the least skilled. It is concerned with determining what facilities and personnel are needed and with providing the educational facilities for the personnel. Although there are some additional care givers such as medical and surgical specialists outside this system and change and conflict and rising medical care costs are no more foreign to this system than to others in our changing world, there is nevertheless a sense of order and wholeness to Denmark's health care system.

In contrast, the supersystem designated the United States of America has a large aggregate of illness care systems, only a few of which articulate with each other. There is, as yet, no specific commitment to either health or illness care on an overall basis, although it has been a major political issue for over a decade. One factor responsible for the fact that the United States is the only major industrialized country today that does not have an identifiable system for delivering health care to every citizen is our traditional emphasis on local decision making and on states' rights and communities' rights to determine their own needs and how they should be met. Although health care is not mentioned in the Constitution, a good case can be made that the well-known and accepted right of each citizen to life, liberty, and the pursuit of happiness cannot be achieved without provision for adequate health care.[10]

Still another factor in the health care dilemma in the United States is the private enterprise concept of operation and the fact that, except for those conditions that affect the health of large segments of the population and thus come under the aegis of public health (e.g., safe drinking water or protection from communicable disease), the delivery of health care has tended to be mainly a service performed for private profit.

Most illness care is provided by physicians in private practice operating on a fee-for-service basis. Many communities within the supersystem have hospitals for care of the ill. A few of these receive some tax support, and many were built with large amounts of federal funds. However, the majority are operated through payment from those they care for (this payment being managed by means of "health" insurance) plus community fund drives and charitable bequests of various kinds. It is these hospitals that presently employ the largest number of registered nurses in the United States. Associated with these hospitals are the largest number of private, practicing physicians. There is at present also a trend toward corporation-owned hospitals, which are operated strictly for private profit.

There are other illness-care systems. The Veterans Administration hospitals and nursing homes are completely tax supported and provide care for veterans of U.S. wars. Some labor unions, such as the United Mine Workers, have provided similar services for their members, supported by dues or company contributions to their welfare funds. Some large communities, such as New York City, have their own tax-supported hospital systems; and most states support hospitals for special problems such as mental illness and chronic disease. Federal hospitals for merchant seamen were among the earliest public facilities of a young U.S. government and formed the nucleus of the U.S. Public Health Service.[10]

Care of the elderly and chronically ill in the United States has gradually assumed a place of major importance as our society has moved to a higher and higher median age. Institutional care for the aged was not greatly needed when the country was younger. Most of the few elderly who did survive to old age lived with their own families. A few unfortunate persons were relegated to "old folks' homes" or poor farms, supported by taxes, where some minimal health care was provided. The major focus of health and illness care was on infants and children and their mothers. A Children's Bureau was established within the federal government. Health care providers for many reasons preferred to devote their knowledge and skills to caring for the young, and the needs of the aging were often ignored.

More people are now living beyond retirement into the seventh, eighth, and ninth decade of life. While less than 5% become institutionalized, the needs of both those living in the community and those needing some type of institutional care are not being met in the same manner that the needs of children were met in the past. The majority of professional health care providers—physicians, nurses, and others—have not been interested in caring for the elderly. There is now some evidence that this attitude is changing as some physicians and many nurses turn to the specialty of gerontology.

For the aging who remain in their own homes or elsewhere in the community, it is evident that additional facilities for their care and well-being, including health care, must be provided. A comparative newcomer on the scene, the day-care center for the chronically ill and the elderly, shows evidence of becoming an important part of the health care scene. In addition, there are a large number of nursing homes for care of the chronically ill, especially the elderly. It is unfortunate that many of these day-care centers and nursing homes are developing as private profit-making enterprises along lines similar to that of private practice medicine and that they often are not closely associated with other health-illness care facilities.

Another very old model of illness care, but one that has an important element of health promoting care, is the Visiting Nurse Association or Public Health Nursing Agency, together referred to as community nursing. Although the original idea was to provide care for illness in the home, health promotion has always been an important focus of these organizations. They may be supported by fees for services, third-party payers, taxes, or voluntary gifts. The term *Home Health Agency* is used to indicate expanded services available to clients in their homes.

All states and many communities have departments of public health, which are supported by tax funds and employ physicians, nurses, and other health care workers. Their primary purpose is to protect the health of the total community; thus they are preventative in focus. Goals and activities of many health departments have been changing and expanding in recent years in response to the changing conditions of our society. In former years communicable disease control was their primary focus; now other environmental threats such as pollution are of greater significance.

Lately a model of health care has emerged that is truly focused on health promotion and illness prevention, at least to the point where the financial advantage to both provider and client is *wellness*. This is the *health maintenance organization (HMO)*. Early models included the Health Insurance Plan of New York, the Ross-Loos plan, and the Kaiser-Permanente Foundation. Employees of Kaiser-Permanente in California were provided with preventive and health maintenance facilities and ambulatory care clinics as fringe benefits of their employment. This model has been adopted by other industries and also by some private medical practices, many of which include nurses. In these systems clients pay a set fee for regular preventive and screening services as well as for illness care. The HMO fares best financially when clients are kept well and out of hospitals. An additional feature, accountability to the public, was built into the HMOs that were financed in their beginning stages by the federal government. Peer review of the quality of care provided was required as a condition of funding.[45]

Despite all of the above resources many of the very poor as well as people with nontraditional life-styles have often felt they did not or could not obtain health care or preventive services from any of the establishment facilities and organizations. In recent years many nurses as well as physicians have worked in so-called *free* or *nontraditional agencies* such as storefronts and other community-based clinics. Many of these were originally funded through federal grants available in the late 1960s and early 1970s and have fallen on hard times in regard to funding. Ideas and lessons learned from such experimental approaches to health care will not be lost, however, and may be built into future health care planning.

In our society individuals and families are responsible for their own health and when concerned about health, or frank illness, are expected to seek the health care provider or agency of their choice. This concept presupposes either the ability to pay the chosen health care provider or possession of insurance to cover the payment. Today many persons do have such insurance; for many it is provided as a fringe benefit of employment. Again, nearly all insurance is directed at coverage for illness. Those who are unemployed or medically indigent are nominally covered for illness care through Medicaid, a plan associated with the welfare systems of each of the 50 states and supplemented by federal funds. But as with other welfare plans, and with Medicare, which is the system for illness care for the elderly and others receiving Social Security benefits, there are many gaps and inadequacies, and many persons do not meet the qualifications set by individual states.

In view of such wide differences of philosophy, ex-

pectations, and objectives, plus much entrenched self-interest in maintaining present systems, national planning for health care delivery has been very difficult. John Bryant has suggested a principle of justice for health care as follows:

Whatever health care is available should be equally available to all. Departures from that equality of distribution are permissible only if those worse off are made better off. . . . There should be a floor, or minimum of health services for all. Resources above the floor should be distributed according to need.[8]

Traditionally, nursing has supported this philosophy. Primary prevention of illness and maintenance of high-level wellness has long been a goal of organized nursing. More recently it has been reiterated by nursing interest groups such as those concerned with maternity and infant nursing, pediatric nursing, gerontologic nursing, and psychiatric and mental health nursing. Still further commitment was made by the establishment of the Commission on Human Rights as a permanent component of the American Nurses Association at the 1976 biennial convention. Nurses have reaffirmed their position that the fulfillment of their national purpose depends on quality health care for every citizen.[32]

The problem of financing such care is one of the major issues that must be faced. The United States presently spends a greater percent of its gross national product (GNP) for illness care than any other country, yet many feel that resources are being wasted and misused. Although there has been increasing financial support for health care, this support has been provided through the existing health care systems. Legislation that provided funding for Medicare and Medicaid continued the use of presently existing models. One outcome of this has been greatly increased costs. As the most conspicuously rising factor in the cost of living within the past decade, health care (illness care) is a target for considerable criticism. Writers outside the health care establishment, for example, Ivan Ilich,[22] as well as many within it believe that only willingness of individual citizens to assume responsibility for their own health, including adopting healthy life-styles and taking preventive measures, can contain health care costs. Nursing has been moving in the direction of promoting and facilitating clients' self-health care. This philosophy has been extensively developed by Orem[38] and other members of the Nursing Development Conference Group.[36]

On the national level the federal government has for many years supported the education and training of health care providers; programs of research and education for certain illnesses, such as heart disease, cancer, and stroke; and considerable basic medical research. More recently systems of delivery of care have been financed on a demonstration basis, such as the HMOs and programs such as those to prepare nurse practitioners and physician assistants. Again, these efforts have served to support and reinforce the existing systems of health care.

In contrast, it is useful to look at a systems model for providing health care to a specific population, for example, to all the people within a given country or state or community (Fig. 4-1). This model would begin by gathering data to determine the needs for service and care of the specified population across a broad spectrum. It would identify those factors relevant for that population and would classify the levels of care appropriate for identified needs. It would next obtain or develop through education and training the providers and the facilities to meet these needs.[3]

Our traditional approach has been exactly the opposite. Especially in medicine, the supersystem has supported the self-determined preparation of increasing numbers of specialists in an increasing array of subspecialty areas and then identified the need for their services. This is not a good economic model for the consumer, although it may be for the provider, and there is increasing evidence that it cannot continue unchecked.[19] In the 1974 Health Planning and Resources Development Act (P.L. 93-641) signed into law in January 1975 the Congress, influenced by constituent dissatisfaction with health care, mandated regional planning. This law lists several national health priorities, including providing for people in underserved areas and the sharing and coordinating of existing facilities. State and local health service planning agencies were set up under the provisions of this law, and consumers as well as health care providers were represented on the planning committees.

Toward the end of the decade concern focused increasingly on costs. Inflation, and especially costs of medical care, greatly alarmed citizens so that once feasible plans for broad-based support (a national health insurance) receded.[12,16] Most analysts now predict only gradual, incremental changes in our systems and methods of delivery of health and illness care for the foreseeable future.[19] The health planning agencies (known as HSAs) have had varying and not always spectacular success; and they are losing fiscal support. National goals at present appear to be in the area of cost control and containment.[19,44]

Nursing within the health care system

Historically, in the United States nursing has been provided in a variety of models. Within institutional settings it has been in acute and chronic care hospitals, in long-term care facilities, and in community nursing agencies. The heyday of private duty nursing was in the early part of this century when it was the major employment opportunity for nurses. In this model of practice nurses were private entrepreneurs. Even though they often depended on the favor and recommendations of specific physicians, they provided service for a fee and were paid directly by the clients they served. From before the turn of the century this service was frequently provided in the homes of the affluent; but as the care of the ill moved into hospitals, so did private duty nursing, still generally for the financially advantaged. It was total patient care and was more art than

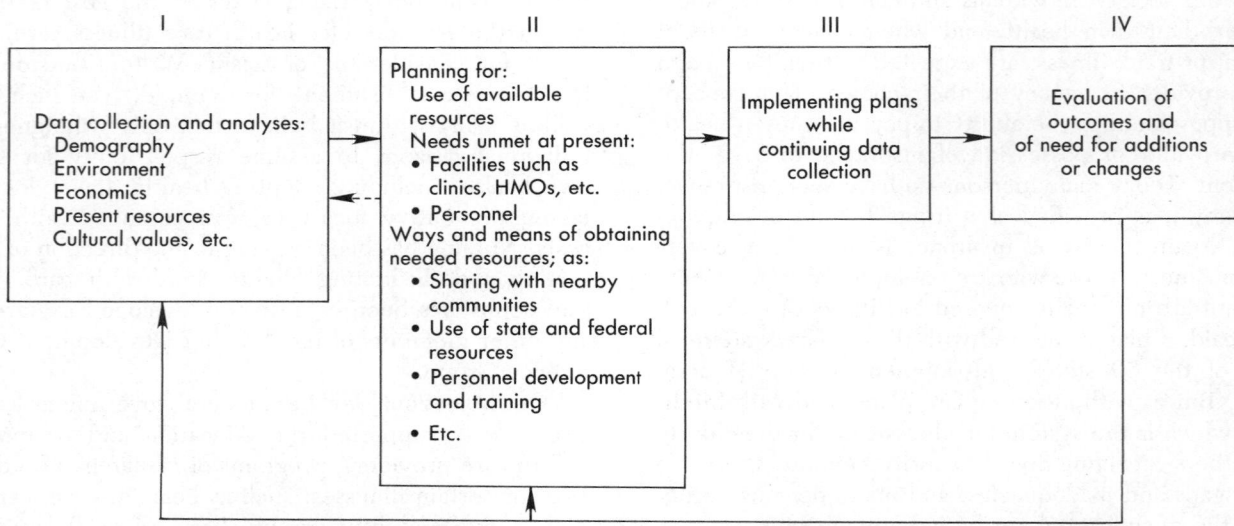

Fig. 4-1. Model for developing health care delivery systems.

science. Even when employed by the hospital, the registered nurse of before World War II usually did everything prescribed for and needed by the patients, since there were few other health care providers. By far the greatest amount of care to those in hospitals was provided by nursing students. Private duty nursing suffered a mortal blow in the Great Depression of the 1930s.

With the shortage of registered nurses during the war years of the 1940s, this total patient care gave way to the functional method of practicing in which each nurse or nursing student in the interest of efficiency of time did a particular task, for example, administering medications to every patient on a unit. This was the beginning of the wide support for and the increasing preparation of licensed practical (vocational) nurses. Although continued long after the war and even into the present, the functional model of nursing care is generally considered both by health care providers and by clients to be unsatisfactory and fragmented. It was succeeded by team nursing, in which a group of health care providers with a variety of preparations (registered nurse, licensed practical [vocational] nurse, and the nursing assistant or aide) cared for a designated group of patients, using the skills of each to best advantage. In concept this was the ideal way to care for patients with a variety of needs. In practice it often did not work as well as conceptualized. One of the main problems seemed to be finding time for the needed team planning and conferences essential for good team nursing. The guidance and coordination of the team by the professional nurse, an essential component of the plan, were often sketchy or completely lacking. There were and still are places where team nursing is felt to be a rewarding and satisfactory way of delivering nursing care, both within acute and chronic hospital settings and in community settings, when the basic concepts and plans can be implemented.

The most recent development in the care of clients in organizational settings (which includes the community health agency) is called *primary nursing*.[29] (This term must be distinguished from primary care, which will be discussed later.) In this model one professional nurse is totally responsible for planning and evaluating the nursing care given to a relatively small number of clients. To those who were active in nursing before World War II this does not appear to be a new method but a coming full circle. The model has been well demonstrated at the Loeb Center for Nursing and Rehabilitation where for many years nurses have been providing care through the primary nursing model.[7] Many agencies are moving or have moved to primary nursing in the belief that it is more satisfying, both to clients and to nurses, and that it is more cost effective than team nursing. More time will be needed, however, to evaluate this model.[6,50]

Thus there have been many attempts to find the ideal way of providing nursing care to groups of clients designated as ill or in need of care. It is likely that all of these will continue to be used in one way or another, even coexisting within the same organization, in accordance with the philosophies of individual health care providers.[6,49]

With the development of scientific and theoretically based nursing within recent years, several distinctive models of professional practice that fit clients' health care needs as currently identified have been developed and tested. Such terms as *extended* and *expanded* roles have been used. The question has been raised: Are these terms accurate, or are client needs expanding and is nursing moving to provide for these needs?[39] The much used terms *nurse clinician* and *nurse practitioner* have also been critically questioned by nursing leaders. If professional nurses are prepared and licensed to practice nursing, are they not in fact nurse practitioners? And if nurses must practice in a clinical setting in order to be practicing at all, must they not be nurse clinicians?

Although the above is undeniably true, the new terms are in vogue and are understood by many to have some specific meaning, even though there may be disagreement about the exact meaning. According to the American Nurses' Association (ANA) definitions of clinician and practitioner, both are skilled in obtaining a health history from clients and in assessing client needs. *Clinicians* manage the care of a case load of clients, usually in a hospital setting such as a coronary care unit, an acute respiratory care unit, or an orthopedic unit. They plan care on the basis of immediate and long-term needs; this care may sometimes be carried out by others. They supervise care given by others and help them perform certain functions and skills in a conceptual frame very closely akin to that of good team nursing. Clinicians also communicate with other disciplines relative to the needs of clients and their families.

Practitioners, in the current definition of the term, usually practice in a broader area than do clinicians, such as an ambulatory care setting or in the community. Thus they may be expected to be aware of even more factors in the larger social systems that impinge on client needs and care. They are expected to be skillful in taking a health history, to be able to do physical assessment, and to recognize abnormal signs and symptoms. They are closely associated with a physician, whether within an institutional setting or in the community. Nurse practitioners usually become members of health care groups such as HMOs, but they may work alone in remote areas with backup of centrally located physicians. The pediatric nurse practitioner is one outstanding example of this model.[53]

According to a survey by the American Nurses Association[4] the majority of pediatric nurse practitioners responding were graduates of baccalaureate nursing programs and had received educational preparation to function as practitioners in short-term continuing education programs. A large number work with high-risk populations such as children in Head Start programs, day-care centers, and neighborhood clinics. Such facilities are often supported by tax funds to provide services to clients who may not normally have access to private physicians.

Other models include practitioners working with adults who have chronic diseases and with aging clients. Many health care systems are presently using nurse practitioners to provide *primary care*. This is the term used to describe the first contact of a client needing care within a health care system. It is also used to describe the care needed by most of the people most of the time. It may be preventive, including identification of health problems at an early stage, or care of minor, noncritical, and chronic illnesses. Most primary care is for those who are ambulatory (not occupying beds in hospitals or other inpatient settings), and most, but not all, ambulatory care is primary care. Several studies have shown that primary care provided by nurses is at least as good as the care provided by physicians and is highly valued by clients.[46] The same positive results have been found when nurse practitioners work with clients who have chronic and long-term health problems.[54]

With additional education leading to a master's degree the nurse may become a *clinical specialist* in a specific area. In contrast to the titles mentioned above, this title is widely accepted, with considerable agreement regarding functions and qualifications. Some examples are the cardiovascular, renal, and oncology nurse specialists, most of whom are employed by hospitals and other health care agencies (Fig. 4-2). Such nurses are well prepared to practice with a great deal of autonomy, and some have set up an independent practice and accept clients, who may contact them on their own initiative or may be referred by physicians.[28]

The issues of responsibility and accountability for one's own professional actions are vital in this type of practice. To some extent it is governed by individual state laws related to medical and nursing practice, although most state laws allow the nurse to practice *nursing* independently. A more telling restriction has been the payment of fees for service. Most third-party payers (Blue Cross/Blue Shield, Medicare, Medicaid, and other insurers) will not directly reimburse nurses for independent nursing services, although there has been some legislative progress made and efforts are continuing.

Mainly because of the fee-for-service problem, it is presently more common to find the nurse clinical specialist in a group practice with other nurses, physicians,

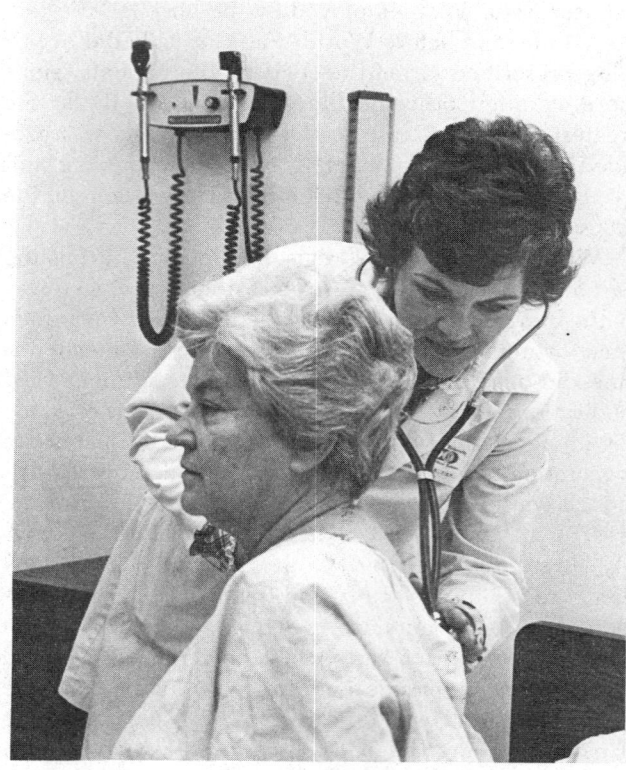

Fig. 4-2. Clinical specialist examines client. Clinical specialist possesses ability to manage case load of clients with needs for clinical expertise in areas such as oncology.

or other professionals. Others are employed in agencies such as a mental health center or a community nursing service. There have been impressive demonstrations, for example, of the effectiveness of pediatric nurse practitioners in a school health program.[41]

Within the United States, nursing has in the past identified populations at risk and set up systems of health care delivery to serve these populations. The educational focus and the broad humanistic approach of caring for individuals and families, with emphasis on primary prevention of illness and disease, led to the establishment of agencies such as the Frontier Nursing Service and the Henry Street Settlement in New York City, which was that city's first community nursing service. These were systems developed by nurses in response to identified needs of clients. Much of the focus in those early days was on children and on the neonatal period. Nurses in these systems expanded their activities to meet the needs of the clients; nurses in the Frontier Nursing Service delivered babies in areas only accessible by horseback. While the needs of mothers, infants, and children remain important, nurses now also identify additional groups of vulnerable persons, notably those with long-term and chronic illness and the aged. Care for such identified populations at risk has become a major concern of specific groups of nurses.

The struggle to bring order out of the confusion among the health care delivery systems and to make access to health care more realistic to all within the supersystem has been greatly enhanced by recent developments in nursing.[43] We might illustrate the activities of the several different nursing models identified above by describing a conference held recently at a community hospital in a medium-sized city in a midwestern state. This hospital is the referral point for clients from the city and the surrounding countryside, which includes several small communities. The conference is held on a regular basis to plan for the continuity of care of clients to be admitted to a rehabilitation unit, either from their homes or from the hospital, or who were returning home from that unit. Among those present were the nurse clinician from a specific hospital unit, the staff physician, the dietitian, the social worker, the occupational therapist, and the physical therapist. Also present was a staff nurse from the community health agency of the city. They discussed Mr. W., who had suffered a stroke 2 weeks previously and had been admitted by way of the emergency room to the hospital.

The nurse clinician from the neurology unit discussed the progress Mr. W. had made and his present status. On that unit the staff practiced primary nursing, and Mr. W. was one of a small number of patients to whom this nurse gave total care. She reported not only on his physical state, which was improving, but on his emotional state and his motivation, both of which were good at that time. She recommended his admission to the special rehabilitation unit for care before returning home.

The staff nurse from the community agency had cared for Mr. W. and his wife in the past. She was familiar with the home situation and offered pertinent data related to the prospect for his continued progress at home. Because of special skills she had acquired in a continuing education course, she had the title of Nurse Practitioner; she had a case load of families in the community for whom she was the primary care provider, the health professional whom they contact first when they need care. She was the person called by Mrs. W. when her husband suffered his stroke, and it was she who referred him to the emergency room of the local hospital.

The nurse who coordinated the rehabilitation unit had a master's degree in rehabilitation nursing. He was a clinical specialist and was expected to be responsible for planning the program for Mr. W. in the rehabilitation unit, arranging for the special services such as physical and occupational therapy and medical care. He also was responsible for communicating with the community nurse practitioner about Mr. W.'s plans to return home.

Familiar modes of nursing practice by which care is given to the ill, injured, and infirm in acute and chronic settings will continue; and demand for the exceptional skills of nurses in critical care areas is expected to remain high and even to increase.[44] In the long range, the proportion of nurses working outside hospitals will probably increase. Client awareness and demand is likely to cause a shift from receiving care in places and settings more convenient for *providers* to those settings that better meet needs of *consumers*. At the same time, cost effectiveness of care in inpatient settings is being compared with cost of care received in clients' own homes and communities.[20] Skilled nurses will increasingly provide care in these settings, meeting health care needs as they have done through the past hundred years and more. Increasingly nurses are preparing themselves to practice in these settings.

Health and the prevention of illness are inexorably joined to the culture and the life-style of an individual. In our present society there are very few diseases or problems, especially in adulthood, for which a totally external cause can be identified and eliminated. Yet people continue to live and to think of health and illness as if this were not true. To some extent the providers of health care have supported this idea, and many have gained great advantage and power in the society from their image as great healers, as possessors of almost magical knowledge and ability.

A majority of nurses have been caught up in this myth for generations. The reasons are many: none of us can escape our own culture, nor are we usually even aware of the culture as more than the way things are ordained to be. The changes that have occurred in nursing's image of itself are enormous and only beginning to be felt in the supersystem.

Few are gifted with sight into the future, but it is impossible to believe that the significant beginnings that have been made will not continue and expand, or that the numbers of well-prepared and assertive young people in professional nursing today will be held back by the existing power structure in health care systems from offering and practicing the skills they have in helping to improve the health of our society.

Thus in an era when citizens and clients, the consumers of health care, are becoming better informed, more critical of existing care, and more active as decision makers in the kind and quality of care they need and want, nurses are being prepared through a variety of models to contribute to that care. The concept that nursing has a unique service to offer the health care consumer has been held by nurses throughout history. Through research and through demonstration, the reality of that concept is presently in evidence and is continuing to be affirmed.

REFERENCES AND SELECTED READINGS
Contemporary

1. Abel-Smith, B.: Health care in a cold economic climate, Lancet **8216**(1):373-376, 1981.
2. American Academy of Nursing: Long-term care in perspective: past, present, and future directions for nursing, American Academy of Nursing papers presented at annual meeting, Sept. 22-23, 1975.
2a. American Nurses Association: A social policy statement, Kansas City, Mo., 1981, The Association.
3. American Nurses Association: A national policy for health care: principles and positions, pub. no. G-130, Kansas City, Mo., 1977, The Association.
4. American Nurses Association: Pediatric nurse practitioners: their practice today, Kansas City, Mo., 1975, The Association.
5. Andreopolis, S., editor: Primary care: where medicine fails, New York, 1974, John Wiley & Sons, Inc.
6. Betz, M.: Some hidden costs of primary nursing, Nurs. Health Care **2**(3):150-154, 1981.
7. *Bower-Ferres, S.: Loeb Center and its philosophy of nursing, Am. J. Nurs. **75**:810-815, 1975.
8. Bryant, J.H.: Some interrelations between the evolving health care system and nursing practice and education, paper presented at Duke University School of Nursing Conference on Distributive Nursing and Mental Health, Durham, N.C., Sept. 20, 1973.
9. Cambridge Research Institute: Trends affecting the U.S. health care system, U.S. Department of Health, Education and Welfare, no. (HRA) 76-14503, vol. 1, 1976.
10. Chapman, C.B., and Talmage, J.M.: The evolution of the right to health concept in the United States, Pharos **34**:31-33, 1971.
11. *Chopoorian, R., and Craig, M.M.: Nursing and health care delivery, Am. J. Nurs. **76**:1988-1989, 1976.
12. Congressional Quarterly, Inc.: Health policy, the legislative agenda, Washington, D.C., 1980, The Quarterly.
13. *Craven, R.G.: Primary health care: six nurses talk about what they do in a variety of settings, Am. J. Nurs. **76**:1958-1968, 1976.
14. Davis, A.J., and Aroskar, M.A.: Ethical dilemmas in nursing practice, New York, 1978, Appleton-Century-Crofts.
15. Donabedian, A.: Issues in national health insurance, Am. J. Public Health **66**:342-350, 1976.
16. Etzioni, A.: Revitalization of the health care system in America, keynote address presented at the National League for Nursing convention, May 1981.
17. Fagin, C.M., and Maraldo, P.: Health policy in the nursing curriculum: why it is needed, Nurs. Health Care **2**(1):24-28, 1981.
18. Ginsberg, E.: The economics of health care and the future of nursing, J. Nurs. Adm. **11**(3):28-32, 1981.
19. Ginsberg, E.: The limits of health reform, New York, 1977, Bantam Books, Inc.
20. Hapgood, D.: What people like you and me are doing to get better health care, The Washington Monthly, Oct. 1976.
21. *Hellman, C.: The making of a clinical specialist, Nurs. Outlook **22**:165-167, 1974.
22. Ilich, I.: Medical nemesis: the expropriation of health, New York, 1976, Pantheon Books, Inc.
23. Isaacs, G.: The family nurse and primary health care in rural areas. In Nolan, R.L., and Schwartz, J.L.: Rural and Appalachian health, Springfield, Ill., 1973, Charles C Thomas, Publisher.
24. Jacox, A., and Norris, C.: Organizing for independent nursing practice, New York, 1977, Appleton-Century-Crofts.
25. Kennedy, E.M.: Congress and the national health policy, Rosenhaus lecture, Am. J. Public Health **68**:241-244, 1978.
26. *Kinlein, M.L.: Independent nursing practice with clients, Philadelphia, 1977, J.B. Lippincott Co.

27. Knowles, J.H., editor: Doing better and feeling worse: health in the United States, New York, 1977, W.W. Norton & Co., Inc.
28. *Lane, H.: Promoting an independent nursing practice, Am. J. Nurs. **75**:1319-1321, 1975.
29. Marram, G.D., Barrett, M.W., and Bevis, E.O.: Primary nursing: a model for individualized care, ed. 2, St. Louis, 1979, The C.V. Mosby Co.
30. *Mauksch, I.G.: On national health insurance, Am. J. Nurs. **78**:1323-1327, 1978.
31. *Mauksch, I.G., and Young, P.R.: Nurse-physician interaction in a family medical care center, Nurs. Outlook **22**:113-119, 1974.
32. Members named to Commission on Human Rights: Editorial, Am. Nurse **8**:11, 1976.
33. Miller, C.A.: Societal change and public health: a rediscovery, Am. J. Public Health **66**:54-60, 1976.
34. Millman, M.L., editor: Nursing personnel and the changing health care system, Cambridge, Mass., 1978, Ballinger Publishing Co.
35. Navarro, V.: A critique of the present and proposed strategies for redistributing resources in the health sector and a discussion of alternatives, Med. Care **12**:721-742, 1974.
36. Nursing Development Conference Group: Concept formalization in nursing: process and product, Boston, 1973, Little, Brown & Co.
37. Olendski, M.C.: Cautionary tales, Wakefield, Mass., 1973, Contemporary Publishing.
38. Orem, D.E.: Nursing: concepts of practice, ed. 2, New York, 1981, McGraw-Hill Book Co.
39. Ozimek, D., and Yura, H.: Who is the nurse practitioner? New York, 1975, National League for Nursing.
40. Porter, P.: The role of the independent nurse practitioner, Nurs. Clin. North Am. **15**:419-428, 1980.
41. Porter, P.J.: The Cambridge story, Am. J. Public Health **71**(suppl.):86-88, 1981.
42. Public Health Service: Forward plan for health, FY 1977-81, U.S. Department of Health, Education and Welfare, no. (OS) 76-50024, Washington, D.C., 1975.
43. Record, J.C., editor: Staffing primary care in 1990, New York, 1981, Springer Publishing Co., Inc.
44. Rorrie, C.C., Jr., and Dearman, F.V.: Health planning: a new phase, Public Health Rep. **95**:177-182, 1980.
45. Saward, E.W., and Greenlick, M.R.: Health policy and the H.M.O. In Leininger, M.: Barriers and facilitators in quality health care: health care dimensions, Philadelphia, 1975, F.A. Davis Co.
46. Spitzer, W.O., et al.: The Burlington randomized trial of the nurse practitioner, N. Engl. J. Med. **290**:251-256, 1974.
47. Starr, R.: Changing the balance of power in American medicine, Milbank Mem. Fund Q. **58**:166-171, 1980.
48. Sultz, H., Zielman, M., and Matthews, J.: Highlights, phase 2, longitudinal study of nurse practitioners. In Millman, M.: Nursing personnel and the changing health care system, Cambridge, Mass., 1978, Ballinger Publishing Co.
49. Vanservellan, G.N.: Primary nursing: variations in practice, J. Nurs. Adm. **11**(9):40-46, 1981.
50. Vanservellan, M.: Primary nursing: the adoption of a nursing care modality, Nurs. Health Care **1**(3):144-147, 1980.
51. Walters, W.J.: State level comprehensive health planning: a retrospect, Am. J. Public Health **66**:139-144, 1976.
52. Yett, D.E.: An economic analysis of the nurse shortage, New York, 1975, Lexington Books.

Classic

53. Silver, H.K., Ford, L.C., and Stearly, S.G.: A program to increase the health care for children: the pediatric nurse practitioner program, Pediatrics **39**:756-760, 1967.
54. Stoeckle, J.D., et al.: Medical nursing clinic for the chronically ill, Am. J. Nurs. **63**:87-89, 1963.

*References preceded by an asterisk are particularly well suited for student reading.

CHAPTER 5

EPIDEMIOLOGY AND HEALTH

NANCY FUGATE WOODS

Concepts of epidemiology have changed markedly over time, reflecting the major health concerns and problems of the day and the level of sophistication of scientists' and practitioners' conceptions of health and disease. Initially, the term *epidemiology* referred to the study of epidemics. During the era in which the discipline was christened, this was quite appropriate inasmuch as the major health problems of the world were outbreaks of infectious diseases. As major health problems have changed, so have the concerns of epidemiologists. The subject matter of journals of epidemiology currently includes studies of infectious diseases, chronic illnesses such as cardiovascular disease, cancer, and metabolic disorders, nutritional problems, occupational health problems, accidents, and even homicide. Epidemiologists' interests have transcended the boundaries of disease and now include such concerns as population dynamics, health and illness behavior, and health program evaluation.[14]

Definitions of epidemiology

Despite the wide-ranging interests of the discipline, there are some commonly accepted definitions of epidemiology. The word epidemiology is literally translated as the study of what comes upon people:

epi = upon
demos = people
logos = study

Omran[14] defines epidemiology as the "study of the occurrence and distribution of health conditions and disease and population change, as well as their determi-

Portions of this chapter appeared in Woods, N.F., and Woods, J.S.: Epidemiology and the study of cancer. In Marino, L.B.: Cancer nursing, St. Louis, 1981, The C.V. Mosby Co.

nants and consequences in population groups." This definition is sufficiently broad to encompass the interests of nurses whose concerns are not only with the etiology of disease and its prevention, but also with the consequences of the disease and related therapy for the quality of life. Other epidemiologists would add that the assessment of outcomes of therapies, their human and economic costs as well as their utility, is an appropriate challenge for the discipline.

Scope of epidemiology

The scope of epidemiology includes the study of a variety of health-related phenomena and the people affected by these phenomena. The phenomena of interest include health and physiologic states, disease and death, health-related behavior and population dynamics, as well as the determinants of an intervention program for each of these. The characteristics of people studied might include group characteristics such as age and sex, behavioral characteristics, risk factors in certain population groups, and environmental settings of the people. While the scope of epidemiology is similar to that of some other disciplines, there are three principal traits that are specific to the way epidemiologists study phenomena:

1. The epidemiologist's primary concern is with a population or an aggregate of people rather than with individuals from that population.
2. Epidemiologists are concerned with comparisons between groups or populations.
3. Epidemiologists are interested not only in asking the question, "Why do those people having a certain condition have it," but also in asking the question, "Why were the people who do not have the condition spared?"[14]

Strategies used in epidemiologic investigations

Epidemiology as a discipline contributes to the *description* and *analysis* of health-related conditions. One common focus of epidemiologists is the description of the natural history of disease, how the course differs in people having different characteristics or environments, and how the disease course may be altered in response to prevention or therapy. Another focus includes the description of patterns of health and disease in communities, often referred to as "community diagnosis." Commonly used descriptive measures of health status are the incidence or prevalence rates of a disease or the mortality associated with it. Description of population dynamics is another important concern of epidemiologists, as is the development of descriptive indices such as the rates and ratios used in describing morbidity and mortality.

Epidemiology has contributed significantly to the understanding of the etiology of disease. These contributions have included the documentation of causal relationships between factors and disease as well as the study of epidemics to identify their origin.

Increasingly, epidemiologic methods are used in experimentation, such as in the clinical trials of new therapies or preventive measures, and even experiments with animal models. Studies of program acceptance and evaluation of health programs are commonly using epidemiologic methods.

With this overview in mind, we shall explore in more detail the descriptive, analytic, and experimental approaches to epidemiology and their application.

Descriptive approaches in epidemiology

Descriptive epidemiologic approaches have yielded important information concerning the etiology of various health problems. The traditional descriptive variables explored by epidemiologists are person, place, and time. By studying the amount and distribution of various diseases within a population according to these three variables, epidemiologists have been able to generate hypotheses to guide more focused investigations of etiology.

Descriptive variables

Person

Although there are numerous characteristics of individuals that may be explored, it is customary for epi-

TABLE 5-1. Risk factors for fatal myocardial infarction in young women 15 to 44 years of age*

	Odds ratio	
Risk factor	White women	Black women
Prior myocardial infarction	48.6	22.5
Other heart disease	6.9	7.4
High cholesterol level	8.2	35.6
Current smoker	2.5	1.9
Obesity	2.0	3.0
Bilateral oophorectomy	1.3	0
Hypertension	3.4	3.8
Diabetes	4.7	5.7
Oral contraceptive use in past month	1.7	0
Thromboembolism	2.4	1.9

*Adapted from Krueger, D., et al.: Am. J. Epidemiol. **113**(4):357-370, 1981.

demiologists to explore the frequency of disease for various age, sex, and ethnic or racial groups. In addition, such variables as religion, social class, occupation, income, education, marital status, family variables (e.g., family size and type, birth order, parental characteristics) and the individual's general health status are explored. Table 5-1 illustrates the relationship between several "person" variables and the incidence of fatal myocardial infarction. Investigation of the frequency with which certain health problems are seen among populations with varying personal characteristics is important for several reasons. First, high-risk groups can be identified, and close surveillance can be planned so that health problems can be detected and treated early in their course. Next, trends in incidence and mortality among high-risk groups can be systematically studied. Third, identification of characteristics associated with these problems can provide a basis for generation of hypotheses regarding their etiology and further etiologic studies.

Place

The frequency of occurrence of various diseases can also be related to the geographic area in which they occur. Place can be described in terms of natural boundaries, political subdivisions, international scope, or rural vs. urban comparisons. In addition, the comparison of rates for people who migrate from one area to another is of assistance in separating the role of genetic from environmental factors in disease incidence. One example in which location has been shown to be closely associated with the occurrence of disease is multiple sclerosis. Indeed, a most striking characteristic of multiple sclerosis is its increasing frequency with increasing latitude in the temperate zones.[16]

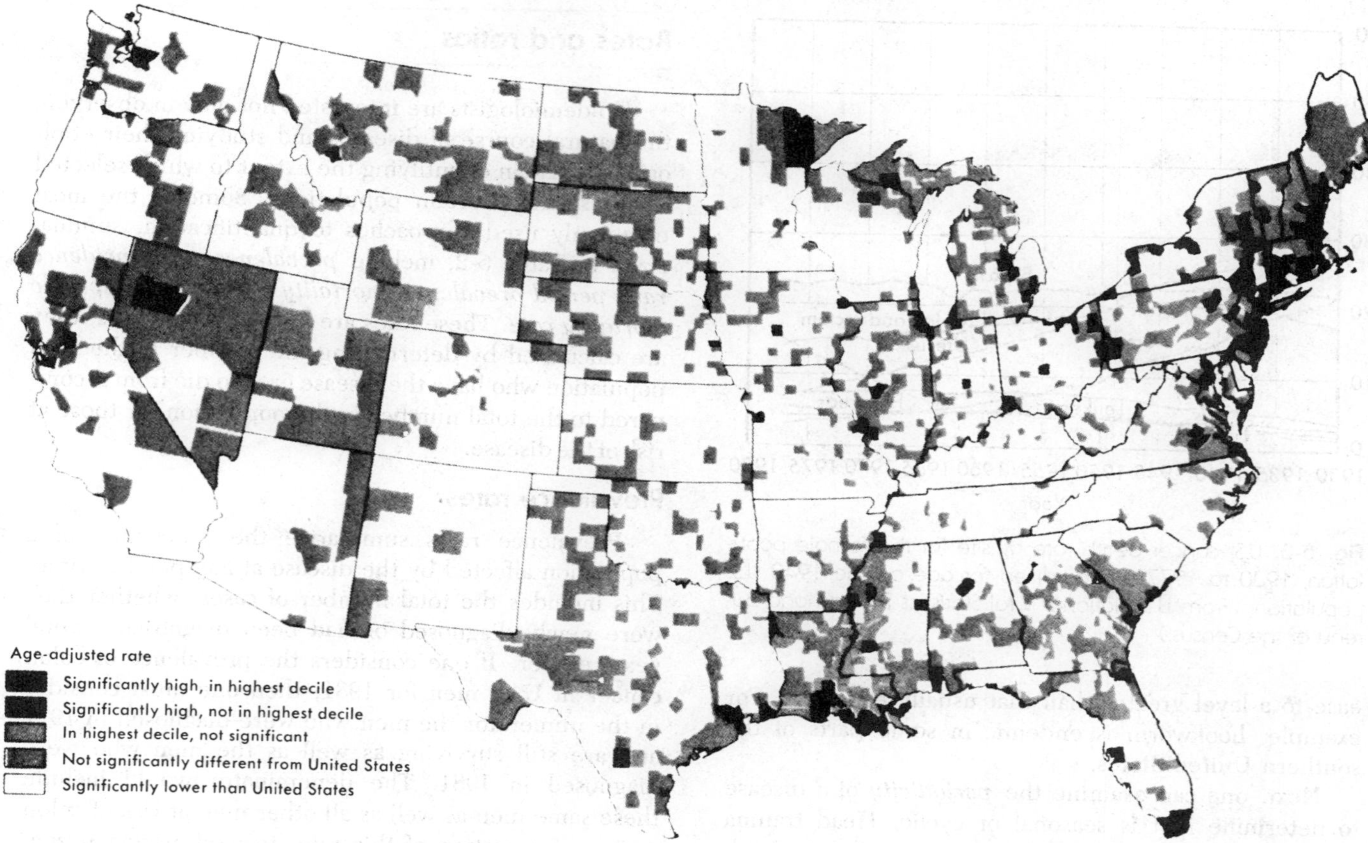

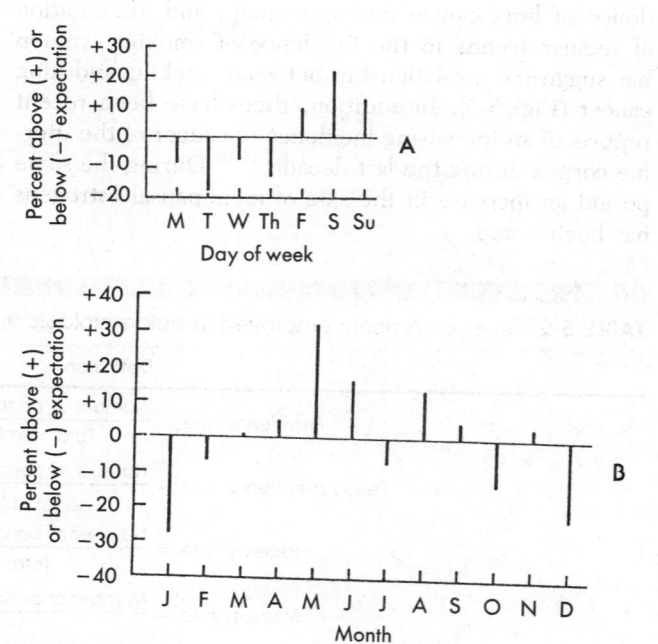

Age-adjusted rate
Significantly high, in highest decile
Significantly high, not in highest decile
In highest decile, not significant
Not significantly different from United States
Significantly lower than United States

Fig. 5-1. Mapping of lung cancer distribution. (From Mason, T.J., and McKay, W.: Atlas of cancer mortality for U.S. counties 1959, Washington, D.C., 1969, U.S. Department of Health, Education and Welfare, p. 76. In Marino, L.B., editor: Cancer nursing, St. Louis, 1981, The C.V. Mosby Co.)

Frequently, mapping techniques are employed in studying the geographic distribution of disease. Maps such as those prepared by the National Cancer Institute (NCI) in their *Atlas of Cancer Mortality of U.S. Counties: 1950-1969* have proven to be particularly useful in this respect. The atlas shows geographic variation of cancer death rates across the United States for 35 anatomic sites of cancer and therefore provides clues as to the geographic location of environmental factors that may be important in cancer etiology. For example, the use of the atlas to identify high rates of lung cancer among male residents of southern U.S. coastal counties led to studies showing a correlation between lung cancer mortality and the heavy industrial characteristics of those counties (Fig. 5-1).

Time

Epidemiologists are concerned not only with the occurrence of disease, but also with changes in its patterns of occurrence over time. Time variations can be described in several ways. First one can differentiate endemic and epidemic disease. *Endemic* conditions are always present in an area in some form, whereas an *epidemic* is a temporary rise in the incidence of a dis-

Percent above (+) or below (−) expectation
+30
+20
+10
0
−10
−20
A
M T W Th F S Su
Day of week
Percent above (+) or below (−) expectation
+40
+30
+20
+10
0
−10
−20
−30
−40
B
J F M A M J J A S O N D
Month

Fig. 5-2. Percent of head injured above or below expectation by day of week, **A**, and month of year, **B.** (From Klauber, M., et al.: The epidemiology of head injury, Am. J. Epidemiol. **113**[5]:500-509, 1981.)

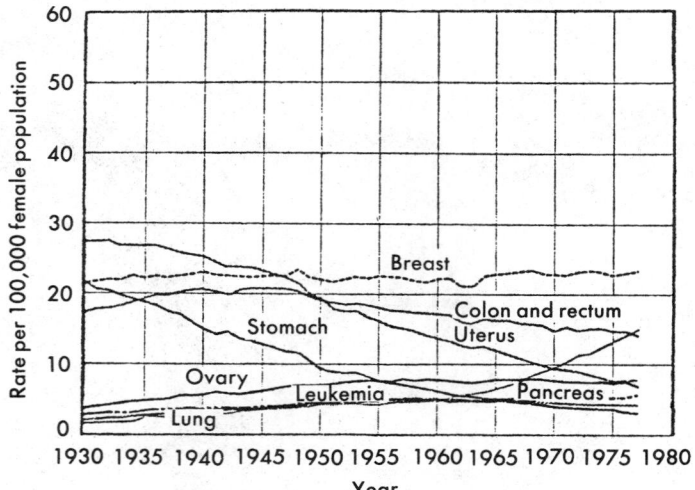

Fig. 5-3. U.S. cancer death rate by site for the female population, 1930 to 1977, standardized for age on the 1940 U.S. population. (From U.S. National Vital Statistics Division and Bureau of the Census.)

ease to a level greater than that usually expected. For example, hookworm is endemic in some parts of the southern United States.

Next, one can examine the *periodicity* of a disease to determine if it is seasonal or cyclic. Head trauma appears to vary temporally in San Diego County, with an excess of injuries occurring on weekends vs. weekdays and during the spring months (Fig. 5-2).

Finally, *secular trends* in disease or mortality can be described. Such a trend has been noted in the incidence of lung cancer among woman, and examination of secular trends in the incidence of smoking women has suggested a relationship between smoking and lung cancer (Fig. 5-3). In addition, there have been recent reports of an increasing incidence of cancer of the uterine corpus during the last decade.[17,18] During the same period an increase in the sale of menopausal estrogens has been noted.

Rates and ratios

Epidemiologists are interested not only in observing the natural course of diseases and studying their etiology, but also in quantifying the extent to which selected diseases affect certain populations. Some of the most commonly used approaches to quantification, summarized in Table 5-2, include *prevalence rate, incidence rate, period prevalence, mortality rate,* and *age-specific mortality rate.* These rates are proportions; that is, they are calculated by determining the number in the total population who have the disease or who die from it compared to the total number in the population, or those at risk of the disease.

Prevalence rates

Prevalence rates summarize the proportion of a population affected by the disease at any point in time. This includes the total number of cases, whether they were newly diagnosed or had been diagnosed several years earlier. If one considers the prevalence of colon cancer in U.S. men for 1981, then one must consider in the numerator the men who were diagnosed in 1971 and are still surviving as well as the men who were diagnosed in 1981. The denominator would include these same men as well as all other men at risk of colon cancer. A variation of this rate, termed *period prevalence,* describes the number of persons with a disease during a period of time, such as from 1975 to 1977, per the total number of persons in the group.

Incidence rates

Incidence rates describe the occurrence of *new* cases of disease over a specified period of time. Incidence rates imply the rate of development of a disease over time. When calculating incidence rates, epidemiologists consider that persons who have already developed diseases of lifelong duration cannot be counted as new cases more than once. Therefore the denomi-

TABLE 5-2. Rates commonly employed in epidemiologic studies

	Definition
Prevalence rate =	$\dfrac{\text{Number of persons with a disease}}{\text{Total number in group}}$
Period prevalence rate =	$\dfrac{\text{Number of persons with a disease during a period of time}}{\text{Total number in group}}$
Incidence rate =	$\dfrac{\text{Number of persons developing a disease}}{\text{Total number at risk}}$ per unit of time
Mortality rate =	$\dfrac{\text{Number of persons dying from a particular cause}}{\text{Total number in group}}$ per unit of time
Age-specific mortality rate =	$\dfrac{\text{Number of persons dying in a particular age group}}{\text{Total number in that age group}}$ per unit of time

nator for incidence rates includes only the population at risk of developing the disease, rather than the total population. In the case of cancer, we find that the estimated incidence for 1980 is about 785,000 new cases, whereas the prevalence of cancer is estimated to be 3 million cases. Thus the incidence rate would be calculated as follows:

Cancer incidence rate =
$$785,000 \text{ (total U.S. population } - 3,000,000)$$

Mortality

In addition to estimating the number of cases of disease compared to the total population, epidemiologists are concerned with rates that reflect the outcomes of disease. Mortality is commonly used to reflect the number of deaths from certain causes as compared to the total population. For example, the death rate per 100,000 population for heart disease in 1977 was 303.4. Rates may refer to special subgroups of the population as well as to the total population. The *age-specific mortality* refers to the number of persons dying in a particular age group compared to the total number of persons in that same age group per unit time. For example, the age-specific mortality for lung cancer for men 35 to 54 years old for 1977 could be calculated by counting all men who died from lung cancer in that age group (10,110) and dividing it by the total number of men who were 35 to 54 years of age in 1977.

Application of rate use

Rates allow for comparison of groups and comparison of phenomena over time. For example, one might compare the rate of lung cancer among smokers to the rate of lung cancer in nonsmokers. One might also compare the incidence rate of lung cancer for a population during one period of time to the same rate for another period.

Rates can also be compared by determining the ratio of one rate to another. For example, the age-adjusted death rate for lung cancer among women in 1950 to 1952 was 3.9, and from 1975 to 1977 it was 14.0. The rates could be compared as follows: 14.0 (rate for 1975 to 1977) − 3.9 (rate for 1950 to 1952) = 10.1. This indicates that the death rate for lung cancer has increased by approximately 0.1 per 100,000, and this represents about a 260% increase. In conjunction with the studies discussed later in this chapter, further application of the use of rates and ratios will be evident.

Cyclic nature of epidemiologic investigations

Although descriptive studies are vitally important in epidemiology, they are usually the first step in a cycle of investigation. The descriptive study frequently gives rise to hypotheses about the relationship between certain characteristics and health conditions; in some cases a causal model might be suggested. Such thinking provides the basis for further studies that are designed to test hypotheses. These studies are commonly referred to as *analytic studies*. Although analytic studies can generate support (or lack of it) for a hypothesis, they do not represent a final point in the search for knowledge. Usually, the analysis of results from these studies suggests further descriptive studies or generates new hypotheses.

Causation and association

Epidemiology as a discipline is concerned with a search for causes, with the ultimate goals of prevention of disease and death and promotion of health. To these ends epidemiologists explore hypotheses linking suspected causes to suspected effects, usually disease.

Criteria for causal associations

A hypothesis of causation asserts that X is a factor that determines Y. In other words, whenever X occurs, Y will follow. It is recognized, however, that conditions often obtain where a single factor is a partial or contributory cause. Furthermore, in epidemiologic studies events are usually viewed in a probabilistic rather than a deterministic way. Our current frameworks for causation of disease recognize that usually a web of causation exists in which multiple variables are involved. Where it was once believed that one could find a single cause that was both necessary and sufficient to produce disease, it is now recognized that most health problems are determined by multiple factors.

There are generally accepted criteria for causal associations: *covariation, causal direction,* and *nonspuriousness*. Covariation means that the dependent variable varies with the independent variable, or that a change in X results in a change in Y. A dose-response relationship implies that for a range of X there is a gradient in the degree of Y. Causal direction implies that the cause must precede the effect in time: X → Y (antecedent-consequent relationship). Nonspuriousness means that we must observe that there are no other variables that cause changes in the dependent variable and are associated with the independent variable.

There are two basic approaches to testing causal hypotheses in epidemiology: observational and experimental. In the *observational* study, the investigator can only perceive and report the natural variation of two variables, whereas in an *experimental* study the investigator can manipulate the causal variable under controlled conditions. The observational study will undoubtedly continue to provide a major contribution to the understanding of disease etiology, although experimentation can establish a causal relationship between a factor and a disease more conclusively than observation. Sometimes groups may be similar in every characteristic except in exposure to a specific factor. In this instance, the conditions for making a causal inference are so favorable that a "natural experiment" may be said to occur. An example of a natural (but unfortunate) experiment was that afforded by the bombing of Japan during World War II. Observation of people who had been exposed to varying amounts of radiation led to the discovery of an increased risk of certain cancers, for example, leukemia.

Because of the need to rely on observational methods in epidemiologic studies, additional considerations in establishing a causal relationship are appropriate. Once the noncausal explanations for the association have been excluded, the following additional criteria can be used to explore the likelihood of a causal association:

1. *Strength of the association*. The stronger the association, the less likely it is that it might be produced by unknown confounding factors.
2. *Consistency of the association*. The relationship is repeatedly observed by different investigators, in different samples, and in different places and times by different research designs.
3. *Coherence*. The relationship does not contradict current knowledge about the phenomenon. The finding is coherent with the body of knowledge.
4. *Experimental confirmation*. Confirming an association in an experiment is a powerful way to establish a causal relationship.[2]

When considering the relationship between two variables, it is important to recognize that they may be:

1. Independent (not statistically associated)
2. Statistically associated
   a. Noncausally associated
   b. Causally associated
      (1) Indirectly causal
      (2) Directly causal

Independence between two variables, for example, a characteristic and a type of cancer, can be established by means of statistical tests of significance. If the two variables are statistically associated, that is, associated not simply by chance, the investigator must then proceed to determine whether the relationship is a noncausal or a causal one.

Noncausal associations

Artifact

Two variables can be statistically but noncausally related simply because of artifact. Such an association would be spurious. It is well known that in a certain proportion of statistical tests, an association will be declared statistically significant when in fact it is not (type I error). In this instance the association may simply be a result of random fluctuation, or *chance*.

A second source of artifact is *bias*, that is, the false labeling of either the characteristic or the condition under study. Bias can occur as a result of lack of reliability or validity in measurement, selective recall of the person being studied, or the reverse bias of the investigator. Selective recall may occur when the person either exaggerates part of a history or fails to recall some characteristic such as exposure. For example, a mother whose child is born with a congenital anomaly will probably remember her behavior during pregnancy more clearly than a mother whose child is born without any problems. Sometimes characteristics or conditions are falsely labeled in a study. For example, statistics may indicate that a disease rate has changed when in reality all that has changed is the ability to diagnose it. Sometimes investigators have strong preconceived notions about the relationship between a characteristic and a condition. This may result in their being more attentive to these characteristics in persons who have the condition. Sometimes reverse bias occurs when the investigator makes a conscious effort to avoid bias; this leads to underdetection; for example, the person with a mild version of the disease is not labeled as a case. Bias can be prevented by measuring concordance between observers or diagnosticians whenever possible and establishing the validity, sensitivity, and specificity of measuring instruments.

Another source of artifact is *selection bias*. This occurs when by some fault in the research design or sampling, it has become easier for people in whom there is an association between the characteristic and disease to be selected into the study or excluded from it. The former results in an inflation of the strength of the association, and the latter leads to an underestimation of the association.

Secondary association

Secondary association occurs when the association between two factors is produced by a third factor, termed a *confounding* factor. Confounding factors are associated both with the characteristic and the condition. An example of a secondary association is that seen between race and birth weight. The incidence of low–birth weight infants is much higher among blacks than whites. Race is associated with both socioeconomic status and birth weight, such that blacks as a group have lower incomes, and lower income is associated with low birth weight. When one controls for the effect of socioeconomic status on birth weight, the effect of race disappears, thus indicating this was a *secondary association*. Fortunately, confounding factors can usually be controlled both in the study design and in analytic approaches.

Causal associations

Causal associations may be classified as indirect or direct. An association is said to be *indirect* when the characteristic and condition are related only because they both are encompassed by the actual case. In other words, if X is causally related to Y, and Y is causally related to Z, there will be a causal relationship between X and Z, but the association is indirect. An example of an indirect association was related to the notion of miasma popular in the early nineteenth century. People believed that foul emanations from the soil and water caused disease. It was not until the germ theory had been popularized and the existence of microorganisms was discovered that the indirect association became evident. The soil and water contained bacteria that caused the disease: soil → microorganisms → disease.

The *direct* causal association occurs when the characteristic can be associated with the condition with some specificity. Usually, however, the distinction between indirect and direct causal associations is a relative one, and assertion of a direct relationship depends on our current level of knowledge.

A final type of causal relationship is known as *configurational association*. This means that one factor is capable of producing a condition only in the presence of another factor. For example, we know that co-carcinogens are involved in the development of certain cancers; certain malignancies are caused by more than one co-carcinogen, and one of these may be capable of producing cancer only in the presence of the other.

Analytic approaches in epidemiology

Analytic approaches to the study of disease have been primarily directed toward elucidating etiologic agents or models. Data sources for these studies include not only persons who have disease and their disease-free counterparts, but also clinical records and studies in laboratories. Generally, the studies take one of two forms: prospective or retrospective (or some variation of these).

Prospective studies

Prospective studies are a very important form of epidemiologic investigation for testing hypotheses about disease causation. The study population for a prospective study consists of people who initially do not have the disease to be studied. From the reference population, people who are free from the disease are selected. They are subsequently classified according to presence or absence of the characteristic or characteristics thought to be related to the disease. The sample (usually termed a *cohort*) is then studied prospectively for a specified period of time (often for several years) to determine what proportion of the comparison groups under study develop the disease. Fig. 5-4 includes an example of a prospective study of the relationship be-

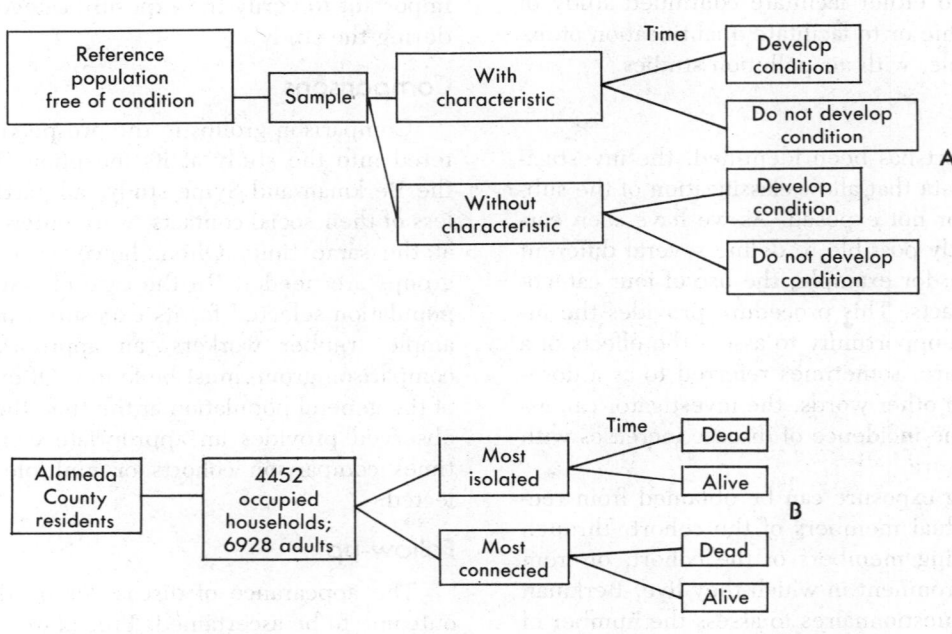

Fig. 5-4. An illustration of a prospective study. **A,** Basic approach. **B,** Example.

tween social networks and mortality. In 1965, 4452 occupied housing units were selected from Alameda County, 6928 adults returned questionnaires.[1] Participants were asked a series of questions regarding the number of social ties they had and their relative importance. In 1974, a follow-up survey was conducted of death records of those people who died within the state and, where records were obtainable, out of state. In addition, all but 302 of the original participants were located. The mortality from all causes was computed for four groups of people who ranged from having the least to the most social connections. As the number of social connections decreased, the mortality increased. With this introduction in mind, let us consider in more detail the process of conducting a prospective study.

Selecting the cohort

The initial cohort can be selected for a number of reasons: (1) they may have been exposed to the particular factor under study; (2) they may belong to a group where follow-up is facilitated; (3) they may be as appropriate as any other cohort for the study. In this study the cohort was originally selected to participate in a large-scale study of health in Alameda County. They were subsequently observed in 1974 to assess mortality outcomes. Other cohorts frequently studied might include special occupational groups exposed to disease-producing agents, such as workers, persons enrolled in prepaid medical plans who will get most of their care through a single source of care, persons taking out life insurance policies, obstetric populations (for neonatal or prenatal experiences), and volunteer groups of subjects, such as persons who volunteer for screening or who are identified by other volunteers. Other cohorts might be selected on the basis of their presence in a single geographic location to either facilitate continued study of the cohort over time or to facilitate quantification of exposure, for example, with air pollution studies.[7]

Exposure

Once the cohort has been identified, the investigator must collect data that allow classification of the subjects as exposed or not exposed. As we have seen earlier, it is frequently possible to define several different levels of exposure, for example, the use of four categories of social contacts. This procedure provides the investigator with an opportunity to assess the effects of a gradient of exposure, sometimes referred to as a dose-response effect. In other words, the investigator can ascertain whether the incidence of disease increases with the grade of exposure.

Data regarding exposure can be obtained from records, from individual members of the cohort, through testing or examining members of the cohort, or from assessing the environment in which they live. Berkman and Syme[1] used questionnaires to assess the number of personal ties.

One of the difficult aspects of obtaining data from individual members of a cohort is that there is frequently nonresponse. When a certain proportion does not provide data regarding exposure, it is possible that the loss of the respondents is biased with respect to either exposure, disease outcome, or both. The effects of bias in exposure or bias in disease or outcome differ from the effects of bias in *both* exposure and disease. When persons with high exposure levels fail to respond, the impression of the distribution of the exposure factor in the population will be inaccurate, but the association between the exposure and the disease will probably be accurate. When the nonresponse is biased with respect to disease (e.g., the most ill do not respond), the disease rates for the cohort will be underestimated, but the ratio of disease rates among the exposed to disease rates among the nonexposed will probably be similar to that in the population as a whole. When persons who do not respond to the study are biased with respect to both the exposure factor and the disease, the true relationship between the factor and the disease will be biased. It is often difficult to ascertain which type of bias is operative. Some approaches include more intense efforts to obtain data about exposure from nonrespondents, such as by sending out a second questionnaire. Comparing the nonrespondents to the respondents on other variables, monitoring outcomes in the nonrespondents, and assessing the disease rates in the cohort over time (normally the effects of selection bias would be most apparent early in the study) may also help.[7]

Another concern in assessing exposure is that people may be exposed to different experiences over time. For example, a person may change jobs and alter industrial exposure to toxic substances. Thus it is often important to verify the exposure categories periodically during the study.

Comparisons

Comparison groups in the prospective study are entered into the study at its inception. For example, in the Berkman and Syme study[1] all participants, regardless of their social contacts, were entered into the study at the same time. Often, however, other comparison groups are needed. In the case of a study of a special population selected for its exposure experience, for example, rubber workers, an appropriate nonexposed comparison group must be found. Often the experience of the general population at the time the cohort is being observed provides an appropriate comparison. Sometimes comparison cohorts or multiple groups are selected.

Follow-up

The appearance of disease or death is usually the outcome to be ascertained. Procedures may include examination of members of the cohort or the surveillance of other data sources such as death certificates. Berkman and Syme used death registry data in ascertaining mortality. There are many difficulties associated with the use of these procedures to assess outcome, not the least of which is migration of members of the cohort, misclassification of disease on death certificates, or changes in diagnostic procedures. When cohort members are examined, there is also the possibility of bias in diagnosis when the examiner is aware of the individual's exposure status. This can be limited by use of objective measures and by keeping information regarding the exposure status from the examiner.

Analysis

Rates. The primary focus of analysis of data from prospective studies is the derivation of rates of an outcome (disease or mortality) for the cohorts studied. The rates are then usually compared across exposure groups.

Because of variability in the number of years during which each person in the cohort is observed, a commonly used denominator for calculating rates is person-years. The concept of person-years considers the number of persons observed and the duration of each observation. For example, let us consider the following distribution:

Years of observation	Number of persons
5	30
10	20
15	10

The person-years denominator for this study would be computed as follows:

$$(5 \times 30) + (10 \times 20) + (15 \times 10) = 500 \text{ person-years}$$

This denominator allows for the variation in entrance dates into the study (e.g., often persons in the cohort are enrolled over several years) as well as for loss of certain individuals from the cohort.

The age distribution of the cohort also changes over time. For this reason, separate calculations of rates are usually made for persons in certain age groups.

When persons are lost to follow-up a situation analogous to failure to obtain exposure information occurs. Losses that are biased with respect to both exposure and outcome will affect the relative rates of disease or death for exposure categories. When losses are large, there may be considerable distortion of estimates of risk. Often investigators compute several estimates based on different sets of assumptions regarding possible biases. For example, the investigator might assume that persons lost to follow-up were lost immediately after entry into the cohort. The investigator then may use only the number of persons examined on each occasion (beginning and end of the study) to compute rates. Another possibility is to make varying assumptions regarding the number of years persons lost to follow-up were actually observed. This may be a useful technique when multiple measures are made of the outcome at varying intervals during the study. Yet another approach might be to calculate a range of rates possible in each exposure category. In this instance the investigator might first assume that none of the persons lost developed the outcome, and second that all of them developed the outcome. The usefulness of the latter option, however, is limited inasmuch as the frequency of the outcome measured is often smaller than the proportion lost to follow-up.[7]

Risk estimates. In addition to calculating rates of disease or death, epidemiologists are concerned about the association between exposure to certain factors and the risk of a particular outcome. Two commonly used measures are the relative risk and the attributable risk. The *relative risk (RR)* is the ratio of the incidence rate in those exposed to the risk factor (or characteristic) to the incidence rate in the population not exposed. One can use as an example the relative risk of death for those who were the most isolated compared to those with the most connections. The age-adjusted mortality associated with each group is given in Table 5-3. Taking the ratio of RR (relative risk) $= I_e/I_o$, where I_e is the incidence in the exposed, or here the least connected to a social network (15.6 for men), and where I_o is the incidence in the nonexposed, or here those with many connections (6.4 for men), we find that RR $= 15.6/6.4 = 2.5$. The relative risk of mortality for those men with few connections compared to those with many is 2.5. *Attributable risk* (AR_e) is another measure of association between risk factors and outcome. AR_e is the rate of the disease in exposed persons that can be attributed to the exposure: $AR_e = I_e - I_o$. Using the Berkman and Syme data, the attributable risk for those with few connections would be $15.6 - 6.4 = 9.2$. In addition, the attributable risk percent can be computed $(AR_e\%)$, where $AR_e\% = (I_e - I_o)/I_e$. The attributable risk percent, also referred to as the etiologic fraction among the exposed, is the proportion of disease in the exposed population that is attributable to the risk factor.

The population-attributable risk (AR_p) is the rate of the disease in the entire population that can be attributed to the risk factor. The population-attributable risk percent $(AR_p\%)$, sometimes referred to as the etiologic

TABLE 5-3. Social isolation and age-adjusted mortality

Social network index	Men	Women
I (fewest connections)	15.6	12.1
II	12.2	7.2
III	8.6	4.9
IV (most connections)	6.4	4.3

fraction in the population, is the proportion of the disease rate in the total population that is attributable to exposure to the risk factor: $AR_p\% = (I_t - I_o)/I_t$.

The comparison of rates can also be achieved for a number of risk factors. Often it is found that two risk factors act synergistically. That is, the joint effect of the two risk factors results in a rate that exceeds the sum of the risks of those exposed to either risk factor individually. Recently, synergistic effects have been observed in workers exposed both to asbestos and smoking.

Interpretation

Results of a cohort study are interpreted in relation to two primary questions: (1) Are there alternative explanations for the association (or lack of association) between risk factors and outcome? (2) Is the association likely to be a causal relationship? In order to answer question 1, the investigator must meticulously review all previous steps in the study. The second question can be answered by considering the criteria for causal relationships discussed earlier in this chapter.

Advantages

The fact that the cohort is drawn from a reference population enables the investigator to generalize from the sample to the reference population with some degree of certainty. In addition, it is clear that the characteristic precedes the development of the condition, one of the necessary conditions for a causal relationship. The investigator can directly quantify the risk of developing a condition in the presence of a risk factor. The likelihood of bias in reporting the relationship between the characteristic and the condition is reduced, since the characteristic is described before the outcome is measured. Selective survival, the survival of only special groups until the study is initiated, is not a problem here as it is for retrospective studies.

Disadvantages

Prospective studies are very costly in time, personnel, and follow-up. They are not feasible when the condition being studied is rare. Attrition of persons in the cohort constitutes a considerable problem in interpretation of results. Likewise, there may be attrition among investigators. Finally, other changes may occur over time in the environment, individuals, or treatment of the condition, and these may affect the outcomes.

Historical or reconstructed cohort study

A variation of the prospective cohort study is the historical cohort study. Here the cohort is reconstructed from records of their exposure, and they are then subsequently observed to see who develops the condition. In this case the investigator has a reference population and proceeds from that point in time with the study.

Retrospective studies

Retrospective studies involve comparisons between groups of individuals who have the disease (cases) and groups who do not have the disease. The cases and comparison groups (commonly referred to as controls or referent group) are then compared with respect to current or past characteristics that the investigator believes have relevance to the particular disease being studied.*

Fig. 5-5 illustrates the approach used in a recent study of smoking and nonfatal myocardial infarction (MI) in women.[19] All married female registered nurses 30 to 55 years of age and residing in 11 of the larger of the United States were polled in 1976. They were asked questions regarding many health-related variables as well as smoking history and whether they had been hospitalized for an MI. All who had MIs were asked for permission to review their hospital records; 173 records were reviewed and 128 diagnoses of acute MI were confirmed. For each woman who had had an MI (case), 20 women who had not had an MI (controls) and were born in the same year as the index case were chosen. The investigators then compared the relative proportion of smokers among the cases and controls.

Selection of cases

In selecting the cases for a case-control study, the criteria for the definition of the disease, the source of cases, and the inclusion of incident or prevalent cases are extremely important considerations. Valid and reliable definitions of the disease are essential. Often the investigator must decide whether or not to include borderline cases or how to cope with differences in pathologists' use of diagnostic categories. One investigator[19] attempted to use a medical record review as the criterion for whether an MI had actually occurred. Other studies might include criteria such as electrocardiogram documentation, enzyme elevation, symptoms, or autopsy results to confirm the diagnosis.[5]

Cases may be obtained from persons being treated for the disease at a certain facility or from persons with the disease from a more general population. Willett et al. tried to identify all the cases of MI from a large study of nurses in 11 states. This approach allows the investigator to avoid problems of bias associated with use of a certain source of medical care, as would have been the case had the cases been selected from a hospital or clinic.

---

*This approach is also commonly referred to as a case-control study. It is apparent, however, that the "controls" in this case are not equivalent to the controls in an experimental study.

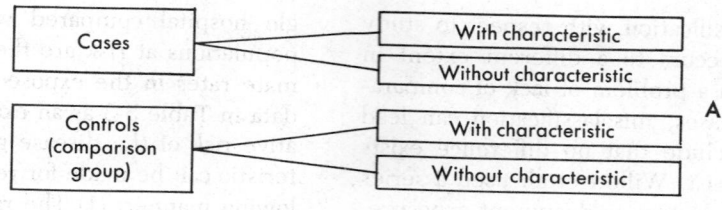

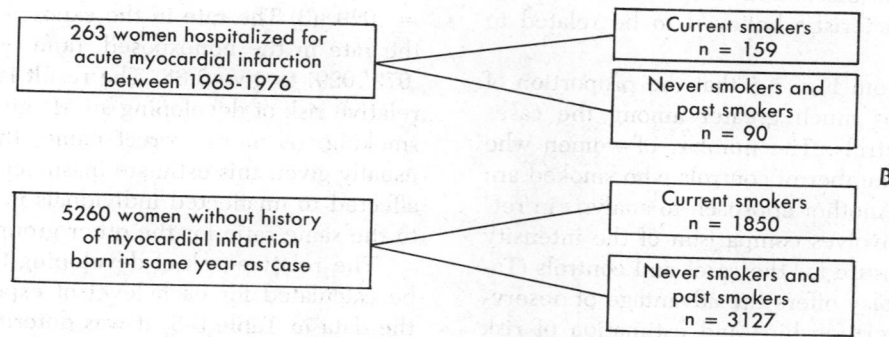

Fig. 5-5. An illustration of a retrospective study. **A,** Basic approach. **B,** Example.

Inclusion of incident or prevalent cases is also an important consideration. Willett et al. studied only those cases occurring from 1965 to 1976.

Selection of controls

Decisions about the source of controls are also important in the conduct of case-control studies. Controls may be obtained from the general population, hospitalized patients, or relatives or associates of the cases. In general, if the cases represent all the affected persons in a defined population, then controls should be selected from that same population. Some of the concerns in the selection of controls relate to whether information on the study factors can be obtained from the control group in a similar manner to that by which it was obtained from the cases, whether to match the controls with the cases to control for a certain confounding factor, whether the controls are similar to the cases in general, and practical and financial considerations. Willett et al. studied 20 women who were the same age as each case. Matching women on age was done to control for the confounding effects of age; that is, age is likely to be associated with both smoking history and MI. If age were not controlled, the proportion of women smoking among the cases might be greater than among the controls simply because the cases were older. The data were obtained by the same questionnaire for cases and controls.

Sampling

Once the source of controls is identified, the investigator must decide whether to study the entire population or a sample from the population. Because of the difficulty encountered in enumeration of everyone in order to draw a random sample from a large population, paired sampling is often used. This means that for each case, one or more controls is selected. This may be accomplished, for example, by asking the cases to identify someone in the same neighborhood of the same age. In this study, controls were obtained from the nurses who had not had an MI.

Information about exposure

Sources of data on exposure include the individual being studied or a relative and records such as hospital charts, birth certificates, and employment records. If the data on exposure differ systematically in completeness or accuracy between cases and controls, the association between exposure and disease will be spurious. The validity of exposure data is extremely important; where possible, information about exposure recorded prior to discovery of the disease is desirable to reduce bias in reporting. Further efforts to ensure validity are the use of similar procedures for cases and controls. Finally, the sensitivity and specificity of classification schemes should be established in advance of the study (these will be discussed in greater detail later in this chapter). When misclassification with respect to study variables occurs, and occurs to a different extent in cases and controls, then a problem of lack of comparability exists. In some cases, misclassification can lead the investigator to conclude that no difference exists when, in fact, it does exist. Willett et al. used a series of questions on smoking history to document exposure.

Analysis

The analysis of a case-control study consists of a comparison between cases and controls of the frequency of the characteristic believed to be related to the condition.

It can be seen from Fig. 5-5 that the proportion of current smokers was much greater among the cases than among the controls. The number of women who had an MI and the number of controls who smoked are given in Table 5-4. Another approach to analysis in retrospective studies involves comparison of the intensity and duration of exposure for the cases and controls (Table 5-5). Such a display offers the advantage of observing dose-response relationships and estimation of risk for a variety of levels of exposure.

In addition to assessing the significance of observed differences between cases and controls, investigators can also estimate the risk of developing the disease associated with the exposure and determine to what extent differences in the two groups might be attributable to a confounding variable.

When cases are referable to a population and controls are also representative of the same population, it is possible to estimate rates of the disease in exposed and nonexposed groups and also to derive relative and attributable risks from these estimates.[7] Procedures similar to those described for calculating relative risk for prospective studies would be appropriate.

Many retrospective studies, however, cannot be related to a defined population, such as cases from a single hospital compared with neighbors. Because the populations at risk are then unknown, one cannot estimate rates in the exposed and nonexposed. Using the data in Table 5-3 as an example, an estimate of the relative risk of the disease given exposure to the characteristic can be made for retrospective studies in the following manner: (1) The rate in exposed persons is calculated. In Table 5-4, the rate in the exposed persons is $a/(a + b)$ or $159/2009 = .079$. (2) The rate in the nonexposed persons is also calculated. In Table 5-4, the rate in the nonexposed persons is $c/(c + d)$ or $90/3127 = .029$. (3) The rate in the exposed is then divided by the rate in the nonexposed, $[a/(a + b)]/[c/(c + d)] = .079/.029$, to give 2.38. The result is an estimate of the relative risk of developing an MI given the exposure to smoking. (A more correct name, the relative odds, is usually given this estimate inasmuch as it is the ratio of affected to unaffected individuals in one group relative to the same ratio for the other group.)

The relative risk of developing the disease can also be calculated for each level of exposure. Referring to the data in Table 5-5, it was determined that the relative risk of developing MI for the group who smoked 1 to 14 cigarettes a day was 2.7; for those who smoked 15 to 20 per day, 2.9; 25 to 34 per day, 2.3; and 35 or more, 5.2. Thus women who smoked 35 or more cigarettes per day had a fivefold increase in the risk of developing an MI when compared to nonsmokers.

The investigators noted that age was related both to having an MI and smoking. It was therefore necessary to take age into account in analyses to prevent any distortion of the association between smoking and age.

Adjustment can be made for confounding variables in the study design or in analysis. One way of controlling for the effects of age was used in this study. Each case was matched with one or more controls of the same or similar age. While this is a useful technique, it is cumbersome and often an appropriate match cannot

---

TABLE 5-4. Number of women who had a myocardial infarction and controls who had reported they were currently smoking*†

Currently smoking	Cases	Controls	Totals
Yes	159 (a)‡	1850 (b)	2009
No	90 (c)	3127 (d)	3217
TOTALS	249	4977	5226

*Data from Willett, W., et al.: Am. J. Epidemiol. **113**(5):572-582, 1981.
†Excludes women for whom smoking status was unknown.
‡Letters refer to further explanation given in the text.

TABLE 5-5. Distribution of women with a myocardial infarction and controls according to cigarettes smoked per day*

Cigarettes per day	Cases (n = 220)	Controls (n = 3991)	Relative risk
Never smoked	61	2141	1
1-14	37	473	2.7
15-24	68	836	2.9
25-34	21	319	2.3
35 +	32	216	5.2
Unknown	1	6	—

*Data from Willett, W., et al.: Am. J. Epidemiol. **113**(5):572-582, 1981.

be found for the cases, or the data for many controls must be ignored. Another approach to controlling for confounding is *stratification analysis*. This implies examining the relationships between the exposure and disease for each of several strata. In the analysis of relative risk, the investigators then would standardize for age. (For further information about stratification analysis, see reference 11, and for further information about matching see reference 7.)

Advantages

There are several advantages associated with retrospective studies. They are short term and relatively cheap when compared to cohort studies. The retrospective study is feasible particularly when the disease occurs only rarely. The problem of attrition often associated with cohort studies is less marked in the retrospective study, although people may refuse to participate in the study. As earlier illustrated, these studies can support the estimation of a dose-response relationship, and they are particularly powerful when the cases and controls were both obtained from a referent population. When a number of retrospective studies conducted by different investigators on different populations confirm one another, confidence can be attached to the conclusions.

Disadvantages

There are, however, some major disadvantages associated with retrospective studies. First, the reference population for the cases and controls is often unknown, whereas the sample drawn for a cohort study is based on a reference population. Therefore generalization to a reference is usually not possible. Because there is often not much information about the population from which those with the disease come, it is difficult to give precise estimates of risk, although such estimates as the relative odds are commonly used. Because of the retrospective nature of the study, it is often not possible to know whether the exposure characteristic is antecedent to the disease or consequent to it.

Often the investigator must be concerned with bias, which may take the form of *selective recall, selection, false labeling* or *reverse bias* (see earlier discussion). A final problem associated with retrospective studies is selective survival. When this type of study is initiated, only persons who have survived the disease are available for the investigation. Survival may be associated with a variable such as income, which in turn influences access to treatment and survival. Thus it is easy to see how the representation of certain groups, such as the wealthy, might be artificially inflated. This in turn might give the impression that the wealthy are at greater risk of developing the disease when in fact it is only that the wealthy who have the disease survive.

Interpretation

MacMahon and Pugh[7] suggest that two important questions to consider in interpreting findings from a case-control study are (1) Do the findings reflect the true situation with respect to the presence or absence of association between the disease and the study factor? and (2) If an association *is* observed, is it a causal one? In considering the first question, the investigator must refer again to all previous steps of the study, attempting to find alternative explanations for the observed association. In addition, the investigator is concerned with the findings as a whole. In considering the differences between cases and controls, one or only a few sharp differences are more compelling than many differences. The second question can be considered in relation to the earlier discussion on causality.

Cross-sectional studies

Another approach used in epidemiologic investigations is the cross-sectional study. A reference population is identified and for a sample of that population both the characteristic and the condition are ascertained simultaneously. Because these studies begin with a reference population, rates such as prevalence can be computed, as well as risk estimates. These studies enable the investigator to generalize to the reference population. Although bias and attrition can present problems, they can be minimized with careful designs. These are short-term, relatively inexpensive studies in comparison to prospective studies. The cross-sectional study does, however, have some disadvantages; it is sometimes impossible to disentangle antecedent-consequent relationships, and selective survival or migration may occur.

Analytic approaches to studying the effectiveness of interventions

Frequently, prevention or treatment programs are conducted with enthusiasm but without careful assessment of their effectiveness and possible undesirable outcomes. Often assumptions about the advisability of a certain therapy dictate the clinical approach rather than the results of careful clinical trials.

An important intervention trial begun in the United States in the 1970s involved the simultaneous intervention on multiple risk factors for myocardial infarction (MI). The Multiple Risk Factor Intervention Trial (MRFIT) includes a population of individuals considered at high risk of MI based on a score developed from the Framingham Study data. The score included data about blood pressure, current cigarette smoking history, and serum cholesterol levels. Individuals eligible

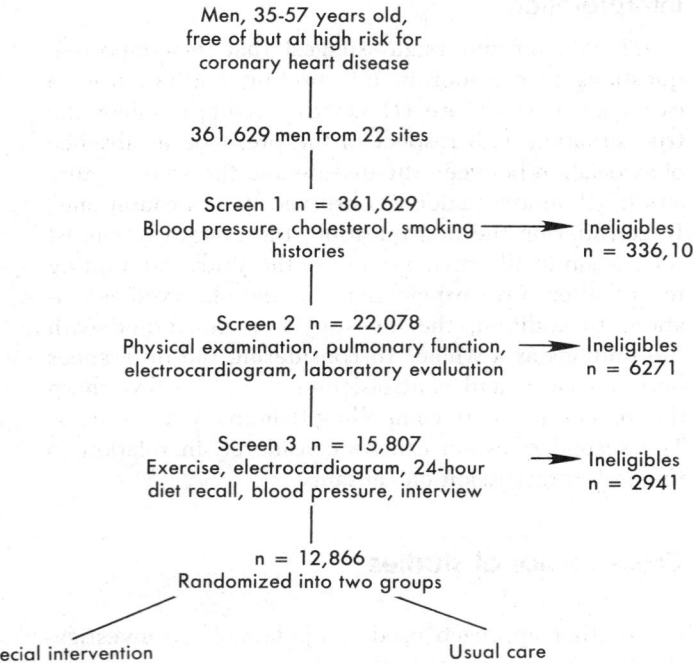

Fig. 5-6. Selection of participants for Multiple Risk Factor Intervention Trial (MRFIT). (From Kuller, L., et al.: Primary prevention of heart attacks: the Multiple Risk Factor Intervention Trial, Am. J. Epidemiol. **112**[2]:185-199, 1980.)

to participate in the study were randomized into two groups, one of which received a special intervention and the other, usual care. The MRFIT project involves the collaboration of 22 centers in the United States. Its goal is to determine whether reduction of serum cholesterol through dietary intervention, decreased cigarette smoking and treatment of hypertension by drugs or diet produces a reduction in arteriosclerotic heart disease mortality, MI, and total mortality over a 6-year period. A total of 12,866 men, 35 to 57 years of age and free of coronary heart disease at entry into the study, was randomized into the two groups, special intervention and usual care (Fig. 5-6).[6]

The intervention trial

In an intervention trial, the investigator manipulates the treatment, which becomes the independent variable, and measures the effect, the dependent variable. The basic strategy involves an application of the experimental method, with some special modifications necessary in view of the concern for the human population being studied.

Study groups

In some studies it is possible to enroll a study group that receives the treatment and a control group or groups that are not given the treatment but perhaps a placebo. In other instances, it would be considered unethical to withhold any treatment at all, such as in the study of breast cancer treatment.

The reference population for the study is the group to which the investigator can ideally generalize results of the study. In the MRFIT project, the reference population would be men between 35 to 57 years of age who are free of coronary heart disease, but who are at high risk of MI. The experimental population is the actual population being studied, in our example, the men actually treated in the 22 centers. Ideally, the experimental population is as similar as possible to the reference population. Convenience and accessibility, incidence of the disease to be prevented (in prophylactic trials), and size of the population needed to detect statistically significant differences are all important considerations in selecting the experimental group. Because humans have the right to refuse involvement in an experiment, the final complement of the experimental population is not in the control of the investigator. Careful assessment of systematic differences between volunteers and refusals should be made when possible. Usually, allocation to the experimental or control group is done *after* the person consents to participate. In an attempt to attain equivalence or similarity of the experimental and control groups, the investigator can randomly allocate participants to one or more treatment or control groups. It is best that a system of randomization be developed in advance of the study to limit the noncomparability between the groups.

The double-blind trial

The double-blind trial includes two safeguards to prevent bias in the ascertainment of the outcome as a result of knowledge of the group to which the participant was assigned: blind assignment is made of the participants to the study groups, and a blind assessment of outcome is achieved. First, neither the study personnel nor the participants know to which group the participants are assigned. While this is feasible in studies of medications, it is clearly impossible in the study of surgical or other procedures where both the staff and the patients are obviously aware of the treatment. The second component involves blind ascertainment of outcome. This might be achieved by keeping knowledge of the treatment group from a pathologist or interviewer measuring disease, survival, or other outcomes and from the statistician or epidemiologist analyzing the data. This was the case in the MRFIT study.

Protocols

In order to ensure that each participant in the experimental and control groups receives the same treatment, study protocols are usually developed that de-

TABLE 5-6. Rates and risk estimates associated with specific study approaches

	Cohort study	Case-control study	Cross-sectional study
Rates	Incidence	Proportion of the cases with the characteristic, unless the cases are from an identifiable reference population; then incidence can be estimated directly	Prevalence
Risk estimate	Relative and attributable risk	Relative odds; when cases and controls are from an identifiable reference population, then relative risk is appropriate	Relative and attributable risk

scribe in detail the types of procedures to be used in both groups. This is particularly important when several investigators from different areas participate in a collaborative trial. In our example a single protocol was used for the people in the special intervention group, including an active program of nutrition counseling, modification of smoking behavior, and treatment of high blood pressure by diet and drugs. Usual care participants were referred to their personal physicians for treatment of risk factors deemed appropriate by that physician.

Ascertaining outcomes

Ascertaining outcome in cases where the outcome does not occur for several years, as in the example above where 6-year outcomes will be measured, presents the same problems that were discussed in conjunction with prospective studies, namely, migration and selective survival. Measures are usually taken to ensure as complete a follow-up as possible, and blind assessment is desirable. A very important concern is the type of outcome measure most appropriate to the study. In MRFIT, several outcome measures, that is, mortality, MI incidence, and total mortality, will be assessed at 6 years. Other measures that could be used are mortality at 10 and 20 years, other cardiovascular morbidity, and quality of life after treatment.

Sequential designs are sometimes employed in intervention studies. This means that data are continuously analyzed during the trial, and as soon as statistically significant differences appear the trial is stopped. It is possible to maintain double-blind procedures and incorporate sequential designs by having investigators not involved in the clinical work analyze the data submitted to them. In MRFIT, ascertainment of myocardial infarction is made by review of an annual electrocardiogram rather than physicians' or hospital records. In addition, data regarding mortality such as death certificates and hospital records are being reviewed by a committee of scientists who are not MRFIT in-

vestigators and are unaware of the person's treatment group.

Analysis

The analysis of an intervention trial is similar to that for a cohort study (Table 5-6). Special attention, however, must be given to those who did not participate in the control group or study group and any systematic differences between those who participate and those who did not. This can be attained by attempting to measure outcome for at least a sample of the nonparticipants. The MRFIT study cannot classify those persons who skipped an annual examination with respect to their myocardial infarction status.

Screening

Screening is an extremely important contribution of epidemiology to detecting disease. It is assumed that by selecting from apparently healthy volunteers those persons who have an increased risk of suffering from a certain disease that treatment will be easier and more effective. It is important to remember that an instrument used for screening a population is not intended to be diagnostic; instead, it is intended only to separate those persons with a high probability of disease from those with a low probability of disease. In turn, the former are subjected to further diagnostic tests and to treatment, if appropriate.

Screening tests must meet several criteria. First, they must be valid and reliable. The *validity* of the test refers to whether it is able to separate those with the disease from those without the disease. In epidemiology the validity of a test is commonly assessed by determining its sensitivity and specificity. *Sensitivity* refers to the test's capacity to identify correctly those with the disease, whereas *specificity* refers to its ability to

DISEASE BY DIAGNOSIS

Screening results	Present	Absent
Positive	True positive (TP)	False positive (FP)
Negative	False negative (FN)	True negative (TN)

$$\text{Sensitivity} = \frac{TP}{TP + FN} \qquad \text{Specificity} = \frac{TN}{TN + FP}$$

PHYSICIANS' GENERAL HEALTH RATINGS FOR WOMEN*

Screening results	I	II	III	IV
Cornell Medical Index $\geq$ 30	23	26	21	8
Cornell Medical Index < 30	54	10	7	1
TOTALS	77	36	28	9

$$\text{Sensitivity}\dagger = \frac{21 + 8}{28 + 9} = .78 \qquad \text{Specificity}\dagger = \frac{54 + 10}{77 + 36} = .57$$

*Data are interpolated from Abramson, J., et al.: Br. J. Prev. Med. **19**:103-110, 1965.
†Using grades III and IV as an indicator of ill health.

identify correctly those who do not have the disease. Such values are determined by comparing results on the screening tool to those derived from a definitive diagnostic procedure. Usually, the sensitivity and specificity can be varied by raising or lowering the level at which the test is considered positive.

The Cornell Medical Index (CMI) is a commonly used measurement of general health status, with the M-R subscales reflecting mental health status. Using the data in the boxes above, we can see that the sensitivity of the CMI, using a cutoff point of a total score over 30, correctly identifies those women who physicians rate as in poor health 78% of the time. The specificity, those who are not ill and have CMI scores less than 30, is only 57%. When the value of the screening tool's results is continuous (e.g., the level in units of an enzyme), the sensitivity and specificity can be adjusted by changing the cutoff point for "positives" on the test. In some instances multiple tests can be used to increase the sensitivity of the screening.

Reliability (precision) of a screening test refers to the reproducibility of its results. Variation in the method and observer error can be sources of inconsistent results. Standardizing procedures and training observers improve reliability.

The *yield* of a screening tool refers to the amount of a previously undiagnosed disease that can be diagnosed and treated as a result of the screening. The yield depends not only on the sensitivity of the test, but also on the prevalence of unrecognized disease, the extent of previous screening in the population, and the degree to which people will participate in the screening.

There are varying opinions regarding what criteria should be used to judge whether to implement a screening program. The criteria suggested by Wilson and Jungner[22] follow:

1. The condition to be screened should constitute an important health problem.
2. For patients with recognized disease there should be an accepted treatment.
3. Facilities for diagnosis and treatment should be available.
4. The disease should have a recognizable latent or early symptomatic stage.
5. A suitable test or examination should exist.
6. The test should be acceptable to the population to whom it is applied.
7. The natural history of the disease, including development from latent to declared disease, should be adequately understood.
8. There should be a policy on whom to treat as patients after they are identified as possible cases.
9. The cost of case finding (including diagnosis and treatment) should be economically balanced in relation to possible expenditures on health care as a whole.
10. Case finding should be a continuing process.

Although screening procedures have become institutionalized without careful adherence to these criteria, it is important to recall that screening itself is not completely risk free, and in some cases could do harm if misapplied, for example, the radiation exposure from mammography.

REFERENCES AND SELECTED READINGS
Contemporary

1. Berkman, L., and Syme, S.: Social networks, host resistance and mortality: a nine year follow-up study of Alameda county residents, Am. J. Epidemiol. **109**(2):186-204, 1979.
2. *Friedman, G.: Primer of epidemiology, New York, 1980, McGraw-Hill Book Co.

* References preceded by an asterisk are particularly well suited for student reading.

3. Holland, W.W., and Wainwright, A.H.: Epidemiology and health policy, Epidemiol. Rev. 1:211-232, 1979.
4. Klauber, M., et al.: The epidemiology of head injury: a prospective study of an entire community, San Diego County, California, 1978, Am. J. Epidemiol. 113(5):500-509, 1981.
5. Krueger, D., et al.: Risk factors for fatal heart attack in young women, Am. J. Epidemiol. 113(4):357-370, 1981.
6. Kuller, L., et al.: Primary prevention of heart attacks: the multiple risk factor intervention trial, Am. J. Epidemiol. 112(2):185-199, 1980.
7. *MacMahon, B., and Pugh, T.: Epidemiology: principles and methods, Boston, 1970, Little, Brown & Co.
8. Mason, R.J., et al.: Atlas of cancer mortality for U.S. counties: 1950-1969, Department of Health, Education and Welfare publication no. (N/W) 75-780, Washington, D.C., 1975.
9. Mason, T.J., et al.: Atlas of cancer mortality among U.S. nonwhites: 1950-1969, Department of Health, Education and Welfare publication no. (N/W) 76-1204, Washington, D.C., 1976.
10. Mason, T.J., and McKay, F.W.: Cancer mortality by county: 1950-1969, Department of Health, Education and Welfare publication no. (N/W) 74-615, Washington, D.C., 1974.
11. Mausner, J., and Bahn, A.: Epidemiology: an introductory text, Philadelphia, 1974, W.B. Saunders Co.
12. Miettenen, O.: Confounding and effect: modification, Am. J. Epidemiol. 100:350-353, 1974.
13. Morris, J.N.: Uses of epidemiology, ed. 3, Edinburgh, 1975, Churchill Livingstone.
14. Omran, A.: Modern concepts of epidemiology. In Omran, A., editor: Community medicine in developing countries, New York, 1974, Springer Publishing Co., Inc.
15. *Susser, M.: Causal thinking in the health sciences: concepts and strategies of epidemiology, New York, 1973, Oxford University Press.
16. Visscher, B.R., et al.: Latitude, migration, and the prevalence of multiple sclerosis, Am. J. Epidemiol. 106:470-475, 1977.
17. Walker, A., and Jick, H.: Cancer of the corpus uteri, Am. J. Epidemiol. 110:47-51, 1979.
18. Weiss, N., Szekeley, D., and Austin, D.: Increasing incidence of endometrial cancer in the United States, N. Engl. J. Med. 294:1259-1261, 1976.
19. Willett, W., et al.: Cigarette smoking and nonfatal myocardial infarction in women, Am. J. Epidemiol. 113(5):575-582, 1981.

Classic

20. Abramson, J., et al.: Cornell Medical Index as a measure in epidemiologic studies: a test of the validity of a health questionnaire, Br. J. Prev. Med. 19:103-110, 1965.
21. Hill, A.B.: The environment and disease: association or causation? Proc. R. Soc. Med. 58:295-302, 1965.
22. Wilson, T., and Jungner, G.: Principles and practices of screening for disease, Public Health Paper no. 34, Geneva, 1968, World Health Organization.

CHAPTER 6

PERSPECTIVES FOR NURSING PRACTICE

MARIE L. LOBO

The practice of modern nursing is based on the use of knowledge of nursing as well as that from other disciplines, such as psychology, biology, physiology, sociology, and philosophy. Within each of these disciplines, including nursing, there are many different perspectives that help one predict and explain the phenomena with which that discipline is concerned. The discipline of nursing is primarily concerned with human health, including its physical and mental components, and the environments that promote or interfere with health. Several nurses have offered unique perspectives about nursing. These perspectives not only help practitioners understand human health and its relationship to the environment, but they also suggest approaches to providing care to clients. These perspectives about nursing serve as frames of reference that guide nurses as they assess health status and implement and evaluate nursing care.

The purpose of this chapter is to describe the perspectives offered by several selected nursing authors. The discussion of these perspectives is ordered historically to enable the reader to appreciate the evolution of nursing thought. Some of these perspectives are broad enough to account for the nursing care of people regardless of their developmental state, their health status, and the environment for care. Some are more useful than others in thinking about adult patients with medical-surgical problems who are receiving care in the hospital or community. All, however, provide a frame of reference that nurses may adapt to guide their practice with specific populations of clients.

Florence Nightingale

Nightingale, the founder of modern nursing, recorded her observations on nursing in *Notes on Nursing*, originally published in 1859. Nightingale observed that symptoms are often the result of impairments in the environment, such as want of fresh air, light, warmth, quiet, or cleanliness in human care. She believed that in a nurturing environment the body could repair itself. Nightingale advocated manipulating the basic environment; providing fresh, odor-free air, pure water, efficient drainage, and cleanliness; eliminating unnecessary noise; and providing variety in colors and forms as a means of stimulating recovery. She proposed the practice of gathering data about the person by observation. From her point of view, nursing ought to signify the proper use of fresh air, light, warmth, cleanliness, quiet, and the proper selection and administration of diet—all at the least expenditure of vital power by the patient.[43]

Nightingale's admonitions would be quite appropriate today. For example, in hospitals, an intensive care syndrome has been identified that includes disorientation caused by noise, light, and lack of recognizable visual cues in the intensive care unit (see p. 1920). Consideration of Nightingale's suggestions for creating a supportive, nurturing environment would be quite appropriate even in the sophisticated environment of a twentieth century hospital.

Lydia Hall

Hall was the first director for the Loeb Center Nursing and Rehabilitation Unit. She provided a basic philosophy that guides the nursing care at Loeb Center, an adult rehabilitation center. Hall's philosophy is indicated by three interlocking circles representing *care*, *core*, and *cure*. The *care circle* represents the nurturing aspects of nursing and is viewed as a property of nursing. The care circle has a strong emphasis on the biologic aspects of the client but includes the psycho-social-spiritual needs as well. The *core circle* involves the therapeutic use of self by the nurse and other members of the health care team. The psycho-social-spiritual needs of the client are stressed. The *cure circle* again is shared with other members of the health care team and focuses on the pathologic and therapeutic sciences. This perspective emphasizes the unique contribution of nursing care, the importance of the nurse's ability to use her or his self, and the collaborative relationships essential for promoting health. Hall's philosophy is particularly applicable to adults who need rehabilitative care.[6]

Virginia Henderson

Early in her career, Henderson recognized two features of nursing: first, that nursing was different from medicine, and, second, that a clear definition of nursing was needed. By 1960, Henderson had evolved the following definition of nursing:

The unique function of the nurse is to assist the individual, sick or well, in the performance of those activities contributing to health or its recovery (or to peaceful death) that he would perform unaided if he had the necessary strength, will or knowledge. And to do this in such a way as to help him gain independence as rapidly as possible.[8]

Henderson identified 14 components of basic nursing care to help the client perform these tasks. These included breathing normally, eating and drinking adequately, eliminating body wastes, moving and maintaining desirable posture, and sleeping and resting. In addition, Henderson emphasized selecting suitable clothing, maintaining body temperature within normal range by adjusting clothing and modifying the environment, keeping the body clean and well groomed and

protecting the integument, avoiding dangers in the environment, avoiding injuring others, and communicating with others in expressing emotions, needs, fears, or opinions. Henderson also emphasized the importance of worshiping according to one's faith, working in such a way that there is a sense of accomplishment, playing or participating in various forms of recreation, and learning, discovering, or satisfying the curiosity that leads to normal development and health and using the available health facilities.[37]

Henderson's perspective of nursing reflects concern for the person's biologic as well as emotional, social, and spiritual well-being. Like Nightingale, she recognized the important influence of the environment on health. Because of the diversity of the components of nursing care, Henderson advocated a solid knowledge base in the biologic sciences as well as the social sciences for nurses in order that they might assess, plan, implement, and evaluate care. Her framework can guide nursing care with clients at any point on the continuum from health to illness and is particularly useful when the goal for the client is maximal independence.

Hildegard Peplau

In 1952, Peplau's text *Interpersonal Relations in Nursing* was published. This book has become a nursing classic, with many of her ideas applicable today. Peplau defines nursing as "a human relationship between an individual who is sick or in need of health services, and a nurse especially educated to recognize and respond to the need for help."[47] She identified and defined characteristics of the nurse and the client as they experience four phases of the nurse-client relationship (Fig. 6-1).

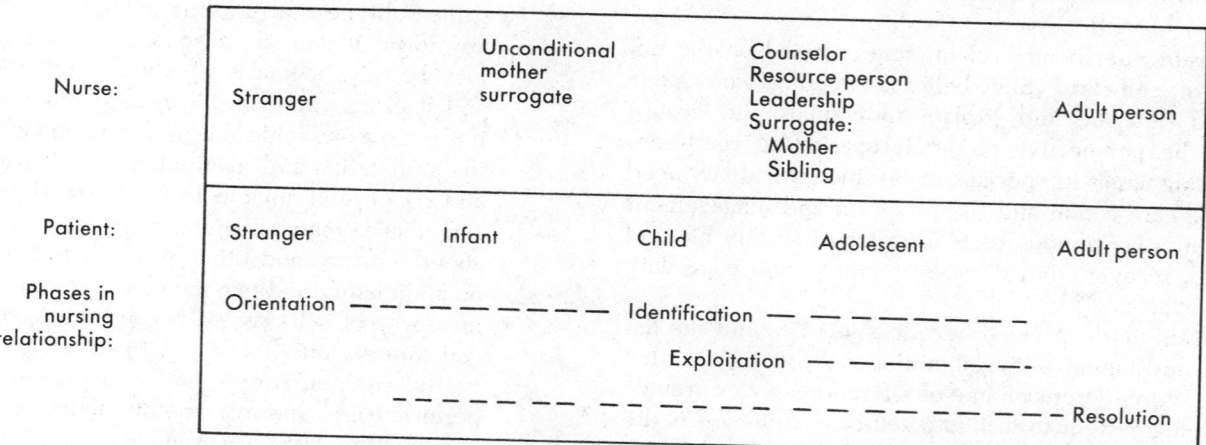

Fig. 6-1. Phases and changing roles in nurse-patient relationships. (From Peplau, H.E.: Interpersonal relations in nursing, New York, 1952, G.P. Putnam's Sons.)

The four phases are *orientation, identification, exploitation,* and *resolution*. In orientation the nurse and the client initially do not know each other and must explore, discovering each other's goals and testing the role each will assume. There is also an orientation phase to each subsequent encounter, as client and nurse explore to find what, if any, changes have occurred since their last encounter. During the first phase, the client attempts to identify difficulties and the amount of nursing help that is needed.

In the identification phase the client responds to the professionals or significant others who can meet the identified needs. Both client and nurse plan together an appropriate program to foster health.

In the exploitation phase the client utilizes all available resources to move toward a goal of maximal health or functioning. He or she may show varying degrees of dependence (on the nurse) during this phase of the nurse-client relationship.

The final stage, resolution, refers to the termination phase of the nurse-client relationship. Resolution occurs when the client's needs are met and he or she can move toward a new goal. Peplau assumes that the nurse-client relationship fosters growth in both the client and the nurse.

Peplau's frame of reference made a unique contribution to nursing thought, namely, a description of the nature of the professional relationship that nurses develop with clients. Although Peplau's text focused on clients with mental or emotional problems, her thinking about the nurse-client relationship is applicable to all clients and patients regardless of their health status, their developmental status, or the environment in which care is provided.

Dorothea Orem

Orem's perspective of nursing is based on the notion of self-care. She believes nursing knowledge should describe and explain individuals and groups from the perspective of the incapacitating condition. "Nursing has as its special concern the individual's need for self-care action and the provision and management of it on a continuous basis in order to sustain life and health, recover from disease or injury, and cope with their effects."[18]

Orem first expressed her ideas in 1958, and she has been developing and elaborating on them since that time. Within Orem's frame of reference, nurses provide a helping system to facilitate self-care. Self-care is defined as the ability for a human to engage in self-care for meeting activities of daily living.[18]

The interrelationships between the client's self-care

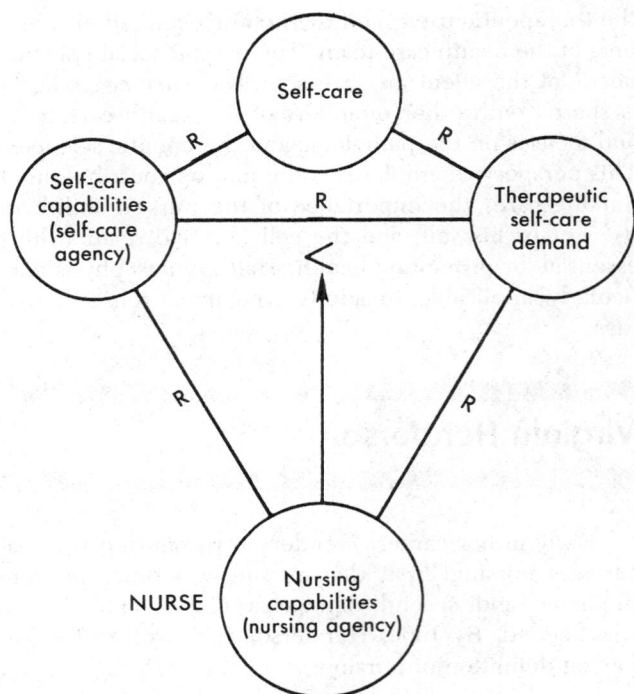

Fig. 6-2. A conceptual framework for nursing. *R*, relationship; <, deficit relationship, current or projected. (From Orem, D.E.: Nursing concepts of practice, ed. 2. Copyright © 1980 by McGraw-Hill Book Co. Used with the permission of the McGraw-Hill Book Co.)

capabilities, therapeutic self-care demand, nursing capabilities, and self-care are shown in Fig. 6-2. Orem views the organization of nursing actions as nursing system and proposes three variations of these systems to promote the self-care agency of the client (Fig. 6-3). The three systems of care are as follows:

1. Wholly compensatory—utilized by the nurse when there is a health care deviation. There are three subtypes: (a) persons unable to engage in any form of deliberate action; (b) persons who may be able to make observations, judgments, and decisions about self-care and other matters but cannot or should not perform actions requiring ambulation and manipulation of movements; and (c) persons unable to attend to themselves and make reasoned judgments and decisions about self-care and other matters, but who can be ambulatory and may be able to perform some measures of self-care with continuous guidance and supervision.

2. Partly compensatory—both nurse and client perform care measures or other actions involving manipulative tasks or ambulation.

3. Supportive-educative—client is able to perform, or can and should learn to perform, required

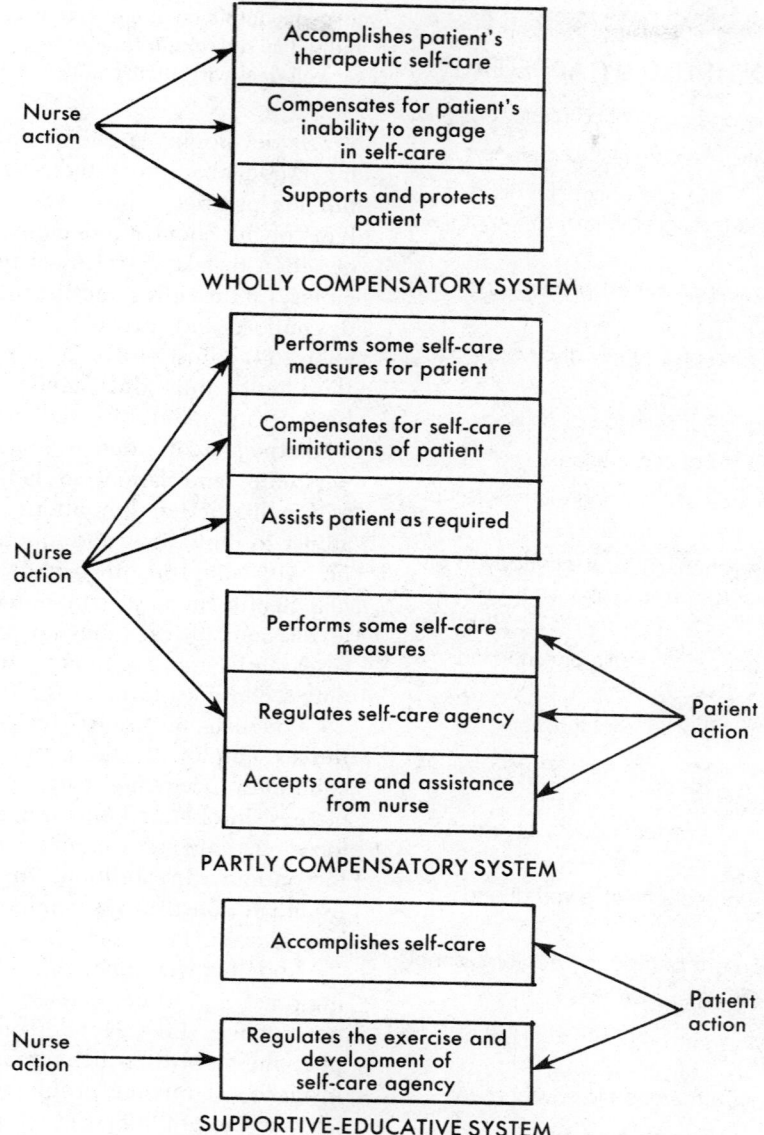

Fig. 6-3. Basic nursing systems. (From Orem, D.E.: Nursing concepts of practice, ed. 2. Copyright © 1980 by McGraw-Hill Book Co. Used with the permission of the McGraw-Hill Book Co.)

measures or externally or internally oriented self-care but needs assistance to do so.[18]

Orem asserts that self-care deficits for dependent care, whether health derived or health related, are predictive of nursing requirements. Thus self-care deficits and deficits for dependent care are the proper object or focus of nursing in society and provide criteria for identifying persons needing nursing care. Moreover, "self-care and dependent care are systematized, deliberate actions that, when continuously and effectively engaged in, regulate structural integrity, human functioning, and human development (sometimes through the control of environmental factors)."[18] Thus these forms of care are essential for the continuance of human life. In

addition, Orem explains how persons can be helped by nurses: "the product of nursing practice is a nursing system(s) through which the capability of patients to engage in self-care is regulated and self-care is continuously produced."[18]

Orem's frame of reference provides useful guidelines for nurses who care for clients, regardless of the nurses' developmental level, health status, or the context in which they practice. Her special contributions to the understanding of nursing include the specification of different systems of nursing care and the relationships between clients' self-care capabilities and the requirements for different systems of nursing care.

NURSING PROBLEMS IDENTIFIED BY ABDELLAH*

1. To maintain good hygiene and physical comfort

2. To promote optimal activity: exercise, rest, and sleep

3. To promote safety through the prevention of accidents, injury, or other trauma and through the prevention of the spread of infection

4. To maintain good body mechanics and prevent and correct deformities

5. To facilitate the maintenance of a supply of oxygen to all body cells

6. To facilitate the maintenance of nutrition of all body cells

7. To facilitate the maintenance of elimination

8. To facilitate the maintenance of fluid and electrolyte balance

9. To recognize the physiologic responses of the body to disease conditions—pathologic, physiologic, and compensatory

10. To facilitate the maintenance of regulatory mechanisms and functions

11. To facilitate the maintenance of sensory function

12. To identify and accept positive and negative expressions, feelings, and reactions

13. To identify and accept the interrelatedness of emotions and organic illness

14. To facilitate the maintenance of effective verbal and nonverbal communication

15. To promote the development of productive interpersonal relationships

16. To facilitate progress toward achievement of personal spiritual growth

17. To create and/or maintain a therapeutic environment

18. To facilitate awareness of self as an individual with varying physical, emotional, and developmental needs

19. To accept the optimum possible goals in the light of limitations, physical and emotional

20. To use community resources as an aid in resolving problems arising from illness

21. To understand the role of social problems as influencing factors in the cause of illness

*From Abdellah, F.G., et al.: Patient-centered approaches to nursing, New York, 1960, Macmillan Publishing Co., Inc.

Faye Abdellah

Abdellah defines nursing as follows:

. . . a service to individuals and to families, therefore to society. It is based upon an art and science which mold the attitude, intellectual competencies and technical skills of the individual nurse into the desire and ability to help people sick or well deal with their health needs.[33]

In developing a client-centered approach to nursing, Abdellah enumerated several processes involved in nursing practice. These were (1) recognizing the problems of the client; (2) deciding the appropriate courses of action to take in terms of the relevant nursing principles; (3) providing continuous care to relieve pain and discomfort and provide immediate security for the client; (4) adjusting the total nursing care plan to meet the client's individual needs; (5) helping the client to become more self-directed in attaining or maintaining a healthy state of mind and body; (6) instructing nursing personnel and family to help the client do for self within his or her limitations; (7) helping the client to adjust to limitations and emotional problems; (8) working with allied health professions in planning for optimal health on local, state, national, and international levels; and (9) carrying out continuous evaluation and research to improve nursing techniques and to develop new techniques to meet the health needs of people.[1]

Abdellah not only described the processes that nurses employ in their practice, but also identified commonly occurring nursing problems. Consideration of these problems helps nurses meet clients' needs by focusing their assessments and thus directing their interventions. In addition, the problems identified by Abdellah constitute a common focus for both nursing care and nursing research.

Abdellah was concerned with the processes in nursing practice, but her primary focus was from the nurse's perspective. Like Henderson, Abdellah specified the phenomena with which nursing is concerned, in this instance, 21 nursing problems (see box at left). Abdellah was one of the first nursing scholars to make explicit that the phenomena that concern nurses in practice should be the phenomena that concern researchers.

Ida Jean Orlando

Orlando contributed one of the first scholarly works specifically aimed at offering "the professional nursing student a theory of effective nursing practice."[45] She identified three elements of the nursing situation: (1) the patient's behavior, (2) the nurse's action and (3) the nurse's reaction as they influence the situation in which the nurse and patient find themselves. Her frame of reference applied to care of "patients" in a hospital situation with the involvement of a physician in the care. Her perspective is the result of 3 years of observation and participation in experiences with patients, students, nursing service, and instructional personnel. She views patients and clients as requiring "help" when their distress stems from (1) physical limitations, (2) adverse reactions to the setting, and (3) experiences that prevent them from communicating their needs. Accordingly, the purpose of nursing is to supply the help patients require for their needs to be met. Nursing is viewed as an interactive process, and the nurse must be sensitive to nonverbal and physiologic manifestations, as well as verbal cues from the client.[45]

The nurse functions in response to a patient's display of distress. There are four practices basic to nursing: *observation*, *reporting*, *recording*, and *action*. Knowledge about the patient comes from indirect sources, such as observations or family member input, or direct sources, such as (1) patient or (2) the feeling the nurse has from experience of the patient's behavior. Observations are then shared with the patient to clarify and validate the nurse's observations. The nurse's reaction consists of (1) perceptions of the patient's behavior, (2) the thoughts stimulated by the perceptions, and (3) feelings in response to these perceptions and thoughts. The nurse does not assume anything about the patient or situation until it is clarified with the patient. The nurse's action can be either deliberative and specific to the situation or automatic, that is, required by the patient but not specific to the immediate problem.[45] Orlando's frame of reference relates to a nurse-patient interaction occurring at a specific point in time.

Her perspective, like that of Peplau, focuses on the interactions between nurse and patient. It may be useful in guiding nursing students and practitioners alike in analyzing what is transmitted in nurse-patient interactions. Orlando's frame of reference is also useful in organizing data about the hospitalized patient's needs for assistance.

Myra Levine

Levine evolved her frame of reference through study of the arts and sciences. She views nursing as a human interaction and proposes four *conservation principles of nursing* based on the holistic nature of human response to the environment.[12] The client is viewed as an adaptive individual in a dynamic state of homeorrhesis rather than homeostasis, which suggests a stable or static relationship (Fig. 6-4). By recognizing the dynamic aspects of human life, the nurse can consider the nature of the changes or adaptation taking place in the client.

The four conservation principles of nursing are concerned with the unity and integrity of the individual:

1. *The principle of the conservation of energy.* The human body, as does every living organism, functions by utilizing energy. The human body needs energy-

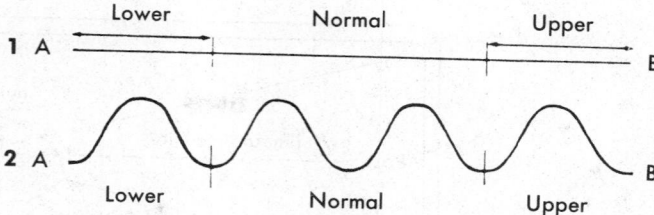

Fig. 6-4. *1*, Homeostasis—a straight line continuum with an upper *(B)* and lower *(A)* limit. *2*, Homeorrhesis—a stable flow retaining an upper and lower limit but also suggesting "normal" variation in response to periodicity of physiologic balance. (From Levine, M.E.: Introduction to clinical nursing, ed. 2, Philadelphia, 1973, F.A. Davis Co.)

producing input, such as food, oxygen, and fluids, to allow energy utilization or output. The balancing of energy input and output is viewed as a critical goal of nursing care.

2. *The principle of the conservation of structural integrity.* The human body has physical boundaries that must be maintained to facilitate health and prevent harmful agents from entering the body. The skin and mucous membranes of the client are the critical barriers to the environment. Nursing care protects or enhances the integrity of the skin and mucous membranes.

3. *The principles of the conservation of personal integrity.* Nursing interventions are based on the conservation of the individual client's personal integrity. Every individual has a sense of identity, self-worth, and self-esteem. It is critical for nurses to guard and care for the self-worth and self-esteem of the client. This includes the clients often treated with moral censure, such as alcoholics and drug abusers.

4. *The principles of conversation of social integrity.* Nursing interventions are based on the conservation of the individual client's social integrity. The social integrity of the client reflects the family and community in which the client functions. Health care institution rules may separate individuals from their family. It is important for nurses to consider the individual in the context of the family.[12]

Levine focuses primarily on the phenomena of nursing, with nursing interventions deriving from the perspective of the client's integrity and unity.

Martha Rogers

Rogers bases her ideas about nursing on a broad background of physical and social sciences. She believes nursing is both an art and a science. Like Nightingale, Rogers emphasizes strongly the importance of environment and environmental factors to nursing. She asserts that the focus of nursing is "unitary man."[21] She further asserts that a human being's wholeness must be per-

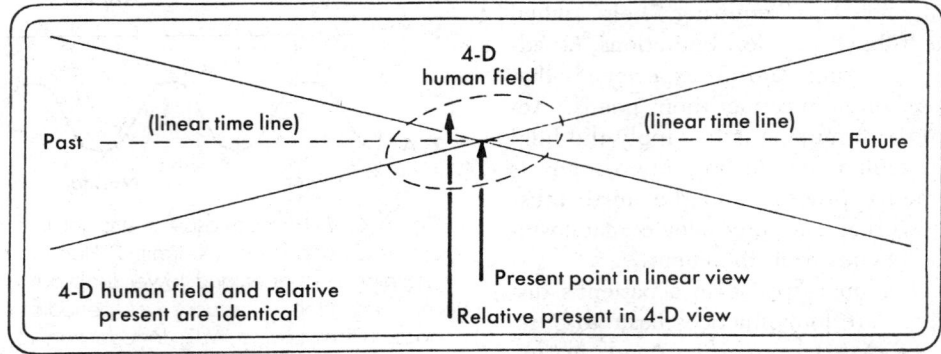

Fig. 6-5. Environmental field. (From Rogers, M.E.: Nursing: a science of unitary man. In Riehl, J.P., and Roy, C.: Conceptual models for nursing practice, ed. 2, New York, 1980, Appleton-Century-Crofts.)

ceived: "Human beings are more than and different from the sum of their parts."[21]

Rogers identifies four "building blocks" essential for understanding her perspective:

energy fields Both humans and environments are energy fields, with energy signifying the dynamic nature of a field and field used as a uniform concept.

universe of open systems Energy fields extend to infinity; human fields are open to exchange energy with the environmental field.

pattern and organization The continuously changing characteristics of an energy field.

four dimensionality The relative present for any individual, characterized by continuously fluctuating imaginary boundaries (Fig. 6-5).

From these building blocks emerge the definitions of unitary man and the environment:

unitary man A four-dimensional, negentropic energy field identified by pattern and organization and manifesting characteristics and behaviors that are different from those of the parts and that cannot be predicted from knowledge of the parts.

environment A four-dimensional, negentropic energy field identified by pattern and organization and encompassing all that outside any given human field.[21]

Rogers evolved her principles of homeodynamics as a way of viewing a human being as unitary man using the concepts above. Her three principles of homeodynamics are as follows:

principle of helicy The nature and direction of human and environmental change are continuously innovative, probabilistic, and characterized by increasing diversity of human field and environmental field pattern and organization, emerging out of the continuous, mutual, simultaneous interaction between the human and environmental fields and manifesting nonrepeating rhythmicities.

principle of resonance The human field and the environmental field are identified by wave pattern and organization manifesting continuous change from lower frequency,

longer wave patterns to higher frequency, shorter wave patterns.

principle of complementarity The interaction between human and environmental fields is continuous, mutual, and simultaneous.[21]

As unitary man, a human being is always changing, progressing forward through space and time and unable to return to an earlier stage. According to Rogers's concepts, an adult portraying "childlike" behaviors has not "regressed" to an earlier stage of development because the events occurring between childhood and the present have irrevocably changed or affected the individual.

Rogers provides a broad perspective that is useful in helping nurses appreciate the interrelationships between humans and their environment, recognizing patterns and organization in these relationships, and appreciating that humans are ever changing as a consequence of their interrelationship with the environment.

Imogene King

King, like other nurse authors, believes that knowledge in the basic sciences is critical for nurses. She views the basic abstraction of nursing as the phenomenon of man and his world.[11] Like many others, she identifies the person-environment interaction as a critical concept for nurses to take into consideration.

King views persons as functioning in social systems through interpersonal relationships in terms of their perceptions that influence their lives and health.[11] The major concepts in her frame of reference are as follows:

social systems Groups of individuals joined together in a network of social relationships to achieve common goals developed about a system of values with an organized set of practices and the methods to regulate practices and administer the rules.

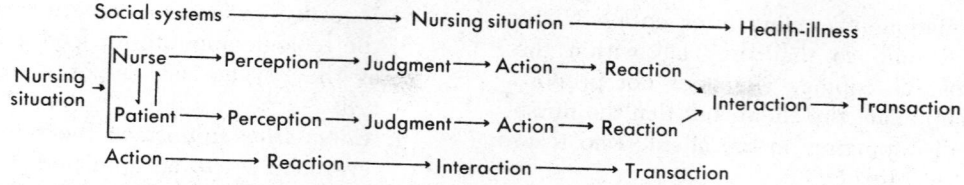

Fig. 6-6. The human process—a method for studying nursing process. (From King, I.M.: Toward a theory for nursing, New York, 1971, John Wiley & Sons, Inc.)

perception Each individual's representation or image of reality; an awareness of objects, persons, and events.

interpersonal relationships The interaction of two or more individuals in the existential moments in time for some purpose or goal.

health A dynamic state in the life cycle of an organism, which implies continuous adaptation to stresses in the internal and external environment through optimum use of one's resources to achieve maximal potential for daily living.[11]

In King's terms:

Nursing is a process of action, reaction, interaction, and transaction, whereby nurses assist individuals of any age and socioeconomic group to meet their basic needs in performing activities of daily living and to cope with health and illness at some particular point in the life cycle.[11]

Her process of action, reaction, interaction, and transaction is viewed as a method of studying the nursing process (Fig. 6-6), particularly the interpersonal relationship aspects of the nursing process. Action occurs when the nurse and client interact, making some type of judgment and decisions about responses to each other. The reaction occurs when observable behavior, a result of the action, occurs. The actions and reactions evolve into an interrelationship between the individuals. Transaction is a higher level of interaction, with mutual goal setting and planning by the client and the nurse. Transaction is particularly critical in the nursing process if maximal benefit of nursing care to the client is to be attained.[11]

King's perspective is useful for nurses considering relationships with any client regardless of health status, developmental stage, or the context in which nursing care is given. Like Peplau and Orlando, King has contributed to the understanding of the nurse-patient relationship and its components. Nursing students and practitioners may find her perspective useful in analyzing interactions and transactions with patients.

Sister Callista Roy

Roy presents an adaptation model of nursing in which the person-environment interaction is a critical notion basic to nursing. There are three essential elements to the Roy model: *the client, the goal,* and *the nursing intervention.*

The nursing client may be a person, a family, a group, a community, or society.[26] These clients or recipients are viewed as "adaptive systems." There are two major components or subsystems of the adaptive system: the regulator and the cognator.

The regulator subsystem is described by the inputs, major parts, process, effectors, and feedback loops. The inputs to the regulator are stimuli from the external environment and from change in the internal state. The major parts of the regulator subsystem are the neural, endocrine, and perception-psychomotor portions. The process is the conscious and unconscious responses occurring within the body. The effectors are neurally controlled glands and muscles responding to the process. Feedback loops provide information about outcomes as a form of input that is reprocessed through the system.

The cognator subsystem is described in terms of its inputs, parts, processes, and effectors. The inputs to the cognator are internal and external stimuli related to psychologic, social, physical, and physiologic factors.

Roy's perspective is in an evolutionary process, and the psychosocial parts of the model are the most developed. These include (1) perceptual/information processing, (2) learning, (3) judgment, and (4) emotion. Discrete processes can be identified within the four separate parts. The effectors for the psychosocial cognator subsystem involve the musculoskeletal subsystem and the psychomotor subsystem, resulting in verbalization.[26]

The client's adaptation is a function of the stimulus to which the client is exposed and the adaptation level. There are three classes of stimuli: (1) focal stimuli, or stimuli immediately confronting the person; (2) contextual stimuli, or all other stimuli present; and (3) residual stimuli, such as beliefs, attitudes, or traits, that have an indeterminate effect on the present situation.[26]

The goal of nursing refers to the outcome of the nursing action and is influenced by the adaptation level of the client. The adaptation level is the region each client has in which stimuli will evoke a positive response. The goal is directed toward the healthy or well end of the health-illness continuum established by Roy.[25] The goal assists in determining whether or not an individual requires nursing to assist with adaptation.

Roy's interpretation of nursing intervention is the manipulation of stimuli so that they fall within the boundaries of positive coping. She does not propose that the nurse manipulate the client, but that the nurse manipulate stimuli impinging on the client, who is an active participant in care.

Roy proposes four modes of adaptation: physiologic needs, self-concept, role function, and interdependence. These modes are viewed as *effectors* of adaptation while cognator and regulator activities are the *means* of adaptation.[26] All nursing activity is aimed at promoting the client's adaptation to physiologic needs, self-concept, role functioning, and interdependence during health and illness.[23]

Roy's perspective fosters an appreciation of the interrelationship between the individual and the environment. Her use of the notions of adaptive subsystems (the cognator and the regulator) helps define the means by which individuals adapt. The modes of adaptation as well as the adaptive subsystems and stimuli impinging on the client may be used in organizing nursing assessment of the client, determining goal setting and conceptualizing nursing interventions. Roy's perspective is unique in that it attempts to account for human adaptative processes as they relate to health and to link adaptation to concepts of nursing practice.

Dorothy Johnson

Johnson's behavioral systems model for nursing has been "developed from a philosophical perspective, supported by a rich, sound and rapidly expanding body of empirical and theoretical knowledge."[9] She published aspects of her concepts and ideas for several years; however, her first published integration of these ideas occurred in 1980. The goal of nursing, for Johnson, is "to assist a person (1) whose behavior is commensurate with social demands, (2) who is able to modify his or her behavior in ways that support biologic imperatives, (3) who is able to benefit to the fullest extent during illness from the physician's knowledge and skill, and (4) whose behavior does not give evidence of unnecessary trauma as a consequence of illness."[9]

Although others have interpreted Johnson's work to have more subsystems, Johnson has identified seven human subsystems:

1. *Attachment or affiliative subsystem:* the first response system to emerge; the basis for all social organization.
2. *Dependency subsystem:* the behavior that has as its consequence approval, attention, and physical assistance, as well as behavior calling for nurturance.

3. *Ingestive subsystem:* appetite satisfaction, both the biologic appetite for food and fluids, as well as the psychosocial appetite for nurturance of self.
4. *Eliminative subsystem:* the removal of both energy and waste accumulated from the ingestive subsystem action. Elimination of biological excess and wastes in urine and feces is concrete and easily understood. Elimination of accumulations from the psychosocial realm is less well understood.
5. *Sexual subsystem:* a subsystem with dual functions of procreation and gratification; originates with gender role identity.
6. *Aggressive subsystem:* self-protection and preservation.
7. *Achievement subsystem:* exploratory behaviors and attempts to manipulate the environment.[9]

Johnson states that the subsystems and the system as a whole tend to be self-maintaining and self-perpetuating so long as conditions in the internal and external environment of the system remain orderly and predictable, the conditions and resources necessary to their functional requirements are met, and the interrelationship among the subsystems are harmonious. Each of the systems or subsystems must be protected, nurtured, and stimulated to grow and develop to their optimal states.[9]

Johnson's thoughts about human functioning may be useful to nurses as an organizing framework for nursing assessment and goal setting. Johnson stipulates that nursing is concerned with the protection, nurturing, and stimulation of growth in these subsystems.

Josephine Paterson and Loretta Zderad

Paterson and Zderad have taken a phenomenologic approach to the study of nursing, which they have extended to a practice theory of humanistic nursing. Knowledge of the concepts basic to existential philosophy is critical to understanding the approach to humanistic nursing. Nursing is viewed as an experience between human beings that has meaning for the existence of all parties involved. Human awareness of the self and of otherness is essential for existential experiences.[19] Each human being is unique and the nurse must be in touch with self to be open to the uniqueness and richness of the individuals with whom interaction is taking place. The experiences of the nurse and the meaning of the reality of experiences are critical components of humanistic nursing.

Humanistic nursing asks that "the nurse describe what she or he comes to know: (1) the nurse's unique perspective and responses, (2) others' knowable responses, and (3) the reciprocal call and response, what goes on between, as they occur in the nursing situation."[19] In humanistic nursing, nursing is defined as "the ability to struggle with other men through peak experiences related to health and suffering in which the participants in the nursing situation *are* and *become* in accordance with their human potential."[19] Humanistic nursing is not a matter solely of doing, but also of being. In the nurse-client situation, the nurse's total being is available and responds to the experience of the situation:

The nursing situation is a particular kind of human situation in which the relating between humans is purposely directed toward nurturing the well-being or the capacity to become more human of a person with perceived needs. The elements of humanistic nursing would include incarnate men (patient and nurse) meeting (being and becoming) in a goal directed (nurturing well-being and more-being) intersubjective transaction (being with and doing with) occurring in time and space (measured and as lived by patient and nurse) in a world of men and things.[19]

Humanistic nursing allows the nurse to approach the client from many angles and to enhance the development of human potential, in both the nurse and the client.

Paterson and Zderad emphasize the importance of understanding oneself as well as the meaning of reality for others. Their approach may be particularly useful to nurses who care for individuals in experiences related to health and suffering.

Rozella Schlotfeldt

Schlotfeldt's frame of reference focuses primarily on health-seeking behaviors and mechanisms of human beings. She defines nursing as assessing and enhancing the health status, health assets, and health potentials of persons with the goal of their optimal health. Health-seeking behaviors are seen as action terms, implying that people are active and seek optimal health. The emphasis is on positive aspects of health assets and health potentials rather than on negative aspects such as deficits or problems. Nursing practice focuses on behaviors and mechanisms actively used by persons in efforts to attain or retain optimal health and function, to overcome threats from intervening variables that affect the mechanisms, and to cope with crises encountered during development, decline, and time of death.[27] Nursing strategies include *compensating, teaching, guiding* and *counseling, supporting, monitoring, motivating,* and *inspiring.*

Although this perspective of nursing has not been developed to the extent of several others, it is useful in its emphasis on clients' health rather than disabilities, problems, or tasks. People are viewed as having health assets to be enhanced even when ill or in decline. Health goals include those leading to self-preservation, comfort, procreation, productivity, and dignified death.

Summary

After reviewing the work of these nurse authors it is apparent that there is no single nursing perspective. Instead, it can help one to appreciate the rich and diverse heritage in nursing thought. Although most nurse scholars address the importance of the individual, human health, the environment, and nursing, each contributes a unique perspective for practice and scholarship.

Use of most of these perspectives can be justified on the basis of the populations for whom nurses care, including their health status, developmental stage, and the context in which health care is delivered, as well as the nurse's own perspective and personal intellectual preferences. For example, in the nursing care of a client in the hospital after emergency surgery, a variety of perspectives might be appropriate. Concepts from Nightingale may be applied during manipulation of the environment to provide a comfortable, odor-free room. Hall provides a care framework emphasizing nurturance of the client. Henderson and Abdellah provide frameworks for assessment and care in the early postanesthesia stage. In Rogers's and King's perspectives, the client's relationships with family and community may be more fully assessed, while Orem provides a framework for assisting the client back to total self-care. Schlotfeldt additionally emphasizes the health assets of the client even during trauma or illness.

This chapter has attempted to highlight some of the best-known nursing perspectives. It was not intended to be all inclusive. Readers are encouraged to explore further the perspectives of those that they find the most useful in caring for the adult client. Students are also encouraged to look at the historical development of the nursing theorists' thoughts and ideas. Reviewing earlier works will assist readers in understanding the evolution of these perspectives. Lastly, readers are encouraged to use aspects of many perspectives, putting together an eclectic framework that is most appropriate for the client-environment situation with which they are involved. There is no "right" frame of reference that applies uniformly in a given situation.

REFERENCES AND SELECTED READINGS
Contemporary

1. Abdellah, F.G., et al.: New directions in patient-centered nursing, New York, 1973, Macmillan Publishing Co., Inc.
2. Ashley, J.: Hospitals, paternalism, and the role of the nurse, New York, 1976, Teachers College Press.
3. Blake, M.: The Peplau developmental model for nursing practice. In Riehl, J.P., and Roy, C., editors: Conceptual models for nursing practice, ed. 2, New York, 1980, Appleton-Century-Crofts.
4. Ehrenreich, B., and English, D.: Witches, midwives and nurses: a history of women healers, Old Westbury, N.Y., 1973, The Feminist Press.
5. Francis, G.M.: This thing called problem solving, In Marriner, A.: The nursing process: a scientific approach to nursing care, ed. 2, St. Louis, 1979, The C.V. Mosby Co.
6. Hale, K., and George, J.B.: Lydia Hall. In The Nursing Theories Conference Group: Nursing theories: the base for professional nursing practice, Englewood Cliffs, N.J., 1980, Prentice-Hall, Inc.
7. Henderson, V.: We've come a long way, but what of direction? Nurs. Res. **26:**163-164, 1977.
8. Henderson, V., and Nite, G.: Principles and practices of nursing, ed. 6, New York, 1978, Macmillan Publishing Co., Inc.
9. Johnson, D.E.: The behavioral system model for nursing. In Riehl, J.P., and Roy, C., editors: Conceptual models for nursing practice, ed. 2, New York, 1980, Appleton-Century-Crofts.
10. Kelly, L.Y.: The eternal fascination with nursing education, Nurs. Outlook **26:**403, 1978.
11. King, I.M.: Toward a theory for nursing, New York, 1971, John Wiley & Sons, Inc.
12. Levine, M.E.: Introduction to clinical nursing, ed. 2, Philadelphia, 1973, F.A. Davis Co.
13. Levine, M.E.: Holistic nursing, Nurs. Clin. North Am. **6:**253-264, 1971.
14. Marriner, A.: The nursing process, ed. 3, St. Louis, 1983, The C.V. Mosby Co.
15. Newman, M: Theory development in nursing, Philadelphia, 1979, F.A. Davis Co.
16. The Nursing Development Conference Group: Concept formalization in nursing: process and product, ed. 2, Boston, 1979, Little, Brown & Co.
17. The Nursing Theories Conference Group: Nursing theories: the base for professional nursing practice, Englewood Cliffs, N.J., 1980, Prentice-Hall, Inc.
18. Orem, D.E.: Nursing: concepts of practice, ed. 2, New York, 1980, McGraw-Hill Book Co.
19. Paterson, J.G., and Zderad, L.T.: Humanistic nursing, New York, 1976, John Wiley & Sons, Inc.
20. Riehl, J.P., and Roy, C.: Conceptual models for nursing practice, ed. 2, New York, 1980, Appleton-Century-Crofts.
21. Rogers, M.E.: Nursing: a science of unitary man. In Riehl, J.P., and Roy, C., editors: Conceptual models for nursing practice, ed. 2, New York, 1980, Appleton-Century-Crofts.
22. Rogers, M.E.: An introduction to the theoretical basis of nursing, Philadelphia, 1970, F.A. Davis Co.
23. Roy, C.: The Roy adaptation model. In Riehl, J.P., and Roy, C., editors: Conceptual models for nursing practice, ed. 2, New York, 1980, Appleton-Century-Crofts.
24. Roy, C.: Adaptation: a basis for nursing practice, Nurs. Outlook **19:**254-257, 1971.
25. Roy, C.: Introduction to nursing: an adaptation model, Englewood Cliffs, N.J., 1976, Prentice-Hall, Inc.
26. Roy C., and Roberts, S.L.: Theory construction in nursing: an adaptational model, Englewood Cliffs, N.J., 1981, Prentice-Hall, Inc.
27. Schlotfeldt, R.M.: The need for a conceptual framework. In Verhonick, P.J.: Nursing research I, Boston, 1975, Little, Brown & Co.
28. Schlotfeldt, R.M.: This I believe . . . nursing is health care, Nurs. Outlook **20:**245-246, 1972.
29. Stevens, B.J.: Nursing theory: analysis, application, evaluation, Boston, 1979, Little, Brown & Co.
30. Sundeen, S.J., et al.: Nurse-client interaction: implementing the nursing process, ed. 2, St. Louis, 1981, The C.V. Mosby Co.
31. Torres, G.: The place of concepts and theories within nursing. In The Nursing Theories Conference Group: Nursing theories: the base for professional nursing practice, Englewood Cliffs, N.J., 1980, Prentice-Hall, Inc.

Classic

32. Abdellah, F.G., et al.: Patient-centered approaches to nursing, New York, 1960, Macmillan Publishing Co., Inc.
33. Abdellah, F.G., and Levine, E.: Better patient care through nursing research, New York, 1965, Macmillan Publishing Co., Inc.
34. Henderson, V.: Excellence in nursing, Am. J. Nurs. **69:**2133-2137, 1969.
35. Henderson, V.: Basic principles of nursing care, Geneva, 1960, International Council of Nurses.
36. Henderson, V.: The nature of nursing, Am. J. Nurs. **69:**64-68, 1964.
37. Henderson, V.: The nature of nursing, New York, 1966, Macmillan, Co., Inc.
38. King, I.: A conceptual frame of reference for nursing, Nurs. Res. **17:**27-31, 1968.
39. King, I.: Nursing theory—problems and prospect, Nurs. Sci. **2:**394-403, 1964.
40. Kopf, E.W.: Florence Nightingale as statistician, Am. Stat. Assoc., pp. 338-405, 1916.
41. Levine, M.E.: The pursuit of wholeness, Am. J. Nurs. **69:**93-98, 1969.
42. Levine, M.E.: The four conservation principles of nursing, Nurs. Forum **6:**45-59, 1967.
43. Nightingale, F.: Notes on nursing, Philadelphia, 1859, J.B. Lippincott Co.
44. Orlando, I.J.: Behind the theory of nursing practice, Am. J. Nurs. **63:**54-55, 1963.
45. Orlando, I.J.: The dynamic nurse-patient relationship, New York, 1961, G.P. Putnam's Sons.
46. Peplau, H.E.: Interpersonal relations and the process of adaptation, Nurs. Sci., pp. 272-279, 1963.
47. Peplau, H.E.: Interpersonal relations in nursing, New York, 1952, G.P. Putnam's Sons.
48. Rogers, M.E.: Educational revolution in nursing, New York, 1969, Macmillan Publishing Co., Inc.
49. Rogers, M.E.: Reveille in nursing, New York, 1965, F.A. Davis Co.

CONCEPTS AND PROCESSES

As nursing practice becomes increasingly sophisticated, nurses are seeking more specialized knowledge as a basis for decision making. Despite increasing specialization, there remains a group of concepts and processes that are common to nursing practice regardless of the clinical practice area.

The focus of this unit is on concepts and processes common to the practice of nursing in a variety of clinical areas. A systematic approach to nursing care, commonly termed *nursing process,* is addressed since this serves as the basic framework for the latter part of the book. The overall process in terms of assessment, intervention, and evaluation is addressed first, followed by a more in-depth discussion of *assessment* with special emphasis on data collection and analysis. Since much of nursing assessment and intervention involves interaction between nurse and client or patient, *nurse-patient relationships* are considered. The last two chapters deal with the use of a *problem-oriented system* for both planning and recording health information and the monitoring of patient/client outcomes by means of *quality assurance programs.*

CHAPTER 7

NURSING PROCESS

JANE E. ANDERSON

KAREN K. YODER

Nursing process is a rational, scientifically based framework for nursing. It provides organization and direction to various elements of nursing practice and an accurate means of predicting outcomes, prescribing action alternatives, and evaluating results. Nursing process is a way of thinking about nursing care. It provides a more rational basis for nursing practice than intuition. Furthermore, nursing process provides a method for establishing standards of nursing care. These standards constitute a means for judging the quality of nursing services given to patients and clients. Thus the quality of nursing care is monitored on the basis of objective data and scientific criteria.[2] In addition, nursing process provides a framework for identifying recurring nursing problems, relationships between data, and various nursing care approaches. This information in turn initiates research that further contributes to the theoretical basis of nursing.

The most commonly designated steps or phases of the nursing process are assessment, planning, intervention, and evaluation. Other formulations stipulate five steps: assessing, analyzing, planning, implementing, and evaluating (see the following outline). In this approach assessing means establishing a data base about a client and analyzing means identifying the client's needs or goals of care. Some experts eliminate planning as a step because they believe planning is essential to all phases of the nursing process. Thus *assessment, intervention,* and *evaluation* appear in all formulations of nursing process as noted in Fig. 7-1.

1. Assessing: establishing a data base about a client
   a. Gathers information relative to the client
   b. Verifies data
   c. Communicates information gained in assessment of client

2. Analyzing: identifying the client's health care needs and selecting goals of care
   a. Interprets data
   b. Identifies client needs
   c. Determines goals of care
3. Planning: designing a strategy to achieve the goals established for client care
   a. Develops and modifies client care plan
   b. Cooperates with other health personnel for delivery of client care
   c. Records information relevant to client management
4. Implementing: initiating and completing actions necessary to accomplish the defined goals
   a. Performs or assists in performing activities of daily living
   b. Counsels and teaches client and/or family
   c. Gives care to achieve therapeutic goals for the client
   d. Gives care to optimize achievement of health goals by the client
   e. Supervises and checks the work of staff for whom responsible
   f. Records and exchanges information
5. Evaluating: determining the extent to which the goals of care have been achieved
   a. Estimates the extent to which objectives of the plan of care are achieved
   b. Evaluates implementation of measures
   c. Investigates compliance with prescribed and/or proscribed therapy
   d. Records client's response to treatment or care

Nursing process has several characteristics. The following attributes should be integral parts of nursing process as a whole and each of its phases.

1. Systematic: characterized by the use of an orderly procedure
2. Purposeful: guided by a definite aim
3. Interactional: involves reciprocal actions between nurse and client
4. Specific: formulated precisely
5. Theoretically based: determined according to an assumed set of facts or principles
6. Based on priorities: established according to preferential rating
7. Validated: well grounded; conclusions reached by the nurse are verified with the client
8. Dynamic: characterized by continuous change
9. Mutually derived: formed by both nurse and client
10. Generalized: rendered applicable to a wide class of clients

Another feature of nursing process is that there are no constraints as to who or what entities are defined as participants in the process or in what setting the process occurs. The client may be defined as an individual, family, group, community, organization, or society. The process may be applied to populations defined on the basis of characteristics such as physical, social, or economic. The process occurs in multiple settings such as homes, schools, clinics, or hospitals.

Assessment

The first phase of the nursing process is assessment, which involves systematic data collection and data analysis. This phase is usually initiated when there is a discrepancy between what is and what should be in relation to optimal health for the client. Either the nurse or the client identifies the discrepancy and provides the impetus for change. The felt need for change, then, provides the initial input to establish a data base derived from a variety of sources.[1]

Collection of data

To provide a comprehensive data base, the information gathered must reflect the perceptions of both the client and the nurse regarding the individual, the subsystem, and the suprasystem. When the client is the family, for example, data are collected about the family (client), each member of the family (subsystems), and the community of the family (suprasystem). The family's self-report of their perceptions is *subjective data*. The data obtained by the nurse is *objective data*. Specific examples of subjective and objective data for each aspect of a client system are listed in Table 7-1.

Primary and *secondary* sources provide data about

TABLE 7-1. Examples of subjective and objective data collected for each aspect of a client system

Client	Subjective data	Objective data
Individual	Results of interview, such as symptoms, feelings about wellness-illness, attitudes toward hospitalization	Results of inspection, palpation, percussion, auscultation
Family	Values, norms, status	Communication patterns, roles
Community	Culture, folkways, customs	Population characteristics, geographic factors, facilities

the client's present and past status. The client provides primary data, and sources related to the client contribute secondary data. The following sources of data are defined as either primary or secondary depending on the client system being considered: significant others, written records about the client, nursing personnel and other members of the health team, and relevant humanistic and scientific literature.

Data are collected through interview, observation, examination, and literature review. Although data may be collected from the client in an informal manner, there is evidence that a systematic approach results in a more complete data base. Since no one method or tool is sufficient to gather all the necessary information, the vehicle for data collection is determined by considering the nature of the situation and the time available to collect the data. Examples of comprehensive data collection forms can be found in Chapters 8 and 10. References providing information on other published forms can be found in the list of references following Chapter 8.

An important feature of the assessment is that it is mutually derived by the nurse and the individual. If nurses do not verify their perceptions with the client system, they are practicing in an automatic, nontherapeutic manner.[8] Nursing assessment conducted in consultation with the individual is more likely to yield effective nursing interventions than if the client is not given opportunity to participate in the assessment.[7]

Analysis of data

Data analysis involves *sorting* and *organizing* the collected data into a logical framework. This procedure makes the accumulated data more meaningful and easier to manage, suggests missing data, prevents omission of relevant data, and saves time and energy for both the nurse and the client.

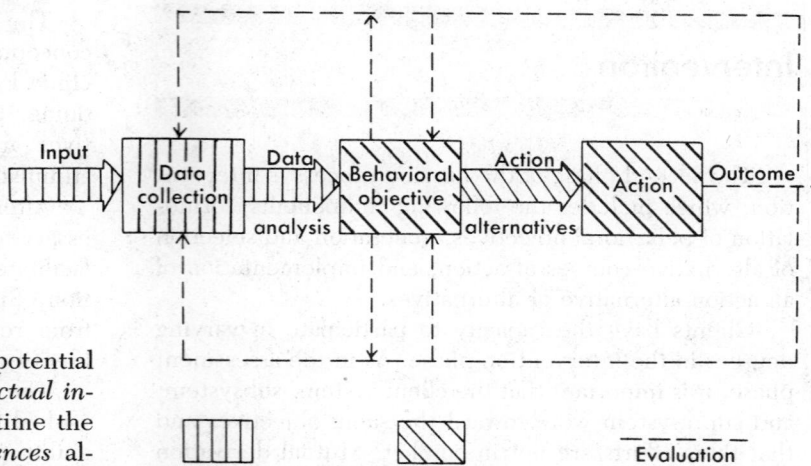

Fig. 7-1. Model of nursing process.

Analysis of the data focuses on actual and potential interferences with the client's health status. *Actual interferences* indicate difficulties present at the time the assessment is made, while *potential interferences* allude to difficulties that the individual is at unusually high risk of developing or experiencing.[4]

The framework utilized for organizing the data is determined by the amount and type of data collected, the client, and the nurse's knowledge and philosophy about nursing. The data may be analyzed according to several approaches. Nursing diagnoses may be made or assets and limitations may be identified (see Chapter 8 for additional discussion). A list of health problems may be generated (see Chapter 10 for additional discussion).

Conclusions from data analysis indicate how well the client is dealing with the situation. The conclusions indicate that the individual is successfully handling the situation or is utilizing preventive measures, needs help but is getting it, or is unable to handle the situation or prevent it with personal resources. If the client is successfully handling the situation alone or by means of other resources, the nurse concludes that nursing intervention is not currently needed. If the individual cannot handle or prevent the situation, the nurse intervenes by determining what help is needed and who can provide it.[5]

Establishment of priorities

After the data have been analyzed, priorities are determined. The establishment of priorities allows the nurse to make rational choices at any given time when several problems or needs compete for attention.[5] Priorities usually reflect differentiation between life-threatening problems and problems of lesser importance or those that are long term in nature.[3]

One hierarchy that can be used in setting priorities for the client follows.[3] Consideration is first given to the problems that threaten the *life, dignity,* and *integrity* of the individual. Examples of such problems for the various client systems are the following:

Individual: Lack of patent airway
Family: Difficulty affecting whole unit that contributes to conflict and breakdown
Community: Epidemic

Secondary consideration is given to the problems that threaten to destructively change the client. Examples of such problems are the following:

Individual: Metabolic imbalance, abnormal cell growth, or retreat from social contacts
Family: Breakdown of communication
Community: Drug abuse

Finally, consideration is given to the problems that affect the normal growth and development of the client. Examples of such problems are the following:

Individual: Nutritional deprivation
Family: Lack of defined rules
Community: Lack of resources

The above hierarchy indicates how priority is given to situations where *illness* is prevalent. Establishment of another priority is necessary in *wellness* situations where the emphasis is on preventive health care. One suggestion is that the priority be reversed in wellness situations. Primary consideration in wellness situations, therefore, pertains to interferences with the normal growth and development of the individual. Secondary consideration in wellness situations is given to interferences in the client's status that have the potential to destructively change the person. Then, at the point where the interferences actually do change the individual's status, the priority indicated in the hierarchy is initiated. While collecting and analyzing the data, the individual may make a request or the nurse may recognize the need for an action. The nurse therefore may be tempted to intervene during the assessment phase. However, if the nurse waits to intervene until the data are analyzed and specific interventions are planned, more complete and accurate conclusions can usually be drawn. The components of the assessment phase are illustrated with vertical lines in Fig. 7-1.

Intervention

The second phase of the nursing process is intervention, which includes the following components: formulation of behavioral objectives, generation and selection of alternative courses of action, and implementation of an action alternative or alternatives.

Clients have the capacity to participate in varying degrees in the intervention phase. As in the assessment phase, it is important that the client system, subsystem, and suprasystem work toward the same objectives and that their efforts are not in conflict. Mutual derivation of objectives and action alternatives enhances the effectiveness of nursing interventions.

Formulation of objectives

The first component of the intervention phase involves the formulation of behavioral objectives. These objectives provide guidelines for determining the aim of intervention, or what is to be accomplished as a result of intervention. When stated behaviorally, objectives indicate desired client outcomes that can be observed, demonstrated, heard, or felt. The desired outcomes, therefore, provide standards for evaluating client progress.

Behavioral objectives contain the following elements: client, action verb, and criterion or condition under which performance occurs. The designated client (individual, family, group, or community) indicates who is to perform the desired behavior. A specific measurable action verb then states what the client needs to do to indicate achievement of the objective. By stating the criterion or condition in relation to a time period or accuracy of performance, the standards for judging the outcome behavior are defined. An example might be that "Mrs. Jones states the procedure for instilling her eye drops with 100% accuracy." Objectives provide the scope and focus for delineation of alternatives for action.

Formulation of action alternatives

The action alternatives are hypothesized solutions that indicate how to achieve the desired outcome. The complexity of the situation and the desired outcome usually influence the number and quality of alternatives. The alternatives proposed for a singular or isolated event, for example, may be decreased in number and quality. If the situation is complex, however, the quantity and quality of the alternatives are likely to be increased.[3]

The determination of action alternatives is based on concepts and principles in the literature, the nurse's clinical experience, observation of what others are doing, and the nurse's creative inclinations. Alternatives are proposed through brainstorming: one idea stimulates the formation of another idea.[1]

After the action alternatives are proposed, it is necessary to select among the alternatives. The selection is facilitated by considering the consequences of each action. Since consequences are conclusions that result from reason, a sound theoretical base is essential to identify all the consequences of the action.

The consequences of proposed alternatives are ranked in relation to probability and desirability. Probability provides an estimate of the likelihood that the consequences of a proposed alternative will occur. This ranking is derived from the subjective experience of self and others and from objective recorded information. The desirability of the consequences of an alternative is also considered. An alternative is considered desirable if the preferred intent is likely to be accomplished, no harmful side effect is apt to occur, and the means for accomplishing the goal are efficient and appropriate.[3] Consideration of the side effect or risk is especially crucial. When considering risk, the negative aspect of the safety issue often becomes the critical criterion for decision making. Safety then tends to assume unrealistic proportions and overrides consideration of other more positive consequences. As a result, the potential outcome for the individual may be compromised at a low level of attainment. In ranking the consequences of alternatives according to risk, factors in addition to safety must be considered to maximize the client's potential. Thus when the consequences of action alternatives are considered, the alternatives selected for implementation usually reflect high probability and desirability.

Implementation of action

The last component of the intervention phase is to implement the selected alternative. During implementation there are potential ramifications and outcomes for all levels of the system (client system, subsystem, and suprasystem). When a family is the client system, for example, actions designed to alleviate family stressors will also have an effect on the individual (subsystem) and the community (suprasystem).

When the action is occurring, several health care providers may be interacting with the individual. The actions taken by these providers of health care may potentially be in conflict and may hinder the individual's progression toward optimal health. The action, therefore, should be sufficiently detailed to provide consistency in the implementation. The components of the intervention phase, formulation of behavioral objectives and action, are illustrated by the diagonal lines in Fig. 7-1.

Evaluation

The last phase of the nursing process is evaluation, which involves appraisal of the actual outcome that results from the action. The actual outcome is compared with the behavioral objective (desired outcome) through the evaluation feedback loop. This comparison yields the following possible results:

1. Objective (desired outcome) successfully accomplished
2. Objective partially accomplished: some of the variables in the objective not accomplished
3. Objective not successfully accomplished and corrective action in the process necessary
4. Objective accomplished and data collected regarding other outcomes

If the actual outcome is consistent with the desired outcome, the actual outcome becomes part of the data collection. However, if there is a discrepancy between actual and desired outcomes, revision of the process is essential. In accordance with the progression of the feedback loop (as indicated by dotted lines in Fig. 7-1), revision may be appropriate at various points. Solutions for the revision therefore may include the following procedures:

1. Redesigning the behavioral objective
2. Selecting and implementing another action alternative
3. Collecting and analyzing more data to evolve new nursing diagnoses (or problems), behavioral objectives, action alternatives, and actions.

For the evaluation process to be successful, the participants must be able and willing to receive the feedback. Therefore from the beginning, plans for evaluation involve the client system, subsystem, and suprasystem. Mechanisms are established to make the evaluation reliable and replicable. For example, a high degree of agreement on evaluation tools is established before they are used by the nursing staff.

This last phase of the nursing process, therefore, is not an end in itself. Evaluation provides a means to facilitate processing and reprocessing by means of corrective mechanisms. The cyclic quality of evaluation contributes to the dynamic nature of nursing process and is shown by the dotted lines in Fig. 7-1.

Relationship of nursing process to other approaches to thinking

Since nursing process is a way of thinking, the elements of the process are inherent in other guidelines for thinking: general systems perspective, scientific method, American Nurses Association Standards of Practice, and problem-oriented record. The common elements of assessment, intervention, and evaluation are evident when comparing the other guidelines to thinking, as noted in Table 7-2.

TABLE 7-2. Comparison of guidelines for thinking with phases of nursing process

Guidelines for thinking	Phases of nursing process		
	Assessment	Intervention	Evaluation
General systems perspective	Input	Throughput	Output, feedback
Scientific method	Identify and define problem, collect data	Formulate a hypothesis; evaluate the hypothesis; test the hypothesis	Form conclusions
ANA Standards of Practice	Collect data systematically and continuously about health status of client; communicate and record data	Implement nursing actions that provide client participation in health promotion, maintenance, and restoration	Reassess, reorder priorities, set new goal, and revise plan based on progress or lack of progress
Problem-oriented record	Collect a data base, derive a problem list	Establish an initial plan	Write progress notes, including: Subjective: what client says Objective: information observed by another or measured by instruments Assessment: interpretation, evaluation Plan: decisions for immediate or future action

Summary

The nursing process provides a rational, scientifically based framework for nursing practice. Each level of the system (client, subsystem, and suprasytem) is considered throughout the process. Input from the nurse or client regarding the need for change initiates the assessment phase. During the assessment phase data are collected and analyzed. During the intervention phase behavioral objectives are formulated to designate the desired outcome and alternative actions are proposed to indicate how the desired outcome may be achieved. After reviewing the proposed alternatives the selected actions are implemented. During the evaluation phase the actual outcome is compared with the behavioral objectives (desired outcome). If the actual outcome is consistent with the desired outcome, the actual outcome becomes part of the data collection. However, if there is a discrepancy between actual and desired outcomes, the process begins anew at assessment or intervention. The nursing process therefore is a means for providing dynamic, scientifically based client care.

Each phase is considered as a separate step; however, in reality the phases occur concurrently. To the beginning nurse practitioner, each phase of the nursing process may seem time consuming. With practice, however, the time involved in utilizing the various phases is minimized.

REFERENCES AND SELECTED READINGS
Contemporary

1. *Bailey, J.T., and Claus, K.E.: Decision making in nursing: tools for change, St. Louis, 1975, The C.V. Mosby Co.
2. *Becknell, E., and Smith, D.: System of nursing practice, Philadelphia, 1975, F.A. Davis Co.
3. *Bower, F.L.: The process of planning nursing care: nursing practice models, ed. 3, St. Louis, 1982, The C.V. Mosby Co.
4. *Mayers, M.: A systematic approach to the nursing care plan, ed. 2, New York, 1978, Appleton-Century-Crofts.
5. *Mitchell P., and Loustau, A.: Concepts basic to nursing, ed. 3, New York, 1981, McGraw-Hill Book Co.
6. *Mundinger, M., and Jauron, G.: Developing a nursing diagnosis, Nurs. Outlook **23**:94-98, 1975.

Classic

7. *Dumas, R., and Leonard, R.C.: The effect of nursing on the incidence of postoperative vomiting, Nurs. Res. **12**:12-15, 1963.
8. *Orlando, I.J.: The dynamic nurse-patient relationship, New York, 1961, G.P. Putnam's Sons.

*References preceded by an asterisk are particularly well suited for student reading.

CHAPTER 8

ASSESSMENT PROCESS: DATA COLLECTION AND ANALYSIS

JANE STEINMAN KAUFMAN

Assessment is the crucial foundation on which the future steps of the nursing process depend. Assessment includes two phases: the collection of data from multiple sources and analysis of the data into nursing care problems or diagnoses. Data are collected systematically, through interview subjectively and objectively through physical examination. A complete data base assures that the nurse will be aware of the patient's problems and will be able to plan care based on the data. When the data base is incomplete, the nurse may assume incorrectly that the client's problems are adequately identified and can be appropriately addressed. In other words, the nursing plan is only as complete and accurate as the data on which it is based.

The process of assessment is a complex one that most beginning practitioners find extremely time consuming. Identifying and analyzing a client's nursing care problems requires a knowledge base on which to make judgments, the ability to compare data with established norms and standards, and the ability to think analytically.

Data collection

Data collection is initiated with the first client contact. During all succeeding contacts the nurse continually collects information relevant to the nursing care of a client. Observations range in complexity from the gross observation that a patient is bleeding to more intricate mental noting of nonverbal cues emitted by a client.

In our everyday lives data collection and observation occur constantly, often in a random pattern: one often observes something by chance. In nursing one collects data systematically in order to improve accuracy, to avoid missing cues, and to ensure a complete data base.

There are three basic components of systematic data collection. First, it is *purposeful*. The nurse has particular reasons for collecting the data. Second, data collection is *planned systematically* with criteria or methodology outlined in advance. For example, if the nurse is assessing the normal growth and development of a 6-month-old child, criteria used to evaluate children of this age need to be available. The data to be collected are also ordered, or organized. Third, systematic data collection requires *accurate observations* in order to draw valid conclusions.

To assess systematically decisions are made concerning (1) the areas of daily living about which information will be sought, (2) the methods of collecting information that are most appropriate to the situation, (3) the priorities for collecting data and for instituting therapy, and (4) the means to be used for organizing and analyzing the data.[50]

Fact vs. inference

When gathering data, facts or descriptive data are collected before meaning is attached to the information. Facts are objective and noncontroversial. Conversely, inference allows one to attach meaning to the information or behavior that is more useful than the information itself. Various inferences can be made from one item of data. The nurse asks, "What could this behavior mean?" Consider a patient who is teary eyed, has a downcast head, and is curled up in bed. Inferences could include: (1) the patient is depressed, (2) the patient is homesick, (3) the patient is in pain.

Inferences must be validated before the nurse acts on them. There are four main approaches to validation. One way to validate is to *refer to an authoritative source*. For example, one might compare findings with an expert nurse clinician or a reference book to determine if the observations are concordant. The nurse may think a newborn baby has a skin infection; however, an obstetrics textbook may reveal that this is a normal characteristic of a newborn called *milia*.

Second, the nurse can determine if all other cues are *consistent*. For example, the patient may be picking at food, not sleeping well at night, and constantly looking downcast. It may be inferred that the client is depressed. However, other cues need to be checked to see if they are consistent with the picture of depression. For example, it should be determined whether the patient has recently experienced some type of loss or has a major physical problem. From the other cues it may be determined whether depression is the correct inference.

Third, the nurse can *clarify inferences* with the client. The nurse asks specific, pointed questions when validating inferences. For example, the nurse may see an elderly man sitting in his room with his food tray out of reach. The nurse may walk into the room and say, "You can't eat?" If the patient says, "No," the nurse may then offer to cut up the patient's food and move the tray closer. However, this man's real problem may be that he cannot eat because of nausea. In this case the nurse made the wrong inference because precise, pointed questions were not used.

Fourth, the nurse can *seek consensus* from the appropriate reference group. For example, the nurse may validate the inferences with other nurses in team conference or with the physical therapist or physicians. However, each of *these* individuals also may have made incorrect inferences. Therefore it is advisable to use other methods of validating an inference before seeking consensus.

Factors affecting data collection

As a nurse observes and collects data about a client, there are a variety of factors, both environmental and personal, that may influence the data collected. Awareness of these factors enhances objectivity in data collection.

One of the most important factors influencing data collection is *selective perception*. Because of our unique perceptual fields, we all see selected aspects of a situation. We may see more detail in familiar than unfamiliar situations. We also tend to see only what we know.

It is much easier to see the superficial aspects of a situation than the more covert aspects.

One also tends to remember items that conform to one's own picture of a situation. One may *stereotype* or distort what is seen because of preconceived ideas or past experiences with a situation. Error or bias may occur because of the invention of items or omission of items. Bias often occurs with random observations; stereotyping often distorts our view. Unfortunately, nurses may stereotype or label individuals. For example, a nurse who equates confusion and senility with old age may label an elderly man who is up walking at night as confused. In actuality, the man may be merely seeking the bathroom or stretching his legs.

Finally, *anxiety* may affect data collection inasmuch as it may narrow one's perceptual field. The hospital and certain areas in the community may contain unfamiliar and frightening situations. These environments may cause nurses to feel anxious and subsequently to omit or invent observations.

The nurse's *biologic, psychologic,* and *sociocultural systems* influence data collection and observation skills. Biologic examples include hunger, illness, or fatigue. The nurse who is tired may overlook significant observations.

The nurse's *mood, beliefs, needs,* or *motivation* may influence the data collected. For example, the nurse may assist the patient with activities of daily living that the patient is capable of doing independently. One inference might be that the patient likes to be dependent. It may be, however, that the nurse has a particular need to be liked or to be seen as helpful.

Numerous *sociocultural factors*, such as language, role, mores, or socioeconomic class, may influence observations. A common sociocultural factor that widely influences new practitioners is *role*. Often the beginning nurse is unsure of the parameters of the nurse role and what can and cannot be done within it. The nurse may be uncomfortable with data collection methods, such as the history, that require asking the patient questions about such things as financial situation, which may be viewed as invasion of privacy. Examining the rash on a patient's buttocks may be seen as too intrusive.

The factors discussed above may be present in the patient as well as the nurse, since a person's biologic and psychologic state does affect the way in which data collection is approached.

The client's level of understanding, ability to remember, fear, or embarrassment may be psychologic factors that influence the data that can be collected. The individual may be extremely afraid to offer information during the nurse's history or examination because of fear of hospitals. Clients may be embarrassed to offer particular information if they think it will reflect poorly on their characters. For example, a middle-aged woman from a middle-class family who fears she may have contracted tuberculosis ,may be reluctant to discuss her symptoms with the nurse. She may be embarrassed because of the stigma that was placed on having tuberculosis when she was a young child.

The client's family and culture also influence the data collected, and the nurse and client may be from very different cultural backgrounds. They may differ in terms of their language, customs, and beliefs. For example, nurses may not realize the importance to the Italian family of having numerous family members in attendance when a patient is admitted to the hospital. The family may be very important to the patient, who may not divulge necessary information without the family members being present.

Data collection roles

The extent of interaction between the nurse and clients affects the accuracy of data collected. Generally, nurses are *participant observers*. That is, the nurse participates in the daily life of clients while simultaneously collecting data. The role of participant observer has advantages and disadvantages. The *advantages* are that the nurse can validate clients' feelings with them and that people are more likely to be themselves when the observer is participating in their care. The nurse is therefore more likely to observe behavior that is characteristic of the client's usual way of behaving.

Participant observation also has *limitations*. It is more difficult to be objective when interacting with a person. The nurse may draw inferences without validating them. Being emotionally involved in the situation may also bias observations, since the nurse's feelings may affect the client's feelings and responses.

It is important to record data as soon as possible after obtaining it. Otherwise, important information may be forgotten and thus omitted. Whenever possible the data should be recorded as close to the source as possible. In certain health care facilities portions of the patient's records where nurses make entries are placed close to the patient's bedside. Thus it is not unusual for flow sheets and even nurse's notes or progress sheets to be placed outside the patient's room or at a minicharting area geographically removed from the nursing station on the division. When this is done the nurse is encouraged to record the data as soon as possible rather than waiting to do it all at the end of the shift.

Nurses can also assume the *nonparticipant observer role*. This role entails observing only, not participating. For example, nurses practicing in nursery schools or elementary schools may observe a particular age group in an unobtrusive way in order to determine stages of growth and development. In this situation the individuals being observed may or may not know that they are being observed.

There are also advantages and limitations to the nonparticipant observer role. One advantage is greater objectivity in data collection. A greater number of cues may be absorbed and more accurate data can be collected without the need to attach meaning to it. Additionally, the observations can be recorded immediately. This should improve the accuracy and validity of the data, since the nurse is performing only one role and thus can concentrate all energies on that role.

A limitation of the nonparticipant observer role is that the nurse is unable to clarify and validate with the individuals being observed. Therefore the nurse cannot investigate the subjective feelings of those observed. The nurse's mere presence in the environment may also influence the behavior of those being observed. For example, the children in the nursery school may behave quite differently when a stranger is present. Therefore data collected may not represent their usual behavior. Finally, because nurses are accustomed to being participants many find the nonparticipant observer role difficult to tolerate.

Data resources

Nurses have begun to expand their data collection methods. The are becoming more sophisticated not only in using themselves but also in using a variety of assessment instruments. The nurse has numerous resources available for the assessment process.

Self

One use of self is in the use of the five senses as a means of data collection. *Sight* is probably the sense that most nurses learn to use first. Using sight to make observations is called *inspection*. Sight is also involved in the use of equipment such as the otoscope and the ophthalmoscope. *Hearing* is employed in listening to patients when they express feelings and when they talk with other persons, such as family members. Environmental noises that nurses hear may be disturbing to patients, and they are often pleased to learn that others are aware of these noises and might be able to do something about them. Another use of hearing is in *auscultation* of sounds through the stethoscope. *Touch* is frequently used to collect data, as in *palpation* in which an area is felt to determine whether body parts are of normal size, contour, and texture. *Percussion* may be used to distinguish the relative density of tissues. Although the sense of *taste* is seldom used, the sense of *smell* can be used to detect fetid wounds or the fruity breath of a person with ketoacidosis.

Various *mechanical instruments* are used by the nurse to expand the scope of data collection and to per-

TABLE 8-1. Types of data obtained with assessment instruments

Instrument	Data obtained
Sphygmomanometer (blood pressure cuff)	Status of respiratory, cardiovascular, and renal systems; psychologic state
Thermometer	Body temperature
Tape measure	Girth of body parts such as abdomen, leg
Light source	Constriction of pupils in response to light; status of oral cavity (e.g., inflamed or obstructed)
Reflex hammer	Presence of and degree of reactivity of reflexes
Oroscope	Status of eardrum and ear canal
Ophthalmoscope	Status of retina (e.g., variations in veins and arteries)
Chemically treated papers or reagent tablets	Presence of chemical substances in blood, urine, stool, and other body fluids (e.g., Clinitest indicates level of glucose in urine)

mit greater accuracy of observations. These instruments and the types of data they are used to obtain are listed in Table 8-1.

Client's family

Another important data source is the client's family. The client is considered a member of the family system, and what affects one part of the family affects all parts. It is often essential to collect information from family members regarding their response to the client's illness. Family members are vital when working with clients who are unable to communicate effectively, such as children or adults who are unable to communicate either because of age or physical impairment.

The nurse may also find that the client and family members do not have the same perceptions, since a question asked of both elicits different information. The family's perception of how the client's life-style may have changed because of an alteration in health may be quite different from that of the client. In addition, family members are often helpful in giving the nurse insight about the client's past behavior and current level of coping with the health alteration

Other resources

The patient's past and present *medical records* often contain data that are helpful in assessment. The nurse uses data from the medical history and other health care workers' notes rather than subjecting the patient to repeated questioning on the same topic.

The physician can provide data about the patient's health alteration and assist the nurse with predicting other potential or existing problems. The beginning nursing student is often somewhat hesitant to contact the physician and collect information. Often this occurs because of preconceived ideas about physicians and perhaps the aloof reception the student expects to receive from them. However, most nursing students find that physicians will respond positively to requests for assistance made of them.

Other health care workers have a wealth of useful information. Nurses who have worked with the client in the past or are currently working with the client are most likely to have relevant information that can add to or clarify the nurse's assessment. In addition, the physical therapist, social worker, respiratory therapist, dietitian, chaplain, and many other health care workers can provide information about the client from the perspective of their own disciplines.

Some hospitals record patient histories in a computer as the patient responds to a series of questions (Fig. 8-1). The patient's answers are stored in the computer, and the nurse or other health care providers can retrieve the data from the computer anytime they need particular information. It is predicted that computers will be used more and more in the future for storage of vital client information, and for this reason nurses can expect to be more involved in using them.

The literature (books, journals, monographs) is a vital source of information. Data can be obtained here to explain or validate information collected from the patient.

Subjective data collection: assessment interview or history

Data collected are both subjective and objective. Subjective data are reported by the client but are not directly observable. Objective data are those items of information that can be gathered by a second party, in this case the nurse. Subjective data are obtained through the *nursing history*, while objective data are obtained by *physical examination* of the client.

In order for a nursing history to be complete and comprehensive it must be well organized and used systematically. The history contains a series of questions designed to obtain information needed to plan nursing care. Questions are asked about the client's present functional abilities and how these compare with previous ability to function. In addition, questions may be asked about how the functions have been impaired[37,69,70] and what *adaptive processes* the client is using to cope with alterations in health. The client should also be asked about *self-perception* of present health status and what effect this has on personal life-style.

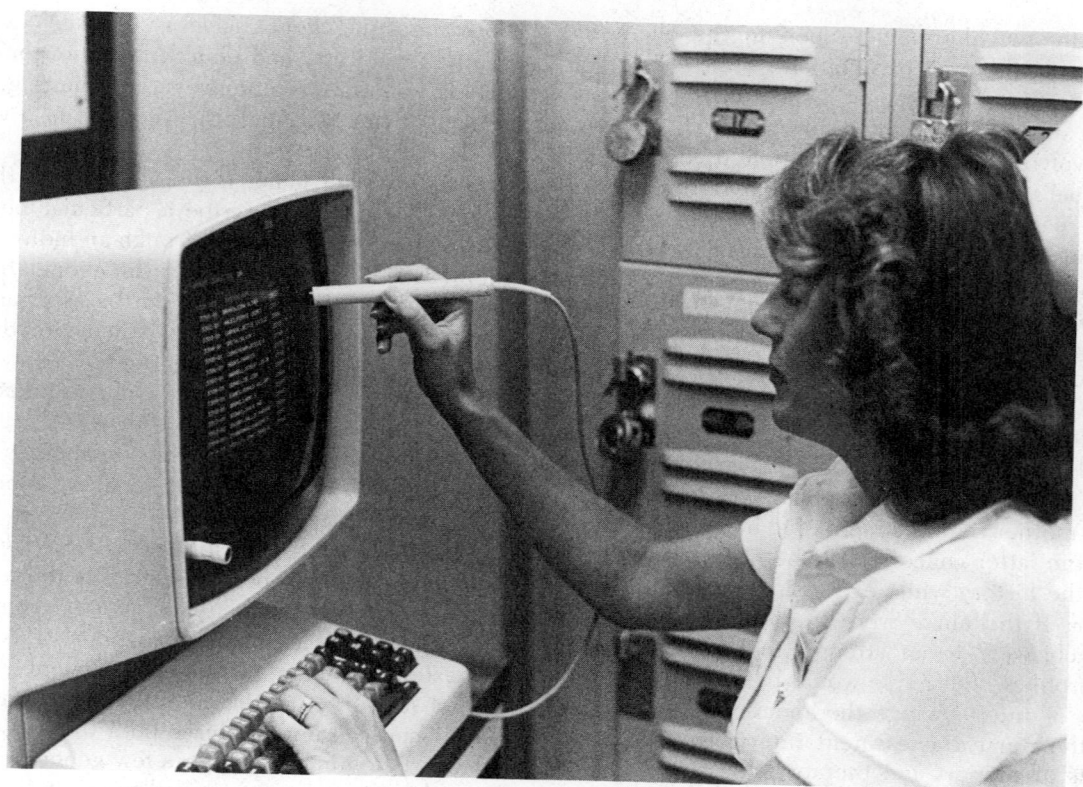

Fig. 8-1. Nurses have access to vast data resource by means of computer.

In summary, the purpose of the nursing history is to obtain data as a basis for determining potential or existing nursing care requirements or client problems, which in turn will guide nursing actions. The nursing history also provides data that enable nurses to personalize care based on the individual's values, life-style, and patterns of living. Thus nurses acquire a unique data base that focuses on the total person and that person's health maintenance.

For example, a nurse may ask questions about the patient's syncope and its frequency, precipitating factors, and time of occurrence. Because the nurse realizes the safety factors necessitated by fainting, the questions determine what changes in the patient's environment need to be made. On the other hand, the physician may also inquire about the syncope but for a different purpose. A diagnosis may be sought about a mitral valve problem with syncope recognized as a symptom.

The type and level of information collected by the nurse depend on numerous factors. The nurse's educational preparation and years of experience will affect the kind of information sought. Other factors influencing the content of the history are the nurse's and employing agency's philosophy about nursing and the nurse's level of practice. If nurses view their practice as fairly autonomous, their data base will emphasize information related to the independent aspects of practice. The clients who are the recipients of health care also dictate the content of the history. For example, an elderly person would be asked different questions than a 5-year-old. Each history should contain questions appropriate to the client's bio-psycho-sociocultural systems and life experience.

Interviewing

Interviewing is a method used to collect information for the history. It is purposeful communication that focuses on specific content. The assessment interview usually occurs early in the nurse-client relationship; therefore the nurse needs to begin to establish a trust relationship with the client and set mutually agreed on goals from the beginning. The process of establishing a relationship with a client is vital to the nursing process (see Chapter 9 for explanation of the process).

Functions of an interview may be to:
1. Assess the client's bio-psycho-sociocultural status and needs
2. Understand the (client's) perceptions of self and others
3. Gain information about teaching needs
4. Assist the client to identify needs, conflicts, or problems
5. Review with the client usual coping mechanisms

6. Identify the alternatives open to the client in managing the present situation.

Assessment interviewing or history taking encompasses each of these functions. However, the primary purpose involves gathering information to determine the individual's bio-psycho-sociocultural status and to identify the patient's unique perception of the present situation and coping mechanisms. Because the subjective data (history) is often obtained in situations where the client is actively seeking help in coping with a problem, he or she may be anxious to have these problems solved. Also, there may be other factors that are affecting coping. For example, a woman may come to a clinic seeking additional treatment to control the pain of rheumatoid arthritis when in reality her major problem is inability to observe rest periods as ordered because her invalid mother requires increasing hours of physical care. It is the latter concern that the client may dwell on during the history while expressing frustration with her mother. If the nurse were to concentrate on this concern exclusively in an attempt to help the client solve the problem, the nurse would be engaging in another type of interviewing, therapeutic interviewing. Although the nurse's assessment interview may have components of support and therapy, the *primary emphasis* of assessment interviewing is to collect data about the patient's current health status. Therapeutic counseling may be offered after the assessment is completed and goals are established for the nurse and client to work together. During the history the nurse needs to acknowledge the patient's concerns and indicate a willingness to discuss them later. In the above example the nurse could acknowledge the individual's concern about her mother and later discuss ways the patient might receive help in caring for her mother. In other words, the nurse needs to keep in mind the primary purpose of the assessment interview while at the same time noting the patient's plea for help.

Guidelines for interviewing. In preparing for the interview the nurse may wish to review mentally the purposes of the interview and the approach to be taken, thus internalizing the *role of interviewer*. The client needs to have a simple explanation of the purpose of the interview and how the nurse will use the information obtained.

The following principles may be used as guidelines for the interview.

1. *Content to be explored is clearly delineated and systematically outlined in advance.* The nurse decides whether the data can be collected best through direct or indirect means. For example, the client may be asked directly, "Does your stomach burn after ingesting spicy foods?" This is an example of a *closed* question requiring little elaboration other than yes or no. Content in the history that is noncontroversial or not open to interpretation can be sought by this method. Ques-

tions about the client's social system such as number of children, address, and church affiliation or items pertaining to certain symptoms such as fainting, headache, or nausea can be appropriately asked in a very direct, or closed, manner.

On the other hand, if the nurse wants the client to express feelings or describe a particular behavior, the information is best sought through an indirect, or *open*, method, since is may uncover the client's true feelings and perceptions, which may not be ascertained by the direct method. If the client is asked directly, "Do you resent your wife's lack of attention?" he may respond in the negative. However, if the client is asked, "Tell me about your relationship with your wife," it is hoped he will express some of the negative feelings as he tells the story. A series of indirect statements may be needed in order to elicit feelings.

2. *Interviewing is facilitated by establishing rapport with the client.* Rapport implies that there are mutual feelings of comfort, confidence, and harmony. A variety of modes can be used to foster rapport. First, the nurse can extend common courtesy to the client. An introduction of self, greeting the client by name, and extending one's hand can initially place both the nurse and client at ease. The nurse can offer a few general comments to help the client be recognized as an individual. Comments on the client's pictures or flowers or even comments about the weather can be phrased to relax both individuals.

3. *The purpose of the interview and examination is clarified with the client.* If clients understand how the obtained data are relevant to care, they are more apt to cooperate. The client may not have previously experienced a nurse asking numerous questions. Therefore the client needs to be informed that the questions are asked in order to provide the best nursing care. It might also be noted that the questions will determine not only health-related difficulties the client is experiencing but also ways to keep the client as healthy as possible. The nurse informs the client that if any aspect of the question is not understood, the nurse will be pleased to clarify the point. The nurse may inquire as to the client's thoughts about notes being taken during the interview. Notes are helpful to the nurse, as specific facts can be recorded immediately and are less biased than on later recall. Most clients will not object to the nurse taking notes as reminders of the content. Taking notes in view of the client helps keep the atmosphere open.

4. *"The climate the nurse creates influences the substance of the interviews."*[63] Climate refers to the immediate conditions, both physical and psychologic, that surround an individual. One component of a climate conducive to effective interviewing is appropriate timing. The initial history is usually taken soon after admission or contact with a health facility. However, the

acuteness of the client's state will affect the timing and type of interview obtained. For example, a nurse would not obtain a lengthy initial history from someone with a ruptured appendix when immediate care is essential.

The length of time needed to complete the history and examination should be communicated to the client. The length of time needed to complete the data collection will depend on a variety of factors, such as the nurse's skill, amount and complexity of assessment, the content covered, and the client's willingness to converse and participate. In any case the nurse allows sufficient uninterrupted time that is as anxiety free as possible for the client. For example, the busy preoperative morning would not be an effective time for an assessment interview.

A comfortable climate is facilitated by creating environmental privacy. Closing the client's door or pulling the curtains between beds will help the interviewer and client feel more at ease. Environmental noise should be kept at a minimum. The nurse may also ask that the client's family leave for certain segments of the history and examination. Frequently, beginning nurses who feel somewhat unsure of their roles will hesitate to ask the family to step out of the room while they proceed. However, families are excellent data resources and can often validate or refute baseline information collected by the nurse *after* the interview has concluded.

Physical comfort of both nurse and client contributes to a positive climate. The nurse can assist the client to the bathroom, have water available, or adjust the bed pillows. The nurse will find that sitting in a chair facing the client will facilitate comfort of both nurse and client (Fig. 8-2). As the chair is placed for the interview, the nurse is aware of the personal space surrounding individuals. Various cultures proscribe different meanings to space surrounding the body. An individual from the Middle East may feel quite comfortable speaking with a stranger at a distance of 6 to 18 inches, whereas an American would consider that improperly close.[67] The nurse observes these distances as the interview proceeds. This is not to say that touch should not be utilized. To the contrary, a touch of the hand can be quite effective in an interview to relay warmth and concern for a client.

5. *The interview is initiated with those topics that are the least threatening to the patient and easiest to discuss.* Questioning that moves from the least personal to the most personal items helps to gain the patient's confidence and cooperation. For example, the nurse might be more effective if the beginning question refers to the patient's occupation rather than bowel habits.

6. *Questions should be brief and limited to a single idea.* Only one question should be asked at a time. If questions are too lengthy the patient may become confused and stop listening. The client may be unsure of the relevant data on which to concentrate. Also, if more than one question is asked the patient will be unsure of which is to be answered.

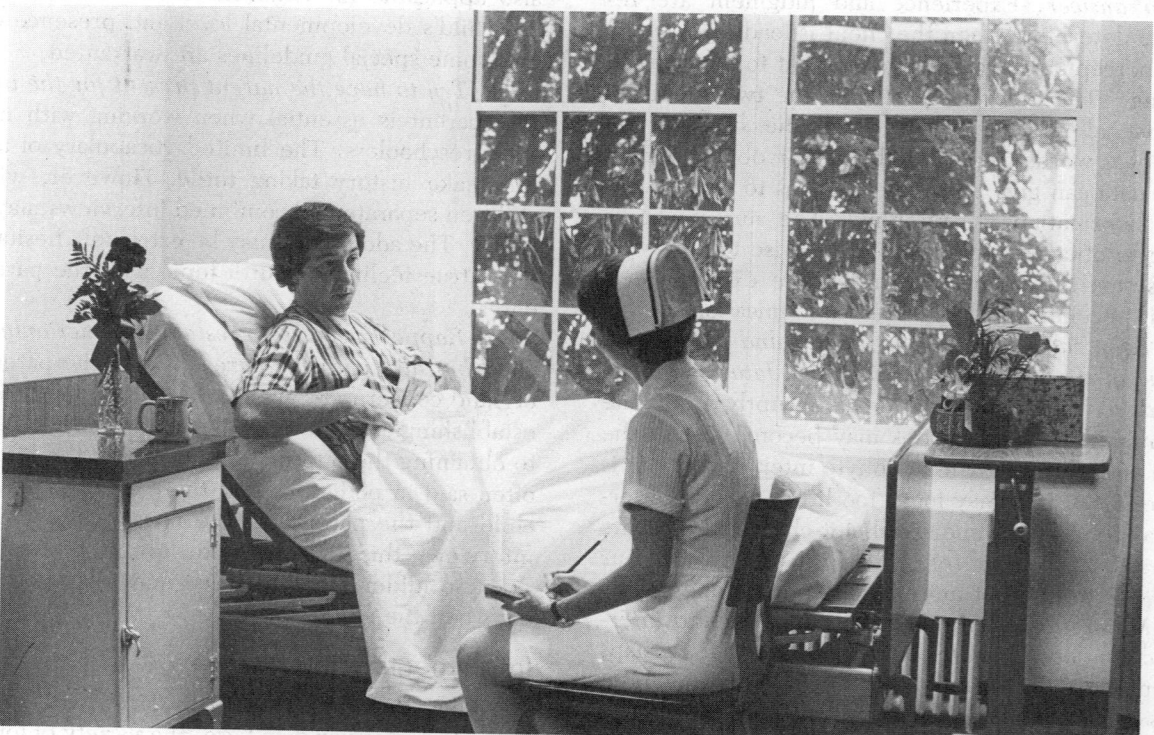

Fig. 8-2. Sitting in chair facing client enhances comfort of both during history taking.

7. *Leading questions should be avoided.* A leading question may place the client in an uncomfortable position and squelch spontaneity. For example, a question such as, "Do you still smoke?" places the client in a double bind in which either a yes or no answer fails to convey that the client never did smoke.

8. *Language used should be understood by the client.* Clients may be too embarrassed to admit they do not understand the words used by the nurse and may give inaccurate information. Medical terminology is a type of jargon that can be quite confusing to the lay person. A man may not comprehend that "up ad lib" means he can be up walking at his liberty. After beginning the interview the nurse will be able to determine major language patterns of the client, noting if the language needs to be simple and concrete or if more complex ideas can be utilized.

Not only does the nurse need to communicate clearly to the client, but the language used by the client needs to be clarified and clearly understood by the nurse. Often words used by clients are quite descriptive or are a play on words, yet may be unfamiliar terms to the nurse. For example, the following terms have been used by clients: "cascading" for vomiting, "avalanche" for ambulance, "falling out" for fainting, "fireballs in the universe" for fibroids of the uterus. (See Robert Whalen's article "Medical Malaprops"[75] for an interesting and humorous history and play on words as told by the client and interpreted by the physician.)

9. *Allow an appropriate amount of time for the client to answer.* Experience and judgment are required to determine when the client is leading into discussing perceptions and feelings relevant to the care vs. "rambling." The difference between the two is subtle. The nurse allows the client to tell the story in the client's own words; repeated themes or obvious omissions of data can give the nurse clues as to what is important information vs. rambling. The nurse who is learning to obtain histories would be wise to allow too great vs. too little rambling until more experience is gained in recognizing themes of communication.

10. *Keep the interview purposeful and focused on the topic of discussion until necessary data have been obtained.* If the interview moves abruptly from one topic to another, both parties may become lost in the maze of conversation. The neophyte interviewer who is insecure in the role may focus too little, and the interview may tend to become social chit-chat. If this occurs the nurse may refocus (e.g., "Before we discuss your job, I'd like to find out more about your dizziness.").

11. *Maintain momentum and move to the next interview section once the data have been obtained.* Perhaps the client has expressed all he or she possibly can about feelings about a job loss. The nurse may lose the client's interest and cooperation if the point is belabored.

12. *Specific answers should be obtained.* Words such as "good," "sometimes," and "regular" have many different interpretations; therefore clarification is sought. Do regular dental checkups mean once or twice a year or every 3 years?

13. *Transitional comments are made when moving from one section of the interview to the next.*[6] This helps the history flow smoothly rather than jumping from one part to another. The patient will also realize that it is time to move to a new topic. For example, the nurse may say, "I have all the information I need about your daily activities. Could we move on to discuss your employment?"

14. *At the end of the history the nurse states that the information needed to plan care has been obtained.*[6] A courteous manner will help the client feel a sense of cooperation in volunteering the needed information. The nurse might say, "Thank you for giving the information I need to plan your care more effectively."

15. *Before leaving the patient the nurse should summarize the major ideas offered by the patient and inform him or her when contact will be made.* The nurse may state, "It sounds like you have most trouble with shortness of breath and decreased physical activity. I will talk with the other nurses about helping you with this. Also, I will be back at 7:00 AM tomorrow and will help you with your care then." This will help the patient clarify any misconceptions gained by the nurse. Also the patient will know when to expect the nurse again.

SPECIAL GUIDELINES FOR INTERVIEWING CHILDREN. For the most part the guidelines previously listed are also applicable for children. However, depending on the child's developmental level and presence of a parent, some special guidelines are warranted.

1. *Try to have the parent present for the interview.* The parent is essential when working with newborns and preschoolers. The limited vocabulary of a toddler can make history taking futile. However, with older children separate and combined interviews may be necessary. The adolescent may be extremely hesitant to express true feelings about a topic with the parent present.

2. *Rapport needs to be established not only with the child but also with the parent.* Often the parent's anxiety and concern are greater than the child's. Therefore establishing a warm, trusting relationship is paramount to obtaining the information needed in the history. It is often said in pediatrics that there are two patients, the child and the parent. As the nurse proceeds with the interview, this phrase needs to be remembered. A quiet, confident tone of voice may allay both the parent's and the child's anxiety.

Implementing the interview

When the nurse is actually faced with obtaining a patient's history or data base, the variety of forms available in texts and articles may be overwhelming. The educational preparation of the nurse, the setting, the psychophysical condition, and the developmental level of the patient influence the type of information collected.

Two basic types of history forms for the data base are found in the literature: the structured and the semistructured. The *structured* format may consist of a *questionnaire* that the patient fills out on entry into the health care system. This format will save the nurse time but allows for little free expression by the patient. However, this format may yield more complete data than an unstructured interview administered by the nurse. The structured format may also be initiated by the nurse and may consist of a list of specific questions related to various bio-psycho-sociocultural, systems where the nurse directly records answers, or client's responses may be typed into a teletypewriter to allow for computerizing the information. In a study comparing the use of a self-completed questionnaire with unstructured interviews conducted by nurses, the nurses made significantly more errors of omission than the patient.[4]

A structured interview may also list *specific topics* about each patient's system. The nurse then decides how to phrase the particular question. This method allows for more individuality in the interview yet assures that certain topics will be covered (see reference 69 for examples).

The other main type of interview method is the *semistructured* interview. Here the nurse will investigate *broad* categories of data. The questions to be asked may be open or closed and are developed by the nurse in the process of interviewing. The nurse may record a few brief notes but usually writes up the data *after* the interview. The main difficulty with this approach is that it is time consuming. It does allow for free expression of the client's feelings but may not be conducive to obtaining specific, precise data necessary for valid inferences. Research has elicited that the structured interview yielded significantly more data than the unstructured and took half the time.[46]

The box in the next column describes data to be collected under one system (gastrointestinal-nutritional habits) and may serve to clarify the differences between the methods of structured (questionnaire and topics) and semistructured data collection.

Systems framework for assessment

As stated in the previous section, the data base, or history, may be collected in a structured or semistructured manner. The important point is to make sure the data are collected in a comprehensive and organized fashion. The approach used in this chapter seeks to obtain objective and subjective data by means of a nurse-initiated, semistructured, bio-psycho-sociocultural systems format. For our purposes the individual is seen as

Structured—questionnaire

1. How many meals do you eat each day?
2. What do you typically eat for breakfast? Lunch? Dinner? Snacks?
3. What foods do you like?
4. What foods do you dislike?
5. How many glasses of fluid do you drink each day?

Structured—topics

1. Number of meals and snacks
2. Amount of basic four food groups daily
3. Amount of daily fluid intake
4. Likes
5. Dislikes

Semistructured

Nutritional habits, food-fluid intake

a system with subsystems or suprasystems (Fig. 8-3, *top row*). However, components other than the individual may be identified as the system, thus shifting the definitions of corresponding subsystems and suprasystems (Fig. 8-3, *middle row*). For example, if the organ system is identified as the system of interest, the individual and higher systems on the continuum become the suprasystems.

Fig. 8-3, *bottom row*, illustrates the subsystems of the individual's bio-psycho-sociocultural systems and where each falls along the continuum. The biologic systems are largely related to organ systems, organs, and cells. The psychologic systems (cognitive and emotional) are related to the individual. The social systems relate to the individual, family, community, and society. Subsystems can be noted in each bio-psycho-sociocultural system. For example, "respiratory" is listed under organ system and biologic systems, whereas "work" is part of community and social system. The placement of these subsystems is somewhat arbitrary since several items involve numerous levels of the individual. For example, sexual development is listed under the individual system and the psychosystem. However, there are certainly biologic and social components of sexual development.

When the nurse utilizes the systems approach, the concept of the individual as an open system needs to be uppermost in the mind. As the nurse collects data within the bio-, psycho-, or social systems, it is assumed that these areas are not isolated but affect and are affected by other named subsystems or suprasystems. The reader will note that the vertical lines between the systems in Fig. 8-3 are dotted and not solid,

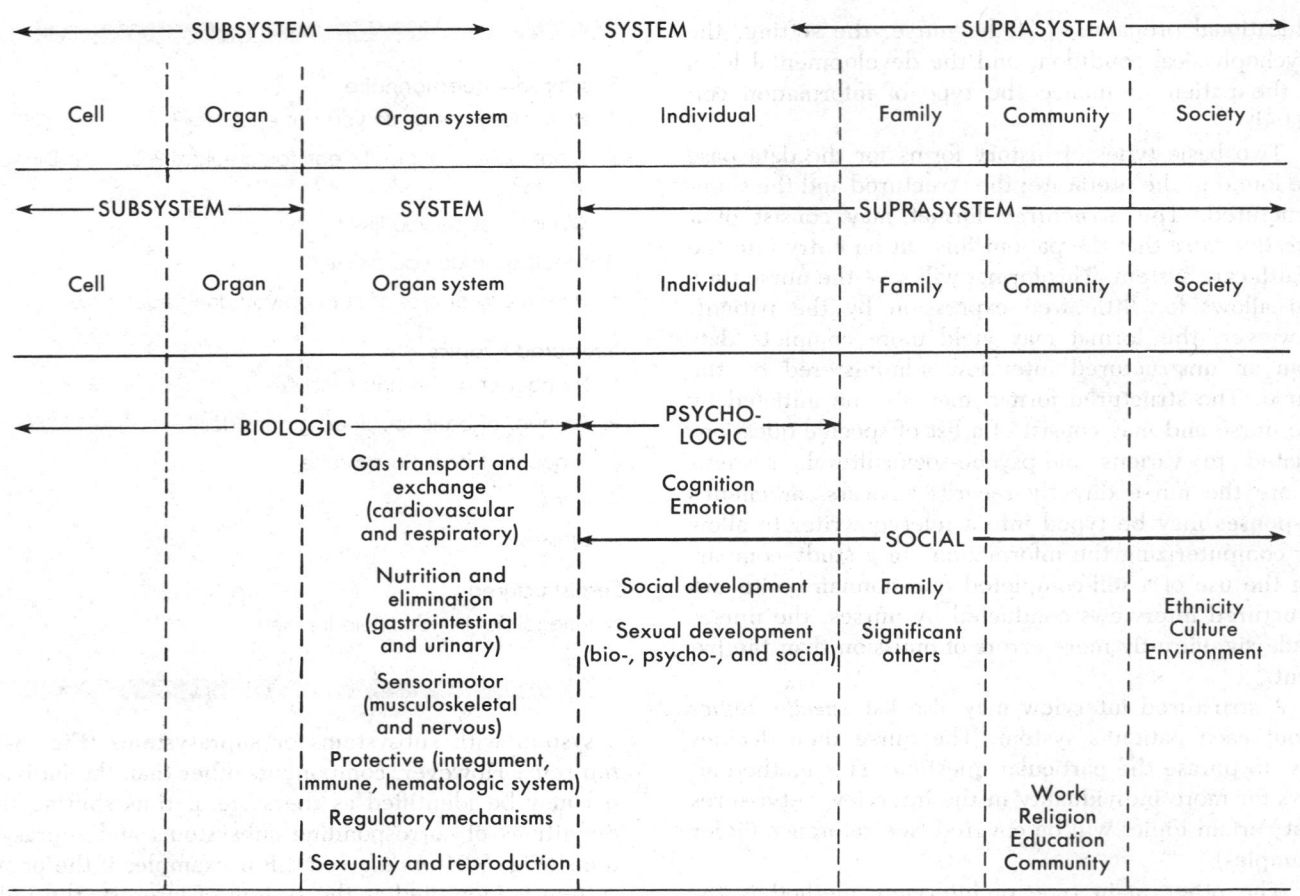

Fig. 8-3. Systems framework for assessment. *Top row,* focal system as individual. *Middle,* focal system as organ system. *Bottom,* individual with corresponding bio-psycho-social subsystems. (Adapted from Byrne, M.L., and Thompson, L.F.: Key concepts for the study and practice of nursing, ed. 2, St. Louis, 1978, The C.V. Mosby Co.)

denoting a constant exchange between systems. As the nurse explores one system, decisions need to be made about which other suprasystems or subsystems also need to be explored. For example, the nurse gathering data about the gastrointestinal system of a patient not only inquires about and examines the biologic system of anatomic organs from the mouth to the stomach to the rectum but also collects data about food intake, a phenomenon largely influenced by the social system, that is, social development, religion, work-economics, and culture.

Using the systems approach, specific topics for a structured interview have been listed for each subsystem of biologic, psychologic, and social systems. Although the format may look overwhelming at first glance, it can be modified to fit the setting, particular client, and experience of the nurse. Since what affects one system affects all systems, data for each of the subsystems need to be collected to prevent missing important information.

A health history is outlined in the box on pp. 99-101. If the data collected via the health history reveals

a dysfunction, further investigation would need to occur within the subsystem. For example, a patient may state that he or she has chronic bronchitis, experiences shortness of breath after walking 100 feet, and coughs up 2 tablespoons of mucus each morning. The nurse may then need to inquire about other data not listed here, such as factors affecting breathing, such as emotion, pollution, and position. Also, during the examination the color of nails and skin and sputum characteristics are noted.

Practice improves the nurse's ability to determine which subsystems require greater investigation with particular clients. Certain health needs may require depth in particular areas of assessment. For example, an elderly individual on bed rest would warrant particular inquiry about the integumentary system to check for dryness, areas of redness, and lesions. In contrast, a young child entering a clinic for a well-child examination would most likely not require as great an inquiry into the same system. The integument of the child might be noted for cleanliness and lesions and little else.

HEALTH HISTORY: A SUBJECTIVE DATA BASE

I. Chief complaint of client
   A. Location
   B. Character
   C. Chronology
   D. Circumstances of occurrence
   E. Aggravating or alleviating factors
   F. Associated complaints
   G. Previous attempts at therapy and their effectiveness
   H. Disability resulting from this complaint
II. Social systems
   A. Social development
      1. Age
      2. Sex
      3. Developmental tasks
      4. Psychosocial personality development (Erickson's eight stages of man)
      5. Diversional, recreational interests (what to do to pass time while ill)
      6. Roles in family, community, work, and perceived performance of them
      7. Child's favorite play activity
      8. Socially oriented habits (include alcohol, drugs), frequency of use, and response to use
   B. Family or significant others
      1. Others in living group
      2. Significant others outside living group
      3. Visiting preferences and who is able to visit
      4. Marital status
      5. Alterations for family's life-style because of ill member
      6. Interaction patterns (observe this also)
      7. History of disease in other family members, especially those diseases with familial tendency
   C. Work
      1. Occupation
      2. Source of income
      3. Insurance (hospitalization)
      4. Changes in work pattern because of illness
      5. Feelings about work and being away from productivity and routine
   D. Religion
      1. Religious affiliation
      2. Desire for chaplain visit
      3. Practices or beliefs that might affect reaction to health care (proscriptions against immunization or blood transfusions, dietary laws, beliefs about disease causation and death)
   E. Education
      1. Formal education
      2. Satisfaction and progress with school
   F. Community
      1. Type of housing
      2. Contacts or previous referrals to social agencies
      3. Availability and pattern of utilization of health care facilities (physician, dentist); frequency and reason for visits
      4. Immunizations (type, date)
   G. Ethnic-cultural system
      1. Factors that may influence reaction to hospitalization, therapy, illness
      2. Food preferences
      3. Response to stress (e.g., pain)
   H. Environment
      1. Effect of present environment on health status and developmental level (e.g., lighting, noise, activity—variation, consistency, excessive or absent)
      2. Arrangement of environment in relation to functional abilities or disabilities
      3. Safety factors
         a. Mobility (arrangement of objects in physical environment)
         b. Use of prosthetic or supportive devices (e.g., crutches, wheelchair)
      4. Infection control
         a. Ready sources of infection
         b. Barriers to infection (isolation technique, handwashing facility)
III. Psychologic systems
   A. Cognition
      1. Level of consciousness (response to sensory stimuli)
      2. Orientation to time, place, person
      3. Mental skills
         a. Ability to read and write
         b. Vocabulary
         c. Ability to comprehend and follow directions
         d. Attention and memory span
      4. Intellectual development relative to chronologic age (e.g., Piaget's formulation)
      5. Understanding of and reaction to health concerns and goals of medical-nursing therapy
      6. Desired information about present tests and treatment
      7. Previous experiences with and reactions to past illnesses and hospitalizations
      8. Name child or adolescent prefers
   B. Emotion
      1. Quality of mood, expression, intensity of reaction
      2. Activity level (active, sluggish, hyperactive)
      3. Effect of illness on life-style and expectation of future effects
      4. Feelings about hospitalization
      5. Coping patterns in stressful situations (describe stressful situations); availability, need for, and effectiveness of internal-external support systems
      6. Special concerns or fears
      7. Patterns of relating to others (e.g., verbal, congenial)
      8. Self-concept (body image before and in relation to current health problem)
      9. Any nervous breakdown
      10. Comfort, rest, and sleep patterns (hours, time, nap periods, feeling of being rested) before and since illness
      11. Aids used to sleep

Include laboratory data (complete blood count, electrolytes, urinalysis, cultures, other relevant values) under appropriate system.

Continued.

HEALTH HISTORY: A SUBJECTIVE DATA BASE—cont'd

12. Presence of pain or discomfort (location, duration, degree, character, precipitating factors, change in pattern)
13. Use of aids to relieve pain

IV. Biologic systems
  A. General
    1. Fatigue
    2. Fever
    3. Weakness
    4. Activity tolerance
    5. Usual weight, recent weight change
  B. Gas transport and exchange
    1. Cardiovascular
      a. Past or present disease of cardiovascular system
      b. Syncope
      c. Dizziness
      d. Chest pain
        (1) Type
        (2) Pattern
        (3) Precipitating factors
        (4) Relief measures
      e. Edematous body parts
      f. Palpitations
      g. Orthopnea
      h. Medications taken to affect cardiovascular system
    2. Respiratory
      a. Past or present diseases of respiratory system
      b. Cough
        (1) Frequency
        (2) Duration
      c. Sputum
        (1) Color
        (2) Odor
        (3) Amount
      d. Shortness of breath
        (1) Precipitating factors
        (2) Frequency
        (3) Effect on activity
      e. Smoking
        (1) Pack-year history
        (2) Attempts and success at stopping
      f. Hemoptysis
      g. Frequency of colds and sore throats
      h. Medications taken to affect respiratory system
  C. Nutrition and elimination
    1. Gastrointestinal
      a. Past or present disease of gastrointestinal system
      b. Dietary habits
        (1) Amount of basic four food groups
        (2) Likes
        (3) Dislikes
        (4) Number of meals and snacks
        (5) Time of meals
        (6) Assistance needed with eating
      c. Appetite, thirst

    d. Factors related to ingestion
      (1) Nonoral intake
      (2) Chewing
      (3) Swallowing
      (4) Oral hygiene habits
    e. Factors related to digestion
      (1) Ease
      (2) Nausea
      (3) Vomiting
      (4) Belching
      (5) Pain in abdomen
    f. Bowel elimination pattern
      (1) Time and frequency of bowel movements
      (2) Degree of child's independence in toileting
      (3) Words used by child regarding elimination
      (4) Character of stools
      (5) Ease (constipation, diarrhea)
      (6) Hemorrhoids
      (7) Passage of flatus, blood
    g. Medicines taken to alter digestion and metabolism of foods
  2. Urinary
    a. Past or present diseases of urinary system
    b. Fluid intake
    c. Urination pattern
      (1) Amount
      (2) Color
      (3) Odor
      (4) Frequency, night or day urgency
      (5) Dysuria, hematuria
    d. Vaginal or urethral discharge
    e. Degree of independence in toileting
    f. Medications taken to alter urinary system
  D. Sensorimotor
    1. Musculoskeletal
      a. Past or present disease of musculoskeletal system
      b. Abnormal innervation to muscles (paralysis, weakness, spasticity)
      c. Method of ambulation
        (1) Assistance needed with dressing, hygiene
        (2) Safety measures needed
      d. Range of motion limitations
      e. Medicines taken to affect musculoskeletal system
    2. Nervous
      a. Past or present diseases of nervous system
      b. Visual status
        (1) Acuity
        (2) Deficits and corrective devices
      c. Auditory status
        (1) Deficits and corrective devices
        (2) Unusual sensations (ringing, buzzing, vertigo, pain)
      d. Olfactory status
      e. Gustatory status

HEALTH HISTORY: A SUBJECTIVE DATA BASE—cont'd

    f. Tactile status (ability to discriminate sharp-dull, light-firm, hot-cold sensations)

    g. Paresthesias

    h. Mobility (coordination, balance)

    i. Medicines taken to affect nervous system

E. Protective mechanisms

  1. Integument

    a. Past or present diseases of integumentary system

    b. Factors predisposing to skin breakdown

    c. Personal hygiene

      (1) Bathing (kind, type, frequency)

      (2) Frequency, time of shaving

      (3) After-bath skin care

    d. Medicines taken to affect integumentary system

  2. Immune mechanism

    a. Past or present allergy

    b. Past or present sensitivities to drugs or other agents (pollens, insect bites)

    c. Past or present high susceptibility to infection

  3. Hematologic

    a. Easy bruiseability

    b. Swelling in neck or groin

    c. Past transfusions

F. Endocrine mechanisms

  1. Abnormal function of endocrine gland or glands and effects; past or present diseases

  2. Growth patterns

  3. Heat or cold intolerance

  4. Excessive thirst, hunger, or urination

  5. Medicines taken to affect endocrine system

G. Sexuality and reproduction

  1. Past or present alterations of reproduction system

  2. Reproductive data

    a. Number of pregnancies

    b. Live births

    c. Living children

    d. Family planning (method used)

    e. Menstrual pattern

    f. Menopause (age of onset and associated factors)

  3. Breast self-examination routine

  4. Frequency of Pap smears

  5. Sexual desire and function

  6. Level of sexual development

  7. Attitudes toward own sexuality

  8. Medicines taken to affect reproductive system

Beginning the interview

As with other aspects of the assessment process, the setting and condition of the client will influence how the interview is begun. The nurse should utilize a specific tool rather than rely on intuition.

The nurse can begin with an open-ended, fairly nondirective statement such as "What brings you to the health care setting?" This is also known as the *chief complaint*. The complaints reflect the patient's subjective perception of the situation. The chief complaint should be noted in a brief statement that includes limited symptoms and their duration.

Within this context the patient should be encouraged to elaborate on the specific symptom, duration, and chronologic history of the problem or a history of present illness. Specific data to investigate about the symptom would include the following:

1. Location in the body and extension to other body parts

2. Character, both quality and quantity (what is it like and how severe is it?)

3. Time chronology (when did it begin and what course has it followed?)

4. Circumstances of occurrence

5. Aggravating or alleviating factors (what makes it better or worse?)

6. Associated complaints

7. Previous clinicians consulted and effects of prescribed therapies

8. Disability rendered by the chief complaint

Many of the above items are asked by the physician. The nurse may also wish to inquire about the details of the patient's main concern, as the version told to the nurse is often quite different from that told to the physician. For example, the patient's chief complaint may be "increasing shortness of breath over the past 6 weeks." The nurse may determine from the patient's elaboration on the shortness of breath a concern about inability to socialize with friends. The nurse may capitalize on this issue and center interventions around increasing the patient's social network. On the other hand, the physician would delve into determining the cause of the breathing difficulty.

If the nurse obtains the history several days after the admission, it should be remembered that what brought the patient to the hospital and the current chief complaint may be different. To illustrate, the patient may have entered the hospital with a complaint of "a red, swollen, painful left lower leg," which was diagnosed as thrombophlebitis. The nurse needs to collect data about this problem but also note that the patient may think of the current main problem as the "bad food."

After inquiry is made into the chief complaint, data about the individual's *social system* are obtained. As noted in the health history, the categories of data are not extremely personal. Information about family, work, and so forth gives one a picture of the patient's suprasystems and allows the patient to be seen in another role, as a person. Often this section of the history facilitates the development of rapport with the patient. Another term for this part of the history is the *patient profile*.

Next the nurse can inquire about data listed under the *psychologic systems*. Direct, open-ended questions are asked about some of the categories; for example, "What feelings do you have about this hospitalization?" However, much of the data about the cognitive and emotional systems, such as mood and attention span, will surface indirectly through the course of questioning in the other systems or during the physical appraisal. Often much of the data in this section are not gained by direct questioning.

The final subjective data to be collected relate to the *biologic systems*. This section is also called the *review of systems*. As one develops skill in the assessment process, parts of the biologic systems history may be done during the physical appraisal. For example, the patient's pharynx may appear erythematous on examination. At that point the nurse may inquire about soreness and difficulty in swallowing. With practice the nurse can determine what questions are effectively asked before and during the physical appraisal.

It is important to note that with increased knowledge and practice the nurse will improve the ability to recognize patients' significant behavior cues. The questioning will also become more precise in areas related to those behavioral cues.

Subjective data collection (history) does not occur only in the initial encounter with the patient but is ongoing. Initially questions are asked to gather information to plan care. In ongoing assessment, questions are asked in those areas where deficits were initially identified, such as a problem with diet. Often as nursing care is given, the patient may develop new complaints. Subsequently, relevant areas within the *subsystem* and *suprasystem* related to the complaint are investigated to increase the data pool. For example, the patient may complain of constipation. Rather than immediately administering a laxative the nurse evaluates factors within the suprasystem of the gastrointestinal system, such as level of exercise and comfort in using a bedpan in a two-bed room. Subsystem factors such as dietary intake, bowel movement frequency, and fluid intake are also assessed.

Objective data collection: physical appraisal

A controversy exists concerning the level and scope of physical assessment skills appropriate to nursing practice. Many basic nursing programs now include these skills as part of the curriculum.

Physical assessment skills are an important adjunct to the assessment process. Even though a thorough history generally yields more data, the physical appraisal (or objective data collection) contributes to the nurse's inferences about the patient's strengths and limitations. These skills also offer measures to evaluate nursing interventions.

Techniques

The four techniques utilized in physical appraisal are inspection, palpation, percussion, and auscultation.

The skill of *inspection,* or visual examination, was alluded to earlier. This examination technique considers the general appearance and specific characteristics of the patient's body. Notations may be made about color, shape, position, size, and symmetry (to name a few). Inspection begins on first meeting the patient and may be integrated with other techniques. Of the four techniques inspection may be the most difficult to use, but it yields the most relevant, important data.

Palpation capitalizes on the sense of touch for the purpose of determining the characteristics of tissues or organs. Characteristics such as movement, pain, edema, consistency, temperature, form, vibration, and texture can be assessed. Different parts of the hands are used for different aspects of the appraisal. The fingertips are the most sensitive part of the hand and are the best for fine, tactile discriminations such as texture of skin and size of lymph nodes. The dorsum of the finger has thin skin and is most sensitive to temperature. The palmar aspects of the hands are the most sensitive to vibration. Palpation is also used to check for symmetry of a body part. Pressure is applied with the warmed hands in a deliberate, gentle manner, first using light palpation then deep palpation.

The skill of *percussion* involves tapping a body surface to produce sounds that determine the position or density of an underlying structure. The usual method is direct percussion. The middle or index finger of the nondominant hand is placed against the body surface with the palm and the other fingers of the same hand on the skin. The tip of the middle finger of the opposite hand strikes the base of the distal phalanx of the finger on the patient's skin. The stroke delivered is sharp, with the wrist flexing and the forearm stationary; the striking finger is immediately removed (Fig. 8-4). The sound is then evaluated to determine the type of substance or location of structure percussed. For example, dense solid tissue such as muscle has a flat sound. Air-filled cavities such as the lungs have a resonant sound. The more dense a tissue, the shorter and softer the sound.

The sense of hearing is used in *auscultation* to delineate the sounds of organs such as heart, lungs, and intestines. Characteristics of sounds, such as frequency, intensity, quality, and duration, are evaluated. The stethoscope is used in auscultation, with the diaphragm evaluating high-pitched sounds and the bell low-

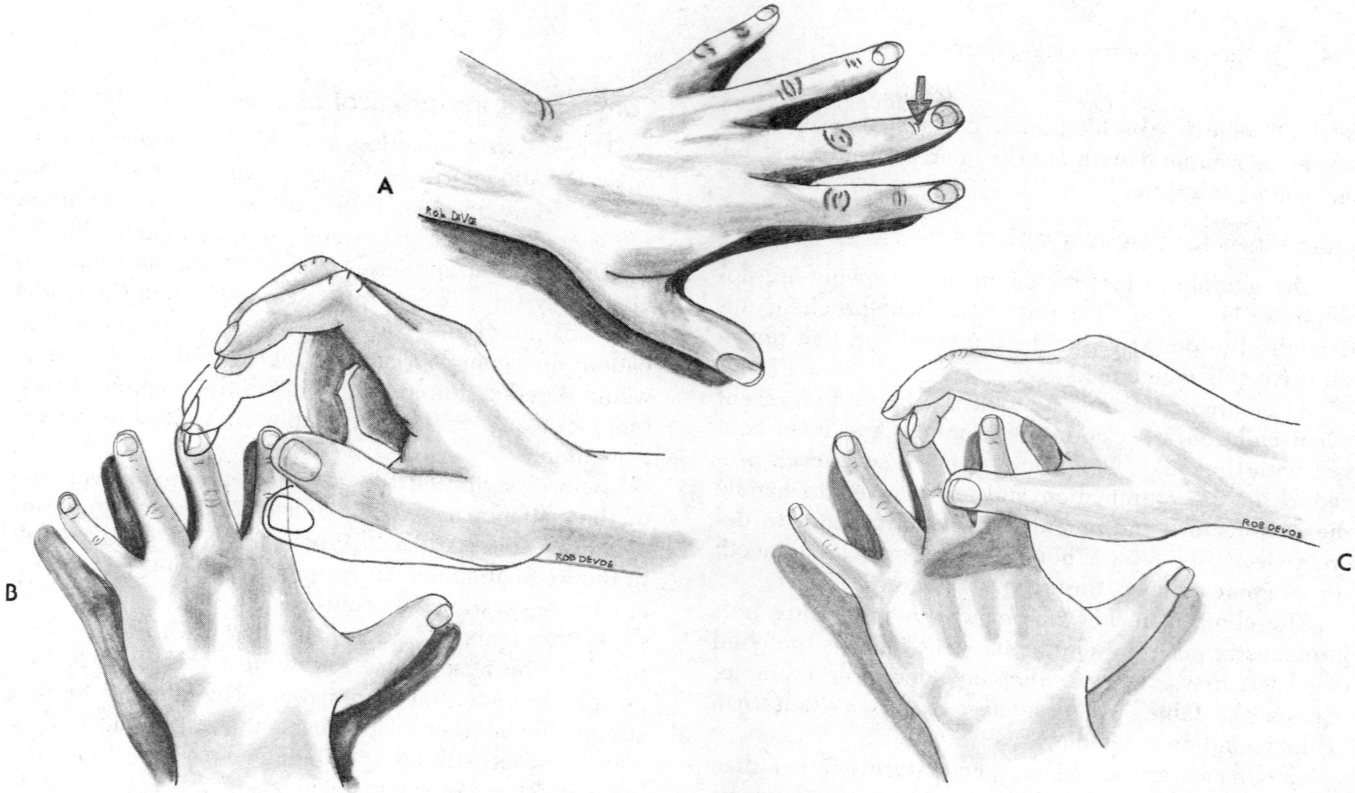

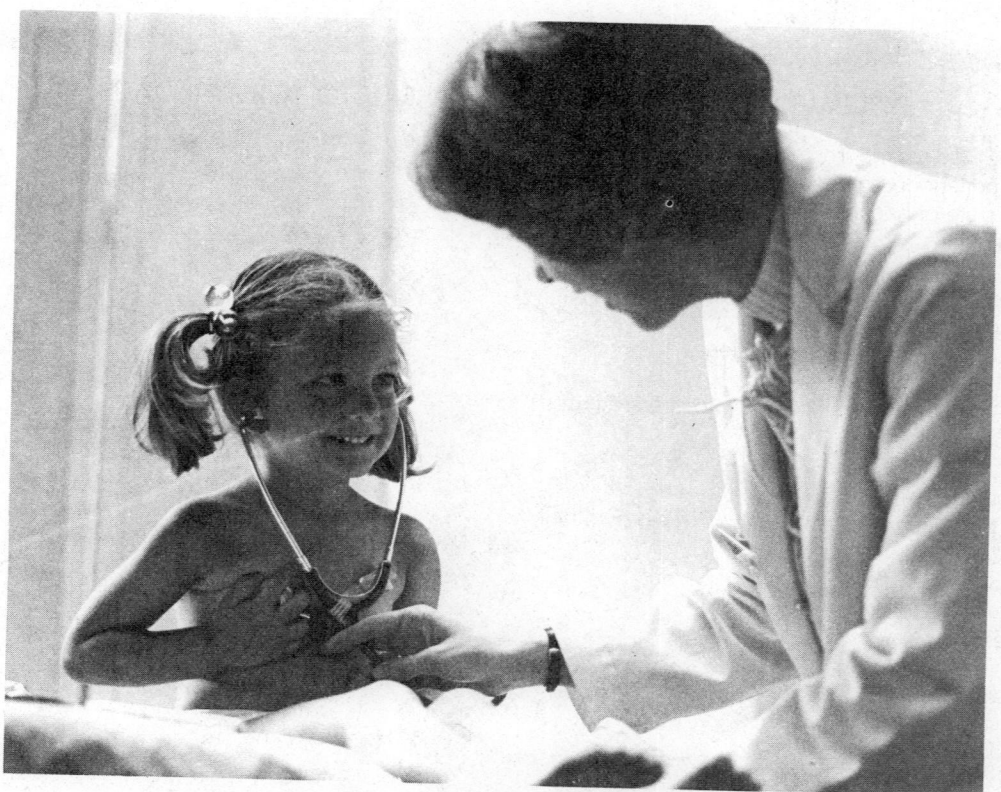

Fig. 8-4. Percussion. **A,** Middle or index finger is placed on body surface with palm and other fingers held away from skin. **B,** Tip of middle finger of opposite hand strikes base of distal portion of finger next to body surface. **C,** Wrist is flexed with forearm in stationary position.

Fig. 8-5. Physical examination of child is enhanced by eye contact, explanation of procedures, and opportunity to handle equipment. Parent's presence is encouraged.

pitched sounds. Auscultation is performed in a quiet, warm environment with the listener concentrating on one sound at a time.

Guidelines for physical appraisal

The guidelines for assessment interviewing are appropriate here also. It is important that the client understand the purposes for the appraisal and that physical privacy is maintained.

As mentioned earlier, the parent should be present when children are examined. Maintain eye level contact with the child. Children are informed of each procedure in the examination and are allowed to handle the examination equipment, when appropriate, to decrease fear (Fig. 8-5). When procedures are announced, the examiner follows through with them.

The clinician makes commands for the child's performance in positive statements. This informs the child of what *can* vs. what *cannot* be done. For example, "Sit on the table" yields a more positive result than "Don't stand on the table!"

Commands are stated in *specific* terms rather than general ones. When the child is asked to perform, be patient and allow time.

The child's participation in the appraisal is encouraged. The bulk of conversation with school-aged and older children is directed toward the child rather than the parent.

Carrying out the physical appraisal

The key to completing a worthwhile appraisal is to be systematic and thorough. For adults, collecting data in a head-to-toe fashion is best utilized during the initial assessment (see box below and on pp. 105 and 106).

The physical appraisal or examination according to biologic systems is best utilized when specific concerns or problems of the patient evolve. For example, the patient may complain of a productive cough. The nurse would then key into data specific to the respiratory system (see Chapter 48) vs. completing a head-to-toe examination.

Before beginning the appraisal a general overview of the patient can yield many clues about significant data to be collected later. Proceeding from head to neck to thorax to abdomen to extremities provides a systematic framework for data collection.

With infants the nurse may start with the feet and move to the head, since they object less strongly to a peripheral-to-central examination. The infant or toddler sits on the mother's lap during the appraisal, as they usually react strongly to being separated from the mother. This age group may resent intrusion of body parts by an unfamiliar person. Therefore the systematic approach may be quite jumbled. Their mouths may not open when you ask but can be examined at an unsuspecting moment or when the child cries. Nurses must be flexible!

SYSTEMATIC PHYSICAL APPRAISAL: A HEAD-TO-TOE APPROACH

I. General survey (60-second impression regarding immediate status of patient on entering room)
  A. Apparent state of health
  B. Signs of distress
  C. Skin color
  D. Stature and body build
  E. Posture, motor activity, and gait
  F. Dress, grooming, and personal hygiene
  G. Odors of body and breath
  H. Manner, mood, and relationship to persons and things around client
  I. Speech
  J. State of awareness, consciousness
  K. Presence of supportive or monitoring devices and their function
  L. Facial expression
II. Vital signs
  A. Blood pressure
  B. Temperature
  C. Radial pulse
    1. Quality
      a. Equal on both sides
      b. Thready, bounding, weak, strong

    2. Rhythm
      a. Regular
      b. Irregular-irregular
      c. Irregular-regular
    3. Rate
  D. Respiration
    1. Rate
    2. Rhythm
    3. Depth
    4. Ease
  E. Height, weight, head circumference
III. Head
  A. Hair, scalp, skull
    1. Texture, cleanliness, quantity, distribution, pattern of loss or gain of hair
    2. Scalp condition (scaly, lumpy, other lesions)
    3. Skull contour, head circumference
    4. Condition of fontanels (infants)
  B. Face
    1. Facial expression
    2. Symmetry, involuntary movements, edema, lesions, masses

C. Eyes
1. Position and alignment of eyes
2. Position of eyelids in relation to eyeballs
3. Eyelid (closed completely [ptosis], edema, lesions)
4. Eyelashes (presence, direction of growth)
5. Eyes
   a. Conjunctiva, sclera, color
   b. Lens
   c. Iris
   d. Pupil (size prestimulation and poststimulation, shape, equality, reaction to light and accommodation)
6. Visual fields by confrontation method
7. Corrective or prosthetic devices
8. Test range of extraocular movement through six cardinal fields of gaze

D. Ears
1. Auricle color, lumps, lesions
2. Patency of canal and color (use otoscope)
3. Weber's and Rinne tests

E. Nares
1. Inhales through nose or mouth
2. Flaring, patency, position of septum
3. Palpate for sinus tenderness

F. Mouth
1. Lips (color, moisture, lumps, ulcers, cracking)
2. Mucous membranes (ulcers, nodules, color, moistness)
3. State of teeth and gums
4. Tongue
   a. Coated
   b. Lesions (including floor of mouth; palpate if found)
   c. Edema
   d. Symmetry of movement
5. Tonsils, uvula
   a. Color, exudate
   b. Edema
   c. Symmetry

IV. Neck
A. Lymph nodes
B. Jugular vein (distention)
C. Carotid pulse (palpate)
D. Trachea (inspect and palpate for deviation)

V. Thorax
A. Inspection: lungs
1. Shape of chest, deformity of thorax, spine contour, symmetry of chest expansion
2. Use of accessory muscles and retraction of intercostal muscles
3. Presence of cough
4. Sputum
   a. Color
   b. Odor
   c. Amount
5. Local lag or impairment of respiratory movement
6. Position of comfort

B. Inspection and palpation: heart
1. Point of maximal intensity (PMI) (location, amplitude)
2. Pulsations over chest wall

C. Inspection: breasts, nipples
1. Female clients
   a. Size, contour
   b. Puckering, dimpling, flattening
   c. Discharge, nipple crusting
   d. Inspect as patient sits, raises arm over head, presses hands against hips
2. Male clients
   a. Nodules, swelling, ulceration

D. Palpation: lungs
1. Distance of chest wall excursion
2. Tenderness around pain or lesions
3. Fremitus

E. Palpation: breast (periphery, tail, areola), nipple
1. Note consistency, induration, tenderness
2. Nodules (size, location, shape, mobility, tenderness, consistency)
3. Elasticity of nipple

F. Percussion: lungs
1. Symmetry of chest wall sounds
2. Abnormal areas (identify, localize, describe)
3. Diaphragmatic excursion

G. Auscultation: lungs (NOTE: Examination of respiratory system is done anteriorly and posteriorly.)
1. Presence and loudness of breath sounds throughout lung fields (symmetry)
2. Breath sounds (quality, intensity)
   a. Vesicular
   b. Bronchial
   c. Bronchovesicular
3. Adventitious sounds
   a. Rales
   b. Rhonchi, including wheezes

H. Auscultation: heart
1. First and second heart sounds at aortic, pulmonic, mitral, tricuspid areas
2. Heart rate, rhythm
3. Apical, radial pulses
4. Extra sounds or murmurs

VI. Abdomen (NOTE: Order of examination: inspection, auscultation, percussion, palpation)
A. Inspection
1. Abdominal contour
2. Scars, striae
3. Umbilicus, contour, signs of inflammation
4. Pulsations
5. Hernia

B. Auscultation
1. Bowel sounds (frequency, character)

C. Percussion
1. Abdominal distention
2. Distended bladder (in suspected individuals)

Continued.

SYSTEMATIC PHYSICAL APPRAISAL: A HEAD-TO-TOE APPROACH—cont'd

D. Palpation
1. Tenderness (including rebound tenderness)
2. Abdominal masses and organs in four quadrants
3. Distended bladder (in suspected individuals)
4. Sacral edema

VII. Perineal area
A. Inspection
1. Vaginal or urethral discharge (amount, color, odor)
2. Indication of bladder or bowel incontinence
3. Presence and size of hemorrhoids
4. Infant/toddler: configuration of genitalia
5. Male clients: penis skin, foreskin, scrotum, hernias
6. Female clients: labia, clitoris, vaginal orifice, perineum

VIII. Extremities
A. Inspection: arms
1. Size, symmetry
2. Color and blanching of nail beds
3. Bilateral hand grasp
4. Movement of limbs on command, symmetry of movement
5. Degree of strength necessary to raise and lower arms against resistance
6. Degree of range of motion
B. Palpation: arms
1. Brachial, ulnar pulses (if arterial insufficiency suspected)
2. Edema
C. Inspection: legs
1. Size, symmetry
2. Hair distribution of legs, feet, toes
3. Color of skin of lower legs and ankles
4. Color, temperature of feet
5. Color of toenails and blanching
6. Degree of range and motion
7. Degree of strength to raise and lower legs and flex and extend feet and legs against resistance
8. Flexor plantar reflex (Babinski)
9. Homans' sign

D. Palpation: legs
1. Tenderness of thigh and calf muscles
2. Varicosities
3. Presence of edema (pretibial, medial malleolus, dorsum of foot)
4. Femoral, popliteal, posterior tibial, dorsalis pedis pulses (normal, diminished, absent)

IX. Skin
A. Inspection
1. Hair distribution
2. Vascularity (bleeding, bruising, varicosities)
3. Mobility, turgor, thickness, texture
4. Color
5. Edema
6. Odor, excretions, cleanliness
7. Moisture, dryness
8. Lesions (color [note nevi], drainage, distribution)
B. Palpation
1. Temperature

X. Concomitant observations
A. Cognitive-emotional systems
1. Restlessness
2. Hostility
3. Apprehension
4. Speech perception, formation
B. Condition of neuromuscular system
1. Level of consciousness (persons, place, time)
2. Muscle mass
3. Abnormal innervation to muscles (paralysis, weakness, spasticity)
4. Ability to discriminate sharp-dull, light-firm, hot-cold sensations
5. Mobility (gait, balance, coordination, method of ambulation)
6. Activity endurance
7. Presence or absence of primitive reflexes (infants)
8. Visual acuity using Snellen chart or news print
9. Romberg's sign
10. Cranial nerve function
C. Laboratory tests relevant to each body system

Data analysis

The second aspect of nursing assessment is data analysis. This component of the nursing process is perhaps the most important yet it was relatively overlooked until the mid-1970s. Also, there has been considerable disagreement in the nursing field as to the labeling of this component. For example, when the nurse analyzes the data, is it called identifying needs, problems, strengths, and liabilities, or is it diagnosis? Regardless of the terminology, this aspect of the nursing process is finally receiving more attention both in the literature and in active investigation by nurses.

Data analysis requires high-level thinking, such as inductive and deductive reasoning, synthesis, and comparison of data with norms and standards to determine their significance. Each data analysis method *must* be substantiated by a sound theoretical rationale. To utilize the above mentioned thinking processes, nurses need a sound knowledge base. Data analysis is closely linked with inference making, described earlier. Data analysis is farther reaching than inference making but permits greater specificity. Whereas the inference might be "patient fearful," the data analysis might be "patient fearful of death, especially of dying alone." The latter was attained by considering a wider range of clinical behaviors and required synthesis. The nurse may utilize the three methods described here for data analysis.

Strengths and liabilities

One method used by nurses is to group the collected raw data into strengths and liabilities according to each system listed on the tool. For example, the history and examination of the integumentary system may reveal strengths and liabilities as follows:

Strengths

1. No past history of problem
2. Clean, intact body skin with pleasant odor
3. Normal hair distribution
4. Bathes self every day (sponge bath)
5. Warm, dry, pink skin

Liabilities

1. Thin, 76-year-old woman requiring bed rest
2. Hair oily with ¼-in. white scaly patches on scalp
3. Dry, flaky skin on extremities

After completing the process with each system, the nurse has a view of the patient's overall status. Plans can be made to correct the liabilities.

This method requires organization rather than synthesis of data. Usually this method is a precursor to further data analysis, which may consider numerous liabilities in diverse systems and produce a broader inference on which to plan care.

Needs and problems

Before beginning to establish patient goals, the nurse critiques the raw data or strengths and liabilities and delineates patient *needs* or *problems*, thus using a second major method of data analysis. The nurse must ask: What kind of needs or problems do the data reflect?

At times needs and problems are used interchangeably. However, a need is a requirement that an individual often defines in relationship to society's norms. Orlando defines need situationally "as a requirement of the patient which, if supplied, relieves or diminishes his immediate distress or improves his immediate sense of adequacy or well-being."[71] Examples might be a need for oxygen, which may be deficient and could relieve distress. There may be a need for a positive self-image, which could improve one's sense of adequacy.

Maslow's hierarchy of needs is very applicable in the clinical setting (see Chapter 1). The nurse may identify liabilities from the data, such as inadequate hydration and loneliness. In Maslow's hierarchy the problem of inadequate hydration would reflect a block in the physiologic need for fluid. Plans are then made to provide fluids for the patient. The difficulty of loneliness reflects inadequate meeting of the need for belongingness and love.

Maslow's hierarchy not only helps the nurse identify needs but also places them in priority, or order of importance. For example, the nurse should meet the patient's need for fluid before concentrating on the need for love. Likewise, if a patient is bleeding, the nurse should attend to that physiologic need before talking to the patient about retirement. In establishing priority of needs the patient should be actively included, as much as possible.

Another aspect of the second method of data analysis is identifying a patient's *problems*. Problems reflect a difficult situation with which the person usually requires outside help for effective coping. Problems may be actual or potential negative alterations in a person's bio-psycho-sociocultural health or steady state. Problems may reflect an unmet need or a conflict between two needs. In the previous example inadequate hydration is the problem and adequate fluid intake is the need. When an individual or family does not realize that a need exists or is meeting the need ineffectively, objective data identifies that a problem exists. A young mother may not realize that her 18-month-old child needs nutritional intake in addition to milk. Therefore the need for food is reflected in the problem of inadequate nutritional intake, namely, vitamins and iron.

Problems may be overt or covert. Overt problems are readily identifiable, such as immobility or inadequate urinary output. Covert problems are more difficult to identify, require greater synthesis of a variety of data, may be masked by other problems, or lack objectivity. A patient's crying may have a variety of meanings. The nurse may need to collect a variety of data to determine that this patient is not crying because of postoperative pain but because of a sense of loss because today is the first anniversary of her mother's death.

Problems may be identified through inductive or deductive reasoning. With induction the nurse critiques the data collected in each system. Then a generalization is made (similar to inference making) that has support from a theoretical base. For example, a postoperative patient may be seen with weak, thready, increasing pulse of 98 beats/min; cool, pale, dry skin;

decreasing blood pressure to 98/40; respiratory rate of 36/min; and apprehension. The nurse may delineate the problem as hemorrhagic shock based on knowledge of its manifestations.

With the deductive method the nurse moves from generalizations to specifics. For example, the patient may be immobile because of a fracture. The nurse then delineates problems indicative of immobility that should be validated such as stasis of pulmonary secretions, constipation, skin breakdown. Then the nurse proceeds to establish goals based on the defined problems.

Nursing diagnosis

The final method of data analysis is nursing diagnosis. Some authors note that nurses have diagnosed since the first century AD.[42] The impetus for a diagnostic classification system, however, has rapidly expanded since the National Group on Classification of Nursing Diagnoses held its first conference in 1973.*

Nursing diagnosis emanated in part from nurses seeking to define and delimit their scope of practice. The diagnostic classification system seeks to move nursing into a more sound theoretical base as actual and potential health problems encountered in nurses' practice are enumerated and studied. Clinical science development requires description of the phenomenon of concern,[27] and the classification of actual and potential health problems diagnosed and treated by nurses is a major and primary step in organizing and building the science. The need to create nursing diagnoses (as shown in the following example) has also evolved from the American Nurses Association Standards of Practice:

Standard II: Nursing diagnoses are derived from health status data

Rationale: The health status of the client/patient is the basis for determining the nursing care needs. Data are analyzed and compared to norms when possible.[2]

An established diagnostic nomenclature would also help standardize the care given by providing a common frame of reference for all nurses. For example, if the diagnosis of "role disturbance" were fully defined, all nurses would have a mind set of the clinical findings expected, the subjective and objective data base to collect, the etiology or etiologies, and the appropriate interventions.

Nursing diagnosis can also lead to clarification of roles by emphasizing areas that nurses treat. To illustrate, nurses would clearly understand what aspects of the diagnosis "respiratory dysfunction" would be appropriate for their treatment and what aspects would be more appropriately met by the physician, respiratory therapist, or physical therapist.

With the movement toward a classification system, more sophisticated definitions of nursing diagnoses have evolved. Gordon defines nursing diagnoses as those "made by professional nurses which describe actual or potential health problems which nurses, by virtue of their education and experience, are capable and licensed to treat."[21] Nursing diagnosis requires that a conclusion be made after interpreting the data and comparing them to theoretical or scientific knowledge. The conclusion usually relates to an actual or potential health problem or unhealthful response, such as lack of knowledge about medications or potential for impaired skin integrity. One should keep in mind that the conclusion reached may not be a problem. Instead, the conclusion reached may be that the patient is in normal health and growth and developmental status, as found on a well-child visit. A person may be free of disease but have health-related needs, such as a new father who feels inadequate in the parenting role.

Identification of the etiology of a problem, in addition to a problem statement, is necessary in the nursing diagnosis since this provides direction for the nursing activities. For example, the diagnosis "potential for injury" could be related to a cluttered room, suicidal gestures, or lack of child proofing. The nursing interventions would be very different depending on the etiology. One problem statement may have multiple etiologies; in addition, one etiology may be the basis for several problems. For example, the diagnosis of "nutritional alteration—undernutrition" may be associated with lack of money, lack of knowledge about proper nutrition, and lack of physical stamina in an elderly person. Conversely, the four diagnoses—anxiety, altered bowel elimination (constipation), altered self-care activities, and impaired skin integrity (pressure necrosis)—could all have a common etiology of immobility secondary to bed rest.

Students beginning nursing study may find it extremely difficult to delineate etiology. Identification of etiology depends on one's repertoire of theoretical and factual knowledge as well as clinical experience. Several etiologies for one problem may be tested until the correct one is found; therefore the diagnostic statement may say "related to" or "associated with" rather than "because of" or "due to" until diagnostic certainty is established. To illustrate, a statement may read "impaired physical mobility *related to* fear of pain" if the etiology is uncertain or "potential for falls *secondary to (due to)* impaired balance" if the etiology is certain.

A nursing diagnostic statement reflects a pattern of signs and symptoms. A diagnosis is not based on just one bit of data but on a cluster of signs and symptoms or other related data. Signs are objective manifestations

*Information can be obtained by subscribing to a newsletter from Clearinghouse for Nursing Diagnoses, St. Louis University, Department of Nursing, 3525 Caroline St., St. Louis, MO 63104.

such as scratching, vomiting, or purulent sputum. Symptoms are subjective manifestations such as itching, pain, and nausea. A nursing diagnosis of impaired mobility implies a grouping of signs and symptoms. The nursing diagnosis is stated in terms of the patient's state rather than the nurse's. For example, "needs to be turned in bed" describes a nursing activity rather than the patient's problem of "impaired mobility, unable to turn in bed."

Nursing diagnosis may be delineated in a PES format.[25,26] *P* refers to the problem, existing or potential, *E* denotes etiology as defined above, and *S* relates to the signs and symptoms that provided the data base on which the problem was developed. The PES method is extremely thorough and identifies all components necessary to determine a diagnosis. The PES method is complementary with problem-oriented medical charting, and recording is readily done in the SOAP format as listed in the box below.

A difference exists between medical and nursing diagnoses. The physician reaches a conclusion concerning abnormalities in structure and function after reviewing signs and symptoms. The nurse usually reaches a conclusion about the patient's ability to function in activities of daily living because of the impairment after reviewing signs and symptoms. The physician diagnoses a medical condition such as multiple sclerosis. The nurse diagnoses problems as a consequence of the disease, such as difficulty ambulating. A medical diagnosis tends to be the same throughout the illness, for example, pancreatitis. The nursing diagnosis problem areas, however, may be multiple and dynamic depending on the patient's state.[59] A patient with pancreatitis may have problems with pain, digestion, and sleep and rest depending on the health state.

Nurses may identify medical problems without engaging in a medical diagnosis. They may observe the signs and symptoms of asthma, ventricular fibrillation, pulmonary edema, or hemorrhagic shock without identifying the disease etiology, and they would refer patients with these problems to the physician for therapy.

Some medical diagnoses are the same as those made by other health professionals, especially in the emergency setting. For example, a cardiac arrest may be identified by a nurse, respiratory therapist, or physician, and appropriate therapy is often initiated by any or all of these professionals. The rapidity with which diagnosis and treatment must occur in life-threatening situations necessitates collaboration of many health professionals, and in these settings diagnoses are often treated by many disciplines.

Little and Carnevali[39] list some helpful guidelines that describe what a nursing diagnosis is *not*:
1. Not the medical diagnosis (e.g., cirrhosis)
2. Not the diagnostic test (e.g., barium enema)
3. Not the medical treatment (e.g., colostomy)
4. Not the equipment (e.g., catheter)
5. Not the nurse's problem with the client (e.g., uncooperative)

Nursing diagnoses may be derived via deductive or inductive modes. In the deductive mode diagnoses are derived from considering a conceptual framework; for example, the National Group on Classification on Nursing Diagnosis decided in 1978 to use the concept of unitary man to delineate diagnoses.[27] Campbell uses Maslow's hierarchy of human needs as a theoretical framework for the process.[12] With the inductive mode patients' problems are identified based on the subjective and objective data collected from clinical practice. The fourth conference on nursing diagnosis, the National Group on Classification, delineated a list of 37 nursing diagnoses (see box on p. 110). The list is not exhaustive, and further refinements and clinical validation are needed.

In summary, nursing diagnoses are derived by (1) collecting an organized, complete subjective and objective data base; (2) analyzing data by cognitive processing and comparing the data base with knowledge or theory to determine healthy or unhealthful states, actual or potential; (3) sorting and organizing data to determine if *patterns* exist and if any of the problems have a common basis; and (4) determining if sufficient data are available and have been collected, if the signs and symptoms are characteristic of a health problem, and if the diagnoses are amenable to independent nurse actions.[53,59]

Nursing diagnosis has received increased emphasis as nurses strive to become more autonomous in practice, as the scope of nursing practice expands, as nurses attain a greater degree of professionalism and equality with other professions, and as the Standards of Practice of the American Nurses Association are implemented. Also, legislation defining the rights and responsibilities of nurses, expectations of better health care by consum-

PES format		SOAP format
P:	Impairment of skin integrity on coccyx	*Problem*
E:	Bed rest, lack of turning, aging (fragile skin), inadequate vitamin intake	*Assessment*
S:	Signs: 2-in. diameter erythematous area on coccyx, warm to touch with oozing serous fluid; 82-year-old woman eating only pudding; remains in semi-Fowler's position 4 hours at a time without turning self	*Objective*
	Symptoms: Doesn't "like to eat" and "I can't move myself"	*Subjective*

NURSING DIAGNOSES ACCEPTED AT THE FOURTH NATIONAL CONFERENCE (1980) OF THE NATIONAL GROUP ON CLASSIFICATION*

Airway clearance, ineffective
Bowel elimination, alteration in: constipation
Bowel elimination, alteration in: diarrhea
Bowel elimination, alteration in: incontinence
Breathing pattern, inneffective
Cardiac output, alteration in: decreased
Comfort, alteration in: pain
Communication, impaired verbal
Coping, ineffective individual
Coping, ineffective family: compromised
Coping, ineffective family: disabling
Coping, family: potential for growth
Diversional activity, deficit
Fear
Fluid volume, deficit, actual†
Fluid volume, deficit, potential
Gas exchange, impaired
Grieving, anticipatory
Grieving, dysfunctional
Home maintenance management, impaired
Injury, potential for; poisoning, potential for; suffocation, potential for; trauma, potential for
Knowledge deficit (specify)
Mobility, impaired physical
Noncompliance (specify)
Nutrition, alteration in: less than body requirements
Nutrition, alteration in: more than body requirements
Nutrition, alteration in: potential for more than body requirements
Parenting, alteration in: actual
Parenting, alteration in: potential
Rape-trauma syndrome: rape trauma, compound reaction, silent reaction

Self-care deficit (specify level): feeding, bathing/hygiene, dressing/grooming, toileting
Self-concepts, disturbance in: body image, self-esteem, role performance, personal identity
Sensory perceptual alteration: visual, auditory, kinesthetic, gustatory, tactile, and olfactory perceptions
Sexual dysfunction
Skin integrity, impairment of: actual
Skin integrity, impairment of: potential
Sleep pattern disturbance
Spiritual distress (distress of the human spirit)
Thought processes, alteration in
Tissue perfusion, alteration in: cerebral, cardiopulmonary, renal, gastrointestinal, peripheral
Urinary elimination, alteration in patterns
Violence, potential for

Diagnoses "accepted" without defining characteristics
The following diagnoses are unacceptable but are to be listed separately as diagnoses to be developed (TBD).
Cognitive dissonance
Decision making, impaired/ineffective (decisions made by client produce results other than or less than desired)
Family dynamics, alteration in‡
1. Family role changes/shifts
2. Dysfunctional coping
3. Stress management patterns
4. Developmental transition
5. Situational transition
Fluid volume, alteration in, excess: potential for memory deficit, rest-activity pattern (ineffective), role disturbance, social isolation

---

*From Kim, J., and Moritz, D.: Classification of nursing diagnoses: proceedings of the third and fourth conferences. Copyright © 1981 by McGraw-Hill Book Co. Used with the permission of McGraw-Hill Book Co.
†Two sets of defining characteristics with two etiologies for the same nursing diagnosis.
‡To be developed further as a set of family-level diagnoses, as opposed to individual diagnosis.

ers, the women's liberation movement, and rapid technologic advances and the increasing complexity of health care encourage further development of nursing diagnoses.

Summary

This chapter has considered how to systematically assess a patient's bio-psycho-sociocultural systems in an effective manner. Both data collection and analysis have been discussed. It is the nurse's responsibility to develop the skills mentioned here in order to provide a data base and problem list that can support individualized nursing care.

REFERENCES AND SELECTED READING
Contemporary

1. Alexander, M.M., and Brown, M.S.: Physical examination: history taking, part 2, Nurs. '73 3:35-39, 1973.
2. American Nurses Association: Standard of nursing practice, Kansas City, Mo., 1973, The Association.
3. Aspinall, M.J.: Nursing diagnosis: the weak link, Nurs. Outlook 24:433-437, 1976.
4. Aspinall, M.J.: Development of a patient completed admission questionnaire and its comparison with the nursing interview, Nurs. Res. 24:377-381, 1975.
5. Bates, B., and Lynaugh, J.: Teaching physical assessment, Nurs. Outlook 23:297-302, 1975.
6. Becknell, E.P., and Smith, D.M.: System of nursing practice, Philadelphia, 1975, F.A. Davis Co.
7. Bircher, A.U.: On the development and classification of diagnosis, Nurs. Forum 14:10-29, 1975.
8. Bower, F.L.: The process of planning nursing care: nursing practice models, ed. 3, St. Louis, 1982, The C.V. Mosby Co.
9. Brill, E.L., and Kilts, D.F.: Foundations for nursing, New York, 1980, Appleton-Century-Crofts.
10. Bruce, J.: Implementation of nursing diagnosis: a nursing administrator's perspective, Nurs. Clin. North Am. 14:509-515, 1979.
11. Byrne, M.L., and Thompson, L.F.: Key concepts for the study and practice of nursing, ed. 2, St. Louis, 1978, The C.V. Mosby Co.
12. Campbell, C.: Nursing diagnosis and intervention in nursing practice, New York, 1978, John Wiley & Sons, Inc.
13. Carrieri, V.K., and Sitzman, J.: Components of the nursing process, Nurs. Clin. North Am. 6:115-124, 1971.
14. Chinn, P.L., and Leitch, C.J.: Handbook for nursing assessment of the child, Salt Lake City, 1973, University of Utah Press.
15. Crane, J.: Physical appraisal: an aspect of the nursing assessment. In Sana, J.M., and Judge, R.D.: Physical appraisal methods in nursing practice, Boston, 1975, Little, Brown & Co.
16. Dossey, B.: Perfecting your skills for systematic patient assessments, Nurs. '79 2:42-45, 1979.
17. Dugas, B.W.: Introduction to patient care, ed. 3, Philadelphia, 1977, W.B. Saunders Co.
18. Field, L.: The implementation of nursing diagnosis in clinical practice, Nurs. Clin. North Am. 14:497-508, 1979.
19. Fortin, J.D., and Rabinow, J.: Legal implications of nursing diagnosis, Nurs. Clin. North Am. 14:553-561, 1979.
20. Fredette, S., and O'Connor, K.: Nursing diagnosis in teaching and curriculum planning, Nurs. Clin. North Am. 14:541-552, 1979.
21. Fuller, D., and Rosenaur, J.A.: A patient assessment guide, Nurs. Outlook 22:460-462, 1974.
22. Garant, C.: A basis for care, Am. J. Nurs. 72:699-701, 1972.
23. Gebbie, K., and Lavin, M.A., editors: Classification of nursing diagnoses, St. Louis, 1975, The C.V. Mosby Co.
24. Gebbie, K., and Lavin, M.A.: Classifying nursing diagnosis, Am. J. Nurs. 74:250-253, 1974.
25. Gordon, M.: The concept of nursing diagnosis, Nurs. Clin. North Am. 14:487-496, 1979.
26. Gordon, M.: Nursing diagnosis and the diagnostic process, Am. J. Nurs. 76:1298-1300, 1976.
27. Gordon, M., and Sweeney, M.A.: Methodological problems and issues in identifying and standardizing nursing diagnoses, Adv. Nurs. Sci. 2:1-15, 1979.
28. Guzetta, C.E., and Forsyth, S.L.: Nursing diagnostic pilot study: psychophysiologic stress, Adv. Nurs. Sci. 2:27-44, 1979.
29. Hamdi, M.E., and Hutelmyer, C.M.: A study of the effectiveness of an assessment tool in the identification of nursing care problems, Nurs. Res. 19:354-358, 1970.
30. Hazzard, M.E.: An overview of systems theory, Nurs. Clin. North Am. 6:385-393, 1971.
31. Helfer, R.E., Black, M.A., and Helfer, M.E.: Pediatric interviewing skills taught by nonphysicians, Am. J. Dis. Child. 129:1053-1057, 1975.
32. Henderson, B.: Nursing diagnosis: theory and practice, Adv. Nurs. Sci. 1:75-83, 1978.
33. Hermone, R.H.: How to get results from an interview, Hosp. Topics 49:88-89, 1971.
34. Johnson, I.: The art of history taking, J. Neurosurg. Nurs. 2:5-17, 1970.
35. Johnson, M.M., and Lawbaugh, A.M.: Problem solving in nursing practice, ed. 3, Dubuque, Iowa, 1980, William C. Brown Co.
36. Jones, P.E.: A terminology for nursing diagnoses, Adv. Nurs. Sci. 2:65-72, 1979.
37. Langer, S.R.: The nursing process and the interview, Occup. Health Nurs. 21:19-23, 1973.
38. Lewis, L.: Planning patient care, ed. 2, Dubuque, Iowa, 1976, William C. Brown Co.
39. Little, D., and Carnevali, D.: Nursing care planning, ed. 2, Philadelphia, 1976, J.B. Lippincott Co.
40. MacFarlane, J.: Pediatric assessment and intervention: some simple-how-to's for ambulatory settings, Nurs. '74 4:66-68, 1974.
41. Mahoney, E., Verdisco, L., and Shortridge, L.: How to collect and record a health history, Philadelphia, 1976, J.B. Lippincott Co.
42. Mahoney, E.A.: Some implications for nursing diagnoses of pain, Nurs. Clin. North Am. 12:613-619, 1977.
43. Malasanos, L., et al.: Health assessment, ed. 2, St. Louis, 1981, The C.V. Mosby Co.
44. Mansell, E., and Stokes, S.: Patient assessment: taking a patient's history, Am. J. Nurs. 74:293-324, 1974.
45. Marriner, A.: The nursing process: a scientific approach to nursing care, ed. 3, St. Louis, 1983, The C.V. Mosby Co.
46. Marshall, J.C., and Feeney, S.: Structured versus intuitive intake interview, Nurs. Res. 21:269-272, 1972.
47. Matthews, C.A., and Gaul, A.L.: Nursing diagnosis from the perspective of concept attainment and critical thinking, Adv. Nurs. Sci. 2:17-26, 1979.
48. McCloskey, J.C.: The nursing care plan: past, present and uncertain future; a review of the literature, Nurs. Forum 14:364-382, 1975.
49. McKeehan, K.M.: Nursing diagnosis in a discharge planning program, Nurs. Clin. North Am. 14:514-524, 1979.

50. Mitchell, P.H., and Loustau, A.: Concepts basic to nursing, ed. 3. New York, 1981, McGraw-Hill Book Co.
51. Mundinger, M.O., and Jouron, G.D.: Developing a nursing diagnosis, Nurs. Outlook 23:94-98, 1975.
52. Murray, M.: Fundamentals of nursing, ed. 2, Englewood Cliffs, N.J., 1980, Prentice-Hall, Inc.
53. Price, M.R.: Nursing diagnosis: making a concept come alive, Am. J. Nurs. 80:668-671, 1980.
54. Roy, Sister C.: Introduction to nursing: an adaptation model, Englewood Cliffs, N.J., 1976, Prentice-Hall, Inc.
55. Roy, Sister C.: A diagnostic classification system for nursing, Nurs. Outlook 23:90-94, 1975.
56. Roy, Sister C.: The impact of nursing diagnosis, A.O.R.M.J. 21:1023-1030, 1975.
57. Ryan, B.J.: Nursing care plans: a systems approach to developing criteria for planning and evaluation, J. Nurs. Adm. 3:50-58, 1973.
58. Seedor, M.M.: The physical assessment: a programmed unit of study for nurses, New York, 1974, Teachers College Press.
59. Shoemaker, J.: How nursing diagnosis helps focus your care, R.N. 42:56-61, 1979.
60. Sobol, E.G., and Robischon, P.: Family nursing: a study guide, St. Louis, 1975, The C.V. Mosby Co.
61. Wesseling, E.: Automating the nursing history and care plan, J. Nurs. Adm. 2:34-38, 1972.
62. Wilson, G.: Nursing diagnosis (assessment) and changing accountability, Aust. Nurses' J. 9:36-38, 1980.

Classic

63. Bermosk, L.S., and Mordan, M.J.: Interviewing in nursing, New York, 1964, Macmillan Publishing Co., Inc.
64. Chambers, W.: Nursing diagnosis, Am. J. Nurs. 62:102-104, 1962.
65. Culver, C.M., and Dunham, F.: The inference process, unpublished paper prepared in conjunction with USPHS Grant no. 81-1362, 1964.
66. Durand, M., and Prince, R.: Nursing diagnosis, process, and decision, Nurs. Forum 5:50-64, 1966.
67. Hall, E.T.: The hidden dimension, New York, 1966, Doubleday & Co., Inc.
68. Maslow, A.: Motivation and personality, New York, 1969, Harper & Row, Publishers.
69. McCain, R.F.: Nursing by assessment—not intuition, Am. J. Nurs. 65:82-84, 1965.
70. McPhetridge, L.M.: Nursing history: one means to personalize care, Am. J. Nurs. 68:68-75, 1968.
71. Orlando, I.J.: The dynamic nurse-patient relationship, New York, 1961, G.P. Putnam's Sons.
72. Pearsall, M.: Participant observation as role and method in behavioral research, Nurs. Res. 14:37-42, 1965.
73. Peplau, H.E.: Talking with patients, Am. J. Nurs. 60:964-966, 1960.
74. Prange, A.J., Jr., and Martin, H.W.: Aids to understanding patients, Am. J. Nurs. 62:98-100, 1962.
75. Whalen, R.: Medical malaprops, J.A.M.A. 177:158-160, 1961.

CHAPTER 9

NURSE-CLIENT INTERACTIONS

LINDA WAGNER CRAIG

Communication theory

The ability to analyze the dynamics of nurse-client interactions is a skill basic to all areas of nursing. This chapter focuses on the dyadic (two-person) interpersonal communication process within these interactions and discusses the elements the nurse needs to understand, namely, the self, the client, and the interactions between self and client. The development, over time, of the nurse-client relationship is also studied.

The concept of communication is difficult to define because of its breadth. Researchers from many fields have viewed communication from various perspectives and have developed different definitions and models. While many of these definitions are complementary, others conflict, especially with regard to the inclusiveness of the concept, the intentions of the communicators, and the success of the messages sent. Some researchers define communication to include all behavior, and others limit the meaning to the *purposive* behavior of persons in *conscious* interactions. There is a disagreement whether intent to send a message is a requirement and whether success of the message is essential to the definition.[8] Success of the message requires that the message sent be the one the sender intended and that the receiver perceive the message correctly.

If dyadic interpersonal communication is defined as *the exchange, with acknowledgment, of messages between two persons*, then the scope is limited to acknowledged behavior, the intent to communicate does not have to be conscious, and the accuracy of the message perception is irrelevant so long as the message is acknowledged. For dyadic interpersonal communication there must be five essential elements: *sender/receiver, message/feedback, encoding/decoding, channels,* and *context*. Fig. 9-1 shows the dyadic interpersonal communication model.

The communication system

Sender/receiver

There is no real separation between the sender and the receiver roles in dyadic interpersonal communication. This is because when two people communicate, they create a communication system. Each person is simultaneously a sender and a receiver. Many messages are being transmitted simultaneously, some at a conscious level, some unconscious. Communication is *dynamic*, involving active response from the receiver, which in turn influences the sender's message. This concept is essential to the understanding of the *circular* or systems model of communication as depicted in Fig. 9-1, as opposed to the earlier *linear* model. In the circular or systems model communication occurs *simultaneously between* persons A and B, whereas in the linear model communication goes *from* person A *to* person B.

Message/feedback

Just as there is no real separation between sender and receiver, there is no real separation between message and feedback. Feedback is a return message. Return messages stimulate further messages and so on. Feedback has traditionally been the term used to indicate *acknowledgment* of a message. A return message, or feedback, is crucial to establishing that communication has occurred. Without feedback we may be whistling in the dark. Without feedback we also often feel a rejection of our message or even a rejection of our presence. Delayed feedback may create similar feelings of rejection. Feedback need only be an acknowledgment of the communication received; it need not be a detailed response or answer to a question. One might respond "I hear you" or "I'm thinking about what you

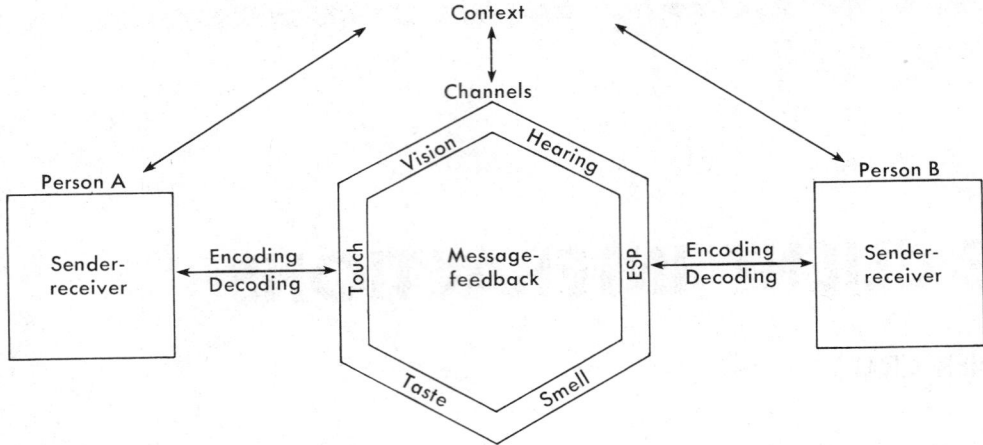

Fig. 9-1. Model of dyadic interpersonal communication.

said" if one desires more time to give a complete response. A prompt acknowledgment of a person's message with some form of return message (feedback) communicates a degree of respect for the other person.

Messages/feedback may be intentional or unintended. They may be sent consciously, or the person may be entirely unaware of sending the message. One message may confirm or contradict another message.

Channels

Messages are sent over a variety of channels or media. All of the sensory (and perhaps extrasensory) channels are used in communicating. A high degree of facility in the use of all channels enables people to be more flexible in their communication. Good judgment in the choice of channels increases the effectiveness of communication and requires knowledge of the total communication system. When the same message is sent over different channels, its effectiveness may be increased. For example, if one is teaching a young child about oranges, one could give a detailed verbal description of an orange and perhaps show a picture. Consider how much more effective the message would be if the child was given an orange to feel and smell and some orange juice to taste.

The channel over which a message comes has a definite effect on the message. Indeed, McLuhan felt the effect was so great that he decided the medium was the message. Certainly the medium or channel reflects a choice or judgment by the sender, which, in itself, can be a message. For example, if a friend wants to communicate love, the friend might write the words "I love you" on a note or say the words "I love you" over the telephone or say the words "I love you" while looking into your eyes. Sometimes written communication is easier than saying the same words face-to-face. It is easier for some people to send and possibly easier for some to receive a written communication. At any rate the

medium or channel does leave the receiver with some inferences about the sender.

Encoding/decoding

Messages are essentially ideas, thoughts, and feelings; they are without substance until encoded. *Encoding* refers to how one symbolizes ideas in order to send them via a channel. This includes the selection of verbal and nonverbal symbols to convey the message. *Decoding* refers to the process of interpreting incoming verbal and nonverbal messages. An example of how the process of encoding/decoding occurs might be helpful.

Julia has an idea about how her 12-month-old daughter, Anna, can get out of the tight space she is stuck in.

Idea: If Anna will first stand up, she could get out of that tight space. She can't fit through if she tries to crawl.

Julia knows that Anna's use of vocabulary (verbal symbols) is limited. She also infers that Anna is frightened or angry because she is crying loudly. Julia and Anna have a good relationship. So Julia approaches Anna confidently, smiles, takes Anna's hand, lifts it upward, and says "Up, Anna."

Julia used several symbols to encode the original idea that she wanted to communicate to Anna. The language symbols (words) were simple and age appropriate: "Up, Anna." Nonverbal symbols of gesture and touch were lifting Anna's hand upward and lifting her own head upward. Julia also unconsciously sends some extra messages to Anna designed to decrease Anna's anxiety level and thereby facilitate her reception of the original idea. These extra messages were all nonverbal:

1. I see you are in a tight place (recognition of child's problem).
2. I want to help you (intention).
3. You will be able to get out (confidence).

What were some of the symbols Julia used to encode

these nonverbal messages? They were symbols such as touch, eye contact, tone of voice, affect, demeanor, and facial expression, to name a few.

Encoding involves selecting symbols that you believe the other person will understand in the way you intended them to be understood. In general, verbal symbols allow more precision in the communication of *ideas* and sophisticated concepts. Nonverbal symbols are used widely for the communication of *feelings*. The eyes, for example, offer a range of nuance of feeling unparalleled by language.

Nonverbal communication is the most basic form of communication. It is also the most primitive form of communication as well as the first form of communication learned by the child. Some have estimated that two thirds of all information transferred between people is nonverbal. Nonverbal communication is continuous when two persons are interacting. It is much less subject to conscious control than verbal communication. Because of this, it tends to reflect more accurately the sender's true thoughts and feelings. Nonverbal symbols include demeanor, gestures, mannerisms, physical appearance, dress, posture, gait, bearing, eye contact, body sounds, intonation of voice, and use of silence and touch.

Nonverbal communication has a greater chance of being misinterpreted. Interpretation of nonverbal symbols varies with the receiver's culture, age, needs, awareness, past experiences, and so on. Past experiences within the family group are especially influential in determining how a person uses and interprets nonverbal symbols. The interpetation the receiver assigns to the nonverbal message determines the manner of response to the message.

Touch is a special kind of nonverbal symbol and one quite necessary to health professionals. Touch is the chief way a person can attempt to communicate love, safety, and security to a little child who does not yet understand words. The infant understands touch directly. However, the adult understands touch more through past associations, connotations, and experiences, especially those related to closeness, sexuality, and comforting, than through the gesture alone. It is well for health professionals to remember that the well-intended use of touch has the potential of decreasing *or* increasing anxiety. For example, touch may be associated with procedures, pain, and the use of restraint in the health profession, as well as with gestures of perceived kindness. Touch, as with other nonverbal symbols, has less chance of being misunderstood when it is accompanied by verbal messages that are congruent with the kind of touch.

Verbal communication involves the use of a highly developed language of word symbols. Effective verbal communication obviously requires knowledge of and facility with the language on the part of the receiver and the sender. Judgment in the choice of verbal symbols, just as with nonverbal symbols, requires sensitive assessment of the receiver's level of use and understanding of the symbols. Many other factors must be assessed also, such as the receiver's needs, attitudes, values, beliefs, and customs. It has long been recognized that the personality of the sender influences effectiveness in communicating. The same words said by two different people may convey two different meanings.

Context

Interpersonal communication always occurs within a context or setting. This refers to the environment around the interaction, including the physical setting, atmosphere, and the presence or absence of other people. The nurse and the client communicate within the context of other systems, for example, the client's family system, the hospital unit administration, the community health care system, the political system, and the ecosystem.

Summary

In *summary*, dyadic interpersonal communication is a complex system comprising five essential elements: *sender/receiver*, *messages/feedback*, *encoding/decoding*, *channels* and *context*. These elements interact to produce an infinity of possibilities in communicating.

Obstacles to effective communication

One common problem in communication is the sending of contradictory messages, such as the verbal-nonverbal split. In this case, the verbal message contradicts the accompanying nonverbal message. If a nurse says to a client that he seems to be angry, and the client scowls and uses a very angry-sounding tone of voice to protest, then the message of anger is nonverbally affirmed while verbally denied. Although there is the option to believe the verbal message, the nurse will probably tend to believe the nonverbal message. We learn as we grow that nonverbal messages are usually accurate reflectors of feelings.

Children, especially, are confused by verbal-nonverbal splits—confused about how to interpret them and how to respond. The possibilities for responding to a verbal-nonverbal split are numerous. One can respond verbally or nonverbally to either the verbal or the nonverbal message or to the verbal and nonverbal messages together, perhaps pointing out the inconsistency. One can also choose *not* to respond. The choice of response will be influenced by the receiver's needs and goals as well as by the receiver's perception of the sender's needs and goals.

The presence of a verbal-nonverbal split is itself a message. One might infer ambivalence or conflict within the sender regarding the message. One wonders which message was probably intended and if the sender is aware of sending both messages. Perhaps the sender is testing to see which message the receiver prefers. An increased anxiety level usually accompanies reception of a verbal-nonverbal split unless or until a comfortable predictable pattern of communication is established. We learn with some people not to argue with their verbal messages but to proceed on the basis of their nonverbal messages when verbal-nonverbal splits are sent. This may become a predictable, workable pattern although certainly it is not a model of clear communication.

The sender may seek to disguise the meaning of a message because of fears of rejection by the receiver or perhaps because the sender finds the message unacceptable or uncomfortable. This might result in the sender actually saying the opposite of what he means. This coping mechanism is called reaction formation. (See Chapter 14.)

Numerous problems exist in the area of encoding and decoding messages. We typically have peculiarities (idiosyncrasies) in these areas that are specific to us as individuals. *The more aware we are of our own peculiarities and the more sensitive we are to the peculiarities of others in the area of encoding and decoding, the better chance we have of successful communication.* For example, some people decode touch from nonintimate friends as being forward or taking liberties, whereas others might interpret that same touch as an indication of warmth and acceptance and perhaps comfort on the part of the sender.

Difficulty in receiving the message constitutes another obstacle to effective communication. This may stem from a number of related problems including distaste for the channel over which the particular message came, unwillingness to accept the content of the message, inability to perceive the message because of a physical handicap such as blindness, or deafness, decreased receptivity to any messages because of fatigue, illness, or preoccupation with other thoughts, and emotional reaction to a message, which interferes with reception of the cognitive content. For example, when strong affect (feeling) such as fear exists, the person may shut out any incoming stimuli that are felt to further increase his or her fear. The need to feel secure causes the person to *selectively inattend* to incoming stimuli.[46] Thus the message may not be decoded or if it is decoded, it will not be acknowledged.

Hidden agendas create another problem area of communication. These agendas are suspected when persons communicating are not straightforward and direct in their purposes or goals for interacting. Their stated or *manifest* reasons for communicating are not their primary reasons. Their messages may be confusing and misunderstood by the receiver because they are not being interpreted with knowledge of the total context. Consider the woman who is unexpectedly praised by her employer and given a small merit raise. A bit bewildered, the employee nevertheless concludes that she must have been doing an outstanding job. A day later the employer asks the employee to do a personal favor that could seriously jeopardize the reputation of the employee. The employee may now interpret the praise and salary increase differently. Obstacles to effective communication may occur as a result or consequence of sending contradictory messages or disguised messages, experiencing encoding and decoding problems or difficulty in receiving messages, or because of hidden agendas.

Nurse-client relationship

As a *relationship*, the nurse-client relationship is more than just an *interaction*. An interaction refers to any contact between two people by which these individuals mutually influence each other. An interaction can be superficial, automatic, helpful, voluntary, or inconsistent. A relationship, however, implies a *series of experiences* between two people, and this experience is *mutually significant.*[33] Moreover, relationships develop over time.

Not all interactions between nurses and clients develop into relationships. Some of these contacts are one-time interactions. This does not imply that they are not therapeutic, as one interaction may be all that is needed by the individual. Often nurse-client interactions are interrupted by unexpected discharge or transfer of the client, change of nurse assignment, nurse vacations, and other circumstances that force premature terminations of relationships or abort the establishment of relationships.

A nurse-client relationship has as a specific purpose to identify the client's needs, to help the client promote his or her health, and to assist the client in preventing or coping with illness and suffering. The latter may include helping the client achieve a peaceful death. A nurse-client relationship differs from a social relationship in that it is designed to meet the needs of the client, not the nurse. A social relationship usually allows for focus on the needs of both persons. While nurse-client relationships may allow for the meeting of nurse needs, they are not designed to focus on the needs of the nurse per se. The nature of the nurse's obligation differs from that of a friend. Nurses are obligated to use their knowledge and skills to assess the client's health care needs and to provide quality nursing care. The very establishment and maintenance of the nurse-client relationship may be the nurse's responsibility alone, since illness may preclude the client from initiating interactions with the nurse.

The *structure* of the nurse-client relationship varies according to the client's needs, nurse and client goals, and the context of the relationship. Structuring an interaction involves making interactions predictable and purposeful; subsequent interactions can be tested, trust can begin to grow, and a relationship becomes established.

The *nature* of the nurse-client relationship varies with the context. The extended role of the nurse has increased the range of contexts within which nursing is practiced. Nursing is no longer practiced primarily within highly structured and controlled environments such as hospitals, where roles are usually well defined for both nurse and client. Nurses may be faced with defining their own employment roles for themselves, their employers, and their clients. Nurses who choose to open new roads for nursing need to be quite skillful at defining their roles in very open, undefined areas of practice. Nurses need to interpret their roles effectively to all people. Clients may be uncomfortable with nurse roles in new contexts, such as the nurse functioning as a primary care practitioner in areas where other health professionals are not readily accessible.

The *context* of the nurse-client relationship differs greatly in inpatient as opposed to outpatient settings. The individual is in a potentially better position to control his or her affairs and make independent decisions as an outpatient. Nurses in outpatient settings function increasingly as consultants and teachers, even though they may give direct physical and psychosocial care. The nurse who enters a client's home is a guest in that home, a status quite different from the status of the nurse who treats clients in a clinic or cares for the patient in a hospital. In the hospital, individuals often feel that they have little or no control and assume very dependent roles. This dependency can foster regression and interfere with physical and psychosocial recovery. Nurses strive to give clients maximal input into planning their care and controlling their immediate environment, for example, their room or area of a room. The issue of control over the environment is thus a significant factor in determining the nature of the nurse-client relationship in different contexts.

The nurse-client relationship involves acceptance of the client's needs, values, rights, and dignity. It is *dynamic* in that it is ever changing, requiring continuous assessment and evaluation. The nurse-client relationship utilizes both *affective* and *cognitive* levels of interaction, since the nurse teaches and provides physical and psychosocial care. The relationship is *time limited* and geared to the time needed to accomplish mutually defined goals. It is *honest* and *responsible*, requiring both nurse and individual to examine their behavior and be accountable to one another.

The nurse-client relationship is a series of *mutually significant* experiences with a specific purpose. It is *structured* to accomplish its purpose in varying contexts.

Phases in nurse-client relationships

A nurse-client relationship develops over time and proceeds through predictable phases or stages. These phases are not discrete but may overlap one another. They are sometimes omitted, and regression to an earlier phase may occur, especially at stressful points.

The basic phases of the nurse-client relationship—*establishment*, *development*, and *termination*—correspond roughly to the beginning, middle, and end of the nurse-client relationship.[44] Each phase will be explained in greater detail.

Establishment phase

As the establishment phase begins, the nurse and the client are strangers. Both nurse and client may be anxious. If anxiety is high, communication may be difficult. Client and nurse may have different ideas of what the client's problem is. There may be a great tendency on the part of the nurse to do something before adequate data collection is accomplished. The nurse may also be overcome with "rescue fantasies."

During the establishment phase the nurse establishes initial structure, making clear the purpose, timing, and context of the relationship. To establish predictability, it is necessary to define certain unknowns. The client needs to know who the nurse is, what the nurse's roles entail, the purpose of the interaction, how long the nurse will stay, if and how often the nurse will return, and where they will meet. Basically, the nurse states "who," "what," "when," "where," and "why", so that realistic mutual expectations can be established. The nurse can give the client a good indication of the probable duration of the relationship. In this way termination is begun from the onset, establishing a valuable foundation for the last phase. This initial structure need not be *announced* to the client but may be *discussed* with the client, while seeking his or her input and suggestions. Thus a climate of mutual respect and flexibility can be created.

The structure of the relationship will, of course, be open to revision when there is agreement by nurse and client that revision is needed. The degree of responsibility the nurse expects from the client in helping to establish and maintain the structure will vary according to the client's abilities and the context of the nurse-client relationship.

During the establishment phase the nurse and client together define the client's problem and set goals to work toward, with some time estimate in mind.

Some authors refer to this as *contracting* with the client. Such contracts are often verbal, but on occasion may be written. The purposes of contracting (or setting goals) with the client are to clarify or reinforce roles and purposes and to facilitate coordinated efforts toward common goals. Otherwise, nurse and client may work at odds, inefficiently, and with limited success toward different goals.

The nurse collects much data about the client during the establishment phase. It is the responsibility of the nurse to respect the client's dignity and rights and to ensure that this information will be treated confidentially. It is also the nurse's responsibility to protect the client's privacy while collecting data. This involves being mindful of others in the environment and being sensitive to the client's feelings and need for privacy.

The following illustrates an episode from the *establishment phase* of a nurse-client relationship.

EPISODE 1. Establishment phase

Mr. Winston, a 58-year-old married man, was admitted to a medical inpatient unit with the complaints of dyspnea, cough, rusty-colored sputum, and pain on inspiration. He is a manager of a local supermarket and had been working until a week ago. At this time he consulted his general practitioner, who told him he must be evaluated in the hospital for possible lung cancer. Mr. Winston is very apprehensive. Under pressure from his wife, he has just given up cigarettes. He is often found pacing in his room and wringing his hands.

Ms. Ames, R.N., met Mr. Winston yesterday when she admitted him to the unit. She and the physician collected appropriate admission data. Ms. Ames will be directly responsible for Mr. Winston's care during his hospitalization. She decides to set aside 15 minutes today to initiate the nurse-client relationship with Mr. Winston. The following interaction takes place.

Dialogue	Analysis
Ms. A.: (*stops at Mr. Winston's door and knocks*) Mr. Winston, I'll have some time to spend with you in about a half hour. I'd like to come in and talk with you for a few minutes then. Will you be in your room?	Ms. A. warns Mr. W. of her presence. She respects his privacy. She explains her plan to speak with him so he can cooperate if he chooses, allowing him some control of his environment. She makes herself predictable, setting up a structure to which she will adhere. This is useful groundwork for the establishment of trust. Yet Ms. A. does not explain the purpose of the interaction. Lack of this element of structure increases anxiety.
Mr. W.: (*pacing the room, frowning, sweating, and wringing his hands*) Where else do you suppose I'd be? (*gruffly and only*	Mr. W. lashes out verbally at Ms. A. He sounds irritated. He implies he has no choice over where he will be. He seems to have been angered

Dialogue	Analysis
glancing up) Do you have a thousand more questions to ask? I told you everything yesterday.	yesterday by all the data collection. He does not seem to want to engage in conversation with the nurse. Perhaps he sees no need to.
Ms. A.: (*feels defensive, attacked, angry*) No, Mr. Winston. I don't have any specific questions, but I wanted to talk with you about how we can work together toward your recovery while you're in the hospital.	Ms. A. does not feel that the attack is justified, so she wonders where the feelings originate. Perhaps if she had clarified her purpose from the start, Mr. W.'s response might have been different. Perhaps not. The nurse accepts Mr. W.'s anger without judgment or retaliation. She explains her purpose. If Mr. W. sees this purpose as fulfilling a need he has, then motivation for the relationship is established.
Mr. W.: (*no response*)	Mr. W. does not acknowledge Ms. A.'s messages. This leaves her feeling rejected.
Ms. A.: (*feels rejected*) I'll be back in a half hour to talk with you.	Ms. A. establishes a basis for predictability. She might have added, "We'll see how you feel then," giving him the chance to change his mind
Mr. W.: (*no response*)	Mr. W. may still be angry—unwilling to accept Ms. A.'s help. He may be testing to see if she cares enough to come despite his lack of enthusiasm.
(*One half hour later*)	
Ms. A.: (*knocks*) Mr. Winston?	It is very important that the nurse returns when she said she would. Ms. A. has been predictable. Again she respects his privacy by knocking.
Mr. W.: Yeah. (*head down, sitting on bed*) **Ms. A.:** May I come in to talk with you?	By asking his permission to talk, Ms. A. gives Mr. W. some sense of control over his immediate environment. Ms. A. remembers that she and the client are still strangers, even though Mr. W. has given her considerable data the day before.
Mr. W.: Umm… **Ms. A.:** (*sits in chair near door*) You seem upset today. I guess yesterday was long and tiring for you and you went for chest x-ray films this morning, right?	Mr. W. is noncommittal. Ms. A. sits at a distance from Mr. W., respecting his body space, allowing him time to get to know her. Ms. A. should have let Mr. W. know of her time limit of 15 minutes today. Ms. A. tries to explore other sources of Mr. W.'s angry feelings. She tries to show understanding of his experiences.

Dialogue	Analysis
Mr. W.: Yeah.	
Ms. A.: How did that go?	Ms. A. again attempts to explore other possible sources for Mr. W.'s feelings.
Mr. W.: Okay. Tomorrow they're gonna operate. *(with emphasis and looking fearful)*	Mr. W. reveals a source of fear.
Ms. A.: *(surprised)* Operate?	
Mr. W.: He said they're gonna take me to the operating room and do a bronchoscopy. What's that anyway? What does that mean—that I have cancer? *(looks worried)*	Mr. W. reveals his misunderstanding of the bronchoscopy. This seems to be his immediate problem.
Ms. A.: A bronchoscopy is a test, Mr. Winston. They are still doing tests to see what you do have. They do this particular test in the operating room. They are prepared there to give you anesthesia and deal with any unforeseen complications. Also, the doctor needs a dark room so he can better see the tissues lighted by the bronchoscope. Did your doctor explain the procedure of the test?	Ms. A. clarifies, explains, collects data about what he knows, and teaches Mr. W. about the procedure.
Mr. W.: Yes, he did. I can't tell you what he said, though.	Mr. W.'s response may indicate that the doctor did not explain well or that the client, being very anxious, used *selective inattention* and did not "hear" the explanation. This factor must always be considered in teaching the client.
Ms. A.: I will go with you for the procedure tomorrow if you like, Mr. Winston.	This is a supportive act designed to reduce Mr. W.'s anxiety.
Mr. W.: *(surprised)* You will?	
Ms. A.: Yes. Would you like that?	
Mr. W.: *(looking quite relieved)* Yes.	Mr. W.'s attitude toward Ms. A. has changed. This could be because his most pressing need was met. It could be because the nurse has accepted his anger and given of herself without requiring anything of him. Also, the client could feel that Ms. A. really cares and can meet some of his needs.

Dialogue	Analysis
Ms. A.: Mr. Winston, I will be responsible for your nursing care during the day shift—7:00 to 3:30—while you are in the hospital. I know this will be a difficult time for you while they are doing many diagnostic tests to find your problem.	Ms. A., taking advantage of her leverage, decides to introduce the nurse-client relationship idea. She defines the nature of the relationship. She says that she is responsible for his care while hs is in the hospital. This is not correct, as her responsibility for him is contingent on his being on this division. She inadvertently promises more than she can deliver.
Mr. W.: Umm . . .	
Ms. A.: You must be very worried about the possibility of having cancer and what can be done.	Ms. A. suggests that Mr. W. has needs and opens up the topic of his feelings about the prospects of cancer.
Mr. W.: Yes . . . it's awful to think about. God! What would I *do?* I had a buddy who died of cancer of the colon. His wife is a wreck now—torn up with grief.	When Mr. W. indicates readiness to explore this right now, Ms. A. has a conflict. Her hidden agenda was to suggest topics they could discuss at another time so as to establish a need for the nurse-client relationship and have Mr. W. agree to the relationship today.
Ms. A.: *(first silent, listening; then, wanting to get back to her task of defining the nurse-client relationship, she shakes her head sadly)* Yes, it is sad and scary to think about. Yet, we don't know for sure whether you have cancer.	Ms. A. tries to respond to his feelings but ends up cutting him off by saying that it isn't time to worry yet. Mr. W. may well have been confused as to her intent. She needs to get her hidden agenda on the table and tell him that she wants to discuss this with him—that today she has limited time but wants to set up times to get together regularly to discuss his problems, feelings, and so on. Then Mr. W. would understand why he was being cut off. Ms. A. could also have helped Mr. W. to see that having cancer does not necessarily mean you will die, as was the case with his friend.
Mr. W.: *(hesitantly)* No . . .	
Ms. A.: Mr. Winston, I'd like to set aside some time each day for us to talk about how things are going and what we can do together to make your stay here as comfortable as possible and . . . just to talk about how you are feeling and what your concerns are.	Now Ms. A. gets her hidden agenda out into the open by telling Mr. W. what she wants. She defines the purpose of the relationship.

Dialogue	Analysis
Mr. W.: Umhm. . .	
Ms. A.: I have some other patients, too, so it would be a good idea if we could agree on a regular time.	Ms. A. asks for Mr. W.'s input as to time.
Mr. W.: Well, yes, but I never know when they'll come take me for tests.	
Ms. A.: That's true. Perhaps we should leave it flexible but agree to save a half hour each day for talking together.	Ms. A. allows her client to participate in the defining of the structure of the relationship. Again, this allows Mr. W. more control and may increase his motivation to adhere to the structure.
Mr. W.: that's okay	
Ms. A.: Do you think we can talk here in your room without disturbing your roommate?	Ms. A. was trying indirectly to ask Mr. W. where he'd prefer to meet, thinking of his need for privacy and confidentiality. This intent did not come through. It sounded more like concern for his roommate. The nurse should have been more direct. She could ask, "Will you be comfortable talking here with your roommate nearby, or would you prefer the privacy of the office down the hall?"
Mr. W.: Oh, yes. He doesn't hear well.	
Ms. A.: Okay.	

Development phase

The next phase of the nurse-client relationship is the development phase. After initial structure has been defined by the client and nurse, both will test to determine the reliability of the other. Both may wonder: "Will he or she do what he or she said?" and "Does the other person refrain from doing what he or she said wouldn't be done?" Through the process of structuring, testing, and consistent behavior, the nurse and client develop mutual trust. The nurse begins to discover whether the client is committed to working on the defined problems and whether the client's part of the contract will be fulfilled. Trust takes time to develop and is established to varying degrees in nurse-client relationships. Without some degree of trust, it is extremely difficult to establish a working relationship. Testing need not be interpreted as an affront to the nurse, but as a chance for the nurse to establish credibility with this client.

The following illustrates an episode from the *development phase*.

EPISODE 2. Development phase

After 5 days of hospitalization, Mr. Winston has been diagnosed as having bronchogenic carcinoma. Ms. Ames has just learned this, and she is quite upset, having learned to like Mr. Winston very much in 5 days. She has supported him through several unpleasant diagnostic procedures, and he has come to rely on her.

Dialogue	Analysis
Mr. W.: (*smoking a cigarette*)	
Ms. A.: Hello, Mr. Winston. (*looks very disapproving*) I see you are smoking.	The nurse's opinion is communicated to Mr. W. nonverbally. She decides not to remind him that smoking is hazardous to his health, as she knows that he must be very upset just now. Thus she sets a priority of present needs.
Mr. W.: Hell, what difference does it make? The damage is done. (*laughs*)	Mr. W. indicates hopelessness and resignation. He may laugh instead of cry—a reaction formation.
Ms. A.: The damage?	Ms. A. prompts him to continue. Mr. W. here shows a typical verbal-nonverbal split. The feeling tone he communicates nonverbally does not coincide with the content of his verbal message. While the nonverbal is usually the truer message, as it is less subject to conscious control, it appears to be a defense here—an attempt to avoid facing his real feelings. Ms. A. infers this because she knows how worried Mr. W. has been about the possibility of cancer.
Mr. W.: The doctor just told me the tests proved I had a cancer . . . tumor . . . . I just couldn't believe it at first. (*laughs*) I kept asking him over . . . to repeat himself.	Mr. W. expresses his initial disbelief and shock, a characteristic initial defensive reaction to a crisis. This is a prime example of one of the obstacles to communication—difficulty receiving the message. The laugh seems to be defensive again, defending against his sadness and grief.
Ms. A.: I'm *very* sorry to hear you do have lung cancer, Mr. Winston.	Ms. A. expresses her own feelings about the diagnosis. Perhaps the nurse model will help Mr. W. express his feelings
Mr. W.: (*silence, smoking, inhaling deeply*)	Mr. W. cannot respond to Ms. A.'s feelings verbally but shows nonverbal signs of increasing anxiety. His sad feelings may be surfacing. Ms. A. allows him time to deal with sad feelings and the anxiety they engender.

Dialogue	Analysis
Ms. A.: *(pause)* What else did the doctor say?	Ms. A. tries to get him to focus on the facts to ascertain his understanding of his condition.
Mr. W.: He thinks he can get it all out if he operates. . . . He doesn't think it's spread.	
Ms. A.: That's hopeful.	Ms. A. comments on the hopeful, partly to reassure herself. She went into this interaction upset by just hearing the news herself, and she is beginning to "catch" Mr. W.'s fear.
Mr. W.: *(staring straight ahead, blank facial expression)* Umm . . .	Mr. W. is not reassured or cheered by the hope. He shows little feeling at all.
Ms. A.: Are you feeling kind of numb from hearing all of this?	Ms. A. interprets this as a defensive withdrawal of feelings to protect the self. She allows him to feel numb—or not to feel.
Mr. W.: Yes. *(pause)* I have to decide soon about surgery.	Ms. A. stays silent during the pause to communicate acceptance of his feelings and give him time to organize his thoughts. Mr. W. now brings up a pressing problem that is also on his mind and perhaps one reason why he hesitates to express his feelings. He may be afraid that his feelings will interfere with his ability to make a very important decision in a rational way.
Ms. A.: What are your thoughts about it now?	Ms. A. encourages him to think about his decision, since it is imminent.
Mr. W.: It's not without risk. I've got heart damage from a heart attack.	
Ms. A.: Yes.	
Mr. W.: But there's not a lot of choice. Untreated, he said I'd have less than a year. . . *(begins to cry)* . . . my poor wife. . .	Mr. W. reveals his concerns and fear of death. With this he begins to express his feelings, yet indicates that it is his wife that he's worried about. Perhaps he feels he should not grieve over his own potential loss, just his wife's. Perhaps he is grieving over the possible separation from his wife.
Ms. A.: *(feeling very sad and hopeless, reaches over and puts her hand on client's hand, pats it briefly)*	Ms. A. uses touch to communicate caring.
Mr. W.: I don't want to die yet. I wanted to work till I was 62, retire and enjoy life. *(crying)*	Mr. W. uses the past tense, "wanted," as if his wishes were no longer possible.

Dialogue	Analysis
Ms. A.: *(weakly)* It is still possible, perhaps.	Ms. A. picks up on this but is not convinced. She is beginning to experience the vacuum-sweeper syndrome. She is losing her objectivity and perspective.
Mr. W.: I feel like I have a death sentence, that I'm rotting inside. Who knows what they'll find when they cut in. Oh, it would be awful to rot away slowly.	Mr. W. continues to express how badly he sees things. He needs the nurse to accept that he sees such a black picture but does not need her to be convinced by him that it *is* necessarily that black.
Ms. A.: *(also feeling hopeless, stays silent; feels like crying; feels afraid for Mr. W.; feels helpless; wants to comfort him; cannot find words; anxiety level very high)* When will your wife be in?	Ms. A. is becoming more distressed; her anxiety level is increasing. She has difficulty coping with her feelings of despair, hopelessness, and helplessness, so she changes the subject.
Mr. W.: *(first silence, then muttering)* Oh God, I don't know—about an hour I guess. What am I gonna tell her?	
Ms. A.: Mr. Winston, I will be back shortly so we can talk about this some more—so much has happened today. *(leaves)*	Ms. A. finally removes herself from the situation, recognizing she cannot meet Mr. W.'s needs until she meets her own. She tries not to do this in a rejecting way, indicating her intent to return and continue the conversation. Considering her needs at the time, she ended the conversation as well as she could. She was able to return later, after she had her feelings under better control, and help the client and is wife with their feelings.

During the development phase the client will begin to depend on the nurse to some degree. The nurse's response to this dependency is crucial to the relationship. The nurse must assess the degree of dependency necessary to help the individual meet the goals of the nurse-client relationship. Allowing too much dependency may frighten the client or lead to a conclusion that the nurse is not confident of the person's ability to be independent. Not allowing dependency may interfere with the development of trust and may lead the individual to conclude that the nurse does not want to help.

During the development phases nurse and client get to know one another better. While they began to set goals in the establishment phase, they now formulate plans around their goals, putting the plans into action and evaluating the results. As the nurse becomes more involved with the client it is often easy to get caught up in the individual's problems. The nurse may begin to experience the individual's feelings of hopelessness and helplessness. This might be termed the *vacuum-sweeper syndrome,* assimilating all the client's feelings with loss of professional objectivity.

When this occurs, it is necessary that objectivity be reestablished. This is accomplished by the nurse's examining his or her own feelings and trying to understand their origins, examining his or her own needs and how these needs are influencing behavior, and revalidating the abilities and limitations of the client.

Development can be a rewarding phase, as the client trusts enough to dare to try new approaches to problem solving. Yet both nurse and client cannot expect all progress and no regression. There will be setbacks in the growth process. Nurse and client should discuss this as they plan, so that they are prepared for problems in implementation. Nurses can help clients learn the problem-solving process so that clients can better solve problems after termination of the relationship.

The following illustrates an episode from the *termination phase.*

EPISODE 3. Termination phase

Ms. A. returned yesterday afternoon and had a long talk with Mr. W. and his wife. They discussed the diagnosis, prognosis, surgery, and their feelings. Mr. W. seemed to be deciding that he should have the surgery. The doctor was to speak with him this morning.

Dialogue	Analysis
Ms. A.: Good morning, Mr. Winston.	
Mr. W.: Good morning, Ms. Ames. *(smiling)* Well, I've decided to have the surgery.	Mr. W. seems proud of his decision. He announces it to Ms. A. immediately.
Ms. A.: You have! *(smiling)* You look as if you feel good about your decision.	Ms. A. acknowledges his message that he is pleased with the decision; that is, she acknowledges his verbal and his nonverbal messages.
Mr. W.: Yes. Can't say I'm not scared, but if there's a possibility of a cure, I guess I should risk it.	Mr. W. admits that not all the scared feelings are gone and that he still has needs.
Ms. A.: I'm glad to hear you are feeling optimistic!	Ms. A. puts a value on his optimism by praising it. This could cause problems. Mr. W. may feel that optimism is more acceptable than fear and hope-

Dialogue	Analysis
	lessness and therefore may be reluctant to express these latter feelings again. He may feel badly about having been so dejected yesterday.
Mr. W.: Yes, I feel better today. I was pretty down yesterday.	This may indicate that Mr. W. does feel bad about being so dejected yesterday.
Ms. A.: So was I. I feel better today too. *(smiles and pats his shoulder; sits down on chair; thinks about client's transfer)* Tell me, did your doctor say when you might have surgery?	Ms. A. alludes to her own "down" feelings yesterday, which is helpful in that Mr. W. may have received that impression from her nonverbal messages yesterday anyway. However, Ms. A. must be careful not to leave Mr. W. feeling guilty for having upset her. Ms. A. uses nonverbal communication to convey her warm feelings. Feelings are more often communicated nonverbally. Ms. A. begins to prepare Mr. W. for termination of their relationship.
Mr. W.: Well, he said that if I felt sure, he could schedule me for this week. I told him to go ahead. I guess the sooner I get the operation, the better it will be.	
Ms. A.: *(feeling very sad to see him leave the unit)* I wish I could go with you, Mr. Winston.	
Mr. W.: Why, what do you mean?	Mr. W. does not seem aware that his surgery will signal the end of the relationship with Ms. A.
Ms. A.: That I would have liked to have gone with you to surgery and stayed with you in the Recovery Room.	Ms. A. is able to express feelings of sadness at Mr. W.'s leaving.
Mr. W.: *(shocked)* You won't be there?	Mr. W. is shocked. He has not expected the termination.
Ms. A.: No. You will be going to a surgical unit for your operation.	Ms. A. assumes he knows the hospital policy of first assigning nurses to divisions and then assigning nurses to clients. Assumptions should be validated with the client.
Mr. W.: I know, but I thought you were my nurse for my whole hospitalization. Wasn't that what you said in the beginning?	Mr. W. reveals the source of his confusion. This also indicates the importance he attached to the initial structure, which is why it is so crucial to structure carefully.

Dialogue	Analysis
Ms. A.: (recalling her initial structure) Yes, I think I did, Mr. Winston. What I meant was during your stay on this unit . . . .I'm sorry that I didn't make that clear. (feeling very guilty, afraid client will lose trust)	Ms. A. admits her mistake and clarifies the structure. Ms. A.'s feelings of guilt over her mistake are increased by her natural feelings of guilt at termination, especially termination without resolution.
Mr. W.: (mumbling) Oh it's okay. (louder) It's just that you've been through a lot with me already, and I'd like to have you there when I go under.	Mr. W. sounds angry. He says he still needs her. His problems are not yet resolved. He indicates his trust in her based on the development of their relationship. His tone communicates an appeal to Ms. A. to come with him anyway.
Ms. A.: (feeling very guilty, like she is abandoning Mr. W., and wondering how he will do without her) Perhaps I could go up and speak to the nurse who will be responsible for your care on the surgical unit. She may want to come down and talk with you before your transfer.	Ms. A.'s guilt leads her to wonder if Mr. W. can manage without her, though cognitively she knows that he can and that another nurse will assist him. Both her guilt and fears and positive concern for Mr. W. motivate her to offer to identify her substitute, which does facilitate continuity of care.
Mr. W.: I guess so. That would be nice. (doctor arrives and tells Mr. W. that a bed is ready for him on the surgical unit and that he will be taken there directly; the situation forces abrupt termination, as is often the case in the hospital; Mr. W's surgery is scheduled for 2 days later)	Ms. A. does not deal with his angry feelings at all. She might have said, "I can see you are upset with me, Mr. W., which is understandable. You expected I would stay with you until you were ready to go home. I'm sorry I misled you." She could then allow him time to respond with his feelings. Feelings are more likely to be left undiscussed and unresolved when the relationship is terminated abruptly. There is not time for resolution of feelings.
Ms. A.: Well, I guess we will not have much time to say our goodbyes.	
Mr. W.: No. Things happen in a hurry around here.	
Ms. A.: Mr. Winston, I've enjoyed getting to know you, and I think you are a fine person.	Ms. A. begins to summarize the relationship briefly and to share her feelings—tasks of termination.
Mr. W.: Why, thank you, Ms. Ames. You've helped me through a lot and have always been willing to listen when I got upset, and I've been a lot of that	Mr. W. is quite able to take part in this process, despite his disappointment and lack of preparation for the termination. He gives Ms. A. quite specific feedback about what
lately. It was nice knowing you were my nurse. You explained things to me— let me know what was going on. That helped.	he liked about the relationship.
Ms. A.: I'm glad it helped. You've been through a lot in a short time. You've coped very well. The surgery won't be easy, but I know you'll cope with that too.	Ms. A. attempts to help him put the relationship in a time perspective—what he's already come through and what he has ahead of him. This is a variation of integration—another task of termination. It is not appropriate at this time to focus on integrating this experience into Mr. W.'s total life experience. Yet this will be crucial after surgery, before hospital discharge.
Mr. W.: Yes.	
Ms. A.: I'll try to get up to visit you when I can during my shift. But I will be a visitor then. You will have another nurse. (feels guilty that she cannot go with Mr. W.)	Ms. A. explains that the nurse-client relationship is terminated, even though she will see the client again. She redefines the nature of the relationship. She might anticipate having to be more specific about what she can and cannot do in the new relationship when she visits Mr. W. later. He may test the new structure. For example, he might say, "My nurse is busy now, Ms. Ames. Would you speak to my doctor about getting me a laxative?" Ms. A. will need to think ahead about how she will define the limits of her new role and establish mutual expectations. Again she will need to be consistent and predictable. As she has already established trust, this process may be shortened. However, it will not be eliminated, as the relationship is new.
Mr. W.: (smiles) I hope she's like you. (feels very sad to leave Ms. A.)	
Ms. A.: Thank you, Mr. W. I hope things work out well for you.	Mr. W.'s new nurse should anticipate that Mr. W. will need to discuss his feelings about terminating with Ms. A. before he is ready to reengage in a new nurse-client relationship. This is one of the side effects of termination without resolution—it interferes, even if briefly, with establishment of subsequent relationships.

Termination phase

Termination, the last phase of the nurse-client relationship, occurs logically when the nurse and client agree that they have accomplished the goals of the relationship. *Termination with resolution* occurs when the client becomes more independent. Both the actual need and the felt need for resolution by the nurse are less. Resolution is a freeing process, freeing the client to manage again without a nurse.[44] In termination with resolution, both the client and the nurse feel that the time has come to end the relationship, even though it may be difficult to give up the relationship. The degree of mutual involvement experienced influences the depth of pain and anxiety felt at separation.

The nurse and client conjointly evaluate the total relationship and the learning that has occurred. Nurses can assist clients to transfer this learning to other aspects of their lives as applicable, helping them to integrate their experiences into their general life experiences. If clients see their learning as isolated events out of the context of general life experiences, they will have difficulty utilizing the learning that has occurred. Nurses and clients benefit from sharing their feelings at termination. Although this may be difficult and uncomfortable, it provides valuable feedback to both nurse and client.

Sometimes, even if feelings are strong, defenses may shelter individuals from their feelings. This may be the case when a client cannot understand why he does not feel sad when he expected he would. Another manifestation of defense is minimizing the importance of the relationship. It may be easier to give up a relationship if its meaning is denied.

Feelings at termination are generally mixed. There may be relief that the relationship is over; joy in the new, more independent position; sadness or anger at giving up the comfortable security of the predictable relationship; pride in accomplishment of goals; or fear and arousal of old insecurities. The latter may produce temporary regressions before termination of the nurse-client relationship.

Unfortunately *termination* often occurs *without resolution*. This occurs when the nurse or client leaves the relationship before resolution; for example, the nurse is transferred, the client is discharged or dies, the client or nurse voluntarily withdraws because of dissatisfaction with the relationship or some other factor. These situations arouse all the feelings of termination and, in addition, frustration. If circumstances of termination are beyond nurse or client control, it is hard to know where to direct the feelings of frustration or anger. Feelings are often displaced; for example, the nurse may become unjustifiably angry with the family of the client if the client dies. Rejection and anger on the part of the person who is "left," guilt on the part of the person "leaving," and perhaps relief on both parts may also occur in this type of termination.

If possible, the nurse and client should summarize and evaluate the relationship, recognizing and dealing with their feelings as time permits. In general, the nurse terminates the relationship by accomplishing all the tasks of the phase that are appropriate.

The nurse in the nurse-client relationship

As should be clear from the discussion of the nurse-client relationship, *one of the nurse's most valuable tools is the self. The self is the part of the health care system over which the nurse has the most control*. The concept of therapeutic use of self is not new to nursing. It refers to the nurse's ability to help the client by the way the nurse interacts and relates as opposed to using such tools as medications and treatments. The nurse consciously makes use of knowledge, communication skills, and a unique personality to bring about a desired client outcome. This outcome is therapeutic when it helps individuals cope with their problems and alleviates their suffering.

To use the self therapeutically the nurse needs a knowledge and awareness of self, the ability to reflect on and analyze own and client behavior, and the ability to alter one's behavior when evaluation indicates the need to do so. The second and third tasks are obviously facilitated by the accomplishment of the first task.

Increasing one's self-awareness is not always easy or pleasant, since not every insight will please the self. Sometimes a person cannot even admit to certain of his or her own characteristics. Sullivan's "good-me," "bad-me," and "not-me" conception of the self serves to elucidate this. The "good-me" is the self a person likes and prefers to identify with, the ideal self. The "bad me" is the part of the self the person has learned to dislike, the part of which he or she is ashamed. The "not me" is the part of the self the person considers to be so bad that he or she cannot admit to it.[46]

One of the purposes of increasing self-awareness is to decrease the percentage of the "not me" so that the person sees more of the total self, thus making it possible to change this part of the self. In order to bring more "not me" into awareness, the person needs an adequate percentage of "good me." Bringing into awareness areas of the self which were so unacceptable that they were blocked out of awareness (not me) increases anxiety. Increasing the percentage of "good me" enables the person to cope with the anxiety generated by recognizing the "not me" and may require the help of another person who can serve as a listener-counselor.

The process of increasing self-awareness takes time and patience; it involves focusing on needs, knowledge and skills, self-concept, roles, beliefs and values, and feelings. Each of these will be discussed in more detail.

Needs

As stated earlier, the nurse-client relationship allows for the meeting of nurse needs but is not designed to *focus* on the nurse's needs, since the primary reason for the nurse-client relationship is to focus on the client's needs. If the nurse happens to meet some needs as a result of helping the client meet his or her needs, there is no problem. Problems do arise when the nurse's needs begin to interfere with helping the client meet his or her needs, especially when this happens outside of the nurse's awareness. A nurse who needs to be needed (loved) may inadvertently encourage inappropriate dependency in the client, whose need is for increased independence (self-esteem and self-actualization). The nurse who needs to be praised may be effectively manipulated by the thankful but demanding client. To reduce such problems to a minimum, it is necessary that nurses gain awareness of their own needs and satisfy them as much as possible outside the nurse-client relationship.

Knowledge and skills

The knowledge required to practice nursing is vast and ever increasing. Nurses cannot acquire in their professional schools all of the knowledge they will need in practice. To keep abreast they must have the desire and ability to continue to learn independently as long as they practice.

Nurses need to assess honestly their level of knowledge and ability. If nurses have learned to value their clients and to practice nursing with integrity, they will make sure that their knowledge and skills are sufficient to the needs of their clients. Of course, practitioners can actively seek to increase their knowledge and skills by engaging the assistance and consultation of colleagues to ensure the quality of their care.

Self-concept: personal and professional

"What kind of person am I?" The self-concept is an important variable in determining the nurse's behavior. For example, nurses with very negative self-concepts will not be able to utilize effectively their knowledge and skills because they lack self-confidence. They may spend considerable energy trying to present a desirable picture of themselves to others. Nurses with positive self-images may find it easier to be closer to others and to share more of themselves.

Both the client and the nurse have their own personal self-concepts, which are largely products of their past experiences. The self-concept is formed early in life and is based on reflected appraisals of significant others as well as the person's own estimate of himself or herself.[46] A self-concept is not static, but fluctuates with daily experiences. In the healthy person, however, it is relatively stable, with smaller fluctuations than those of the more vulnerable or less healthy person. A stable self-concept that is realistic and generally positive is perhaps the nurse's most valuable resource. It sustains the nurse through problems, disappointments, and failures and allows the nurse to use more energy for learning and self-growth.

Closely related to the personal self-concept is the professional self-concept—the evaluation of one's performance in the professional role. What is my professional ideal, and how do I measure up to that ideal? Nurses' ideas about the role of the nurse undergo much growth and development during their basic educational preparation. As nurses begin to bring their ideal closer to reality, they might begin to discover that they do not like all of their clients, that some of their clients do not want their help, or that they are unable to help some of their clients. Often, nurses then begin to identify and define their strengths, their limitations, and their potential for growth.

Striking a good balance between reality and the ideal is crucial for the nurse, especially during the first year of employment, a period termed reality shock.[21] Many nurses withdraw from active nursing practice because they cannot sustain a very idealistic professional self-concept in the reality of initial employment. They lack the supervision and support systems necessary to sustain their positive professional self-concept as it is undergoing a stressful test. However, most nurses do survive and continue in nursing.

Roles

The roles nurses assume in their work depend on the context of the health care system, the clients' abilities and concept of their client role, and the nurses' abilities and concept of the nurse role. Nurses' personalities influence the types of roles they assume most comfortably or successfully. The reticent nurse who desires to please others and who prefers to avoid conflict rather than problem solve probably will not function well as a team leader, whereas the more assertive nurse may function well as a team leader. It is important to remember that new behavior patterns can be learned.

Just as the nurse has certain expectations of self in

the nurse role (such as to be kind, patient, understanding, sensitive, and fair), the nurse has certain expectations of the client in the client role (such as to be appreciative, able to define own problem, to help in own care, and to want to get well). It is very helpful for nurses to examine just what they expect from their clients, how the clients meet these expectations, how this affects abilities to function in the nurse role, and their feelings in this regard.

Beliefs and values

One's expectations of self and others are influenced strongly by one's beliefs and values. Culture has a decided impact on one's beliefs and values. Common values in the United States include the value of work, individuality, social welfare, status, material wealth, and youth. Since values often conflict, priorities must be established. A nurse who values life as well as individual freedom must struggle with conflicting values when working with a suicidal client.

The nurse's social class also influences values and beliefs. Health workers typically come from the middle class and are often accused of imposing their middle-class values on clients. A community health nurse committed to zero population growth might urge a postpartum client to consider tubal ligation, although the woman may desire a third child.

Nurses can become aware of their own beliefs and values and be alert to the ways in which these influence clinical inferences and behavior. It is necessary to evaluate one's own value system as well as to gain an appreciation of and respect for the values of others.

Feelings

All of the variables mentioned (needs, knowledge and skills, self-concept, roles, and beliefs and values) influence the nurse's feelings. Nurses can examine their feelings in general (e.g., happy, excited, disappointed, depressed, angry) as well as their feelings about particular clients (e.g., like them or feel uneasy about them). Awareness and acceptance of feelings can facilitate a nurse's understanding of how feelings may color perceptions. Acknowledging these feelings should increase the nurse's objectivity.

The nurse's increased self-awareness results in an increased capacity to understand the client. Since the nurse's perception is influenced by past experience, knowledge, needs, and expectations, it follows that *the more the nurse knows about these aspects of the self, the greater can be the reliability of the nurse's inferences about the client*. In systems terms, the more var-

iables that can be defined in the communication network (the nurse, message, channel, and context), the easier it will be to identify what aspects of the systems' process are caused by the undefined variable (the client). If an interpersonal problem arises in the nurse-client relationship, the nurse will be better able to differentiate between the parts played by the client and the nurse.

One's knowledge of self is not akin to knowledge of a fixed variable. An individual is dynamic and changing and, it is hoped, ever growing. Therefore knowledge of the self is not static. Personality patterns, typical defense mechanisms, areas of perceptual blindness, and areas of vulnerability in self-concept can be anticipated, and their effects on the nurse-client relationship can be recognized more quickly with increased self-awareness.

The client in the nurse-client relationship

Like nurses, clients have needs, knowledge and skills, self-concepts, roles, beliefs and values, and feelings. These client variables influence clients' behavior and nurses' behavior.

Needs

One of the first steps in the nursing process is assessment of client needs. Clients cannot always verbalize what their needs are, but they may indicate their needs by their behavior. The nurse collects data and makes inferences, which can then be validated with the client. The client who is *unusually* irritable, complaining, unhappy, and sarcastic could be expressing fear of his or her diagnosis, prognosis, treatment, decreased mobility, or any number of things. The client may be unaware of his or her fear, being preoccupied with the symptoms as opposed to his or her actual problem. The nurse might attempt to clarify the problem source by saying, "Mr. Jones, you seem out of sorts this morning. Are you worried about the outcome of your tests?" This gives the client a chance to reflect on his feelings and validate (or refute) the nurse's inference. In general, the nurse's goal is to define the individual's needs and help him or her meet them, not necessarily to increase the client's insight into how needs influence his or her behavior, although this may be a therapeutic side effect. (When working with clients with special communication problems, the nurse's goal may be to increase the client's insight into his or her behavior.)

Knowledge and skills

Clients differ in their knowledge levels—knowledge of the health care system, of daily hygiene, of illnesses, of treatments, of diets, and of medications. The client's present level of knowledge is assessed before teaching begins. Increased knowledge about illness can serve to increase *or decrease* the client's ability to cope with illness. Lack of knowledge of an illness usually will increase a client's anxiety because of fear of the unknown. This varies with the client. Therefore the nurse assesses carefully what to teach the client and when to teach it. Learning goals for the client need to be clear and related directly to the promotion of the client's health. For example, the nurse preparing to do preoperative teaching will need to assess the client's readiness for learning. This will include (1) assessing the client's anxiety, (2) determining the present level of knowledge, (3) deciding on any further knowledge the client needs, (4) determining the best time for teaching, (5) choosing the best method, (6) teaching, and (7) evaluating the teaching process, the client's level of learning, and any observable effect of the learning on the client. The same process applies to the client's learning of skills, such as the person who is newly diagnosed as being diabetic learning to give his or her own insulin.

The nurse is cognizant of the client's coping abilities, present as well as *potential*. The client's abilities and limitations may well differ from preillness status and recovery status. In some instances illness accentuates limitations. In others, crisis may increase the client's capabilities.

Self-concept

The client's self-concept will influence the ability to request and accept help from another person. A client who has a poor self-concept may feel unworthy of attention and decline to make requests. Thus such a client may deny his or her own needs or attempt to meet them without seeking help. This may consume unnecessarily the energy needed for recovery. The client whose self-concept is threatened by an illness (and its implications for changes in the person's life-style) may be demanding of help, may stubbornly refuse help, or may accept help reluctantly. Clients often fear the dependency of forced immobility, especially if their former independence contributed strongly to their positive self-concepts. Clients may also fear change of body image because of surgery or loss of bodily function. These clients need help accepting their altered bodies while still maintaining self-esteem. Other strengths can be identified and developed to help compensate for the loss, thus broadening the basis of self-esteem.

Roles

The client may have a preconceived notion of the "client role." For instance, a client may expect to present a problem to the nurse and expect the nurse to take care of it. The idea of mutual problem solving and the enlisting of the nurse as a resource person may be foreign to the client, so he or she may resist interacting with the nurse in this manner. Clarification of this issue will avert many problems if the nurse can learn about the client's role perceptions by clarifying mutual expectations during the establishment phase of the nurse-client relationship.

Beliefs and values

The client's beliefs and values influence the reactions to illness and treatment. A client could have the religious belief that God is using illness as a means of bringing the client into contact with a hospital roommate whose needs are great. Thus the client may have images of self as an instrument of God and illness as a means to God's ends. There is nothing to be gained by the nurse's countering the client's beliefs, especially if the client's beliefs do not interfere with meeting the client's other needs (or with meeting the roommate's needs). Even when the client's beliefs interfere with meeting health needs, such as might be the case when a Christian Scientist refuses emergency treatment, the client has the right to refuse individual treatment. Other values that influence the client's response to illness include independence, youth, productivity, family life, and socioeconomic status. The nurse can be instrumental in helping the client define how illness will affect the individual's life-style and values and how to make the best adjustment, considering the realities of the situation.

Feelings

The client's feelings are influenced by all of the previously mentioned factors. The client has feelings about illness, prognosis, treatment, the health care facility, the health team members, the family, and so on. The client's feelings about the nurse may stem from past experiences with nurses or attitudes about the health professions. These feelings will color perception of the nurse-client relationship and attitudes about cooperation. The client may displace feelings about his or her general situation onto the nurse because the nurse is a convenient target. The client may scream at the nurse upon learning that the exploratory laparotomy uncovered cancerous tissue.

Even when feelings seem irrational, the nurse tries to accept them and seeks to help the client express and resolve them. The nurse's judgment and sense of timing are crucial. The nurse would not encourage a previously anxious client to explore feelings immediately before going to the operating room. The nurse would instead seek to alleviate anxiety by reassuring and staying with the client, using touch, structuring, and listening. However, the nurse recognizes this as a stopgap measure and would try to discuss the client's feelings after the operation and initial recovery. In this way the client is given an opportunity to review feelings in a less threatening situation and to understand their origin. This is valuable preparation for future crises that may arouse similar feelings.

Conclusion

Nurses very often engage in short-term nurse-client relationships, especially in inpatient medical and surgical divisions. While short-term relationships have their frustrations, they can be highly rewarding for client and nurse. Hospitalization can be a very stressful experience for clients. To have a nurse interested enough to become therapeutically involved can have a major impact on the client's physical and psychologic status. Nurses can remember that they are their own best tools, especially when some might be inclined to say, "There is nothing I can do." Nursing involves, most crucially, the ability to comfort, to lend strength, and to help clients cope with problems, including terminal illness and death. Realizing one's potential in therapeutic use of self requires time, experience, and flexibility, and the ability to assume for the moment the other person's perspective, without completely losing one's own. Sharing another person's fears, sorrows, joys, and hopes has a humbling effect that most health workers find therapeutic for themselves.

REFERENCES AND SELECTED READINGS
Contemporary

1. Bird, B.: Talking with patients, ed. 2, Philadelphia, 1973, J.B. Lippincott Co.
2. Birdwhistell, R.L.: Kinesics and context: essays on body motion communication, New York, 1970, Ballantine Books, Inc.
3. *Bothamley, V.A.: Communication and the ventilated patient, Nurs. Times 71:628-630, 1975.
4. *Brill, N.: Working with people: the helping process, Philadelphia, 1973, J.B. Lippincott Co.

5. *Carlson, C.E., coordinator: Behavioral concepts and nursing intervention, ed. 2, Philadelphia, 1978, J.B. Lippincott Co.
6. *Carter, F.M.: Psychosocial nursing, ed. 2, New York, 1976, Macmillan Publishing Co., Inc.
7. Chapman, J.E., and Chapman, H.H.: Behavior and health care: a humanistic helping process, St. Louis, 1975, The C.V. Mosby Co.
8. Dance, F.E.X.: The "concept" of communication, J. Commun. 20:201-210, 1970.
9. Darnell, D.K., and Brockriede, W.: Persons communicating, Englewood Cliffs, N.J., 1976, Prentice-Hall, Inc.
10. *Dorroh, T.L.: Between patient and health worker, New York, 1974, McGraw-Hill Book Co.
11. *Eisenberg, A.M.: Living communication, Englewood Cliffs, N.J., 1975, Prentice-Hall, Inc.
12. Finkelman, A.: Commitment and responsibility in the therapeutic relationship, J. Psychiatr. Nurs. 13:10-14, 1975.
13. Fisher, S.: Body consciousness: you are what you feel, Englewood Cliffs, N.J., 1973, Prentice-Hall, Inc.
14. Florer, R.M.: Nurse-patient relationships in general nursing, Nurs. Mirror 136:41-43, 1973.
15. *Francis, G., and Munjas, B.: Manual of social psychologic assessment, New York, 1976, Appleton-Century-Crofts.
16. *Garnett, A.: Interviewing: its principles and methods, ed. 2, New York, 1972, Family Service Association of America.
17. *Hagerty, B.K.: Denial isn't all bad: sometimes not facing facts is helpful, Nurs. '80 10(10):58-60, 1980.
18. Hall, E.T.: The silent language, New York, 1973, Anchor Books.
19. Hollister, W.G., and Edgerton, J.W.: Teaching relationship: building skills, Am. J. Public Health 64:41-46, 1974.
20. *Johnson, M.N.: Self-disclosure: a variable in the client relationship, J. Psychiatr. Nurs. 18(1):17-20, 1980.
21. Kramer, M.: Reality shock: why nurses leave nursing, St. Louis, 1974, The C.V. Mosby Co.
22. McCann, J.: Termination of the psychotherapeutic relationship, J. Psychiatr. Nurs. 17(10):37-46, 1979.
23. Mercer, L.S., and O'Connor, P.: Fundamental skills in the nurse-patient relationship: a programmed text, ed. 2, Philadelphia, 1974, W.B. Saunders Co.
24. Mitchell, P.H.: Concepts basic to nursing, ed. 3, New York, 1981, McGraw-Hill Book Co.
25. *O'Brien, M.J.: Communications and relationships in nursing, ed. 2, St. Louis, 1978, The C.V. Mosby Co.
26. *Pasquali, E.: East meets West: a transcultural aspect of the nurse-patient relationship, J. Psychiatr. Nurs. 12:20-22, 1974.
27. Pearce, W.B., and Sharp, S.M.: Self-disclosing communication, J. Commun. 23:409-425, 1973.
28. *Rawnsley, M.M.: Toward a conceptual base for affective nursing, Nurs. Outlook 28:244-247, 1980.
29. Scheflen, A.E.: How behavior means, New York, 1974, Anchor Books.
30. Smoyak, S.: A strategy for change: nurse and client ethnicity and its effect upon interaction, no. M-27, Kansas City, Mo., 1979, ANA Publication Commission on Human Rights.
31. Spiegel, J.P.: Messages of the body, New York, 1974, The Free Press.
32. Ticho, E.A.: Donald Winnicott, Martin Buber and the theory of personal relationship, Psychiatry 37:240-253, 1974.
33. *Travelbee, J.: Interpersonal aspects of nursing, ed. 2, Philadelphia, 1971, F.A. Davis Co.
34. Ujhely, G.B.: Current technological advances and the nurse-patient relationship, J. N.Y. State Nurses Assoc. 5:25-28, 1974.
35. Wallston, K.A., and Wallston, B.S.: Nurses' decisions to listen to patients, Nurs. Res. 24:16-22, 1975.
36. Zefron, L.J.: The history of the laying-on of hands in nursing, Nurs. Forum 14:350-363, 1975.

*References preceded by an asterisk are particularly well suited for student reading.

Classic

37. Buber, M.: I and thou, ed. 2, New York, 1958, Charles Scribner's Sons. (Translated by R.G. Smith.)
38. *Carson, R.C.: Interaction concepts of personality, Chicago, 1969, Aldine Publishing Co.
39. Goffman, E.: Strategic interaction, Philadelphia, 1969, University of Pennsylvania Press.
40. Goffman, E.: Interaction ritual: essays on face-to-face behavior, New York, 1967, Doubleday & Co., Inc.
41. Laing, R.D., Phillipson, H., and Lee, A.R.: Interpersonal perception: a theory and a method of research, New York, 1966, Harper & Row, Publishers.
42. Maslow, A.: Motivation and personality, New York, 1969, Harper & Row, Publishers.
43. Minter, R.L.: A denotative and connotative study in communication, J. Commun. **18:**26-36, 1968.
44. Peplau, H.E.: Interpersonal relations in nursing, New York, 1952, G.P. Putnam's Sons.
45. Ruesch, J., and Bateson, G.: Communication: the social matrix of psychiatry, New York, 1968, W.W. Norton & Co., Inc.
46. Sullivan, H.S.: The interpersonal theory of psychiatry, New York, 1953, W.W. Norton & Co., Inc.

AUDIOVISUAL RESOURCE

*Concept Media: Nurse-patient interaction series, slide cassettes, Costa Mesa, Calif., Concept Media.

CHAPTER 10

THE PROBLEM-ORIENTED SYSTEM

GRETCHEN KRAMER DERY

Professional nursing practice uses a problem-solving process, commonly referred to intraprofessionally as the "nursing process." This problem-solving process originated in the scientific method that has been used successfully by many professions for decades.

The purpose of this chapter is to explore a specific method of recording client health and illness data within the context of the problem-solving method. Problem-oriented record keeping is not merely a mechanism for preserving specific data, although this is indeed part of the system. The problem-oriented system stipulates a defined and structured manner of procuring and communicating information and will ultimately influence and mold the system of health care provided.

Within the traditional hospital setting, nurses, physicians, social workers, physical therapists, and others have labored to provide illness care for those in need. There has been a tendency for the care provided to be fragmented, divided, and delivered within the context of departments or professions within the bureaucratic setting. Even with the best intentions, there is a lack of communication between health and illness care personnel. Nurses identify and work with nursing problems, the physician defines medical problems, and other groups define problems from other perspectives. There has recently been a trend to attempt to define health and illness care problems from the client's perspective, since in fact the problems *are* the client's. The problem-oriented system allows different professions to identify, from their particular frame of reference, problems relating to the client's past, present, and future situation. It additionally allows the client and professionals involved in the client's care to plan and problem solve together. Because of increasing complexity and specialization, health and illness professionals must develop some understanding of each other's skills and abilities, learn to value the contributions of differing professions, and develop an effective method of communication.

The nursing process consists of three steps: assessing, intervening, and evaluation (see Chapter 7). The problem-oriented system is easily incorporated into the nursing process and complements the traditional problem-solving approach to client care.[46] Its use can facilitate understanding and application of the nursing process by adding specific form to parts of the process.[42] As specific components of the problem-oriented record are presented and discussed, articulation with the nursing process will be highlighted.

Each profession tends to develop its own language, which facilitates intraprofessional communication, but this can be a formidable barrier to interprofessional communication. Unless this communication barrier is minimized, it may be impossible for the client or other professionals to understand what is being said.

Traditional charting reflects a separatist philosophy. It is "source oriented"; that is, information is recorded according to where it originated. Nurses write on "nurse' notes" or "progress notes"; physicians write on physicians' "order sheets" and "progress notes"; radiologists report on "x-ray sheets"; the laboratory personnel report in the "lab report" section. This system illustrates the communication barriers between and among disciplines.[66]

Nursing has used both written and verbal mechanisms for communication but has relied more heavily on verbal means.[9] Verbal communication has some drawbacks as a primary mode of communication: it can be time consuming because of frequent repetition; it is not highly organized; it cannot easily be retrieved; it is more subject to misinterpretation; and it has no value in the courtroom situation.[2]

Is there a need for written records? In the hospital setting the increasing complexity of care, the increasing amount of data collected about each patient, and the increasing number of personnel caring for patients necessitates written means of communication. Written records serve to communicate information, document the patient's status, allow for measurement of change, record interventions that might account for changes in the client's status, describe what is done in a way that makes the logic apparent to others, serve as a means for storing information, and allow for auditing.[65]

To a great extent, nursing notes have been an exercise in futility. Nurses have in the past been socialized not to analyze the data collected but merely to act as a vehicle for data transmission, especially in the written record. Most notations were preceded by qualifiers, giving the observation, but not risking an inference. A typical situation might involve a patient grimacing, groaning, moaning, and holding her operative side. The nurse's note would read: "Ms. Thompson is holding her operative site and moaning and groaning." To say that the patient was in pain was considered paramount to making a medical diagnosis and was not encouraged.

Thus charting became a routinized task and suffered from many shortcomings. Notes were disorganized, disconnected, long, random, dissociated, and written in terms of specific events that occurred rather than an overall scheme or plan. Additionally, they were repetitious and unused by other professional colleagues. Attempts were made to minimize the repetition by charting only significant data and omitting all other data; thus practically no charting was done. Perhaps the most significant difficulty was, and still is, the fact that nurses' notes reflected written response *only* to delegated medical interventions rather than nursing interventions. Such things as administering prescribed medications and carrying out prescribed treatments were and are well documented, but *nursing* functions were not.

The nursing care plan, a close ally to the nursing note, suffers from another set of difficulties, and there has been a growing disenchantment with its use.[42] Common criticisms of nursing care plans include the following complaints: they are limited in physical size, they are unused, they do not individualize care, and they are too difficult to write and maintain. There are two features of nursing care plans that are problematic. The nursing care plan is often separate from the remainder of the patient's record (i.e., in a Kardex) and is relatively inaccessible or unused rather than visible and available to other health and illness professionals. Data can only be useful if it can be used. The second feature is that nursing care plans are written in pencil, updated by erasures, and destroyed when the patient is discharged from the institution. The nursing care plan never becomes a permanent part of the patient's record, and one cannot retrospectively use the data for a subsequent admission or for evaluation of outcomes of nursing care. Thus nursing care plans are disposable and transient—certainly not the material from which accountability is made. However, saying that nursing care plans may not be the best tool to accomplish

client-care planning does in no way negate the value of the nursing process per se.[42]

If the nursing care plan and traditional mechanisms for charting have been ineffective methods for communication, what are the alternatives? One alternative, based specifically on the writings of Weed, advocates the use of the "problem-oriented" record.[62] The problem-oriented record is a method of record keeping that requires several ongoing processes to be operant. The components of the problem-oriented record include a data base, problem list, initial plans, progress notes, flow sheets, and periodic summaries (including a discharge summary for institutions that do not provide for ongoing health and illness care for clients). All professionals contributing to health or illness care for clients can successfully utilize this method, and its use is not restricted to hospitals or institutions. The method has been used by health and illness care professionals in a variety of settings including federally operated hospitals, community hospitals,[30] physicians' practices, and public health agencies.[29] The method encourages a multidisciplinary approach, which has led to use by nurses, social workers, dietitians, physical therapists, pharmacists, and physicians.[37,45] The problem-oriented record has been successfully utilized in a variety of health and illness care settings.[22,48,50]

In the discussion of the problem-oriented record, each of the component parts will be defined and discussed, and the relationship between the problem-oriented record and the nursing process will be detailed. Because of the nature of the illness problems presented within this text, the example used to illustrate these component parts will be one exemplifying the stressors commonly found in a medical-surgical hospital setting.

Data base

The data base is the information gathered about a client and is one part of the assessment component of the nursing process. The data base is acquired *before* the identification of client problems begins. It consists of all information necessary to begin to determine the client's health or illness status. A data base provides a nurse with information that will serve as a beginning point for planning nursing interventions. Those concerned with the delivery of specified care to a selected population need to identify the components of the data base before the method is instituted.[53] Weed suggests that the initial data base be as complete as possible and only be constrained by three factors: expense, discomfort, and possible hazard.[62] Gathering a data base generally includes three basic processes: interviewing, physical examination, and laboratory tests.

One frequently asked question is "Who collects the data base?" The answer may vary from situation to situation, but in the hospital setting it seems imperative that a minumum of four people be involved. These four people would include employees from the *admitting office* (to help with insurance and other very real necessities involved in the process of hospitalization in the United States), the *physician* (who must be involved to a greater or lesser extent to ascertain that the information needed to make a medical diagnosis is available), and a *nurse* (to ascertain that the information needed to make a nursing diagnosis is available). For a hospitalized patient this is the minimum involvement. In addition, the *patient* (or other substitute) should be *actively* involved in the gathering of the data base.[66] In many situations in the community the private practitioner (nurse or physician) and the client will be the primary persons involved.

Perhaps the most important issue is not necessarily who collects the data base. In some hospitals nurse practitioners collect the majority of the data base, and in some the task is more equally shared. The crucial issue is *what* information *is* gathered, and whether it is sufficient for the professions involved to formulate a problem list.

Different groups or institutions have a variety of forms or mechanisms that assist in the data-collection process. In some instances a one-to-one interview is done, in some instances a computer "interviews" a client, and in some instances the patient simply responds to a paper and pencil tool. In the majority of cases several of the above options are combined.

A hospital-defined data base usually contains three major categories of information: the patient's *history* (including a review of systems), a *physical examination,* and *laboratory findings*. The patient's history has several components: (1) reason for contact, (2) patient's profile, (3) family illness history, (4) patient's present illness history, (5) patient's past illness history, and (6) patient's current health practices. The patient's significant others, such as spouse, family, or friends, can help supply the history component of the data base.

The *reason for contact*, the first part of the defined data base, is generally simply stated in the patient's own words. Throughout the following discussion, an example of the component parts of a problem-oriented record for a patient entering a small community hospital will be used for illustration.

Date: July 1, 1982

I. PATIENT HISTORY
A. Reason for contact
"I have been having stomach pains and upsets."

The second section of the patient history, the *pa-

tient profile, might include data related to name, age, sex, race, occupation, place of residence, admitting physician, number of children and their state of health, marital history, significant others, financial matters, living conditions, education, dietary habits, interests, future plans, fears, handicaps, and response to illness.

B. Patient profile
Ms. Melissa Smith is a 45-year-old white woman. She presently does not work outside the home but was an elementary school teacher. She has not been actively involved in teaching for 12 years. She lives in the immediate suburban area. Dr. Mary Jane Long is her admitting physician. Ms. Smith has daughters, ages 21 and 23. Both children are in college out of state.

Ms. Smith has been recently widowed (6 months ago). She has no present financial difficulties and owns her own four-bedroom home. Her late husband's insurance provides her with a continued adequate income to maintain her present life-style, and she possesses comprehensive health insurance. Money had been secured for the children's education before her husband's death. She feels she has "no financial concerns at the present." Ms. Smith is a college graduate. She is a "Protestant," but "religion does not serve a significant function in my life."

She spends an "average day" in the following manner: She wakes up early but arises around 10:00 AM. She does not eat breakfast or lunch, but watches TV or reads. She takes a walk in the afternoon or goes to the movies occasionally. She fixes supper, generally convenience foods, retires about 1:00 AM, but has trouble "falling asleep and never feels rested." She used to be interested in growing plants, needlework, and painting landscapes. She states she "has not felt like doing anything" since her husband's death. She "has no future plans, finds it enough of a challenge to get through one day at a time." She voices no fears at the present time, but is "concerned about her stomach upsets." She has not been hospitalized since her last childbirth experience and does not know what the "rules and regulations" are for this hospital.

Ms. Smith has no visible handicaps.

A *family illness history* could include data about ages and illness or cause of death in parents, siblings, and children. Some information about diseases such as diabetes, heart disease, hypertension, stroke, renal disease, cancer, arthritis, tuberculosis, drug or alcohol abuse, epilepsy, and mental disorders is usually collected. This gives information that could be related to genetic transmission or exposure or problems that have increased "familial occurrence."

C. Family illness history
Parents

Mother:	Age 68—living—arthritis
Father:	Age 70—deceased—coronary heart disease

Siblings
Brother: Age 45—living and well
Children
Daughter: Age 23—living and well
Daughter: Age 21—living and well

The *current illness status* generally includes information related to each current illness problem perceived by the client. Data are gathered around such parameters as onset, progression, signs and symptoms, any attempts by the client to treat the problem, and the client's understanding of the problem.

D. Current illness status

Ms. Smith states that she has had an "upset stomach" for the past 3 months. It began gradually, but now she feels nauseated, especially on arising. She vomits occasionally, that is, four or five times a week. This almost always occurs in the morning. She has noticed a recent change in her bowel habits alternating between diarrhea and constipation. This has occurred in the last 2 weeks. Also during the last 2 weeks she has been having "burning" pain in her stomach. She has been taking aspirin for her stomach pain, 0.64 g, three or four times daily. She feels that she is "not well" and states that "it may be due to the fact that I have not been taking care of myself lately."

The patient's *past illness history* generally includes any significant illness episodes, a description of all illnesses requiring hospitalization, any major surgical procedures, previous developmental problems, and information related to foreign travel, which may be implicated in the etiology of certain diseases such as malaria that are not commonly found in the United States.

E. Past illness history

Ms. Smith has had the following childhood diseases: mumps, rubella, and chicken pox. No noted sequelae. She has been hospitalized twice for childbirth, both uncomplicated. She has had no major surgical procedures, and has not traveled out of the country in the past 5 years. Ms. Smith is in her middle-adult period and appears to have had an unremarkable growth and development until the present period.

The *current health practices* section describes health maintenance or preventative health behaviors undertaken by the patient either to increase the level of wellness or prevent illness episodes.

F. Current health practices

Ms. Smith has had her personal and family primary health care needs met by Dr. Long for the past 10 years. She has a physical examination, including Pap smear, every year. She performs a monthly self-breast examination. She sees the dentist routinely every 6 months.

The next section of most hospital-based patient histories in the *review of systems*. The review of systems is the patient's verbal or written response to an orderly systematic group of questions primarily related to the body's biosystems. The specific details of a review of systems may vary, but the overall characteristics are generally similar from setting to setting. The reader will note that although the general topics included in the review of systems in Chapter 8 are similar to these, the specific bits of data vary.

II. SYSTEM REVIEW

Please check (√) "yes" or "no." If "yes," give further data in "Comments" section.

A. General	Yes	No	Comments
1. Weight loss or gain	√		Past 3 to 6 months (20 lb)
2. Fever or chills		√	
3. Weakness		√	
4. Malaise	√		Past 3 months

B. Integument—skin	Yes	No	Comments
1. Color changes		√	
2. Pigmentation		√	
3. Temperature changes		√	
4. Dryness		√	
5. Bruising		√	
6. Pruritus		√	
7. Scaling		√	
8. Abnormal perspiration		√	

Integument—hair	Yes	No	Comments
1. Color			
2. Texture		√	
3. Distribution		√	
4. Abnormal growth or loss		√	

Integument—nails	Yes	No	Comments
1. Color changes		√	
2. Brittleness		√	
3. Ridging		√	
4. Pitting		√	
5. Curvature		√	

C. Head	Yes	No	Comments
1. Headache		√	
2. Migraine		√	
3. Trauma		√	
4. Syncope		√	
5. Seizures		√	

D. Eyes	Yes	No	Comments
1. Pain		√	
2. Discharge		√	
3. Visual loss		√	
4. Color blindness		√	
5. Trauma		√	
6. Diplopia		√	

D. Eyes—cont'd	Yes	No	Comments
7. Glasses or contacts (date of refraction)	✓		

E. Ears

	Yes	No	Comments
1. Pain		✓	
2. Discharge		✓	
3. Hearing changes		✓	
4. Vertigo		✓	
5. Tinnitus		✓	

F. Nose

	Yes	No	Comments
1. Pain		✓	
2. Epistaxis		✓	
3. Discharge		✓	
4. Obstruction		✓	

G. Throat

	Yes	No	Comments
1. Pain		✓	
2. Soreness		✓	
3. Voice changes		✓	
4. Hoarseness		✓	

H. Mouth

	Yes	No	Comments
1. Sore throat		✓	
2. Sore tongue		✓	
3. Bleeding gums		✓	
4. Dentures		✓	

I. Neck

	Yes	No	Comments
1. Swelling		✓	
2. Pain		✓	
3. Limitation of motion		✓	
4. Enlargement of lymph nodes		✓	

J. Breasts

	Yes	No	Comments
1. Lumps		✓	
2. Pain or tenderness		✓	
3. Nipple discharge		✓	
4. Gynecomastia		✓	
5. Nipple change		✓	
6. Normal development and lactation history	✓		Breast-fed both children for 12-month period
7. Dimples		✓	

K. Respiratory system

	Yes	No	Comments
1. Cough		✓	
2. Sputum		✓	
3. Dyspnea		✓	
4. Shortness of breath		✓	
5. Orthopnea		✓	
6. Wheezing		✓	
7. Pain		✓	
8. Hemoptysis		✓	

L. Cardiovascular system

	Yes	No	Comments
1. Claudication		✓	
2. Palpitations		✓	

L. Cardiovascular system	Yes	No	Comments
3. Edema		✓	
4. Chest pain/discomfort		✓	
5. Tachycardia		✓	
6. Irregularities of rhythm		✓	

M. Gastrointestinal system

	Yes	No	Comments
1. Change in appetite	✓		Decreased appetite since husband's death—past 6 months
2. Dysphagia		✓	
3. Heartburn		✓	
4. Nausea and vomiting	✓		Especially in early morning and with increased frequency
5. Hematemesis		✓	
6. Melena		✓	
7. Jaundice		✓	
8. Food intolerance		✓	
9. Abdominal pain	✓		Burning in epigastrium
10. Changes in bowel habits	✓		Alternating diarrhea and constipation

N. Genitourinary system

	Yes	No	Comments
1. Frequency		✓	
2. Nocturia		✓	
3. Dysuria		✓	
4. Incontinence		✓	
5. Polyuria		✓	
6. Hematuria		✓	
7. Pyuria		✓	
8. Urinary retention		✓	
9. Passage of stones		✓	

O. Genitourinary system—menstruation

Last menstrual period: 5/20/81
Gravida/para/abortion: 2/2/0
Age at onset of menses: 12
Last Pap smear: _____ Positive __✓__ Negative

	Yes	No	Comments
1. Abnormal menses		✓	
2. Vaginal discharge		✓	
3. Dyspareunia		✓	
4. Pelvic pain		✓	
5. Itching		✓	
6. Burning		✓	
7. Menorrhagia		✓	
8. Metrorrhagia		✓	
9. Contraception	✓		Has diaphragm
10. Menopause		✓	

P. Musculoskeletal system

	Yes	No	Comments
1. Backache		✓	
2. Joint pain		✓	
3. Stiffness		✓	

P. **Musculoskeletal system—cont'd**

	Yes	No	Comments
4. Joint swelling		✓	
5. Muscle weakness		✓	

Q. **Neurologic system**

Cranial nerves

	Yes	No	Comments
1. Changes in smell (I)		✓	
2. Changes in vision (II, III, IV, VI)		✓	
3. Orofacial parathesias or chewing difficulties (V)		✓	
4. Facial weakness or taste disturbances (VII)		✓	
5. Disturbances in hearing or equilibrium (VIII)		✓	
6. Disturbances in speech, swallowing, and taste (IX, X, XII)		✓	
7. Limitation in neck motion (XI)		✓	

Sensory nerves

	Yes	No	Comments
1. Paresthesia		✓	
2. Hyperesthesia		✓	
3. Hypesthesia		✓	
4. Anesthesia		✓	

Motor nerves

	Yes	No	Comments
1. Paralysis		✓	
2. Atrophy		✓	
3. Involuntary movements		✓	
4. Incoordination		✓	
5. Gait disturbances		✓	
6. Convulsions		✓	

R. **Mental status**

	Yes	No	Comments
1. Memory change		✓	
2. Sleep disturbance	✓		As in history
3. Crying spells	✓		Cries easily—almost every day
4. Anxiety		✓	
5. Depression	✓		Feels "down" almost all the time
6. Hallucinations		✓	
7. Social withdrawal	✓		"Doesn't fit in well" without husband
8. Difficulties with sex life	✓		No interest in sex since husband's death

The physical examination makes up the second major part of the data base. It can be performed in a manner similar to the review of systems, that is, either a head-to-toe or body-systems fashion. The extent and depth of the physical examination will also vary from setting to setting, based on the types of services offered.

III. **Physical examination**

A. **General**

1. Height:	5'8''
2. Weight:	115 lb (Normal weight: 135 lb)
3. Temperature:	37° C (98.6° F)
4. Pulse:	84
5. Blood pressure:	100/80
6. Respiration:	14

Check all examined areas normal or abnormal. If abnormal, please explain under "Comments."

B. **Integument**

	Normal	Abnormal	Comments
1. Turgor	✓		
2. Lesions	✓		
3. Hair	✓		
4. Nails	✓		

C. **Head**

	Normal	Abnormal	Comments
1. Skull	✓		
2. Scalp	✓		

D. **Eyes**

	Normal	Abnormal	Comments
1. Vision (Snellen test)	✓		
2. Extraocular movements	✓		
3. Eyelids	✓		
4. Conjunctivae	✓		
5. Cornea	✓		
6. Sclera	✓		
7. Lens			
8. Pupils	✓		
9. Fundi	✓		

E. **Ears**

	Normal	Abnormal	Comments
1. Auditory acuity	✓		
2. External ear	✓		
3. Canals, drums	✓		

F. **Nose**

	Normal	Abnormal	Comments
1. External	✓		
2. Mucosa	✓		
3. Septum	✓		
4. Turbinates	✓		

G. **Mouth and throat**

	Normal	Abnormal	Comments
1. Lips	✓		
2. Breath	✓		
3. Teeth, gums	✓		
4. Tongue	✓		
5. Mucosa	✓		
6. Tonsils	✓		
7. Pharynx	✓		

G. Mouth and throat	Normal	Abnormal	Comments
8. Speech	✓		
9. Salivary glands	✓		

H. Neck

1. Range of motion	✓		
2. Appearance	✓		
3. Trachea	✓		
4. Thyroid	✓		
5. Masses	✓		

I. Breasts

1. Masses	✓		
2. Nipples	✓		

J. Nodes

1. Cervical	✓		
2. Axillary	✓		
3. Inguinal	✓		

K. Chest

1. Configuration of thorax	✓		
2. Respiratory movements	✓		
3. Percussion	✓		
4. Inspiratory breath sounds	✓		
5. Expiratory breath sounds	✓		

L. Vascular

1. Carotid pulse	✓		
2. Radial pulse	✓		
3. Femoral pulse	✓		
4. Posterior tibial pulse	✓		
5. Dorsal pedal pulse	✓		
6. Popliteal pulse	✓		
7. Neck veins	✓		
8. Peripheral veins	✓		

M. Heart

1. Impulse	✓		
2. Palpation	✓		
3. Rhythm	✓		
4. Auscultation	✓		

N. Abdomen

1. Abdominal wall	✓		
2. Distention	✓		
3. Tenderness		✓	Abdominal tenderness noted over epigastrium
4. Liver	✓		

N. Abdomen—cont'd	Normal	Abnormal	Comments
5. Spleen	✓		
6. Kidneys	✓		
7. Other masses	✓		
8. Bowel sounds	✓		

O. Rectal

1. Anus and sphincter	✓		
2. Rectum	✓		
3. Prostate	N/A	N/A	

P. Genitalia

Male

1. Penis	N/A	N/A	
2. Scrotum	N/A	N/A	
3. Testes	N/A	N/A	
4. Epididymis	N/A	N/A	
5. Inguinal canal	N/A	N/A	

Female

6. External genitalia	✓		
7. Urethra	✓		
8. Vagina	✓		
9. Cervix	✓		
10. Uterus	✓		
11. Adnexa	✓		

Q. Extremities

1. Muscles	✓		
2. Joints	✓		
3. Edema	✓		
4. Ambulation	✓		
5. Coordination	✓		
6. Amputation; deformities	✓		

R. Spine

1. Configuration	✓		
2. Mobility	✓		
3. Tenderness	✓		

S. Neurologic system

1. Cranial nerves	✓		
2. Gait	✓		
3. Biceps reflex	✓		
4. Triceps reflex	✓		
5. Patellar reflex	✓		
6. Achilles reflex	✓		
7. Plantar response	✓		
8. Peripheral nerves	✓		
9. Sensory	✓		

T. Mental status

1. Orientation	✓		
2. Memory	✓		
3. Mood		✓	Has been very "depressed" since husband's death,

T. Mental status—cont'd   Normal   Abnormal   Comments

	Normal	Abnormal	Comments
			which coincided with youngest daughter's departure for college
4. Consciousness	√		

The last section of most data bases for hospitalized patients is *routine admission laboratory work*. In most settings this will minimally include a urinalysis and a complete blood count.

IV. Laboratory reports

CBC and urinalysis to laboratory.

Master problem list

The next section of a problem-oriented record is the *master problem list*. The problems are derived from the data base, and the more adequate the data base, the more comprehensive the problem list.

The formulation of problems is similar to the assessment phase of the nursing process. The problems are not just a numbering of information contained in the data base, but a conclusion or decision resulting after careful investigation, examination, and analysis of the data.[6]

Problems can be defined as anything that causes concern to the client or those professionals providing care.[65] They can include any situation or condition in which a person requires help to maintain or regain a state of health or achieve a peaceful death.[6]

Problems can include physical abnormalities, symptoms, physical findings, laboratory abnormalities, psychologic disequilibrium, socioeconomic difficulties, demographic variables, past illnesses, potential problems, or incomplete data.[4]

Every problem identified may not be treated, but it can be identified and examined in relation to its effect on the patient's situation. Since the focus of the patient and the providers of illness care can differ, what constitutes a problem may differ, depending on the perspective involved. But all problems that belong on the problem list *are* the patient's problems, and it is gen-

erally important when several professions are involved with providing care for an individual that their perspective be shared *interprofessionally* and *with the patient*. This helps to avoid having those involved working in isolation and at differing purposes. Thus all involved are responsible for identifying and adding problems to the problem list.

Several general categories of problems can be defined. *Active problems* are those problems that require attention or treatment at the present time. *Inactive or resolved problems* are those that have caused previous significant difficulties and may recur or lead to other problems.[62] Minor problems of short duration can be identified as *temporary problems*. Later, if they prove to be of significant magnitude, they can be added to the permanent problem list. *Potential problems* are those that have an increased likelihood of occurring because of the characteristics and number of factors present in the situation.

Problems should be worded at the level of sophistication that the data support. Problems are not defined as a probable or possible medical diagnosis. Until the medical diagnosis is confirmed, the problem is stated in

MASTER PROBLEM LIST

Active problems	Date of onset	Date of resolution	Inactive or resolved problems
Gastrointestinal symptoms	3/1/82		
Nausea and vomiting	3/1/82		
Decreased appetite	3/1/82		
Burning pain in stomach	1/1/82		
Change in bowel habits	1/1/82		
Weight loss	3/1/82		
Sleep difficulties and lethargy	3/1/82		
Lack of future orientation	3/1/82		
Social withdrawal	3/1/82		
Poor dietary habits	3/1/82		

terms reflecting the health team's level of certainty. Once the diagnosis is confirmed, it is entered as a problem. For an active or current problem, the date of onset should be recorded, and the date of resolution should be recorded for resolved or inactive problems.

One format for recording problems is to title, number, and list permanent active and inactive problems at the front of the chart on a master problem list. However, some persons feel numbering problems quickly becomes cumbersome in multiproblem patients, and they prefer to list problems by title alone.

The problem list must be dynamic if it is to serve its purpose of structuring communication between professionals. It is updated by any professional member of the patient care team as new information is obtained, new problems are identified, and as active problems become inactive.[53]

Plan

The third major section of the problem-oriented record is the initial plan. The initial plan is formulated through the description and assessment of each problem and a proposed action to be taken in relation to the problem. These actions are usually described as diagnostic, therapeutic, or educational. An additional category of actions is seeking further information. This part of the problem-oriented process incorporates aspects from the assessment and intervention phases of the nursing process.

The initial plan is written on the progress note. The "SOAP" format is used in formulating the initial and all

INITIAL PLAN

Date: July 1, 1982 (admission day)

Problem 1: GI symptoms

S: Early morning nausea and vomiting; lack of appetite, burning pain in stomach; weight loss; bowel function changes

O: Tenderness in epigastric area on palpation; thin

A: Gastrointestinal distress

P: Regular diet with no spicy foods; record types and amounts of foods eaten; weigh daily in early morning before breakfast; note frequency, color, and consistency of stools; Maalox, 1 oz, q 2 to 3 hr prn for burning; stool for guaiac; upper and lower GI series

Problem 2: Sleep difficulties and lethargy

S: Unable to sleep well at night, feels tired all day

O: Looks and acts lethargic

A: Inadequate sleep

P: Talk further with patient about her usual sleep patterns and routines; try to keep active during daytime; observe but do not awaken at night; schedule interventions for time when patient is awake

Problem 3: Lack of future plans or goals

S: "It seems as if I am no use to anyone any more—no one needs me."

O: None

A: Situational crisis—husband's death and daughter's leaving home; still grieving loss of husband and children

P: Let patient verbalize her feelings about her present situation and changes it has made in her life-style; assess her readiness or ability and motivation to explore new directions for her life

Problem 4: Social withdrawal

S: "My husband's gone, my daughters don't need me. I don't fit in with my friends anymore. I tried to go out when my friends invited me—but they are couples and I am alone."

O: Tearful, sad

A: Separation from "significant others"; self-isolation

P: Allow one consistent nurse to care for Ms. Smith to allow for establishment of solid relationship; in light of problems 2 and 3, might consider the nurse clinician for this

Problem 5: Poor dietary habits

S: Eats only one meal per day, usually convenience foods

O: None

A: May be secondary to problem 1, lack of appetite, or may be result of other factors

P: Schedule interview with dietitian sometime this week for purpose of gathering more data

Temporary problem: Unfamiliar with hospital routine

S: "I don't know the rules and regulations."

O: Appears to be anxious lest she do something "against the rules"

A: None

P: Thorough orientation today regarding visiting hours, mealtimes, physical layout, access to other areas of hospital, and her upcoming activities

M.J. Long, M.D.
J. Gelein, R.N., Primary Nurse

subsequent plans. The "S" represents subjective data and is a description of the problem from the patient's view. The "O" represents objective data and includes information gathered from inspection, percussion, auscultation, and laboratory and other tests. The "A" represents assessment and is the analysis of the subjective and objective components. The "P" represents the plan and can include diagnostic plans, therapeutic plans, and patient education plans.

From this point forward all subsequent data are recorded in the body of the record under the specific related problem. Thus all further assessment and interventions will be related to the appropriate problem in the progress note or will be the stimulus for the definition of a new problem.

Laboratory work, medications, diet, activity modification, and procedures all are related to the specific problems. Unchanged unremarkable events are not recorded in the problem-oriented system.

The initial statement of plans establishes the need for further data and the type of treatment to be given. Nursing and medical and other plans need to be complementary, and plans of the involved professions should be integrated and written as notes under the specific problems.[66] The patient's profile and the complete problem list need to be reviewed before any discipline makes plans for a single problem. Plans made without understanding of overall problems and the patient's life-style are likely to be ineffective, even though they might seem appropriate when related to a single isolated problem.[62]

Progress notes

After the initial plan for each problem is formulated and recorded, the next section for the problem-oriented record is what has been traditionally called "progress notes." In the problem-oriented record there are three types of progress notes: the *narrative note*, the *flow sheet*, and the *discharge summary*.

Each *narrative note* should relate directly to a problem and should be titled (or numbered) accordingly. Progress notes can be used to record the patient's progress, resolution of old problems, and development of new problems.[44] Progress notes follow the same SOAP format as the initial plan.[44] Nurses, social workers, physical therapists, physicians, and all other professions providing care for the client record their data in relation to a specific problem and in sequence with all other data related to that problem. Thus the helping professions assume an integrated role in the solution of patient problems, and each profession avoids establishing the kind of identity that permits or encourages the possibility of dealing with problems out of context.

Narrative notes do not need to be made on each problem daily, only when indicated. Two problems can be combined in a progress note, as long as it is clearly noted that this is being done. If this happens frequently, it may indicate that the two problems are actually subparts of another problem. And it is not always necessary to use each step of the SOAP formula with each note.

Progress notes contain the ongoing elements of evaluation—the final phase of the nursing process. As plans for particular problems are executed, the ongoing results should be visible in the data collected in the progress notes.

Flow sheets, the second form of the progress note, are used to record significant data in a tabular or graphic manner. Flow sheets are predesigned and variable. They help to facilitate interpretation of rapidly changing interrelated variables. Flow sheets also serve as a place to record everyday activities, such as mouth care, bathing, and ambulation, that need documentation but require no other comment (p. 141).

Flow sheets are a permanent part of the patient's record. All entries on the sheet are signed and dated. They have several advantages. Specifically, they prevent overlooking important items of information. Once designed, they cause a series of actions to be completed automatically rather than requiring a person to plan each action. They may be the only record for certain rapidly changing variables. They save a tremendous amount of time trying to unravel and assemble disorganized data. Flow sheets can be used as an evaluative tool for certain interventions by outlining results, and they allow for some consistency of data gathered from patient to patient by allowing analysis of data for more than one patient. They can also provide structure for new persons giving care to the patient.

Common examples of flow sheets are vital sign sheets, intake and output records, medication sheets, diabetic records, and treatment records. In some situations (i.e., ICU, CCU) a great variety of data is kept on a very large flow sheet that shows several interrelated variables for 15-minute time spans (see Chapter 74). Thus such parameters as drugs, intravenous fluids, laboratory work, vital signs, and urinary output can be easily visualized almost on a minute-to-minute basis, and changes in one variable can be related to changes in others.

The third and final section of the progress note is the *discharge planning summary*. Discharge summary notes from the hospital are merely final narrative notes that relate the overall assessment of progress while hospitalized and plans for the patient's continued follow-up or referral. The SOAP format provides a systematic method for reviewing what was identified (subjective

PROGRESS NOTES

2nd hospital day
Monday: 2 PM

Problem: Unfamiliar with hospital routine

S: "I feel more comfortable here now—I know visiting hours, mealtimes, physicians' visiting times, and the plans for the next 2 days."

O: Nervous movement of hands; anxious look of face

A: Appears more comfortable with hospitalization routine; still somewhat apprehensive

P: Continue to be alert for need to inform patient of varying aspects of her care

J. Gelein, R.N., Primary Nurse

2nd hospital day
Monday: 8 PM

Problem: Sleep difficulties and lethargy

S: Unable to sleep last night, even after two sleeping pills

O: Patient awake all night, even after repeated dose of Seconal; had not napped during day

A: May be due to first night in strange place; seems to have unusual tolerance to sedatives

P: Talk again with patient about current medications being taken; observe again this evening for response

N. Yates, R.N.

2nd hospital day
Monday: 8 PM

New problem: Anxious, irritable, hallucinating

S: "I am very nervous. I hear my daughters. I need a drink."

O: Patient's face and body tense; answers questions in tense manner; hearing voices of persons not present; blood pressure 114/110, pulse 128, respirations 26; nauseated and vomiting

A: Possible drug withdrawal

P: 1. Notify Dr. Long immediately; request prn sedation orders
2. Observe for changes (↑) in V.S.

3. Establish a relaxed atmosphere—prevent excessive fear and anxiety
   a. Medicate patient per physician's orders
   b. Remain with patient
   c. Assure patient that "voices" are only her mind playing tricks on her
   d. Keep the room well lighted and avoid shadows
   e. Keep out loud noises and unnecessary traffic
   f. Calm patient by lowering voice, speaking slowly, and moving deliberately
   g. Remain firm with patient and assure her that she can be responsible for her behavior
   h. Encourage patient to drink 8 oz. fluid (juices) to maintain blood sugar and electrolytes
   i. Offer small high-protein snacks q 4 hr after nausea and vomiting abate
   j. Encourage ambulation with assistance q 1 to 2 hr to bathroom; change position in bed frequently
   k. Use touch as in backrubs for comfort
   l. Frequent mouth care
   m. Seizure precautions

P. Craig, R.N.

2nd hospital day
Monday: 11 PM

Problem: Anxious; irritable; hallucinating; increase in blood pressure, pulse, and respirations; and nausea and vomiting

S: Hallucinating, feels very nervous, admits to drinking 5 to 10 drinks per day since husband died

O: Agitated; increased blood pressure, pulse, and respirations; vomiting

A: Acute alcohol withdrawal

P: 1. Chlordiazepoxide (Librium), 75-100 mg IV stat, then q 2-3 h prn, not to exceed 300 mg in 24 hr; may give PO after nausea subsides
2. Thiamine, 100 mg IM daily × 3 days
3. Magnesium sulfate 50% solution, 2 ml IM q 12 hr × 3 days
4. Stat chemistry 6, amylase, and blood alcohol level

M.J. Long, M.D.

FLOW SHEET

Name: Ms. Smith
Date:

Parameter observed	3rd hospital day		4th hospital day		5th hospital day
	Hour				
	9 PM	11 PM	1 AM	3 AM	4 PM
Vital signs					
Blood pressure	140/100	130/100	128/98	130/100	110/80
Pulse	126	120	118	122	80
Respirations	26	24	24	22	16
Fluid intake					
PO	Refused	120 ml OJ	Refused	150 ml	240 ml OJ
IV	—	—			
Protein snacks	Nauseated	Nauseated		One cheese cracker	Peanut butter crackers
Fluid output					
Urine	—	100 ml			400 ml
Emesis	50 ml	—	—	200 ml	
Other	—	—	—	100 ml	—
Patient's behavior state	Hearing voices; moving nervously about in bed	Somewhat calmer; still having auditory hallucinations	Unchanged	Increased restlessness; visual hallucinations	Some tremulousness; embarrassed
Activity	Position changed	Up with assistance to bathroom	Turned	Turned	Up walking and in chair
Sedation	Chlordiazepoxide, 100 mg IM	—		—	—
Mouth care	Done	Done	Done	Done	Self-care
	P. Craig, R.N.	P. Craig, R.N.	J. Fugare, R.N.	N. Yates, R.N.	J. Gelein, R.N.

and objective), what interventions were planned (assessment), and what must still be done (plan). The discharge summary should be problem oriented and should include only that information from the data base necessary for ongoing management of a problem.[62] Discharge summaries can help facilitate continuity of care from the hospital to other agencies or professionals who will continue to provide care for the patient or client (p. 142).

Conclusion

Are there advantages to using the problem-oriented process? Are there disadvantages? What threats to professionals are implicit in this process? And what, if any, are the long-term implications for clients and professionals?

There are several suggested advantages to using the problem-oriented record. It is well established that this type of record keeping provides a means for permanent documentation of the thinking process of those involved in health and illness care. It can be and has been used as an evaluative tool for the peer review process and as a means for auditing for quality control; thus it logically should lead to provision of improved quality of care.[16,28,51,59]

Quality of care, however, is a very nebulous phenomenon and lacks adequate definition. A distinctly causal relationship between using the problem-oriented record and subsequent improvement in patient care is at best difficult to prove.[43,56] Neither the traditional record nor the problem-oriented record can ensure the concern, compassion, and understanding that are crucial components of patient care.[19]

The problem-oriented record allows for several modifications that facilitate the teaching-learning pro-

DISCHARGE PLANNING SUMMARY

Tuesday: 10th hospital day

Problem: Acute/chronic alcoholism (GI symptoms, sleep difficulties, and poor dietary habits)

S: "I feel much better now. I know I have to work through several problems, but at least I am beginning to realize that drinking has not helped me solve anything."

O: Patient suffered withdrawal symptoms 28 hr after admission for GI distress; tolerated withdrawal with no untoward effects; blood chemistries and vital signs now within normal limits; stool guaiac negative and back to her normal routine; eating three meals per day with snacks; weight gain of 8 lb; occasional burning in stomach controlled with Maalox; minimal nausea; no vomiting; taking no medication except Maalox prn; able to sleep most of the night with relaxation techniques

A: Has made considerable progress; recognizes and admits her dependence on alcohol; feel future prognosis is guarded, but she is an excellent candidate for rehabilitation; needs to increase her self-esteem

P: 1. Return appointment with Dr. Long in 2 wk
2. Refer to Dr. Ann Spencer, psychiatrist, for follow-up
3. Continue emphasis on diet; have dietitian who has been following Ms. Smith review diet before she completes discharge; she is going to keep a diet history to help keep her nutrition needs foremost in her mind; she has an adequate knowledge base about good nutrition and seems to be motivated

Problem: Social withdrawal

S: "Perhaps I have been overly sensitive about not having a partner. My friends have shown their concern throughout my hospital stay. If I still feel strange in some social situations, perhaps I need to make some new friends who won't always think of me as John's wife. I know my daughters can't stay home with me."

O: Patient able be verbalize concerns and feelings

A: Still actively grieving loss of husband, daughters (to college), and life-style; will need continued support to complete the grief process, since losses involve so many of previous valued ways

P: 1. Suggest possibility of going to "widows' group" as additional social support
2. Work with Dr. Spencer on this problem

Problem: Lack of future orientation

S: I know I felt I had no future. I still do not know if I can find an important reason for being other than my husband and children, but I was a whole person before I had them and perhaps I can be again. I realize I either have to take control of my life or just let things happen."

O: Patient had previous marketable skills, is intelligent, and able to recognize the possibility of functioning in different manner than before—but still have a satisfying situation

A: Alcohol noneffective coping mechanism for empty-nest syndrome and grieving process; new awareness on Ms. Smith's part that she is not the only person who has ever experienced these problems or sought a similar solution; support needed to assume active life-style built around some aspect other than nuclear family

P: 1. Dr. Spencer to help with further development of self-concept separate from deceased husband and living children
2. After return appointment with Dr. Long, Ms. Smith is going to "tutor" students with long-term goal of returning full time to the teaching profession

Mary Jane Long, M.D.
Janet Gelein, R.N., Primary Nurse

---

cess. Since the problem-oriented record reflects problem-solving behavior, one can use it to evaluate students' knowledge and understanding. It allows for self-teaching in that a learner can review in depth one patient's record or several records cross sectionally. Because of its inherent logic and flow, it facilitates learning by making explicit the decision-making process used in giving patient care.

The problem-oriented record allows for another person to grasp easily the important aspects of a patient's situation and to see quickly the plans in progress for each person. Thus when a person must substitute temporarily or permanently for a specified care giver, the transition is eased. Such substitutions result from many types of situations in the daily lives of professionals, such as illness, vacations, and moving.

Another presumed benefit resulting from this process is increased collaboration among professionals.[11] This in turn is significant primarily if it results in improved patient care. In a situation involving several different health and illness care professions, each practitioner can advantageously utilize the problem-oriented method to document his or her particular contribution to the patient's progress and plan of care, or it is possible for the method to be used as traditional charting has been—only to document the client's response to medical intervention.

A significant positive benefit resulting from the use of the problem-oriented format is the regular inclusion of subjective data. This promotes the possibility that the client's point of view is being solicited and considered. In practice, this has been the basis for a process called record sharing, where clients are asked not only to read their records but also to comment on the accuracy, thoroughness, and clarity and to express their opinions about the problem statements and goals.[10,52]

One overriding limitation of the problem-oriented record is its tendency toward reductionism. The problem-oriented system, while attempting to encourage a patient-oriented approach to assessment, lacks the ability to provide whole-person descriptions of illness. Lists of physical, sociocultural, and psychological problems are not holistic statements.[21]

Another major shortcoming of the problem-oriented process and record is its exclusive focus on problems. It appears that there is little room for careful assessment of the strengths of the client or patient in relation to the problem-solving process. The management of a problem from the client's perspective will depend heavily on what strengths and assets this person brings to the situation, and building on those assets may be a crucial function of health and illness care professionals. Additionally, attempts to help clients attain a higher level of wellness do not appropriately appear to fall into a "problem" category.

Another shortcoming of the problem-oriented record is redundancy in data recording. A single piece of information may be pertinent to several problems and it will have to be noted in the record in several different locations.[1,19]

The one inherent threat for professionals in the use of the problem-oriented record is that it exposes the practitioner to criticism. Information collected is explicit and easily retrieved. Lack of judgment or ignorance is readily apparent. Inadequacies become obvious, and practitioners have to admit when they lack knowledge or understanding. While exposure is an inherent threat in this system, it also can be viewed as having a positive aspect in its tremendous potential for growth.

One possible threat to clients that is inherent in the use of this system is the permanent keeping of easily retrievable, confidential information related to a person. This method of record keeping has the potential of being and in some instances has been computerized. Information could be collected and stored from birth to death in a well-organized fashion. In one manner this could provide for the possibility of continuity of care throughout a lifetime. On the other hand, the potential for possible invasion of privacy and use of data for reasons other than those specifically requested by the client presents possible abuses.[54]

Other implications for the use of the problem-oriented record revolve around the areas of research, licensure, and third-party payment. The need for research in education and practice is obvious. Adequate record keeping is a prerequisite to all forms of research, including nursing. A format that outlines problems and assigns names to them can easily serve as a source of statistical data in reviewing care from records. Additionally, problems can be categorized and used to study the complementary care given by various health and illness care personnel. A review of multiple records might reveal common client problems, effective vs. ineffective approaches used in meeting them, and the complementary roles of the varying professionals contributing to the care. Predictive outcomes of approaches to clients' problems can then be made in various situations. Yet the fact remains that at this time there is no universally accepted taxonomy of problems. Since there is no standardization for the names given to problems, the retrieval of data according to problem definition becomes formidable.[19,25]

The problem-oriented record has implications for licensure. The potential for peer review and audit may contain the essence of a more valid approach for determining licensure or certification. The possibility of evaluation based on documented performance, with or without other "tests," may allow for more definite and well-defined evaluation criteria.

Another possible implication for the problem-oriented record involves third-party payment systems. The thorough documentation of the skilled contributions made by the participating health care personnel may allow for more equitable distribution of health-insurance remunerations. Nursing especially has not been visible in this area and has generally been unable to seek remuneration for services rendered. This may be a crucial issue with the potential advent of some type of national health insurance.

In conclusion, Weed has stated that form leads to economy of time in almost all human endeavors.[62] While this cannot be denied, it must also be remembered that form is restrictive and any form is derived from the basis of a set of assumptions. In this particular case the assumptions are influenced by a person's background of knowledge, past experiences, and definition of health and illness care. If one can recognize the assumptions underlying this process of thinking and method of record keeping, then one can intelligently accept or reject the problem-oriented record as a mechanism for improving health and illness care.[18]

REFERENCES AND SELECTED READINGS
Contemporary

1. Antoniore, A.G., Sever, E.D., and Toby, J.P.: Problem-oriented medical records—all or none? Med. Educ. 13:217-218, 1979.
2. *Atwood, J., Mitchell, P.H., and Yarnall, S.R.: The problem-oriented record: a system for communication, Nurs. Clin. North Am. 9: 229-234, 1974.
3. Baum, R., and Iber, F.L.: Initial treatment of the alcoholic patient. In Gitlon, S.E., and Peyser, H.S., editors: Alcoholism: a

*References preceded by an asterisk are particularly well suited for student reading.

practical treatment guide, New York, 1980, Grune & Stratton, Inc.

4. Bauman, K.: The problem-oriented medical record: a self-instructional manual for nurses, Chapel Hill, N.C., 1975, University of North Carolina.

5. Beckman, L.J.: Alcoholism problems and women: an overview. In Greenblatt, M., and Schuckit, M.: Alcoholism problems in women and children, New York, 1976, Grune & Stratton, Inc.

6. Becknell, E.P., and Smith, D.M.: System of nursing practice: a clinical assessment tool, Philadelphia, 1975, F.A. Davis Co.

7. *Berni, R., and Nicholson, C.: The POR as a tool in rehabilitation and patient teaching, Nurs. Clin. North Am. 9:265-270, 1974.

8. *Bloom, J.: Problem oriented charting, Am. J. Nurs. 71:2144-2148, 1971.

9. Bronkowski, M.S.: Adapting the POMR to community for health care, Nurs. Outlook 20:515-518, 1972.

10. Bronson, D.L., Rubin, A.S., and Tufo, H.M.: Patient education through record sharing, Quality Review Bulletin, Dec., 1978.

11. Calder, M.: How we won the team's support for POMP, Nurs. '81 11:27-29, 1981.

12. Calobrisi, A.: Treatment programs for alcoholic women. In Greenblatt, M., and Schuckit, M.: Alcoholism problems in women and children, New York, 1976, Grune & Stratton, Inc.

13. Carroll, J.F.: "Mental illness" and "disease": outmoded concepts in alcohol and drug rehabilitation, Community Ment. Health J. 11:418-429, 1975.

14. Chavigny, C.: Self-esteem for the alcoholic: an epidemiologic approach, Nurs. Outlook 24:636-639, 1976.

15. Conn, H., editor: Current therapy: latest approved methods of treatment for the practicing physician, Philadelphia, 1980, W.B. Saunders Co.

16. Dickie, G.L., and Bass, M.J.: Improving problem-oriented medical records through self-audit, Nurs. '80 10:487-490, 1980.

17. Ditzler, J.: Rehabilitation for alcoholics, Am. J. Nurs. 76:1772-1775, 1976.

18. Dunea, G.: Confusion oriented medical records, Int. J. Biomed. Comput. 10:91-95, 1979.

19. Feinstein, A.R.: The problems of the "problem-oriented medical record," Ann. Intern. Med. 78:751-762, 1973.

20. Field, F.W.: Communication between nurse and physician, Nurs. Outlook 20:722-725, 1972.

21. Freer, C.B.: Description of illness: limitations and approaches, J. Fam. Pract. 10:867-870, 1980.

22. Froom, J.: The problem-oriented medical record, part VI, J. Fam. Pract. 1:48-51, 1974.

23. *Gane, D.: Sparky: a success story, Am. J. Nurs. 73:1176-1177, 1973.

24. Gerken, B., Molitor, A.M., and Reardon, J.: Problem-oriented reocrds in psychiatry, Nurs. Clin. North Am. 9:289-300, 1974.

25. Goldfinger, S.E.: The problem-oriented record: a critique from a believer, N. Engl. J. Med. 288:606-607, 1973.

26. Heinemann, E., and Estes, N.: Assessing alcoholic patients, Am. J. Nurs. 76:785-789, 1976.

27. Henneke, L., and Fox, V.: The woman with alcoholism. In Gitlon, S.E., and Peyser, H.S., editors: Alcoholism: a practical treatment guide, New York, 1980, Grune & Stratton, Inc.

28. Hofing, A.L., et al.: The importance of maintenance in implementing change: an experience with problem-oriented recording, J. Nurs. Adm. 9:43-48, 1979.

29. *Kelly, M.E., and McNutt, H.: Implementation of problem-oriented charting in a public health agency, Nurs. Clin. North Am. 9:281-287, 1974.

30. *Kinney, S., Smith, C., and Barnes, R.H.: The problem-oriented record: a community hospital approach, Nurs. Clin. North Am. 9:247-254, 1974.

31. Kurose, K., et al.: A standard care plan for alcoholism, Am. J. Nurs. 81:1001-1006, 1981.

32. Larkin, P.D., and Backer, B.A.: Problem-oriented nursing assessment, New York, 1977, McGraw-Hill Book Co.

33. Leitzell, J.D.: Patient and MD: is either objective? N. Engl. J. Med. 296:1070, 1977.

34. Leonard, P., Cowan, D.B., and Mattingly, P.H.: The POR as a means of collaboration between pediatric nursing practitioner and other health team members, Nurs. Clin. North Am. 9:271-279, 1974.

35. Lewis, L. Recognizing the alcoholic, Nurs. '77 7:59-61, 1977.

36. Lewis, L.: The hidden alcoholic: a nursing dilemma, Nurs. '75 5(7):20-30, 1975.

37. Longbaugh, R., et al.: Focus on patient problems: use of the problem-oriented record in a proposed evaluation study of social isolation, Quality Review Bulletin 4:4-7, 1978.

38. Luke, B.: The nutritional implications of alcohol abuse, R.N. 39(4):32-34, 1976.

39. Mahoney, E.A., Verdisco, L., and Shortridge, L.: How to record a health history, Philadelphia, 1976, J.B. Lippincott Co.

40. Malloy, J.L.: Taking exception to problem-oriented nursing care, Am. J. Nurs. 76:582-583, 1976.

41. *Marshall, J.C., and Feeney, S.: Structural versus intuitive intake interview, Nurs. Res. 21:269-272, 1972.

42. *McCloskey, J.C.: The problem-oriented record vs. the nursing care plan: a proposal, Nurs. Outlook 23:492-495, 1975.

43. Merkel, S.I., McGugin, M.B., and Hofing, A.L.: Evaluation: the often neglected aspect of POR education, Superv. Nurse 11:68-71, 1980.

44. *Mitchell, P.H.: A systematic nursing progress record: the problem-oriented approch, Nurs. Forum 12:187-210, 1973.

45. National League for Nursing: The problem-oriented system: a multidisciplinary approach, NLN no. 20-1546, New York, 1974, Department of Hospital and Related Institutional Nursing Services.

46. *Niland, M.B., and Bentz, P.M.: A problem-oriented approach to planning nursing care, Nurs. Clin. North Am. 9:235-245, 1974.

47. Nursing grand rounds: the alcoholic surgical patient, Nurs. '77 7:56-61, 1977.

48. Palomaki, J.F.: Organization of medical care in obstetrics and gynecology, Obstet. Gynecol. Annu. 9:357-382, 1980.

49. *Payne, S., McBarron, R.A., and O'Connor, E.J.: Implementation of a problem-oriented system in a CCU, Nurs. Clin. North Am. 9:255-263, 1974.

50. Pollak, V.E.: On-line computerized data handling system for treating patients with renal disease, Arch. Intern. Med. 137:446-456, 1977.

51. *Rieder, K.A., and Wood, M.J.: Problem orientation: an experimental study to test its heuristic value, Nurs. Res. 27:25-29, 1978.

52. Rubin, A.S., and Bronson, D.L.: Patients who read their hospital charts, N. Engl. J. Med. 302:1482-1483, 1980.

53. Schell, P.L., and Campbell, A.T.: POMR—not just another way to chart, Nurs. Outlook 20:510-514, 1972.

54. Schuchman, H.: Toward assuring confidentiality of records in large-scale assessment programs, Am. J. Orthopsychiatry 48:71-76, 1978.

55. *Stevens, B.J.: Why won't nurses write nursing care plans? J. Nurs. Adm. 2(5):6-7, 91-92, 1972.

56. Stratmann, W.C.: Assessing the problem-oriented approach to care delivery, Med. Care 18:456-464, 1980.

57. Strong, M.L.: Evaluation of problem-oriented nursing notes, J. Nurs. Adm. 2(3):50-58, 1972.

58. Thoma, D., and Pittman, K.: Threats of the WEED system, N. Engl. J. Med. 284:925, 1971.

59. Tufo, H.M., et al.: Problem-oriented approach to practice: de-

velopment of the system through audit and implication, J.A.M.A. **238:**502-505, 1977.

60. *Walker, H.K., Hurst, J.W., and Woody, M.F.: Applying the problem-oriented system, New York, 1973, Medcom Books, Inc.

61. Walter, J.B., Pardee, G.P., and Molbo, D.M.: Dynamics of problem-oriented approaches: patient care and documentation, Philadelphia, 1976, J.B. Lippincott Co.

62. *Weed, L.L.: Medical records, medical education, and patient care, Cleveland, 1971, Case Western Reserve University Press.

63. Wooddell, W.J.: The alcohol withdrawal syndrome, Fam. Community Health **2:**23-30, 1979.

64. *Woody, M., and Mallison, M.: The problem-oriented system for patient-centered care, Am. J. Nurs. **73:**1168-1175, 1973.

65. Woolley, F., et al.: Problem-oriented nursing, New York, 1974, Springer Publishing Co., Inc.

66. *Yarnall, S., and Atwood, J.: Problem-oriented practice for nurses and physicians: general concepts, Nurs. Clin. North Am. **9:**215-228, 1974.

67. Zelechowski, G.P.: Helping your patient sleep: planning instead of pills, Nurs. '77 **7:**62-65, 1977.

Classic

68. Degowin, E.L., and Degowin, R.L.: Bedside diagnostic examination, New York, 1969, Macmillan Publishing Co., Inc.

CHAPTER 11

QUALITY ASSURANCE AND NURSING

MARY LOU MONAHAN

Impetus for quality assurance

Concern with defining and measuring nursing care efficiency has arisen from a variety of sources. Indeed, no study of quality assurance can proceed far without at least some attention being given to these origins.

Historically, the impetus for accountability in nursing came from four major sources: (1) legislation, (2) third-party rules for reimbursement, (3) societal economic conditions, and (4) the responsibility held by the nursing profession to society as a whole.

Legislation

Since 1965 the federal government has been increasingly involved as a major purchaser of health care—mainly through its Medicare and Medicaid programs. Given this increasing financial commitment, Congress and governmental officials at all levels are themselves under pressure to ensure (1) that the services rendered are necessary, (2) that they meet professionally recognized standards of care, and (3) that they contain costs. This concern on the part of the legislators is naturally passed on to the providers of those services.

Third-party reimbursement

In effect, the federal government has become the country's largest third-party health care payment source. To establish some mechanism for accountability over this activity, Congress created a system for reviewing the expenditures of these monies as part of

P.L. 92-603, the Social Security Amendments of 1972. This legislation established a nationwide network of organizations, known as *professional standards review organizations* (PSROs), for review of patient care financed by the federal government. The stated purpose of PSRO review was to determine if medical services were necessary, if they met certain standards, and if maximal effective utilization was being made of available services. The government, however, is not alone in these concerns. In certain areas of the country, third-party payers such as Blue Cross and other private insurance companies have also established standards by which they review the care for which they make payment.

Studies since 1973, however, have shown that in general attempts to control utilization have been unsuccessful.[36] Critics of PSROs, in particular, contend that where there is compliance, it is compliance on paper only, that such programs are very expensive to initiate and maintain, and, most importantly, that the quality of health care has not changed.

Despite these limitations, the requirement for public accountability of the health professional nevertheless remains, and it remains for one overriding and understandable reason. Society, which gives the health professionals the authority and the money to deliver a human service, is simply asking for an accounting of the outcomes and benefits of health care services. If health care agencies and providers agree to accept these monies, then they have an obligation to be accountable to those providing this financial support.

Economic factors

Health care is one of the largest industries in the United States. Each year it claims an increasing share of the gross national product (GNP). In an era of cost consciousness and "small is beautiful" economic thinking, budgetary cutbacks have become routine. For nursing this means that the profession must, more than ever, demonstrate the value and benefits of its services if it wishes to maintain governmental and consumer support.

Professionalism

Last but certainly not least is the professional and ethical concern that the profession places on itself for quality care. In 1973 the American Nurses Association (ANA) published generic *Standards of Nursing Practice* for the purpose of ensuring quality nursing care to the public. The primary responsibility for implementing these standards, however, rests with the individual nurse who bears the responsibility for ensuring that these criteria are met in his or her own practice setting. To fulfill this responsibility, professional nurses must be familiar with both the generic (general) and the specific standards pertinent to the care of the patient population for whom the nurse is responsible. These standards identify the elements of nursing care that must be met to ensure quality care and to provide a baseline for measuring that quality.

Three other sets of professional standards must also be considered: the nurse practice acts, the medical practice acts, and the standards set by the Joint Commission on Accreditation of Hospitals. Presently, almost every state has a nurse practice act and a medical practice act. Both of these constitute external sources of standards for nursing practice. Taken together they define and delineate from a legal standpoint the content and practice of nursing.

The *nurse practice acts* define nursing practice and identify those activities that fall within the province of nursing. The *medical practice acts* further delineate nursing practice by outlining those areas that constitute the exclusive province of the physician. Such exclusions restrict the activities in which nurses may engage. Neither type of act sets actual standards for practice; rather the acts designate general areas of activity for both professions, and they establish the legal relationship of the nurse to society and to other related professions.

The *Joint Commission on Accreditation of Hospitals* (JCAH) is another highly influential external source of nursing standards. In 1976 the Joint Commission added a section on quality of professional services to the *JCAH Accreditation Manual for Hospitals*. This standard delineates the characteristics of patient care evaluation programs. As a result, *patient care audits* have become commonplace in most hospitals, with the number of audits performed at each institution related to the number of hospital admissions. In 1979 this stan-

dard was revised, and the numerical requirement for a specific number of audits was removed.

The 1982 *Quality Assurance Nursing Standard* of the JCAH requires a problem-focused, effective review and evaluation of the quality appropriateness of patient care.[19] This standard includes the following components:

1. A designated person responsible for the quality assurance activities
2. A written quality assurance plan (might include a statement of purpose, a statement of scope, the problem-solving focus including a description of how the priorities for problems are determined, the administration and coordination of the program, and an evaluation mechanism to assess the program's impact)
3. Evidence that there is progress toward coordination and integration of all quality assurance activities in the hospital

Definition of quality assurance

The definition of *quality* when applied to nursing care is complex and multidimensional. Wandelt and Stewart[32] define quality as "a characteristic or attribute of something." Phaneuf[24] defines quality as "the essential character of care considered within the context of degree or merit." Zimmer[37] postulates that quality of care is "the observable characteristics that describe a desired and valued degree of excellence and the expected, observed variations." *Assurance* is defined as "safeguarding a quality by instituting a systematic evaluation to be sure that the care that is delivered meets the standard that is set."[28]

Quality assurance therefore is defined as a *process that involves evaluating the degree of excellence of the observable and measurable characteristics of delivered nursing care*. Components of the quality assurance process are delineated in Fig. 11-1.

In health care delivery the purpose of quality assurance evaluation is always twofold. The first part determines the extent to which the predetermined standards are being met by a particular nursing program. Second, these findings are used to make decisions about changes that are to be implemented by the persons carrying out the program of care. These two parts must be in place if nursing is to ensure its accountability to the consumer. Although the specific target of each evaluation may differ depending on what information about quality is desired, the purpose of the evaluation is always the same.

Nurses who are engaged in the delivery of health care cannot escape inclusion of quality assurance reviews in their practice responsibilities. Indeed, proficiency in evaluation must become part of a modern nurse's basic repertoire of skills. Corresponding to this responsibility on the part of the individual nurse is also a responsibility on the part of nurse evaluators to ensure that this skill is an ongoing part of nursing education and practice.

The process is fortunately not a mysterious one. Indeed, most nurses are more than halfway toward expertise in this area by virtue of their basic education and experience. Nurses who are expert in the care of a specific patient population, by definition, possess the knowledge necessary to determine desired *health* and *wellness outcomes* for that population. These nurses already know what direct care processes to employ in assisting clients toward health and wellness. They also know what observable changes in clients' problems should occur at certain time intervals.

Unfortunately, most nurses are not expert in the methods that are needed to conduct these evaluation reviews. This is the one remaining critical piece that nurses can learn from staff development programs in employing agencies or from other continuing education programs in the community.

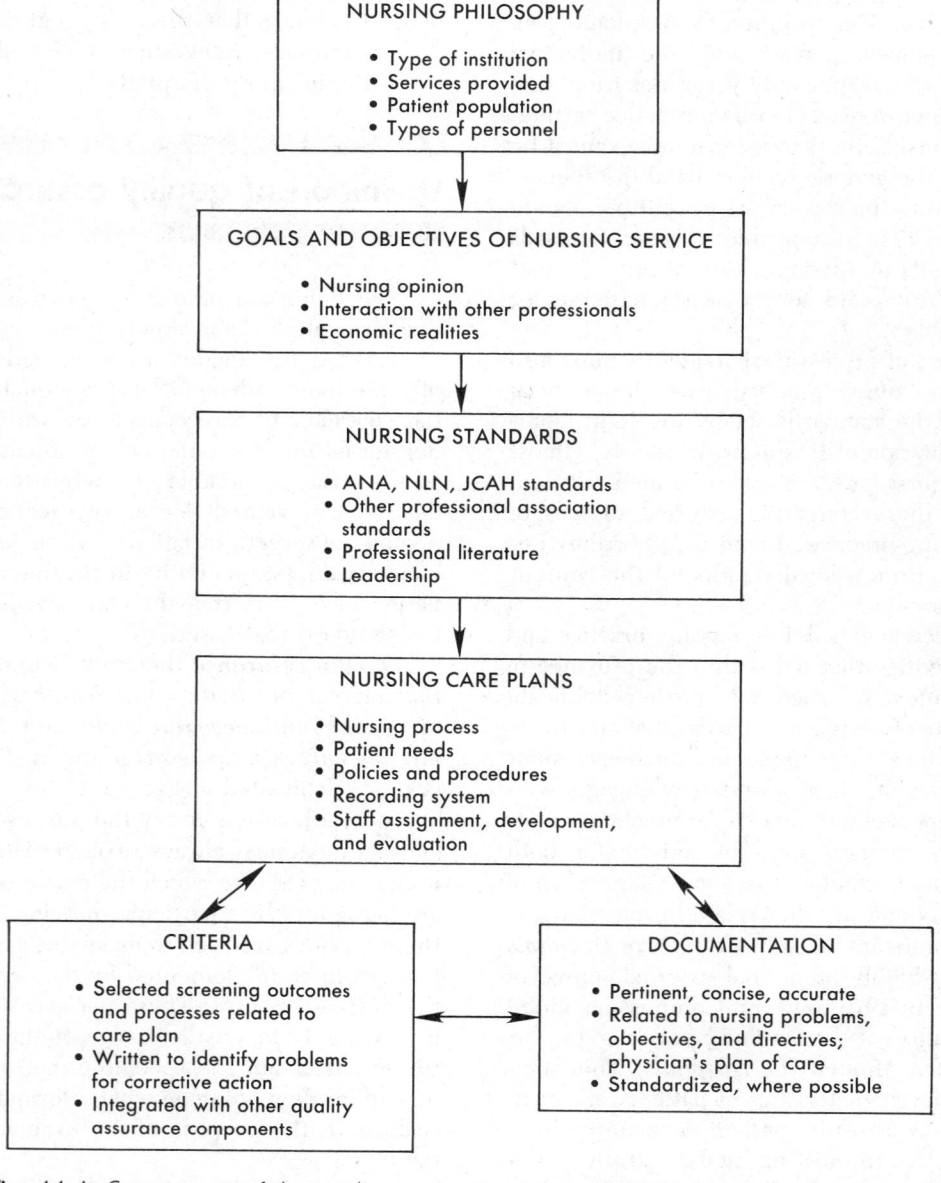

Fig. 11-1. Components of the quality assurance process. (From Interqual: Quality assurance in nursing seminar manual, Chicago, 1980, InterQual, Inc.)

Quality assurance review

A variety of models have been proposed to describe the quality assurance review process. Presented here will be the model devised by the American Nurses Association (ANA).[2] This model is a problem-solving process that utilizes *structure, process,* and *outcome criteria* as the primary tools of inquiry. As illustrated in Fig. 11-2, the model contains the following eight steps:

1. Identification of values
2. Identification of structure, process, outcome standards, and criteria
3. Collection of data necessary to measure degree of attainment of standards and criteria
4. Interpretation of the data in terms of the strengths and weaknesses of the program
5. Identification of possible courses of action
6. Choosing a course of action
7. Taking action
8. Reevaluation

Each of these steps is discussed below.

Identification of values

Before the implementation of this or any other quality assurance review model, there must be an examination of the *societal, professional,* and *individual values* that guide the activities of the health care agency.

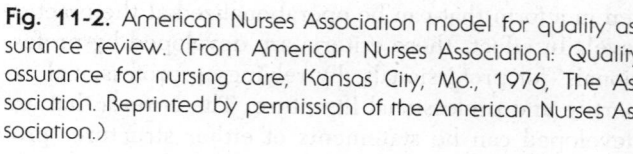

Fig. 11-2. American Nurses Association model for quality assurance review. (From American Nurses Association: Quality assurance for nursing care, Kansas City, Mo., 1976, The Association. Reprinted by permission of the American Nurses Association.)

Such a process is unavoidably inherent in the word *quality.* The very word *quality* implies that somewhere, someone has determined that certain outcomes have more value than other outcomes. As the term *value* applies to nursing care, it means that the individual nursing department, hospital, or health care agency, as well as the surrounding community, will interact to influence the development of criteria that will be used in the review process.

To cite some obvious examples, in most Catholic hospitals a high value is placed on human life from the moment of conception; therefore in Catholic institutions no abortions will be performed. In another hospital a prevailing societal or cultural value may have influenced it to favor a youth orientation. The emphasis in health care at that institution may therefore be oriented toward teen and young adult programs as opposed to geriatric programs. In whatever setting the nurse happens to be, that setting operates under a set of values that must be identified and understood if the quality assurance review is to be fair and accurate.

Identification of structure, process, outcome standards, and criteria

The priority of topics for a quality assurance review is usually determined by its real or potential impact on patient care.[20] The review may have impact on either the *effectiveness* of care, the *efficiency* with which care is delivered, or both. If a nursing care problem has

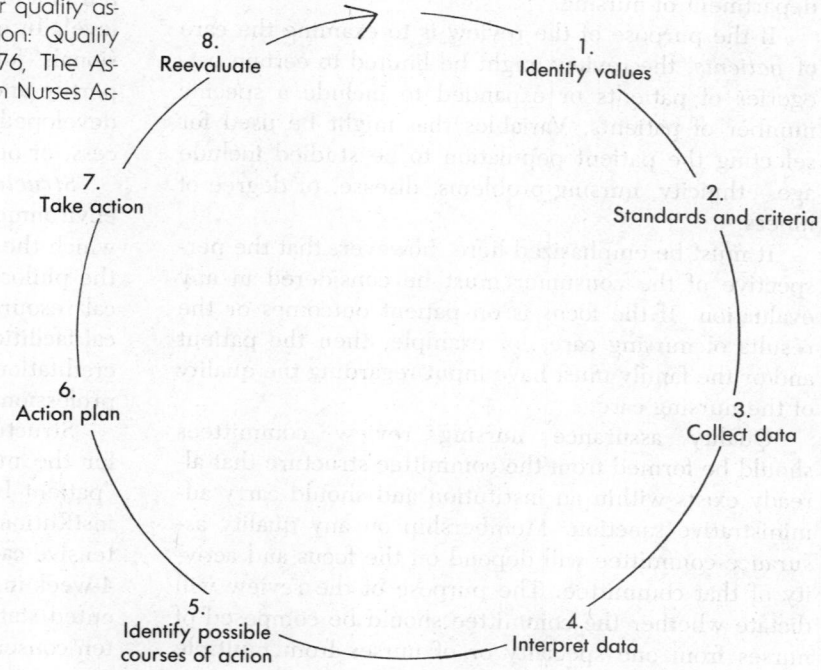

8. Reevaluate
1. Identify values
2. Standards and criteria
3. Collect data
4. Interpret data
5. Identify possible courses of action
6. Action plan
7. Take action

been identified with some frequency, it is, of course, given a higher priority.

Identification of the focus of the review. The focus of the evaluation can be the institution, the nurses, the patient, or a combination of all three of these. Selection of the exact focus will vary depending on individual and institutional values.

If the quality assurance review focuses on the *institution*, it may examine the types of services delivered, the administrative structure, or features of the health care setting such as the physical plant, equipment, organization, or staffing. A quality assurance review could also be employed if one wanted to measure the institution's adherence to external standards, selected personnel policies, or the qualifications of nursing staff assigned to special care areas, such as intensive care units.

If the focus of the review is *the nurse*, an area of nursing practice will be selected for review. The review could examine almost any aspect of nursing activity. It might be utilized if the objective of the evaluation is to measure adherence to nursing department policies and procedures or it might be employed if the objective were to evaluate whether the most appropriate nursing care methods were being used.

Specific examples of measures that focus on the nurse might include criteria that assess frequency of vital sign monitoring in the immediate postoperative period, criteria that establish content and time frames for completion of the nursing assessment form, or criteria that the nurse uses to assess the patient's intravenous needle puncture site. Measures that focus on nursing can therefore include activities of a single nurse, of all nurses assigned to a specific unit, or of all nurses in the department of nursing.

If the purpose of the review is to examine the care of *patients*, the review might be limited to certain categories of patients or expanded to include a specific number of patients. Variables that might be used for selecting the patient population to be studied include age, ethnicity, nursing problems, disease, or degree of illness.

It must be emphasized here, however, that the perspective of the consumer must be considered in any evaluation. If the focus is on patient outcomes or the results of nursing care, for example, then the patient and/or the family must have input regarding the quality of the nursing care.

Quality assurance nursing review committees should be formed from the committee structure that already exists within an institution and should carry administrative sanction. Membership on any quality assurance committee will depend on the focus and activity of that committee. The purpose of the review will dictate whether the committee should be composed of nurses from one specialty or of nurses from multiple specialties. A committee that is composed only of surgical nurses, for example, would review nursing care only for surgical patients. On the other hand, a committee composed of nurses from multiple specialties might review the nursing care of an entire institution.

Multidisciplinary committees might also be formed. These would be composed of representatives from several health professions, such as medicine, nursing, dietetics, social work, occupational therapy, physical therapy, and pharmacy. A multidisciplinary committee would have as its focus the total care that a patient or population of patients received during hospitalization. In these circumstances, committee members would develop jointly the criteria to be used in the patient care review.

Identification of criteria and standards. After selecting the focus of the review, the next step in the ANA model is to specify the criteria and standards that are appropriate to evaluating care.

A *standard* is defined as the desired or achievable level or range of performance of a certain criterion, or as a framework against which performance is compared.[12] A *criterion measure* is defined as the variable that is believed to be an indicator of the quality of care.[12] Thus the statement that "every patient will have a plan of care recorded on the nursing care plan" would be a standard, whereas the statement that "a nursing care plan will be developed by a registered nurse within 12 hours of admission" would be a criterion measure.

The task of the *quality assurance review committee* is to develop *criteria* that will be used in the actual evaluation. The *standards* for nursing practice are usually developed by clinical nursing leaders and are written in a form that can be operationalized at the practice level. In effect, these criteria are developed by professionals, for professionals, by relying on professional expertise and professional literature. The criteria that are developed can be statements of either structure, process, or outcome.

Structure criteria are statements that describe the environmental elements, setting, and conditions under which the nurse-patient relationship occurs. It includes the philosophy and objectives of the institution, its fiscal resources, legal responsibilities, equipment, physical facilities, management structure, licensure, and accreditation, as well as the quality and characteristics of professional, nonprofessional, and technical employees.

Structure criteria can be written for the institution, for the nurse, or for the patient. The statement that "patient beds must be 3 feet from one another" is an institutional statement. "Any nurse assigned to the intensive care unit must have satisfactorily completed the 4-week intensive care orientation course" is a nurse-oriented statement. And, "All patients are to sign a written consent form before any surgical or invasive radiological procedure" is a patient-oriented statement.

Process criteria focus on the nature and sequence of health care activities. They focus on the activities that the nurse engages in to respond to the patient's illness. For example, process criteria might describe the communication patterns that a nurse has with a dying patient or the preoperative teaching plan for the cardiac patient scheduled for surgery.

Outcome criteria focus on the results of the processes of health care. They are considered by many to be the ultimate indicators of the quality of patient care.[15,37] For the patient *the measurable outcome could be a change in health, knowledge, or functional status*. In addition, these outcomes can be either positive or negative. Examples of outcome measures might include the following: "The patient can state the name, dose, and side effects of his prescribed medication" (positive outcome) or "The patient has not developed any decubiti during the period of immobilization" (negative outcome).

After the criteria have been developed, they need to be validated before being used in a quality review process. This *validation* process is usually performed by a "consensus among peers." The rationale for this validation step is to be certain that the selected criteria are accurate and relevant and that they reflect the realities of nursing practice at that particular institution. The nurses who work daily with the topic chosen for the review are usually in the best position to make these determinations.

Following criteria development and validation, the next step is for the committee to establish a specific observable and measurable level of performance for each criteria; for example, "At discharge 100% of the patients should be afebrile" or "By the time of discharge, 75% of all ostomy patients should be able to apply their own bags."

Not all criteria, however, necessarily carry a 100% level of performance. In the second example mentioned above, a 75% compliance level was selected because many of the patients may be discharged to extended care facilities for further care and are not expected to be fully independent by the time of discharge.

Measurement of degree of attainment of standards and criteria

A wide variety of methods can be used to gather data on nursing performance. The degree to which actual practice meets or exceeds the validated criteria in turn provides the data necessary to evaluate the strengths and weaknesses of the nursing care program. These data gathering methods might include *self-assessment, supervisor evaluation, performance observation, utilization review, audits, review of patient records, staff surveys,* or *patient/medical staff/employee complaints*.

Whatever method of review is chosen, the data should be easily accessible and retrievable. The review may be looking at activities that happened in the past, or it may be examining current nursing activities. A review that examines past happenings is called a *retrospective review*. A *concurrent review* looks at what is happening in the present, while the patient is receiving care.

Specific questions that the quality assurance review committee needs to answer at this point include:

- Who will collect the data?
- What will be the source of the data?
- Where will the data be collected?
- When will the data be collected?
- How will the data be collected?

The answers to these questions will assist the committee in deciding whether the review can be accomplished as planned given the inherent requirements for efficiency and accuracy. As a final check, the committee should be certain that each criterion measure is written so that a decision can be easily made as to whether or not the standard has been met.

Once the data collection has occurred, the results are tabulated, and it is determined whether the percent of yes and no answers corresponds to the previously established level of performance (i.e., percent compliance) for each criterion. If the level of performance does not achieve the expectations, the criterion for this evaluation item has not been met.

Table 11-1 illustrates one method of keeping track of a multicriterion evaluation process.

Interpretation of strengths and weaknesses of program

The degree to which the levels of performance have been met serves as a basis for describing the strengths and weaknesses of the nursing care program or practice. But in addition to this obvious analysis there are other factors that are frequently overlooked. These include factors that might be related to the degree of success in achieving certain outcomes. Consider the following case:

On Nursing Unit A there was 100% compliance with the criterion that all ostomy patients would be able to apply their own ostomy bag by the time of discharge. However, on Unit B the compliance was only 65%. A comparison of the procedures and practices on the two units revealed that the ages of the patients on Unit B were significantly higher than those on Unit A and that the majority of Unit B patients were discharged to extended care facilities instead of to their homes.

TABLE 11-1. Criteria tracking form

Outcome criteria for person with colostomy	Expected level of performance (percent compliance)*	Identified problems, strengths, and weaknesses
Patient or significant others can:		
Demonstrate how to measure the stoma for an appliance.	85%	One patient was blind; no documentation on two patients.
Demonstrate proper application of the appliance.	85%	Two patients stated it would have been helpful to have a mirror provided; one patient was blind.
State plans for follow-up care.	60%	Forty percent of patients were being transferred to an extended care facility.
State community resources available for purchase of permanent appliances, for financial assistance, and support groups.	80%	Twenty percent of charts audited had one of these components missing.
State need to observe stoma and skin around it for redness and excoriation.	75%	No documentation of this being done on 25% of charts.
Patient or significant others have ostomy informational booklet, which has been reviewed with nurse.	100%	

*Expected compliance in these areas is 100%.

This comparison provides insight into reasons for the differences in these two units and would have been missed had not the evaluator been careful to look for extenuating factors.

In some instances the cause of the identified problem may lie outside the control of nursing and fall within the purview of medicine or hospital administration. For example, an evaluation of the nursing management of postoperative pain at one hospital revealed that the physician staff was ordering almost identical pain relief medication for all patients. The consequence of this lack of individualized patient assessment regarding pain relief measures by the physicians caused frequent patient complaints as well as frequent calls to the physicians by the nursing staff. These results were shared with the physician staff who agreed that an educational program for physicians and corrective measures were needed in this area.

Identification of possible courses of action

After identification of strengths and weaknesses, possible courses of action are developed. They will have as their primary focus the reduction or elimination of the weaknesses and reinforcement of the strengths of the existing program and practices. Consideration must also be given to the best means of motivating the nursing staff to accomplish the needed changes. Indeed, the best results are usually obtained when the persons most affected by the quality assurance review are involved in the process of planning the subsequent course of action. The eventual attainment of the preset levels of performance coupled with appropriate availability of resources and cooperative relationships between evaluators and those affected by the evaluation generally serve as the basis for most successful changes in nursing practice.

Alternative solutions to an identified problem can be numerous. Frequently, these actions include administrative changes, further clinical research into the problem, continuing education, changes in practice, environmental changes, a reward system for improved compliance, or even the organization of peer pressure.

Each of the above alternatives has advantages and disadvantages and each must be weighed by the peer group in terms of how efficiently and effectively the problem can be solved. At times the involvement of nurses in the development of criteria is all that is needed to bring about changes in practice.

Selection of a course of action

After examination of the alternatives, the course of action that is felt to be best by the nurse peer group is selected. The specific course of action will generally depend on the identified problem, the availability of resources, and the inherent organizational structure of the institution. In certain cases there may be multiple causes for an identified problem, and many possible solutions may have to be explored.

After a decision is made, the individual institution will vary as to how the plan for change is presented to the administration and in how the change is to be implemented. In the case of a nursing practice change the director of nursing may wish to make the final decision. At other institutions the director of nursing may only wish to be informed of the findings, and the committee will be charged with making appropriate changes.

Taking action

Attempting to improve the quality of nursing care implies change. This in turn implies that the persons making decisions about changes will somehow find a way to execute their decisions. If it is felt that the information has been inadequate, the action taken may be to gather more information systematically. Sooner or later, however, *action must be taken*. This is a critical point. Without this step the entire quality assurance review process becomes a hollow, futile exercise.

Reevaluation

At this point the cycle begins again. If a change has been made, the progress of nursing practice needs to be reassessed and remeasured to determine the effectiveness of that action.

Monitoring activities and instruments

Periodic monitoring must be a part of the continual and routine reevaluation of nursing practice. As described earlier, this monitoring is performed using established criteria and levels of performance. It indicates how well the change is progressing and whether the actions taken have been effective. It is especially important to evaluate and monitor new programs and changes in practice. Only through this sort of systematic evaluation and analysis can nursing assure continued improvement in the quality of nursing care.

A variety of methods have been developed to provide an ongoing monitoring of nursing activities. A brief description of some of the more frequently used methods follows.

Nursing audit. The traditional emphasis in quality assurance review has been on the audit. However, the nursing audit is only one part of a total evaluation process. The term is generally employed when one wishes to compare predetermined criteria with the documen-

tation found in the patient record. There are basically two types of nursing audit. The first is called a retrospective audit and the second, a concurrent audit.

The *retrospective audit* is a critical examination of nursing actions with a view toward improvement in practice. A retrospective audit has the advantages of using data for the full continuum of nursing care from admission to discharge and of evaluating the results of that care for a large series of comparable cases. Practitioners may at times gain impressions from single cases in which they are personally involved. These impressions, however, are generally not reliable and may or may not be borne out by later systematic study of a large number of similar cases.

A *concurrent audit* is a critical examination of the patient's progress toward the desired health status (outcome) and patient care management activities (processes) while the patient care is still in progress. Documentation in the patient's record, interviews, observations, questionnaires, and direct inspection of the patient are possible sources of data. Concurrent review is another dimension of quality assurance activity and has the advantage of providing opportunities for making changes in the ongoing care program. While both retrospective and concurrent reviews have different advantages, both can be used separately or together in a quality assurance review.

Audits that have as their objective some assessment of the quality of care generally deal with one or more of the structure-process-outcome measures described earlier. These types of audits are based on the assumption that adequate resources (structure) contribute to adequate nursing problem identification and intervention (process), which in turn result in favorable health (outcome).

Peer review. Expert professional nurses and clinicians are essential components in the quality assurance review program. These are the persons who are not only involved with the daily care of patients but also are accountable for the care that the patients receive. As previously described, they are the persons who write the nursing standards and criteria, set expected levels of compliance, identify causes for less than optimal performance, and recommend and implement action plans to improve nursing care outcomes.

Patient satisfaction questionnaires. Patient satisfaction questionnaires are frequently employed if written data are desired regarding patient's perceptions of their hospitalization experiences. Many hospitals distribute such questionnaires to patients as part of the admission procedures and request that the patients complete and return the forms at the end of their hospitalizations. Other hospitals have initiated patient ombudsman programs. In these programs the ombudsman visits the majority of inpatients, questions them regarding their perceptions of their hospitalization experiences, and intervenes in their behalf when it is appropriate.

Staff satisfaction questionnaire or interview. A staff satisfaction questionnaire or interview is generally employed by administration to assess organizational changes, policies, or the general satisfaction that might

be experienced in a specific work setting.

Utilization review. The utilization review program was mandated by the JCAH in 1978. It has as its primary goal the appropriate allocation of a hospital's resources. While a utilization review program is not ori-

TABLE 11-2. Comparison of eight nursing assessment instruments*

Name of assessment tool	Theoretical basis for tool	Focus	Type/number of criteria/items	Time frame for review	Data collection	Use of tools
JCAH's *Pep Patient Care Evaluation*	Problem-solving process	Nursing process and/or patient outcomes	Varies by study	Concurrent and/or retrospective	Usually medical record review	Review of quality of nursing care in any setting
ANA's *Guidelines for Review of Nursing Care at Local Level*	Problem-solving process	Patient outcomes	Sample sets of outcome criteria (15 topics)	Retrospective	Usually medical record review	PSRO screening of quality, necessity, appropriateness of nursing care in variety of settings
HEW's *Methodology for Monitoring Quality of Nursing Care*	Nursing process plus patient classification	Nursing process	Master list of 216 process criteria/subset of 56 criteria per study	Concurrent	Nurse observer completes work sheet	Review of medical, surgical, pediatric, intensive care nursing in acute care setting
Slater Nursing Competencies Rating Scale	Six primary scientific and cultural bases for nursing care actions	Nursing performance	84 process items	Concurrent	Nurse observer completes scale	Evaluation of nursing personnel, review of care as it relates to performance
Quality Patient Care Scale (QualPacs)	Six primary scientific and cultural bases for nursing care actions	Nursing process	68 process items (subset of Slater)	Concurrent	Nurse observer completes scale	Measure of quality of nursing care in any setting
Phaneuf Nursing Audit	Seven functions of professional nursing	Nursing process	50 process items	Retrospective (portions could be concurrent)	Medical record review	Review of quality of nursing care in hospitals, nursing homes, home health agencies
Rush-Medicus Nursing Process Instrument	Process model of patient care	Nursing process	Master list of 220 process criteria/subsets of 30-50 criteria per study	Concurrent	Nurse observer completes work sheet based on observations plus documentation review	Review of quality of medical, surgical, pediatric nursing care in acute care settings
Horn-Swain Criteria/ Measures of Nursing Care Quality	Orem's self-care theory of nursing	Patient outcomes	Master list of 539 outcome criteria/subsets available for individual study	Concurrent	Nurse observer/ interviewer completes work sheet	Research on models for delivery of nursing care; subsets assess quality of care

*From InterQual: Quality assurance in nursing seminar manual, Chicago, 1980, Interqual, Inc.

ented specifically toward nursing, the monitoring activities of this program occasionally identify nursing areas that may need to be evaluated further.

Infection control report. Because of their direct contact with patients, the nursing staff is frequently involved in programs to monitor and control infection rates. An infection control report provides monthly data on the number and types of nosocomial infections on a given hospital unit. Questions can then be raised about nursing procedures or practices that may influence the number or types of infections. See Chapter 22 for details about infection control studies.

Incident reports. Whenever an untoward event occurs to patients, personnel, or visitors, an incident report should be completed. A statistical analysis of these reports comparing year-to-date and monthly statistics is generally compiled by a hospital or by the hospital's liability insurance carrier. Increases in certain types of incidents, such as medication errors, would be a signal to the quality assurance committee that it should begin a review of the entire medication delivery system.

Additionally, there are a variety of other instruments that have been developed by nurses to assess various aspects of nursing practice. Table 11-2 contains a brief description of a number of these instruments.

Summary

The political climate in the United States today suggests that concerns about the quality of health care may well become secondary to concerns about health care costs. Quality assessments, however, allow nursing to define and describe more thoroughly the fundamental efficacy and importance of nursing care, and because of this they will become even more critical in the decades ahead.

Nursing has made enormous strides in recent years. It has done so largely because of the demonstrable effectiveness, quality, and utility of the care it has provided. Nursing cannot afford to stop this progress now. Patients deserve it, communities in which nurses practice deserve it, and nurses owe it to themselves and to their profession to constantly monitor the effectiveness of their actions.

Properly designed and executed quality assurance reviews are the irreplaceable feedback devices needed to ensure that this progress continues. The reader will note that specific outcome criteria are presented in chapters throughout this book. It is hoped that these outcome criteria will help the reader become more aware of desired patient outcomes and that this knowledge will be used as nursing care is planned and delivered.

REFERENCES AND SUGGESTED READINGS

1. Aldhizer, T., et al.: A multidisciplinary audit of diabetes mellitus, J. Fam. Pract. 8:947-950, 1979.
2. *American Nurses Association: Quality assurance for nursing care, Kansas City, Mo., 1976, The Association.
3. *American Nurses Association: Standards of nursing practice, Kansas City, Mo., 1973, The Association.
4. Atwood, J.: A research perspective, Nurs. Res. 29:104-108, 1980.
5. Bellinger, A.: Evaluation research: a total health care system perspective, Nurs. Res. 29:119-122, 1980.
6. *Blake, B.: Quality assurance: an ethical responsibility, Superv. Nurse 12:32-38, 1981.
7. Bloch, D.: Criteria, standards, norms: crucial terms in quality assurance, J. Nurs. Adm. 7:20-29, 1977.
8. Bloch, D.: Interrelated issues in evaluation and evaluation research: a researcher's perspective, Nurs. Res. 29:69-73, 1980.
9. Brook, R., et al.: Selected reflections on quality of medical care evaluation in the 1980's, Nurs. Res. 29:127-133, 1980.
10. Chance, K.: The quest for quality, Image 12:41-45, 1980.
11. Clinton, J., et al.: Developing criterion measures of nursing care: case study of a process, J. Nurs. Adm. 7:41-45, 1977.
12. *Donabedian, A.: Criteria, norms and standards of quality: what do they mean? Am. J. Public Health 71:409-412, 1981.
13. Downs, F.: Relationship of findings of clinical research and development of criteria: a researcher's perspective, Nurs. Res. 29:94-97, 1980.
14. Egelston, E.: New JCAH standards on quality assurance, Nurs. Res. 29:113-114, 1980.
15. *Given, B., Given, W., and Simmoni, L.: Relationship of process of care to patient outcomes, Nurs. Res. 28:85-93, 1979.
16. Gordon, M.: Determining study topics, Nurs. Res. 29:83-87, 1980.
17. Horn, B.: Establishing valid and reliable criteria: a researcher's perspective, Nurs. Res. 29:88-90, 1980.
18. *Howe, M.: Developing instruments for measurement of criteria: a clinical nursing perspective, Nurs. Res. 29:100-103, 1980.
19. Joint Commission on Accreditation of Hospitals: Accreditation manual for hospitals, 1982 edition, Chicago, 1982, The Commission.
20. Kaplan, K., and Hopkins, J.: The q a guide, Chicago, 1980, Joint Commission on Accreditation of Hospitals.
21. Krueger, J.: Establishing priorities for evaluation and evaluation research, Nurs. Res. 29:115-118, 1980.
22. *Marriner, A.: The research process in quality assurance, Am. J. Nurs. 79:2158-2161, 1979.
23. *Moore, K.: What nurses learn from nursing audit, Nurs. Outlook 27:254-258, 1979.
24. *Phaneuf, M.: Future direction for evaluation and evaluation research in health care, Nurs. Res. 29:123-126, 1980.
25. Phaneuf, M.: The nursing audit, ed. 2, New York, 1976, Appleton-Century-Crofts.
26. Rinaldi, L.: Quality assurance 1981—satisfying JCAH, Nurs. Management 12:23-25, 1981.
27. Rowland, H., and Rowland, B.: Nursing administration handbook, Rockville, 1980, Aspen Systems Corp.
28. *Schmadl, J.: QA examination of the concepts, Nurs. Outlook 27:462-465, 1979.
29. Tan, M.: Quality assurance in nursing, Chicago, 1980, InterQual.
30. Tucker, S., et al.: Patient care standards, ed. 2, St. Louis, 1980, The C.V. Mosby Co.
31. VanMaarem, H.M.: Improvement in the quality of nursing care: a goal to challenge in the 1980's, J. Adv. Nurs. 6:3-6, 1981.

*References preceded by an asterisk are particularly well suited for student reading.

32. Wandelt, M.A., and Stewart, D.: Slater nursing competencies rating scale, New York, 1975, Appleton-Century-Crofts.
33. Weinstein, E.: Developing a measure of the quality of nursing care, J. Nurs. Adm. 7:1-3, 1976.
34. Williamson, J.: Information management in quality assurance, Nurs. Res. 29:78-81, 1980.
35. Woody, M.: An evaluator's perspective, Nurs. Res. 29:74-77, 1980.
36. *Zimmer, M.: Quality of care assessment: its role in the 80's, Am. J. Public Health 71:681-682, 1981.
37. *Zimmer, M.: Quality assurance for outcomes of patient care, Nurs. Clin. North Am. 9:305-315, 1974.

PART TWO

STRESS
AND
ADAPTATION

ADAPTATION

Individuals with medical-surgical problems are exposed to multiple stressful events in the course of their illnesses and therapy. Exposure to these stressors may enhance their growth or be detrimental to their health. It is important for nurses to identify those variables that foster positive outcomes as well as those that may intensify the individual's response to a stressor.

This unit begins with a framework for examining the concepts of *stress*, *coping*, and *adaptation*, which is followed by a discussion of methods of *stress management*. *Adaptive behavior* with an emphasis on cognitive and noncognitive coping mechanisms and *maladaptive behavior*, or inadequate coping, are addressed. *Adaptation throughout the life cycle* follows with emphasis on age-specific adaptations required of the individual. Ways in which the nurse can maximize the coping processes of the *dying* person to promote an appropriate *death* are also explored.

The final three chapters of the unit explore the physiologic responses of the body to stressors. Maintenance of a stable internal environment requires adequate functioning of *regulatory* and *integrative* mechanisms; factors that mediate the effects of stressors are discussed. *Biologic* defense mechanisms, both nonspecific and specific (immunologic), must also be intact to protect the body from external or internal threats. The processes involved in maintaining a relatively constant internal environment (*dynamic equilibrium*) necessary for cellular growth and functioning are discussed with emphasis on the mechanisms regulating fluid and electrolyte balance.

CHAPTER 12

ADAPTATION, STRESS, AND COPING

PAMELA HOLSCLAW MITCHELL

Adaptation, stress, and coping are words commonly used in both lay and professional writings to refer to problematic life situations and the ways of dealing with them. These terms are entrenched in nursing writings to the extent that it is now common knowledge that a major function of nursing is to help people cope with stress and adapt to stressful situations.

Yet, when attempting to define these terms in order to study and understand them better, we find that there is no scientific consensus as to their meanings. Since this is the case, how can these terms be used professionally to understand the nature of human problem-solving behavior? Why have they come to such prominence in the helping professions? Is there a set of related phenomena that these terms describe, or should they be abandoned as bad jargon?

The position is taken here that these terms are in the literature to stay and that they describe similar phenomena regarding the ways humans and nonhumans deal with life's changing events. The terms each provide a general reference point to approach common experiences of living systems interacting with their environments even though precise definitions acceptable to most investigators have been elusive. At best, one may recognize common themes that emerge from the multiple perspectives of those who have tried to define these terms precisely. Thus in this chapter the common themes that have emerged from the scientific study of adaptation, stress, and coping will be presented. These themes will then be applied in a framework useful for helping people in health, in acute illnesses, and in chronic illnesses throughout the life cycle.

Adaptation

Adaptation is a term that implies a variety of processes, depending on the differing perspectives of the discipline defining the term. In the colloquial or common meaning, adaptation connotes individual adjustments or compromises to meet the demands of a situation. To anthropologists adaptation is defined in terms of the evolution of populations or groups to meet changing environmental demands—the survival of species.[35] Biologists tend to view adaptation as those processes that restore homeostasis or balance to internal environmental systems when the system is perturbed.[5] Grinker suggests classification of adaptation by levels of the biopsychosocial system. At the *biologic* level adaptation is directed toward survival or stability of internal processes. At the *psychologic* level the goal of adaptation is preservation of self-identity and self-esteem,[5] and at the *social* level, adaptations provide for (1) definition of modes of adaptation for individuals, (2) support systems for coping endeavors, and (3) anticipation of common developmental tasks.[3]

Adaptation as a concept in nursing is tied most closely to Roy's conceptualization.[18] In Roy's view, adaptation is defined as those processes, in interaction with environmental demands, that promote health. Conversely, those responses that promote ill health are termed *maladaptation*. (Note that values were not attached to adaptive processes in relation to outcome in the conceptualizations discussed previously.) Roy describes levels of adaptive modes that are similar to Grinker's levels. Roy's adaptive modes consist of physiologic needs, self-concept, role function, and interdependence relations. Growth or development to a higher level is not explicitly addressed by Roy as a part of adaptation, but it is implicit in the notion of positive or health-promoting adaptation.

The literature regarding adaptation is extensive and often seems to be describing quite different phenomena, depending on the unit of analysis (group, individual, organ system, cell), the disciplinary perspective of the investigator (anthropologist, sociologist, psychologist, physician, nurse), or the definition of adaptation as process or end point. Common threads do emerge, however, and these can guide health workers as they seek to help individuals, groups, and populations in interaction with their environments.

1. Adaptation is a process that characterizes living systems in interaction with their environments.
2. These environments may be internal or external to the living system.
3. Stimuli resulting in adaptation may be developmental (or maturational) events or situational crises that occur in day-to-day living.
4. The processes of adaptation lead to growth and autonomy as well as to preservation and stability.
5. Coping and stress are concepts related to adaptation; coping suggests the *strategies* of adaptation, and stress often connotes *responses* that tax adaptive capacities.

Adaptation as interaction with the environment

Adaptation was defined by Simpson[35] as both the processes and the outcome (end point) that create and maintain useful relationships between an organism or population of organisms and the environment.[35] Nonliving systems are not regarded as adapting because they do not change or grow to meet the demands of changing environments. Living systems, in contrast, are capable of seeking and using information, both biologically and cognitively, to effect change in response to changing environments.[23] Living systems are not only acted on by external environments, but also can act on the environment to further adaptation. As a simple example, humans in northern climates create more comfortable winter environments by building shelters, making clothing, and using parts of the environment for fuel to warm the shelters. To the extent that these components of the environment are not renewable, people may be faced in the near future with the need to adapt life-styles to a markedly changing environment.

Human beings and other organisms adapt biologically and socially as well as technologically to changing environments. The Tierra del Fuegans, the inhabitants of the tip of South America, startled Darwin by their seeming imperviousness to severe cold and snow. More modern scientists have found that these people conserve heat far more efficiently than persons adapted to more temperate climates.[4] Various species of monkeys have adapted anatomically as well as biologically to their environments. For example, the gibbon has long, very strong arms that are well suited to swinging through the dense forests in which it lives. In contrast, the patas monkey has developed protective coloration to camouflage itself in the grasslands and social habits that allow quick dispersion should there be an attack in so open a place.[20]

If humans are constantly interacting with their environments, it follows that adaptation must be a constant and dynamic factor of living. If adaptation is viewed as including growth as well as maintenance, it becomes a central concept in understanding living systems. All life processes then support the person-environment interaction. In the framework of adaptation, all person-environment interactions are intimately tied to interactions with successively larger environments (Fig. 12-1).

Environments: internal and external

Nurses frequently work with individuals, families, or small groups. Consequently, the interaction of these entities with their immediate environments becomes the most common unit of analysis for nursing.[18] However, in living systems, including human beings, there are many environments, both internal and external to the whole organism.[14] The cell, which is often considered a fundamental unit of analysis, has an internal environment—the mitochondria, ribosomes, and other machinery of replication and metabolism. It also has many external environments—the immediate fluid environment, the organ and organ system of which it is a part, and the whole organism in which it resides. This organism in turn has the cell, its organ and organ systems, and integrating mechanisms as an internal environment, and an external environment consisting of all the animate and inanimate entities outside its skin. These entities may constitute a physical environment of such elements as heat, light, sound, form, and motion and a sociocultural environment composed of the social groupings, institutions, and cultures through which many adaptive strategies are transmitted. Finally, one may consider cultures or nations as the systems of analysis, with terrestrial and supranational environments as external to the system and nations, economic cartels, and racial subgroups as the internal environments.

For the most part, the medical-surgical nurse is concerned with an individual or a family attempting to maintain health or to adapt to an episode of acute

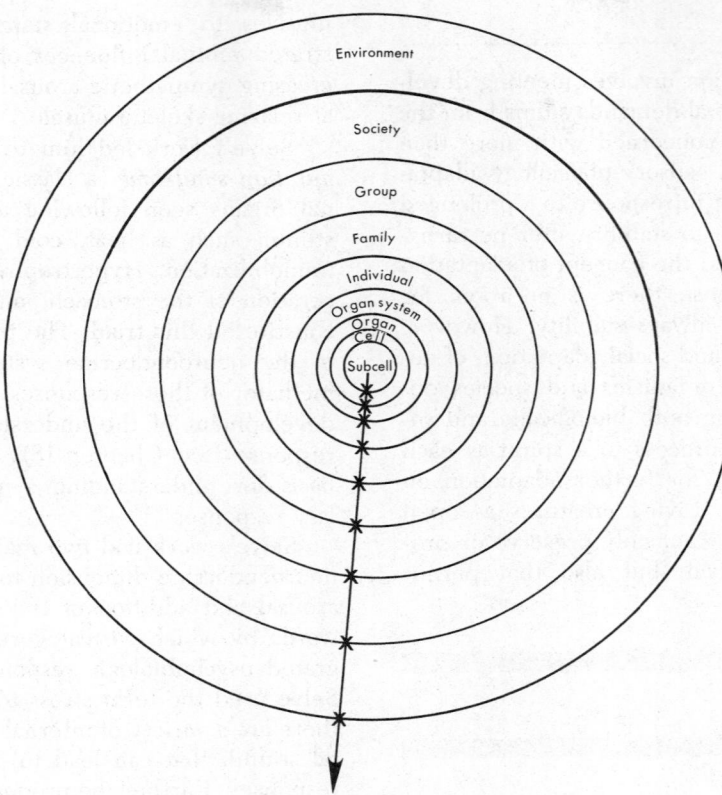

Fig. 12-1. Person-environment interactions. There are many environments, both inside and outside an individual, with which the person interacts. Each environment could be considered internal to the larger environment of which it is a part.

or chronic illness. Consequently, evaluation of adaptive demands and strategies will most often occur in relation to an individual and his or her immediate physical and sociocultural environment. It is important, however, to be aware that these immediate environments are influenced by considerably larger environments.

Adaptive stimuli: developmental and situational

Although by definition any changing environmental stimulus initiates adaptive processes, two classes of events create major adaptive demands for individuals or groups. These have been termed *developmental crises* and *situational crises*.[3] Adams and Lindeman[1] define a crisis as any situation that requires an individual or a group to mobilize new resources or master new skills. Developmental demands are those that predictably occur in a given culture as the individual moves from one state of development to another; for example, the transition from childhood to adolescence or from early to middle adulthood. Many of these transitions are

marked by biologic as well as psychologic changes accompanying maturation (see Chapter 16).

Situational crises, in contrast, do not occur predictably in relation to the maturational development of people (although most people face many situational crises at some times during their lives). Illness, accidents, loss, divorce, a new job, and fame are all examples of events that can produce situational adaptive demands. Note that not all the examples are negative or "bad" events; the common denominator is the demand for new resources or mastery of new skills.

For a given individual or family, situational crises will interact with the state of development or maturation of the individual or family. The biologic and social capacity to cope with the demands of the situation depend in part on (1) the state of maturation and (2) the social and physical support systems available in the environment. For example, short-term malnutrition may permanently alter the intellectual capacity of the child whose brain is still developing but cause only temporary apathy in an adult. That same child, however, may become a contributing member of society, with appropriate social support systems such as sheltered workshops and special education.

Stability and growth

The notion that adaptation involves meeting developmental as well as situational demands stems from the concept that adaptation is concerned with more than just organismic stability. In sensory physiology adaptation refers to the decrement in response to a prolonged stimulus, implying a return to stability after perturbation.[12] Rogers[17] has criticized the concept of adaptation as being too limited because there is no room for growth if the end result is always stability. However, all accounts of evolutionary and social adaptation, of necessity, include growth as organisms and species develop new ways of behaving both biologically and socially. Dubos[26] likens this process to a spiral as each adaptation creates demands for further adaptation on successively higher planes. Living creatures as open systems behave in ways that not only preserve or protect their existence (survival) but also that permit growth and striving.[23]

Stress

Historical perspective

The term *stress* has been used colloquially for centuries to refer to mental and emotional strain or pressure. In physics stress has a precise mechanical meaning—the force put on an object. The resulting deformation or response is designated as *strain*. Selye[33] was the first to use the term stress in a biologic context—the nonspecific response of the body to a variety of noxious stimuli. He termed the stimulus the *stressor*. Initially, Selye avoided the term stress because of its common use in connoting emotional turmoil.[34] However, as he came to see that many strong stimuli were capable of provoking the general adaptation syndrome (discussed below), he postulated that emotional stimuli were equivalent to physical stressors (e.g., heat, cold, trauma) in evoking the response, and he began to use stress as synonymous with the general adaptation syndrome.[33]

The notion of a general integrated and mutually interacting biologic and psychologic response to a variety of environmental stimuli was not unique to Selye. In fact, his work was preceded by the philosophic writings of James[29] and Lange,[9] who proposed that the perception of visceral responses to emotional events *was* the emotion, by the experiments of Cannon,[25] who observed the similarity of physiologic responses of the sympathetic nervous system during a variety of emotional states, and by Jacobsen,[28] who documented responses of the sympathetic nervous system and skeletal

muscles to emotional states. Jacobsen also demonstrated mutual influences of these subsystems by decreasing sympathetic arousal through therapy directed at relaxing skeletal muscle.

Selye's work led him to describe the *general adaptation syndrome*, a classic triad of changes in internal organs seen following a wide variety of noxious stimuli such as heat, cold, skin trauma, and forced immobilization. Hypertrophy of the adrenal gland, ulceration of the stomach, and atrophy of the thymus constituted this triad. The pituitary-adrenocortical axis of the neuroendocrine system was found to be the mediator of these responses, thus setting the stage for development of the understanding of neuroendocrine response (see Chapter 18). Cannon's work forms the basis for understanding sympathetic–adrenal medullary responses.

Selye's work had two major effects: addition of the neuroendocrine dimension to biologic manifestations of arousal and addition of the term stress to the list of words by which we categorize knowledge about integrated psychobiologic responses to our environments. Selye used the term stress to present the concept that there are a variety of internal and external environmental stimuli that can lead to similar protective biologic responses. Further, he proposed that continued intense stimulation would lead to depletion of the biologic ability to respond and to diminished ability to respond to additional challenges.

Conceptualizations of stress

These early ideas have led to a vast research and clinical literature regarding stress as a common denominator in causation of illness and as an impediment to recovery from illness. Despite the nearly 50 years that stress has been used as a research concept, investigators do not agree on its definition or measurement. Some suggest discarding the term altogether.[8] Overlapping of concepts is evident in the multiple headings under which one may find studies and reviews relevant to the phenomenon: emotion, anxiety, stress, psychophysiology, arousal, activation, and adaptation.

Early workers in the area of psychologic stress tended to view events or stimuli as stressful in themselves; however, it has become increasingly evident that the critical factor is the psychologic meaning attached to the stimulus.[13] Some theorists contend that the stimulus must symbolize threat to be stressful, thus emphasizing the stimulus and its appraisal.[6,31] Others note similar biologic responses to both threat and pleasure, thus defining stress from the standpoint of biologic response.[11] Lazarus, Averill, and Opton[10] integrate these approaches by suggesting that the key is the psychobiologic appraisal of stimuli that are highly relevant to one's welfare, whether this relevance be positive or negative.[10]

A third approach is to define stress as existing when adaptive capacities are exceeded, thus suggesting an interactive state between stimulus and response.[27] The more complete theories in this perspective emphasize biologic as well as psychosocial responses and initiating stimuli. Examples of events that exceed adaptive capacity in most people are widespread infection, trauma, and surgery.

Distinguishing the different ways in which stress is conceptualized is important because the way we think about stress influences the way we use the concept in clinical work with both well and ill people. If we think of stress as a defined set of biologic events happening *to* people, we may not appreciate gradations of response or the influence of an individual's perceptions on the intensity or even presence of the response. Further, if we consider stress as external to the person, we may not consider using measures that help people manage their own perceptions and responses to the changing environment.

Integrated psychobiologic response

There are some commonalities that emerge, however, from the differing perspectives from which stress has been approached. First, Selye's observation that many different stimuli are capable of producing a common physiologic response has stood the test of time. There are, however, important qualifiers regarding when and to what degree diverse stimuli elicit this response.

Mason[13,32] has presented convincing evidence that psychologic appraisal of any stimulus as challenging or threatening is the key mediator of the multiple neuroendocrine responses to stimuli. If stimuli such as heat, cold, or even trauma can be introduced in such a way that the organism is unaware of the change,* only the response specific to the stimulus is elicited and not the multiple endocrine stress response. The biologic responses of sympathetic–adrenal medullary, pituitary-adrenocortical, and hypothalamic-endocrine systems are described in Chapter 18. Physical immobility, surgery, fear, anger, and inescapable noxious stimuli have all been shown to be capable of eliciting this multisystem response. The intensity of response depends on a combination of (1) intensity of stimulus, (2) duration of stimulus, and (3) perception of control over the stimulus.

---

*Trauma can be introduced so that an experimental animal is unaware of it by injuring a limb that has no nervous connections to the rest of the body (a denervated limb).

Intensity of stimulus

Intense physical and psychologic stimuli such as trauma, forceful immobilization, and strong fear lead to stress responses in most organisms—human and non-human. In experimental situations in which intense stimuli can be gradated, as in trauma or burns, the intensity of the multisystem response is also gradated in proportion to the stimulus.[24] A similar graded response is at least partially evident in human response to various traumas and surgical procedures. For example, the metabolic response to a burn over 40% of the body area is considerably greater than that to a hernia repair. The psychologic component (threat, fear, inescapability, lack of control) is also greater for the patient with a burn than for the person experiencing elective surgery.

Duration of stimulus

Some investigators have suggested that while most organisms may have similar emergency responses to acute and intense stimuli, ongoing stimuli may elicit different individual responses. The adaptive response of one organism to ongoing stimuli may either resemble or differ from the response of another organism. Henry's work with colonies of mice is the most extensive long-term investigation of the physiologic responses of animals to their ordinary social interactions.[7] As these animals established their social dominance hierarchy, those who became the dominant animals exhibited primarily sympathetic–adrenal medullary activation, characterized biochemically by elevated catecholamine levels, behaviorally by muscular activity, and symptomatically by hypertension. In contrast, the animals at the bottom of the social hierarchy showed primarily a pituitary-adrenocortical response: elevated corticosteroid levels, withdrawn behavior, and ultimately enlarged adrenal glands and stomach ulcers. The animals who challenged the dominant animals had profiles midway between the two groups. While this study is not presented to suggest that socially dominant people will become hypertensive, it does support the notion that in ordinary daily living organisms, including humans, tend to respond in a characteristic mode. This mode is partially dependent on genetic factors, social position, and learned modes of coping with or responding to everyday events.

Perception of control

Perception of control over a situation and relevant feedback regarding the effect of one's behavior on the stimulus appear to be potent factors regulating the multihormonal stress response. When a dominant animal from Henry's mouse colony was put into a colony in which dominance had already been established, the previously dominant mouse became submissive, and its behavior and physiologic response became that of the submissive mice. One could argue that the mouse perceived itself as no longer being in control. Parachutists in training in Norway exhibited all the characteristic neuroendocrine stress responses before their first jump but rapidly returned to baseline values in subsequent jumps. Their subjective fear decreased as their sense of mastery and control over the task increased.[12] Weiss[22] presents an excellent summary of animal research demonstrating that control over aversive stimuli (shock) and relevant feedback regarding one's efforts reduced and even prevented pathologic physiologic stress responses in a variety of situations.

Stress has been linked both in the popular press and in scientific literature with disease, presumably caused by prolonged or excessive physiologic responses to a variety of situations. It should be evident from the foregoing, however, that it is not the situations by themselves that create the stress response, but rather the combination of psychologic appraisal and sense of control. These concepts lead logically to the notion of coping with change: the perception and appraisal of some relevant but challenging situation, and the psychobiologic responses emanating from that perception.

Coping

The definitions of coping are as many and varied as were those for adaptation and stress. White[23] considers coping the *strategies* of adaptation—the means by which adaptation takes place. Many authorities identify coping most easily in the context of crisis or in adjustment to adverse circumstances. It is often defined as involving problem-solving efforts in situations that are perceived as being highly relevant to the individual and that tax adaptive resources.[10,27] While many persons explicitly or implicitly consider coping to be primarily a cognitive process, some authors recognize the interrelationship between physiologic and cognitive responses to adverse circumstances. Levine, Weinburg, and Ursin[12] define the ultimate goal of coping processes to be reduction of physiologic activation, whereas Murphy[16] divides coping processes into Coping I, the capacity to deal with the changing environment (action and cognition), and Coping II, the capacity to maintain the internal environment.

In general, then, coping refers to processes or skills that individuals use to deal with events, circumstances, or situations that are out of the ordinary. It is an integrated psychobiologic process in which "gut" feelings influence cognition of the need to cope and coping efforts influence the state of arousal of the internal environment. Stimuli to coping may arise in the external environment in the form of physical stimuli, interpersonal relationships, or community and international events. Similarly, stimuli may arise in the internal environment in terms of thoughts, feelings, and physical illness.

General themes in coping

Coping processes enable us to learn from new situations strategies that may be useful in the future, and they arise from what has been learned in the past. Coping processes may thus be considered the major means for growth in the continual process of adaptation. When various perspectives on coping are evaluated, recurrent themes are evident: (1) coping stems from appraisal of relevant situations; (2) there is motivation to change; (3) information must be sought and used; (4) either action is practiced and tried or attitudes are changed; (5) there must be relevant feedback regarding coping efforts; and (6) coping takes place in a social context that defines appropriate and inappropriate coping and that transmits coping strategies from one generation to the next.[3] People tend, over time, to develop coping styles, using strategies that have served them well in the past, to reduce physiologic arousal and to meet the developmental challenges of maturation.

Coping strategies have been categorized as those involving direct action on oneself or on the environment or involving intrapsychic processes.[10,31] With direct action one may change the environment or oneself or in some way directly confront, avoid, or sidestep the situation out of which the need to cope arises. Intrapsychic processes are largely cognitive ways of changing the meaning of the situation or of dealing with the emotions that arise from the situation. Many investigators have found that those who are judged as coping most successfully with a variety of situations are flexible in using strategies from both categories rather than rigidly repeating the same strategies in each new situation.[21]

Coping in illness and disability

Illness often represents a crisis that challenges comfortable coping styles. Chronic illness and physical disability demand the development of new coping skills. As with all coping the individual's appraisal of the meaning of the illness and disability determines the extent to which these situations represent a crisis. However, the characteristics of a given illness or disability together with societal expectations of related behaviors add a new dimension to previously learned coping skills.

Adams and Lindemann[1] define four mechanisms fundamental to successful coping with the environment: movement, sensing, energy production, and cerebral integration. Impairment of any of these leaves an individual with a diminished capacity to cope with the environment and thus with a disability. All acute and chronic illnesses affect one or more of these fundamental functions and thus by their nature diminish the available capacity for coping. When experiencing acute or chronic illness, people have two sets of adaptive tasks, as defined by Moos[15]: general tasks, as in any life crisis, and illness-related tasks. The *general tasks* defined by many authors include maintaining a sense of personal worth or self-esteem, maintaining a reasonable emotional balance, maintaining or restoring relationships with significant persons, and preparing for an uncertain future. *Illness-related tasks* include dealing with pain and incapacitation, enhancing the recovery of body functions, dealing with the hospital environment, and developing adequate relationships with hospital personnel.[1,15] The latter two are integral to increasing the likelihood of the individual's return to a valued and socially accepted life-style after maximal physical recovery. These tasks are quite similar to the appropriate "sick role" behavior described by Parsons (see Chapter 1).

Chronic illness or *disability* imposes additional adaptive tasks.[19] These tasks include the prevention of medical crises, control of ongoing symptoms, carrying out treatment regimens, adjustment to changes in the disease course, obtaining funding for survival and ongoing treatment, adapting to or preventing social isolation, and normalizing relationships with others (see Chapter 29).

A number of coping skills are as relevant to dealing with illness and disability as they are to general crisis situations. They relate to both action (problem-focused) or intrapsychic (emotion-focused) strategies.

Action-focused strategies include seeking relevant information about the illness or disability, learning procedures or tasks specifically related to it, setting concrete and realistic goals, and rehearsing alternative outcomes.[15] For example, a person faced with long-term hemodialysis for renal failure may cope with this major change in life-style and threat to life by learning everything possible about home dialysis and how others have managed and about the procedures that must be mastered to safely accomplish it. Information regarding expected energy levels, time required for dialysis, and duration between treatments may help the individual set realistic goals for employment or education. While the intended goal of home dialysis is to allow continued life and reasonable functioning, it is possible that the condition will worsen and less and less time off dialysis will be possible. Rehearsal of alternative outcomes is a strategy by which such possible outcomes are thought about, discussed, and possible options considered (e.g., kidney transplant or death). Rehearsal is one strategy by which all of us "practice" behaviors for anticipated circumstances.

Coping strategies are not entirely rational, however. Emotional responses to crises are dominant and interact with action responses at all points. *Emotional strategies* that serve to protect us, consciously or unconsciously, from severe distress or anxiety have often been called defense mechanisms. Denying, minimizing, and dissociating oneself from situations are mechanisms that serve to reduce anxiety and often are helpful in buying time as one prepares to face the situation (see Chapter 14). However, when such strategies are prolonged, they may serve to prevent the gaining of needed information or learning necessary skills.

Other *intrapsychic strategies* include reframing the problem or finding some meaning or general purpose in it. If the event is explicable in the context of some larger purpose or understanding of life, distressing emotions may become more manageable and energy can be freed to focus on the problem itself. Simultaneously, one may be requesting reassurance and emotional support from others in the environment. Such support helps reaffirm a sense of personal worth in the face of major change.

There is no one specific or best way to cope with any given situation. What is useful to one individual may be inappropriate for another. The nature of the particular illness, the state of development of the individual, the social and cultural environment, and the physical and interpersonal resources available all influence the style and effectiveness of coping strategies. In nursing, as in other helping relationships, it is most useful to assist a person to cope in ways that are congruent with previously established styles. Weisman[21] suggests seven simple questions that can garner a great deal of information about coping strategies:

1. What problems, if any, do you see this illness creating?
2. How do you plan to deal with them?
3. When faced with a problem you must do something about, what do you do?
4. How does it usually work out?
5. To whom do you turn when you need help?
6. What has happened in the past when you have asked for help?
7. What kinds of problems usually tend to get you upset or down?

These questions establish perception of the current problem (numbers 1 and 2), usual style of dealing with problems (numbers 2, 3, and 4), sources of help and response to help (numbers 5 and 6), and recurrent trouble areas (number 7).

Adaptation, stress, and coping: application to nursing

Adaptation, stress, and coping are related concepts pervasive in everyday life. In *health* people turn to the helping professions most often when they desire assistance in developing new coping strategies for developmental crises. For example, prospective parents are taught information and specific skills in childbirth education classes or parenting skills and tactics for coping with difficult ages in rearing children. Physical fitness classes and stress management classes are other examples of help provided to people who are not ill. Nursing roles with respect to coping and stress in the well person are primarily educative, facilitating the ability of individuals and groups to identify sources of and to manage stress by themselves, to identify common crises in ordinary living, and to facilitate coping.

In *acute illness* the illness itself poses a major crisis for the person. Nursing roles are twofold: managing the environment to prevent the addition of further challenges to the person's equilibrium and supplementing, insofar as possible, the person's own adaptive responses. This supplementation may consist of care and comfort measures designed to reduce fear, pain, and anxiety as well as therapeutic activity within the patient's adaptive tolerance.

Chronic illness implies reduced adaptive capacity in one or more areas. Thus while the individual may cope adequately with ordinary living demands, the compensatory reserve for adjusting to unusual circumstances may not be available. For example, persons with compensated congestive heart failure may have no difficulty doing their own laundry when the equipment is all on the same floor as the living areas. However, they might be unable to cope with this simple part of living if forced to use a laundromat located down one flight of stairs. Nursing roles in chronic illness are both supportive and educative: helping the person identify usual limits of adaptive capacity, helping the person learn ways to reach goals within adaptive limits, and locating resources to supplement the person's capacities.

REFERENCES AND SELECTED READINGS
Contemporary

1. Adams, J., and Lindemann, E.: Coping with long-term disability. In Coehlo, G.V., Hamburg, D.A., and Adams, J.E., editors: Coping and adaptation, New York, 1974, Basic Books, Inc., Publishers.
2. Burchfeld, S.: The stress response: a reappraisal, Psychosom. Med. **41:**661-672, 1979.
3. Coehlo, G.V., Hamburg, D.A., and Adams, J.E.: Coping and adaptation, New York, 1974, Basic Books, Inc., Publishers.
4. Follinsbee, F.J.: Environmental stress, New York, 1978, Academic Press, Inc.
5. Grinker, R.R.: Forward. In Coehlo, G.V., Hamburg, D.A., and Adams, J.E.: Coping and adaptation, New York, 1974, Basic Books, Inc., Publishers.
6. Gross, E.: Work, organization and stress. In Levine, S., and Scotch, N.A.: Social stress, Chicago, 1970, Aldine Publishing Co.
7. Henry, J.P.: Mechanisms of psychosomatic disease in animals, Adv. Vet. Sci. **20:**115-145, 1976.
8. Hinkle, L.E.: The concept of stress in the biological and social sciences, Int. J. Psychiatr. Med. **5:**335-337, 1974.
9. Lader, M., and Tyer, P.: Vegetative system and emotion. In Levi, L.: Emotions: their parameters and measurement, New York, 1975, Raven Press.
10. Lazarus, R.A., Averill, J.R., and Opton, E.M.: The psychology of coping: issues of research and assessment. In Coehlo, G.V., Hamburg, D.A., and Adams, J.E.: Coping and adaptation, New York, 1974, Basic Books, Inc., Publishers.
11. Levi, L.: Stress and distress in response to psychosocial stimuli, Int. Ser. Monographs Exp. Psych., vol. 17, 1972.
12. Levine, S., Weinberg, J., and Ursin, H.: Definition of the coping process and statement of the problem. In Ursin, H., Baade, E., and Levine, S.: Psychobiology of stress: a study of coping men, New York, 1978, Academic Press, Inc.
13. Mason, J.W.: A historical view of the stress field, J. Human Stress **1**(1):6–12, **1**(2):22-36, 1975.
14. Miller, J.: Living systems, New York, 1979, McGraw-Hill Book Co.
15. Moos, R.: Coping with physical illness, New York, 1977, Plenum Publishing Corp.
16. Murphy, L.P.: Coping, vulnerability and resilience in childhood. In Coehlo, G.V., Hamburg, D.A., and Adams, J.E.: Coping and adaptation, New York, 1974, Basic Books, Inc., Publishers.
17. Rogers, M.: An introduction to the theoretical basis of nursing, Philadelphia, 1970, F.A. Davis Co.
18. Roy, Sr. C.: The Roy adaptation model. In Riehl, J., and Roy, Sr. C.: Conceptual models for nursing practice, ed. 2, New York, 1980, Appleton-Century-Crofts, Inc.
19. Strauss, A., and Glaser, B.: Chronic illness and the quality of life, St. Louis, 1975, The C.V. Mosby Co.
20. Washburn, S.L., Hamburg, D.A., and Bishop, N.H.: Social adaptation in nonhuman primates. In Coehlo, G.V., Hamburg, D.A., and Adams, J.E.: Coping and adaptation, New York, 1974, Basic Books, Inc., Publishers.
21. Weisman, A.: Coping with cancer, New York, 1979, McGraw-Hill Book Co.
22. Weiss, J.M.: Psychological factors in stress and disease, Sci. Amer. **226**(6):104-113, 1972.
23. White, R.D.: Strategies of adaptation: an attempt at systematic description. In Coehlo, G.V., Hamburg, D.A., and Adams, J.E.: Coping and adaptation, New York, 1974, Basic Books, Inc., Publishers.
24. Wilmore, D., et al.: Stress in surgical patients as a neurophysiologic reflex response, Surg. Gynecol. Obstet. **142:**257-269, 1976.

Classic

25. Cannon, W.B.: The wisdom of the body, New York, 1939, W.W. Norton & Co., Inc.
26. Dubos, R.: Man adapting, New Haven, Conn., 1965, Yale University Press.
27. Howard, A., and Scott, R.A.: A proposed framework for the analysis of stress in the human organism, Behav. Sci. **10:**141–160, 1965.
28. Jacobsen, E.: Anxiety and tension control, Philadelphia, 1964, J.B. Lippincott Co.

29. James, W.: What is emotion? Mind **19**:188-205, 1884.
30. Janis, I.: Psychological stress, New York, 1958, John Wiley & Sons, Inc.
31. Lazarus, R.A.: Psychological stress and the coping process, New York, 1966, McGraw-Hill Book Co.
32. Mason, J.W.: Organization of the multiple endocrine responses to avoidance in the monkey, Psychosom. Med. **30**(suppl.):774-790, 1968.
33. Selye, H.: The stress of life, New York, 1956, McGraw-Hill Book Co.
34. Selye, H.: A syndrome produced by diverse noxious agents, Nature **138**:32-35, 1936.
35. Simpson, G.G.: Behavior and evolution. In Roe, A.R., and Simpson, G.G.: Behavior and evolution, New Haven, Conn., 1958, Yale University Press.

CHAPTER 13

STRESS MANAGEMENT

PATRICIA A. BETRUS

An old adage suggests that in the course of an individual's lifetime three events will occur: birth, death, and taxes. Perhaps this adage is outdated and a fourth category needs to be included: stress. Stress is present in all aspects of our daily life. It is a normal part of the homeostatic process that maintains the relative constancy of the external environment. Stress motivates and challenges us. In response to stress, individuals are activated to learn and test new responses and coping behaviors. Life without stress would be a life without challenge, a continual state of nonarousal. Stress is necessary for our existence.

Although stress is essential for being and part of the normal homeostatic process, it can also be disruptive to this process. When stress occurs too frequently, is too long lasting, or is of great intensity, the individual's ability to continuously cope or adapt is exhausted. Also, if stress is chronic, the homeostatic mechanism can reset to a new level, often abnormal, and this new level is maintained even when stress is reduced.[8]

Every individual has a baseline of stress within which the homeostatic process operates normally. The boundaries of normal homeostasis are ubiquitous to the individual and are defined by the individual's genetic background, environment, and appraisal of events.[5] Fig. 13-1 illustrates the relationship between stress and the homeostatic process.

It has been estimated that 50% to 85% of all illnesses are stress aided or stress induced.[6] Traditionally, stress and its effects have been treated within the framework of the medical model. Within this framework, amelioration of the effects of stress is achieved by the use of drugs. For example, insomnia, an affliction linked to stress, is often treated by the prescription of sleep medications. A survey of persons with insomnia in the San Francisco area indicated that 40% used sleep drugs nightly, and another 26% used sleep drugs occa-

sionally. It was also found that in this sample 33% used alcohol to induce sleep, and yet another 14% used a combination of drugs and alcohol to get to sleep.[4]

Often when medications are used to diminish the stress response, the medications become new stressors to the individual. Many medications have side effects that are stressful to the individual. The iatrogenic effects of medical treatment for stress (side effects) are often controlled by prescribing additional medications to contain the side effects. The use of drugs to control the side effects of drugs used to diminish the effects of stress has been referred to as the domino theory approach to managing stress.[13]

The use of medications to diminish the effects of the stress response is not always inappropriate. Drugs can be of use, especially for short-term intervention. Drug usage for stress becomes problematic when used chronically and physiologic or psychologic dependence results. Dependence on drugs, with all the accompanying medical problems, also prevents the individual from exploring new coping strategies and utilizing internal resources.[13]

Stress management as a therapy

In response to the problems inherent in the traditional approach to stress reduction, alternative strategies have been developed. These strategies utilize physiologic, cognitive, or behavioral techniques to diminish the effects of stress. Stress management as a therapeutic process has proliferated in the past 2 decades. Many of its techniques have been scrutinized carefully, and research documents the efficacy of these procedures in the management of stress.

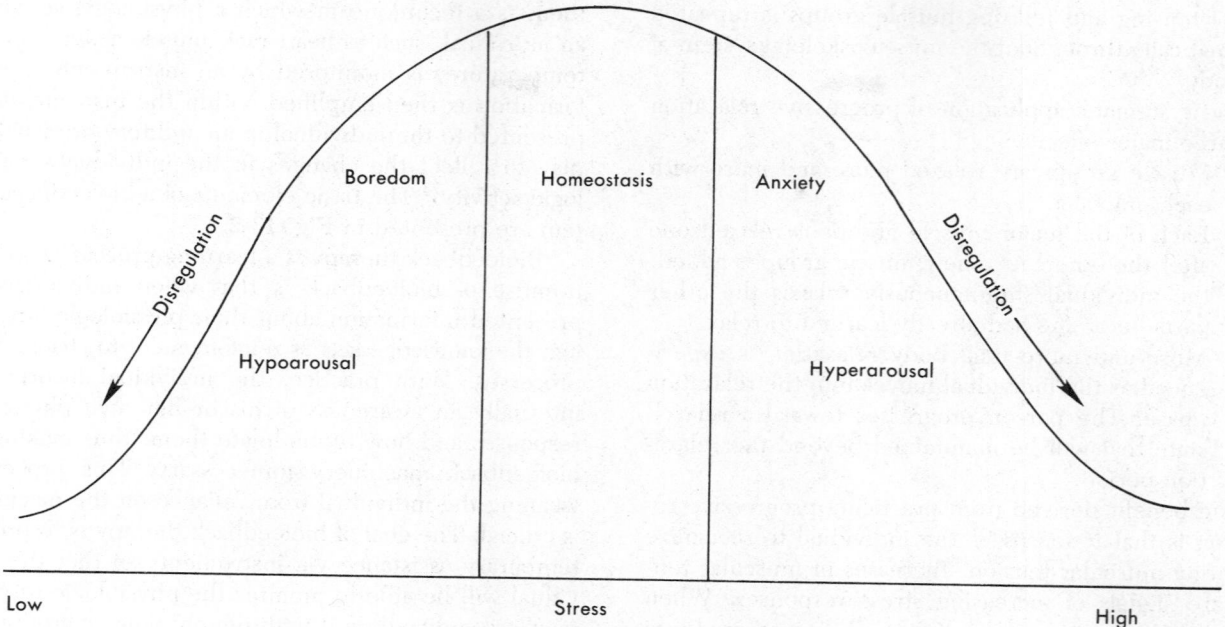

Fig. 13-1. Stress and the homeostasis process.

Stress management embraces a self-management orientation, emphasizing individual responsibility and participation in treatment.[10] The goal of treatment for the therapist is to provide the behavioral, cognitive, and psychophysiologic skills necessary for individuals to manage their own stress responses. In contrast to the traditional relationship between the individual and health care practitioner, which focuses on "compliance," individuals receiving stress management are active change agents. The stress management therapist, adhering to the self-management model, is cognizant of the limitations of his or her own therapeutic role. Ideally, the stress management therapist is a proficient therapist who acts as an instigator, facilitator, and model in order to assist the individual in the acquisition of relaxation and related stress management skills. The stress management therapist assumes the responsibility for designing a structured, realistic program of change, but it is the individual's responsibility to implement and maintain the program.[11]

The specific goals of a comprehensive stress management program are to assist the individual in the following ways:

1. Developing an awareness of the stressors present in the environment
2. Recognizing his or her own specific response to stress
3 Developing and testing new coping behaviors
4. Gaining voluntary self-control over physiologic processes

Self-management training does not make any at-
tempt to eliminate stress from the life of the individual. As stated earlier, stress is essential for life, and stress management training is designed to enhance the individual's ability to take charge of his or her own wellness-illness behaviors.

Psychophysiologic stress management strategies

Progressive relaxation

Progressive relaxation was developed by Jacobson and described in *Progressive Relaxation,* his classic book of 1938. The major premise of the progressive relaxation strategy is that anxiety and muscular relaxation are mutually exclusive events. Thus anxiety does not and cannot exist when the muscles of the body are relaxed.[3]

The procedures involved in Jacobson's progressive relaxation are fundamentally simple. People typically have little or no awareness of the sensation of relaxation. In progressive relaxation the individual first tenses a specific set of muscles as hard as possible and acknowledges the feelings of tenderness, tension, and even pain in those muscles. Then the person relaxes the muscle group as much as possible and focuses on the feelings of relaxation. Furthermore, the individual is taught to recognize the difference in sensations between the tension and the relaxation states. This pattern of tensing and relaxing muscle groups is repeated systematically throughout the musculoskeletal system of the body.

The systematic application of progressive relaxation has three major effects:

1. Muscle groups are relaxed more and more with each practice.
2. Each of the major muscle groups is relaxed one after the other. As a new muscle group is added, the individual simultaneously relaxes the other parts he or she had already learned to relax.
3. More and more total body relaxation is experienced as the individual moves into the relaxation phase. The person progresses toward a relaxed state that will be maintained beyond the relaxation period.[5]

The benefit derived from practicing progressive relaxation is that it sensitizes the individual to recognize mounting muscular tension. Increases in muscular tension are signals of increasing stress responses. When progressive relaxation is practiced and incorporated into the individual's life-style, it can help neutralize the stress response.

Biofeedback

Biofeedback arose from a debate between classical and operant conditioning theorists. Classical conditioning, introduced by Pavlov, refers to learning that takes place when a conditioning stimulus is paired with an unconditioned stimulus. Operant conditioning, introduced by Skinner, refers to learning that occurs without a known stimulus, usually through the receiving of rewards. The debate between the theorists focused on how many kinds of learning there were. Skinnerians claimed that only operant learning existed and that it involved voluntary processes. Other theorists stated that operant learning could also involve the involuntary processes of the autonomic nervous system. Miller, in his classic experiments, taught curarized rats to raise and lower their heart rates, blood pressure, renal blood flow, and so on through operant rewards.[9] This initial research was rapidly expanded and applied to humans experiencing psychophysiologic disregulation caused by stress.

Biofeedback, simply stated, is a process for learning voluntary control over autonomically regulated body functions. We have all received biofeedback in its simplest form during our lives. When we step on a bathroom scale, we get direct feedback regarding our weight. When we think we have a fever and place a thermometer in our mouths, the reading (feedback) tells us something of what is going on inside us.[6]

Biofeedback as a strategy for stress management is used to reduce tensions and anxiety that are manifested in increased sympathetic arousal. Biofeedback therapy, then, is a technique in which a physiologic activity of an individual, such as heart rate, muscle activity, or skin temperature, is monitored by an instrument. This information is then amplified within the instrument and presented to the individual in an auditory or visual display to reflect the changes in the individual's physiologic activity.[3] The basic elements of a biofeedback system are presented in Fig. 13-2.

Biofeedback therapy is a learning process. The basic premise of biofeedback is that when individuals are presented information about their physiologic functioning, the knowledge acts as reinforcement to change those processes. With practice, the individual incorporates internally an awareness of his or her own physiologic responses and how to modulate them, thus making the biofeedback machinery unnecessary. This process of weaning the individual from reliance on the machinery is crucial. The goal of biofeedback therapy is to provide temporary assistance via instruments so that the individual will be able to monitor the physiologic response to stress and replace it with nonphysiologic arousal.[8]

Methods of biofeedback

EMG biofeedback. Muscle activity is monitored and measured by an electromyograph (EMG). Electrodes are placed on the skin over the selected muscle group. These electrodes monitor the electrical activity of the underlying muscle group and send this information to the biofeedback instrument. The instrument converts the raw signal into a display that is then fed back to the individual in the form of visual or auditory information. Muscle tension is an indication of stress. Utilizing the EMG biofeedback information, individuals are able to reduce muscle tension and replace it with muscular relaxation.

Peripheral skin temperature biofeedback. Peripheral skin temperature reflects patterns of vascular constriction and dilation. A thermistor or sensor is placed on an area of skin (generally a finger or toe) to measure changes in temperature. Absolute temperature or a change in temperature is then fed back to the individual. Low skin temperatures are associated with stress; increasing skin temperature reflects relaxation.

Skin conductance levels biofeedback. Skin conductance measures sweat level activity. Two electrodes are placed on hairless skin (typically the palm of the hand or fingers) and a tiny electrical current is passed between the two electrodes. When an individual becomes stressed, perspiration tends to increase. The increased moisture heightens the electrical conductance between the electrodes. When an individual relaxes, there is decreased conductance. These changes in conductance are fed back to the individual.

Other forms of biofeedback. Other physiologic forms of feedback that are used clinically and for research purposes are heart rate, blood pressure, pulse wave ve-

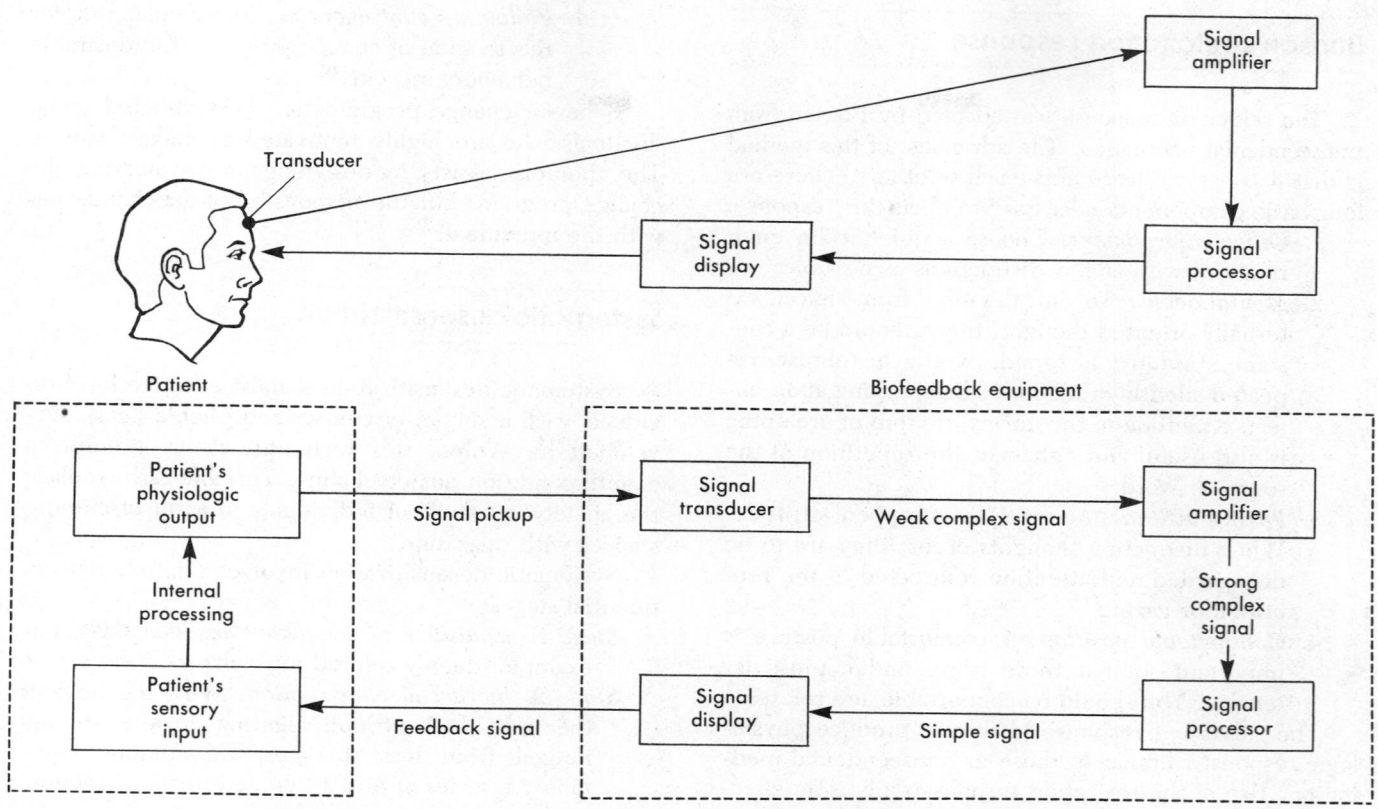

Fig. 13-2. Elements of biofeedback system. (From Gaarder, K., and Montgomery, P.: Clinical biofeedback: a procedural manual, Baltimore, 1977, The Williams & Wilkins Co. © 1977, The Williams & Wilkins Co., Baltimore.)

locity, stomach acidity levels, and respiration feedback.[6]

Biofeedback program

In stress management training the aim of biofeedback is to produce the physiology of relaxation. Merely presenting feedback in a selected system (i.e., muscle) or in a specific site does not guarantee generalization to other systems or sites. A comprehensive biofeedback training program includes monitoring and providing feedback of multiple systems and sites. Only through the use of multimodal sequencing of biofeedback can the acquisition of total body relaxation be accomplished.[11]

Cognitive-behavioral stress management strategies

Meditation

For centuries the art of meditation has been practiced in the East. Proponents of meditation techniques claim that meditators can control physiologic processes, some as dramatic as voluntarily stopping heart beats.[1] There are many different types of meditation with differing goals and foci, including Zen Buddhism, Yoga, and transcendental meditation. Research has focused on transcendental meditation (TM) because it is one of the most practiced forms of meditation in the West.

Meditation produces a hypometabolic response in an individual. Experienced meditators are able to reduce oxygen consumption and blood lactate levels and increase alpha-electroencephalogram (EEG) production following periods of meditation.[1] This response is in direct opposition to the sympathetic activation of stress.

TM is not a complicated process. The individual is given a word, a mantra, which is to be repeated silently by the individual. The individual sits in a comfortable position and focuses attention on breathing and repeating the mantra. The purpose of the mantra is to enhance a passive attitude and prevent distracting thoughts. Meditators are instructed to practice twice daily for at least 20 minutes. The physiologic relaxation that is produced during meditation generalizes to the individual's life as a protection against the effects of stress.

Benson's relaxation response

The relaxation response was adapted by Benson from transcendental meditation. The advantage of this method is that it is easy to learn and teach to others. There are four basic components necessary to elicit this response:

1. *Quiet environment*. Choose a quiet, calm environment with as few distractions as possible.
2. *Mental device*. To shift the mind from logical, externally oriented thought, there should be a constant stimulus: a sound, word, or phrase repeated silently or aloud; or fixed gaxing at an object. Attention to the normal rhythm of breathing is also useful and enhances the repetition of the sound or word.
3. *Passive attitude*. Adopt a "let it happen" attitude. When distracting thoughts occur, they are to be disregarded and attention redirected to the repetition or gazing.
4. *Comfortable position*. A comfortable posture is important so that there is no undue muscular tension. You should be comfortable and relaxed.[1]

The relaxation response is able to produce physiologic responses similar to those in transcendental meditation. Use of the relaxation response daily is an effective mechanism to counteract the effects of stress.

Behavioral change programs

Behavioral change programs typically focus on eliminating a specific stress-related symptom, such as smoking or overeating. The specific components of a behavioral program are as follows:

1. *Self-monitoring of behaviors*. Monitoring of behaviors involves determining the frequency, duration, and intensity of the behavior. Furthermore, any antecedent behaviors or situations associated with the behaviors are recorded.
2. *Target behavior*. Identify in precise measurable terms the final outcome behavior that is desired.
3. *Contracting*. A formal (usually written) contract between the individual and therapist. The contract should include:
   a. *Goals*. Time-limited goals (daily/weekly) related to the target behavior.
   b. *Contingency management*. The selected application of rewards and punishments used to increase or decrease behaviors. Also, the use of operant procedures, such as stimulus control and shaping.
   c. *Evaluation*. Established points of time used to evaluate progress of the change project. At these preset evaluations, the contract can be redesigned if it is found lacking.

   d. *Follow-up contingencies*. Future planning for reactivation of change program if undesirable behaviors reoccur.[10]

Behavior change programs are best directed to individuals who are highly motivated to make changes. The therapist assists in designing and evaluating the change program, but the responsibility for change lies with the individual.[10]

Systematic desensitization

Systematic desensitization is most effective for individuals with a single, circumscribed phobia (fear). Developed by Wolpe, this technique is an attempt to countercondition anxiety habits. The aim is to replace the anxiety reactions of individuals to a set of circumstances with relaxation.

Systematic desensitization involves a number of sequential stages:

Stage 1: acquisition of adequate relaxation skills. For example, deeply relaxed musculature.

Stage 2: hierarchy construction. With the help of the individual, stimuli eliciting anxiety are arranged from least to most threatening; commonly a series of 8 to 12 graded images is generated.

Stage 3: systematic desensitization proper. The person is instructed to relax while imagining progressively more threatening circumstances.

The efficacy of this technique rests on the concept of a "competing response," a basic principle of behavior therapy. Here an individual is asked to engage in a behavior that is incompatible with a given problem behavior. For example, an individual cannot be anxious and relaxed at the same time; relaxation "competes" with the phobic anxiety.[11]

Attitudinal restructuring

The basic premise of rational-emotive therapy, developed by Ellis, is that much if not all emotional suffering (stress) is due to the irrational ways people perceive the world. The assumptions that people make lead to self-defeating internal dialogues or negative self-talk.[12] The goal of therapy is to replace negative self-statements with positive self-statements. Changing self-talk involves three steps: identifying our self-talk, evaluating it, and replacing it with more appropriate self-talk.

Detection of self-talk may be difficult at first because it is "inaudible." Detection of self-talk usually involves keeping a daily log to identify specific thoughts and feelings.

Self-talk often distorts reality or arrives at false conclusions. The following five questions are useful in examining self-talk and the situations that are antecedent to it:

1. Have I disregarded an important aspect of the situation?
2. Have I exaggerated the meaning of an event?
3. Are my perceptions of the situation overly simplified or rigid?
4. Have I drawn conclusions where evidence is lacking or where evidence supports a contrary conclusion?
5. Have I overgeneralized or generated a false conclusion?

The answers to the five questions will probably reveal when self-talk is inappropriate and how to restructure it. Negative internal dialogues are probably a major source of stress to many individuals.[2]

Autogenic training

Autogenic training, developed by Schultz and Luthe, teaches cognitive behavior change simultaneously with physiologic behavior change. The autogenic state involves a significant reduction in sympathetic nervous system activity. The procedure applies the principles of self-management and training in passive concentration (not unlike transcendental meditation) through six standard physiologically oriented steps (see box below).[2,6]

Physiologic states	Repeated statement
1. Heaviness in extremities	"My right arm is heavy."
2. Warmth in extremities	"My right arm is warm."
3. Regulation of cardiac activity	"My heart beat is calm and regular."
4. Regulation of respiration	"My breathing is calm and regular."
5. Abdominal warmth	"My solar plexus is warm."
6. Cooling of forehead	"My forehead is cool."

It generally takes 3 to 6 months to go through the six phases of autogenic training. An accomplished practitioner of autogenics should be able to induce a state of relaxation in any environment or situation.

Stress inoculation

Individuals who undergo stress inoculation are provided with a prospective defense or a set of skills to deal with future stressful situations.[7] Stress inoculation training involves three phases:

I. Educational phase. This phase is designed to provide the individual with a conceptual framework for understanding stressful situations. The individual is provided with an explanatory scheme for understanding his or her specific responses to stress.

II. Rehearsal phase. During this phase individuals are provided with a variety of coping techniques. These coping techniques include both direct action and cognitive coping skills.

III. Application training. The individual tests out and practices the coping skills by actually employing them under stress situations.

Stress inoculation therapy has proved to be useful, especially in situations of extreme stress or anxiety.[7]

Obstacles to and benefits of successful stress management

Several factors may impede the progress of stress management training. Recognition of these factors assists the therapist in selecting the appropriate stress management technique. The common obstacles to change are as follows:

1. *Secondary gain.* The individual may have been or may currently be rewarded for maintaining stress symptomatology; for example, by significant others or by monetary reward.
2. *Family dynamics.* One or more family members may have a vested interest in the maintenance of a particular illness behavior in another family member.
3. *Life-style habit patterns.* A client's occupation or leisure pursuits may have inherent stressors. That is, of course, a relevant topic for stress counseling.
4. *Change represents the unknown.* Therefore it is somehow frightening. There is often a cognitive and emotional reluctance to change because of this fear.
5. *Relevancy.* The therapy may not be seen as relevant to the problem at hand. An alcoholic, for example, may wonder what EMG training has to do with abstinence.[11]

Stress management has rapidly been gaining popularity as a training modality in recent years. Research has demonstrated its effectiveness in alleviating discomfort in a number of illnesses. The box on p. 176 lists several of the effective applications of stress management.

No one strategy or technique should be viewed as a panacea for stress reduction. Rather, a comprehensive stress management program recognizes the ubiquitous

STRESS-RELATED ILLNESSES FOR WHICH STRESS MANAGEMENT HAS BEEN EFFECTIVE

Muscle tension	Gastrointestinal distress
Insomnia	Anxiety
Hypertension	Phobias
Stuttering	Dysmenorrhea
Asthma	Menopausal hot flashes
Raynaud's disease	Tension headaches
Migraine headaches	Bruxism
Colitis	Chronic pain
Ulcers	Arthritis
Neuromuscular tics	

nature of stress, and a program should be individually tailored. Many individuals benefit from a combination of several stress management strategies. Furthermore, stress management strategies are often enhanced by adjunctive techniques such as imagery, directed fantasy, catharsis, thought stopping, and insight. The decision as to which strategies are likely to be effective is determined by the therapist after a complete assessment of the individual and his or her response to stress has been made.

REFERENCES AND SELECTED READINGS
Contemporary

1. Benson, H.: The relaxation response, New York, 1975, William Morrow & Co., Inc.
2. Betrus, P., and Logan, H.N.: Stressors in nursing: causes, results and interventions. In Stressors in nursing: responses and resolutions, Seattle, 1981, University of Washington.
3. Brown, B.: Stress and the art of biofeedback, New York, 1977, Harper & Row, Publishers.
4. Coates, T., and Thoresen, C.: How to sleep better, Englewood Cliffs, N.J., 1977, Prentice-Hall, Inc.
5. Curtis, J., and Detert, R.: How to relax, Palo Alto, Calif., 1981, Mayfield Publishing Co.
6. Danskin, D., and Crow, M.: Biofeedback: an introduction and guide, Palo Alto, Calif., 1981, Mayfield Publishing Co.
7. Davidson, P.: Behavioral management of anxiety, depression and pain, New York, 1976, Brunner/Mazel Inc.
8. Gaarder, K., and Montgomery, P.: Clinical biofeedback: a procedural manual, Baltimore, 1977, The Williams & Wilkins Co.
9. Hassett, J.: A primer of psychophysiology, San Francisco, 1978, W.H. Freeman & Co., Publishers.
10. Kanfer, F., and Goldstein, A.: Helping people change, New York, 1975, Pergamon Press, Inc.
11. Kogan, H., et al.: Therapeutic manual for the management of stress response, Seattle, 1980, University of Washington.
12. Meichenbaum, D.: Cognitive-behavior modification: an integrative approach, New York, 1977, Plenum Publishing Corp.
13. Sutterley, D.C., and Donnelly, G.S.: Stress management, Top. Clin. Nurs. 1(1):1-104, 1979.

Classic

14. Ellis, A.: Reason and emotion in psychotherapy, New York, 1962, Lyle Stuart, Inc.
15. Jacobsen, E.: Progressive relaxation, Chicago, 1938, University of Chicago Press.
16. Miller, N.E.: Learning of visceral and glandular responses, Science 163:434-445, 1969.
17. Schultz, J.H., and Luthe, W.: Autogenic training: a psychophysiologic approach in psychotherapy, New York, 1959, Grune & Stratton, Inc.
18. Wolpe, J.: Psychotherapy by reciprocal inhibition, Stanford, Calif., 1958, Stanford University Press.

CHAPTER 14

ADAPTIVE BEHAVIOR

MAY WYKLE

Personality and behavior

Personality refers to all that a person is, feels, and does, either consciously or unconsciously, as manifested in interactions with the environment. Behavior is an expression of personality and is defined as all the activity of which a human being is capable. It is a person's never-ending attempt at adjustment to the environment and is determined by unmet needs. Thus according to the humanists, all behavior is motivated, purposeful, and meaningful.

Behavior is the manner in which an organism responds to a need stimulus. Once the stimulus is gratified, the organism changes its behavior. Unmet needs create frustration, which leads to increased anxiety. This anxiety is then released as behavior.

If the behavior is such that anxiety is resolved in an acceptable manner to the person and to others in the environment, it is termed *adaptive*. Persons who display adaptive behavior are those who make appropriate use of their coping mechanisms and do not resort to symptoms for relief of anxiety. Those with *maladaptive* behavior are at the other end of the spectrum (Fig. 14-1) and use psychiatric symptoms to deal with increased stress.

Humans are social beings, and one of their basic needs is to feel secure and accepted by others in a social group. An individual's entire life from birth to death consists of a series of adjustments to meet biologic and emotional needs in socially acceptable ways. Because human behavior is characterized by a powerful tendency to repeat itself, especially if the behavior is rewarded, it is essential that health care professionals possess a thorough knowledge of human behavior and factors that influence it. Not only must care givers un-derstand client behavior, but also they need to have reasonable insight into their own behavior. Responses to people are influenced by many factors, particularly early life experiences with significant others. Parents, teachers, neighbors, heroes, and peers all have had a part in shaping a person's behavior and have had some effect on why people behave as they do.

Personal problems and feelings of health care providers also produce conflict in the work setting. Sometimes it is necessary for an outsider (client, friend, coworker) to point this out. Yet the more individuals know about themselves, the more capable they become in establishing working relationships with co-workers and clients. An awareness of what shapes their own behavior, how they manage stress, and how their behavior affects others will facilitate care givers' effectiveness in implementing nursing interventions.

Illness and behavior

It is essential that nurses not underestimate the psychosocial aspects of health care. Emotional stress may accentuate physical symptoms in patients. Because of this effect alone, nurses need to have a working knowledge of the dynamics of behavioral responses to illness.

Illness stimulates certain kinds of behavior based on the person's previous adjustment patterns, degree of physical impairment, abruptness of illness onset, prognosis, and meaning of the part of the body affected. All illness is a threat to self and evokes some anxiety, but an acute illness can create a crisis situation for the patient. A necessary part of total care therefore is to support the person's adaptive behaviors and prevent further decompensation.

The anxiety resulting from the stress of illness is manifested as an energy that must be discharged in order to restore equilibrium of the individual. This en-

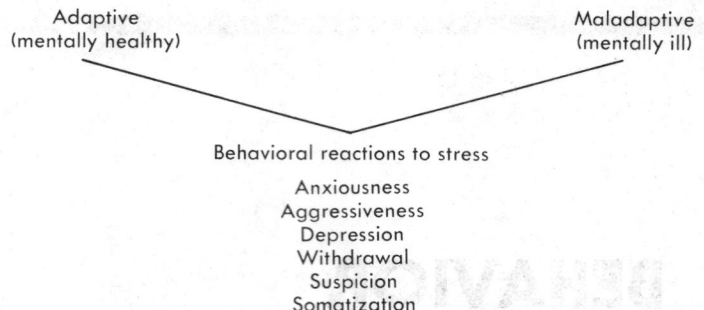

Fig. 14-1. Behavioral responses of persons experiencing anxiety from stress such as illness range from behavior that is adaptive to that which is maladaptive.

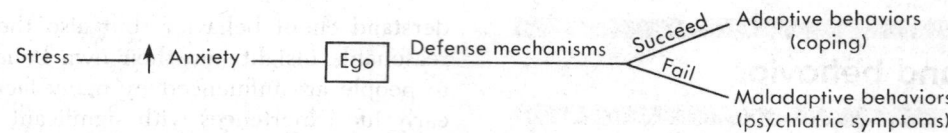

Fig. 14-2. When increased anxiety occurs from stress such as illness, the ego attempts to decrease anxiety by means of defense mechanisms. If these mechanisms fail, the ego resorts to psychiatric symptoms (maladaptive behaviors) as a means of coping.

ergy is discharged through behavioral reactions (Fig. 14-1). The type of behavioral reaction that occurs is influenced by psychosociocultural factors such as basic personality development, past experiences, values, and economic status.

When anxiety is markedly increased, the ego attempts to manage the disequilibrium through coping behaviors that will either reduce the anxiety or make the tension tolerable to the individual. The organism can handle the stress by fight, flight, or immobility. The increase in anxiety initially calls for the use of defense mechanisms (p. 179). Failure of these mechanisms to solve conflict may lead the ego to utilize psychiatric symptoms, which are considered to be maladaptive (Fig. 14-2).

The capacity to tolerate stress varies among individuals. Whether behavior is adaptive or maladaptive will depend on the amount of stress, the strength of the ego, and its ability to use coping mechanisms. Since behaviors reflect how well stress is being managed, an assessment of behavioral reactions is essential for planning nursing care. Nursing intervention is geared toward support of the person's coping mechanisms, which prevents further escalation of anxiety.

Defense mechanisms

Defense mechanisms are unconscious processes used by individuals in adjustment to life stresses. They evolve during personality development and serve to protect the personality, to satisfy emotional needs, to maintain harmony between conflicting tendencies, and to reduce tension of anxiety by modifying reality to make it more acceptable. Defense mechanisms are compromise solutions.

There are two levels of defense mechanisms: those that are considered more primitive and those that are of a higher level (see box, p. 179). Defense mechanisms are used by mentally healthy people as well as by those who are neurotic or psychotic. In the mentally healthy the mechanisms are used less frequently and those mechanisms of a more primitive kind are avoided. Defense mechanisms become pathologic when they are overused.

A defense mechanism is effective when it succeeds in easing intrapsychic tension. When lower level defense mechanisms fail, a more pathologic process evolves and the person exhibits psychiatric symptoms. All defense mechanisms are unconscious with the exception of suppression. Two defense mechanisms, denial and repression, that are frequently manifested by the hospitalized patient are discussed in more detail.

Denial

One of the defense mechanisms used frequently in dealing with the stress of illness is denial. This mechanism occurs during the early stages of crisis after the initial stressful impact. Denial of the illness helps the person deal with increased tension by protecting the

DEFENSE MECHANISMS

Higher level: less primitive mechanisms

repression Ideas painful to consciousness are forced into the unconscious.

suppression Thoughts or desires are consciously inhibited.

sublimation Energy of repressed tendencies is transformed and directed to socially acceptable goals.

identification Person assumes the personal qualities or elements of the personality of another.

compensation Person makes up, covers up, or disguises real or fancied inadequacies in another area.

displacement An emotion is transferred or displaced from its original object to a more acceptable substitute that is less threatening.

rationalization Plausible explanations are given to account for a belief or behavior motivated from unconscious sources.

Lower level: more primitive mechanisms

denial The disavowal of intolerable thoughts, feelings, or wishes. Person refutes external elements of reality that are unpleasant or painful.

regression Person reverts to a pattern of behavior belonging to an earlier stage of development.

conversion Painful emotional experience is repressed and later is expressed in the form of a physical symptom.

projection That which is emotionally unacceptable within the self is rejected and attributed to others.

introjection Person absorbs the emotional attitudes, wishes, ideals, or personality of others into oneself; the aspirations and self restraints of others are incorporated into the personality.

reaction formation Person adopts attitudes and behavior that are opposites of the impulses to which the individual is reacting.

---

ego (self) from reality. The pattern used by the person is similar to games played by children when they close their eyes and believe no one can see them. "It's not there because I don't see it." That which cannot be perceived is therefore not painful.

During denial intolerable thoughts are disowned. The ego gets rid of unwelcome facts (such as an illness) while still retaining its faculty for reality testing. The patient manifests denial by disowning any body changes. For example, patients with coronary disease may deny they have had heart attacks and will blame their discomfort on indigestion. Patients may even deny the severity of the pain and act as though the pain was not present.

Denial works well for the person who has been independent and has a self-image of a strong, self-made individual or who views sickness as a sign of weakness. Denial can be complete or partial and includes a "splitting" of thoughts, feelings, and actions; for example, the patient may own the thoughts but deny the feelings.

Intervention for denial is vital if improvement in the physiologic condition of patients depends on their gaining some awareness of the seriousness of the illness or at least enough insight so that they can participate in nursing care. At one time it was believed necessary to confront the patient's denial; however, *direct* attack usually makes the patient more defensive. Patients will give up the need to deny once they feel supported by others and the anxiety is lessened. Denial, although a more primitive mechanism, can be very useful to the person in the face of sudden crisis. Patients should be given reasons for their needed cooperation, but the nurse does not dwell on the patients' dependency or fearfulness. Patients need not agree that the treatment procedures are necessary for them, but neither can their participation cause any harm.

Limits are set firmly but kindly when denial behavior interferes with treatment. Persons experiencing denial need control over those routines not vital to their care and need reassurance that it is all right to ask for help because the nurse is there for assistance. Nursing care is given in a manner that emphasizes the patient's worthwhileness as a human being although in a dependent state. When patients get enough support and reassurance, they will be able to give up some of the denial and face reality.

Regression

Regression is a defense mechanism often seen in persons who are ill since regression facilitates acceptance of the patient role. The ego is acted on rather than doing the action. Regression makes a dependency relationship possible because of the individual's reversion to behavior patterns of an earlier level of development. Illness necessitates that patients place themselves in the hands of competent others. They often become self-centered and concerned only with their own needs and interests. These interests focus on what is happening to the person and on their acceptance or rejection by care givers. Often regression is a help to patients in that it promotes conservation of energy.

Behavioral responses to stress

Anxiety

The state of anxiousness is the behavioral manifestation of anxiety. Although the ego attempts to deal with anxiety through defense mechanisms, a certain amount of anxiety manifests itself through anxious behavior. This behavior is usually seen following the initial impact of an acute illness. The level of anxiety engendered and its manifestations will depend on the individual's maturity, understanding of the illness, level of self-esteem, and coping mechanisms.

There are four levels of anxiety according to Peplau.[21] The *mildly* anxious person is more alert, exhibits quick eye movements, and has increased hearing ability. The field of awareness is enlarged, and the person sees, hears, and grasps more of the environment than usual. As anxiety increases to the second stage, *moderate* anxiety, the person sees, hears, and grasps less detail of the surroundings. Patients may focus on a few details of their illnesses and ignore the rest. They are able to recall only with clues from the nurse. In the third stage, *severe* anxiety, the nurse may notice disturbances in the person's thought patterns. Thoughts, feelings, and actions may not be congruent; for example, patients may know they are supposed to stay in bed but may still get out of bed and go to the bathroom or walk in the hall. The fourth stage of anxiety is one of pure *panic*. Perceptions of what is actually happening to the person are blown out of proportion, and patients may be described as "climbing the walls." Persons can vacillate between several stages of anxiety.

Since anxiety is felt empathetically and communicated interpersonally, it is imperative that the nurse take steps to reduce a patient's anxiety to a lower stage. If anxiety is not lowered, other patients and staff are caught up in the tension. Recognition of the effects that the patient's anxiety is having on the nurse, followed by problem-solving steps to reduce anxiety in self, will in turn help to reduce some of the patient's anxiety.

Assessment of anxiety level

In assessing a patient, the nurse observes appearance, behavior, and conversation for signs of anxiety (see boxed material). The conclusion that the patient is demonstrating anxious behavior can be made when several of the signs of anxiety are present. With mild anxiety the signs are fewer and less prominent, and it is important to validate the conclusion with the patient. Signs of anxiety will be more overt in persons who are experiencing severe anxiety or who are in a state of panic.

Intervention to prevent and release anxiety

The type of intervention used by the nurse will depend on the level of the patient's anxiety and include explanations, exploration of feelings, and intervention for severe anxiety.

Explanations. Structure decreases anxiety. Explanations are one method of providing structure, which is helpful for the person experiencing mild or moderate anxiety. Newly admitted patients are usually anxious; therefore orienting them (and their families) to the hospital environment and routines tends to minimize anxiety. Each new experience should be explained to pa-

SIGNS OF ANXIETY

Appearance
↑ Muscle tension (rigidity)
Skin blanches, pales
↑ Perspiration, clammy skin
Fatigue
↑ Small motor activity (e.g., restlessness, tremor)

Behavior
↓ Attention span
↓ Ability to follow directions
↑ Acting out
↑ Somatizing
↑ Immobility

Conversation
↑ Number of questions
Constant seeking of reassurance
Frequent shifting of topics of conversation
Describes fears with sense of helplessness
Avoids focusing on feelings
Focuses on equipment or procedures

Physiologic signs mediated through autonomic nervous system
↑ Heart rate
↑ Rate or depth of respirations
Rapid extreme shifts in body temperature, blood pressure, menstrual flow
Diarrhea
Urinary urgency
Dryness of mouth
↓ Appetite
↑ Perspiration
Dilation of pupils

Signs of anxiety are dependent on the degree of anxiety. Mild anxiety heightens the use of capacities, whereas severe and panic states severely paralyze or overwork capacities.

tients and, if possible, related to familiar experiences. It is helpful to inform patients as to how to call the nurse, when they will see the physician, the hours the religious adviser is available, and how they may contact their family. In addition, the family should be told how to obtain information concerning the patient, when they may visit, and any immediate plans for the patient.

If patients are to have treatments or tests they must be given some idea of what will be done, the preparation involved, and the reasons why the procedure is necessary. To remove the water pitcher and inform patients that they cannot have any more water until after the x-ray examination can generate many anxious thoughts: "What x-ray examination?" "I wonder when it is?" "What will it be like?" "It must be something special if I can't have any water." Lack of knowledge as a cause of anxiety reflects the nurse's lack of consideration for the patient's rights as an individual.

Explanations should be given in the patient's own terms at appropriate times and repeated as necessary. If the patient is very anxious, repeated explanation may be necessary, since extreme anxiety reduces intellectual function. It is useless to give detailed explanations to patients who are severely anxious or sedated or to those who have high temperatures or severe pain. Repetition is often required for older persons and children because they may have short memory spans.

Time spent in giving explanations to relatives is not wasted. Not only does it relieve their anxieties, which may be transmitted to the patient, but it also saves having to untangle misinformation. Often the family is helpful in interpreting necessary instructions to the patient in a manner that the patient understands and accepts.

Exploration of feelings. In most instances a large part of the nurse's work is to encourage patients to express anxieties, to help patients see the universality of fear in their situation, to help them seek outlets for their fears and tensions, and to allay them whenever possible. Nurses should provide opportunities for the patient to talk, but they should not probe. There is a difference between prying into a patient's thoughts and beliefs and eliciting information that will aid in the understanding of behavior and in planning for care. Without seeming unduly curious, one can usually find some topic of personal interest to the patient that will provide an opening. A picture on the bedside table may create such an opening. Nurses who listen with sincere interest and without making judgments about the patient may begin to gain insight into the patient as a person. And more important, the patient may begin to speak about personal fears.

As soon as the patient begins to talk about feelings, the nurse should proceed with conversation, taking cues from what the patient offers. The nurse who feels inadequate or anxious may cut off the conversation. For instance, if a patient says, "You know, I don't think I'll ever get to see my little boy again," a common response is "Oh, don't say that, certainly you will; you're going to be all right." The patient may very well not be all right. Would it not be better to respond, "What makes you feel this way?" Such a response helps the patient explore the subject and leaves opportunity for the pa-

tient to examine this fear. It also gives the nurse a chance to find out what the patient fears. The nurse who is willing to listen to patients, to be guided by their reactions, and to work with them rather than to make decisions for them will give them needed emotional support. Solving patients' problems for them, even if it were possible, is not the aim of nursing. Indeed it would tend to make patients less healthy psychologically.

The art of meaningful communication involves more than just listening; it includes moving the conversation so that the patient's attempts to communicate are assisted. Observing the patient for facial changes and general body movements provides opportunities for the nurse to discover from the individual the full meaning of the situation. For example, consider the patient who sucks in air while talking. The mouth becomes drier and drier as the tongue seems to stick in the mouth. These patients are not at ease and show anxiety even though their words may be quite innocuous. A simple statement such as, "Your mouth seems very dry. Would a glass of water help?" allows the nurse to clarify observations. Such an approach gives the patient a chance to tell what is being experienced, and to gain understanding by talking about it.

The nurse helps patients examine those problems that they are able to bring into awareness. Underlying problems should be handled by people trained in psychotherapy. A nurse needs to be able to recognize normal anxiety reactions and to report exaggerated reactions that may indicate the need for psychiatric referral. Stuttering and blocking of words may indicate increasing tension.

Intervention for severe anxiety

When any patient's anxiety increases to a high level, the nurse may need to sit with the patient. The nurse's very presence is often reassuring. If possible, the patient is helped to recognize the anxiety by the nurse asking, "Are you uncomfortable?" or "What are you feeling?" In severe anxiety and panic, being there is most important, and touch may be used as a means of reassurance. Some severely anxious persons, however, view touching as an intrusion of their personal boundary, and the nurse needs to keep this in mind. When the patient is able to talk, the nurse helps the patient to describe what is happening, what has happened, and what is expected to happen.

Crisis model

Overwhelming anxiety may be indicative of a crisis situation that demands specific intervention. Nurses may be confronted with clients in crisis in a variety of settings: emergency rooms, intensive care units, cardiac or surgery units, community health centers, and clinics.

Awareness of what occurs during a crisis helps the nurse understand the behavior occurring when a person experiences a crisis.

When the *ego* is met with overwhelming anxiety created by biologic, physiologic, or social threats to the *self*, a crisis ensues. The ego is not able to cope successfully with the sudden disequilibrium. Several authors[1,8,17] have described what occurs during crisis and what is involved in assisting the client to utilize the situation as a growth experience.

A crisis occurs when a person is unable to utilize customary methods of coping when faced for a time with what seems to be an unsurmountable obstacle to an important life goal.[17] A period of disorganization ensues, a period of upset during which many abortive attempts at solutions are made.

Phases of crisis

Shontz describes several phases or stages that occur during crisis.[12] These stages are similar to the stages of death and dying as described by Kübler-Ross.

1. *Initial impact*. During this phase the client experiences shock and depersonalization as reality is clearly perceived. Functioning is organized and automatic with individual centering and docility.

2. *Realization*. In the second phase there is a collapse of the existing self-structure. Reality seems overwhelming, and the person experiences high anxiety, panic, and helplessness. There is inability to plan, reason, or understand the situation.

3. *Defensive retreat*. The third phase is one of regression in which there is an attempt to establish previous identity, to return to better times. There is an avoidance of reality, and denial and wishful thinking may ensue to relieve the anxiety. When challenged the ego reacts with anger and may experience rage and disorientation. Thinking is situation-bound, and there is a resistance to change.

4. *Acknowledgment*. This is the "yes" stage: "It has happened to me." The individual experiences depression and self-depreciation. Reality imposes itself again and looms large in relating the event to one's life. Without intervention the client may become more disorganized, depressed, and suicidal.

5. *Adaptation*. This is the stage when change occurs if help is adequate. New identity appears along with hope and renewed sense of personal worth. There is a subsequent decrease in anxiety and an increase in satisfaction due to the stabilization and reorganization. Functional improvement is noted without actual change in disability status.

The above model is a useful approach for explaining what a patient experiences during an illness crisis, even though reactions to crisis are individual. Patients are not equally vulnerable to all categories of stress, but there is thought to be some commonality in the reactions. Knowledge about the commonalities can facilitate plans for nursing intervention.

Crisis intervention

The essential element of crisis intervention is the intensive nature of support required to help the ego maintain its integrity and its ability to use coping mechanisms. Crisis, according to Caplan,[17] is self-limiting. Early intervention can prevent maladaptive behavior, and the individual can emerge a stronger person. Acute illness or catastrophic illness often precipitates a crisis reaction. The outcome of a crisis is governed by the kind of interaction that takes place between the individual and key figures in the environment during the time of crisis.

Often because of changes in society, previous guidelines for behavior in stressful situations render the individual helpless. In crisis the individual is helped to find ways to facilitate efforts to enlarge on the experience. A state of disequilibrium produces a felt need to reduce anxiety. The following balancing factors have been identified as being necessary to resolve the problem and to avert crisis: (1) a realistic perception of the event, (2) adequate situational support (staff and family), and (3) adequate coping mechanisms.[1] When one or more of these balancing factors are absent, the result is an increase in anxiety, with immobilization and an inability to avert the crisis (Fig. 14-3).

In crisis, help should be immediate. Staying with the person, talking through the situation, and encouraging catharsis facilitate recognition of feelings, expression of feelings, and subsequent relief of guilt. Strengthening of coping mechanisms is crucial in preventing the formation of symptoms. Growth in the client is facilitated by using problem-solving skills and a hierarchy of needs framework to help the client set priorities. Nurses are in strategic positions to observe clients in crises and add to a theory of behavioral reactions to illness and to the prevention of maladaptive behavior.

Intervention to aid normal behavioral responses to stress

Many persons are able with the added support from health professionals to maintain behavior within the adaptive range when subjected to the stress of illness. In order for support to be provided, for the ego to achieve balance, the client's coping mechanisms and dependency needs are assessed. By reinforcing existing coping mechanisms that are appropriate to the reduction of anxiety and by supporting problem-solving skills,

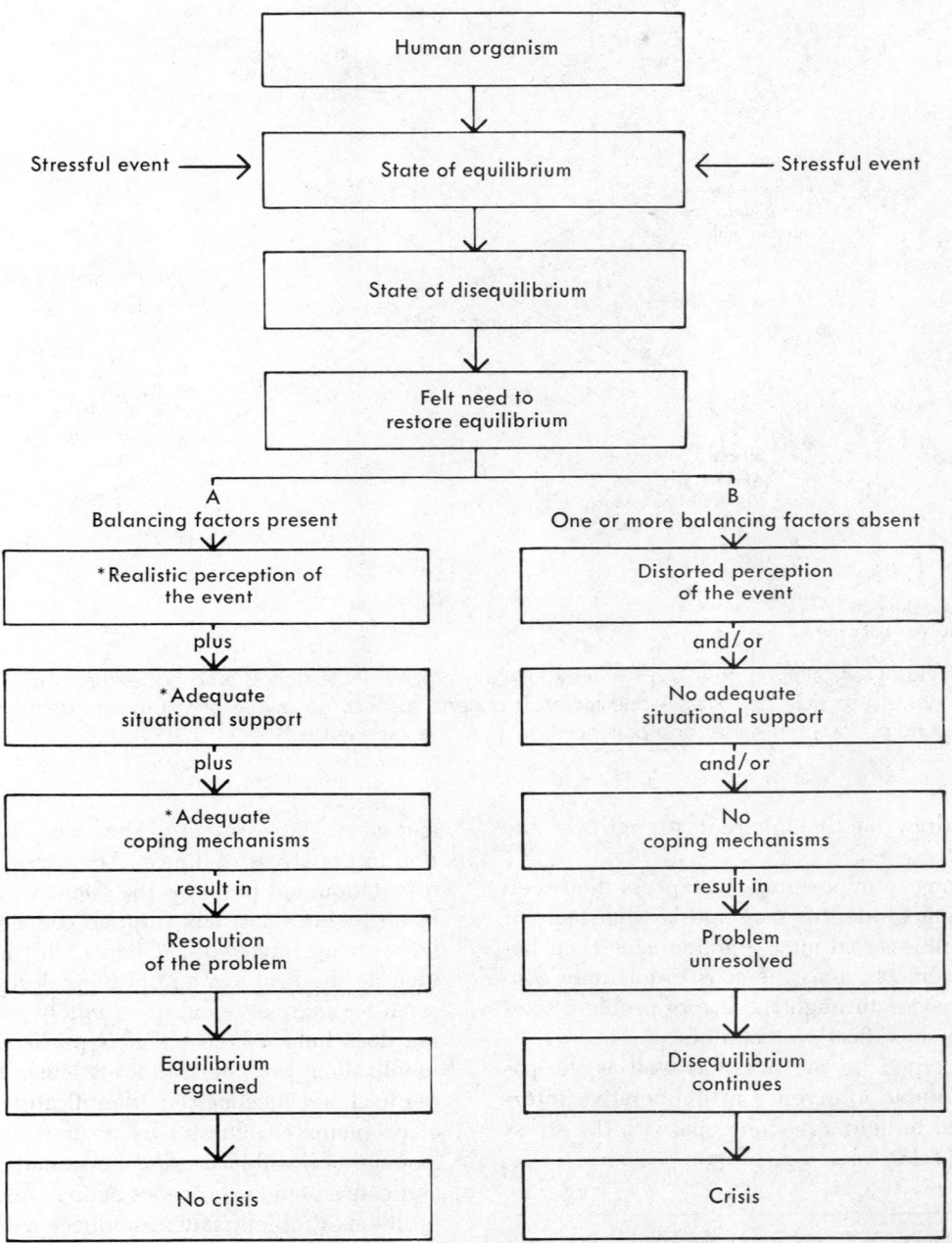

*Balancing factors.

Fig. 14-3. Paradigm: effect of balancing factors in stressful event. (From Aguilera, D.C., and Messick, J.M.: Crisis intervention: theory and methodology, ed. 4, St. Louis, 1981, The C.V. Mosby Co.)

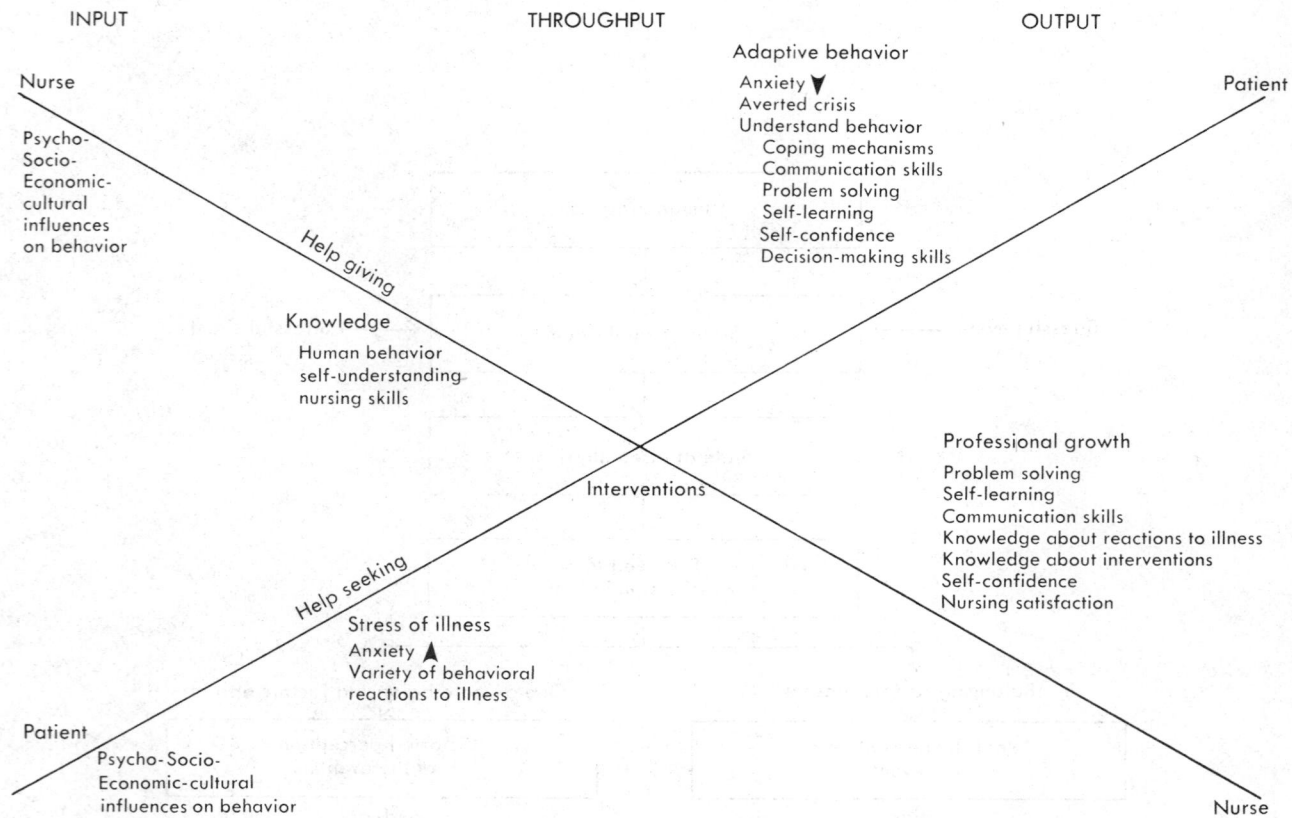

INPUT   THROUGHPUT   OUTPUT

Nurse   Adaptive behavior   Patient

Psycho-   Anxiety ▼
Socio-   Averted crisis
Economic-   Understand behavior
cultural   Coping mechanisms
influences   Communication skills
on behavior   Problem solving
                                               Self-learning
                   Help giving   Self-confidence
                                               Decision-making skills
              Knowledge

                Human behavior
                self-understanding
                nursing skills

                                                         Professional growth

                                                           Problem solving
                                                           Self-learning
                          Interventions   Communication skills
                                                           Knowledge about reactions to illness
                                                           Knowledge about interventions
                                                           Self-confidence
                   Help seeking   Nursing satisfaction

                Stress of illness

                Anxiety ▲
                Variety of behavioral
                reactions to illness

Patient   Nurse

        Psycho-Socio-
        Economic-cultural
        influences on behavior

Fig. 14-4. Nursing care is a two-way learning process. Professionals who understand themselves use skills and knowledge to teach patients to become aware of self, assets, deficits,
and needs. Both nurses and patients grow from the experience.

the nurse can draw on the inherent strengths of the person.

Giving persons an opportunity to express their feelings enables them to identify consciously their fears or concerns about illness that may be influencing their behavior. Care givers can assist persons to maintain control of their behavior through the use of problem-solving and behavior modification techniques.

Gains are accrued by the nurse as well as the patient when the nurse intervenes in deliberative interventions planned to help a person cope with the stress of illness (Fig. 14-4).

Problem solving

The problem-solving approach is a useful nursing intervention for behavioral reactions to illness and during crisis. A crucial aid in problem solving is the establishment of a nurse-client relationship (for further information see Chapter 9). The nurse's approach is one of openness, warmth, and nonjudgmental, sensitive caring.

The first step of problem solving includes the nurse's

and client's assessment of the stage of the client's reaction to the stress of illness. The nurse promotes reality orientation and provides the client with an opportunity to air feelings and talk through concerns using a problem-solving framework. Clients vary in their ability to identify the problem and in their desire to discuss personal feelings, although it is widely accepted that talking does help. If the client is pushed indiscriminately to talk about problems, the relationship will become superficial and mechanical. Identification and description of problems is followed by analysis, which consists of looking at possible causes. Formulation of alternatives and consequences precedes action aimed at solving the problem. Problem solving reduces ambiguity and feelings of loss of control; the way back to health is a learning process.

When using the problem-solving approach with patients, nurses need to consider the patient's family and others in the support system. Assessment of the family network often provides the patient with avenues of support previously neglected. In addition, attention given to families, who often have similar behavioral reactions as the client, will prevent potential conflicts between client and family.

Behavior modification

Behavior modification principles may be useful in planning nursing interventions related to emotional aspects of illness. The focus of this approach is to change the behavior of the patient. Thoughts, feelings, and actions normally are syntonic, and therefore a change in one affects the other two. Behavior modification provides a meaningful approach to growth in patients.

Essentially behavior modification consists of deciding which behaviors exhibited by a particular client are desirable and which are undesirable; actions are then taken to increase the frequency of the desirable behaviors and to decrease the frequency of the undesirable behaviors. Basically people behave in ways that will fulfill their needs; the task is to help select those behaviors that are most helpful and most socially acceptable. For example, the patient who becomes demanding and puts on the call light every 5 minutes would benefit from the use of the principle of saturation. In this situation, if the call light is consistently answered each time it is put on or the patient is seen before he puts on the light, the patient's needs are anticipated and the demanding behavior will cease. The patient's need for attention through turning on the light becomes saturated. The behavior must be tolerated and handled in a nonhostile manner. Interacting with the patient before he puts the light on becomes a reward for positive behavior. The focus of intervention is on building up desirable behavior and not on why the patient is hostile. Saturation works well with overdependency. Once dependency needs are saturated, the patient will be able to give up overdependent behavior.

Behavior modification focuses on reinforcing behaviors that are curative for patients. The nurse can plan with the patient and agree on which behaviors should be strengthened. For example, weight reduction through behavior modification using positive and negative reinforcement is beginning to gain popularity as a successful, nonharmful way to lose weight. (For more information see reference 16 at the end of this chapter.)

Intervention for specific behavioral reactions to illness

The five behaviors presented in this section are all adaptive behaviors that are normal reactions to illness, both acute and chronic (Fig. 14-1). Anxious behavior is discussed on p. 179. Intervention is aimed at preventing further disintegration and crisis.

Aggressive behavior

Whenever there is a threat to self-concept, such as occurs with illness, the individuals may respond by aggression, a way that makes them feel less helpless and more powerful. Aggression is another way of handling anxiety. People are often angry at the loss of health status and question what is happening. They become irritable and uncooperative and may project their anger onto the staff and become demanding. It is important that staff accept patients' hostility without retaliation and that patients not be made to feel guilty. Limits should be set and the patient's demands anticipated. Expression of anger in socially acceptable ways prevents anger from being turned inward, causing depression. Patients should be given reasonable control of their environment and the opportunity to participate in planning and implementing their own care.

Depressed behavior

Depression is a normal response to illness, once the illness has been accepted. In making an assessment of the person who is depressed, the nurse needs to be aware of the clinical signs of depression. These patients are quiet and may show some confusion. They are apt to lack interest in the surroundings or activities around them. They may voice concern about the illness or the amount of care the illness requires and may express wishes or concerns about dying. The patient's behavior may be extremely dependent and activity and conversation are slowed. Complaints of weakness and fatigue are common.

Intervention requires that the nurse approach the patient in a serious mood, conveying through actions and communication an understanding of what the patient must feel. The nurse helps the patient express feelings and conveys acceptance of the right to feel sad. When patients show signs of readiness, they are helped to focus on interested areas outside the illness. These patients may need to talk about activities that they were involved in prior to hospitalization. This is particularly true for persons who have chronic illnesses. It is important to *listen* to the person who is depressed complain about problems so that the anger may be turned outward.

Dependency, a common behavior of the depressed patient, is a reaction that may follow the stage of accepting an illness. Patients readily place themselves in the hands of others. While dependency is a form of regression, it is also a part of learning to trust. These patients do not want to do much for themselves and accept total care, although they may not demand it. Supportive care is indicated in the early stages with gradual advancement from doing *for* the patient to doing *with* the patient, and then facilitating patient self-care. Thus patients return gradually to helping themselves.

Overdependency exists when the patient shows physical readiness to progress but prefers to remain dependent. Nurses need to assess the difference through deliberate observation and then set limits kindly on those nursing interventions that continue to promote the dependency. Appropriate interventions at this time include the use of saturation along with helping these patients develop cognitive awareness of their physical ability to do more for themselves. The nurse also makes it clear that patients will not be abandoned and that support in the form of the presence of a member of the nursing staff will be available as they do more for themselves.

Withdrawn behavior

Withdrawn patients usually do not pose as many problems and are apt to be labeled "good" patients. They demand little from others and thus may be overlooked. Withdrawn patients regress more easily to earlier levels of behavior at which they can accept the patient role. Withdrawn patients need gentle encouragement to talk, to express feelings, and to relate to the staff. Spending time sitting with these patients, often in silence, does much to increase their sense of self-worth.

Suspicious behavior

Suspicious patients have difficulty with trust and may have had previous experiences in which they learned to distrust care givers. They are often suspicious of staff, the routines, the medicine, and the procedures. They need to talk about these concerns but should not be forced to do so. It is imperative that staff keep promises made to these patients and avoid an overzealous approach. Explanations of procedures and establishment of expected routines are helpful. Whispering and talking about patients within their field of hearing are avoided as the communication may be misinterpreted.

Somatic behavior

A familiar reaction to illness is one that can be labeled flight into illness. Patients somatize their concerns; that is, they have learned to express anxiety through complaints about a variety of physical symptoms. They may be preoccupied with bodily functions and feelings of pain. Vague complaints of backache, headache, or fatigue are expressed in order to legitimize the attention needed. Support and acceptance by allowing patients to talk about their symptoms with some limit setting will decrease the anxiety.

Staff often become angry at patients who utilize so-matic behavior because of the vague symptomatic complaints and because staff members feel "caught" if they "play down" the symptoms, since there is always the possibility that the complaints are truly connected with an illness. Guilt on the part of staff prevails for some time if a complaining patient who was ignored is diagnosed as having a physical illness. It is wise for the staff to accept all symptoms and report them. Time spent with these patients, listening to their complaints and using a saturation technique (p. 185), will help lessen this behavior.

REFERENCES AND SELECTED READINGS
Contemporary

1. *Aguilera, D.C., and Messick, J.M.: Crisis intervention: theory and methodology, ed. 4, St. Louis, 1981, The C.V. Mosby Co.
2. Bailey, D.S., and Dreyer, S.O.: Therapeutic approaches to the care of the mentally ill, Philadelphia, 1977, F.A. Davis Co.
3. *Carlson, C.E., editor: Behavioral concepts and nursing interventions, ed. 2, Philadelphia, 1978, W.B. Saunders Co.
4. *Harris, E.: Mental status assessment, Am. J. Nurs. 81:1493-1518, 1981.
5. Lambert, V.A., and Lambert, C.E.: The impact of physical illness and related mental health concepts, Englewood Cliffs, N.J., 1979, Prentice-Hall, Inc.
6. Pasquali, E.A., Alesi, E.G., Arnold, H.M., and DeBasio, N.: Mental health nursing: a bio-psycho-cultural approach, St. Louis, 1981, The C.V. Mosby Co.
7. Programmed instruction: helping depressed patient in general nursing practice, Am. J. Nurs. 77(suppl.):1-32, June 1977.
8. Rappaport, L.: The state of crisis: some theoretical considerations, Chicago, 1972, University of Chicago Press.
9. *Reynolds, J.I., and Logsdon, J.B.: Assessing your patient's mental status, Nurs. '79 9(8):27-32, 1979.
10. *Robinson, L.: Liaison nursing: psychological approach to total care, Philadelphia, 1974, F.A. Davis Co.
11. Schwartz, L.H., and Schwartz, J.L.: The psychodynamics of patient care, Englewood Cliffs, N.J., 1972, Prentice-Hall, Inc.
12. *Shontz, F.: The psychological aspects of physical illness and disability, New York, 1975, Macmillan Publishing Co., Inc.
13. Simmons, J.A.: The nurse-client relationship in mental health nursing, Philadelphia, 1976, W.B. Saunders Co.
14. *Snyder, J.C., and Wilson, M.F.: Elements of psychological assessment, Am. J. Nurs. 77:235-239, 1977.
15. Strain, S.: Psychological care of the medically ill, New York, 1975, Appleton-Century-Crofts.
16. *Stuart, R.B., and Davis, B.: Slim chance in a fat world: behavioral control of obesity, Champaign, Ill., 1972, Research Press.

Classic

17. Caplan, G.: Principles of preventative psychiatry, New York, 1964, Basic Books Inc., Publishers.
18. Erickson, E.H.: Childhood and society, New York, 1963, W.W. Norton & Co., Inc.
19. Janis, I.: Psychological stress: psychoanalytical behavioral studies of surgical patients, New York, 1958, John Wiley & Sons, Inc.
20. Maslow, A.H.: Toward a psychology of being, New York, 1968, D. Van Nostrand Co.
21. *Peplau, H.: A working definition of anxiety. In Burd, S., and Marshall, M., editors: Some clinical approaches to psychiatric nursing, New York, 1963, Macmillan Publishing Co., Inc.

*References preceded by an asterisk are particularly well suited for student reading.

CHAPTER 15

MALADAPTIVE BEHAVIOR

MAY WYKLE

The individual with a well-integrated personality has learned to live in relative harmony with the environment. Poor adjustment leads to difficulty in interpersonal relationships. Maladjustments vary in degree from occasional withdrawal to overt psychosis. Many individuals with such emotional problems have nevertheless made marginal adjustments within a particular environment. The additional stress accompanying illness may threaten their security enough to disrupt their personalities, causing personality disorganization and disintegration. This disintegration has been referred to over the years as a "nervous breakdown" by most people and is classified *medically* as mental illness.

It is important to remember that the well-integrated person may have intense emotional responses to illness. The main difference is that these reactions are usually reversible, while the maladaptive individual has an underlying problem that has been "instigated" by stress. Removal of the stress may stop the specific difficulty, but it will seldom if ever change the basic maladaptive behavior pattern.

Since the signing of the community Mental Health Centers Act in 1963 the number of patients in public mental hospitals declined from 558,922 to 215,566 in ten years. The National Institute of Mental Health has helped fund some 600 community centers, increasing services available to 41% of the nation's population. Nevertheless, over 50% of hospital beds in the United States are occupied by patients with a diagnosis of mental illness. Another 25% are taken by patients with psychophysiologic diseases such as peptic ulcers, colitis, and asthma; some experts include essential hypertension, arthritis, and other somatic complaints in this classification. Drug abuse and alcoholism, often seen in persons with maladaptive behaviors, frequently cause physical illness severe enough to require hospitalization.

It is sometimes difficult to differentiate maladaptive behavior from physical illness because of the intimate relationship between the mind and the body. Illness of one always affects the other. Physical illness is usually organic, while mental illness is termed functional. These terms are used when trying to determine the cause of behavior. For example, there may be similarity in the behavior of the patient with an adrenal tumor and the individual with schizophrenia, as can be seen in the following case history.

An 18-year-old high school student had been in a general hospital for diagnosis and treatment of "blackout spells." No organic basis for these spells was found. She was transferred to a private psychiatric hospital with a diagnosis of schizophrenic reaction, catatonic type. She appeared somewhat shy, especially with her peer group. Occasionally she was difficult to rouse in the morning, and she took frequent naps. One morning the nurses decided to try some TLC while attempting to wake her. She was brought a glass of chocolate milk and fed with a spoon, being assured that people cared about her and wanted to help her face the day. Her response was much more rapid than usual, and the nurses felt they had hit on a solution to her problem. The psychiatrist was impressed with their reports but questioned whether the response to the milk was psychologic or physiologic and ordered blood to be drawn for blood sugar level testing the next time she was "catatonic." This was done. The sugar level was 37 mg/100 ml serum (normal 75 to 105 mg/100 ml serum). The patient was transferred to a general hospital for further diagnostic workup. It was determined that she had a left adrenal tumor. This was surgically removed, and she took up life as a relatively normal, healthy young woman.

This case history demonstrates that careful observation, laboratory studies, and even surgery may be necessary to determine the cause of a disease.

Naturally, maladaptive individuals are subject to injury and physical illness, and when they are sick they may need treatment in a general hospital. Many general and community hospitals have set aside a few rooms with special safety provisions to meet the particular needs of clients who are emotionally disturbed.

Basic courses in personality development provide an understanding of normal behavior of patients, but specialized help may be necessary when caring for persons with maladaptive behavior. If the hospital has a psychiatric division, it may be possible for the psychiatric nurses to consult with the medical and surgical nurses regarding the care of patients who are mentally ill. Many hospitals do not have such experts available, however, and nurses must depend largely on their own integrated knowledge and resources. When a nurse is assigned to care for patients with severe emotional problems, textbooks, journal articles, audiovisual resources, and other materials on psychiatric nursing provide excellent information. This chapter contains only a brief discussion of a few important principles or criteria to follow in caring for clients with maladaptive behavior.

Maladaptive behavior

The behavior of the maladjusted individual does not differ in kind from that of the defined normal person; it *differs only in degree*.[24] Many clients with maladaptive behavior appear quite normal on casual observation and conversation, and it is only on more prolonged contact that abnormalities of personality may be evident. Consequently, the nurse needs to take time to assess the patient. On the other hand, patients' interactions with others and their self-control may have deteriorated to a point where they are conspicuous. This type of behavior is often manifested during an acute psychotic episode.

The nurse who for the first time encounters a patient in an acute psychotic episode may be unprepared for the behavior demonstrated. Nurses have been accustomed in their daily living and in their dealings with patients to meeting persons who are able to face challenges to their security with a normal amount of assurance, thus keeping themselves in harmonious association with others. In the hospital the client is often expected to repress fears, irritations, and aggressive impulses to a socially acceptable degree and to be a "good" patient. Because normal patients have a reasonably well-integrated personality and anticipate a short stay in the hospital, they are usually able to live up to these expectations. Patients who have severe emotional disturbances may be unable to control emotional responses and may react freely and impulsively. They may be out of contact with reality at times, expressing bizarre ideas *(delusions)*, and may have false sensory perceptions *(hallucinations)*. Hallucinations are usually auditory or

visual, but they may be tactile, olfactory, or gustatory. The individual may also feel pain for no apparent physical reason. Regardless of the unreality of these sensations, they are real to the patient. Hearing voices is very common, and patients often answer the voices or respond to the directions given by them. Tactile sensations usually are of crawling objects, and patients may try to flick them away or to run from them.

Depressed behavior

It is common for emotionally disturbed persons to be severely depressed. This depression is much deeper than that experienced in varying degrees by normal people. It is described as a feeling of utter hopelessness or as a living death. These persons feel exhausted and are dejected in posture, facial expression, gait, and verbal reactions. They lose interest in physical surroundings and personal appearance. Appetite is poor, and constipation may develop. Depressed persons seldom enter a deep-sleep state although they may be quiet and lie for hours with their eyes closed. At times they may become quite tense and restless, showing signs of agitation such as pacing the floor and wringing their hands. They may be tearful and express feelings of inadequacy, unworthiness, and guilt. Depressed persons may mention and often contemplate suicide. Severely depressed persons who suddenly seem much better should be watched carefully, since this improvement often means only that they have decided on suicide as a means of escape.

Research has shown that individuals contemplating suicide almost always show warning symptoms in a desperate plea for help. They may talk about death or dying; get their affairs in order; ask to see business associates, family members, or friends; and if hospitalized often make a point of bidding good-bye to nurses at night or when the nurse is leaving.

For the last several years suicide has been among the ten leading causes of death in the United States. In recent years there have been over 23,000 reported suicides each year. Suicide accounts for deaths in 11 out of 10,000 people in the United States.[23] Interesting studies have shown that by the mid 1980s the fastest growing rate of suicide will be among teenagers and the elderly. The actual number of suicides is probably much higher than figures indicate, since many experts consider many automobile accidents and other accidental deaths as possible suicides (e.g., drownings and carbon monoxide poisonings).

Hyperactive behavior

Emotionally disturbed patients may be hyperactive (manic) or aggressive in their behavior. They may flit from one activity or one subject of conversation to another, and it may be impossible to hold their attention for more than an instant. Profanity and vulgarity are common, and these patients may be critical of the hospital and personnel as well as sarcastic, caustic, and domineering. The manic patient has the exaggerated behavior of the noisy, demanding patient and may become irritated easily and express irritation in assaultive behavior. Hyperactivity may become so pronounced as to cause exhaustion.

Suspicious behavior

Suspicion (paranoid reactions) may be exhibited by some maladjusted persons. They may appear suspicious, critical, and watchful of every move others make, and they may question activities and refuse medications, treatment, and even food. At the same time, they may feel persecuted and neglected if left out of an activity.

Obsessive-compulsive behavior

Some people with maladaptive behavior are compelled to follow certain rituals or behavior patterns that are far beyond normal but that in some ways serve to relieve inner tensions. For example, it is normal for many persons to count fence posts as they walk down the road. However, a compulsion neurosis is evident when a person cannot ever walk down a road without counting and touching each post. Ritualistic compulsions in such matters as bathing, washing hands, and dressing in certain sequence are common and, even when carried to great extremes, may sometimes be successfully concealed from the outside world.

Hysteria

Hysteria is an abnormal behavior pattern that has been recognized for centuries. Despite the lack of physical cause, these persons may not be able to do such things as void or move a particular limb. They may have areas of numbness, lack of one of the special senses, or a variety of other physical complaints. They may have apparent convulsive seizures, although unlike patients with true convulsive disorders, they are not likely to injure themselves during an attack.

Anxiety states

Anxiety states are common among emotionally disturbed persons. These individuals may have an abnormal fear of impending disaster, and this fear may be expressed in bodily signs such as flushing, tachycardia, and excessive perspiration. Although there may be no rational basis for the fear, it is very real to the person and cannot be dissipated by rational explanation. A word or two picked out of a statement made by the physician may serve as a basis for worries and fears.

If anxiety becomes too great, *panic*—complete disorganization of behavior in the face of overwhelming terror—may result. There is complete loss of control, and the person is unable to perceive, communicate, or control motor actions. The environment is often misinterpreted, and the person may try to escape from what is imagined as immediate acute danger. This behavior may lead to physical injury such as may be sustained from disconnecting intravenous tubes, removing drainage tubes, or falling out of bed. These patients may not be intent on suicide but may destroy themselves as they attempt to flee from the imagined danger unless special precautions are taken for their safety. Persons in panic may attack hospital personnel in the belief that they are a source of danger. These patients may act quickly and impulsively, and therefore should be observed and assessed carefully.

Intervention for patients with maladaptive behaviors

General principles for nursing care

The care needed by patients with maladaptive behaviors on a medical or surgical unit is no different from that needed by any other patient. They need acceptance as persons, provision for physical needs, and provision for safety. Bizarre, socially unacceptable behavior can often be handled by a clear statement of recognition of the behavior and its importance to the patient. This will not necessarily change the behavior, but it will often help prevent further disintegration. It is important that patients not lose self-esteem; therefore they should be protected from the curious eyes of staff and other patients. Many drugs are available that can help disturbed patients be more comfortable, and when they are more comfortable, they will be more cooperative. The nurse who approaches the disturbed patient with an objective, nonprejudiced attitude communicates acceptance and concern. A positive, assertive, expectant manner will shore up patients' self-respect and help them be less fearful in a foreign environment.

Emotional care

Patients with maladaptive behavior benefit from calmness, consistency, and uniformity in the environment. Procedures should be explained calmly and sometimes repeatedly, even though the individual may not appear attentive or concerned. Even the smallest details of necessary medical or surgical treatment should be explained before they are undertaken. The equipment used for procedures should be reduced to a minimum, but basic principles such as aseptic technique used in changing dressings should not differ from those used in safe nursing anywhere. The patient must also be prepared for routine nursing measures; for example, when lights are to be turned out, a meal is to be presented, or a visit to the bathroom is to be made, the patient should be told what is going to occur.

Anything that increases anxiety may be harmful to the person. The use of technical language and discussion of disease and technical procedures should be avoided. Subjects that appear to increase the patient's anxiety are assessed carefully, and mention of them should be made in the nurse's records. Religion is commonly associated with anxiety or feeling of guilt. Also sexual maladjustment is common in persons who are maladaptive. Discussion of close members of the family may also produce anxiety. Often the final failure in interpersonal relationships occurs in the family environment, among those whose acceptance is most valued by the patient. It is safest to let patients volunteer information. If they share personal information, the nurse must let them know that their confidences will be kept and that the disclosures, regardless of their nature, will not be judged.

The nurse assesses change in behavior indicating that anxiety is increasing and panic may develop. These may include failure to hear people speaking, muscular tension, perspiring for no observable reason, failure to make connections between details in conversation or conduct, headaches, nausea, trembling, and weakness. At this time intervention should be taken to help the patient release tension. The patient is constantly assessed, and, if possible, should be removed from the situation that induces the increased anxiety. Activities such as walking, talking, counting, describing something, or playing a simple game reduce anxiety. It also helps to increase the patient's awareness of the surroundings.

If panic does occur, the best approach is by two people calmly approaching the patient, speaking firmly but slowly, and leading the person away from the situation. Large groups should not suddenly approach a greatly disturbed or active patient unless emergency measures are needed to protect either the person or others. The person is then placed in an environment as free from stimuli as possible and is assessed constantly by a practitioner until panic subsides. When left alone again, the patient should be assured of immediate response if help should be needed.

It is useless to argue with maladaptive persons or to attempt to talk them out of their delusions by reasoning. These persons have lost the ability to understand the psychotic nature of their ideas or to see the fallacies

in them. No attempt should be made to explain their behavior to them. Many patients become confused and disoriented and may be terrified by their delusions or hallucinations. The nurse can best support the patient by confirming what is real to the individual. For example, the most bizarre concept usually has some element of reality in it. Listening and reflection of the real portion of the patient's experience will help the patient with reality testing. It is useless to ask confused persons such questions as time and place. It is better to tell them in a general, conversant manner, "It is 3:00 PM. I'll be leaving at 3:30, and I wanted to see if you would like to sit up for a while before I go."

Nonspecific reassurance should be avoided. Simply telling patients that they are not going to die or that they are worthy of their family may do more harm than good, since it may destroy a picture of themselves that is necessary to maintain at the moment. Specific reassurance that produces a calm, quiet, accepting environment is always of value. Patients should feel that they will not be censured or rejected because of their behavior. They should be given security by assurance of consistency in routine, of the conduct of others toward them. They may gain reassurance from consistency in the way in which they are encouraged to express negative feelings. They may show such feelings by disliking the nurse, for example. They may dislike the nurse without fear of retaliation that would be present if they disliked their spouse or any other close member of the family. Thus hostility toward personnel may be a healthy sign and is to be accepted as such by the nurse. Efforts are made to have patients feel that their behavior is understood even though it may not be approved. The right of patients to want to behave as they do is acknowledged. For example, patients may have the right to want to hurl a water pitcher, but they should know that the staff will continue to prevent them from harming themselves or others.

Drug therapy

Adequate control of behavior can usually be maintained by the use of antipsychotic drugs (Table 15-1). Drugs that are in the phenothiazine group have side effects such as dry mouth, blurred vision, and photophobia that may be uncomfortable to the patient. It is especially important to observe patients for extrapyramidal reactions such as tremors, shuffling gait, masklike face, drooling, and restlessness. Severe reactions (dystonias) may cause extreme muscle spasm, particularly of the upper body and frequently limited to one side. This reaction can be quickly alleviated by the use of antiparkinsonian drugs such as diphenhydramine (Benadryl), benztropine mesylate (Cogentin), biperiden (Akineton), or trihexyphenidyl hydrochloride (Artane) administered intramuscularly or intravenously. In psychiatric facilities patients receiving phenothiazines often

TABLE 15-1. Drugs commonly used with persons exhibiting maladaptive behavior

Type of agent	Generic name	Trade name	Average daily dosage (mg)
Antipsychotic agents	Chlorpromazine hydrochloride	Thorazine	30-1200
	Thioridazine hydrochloride	Mellaril	30-800
	Fluphenazine dihydrochloride	Prolixin	1-20
	Trifluoperazine hydrochloride	Stelazine	2-20
	Prochlorperazine	Compazine	15-150
	Haloperidol	Haldol	4-15
Antianxiety agents	Chlordiazepoxide hydrochloride	Librium	15-300
	Diazepam	Valium	4-10
	Meprobamate	Equanil, Miltown	200-1200
Antidepressant agents	Amitriptyline	Elavil	75-150
	Imipramine hydrochloride	Tofranil	100-300
	Phenelzine sulfate	Nardil	15-75

are given anticholinergic drugs prophylactically. The appearance of side effects may necessitate changing the dosage or even the drug. Intolerance to one drug does not necessarily indicate intolerance to other tranquilizers. Tranquilizers derived from compounds other than phenothiazines and used for mild to moderate anxiety states include chlordiazepoxide hydrochloride (Librium), diazepam (Valium), and meprobamate (Equanil, Miltown).

Antidepressant drugs, often referred to as psychic energizers, produce feelings of well-being in depressed persons. Amitriptyline (Elavil), imipramine hydrochloride (Tofranil), and phenelzine sulfate (Nardil) are some of the common ones prescribed. Antidepressant drugs may produce any of the more severe as well as the less severe side effects that are observed in patients taking tranquilizers. Since all of these drugs can produce serious side effects, the nurse is cautioned to be aware of average doses and individual tolerance to the drugs. Patients are taught the purpose, dosage, and side effects of medications prescribed.

Medications are often refused by the maladaptive patient, who may be exceedingly clever at concealing drugs not swallowed. When staff have reason to believe the patient is not taking the medication, pills may be crushed and dissolved unless their bitter taste precludes this measure. Serious problems in giving medications orally are reported to the physician so that another method of administration may be ordered.

Safety needs

The confused or psychotic patient may be unable to comprehend medical orders such as bed rest or intravenous feedings. Repeated clear explanation of treatments and, most important, frequent short contacts with the patient will do much to gain cooperation. If patients are unable to comply with medical orders, it may be

necessary to restrain them. For instance, if a catheter is in place and the patient repeatedly pulls it out, there is a danger of injury to the bladder and urethra. In this instance soft restraints may be enough of a reminder to prevent the patient from removing the catheter.

Severe restriction of motion such as by leather restraints should be avoided unless there is real danger to the patient or others. Restraining patients often causes increased anxiety, and increased anxiety decreases the patient's ability to deal rationally with the environment. A family member, friend, or staff member who can stay with the patient provides the best way to help the agitated patient adjust to the hospital.

Physical needs

When the patient's behavior in a general hospital becomes maladaptive, there is a tendency to become overconcerned with the behavior and to neglect the physical needs. It must be remembered that these patients need good general nursing care, including mouth care and attention to hygiene. Even if these patients are physically able to carry out these tasks for themselves, they often need help since they may be too preoccupied with thoughts or with other activities to care for themselves completely or safely. Patients have been known to lean against a hot radiator and sustain a severe burn or to step into a tubful of very hot water without flinching. Treatments need to be given as ordered. Often patients will not even ask for a bedpan or urinal or for medication for pain, and the nurse is responsible for assessing and providing for these needs.

For some time before hospitalization, nutritional intake of depressed patients may have been inadequate. Patients may refuse to eat or they may hide their food to give the impression that they have eaten. Hyperactive patients may be too frightened or preoccupied to eat, yet they may require more than the usual amount of food. Food and fluid intake as well as urinary and bowel output should be monitored for patients with maladaptive behavior. Patients who are depressed often suffer from constipation, and hyperactive patients may delay going to the bathroom because of their many preoccupations.

Sleep is necessary for mentally ill patients but is sometimes hard to achieve. Adequate sleep and good general physical health make it easier to face problems and attempt to solve them. Patients with acute mental illness may require large doses of sedatives or tranquilizers to control daytime behavior, although these drugs may actually interfere with sleep, particularly dream (REM, or rapid eye movement) sleep. Exercise outdoors, a quiet environment, a back rub or warm bath, and warm drinks are often surprisingly helpful.

Observations and recordings

The nurse's records are very important to the care of maladaptive patients. The nurse is around the patients more than any other professional person and may be the only one who observes and assesses them during the evening and night hours. Recorded observations can be of great help to the staff in management of patients. These notes should be remarkable for their quality rather than their length, but it is best to err on the side of length than of brevity. They may contain actual expressions of the patient, using quotation marks and taking care that the words recorded are exactly those of the patient. Notes should be recorded immediately after significant conversation or behavior has been observed and assessed. Although the specialty of psychiatry has a complete vocabulary of its own, it is wiser to clearly record actual statements and situations rather than label the patient's symptoms as delusions or hallucinations. Factual statements such as "States over and over, 'I see men at the window, they are wearing red, they have come to kill me'" can provide a clearer understanding of the patient's mental state. The nurse's notes should also contain accounts of what the patient does and the nursing interventions.

Special needs of depressed patients

Deeply depressed patients may require almost complete physical care, and they may be almost totally unresponsive to any attempts at communication. Nevertheless, these patients need human contact both physically and interpersonally even though they may seem oblivious to it. Observant nurses usually will be able to determine to some extent what type of activity or conversation seems to help a particular patient and try to provide it. Overcheerfulness, overt solicitude, abruptness, or a dictatorial manner on the part of personnel is particularly upsetting to depressed patients. Deeply

disturbed patients may be depressing to the nurse or other personnel caring for them. If so, personnel should plan their contacts with the patients so that they can provide continuity of care, prevent evident avoidance of the patients, and still retain reasonable emotional personal comfort.

If there is just one person who consistently demonstrates caring about the patient, this may be sufficient to prevent consideration of suicide as the only means of escape from an untenable situation. Depressed persons want someone to be concerned about their welfare, even though they are unable to ask for help openly. They wish to be protected from themselves and their impulsive behavior. In contemplating suicide they do not necessarily want to die but rather want to express the urgency of the need to escape from an unbearable situation.

It is not true that persons who talk about suicide rarely attempt it. At least a third of those committing suicide talk about it or give some indirect indication of their intent. Mention of suicide intent by the patient should be taken calmly by the nurse but reported to the physician at once and recorded in the patient's record. The patient should immediately be given increased attention, with sympathetic and serious concern. By showing more concern, the nurse indicates that the person really matters. It is exceedingly important that the nurse not answer suicidal patients in a way that appears to dare them to carry out their threat. A comment such as, "I know you don't mean that" leaves the patient with the possible choice of carrying out the threat to prove the seriousness of the statement.

Prevention of suicide or other injury requires alert observations and assessment of the patient on the part of the nurse. Pocketknives and objects such as nail files, razor blades, belts, drugs, and any pieces of equipment that might be used either impulsively or with premeditation are removed. If the patient is known to be suffering from maladaptive behavior, such belongings should obviously be removed on admission. If windows can be raised enough so that the patient could crawl through them, they must be equipped with stop devises to prevent complete opening, and occasionally protection over the glass is necessary. Doors should be fitted with locks that cannot be turned from the inside. Electrical fixtures must be out of reach of patients who might attempt to electrocute themselves by tampering with the socket or who might injure themselves with glass from bulbs.

The physician is responsible for ordering constant observation if it is necessary because of the danger of suicide or injury to others. The newspapers bear testimony to many instances of patients leaping from windows or otherwise destroying themselves in the few brief moments when the care giver's back was turned. A decrease in the patient's tension should not cause a relaxation of observation, since decision on a plan of action may be its cause.

Suicidal patients are observed and assessed carefully and sympathetically without making them feel that they are under constant scrutiny. Patients may resent constant observation, believing that they are being spied upon or that they are in danger from the observer. The least conspicuous way to observe patients is by observing them in a group, but such an arrangement may not be feasible on the medical-surgical unit. The nurse may appear to be busy with a patient in an adjoining room while watching the maladaptive patient. Sometimes locating the observer outside the patient's room may cause the least annoyance. Efforts should be made to convey to depressed patients that they are being given special attention because the nurse cares about them and feels they need this attention.

Individuals who have made unsuccessful suicide attempts are often admitted to general hospitals for emergency care by means of community rescue services, mobile intensive care units, or private ambulance services. The immediate care depends on the attempts made and the physical emergency care provided at the scene. Patients are frequently treated for drug overdose and other poisoning, severed arteries, and gunshot wounds. They then face not only the original problem that precipitated the suicide attempt but the consequences of the act. Special care needs to be taken to avoid a repeated attempt, and psychotherapy usually is instituted. Family members, too, often need help in understanding and accepting the patient's problems. Sometimes families need the help of the physician, mental health consultant, nurse, social worker, or member of the clergy in planning for the role they will take in the future in helping the patient.

Special needs of aggressive patients

Patients with aggressive behavior are often overactive and fare best in a nonchallenging and nonstimulating environment. Noise should be kept at a minimum, and distraction and irritations of all kinds should be avoided.

Aggressive patients need to be allowed to express their feelings in a calm, accepting atmosphere. Although they may be most annoying, they are not allowed to feel that they are a nuisance or are unliked. They should not be prevented from verbalizing annoyances, and no attempt is made to talk them out of their attacks or to defend the person or situation being verbally attacked. The patient is never compared with other patients or with past behavior as the comparison may lead to feelings of rejection. Answers to questions should be simple and direct. The nurse avoids encouraging stimulating conversation, while still conferring a feeling of warmth and interest. Such encouragement may lead to provocation of aggression when the interaction is ended and the patient assumes rejection.

Aggressive patients may not respond favorably to direct requests. They usually are happier associating with quiet patients, since their aggressiveness often calls forth aggression in others. Attempts should be made to channel their energy into constructive activities, but they are observed carefully to detect signs of approaching exhaustion and to prevent upsetting situations from arising because of the possibility of injury to themselves or to others. Establishing a relaxed atmosphere in a darkened, quiet room may be helpful for the overactive, aggressive patient, and a sedative may also be given.

Special needs of patients who focus on physical symptoms

Persons with a psychoneurosis concerning physical symptoms require infinite patience and understanding. They also need firm and thoughtful management. Usually they have told their physical symptoms endless times to numerous people and have worn out their welcome with all. The nurse listens attentively for a reasonable time and should then try to redirect conversation away from the patient. The nurse should not be trapped into implying that there is nothing wrong with the patient, and it is well to avoid discussion of any medical subject. Activity therapy that can be undertaken at the bedside often helps divert conversation away from the patient and also may result in creativity that earns self-recognition.

The nurse watches for any attempts patients may make to aggravate the physical ailment or to produce symptoms. So great may be their need to maintain an acceptable outlet for problems through illness that they may go to surprising lengths to delay a cure. Patients have been known to hold their thermometers against light bulbs, add water to urine collection bottles, tamper with their wounds to cause infection, and even subject themselves to needless surgery. The nurse has the responsibility to report to the physician if there is reason to believe that a patient is attempting to falsify the clinical picture. An example of such behavior is seen in the following case history.

A 39-year-old unmarried woman who resided with her mother was admitted to the medical service for severe diarrhea and blood loss through her ileostomy. Initially the staff was concerned about fluid loss and dehydration although there was no clinical evidence such as weight loss, poor skin turgor, or changes in laboratory findings. The patient kept her own intake and output record. In one 24-hour period she recorded 450 ml intake and 4,700 ml output, including 28 loose stools, none of which was observed by a staff member. The ileostomy site was reddened and bleeding. The patient in the next bed reported seeing her using a rat-tail comb to irritate the site.

In an attempt to provide more healthy attention-getting activities, a very active occupational therapy program was initiated. The patient was quite talented artistically and received many honest compliments on her work. She accepted an invitation to work as a volunteer in the children's ward. Since the intake-output record served no purpose, it was discontinued. No questions were asked about loose stools. She was weighed routinely and without comment about her weight. The patient was most responsive to this regimen and after discharge returned to the hospital weekly for occupational and group therapy. She also entered therapy with a psychologist. The improvement was maintained for 3 months, at which time her mother had a serious fall. The patient was admitted to a surgical floor with an acute exacerbation of symptoms. (The patient had had 27 prior surgical procedures in over 40 hospital admissions.)

To assure reasonable success of this type of approach, each staff member must be well informed about what is being done and why. This prevents patients from "using" one staff member against another to defeat the program and thus themselves.

Disorders not related to maladjusted personality

Organic psychoses are due to disease processes that have produced physical changes. Among the common causes of organic psychoses are neurologic syphilis, arteriosclerosis, and epilepsy with deterioration. Brain tumors, brain trauma, Huntington's chorea, and encephalitis are other examples of organic origins of mental illness.

Toxic reactions or *toxic delirium* may occur when high temperature is present or when toxins have accumulated in the body from disease (for example, uremia). When such factors are the cause, the toxic reaction is *endogenous*. When psychosis results from a reaction to drugs such as bromides, anesthetics, and alcohol, the reaction is *exogenous*.

Toxic reactions are the most common of the psychoses seen in general hospitals. They usually come on suddenly and may disappear as quickly, particularly if the cause can be found and eliminated. Patients with toxic reactions almost always suffer from confusion, hallucinations, and delusions that usually cause fear and sometimes panic.

Specific disorders related to maladjusted personality

Functional psychoses

Functional psychoses have no demonstrable organic cause, although it is suspected that eventually one may be found. The emotional disorders commonly classified as functional psychoses include involutional psychotic reaction (involutional melancholia), manic-depressive reaction, schizophrenia (dementia praecox), and paranoia. Functional psychoses are rarely classified as distinct entities, since most patients have a mixture of reactions. Both schizophrenia and paranoia are serious mental illnesses for which the patient often needs long-term care in a special psychiatric facility. Patients with involutional melancholia and manic-depressive reactions have a fairly good prognosis for recovery from an attack, but attacks tend to recur. If it is known that a patient has suffered from a functional psychosis, the nurse should be alert for early signs of recurring emotional illness, since mental health is taxed by physical illness.

Psychoneuroses

Patients with psychoneuroses are seen most often in general hospitals. This is because their behavior, although exasperating to all who must help them solve their health problems, is seldom such that care in a mental hospital is necessary. Patients suffering from psychoneurosis conform to social standards and are able to appreciate the rights of others in a general sense. They are oriented as to time and place. However, in compromising their desires with social demands they have failed to make a satisfactory emotional adjustment and have escaped from the untenable demands of living by developing psychoneurotic behavior. This behavior may take the form of hypochondriasis, anxiety states, hysteria, or obsessive compulsive behavior. Although the patient may have a physical disease that may or may not be related to the basic emotional disturbance, the emotional problem is predominant and is the one that is really important to the patient. These patients are less upset by symptoms than would be expected, and even when extensive diagnostic procedures and surgery are performed, they are usually surprisingly philosophic about the whole experience.

The nurse or anyone else caring for psychoneurotic patients should not assume that these patients are willfully sick. Unfortunately, they are too often considered problems by members of the staff who lack the insight to recognize their need to be ill. The patient does feel real pain and discomfort even though no physical cause may be found. Psychoneurotic patients are large consumers of medical care and all related services. It is probable that the economic cost to society of this group of patients is greater than the cost for all the psychoses combined.

Alcoholism

Alcoholism is very common and may compound the problems of a person experiencing other health disorders. Excessive alcohol intake may lead to coma or near death from acute alcohol poisoning, or if it occurs over a period of time may lead to numerous other health disorders. Alcoholism is recognized today as a treatable entity. Significant changes in the identification and treatment of alcoholism point toward advances that are having an important impact on this major health problem.

Epidemiology

Alcoholism in the United States is on the increase. Conservative estimates are that 90 million people use alcohol and about 9 million people are afflicted with alcoholism. Alcoholism is defined as a continuing problem (with alcohol) that affects the person's life, such as family, work, and social activities. Also, alcoholics cannot predict with 100% accuracy what their behavior will be after the first drink. The second definition has to do with the individual's control of the amount that is drunk. Nonalcoholics can say they will have one or two drinks and stick to the plan, whereas the alcoholic may not be able to do so. In defining alcoholism one can extrapolate from the quantity-frequency-variability information on alcohol intake, on the presence or absence of physical addiction, or the presence of alcohol-related life problems.[13]

Industries lose at least $10 billion yearly because of alcoholism. This figure includes the cost of time lost, misjudgments, spoiled materials, broken machines, and other factors. Many companies have special programs for the treatment and rehabilitation of employees with alcoholism. Referrals are made by supervisors and managers on the basis of decreased productivity, thus eliminating the need for them to make a diagnosis.

Recent court rulings have declared that the alcoholic is sick and entitled to medical treatment, not imprisonment. Unfortunately, there are not enough facilities to treat the alcoholic; treatment is long, expensive, and often unsuccessful.

Etiology

There is no one cause of alcoholism, but alcoholics have been classified empirically into three groups: those whose alcoholism is a symptom of mental disease, those for whom alcohol is a physiologic poison, and those who develop from social drinkers. Persons in the latter group may appear well adjusted until some trouble arises to cause excessive drinking, or they may drift slowly and unknowingly into alcoholism. The alcoholic is likely to be basically insecure and to face realities with difficulty. Alcohol may become a means of escaping the demands of life. Persons who are becoming alcoholics tend to be untruthful about their drinking and to defend themselves by rationalizations and pretenses. Alcoholism, like mental illness, is in no way related to social or economic class. It is equally common among the rich and the poor, the intelligent and the mentally limited, the successful and the unsuccessful.

Pathophysiology

Alcohol does not require digestion and is absorbed in both the stomach and intestine. Absorption is accelerated by increased alcohol concentrations and an empty stomach. After absorption, alcohol is distributed equally throughout body fluids, passing across all membranes. Blood alcohol levels depend on the amount ingested and the size of the individual. Most laws designate blood alcohol serum levels of 100 mg/100 ml (0.10%) as the legal limit for driving a motor vehicle. Increasing blood alcohol levels have increasingly more serious effects (see box below).

Alcohol also has a diuretic effect, partly due to the increased amount of fluids ingested. Increased amounts of electrolytes, particularly potassium, magnesium, and zinc, may be excreted in the urine of the heavy drinker. Prolonged use of alcohol has a toxic effect on the intestinal mucosa resulting in decreased absorption of thiamin, folic acid, and vitamin B_{12}.

Since alcohol is not converted to glycogen, it cannot be stored, and it provides calories but no minerals or

EFFECTS OF BLOOD ALCOHOL LEVELS ON AVERAGE-SIZED, NONTOLERANT ADULT

Blood alcohol levels (per 100 ml blood)	Effects
50-75 mg	Pleasant relaxed state, mild sedation, loosening of inhibitions
100-200 mg	Overt signs of intoxication: loosening of tongue, clumsiness, beginning emotional changes
200-400 mg	Severe intoxication: difficulty speaking, stumbling, emotional lability
400-500 mg	Stupor, coma
Over 500 mg	Usually fatal

vitamins. One ounce (30 ml) of alcohol provides about 200 kcal. Most of the ingested alcohol is metabolized in the liver at a rate of about 10 g/hr. The excess remains in the bloodstream where it acts as a depressant and an anesthetic, which in turn slows down cellular metabolism. The anesthetic action of alcohol can have serious consequences. The margin of safety for the person anesthetized by alcohol is very small. Unless stimulants are given, alcohol is removed from the stomach, and attention is paid to respiratory function, death may occur.

Assessment

Habitual drunkenness is the main symptom of the disease of alcoholism. Usually alcoholism develops slowly, over a period of 10 to 20 years, until the persons reach a point where they "drink to live and live to drink." At this point they tend to be irritable and unreasonable. They may lack judgment and develop physical as well as mental ailments.

The true alcoholic is more interested in alcohol than in food. Persons who drink a great deal may get as much as a third of their daily intake of calories from alcohol, and alcoholics may get more calories from alcohol than from any other source. When they obtain the alcohol they wish, they may be too intoxicated to eat or they may have no appetite for normal food. Alcohol is also the most common cause of acute gastritis that results in severe vomiting, which contributes to poor nutrition. Malnutrition may therefore contribute greatly to the alcoholic's physical and mental decline. Alcoholics may be in a general state of poor health with vitamin deficiency, anemia, liver changes, and debility. Resistance to infectious disease is low, and contact with infection is likely during severe bouts of drinking. Consequently, alcoholics are often admitted to the hospital with infectious diseases such as pneumonia or tuberculosis (see box in next column).

Many alcoholics have neurologic symptoms (polyneuropathy) that may include severe pain in the legs and arms and burning of the soles of the feet. Foot drop and wrist drop may develop, and walking and use of the hands may be seriously limited or made impossible. Many alcoholics develop pellagra with its characteristic skin changes of redness, dryness, scaling, and edema. Both pellagra and polyneuropathy are due to vitamin deficiency and are treated with massive doses of vitamin B complex. Weakening of the heart muscle and resultant heart enlargement ("beer heart") is believed to be caused largely by vitamin deficiency. Symptoms of acute heart failure may bring the patient to the hospital. Cirrhosis of the liver occurs often in persons who are alcoholic, and it is believed that the cause is primarily malnutrition—a lack of protein and perhaps other food constituents that are not contained in alcohol.

Chronic alcoholics often exhibit personality changes

DISORDERS ASSOCIATED WITH ALCOHOLISM

Hepatic	Alcoholic hepatitis, Laennec's cirrhosis, fatty liver
Gastrointestinal	Gastritis, pancreatitis, duodenal ulcers, malabsorption syndromes, cancer of mouth and esophagus
Neurologic	Peripheral neuropathy, Wernicke-Korsakoff's syndrome, organic brain disease
Cardiovascular, hematologic	Cardiomyopathy, hypertension, familial type IV hyperlipidemia, hypoglycemia, anemia, hyperuricemia
Musculoskeletal	Skeletal myopathies
Immunologic	Increased susceptibility to infections

and general deterioration of thinking processes. They may be emotionally unstable, suspicious, quick to take offense, and unpredictable in social and related situations. Serious impairment of memory may occur. Severe tremor, visual hallucinations, and loss of memory may develop even if nutrition has been adequate.

Any hospitalized patient who is not known to be an alcoholic but who does not respond normally to preoperative medication, to anesthetics, or to sedatives should be observed carefully for signs of alcoholism. Alcoholic patients usually require large doses of sedatives and anesthetic agents for effect and are likely to be overly excited and active as they react from anesthesia. The most apparent signs of chronic alcoholism that may be noted by the nurse are a tremor that is worse in the morning and morning nausea. These patients feel "jittery," and if alcohol is available, they will have one or two drinks to "steady the nerves" before eating.

Intervention

Care of hospitalized alcoholic persons. Alcohol may be prescribed for alcoholic patients during their hospitalization, particularly during an acute illness when reaction to deprivation is severe. However, close observation is necessary because even the patient receiving alcohol as prescribed may be extremely resourceful in obtaining an additional supply. If a patient appears to be obtaining unauthorized alcohol, the physician is notified, since additional alcohol may interfere with the medical regimen. Any alcoholic patient admitted to the general hospital for an acute medical or surgical condition is observed closely for signs of impending delirium tremens. Early treatment may prevent the development of an acute psychosis.

Regardless of the circumstances surrounding hospitalization, alcoholic patients often feel hopeless, guilty, and apprehensive. If their physical ailment is related directly to alcoholism, they are usually quite ill before they consent to be hospitalized. Often they wish to talk to someone, but the person must be one who seems to accept them as they are and to understand their problems. Nurses providing care to alcoholic patients need to be calm and willing to listen. They should not appear critical of the patients or offer specific advice but should try to make the patients feel that they are ill and that help is available. Patients are more likely to be able to accept help if they feel that they still have their self-respect.

Alcohol withdrawal. Persons with a physical dependence (see box at right) to alcohol experience varying symptoms ranging from mild tremors to severe agitation and hallucinations (delirium tremens) when alcohol intake is withheld. The type and severity of symptoms depend on several factors. Alcoholics at higher risk of experiencing severe withdrawal symptoms are older aged persons, those who have had previous convulsive seizures or delirium tremens with withdrawal, and those with coexisting acute illnesses or nutritional deficiencies. The amount of alcohol consumed and the duration of the drinking episode also influence the severity of withdrawal symptoms.

Tremors may be observed 6 to 48 hours after withdrawal of alcohol and persist for 3 to 5 days. The hands are involved first, but the tremors may become generalized with involvement of the extremities, tongue, and trunk. Chlordiazepoxide (Librium) is useful in reducing tremors without affecting the person's ability to eat and drink.

Seizure disorders may occur 12 to 24 hours after abstinence. Usually auras do not precede the grand mal seizures, but postictal stupor usually follows them. Dilantin is of questionable value in controlling seizures. Chlordiazepoxide may be helpful, and measures are taken to protect the patient's safety.

Delirium tremens, an acute alcoholic psychosis, is more rare and usually occurs 3 to 4 days after abstinence. It can occur when the confirmed alcoholic is denied a regular supply of alcohol, or it may develop when the patient is taking alcohol regularly. It may follow injury, infectious disease, anesthesia, or surgery and may develop in patients who have not revealed their alcoholic status to the physician. Delirium tremens is a serious mental illness and may cause the death of the patient. Signs of acute alcoholic psychosis include severe uncontrollable shaking and hallucinations. These patients often say that they see insects on the wall and that rats or mice are on the bed and sometimes that they are biting. They become extremely restless and apprehensive and perspire freely; sometimes true panic occurs. The treatment consists of tranquilizing drugs such as chlordiazepoxide; sedatives such as paraldehyde given

TERMS USED TO DESCRIBE RESPONSES TO DRUGS/ALCOHOL

Tolerance	Decreased susceptibility to effects because of long-term ingestion of drug/alcohol
Behavioral tolerance	Few changes in social behavior or activities despite ingestion of large amounts of drug/alcohol
Pharmacologic tolerance	Adaptive metabolic changes despite ingestion of large amounts of drug/alcohol
Cross tolerance	Decreased sensitivity to other drugs as a result of tolerance to drug/alcohol
Dependence	Need to continue use of drug/alcohol to prevent symptoms
Physical dependence	Withdrawal symptoms occur when the drug/alcohol is withheld
Psychologic dependence	Person feels the need to take the drug/alcohol to prevent occurrence of symptoms
Cross dependence	Suppression of abstinence symptoms by withdrawal of another drug

rectally, intramuscularly, or orally; and a high-caloric and high-vitamin diet that may have to be given by nasogastric tube. The patient must be protected from physical injury and observed carefully for signs of cardiac failure. Corticosteroids may be given. Recovery usually takes from 1 to 2 weeks.

Long-term care. It is only when alcoholic patients truly desire and seek help with their alcohol problem that treatment is useful. The nurse frequently is the person present at the time patients are most ready for help—when they have "reached the bottom" and are suffering from the embarrassment and discomfort of a physical misfortune brought on by drinking. It may be at this time that they are a little more ready to face reality than they have been for some time in the recent past. Nurses' attitudes toward patients and their knowledge of facilities for treatment of alcoholism may be crucial to the life of patients and their families.

The objective of all treatment is to induce patients to stop drinking alcohol. When alcoholics do stop drinking, they can *never take one single drink* on any occasion without serious danger of relapsing. They are never considered cured, and abstinence is their major course. Sedatives and tranquilizers may be administered until they recover from the nervous agitation and insomnia caused by the withdrawal of alcohol. Vitamins and a diet high in calories, proteins, and carbohydrates may be prescribed to improve nutrition and to help overcome weakness and fatigue. Psychotherapy may be helpful to patients in overcoming the desire to drink.

Because alcoholism is a major health concern, nurses need to be aware of community efforts and resources for its treatment. Most facilities do not require a physician's referral; patients simply present themselves. If the nurse encounters alcoholic persons in the community who are seeking help, they should be directed to sources of help. If the patient is hospitalized, the nurse would work with the physician in charge and often with the social worker. Alcoholics Anonymous (AA) is a group of self-acknowledged alcoholics whose aim is to stay sober and to help other alcoholics gain sobriety. There are AA groups in most communities, and usually regular meetings are held. These groups are open to anyone who has a problem with alcohol, and there are no charges involved. Local groups are listed in the telephone directory for each community. A phone call at any hour of the day or night will bring an AA member to see any alcoholic desiring help. Some communities have subgroups of AA that also hold regular meetings. They include Al-Anon for relatives and friends of alcoholics and Al-Ateen for children of alcoholics. Many communities have alcoholic clinics where medical and psychiatric help are available, and many industries now have medical and rehabilitation programs for alcoholics. Information on alcoholism and programs for alcoholics and others are available for interested individuals and groups.*

Drug abuse

In recent years drug abuse has risen sharply. There are no reliable statistics on drug abusers, and experts disagree as to what actually constitutes drug abuse. Some would include repeated use of any drug, while others limit it to those drugs that used repeatedly lead to habituation or addiction. The Alcohol, Drug Abuse and Mental Health Administration estimates that there are 25 million narcotic addicts and drug abusers in the United States.[25]

Drug traffic has particularly increased among adolescents and young adults, and drugs are readily available on most elementary and secondary school and college campuses. The use of marijuana is widespread. There is much controversy as to whether it is addicting; many experts say that it is not. There have been many

---

*National Council on Alcoholism, 733 Third Ave., New York, NY 10017; North American Association of Alcoholism Programs, 1101 15th St. N.W., Washington, DC 20036; Alcoholics Anonymous General Services Board, 468 Park Ave. S., New York, NY 10016; Al-Anon Family Group Headquarters, 1 Park Ave., New York, NY 10016.

reports of actual psychotic episodes following the use of drugs such as LSD (lysergic acid diethylamide) or other hallucinogenic drugs such as peyote or mescaline. It must be remembered that the person using drugs may have an underlying personality problem that is aggravated by the drug, not necessarily caused by it. Drugs commonly taken in an attempt to "get high" include barbiturates, sedatives, amphetamines, synthetic analgesics, and cough syrups.

While there is no general agreement on a definition for drug addiction, the World Health Organization has suggested the following:

Drug addiction is a state of periodic or chronic intoxication produced by the repeated consumption of a drug (natural or synthetic). Its characteristics include an overpowering desire or need (compulsion) to continue taking the drug or to obtain it by any means; a tendency to increase the dose; a psychological and gradually a physical dependence on the effects of the drug; and a detrimental effect on the individual and on society.*

The tolerance and dependence effects of mind-altering drugs that are frequently abused are listed in Table 15-2.

Heroin, an opium derivative that quickly produces addiction, is the drug used most often by American addicts today. There is uncertainty as to the extent of the

---

*From Expert Committee on Addiction-Producing Drugs: Seventh report, Technical report series no. 116, Geneva, 1957, World Health Organization.

TABLE 15-2. Effects of mind-altering drugs

Drug	Tolerance	Physical dependence	Psychologic dependence
CNS depressants			
Narcotics	High	High	High
Barbiturates	Moderate	High	High
Glutethimide (Doriden)	Moderate	High	High
Methaqualone (Quaalude, Sopor)	Moderate	High	High
Tranquilizers	Moderate	Moderate	High
CNS stimulants			
Amphetamine	High	Low to moderate	High
Cocaine	Low	Low to moderate	High
Hallucinogens			
LSD	Moderate	None	Moderate
Mescaline	Low	None	Moderate
Phencyclidine (PCP, angel dust)	Low	None	Low
Cannabis			
Marijuana	Low	None	Moderate

narcotic problem because many narcotic users are not known. In New York City alone it is believed that there are over 100,000 heroin addicts. Federal agents estimate that heroin addiction in persons below age 25 years rose by 40% from 1968 to 1969 in the United States.[16] There are many reported cases of children aged 12 years and under who admit to heroin addiction. There has been a shift toward younger addicts and an increase in the percentage of whites using heroin. In 1975, 51% of addicts in the United States were white, compared with 44% in 1959. The average age has dropped from 35 years in 1950 to 23 in 1975.

The use of drugs is not limited to any socioeconomic group. The problem has long existed in the ghetto, and today it has spread to the affluent suburbs and homes of middle-class Americans. Increased social pressures, stresses of puberty and the search for self, frustration, and even boredom can lead adolescents to try drugs as they seek something to ease the pain of growing up.

One of the obstacles to early detection and treatment of addiction is the reluctance of parents to admit that their son or daughter is a drug user. Even members of the health professions "overlook" the often obvious symptoms of drug addiction or, having confronted the user, fail to report their findings to the parents or authorities. The incidence of drug addiction is high also among health care professionals, probably because drugs are more available to them than to other groups of people. Occasionally a patient who must be given narcotics to control pain over a long period of time becomes an addict. It is rare, however, that addiction develops in those given narcotics for real pain, and nurses should not let fear of the development of addiction keep them from administering prescribed narcotics to patients hospitalized and in severe pain.

Assessment

Early indications of drug use vary with the individual but frequently include (1) abrupt changes in behavior, mood swings; (2) loss of interest in school, sports, dates, other activities; (3) frequent talking and reading about drugs; and (4) loss of appetite, increased thirst, and constipation. When the drug is actually present in the body, the user may seem drowsy or inebriated and be unconcerned about painful stimuli; the pupils of the eyes may be constricted to pinpoints.

After persons have developed a tolerance, they may appear quite normal, converse easily, and carry on activities. Constipation and appetite loss persist, and the person may look undernourished. If the person has been "mainlining" (injecting the drug directly into the vein), needle marks, scars, or small scabs can be seen on the hands and forearms or the instep. Addicts often wear long sleeves to hide such marks. However, many other veins are used as points of entry to conceal addiction, including such inconspicuous areas as the dorsal vein of

the penis or the conjunctival artery of the eyelid.

Persons who are drug abusers may develop toxic effects from high doses taken accidentally or in efforts to achieve desired mind-altering effects, especially when tolerance to lower doses develop (Table 15-3). Different symptoms result from withdrawal of the drug. Complete withdrawal of the drug without the substitution of another drug is called "cold turkey" and is a very uncomfortable physical and psychologic condition that may last up to 3 days.

Because of the expense involved, users often sell their belongings or steal to get the money to buy a "fix." Each day abuse of drugs in the United States costs the economy millions of dollars. Property loss through crimes connected with drugs can be extensive. The disappearance of such items as radios, watches, jewelry, and other similar objects from the home should arouse the suspicion of parents and friends.

Intervention

In the United States the addiction to narcotics has been considered a crime ever since the passage of the Harrison Narcotic Act in 1914. The general feeling of the Council on Mental Health of the American Medical Association is that narcotic addiction should be considered and treated as an illness. The present methods of treating narcotic addicts are not satisfactory, and the incidence of relapse is high.

One approach to the treatment of narcotic addiction is the methadone maintenance program. Methadone is a synthetic drug, and the average narcotic user's daily dose is inexpensive. The drug is given legally as a part of a rehabilitation program that includes group or individual therapy or both. The drug reduces the severity of the heroin withdrawal, and the user can often maintain employment while undergoing treatment. Methadone itself is addictive and must be tapered off or the user may continue the habit the rest of his life. Because this drug is easily available through legal channels and permits the person to work, methadone advocates feel its use is essentially the same as that of the diabetic taking insulin or that of persons on maintenance doses of other drugs such as steroids or digitalis. A newer drug, acetylmethadol, may prove to be superior to methadone.

One of the most effective means of treatment to evolve recently is the use of residential communities, usually run by ex-addicts, with or without professionals. Synanon is such a community. It was founded in California in 1958, and there are now several chapters across the country. In New York there are the Phoenix and Horizon Houses. Marathon House serves the Rhode Island–Massachusetts area. In Chicago the program is available under the name of Gateway Houses. Such services are usually listed in local telephone directories, and the organizations often have literature for distribu-

TABLE 15-3. Acute intoxication and withdrawal of mind-altering drugs

| Drug group | Acute intoxication | | Withdrawal symptoms |
	Symptoms	Treatment	
Narcotics	Respiratory depression, bradycardia, hypotension, cold clammy skin, decreased body temperature; deep sleep, stupor, or coma; pinpoint pupils	Maintain ventilation, provide oxygen Give narcotic antagonist: naloxone (Narcan) 0.4 mg IV Monitor vital signs every 15-30 min until patient is conscious Treat for shock	(Not life threatening) Early: restlessness, irritability, drug craving, yawning, lacrimation, diaphoresis, rhinorrhea; followed by "yen" sleep (intense desire to sleep; sleeps restlessly) Later: awakens with more severe symptoms, nausea, vomiting, anorexia, abdominal cramps, bone and muscle pain, tremors, piloerection ("gooseflesh")
Other CNS depressants	Same as narcotics (above)	Lavage if recent oral ingestion Maintain ventilation, provide oxygen Monitor vital signs every 15-30 min until patient is conscious Position patient side-lying or prone, not supine Treat for shock Hemodialysis for renal shutdown	(May be life threatening) Insomnia, restlessness, tremors, anorexia, followed by convulsions, and symptoms similar to delirium tremens (confusion, visual and auditory hallucinations), fever, dehydration
CNS stimulants	Labile cardiovascular symptoms (flushing or pallor, pulse and blood pressure changes, arrhythmias), hyperpyrexia, mental disturbances (agitation, paranoia, hallucinations), convulsions, circulatory collapse	Give chlorpromazine, 25-50 mg IM Provide a quiet environment Orient patient to reality Monitor vital signs until stable	(Withdrawal is not severe) Somnolence, apathy, irritability, depression, fatigue
Hallucinogens	Physiologic toxicity low at doses that produce strong psychologic effects Acute panic reaction ("bad trip") may lead to suicide "Flashback" episodes Prolonged psychotic disorders (paranoia, depression) Phencyclidine: CNS depression or stimulation may lead to death	Provide quiet, supportive environment and constant attention Give diazepam (Valium), 2-10 mg IM for severe anxiety	No evidence of withdrawal symptoms
Cannabis	Adverse reactions infrequent Simple depression, paranoid ideation, confusion, disorientation, hallucinations	Provide support and reassurance Give tranquilizer for agitation	(Withdrawal symptoms rare) Insomnia, anorexia

tion and will provide speakers for groups.* The treatment in such communities consists of helping individuals through the withdrawal state and then attempting to help them increase self-understanding and to change their life pattern. Therapy is provided by the group. Rules of the community are strict, and breaking them results in severe consequences. The programs range in length from 18 to 36 months. Many addicts stay in the community after they no longer use the drug and help to rehabilitate other addicts. This provides support, and a good number of former users can "stay clean." Of those who leave the community, many return to drug use.

*Additional information on drugs and drug abuse can be obtained from the National Institute of Mental Health, 5600 Fishers Lane, Rockville, Md. 20857.

There are two federal narcotics hospitals, one in Lexington, Kentucky, and the other in Fort Worth, Texas. Most of the patients in these institutions are there by court order and have little motivation for giving up drugs. Treatment is conservative. More than 90% of these patients return to heroin use. There is much controversy as to the merits of the various programs. Financial problems are serious, and there is much competition for the limited available funds.

Although patients receiving treatment for drug addiction usually are housed in special units of psychiatric facilities, medical or surgical units may have patients who are drug addicts. The drug addict may develop any of the medical and surgical ailments that any other person may have. Because of their poor nutritional state, many addicts have lowered resistance to disease and infection. The use of contaminated syringes and needles often causes hepatitis. In addition, drug addicts, in an attempt to get drugs, may seek admission to a general hospital. They may complain of severe pain such as that from renal colic or back strain, since these are disorders for which narcotics often are given even before a specific diagnosis is made. Thus complaints of the drug addict stem from either acute drug toxicity or an abstinence syndrome.[23] These persons need to learn new ways of handling stress and to learn to develop satisfying interpersonal relationships. Education is an important part of their management.[23]

REFERENCES AND SELECTED READINGS
Contemporary

1. *Bahra, R.: The potential for suicide, Am. J. Nurs. **75:**1782-1788, 1975.
2. Bailey, D., and Dryer, S.: Therapeutic approaches to the care of the mentally ill, Philadelphia, 1977, F.A. Davis Co.
3. Beck, A.R.: The diagnosis and management of depression, Philadelphia, 1973, University of Pennsylvania Press.
4. Carter, R.M.: Psychosocial nursing, New York, 1971, Macmillan, Inc.
5. Corsini, R.: Current psychotherapies, Itasca, Illinois, 1978, F.E. Peacock Publishers, Inc.
6. *DeGennaro, M.D., Hymen, R., Cranwell, A., and Mansky, P.A.: Antidepressant drug therapy, Am. J. Nurs. **81:**1304-1308, 1981.
7. *Ditzler, J.: Rehabilitation for alcoholics, Am. J. Nurs. **76:**1772-1775, 1976.
8. Finkel, N.S.: Mental illness and health, New York, 1976, MacMillan Co.
9. *Haber, J., et al.: Comprehensive psychiatric nursing, New York, 1978, McGraw-Hill Book Co.
10. *Harris, E.: Antipsychotic medications, Am. J. Nurs. **81:**1316-1328, 1981.
11. *Harris, E.: Lithium, Am. J. Nurs. **81:**1310-1315, 1981.
12. *Harris, E.: Sedative and hypnotic drugs, Am. J. Nurs. **81:**1329-1334, 1981.
13. *Heinemann, E., and Estes, N.: Assessing alcoholic patients, Am. J. Nurs. **76:**785-789, 1976.
14. *Jourard, S.M.: Living and dying, suicide: the invitation to die, Am. J. Nurs. **70:**273-275, 1970.
15. Kaufman, R., and Levy, S.B.: Overdose treatment, J.A.M.A. **227:**411-413, 1974.
16. *Kids and heroin: the adolescent epidemic, Time, pp. 16-25, March 16, 1970.
17. *Kline, N., and Davis, J.M.: Psychotropic drugs, Am. J. Nurs. **73:**54-62, 1973.
18. Lancaster, J.: Community mental health nursing, St. Louis, 1980, The C.V. Mosby Co.
19. Manfredo, L., and Krampetz, S.: Psychiatric nursing, Philadelphia, 1977, F.A. Davis Co.
20. Mereness, D.A., and Taylor, C.M.: Essentials of psychiatric nursing, ed. 10, St. Louis, 1978, The C.V. Mosby Co.
21. *Mueller, J.F.: Treatment for the alcoholic: cursing or nursing, Am. J. Nurs. **74:**245-247, 1974.
22. *Nelson, K.: The nurse in a methadone maintenance program, Am. J. Nurs. **73:**870-874, 1973.
23. Rosenbaum, C.P., and Beebe, J.E.: Psychiatric treatment: crisis, clinic, consultation, New York, 1975, McGraw-Hill Book Co.
24. Topalis, M., and Aguilera, D.: Psychiatric nursing, ed. 7, St. Louis, 1978, The C.V. Mosby Co.
25. U.S. Department of Health, Education and Welfare: Meeting America's needs, Alcohol, Drug Abuse and Mental Health Administration, Washington, D.C., 1975, U.S. Government Printing Office.
26. *Vaillot, Sister M.C.: Living and dying: hope, the restoration of being, Am. J. Nurs. **70:**268,270-273, 1970.
27. Wilson, H.S., and Kneisl, C.R.: Psychiatric nursing, Menlo Park, California, 1979, Addison-Wesley Co.

Classic

28. *Bowles, C.: Children of alcoholic parents, Am. J. Nurs. **68:**1062-1064, 1968.
29. *Burd, S.R., and Marshall, M.A.: Some clinical approaches to psychiatric nursing, New York, 1963, Macmillan, Inc.
30. *Farberow, N., and Schneidman, E.S.: The cry for help, New York, 1961, McGraw-Hill Book Co.
31. *Long, B.: Sleep, Am. J. Nurs. **69:**1896-1899, 1969.
32. *Peplau, H.: Interpersonal techniques: the crux of psychiatric nursing, Am. J. Nurs. **62:**111-116, 1965.
33. *Thomas, B.J.: Clues to patients' behavior, Am. J. Nurs. **63:**100-102, 1963.
34. *Umscheid, Sister T.: With suicidal patients caring for is caring about, Am. J. Nurs. **67:**1230-1232, 1967.
35. Wilner, D.M., and Kassebaum, G.G., editors: Narcotics, New York, 1965, McGraw-Hill Book Co.

*References preceded by an asterisk are particularly well suited for student reading.

CHAPTER 16

ADAPTATION THROUGHOUT THE LIFE CYCLE

PATRICIA HUMPHREY
DONNA WILLIAMS HEWITT
RUTH F. CRAVEN

Each client that the nurse meets in any setting is engaged in the process of growth, from the pregnant mother and her growing fetus to the toddler, the adolescent, and the aged grandmother. Growth encompasses physical, mental, and emotional spheres; therefore in planning nursing care it is just as important to provide for the patient's growth and development needs as it is to meet needs generated by the client's illness. Each contact that a nurse has with a child or a family is an opportunity for developmental assessment.

Diseases and disorders requiring medical or surgical treatment afflict persons of all ages, from newborn infants to octogenarians. The age of a patient influences nursing needs and must always be considered in planning and providing care. Each person, regardless of age and whether sick or well, has needs related to physical and emotional welfare. These include being fed, clothed, and housed, being safe and comfortable both physically and spiritually, and being important to others.

In the United States two age groups have received a great deal of society's attention: children and the elderly. These groups of people were easy to study because they were in institutions such as schools or rest homes. The adult population has not been quite so easy to study. It is only in recent years that we are seeing more information in the literature regarding young adults and middle-aged persons. The number of elderly people in the United States has increased steadily over the past 50 years. Approximately 21.8 million persons are 65 years of age or over.[25] By 2000 it is estimated that this number will reach or surpass 31 million.[44] At present those persons 75 years of age or over are increasing proportionately faster than the total age group who are over 65. The increasing number of elderly persons has come about primarily through the decrease in infant mortality, the prevention and control of communicable disease during childhood, the improved treatment of adult acute and chronic disease, and improvements in medical care in general. At the same time the birth rate in the United States is declining; in 1973 it was slightly above the zero population growth level.

The growth rate of the older population has been consistently faster than that of persons under 65. Every day approximately 4000 Americans turn 65; every day 3000 Americans 65 years or older die. Thus every day there is a net increase of 1000 persons in the older population.[25]

Cycles of human growth

Growth may be defined as a change in body structure or size. Physical growth is a continuous process from the moment of conception until the organism reaches adulthood. Growth takes place by the development and integration of differentiated cells and tissues. *Development* denotes increases in functional capacity evolved from maturation of physical and mental capacities and learning. *Maturation* implies the replacement or rejection of a previously learned appropriate behavior with one more appropriate to the age of the changing individual. In all children development takes place as growth takes place—regularly and in a predictable, continuous pattern. Every child moves

TABLE 16-1. Cephalocaudal development during first year of life

First year	Development
First quarter	Control of eyes and head
Second quarter	Control of upper trunk and arms
Third quarter	Control of lower trunk and fine prehensile grip
Fourth quarter	Erect posture and bipedal locomotion begin

through the same developmental stages in a characteristic human way. As mentioned, development is dependent on physical maturation. The organism must reach a certain level of physical growth before certain developmental tasks are possible. One illustration is that infants can make primitive stepping motions but cannot walk because the bones and muscles of the legs are not physically mature enough to support the body weight.

While allowing for individual variations, development is always governed by a few principles. There is a cephalocaudal (from head to toe) and proximodistal (from the midline of the body outward) progression of development (Table 16-1).

Development also proceeds from the general to the specific. The infant possesses the gross or large muscle movements long before fine motor skills are developed.

Predictable patterns of physical growth and psychosocial development occurring at different age periods are described in this chapter. Infancy (birth to 12 months) is a time of rapid physical growth and sensorimotor development. Childhood can be divided into toddlerhood (1 to 3 years), preschool years (3 to 5 years), and middle childhood (6 years to puberty). During these years the child grows rapidly, learns to communicate with others, develops a sense of "self," becomes enculturated, and emerges as a social being. Adolescence (the "teen" years) is a time of transition from childhood to adulthood—a time of physiologic, psychosocial, and cognitive maturation. The adolescent develops emotional independence from the family with development of ego identity.

Adulthood is one of the most stable periods in the life span. Even though various physical and psychologic changes occur during these years, there is relative stability in values, attitudes, and feelings about the self and others. The adult has developed a sense of self-utilization to achieve desired goals as contrasted with the self-consciousness of the adolescent.[47]

While dramatic changes in physical development are few, the main physiologic event of the adult years is the menopause. The psychologic changes that may occur are largely responses to changing life events.

Early and middle adulthood covers a long period of life, extending approximately from ages 20 to 65. Because circumstances and expectations are not the same in the first 25 years as they are in the second 20 years, adulthood is separated into three stages: young adulthood, middle adulthood, and late adulthood.

Infancy

The greatest risk of death is in the period immediately following birth when the transition must be made from intrauterine symbiotic existence to extrauterine independent life.[40] Neonates must make several adaptations in order to survive. They must establish respiration and adapt their circulatory system to function independently of the placenta.

On the other hand, some systems are able to function very well at birth. For example, the gastrointestinal system is able to handle complex sugars in human milk. The infant can digest carbohydrates for energy in the first 5 hours of life, and fat becomes an important source of energy by the second day. It is not until the third day that protein metabolism begins.[5] The liver is immature at birth and has limited ability to conjugate bilirubin and corticosteroid. The nervous system of the newborn, even though it functions primarily at a reflex level, is fully functional in a life-sustaining sense.

Assessment of the neonate

Assessment begins at birth. Apgar scoring charts available in most delivery rooms evaluate five signs of a healthy neonate: a heart rate of 120 to 160 beats per minute, a good strong cry, well-flexed extremities, irritable reflexes, and a healthy pink color. An initial assessment is made at 60 seconds, and a second assessment, which gives some measure of the infant's adjustment to extrauterine life, is made at 5 minutes (Table 16-2). In addition to Apgar ratings, newborns are given a maturity rating and classification based on physical and neuromuscular maturity.[1] This examination is usually done shortly after birth and repeated again before discharge. It allows the health care provider to determine if the newborn is small for gestational age (SGA), appropriate for gestational age (AGA), or large for gestational age (LGA). Such classifications alert health care providers to potential problems of the neonate.

Gross physical anomalies such as cleft lip or palate, omphalocele, or club foot may be observed on initial examination at birth.

More detailed assessment of the infant may be conducted at this time if the infant is stable, or it may be

TABLE 16-2. Apgar scoring

Sign	Score		
	0	1	2
Heart rate	Absent	Slow (below 100)	Over 100
Respiratory effort	Absent	Weak cry, hypoventilation	Good; strong cry
Muscle tone	Limp	Some flexion of extremities	Active motion, extremities well flexed
Reflex irritability	No response	Grimace	Cry
Color	Blue, pale	Body pink, extremities blue	Completely pink

TABLE 16-3. Feeding schedule for the first year

Age	Food or supplement
Birth to 11-12 mo	Breast milk or fortified formula
Birth to 4 mo	Supplements of vitamin C, vitamin D, and fluoride may be required depending on fluoride content of water
5-6 mo	Introduce commercially prepared infant cereal (iron fortified); begin with a single grain cereal such as rice, which is the least allergenic grain; never use mixed cereals until all grains have been introduced individually and allergy ruled out
6 mo	Introduce strained fruits; start with bland fruits such as applesauce or pears; offer the same fruit for 3 days to rule out allergies; the more tart and acid fruits are added last
6-8 mo	Introduce strained vegetables and strained meats, egg yolks, and firmer textured foods; finger foods such as zwieback, hard toast, crackers, and raw apples may be introduced as tooth eruption occurs; foods are always introduced one at a time to rule out allergies
8-12 mo	Introduce firmer textured foods; whole egg may be introduced toward the end of the first year; iron-fortified formula is continued; introduce to cup towards end of first year; breast-feeding may continue until baby initiates weaning

delayed until a later time. Nursing care during the immediate postnatal period is directed toward provision of warmth, safety, adequate respiration, and nutrition.

Assessment of the infant

Length and weight

Infancy is the most rapid period of physical growth during life. The average infant increases in length by 50% during the first year. Most infants double their birth weight by 6 months and triple their birth weight by 1 year. Infants are usually weighed at each visit to the health care provider, as a steady weight gain is one indication that the infant is progressing satisfactorily with regard to physical growth. Failure to gain weight over several months is a clue to health care providers that something is wrong either with the internal or external environment. Of equal concern today is the problem of too rapid a weight gain. When weight gain appears to be too rapid, the nurse needs to assess the quantity and quality of the diet.

Head circumference

Head size increases rapidly during infancy. Head circumference is measured at birth and at frequent intervals during infancy. This information along with height and weight is usually plotted on a standardized growth chart. Measurements allow the health care provider to evaluate whether the head is growing too rapidly or too slowly; either situation can lead to brain damage or in extreme cases even death. Head circumference is usually about 2.5 cm (1 in.) larger than chest circumference at birth.

Fontanelles

The two fontanelles, sometimes referred to as soft spots, are membrane-covered spaces remaining in the incompletely ossified skull. The anterior fontanelle is

diamond shaped and is located at the juncture of the parietal and frontal bones; it is normally 3 to 4 cm long and 2 to 3 cm wide. Closure of the anterior fontanelle at about 18 months is caused by gradual growth of the cranial bones. The posterior fontanelle, which is triangular in shape, is located at the junction of the parietal and occipital bones. The posterior fontanelle is quite small, approximately 0.5 to 1 cm, and usually closes sometime in the third month. The anterior fontanelle normally pulsates with the heart beat and bulges slightly during periods of crying.

Fontanelles are checked frequently during the first few months of life. Too rapid or delayed closure may signal abnormal cranial processes.

Physiologic growth of the neonate and infant

Gastrointestinal system

The relatively immature gastrointestinal tract of the neonate matures, and the rapid emptying time begins to slow by the end of infancy. At birth the gastrointestinal tract is capable of digesting breast milk or an equivalent formula. By the end of the first year the gastrointestinal tract has matured sufficiently to allow for digestion of more complex foods (Table 16-3).

DAILY NUTRITIONAL NEEDS OF INFANTS*

Calories	115 cal/kg body weight
Protein	2-2.2 g/kg body weight
Vitamin A	420 μg RE†
Thiamine	0.3-0.5 mg
Riboflavin	0.4-0.6 mg
Niacin	6-8 mg
Vitamin C	35 mg
Vitamin D	400 IU
Calcium	360-540 mg

*From Food and Nutrition Board, National Academy of Sciences—National Research Council: Recommended daily dietary allowances, revised 1979, Washington, D.C.
†RE = Retinal equivalent.

DISAPPEARANCE OF INFANTILE REFLEXES

Sucking	Persists throughout infancy, particularly during sleep
Rooting	3-4 mo while awake; many persist during sleep for 9-12 mo
Palmar grasp	5-6 mo
Plantar grasp	9-12 mo
Moro reflex	4-7 mo
Stepping	3-4 mo
Placing	10-12 mo
Incurvation of trunk	2-3 mo

The infant's large intestine is initially immature in water absorption, resulting in stools which contain great amounts of water and which are loose in consistency. Because the rate of water turnover is great during infancy, an increased amount of fluid must be ingested each day to keep pace with normal fluid loss. Water needs are generally met if the infant is fed properly, as most sources of food for infants are very dilute. The infant's need for calories, fluids, and all nutrients is greater proportionately than that of persons of other age groups (see box above). Due to limited reserves of fat, glycogen, and extracellular water, the infant cannot tolerate loss of fluid or omission of food or fluids for more than a few hours without experiencing acidosis and dehydration.

The infant generates large amounts of heat because of an active metabolism. However, infants lose proportionately larger amounts of fluid than older persons when dissipating heat. Thus there is a danger of rapid dehydration when the infant is febrile. In addition, the infant's poor control of vascular dilation and constriction interferes with body heat retention. Thus the infant chills easily. Both fluid balance and temperature control warrant special concern by those providing infant care.

Neurologic system

During infancy neurologic development proceeds from reflexive behavior, which is normal during the early months of infancy, to voluntary control as association pathways begin to develop (see box above, at right). Brain growth is rapid during infancy and reaches about two thirds of eventual adult weight by the end of the first year.

The sense organs

Vision. At birth the eye is structurally incomplete, and the neonate sees little. Pupillary and corneal reflexes are present at birth, and the neonate can fixate on an object at very close range (8 to 10 in.). Visual acuity gradually improves during infancy, and by 4 months the infant can focus on the parent as he or she speaks. Binocular vision is well established by 4 months. By 6 months infants can distinguish between familiar and strange faces. By the twelfth month the infant is able to recognize familiar objects such as the bottle or a favorite toy.

Hearing. Hearing is more developed than vision at birth; the neonate responds to loud noises close to the ear by the startle reflex, while low-pitched sounds, such as a heartbeat, have a quieting effect. Between 8 to 12 months the infant responds to sound by turning the head to the side when sound is made at ear level.[18]

Cardiorespiratory system

The normal neonate is an abdominal breather; respiratory rates are between 30 and 50 breaths/min. Growth of the respiratory system is gradual, and during infancy the rate slows to about 30 breaths/min and becomes more regular.

Dramatic changes occur in the circulatory system at birth; complete closure of some of these fetal structures may not occur until late infancy, which results in as many as 50% of children having innocent murmurs beyond the neonatal period. While the heart does not grow as rapidly as some other parts of the body, it usually doubles in weight in the first year. At birth the heart lies in an almost horizontal position but gradually shifts to a permanent vertical position as the infant grows older. The heart rate averages 120 to 130 beats/min during the first year; normal blood pressure is 60/90.

Hemopoietic changes during the first year of life reflect the infant's increasing ability to produce hemoglobin. During the first 5 months fetal hemoglobin is dominant; adult hemoglobin begins to appear around 13 weeks of age. Maternal iron stores are sufficient for the first 5 to 6 months; as they gradually diminish, infants must ingest their own iron. During infancy the normal hemoglobin value should be 10 to 15 g/100 ml; hematocrit (PVC) 30% to 40%.[52]

Genitourinary system

The genital organs remain relatively immature during infancy. The renal structures also remain immature during infancy, which predisposes infants to dehydration. The young infant's ability to reabsorb urinary filtrates for body use is not well developed; therefore the infant's fluid needs are relatively greater than the adult's.

Dentition

Tooth formation and placement are in process at birth. The lower central incisors are usually the first to erupt at or around 5 to 6 months.

Psychosocial development

Infants are primarily egocentric beings and are concerned only with themselves and the satisfaction of their own needs and desires. Most of their reactions are based on the "pleasure principle."

Basic to emotional development during infancy is the acquisition of a *sense of trust* (Fig. 16-1). Most often the mother, who is the primary caretaker, is the most significant person involved in the achievement of basic trust. When the mother provides nurturance, familiarity, security, and continuity of experience, the infant is able to develop a sense of trust of the world around him or her and the people in it. A sense of mistrust of the environment and the people in it may result if an inadequate parenting relationship is present. Erikson feels this experience is irrevocable and influences the way subsequent stages evolve.[10]

Research in learning indicates that early stimulation during infancy is important for the future learning capacity of the individual.[61] According to Piaget's theory of cognitive development, the period of infancy is termed the period of *sensorimotor development*. During the first month of life the infant acts on the ready-made sensorimotor schemata consisting primarily of reflexes and the innate capacities for performance. From 1 to 4 months infants act primarily on events that are centered around their own bodies. They begin sucking as the bottle approaches, show signs of recognition, and may respond to a familiar toy. Objects have no permanence as attested to by the fact that an infant makes no search when a toy disappears from the visual field. Be-

---

TASKS OF THE INFANT

Stabilization of newly independent physiologic processes

Developing control of muscular and nervous sytem

Learning to understand and control the physical world through exploration

Beginning to acquire language

Establishing self as separate entity

Learning to trust

Developing independent emotional relationships with others

---

tween 4 and 8 months, building on the schemata of the first two periods, infants develop the ability to perceive objects as separate from themselves and become more active in causing events to happen. In the last 4 months of the first year of life the infant continues refinement of characteristics acquired during the third period. They begin to develop a more mature notion of causality and of the concept of means-end relationships.

Language development begins shortly after birth with the ability to cry. Infants develop different cries to communicate specific needs such as hunger, pain, or being wet. By 3 months of age most infants develop the beginnings of prelanguage, vocalizing by babbling and cooing. Before the age of 6 months infants respond to their names and begin to respond to simple instructions such as "Come here." At 7 months of age the infant is able to vocalize four different syllables and makes talking sounds in response to the talking of others. The 8-month-old babbles to produce consonant sounds and says "dada" or "mama." By 11 months the infant initiates definite speech sounds and uses jargon. At this age he communicates a great deal by pointing at objects. By the end of the first year the child can say a few simple words and jabbers expressively. The tasks to be mastered during infancy are shown in the box above.

Health concerns

During the first year or two of life the infant's endocrine functions are sluggish. Their fluid and electrolyte balance is easily upset, and they have little resistance to infection or stressors of any kind. Babies therefore respond quickly and critically to illness. They may be apparently well one moment and an hour later seriously ill. The younger the child, the more pronounced is this response.

Hydration

Because of the immature system, loss of fluids and the accompanying loss of electrolytes present a serious

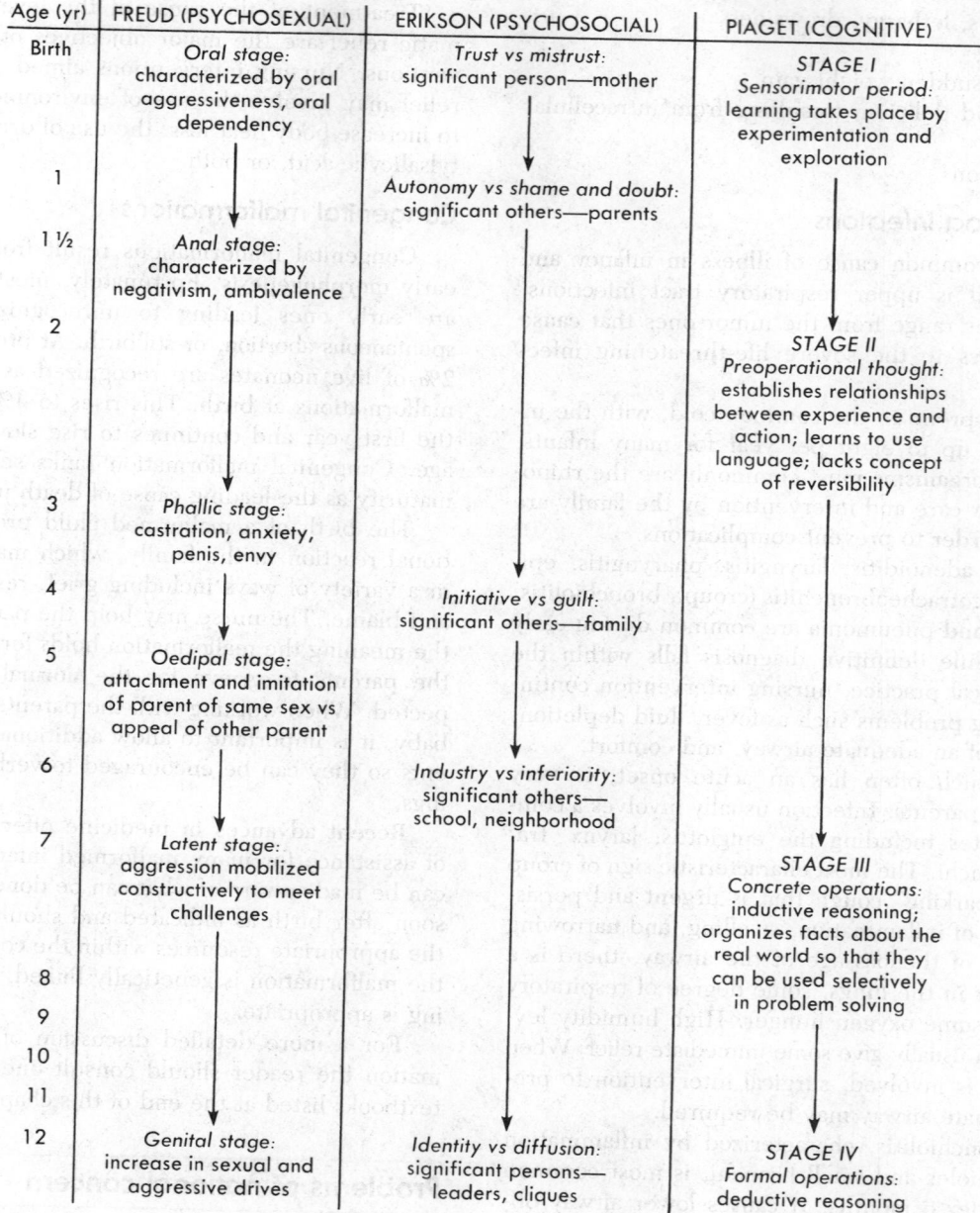

Age (yr)	FREUD (PSYCHOSEXUAL)	ERIKSON (PSYCHOSOCIAL)	PIAGET (COGNITIVE)
Birth	*Oral stage:* characterized by oral aggressiveness, oral dependency	*Trust vs mistrust:* significant person—mother	STAGE I *Sensorimotor period:* learning takes place by experimentation and exploration
1		*Autonomy vs shame and doubt:* significant others—parents	
1½	*Anal stage:* characterized by negativism, ambivalence		
2			STAGE II *Preoperational thought:* establishes relationships between experience and action; learns to use language; lacks concept of reversibility
3	*Phallic stage:* castration, anxiety, penis, envy		
4		*Initiative vs guilt:* significant others—family	
5	*Oedipal stage:* attachment and imitation of parent of same sex vs appeal of other parent		
6		*Industry vs inferiority:* significant others—school, neighborhood	
7	*Latent stage:* aggression mobilized constructively to meet challenges		STAGE III *Concrete operations:* inductive reasoning; organizes facts about the real world so that they can be used selectively in problem solving
8			
9			
10			
11			
12	*Genital stage:* increase in sexual and aggressive drives	*Identity vs diffusion:* significant persons— leaders, cliques	STAGE IV *Formal operations:* deductive reasoning

Fig. 16-1. Summary of psychosocial development in early life.

hazard for the infant. During infancy and early childhood there is an increased percentage of fluid in the extracellular spaces, which makes the infant more vulnerable to fluid losses. The resulting imbalance in fluid and electrolyte composition of the interstitial and intracellular spaces presents serious threat. Fluid loss in infants and young children from diarrhea and vomiting, which may occur in association with many illnesses during infancy, is initially assumed to be isotonic for purposes of immediate therapy. Since electrolyte composition of the extracellular spaces of the infant and young child differs significantly from that of the older child and adult, replacement needs must be estimated cor-

rectly. Care must be taken not to cause overhydration.

The clinical signs of the state of hydration in the young infant may be difficult to determine. Chinn[5] lists the following signs of dehydration for the infant and young child:

1. Dry skin, parched tongue, sunken eyeballs, sunken fontanelle
2. Decreased urinary output
3. Specific gravity of urine greater than 1.030
4. Recent weight loss of over 6% of initial body weight

Signs of overhydration include:

1. Increased urinary output

2. Weakness, lethargy, drowsiness
3. Vomiting
4. Edema, sudden weight gain
5. Coma and delirium (resulting from intracellular edema)
6. Convulsions[5]

Respiratory tract infections

The most common cause of illness in infancy and early childhood is upper respiratory tract infections. These infections range from the minor ones that cause minimal distress to the severe life-threatening infections.

Infants are prone to the common cold, with the incidence being up to eight per year for many infants. The invading organisms most commonly are the rhinoviruses. Proper care and intervention by the family are important in order to prevent complications.

Tonsillitis, adenoiditis, laryngitis, pharyngitis, epiglottitis, laryngotracheobronchitis (croup), bronchiolitis, pneumonitis, and pneumonia are common during early childhood. While definitive diagnosis falls within the realm of medical practice, nursing intervention continues for nursing problems such as fever, fluid depletion, maintenance of an adequate airway, and comfort.

Croup, which often has an acute onset, is very frightening to parents. Infection usually involves a combination of sites including the epiglottis, larynx, trachea, and bronchi. The most characteristic sign of croup is a hoarse "barking" cough that is urgent and persistent. Because of inflammation, swelling, and narrowing of the lumen of the passage of the airway, there is a trapping of air in the lungs, some degree of respiratory distress, and some oxygen hunger. High humidity levels and oxygen usually give some immediate relief. When the epiglottis is involved, surgical intervention to provide an adequate airway may be required.

Acute bronchiolitis, characterized by inflammation of the bronchioles and small bronchi, is most common in infants under 6 months. It causes lower airway obstruction. This infection most commonly occurs in epidemics during the winter and spring.

Supportive measures including fluids to prevent dehydration and to liquefy mucus in the lower respiratory tract are usually successful. If significant respiratory distress is present, hospitalization may be necessary to provide humidified oxygen. Careful attention should be given to infants with bronchiolitis in order to prevent complications such as pneumonia.

Fever

Fever often accompanies illness during infancy and childhood. The hypothalamus, which is the center for temperature control, is immature during early life. A temperature of 42.5° C (104° F) carries critical risk of febrile convulsions.

Treatment of the cause of the fever and symptomatic relief are the major objectives of nursing interventions. Nursing interventions aimed at symptomatic relief may involve the use of environmental measures to increase body heat loss, the use of drugs such as acetylsalicylic acid, or both.

Congenital malformations

Congenital malformations result from problems in early morphogenesis. Fortunately, most malformations are early ones leading to unrecognized pregnancy, spontaneous abortion, or stillbirth. At present only about 2% of live neonates are recognized as having serious malformations at birth. This rises to 4% by the end of the first year and continues to rise slowly until school age. Congenital malformation ranks second after prematurity as the leading cause of death in infants.

The birth of a malformed child produces an emotional reaction in the family, which may be expressed in a variety of ways including grief, resentment, guilt, and blame. The nurse may help the parents to identify the meaning the malformation holds for them and allow the parents to grieve for the normal child they expected. When working with the parents of a malformed baby, it is important to allow additional time with parents so they can be encouraged to verbalize their feelings.

Recent advances in medicine offer increased hope of assistance for many malformed infants. The parents can be made aware of what can be done for the child as soon after birth as indicated and should be directed to the appropriate resources within the community. When the malformation is genetically linked, genetic counseling is appropriate.

For a more detailed discussion of specific malformation the reader should consult one of the pediatric textbooks listed at the end of this chapter.

Problems of national concern

Sudden infant death syndrome

Sudden infant death syndrome (SIDS) is the leading cause of death between the ages of 1 and 12 months and accounts for up to 10,000 infant deaths per year in the United States.[29] Until recently physicians had no idea what caused the sudden death of these apparently healthy babies. Recent studies indicate that the victims of crib death are not completely normal, as once was thought. There is evidence that these infants have subtle physiologic defects, probably in mechanisms that control breathing.[29] Many adults and infants have periods of apnea during sleep, and the question of what constitutes a dangerously long apneic episode is as yet unanswered. It is hypothesized that infants who die of crib death may be prone to prolonged periods of apnea during sleep. Other investigators have found that the formation of certain chemicals involved in the transmission of nerve impulses that control breathing are impaired in premature infants with apnea, and this may be a contributing factor to SIDS in these infants. Most investigators believe that there is more than one cause of SIDS. At present major efforts are being directed toward applying this new information to devise tests that will predict which infants are at risk of SIDS. The National Sudden Infant Death Syndrome Foundation (NSIDSF)* serves as a clearinghouse of information for parents and health professionals.

Nurses are concerned primarily with preventive mental health care and family advocacy. In order to work effectively with these families, the nurse must have adequate knowledge of the concepts of grief and loss and counseling skills and be willing to become involved.

Child abuse

In 1961 Kempe coined the phrase "battered child" and began a campaign that brought national attention to the problem of child abuse. While it may be due in part to better reporting and an increased awareness of the problem, child abuse appears to be on the incline in the United States. The problem of child abuse is multifactorial. Numerous studies of the late 1960s and early 1970s provide health professionals with better guidelines for identifying potential child abusers and abused children (see box at right).

Health care personnel need to be alert to the clinical pathology of the battered child such as surface marks (e.g., abrasions, bruises, burns), musculoskeletal injuries (e.g., multiple fractures in varying stages of repair), and visceral injuries (e.g., head injury, ruptured liver or spleen).[4]

For treatment to be effective health personnel must regard the family as a unit, and rehabilitation of the family as a viable unit must be the aim of intervention. Unless the abusive cycle is broken completely, one can expect the act to be repeated. Studies show that approximately one-half of the small children who are abused will be brain injured or dead within 1 year if returned to unchanged environments.[43]

Health workers and others in society must exercise care not to exhibit feelings of disgust and repulsion toward abusive parents. Abusive parents are often frightened, defensive, and angry. They need help and most often want help but do not know how to face the reality of the problem. Many communities now have Parents Anonymous and other groups that both potential abusers and abusers find to be a great source of help. Information about local groups can be obtained from child

---

GUIDELINES FOR IDENTIFYING POTENTIAL CHILD ABUSERS

One or both parents were often abused as children. Studies indicate over 90% of abusive parents were abused children.

Parents tend to be lonely adults, attracted to each other as they search for loving parent figures.

Extreme personal and social isolation. These parents lack group and community integration and most often lack family support.

Unstable marital relationship. Parents lack positive feedback and support.

Low self-esteem.

Parent-child role reversal. The parents want the infant to meet their unfulfilled needs for mothering.

Unrealistic expectations of infants. Parents expect children to act older.

Parents unable to reach out and ask for help.

SPECIAL TRAITS THAT MAKE A CHILD VULNERABLE TO ABUSE

Usually young child, under 3 years of age.

Something different about child (i.e., pregnancy or delivery uncomfortable, child unwanted, premature birth).

Child is extremely irritable or cries often.

Birth order. Most often it is the first or last child who is abused.

---

welfare agencies. One such group is CALM (Child Abuse and Listening Mediation, Inc.).*

Maternal deprivation

Early in the nineteenth century astute physicians wrote about children who suffered under institutional conditions. By the late 1950s and the 1960s recognition of the problem of maternal deprivation became more apparent. Maternal deprivation exists when an infant is deprived of the opportunity of forming an initial tie with a mother figure or when an infant is deprived of the mother figure after a meaningful tie has been formed.

While many of the studies done in this area are beset with methodologic difficulties, the majority of studies point out the damaging effects to the infant in motor, intellectual, and emotional development resulting from separation from the mother figure during the early years (see Chapter 26). The extent of damage depends on the degree of emotional and sensory deprivation, the stage of development of the child, and the quality of the relationship with the mother prior to separation.

Such studies indicate the need for continuity of the

---

*National Sudden Infant Death Syndrome Foundation, 310 S. Michigan Ave., Suite 1904, Chicago, IL 60604.

*P.O. Box 718, Santa Barbara, CA 93102.

relationship and emphasize the desirability of rooming-in for mothers with sick infants or young children.

Nursing assessment and intervention

Whenever possible, facilities for rooming-in should be available for mothers of hospitalized infants. When the mother is present, she is encouraged to participate in the infant's care as much as possible, which makes the infant more secure and helps the mother to become more comfortable with a sick child. When possible one staff member should work consistently with the mother and the child. Such a plan helps the mother to continue her mothering responsibilities under stress and will make her more comfortable if it is necessary for her to leave the infant. When the mother is unable to be present, the staff member should take over the mothering. Infants need cuddling, verbalization, and stimulation.

The nursing assessment may include questions relative to eating habits, the home routine, and methods of comforting the baby. The home routine should be followed as much as possible to facilitate the development of the infant's sense of trust. If the infant has a favorite blanket or toy, parents should be encouraged to bring it to the hospital.

The hospital staff can make certain the parents are informed relative to the care of their infant. All procedures need to be carefully explained to the parents.

Toddlerhood (1 to 3 years)

Physical growth

Probably one of the most significant occurrences during the toddler stage is that the child develops the ability to move about unassisted. Physically the musculoskeletal system expands and matures to allow the child to develop a standing posture and to walk. Previously the child could only lie or sit. The world now contains a new facet. Locomotion allows for development in a variety of ways including running and jumping and a variety of other motor skills.

Growth of the nervous system continues at a steady rate during toddlerhood. The brain has reached three quarters of adult size by 3 years of age. Maturation of the brain combined with increasing opportunities to experience more of the world contributes to the child's cognitive growth. The hypothalamus, the temperature regulating center of the brain, becomes more mature; thus the child is less subject to the temperature fluctuations common in infancy. Myelinization of the central nervous systems continues to be rapid until 2 years of age and then slows, reaching completion at puberty.

The corticospinal tract is sufficiently myelinated by 2 years of age to allow the child to perform most movements.[39]

Self-regulatory activities such as bowel-bladder control, eating, sleeping, and physical manipulative skills become important during the toddler period. Neurologic maturation of the bowels and bladder, occurring between 18 and 24 months, allows the toddler to develop an awareness of the sensations related to elimination. Not until neurologic maturation is complete will toilet training be successful or meaningful to the child. By 2½ years daytime bowel and bladder control is usually possible, but nighttime control is more difficult to master.

After the first year of life the growth rate slows and stabilizes, with gains in height and weight occurring slowly. There are also proportional changes in the body contour as the child loses subcutaneous fat. The arms and legs grow longer as ossification and growth in the epiphyseal centers of the long bones occur. The trunk and head grow at a slower rate. Toward the end of the toddler period the protruding abdomen and lumbar lordosis disappear.

Development of motor skills

Both gross and fine motor skills develop rapidly during the toddler period. Maturation of the CNS, along with the repetitive activities of this age group, contributes to improvement in motor skills.

Psychosocial development

Language development

During the toddler stage the child makes rapid strides toward becoming a social being. The ability to communicate increases as the toddler acquires language. The voice structures develop to a point that allows for the formation of words. As the brain structures mature, new behavior patterns are possible and the child begins to build a vocabulary. Two-year-olds commonly have a vocabulary of 200 to 300 words consisting mostly of nouns and verbs, while 3-year-olds have a vocabulary of 900 words consisting of verbs, nouns, pronouns, and adjectives. By 3 years of age approximately 90% of the child's speech should be intelligible.

Cognitive development

The child continues to operate on a sensorimotor level until about 2 years of age (Fig. 16-1). The next stage of cognitive development, the period of preconceptual thought, is a period of preparation for conceptual thought. The child begins to understand simple abstractions, but thinking remains basically concrete and literal. The child begins to associate certain objects as being representative of other objects. This is easily seen

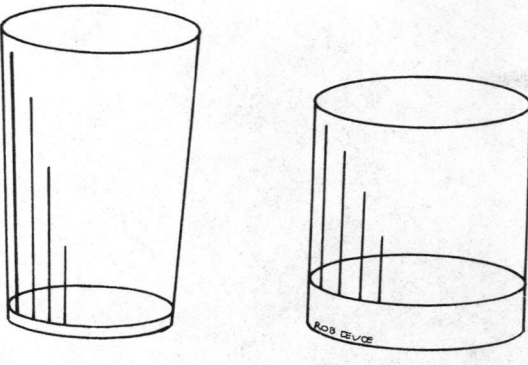

Fig. 16-2. Which is more? Child of 2 or 3 years is likely to choose taller glass on left rather than shorter glass on right, even though glasses hold same volume.

in symbolic play where dolls are given the roles of babies or mothers and where the sandbucket becomes the garbage can as the child plays at being the garbage collector.

The child has no clear conception of quantity but operates on the principle that if it looks like more, it is more. The child of 2 or 3 years is likely to think 100 ml of orange juice in a tall glass is more than 100 ml of juice in a shorter, wider container. The child has not yet mastered the concept of conservation of matter (Fig. 16-2).

The child of this age has not yet formed concepts of time and space. Time is now and space is what is seen at this moment. Children's stories begin with "once upon a time" or "long, long ago" because time and space are felt by the young child, not measured.

Emotional development

Egocentrism remains a major characteristic of early childhood. Toddlers are very much concerned with their own importance, constantly seeking attention, approval, and their own goals. They are only poorly able to take another person's point of view. At this age they exhibit a great deal of testing behavior in their quest for independence. They lack any self-control over exploratory impulses and rely on their parents to help them develop safe and socially acceptable behaviors. They require the attention and approval of parents, as it is one of the main motivational forces in socialization and ego development.

According to Erikson, the developmental crisis of this age level is achieving *autonomy vs. shame and doubt*. Autonomy is achieved as the toddler gains self control over motor abilities and sphincter muscles. It can be seen as the child develops some measure of control over self and learns to make and carry out decisions, to cope with small problems, to wait patiently, and to share.[10]

Rituals in activities performed are at a peak at 2½ to 3 years, especially those associated with feeding and

bedtime. Rituals contribute to developing autonomy because the child learns to master tasks through rituals.

Negativism and dawdling are ways toddlers learn to control their own bodies. They often continue in an activity over parents' objections or say no even as they are doing what they have been asked to do.

If the child fails to develop a positive self-concept and a sense of autonomy, shame and doubt predominate. It is important that parents create an atmosphere in which expectations are reasonable and in which criticism, blame, and punishment are not excessive. The major developmental tasks of the toddler are outlined in the box above.

TASKS OF THE TODDLER

Learning to control socially unacceptable emotional impulses

Learning appropriate sex role distinction

Tolerating separation from the mother

Learning to differentiate self from other people and things

Reaching a stable physiologic state

Becoming enculturated

Nursing assessment and intervention

With the well child the nurse's role is primarily one of assessing and evaluating to determine whether growth and development are proceeding in a normal pattern. The nurse serves as a resource person providing anticipatory guidance and teaching. Intervention can be undertaken when needed to promote and foster the child's developmental potential. Another vital role the nurse plays is serving as a sounding board for parents who have concerns about their child's behaviors or just need to ventilate their feelings.

Special needs of the hospitalized child

If hospitalization is necessary, children of any age should be prepared for the experience by the parents. The nurse in the physician's office or clinic should be sure the parents know how to prepare them. Parents should tell children truthfully about the hospital and why they must go there. Children should not be frightened about the experience, but neither should they be led to expect the experience to be completely pleasant. They should be told about the high beds, bedpans, urinals, bed baths, eating in bed, the attire of nurses and physicians, and the play facilities in a matter-of-fact and reassuring way. If possible, the preparation for hospitalization should be done gradually. Well-written sto-

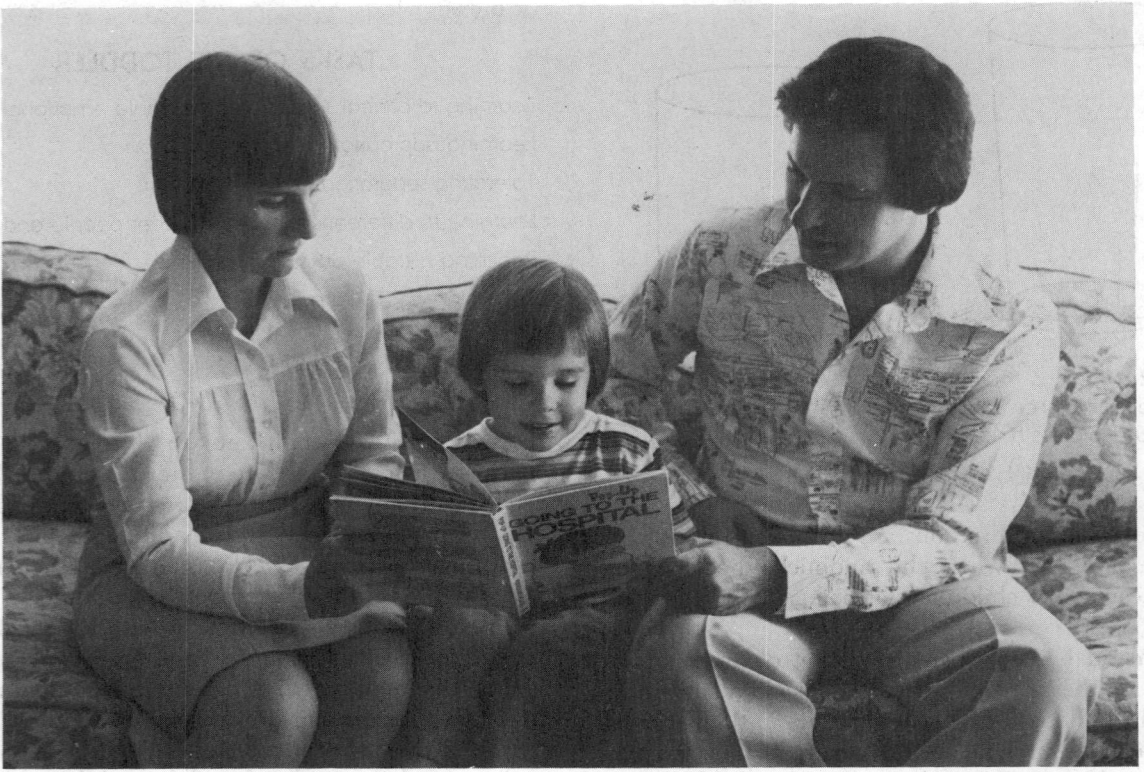

Fig. 16-3. Parents preparing child for hospitalization. Parents can make important contribution to child's hospitalization by proper preparation.

rybooks concerning hospitalization are available in bookstores and may be helpful in introducing the topic (Fig. 16-3). In addition, many children's hospitals have written their own books for patients.

Children, especially those between 2 and 5 years of age, tend to form attachments to inanimate objects such as well-loved toys or blankets. Such an object, whatever it may be, gives the child comfort and security. Even sick children of school age may want to bring some favorite object to the hospital. They should be allowed to do so, and no one should worry if it is old or ragged. The object is a link with home, and the child should be free to take it everywhere, even to treatment rooms and to the operating room.

It is important too for parents to allow children of any age, prior to their departure for the hospital, to help prepare for their return home again. Often children can pack bags with clothes that will be worn upon discharge from the hospital or they may help prepare the room where they will stay while recuperating.

During the toddler stage attachment to the mother is quite strong, and this group experiences the greatest amount of regression due to separation anxiety. The effects of hospitalization and illness can be severe. Health care providers, especially nurses, can make every effort

to make hospitalization as pleasant an experience as possible and to minimize emotional trauma.

Parents need to leave their children. They should be given permission to leave the child and help in separating from him. They should not try to sneak out but should tell the child they are leaving and when they will return. Leaving personal articles with the children helps to assure them that parents will return. The clinging behavior generally subsides after the parents set up a pattern of reappearance and keep promises.

The initial nursing history should include assessment data relative to toilet training, and every effort should be made to continue the routine carried out at home. Potty chairs should be available for the child who is trained.

If the 2- or 3-year-old is still drinking from a bottle, do not attempt to change these habits while the child is in the hospital.

If the procedure will be uncomfortable, a parent or a nurse who is well liked by the child should be present to comfort and firmly hold the child as necessary. Children of any age should be told truthfully what type of sensation they may expect, and it usually is advisable to tell them when they are about to be hurt. Restraining techniques such as "mummying" (use of blanket re-

TABLE 16-4. Recommended daily dietary allowances for children*

Age (yr)	Calories (cal)	Protein (g)	Vitamin A (μg RE†)	Thiamine (mg)	Riboflavin (mg)	Niacin (mg NE‡)	Vitamin C (mg)	Vitamin D (μg)	Calcium (mg)
1-3	1300	23	400	0.7	0.8	9	45	10	800
4-6	1700	30	500	0.9	1.0	11	45	10	800
7-10	2400	34	700	1.2	1.4	16	45	10	800

*From Food and Nutrition Board, National Academy of Sciences—National Research Council: Recommended daily dietary allowances, revised 1979, Washington, D.C.
†RE = Retinal equivalent.
‡NE = Niacin equivalent.

straints) occasionally must be used for the safety of a toddler who is overactive, but usually just talking to the child and holding firmly is all that is needed.

Health concerns

Nutrition

As the growth rate slows, the appetite decreases and the child loses subcutaneous fat. The actual number of calories needed per day decreases from infancy as the child is growing less rapidly. Table 16-4 summarizes the daily dietary requirements for toddlers. Mothers often express concern about this behavior and feel the child is not healthy. Anticipatory guidance can prepare mothers for this change in eating habits and alleviate much of their worry. Toddlers are finicky eaters and are given to food jags. When they are hospitalized, special care should be taken to see that they are served familiar foods. It is most unlikely they will eat unfamiliar foods or foods that do not resemble those served at home. They often dawdle and play with their food.

Injuries

Accidents are the leading cause of death in children from 1 to 14 years of age. Some 15 million children are brought for treatment for accident-related injuries each year. Automobile accidents account for the largest number of deaths. Many smaller children are hit by cars and trucks while playing or crossing streets. The most frequent injuries are fractures and concussions.

Burns are a significant cause of mortality and morbidity in children. Unfortunately, it is often the action of the child that causes the injury. As concerned citizens nurses must push for better education of the public relative to fire prevention. Care of the burned client is discussed in Chapter 70.

Poisoning

The 2-year-old is the most common victim of accidental ingestion of *poisons*. Most often the poison is a drug or household product. These products should be kept in their original containers and locked up or placed on high shelves out of reach of toddlers. Care of the person who has ingested poisons is discussed in Chapter 73.

Illnesses

Respiratory tract infections remain a problem during the toddler years. Otitis media (see Chapter 50) is seen most commonly in young children because their eustachian tubes are short and straight, permitting easier passage of bacteria from the nasopharynx to the middle ear. The use of antibiotics has markedly decreased the incidence of mastoiditis frequently seen in young children in previous decades.

Recognition and treatment of otitis media are extremely important to prevent hearing loss and subsequent emotional and learning difficulties. Unrecognized otitis media results in persistent fluid in the middle ear, which leads to glue-ear syndrome (sequelae of serous otitis media often leading to hearing loss).

Preschool years (3 to 5 years)

The refinement of motor skills occurs during the preschool years and allows the child to do progressively more difficult things and to achieve integrated motor and perceptual control. Physical activity becomes goal directed. The child makes rapid progress toward the perfection of certain skills such as improving the ability to comprehend and communicate, forming simple concepts of social and physical reality, learning how to behave toward persons and things, learning to distinguish right from wrong, and developing a value judgment system (conscience).

Physical growth

Physical growth remains slow and steady; average weight gain is about 2.3 kg (5 lb) per year, while gain in height is about 6.75 to 7.5 cm (2.5 to 3 in.). The gain in height is usually the result of elongation of the legs rather than of the trunk. The gain in height is faster than the weight gain; thus the child changes from a chubby toddler to a thinner, sturdier child. The child is also losing the baby look and maturing into the kind of person he or she is going to be in later life.

The lungs gradually increase in size and volume, and their capacity for oxygenation increases. The respiratory rate decreases to approximately 24 breaths/min. Diaphragmatic respiration predominates until the fifth or sixth year. As the heart continues slowly to increase in size, a gradual reduction in heart rate (pulse) occurs and blood pressure rises slightly.

By 5 years of age the child may begin to lose the deciduous teeth, and the first permanent teeth may erupt. If eruption of permanent teeth does not closely follow shedding of decidious teeth, dental consultation should be sought as alignment of the permanent teeth may be affected. Vision is improving; however, the preschooler remains far-sighted. It is normal for a 5-year-old to have 20/50 or 20/40 vision on Snellen chart testing. It is very important that vision screening be done during the preschool years so that defects such as strabismus and amblyopia can be identified and corrected so that permanent damage can be prevented or minimized.

Nutrition

Preschool children become more selective and independent in their eating habits. The desire to eat varies over the time span, and there is a noticeable decrease in the amount of food eaten between the second and third years. Attempts to force or bribe the child to eat may only create anxieties in child and parents. If the diet during this period is deficient (Table 16-4), supplements may be given. Preschool children usually prefer simple foods that can be handled and often will eat only a few selected foods exclusively between ages 4 and 5. By the time the child starts school, appetite and food selection have increased.

Psychosocial development

A major developmental task of the preschool period is the *emergence* of the *child* as a *social being*. The child now spends more time in association with his peers. The 4-year-old child is imaginative and creative, often talking and playing with imaginary companions. These children are struggling with fact and fantasy and are fond of telling long and elaborate stories, which are mostly imaginary. During this period the child changes from a self-centered being to a person who can relate to others in play and is ready for group experiences such as nursery school, playgroups, and kindergarten (see box, at right).

Another important task of this period is the process of *identification* and gender identity. During the phallic stage children become aware of anatomic differences between the sexes (Fig. 16-1). Development of sexuality comes to the forefront during the oedipal stage. Children become interested in the appearance and function of their bodies. The child first assigns sex on the basis of the appearance of men and women.

Identification is imitation of behavior of the parent of the same sex. The child tries to imitate the role of mother or father. Identification is influenced by the attitudes about sexual, moral, social, and occupational roles and values dominant in the culture.

Erikson's developmental task of *initiative vs. guilt* is dominant during the preschool period. Children who do not develop a sense of initiative, the ability to assure themselves, to plan and control their own activity, are likely to feel a sense of anger or defeatism. If the guilt and anger persist, the child develops a rigid superego.

Cognitive development remains in stage II, *preoperational thought*. The intuitive phase, beginning at age 4, is a period during which children begin to think more completely and elaborate their concepts more. A concept is formed when a word comes to define an area of experience. At this age children become more flexible in use of language; they use the word "because" and make simple associations between ideas. "Centering" is still very characteristic, with the child's attention being centered on one detail of an event to the exclusion of other parts of the event. Children of this age are unable to cope intellectually with problems of time, space, causality, measurement, numbers, quantity, or movement. They think everything is just as it appears.

Language development continues during the preschool years with increasing use of more complex words and sentences. By 5 years of age most children have a vocabulary of approximately 2500 words.

Children of this age sometimes project their own feelings onto their playthings; toys are used as safety valves for aggressive feelings. Parents are sometimes distressed at this behavior and need to understand that it is normal.

In summary, the preschool age is a period of rela-

TASKS OF THE PRESCHOOL CHILD

Achieving integrated motor and perceptual control

Forming concepts of social and physical reality

Emerging as a social being

Identifying sex differences

Learning right from wrong

tive calm with a steady gain in height and weight, refinement of motor skills with increasing control over the body, and development of social relationships with peers. Self-care activities greatly improve as a result of improved physical skills. The human organism is transformed in 5 short years from a helpless infant to a sturdy and complicated being capable of communication, conceptualization, and complex social and motor behavior.

Nursing intervention

As with younger children, it is desirable to have one nurse assigned to the hospitalized child as consistently as possible. Mothers should be encouraged to participate in the child's care, as this indicates to the child that mother approves of hospital routine.

Castration and mutilation fantasies are common to this age group. Preschoolers often feels that they are in the hospital as punishment for something bad that they did. It is important to offer frequent reassurance that the child is not to blame for the illness or hospitalization. The fears commonly expressed before age 5 include abandonment, loss of control over usual routines, pain, and invasion of body orifices.

Play is extremely helpful with this age group. Dolls may be used to demonstrate the external appearance postoperatively. Children of this age enjoy the opportunity to manipulate equipment and will often act out their feelings with toys. Storytelling and puppet play are also useful in teaching preschoolers to express their feelings.

The 5-year-old is just mastering self-care activities and should be encouraged to take care of self-hygiene as much as possible. This sense of accomplishment is threatened when the child must relinquish self-care activities to others.

Health concerns

Upper respiratory tract infections continue to be the most common cause of illness in children between 3 and 5 years of age. Toward the end of the preschool years the child's respiratory tract matures, and infections are localized to a greater degree.

Entrance into nursery school and kindergarten exposes the child to a variety of infections, particularly the common communicable diseases of chickenpox, measles, and mumps. All children should receive early immunization against measles because of its severe complications (see Chapter 19).

Accidents and burns continue to remain a major health concern during the preschool years as the child gains greater mobility and moves into new environments. The preschooler should be taught some very basic rules of safety and what to do should there be an accident on the playground.

Middle childhood

The period between 6 years and the onset of puberty is a phase of gradual growth and development. It is a steady period in both physical and emotional aspects (see box below).

Physical growth

During the first few years of school, the gross motor activities such as running and climbing of the earlier years become increasingly directed to more specialized activities and games requiring particular motor and muscular skills. The child refines skills, especially those dealing with neuromotor coordination; that is, those involving fine coordination of the hands, eyes, and cerebral cortex.

Development of the facial bones continues actively during the school years, particularly with enlargement of the sinuses. The frontal sinuses have usually made their appearance by the seventh year. The face begins to change, taking on a more adult appearance.

The first of the permanent teeth, the first-year molars, most often erupt during the sixth year. With the so-called *six-year molars* in place, the shedding of the deciduous teeth begins, following approximately the same sequence as their acquisition. They are replaced at a rate of about four teeth a year over the next 7 years. The second permanent molars are commonly erupted by the fourteenth year, and the third molars, irregular in occurrence and time of eruption, may not appear until the early twenties.

TASKS OF MIDDLE CHILDHOOD

Acquiring motor and muscular skills for specialized activities and games

Developing independence from family with socialization into peer groups

Developing concepts and systematic reasoning

Learning fundamental skills in reading, writing, and calculating

Developing value systems of self as related to others

Developing self-control

Lymphatic tissues are at the peak of their development during these years and generally exceed the amount of such tissue present in adults.

Visual development should be completed by the sixth or seventh year. The child should have fully developed peripheral vision and be able to discriminate fine differences in shades of colors. A maximum level of acuity, at least 20/30 in each eye by Snellen chart testing, is normal by 7 years of age. The child learns to coordinate eye movements, to see a single image, and to associate incoming visual stimuli with past and present mental images and functions.

The lungs achieve adult maturity, and lung capacity is proportional to body size. The respiratory rate continues to decrease, average respiratory rates being 19 to 20 breaths/min. Cardiac growth continues, and the heart assumes a more vertical position within the thoracic cavity. The increased cardiac function allows the heart to meet the oxygen and circulatory needs of the growing body. The pulse rate continues to decrease (average rate 70 beats/min) as the heartbeat gradually comes under the influence of the vagus nerve.[40] As the left ventricle of the heart develops, the blood pressure increases.

The physical growth rate is slow and steady. There may be considerable variation in height and weight among children, depending on genetic and environmental influences. During the early school years the child gains an average of 3 kg (6 to 7 lb) yearly and increases in height by about 6 cm (2½ in.) yearly.

Nutrition

The nutritional requirements of the schoolchild remain relatively greater than the adult's. Approximately 80 cal/kg body weight daily are required by the young schoolchild. This gradually decreases to 70 cal/kg body weight daily by age 12 years. The caloric needs for a child can be calculated as 1000 calories for the first year and 100 calories for each additional year.[30] The recommended dietary allowances for the school-aged child are presented in Table 16-4.

Psychosocial development

Middle childhood is characterized by three great outward pushes:

1. Socially the child makes a way out of the family environment into a peer group society.

2. Physically the child moves into a world of games and activities requiring neuromuscular skills.

3. Mentally the child is thrust into school and a world of concepts, symbols, logic, and communication.

Influence of school

The school is the one agency in the United States that reaches, by compulsion of law, all the community's children. The objectives of schools are the teaching of certain subject matter, the promotion of health, the development of character, and preparation for citizenship. It may be said that school is the child's business or job and that attitudes about school are very important in later life.

Children begin increasingly to live independently and to look outside the home for goals and standards of behavior. They find new role models, such as their school teachers.

Emergence of peer groups

During the school years there is a tendency for children to form into groups or clubs. This is the child's first experience with a society of his own making. During the early school years these groups are characteristically limited to members of the same sex. Being accepted and being active with the peer group is very important for healthy development. Around the age of 9 or 10 years the chum stage emerges, when the affection shifts from the peer group to a special friend of the same sex and age.

Emotional development

The developmental crisis of the school-aged child is that of industry versus inferiority. *Industry* is achieved as the child successfully learns to problem solve, develops reasonable work habits and attitudes, and masters age-appropriate tasks. Children compare themselves with peers, and if they cannot perform as well as others, they will eventually perceive themselves in a negative manner. If this continues and age-appropriate tasks are not mastered, a sense of inferiority will develop.

Cognitive development

By 6 years of age most children are able to understand the use of abstract concepts, permitting the beginning contact with the subjects of reading, writing, and arithmetic. Academic education is also made possible by the child's progress in the emotional aspects of development.

Intellectual behavior evolves descriptively from activity without thought to thought with less emphasis on activity. Cognitive behavior evolves from doing to doing knowingly. In earlier years when told, "Don't touch the stove" or, "Wash your hands" the child performs the task because of commands to do so. By 6 years of age there is learning of the whys behind these activities.

By 7 years of age the child is in stage III (Fig. 16-1), the period of concrete operations, which is characterized by the ability to solve concrete problems. Systematic reasoning about actual or imagined situations is now possible. Classification, seriation, and multiplication are characteristic operations during this stage. *Classification* involves the placement of objects in groups depending on their attributes such as size, shape, or color. *Seriation* involves the placement of objects in an increasing series relative to characteristics such as height and weight. *Multiplication* involves simultaneous classification and seriation, or the use of two attributes together. During stage III, *reversibility*, the performance of operations or actions with the same problem or situation becomes possible. This allows the child to move into mathematics.

At this age, children recognize that other people see things differently from the way they do. A value system and social interaction are necessary; children must interact socially to grow intellectually because without social life they will never succeed in understanding the viewpoints of others.

Language

During the school years vocabulary is increased and more complex sentences are used. Consensual or syntactic communication is used when cause-and-effect relationships are seen in an objective logical way. Observations are validated by others.

Male-female differences

In latency girls are likely to be a year or two ahead of boys in social and emotional maturity and perhaps in the capacity to use intellectual abilities. Schools in the United States have been accused of fostering this and being female oriented. Looking at school performance, one finds that girls generally are better achievers in the early years of school when language development, reading, and writing are heavily stressed. In the latter years when the concepts of mathematics and science are introduced, boys improve in performance. To what extent these differences are fostered by the socialization process is open to question.

To summarize middle childhood:

1. It is a period of steady growth and steady emotions; the child is developing *self-control*.

2. There is an outward shift, and school and peer groups become very important; the child is developing *increased independence*.

3. It is a time for building a wholesome concept of the self; the child is developing a sense of *self-worth*.

Health and middle childhood

Middle childhood is ordinarily characterized by health and well-being. Many of the problems encountered during the school years are preventable and subject to nursing intervention. Nurses are most likely to have contacts with the well child of this age through the schools, in pediatrician's offices, and in well-child nurse clinics. As with the younger child, assessment of the pattern of growth and development is an important factor. Vision, speech, hearing, and dental problems appear during these years and should be identified as early as possible for correction to be most effective. Screen-

ing programs for such defects should be part of all school health programs and should be included in assessment during routine physical examinations.

Nursing intervention

Hospitalization apparently is not too psychologically traumatic for school children, especially if they have been adequately prepared for it. Unless the child is acutely ill or will be having an operation, the constant attendance of the mother is rarely necessary. However, parents should be urged to visit regularly or if frequent visits are not possible, to keep in regular contact by telephone or letter.

When preparation has been adequate, hospitalization can be an educational and social experience. By middle childhood the child is capable of learning a great deal from contacts with staff and other children. Children of this age are capable of verbalizing their feelings and concerns. These children can be reasoned with, since they are capable of understanding cause-and-effect relationships.

Preoperative teaching and preparation for diagnostic procedures are important. The child of this age is interested in the scientific approach and likes to learn scientific terminology for body parts and medical procedures. Useful guidelines for teaching the school-aged child are available.[36]

If a child of school age is hospitalized or is sick at home for a long period of time (usually over 2 weeks), most boards of education provide visiting teachers. Parents need to be reminded of this service. Continuing with schoolwork not only provides diversion for the child but also assures keeping up with classmates.

The school-aged child may be interested in reading, listening to records, observing and caring for birds or fish, making such objects as model planes or jewelry, painting, or taking part in competitive activities. Playing with others usually is possible even for the bedridden child. Care should be taken that the child does not overexert or become overtired. Educational play activity and play with others are especially important for the child who has a prolonged illness because they assure continued mental and social development.

Health concerns

Respiratory tract disease

Minor respiratory tract diseases spread rapidly among children in the close proximity of classrooms. Many of the respiratory tract illnesses discussed with previous age groups continue to occur frequently during middle childhood. The more mature structures of the respiratory tract are not as prone to communicate infection from one area of the system to another; thus the older child has increased capacity to localize infection. The anatomy of the ear now begins to approach adultlike proportions, resulting in a decline in the incidence of otitis media. Colds occur 3 or 4 times a year.

Communicable diseases

The incidence of many of the communicable diseases has greatly decreased due to immunizations. Public health officials are concerned, however, with the breakdown in immunizations occurring in the United States in recent years. Small epidemics of childhood diseases have occurred in some areas of the United States, and the Public Health Service has launched a massive program to increase the level of immunization. Some states have passed laws barring children who are not immunized from school in order to emphasize the seriousness of the problem. The National League for Nursing (NLN) and its constituent members sponsored immunization clinics in many areas of the United States in 1977.

Streptococcal infections are a major health problem among school-aged children, with the highest incidence occurring between 6 and 12 years of age. Incidence is highest in areas where the weather is temperate and during the winter months. Transmission occurs primarily by direct contact with an infected person. Serious sequelae can result as a response to streptococcal infection; therefore prevention and control of the spread of this infection among children is very important.

Tonsillitis, pharyngitis, scarlet fever, and skin eruptions such as impetigo are the primary forms of streptococcal infections. Streptococcal infection is characterized by an abrupt onset, which may be accompanied by fever, abdominal pain and vomiting, headaches, and chills. With scarlet fever the typical skin rash appears within 12 to 48 hours after the onset of throat and constitutional symptoms.

An accurate diagnosis depends on positive throat culture results. Nurses working in settings with children may carry supplies for collecting throat cultures. Many school systems have developed plans for obtaining cultures from the entire student body when the incidence of streptococcal infections is high. Antibiotic (penicillin) therapy should be instituted within 7 days of onset to prevent deleterious sequelae. In order to effectively prevent rheumatic and renal sequelae the antibiotic must be administered for at least 10 days.

For a detailed discussion of rheumatic fever and renal sequelae the reader is referred to a pediatric text on communicable disease.

Skin and skeletal injuries

As the child becomes increasingly mobile, active, and more daring and is exposed to greater danger, injuries to the skin and skeletal system increase. Broken bones, dislocated joints, and muscle and ligamentous injuries are prevalent. The nature of the injury should be carefully assessed, and measures should be taken to prevent bleeding, promote comfort, and protect the injured area from further insult during efforts to move or reposition. The child should receive treatment from a specialist in skeletal trauma care.

Adolescence

Following World War II the American public became increasingly conscious of adolescents. It was during this period that the word "teenager" was coined and became popular. The adolescent, who is no longer a child but not yet adequately prepared for the adult world, is searching for emotional and social maturity on his own terms. Adolescents have acquired specific identity as a population in the United States. Adolescence varies depending on the culture. In the United States the length of this period has extended even more than formerly. Adolescence is seen in most countries in which the level of affluence permits a prolongation of dependent behavior beyond puberty.

The U.S. Bureau of the Census estimates for 1972 show 42 million people between the ages of 10 and 19 who can be labeled adolescents. If present trends continue, it is projected that by the year 2000 the number of adolescents in the United States will reach 54 million.[49]

It may be said that adolescence begins in biology and ends in culture. Many people have proposed various definitions for the adolescent. One nurse-author comments that a friend of hers defines an adolescent as "someone who doesn't have his act together yet."[12] In many ways this is an appropriate definition.

Adolescence refers to a specific stage or period in the life cycle. It is the outgrowth of childhood and the prelude to adulthood. It consists of the psychologic, social, and cognitive maturational processes initiated by puberty. Puberty may be defined as the biologic stage of sexual development at which one is able to bear or beget children.

Adolescence is a developmental phenomenon unique to the higher primates. Our nature as interdependent social animals, with unique adaptations of culture and society, has its basis in a specifically human pattern of biologic maturation. The delay in attainment of full growth and sexual maturity in humankind would appear to be essential to our longer and richer development, and on this basis it has been suggested that adolescence is an important evolutionary trait.

Physical growth

The most important concept to remember when dealing with the adolescent is *individuality of growth*.

Biologic changes

Puberty refers to maturational, hormonal, and growth processes occurring within the body. Sexual maturation becomes evident in the first phase of adolescence. Puberty is initiated by the liberation of hormonal secretions in response to hypothalamic stimuli. The pituitary gland (master gland) sends out messages to certain parts of the body causing activation of TSH, ACTH, gonadotropic, and growth hormones. These in turn stimulate other endocrine glands activating their own growth-related hormones. Fig. 16-4 illustrates the hormonal pathways believed to be involved at adolescence.

The sequence of events occurring at adolescence has been well documented by the work of Tanner and others (see box, p. 220). All humans seem to follow this sequence of development of breasts, genitalia, and pubic hair. The age at which these physical changes occur varies by sex. By comparing the ages of development one notes that physical changes in adolescent girls precede those of boys (Fig. 16-5). Both are considered reproductively mature, however, at almost the same age.

Changes in body dimensions

Virtually all parts of the skeletal and muscular structures take part in the growth spurt. The head, hands, and feet achieve adult form earliest; this is why one often thinks junior high school basketball players are all hands and feet. The arms and legs achieve adult form next. Adult trunk length is achieved last but accounts for the greatest proportion of the increase in height; adolescent boys often outgrow the coat of a suit while the pants still fit.

Ossification of bones

During adolescence a great deal of the cartilage in the body calcifies. This process is speeded up during the growth spurt and is completed more rapidly by girls.

By 17 years of age an average girl's bones are mature in size and ossification. Boys do not complete bone growth until late adolescence or early adulthood.

Differential development of muscle and fat

Increased muscular development occurs in both sexes. The overall gain, however, is greater for boys and remains so during the adult years.

During adolescence there is an overall decrease in the *rate* of development of fat. In girls this decrease in the rate is not so great as to eliminate a modest gain in fat. In boys the rate of decline is so great that it produces an actual, though temporary, loss of fat in the months preceding and following the point of peak velocity in height.

Changes in strength and exercise tolerance

The increase in strength and exercise tolerance is greater for boys than for girls. Relative to size, boys develop larger hearts and lungs, an increase in systolic blood pressure, a greater capacity for carrying oxygen in the blood, a decreased heart rate at rest, and a greater power for neutralizing the chemical products of muscular exercise such as lactic acid, which manifests itself in fatigue. Since women have had the opportunity to participate in sports activities we have begun to question the physiologic basis for greater strength and exercise tolerance of males. Females may have equal potential for the development of increased strength and exercise tolerance, given the opportunity to participate equally in sports and exercise programs. Many of the outstanding female athletes appear to have a capacity equal to that of their male counterparts.

Basal metabolic rate

The basal metabolic rate (BMR) declines during adolescence. This decline is less in boys, probably due

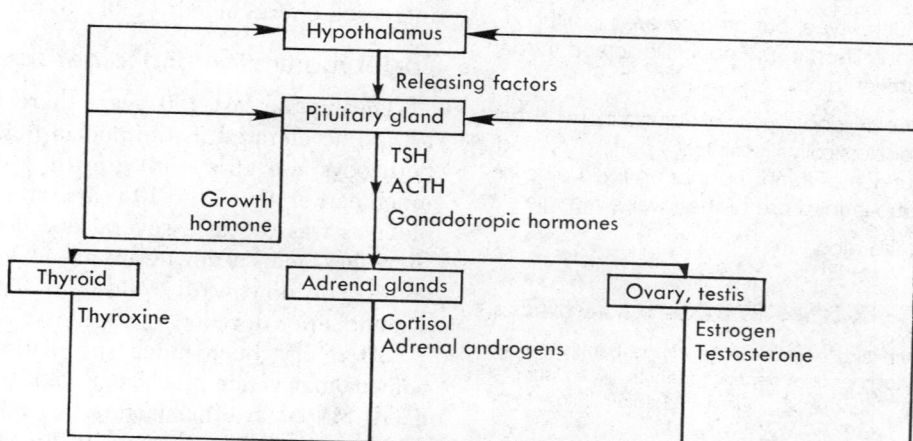

Fig. 16-4. Endocrine control at adolescence. Activating hormones from pituitary gland stimulate other endocrine glands, activating their own growth-related hormones. These hormones in turn provide for orderly and progressive physical and psychologic changes of adolescence.

PUBERTAL STAGES ACCORDING TO TANNER

Boys: genital development

Stage 1 Preadolescent: testes, scrotum, and penis are about the same size and proportion as in early childhood.

Stage 2 Scrotum and testes are enlarged. Skin of scrotum reddened and changed in texture. Little or no enlargement of penis is present at this stage.

Stage 3 Penis is slightly enlarged, which occurs at first mainly in length. Testes and scrotum are further enlarged.

Stage 4 Increased size of penis with growth in breadth and development of glands is present. Testes and scrotum larger; scrotal skin darker than in earlier stages.

Stage 5 Genital adult in size and shape.

Girls: breast development

Stage 1 Preadolescent: elevation of papilla only.

Stage 2 Breast bud stage. Elevation of breast and papilla as small mound. Enlargement of areola diameter.

Stage 3 Further enlargement and elevation of breast and areola with no separation of their contours.

Stage 4 Projection of areola and papilla to form a secondary mound above the level of the breast.

Stage 5 Mature stage: projection of papilla only, due to recession of the areola to the general contour of the breast.

Both sexes: pubic hair

Stage 1 Preadolescent: vellus over the pubes is not further developed than that over the abdominal wall (i.e., no pubic hair).

Stage 2 Sparse growth of long, slightly pigmented downy hair, straight or curled, chiefly at the base of the penis or along labia.

Stage 3 Considerably darker, coarser, and more curled. The hair spreads sparsely over the junction of the pubes.

Stage 4 Hair now adult in type, but area covered is still considerably smaller than in the adult. No spread to the medial surface of thighs.

Stage 5 Adult in quantity and type with distribution of the horizontal (or classically "feminine") pattern. Spread to medial surface of thighs but not up linea alba or elsewhere above the base of the inverse triangle.

Stage 6 Spread up linea alba.

From Tanner, J.M.: Growth and endocrinology of the adolescent. In Gardner, L.I., editor: Endocrine and genetic diseases of childhood, Philadelphia, 1969, W.B. Saunders Co. Cited in Pediatr. Clin. North Am. **20**:4, 1973.

to greater muscular development, which requires greater oxygen consumption, and because of hormonal differences.

Cardiorespiratory changes

Growth of the heart continues until age 17 or 18 when it reaches full adult size. The pulse rate continues to slow; mean pulse rate during adolescence is 82. The mean blood pressure during adolescence is 120/65 mm Hg.

The lungs reach adult weight by 17 years, and vital capacity of the lungs increases rapidly. The respiratory rate continues to decline with increased efficiency of the lungs; the respiratory rate averages 17 to 20 breaths/min in early adolescence and reaches adult levels of 15 to 20/min between 15 and 19 years.[21]

Types of physical growth

The four chief types of physical growth are as follows:
1. *Lymphoid:* reaches peak between 10 and 12 years. Gradually declines to steady point by 20 years.
2. *Brain and head:* reaches peak at 6 years with small gradual increase up to 20 years.
3. *General:* increases to 6 years then levels off until 12 years. Increases steadily until 20 years, then reaches steady point.
4. *Reproductive:* gradual increase until 11 to 12 years, then rises rapidly until age 20 years.

Nutrition

Nutritional needs are greatly accelerated during this period of rapid growth. The need for increased calories is greater than for any period of life except for during pregnancy and lactation. The increased need for protein, calcium, and iron is especially important for building of bones and muscles. There is increased need for calories, especially carbohydrates, to provide fuel for the increased energy needs (Table 16-5).

Earlier maturation and larger size

During the last 100 years there has been a trend toward accelerated maturation in height and weight in both boys and girls. Full growth is now achieved at a much earlier age: 18 to 19 years rather than 25 years or older as was the case several decades ago. Since 1850 there has been a downward trend in the age of menarche. This downward trend occurs at the rate of about 4 months per decade.

There has been much speculation that these phenomena may create psychologic and social problems. One needs to look at other factors that influence this downward trend. When the age of menarche is compared across generations reared under nearly identical conditions, no dramatic continuing downward trend in menarcheal age is found. In the United States it appears

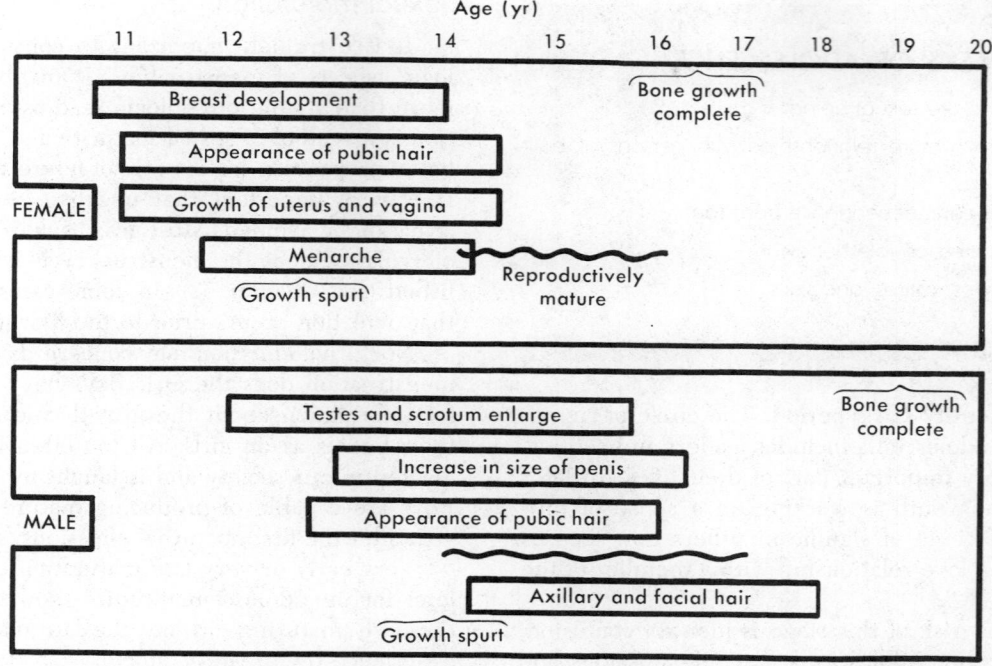

Fig. 16-5. Physical changes of adolescence by age and sex.

TABLE 16-5. Recommended daily dietary allowances for adolescents*

	Age (yr)	Calories (cal)	Protein (g)	Vitamin A (µg RE†)	Thiamine (mg)	Riboflavin (mg)	Niacin (mg NE‡)	Vitamin C (mg)	Vitamin D (µg)	Calcium (mg)	Iron (mg)
Male ♂	11-14	2700 (range: 2000-3700)	45	1000	1.4	1.6	18	50	10	1200	10
	15-18	2800 (range: 2100-3900)	56	1000	1.4	1.7	18	60	10	1200	18
Female ♀	11-14	2200 (range: 1500-3000)	46	800	1.1	1.3	15	50	10	1200	18
	15-18	2100 (range: 1200-3000)	46	800	1.1	1.3	14	60	10	1200	18

*From Food and Nutrition Board, National Academy of Sciences—National Research Council: Recommended daily dietary allowances, revised 1979, Washington, D.C.
†RE = Retinal equivalent.
‡NE = Niacin equivalent.

that there has been a tapering off of this downward trend in the last 20 years; that is, it has reached a plateau.

Apparently nutrition plays an important part in determining when menarche occurs. During and following World War II when many countries experienced periods of nutritional deprivation, a number of European countries reported that the age of menarche was significantly retarded. Contrary to myth, there is no evidence to support the direct influence of climate on maturational rate; however, maturational age may be related to genetic factors that vary from one individual or group to another.

Psychosocial development

Ego identity

The central problem in adolescence is Erikson's *ego identity,* or the development of one's identity as a person. This requires a perception of the self as *separate* from others, hence the breaking away from the family (see box, p. 222). Ego identity is a feeling of wholeness and of self-consistency. Erickson theorizes that the youth culture has developed in technologic societies as an attempt to establish identity formation. Dedication to the adolescent culture provides a means of moving into and

TASKS OF ADOLESCENCE

Emerging as a mature sexual being

Developing more mature relationships with persons of both sexes

Achieving emotional independence from family

Achieving socially responsible behavior

Redefining attitudes, values, and skills

through the identity crisis period. The circle of significant others for adolescents includes leaders and cliques, which are a very important part of their lives. In later adolescence the youth is working on a sense of intimacy, and the circle of significant others now focuses on developing a love relationship with a member of the opposite sex.

The primary risk of this stage is identity confusion, which occurs when adolescents feel self-conscious and have doubts about themselves as human beings and their roles in life. When identity confusion is great, delinquent behavior or borderline psychotic episodes may occur.

In a sense the identity crisis involves a restaging of each of the previous stages of development. The extent to which the earlier tasks were successfully resolved influences the adolescent's success in finding identity.

Accelerated outward shift

With the onset of adolescence there is an accelerated shift from dependence on the family to dependence on the peer group as a major source of security and status.

Many authorities have described the adolescent group as a marginal group with the characteristic of being uncertain in itself. As a marginal group there is much emphasis on conformity. Adolescents have highly idealized norms for physical appearance and skills associated with male and female roles. These roles conform largely to culturally determined stereotypes of males and females.

Intellectual and cognitive development

According to Piaget the *formal operation stage* begins at around 12 years of age. At this stage thought proceeds from combination of possibility, hypothesis, and deductive reasoning. By this age the person can deal with problems not related to real or current situations. Purely abstract and verbal problems can be solved without the presence of actual referents.

There are also quantitative gains. The adolescent is capable of accomplishing more easily, more quickly, and more efficiently intellectual tasks that as a child or preadolescent were accomplished only slowly.

Sexual maturation

It is extremely important to consider the psychologic aspects of menstruation. It involves a great deal more than simple physiologic readjustment. Menstruation is a symbol of sexual maturity and for some a symbol of preparation for the role of future wife and mother. It is very important that negative reactions to menstruation be avoided. Most girls usually become capable of ovulating once the menstrual cycle is regularly established (see Chapter 63). In some cases it is suspected that ovulation occurs prior to the first menstrual flow.

Nocturnal emission may concern the boy as much as menstruation does the girl. Boys have as great a need for information about the growth and development of their bodies as do girls. All too often this may be neglected in our society and is taught by the peer group. Boys are capable of producing mature sperm about a year after the first nocturnal emissions (see Chapter 63).

Very early or very late maturation can create problems for the adolescent. Studies show that it is usually the early maturing girl and the late maturing boy who experience the greatest difficulty.

Body image changes

Adolescence is a time of change in body image (see Chapter 28). Rapid growth in height, weight, and sexual maturation demands that the adolescent deal with a changing body image. Adolescents are very much aware of and concerned about their changing bodies. One way they integrate this change in body image is by spending a long time in front of mirrors, in personal hygiene, and in grooming and dressing.

Adolescents are very sensitive and are often upset by their clumsy movements, acne, and early signs of sexual development. They need the support of the adults around them, especially their parents. They need help in accepting the positive and negative aspects of their bodies so that they can develop a healthy body image.

Influence of family, society, and culture on adolescents

The psychosocial implications of adolescence are greatly influenced by the culture in which one lives. The culture determines whether the period of adolescence is long or short, whether the social demands represent an abrupt change or only a gradual transition from earlier stages of development. In many of the more traditional cultures where people are still taught by apprenticeship, adolescence simply represents a gradual change with an increase in responsibilities and work expectations. The culture may also influence whether these changes become a source of pride or a source of anxiety and confusion. Many cultures practice puberty rites or rites of passage to adulthood. The Bar and Bas Mitzvah ceremonies, graduation from high school, and the Debutante Ball may be viewed as rites of passage.

In the United States the difference between a child

and an adult is emphasized sharply by social and legal institutions. The Twenty-sixth Amendment gives 18-year-olds the right to vote, and many states have redefined the beginning of adulthood as 18 years of age.

The change from one mode of interpersonal relationship to another creates discontinuity in the growth process. Attitudes, values, and skills learned as a child must be redefined as an adult. For example, sexual taboos must be unlearned, and the way one relates to parents of the opposite sex is changed.

In Western society the major changes that occur during adolescence are (1) responsible versus nonresponsible status role, (2) dominance versus submission, and (3) contrasted sexual role.

In terms of the influence of the modern family and society on adolescence, the greater the rate of social change the larger the generational gap. In the developed countries the rate of social change in the past 25 years has been greater than at any other period in history. In the previous generation the extended family and neighborhood ties were very prevalent and important. Geographic mobility was limited. Today families are quite mobile, with one in three moving every 5 years. Nuclear families and single-parent families are more common. Families of the adolescent's peers are unlikely to know one another, much less be friends. Parents are less likely to be united in rules for the conduct of adolescents.

Health and adolescence

It was not until the 1950s that the special health needs of adolescents gained recognition. Dr. Rosewell Gallagher of Boston called attention in his writings to the medical problems peculiar to adolescents. He advocated special support and companionship for adolescents needing health care. In response to his suggestions several health agencies opened adolescent outpatient clinics centered around diseases prevalent in this age group. These clinics met with much success.

Before the late 1950s adolescence had been viewed as a relatively healthy period with few true "medical" illnesses or diseases. Between 1965 and 1975 the existing health facilities were not prepared to deal with the health needs of adolescents, either in number or scope. Few adolescents receive adequate or appropriate health care, yet every adolescent deserves the best possible health care.

Nursing assessment and intervention

The role of the nurse varies and includes assessment of normal growth and development with appropriate intervention when needed, counseling and teaching in areas such as nutrition, health habits, sexuality, and family planning, and caring for the pregnant adolescent or the hospitalized adolescent. Adolescent clients must be accepted and understood as individuals and allowed as much independence as they can handle. Although some limits must be imposed due to hospitalization, whenever possible choices should be allowed. It is most important to be alert to adolescent patients' concerns about their bodies and to give thorough explanations about procedures. A working knowledge of the theories of cognitive development enables nurses to plan for teaching that is age appropriate.

The teenager's relative maturity must be acknowledged by nurses. The adolescent is likely to be flattered by being talked to as an adult and usually responds well. Teenagers are usually interested in their health problems even though they may appear very blasé and even disinterested. Unless nurses make a deliberate effort, this kind of attitude may cause nurses to be negligent about exploring the true reaction of adolescent patients to their condition and even about explaining procedures. Actually, the teenager usually is eager for health teaching and is likely to accept it well and often enjoys discussions of a scientific nature.

Health concerns during adolescence

Acne

Acne is the most common skin disease of adolescence, and almost every adolescent experiences some skin eruption. A very common, minor ailment, it is of great significance to the adolescent who has it. Acne can affect popularity, decrease self-confidence, and keep the individual from activities that might bring friends and success. Acne is thought to be associated with an increased androgen level. It is important for health care professionals to remember that no matter how insignificant the acne appears, it is a major concern to the adolescent (see Chapter 71 for a further discussion of acne).

Fatigue

Adolescents use their energy for activity and growth. Activity includes daily work and play. When energy is used rapidly for growth, as occurs during adolescence, there is less energy for activity and the adolescent shows signs of fatigue. The nurse can help the adolescent make changes in the daily schedule to allow for more rest. The adolescent should be reassured that the fatigue is normal and does not indicate that one is in poor health.

Faulty nutrition

Much has been written about the poor eating habits of the adolescent population. Studies show that many adolescents have adequate knowledge of what foods are good for them but are often too busy to eat or they eat on the run and rely on the foods available. Often the most readily available foods are obtained from vending machines. There is a need for concerned citizens and health professionals to encourage vending companies to make good, healthful foods available instead of junk foods.

Both consistent overeating (obesity) and chronic loss of appetite (anorexia nervosa) may result from emotional problems during the adolescent years. These behaviors may be conditioned by the culture in which one is reared.

Obesity (overnourishment)

Obesity is common among adolescents who live in societies where food availability is not severely limited by costs or scarcity. Obesity is defined as an excess of body fat. The male with 20% to 25% excess body fat and the female with 25% to 30% excess body fat are classified as obese.[2]

Obesity prevalence rates range from 11% to 30% in high school populations according to several recent studies. It is estimated that between 80% to 90% of obese children become obese adults.

Obesity is multifactorial in etiology. Factors contributing to obesity operate in varying degrees and combinations. Some factors that have been identified include:

1. Constitutional factors such as genetic and structural makeup
2. Cultural factors such as reactions to food and being fat
3. Psychologic factors such as the values of food and obesity to the person
4. Activity level of the individual

The earlier one can identify the obese state and institute treatment, the better the hope for a rational program of dietary control. Adolescent obesity is best managed with a combination of moderate diet and exercise. Rigid restrictions of food or crash diets should be discouraged because the rapid growth process at this time requires a high caloric intake and rigid dietary restrictions could interfere with growth.

Motivation, which is difficult to achieve, may be provided with group counseling and group activities with other overweight adolescents. Cooperation and understanding from the parents is essential. A family history of obesity suggests that eating habits may be firmly entrenched, and weight loss will be much more difficult.

Undernutrition may be due to a rapidly increasing basal metabolism rate. These children may not be eating enough to meet all the body's needs during this period of rapid growth. The underweight adolescent may need to slow down and get more rest. Mammer and Eddy found that approximately 20% of teenagers are underweight.[2]

Orthopedic problems

While orthopedic problems may show up during the school years, many tend to surface during adolescence.

Abnormal curvatures of spine. Kyphosis, lordosis, and scoliosis are the most commonly encountered disorders of the spine. *Kyphosis*, a fixed flexion deformity, most often occurs in the thoracic and upper lumbar parts of the spine. Adolescent kyphosis is a self-limiting process and often goes undiagnosed, with the child being accused of having "poor posture" or "round shoulders." Should the curvature progress, moderate back pain will be felt. Treatment is usually conservative and includes spine-stretching exercises and sleeping without a pillow and with a board under the mattress. In severe cases the Milwaukee brace may be modified to treat kyphosis. In rare cases spinal fusion may be necessary.

Lordosis, a fixed extension deformity, often forms to compensate for other abnormalities. It is often present with kyphosis. Treatment is generally conservative.

Structural scoliosis is caused by changes in the vertebral bodies. *Idiopathic scoliosis*, which accounts for 80% of scoliosis, is a hereditary condition occurring five to six times more often in girls. It is most commonly seen between the ages of 8 and 15 years, and most often a right thoracic curve occurs.

Treatment must be instituted to prevent progression of mild scoliosis and to stabilize or correct the more severe curvature. Without treatment pulmonary function may be impaired and back pain may be a problem in later life. The older the age at which the curvature begins and the milder the curvature at initial diagnosis and treatment, the better the prognosis.

Conservative treatment with the Milwaukee brace and exercise is the preferred treatment. Surgical intervention is required when the deformity is progressive and does not respond to conservative measures. The aim of surgery is to correct the curvature and stabilize that area of the spine. A variety of surgical procedures including Harrington's rod or other instrumentation, spinal fusion, and immobilization in a body cast for several months may be employed.

The nursing care of these patients is similar in many cases to the care of adult patients having spinal fusions (see Chapter 42). The psychosocial implications of scoliosis are most important. The alteration in body image caused by the disease and by most modes of treatment creates anxiety and concern for most adolescents. Treatment may also impose restrictions on the activities of adolescents, and they may feel left out. It is important to help the adolescent devise ways to remain active with his peer group. Kalafitch[22] presents an excellent case history dealing with the management of an adolescent hospitalized with scoliosis.

Slipped femoral epiphysis. In *slipped femoral epiphysis* a weakness of the epiphyseal plate allows the epiphysis to slip off the femoral neck in reaction to force. It is more common in boys than in girls and occurs between the ages of 10 and 16 years. Treatment consists of internal fixation with an epiphyseal plate. Without treatment a permanent limp and degenerative hip disease in adulthood may result.

Athletic injuries. A variety of orthopedic injuries may result from athletic injuries caused by either internal or external forces. Many of these injuries are preventable by proper conditioning and training of athletes, and many occur during unsupervised sports activities. In 1973 adolescents sustained 12,591 football-related injuries.[12] It is important to teach young people the principles of first aid to be employed in case of injuries. Another source of sport-related injuries is bicycle accidents, which numbered 17,411 in 1973.[12] Good preventive care demands that young people be taught the basics of bicycle safety and maintenance of the bicycle, as many accidents are the results of defective brakes or other mechanical failures.

Accidents

Between the ages of 15 to 24 years, accidents are the leading cause of death, with motor vehicles being the major problem. In 1975, 24,121 motor vehicle accidents involving persons 15 to 24 years old were reported.[51] Poor coordination, carelessness, alcohol, and drug abuse as well as increased risk-taking contribute to the high rate of accidents among adolescents. In addition to these factors, there is also concern that many automobile accidents may be the result of suicide attempts. Many adolescents injured in automobile accidents must be hospitalized for extended periods of time due to orthopedic injuries (see Chapter 42 for discussion of nursing care). If a friend or relative is killed in the accident, the nursing staff are often the ones who must help the adolescent deal with grief and guilt. It is important to allow the adolescent to express feelings about loss and death and to assist the individual to vent feelings.

Earlier sexual activity

Research data indicates that more adolescents are sexually active, and many are sexually active at an earlier age than was the case in the past.[17] A recent study showed that 50% of teenagers in metropolitan areas are sexually active before marriage.[55] While adolescents may become sexually active for a variety of reasons, they may also feel guilty about having sex. The decision about sexual activity is often one of the most difficult decisions an adolescent has to make. Adolescents need an understanding person with whom they can discuss their feelings and concerns. The health care provider can be that person if he or she creates the appropriate environment.

Frequently adults, even health care providers, have difficulty understanding why adolescents do not use contraceptives. The reasons include lack of availability and acceptability, ignorance, fear, and finally the inability of many females to see themselves as capable of reproduction. Even with teens who do have access to contraceptives, insufficient motivation often leads to noncompliance.

Pregnancy

If pregnancy occurs before a girl completes her own physical growth, she is at increased risk both biologically and emotionally. According to recent studies pregnant adolescents have higher rates for toxemia, prolonged labor, pelvic disproportion, and cesarean section. Mortality is much higher for infants born to very young mothers.[46]

The pregnant adolescent requires more intensive maternity care than older women. While she is still dealing with the crisis of adolescence, she is thrust into another crisis situation, that of pregnancy. The pregnant teenager has all the needs and wants of any adolescent. At a time when she is trying to deal with her recent growth and body image change, pregnancy creates yet another disturbance in the self-concept. At a time when peer association is at a peak, the pregnant teenager is often isolated from her peers by school regulations or social sanctions. As mentioned earlier, nutrition is often less than ideal among adolescents, and this is of special concern during pregnancy because the girl's own physical growth is incomplete. Her nutritional needs may suffer if nutritional intake is not sufficient to meet both her needs and those of the fetus.

Progressing through her pregnancy the adolescent will experience all the physical and emotional changes that the adult pregnant woman experiences. The teenager most often has less knowledge and understanding about these changes, and the need for prenatal teaching is especially important.

To prevent future unwanted pregnancies it is important that the pregnant adolescent have adequate information regarding contraception. Acceptable family planning services should be available to and used by the sexually active teenager. For more detailed information on contraceptive devices the reader is referred to Chapter 64.

Sexually transmitted diseases

The incidence of sexually transmitted diseases (STD) among the adolescent population in the last decade has been frightening. Both gonorrhea and syphilis have reached epidemic proportions. It is estimated that one adolescent is infected with gonorrhea or syphilis every minute in the United States; over one-half million infections are reported yearly.[39]

Teenagers who suspect that they have contracted a sexually transmitted disease should be encouraged to seek medical help as soon as possible. Most cities have free STD clinics, and emergency departments in general hospitals screen for STD. Adolescents need to understand that in many states they do not need parental consent to be treated, and that information about their disease will be kept confidential and their parents will not be informed by those treating them. See Chapter 65 for further information about STD.

Drug abuse

Since the late 1960s there has been a growing concern about drug abuse among adolescents. While there is some evidence to indicate a decrease in the use of hard drugs by older adolescents, there is evidence to indicate that adolescents are experimenting with some form of drugs at earlier ages than was true in the past decade. Like many other problems among teenagers the explanations for the use of drugs are varied and include experimentation, escapism, rebellion, and pursuit of new meanings for human existence.

There is a high rate of recidivism (recurrence of the problem), and rehabilitation for drug addicts is expensive. Rehabilitative and preventive programs developed with the cooperation of young people appear to be the most promising avenue for combating drug abuse.

According to a national survey conducted among 14,000 American seventh through twelfth graders in 1975, most adolescents had some experience with alcoholic beverages; one in three adolescents can be classified as an infrequent or light drinker, but one of four is a moderately heavy or heavy drinker.[37] It appears that the young are switching from drugs to alcohol, which is more readily available and has less severe legal penalties for illegal use. Alcohol problems among teenagers have resulted in development of many Alcoholics Anonymous groups for teenagers in this country.

While many adults in the United States struggle to quit smoking, adolescents increasingly are taking up the habit. One out of four teenagers smokes. A 1972 survey revealed that boys were less likely to smoke in 1972 than in 1970, but girls were taking up the habit at a much more rapid rate.[32]

Mental health

There appears to be an increase in mental health disorders among adolescents. Many of the complaints of clients attending adolescent clinics have an emotional cause.[49]

Probably the most dramatic indicator of emotional instability is the increasing incidence of suicide. The adolescent suicide rate doubled in the last decade and tripled in the past 20 years, while the nation's overall suicide rate remained stable.[31] Suicide is the third leading cause of death in older adolescents.

To combat the high morbidity and mortality, there is a need for preventive mental health programs that include early identification and surveillance of those most likely to be susceptible to stresses within the environment. Patient assessment should include questions about the adolescent's emotional state. Other clues are a fam-

ily history of mental illness, alcoholism, or drug abuse. Difficulty with interpersonal relationships and a preference for solitary pursuits are also clues that the adolescent may need special help.

Young adulthood

The young adult years, extending from approximately 20 to 45, is a complex period of life, a time in which the achievement of personal goals is the primary focus. The young adult years are referred to as the expansion years in which energies are directed toward career fulfillment, social involvement, and the initiation and maintenance of a family.[47]

Physical development

Full growth and development are completed by the mid-twenties, and most body systems are functioning at maximum levels. Of those changes that occur in adulthood, some begin early and others not until later in middle age; some are abrupt and some are gradual.

Psychosocial development

Adulthood is often equated with maturity and is characterized by a sense of responsibility, maintenance of appropriate impulse control, ability to plan and implement realistic goals, and the capacity to enter into intimate relationships.

The nurse needs to understand that everyone does not arrive at young adulthood with the same level of maturity. Emotional maturity varies from person to person, as do intellectual ability and physical characteristics. In addition, an adult who appears reasonably mature under usual circumstances may, when under stress, exhibit certain immature behavior. For example, a person may become more demanding or very critical or lose his temper.

In Erikson's *eight ages of man*, the first adult stage is characterized by *intimacy vs. isolation* (Fig. 16-6). Intimacy is seen as sharing the self to form a commitment to an intense lasting relationship with another person, a cause, or a creative effort without fearing the loss of identity. Intimacy requires responsibility, impulse control, the ability to plan, and also the ability to trust. The inability to develop some form of intimacy draws the person into increasing feelings of isolation, alienation, and self-absorption.

The successful resolution of this phase of the life cycle is dependent on a positive self-concept. How per-

Age	FREUD (PSYCHOSEXUAL)	ERIKSON (PSYCHOSOCIAL)	PIAGET (COGNITIVE)
Young adulthood	Young adulthood	Intimacy vs isolation: significant objects— persons, causes	STAGE IV continued formal operations: development beyond this stage has not been studied
Adulthood	Adulthood	Generativity vs stagnation: Significant persons— spouse, grandchildren, friends	
Maturity	Maturity	Integrity vs disgust, despair: significant persons— spouse, family members, friends	

Fig. 16-6. Summary of psychosocial development in later life.

sons feel about themselves affects relationships as well as the choices made during this period. A person who feels adequate and competent in setting and achieving goals tends to experience more positive outcomes than one whose self-concept is that of inadequacy and incompetency. These negative feelings tend to foster withdrawal and the inability to mobilize resources for positive gains. When caring for the young adult it is therefore important to assess the individual's self-perception. These data not only provide information as to motivation potential but are a basis for nursing intervention to help increase the individual's self-esteem.

Body image, an important aspect of self-concept, is a mental picture of the body's appearance as well as the attitudes, emotions, and personality of the individual. At a period of life when acceptance by others is most important, and with society's emphasis on youth, beauty, and physical fitness, any alteration in body function or structure poses a threat to a positive body image. Adaptation to these alterations depends on the nature and meaning of the threat, coping mechanisms, and available support systems.

Therefore nursing intervention to help someone deal with a threat to or change of body image involves (1) careful assessment of the individual's perception of the condition, (2) assistance in helping the individual maintain a realistic perception of the threat in relation to the person's total self-image, (3) assistance in identifying useful coping mechanisms, and (4) identification of support systems (see Chapter 28).

Intellectual development

Cross-sectional studies have shown that the highest overall intelligence test performance occurs at some time between the late teens and late twenties. People in their thirties, forties, and fifties tend to score somewhat lower. Longitudinal evidence has shown that general intelligence either remains the same or increases slightly during the adult years.[48] Certain factors may influence intellectual development and performance, such as education and other sociocultural factors.

Sexuality in young adulthood

Sexuality is an integral part of self-concept. Competence in the area of one's sexuality is of prime importance during the adult years. Sexuality may be defined as a "deep pervasive aspect of the total person, the sum total of one's feelings and behavior as a male or female, the expression of which goes beyond genital response."[31] Young adulthood is normally the time when the body's sexual response is powerful and there is a need to find adequate and satisfactory expression. It is known that a man reaches his peak sexual capacity at about 18 years of age. Women, however, reach their peak of sexual capacity in their early thirties.

If the expression of sexual feelings is restricted, perhaps because of illness or injury, causing a felt or imagined change in body image, sexual concerns may become paramount. Nurses frequently are asked by young adults for assistance with marital or sexual concerns. Unless the nurse is secure in his or her own sexual identity and has had adequate preparation to deal with such matters, clients should be referred to appropriate persons who can deal with these concerns (see Chapters 63 and 64).

Developmental tasks

Other psychologic and social aspects of the young adult's development can be gleaned from the developmental tasks common to this period (see box, p. 228).

TASKS OF YOUNG ADULTHOOD

Developing a sense of social responsibility

Choosing a vocation

Choosing a life-style

Choosing a marriage partner and raising children

The developmental tasks of early adulthood, most concretely seen in the choice of a vocation and a marriage partner, clearly involve a certain choice of life style. While fairly clear boundaries have been established between self and parents by this time, parental attitudes and value systems have been internalized in young adults to become a salient part of their identity, thus affecting their future life choices. Inherent in these choices is the quest for independence from family, social, and economic dependence.

Occupational choice. An occupation represents much more than a set of skills and functions. It is a way of life that determines much of the environment, both physical and social, in which a person lives.[26] Occupational choice plays a significant part in further shaping the personality by providing a social system, status, roles, and a life style. The choice of an occupational role often necessitates consideration of appropriate educational preparation, and thus educational goals and achievements become a very important part of this choice.

At a time in life when involvement in an occupation is of prime importance, unemployment may cause the individual to feel that he or she is not needed or wanted, thus breeding feelings of inadequacy and failure. When caring for an individual it is very important for the nurse to be as sensitive to the concerns and anxieties of those who are employed and face many pressures as to those who are faced with the problems of unemployment.

The women's liberation movement has exerted a significant influence on women relative to occupational choices. As a result, it is now more socially acceptable for a women to choose a career goal as an alternative or as a supplement to the traditional housewife-mother roles. Among married young adults there is a growing tendency to delay having children until career goals are more solidified. Some married women in this age group may choose to have an abortion if they become pregnant at a time that is not convenient relative to their career or other anticipated goals or when children are not desired.

Marital choice. Another major decision of early adulthood is whether to marry or not to marry. Our society continues to support strongly marital status among young adults. However, some people are choosing not to marry, enjoying the independence and freedom of single living. While there may be many reasons for entering into the marital relationship, marriage is generally recognized as a close and loving partnership between two people where intimacy and affection exist in a free and equal relationship as opposed to only a social institution where the man is the undisputed head of the house and the wife is the childbearer.[31]

The arrival of the first child transforms the spouses into parents as they take on the roles and parenting behavior learned from parents. Parenthood is experienced as a joy as well as a crisis: a joy because a child is the product of their common bond and fulfillment of goals; a crisis because the child necessitates adjustments in daily routine and life-style, which is often seen as a burden. Preparation for parenthood has not been widespread in our society. It is therefore difficult for an individual to anticipate many of the stresses of being a parent and the changes required in themselves and their marital relationship. If the nurse assesses that an individual is experiencing undue stress and an inability to cope, resources for this kind of assistance can be made available.

While personality characteristics and interpersonal problems are primary sources of difficulties in adjustment to marriage and parenthood, cultural and societal variables often make these adjustments difficult. For instance, the mobility of our society results in a dispersal of family members and close relatives, with less available help from these significant others in times of need and stress.

While the institutions of marriage and family are the most socially acceptable, there is an increasing tolerance for diversity relative to optional living patterns such as communes as a temporary way of life, living together, staying single, becoming a bachelor mother or remaining a childless couple, and experimenting with bisexuality or homosexuality.[41] It is important that the nurses be in touch with their attitudes about varying life-styles and choices and remain nonjudgmental, refraining from imposing their own values on others.

Health needs

The cessation of physical growth and development by the time a person reaches the young adulthood period of life, together with the changes in life styles, necessitates certain alterations in physical and psychosocial needs.

Three aspects of physical needs dealt with here relate to nutrition, exercise, and rest and sleep.

Nutrition

The young adult's nutritional needs are not the same as those of adolescents. The cessation of physical maturation necessitates a reduction in some nutritional requirements such as calcium and protein, while an increase in some nutrients is needed. Young men should increase their consumption of foods high in vitamin C, E, B_6, and riboflavin. In young women the needs for protein, vitamins A, E, B_6, B_{12}, and riboflavin remain about the same, but the need for vitamin C increases. In relation to the need for iron in the diet, the man needs only 10 mg of iron daily and the woman 18 mg. Sometimes dietary modifications are indicated, especially for young adults at risk of heart disease. Foods high in cholesterol and saturated fats should be limited in the diet of the young adult, since they contribute to the formation of atheromatous plaques in the blood vessels, resulting in cardiovascular problems.[6] Nutritional problems of young adults frequently stem directly from their life styles, such as busy schedules, limited income, and job or educational demands. The increased demands placed on the young adult (job, home, children, economics) often lead to poor nutritional choices and habits.

The nurse can help the young adult understand the importance of adequate nutrition and of adjusting schedules to allow more time for meals. An understanding of how illnesses and prolonged recovery periods can be related to inadequate nutritional intake is important. Young wives may need suggestions about planning nutritionally adequate meals that are as economical as possible.

Exercise

Exercise serves several functions in the young adult. It helps to regulate appetite, release tension, aid sleep, retard aging, and keep body muscles firm and it protects the heart. It is important to note that exercise should be regular and appropriate to the individual's physical condition. Too often adults think they have worked hard all day and feel they have gained the necessary exercise. Many sport activities such as tennis, horseback riding, and swimming provide physical exercise and exertion. However, sporadic involvement in these activities is not as effective as a regularly planned physical exercise program.[31] Sporadic exertion often produces sudden demands on body systems, not allowing the body to compensate adequately and adjust to the demands. A gradual increase in the intensity of exertion allows the body to adapt to the physical demands, while regularity contributes to sustained maintenance and optimal functioning of body systems.

Rest and sleep

As the demands of jobs, social activities, responsibilities, and educational pursuits increase, the young adult's need for adequate rest and sleep also increases, but in actuality the young adult often goes without proper rest and sleep. While an individual can adjust to a lack of sleep for a length of time, prolonged periods of lack of sleep and rest can contribute to altered mental and physical functions resulting in illness and slowed recovery periods.

Health concerns

Research has shown relationships between physical adaptation and illness and sociocultural experiences. Death rates from cancer, diabetes, tuberculosis, heart disease, and multiple sclerosis in urban populations are inversely proportional to income, implying that stresses of poverty may be determinants of such diseases. Accidents are the leading cause of death of young adults.[31] Many injuries and illnesses require restriction of activity, which presents the young adult with social and economic problems.[31] Injury and illness may also necessitate some dependence, creating conflict with the young adult's quest for independence.

Acute conditions such as upper respiratory tract infection and influenza occur more frequently in the young adult than do other acute illnesses. With young adults the primary responsibility of the nurse lies in the teaching of preventive measures. Prevention is directed at supporting the body defenses and reducing the person's susceptibility. Avoiding environmental pollutants, including cigarette smoke, as much as possible and keeping alcohol intake at an acceptable level as well as observing basic health practices (adequate rest, sleep, exercise, and nutrious diet) should be stressed.

Physiologic and psychologic changes resulting in unusual or disturbed adaptive behavior patterns occur when the young adult is unable to cope with the newly acquired tasks and responsibilities. Mate selection, marriage, childbearing, college, job demands, social expectations, and independent decision making are all stressors, carrying the threats of insecurity and possibly some degree of failure. Some of these stress reactions take the form of physical illness. Related to the stresses of achievement in the young adult years is the occurrence of gastric and duodenal ulcers. Prevention here is directed at reinforcement of appropriate diet, exercise, and rest. When stressors are perceived as overwhelming, they may result in self-destructive behavior such as drug abuse and addiction, alcoholism, excessive smoking, and suicide (ranking as one of the leading causes of death among this age group).

Sensitivity to the many pressures and responsibilities facing the young adult is vital to good nursing care. The patient's major concern often is not about himself. He or she may be the breadwinner of a family. How is the family being supported during the illness? How are the medical bills to be paid? The patient may be a mother of small children. Who will care for them? If she is hospitalized, she is often concerned about how her family is getting along at home. The patient may have no family. Who will look in on him if he is ill at home? Who will care for him during convalescence? These are only a few of the problems frequently facing the young adult patient. Some problems of hospitalized patients may be alleviated by providing the use of a telephone or by arranging a visit with a family member, friend, or business associate. Help needed by the patient may be available through other support systems such as social services in the hospital or through family service or public health agencies. It is important also for the nurse in a physician's office or clinic to be alert for clients who need this kind of assistance.

The adult patient is often expected "to act like an adult," and this is especially true if he is a man. Social expectations have made it difficult for men to cry or reveal their emotions. Thus when ill they may become irritable, withdrawn, and depressed because they may be concealing their true feelings. The nurse needs to be able to convey sincere interest in the patient as a unique human being and acceptance of his behavior.

Middle adulthood

While the transition from young adulthood to the middle years involves more of a state of mind than some dramatic bodily change, it is generally agreed that middle adulthood comprises those years between 45 and 65 years of age. As the young adulthood phase begins to taper off in the middle to late thirties, a change begins to occur in the perceptions of time left to live, productivity, self, and others. The middle years are approached with a sharpened sense of awareness as the individual begins to take stock of life. Has it been fulfilling? Am I doing what I really want to be doing? What are my goals from now on? How the individual evaluates the quality of life already lived and the potential outlook for the future may have a significant influence on further adaptation in the succeeding years.

Erikson has described adaptation to this stage in terms of the resolution of the crisis, *generativity vs. stagnation* (Fig. 16-6). He sees generativity as "primarily the concern in establishing and guiding the next generation."[60] Generativity also includes productivity, creativity, and concern for others in the broadest sense. When this enrichment and fulfillment is not experienced, stagnation and personal impoverishment occur to the point of isolation and preoccupation with self.[41]

Many variables affect the degree to which one experiences productivity or stagnation. The discussion that follows focuses on some of those physiologic and psychosocial variables that influence one's adaptation to this stage of the life cycle.

Physical development

The adult usually approaches this phase of life functioning at near peak efficiency. As the middle years progress gradual physiologic changes occur. The individual becomes aware of the appearance of gray hairs, small creases or lines, and dry skin that begins to show signs of decreasing elasticity. There is a redistribution of fatty tissue regardless of a change in diet or exercise patterns. The skeletal muscles increase in bulk until about the age of 50 and do not begin to degenerate until approximately 60 years of age. Smooth muscles, on the other hand, change very little with age; therefore the vital organs can, by and large, be kept healthy until death.[23]

The sense organs undergo change in the middle years, one of the most noticeable being the eyes. The necessity to wear bifocals, trifocals, or reading glasses is brought on by a condition called presbyopia, characterized by a reduction in the elasticity of the lens of the eye resulting in decreased accommodation for near points of vision. During the middle years there is a gradual deterioration and hardening of the auditory cells and nerves resulting in some loss of auditory acuity.

Hormonal deficiencies associated with menopausal changes in women take place, on the average, between 40 and 55 years of age. As ovarian function gradually diminishes, decreased amounts of estrogen and progesterone are produced by the ovaries, while other body tissues continue to produce small amounts of estrogen for several years after ovarian function ceases. Some of the symptoms associated with menopause are "hot flashes," the cause of which is unknown; atrophic vaginitis in which the vaginal mucosa becomes thin and dry, contributing to itching, burning, and possible discharge; and osteoporosis, which is not necessarily a product of menopause but often accompanies or follows menopause as bone demineralization is accelerated in the absence of estrogens.[11]

The psychologic changes that often accompany menopause may not be precipitated by the hormonal deficiency but may be more appropriately related to the adjustments and adaptations of the middle years.[11] Mood swings may be apparent. The middle-aged woman can be laughing one minute and crying the next. Nervousness, insomnia, and fatique are common complaints at this time. There may be mild depression, but this is usually transitory. This depression may be a reaction to the loss of generativity, at which times stages of the grief process may be observed.[11]

There are no physical changes in men comparable to the menopausal changes in women, although some emotional changes occur in men during this period of life. This is not believed to be the result of hormonal deficiency, as androgen levels decline very slowly.[25] Reproductive capabilities continue into the later years, and any loss of sex drive or potency may be more a state of mind than a result of some physical change.

As activity and metabolism slow down during this period, the weight gain that often results may have detrimental effects on other body systems. The incidence of diabetes, kidney disease, and gallstones increases during this period. While adults get fewer respiratory tract infections than children do, the decreased elasticity of the lungs results in certain chronic respiratory diseases. The loss of elasticity and changes in the structure of the arteries lead to many cardiovascular problems. The middle-aged adult needs more time for recovery from both minor and serious ailments.[23]

Patient education about these potential threats to health and knowledge of how these problems may be prevented is a necessary part of nursing care of the middle-aged adult. It is important to encourage these individuals to receive physical examinations yearly in order that sound health might be maintained throughout the remaining years of their lives.

Psychosocial development

Intellectual development

Contrary to some popular beliefs, mental capacity if used is unimpaired in the middle years. Data suggests that there is little or no decrement in learning capability and memory function.[48] Cerebral capacity deteriorates slowly and only begins to weaken at about the age of 70 years.[23] Active utilization of mental capacity throughout the years will contribute to mental productivity in the later years. It is therefore important that the nurse provide mental stimulation as a part of nursing care and encourage the middle-aged adult to continue with involvement in activities that will facilitate mental productivity.

Sexuality in middle adulthood

The physical aspects of aging, together with the many pressures that are common to this stage of life, affect the attitudes about one's sexuality and sexual functioning.

Some adults expect that with middle age (particularly after menopause) comes the end of their physical attractiveness and thus a decline in sexual interest and the capacity for competent sexual functioning. It has been found that this is more a psychologic phenomenon than an actual physical occurrence. It seems that cultural influences have been significant in perpetuating the idea that with the aging process comes decline of sexual interest and activity. Ambivalence about oneself growing older in a youth-oriented society often breeds feelings of inadequacy relative to one's sexuality. As a result some adults may become depressed and sexually unresponsive. Others may feel a need to retrieve that sense of youthfulness by behaving and dressing in a youthful manner or by having an affair with a younger person.

The middle-aged adult who approaches these years with self-acceptance and appreciation is apt to continue into the later years with a satisfying and fulfilling sexual life.

Some of the physical changes that accompany the menopause may affect the pleasure of sexual intercourse. For example, delay in the production of vaginal lubrication caused by the decrease in steroids may result in some discomfort during intercourse, and on occasion the irritation may cause cystitis. There may be a tendency to refrain from sexual activity because of discomfort. If such problems exist the nurse can explain their causes, suggest use of a water-soluble lubricant during intercourse, and advise the woman to consult her physician.

As men age, certain social and psychologic factors influence their sexual responsiveness. Masters and Johnson noted several recurrent themes in interviews about waning sexual responsiveness: monotony in the sexual relationship or a feeling of being taken for granted, concerns with economic or career pursuits, mental and physical fatigue, physical or mental illness of the individual or spouse, overindulgence in food or drink, and fear of failure. They suggest that practice of sexual activity contributes to quality of the sexual relationship as well as to the continuation of sexual activity into the later years.[54]

In another study of persons aged 45 to 69 years, previous sexual experience was the most significant contributing factor to current sexual functioning, including interest in, frequency, and enjoyment of sexual relations.[9]

Because of prevailing cultural attitudes about waning sexual interest in the middle years, sexual concerns are often ignored in the care and rehabilitation of the middle-aged adult. It is very important therefore that health care providers become knowledgeable about and sensitive to the sexual needs of patients, particularly those who experience injury or illness that restricts physical activity. The nurse can help the patient deal with these anxieties by providing the opportunity to discuss these concerns. If the nurse does not feel competent to discuss such matters, someone with more proficiency in this area can be sought (see Chapter 64).

Developmental tasks

The psychologic and social development of an individual in the middle years is best exemplified in the various developmental tasks that are common to this stage of life (see box, p. 232).

Many of the developmental tasks associated with the middle years involve role transitions, which may involve some alteration in self-image, life style, values and attitudes.

TASKS OF MIDDLE ADULTHOOD

Assisting children to become responsible adults

Coping with role transition

Renewing and redeveloping earlier relationships

Adjusting to aging parents

Reevaluating life's goals

Developing adult leisure-time activities

The ability to shed roles and take on new roles smoothly contributes to a creative and productive life during the middle years. With the maturation of children comes the transition of parental attitudes, values, and actions that formerly were child oriented to those more appropriate to an adult relationship. In those instances where the focus of life revolved solely around the children, the outcome of their departure from home may be an experience of loss. Often referred to as the "empty nest syndrome," this sudden loss frequently leads to depression in women. What is lost is not only the grown child but all the attachments associated with the mother role, resulting in altered perceptions of the self as being needed.[35]

Not only is the role transition relative to one's offspring complex, but this may also be a time when the health status of one's parents is changing. Illnesses and perhaps impending death often necessitate assuming the role of parent to one's own parent(s). The decision making regarding the care of aging parents may necessitate changes in life style if the parents come to live in the home.

While the adult must deal with many changes and alterations during these middle years, this is the time when renewal and full development of relationships can occur. It is a time of altering the patterns of child-centered days and of nurturing the intimate relationship of husband and wife. If throughout previous years a couple has not developed mutual support, open communication, and awareness of each other's needs, the development of an enriching relationship may be difficult if not impossible to achieve.

At the same time that the individual may be enjoying the enrichment of new and renewed relationships and a new sense of freedom, there is the inevitable experience of loss of significant others. Death begins to take friends, parents, and spouse, necessitating alterations in relationships and life styles.

For some adults the middle years are a time when peak social influence, prosperity, economic success, and stability are experienced. But for many the middle years are approached with a sense of frustration and failure if goals and expectations set in earlier years have not been reached and are not realistically attainable. The realization that the time has passed for significant achievement of status and success is often a crisis-producing situation. For example, limited upward career mobility is experienced as younger individuals move up more quickly and are selected for the more choice positions and jobs.

Stock taking and reevaluation often result in ambivalence and uncertainties associated with everyday tasks, reflecting a change in values and attitudes. The adult who previously perceived daily responsibilities to be fulfilling and enjoyable may at this time begin to complain about being trapped and hemmed in, with few rewards. It may not be, however, the job or situation that has changed, but the individual.

Wives who perceived their status relative to the success of their husbands may become dissatisfied with themselves for not being involved in self-fulfilling activities. At this time many wives previously linked only to the home embark on new careers in search of self-fulfillment and satisfaction. The women's movement has contributed much to women's motivation to seek heightened self-fulfillment, satisfaction, and usefulness.

Development of creativity may have been impeded during the childrearing and career development days. Productive use of leisure may be a source of contentment for some adults with the exploration and development of new hobbies and areas of talent and skill. The adult may now have more time to invest in outside activities such as clubs, organizations, church, and politics.

The new and renewed relationships and increased involvement in outside activities is demonstrative of the external orientation to those things outside the individual characteristic of this period of life. This is compared with the internal orientation of the young adult years in which the individual is more preoccupied with achieving mastery of goals and responsibilities and gaining approval from the outside world.

When there is a lack in the cultivation of various relationships and areas of interest that contribute to the meaningfulness and satisfaction of life, stagnation and immobilization often occur. It is the mobilization of one's inner resources that generates the kind of creativity and productivity that facilitate continued growth throughout the remaining years.

Health needs

One important reason for studying growth and development is to gain a better understanding of those physical and psychosocial variables that determine the health needs of individuals as they progress through life. For as individuals change, so do their health needs.

Consideration of the needs of proper nutrition, rest, and exercise are most important during these middle years.

Nutrition

Reduced energy requirements together with reduced physical activity dictate a lesser demand for calories. Improper nutrition, excessive to the physical demands, may result in obesity and atherosclerosis, which are risk factors for such diseases as coronary artery disease, chronic hypertension, renal failure, and diabetes. Thus the middle-aged adult needs to be aware of the fact that biophysical changes necessitate a reduction in calories, saturated fats, and cholesterol. The diet should contain the basic four food groups with an emphasis on protein, minerals, and vitamins; the caloric intake should be based on age, body build, size, and activity patterns. Diet counseling should include specific examples of polyunsaturated oils, dairy products, and meats that can be substituted for those that are high in saturated fats and cholesterol.[20] Adequate fluid intake and an appropriate diet help prevent constipation, and dietary discretion will help maintain weight control.

Exercise

Changes in life-style may result in mental strain and frustration and a lack of exercise, restful sleep, and relaxation. It is important that rest and sleep be balanced with physical activity in order to keep the body functioning at its optimum. Exercise helps to promote relaxation and improves muscle tone, strength, and coordination. It improves work performance, reduces chronic fatigue, and improves the efficiency of the cardiopulmonary system. An assessment of daily activities may give some indication as to the kind and amount of exercise necessary. Exercise activities that are performed incorrectly and cause overexertion can be detrimental to one's health. The regularity of exercise is of great importance; sporadic exercising is not as effective. Middle-aged individuals should take certain precautions: (1) increase exercise gradually, (2) exercise consistently, and (3) avoid overexertion. Ten minutes after exercising, the heart rate and respirations should return to their normal status. Prior to instigating any exercise program a physician should be consulted if the person is overweight, has a personal or family history of cardiovascular or respiratory tract disease, or has led a physically inactive life.

Health assessment

Middle-aged adults should be encouraged to have a thorough medical examination that includes not only a careful medical history and physical assessment of body systems but also blood and urine tests, electrocardiogram, chest x-ray examination, and rectal or proctoscopic examination; women should have Pap smear tests.

Routine dental, vision, and hearing examinations should also be done because periodontal disease, glaucoma, and hearing loss may be prevented or treated if detected early.[20]

Health concerns

The gradual changing physical characteristics may account for the high incidence of accidents among middle-aged adults. Fractures and dislocations are leading causes of injuries to both sexes.[31] Motor vehicle accidents, occupation-related accidents, and falls in the home are leading causes of death.[32] Respiratory conditions are frequent causes of absenteeism from work. Generally, middle-aged women have more disability days from work because of respiratory and other acute disorders, while men have more disability days from injury.[31]

The main health problems of this age group are cardiovascular disease, cancer, pulmonary disease, rheumatoid arthritis, diabetes, obesity, alcoholism, anxiety, and depression. Mounting statistical evidence points to excessive smoking as an influence in lung cancer, cardiovascular disease, chronic obstructive pulmonary disease, and peptic ulcer.

The close interrelationship between physical and psychologic makeup of the human body is exemplified in the climacteric (change of life) phase. How a woman reacts to the menopause depends a great deal on her feelings about herself and her womanhood. If over the years procreation and motherhood have been her major sources of self-esteem, equated with youth and femininity, she may have a much more severe reaction to menopause than a woman who has other sources of self-esteem. Some women who cannot adapt to their physical changes and changing life circumstances may become severely depressed (involutional melancholia) and may need treatment, as the danger of suicide is great. Reactions to menopause may vary depending on the woman's past use of measures to control reproduction. If sterilization occurred earlier in her life, the woman may not perceive menopause as the loss of her femininity.

It is helpful to allow the client to discuss her feelings about herself and this phase of her life. It is also important to help the client identify those strengths and inner resources on which she can focus and build up her self-esteem.

While men do not experience the same physiologic menopausal phenomena as women, they often go through a kind of psychologic "change of life." Symptoms may include fatigue, headaches, increased moodiness, impatience, worry, and psychosomatic complaints such as indigestion, heartburn, rapid or irregular heart beat, urinary problems, respiratory difficulties, and insomnia. Many of these symptoms are often related to emotional depression and anxiety that may be associated with preoccupation with thoughts of aging, anticipation of retirement, loss of career status, and a general feeling of worthlessness.

For the middle-aged person who feels depressed, trapped, frustrated, or isolated, easily accessible escapes may be alcoholism, drugs, or excess food intake. Illness or accident proneness may also become escape mechanisms as a means of avoiding responsibility or resolving serious difficulties. Hypochondriasis is a common symptom of the self-absorbed adult and may become a means of getting attention. Suicide is a leading cause of death among the middle aged. The nurse therefore should be alert and sensitive to any communication that might be suggestive of suicidal thoughts.

Nursing assessment and intervention

When encountering the adult individual experiencing physical or emotional stress, it is important to make a careful assessment not only of the major problem at hand but also of the physical, psychologic, and situational variables relative to the individual's current developmental status. These data are important in that they provide guidance in understanding those factors that may be affecting the individual's response to stress as well as feelings and attitudes about recovery. For example, if an individual unconsciously uses injury, disability, or illness as a way to escape problems or responsibility, progress and treatment may be slowed. Again, the self-absorbed individual is likely to demonstrate regressed, immature behavior resulting in increased dependency needs. Situations such as these are often frustrating for the nurse because there is the tendency to think that adults should react to situations in a mature, logical manner, making appropriate decisions about their welfare. When adults do not react according to our expectations, there is the danger of treating them as children, thereby reinforcing dependency and regression. It is important that the nurse demonstrate acceptance of the adult's behaviors and attitudes, realizing that this may be the individual's manner of coping with stress. Usually when certain needs are met or problems are resolved or dealt with, the individual returns to more mature behavior patterns. Thus facilitating the individual's expression of fears, anxieties, and concerns is often very therapeutic relative to emotional as well as physical healing.

Adulthood is a time when productivity, achievement, and responsibilities are dominant concerns in the individual's life. When goals and expectations are thwarted by illness or disability a crisis often results. This crisis may not affect just a single individual but the family as well. When stress is intense, problem solving may be diminished. The nurse can be helpful at this time by assisting the individual or family in making some decisions by offering options and resources that will help meet their needs, while at the same time being careful to foster and maintain independence by facilitating the client's participation in care planning and decision making.

Sensitivity to the concerns and anxieties brought about by illness or disability is of utmost importance. For example, the paraplegic who is impotent as a result of a spinal cord injury is concerned about his sexuality and adequacy as a man. The woman who must have a mastectomy or hysterectomy is also concerned about her self-image and sexuality. The adult who must be hospitalized for a long period of time may worry about financial support for the family or child care. Coping, like healing, is more than a physical process. Thus genuine acceptance and enlightened concern rather than indifference or pity can be of incalculable benefit to the patient.

While it is a fact that the nurse cannot meet all of an individual's needs, it should be emphasized that nursing is concerned with the total picture of a person's needs. Therefore the nurse who is knowledgeable about all aspects of growth and development and incorporates that knowledge into nursing care planning and intervention is better able to deal with more of the individual's needs and concerns.

Late adulthood

Although 65 years of age is usually considered the beginning of late adulthood or old age, tremendous individual variation exists. Age is really a sociocultural concept and not wholly physiologic and chronologic. Chronologic age is related to but not identical with aging because individual and personal variables enter the picture. The three main components of the aging process are biologic age (a person's position in time relative to potential life span), psychologic age (the individual's capacity for adapting to the environment), and social age (a person's role in the family, at work, and in the community as well as the person's interests and activities). Some people may be old at 45 years of age, while others are not old at 80.

Physical development

Aging is a normal developmental process in which certain *anatomic* and *physiologic changes* take place. Criteria for distinguishing normal aging from other abnormal changes were proposed by Strehler[66] in 1962. According to his criteria, normal changes are (1) *univer-*

sal in all members of the species; (2) *intrinsic* to the organism; (3) *progressive* and cumulative; and (4) *deleterious* to the organism as a whole and associated with an increased mortality rate.

The speed with which aging occurs varies and depends on hereditary factors and the stresses of life. The genetic factor in these biologic processes determines the time of onset, the course and direction, and the time sequences of the various aging processes.

Aging is now being explored by many researchers. Many models of aging have been hypothesized. These models are generally divided into two classes, programmed aging and random deterioration. Programmed-aging theories attribute aging to a sequential program, which results in a predetermined series of events leading to aging and eventual death of the individual. The sequential program may be contained within the DNA of the cell of a "biological clock," possibly located in the central nervous system. Random-deterioration theories incorporate the wear-and-tear hypothesis, error and mutation theories, accumulation of free radicals/waste products theories, and collagen cross-linkages theories. The basic mechanism in this class of theories is an interference with proper functioning of the cells due to errors, waste products, or other biological changes.

Biologic aging leads to some general responses in the older person. There is a gradual decline in functional ability, particularly where multisystem coordination is required. Age decrements are greater in performances that require more complex functioning than with those involving individual system functions. There seems to be growing evidence that some effects of aging are related to decreased effectiveness of control mechanisms in maintaining homeostasis. These concepts undergird the readily recognized fact that the elderly have increased vulnerability to pathophysiologic occurrences.

Cardiovascular changes that started during middle age begin to present symptoms in the older years. The elasticity of the blood vessels lessens, and the cardiac output decreases as the cardiac muscle strength is less; thus the heart in the elderly person must work harder to provide adequate oxygenation. Consequently, diminished regional perfusion to some organs along with arteriosclerosis and atherosclerosis, prevalent in the elderly, may result in ischemia and eventually in death of the tissue in one or more organ systems.

Peripheral resistance increases with age as a result of diminished vascular flexibility. To overcome the increased peripheral resistance, blood pressure may increase markedly both in systolic and diastolic readings. The effects of these age-influenced changes are that the circulatory dynamics are less efficient. The actual circulation time lengthens,[58] and when the heart rate increases to meet demands, it requires a longer period of time to return to its resting rate. With prolonged standing, decreased efficiency of valves in veins of lower extremities may result in accumulation of blood so that not enough is provided for cerebral perfusion. Dizziness and accidents may follow.

The lungs are capable of providing adequate gas exchange throughout the life span in the absence of disease. The structures of the *respiratory system* do undergo changes, however, that lead to decreased elasticity and increased rigidity. Chest wall stiffness results from the increased calcification of costal cartilage and the decreased strength of intercostal and accessory muscles and the diaphragm. The chest wall stiffness, combined with reduced elasticity and recoil pressure of the lungs, results in increased residual volume and decreased forced expiratory volume (FEV_1) with age. The arterial oxygen (PaO_2) decreases about 4mm Hg per decade, while the arterial carbon dioxide ($PaCO_2$) and pH remain unchanged. The diminished defense mechanisms of airway clearance and of humoral and cellular immunity combine with the previously described changes to increase susceptibility to lung congestion and infections.

Aging changes in the *nervous system* include gradual degeneration and atrophy, leading to lessened nerve acuity and impaired sensation. There is generalized loss of neurons with age and a progressive decrease in the weight of the brain. The older person's gag reflex may be less acute than that of a younger person, and therefore aspiration of mucus or other foreign material such as food may occur easily. The person may be unaware of burning himself or of pressure on soft tissues. Bed rest causes the elderly person's circulation to slow; consequently many elderly people become confused when they must stay in bed. This is noticeable in some even after several hours of sleep. Loss of interest in life may also make an elderly person appear dull mentally. Oftentimes these individuals will become more bright and alert when stimuli are increased by contact with others; therefore it is often preferable to put the elderly person in a room with others rather than in a single room.

The acuity of the senses begins to decline with old age. As with all the changes associated with the aging process, the amount of decline varies with the individual. One in four persons over 65 years of age has some type of hearing problem.[3] Sensitivity to sound decreases with age, and there is some selective loss of hearing of the higher pitches. Such changes are usually not reversible because they are due to neurologic decline. If the loss is due to ossification of the bones of articulation in the middle ear, some hearing may return following surgery and the use of a hearing aid (see Chapter 38 for information about hearing aids).

More light is required for the aged retina to produce the same physiologic sensation as was produced in the younger years. Adaptation to light and dark requires more time. Visual acuity, especially for close reading, is impaired as a result of changes in the structure of the eyeball and its muscles. Twice as many elderly people have visual impairments as have hearing loss.

The sense of taste appears to decline with age, which is often one explanation for the aging person's lack of appetite or loss of interest in foods that were once favorites.

The senses of touch and smell also decline as a part of the aging process. Since aromas often stimulate eating, the decline in the sense of smell contributes to the appetite decline in many aging persons. Decline in the senses of touch and smell present certain safety hazards that need to be discussed with the aging individual and his family.

The *liver, heart, kidneys,* and other vital organs of many elderly people may be working hard to maintain normal function with little margin available for adaptability to stress. Any additional burden may be enough to tip the balance unfavorably unless particular care is given. The physiologic controls of fluid and electolyte balance provided by the kidney are altered with aging, as reduced renal flow leads to a progressive decrease in the glomerular filtration rate. One consequence of this age change is the potentiation of the half-life of many drugs that are excreted by the kidneys. Additionally, faintness and shock may follow relatively short periods without food and fluid because of fluid and electrolyte imbalances. Therefore the elderly person should receive medical attention for even apparently slight indispositions.

In the *musculoskeletal system* there is a decrease in lean muscle mass and an increase in body fat. This loss of muscle fiber leads to decreased muscular strength and function. The bones lose density through demineralization. This change is particularly noticeable in the vertebral bodies, through gradual decrease in body stature and posture changes, and in the femur, which has a greater propensity for fracture. The movable joints have less mobility with the large weight-bearing joints showing greater wear, friction, and stiffness. Maintaining activity and encouraging a diet with necessary nutrients helps preserve muscle tone and decrease the rate of bone demineralization. As one ages, muscular tone is also reflected in the *gastrointestinal* and *genitourinary systems,* contributing to increased problems of constipation and incontinence.

Psychosocial development

Psychologic and social development continue during maturity. Psychologic and socioeconomic concepts of aging are most important for all who work with the aged. A knowledge of the crises occurring in this stage of life

---

TASKS OF THE OLDER ADULT

Accepting life with serenity

Adjusting to new limitations of declining physical strength and declining health

Adjusting to retirement and changed financial status

Adjusting to reorganized family patterns

Adjusting to a new pattern of social and civic responsibilities

Adjusting to death of spouse and other loved ones

Establishing affiliation with one's age group

Maintaining satisfactory living arrangements

Accepting death with serenity and assisting others to accept death

---

is useful if one is to assist clients and their families in attainment of developmental tasks (see box above). These tasks are illustrative of the components of Maslow's hierarchy of needs (see p. 7). As these tasks demonstrate, the five levels of human need as defined by Maslow[63] are dynamic, and an individual is frequently in the process of moving among the levels. This is particularly true for the elderly person, who may be making frequent adjustments for reasons of health, loneliness, or other adaptations.

Emotional development is reflected in Erikson's description of the mature years, *integrity vs. disgust or despair*.[60] As the individual looks back and perceives life to have been rich and fulfilling, with purpose and meaning, that individual will experience a sense of satisfaction and contentment in the remaining years. If one does not evaluate his life as such, the final years will be faced with despair.

Another kind of emotional and psychologic response is often seen as the elderly individual looks forward to contemplate the subsequent brevity of and end to life. Cummings described this response as *disengagement*, characterized by a "mutual withdrawal or disengagement" when the individual perceives the reality of being mortal and death.[58] This behavioral response may be initiated by the individual or by others in the social system, with the outcome being a movement away from involvement, achievement, and productivity on the part of the mature individual.[45]

Conversely, activity theorists propose the belief that social involvement, not disengagement, facilitates successful adaptation to aging.[62] The concept involves the substitution of new social roles and activities for those that were lost (work, parenting). In actuality, there are probably aspects of both activity and disengagement behaviors in all elderly persons to a greater or lesser degree as determined by their personalities throughout life.

Many younger people falsely assume that older people have no interest in sex and lack the ability to perform sexually. Men and women of all ages are capable of sexual arousal and orgasm. Masters and Johnson emphasize the consistency of sexual behavior for the maintenance of sexual activity in old age.[45] Studies conducted at the Duke University Center for the Study of Aging revealed sexual activity in the eighth and ninth decades. Often the aged person becomes sexually inactive due only to a lack of an acceptable partner.[54]

The basic *psychologic needs* of the elderly are no different from those of adults. In one survey,[15] elderly persons were asked what they considered essential for their happiness. They mentioned good health, a place to live, enough money to live comfortably, recognition by others, participation with others, and opportunity for a variety of experiences. However, the elderly typically have greater difficulty obtaining their desires than do younger adults. Both their desires and the difficulties that must be overcome to obtain them should be considered in planning the nursing care of elderly people. The primary objective in caring for elderly persons is to help them make the adjustments necessary to make life worth living. Each patient has different limitations and frustrations, and each will react to them differently. In general, elderly persons will react essentially as they have reacted to other stresses throughout their lives.

Health needs

In assessing the health needs of the elderly, some general factors must be recognized. First, age-related decline in immune function results in less rapid and less effective response to infections and to an increased incidence of autoimmunity and malignancy.[28] Second, stress situations (either physiologic or psychosocial) produce more pronounced reactions in the aged and require a longer period of time for readjustment. Third, complex functions which require multisystem coordination show the most obvious decline and require the greatest compensation and support. Fourth, the elderly very frequently have an atypical presentation of an illness. Pain may be less pronounced, and some typical symptoms may be either missing or the opposite of what is expected. Confusion, restlessness, or other altered mentation are common occurrences in the presence of illness. Obscure or unexplained deterioration of health or function should not be accepted as normal aging and needs to be carefully evaluated.

Multiplicity and chronicity of diseases are not uncommon among the elderly and most patients have several chronic ailments. Some of these ailments are not particularly troublesome. Most have developed slowly

and usually take time to alleviate. Heart disease, cancer, renal disease, vascular disease such as cerebrovascular accident, chronic obstructive pulmonary disease such as emphysema, and accidents are the most common problems that bring older patients to the hospital. Other common chronic ailments such as arthritis, skin disorders, and mild neuromuscular conditions are usually cared for while the client is ambulatory. The most prevalent acute illnesses of later life are acute respiratory conditions such as pneumonia and pulmonary edema.

Elderly persons who become ill may be particularly apprehensive and worried, probably because their security is more profoundly affected by illness than that of younger persons. They often fear helplessness and physical dependence on others. Elderly patients may face many adjustments that make it difficult and sometimes impossible for basic emotional needs to be met. In addition to illness and the depleted physical energy which almost always accompanies it, they may have no family and few friends, or the spouse may be ill also. They often have an inadequate income and housing problems. Even before the illness, they may have been depressed because of feeling unwanted and useless.

Illness may break down psychologic defenses that have been built up over a lifetime. Aged individuals may be overwhelmed with fear of increased dependency needs or other problems to which they may react with extreme irritability. If self-esteem is low due to years of suffering from economic or emotional deprivation, they may use illness aggressively as a means of revolt. A trivial and purely incidental event may precipitate irritability. Other individuals, even those who had been quite active, may develop excessive lethargy with the onset of illness and may seem to give up all hope and desire to live.

Similarities between childhood and old age should not be assumed, because they are not valid. Even in the matter of helplessness there is no similarity. Children are in ascendance; they are developing new power daily and marking up achievements over the environment. The aged person's helplessness is infinitely more frustrating because it is increasing rather than decreasing.

Nursing intervention

The goal of medical and nursing care is to keep people functioning at the highest possible level for their age. This includes living with chronic ailments and continuing degenerative changes. The nurse who views aging as a normal, inevitable process, one requiring adjustments in living patterns but not a withdrawal from life, is best prepared to work with the aging patient. The nurse's philosophy of aging can be one of ever-

TYPES OF COMMUNITY SUPPORT SERVICES FOR OLDER PERSONS

Senior citizen centers	Social, nutritional, educational, and counseling services at a center
Geriatric day care centers	Assistive daytime nursing care; social, nutritional, and rehabilitative services may be available
Adult foster home care	Care in another private home when older person unable to live alone
Meals on wheels	Meals delivered to the person's home
Homemaking service	Household chores, shopping, etc.
Transportation service	Arranged pick-up by public transportation system
Home health service	Skilled home nursing care

changing life that eventually will end in death, not one of approaching death.

Necessary nursing care depends on the physiologic and anatomic changes that have taken place, the diseases which are present, and the person's own emotional makeup and apparent adjustment to the particular situation. In planning nursing care for elderly patients, consideration is given to each patient's physical, social, economic, and psychologic capacities and limitations. Older patients frequently talk at length about their families and the past to the nurse who is willing to listen. Their conversations may give clues to interests that should be encouraged and of problems that are confronting them. These clues are evaluated and plans made to help patients maintain as much independence as possible despite their limitations. Different types of resources (see box above) are available in communities to assist older persons maintain independence and meet their social needs.

Cognitive impairment

Changes in mental functioning seen in some older persons may be due to several causes, some of which are reversible. Cognitive functioning may be impaired by acute or chronic organic brain syndromes or by depression. *Acute organic brain syndrome,* which is potentially reversible, may be caused by fluid and electrolyte imbalances, malnutrition, metabolic imbalances, toxic states, trauma, infections, decreased cardiac or renal function, drugs, or overwhelming stress. The person is physically ill, is confused and delirious, and experiences hallucinations.

Chronic organic brain syndromes, which include

Alzheimer's disease and vascular brain disease, are irreversible. *Alzheimer's disease* (presenile dementia) is a disease of the brain parenchyma, is thought to be an inherited tendency, and occurs in about 50% of the chronic disorders. Approximately 6% of persons over 65 years of age develop dementia, and it occurs primarily among women. The dementia is characterized by a defect in memory and orientation, deterioration of intellectual functioning, and alterations in judgment and affect.[53] It is chronic and progressive and may lead to institutionalization of the person. Early signs include irritability, subtle changes in personality, moderate anxiety, and depression. Eventually the person becomes disoriented in all spheres, has illogical or incoherent communication, and is incontinent.

Vascular brain disease originates in the vascular system of the brain and may result from closure of the vessels by arteriosclerotic plaques or emboli or from insufficient perfusion to the brain. The onset is abrupt, and there are periods of remission and exacerbation. During remission personality remains intact and the person has some awareness of the problems. Early signs include symptoms of decreased oxygenation of the brain: blackouts, falls, seizures, and transient ischemic attacks. As the disease progresses, there is memory loss, emotional lability, and depression.

Depression is often confused with dementia and can occur with true dementia; therefore, many elderly persons with a treatable depression are not recognized. Depression is a dysphoric mood causing loss of interest in usual activities and is of acute onset. It is characterized by at least four of the following symptoms: (1) altered appetite or weight, (2) altered sleep patterns, (3) expressions of self-reproach, guilt, hopelessness, (4) lack of energy, (5) psychomotor retardation or agitation, (6) loss of interest or pleasure in usual activities, and (7) recurrent thoughts of suicide. If there is any possibility of the existence of depression, the older person should receive treatment.[53]

Promoting self-worth

When giving nursing care to elderly patients, it is necessary to take special care *to build up and protect their sense of worth and their feelings of adequacy.* Remembering the names of patients and calling them by name instead of using such terms as "grandma" or "grandpa" helps. Giving clear and slow explanations to the patient may spare him the embarrassment of mistakes caused by misunderstanding. Since many elderly patients experience some loss of hearing, special care must be taken to be sure the patient has heard the explanation. The nurse should always face elderly patients when speaking and speak distinctly so that they can lip-read inconspicuously if necessary. If hearing is better in one ear than the other, the nurse should talk into the good ear. It usually does no good to shout in an attempt to help the elderly person to hear, since shouting increases the voice frequency and the elderly have the greatest difficulty hearing sounds in the higher frequency range. If the patient uses a hearing aid, care should be taken to assure that it is working properly. Written instructions are helpful for some elderly patients. The nurse should also be thoughtful about repeating instructions because the short-term memory span decreases with age.

Promoting self-care

Placing equipment conveniently so that assistance need not be requested also makes elderly patients feel more adequate. Self-help devices may help him maintain some degree of independence. For example, an overbed trapeze or side rails on the bed may facilitate movement in bed. Handrails along hallways and in the bathroom or a walkerette may make it possible to walk alone. Sturdy chairs with arms and wooden seats make it easier for many elderly patients to get into and out of chairs themselves. Electric beds also allow them to be more independent. If the patient uses a cane, glasses, hearing aid, or dentures, these devices should be readily available. Showers or bathtubs equipped with handrails and with nonskid strips may make it possible for some patient to bathe independently.

Many adjustments can be made to help the patient who is confined to a wheelchair retain some measure of independence. If the patient is able to transfer onto the toilet, arranging a bathroom to facilitate this maneuver is desirable. Some patients, especially if they have urinary frequency or incontinence, appreciate their wheelchair or chair being fixed as a commode. Removal of door sills may make is possible for an elderly patient confined to a wheelchair to move about the house. If elderly patients are unable to propel their chair manually, they may be able to use a motorized wheelchair.

Elderly patients often need help with personal care such as arranging the hair, applying cosmetics, shaving, and dressing. Personal appearance is important to everyone's morale.

Many elderly patients can give most or all necessary *physical care* to themselves. Some may need encouragement to do so; others resent not being allowed to care for themselves. The nurse or the family member caring for them, however, must be patient and give them adequate time. The older patient often is exceptionally slow in the morning and, in fact, geriatricians instruct their patients to take twice the usual time to shave, to dress slowly, and to avoid hurry of any kind, particularly in the morning hours. Since elderly patients may tire easily, the nurse should ascertain that individuals are physically able to give their own care.

If the patient is in a general hospital, a slow pace is often hard to assume. For example, many diagnostic procedures must be carried out in the morning, and breakfast must usually be served with that of other patients. When possible many hospital routines can be adjusted for elderly patients. For instance, they may prefer to bathe and shave in the afternoon or early evening. The nursing care plan for physical care of each elderly patient should include what self-care is possible, what assistance is needed, the method used, and the schedule the patient follows. Most elderly patients find comfort in familiar things and processes. Therefore it is important to maintain routine as much as possible. The elderly are not unable to make changes but require more time to adjust to new routines. The patient should participate in planning the schedule, and whenever possible it should parallel the pattern of care at home.

Providing skin care

Since *physical change* occurs in the aging process, elderly people need to use somewhat different hygienic practices than an adult uses to maintain an optimum physical condition. The *skin* of an elderly person is usually thin, delicate, and sensitive to pressure and trauma. The loss of subcutaneous fat and the hardening of the tiny arterioles near the surface cause the skin to be wrinkled, sagging, and sallow. Sweat glands atrophy and the excretory function of the skin is lessened, making the skin dry and flaky and sometimes causing it to itch. Color changes occur in the skin with aging. Seborrheic keratoses, which are lesions resembling darkened, greasy warts, are common. These lesions are nonmalignant but should be inspected frequently for signs of any irritation or change.

Because the skin is likely to be very dry, daily bathing is often contraindicated for the elderly. Usually one or two baths a week are sufficient, although the patient who is incontinent needs local sponging at frequent intervals and perhaps more frequent baths. Because regular soaps can be irritating, mild superfatted soaps are preferred. Bath oils may be used, or lanolin or body lotions can be applied after bathing to promote water retention in the skin.

If the patient is confined to bed, an alternating pressure mattress, flotation pad, or flotation mattress may be extremely helpful in maintaining the skin in good condition. Above all, the patient's position should be changed frequently, and bony prominences and weight-bearing areas should be massaged at least every 2 hours. Sheepskin pads placed under bony prominences are also used to relieve pressure and to prevent irritation of the skin. Every effort should be made to get the elderly out of bed as much as possible. This not only helps to redistribute pressure over the body and improve circulation but can also give patients a psychologic boost.

Because of dryness, poor circulation, and low resistance to infection, the skin of elderly persons readily becomes infected. Elderly persons often need assistance in drying their feet after bathing and in cutting and caring for their toenails. Nails are often hard and scaly; soaking the feet in warm water or applying oil to the nails for a day or two prior to cutting softens them and makes cutting easier and safer. A podiatrist should be asked to care for very hard nails and other conditions such as calluses, corns, and bunions.

As the tissues age and circulation becomes sluggish, the *hair*, becomes thin, dry, and colorless. Massage of the scalp and daily brushing with a soft-bristled brush help to preserve its beauty. Frequent shampooing should be avoided, although some people who have washed their hair more frequently throughout their lives may wish to continue to do so.

Providing eye care

Changes occur in the *eyes* with aging. There is a decrease in the conjunctival secretions, and sometimes the lower lid droops (ectropion), causing the moistening fluid of the eye to be lost. Therefore irritation of the conjunctivae and tearing are common complaints of the aged. Smoke also may be more irritating to their eyes than to those of younger persons. Isotonic solution eye-drops are frequently ordered as a comfort measure.

An accumulation of secretions at the inner canthus of the eye may be present, particularly on awakening, and may be uncomfortable and unsightly. A sterile cotton sponge moistened with a physiologic solution of sodium chloride can be used to cleanse the eyes. Care must be taken not to press on the eyeballs or to irritate any exposed conjunctiva.

The lens of the eye loses its ability to accommodate effectively as aging progresses. Most people over 50 years of age need glasses, at least for reading. Care of glasses, making certain that they are not lost or broken, is important in the nursing care of the elderly. It is advisable to label glasses with the patient's name. They should also be kept clean. Smudged glasses rather than failing vision may be the cause of difficulty in seeing. The patient should have the glasses available at all times, since confusion and inability to deal with situations in an adequate fashion may result if they become misplaced. The eyes of older people also accommodate more slowly to changes in light. Bright lights or sunlight may be almost unbearable to some elderly people. Many elderly persons see very poorly in the dark; therefore nightlights should always be used to reduce confusion in patients and to prevent those who get up during the night from having accidents. Cataracts, failing vision, and actual blindness are common in the aged (see p. 860 for care of the patient with visual impairment).

Care of mouth and teeth

The elderly person should be urged to give special attention to the care of the *mouth* and *teeth*. The gums become less elastic and less vascular. They may recede from the remaining teeth, exposing areas of a tooth not covered with enamel. These areas are sensitive to injury from brushes and coarse dentrifices. In addition, diseases of the gum that may have been progressing symptom free for years may cause loss of teeth. Many elderly persons have decayed, broken, or missing teeth. This leads them to avoid foods that are difficult to eat but that may be necessary for the health. The effect of oral health on nutrition is very real; definite improvement in appetite has followed correction of unhealthy conditions in the mouth.

By 70 years of age, the loss of teeth is common, frequently necessitating dentures. Many individuals over 65 years of age have oral lesions of which they are unaware. Some of these lesions are potentially malignant.[57] Consequently, care of dentures and prevention of their loss are part of the general nursing care of most elderly patients. Patients may be encouraged by their dentists to keep dentures in place while they sleep as well as when they are awake, since this helps to preserve the normal contours of the face. One must be aware, however, of the potential danger of dentures dislodging which could cause respiratory problems. Dentures should be cleansed following each meal. Because dental plates may be conductors of heat and since the mouths of aged patients are often not very sensitive to excessive heat, these persons should be urged not to consume very hot food or fluids. Care should be taken that dentures are not lost, as they are costly. Dentures can also be easily mixed up, especially if the patient removes them frequently and then forgets where they were placed. Dentures should be marked, and there is equipment now available to do this.

Promoting activity

The feet and legs usually show the results of limitation in peripheral circulation before any other body part. Therefore it is important for the aging person to *exercise the feet and legs regularly,* to avoid constriction or stasis of the circulation to their lower extremities, and to avoid injury and infections of their feet and legs. Precautions similar to those described for the patient who has peripheral vascular disease (p. 1146) should be taken by all elderly people.

As the muscles become less active in age, slumped posture may result. The abdomen may sag, the spine becomes rounded, and the chest and shoulders droops forward. Lessened elasticity of tissue tends to make these changes fixed. Attention to preventive posture is therefore essential. Although corrective postural exercises and general exercise must be prescribed carefully by a physician, teaching good posture and encouraging deep breathing are part of the daily nursing care of all elderly patients. Any improvement in posture will enable the elderly person to use diminishing resources to better advantage. Proper body alignment adds to the comfort of the patient confined to bed as well as decreasing the need for corrective exercises later. A firm mattress is usually preferable and helps to make the use of pillows more effective. If greater stability is needed, a fracture board can be placed under the mattress. Bedcovers should be light and warm and should be tucked loosely, giving sufficient room for the patient to move about in bed. A block or board placed at the foot of the bed helps to keep covers off the toes and provides something firm against which the patient may press the feet and thereby get some exercise. A pillow placed lengthwise under the head and shoulders helps to bring the chest forward, thereby permitting good chest expansion. Pillows placed under the arms support the muscles of the shoulder girdle and provide comfort for the patient who must have the head of the bed raised for long periods of time.

Unless there is some particular contraindication, exercises for the arms and legs, exercises to keep abdominal and gluteal muscles in good tone, and exercises to strengthen the extensor muscles of the spine should be performed several times each day by every bed patient. The patient is taught to flex, abduct, adduct, and extend each leg separately and both legs simultaneously. The heel of one foot can be placed on the knee of the opposite leg and then the heel passed slowly down the leg to the ankle. This can then be repeated, alternating the legs. Arm, hand, neck, and shoulder movements can be encouraged by having the patient first raise and lower the head, neck, and shoulders from a flat supine position without a pillow and then by having the patient extend the arms in front of the chest, followed by raising them above the head. Each of these exercises should be done, if possible and if not contraindicated, in time to regular, deep respiration to encourage deep breathing while bedfast. These exercises should be taught to the patient by the nurse, and they should be supervised daily by the nurse or the family member caring for the patient. The regular performance of exercises will help to prevent the loss of muscle tone that occurs in all bed patients, regardless of age, unless activity is continued. If the elderly person is unable to do active range-of-motion exercises independently, the nurse should assist with them or do passive range of motion exercises.

Promoting comfort

Elderly persons should wear *clothing* that is comfortable. They often feel cold and may wear woolen clothing even when it seems very warm to others. Hospitalized patients often wish to wear socks, woolen underwear, a bed jacket, a cap, or other items of clothing to which they are accustomed. Some provision must be made for the care of this clothing. Sometimes members of the family are glad to care for special clothing that the patient needs.

Elderly women often appreciate assistance with altering their clothes. They may be unable to afford new ones, but they are often interested in remaining stylish. Wearing a well-fitted brassiere and corset not only improves the elderly woman's appearance, but the support given to sagging tissues may make her more comfortable.

The elderly person should be encouraged to wear firm well-fitted shoes with good support to prevent damage to the arches of the feet, since the muscles are often weak. Hospitalized patients should have their shoes and should wear them when they are up. If an elderly person wears slippers, they should also fit well and be firm, since the person is less likely to slip or stumble and fall.

Fresh air is especially necessary for the elderly person because with his diminished chest expansion poorly oxygenated air may not provide a sufficient blood level of oxygen. The aged, however, may be susceptible to drafts not even noticed by younger persons; consequently, they may dislike open windows.

Protective adipose tissue under the skin disappears with age, and the volume of circulating blood, particularly to the small outer arteries, may be diminished, thus affecting the ability to withstand chilling without discomfort. Decreased activity also lessens circulatory function, resulting in lowering of skin temperature and susceptibility to chilling. Many elderly people suffer from mild arthritis and fibrositis, which produce vague muscle and joint pains, and these conditions are aggravated by chilling. Measures to provide fresh air but to avoid drafts and chilling are essential.

Promoting rest and sleep

Rest is essential for the aged. However, confusion, decubitus ulcers, lung congestion, and general deterioration may result from prolonged bed rest. It is undesirable for an elderly patient to be confined to bed, and even acutely ill elderly people may often be up in a chair for most of the day and may even be encouraged to walk. When the patient is being cared for by the family, the nurse should try to impress on them the great importance of keeping the patient active, since they may be oversolicitous of the patient or it may seem to require too much effort to get the patient in and out of bed.

Elderly people usually *sleep* lightly and intermittently with frequent waking. At home the aged person may get out of bed, read, wander about the house, and even prepare something to eat at odd hours. Actually this activity is probably good, since it prevents excessive slowing of circulation. Some wakefulness, therefore, can be expected in the elderly patient who is hospitalized. If the patient is allowed out of bed, it probably is best for home activity patterns to be followed. However, a low bed, nightlights, and adequate supervision should be employed to avoid accidents, and the nurse should be sure that the patient is not constantly wakeful. Elderly patients, similar to all others, may be unable to sleep. Sedation has limited usefulness in the elderly and other methods for inducing sleep are preferable. Altered sleep patterns that are normal in aging need to be differentiated from depression and dementia (see p. 238).

Promoting nutrition

Many elderly people are undernourished, and for this reason a great deal of emphasis is placed on *nutrition* for the aged. Other than acute and chronic illness, possible causes of malnutrition in the elderly are limited financial resources, psychologic factors such as boredom and lack of companionship when eating, edentia, lifelong faulty eating patterns, fads and notions regarding certain foods, lack of energy to prepare foods, and lack of sufficient knowledge of the essentials of a well-balanced diet. Many elderly persons, particularly those living alone, subsist on a diet high in carbohydrates and low in vitamins, minerals, and protein. Often they think that because they are elderly they do not need much food. A diet composed largely of tea and toast may seem sufficient to them.

The nurse should instruct the patients and those responsible for their care in the essentials of a well-balanced diet (Chapter 52). Qualitative nutritional needs of the elderly are essentially the same as for other adults except that caloric needs diminish. Increased fiber is beneficial to the gastrointestinal system. Fluid intake is important, yet many do not drink much water. Tea, coffee, and other beverages are usually preferred. Drinks prepared with dry skim milk supply essential protein and are useful in helping to meet the protein and calcium needs of older patients without supplying too many calories.

Some elderly persons are obese even though they may be undernourished. Excess weight burdens the heart, liver, kidneys, and musculoskeletal system and should be avoided. Weight reduction for the aged person, however, should be gradual and must be supervised by a physician. Sudden loss of weight is poorly tolerated by many elderly persons whose vascular system has become adjusted to the excess weight. Sudden weight reduction may lead to serious consequences, including confusion associated with lowered blood pressure, exhaustion, and vasomotor collapse.

Promoting elimination

Elderly patients may worry about their *bowel function*. They tend to forget that less food and less activity will result in reduced bowel function. Any marked change in bowel habits, however, and any unusual reactions to normal doses of laxatives should be reported, since malignancies of the large bowel and diverticulitis are fairly common among this age group.

Regularity in going to the toilet is important, since it provides stimulus to evacuate the bowel. Motor activity of the intestinal musculature may be decreased with age, and supportive structures in the intestinal walls become weakened. Sense perception is less acute, so that the signal for bowel elimination may be missed. Constipation may occur and in turn lead to impactions. The very elderly and somewhat confused patient should be reminded to go to the bathroom following meals. The addition of bran to a person's daily food intake has been found to be helpful in preventing constipation. If the patient is constipated, it may be necessary occasionally to carefully insert a gloved finger into the rectum to be certain impaction has not occurred.

Frequency of voiding is common with aging and becomes a problem during illness. The glomerular filtration rate and the renal blood flow decrease gradually with age. In addition, decreased muscle tone in the bladder with resultant impairment of emptying capacity may result in residual urine in the bladder and subsequent infection. It may be necessary to catheterize the patient to check for residual urine. One of the first signs of diminishing or failing kidney function is frequency of micturition during the night. Frequency and slight burning on urination are symptions of bladder infection.

Elderly women have relaxation of perineal structures, which may also interfere with complete emptying of the bladder and predispose to bladder infection. Some elderly patients have decreased sensation and do not realize when the bladder must be emptied. Periodic dribbling of urine suggests that the bladder is not being emptied completely. The nurse should observe the very elderly patient for distention of the bladder and consult the physician about it.

Unless there is a definite contraindication to high fluid intake, the elderly patient should be urged to take sufficient fluids to dilute urine and decrease its irritating properties. Fluids may be limited in the evening if nocturia is troublesome and is interfering with sleep. If the patient is quite feeble, it is well to offer a urinal or bedpan during the night.

Involutional changes in the lining of the vagina lead to lessened resistance to invasion of organisms. Mild infections with troublesome discharge are not unusual in elderly women. This condition should be reported to the physician, who may order specific therapy for it. Frequent local bathing may be helpful in allaying itching. Application of cornstarch also relieves itching. Embarrassment may prevent the elderly patient from reporting symptoms. The nurse should be aware of the symptoms of this condition and watch for them.

Almost all elderly men have hypertrophy of the prostate gland, which makes urination difficult. The nurse must report or must urge the patient to report such complaints to his physician because specific treatment is often necessary and can be safely administered even when the patient is far advanced in years.

Incontinence of urine or feces is twice as common among women as men. It is a particularly upsetting problem not only to the patient and family but also to the nursing staff. Every effort should be made to institute and maintain the patient on a bowel and bladder training regimen. Specific details about bladder and bowel training can be found in Chapters 58 and 61.

Meeting psychosocial needs

An important part of nursing care for the elderly is helping to meet their *emotional needs*. Elderly patients are often lonely and individual attention should be given to them. They often appreciate just talking with others. If possible the nurse should plan time to visit with them daily. Volunteers may also be used to visit the elderly. Many patients appreciate visits with a clergyman.

When visiting with elderly patients, one should remember that, although they commonly talk about events and activities in their own past, they usually are interested in the activities of young people and of the world about them. These interests often must be satisfied for them through the eyes and ears of others. If the patients are unable to see well enough to read they may enjoy being read to by others.

Provisions should be made for the patient who requires long hospitalization to maintain family contacts. A grandfather or grandmother often wishes to see a grandchild, and a visit should be arranged, if possible. Sometimes plans can be made for the patient to make a short visit outside the hospital. This is especially important if a wife or husband is physically unable to visit the patient. Arranging for telephone conversations with family members also is desirable.

If elderly patients like to read, reading materials should be provided. If they are unable to see to read, talking books available through public libraries may be appreciated. It is also possible to get books and magazines with large print for persons with reduced vision. Television and radio also provide desirable diversion and stimulation.

Elderly people often are interested in doing useful tasks. There are many tasks in which even the elderly person who is ill may be able to participate. If they are at home they may be able to help with dishes or meal preparation. They may be interested in crafts such as knitting, repairing toys, or making useful gadgets for the house. Many elderly persons enjoy painting. The older person may be quite slow in all activities, and great care must be taken not to show impatience, which may discourage further participation.

Elderly patients are usually aware of death as an imminent possibility and sometimes see it as a welcome event. The nurse should not avoid this issue. If the nurse senses that there is genuine concern about death, the patient can be urged to discuss feelings about it (see Chapter 17). They may also wish to see a clergyman, a family member, or the physician or perhaps to arrange to transact some unfinished business. The nurse must always be responsive to such requests, since they frequently are more important for the patient's peace of mind than the medical treatment. The feelings of the family of the elderly person must also be considered in dealing with the question of death. They may find it a very uncomfortable subject.

Special precautions related to diagnosis and treatment

Medications

Elderly persons consume disproportionately more of all kinds of drugs than middle-aged adults as a result of increased frequency of illness, especially chronic illness, among the aged. These drugs may not be well tolerated, may have adverse reactions and interactions, and may have unpredictable responses in the elderly. Age-related physiologic changes contribute to altered responses to drugs in the elderly.

The *absorption* of drugs may be altered because of the decrease of hydrochloric acid that normally occurs with aging. Drugs that depend on an acid medium may be absorbed less effectively. Absorption may also be altered by the rate of transit through the gastrointestinal system.

The *distribution* of drugs is affected by the loss of lean body mass and the increased proportion of body fat. Fat-soluble drugs tend to be stored in fat, thereby decreasing the intensity of the reaction while increasing the duration. Within the bloodstream the distribution of drugs is affected by the amount of serum protein, specifically the albumin, available as binding sites for drugs. In aging the serum albumin levels tend to be lower, resulting in altered concentrations of bound (inactive) and unbound (active) drugs. Unbound drugs in the circulation are active in producing the effects of the drug, and it is these drugs that can be excreted by the kidney. A principal mechanism of drug interaction seems to be the displacement of one drug by another from these protein-binding sites. For example, warfarin may be displaced by aspirin, indomethacin, and other drugs, causing increased anticoagulant activity.

The *metabolism* of drugs in the elderly may be altered by lower levels of enzyme activity in the liver. The result of prolonged or incomplete metabolism is an increase in the half-life of some drugs, which allows the drug to exert its effect over a longer period of time.

The kidney is the primary route of *excretion* of drugs. The aging changes of decreased renal plasma flow to the kidney, the decreased glomerular filtration rate, and the decreased number of functional tubules combine to result in inefficient excretion of active drug. This effect increases the risk of accumulation of drugs to potentially toxic levels due to decreased renal clearance. The decreased rate of excretion along with the changes in binding sites in the blood unite to prolong the elevated blood level and activity of many drugs. Digoxin has a narrow margin of safety and is an example of a drug that is critically affected by the change in renal excretion.

Drug treatment in the elderly has its definite place in the therapeutic regimen, but it must be handled carefully. One general principle in treatment of the elderly with medication is that the drug level should be built up gradually and that the fewest possible number of drugs should be used.

The nurse should carefully check for untoward reactions from medications and report them to the physician. If the patient is emaciated or of very advanced years, the use of full adult doses of drugs should be questioned.

Many elderly patients must administer medicines to themselves. The nurse should carefully determine their ability to do so and should report to the physician if the practice does not seem to be safe so that other plans can be made. In planning self-administration of drugs with the elderly patient, it is frequently helpful to determine the easiest time for the person to remember to take medication. This time is usually tied in with some incident of daily living such as arising or taking meals. The use of a medication check sheet is helpful in reminding some patients. Plans may also include placement of the medication so that seeing it will be a reminder. Special care needs to be taken, however, to put it where it will not accidentally be taken in place of another drug or where other family members such as small children may take it. Some elderly persons have found it helpful to use something such as an egg carton with the days marked. One dose is put into each hole, and it is easy to know if the medication has been taken.

Elderly persons should understand the medications they are taking. They should be cautioned against taking extra doses of the medication because some believe that if one tablet or pill helps, two will be better.

Diagnostic tests

Elderly patients who are undergoing diagnostic tests requiring withholding of meals or the use of enemas or cathartics should be attended unless they are in their beds because they often become quite weak and dizzy. No elderly patient should ever be left unattended on a treatment table and such patients should be helped on and off the table. Since the person often is quite dizzy, it is advisable to arise slowly and sit on the edge of the table for a few moments before standing. The dizziness is caused by the slow compensation of inelastic blood vessels. Older patients with cardiovascular disease may also be orthopneic and cannot tolerate lying flat for examinations.

Because of the rapidity with which they develop pressure ulcers, elderly patients who must lie on x-ray, treatment, or operating room tables for lengthy periods of time need pads placed under the normal curves of their backs and a pad of material such as sponge rubber placed under bony prominences. Skin over bony prominences should be rubbed occasionally to improve the circulation to the area. On return to the unit the patient's skin should always be checked for pressure areas, and if any signs of pressure are evident, these areas should be massaged frequently until the tissue appears normal in color. If possible the patient should be kept off these areas until signs of pressure disappear. If the patient is placed in lithotomy position, care must be taken to place both legs in the stirrups at the same time to prevent undue pull on unresilient muscles. The same principle applies when removing the legs from the stirrups. Care must also be taken to prevent hyperextension and hyperflexion of the joints, since many elderly patients have arthritis and reduced flexibility.

The kind of nursing care given to the elderly may be influenced by the attitudes one has toward the elderly and aging. Societal attitudes have yielded a stereotype of the elderly that says that they are slow, cannot think as well as in earlier years, are consumed by mental confusion, do not want to learn anything new, are plagued by disease, are most dependent, behave in a childlike manner, and are burdens to family and society. If these attitudes are also held by the nurse, the elderly individual may be approached with condescending tolerance, thereby reinforcing often felt feelings of inferiority.

It is most helpful when the nurse can deal with the individual in an empathetic manner, demonstrating a willingness to listen, explain, comfort, and support independent functioning. Accepting elderly individuals as they are and where they are in terms of their developmental status as well as suspending youth-oriented attitudes and standards that may be inappropriate are essential elements in adequately meeting the elderly person's needs and fostering a better quality of life.

While many of the changes discussed above do necessitate special nursing approaches for the elderly, it should be emphasized that not all of these changes occur with all aging persons. Indeed many older persons are very healthy and actively engaged in the world around them.

REFERENCES AND SELECTED READINGS
Contemporary

1. Ballard, J.L., et al.: A simplified assessment of gestational age, Pediatr. Res. **11**:374-376, 1977.
2. Berengerg, S.R., editor: Puberty: biologic and psychosocial components, Netherlands, 1974.
3. Burnside, I.: Nursing and the aged, ed. 2, New York, 1981, McGraw-Hill Book Co.

4. *Cameron, J.M.: The battered baby, Nurs. Mirror **9**:32-37, 1972.
5. Chinn, P.: Child health maintenance concepts in family centered care, ed. 2, St. Louis, 1979, The C.V. Mosby Co.
6. *Dickelman, N.L.: The young adult: the choice is health or illness, Am. J. Nurs. **75**:1272-1277, 1976.
7. *Dickelman, N.L.: The middle years: emotional tasks of the middle adult, Am. J. Nurs. **75**:997-1001, 1975.
8. *Dickelman, N.L., and Galloway, K.: The middle years: a time of change, Am. J. Nurs. **75**:994-996, 1975.
9. *Dresen, S.E.: The middle years: the sexually active middle adult, Am. J. Nurs. **75**:1001-1005, 1975.
10. Erickson, M.L.: Assessment and management of developmental changes in children, St. Louis, 1976, The C.V. Mosby Co.
11. *Galloway, K.: The middle years: the change of life, Am. J. Nurs. **75**:1006-1011, 1975.
12. *Giffra, M.: Demystifying adolescent behavior, Am. J. Nurs. **75**:1724-1727, 1975.
13. Gould, R.: Adult life stages: growth toward self-tolerance, Psychology Today, pp. 74-78, Feb. 1975.
14. *Hargreaves, A.G.: Life in the middle years: making the most of the middle years, Am. J. Nurs. **75**:1772-1776, 1975.
15. Havighurst, R.J.: Perspectives on health care for the elderly, J. Gerontol. Nurs. **3**(2):21-24, 1977.
16. Howells, J.G., editor: Modern perspectives in the psychiatry of middle age, New York, 1981, Brunner/Mazel, Inc.
17. Hunt, M.: Sexual behavior in the 1970's, New York, 1974, Dell Publ. Co.
18. Illingworth, R.S.: The development of the infant and young child, New York, 1975, Churchill Livingstone.
19. Ivey, M.: Drug use. In Carnevali, D., and Patrick, M.: Nursing management for the elderly, Philadelphia, 1979, J. B. Lippincott Co.
20. *Johnson, L.: The middle years: living sensibly, Am. J. Nurs. **75**:1012-1016, 1975.
21. Johnson, T.R., Moore, W.M., and Jeffries, J.E.: Children are different: developmental physiology, ed. 2, Columbus, Ohio, 1978, Ross Laboratories.
22. Kalafitch, A.: Approaches to care of adolescents, Englewood Cliffs, New Jersey, 1975, Appleton-Century-Crofts.
23. Kaluger, G., and Kaluger, M.F.: Human development: the span of life, ed. 2, St. Louis, 1979, The C. V. Mosby Co.
24. Knox, A.B.: Adult development and learning, San Francisco, 1977, Jossey-Bass, Inc., Publishers.
25. Lawton, M.P., et al.: Community planning for an aging society, Stroudsburg, Pa., 1976, Dowden, Hutchinson & Ross, Inc.
26. Lidz, T.: The person: his and her development throughout the life cycle, rev. ed., New York, 1976, Basic Books, Inc., Publishers.
27. Lowery, G.H.: Growth and development of children, ed. 7, Chicago, 1978, Year Book Medical Publishers, Inc.
28. Makinodan, T., editor: Handbook of the biology of aging, New York, 1977, Van Nostrand Reinhold Co.
29. *Marx, J.: Crib death: some promising leads but no solution yet, Nurs. Digest **4**:12-15, 1975.
30. McKenny, P.C., Tishler, C.T., and Christman, K.L.: Adolescent suicide and the classroom teacher, J. Sch. Health **50**(3):130-132, 1980.
31. Murray, R., and Zentner, J.: Nursing assessment and health promotion through the life span, ed. 2, Englewood Cliffs, N.J., 1979, Prentice-Hall, Inc.
32. National Clearinghouse for Smoking and Health: Patterns and prevalence of teenage cigarette smoking: 1968, 1970, and 1972, pub. no. 919-684-3786, U.S. Department of Health, Education, and Welfare, Aug. 6, 1972.

33. Norman, W.H., and Scaramella, T.J., editors: Mid-life: developmental and clinical issues, New York, 1980, Brunner/Mazel, Inc.
34. Oill, P.A., and Mistell, D.R.: Symposium on adolescent gynecology and endocrinology: venereal disease in adolescents and contraception in teenagers, West. J. Med. **132**:39-48, 1980.
35. *Peplau, H.E.: Life in the middle years: mid-life crises, Am. J. Nurs. **75**:1761-1765, 1975.
36. Petrillo, M., and Sanger, S.: Emotional care of hospitalized children, ed. 2, Philadelphia, 1980, J.B. Lippincott Co.
37. Rachal, J.V., et al.: A national survey of adolescent drinking, behavior, attitudes, and correlates, National Institute of Alcohol Abuse and Alcoholism, U.S. Department of Health, Education, and Welfare, no. HSM 42-73-80 (HIA), April 1975.
38. *Roznoy, M.S.: The young adult: taking a sexual history, Am. J. Nurs. **76**:1279-1282, 1976.
39. Schuster, C.S., and Ashburn, S.: The process of human development, Boston, 1980, Little, Brown & Co.
40. Scipien, G., et al.: Comprehensive pediatric nursing, ed. 2, New York, 1981, McGraw-Hill-Book Co.
41. *Sheehy, G.: Passages, New York, 1976, E.P. Dutton & Co., Inc.
42. Shock, N.W.: Systemic physiology and aging: introduction. Fed. Proc. **38**(2):161-162, 1979.
43. *Shydro, J.: Child abuse, Nursing '72 **2**:37-41, 1972.
44. Starr, B.D., and Goldstein, H.S.: Human behavior and development, New York, 1975, Springer Publishing Co.
45. Source book on Aging, ed. 2, Marquis Academic Media, Chicago, 1979, Marquis Who's Who, Inc.
46. Stevenson, J.S.: Issues and crises during middlescence, New York, 1977, Appleton-Century-Crofts, Inc.
47. Sze, W.C.: Human life cycle, New York, 1975, Jason Aronson, Inc.
48. Troll, L.E.: Early and middle adulthood, Monterey, Calif., 1975, Brooks/Cole Publishing Co.
49. U.S. Department of Health, Education and Welfare: Approaches to adolescent health care in the 1970's, no. (HSA) 75-5014, 1975.
50. U.S. Department of Health, Education and Welfare: Working with older people, Public Health Service, no. 1459, vol. 2, Washington, D.C., 1970, U.S. Government Printing Office.
51. U.S. Department of Health, Education, and Welfare, Public Health Service, National Center for Health Statistics, 1975.
52. Whaley, L.F., and Wong, D.L.: Nursing care of infants and children, St. Louis, 1979, The C.V. Mosby Co.
53. Wolanin, M.D., and Phillips, L.R.F.: Confusion: prevention and care, St. Louis, 1981, The C.V. Mosby Co.
54. Woods, N.F.: Human sexuality in health and illness, St. Louis, 1978, The C.V. Mosby Co.
55. Zelnik, M., and Kantner, J.K.: Sexual activity, contraceptive use and pregnancy among metropolitan-area teenagers: 1971-1979, Fam. Plann. Perspect. **12**(5):230-231, 1980.
56. Zlatnik, F.G., and Burmeister, L.F.: Low gynecological age: an obstetric risk factor, Am. J. Obstet Gynecol. **128**:183-186, 1977.

Classic

57. Bhaskar, S.: Oral lesions of the aged population, Geriatrics **23**:137-149, 1968.
58. Cummings, E., and Henry, W.E.: Growing old, New York, 1955, Basic Book Co.
59. Diettert, G.: Circulation time in the aged, J.A.M.A. **183**:1037, 1963.
60. Erickson, E.H.: Childhood and society, ed. 2, New York, 1963, W.W. Norton & Co., Inc.
61. Goldfarb, W.: Effects of psychological deprivation in infancy and subsequent stimulation, Am. J. Psychiatr. **102**:18-23, 1945.
62. Havighurst, R.J., et al.: Psychology of aging, Bethesda Conference, Public Health Rep. **70**:837-856, 1955.

---

*References preceded by an asterisk are particularly well suited for student reading.

63. Maslow, A.: Motivation and personality, New York, 1954, Harper & Row.
64. Neugarten, B.L., editor: Middle age and aging, Chicago, 1968, The University of Chicago Press.
65. Neugarten, B.L.: Personality in middle and late life, New York, 1964, Atherton Press.
66. Strehler, B.L.: Time, cells and aging, New York, 1962, Academic Press.

AUDIOVISUAL RESOURCES

A visit with Clipper: Media Center, Children's Hospital National Medical Center, Washington, DC 20009.

Aging: 16-mm color film, CRM educational films, 1104 Camino Del Mar, Del Mar, CA 92014.

Denver developmental screening test: Series of films, Ladoca films, Denver, CO.

Patient mental health, psychological growth and adjustment: Color filmstrip and audiotape, Westinghouse Learning Corp., Oakland, IL 60453.

Perspectives on aging, Costa Mesa, Calif., Concept media.

Play in hospital: 16-mm color film, Campus Film Distributors Corp., 2 Overhill Road, Scarsdale, NY 10583.

To prepare a child: 16-mm color films, Media Center, Children's Hospital National Medical Center, Washington, DC 20009.

CHAPTER 17

DEATH AND DYING

JANET LARSON GELEIN

This chapter is about death and the process of dying in America. Birth and death are two processes that are inevitable to all people. Birth is generally perceived as a joyous, exciting event in our society; death is often something dreaded, feared, and denied. For nurses who have the responsibility of assisting individuals with the event of death, an assessment of their own feelings and reactions is as important as the assessment of the individual who is facing death. Only after nurses acquire an awareness of and appreciation for their own values and beliefs can they reach out to help others. An examination of the factors in American society that affect attitudes toward dying can help nurses gain an awareness of not only their own, but also their clients' beliefs about death and dying.

Factors affecting attitudes about death and dying

A newspaper revealed the following account:

Mr. S.'s son died November 8 of injuries suffered in an auto accident. He won't be buried. Instead, Mr. S. said, the body will remain in a casket with a clear plastic top in a room off the family's kitchen. Mr. S. went on to say: "There are three especially painful moments at the death of a loved one. The first is at the news of the death, the second when you see the body in the casket at the funeral home, and the third and most difficult is when you have to turn away from the grave site and know you'll never see that person again. We simply decided not to go through that last step."*

*From *Durham Morning Herald*, July 25, 1975, Louisville, Ky. Printed with permission of The Associated Press.

In the following pages, four characteristics of life in America that may have influenced the attitudes and behaviors of Mr. S. and his family will be explored. The four factors implied by the acronym LIFE are *L*ongevity, *I*solation, *F*amily life, and *E*nvironment for the dying. This discussion will consider how these social phenomena influence those persons and their families who are confronting death, as well as those who care for the dying.

Longevity

The United States may be described as a nation of aging citizens. Today the average life expectancy is 72 years, as compared to 1900 when it was 47 years. Low infant mortality, control of infectious diseases, and improved socioeconomic conditions have prolonged life. A decreasing birthrate has produced an increased proportion of older persons in our society.

Mortality control has been facilitated by technology and modernized American society. Medical sciences have developed the technology for extending life. Intensive care units, kidney dialysis, heart-lung machines, respirators, artificial pacemakers, and transplanted organs have all prolonged lives. These technologies have created a dilemma for nursing and medicine: no longer can clinical death be clearly defined. Although technologies directed toward prolongation of life have received much emphasis in medical research, there have been few investigations of the quality of the lives our technologies have extended.

The "modernization" of our society implies career specialization and social mobility.[15] Long-term planning is demanded of modern economies; as a consequence, society values youth and invests energy and resources

TABLE 17-1. Nursing care homes and related care facilities: 1939 to 1978*

Measurement criteria	1939	1963	1969	1973	1976	1978
Facilities	1200	16,701	18,910	21,834	20,468	18,722
Beds (1000)	25	569	944	1328	1415	1349

*From U.S. National Center for Health Statistics: Health Resources Statistics, Washington, D.C., 1980, Public Health Service.

in the education of children to prepare for the specialized careers and leadership positions of tomorrow. The modernization of an aging American society, with an emphasis on youth, has evolved—but not without consequences.

The aged, who in many ways provide us with physical proof of our own mortality, are frequently relegated to institutions or retirement villages that shield us from the realities of aging and approaching death.[12] The number of nursing care homes and homes for the aged grew considerably until 1973. Since then the numbers have gradually decreased (Table 17-1).

Decreased mortality and increased segregation of the elderly reduce regular confrontations with death. "When death is confined largely to the elderly—those retired from work, finished with direct parental responsibilities—and handled within specialized bureaucracies, mortality becomes removed from the daily business of social life. The 'nonpresence' of death in modern societies physically and socially removes the death of man from the life of society."[12] According to one author, the modern emphasis on youth, health, sports cars, long vacations, and longevity has led people to see death as an infringement on their basic rights to both life and the pursuit of happiness.[57]

Isolation

Americans live in a culture that in many ways isolates them from direct confrontation with death. Recent national data indicate that over half of all deaths in this country occur in institutions, either hospitals, convalescent homes, nursing homes, or other domiciliary institutions.[23]

Contemporary burial customs also isolate individuals from the dead. Mittford[72] provides insight into the burial customs and practices in America. What one may assume to be accepted custom, elaborate funeral arrangements, commercially prepared flowers, and so on, may be designed for profit of the funeral director, rather than for support of the next-of-kin. There is little resemblance between the funeral practices of today and those of even 50 to 100 years ago.

From colonial times to the nineteenth century, funeral practices were almost exclusively a family affair.

Friends of the family and family members were responsible for the body after death. After washing, wrapping, and placing the body in a wooden casket, they placed it in the family parlor for all mourners to grieve over. What today is viewed as the funeral director's responsibility was yesterday largely the task of the family and close friends.

This observed change in family responsibility for care after death is only one outcome of the changes in the structure of family life over the past century. Several other features of the family in modern society have changed our relationship to the dying and beliefs and attitudes about death.

Family life

Families, as a unit of American society, provide an environment for their young members to learn social roles and acquire values. Some changes in family life in our society that have influenced value systems and role relationships within the family are the size of the family unit, mobility, and the decline in the influence of religion.

In societies with high mortalities, social organization and identification are around kinship units. Extended families are necessary for survival; they function to allocate status, distribute goods, and exercise power. With the immediate threat of death always present, isolated individuals without support are prone to a precarious existence. In American society, families are often isolated from extended kin and lack their close support when confronting death.

In traditional, early American society an extended family provided multiple resources for a single family member facing death. The dying individual and family were often supported by grandparents, aunts, uncles, and other relatives. This extended family provided a system of relationships that drew together resources in times of need. Today family members must depend on each other for assistance, manage by themselves, or cope with a crisis through the utilization of resources provided within the community. For some single persons, friends become the significant others and serve in lieu of the family.

A family's ability to utilize community resources depends somewhat on its familiarity with available resources and its knowledge and skill in using them. Rapid social mobility of families has influenced these skills. With a change in residence comes the need for developing new social relationships and the ability to orient oneself quickly to the resources within a community. If the family lacks these relationships or abilities to allocate and procure supports, they may cope with death or dying in relative isolation. To some families, their religion and church may be support in such times of need.

Studies of American cultures tend to reflect an emerging secular attitude toward death. Today death has become a subject for scientific investigation and rationalization. The decline of religious influence has been cited as one of the factors contributing to the fragmentation of caring for the dying and their significant others.[17] One writer suggests that the decline of religions and the emergence of secularism is related to the needs that religion satisfies in American society. If a society is confronted with frequent deaths and life is precarious, social institutions are needed to explain death. When mortality is decreased and concentrated among the elderly, as it is in American society, the need to explain why we should die is decreased.[49]

Recent literature suggests a return to more spiritual and, in some instances, mystical concerns. Moody[28] has documented the religious experiences of those who have survived life-threatening events. Descriptions of those persons have included "life-after-life" or "out-of-body" experiences. These persons reported observing events surrounding their "deaths" and related feelings of moving toward a deity toward a peaceful "out-of-body" existence. The lay literature also contains references to faith healing and therapies that transcend clinical sciences. Perhaps literature such as this indicates a trend away from the secularization of death and a movement toward a more spiritual orientation toward death.

Environment for dying

Increasingly, people are dying in health care institutions. More than half of the deaths in America occur within an institutional setting. Removed from a familiar home dwelling, individuals facing death are often subjected to a mechanical, dehumanized environment in an institutional setting. Kübler-Ross speaks about the person dying in an institutional environment and the reactions of health care providers:

He may cry for rest, peace, and dignity, but he will get transfusions, a heart machine, or tracheostomy if necessary. He may want one single person to stop for one single minute so that he can ask one single question—but he will get a dozen people around the clock, all busily preoccupied with his heart rate, pulse, electrocardiogram or pulmonary functions, his se-

cretions or excretions but not with him as a human being. He may wish to fight since all this is done in the fight for his life, and if they can save his life they can consider the person afterwards. Those who consider the person first may lose precious time to save his life! At least this seems to be the rationale or justification behind all this—or is it? Is the reason for this increasingly mechanical, depersonalized approach our own defensiveness? Is this approach our own way to cope with and repress the anxieties that a terminally or critically ill patient evokes in us? Is our concentration on equipment, on blood pressure our desperate attempt to deny the impending death which is so frightening and discomforting to us that we displace all our knowledge onto machines, since they are less close to us than the suffering face of another human being which would remind us once more of our lack of omnipotence, our own limits and failure, and last but not least perhaps our own mortality?*

Confrontation with death: a holistic approach

The primary goal of the nurse assisting an individual who is confronting death is to *maximize the coping processes of the dying person in order to promote an appropriate death*. An appropriate death implies that the individual completes the act of dying in a manner that is meaningful to that person's existence. This goal protects an individual's autonomy and personal dignity and provides a climate for persons to express their needs and control their own destiny. The following discussion may assist the nurse with an assessment of factors influencing the coping processes in individuals confronting death.

Coping processes

Death may occur at various ages, at different rates, and with a different degree of participation from the individual involved. Coping processes are the strategies used by an individual when confronting a crisis such as death. The strategy used will depend on the individual's perception of death and the anticipated threat or harm associated with death. Unless death is perceived as an agent of harm, direct forms of coping, such as avoidance or attack, are not possible—one must be able to identify the threat if one is to avoid or attack it.[67]

In some circumstances death is not a threat but a release or welcome relief from a painful existence.

*From Kübler-Ross, E.: On death and dying, New York, 1969, Macmillan Publishing Co., Inc. Copyright © 1969 by Elisabeth Kübler-Ross.

To the person contemplating suicide, life may be more painful than the prospect of death itself. However, for the individual who appraises death and defines it as threatening, the process of coping is initiated to reduce, eliminate, or master the anticipated harm. Coping is mobilized by the realization that life, health, cherished relationships, or wealth is in danger.

One nurse author[25] states that in general people respond to dying in the same way they have responded to stresses and crises throughout their lives. Some persons will continue to prefer making decisions regarding their own lives if possible, whereas others will prefer having decisions made for them, patterns that were established during their lifetimes. Some individuals will continue to protect their privacy, whereas others will share their thoughts; some will confront issues and others will avoid them, and so forth. Coping styles used during life will usually continue to be used when living through the dying period.

The individual's response to death may be influenced by perception, beliefs and value systems, developmental level, sex and social role, education and intellectual resources, ego strength and coping style, and time and mode of dying along with situational supports and the social structural setting in which the individual dies. An assessment of each of these variables and their influence on the person facing death can provide the nurse with insight into the coping processes available to a person who is dying.

In caring for the individual who is confronting death, it is useful to consider three sets of variables: (1) factors related to the *configuration of death*, (2) elements within the *psychologic structure of the individual*, and (3) characteristics of the *situational and social structural setting* in which the individual is facing death. These variables may influence the coping process in the individual confronting death (Fig. 17-1).

Configuration of death

The configuration of death or the stimulus that promotes confrontation with death may be *external* or *internal* in nature. For example, an individual may confront death through an accident, homicide, or suicide (situational—external in nature) or through genetic factors or illness (biologic—organic or internal in nature). These two classifications are not mutually exclusive, and often situational and organic processes interact simultaneously to promote death. For example, an individual with a terminal illness may be experiencing such intense pain and turmoil that the person commits suicide to hasten dying.

Another factor related to the configuration of death is the *temporal aspect of dying*, which refers to the time when certain death will occur, or when uncertain death will be resolved. Glaser and Strauss, who have studied the temporal features of dying in hospitals, have identified four types of death expectations associated with dying. These death expectations refer to the "degree of certainty" or the degree to which the defining person is convinced the patient will die and the time expectations related to this certainty, which may vary from minutes to months. Four types of death expectations based on certainty and time are (1) certain death at a known time, (2) certain death at an unknown time, (3) uncertain death but a known time when certainty will be established, and (4) uncertain death and an unknown time when the question will be resolved.[59] These time variables, along with expectations of persons confronting death, may affect the interactions and coping mechanisms of the dying individual.

Psychologic structure of the individual

Aspects of the psychologic structure of an individual that may influence coping and behavior when confronting death are perception, beliefs and value systems, de-

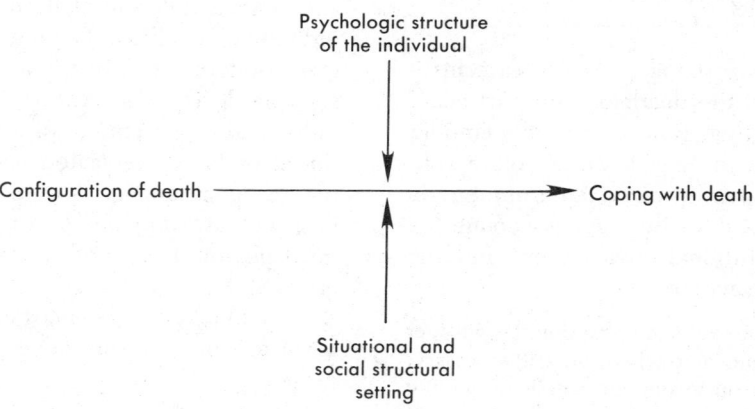

Fig. 17-1. Coping with death.

velopmental level, ego strength and coping style, education and intellectual resources, and sex and social role. Selected aspects of these will be discussed next.

Perceptions. Perceptions vary when one examines confrontations with death. Cognitive appraisal of the configuration of death involves an interaction between the individual, judgment about the meaning and future significance of death or dying, and the properties of the situation in which the person confronts death. Coping processes are initiated first through perception and then mediated through situational-environmental elements that result in an observable behavioral response. The nurse interacting with an individual coping with death, and concerned with maximizing this individual's resources in this confrontation, will be cognizant of those factors believed to influence perception of death.

Perception involves the process of appraisal, which requires the cognitive activities of choice, discrimination, and judgment. The statement "I will die" implies the ability to formulate concepts such as the following:

1. I am an individual with a life of my own, a personal existence.
2. I belong to a class of beings, one of whose attributes is mortality.
3. Using the intellectual process of logical deduction, I arrive at the conclusion that my personal death is a certainty.
4. There are many possible causes of my death, and these causes might operate in many different combinations. Although I might evade or escape one particular cause, I cannot evade all causes.
5. My death will occur in the future. By the future, I mean a time-to-live that has not yet elapsed.
6. But I do not know when in the future my death will occur. The event is certain; the timing is uncertain.
7. Death is a final event. My life ceases. This means that I will never again experience, think, or act, at least as a human being on this earth.
8. Accordingly death is the ultimate separation of myself from the world.*

How an individual perceives a confrontation with death will partially depend on his appraisal of this constellation of abstract concepts. One factor influencing this appraisal is the developmental level of the individual.

Developmental level. Appraisals of death seem to vary throughout the life span. The examination of perceptions and the development of death conceptions will be reviewed by considering three broad areas of growth and development: childhood, adulthood, and late maturity. Perceptions of death or deathlike attributes are considered to be the forerunners of death conceptions.

INFANCY AND EARLY CHILDHOOD. Conceptions of death in childhood may be roughly divided into three

broad age categories: infancy and early childhood (birth to 5 years), middle and late childhood (5 to 10 years), and adolescence (10 to 20 years). Mauer has proposed that selected processes associated with being and nonbeing are evident even in the *newborn infant*. Periodic sleeping and waking cycles are considered to be the first introduction to an appreciation of being and nonbeing. This phenomenon is followed by infant experimentation involving a variety of disappearance-and-return games such as "peekaboo" and "all-gone." (Peekaboo is believed to have originated from an Old English phrase meaning "alive or dead.") Through such activities the infant begins to develop a conception of self and organismically becomes involved in states of being and nonbeing.[68]

The *infant* and *young child* are exposed to a variety of feelings toward death; however, it is generally accepted that a child of this age does not have a conception of personal mortality.[1,8] Nagy, in her studies on Hungarian children, made one of the most important contributions to the psychology of children and their conceptions of death. Her work considered children from 3 to 10 years of age. The first stage she described, from 3 to 5 years, is a time when the child views death as continuous with life. Death is not recognized as final; rather, the child in this stage explains death as a reversible or temporary departure. Even though the child may recognize death as a physical event, he cannot separate it from life; he considers death as gradual or temporary.[72]

MIDDLE AND LATE CHILDHOOD. Sometime between the ages of 5 and 10 the child begins to comprehend that death is final. Death to a child at the beginning of this stage of development is often metaphorically personified as a "death man" or person. Children may describe death as the bogeyman, a skeleton, angel, or witch. Generally, death is conceived as reversible and some-

---

DEVELOPMENTAL STAGES AND SELECTED RESPONSES OF CHILD TO DEATH

Developmental stage	Selected response to death
Birth	Physiologic reaction to "death agony"
5 to 6 mo	Reacts to disease symptoms and treatment procedures
2 to 4 yr	Aware of changes in personal self: separateness, "me," "I," "not me"
5 to 7 yr	Appreciates death as a final separation from life; reacts to prognosis; changes in social role and relationships

---

*From Kastenbaum, R., and Aisenburg, R.: The psychology of death, New York, 1972, Springer Publishing Co., Inc.

thing that can be avoided. To the child in middle childhood, death is still something separate from his own being. "Run faster than the death-man, lock the door, trick him, somehow, elude Mr. Death and you will not die."[17]

In later childhood, around age 9 or 10, children come to develop the conception of death as final, universal, and inevitable.[71] Anthony found two dominant themes in a child's conceptions of death at this age: sorrowful separation and the ultimate result of aggression.[47] Children in late childhood may be concerned about their own deaths and the death of parents or pets. Zeligs believes that children around this age fear death and keep it at a distance.[82]

A child's perception of death is influenced by the developmental capacity to conceive the meaning of death; however, the child responds to selected aspects of death long before conceptualizing "I will die" (see box, p. 251). Since the young child does not conceptualize death, perceptions of confronting death are often associated with the reactions of others, bodily instincts, and sensations. As one advances up the scale of growth and development, behavior increasingly depends on learning rather than instinct.

ADOLESCENCE. One particularly relevant conception about death acquired during this age span is the conception of time. An adult conception of time is achieved around age 13 to 15; however, *adolescents* seem to prefer to limit their conceptions of time to the immediate future.[63,78] To adolescents the prospect of death is a threat to future identity; in an attempt to deny this possibility, they prefer to live in the present or near future. The rationale for this orientation may be that death threatens the adolescent's possibility of becoming the self that he or she values and seeks to become. Adolescents cannot bolster a sense of identity by looking back on a lifetime, nor are they at a stable point in their current existence. Instead, they are emerging.[17]

To adolescents, death is something that exists in the future. Through extending the time between life today and death sometime in the distant future, adolescents successfully create a psychologic distance between themselves and death. One study indicated that adolescents who displayed high manifest concern over death were limited in their abilities to project into the future.[52] Time appears to serve as an insulation between the adolescent's present self and eventual death. A direct confrontation with death in adolescence may promote one of several responses. The early adolescent (ages 10 to 14) with a growing need for independence is vulnerable to rejection and loneliness when confronting death. Growing away from parental and family ties and moving toward peer groups, gangs, and crowds for support, the dying adolescent may feel rejected by parents and isolated from peers. Midadolescence (ages 14 to 16) brings increased self-confidence and an achievement of

self-identity: adolescents now follow their own standards. To the competent adolescent who has just begun to feel mastery, death represents defeat.[8] Finally, approaching adulthood, late adolescents (ages 17 to 20), alive and in love with the world, are likely to perceive death as the loss of a rich and meaningful relationship that they have just attained.[8]

ADULTHOOD. Erikson[54] suggests that young adulthood is a time of intimacy in which individuals emerge from the search for and insistence on identity and are ready to fuse their identity with that of another. It is also a period when physical and mental vigor are at the peak of development. To the adult who has expanded the ego and become less egocentric, and who may have a spouse and family, confrontation with death may intensify feelings about loss of physical and mental control, body image disturbances, and role expectations.

Another author describes a crisis of midadulthood that accompanies the realization that one is growing old and approaching the latter half of life. Paradoxically, the adult is at a midpoint in life: he simultaneously enters the prime of life and a stage of fulfillment and recognizes that death lies beyond.[16]

There is relatively little literature about the adult confronting death in comparison to the literature on children and the elderly. Perhaps the dying adult is too close to the lives of those who are involved in the research on death. Choron[50] suggests that humans tend to suppress the part of reality emphasizing finitude rather than adjusting to death. One of the early studies on adult attitudes toward death demonstrated that the adult considers death in much the same way as a child. This study revealed that the adult conceived of death as an unnatural end of life: the result of a violent act, either an accident or catastrophe.[49]

Kastenbaum and Aisenburg describe a contemporary personification of death in adults. The automaton is an image of death, an unfeeling instrument in the guise of a human. The automaton advances an automatic or soulless apparatus devoid of emotion.[17] If personifications tell us something about an individual's conception of his place in the universe and the meaning of life, there is something rather absurd about the personification of death as a nonperson. The automaton may be part of a broader image of the universe—a vast chamber whose design is indifferent to the feelings and purposes of humans.[17] Perhaps this orientation to humans accounts for some of the dehumanized, mechanical care the dying often receive from adult health care professionals in an institutional setting.

LATE MATURITY. From a developmental perspective, the unique feature of old age is the inevitability of death, bringing with it the task of integrating one's past life and the acceptance of one's own death. To the elderly person who has formed basic values, achieved life goals, and developed a conception of self, one of the final tasks of life is the achievement of integrity. Elderly individuals with a sense of integrity are ready to defend the dignity of their own life-styles against physical and economic threats. In such final consolidation, Erikson notes that death loses its sting.[54] Several studies on the attitudes of elderly people toward death indicate that only a small number of old people fear death.[56,61,71]

The meaning given to aging and approaching death depends to a great extent on one's interpretation of the immediate and total life situation. Elderly persons who do not develop or socially inherit adequate modes for shaping experience may experience aging as a marking of time that is devoid of purpose; losses and impairments appear without pattern from both the self and environment.[62] In one context the distinction between modes of relating potentialities is referred to as the "clinging person" and the "letting-go person." The "clinging persons" are secretly frightened by the passage of time and their own mortality. These are events that they cannot personally subdue or control. The "letting-go persons" allow themselves to experience the passage of time and their own aging, with its bodily manifestations. Their feeling life, unlike their aging limbs, need not become rigid and arthritic.[83]

The possible importance of one's ability to grasp the concept of a future and, with this, death, may play more of a role in present behavior than we now assume. A contemporary novel about the lives and deaths of several aging individuals depicts how some elderly individuals reflect anxiety toward approaching death while others recount that to remember one's death is in short, a way of life.[77] Death, a universal and inevitable experience, is a fact of human existence.

Sequential responses to death. Coping processes used by individuals confronting death have been described by authors, poets, clinicians, and investigators involved with various aspects of death and dying. Generally, the processes used by individuals facing death have been analyzed from two perspectives: as *sequential* responses to death and as *tactics* unique to the life-style of the person confronting death. Examples of the sequential responses to coping with death include the theories of Kübler-Ross, Engel, and Weisman.

Kübler-Ross has delineated five psychologic stages related to the process of dying. Stage one is characterized by *shock* and *denial:* "No, not me." The second stage involves *anger* and *rage:* "Why me?" During the third stage, *bargaining* occurs: "Yes, me, but. . . ." Stage four is characterized by *depression* and *preparatory grief:* "It *is* me. . . .what's the use?" Stage five, *acceptance*, could be characterized by "I am ready"; it is seen as a final rest before the long journey.[66] Kübler-Ross has stimulated deep concern among many health care professionals for a humanistic approach in the care of the dying. However, clinical research on the process

of dying has not supported a predictable order to the five stages described by her theory.[37] Rather, it has been observed that these stages may vary in their order and may even recur in a cyclic fashion. In any case, her work has provided health professionals with a heightened awareness of the way people adapt to impending death, and the fact that *hope* may be the single most important factor in this process.

Weisman, who examined the psychodynamics of death, found that denial occurred in four sequential steps. First, the person accepts the public perception that death may occur. Next, a portion of the shared meaning of that public perception is repudiated. Third, the dying person replaces the repudiated meaning with a more congenial version that is acceptable. Finally, the individual reorients himself or herself within the scope of the total meaning in order to accommodate a revised reality.[43] These steps in the development of denial seem to result in the constant interplay between disbelief and hope. Interactions between acceptance and denial, understanding that one is dying and magically disbelieving it, may reflect a deeper dialogue of the human mind that involves different layers of the conscious awareness: knowing, yet needing not to know.[76]

Engel provides a framework for viewing those who are *bereaved*. The sequence of events comprising normal grief reactions include shock and disbelief, developing awareness, and restitution. The first reaction, *shock and disbelief*, helps the bereaved gradually become aware of the loss. It can be characterized as "numbness." As *awareness* develops, the bereaved demonstrates sadness and anger in ways modulated by culture. Finally, *restitution* involves resolving the loss and idealizing the person who was lost.[53] *Mourning* may continue for several years, and the process cannot be accelerated.

Furthermore, it is important for nurses to recognize that just as the individual's response to the threat of death varies, so does the family's response. It is also important to bear in mind that the individual's and family's responses may be at variance with one another; the family may have accepted the individual's death as inevitable whereas the individual is still denying it. This is illustrated well by the family who has accepted the inevitable death of their loved one and subsequently has their hopes resurrected by remission of a terminal illness. The individual may continue to live with a family who is mourning his or her loss.

These sequential responses to death that incorporate the defense mechanisms of anger, denial, shock, and depression provide useful frameworks for the assessment of coping activity. However, nurses must also consider several other factors related to the individual that are equally influential in the process of coping.

Life-style approach. An alternative perspective of coping activity and death is termed the life-style approach. Life-style, a term that has been popularized in the gerontology literature, refers to a general attribute of the social system of individuals, governing the person's investment and involvement in areas of living.[81] It is believed that all people develop a primary style of living that influences their expectations and interactions with others. One's life-style affects attitudes and beliefs about living and may influence choices related to the process of dying.

McCoy explores the relationship between life-style and the final achievement of death. She describes the following styles of living: *accepting, defiant, sensual, humorous, tragic,* and *questing.* Each life-style has positive and negative aspects. Each individual prepares for death in much the same manner as he or she participates in life. This does not mean that individuals cannot change their life-style or process of coping, or that they have a predestined style of dying. Rather, each person, through being aware of the self, expresses a style of living that has implications for his or her death. Although one cannot choose to avoid death indefinitely, one may be able to make choices about how to die and to die in one's own style.[27]

Social structural setting

Humans, when confronting death, are influenced by their environment—social structural setting, family, community, society, and culture—and likewise affect their environment through behavioral responses. Structures unique to the individual and external structures affect the coping process and resultant behavior. This discussion explores the social structural setting as a factor in the individual's confrontation with death.

The social structural setting where a person dies will influence coping and behavior in the process of dying. A major factor influencing the person who is dying in an institutional environment is the *loss of control:* the power to influence awareness, the information received about one's health or illness, and the means to relieve pain, suffering, isolation, and loneliness.

Awareness. Many physicians believe in being reticent with the dying. Studies report that 69% to 90% of physicians are opposed to telling a patient the truth, while 77% to 89% of all patients with a terminal illness want to be told.[55] In a sample of 52 terminally ill patients, one author found that 82% wanted to be informed about their condition for such reasons as "to settle affairs," "to make various financial and family arrangements," because they "don't want to be denied the experience of realizing that I am dying," and because they want to "have time to come to live with the idea, and to learn to die."[55]

Two sociologists have examined information given to terminal patients and the resultant patterns of interaction between staff and patients in an institutional setting. They use the term *awareness context* to describe what each interacting person knows of the patient's defined status, as well as each person's perception of the others' awareness of his or her definition. The total picture of an awareness context is complex and changes over time. The following types of awareness are described: *closed awareness, suspicion awareness, mutual pretense,* and *open awareness.* Each awareness context includes tactics for interaction that guide communication and behavior based on what each person knows and with what degree of certainty.[55]

In a *closed awareness* context the patient does not recognize impending death even though hospital personnel have this information. Initially, these patients believe they will recover and continue to live as though they had a temporary illness; however, as new symptoms develop and continued treatment and medication are required, these persons begin to question their diagnoses. The potential consequence of this context is a feeling of betrayal and a loss of trust in care givers when and if the truth is revealed.

Suspicion awareness is the situation that exists when patients do not know but suspect in varying degrees that others believe them to be dying. Continued therapy along with deteriorating bodily changes arouse suspicions of terminality. This context becomes a fencing match with the patient on the offensive and the health team on the defensive. The staff will determine whether the patient will play a mutual pretense game or move to an open awareness context.

Mutual pretense is the context in which both staff and patient are aware that the patient is dying but choose to pretend otherwise. This context is the most predominant one seen in an institutional setting. In some ways this pretense may yield a measure of dignity or privacy for the patient, since it minimizes the interactional strain that could exist in an open awareness between staff, patient, and family. Since many staff members are uncomfortable in their interactions with dying patients and their families, this context is one that promotes safe topics of discussion—conversation about most anything but death. The consequence of this context is that it does not allow the patient to express needs or share feelings related to dying. Observations of terminally ill, institutionalized elderly persons suggest that they wish to express their thoughts about death but do not have anyone to listen to them.[59]

Open awareness exists when both staff and patient know that the patient is dying and acknowledge it in their actions. This context provides patients an opportunity to close their lives according to their own ideas of dying. However, open awareness is not a context that necessarily promotes adaptation. Certain potential consequences also exist, since once patients are aware of their diagnoses, they are held responsible for their actions as dying persons. Glaser and Strauss observed that health professionals perceive certain standards of proper conduct for dying such as courageous, decent behavior, relative composure, and cheerfulness.[59]

Should nurses expect all people to accept death with courage and composure? How do nurses react to patients who fear death or who rage with anger when death draws near? Nurses who promote a social structural setting for an appropriate death do not assume that all individuals will accept death. A nurse who shared some lessons from a dying patient revealed: "And the question must still remain: Must there be a 'happy' ending, or isn't the struggle not to die as much a successful adjustment for some as is a peaceful death for others?"[76]

The social structural setting that provides for an appropriate death is one that enhances individuals' rights to express emotions and feelings as they choose. A closed or *suspicion awareness* context does not enhance the expression of needs; in these contexts those around the patient are in control. They have decided to withhold selected information about the individual, and through making such a decision, the individual does not have the right to control the last phase of life. However, information about health or illness is not a sole prerequisite for the expression of needs related to dying. The individual confronting death may elect to establish a *mutual pretense* context and feel most comfortable discussing topics unrelated to illness or approaching death. The nurse does not assume that all people will be open with their feelings about dying. "Tacit communication can actually be quite successful: the patient is grateful for being spared the emotional pain of discussing his fate."[80] Nurses participating in a *mutual pretense* context, however, must be comfortable enough with their own feelings and beliefs about death to be attuned to cues that a patient desires to change the context from mutual pretense to open awareness. Often a nurse's own anxiety about dying patients prevents the establishment of an open awareness context. Hackett and Weisman[60] have observed that some patients prefer to avoid the truth rather than risk the withdrawal of those who cannot confront death.

Pain and suffering. Chapter 23 describes the assessment of pain and nursing interventions for pain. This discussion will review selected issues related to the form of suffering we call pain as it is experienced by the dying. Pain accompanies birth, growth, disease, and death and thus is intertwined with most of human existence.[48] Pain is an individual experience; and like death, pain can only be defined introspectively, as each person defines it for himself or herself.

Although pain is an individual experience, the social structural setting in which the individual experiences pain may influence perception and response to pain. Saunders,[35] an authority on the nature and management of pain in the terminally ill, advocates constant pain control to permit dying persons to take part in suitable activities and enjoy open visiting hours with their families. One of the most difficult aspects of pain in the terminally ill is that it appears to be meaningless as well as endless, often bringing a sense of isolation and despair. Regular doses of analgesics seem to decrease the threat and anxiety associated with this pain and reduce the guilt and despair of family members.[36]

When an individual is in an institution that discourages self-control of pain, pain relief is frequently in the form of a "demand schedule." The demand schedule is usually referred to as prn medication for pain, meaning "whenever the nurse judges the patient needs pain relief." A demand schedule can constitute a very demoralizing experience for both the patient and the nurse. The nurse must watch for symptoms of pain; the patient must withstand more pain before it is reduced by the nurse's action.[59] Alternatives to this demand schedule are self-administration of pain medication or a regimen that provides constant control of pain, such as that advocated by Saunders.

Suffering is a response to pain. Pain has been conceived of as a universal language: it produces an outcry that evokes help from others.[48] The nature of this help may influence the perception of pain and suffering. Sometimes the inability of helpers to relate to those who are dying and to ease pain through the therapeutic use of self results in the oversedation and tranquilization of those in need of help. Kübler-Ross, in discussing the use of psychopharmacologic agents for the dying patient and the bereaved, expressed the belief that the dosage and number of drugs prescribed might be used as an index of the comfort (or discomfort) of the prescribing physician. She equates sedation of the dying with the health professional's discomfort in caring for them.[20] Perhaps if nurses gave more of themselves, rather than of sedatives and tranquilizers, the pain and suffering that accompany some dying could be eased. As the next discussion on loneliness and isolation will explore, the art of caring may decrease suffering.

Loneliness and isolation. The beginning of this chapter explored characteristics of American society that influence attitudes and behaviors toward death and dying. The following discussion will consider how the dying individual perceives the actions of others. A dying professor shared these perceptions: "The nonverbal response, the avoidance itself, generates considerable anxiety, fear, and confusion on the part of any patient in that kind of situation."[32] Another young girl dying of cancer expressed these feelings, "I don't think dying would be so tough if it could be shared with those around you. There are times when I feel people are really avoiding me and it is a sinking sensation to feel you are being isolated." It is widely accepted that for many who confront death, death itself is often less of a threat than the process of dying and the perception of loneliness and isolation.

The perception of loneliness and isolation is enhanced by many rituals that exist within an institutional setting. Hospital practices such as limiting visitors, moving the dying to single rooms, rotating assignments of personnel, closing doors, and "hushing" discussions on deaths of patients are all strategies for decreasing the anxiety associated with dying. These practices limit interaction between the dying individual, family, and staff. They also decrease the possibility of threatening questions to the staff. As the father of a dying child revealed, "Death always brings one suddenly face to face with life. . . . It raises all the infinite questions, each answer ending in another question.[74] Inability to feel at ease with these questions is one reason for isolation of the dying—rituals and formalities in hospitals promote a comfortable distance between the nurse and death.

Isolation of the dying creates feelings of loneliness. The basic reason for loneliness is that human beings experience the self out of their relatedness to other persons; without other persons, they fear they will lose the experience of being a self.[69] Loneliness has been described as a response to a relational deficit and the product of emotional or social isolation.[44] If the process of dying results in the loss of a truly intimate tie, such as the lack of relationships with a child, parent, spouse, or lover, the individual may experience *emotional isolation*. The loneliness of *social isolation* is a consequence of the lack of a network of involvement with peers, fellow workers, kinfolk, neighbors, or friends.[43] Loneliness that results from social or emotional isolation has been decreased in some settings that provide care for the terminally ill. St. Christopher's Hospice in Sydenham, England, is probably best known for the care given there to dying persons.

The hospice, unlike the hospital that treats sick people, is a place where people come to die. This concept of a hospice is just beginning to develop in the United States. St. Christopher's Hospice, of which Dr. Cicely Saunders is the founder and medical director, has few rituals and institutional rules. To decrease social and emotional isolation and loneliness, visiting hours are unlimited, except for Monday—the "family day off." Children are welcomed as visitors, and there is no age limit on visitations. Family pets also frequent the hospice. Families are encouraged and helped to care for their loved ones.[13]

At St. Christopher's the staff understands and practices the concept of caring. One nurse who visited the setting reflected, "The secret of the care of patients is still caring."[16] Patients are encouraged to have as much control over their daily lives as possible. When a resident dies, the staff makes a point of giving the others in a ward the chance to talk about it. Things do not take precedence over people; the nurse takes time to care, to see the person as an individual, and to hear and respond to questions of worried families. This caring part of St. Christopher's can be emulated in any setting. For

the individual confronting death, the issue seems to be not *how many days*, but *what kind of days* are left.

Health professionals. Several studies indicate that not all nurses respond in the most supportive manner with dying patients. One psychologist who examined the amount of time required to respond to call bells at the bedside of hospitalized patients found that nurses took longer to respond to requests for help from patients with terminal prognoses.[62] Another study found that nurses displayed a variety of behavioral strategies to maintain "professional demeanor" in work situations with the dying.[64] Yet another study demonstrated that nursing students with the least experience in caring for dying persons were actually better able to provide human comfort during lengthy assignments to dying patients than those with more experience.[73] Nurses need to ask themselves if, rather than providing humanistic care, they become less human with continued personal contact with the institutionalized dying individual. Also, they need to discern whether their own anxieties and concerns about death are preventing them from humanely caring for those most often dependent on them for their needs—those who are dying.

Caring. If nurses are attuned to their own beliefs and feelings as well as those of the individual who is dying, they will create a social structural setting that facilitates an appropriate death. Such a setting would be one in which the nurse cares enough to help the person die in a manner than is meaningful to existence. This element of caring was succinctly summarized by a dying student nurse: "Please believe me, if you care, you can't go wrong. Just admit that you care. That is really for what we search. We may ask for why's and wherefore's, but we really don't expect answers. Don't run away . . . wait . . . all I want to know is that there is someone to hold my hand when I need it. . . . Then, it might not be so hard to die . . . in a hospital . . . with friends close by."[6]

Caring for another person is a process that involves development such as that involved as a friendship emerges: through mutual trust and through a deepening and qualitative transforming of the relationship.[26] Mayeroff[26] describes eight major ingredients of caring: *knowing, alternating rhythms, patience, honesty, truth, humility, hope,* and *courage*. These ingredients can be applied to the nurse who cares for the dying in the following ways:

1. *Knowing*. To respond to another who is in need and to care, I must first know myself. I continue to refine my philosophy of life and death and recognize my powers and limitations. I also understand the necessity of knowing the beliefs, values, and needs of those I care for, along with their limitations and strengths.
2. *Alternating rhythms*. I invest my energy in caring for another in a way that meets that person's

needs, maintaining or modifying my behaviors to better help.

3. *Patience*. I patiently participate with another in the process of caring, believing that that person will grow in a way that is meaningful to existence. Patience also allows for growth of myself.

4. *Honesty*. I care for the other in a way that facilitates an appropriate death: one that is defined by the individual, a death that gives meaning to existence. I am honest with myself in that I do not believe that another should die in a manner that I define. "In caring I am honest in trying to truly see."

5. *Trust*. Trust allows me to give the type of care that enables the other to grow in his or her own way and time. Besides trusting the other, it involves the courage to believe and trust in my own capacity to care.

6. *Humility*. I believe that each encounter with a dying person or family brings a new, novel learning experience. Each encounter requires the readiness and willingness to learn and care. Humility also means accepting myself, being open to others, and recognizing that others have an integrity of their own.

7. *Hope*. Hope is an expression of belief in "now," the plentitude of the moment, alive with a sense of the possible. Hope also implies that my caring for another is a commitment: a commitment to a relationship that exists in this moment for the realization of the other through my caring.

8. *Courage*. I communicate courage when I take existential anxiety on myself. The anxiety associated with death and the unknown belongs to existence. Courage takes the anxiety of nonbeing into itself: "The courage to be enrooted in the God who appears when God has disappeared in the anxiety of doubt."[79] "Courage gives me the trust I have in myself to care, and the trust I have in the belief that the other who is confronting death will grow."*

Summary

Implementation of humanistic caring for the dying requires not only an awareness of those actions fostering death with dignity, but also introspection on the part of the practitioner. Examination of one's own feelings, attitudes, and values about death and dying contributes to one's abilities to care and grow. Just as the dying may suffer from isolation and grow by sharing their experiences with others, so do nurses suffer when they are unable to share their losses with colleagues. Practitioners often find it helpful, if not essential, to share their feelings about death and their dying patients with others who can listen supportively.

REFERENCES AND SELECTED READINGS
Contemporary

1. Anthony, S.: The discovery of death in childhood and after, London, 1971, Penguin Publishing Co. Ltd.
2. Aries, P.: Western attitudes toward death: from the middle ages to the present, Baltimore, 1974, The Johns Hopkins University Press.
3. *Bunch, B., and Zahra, D.: Dealing with death: the unlearned role, Am. J. Nurs. 76:1486-1488, 1976.
4. *Craven, J., and Wald, F.: Hospice care for dying patients, Am. J. Nurs. 75:1816-1822, 1975.
5. *Craven, M.: I heard the owl call my name, New York, 1973, Dell Publishing Co., Inc.
6. *Death in the first person, Am. J. Nurs. 70:336, 1970.
7. Denton, J., and Wisenbaker, V., Jr.: Death experience and death anxiety among nurses and nursing students, Nurs. Res. 26(1):61-64, 1977.
8. Easson, W.: The dying child, Springfield, Ill., 1970, Charles C Thomas, Publisher.
9. Epstein, C.: Nursing the dying patient, Reston, Va., 1975, Reston Publishing Co.
10. Family balking at "last step," *Durham Morning Herald*, July 25, 1975, Louisville, Ky.
11. Gaston, S.: Death and midlife crisis, J.P.N. Ment. Health Serv. 18:31-35, 1980.
12. Goldscheider, C.: The mortality revolution. In Shneidman, E.S.: Death: current perspectives, Palo Alto, Calif. 1976, Mayfield Publishing Co.
13. *Ingles, T.: St. Christopher's hospice, Nurs. Outlook 74:759-763, 1974.
14. International Work Group in Death, Dying, and Bereavement: Assumptions and principles underlying standards for terminal care, Am. J. Nurs. 79:296-297, 1979.
15. Jackson, C.: Death shall have no dominion: the passing of the dead in America, Omega 8:195-203, 1977.
16. Jaques, E.: Death and the midlife crisis. In Ruitenbeck, H.: The interpretation of death, New York, 1973, Jason Aronson, Inc.
17. Kastenbaum, R., and Aisenburg, R.: The psychology of death, New York, 1972, Springer Publishing Co., Inc.
18. Keck, V., and Walther, L.: Nurse encounters with dying and nondying patients, Nurs. Res. 26:465-469, 1977.
19. Kübler-Ross, E.: Death: the final stage of growth, Englewood Cliffs, N.J., 1975, Prentice-Hall, Inc.
20. Kübler-Ross, E.: On the use of psychopharmacologic agents for the dying patient and the bereaved. In Goldberg, I., Malitz, D., and Kutscher, A.: Psychopharmacological agents for the terminally ill and bereaved, New York, 1973, Columbia University Press.
21. Lamers, W.M., Jr.: The changing American way of death, Hosp. Forum 23(1):5-6, 1980.

---

*Abridged and adapted from pp. 9-20 of On caring, by Milton Mayeroff, vol. 43 of World Perspectives series. Planned and edited by Ruth Nanda Anshen. Copyright © 1971 by Milton Mayeroff. By permission of Harper & Row, Publishers, Inc.

---

*References preceded by an asterisk are particularly well suited for student reading.

22. *Lande, S.: A gift of hope, Am. J. Nurs. **77**:639-640, 1977.
23. Lerner, M.: When, why and where people die. In Shneidman, E.S.: Death: current perspectives, Palo Alto, Calif., 1976, Mayfield Publishing Co.
24. *Mandel, H.R.: Nurses' feelings about working with the dying, Am. J. Nurs. **81**:1194-1197, 1981.
25. *Martocchio, B.: Living while dying, Bowie, Md., 1982, Prentice-Hall, Inc.
26. Mayeroff, M.: On caring, New York, 1971, Harper & Row, Publishers.
27. McCoy, M.: To die with style, Nashville, Tenn., 1974, Abingdon Press.
28. Moody, R.: Life after life, New York, 1976, Stockpole Books.
29. Moroney, R., and Kurtz, H.: The evolution of long-term care institutions. In Sherwood, S.: Long-term care, New York, 1975, Spectrum Publications Inc.
30. Mullins, L.: A humanistic view of the nurse and the dying patient, J. Gerontol. Nurs. **7**:148-152, 1981.
31. Nash, M.: Dignity of person in the final stages of life: an exploratory study, Omega **8**:71-81, 1977.
32. *Notes on a dying professor, Nurs. Outlook **23**:503-506, 1972.
33. *Paige, R.L.: Living and dying, Am. J. Nurs. **79**:2171-2172, 1979.
34. Pattison, E.M., editor: The experience of dying, Englewood Cliffs, N.J., 1977, Prentice-Hall, Inc.
35. Saunders, C.: A therapeutic community: St. Christopher's Hospice. In Schoenberg, B., et al.: Psychosocial aspects of terminal care, New York, 1972, New York University Press.
36. Saunders, C.: The nature and management of terminal pain. In Shotter, E.: Matters of life and death, London, 1970, Darton, Longman & Todd Ltd.
37. Schulz, R., and Aderman, D.: Clinical research on the stages of dying, Omega **5**:137-143, 1974.
38. Shneidman, E.S.: Voices of death, New York, 1980, Harper & Row, Publishers.
39. Shneidman, E.S.: Death work and stages of dying. In Shneidman, E.S.: Death: current perspectives, Palo Alto, Calif., 1976, Mayfield Publishing Co.
40. Statistical abstracts for the United States, 1981, Washington, D.C., 1981, U.S. Bureau of Census.
41. Stoller, E.P.: Effect of experience on nurses' responses to dying and death in the hospital setting, Nurs. Res. **29**:35-38, 1980.
42. Strauss, A., and Glaser, B.: Anguish: a case history of a dying trajectory, Mill Valley, Calif., 1970, The Sociology Press.
43. Weisman, A.: On dying and denying, New York, 1972, Behavioral Publications, Inc.
44. Weiss, R.: Loneliness: the experience of emotional and social isolation, Cambridge, Mass., 1973, The MIT Press.
45. *Wentzel, K.: The dying are the living, Am. J. Nurs. **76**:956-957, 1976.
46. Williams, J.: Understanding the feelings of the dying, Nurs. '76 **6**(3):51-56, 1976.

Classic

47. Anthony, S.: The child's discovery of death, New York, 1940, Harcourt Brace Jovanovich, Inc.
48. Bakan, K.: Disease, pain and sacrifice: toward a psychology of suffering, Chicago, 1968, The University of Chicago Press.
49. Bromberg, W., and Schilder, P.: Attitudes to death and dying, Psychoanal. Rev. **20**:133-185, 1933.
50. Choron, J.: Modern man and mortality, New York, 1964, Macmillan Publishing Co., Inc.
51. *Craytor, J.: Talking with the persons who have cancer, Am. J. Nurs. **69**:744-748, 1969.
52. Dickenstein, L., and Blatt, S.: Death concern; futurity and anticipation, J. Consult. Clin. Psychol. **30**:11-17, 1966.
53. *Engel, G.: Grief and grieving, Am. J. Nurs. **64**:93-98, 1964.
54. Erikson, E.: Childhood and society, ed. 2, New York, 1950, W.W. Norton & Co., Inc.
55. Feifel, H.: The function of attitudes toward death, J. Long Island Cons. Center **5**:26-29, 1967.
56. Feifel, H.: Older persons look at death, Geriatrics **11**:127-130, 1956.
57. Fulton, R.: Attitudes of American public toward death. In Fulton, R.: Death and identity, New York, 1965, John Wiley & Sons, Inc.
58. Glaser, B., and Strauss, A.: Time for dying, Chicago, 1968, Aldine Publishing Co.
59. Glaser, B., and Strauss, A.: Awareness of dying, Chicago, 1965, Aldine Publishing Co.
60. Hackett, R., and Weisman, A.: Reactions to the imminence of death. In Grosser, H.G., Wechsler, H., and Greenblatt, H.: The threat of impending disaster, Cambridge, Mass., 1964, The MIT Press.
61. Jeffers, F., Nichols, C., and Eisdorfer, C.: Attitudes of older persons toward death: a preliminary study, J. Gerontol. **16**:53-56, 1961.
62. Kastenbaum, R.: Theories of human aging: the search for a conceptual framework, J. Soc. Issues **21**:13-36, 1965.
63. Kastenbaum, R.: Time and death in adolescence. In Feifel, H.: The meaning of death, New York, 1959, McGraw-Hill Book Co.
64. Kastenbaum, R., and Weisman, A.: The psychological autopsy: a study of the terminal phase of life, Monograph series No. 4, Comm. Ment. Health J., New York, 1968, Behavioral Publications, Inc.
65. *Kneisal, D.: Thoughtful care of the dying, Am. J. Nurs. **68**:550-553, 1968.
66. *Kübler-Ross, E.: On death and dying, New York, 1969, Macmillan Publishing Co., Inc.
67. Lazarus, R.: Psychological stress and the coping process, New York, 1966, McGraw-Hill Book Co.
68. Maurer, A.: Maturation of concepts of death, Br. J. Med. Psychol. **39**:35-41, 1966.
69. May, R.: Man's search for himself, New York, 1953, W.W. Norton & Co., Inc.
70. *Mittford, J.: The American way of death, New York, 1963, Simon & Schuster, Inc.
71. Munnichs, J.: Old age and finitude, Basel, Switzerland, 1966, S. Karger AG.
72. Nagy, M.: The child's view of death. In Feifel, H.: The meaning of death, New York, 1959, McGraw-Hill Book Co.
73. *Quint, J.: The nurse and the dying patient, New York, 1967, Macmillan Publishing Co., Inc.
74. *Quint, J.: Obstacles to helping the dying, Am. J. Nurs. **66**:1568-1571, 1966.
75. *Roose, L.: To die alone, Ment. Hyg. **53**:321-326, 1969.
76. *Sharp, D.: Lessons from a dying patient, Am. J. Nurs. **68**:1517-1520, 1968.
77. Spark, M.: Momento mori, New York, 1964, Meridian Books.
78. Sturt, M.: The psychology of time, New York, 1925, Harcourt Brace Jovanovich Inc.
79. Tillich, P.: The courage to be, New Haven, Conn., 1952, Yale University Press.
80. *Verwoerdt, A., and Wilson, R.: Communication with fatally ill patients: tacit or explicit? Am. J. Nurs. **67**:2307-2310, 1967.
81. Williams, R., and Wirths, C.: Lives through the years, New York, 1965, Atherton Press, Inc.
82. Zeligs, R.: Children's attitudes toward death, Ment. Hyg. **51**:393-396, 1967.
83. Zinker, J., and Hollenback, C.: Notes on loss, crises and growth, J. Gen. Psychol. **73**:347-354, 1965.

CHAPTER 18

NEUROENDOCRINE INTEGRATING MECHANISMS

VIRGINIA L. CASSMEYER

The human body is made up of billions of cells. For these cells to stay healthy and function properly they must have a stable internal environment that supplies adequate oxygen, nutrients, water, and electrolytes and a constant temperature. The maintenance of a stable internal environment requires the integrated functioning of all body systems. The body systems must be integrated in such a manner that any change in the internal environment, no matter how minute, is recognized and automatic reactions that make corrective changes occur.

In times of health the internal environment is constantly changing. In addition, every disease state has associated with it physical or psychologic stressors that change the internal environment. The body systems that function in the maintenance of a stable internal environment are under the control of the nervous and endocrine systems. These two systems can function dependently, independently, and interdependently. The nervous and endocrine systems have other complex functions, which will be discussed in Units V and VI.

This chapter focuses on the parts of the systems involved in integrating body functions necessary to maintain a stable internal environment. The first section describes the physiologic concepts and the component parts involved in the integration of body systems; the second section describes how the neuroendocrine integrating mechanisms maintain energy, water, electrolytes, oxygen, and temperature balance on a minute-to-minute basis; and the third section describes the neuroendocrine integrating mechanisms' responses to major stressors.

Physiologic concepts

The parts of the nervous and endocrine systems responsible for integrating the body functions necessary to the maintenance of a stable internal environment are (1) the hypothalamus, (2) the medulla oblongata, (3) the sympathetic nervous system, (4) the adrenal medulla and its catecholamines, and (5) the pituitary gland, adrenal cortex, and thyroid gland and their respective hormones (adrenocorticotropic hormone [ACTH], glucocorticoids, aldosterone, antidiuretic hormone [ADH], growth hormone [GH], and thyroid hormones).

Components of the nervous system

Hypothalamus

The hypothalamus develops from the neural tube, which is a strip of ectoderm. In embryonic development the neural tube gives rise to three primary vesicles: the forebrain, midbrain, and hindbrain. As it grows the forebrain divides into the telencephalon and diencephalon. The *diencephalon* is made up of the thalamus and hypothalamus. The hypothalamus forms the floor and the lower parts of the wall of the third ventricle. The *optic chiasm* lies in the front of the hypothalamus, and the cerebral peduncles lie on the posterior basal surface of the hypothalamus. The hypophysis (pituitary gland) is connected to the hypothalamus by the infundibulum. The hypothalamus is gray matter and is made up of many nuclei that are concerned with integration of body functions and the regulation of visceral activities. Although the hypothalamus is a relatively small area, it receives input directly and indirectly from almost all parts of the brain.[20]

Medulla oblongata

The medulla oblongata arises from the hindbrain. During development the hindbrain divides into the metencephalon and myelencephalon. The myelencephalon part of the hindbrain is the medulla oblongata. The myelencephalon, metencephalon, and midbrain (mesencephalon) make up the brain stem.

The medulla oblongata is cone shaped and extends from the pons to the spinal cord. All ascending and descending tracts to and from the cerebral cortex and other centers above the medulla pass through, cross over, or terminate in the medulla. Cranial nerves VIII to XII emerge from the medulla. The medulla contains abundant reticular formation. The nuclei of the vital cardiac, vasomotor, and respiratory centers are located in the medulla. Ascending and descending connections from the rest of the brain stem, the cortex, and the cerebellum are connected to the medulla.

The body has multiple receptors, which monitor blood levels of oxygen, carbon dioxide, sodium, and water. They also monitor the pressure within the vascular bed, the blood level of glucose, and body temperature. Increases or decreases in any of these are transmitted directly to the hypothalamus or indirectly via the medulla to the hypothalamus. Once the hypothalamus is stimulated, it activates the endocrine system while the medulla activates the autonomic nervous system. The *somatic neural efferent system* may also be involved. The two mechanisms that are stimulated by the hypothalamus or the medulla oblongata and are involved in the body's response to stressors are the sympathetic–adrenal medullary mechanism and parts of the endocrine system.

Sympathetic–adrenal medullary mechanism

The sympathetic nervous system is part of the autonomic nervous system. The autonomic nervous system contains two divisions: the parasympathetic division, which is concerned with conservative and restorative functions, and the sympathetic division, which is concerned with body defense and provision of energy and maintenance of stability in stress situations.

All sympathetic fibers have two neurons. The primary neuron (preganglionic neuron) is located in the intermediolateral gray column of the thoracic and lumbar spinal cord. These preganglionic neurons give rise to axons that emerge from the thoracic and lumbar spinal cord in the ventral root. These axons branch off toward an autonomic ganglion. Since the preganglionic fibers are myelinated, they are white, and thus this bundle of fibers is known as the *white ramus communicans*.

The white ramus communicans enters the paravertebral (chain) ganglia. Some of the axons synapse with postganglionic neurons immediately on entering the ganglia. Other preganglionic fibers pass up and down the paravertebral ganglia to synapse at higher or lower levels. The paravertebral (chain) ganglia lie along all levels of the spinal cord on both sides of the vertebral bodies. Once the preganglionic fibers synapse with the postganglionic fibers in the chain ganglia, the postganglionic fibers can directly travel to effector organs such as the eyes, the cardiac system, or the respiratory system, or the postganglionic fibers may travel back toward the spinal cord through the gray ramus communicans (so named because the postganglionic fibers are unmyelinated and gray in color) to travel with spinal nerves. The postganglionic fibers that travel with spinal nerves innervate sweat glands, peripheral vessels, and hair follicles.

Some of the preganglionic fibers from the spinal cord pass through the paravertebral ganglia to synapse with cell bodies of postganglionic fibers in prevertebral ganglia. The prevertebral ganglia are more peripheral and the postganglionic fibers emerging from these ganglia innervate abdominal and pelvic organs. These prevertebral ganglia are also called preaortic ganglia because they lie close to main branches of the aorta. Examples of these ganglia are the celiac, superior mesenteric, and inferior mesenteric ganglia.

Sympathetic innervation of the adrenal medulla differs from sympathetic innervation of other organs. The preganglionic fiber travels, without synapsing at any ganglia, directly to receptors on the adrenal medulla, where it synapses. The adrenal medulla embryonically arises from ectodermal cells that also give rise to sympathetic ganglia. The adrenal medulla itself acts as the postganglionic neuron. Fig. 18-1 diagrams the sympathetic nervous system.

Chemical transmission of acetylcholine and norepinephrine. At the synapses neurotransmitters are released from the presynaptic fibers to allow the impulse to travel to postsynaptic sites. The neurotransmitter released at the preganglionic-postganglionic junction is acetylcholine, whereas the neurotransmitter released from most postganglionic sympathetic fibers is norepinephrine (noradrenalin). The postganglionic fibers innervating most sweat glands and some blood vessels in the lower extremities release acetylcholine, whereas the adrenal medulla releases both norepinephrine and epinephrine.

All organs receiving sympathetic innervation have specialized receptors. These receptors have been classified into two major types: alpha-adrenergic (α-adrenergic) receptors and beta-adrenergic (β-adrenergic) receptors.

β-Receptors can be subdivided into β_1- and β_2-re-

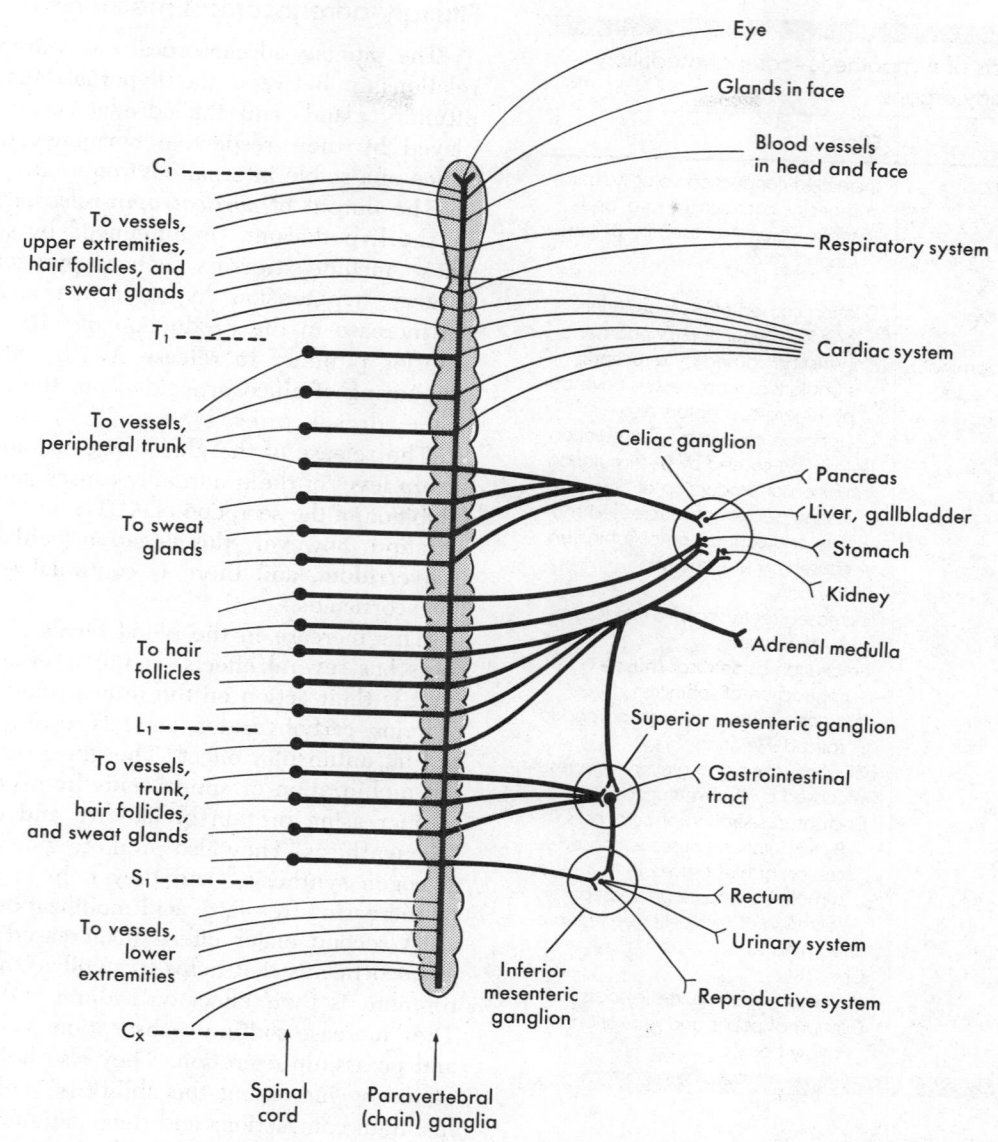

Fig. 18-1. Sympathetic nervous system. Preganglionic fibers (dark lines) leave spinal cord at T1 to T12 and L1 to L5 and travel through white ramus communicans to paravertebral (chain) ganglia. Once fibers reach paravertebral ganglia they may synapse immediately, pass up or down ganglia, or pass through paravertebral ganglia to prevertebral ganglia. Once preganglionic fiber synapses in paravertebral ganglia, postganglionic fibers (light lines) can either pass to effector organs such as eye or cardiac system or pass back toward spinal cord through gray ramus communicans and leave with spinal nerves to innervate peripheral vessels, hair follicles, and sweat glands. Ganglionic fibers originating in the prevertebral ganglia innervate effector organs in the abdominal and pelvic cavities.

ceptors. β_1-Receptors are located primarily in the heart, and β_2-receptors occur elsewhere in the body. There may be other types of β-receptors and these are currently under investigation. There also appear to be two types of α-receptors, α_1-receptors, which are excitatory, and α_2-receptors, which inhibit norepinephrine release.[10] Stimulation of β- and α-receptors leads to different effects. Various drugs used in clinical practice have the ability to selectively stimulate only one type of receptor. These drug effects are discussed on p. 317.

As Fig. 18-1 shows, sympathetic fibers have many branches and terminate in a very dispersed manner. Because of this, when almost any portion of the sympathetic system is stimulated, the whole system responds. Since the purpose of the sympathetic system is to prepare for defense or assist in returning the internal

TABLE 18-1. Effects of sympathetic–adrenal medullary stimulation on body organs

Organ	Effect
Heart	Increased conduction velocity, automaticity, contractility, rate, and stroke volume caused by β_1-stimulation
Blood vessels	
Coronary vessels, brain, lungs	Dilation caused by β_2-stimulation and autoregulatory phenomena
Skin, mucosa, abdominal viscera, renal and salivary gland vessels	Constriction caused by α-receptor stimulation; renal vessels have dopaminergic receptors also
Veins	Constriction caused by α-stimulation
Bronchial muscles	Relaxation caused by β_2-stimulation
Gastrointestinal tract	Inhibition of production of gastrointestinal secretions; decreased motility and contraction of sphincters caused by β_2-stimulation
Gallbladder	Relaxation
Kidney	Increased renin secretion caused by β_2-stimulation
Urinary bladder	Relaxation of detrusor muscle and contraction of sphincter
Skin	Pilomotor muscle contraction and localized sweating
Liver	Glycogenolysis and gluconeogenesis caused by β_2-stimulation
Pancreas	Decreased secretion of acini cells; β_2 stimulation causes increased secretion of islet beta-cells, but α-stimulation causes decreased secretion of islet cells; α-effect predominates
Fat cells	Lipolysis
Brain	Increased alertness, restlessness
Eyes	Dilation of pupils and relaxation of ciliary bodies

environment to normal, and because these activities require the integration of many body systems, the total response of the system to any stimuli is what is desired. The effects of stimulation of the sympathetic system are summarized in Table 18-1. In general, complete stimulation suppresses functions that are not essential for life and augments functions essential for life.

Components of the endocrine system

The second system involved in integration of body systems and the maintenance of a stable internal environment is the endocrine system. In this section only those endocrine glands and glandular functions specific to the maintenance of a stable internal environment will be discussed. The relationship among the hypothalamus, pituitary, and other endocrine glands and the overall function of all endocrine glands are described in Chapter 30.

Pituitary-adrenocortical mechanism

The pituitary-adrenocortical mechanism refers to the relationship between the hypothalamus, the anterior pituitary gland, and the adrenal cortex and the role played by their respective hormones in the maintenance of a stable internal environment.

The output of *corticotropin-releasing factor* (CRF) by the hypothalamus is influenced by several stimuli. These include stressors such as pyrogenic infections, surgery, hypotension, hypoglycemia, anxiety, and fear. An increase in the production of CRF stimulates the anterior pituitary to release *ACTH*, which causes an outpouring of glucocorticoids from the zona fasciculata of the adrenal cortex.

The release of the glucocorticoids and an increased serum level of them normally causes *negative feedback* inhibition of the secretion of ACTH and CRF. In a stress situation, however, this negative feedback mechanism is overridden and there is continual secretion of the glucocorticoids.

This increase in the blood levels of the glucocorticoids has several effects on the internal environment. First is their action on the intermediary metabolism of proteins, carbohydrates, and fats resulting in catabolism and an antiinsulin effect. The glucocorticoids promote the mobilization of amino acids from peripheral tissue by increasing protein breakdown and decreasing protein synthesis. They also promote gluconeogenesis and glycogen synthesis,[3] and they help to provide energy by increasing free fatty acid mobilization.

A second major effect of increased blood levels of glucocorticoids that helps to stabilize the internal environment is their effect on sodium and water balance. They increase sodium reabsorption, volume expansion, and potassium excretion. They also help in stress situations by increasing the ability of skeletal muscles to maintain contractions and delay fatigue, thus helping a person to escape from danger.

The glucocorticoids also assist in combating stressors by their influence on other hormones and catecholamines. They stimulate glucagon, which is necessary for gluconeogenesis.[18] Their catabolic effects require decreased insulin, and they depress insulin secretion. In addition, the glucocorticoids increase the α- and β-adrenergic effects of the catecholamines and the synthesis of catecholamines.[8] This action helps maintain adequate blood pressure and heart rate. Finally, the glucocorticoids are used in the treatment of physiologic shock and may play a role in maintaining a stable internal environment by stabilizing lysosome membranes and preventing cell death, increasing oxygen transport, decreasing lactic acidosis, and increasing microcirculatory flow.[26]

Additional hormones

Although the major endocrine effects on maintenance of a stable internal environment are due to the effects of stimulation of the pituitary-adrenocortical mechanism, other hormones also play important roles. These hormones are *aldosterone, ADH, growth hormone,* and *thyroid hormone*.

Aldosterone. Aldosterone is a mineralocorticoid produced by the zona glomerulosa of the adrenal cortex. Although high levels of ACTH possibly stimulate the adrenal cortex to secrete high levels of aldosterone, the major stimulus is the *renin-angiotensinogen system*. Diminished blood flow to the kidneys or decreased blood levels of sodium are sensed by the macula densa of the kidney. The macula densa signals the juxtaglomerular apparatus to release renin. The juxtaglomerular apparatus may also be stimulated directly by β-adrenergic stimulation. Renin acts on a serum protein, angiotensinogen, to convert it to angiotensin I. *Angiotensin I* is converted by the effect of a second enzyme to *angiotensin II*. Angiotensin II stimulates the adrenal cortex to secrete aldosterone. In addition, angiotensin II is a potent vasoconstrictor that can act directly on renal arterioles causing vasoconstriction, leading to a decreased glomerular filtration rate (GFR) and the reabsorption of sodium and water.

Aldosterone aids in the body's response to stress by stimulating sodium reabsorption, especially in the distal tubules, and water reabsorption and the excretion of potassium, ammonium, and magnesium ions.

Antidiuretic hormone. Antidiuretic hormone (ADH) is a hormone produced by the supraoptic nuclei and paraventricular nuclei of the hypothalamus.[20] It is carried down neural axons to the posterior pituitary, where it is stored and from which it is released. With changes in the internal environment, such as increased osmolality, decreased vascular volume, and decreased blood pressure, or other stressors, such as pain, exercise, or β-adrenergic stimulation, the posterior pituitary releases ADH.

ADH aids in maintenance of a stable internal environment by causing water reabsorption in the distal tubules and collecting ducts. The presence of ADH results in the excretion of a concentrated urine.

Growth hormone. Growth hormone (GH) is secreted by the anterior pituitary under the control of the hypothalamus. The hypothalamus releases growth hormone releasing factor and depresses the release of somatostatin, thus stimulating the release of growth hormone. Growth hormone helps to maintain adequate energy by mobilizing fatty acids and increasing fatty acid oxidation. It also causes increased gluconeogenesis and decreased utilization of glucose by fat cells and muscles.

Thyroid hormones. Thyroid hormones are secreted by the thyroid gland under hypothalamic-pituitary control. Psychologic stress and cold are known to stimulate the hypothalamus to secrete thyroid releasing hormone

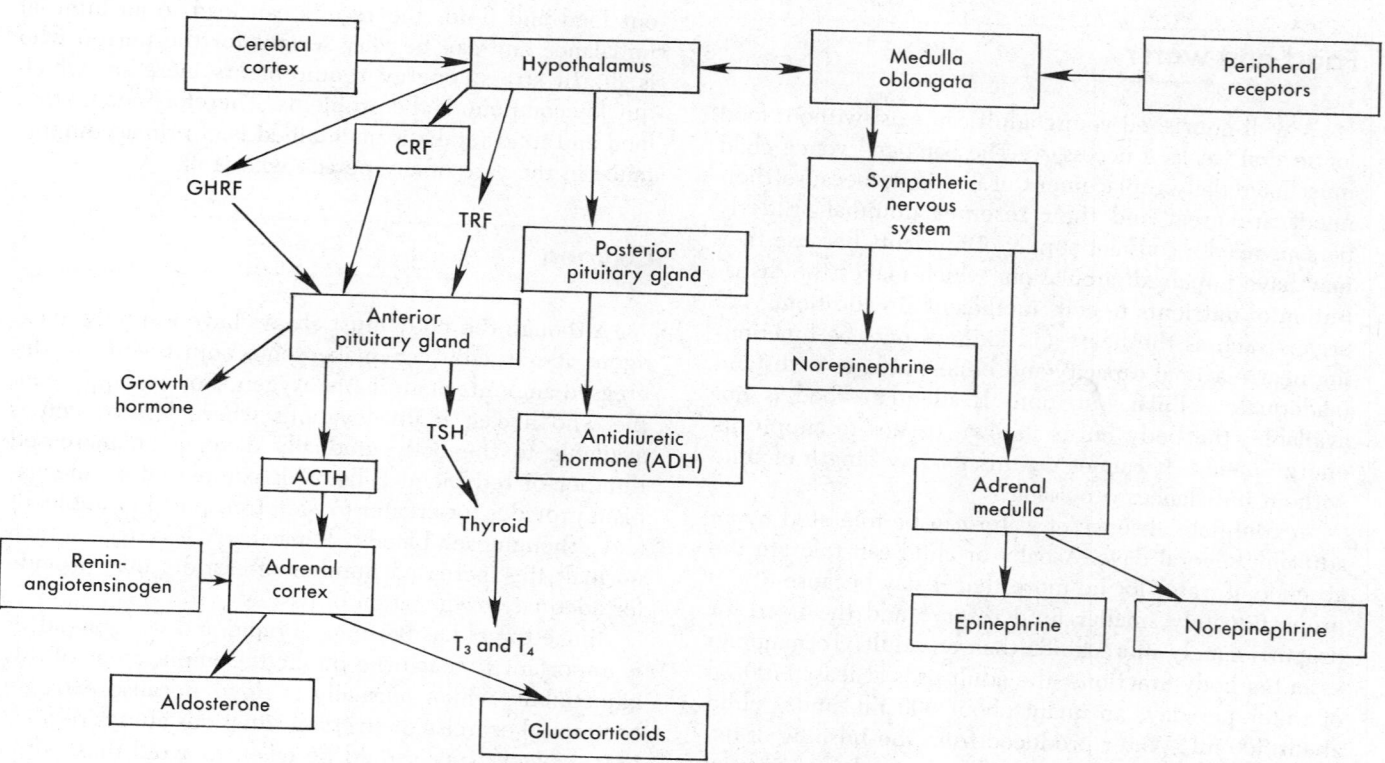

Fig. 18-2. Relationship among hypothalamus, sympathetic–adrenal medullary system, and various endocrine glands involved in body's reponse to stress. Principal hormonal and nervous components are boxed.

(TRH). TRH stimulates the anterior pituitary to secrete thyroid stimulating hormone (TSH). TSH stimulates the thyroid gland to secrete *thyroxine* (T_4) and *triiodothyronine* (T_3). T_4 and T_3 aid in the maintenance of a stable internal environment by maintaining a stable temperature and by aiding in the maintenance of an adequate energy supply.

The relationship between the hypothalamus, sympathetic—adrenal medullary system, and various endocrine glands involved in the body's response to stress is depicted in Fig. 18-2.

Nutrients, water, oxygen, and temperature balance

Even in states of health the body has a very limited ability to withstand inadequate replacement of nutrients, water, and oxygen or variations in the temperature of the body. In everyday life the integrative mechanisms are frequently called into action to maintain internal balance when deviations occur. The following section describes what happens when nutrients, water, oxygen, and temperature needs are not being adequately met.

Food and water

A well-nourished young adult can exist without food for several weeks if necessary. The baby and young child must have daily replacement of nutrients because their needs are great and their reserves minimal. Elderly persons need a constant supply of nutrients because they may have impaired circulation, which makes the distribution of nutrients to cells inefficient. In addition, vital organs such as the heart and kidneys may be functioning near maximal capacity and be less able to withstand inadequate cellular nutrition. If adequate food is not available, the body burns its own tissues to supply its energy needs. It cannot do this for any length of time without imbalances occurring.

A complete absence of water can be tolerated by an adult for several days. A baby or child can tolerate the absence of water for no more than 1 day because of the proportionately smaller fluid reserve and the need for proportionately more fluids than an adult. To maintain essential body functions, the adult uses at least 1700 ml of water per day, an infant about 300 ml, and a child about 500 ml. Water produced from the burning of tissues (oxidation) and water pulled from the interstitial spaces can be used to maintain the body's needs for a short time. The kidneys too can conserve some water.

However, since only 150 ml per day is produced by oxidation (proportionately less in infants and children despite their higher metabolic rate), the available supply is rapidly depleted and the person can become seriously ill.

Lack of adequate food and water is a stressor. The perception of lack of water and food by the body leads to the stimulation of the hypothalamus and a resultant stimulation of the sympathetic—adrenal medullary mechanism and the endocrine system. To supply its energy needs the body first burns its glycogen stores, and then body proteins are mobilized and burned for energy and fats are oxidized. The burning of body fats produces ketones, and as proteins are burned nitrogen and potassium are liberated. The stimulation of the sympathetic—adrenal medullary mechanisms and the endocrine mechanisms leads to a conservation of sodium and water. If this occurs at the same time that a lack of fluid is present, the end-products of metabolism will build up since they cannot be adequately excreted.

The release of norepinephrine, epinephrine, glucocorticoids, GH, thyroid hormone, aldosterone, and ADH provide needed energy and water for a short time; however, symptoms of fluid and electrolyte imbalance will occur. The ketones produced will lead to metabolic acidosis (p. 355), the blood urea nitrogen level will rise (p. 601), and symptoms of hyperkalemia (p. 338) and hypernatremia (p. 336) can result.

Although it is possible to live for short periods without food and fluid, the results can lead to an internal imbalance and can be very serious for the person who is ill. In stress, energy requirements increase, which quickly compounds the problems. Therefore seeing that food and fluid intake is maintained is of primary importance in the care of any person who is ill.

Oxygen

Although the body must always have a supply of oxygen, it normally can make some adjustments to decreased amounts of available oxygen. For example, people who live at high elevations where less oxygen is available to the body gradually develop an increased number of red blood cells. This compensatory mechanism provides for greater oxygen transport in the blood, and although each blood cell may carry less oxygen than normal, the increased number of carriers may provide for adequate oxygenation of tissues.

Since travel has become so rapid and widespread, it is important to teach the public the implications of this adjustment, which normally is slow. Because extreme or unusual exercise or stressful situations always require extra oxygen, care should be taken to avoid these situations for several days after arriving in a place where the altitude is higher than that to which a person is accustomed. In high altitudes the atmospheric pressure is low, and at low atmospheric pressures less oxygen diffuses across the alveoli into the blood, while carbon dioxide diffuses more rapidly than usual from the blood, causing respiratory alkalosis. If precautions are not taken before the body has had an opportunity to compensate by increasing the number of red blood cells, the tissues may not receive enough oxygen. Persons whose work takes them to places where the altitude is high are likely to have serious difficulty if they contract a respiratory illness. They also need to avoid strenuous physical activity for several days after arrival.

Because of the dangers accompanying atmospheric pressure changes, most airplanes now have pressurized cabins as well as additional oxygen supplies. It is unwise for anyone who would be susceptible to the development of problems caused by a low concentration of oxygen to travel in an airplane without these protections. Elderly persons and those persons who have circulatory or respiratory diseases often tolerate atmospheric pressure changes poorly. They should be advised to consult their physician before planning a trip that entails going to mountainous regions.

A precipitous change from an area of high pressure to one of low pressure can cause rupture of the alveoli because of the expansion of the gases in the alveoli. This type of pressure change also causes a decrease in the solubility of the nitrogen in the blood, causing the nitrogen to form bubbles that obstruct blood flow. This condition is commonly known as "the bends" (*decompression sickness* or *caisson disease*) and may be a problem for pilots, divers, and others, such as "sand hogs," who work underwater for long periods of time. Unless pressurized cabins or tanks are used, descent from airplanes or ascent from diving should be gradual enough to allow time for accommodation to pressure changes. Informing the public about this reaction is very important because many people today engage in flying and diving for recreation.

The preceding discussion shows that if given time the body can make some adjustments to decreased amounts of available oxygen. But in everyday life, situations leading to an inadequate supply of oxygen or a buildup of carbon dioxide can occur quickly. In addition, in stress situations there is a need for a rapid exchange of oxygen and carbon dioxide. In these instances the respiratory center in the medulla oblongata is directly or indirectly stimulated to fire more rapidly. The multiple influences on the respiratory center are described in Chapter 20. Increased firing by the respiratory center leads to increased rate and depth of respiration. Respiration may become gasping, allowing more air to be inspired. In stress situations, the stimulation of the sympathetic–adrenal medullary mechanism causes the bronchioles to dilate to enhance the exchange of oxygen and carbon dioxide (unless disease prevents di-

lation) and the heart rate to increase to provide for more rapid transport of oxygen to the vital organs.

Although the body has mechanisms to help ensure an adequate supply of oxygen, the person suffering from an oxygen deficit should be protected from any additional stressors. The body may be functioning at maximal capacity, and stress will increase oxygen needs further.

If the body is unable to accommodate to an inadequate oxygen supply in the external environment or if, even though oxygen is available, the blood is unable to carry adequate amounts of it because of a low hemoglobin level (anemia), oxygen may be administered. Usually adequate amounts can be provided by face mask, nasal catheter, or cannula. Occasionally, oxygen must be administered under positive pressure, and in some instances hyperbaric oxygen chambers may be used.

Temperature

For normal body function the body temperature must be maintained around 37° C (98.6° F). Various parts of the body have different temperatures. The extremities are generally cooler than the rest of the body. The magnitude of the temperature difference between body parts varies with the environmental temperature. The rectal temperature is representative of the temperature at the core of the body and varies least with the environmental temperature.

There is a clear *circadian rhythm* in body temperature. The normal human core temperature undergoes a regular *diurnal fluctuation*, being lowest during sleep and highest during the waking state. In women the temperature pattern also follows the menstrual cycle, with a rather sharp rise in temperature occurring at the time of ovulation (see Chapter 63).

The body produces heat as a result of a variety of basic chemical reactions that include metabolic processes and the ingestion and metabolism of food. The major source of heat, however, is from the contraction of skeletal muscles. *Epinephrine* and *norepinephrine* produce a rapid but transient increase in heat production; *thyroxine* causes a slowly developing but prolonged increase in heat production. Body heat is lost by various processes, such as radiation, conduction, and vaporization from perspiration, respiration, urination, and defecation.

The maintenance of normal body temperature depends on maintaining a balance between heat production and heat loss. The primary integrating area for temperature regulation is located in the hypothalamus. There are two neural pathways to the hypothalamus: the skin receptors and the thermoreceptive properties of the hypothalamus itself. The stimulation of the hypothalamus results in efferent output from the hypo-

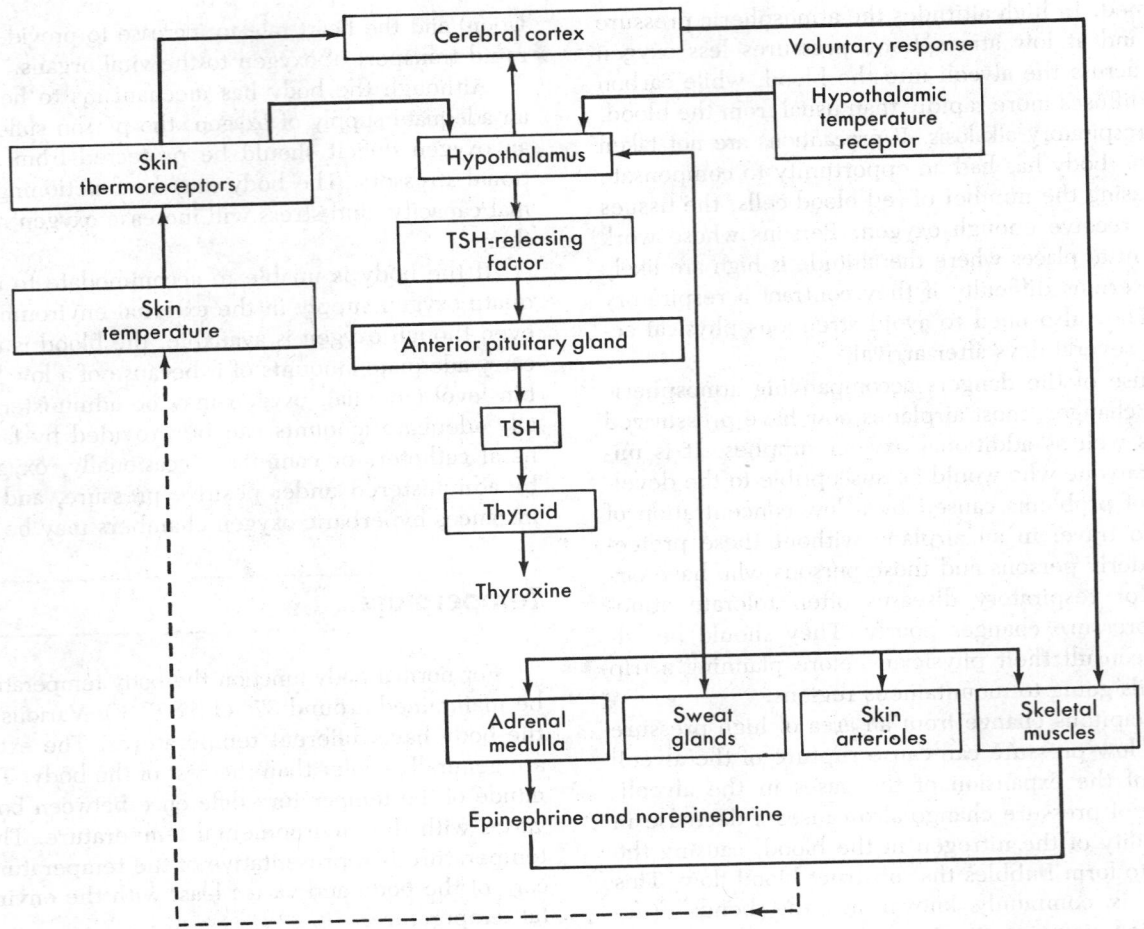

Fig. 18-3. Summary of temperature-regulating mechanisms in body. (Adapted from Vander, A.J., et al.: Human physiology: the mechanisms of body functions, New York, 1975, McGraw-Hill Book Co.)

thalamus to bring about appropriate responses. Fig. 18-3 summarizes the temperature-regulating mechanisms in the body. As can be seen from the figure, in addition to the control exerted by the hypothalamus, humans exert voluntary control by increasing skeletal muscle activity when cold and decreasing skeletal muscle activity when hot.

When the environment is hot, body temperature rises. Skin receptors and the hypothalamic thermoreceptors are stimulated by the increased temperature. This information is transmitted to the hypothalamus by afferent fibers. The efferent output from the hypothalamus leads to dilation of blood vessels in the skin so that heat can be released. Sweat is produced, and as the moisture evaporates the air enveloping the skin is cooled so body heat can radiate to the environment. Respirations increase, with a resultant release of heat and moisture. When the body temperature is decreased to normal this information is sensed by the skin receptors and the hypothalamic thermoreceptors. This infor-

mation is transmitted by afferent fibers to the hypothalamus, and measures leading to heat loss are stopped.

When the internal environment is cold, body temperature begins to drop. Skin receptors and the hypothalamic thermoreceptors are stimulated. This information is transmitted to the hypothalamus by afferent fibers. The efferent output from the hypothalamus leads to constrictions of blood vessels so that heat is retained. If too much heat is still being lost, shivering occurs. Shivering increases heat production. In some cases epinephrine, norepinephrine, and thyroxine may be secreted, causing an elevation in the basal metabolic rate and increasing heat production. When the body temperature is increased to normal, this information is sensed by the skin receptors and the hypothalamic thermoreceptors. The information is transmitted to the hypothalamus and measures leading to heat conservation and production are stopped.

Another mechanism of heat production found in many animals when they are chronically exposed to cold is nonshivering thermogenesis. *Nonshivering thermogenesis* refers to an increase in metabolic rate over and above the basal metabolic rate (BMR) that is not due to mechanical activity.[13] Nonshivering thermogenesis can be differentiated from thyroid-induced thermogenesis in that it can be quickly switched on and off. The rapid switching on and off is mediated by the sympathetic nervous system.[13] The site of nonshivering thermogenesis seems to be *brown adipose tissue* (BAT) and skeletal muscles. The role of nonshivering thermogenesis in heat production in adults is unknown, although brown fat cells have been found in men in their forties.[12]

The ability to regulate body temperature varies with age. Infants have no difficulty with the production of heat but do have difficulty regulating heat loss. This difficulty is due to their scanty layer of insulating fat, smaller size, and greater surface–to–body weight ratio as compared with adults. The elderly are capable of maintaining constancy of their internal temperature under conditions of favorable environmental temperature, but their response to extreme environmental temperatures is less efficient than in younger adults. The reasons for this are believed to be a slowing of the circulation and structural and functional changes that occur in the skin as the result of aging. Even the normal person may be unable to compensate for extremely high or extremely low environmental temperatures. If compensatory mechanisms are ineffective, heat syncope, heat exhaustion, sunstroke, or freezing may occur (see Chapter 73). Heat syncope results when extensive peripheral vasodilation combined with orthostatic hypotension produces cerebral ischemia. Drugs that cause vasodilation, such as those used to lower blood pressure, may predispose an individual to heat syncope. In addition, sedative and tranquilizing drugs suppress or interfere with temperature regulation.

Temperature regulation is affected by diseases that cause pathologic changes in blood flow, including congestive heart failure (p. 1127), Raynaud's disease (p. 1157), Buerger's disease (p. 1157), other arteriosclerotic diseases, dysfunction of the autonomic nervous system caused by drugs, surgery, or injury, and diseases of the hypothalamus or medulla.

Fever

Fever is a state of *hyperthermia*. It may result from faulty regulation of body temperature because of age, circulatory disturbances, or dysfunction of the autonomic nervous system, hypothalamus, or medulla from injury, disease, or drugs. Fever also can occur even though regulatory mechanisms are normal. It is a cardinal sign of many diseases. The cause of fever in these situations is thought to be a "resetting" of the hypothalamic thermostat. The patient regulates body temperature in response to heat and cold but at a higher level. The "resetting" of the hypothalamic thermostat is thought to be caused by effects on it by endogenous pyrogens released by injured body cells.

Measures may need to be taken with some patients to help the body regulate its temperature. Persons who have a tendency to lose body heat can be protected against the cold by light, warm clothing, and bed coverings. Persons who may have ineffective temperature regulatory mechanisms because of age or disease need to have their temperatures carefully checked at frequent intervals.

In giving nursing care to patients it is important to avoid measures that counteract the natural defenses for heat control. For example, providing too much warmth for a patient who has a fever yet feels chilly may cause the temperature to rise higher. However, if the patient is not protected enough to prevent shivering, the temperature also will be increased. If shivering occurs as a result of the "resetting" of the hypothalamic thermostat, adding warmth will not stop the shivering. Sudden warming of a person whose body temperature has been markedly lowered may actually cause it to drop further because unless the environment is very warm, the heat is lost through the dilated vessels. The temperature control mechanisms are especially ineffective when there is a wide swing in environmental temperature or when a fever-producing disease is present. The temperature of the external environment needs to be carefully controlled when giving care to any patient with the above problems, and treatment to reduce fever needs to be instituted promptly (see Chapter 22).

Generalized response to major stressors

The body responses essential for life and controlled by the neuroendocrine integrating mechanisms will be activated in the presence of any major stressor. Examples of major stressors include trauma, surgery, disease, anger, frustration, or fear. It is important to remember that what is a minor occurrence to one person may be seen as a frustrating, fearful, or anxiety-provoking stressor by another person. Inadequate supplies of water, nutrients, and oxygen also serve as major stressors. Any of these situations if perceived as a stressor will lead to the activation of the sympathetic–adrenal medullary mechanism and the endocrine mechanisms.

The intensity of the response to the stressor is related to the extent and severity of the stressor. The response activated by the neuroendocrine integrating mechanisms is a generalized nonspecific response to the stressor. This means that the same response occurs regardless of the initiating event. The body's response in most instances does not eradicate the stressor but only allows the body to contain or resist the stressor until it is alleviated naturally or by outside interventions.

First described by Selye in 1936, this defense mechanism is referred to as the stress syndrome or the *general adaptation syndrome* (GAS).[31] Three stages were identified in the general adaptation syndrome. The first stage is called the *alarm reaction*. During this stage the nervous and endocrine mechanisms are activated and the body's response to this activation is initiated. Stage two is the *stage of resistance*. During this stage the body has reached its full ability to fight or resist the stressor, and the stressor is contained by the body's response. Stage three is the *stage of exhaustion*. If the stressor continues, the body's ability to fight or contain it is depleted. The stressor overrides all the efforts of the neural and endocrine mechanisms to contain or resist it. Death may ensue.

In addition to adapting to general systemic stressors, the body is able to adapt to localized stressors. This is called the *local adaptation syndrome* (LAS). Inflammatory response is an example of the local adaptation syndrome.

Assessment

The signs and symptoms seen in the presence of major stressors are caused by both the stressor and the neural and hormonal activation of body responses. The person appears pale, the skin is cool and moist, the pupils are dilated, the pulse is full and rapid, and if the body's response to the stressors is effective, the systolic blood pressure is elevated (otherwise it may be decreased). Respirations are deep, and their rate is increased if the patient has no underlying respiratory deficiencies preventing this compensatory reaction. The person may be keenly alert and have tense muscles. Restlessness may be present. These changes are caused by increased *sympathetic–adrenal medullary stimulation*. The person may have abdominal distention, be nauseated, vomit, and have diarrhea because of decreased parasympathetic stimulation and increased sympathetic stimulation. Other signs and symptoms are related to the activation of the endocrine mechanisms.

One sign is decreased urine output resulting from increased levels of glucocorticoids, aldosterone, and ADH and arteriole vasoconstriction. The urine is very concentrated and shows an increased specific gravity and increased osmolality because of water reabsorption. Urine sodium content will be decreased because of sodium reabsorption. Blood glucose levels, fatty acids, and proteins may be elevated as a result of the effects of the glucocorticoids and GH. Muscle wasting will occur in long-term stress situations secondary to increased protein breakdown and decreased protein synthesis. Over-

all, the person is ready for "flight or fight." In times of minor stressors or danger the body's response may be minimal or so short lived as not to produce any symptoms. Fig. 18-4 diagrams the body's response to major stressors and the signs and symptoms that would be manifested in patients.

Intervention

Any hospitalized patient may show signs and symptoms associated with the body's response to stressors because of the stress of illness or the fears associated with the illness. Without an understanding of the body's mechanisms for handling stressors, nursing actions may impede rather than complement or supplement the protective mechanisms. It should be remembered that the purpose of the initial response to stressors is to help the person escape the stress-producing situation or mobilize all defenses to resist it. Nursing measures designed to support the protective mechanisms are necessary. Rest is absolutely essential, since activity can impede maintenance of body functions essential to life. The patient is kept comfortably warm but never overly warm, because overheating causes vasodilation and counteracts arteriolar constriction necessary to ensure an adequate blood supply to the vital organs.

Measures to prevent additional physical or emotional stress are necessary, because although the patient may be able to cope with one stress-producing situation, his or her body may not be able to adapt to further stressors. Special care needs to be taken to prevent further trauma, superimposed infection, anxiety, or fear. Extraordinary thoughtfulness is necessary, since the patient is likely to be very alert. Anxiety-producing conversations with the patient or in the vicinity of the patient are to be avoided. Noise, bright lights, and disturbances should be kept to a minimum. Pain should be alleviated as much as possible.

Even minor stress reactions cause annoying discomforts such as backache, generalized muscle tension, and headache. These discomforts can act as additional stressors, and comfort measures such as back rubs, position changes, and back support to relax the muscles are indicated. During severe stress oral food and fluids may need to be withheld until nausea subsides and gastrointestinal tract activity returns to normal.

While caring for a patient who is facing a stressful event or is experiencing a major stressor, the nurse should be alert to symptoms and signs of stress. The sudden appearance or the worsening of these signs and symptoms may be the first indication that the patient's condition is deteriorating. Transitory signs and symptoms of stress, such as a temporary rise in systolic blood pressure and pulse rate and periodic deep breathing, may be signals that there is an increase in

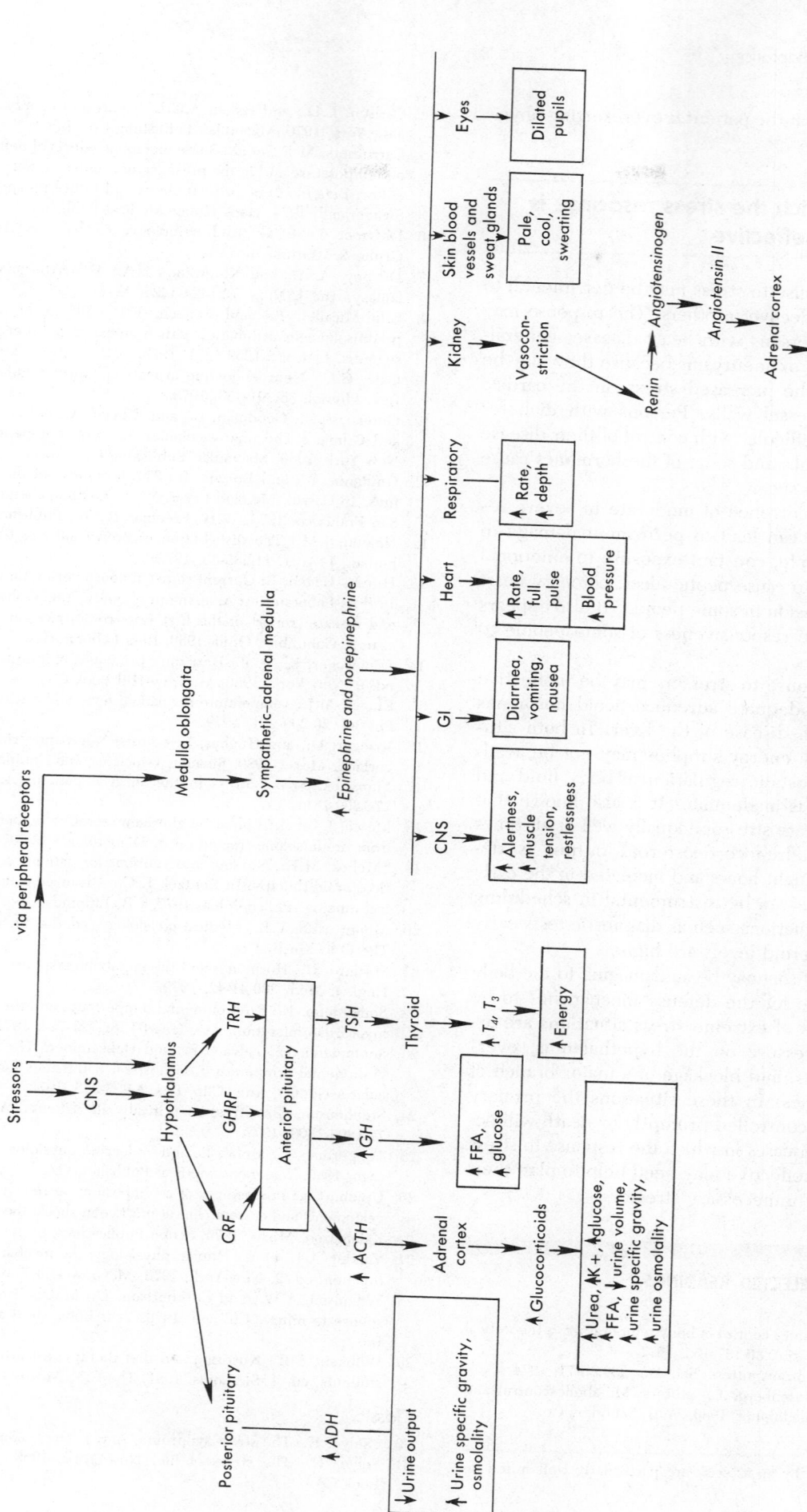

Fig. 18-4. Neuroendocrine integrating mechanisms in stress and resultant signs and symptoms. Resultant signs and symptoms from stimulation of various parts of neuroendocrine integrating mechanisms are in boxes. Hormones and catecholamines are in italics.

emotional stress or that the patient is overexerting physically.

Conditions in which the stress response is detrimental or ineffective

The body's response to stress may be detrimental to some persons or ineffective in others. The response may be detrimental in persons with heart disease, generalized arteriosclerosis, or aneurysms because they may be unable to tolerate the increased stress on the cardiac muscles or blood vessel walls. Persons with diabetes mellitus may have difficulty with control of their disease because catecholamines and some of the hormones cause an increase in blood sugar.

The frequent occurrence of moderate to severe responses to stressors can lead to permanent damage to the body. For example, constant exposure to emotional stressors is thought to cause peptic ulcer, coronary heart disease, or hypertension in some people. It also appears to play a part in the responsiveness of some people to allergenic substances.

The body's response to stressors may be ineffective in patients with inadequate adrenocorticoid hormones and in patients with disease of the liver. In both situations the necessary energy supplies may not be available and the homeostatic regulation of body fluid and electrolyte balance is inadequate. It is also known that persons do not tolerate stressors equally well at all times of the day. The adrenocorticosteroid output is decreased during the night hours and increased in the early morning. The nurse can be instrumental in scheduling stress-producing situations such as diagnostic tests early in the day when steroid levels are higher.

The original stressor may be so damaging to the body that it is impossible for the defense mechanisms to be effective. Examples of extreme stress situations are arterial bleeding, pressure on the hypothalamus, overwhelming infections, and blockage of a major branch of the coronary arteries. In these situations the primary condition must be controlled promptly or death will occur. Persons with diseases in which the response to stress is detrimental or ineffective may need help to plan their lives so as to avoid unnecessary stressors.

REFERENCES AND SELECTED READINGS
Contemporary

1. Albers, C.: Respiratory control of body temperature: a theoretical model, Respir. Physiol. **30:**137-155, 1977.
2. *Axelrod, J.: Neurotransmitters, Sci. Am. **230:**58-71, 1974.
3. Bondy, P., and Rosenberg, L., editors: Metabolic control and disease, ed. 8, Philadelphia, 1980, W.B. Saunders Co.

4. Carlson, L.D., and Hsieh, A.C.L.: Control of energy exchange, New York, 1970, Macmillan Publishing Co., Inc.
5. Carruthers, M.E., et al.: Some metabolic effects of beta-blockade on temperature and in the presence of trauma. In Schweizer, E., editor: Beta-blockers' present status and future prospects, Bern, Switzerland, 1974, Hans Huber Medical Publisher.
6. DeGroot, L., et al.: Endrocrinology, 3 vols., New York, 1979, Grune & Stratton, Inc.
7. Devney, A.M., and Kingsbury, B.A.: Hyperthermia: fact and fantasy, Am. J. Nurs. **72:**1424-1425, 1972.
8. Ellul-Micallef, R., and Fenech, F.F.: Effects of intravenous prednisolone in asthmatics with diminished adrenergic responsiveness, Lancet **2:**1269-1271, 1975.
9. Gale, C.C.: Neuroendocrine aspects of thermoregulation, Ann. Rev. Physiol. **35:**391-430, 1973.
10. Gilman, A.G., Goodman, L., and Gilman, A., editors: Goodman and Gilman's The pharmacological basis of therapeutics, ed. 6, New York, 1980. Macmillan Publishing Co., Inc.
11. Guillenin, R., and Burgus, R.: The hormones of the hypothalamus. In Calvin, M., and Pryor, W.A.: Organic chemistry of life, San Francisco, 1973, W.H. Freeman & Co., Publishers.
12. Heaton, J.M.: The distribution of brown adipose tissue in the human, J. Anat. **112:**35-39, 1972.
13. Himms-Hagen, J.: Current status of nonshivering thermogenesis. In Ross Laboratories: Assessment of energy metabolism in health and disease: report of the first Ross conference on medical research, Columbus, Ohio, 1980, Ross Laboratories.
14. Isselbacher, K., et al.: Harrison's principles of internal medicine, ed. 9, New York, 1980, McGraw-Hill Book Co.
15. Kluger, M.J.: Temperature regulation, fever and disease, Int. Rev. Physiol. **20:**209-251, 1979.
16. Krieger, D., and Hughes, J., editors: Neuroendocrinology, Sungerland, Mass., 1980, Sinauer Associates, Inc., Publishers.
17. Marcinek, M.B.: Stress in the surgical patient, Am. J. Nurs. **77:**1809-1811, 1977.
18. Marco, J., et al.: Enhanced glucagon secretion by pancreatic islet from prednisolone-treated mice, Diabetologia **12:**307-311, 1976.
19. *Melick, M.E.: Nursing interventions for patients receiving corticosteroid therapy. In Kentzel, K.C.: Advanced concepts in clinical nursing, Philadelphia, 1977, J.B. Lippincott Co.
20. Mountcastle, V.B.: Medical physiology, ed. 14, St. Louis, 1979, The C.V. Mosby Co.
21. *Munro, H.: Hormones and the metabolic response to injury, N. Engl. J. Med. **300:**41-42, 1979.
22. Sontaniemi, E.: Environmental temperature and the incidence of myocardial infarction, Am. Heart J. **82:**723-724, 1971.
23. Sontaniemi, E., Palva, I.P., and Hakkarainen, H.: Effect of environmental temperature on hospital admissions for cerebrovascular accidents, Ann. Clin. Res. **4:**233-235, 1972.
24. Stephenson, C.: Stress in critically ill patients, Am. J. Nurs. **77:**1806-1808, 1977.
25. Tepperman, J.: Metabolic and endocrine physiology, ed. 4, Chicago, 1980, Year Book Medical Publishers, Inc.
26. Upjohn Co.: Proceedings of a symposium on recent research developments and current clinical practice in shock: the cell in shock, Kalamazoo, Mich., 1974, Scope Publications.
27. Vander, A.J., et al.: Human physiology: the mechanisms of body function, ed. 2, New York, 1975, McGraw-Hill Book Co.
28. Wilkinson, A.W., and Cuthbertson, D.: Metabolism and the response to injury, Chicago, 1978, Year Book Medical Publishers, Inc.
29. Williams, S.R.: Nutrition and diet therapy: a learning guide for students, ed. 4, St. Louis, 1981, The C.V. Mosby Co.

Classic

30. *Selye, H.: The stress syndrome, Am. J. Nurs. **65:**97-99, 1965.
31. Selye, H.: The stress of life, New York, 1956, McGraw-Hill Book Co.

*References preceded by an asterisk are particularly well suited for student reading.

CHAPTER 19

BIOLOGIC DEFENSE MECHANISMS

E. RONALD WRIGHT

Concept of biologic defense

The human body exists within a milieu of antagonistic environmental forces that are constantly attacking and threatening the integrity of the individual. In response to these onslaughts, the body exhibits a wide array of adaptations (structures, mechanisms, and responses) designed to provide a defense against these encroachments. These mechanisms serve to protect the body from both external and internal deleterious agents. This chapter deals with those anatomic and biologic mechanisms that provide protection against environmental factors that physically threaten the client's body. The implications and applications of the functions of these systems are also discussed.

Knowledge of the basic structures and mechanisms that provide this protection helps in the understanding of (1) resistance to infectious disease, (2) diagnosis of disease and physiologic state, (3) rejection of tissue transplants, (4) prevention of the development of malignancies, (5) adaptations in the aging process, (6) immunization against infectious disease, (7) expression of disease of autoimmunity or immunodeficiency, (8) development of allergic reaction, and (9) significance of the localized or systemic inflammatory response. Much of preventive and restorative nursing practice is built on the maintenance or restoration of the cells, systems, and mechanisms that provide defenses against harmful factors in the external environment.

Self vs. nonself

Each human being can be regarded as a genetically and immunologically unique collection of cells and mol-
ecules that make up a biologic unit of *self*. It is the function of the biologic defense mechanisms of the body to protect the integrity of self from encroachment by *nonself* (or foreign) materials. These mechanisms (Fig. 19-1) serve to protect self from both external and internal destructive agents in the following ways:

1. *Exclusion* of harmful agents from the body
2. *Recognition* of harmful agents within the body
3. *Response* designed to rid the body of the harmful agents that do gain access

The sources of these harmful nonself materials are generally external. These external agents include nonliving materials of the environment such as potentially harmful inorganic chemicals and compounds produced by other living organisms. The most serious external threats to biologic integrity, however, come from the living organisms that constantly surround the body. Some of these organisms pose no real threat because the mechanical, biochemical, and metabolic processes of the human body will not support them or offer them shelter. There are a myriad of living forms, on the other hand, for which the human body is an ideal haven for growth and survival. Most of these organisms, if allowed to penetrate the body, would wreak havoc on the normal functionings of the body. The living forms that come to mind in this regard are the organisms classified as pathogenic (disease causing). While it is true that the progress of these organisms in the body can be altered by external agents such as antibiotics, the eradication of the offending organism from the body must be accomplished by the host's own adaptive mechanisms.

In addition to protection against external agents, the defense mechanisms also protect against the accumulation of damaged or dysfunctional self-material. If it were not for these processes that carry out the systematic, specific removal of damaged or worn out cellular material, the body would become clogged with debris. Still another general function of these systems is that of rec-

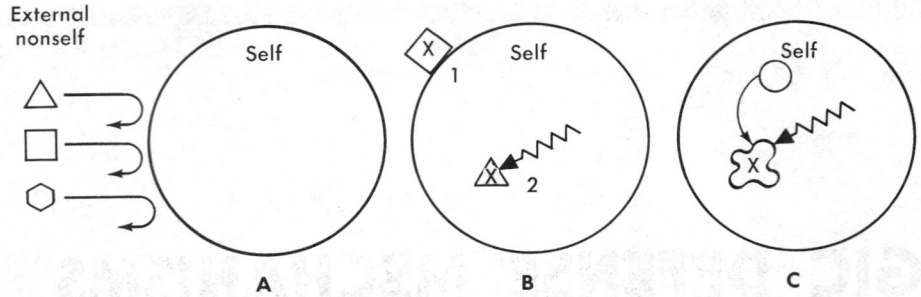

Fig. 19-1. Mechanisms of biologic defense in human body. **A,** Exclusion of external nonself. **B,** Destruction of external nonself by *(1)* nonspecific external mechanisms and *(2)* nonspecific or specific internal mechanisms. **C,** Destruction of altered self. *X* indicates nonspecific mechanisms; ↝ indicates specific mechanisms.

TABLE 19-1. Biologic defense mechanisms

Nonspecific mechanisms	Specific mechanisms
External	
Mechanical exclusion	Immunoglobulin A
Physical structures	In mucosal secretions
Skin	In mucosal cells
Mucous membranes	
Specialized structures	
Physical actions	
Biochemical factors	
Body secretions	
pH	
Lysozyme	
Microbial antagonism	
Internal	
Reticuloendothelial system	Antigen processing by macro-
Blood	phage
Cellular components	Primary immune response
Fluid components	Humoral immune response
Opsonins	Synthesis of circulating anti-
Complement	bodies by B cells
Properdin	Interaction of antibodies with
C-reactive protein	antigen
Phagocytosis	Cell-mediated immune response
Inflammatory response	Sensitization of T cells
Interferon	Lymphokines
	Combined immune response
	Secondary immune response

ble and complex. For the sake of orderly presentation they may be divided into *nonspecific* and *specific* mechanisms (Table 19-1). The specific and nonspecific mechanisms can be further divided on the basis of where the lines of defense are formed, that is, *external* for the mechanisms of mechanical exclusion, biochemical destruction, and microbial competition and *internal* for the physiologic reactions. The nonspecific mechanisms are nonselectively directed against *any* foreign substance. The specific mechanisms are specifically elicited by *unique* substances to which the body has *acquired* the ability to respond.

Concept of immunity

The objective of the biologic defense mechanisms is to provide the host with protection. The ultimate protection would be total resistance to encroachment or damage by an organism or agent; this is usually termed *absolute immunity*. Absence of such protective barriers is called *susceptibility*. Although these terms are generally applied to immunity from infectious organisms, they can be used to describe the relative susceptibility to encroachment by any external agent. *Nonspecific immunity* (or *innate immunity*) is provided when the external and internal nonspecific defense mechanisms serve as the barrier excluding or destroying the invading agent. *Specific immunity* protects against a single unique agent through the development of specific antibodies (Ab) or responsive cells in the body. It is *acquired* from prior contact with that agent (antigen [Ag]) or through the introduction of specifically protective antibodies or cells into the body.

The acquisition of specific immunity may result from *natural* encounter or *artificial* introduction. Immunity acquired naturally means under natural conditions, such as recovery from a disease. Immunity acquired artificially means that the antigen or protective antibodies were purposely introduced into the body (e.g., by vac-

ognition of the alteration of self to a potentially dangerous state. When this defense function falters, the tragedy of malignancy (cancer) results.

Scope of defense mechanisms

The array of defense mechanisms that have been adapted to protect the normal human body is formida-

TABLE 19-2. Types of acquired specific immunity

Type of immunity	Acquisition of immunity	Protection	Examples
Active: antibodies synthesized by body in response to antigenic stimulation	*Natural:* natural contact with antigen through clinical or subclinical case	*Development:* develops slowly; protective levels reached in a few weeks *Duration:* long term; often lifetime *Spectrum:* specific to antigen contacted	Recovery from childhood diseases (e.g., chickenpox, measles, mumps)
	Artificial: immunization with antigen	*Development:* develops slowly; protective levels reached in a few weeks *Duration:* several years; extended protection with "booster" doses *Spectrum:* specific to antigen immunized against	Immunization with live or killed vaccines; toxoid immunization
Passive: antibodies produced in one individual are transferred to another	*Natural:* transplacental and colostrum transfer from mother to child	*Development:* immediate *Duration:* temporary; several months *Spectrum:* to all antigens that mother has immunity	Maternal immunoglobulins in neonate
	Artificial: injection of serum from immune human or animal	*Development:* immediate *Duration:* temporary; several weeks *Spectrum:* to all antigens that source has immunity	Injection of pooled human gamma globulin; injection of animal hyperimmune sera

cination). The immunity may be an *active* or *passive* immunity. When an individual is producing the antibodies within his or her own body, the immunity is termed active. When an individual receives the protective antibodies from some other source, the immunity is termed passive. Thus when antibodies are transferred from the mother across the placenta, the child is said to have a natural passive immunity; or when a vaccine is given, so that antibodies are produced within the body, the immunized individual is characterized as having an artificial active immunity. Table 19-2 summarizes the different types of specific acquired immunities.

Specific or nonspecific immunity to harmful agents is a relative state. The effect of different dosages of an infectious organism or the toxic products of such organisms in experimental studies clearly demonstrate that administration of sufficiently large numbers of an organism or high dosages of a toxin can overwhelm even the most highly immunized animal. Further, when the normal mechanisms of defense are breached, even in the highly resistant host, disease can result. Thus acquired immunity to infection is not always an absolute condition but depends on a large number of complex variables. These include not only the defense mechanisms

of the host but also the dosage, route of contact, and virulence of the harmful agent.

External nonspecific defense mechanisms

Anatomic structures and mechanical actions

Skin and mucous membranes

The first line of defense against penetration by foreign materials, including pathogenic microorganisms, is the skin. When the skin is intact it serves as an extremely efficient physical barrier to harmful agents and environmental forces such as heat, cold, and trauma. This protection is afforded by the keratinized surface cells, which provide a tough, dense, waterproof covering. Beneath this outermost layer is a dense layer of highly vascularized connective tissue (see Fig. 68-1).

Even though some of the fatty acids derived from sebaceous gland secretions have antimicrobial activity, the environment provided by the skin does allow the growth of microorganisms on its upper layers and within hair follicles and sweat glands. For the most part these resident microorganisms are nonpathogenic; however, when these organisms gain entrance to the tissues of a host exhibiting reduced resistance, they may cause significant problems. Because even thorough scrubbing with soap and water removes only the surface organisms, the skin can never be considered sterile.

Any time the physical integrity of the skin is broken, such as in surgery, indwelling venous catheterization, or physical irritation or trauma, there is significant risk of microorganisms gaining entrance to the body. The skin must be kept relatively dry, since the continued presence of moisture tends to cause maceration of the skin. Further, when essential oils are lost from the skin surface they should be supplemented by lotions to maintain the resilience and unbroken texture of the surface cells. Adequate care of the skin of the hospitalized patient is not just a luxury but a necessity for the provision of an extremely important aspect of biologic defense.

Mucous membranes protect the eye and line all body tracts that have external openings. When intact, the mucous membranes, like the skin, are basically impervious to foreign materials and microorganisms. The surfaces are covered by a viscous secretion that tends to trap and inactivate microorganisms. The mucous membrane of the respiratory tract is further protected by the surface activity of the ciliated epithelial cells, which sweep foreign material out of the tract. The mucous membranes are highly vascularized so that the internal defense mechanisms are readily available to attack any microorganisms that do gain access to the surface of these cells.

Also found in the mucosal secretions and in high concentration within the secretory mucosal cells of the respiratory and intestinal tracts are a specific class of immunoglobulins (antibodies) known as immunoglobulin A (IgA). These specific antibodies are secreted from the mucosal cells and have antibacterial, antiviral, and antitoxic properties. These antibodies serve to prevent microbial adherence and colonization of these tracts by pathogens.

Specialized structures and mechanical functions

Other structures and functions of the human body that are generally taken for granted actually serve extremely important roles in defense. The filtration action of the nasal hairs serves to trap particles and microorganisms. The flushing action of saliva and urine prevents the buildup of organisms. The eyes are protected from the entrance of dirt particles and organisms by the lids and lashes. Foreign material that does gain entrance to the eye tends to be washed out by tears. The constant movement of foods through the stomach and intestines prevents the buildup of organisms or toxic waste products. Even the action of vomiting and the

watery stools of diarrhea are active mechanisms of removal of harmful products from the gastrointestinal tract. Dysfunction or blockage of any of these processes means that special measures must be taken to protect against the establishment of pathogenic organisms and the buildup of toxic materials.

Biochemical factors

Many areas of the body are protected not only by mechanical barriers but also by the presence of specific antimicrobial chemicals that provide added protection.

Skin

The acetic acid and salt concentration of perspiration is toxic to many pathogenic microorganisms. Some of the fatty acids released to the skin surface by the sebaceous glands also serve to inhibit the growth of some microorganisms.

Gastrointestinal tract

In the stomach the acidity (approximate pH 2) of the gastric juice kills many organisms and detoxifies certain potentially toxic substances. For this reason, when gastric acidity is low special precautions must be taken to avoid introduction of organisms through the nose and mouth. Low gastric acidity is characteristically encountered in neonates; therefore special care should be taken in feeding and handling babies to prevent exposure to pathogens by the oral route. The upper intestine is generally freed of organisms by the action of bile and other proteolytic enzymes.

Vagina

Vaginal secretions allow certain harmless acid-producing bacteria to colonize the vagina and create an acidic environment. This reduces the chance of the colonization of the vagina by pathogens. When either the amount or acidity of the vaginal secretions is reduced, there is a much greater chance that a vaginal infection will develop. Since vaginal secretions are not present before puberty and are greatly reduced after menopause, both young girls and older women are more prone to vaginitis. The use of birth control pills causes a shift in the composition and pH of the vaginal secretions, which increases the possibility of colonization of the vagina, especially by the causative agent of gonorrhea, *Neisseria gonorrhoeae*.

Lysozyme

The most ubiquitous antimicrobial factor in the body is the enzyme lysozyme. It is capable of lysing (splitting) the bacterial cell wall of many gram-positive organisms, causing their destruction. The enzyme is present in mucus, tears, saliva, and skin secretions and is also found in many of the internal fluids and cells of the

TABLE 19-3. Distribution of normal microbic flora

Region of body	Sterile areas	Nonsterile areas	Microorganisms
Skin	None	All skin	*Staphylococcus, Bacillus, Corynebacterium, Mycobacterium, Streptococcus,* transient environmental organisms
Respiratory tract	Larynx, trachea, bronchi, bronchioles, alveoli, sinuses	Nose, throat, mouth	*Staphyloccus, Candida, Streptococcus, Neisseria, Pneumococcus,* oral organisms
Gastrointestinal tract	Esophagus, stomach, upper small intestine	Esophagus and stomach (transiently), large intestine	Gram-negative rods, *Streptococcus, Bacteroides, Proteus, Clostridium, Lactobacillus*
Genitourinary tract	Cervix, uterus, fallopian tubes, ovaries, prostate gland, epididymis, testes, bladder, kidney	External genitalia, anterior urethra, vagina	Skin organisms, *Lactobacillus, Bacteroides*
Body fluids and cavities	Blood pleural fluid, synovial fluid, spinal fluid, lymph, etc.	None	

body. Within the body it tends to work in combination with complement and other blood factors to destroy bacteria directly.

Microbial antagonism

The skin and mucosal surfaces offer varying nutritional and environmental conditions for the growth and multiplication of certain microbial cells. Although the surfaces of the body are constantly exposed to temporary contamination by organisms from the environment, most of these organisms, known as *transient flora*, do not find conditions suitable for the colonization of the body; however, there are many microorganisms that do colonize the skin and mucosal surfaces. These organisms make up what is known as the *normal microbic flora*. Although this normal flora varies from site to site within the body and may vary in response to environmental, hygienic, and physiologic changes, it is capable of reestablishment and reflects a fairly predictable pattern. Table 19-3 provides an overview of the body areas normally colonized and shows which organisms most often make up the normal flora of the various areas.

The maintenance of this balanced microbic flora serves to make it difficult for pathogenic organisms to establish themselves on the body surfaces. Since the normal flora have a selective advantage in their environmental niche, they compete for nutrients and space. Some release antimicrobial substances to retard the growth of transient organisms seeking to occupy the same site. These microbial interferences are known as *microbial antagonism*.

Most of the normal microbic flora are basically nonpathogenic; however, some overtly pathogenic organisms, such as *Staphylococcus aureus* and *Streptococcus pyogenes*, can be part of the normal flora. The individual who harbors such organisms without demonstrating any symptoms of disease is known as a *carrier*. This carrier state is of significance because the carrier may be unknowingly shedding organisms into the environment and infecting others.

The protective effects of the normal microbic flora become most apparent when something upsets the microbic balance within the body. The use of broad-spectrum antibiotics sometimes creates such an effect. The imbalance may allow a segment of the normal flora to gain ascendency, causing adverse reactions. An example of this phenomenon is seen when certain oral antibiotics induce marked shifts in the normal intestinal flora, allowing organisms that are generally suppressed by the growth of competitors to thrive to an unusual degree. This imbalance may induce uncomfortable gastrointestinal tract problems or even allow gastroenteritis to develop.

Internal nonspecific defense mechanisms

Once a foreign agent (living or nonliving) penetrates the external resistance barriers, it is met by an even more complex array of defense mechanisms, which provides for the recognition, capture, and disposal of the foreign material. The key to this process is the specific recognition and vigorous action taken against the foreign material while at the same time protecting the host tissues from extensive damage. The physiologic reactions that serve to contain and inactivate the foreign agent are carried out through interactions of cells and molecules of the blood, reticuloendothelial system, vascular system, and body tissues.

Reticuloendothelial system

The reticuloendothelial system (RES) is a widespread system of phagocytic cells (devouring cells) scattered throughout various body tissues (Fig. 19-2). The role of these cells is to ingest foreign particulate matter and damaged host tissues. Some of the phagocytic cells are *fixed* in a variety of tissues, such as lymphoid tissue, liver, spleen, bone marrow, lungs, and blood vessels. Within the different tissues these anchored cells have been given unique names (Table 19-4). It is the function of the fixed cells to capture and destroy foreign materials found in the fluids of their environment.

Other cells making up the reticuloendothelial network are not stationary and are given the name *wandering macrophages*. Depending on where they are found, they may be known as monocytes (in the bloodstream) or histiocytes (in loose connective tissues). The wandering macrophages carry out the important role of final cleanup of a damaged site in preparation for repair. The cells have the capacity to engulf and destroy virtually any type of foreign material or debris within the body. The macrophages also play an important role in the specific response mechanisms.

Blood

Blood is one of the primary sources of elements designed to provide protection against injurious agents. The blood transports these active factors to the site of an injury or intrusion and through specific vascular changes concentrates these materials at the site. Both the fluid and cellular constituents of blood contain these factors.

Cellular components

The cellular components of blood that are of importance in this nonspecific response include granulocytes, lymphocytes, monocytes, and thrombocytes (platelets). The granulocytes, also referred to as polymorphonuclear leukocytes (PMNs), and the monocytes are of the most importance because of their phagocytic activity.

One of the key methods of nonspecific defense is the ingestion of microorganisms and other particulate matter by the phagocytic white blood cells. The phagocytes carry out the process of *phagocytosis* in several discrete steps (Fig. 19-3). Most infecting microbes are quickly and efficiently destroyed by phagocytosis; however, some pathogens exhibit methods of escape from this destruction. Some bacteria, such as strains of the

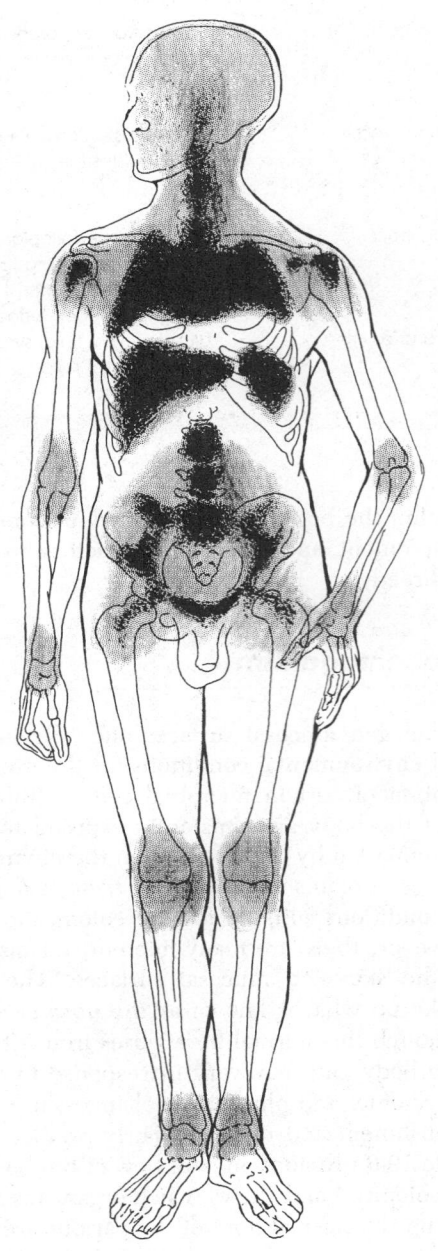

Fig. 19-2. Reticuloendothelial system. Note anatomic distribution of maximal activity in system, as indicated by black areas over body. To produce such an image certain radioactive colloidal particles are given to subject, and radiation detection techniques delineate tissue uptake. Note definition of liver, spleen, and active bone marrow in axial skeleton and proximal parts of long bones. (From Smith, A.L.: Microbiology and pathology, ed. 12, St. Louis, 1980, The C.V. Mosby Co.)

streptococci and staphylococci and *Bacillus anthracis* (anthrax), actually produce factors that will kill the phagocyte. Other organisms resist ingestion or digestion. Some organisms may survive within the phagocytes or reticuloendothelial cells and multiply there. This may lead to the transport of the organism to other sites in the body or serve as a chronic focus of continued infection.

The granulocytes can be divided on the basis of their structure and function into neutrophils, eosinophils, and basophils. The "granules" found within these cells represent discrete packets of degradative enzymes used to digest the ingested materials. The neutrophils are the most numerous in circulation and are the most efficient and responsive phagocytic cells involved in the inflammatory process. Where there is adequate blood supply to a region, the phagocytes are constantly available to move from the blood vessels to the site of injury or infection. The neutrophils and monocytes are actually attracted to the scene by chemicals released during infection or injury. This cellular response to chemical attractants is known as *chemotaxis*, and the substances released are called *chemotactic substances*.

Fluid factors

The fluid portion of uncoagulated blood is called *plasma*. Some of the components of plasma provide important constituents for the internal defense mechanisms. Plasma transports the *circulating antibodies* pro-

TABLE 19-4. Distribution and names of macrophages in various tissue sites

Tissue	Name
Peripheral blood	Monocyte
Loose connective tissue	Histiocyte
Liver	Kupffer's cells
Spleen and reticuloendothelial system	Wandering or fixed macrophage
Lung	Alveolar macrophage or dust cell
Granulomatous tissue	Epithelioid and giant cells
Peritoneal cavity, pleural cavity, and bone	Macrophages

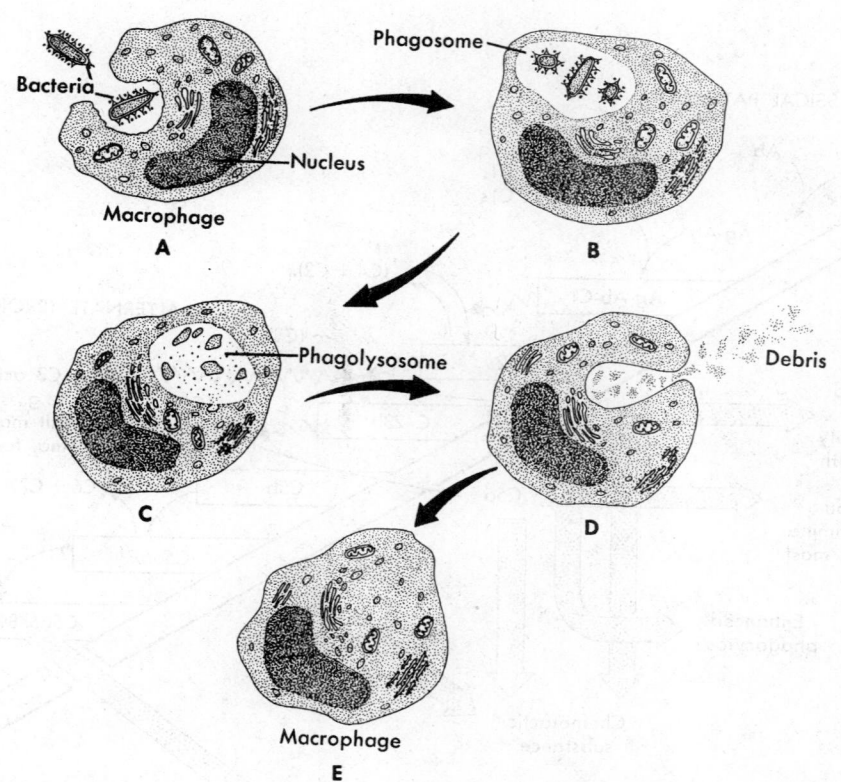

Fig. 19-3. Phagocytosis sketched in macrophage. **A,** Opsonized bacteria engulfed by phagocyte (macrophage). **B,** Phagosome formed. **C,** Phagosome becomes phagolysosome; bacteria digested. (to this point process of phagocytosis is comparable in either macrophage or neutrophil, not shown.) **D,** Debris is egested. (Neutrophil would succumb here.) **E,** Macrophage returns to resting state. (From Smith, A.L.: Microbiology and pathology, ed. 12, St. Louis, 1980, The C.V. Mosby Co.)

duced in specific response to antigenic stimulation. These antibodies, when bound to their specific antigens, enhance the ability of white blood cells to engulf the clumped and sticky antigens. The antibodies of the blood that create this coating effect are known as *opsonins*. Another plasma constituent, *fibrin*, may create a meshwork around the injured area causing the sealing off of the area. Microorganisms may also become trapped within this meshwork where they are more easily captured by the phagocytic cells.

One of the most important constituents of plasma is a complex series of 11 proteins known by the singular name of *complement*. The primary role of complement is to provide specific lysis (rupturing) of cell membranes. The initiation of the "complement cascade" is most often triggered by the binding of the first complement protein to complement binding antibodies that have already bound to their antigens. Thus complement serves to accentuate or complete the action of an antibody. The antibody by itself cannot produce cell lysis, but with the recruitment of complement to join in the reaction the cell may be ruptured. However, other substances of a nonimmune nature can also activate complement. Complement is considered a nonspecific component of

the plasma because it is not increased by immunization. In addition to its cytolytic effects, complement is involved in leukocyte chemotaxis, release of histamines, enhancement of phagocytosis by PMNs, viral neutralization, and bactericidal activity.

The classical activities ascribed to complement depend on the sequential interaction of nine protein subunits (C1 to C9), the first component of which consists of three subfractions termed C1q, C1r, and C1s (thereby accounting for the 11 separate proteins mentioned above). When the first component, C1, is bound by an antigen-antibody complex on the surface of a cell, it acquires the enzymatic ability to activate several molecules of the next components in the sequence, C4 and C2, to form an active C42 complex (Fig. 19-4). (Unfortunately, the numbering system of the complement components reflects their order of discovery and not their sequential additive pattern.) Each of the activated C42 complexes is then able to act on the next component, and so on, producing both a cascade effect and greatly amplifying the reaction. As each component is added there is created new enzymatic activity to initiate the next step. The final component, C89, has the ability to create a lesion in the cell membrane, and if enough lesions are

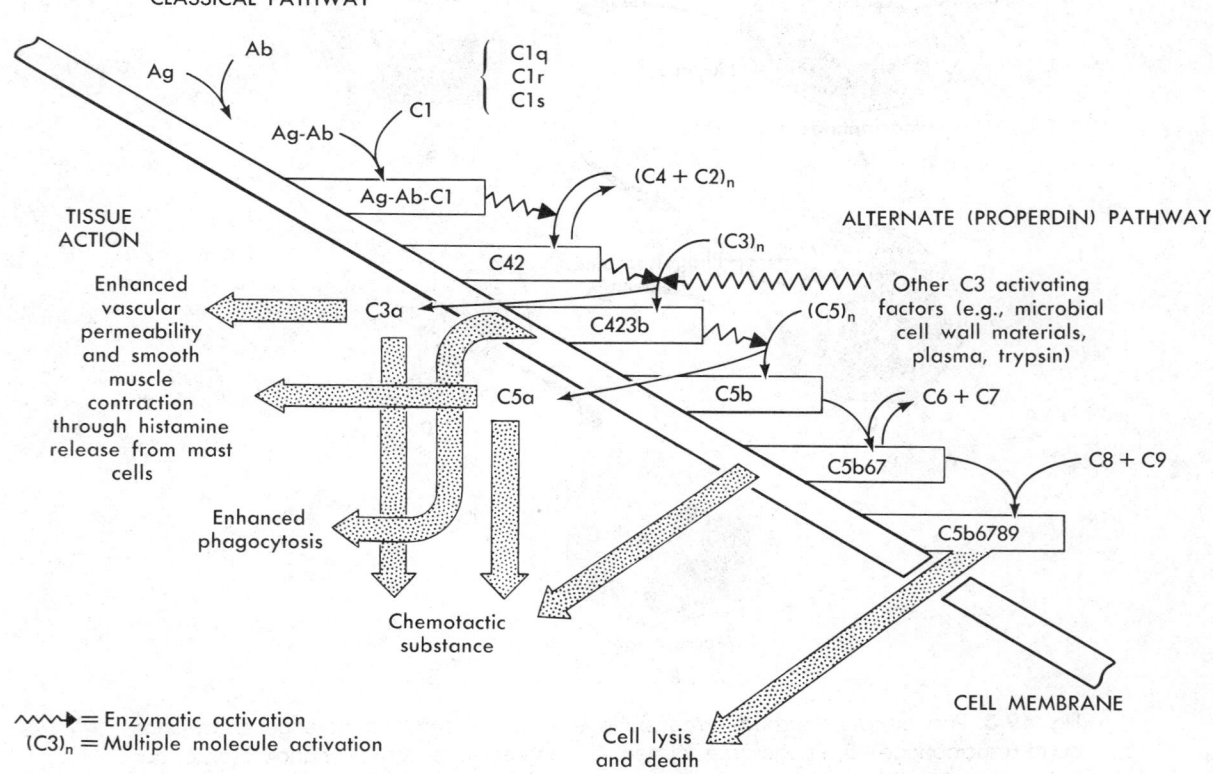

Fig. 19-4. Classical and alternate complement cascade. Sequence of complement activation generates multiple biologically active intermediate molecules, which are active in inflammatory response.

created on the membrane, cell death results. The intermediate stages in the complement sequence also give rise to complexes and fragments with other significant biologic activities. Fig. 19-4 depicts the generation of some of these activities. These include the following:

1. *Histamine release*. Histamines cause an extreme increase in vascular permeability and contraction of smooth muscle. A fragment (C3a) split off during the activation of C3 and another fragment (C5a) created by the activation of C5 are released into the surrounding tissues, where they cause the release of histamine from mast cells. The histamines in turn exert their physiologic effects on the smooth-muscle tissues and vascular system. Because these histamine-mediated reactions are the same as those created during anaphylactic shock (p. 1863), these fragments are called *anaphylatoxins*.

2. *Enhanced phagocytosis*. One of the intermediate activators in the cascade, C423b, makes the labeled antigen tend to stick to the surface of cells so that it is more easily phagocytosed.

3. *Chemotactic substance formation*. Several of the fragments and intermediate factors serve as chemotactic substances to attract phagocytes to the site of the reaction.

All of these activities are central to the inflammatory response.

The plasma fraction contains several proteins that inhibit the action of the activated components of complement in the fluid phase, that is, off of the membrane surface. Such inhibitors serve to localize the effects of the membrane surface and thereby to protect the "innocent bystander" membranes.

In addition to the activated C42 complement complex, a number of other enzymes exhibit *C3 convertase* activity. These include trypsin, plasmin, and thrombin as well as bacterial endotoxins and a factor derived from cobra venom. Each leads to alterations of C3, which are similar to if not identical with those produced by the complement cascade–derived C3 convertase. These activations are mediated through a plasma component known as *properdin* and are referred to as the *alternative*, or *properdin*, *pathway*.

C-reactive protein is a beta-globulin (β-globulin) found in the serum of individuals suffering from any type of severe inflammatory process. Both infectious and noninfectious inflammations will elicit the formation of this protein in the plasma. The protein will form a precipitate with a consituent of the cell wall of *Streptococcus pneumoniae* known as the C polysaccharide; hence its name. The amount of C-reactive protein found in the serum is roughly proportional to the severity of the inflammation; therefore a test for this protein is useful in the diagnosis and management of hard to differentiate diseases that have a hidden inflammatory aspect, such as bacterial endocarditis, cryptic abscesses, rheumatic fever, and certain types of cancer.

Interferon

Interferon is a low–molecular weight protein produced by certain virally infected cells. The protein is released into the extracellular environment, and when taken up by uninfected cells, it can protect those cells from viral multiplication. This antiviral action is exerted before the antibody levels can reach protective levels. The interferons are synthesized by the cells of many different animal species, but they are species specific; that is, bovine interferon will not protect human cells. In general, the product of a viral infection is the same regardless of the viral agent that initiated its formation. Therefore interferons can be described as being host specific but viral nonspecific.

Interferons are produced by cells infected with infectious viral particles, infectious inactivated viruses, or even laboratory-synthesized double-stranded polynucleotides. Virtually all tissue cells are capable of producing interferons when properly stimulated. The stimulation seems to be tied to the recognition of the "foreign" nucleic acid, which signals the infected cells to synthesize and liberate interferon for a few hours (up to about 24 hours). The interferon acts on the uninfected cells, causing them to synthesize another protein that remains within the protected cell. This protein inhibits the synthesis of the viral particle without blocking normal cell synthetic functions (Fig. 19-5). The interferon itself has no direct effect on the viral particles, nor does it interfere with the entry of the viral particle into the interferon-protected cell. This interferon-mediated protection lasts for only about 24 hours.

While viruses seem to be the most potent inducers of interferon production, other microorganisms also stimulate its synthesis. Included in this group are the causative agents of malaria, rickettsial diseases, brucellosis, and tularemia.

Interferon does not inhibit all viruses equally; some are more readily inhibited than are others. Among the viruses that seem to be especially sensitive are the arboviruses, influenza, and smallpox viruses.

That interferon plays a significant role in the recovery from viral infections seems inescapable; however, it has never been shown conclusively that interferon is a necessary part of defense against viral infection. Since naturally occurring deficiencies have never been demonstrated and since there is no mechanism for selective inhibition in experimental animals, it is not possible to evaluate specifically the role of interferon as a defense mechanism.

Because of its general protective effect against a wide range of viruses and its low toxicity and antigenicity,

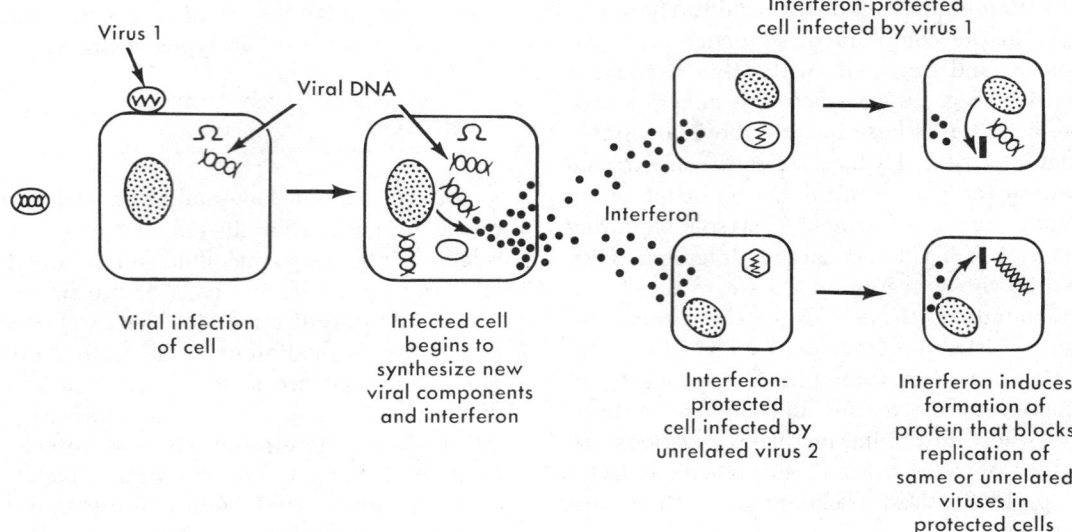

Fig. 19-5. Mechanism of interferon action.

interferon has great potential as a prophylactic and therapeutic agent. At the present time, however, its limitations make it of little clinical significance. These limitations include (1) its species specificity, which means that it would have to be produced in tissue cultures of human cell lines, which is both difficult and expensive; (2) the difficulty in purification, which makes the recovery of large enough quantities impractical; (3) the lack of any effect on viral synthesis already in progress; (4) the inability to deliver protective doses to susceptible host cells; and (5) its short duration of activity. If some means can be found to stimulate interferon production within the host to maintain effectively protective levels, the control of a number of viral infections might be obtained.

Additional areas of interest in interferon currently being widely researched are the use of interferon or interferon inducers as chemotherapeutic agents against certain cancers and as protective agents in immunosuppressed patients. Some tumors have shown regression patterns in clinical field trials utilizing interferon therapy. Protection of immunosuppressed patients, such as those receiving tissue transplants or immunodeficient children, from certain viruses (herpesviruses, influenza virus) has been achieved by interferon therapy.

Inflammatory response

When injury occurs in the body, all of the nonspecific and to some degree the specific defense mechanisms are directed toward localizing the effects of the injury, protecting against microbial invasion at the site, and preparing the site for repair. This process is called *inflammation*. When an inflammation occurs at a partic-

ular site in the body, the addition of the suffix *-itis* is added to the site designation to indicate the pathologic state; for example, an inflammatory response on the pericardium is termed pericarditis; of the bladder, cystitis.

The inflammatory response can be initiated by any type of injury: heat, cold, irradiation, chemicals, trauma, infection, immunologic injury, or neoplasia. Whatever the stimulus, the response of the body is the same, but the extent of the involvement of the various facets of the nonspecific response system depends on the extent and severity of the injury.

Three major physiologic responses occur during the inflammatory process: vascular response, fluid exudation, and cellular exudation (Table 19-5). The *vascular response* consists of a transitory vasoconstriction (stress response) followed immediately by vasodilation. This occurs as a result of chemical substances such as histamine or kinins released at the site of injury or invasion. The amount of blood flow to the area is thus increased (*hyperemia*), causing redness and heat. Blood flow slows as the capillaries dilate. There is increased permeability of the capillary walls facilitating fluid and cellular exudation. *Fluid exudation* from the capillaries into the interstitial spaces begins immediately and is most active during the first 24 hours after injury or invasion. Initially, the fluid exudate is primarily serous fluid, but as the capillary wall becomes more permeable, protein (albumin) is lost into the interstitial spaces. This increases the colloid osmotic pressure in the interstitial spaces, which enourages more fluid exudation. The swelling of the tissue from the fluid in the interstitial spaces is called *edema* (p. 331). *Cellular exudation* refers to the migration of white blood cells (leukocytes) through the capillary walls into the affected tissue. An increased number

TABLE 19-5. Summary of the steps of the inflammatory response

Steps	Mediators	Outcome
1. Injury	Physical, chemical, biologic, immunologic stimulus	Cell and tissue injury
2. Vascular response		
a. Vascular dilation	Histamine, plasmin, serotonin, kinins, prostaglandins released or activated by injury	Dilation of vessels causing stasis of blood and margination of leukocytes
b. Fibrin clot formation	Activation of clotting mechanism	Containment of irritants
3. Fluid exudation	Histamine, kinins, prostaglandins cause opening of venule—endothelial cell junction	Fluid exudation into tissues
4. Cellular exudation		
a. Leukocyte exudation	Chemotactic substances released by complement activation, clot formation, and injured cells	Passage of leukocytes from blood to site of injury and accumulation there
b. Attack and engulfment of foreign materials	Neutrophils and macrophages	Removal and digestion of bacteria, foreign particles, and damaged tissues
5. Healing	Fibroblasts produce collagen fibers and tissue regeneration	Resolution of inflammation and formation of scar tissue

of white blood cells are attracted to the vessels in the affected area as a result of chemotactic substances being released from the tissues by cell injury and complement activation. The white blood cells adhere to the capillary wall and then pass ameboid fashion through the widened endothelial junctions of the capillary wall. Neutrophils (polymorphonuclear leukocytes), which make up about 60% of the circulating white blood cells, are the first leukocytes to respond, usually within the first few hours. The neutrophils ingest the bacteria and dead tissue cells (*phagocytosis*); then they die, releasing proteolytic enzymes that liquefy the dead neutrophils, dead bacteria, and other dead cells (pus). Monocytes and lymphocytes appear later. The macrophages continue the phagocytosis, and the lymphocytes play a role in the antigen-antibody response at the site.

The five cardinal symptoms of inflammation were identified many centuries ago. These are redness (*rubor*) and heat (*calor*) caused by the hyperemia, swelling (*tumor*) caused by the fluid exudate, pain (*dolor*) caused by the pressure of the fluid exudate and by chemical (bradykinin) irritation of the nerve endings, and loss of function of the affected part caused by the swelling and pain.

The inflammatory response serves to prepare the tissue for healing and to contain the spread of bacterial invasion. To prevent the spread of bacteria, fibroblasts are attracted to the area and secrete fibrin, a threadlike substance that encircles the affected area to wall it off from healthy tissue. If there is interference with this

walling-off process, bacteria can spread into the surrounding tissue. This explains why an abscess should not be incised and drained until it has "come to a head" or until the walling-off process is completed.

Bacteria may fail to be contained locally and spread to other parts of the body by means of the lymph system or bloodstream. If picked up by the lymph stream, the bacteria will be carried to the nearest lymph node. These nodes are located along the course of all lymph channels, and here too bacteria can be ingested and destroyed. If the bacteria are virulent enough to resist the action in the lymph nodes, leukocytes are brought in by the bloodstream to attack and engulf the bacteria in the node. The node then becomes swollen and tender because of the accumulation of phagocytes, bacteria, and destroyed lymphoid tissue. This is known as *lymphadenitis*. Swollen lymph nodes can be palpated primarily in the neck, axilla, and groin.

Moderate to severe inflammatory responses can produce generalized systemic effects. Products from the breakdown of bacteria and white blood cells can affect the temperature-regulating center in the hypothalamus and produce fever. A severe infection without an accompanying fever may suggest a poor prognosis. Loss of appetite (anorexia) and fatigue may be caused by conservation of body energy needed to resist the infection. The body increases the production of white blood cells to help fight the infection, and *leukocytosis* (serum white blood cell levels greater than 10,000/cu mm) may occur. With infection there is also an increased blood sedimentation rate; that is, when an anticoagulant is added to the blood in the laboratory, the red blood cells settle to the bottom of a test tube more rapidly than normal. This increase in the sedimentation rate is believed to be caused by an increase in fibrinogen (a blood protein essential to the healing process). The sedimentation rate is elevated during the acute inflammatory stage of infection. Its elevation is an indication that the body's defense mechanism for the repair of damaged tissue is operating. Because the sedimentation rate gradually returns to normal as tissues heal, it also is used to determine when physical activity can be safely resumed following an acute infection.

Inflammations can be classified as acute or chronic. *Acute* inflammations are characterized by a sudden onset and an increase in the fluid exudative response. *Chronic* inflammations have a slower, more insidious onset and are characterized by increased cellular exudation.

Knowledge of the physiologic changes that occur during the inflammatory process helps the nurse to understand the changes that occur in a wide variety of diseases. For example, whenever cells die as a result of injury or disease *(necrosis)*, such as during a myocardial infarction (p. 1118), the inflammatory process will occur. Fat deposits (atheromas) on blood vessel walls cause injury to the lining of the vessel wall and initiate an inflammatory response. Irritation of the peritoneum by trauma or bacterial invasion can cause inflammation of the peritoneum *(peritonitis)*.

No healing will occur until inflammation has subsided and pus and dead tissue have been removed. Pus is a local accumulation of dead phagocytes, dead bacteria, and dead tissue. The bacteria most commonly causing this reaction are the staphylococci, streptococci,

Neisseria, and *Pseudomonas aeruginosa (pyocyanea)*. A collection of pus that is localized by a zone of inflamed tissue is called an *abscess* (Fig. 19-6). An inflammation that involves cellular or connective tissue is called *cellulitis*, whereas an inflammation in which pus collects in a preexisting cavity such as the pleura or gallbladder is called *empyema*. When infection forms an abscess within the body, develops a suppurating channel, and ruptures onto the surface or into a body cavity, it is called a *sinus*. If the infection forms a tubelike passage from an epithelium-lined organ or normal body cavity to the surface or to another organ or cavity, it is called a *fistula*.

After the infected area is clean, new cells are produced to fill in the space left by the injury. They may be the normal structural cells, or they may be fibrotic tissue cells known as *scar tissue*. If they are fibrotic cells, they will not function as formerly but only serve to fill in the injured area. Some body cells readily regenerate; for instance, after the bowel has healed it is almost impossible to find the injured area. The respiratory tract also regenerates its tissues readily. Liver tissue has the capacity to regenerate its tissue, but over a longer period of time. Some nerve cells are always replaced with fibrous tissue. If a large amount of tissue is destroyed, structural cells may not be replaced, regardless of the type of tissue. (See Chapter 24 for discussion of wound healing.)

Some people, especially those with brown or black skin, are prone to excessive scar formation. Such tissue formation, known as a *keloid*, is hard and shiny in appearance and may enlarge to a surprising degree. It may cause disfigurement or undergo malignant degeneration and for this reason is usually excised surgically. Serous membranes sometimes become adherent during inflam-

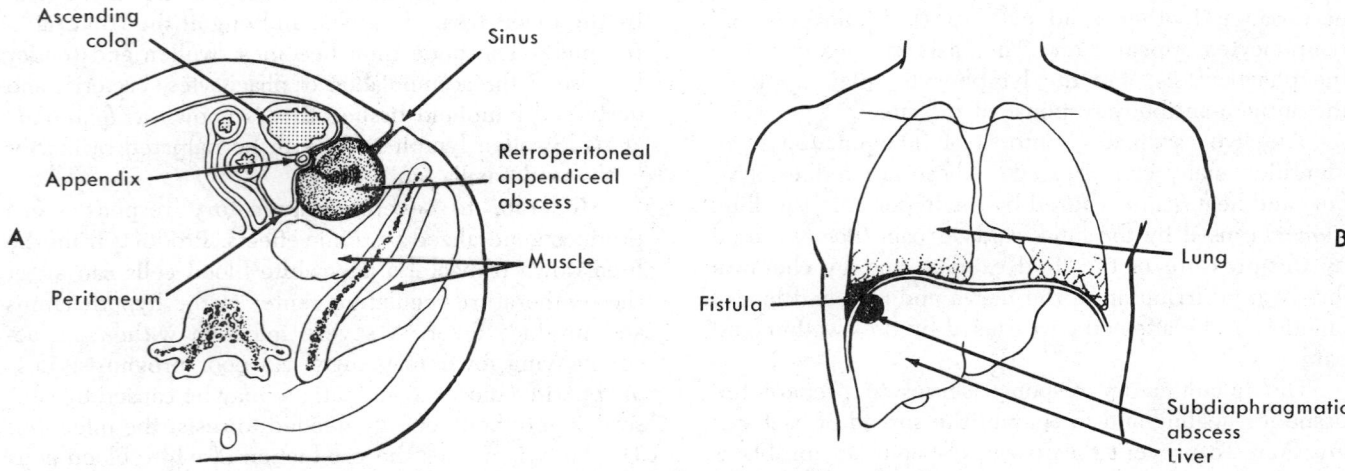

Fig. 19-6. A, Cross section of torso showing appendiceal abscess with sinus that has developed through abdominal wall. **B,** Subdiaphragmatic abscess that has developed fistula opening into pleural cavity.

matory and healing processes, and as the inflammation subsides, fibrous tissue forms, holding the membranes together. This fibrous tissue is called an *adhesion*. Adhesions may occur in the pleura, in the pericardium, about the pelvic organs, and in many other parts of the body. They often occur in and about the intestinal tract, where they may cause an obstruction.

Instead of healing there may be necrosis, or death of the tissue. Bacteria, both pathogens and nonpathogens, often invade the necrotic tissue and cause decomposition, which is called *gangrene*. The body defenses are useless in preventing or curing gangrene because no blood can get to the area. Gangrenous tissue must be completely removed before healing can occur.

Specific defense mechanisms

Concept of an adaptive specific immune system

Specific defense mechanisms within the body provide specific protection against a particular microorganism or molecular entity. This mechanism of protection leads to what is termed *immunity*. Depending on the relative levels of protection, the body may be able to defend itself totally or only partially from damage by the agent. The *immune system,* which is composed of many of the same organs, cells, and molecular entities that are operative in providing nonspecific defense, works in concert with the nonspecific mechanisms to focus and amplify the general mechanisms of defense against specifically recognized foreign materials.

The fundamental nature of the specific immune response is characterized by diversity, specificity, recognition, memory, and action. Among the most intriguing aspects of immune response is its *diversity of ability to respond* while at the same time responding with *specificity of action*. Almost any conceivable organic molecular array on the surface of a molecule has been shown to be able to induce a series of cellular events culminating in the production of *antibodies*. These antibodies combine with the inducing *antigen* by virtue of combining sites on the antibody molecule, which exhibit an extremely narrow specificity. The remainder of the antibody molecule is chemically and structurally quite similar to all other antibody molecules with distinctly different combining site specificities. *Recognition* and *memory* are two other aspects of this system that make it unique. The normal organism recognizes its own antigenic makeup and will not produce antibodies against its own antigens. This is known as *recognition of self*. At the same time this intricate system of self-recognition must be able to recognize extremely subtle changes

in its own cells when incipient tumors that differ only slightly in antigenic constitution are forming. Further, once the immune system has responded to an antigen, subsequent encounters with that antigen will produce an even more vigorous and rapid response. This response includes a wide variety of mechanisms designed to take *action* against the offending agent. Many of these actions are among the most potent biochemical and cellular reactions that the body can produce, yet they are focused so discretely that the foreign agent is rapidly destroyed with a minimum of damage to the host.

Antigens and antibodies

Antigens

An antigen is defined as a substance that when introduced into an animal elicits the formation of antibodies, or specifically sensitized cells. The antigen must be recognized as "nonself" or "foreign" material within the body. While most antigens are naturally occurring proteins of at least 10,000 molecular weight, other substances such as polysaccharides, nucleoproteins, lipoproteins, and glycoproteins may also serve as antigens. The bulk of the antigen consists of subsurface molecular structures that do not elicit an immune response but do serve as carrier for the multiple *antigenic determinants* on the surface. Most antigens have multiple antigenic determinants and are termed *multivalent antigens;* however, some molecules may be monovalent.

Certain molecules because of their small size cannot by themselves induce the synthesis of antibodies; however, when coupled with a high–molecular weight carrier, they can serve as antigenic determinants. These molecules are *incomplete antigens,* or *haptens*. These molecules take on special significance in the consideration of hypersensitivities (allergies to low–molecular weight compounds such as certain drugs and antibiotics) (p. 1871).

Antibodies

The body's response to the introduction of an antigenic substance is the production of a specific, soluble *antibody* or a sensitized (antigen reactive) lymphocyte population. The type of antigen introduced will determine the immune response: antibody synthesis, antigen-reactive lymphocyte, or a combination of both.

The circulating antibodies represent modified (i.e., antigen specific) globulin proteins found in blood serum. The serum contains several distinct protein fractions, which are separable on the basis of their net electrical charge, molecular size, and molecular conformation into several fractions: albumin, alpha-globulins (α-globulins), beta-globulins (β-globulins), and gamma-globulins (γ-globulins) (Fig. 19-7). The antibody activity of the serum is characteristically associated with the γ-globu-

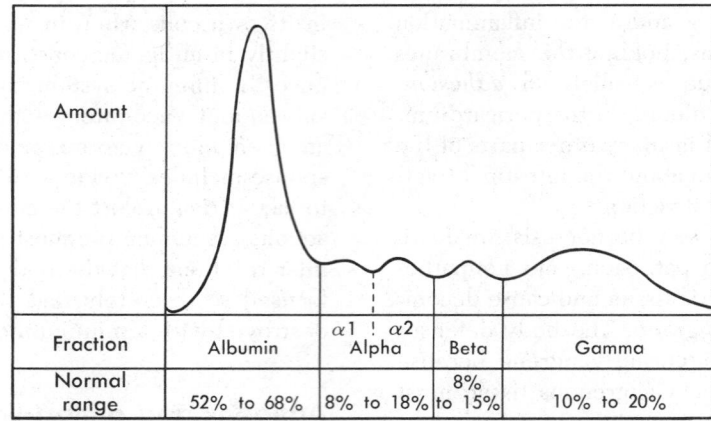

Fig. 19-7. Electrophoretic separation of major serum proteins. Majority of antibody activity lies within γ-globulin fraction. γ-Globulin fraction will rise with active synthesis of antibodies in response to antigenic stimulation.

TABLE 19-6. Properties of immunoglobulin classes

Property	Immunoglobulin class				
	IgG	IgM	IgA	IgE	IgD
Physiochemical					
Percent of Ig	82	7	10	0.002	1
Configuration	Monomer	Pentamer	Monomer, dimer	Monomer	Monomer
Half-life in serum (days)	23	5	6	2	3
Functional antigen-binding sites	2	5	2	2	?
Biologic					
Principal site found	Internal body fluids	Serum	Serum and exocrine secretions	Tissue bound	?
Fixed complement	Yes	Yes	No	No	No
Crosses placenta	Yes	No	No	No	No
Principal functions	Agglutination, detoxification, virus neutralization; enhances phagocytosis	Agglutination, cytolysis; enhances phagocytosis	Protection of mucosal surfaces	Mediates immediate-type hypersensitivity	?

lin fraction. Those γ-globulins with the ability to bind antigens are called *immunoglobulins*. The immunoglobulins can be further subdivided into different *classes* on the basis of structure and function of the molecules. The generic symbol for immunoglobulins is Ig, and each of the classes is designated by a letter of the alphabet: IgA, IgD, IgE, IgG, and IgM (Table 19-6).

The basic pattern of structure for all immunoglobulins is based on a four–peptide chain monomeric unit (Fig. 19-8). Two of the chains are of higher molecular weight and are termed *heavy* (H) *chains;* two are of lower molecular weight and are called *light* (L) *chains*. Each

L chain is linked by disulfide (—ss—) bonds to an H chain, and in turn the H chains are linked to each other by a disulfide bond. When immunoglobulin monomers are visualized by electron microscopy, they are seen to have a Y-shaped structure. At the ends of the two arms of the Y are the sites where antigen is bound. Both the H and L chains participate in the formation of these *antigen-binding* sites. Thus most monomers of immunoglobulin have two antigen-binding sites and are termed *bivalent*. The two arms of the Y are designated the *Fab* (for fragment, antigen-binding) *regions*. The base of the Y is called the *Fc region* (for fragment, crystallizable).

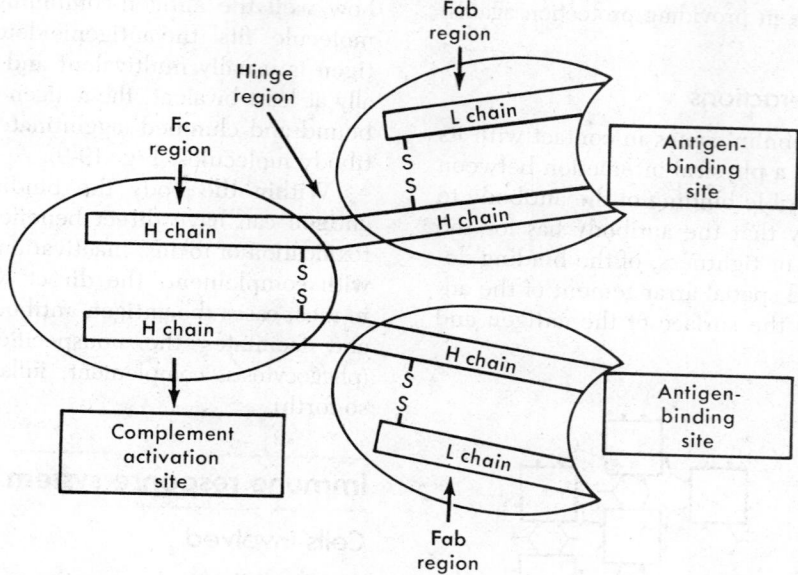

Fig. 19-8. Basic structure of IgG immunoglobulin monomer. All immunoglobulin classes are composed of variations of this basic structure with combination to form dimers (IgA) or pentamers (IgM).

In the region of the disulfide bond joining the H chains the molecule seems to be flexible, and this region is known as the *hinge region.*

The predominant class of immunoglobulins in normal adult serum is *IgG.* It makes up about 75% to 85% of the immunoglobulin fraction. Because of its structure and biologic activity, it is also found in the extravascular fluids of the body (Table 19-6). IgG is capable of crossing the placenta to provide the newborn with temporary natural passive immunity to those diseases against which the mother has circulating antibodies. It functions in the processes of toxin neutralization and virus and bacterial inactivation and in the formation of antigen-antibody-complement immune complexes associated with certain types of hypersensitivity (p. 1871). IgG is the immunoglobulin class primarily responsible for the rise in serum antibodies during a secondary (anamnestic, booster) response (p. 290).

IgM structurally is composed of five monomeric units attached to each other at the Fc region. Thus the star-shaped molecule with the antigen-binding sites pointed outward that results from this macromolecular arrangement is termed a *pentamer.* Sometimes this immunoglobulin class, which constitutes about 7% of the immunoglobulin in serum, is called the *macroglobulins* because of its molecular size. As a result of its size it is confined primarily to the intravascular fluids. IgM, like IgG, is capable of binding the C1 component of complement and initiating the complement cascade. In each antigenic stimulation IgM antibodies are the first to appear, but they do not reach the levels of IgG, nor do

they exhibit an anamnestic response on subsequent antigen contact. They are primarily involved in providing protection against viral and bacterial invaders in the blood. Because of their ability to bind complement, they too are responsible for certain immune complex hypersensitivities and autoimmune diseases, such as rheumatoid arthritis.

IgA constitutes about 10% of the total immunoglobulin in serum. It can be found in a variety of polymeric forms (primarily monomer in serum and dimer in exocrine secretions). IgA is also termed the *secretory immunoglobulin* because it is found in the exocrine secretions of the body (milk, mucin, saliva, tears). Within these secretions IgA provides specific protection of the mucosal surfaces of the respiratory, digestive, and genital tracts from pathogenic invasion.

IgD makes up only about 1% of the immunoglobulin fraction of serum. Its biologic functions are unknown. It may be an early receptor or precursor necessary for the later development of IgM and IgG.

IgE is present in the serum in extremely small amounts (0.002%). This is the result of the predilection this immunoglobulin class has for attachment to the surface of mast cells and basophils. Once bound by the Fc region of the monomer to the surface of these cells, which are rich in the potent physiologically active substances histamine, kinins, and serotonin, IgE serves to mediate the severe and occasionally fatal anaphylactic type of hypersensitivities. These include anaphylactic shock, allergic asthma, and hay fever (p. 1862). The protective role of these immunoglobulins is not clear, but they may be effective in providing protection against certain parasitic worms.

Antigen-antibody interactions

When an immunoglobulin comes in contact with its specific antigen, there is a physical interaction between the two, causing a reversible binding of the antibody to the antigen. The affinity that the antibody has for the antigen and the avidity, or tightness, of the binding depend on the location and spatial arrangement of the antigenic determinants on the surface of the antigen and how well the antigen-combining site on the antibody molecule "fits" the antigenic determinant. Since the antigen is usually multivalent and the antibody is generally at least bivalent, the antigen molecules may be cross bound and clumped (agglutinated, precipitated) by antibody molecules (Fig. 19-9).

Within the body the binding of antibody to the antigen can have direct beneficial effects, such as detoxification of toxins, inactivation of viruses, or, coupled with complement, the direct lysis of cells. However, in most cases the antigen-antibody combination initiates and facilitates the nonspecific defense mechanisms (phagocytosis, complement, inflammatory response, and so forth).

Immune response system

Cells involved

The cells involved in the specific immune response are all derived from the original undifferentiated stem cells of the bone marrow. The stem cell has the possibility of developing into any of the blood cells of the body depending on various signals and influences. The primary cells of the immune response system develop from the lymphocytic cell population (Fig. 19-10). One

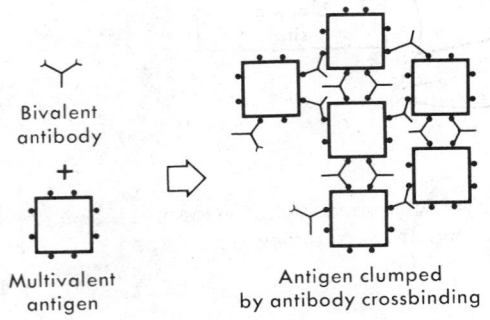

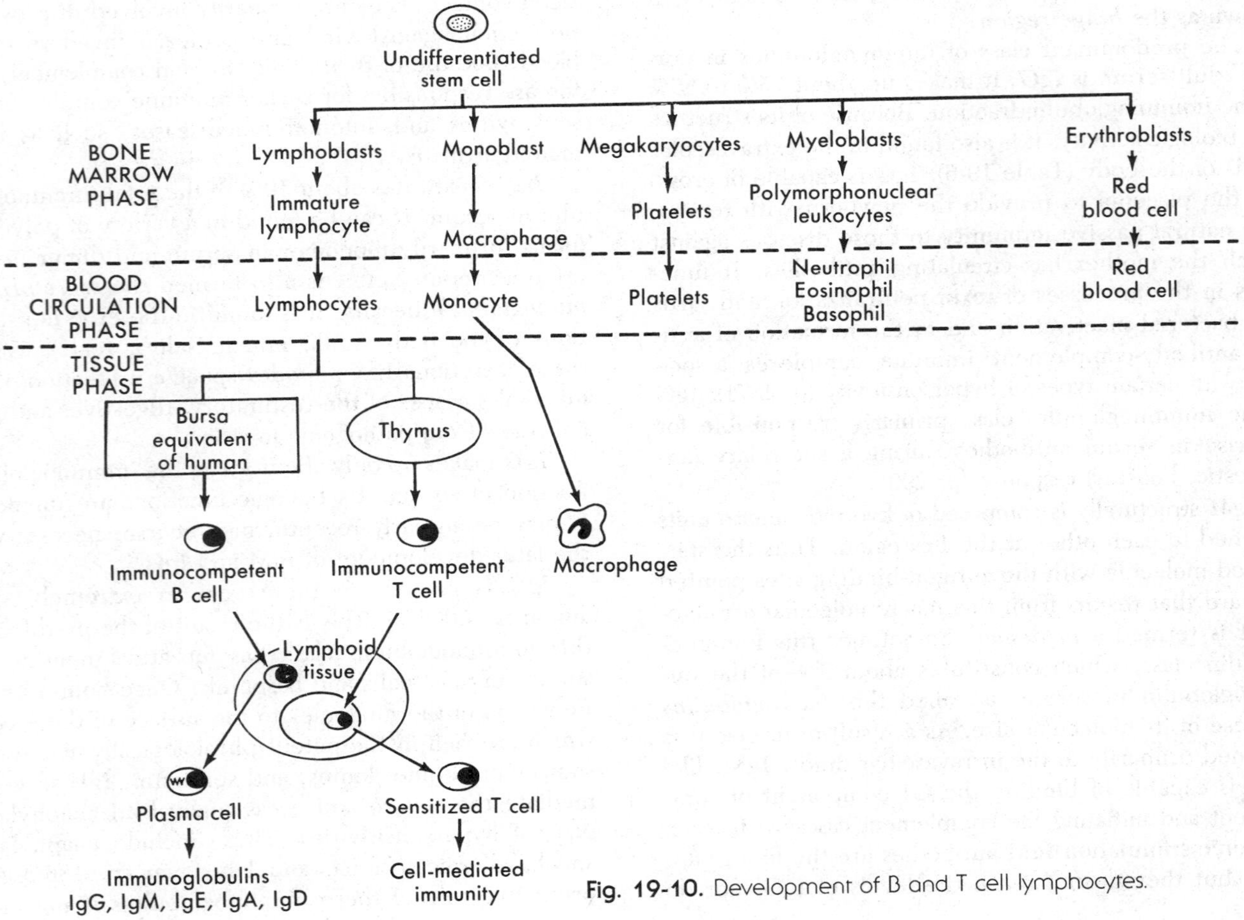

Fig. 19-9. Clumping of multivalent antigen by its specific antibody.

Fig. 19-10. Development of B and T cell lymphocytes.

population of lymphocytic cells undergoes differentiation under the influence of the thymus gland and becomes known as *thymus-dependent lymphocytes,* or *T cells.* These cells become responsible for mediating the *cell-mediated immune responses* (CMI). Another population of lymphocytes matures in the lymphoid tissues and is referred to as *thymus-independent lymphocytes,* or *B cells.* The designation B cell comes from the fact that in the chicken, where this process was first detected, there is a single site where this differentiation occurs, the *bursa of Fabricius.* No such singular lymphoid organ is found in humans, but it is believed that the gut-associated lymphoid tissues, such as tonsils, Peyer's patches of the intestine, and appendix, serve as the equivalent sites in humans. The B cells are responsible for the production of the immunoglobulins and the provision of the *humoral immune response.*

The role of the lymphocytes (B or T cells) is to recognize the presence of an antigen and to initiate specific mechanisms of disposal. Just as important, the lymphocyte must recognize a component of host tissues as *self* and protect that tissue from immunologic response reactions.

The *macrophage* appears to act nonspecifically, but its role in the immune response is critical. First, the macrophage seems to be responsible for initially capturing, processing, and presenting the antigen to the lymphocytes. Capture of the antigen occurs by phagocytosis as described earlier in this chapter. The processing of the antigen is a poorly understood mechanism, but there is evidence that the macrophage digests and concentrates the antigen and then couples the antigen to RNA. This processed signal is transferred to the surface of the macrophage for presentation to lymphocytes. Antigen presented to lymphocytes in this manner triggers the series of events within the lymphocytes that leads to full immunologic response. Antigen that escapes this macrophage processing will stimulate only a weak immune response or no response at all.

At the other end of the immune response the macrophage is activated to its maximum of phagocytic efficiency by the release of stimulatory, soluble substances, known as *lymphokines,* by activated lymphocytes (Table 19-7). In this way the macrophage is stimulated at the site of an immune reaction. Other of the soluble lymphokines serve to attract the macrophages to the site by chemotaxis.

Organs and tissues involved

The organs and tissues of the specific immune response system include the central organs (bone marrow, thymus, and gut-associated lymphoid tissues) and the peripheral organs (lymph nodes, spleen, and lymphatic vessels). Within the central organs the immune response cells are synthesized and matured, while within the peripheral organs the mature cells are concentrated.

The *thymus* serves as the control organ of the immune system. It is the site of differentiation of the T cell lymphocytic populations and through certain soluble thymic hormones serves to regulate the overall immune system. The activity of the thymus reaches it peak in childhood, and the organ begins to shrink in size after puberty. If the thymus is removed (thymectomy) very early in the life of an animal, a severe state of immunodeficiency is induced and T cell–mediated immunity never develops. The thymectomized animal develops a wasting disease characterized by stunted growth, diarrhea, and death from massive infection by intestinal or respiratory tract normal flora. The B cell function is also reduced, pointing to a cooperative effect between the two basic systems. The loss of the thymus from the adult animal creates less severe reactions. This is probably due to the establishment of an already functional, long-lived population of T cells.

The *lymph nodes* and *spleen* serve as the primary sites of localization of the immune response cells. The lymph node serves to filter the lymph drained from a region of tissue. The structure of the lymph node (Fig. 19-11) consists of an inner medullary and paracortical region made up primarily of T cells and an outer cortex composed of clusters, or germinal centers, of B cells known as follicles. The spleen is structured on somewhat the same pattern with diffusely packed T cell areas and germinal centers of tightly packed B cells. In certain types of antigenic stimulation, either the T cell areas or the B cell areas will show tissue proliferation, while the other area remains quiescent. By the same principle, if a person is suffering a basic primary immunodeficiency of one system, the corresponding area of lymph nodes and spleen may degenerate.

During the course of the immune response reaction, within the lymph nodes there is significant proliferation of specific cells and migration of phagocytic cells to the site, which may lead to lymph node enlargement. Enlargement of the lymph nodes in a region may be the

TABLE 19-7. Lymphokines liberated by activated T cell lymphocytes

Lymphokine	Function
Lymphocyte-derived chemotactic factors	Chemotactic for macrophages
Lymphocytotoxins	Nonspecific lysis of cells
Macrophage inhibition-activation factors	Maintains macrophage at site and activates it
Interferon	Inhibits replication of viruses
Lymphocyte-activating factors	Activates nonsensitized lymphocytes

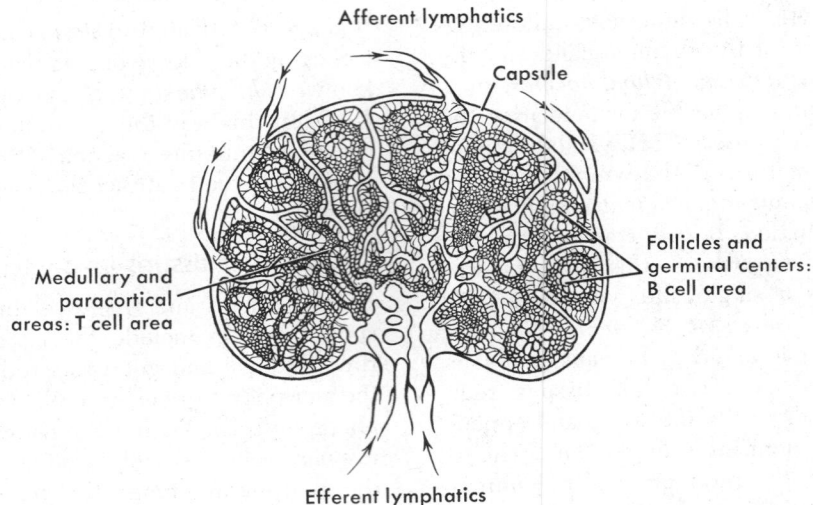

Fig. 19-11. B and T cell areas of lymph node.

result of (1) infections, (2) immune diseases, (3) intrinsic neoplasms of the lymph node itself, or (4) metastatic spread of malignant cells to the node. The presence of an enlarged spleen or enlarged lymph nodes is virtually always an important clinical finding.

Immune response

Primary immune response

Antigenic challenge. When an antigen is introduced into the body, it can trigger a wide or narrow spectrum of response mechanisms. The specific pattern of response depends on (1) the amount of antigen introduced, (2) the site of introduction, and (3) the type of antigen introduced.

Small amounts of a noninvasive, large, particular antigen introduced at a single body site are quickly and efficiently handled at a local site with little or no systemic involvement beyond the local lymph node. Since the inflammatory response and local lymph node can localize the spread of the antigen, the immune response may go completely unnoticed by the host organism. Larger, particulate antigens are readily cleared, but small, soluble antigens are more difficult to clear from the circulation.

Large amounts of an antigen may allow the antigen to escape from the local site by simply overwhelming the local defense mechanisms. Even though the lymph nodes and reticuloendothelial organs can clear 80% to 90% of an antigen on a single pass, if the amount of the antigen is extremely large some antigen may escape the local site. An excessively large, sustained antigen dose can exhaust not only the local site but the entire reticuloendothelial system as well. This greatly reduces the body's ability to respond to even minor invasive challenges and renders the host vulnerable to secondary infections.

Highly invasive antigens (e.g., bacteria such as *Staphylococcus aureus* or *Streptococcus pyogenes*) or those introduced directly into the bloodstream by blood transfusion, intravenous catheterization, or injection can immediately establish a systemic type of immune response. This is why extreme care must be exercised in the use of any type of medical procedure that would allow the introduction of organisms into the general circulation. The localization action of the immune response is critical to efficient functioning of the response.

Humoral response. When the antigen is introduced for the first time, one of three basic mechanisms of response will be elicited: (1) a response mediated primarily by B cells, the humoral response; (2) a response in which the T cells are primarily involved, the cell-mediated response; or (3) a combined type of response.

If the antigen is of the type that triggers a humoral response, the first time the body is exposed to the antigen the B cell system responds with the synthesis of circulating immunoglobulins (Fig. 19-12). The encroaching antigen is phagocytosed by a lymph node macrophage or tissue-active macrophage. The macrophage processes the antigen and presents the antigenic stimulus to a B cell, which has been preprogramed to respond to the introduced antigen. These antigen-specific B cells bear receptors on their surface, which allow them to recognize their antigenic stimulant. Only a few lymphocytes within a lymph node have the ability to respond to the antigen. The stimulated B cell then begins a process of proliferation (increase in number) and differentiation (change in structure and function). The progeny of the stimulated cell increase in number within the lymph node, forming *clones* of specifically adapted lympho-

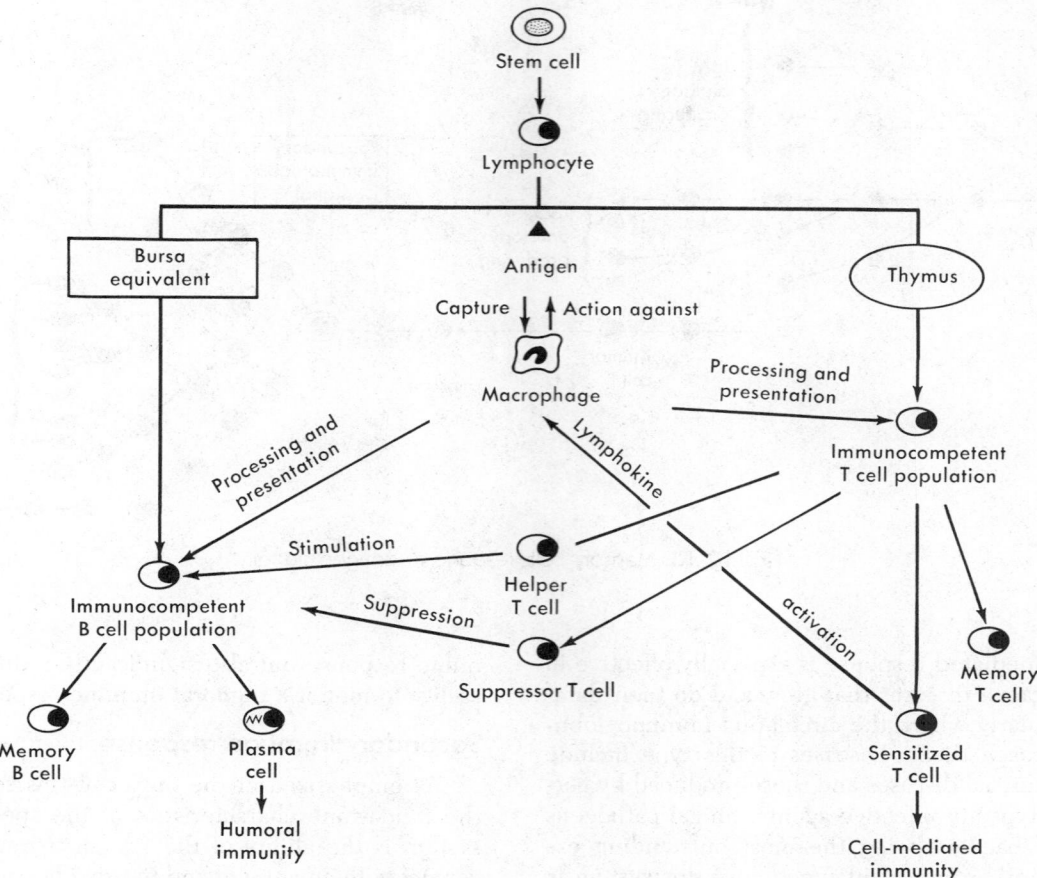

Fig. 19-12. Combined response of B and T cell systems.

cytes. With each generation of new cells within the clone, the lymphocytes become more differentiated toward a cell population ideally suited for the synthesis and release of immunoglobulin. These cells are known as *plasma cells*. With the development of this cell population in the lymph node (several days after the introduction of the antigen), antibodies can be detected in the lymph node. However, it is not until about 1 to 2 weeks after the antigenic challenge that detectable levels of specific antibodies appear in the serum. The plasma cell population of the lymph node and the levels of antibody in the blood continue to increase for another 2 to 3 weeks, and then both begin to retreat. Some of the lymphocytes of the activated clone become "memory cells," which are much more responsive, both in time of reaction and efficiency of antibody synthesis, to subsequent contact with the antigen (Fig. 19-13).

The humoral response serves to protect the body from such agents as microbial toxins, bacteria within the extravascular spaces in the blood and on mucosal surfaces, and viruses that must pass through the circulatory system to reach their site of infection (e.g., poliomyelitis virus).

Cell-mediated response. Certain antigens trigger a response mediated by T cell proliferation and reaction. A T cell that has received its antigenic stimulus is referred to as a *sensitized T cell lymphocyte* (Fig. 19-12).

The initial steps of the cell-mediated response, those involving the antigen processing by the macrophage, seem to be the same as in the humoral response. Following the presentation of the antigenic stimulus to lymph node T cells, there is proliferation in the T cell domain. There is no release of circulatory antibodies; rather, sensitized lymphocytes are released into the circulation. These cells migrate to the site of the entrance of the antigen into the body where the invading agent or residual antigen is found. These activated lymphocytes along with macrophages infiltrate the regions of the tissue and begin a direct attack on the antigen or tissue cells labeled with the antigen. The T cells participating in this direct attack are known as *killer T cells*.

To amplify the site reaction further, the sensitized lymphocytes activate the nonspecific phagocytotic cells (macrophages, PMNs, and noncommitted lymphocytes) in the region of the antigen. This is accomplished through the release of the soluble lymphokines (Table 19-7), which marshall this additional cellular involvement to attack the antigenic materials.

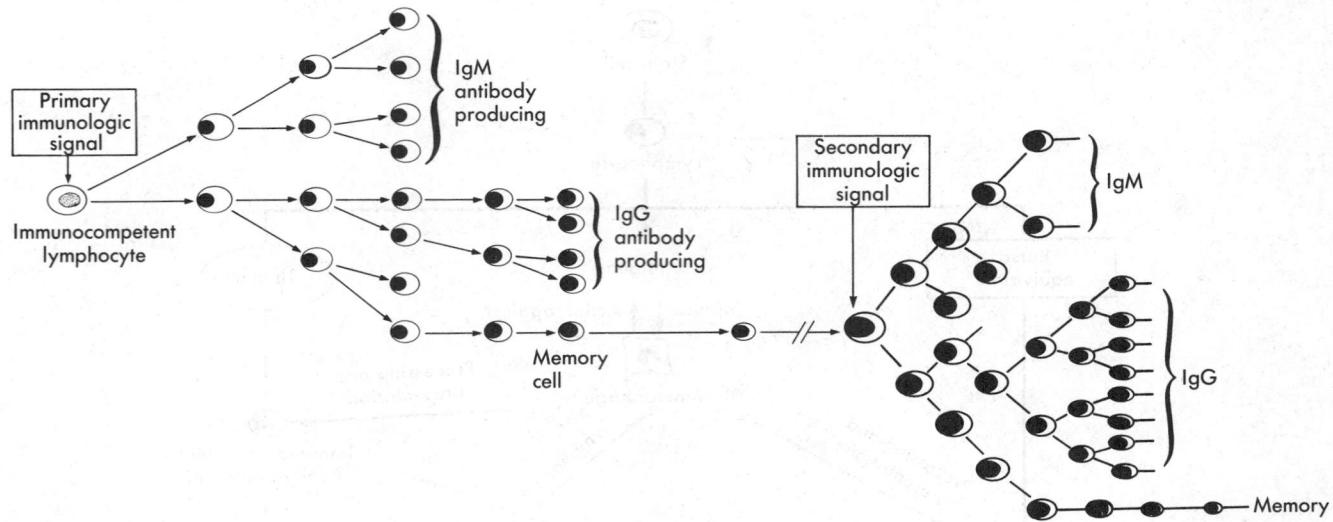

Fig. 19-13. Memory cells respond to antigen signal.

The cell-mediated response is especially effective in protection against diseases that grow and do their damage intracellularly where the circulating immunoglobulins cannot reach them. Diseases of this type include viral and rickettsial diseases and those produced by certain chronic types of infective agents, fungal pathogens and tubercle bacillus being the most outstanding examples. One other important function of this system is the provision of *cancer cell surveillance* (p. 293).

Combined immune response. Most antigens do not cause a purely humoral or purely cell-mediated response; rather, both types of response are evoked. Likewise, our protection against most harmful antigens is the result of both of these specific response systems being brought to bear on the antigen involved. In the *combined type of response* there is an initial perturbation within the T cell areas of the lymph node. This becomes obvious within about 2 days after the introduction of the antigen. About 3 to 5 days later the B cell areas begin to proliferate.

To mount a maximal immune response, the cooperative action of the three central cell types is necessary. The macrophage serves to capture, process, and present the antigen to immunocompetent cells of both T and B cell ancestry. The T cells aid in the direct cell-mediated response, but there also seems to be a population of T cells that serves to interact with the B cell population to control the development of an effective immune response. A *helper T cell* population cooperates with the B cells by some as yet undefined mechanism to enhance the activation and proliferation of the immunoglobulin synthesizing cells. The existence of the helper T cell explains the observation noted earlier in this chapter that the removal of the thymus from the neonate not only compromises the cell-mediated immune response but also significantly reduces the host's ability to mount a humoral immune response.

Secondary immune response

As emphasized at the outset of this section, one of the touchstone characteristics of the specific response system is the ability of the system to remember prior contact with an antigen and to provide a more complete protective reaction on subsequent contact. The first contact between the immune response system and an antigen leads to what is termed the *primary response,* the events of which have been laid out in the preceding paragraphs. When antibody synthesis is measured in a primary response, there is a significant lag time to the appearance of antibodies in the circulation (Fig. 19-14). Immunoglobulins of the IgM class are the first to appear, but they maintain protective levels for only a short period. Specific IgG antibodies follow and reach protective levels within 12 to 14 days, but they too fall off fairly quickly with only this initial exposure. When the "primed" immune response system encounters the antigen again, a *secondary response* ensues, which is more rapid, of greater intensity, and longer lasting than the primary response. This secondary response is also termed an *anamnestic response.* This "remembered" response is a characteristic of both the B and T cell systems. The prior contact with the antigen is stored in special memory cells of both cell lines. As illustrated in Fig. 19-13, the memory cells respond immediately to the antigenic signal, so that the lag time between exposure to the antigen and production of protective antibody levels is greatly reduced. This phenomenon provides the basis for active immunization and "booster" doses to maintain the protective levels of immunity. In an immunized individual the memory cells elicit the rapid response in

Fig. 19-14. Primary and secondary humoral responses.

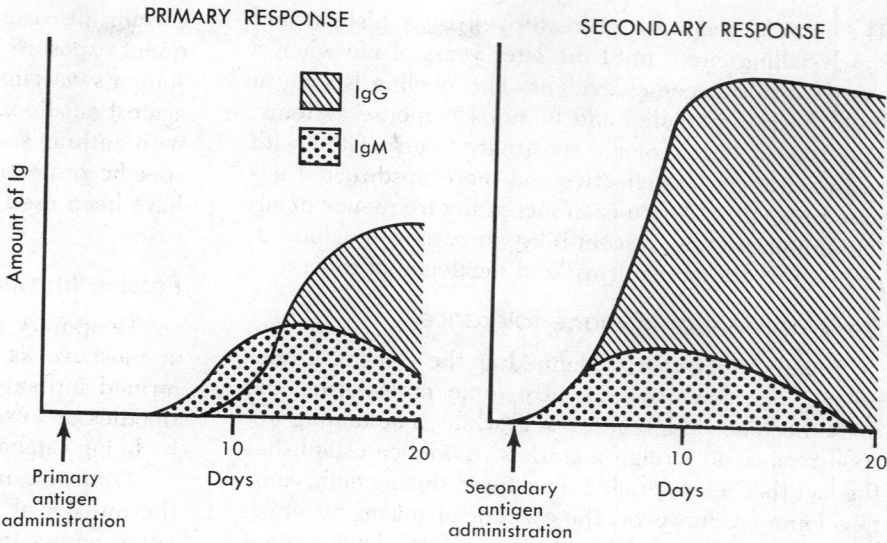

Fig. 19-15. Immunoglobulin levels in fetus and neonate.

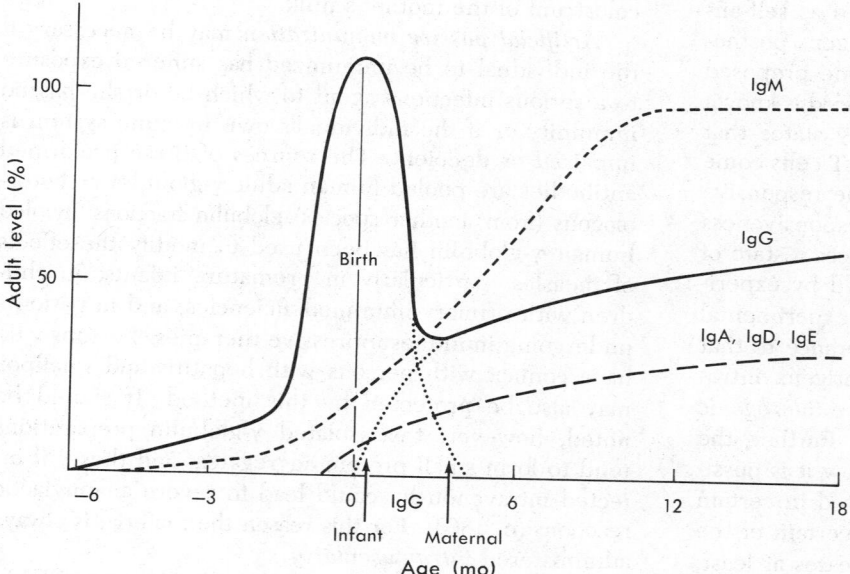

time for the immune system to overwhelm the pathogen or toxin before it can produce its damage.

Developmental aspects of the immune response

Lymphoid cells first appear in the fetus as stem cells in the fetal liver at about the end of the first trimester. The lymphoid tissues of the thymus also develop fairly early in the fetus. At birth, however, the lymph nodes and spleen are still underdeveloped, but T and B cell responsiveness is fully functional. The fetus is capable of some immune response if challenged by an in utero (within the uterus) infection such as in the case of congenital syphilis or rubella. Unless the fetus has been exposed to a congenital infection, at birth the neonate-synthesized immunoglobulin levels are low (Fig. 19-15).

The child does have high levels of transplacentally acquired maternal IgG antibodies. These maternal antibodies have a half-life of about 30 days in the child, and this coupled with the increase in blood volume in the growing infant leads to a drop in the IgG levels of the blood over the first 3 months. Thereafter the rate of the child's own synthesis of IgG provides for a steady increase in the immunoglobulin concentration within the serum. IgM levels reach adult concentrations by about the age of 9 months.

Numerous studies in both animals and humans have shown that during the aging process there is a progressive loss of immunologic vigor. The prime immunologic age probably is achieved during the late teen years when virtually the full complement of immunities have been developed and the responsiveness of the system peaks.

The middle years are characterized by a plateau and slowly falling curve until the later years of life when a sharp decline becomes evident. This decline is seen in both the cell-mediated and humoral response systems. This loss in immunologic sensitivity is associated with an increasingly less effective and more misdirected immune response. There is an increasing frequency of autoimmune disease, susceptibility to pathogenic and opportunistic microorganisms, and incidence of cancer.

Development of immune tolerance

Immune tolerance is defined as the state of immunologic nonresponsiveness. By some mechanisms the body becomes tolerant to self while maintaining responsiveness to foreign materials. Evidence establishes the fact that self-tolerance is acquired during embryonic development; however, the exact mechanisms by which it develops remain an issue. During fetal development the immune system is presented with antigens from the developing tissues; these become identified as self-antigens, so that when exposed to these antigens postnatally the individual is tolerant of them. One proposed mechanism by which this state could be induced is known as the *clonal selection theory*. This theory states that when potentially responsive clones of B or T cells come into contact with an antigen prenatally, the responsive cell line is killed, thus eliminating the responsiveness to that antigen from the body. This produces a state of *natural tolerance*. This theory is supported by experimental data that show that by exposing experimental animals to foreign antigens in utero a tolerance to that antigen is developed; however, some antigens introduced in this manner are found to be more *tolerogenic* (capable of inducing tolerance) than others. Further, the clonal selection theory does not explain how it is possible to break tolerance in adults as indicated in certain experimental studies or as in the case of certain of the autoimmune diseases (p. 1874). In some cases at least, tolerance is not due to the total elimination of specifically reactive cells but to the blocking of expression or temporary inactivation of the responsive cells. The action of suppressor T cells or the failure of mobilization by helper T cells may play a significant role in maintaining the state of self-tolerance.

Applications and implications of immune response

Immunization

Long before the mechanisms of immune response were worked out, it was recognized that recovery from certain diseases conferred protection against subsequent exposure to that disease. Dating from the days of Jenner's vaccination with cowpox exudate to protect against smallpox (1798), through the success of Pasteur with anthrax and rabies (1880s), up to the present, the specific protective mechanisms of the immune system have been used to protect against serious infectious diseases.

Passive immunization

Temporary protection, usually measured in days or at most weeks, is afforded by the acquisition of preformed antibody from another host. As the acquired antibodies are used up through binding with antigen or by being catabolized, the protection is lost.

Transplacental passive immunization occurs through the transfer of IgG antibodies from the maternal circulation across the placenta to the fetal blood. There is also some acquisition of immunoglobulins through the colostrum of the mother's milk.

Artificial passive immunization may be necessary if the individual to be immunized has suffered exposure to a serious infectious agent to which he or she has no immunity or if the individual's own immune system is impaired or deficient. The sources of these preformed antibodies are pooled human adult γ-globulin or heterologous (from another species) globulin fractions. Pooled human γ-globulin has been used to modify the effects of measles, particularly in premature infants, in children with primary immunodeficiencies, and in patients undergoing immunosuppressive therapies. Persons who have contact with persons with hepatitis and smallpox may also be protected by this method. It should be noted, however, that isolated γ-globulin preparations tend to form small protein aggregates, and these, if injected intravenously, could lead to severe anaphylactic reactions (p. 1863). For this reason the material is always administered *intramuscularly*.

The most commonly used heterologous antibody fractions are antitetanus and antidiphtheria antisera derived from horse globulins. Since these are foreign proteins, they can lead to the development of serum sickness (p. 1871). Serum sickness is more likely to occur in subjects already primed by previous contact with horse globulin; thus multiple use of heterologous sera is to be avoided.

Active immunization

The objective of active immunization is to provide effective long-term immunity by establishing within the individual's own body the capacity to produce effective levels of immune response and to establish a population of sensitive cells that can respond to a subsequent antigenic contact.

Immunizing agents ideally should be noninjurious to the individual being immunized. To accomplish this the pathogenic effects must be modified while at the same time maintaining the antigenicity of the agent. Bacteria exotoxins such as those produced by the diphtheria and tetanus bacteria can be successfully detoxified by formaldehyde treatment without destroying the major antigenic determinants on the protein molecule. Such detoxified antigenic materials are called *toxoids*. The use of *killed vaccines* of viruses and bacteria can also provide a safe antigen for immunization. Killed vaccines include those for pertussis (whooping cough), typhoid and cholera, and the Salk poliomyelitis vaccine. The protection conferred by these vaccines is generally inferior to that produced by live vaccines. A number of the most successful vaccines consist of living organisms that have been modified so that they are nonvirulent. The *attenuated live vaccines* provide excellent protection, but there is some risk in their use because of the possibility of reversion to the virulent form of the organism. Live vaccines of importance are those for measles, mumps, and tuberculosis (BCG) and the Sabin poliomyelitis vaccine.

The provision of protective levels of residual immunity depends on the inducement of (1) the right type of response (i.e., cell mediated or humoral), (2) in sufficient amounts, (3) at the right place (i.e., where the immune response can contact the antigen), and (4) against the right antigenic determinants (i.e., the antibodies formed produce an inactivating effect). Simply the induction of an immune response is not sufficient to provide protection. For example, the early killed virus measles vaccines elicited a splendid production of circulating antibodies against the measles virus, but protection against measles is most effectively mediated by cellular immune responses. The humoral protection did not prevent infection.

Another problem of immunization for which provision must be made is the *interference* that one antigen may have with another if the two are given simultaneously. The live virus vaccines occasionally interfere with each other; when measles and smallpox vaccines are administered at the same time, they each interfere with the development of immunity by the other. This is probably the result of interferon production. Some live virus vaccines contain more than one strain of the virus and these can cross-inhibit. In the case of the Sabin oral polio vaccine three separate doses are required because there are three strains within the same vaccine. With the initial dose, immunity to only one strain may develop if the strain interferes with the other two.

Complications of immunization

Although immunization is the most successful approach to the control of many infectious diseases, there are small but still real risks involved. The development of postvaccination encephalitis or other neural autoimmune complications is a serious risk with such vaccines as those for smallpox or rabies. Children with immunodeficiencies may be overwhelmed by vaccination with live vaccine. With viral vaccines, which are produced in monkey kidney of human cell culture, there is a slight risk of the introduction of oncogenic (cancer causing) viruses. A fetus may be significantly at risk if the mother receives a live virus vaccine during pregnancy. Such vaccines as smallpox and live influenza should never be administered to a pregnant woman. It is still unclear whether the rubella virus vaccine harms the fetus or not, so it too should be avoided. Besides these rather serious risks, general discomfort is to be expected from some forms of immunization. The typhoid vaccine, for instance, is composed of large numbers of killed salmonella bacteria; since the endotoxic cell wall materials of these cells is a pyrogenic (fever producing) substance, fever and malaise are not uncommon sequelae. The influenza vaccines often produce febrile reactions in children.

Cancer immunology

One of the primary functions of the cell-mediated immune response system seems to be the recognition and destruction of cancer cells within the body. By the same mechanisms that are operative in allograft rejection, it is postulated that the immune system continually protects against the establishment of tumor growths. The recognition of these cells as nonself is based on the appearance of "new" surface antigens that allow identification. There is a growing body of evidence to support the view that this is a vital function of the immune system. Patients in whom the cellular immune system is impaired (immunosuppressed) or defective (immunodeficient) for significant periods are at especially high risk of certain neoplastic diseases. To these data is coupled the observation that cancers are most prone to appear early in life before the immune system is fully functional or in later life as the system becomes less effective.

Cancers may become established in the body by escaping the surveillance mechanisms or by growing so rapidly that they outdistance the immune system's ability to respond. Experimentally, if a few thousand tumor cells are transferred from a cancerous animal to a noncancerous animal, the latter is capable of responding and destroying the tumor; however, if the tumor cell load is increased to several billion cells, the tumor may become established. The humoral immune system may actually serve to protect the developing cancer by producing noncytotoxic antibodies (*enhancing antibodies*) that coat the tumor cell surfaces and mask the surface from recognition by sensitized lymphocytes. As a tumor grows it is capable of both specific and nonspecific suppression of the immune system. This further reduces the effectiveness of a response.

Some of the new surface antigens (known as *tumor-specific transplantation antigens* [TSTA]) appearing on the cancerous cell are shed into the circulation and can be immunologically detected there. Some of these antigens, such as carcinoembryonic antigen (CEA) and alpha-fetoprotein (α-FP), are present during fetal development but are not expressed in the adult. Their reappearance lends support to the theory that cancer represents a dedifferentiation to a more primitive cell. These antigens, termed *oncofetal antigens* (OFA), are of some significance in early detection, diagnostic confirmation, and determination of malignant disease progress.

Some very early progress has been made in stimulating, both specifically and nonspecifically, the body's immunologic response to cancers in the hope of preventing further growth of the tumors. With further knowledge of both the cancer process and the immune response mechanisms, the possibility of utilizing immunotherapy, immunoprophylaxis, and immunodiagnosis as specific tools against malignancies seems quite realistic.

REFERENCES AND SELECTED READINGS
Contemporary

1. Abdou, N.I., et al.: The thymus in myasthenia gravis: evidence for altered cell populations, N. Engl. J. Med. **291**:1271, 1975.
2. *Alexander, J.W., and Good, R.A.: Fundamentals of clinical immunology, Philadelphia, 1977, W.B. Saunders Co.
3. *Allen, J.C.: Infection and the compromised host, Baltimore, 1976, The Williams & Wilkins Co.
4. American Academy of Pediatrics: Report of the Committee on Infectious Disease, ed. 17, Evanston, Ill., 1974, The Academy.
5. Barrett, J.T.: Textbook of immunology: an introduction to immunochemistry and immunobiology, ed. 3, St. Louis, 1978, The C.V. Mosby Co.
6. Bernstein, I.D.: Immunologic defenses against cancer, J. Pediatr. **83**:906, 1973.
7. Buckley, C.E., III, and Roseman, J.M.: Immunity and survival, J. Am. Geriatr. Soc. **24**:241, 1976.
8. *Bunting, F.W.: Immunity against infectious disease, Nurs. Times **67**:634, 1971.
9. *Burke, D.C.: The status of interferon, Sci. Am. **236**:42, 1977.
10. *Burnet, F.M.: Immunology, aging, and cancer, San Francisco, 1976, W.H. Freeman & Co., Publishers.
11. Butterworth, A.E., and David, J.R.: Eosinophil function, N. Engl. J. Med. **304**:154-157, 1981.
12. Cohen, S., Pick, E., and Oppenheim, J.J.: Biology of the lymphokines, New York, 1979, Academic Press, Inc.
13. Edelman, G.M.: Antibody structure and molecular immunology, Science **180**:290, 1973.
14. Eisen, H.N.: Immunology, New York, 1974, Harper & Row, Publishers, Inc.
15. Evans, H.E., et al.: Flora in newborn infants: annual variation in prevalence of *Staphylococcus aureus, Escherichia coli,* and streptococci, Arch. Environ. Health **26**:275, 1973.
16. Fahey, J.L., et al.: Immunotherapy and human tumor immunology, Ann. Intern. Med. **84**:454, 1976.
17. *Faulk, W.P., Demaeyer, E.M., and Davies, A.J.: Some effects of malnutrition on immune response in man, Am. J. Clin. Nutr. **27**:638, 1974.
18. *Francis, B.J.: Current concepts in immunization, Am. J. Nurs. **73**:646, 1973.
19. Gell, P.G.H., et al.: Clinical aspects of immunology, ed. 3, Oxford, England, 1975, Blackwell Scientific Publications Ltd.
20. Gordon, B.L.: Essentials of immunology, ed. 2, Philadelphia, 1974, F.A. Davis Co.
21. *Hardy, C.S.: Infection control: what can one nurse do? Nurs. '73 **3**:18, 1973.
22. Kaplan, M.M., and Webster, R.G.: The epidemiology of influenza, Sci. Am. **237**:88, 1977.
23. Makinodan, T.: Immunobiology of aging, J. Am. Geriatr. **24**:249, 1976.
24. Marx, J.L.: Tumor immunology: the host's response to cancer, Science **184**:552, 1974.
25. *Maugh, T.H.: Leukemia: much is known but the picture is still confused, Science **185**:48, 1974.
26. Medawar, P.B.: The new immunology, Hosp. Pract. **9**:48, 1974.
27. Metz, D.H.: The mechanism of action of interferon, Cell **6**:429, 1975.
28. *Mims, C.A.: The pathogenesis of infectious disease, New York, 1977, Academic Press, Inc.
29. Murillo, G.J.: Synthesis of secretory IgA by human colostral cells, South. Med. J. **64**:1333, 1971.
30. Nathan, C.F., Murray, H.W., and Cohn, Z.A.: The macrophage as an effector cell, N. Engl. J. Med. **303**:622-625, 1980.
31. *Nysather, J.O., Katz, A.E., and Lenth, J.L.: The immune system: its development and function, Am. J. Nurs. **76**:1614, 1976.
32. *Oettgen, H.F.: Immunotherapy of cancer, N. Engl. J. Med. **297**:484, 1977.
33. *Old, L.J.: Cancer immunology, Sci. Am. **236**:62, 1977.
34. Park, A.K., et al.: Immunosuppressive effect of surgery, Lancet **1**:53, 1971.
35. Pierce, J.C., et al.: Lymphoma, a complication of renal allotransplantation in man, J.A.M.A. **219**:1593, 1972.
36. Reinherz, E., and Schlossman, S.F.: Regulation of the immune response—inducer and suppressor T-lymphocyte subsets in human beings, N. Engl. J. Med. **303**:370-377, 1980.
37. Remington, J.S.: The compromised host, Hosp. Pract. **7**:59, 1972.
38. Richards, F.F., et al.: On the specificity of antibodies, Science **187**:130, 1975.
39. Roberts-Thomson, I.C., et al.: Aging, immune response and mortality, Lancet **2**:368, 1974.
40. *Roitt, I.M.: Essential immunology, ed. 3, Oxford, England, 1979, Blackwell Scientific Publications Ltd.
41. Rose, N.R., and Friedman, H.: Manual of clinical immunology, Washington, 1976, American Society for Microbiology.
42. *Rosenberg, L.E., and Kidd, K.K.: HLA and disease susceptibility, N. Engl. J. Med. **297**:1060, 1977.
43. Sell, S.: Immunology, immunopathology, and immunity, ed. 3, New York, 1980, Harper & Row, Publishers, Inc.
44. Smith, A.L.: Microbiology and pathology, ed. 12, St. Louis, 1980, The C.V. Mosby Co.
45. Solomon, G.F., and Amkraut, A.A.: Emotions, stress and immunity, Front. Radiat. Ther. Oncol. **7**:84, 1974.
46. Stossel, T.P.: Phagocytosis, N. Engl. J. Med. **290**:833, 1974.
47. Tarnawski, A., and Balko, B.: Antibiotics and immune processes, Lancet **1**:674, 1973.

---

*Readings preceded by an asterisk are particularly well suited for student reading.

48. Thaler, M.S., et al.: Medical immunology, Philadelphia, 1977, J.B. Lippincott Co.
49. Unanue, E.R.: Cooperation between mononuclear phagocytes and lymphocytes in immunity, N. Engl. J. Med. 303:977-981, 1980.
50. Weiss, H.J.: Aspirin: a dangerous drug? J.A.M.A. 229:1221, 1974.
51. Yunis, E.J., Fernandes, G., and Greenberg, L.J.: Tumor immunology, autoimmunity and aging, J. Am. Geriatr. 24:253, 1976.
52. Zweifach, B.W., et al.: The inflammatory process, ed. 2, New York, 1974, Academic Press, Inc.

AUDIOVISUAL RESOURCES

Immunology, Kalamazoo, Mich. 1976, Upjohn Co. (Color slides and text.)
Immunology, Philadelphia, 1978, W.B. Saunders Co. (Slides.)
Man's response to pathogens, Costa Mesa, Calif., 1974, Concept Media. (Color sound filmstrip.)
A question of immunity, San Francisco, 1976, Alternatives on Film. (Color 13-min. 16mm film.)

CHAPTER 20

MECHANISMS FOR MAINTAINING DYNAMIC EQUILIBRIUM

VIRGINIA L. CASSMEYER

Humans live in two environments, an external one that is changing constantly and a much more stable internal one. The human machinery, steered by the neuroendocrine integrating mechanisms (see Chapter 18), is constantly adapting to changes on the cellular level to maintain a stable environment. Cellular growth and functioning can occur only when the internal environment has an adequate supply of oxygen, nutrients, and electrolytes. The amount and characteristics of body fluid bathing the cells must be kept relatively stable to provide the cells with the requirements necessary for survival and growth. The process of maintaining this relatively constant environment is called *dynamic equilibrium*. Functioning body systems that can provide oxygen and remove carbon dioxide, provide nutrients, maintain fluid and electrolyte balance, excrete waste, and transport needed products to cells and waste products to elimination sites are necessary to maintain dynamic equilibrium.

The nurse must know how body systems function to maintain dynamic equilibrium in order to help persons maintain health and to give supportive nursing care when disease or injury upsets the body's ability to maintain its checks and balances.

Maintenance of adequate oxygen– carbon dioxide exchange

Cellular need for oxygen

Maintenance of adequate oxygen–carbon dioxide exchange is dependent on the process of respiration. Of all body functions involved in maintaining cellular growth and functioning, the maintenance of normal respiration probably has the greatest immediate significance. All body functions require energy. The most important energy component in cellular work is adenosine triphosphate (ATP).

ATP is formed from the metabolism of carbohydrates (CHO), fats, and proteins. Carbohydrates, fats, and proteins are catabolized completely to carbon dioxide, water, and ATP only if there is an adequate supply of oxygen. For example, in the absence of oxygen, glucose can only be metabolized to pyruvic acid or lactic acid in the glycolytic pathway (Embden-Meyerhof pathway) yielding only two molecules of ATP. When oxygen is present, the glycolytic pathway contributes six additional molecules of ATP. In addition, pyruvic acid can enter the Krebs cycle (citric acid or tricarboxylic acid cycle) yielding 30 molecules of ATP, for a total of 36 additional molecules of ATP for each molecule of glucose.

The metabolism of neutral fat to produce ATP also requires oxygen. Neutral fat is first broken down into glycerol and fatty acids. The glycerol enters the glycolytic pathway, and the fatty acid is then broken down to acetyl coenzyme A (acetyl CoA) and carrier—H_2 molecule.[91] The acetyl CoA enters the Krebs cycle and in the presence of oxygen releases ATP. The carrier— H_2 molecule in the presence of oxygen transfers hydrogen to the electron transport chain and ATP is synthesized. Each molecule of neutral fat (C_{18}) can be metabolized to 463 molecules of ATP.

Proteins not necessary for growth and repair of body tissues are broken down into intermediary metabolites that enter the Krebs cycle and release ATP. As is true with carbohydrate and fat metabolism, oxygen is necessary for this synthesis to occur. The reader is advised to consult physiology and biochemistry texts for more detailed information.

Mechanisms for providing oxygen

The oxygen necessary to maintain adequate levels of ATP for energy and thus for cellular function must be obtained from the environment and be transported to the cells. This is accomplished through the process of *respiration*. Respiration is defined as the gas exchange (O_2 and CO_2) between an organism and its environment. There are three components of respiration: *ventilation*, *perfusion*, and *diffusion*.

Ventilation

Ventilation is a mechanical process by which air is moved in and out of the lungs. There are two phases to ventilation: inspiration and expiration, which occur because of the integration of many neural and chemical factors.

Neural control of ventilation. Two respiratory centers are located in the reticular formation of the medulla. One set of neurons is associated with inspiration (inspiratory center) and the other set with expiration (expiratory center). These two centers have interconnections that are inhibitory in nature.[91] The inherent rhythmicity of the medullary respiratory center is probably the result of these interconnections.[94] The medullary respiratory center also has connections with the respiratory center in the pons and with the cerebral cortex.

Inspiration occurs because of rhythmic impulses arising from the inspiratory center in the medulla that stimulate the phrenic and intercostal nerves. Stimulation of the phrenic nerves causes the diaphragm to contract and move downward. Stimulation of the intercostal nerves causes the external intercostal muscles to contract, moving the ribs upward and out. The net result is an enlarged thoracic cavity and a decrease in the intraalveolar (intrapulmonary) pressure to less than atmospheric pressure (760 mm Hg), and air moves into the lungs.

Expiration occurs primarily because of inhibition of the inspiratory center. After inspiration reaches a certain point, the pons sends impulses to the inspiratory center that inhibit inspiration.[94] When the inspiratory center is inhibited by the pons, the expiratory center is released from inhibition and it also then helps to terminate inspiration by sending inhibitory impulses to the inspiratory center. With inhibition of the inspiratory center stimulation of the phrenic and intercostal nerves ceases, the diaphragm and external intercostal muscles relax, and the thoracic cavity decreases in size. The net result is an intraalveolar (intrapulmonary) pressure greater

than that of atmospheric pressure, and air moves out of the lungs. Expiration is usually a passive event but in certain conditions involving active expiration, the expiratory center can send impulses to expiratory muscles.[94]

During inspiration the Hering-Breuer stretch receptors are stimulated. Impulses from the stretch receptors are transmitted by the vagus nerve to the inspiratory center, thus further inhibiting inspiration. At one time this reflex was thought to play a major role in the control of ventilation. However, this reflex seems to be largely inactive in adult men unless the tidal volume exceeds 1 L.[94]

Chemical control of ventilation. In addition to the neural controls described above, breathing is influenced by the levels of CO_2, O_2, and pH in arterial blood and cerebrospinal fluid and by changes in blood pressure. The normal stimulus for respiration is the cerebral CO_2. This control is so sensitive that during periods of rest and exercise, the arterial P_{CO_2} is held within 3 mm Hg.[94] The chemoreceptors in the medulla are bathed in CSF allowing CO_2 to readily diffuse from the blood to the spinal fluid. As the level of arterial CO_2 increases, the level of CO_2 in the cerebrospinal fluid also increases and the medulla is stimulated.

Other chemical factors that stimulate respiration are O_2 and pH. Chemoreceptors located in the carotid and aortic bodies respond to decreased blood levels of P_{O_2}, decreases in pH, and increases in P_{CO_2}. These peripheral chemoreceptors are most sensitive to changes in P_{O_2}. A decrease in blood pressure also affects respiration. These changes are sensed by the baroreceptors located in the carotid and aortic sinuses.

Fig. 20-1 summarizes these neural and chemical influences on the medullary respiratory center.

Although CO_2 is normally the stimulus for respiration, when CO_2 retention of long standing occurs, as in patients with chronic lung disease, the respiratory center can become depressed by excessive levels of CO_2, resulting in a condition known as *CO_2 narcosis*. In this situation the *peripheral chemoreceptors* in the carotid and aortic bodies, which are sensitive to decreases in arterial oxygen tension, stimulate the respiratory center to maintain breathing. Since respiration in this situation is being maintained by a decrease in the P_{O_2}, it is important that high levels of oxygen not be administered to these patients or the mechanism that is keeping them breathing will be removed. In patients with the potential for developing CO_2 narcosis, only low-flow oxygen (1 to 3 L/min) is administered (p. 1332). If the oxygen needs cannot be met with low-flow oxygen, mechanical ventilation is necessary (p. 1244).

Perfusion

Perfusion is the movement of blood to and from the alveolar capillary bed. The pulmonary circulation is de-

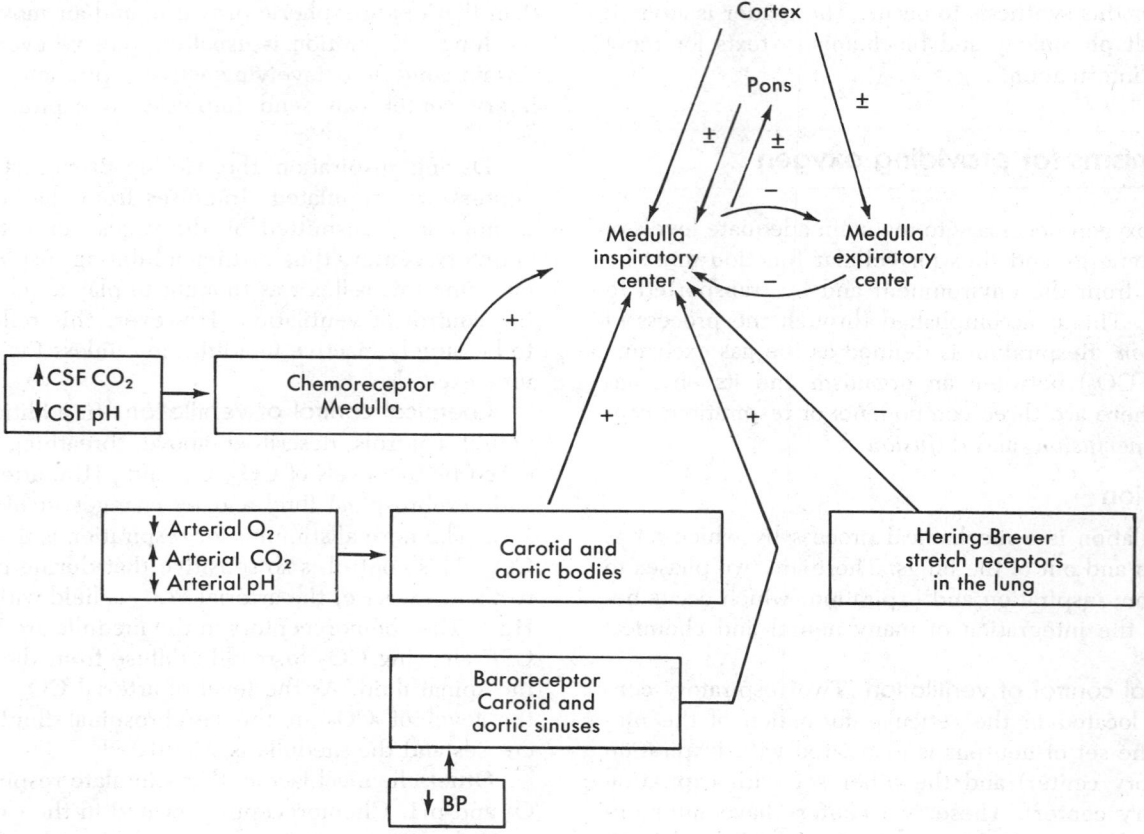

Fig. 20-1. Neural and chemical influences on medullary center. +, Stimulates; −, inhibits.

rived from the main pulmonary trunk, which receives venous blood from the *right* ventricle. The pulmonary trunk divides into the right and left pulmonary arteries. The pulmonary arteries branch following the bronchial tree to form the capillary plexus surrounding the alveoli. The capillary plexus reunites to form the pulmonary veins, which return blood to the *left* side of the heart.

The pulmonary vascular bed is a low-pressure system as compared with the systemic circulation. The pulmonary capillaries are surrounded only by gas, and they collapse or distend if the pressure within or outside of them changes. The pulmonary capillary vascular bed is responsive to changes in alveolar oxygen levels, blood pH, and sympathetic outflow. The perfusion of all the alveoli is not uniform, and at any one time not all alveoli are being perfused. The important determinant of oxygen–carbon dioxide exchange is the ratio of alveolar ventilation to capillary perfusion. This ratio is usually designated by symbols: alveolar ventilation by $\dot{V}_a$ (alveolar gas volume per unit of time) and pulmonary capillary perfusion by $\dot{Q}_c$ (pulmonary capillary blood flow per unit of time). The normal $\dot{V}_a/\dot{Q}_c$ is approximately 0.8 (or 1.0). This is derived from the fact that $\dot{V}_a$ is 4200 ml/min (tidal volume of 500 ml/breath − 150 ml/breath

of dead space × 12 breaths/min) and $\dot{Q}_c$ is about 5400 ml/min. Certain disease processes cause changes in ventilation, perfusion, or both (see Chapter 51 for further discussion).

Diffusion

Diffusion is the process by which oxygen and carbon dioxide are exchanged across the alveolar-capillary membrane. Oxygen and carbon dioxide diffusion is passive, since the two gases diffuse with a pressure gradient (from greater pressure to lesser pressure). Fig. 20-2 shows the PO_2 and PCO_2 levels in the alveolus and the capillary. Diffusion is a rapid process, and oxygen enters the red blood cell in less than 1 second.[94] Carbon dioxide diffuses about 20 times faster than oxygen. The diffusion of oxygen into blood is limited only by the amount of perfusion. After oxygen diffuses into the blood it reacts with hemoglobin to form oxyhemoglobin. It is in this manner that the majority of oxygen is carried to the tissue.

Oxygen deficit or carbon dioxide excess or both can be caused by a variety of conditions that interfere with ventilation, perfusion, or diffusion (see box on p. 299). In addition, anemia can lead to oxygen deficit, since the amount of hemoglobin present is inadequate to carry

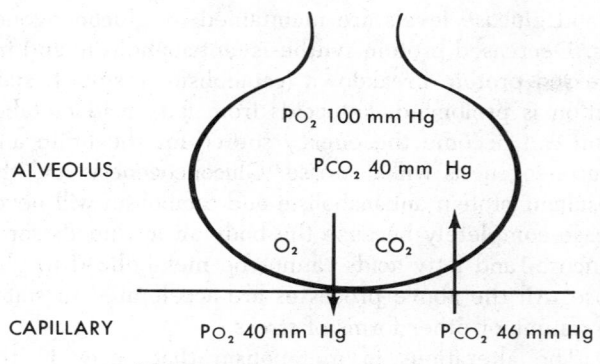

Fig. 20-2. Oxygen and carbon dioxide levels in alveolus and pulmonary capillaries.

CAUSES OF OXYGEN DEFICIT OR CARBON DIOXIDE EXCESS FROM INTERFERENCE WITH VENTILATION, PERFUSION, OR DIFFUSION

Ventilation

Inhibition of thorax or lung (bronchioles, alveoli) expansion

Decrease in elastic recoil

Perfusion

Circulatory collapse, shock

Blockage of pulmonary capillaries (emboli)

Compression of pulmonary capillary bed (increase in alveolar pressure)

Vasoconstriction from alveolar hypoxia

Decrease in blood pH

Destruction of capillary bed

Diffusion

Decrease in alveolar surface area; thickening of alveolar membrane

Increase in fluid/secretions in interstitial space or alveoli

the amount of oxygen necessary for cellular metabolism.

Early signs of inadequate oxygenation include restlessness, dyspnea, tachycardia, and confusion. Although cyanosis is a classic sign of hypoxia, it is unreliable because it does not occur until there are 5 g or more of reduced hemoglobin in the blood. Also, severe cyanosis may be present even when arterial oxygen level is satisfactory, as occurs in polycythemia. In the presence of hypoxia the nurse carries out measures to enhance optimal oxygenation, such as positioning to facilitate

breathing and assisting the patient to clear and maintain the airway and to perform appropriate breathing exercises. When these measures are not effective, nasotracheal suctioning (p. 1246) and ventilatory support (p. 1244) may be necessary.

Adequate respiration is necessary not only to maintain adequate oxygen levels but also to maintain acid-base balance. The respiratory system helps eliminate acid by the excretion of carbon dioxide. In conditions leading to hyperventilation the level of carbon dioxide and thus the hydrogen ion level decrease, causing respiratory alkalosis. In some diseases carbon dioxide is trapped in the alveoli, and the serum level of carbon dioxide and hydrogen ions increases, causing respiratory acidosis. The relationship between alveolar ventilation $\dot{V}_a$ and P_{CO_2} is given by the following formula:

$$P_{CO_2} = \frac{\dot{V}_{CO_2}}{\dot{V}_a} \times K$$

where $\dot{V}_{CO_2}$ is the CO_2 production and K is a constant.[94] This formula demonstrates that if alveolar ventilation is halved, the P_{CO_2} is doubled.[94]

The respiratory system also serves as a compensatory mechanism for metabolic acid-base imbalances. In metabolic acidosis the respiratory system can excrete increased amounts of hydrogen ions in the form of carbon dioxide. Respirations will be deep and rapid (Kussmaul's breathing). In metabolic alkalosis the respiratory system can conserve increased amounts of hydrogen in the form of carbon dioxide. Respirations will then be slow and shallow.

Maintenance of adequate nutrient levels

Adequate energy production requires adequate nutrients such as carbohydrates, fats, and proteins in addition to its oxygen requirements. Minerals and vitamins are also needed to build body tissue and to carry out the metabolic processes of the cells. Thus for adequate energy production all nutrients must be available.

Basal metabolic needs and energy stores

The healthy man of average size who lives in a moderate climate needs 1500 calories and 0.5 to 1 g of protein per kilogram of body weight a day to maintain the basic functions essential to life, that is, those functions that continue even while a person is at rest. Basic caloric needs vary with age, sex, body size, climate, genetic factors, physical activity, and body temperature. Additional physical activities require additional calories. Normally, an adequate diet with selections of food from the various food groups will supply the energy needs and provide nutrients for cell growth.

Because energy and glucose are constantly needed the body has energy reserves of fats and carbohydrates that can be used in times of fasting. A 70 kg nonobese man has approximately 135,000 calories stored as triglycerides in adipose tissue.[82] Carbohydrates are stored in the form of glycogen in the liver and muscles. The liver glycogen content is about 75 g and can provide 250 to 300 calories. There are 200 to 400 g of glycogen stored in muscles. For all practical purposes it can be assumed that there are no reserves of protein in the body, since all protein in the body serves some functional purpose and protein depletion leads to dysfunction.

Although all proteins are functional, they are not static and are constantly being resynthesized. The amino acids from ingested proteins and those resulting from endogenous breakdown (approximately 3 to 4 g/kg of body weight/day) enter a hypothetical pool from which new proteins are synthesized. Approximately 10% of the amino acids are lost during resynthesis, and this is the amount of protein that needs to be replaced daily to meet basal metabolic needs.[82]

Glucose is needed consistently even in times that are free of stressors. For example, the central nervous system requires glucose unless it adapts to using ketones from fat breakdown. Red blood cells also need glucose since they do not have the mitochondria necessary to metabolize fatty acids. Leukocytes also require glucose since they primarily obtain their energy by anaerobic metabolism.

Effects of stressors on nutrient needs

In the presence of stressors there is an increased need for energy, proteins, and glucose. For example, each degree Fahrenheit rise in temperature increases energy needs by 7% to 8%. Surgery increases energy needs at least 5% above basal level, and severe stressors such as burns and trauma can increase needs as much as 650%.[16] If the patient has a large tumor that is unchecked in growth, the tumor growth and metabolism may require energy that is greater than 100% of basal needs.[82]

Therefore it can be seen that the body needs a continual supply of energy, proteins, and glucose in times of health and increasing amounts in the presence of stressors. In a healthy person the liver glycogen can be broken down to meet the glucose needs during overnight fasting and for a few additional hours. If fasting continues longer or unmet metabolic needs are present,

blood glucose levels are maintained by gluconeogenesis. Decreased protein synthesis (antianabolism) and increased protein breakdown (catabolism) result. If starvation is prolonged, ketoacids from fatty acid metabolism can become the energy source for the brain and gluconeogenesis will decrease. Gluconeogenesis and the resultant protein antianabolism and catabolism will never cease completely because the body always needs some glucose, and fatty acids cannot be metabolized to glucose. All the above processes are accelerated in states of trauma or other forms of stress.

The alterations in metabolism that occur in the presence of stress continue for some time after the stress is relieved. For example, Beisel, Wannemacker, and Neufeld[5] found that, in persons with a mild febrile illness, decreased protein synthesis and increased protein catabolism and nitrogen loss continued for approximately 1 to 2 weeks after their temperatures returned to normal. After uncomplicated major surgery the protein antianabolism and catabolism may continue for up to 6 weeks. This continual acceleration in metabolic processes is probably caused by the presence of adrenocortical hormones.

Accelerated protein breakdown and decreased protein synthesis can have many devastating effects, including decreased skeletal and cardiac muscle mass, decreased visceral and plasma proteins, and impaired immune response, wound healing, and organ function. In addition, the breakdown of protein can cause a serious chemical imbalance.

Protein breakdown causes the release of large amounts of nitrogen and potassium, which must be excreted by the kidneys. The excretion of these products requires an increased fluid intake, which presents problems for patients with renal or cardiac failure who cannot tolerate an increase in fluid intake.

The resultant effects of stressors may be even more damaging if the person has a chronic disease. For example, in diabetes mellitus there may be inadequate supplies of glycogen causing decreased protein synthesis and increased protein breakdown. Also, since the person with diabetes mellitus does not metabolize glucose effectively, ketogenesis may occur and be more severe. In other diseases such as renal and hepatic failure, the body may not have the ability to handle the nitrogen waste products that accumulate with the accelerated gluconeogenesis. The excess nitrogen buildup in these patients can lead to uremia or hepatic coma, respectively.

Intervention

Intervention to maintain adequate nutrient levels varies depending on the patient's ability to take nutrients orally.

When calories cannot be taken by the alimentary route, calories are provided parenterally. It is not possible to meet even the basic energy requirements of a person by the administration of glucose alone. For example, 1000 ml of 5% dextrose in water contains 50 g of glucose, or the equivalent of 200 calories. To provide even basic caloric needs for the average man 7500 ml of fluid would be needed. This amount of fluid would severely compromise the circulatory system.

For this reason total parenteral nutrition (TPN) is being widely used for persons who cannot take nutrition by mouth for prolonged periods. Total parenteral nutrition can be provided in several ways. Hyperalimentation is one way of providing total parenteral nutrition. In this technique, first developed by Dudrick in 1968, hypertonic solutions of dextrose, amino acids, vitamins, and electrolytes are delivered through a central venous catheter. In other instances TPN may employ glucose, amino acids, vitamins, electrolytes, and fat emulsion given by a peripheral or central vein depending on the glucose and amino acid concentration. Ten percent fat emulsion has one advantage as a caloric source, in that it is isotonic and can be given through a peripheral vein. With the methods described above, a positive nitrogen balance and normal growth and development can be maintained.

At times total parenteral nutrition may not be used, and isotonic solutions of amino acids with or without dextrose may be given. This form of therapy is not adequate to prevent nitrogen wasting, but it will help to minimize nitrogen loss.

Although TPN can provide all the nutrients needed for normal growth and development, oral feedings should be resumed as soon as the patient is able to tolerate them. The diet needs to be relatively high in calories (2000 to 3000 calories per day) despite limited physical activity because extra energy is being expended by the increased metabolism secondary to stressors (early) and tissue repair (later). The diet should also be high in protein. Persons who are ill at home or are returning home after an illness are instructed to continue this high-calorie diet until they regain their normal weight. Caloric and protein intake should then be reduced to normal. When it is expected that someone will be unable to eat for several days, as after certain surgical procedures, special emphasis is placed on maximizing nutritional status preoperatively (see Chapter 24).

Maintenance of fluid and electrolyte balance

In order for survival, fluid and electrolyte balance must be maintained. In health, fluid and electrolyte balance is maintained without difficulty by multiple body systems. As mentioned (p. 300), any stressor and the resultant stress response can cause some fluid and electrolyte imbalance. Normal fluid and electrolyte *balance* is discussed next; fluid and electrolyte *imbalance* is discussed in Chapter 21.

Body fluid and electrolyte compartments, distribution, and functions

Fluid and electrolytes are found in the body either within the cell (*intracellular*) or outside the cell (*extracellular*). The extracellular fluid is contained in two compartments: the *interstitial* fluid (fluid between the cells) and the *intravascular* fluid (fluid in the blood vessels). A third type of fluid, *transcellular*, denotes fluid separated by a layer of epithelial cells from other extracellular fluid.[56] Transcellular fluid includes digestive juices, water, and solutes in the renal tubules and bladder, intraocular fluid, and cerebrospinal fluid. Some authorities consider this to be a part of the extracellular compartment, and others consider it to be a separate compartment. Transcellular fluid makes up 1% to 3% of body weight.

Body water is the largest single constituent of the body, representing 45% to 75% of body weight. The volume and distribution of body water vary with age and sex (Fig. 20-3). In the newborn infant almost three fourths of the body weight is water, with the greatest percentage found in the extracellular compartment. The volume and distribution change over time, and by adulthood in the young male only 60% of body weight is water and two thirds of this is in the intracellular compartment. In the average young female only approximately 50% of body weight is water. This difference between men and women is due to an increased

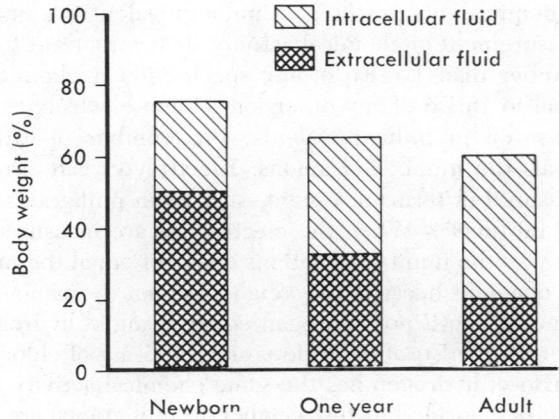

Fig. 20-3. In newborn more than half of total body fluid is extracellular. As the child grows, proportions gradually approximate adult levels.

TABLE 20-1. Normal electrolyte content of body fluids*

Electrolytes (anions and cations)	Extracellular		Intracellular (mEq/L)
	Intravascular (mEq/L)	Interstitial (mEq/L)	
Sodium (Na$^+$)	142	146	15
Potassium (K$^+$)	5	5	150
Calcium (Ca^{++})	5	3	2
Magnesium (Mg^{++})	2	1	27
Chloride (Cl$^-$)	102	114	1
Bicarbonate (HCO$_3^-$)	27	30	10
Protein (Prot$^-$)	16	1	63
Phosphate (HPO$_4^=$)	2	2	100
Sulfate (SO$_4^=$)	1	1	20
Organic acids	5	8	0

*Note that the electrolyte level of the intravascular and interstitial fluids (extracellular) is approximately the same and that sodium and chloride contents are markedly higher in these fluids, whereas potassium, phosphate, and protein contents are markedly higher in intracellular fluid.

amount of fat in women. Fat is essentially water free.

Body water has multiple functions. The extracellular water maintains blood volume and serves as the body's transport system to and from cells. Intracellular fluid provides the internal aqueous medium for cellular chemical function. Adequate body water balance is also necessary for the maintenance of normal body temperature and for the elimination of waste products.

All body fluids contain electrolytes, electrolytes are chemical compounds in solution that have the ability to conduct an electrical current. In solution electrolytes break into charged particles called *ions*. Positively charged ions are called *cations,* and negatively charged ions are called *anions*. Electrolytes are distributed in different concentrations in the intracellular, intravascular, and interstitial compartments (Table 20-1).

The electrolyte quantities given in Table 20-1 are in milliequivalents per liter. A milliequivalent is a unit of measurement of chemical activity. It is important to remember than 1 mEq of any specific ion is chemically equal to 1mEq of any other ion. When electrolytes are measured in milliequivalents, the number of cations equals the number of anions. Electrolytes can also be measured in terms of weight, such as in milligrams per 100 ml (mg%). When the electrolytes are measured in this way the number of cations does not equal the number of anions because the weights are not the same. For example, 1 mEq of hydrogen equals 1 mg of hydrogen, whereas 1 mEq of chloride equals 35.5 mg of chloride; 1 mEq of hydrogen has the same chemical activity as 1 mEq of chloride but the weights (in milligrams) are different. At times nurses need to be able to make conversions between the two systems of measurement. The box above gives the formulas for these conversions.

FORMULAS FOR CALCULATING MILLIEQUIVALENT QUANTITY OF AN ION AND OF A SALT FROM WEIGHT (IN MILLIGRAMS) AND CONVERSION BETWEEN MILLIEQUIVALENTS PER LITER AND MILLIGRAMS PER 100 ML

Calculation of milliequivalent quantity of an ion

$$mEq = \frac{\text{Atomic weight of ion}}{\text{Valence}}$$

Calculation of milliequivalent quantity of a salt from weight in milligrams

$$mEq = \frac{\text{Weight in milligrams}}{\text{Atomic weight}} \times \text{Valence}$$

Example: 0.5 g of NaCl = 500 mg. Molecular weight of NaCl = 23 (atomic weight of Na$^+$) + 35.5 (atomic weight of Cl$^-$) = 58.5. Valence = 1.

Thus $\frac{500}{58.5} \times 1$ = 8.5, or 500 mg of NaCl = 8.5 mEq of NaCl.

Conversion of milliequivalents per liter to milligrams per 100 ml

$$mg/100 \text{ ml} = \frac{\text{mEq/L} \times \text{Atomic weight}}{10 \times \text{Valence}}$$

Conversion of milligrams per 100 ml to milliequivalents per liter

$$mEq/L = \frac{\text{mg/100 ml} \times 10 \times \text{Valence}}{\text{Atomic weight}}$$

Transcellular fluids have very distinct patterns of electrolyte concentration. For example, gastric secretions have a high hydrogen ion concentration, pancreatic secretions have a high bicarbonate concentration, and renal tubular and bladder fluids vary on a daily basis. Gastric, pancreatic, and intestinal juices and bile all contain high concentrations of sodium. In all fluid compartments, although the concentration of electrolytes will vary, electrical neutrality will be maintained; that is, the solution will contain equal quantities in terms of chemical activity (milliequivalents per liter) of anions and cations.

Each electrolyte has specific functions. The general functions of all electrolytes are to (1) promote neuromuscular irritability, (2) maintain body fluid volume and osmolality, (3) distribute body water between fluid compartments, and (4) regulate acid-base balance.

Before discussing normal fluid and electrolyte balance, the terms *osmolality* and *osmolarity* need to be defined even though they are frequently used interchangeably when discussing body fluids. Osmolality is an expression of the concentration of solution in terms of 1000 g of water. Neither the temperature (which can affect volume) nor the amount of solute has an effect on the osmolality of a solution. A 1 osmol solution is made by adding 1 g mole of solute to exactly 1000 g of water. The volume of the solution will then be greater than 1 L.

Osmolarity is an expression of concentration in terms of 1000 ml of solution. Temperature and the amount of solute will affect the amount of water in 1000 ml of solution. A 1 osmolar solution is made by placing 1 g mole of solute in a container and then adding water sufficient to make exactly 1 L of solution.

From the above, it can be seen that 1 osmolar solution and 1 osmol solution are not exactly the same. However, if the concentration of solute is small and the temperature is within normal body temperature range, the difference is negligible. This is why the difference between osmolarity and osmolality is negligible in normal body fluids.

Normal exchange of fluid and electrolytes

In health, body fluids (water and electrolytes) are constantly being lost and must be replaced in order to maintain normal processes. The fluid that is lost is not "pure water" but always contains some electrolytes; thus both water and electrolytes must be replaced daily. By knowing the concentration of fluid and electrolytes in the various compartments, the nurse can anticipate which fluid and electrolyte imbalance will most probably occur if abnormal losses occur from any particular site.

In a state of health body fluids are lost daily from the kidneys, lungs, gastrointestinal tract, and skin, with negligible amounts being lost in saliva and tears. Two processes demand continual expenditure of water: control of body heat and excretion of metabolic waste products. The volume of fluid used in these processes depends on such things as external temperature, humidity, metabolic rate, and physical activities. In normal fluid balance the output of fluid equals the intake of fluid. In addition, a balanced diet (see Chapter 52) provides excess amounts of electrolytes; the excess is excreted, and electrolyte balance is maintained.

Table 20-2 summarizes the normal routes of gains and losses in an adult eating approximately 2500 calories per day. It shoud be noted that approximately two fifths of the normal fluid intake is obtained from water in food, or "preformed water." Solid foods such as meat and vegetables are 60% to 90% water. The fact that a large quantity of water is obtained from food has important implications if a person's food intake decreases substantially.

Approximately two fifths of the fluid lost daily is lost through the insensible route (skin, lungs, and gastroin-

TABLE 20-2. Normal fluid intake and loss in an adult eating 2500 calories per day (approximate figures)

Intake		Output	
Route	Amount of gain (ml)	Route	Amount of loss (ml)
Water in food	1000	Skin	500
Water from oxidation	300	Lungs	350
Water as liquid	1200	Feces	150
		Kidney	1500
TOTAL	2500	TOTAL	2500

testinal tract). Insensible loss through the skin refers to invisible perspiration. When visible perspiration occurs, such as that following heavy physical activities or with shock, the loss of water through the skin is greater than the normal 500 ml. Fecal loss increases in the presence of diarrhea or watery stools. Persons with certain pulmonary problems lose more than the normal amount of fluid (350 ml) from the lungs. Increased loss of fluids through these insensible routes also results in the loss of electrolytes.

Internal regulation of body water and electrolytes

Fluid and electrolyte balance depends on an adequate intake and output. This means that the intake must equal the output. The control of intake and output is regulated by various internal mechanisms. In this section the regulation of body water and major electrolytes is discussed. The reader is referred to physiology texts for a more in-depth review.

Sodium and water

Thirst. The major control of actual fluid intake is thirst. The thirst center is located in the ventromedial nucleus of the hypothalamus. Impulses from this center can stimulate the cerebral cortex, which then interprets this stimulation as the preception of thirst. The thirst center is stimulated by hypertonic body fluid, isoosmotic contraction, decreased blood pressure, decreased cardiac output, dryness of the mouth, and angiotensin (p. 305). How these factors cause the thirst center to be stimulated is not fully understood. It is felt that when the cells in the thirst center become dehydrated (shrink), this causes stimulation of the neurons, which transmit the impulse to the cerebral cortex, which translates the sensation to that of thirst. Most of the time thirst is not thought of as a control because social and cultural habits greatly influence the quantity of liquid humans drink.

Persons who are dependent on others to supply their intake of fluid or persons who have a sudden increase in fluid loss (bleeding, increased sweating) will complain of being thirsty. Also there is some evidence that humans have a salt appetite; that is, when persons are deprived of or have a deficit in salt, they will have a craving for salt.

Kidney. The major organ controlling output is the kidney, which is under the influence of several control mechanisms. The kidney is responsible for regulating the volume and osmolality of body fluids. The osmolality of body fluids is predominantly dependent on sodium and its associate anions. The maintenance of water and sodium balance depends on glomerular filtration rate (GFR), antidiuretic hormone (ADH), and the aldosterone-renin-angiotensin system.

Glomerular filtration. Glomerular filtration is an involved topic, and the reader is urged to consult references 56, 90, 91, and Chapter 60 for more information. Three factors determine glomerular filtration: glomerular capillary blood pressure, Bowman's capsule hydrostatic pressure, and plasma protein concentration. Many factors and pathophysiologic states can affect these three factors and thus change glomerular filtration. Conditions such as shock and hypertension change glomerular capillary blood pressure. Changes in Bowman's capsule pressure can be caused by urinary obstruction. A decrease in plasma protein concentration can occur with increased loss, decreased intake, or decreased production of proteins.

Antidiuretic hormone. ADH is a hormone produced by the supraoptic and paraventricular nuclei of the hypothalamus and released from the posterior pituitary gland. The neurons in the hypothalamus receive input from volume receptors in the left atrium and great veins and from osmoreceptors in the hypothalamus. Volume receptors are stimulated by changes in atrial blood volume or blood pressure. Impulses from the volume receptors are transmitted by afferent nerve fibers to the hypothalamus. Increased blood volume or increased blood pressure increases the firing of the volume receptors, stimulates the hypothalamus, and inhibits ADH production. Conversely, decreased blood volume or blood pressure decreases the firing of the volume receptors and increases ADH production.

Osmoreceptors are stimulated by changes in cell size. If pure water is added to the body fluids, this increases the size of the cells in the osmoreceptors and leads to the inhibition of ADH production. A loss of pure water causes the cells to shrink and stimulates the secretion of ADH. ADH secretion is also stimulated by angiotensin, narcotics, stress, heat, nicotine, antineoplastic agents, and anesthetic agents. Fig. 20-4 depicts the factors and mechanisms involved in ADH production and the results of ADH production.

ADH acts on the kidney cells by stimulating 3'5'-cyclic AMP release, and the cyclic AMP causes appropriate cellular metabolism. In the kidney, ADH causes increased water reabsorption in the distal convoluted tubules and collecting ducts. It also may stimulate the pumping of sodium in the loop of Henle and regulate the rate of blood perfusion, both of which would lead to increased water reabsorption. In the presence of ADH, the kidney can concentrate urine to 1200 mOsm/kg H_2O.

The conservation of water increases blood volume and blood pressure and decreases osmolality. Since ADH can be secreted in response to factors other than a deficit of water (narcotics, anesthetic agents, stress) fluid overload can occur. Patients who are at high risk of inappropriate ADH secretion need to be monitored closely by the nurse. This would include postoperative patients (see Chapter 24).

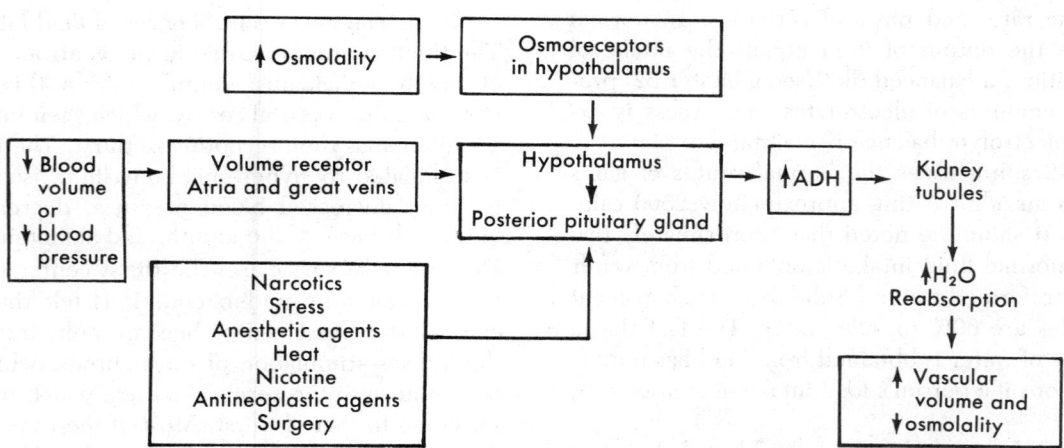

Fig. 20-4. Factors and mechanisms involved in ADH production and effect of ADH.

Aldosterone-renin-angiotensin system. Aldosterone is a hormone produced by the zona glomerulosa of the adrenal cortex. It increases the kidney's reabsorption of sodium and thus water in the proximal tubules and the distal convoluted tubules. In the complete absence of aldosterone a person may excrete 25 g of sodium per day, whereas if large quantities of aldosterone are present no sodium will be excreted.

The major stimulus for aldosterone production is a reflex initiated by the kidney. Cells in the kidney monitor sodium levels and blood volume. When the serum sodium level or the blood volume decreases, the juxtaglomerular cells in the kidney secrete a protein, *renin*. Renin acts on *angiotensinogen*, a plasma protein formed in the liver, to form *angiotensin I*. Angiotensin I is converted to angiotensin II by another enzyme (p. 1178).

Angiotensin II stimulates the adrenal cortex to secrete aldosterone. Aldosterone causes the retention of sodium by the kidneys, intestines, and sweat and salivary glands. In addition, angiotensin II causes vasoconstriction of arterial smooth muscles, thus decreasing the glomerular filtration rate. Some aldosterone may be secreted in response to ACTH (p. 262). Another important fact is that aldosterone is catabolized by the liver, and with liver failure inappropriate amounts of aldosterone may lead to sodium and water retention because of ineffective catabolism. Fig. 20-5 depicts the factors and mechanisms involved in aldosterone production and the effects of aldosterone production.

Third factor. Glomerular filtration, ADH, and the aldosterone-renin-angiotensin system do not explain the kidney's complete control of sodium and water reabsorption and excretion. It is hypothesized that a "third factor" is involved in the control of sodium and water

balance.[90,91] The term *third factor* is used because there is little known about this mechanism. At present there seem to be three other factors that assist in the control of sodium and water: (1) a natriuretic hormone, (2) intrarenal physical factors, and (3) redistribution of blood flow. Research is ongoing in this area.

Potassium

Potassium (K^+) is the major intracellular cation and regulates intracellular osmolality. Potassium is very important in conduction of nerve impulses and promotion of proper skeletal and cardiac muscle activity. Because of potassium's role in the excitability of nerves and muscles, it is important that the extracellular concentration of potassium be maintained within the normal range.

The major excretion site of excess potassium is the kidney. The majority of excess potassium (80% to 90%) is excreted in the urine, and the remainder is excreted by the gastrointestinal tract. Potassium is completely filtered by the kidney, but most of the potassium filtered is reabsorbed in the proximal tubules and the loop of Henle. Glomerular filtration of potassium plays only a minimal role in normal potassium excretion. The control of renal excretion of potassium resides in the distal tubular cells' ability to secrete potassium into tubular fluid. As extracellular potassium levels rise, more potassium moves into all cells including the distal tubular cells. This higher concentration in the cells facilitates potassium secretion into tubular fluid because of the gradient difference between the distal tubular cells and the fluid in the tubular lumen. Conversely, if potassium intake is low or if there is increased loss of potassium through the gastrointestinal tract, the potassium level

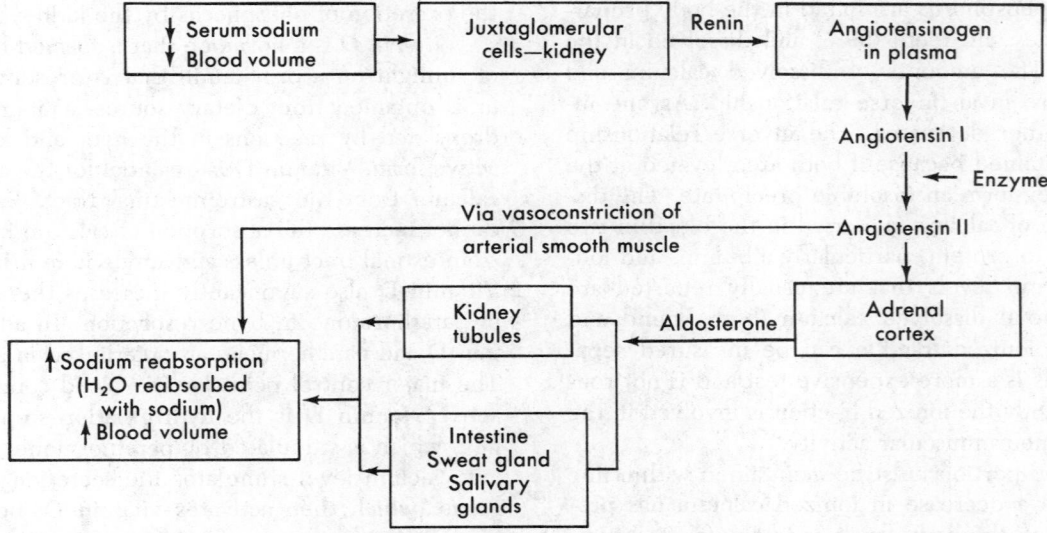

Fig. 20-5. Factors and mechanisms involved in aldosterone production and effects of aldosterone production.

in the distal tubular cells is decreased. This causes a decrease in the gradient, and less potassium is secreted.

Even though glomerular filtration plays only a minimal role in the amount of potassium excreted in the urine, it is an important point to remember. Certain situations interefere with the reabsorption of the filtered potassium in the proximal tubules, and this can lead to an increased loss of potassium. Osmotic diuretics and disease states that produce osmotic diuresis are examples of situations in which there is interference with the reabsorption of potassium in the proximal tubules.

Aldosterone can increase the amount of potassium secreted by the distal tubules. The aldosterone-secreting cells of the adrenal cortex are sensitive to the extracellular concentration of potassium. If the extracellular concentration of potassium increases, aldosterone is produced and stimulates the distal tubular cells to secrete more potassium. The renin-angiotensin system is not involved in this stimulation of aldosterone.

It is apparent that a conflict arises when potassium levels and sodium levels are high, since these changes stimulate aldosterone production to move in different ways. What happens in such a situation is unknown. This is not the only conflict that can arise between different electrolytes. Hydrogen ion concentration affects potassium levels. The existence of a low hydrogen ion concentration increases potassium excretion and leads to potassium depletion (hypokalemia). The presence of a high hydrogen ion concentration decreases potassium excretion and can cause potassium excess (hyperkalemia).

Calcium and phosphorus

Calcium (Ca^{++}) plays a major role in the promotion of neuromuscular irritability and muscular contractions. Calcium and phosphorus are found in the body primarily in the bones and teeth (99%) and dissolved in the blood (1%). The amounts of dissolved calcium and phosphorus are in an inverse relationship. As one increases the other decreases. The inverse relationship must be maintained because if both are elevated at the same time they form an insoluble precipitate. The dissolved portion of calcium is carried in the blood in two forms: bound to protein, particularly albumin, and ionized. The serum levels that are usually reported are measures of total dissolved calcium (both bound and ionized). The ionized fraction can be measured separately, but this is a more expensive test and is not routinely done. Only the ionized fraction is involved in the promotion of neuromuscular activity.

The ionized portion must be maintained within fine limits because a decrease in ionized calcium has profound effects on the body, such as *tetany* (p. 341). In a person with a normal serum protein and albumin level and a normal calcium level, the ionized fraction is usu-

ally a little greater than 50% of the total dissolved level. Since part of the dissolved calcium is bound to protein, the concentration of serum calcium will vary as the protein level varies. If the total protein and albumin levels fall, the total serum calcium level will fall. Many times persons with serum calcium levels below normal exhibit no symptoms of *hypocalcemia* because although their total calcium level is low, the ionized fraction may still be within normal limits. However, a decrease in protein and albumin will cause a decrease in the bound fraction.

The ratio between the dissolved calcium that is bound and the ionized fraction is affected by acid-base status. Acidosis causes more calcium to be ionized, whereas alkalosis causes more of the ionized fraction to become bound. These changes are probably not detrimental to persons with a normal serum calcium level, but alkalosis in a person who already has a low serum calcium can lead to tetany. Calcium also binds to other agents, such as citrate, which is normally metabolized by the liver. Since citrate is commonly used as an anticoagulant in stored blood, persons receiving a large number of transfusions rapidly should be watched carefully for signs of hypocalcemia. Some authoritites recommend that for every 3 to 4 units of blood given rapidly, the patient should receive 10 ml of calcium gluconate.[33]

The level of calcium is dependent on three hormones: parathormone, vitamin D, and calcitonin. *Parathormone* is a hormone produced by the parathyroid gland, and decreased calcium and possibly increased phosphorus levels stimulate the production of it. Parathormone causes increased movement of calcium from the bone, increased absorption of calcium from the gastrointestinal tract, and increased reabsorption of calcium in the renal tubules, all of which lead to an increase in calcium levels. Parathormone also increases the excretion of phosphorus by the kidneys.

Vitamin D is a hormone that is formed by the action of sunlight on a provitamin that is present in the skin or is obtained from dietary sources. Vitamin D is hydroxylated by reactions in the liver and kidney to its active form. Vitamin D is essential for the absorption of calcium from the gastrointestinal tract. Parathormone cannot increase the absorption of calcium from the gastrointestinal tract unless activated vitamin D is present. Vitamin D also significantly increases the effectiveness of parathormone in bone resorption. In addition, vitamin D and parathormone are interlinked in another way. The major control point for the blood concentration of active vitamin D is the hydroxylation step in the kidney, which is stimulated by parathormone. Therefore a low calcium level stimulates the secretion of parathormone, which then activates vitamin D; both then increase the absorption of calcium from the gastrointestinal tract and the resorption of calcium from the bone.

Calcitonin, a hormone produced by the thyroid gland,

decreases calcium levels by preventing bone resorption of calcium. It opposes the effects of parathormone and vitamin D on bones. High calcium levels stimulate the thyroid gland to release calcitonin, which inhibits the release of calcium from the bone and thus lowers serum calcium levels.

Acid-base status

Hydrogen ions are vital to life and health. The concentration of hydrogen in the body is less than that of other ions (0.00004 mEq/L). Hydrogen ion concentration is expressed as pH. Normal arterial body pH is 7.35 to 7.45. A reading less than 7.35 is present in acidosis, and a reading greater than 7.45 is present in alkalosis. Limits of pH compatible with life are 7.0 to 7.8.

Hydrogen circulates throughout the body fluids in two forms: the volatile hydrogen of carbonic acid and the nonvolatile form of hydrogen in organic acids such as sulfuric, pyruvic, phosphoric, and lactic acids. In a day's time many acids are produced as the end products of metabolism. In the normal person, the lungs excrete 13,000 to 30,000 mEq/day of the volatile hydrogen in carbonic acid (H_2CO_3) as CO_2, and the kidneys excrete approximately 50 mEq/day of nonvolatile acids.

Buffer systems. The body cells are very sensitive to changes in hydrogen ion concentration (pH), and the pH is kept relatively constant by the *buffer systems* in the body. A buffer is a substance that can act as a chemical sponge, either soaking up or releasing hydrogen ions so that the pH remains stable. The main buffer systems of the extracellular fluid are hemoglobin, protein, and the carbonic acid–bicarbonate buffer system. The carbonic acid–bicarbonate buffer system is the system that is monitored clinically. If this buffer system is stable the other buffer systems are stable.

The ability to maintain a stable pH relies essentially on maintenance of the normal ratio of 20 parts bicarbonate to 1 part carbonic acid. The normal serum bicarbonate is 24 to 28 mEq/L. The carbonic acid level is determined by taking the P_{CO_2} (normally 40 mm Hg) and multiplying it by the constant 0.03. This constant is the dissolvability factor of CO_2. This computation gives an approximate figure of 1.2. From these figures it can be seen that the normal bicarbonate–carbonic acid ratio is 20:1 (Fig. 20-6).

This ratio of 20:1 is maintained by the lungs and the kidneys. The carbonic acid concentration is controlled by the lungs' excretion of the gas carbon dioxide. The depth and rate of respiration change in response to changes in carbon dioxide (p. 297). The bicarbonate concentration is controlled by the kidneys, which selectively retain or excrete bicarbonate in response to the body's needs.

Compensation. The kidneys and lungs serve a compensatory function in relation to maintaining acid-base balance. Many disease conditions can affect the excre-

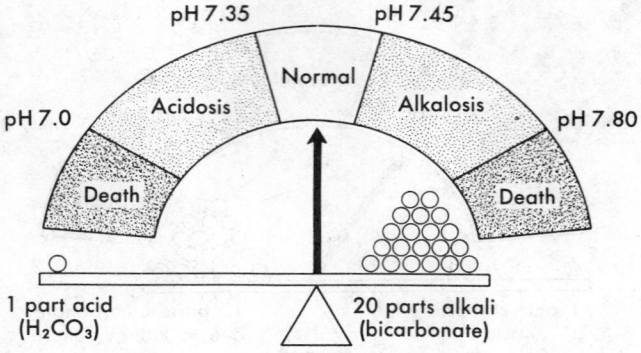

Carbonic acid–base bicarbonate balance

Fig. 20-6. Note that relationship of 1 part carbonic acid to 20 parts bicarbonate will maintain hydrogen ion concentration (pH) within normal limits. Increase in H_2CO_3 or decrease in HCO_3 will cause acidosis; similarly, decrease in H_2CO_3 or increase in HCO_3 will cause alkalosis. (Redrawn from Abbott Laboratories: Fluid and electrolytes, North Chicago, Ill., 1970, Abbott Laboratories.)

tion and retention of carbon dioxide and bicarbonate (see Chapter 21). In a disease state that leads to an acid-base imbalance the normal ratio of 20:1 will be lost. In compensation the system not involved (kidneys or lungs) will conserve or excrete the products it controls to bring the ratio back to normal. Fig. 20-7 illustrates what happens in metabolic acidosis and how compensation of acid-base imbalance can occur.

Another compensatory mechanism that can be employed by the body in the presence of *acid-base* problems is the shifting of hydrogen ions from the extracellular to the intracellular compartment or vice versa. When there is an increased level of hydrogen ions they can be shifted into the intracellular compartment in exchange for potassium. This shift alone increases the pH. In addition, since the hydrogen ion concentration is now higher in the renal tubule cells, hydrogen will be excreted in exchange for the sodium reabsorbed. In *metabolic alkalosis*, hydrogen ions will be pulled from the intracellular compartment and potassium ions will be shifted into the intracellular compartment. Again, this shift alone will help to lower the pH. Also, since potassium ion concentration is now higher in the renal tubule cells, potassium will be excreted for the sodium conserved and hydrogen ions will also be conserved. These compensatory mechanisms can lead to hyperkalemia when metabolic acidosis is present and hypokalemia when metabolic alkalosis is present. It must be remembered that the buffer systems and the compensatory mechanisms provide for only temporary adjustment and the underlying cause of the disturbance must be identified and corrected. However, the kidney can make permanent adjustments as seen in persons who

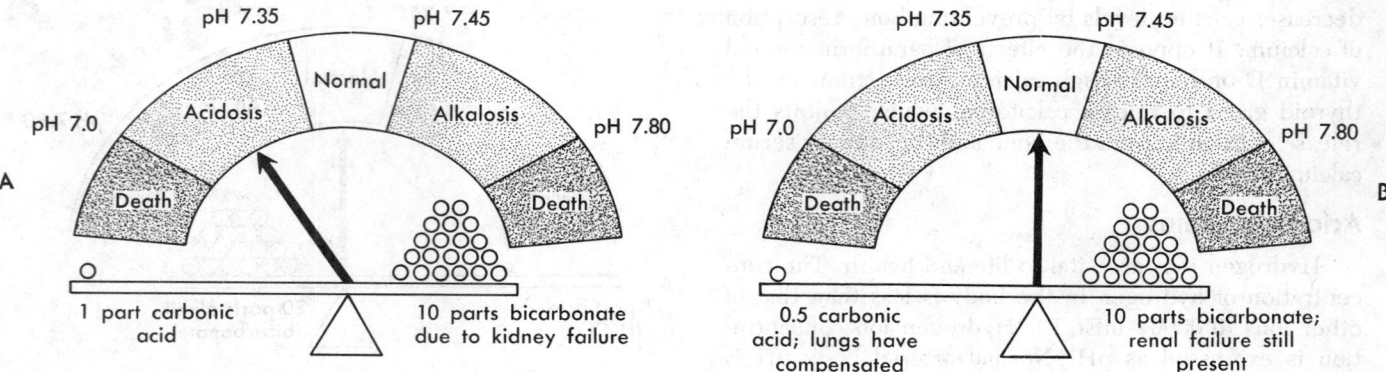

Fig. 20-7. A, Example of metabolic acidosis. Bicarbonate decreased because of renal failure. Carbonic acid to bicarbonate ratio is 10:1; acidosis is present. **B,** Example of compensation. Note bicarbonate is still decreased, but now carbonic acid is also decreased. Ratio returned to 20:1; pH is normal.

have respiratory acidosis as a result of chronic obstructive pulmonary disease (p. 1320).

Movement of fluids between compartments

The preceding discussion has referred to the fact that water and solutes are in various compartments. The water and solutes in these compartments are not static but are constantly moving between compartments. The movement of water and solutes is how needed materials are carried to the cells and waste products are removed from the cells.

Fluid and solute transport between extracellular and intracellular compartments

Fluids and electrolytes flow between the extracellular and intracellular compartments by passive or facilitated *diffusion, osmosis,* and *active transport.* Some electrolytes and other solutes flow between the two compartments with a concentration gradient by the process of passive or facilitated diffusion. Other solutes, to move into the cell, must flow against a concentration gradient by active transport. Active transport is not well understood but implies that solutes are moving against a concentration gradient or an electrical potential gradient. The mechanism involves the expenditure of energy. It has been shown that with the expenditure of one high-energy phosphate bond from adenosine triphosphate (ATP) (p. 296), three sodium ions move out of the cell and two potassium ions move into the cell. Active transport uses a large percentage of the energy formed each day because sodium is constantly diffusing into the cell and potassium is constantly diffusing out of the cell. Active transport is required to keep the concentration of the two electrolytes in the appropriate amounts within the cell.

Water, like solutes, moves between the extracellular compartment and the intracellular compartment. The movement of water is controlled by the osmolality of the two compartments. Sodium is the main regulator of extracellular osmolality, and potassium is the main regulator of intracellular osmolality.

Water moves from an area of high concentration of water (low concentration of solutes) to an area of low concentration of water (high concentration of solutes). This process is called osmosis. The movement of water will continue until the osmolality between the two compartments is approximately equal. Therefore if the water content increases in the extracellular compartment or the solute concentration decreases in the extracellular compartment, water moves into the cells to equalize the osmolality. Likewise, if the water content decreases in the extracellular compartment or the solute concentration increases in the extracellular compartment, water moves from the cells to equalize osmolality. Solutes are moving back and forth between the two compartments, but the cell membrane is more permeable to water than it is to solutes.

The mechanisms that control water and sodium levels control osmolality and thus the movement of fluid between the extracellular compartment and the intracellular compartment. Various disease states can change the osmolality and cause cellular edema or cellular dehydration. These processes are discussed in Chapter 21.

Fluid transport between vascular and interstitial spaces

The control of fluid movement between the vascular and interstitial spaces is governed by Starling's law of the capillaries. Two different types of pressures influence the flow of fluid between the vascular space and the interstitial space. These are hydrostatic pressure and colloid osmotic pressure (oncotic pressure). *Hydrostatic*

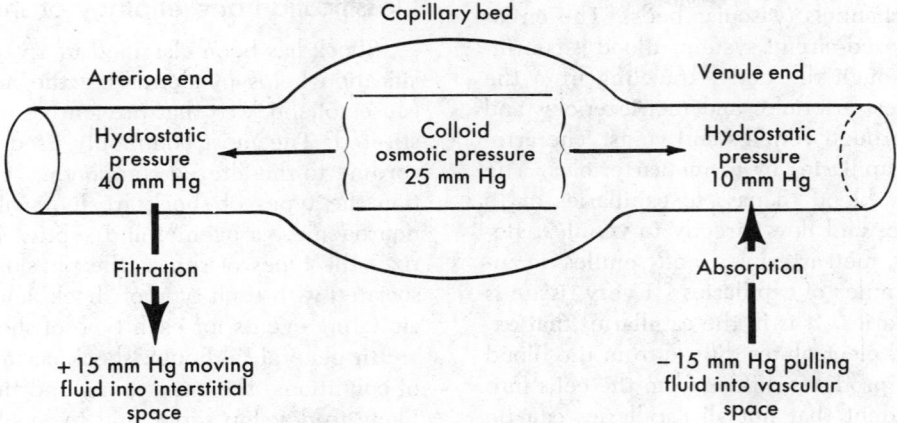

Fig. 20-8. Pressure difference across capillary provides for movement of fluid, nutrients, and waste between interstitial and vascular space.

pressure is that pressure caused by the blood pressing against the walls of the blood vessels. Hydrostatic pressure also exists in the tissue but is minimal (5 mm Hg or less) and some authorities believe that the hydrostatic pressure in the tissue is actually a negative pressure.[35] Hydrostatic pressure effectively pushes fluid out of the vascular bed into the interstitial space.

Colloid osmotic pressure is the pressure needed to overcome the pull of the proteins in the blood. The proteins do not pass freely through the walls of the capillaries because of their size. There are a few proteins in the interstitial space but a much larger concentration is in the vascular space. The colloid osmotic pressure within the vascular space serves as a force to *pull* or *absorb* fluid from the interstitial space.

The difference between the vascular hydrostatic pressure and the vascular colloid osmotic pressure determines the movement of fluid between the vascular and interstitial spaces. For example, in Fig. 20-8, the tissue hydrostatic pressure and tissue colloid osmotic pressure would be zero. The hydrostatic pressure at the arteriole end of the capillary (approximately 40 mm Hg) is greater than the hydrostatic pressure at the venule end of the capillary (approximately 10 mm Hg). The colloid osmotic pressure stays approximately the same throughout the vascular bed and equals about 25 mm Hg.

The difference between the hydrostatic pressure and colloid osmotic pressure at the arteriole end of the capillary is +15 mm Hg (40 mm Hg − 25 mm Hg = 15 mm Hg) and favors the movements of fluid out of the vascular compartment. The difference between the hydrostatic pressure and colloid osmotic pressure at the venule end of the capillary is −15 mm Hg (10 mm Hg − 25 mm Hg = −15 mm Hg) and favors the movement of fluid into the vascular compartment (Fig. 20-8).

Overall, this system allows fluids high in nutrients

and oxygen to diffuse out of the vascular bed at the arteriole end of the capillary and fluids containing waste products to move back into the vascular bed at the venule end of the capillaries. The system is not perfect, however, and some excess fluid will be left in the interstitial space. In addition, some proteins may escape from the vascular bed and, if allowed to accumulate, will act as a force to pull even more fluids from the vascular bed. The lymphatic system picks up the excess fluid and the escaped proteins and returns them to the vascular space.

Multiple factors affect the hydrostatic pressure. At the arteriole end of the capillary the hydrostatic pressure is dependent on the volume of blood, viscosity of the blood, force of the heart, and resistance of the blood vessels. Hydrostatic pressure at the venous end is dependent on the venous pressure. The venous pressure in turn is dependent on the condition of the veins, respiration, and skeletal muscle contractions. The colloid osmotic pressure is dependent on the protein level, which is dependent on the dietary intake, the liver's ability to produce proteins, and the fact that excess proteins are not lost from the body. Various disease states can interfere with any of these multiple factors and result in edema. Damage to the lymphatic system can also cause edema. Edema is discussed in detail in Chapter 21.

Maintenance of adequate circulation

The delivery of oxygen, nutrients, and electrolytes to cells and the delivery of waste products to elimination sites depend on an adequate circulatory system. Adequate circulation requires a functioning pump (the heart) to propel approximately 5 L of fluid (blood) continuously through channels (vascular beds). The circulatory system is a closed-circuit system. Blood is continuously perfused through the body, traveling from the heart through arteries, arterioles and metaarterioles and back to the heart through venules and veins. The arterioles give rise to capillaries or to metaarterioles. The metaarterioles allow blood to pass to capillaries or to bypass the capillaries and flow directly to venules. Between the arterioles, metaarterioles, and venules lie approximately 60,000 miles of capillaries.[91] Every tissue is permeated by capillaries. It is in the capillaries that oxygen, nutrients, and electrolytes diffuse from the blood into cells and waste products diffuse from the cells into the blood. It is evident that not all capillaries can be perfused at the same time. At the junction between arterioles and capillaries and between metaarterioles and capillaries precapillary sphincters are found. The precapillary sphincters open and close to shunt blood to the capillary beds that need blood. The arterioles and precapillary sphincters are under the control of neural, vasomotor, and metabolic factors.

The survival of cells depends on a circulatory system that has an adequate pump, an adequate vascular volume, and a vascular bed that constricts and dilates as necessary. Severe malfunction of any of these components can lead to a state of shock.

Interference with maintenance of cellular metabolism

Shock

Although shock has been a clinical problem for centuries, it still is not well defined. In the past shock was thought to be totally the result of an inadequate pump, inadequate fluid volume, or inadequate vascular bed. But not all patients, particularily those in septic shock, have inadequacies in one of these three components. The following definition seems to better define shock as it is now understood.

Shock is a pathologic syndrome characterized by abnormal cell metabolism that results from inadequate perfusion and oxygenation or cellular dysfunction. Shock is seen in a wide variety of patients with different clinical problems. Conditions such as severe cardiac and pulmonary disease, burns, dehydration, hemorrhage, anaphylaxis, and spinal injury interfere with one of the components of the circulatory system causing altered cellular metabolism secondary to inadequate perfusion and oxygenation. When infection and sepsis are present, shock may be present even though all components of the circulatory system are adequate.

Classification and etiology of shock

Shock has been classified in a variety of ways. Classification helps in identifying the most likely cause or causes of shock so that preventive measures can be instituted. The most commonly used classification is according to the altered component. Using this classification the types of shock are hypovolemic, cardiogenic, neurogenic, vasogenic, and septic. Table 20-3 summarizes the types of shock, the physiologic alterations associated with each type of shock, and the common precipitating events for each type of shock.

In general, although shock occurs in a wide variety of conditions, the very young and the elderly are more likely to develop septic and hypovolemic shock following surgery or trauma than the young healthy adult. The person with a chronic disease such as diabetes mellitus or cardiovascular disease also is at increased risk of developing shock. Persons with diseases of the immune system or intentional depression of the immune system from drug therapy, persons receiving glucocorticoids for replacement therapy or for their therapeutic effect, and persons who have had glucocorticoids discontinued recently are at increased risk of developing septic shock because of an actual or potential depression of immune response. In addition, persons receiving glucocorticoids are at higher risk for developing shock following any injury or surgery because they may have decreased compensatory mechanisms.

Pathophysiology and signs and symptoms of shock

Shock is a dynamic state that moves through various stages and eventually, if not treated effectively, proceeds to an irreversible stage. The pathophysiology and signs and symptoms vary depending on the stage of shock. In the following sections changes seen in early and late stages of shock will be discussed.

Early stage. In the early stage of shock signs and symptoms may be minimal. The classic signs of shock, such as decreased blood pressure, cold, clammy skin, and oliguria, are seen only after the shock syndrome has progressed. Early in shock the neuroendocrine integrating mechanisms (see Chapter 18) may prevent many of the signs and symptoms of shock from being obvious. Although the initiating event may be one of a vast number of insults, the neuroendocrine integrating mechanisms are stimulated.

Early signs and symptoms include hyperventilation with a minute volume 1.5 to 2 times normal.[101] As a result of the hyperventilation, respiratory alkalosis occurs. The PCO_2 may fall to less than 25 mm Hg while the PO_2 may remain normal. The blood pressure may remain normal or be only slightly decreased. These findings are the result of stimulation of the sympathetic adrenal medullary mechanism and other compensatory mechanisms. The changes in blood pressure that are

TABLE 20-3. Physiologic alterations and common precipitating events associated with types of shock

Type of shock	Physiologic alteration	Common precipitating events
Hypovolemic	Depletion of vascular volume, signs of shock occur when volume depleted 15-25%	Blood loss resulting from trauma; surgery; erosion of blood vessel by drainage tubes, tumor, or infections; gastrointestinal bleeding; hemorrhage at various sites caused by clotting defects; or fluid loss from burns, severe vomiting or diarrhea, or fistulas
Cardiogenic	Inadequate pump and thus ↓ cardiac output	Myocardial infarction (15% of patients develop cardiogenic shock) Secondary to ventricular failure resulting from cardiac tamponade or massive pulmonary emboli
Neurogenic	Sudden vasodilation of arterioles and precapillary sphincters because of interference with sympathetic nervous system; vascular capacity increases and a relative hypovolemia results	Sympathetic nervous system damage or depression from spinal cord injury, anesthesia, and drugs such as ganglionic blocking agents and barbiturates; fainting is sometimes classified as neurogenic shock; brain damage is a very rare cause
Vasogenic	Sudden vasodilation of arterioles and precapillary sphincter because of direct action of toxic products on vascular smooth muscles; vascular capacity increases and a relative hypovolemia results	Anaphylactic reaction to drugs, insect venom, blood transfusions, or food
Septic	Alteration in physiology not fully understood; several factors may be involved: impairment of cell membrane preventing cells from absorbing oxygen, nutrients, electrolytes, etc.; shunting of blood around capillary beds through arteriovenous (A-V) shunts; relative hypovolemia because of leakage of blood and plasma into infected area; relative hypovolemia caused by vasodilation	Infections in any organ with any organism can precipitate septic shock; most frequently seen in elderly and immunosuppressed persons who develop *gram-negative* infections; common organisms are *Escherichia coli, Klebsiella, Aerobacter, Pseudomonas, Proteus,* or coliform species

more likely to be seen are an increased diastolic reading and a decreased pulse pressure because of increased arteriole vasoconstriction. Blood pressure and cardiac output are also maintained because of the cardiovascular stimulation that results from stimulation of the sympathetic adrenal medullary mechanism. Tachycardia will usually be present.

Fluid shifts occur in the early stage of shock. Fluid enters the vascular space from the interstitial space. This may stimulate *thirst*. Volume replacement also occurs because of the effects of various hormones released when the neuroendocrine integrating mechanisms are stimulated. Red blood cells are released from the bone marrow and vascular beds of the liver and spleen, helping to increase volume. The vasoconstriction that occurs as a compensatory mechanism may result in some oliguria. But urine output may not drop significantly because of the increased volume that results from stimulation of the neuroendocrine integrating mechanisms. Urine osmolality is increased, and urinary sodium is decreased.

Another phenomenon that occurs early in shock is platelet aggregation. These aggregates can occur anywhere in the body and may lead to emboli formation. In early shock the patient is usually restless and very alert and may become confused or disoriented. Skin temperature changes may not be prominent in early

stages of either hypovolemic or cardiogenic shock. In septic, neurogenic, and vasogenic shock the skin may be flushed and warm.

Late stage. If the shock state progresses to the late stage, additional signs and symptoms will be seen. The neuroendocrine integrating mechanisms will no longer be able to maintain blood pressure and the blood pressure will fall. Respiratory function will decrease, and respirations will be shallow and rapid. Breath sounds will reveal lung congestion. Vasoconstriction may become more severe in an effort to maintain adequate perfusion. Oliguria or complete renal shutdown may be seen, and waste products normally excreted by the kidney will be retained. Perfusion to the liver and gastrointestinal tract decreases, and diminished bowel sounds may be present. The skin will become cool and clammy in hypovolemic, cardiogenic, or septic shock, and it may become cool and mottled in neurogenic or vasogenic shock.

When the shock state persists, metabolic pathways are changed and cells switch to anaerobic metabolism. This results in significantly less ATP production and a buildup of lactic and pyruvic acids. *Metabolic acidosis* results from the anaerobic metabolism and the renal decompensation. Respiratory acidosis results from the decreased respiratory function and further complicates the metabolic acidosis that is already present.

Fluid shifts occur in the late stages of shock. These shifts are opposite those seen in early shock. Capillary permeability increases, allowing fluids and proteins to leak into the interstitial space. The sodium pump is no longer effective because of lack of ATP. Sodium and water enter the cells, resulting in intracellular edema.

The continued sluggish blood flow, the vasoactive substance released from damaged tissue, and the accumulation of metabolic acids may cause disseminated intravascular coagulation (DIC) (p. 1201) to occur. If DIC results, the patient may develop thrombi and may bleed from many sites. Table 20-4 compares the signs and symptoms seen in the various body systems in early and late shock.

The common element in all types of shock in the late stage is cell death. Schumer[72] summarized the cause of cell death as follows. First there is decreased oxygen to the cells, which then causes a disarrangement of metabolic pathways resulting in decreased adenosine triphosphate (ATP) production and increased acid production. The decreased production of ATP causes malfunction of the sodium and potassium pump with sodium entering the cell and potassium leaving the cell. The influx of sodium and water into the cell causes cellular edema and further interferes with cellular function. The increased acid end products cause intracellular acidemia, which causes lysosomal membranes to rupture and lytic enzymes to be released. The lytic enzymes degrade protein, carbohydrate, and fat, and death of the cell occurs. With cellular death multiple substances are released into the bloodstream that can destroy other cells directly or increase the degree of cellular hypoxia.

The progression of shock will vary with the underlying disease, the health status of the patient, and the type of shock. The compensatory mechanisms activated by the neuroendocrine integrating mechanisms are not equally effective in maintaining essential body functions in all types of shock. The best compensation occurs in hypovolemic shock. It must be remembered that although the compensatory mechanisms can be beneficial in early shock, if allowed to persist they can increase the degree of tissue anoxia and lead to cellular death in the same manner as that of the original insult.

Organ damage in shock

Organ damage in shock occurs from the original insult and because of the hypoperfusion associated with the shunting and pooling of blood and vasoconstriction. As a result organ hypoxia and cell death occur. Most prone to damage in shock are the kidneys, lungs, and liver. The damage to these organs and the damage that occurs in the intestines and heart are discussed below.

Kidney damage. In early stages of shock, signs and symptoms of renal failure, such as oliguria, increased BUN and creatinine, decreased excretion of other waste

TABLE 20-4. Comparison of signs and symptoms in early and late shock by body systems

	Early shock	Late shock
Respiratory system	Hyperventilation; ↑ minute volume; ↓ Pco₂; normal Po₂	Respirations shallow; breath sounds may suggest congestion; ↑ Pco₂; ↓ Po₂
Cardiovascular system	Blood pressure normal to slightly lowered; ↑ diastolic pressure; ↓ pulse pressure; cardiac output normal; tachycardia; mild vasoconstriction in hypovolemic and cardiogenic shock	↓ Blood pressure; ↓ cardiac output; tachycardia continues; vasoconstriction worsens in hypovolemic, cardiogenic, and septic shock
Renal system	Normal to slightly depressed urine output; ↑ urine osmolality; ↓ urine sodium	Oliguria or complete renal shutdown; buildup of waste products
Acid-base balance	Respiratory alkalosis	Metabolic acidosis; respiratory acidosis
Vascular compartment	Fluids shift from interstitial space to vascular compartment; thirst occurs	Fluids shift from vascular space to interstitial and intracellular space, causing edema
Skin	Minimal to no change in hypovolemic and cardiogenic shock; warm, flushed skin in nuerogenic, vasogenic, and septic shock	Cool, clammy skin in hypovolemic, cardiogenic, and septic shock; cool and mottled skin in neurogenic and vasogenic shock
Hematologic system	Release of red blood cells from bone marrow to increase vascular volume; platelet aggregation	Disseminated intravascular coagulation (DIC)
Mental-neurologic system	Restless; alert; confused	Lethargic; unconsciousness
Gastrointestinal-hepatic system	No obvious changes	Perfusion decreases and bowel sounds may be diminished

products, and excess electrolytes, may be seen, although no actual renal damage is present. This is due to the vasoconstriction and the stimulation of glucocorticoids, ADH, and aldosterone. The continual shunting of blood from the kidneys can lead to acute tubular necrosis.

Lung damage. Damage to the lungs begins very early in shock and results in a variety of problems. These include atelectasis, pulmonary edema, and adult respiratory distress syndrome (ARDS). The pulmonary vascular system may become plugged with white blood cells, red blood cells, and platelets. Very early in shock, anoxia causes damage to the epithelial cells of the alveoli and capillaries and fluid leaks out of the capillaries into the alveoli. The leakage of fluid and decreased blood flow can cause a <u>decrease</u> in <u>surfactant</u>. Surfactant is a lipoprotein secreted by the alveoli epithelium cells (type II cells). It is important in normal pulmonary function because it decreases the work of expanding the lung and helps to maintain stability of the alveoli. When there is a decrease in surfactant the alveoli may collapse. This along with other factors may result in adult respiratory distress syndrome (see Chapter 51).

Pulmonary edema resulting from overhydration and a decrease in ventricular function can also be present. Decreased frequency of deep breathing and sighing can result in atelectasis. The pulmonary damage increases tissue hypoxia, since the amount of oxygen that can be diffused across the alveolar-capillary membrane is decreased.

Liver damage. The tissue hypoxia occurring during shock leads to liver damage. Normally, the reticuloendothelial system (RES) of the liver rapidly and effectively picks up toxic elements from the blood. In shock this does not occur. The loss of the RES in the liver increases susceptibility to all types of infections and may result in a septic component being added to the original shock. Loss of liver function also prevents lactic acid conversion to glycogen, which further compounds the metabolic acidosis.

Intestinal damage. In shock the gastrointestinal tract seems to be exceptionally susceptible to vasoconstriction, which leads to ischemic damage and loss of the bowel integrity. The loss of intestinal integrity allows the bacteria normally present in the gastrointestinal tract to be released into the general circulation. The seeding of the circulatory system by bacteria from the gastrointestinal tract is believed to play a role in the shock state moving to an irreversible stage. Another consequence of shock is gastrointestinal tract <u>bleeding</u>, which may be secondary to a destruction of the gastric mucosal barrier secondary to ischemia, increased acid production, or decreased clotting factors.

Cardiac damage. In shock the myocardium is depressed and the coronary vascular bed seems to lose its autoregulatory ability and becomes entirely pressure dependent.[87] This loss easily leads to ischemic changes, arrhythmias, and cardiac failure. The myocardial depression decreases cardiac output further and may be responsible for shock entering the irreversible stage. The organ damage described above increases cardiac decompensation and worsens the shock state. Additional signs and symptoms such as those seen in renal failure, respiratory insufficiency, gastrointestinal bleeding, and myocardial damage may be present.

Assessment

The management of shock will depend on the data obtained from continuous monitoring of the status of the patient. To pick up subtle changes, a flow sheet on which data from all parameters can be recorded should be used. The box above lists parameters to be moni-

PARAMETERS FOR ASSESSING STATUS OF PATIENT IN SHOCK

Hemodynamic monitoring
Blood pressure (cuff and/or intraarterial)
Pulse
Central venous pressure (CVP)
Pulmonary artery pressure (PAP)
Pulmonary wedge pressure (PWP)
Cardiac output (CO)
Electrocardiogram

Respiratory monitoring
Respiratory rate, depth
Breath sounds
Blood gases
  pH
  PO_2
  PCO_2
Percent saturation

Fluid and electrolyte monitoring
Serum electrolytes
Blood lactate and pyruvate levels
Intake
  By mouth (P.O.)
  Intravenous (I.V.)
  Nasogastric (N.G.)
  Irrigation solutions
  Solution in medications

Output
  Urinary
  Gastrointestinal tract
  Sweating
  Dressings
Weight
Serum creatinine level
Blood urea nitrogen (BUN) level
Serum and urinary osmolality
Urinary specific gravity

Neurologic monitoring
Alertness
Orientation
Confusion

Hematologic monitoring
Erythrocytes
Hematocrit and hemoglobin levels
Leukocytes
Platelets
Prothrombin and partial thromboplastin time
Clotting time

Other monitoring
Bowel sounds
Skin temperature

tored. The assessment of multiple parameters is necessary to obtain an adequate evaluation of the adequacy of tissue perfusion. Not all parameters will necessarily be measured on any one person. The following section discusses some of the special monitoring techniques that may be used.

Hemodynamic monitoring. The *blood pressure* may be monitored by auscultation; however, auscultation may give inaccurate results because of the vasoconstriction or the poor stroke volume that occurs with shock. The vibration produced by the blood may be too minimal to produce audible sounds. Other methods may be necessary to monitor the blood pressure. Intraarterial monitoring is used often (Fig. 20-9). An intraarterial line is inserted into the radial, brachial, or femoral artery and attached to a transducer and monitor. If transducers are not available, there is another simple way of measuring

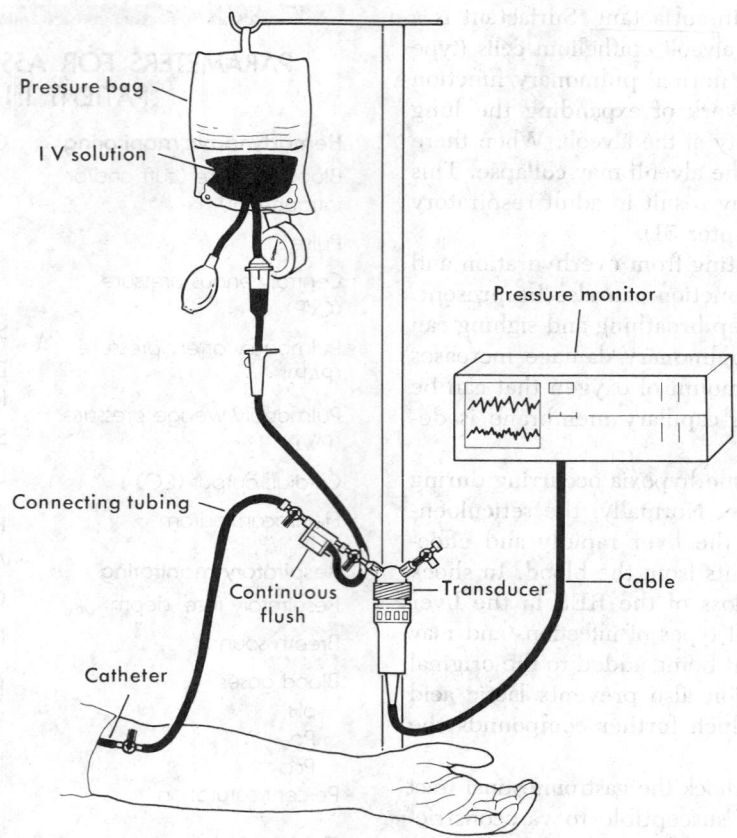

Pressure bag

I V solution

Pressure monitor

Connecting tubing

Continuous flush

Transducer

Cable

Catheter

Fig. 20-9. Connections between intraarterial catheter, transducer, monitor, and fluid. (From Daily, E.K., and Schroeder, J.: Techniques in bedside hemodynamic monitoring, ed. 2, St. Louis, 1981, The C.V. Mosby Co.)

intraarterial pressure, as described in other literature.[87]

Intraarterial monitoring is not without its hazards. One problem encountered involves maintenance of catheter patency. A pressure bag over the IV solution and the use of a continuous flush device help to control this problem. Insertion of a catheter into an artery may interfere with circulation to the body area distal to the insertion site. The catheter may cause arterial spasms and thrombosis formation. The area distal to the insertion site should be checked for adequate perfusion immediately after insertion and every hour thereafter. The checks should include observation of pulse, skin temperature, color, capillary refill, and sensory and motor function. Hemorrhage may occur through loose connections and from the insertion site after removal of the catheter. All connections should be visible and should be checked for tightness frequently. Following removal of the catheter, manual pressure is maintained over the insertion site for 5 to 15 minutes and a pressure dressing is applied for several hours. Infection and sepsis may occur. The catheter is inserted with aseptic technique and the site is observed, cleansed with antiseptic solu-

tion, and dressed with a sterile dressing every 24 hours. The flush solution and tubing are changed every 24 to 48 hours. All tubing, transducers, and solutions should be handled with aseptic technique, and stopcocks should have protective caps. Aseptic technique is used when flushing the catheter or withdrawing blood. Catheters are usually not left in place longer than 72 to 96 hours.

Central venous pressure (CVP) may be monitored in all types of shock but is most helpful in hypovolemic shock. The CVP assists in assessing the adequacy of the vascular volume, the function of the right ventricle, and venous return. There are several pointers that must be remembered to gain the most information from CVP monitoring. The technique and important points in obtaining an accurate CVP reading are discussed on p. 1055. Normally, the function of the right and left ventricles is similar, but in shock the left ventricle may be deficient, and this deficiency will not be picked up by monitoring the CVP.

Accurate information about left ventricular function is obtained by measuring the *pulmonary artery pressure* (PAP) and the *pulmonary wedge pressure* (PWP). To obtain the PAP a Swan-Ganz catheter is inserted

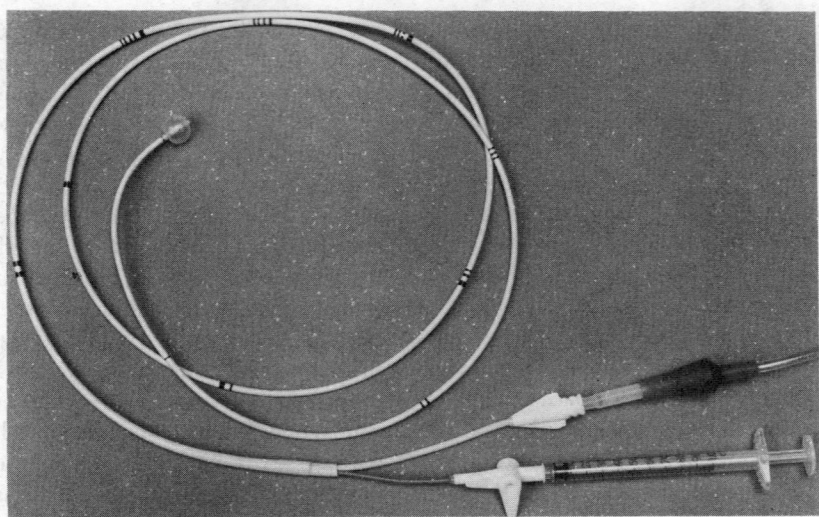

Fig. 20-10. Swan-Ganz flow-directed, balloon-tipped catheter for PA pressure monitoring. The tuberculin syringe is used for inflating balloon with air. IV tubing is attached to other lumen for infusion of fluid or pressure measurement at catheter tip. (From Daily, E., and Schroeder, J.: Techniques in bedside hemodynamic monitoring, ed. 2, St. Louis, 1981, The C.V. Mosby Co.)

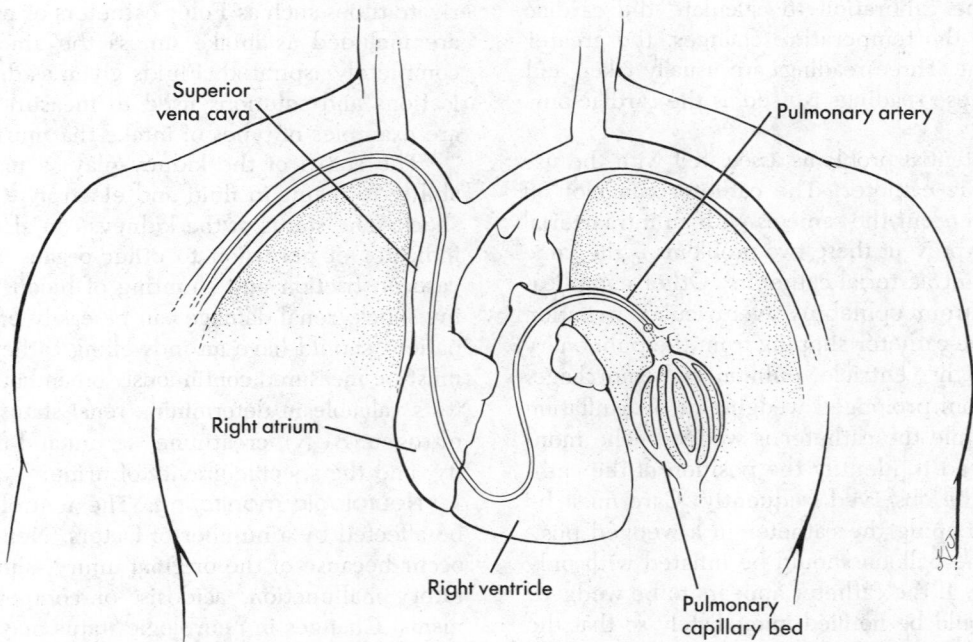

Fig. 20-11. Position of Swan-Ganz catheter. Catheter is passed into pulmonary artery from superior vena cava. Normally catheter is floating freely in pulmonary artery with balloon deflated. For PWP reading, balloon is inflated and will wedge into position (shown in dotted lines).

into the pulmonary artery by way of the superior vena cava from a more peripheral vein. The Swan-Ganz catheter is a multilumen tube with an inflatable balloon. An example of a two-lumen tube is shown in Fig. 20-10. A third lumen and a fourth lumen are present on some catheters. Normally, the catheter floats in the pulmo-

nary artery, but it can be advanced with the balloon inflated into the wedged position to give the PWP (Fig. 20-11). The catheter is attached to a transducer and recorder, which gives constant pressure readings. The setup is similar to that shown in Fig. 20-9. The exact location of the catheter is determined by the pressure readings. The normal systolic pulmonary artery pressure is 20 to 30 mm Hg with a diastolic pressure less than 12 mm Hg and a mean pressure less than 20 mm Hg.[20] The normal PWP is approximately 4 to 12 mm Hg. If left ventricular failure is suspected, PWP monitoring is necessary because the PWP can be dangerously elevated even though the CVP is low or normal. This is discussed further in Chapter 51.

Cardiac output measurements can assist in the assessment of the status of the patient and in evaluating the effectiveness of therapy. Cardiac output can be measured in several ways. A common way is the thermodilution technique. In this method a quadruple-lumen Swan-Ganz catheter with a thermistor electrode on the tip is placed in the pulmonary artery. The lumen from the thermistor is attached to a cardiac output computer. The computer is calibrated for the amount and temperature of solution that is going to be injected. The solution is injected rapidly and evenly through the proximal lumen of the quadruple catheter into the right atrium. The thermistor, which is positioned in the pulmonary artery, picks up the temperature of the solution when it reaches that area. The computer uses this temperature plus the calibration to calculate the cardiac output. The less the temperature changes, the greater the cardiac output. Three readings are usually taken and the average of these readings is used as the cardiac output.

There are potential problems associated with the use of the Swan-Ganz catheter. The catheter can clot off and infection can occur the same as with an intraarterial catheter. Care to prevent these two problems is the same as that used for intraarterial catheters. Other complications include thrombophlebitis, ventricular irritation resulting from the catheter slipping from the pulmonary artery into the right ventricle, pulmonary hemorrhage, and infarction from prolonged wedging or overinflation of the balloon while the catheter is wedged. The monitor pattern is used to identify the position of the catheter and should be observed frequently. Care must be taken to avoid keeping the catheter in a wedged position too long. The balloon should be inflated with only 0.8 to 1 ml of air. If the catheter appears to be wedged, the physician should be notified immediately so that the catheter can be removed.

Respiratory monitoring. The importance of an adequately functioning respiratory system has been discussed. The person in shock is susceptible to a wide variety of pulmonary problems, and pulmonary status must be continually assessed. This is accomplished by evaluating breath sounds (p. 1216), measuring blood gas levels (p. 1221), determining lung compliance and airway resistance (p. 1289), and measuring pulmonary shunting.

The passage of blood from the pulmonary artery to the pulmonary vein without being oxygenated is called pulmonary shunting. A certain amount of shunting oc-

curs normally, but an increased amount of shunting can occur in shock because of lung damage. The amount of shunting can be determined by use of a special formula.

Fluid and electrolyte monitoring. Some of the parameters discussed under hemodynamic monitoring also assess fluid status. In addition to the previously described monitoring elements, the serum and urine osmolalities are measured frequently. The presence of injuries, wounds, trauma, or internal bleeding can result in significant amounts of undetected fluid loss. The patient in shock cannot tolerate even minute changes in fluid balance. All potential sites of fluid loss must be monitored, dressings are weighed, and the number of times bed linens or gowns need to be changed is recorded. This will help approximate fluid loss by perspiration. The output from the gastrointestinal tract (nasogastric drainage, diarrhea, and vomitus) is also measured. Since some fluid losses can only be approximated, accurate body weights are necessary.

Fluid intake must be carefully monitored. All fluids the patient receives are recorded. The patient may receive fluids in many ways other than those given as replacement therapy or orally. Fluids that are used to irrigate tubes such as Foley catheters or nasogastric tubes are included as intake unless the amount injected is completely aspirated. Fluids given as diluents for medications and solutions used to measure cardiac output are examples of types of intake that must be recorded.

The status of the kidney plays a major role in the ability to maintain fluid and electrolyte balance during shock. The status of the kidneys can also be used as an indicator of perfusion to other organs. Because of the vasoconstriction and shunting of blood that occur during shock, renal damage can be easily precipitated. The patient should have an indwelling catheter, and output must be measured continuously on an hourly basis. Other tests valuable in determining renal status are blood urea nitrogen (BUN), creatinine, serum and urinary osmolality, and the specific gravity of urine.

Neurologic monitoring. The neurologic status can be affected by a number of factors. Neurologic changes occur because of the original injury, shock state, respiratory malfunction, acidosis, or compensatory mechanisms. Changes in neurologic status may be the earliest signs of shock and should be assessed on a continual basis to judge the adequacy of cerebral blood flow.

Hematologic monitoring. Hematologic changes can occur because of blood loss, hemodilution and concentration, and disseminated intravascular coagulation (DIC) (p. 1201). The red blood cell count and hematocrit and hemoglobin levels are used as guides to fluid status and need for blood replacement. Leukocyte counts assist in detecting the onset of an infection. The other factors listed in the box on p. 313 will assist in detecting the onset of DIC or other possible causes of continuous blood loss.

Other monitoring. Skin temperature will vary depending on the type and stage of shock, the amount of physiologic compensation, and the treatment. Changes in skin temperature may help to assess the limited or improved state of tissue perfusion. With continual sympathetic stimuli, vasoconstriction, and the shunting of blood, the normal peristaltic movement of the gastrointestinal tract is decreased. Assessment of bowel sounds helps determine adequacy of blood flow to the gastrointestinal tract.

Intervention

Interventions for every patient in shock are unique and depend on the patient's status as determined by the data gathered from continuous assessment. There is no single type of management, but there are general principles of management. The patient's care is guided by four major outcomes:

1. The patient's tissue perfusion, cellular oxygenation, and cellular metabolism will return to normal.
2. The patient will have decreased metabolic needs.
3. The patient and significant others will be free of avoidable anxiety.
4. The patient will be free of avoidable injuries.

The particular criteria used by the health team to measure the effectiveness of therapy will depend on the individual patient. Each of the above outcomes is discussed in detail below.

OUTCOME: Tissue perfusion, cellular oxygenation, and cellular metabolism will be normal.

Fluid replacement. Almost all patients in shock, no matter what type, will require some fluid replacement because of the pooling of vascular fluid in the microcirculation. The type of fluid replaced depends on the type and amount lost. Blood, plasma, albumin, hydroxyethyl starch, dextran, 5% dextrose, and electrolyte solutions are used.

Most persons can tolerate blood losses of 500 to 1000 ml without difficulty. Blood is replaced if the loss exceeds this amount. In addition, the etiology of the blood loss must be identified and corrected. Measures to control hemorrhage are discussed on p. 321.

Plasma, dextran, hydroxyethyl starch, or albumin is used if the initiating event is a disorder such as pancreatitis, peritonitis, or severe burns where there is an excessive loss of plasma. These solutions are preferred over glucose solutions because the molecules are larger and will remain in the vascular bed longer. These solutions also are used to expand the vascular volume while waiting for blood to be typed and cross matched. They are not without risk, however. Viral hepatitis can be transmitted by plasma; normal human-weight dextran causes red blood cell aggregation; and high– and low–

molecular weight dextran and hydoxyethyl starch can interfere with clotting mechanisms. Albumin is the safest plasma expander but is ten times as expensive as the commercially made plasma expanders.[88]

The type of solution used will depend on the patient's serum and electrolyte levels. Bicarbonate solutions may be used to correct metabolic acidosis, and dextrose is given to provide some of the needed calories. Saline solutions may have to be limited if cardiac disorders are present.

Most patients will receive a combination of fluids, blood, and plasma expanders. The amount of fluid given will depend on the CVP and the PWP. Patients require sufficient fluids to make up for vasodilation, pooling, and extravasation of fluids out of the vascular bed. With adequate fluid replacement a gradual but not extreme rise in CVP and PWP will occur. Care must be taken to prevent hypervolemia and pulmonary edema.

Drug therapy for cardiovascular support. If fluid replacement, correction of electrolyte and acid-base balance, and improvement of oxygenation do not succeed in increasing cardiac output and perfusion, and in maintaining blood pressure at an adequate level, drug therapy will be used. The first line of therapy is directed toward maximizing cardiac function. Arrhythmias need to be controlled with use of antiarrhythmic agents. Cardiac glycosides may be given to strengthen cardiac contractility if signs of failure are present.

SYMPATHOMIMETIC THERAPY. If blood pressure is still inadequate or has dropped to a lethal level before measures listed above are effective, sympathomimetic agents will be used. A mean blood pressure of 60 is necessary to maintain adequate cerebral perfusion. Sympathomimetic drugs are potentially lethal and have many side effects. They can be classified according to the adrenergic receptors they stimulate. The effects of the drug vary depending on the receptors stimulated.

Alpha-adrenergic stimulators. Two pure *alpha-adrenergic (α-adrenergic) stimulators* are methoxamine (Vasoxyl) and phenylephrine (Neo-Synephrine). These drugs will cause a significant rise in blood pressure by their effect on α-adrenergic receptors. They cause massive vasoconstriction and increased peripheral resistance. Their use may cause a worsening of the shock state by potentiating end-organ damage. They are not used as frequently as some of other sympathomimetic drugs because of their severe vasoconstrictive effects.

Beta-adrenergic stimulators. Isoproterenol (Isuprel) is a pure *beta-adrenergic (β-adrenergic) stimulator*. It increases blood pressure by its cardiac stimulant effects. Increased heart rate and contractility will occur. Isoproterenol also causes vasodilation of arterial vascular beds, although blood pressure will usually be maintained because of the effect on heart rate. Its use in shock states is limited because it increases myocardial oxygen needs[64] and causes tachyarrhythmias. The usual dose is 1 to 8 μg/min by continuous intravenous infusion.[4]

Mixed alpha- and beta-stimulators. Mixed α- *and* β-*stimulators* commonly used are norephinephrine, levarterenol bitartrate (Levophed Bitartrate), metaraminol bitartrate (Aramine), epinephrine (Adrenalin), dopamine (Intropin), and dobutamine (Dobutrex). These drugs all have varying affects on β- and α-receptors.

Norepinephrine is primarily an α-adrenergic stimulator with less potent β- effects.[32] It increases blood pressure, stroke volume, and peripheral vascular resistance. It increases coronary blood flow but decreases blood flow to the kidney, liver, and skeletal muscles, and its vasoconstrictor effects increase as the dosage increases. The oxygen consumption of the heart and the work load of the heart may be increased because there is increased peripheral resistance.[64] Extravasation of norepinephrine solution into tissue can cause local tissue necrosis. The infusion site should be observed carefully and if infiltration is thought to have occurred, the drug is discontinued and the IV site is injected with an α-blocker such as phentolamine. The initial dosage is usually 1 μg/min by continuous IV infusion. The dosage is increased or decreased as necessary, depending on the patient's response.

Metaraminol is very similar to norepinephrine. Although slightly less potent, it has a much longer duration of action.[32] It acts directly on the vessels and indirectly by stimulating the release of endogenous norepinephrine. If the patient's body store of norepinephrine is depleted, this drug will not be as effective as other sympathomimetic agents.

Epinephrine stimulates both α- and β-adrenergic receptors. It is a strong inotropic and chronotropic drug, increasing heart rate and contractility. It has two effects on peripheral vasoconstriction. At very low doses (0.1 μg/kg) it causes decreased vascular resistance and can cause a decrease in blood pressure. As the dosage is increased, generalized vasoconstriction occurs with a resultant increase in blood pressure. Epinephrine can cause tachyarrhythmias and end-organ damage, particularly in the kidney because of the vasoconstricting effect. The normal initial dosage is 1.0 μg/min by continuous intravenous infusion. The dose is increased or decreased as necessary, depending on the patient's response.

Dopamine stimulates both α- and β-receptors and also stimulates dopaminergic receptors located in renal, mesenteric, and splanchnic vascular beds. At low infusion rates (5 μg/kg/min or less)[64] the dopaminergic effect is maintained and some β-receptors are stimulated, causing increased heart rate and increased blood pressure. At higher dosage levels (greater than 10 μg/kg/min)[64] α-receptors are stimulated and generalized vasoconstriction occurs, although the vascular beds with dopaminergic receptors will be less vasoconstricted than other beds.[64] An increase in dosage to greater than 20

μg/kg/min blocks all dopaminergic effects and the effect is similar to that of norepinephrine.[106] The initial starting dosage is at low levels with changes dependent on the patient's response to the drug.

Dobutamine is a new agent that is sometimes used to treat shock. It stimulates β-adrenergic receptors and is similar to epinephrine and isoproterenol in its activity. It does not seem to cause tachycardia and arrhythmias as frequently[40] as some other adrenergic drugs. It has a weak effect on α- and β-receptors.[64] Dosages ranging from 2.5 to 15 μg/kg/min produce decreased pulmonary wedge pressure, increased cardiac output, increased urinary output, and little change in peripheral resistance. It is being used to treat patients with acute myocardial infarction and heart failure and patients emerging from cardiopulmonary bypass surgery.[32] The exact role of this drug in shock states is unknown. The initial infusion rate is 2 to 4 μg/kg/min with dosage changes as necessary.[40]

VASODILATORS. In some instances when patients show excessive vasoconstriction with abnormal blood pressure, vasodilators may be used to improve tissue perfusion. It is *imperative that a patient have adequate volume replacement before a vasodilator is given because these drugs increase vascular capacity*. The blood pressure often drops 5 to 10 mm even if the patient is adequately hydrated. In the past, small intravenous doses of chlorpromazine hydrochloride (Thorazine) were used as a vasodilator. Other vasodilators are phenoxybenzamine (Dibenzyline) and phentolamine mesylate (Regitine). The drug most frequently used now is sodium nitroprusside (Nipride). Nitroprusside relaxes smooth muscles, thus increasing the dilation of the arterial vascular bed. It also increases dilation of the venous system. Nitroprusside is given by continuous intravenous infusion and the dose is regulated on a continual basis depending on the patient's response. In some instances combination therapy using both a sympathomimetic drug and a vasodilator is used. The two drugs are regulated together to maintain adequate perfusion, cardiac output, and blood pressure.

MONITORING OF PATIENTS RECEIVING SYMPATHOMIMETICS AND VASOPRESSORS. The vasopressors and sympathomimetics have other actions, uses, side effects, and potential hazards. The reader should consult appropriate references for a complete understanding of these drugs. These drugs all have dynamic effects on the patient's cardiovascular status and the patient receiving them requires very close monitoring. The patient should be attached to a cardiac monitor so abnormal rhythms can be identified rapidly. The dosage is titrated to keep the mean blood pressure at a prescribed level, usually 80 mm Hg. The blood pressure should be checked every 5 to 15 minutes at the beginning of the infusion and every 15 minutes thereafter. If the blood pressure is being measured by both cuff and intraarterial line, the two readings may vary. *It is imperative that everyone working with the patient use the same measurements in adjusting the rate of infusion of the drugs.* These patients may also need to be monitored with a Swan-Ganz catheter to collect data on PAP, PWP, and cardiac output, since these parameters are also affected by these drugs. It is also imperative that an intravenous infusion pump be used when these drugs are being given to ensure that the correct dose is being administered. The amount of drug the patient is receiving should be documented carefully in micrograms (μg) per minute or per kilogram per minute. When the drugs are to be discontined they are tapered off slowly with the blood pressure being checked every 15 minutes.

GLUCOCORTICOIDS. Glucocorticoids are used in some patients with shock, although their use is still controversial. Several beneficial effects of the glucocorticoids have been hypothesized. Glucocorticoids stabilize mitochondrial lysosomal membranes. They seem to strengthen cardiac contractility, and they have a mild α-adrenergic blocking effect, thus causing some vasodilation and improvment in tissue perfusion. Glucocorticoids also increase lactic acid conversion to glycogen and increase ATP production.

Cardiac support. Other measures to augment tissue perfusion and oxygenation may be used. If severe left ventricular dysfunction is present, an intraaortic counterpulsation balloon may be used. The catheter with balloon is inserted into the femoral artery and threaded into the aorta to the approximate level of the thoracic aorta. The balloon inflates at the beginning of diastole and deflates just before systole. The inflation at the beginning of diastole pushes blood into the coronary arteries and into the periphery. The deflation just before systole decreases the resistance in the aorta so that the ventricle does not have as much resistance to overcome. *Antishock trousers* may be used in emergency situations when it is known that shock is of a hypovolemic or neurogenic nature. See Chapter 73 and reference 23 for additional information on antishock trousers.

Respiratory support. To ensure adequate oxygenation, oxygen administered by mask or catheter will be needed. If an adequate PO_2 level cannot be maintained, the patient may need to be placed on a respirator. PO_2 should be maintained at a minimum of 60 mm Hg. Respiratory support may also be necessary to prevent or treat acid-base imbalance.

Oxygen in high levels can cause alveolar damage; therefore only the amount of oxygen necessary to maintain a PO_2 of 60 is given. If a high fraction of forced inspiratory oxygen (FIO_2) is necessary to maintain a PO_2 of 60, when the patient is on a respirator added ventilatory support such as positive end-expiratory pressure (PEEP) may be necessary (p. 1332).

The nurse must remember that oxygen is very drying, and adequate humidity must always be provided. In addition to supplemental oxygen, good respiratory care consisting of turning the patient and helping the patient to cough and deep breathe is necessary. If the patient is unable to cough effectively, nasotracheal suctioning is necessary. If the patient is intubated or has a tracheostomy, endotracheal and tracheostomy suctioning will be necessary. (See p. 1232 for technique.)

Renal support. One of the primary organs affected by the vasoconstrictive effects of the compensatory mechanisms and administration of vasopressor drugs is the kidneys. Adequate renal function is necessary to prevent major fluid, electrolyte, and acid-base imbalance. If fluid replacement and establishment of adequate blood pressure do not increase urinary output to an adequate level, diuretics may be given. Urinary output should be at least 25 to 30 ml/hr. Commonly used diuretics are mannitol (Osmitrol) and furosemide (Lasix).

Reticuloendothelial support. In septic shock and in almost all other types of shock, broad-spectrum antibiotics are used. A combination of antibiotics to cover both gram-positive and gram-negative organisms is given. In sepsis, cultures of urine, sputum, blood, and secretions from any other orifice that is a possible site for sepsis are obtained before instituting antibiotic therapy.

Positioning. A measure that assists in promoting adequate tissue perfusion, oxygenation, and metabolism is positioning of the patient. In the past the Trendelenburg position (head-low position) often was used to increase the flow of blood to the brain. However, this position has been found to inhibit cardiac output and respirations because the visceral organs push up against the diaphragm. Many physicians now prefer that the lower extremities be elevated at a 45-degree angle from the hip, with the knees straight and the head level with or slightly higher than the chest. This position promotes increased venous return from the legs without interfering with the cardiac output. The nurse should assess each situation to determine the position of maximal physiologic effect and comfort. In some settings in which the nurse is functioning there may be policies concerning positioning of the patient in shock; nevertheless, the nurse should assess the patient's response to such positioning and take appropriate action as necessary.

OUTCOME: Metabolic needs will be decreased.

To achieve this outcome, all the necessary interventions must be carried out, yet rest periods must be provided for the patient. Only the essential physical care needs should be met. Unnecessary activities should be eliminated and sedatives may be given to increase rest and comfort. Pain and discomfort increase restlessness and thus metabolism. Morphine sulfate may be used to decrease pain. It should be given intravenously, since in shock it may be absorbed too slowly or may accumulate in the tissues.

The patient is kept warm, not hot or cold. Decreased temperature causes chilling and shivering and thus increases metabolic needs. Increased temperature leads to vasodilation, which can cause hypoperfusion because of movement of blood to the body surface. Sweating accompanies increased temperature and also increases metabolic needs.

OUTCOME: The person or significant other will be free of avoidable anxiety.

Measures to decrease or eliminate anxiety must be incorporated into the care of the patient. Questions from the patient or significant others should be answered and all interventions should be explained. Talking around the patient should be eliminated. Time to sit down and talk with the patient and family should be planned for so that they have an opportunity to verbalize their fears. The nurse must remember that anxiety can stimulate the body's compensatory mechanisms and increase metabolic needs. The environment of an intensive care unit (ICU) increases anxiety (p. 1921), and the nurse plays a major role in controlling the environment and in eliminating anxiety insofar as possible.

OUTCOME: The person will be free of avoidable injuries.

The person in shock has the potential of developing multiple injuries. Three common avoidable injuries are those caused by infection from invasive procedures, those caused by the accidental dislodgement of tubes and lines, and those caused by immobility.

These patients have decreased resistance to infection. In addition, the presence of multiple tubes (intravenous, intraarterial, nasogastric, urinary, and endotracheal) increases the risk of infection. Sterile handling of all tubes is of primary importance. Suctioning, if necessary, must be done with sterile technique (p. 1232). Intraarterial and intravenous tubing should be changed on a regular basis. A routine for appropriate care of intravenous and intraarterial insertion sites should be planned and instituted on a continuous basis.

The patient in shock may be confused and often is restless and anxious. These behavioral changes make the patient very vulnerable to accidents. The patient can easily fall if side rails are not in place. A more frequent injury results from dislodgement of the various lines and tubes by the patient. The tubes and lines are irritating, and the patient may not be able to understand the purpose of them and may accidently or intentionally remove them.

Soft restraints or mittens may be necessary. They should only be used if the patient's cooperation cannot be obtained. Usually if restraints or mittens are used they can be removed while the staff is with the patient. They should be removed at least every 4 to 8 hours so that the extremities can be moved and inspected.

Care to prevent pulmonary stasis, thrombophlebitis, urinary stasis, and decubitus ulcers must be incorporated into the care plan. All these problems can result from immobility.

Outcome criteria for the person in shock

1. Tissue perfusion, cellular oxygenation, and cellular metabolism will return to normal.
   a. Mean BP will be >80 mm Hg.
   b. Pulse will not be >10 of preshock baseline.
   c. Cardiac arrhythmias will be controlled.
   d. Cardiac output will be normal.
   e. CVP will be >6 cm of H_2O and <15 cm of H_2O.
   f. PWP will be >10 mm Hg and <12 mm Hg.
   g. Urinary osmolality will be >serum osmolality.
   h. Urinary output will be ≥25 ml/hr.
   i. Serum electrolytes will be within normal limits.
   j. BUN and creatinine levels will not increase and will decrease toward normal.
   k. Serum lactic acid will return to normal.
   l. Temperature will be normal.
   m. Skin will be warm and dry without cyanosis or mottling.
   n. Blood gas results will be:
      (1) Po_2 60 to 100 mm Hg.
      (2) Pco_2 38 to 42 mm Hg.
      (3) CO_2 content (plasma) 25 to 32 mEq/L.
      (4) HCO_3^- 23 to 25 mEq/L.
      (5) pH 7.38 to 7.42.
      (6) O_2 saturation 97%.
   o. Mental status will return to preshock state.
   p. Respiratory rate will be 12 to 22/min, regular, deep.
   q. Breath sounds will be clear in all lobes.
   r. Physiologic shunting will be <15%.
   s. Red blood cell count and hematocrit and hemoglobin levels will be normal or at least at the preshock levels.
   t. Coagulation factors and platelets will be within normal range.
   u. White blood cell count will be normal or returning to normal.
2. The patient will have decreased metabolic needs.
   a. Will have periods of REM sleep.
   b. Will be free of discomfort.
   c. Will be warm, not hot or cold.
3. The patient or significant others will be free of avoidable anxiety.
   a. Will receive explanations of all interventions.

   b. Will be informed of the client's status.

   c. Will not exhibit behavior showing anxiety (e.g., restlessness, inappropriate movements).

   d. Will be able to verbalize fears and feelings.

4. The patient will be free of avoidable injuries.

   a. Will not develop a nosocomial infection from venous or arterial lines; from the presence of an indwelling catheter, endotracheal or tracheostomy tubes, or ventilator; or from suctioning.

   b. Will not develop deleterious effects of immobility (e.g., foot drop, contractures, atelectasis).

   c. Will not injure self (e.g., by pulling out tubes, developing skin abrasions).

Hemorrhage

A second major insult to the circulatory system is hemorrhage. If not controlled, hemorrhage can lead to shock, discussed above. This section deals with measures to control blood loss.

Hemorrhage is the loss of a large amount of blood from the bloodstream as a result of rupture or injury of a blood vessel; slipping of a ligature from a blood vessel postoperatively; erosion of a vessel by a drainage tube, tumor, or infection; or some interference with the clotting mechanism of the blood such as occurs in hemophilia. A person may lose small amounts of blood over a long period or may lose a large amount of blood in a short period. The bleeding may be arterial (bright red and spurting), venous (continuous flow of dark red blood), or capillary (oozing). The blood may be expelled from any body orifice, from an incision, or from the site of an injury, or it may collect under the subcutaneous tissues as a tumor mass (*hematoma*) or in a body cavity such as the peritoneal cavity.

Assessment

Symptoms of massive hemorrhage, both internal and external, are apprehension, restlessness, thirst, pallor, cold moist skin, drop in blood pressure, increased pulse rate, subnormal temperature, and rapid respirations. As hemorrhage continues, the lips and conjunctivae become pale and the patient may complain of spots before the eyes, ringing in the ears, and extreme weakness. If the hemorrhage is not controlled, shock and finally death will occur.

Intervention

The treatment of hemorrhage is directed toward stopping the bleeding if possible and replacing blood loss. When bleeding occurs, the vessel walls constrict, narrowing the lumen of the vessels, and a clot forms over the end of the bleeding vessel. Clotting usually occurs much earlier in the child and very young person than in older persons because the blood vessels of children and young persons are more elastic. In arterial bleeding the clotting phenomenon is not possible until there has been enough blood loss to decrease the pressure of the blood circulating through the bleeding vessel. However, pressure against the artery proximal to the bleeding point decreases the flow of blood through it and permits clotting to take place. Elevation of the part also may decrease arterial bleeding. *Direct pressure* at the site of the bleeding also decreases the blood flow and encourages clotting. This method is frequently used in superficial wounds, and a gelatin sponge (Gelfoam) also may be applied to help form a clot. The principle of direct pressure may also be used to control hemorrhage from esophageal varices. An esophageal balloon is inserted and then inflated until it compresses the bleeding vessels. In a similar way bleeding from the prostrate gland such as may occur following prostatectomy is controlled by direct pressure. A Foley catheter is inserted and the balloon inflated to compress bleeding vessels.

Cold applications are often used to control bleeding into tissues or into body cavities, since the cold causes the small vessels to constrict. In uterine hemorrhage an ice bag may be applied to the abdomen over the uterus. In gastric hemorrhage cold can be applied by irrigating the stomach with iced solution through a gastric tube. (See p. 1424 for additional information.)

Very *hot applications* cause reflex vasoconstriction and control bleeding temporarily. This method is often used during surgery in which there is considerable vascular oozing. To control the bleeding permanently, large vessels usually have to be ligated, and smaller ones may be electrically cauterized. A ruptured organ such as the spleen may have to be removed to control bleeding. Removal of the spleen also may be necessary to control bleeding caused by a blood dyscrasia such as idiopathic thrombocytopenic purpura.

When the bleeding is caused by a prothrombin deficiency, such as occurs in liver diseases in which hepatic ducts are obstructed or in biliary duct obstruction, *vitamin K_1* is given parenterally. Vitamin K_1 is helpful in controlling hemorrhage following overdoses of bishydroxycoumarin (Dicumarol). Protamine sulfate is given after overdoses of heparin.

If possible the blood loss should be measured so that the physician can prescribe replacement more accurately. Dressings saturated with blood can be weighed, and bloody vomitus, which may be bright red or coffee-ground color, and drainage from gastric tubes should be measured. Whenever possible tarry stools and bright blood discharged from the rectum should be measured. If this is not feasible the amount should be estimated, although it has been shown that estimates are often incorrect.[18] The physician often will want to see evidence of bleeding, such as bloody stools or urine, vaginal clots, and bloody vomitus.

Blood replacement usually is started before complete hemostasis has been accomplished, since the restoration of blood volume is imperative in preventing the occurence of irreversible shock. Blood plasma or a plasma expander may be given until whole blood is available. The physician's determination of the amount of blood to be given depends on the amount of blood loss, the central venous pressure, and the condition of the patient. When large amounts of blood must be given rapidly, the blood should be warmed to body temperature, since cold blood can act as a hypothermic agent. A decrease in the body temperature may cause cardiac slowing, with decreased cardiac output or the development of ventricular fibrillation. The speed at which blood is given depends on the patient's condition. If the blood pressure is very low, the blood may be given very rapidly and may even be pumped in under pressure by the physician.

During blood transfusions the patient should be observed carefully for signs of reaction. The patient may develop an allergic or febrile reaction or a reaction caused by incompatibility of the blood. Circulatory failure can occur particularly in patients with underlying cardiac problems. Other risks associated with blood transfusions are hyperkalemia, transmission of hepatitis or other infections, and air embolism. During the infusion of the first 50 ml, the patient should be observed continuously. A routine for monitoring of vital signs and other observations should be established and implemented.

The patient is usually very apprehensive because of the hemorrhage and because of the emergency measures that follow it. Every attempt should be made to keep the patient quiet, reassured, and comfortable. The patient should never, under any circumstances, be left alone while a hemorrhage is occurring. Morphine sulfate is often ordered as a sedative. Evidences of bleeding should be removed from the bedside, and stained linen and clothing should be replaced. Noise and excitement should be kept to a minimum, and all treatments and procedures, such as frequent blood pressure readings, transfusions, the use of unusual positions, and, if necessary, restriction of food and fluids, should be explained to the patient and family. The patient with a massive hemorrhage usually is given nothing to eat or drink until the hemorrhage is controlled, since surgery may be necessary. Food and fluid also are often withheld when the bleeding is from the gastrointestinal tract.

REFERENCES AND SELECTED READINGS
Contemporary

1. Andersson, B.: Thirst and brain control of water balance, Am. Sci. **59:**408-415, 1971.
2. *Andreoli, K.G., et al.: Comprehensive cardiac care: a text for nurses, physicians, and other health practitioners, ed. 4, St. Louis, 1979, The C.V. Mosby Co.
3. *Armstrong, P., and Baigrie, R.: Hemodynamic monitoring in critically ill patients, Heart Lung **9:**1060-1062, 1980.
4. Beck, J.L.: Vasoactive drugs in the treatment of shock, Surg. Clin. North Am. **55:**721-728, 1975.
5. Beisel, W., Wannemacker, R., and Neufeld, H.: Relation of fever to energy expenditure. In Assessment of energy-metabolism in health and disease. Report of the first Ross Conference on Medical Research, Columbus, Ohio, 1980, Ross Laboratories.
6. Beland, I.L., and Passos, J.Y.: Clinical nursing: pathophysiological and psychosocial approaches, ed. 4, New York, 1980, Macmillan Publishing Co., Inc.
7. Bergersen, B.S., and Goth, A.: Pharmacology in nursing, ed. 14, St. Louis, 1979, The C.V. Mosby Co.
8. Berne, R.M., and Levy, M.N.: Cardiovascular physiology, ed. 4, St. Louis, 1981, The C.V. Mosby Co.
9. *Bordicks, K.: Patterns of shock. Implication for nursing, ed. 2, New York, 1980, Macmillian Publishing Co., Inc.
10. Brand, L.: A practical approach to infection surveillance in the intensive care unit, Heart Lung **5:**788-790, 1976.
11. *Brand, L., and Wilson, R.F.: Shock. In Meltzer, L. E., et al.: Concepts and practices of intensive care for nurse specialists, Bowie, Md., 1976, The Charles Press.
12. Brodows, R., Pi-Sunyer, F., and Campbell, R.: Neural control of counter-regulatory events during glucopenia in man, J. Clin. Invest. **52:**1841-1844, 1973.
13. Brooks, S.M.: Basic facts of body water and ions, ed. 3, New York, 1977, Springer Publishing Co., Inc.
14. Brown, W.J.: A classification of microorganisms frequently causing sepsis, Heart Lung **5:**397-405, 1976.
15. Brown, W.J.: The increasing incidence of sepsis and antibiotic resistance, Heart Lung **5:**593-597, 1976.
16. Cahill, G.F., and Aoki, T.: Partial and total starvation. In Assessment of energy metabolism in health and disease. Report of the First Ross Conference on Medical Research, Columbus, Ohio, 1980, Ross Laboratories.
17. Cell in shock. Proceedings of a synposium on recent research developments and current clinical practice in shock (Upjohn), Kalamazoo, Mich., 1974, Scope Publication.
18. *Clough, D.H., and Higgins, P.: Discrepancies in estimating blood loss. Am. J. Nurs. **81:**331-333, 1981.
19. Cushing, R.: Pulmonary infection, Heart Lung **5:**611-613, 1976.
20. Daily, E., and Schroeder, J.: Techniques in bedside hemodynamic monitoring, ed. 2, St. Louis, 1981, The C.V. Mosby Co.
21. Davis, B.D., et al.: Microbiology, ed. 2, New York, 1973, Harper & Row, Publishers, Inc.
22. Denny, M.: Septic shock, J. E.N. **3:**19-23, 1977.
23. Dillman, P.: The bio-physical response to shock trousers, J.E.N. **3:**21-25, 1977.
24. *Duff, J.H.: Cardiovascular changes in sepsis, Heart Lung **5:**773-776, 1976.
25. Dutcher, I.E., and Hardenburg, H.C., Jr.: Water and electrolyte imbalances. In Meltzer, L.E., et al.: Concepts and practices of intensive care for nurse specialists, Bowie, Md., 1976, The Charles Press.

*References preceded by an asterisk are particularly well suited for student reading.

26. Elenbass, R.: Anaphylactic shock, Crit. Care Q. **2**:85-90, 1980.

27. Eskridge, R.: Septic shock, Crit. Care Q. **2**:55-76, 1980.

28. Fisher, E.J.: Antimicrobial therapy: some guidelines, Heart Lung **5**:437-448, 1976.

29. Fisher, E.J.: Surveillance and management of hospital-acquired infections, Heart Lung **5**:784-787, 1976.

30. Frienkel, N.: The role of nutrition in medicine, J.A.M.A. **239**:1868-1875, 1978.

31. Gale, C.C.: Neuroendocrine aspects of thermoregulation, Annu. Rev. Physiol. **35**:391-398, 1973.

32. Gilman, A.G., Goodman, L., and Gilman, A., editors: Goodman and Gilman's the pharmacological basis of therapeutics, ed. 6, New York, 1980, MacMillan Publishing Co., Inc.

33. Golderger, E.: A primer of water, electrolyte and acid-base syndromes, ed. 6, Philadelphia, 1979, Lea & Febiger.

34. Goldmann, D.A., and Maki, D.G.: Infection control in total parenteral nutrition, J.A.M.A. **223**:1360-1364, 1973.

35. Guyton, A.: Textbook of medical physiology, ed. 6, Philadelphia, 1981, W.B. Saunders Co.

36. Harmon, A., and Harmon, D.: Anaphylaxis: sudden death anytime, Nurs. '80 **10**(10):40-43, 1980.

37. *Hathaway, R.: Hemodynamic monitoring in shock, J.E.N. **3**:37-42, 1977.

38. Holliday, R.L.: Intra-abdominal sepsis, Heart Lung **5**:781-783, 1976.

39. *Hoshal, V.L., Jr.: Intravenous catheters and infection, Surg. Clin. North Am. **52**:1407-1417, 1972.

40. Huss, P., et al.: The new inotropic drug, dobutamine, Heart Lung **10**(1):121-126, 1981.

41. Isselbacher, K., et al.: Harrison's principles of internal medicine, ed. 9, New York, 1980, McGraw Hill Book Co.

42. *Jahre, J.N.: Medical approach to the hypotensive patient and the patient in shock, Heart Lung **4**:577-587, 1975.

43. Kee, J.L.: Fluids and electrolytes with clinical applications: a programmed approach, New York, 1976, John Wiley & Sons, Inc.

44. King, O.M.: Care of the cardiac surgical patient, St. Louis, 1975, The C.V. Mosby Co.

45. Kluger, M.: Temperature regulation, fever, and disease, Int. Rev. Physiol. **20**:209-251, 1979.

46. Lauter, C.B.: Opportunistic infections, Heart Lung **5**:601-606, 1976.

47. Ledgerwood, A.: Hepatobiliary complications of sepsis, Heart Lung **5**:621-623, 1976.

48. Lefer, A., Saba, T., and Mela, L.: Advances in shock research, vol. I, New York, 1979, Alan R. Liss, Inc.

49. Lillehei, R.C., and Dietzman, D.H.: Circulatory collapse and shock. In Schwartz, S.I., et al.: Principles of surgery, New York, 1974, McGraw-Hill Book Co.

50. Linton, A.L.: Diagnosis and treatment of infections of the urinary tract, Heart Lung **5**:607-610, 1976.

51. Long, C.L., and Blakemore, W.S.: Energy and protein requirement in the hospital patient, J.P.E.N. **3**:69-71, 1979.

52. McGarry, J., and Foster, D.: Hormonal control of ketogenesis, Arch. Intern. Med. **137**:495-501, 1977.

53. Meltzer, L.E., et al.: Concepts and practices of intensive care for nurse specialists, Bowie, Md., 1976, The Charles Press.

54. Metheny, N., and Snively, W.D.: Nurses handbook of fluid balance, ed. 3, Philadelphia, 1979, J.B. Lippincott Co.

55. Millward, D., and Waterlow, J.C.: Effects of nutrition on protein turnover in skeletal muscles, Fed. Proc. **37**:2283-2290, 1977.

56. Mountcastle, V.B.: Medical physiology, ed. 14, St. Louis, 1979, The C.V. Mosby Co.

57. Munro, H.: Energy intake and nitrogen metabolism. In Assessment of energy metabolism in health and disease. Report of the first Ross Conference on Medical Research, Columbus, Ohio, 1980, Ross Laboratories.

58. *Munro, H.: Hormones and the metabolic response to injury, N. Engl. J. Med. **300**:41-42, 1979.

59. Munro, H.: Nutrition and muscle protein metabolism. Fed. Proc. **37**:2281-2282, 1977.

60. *Murray, J., and Smallwood, J.: CVP monitoring, Nurs. '77 **7**(1):42-47, 1977.

61. Park, G.: Cardiogenic shock, Crit. Care Q. **2**:43-54, 1980.

62. *Phipps, W.J., et al.: Respiratory insufficiency and failure. In Meltzer, L.E., et al.: Concepts and practices of intensive care for nurse specialists, Bowie, Md., 1976, The Charles Press.

63. Pitts, R.F.: Physiology of the kidney and body fluids, ed. 3, Chicago, 1974, Year Book Medical Publishers, Inc.

64. *Plachetka, J.R.: Sympathomimetic pharmacology, Crit. Care Q. **2**:27-35, 1980.

65. Reed, L.: Intra-aortic balloon pump, A.O.R.N. J. **23**:995-1001, 1976.

66. Roberts, A.: Body fluids. 18. Body water and its control, Nurs. Times **74**(suppl.):69-72, 1978.

67. Roellig, S.: Management of patients with contagious illness, Heart Lung **5**:596-600, 1976.

68. *Rosenberg, I.K.: Renal hemodynamic effects of sepsis, Heart Lung **5**:777-780, 1976.

69. Sargis, N.M.: Cardiogenic shock, J. N.Y. State Nurs. Assoc. **3**:22-28, 1972.

70. *Schaag, H.: Special problems in critical care: septic shock. In Daly, B.: Intensive care nursing, New York, 1980, Medical Examination Publishing Co., Inc.

71. Schuler, J.J., Erve, P.R., and Schumer, W.: Glucocorticoid effect on hepatic carbohydrate metabolism in the endotoxin-shocked monkey, Ann. Surg. **183**:345-354, 1976.

72. *Schumer, W.: Metabolism during shock and sepsis, Heart Lung **5**:416-421, 1976.

73. Schumer, W., and Sperling, R.: Steroids in the treatment of clinical septic shock, Ann. Surg. **184**:333-341, 1976.

74. Schumer, W., Spitzer, J., and Marshall, B.: Advances in shock research, vol. 2, New York, 1979, Alan R. Liss, Inc.

75. Schwartz, S.I., et al.: Principles of surgery, ed. 2, New York, 1974, McGraw-Hill Book Co.

76. Shubin, H., and Weill, M.H.: Touchstones in critical care medicine: an introduction, Crit. Care Med. **2**:281-282, 1974.

77. Sibbald, W.J.: Bacteremia and endotoxemia: a discussion of their roles in the pathophysiology of gram-negative sepsis, Heart Lung **5**:765-771, 1976.

78. Silva, J.: Anaerobic infections, Heart Lung **5**:406-410, 1976.

79. *Snively, W., and Roberts, K.T.: The clinical picture as an aid to understanding body fluid disturbances, Nurs. Forum **12**:132-159, 1973.

80. Sodeman, W.A., Jr., and Sodeman, W.A.: Pathologic physiology: mechanisms of disease, ed. 5, Philadelphia, 1974, W.B. Saunders Co.

81. Spinella, J.: Clinical assessment of the shock patient, J.E.N. **5**:34-45, 1979.

82. *Steffee, W.: Malnutrition in hospitalized patient, J.A.M.A. **244**:2630-2635, 1980.

83. Stroot, V., et al.: Fluid and electrolytes: a practical approach, ed. 2, Philadelphia, 1977, F.A. Davis Co.

84. Strouth, C.: Some common ions: how well do you know them: chemical bases of electrolyte balance, J. Nurs. Care **12**:21-22, 1979.

85. *Taylor, C.M.: When to anticipate septic shock, Nurs. '75 **5**(4):34-38, 1975.

86. Tepperman, J.: Metabolic and endocrine physiology, ed. 3, Chicago, 1973, Year Book Medical Publishers, Inc.

87. Thal, A.P., et al.: Shock: a physiologic basis for treatment, Chicago, 1971, Year Book Medical Publishers, Inc.

88. Thompson, L.: Management of shock: rational use of plasma

substitutes, vols. 1 and 2. In therapeutic topics, Cleveland, 1975, University Hospitals of Cleveland.

89. *Urrows, S.T.: Physiology of body fluids, Nurs. Clin. North Am. **15:**537-548, 1980.

90. Vander, A.J.: Renal physiology, New York, 1975, McGraw-Hill Book Co.

91. Vander, A.J., et al.: Human physiology: the mechanisms of body function, ed. 2, New York, 1975, McGraw-Hill Book Co.

92. *Visalli, F., and Evans, P.: The Swan-Ganz catheter: a program for teaching safe, effective care, Nurs. '81 **11**(1):42-47, 1981.

93. Wade, J.F.: Respiratory nursing care: physiology and technique, ed. 3, St. Louis, 1982, The C.V. Mosby Co.

94. West, J.B.: Respiratory physiology: the essentials, ed. 2, Baltimore, 1979, The Williams & Wilkins Co.

95. Williams, S.R.: Nutrition and diet therapy, ed. 4, St. Louis, 1981, The C.V. Mosby Co.

96. Wilmore, D.W.: Alimentation in injured and septic patients, Heart Lung **5:**791-792, 1976.

97. Wilson, J.A.: Infection control in intravenous therapy, Heart Lung **5:**430-436, 1976.

98. Wilson, R.F.: Endocrine changes in sepsis, Heart Lung **5:**411-415, 1976.

99. *Wilson, R.F.: The diagnosis and management of severe sepsis and septic shock, Heart Lung **5:**422-429, 1976.

100. *Wilson, R.F.: The diagnosis and treatment of acute respiratory failure in sepsis, Heart Lung **5:**614-620, 1976.

101. *Wilson, R., and Wilson, J.: Pathophysiology, diagnosis and treatment of shock, J.E.N. **3:**11-26, 1977.

102. Woods, M., and Mazza, I.: Blood and component therapy, Nurs. Clin. North Am. **15:**629-646, 1980.

103. Young, U., and Scremshaw, N.: Genetic and biological variability in human nutrient requirements, Am. J. Clin. Nutr. **32:**486-500, 1979.

Classic

104. Ando, S., Guze, L.B., and Gold, E.M.: ACTH release in vivo and in vitro: extrapituitary mediation during *Escherichia coli* bacteremia, Endocrinology **74:**894-901, 1964.

105. Dudrick, S.J., et al.: Can intravenous feedings as the sole method of nutrition support growth in the child and restore weight loss in an adult? An affirmative answer, Ann. Surg. **169:**974-985, 1969.

106. Lands, A.M., et al.: Differentiation of receptor systems activated by sympathomimetics amines, Nature **214:**597-598, 1967.

107. *Schumer, W.: Shock and its effect on the cell, J.A.M.A. **205:**75-79, 1968.

108. Schumer, W., et al.: Endotoxin effect on respiration of rat liver mitochondria, J. Surg. Res. **10:**609-612, 1970.

AUDIOVISUAL RESOURCES

Thomas, L.A.: Shock, Bowie, Md., 1980, Robert J. Brady Co. (Film strips, 6 modules.)

Trainex Corp.: Fluids and electrolytes: clinical application. Garden Grove, Calif., 1970, Trainex Corp. (Film strips, PC261-PC264.)

COMMON STRESSORS AND THEIR MANAGEMENT

Persons with medical-surgical problems encounter many stressful situations in conjunction with their illnesses and the interventions necessary to their treatment. This unit explores common stressors that occur regardless of the pathologic entity or biologic system involved. Emphasis is placed on the effects of the stressors and on nursing interventions to modify effects that are detrimental to health.

Fluid and electrolyte imbalance considers such stressors as excesses and deficiencies of water and electrolytes. In the chapter on *infectious agents* and the adaptive responses, emphasis is placed on infection control, and persons with minimal adaptive potential are identified. *Pain* is explored as a stressor, and adaptation is discussed from biologic as well as psychosocial perspectives. Nursing measures for pain relief are emphasized. Surgery is a threat to the integrity of the body and the self. Implications for nursing are considered for the preoperative, intraoperative, and postoperative phases of surgery. The effects of having a malignant disease regardless of location are discussed in the chapter on *neoplasia*. Information relative to specific malignant diseases is dealt with in later chapters.

Sensory deprivation and overload are also common stressors and are discussed in terms of assessment and management. Changes in *level of consciousness* are explored, emphasizing the protective interventions necessary for the dependent unconscious patient. Many of the diseases seen in persons with medical-surgical problems or interventions to treat these problems result in alteration in *body image,* and the adaptive responses this elicits are discussed. The experience of having a *prolonged illness,* of being chronically ill, including altered roles and adaptation to long-term impairments, is also explored.

CHAPTER 21

FLUID AND ELECTROLYTE IMBALANCE

BARBARA SOLTIS

Almost all medical and surgical conditions threaten fluid and electrolyte equilibrium. In some instances, imbalances are minor and can be corrected by merely adjusting a patient's food and fluid intake. In other instances; imbalances are life threatening and require prompt medical treatment to prevent death.

Although a physician prescribes medical therapy to prevent and treat imbalances, nurses have many vital functions to carry out in this area: (1) recognition of situations that are likely to cause imbalances; (2) intervention to prevent imbalances from developing; (3) carrying out preventive and therapeutic measures ordered by the physician and monitoring patients' responses to these measures; (4) recognition of signs and symptoms of fluid, electrolyte, and acid-base disturbances; (5) monitoring patients to prevent and recognize imbalances related to their specific conditions or treatments; and (6) alleviation of the effects of disturbances on patients' comfort and safety.

The reader is referred to Chapter 20 for a description of normal fluid and electrolyte balance and some of the control mechanisms that maintain this balance. This chapter deals with the causes, prevention, assessment, and management of imbalances of body fluids, sodium, potassium, calcium, magnesium, and hydrogen ions. Each imbalance will be discussed separately, although in most instances a disturbance in one is accompanied by a disturbance in the balance of one or more of the others.

Normally, the body receives oxygen through the lungs, and water and various organic and inorganic substances through the gastrointestinal tract. After utilizing what is needed for healthful functioning, any excesses are excreted along with the waste products of metabolism through the body's excretory organs, the skin, lungs, kidneys, and gastrointestinal tract (see Chapter 20). When these normal processes of intake, utilization, and excretion are disrupted, fluid, electrolyte, and acid-base imbalances result. These imbalances are manifest as excesses, deficits, or abnormal shifts among body compartments.

Excesses result from increased intake or decreased loss, and deficits result from decreased intake or excess loss of fluids or electrolytes. Either an excess or a deficit can result from abnormal shifts of fluids or electrolytes among the body compartments. For example, *excesses* occur when the intake of fluids and electrolytes exceeds the ability of the body's control and excretory mechanisms to eliminate the amounts that are not needed. Fluids, electrolytes, and metabolic wastes are retained when kidney function is impaired. An excess of carbon dioxide accumulates when there is inadequate respiratory function.

On the other hand, *deficits* develop when an individual is unwilling or unable for some reason to take in adequate fluids and food. Excessive amounts of fluids and electrolytes are lost through the skin as a result of diaphoresis or oozing from severe wounds or burns. Fluids and electrolytes are lost from the gastrointestinal tract when profuse diarrhea or vomiting occurs and when the gastrointestinal tract is drained by intubation or purged with cathartics or enemas. In hemorrhage, body fluids and electrolytes are always lost.

Deficits may also result from the inability to utilize needed substances, such as when fluids with their electrolyte constituents are trapped in the body by edema or intestinal obstruction. They are therefore not available for normal processes.

Fluid imbalance

Osmotic pressure of the extracellular fluid (ECF) varies proportionately with its sodium concentration.

TABLE 21-1. Water and sodium imbalances

Osmolar imbalances				Isotonic volume imbalances	
Hyperosmolar		Hyposmolar		Volume excess	Volume deficit
Water deficit: water ↓ in relation to sodium and other solutes	Sodium or solute excess: sodium or other solutes ↑ in relation to water	Water excess: water ↑ in relation to sodium and other solutes	Sodium deficit: sodium ↓ in relation to water	ECF volume excess (edema): water and sodium ↑ proportionately	ECF volume deficit: water and sodium ↓ proportionately

Sodium and its anions (chloride and bicarbonate) make up 90% to 95% of the total solute in the ECF.[28] When there is a change in the sodium-to-water ratio, a disturbance in osmolality (p. 302) results; that is, the extracellular fluid becomes more dilute (*hyposmolar*) or more concentrated (*hyperosmolar*) than normal. A considerable change in the concentration of solutes other than sodium in the extracellular fluid can also effect osmolar disturbances.

Hyposmolality of the extracellular fluid causes water to move into body cells by osmosis to equalize the concentration of fluid on both sides of the cell membrane. Hyperosmolality of the extracellular fluid causes water to move out of the cells to dilute the extracellular fluid and to equalize concentration in both compartments.

When there are changes in the volume of extracellular fluid but no change in osmolality, an *isotonic* volume disturbance results. There is no significant change in the sodium-to-water ratio; sodium deficits or excesses are accompanied by proportional water deficits or excesses. There is no appreciable movement of water between the intracellular fluid (ICF) and extracellular fluid compartments, and the imbalance is essentially restricted to the extracellular fluid compartment. Table 21-1 shows the types of fluid imbalances that are likely to occur.

Hyperosmolar imbalance: extracellular water deficit and solute excess

An extracellular water deficit occurs when the amount of extracellular water is diminished in proportion to the amount of solute contained therein. The solute excess raises the osmolality to above the normal 300 mOsm/L.

Etiology

Imbalances may originate in either the fluid or the solute portion of the extracellular fluid. There may be (1) decreased intake of water, (2) excess loss of water without proportionate loss of solutes, (3) increased solute intake without sufficient water, and (4) excess accumulation of solutes secondary to a particular disease condition.

Any person who does not have fluids available to drink, who cannot take fluids independently, or who does not respond to thirst will be likely to develop a water deficit.

In a disaster such as a flood or an earthquake, a supply of drinkable water may not be available. Any patient who is unable to ask for fluids, to identify his own need for fluid, or to swallow easily may develop a fluid deficit. Thus a patient with a cerebral vascular accident and aphasia may not be able to communicate a desire for fluids or may have difficulty swallowing fluids that are offered. A confused or disoriented patient may not be aware of thirst. Patients who are comatose, weak, or catatonic may also develop fluid deficits.

Although loss of body water is usually accompanied by loss of electrolytes, there are a number of conditions in which water is lost in excess of electrolytes. These include increased loss through the lungs in hyperventilation or in secretions from a tracheostomy, through the skin with a high fever, through the gastrointestinal tract when there is watery diarrhea, or in urine when the kidneys fail to concentrate solutes.

Pathophysiology

When solutes are taken in without sufficient water, hyperosmolality results, such as occurs with intake of tube feeding solutions, which are high in protein, dextrose, and electrolytes. The excess of solutes causes an *osmotic diuresis*, the body's attempt to excrete a solute load through the kidneys by excreting a large volume of urine. Formation of the urine in this process requires the use of a great deal of water and interferes with the normal water conservation mechanisms resulting in a water deficit.

Several conditions lead to endogenous (internal) addition of excess solutes—large amounts of glucose can accumulate in the blood in diabetes mellitus, and glucose and ketone bodies can accumulate in the blood in diabetic ketoacidosis (p. 662). A large volume of nitrogenous waste products results from metabolism of a high-protein diet. All of these solute excesses cause large water losses during osmotic diuresis.

When an extracellular water deficit occurs, water moves out of the cells to replace water lost from the extracellular compartment, thus maintaining an adequate circulating blood volume. If the water deficit is not corrected, the cells eventually become unable to compensate for extracellular losses, and circulation begins to fail. As both intracellular and extracellular fluids decrease, cell function is impaired because food, oxygen, and waste products are diffused inadequately. Brain cells are particularly sensitive to these changes and a disruption of brain cell function develops, manifested as mental changes in the patient.

Prevention

Prevention is crucial in the nursing care of patients who are at risk of developing a water deficit. The nurse is alert to those patients who may not be receiving adequate fluid intake, monitors their intake and output, and plans a schedule for offering fluids to them. Patients who are hyperventilating for long periods of time, regardless of the reason, should have their fluid intake increased somewhat because they are losing more fluid than usual through the lungs. Those receiving high-protein tube feedings need sufficient water to prevent water deficit and osmotic diuresis.

Clinical picture

Thirst and weight loss are early symptoms of water deficit and become more pronounced as the deficit increases. Body temperature begins to rise as less water is available for temperature regulation. When cells are not able to continue providing water to replace extracellular fluid losses, signs of collapse of the circulatory system appear. Signs and symptoms of water deficit are shown in Table 21-2.

Intervention

Goals of treatment are to treat the underlying causes to prevent further water loss and to replace lost fluid.

The physician can use several methods, such as those based on serum sodium concentration or change in the patient's weight, to calculate the volume of water loss.[12] For instance, if a patient has lost 4 kg of body weight, the fluid deficit equals 4 L (1 kg weighs 1 L). Therapy will require replacement of the volume lost plus about 1.5 L of fluid to supply current daily need. Often the replacement is administered over a period of several days, since too rapid infusion of fluid may cause sudden intercompartmental shifts of water and pulmonary edema.

When water deficit is not severe, fluids can be replaced orally if the patient is able to drink fluids. Otherwise, intravenous fluids are given.

Intravenous glucose and water are usually given first to replace the water loss and increase urinary flow. Urinary output must be adequate so that electrolytes in excess of body needs can be excreted. Solutions containing electrolytes are therefore not given until renal function is established. Normal saline or half-strength

TABLE 21-2. Signs and symptoms of water deficit

	Moderate deficit	Severe deficit
Skin	Flushed, dry	Cold, clammy
Mouth	Dry mucous membranes	Dry, cracked tongue
Eyes	Decrease in tears	Soft, sunken eyeballs
Cardiovascular system	—	Tachycardia, low blood pressure, rapid respirations
CNS	Apprehension, restlessness	Lethargy, coma
Blood	—	Hemoconcentration, increase in hematocrit, BUN, electrolytes
Urine	High specific gravity, scant amount (except with osmotic diuresis)	Oliguria
Other	Thirst, weight loss	Thirst, weight loss, fever

saline (0.45%) can be given with other ions—potassium, calcium, and lactate—as needed.

In addition to providing fluids and participating in the treatment of conditions underlying water loss, nurses employ measures to decrease discomfort and ensure patient safety. Mouth care is especially important to relieve dryness and remove sordes (foul debris on lips and teeth) from oral mucous membranes. Safety measures such as side rails on beds are necessary for patients who have developed restlessness, confusion, lethargy, or other mental changes as a result of water deficit. Monitoring intake and output and changes in the patient's weight and vital signs will indicate whether the patient's condition is improving or deteriorating.

A state of adequate hydration will be evidenced by mental alertness, moist mucous membranes, and urinary output that is approximately equal to fluid intake.

Hyposmolar imbalance: water excess or water intoxication

When there is an excess of water in relation to solutes in the extracellular fluid, a hyposmolar imbalance known as *water excess* or *water intoxication* exists. Although this imbalance is not common, it can develop when water intake exceeds the ability of the kidneys to excrete it. Usually there is a concomitant increase in secretion of ADH, which promotes water retention and aggravates the water excess.

Under normal conditions, a decrease in osmotic pressure suppresses ADH production and permits free water to be excreted by the kidneys.

Etiology

One or more of the following conditions exist when water intoxication develops: (1) excess intake of electrolyte-free fluid, (2) increased secretion of ADH, or (3) decreased or inadequate output of urine.

Water excess can be caused by ingestion of large amounts of tap water by a person who is hysterical or psychotic. This behavior is called *psychogenic polydipsia*. The ingestion of frequent sips of tap water by one who is not able to tolerate food or other fluids because of illness can also lead to water excess. Some treatments that lead to excessive water intake are multiple tap water enemas and absorption of water from irrigating solutions during transurethral resection of the prostate gland.

Excess or inappropriate secretion of ADH occurs in response to stress, drugs, and anesthetics. (See Chapter 20 for more information on ADH.) It can also accompany inflammatory conditions of the lung (tuberculosis, pneumonia) and brain (encephalitis, meningitis), endocrine disturbances and tumors in the lungs (especially oat cell carcinoma), pancreas, duodenum, and other body organs.[12] Inadequate kidney function or renal failure will potentiate the development of water excess.

A low serum sodium or sodium deficit can also produce a hyposmolar imbalance. This condition is discussed under sodium deficit (p. 334).

Pathophysiology

When water intoxication occurs, hyposmolar water excess in the extracellular compartment quickly becomes an *intracellular water excess*. There is a lesser concentration of solutes in the extracellular fluid as compared to the intracellular fluid; therefore water moves into the cell to equalize concentration on both sides of the cell membrane causing the cell to swell.

Prevention

Water intoxication can be anticipated by identifying patients who present one or more risk factors. Daily weights and careful monitoring of intake and output will help to detect the developing problem before it becomes severe.

Clinical picture

Since brain cells are particularly sensitive to the increase in intracellular water, the most common symptoms are manifestations of changes in the patient's mental status.

In acute water intoxication there is swelling of the cells, which may develop rapidly and dramatically. Signs of water intoxication include changes in behavior, confusion, incoordination, convulsions, hyperventilation, sudden weight gain, and warm, moist skin. When the condition develops more slowly, there may be apathy, sleepiness, anorexia, nausea, and vomiting. A low serum sodium concentration is a usual finding. Signs of increasing intracranial pressure may develop—slow, bounding pulse and rising pulse pressure as the systolic blood pressure rises and the diastolic pressure falls. Some peripheral edema may be present, but it is not marked.

Intervention

The patient will usually recover with only careful water restriction. When severe symptoms (coma and convulsions) develop, a small amount of intravenous hypertonic saline, along with the fluid restriction, will hasten the return to normal water balance.

Providing for the safety of patients with this imbalance is a priority nursing function because of the confusion and other mental changes that exist. Any patient who is receiving a large amount of water orally, rectally, or intravenously needs to be monitored carefully for signs of water intoxication, especially if a condition of excess ADH prevails.

Isotonic volume deficit: extracellular fluid deficit

Conditions causing a loss of water together with a loss of electrolytes lead to *isotonic volume deficit*, also known as *extracellular fluid depletion*.

Etiology

Water and electrolytes are lost in hemorrhage and profuse sweating. About 8 L of fluid circulate through the gastrointestinal tract per day (Table 21-3). These fluids are derived from the ECF; therefore vomiting, diarrhea, draining intestinal fistulas, and surgical openings such as ileostomy and cecostomy result in ECF loss. Severe losses can deplete the extracellular compartment rapidly.

Pathophysiology

In isotonic volume deficit the extracellular osmolality does not change because sodium, the chief contributor to extracellular osmolality, is lost along with water. Consequently, water content of the cells is not affected, and the deficit remains restricted to the extracellular compartment. Fluid movement is from the extracellular compartment to outside the body, depleting blood and interstitial volume.

Prevention

Nurses are responsible for identifying and monitoring patients who are likely to develop isotonic fluid deficit. Taking postural (orthostatic) blood pressures helps to detect this deficit before more severe cardiovascular symptoms develop. *Postural blood pressures* are a comparison of a patient's blood pressure measured first in a lying position and then in a sitting or standing position.

TABLE 21-3. Fluid composition of total internal secretions*

	Approximate ml of fluid (daily)
Saliva	1500
Gastric juice	2500
Intestinal juice	2000
Pancreatic juice	1500
Bile	500
TOTAL	8000 ml/24 hr

*Note that approximately 8 L of fluid are used daily for digestive purposes. Normally, most of this fluid is reabsorbed. Some of each of the ions found in blood plasma are present in each of the fluids listed, but the individual concentration varies with each fluid.

A drop in blood pressure of 10 mm Hg or more in the upright position is significant.

The healthy person who is perspiring profusely needs extra dietary salt and should drink extra fluids. Patients on low sodium diets and those with draining gastrointestinal fistulas are prone to develop sodium depletion. They should always be taught to increase their salt intake slightly whenever they perspire profusely. Patients who have hot packs applied to large areas of the body also lose sodium and water, although the loss may not be readily noticeable as perspiration. Attention to ingesting more salt and water than usual in situations of excessive heat may prevent heat exhaustion.

Clinical picture

The most prominent symptoms are manifest in the cardiovascular system as a result of volume depletion. Following is a listing of the symptoms of extracellular fluid depletion:
1. Skin: poor turgor
2. Mouth: dry mucous membranes
3. Cardiovascular: postural hypotension (early), low blood pressure, tachycardia, increased respiration, decreased vein filling
4. Weight: loss
5. Urine: low output, increased specific gravity

Intervention

Treatment consists of identifying and correcting the underlying cause to prevent further fluid and electrolyte loss and replacing those fluids and electrolytes that have been lost. Hemorrhage must be controlled (see Chapter 20). Vomiting may be treated with antiemetics, such as trimethobenzamide hydrochloride (Tigan) and prochlorperazine (Compazine), and diarrhea with antidiarrheal drugs (Lomotil, paregoric, Kaopectate).

Any patient who is losing body fluids through perspiration, fever, or loss of gastrointestinal fluid should be given salty fluids to drink. Meticulous mouth care will relieve the discomfort of dry mucous membranes.

As blood volume decreases, postural hypotension develops, and the patient's safety may be threatened by the resultant weakness, dizziness, or fainting on standing upright.

Isotonic volume excess: extracellular fluid excess and edema

If there is an excess of body water with a concomitant increase in sodium, the excess fluid will be retained in the *extracellular* compartments and lead to the formation of edema. *Edema* is the accumulation of fluid in the interstitial spaces.

Etiology

Edema can be produced by any of the following: increase in capillary fluid pressure, decrease in capillary oncotic pressure, increase in interstitial oncotic pressure, and any condition that increases the amount of aldosterone circulating in the blood. Causes of edema with clinical examples are shown in Table 21-4.

Pathophysiology

In the normal tissue there is a minimally positive interstitial fluid or possibly a negative interstitial fluid pressure[15] and cells are held in close approximation to facilitate the exchange of gases, nutrients, and waste products between the cells and capillaries. If fluid accumulates in the interstitial space and is not removed either by direct return to the blood vessel or through the lymph system, a more positive interstitial fluid pressure develops, and cells are pushed further apart. In the healthy individual, edema does not develop immediately after the initial inflow of fluid into the interstitial spaces because of the body's compensatory mechanisms, which include the existing low interstitial fluid pressure and the lymph system, which removes excess fluids and proteins.

A review of normal capillary dynamics will facilitate understanding of the various factors that can cause the development of edema. Two different types of pressures influence the flow of fluid across a capillary membrane: *fluid pressure* (pressure resulting from the hydrostatic force of fluid) and the colloid osmotic pressure, or *oncotic pressure* (pressure resulting from the presence of the proteins that do not diffuse across the membrane wall). Fluid pressure within the capillary at the arterial end of the capillary is greater than the tissue hydrostatic pressure and greater than the colloid osmotic pressure; thus fluid is forced out of the capillary (filtration). The colloid osmotic pressure within the capillary bed is greater than the fluid pressure at the venule end of the capillary and the tissue oncotic pressure; thus fluid is absorbed. According to Starling's law of the capillaries, there is equilibrium between the forces fil-

TABLE 21-4. Causes of edema according to underlying physiologic mechanism

Fluid pressure	Oncotic pressure
Increased capillary fluid pressure	**Decreased capillary oncotic pressure**
Increased venous pressure	*Loss of serum protein*
Vein obstruction	Burns, draining wounds, fistulas
Varicose veins	Hemorrhage
Thrombophlebitis	Nephrotic syndrome
Pressure on veins from casts, tight bandages, or garters	Chronic diarrhea
Increased total volume with decreased cardiac output	*Decreased intake of protein*
Congestive heart failure	Malnutrition
Fluid overloading	Kwashiorkor
Sodium and water retention: increased aldosterone from:	*Decreased production of albumin*
Decreased renal blood flow	Liver disease
Congestive heart failure	
Renal failure	**Increased interstitial oncotic pressure**
Increased production of aldosterone	*Increased capillary permeability to protein*
Cushing's syndrome	Burns
Aldosterone added to system	Inflammatory reactions
Corticosteroid therapy	Trauma
Inability to destroy aldosterone	Infections
Cirrhosis of liver	Allergic reactions (hives)
	Blocked lymphatics: decreased removal of tissue fluid and protein
	Malignant diseases
	Surgical removal of lymph nodes
	Elephantiasis

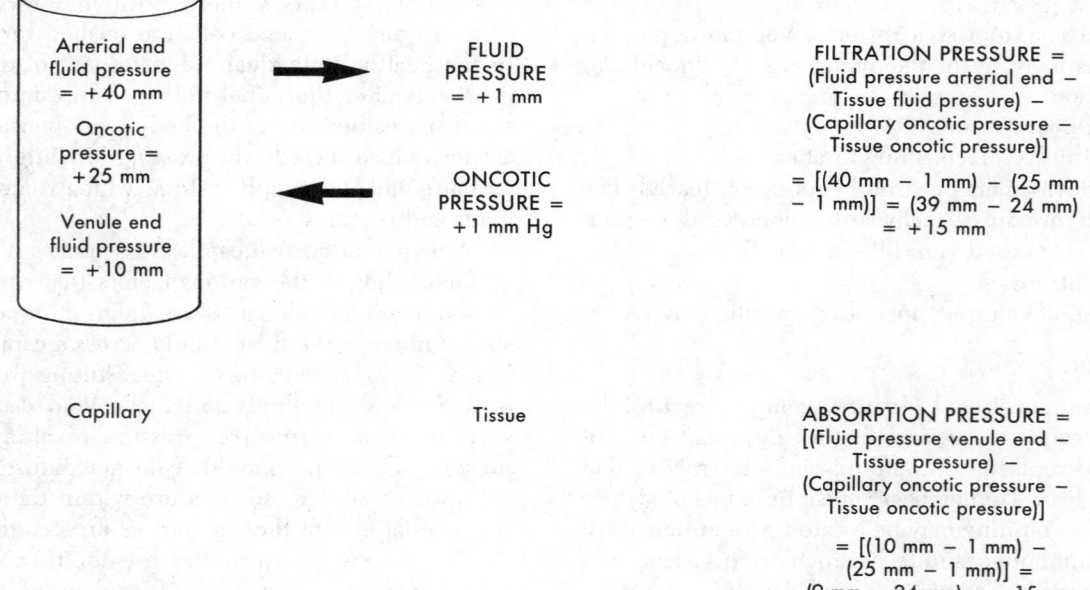

Fig. 21-1. Starling's law of capillaries. An equilibrium exists between forces filtering fluid out of capillary and forces absorbing fluid back into capillary. Note that fluid pressure within capillary is greater than fluid pressure in tissue. This differential (fluid pressure gradient) serves as a filtering force. Note also that oncotic pressure (colloid osmotic pressure) is greater within capillary. This serves as an absorbing force.

tering fluid out of the capillary and the forces absorbing fluid back into the capillary (Fig. 21-1). If there is a change in the oncotic pressure in or out of the capillary or in the capillary fluid pressure, there will be a rapid fluid flow across the capillary membrane, creating a change in the interstitial fluid pressure.*

The same mechanisms that create edema in the interstitial spaces can create fluid collection in *potential fluid spaces*, spaces between two membranes that normally contain only traces of fluid. The main potential fluid spaces are *intrapleural* (lung and chest wall), *pericardial* (heart and pericardial sac), *peritoneal* (intestines and abdominal wall), and joint capsules. The symptoms of fluid collection in these spaces are caused by the pressure of the collected fluid on adjoining organs or walls. Large amounts of fluid can collect in an operative site and in tissues surrounding an injury. Fluid that collects in the intrapleural space is termed *pleural effusion*, and in the pericardial space, *pericardial effusion*. Fluid high in protein and electrolytes that accumulates in the peritoneal space is termed *ascites*. An accumulation of fluid in all body tissues is a generalized edema or *anasarca*.

Overloading of the vascular system with fluid causes an increase in the hydrostatic pressure of the blood, resulting in generalized tissue edema. More important, if the increase in hydrostatic pressure is great enough, large amounts of fluid will be pushed across the alveolar-capillary membrane into the alveoli of the lungs. *Pulmonary edema* can occur unless it is rapidly treated and the process reversed.

Overloading of the vascular system may be caused by giving too much fluid within a short period of time to a person who, because of circulatory or renal disease, cannot dispose of the surplus. Infants and young children can also be overloaded easily because they normally have little extravascular fluid reserve. Elderly people tolerate increases in blood volume very poorly, since with inelastic vessels only relatively small increases in volume are needed to markedly increase the hydrostatic pressure. Monitoring the central venous pressure is one method used to determine if overloading is occurring.

Overloading of the vascular system also may be caused by increasing the oncotic (pull) pressure of the intravascular fluid by giving proteins so rapidly that the body cannot dispose of those that are in excess of its need. This overloading causes fluids to be pulled into the intravascular compartment from other body fluid compartments. The blood volume increases rapidly, neutralizing the oncotic pressure but increasing the hydrostatic pressure of the vascular system and the oncotic pressure of the interstitial fluid compartment. Fluid is then pushed into the tissues. Overloading the vascular system is a risk when fluids such as plasma, plasma expanders, albumin, or blood are given to any patient regardless of age or state of health.

Prevention

Overhydration is considered whenever intravenous fluids are being given and during planning of "forced fluid" regimens. Patients with renal or circulatory impairment can easily be overhydrated. Such patients usually must restrict fluid and sodium intake.

Patients on a low sodium diet need to know which foods to avoid. They should read labels on all prepared foods because many contain large amounts of sodium. They may need assistance in planning ways of adhering to a specified fluid restriction regimen. If medications are to be taken with minimal medical supervision over a period of time, patients should know the purpose of each drug and its usual side effects. They should also record the fluid taken with medications, monitor their own weight daily at home, and notify the physician if there is a significant change.

Clinical picture

In general, *weight gain* is the best indicator of an extracellular volume excess, since several liters of fluid can be retained without visible evidence of edema. Because hydrostatic pressure in the capillaries is greatest at the lowest parts of the body, edema will collect in these areas. This is called *dependent* edema. When one is standing, or sitting with feet on the floor, edema develops in the ankles and feet; when in a supine position edema fluid collects in the sacral area of the back.

If a finger is pressed over an edematous area, the indentation made by the finger will remain briefly as the fluid is pushed to another area; this is called *pitting edema*. Fluid refills the interstitial place in the "pit" area gradually. A subjective measure is sometimes used to describe pitting edema on a scale from "one plus" (+) to "four plus" (+ + + +), with the latter indicating severe pitting edema because it takes longer for fluid to move into the pit area. Skin over parts of the body with marked edema is usually tight, smooth, and shiny. It is cool and pale because of poor circulation. If edema is very severe, fluid will leak out of pores when the skin is pressed. This is called *weeping* edema.

Overhydration causes neck vein engorgement, so that these veins will appear distended even when the patient is in an upright position. Pulmonary edema is a medical emergency requiring rapid and knowledgeable treatment (p. 1135). In pulmonary edema the symptoms are dramatic—the patient gasps for air, is anxious

---

*For example, a decrease in capillary oncotic pressure to 20 mm Hg would produce the following (Fig. 21-1): (40 mm − 1 mm) − (20 mm − 1 mm) = 39 mm − 19 mm = 20 mm of filtration pressure at arterial end; and, (10 mm − 1 mm) − (20 mm − 1 mm) = 9 mm − 19 mm = −10 mm absorption pressure at venule end. Filtration pressure would be 10 mm Hg greater than absorption pressure and fluid would accumulate in the interstitial space.

and frightened, has moist "gurgling" respirations, coughs up frothy sputum, and shows signs of cyanosis. The symptoms are related to the fact that the alveoli are filled with fluid and oxygen is unable to diffuse across the alveolar-capillary membrane.

Intervention

The treatment of edema depends on the condition that has caused it. Congestive heart failure is usually treated with digitalis, diuretics, and sodium and fluid restriction (p. 1127). Cirrhosis of the liver is also treated with diuretics and sodium and fluid restriction (p. 687), and renal failure requires severe restrictions of water and electrolytes (p. 1570).

Reducing sodium intake alone may reduce edema because the supply of body sodium is reduced, and that which remains appears to be needed to maintain isotonicity of the blood.

Malnutritional edema responds to adequate dietary intake, especially the addition of protein to the diet, unless the condition is far advanced, as occurs in starving children and adults in famine areas where kwashiorkor is a common cause of death. Edema associated with infection and burns resolves over time as the underlying cause responds to treatment.

Excess fluid in the tissues results in poor cellular nutrition as cells are pushed further apart and away from capillaries. Normal exchange of nutrients and wastes is interrupted. Edematous tissues therefore are poorly nourished, susceptible to trauma and infection, and heal poorly.

Caution must be taken to protect edematous parts of the body from prolonged pressure, injury, and extremes of heat and cold. Skin over these parts should be kept well lubricated to prevent dryness. If edematous areas are exposed to extensive moisture from incontinence or perspiration, they should be kept dry to prevent maceration. When edema is caused by venous stasis, elevating dependent body parts and applying supportive stockings to the legs helps promote venous return. Extremities that become edematous as a result of surgery or trauma should also be elevated and supported.

Diuretics. Edema is often treated with diuretics that act on the kidneys. Thiazide diuretics, the most commonly used, inhibit reabsorption of sodium and chloride in the proximal renal tubules, thus promoting excretion of sodium and water, or *diuresis*. Potassium is usually lost along with sodium and water unless a potassium-sparing diuretic is used. Fluid and electrolyte imbalances are undesirable but are rather common side effects of diuretic therapy. When diuretics are given, a large amount of fluid is lost from the vascular compartment, decreasing its hydrostatic pressure and causing fluid to be pulled back into it from the tissues.

Before excess fluid in the interstitial spaces can be excreted, it must be moved back into the vascular compartment; otherwise, diuresis causes serious vascular depletion. Table 21-5 shows some diuretics and their effects.

Electrolyte imbalance

No single electrolyte can be out of balance without causing other electrolytes to be out of balance also. This fact should be kept in mind while reading this section.

Sodium, potassium, and calcium are all essential for the passage of nerve impulses. Whenever the concentration of any of these cations is increased or decreased in body fluids, the increase or decrease is reflected in the stimulation of muscles by nerves. The muscles may become weak and atonic because of inadequate stimulation, or they may become somewhat spastic because of excess stimulation. A decrease in calcium concentration in body fluids may cause the stimulus to be irregular, and muscle spasms result. Gastrointestinal and cardiac symptoms so often produced by electrolyte imbalances result in part from changes in neural stimulation of the muscles of these systems.

With cation imbalances, the distribution of body fluids frequently is upset. Abnormal collections of fluid may cause gastrointestinal symptoms such as nausea, vomiting, and diarrhea. Decreased amounts of fluid may cause anorexia, dyspepsia, and constipation. It is thought that edema of cerebral tissues may be responsible for headache, convulsions, and coma.

Sodium

The normal concentration of sodium in the blood is 138 to 145 mEq/L. Sodium is the most prevalent cation in the extracellular fluid and controls the osmotic pressure of this compartment. It is essential for neuromuscular functioning, for many intracellular chemical reactions, and for helping to maintain acid-base balance in the body. The sodium gradient theory states that sodium must be present in order for glucose to be transported into cells.[13]

As previously mentioned, aldosterone causes reabsorption of sodium in the kidney tubules (p. 305). When sodium supply becomes low, renal loss of sodium drops to zero. Aldosterone does not greatly influence sodium *concentration*, however, because as sodium is reabsorbed, water is also reabsorbed in equal proportions.

Deficit

A low sodium level in the blood, *hyponatremia*, can result from either a sodium loss or a water excess.

Table 21-5. Common diuretics and their effect on fluid and electrolyte balance

Generic name	Trade name	Method of administration	Peak effect	Probable effects on fluid and electrolyte balance
Thiazides				
Chlorothiazide	Diuril	Oral	4 hr	Hyponatremia Hypokalemia ↓ ECF volume Hyperglycemia Hyperuricemia
Hydrochlorothiazide	Esidrix HydroDiuril	Oral	3-4 hr	Hypomagnesemia
Loop diuretics (act mainly on ascending loop of Henle)				
Furosemide	Lasix	IM or IV Oral	½ hr 2-4 hr	Hypokalemia Hyperuricemia ↓ ECF volume
Ethacrynic acid	Edecrin	Oral IV	2-4 hr ½ hr	Hyponatremia
Aldosterone antagonist (opposes potassium-losing action of aldosterone)				
Spironolactone	Aldactone	Oral	72 hr	Hyperkalemia Hyponatremia
Potassium-conserving action				
Triamterene	Dyrenium	Oral	4-8 hr	Hyperkalemia
Osmotic agent				
Mannitol	Osmitrol	IV infused over 24-hr period	—	Hyponatremia Hypochloremia ↑ ECF volume

Pathophysiology. Sodium loss from the intravascular compartment causes fluid from the blood to diffuse into the interstitial spaces. As a result, the sodium in the interstitial fluid is diluted. In response to this reduction in sodium concentration in the extracellular fluid, potassium moves out of the intracellular fluid. Therefore the patient with a sodium imbalance is also likely to have a potassium imbalance.

The decreased osmolality of extracellular fluid that exists with sodium loss creates a condition similar to water excess; water moves into the cells by osmosis and leaves the extracellular compartment depleted. It differs from water intoxication because there is not an excess of total body water, but an intercompartmental movement of water and depletion of the extracellular compartment.

The laboratory test for plasma sodium does not always give an accurate indication of total body sodium. Some clinical conditions in which the level of serum sodium is not an accurate indicator of total body sodium can be seen in Table 21-6.

Etiology. Sodium depletion results most often from the loss of gastrointestinal secretions. This can occur through vomiting, diarrhea, gastrointestinal or biliary drainage, or fistulas. Symptoms of sodium depletion appear rapidly in patients with profuse ileostomy drain-

TABLE 21-6. Comparison of serum sodium levels with total body sodium*

Condition	Serum sodium	Total body sodium
Prolonged sweating	Low (hyponatremia)	Low
Diuretics and low sodium diets	Low	Low
Addison's disease	Low	Low
Edema (cardiac, renal, hepatic disease)	Low or normal	High
Excretion of dilute urine, early stages of gastrointestinal sodium loss	Normal	Low
Excess oral or IV sodium intake	High (hypernatremia)	High
Water and sodium loss with water loss > sodium loss	High	Low

*Note that a low or high serum level does not necessarily correspond with total body sodium.

age. Diarrhea in infants is extremely dangerous. Infants normally have large sodium losses through the skin; therefore when large amounts of sodium are lost through the bowels as well, their sodium supply quickly becomes depleted. Sodium depletion can also occur in the shifting of body fluids so that the sodium and water are "trapped" in certain body areas and are not accessible for use. This can occur in massive edema, ascites, burns, or small bowel obstruction.

Anyone who is perspiring profusely because of climate, exercise, or fever is losing large amounts of both sodium and water. A form of chronic renal disease, "salt-wasting nephritis," also causes large daily losses of sodium ions. Sodium depletion caused by any of the above conditions is aggravated by a low sodium diet.

Prevention. Athletes and persons who work in very hot environments are advised to ingest fluids containing sodium and to add some salty foods to their diets. If salt is not replaced with water, such as when thirst is quenched by drinking large amounts of tap water, water intoxication can occur. Salt tablets may be taken during the period of adaptation to an exceptionally hot environment. Diuretics such as the thiazides eventually may cause sodium depletion; therefore the patient who is receiving extensive diuretic treatment should be observed for symptoms of sodium depletion. Since many patients receiving diuretics are at home, they should be taught to report symptoms of sodium depletion to the physician. These patients should not be on severely restricted sodium diets.

Clinical picture. The symptoms of sodium depletion are headache, muscle weakness, fatigue, apathy, postural hypotension, anorexia, nausea and vomiting, and abdominal cramps. In contrast to water excess, in which there is a weight gain, with sodium deficit there is a loss of weight. As the sodium loss becomes more severe, the increase in intracellular fluid and decrease in circulating blood volume produce symptoms of mental confusion, delirium, coma, and shock. If the onset of sodium depletion is rapid, shock can ensue quickly from the sudden decrease in blood volume.

Intervention. Treatment of shock, if present, is the first concern of the physician. Saline solution, usually 0.9% sodium chloride, is given intravenously at a rapid rate. Plasma expanders may also be infused.

If other electrolytes (potassium, calcium, bicarbonate) have been depleted, these also need to be replaced. Treatment that alleviates the underlying cause will prevent further sodium loss. Salt or salty foods are added to the diet for sodium depletion, which develops slowly or follows profuse perspiration (diaphoresis) or vomiting. (See Chapter 20 for a more detailed description of the treatment.)

Safety measures, such as the use of side rails on the bed, supervision of ambulation, and frequent observation, are necessary if the patient becomes weak or confused or experiences marked hypotension.

Excess

A serum sodium level greater than 145 mEq/L is known as *hypernatremia*. There are actually two kinds of sodium excess, edema or hypernatremia. When there is a sodium and water excess, edema exists; when there is an excess of sodium in relation to water in the extracellular compartment, hypernatremia exists. As seen in Table 21-6, hypernatremia does not necessarily indicate an excess of total body sodium.

Pathophysiology. If sodium becomes concentrated in the extracellular fluid, osmolality rises, water leaves the cells by osmosis and enters the extracellular compartment to dilute fluids there, and the cells are water depleted. The presence of hypernatremia will suppress aldosterone secretion, and sodium will be excreted in the urine.

Etiology. Hypernatremia occurs when more water than sodium is lost from the body and sodium concentration in the blood rises. It can also result from an abnormally large oral intake of sodium, such as when a child accidentally eats many salt tablets, or when intravenous saline is infused so rapidly that the body cannot excrete the amount not needed.

Prevention. Sodium excess can be prevented in persons whose ability to excrete it is impaired. Persons with kidney failure, congestive heart failure, or increased aldosterone production need to have sodium intake restricted. Whenever intravenous electrolyte solutions are being given, the urinary output must be adequate so that portions of the electrolytes not needed by the body can be excreted. This usually means that fluid intake should not exceed urinary output.

Clinical picture. Hypernatremia causes dry, sticky mucous membranes, low urinary output, and firm, "rubbery" tissue turgor. If adequate fluid is not given to dilute the sodium, and if excretion of sodium is not increased, severe fluid and electrolyte imbalances will occur, and manic excitement, tachycardia, and eventual death will ensue.

Intervention. Water alone is given in the treatment of sodium excess. If cardiac and renal function are normal, a liberal amount of water is administered orally or 5% dextrose in water is given intravenously. In the absence of normal cardiac and renal function, hydration must be carried out with caution to prevent fluid overloading in the patient.

Diuretics are of value in removing sodium. If sodium excess is severe, with or without excess water retention, and does not respond to other treatment, renal dialysis may be necessary.

Potassium

The normal concentration of potassium in the blood is 3.5 to 5.0 mEq/L. Because most of the potassium in the body is intracellular, the serum potassium level does not necessarily indicate the total body potassium content. Maintenance of serum potassium within normal range, however, is vital to normal body functions.

Potassium has a direct effect on the excitability of nerves and muscles, contributes most to the intracellular osmotic pressure, and helps maintain acid-base balance and normal kidney function. A potassium deficit is associated with excess alkalinity (alkalosis) of the body fluids, and a potassium excess accompanies an excess of acid (acidosis). These conditions are discussed later in this chapter.

Potassium is the major cation of the cells. During the formation of new tissues (anabolism) or when glucose is converted to glycogen, potassium enters the cell. With tissue breakdown (catabolism) such as occurs with trauma, dehydration, or starvation, potassium leaves the cell. The body conserves potassium less effectively than it conserves sodium, and the kidneys excrete potassium even when the body needs it. Normally about 5% of the total body potassium is excreted each day.

Deficit

A low level of serum potassium, below 3.5 mEq/L, is known as *hypokalemia*.

Pathophysiology. Movement of sodium (inward) and potassium (outward) across the cell membrane causes depolarization of the membrane and initiates an action potential creating nerve and muscle activity. When extracellular potassium is low, the resting membrane potential increases (hyperpolarization) and the cell becomes less excitable. For this reason the major symptoms of hypokalemia are muscle weakness and atony.

Potassium is involved in acid-base balance because it moves out of the cells when hydrogen ions move to the intracellular compartment in acidosis; therefore hyperkalemia accompanies acidosis. As the acidosis is treated, potassium moves back into the cells and hypokalemia may develop. In alkalosis, hypokalemia usually develops because of movement of potassium into cells and also because potassium is excreted by the kidneys while hydrogen ions are being retained.

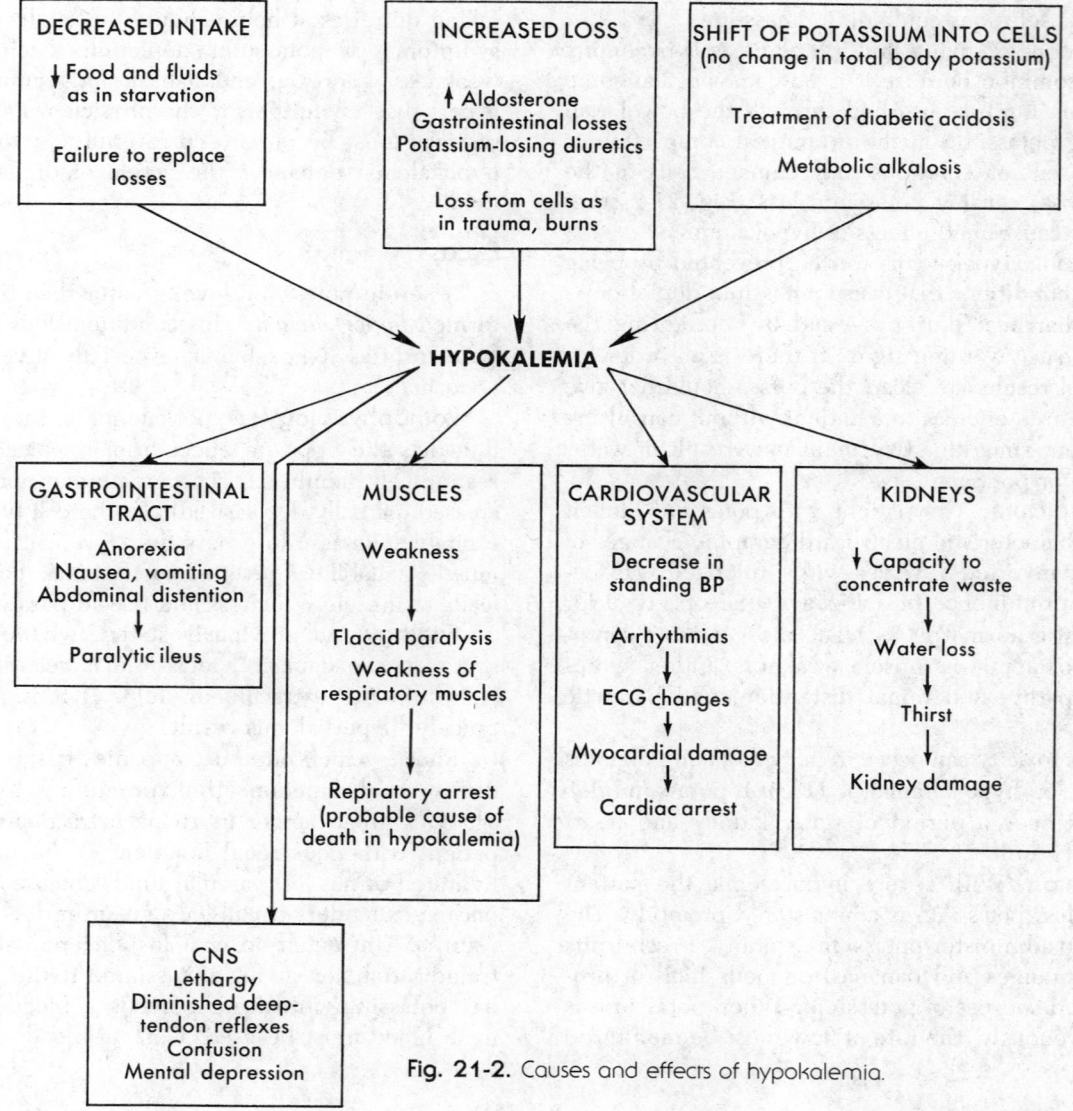

Fig. 21-2. Causes and effects of hypokalemia.

Whenever sodium is being retained in the body through reabsorption by the kidney tubules, potassium is excreted. Thus whenever aldosterone secretion is increased such as in stress, potassium will be excreted. Potassium may also be lost in the urine when there is considerable urinary output and as a result of certain diuretics such as the thiazide derivatives, the latter being the most common cause of hypokalemia.

Etiology. The patient who has food withheld for several days, is dehydrated, or is given large amounts of parenteral fluids with no replacement of potassium develops potassium depletion. The parenteral administration of 5% dextrose in water without the addition of potassium tends to dilute the potassium in the extracellular tissues. This dilution, in addition to the lack of a balanced diet and to potassium loss caused by catabolism of body proteins, accounts for many instances of electrolyte imbalance in the postoperative patient. Patients who eat an inadequate diet, who take no food for an extended period of time, or who are losing large amounts of fluid from the gastrointestinal tract through diarrhea or a draining fistula usually are given intravenous glucose solutions containing potassium.

The practice of giving multiple enemas is becoming much less common because it is now known that some of the enema fluid is absorbed through the bowel wall diluting the potassium in the interstitial compartment. Hypertonic enema solutions may damage cells in the bowel mucosa, causing potassium loss. Fig. 21-2 summarizes the causes and effects of hypokalemia.

Prevention. Hypokalemia can be prevented by being alert to the conditions that cause potassium depletion—vomiting, diarrhea, diuretics—and by monitoring the patient for early warning signs. If there is an order for enemas until results are clear, the nurse should not give more than three enemas to a patient without consulting the physician, since this treatment may result in water intoxication or potassium loss.

Clinical picture. The patient with potassium deficit will show characteristic electrocardiographic changes of flattened or inverted T waves with prolonged QT segments and prominence of a U wave. (See p. 1049 for discussion of a normal ECG.) The most striking symptom of hypokalemia is muscle weakness. Other symptoms are apathy, abdominal distention, and paralytic ileus.

Digitalis toxicity can occur in persons taking digitalis if they develop hypokalemia (p. 1133). If potassium deficit persists over a period of time, kidney and heart damage will result.

Interventon. With severe hypokalemia the patient may die unless potassium is administered promptly. The safest way to administer potassium is orally. Fresh fruits (especially oranges and bananas) or foods high in protein are good sources of potassium. When potassium is given intravenously, the rate of flow must be monitored

closely in order to prevent hyperkalemia and atrial arrest. The usual rate of infusion should not exceed 20 mEq/L of potassium per hour. Since potassium is irritating to the veins, it is given very diluted, usually 20 to 40 mEq/L of intravenous solution. In some instances potassium will be given at a greater concentration (40 mEq/100 ml) per 4 hours. When potassium is administered in this concentration it must be given through a central vein and must be delivered by a controlled infusion pump such as an IVAC. Because of the potential cardiovascular complications that can occur with this concentration of potassium, the patient must be on a cardiac monitor so that changes in cardiac status will be identified immediately.

Persons who are receiving potassium-losing diuretics (p. 335) should be instructed to include foods high in potassium in their diet (Table 21-7). If low serum potassium levels are shown to result from diuretic therapy, a potassium supplement may be ordered by the physician, usually in the form of potassium chloride (elixir of potassium chloride), or a potassium-sparing diuretic such as triamterene (Dyrenium) may be used. Persons taking diuretics at home should be taught to recognize symptoms of potassium depletion, such as muscle weakness, anorexia, and nausea and vomiting, and to report these symptoms to the physician. Patients taking digitalis must be monitored carefully for toxicity, since hypokalemia enhances the action of digitalis preparations.

Excess

A serum potassium level greater than 5.0 mEq/L is termed *hyperkalemia*. This condition does not occur as frequently as hypokalemia, especially if renal function is normal.

Pathophysiology. Hyperkalemia in the extracellular fluid has the opposite effect from hypokalemia on the resting cell membrane. The membrane potential is decreased (partially depolarized) and the cell becomes more excitable. Potassium excess therefore causes nerve and muscle irritability. Severe hyperkalemia, however, soon leads to muscle weakness and flaccid paralysis.

Etiology. As previously stated, whenever there is severe tissue damage, potassium is released from the cells into the extracellular fluid. If it is not excreted quickly, hyperkalemia results.

Shock, which often accompanies tissue damage, reduces renal function, thus promoting hyperkalemia. There is great danger in giving extra potassium to any patient with poor renal function. If the patient is dehydrated or has lost vascular fluid, glucose and water or plasma expanders usually are given until renal function returns. Untreated adrenal insufficiency also is a contraindication for giving potassium. If the patient who has potassium intoxication needs a blood transfusion, fresh blood must be used. Cells in blood that has been

TABLE 21-7. Foods high in potassium

Food	Approximate amount	Potassium (mEq)	Food	Approximate amount	Potassium (mEq)
Fruits			Buttermilk	1 cup	8.5
Apricots			Skim	1 cup	8.8
Canned	½ cup	6.0	Powdered, skim	¼ cup	13.5
Dried	4 halves	5.0	Vegetables*		
Fresh	3 small	8.0	Asparagus		
Banana	1 small	9.6	Fresh	½ cup	4.7
Strawberries	1 cup	6.3	Frozen	½ cup	5.5
Grapefruit sections	¾ cup	5.1	Beans		
Melon			Dried, cooked	½ cup	10.0
Cantaloupe	½ small	13.0	Lima	½ cup	9.5
Honeydew	¼ medium	13.0	Beet greens	½ cup	8.5
Watermelon	½ slice	5.0	Broccoli	½ cup	7.0
Nectarine	1 medium	6.0	Cabbage, raw	1 cup	6.0
Orange	1 medium	5.1	Carrots, raw	1 large	8.8
Orange juice	½ cup	5.7	Celery, raw	1 cup	9.0
Peach			Collards	½ cup	6.0
Dried	2 halves	5.0	Mushrooms, raw	4 large	10.6
Fresh	1 medium	6.2	Mustard greens	½ cup	5.5
Protein foods			Peas, dried	½ cup	6.8
Beef	3 oz	8.4	Potato		
Chicken	3 oz	9.0	Baked, white	½ cup	13.0
Frankfurters	1	3.0	Boiled, white	½ cup	7.3
Liver	3 oz	9.6	Baked, sweet	½ cup	8.0
Pork	3 oz	9.0	Spinach	½ cup	8.5
Veal	3 oz	11.4	Tomatoes	½ cup	6.5
Scallops	1 large	6.0	Brussels sprouts	⅔ cup	7.6
Turkey	3 oz	8.4	Squash, winter, baked	½ cup	12.0
Milk			Miscellaneous†		
Whole	1 cup	8.8	Peanut butter	2 tbsp	5.0
Powdered, whole	¼ cup		Nuts, unsalted	25	4.5

*Most raw vegetables contain potassium, much of which is lost during cooking.
†Beverages that contain large amounts of potassium are cocoa, cola drinks, and dry, instant coffee and tea.

kept for several days tend to release potassium during storage. Administration of stored blood may increase the patient's blood potassium level still further. Fig. 21-3 shows the causes and effects of hyperkalemia.

Prevention. Hyperkalemia can be anticipated and prevented in patients who for any reason have a significant decrease in urinary output, especially if they are receiving oral or intravenous potassium preparations.

Clinical picture. The patient with potassium intoxication develops spasticity of muscles because of their overstimulation by nerve impulses. The patient complains of nausea, colic, diarrhea, and skeletal muscle spasms. The muscles later become weak because overstimulation produces an accumulation of lactic acid and because potassium is lost from the muscle cells.

If the condition is not controlled, overstimulation of the cardiac muscle will cause the heartbeat to become irregular and eventually stop. ECG evidence of potassium elevation includes tall, peaked, symmetric, or tented T waves with a short QT segment. As the blood potassium level increases further, the QRS complex spreads and atrial arrest occurs.[1]

Intervention. When potassium intoxication occurs, the patient is allowed nothing orally, and an infusion of 10% glucose with 50 units of insulin is often given to induce transfer of potassium from the serum to the intracellular fluid. If the patient is in acidosis, correction of the acidosis will result in movement of potassium back into the cell (p. 356). Cation exchange resins such as sodium polystyrene sulfonate (Kayexalate) may also be given. If the patient is in acute renal failure, dialysis may be necessary. Calcium, given intravenously, will antagonize the effect of potassium on the heart.

The patient with potassium excess is placed on bed rest and receives complete nursing care until the potassium blood level returns to normal.

Patients who retain potassium secondary to renal failure or a decrease in aldosterone will need instruc-

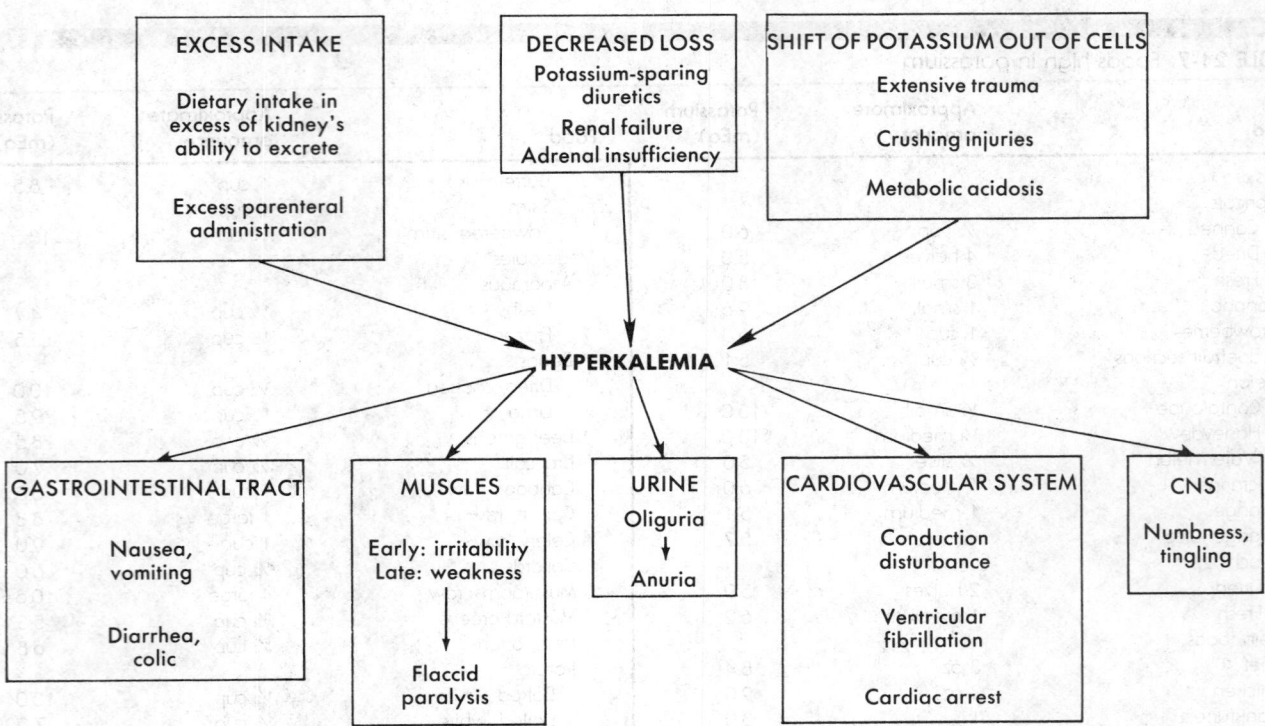

Fig. 21-3. Causes and effects of hyperkalemia.

tion in restricting foods high in potassium (Table 21-7). If salt substitutes are being used, patients need to be aware that these usually contain potassium as a substitute for sodium.

Cation exchange resins act by exchanging other cations in the resin for potassium in the intestine; the potassium is then excreted in the stool. Maintenance of good bowel function is necessary for this therapy to be effective.

Calcium

The normal calcium level in the blood is 4.5 to 5.8 mEq/L. Calcium in the blood is in two forms: ionized and bound to plasma proteins. Free, ionized calcium is needed for (1) blood coagulation; (2) smooth, skeletal, and cardiac muscle function; (3) nerve functions; and (4) bone and teeth formation. Only the ionized calcium is physiologically active. *Vitamin D* is necessary for absorption of calcium from the gastrointestinal tract and in mobilization of calcium from bones.

Both vitamin D and parathyroid hormone must be present for calcium absorption from the gastrointestinal tract (p. 306). Calcium is excreted principally through the gastrointestinal tract, with very small amounts being lost in the urine.

Deficit

Hypocalcemia is a decrease of the serum calcium level to below 4.5 mEq/L.

Pathophysiology. It is thought that calcium ions line the pores of cell membranes. Since both calcium and sodium ions carry a positive charge, they tend to repel each other. The presence of calcium in the pores of cells (especially neurons) through which sodium must pass for depolarization to take place has a blocking effect on this permeability to sodium. When calcium levels in the blood are low, this blocking effect is minimized, sodium moves more easily into the cell, and depolarization with resulting action potential takes place more readily.[13] The result is increased excitability of the nervous system leading to muscle spasm, tingling sensations, and if severe, to convulsions and tetany. Skeletal, smooth, and cardiac muscle function are all affected by overstimulation.

Etiology. Calcium deficit results from inadequate intake, vitamin D deficiency, hypoparathyroidism, interruption of normal calcium absorption from the gastrointestinal tract, and excess loss of calcium through the kidneys.

Patients with pancreatic disease or disease of the small intestine may fail to absorb calcium normally from the gastrointestinal tract, and they may excrete large amounts of calcium in the feces. Persons with chronic pancreati-

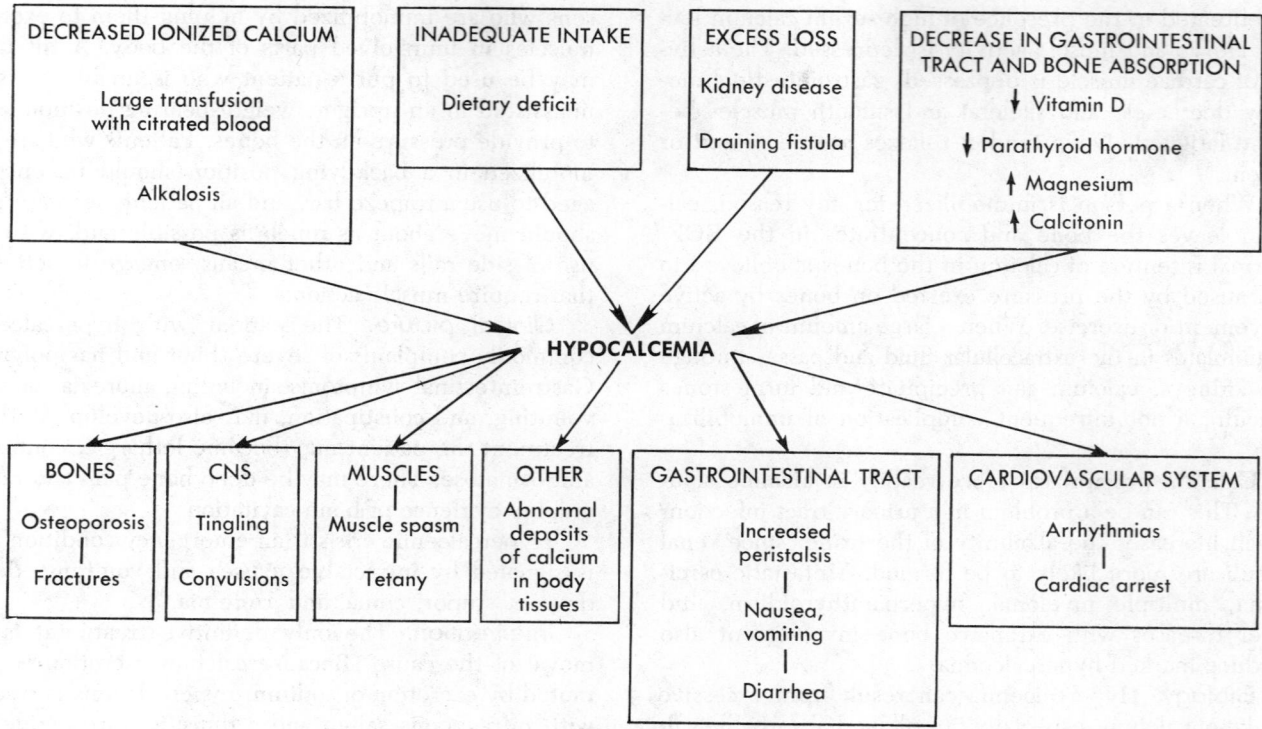

Fig. 21-4. Causes and effects of hypocalcemia.

tis have persistent hypocalcemia. Draining intestinal fistulas also cause excess calcium loss. These causes and effects are shown in Fig. 21-4.

Prevention. Calcium deficiency can be prevented by alertness to conditions of inadequate intake, excess calcium loss, or vitamin D deficiency. Patients who are on extremely poor diets or who have calcium-depleting conditions should be monitored for signs of hypocalcemia. Teaching persons with low calcium and vitamin D intake to include more of these nutrients in the diet is an important nursing action.

Clinical picture. Tetany is the most characteristic sign of severe hypocalcemia. The patient who has calcium deficiency usually complains first of numbness and tingling of the nose, ears, fingertips, or toes. If calcium is not given at this time, painful muscular spasms (tetany), especially of the feet and hands, muscle twitching, and convulsions may follow.

There are two tests used to elicit signs of calcium deficiency. *Trousseau's sign* is elicited by grasping the patient's wrist or inflating a blood pressure cuff on the upper arm to constrict the circulation for a few minutes. If the hand goes into a position of palmar flexion (carpopedal spasm), the person probably has a serious calcium deficit. *Chvostek's sign* is elicited by tapping the patient's face lightly over the facial nerve (just below the temple). A calcium deficit is probably present if the facial muscles twitch.

Intervention. The drug of choice in treating calcium deficiency is a 10% solution of calcium gluconate given slowly.[2] In milder cases, high calcium diet or oral calcium salts may be sufficient. When decreased parathyroid hormone or vitamin D is the causative factor, these substances must be supplied. When the serum phosphorus level rises, the calcium level falls; aluminum hydroxide gel can be given to lower a high serum phosphorus concentration.

Any patient who has had thyroid surgery must be watched very closely for symptoms of calcium deficiency (tetany), since there is a possibility that parathyroid glands may have been inadvertently removed with the thyroid tissue or may be temporarily suppressed by local edema.

Since chronic hypocalcemia can result in loss of calcium from bone to replenish low serum calcium, persons with this condition must be carefully moved, turned, or ambulated to prevent fractures of the demineralized bone. Calcium preparations must be given with caution to cardiac patients, since calcium has an effect on the heart similar to digitalis.

Excess

A serum calcium level above 5.8 mEq/L is called *hypercalcemia*.

Pathophysiology. The blocking effect of calcium on cell membrane permeability, as previously discussed, is accentuated in the presence of high serum calcium levels. Nerve and muscle activity is depressed. The activity of cardiac muscle is depressed, gastrointestinal motility decreases, and skeletal and smooth muscles become fatigued. Deep tendon reflexes are decreased or absent.[45]

When a person is immobilized for any reason, calcium leaves the bone and concentrates in the ECF. Normal retention of calcium in the bones is believed to be caused by the pressure exerted on bones by active movement or exercise. When a large amount of calcium accumulates in the extracellular fluid and passes through the kidneys, calcium can precipitate and form stones (calculi), a not infrequent complication of immobilization.

Calcium precipitates more readily in alkaline solution. This can be a problem in a urinary tract infection, which increases the alkalinity of the urine, since renal calculi are more likely to be formed. Metastatic carcinoma, multiple myeloma, hyperparathyroidism, and other diseases with extensive bone involvement also produce marked hypercalcemia.

Etiology. Hypercalcemia can result from excessive intake of calcium, especially in milk and absorbable calcium-containing antacids (milk-alkali syndrome), from excessive vitamin D intake, and from conditions that promote release of calcium from the bones into the extracellular fluid. These causes and their effects are shown in Fig. 21-5.

Prevention. Hypercalcemia can be alleviated in persons who are immobilized by helping them to exercise muscles in uninvolved parts of the body. A tilt table may be used to put a patient who is unable to stand unassisted in an upright, weight-bearing position so as to provide pressure on the bones. Patients who are immobilized in a back-lying position should be encouraged to use a trapeze bar, and all patients who are able should move about as much as possible and, with the use of side rails and other means, engage in activities that require muscle action.

Clinical picture. The patient with hypercalcemia commonly complains of severe thirst and has polyuria. Gastrointestinal symptoms, including anorexia, nausea, vomiting, and constipation, may also develop. Without treatment the patient may become lethargic, confused, and comatose. There may be deep bone pain and radiographic evidence of bone cavitation.

Hypercalcemic crisis is an emergency condition that is signaled by intractable nausea and vomiting, dehydration, stupor, coma, and azotemia.[36]

Intervention. The only definitive treatment is removal of the cause. Because calcium excretion is promoted by excretion of sodium, hypercalcemia is treated with intravenous saline and a diuretic (furosemide). If this treatment fails, inorganic phosphate preparations given orally or intravenously may be effective. Mithramycin (Mithracin), a potent antitumor drug, has been used successfully to reduce serum calcium. If the hypercalcemia is caused by multiple myeloma or other cancers, glucocorticoids may be effective in reducing

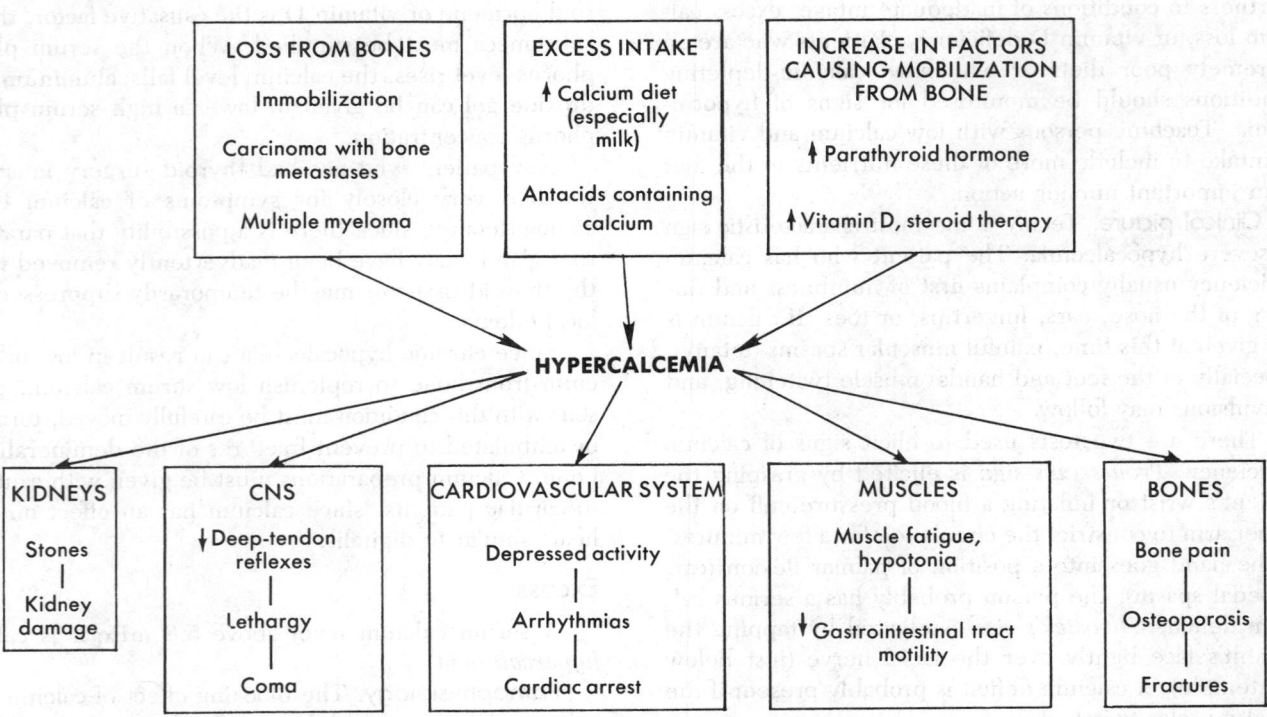

Fig. 21-5. Causes and effects of hypercalcemia.

hypercalcemia either because they decrease the size of the tumor or because the effect of the tumor on bone is reduced.

Because persons with marked hypercalcemia often are losing calcium from their bones or have malignant involvement of bone, special care should be taken to prevent pathologic fractures. Even the pressure used in giving a back rub must sometimes be avoided.

Careful attention must be directed to the prevention of calcium stone formation in the kidneys. Acid-ash fruit juices, cranberry and prune juice, or ascorbic acid can be given to promote urinary acidification and discourage stone formation. Urinary tract infections must be avoided. Good perineal care and meticulous technique in caring for Foley catheters are mandatory.

Unless contraindicated, persons with hypercalcemia are encouraged to drink 3000 to 4000 ml of fluids per day to reduce the possibility of renal calculi and to overcome the thirst that accompanies hypercalcemia.

Magnesium

The normal serum magnesium level is within the range of 1.5 to 2.5 mEq/L. About 50% of magnesium is located in bones, 5% in extracellular fluid, and the remaining 45% in the intracellular compartment. It functions in the activation of enzymatic reactions, especially in carbohydrate metabolism. Magnesium has a sedative effect on the central nervous system similar to that of calcium. It has been used successfully to prevent convulsions in toxemia of pregnancy. High serum levels result in vasodilation with lowering of blood pressure.

Deficit

Hypomagnesemia is a serum magnesium level below 1.5 mEq/L.

Pathophysiology. A low serum magnesium level leads to increased neuromuscular irritability by increasing acetylcholine release, increasing the sensitivity of the myoneural junction to acetylcholine, diminishing the threshold of excitation of the motor nerve, and enhancing the force of contraction of the myofibril.[25]

In the presence of a large amount of calcium in the gastrointestinal tract, calcium is absorbed in preference to magnesium and the magnesium is excreted. Conversely, low calcium levels increase magnesium absorption. The kidneys effectively conserve magnesium when intake is low. Hypocalcemia and hypokalemia that are unresponsive to therapy may indicate hypomagnesemia.[10] Metabolically, magnesium is closely interrelated with both calcium and potassium.

Etiology. Hypomagnesemia may be caused by impaired absorption from the gastrointestinal tract, excess loss through the kidneys, or prolonged malnutrition states. Patients in withdrawal from alcohol are frequently hypomagnesemic. Fig. 21-6 shows some of the causes and effects of magnesium deficit.

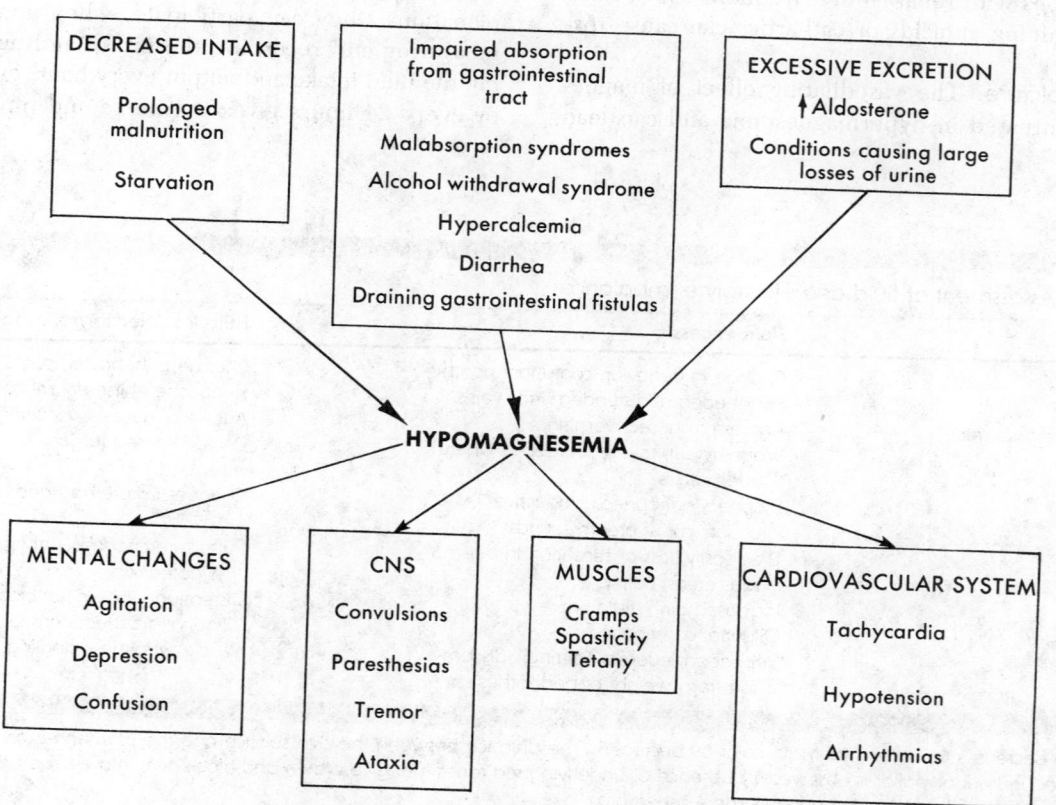

Fig. 21-6. Causes and effects of hypomagnesemia.

Prevention. Dietary teaching and management can help to prevent magnesium deficit, especially in persons with magnesium-depleting conditions. Fruits, green vegetables, whole grain cereals, milk, meats, and nuts are good dietary sources of magnesium.

Clinical picture. Hypomagnesemia is usually manifested by behavioral and neurologic symptoms such as confusion, hallucinations, convulsions, increased reflexes, tremors, muscle spasms, and paresthesias.

Intervention. Treatment of magnesium deficit consists of correction of the underlying cause and the administration of magnesium salts orally or parenterally. Providing for patients' safety until the magnesium deficit is corrected is the prime nursing responsibility. Careful observation and supervision of the patient who is confused or hallucinating and protective measures for patients who develop convulsions will prevent injury.

Excess

Hypermagnesemia is a serum magnesium level greater than 2.5 mEq/L.

Pathophysiology. The action of magnesium is on the myoneural junction where a high magnesium level blocks acetylcholine release, decreasing the excitability of the muscle cells.

Etiology. Hypermagnesemia seldom develops unless there is renal failure, although it has been identified in diabetic ketoacidosis where there is severe water loss. In persons with renal failure, frequent use of magnesium-containing antacids or cathartics can cause toxicity.

Clinical picture. The vasodilating effect of magnesium is accentuated in hypermagnesemia and can lead to hypotension. A very high magnesium level can cause loss of deep tendon reflexes, respiratory depression, and cardiac arrest.[10]

Intervention. Correction of the underlying cause will correct the magnesium excess. If renal failure is present, dialysis will be necessary. Intravenous calcium gluconate may be a useful temporary treatment, since calcium has an antagonistic effect on magnesium.

Assessment of fluid and electrolyte imbalance

The nurse needs to recognize the symptoms of fluid and electrolyte imbalance and make ongoing physical assessments of those patients who have a potential for fluid and electrolyte imbalances (Table 21-8). For subjective data such as headache, thirst, nausea, or dyspnea, time of onset and extent of symptoms are ascertained. Objective data can be compared to baseline assessments made at the time of the patient's entry into the health system.

Data of particular importance in assessing fluid and electrolyte imbalance are comparison of fluid intake to output and changes in the patient's weight. Acutely ill medical patients and patients undergoing major surgery should have their fluid intake and output and daily weight closely monitored. If patients and families are given explanations, they can participate, when appropriate, in measuring and recording the intake and output. Totaling the fluid intake and output every hour, every 8 hours, or every 24 hours gives the nurse and physician addi-

TABLE 21-8. Assessment of fluid and electrolyte imbalance

	Fluid excess	Fluid loss/electrolyte imbalance
Behavior	Change in behavior, confusion, apathy	Change in behavior, confusion, apathy
Head, neck	Facial edema, distended neck veins.	Headache, thirst, dry mucous membranes
Upper gastrointestinal tract	Anorexia, nausea, vomiting	Anorexia, nausea, vomiting
Skin	Warm, moist, taut, cool feeling where edematous	Dry, decreased turgor
Respiration	Dyspnea, orthopnea, productive cough, moist breath sounds	Changes in rate and depth of breathing
Circulation	Tires easily, loss of sensation in edematous areas, pallor*	Pulse rate changes, arrhythmias, postural hypotension
Abdomen	Increased girth, fluid wave	Distention, abdominal cramps
Elimination	Oliguria, constipation	Oliguria, diarrhea, constipation
Extremities	Dependent edema, "pitting," discomfort from weight of bedclothes	Muscle weakness, tingling, tetany

*Pallor-edema decreases the intensity of skin color by decreasing the distance between the skin surface and the pigmented or vascular areas. In the dark-skinned individual, pallor is observed by absence of underlying red tones that give brown and black skin "glow." The brown skin appears more yellow-brown and the black skin appears more ashen gray.[40]

tional data for determining if the patient may have a fluid imbalance.

Since symptoms of fluid and electrolyte imbalance are sometimes not very specific, a good rule is to be alert for any changes in behavior, level of consciousness, vital signs, skin turgor, muscle strength, and condition of mucous membranes. Baseline obervations made during the first encounter with a patient are essential for comparison with subsequent observations in order to be able to detect changes.

Intake record

The intake record should show the type and amount of all fluids the patient has received and the route by which these were administered. This includes fluids given orally, parenterally, rectally, or fluids administered by tubes. A record of solid food intake is sometimes necessary, especially with very young children. Foods that are eaten in a semisolid state but which are basically liquid, such as gelatin or ice cream, are recorded as fluids. Ice chips are recorded by dividing the amount of chips by one half (60 ml of chips would equal 30 ml of water). Patients may receive a considerable amount of fluid intake through the frequent sucking of ice chips.

Urinary output

Urinary output is recorded as to time and amount of each voiding. If renal function is a major concern, as in a severely burned patient, an indwelling catheter is used so that the amount of urinary drainage can be recorded every hour and fluid intake regulated accordingly. It has been said that nothing is more difficult to obtain in a modern hospital than an accurate record of urinary output, and unfortunately this statement is often true. Conspicuous signs posted on the patient's chart and in the utility room and bathrooms will help to prevent the discarding of urine before it is measured. Flow sheets kept close to the patient's room facilitate the recording of intake and output and other patient data.

Wound drainage

All drainage from body orifices or artificial openings should be measured. This would include such drainage as that from an ileostomy, from a T tube following exploration of the common bile duct, or from any catheter draining a surgical area. If there is excessive drainage from a wound, it may be necessary to weigh the dressings. Fluid loss is the difference between the wet weight and the dry weight of the dressing.

Gastrointestinal output

Vomitus, gastrointestinal drainage, and liquid stools are measured as accurately as possible and are described as to color, content, and odor. Gastric secretions are watery and a pale yellowish green; they usually have a sour odor. However, if the acid-base balance has been upset, gastric secretions may have a fruity odor because of the presence of ketone bodies (acetone). Bile is somewhat thicker than gastric juice and may vary from bright yellow to dark green in color. It has a bitter taste and acrid odor. Intestinal contents vary from dark green to brown in color, are likely to be quite thick, and have a fecal odor. The amount of fluid retained during irrigation of nasogastric tubes is added to "intake" and needs to be subtracted from total drainage before it is recorded.

It is difficult to determine accurately the amount of water lost in the stools, but a description of their consistency and a record of the number of stools passed gives a good estimate. The color of stools is also recorded. Because infants are likely to lose large amounts of water in their stools, daily records usually are kept for any baby who is ill.

Other output

Fluid aspirated from any body cavity such as the abdomen (paracentesis) or pleural spaces (thoracentesis) must be measured. The fluid contains not only electrolytes and water but also proteins. Blood loss from any part of the body is measured carefully.

Diaphoresis is difficult to measure without special laboratory equipment; however, it may be important to estimate the loss of fluid by this route in some patients. Careful note of "excessive" perspiration and its duration is made. If the clothing and linen become saturated, dry and wet weights may be taken. Accurate recording of body temperature helps the physician to determine how much fluid should be replaced, since fluid loss through the skin and lungs increases as the temperature rises. A patient with a high fever and who is breathing rapidly can lose as much as 2500 ml/day through the lungs.[12]

Daily weight

The daily weight record is often the best way to determine the onset of dehydration or the accumulation of fluid either as generalized edema or as "hidden" fluid in body cavities. An increase of 1 kg in weight is equal to the retention of 1 L (1000 ml) of fluid in the edematous patient. If the weight record is to be accurate, the patient must be weighed on the same scale and at the same hour each day and must be wearing the same amount of clothing. Circumstances that may affect the weight should be kept as nearly identical as possible from day to day. Usually weights are taken in the early morning before the patient has eaten or defecated, but after voiding. When extremely accurate measurements are needed, all clothing and even wound dressings are removed before the patient is weighed. A person maintained on intravenous fluids alone can be expected to lose approximately 0.2 to 0.5 kg/day (p. 301).

Laboratory values

Laboratory determinations of serum levels of the specific electrolytes help in making decisions concerning electrolyte excesses or deficits. When there is water excess, hemodilution will occur and the hematocrit, hemoglobin, BUN, and electrolyte levels will be decreased. With excessive fluid loss there will be hemoconcentration, and the hematocrit, hemoglobin, BUN, and electrolyte levels will be increased.

Replacement and maintenance of water, electrolytes, and nutrients

Replacement of the water and electrolyte losses from the body and the necessary daily intake of these substances and other nutrients are usually accomplished by one of the following methods: (1) oral intake, (2) tube feeding (gavage), (3) intravenous infusion, and (4) parenteral hyperalimentation.

The best way to administer water, electrolytes, and nutrients is to give them orally. When fluids can be tolerated by the stomach but cannot be swallowed, a nasogastric tube may be passed, and fluids containing all the essentials of a balanced diet may be given through it. Normal saline solution or plain water also may be given by slow drip through the tube to replace fluid loss and provide for daily fluid needs.

If it is not possible for a patient to take food or fluid through the alimentary tract, the most common method of replacement is by intravenous infusion. In adults a vein in the leg or arm is commonly used, but in infants a vein in the scalp or the femoral or jugular vein may be used. An intravenous infusion may be given by introducing a needle or intracatheter into a vein and tapping the needle in place or by making an incision (cutdown) and threading a polyethylene catheter (intracatheter) into the vein. The intracatheter is the method of choice for parenteral hyperalimentation in which a concentrated nutrient solution is infused into the superior vena cava.

Fluids given by any route should be spaced throughout the 24-hour period. Not only does this practice help to maintain normal body fluid levels, but it also provides for better regulation of the electrolyte balance by the kidneys and prevents the end products of metabolism and toxic materials from being excreted in concentrated form. In this way the danger of renal damage, formation of calculi, and irritation of the lower urinary tract is reduced. In addition, fluid spacing prevents overloading of the circulation, which may result in dilution of body fluids, with resultant fluid and electrolyte shifts, the most serious of which causes pulmonary edema (p. 1135).

Concentrated solutions of sugar or protein should always be given slowly and in small amounts at a time because they require body fluids for dilution. Hypertonic saline solutions may cause fluid to diffuse from the tissues to equalize the concentration of salt in the vascular compartment; therefore it too should be given slowly and in small amounts. The superior vena cava is the preferred site for infusions of hypertonic solutions given by parenteral hyperalimentation because of the rapid dilution by the larger amount of blood at this site. If any of these concentrated solutions flows too rapidly into the vascular system, pulmonary edema can develop.

Giving concentrated solutions rapidly and in large amounts into the alimentary tract causes a rapid shift of fluid from the vascular compartment into the intestinal lumen and a resultant decrease in blood volume, which can lead to shock. The "dumping syndrome," which sometimes occurs after a gastric resection, is caused by this abnormal shift of fluid. Concentrated solutions sometimes are given intentionally to reduce cerebral edema (p. 757). Giving large amounts of fluid either orally or parenterally is potentially dangerous even in a healthy person, and therefore fluids of any kind should never be replaced faster than they are lost.

The size of the patient should be considered when administering fluids. The small adult normally has less fluid in each body compartment, especially in the intravascular system. This person therefore becomes seriously dehydrated more quickly than a larger adult and needs fluid losses replaced more promptly. Prompt replacement is even more important in infants and young children. Because so much of their body fluid normally is extracellular, they have proportionately less reserve fluid in the cells from which to pull than has a small adult (see Fig. 20-3). People with small or inelastic vascular systems also become overhydrated easily. It is important to remember that the vascular system of a person who has had a large portion of the body such as a limb removed either by surgery or trauma is not the same size as previously.

Oral intake

Adults who have no circulatory or renal malfunction usually are given between 2500 and 3000 ml/day. Precautions should be taken so that the overzealous patient does not drink too much fluid in a day or does not take too much (3 to 4 glasses) at one time. Excessive water intake may cause water intoxication.

Many persons, when ill, find it difficult to eat or drink even though they are allowed to do so. There are many ways that the nurse can help the patient take adequate food and fluids orally and thus avoid the need for parenteral fluids. Fruit drinks, tea, coffee, ginger ale, or other soft drinks may be substituted for part of the water. Soup, bouillon, milk, eggnog, and cocoa provide both fluid and nutrients. Juicy fruits and other semisolid foods with a high fluid and nutrient content, such as custard, ice cream, or gelatin, may be more palatable than regular meals and tap water. Care must be taken, of course, that any substitutions are allowed on the diet prescribed for the patient. If a fluid record is needed, the amount of fluid given in semisolid form is estimated and recorded. A juicy orange, for example, contains about 50 ml of fluid.

The methods used in presenting food and fluids to patients may influence their consumption; often a small amount of either food or fluid offered at frequent intervals is more acceptable than is a large amount presented less often. Serving foods that the patient likes may improve appetite. For example, carbonated beverages may be better tolerated by patients who are nauseated. Consideration should always be given to the cultural and esthetic aspects of eating.

Vomiting and diarrhea are common symptoms of many illnesses, and most people suffer from them from time to time. Sodium and some potassium are lost in vomiting and diarrhea, while chloride is lost only in vomitus. As soon as fluids are tolerated, the patient who has vomiting or diarrhea should be served salty broth and tea or another fluid high in potassium (see Table 21-7) in order to replace the losses. This measure often keeps the patient from feeling so weak and exhausted. Dry soda crackers often are tolerated when fluids are not and can be used to replace sodium. If vomiting or diarrhea persists for even a few hours and oral foods are not tolerated, infants should have medical attention, since they may need intravenous replacement of losses.

A patient with a draining fistula from any portion of the gastrointestinal tract loses sodium, calcium, and potassium, and dietary supplements are necessary. Extra milk will replace all the losses, and the patient is instructed to increase milk intake somewhat above normal levels. For the body to use the calcium, vitamin D also must be available, but most milk is now fortified with vitamin D. Persons with a permanent fistulous opening, such as an ileostomy, need to be especially careful to supplement sodium and potassium when vomiting, diarrhea, or fever add to their already unusually large loss of electrolytes.

The nurse needs to know which foods contain large and small amounts of various essential nutrients, minerals, and vitamins (see Chapter 52). When losses must be restored, the patient needs more than is required in the usual adequate diet. It is especially important to know which foods and fluids are high or low in potassium and sodium and which foods are complete proteins. Bananas, citrus fruits, all fruit juices, many fresh vegetables, coffee, and tea are relatively high in potassium and low in sodium content. Salty broths and tomato juice provide extra sodium but have a high potassium content. Meat, milk, and eggs are all complete protein foods and contain relatively large quantities of both sodium and potassium. Current nutrition literature and the dietitian or nutritionist should be consulted as necessary.

The nurse frequently has an order to "force fluids." Since the amount required depends on the size of the patient, the amount of fluid loss, and the patient's circulatory and renal status, no standard amount can be given. The nurse must therefore make a judgment as to the desirable amount and inform members of the nursing team or family members who will care for the patient. If there is any question, the physician is consulted.

If an elderly person living at home complains of pronounced weakness without apparent cause, the nurse should ask whether cathartics or enemas have been taken. If so, stopping this procedure, eating foods with high sodium and potassium content, and increasing the fluid intake may relieve the symptoms. Methods to combat constipation without purging should be taught.

Any patient with renal or circulatory impairment, as may occur in shock, cardiac decompensation, or constriction of blood vessels because of disease, may develop electrolyte imbalance. Sodium and water may be held in the tissues, the potassium level of the blood may rise, acidosis may develop from inadequate tissue oxygenation, or the kidneys may be unable to excrete waste products properly. Patients with cardiac and renal impairment are instructed to avoid taking too much food containing sodium, potassium, or bicarbonate.

Gavage (feeding by tube)

Water, a physiologic solution of sodium chloride, high-protein liquids, or a regular diet that has been passed through a blender and diluted is often given by gavage to older children and adults (see Chapter 53). As previously mentioned, high-protein tube feeding can cause water deficit through osmotic diuresis. A need to increase water intake along with the tube feeding should be considered when (1) the patient complains of thirst; (2) protein content of the tube feeding is high; (3) the patient has a fever; (4) urinary output is decreased or very concentrated; and (5) signs of water deficit develop.[26]

Parenteral fluids

The nurse needs to know the common solutions used parenterally (Table 21-9). A solution of 5% dextrose in distilled water is often used to maintain fluid intake or to reestablish blood volume. Ascorbic acid and vitamin B (Solu-B) are frequently added. Dextrose, 5%, in saline solution may be given depending on the serum levels of sodium, and potassium chloride may be added to meet normal intake needs of potassium and to replace losses. A physiologic solution of sodium chloride is given primarily when sodium chloride has been lost in large amounts such as in loss of gastrointestinal fluids or in burns. A one-sixth molar lactate solution may be ordered when sodium, but not chloride, needs replacement; ammonium chloride solution may be used to replace chlorides when added sodium is undesirable. Balanced solutions containing several electrolytes may be used. Ringer's solution and lactated Ringer's solution are examples.

Body needs for carbohydrates may be partially met by giving fructose or 10% or 20% glucose in distilled water, but these solutions are hypertonic and require additional water for excretion.

Amino acid preparations (Aminosol) are seldom given by standard intravenous methods. Whole blood is the fluid of choice to replace blood loss, but plasma, 25% salt-poor albumin, or plasma volume expanders can be given to substitute for blood protein loss and are used to reestablish normal blood volume and prevent shock. Dextran is the most generally accepted plasma volume expander. It increases the oncotic pressure of the blood, thus increasing the reabsorption of fluid from interstitial spaces and increasing plasma volume. Low–molecular weight dextran decreases the viscosity of the blood, allowing greater flow of blood through the capillaries; thus is it useful in treating cardiogenic, hemorrhagic, or septic shock (see Chapter 20). It may cause a prolonged bleeding time and should not be used if renal disease with severe oliguria or anuria is present or during pregnancy.[12]

Intervention

Intravenous fluids containing electrolytes should be run slowly to allow the body to regulate their use. The patient is watched carefully for untoward signs (excess of fluids or electrolytes). Increased serum potassium (hyperkalemia) can be particularly dangerous, since it may cause cardiac arrest. When solutions containing electrolytes are given, the nurse monitors the urinary output carefully and reports any marked decrease in the amount to the physician. Because the kidneys select the ions needed and excrete surplus ones, a normal output is essential. If the nurse is planning the sequence of intravenous fluids, hydrating fluids such as one-half strength physiologic solution of sodium chloride or glucose in water solution should be given first. Renal failure and untreated adrenal insufficiency are contraindications for the use of potassium. If these conditions are known or suspected to exist, the nurse should verify orders for its administration. Many physicians do not start intravenous therapy for the day until blood chemistry results have been reported.

TABLE 21-9. Solutions for intravenous use

Type of solution	Contents of solutions								
	Cations (mEq/L)					Anions (mEq/L)			
	Na^+	K^+	Ca^{++}	Mg^{++}	NH_4^+	Cl^-	HCO_3^- lactate	PO_4^-	Glucose (g/L)
5% Dextrose in water									50
10% Dextrose in water									100
Normal saline (0.9%)	154					154			
3% saline	513					513			
Ringer's solution	147	4	4			155			
5% Dextrose in Ringer's lactate	130	4	3			109	28		50
Ringer's lactate	130	4	3			109	28		
Ammonium chloride (0.9%)					170	170			
Sodium lactate ⅙ molar	167						167		
5% Dextrose in 0.2% saline	34					34			50
5% Dextrose in 0.45% saline	77					77			50

Usually the rate of administration of fluids is ordered by the physican and will depend on the patient's illness, the kind of fluid given, and the patient's age. An infusion is rarely run at a rate faster than 4 ml/min. If it is given continuously or if it is given when there is impaired renal function or impaired cardiac function, it is rarely run faster than 2 ml/min. The usual rate for replacement of fluid loss is 3 ml/min. This rate allows time for the fluid to diffuse into the extracellular fluid compartments and avoids overloading the circulation or raising the blood volume high enough to produce a diuretic effect. The equipment used for fluid administration may have varying numbers of drops per milliliters, and the nurse needs to check the equipment used to determine the rate of delivery, since it is not the drops per minute but the milliliters per minute that is important.

Nurses should question the advisability of the rather common practice of speeding up the rate of flow of solutions given intravenously primarily to complete the treatment at a specified time. Every nurse should recognize the initial signs of pulmonary edema (bounding pulse, engorged peripheral veins, hoarseness, dyspnea, cough, or pulmonary rales) and should observe closely for them in those patients who are receiving concentrated solutions, those who must be given any intravenous solution rapidly, and those whose age or physical condition makes them special risks. At the first signs of increased blood volume the rate of flow of the infusion should be reduced to a "keep open" rate or barely running at 5 to 6 drops/min and the physician notified. Special care needs to be taken in giving fluids to infants, elderly patients with circulatory impairment, patients whose hearts are decompensated, those with renal impairment, those who have had plasma shifts such as

burned patients, and those with extensive tissue trauma for other causes. Patients whose plasma has shifted need to be watched especially carefully because after a few days the plasma tends to shift back suddenly from the interstitial tissue to the blood, producing an increase in blood volume with resulting pulmonary edema.

It is imperative that the nurse check the labels of fluid bottles carefully for correctness of content and record accurately the fluids given. (For details of equipment and nursing techniques needed in parenteral fluid administration refer to a textbook on fundamentals of nursing.)

Patients who are receiving fluids intravenously are observed frequently so that symptoms indicating the need to slow down, speed up, or stop the infusion may be noted (Table 21-10). The tissue at the site of the inserted needle is checked at intervals for signs of infiltration or inflammatory reaction. If infiltration occurs, the infusion should be stopped at once and plans made to restart it. Solutions containing potassium are very irritating, and extravasation may cause tissue necrosis. When dextran or other protein solutions are being given, the patient is observed for signs of anaphylactic reaction (apprehension, dyspnea, wheezing respirations, tightness of chest, itching, hypotension) (p. 1863).

Parenteral hyperalimentation

Parental hyperalimentation, also known as total parenteral nutrition (TPN), is a method of giving highly concentrated solutions intravenously to maintain the nutritional purpose of protein synthesis (Fig. 21-7). Indications for this therapy are (1) major gastrointestinal diseases, fistulas, or inflammatory diseases; (2) exten-

TABLE 21-10. Complications of intravenous fluid therapy

Complication	Observations	Nursing actions
Circulatory overload	Bounding pulse, venous distention, hoarseness, dyspnea, cough, pulmonary rales, restlessness	Notify physician Reduce flow to "keep open" rate Raise head of bed to facilitate breathing
Local infiltration	Decreased rate or cessation of fluid flow Tissue around needle site cold, pale, swollen, hard Complaint of local pain	Stop infusion Arrange to restart infusion at another site Apply moist heat Elevate lower arm
Thrombophlebitis	Pain, redness, warmth, edema along vein	Same as for local infiltration Cold compresses may be applied initially
Pyrogenic reaction	Fever, chills, general malaise, nausea and vomiting 30 min after infusion started Hypotension (if severe)	Stop infusion Notify physician Monitor vital signs Save infusion fluid for culture
Anaphylactic reaction (with proteins)	Apprehension, dyspnea, wheezing, tightness of chest, itching, hypotension	Slow infusion to "keep open" rate Notify physician Monitor vital signs

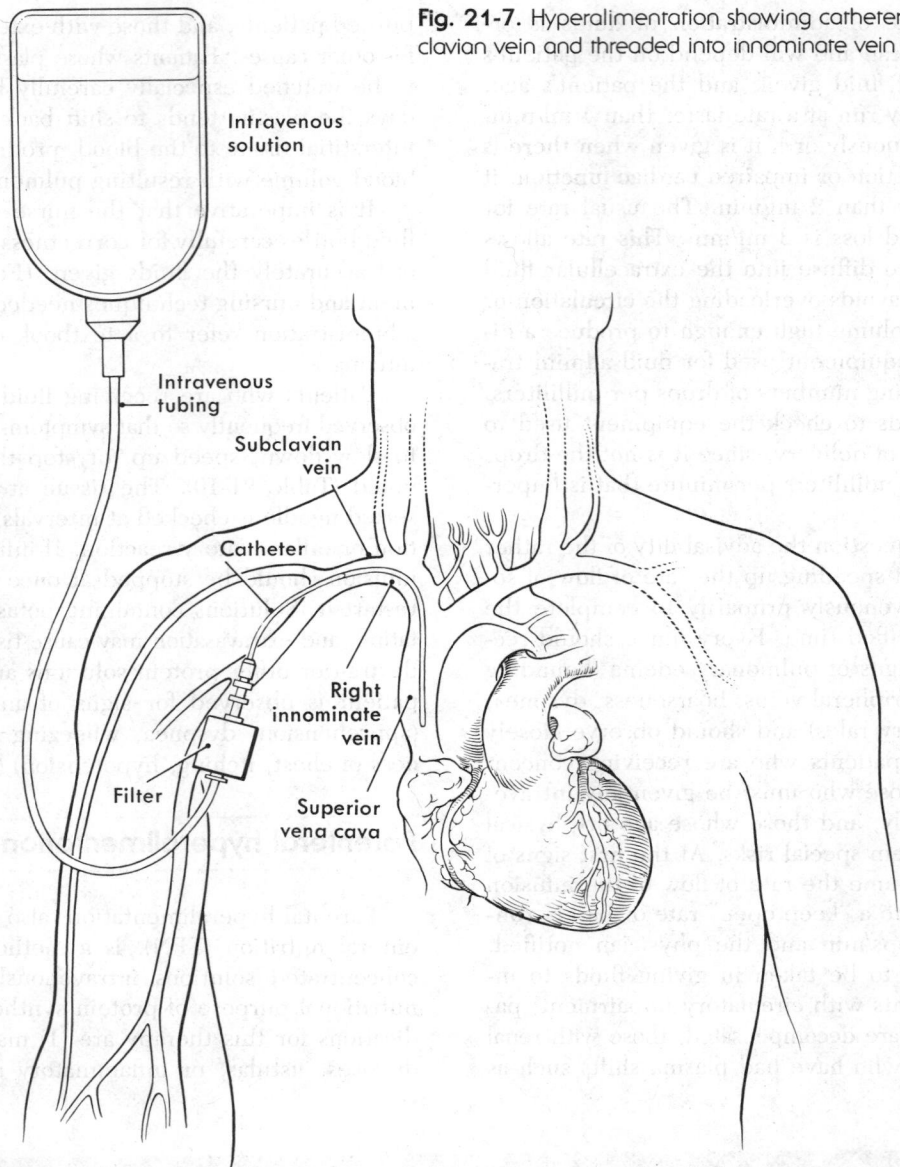

Fig. 21-7. Hyperalimentation showing catheter placed directly into subclavian vein and threaded into innominate vein and superior vena cava.

Intravenous solution

Intravenous tubing

Subclavian vein

Catheter

Right innominate vein

Filter

Superior vena cava

sive negative nitrogen balance such as occurs with major body burns, extensive wounds, or starvation; and (3) gastrointestinal side effects from radiation therapy.

The physician initiates the infusion by inserting an intracatheter either into the basilic vein and into the subclavian vein or directly into the subclavian vein and threading it through the innominate vein into the superior vena cava. The large amount of blood in the superior vena cava helps to dilute the highly concentrated solution rapidly and thus prevent phlebitis or vein occlusion. The jugular vein is preferred in infants for ease of insertion but is too close to hair-growing areas in adults (possibility of sepsis) and is more restricting of neck movements.

Experts recommend that the patient be taken to the operating room for insertion of the intracatheter in order to maintain sterility. The insertion of the intracath-

eter is not painful, but the patient may experience a feeling of pressure. The intracatheter is sutured with one suture and covered by an air-occlusive dressing. The infusion is started with a standard intravenous fluid (5% dextrose) until a radiograph confirms the location of the catheter tip in the superior vena cava.

Solutions for parenteral hyperalimentation are good culture media and should be prepared under strict aseptic conditions, preferably in the pharmacy under a laminar airflow hood. The physician orders the solution contents based on the patient's nutritional needs. A sufficient amount of glucose to meet energy needs is necessary so that the amino acids are used for protein synthesis rather than for energy. The basic nutrient solution usually contains 20% to 25% glucose to which amino acids, minerals, electrolytes, and vitamins are added. The commercial preparations are relatively trouble free, but some patients do demonstrate sensitivity reactions (headache, fever, myalgia, chills, nausea and vomiting, rash, vasodilation, abdominal pain, convulsions). Prepared solutions must be kept refrigerated and should be warmed to room temperature just before infusion. Solutions should not be hung for longer than a 12-hour period.

Broviac and Hickman catheters are two types of central venous catheters that can be used for intermittent infusions of chemotherapy and antibiotic drugs, blood, blood components, and bone marrow transfusions, as well as for TPN solution. They are designed so that the end of the catheter can be capped between infusions. At the completion of an infusion, the catheter is filled with heparinized saline to prevent clotting and is capped until time for the next infusion.

TPN solutions may consist of glucose, amino acids, electrolytes, minerals, and vitamins in various concentrations plus fat emulsions. If the amino acid and glucose concentrations are not hypertonic, the infusions can be given by peripheral veins. The nursing interventions with this type of infusion are similar to that described below, except that the problems with fluid and electrolyte balance are not as likely to occur.

Intervention

Prevention of infection. Strict aseptic technique is mandatory during changing of bottles, tubings, or dressings. The nurse should be knowledgeable concerning the frequency and method of dressing changes being utilized. Some medical centers have a hyperalimentation team, and one nurse changes the dressings for all patients, usually three times weekly. The purpose of having only one nurse involved in changing the dressings is to ensure consistency of technique and to reduce the chance of infection. If a dressing becomes wet, it is changed immediately to prevent transmission of bacteria by capillary action. The dressing should be air occlusive. Presence of an elevated temperature is reported immediately to the physician, and cultures are taken of the insertion site, tubing, and solutions for fungal as well as bacterial studies. Patients who experience itching under the dressing are cautioned not to scratch or disturb the dressing.

Prevention of air embolism. The possibility of air embolism is greater with use of the superior vena cava than with a peripheral vein because the decreased venous pressure as the blood approaches the heart can cause air to be sucked into the hyperalimentation tubing. All connections in the parenteral hyperalimentation setup are taped to prevent accidental separation. Tubing changes are made quickly with the patient lying flat in bed. The patient may be asked to perform the Valsalva maneuver (forced expiration against a closed glottis) while the tube is disconnected. Filters are useful for trapping air as well as bacteria.

Maintenance of fluid and electrolyte balance. The goal of parenteral hyperalimentation is a continued and uniform infusion rate of the hypertonic solution. Frequent checking (every 30 to 60 minutes) of the established drip rate and patency of the infusion is important. A decreased flow rate may be caused by a plugged filter. Changes in body position will also alter the flow rate. If the rate becomes too slow, hypoglycemia may develop. The flow rate should be maintained as ordered and never "speeded up," since overload of the hypertonic solution can cause hyperglycemia and massive dehydration of body cells. Daily weights and recording of intake and output help in monitoring fluid balance. The patient is observed for signs of fluid overload (p. 333). Hyperglycemia can be identified by presence of sugar in the urine. Serum electrolytes, glucose, and BUN levels are usually monitored daily initially and then at longer intervals.

Promotion of health. The patient should be encouraged to assume activities of daily living. Initially, the person is likely to be in a catabolic state, which increases the susceptibility to infections of the mouth and respiratory tract. Good mouth care is essential if food and fluids are not permitted orally. Ambulation should be encouraged, if possible, since inactivity promotes catabolism and negative nitrogen balance.

Emotional support. Patients may have many fears and concerns about being fed by intravenous fluids over a long period of time. They should have an understanding of what is occurring and the reason for the frequent dressing changes. If not permitted food orally, they may need aid in coping with stress incurred by the smell of food or watching others eat. If receiving parenteral hyperalimentation over an extended period of time, they may be concerned about regaining appetite, taste, or normal eating patterns.[9] Being fed only by tube, even though temporary, may create stress from a change in body image.

Relief of symptoms

Patients with fluid and electrolyte imbalance often have extreme thirst, nausea, and vomiting. These symptoms are distressing, and the nurse should know measures that can be used to give the patient relief.

Thirst

Thirst, the first and most insistent sign of dehydration, sometimes causes the patient more misery than surgery or the symptoms of a disease. It may develop even when fluids have been withheld only for a number of hours. If fluids are being withheld intentionally, thirst often is made more bearable by explaining to the patient why the fluids are being withheld and when they will be reinstituted.

Usually, thirst is relieved readily by taking fluids. When fluids cannot be taken orally, the administration of fluids parenterally usually gives relief. This is often helpful to explain to the patient. Mouth care will allay some of the discomfort from thirst. This care includes cleansing the tongue, teeth, and mucous membranes lining the oral cavity. It may be necessary to repeat the procedure every hour. Cleansing the mouth with lemon and glycerine swabs is usually helpful. A patient who can be trusted not to swallow may be given mouthwash, water, or ice chips to be held in the mouth and then expelled. Hard lemon candies (sour balls) often give relief even though they must be expelled. The chewing of gum helps some patients.

When fluids are not permitted, the water pitcher at the bedside is removed, and if the patient cannot be relied on not to get up and drink at a water tap, special provisions such as constant attendance or insistence on bed rest may be necessary. Thirst sometimes compels the patient to obtain water in any way possible.

Pronounced and continued thirst, despite the administration of fluids, is not normal and should be reported. In the immediate postoperative period, this kind of thirst suggests internal hemorrhage, elevation of temperature, or some other untoward development. In the chronically ill patient it may indicate the onset of disease such as diabetes mellitus in which extra water is used by the kidneys to eliminate glucose in the urine. It also is a symptom of hypercalcemia.

Nausea and vomiting

Fluid and electrolyte imbalances may cause nausea and vomiting. Vomiting in turn frequently leads to further fluid and electrolyte imbalances as a result of the loss of gastric secretions. A vicious cycle may be set up:

Vomiting → Losses → Vomiting → (etc.)

Treatment of severe nausea and vomiting is by replacement of the fluids and electrolytes by parenteral methods and by the use of antiemetic medications. The care of the person experiencing nausea and vomiting is described on p. 1390.

Acid-base imbalances

Control of acid-base balance in the body is accomplished by regulation of hydrogen ions in body fluids (p. 307). The pH of body fluids is normally maintained within a range of pH 7.35 to 7.45, or slightly alkaline. When pH of the blood drops below 7.35, a state of *acidosis* exists; above 7.45 a state of *alkalosis* exists. A pH below 6.8 or above 7.8 is incompatible with life (see Fig. 20-6).

The major effect of acidosis is depression of the central nervous system as evidenced by disorientation followed by coma. Alkalosis is characterized by overexcitability of the nervous system, and the muscles may go into a state of tetany and convulsions. Acid-base imbalance always produces an imbalance of the body's other cations as well; therefore symptoms of these imbalances will also occur.

Pathophysiology

Regulation of pH is vital because even slight deviations from the normal range will cause marked changes in the rate of cellular chemical reactions. Acid-base balance is controlled by several regulatory mechanisms shown in Table 21-11. (See p. 307 for further information on regulatory mechanisms.)

Chemical buffer systems

There are three major buffer systems in cells and extracellular fluid, carbonic acid–bicarbonate, phosphate, and protein buffer systems, that act very rapidly to prevent minute-to-minute changes in pH.

Carbonic acid–bicarbonate. The carbonic acid–bicarbonate system is present in extracellular fluids. Carbonic acid is formed by the combination of carbon dioxide and water: $CO_2 + H_2O \rightleftharpoons H_2CO_3$. When a strong base is added to the body fluids, it is buffered by carbonic acid to a bicarbonate salt and water: $H_2CO_3 + NaOH \rightarrow NaH CO_3 + H_2O$. When a strong acid is added to the system, a bicarbonate buffer changes it to a salt and carbonic acid: $HCl + NaH CO_3 \rightarrow NaCl + H_2CO_3$. The carbonic acid then dissociates into carbon dioxide and water and can be excreted by the lungs and kidneys.

Bicarbonate and carbonic acid normally exist in the extracellular fluid in a ratio of 20:1, respectively (or 27:1.34). This ratio is more vital to maintenance of acid-base balance than the actual amounts of the two substances. For instance, if the amount of carbonic acid increases, an increase in bicarbonate, which keeps the 20:1 ratio intact, will prevent a change from normal pH.

The carbonic acid–bicarbonate buffer system is important because concentrations of these two substances can be controlled by the respiratory and renal systems (discussed later in this chapter).

Phosphate buffer system. The phosphate buffer system is present in cells and extracellular fluids; it is especially active in the kidneys. This system is com-

TABLE 21-11. Mechanisms regulating acid-base balance

	Action time	Effect
Chemical buffers in cells and extracellular fluid	Instantaneous	Combine with acids or bases added to the system to prevent marked changes in pH
Respiratory system	Minutes to hours	Controls CO_2 concentration in extracellular fluid by changes in rate and depth of respiration
Kidneys	Hours to days	Increases or decreases quantity of $NaHCO_3$ in extracellular fluid Combines HCO_3^- or H^+ with other substances and excretes them in urine

posed of sodium and other cations in combination with $H_2PO_4^-$ and $HPO_4^=$. When a strong acid is present, the following action takes place: $Na_2HPO_4 + HCl \rightarrow NaCl + NaH_2PO_4$. A hydrogen ion is excreted via the urine in the NaH_2PO_4. A strong base is buffered in the following reaction: $NaOH + NaH_2PO_4 \rightarrow Na_2HPO_4 + H_2O$. The NaH_2PO_4 is a weak base and minimizes the pH change.[15]

Protein buffer system. The protein buffer system is located in the plasma and inside cells; the protein hemoglobin in red blood cells is one of the proteins involved. Although most protein buffers are intracellular, they assist in buffering extracellular fluid. Some of the amino acids in proteins contain free acid radicals, —COOH, which can dissociate into CO_2 + H, thus adding a hydrogen ion. Other proteins have basic radicals, —NH_3OH, which can dissociate into —NH_3^+ and OH^-; the OH^- combines with a hydrogen ion to form water, thus removing one hydrogen ion from body fluid. The protein buffer system is the most plentiful buffer system in the body.[15]

Respiratory control of pH

The respiratory control center in the brain responds to increases of carbon dioxide and hydrogen ions in body fluids. Rate and depth of respiration are in turn controlled by the respiratory control of pH as follows: (1) when pH decreases (more acid), respiratory rate and depth are increased, and there is greater excretion of carbon dioxide through the lungs; thus less carbon dioxide is present to produce carbonic acid by the reaction: $CO_2 + H_2O \rightleftharpoons H_2CO_3$, and the pH increases toward alkalinity; and (2) when pH rises above the normal range (more alkaline), the respiratory center is depressed, rate and depth of respiration decrease, carbon dioxide is retained, and more carbonic acid is formed, moving the pH toward acidity.

Because carbon dioxide is constantly being formed as a product of metabolism, the concentration of carbon dioxide in ECFs must be continuously balanced between the rate of metabolism and the rate of pulmonary excretion. The buffering capacity of the respiratory system is more than double that of all the chemical buffers combined.

Renal regulation of pH

Both chemical buffers and respiratory regulation have limited ability to make complete adjustments in pH, and it remains for the kidneys to make permanent adjustments in the pH of body fluids. The renal regulation of pH is effected by control of the retention or excretion of bicarbonate and hydrogen ions. The kidneys usually excrete an acid urine because of the excess of acid metabolic products (nonvolatile acids), which must be eliminated by the renal route. Normally, almost all of the bicarbonate formed by the kidneys is retained.

Hydrogen ions, secreted by kidney tubule cells, and bicarbonate, filtered into the glomerular filtrate, combine in the kidney tubules to form carbon dioxide and water, which is excreted through exhalation (CO_2) and in urine (H_2O). In acidosis, excess hydrogen ions are secreted into the kidney tubules, where they combine with buffers and are excreted in the urine. In alkalosis, bicarbonate ions enter the tubules, where there exists a lack of the hydrogen ions with which they normally combine to form carbonic acid; the bicarbonate ions combine instead with sodium or other cations and are excreted in the urine. Hydrogen ions can be exchanged for sodium and potassium ions in the kidney tubules; therefore conservation of hydrogen ions can result in imbalances of sodium and potassium.

Compensation

Compensation is a response that tends to reverse an abnormal trend in pH. The kidneys attempt to compensate for changes in blood CO_2 by making a corresponding change in blood bicarbonate, and the lungs attempt to compensate for abnormal changes in blood bicarbonate by making corresponding changes in blood CO_2. Compensation is an effort to maintain the normal 20:1 ratio between bicarbonate and carbonic acid that is necessary to maintain the pH within normal range.

TABLE 21-12. Types of acid-base disturbances and compensatory mechanisms

Disturbance	Physiologic causes	Method of compensation
Respiratory acidosis	Carbonic acid excess: lungs not removing sufficient CO_2 (hypoventilation)	Bicarbonate production by kidneys increased; bicarbonate retained and chloride excreted instead by kidneys; secretion and excretion of hydrogen ions in urine increased
Respiratory alkalosis	Carbonic acid deficit: lungs removing too much CO_2 (hyperventilation)	Kidneys increase excretion of bicarbonate ions
Metabolic acidosis	Bicarbonate deficit: retention of acid metabolites, diabetic ketoacidosis, excess acid intake (salicylate poisoning), or loss of bicarbonate	Increased rate and depth of respiration cause increased excretion of CO_2 by lungs; formation of bicarbonate ions in the kidneys increased
Metabolic alkalosis	Bicarbonate excess: excess intake (sodium bicarbonate, carbonated drinks) or retention of bicarbonate; Potassium depletion; Loss of acid	Rate and depth of respiration decreased; lungs retain more CO_2; kidneys excrete bicarbonate

Types of acid-base disturbances

Table 21-12 shows the four types of acid-base disturbances that occur and their compensatory mechanisms.

Following are the laboratory values used in diagnosing and monitoring acid-base disturbances: pH, 7.35 to 7.45; PCO_2, 38 to 42 mm Hg; and plasma bicarbonate, 23 to 25 mEq/L.

Bicarbonate is sometimes expressed as a CO_2 content value, which is actually the sum of all carbon dioxide dissolved in the plasma. Actual bicarbonate can be calculated from a CO_2 content value by the following formula: Bicarbonate = CO_2 content − (0.03 × PCO_2). Both pH and PCO_2 are determined from a sample of arterial blood, a blood gas analysis.

Table 21-13 shows whether laboratory values characteristic of the four types of acid-base disturbances are increased or decreased and the results of the body's compensatory efforts.

Respiratory acidosis: carbonic acid excess

Any factor that decreases the rate of pulmonary ventilation increases the concentration of dissolved carbon dioxide, carbonic acid, and hydrogen ions and results in *respiratory acidosis*. An excess of carbon dioxide (hypercapnia) can cause carbon dioxide narcosis. In this condition carbon dioxide levels are so high that they no longer stimulate respirations but depress them. Associated with the decreased respiratory rate are lack of oxygen and hypoxia. During respiratory acidosis, potassium moves out of the cells, producing hyperkalemia.

Ventricular fibrillation may occur if the blood potassium levels are greatly increased.

Etiology. Respiratory acidosis can result from a number of pathologic conditions: (1) damage to the respiratory center in the medulla, (2) obstruction of respiratory passages (e.g., pneumonia, chronic bronchitis), (3) loss of lung surface for ventilation (e.g., atelectasis, pneumothorax, emphysema, pulmonary fibrosis), (4) weakness of respiratory muscles (e.g., poliomyelitis, hypokalemia), and (5) severe depression of respirations (e.g., overdose of respiratory depressant drugs).

Prevention. Patients with diseases such as emphysema that limit lung excursion and therefore limit gaseous exchange should not take carbonated beverages or bicarbonate of soda. These substances tend to make the blood more alkaline than normal, and respirations are depressed in an effort to correct this imbalance. Depression of respirations is highly undesirable for these patients.

Any patient with symptoms of inadequate oxygenation or carbon dioxide retention requires medical treatment. Early recognition and treatment of the primary condition often prevent its becoming complicated by acid-base imbalance. Therefore any person with symptoms suggestive of anemia, cardiac insufficiency, chronic bronchitis, emphysema, asthma, or other obstructive diseases of the bronchioles should receive medical attention. These conditions are discussed in detail in the latter half of this book.

Clinical picture. Signs and symptoms of respiratory acidosis include hyperpnea, visual disturbances, and headache. Later, confusion, drowsiness, and coma can

TABLE 21-13. Laboratory values in uncompensated and partially compensated acid-base disturbances

	pH	Pco$_2$	HCO
Respiratory acidosis			
Uncompensated	Below 7.35	↑	Normal
Partially compensated	Move toward normal, but still ↓	↑	↑
Respiratory alkalosis			
Uncompensated	Above 7.45	↓	Normal
Partially compensated	Move toward normal, but still ↑	↓	↓
Metabolic acidosis			
Uncompensated	Below 7.35	Normal	↓
Partially compensated	Move toward normal, but still ↓	↓	↓
Metabolic alkalosis			
Uncompensated	Above 7.45	Normal	↑
Partially compensated	Move toward normal, but still ↑	↑	↑

ensue. Ventricular fibrillation may be the first sign noted in some cases.

Intervention. Treatment is aimed at increasing the alveolar ventilation rate in order to improve the exchange of carbon dioxide and oxygen. This objective is accomplished by using an intermittent positive pressure breathing (IPPB) machine to assist the patient to exhale carbon dioxide. Because the respiratory center is narcotized by the increased amounts of carbon dioxide, the lowered oxygen tension of the blood is the stimulus for respiration. If a patient whose respiratory drive is dependent on a low Po$_2$ is given large amounts of oxygen, the stimulus for breathing is removed and respirations will cease. For this reason, oxygen is never given to patients with carbon dioxide narcosis. Low flow oxygen (1 to 3 L/min) is given to a patient with chronic pulmonary disease who maintains a chronically high Pco$_2$. IPPB treatments are usually given using compressed air or room air instead of oxygen in these situations (p. 1332).

If ventricular fibrillation or severe potassium excess exists, it may be necessary to administer sodium bicarbonate intravenously.

The major nursing responsibility is to recognize patients who have the potential for developing respiratory acidosis because of conditions that interefere with normal respiratory gas exchange. A patient whose airway is compromised by the presence of secretions must be encouraged to cough frequently or may need to have nasopharyngeal or tracheal suctioning.

Respiratory alkalosis: carbonic acid deficit

Etiology. Excessive pulmonary ventilation will decrease hydrogen ion concentration and thus cause *respiratory alkalosis*. A common cause of respiratory alkalosis is *hyperventilation*. A person who hyperventilates blows off large amounts of carbon dioxide. Hyperventilation may be caused by anxiety, hysteria, or lesions

affecting the respiratory center in the medulla (brain tumor, encephalitis). Some other causes of respiratory alkalosis are conditions that greatly increase metabolism (hyperthyroidism) and the overventilation of patients with mechanical respirators.

Prevention. Respiratory alkalosis can be prevented in a person who is hyperventilating by administering a few whiffs of carbon dioxide or by having the person breathe into a paper bag and then rebreathe his own exhaled carbon dioxide. Care should be taken in adjusting mechanical respirators so that the patient is not being breathed too deeply or rapidly.

Clinical picture. The patient may complain of light-headedness and numbness or tingling of the fingers and toes. If the alkalosis becomes more severe, tetany and convulsions may be present. Serum potassium levels will be decreased because the kidneys retain hydrogen ions and excrete potassium instead.

Intervention. Treating the underlying condition usually effectively resolves the respiratory alkalosis. Respiratory alkalosis becomes especially dangerous when it leads to cardiac arrhythmias caused partly by a decreased serum potassium level. If a patient who is receiving assisted ventilation complains of dizziness or shows any signs of muscle irritability, it is likely that the depth of respiration is too great, and the respiratory rate of the machine should be decreased. If tetany is present, calcium gluconate is given intravenously (p. 341). Renal function must be maintained to promote renal compensation of the disturbance.

Metabolic acidosis: bicarbonate deficit

When excess acids are added to the body fluids, or when bicarbonate is lost, a *metabolic acidosis*, or nonrespiratory acidosis, results.

Etiology. In some conditions, such as uncontrolled diabetes mellitus or starvation, glucose either cannot be utilized or is not available for oxidation. The body compensates for this by using body fat for energy, producing abnormal amounts of ketone bodies in the process. In an effort to neutralize the ketones and maintain the acid-base balance of the body, plasma bicarbonate is exhausted. The resultant acid-base imbalance is called metabolic acidosis or *ketoacidosis*. This condition can develop whenever the person does not eat an adequate diet and body fat must be burned for energy. It is the reason why extremely low-carbohydrate or high-protein–no-carbohydrate reduction diets are criticized by nutrition experts.

Ketoacidosis develops more rapidly in infants than in adults because they have fewer glycogen reserves. It also can develop whenever excessive amounts of lactic acid are produced, such as in prolonged strenuous muscle exercise, or when oxidation takes place in cells without adequate oxygen, such as occurs in heart failure and shock. Loss of large amounts of alkaline intestinal secretions, such as in severe diarrhea or through fistulas, can also create a bicarbonate deficit.

The normal functioning kidney excretes an excess of hydrogen ions in conditions of acidosis and, in so doing, retains potassium so that hyperkalemia as well as acidosis is present. In kidney failure, metabolic acids accumulate in the bloodstream. Following is a listing of the many causes of metabolic acidosis:

1. Diarrhea or draining intestinal fistulas (loss of bicarbonate)
2. Renal failure
3. Ureteroenterostomy (retention of Cl^- ions)
4. Diabetic ketoacidosis
5. Lactic acidosis
6. Salicylate intoxication
7. Starvation (increased breakdown of body fat or protein)
8. Surgical anesthesia
9. Conditions that greatly increase the body's metabolic needs (high fever, infectious disease, thyrotoxicosis)
10. Shock
11. Convulsions

Prevention. Metabolic acidosis can be prevented by careful medical management or, when possible, prevention of the conditions that lead to acidosis.

Clinical picture. Headache and mental dullness are early signs of acidosis. The patient in acidosis is hyperpneic and has deep respirations (Kussmaul's respirations). This breathing pattern represents an attempt to blow off carbon dioxide, thus compensating for the acidosis. If the condition is untreated, disorientation, stupor, coma, and death will occur.

Hyperkalemia results from the movement of potassium out of the cells as hydrogen ions move in and from the retention of potassium by the kidneys. Aside from laboratory evidence, there may be few indications of the acidosis until the pH falls to 7.1 or lower.

Intervention. Treatment of acidosis is directed toward treating the underlying cause and restoration of electrolyte balance. If the acidosis is severe, intravenous sodium bicarbonate is given. In milder cases, sodium bicarbonate may be given orally if the patient is able to retain it. Bicarbonate preparations must be administered with caution because they can induce a metabolic alkalosis and lead to tetany and convulsions. When acidosis is caused by renal failure, renal dialysis is necessary.

As the acidosis is corrected, potassium moves back into cells and hypokalemia develops. If a patient being treated for acidosis needs to receive potassium, it is given after the acidosis has been partially corrected and as pH is returning to normal. It is important to bear in mind that even though acidosis is accompanied by hyperkalemia, the patient may be potassium depleted. The potassium leaves the cells in exchange for the hydrogen ions, and much of it is excreted.

Maintenance of good respiratory function in a patient with metabolic acidosis will facilitate the excretion of carbon dioxide. If the kidneys are functioning well, they can help correct the acidosis by producing more bicarbonate. Since many conditions that lead to this imbalance are hyperosmolar as well, osmotic diuresis will take place and the patient will need fluid replacement along with careful monitoring of intake and output. If changes in the sensorium have resulted, safety precautions are instituted.

Metabolic alkalosis: bicarbonate excess

When excessive amounts of acid substance and hydrogen ions are lost from the body, or when large amounts of bicarbonate or lactate are added orally or intravenously, the result is an imbalance in which there is an excess of base elements, *metabolic alkalosis*. This type of imbalance does not occur as often as metabolic acidosis. In alkalosis, potassium enters the cells and hypokalemia results. A potassium loss causes a metabolic alkalosis, while an alkalosis causes hypokalemia.[12] An excess of bicarbonate in distal tubular fluid causes obligatory potassium loss.

Etiology. Metabolic alkalosis can occur in the following conditions: (1) loss of hydrochloric acid from the stomach caused by vomiting or gastric drainage from a nasogastric tube (loss of chloride leaves more sodium to combine with and retain bicarbonate in the kidneys); (2) loss of potassium ions through intestinal fistulas, diarrhea, or in the urine; (3) ingestion of large amounts of sodium bicarbonate or antacids to treat indigestion or ulcers; (4) infusion of excessive amounts of bicarbonate or lactate intravenously; (5) diuretic therapy; and (6) excessive mineralocorticoids.

Prevention. Persons must be cautioned against the excessive use of sodium bicarbonate to alleviate indigestion. Controlling the conditions that can cause metabolic alkalosis can prevent this imbalance from developing. If drug therapy is causing the alkalosis, these drugs should be discontinued and others substituted where possible.

Clinical picture. In metabolic alkalosis, breathing becomes depressed in an effort to conserve carbon dioxide for combination with hydrogen ions in the blood to raise the blood level of carbonic acid. Symptoms that can occur are mental confusion, dizziness, numbness and tingling in extremities, muscle twitching, and later, tetany and convulsions. There may be electrocardiographic changes consistent with hypokalemia.

Intervention. Treatment is aimed at correcting the cause of the metabolic alkalosis. Sodium chloride or ammonium chloride may be given orally or intravenously. If the condition is associated with loss of sodium chloride, potassium must be restored because it is lost with the sodium. It is given in the form of potassium chloride. A diuretic that acts as a carbonic anhydrase inhibitor (Diamox) may help relieve the alkalosis by increasing excretion of bicarbonate by the kidneys.

The nurse assists in maintenance of good respiratory function so that compensation can take place through this mechanism. Careful monitoring of the patient for adequate renal function and safety precautions are important in the nursing care of patients with metabolic alkalosis. Since convulsions may occur, precautions are taken for the patient's protection.

REFERENCES AND SELECTED READINGS

1. Beeson, P.B., McDermott, W., and Wyngaarden, J.B.: Textbook of medicine, ed. 15, Philadelphia, 1979, W.B. Saunders Co.
2. Bergersen, B.S.: Pharmacology in nursing, ed. 14, St. Louis, 1979, The C.V. Mosby Co.
3. *Bjeletich, J., and Hickman, R.: The Hickman indwelling catheter, Am. J. Nurs. **80**:1591-1599, 1980.
4. *Blood gas and acid-base concepts in respiratory care; a programmed instruction, Am. J. Nurs. **76**:1-30, 1976.
5. Brobeck, J.R., editor: Best and Taylor's physiological basis of medical practice, ed. 10, Baltimore, 1979, The Williams & Wilkins Co.
6. *Brooks, S.M.: Basic facts of body water and ions, ed. 3, New York, 1973, Springer Publishing Co., Inc.
7. *Butts, P.: Magnesium sulfate in the treatment of toxemia, Am. J. Nurs. **77**:1294-1298, 1977.
8. Davis, L., editor: Christopher's textbook of surgery, ed. 11, Philadelphia, 1977, W.B. Saunders Co.
9. *Dudrick, S.J., and Rhoads, J.E.: Total intravenous feeding, Sci. Am. **226**:73-80, 1972.
10. *Elbaum, N.: Detecting and correcting magnesium imbalance, Nurs. '77 **7**:34-35, 1977.
11. *Felver, L.: Understanding the electrolyte maze, Am. J. Nurs. **80**:1591-1599, 1980.
12. *Goldberger, E.: A primer of water, electrolytes and acid-base syndromes, ed. 6, Philadelphia, 1980, Lea & Febiger.
13. *Grant, M., and Kubo, W.: Assessing a patient's hydration status, Am. J. Nurs. **75**:1306-1311, 1975.
14. Groër, M.: Physiology and pathophysiology of the body fluids, St. Louis, 1981, The C.V. Mosby Co.
15. Guyton, A.: Textbook of medical physiology, ed. 6, Philadelphia, 1981, W.B. Saunders Co.
16. *Haughey, E., and Sica, F.: Diuretics: how safe can you make them? Nurs. '77 **7**:34-39, 1977.
17. Humes, D., et al.: Disorders of water balance, Hosp. Pract. **13**:95-106, 1978.
18. *Kee, J.: Fluids and electrolytes with clinical applications: a programmed approach, ed. 2, New York, 1978, John Wiley & Sons, Inc.
19. *Kee, J.: Fluid imbalances in elderly patients, Nurs. '73 **3**:40-43, 1973.
20. *Kee, J.: The critically ill patient and possible fluid and electrolyte imbalances, Nurs. '72 **2**:6-11, 1972.
21. Kettel, L.: Acute respiratory acidosis, Hosp. Med. **12**:31-33, 1976.
22. Keyes, J.: Basic mechanisms in acid-base homeostasis, Heart Lung **5**:239-245, 1976.
23. Keyes, J.: Blood gas analysis and the assessment of acid-base status, Heart Lung **5**:247-255, 1976.
24. Krause, M.V., and Mahan, L.K.: Food, nutrition and diet therapy, ed. 6, Philadelphia, 1979, W.B. Saunders Co.
25. Krupp, M., and Chatton, M.: Current medical diagnosis and treatment ed. 17, Los Altos, Calif., 1981, Lange Medical Publications.
26. *Kubo, W., et al.: Fluid and electrolyte problems of tube-fed patients, Am. J. Nurs. **76**:912-916, 1976.
27. *Lawson, M., et al.: Long-term I.V. therapy: a new approach, Am. J. Nurs. **79**:1100-1103, 1979.
28. Levy, M.: The pathophysiology of water balance, Hosp. Pract. **13**:95-106, 1978.
29. Lumb, P., et al.: Aggressive approach to intravenous feeding of the critically ill patient, Heart Lung **8**:71-80, 1979.
30. *MacLeod, S.: The rational use of potassium supplements, Postgrad. Med. **57**:123-127, 1975.
31. *Manzi, C.: Edema, how to tell if it's a danger signal, Nurs. '77 **7**:66-70, 1977.
32. *McGann, M.: Secondary hyperaldosteronism, Am J. Nurs. **76**:634-637, 1976.
33. *Metabolic acid-base disorders: programmed instruction, part I, Am. J. Nurs. **77**:1-32, 1977.
34. *Metabolic acid-base disorders: programmed instruction, part II, Am. J. Nurs. **78**:1-20, 1978.
35. *Metheny, N.: Water and electrolyte balance in the postoperative patient, Nurs. Clin. North Am. **10**:49-57, 1975.
36. *Metheny, N., and Snively, W.: Nurses handbook of fluid balance, ed. 3, Philadelphia, 1979, J.B. Lippincott Co.
37. *Metheny, N., and Snively, W.D.: Perioperative fluids and electrolytes, Am. J. Nurs. **78**:840-845, 1978.
38. Newmark, S., and Dluhy, R.: Hyperkalemia and hypokalemia, J.A.M.A. **231**:631-633, 1975.
39. Reed, G.M., and Sheppard, V.: Regulation of fluid and electrolyte balance, ed. 2, Philadelphia, 1977, W.B. Saunders Co.
40. *Roach, F.B.: Color changes in dark skin, Nurs. '72 **2**:20-22, 1972.
41. Robinson, C., and Lawler, M.R.: Normal and therapeutic nutrition, ed. 15, New York, 1977, Macmillan Publishing Co., Inc.
42. *Sharer, J.: Reviewing acid-base balance, Am. J. Nurs. **75**:980-983, 1975.
43. *Snively, V., and Roberts, K.: The clinical picture as an aid to understanding body fluid disturbances, Nurs. Forum **12**:132-159, 1973.
44. Stroot, V., Lee, C., and Schaper, C.: Fluids and electrolytes: a practical approach, ed. 2, Philadelphia, 1977, F.A. Davis Co.
45. *Tripp, A.: Hyper- and hypocalcemia, Am. J. Nurs. **76**:1142-1145, 1976.

---

*References preceded by an asterisk are particularly well suited for student reading.

46. *Wade, J.F.: Respiratory nursing care: physiology and technique, ed. 2, St. Louis, 1977, The C.V. Mosby Co.
47. Widman, F., editor: Goodale's clinical interpretation of laboratory tests, ed. 8, Philadelphia, 1979, F.A. Davis Co.
48. *Wilson, J., and Colley, R.: Meeting patients' nutritional needs with hyperalimentation, Nurs. '79 9:56-63, 1979.
49. Zeluff, G., et al.: Hypokalemia: cause and treatment, Heart Lung 7:854-860, 1978.

AUDIOVISUAL RESOURCES

Trainex Corp.: Fluid loss, Garden Grove, Calif., 1972, Trainex Corp. (Filmstrip and audiotape.)
Trainex Corp. : Rapid fluid gain, Garden Grove, Calif., 1972, Trainex Corp. (Filmstrip and audiotape.)
Trainex Corp.: Parenteral hyperalimentation, Garden Grove, Calif., 1971, Trainex Corp. (Filmstrip and audiotape.)
Trainex Corp.: Compensation of imbalances, Garden Grove, Calif., 1970, Trainex Corp. (Filmstrip and audiotape.)

CHAPTER 22

INFECTIOUS DISEASE

ELIZABETH CAMERON ECKSTEIN

Historical perspective

Infection control has become a recognized discipline only in the last decade, although the principles governing it have been in existence for some time. In the middle of the nineteenth century Semmelweiss, an obstetrician in Vienna, demonstrated the significance of hand washing in combating the transmission of infection. He observed that the incidence of puerperal fever, a major cause of postpartum mortality, was much higher on the ward where the medical students trained than on the ward attended by the midwives. Although the role of microorganisms in causing infection was not yet realized, Semmelweiss felt that somehow the medical students could be transmitting disease from the autopsy suite to maternity patients. He showed that when the students and physicians were required to wash their hands and rinse them in a chlorinated lime solution before a delivery, the incidence of puerperal fever decreased markedly. The idea that hand washing alone could prevent the spread of disease met with much opposition by his colleagues. Better acceptance came after Pasteur, Lister, and Koch developed the germ theory of disease and related asepsis to the prevention of the spread of disease. At about the same time, Nightingale made significant contributions to sanitation and isolation practices. From this evolved an era in which medical asepsis was practiced more by ritual than with the true understanding of the scientific principles on which it was based.

A turning point came during World War II when the sulfonamides and penicillin were first used successfully to treat infections. As new antibiotics were developed, a false sense of security developed about infection control. It soon became apparent, however, that antibiotics were not the sole answer to infection control. Once well controlled by antibiotics, organisms demonstrated the ability to develop resistant strains. In the late 1950s and the 1960s outbreaks of penicillin-resistant *Staphylococcus aureus* infections were common, and gram-negative organisms such as *Psuedomonas*, which were previously considered nonpathogenic (incapable of producing disease), were suddenly implicated as the cause of infections acquired in the hospital. Along with drug resistance and the emergence of newly recognized pathogens came an increase in the number of persons at risk of secondary infections. An increase in life expectancy, the use of immunosuppressive agents, and an increase in the use of invasive procedures to diagnose and treat disease all increased the risk of infection in certain persons.

The rise in the number of hospital infections made apparent the need to examine preventive and control measures, including a reemphasis on aseptic techniques. In 1970 an international conference to address the problem of hospital-acquired infections was held in Atlanta. As a result, the Centers for Disease Control (CDC) in Atlanta set forth guidelines for prevention and control of infections in hospitals. The CDC is constantly updating and revising its recommendations based on epidemiologic studies and research findings. The American Hospital Association (AHA) and the Joint Commission on Accreditation of Hospitals (JCAH), a major private accrediting agency, looked at the ethical and economic issues concerning hospital-acquired (nosocomial) infections and established standards for programs in infection control. The purpose of these programs was to decrease morbidity and mortality of infections as well as to reduce the cost of infections that could have been prevented. Consumer awareness of the problem also contributed to the attention given the issue of infection control. In the early 1970s only 10% of United States hospitals had infection surveillance and control programs, while by the end of the decade nearly all had them.

The field of infection control is a challenging one, with the identification of new pathogens (e.g., *Legionella pneumophila*) and advances in research uncovering new information that may change current thinking and practices. Infection control practitioners (ICPs) serve as a valuable resource since they interact with virtually every department in a hospital as they survey for infections and teach prevention and control of infection. The ICP is an important link between personnel from various hospital departments. When there is a question or problem regarding infection control, the ICP should be called on without hesitation.

This chapter presents an overview of the role of the nurse in the prevention and control of infection. For further information regarding a specific infectious disease, the reader should consult the chapter in which the site of the disease is discussed; for example, Chapter 33 for hepatitis, Chapter 51 for tuberculosis, and so on.

The infectious disease process

Definitions

A *pathogen* is a microorganism or substance that is capable of producing disease. This discussion will be concerned with microorganisms as pathogens. Factors that affect the microorganism's *pathogenicity*, or capacity to infect and produce disease, include the ability of the pathogen to survive and multiply outside its host, its virulence, its host specificity, and the resistance of the host.

Infection is the presence in the body of a pathogen that multiplies and produces effects that are injurious to the host. This injury may be the result of the presence and spread of the microorganism through the body tissues, known as the pathogen's *invasiveness*, or the injury may be due to the effects on the body of toxins produced by the microorganism; this is known as its *toxigenicity*. Some organisms, such as pneumococci, are highly invasive and virtually nontoxigenic, whereas others, such as *Clostridium tetani*, present the other extreme of high toxicity but low invasiveness. An infection may be *apparent*, thus causing clinical signs and symptoms, or *inapparent*, in which case there are not perceivable signs or symptoms (asymptomatic).

Pathogenic organisms that are present in the body but that do not produce injury to the body or incite an injurious body response are said to be colonizing the body. Patients who have an endotracheal tube or tracheostomy often have *colonization* with microorga-

nisms. Another example is the person whose nasal passages or skin surfaces are colonized with *Staphylococcus aureus*. The question of whether a person has an infection or colonization can be a difficult one to answer. What is important to realize is that persons who are colonized, as well as infected persons, can easily serve as a source of infection to themselves and to others who are at risk.

Chain of infection

Essential to appropriate intervention in the prevention and control of infection is an understanding of the infectious disease process. With all infectious diseases, a common sequence of events occurs (Fig. 22-1). First there must be a *causative agent*, or pathogen. This can be a bacterium, virus, fungus, rickettsiae, protozoa, or helminth (worm). There must be a *reservoir* where the agent can be found. The reservoir can be animate (human or animal) or inanimate (soil, water, intravenous solutions, equipment, etc.) Human reservoirs can be either persons with an acute clinical infection or persons who are asymptomatic *carriers*, who harbor the infectious agent but do not develop the infection. Carriers can (1) be *incubating* the agent before the onset of signs and symptoms, (2) have an *inapparent infection (subclinical)*, (3) be in the *convalescent stage* of an infection, or (4) be *chronic carriers* of the agent. Viral hepatitis B is an example of an infectious disease that can be transmitted by human carriers in all of the above mentioned stages. Often the reservoir for an agent responsible for an outbreak of an infection is not readily apparent and, in fact, may never be identified. If the process of infection is well understood, however, appropriate and effective control measures can be instituted even though the original source of the causative agent is not known.

The agent must have a *means of exit* from the reservoir. If the *reservoir* is human, the exit can be (1) the respiratory tract, (2) the gastrointestinal tract, (3) the genitourinary tract, (4) open lesions on the skin, or (5) across the placenta.

Once the agent has left the reservoir, it needs a *mode of transmission* to a host. Transmission can be by direct contact, by airborne vehicle, or by vectors. *Contact transmission* includes *direct, indirect* or *droplet* contact. Direct contact transmission occurs when there is spread of infection from the source to the host without the presence of an intermediate object. This happens when there is physical contact with or skin shedding onto the host. Gonorrhea is an example of a disease transmitted by direct contact.

Indirect contact transmission has an intermediate object that serves as the go-between the source and the host. This intermediary can be the contaminated hands

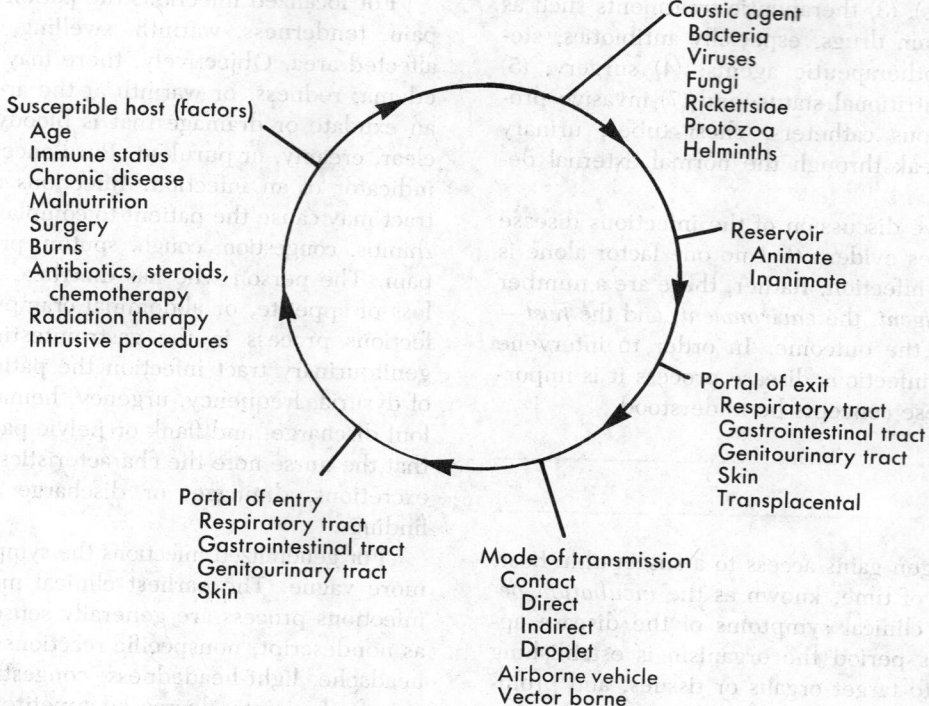

Fig. 22-1. The infectious disease process.

Susceptible host (factors)
Age
Immune status
Chronic disease
Malnutrition
Surgery
Burns
Antibiotics, steroids, chemotherapy
Radiation therapy
Intrusive procedures

Caustic agent
Bacteria
Viruses
Fungi
Rickettsiae
Protozoa
Helminths

Reservoir
Animate
Inanimate

Portal of exit
Respiratory tract
Gastrointestinal tract
Genitourinary tract
Skin
Transplacental

Portal of entry
Respiratory tract
Gastrointestinal tract
Genitourinary tract
Skin

Mode of transmission
Contact
Direct
Indirect
Droplet
Airborne vehicle
Vector borne

of a person who has had contact with an infected source and then proceeds to touch a susceptible host without washing the hands.

An inanimate object that has been contaminated by an infectious source is known as a *fomite*. Bed linen, respiratory therapy equipment, tissues, and silverware are examples of fomites that can be responsible for the indirect transmission of an infectious agent. *Droplet transmission* occurs when the infectious agent is expelled from the reservoir in the form of droplets, as happens with a sneeze or cough, to a recipient who is within a few feet. These droplets do not become airborne but settle on surfaces about 3 to 4 ft from their source. Meningococcal meningitis and influenza are examples of diseases transmitted in this manner.

Airborne transmission occurs when the infectious agent expelled from the source remains suspended in the form of droplet nuclei or dust in the air. The agent is then inhaled by a host. These droplet nuclei are 1 to 5 μm in size and are smaller than the droplets discussed in droplet transmission, and they can thus be carried by air currents. Chickenpox (varicella zoster) and tuberculosis are diseases that can be spread by this route.

Common vehicle transmission occurs when a contaminated inanimate vehicle acts as the intermediary for the infectious agent from the source to multiple hosts. Contaminated water, food, and intravenous fluids can be common vehicles. Salmonellosis and hepatitis B are

examples of diseases that can be transmitted in this manner.

Vector-borne transmission occurs when there is an animate intermediary from the source to the recipient. For example, mosquitos are the intermediary in the transmission of malaria, and ticks serve as the intermediary in the spread of Rocky Mountain spotted fever.

Once the infectious agent has been transmitted to a host, it must gain entry into the host. The *portals of entry* are similar to the modes of exit from the human reservoir mentioned previously and include the respiratory tract, the gastrointestinal tract, the genitourinary tract, and breaks in the skin or mucous membranes.

The final step in the process after the inoculation of the host is the maturation and multiplication of the infectious agent. Entry of an infectious agent into a host does not mean that the agent will proliferate and cause infection. Infection depends on the dose of the agent and the *susceptibility of the host*. The healthy human body is extremely resistant to infection; however, when the basic biologic defense mechanisms of the body are compromised, an infectious organism has a much greater chance of causing an infection. Chapter 19 deals with many of the factors of biologic defense exhibited by the host to prevent infection and injury. Some of the factors that affect host susceptibility to infection include (1) age (the very young and the very old being more susceptible); (2) immune status (certain disease states such as diabetes, cancer, or other chronic diseases can impair the immune status); (3) therapeutic treatments such as radiation and certain drugs, especially antibiotics, steroids, and chemotherapeutic agents; (4) surgery; (5) burns; (6) poor nutritional status; and (7) invasive procedures (intravenous catheters, chest tubes, urinary catheters) that break through the normal external defense barriers.

From the above discussion of the infectious disease process, it becomes evident that no one factor alone is responsible for an infection. Rather, there are a number of variables—the *agent*, the *environment*, and the *host*—which determine the outcome. In order to intervene effectively in the infectious disease process it is important that all of these concepts be understood.

Assessment

Once a pathogen gains access to a susceptible host, there is a period of time, known as the *incubation period*, before the clinical symptoms of the disease appear. During this period the organism is establishing itself, spreading to target organs or tissues, and proliferating within various body sites. This incubation period is variable depending upon the condition of the host but is often predictable and diagnostically significant. The appearance of the symptoms will depend upon the type of injury elicited by the virulent pathogen and the site of the organism within the body. The disease may be described as being *localized* (a focal point of symptoms or injury) or *generalized* (systemic involvement). The course of the disease may be *acute* or *chronic*. An acute disease often incites an immediate violent host response. The outcome of the infection (pathogen over host or host over pathogen) is determined within a relatively short span of time, as seen in mumps, plague, or smallpox. Conversely, in a chronic infection the pathogen establishes itself more insidiously within the host, does not cause immediate damage, and tends to provoke less of a host response, as in tuberculosis and aspergillosis. Although the terms chronic and acute are generally useful in describing the relationship between the host and a pathogen, there are many examples of acute infections becoming chronic and vice versa.

The establishment of an infection within the human body leads to a number of specific and generalized manifestations. The exact signs and symptoms elicited in the host depend on the agent responsible for the infection and the site of the infection. (For details on host response to specific infectious disease, see the particular chapter that discusses the disease site.) There are some general subjective, objective, and diagnostic findings that can alert the nurse to suspect an infection, even if the causative agent is not known. Recognition of the patient with a suspected infection is a crucial step in initiating early prevention and control measures.

For localized infections the patient may complain of pain, tenderness, warmth, swelling, or itching at the affected area. Objectively, there may be inflammation, edema, redness, or warmth at the area. There may be an exudate or drainage that is bloody, serous, cloudy, clear, creamy, or purulent. Purulence is a fairly reliable indicator of an infection. Infections of the respiratory tract may cause the patient to complain of a sore throat, rhinitis, congestion, cough, sputum production, or chest pain. The person who has diarrhea, nausea, vomiting, loss of appetite, or abdominal cramps may have an infectious process in the gastrointestinal tract. With a genitourinary tract infection the patient may complain of dysuria, frequency, urgency, hematuria, purulent or foul discharge, and flank or pelvic pain. It is important that the nurse note the characteristics of any secretions, excretions, drainage, or discharge and record these findings.

For generalized infections the symptoms may be even more vague. The earliest clinical manifestations of an infectious process are generally sensed within the host as nondescript, nonspecific reactions such as weakness, headache, light-headedness, congestion, muscle aches, pain in the joints, decreased appetite, or malaise. These sensations are broadly referred to as *prodromal symptoms* (preceeding the infection). As the infection progresses, other manifestations develop. These include fever, increased pulse rate, hypotension, altered mental status, or even jaundice, shock, confusion, and convulsions.

Of all the clinical symptoms mentioned, fever is one of the most valuable diagnostic indicators of infection, although not all fevers are the result of an infectious process. Most persons with an infectious disease develop fever (pyrexia) as a generalized response of the body to the infectious agent.

Another systemic response to infection is the variation in leukocytes (white blood cells [WBCs]) in peripheral circulation. The normal WBC count in blood is 5000 to 10,000 WBC/cu mm. With the presence of a serious infection the number of WBCs rises above 10,000/cu mm in response to the infectious inflammation. Leukocyte values between 10,000 and 20,000 are considered slightly elevated; 20,000 to 40,000 moderately elevated; and greater than 40,000 greatly elevated. In a few infectious diseases the number of WBCs in circulation actually drops, which is also a significant piece of diagnostic data.

Five types of mature WBCs are found in circulation: *neutrophils*, *eosinophils*, *basophils*, *lymphocytes*, and *monocytes*. Each type of WBC plays a more or less specific role in body defense (see Chapter 19); therefore different diseases produce different reactions among the white cell populations in the blood. These changes in patterns of distribution are detected not just by counting the total number of WBCs in a stained blood smear

TABLE 22-1. White blood cell response to infections

Leukocyte response	Associated infectious process
Increase in neutrophils (neutrophilia)	Usual in a large number of acute local and systemic infections caused by bacteria (especially pyogenic bacteria), rickettsia, some viruses, and a few protozoa
Decrease in neutrophils (neutropenia)	Frequent in salmonellosis, brucellosis, whooping cough, overwhelming bacterial infections, influenza, infectious mononucleosis, infectious hepatitis, mumps, rubella, rubeola, and some rickettsial and protozoan diseases
Increase in eosinophils (eosinophilia)	Frequent in allergic reactions, chronic skin disease, helminthic infections, and scarlet fever
Increase in lymphocytes (lymphocytosis)	Frequent in chickenpox, mumps, measles, infectious mononucleosis, influenza, whooping cough, syphilis, tuberculosis, salmonellosis, viral hepatitis, and viral pneumonia; sometimes in convalescence from actue bacterial infection
Increase in monocytes (monocytosis)	Common in tuberculosis, chickenpox, brucellosis, mumps, syphilis, and certain rickettsial diseases; may occur in certain viral and protozoan diseases and in convalescent phase of acute bacterial infections

but also by classifying them according to morphology and calculating the relative percentage of each cell type present. This type of count is known as a differential count. The differential count may provide information that can be correlated with other clinical data to help diagnose a situation. Table 22-1 provides some general correlations between leukocyte response and infectious diseases.

None of the signs and symptoms present in localized or generalized infections are diagnostic in themselves. Many can be demonstrated by other disease processes. They can, however, serve as helpful clues in the diagnosis of a suspected infectious process.

Diagnostic tests

Diagnostic tests are an important adjunct in the diagnosis of an infection. Some of the diagnostic tests used to obtain data include *skin tests, radiologic tests, gallium scans, ultrasound,* and *computed tomography (CT scan)* of various body sites. Examples of data obtainable from such tests include leukocytosis; anemia; increase in erythrocyte sedimentation rate (p. 281); appearance of C-reactive protein (p. 279); proteinemia; positive bacterial, viral, and fungal cultures; and positive radio-

logic findings, all of which may indicate the presence of an infection.

Proper collection and handling of laboratory specimens are essential to ensure accurate laboratory results. Inappropriate collection or handling of specimens may lead to unnecessary delays in test results or to inaccurate results, thus affecting the therapy given to the patient. When an infection is suspected, cultures are taken of the suspected site. In the patient who has a fever and in whom the site of infection is unknown, cultures are commonly taken of the blood, urine, sputum, and any other possible sites of infection. This may include spinal fluid cultures, aspirates of body fluid, or intravenous catheter tips. *It is imperative that these cultures be obtained before the initiation of antibiotic therapy, since antibiotics can suppress any bacteria that are present and give inaccurate or false-negative culture results.* Cultures should be obtained in a manner that avoids contamination. Aseptic preparation of the site to be cultured, observance of aseptic technique, and placing specimens in an appropriate container are crucial factors to be observed in ensuring the best sample. Once obtained, the specimen must be properly stored and transported promptly to the laboratory. Each institution should have guidelines for the proper method for collecting and handling specimens for the laboratory. All specimens must be accompanied by the correct requisition and include the following information: (1) patient's name, (2) date and time of collection, (3) test requested, (4) type of specimen, (5) how specimen was obtained (i.e., clean void or catheter urine, expectorated sputum, or tracheal aspirate), and (6) where the results are to be sent. A record of all tests is kept to avoid unnecessary duplication of tests.

Interpretation of laboratory results is sometimes difficult. Certain body sites have bacteria known as *normal flora,* which reside there in a commensalistic (intimate) relationship with the host. The skin, upper respiratory tract, vagina, urethra, and bowel are examples of body sites in which normal bacterial flora can be found. The bacteria found vary from site to site, and knowing the normal flora is helpful in discerning the significance of laboratory culture results. *A Clinician's Dictionary Guide to Bacteria and Fungi*[24] is an excellent publication that lists in detail the normal flora of various sites. It must be emphasized that laboratory results alone cannot be used to make diagnostic and therapeutic decisions. Rather, they are used in conjunction with the clinical status of the patient to make appropriate diagnostic and therapeutic decisions.

Knowledge about the infectious disease process and about how to recognize or suspect an infectious process is vital to the prevention and control of infectious diseases in both community and hospital settings. Prevention and control of disease are addressed in the remainder of this chapter.

Infection control in the community

An infectious disease is termed a *communicable disease* when it is highly transmissible to other persons (p. 360). Smallpox is an example of a communicable disease, which, through cooperative efforts worldwide, has been successfully eradicated from the world.[20] The methods used to eradicate smallpox throughout the world can serve as a model of how to eliminate other communicable diseases. The eradication of smallpox also demonstrates the importance of accurate reporting of communicable diseases to the proper authorities so that appropriate prevention and control measures can be instituted.

On the international level the World Health Organization (WHO), a special agency of the United Nations, has as its primary purpose the improvement and standardization of measures to prevent and control disease throughout the world. Its Epidemiological Intelligence Service in Geneva receives immediate notification of large-scale outbreaks of infectious diseases throughout the world and advises the world community of impending epidemics. The *Weekly Epidemiological Record* is an official publication of the agency.

On the national level the Centers for Disease Control (CDC) of the Public Health Service, located in Atlanta, is responsible for programs for the prevention and control of communicable and other preventable disease in the United States. The CDC provides epidemiologic and laboratory services to state health facilities on request. It enforces quarantine regulations, conducts foreign quarantine activities, administers international activities for the control of malaria, smallpox, and measles, and provides consultation to other nations in the control of preventable diseases. It also collects, tabulates, and assesses data on reportable diseases from state health departments and publishes the findings in the *Morbidity and Mortality Weekly Report*. Through its continuous surveillance, the CDC is able to detect new cases of diseases and to intervene to control disease outbreaks. In addition, the CDC is instrumental in providing guidelines and recommendations for infection control.

In the United States the control of infectious diseases is the responsibility of each state. State health officers usually delegate this responsibility to a division of communicable diseases. A staff of physicians, nurses, veterinarians, and sanitary engineers works closely with a state epidemiologist in detection, assessment, and control of specific reportable diseases.

Local public health departments work in conjunction with their state health departments in this effort. The community health nurse plays a vital role in the collection of data, surveillance activities, immunization programs, education, and other control measures. Physicians and health care facilities have a responsibility to report communicable diseases promptly to the health department. Health agencies in the community can use the reported data to determine potential or real problems, to identify the causative agent and hopefully its source, and to identify the population at risk. A method to control the problem, care for the exposed, and protect the population at risk can then be devised and implemented.

Prevention and control measures

One method of prevention and control of disease in the community involves environmental control measures such as sanitation techniques that ensure a pure water supply and proper disposal of sewage and other potentially infectious materials. These measures have been legislated into building codes, state laws, and federal regulations. Similarly, there are regulations regarding health practices in institutions that handle, package, and prepare foods. Another example of an environmental control measure is the spraying of a designated area to kill mosquitos, which are implicated in the spread of viral encephalitis. Spraying usually is done only after an outbreak has been identified.

Depending on the communicable disease, care of exposed persons and protection of the population at risk for contracting the disease may entail prophylaxis, immunization, or only careful monitoring of new cases. Often, simple adherence to basic principles of hygiene is sufficient. Determination of additional required measures should be made by the local or state health department. Attempts are made to reach those at risk and inform them of the preventive measures. Education of the public is a key component of these efforts.

In the United States there has been a marked reduction in recent years in the incidence of infectious diseases, such as measles, whooping cough, and poliomyelitis, which can be prevented by immunization. Concern is being expressed, however, about the decrease in the number of children presently being immunized, despite the fact that these immunizations can often be obtained free of cost. Additionally, concern is being expressed that federal monies used to support local immunization efforts may be reduced to such a level that free immunizations will no longer be equally available in all 50 states. Infections formerly seen only in children are now being seen more frequently in adults because of the failure of the population to develop acquired immunity during early childhood. This reduction in childhood infections is believed to be directly related to improved sanitary conditions.

A more recent concern is the elimination because of

air travel of the barriers of time and distance and the possibility of a person with an infectious disease being brought from a remote area of the world to a major population center where the disease can be readily spread to a susceptible public.

The dramatic control of several infectious diseases has been caused by the development and use of a variety of *inactivated vaccines* and *live attenuated antigens*. The potential for eradication of common infectious diseases brings with it major responsibilities for public health agencies, physicians, and nurses. Ways must be found not only to carry out planned programs of immunization, but also to educate the public to the hazards of apathy and failure to maintain proper levels of immunization. Continued progress in control and eradication requires that there be commitment to continue to add to knowledge about immunization patterns, to evaluate effectiveness and risks of antigens used, and to monitor the levels of protection present in a population.

Immunization programs

Immunization programs have played and continue to play a primary role in the control of infectious disease throughout the world. The body can be stimulated to produce antibodies against some specific diseases without actually having the disease (*active artificial immunity*). Temporary protection sometimes can be provided by injecting antibodies produced by other persons or other animals into the bloodstream of a human being (*passive artificial immunity*).

Recommendations concerning current immunization schedules are found in the *Red Book* published by the Committee on Infectious Diseases of The American Academy of Pediatrics and in *Morbidity and Mortality Weekly Reports*, which present recommendations of the United States Public Health Service's Advisory Committee on Immunization Practices (ACIP). The reader should refer to these resources when there are questions about proper immunization practices, prophylaxis, interruption in immunization schedules, or adverse reactions and side effects.

Active immunization

Active immunity can be acquired by artificially injecting small numbers of attenuated (weakened) or dead organisms of specific types or modified toxins from the organisms (toxoids) into the body (p. 273). This procedure is known as *inoculation*. If 90% of the population is protected against organisms that require continued passage through human beings in order to reproduce and live, the disease caused by the organism can be virtually eliminated because there are too few susceptible hosts for organism spread. Smallpox has been eliminated from the world in this way. This type of protection of a group is called *herd immunity*. It is ineffectual, however, against organisms such as tetanus bacilli that can exist indefinitely (in the soil,) and in this instance each person must be immunized to be protected. If the disease is one not prevalent in the environment, such as diptheria in the United States, or is not spread from person to person by direct contact, such as tetanus, the inoculation must be repeated at regular intervals to maintain protection. This inoculation is called a *booster dose*, and usually one tenth of the original inoculating dose is sufficient.

An inoculation often causes a local tissue response. Symptoms of inflammation (redness, tenderness, swelling, sometimes ulcerations) appear at the site of the injection, and symptoms of widespread tissue involvement (slight febrile reactions, general malaise, muscle aching) for a day or two are common. The initial inoculation produces delayed symptoms because the immune response system must become sensitized to the antigen. There usually is an accelerated and less severe systemic reaction to subsequent inoculations because the immune response is stimulated at once. The local reaction also is less severe than that which occurs following the initial inoculation because the organisms have less opportunity to produce inflammation.

Active artificial immunization against many bacilli and viruses is now available. All persons should be encouraged to avail themselves of the protection advised by health officials in their local area. They also should be advised to keep a permanent record of the date of each immunization.

In the United States the ACIP recommends that all children be immunized against diphtheria, pertussis (whooping cough), tetanus, mumps, rubella, poliomyelitis, and measles.

Primary immunization schedules. The immunization schedule for *diphtheria, pertussis,* and *tetanus* (DPT) begins with one dose of combined toxoid and vaccine when an infant is 6 weeks to 2 months old. The next two doses are given at 4- to 8-week intervals thereafter. The fourth dose is administered about 1 year after the third dose. This schedule maintains adequate antibody levels until the child enters kindergarten, when a booster immunization is given. Thereafter, booster doses of tetanus and diphtheria only are given every 10 years.

Trivalent oral poliomyelitis vaccine (TOPV) is a live attenuated vaccine combining all three strains of poliomyelitis virus. One dose consists of 2 drops of vaccine on a cube of sugar, in a small amount of distilled water, or in a spoonful of corn syrup. TOPV is the vaccine of choice for primary immunization of children, although inactivated polio vaccine (IPV) is also effective. Parents of the child receiving the vaccine should be made aware of the advantages and disadvantages of each vaccine. The primary series of TOPV consists of three doses. The first is usually given at the same time the DPT series is begun (6 to 12 weeks of age). The next dose is given 6 to 8 weeks later, and the third dose is given at least 6 weeks and preferably 8 to 12 months after that. A fourth dose is given just before entry into school.

A single dose of live attenuated *measles (rubeola) vaccine* is given when the child is 15 months old for maximal seroconversion. Before 15 months of age the mother's antibodies transmitted in utero give adequate protection and may also interfere with the infant's seroconversion. Children who have not been immunized as infants can be vaccinated at any age. Surveillance has shown an upward shift in the age distribution of reported cases of measles, indicating a need for better immunization of susceptible adolescents and young adults.[22]

Mumps vaccine (also a live attenuated vaccine) is given as a single dose at any age after 12 months. It should not be given before 12 months of age because of the persistence of maternal antibodies, which may interfere with seroconversion. Mumps vaccine is usually given in a combined vaccine with measles and rubella at 15 months of age. All susceptible children, adolescents, and adults should be vaccinated unless contraindicated.

A single dose of live *rubella vaccine* is recommended for children after 12 months of age for maximal seroconversion. As mentioned earlier, it can be given in a combined form with measles and mumps vaccines. As with measles, most cases of rubella are now being seen in adolescents and young adults, whereas before the vaccine became available in 1969, most cases were in school-aged children. Thus increased surveillance and vaccination of children need to be undertaken for better prevention and control. As a preventive measure, women in childbearing years should be tested for rubella antibodies, since rubella infection during the first trimester of pregnancy is associated with neonatal morbidity and mortality. If antibodies are not present, vaccination is recommended. *Because of the theoretical risk of the vaccine to the fetus, females of childbearing age are vaccinated only if they are not pregnant and they are counseled not to become pregnant for 3 months following vaccination.*

Routine vaccination against smallpox is no longer recommended by the Public Health Service since the side effects and complications of the vaccine are greater than the danger of acquiring the disease. The vaccine is indicated only for laboratory workers who are directly involved with smallpox or closely related orthopox viruses.

At the present time, immunization against typhoid fever is recommended only when there is exposure to a typhoid carrier in the household, when there is an outbreak of typhoid in a community, or when traveling to countries where typhoid is endemic (always present). Immunization to protect against other diseases is given on a selective basis; that is, groups at a high risk are immunized. Because of the prevalence of *influenza* and its potential for causing death, the ACIP recommends immunization against influenza for all individuals at increased risk of adverse consequences from infection of the lower respiratory tract. This includes persons over 60 years of age and persons over 2 years of age who have chronic cardiac, respiratory, metabolic, or renal disease or diseases that impair the person's immune system. Initial protection is obtained by giving two injections of influenza vaccine 4 weeks apart beginning in October or November. Infants and children up to 6 years old who are at risk are given a subviron, split-virus vaccine in two doses 4 weeks apart. A yearly booster dose is needed to maintain and update immunity. Persons who are allergic to eggs or egg products may not be immunized because of the danger of hypersensitivity reactions.

The use of pneumococcal vaccine against *Streptococcus pneumoniae* is under investigation. There is not yet enough data for the ACIP to formulate formal recommendations about the routine use of the vaccine for immunization in the general population. It is currently being administered to adults and children over 2 years of age with chronic illnesses who are at increased risk of complications associated with pneumonoccal infections. A single dose is given only once. The duration of protection is unknown. Further investigation of the use of vaccines for protection against other bacterial infections is under way and could offer promise in improving immune defenses in immunocompromised patients.

Passive immunization

Antibodies produced by other persons or by other animals such as the horse, cow, and rabbit can be introduced into the bloodstream of a person for protection against attack by a pathogen. This protection is *temporary,* usually lasting only a few weeks, and stimulates no production of antibodies by the recipient. It is called *artificial passive acquired immunity.* Artificial passive immunization is given to a person who has been exposed to a disease and has no natural or artificial active immunity. It usually is given before the disease develops, but it may be given to modify the symptoms of a disease. However, for effectiveness after the disease has developed, it must be administered early, before extensive damage to body tissue has occurred.

Passive immunization usually is reserved for situations in which the disease would be detrimental to the person. For example, it is rarely given to prevent a disease such as chickenpox or mumps in children because they are at an optimal age for the body to respond immunologically with minimal inflammatory response. On the other hand, an adult exposed to the same diseases often would be given antibodies because adults may have a severe pathologic response. Immunization is given to all age groups exposed to pathogens that cause serious diseases such as hepatitis, poliomyelitis, diphtheria, tetanus, or rabies. Antivenins, which are given to people bitten by poisonous snakes or black widow spiders, are other examples of passive immunologic products.

Products used for passive immunization may be specific to the disease. Antitoxins and immune animal and human sera are examples. These materials contain elevated levels of immune globulins, which can specifically detoxify the toxin, neutralize the virus, or inactivate the bacterium. The whole blood of a patient who has recently recovered from a disease against which antibodies are produced also may be used. Antitoxins are available for diphtheria, tetanus, botulism, gas gangrene, and the venom of snakes. *Immune animal serum* is available against rabies; *human immune serum* is available for mumps, measles, pertussis, poliomyelitis, and tetanus.

Immune serum globulin (ISG), or gamma globulin (γ-globulin), is an antibody-rich fraction of pooled plasma from normal donors. The rationale for pooling plasma is that someone among the donors will have had the diseases and will have developed antibodies against them. The *globulin fraction* of the plasma carries the *antibodies,* and because it is known not to transmit the virus of hepatitis, it is considered safe to use. Because of occasional side effects, it is now recommended that the use of immune serum globulin be limited to those disorders in which its efficacy has been definitely established. These are measles prophylaxis or modification, viral hepatitis type A prophylaxis or modification, and immune deficiency diseases. Immune serum globulin is considered to be of questionable value in the following situations: (1) prevention of rubella in the first trimester of pregnancy, (2) prevention or modification of varicella in certain high-risk patients, (3) prevention or modification of viral hepatitis type B (serum hepatitis) after accidental inoculation, and (4) life-threatening bacterial infections.

Special human immune serum globulins are derived from the sera of persons previously immunized or convalescing from specific diseases. Tetanus immune globulin (human) is of value in prophylaxis and treatment of tetanus in persons who have not received prior immunization. Pertussis immune globulin (human) and mumps immune globulin (human) are of uncertain or unproved value in the prevention and treatment of pertussis and mumps, respectively. Hepatitis B immune globulin (human) is available for prophylaxis after exposure to hepatitis B. Zoster immune globulin (human) is available for restricted use for prophylaxis against chickenpox.

Nursing responsibilities in immunization

Probably the greatest responsibility of the nurse in immunization programs is to teach the public the ad-

vantages of immunization and encourage widespread participation in programs recommended by the local public health officer.

Teaching. In teaching it is advisable to provide the public with the following information: against what disease protection is being given, why immunization is desirable, and when booster doses should be obtained. The relative safety of the immunization and the advantages of immunization early in life should be stressed.

The nurse is responsible for assessing persons before immunization because there are some contraindications to receiving certain immunizing substances. Those that are prepared in chicken or duck embryos may cause an allergic reaction in persons who are allergic to eggs. Many people are allergic to horse serum, and substances containing horse serum, such as tetanus antitoxin, should never be given unless a small amount of the substance has been injected intradermally (a sensitivity test) and after 20 minutes produces no "hive" reaction about the injection site. *Active immunologic products* should not be given while a person has a cold or other infection because the inflammatory reaction from the immunization will be greater than usual.

Children with histories of allergy often are *not* given routine immunization against diseases for which there is *herd immunity* because the danger of severe allergic response to the immunization is greater than the danger of contracting the disease. These children should be immunized against diseases such as tetanus, however, and immunization is achieved by giving the vaccine or toxoid in small doses over a period of several weeks or months. The package inserts accompanying the immunologic product should always be read carefully to determine the indications, precautions, and side effects.

Live attenuated virus vaccines should not be given to persons with alterations in their immune status, since virus replication after administration may be unchecked in these individuals. TOPV viruses are excreted by the recipient of the vaccine and are communicable to other persons, so individuals who live with an immunocompromised person should not receive TOPV. If a person has a febrile illness, it is usually best to wait until recovery before vaccination is given. Pregnant women should not receive *live attenuated virus* vaccines because of the theoretical risk to the fetus. Live attenuated virus vaccines should not be given at the same time as passive immunization since passively acquired antibodies can interfere with the response to live attenuated virus vaccines.[20]

Before leaving the clinic, the person or family members should be instructed as to the expected effects of an inoculation and told to contact the physician or to report to a hospital emergency room if any other symptoms develop. The person is cautioned not to scratch any lesion produced by an inoculation. If a severe local reaction with redness, swelling, and tenderness occurs, the physician may order the application of hot, wet dressings. If the lesion is open, these dressings should be sterile.

When antitoxins, antisera, or antivenins are given, the patient is kept under observation for 20 to 30 minutes. Symptoms of severe allergic response usually will appear within that period of time.

Persons employed in health care facilities should maintain their immune status against poliomyelitis, diphtheria, and tetanus. Persons with negative tuberculin tests should be retested every 6 months, and those with positive tuberculin tests should have a yearly chest x-ray film taken. Persons working in dialysis units and blood processing areas (laboratories, blood banks) need to guard against infection with hepatitis B virus.

Home care. Persons with communicable diseases are frequently cared for at home. The community health nurse is often asked to teach family members how to care for the patient and how to protect family members, friends, and neighbors. The same principles apply in the home as in the hospital. It must be emphasized that the extent of the care measures depends on the communicable disease involved. The local health department should be consulted for full information regarding specific communicable diseases. Some general principles for home care of persons with communicable diseases follow: A smock or coverall may be used to protect the clothes. A mask, if indicated, can be improvised from any closely woven, absorbable material, or disposable ones can be purchased at a pharmacy. All liquid wastes can be flushed down the toilet. Garbage and other wastes from the room can be wrapped in several layers of newspaper, placed in a plastic bag, and tied securely before discarding in a rubbish container. Dishes that are not disposable should be boiled for 10 minutes before washing. If a dishwasher is available, boiling of dishes is unnecessary. Laundry should be washed in the washing machine in hot water with a detergent and chlorine bleach or a disinfectant to disinfect it. When the patient has recovered, the room should be thoroughly aired. Depending on the type of illness, the walls, floors, and furniture may need to be washed well with a detergent or a disinfectant and warm water. If materials that cannot be washed, such as books or toys, have been contaminated, exposing them to the sun and air for 24 to 48 hours usually provides sufficient protection. *Regardless of the disease, good hand washing should be practiced following contact with any excretions, secretions, or drainage.*

The person who is discharged from the hospital with an infection that may be apparent or incubating at the time of discharge is also a public health concern. This person should be cared for similarly to those with known infections using the guidelines mentioned above. Likewise, the person who is admitted to the hospital from the community with an infection poses a potential problem in the hospital as well. This person can serve as a source of infection to other patients and personnel and it would be best to treat such a person at home, if possible. The special problems the nurse encounters in controlling *hospital-acquired infections* will be the focus of the remainder of this chapter.

Infection control in the hospital

Scope of the problem

A *nosocomial* infection is one that is not present or incubating at the time a person is admitted to the hospital but develops after admission. A *community-acquired infection* is one that is present or incubating at the time of admission to the hospital. The nurse should be aware of the problem of nosocomial infections; their effects on patient morbidity, mortality, and increased hospital costs; as well as the legal aspects concerning them. The nurse also should be knowledgeable about the types of infections seen most often, the common pathogens and how they are transmitted, factors that predispose a patient to a nosocomial infection, how to recognize persons at risk of infection, and the prevention and control measures necessary to decrease the incidence of nosocomial infections.

At least 2 million persons, or about 5% of all patients admitted to United States hospitals each year, develop nosocomial infections. In addition to the considerable morbidity and mortality caused by these infections, their diagnoses and treatment (including additional days of hospitalization) cost more than 1 billion dollars per year.[26] The JCAH requires that those institutions seeking accreditation have a program of infection control centered around *monitoring* (1) patients with infections, (2) patient care practices, (3) antibiotic usage, (4) health of personnel, and (5) the environment of the institution. The AHA and the CDC have developed guidelines for the prevention and control of infectious diseases for use in patient care centers. Because of these external forces, as well as to provide the best possible care for their patients, hospitals are recognizing the need to increase infection surveillance and to upgrade programs to prevent nosocomial infections.

As seen in Table 22-2, the incidence of *nosocomial* infections varies with the type of hospital, and this can be attributed to differences in the size of hospitals, the severity of illness in the patient population, susceptibility of the patient population, and the number of personnel who have hands-on contact with the patients. The patient with the greatest risk of developing a nosocomial infection is one with a chronic illness, a prolonged hospital stay, and the most direct contact with various hospital personnel (i.e., physicians, students, nurses, therapists, etc.). These factors hold true not only for variations of infection rates from institution to institution, but also for variations in infection rates within an institution. Certain patient care areas are considered to be *high-risk areas* for developing nosocomial infections. These areas understandably are those that care for patients who have decreased host defenses or in whom invasive procedures and devices are common. Areas generally considered to be high risk are (1) intensive care units (including neonatal units), (2) burn units, (3) dialysis units, and (4) oncology units. The infection rate in these areas may be well over 20%.

Persons at risk

The nurse needs to be able to recognize those patients who are at the greatest risk of a nosocomial infection. Some of the factors that predispose a person to infection were mentioned previously; briefly, they include (1) the age of the patient, the very young and the very old being the most susceptible; (2) impairment of normal immune defenses because of an underlying disease process such as cancer, chronic renal disease, chronic lung disease, diabetes, and so on; (3) impairment of the normal immune defenses because of the therapy being given, such as radiation, steroids, or chemotherapy; (4) use of antibiotics, which can eliminate the patient's normal flora, providing opportunity for colonization with pathogenic and drug-resistant organisms that may then progress to cause infection; (5) use of invasive diagnostic and therapeutic procedures and devices (which bypass the patient's normal defense barriers and thus provide a portal of entry into the body, e.g., use of indwelling urinary catheters, monitoring devices, intravenous catheters, and respiratory assistive devices); (6) surgery; (7) burns; and (8) length of hospitalization. Probably the single most important factor predisposing a patient to acquiring a nosocomial infection is the severity of the patient's underlying disease.

A patient admitted to the hospital with an infection may during the hospitalization develop a *superinfection* with another organism. Often this superinfection is with a more virulent or drug-resistant organism. For example, a patient admitted with a leg ulcer infected with *Staphylococcus aureus* may develop further infection (not colonization) with *Pseudomonas aeruginosa*. Furthermore, if this infection progresses to involve the bloodstream, then a *secondary bacteremia* has occurred. Infection can occur secondary to (1) an existing infection, (2) an underlying disease process, or (3) an anatomic defect that may be causing obstruction. An example of this is the man who has benign prostrate hypertrophy (BPH) and who develops a urinary tract infection secondary to the obstruction caused by the BPH. These are the concepts that are the most helpful when seeking to determine the etiology of a particular infection.

The most common site for a nosocomial infection is the urinary tract; 75% of these infections are related to instrumentation, including indwelling urinary catheters, catheterizations, and urologic procedures. Infected surgical wounds, followed by lower respiratory tract infections, and then bloodstream infections (some associated with the use of intravascular lines) are the next most frequently encountered types of nosocomial infections. Together these sites account for about 85% of all nosocomial infections (Fig. 22-2).

TABLE 22-2. Nosocomial infection rates by category of hospital*

Category of hospital	Percent of patients with nosocomial infections†
Community	2.5
Community-reaching	3.3
Federal	4.6
Municipal or county	4.4
University	4.2
All hospitals	3.4

*From Centers for Disease Control: National nosocomial infections study report: annual summary 1978, issued March 1981, Atlanta, 1981, The Centers.
†Rate per 100 patient discharges.

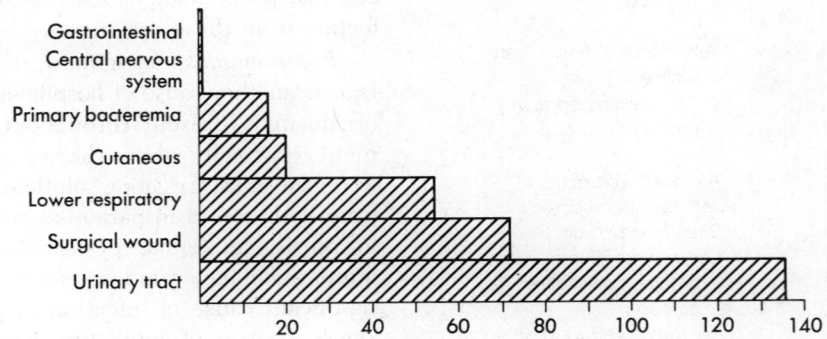

Fig. 22-2. Nosocomial infection rates per 10,000 patients discharged by site of infection. (From Centers for Disease Control: National nosocomial infections study report. Annual summary 1978, issued March 1981, U.S. Department of Health and Human Services.)

Pathogens causing nosocomial infections

The different types of pathogens commonly responsible for nosocomial infections and their most common reservoirs are listed in Table 22-3. In the past 2 decades there has been a decline in the number of nosocomial infections caused by gram-positive bacteria, especially staphylococci and streptococci; however, *Staphylococcus aureus* is still the single most common organism causing nosocomial surgical wound infections. At the same time, there has been an increase in the incidence of nosocomial infection caused by gram-negative bacteria, particularly members of the family enterobacteriaceae and the genus *Pseudomonas*, which now cause 60% to 65% of all nosocomial infections. These gram-negative organisms collectively are responsible for nearly all nosocomial urinary tract infections, 70% of the bacteremias, and the majority of respiratory tract and surgical wound infections.

TABLE 22-3. Modes of transmission of some common pathogens

Pathogen	Common reservoir
Gram-positive cocci	
Staphylococcus aureus	Contaminated objects, *hands* and nasal tracts of health care workers, air, self
Group A *Streptococcus* organisms	Direct contact, air, *hands*, rarely objects
Enterococcus organisms	Self, *hands* of health care workers, environmental surfaces
Gram-negative rods	
Escherichia, Klebsiella, Enterobacter	Self, *hands* of health care workers, contaminated solutions
Proteus, Salmonella, Providencia, Serratia, Citrobacter	Contaminated food and water, *hands* of health care workers, self
Pseudomonas	Contaminated environment, *hands*, self
Anaerobic bacteria	
Clostridium, Bacteroides	Self, contaminated environment, *hands*
Fungal organisms	
Yeasts	Self, *hands* of health care workers
Fungi	Air, contaminated environment
Viruses	
Varicella	Air, direct contact
Herpes	Self, direct contact, air
Rubella	Direct contact, air
Hepatitis B	Contaminated instruments or injectables, direct contact
Poliomyelitis	Contaminated food or water

The reservoir for *Staphylococcus aureus* is the respiratory tract and skin. Ten to fifteen percent of the general population can be persistent carriers of this organism, which is harbored in the anterior nares. Among individuals working in hospitals the carrier rate may be as high as 25% to 30%. Nasal carriers, especially those with respiratory tract infections, are potential sources of environmental and human contact contamination. *Careful attention to hand washing before and after contact with patients, and the institution of appropriate isolation for patients with known Staphylococcus aureus infections are the most effective means of preventing cross-infection.*

Group A streptococci (*Streptococcus pyogenes*) are also gram-positive organisms that are seen in nosocomial infections. Strains of these organisms cause streptococcal sore throat, scarlet fever, and streptococcal skin infections. Streptococci are found in animate reservoirs, particularly the pharynx and nares of personnel and patients.

Other organisms involved in nosocomial infections include gram-negative coliforms, *Escherichia, Klebsiella*, and *Enterobacter*, which live in the human intestinal tract. Although these organisms are usually susceptible to antibiotics, they have the capacity to develop antibiotic resistance. The large reservoir of coliform organisms within the general population can be a source for self-infection or for cross-infection from the hands of hospital personnel through the ingestion of foods or through the contamination of other materials. Some strains of these organisms are more likely to produce infection than are other strains. The more pathogenic strains seem to gain the ascendency in patients who are receiving antibiotic therapy; immune-deficient patients are particularly susceptible to infection by the coliforms.

Although *Salmonella* organisms are usually acquired outside the hospital, the organism is readily transmissible and can be the cause of nosocomial infection. It is transmitted by direct or indirect contact with an infected person or through food, dairy products, or water contaminated with the organism. Patients with sickle cell disease or malignancies are more vulnerable to infection from these organisms.

Pseudomonas aeruginosa, a gram-negative organism, is another cause of hospital-associated infection. The organism is present throughout the hospital environment, especially where there is a persistent presence of water (in sinks, irrigating solutions, nebulizers). It is more frequently found in patients with *leukopenia* secondary to burns, leukemia, cystic fibrosis, and various immune-deficiency syndromes. It is also known to be a significant cause of infection in patients receiving prolonged courses of antibiotics, immunosuppressive drugs, and inhalation therapy. It can be a threat to patients undergoing instrumentation (tracheostomy, urinary tract catheterization) and to recipients of renal transplants. Newborns, particularly premature infants, as well as the elderly and the debilitated are the most vulnerable.

Serratia marcescens and *Serratia liquefaciens* are gram-negative organisms that are being seen with increased frequency in nosocomial infections. The reservoirs for these organisms are soil and water, and they are found in the hospital in similar reservoirs as *Pseudomonas*. Previously thought to be non-pathogenic, *Serratia marcescens* was used because of its red pigmentation to mark air flow and settling patterns of bacteria. It is now recognized as a pathogen that can cause severe infection in a susceptible host. One problem with *Serratia* has been its ability to develop resistance to antibiotics rapidly. This can have devastating consequences in an intensive care or burn unit when an outbreak occurs. Because its mode of transmission is through direct or indirect contact on the hands of personnel or on contaminated articles, good hand-washing and aseptic techniques are the most effective measures to prevent outbreaks of infection.

Candida albicans is a yeastlike fungus that can cause infection, especially in immunocompromised patients or in patients receiving antibiotics. These patients have a decrease in their normal flora, which provides a niche for the *Candida* to settle in and proliferate. Antibiotics suppress bacterial growth but do not affect fungal growth; special antifungal agents are necessary to control these infections unless there is a return of the normal flora following discontinuance of the antibiotics.

Prevention and control measures

In the hospital there are many potential sources of infection, including patients, personnel, visitors, equipment, linen, and so on. The patient may become infected with organisms from either the external environment (*exogenous*) or, as is often seen in the severely immunocompromised host, from their own internal organisms (*endogenous*). Virtually any microorganism can be a potential pathogen to the immunocompromised patient. Most of the causative organisms are present in the external environment of the patient and are introduced into the body through direct contact or contaminated materials. In many instances nosocomial infections could be prevented by strict aseptic technique when giving care to the patient and by using greater restraint in the use of invasive procedures and antibiotics. Some specific infection control measures follow.

Control of external environment

Health care providers should be in good health and keep their immunization status up to date. They should report to the employee health service when they feel ill. Visitors, too, should be in good health and should be limited in numbers to prevent overcrowding in the patient's room. Personnel should wear clean clothing and observe good personal hygiene practices, especially thorough hand washing, which decreases transient and resident flora on the hands and thus acts as a deterrent to cross-infection via the hands. Friction and rinsing are the two most important components of good hand washing. Ample hand-washing facilities are necessary throughout the hospital and should be used by all personnel before and after patient contact, after contact with excretions, secretions, wound drainage, or any contaminated articles; and before any clean or sterile procedure or contact with clean or sterile equipment. *Hand washing is the single most effective method for preventing nosocomial infection.*[28] Dermatologic conditions of the hands should be corrected, since dry, cracked skin can more readily become colonized with pathogens and broken skin is more difficult to rid of transient and resident flora. The person with a skin problem on the hands also tends to avoid proper hand washing, since it can further increase dryness and irritation. The person with active herpes simplex infection of the hand (herpetic whitlow) should not give direct patient care until the lesion has healed.

Housekeeping and sanitation practices should be strictly observed to reduce dust and environmental reservoirs of organisms, especially in high-risk areas such as nurseries, operating rooms, and intensive care units. Linens should be changed with as little contact with the nurse's uniform as possible; linen should not be thrown on the floor or shaken in the air, since this not only will further contaminate the linen but also will stir up dust particles and create air currents that can transmit pathogens. Waste products should be disposed of in the appropriate receptacle. Proper cleaning and sterilization of contaminated articles and equipment are essential. There should be a program to monitor the effectiveness of these practices; however, routine culturing of the environment is not advocated. Proper ventilation of patients' rooms is necessary to provide adequate air exchange and to decrease the concentration of organisms in the air. Most patient rooms in modern hospitals are under negative pressure, which means air will move into the room from the hallway instead of vice versa.

Control of internal environment

Reducing the *endogenous* sources of infection is more difficult than control of the external environment. Often the source is the patient's own normal flora, and these infections are not directly preventable by the nurse. Preventive measures are aimed at increasing the patient's defense mechanisms and thus decreasing the risk of the infection. Teaching the patient about good nutrition and personal hygiene is a practical measure that is part of nursing care. Maintaining the patient's normal flora and preventing colonization with pathogens that can serve as a source of infection are other effective measures. These, however, are not always possible when patients are receiving antibiotics or undergoing chemotherapy, since these measures may disrupt the normal flora and provide for colonization. Appropriate use of antibiotics for prophylaxis and treatment helps to prevent colonization with pathogens and decreases the incidence of infection with drug-resistant organisms. Good hand washing by all who have contact with the patient will decrease the possibility of inoculation of the patient with pathogenic organisms. Personnel should develop the habit of working from clean procedures to dirty procedures when delivering patient care. For example, the nurse should adjust the intravenous infusion rate and check the intravenous site *before* changing the bed of an incontinent patient.

Prevention of urinary tract infections

As mentioned previously, *urinary tract infections* (UTIs) are the most common nosocomial infections seen in the hospital. The majority of these infections are associated with catheterization and instrumentation of the urinary tract. Urinary catheters should be used only when absolutely necessary. If a catheter must be used, it should be discontinued as soon as medically feasible, since the longer the catheter is in place, the greater the risk of developing an infection. Strict aseptic technique is necessary when inserting the catheter to prevent transmission of bacteria into the bladder. Bacteria that are present around the catheter-meatal junction can also be transmitted on the tip of the catheter into the bladder along the thin layer of mucus that surrounds the catheter in the urethra. For this reason, the catheter should be securely anchored to prevent it from moving in and out of the urethra. Movement of the catheter can track bacteria into the urethra and up into the bladder along the mucous sheath. Furthermore, the catheter-meatal junction should be kept clean; the patient incontinent of stool can pose a problem in this regard. In some institutions antiseptic agents are used to cleanse the meatus and antimicrobial agents are applied around the catheter-meatal junction. *Both of these practices are considered controversial.* Good hand-washing techniques by personnel, cleansing of the patient's meatal area with soap and water, and proper anchoring of the catheter are considered to be effective ways to reduce the incidence of UTIs in patients with indwelling catheters.

Another portal of entry for bacteria is through the distal catheter–proximal drainage tube junction. Every time the system is disconnected there is an increased risk of introducing bacteria into the system. For this reason a closed drainage system should be maintained. Bladder irrigations should not be a routine practice. If irrigation is necessary, a sterile disposable syringe and sterile solution should be used. If frequent irrigations

are necessary, such as in patients who have had a transurethral prostatectomy (TURP) in which blood clots are common, a three-way catheter drainage system with continuous bladder irrigation is recommended. In this way a closed system is maintained. Urine specimens should be obtained from the rubber portal on the drainage tubing (see Fig. 61-3). The portal should be cleansed with an antiseptic before insertion of the needle into the portal. Another portal of entry of bacteria into the system is through the collection bag. The bag should be kept below the bladder level at all times to prevent reflux of urine into the bladder. It also should be kept off the floor and the emptying spout should be cleansed with an antiseptic before and after the urine is emptied from the bag. The container used to collect the urine from the bag must be used for only one patient; it should not be shared between patients. A final control measure in preventing nosocomial UTIs is to place patients with urinary catheters in separate rooms. This is helpful in preventing cross-infection between patients.

Prevention of surgical wound infections

Surgical wounds often are inoculated with bacteria at the time of surgery. The operating room nurse is responsible for maintaining surgical asepsis during surgery. On the patient care units nurses continue to play vital roles in ensuring that aseptic technique is maintained by all who have contact with the patient's wound or dressing. Again, hand washing is the major measure to prevent nosocomial surgical wound infections. Appropriate use of antibiotics both preoperatively and postoperatively is also a concern because of their effect on the patient's own flora.

Prevention of respiratory tract infections

Pneumonia is the most common nosocomial infection of the lower respiratory tract. Preventive measures include proper maintenance and decontamination of respiratory therapy equipment and respiratory assistive devices. Special attention should be given to nebulizers, which contain moisture and are ideal reservoirs for organisms, especially gram-negative organisms such as *Pseudomonas* and *Serratia*. The patient who has a tracheostomy or is intubated is at great risk because these tubes bypass the patient's normal oropharyngeal defense mechanisms. Suctioning should be performed using aseptic technique and sterile irrigants (p. 1231). Inappropriate use of antibiotics should be avoided to minimize oropharyngeal colonization with pathogens that could be aspirated and lead to pneumonia. Patients should be taught the importance of pulmonary toilet and should be instructed how to cough, take deep breaths, and use respiratory therapy equipment properly. Debilitated patients should be protected from the hazards of aspiration, especially while eating.

Prevention of bacteremias

Many blood infections (bacteremias) occur secondary to infections at another site; thus prevention may depend a great deal on control of the underlying infection. Some bacteremias are the result of the use of intravascular devices and systems. The sources of infection in these instances are the hands of personnel, the patient's skin, or infusions that are contaminated either from mishandling by hospital personnel or, less commonly, at the time of manufacture. Intravenous and intraarterial catheters should be inserted under aseptic conditions, and catheter insertion sites should be cared for aseptically. The insertion site is treated like an open wound and is inspected frequently for any sign of infection, such as redness, swelling, exudate, purulence, or warmth. The patient may also complain of pain at the site. Central lines should have an occlusive dressing to prevent contamination. Peripheral catheters should be changed every 48 to 72 hours or more often if there is a complication such as infiltration or phlebitis. The catheter is secured to prevent in-and-out movement and tracking of bacteria into the cannula site. Aseptic technique should be followed when mixing and adding drugs, changing the infusion, or manipulating connections or stopcocks. It is recommended that the tubing be changed every 24 to 48 hours. Before hanging a solution, the nurse should check it for turbidity and particulate matter and for leaks in the system. Solutions should be discarded after 24 hours. Hyperalimentation solutions require special adherence to these practices since they are composed of nutrients that are an excellent culture media for organisms. *Candida* infections are commonly seen in patients receiving hyperalimentation, particularly those who are immunocompromised.

Protection by isolation

When a person is admitted to the hospital with an infection or develops a nosocomial infection, other patients and personnel should be protected against possible infection from this person. This is accomplished by isolation. In planning care the nurse determines the *site of the infection* and the *characteristics of the pathogen involved* in deciding whether isolation is indicated and, if so, what type is required. Factors that affect the decision include the *virulence of the organism* and its *mode of transmission*. The nurse must correlate the clinical status of the patient with the laboratory results to ascertain whether the patient has an infection or is merely colonized. This facilitates making an intelligent decision about the appropriate isolation measures. There are five major types of isolation—*strict, respiratory, wound and skin, enteric,* and *protective*. Each institution should have its own policies for the use of each type of isolation. The CDC has explicit guidelines and recommendations published in *Isolation Techniques for Use in Hospitals*.[53] This is a valuable resource for nurses.

General principles of isolation. Some general principles apply regardless of the type of isolation. Gowns, gloves, and masks should be used only once and then discarded in an appropriate receptacle before leaving the patient's room. Clean gowns, gloves, and masks are kept on a table or cart outside the door of the contaminated room. Hands must be washed before and after patient contact, even when gloves are a required part of the isolation procedure. Masks become ineffective when they are moist and therefore should never be reused. They should be worn over the nose and mouth and should not hang around the neck and then be reused. Contaminated articles should be placed in an impervious clean bag in the contaminated area, closed securely, placed into a second clean bag outside the contaminated area, sealed, and labeled "contaminated". Mattresses and pillows should be covered with impervious plastic.

Strict isolation. Strict isolation is recommended only for highly transmissible diseases that are spread by direct contact and airborne routes of transmission. Some examples of disease requiring strict isolation are burn or skin wounds infected with *Staphylococcus aureus* or Group A *Streptococcus* organisms in which the wound drainage cannot be adequately contained by a dressing, diphtheria, disseminated herpes zoster, and staphylococcal pneumonia. Strict isolation requires that the patient be in a private room with the door kept closed; gowns, masks, and gloves are worn by all persons entering the room; hands are washed on entering and leaving the room; and all articles in the room must be placed in impervious plastic or paper bags and double-bagged for disinfection or sterilization.

Respiratory isolation. Respiratory isolation is recommended to prevent transmission of organisms by droplets or droplet nuclei that are coughed, sneezed, or breathed into the environment. Some of the diseases for which respiratory isolation is recommended are measles, meningococcal meningitis, meningococcemia, mumps, whooping cough, and German measles. (See Chapter 51 for discussion of care of the patient with pulmonary tuberculosis.)

The precautions to be practiced in respiratory isolation include placing the patient in a private room with the door closed. Masks are worn only by persons susceptible to the disease; gowns and gloves are not necessary. Tissues and dressings are placed in a paper or plastic bag, sealed, and then placed in an impervious plastic or paper bag before removal from the room.

Wound and skin precautions. Wound and skin precautions are used to prevent cross-infection where infective material is present in wounds, on body surfaces, or on heavily contaminated articles. It is recommended for infected burn wounds except those infected with *Staphylococcus aureus* or Group A *Streptococcus* organisms, which require strict isolation as described above.

Other infections requiring wound and skin precautions are gas gangrene (*Clostridium perfringens*), localized herpes zoster, bubonic plague, and puerperal sepsis with Group A *Streptococcus* organisms isolated from the vaginal discharge. In addition, any wound or skin infection that is not covered by a dressing or where there is copious drainage that seeps through the dressing requires these precautions.

Wound and skin precautions are also used for patients who have infections caused by multidrug-resistant organisms or when an epidemic strain of these organisms is present. For example, a patient with a urinary catheter who has a urinary tract infection with multidrug-resistant *Pseudomonas* should be placed on wound and skin precautions. The urinary catheter is then regarded as the "infected" wound, and gloves should be worn during perineal care and urinary catheter manipulation. General recommendations for wound and skin precautions include proper hand washing before and after patient contact; gowns and gloves should be worn during direct contact with the infected area, as when changing dressings. A mask is necessary only if the infecting organism is spread by airborne transmission. Soiled linen and dressings should be double-bagged. A private room is desirable but not required.

Enteric precautions. Enteric precautions are recommended for patients with cholera, viral hepatitis (A and B), salmonellosis (including typhoid fever), shigellosis, staphylococcal enterocolitis, and diarrhea associated with an acute illness of suspected infectious etiology. The purpose of enteric precautions is to prevent transmission of disease through direct or indirect contact with infected feces or heavily contaminated articles. Pathogens are spread from infected hands to the mouth, where they are ingested. In this type of isolation the emphasis is placed on proper hand washing, gown technique, and excreta precautions. Gloves are recommended by some experts because of the fear that proper hand washing will not be practiced consistently.

Protective isolation. Protective isolation (reverse isolation) is used to prevent contact between potentially pathogenic organisms and uninfected persons who have seriously impaired resistance. Patients with agranulocytosis, extensive burns, or with leukemia or lymphoma receiving radiation, steroid, or antimetabolite therapy are much more susceptible to infections than other patients, and they may need to be protected from other people and the environment. The patient should be placed in a single room with the door kept closed, and there should be provision for air flow from the room into the hall (positive pressure). Air should not be recirculated from other hospital areas unless it has been filtered through a high-efficiency filter. Meticulous hand washing and use of gowns, gloves, and masks are essential during each patient contact. Only procedures that are essential should be done in order to avert possible exposure to pathogenic organisms. A procedure such as a catheterization is avoided, since it could result in a fatal infection. Patients whose immune response has been severely compromised must even be protected from their own body flora. The degree to which sterility of certain items such as bed linen needs to be ensured depends on the level of protection required. The benefits of using simple protective isolation as described above is a controversial issue. Some studies conclude that it offers no significant benefit to granulocytopenic patients.[56] These patients are thought to infect themselves with their own normal flora. Many hospitals leave the decision as to the extent of isolation indicated to the discretion of the physician or the nurse in charge of the patient division.

Conclusion

The goals of infection control should be to keep the institution as germ free as possible, to control the sources of contamination, to prevent transmission of infectious agents, and to protect those at risk of acquiring infection. All personnel have a responsibility to help attain these goals. The importance of proper hand washing cannot be overemphasized. Personnel should also utilize the infection control nurse, the hospital epidemiologist, and the infection control committee in their institutions to address problems concerning any of the many aspects of infection control.

REFERENCES AND SELECTED READINGS

1. Aach, R.D., and Kahn, R.A.: Posttransfusion hepatitis: current perspectives, Ann. Intern. Med. **92:**539-546, 1980.
2. Albert, R.K., and Condie, F.: Handwashing patterns in medical intensive care units, N. Engl. J. Med. **304:**1465-1466, 1981.
3. Altemeier, W.A., et al.: Studies of the staphylococcal causation of toxic shock syndrome, Surg. Gynecol. Obstet. **153:**481-485, 1981.
4. Ambinder, E.: The growing role of granulocyte replacement therapy, Drug. Ther. Hosp. **6:**311-40, 1981.
5. American Academy of Pediatrics: Report of the Committee on the Control of Infectious Diseases, ed. 18, Evanston, Ill., 1977, The Academy.
6. American Hospital Association: Infection control in the hospital, ed. 4, Chicago, 1979, The Association.
7. American Public Health Association: Control of communicable disease in man, ed. 13, New York, 1975, The Association.
8. Band, J.D., and Maki, D.G.: Infections caused by arterial catheters used for hemodynamic monitoring, Am. J. Med. **67:**735-741, 1979.
9. Band, J.D., and Maki, D.G.: Safety of changing intravenous delivery systems at intervals longer than 24 hours, Ann. Intern. Med. **91:**173, 1979.
10. Barrett-Connor, E., et al.: Epidemiology for the infection control nurse, St. Louis, 1978, The C.V. Mosby Co.
11. Bennett, J.V., and Brachman, P.S., editors: Hospital infections, Boston, 1979, Little, Brown & Co.
12. Breman, J.G., and Arita, I.: The confirmation and maintenance of smallpox prediction, N. Engl. J. Med. **303:**1263-1273, 1980.

13. Bryan, J.A.: Viral hepatitis. I. Clinical and laboratory aspects and epidemiology, Postgrad. Med. **58**:66-76, 1980.

14. Bryan, J.A.: Viral hepatitis. II. Prevention and control, Postgrad. Med. **58**:81-86, 1980.

15. Buxton, J., et al.: Contamination of intravenous infusion fluid: effects of changing administration sets, Ann. Intern. Med. **90**:764, 1979.

16. Centers for Disease Control: National nosocomial infections study report. Annual summary 1978, issued March 1981, U.S. Department of Health and Human Services.

17. Centers for Disease Control: Recommendation of the Immunization Practices Advisory Committee (ACIP): diphtheria, tetanus, and pertussis: guidelines for vaccine prophylaxis and other preventive measures, Morbid. Mortal. Week. Rep. **30**:32, 1981.

18. Centers for Disease Control: Recommendation of the Immunization Practices Advisory Committee (ACIP): rubella prevention, Morbid. Mortal. Re. **30**:37-47, 1981.

19. Centers for Disease Control: Mumps vaccine: recommendations of the Immunization Practice Advisory Committee, Ann. Intern. Med. **92**:803-804, 1980.

20. Centers for Disease Control: Recommendation of the Immunization Practices Advisory Committee (ACIP): general recommendations on immunization, Morbid. Mortal. Week. Rep. **29**:76-83, 1980.

21. Centers for Disease Control: Recommendation of the Immunization Practices Advisory Committee (ACIP): smallpox vaccine, Morbid. Mortal. Week. Rep. **29**:417-420, 1980.

22. Centers for Disease Control: Recommendation of the Immunization Practices Advisory Committee (ACIP): rubeolla vaccine, Morbid. Mortal. Week. Rep. **27**:427-430, 435-437, 1978.

23. Centers for Disease Control: National nosocomial infections study report: U.S. Department of Health, Education & Welfare pub. no. (CDC)78-8257, Washington, D.C., 1976, U.S. Government Printing Office.

24. A clinician's dictionary guide to bacteria and fungi, ed. 4, Indianapolis, 1981, Eli Lilly Co.

25. Crossley, K.: Changing patterns of antibiotic resistance, Int. Med. Specialist **2**:56-63, 1981.

26. Dixon, R.E., editor: Nosocomial infections, New York, 1981, Yorke Medical Books.

27. Downer, D.J.: Infection precautions for pregnant ICU personnel, Crit. Care Med. **7**:225-226, 1979.

28. Farke, B.F., Kaiser, D.L., and Wenzel, R.P.: Relationship between surgical volume and incidence of postoperative wound infection, N. Engl. J. Med. **305**:200-204, 1981.

29. Favero, M.S., et al.: Guidelines for the care of patients hospitalized with viral hepatitis, Ann. Intern. Med. **91**:872-876, 1979.

30. Fekety, R.: Prevention and treatment of viral infection, Postgrad. Med. **69**:133-141, 1981.

31. Garibaldi, R.A., et al.: Meatal colonization and catheter-associated bacteremia, N. Engl. J. Med. **303**:316-318, 1980.

32. Garibaldi, R., Brodine, S., and Matsmuja, S.: Infections among patients in nursing homes. N. Engl. J. Med. **305**:731-735, 1981.

33. Goldmann, D.A., et al.: Guidelines for infection control in intravenous therapy, Ann. Intern. Med. **79**:848-850, 1973.

34. Haley, R.W., et al.: Extra charges and prolongation of stay attributable to nosocomial infections: a prospective interhospital comparison, Am. J. Med. **70**:51-58, 1981.

35. Infection control: topics in clinical nursing, vol. 1, no. 2, Germantown, Md., 1979, Aspen Systems Corp.

36. Joseph, P.: Zeroing in on the causes of pneumonia, Consultant **21**:47-64, 1981.

37. Knittle, M.A., Eitzman, D.V., and Baer, H.: Role of hand contamination of personnel in epidemiology of gram negative nosocomial infections, J. Pediatr. **86**:433-437, 1976.

38. Kunin, C.: Detection, prevention, and management of urinary tract infections, ed. 3, Philadelphia, 1979, Lea & Febiger.

39. Labet, C., and Roderick, M.: Infection control in the use of intravascular devices, Crit. Care Q. **3**:67-80, 1981.

40. Maki, D.G.: Nosocomial bacteremia: an epidemiologic overview, Am. J. Med. **70**:719, 1981.

41. Maki, D.G., Goldmann, D.A., and Rhane, F.J.: Infection control in intravenous therapy, Ann. Intern. Med. **79**:867, 1973.

42. Mallison, G.F.: Monitoring of sterility and environmental sampling in programs for control of nosocomial infections. In Cundy, K., and Ball, W.: Infection control in health care facilities: microbiological surveillance, Baltimore, 1977, University Park Press.

43. Masten, J.: Pathogens: their sources and control. Hospitals, J.A.M.A. **49**:63-65, 1975.

44. Masten, J.: Pathogens: their sources and control. Hospitals, J.A.M.A. **48**:71-76, 1974.

45. McHenry, M.C.: The infectious pneumonias, Hosp. Pract. **15**:41-52, 1980.

46. Meers, P.D., et al.: Cross infection with *Serratia marcescens,* Br. Med. J. **1**:238-239, 1978.

47. Miller, T.E., and North, D.K.: Clinical infections, antibiotics, and immunosuppression: a puzzling relationship, Am. J. Med. **71**:334-336, 1981.

48. Mufson, M.A.: The new vaccines, Drug Ther. **10**:39-48, 1980.

49. Palmer, D.L.: Understanding and treating infections in the elderly, Consultant **21**:201-213, 1981.

50. Pierson, C.L.: Infection control in burn care facilities, Crit. Care Q. **3**:81-92, 1981.

51. Pizzo, P.: The value of protective isolation in preventing nosocomial infections in high risk patients, Am. J. Med. **70**:631-637, 1981.

52. Polk, F.B., et al.: An outbreak of rubella among hospital personnel, N. Engl. J. Med. **303**:541-545, 1980.

53. Public Health Service, Center for Disease Control: Isolation techniques for use in hospitals, ed. 2, U.S. Department of Health, Education and Welfare pub. no. (CDC) 76-8314, 1975.

54. Rose, R. M., and Weiss, S.T.: Management of pneumonia in the compromised host, Drug Ther. Hosp. **6**:17-30, 1981.

55. Rutstein, D.P.: Controlling the communicable and the man-made diseases, N. Engl. J. Med. **304**:1422-1424, 1981.

56. Schimpff, S.C.: Infection prevention during profound granulocytopenia—new approaches to alimentary canal microbial suppression, Ann. Intern. Med. **93**:358-361, 1980.

57. Schoberg, D.R., et al.: An outbreak of hospital infections due to multiply resistant *Serratia marcescens*: evidence of interhospital spread, J. Infect. Dis. **134**:181-188, 1976.

58. Stamm, W.E.: Nosocomial infections: etiologic changes, therapeutic challenges, Hosp. Pract. **16**:75-88, 1981.

59. Stamm, W.E.: Guidelines for prevention of catheter associated urinary tract infection, Ann. Intern. Med. **82**:386-390, 1975.

60. Steere, A.C., and Mallison, G.F.: Handwashing practices for the prevention of nosocomial infections, Ann. Intern. Med. **83**:683-690, 1975.

61. Symposium on Infection Control: Nursing Clinics of North America, vol. 15, no. 4, Philadelphia, 1980, W.B. Saunders Co.

62. Symposium on Nosocomial Infections: Part I, Am. J. Med. **70**:379-473, 1981.

63. Symposium on Nosocomial Infections: Part II, Am. J. Med. **70**:631-744, 1981.

64. Symposium on Nosocomial Infections: Part III, Am. J. Med. **70**:899-986, 1981.

65. Wallace, R.B.: How to recognize and deal with outbreaks of communicable disease, Consultant **20**:129-138, 1980.

66. White, F.M.: Nosocomial infection control: scope and implications for health care, Am. J. Infect. Control **9**:61-69, 1981.

67. Youmans, G.P.: The biological and clinical basis of infectious diseases, ed. 2, Philadelphia, 1980, W.B. Saunders Co.

68. Ziment, I.: Common errors in sputum collection and evaluation, Practical Cardiol. **6**:93-113, 1980.

CHAPTER 23

PAIN

VIRGINIA BURKE KARB

Pain is a two-edged sword. On the one hand, it warns us to move away from heat, cold, and sharp objects before injury occurs and makes us aware of the presence of disease and tissue damage; thus it usually influences us to seek medical attention. On the other hand, fear of pain may cause us to delay medical treatment, and if its cause cannot be located and relieved, its presence serves no useful purpose and it becomes harmful. Continuous, severe pain eventually causes physical and mental exhaustion and prevents the individual from functioning productively. Pain accompanies almost all illnesses, and perhaps no sensation is more dreaded by patients undergoing medical treatment or surgery.

Pain has never been satisfactorily defined or understood. It is an unpleasant feeling, entirely subjective, that only the person experiencing it can describe. It can be evoked by a multiplicity of stimuli (chemical, thermal, electrical, mechanical), but the reaction to it cannot be measured objectively. Pain is a learned experience that is influenced by the entire life situation of each person. What is perceived as pain and the reaction to that pain differ among people and sometimes differ in the same person from one time to another.

Care of patients suffering pain demands skill in both the science and the art of nursing. The nurse's responsibility is to make the patient as comfortable as possible and to observe and report findings so that they may help the physician make a correct diagnosis and prescribe appropriate treatment.[22,101]

Concepts of pain

Definition of pain

Sternback[104] describes pain as an abstract concept that refers to sensation, stimulus, and response. An-other author points out that there is an emotion of pain in addition to the sensation of pain.[97] It is probably not necessary to have an elaborate definition of pain in order to provide nursing care to a patient in pain. Mc-Caffery states that "pain is whatever the experiencing person says it is and exists whenever he says it does."[57] The nurse therefore will see persons in pain frequently and must learn to assist each individual to deal as effectively as possible with it.

Significance and frequency of pain

Pain serves a major function by alerting us to possible harm or damage. It may or may not influence us to seek medical attention. Pain may have other meanings for an individual: the possible loss of mobility or activity, the recurrence of a particular disease, the reminder that the individual may be aging. Pain may precipitate feelings of fear, anger, uneasiness, challenge, or punishment. Other individuals may see pain as an opportunity for creative expression, for self-searching, for self-testing, or for fostering an appreciation of what less fortunate patients have gone through.

In general, however, most persons view pain as a negative experience. Below is a list of the top 20 words used to describe pain as listed by 148 patients:

Treacherous	Hidden	Variety of words
Mean	Obnoxious	meaning satanic
Hateful	Faceless	Nasty
Detestable	Degrading	Sharp
Sneaky	Cruel	Cunning
Intense	Inconsiderate	Nervous
Dark	Invading	Persistent[17]

Factors that influence the meaning of pain to an individual are many and varied. Some of these include age,[7,29] sex, cultural background,[22,101] psychosocial factors,[62] environmental factors, expected response, and other assorted problems and diagnoses. The setting in which pain occurs may be important. For example, a professional athlete injured in an athletic event may be in such pain that he has to withdraw from the event. A soldier injured in wartime activities may see injury and concomitant pain as relatively minor if the injury also means relief from the pressure of battle and possible return home.[100]

Pain is experienced by most individuals at various times throughout life. It may be the result of or associated with trauma, exposure to excessive heat or cold, excessive strain or use of body parts (as in the person who exercises vigorously), normal body functions such as labor and delivery, surgical intervention, and so on. Most individuals try to avoid pain but at the same time expect that it will occur with various activities.

Pain threshold

Pain threshold refers to the intensity of the noxious stimulus necessary for the person to perceive pain. For many years it was felt that the pain threshold was approximately the same for all individuals. This belief has come under criticism recently.[12,56] It is important to note that the intensity of the pain is not related to the intensity of the noxious stimulus, and furthermore most experts in the field agree that pain can exist without tissue damage or demonstrable noxious stimulation.[37,50] As an example, the severe pain of *tic douloureux* can be initiated by only a light touch on the face. The tolerance for pain, on the other hand, refers to "the duration of time or the intensity of which a subject accepts a stimulus above the pain threshold before making a verbal or overt pain response."[104] McCaffery defines tolerance for pain as "the duration or intensity of pain the patient is *willing* to endure."[56]

The tolerance for pain may be raised by alcohol, drugs, hypnosis, warmth, rubbing, or distracting activities. Strong beliefs and faith seem to increase tolerance for pain, and it is sometimes difficult to judge how much pain a patient with deep religious faith is actually experiencing. Fatigue, anger, boredom, and apprehension may decrease one's ability to tolerate pain. Pain tolerance also is lowered by persistent pain such as that sometimes experienced by patients with far-advanced carcinoma. A weak, debilitated patient usually tolerates pain less well than a healthy person, although increasing debility will eventually cause mental dulling with a resultant decrease in pain perception.

Perception of pain

The perception of pain, or the actual feeling of pain, takes place in the cerebral cortex. It is known that a functioning frontal lobe of the brain is required to experience the full suffering and worry that result from pain. The reaction to the same stimuli differs widely among people and in the same person from one time to another because the final perception of pain depends more on the interpretation in the cerebral cortex than on the characteristics of the original stimuli. What the cerebral cortex interprets as pain will depend on childhood training, previous experience, cultural values, religious beliefs, physical and mental health, knowledge and understanding, attention and distraction, fatigue, anxiety, tension, fear, state of consciousness, and the frequency and intensity of pain impulses.

Atrophy of nerve endings, degenerative changes in the pain-bearing pathways, and decreased alertness may reduce the perception of pain in the elderly, and more stimulation may be required to evoke a response. Elderly persons therefore may fail to perceive tissue damage that normally would cause pain and thus alert a younger person.

The perception of a pain stimulus may be altered at many points by both normal and abnormal conditions. A pleasant environment, an enjoyable book, stimulating conversation, or other distracting activity of a pleasing nature may serve to lessen the sensation of pain. Tissue damage or inflammatory conditions at the site where the stimuli originate may increase or decrease the impulse. For example, slapping a person who has a sunburn may set off a far greater impulse than if the person were not sunburned. On the other hand, if the local nerve endings have been damaged by a severe burn, the patient may not respond at all to what would ordinarily be painful stimuli. Abnormal conditions within the spinal cord such as inflammatory diseases, tumors, or injuries may prevent transmission of nerve impulses. This may occur at either the spinal or the thalamic relay stations. The impulse may also be altered at either of these two relay stations by other activity going on simultaneously within the spinal cord. This probably accounts for the fact that sometimes bruises and cuts sustained during absorbing activities go unnoticed until the activity is over. Perception in the cortex may be influenced by abnormal conditions such as inflammatory processes, degenerative changes, and depression of brain function, which may alter the original signal pattern. Anesthesia and analgesia also cause depression of sensory perceptions.

Reaction to pain

Meaning and perception of pain are accompanied by reaction to pain. Reaction to pain also is influenced by such factors as past experience, conditioning, cultural values, and physical and mental health. Consequently, people will respond differently to the same stimuli. Some may be fearful, apprehensive, and anxious, while others are tolerant and optimistic. Some weep, moan, scream, beg for relief or help, threaten to destroy themselves, thrash about in bed, or move about aimlessly while they are in severe pain. Others lie quietly in bed and may only close their eyes, grit their teeth, bite their lips, clench their hands, or perspire profusely when experiencing pain.

Some people, by training and example, are taught to endure severe pain without reacting outwardly. American Indian men have rites in which they show their strength by the amount of pain they can endure. Such individuals probably would tolerate pain from disease or injury better than those from a culture in which free expression of feelings is encouraged. Persons from cultures in which health teaching and disease prevention are emphasized tend to accept pain as a warning to seek help and expect the cause of pain will be found and cured.

Parents' attitudes toward pain may determine their children's lifelong reaction to pain. In the American culture parents usually begin to teach their children what is expected of them in regard to courage and self-control at about the age of 2 or 3 years. They try not to appear too concerned about minor injuries and usually encourage their children not to cry when they are hurt. Children try very hard to be brave, especially in the presence of other children.

The setting in which injury occurs may influence the external response to pain. A child may feel, for example, that the pain suffered from injury during a hockey game, although perhaps severe, should nevertheless be born quietly because of its personal meaning, whereas pain resulting from an automobile accident may be expressed freely.

Influence of fear

Morbid fear of a disease may intensify pain caused by it, or it may lead the individual to deny pain in his or her eagerness to believe that nothing is wrong. Anticipation of pain based on past experience often intensifies pain. For example, a boy who enters the hospital for the last of several operations may react more vigorously to postoperative pain than he did on his first encounter with the sensation.

One's personality also influences reaction to pain. A person who reacts hysterically to trying situations may find even a small amount of pain intolerable. People may sometimes use moderate pain as an escape from unacceptable life situations, or they may try to use it to control situations around them. This latter reaction is often demonstrated both in the hospital and at home.

There is more reaction to pain during the night and early morning hours when the person's physiologic processes are at low ebb and there is little distracting activity. Patients' thoughts may easily turn to concern for themselves and loved ones, and worrying may may increase their reaction to pain.

Age affects the reaction to pain. The young fear it because it may represent an unfamiliar experience, and they frequently respond to it by crying. Older persons may know what to expect and accept it, or they may be withdrawn and quiet while experiencing it because of emotional exhaustion.

Theories of pain transmission

People have been studying pain and attempting to develop theories of pain transmission for centuries. Four major theories are mentioned briefly: the specificity theory, the intensive theory, the pattern theory, and the gate control theory. None of these provides all the answers to explain pain transmission, but many recent experiments in pain therapy have been based on the gate control theory.

The *specificity theory* holds that there are certain specific nerve receptors that respond to noxious stimuli and that these noxious stimuli are always interpreted as pain. In addition, this theory states that pain impulses are carried by pain fibers—fast, myelinated A-delta (A-δ) fibers and more slowly conducting unmyelinated C fibers—to the lateral spinothalamic tract in the spinal cord to a pain center in the thalamus. Impulses are then sent to the cerebral cortex by way of the corticothalamic tract where the actual perception of pain takes place (Fig. 23-1). Opponents of this theory point out that specific pain receptors have not been identified, nor does the body always interpret certain stimuli as noxious.[12,43,102]

The *intensive theory* suggests that pain is produced by intense stimulation of nonspecific fiber receptors. In other words, any stimulus could be perceived as painful if the stimulation were intense enough.[12] This model does not explain, for example, the functioning of the spinal cord in pain transmission and thus does not explain the pain relief provided by many neurosurgical therapies.

In the *pattern* theory it is felt that pain results from the combined effects of stimulus intensity and a critical summation of these impulses in the dorsal horns of the spinal cord. In other words, a pattern of impulses is transmitted to the cortex and is there perceived as pain.[12,37,43,99] This theory is considered to be vague.[12]

In 1965 Melzack and Wall[102] proposed the *gate control theory*, and Wall[94] revised it in 1978. This theory proposes that pain and its perception depend on the interaction of three systems: the substantia gelatinosa in the dorsal horn of the spinal cord, which modulates impulses entering the spinal cord; a central control system in the cortex and thalamus, which influences the impulses reaching the brain; and the neural system associated with perception of pain. The theory proposes that pain impulses are conducted over small-diameter fibers to the spinal cord, travel across an "opened gate" in the substantia gelatinosa to the anterolateral spinothalamic tract, and then ascend the tract to the thalamus and cortex where pain perception and interpretation occur.

The "gate" in the substantia gelatinosa can be "closed" (Fig. 23-2) so that the contact is not made, thus interrupting the pain impulse. This gate can be closed by conflicting impulses from the skin conducted over large-diameter fibers, by impulses from the reticular formation in the brain stem, or by impulses from the entire cortex or thalamus (central control system).[82] Thus impulses from the peripheral fibers, brain stem, thalamus, or cortex can effectively block the transmission of pain impulses or can intensify the impulse. In this manner, thoughts (cognition), attitudes, past experiences, and so forth can modify or intensify the pain experience.

Not all scientists accept the gate control theory, and in fact new theories are still being proposed. It would seem, though, that most new theories take as their starting point the gate control theory, and it is still the most widely accepted theory.*

Endorphins

The brain and spinal cord contain receptors to which morphine binds. Discovery of these receptors led researchers to seek endogenous substances resembling morphine that would also bind to these receptors. In 1975 researchers discovered small polypeptides called enkephalins that appeared to have morphinelike action. Further research led to the discovery of larger peptides labeled endorphins (a combination of the words *endogenous* and *morphine*). Another substance with opiate

*References 12, 19, 37, 43, 57, 65, 94, 95, 99, 102.

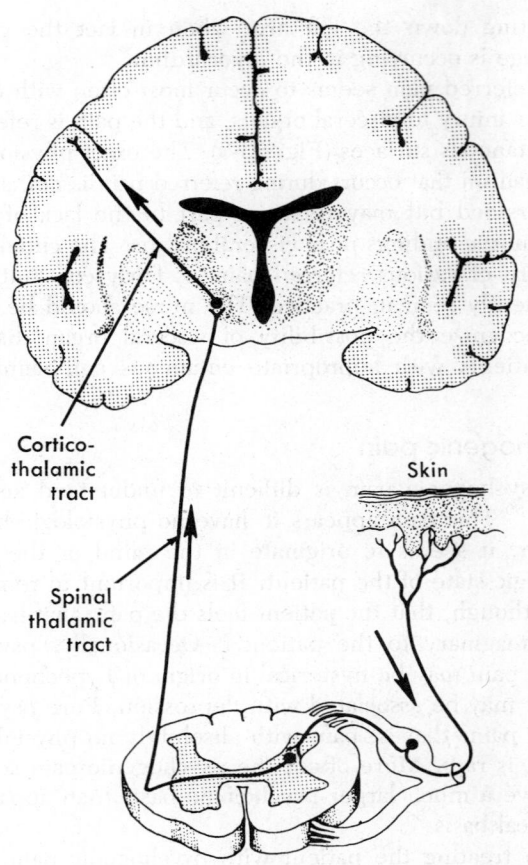

Fig. 23-1. Pathways of pain transmission according to specificity theory.

Cortico-thalamic tract

Spinal thalamic tract

Skin

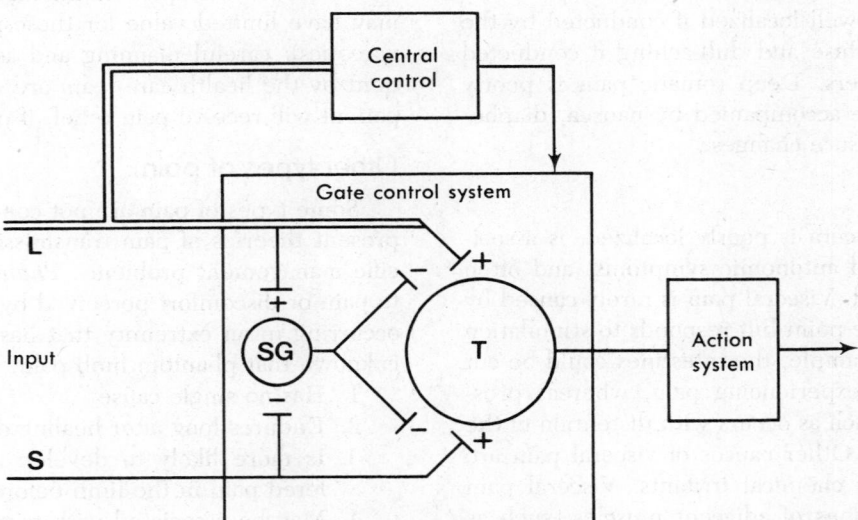

Fig. 23-2. Schema of gate control theory of pain mechanisms. *L,* Large-diameter fibers; *S,* small-diameter fibers. Fibers project to *SG,* substantia gelatinosa, and *T,* first central transmission cells. Inhibitory effect exerted by SG on afferent fiber terminals is increased by activity in L fibers and decreased by activity in S fibers. Central control processes project to gate control system. They include fibers from brain stem, which have predominantly inhibitory effect, as well as fibers from cortex. T cells project to entry cells of actions system. +, Excitation; −, inhibition. (From Weisenberg, M.: Pain: clinical and experimental perspectives, St. Louis, 1975, The C.V. Mosby Co.; after Melzack and Wall.)

activity has been found in the pituitary gland and is called a beta-endorphin (β-endorphin).

Opiate receptors and endorphins are found in high concentration in the brain stem, specifically in the periaqueductal gray (PAG), which is the gray matter surrounding the aqueduct of Sylvius (see Fig. 34-4), and in the substantia gelatinosa of the spinal cord. It is now hypothesized that there is a *descending pathway* from the brain that can *inhibit pain transmission*. Cells in the PAG are activated by a noxious stimulus sending a stimulus to the raphe neurons in the medulla, effecting release of a neurotransmitter, serotonin. The impulse is then transmitted to the dorsal horn of the spinal cord, where the pain stimulus is inhibited by action of the endorphins. The PAG can be activated by systemic opiates, by electrical stimulation, and by ascending pain transmission pathways.

The complete significance of the endorphins is still unclear, but studies show that they may influence or be associated with pain relief from analgesics, electrical stimulators, acupuncture, and other methods. Patients with chronic pain may have lower levels of endorphins.[96]

Types of pain

Somatic pain

Pain may originate in superficial structures, such as the skin and subcutaneous tissue, or in deeper structures, such as muscles or bones. Cutaneous pain may be either sharp and well localized if conducted by the fast A-δ fibers or diffuse and dull-aching if conducted by the slower C fibers. Deep somatic pain is poorly localized and may be accompanied by nausea, diaphoresis, and blood pressure changes.

Visceral pain

Pain from the viscera is poorly localized, is associated with nausea and autonomic symptoms, and often radiates or is referred. Visceral pain is rarely caused by stimulation at a single point but responds to stimulation at many sites. For example, the intestines could be cut without the person experiencing pain, whereas pressure at many sites, such as occurs with distention of the viscera, causes pain. Other causes of visceral pain are ischemia, spasms, or chemical irritants. Visceral pain may initiate contractions of adjacent muscles, such as the abdominal wall; thus abdominal rigidity may be observed with inflammation of abdominal viscera.

Referred pain

Referred pain is that pain felt in areas other than those stimulated. It may occur when stimulation is not perceived in the primary area. For example, the person experiencing a heart attack may complain only of pain radiating down the left arm when in fact the tissue damage is occurring in the myocardium.

Referred pain seems to occur most often with damage or injury to visceral organs, and the pain is referred to cutaneous surfaces (Fig. 23-3). The exact physiologic mechanism that occurs during referred pain is not clearly understood but may relate in part to the lack of sensory nerve endings near visceral organs. The cutaneous pattern of various referred pains is fairly constant and frequently seen in practice. The nurse should be able to recognize the possibility of visceral organ disease in patients with appropriate cutaneous complaints of pain.

Psychogenic pain

Psychogenic pain is difficult to understand and to treat.[50] This pain appears to have no physiologic basis; rather, it seems to originate in the mind or the psychologic state of the patient. It is important to remember, though, that the patient feels the pain; that is, it is not imaginary to the patient.[57] Occasionally, psychogenic pain may be hysterical in origin or hypochondriacal; it may be associated with depression. Pure psychogenic pain, that is, pain with absolutely no physiologic basis, is rare. More often, the psychogenic pain seems to have a much larger psychologic basis than apparent physical basis.[56]

In treating the patient with psychogenic pain, the nurse should remember what McCaffery points out: "Calling pain imaginary does not make it go away."[56] While certain therapies traditionally used for pain relief may have limited value for these patients (e.g., use of narcotics), careful planning and assessment of the patient by the health care team are necessary so that the patient will receive pain relief, if possible.

Other types of pain

Some types of pain are not completely explained by present theories of pain transmission and present specific management problems. *Phantom limb* pain refers to pain or discomfort perceived by the individual to be occurring in an extremity that has been amputated. It is known that phantom limb pain:

1. Has no single cause
2. Endures long after healing of the injured tissues
3. Is more likely to develop in patients who suffered pain in the limb before amputation
4. May be associated with trigger zones that when stimulated will result in the perception of this pain; the trigger zones may spread to healthy areas on the same or opposite sides of the body
5. Is influenced by emotional factors and sympathetic nervous system, but neither cause it[65]

Phantom limb pain may be very difficult to treat, probably because it is not clearly understood.

Another unusual type of pain is *causalgia,* which is

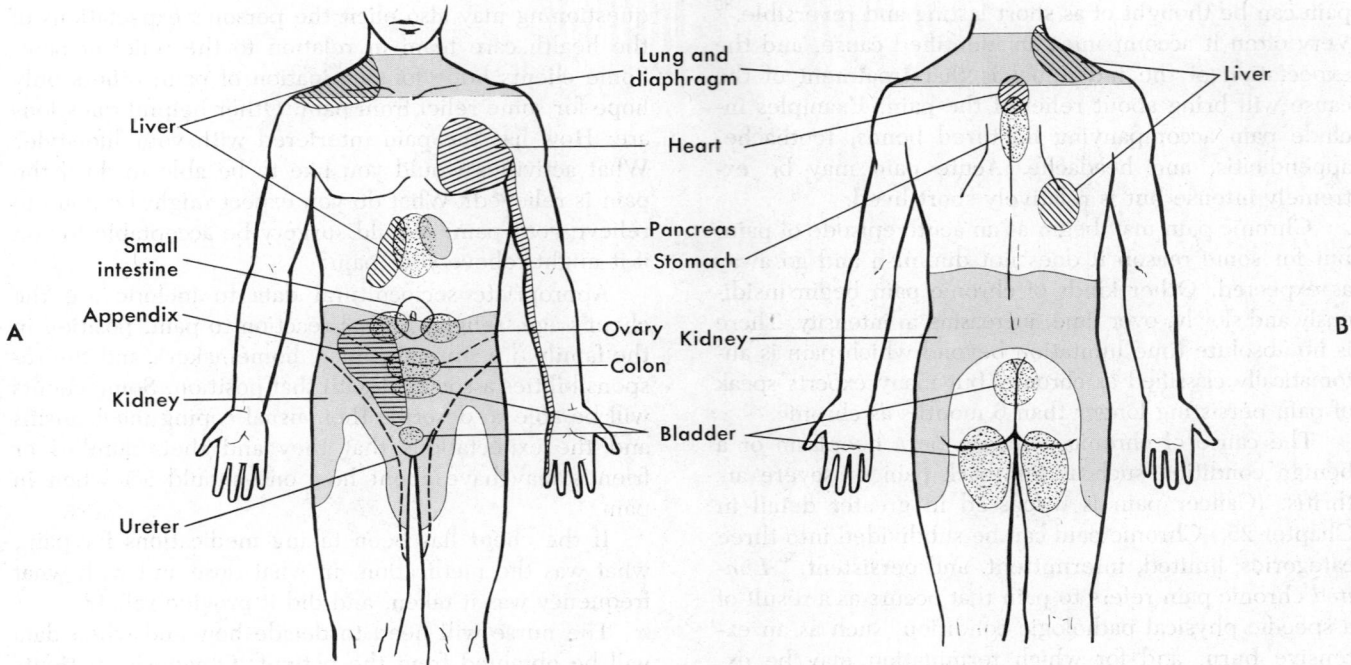

Fig. 23-3. Referred pain. **A,** Front. **B,** Back.

a severe, burning pain sometimes associated with nerve injuries. This type of pain may gradually disappear, but a significant number of patients may still be complaining of pain a year after injury. An unusual feature of this type of pain is that it may sometimes be triggered by normally nonnoxious stimuli such as the noise created when planes fly overhead.[65]

Neuralgia refers to pain or discomfort that occurs as a result of infection or disease that damages peripheral nerves. Causalgia may be thought of as a type of neuralgia, but the converse is not true.

Headache is another type of pain that may vary sig-

nificantly from one individual to another. The causes of certain headaches are fairly well understood: tension, increasing intracranial pressure as a result of a mass lesion, infection, and so on. The migraine headache is less clearly understood, as is the cluster headache characterized by severe localized pain that is intense, of short duration, and difficult to treat (see Chapter 35 and reference 4).

Acute and chronic pain

Recent attention has been focused on the differences between acute and chronic pain (Table 23-1). Acute

TABLE 23-1. Comparison of acute and chronic pain

Characteristic	Acute pain	Chronic pain
Experience	An event	A situation, state of existence
Source	External agent or internal disease	Unknown; or if known, changes cannot occur or treatment is prolonged or ineffective
Onset	Usually sudden	May be sudden or develop insidiously
Duration	Transient (up to 6 months)	Prolonged (months to years)
Pain identification	Pain vs. nonpain areas generally well identified	Pain vs. nonpain areas less easily differentiated; intensity becomes more difficult to evaluate (change in sensations)
Clinical signs	Typical response pattern with more visible signs	Response patterns vary; fewer overt signs (adaptation)
Meaning	Meaningful (informs person something is wrong)	Meaningless; person looks for meanings
Pattern	Self-limiting or readily corrected	Continuous or intermittent; intensity may vary or remain constant
Course	Suffering usually decreases over time	Suffering usually increases over time
Actions	Leads to actions to relieve pain	Leads to actions to modify pain experience
Prognosis	Likelihood of eventual complete relief	Complete relief usually not possible

pain can be thought of as short lasting and reversible.[86] Very often it accompanies an identified cause, and the expectation of the individual is that treatment of the cause will bring about relief of the pain. Examples include pain accompanying fractured bones, toothache, appendicitis, and headache. Acute pain may be extremely intense but is relatively short lived.

Chronic pain may begin as an acute episode of pain, but for some reason it does not diminish and go away as expected. Other kinds of chronic pain begin insidiously and slowly, over time, increasing in intensity. There is no absolute time limitation beyond which pain is automatically classified as chronic, but many experts speak of pain persisting longer than 6 months as chronic.

The cause of chronic pain can be a neoplasm or a benign condition such as low back pain or severe arthritis. (Cancer pain is discussed in greater detail in Chapter 25.) Chronic pain can be subdivided into three categories: limited, intermittent, and persistent.[56] *Limited* chronic pain refers to pain that occurs as a result of a specific physical pathologic condition, such as an extensive burn, and for which termination may be expected. The person with *intermittent* chronic pain, such as from migraine headaches, experiences pain only at certain times, but the situations recur over a long period. Low-back-pain syndrome is an example of *persistent* pain that continues without interruption.

It is not clear whether there are different physiologic processes accompanying acute and chronic pain.[6,13] It does seem that the patient with chronic pain manifests different problems than the individual with acute pain. Some of these characteristics may include a long history of repeated physician contacts and multiple diagnostic studies or surgeries, preoccupation with the pain, despair, depression, anxiety, and altered sleep patterns.* The nurse may need to develop completely different plans of care for two patients who may both be in pain, if one has acute and the other chronic pain.

Assessment of the client with pain

Subjective data

Assessment of the client undergoing a pain experience begins with a careful history. Information to elicit includes characteristics and description of the pain. The client is asked to describe the pain, and the nurse should take care to validate with the client the exact meaning if it is unclear to the nurse. The characteristics may include the site, severity, duration, and location of pain. If the client is asked what may be causing the pain, some light may be shed on other possible topics for further elaboration.

The client also should be asked what relieves the pain and what does not help relieve the pain. Careful questioning may also elicit the person's expectations of the health care team in relation to the relief of pain. Some clients hope for elimination of pain; others only hope for some relief from pain. Other helpful questions are: How has the pain interfered with your life-style? What activities would you like to be able to do if the pain is relieved? What do you expect might be done to relieve your pain? Would surgery be acceptable to you if it might relieve your pain?

Appropriate sociocultural data to include are the client's age, religion, usual reaction to pain, position in the family (i.e., breadwinner, homemaker), and the responsibilities associated with that position. Some clients will be able to describe their usual coping mechanisms and the expectations that they and their families or friends may have about how one should act when in pain.

If the client has been taking medications for pain, what was the medication, in what dose and with what frequency was it taken, and did it provide relief?

The nurse will need to decide how and when data will be obtained from the patient. Obviously, patients who are critically ill should be asked only a few key questions rather than subjected to a long list of questions at one time.

The nurse who has an opportunity to work with the patient on an ongoing basis can easily assess the patient's pain and response to it over time and during various circumstances. The ongoing assessment should still include subjective data about the location, duration, and intensity of pain. The nurse and patient may also determine that there are factors associated with the pain experience: time of day, week, or month; certain body positions or actions; certain environmental situations; and so on. In every case the nurse needs to convey trust and interest so that the patient will feel free to discuss concerns with the nurse.

There has been interest recently in developing tools specifically for assessment of pain.* Nurses who are frequently faced with difficulties in assessing pain may wish to use one of the currently available tools or to develop one. One effective method of identifying pain intensity is the McGill Pain Scale.[64] The person is asked to rate the pain on a scale of 0 to 5 as described below:

0 No pain
1 Mild pain
2 Discomforting
3 Distressing
4 Horrible
5 Excruciating

Visual analog scales can also be used (Fig. 23-4) and may be helpful for comparison of a person's concept of the pain intensity over time.

---

*References 10, 16, 20, 28, 48, 86.

*References 36, 56, 60, 63, 64, 73.

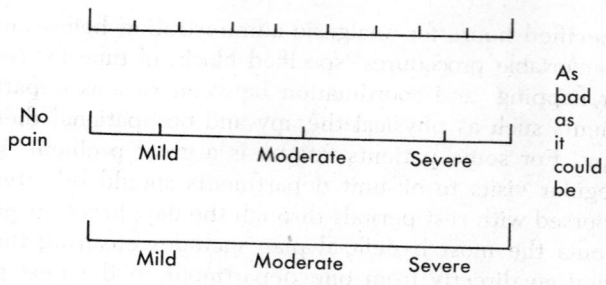

Fig. 23-4. Visual analog pain scales. Person marks line describing intensity of pain.

Objective data

The nurse needs to make careful objective observations of all clients. The objective data may help clarify the subjective response, or it may be the only way the nurse becomes aware of the client's pain.

Physiologic signs of pain may include increased heart rate, increased frequency or depth of respiration or both, diaphoresis, increased systolic and diastolic blood pressure, pallor, dilated pupils, increased muscle tension, and piloerection (goose bumps). The client may complain of nausea or of feeling weak or sick.

If the pain is chronic or less severe, the physiologic manifestations may be less prominent and less severe. Instead, the nurse may notice changes in facial expression, such as frowning or gritting of teeth. Some persons clench their fists and withdraw inwardly when in pain. Others may complain bitterly, cry, moan, toss about in bed, assume a fetal position, or clutch at the affected body part. Still others will pace up and down if they have the energy to do so. Some patients in pain want someone in constant attendance, whereas others want to be left alone.

Observing the behavior of young children who cannot yet talk is the only way to determine if they are in pain and where it may be located. Some children tug at the ear that is aching or double over to relieve abdominal pain. They also may not let anyone touch the part that hurts. Irritability and continuous crying that is unrelieved by the usual comfort measures may mean that the child is in pain. Parents may be asked about activities they have observed that appear to cause discomfort. When signs of pain are apparent, a close examination of the child's body should be made to rule out an injury or other obvious cause of distress.

Nurses must be able to assess patients' pain and their emotional responses to it in a nonjudgmental manner. The way patients act when in pain is influenced by their life experiences and cannot be voluntarily modified with ease. Regardless of the cause of the pain or the patient's behavior, the immediate goal is to relieve or modify the pain. Knowing how the patient feels about pain helps

the nurse initiate appropriate comfort measures.

There are times when the patient's subjective response to questions about pain differ from the objective signs the nurse might expect to see. For example, the patient may request an analgesic, a back rub, or other measures to relieve pain. As the nurse arrives to carry out the request, the patient is found to be asleep. Some nurses feel that sleeping (or laughing or reading) or other behaviors indicate that the patient is not really in pain. It is important to reiterate that pain is what the patient says it is, and while objective data may assist in confirming the existence of pain, the nurse should not believe that there is a certain way the patient ought to behave when in pain. In the above example, a possible explanation is that the patient is exhausted by the pain and thus falls asleep, but the sleeping may be totally unrelated to the continuing presence of pain.

The need to assess the person with pain is ongoing, yet the nurse must begin to plan an approach to the person and the pain. The nurse is able to function independently with many interventions, but careful planning with other members of the health care team should ensure that all have the same patient outcomes or goals in mind.

Intervention for relief or alteration of pain

The first step in developing and implementing the plan of care is to obtain the patient's trust. Ideally, the nurse would have begun the initial assessment of the person with this need for trust in mind. To convey trust and interest, the nurse needs to remember that the pain is whatever the experiencing person says it is and that it exists whenever the person says it does.[57] Thus the nurse may not always know when to anticipate that the patient will manifest pain. Patience, conveying an interest, being willing to help, and avoiding prejudging the patient are helpful. Prejudging implies tending to look for behavior associated with acute pain.

Careful patient assessment and planning should help the nurse to choose among many possible ways to relieve pain and to try them systematically. One aspect of the treatment plan that is often forgotten or omitted is the incorporation of measures the patient thinks may help relieve the pain, even if these measures are different from those usually employed or carried out in that institution. Without the nurse's encouragement, the patient may hesitate to mention these possible remedies. Examples might include nonprescription liniments, special applications of heat or cold, unusual positioning, or favorite homemade foods or drinks. As long as there are no contraindications to the remedy the patient wishes to try, the health care team may consider using it before trying other relief measures to relieve pain.

Interventions for pain relief fall into three categories: (1) those that modify the pain stimulus, (2) those that alter the mode of transmission, or (3) those that modify the reaction to pain.

Modification of the stimulus: changing the cognitive or sensory input

Explanation of the problem

As the result of the nursing assessment, it may become clear that the patient's response to pain is really the manifestation of a lack of knowledge about the cause of the pain. Sometimes a simple explanation about what is causing the pain and how long it will last is all that is necessary. Understanding that pain or discomfort is to be expected may relieve anxiety or help the patient to alter expectations and be better prepared for what will happen. In all cases an explanation that includes information about pain is given before each diagnostic test. An example might be the pain associated with a lumbar puncture or bone marrow biopsy.

Decision making

Allowing the individual to retain some control over daily activities may allow for better control over pain. If possible and within limits, the patient should be allowed to make decisions about the frequency of certain tasks such as exercises and turning and the order of such daily events as the bath, getting out of bed, and so on. If the patient has delineated the least painful way of doing a certain activity, such as turning, this method is recorded on the plan of care and everyone working with the patient is expected to follow this method.

In some situations it may be appropriate for the patient to help plan the use of pain relief measures. An example would be the patient with cancer who wishes to receive parenteral analgesics at bedtime to improve sleep and to receive a less potent medication that causes less drowsiness before family members visit. Consult Chapter 25 about management of pain in the terminally ill patient with cancer.

Consistency and careful planning

Planning for the same health care team members to care for the patient regularly should result in a more consistent approach and plan of care. Between the small group of health care team members and the patient, a plan of care can be developed in which the patient's decisions are honored, the day-to-day activities are put in order, and a daily routine can be devised that will reduce anxiety and frustration about constant changes. This plan should include, if appropriate, such items as

specified hours for analgesic administration before uncomfortable procedures, specified blocks of time for rest or napping, and coordination between various departments such as physical therapy and occupational therapy. For some patients fatigue is a great problem, so regular visits to off-unit departments should be interspersed with rest periods through the day; for other patients the most beneficial plan includes ensuring that they go directly from one department to the next so that time is not wasted getting in and out of bed or performing other painful maneuvers.

Distraction

Many individuals can be distracted from constant preoccupation with discomfort. Distraction interferes with the pain stimulus, thereby modifying the awareness of the pain. Mild or moderate pain can be modified by focusing on activity in the environment. A very quiet environment providing little or no sensory input can actually intensify the pain experience because the individual has nothing to focus on but the painful stimulus.

Severe pain requires more active participation by the individual in an effort to block out the painful stimulus. This can be enhanced by involving two or more sensory modalities such as vision, hearing, touch, or movement.[57] The distracters must be powerful enough to involve the individual's total interest without resulting in fatigue. Pain of long duration requires a variety of meaningful distracters.

Careful assessment may indicate ways in which the patient can be distracted, for example, playing games such as chess or checkers, watching television, or getting away from a particular setting. Simply talking with someone may be a sufficient distraction for some persons, and allowing time for this in a patient's daily routine may be very helpful. This same intervention can easily be used during some diagnostic procedures. With careful goal-directed questions and comments, the nurse may be able to take the patient's mind off the test. Discomfort will probably still occur, but preoccupation with the pain may be lessened.

Another form of distraction that may help involves the use of rhythmic breathing. To clarify, the nurse may assist the patient to concentrate on respirations, breathing more slowly and more deeply with each respiration. The patient might practice inhaling through the nose and exhaling through the mouth. Pain reduction is enhanced by keeping the eyes open and focusing on one object.[57] This in combination with efforts to relax and breathe may help the person focus on something other than pain.

Exercise

In selected situations exercise is prescribed to assist in the alleviation of discomfort. The individual may need frequent encouragement to do what may actually be painful or what may not seem to be working as well or as quickly as anticipated. The patient should be supervised occasionally while doing the exercises to ensure that they are being done correctly and are not causing unnecessary difficulty.

Working, dressing, and eating may be strenuous exercises for someone who has been unable to do these and other activities of daily living. Reasonable expectations should be determined for the rate and frequency of exercising. Actually doing the exercises may serve as a form of distraction. Patients may volunteer to accept responsibility for remembering to do them, which will increase their independence and control.

Rest, relaxation, and sleep

If the patient has not been able to sleep because of pain or if daily activities are so strenuous or hectic as not to allow rest periods, the response to the pain may reflect exhaustion or fatigue. The nurse may be able to assist in several ways. Determine the patient's usual rest and sleep patterns, decide if they are adequate now, and analyze why the patient is not getting sufficient rest. Develop a plan in consultation with the patient to provide for more rest. This plan might include decreasing the number of interruptions during the night to check vital signs and for other activities, ensuring that the environment is quiet after a certain hour, providing a warm, noncaffeinated drink before sleep, providing rest periods during the day, and administering a sleeping medication or analgesic at a regular time each night.

The nurse may need to assist the client to relax. The approach will be different with each individual but may include the following. Direct the client to assume a comfortable position (the nurse may have to assist). Make certain that this position is one the client can remain in for 2 to 3 hours. Also make certain the sheets are not constricting, the client is warm enough, and so on. Instruct the client to concentrate on each extremity, one at a time, to focus on how light and relaxed each extremity is, and to begin to breathe slowly but fully, allowing no other thoughts to enter the mind. With practice the client may be able to use the above approach when going to sleep.

The Lamaze method of childbirth and other forms of relaxation combined with exercise are examples of ways the patient may be assisted to relax. Just as success with Lamaze depends partly on how well the woman has practiced the exercises and relaxation, the same will be true of the person in pain. The patient should not be led to expect success on the first couple of tries; the nurse and the patient may have to work together for a period of time before the best method for relaxation is achieved. A variety of specific relaxation techniques are now described in the literature.[23,54,56,58]

Waking-imagined analgesia

Waking-imagined analgesia[57] is defined as "imagining a pleasant situation when a noxious stimulus is ap-

plied." This intervention is similar to distraction except that with this approach the person concentrates on trying to relive the sensations that occurred during a previous pleasant experience rather than only on enumerating the events that took place. McCaffery points out that only a small percentage of the population in pain can actually use this method of analgesia; more can derive benefit from distraction alone.

Reduction of social isolation

Social isolation may occur for the patient in pain for a variety of reasons: the serious nature of a patient's disease may necessitate being in a private room for an extended period; isolation to prevent spread of infection may have confined the patient to a single room; hospitalization far away from home may mean few family members and friends can visit; extended periods of hospitalization may result in friends losing interest in visiting; or the patient may complain so much that no one cares to visit to hear this monologue repeated.

Each of the above causes of isolation may have a different solution. In any event, careful assessment by the nurse may indicate that social isolation is a problem for the patient. Before determining the plan for addressing this problem, the patient should be consulted about the desire and need to alter the present situation.

In the hospital careful selection of roommates may provide mutual support for any two or more patients. The need for actual isolation cannot be ignored, but perhaps more frequent visits by the health care team members would help. The nurse might assist a patient to write or telephone often to family and friends so they will keep in close touch. In many cases the hospital staff almost becomes the family for the patient; each day a staff member fails to stop in to talk may contribute to feelings of loneliness for the patient.

Whether the person is hospitalized or at home, it may be possible to contact friends and arrange a time for them to visit regularly or even occasionally. It may be that certain friends are reluctant to come because they feel unsure of their role; the nurse may be able to reassure them or clarify expectations with them before their visits.

A careful but frank discussion with the patient about behavior around guests and family may be necessary. The nurse may be able to help the patient develop new methods for coping with constant pain, and this coupled with genuine interest and support of the nurse may help reduce the patient's social isolation.

Counterirritants and cutaneous stimulation

For some individuals a change in the type of stimulation at the site of pain may result in pain relief. For example, lightly rubbing the affected area may cause significant pain reduction. The *gate control theory* would support changing the amount and type of sensory receptor stimulation, and the nurse with the help of the patient may be able to find a satisfactory and relatively simple stimulus modification to ease the patient's discomfort.

Associated with sensory input modification at the site of discomfort are other forms of cutaneous stimulation. Depending on the individual, various forms of touch may be helpful to diminish pain or distract the client, such as a back rub, application of heat or cold to various body parts, or simply holding the client's hand. A gentle, cool sponge bath or whirlpool massage of a body part may be helpful.

Reduction of painful stimuli

With skill and adequate help the nurse usually can move the patient without causing excessive pain. Proper technique when handling the patient with generalized pain or a painful limb or other body part is important. Support to painful parts of the body is essential. Supporting the trunk and limbs in good body alignment will prevent increasing the pain by unnatural pulling on muscles, joints, and ligaments. A "turning sheet" is often useful in preventing uneven lifting or pull on patients with severe neck, back, or general trunk pain. Painful joints may be moved with less discomfort if they are placed on a pillow or otherwise supported rather than being lifted directly. If there is tenderness or pain in the shaft of the bone, in muscles, or in large skin areas, the limb should be supported at the joints when the patient moves to prevent additional pain.

Binders, surgical belts, and girdles give support to the abdomen. Body casts, corsets, and braces are used to immobilize the vertebral column and thus decrease pain. A firm bed gives support and thereby lessens pain both when the patient is at rest and when moving about in bed. Traction, splints, casts, and braces are used to immobilize a painful part of the body such as an ankle. Special beds (e.g., Stryker frame, Foster bed, Circ-Olectric bed, and Bradford frame) allow movement with minimal handling of the body and thereby help lessen pain. If the nurse in caring for a patient in pain feels that any of these mechanical devices would be of benefit, the problem can be discussed with the physician.

Reduction of noise and visual stimulation

The patient may be suffering from sensory overload. If nurses could stand still for 5 minutes in the patient's environment and watch and listen, they might understand that some patients are simply bombarded with noise and visual stimulation. If these are problems, it may be possible to change the environment. Changes include moving the individual away from a busy nurses' station or, in the home, away from a busy family room. Try to ensure that the lights are turned out or at least significantly dimmed at night. In the home or in the hospital, those around the individual's room may need to be reminded to talk and move more quietly at night.

Television and radio can serve as wonderful distracters, but most individuals tire of them after 14 to 18 consecutive hours. It may be possible to determine a schedule based on the likes and dislikes of family members or roommates that would include periods of silence during the day. Radio and television volume should be at a level comfortable for listening.

Overtalkativeness and overoptimism are often annoying to the person in pain. This is particularly true when the patient knows or suspects that the prognosis is poor. Florence Nightingale gave the following advice on this subject:

But the long chronic case, who knows too well himself, and who has been told by his physician that he will never enter active life again, who feels that every month he has to give up something he could do the month before—oh! spare such sufferers your chattering hopes. You do not know how you worry and weary them. Such real sufferers cannot bear to talk of themselves, still less to hope for what they cannot at all expect.[103]

Plans should be made so that a minimal number of persons enter the room of the patient in severe pain. The patient cannot possibly learn to know and trust all the individuals who enter the hospital room each day. Unless some effort is made to control traffic in and out of the room, the patient may be unable to relax and rest. The same principle applies to care of the individual at home where the problem of too many visitors is frequently a real one. The nurse, of all members of the health care team, is in the best position to give attention to this real need of the patient. Some patients in pain welcome interruptions and distractions, whereas others prefer privacy and seclusion. The nurse should see that the patient's wishes are respected.

Therapeutic touch

A less traditional therapy, that of therapeutic touch, may be helpful to patients in pain.[11] The rationale for the success of this therapy is not clearly understood. The nurse trained in therapeutic touch undergoes a brief period of meditation before coming in contact with the patient. During this period the nurse quiets the energy levels within herself or himself and then goes on to touch the patient and to "transduce and transmit the universal healing energies to the one in need."[11] Few nurses are trained in the use of therapeutic touch as described here. It does seem to be helpful for some patients and some kinds of pain; it certainly seems to do no harm.[56]

Alteration of pain transmission

Medications to alter pain

The nurse needs to know the precise effect on the body of medications used to treat pain (Table 23-2). The time curve of beginning effect, the height of effective-

TABLE 23-2. Commonly used analgesics

Generic name	Trade name	Usual dosage	Route	Onset	Peak	Duration
Narcotics						
Morphine sulfate	—	5-20 mg q 3-4 hr	SC, IM	5-10 min	60 min	4-6 hr
Codeine sulfate	—	15-60 mg q 3-4 hr	SC, PO	5-30 min	30-60 min	3-4 hr
Hydromorphone hydrochloride	Dilaudid	2-4 mg q 4-6 hr	IV, IM, SC, PO	5-15 min	1 hr	4-6 hr
Meperidine hydro-chloride	Demerol	50-150 mg q 3-4 hr	IV, IM, SC, PO	10-15 min	30-60 min	2-4 hr
Methadone	Dolophine	2.5-10 mg q 3-4 hr	IM, SC, PO	10 min	1-2 hr	4-6 hr
Pentazocine	Talwin	15-30 mg q 3-4 hr	IM, SC	10-30 min	1 hr	2-3 hr
		50-100 mg q 3-4 hr	PO			
Nonnarcotics						
Acetylsalicylic acid	Aspirin	300-1000 mg q 3-4 hr	PO	15-30 min	1 hr	3-4 hr
Acetaminophen	Tylenol; Datril	325-650 mg q 4-6 hr	PO	15-30 min	1-2 hr	4-6 hr
Ethoheptazine citrate	Zactane	75-150 mg 3 to 4 times per day	PO	15-30 min	1 hr	3-6 hr

ness, and the time of declining effect must be understood. In addition, the effects of the medication may vary according to the time of day it is administered and the physiologic status of the individual. A brief summary of several categories of drugs is presented here; for a more definitive discussion and elaboration of appropriate nursing measures, refer to pharmacology texts.

Medication to relieve the cause of pain. Pain may be treated by drugs that help to relieve the cause of pain. For example, the belladonna group of drugs (atropine) or synthetic substitutes such as propantheline bromide (Pro-Banthine), which cause relaxation of smooth muscle, may diminish the pain caused by spasm of the smooth muscles. If pain is caused by impaired circulation, drugs that dilate the blood vessels such as papaverine hydrochloride, nitroglycerin, and tolazoline hydrochloride (Priscoline) may do more good than analgesic drugs. A final example includes antibiotics used to treat an infection that may be causing pain. Specific drugs are chosen based on the nature of the infection, the sensitivity of the organism to the antibiotic, and the general condition of the patient.

Salicylates. One of the most widely used analgesic drugs is acetylsalicylic acid (aspirin). This is the safest of the coal-tar products; it usually relieves headache, muscle ache, and arthritic pain. The specific action of aspirin on pain is not known, but it does block *prostaglandin* production and thus may decrease the pain associated with inflammation. Aspirin does not cloud the

sensorium and this is an advantage over many other analgesics. Aspirin is highly effective when given with codeine, the combined effect being much superior to the use of either drug alone. The nurse needs to be constantly aware that some persons are allergic to aspirin. Death can occur when aspirin is given to such individuals. Common side effects of acetylsalicylic acid are irritation of the gastric mucosa, ulceration of the gastric mucosa, and reactivation of peptic ulcers. For these reasons aspirin should never be taken on an empty stomach. It should be taken after meals or with a snack such as a glass of milk. Salicylism can occur in persons who take large doses of aspirin over long periods of time. Nausea, vomiting, ringing in the ears, deafness, and severe headache are common manifestations. A decreased prothrombin level and inhibition of platelet aggregation may also occur, depending on the dose, and may contribute to bleeding manifestations.

Aspirin products are available in a variety of combinations and forms such as timed-relief aspirin, enteric-coated aspirin, and aspirin with phenacetin or caffeine. Individuals vary widely in their response to these, but there has been little conclusive data to indicate that any form or combination is best. Aspirin is also widely used to reduce fever and inflammation.

Acetaminophen (Tylenol, Datril), a para-aminophenol derivative with salicylate-like analgesic effects, has achieved wide popularity because it causes less alteration of the prothrombin level and fewer side effects.

It can, however, cause severe liver damage and should not be used indiscriminately. This drug also has antipyretic action and antiinflammatory action. It is frequently prescribed for persons for whom aspirin is contraindicated.

Other coal-tar analgesics such as phenacetin and acetanilid may produce toxic effects after prolonged use. They should be used only under the direction of a physician despite the fact that they can be purchased without medical prescription.

Nonsteroidal antiinflammatory agents. *Phenylbutazone* (Butazolidin) is prescribed to relieve symptoms of an acute episode of gout. It has some antiinflammatory properties but is poorly tolerated by many individuals and has numerous side effects including hematologic changes, gastric irritation, and fluid and electrolyte disturbances.

Indomethacin (Indocin) also is an effective antiinflammatory drug with antipyretic action. It has many side effects but may be helpful in decreasing pain in individuals with rheumatoid arthritis, osteoarthrosis, and ankylosing spondylosis.

Fenoprofen calcium (Nalfon) and Ibuprofen (Motrin) are chemically related drugs with analgesic, antipyretic, and antiinflammatory properties. They are used in rheumatoid arthritis, osteoarthritis, and in other orthopedic or arthritis-type conditions. As with other drugs in this category, gastric irritation is common, as are changes in hematologic values. The drugs just cited are but a few of the drugs available in this category.

Counterirritants. Ointments, emollients, and liniments such as ethyl aminobenzoate and methyl salicylate (oil of wintergreen) are counterirritants that may be applied locally to alleviate pain. Oil of clove, used for toothaches, is another example.

Medications to control pain

Other types of pain medications are effective through modification of the response of the person experiencing the pain rather than altering the transmission of the pain stimuli. Many of these are thought to act at opiate receptor sites in the brain; these drugs are the exogenous morphines (see discussion of endorphins, p. 379). These medications are discussed in order to serve as a useful reference source for the reader.

Narcotics. The opiates are drugs most widely recognized and used for the control of pain. Morphine and codeine are examples of opium alkaloids commonly used. Synthetic narcotic drugs such as meperidine hydrochloride (Demerol) and methadone hydrochloride (Dolophine) are also widely used. All of these drugs just mentioned are termed *narcotic agonists*; that is, they have affinity for certain receptors, and are efficacious in producing the effects desired of narcotics. When given in therapeutic doses, narcotics act by depressing brain cells involved in pain perception without seriously impairing other sensory perceptions. They also affect to some extent the patient's feeling about pain and thus affect both physical pain and the reaction to it. In addition, the synthetic narcotic drugs have some antispasmodic action and thereby encourage relaxation.

The effects of narcotics vary with the physiologic state of the patient. The very young and the very old are quite sensitive to the effects of narcotics and require smaller doses to obtain relief from pain. A person of any age may be more depressed physically and emotionally by narcotics during the early morning hours (1 to 6 AM) than at any other time of the day and therefore should be watched carefully for untoward effects.

Narcotics can cause lowering of the blood pressure and general depression of vital functions, including respiratory depression, bradycardia, and drowsiness. Some of these reactions can be an advantage in treating a condition such as hemorrhage in which some lowering of blood pressure may be desirable. Hypotension may be a disadvantage in treating the debilitated patient, who may go into shock from an excessive dosage of a drug. The narcotic drugs are less likely to cause shock if the patient is up and moving about and taking food and fluids, since these activities tend to maintain the blood pressure at a safe level. Other common side effects include nausea, vomiting, constipation, and occasionally allergic-type reactions. The appearance of side effects is influenced by such things as dose, route of administration, relation to meals, other medications, and drug idiosyncrasy.

So much emphasis has been placed on the danger of drug addiction (and to be sure, the danger is very real) that nurses sometimes withhold narcotic drugs and allow patients to suffer more than is advisable. The patient in severe pain will not become addicted to narcotic drugs even if they are given at frequent intervals for several days. However, before giving any patient an analgesic drug, the nurse should always determine whether the patient's pain is that for which the drug was ordered. If it is a "new" pain, analgesics may mask symptoms of undiagnosed disease.

It is important that the nurse understand the goals of analgesic therapy with each patient, as there is wide variation in how analgesic drugs should appropriately be used. For example, in postoperative patients, the best pain relief is usually achieved by giving an ordered narcotic every 3 to 4 hours (as often as permitted) around the clock for 24 to 48 hours before slowing the frequency to when the patient requests the drug. This method takes advantage of the fact that it is easier to prevent pain than to treat it after it has become severe. In addition, the patient may be more willing to cooperate with necessary postoperative routines if not in severe pain. This procedure does not increase the incidence of narcotic addiction.

A completely different situation would be the use of

narcotic analgesics with the patient with advanced terminal cancer. In this patient fears of addiction are irrelevant. Some of these patients may require narcotics as often as every hour or even via continuous intravenous infusion.

A commonly used synthetic analgesic is pentazocine (Talwin). The structure of pentazocine is different from morphine and related drugs, causing it to be classified as a weak narcotic antagonist, although it has some morphinelike analgesic properties. The significance of this classification is that pentazocine or any narcotic antagonist should not be given simultaneously with a narcotic agonist, as the analgesic effects of the two drugs may be cancelled. (For further discussion of narcotic antagonists see a pharmacology text.) Pentazocine is often prescribed in place of morphine or meperidine for the relief of moderate to severe pain. It is given orally or parenterally. The most commonly occurring reactions are vertigo, nausea, and euphoria. Since sedation and dizziness have been noted in some instances, clients receiving pentazocine should be warned not to operate machinery, drive cars, or unnecessarily expose themselves to hazards. Pentazocine is contraindicated in persons with increased intracranial pressure, head injury, or pathologic brain conditions in which clouding of the sensorium is particularly undesirable. When first marketed, pentazocine was thought to have little addicting potential. However, dependence can develop with prolonged use.

Propoxyphene hydrochloride (Darvon) and propoxyphene napsylate (Darvon-N) are related chemically to methadone, and are widely used analgesics. They are said to be as potent as codeine, but some trials have indicated that they have little more than placebo effect. Propoxyphene is considered nonaddictive, but dependence may occur after repeated use of high doses. Side effects include dizziness, headache, gastrointestinal disturbances, and rashes. The effectiveness of either drug may be enhanced by use of combination preparations containing propoxyphene.

Recently, there has been an increased interest in looking at the way in which analgesics are actually administered and at their effectiveness. Although probably for a variety of reasons including fear of addicting the patient, lack of adequate understanding of pain or of the action of analgesics, and incorrect assessment and assumptions about the patient's pain, it would seem that often there is a difference between the degree of pain relief the doctor or nurse thinks a patient has and what the patient reports. The reader is referred to indicated references at the end of the chapter.*

Sedatives. Sometimes the patient needs a sedative drug instead of additional analgesics. This type of drug may permit drowsiness and relaxation enough for the

analgesic to be effective. Phenobarbital, for example, often enables the patient to be comfortable with a lower narcotic dose than might otherwise be necessary. The patient with a severe emotional reaction to illness will often get relief when analgesic drugs are interspersed with sedative drugs. This arrangement has been found useful when the narcotic or other analgesic drug does not seem to quite "hold" the patient for the desired interval. Small doses of phenobarbital appear to relieve most of the discomfort expressed by infants and small children when they have pain. The effect of sedative drugs, similar to narcotics, may be increased by the slowing down of physiologic response. In the presence of fever they sometimes produce excitement rather than relaxation. This effect may occur in older patients as well. Because barbiturates may make some patients less aware of their surroundings, side rails and constant nursing supervision may be necessary to protect them from injuries such as from falls.

Ataractic drugs. Ataractic drugs, or so-called tranquilizers, which affect the mood of the patient, have been found helpful in the treatment of pain, particularly when given in combination with narcotics. This combination of drugs tends to separate the perception of pain from the reaction to pain. The sensation of pain appears less acute and therefore the reaction to it becomes less severe. When fear and apprehension appear to be the most striking features of the patient's reaction, tranquilizers alone may be sufficient to cause relaxation. Diazepam (Valium), prochlorperazine (Compazine), and chlordiazepoxide hydrochloride (Librium) are examples of commonly used tranquilizers. If these drugs cause lethargy and failure of normal response, this should be reported to the physician at once. The physiologic state of the person may cause a variance in response to these drugs similar to that seen with narcotics.

Antiemetics. Antiemetics, particularly of the phenothiazine group (haloperidol [Haldol], prochlorperazine [Compazine]) and the antihistaminic group (hydroxyzine [Vistaril] and promethazine [Phenergan]) are often ordered to be administered concomitantly with parenteral analgesics or they may be ordered on a prn basis for the patient. Generally speaking, the antiemetics are not potentiators of analgesic activity.[56] They do, however, have additive effects in producing sedation and central nervous system depression. In addition, the antiemetics may help prevent or reduce nausea and vomiting, frequent side effects of narcotic analgesics.

McCaffery points out that the sedated or sleeping patient should not be equated with the pain-free patient.[53,56] On the other hand, severe pain may contribute to overwhelming fatigue, and sleep, when it occurs, may be most welcome by the patient and family. In some patients nausea may be the only subjective complaint when the problem is actually one of pain. This

*References 5, 37, 49, 53, 56-58, 61.

reinforces the need for individualized patient assessment and care.

Side effects of the antiemetics vary with individual drugs, but usually include sedation, hypotension, dry mouth, hematologic changes, and extrapyramidal side effects.

Placebos. Placebos are sometimes used for their psychogenic effect in relieving pain, but they should never be given without a physician's order. Although the most usual response to a placebo is positive, some persons have negative reactions and may report intensified pain or other symptoms. Therefore when a placebo is being used, the nurse should observe the patient carefully and share with the physician any information that will help determine the best treatment for the patient. Favorable response to a placebo should not lead the nurse to ignore complaints of pain, for the individual who responds to placebos is as much in need of the nurse's interest and support as any other patient. Furthermore, the patient may have a new physical pain that needs to be evaluated.

Nurses and physicians often tend to underestimate how many patients will have a positive response to a placebo and instead reserve the use of placebos for patients who are disliked, thought to be suffering from primarily psychogenic pain, who exaggerate their pain, or who are otherwise atypical in their response to pain.[31] It is important for the nurse to remember that a positive response to a placebo is not related to the cause of the patient's pain or to the patient's subjective feelings about the pain.[8,31,41,71]

Transcutaneous electrical nerve stimulators

A transcutaneous electrical nerve stimulator, or TENS unit, is a battery-powered stimulator worn externally by the patient. Two or more electrodes attached to the battery box are applied on, around, or near the site of pain, and the client then manually regulates the power source to vary the amplitude and frequency of electrical stimulation passing between the electrodes. The goal of the device is to modify the sensory input by blocking or changing the painful stimulation with stimulation perceived as less painful or nonpainful. Success with this device may come only after repeated trials with various electrode placements or battery-box manipulations. The nurse may be very valuable in encouraging patients and assisting them to make these small manipulations.

Because the transcutaneous electrical stimulator is noninvasive in its application, it may be particularly useful for the person who cannot tolerate more extensive procedures.[56,59]

Dorsal column stimulators

The dorsal column stimulator is similar to the transcutaneous electrical stimulator except that an electrode is surgically implanted over the dorsal column of the spinal column through laminectomy and the transmitter is worn externally. The low-voltage pulses produced by the stimulator are thought to block transmission of pain by stimulating large sensory fibers.[33] The success of this therapy and the transcutaneous stimulator is thought to be explained by the gate control theory of pain transmission.

In many institutions where dorsal column stimulators are implanted, candidates for this surgery are chosen only after they demonstrate success with the use of the transcutaneous stimulator or with a temporary percutaneous epidural dorsal column stimulator. The nurse needs to be alert to postoperative complications associated with spinal cord surgery, especially infection and cerebrospinal fluid leak.

The PISCES (percutaneous implanted spinal cord epidural stimulation) system is a newer, less intrusive approach to spinal cord stimulation. The leads are inserted percutaneously into the epidural space with the patient under local anesthesia (Fig. 23-5).

Neurosurgical procedures

Constant, relentless pain that cannot be controlled by analgesics (intractable pain) may be reduced or abolished by one of various neurosurgical procedures.

Neurectomy. When pain is localized to one part of the body it can sometimes be relieved by interruption of the peripheral or cranial nerves supplying the area. The nerve fibers to the affected area are severed from the cord (cell body) in an operation known as neurectomy. Not only pain fibers are interrupted by these procedures but also fibers controlling movement and position sense. Therefore this type of treatment cannot be used to control pain in the extremities. A neurectomy probably is most often performed to relieve the pain of persons with trigeminal neuralgia, in which case it is referred to as a *fifth-nerve resection*. A neurectomy may also be performed to control incapacitating dysmenorrhea and is called a *presacral neurectomy*. One of the difficulties with a neurectomy is that peripheral nerves regenerate, making this type of surgery questionable at times.

Rhizotomy. Resection of a posterior nerve root just before it enters the spinal cord is known as a rhizotomy (Fig. 23-6). This procedure frequently is useful in controlling severe pain in the upper trunk such as that caused by carcinoma of the lung. It is also done to relieve severe spasticity in persons with paraplegia. However, it cannot be used to relieve pain in the extremities, since position sense is lost. The incision is made high in the thoracic or low in the cervical area and involves a laminectomy. Rhizotomy may be carried out lower in the cord, but when this is done bowel, bladder, and sexual function problems are frequent complications.

The postoperative observations and care are similar

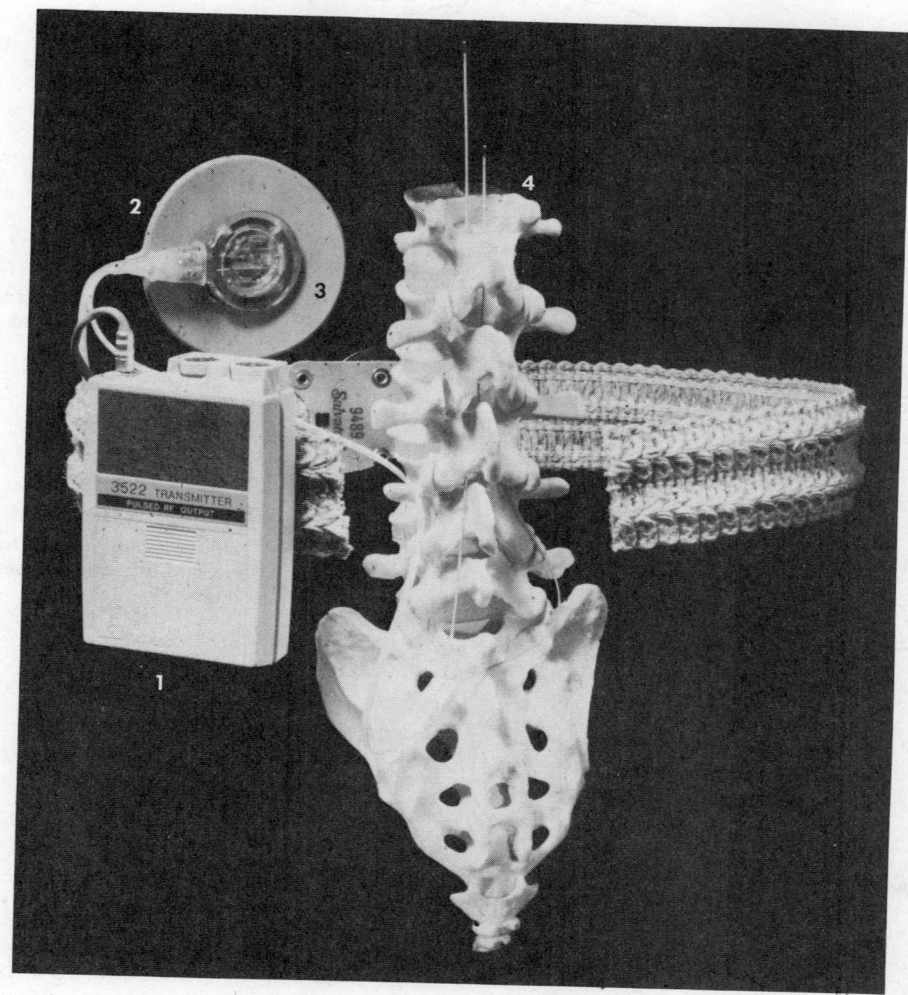

Fig. 23-5. PISCES spinal cord stimulator. *1,* Stimulation transmitter. *2,* Receiver-extension. *3,* Antenna. *4,* Leads. (Courtesy Medtronic, Inc., Minneapolis.)

to that necessary for any patient who has had a laminectomy (p. 820), except that the patient who has had a rhizotomy is usually a poorer operative risk and may be suffering from a severe debilitating disease and therefore develops complications such as decubiti more easily. It is important for both the patient and the nurse to realize that this operation will not prevent pain at the level of the incision because the resected nerves affect only the area below the incision. Nursing intervention involves the usual postlaminectomy care. Teaching the patient what to expect is important so that he or she can adjust expectations accordingly. The patient must understand that the loss of sensory transmission from the area of the rhizotomy interferes with the ability to perceive heat and cold. Care must be taken when the affected area is exposed to extremes in temperature (e.g., heat used for cooking and baking).

Cordotomy. A cordotomy is an operation performed to relieve intractable pain. The advantages of cordot-

omy include a wide sense of analgesia below the surgical site while other sensory and motor functions are preserved. Cordotomy is most often performed on patients with extensive carcinoma of the pelvis. The incision is made high in the thoracic area, two laminae are removed, and the pain pathways in the spinothalamic tract (anterior and lateral aspect of the cord) on the side opposite the pain are severed (Fig. 23-6). If the pain is in the midline, the interruption must be made bilaterally. However, the two operations must be performed separately to avoid extensive damage to the cord from edema.

Following surgery, nursing care is similar to that given a patient who has had a cervical laminectomy for removal of a protruded nucleus pulposus. Frequently, temporary paralysis, or at least leg weakness, and loss of bowel and bladder control follow a cordotomy; these result from edema of the cord and will gradually disappear in about 2 weeks. During the period of paralysis

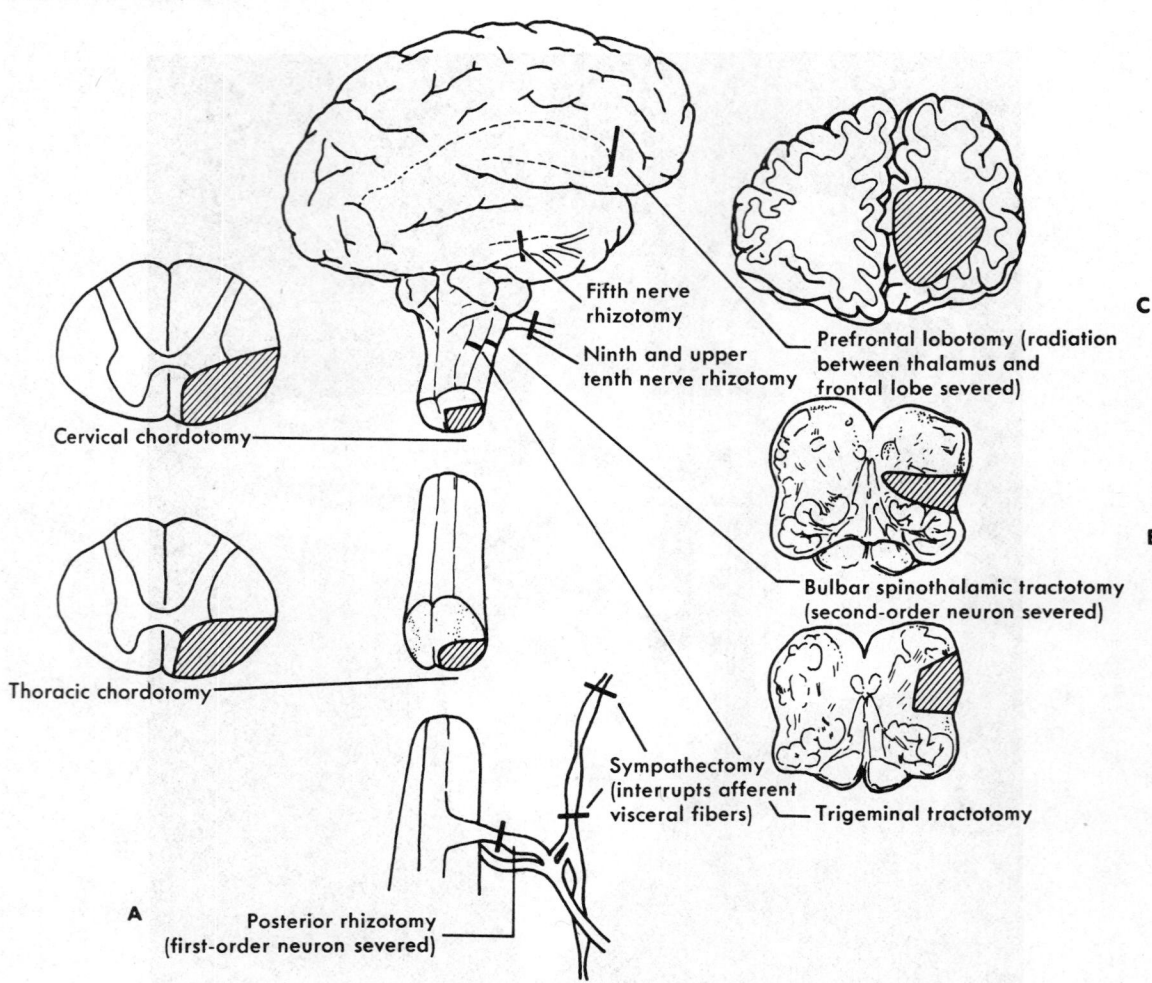

Fifth nerve rhizotomy

Ninth and upper tenth nerve rhizotomy

Cervical chordotomy

Thoracic chordotomy

Sympathectomy (interrupts afferent visceral fibers)

A Posterior rhizotomy (first-order neuron severed)

C Prefrontal lobotomy (radiation between thalamus and frontal lobe severed)

B Bulbar spinothalamic tractotomy (second-order neuron severed)

Trigeminal tractotomy

Fig. 23-6. Neurosurgical procedures for pain relief: **A,** rhizotomy; sympathectomy; cordotomy; **B,** tractotomy; and **C,** prefrontal lobotomy. (From Conway-Rutkowski, B.L.: Carini and Owens' neurological and neurosurgical nursing, ed. 8, St. Louis, 1982, The C.V. Mosby Co.)

the patient may be helped out of bed by using a hydraulic lift (Fig. 23-7). Back care with special attention to pressure points should be given every 2 or 3 hours, since position sense is lessened and the patient is often debilitated. It is advisable to use an alternating-air-pressure mattress, water mattress, or some other measure to reduce pressure until the patient is allowed out of bed. Sometimes a Foster bed or a Stryker frame enables the nurse to give the patient better care. Because of the decreased position sense, special attention needs to be given to placing the patient in proper body alignment. If quadriceps-setting exercises are begun in the early postoperative period, retraining in walking will be less difficult. It is usually easier for patients to use a walker when they begin ambulation and then progress to a cane. Physical therapy activities, such as riding a stationary bicycle, which provide for hip and knee flexion may be used to strengthen leg muscles. Therapy can be started as soon as the patient can be out of bed comfortably for at least 2 hours at a time.

Because temperature sensation is permanently lost,

the nurse must be careful to avoid burning or otherwise injuring the patient's trunk and legs and must teach the patient and family how to avoid injury. The lower portions of the body, especially the feet, are inspected routinely for any breaks in the skin or unnoticed infection.

Percutaneous cordotomy, which permits more precise control of the size and site of the surgical lesion, may be used instead of the direct thoracic approach. It is less traumatic surgically for the debilitated person who has often been on continuous analgesic therapy for long periods.

The procedure consists of inserting a spinal lumbar puncture needle laterally between the cervical (C1 and C2) level. A wire electrode is then inserted into the anterior cord and a lesion is made at a designated site, under radiologic and stereotactic control, in order to destroy the ascending pain fibers. The procedure is performed with the patient under local anesthesia, and a sensation of tingling in the corresponding body area will be noticed when the electrode is stimulated mini-

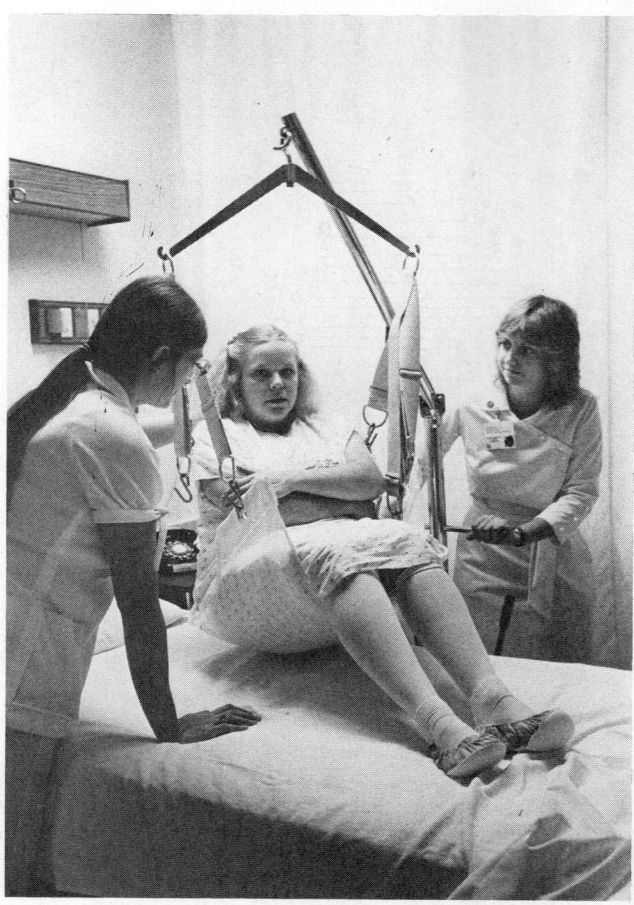

Fig. 23-7. Hydraulic lift can be used to move paralyzed patient from bed to chair.

mally. This assists the surgeon in locating the exact site for the surgical lesion.

Preoperatively, patients are evaluated carefully as to their candidacy for this type of surgery and to establish baseline data. It is important to identify and exclude individuals whose pain is more functionally based. Cordotomy in this instance would not be successful in relief of the pain. Pulmonary function is also carefully evaluated to establish a baseline to be used for comparison postoperatively. The risk of respiratory complications, especially in patients who undergo *bilateral* percutaneous cordotomy, is great. Regional anesthetic blocks (with an epidural catheter) are often evaluated prior to surgery for a 24-hour period or longer in order to test the benefits to the person. Placebo blocks with normal saline solution are also done and the results compared with the anesthetic block. The patient is carefully monitored by the nurse during the regional blocks for hypalgesia and analgesia responses.

Postoperatively, the patient is observed closely for postural hypotension when initially ambulated. The sympathetic fibers in the cord controlling blood pressure may be affected for a period of time. Temperature

sensation is also expected to be lost after this type of surgery. Bladder function and motor function may also be affected and should be observed carefully by the nurse following surgery. Usually such deficits do not increase following unilateral cordotomy but may after bilateral cordotomy. The value of accurate presurgical baseline data of all components is particularly necessary for good postsurgical care of the patient with a cordotomy.

Interruption of nerve pathways in the brain. Numerous attempts have been made to alter the transmission of pain and the response to pain by surgical or stereotactic interruption of pathways in the brain. Lesions have been placed in the thalamus, the cingulum, the mesencephalon, the medulla, and the frontal lobe. The success rate has varied considerably depending on the skill of the surgeon, the type of pain, and the patient's general physical and emotional condition.

These surgeries may have complications, particularly changes in the personality of the patient. Although the assistance of a psychiatrist is helpful in managing all patients with chronic pain, it is highly recommended for any surgery that may change the patient's personality.

A variety of other neurosurgical procedures may be helpful for specific problems. *Hypophysectomy* (destruction or removal of the pituitary gland) is sometimes helpful in patients with pain, particularly bone pain, caused by cancer of the breast or prostate gland.[47] *Sympathectomy* (excision or destruction of one or more sympathetic ganglia or nerves) is useful in cases of true causalgia and pain which is secondary to vascular insufficiency of the extremities.[48]

Intrathecal phenol or alcohol

Another medical intervention used at some institutions is the injection of hyperbaric phenol or hypobaric alcohol into the subarachnoid space via lumbar puncture. The patient is positioned carefully, the desired substance is injected, and the nerve roots involved in the pain transmission are destroyed. The effect is analogous to a chemical posterior rhizotomy, and effects may last several weeks to months.[47,48] Side effects are common and include bladder and bowel dysfunction and various degrees of lower extremity weakness. The value of this intervention is that no major surgery is required, but its use is limited to pain in the trunk, abdomen, and lower extremities. Nursing intervention includes that given a patient undergoing lumbar puncture.

Neuroaugmentation

The term *neuroaugmentation* is a broad one that would include the use of dorsal column stimulators. In neuroaugmentation procedures electrical stimulation is used to produce pain relief, but destruction of nerve function does not occur.[44,48] In addition to spinal cord stimulation, electrodes have also been stereotactically placed in the thalamus. Although apparently similar to dorsal column stimulators in action, in fact, the use of electrodes in the thalamus may work by stimulating production of endorphins.[91]

Nerve block

A nerve block involves the injection of substances such as local anesthetics or neurolytic agents (e.g., alcohol or phenol) close to nerves to block the conduction of impulses over the nerves. Nerve blocks are frequently used for the symptomatic relief of pain. They are used to treat chronic pain associated with peripheral vascular disease, trigeminal neuralgia, causalgia, and cancer. The anesthetic or neurolytic agent can be injected into the appropriate site to block conductivity through peripheral fibers of spinal or cranial nerves, somatic or autonomic ganglia, or the posterior nerve root. A nerve block may be unsuccessful because of difficulty in locating the correct nerve fiber and the complexity of the pain itself. Since the nerve fibers, ganglia, and roots being injected contain other fibers than those for pain and because some of the injected agents may leak out of the injection site and affect other nerves, the recipient of the nerve block will usually experience some other type of neurological deficit.

Acupuncture

Acupuncture is an ancient form of disease treatment that can be used for pain relief. Only recently, however, has the method been used in Western countries. Small needles are skillfully inserted and manipulated at specific body points, depending on the type and location of pain, producing often immediate and continued relief of pain (Fig. 23-8). The gate control theory provides the best explanation for the success of acupuncture: the local stimulation of large-diameter fibers by the needles "closes the gate" to pain. It is not known to what extent the psyche and the power of suggestion contribute to effectiveness of this therapy. Nursing intervention includes careful client assessment and teaching.[1,84]

Modification of the response to pain

Decreasing the anxiety of the patient and family

The patient in pain is often afraid. Fear may be allayed in part by the nurse's calm, quiet manner and particularly by a demonstration of competence. Confidence in the persons who care for them is a tremendous help to patients. It is a great comfort to the patient to know, for example, that the nurse will not hurry while giving nursing care, thus increasing pain, or be so "busy" that pain medication is not given at the prescribed intervals.

Sometimes preparation for pain helps to increase acceptance of it and in turn produces relaxation, which will decrease pain. An example is the benefit derived

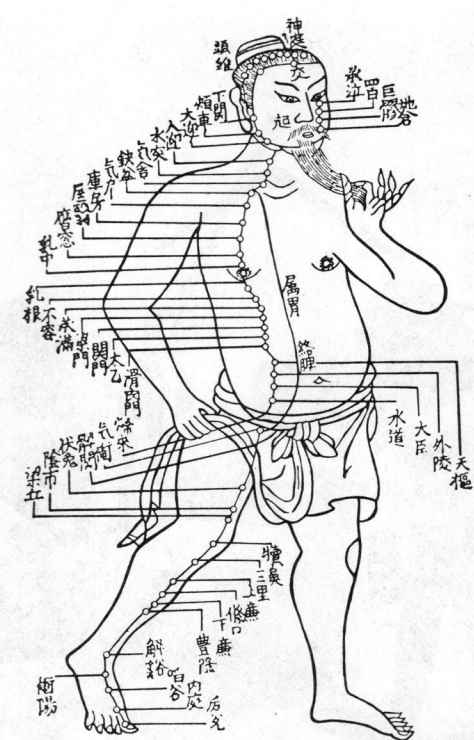

Fig. 23-8. Typical acupuncture chart showing sites for insertion of needles along several body meridians. After two or more needles are inserted, electrical current is usually passed through needles for about 20 minutes. Resulting analgesia can permit major surgery. (From Weisenberg, M.: Pain: clinical and experimental perspectives, St. Louis, 1975, The C.V. Mosby Co.; courtesy *Abbottempo*, vol. X, no. 1.)

from special preparation for childbirth. Fear and irritability can sometimes be allayed by explaining to patients why they have pain. This knowledge may let them relax somewhat and thereby lessen their discomfort. If patients can be told honestly that the pain will probably be of short duration, this should be done. Postoperative pain is often aggravated by movement. Therefore, when certain activities such as turning and coughing are necessary to prevent complications, the nurse explains this to the patient. The nurse may be able to comfort children who are frightened by pain by holding them, rocking them, or talking to them. Older patients also may be comforted by having someone sit quietly with them, and some patients benefit from the personal contact of holding another's hand.

It is understandable that the family will be upset when the patient is in pain. Prompt attention to the patient's needs helps reduce the family's concern, and the patient's behavior should be interpreted as necessary to family and friends with simple, clear explanations. Regardless of explanations, persons who are emotionally close to the patient may need time to accept changes in the patient's behavior. Reassurance of family members is an essential part of nursing care because it may prevent them from communicating their concern to the patient. Expressions of concern by others may make the patient increasingly tense, which in turn lowers tolerance to pain. Helping the family understand the patient's behavior often reduces their demands for the patient to relate to them as usual and may help the patient feel less guilty about not being able to respond to them in the usual way.

Teaching

Teaching as a nursing role has been mentioned frequently in relation to helping the person who has pain. Just as each client's plan of care should be individualized so should the teaching within that plan of care. Careful assessment of the client's willingness and interest in learning and mental and physical ability to tolerate teaching should be made before teaching is initiated. Teaching varies with each client but may include the cause of the pain, even at the physiologic level if the patient wishes to know, why or how various attempts at pain relief could or should work, and alternate ways to do daily activities that might be less painful or consume less energy. Various nursing measures, even if not primarily for pain relief, are explained.

In preparation for surgery or diagnostic procedures, the patient should be told honestly what to expect in terms of duration and intensity of pain *usually* experienced and what measures will be available to assist with this discomfort. If the patient must actually perform certain maneuvers or treatments, it is helpful for the patient to practice these before the procedure, for example, to cough and deep breathe preoperatively. If at all possible the family should be included in these teaching sessions, not only so they can support and assist the patient but also so they will understand what the patient will be expected to do.

Spiritual assistance

Even if no estimate can be made as to the duration of pain, patients should be given encouragement that the problem will not become too great for them to accept with the assistance that is available. Many patients who have prolonged pain with no hope of relief can and do derive benefit from their religious faith. This may help them to consider pain in a more positive way and thus make it more bearable for them. The nurse can arrange for the appropriate religious advisor to be available to the patient who indicates such a desire.

In addition, the nurse may become involved in doing such things as sharing in a prayer with the patient, reading from the Bible or other meaningful book, ensuring that meaningful religious medals or statues are within reach or sight, and so on.

Psychiatric assistance

In some situations the medical team will ask a psychiatrist to evaluate the client and perhaps begin ongoing psychiatric care. The individual suffering from chronic or intractable pain may appear sad, hostile, anxious, and so on. These persons often have spent years undergoing various diagnostic and surgical procedures and have seen many different physicians without significant pain relief.[10,65]

For many individuals psychiatric care is still not as acceptable as other kinds of medical care. The nurse should be supportive to them and help them understand why this type of therapy may be helpful. The nurse's role also includes the careful recording and reporting of objective data about the patient's behavior including interactions with family and others.

Behavior modification

Whether used as part of the psychiatrist's plan of care or not, the nursing plan of care may outline a program designed to increase more acceptable or pleasing behavior or performance in the patient and reduce unpleasant or desired behavior. The basis for this therapy is the idea that "a behavior will tend to occur more frequently if it is consistently followed by a reward such as praise."[57] Forms of this behavior therapy are used unconsciously all the time: a young boy "throwing a tantrum" may be ignored, but as his behavior becomes more appropriate his mother may point this out and reward him with her time and attention.

Behavior modification can be used frequently with persons in pain. For example, the nurse may praise and congratulate a patient for performing postoperative exercises. If the patient is being encouraged to try a new pain relief measure such as relaxation, it is hoped the ultimate reward will come in the form of pain relief. During the practice and learning phase, however, positive reinforcement and verbal praise and encouragement by the nurse when the patient does try relaxation should stimulate the patient to practice the new method regularly.

In using behavioral methods in altering pain-associated behavior or in encouraging patient activities, success will occur only with a consistent approach on the part of the nurses and the health care team. While patients should always be praised for their efforts to comply with or assist with treatment regimens, a true behavior modification program requires careful analysis of patient behavior and the development of a specific and comprehensive treatment plan.[28]

Biofeedback and autogenic training

Some persons are able to alter their body functions through mental concentration.[80] In biofeedback training the individual is repeatedly attached to a machine that monitors brain wave activity (electroencephalograph). The individual then concentrates and tries to slow his or her brain wave activity to rates at which pain and distress are unlikely to cause discomfort (i.e., complete relaxation). Normal waking brain activity is in the beta (β) range, 14 to 22 pulses per second. The goal of biofeedback is to reduce this activity to 8 to 13 pulses per second (alpha [α]) or even slower, 4 to 7 pulses per second (theta [θ]). The biofeedback machine is regulated so that when alpha or theta ranges are reached a signal will sound to indicate success. The goal is to become adept at reaching the alpha or theta range at will and thus suppressing pain. It may take many months of regular practice to achieve the desired level of control. The nurse can be very helpful in encouraging and praising the individual's efforts.[80]

In autogenic training the same type of self-regulation is used to alter various autonomic nervous system functions such as pulse, blood pressure, and muscle tension. Practiced use of transcendental meditation and other methods of concentration and self-control may achieve the same degree of autoregulation without the use of sophisticated physiologic monitoring equipment. As can be seen from the discussion, many of the pain relief therapies combine distraction, relaxation, self-control, and forms of behavior modification.

Hypnosis

Hypnosis has been used for decades in the treatment of various conditions, particularly when these conditions are aggravated by tension and stress. This therapy helps individuals to alter their perception of pain through the acceptance of positive suggestions made to the subconscious, and many patients are able to learn the technique of self-hypnosis.[13] In addition to improved control of pain, some patients may be able to use hypnosis to help reduce nausea, improve appetite, or assist in controlling other problems. Individuals vary in their suggestibility and readiness to try this approach. The skill of the hypnotist is also important. The nurse's most helpful role may be to support the patient's desire to make hypnotism work.

Nutrition

Appetite is affected by pain. When one is in continuous pain nothing, including meals, seems quite right. Care should be taken that foods the patient likes are prepared in a desired way. Appetite may be improved by small, attractive servings and by a sincere interest in the patient's reactions to food. Foods that patients do not like or that they believe disagree with them should not be offered. Very gratifying improvement in appetite has followed the control of intractable pain by surgical procedures that interrupt sensory pathways that transmit the painful sensation.

Suicide prevention

When caring for the patient who is experiencing severe, continuous, or intractable pain, the nurse must keep in mind the possibility of suicide. Pain is wearing and demoralizing, especially when it is difficult to control with medications and when the individual knows or suspects that no permanent relief will be forthcoming. Patients may dread the danger of growing dependence on drugs, they may fear that drugs will no longer help, and they may be depressed by thoughts of being a burden and an expense to their families. They may appear to tolerate pain quite well but at the same time may be planning their own destruction. Plans for protection should be individualized for each patient and will depend on such factors as whether the patient is confined to bed. (For further discussion on patients who commit suicide, see p. 192.)

Pain clinics

In recent years the knowledge that pain has both a physical and an emotional component, combined with increased understanding of client's needs and the treatments available, has resulted in the establishment of pain clinics. Most pain clinics or rehabilitation centers use a team approach. Physicians including internists, dolorologists (specialists in pain), surgeons and psychiatrists, nurses, physical and occupational therapists, social workers, psychologists, vocational rehabilitation counselors, and others may be available to help the client. Treatment may be on an inpatient or outpatient basis, with family members encouraged to participate in various aspects of the program.

At the Pain Rehabilitation Center in LaCrosse, Wisconsin, there are four major goals of therapy for the client: withdrawal from drugs, increased physical activity, improved emotional well-being, and a reduction in pain by 50% to 100%.[80] Each client is assessed individually, and a unique plan of care based on the needs and goals of that client is established. The plan involves most if not all of the following: progressive exercise, massage, application of heat and cold, acupuncture, external electrical stimulation, counseling, and autogenic biofeedback training.

Each pain clinic is organized slightly differently, placing greater emphasis on various aspects of pain relief and manifestation. Many of the clinics with inpatient services employ various forms of behavior modification.

The responsibility of the nurse may vary according to the team members available but often includes assisting in assessment of the patient, documenting observations, creating and maintaining a therapeutic milieu, providing emotional support to the patient and family, and teaching the patient, family, and other nursing team members about the interventions planned for the patient. Nurses who work in pain clinics need to be skilled in nurse-client interactions, be knowledgeable about the mechanisms of pain and the effectiveness of various treatment modalities, and possess patience and understanding as they assist patients to reach their goals.

In-patient chronic pain teams

In-patient protocols* for patients with chronic pain are similar to pain clinics in their organization, use of resources, and goals, but are specific to one type of chronic pain syndrome. The protocol is likely to be employed in the setting of a general medical-surgical nursing division. The purpose of a particular protocol may either be that of evaluation, treatment, or a combination of both with one of the two predominating. The purpose of the protocol will, to a large extent, determine the length of hospital stay. For example, a protocol for the sole purpose of evaluation may be of 1 week's duration. On the other hand, a protocol that employs various modalities for the treatment of chronic pain, particularly behavior modification, is likely to require 4 to 6 weeks of hospitalization.

The chronic back pain protocol used at one large medical center is primarily aimed at accomplishing a comprehensive multidisciplinary evaluation of patients who present with long-standing back pain problems. The protocol is 14 days in duration. The chronic back pain team is composed of medical-surgical nurses, a psychiatric nurse clinician, a physical therapist, an occupational therapist, an orthopedic surgeon, a dietitian, a neurologist, two psychiatrists, three psychologists, a social worker, and a clinical pharmacist. Each of these persons participates in the complete examination and evaluation of every patient. At regularly scheduled multidisciplinary conferences the team discusses their individual evaluations and then decides on a specific plan of treatment for each patient. Other medical specialties may be consulted if they are felt to be relevant to a particular patient's clinical picture.

The diagnostic procedures performed during hospitalization include roentgenograms, myelogram, computed tomography (CT) scan using metrizamide contrast material (p. 740), electromyography (EMG) (p. 745), nerve conduction velocity studies, bone scan, and the Minnesota Multiphasic Personality Inventory (MMPI). Other procedures may be performed (e.g.,

*This section was written by Cheryl Patterson, R.N., M.S.N.

angiograms, muscle biopsy, nerve root or facet injection, intravenous pyelography depending upon the specific signs and symptoms with which the patient presents, as well as the findings of previous procedures. The culmination of the hospitalization is a discharge conference with the patient and the family members where the future treatment plan and recommendations are presented and discussed.

The protocol is divided into two phases: (1) immobilization and (2) mobilization. The *immobilization phase* consists of 5 days on bed rest in pelvic traction. Patients are instructed to move as little as possible, such as eating in a side-lying position without sitting up. The *mobilization phase* is a period of maximal activity. Patients walk to and from physical therapy and occupational therapy appointments and any other tests and appointments unless contraindicated. Patients also walk to the cafeteria for meals and to the nurses' station for all medications. In addition, the patients make their own beds, utilizing principles taught by the occupational therapist. Each day patients record their level of pain on a 10-point pain scale, with 10 indicating "the worst possible pain." The influence of immobilization and mobilization on patients' pain levels is assessed and incorporated into their treatment recommendations.

Some behavior modification techniques are employed during this protocol. One example is a daily 10-minute limit on patients' discussion of their pain experience (with the exception of interviews by various back team health professionals). Patients are also assisted in disassociating the feeling of pain with inappropriate use (reward) of analgesics or other unhealthy behaviors. This is accomplished by putting pain medications on a regular schedule rather than on a prn basis. Zomax, 100 mg PO, and hydroxyzine, 25 mg PO, are given at 6 AM, 11 AM, 4 PM, and 11 PM regardless of patients' pain levels at those times. Patients may refuse the medication but are not given any additional or stronger medication except acetaminophen every 4 hours. During the mobilization period it is the patient's responsibility to come to the nurse's station between ½ hour before or after the designated hour of administration and ask for the medication.

Special treatment plans may be necessary for those patients who have developed a psychologic or physiologic dependence on analgesics or sedatives. An individualized medication regimen, usually involving the use of methadone, is established with the consultation of the clinical pharmacist, and the methadone is administered every 4 or 6 hours with the dose being reduced gradually over time until the patient is completely weaned from narcotics. In addition, such patients receive Zomax and hydroxyzine in the same dose as described above. After methadone is withdrawn, the patients continue to receive the Zomax and hydroxyzine.

During hospitalization patients are taught (1) principles of body mechanics and energy conservation, (2) strengthening exercises for the back and abdominal muscles, (3) relaxation techniques, and (4) nutritional requirements necessary to regain or maintain optimal body weight. All these measures help to reduce back strain. Transcutaneous electrical nerve stimulation (TENS) (p. 390) is applied on a trial basis to determine its effect on the patient's pain. Biofeedback is used with those persons who are felt to be good candidates. It is most successful in persons of above average intelligence who are not deriving considerable secondary gain from being in chronic pain.

Orthotic appliances (e.g., braces, corsets) may be prescribed or it may be decided that surgery is indicated. Surgery is almost always performed during a separate hospitalization at a later date. Ongoing psychologic or psychiatric treatment, if recommended, is continued on an outpatient basis.

Outcome criteria for the person with pain

1. The person states that comfort has improved.
2. The person or significant others can:
   a. Describe general measures for relief of pain:
      (1) State rationale for therapy.
      (2) Demonstrate exercises or other activities that have proved successful in pain control (e.g., satisfactory biofeedback or self-hypnosis).
      (3) Describe method and frequency of specific measures.
   b. Explain prescribed medications:
      (1) State actions, dosage, frequency, and side effects.
      (2) Describe when to seek medical assistance if pain is not relieved as expected.
   c. Demonstrate correct use of transcutaneous electrical stimulator, if prescribed:
      (1) State method and location for applying electrode.
      (2) Describe how to adjust the frequency and amplitude controls.
      (3) Demonstrate how to clean electrodes, how to change electrodes or batteries.
      (4) Explain safety measures (e.g., checking for loose wire connections, not bathing while apparatus is in use).
3. The person demonstrates increased tolerance for pain as manifested by return to full- or part-time employment, decreased analgesic consumption, and independence in activities of daily living.

REFERENCES AND SELECTED READINGS
Contemporary

1. Armstrong, M.E.: Current concepts in pain, A.O.R.N. J. 32:383-390, 1980.
2. *Armstrong, M.E.: Acupuncture, Am. J. Nurs. 72:1582-1588, 1972.
3. Barber, J.: Cancer pain: psychological management using hypnosis, CA. 30:130-136, 1980.
4. *Barrett-Griesemer, P., Meisel, S., and Rate, R.: A guide to headaches—and how to relieve them, Nurs. '81 11:50-57, April 1981.
5. Beaver, W.T.: Management of cancer pain with parenteral medication, J.A.M.A. 244:2653-2657, 1980.
6. Beers, R.F. and Bassett, E.G., editors: Mechanisms of pain and analgesic compounds, New York, 1979, Raven Press.
7. Bellville, J.W., et al.: Influence of age on pain relief from analgesics, J.A.M.A. 217:1835-1841, 1971.
8. *Benson, H., and Epstein, M.D.: The placebo effect: a neglected asset in the care of patients, J.A.M.A. 232:1225, 1975.
9. Black, P.: Management of cancer pain: an overview, Neurosurgery 5:507-518, 1979.
10. Black, R.G.: The chronic pain syndrome, Surg. Clin. North Am. 55:999-1011, 1975.
11. Boguslawski, M.: Therapeutic touch: a facilitator of pain relief, Top. Clin. Nurs. 2:27-37, 1980.
12. Bonica, J.J., editor: Pain. Research Publications—Association for Research in Nervous and Mental Disease, vol. 58, New York, 1980, Raven Press.
13. Bonica, J.J., editor: International symposium on pain. Advances in neurology, vol. 4, New York, 1974, Raven Press.
14. Bonica, J.J., and Albe-Fessard, D., editors: Advances in pain research and therapy, vol. 1. Proceedings of the First World Congress on Pain, New York, 1976, Raven Press.
15. Bonica, J.J., and Ventafridda, V. editors: Advances in pain research and therapy, vol. 2. International Symposium on Pain of Advanced Cancer, New York, 1979, Raven Press.
16. Brena, S.F., editor: Chronic pain: America's hidden epidemic, New York, 1978, Atheneum Publishers.
17. *Copp, L.A.: The spectrum of suffering, Am. J. Nurs. 74:491-495, 1974.
18. *Coyle, N.: Analgesics at the bedside, Am. J. Nurs. 79:1554-1557, 1979.
19. Crue, B.L., Jr., editor: Pain : research and treatment, New York, 1975, Academic Press, Inc.
20. Crue, B.L., Jr., editor: Chronic pain: further observations from the City of Hope National Medical Center, New York, 1979, SP Medical and Scientific Books.
21. *Cummings, C.: Stopping chronic pain before it starts, Nurs. '81 11:60-62, Jan. 1981.
22. Davitz, L.J., Sameshima, Y., and Davitz, J.: Suffering as viewed in six different cultures, Am. J. Nurs. 76:1296-1297, 1976.
23. Degenaar, J.J.: Some philosophical considerations on pain, Pain 7:281-304, 1979.
24. *Diers, D., et al.: The effect of nursing interactions on patients in pain, Nurs. Res. 21:419-428, 1972.
25. *Donovan, M.I.: Relaxation with guided imagery: a useful technique, Cancer Nurs. 3:27-32, 1980.
26. *Fagerhaugh, S.Y., and Strauss, A.: How to manage your patient's pain . . . and how not to, Nurs. '80 10:44-47, Feb. 1980.
27. Fagerhaugh, S.Y., and Strauss, A.: Politics of pain management:

*References preceded by an asterisk are particularly well suited for student reading.

staff-patient interactions, Menlo Park, Calif. 1977, Addison-Wesley Publishing Co., Inc.

28. Fordyce, W.E.: Behavioral methods for chronic pain and illness, St. Louis, 1976, The C.V. Mosby Co.
29. Gildea, J.H.: Assessing the pain experience in children, Nurs. Clin. North Am. **12**:631-637, 1977.
30. Glynn, C.J.: The diurnal variation in perception of pain, Proc. R. Soc. Med. **69**:369-372, 1976.
31. *Goodwin, J.S., Goodwin, J.M., and Vogel, A.V.: Knowledge and use of placebos by house officers and nurses, Ann. Intern. Med. **91**:106-110, 1979.
32. Gowell, E.C.: Transactional analysis strategies for dealing with pain, J. Psychiatr. Nurs. **12**:25-30, 1974.
33. *Gramse, C.A.: Dorsal column stimulation, Am. J. Nurs. **78**:1022-1025, 1978.
34. Hannington-Kiff, J.G.: Pain relief, Philadelphia, 1974, J.B. Lippincott Co.
35. Isler, C.: New approach to intractable pain . . . , R.N. **38**:17-21, 1975.
36. *Jacox, A.K.: Assessing pain, Am. J. Nurs. **79**:895-900, 1979.
37. *Jacox, A.K., editor: Pain: a sourcebook for nurses and other professionals, Boston, 1978, Little, Brown & Co.
38. Johnson, I.: Radiofrequency percutaneous facet rhizotomy, J. Neurosurg. Nurs. **6**:92-96, 1974.
39. Johnson, J.E., and Rice, V.H.: Sensory and distress components of pain: implications for the study of clinical pain, Nurs. Res. **23**:203-209, 1974.
40. Johnson, M.: Pain: how do you know it's there and what do you do? Nurs. '76 **6**:48-50, Sept. 1976.
41. Jourard, S.M.: The transparent self, New York, 1971, Van Nostrand.
42. Kerr, F.W.L.: Pain: A central inhibitory balance theory, Mayo Clin. Proc. **50**:685-690, 1975.
43. *Kim, S.: Pain: theory, research and nursing practice, Adv. Nurs. Sci. **2**:43-59, 1980.
44. Lamb, S.: Neuroaugmentation for the chronic pain patient, J. Neurosurg. Nurs. **11**:215-220, 1979.
45. Lipman, A.G.: Drug therapy in cancer pain, Cancer Nurs. **3**:39-46, 1980.
46. Lipton, S.: Current topics in anesthesia, vol. 2. The control of chronic pain, Chicago, 1979, Year Book Medical Publishers, Inc.
47. *Long, D.M.: Relief of cancer pain by surgical and nerve blocking procedures, J.A.M.A. **244**:2759-2761, 1980.
48. *Long, D.M.: Surgical therapy of chronic pain, Neurosurgery **6**:317-328, 1980.
49. *Marks, R.M., and Sachar, E.J.: Undertreatment of medical inpatients with narcotic analgesics, Ann. Intern. Med. **78**:173, 1973.
50. *Mastrovito, R.C.: Psychogenic pain, Am. J. Nurs. **74**:514, 1974.
51. Maxwell, M.M.: How to use methadone for the cancer patient's pain, Am. J. Nurs. **80**:1606-1609, 1980.
52. *McCaffery, M.: How to relieve your patient's pain. Fast and effectively . . . with oral analgesics, Nurs. '80 **10**:58-63, Nov. 1980.
53. *McCaffery, M.: Patients shouldn't have to suffer. How to relieve pain with injectable narcotics, Nurs. '80 **10**:34-39, Oct. 1980.
54. *McCaffery, M.: Relieving pain with noninvasive techniques, Nurs. '80 **10**:54-57, Dec. 1980.
55. *McCaffery, M.: Understanding your patient's pain, Nurs. '80 **10**:26-31, Sept. 1980.
56. *McCaffery, M.: Nursing management of the patient with pain, ed. 2, Philadelphia, 1979, J.B. Lippincott Co.
57. *McCaffery, M.: Nursing management of the patient with pain, Philadelphia, 1972, J.B. Lippincott Co.
58. *McCaffery, M., and Hart, L.: Undertreatment of acute pain with narcotics, Am. J. Nurs. **76**:1586-1591, 1976.
59. *McDonnell, D.E.: TENS in treating chronic pain, A.O.R.N. J. **32**:401-410, 1980.
60. *McGuire, L.: A short, simple tool for assessing your patient's pain, Nurs. '81 **11**:48-49, March 1981.
61. *McLachlan, E.: Recognizing pain, Am. J. Nurs. **74**:496-497, 1974.
62. McMahon, M.A., and Miller, Sr. P.: Pain response: the influence of psycho-social-cultural factors, Nurs. Forum, **17**:58-71, No. 1, 1978.
63. *Meissner, J.E.: McGill-Melzack pain questionnaire, Nurs. '80 **10**:50-51, Jan. 1980.
64. Melzack, R.: The McGill pain questionnaire: major properties and scoring methods, Pain **1**:277-299, 1975.
65. Melzack, R.: The puzzle of pain, New York, 1973, Basic Books, Inc.
66. Melzack, R., and Chapman, C.R.: Psychologic aspects of pain, Postgrad. Med. **53**:69-75, 1973.
67. Melzack, R., and Loesser, J.D.: Phantom body pain in paraplegics: evidence for a central "pattern generating mechanism" for pain, Pain **4**:195-210, 1978.
68. Neal, H.: The politics of pain, New York, 1978, McGraw-Hill Book Co.
69. *O'Connor, A.B., editor: Nursing: patients in pain, New York, 1979, American Journal of Nursing Co.
70. Perret, G.: Neurosurgical control of pain in the patient with cancer, Curr. Probl. Cancer **1**:1-27, 1977.
71. *Perry, S.W., and Heidrich, G.: Placebo response: myth and matter, Am. J. Nurs. **81**:720-725, 1981.
72. Rankin, M.: The progressive pain of cancer, Top. Clin. Nurs. **2**:57-73, 1980.
73. Reading, A.E.: A comparison of pain rating scales, J. Psychosom. Res. **24**:119-124, 1980.
74. Reuler, J.B., et al.: The chronic pain syndrome: misconceptions and management, Ann. Intern. Med. **93**:588-596, 1980.
75. Rigby, R.: Transcendental meditation, Nurs. Times **71**:1240-1242, 1975.
76. Rogers, A.G.: Pharmacology of analgesics, J. Neurosurg. Nurs. **10**:180-184, 1978.
77. *Sanders, S.H.: Analysis of nurses' knowledge of behavioral methods applied to chronic and acute pain patients, J. Nurs. Educ. **19**:46-50, 1980.
78. Schmitt, M.: The nature of pain, Nurs. Clin. North Am. **12**:621-629, 1977.
79. Shealy, C.N.: Holistic management of chronic pain, Top. Clin. Nurs. **2**:1-8, 1980.
80. Shealy, C.N.: The pain game, Millbrae, Calif., 1976, Celestial Arts.
81. Shimm, D.S., et al.: Medical management of chronic cancer pain, J.A.M.A. **241**:2408-2412, 1979.
82. *Siegele, D.S.: The gate control theory, Am. J. Nurs. **74**:498-502, 1974.
83. Silman, J.: The management of pain: reference guide to analgesics, Am. J. Nurs. **79**:74-78, 1979.
84. Smith, W.L., Merskey, H., and Gross, S.C., editors: Pain, meaning and management, Jamaica, N.Y., 1980, Spectrum Publications.
85. Sternbach, R.A., editor: The psychology of pain, New York, 1978, Raven Press.
86. Sternbach, R.A.: Pain patients: traits and treatment, New York, 1974, Academic Press, Inc.
87. Stiller, R.: Pain—why it hurts, where it hurts, when it hurts, Nashville, Tenn., 1975, Thomas Nelson, Inc.
88. Storlie, F.: Pointers for assessing pain, Nurs. '78 **8**:37-39, 1978.
89. Strauss, A., Fagerhaugh, S.Y., and Glaser, B.: Pain: an organizational-work-interactional perspective, Nurs. Outlook **22**:560-566, 1974.

90. Swerdlow, M., editor: Relief of intractable pain, ed. 2, New York, 1978, Excerpta Medica.

91. *Terzian, M.P.: Neurosurgical interventions for the management of chronic intractable pain, Top. Clin. Nurs. **2**:75-88, 1980.

92. Valentine, A.S., Steckel, S., and Weintraub, M.: Pain relief for cancer patients, Am. J. Nurs. **78**:2054-2056, 1978.

93. Wall, P.D.: On the relation of injury to pain: The John J. Bonica Lecture, Pain **6**:253-264, 1979.

94. Wall, P.D.: The gate control theory of pain mechanisms: A re-examination and re-statement, Brain **101**:1-18, 1978.

95. Weisenberg, M.: Pain: clinical and experimental perspectives, St. Louis, 1975, The C.V. Mosby Co.

96. *West, B.A.: Understanding endorphins: our natural pain relief system, Nurs. '81 **11**:50-53, Feb. 1981.

97. Wilson, W.P., Blazer, D.G., and Nashold, B.S.: Observations on pain and suffering, Psychosomatics **17**:73-76, 1976.

98. *Wilson, R.W., and Elmassian, B.J.: Endorphins, Am. J. Nurs. **81**:722-725, 1981.

99. *Wolf, Z.R.: Pain theories: an overview, Top. Clin. Nurs. **2**:9-18, 1980.

Classic

100. Beecher, H.K.: Relationship of significance of wound to pain experienced, J.A.M.A. **161**:1609-1613, 1956.

101. Blaylock, J.: The psychological and cultural influences on the reaction to pain: a review of the literature, Nurs. Forum **7**:262-274, 1968.

102. Melzack, R., and Wall, P.D.: Pain mechanisms: a new theory, Science **150**:971-979, 1965.

103. *Nightingale, F.: Notes on nursing: what it is, and what it is not, London, 1859, Harrison; Philadelphia, 1957, J.B. Lippincott Co.

104. Sternbach, R.A.: Pain: a psychophysiological analysis, New York, 1968, Acadmic Press, Inc.

105. Zborowski, M.: People in pain, San Francisco, 1969, Jossey-Bass, Inc.

AUDIOVISUAL RESOURCES

Is my patient in pain? Hamilton, Ontario, 1979, McMaster University School of Nursing, Faculty of Health Sciences. (Thirty-three slides in color, cassette tape, and script.)

Management of pain, Bowie, Md., 1979, Robert J. Brady Co. (Four hundred and seventy-one color slides, five cassette tapes, and instructor's guide.) The five topics in the package include neurophysiology of pain (100 slides), assessment of pain (91 slides), pain control through behavior modification (97 slides) psychodynamics of pain (87 slides); and psychologic modulation of pain (96 slides).

The nature of pain, Costa Mesa, Calif., 1971, Concept Media. (Two filmstrips, two cassette tapes, and instructor's manual.)

Pain and its alleviation, Berkeley, Calif., 1962, University of California. (Videorecording, one cassette, and guide.)

Pain and its alleviation, New York, 1976, American Journal of Nursing Co., Educational Services Division. (Videorecording and five cassettes.)

Pain management, Seattle, 1974, Universtiy of Washington Press. (Videorecording, one cassette, and booklet.)

Pain: nursing action, Costa Mesa, Calif., 1971, Concept Media. (Two filmstrips, two cassette tapes, and instructor's manual.)

Patterns of pain, New York, 1977, Filmaker's Library. (Videocassetts and one cassette.)

CHAPTER 24

SURGICAL INTERVENTION

BARBARA C. LONG
C. JOAN GOWIN
MARY E. BUSHONG

Persons experiencing surgery share some common experiences during the preoperative, intraoperative, and postoperative phases. This chapter deals with these commonalities and with the nurse's role in assisting patients to regain their optimal level of functioning after surgery. Patient needs and interventions specific to the types of surgery performed are described elsewhere.

Surgery as a stressor

Although some operations are considered minor procedures by hospital personnel, surgery is always a major experience for the patient and family. Trauma is a stressor and produces both psychologic stress reactions (anxiety) and physiologic stress reactions (neuroendocrine responses). Surgery is a potential or actual threat to a person's integrity and can interfere with need gratification during any of the phases of surgery.

Anxiety is a normal adaptive response to the stress of surgery. Anxiety occurs in the preoperative phase as the patient anticipates the surgery and in the postoperative phase as the patient anticipates or deals with problems such as pain and discomfort, changes in body image or function, increased dependency, loss of control, family concerns, or potential changes in life-style.

The functions of the nurse in assisting the patient to cope with the stress of surgery are to assess the patient's anxiety level and adequacy of coping responses, to prepare the person physically and psychologically for surgery, to provide support during the intraoperative

phase, and to assist in meeting psychologic and physical needs during the postoperative phase.

Pathophysiology

Neuroendocrine responses to surgery

The neuroendocrine responses to stress are described in considerable detail in Chapter 18. It is important to remember that these responses play a major role in the reaction of a patient to the stress of trauma occurring as an accidental injury or as planned surgery (Table 24-1).

Sympathetic nervous system

Stimulation of the sympathetic nervous system serves to protect the body from further damage. Vasoconstriction of peripheral blood vessels enables the body to compensate for blood loss and redirect blood flow to critical areas such as the heart and brain. Increased cardiac output also helps to maintain blood flow. Severe trauma or excessive blood loss, however, will overwhelm the compensatory mechanisms and blood pressure will fall. Certain types of anesthetics or high spinal anesthesia may also interfere with the compensatory vasoconstriction, producing hypotension. The patient's blood pressure is therefore monitored closely during the intraoperative and early postoperative phases.

One aspect of the sympathetic response that may produce undesirable effects is the decrease in gastroin-

TABLE 24-1. Effects of endocrine changes associated with surgery

Physiologic changes	Results	Effect on surgical patient
↑ Norepinephrine secretion	Peripheral vaso-constriction	Helps maintain blood pressure when circulating volume is decreased
	↓ Gastrointestinal activity	May lead to anorexia or constipation
↑ Aldosterone se-cretion	Sodium retention	Maintains blood circulating volume
		Causes ↑ susceptibility to fluid overload
		Decreases urinary output
↑ Glucocorticoid secretion	Gluconeogenesis	Provides energy to meet stress of surgery
	↑ Protein catabo-lism	Provides an additional energy source
		Provides amino acids for cell synthesis following tissue destruction
	Ketogenic effect	Provides fat as an energy source
	Antiinflammatory effect	Causes ↑ susceptibility to infection
	↑ Platelet pro-duction	Promotes clotting to prevent bleeding
		Contributes to development of thrombophlebitis
↑ ADH secretion	Water reabsorp-tion in the kidney tubules	Maintains blood circulating volume
		Causes ↑ susceptibility to fluid overload
		Decreases urinary output

testinal activity. Psychologic stress in the preoperative period may lead to anorexia and constipation. Following the trauma of surgery the patient may experience anorexia, gas pains, and constipation from diminished peristalsis in the gastrointestinal tract. Peristalsis may cease completely after abdominal surgery following manipulation of abdominal organs.

Hormonal response

Adrenocortical activity is increased, producing greater amounts of aldosterone and glucocorticoids. Aldosterone enhances sodium reabsorption by the kidney. This serves to retain fluid to compensate for fluid lost through blood loss, diaphoresis, and respirations. When sodium is reabsorbed by the kidneys, potassium is excreted; thus after surgery there is a loss of potassium. The potassium is excreted regardless of the body's need for it.

The increase in the amount of glucocorticoid from the adrenal cortex is thought to mobilize cellular stores of fats and amino acids for energy and protein synthesis.[62] Healing tissues require protein. Glucose is re-

leased for energy with resultant hyperglycemia and glycosuria. Patients who have diabetes must be carefully monitored during the early postoperative phase for signs of ketosis.

In addition to the increase in adrenocortical hormones, there is an increase in antidiuretic hormone (ADH) by the neurohypophysis (posterior pituitary gland) during the first 24 to 48 hours after surgery. Water is reabsorbed by the kidney, and renal output is decreased. Following surgery the increased production of aldosterone and ADH is evidenced by a decreased urinary output as compared with fluid intake. Spontaneous diuresis occurs as the amount of ADH is decreased, usually in about 24 to 48 hours.

Metabolic responses to surgery

It can be said that after surgery the patient is in a relative state of starvation; metabolism is increased, while nutrient intake is decreased.

Carbohydrate metabolism

As a result of the increased production of glucocorticoid hormones, there is an increase in the carbohydrate metabolism following the stress of surgery. With major surgery there are periods when the patient is not permitted to eat and is given dextrose by intravenous fluids. This is not adequate to meet the body's energy needs (p. 301). Anorexia may also occur as part of the stress response, thus adding to the problem of inadequate carbohydrate intake even if food is permitted by mouth.

Fat metabolism

Glucocorticoids also have a ketogenic effect; that is, they increase the rate of mobilization of fat from the cells to make fat available as an energy source. With the decreased intake of carbohydrates and fats after surgery, body fats are metabolized for energy and the patient loses weight.

Protein metabolism

Body proteins consist of combinations of the essential amino acids, of which nitrogen is an essential component. When tissues break down during catabolism following surgery, some of the nitrogen is lost. As new tissue is formed essential amino acids are needed. If none of these amino acids are taken in, as by ingestion, the body will continue to break down some existing tissue proteins to obtain the amino acids that it needs for healing. The "leftover" amino acids not used at that time are broken down to the nitrogen end products such as urea and are excreted. A *negative nitrogen balance* results; nitrogen loss exceeds nitrogen intake. If there is little or no protein intake following surgery, nitrogen balance will be further compromised; the patient will

TABLE 24-2. Physiologic changes related to aging process that can affect surgery

Physiologic changes	Result	Potential postoperative complications
Cardiovascular		
↓ Elasticity of blood vessels	↓ Circulation	Shock (hypotension), wound infection, thrombophlebitis
↓ Cardiac output		
↓ Peripheral circulation		
Renal		
↓ Blood flow in kidney	↓ Kidney function	Prolonged response to anesthetic, fluid and electrolyte imbalance (especially overhydration)
Respiratory		
↓ Lung expansion	↓ Ability to cough and deep breathe	Atelectasis, pneumonia
Musculoskeletal		
↓ Muscle strength	↓ Activity	Atelectasis, pneumonia, thrombophlebitis, constipation or fecal impaction
Limitation of motion		

continue to lose weight and healing will be delayed. Nitrogen is also needed for production of white blood cells and fibroblasts needed to resist infection and to repair tissue.

Factors affecting patient responses to surgery

No two persons respond to surgery in exactly the same way. A number of variables influence physiologic and psychologic responses throughout the entire surgical experience. These include age, nutritional status, effectiveness of neuroendocrine responses, presence of disease or limiting conditions, surgical procedure performed, complications, and psychologic factors.

Age

Surgery can be performed on persons of any age, from the newborn to the very elderly. Persons at the extremes of age are less able to tolerate stress such as tissue trauma (surgery) or infection.

Children

The very young infant has decreased resistance to stress because of immature development (see Chapter 16). Endocrine functions are sluggish, and reserves of fat, glycogen, and extracellular water are limited. Fluid and electrolyte balance is easily upset and must therefore be monitored very carefully during the postoperative period. Resistance to infection is also limited, and

measures to prevent respiratory and wound infections must be instituted.

The young child tolerates surgery well, and the postoperative course is usually rapid if no complications occur and if the child was essentially well before surgery. The tendency of the child to be active helps to prevent postoperative respiratory and circulatory complications. Young children, however, are sensitive to chilling and rough handling because of body size and immature development.

Elderly persons

The ability of the elderly patient to tolerate surgery depends on the extent of physiologic changes that have occurred with the aging process, the duration of the surgical procedure, and the presence of one or more chronic diseases.

Elderly persons vary greatly in the extent to which physiologic changes occur. The changes that affect responses to surgery are cardiovascular, renal, pulmonary, and musculoskeletal (Table 24-2). The greater the number of changes present, the greater the potential for the patient to develop a postoperative complication. The cardiovascular changes affect mechanisms that help the body compensate for the sympathetic nervous system response to stress. Since heart rate changes in the elderly occur more slowly than in younger persons, pulse rates may not be a good index in assessment of shock, and a longer period of time may be necessary to wait for pulse stabilization after activity.[113] Careful monitoring of the elderly person receiving fluids parenterally is important in order to prevent overhydration (either water intoxication or pulmonary edema).

Since elderly persons tolerate stress less effectively, the duration of the surgical experience can affect the response. Surgery of short duration is more easily tolerated. Presence of chronic diseases such as pulmonary, cardiac, or central nervous system disease limits the elderly person by prolonging recovery or increasing the risk of mortality.[35]

Certain types of surgery, such as thoracic surgery, radical head and neck surgery, closure of a wound dehiscence, colostomy because of obstruction, or surgery for a perforated ulcer, present high risk for the elderly person. The safest type of surgery is elective surgery, surgery away from the diaphragm, surgery not involving suppurative diseases, surgery in which early mobilization is allowed, and surgery requiring a minimal amount of postoperative sedation or narcotics.[44]

Nutrition

Malnourished persons (nutrition deficits or excess) are poorer surgical risks than the well nourished and are more likely to develop postoperative complications.

Nutritional deficiency

Persons most likely to have nutritional deficiencies are the aged and the chronically ill, particularly those with gastrointestinal tract conditions or malignancies. The person who is emaciated or cachectic or who has lost considerable weight below an acceptable level usually has a prolonged postoperative recovery.

The undernourished person already has diminished reserves of carbohydrates and fats. Body proteins will be utilized to provide the necessary energy requirement to maintain metabolic functioning of cells. Nitrogen imbalances (p. 402) will be greater than normal, and less protein will be available for healing. Collagen, the connective tissue that is the substance of scar tissue, is a protein. Wound healing therefore becomes considerably delayed, and wound separation and infection may occur.

If the surgery is not an emergency and can be delayed for several weeks, the undernourished patient is placed on a high-protein, high-carbohydrate diet preoperatively. In the preoperative or postoperative period total parenteral nutrition (hyperalimentation) may be given until the patient is able to tolerate a high-protein, high-carbohydrate diet by mouth. High-protein intake will not result in increased body protein unless there is sufficient carbohydrate to provide the necessary energy. Activity or exercise also is required for protein synthesis (p. 1359).

Nutrition-depleted patients usually have a deficiency of vitamins. Vitamins B_1, C, and K are necessary for wound healing and clot formation, and supplemental vitamins will be prescribed.

Nutritional excess

The obese patient presents several risk factors for surgery, including enlarged organs such as heart, kidneys, liver. During surgery fluctuations of vital signs are more common in the obese person, resulting from the excessive demands on the cardiovascular system.[125] The surgeon incising through layers of fatty tissue has to exert more traction on the tissues to expose the surgical site; this increases trauma to the tissues. Incisional hernias may occur at a later date.

During the immediate postoperative period these patients often require more assistance with turning, coughing, and deep breathing. Excess fat deposits often limit movement of the diaphragm, thereby decreasing ventilation. It is also more difficult for obese persons to move about with ease, and they may require additional assistance. Both decreased activity and decreased diaphragm expansion are contributing factors to development of postoperative pulmonary complications. Decreased activity also predisposes to thrombophlebitis.

The obese person is more likely to develop wound separation and infection. Good circulation is important for the healing process to bring to the wound the white blood cells, fibrocytes, and nutrients necessary for healing. Since fatty tissue has a decreased number of blood vessels, wound healing may be impaired.

Neuroendocrine response ineffectiveness

The neuroendocrine response assists the person to cope with the stress of surgery. If this response is ineffective, postoperative complications such as shock and delayed wound healing may occur. In addition, anesthesia may be tolerated poorly, and fluid and electrolyte imbalances are more likely to occur. Persons with diseases of the adrenal gland or the sympathetic nervous system or those who are under a great deal of stress before surgery may do less well postoperatively. Infants and the elderly also have diminished neuroendocrine response (p. 403).

Chronic diseases or disabilities

The existence of one or more chronic diseases does not necessarily increase surgical risk. The nature and extent of the disease or diseases and the degree to which they are under control are the important variables.

Pulmonary disease, such as chronic obstructive pulmonary disease (COPD), may affect the person's response to the anesthetic and ability to cope with respiratory problems after surgery (see Chapter 51). In preparation for surgery the pulmonary status of persons with COPD will be carefully evaluated and measures will be instituted to improve ventilation. In persons with a history of recent respiratory infection surgery will be delayed until they are in optimal condition. Most surgeons prefer that persons who are heavy smokers decrease their smoking for a period of time before surgery, since smoke irritates the tracheobronchial tree, resulting in increased secretions that impinge on the airway and decrease ventilation.

Persons with chronic pulmonary problems must be monitored very carefully during surgery and in the early postoperative period to prevent atelectasis, respiratory insufficiency, and respiratory acidosis.

Cardiovascular disease can affect the individual's response to surgery. A heart that pumps effectively and blood vessels that constrict effectively are necessary for the prevention of shock and of fluid imbalances. Body responses to hemorrhage and inflammation depend on an adequate supply of red and white blood cells. Surgery is usually postponed if possible when the cardiovascular status of the patient is not at the optimal level of functioning. Measures are instituted to improve the cardiovascular status and reduce the risk of surgery. Careful monitoring for potential problems is carried out by both physician and nurse during the intraoperative and postoperative phases.

Renal insufficiency can increase the risk of surgery because of difficulty in the removal of increased amounts of electrolytes, especially potassium, and waste products from catabolism. Persons with renal disease are prone to develop fluid overload from parenteral fluids if urine production is not adequate.

Endocrine diseases that are influenced by hormonal changes occurring with the stress response can affect the patient's response to surgery. The patient with diabetes mellitus should be well controlled before surgery and monitored closely during and after surgery. Glucocorticoid activity and potassium changes following surgery can influence insulin utilization (see Chapter 32). If the wound is in an area where the patient may have impaired circulation, such as legs and feet, healing may be delayed. In persons who have increased levels of adrenocortical hormones such as occurs in pituitary or adrenocortical disease or who are receiving exogenous hormones, healing may be delayed because of an antiinflammatory response. In contrast the patient with Addison's disease (hypofunction of the adrenal cortex) or patients receiving hormonal replacement will require additional replacement therapy because of the stress of surgery.

Disabilities that can influence response to surgery include those that affect or limit activity. Inability to ambulate, to exercise, or to move about freely in bed increases the risk of atelectasis, pneumonia, or thrombophlebitis postoperatively.

Surgical procedure

The site of the surgical procedure, the type and extent of surgery performed, and the reason for doing the surgery can all influence the patient's response.

Site

Surgery that is performed on body areas that are visible to others may leave scars that are perceived by the patient or significant others as disfiguring. Surgery of vital organs such as the heart, lungs, and kidneys may be threatening to the patient in terms of survival. Surgery of the mouth or throat may create temporary breathing problems that can be perceived as a threat. Surgery of the extremities may create permanent changes or be perceived as creating changes in life-style, especially in activities of daily living (eating, bathing, dressing, walking). Surgery on body areas that have special meaning to the person such as breast, genitalia, or reproductive organs will have differing effects and responses.

Type and extent of surgery

Removal of organs can be perceived as a threat (especially if there is considerable meaning attached to the organ by the patient) or can create changes in life-style. Surgery that creates artificial openings, such as a colostomy, is highly stressful to the patient and produces differing responses. The more extensive the surgery, the greater the physiologic responses that will occur. Psychologic responses are not directly related to the extent of the surgery, since they are influenced by the patient's past experiences, perceptions of what the surgery means to self-image, and possible changes in life-style.

Reasons for surgery

There are a number of reasons why surgery is done (see box below). Anxiety may be decreased if the patient perceives the surgery as a positive experience such as curing disease, relieving discomfort, or creating a more attractive physical appearance. On the other hand, anxiety is usually increased when the underlying pathologic condition is or is believed to be a malignancy or life threatening (e.g., open heart surgery).

REASONS FOR SURGERY

Diagnostic: to determine cause of symptoms (e.g., biopsy, exploratory laparotomy)

Curative: to remove diseased part (e.g., appendectomy)

Restorative: to strengthen weakened area (e.g., herniorrhaphy); to rejoin disconnected or injured area (e.g., hip pinning); to correct deformities (e.g., mitral valve replacement)

Palliative: to relieve symptoms without curing disease (e.g., sympathectomy, total hip arthroplasty)

Cosmetic: to improve appearance (e.g., plastic surgery)

Postoperative complications

Occurrence of complications in the postoperative period will delay recovery. Wounds that separate or become infected may take considerable time to heal, especially if other complicating factors such as inadequate nutrition are also present. Shock, cardiac aberrations, fluid and electrolyte imbalances, atelectasis or pneumonia, or thombophlebitis can all prolong the postoperative course. These complications are discussed in more detail later in this chapter and in later chapters of this book.

Previous experiences with surgery

The patient who has had previous experience with surgery may respond either positively or negatively to the present surgery. A previous negative experience can be transferred to the present experience and increase anxiety. On the other hand, a previous negative experience is sometimes viewed by the patient as an entirely separate event that happened under different circumstances and thus may not influence the present experience.

Anxiety and coping responses

One of the major factors that creates variations in responses to surgery is the extent of anxiety that the patient experiences and the effectiveness of coping responses utilized by the patient to deal with the anxiety (see Chapter 14). Some degree of anxiety before surgery is normal. The degree of anxiety may range from minimal to severe and may not be directly related to the severity of the surgery. Existing and perceived factors in the environment and within the patient all influence the extent of the anxiety and the patient's responses to it.

Preoperative phase

The preoperative phase actually begins when the client first visits a physician or primary nurse for examination. The client may already have some symptoms that led to the seeking of medical advice, or the need for surgery may have been identified during a routine physical examination. There may be a period of time before surgery during which tests are carried out to determine the necessity for surgery. Surgery that follows trauma or sudden onset of acute symptoms, such as acute

TABLE 24-3. Preoperative management

Physician	Nurse
Collect data	
Aid in medical diagnosis	Identify psychologic readiness for surgery
Determine need, type, and extent of surgery	Identify knowledge of events that will occur
Identify potential complications requiring medical intervention	Identify potential complications requiring nursing intervention
Obtain baseline data for future comparison	Obtain baseline data for future comparison
Psychologic preparation	
Explain need, type, and extent of surgery to patient and significant others	Verify patient's understanding and clarify as indicated
	Give explanations about tests
	Give opportunities to express feelings and concerns
	Support significant others
Physical preparation	
Prescribe and/or carry out tests	Assist patient and physician in carrying out tests
Prescribe diet, drugs	Assist patient to meet basic needs in preparation for surgery
Prescribe actions to ensure safety and comfort during surgery	Assist patient in carrying out physician's orders

appendicitis, may take place shortly after the initial medical contact. In this situation there is less time for psychologic and physiologic preparation for surgery. Preoperative intervention by both physician and nurse is directed toward making the surgical experience safe and comfortable for the patient (Table 24-3).

The preoperative phase extends until the patient is transferred to the operating room for surgery.

Psychologic preparation for surgery

Common fears related to surgery

The person facing surgery has numerous decisions to make that involve threat and are therefore anxiety provoking. The first decision may be whether to seek medical advice (fear of the unknown). Decisions may have to be made concerning having specific tests made (fear of discomfort, fear of unknown). The decision to have surgery may be the most difficult. Having major surgery involves putting one's life under the control of others and subjecting oneself to the intrusion of the body and possible pain. It may also involve permanent changes in life-style.

Some of the fears underlying preoperative anxiety are elusive, and the person may not be able to identify

FEARS RELATED TO SURGERY

General	Specific
Fear of unknown	Diagnosis of malignancy
Loss of control	Anesthesia
Loss of love from significant others	Dying
	Pain
Threat to sexuality	Disfigurement
	Permanent limitations

ASSESSMENT OF PREOPERATIVE ANXIETY

Subjective data
1. Understanding of proposed surgery
   a. Site
   b. Type of surgery to be done
   c. Information from surgeon regarding extent of hospitalization, postoperative limitations
   d. Preoperative routines
   e. Postoperative routines
   f. Tests
2. Previous surgical experiences
   a. Type, nature, time interval
3. Any specific concerns or feelings about present surgery
4. Religion
   a. Meaning for patient
5. Significant others
   a. Geographic distance
   b. Perception as source of support
6. Changes in sleep patterns

Objective data
1. Speech patterns
   a. Repetition of themes
   b. Change of topic
   c. Avoidance of topics related to feelings
2. Degree of interaction with others
3. Physical
   a. Pulse and respiratory rates
   b. Hand movements and perspiration
   c. Activity level
   d. Voiding frequency

the cause. Others are more specific (see box above). Fear of the unknown is the most common. If the diagnosis is uncertain, fear of malignancy is frequent regardless of the probability of this being so. Fears concerning anesthesia are usually related to dying, "going to sleep and never waking up." Fears concerning pain, disfigurement, or permanent disability may be realistic or may be influenced by myths, lack of information, or lurid stories recited by friends. The patient may also have other concerns related to hospitalization, such as job security, income, and care of family.

Assessment of psychologic readiness for surgery

If the person facing possible surgery has contact during the prehospitalization period with a professional nurse, data should be collected at that time to identify potential or actual sources of preoperative anxiety and to begin interventions to assist the person in coping with the threat of surgery. Communication of the data to the nurse in the hospital can provide for continuity of care. If preadmission data are not available, the hospital admission or primary care nurse assesses the person's psychologic readiness for surgery.

Subjective data. Much of the data concerning knowledge and perceptions of the coming event will be obtained directly from the patient (see box above at right). It is necessary to know the level of the patient's understanding of the surgical event before any teaching can take place. Since persons respond on the basis of their perceptions, it is important to find out exactly how the surgery is perceived. They may not be able to identify specific concerns, and further exploration may be indicated. If the nurse has identified cues on which conclusions are drawn, these conclusions should be validated with the patient.

Knowledge of the meaning of religion for the patient can help the nurse identify a possible source of support. The effect of family members or significant others on the patient's level of anxiety needs to be determined. Some significant others increase the patient's anxiety by

transmission of their own anxiety by hovering over the patient, displaying anxious behaviors, or by offering false reassurances. Others are calm, and it is observed that the patient's anxiety is reduced when they are present.

Changes in sleep patterns also provide clues about increased anxiety. Major causes of insomnia are worry, fear, and concerns about the future.

Objective data. Signs of anxiety in the presurgical patient are no different than in other persons. Signs vary from person to person and can be observed in a number of ways. Highly anxious persons may talk rapidly, ask many questions without waiting for answers, repeat the same questions, or change topics frequently during the interaction. They may deny that they have any worries or fears, but their actions belie this. Some persons will not talk about the forthcoming surgery, responding only in monosyllables, while others cry and display anger; both behaviors are overt signs of anxiety. Physical signs include an increased pulse and respiratory rate, moist palms, constant hand movements, and restlessness.

Analysis of data. The degree of anxiety experienced by the patient needs to be assessed. Most surgeons will cancel surgery for a patient who is extremely anxious. Persons with anxiety levels so high that they cannot talk about and begin to cope with their anxiety before surgery frequently experience difficulty in the postoperative period. They are more apt to be angry, resentful, confused, or depressed. They are also more vulnerable to psychotic reactions than are persons with lower levels of anxiety.[124]

Lack of any emotional response to surgery may indicate denial; this precludes dealing with and coping with the anxiety before surgery. A moderate amount of anxiety enables the individual to identify and begin to cope with feelings. These persons usually experience a smoother postoperative course.

Intervention

OUTCOME: The person identifies concerns related to surgery and is relaxed; signs of anxiety are decreased.

Having opportunities to talk with a supportive, knowledgeable person will help persons begin to identify the reasons for their anxiety and to marshal coping responses. It is helpful for the nurse to plan for a quiet unhurried time to sit down with the person and give an opportunity to ask questions and talk about concerns. Touch is often a helpful form of communication, sending the message, "I care," and some persons will talk more readily while receiving a back rub. Knowing that a nurse is interested and cares helps to reduce anxiety. If the person knows also that anxiety is a normal reaction to the threat of surgery, it may help to remove the often self-imposed expectation, "I shouldn't be nervous." Emphasis should be on accentuating the positive and helping persons identify their own strengths and coping responses.

Loss of control is one of the fears associated with surgery. Allowing persons to participate in decision making concerning care when feasible helps them partially meet the need for control. Identifying and carrying out measures to help the person meet physical needs in the preoperative phase may help to provide a feeling of security about having postoperative needs met and thus allay some anxiety. Protection of the patient's privacy and modesty may also help.

OUTCOME: The person can explain events that will occur.

Fear of the unknown can be partly relieved by knowledge about what to expect. Too much detail or information can have an opposite effect and serve to increase anxiety. The amount of information to give preoperatively depends on the background, interest, and stress level of the patient. A good rule to follow is to ask patients what they would like to know about forthcoming surgery and to base responses on the types of questions asked. Persons under considerable stress, such as those in considerable pain, cannot cope with much added stimuli, and simple explanations would be indicated. A highly anxious person has a narrow perceptual field and may not perceive events occurring around him or information being given. It is also important to remember that giving someone information does not necessarily mean that the information has been perceived or understood.

The information helpful to most persons preoperatively relates to preoperative tests and activities, events related to surgery to be performed, and expectations about what will happen postoperatively. Most persons are less anxious and participate more effectively if they know the reasons for the tests and preoperative activities. If discomfort is a probability, foreknowledge of the pain and that medication will be given to relieve it helps to decrease the stress response when the discomfort does occur, and the person is better prepared to cope with the discomfort.

Preoperative visits by the operating room nurse are helpful in many instances, especially in those situations when a great deal of anxiety may be expected, such as in open heart surgery (Fig. 24-1). The visit promotes the feeling that "someone in surgery knows me as an individual and will look after me." If it is known that the patient will be in intensive care for a period of time after surgery, a visit by a nurse from the intensive care unit may also help to allay anxiety. Most persons find it helpful to know when they will be taken to surgery, the length of time they will be in surgery, where they will awaken (recovery room), when they will return to their room, and where their family can wait to receive information.

Preparation of the child for surgery depends on the age and developmental level. Some 3-year-olds can be prepared ahead of time for surgery. Up to the age of 7 years, information should be given not more than a week in advance, and after age 7, as soon as the need for surgery is established or about 2 weeks before admission.[76]

The child should be told in language appropriate to age and development level what to expect before and after the operation and what the operative procedure will be (Fig. 24-2). The child, like the adult, should have individualized instruction. Sometimes the preparation should be gradual, and storybooks about hospitalization and anesthesia are available and are useful for parents to use. Unless the child is old enough to have developed a perspective as to time, a small amount of factual information given shortly before the operation is best. Knowing too far ahead may only confuse the child, since his concept of time is immediate and he does not grasp the significance of a waiting period. Parental par-

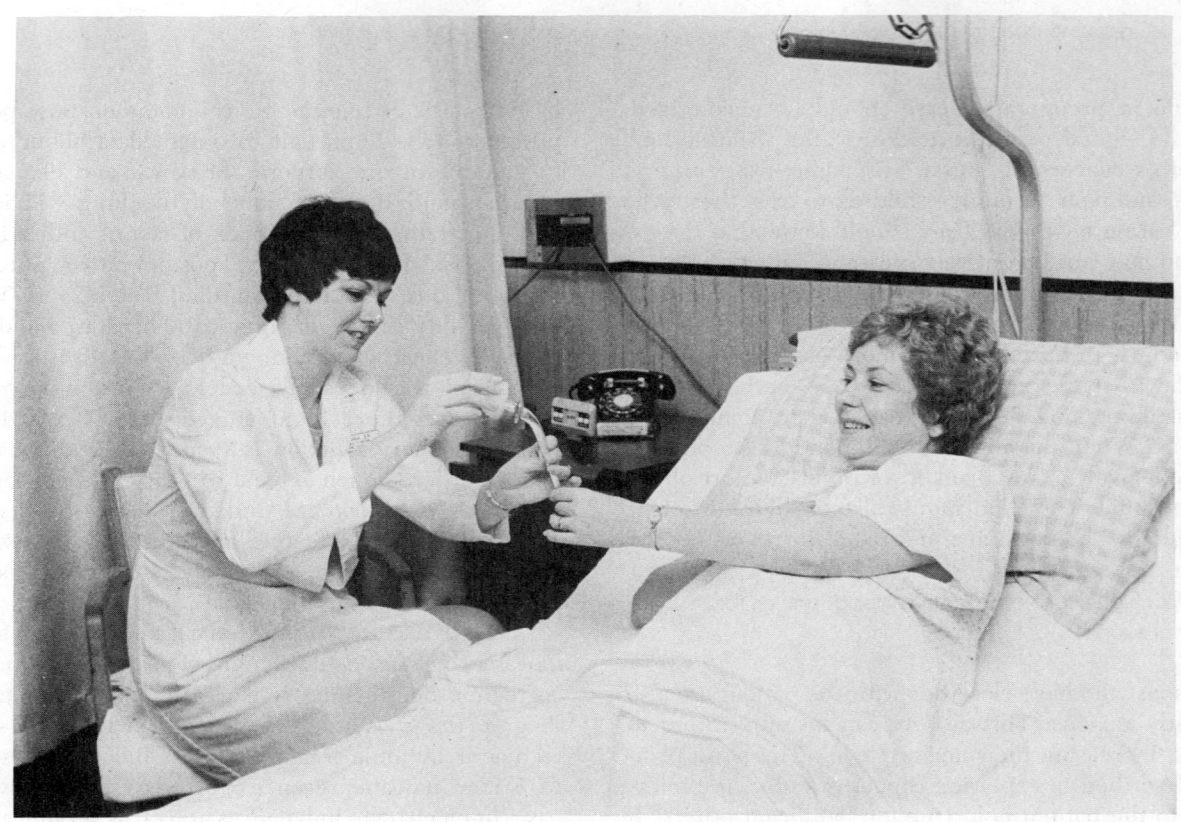

Fig. 24-1. Operating room nurse makes preoperative visit to prepare patient for joint replacement surgery.

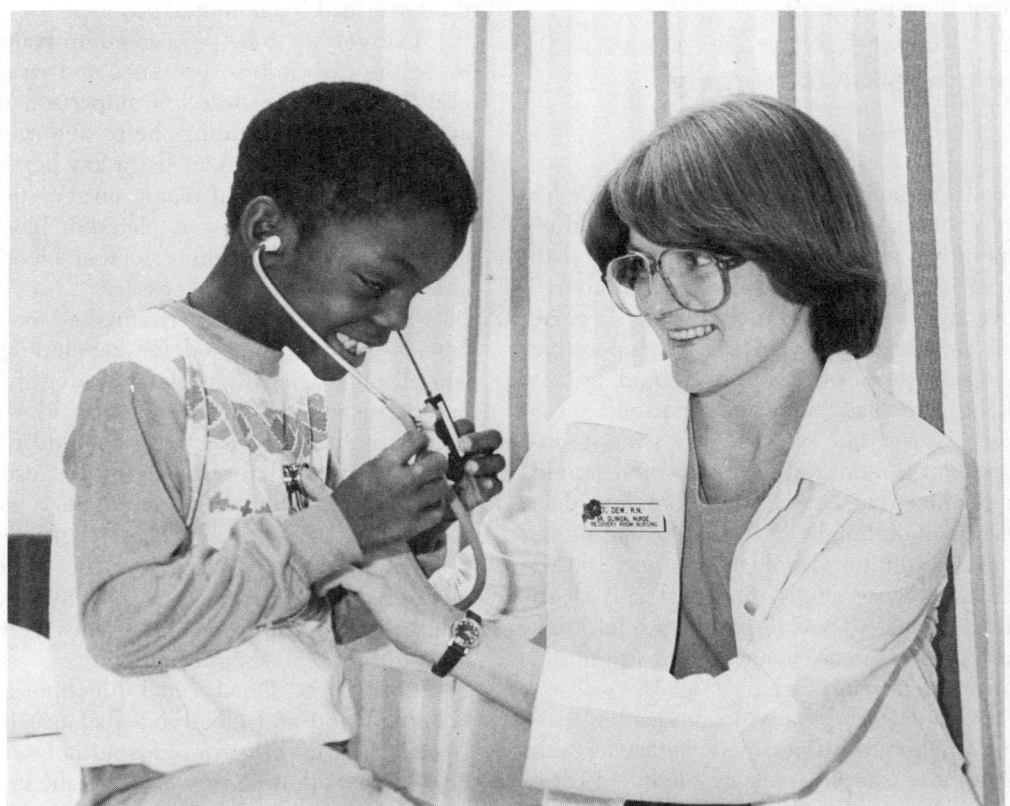

Fig. 24-2. Preoperative teaching familiarizes child with what he can expect during surgical experience.

ticipation in preoperative care should be encouraged. The child should never be told untruths. Honesty and simplicity concerning tests, preparations, surgery, stitches, and pain encourage children to trust those who will be caring for them. They should know that the experience may not be entirely pleasant, but the positive aspects of the situation should be stressed. Placing a child in a room with other children usually helps him or her adjust to hospitalization more easily, and telling the child (if it is true) that his or her mother will be there at awakening helps a great deal to comfort and allay fear. When possible, the child should be allowed to bring a favorite toy, blanket, or other comfort object to the hospital. The child should also be allowed to take this object to the operating and recovery rooms.

OUTCOME: Significant others have opportunities for emotional support.

Persons who have close ties with the patient are also frequently anxious. This anxiety can be transmitted to patients, increasing their anxiety level. The same principles described in exploring concerns and giving information to the patient hold true for significant others. If the patient needs assistance in meeting physical needs, receptive family members can be shown how they can effectively participate if they so desire. This can serve to reduce some of their own anxiety.

Physiologic preparation for surgery

Assessment

The nurse collects data in the preoperative phase for two reasons: to obtain baseline data for comparison during the intraoperative and postoperative phases and to identify potential postoperative problems that may require preventive nursing interventions before surgery. Data of special significance during the intraoperative phase such as blood pressure readings should be recorded so that they are available for comparison.

The nursing history and physical assessment obtained when a patient is admitted to the hospital should contain pertinent data that can serve as baseline data for surgery. Data include height and weight, vital signs, sensory abilities, respiratory and circulatory status, elimination habits, activity status, and rest and sleep habits. Recording of these data is important so that they are available for comparison as changes occur in the patient and for planning nursing care.

Some operative and postoperative complications can be prevented or ameliorated if persons who are at high risk of developing these complications are identified early and measures are taken to try to prevent the complications.

Respiratory status. Decreased ventilation resulting in atelectasis or pneumonia is a common postoperative problem. It is important to obtain data about ventilatory status before surgery. Presence and character of breath sounds for each lobe of the lung will identify baseline status. The presence of factors indicating potential risk for developing postoperative pulmonary complications should be identified (Table 24-4). The patient's ability to use diaphragmatic breathing and to expand the chest when taking a deep breath is assessed.

The physician usually orders a chest radiograph to be sure that there is no lung disease. If interference with pulmonary function is suspected, additional tests will be ordered such as vital capacity, pulmonary function tests, and blood gas studies (Table 24-5). If signs of upper respiratory infection are present (rhinitis, pharyngitis, sore throat, fever, cough), surgery will be postponed until the symptoms abate.

Cardiovascular status. Medical assessment of the cardiovascular status identifies signs of heart disease that need correction before surgery is carried out. An electrocardiogram (ECG) is ordered routinely on adults for signs of cardiac arrhythmia or heart damage. Blood studies (Table 24-5) may indicate presence of blood dyscrasias, liver disease, or electrolyte imbalances as well as serving as baseline data. Blood volume studies or central venous pressure measurements may be ordered when there is known or suspected heart disease or if the patient is elderly and fluid overload is a potential problem.

If surgery is to be performed on major blood vessels or on the extremities, presence and strength of peripheral pulses are recorded. Comparison of preoperative and postoperative findings helps determine adequacy of circulation. If the patient has a low hematocrit or blood hemoglobin level or if major surgery that may involve considerable blood loss is planned, blood is drawn for typing and cross-matching so that blood will be available for transfusion as necessary.

Nutrition. Since undernourished or obese persons have a greater potential for developing postoperative complications, it is important to identify these patients before surgery. Weight is compared with height and bone structure. Diet histories should be taken for high-risk patients to determine likes and usual food habits. (For further information on dietary assessment, see Chapter 52.) Presence of excessive nausea and vomiting preoperatively will dehydrate the patient and cause electrolyte imbalance. Signs of dehydration (decreased skin turgor, dry mucous membranes, soft eyeballs, high hematocrit level) should be noted.

Elimination. Good renal function is necessary to maintain fluid and electrolyte balance postoperatively. Urinalysis will be ordered routinely on all patients. Presence of albumin or a low specific gravity may indicate the possibility of kidney disease, and further evaluation will be necessary. Sugar may indicate diabetes mellitus; thus blood sugar level is also obtained. Ace-

TABLE 24-4. Risk factors in development of postoperative pulmonary complications

Risk factors	Effect
Increased respiratory secretions	
Smoking	Irritation of lining of tra-
Intubation	cheobronchial passages
Inhalant anesthetics	Decreased ciliary action to
Chronic lung disease	remove secretions
Upper respiratory infection	Secretions will block bron-
	chial passages or alveoli
Dry sticky secretions	
Chronic lung disease	Difficult to cough up secre-
Dehydration	tions
	Secretions will block bron-
	chial passages
Decreased thorax expansion	
Pain (chest, upper	Lung does not expand
abdomen)	fully, resulting in hypo-
Obesity	ventilation of alveoli
Age	
Tight binders or casts	
Skeletal abnormalities (e.g., sco-	
liosis)	
Decreased diaphragm mobility	
Abdominal distention	Decreased lung
Surgery of chest or upper	expansion, leading to
abdomen	hypoventilation
Muscle relaxants	
Neurologic deficit	
Depression of respiratory center	
Sedatives	Depressed respirations result
Narcotics	in hypoventilation
Acid-base imbalance	
Aspiration of gastric contents	
Vomiting	Causes aspiration pneumo-
	nia

TABLE 24-5. Preoperative tests to establish baselines and detect presence of diseases that can affect patient responses in intraoperative or postoperative phases

System	Test	Disease or condition
Respiratory	Chest radiograph	Tuberculosis or other
	Vital capacity	pulmonary disease
	Pulmonary function	Tuberculosis, chronic
	Blood gas studies	obstructive lung dis-
		ease, bronchitis,
		asthma
Circulatory	Electrocardiogram	Cardiac arrhythmias,
		myocardial
	Blood studies	damage
	WBC and differential	Chronic infection
	RBC, hemoglobin, he-	Anemia
	matocrit	
	Electrolytes	Electrolyte imbalances
	Platelet count, bleed-	Liver disease, blood
	ing and clotting	dyscrasias
	times, prothrombin	
	Typing and cross-match-	Compatibility for trans-
	ing	fusion
	Blood volume	Heart disease
Renal	Urine studies	
	Bacteria	Urinary tract infection
	Albumin, specific grav-	Kidney disease
	ity	
	Blood studies	
	Creatinine, BUN, NPN,	Kidney disease
	electrolytes	
Metabolic	Blood sugar, urine	Diabetes mellitus
	sugar, acetone	Starvation

tone may indicate diabetes mellitus or starvation. Signs of urinary tract infection include bacteriuria, fever, urgency, frequency, and burning on voiding. Urinary tract infection is treated with antibiotics before surgery if possible. Men with a history of prostatic enlargement may have difficulty voiding postoperatively.

A history of chronic constipation should be noted for vigorous follow-up in the postoperative period when decreased activity may further complicate the problem. Methods that the patient has found effective in the past to control constipation are noted. The presence of diarrhea is reported, since this may lead to dehydration and electrolyte imbalances (p. 334).

Activity. Any limitations that affect the patient's ability to ambulate in the postoperative period are noted.

Comfort, rest, and sleep. The patient's perception of expected discomfort related to the surgery is explored as well as expectations concerning relief of pain. Existing discomforts or limitations in achieving rest or sleep are assessed. Insomnia may be related to anxiety concerning the forthcoming surgery.

Medications. The patient may be taking certain medications that can interfere with anesthesia or contribute to postoperative complications (Table 24-6). Some medications may need to be discontinued for a time before surgery.

Prevention of postoperative difficulties

Correction of existing deficiencies. Postoperative complications can be minimized if existing medical conditions are treated or under good control before surgery. Measures to treat wound infections are carried out before secondary closure or skin grafting. Dehydration from vomiting and diarrhea is treated with parenteral fluids to reestablish fluid and electrolyte balance.

Patients with chronic diseases should be at their optimal health level before surgery. The undernourished patient is placed on a high-protein, high-carbohydrate

TABLE 24-6. Medications that can adversely affect anesthesia or surgery

Medication	Effect
Antibiotics	Potentiate muscle relaxants
Anticoagulants	Increase bleeding and hemorrhage
Antihypertensives	Affect anesthesia and compensatory ability (hypotension may occur)
Aspirin	↓ Platelet aggregation
	Potentiates effect of anticoagulants
Diuretics (thiazides)	Possible potassium imbalance
Steroids	↓ Neuroendocrine response
	Antiinflammatory effect, may delay wound healing
Tranquilizers	Potentiate effect of narcotics and barbiturates
	Hypotension

diet rich in vitamins B_1, C, and K. Supplementary vitamins may be ordered. The obese patient is placed on a weight-reducing diet. Both the undernourished and the obese patient should understand the rationale for the diets, and they may need considerable support and encouragement to maintain the diets.

Patients with chronic obstructive pulmonary disease (COPD) are frequently placed on vigorous respiratory therapy to ensure maximal ventilation and to decrease postoperative respiratory complications. This therapy usually includes postural drainage, aerosol inhalations, and antibiotics. Smoking should be discouraged for all patients preoperatively and especially for patients with COPD. Diabetes mellitus should be under good control.

Teaching. Teaching is an important function of the nurse in the preoperative phase. If persons are to move toward self-care and independence, they need to know early the what, why, and how of activities that will help regain an optimal level of functioning after surgery. Preparation for discharge begins at the time of admission. An assessment that identifies teaching needs should be followed with a teaching plan that starts in the preoperative period and is modified and continued in the postoperative period. Waiting until the patient has sufficiently recovered from the insult of surgery before teaching is started means considerable loss of time, and learning may be less effective. In addition, the patient may be discharged before teaching is completed.

One purpose of teaching is the giving of information related to the forthcoming surgical experience (p. 408). Its goal is to decrease anxiety in the preoperative and intraoperative phases. A second purpose of teaching is to decrease postoperative discomforts or complications.

Principles of teaching and learning should be used. It is important to find out first what the patient already knows. Previous experiences, level of understanding, level of anxiety, and presence of distractors such as pain are assessed. Explanations are kept simple, but the rationale for what is being taught and how it will affect the patient later on is given. Planning ahead may be necessary so that a quiet area conducive to teaching is available. Patients are asked to repeat in their own words what they have learned, or they may be asked to demonstrate how to do an activity such as coughing or arm exercises.

Teaching content should include what patients can expect to occur and what will be expected of them after they awaken from anesthesia. They should know whether they will return to their own room or be in a recovery room or an intensive care unit. Special equipment such as monitors, tubes, and suction equipment that will be used postoperatively should be explained to the patient.

OUTCOME: Persons will explain and carry out exercises to prevent postoperative complications.

All persons potentially at risk of developing postoperative pulmonary complications (Table 24-4) should be taught deep-breathing and coughing exercises before surgery. Waiting to do so until the person is awakening from anesthesia decreases the possibility that these exercises will be carried out effectively; anesthesia and pain decrease ability to retain information. The person should practice deep breathing using diaphragmatic breathing (p. 1242) and should be shown how the incision can be splinted with a pillow, towel, or hands to decrease pain when coughing.

Pain is usually a source of concern for the person. Many persons do not know that medication for pain can be given when necessary, and it is helpful for them to know that they can ask for medication if none has been offered and they are experiencing discomfort. The patient can be taught how to decrease pain by changing position frequently in bed. It is helpful to learn how to use the side rails to turn in bed. The nurse can help the patient role play, first how to sit up on the side of the bed and then how to stand without placing undue strain on the site where the incision will be located. Knowing beforehand what to expect can help the patient feel in control of the situation.

Muscle activity and ambulation help to prevent many postoperative complications. Persons should know that they may be sitting up on the side of the bed and possibly standing and walking the evening after surgery (except in conditions such as orthopedic surgery). Teaching should include bed exercises to strengthen leg muscles for walking and to prevent venous thrombus

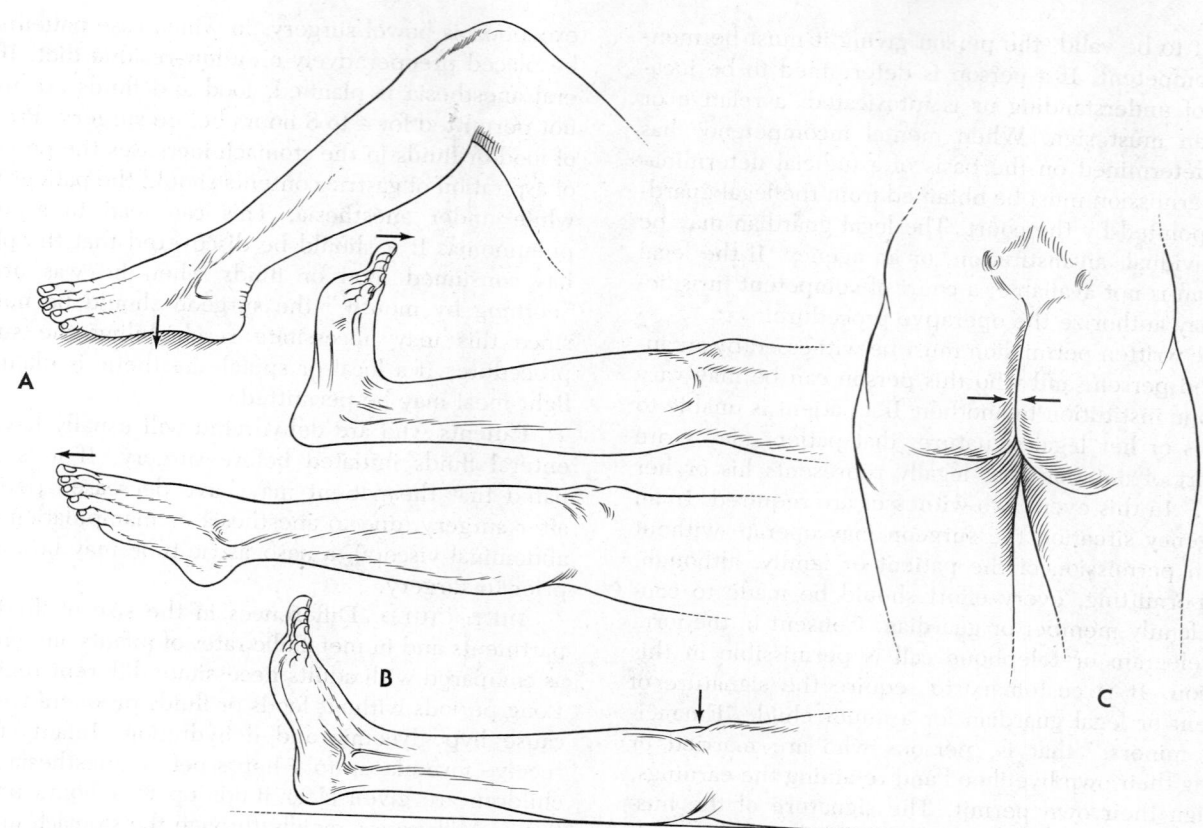

Fig. 24-3. Exercises to strengthen muscles for ambulation and to prevent thrombus formation. **A,** Knees and ankles are flexed and extended. **B,** Knee is pressed against bed and heel is lifted off bed (quadriceps setting). **C,** Buttocks are pinched together and relaxed (gluteal setting).

formation (Fig. 24-3). Flexing the ankle and leg utilizes the muscles as pumps to prevent venous stasis. Quadriceps and gluteal setting exercises strengthen the muscles used for walking.

If the person is scheduled to remain in the hospital for only a few hours postoperatively, instructions for postoperative care are best given before admission to the hospital. At this time the person has not received medication and a family member may be present. If not done before admission, instructions should be given before premedication for surgery. The instructions should be reviewed with the patient and family postoperatively.

Preoperative intervention

Operative permit: informed consent. The patient will be asked to sign a statement indicating consent to have the operative procedure performed. This consent implies that the patient has been provided with the knowledge necessary to understand the nature of the procedure to be carried out as well as the known and possible consequences of the procedure. The individual is informed of the options available and the risks asso-

ciated with each. The patient has thus given an "informed consent" for the procedure to be carried out when the permit is signed. The signed consent protects the hospital and the surgeon against claims that unauthorized surgery has been performed and that the patient was unaware of the potential risks of complication involved. The permit protects the patient from undergoing unauthorized surgery.

Sometimes patients wish to talk to a close family member before signing an operative permit. If so, the nurse should assist them in contacting the relative. If serious, extensive, or disfiguring surgery must be anticipated, the patient may wish to leave the hospital for a short time to confer with relatives or attend to business affairs before signing the operative permit. The nurse should realize that signing the operative permit is a very serious step for the patient and one that is taken much more easily when the nurse conveys warmth, friendliness, and sympathy at this time of decision.

Permission must be obtained for each operation performed and is usually obtained for major diagnostic procedures that involve entering a body cavity such as thoracentesis, cystoscopy, and bronchoscopy. For the consent to be valid, the person giving it must be mentally competent. If a person is determined to be incapable of understanding or is intoxicated, a relative or guardian must sign. When mental incompetence has been determined on the basis of a judicial determination, permission must be obtained from the legal guardian appointed by the court. The legal guardian may be an individual, an institution, or an agency. If the legal guardian is not available, a court of competent jurisdiction may authorize the operative procedure.

The written permission must be witnessed by an authorized person, and who this person can be may vary from one institution to another. If a patient is unable to sign his or her legal signature, that patient may write any sort of notation that legally represents his or her "mark." In this event two witnesses are required. In an emergency situation the surgeon may operate without written permission of the patient or family, although, time permitting, every effort should be made to contact a family member or guardian. Consent in the form of a telegram or telephone call is permissible in this situation. It is customary to require the signature of a parent or legal guardian for a minor child. "Emancipated minors," that is, persons who are married or earning their own livelihood and retaining the earnings, can sign their own permit. The signature of the husband or wife of a married minor is also acceptable. Parenthood alone does not emancipate a minor. Consent for a procedure on the child of an unwed minor parent must be obtained from the adult who is next of kin to the unwed parent.

The nurse is usually responsible for seeing that the operative permit has been signed and attached to the patient's chart before surgery. The signature should be obtained without pressure and before the patient receives sedation. Patients may refuse to undergo an operation, and it is their privilege to do so. The nurse should note whether a permit has been signed at least a day before an elective operation is scheduled. The responsibility for obtaining the necessary permission for an operation rests with the surgeon.

Preoperative medical orders. When the patient is ready for surgery, the surgeon writes orders pertaining to gastrointestinal tract preparation, skin preparation, and medications. All preoperative medical orders are automatically cancelled when the patient leaves the unit for surgery. Following the surgical procedure the physician will write new orders. All medical orders should be written clearly and completely to prevent errors.

OUTCOME: Complications related to gastrointestinal tract (aspiration, bowel obstruction, bowel trauma) are avoided.

DIET: ADULT. On the day before surgery there is usually no change in the patient's dietary intake. One

exception is bowel surgery, in which case patients may be placed preoperatively on a low-residue diet. If general anesthesia is planned, food and fluids are usually not permitted for 4 to 8 hours before surgery. Presence of food or fluids in the stomach increases the possibility of aspiration of gastric contents should the patient vomit while under anesthesia. This can lead to aspiration pneumonia. If it should be discovered that the patient has consumed food or fluids when he was ordered "nothing by mouth," the surgeon should be notified, since this may necessitate rescheduling the surgical procedure. If a local or spinal anesthetic is planned, a light meal may be permitted.

Patients who are dehydrated will usually have parenteral fluids initiated before surgery. If it is anticipated that the patient may have decreased peristalsis after surgery (due to anesthesia or manipulation of the abdominal viscera), a nasogastric tube may be inserted prior to surgery.

DIET: CHILD. Differences in the size of fluid compartments and in metabolic rates of infants and children as compared with adults necessitate different regimens. Long periods without foods or fluids preoperatively can cause hypoglycemia and dehydration. Infants usually receive formula up to 4 hours before anesthesia. Small children are given clear fluids up to 4 hours preanesthesia. Milk passes rapidly through the stomach in young children and is sometimes permitted in preference to clear fluids since it helps to prevent hypoglycemia.[123] No child under 8 years of age should be without supplemental glucose for more than 6 hours preoperatively. If glucose cannot be given orally, parental fluids are started.

BOWEL PREPARATION. Cleansing the bowel preoperatively by means of enemas is not a routine procedure. The surgeon makes the decision based on the surgical site and type of surgery to be performed. Preoperative enemas are frequently ordered before gastrointestinal tract surgery or surgery on the pelvic, perineal, or perianal areas. The purpose of the preoperative enema is to prevent injury to the colon and to provide better visualization of the surgical area. Enemas are seldom ordered for children. Enemas should be given if a patient has had radiographic studies involving barium immediately before surgery. Barium remaining in the intestinal tract may predispose to fecal impactions postoperatively. Enemas given preoperatively should be effective.

If enemas are to be given until the returns are clear, it is important to remember that fluid excess and potassium deficits can occur with repeated enemas. It is common practice to check with the physician if returns are not clear after the third enema. One method is to give up to three enemas the evening before surgery, and then if the returns are still not clear to repeat the enemas the following morning. Repeated enemas are very tiring to the patient and may irritate rectal and bowel mucosa. If antibiotic enemas are ordered for the purpose of decreasing intestinal bacteria before intestinal surgery, synthesis of vitamin K by the intestinal bacteria may be inhibited. Supplementary vitamin K may be given to prevent increased bleeding after surgery.

When a preoperative enema is not ordered it is important to determine that the patient has had a bowel movement in the last day or two. If he has not had a bowel movement, a mild laxative is often given. This prevents fecal impaction after surgery.

OUTCOME: Wound infection caused by the presence of pathogenic organisms on the skin before surgery does not occur.

The skin is the body's first line of defense against invading microorganisms. Any break in the continuity of the skin presents the potential for an infection. The purpose of preoperative skin preparation is to free the operative site of as many microorganisms as possible. The normal flora of even very clean skin contains several types of microorganisms, including staphylococcus and streptococcus.

The skin can never be completely rid of microorganisms, but the numbers can be considerably reduced by thorough cleansing, especially with hexachlorophene preparations. In many instances showering well with a hexachlorophene soap will suffice. In certain types of surgery such as orthopedic surgery where infections can lead to permanent dysfunction, a special cleansing routine with hexachlorophene preparations is often indicated. Hexachlorophene is freely soluble in organic solvents such as alcohol or soap but is insoluble in water. To retain the antiseptic properties of the hexachlorophene solution on the skin, therefore, no soap, alcohol, or alcohol-based solutions should be used in conjunction with the hexachlorophene solutions.

The presence of hair close to the surgical incision can contribute to wound infection because of the microorganisms that cling to the hair. If the patient is not sensitive to depilatories, a depilatory can be used to remove hair from the operative area.[132] Irritation of the skin in the operative area must be avoided since this leads to a break in the body's first line of defense against microorganisms.

There is considerable difference of opinion concerning shaving of hair before surgery. When hair is shaved there is an increased possibility of the skin being abraded or cut by the razor. This destroys the continuity of the skin and provides a site for growth of microorganisms. When the incision is made at the time of surgery, the microorganisms are introduced into the wound. Some surgeons advocate that hair be shaved only when there is excess hair that can interfere with the surgical procedure. Ideally, if hair is shaved, it should be done as close to the time of making the incision as possible such

as in a private section of the holding area of the operating room. Shaving of hair should be carried out by a skilled person with extreme care with a sharp blade to prevent scratching or nicking the skin. Most hospitals use disposable skin preparation sets that are discarded after use. Shaving of the infant or young child is usually not done.

Shaving of hair on certain areas of the body may have a special meaning for some persons. These areas include face, head, and pubic area. If the entire head is to be shaved, this is frequently carried out after the patient has been anesthetized. The eyebrows are not shaved. Pubic hair is shaved only when necessary; the regrowth of this hair is uncomfortable to many patients.

Before carrying out any preoperative shaving, an explanation is given to the patient. The privacy of the patient is protected as much as possible. Every effort should be made to minimize discomfort and embarrassment of the patient by carrying out the skin preparation in a considerate, competent, and professional manner.

Most hospitals have specified procedures delineating the size of the area to be shaved. The surgeon usually specifies which of the areas is to be shaved. An area larger than the anticipated incision is shaved to permit flexibility in location and size of incision.

OUTCOME: The person sleeps the night before surgery.

Anxiety often causes sleeplessness and restlessness. If the patient is extremely restless, a tranquilizer may be given for 1 to 2 days before surgery. Ambulation is encouraged before surgery in order to give the patient a feeling of well-being, to stimulate circulation and ventilation, and to maintain muscle tone. Fatigue is to be avoided, and patients with chronic illnesses may need planned periods of rest.

A sedative is usually ordered on the night before surgery to ensure a good night's rest. If additional sedation or medication for pain is given during the night, it must be given at least 4 hours before the preoperative medication.

Measures to decrease anxiety, as described earlier, are important nursing interventions. An elderly patient who has received a barbiturate or other sedative should be assessed frequently during the night for signs of confusion, and measures should be instituted to protect the patient from injury.

Care of patient on operative day

OUTCOME: The person feels comfortable.

The person should be permitted to sleep on the morning of surgery for as long as possible and to rest undisturbed until shortly before administration of the preanesthetic medication. Many persons therefore prefer to take their bath or shower the evening before surgery rather than in the morning. The person who has bathed the night before is given an opportunity to wash hands and face and to perform mouth care. The person should be reminded not to swallow water if fluids by mouth are not permitted. A hospital gown is worn to surgery.

Comfort also implies readiness for surgery and that the patient is able to marshal effective coping mechanisms. The patient should have an opportunity to have last-minute questions answered. Explanations for last-minute routines are given if not done previously. If the surgery is to be delayed even for a short time, both the person and family should be informed.

It is advisable that the person not be unduly stimulated by visitors before surgery. The person's choice of who he or she wants to see should be taken into consideration whether it be family members or a close friend. The nurse should arrange a short time of privacy for the person and the visitors. A parent is usually encouraged to remain with a child. The person may also desire a visit from a chaplain on the morning of surgery.

OUTCOME: The person is protected preoperatively from potential operative hazards.

A number of interventions are carried out before the person's transfer to the operating room that help to promote patient safety during the intraoperative phase.

1. *Final assessment is made.* Vital signs are taken for identification of significant changes. It is normal for the pulse rate and systolic blood pressure to be increased from baseline levels as a result of the immediacy of the stressful situation; however, marked changes should be reported to the surgeon. Other data to be reported are temperature elevation (possible infection), signs of upper respiratory tract infection, or expressions of new or a different type of pain.
2. *Identification band is checked.* The band should be legible and secured firmly to the person. The identification band is checked in the operative suite to ensure that surgery is performed on the right patient.
3. *Hairpins are removed; hair is protected.* Hairpins may become dislodged and injure the scalp. Hair may become tangled or interfere with equipment used for anesthetic. If the hair is long or bulky, braiding is useful. Wigs are removed since they may become lost. A disposable cap is worn by the patient during surgery to protect the hair should the patient vomit.
4. *Nail polish is removed.* The nail beds are used to observe for signs of hypoxia.
5. *Dentures are removed.* Muscles of the jaw relax under anesthesia, and dentures may fall away from the gums and drop back into the pharynx causing respiratory obstruction.
6. *Hearing aid is left in place.* It is important that the operating room staff be able to communicate with the patient in the crucial minutes before surgery. The operating room nurse should be informed that the hearing aid is in place. If the patient does not speak English, an attempt should be made to locate an interpreter who can accompany the patient to the operating room and remain until anesthesia is induced. Many larger hospitals have foreign language registries of employees who can be called on for such assistance.
7. *Antiembolic stockings or bandages are applied to legs of high-risk persons.* The surgeon may order antiembolic stockings or bandages for patients who are elderly, who have marked varicosities, or who are to have surgical procedures that involve the pelvic area, surgery that will be time consuming, or surgery that will prevent ambulation for a time postoperatively. The stockings or bandages compress superficial veins and increase blood flow through deep veins by pressure, preventing venous stasis. This in turn helps to prevent thromboembolism and shock.
8. *Person's bladder is emptied.* The person is asked to void immediately before leaving for the operating room. An empty bladder permits better visualization of abdominal organs and decreases the chances of inadvertent injury to the bladder. A person who has voided shortly before being asked to do so may not be able to void again because of the fluid restrictions. If the bladder must be kept in a collapsed state throughout the surgery or if the patient has a condition that will interfere with urination postoperatively, an indwelling catheter is inserted and attached by tubing to a closed drainage system. This is frequently carried out in the operating room to ensure asepsis.
9. *Safety measures are instituted after preanesthetic medication.* After the preanesthetic medications are administered, the patient should stay in bed since drowsiness, light-headedness, or unsteadiness on the feet may occur. The patient should be reminded not to smoke and be told to call the nurse for any needs.

OUTCOME: Loss or damage of valuable objects is prevented.

Objects or prostheses taken to the operating room with the patient may become lost or damaged. Prostheses such as dentures, false limbs or false eyes, or wigs should be removed, labeled, and placed in safekeeping. Patients who desire to take religious medals to the operating room can be advised that in many instances paper emblems may be obtained from their priest. All jewelry and money should be sent home with the family if possible or removed from the bedside and locked up. The patient is permitted to wear a wedding ring, but it should be taped or tied securely to the hand.

Preanesthetic medications. The term *premedication* is used to signify medications that are given immediately before the patient's transfer to surgery for the purpose of allaying anxiety and permitting a smoother induction of anesthesia. Some medications also serve to minimize some of the effects of anesthetic agents. The preanesthetic medications most commonly used are barbiturates, narcotics, and tranquilizers (Table 24-7).

The combination and dosages of the premedication vary based on factors identified by the anesthesiologist.

Age is an important factor. The infant is usually given only atropine. Adults frequently receive a combination of drugs, the dosage depending on body size. Dosages are frequently decreased for the elderly.[32] The more commonly used preanesthetic medications for adults are the sedatives and narcotics combined with a tranquilizer such as promethazine hydrochloride (Phenergan).

Narcotics are not given preoperatively to reduce postoperative pain since the desired effect will have worn off before the patient awakens from anesthesia. Narcotics have a number of disadvantages that give rise to some disagreement as to their use as preanesthetic medications. The neuroleptanalgesic agents are newer preparations and are being used with more frequency. Vagolytic drugs are used less frequently now because secretions present less of a problem than formerly because of the more effective techniques of administering anesthetics and the more rapid inductions.

TABLE 24-7. Commonly used preanesthetic medications

Generic name	Trade name	Dose	Desired effects	Undesired effects
Sedative-hypnotics				
Pentobarbital sodium	Nembutal Sodium	50-200 mg	Reduces anxiety; promotes relaxation and sleep	May cause excitement or confusion in elderly persons or those with severe pain
Secobarbital sodium	Seconal Sodium	50-200 mg	Same as for pentobarbital sodium	Same as for pentobarbital sodium
Flurazepam hydrochloride	Dalmane	50 mg	Promotes relaxation and sleep	
Chloral hydrate	—	0.5-1.0 g	Same as for flurazepam hydrochloride	
Narcotics				
Morphine sulfate	—	5-15 mg	Reduces anxiety; promotes relaxation; decreases preoperative pain; decreases amount of anesthetic needed	Depresses respiration, circulation, and gastric motility; may cause nausea and vomiting
Meperidine hydrochloride	Demerol	50-100 mg	Same as for morphine sulfate	Same as for morphine sulfate
Tranquilizers				
Promethazine hydrochloride	Phenergan	12.5-25 mg (children) 25-50 mg (adults)	Reduces anxiety; antiemetic	Postoperative hypotension
Chlorpromazine	Thorazine	12.5-25 mg	Same as for promethazine hydrochloride	Same as for promethazine hydrochloride
Neuroleptanalgesic agent				
Fentanyl and droperidol	Innovar	0.5-2.0 ml	General quiescence; state of indifference; decreased motor activity; analgesia; antiemetic	Respiratory depression; muscle rigidity; hypotension
Vagolytic agents				
Atropine sulfate	—	0.4-0.6 mg	Decreased secretions; prevention of laryngospasms	Excessive dryness of mouth; tachycardia
Scopolamine hydrobromide	Hyoscine	0.3-0.6 mg	Decreased secretions; amnesia; state of indifference; sedation	Excessive dryness of mouth

Preanesthetic medications are usually administered intramuscularly 60 to 90 minutes before the induction of anesthesia so that the maximal effect takes place. Any delay in giving the medication should be reported to the anesthesiologist. All preoperative routines should be completed before the preanesthetic medication is given. Noise and confusion are avoided in order to achieve maximal effect. It must be reemphasized that psychologic preparation of the patient for surgery is the most effective approach to help allay anxiety. Studies have shown that the administration of preanesthetic medication without any attempt at psychologic preparation may render the patient drowsy but does not reduce anxiety.

Patient's family. The patient's family or close friends who plan to be present the day of surgery should be made aware of the schedule and plans for the day. The nurse shares with the patient and family the time the patient is scheduled for surgery, the time the patient will leave for surgery, where the family should wait while the patient is in the operating and postanesthesia recovery rooms, how they will receive information about the patient after surgery is completed, the length of time the patient is expected to be in the recovery room, policies related to recovery room visitation, and plans for the patient if transfer to an intensive care unit is anticipated postoperatively. If the family does not plan to stay in the hospital during the operative period, they should be made aware of the importance of leaving a phone number where they can be reached.

The patient and family should be prepared for the use of any special equipment or devices that may be used in the care of the patient postoperatively (e.g., oxygen, drainage tubes from catheters, intravenous fluids, monitors). If they are prepared for these nursing care activities, the anxiety levels of both the patient and family in the immediate postoperative period will be lessened.

Recording. Before the patient is transported to the operating room all pertinent data should be recorded accurately and completely. It is helpful to have a form that contains space for baseline data and specific data that will be useful during the intraoperative phase (see box above). Having a form with the important data highly visible and accessible facilitates continuity of care and easy retrieval of data for later use. When such a form is not available, it is important that all the data listed be put in a summary note in the nurse's notes. A checklist identifying completion of last minute routines helps to avoid neglecting an important action.

The patient's chart must contain all the necessary information for use by the anesthesiologist and surgeon. The signed operative permit must be attached to the chart. Results of all laboratory tests, x-ray studies, and electrocardiograms should be available and any abnormal findings on late returns reported to the surgeon. It is essential that the nurse record the latest vital signs, the time premedication was given, the time that the

---

DATA TO BE SENT WITH PATIENT TO SURGERY

The following data are useful for operating and recovery room nurses as baseline data for comparison during surgery and identification of potential problems:

Name	Hearing
Age	Vision
Height and weight	Respiratory status
Consciousness level	Drainage systems
Anxiety level	Allergies
Language and speech	Special problems

---

patient voided, removal of prostheses, and the emotional response of the patient before surgery.

Transportation to operating room. The surgical patient is usually transported to the operating room on a mobile stretcher unit or in some instances in bed. To protect the patient from falling each stretcher has body restraint straps and side rails. Stretchers used for transporting children have head and foot rails in addition to side rails. For the tiny infant the Isolette incubator may be used. Foot extensions must be available for use with the patient who is over 6 ft tall and extends beyond the end of the stretcher.

Personnel transporting the surgical patient identify themselves to the clinical unit nursing staff and request assistance. The unit nurse assigned to prepare the patient for surgery checks the patient record, accompanies the transportation attendant to the patient's bedside, and signs the patient identification form. Before the patient is transported from the room the patient identification form is attached to the stretcher or bed. The patient is made comfortable with a pillow under the head and a blanket as a cover. Woolen or synthetic blankets should never be sent to the operating room because they are a source of static electricity. All patients should be protected from drafts, and if the patient holding area in the operating room is kept cool, additional blankets may be needed.

Outcome criteria for person to be transferred to operating room

The person:
1. Demonstrates no more than moderate anxiety.
2. Can explain (if conscious) the surgery to be performed and has signed the operative consent form (consent form on chart).
3. Can explain sequence of events and physical activities expected of him or her in the early post-

operative period (turning, deep breathing and coughing, etc.).

4. Has had a baseline assessment and current vital signs taken and recorded on chart.
5. Has had any significant physical or psychologic changes reported to the surgeon.
6. Is wearing a legible identification band, which has been checked.
7. Is not wearing nail polish, hairpins or wigs, dentures, or jewelry. (Articles have been stored for safekeeping.)
8. Has voided.
9. Has received preanesthetic medication as ordered.

Outcome criteria for family or significant others of person going to surgery

The family or significant others:
1. Know when surgery is scheduled and when they should arrive to see the person before surgery.
2. Know expected length of surgery and stay in the recovery room.
3. Know where they may wait while person is in the operating room, or recognize the need to leave a telephone number where they may be reached.
4. Are informed if surgery is delayed or prolonged.
5. Are prepared for any special condition of the person or equipment that will be used postoperatively.

Intraoperative phase

Anesthesia

Usage

Anesthetics must be given by an experienced person who has been trained in the administration of anesthetic agents. Although surgical nurses do not administer anesthetics agents, they may be called on to assist the physician on the clinical unit or in a specialized area of the hospital such as the emergency room. Therefore nurses should understand anesthetic agents and their purposes and effects. The nurse should also be able to answer questions the patient may have regarding the anesthetic to be administered during surgery. It is essential for the nurse to have an understanding of drug interactions and the preanesthetic preparation of the patient and the effects of anesthetic agents given during the operative phase in order to provide effective nursing care in the postoperative period.

Anesthesia implies amnesia (loss of memory), analgesia (insensibility to pain), hypnosis (artificially produced sleep), and relaxation (rendering a part of the body less firm or rigid). Anesthetic agents may be given to produce unconsciousness (general anesthesia) or to produce loss of sensation in specific body areas (regional anesthesia). "Local" anesthesia is a form of regional anesthesia (Table 24-8).

Choice

The choice of anesthetic is based on many factors: the physical condition and age of the patient; the presence of coexisting diseases; the type, site, and duration of the operation; and the personal preferences of the anesthetist. The anesthesiologist evaluates each patient carefully and selects the anesthetic agents best suited for that individual and the individual's condition. Within limits of feasibility, an important factor to consider when selecting the anesthetic to be administered is the preference of the patient; that is, many patients may have a preference for spinal, local, or general anesthesia. An apprehensive patient may not respond well to a regional anesthetic. Regional anesthetics are not practical for children since they have difficulty in holding still. It should be noted that anesthesiology is a complex and delicate discipline, and a strong knowledge of drug interaction and basic pharmacology is paramount.

TABLE 24-8. Types of anesthesia

Type	Action	Methods of administration	Effect
General	Blocks awareness centers in brain	Inhalation; intravenous; rectal	Unconsciousness, body relaxation, loss of sensation
Regional	Blocks transmission of all nerve impulses along nerve	Nerve infiltration; extradural; spinal	Analgesia over a specific body area (wider than local application), consciousness retained
	Blocks transmission of nerve impulses at site of origin (local)	Topical; local infiltration	Analgesia over a limited tissue area, consciousness retained

Anxiety about anesthesia

Patients have many anxieties related to anesthesia. They may fear going to sleep and not waking up, or they may simply have a fear of the unknown. They frequently express a dislike of ether because of a previous experience and the pungent odor of the agent. They may be apprehensive regarding the effectiveness of the anesthetic and fearful of experiencing pain during the surgical procedure. Patients frequently have concern about nausea and vomiting that may occur postoperatively as a result of anesthesia. Other fears associated with anesthesia may relate to talking and revealing personal information, anticipation of a mask being placed over the face, or receiving an anesthetic that will not induce unconsciousness, that is, spinal anesthesia.

Most anxieties can be dispelled if the patient and family are well informed about the anesthetic selected for use and the care taken by the physician and nurse in assessing the patient's physical condition. The patient should be encouraged to discuss any questions or concerns about the anesthetic with either the anesthesiologist or the surgeon.

The nurse should make the patient and family aware that the patient is under close surveillance while under anesthesia and in the immediate postoperative period. The nurse can reassure patients that they will not be left alone until they have fully recovered from the effects of anesthesia. Very few patients talk while under anesthesia, and what is said is usually unintelligible so that talking need not be of great concern to the patient. Persistent anxiety on the part of the patient regarding the anesthetic should be discussed with the surgeon and the anesthesiologist.

General anesthesia

General anesthesia is produced by inhalation of gases or vapors of highly volatile liquids or by injection into the bloodstream of anesthetic drugs in solution. Certain drugs that produce general anesthesia, such as thiopental sodium (Pentothal sodium), are used to put the patient to sleep and are almost always supplemented with other agents to produce surgical anesthesia.

Frequently, a combination of inhalation anesthetic agents such as nitrous oxide and oxygen may be used with muscle relaxants and narcotics. The choice of agents will depend on the anesthesiologist's judgment and the individual patient's needs (Table 24-9).

General anesthesia affects all the physiologic systems of the body to some degree. It affects chiefly the central nervous, respiratory, and circulatory systems. The anesthesiologist judges the depth of anesthesia by the changes produced in these systems. These changes are observed by monitoring heart rate (with stethoscope and ECG), blood pressure, and respiratory rate.

Stages of general anesthesia. Stages of anesthesia are best seen with diethyl ether. *Stage I* extends from the beginning of the administration of an anesthetic to the beginning of the loss of consciousness. *Stage II*, often called the stage of excitement or delirium, extends from the loss of consciousness to the loss of eyelid reflexes. If the patient is very apprehensive or was not given premedication correctly or on time, this stage, usually of short duration, may last longer. The patient may become excited and struggle, shout, talk, laugh, or cry. *Stage III*, the stage of surgical anesthesia, extends from the loss of the lid reflex to cessation of respiratory effort. The patient is unconscious, the muscles are relaxed, and most of the reflexes have been abolished. *Stage IV* is the stage of overdose or the stage of danger. It is complicated by respiratory and circulatory failure. Death will follow unless the anesthetic is immediately discontinued, possibly counteracting drugs are administered, and artificial respiration is performed. Some patients recovering from the effects of general inhalation anesthesia pass through stage II before becoming fully conscious and are noisy and restless.

Inhalation anesthesia. Inhalation anesthesia is produced by having the patient inhale the vapors of certain liquids or gases. Oxygen is always given with these anesthetic agents. The gas mixture may be administered by mask or it may be delivered into the lungs through an endotracheal tube inserted into the trachea. The use of endotracheal intubation ensures an airway can be maintained when the chest wall is open. The endotracheal tube may have a balloon that is inflated after insertion. The balloon fills the tracheal space, lessening the chance of aspiration of gastric contents. Regardless of the skill of the anesthesiologist, an endotracheal tube cannot help causing some irritation to the trachea and subsequent edema. Because the child's trachea is smaller, edema may more easily obstruct the lumen. Therefore signs of sudden respiratory difficulty are more likely to occur postoperatively in the child than in the adult. The child's respiratory pattern must be observed carefully when an endotracheal tube has been used. Signs of respiratory embarrassment such as cyanosis or difficulty in inspiring must be reported to the surgeon at once.

ETHER. Ether is a volatile, flammable liquid. It has a very pungent odor that is disagreeable to many patients. It is irritating to the mucous membranes of the pulmonary tract, and the first and second stages of anesthesia are prolonged. For this reason a rapid-acting, nonirritating drug such as thiopental sodium may be used to produce sleep before ether is administered. Ether is a relatively inexpensive drug. Although it provides excellent muscle relaxation and has a greater margin of safety than some of the other anesthetic agents, it is flammable and is seldom used in the United States today.

Recovery from anesthesia with ether may be prolonged, especially if a large amount of the drug was used.

TABLE 24-9. Comparison of selected anesthetic agents

Name	Method of administration	Advantages	Disadvantages	Special postoperative care
Nitrous oxide	Inhalation	Rapid induction and recovery; nonirritating; nonflammable but supports combustion	Possible hypoxia with excessive amounts	Monitor for signs of hypoxia
Halothane (Fluothane)	Inhalation	Rapid induction; low incidence of postoperative nausea or vomiting; nonirritating; nonflammable	Shivering with emergence; circulatory-respiratory depressant	Monitor vital signs closely
Methoxyflurane (Penthrane)	Inhalation	Decreased need for analgesics in immediate postoperative period; nonflammable	Prolonged induction; renal toxicity (dose dependent); postoperative nausea or vomiting	Position to prevent aspiration if vomiting occurs
Enflurane (Ethrane)	Inhalation	Rapid induction and recovery; some muscle relaxation on its own; nonflammable	Circulatory-respiratory depression (dose dependent); expensive; shivering with emergence	Monitor vital signs frequently
Cyclopropane	Inhalation	Rapid induction; adequate muscle relaxation	Highly flammable; possible cardiac irritability and arrhythmias; emergence excitement; postoperative nausea, vomiting, headache	Monitor pulse frequently for irregularities; position to prevent aspiration with vomiting
Ether	Inhalation	Inexpensive; good muscle relaxation; decreased need for postoperative analgesia	Irritating to mucous membranes; prolongation of anesthesia; postoperative nausea or vomiting; flammable	Supervise constantly in early postoperative period; position to prevent aspiration; suction if large amounts of mucus present; inspect face and eyes for blistering or irritation
Thiopental sodium (Pentothal Sodium)	IV	Rapid smooth induction and recovery	Laryngospasm with stimulation of larynx; respiratory depression with high doses; blood pressure may drop suddenly	Monitor for signs of stridor, neck tissue retraction, cyanosis; monitor vital signs for ↓ respiratory depth or ↓ blood pressure
Droperidol and fentanyl	IV	Rapid smooth induction and recovery; nontoxic to liver, kidneys, or heart; less analgesia required postoperatively	Hypoventilation	Monitor for ↓ respiratory rate or depth; decrease postoperative narcotics to one third to one fourth usual dose
Ketamine	IV	Profound analgesia with no loss of consciousness; amnesia for surgical event	Unpleasant dreams in early postoperative period and sometimes later; does not block visceral pain	Maintain quiet environment postoperatively
d-Tubocurarine chloride Succinylcholine chloride Pancuronium bromide Gallamine triethiodide	IV	Profound muscle relaxation	Respiratory depression or paralysis	Monitor for signs of respiratory depression
Procaine Cocaine Tetracaine Dibucaine Lidocaine Carbocaine Bupivacaine Chloroprocaine	Tissue injection (local); spray	No loss of consciousness	CNS stimulation or seizures; cardiac depression; absorbed into bloodstream	Monitor for excitability, twitching, pulse, or blood pressure changes, pallor, respiratory difficulty

The patient will require constant supervision until completely awake. Because of ether's irritating qualities, large amounts of mucus may be present, in which case the patient must be suctioned frequently. Since vomiting often occurs after the administration of ether, the patient should be in a side-lying position after surgery to prevent aspiration of any vomitus. If the foot of the bed is elevated, gravity will aid the flow of mucus and vomitus from the throat and mouth. Before anesthesia is started, an isotonic eye ointment in a petroleum base is frequently instilled into the eyes to prevent irritation. If an irritation does occur it should be immediately checked and, if serious, an ophthalmologist consulted. Redness or blistering of the skin, which sometimes occurs around the site of the mask, is caused by the combination of ether, moisture, and pressure. This condition can be unsightly and uncomfortable for the patient. Petroleum jelly or other ointments may be applied as ordered to relieve discomfort.

NITROUS OXIDE. Nitrous oxide is a nonirritating, odorless, colorless, nonflammable gas. The patient becomes anesthetized quickly and recovers rapidly. This gas may be used for dental surgery and as a supplemental agent when ether is to be administered.

Nitrous oxide is also used extensively with halothane and enflurane to supplement their actions. In low concentrations nitrous oxide may provide adequate anesthesia even for intraabdominal procedures in patients who are in profound shock, debilitated, or who are critically ill and cannot tolerate other anesthetic agents. If an excessive amount of this gas is administered there is the possibility of hypoxia.

CYCLOPROPANE. Cyclopropane is a highly flammable and pleasant-smelling gas that quickly produces unconsciousness and produces adequate relaxation for most abdominal surgery. Because it is associated with cardiac irritability and causes arrhythmias, it should be used with caution in patients with cardiac diseases. Postoperatively, the patient's pulse rate and cardiac rhythm should be checked frequently for any irregularities that might occur as a result of receiving cyclopropane gas. Emergence excitement is common. Nausea, vomiting, and headache may also occur in the postoperative period. During the administration of this gas, extreme care must be taken to prevent the production of any electric charge that might cause it to be ignited. Due to its flammability, operating room procedures should be consistent with those for other hazardous environments.

HALOTHANE. Halothane (Fluothane) is a highly potent, nonflammable, colorless liquid with a sweet smell somewhat resembling chloroform. It is easily inhaled and usually administered through special vaporizers with nitrous oxide and oxygen. Halothane is nonirritating; thus irritation to the larynx is reduced and laryngospasm is infrequent. Induction of anesthesia is usually much faster than with ether, and the rate of emergence is more rapid.[57] An important clinical feature of halothane is the low incidence of postoperative nausea and vomiting. Emergence from anesthesia may be accompanied by shivering, probably of neurologic origin rather than the lowered body temperature commonly found.[38] Disadvantages are that it tends to depress respiration and circulation. There is some evidence that in certain very rare individuals exposure to halothane may lead to sensitization so that subsequent halothane anesthesia may be followed by severe, and indeed fatal, jaundice. Some authorities recommend omitting halothane from the anesthesia sequence if multiple administrations for the same patient are anticipated.[139]

METHOXYFLURANE. Methoxyflurane (Penthrane) is a clear, colorless liquid with a characteristic fruity odor. It is a nonflammable agent under normal conditions of clinical anesthesia. It is a halogenated ether, and induction is prolonged. This may be overcome by injecting a quick-acting drug such as thiopental sodium before administration of methoxyflurane. Emergence from anesthesia is slow, and the need for analgesic drugs in the immediate postanesthesia period may be lessened. Methoxyflurane is associated with renal toxicity in a dose-related manner. Nausea and vomiting may occur postoperatively but to a lesser degree than after cyclopropane or ether.

ENFLURANE. Enflurane (Ethrane) is a clear, colorless, nonflammable liquid that has a mild, sweet odor. It is fluorinated ether used for inhalation anesthesia. Induction and recovery from anesthesia with enflurane are rapid. It does not appear to stimulate excess salivation or tracheobronchial secretions, and pharyngeal and laryngeal reflexes are readily deadened. Enflurane reduces ventilation and decreases blood pressure as the depth of anesthesia increases. It provokes a sigh response reminiscent of that seen with diethyl ether. Heart rate remains relatively constant. All commonly used muscle relaxants are compatible with enflurane.

Intravenous anesthesia

THIOPENTAL SODIUM. Thiopental sodium (Pentothal Sodium) is the drug used most frequently for induction of anesthesia. It produces unconsciousness quickly. Recovery is rapid if the total dose is small. Thiopental may also be given to relieve severe, prolonged convulsive states. Laryngeal reflexes are not depressed at light levels of narcosis, and laryngospasm may occur with stimulation of the larynx. Signs of laryngospasm are apprehension, stridor (a harsh whistling sound), retraction of the soft tissue about the neck, and cyanosis. If these signs appear in the postanesthesia period, the nurse should notify the physician immediately. If large doses of thiopental have been used, the patient may sleep for a long time and should be observed for signs of respiratory depression. Some individuals appear to awaken quickly only to return to the anesthetized state when undisturbed.[38] The blood pressure may drop suddenly and should be checked frequently. Thiopental is detoxified in the liver and excreted by the kidneys. Therefore in patients with liver or kidney disease this drug may be eliminated more slowly.

Thiopental is used primarily to produce sleep before an inhalation anesthetic is administered. The major advantage of this agent is the smooth induction afforded the patient. This anesthetic agent may be used for brief surgical procedures such as closed reduction of a fracture or a dislocation or incision and drainage of an abscess.

DROPERIDOL AND FENTANYL. Droperidol and fentanyl (Innovar) are the combination of a potent tranquilizer (droperidol) and a powerful narcotic analgesic (fentanyl). Surgical anesthesia is produced quickly, and recovery is smooth and rapid. In most patients orientation returns quickly without restlessness or emergence delirium. Incorporating droperidol into the anesthetic regimen will usually result in a lower incidence of postoperative nausea and vomiting. It can be given intermittently throughout a surgical procedure. Because of the tranquilizing component, droperidol, the patient requires less analgesia in the postanesthesia recovery room. Patients should be observed for hypoventilation during the immediate recovery period and may need to be urged to breathe. Postoperative narcotic orders should be reduced to one third or one fourth the usual amount. Droperidol and fentanyl may be used as premedication, as an adjunct to general anesthesia, alone, or with regional anesthesia. They may be used in combination or separately.

KETAMINE. Ketamine is a nonbarbiturate, parenteral anesthetic agent. The anesthetic state characterized by ketamine is termed *dissociative anesthesia*. It is a substance permitting surgical operations on patients who may appear to be awake, since movement may occur and the eyes remain open. However, the individuals are anesthetized so far as recollection or awareness is concerned. Ketamine is chemically related to the hallucinogens, and unpleasant dreams during awakening and extending into the postoperative period may constitute a drawback. To help overcome these effects a small dose of diazepam (Valium) may be given, or more important the patient is left undisturbed during the emergence phase.

Ketamine produces profound analgesia but does little to block visceral pain, which eliminates its usefulness for intraabdominal or intrathoracic procedures unless supplemented by an inhalation agent.[38] It is useful in diagnostic procedures such as neuroradiology and for superficial procedures of short duration. Ketamine has been most valuable in the anesthetic management of children. Contraindications for the use of ketamine include patients with upper respiratory tract infections, prior cerebrovascular accident, hypertension, psychiatric disorders, and increased intracranial pressure.

Muscle relaxants. Certain drugs such as *d*-tubocurarine chloride (curare), succinylcholine chloride (Anectine), pancuronium bromide (Pavulon), and gallamine triethiodide (Flaxedil) are neuromuscular blocking agents used to provide muscle relaxation. They are employed for facilitating endotracheal intubation and may be given as adjuncts to provide sufficient relaxation of skeletal muscles.

These agents cause respiratory depression or paralysis; thus the patient must be observed closely for signs of respiratory distress during and after administration of the drug. Patients developing respiratory problems will require intubation and mechanical ventilatory assistance. All patients who are paralyzed with muscle relaxants require skilled airway management with the capability of endotracheal intubation until the patient is able to maintain respirations.

The drug *d*-tubocurarine is injected intravenously. About one third of the amount administered is excreted unchanged in the urine, whereas the rest is metabolically altered. It is probably still the most important competitive neuromuscular blocking agent.[57]

Succinylcholine chloride is a valuable agent for producing short periods of muscular relaxation. The short duration of action of succinylcholine may be attributed to its rapid metabolic degradation. Facilities for artificial respiration are essential, since this appears to be the only effective antidotal measure to apnea.[57]

Pancuronium bromide is approximately 5 times as potent as *d*-tubocurarine chloride. It has little effect on the circulatory system. The most frequently reported observation is a slight rise in pulse rate. A major portion of administered pancuronium bromide is excreted unchanged in the urine.

Gallamine triethiodide is a synthetic drug that has an atropinelike effect on the cardiac branch of the vagus nerve and can produce considerable tachycardia. It is excreted unchanged in the urine and is not the agent of choice in the presence of poor renal function.

Regional anesthesia

Regional anesthesia is produced by the injection or application of a local anesthetic agent along the course of a nerve or at the site of the stimulus, thus abolishing the conduction of all impulses to and from the area supplied by that nerve. The patient experiences no pain in the operative area and remains awake during the entire procedure because the anesthetic affects a particular region only; it does not affect cortical functions.

Regional anesthesia is used for treatments, diagnostic measures, examinations, and surgery. The nurse usually assembles the equipment necessary for the administration of the drugs used to produce anesthesia, assists the physician during the procedure, and observes the patient for reactions to the anesthetic or to the procedure.

The drugs used to produce regional anesthesia are usually called local anesthetics. Examples are procaine (Novocain), cocaine, tetracaine (Pontocaine), dibucaine (Nupercaine), and lidocaine (Xylocaine). When these drugs are absorbed into the bloodstream they cause stimulation of the central nervous system and depression of the heart. Therefore care is taken that they are given in a localized area and in the smallest dose necessary to produce anesthesia. Epinephrine may be added to the solution of local anesthetic drugs to produce vasoconstriction in the area of the injection. Vasoconstriction tends to reduce the rate of absorption, to extend the length of anesthesia, and to reduce hemorrhage. Epinephrine should not be added to solutions when nerve block of the digits is contemplated.

The patient is observed for signs of excitability (laughing, crying, excessive talking), twitching, pulse or blood pressure changes, pallor of the skin, and respiratory difficulties. At the first sign of these toxic reactions an intravenous injection of a short-acting barbiturate such as thiopental sodium should be ready for the physician to administer. Oxygen may also be necessary, and it is important that a patent airway be maintained. If the reaction is due to an idiosyncrasy to the drug, circulatory failure may occur, and emergency measures such as artificial respiration must be started. Patients should be questioned regarding any previous sensitivity to these drugs, and skin tests are usually advocated before their administration.

Regional anesthesia of the limbs can be achieved by injecting an anesthetizing agent such as lidocaine into a vein in the limb to be anesthetized. A tourniquet is applied to the limb to prevent the distribution of the anesthetizing agent throughout the body.

Topical anesthesia. Topical anesthesia is accomplished by applying or spraying a local anesthetic drug such as cocaine or lidocaine directly on the part to be anesthetized. It is used for surgical procedures on the nose and throat and to eliminate pharyngeal and tracheal reflexes during bronchoscopy and similar procedures. Topical anesthesia may be used in genitourinary procedures (urethral meatotomy, cystoscopy) and to provide anesthesia of the lower urethra.

Infiltration anesthesia. Infiltration anesthesia is accomplished by the injection of the anesthetic drug directly into the area to be incised or manipulated. This method is used for minor procedures (incision and drainage, thoracentesis). Nerve block is regional anesthesia in which the drug is injected into or around the nerve a short distance from the site of the operation. This method may be employed for patients having tonsillectomies, dental procedures, or plastic surgery.

In a pudendal block a long 20- or 22-gauge spinal needle attached to a Luer syringe is passed just below and beyond the ischial spine. Solution is then injected to anesthetize the internal pudendal nerve. The needle is partially withdrawn and then inserted laterally toward the ischial tuberosity, where more solution is injected, followed by infiltration of the labia in the same manner, which is repeated on the opposite side. Perineal muscles relax in a few minutes and the skin of the perineum is anesthetized.

Extradural anesthesia. In an epidural block the drug is injected into the epidural space and affects a band around the body, depending on the site of injection and the dose of the drug. When a caudal block is performed, the drug is injected into the caudal canal lying below the cord and affects the nerve trunks that supply the perineal area.

Spinal anesthesia. Spinal anesthesia is accomplished by the injection of a local anesthetic drug into the subarachnoid space, which contains spinal fluid (Fig. 24-4). The anesthetic drug acts on the nerves as they emerge from the spinal cord. Depending on the type of

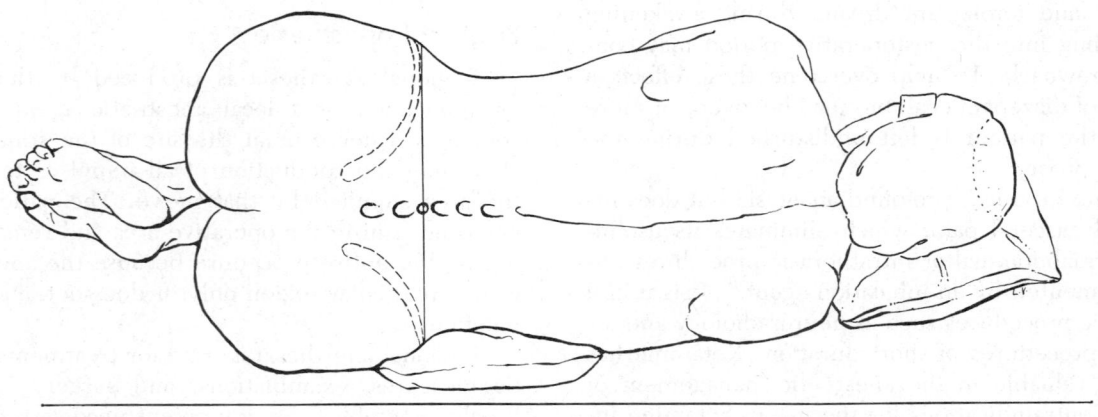

Fig. 24-4. Patient in lateral position for spinal anesthesia.

anesthesia desired, the injection is made through the second, third, or fourth interspace of the lumbar vertebrae. Anesthesia is quickly produced and provides good relaxation of muscles.

Spinal anesthesia is used for surgery of the lower limbs, perineum, and lower abdomen and sometimes for surgery in the upper abdomen such as removal of the gallbladder. It is not used for operations on the upper part of the body because it causes paralysis of the diaphragm and the intercostal muscles used in respiration. A "saddle block" is a low spinal block commonly used in vaginal deliveries. With this block, analgesia rarely extends above the tenth dermatome. The patient may be unable to move her legs for 2 to 8 hours following induction of the anesthetic. With spinal anesthesia the patient may be conscious of pulling sensations throughout the operation but experiences no pain. Occasionally, a feeling of faintness and nausea occurs because of these sensations.

One of the limitations of spinal anesthesia is that the patient may be awake during the operation, although the preoperative medication may decrease awareness of the surroundings. A screen restricts the patient's vision in the operating room, and a towel may be placed over the eyes. The conversation and activities of the members of the operating room staff should be carried on with the patient's consciousness in mind. It is a nursing responsibility to remind other members of the surgical team that the patient is awake and that some topics of conversation may be upsetting. In some hospitals a "Patient is Awake" sign is posted both in the operating room and outside the door.

Because of the sympathetic blockade, hypotension may occur with these anesthetic techniques. Vasopressor drugs such as epinephrine hydrochloride may be given if a drop in blood pressure occurs. This may also be seen with epidural anesthesia.

Following spinal anesthesia the patient should be quiet in bed in a supine position. Safety needs must be considered since sensation may not return to the anesthetized area for 1 or 2 hours. Tissue injuries such as burns from hot water bottles can occur. The patient is monitored for signs of respiratory or circulatory depression and vital signs are checked frequently. Hypotension may occur as a result of relaxation of the vascular bed.

Headache following spinal anesthesia will be reduced if the patient does not sit up or assume the erect position for 8 hours. Spinal headache is thought to be due to leakage of spinal fluid from the puncture in the dura or to sterile chemical meningitis. It usually occurs 24 hours after the puncture and is more common in women than in men. It may last several days, and occasionally it persists for weeks or months. The possibility of this complication is not suggested to the patient. If it does occur, the patient complains of a throbbing, pulsating headache that is aggravated by a change to the upright position or by merely coughing or sneezing; an ice bag may bring relief. To lessen discomfort, analgesics and sedatives should be given as ordered. Hydration of the patient is of great importance, since it will aid in the replacement of spinal fluid. Increased oral intake is encouraged. If the patient is receiving nothing orally, intravenous fluids will be ordered.

When the effects of the anesthetic wear off, the patient occasionally complains of a backache. The pain may be the result of the position in which the patient was placed on the operating table or of the insertion of the needle at the time of the puncture. The complaint is treated symptomatically, and heat applied locally often brings relief.

Fire, explosion, and electrical safety

Certain anesthetizing agents such as ether and cyclopropane are flammable and explosive, therefore extreme caution must be taken at all times to eliminate electric charges that could ignite or explode these agents. Fire and explosion hazards have decreased in recent years as new nonflammable anesthetic agents have been developed, and flammable agents are used with much less frequency. All personnel entering the operating room must strictly adhere to the dress code regulations. Conductive shoes or boots are worn in this area.

Today the greatest hazard to the life of the surgical patient is the electrical one. The present concerns revolve around the grounding systems in operating and recovery rooms and the increasing use of electrical monitoring equipment.

Induced hypothermia

Local hypothermia. Induced local hypothermia refers to the lowering of the temperature of only a part of the body such as a limb. It is used largely to produce surgical anesthesia before amputation of a limb affected by arteriosclerotic gangrene. Elderly, debilitated patients and patients who have diabetes are most likely to be treated with this anesthesia. Advantages of this method are that physical shock to the patient is minimal, no inhalation anesthesia is required, and the lowered temperature reduces cell metabolism.

The extremity is packed in ice and anesthesia is usually obtained in 1½ to 3 hours. The duration of anesthesia produced by this method is approximately 60 minutes. The patient may be experiencing pain from the diseased limb and the weight of the ice causes more discomfort; thus there is a need to administer a barbiturate or narcotic before initiating the procedure.

Another method for producing hypothermia in an extremity is through the use of a blanketlike device consisting of coils that contain circulating water. Thus the temperature of the water can be lowered to produce hypothermia and raised when the limb is to be rewarmed.

General hypothermia. General hypothermia for the patient in surgery is rarely used today. It refers to the reduction of body temperature below normal to reduce oxygen and metabolic requirements. Hypothermia may be used for a variety of illnesses when extremely high temperatures occur. For example, patients with neurologic disease causing a high temperature may be kept in a state of relatively mild hypothermia (30.6° to 35° C [87° to 95° F]) for as long as 5 days.

If hypothermia is to be used as an adjunct to anesthesia during surgery, the patient usually is given meperidine hydrochloride and atropine sulfate 45 minutes to 1 hour before the procedure is to begin. Provision is made for monitoring temperature readings from different parts of the body, preferably the esophagus and rectum, by placing electric thermometers in these areas. In addition, the heart is monitored with an electrocardiograph to detect cardiac arrhythmias produced by lowered temperature and the brain is monitored with an electroencephalograph to detect cerebral anoxia. The care of the patient at this time is under the supervision of the operating room team. The temperature is lowered by one of the following methods.

External hypothermia may be produced by applying crushed ice around the patient, by totally immersing the patient in ice water, or by exposure to the cooling effects of special blankets. The most widely accepted method of hypothermia today is the use of cooling blankets. The patient is placed on and may be covered by body-sized vinyl pads containing many coils. The pads are connected to a reservoir filled with alcohol and water. A pump fills the coils and circulates the solution through the coils in the pad. A recording thermometer monitors the patient's temperature, and an electric unit heats or cools the solution to a preset temperature (Fig. 24-5).

Extracorporeal cooling, a method of bloodstream cooling, consists of removing the blood from a major vessel, circulating it through coils immersed in a refrigerant, and returning it to the body through another vessel. Bloodstream cooling is the fastest method for producing hypothermia and is used primarily for patients who are undergoing surgery. The patient is given heparin to prevent the blood from clotting during the procedure.

Intervention during prolonged hypothermia. The conscious patient who is to undergo hypothermia for an elevated temperature needs reassurance that the procedure will not be too uncomfortable. Because the treatment is often erroneously conceived by the laity, the patient may have fears and apprehension that should be reported to the physician so that specific questions that may be causing worry can be answered. When hypothermia is to be continued for several days, any of the external methods for producing hypothermia may be used. Before the procedure is started the patient is given a complete bath and a thin coating of oil or cream may be applied to the skin; a cleansing enema may also be ordered.

While the temperature is being lowered to the desired level and for as long as the procedure is continued, the patient is observed closely. Any irregularities of pulse, temperature, or blood pressure must be reported at once. It is expected that all of these vital signs will lower gradually. If they rise, drop too suddenly, or fluctuate, the physician is notified. The temperature is monitored by a rectal thermometer probe to determine whether a desired temperature (usually between 30° and 32° C [86° and 89.6° F]) is maintained throughout the treatment.

Shivering is a complication of hypothermia that must be avoided because peripheral vasoconstriction is accompanied by an increase in body temperature, circulation rate, and oxygen consumption. Usually shivering occurs when the temperature is lowered to 30° C (86° F). To prevent shivering, chlorpromazine hydrochloride (Thorazine) usually is administered intravenously before the treatment is started and is repeated as often as every 2 hours if shivering continues.

Since urinary output is decreased when the body temperature is reduced to 32° C (89° F), a retention catheter (Foley type) is inserted before hypothermia is started so that output can be measured carefully and recorded. The gag reflex and other reflexes may be depressed; thus food and fluids are not given orally. Fluids containing glucose and electrolytes are given intravenously and usually through a polyethylene catheter that has been sutured into a vein. Depending on the method being used to produce hypothermia, the patient may be fed by means of a nasogastric tube.

The patient's skin must be observed for signs of pressure, edema, and discoloration. The patient is turned at least every 2 hours, and footboards and pillows should be used to prevent strain on joints and to maintain proper body alignment. Often the patient is placed on a CircOlectric bed to make possible a complete change in position. Good oral hygiene is necessary, and dried secretions are removed from the nares. If corneal reflexes are diminished and eye secretions reduced, the eyes may need to be cleansed and covered to protect them (p. 763).

The cooling agent or blankets are removed at the termination of hypothermia and regular blankets are applied. The temperature must be observed carefully as it approaches normal, and blankets must then be removed. The thermometer probe is removed when the temperature becomes stable.

Induced hypotension

Hypotension may be induced for the purpose of decreasing bleeding at the operative site in selected instances such as radical head and neck or pelvic surgery.

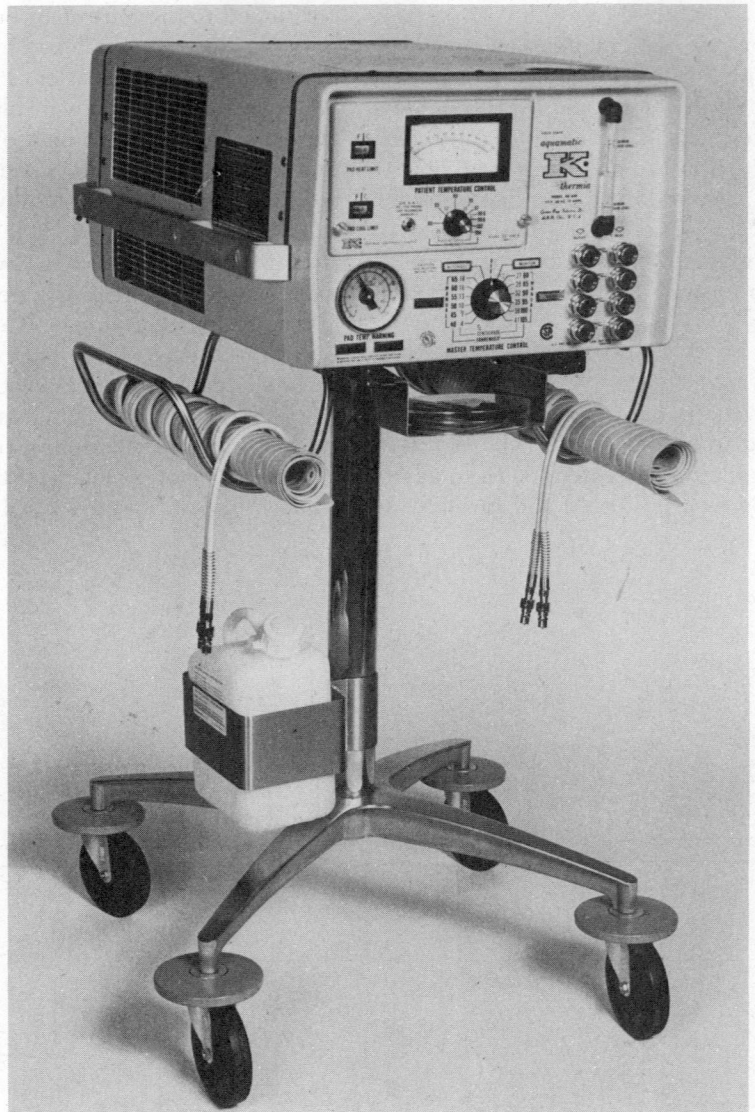

Fig. 24-5. Hypothermia can be produced by means of cooling blanket. Cold alcohol and water are circulated through coils by pressure pump.

Hypotension can be induced by deep anesthesia with an inhalant anesthetic such as halothane or by an intravenous anesthetic that affects the autonomic nervous system. Vital signs are monitored closely in the early postoperative period.

Positioning patient for surgery

The responsibility for positioning the patient on the operating room table is one shared by the nurse, surgeon, and anesthesiologist. The nurse must be aware of the position required for each surgical procedure and understand the many physiologic changes that occur as the anesthetized patient is placed in a particular operative position.

No matter what position is to be assumed, good positioning is important to (1) adequately expose the operative area; (2) make the patient accessible for induction of anesthesia and administration of intravenous solutions or drugs; (3) minimize interference with circulation as a result of pressure on a body part; (4) provide protection from injury to nerves as a result of improper positioning of arms, hands, legs, or feet; (5) provide for the maintenance of respiratory function by avoiding pressure on the chest to allow for adequate ventilation of the lungs and by holding the jaw forward to keep it from dropping on the chest; and (6) provide for the patient's individuality and privacy by proper draping. A brief discussion of the commonly used operative positions and some of the precautions that are necessary follow.

Supine position

In the supine position the patient lies flat on the back with arms at the side, palms down with fingers extended and free to rest on the table, and legs straight with feet slightly separated (Fig. 24-6, *A*). This is the most commonly used position in the operating room and is used for hernia repair, exploratory laparotomy, cholecystectomy, gastric and bowel resection, and mastectomy. Attention must be given to proper support of the patient's neck and jaw to ensure the maintenance of a patent airway.

Prone position

In the prone position the patient lies on the abdomen with the face turned to one side and arms at the side with palms pronated and fingers extended (Fig. 24-6, *B*). The arms should be well protected and carefully positioned to prevent ulnar or radial nerve damage. Elbows may be slightly flexed to prevent overextension of the shoulders. The patient's feet are elevated off the table with a small pillow or blanket roll to prevent plantar flexion and pressure on the toes. Body rolls are placed under each side of the patient to raise the chest and permit the diaphragm to move freely and the lungs to expand. When the patient is in the prone position the restraint strap is placed below the knee. It is important that the patient's head and neck be positioned properly to ensure a patent airway. This position is used for surgery on the back, spine, and rectal area. The patient is anesthetized in the supine position and then placed in the prone position. This position should be assumed gradually and usually four persons are required to turn the patient safely. Details of the turning process can be found in specialized texts and articles.[60]

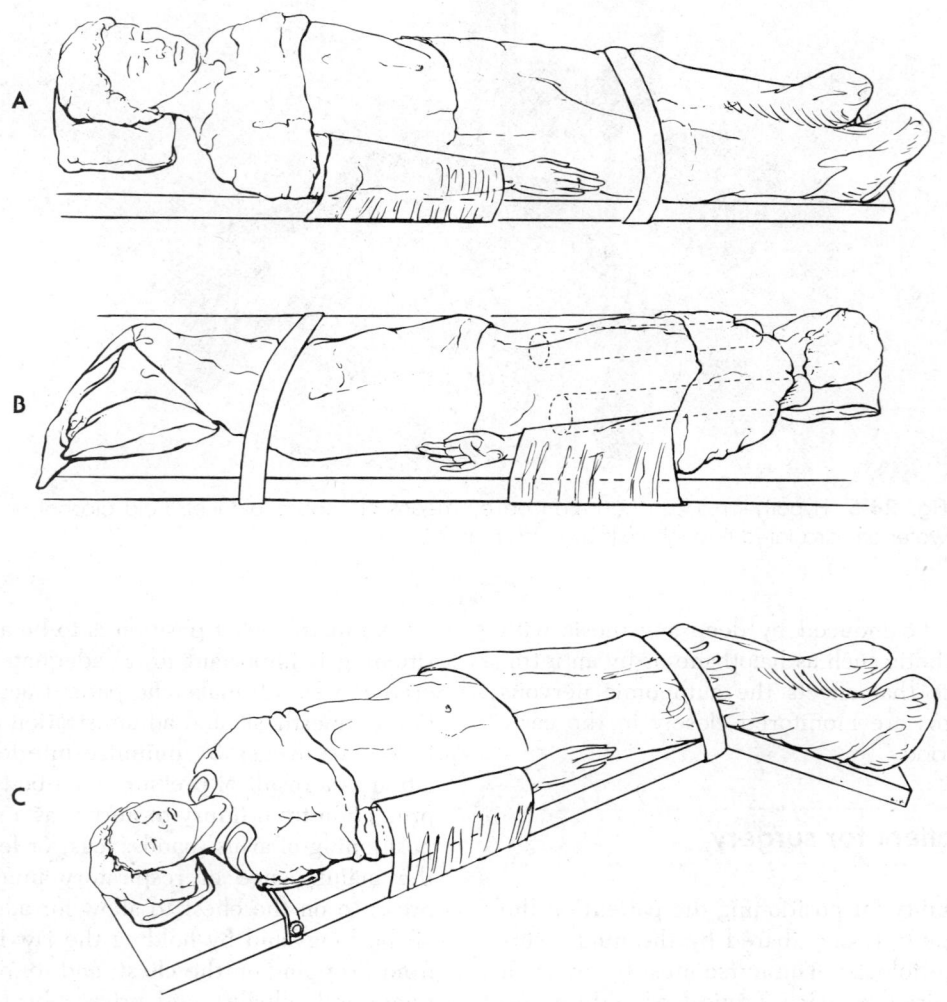

Fig. 24-6. Three commonly used operative positions. **A,** Supine. **B,** Prone. **C,** Trendelenburg's.

When the surgery is completed, the patient will be returned to the supine position. This should be done gradually and slowly to allow the patient's cardiovascular system to adjust to the change in position. Rapid turning of the patient can cause a precipitous drop in the blood pressure.

Trendelenburg's position

In Trendelenburg's position the patient's head and body are lowered into a head-down position. The knees are flexed by "breaking" the table, and the patient is held in position by padded shoulder braces (Fig. 24-6, C). This position is used for operations on the lower abdomen and the pelvis to obtain good exposure by a displacement of the intestines into the upper abdomen. The upward position of the viscera decreases the movement of the diaphragm and interferes with respiratory excursion. For this reason this position is not maintained any longer than necessary. The operating room table should be returned to a normal position very slowly so that the patient's cardiovascular system has time to adjust to the shift in position. When the patient is in Trendelenburg's position, blood pools in the upper torso and the blood pressure rises. As the patient is lowered to a normal position, the venous supply is shunted to the legs and a sudden drop in blood pressure may occur.

Reverse Trendelenburg's position

As the name implies, in reverse Trendelenburg's position the head is elevated and the feet are lowered. This position may be used to obtain better visualization of the biliary tract in surgery. The patient must be properly supported by a footboard, body restraints, and a lift sheet around the arms. Since blood will tend to pool in the lower extremities, caution should be used in slowly returning the patient to a normal position. A sudden influx of the pooled blood from the feet can cause an overloading of the cardiovascular system. Obviously this would be of most concern in elderly patients or in those with preexisting cardiovascular problems.

Lithotomy position

In the lithotomy position the patient lies on the back with the buttocks to the break in the operating table. After the patient is anesthetized the thighs and legs are flexed at right angles and then simultaneously placed in stirrups (Fig. 24-7, A). This prevents injury, which can occur to the muscle if each leg is flexed and placed in the stirrup separately. The hands and arms may be placed over the patient's chest and secured by the gown or positioned on armboards at the side. They should not extend beyond the break in the table since they may be injured when the table is manipulated. The lower

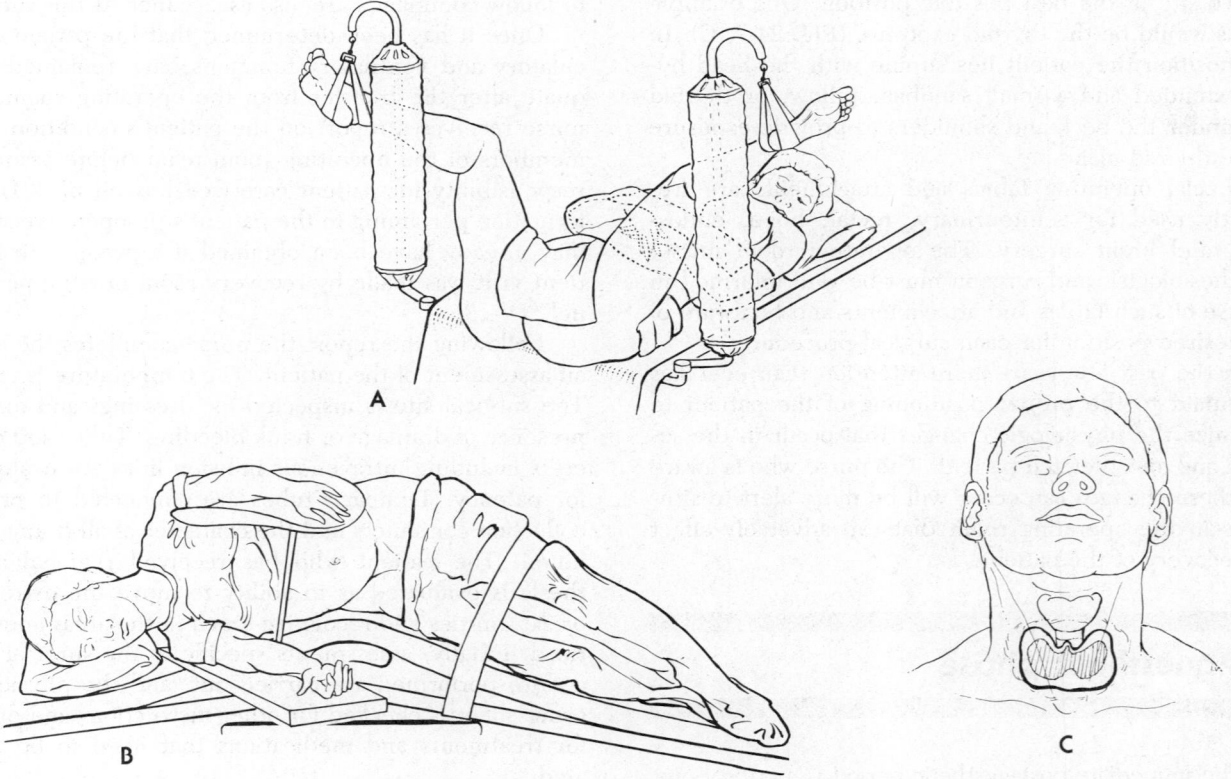

Fig. 24-7. Three operative positions for specialized surgery. **A,** Lithotomy. **B,** Lateral. **C,** Thyroid gland exposure.

section of the table is then lowered. This position is used in perineal, rectal, and vaginal surgery.

In this position the patient has blood from the legs shunted into the torso and upper extremities. If the patient must remain in the lithotomy positon any period of time, Ace bandages are often wrapped around each leg before surgery to lessen pooling and thrombus formation. Because of increased pressure on the sacral area, these patients may also develop pressure areas with redness and maceration of the skin.

When the surgery is completed, the patient's legs must be gradually returned to a normal position. As in Trendelenburg's position, rapid lowering of the legs may cause a sudden drop in blood pressure as part of the total blood volume is shunted back into the legs.

Lateral positions

Various versions of the lateral position are used for surgery on the kidney and the chest. The kidney position (Fig. 24-7, *B*) is used for nephrectomy and pyelolithotomy. As can be seen, this position puts pressure on the lower arm and leg and blood pools in these areas. The position of the chest allows the upper lung to move more freely than the lower lung interfering with pulmonary ventilation.

Other positions

Special positions may be necessary to place the operative site in the best possible position. One example of this would be the thyroid exposure (Fig. 24-7, *C*). In this position the patient lies supine with the head hyper-extended and a small sandbag, pillow, or thyroid rest under the neck and shoulders to provide exposure of the thyroid gland.

Special operating tables and attachments are frequently used for genitourinary, rectal, bone, endoscopy, and brain surgery. The operating room nurse, anesthesiologist, and surgeon must be well informed in the use of such tables and attachments and be aware of the desired position for each surgical procedure.

In the past few years more attention than ever has been paid to the proper positioning of the patient to minimize the physiologic changes that occur in the sedated and anesthetized patient. The nurse who is aware that these changes can occur will be more alert to situations in the operating room that can adversely affect the recovery of the patient.

Postanesthetic phase

The immediate postanesthetic period is a critical one. The patient must be observed diligently and must receive intensive physical and psychologic support until the major effects of the anesthetic have worn off and the overall condition stabilizes. The nurse is largely responsible for the care of the patient at this time.

It is the practice in most hospitals that any patient who has received general, dissociative, or regional anesthesia is taken to a postanesthesia recovery room after surgery where continuous attention can be given for a period of time. In some instances the patient who has had local anesthesia but who requires close observation in the immediate postoperative period may also be cared for in the recovery room. In such an area, specially prepared nursing personnel and all the equipment that may be necessary for the care of the patient in the postanesthetic phase are readily available. Ideally, the recovery room is located on the same floor as the operating rooms or in the immediate vicinity.

Assessment

The patient should be accompanied to the recovery room or to the clinical unit by the anesthesiologist and another member of the operating room professional staff. While the anesthesiologist remains at the bedside, the nurse begins assessment of the patient by obtaining vital signs (blood pressure, pulse rate, respiratory rate). Measuring the vital signs also includes evaluation of the pulse volume and regularity, airway patency, symmetry of chest expansion, depth of respirations, and color of the skin. The patient's level of consciousness and ability to follow commands are also ascertained at this time.

Once it has been determined that the patient's circulatory and ventilatory functions have remained adequate after the transfer from the operating room, the nurse receives a report on the patient's condition from members of the operating room team before assuming responsibility for patient care (see box on p. 431). Information pertaining to the patient's preoperative status may already have been obtained if a preoperative patient visit was made by recovery room nursing personnel.

Following the report the nurse completes the overall assessment of the patient. The temperature is taken. The surgical site is inspected for dressings and for the presence of drainage or frank bleeding. Tubes and catheters including intravenous infusion lines are evaluated for patency. Drainage tubes are connected to proper collection containers and the character of all drainage is noted. The patient who has received regional anesthesia is evaluated as to ability to move the extremity or extremities and recognize touch in the areas anesthetized. Finally, assessments specific to the surgical procedure performed are carried out, and the physician's order sheet is checked for other instructions and orders for treatments and medications that need to be initiated.

It is essential that there is complete and accurate recording of the immediate postanesthetic course so that

DATA TO BE OBTAINED WHEN PATIENT IS ADMITTED TO THE RECOVERY ROOM

Current medical diagnosis

Surgical procedure performed

What, why

Agents administered

Anesthetic

Narcotic

Muscle relaxant

Muscle relaxant reversal agent

Antibiotic

Other (e.g., digitalis preparation, diuretic)

Complications during surgery

Type

Treatment instituted

Fluids

Estimated blood loss (EBL)

Blood and fluid administered

Pertinent preoperative problems

Physical

Psychologic

those who continue management of the patient have a thorough picture to refer to as necessary. The recording should start with a summary of the patient's status when admitted from the operating room, that is, the baseline assessment. Thereafter, changes in the patient's status as determined by frequent reassessments need to be noted. All medications, fluids, and treatments the patient receives during this time must be recorded so that there will be no duplication that might prove harmful to the patient.

Intervention

Much of the ongoing nursing care provided in the immediate postanesthetic period depends on the particular surgical procedure performed and is discussed elsewhere in this text (see specific disease entities and surgical procedures). Some outcomes, however, are the same for all postanesthetic patients: pulmonary ventilation and circulation are maintained, fluid and electrolyte balance is maintained, injury is prevented, and comfort is promoted.

OUTCOME: Pulmonary ventilation is maintained.

The goal of respiratory care for the postoperative patient is to maintain pulmonary ventilation that is adequate to prevent hypoxemia (a deficiency of oxygen in the blood) and hypercapnia (an excess of carbon dioxide in the blood). In the immediate postanesthetic period two of the most common causes of inadequate pulmonary exchange are airway obstruction and hypoventilation.

Airway patency. Airway obstruction most frequently occurs as a result of the tongue, which is relaxed from anesthesia, falling back against the pharynx or as a result of secretions or other fluids collecting in the pharynx, trachea, or bronchial tree. While caring for the postanesthetic patient it is essential for the nurse to recognize that all noisy breathing (e.g., snoring, gurgling, wheezing, crowing) is indicative of some type of airway obstruction. It is equally important, however, for the nurse to realize that obstruction can occur without being accompanied by noise.

POSITIONING. The most desirable position to ensure maintenance of a patent airway depends on the size and condition of the patient, the anesthesia used, the surgery performed, and the amount of experienced nursing care that is available. Ideally, the patient should be in a position to breathe normally with full use of all portions of the lungs and so that vomitus, blood, and mucus can drain out and will not be aspirated. Until protective reflexes have returned, the best position for the majority of patients is a *side-lying* or *semiprone* position with the head tilted back and the jaw supported forward. It is important to remember that aspiration can occur unless the *whole body* is turned. Turning the patient's head when the chest and shoulders remain in the back-lying position is useless. Although the side lying position somewhat diminishes chest expansion, it has the advantages of helping to keep the tongue forward and promoting the drainage of secretions and other fluids outside the mouth. The disadvantage related to chest expansion can be minimized by turning the patient frequently and by raising the flexed upper arm and placing it on a pillow. The supine position with head hyperextended permits fullest expansion of the lungs, but as noted it is dangerous because of its potential for aspiration or obstruction from secretions. Unless absolutely necessary this position should not be used before pharyngeal reflexes have returned and the patient is able to manage secretions. When the supine position must be used, all supplies for suctioning as well as personnel to perform the procedure must be available at the bedside at all times.

ARTIFICIAL AIRWAY. An oropharyngeal or nasopharyngeal airway is often left in place following the administration of a general anesthetic to keep the passage open and the tongue forward until pharyngeal reflexes have returned. These artificial airways are made of rubber, plastic, or metal. They should be removed as soon as the patient begins to awaken and has regained cough and swallowing reflexes. After this time their presence can be irritating and can stimulate vomiting or laryngospasm. If an artificial airway is ineffective or if one is not in place, the majority of obstructions due to the tongue falling back can be alleviated by holding the patient's jaw up and forward or by the side-lying position described previously. When absolutely necessary to clear the airway, the nurse can open the patient's mouth by pushing at the angle of the jaw with the thumbs and have someone insert a padded tongue depressor between the back teeth. The tongue can then be brought forward by grasping it with a piece of gauze. An endotracheal tube may need to be inserted by the physician if there is considerable difficulty maintaining a patent airway.

REMOVAL OF SECRETIONS. Excessive secretions from the nasopharynx or tracheobronchial mucosa can also lead to partial or complete airway obstruction. Unless the patient can manage these secretions by coughing them up and expectorating them, they must be removed by suctioning. Pharyngeal suctioning is often all that must be done. If intratracheal suctioning is necessary, sterile technique should be used and the patient should be hyperventilated with 100% oxygen before and after each introduction of the catheter into the trachea. Rarely, but occasionally, a bronchoscopy may be needed to remove secretions, especially if they are very inspissated. When thick secretions are a problem or potential problem, the humidity of the air breathed should be increased to keep secretions as thin as possible and to prevent dry air from further irritating the already irritated respiratory passages.

Adequate ventilation. Postoperative hypoventilation results from numerous causes. Respirations can be directly depressed by drugs, which may have been administered preoperatively, intraoperatively, or postoperatively. These drugs include inhalation and intravenous anesthetic agents, narcotics, tranquilizers, and sedatives. The residual effects of muscle relaxants and of high spinal or epidural anesthesia in which paralysis of the lower rib cage muscles results can limit the patient's power to breathe. Incisional pain, obesity, chronic lung disease, gastric dilation, and constrictive surgical dressings, also can interfere with lung expansion and thus with respiratory exchange.

OXYGEN THERAPY. Oxygen is usually given postoperatively because after anesthesia almost all patients have decreased pulmonary expansion and areas of atelectasis, both of which result in hypoxemia. Oxygen is administered by nasal cannula or catheter, disposable face mask or shield, or endotracheal or tracheostomy tube if one is in place. How long postoperative oxygen therapy should be continued depends on the individual patient. As a general rule all patients should receive oxygen at least until they are conscious and able to take deep breaths on command. Prolonged oxygen therapy should be guided by arterial blood gas determinations. Patients with thoracic or upper abdominal incisions or with preexisting pulmonary disease may be given oxygen for several hours, perhaps until the next day. Special care must be taken when administering oxygen to patients with chronic obstructive pulmonary disease so that hypoxemia, which is their stimulus to breathe, is not entirely removed (p. 1332). Any patient experiencing shivering, which increases oxygen consumption, should receive oxygen therapy until the shivering has ceased.

BREATHING EXERCISES. To help maintain normal levels of arterial blood gases and to counteract hypoventilation, all patients need to be encouraged to breathe deeply at frequent intervals. Ideally, the patient will take three or four deep inhalations every 10 to 15 minutes. If the patient is unconscious or will not breathe deeply when stimulated, the nurse can hyperventilate the lungs passively using a breathing bag and mask.

OTHER THERAPIES. When hypoventilation exists to the extent that hypercapnia is present, the patient must have respiratory assistance. Drug therapies that might be indicated include narcotic antagonists such as nalorphine or naloxone to counteract the respiratory depressant effects of the opiate, reversal agents such as neostigmine or edrophonium to counteract the effects of nondepolarizing muscle relaxants, and narcotics themselves if pain is causing the patient to splint respirations. With obese patients elevation of the head of the bed is often helpful in relieving pressure on the diaphragm. Nasogastric tubes may be inserted to relieve gastric distention. Constrictive dressings must be loosened. When these measures are ineffective in improving ventilation and in instances of excessive respiratory depression from depolarizing muscle relaxant drugs or from high spinal anesthesia, the patient may need to be intubated and receive mechanical ventilator assistance.

OUTCOME: Circulation is maintained.

Hypotension and *cardiac arrhythmias* are the most commonly encountered cardiovascular complications of the immediate postanesthetic period. Early recognition and management of these complications before they become serious enough to diminish cardiac output depend on frequent assessment of the patient's vital signs. The blood pressure, pulse, and respirations are usually taken every 15 minutes until stable, then every half hour for 2 hours, and then every 4 hours until ordered otherwise. In many hospitals the monitoring of vital signs every 15 minutes extends for as long as the patient is in the recovery room and for at least 1 hour after leaving the recovery room. The rate, volume, and rhythm of the pulse are carefully observed and the character and rate of respiration noted.

Hypotension. Moving the patient from the operating room table to the bed, jarring during transport, reactions to drugs and anesthesia, loss of blood and other body fluids, cardiac arrhythmias, cardiac failure, inadequate ventilation, pain, and residual sympathectomy from conductive anesthesia are among the many factors that will cause circulatory changes that may result in lowering the blood pressure. A mild decrease in the patient's blood pressure from the normal preoperative range is not uncommon during the early postoperative period. It is usually well tolerated in healthy patients and does not require treatment.

Shock, however, must be prevented because the brain, heart, kidneys, and other vital organs do not tolerate long periods of hypoxemia. A weak, thready pulse with a significant drop in blood pressure may indicate hemorrhage or circulatory failure. The surgeon, anesthesiologist or both should be notified at once if any of these signs occur, especially if the skin becomes cold, moist, pale, or cyanotic or the patient suddenly becomes restless or apprehensive. Oxygen therapy should be started to increase the oxygen saturation of the circulating blood. Unless contraindicated, the patient's legs are elevated to facilitate venous return. Blood plasma, or other intravenous fluids usually are ordered to increase the blood volume when the hypotension is a result of hypovolemia. Vasopressor agents may be used when vasodilation is apparent. Digitalis preparations or other inotropic agents may be administered if the decrease in blood pressure is a result of cardiac failure.

Cardiac arrhythmias. When a cardiac arrhythmia is detected, it is important for the nurse to ascertain if the patient has a history of such a disturbance. Arrhythmias unchanged from those that existed preoperatively usually do not require treatment. When there is no history of a cardiac irregularity but one has developed postoperatively, the nurse immediately assesses the patient to determine if ventilation is adequate. Oxygen should be started while the physician is being notified. A patient who is exchanging gases poorly should receive ventilatory assistance with a bag and mask.

Hypoxemia and hypercapnia are common causes of postoperative cardiac arrhythmias, especially premature beats and sinus tachycardia. These arrhythmias often can be suppressed by adequate ventilation. Frequent premature beats of ventricular origin, which are not decreased by oxygen therapy, are usually treated with drugs such as intravenous lidocaine (Xylocaine) or procainamide (Pronestyl). The sinus bradycardia that may follow the administration of neostigmine (Prostigmine) or edrophonium (Tensilon) is counteracted by the administration of atropine. Other common causes of postoperative cardiac arrhythmias include pain, hypovolemia, gastric distention, and acidosis. In the event that a life-threatening arrhythmia such as ventricular fibrillation or cardiac asystole occurs, resuscitation efforts must be started immediately.

OUTCOME: Fluid and electrolyte balance is maintained.

Most patients admitted to the recovery room will be receiving intravenous fluids as their immediate postoperative means of maintaining fluid and electrolyte balance. To compensate for urinary output and insensible fluid loss, the average postoperative adult requires at least 2000 ml of water per day. The exact amount and type of fluid administered will depend on the patient's surgical procedure as well as preoperative status, intraoperative course, and individual response to stress. Careful monitoring of the patient's intravenous fluid administration is essential to ensure adequacy of replacement and prevention of fluid overload (p. 333).

OUTCOME: Injury is prevented.

Following anesthesia, side rails on the stretcher or bed are generally raised and are left so until the patient is fully awake. Although the patient is constantly watched, it is possible for him or her to turn suddenly and be thrown from the bed. Physical restraints are seldom used. Restraints can be frightening to the semiconscious individual and may stimulate violent struggling to get away from them.

The patient is turned frequently and placed in good body alignment to prevent nerve damage from pressure and muscle and joint strain from lying in one position for a long time. The nurse must be constantly aware that unconscious patients and those recovering from spinal or epidural anesthesia have loss of sensation and are unable to indicate discomfort. Heating pads, heat lamps, or cast driers must be used with great care while the patient is unconscious or semiconscious so that burns do not occur. When infusions are being given, the patient's arm should be secured on an armboard if the needle is in an area where it could be easily dislodged.

OUTCOME: Comfort is promoted.

The immediate postanesthetic period is often a frightening time for the patient. Psychologic support is imperative for physical as well as emotional well-being. While awakening from anesthesia, the patient needs frequent orientation to place and reassurance of not being alone. The patient also needs to know that the operation is over and that recovery from anesthesia is satisfactory. Careful explanations of procedures being carried out are given even when it appears that the patient is not alert. The need for privacy should be considered at all times. Patients who receive this type of support frequently recover from anesthesia faster, with fewer complications, and with less incisional pain. The patient who has had regional anesthesia needs the same information and needs to be reassured that the sensation and movement in the extremities will return.

It is also important that the patient's routine hygiene needs are not overlooked. The skin is inspected; excess tape, electrode paste, and skin preparations are removed; and soiled areas are washed. Mouth care should be provided. Meeting these hygiene needs enhances the patient's comfort as well as assisting in maintenance of dignity as a human being.

Incisional pain is a common complaint after surgery, and from the patient's point of view it is probably the most significant postoperative complication. In the immediate postanesthetic period narcotic analgesics should be given for pain when warranted but should be done so with the realization that pronounced depression of the respiratory, circulatory, or central nervous systems may follow. Because the patient generally has not completely recovered from the effects of anesthetic agents, the first postoperative dose of a narcotic is usually reduced to about *one half* the dose to be received after full recovery from anesthesia. Pain medication for restlessness should be given only after it has been determined that the restlessness is not a result of hypoxia.

Discharge from recovery room

Multiple criteria are used to determine when a patient has sufficiently recovered from anesthesia to be transferred from the recovery room (see below). Complications that must be under control include excessive wound drainage, vomiting, fever, pain, or inadequate urinary output as well as complications specific to the type of surgery performed. Acutely ill patients who cannot adequately fulfill these criteria are usually transferred to an intensive care unit.

Before discharging a patient the recovery room nurse needs to determine that there is adequate nursing staff available on the clinical unit to receive and care for the patient. All pertinent information concerning the patient's status must be communicated to the nurse who will be continuing to provide postoperative nursing care.

Outcome criteria for person discharged from recovery room

1. Vital signs are stable and indicate adequate respiratory and circulatory function.
2. Person is awake or easily aroused and can call for assistance if needed.
3. Postsurgical complications have been thoroughly evaluated and are under control.
4. The person who has had regional anesthesia has motor as well as partial sensory return to all anesthetized areas.

Postoperative phase

Preparation for return of patient to clinical unit

Equipment

Before the patient returns to the clinical unit from the postanesthesia recovery room, the patient's room is prepared to facilitate meeting the patient's needs in the immediate postoperative period. The bed is made so that the patient can be moved easily from stretcher to bed. The bed should have added protection in areas where drainage may be expected to occur and sufficient covers to ensure patient warmth.

The patient's room is cleared of any unnecessary equipment and a clear passageway provided for approach to the bed by the stretcher. Equipment that will be needed is placed in readiness. This equipment will depend on the type of surgery and might include such items as an intravenous pole, emesis basin, tissues, sphygmomanometer, and stethoscope. The recovery room nurse alerts the unit staff of any specialized equipment such as for suction or oxygen that may be needed.

Family

The family is kept informed of the patient's progress while in the recovery room, particularly when the patient's return to the unit has been delayed. Information that can be shared with the patient's family helps to lessen their anxiety.

Most surgeons discuss the results of the operation with the family immediately after the surgery and also visit the patient, telling briefly what was found and providing reassurance. The family is frequently highly anxious concerning the patient's condition and may not perceive or understand all that the surgeon tells them. Patients frequently experience periods of amnesia during the hours when they first regain consciousness and may not remember what they have been told. The nurse needs to know what information was given to the patient and family to be able to answer their questions. The family also needs to know what to expect when the patient returns to the unit.

Return of patient to clinical unit

Initial assessment and interventions

The recovery room nurse generally calls the unit when the patient is ready to be transferred and reports on the patient's condition. When the patient arrives the unit nurse accompanies the patient to the room to facilitate a smooth transfer, to make an initial assessment of

PATIENT ASSESSMENT ON RETURN FROM RECOVERY ROOM

Respiratory status

Patency of airway

Respirations: depth, rate, character

Breath sounds: presence, character

Circulatory status

Pulse, blood pressure, temperature

Skin color, temperature

Capillary filling

Neurologic status

Level of consciousness

Dressing

Presence of drainage

Presence of tubes to be connected to drainage systems

Comfort

Presence of pain, nausea, vomiting

Patient position: position of comfort, position to facilitate ventilation

Safety

Necessity for side rails

Call cord within reach

Equipment

Monitors connected and functioning

Intravenous fluids: rate, amount in bag, patency of tubing

Drainage systems (e.g., nasogastric, chest, urinary): type, patency of tubing, connection of appropriate container, character and amount of drainage

TABLE 24-10. Some causes of vital sign changes in early postoperative phase

Vital sign	Increase	Decrease
Temperature	Stress reaction (low-grade fever)	Cold operating room and recovery room
Pulse rate	Jarring during transfer Shock, hemorrhage Hypoventilation Acute gastric dilation Pain Anxiety Cardiac arrythmias	Digitalis overdose Cardiac arrhythmias
Respiratory rate	Hypoventilation: poor positioning, tight chest or upper abdominal dressing, obesity, gastric dilation	Drugs: anesthetics, narcotics, sedatives
Blood pressure	Anxiety ($\uparrow$ systolic) Pain	Jarring during transfer Severe pain Cardiac arrhythmias Shock: fluid loss, hemorrhage, acute gastric dilation

the patient's status (see box above), and to carry out immediate nursing interventions.

Subjective data. The patient is asked for symptoms of discomfort after having been transferred to the bed and positioned in supportive body alignment. This gives the nurse a quick indication of the level of alertness as well as symptoms of discomfort. An indirect question such as, "How do you feel?" will elicit data concerning nausea or pain without focusing on a specific area where there may be no discomfort. There is frequently an increase in pain perception at this time because of the movement from stretcher to bed. It is important to seek specific data concerning location, onset, and change in pain intensity and not to assume that the pain is incisional in nature.

Nausea occurs less frequently postoperatively with the use of newer anesthetics. There is greater possibility of nausea when the stomach has been manipulated

extensively during the surgical procedure or if considerable amounts of narcotics have been administered. The emesis basin should be easily available but not in sight if vomiting is a possibility.

Objective data

RESPIRATORY STATUS. The patient's respiratory status is assessed immediately on return to the unit. A patent airway is of primary importance during the early postoperative period until the patient is fully alert. Respirations are assessed for rate, depth, and sounds. Slow respirations may occur as a result of drugs given intraoperatively or postoperatively. Shallow rapid respirations may be caused by pain, constrictive chest or abdominal dressings, obesity, or gastric dilation. If a nasal catheter is in place, oxygen should be started.

If respirations are very noisy they may be heard without the aid of a stethoscope. Noisy respirations may be caused by airway obstruction from the tongue falling back against the pharynx (Fig. 24-8) or from secretions. The patient with noisy respirations should be assisted to cough and then positioned side lying if possible. Suctioning may be indicated if coughing does not clear the airway.

If the respirations are not noisy, the lungs are auscultated to establish a baseline for future comparison and to identify adventitious sounds (see Chapter 48 for assessment of breath sounds). Absent breath sounds indicate hypoventilation of that lobe (Table 24-10). Coarse rales indicate secretions in air passages. Presence of adventitious sounds indicates the need for energetic ven-

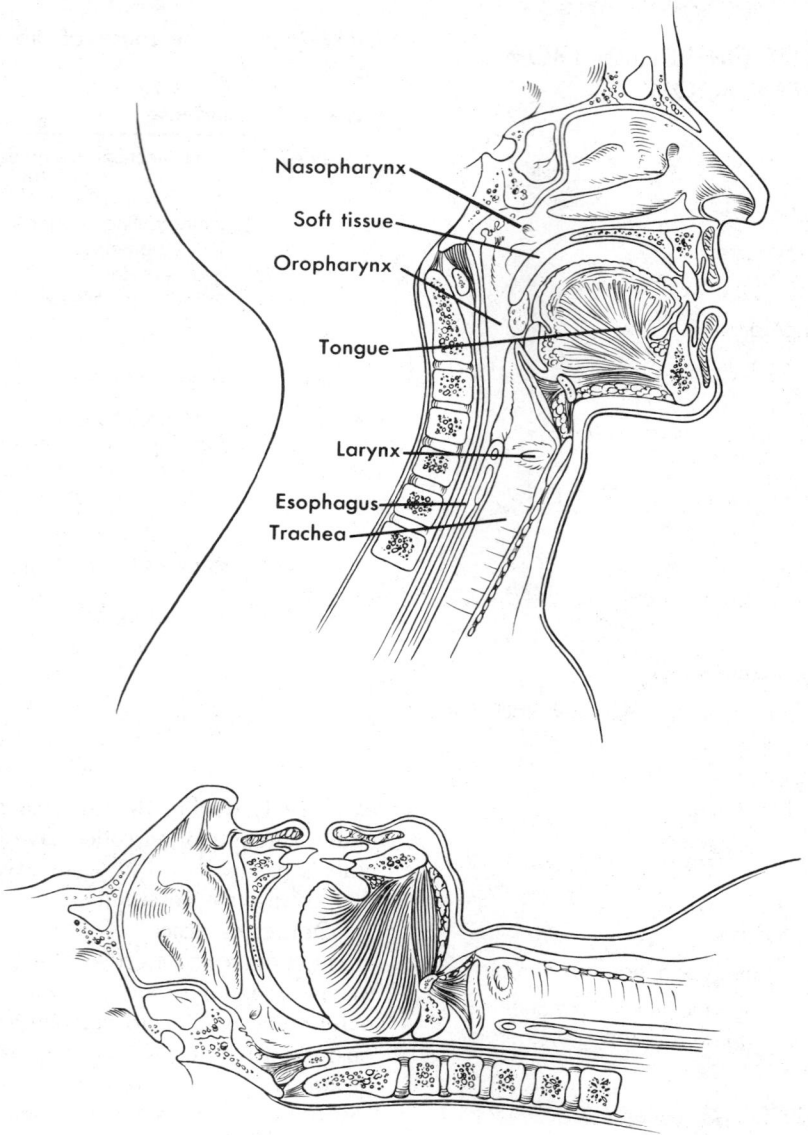

Fig. 24-8. Obstruction of airway by tongue in unconscious patient. Note how back of tongue can obstruct oropharynx in unconscious patient in supine position.

tilatory exercises. Deep-breathing and coughing measures are instituted immediately for all patients who have had general anesthesia.

CIRCULATORY STATUS

Pulse. The pulse is assessed for rate and quality. An increased rate usually occurs during the transfer to the bed, but the rate should return to the patient's usual range. A rapid, weak, thready pulse may indicate increased bleeding. If this is a change from the recovery room status, other signs of shock and evidence of bleeding are assessed and reported to the physician. Tachycardia may also indicate anxiety, hypoxemia, dehydration, overhydration, or acidosis. Bradycardia is usually caused by medications.

The presence and strength of peripheral pulses distal to plaster casts or the operative site on an extremity are used to measure adequacy of circulation. If the dressing is too tight it should be loosened, if this is permissible, or reported at once to the physician.

Temperature. A slight rise in body temperature to about 38° C (100° F) is commonly observed during the first 24 hours after surgery as a result of the stress reaction to the trauma of surgery. A subnormal temperature may be related to the cool air-conditioning found in most operating room and recovery room suites. A light blanket will usually provide sufficient warmth.

Blood pressure. Although the blood pressure has usually reached a stable level before the patient is dis-

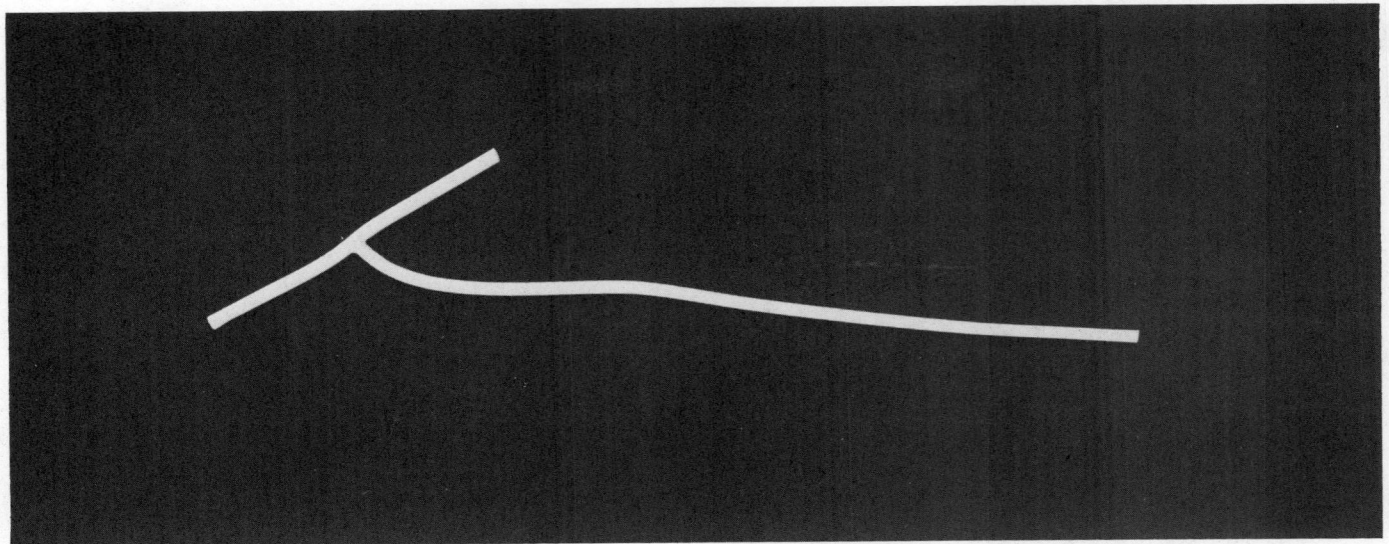

Fig. 24-9. T tube for draining common bile duct.

charged from the recovery room, changes may occur as a result of the transfer to the clinical unit. An increase in systolic pressure may be related to anxiety concerning the transfer or to pain. Hypotensive changes may be due to shock, although other signs of shock usually appear before changes in blood pressure occur. The patient's blood pressure is taken immediately on return to the room and comparisons are made with readings made in the recovery room.

Skin color and temperature. Pallor indicates decreased circulation to the skin. This is difficult to observe in dark-skinned individuals and is usually indicated by a dullness or decrease in the red tones. Pallor in dark-skinned persons may be more easily assessed by examining the mucous membranes of the mouth. Vasoconstriction may result from the coolness of the recovery room suite, from a decrease in the amount of circulating blood as a result of blood loss, or from the neuroendocrine response to stress. Blueness of the lips, mucous membranes, or nail beds may be caused by cold or inadequate oxygenation of the blood. The nail beds are checked for capillary return. If circulation is adequate, pinkness should return to the nail after it is "flicked" by the nurse's finger.

Skin usually feels cool to the touch after surgery because of exposure to a cool environment. Coolness may also be due to vasoconstriction from blood loss or stress reaction. Warm moist skin may be secondary to vasodilation from excessive warmth applied after surgery or to overhydration from excess fluid replacement. The intravenous solution may be running at an excessively rapid rate, and this should be checked if overhydration is a possibility.

LEVEL OF CONSCIOUSNESS. Level of consciousness can be ascertained by asking the patient to respond to simple questions or commands. Variations in consciousness level from alertness to drowsiness will be observed. If the patient is not easily aroused, these data are compared with the patient's consciousness status at the time of discharge from the recovery room. A decrease in consciousness level may indicate shock (from jarring motions during the transfer) and should be reported to the surgeon at once along with any other pertinent data.

DRESSING. For psychologic reasons and to prevent trauma the wound is covered in the operating room with a dry sterile dressing. The entire dressing is inspected with the covers pulled back or the patient turned as necessary. A dressing applied to the side such as for kidney surgery may appear dry on the top visible area if the patient is supine but may have excess drainage on the lower portion as a result of gravity. An excess amount of drainage is reported immediately.

Whenever it is anticipated that fluid may collect in a body area postoperatively, thus leading to delay of healing, the surgeon usually inserts a tube or drain to permit escape of the fluid. One end of the tube or drain is placed in or near the organ or cavity to be drained and the other end passed through the body wall either through a separate "stab wound" or occasionally through the incision. *Tubes* are usually inserted to prevent blockage of a passageway, such as the common bile duct (Fig. 24-9), or when suction is desired (Fig. 24-10); therefore these tubes are connected immediately to a drainage system. *Drains* are made of soft rubber material and the ends are left bound within the dressing. The two most commonly used drains are the *Penrose drain* and the *cigarette drain* (a gauze wick covered by a Penrose drain) (Fig. 24-11). A safety pin is pinned to the external end of the soft rubber drain to prevent the

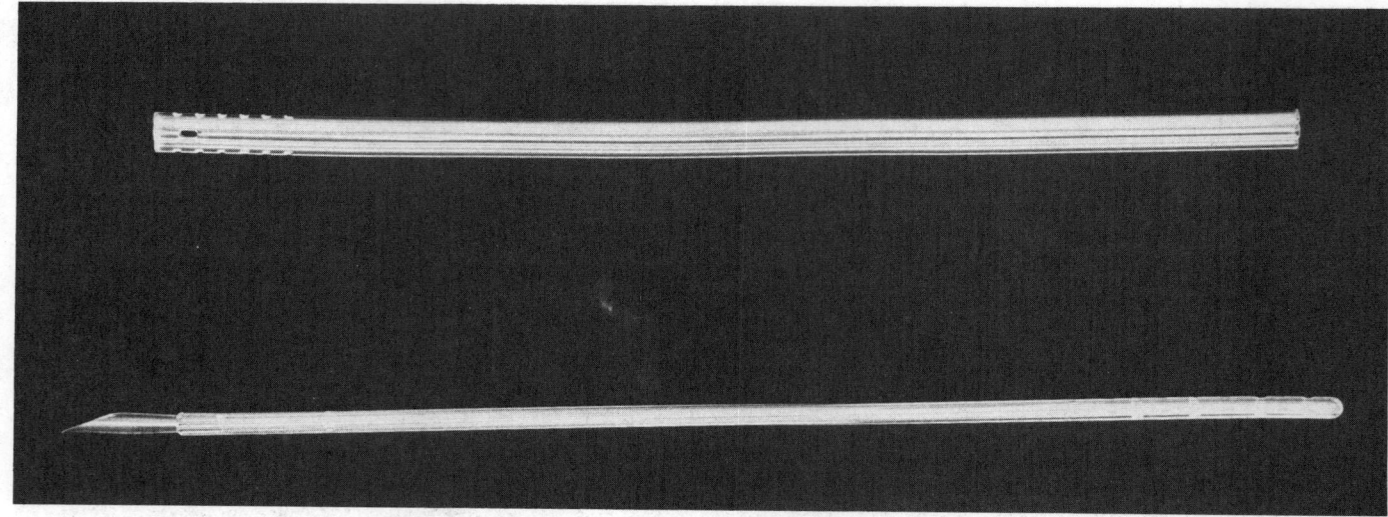

Fig. 24-10. Surgical drain tubes. *Top,* Abramson all-purpose drain has three lumens: for aspiration, irrigation, and instillation. *Bottom,* Saratoga sump drain has a tube within a tube for low-pressure suction.

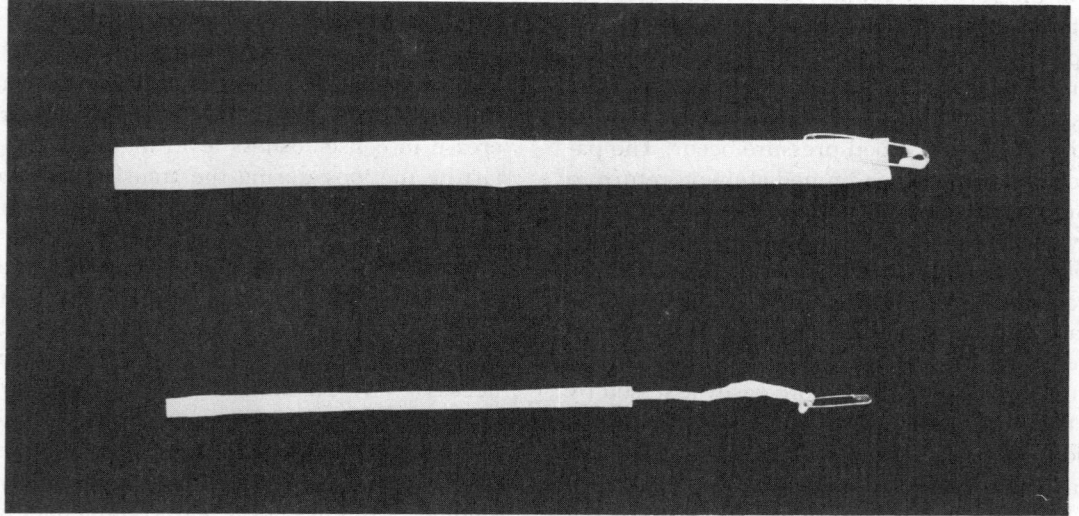

Fig. 24-11. Wound drains. *Top,* Penrose drain. *Bottom,* Cigarette drain.

drain from sliding back into the abdomen. If a large amount of drainage onto the dressing is expected after surgery, such as occurs with certain types of urinary surgery, Montgomery straps will have been applied after surgery so that the dressing can be changed frequently.

After most types of surgery, the surgeon usually changes the dressing for the first time. If small amounts of unexpected drainage occur, especially bright red drainage, the area can be outlined with a pen on the dressing so that the rate of increase can be easily determined. Dressings that *cannot* be changed by the nurse are reinforced with dry dressings if drainage penetrates the outer layer; this prevents bacterial contamination

by capillary action through the wet dressings. If these additional dressings become wet, they are removed and replaced with new dressings, leaving the original dressing intact. Dressings that *can* be changed by the nurse are changed as often as necessary to prevent maceration of the skin and to promote patient comfort. If a drain is present, the end of the drain is placed over a dry dressing then covered by additional dressings. The drain is not permitted to drain directly onto the skin, since this contributes to skin maceration.

Medicated sprays forming a transparent film on the skin may be used as a dressing over clean incisions. The film lasts 3 to 4 days; it may be removed with acetone or will flake and peel off eventually. This type of dress-

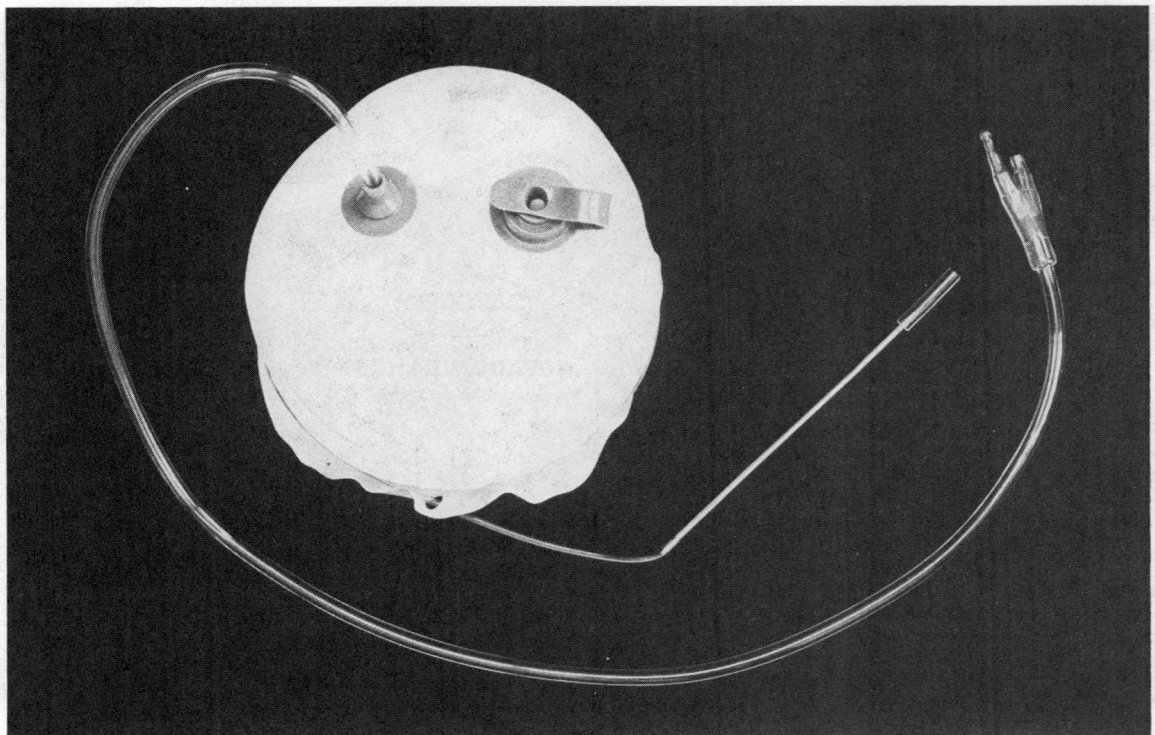

Fig. 24-12. Hemovac apparatus. Top and bottom are pressed together with pouring spout open. When spout is closed, an inner spring slowly expands unit, creating low-pressure suction through tube.

ing is particularly useful in covering wounds in children. Occasionally, surgeons leave an operative wound uncovered, believing that healing progresses best when the wound is exposed to the air.

The nurse should assess the need for restraints with a small child who may be tampering with the wound or dressing. The age of the child, ability to reason, presence and anxiety level of family members, type of surgery, actions of medications given, and safety of the child are factors utilized by the nurse in assessing the need for any type of restraint.

BODY POSITION. The patient is placed in a position of comfort and one that facilitates good ventilation. Except after spinal anesthesia or in certain types of eye surgery or neurosurgery when the bed must remain flat, most patients prefer the head of the bed slightly elevated. The patient who is not very alert needs to be placed in a position of good alignment. There should not be any strain placed on the area surrounding the incision. Pillows should *not* exert pressure on the popliteal area (behind the knee), since this leads to venous obstruction. A side-lying position is used for the unconscious patient to prevent airway obstruction.

Assessment of environmental factors

Equipment. All equipment at the bedside is checked for functioning. Monitors are connected to the patient

and visual patterns should be in working order. Fluids may be ordered to be given to the patient intravenously or instilled in body cavities for irrigation such as in the bladder. The contents of the fluid containers, the patency of the tubing, and the rate of fluid administration are checked. Intravenous fluids are usually given at rates ranging from minimal (to keep the line open, K/O) to 3 ml/min. If the rate is greater than 3 ml/min, and if the physician's order sheet is not available in the patient's room, the rate should be slowed, the order checked immediately, and the rate adjusted appropriately. Rate of administration varies with the amount of fluid lost, size and age of the patient, and the underlying illness (see Chapter 21). The patient and family should be instructed early concerning permissibility of fluids taken orally.

Drainage from tubes can be accomplished by either gravity or suction. Urinary bags are filled by direct gravity (see p. 1521 for care of the patient with urinary drainage). Intermittent or continuous suction may be used for nasogastric drainage. Constant suction under low negative pressure can be accomplished by a Hemovac (Fig. 24-12), a Jackson-Pratt apparatus (Fig. 24-13), or electric suction. These pumps are used for drainage of incisional areas when large amounts of drainage are anticipated (urologic surgery) or when smaller amounts may delay healing (mastectomy, arthroplasty, radical neck

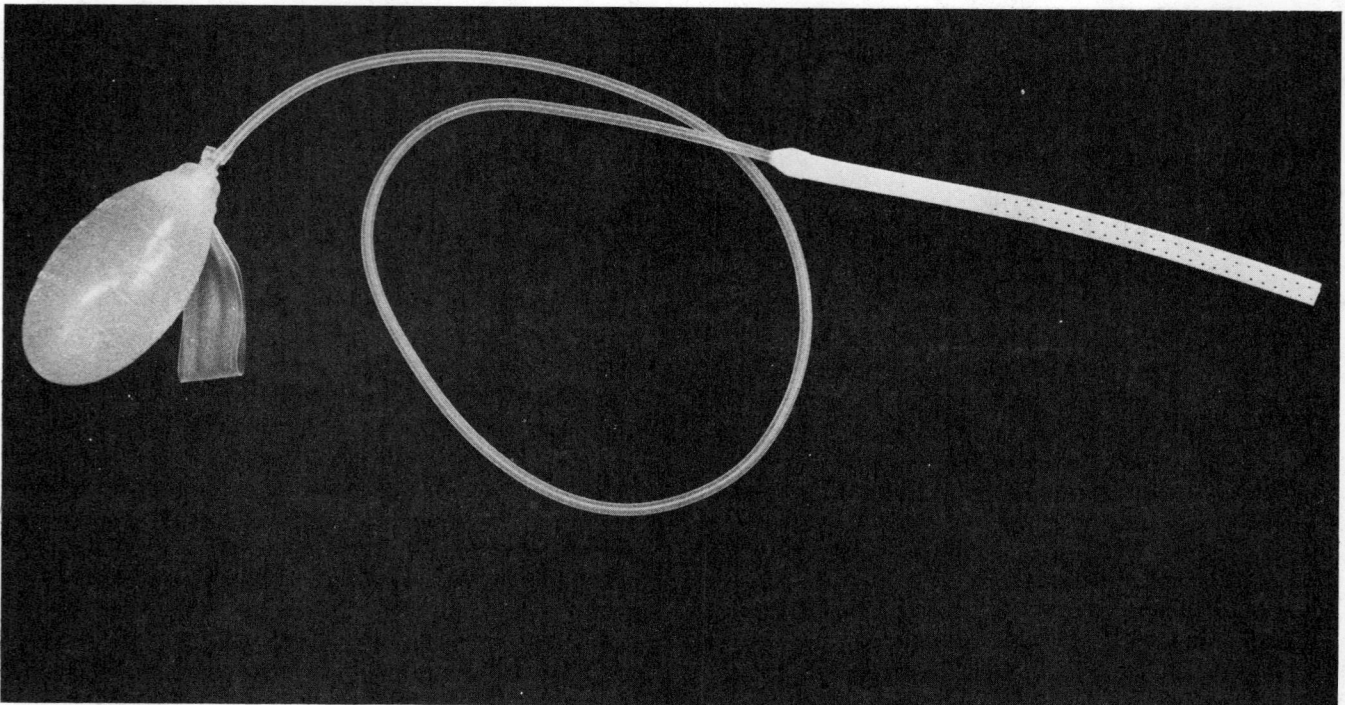

Fig. 24-13. Jackson-Pratt wound suction apparatus. After emptying through spout, reservoir bulb is kept compressed until spout is closed. Slow expansion of bulb creates low-pressure suction.

dissection, amputation). Chest tubes drain by means of a water-seal drainage system by gravity or with added suction. The nurse must be familiar with this type of drainage system before making any connections. All tubing is connected to the drainage receptacle and checked for patency. The amount of fluid in each receptacle is marked on the receptacle and recorded as a baseline for future comparison.

Safety. Side rails of the bed should be kept raised until the patient is fully awake and responding or, if heavily medicated, to prevent falls. There should be easy access to the bed and patient. The patient is instructed early regarding permissibility of ambulation and the need to call for assistance for initial attempts. The call cord should be easily accessible to the patient.

Family members. If the family members are present in the room when the patient returns they may be asked to step outside until the patient has been transferred and assessed. Before leaving the patient the nurse invites the family to return, explains equipment, and describes the patient's state of awareness and comfort. Family members who understand what is occurring can offer support to the patient. Explanations should be simple but concrete and accurate.

Data from patient's chart

Once the initial patient assessment and interventions are completed, the nurse collects the following data from the patient's chart.

Surgeon's orders

1. *Activity.* Range can be from strict bed rest to up as desired. The order should state clearly the extent of activity allowed.
2. *Fluids, food.* Orders for fluids to be given intravenously should include type, amount, and rate. Orders for fluid or food to be taken orally should include type and time these can be started.
3. *Medications.* An order for a pain medication to be given as needed should be included if pain is a possibility. Other medications that need to be reinstituted or started immediately are noted.
4. *Other orders.* These depend on the type of surgery and anesthesia. The nurse should understand the rationale for each order.

Surgical notes

1. *Postoperative diagnosis.* For interpretation to patient or family regarding what the surgeon has told them.
2. *Type of surgery.* For interpretation to patient or family; for direction of specific nursing care.
3. *Anesthetic.* For direction of specific nursing care:
   a. Inhalants: need for active deep-breathing measures.
   b. Muscle relaxants: assessment for respiratory distress.
   c. Spinal: supine position postoperatively; headaches may occur.
4. *Estimated blood loss and fluid replacement.* Po-

tential for fluid and electrolyte imbalance or delayed transfusion reactions.

5. *Drains*. Drainage on the dressing can be expected if a soft Penrose drain is in place.

Recovery room summary

1. *Vital signs before discharge*. Identification of changes in vital signs.
2. *Patient progress*. Identification of problems that may persist.
3. *Medications given*. Identification of time span before next dosage permissible for prn drugs and response by the patient and other medications that have been started.
4. *Urinary output*. Identification of when and how much patient has voided. Urinary suppression may occur with shock; urinary retention may occur from the effects of anesthesia or surgery and may create pressure on abdominal organs or the incision.

Planning patient care

The collected data are recorded in the nursing admission note and utilized to identify the specific needs of the patient in the postoperative period. The preoperative condition of the patient, type of surgery performed, and strengths and resources of the patient are determining factors influencing the occurrence of postoperative discomforts or complications. In planning the patient's care, therefore, the nurse needs to utilize previously collected data, present data, knowledge of factors related to specific types of surgery (as illustrated in succeeding chapters of this text), and specific postoperative needs and possible postoperative complications. Identified problems and specific plans for care are written in the appropriate place on the chart or nursing care plan.

Needs of postoperative patient

All of the individual's basic needs can be affected by the trauma of surgery. Nursing care is directed toward achievement of specific outcomes so that each need is met and the patient has been helped to move toward an optimal level of functioning.

Safety needs

OUTCOME: The person does not fall.

Contributing factors. Next to errors in medication, falls by patients constitute the major reason for incident reports in hospitals. Patients with an increased potential for falls are those who have had extensive surgery or who have had surgery of the extremities. Elderly persons may become confused, especially on the first postoperative night, and may try to get out of bed. Each postoperative patient is assessed to determine the potential for falling.

Assessment. Areas of assessment include level of consciousness, medications given, circulatory adaptability, and physical environment.

LEVEL OF CONSCIOUSNESS. The more alert the patient, the less the possibility of a fall. Decreased alertness may be caused by cerebral hypoxia from blood loss, fluid overload, acid-base imbalances, respiratory insufficiency, shock, hypoglycemia, or chronic brain syndrome.

MEDICATIONS. Many analgesics, sedatives, or tranquilizers produce a feeling of well-being, and the patient may disregard the possibility of weakness and attempt ambulation without assistance. Narcotics may also produce dizziness, and the patient may fall while walking or sitting up in a chair.

CIRCULATORY ADAPTABILITY. The circulatory system is under considerable stress during surgery, and wide fluctuations in vital signs during surgery are common. Orthostatic hypotension (a temporary drop in blood pressure when assuming an upright position) can occur when the patient has been lying flat and inactive for a time. The patient complains of dizziness; pallor and tachycardia can be observed. The patient may fall if ambulating before the blood pressure stabilizes.

MUSCLE STRENGTH. If the patient has been in bed for a time, some muscle strength and tone may be lost. The quadriceps muscles of the legs should be tested for general strength before the patient gets out of bed for the first time. The patient lies flat and flexes the knee with the foot resting on the bed. The nurse places a hand on the lower leg. The patient is then requested to raise the lower leg while the nurse presents resistance. Weak quadriceps muscles indicate decreased ability to stand and walk.

PHYSICAL ENVIRONMENT. The room must be examined for possible physical causes for falls such as equipment or footstools in the path of ambulation to the patient's chair, door, or bathroom, or water spilled on the floor.

Intervention

PATIENT WEAKNESS. If the patient is not alert or is very weak, side rails are kept raised at all times. Patients who attempt to climb over the side rails may need constant attention by a family member. The call cord can be pinned to the gown of a confused patient so that excessive movements can be checked readily. Restraints should be used judiciously and only when really necessary. A Hi-Lo bed may be left in low position to decrease the distance to the floor. An ambulatory patient who has difficulty moving because of an incision can get out of bed more easily and safely if the bed is at chair level. Patients who are receiving parenteral narcotics for pain should not ambulate alone.

Patients sitting up to "dangle" or to get up for the first time after surgery should assume a sitting position gradually, with assistance as necessary, and not be permitted to stand until the pulse has essentially stabilized to the baseline level and the patient no longer feels faint. The pulse is taken *before* the patient sits up as well as after sitting on the side of the bed.

Leg exercises should be carried out by the bedfast patient to prevent loss of muscle tone and to strengthen weakened muscles (Fig. 24-3). Patients with weak leg muscles will need greater support during standing and walking in order to prevent a fall.

PHYSICAL ENVIRONMENT. The equipment and furniture in the room are arranged to promote large open spaces for safe ambulation. Electrical cords should be against the walls or under the bed if posssible. Footstools are used only if needed and kept under the bed when not in use. Portable poles for holding intravenous fluids should have large easily movable wheels. During early ambulation or if the patient is weak, he should not hold onto the pole when ambulating. The floor should be free of debris and water.

Promotion of wound healing

OUTCOME: Incision heals normally; there is no purulent discharge.

Pathophysiology of wound healing

RESULT OF WOUND HEALING. Wounds may heal by *regeneration* of the tissue or by *scar formation*. The type of cells that constitute the tissue determines the end result. There are three types of cells: labile cells, stable cells, and permanent cells. *Labile* cells multiply throughout life, constantly replacing similar cells being destroyed. Regrowth is through regeneration of marginal cells. Examples of labile cells are those of the skin and mucous membranes and the blood cells. *Stable* cells, occurring in bone or functional cells of glandular organs, do not usually multiply vigorously but will do so if injured. Both labile and stable cells necessitate an underlying structure; they will not grow across an empty space. Thus if the framework is intact, there will be regeneration of normal structure. If the framework is destroyed, scarring will occur.

Permanent cells are the main constituents of muscle and nerve tissues. These cells rarely undergo mitotic division and are unable to regenerate. Muscle cells in striated, smooth, and cardiac muscles therefore do not regenerate. Satisfactory performance may result by hypertrophy of the preserved marginal cells. Nerve cells of the central nervous system do not regenerate. In the peripheral nervous system there is no regeneration if the cell body is destroyed. If the axon is injured there is degeneration of the injured part to the closest node of Ranvier; then regeneration will occur. Destruction of permanent cells results in scarring. A typical surgical incision cuts into muscle tissue. Although the epithelial cells regenerate over the scar tissue, the epithelial layer is so thin that the scar tissue is visible.

TYPES OF WOUND HEALING. Tissues may heal by one of three ways: primary, secondary, or tertiary intention. Most surgical wounds heal by *primary intention;* the incision is a clean straight line and all layers of the wound (muscle, subcutaneous tissue, and epithelial tissue) are well approximated by suturing. These wounds, if they remain free of infection and do not separate, heal quickly with a minimum of scarring. Wounds such as ulcers have edges that cannot be approximated; healing occurs by a filling in of the wound by granulation tissue over a larger area. This is healing by *secondary intention*. Because these wounds are more open they have a greater possibility for infection. More granulation tissue is formed than in healing by primary intention; therefore more scarring occurs. Healing by *tertiary intention* occurs when there is a delay between injury and suturing; greater granulation tissue will be formed than with primary intention but less than with secondary intention.

PROCESS OF WOUND HEALING. Regardless of the type of wound healing, the process is the same. The difference is in the length of time for each phase of healing and the extent of granulation tissue formed.

When there is injury to tissue, two major responses occur: the stress response (see Chapter 18) and the inflammatory response (see Chapter 19). The inflammatory response serves to prepare the tissue so that wound healing can take place (Fig. 24-14). During the cellular exudation, leukocytes (white blood cells) invade the injured area to ingest bacteria and debris (phagocytosis). Fibroblasts also migrate from the blood vessesls and deposit fibrin, a threadlike substance that stretches through the clot that has sealed the wound. Adjacent blood vessels begin to develop buds that stretch across the wound using the fibrin for support. When the capillary buds reach across the wound they cannulize, establishing blood flow across the wound. A thin layer of epithelial cells migrate across the wound and help to seal the wound. This is *phase I;* the wound strength is low, although sutured wounds will hold together if sutured correctly. With major surgery the patient looks and feels ill during phase I.

Phase II lasts approximately from day 3 to day 14 in surgical wounds. The leukocytes start disappearing and the fibroblasts start filling in spaces in the network with *collagen*, a white protein fiber. All layers of epithelial cells are completely regenerated in about 1 week. The new tissue is a highly vascular connective tissue, reddish in color from the numerous blood vessels, and is called *granulation tissue*. If scraped, this tissue will bleed readily. The patient begins to look and feel better.

The collagen that is deposited will provide good support for the wound in 6 to 7 days so that stitches can

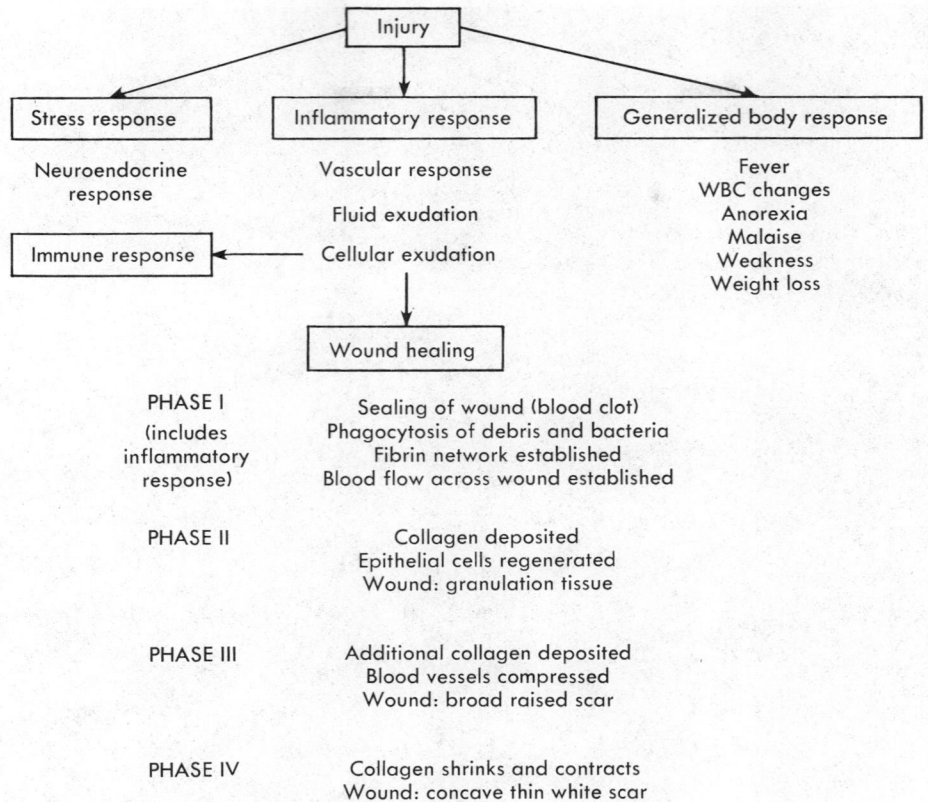

Fig. 24-14. Response of body to injury.

be removed, and there will be normal tissue strength by 2 weeks. Commonly used skin sutures include black silk, metal staples, fine wire, or metal skin clips. Stapling is the newest approach and consists of stapling a superficial layer of the wound edges (Fig. 24-15) by the use of a special skin stapler (Fig. 24-16). The staples do not penetrate deeper tissue layers. Although wound union is weak until after the sixth postoperative day, the sutures permit the patient to deep breathe, cough, and move around or ambulate without danger of wound separation. It is important for patients to know this; otherwise, they may be reluctant to carry out these activities.

Skin sutures are removed from abdominal wounds on about the seventh postoperative day, from neck and face wounds on about the third to the fifth postoperative day, and from wounds of the extremities on the eighth to tenth postoperative day. Retention sutures made of heavy wire and placed deep into muscle tissue usually are not removed until the fourteenth to the twenty-first postoperative day. Most patients become apprehensive when they know the sutures are to be removed. It is helpful to tell them that they will have little if any pain during the procedure; the deeper retention sutures do cause discomfort. Unless there is some seepage of fluid after the sutures are removed, a dressing is not necessary and the area may be washed.

During *phase III* collagen continues to be deposited. This compresses the new blood vessels and blood flow decreases. The wound at this time looks like a broad pinkish raised scar. During this phase, which lasts from about the second to the sixth week after surgery, the patient should avoid heavy use of the affected muscles.

The final phase, *phase IV*, lasts for several months after surgery. The patient may complain of itching around the wound. Although collagen continues to be deposited during this time, there is shrinkage and contraction of the wound. If the wound is near a joint, contractures may occur. Because of the shrinkage the wound becomes a concave thin white line. Scar tissue is acellular, avascular collagen tissue. It will not tan with sunlight nor will it sweat or produce hair.

Factors influencing wound healing. Some of the factors that affect patient responses to surgery (p. 403) are directly related to wound healing. Research to date has not discovered anything that will hasten wound healing. There are, however, a number of factors that can prolong the healing process.

AGE. Wounds in children normally heal more rapidly than in adults. Children have increased metabolism and good circulation. Wounds in the elderly often heal more slowly because of decreased fibroblastic activity and impaired circulation.

NUTRITION. Persons with inadequate vitamin C or

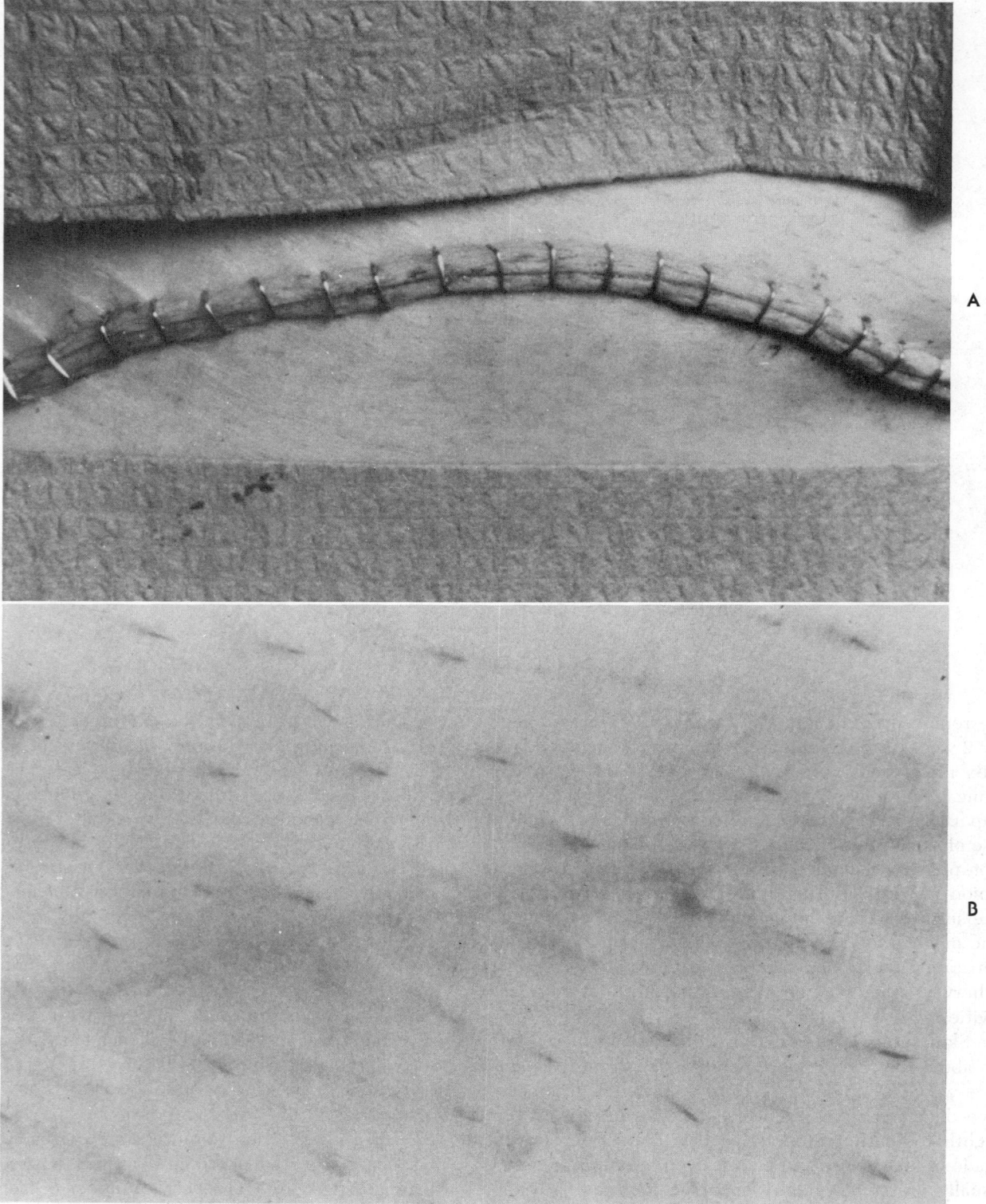

Fig. 24-15. Skin staples used for wound closure. **A,** Immediately after surgery. Note staples grasping only superficial layer of skin. **B,** Same site 6 months later. (Courtesy Ethicon Inc., Somerville, N.J.)

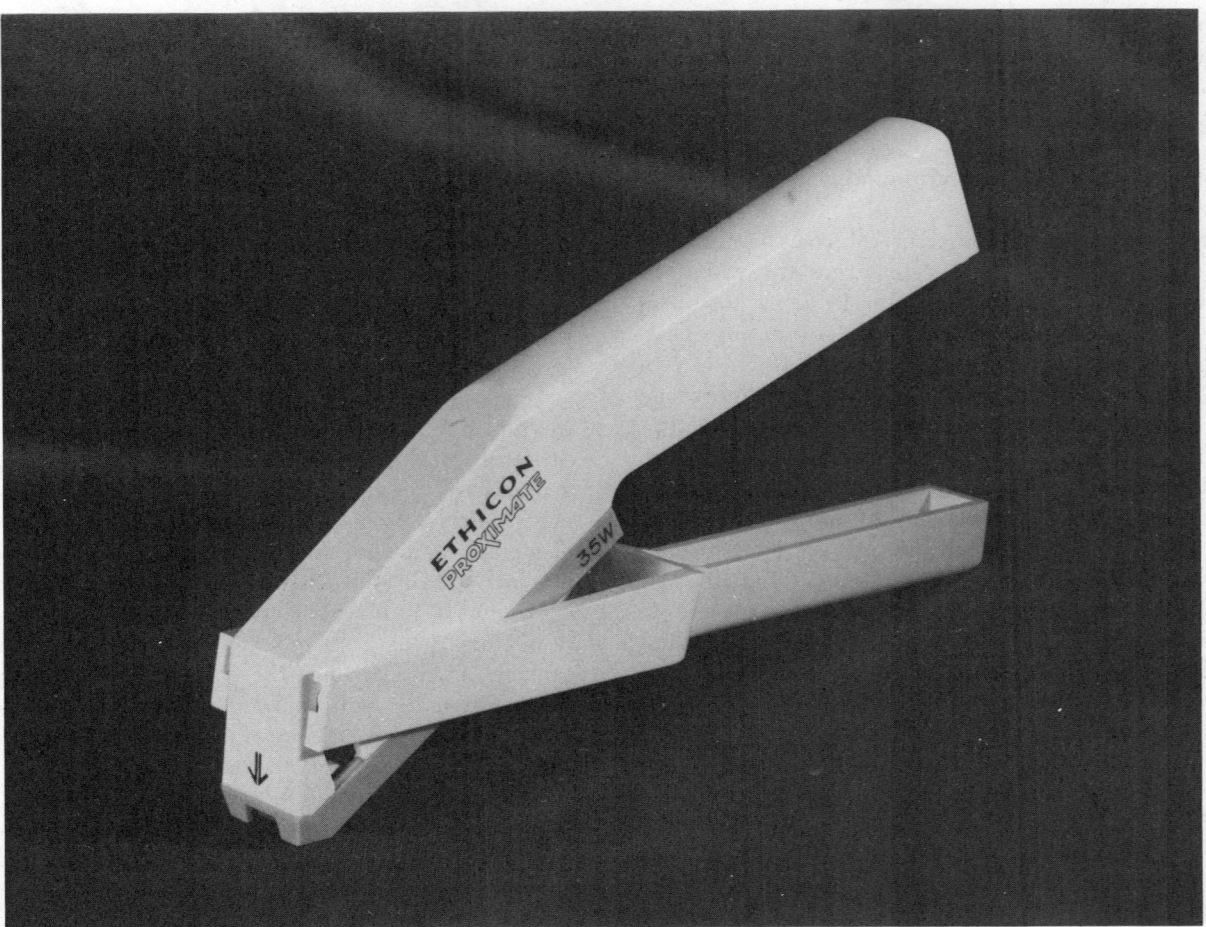

Fig. 24-16. Disposable skin stapler. (Courtesy Ethicon Inc., Somerville, N.J.)

protein intake will have delayed healing. Vitamin C is necessary for collagen formation. It is also necessary to maintain the integrity of the capillary walls. Protein is the major constituent of collagen.

CIRCULATION. Adequate circulation to the injured tissue is important to provide the white blood cells, fibroblasts, and nutrients needed for healing and to remove the debris after phagocytosis. Subcutaneous tissue is poorly supplied with blood vessels; therefore wounds of obese patients may heal more slowly. Patients with peripheral vascular disease will have impaired circulation to the legs causing delayed healing of leg ulcers.

ENDOCRINE FUNCTION. Steroids have an antiinflammatory effect and delay healing by depressing the inflammatory reaction that precedes wound healing. Cortisone also interferes with collagen formation. Patients with diabetes mellitus have decreased movement of leukocytes to the site and may have impaired circulation, which will delay healing.

PRESENCE OF FOREIGN BODIES. Most foreign bodies are not sterile and create an excessive inflammatory re-

action and infection when present in a wound. Foreign bodies are usually removed unless removing them will cause more damage than their being left in the tissue.

INFECTION. A contaminated wound usually becomes infected. There is a greater inflammatory response as the white blood cells fight the invading microorganisms. A wound that is infected will not heal until the infection is cleared up. The greater the number of bacteria or amount of necrotic tissue present, the longer healing will be delayed.

DEAD SPACE. If fluid collects in a closed area where tissue has been removed, a space will occur where tissue healing does not take place. Cells above this dead space may break down in the absence of underlying support. This occurs in surgery such as mastectomy, radical neck dissection, or arthroplasty. Low-pressure suction is often used to remove the fluid so that healing will not be delayed.

RADIATION. Direct radiation of the wound after surgery may slow the development of blood vessels through the wound. Heavy radiation may cause necrosis of the wound.

WOUND SEPARATION. When dehiscence (separation of previously joined edges) occurs, the wound is resutured if infection is not present. The separated area must restart the healing process, and healing occurs by tertiary intention.

Complications of wound healing

HEMORRHAGE

Pathophysiology. External or internal hemorrhage may occur. Although hemorrhage from the wound is most likely to occur within the first 48 hours postoperatively, it may occur as late as the sixth or seventh postoperative day in apparently normal wounds and after a much longer time if the wound is infected. Hemorrhage occurring soon after operation may be due to the slipping of a ligature or the mechanical dislodging of a clot, caused, for example, by vomiting after a tonsillectomy. During surgery small vessels may go unnoticed because of decreased blood pressure or use of a tourniquet. These vessels will not be properly obliterated and hemorrhage may occur with the reestablishment of blood flow. Hemorrhage after a few days may be due to sloughing of a clot or of tissue, to infection, or to erosion of a blood vessel by a drainage tube.

Assessment. Dressings are checked at frequent intervals during the first 48 hours and at least once every 8 hours thereafter. Subjectively, the patient may complain of a wet sensation on the skin or dressing or of feeling restless or weak. Any postoperative patient who complains of an uneasy, restless feeling, such as "Something is wrong, but I don't know what," should be checked for signs of hemorrhage.

Objective data would include signs of shock (tachycardia, weak thready pulse, cold clammy skin, fall in blood pressure or central venous pressure or decreased urinary output). Bright red blood may be present on the dressing or coming from a drainage tube.

Intervention. The physician is notified of any signs of increased bleeding or shock. A small amount of bleeding on the dressing is outlined with a pen and rechecked at 10- to 15-minute intervals for signs of change. If there is bleeding from a tube into a container, the drainage is marked with the time and the amount so that the rapidity of bleeding can be determined at frequent intervals. If the bleeding is profuse, measures to control bleeding are instituted if possible; for example, a pressure dressing is applied over the existing dressing and measures to treat shock are started immediately (p. 317). Constant monitoring of vital signs is important. A calm environment is necessary so that increased anxiety does not add further stress to the patient's system.

If the bleeding is from an open cavity such as the nose, the cavity may be packed or an exposed bleeder cauterized by the surgeon. The patient who is bleeding internally or in profuse amounts externally is usually returned immediately to surgery where the incision is opened and the bleeding vessel is ligated. Intravenous fluids will be started and the patient's blood typed and cross-matched for transfusion before surgery. If a preanesthetic medication is ordered, the time when the last narcotic was given should be checked. Under pressure of the emergency there is danger of the patient receiving an overdose of narcotics. It should also be remembered that during shock peripheral circulation is decreased, resulting in poor absorption of medication from the tissue. Respiratory depression can occur when the shock is corrected and narcotics in the tissue from previous injections are rapidly absorbed.

INFECTION

Pathophysiology. Surgical wound infections are caused by introduction of organisms into the open wound. Streptococcus, staphylococcus, and *Pseudomonas* organisms are the most frequent causes of infection. Modern surgical suites are designed to minimize the entry of organisms during the surgical procedure. Dry dressings are usually not disturbed until the sutures are to be removed, to prevent contamination during phase I of healing. Wet dressings have a greater potential for causing infections, since the bacteria can travel by capillary action through the wet dressing to the wound. Whether a wound becomes infected depends on factors intrinsic to the patient, factors that can delay healing, and the aseptic technique utilized by health personnel (physician, nurse). Whenever there is an open or draining wound, aseptic technique must be scrupulously followed. Infection control teams in hospitals are responsible for monitoring the incidence of wound infections (see Chapter 22).

Assessment. The patient may complain of persistent pain in the incisional area and a feeling of general malaise. Pain is caused by stimulation of the nerve endings from the increased inflammation and by pressure from edema. The malaise is a systemic reaction to infection.

Objective signs include fever after the third postoperative day, increased white blood cell count (leukocytosis), incisional swelling, and erythema. There may be purulent drainage on the dressing. Wound culture and sensitivity studies should be obtained from the infected wound to determine the causative organism.

Intervention. Some patients are at high risk of developing a postoperative infection, either because of the presence of intrinsic factors that may delay healing or because of the type of surgery in which there is an increased number of bacteria present, such as with intestinal, pharyngeal, or biliary surgery. The end result of other surgeries, such as total hip replacement or vascular grafts, may be severely compromised if an infection does occur. In these situations antimicrobial prophylaxis may be instituted *preoperatively* so that adequate antibiotic levels are achieved before contamination occurs. The antimicrobial therapy is terminated either during surgery or within the first 24 hours after surgery to lessen the possibility of resistant bacterial strains. The more commonly used antimicrobials are the cephalosporins, the semisynthetic penicillins, erythromycin, and clindamycin.

Prevention of wound infection is an important nursing measure. All open wound dressing changes are carried out under sterile conditions. Sterile gloves or instruments are used when cleaning an open wound and applying the sterile dressings. Soiled wet dressings should be changed immediately to prevent tissue breakdown from maceration and infection. Sterile moist dressings are covered with a dry sterile cover. The nutritional needs of the patient are assessed and interventions carried out when a deficiency is present that may delay healing.

If a wound infection does occur, the physician may open the wound to facilitate drainage if spontaneous drainage has not already taken place. Wound discomfort usually disappears after the wound has drained. A small drain may be placed in the wound to facilitate drainage, and irrigations may be ordered to wash away debris of infection. Purulent drainage is cleansed from the skin since pus contains proteolytic enzymes that can cause skin breakdown. The pus is sent to the laboratory for culture and sensitivity studies before antibiotics are given to control the infection. To maintain adequate blood levels the antibiotics must be given at the scheduled times.

WOUND DEHISCENCE AND EVISCERATION

Pathophysiology. Wound disruption (dehiscence) is a partial to complete separation of the wound edges. Wound evisceration is protrusion of abdominal viscera through the incision and onto the abdominal wall (Fig. 24-17).

Wound separation that occurs during phase I (first 3 days) is usually related to technical factors such as the suturing. During phase II (3 to 14 days) it is usually associated with postoperative complications such as distention, vomiting, excessive coughing, dehydration, or infection. Many of these complications can be prevented by careful assessment and continued monitoring and by the institution of vigorous preventive measures (ventilatory exercises, ambulation, adequate fluid intake, aseptic technique) on the part of the nurse. Wound separation during phase III (after 2 weeks) is usually associated with metabolic factors such as cachexia, hypoproteinemia or avitaminosis, increased age, decreased resistance to infection, malignancy, multiple trauma, or hypothermia. These factors can also cause wound separation at an earlier time.

Assessment. Subjectively, the patient may complain of a "giving" sensation at the incision or a feeling of wetness. If evisceration has occurred and if a loop of bowel has obstructed, the patient will complain of severe localized pain at the incision. On inspection the dressing will be found to be saturated with clear pink drainage. The wound edges may be partially or entirely

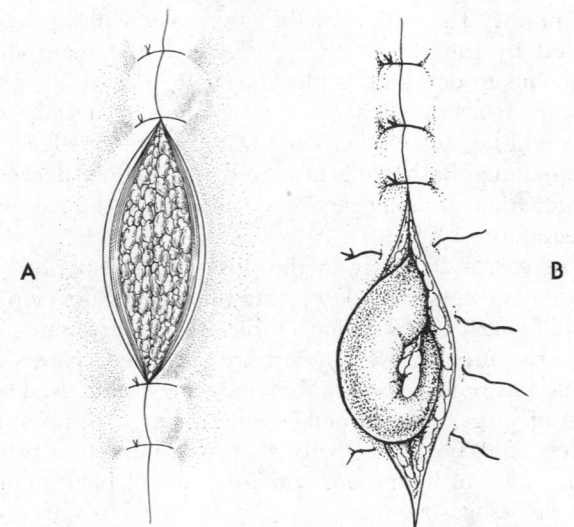

Fig. 24-17. A, Wound dehiscence. Wound edges are partially separated. **B,** Wound evisceration. Viscera protrude through incision.

separated, and loops of intestine may be lying on the abdominal wall. Signs of shock may be present.

Intervention. A patient who experiences either a wound dehiscence or wound evisceration is put to bed in low Fowler's position and told to remain quiet, not to cough, and not to eat or drink anything until the surgeon arrives. Protruding viscera are covered, preferably with a warm, sterile saline dressing. Interventions for shock are initiated if signs of shock are present. The surgeon will cover the wound after inspection.

The treatment for wound dehiscence and wound evisceration is immediate closure of the wound under local or general anesthesia. If the patient is in shock, the preanesthetic medication may be omitted. Convalescence is usually prolonged, although the wound usually heals surprisingly well after secondary closure.

Oxygen needs

OUTCOME: Pulmonary complications do not occur; breath sounds are clear.

Pathophysiology. Many of the respiratory complications that occur in the postoperative patient can be prevented by nursing management. The most common respiratory complications are atelectasis and hypostatic pneumonia. In atelectasis a bronchiole becomes blocked by secretions and the distal alveoli collapse as the existing air is absorbed. This produces hypoventilation. A major bronchus (indicating the main stem bronchus) or many small bronchioles may be involved. The latter situation is frequently undetected because there are few symptoms. The extent of the atelectasis will be determined by the site of the blockage; if the main stem bronchus to one lung is blocked, that lung will be atelectatic. If a bronchus going to a lobe is blocked, that lobe will be atelectatic. Stasis of the secretions leads to pneumonia. Both atelectasis and pneumonia decrease oxygenation, prolong recovery, and add to the patient's discomfort.

Assessment. Early in the postoperative period the patient is assessed to determine the risk for developing a pulmonary complication (Table 24-3). Pertinent data from the preoperative period are reviewed. New data in the postoperative period include anesthetic used and type of surgery performed, medications given preoperatively and postoperatively that will influence secretions, state of hydration, and presence of pain, vomiting, or nasogastric tube.

Inspection of the patient will determine the amount of activity being carried out (movement in bed, ambulation) and position in bed. Respirations are monitored closely. Hypoventilation is indicated by rapid shallow respirations and absent or diminished breath sounds in the lower lobes. Depth of respirations is an important criterion because the alveoli are poorly ventilated when respirations are shallow. Chest expansion is observed during inspiration; if the chest is held fairly rigid, there will be decreased ventilation.

Auscultation of the lungs allows the nurse to detect both hypoventilation of specific lobes (breath sounds will be diminished) and the presence of secretions (rales will be heard). The lungs should be free of rales, but diminished breath sounds may be present during the first 24 hours after surgery.[71]

Presence of a productive cough during the first few days postoperatively is a positive sign that the patient is able to clear the bronchial secretions that might otherwise block the bronchioles. The productiveness of the cough usually decreases as secretions diminish.

An unexplained rise in temperature is often the first sign of atelectasis. Pulse and respiratory rates increase. If a large bronchus is blocked, the patient may exhibit dyspnea and cyanosis and signs of shock. Diagnosis is confirmed by chest radiography. Pneumonia also produces fever, dyspnea, chest pain, and a cough productive of mucopurulent sputum.

Intervention. Prevention of respiratory complications is an area where nursing care provides a key to a smooth postoperative recovery. The use of "routines," however, is not the answer. It is common to find postoperative routines that read "Turn, cough, and deep breath every 2 hours"; the order is never changed. In reality, some patients need ventilatory exercises more often than every 2 hours, others less. Most patients after general anesthesia will need to ventilate their lungs well at least every 1 to 2 hours the first postoperative day, and then every 3 to 4 hours while awake for sev-

eral days if not active. The decision for the type and frequency of preventive respiratory measures should be based on each patient's risk factors and hour-by-hour and day-by-day response. Measures that work effectively in increasing ventilation in one patient may be less effective in another.

A plan should be developed for each patient that best meets oxygen needs. For example, an elderly patient with a history of lung disease, who smokes and has just had high abdominal surgery with an inhalant anesthetic, may need to carry out ventilatory maneuvers as often as every 30 to 60 minutes during the first few hours postoperatively. A young patient with no history of smoking or lung disease, who had preoperative medication and an inhalant anesthetic and who is up ambulating frequently after surgery, may need breathing exercises only every 2 to 3 hours the first day and none thereafter. Reassessment is important, and the plan of care should be updated as the risk factors change.

VENTILATORY MEASURES. There are a number of ventilatory maneuvers that can be used in the postoperative period to prevent atelectasis by inflating the alveoli as fully as possible. Once the alveoli are fully inflated they will remain open for at least 1 hour.[64] The two most effective ventilatory maneuvers that lead to maximal alveolar inflation are the yawn maneuver and the incentive spirometer.

The initiation of the *yawn maneuver* by the patient is easy, especially if demonstrated by the nurse since a yawn is often initiated by seeing another person do it. The patient is asked to take a deep breath with the mouth open and to hold the breath for more than 3 seconds.[21] The yawn is spontaneous and once the yawn starts, it is difficult to stop from taking a deep inspiration. *Deep-breathing exercises* using diaphragmatic breathing (p. 1242) are also useful, but the effectiveness depends on the depth of respiration taken by the patient. Patients with chest or abdominal incisions tend to restrict respiratory excursion, which limits the extent of alveolar inflation.

Patients who use an *incentive spirometer* have significantly fewer and milder respiratory problems than those who use blow bottles or intermittent positive pressure machines.[64] The incentive spirometer is a mechanical device that promotes sustained maximal inspiration. Maximal effect occurs when the full inspiration is held for at least 3 seconds.[126] Only minimal patient instruction is required. The patient breathes in through the mouth piece as deeply as possible and holds the breath for at least 3 seconds if possible. Expiration is passive. There are several incentive spirometers on the market, and each has some way of demonstrating to the patient how much volume has been inspired to serve as an encouragement for the patient to achieve greater inspiratory effort (Fig. 24-18). The patient should take three to five normal breaths between each deep breath to

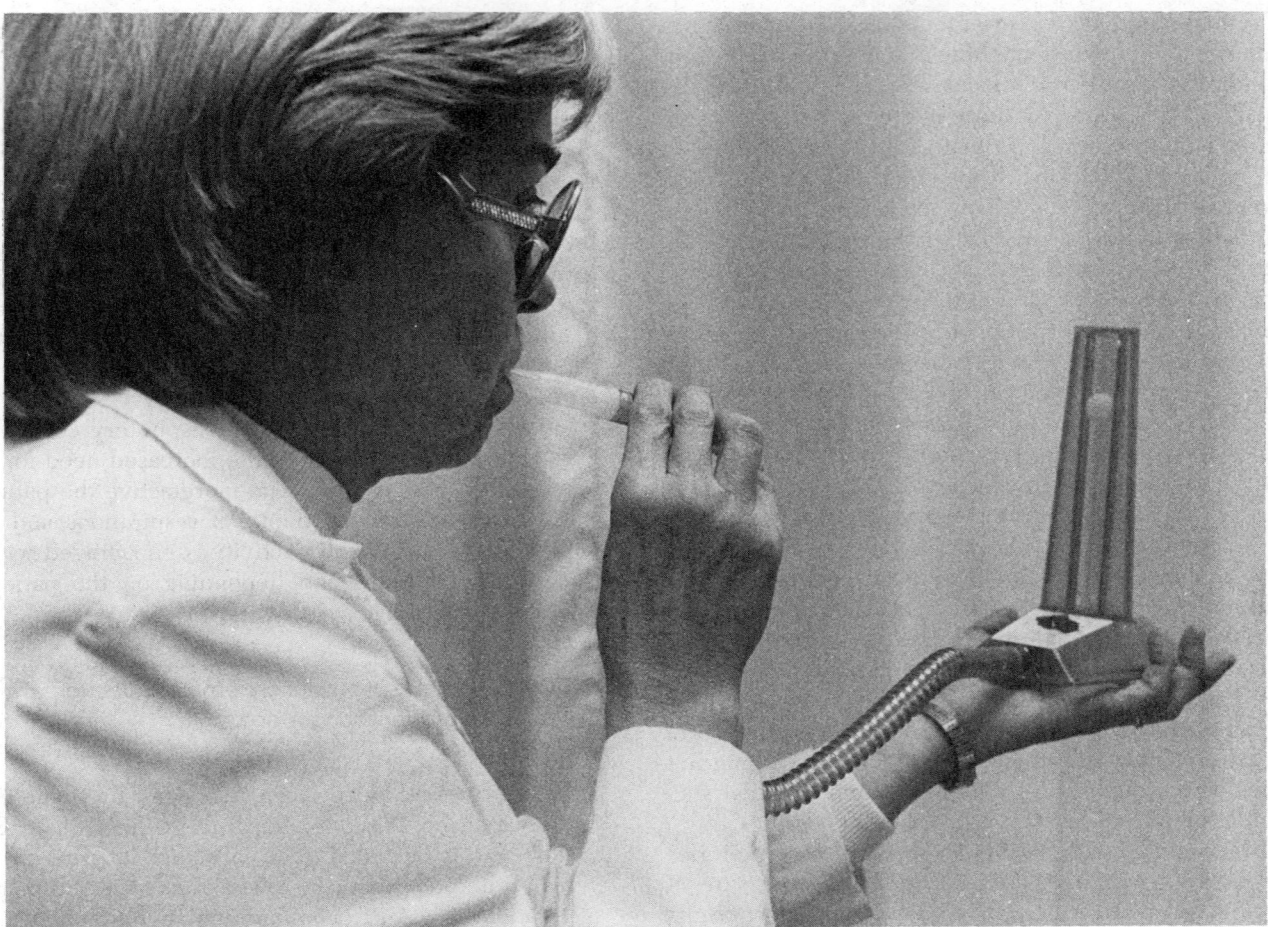

Fig. 24-18. Incentive spirometer. Ball rising with inspiration is a visual cue for patient. Ball remains up as patient holds breath for 3 seconds.

prevent dizziness and light-headedness. Use of the incentive spirometer at mealtimes may cause nausea.

Blow bottles (p. 1243) have been used for a number of years but are less effective than the incentive spirometer. Since the use of blow bottles results in forced expiration against a closed glottis (Valsalva's maneuver), blow bottles should be avoided for persons with known cardiac problems. During Valsalva's maneuver, intrathoracic pressure is increased, interfering with venous return to the heart and lowering blood pressure. When the intrathoracic pressure returns to normal at the end of the forced expiration, there is a sudden surge of venous return to the heart increasing the cardiac work load and raising blood pressure beyond the usual range. Blood pressure then returns to normal.

Rebreathing tubes are used less frequently since the advent of the newer more effective measures, but they are an alternative method to encourage deep breathing. The patient breathes in and out of a long coiled tube that is open at the opposite end. If breathing is shallow,

the air in the tube is not replaced by fresh air and the increased accumulation of carbon dioxide in the tube stimulates the patient to breathe deeper. With deep inspiration the air in the tube is replaced by fresh air.

Intermittent positive pressure breathing (IPPB) is much more difficult for the patient, and it has failed to demonstrate effectiveness in preventing postoperative atelectasis or promoting more rapid clearing of pneumonia.

The nurse may institute any of the ventilatory measures and should be familiar with the advantages and disadvantages of each. It is important to remember that many patients are drowsy or have periods of amnesia during the early postoperative period, so that frequently the *instructions must be repeated*. Persons who have had good instruction in the preoperative phase are usually better able to carry out the measures postoperatively.

All of the ventilatory measures used by the surgical patient are followed by *deep coughing* to remove any secretions that have been loosened. Deep breathing in itself often stimulates coughing. Coughing may be contraindicated in a few instances such as following brain, spinal, or eye surgery because of the increased intracranial or intraocular pressure that can result. Patients with incisions can be told that it may be painful to cough but that assistance will be given. Narcotics given before ventilation exercises may facilitate cooperation of the patient; on the other hand, narcotics decrease the cough reflex and depress respirations. Some patients are afraid that the incision will split open while they are coughing and should be told that the incision can be splinted during coughing. Splinting of the incision can be accomplished by means of a drawsheet or towel, small pillow, or placement of the hands firmly on either side of the incision and with exertion of slight pressure (see Fig. 49-15). Such splinting prevents excessive muscular strain around the incision.

A shallow cough is ineffective in mobilizing secretions and produces fatigue; therefore the patient should be encouraged to cough deeply and productively. If the first attempt is not successful, the patient should rest, then try again. Auscultation of the lungs before and after ventilatory measures provides data for evaluation of the effectiveness. If the patient has noisy breathing but is unable to cough up secretions, respiratory tract suctioning may be required.

The most effective position for ventilatory exercises is high Fowler's, since this decreases the pressure of the abdominal contents on the diaphragm and permits better thorax expansion. If the patient must remain flat in bed, restraining bedclothes and pillows are removed from around the chest.

POSITIONING AND TURNING. If the patient lies in one position with continuous pressure from body weight against the chest wall, proper ventilation and drainage of secretions on that side of the chest are not possible and atelectasis can develop (Fig. 24-19). Turning and changing of position frequently (at least every 2 to 3 hours) provide for better ventilation of the lungs. The patient should be encouraged to help in turning. Most patients assume a supine position and are not eager to change position because of the increased pain during movement. They may find side rails useful for turning during the early postoperative period. Assistance can be given by supporting a limb or helping the patient to turn in one smooth movement. Alternating the height of the bed is useful: high Fowler's position facilitates diaphragm movement; low Fowler's or a flat position facilitates drainage and expectoration of respiratory secretions.

ACTIVITY. Stimulation of the respiratory center occurs with activity because of the increased need for oxygen at the cellular level. The more active the patient, the greater will be the depth of respirations and the ventilation of the alveoli. Activity is encouraged within the prescribed limits and depending on the patient's tolerance to activity.

OUTCOME: Peripheral circulation remains adequate; no calf pain or vascular changes occur.

Pathophysiology. Oxygen is needed by tissue cells for metabolism. It cannot reach the cells if blood flow to the part is curtailed. The formation of clots in the veins of the pelvis and the lower extremities, impairing circulation, is a fairly common and potentially serious postoperative complication.

Blood clots develop because of a roughness in the vessel wall such as occurs with trauma from venous stasis (slowing of blood flow), and from hypercoagulability. Platelets adhere to the vessel wall, and the resulting inflammatory response stimulates blood coagulation and fibrin development, resulting in a blood clot on the vessel wall (thrombophlebitis) (Fig. 24-20). Postopera-

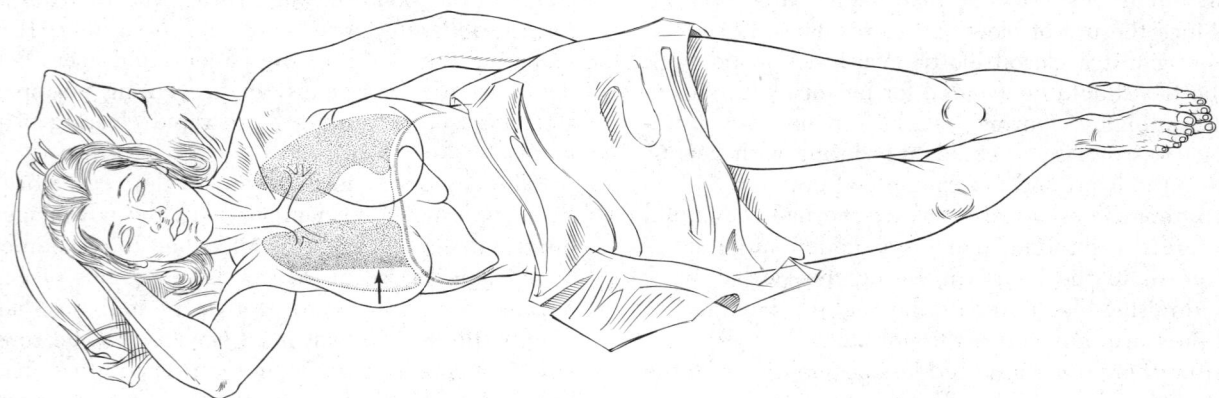

Fig. 24-19. Gravity will facilitate drainage of secretions from upper lung. In lower lung next to bed, secretions will pool in alveoli as a result of gravity and decreased chest expansion. Frequent turning will facilitate drainage from both lungs.

tively, the clot often forms in a vein of the foot, calf, thigh, or pelvis. The clot grows, usually in the direction of the slow-moving blood. It can occur in either a deep or superficial vein. In about 1 of every 10 instances[62] the clot or a portion of it breaks away and flows through the heart into the pulmonary circulation until it occludes a pulmonary vessel (pulmonary embolism) (p. 1320).

Venous stasis occurs postoperatively for a number of reasons (see box at right). A major contribution to venous stasis is inactivity of the legs. Every time the leg is moved the muscle compresses the vein pushing the blood toward the heart (venous pump); valves prevent the blood from moving backward. Exercise therefore promotes return of venous blood to the heart and prevention of venous stasis.

Assessment. A venous blood clot may develop without any local symptoms (*phlebothrombosis*), and the first indication of difficulty may be a pulmonary embolism. Homan's sign, pain on dorsiflexion of the foot, indicates a phlebothrombosis, but this may not always be present. Pain and local tenderness in the leg are signs of thrombophlebitis.

If a superficial vein is involved, *thrombophlebitis* can be noted as a reddened line along the vessel route, which feels firm on gentle palpation. If it forms in the femoral or iliac veins, the entire limb becomes swollen, pale, and cold. There is usually exquisite tenderness along the course of the vein. The swelling and coldness are caused by lymphatic obstruction and arterial spasm. The body temperature often rises. If the thrombophlebitis is confined to the saphenous vein, the accompanying edema is not so marked, but pain and tenderness are just as severe, and heat and redness can be noted along the inflamed vein.

Signs of a *pulmonary embolism* depend on the size

RISK FACTORS FOR DEVELOPMENT OF POSTOPERATIVE VENOUS THROMBOSIS

Intrinsic factors

Older age

Obesity

Malnutrition

Contraceptive use

Pathologic conditions

Malignancy

Congestive heart failure

History of previous deep vein thrombosis

Polycythemia

Type of surgery

Pelvic surgery

Abdominal or thoracic surgery

Fracture of hip or lower extremities

Effects of surgery

Anesthesia

Shock

Decreased mobility

Prolonged sitting with legs dependent

Pressure on popliteal area (pillows, chair)

Intestinal distention

Tight dressings or cast on lower extremities

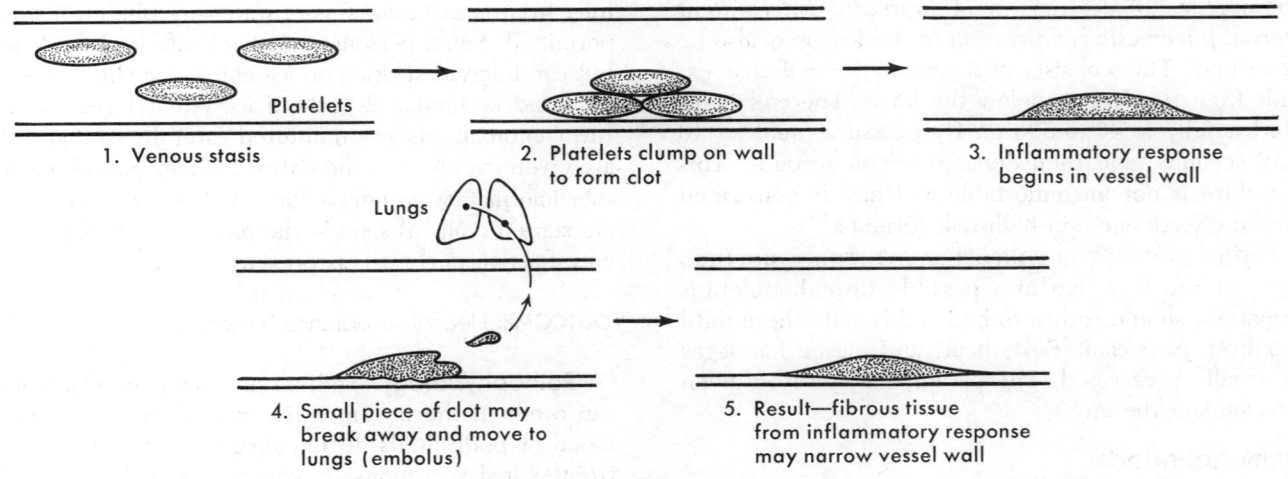

1. Venous stasis
2. Platelets clump on wall to form clot
3. Inflammatory response begins in vessel wall
4. Small piece of clot may break away and move to lungs (embolus)
5. Result—fibrous tissue from inflammatory response may narrow vessel wall

Fig. 24-20. Diagram illustrating formation of thrombus on wall of vein following venous stasis resulting in narrowing of blood vessel.

of the blood vessel that has been occluded. Any complaints of sudden sharp thoracic or upper abdominal pain or dyspnea or any signs of shock are reported immediately to the physician.

Intervention

PREVENTION. Many circulatory postoperative complications can be prevented by nursing management. Patient education in the causes of thrombophlebitis will help ensure greater participation in preventive measures. Elastic stockings or bandages should be worn both in and out of bed by high-risk patients. These stockings compress superficial veins, increase blood flow through deep veins by pressure, and prevent venous pooling. The stockings are removed at least once daily to permit washing and inspection of the legs.

Patients should not sit in one position for a long time and should elevate their feet on a stool to facilitate venous return by gravity. No pressure should be permitted on the popliteal area such as by pillows. When supporting legs on pillows, pressure should be equally distributed along the entire leg. Because of the danger of dislodging a clot, the muscle portion of a patient's leg should not be massaged postoperatively. A patient who is noted to be rubbing a leg should be questioned about discomfort.

Bed exercises (Fig. 24-3) and early ambulation are known to minimize the effects of venous stasis caused by bed rest, and they usually are contraindicated only in the presence of thromboembolic diseases or after vascular surgery such as anastomosis of a blood vessel. Specific exercises for the upper extremities are not usually necessary, since the patient uses the arms in eating, bathing, combing hair, and reaching for articles on the bedside stand or overbed table.

Medical preventive measures in high-risk patients include (1) heparin prophylaxis given 2 hours preoperatively and 8 to 12 hours postoperatively, (2) aspirin in instances when heparin is contraindicated such as for hip surgery, (3) dextran, or (4) warfarin. *Intermittent external pneumatic compression* to the legs may also be prescribed. This consists of a pneumatic cuff that extends from the feet to below the knee. The cuff is inflated rapidly to 40 to 50 mm Hg pressure, held for 10 to 12 seconds, and then deflated for 45 seconds. This procedure is not uncomfortable and has demonstrated marked effectiveness in high-risk patients.[106]

INTERVENTION FOR POSTOPERATIVE THROMBOPHLEBITIS. At the first sign of a possible thrombophlebitis the patient should return to bed and remain there until seen by a physician. Rest, heat, and elastic bandages are usually prescribed. The patient may also be given anticoagulant therapy.

Nutritional needs

OUTCOME: Fluid balance is maintained.

Pathophysiology. Fluid is lost during surgery through blood loss and increased insensible fluid loss through the lungs and skin. During the surgical procedure the blood loss is estimated and fluids are replaced intravenously. Gastrointestinal tract function may be slowed. Surgery of the gastrointestinal tract or on closely related organs within the abdomen usually decreases peristalsis, and paralytic ileus (intestinal obstruction as a result of cessation of peristalsis) may occur.

For at least the first 24 to 48 hours after surgery, fluids are retained by the body because of the stimulation of antidiuretic hormone (ADH) as part of the stress response to trauma and the effect of anesthesia. During surgery there is also renal vasoconstriction and increased aldosterone activity leading to increased sodium retention with subsequent water retention. Overhydration can occur with vigorous fluid replacement, especially in the infant or small elderly person. Both water intoxication and pulmonary edema can occur depending on the type and amount of fluids given (for further information on fluid overload see p. 333).

Assessment. All patients who have had major surgery and those receiving fluids intravenously after surgery need careful monitoring of fluid balance. Fluid intake will exceed fluid output during the first 24 to 48 hours. After this initial period fluid intake should essentially equal fluid output for the patient taking solid foods. The patient receiving fluids intravenously is monitored for signs of pulmonary edema (dyspnea, cough) or water intoxication (change in behavior, confusion, warm moist skin). Weight is monitored in those patients receiving fluid intravenously over a period of several days postoperatively. Sudden weight gain indicates fluid retention. Small elderly persons may need central venous pressure monitoring of fluid volume. The presence of bowel sounds, passing of flatus, or belching indicates the return of peristalsis.

Intervention. As soon as the patient has recovered fully from anesthesia, sips of water are offered if this is permitted. Some persons cannot tolerate iced fluids well but can tolerate sucking on ice chips. Ice chips must be recorded as intake (2 parts of ice equal 1 part water). Intravenous fluids are monitored carefully so that fluids are given evenly over the entire 24-hour period (for further information on intravenous fluids see p. 348). Fluids are started orally as soon as the patient can tolerate them and if active peristalsis is present.

OUTCOME: Electrolyte balance is monitored.

Pathophysiology. Sodium and potassium depletion can occur in the postoperative patient with the loss of blood or body fluids during surgery or the loss of gastrointestinal secretions by vomiting and through nasogastric tubes. Potassium is also lost during catabolism (tissue breakdown) especially following severe trauma or crush injuries. Loss of gastric secretions can result in chloride loss producing a base-bicarbonate excess (metabolic alkalosis).

Assessment and intervention. The patient is monitored for signs of sodium and potassium deficit (p. 337). Potassium is usually added to intravenous fluids of postoperative patients. High-protein foods and fresh fruits, high in potassium, are encouraged when foods are permitted by mouth.

OUTCOME: The person's normal weight is maintained; protein and vitamin C intake is enhanced.

Pathophysiology. The best way to supply essential foods is orally. Solid food can promote the flow of saliva during mastication, aiding digestion and encouraging the stomach to empty. This process in turn stimulates peristalsis of the lower gastrointestinal tract. Ingestion of solid food also helps to prevent the occurrence of nonepidemic parotitis, an inflammation of the salivary glands that occurs occasionally in debilitated patients who have poor oral hygiene and who also may be dehydrated.

Two food substances of special importance in wound healing are protein and vitamin C. During catabolism in the early postoperative period, a negative nitrogen balance occurs; more nitrogen is lost than is taken in (p. 402). Protein intake is necessary to restore nitrogen balance and to provide the necessary amino acids for anabolism. Vitamin C is necessary for tissue healing (p. 445).

Assessment. Daily weight measurement for patients not eating a full meal at least three times a day will give an indication of the degree of tissue loss. Rapid weight gain indicates fluid retention; rapid loss indicates dehydration. A gradual loss of about 0.15 to 0.25 kg (⅓ to ½ lb) per day indicates tissue loss.[88] There is usually an increase in blood urea nitrogen (BUN) levels during catabolism, but unless the patient has renal insufficiency the excess urea is excreted in the urine. Meal trays of surgical patients should be inspected to identify those patients who are not eating foods high in protein and vitamin C.

Intervention. Patients receiving standard intravenous fluids containing dextrose do not have sufficient caloric intake. This is essentially a "starvation diet." As soon as fluids can be tolerated foods are started. Most patients quickly resume their usual diet. Elderly persons or persons who have had stomach surgery may tolerate a soft diet and six small feedings more easily than a standard diet. Urging solid food when the patient has no appetite may induce vomiting and may lessen the desire to eat. The anorexic patient is encouraged to select preferred foods that are high in protein. Carbohydrate is also needed to provide energy expended in early ambulation. After even a few days of enforced starvation the patient may be somewhat indifferent to food, and it may take 2 to 3 days on a well-balanced diet to overcome this. The patient who was malnourished before surgery and who has extensive gastrointestinal surgery is a candidate for total parenteral nutrition.

The usual home diet of elderly persons living alone is frequently low in protein and vitamins. Patient education concerning the increased need for these food substances in the weeks following surgery may be indicated.

Elimination needs

OUTCOME: Urinary output resumes normal pattern; urinary tract infection does not develop.

Pathophysiology. A patient who is well hydrated usually voids within 6 to 8 hours after surgery. Although 2000 to 3000 ml of intravenous solution usually is given on the operative day, the first voiding may not be more than 200 ml and the total urinary output for the operative day may be less than 1500 ml. The small amount of urinary output results from the loss of body fluid during surgery, increased insensible fluid loss, vomiting, and increased secretion of ADH. As body functions stabilize, fluid and electrolyte balance returns to normal in about 48 hours.

Urinary retention, or the inability to void, may occur in the early postoperative period. The difficulty may be due to the recumbent position, nervous tension, the effects of anesthetics that interfere with bladder sensation and the ability to void, the use of narcotics that reduce the sensation of bladder distention, the pain caused by movement onto the bedpan, or pain at the site of operation if it is near the bladder or urethra. Inability to void is a common occurrence following surgery of the rectum or colon and following gynecologic procedures, since the innervation of the bladder musculature may be temporarily disturbed, and local edema may increase the difficulty.

Urinary tract infections may occur in patients who must be on prolonged bed rest after surgery, who have a history of urinary tract infections, who have had pelvic surgery, or who have indwelling catheters.

Assessment. Urinary output is closely monitored after surgery until normal urinary function is reestablished. During the oliguric phase the specific gravity is high since the usual amount of solutes are excreted in less water. The bladder is palpated for distention when output is low to identify urinary retention. The distended bladder rises out of the pelvis just above the symphysis pubis. This may be difficult to palpate when the patient is obese. Occasionally, the overdistended bladder expels just enough urine to relieve the pressure within it temporarily and the patient voids frequently in small amounts. This is known as retention with overflow and differs from frequency seen in urinary tract infections; in the latter the bladder is not distended, and the patient complains of burning on urination and may have fever.

Intervention. Suppression of urine after the initial oliguric phase postoperatively requires medical intervention (p. 1570). If the patient is well hydrated and has no cardiovascular or renal problems, the inability to void past the first 6 to 8 hours is usually the result of urinary retention. This requires nursing intervention. Voiding may be facilitated by measures such as offering fluids, placing the patient on the bedpan frequently or getting the patient up to the bathroom or commode if possible, running water in the bathroom, pouring water over the perineum, and assuring the patient of time and privacy. Many men can void if they are allowed to stand at the side of the bed. If these measures are not effective, the physician may order catheterization. Because of the emotional trauma to the young child, the possibility of reproductive tract infections in men, and the danger of urinary infection in all patients, catheterization may be delayed longer than the usual 8 hours postoperatively in the hope that the patient will void normally. Bethanechol chloride (Urecholine) may be ordered by the physician for acute postoperative retention. It may be given orally or subcutaneously but not by intramuscular injection since this may induce circulatory collapse.

If the patient must be catheterized repeatedly after surgery, an indwelling catheter may be inserted and fluids forced. Good perineal care of a patient with an indwelling catheter will help to prevent ascending infection. Bacteria can move up the outside of the catheter by means of capillary action. Patients who exhibit signs of urinary tract infection should have a urine specimen sent to the laboratory for culture and sensitivity. Fluids are encouraged up to 3000 ml, unless contraindicated, to prevent urinary stasis.

OUTCOME: Bowel patterns are reestablished.

Pathophysiology. Decreased peristalsis from the neuroendocrine response to the stress of surgery and from the effect of anesthesia and narcotics or from hypokalemia may lead to constipation in the early postoperative period. Inactivity and decreased intake of foods that provide roughage are contributing factors. Peristalsis will be decreased in all patients with abdominal or pelvic surgery for at least 24 hours and will be delayed for several days if the patient had surgery of the gastrointestinal tract. For some surgical patients, having a bowel movement may be painful and the patient may be reluctant to pass stool.

A patient receiving therapy intravenously may have bowel movements if peristalsis is present. Stool is composed of 75% water plus waste products, both of which are present in the hydrated patient. Because of the lack of ingested roughage, stools will occur less frequently and may be hard. The longer stool remains in the colon, the more water is reabsorbed and the harder the stool becomes.

Assessment. Return of peristalsis of the lower gastrointestinal tract is indicated by presence of bowel sounds, gas pains, and passing of flatus. Absence of bowel sounds does not indicate absence of peristalsis because the sounds may be occurring only occasionally and may be missed. On the contrary, the presence of bowel sounds does not indicate active peristalsis but may only be gas moving in segments of bowel.

Stool is examined for amount and consistency; small, dry, hard stool indicates constipation. A small amount of diarrhea may be indicative of a fecal impaction, which can be identified by digital examination; this is contraindicated following surgery of the rectum.

Assessment should also be made of the frequency with which narcotics are given, extent of activity, amount of fluid intake, and previous bowel problems to determine the patient's potential for developing constipation.

Intervention. Signs indicating the return of intestinal peristalsis are recorded after abdominal surgery. No attempt is made to hasten bowel evacuation for the first 2 to 3 days after peristalsis fully returns, but preventive measures should be instituted. Fluids are encouraged to 2000 to 3000 ml per day unless contraindicated. Maximal activity is encouraged within the prescribed limits. Bathroom privileges are provided as early as possible.

If there are no results after 3 to 4 days, a mild laxative may help reestablish function. Fruit juices, especially prune juice, may be effective. If these are not effective, a hypertonic (Fleet) enema or small soapsuds enema will usually stimulate defecation. If a fecal impaction is suspected, a mineral oil enema may precede a soapsuds enema to soften the stool. A bowel movement may be intentionally delayed following burns of the buttocks or extensive rectal surgery by the administration of paregoric orally.

Comfort needs

OUTCOME: General discomforts are minimized.

Vomiting

ETIOLOGY. Nausea and vomiting in the postoperative patient may be related to a number of factors: effect of certain anesthetics on the stomach, decreased peristalsis producing a collection of fluid and gas in the stomach, drinking fluids before peristalsis returns, psychologic factors in patients who anticipate postoperative vomiting, drug idiosyncrasies, pain, or disturbances in electrolyte balance.

Persistent postoperative vomiting is usually a symptom of pyloric obstruction, intestinal obstruction, or peritonitis. Vomiting tires the patient, puts a strain on the incision, and causes excessive loss of fluids and electrolytes. Choking while vomiting may lead to aspiration pneumonia.

INTERVENTION. Postoperative vomiting is one of the most distressing problems that a patient encounters. To prevent possible aspiration the patient who is vomiting should lie on the side. Food and fluid are omitted for several hours, and the patient is advised to lie quietly in bed. The emesis basin and soiled linen are cleaned and changed. Frequent oral care is provided. When vomiting has subsided, and unless contraindicated, sucking on ice chips, taking sips of ginger ale or hot tea, or eating small amounts of dry solid food may relieve nausea. Antiemetics such as trimethobenzamide hydrochloride (Tigan) or prochlorperazine dimaleate (Compazine) may be administered by injection. Since vomiting can be a sign of drug idiosyncrasy, presence of other side effects should be observed and the pattern of vomiting in relation to administration of drugs noted. Accurate recording of intake and output of fluids and electrolyte balance is important.

Hiccoughs

ETIOLOGY. Hiccoughs interfere with eating and sleeping and are among the most exhausting postoperative complications. The exact cause of postoperative hiccoughs is not known, but it is known that dilation of the stomach, irritation of the diaphragm, peritonitis, and uremia cause either reflex or central nervous system stimulation of the phrenic nerve. Fortunately, hiccoughs are not a common postoperative complaint. They usually disappear within a few hours.

INTERVENTION. Hiccoughs may be relieved by such a simple measure as having the patient rebreathe carbon dioxide at 5-minute intervals by inhaling and exhaling into a paper bag held tightly over the nose and mouth. Carbon dioxide inhalations, using 5% carbon dioxide and 95% oxygen, may also be ordered for 5 minutes every hour. If dizziness occurs they should be discontinued, since an overdose of carbon dioxide may cause convulsions and coma. Aspiration of the stomach will stop hiccoughs caused by gastric dilation. Chlorpromazine hydrochloride is used to treat mild cases of hiccoughs. If the hiccoughs are persistent and do not respond to these treatments, local infiltration of the phrenic nerve with 1% procaine may be necessary, or in extreme cases surgical crushing of the phrenic nerve may be done.

Abdominal distention and gas pains

PATHOPHYSIOLOGY. Postoperative distention is a result of an accumulation of nonabsorbable gas in the intestines caused by a reaction to the handling of the bowel during surgery, by swallowing of air during recovery from anesthesia and as the patient attempts to overcome nausea, and by passing of gases from the bloodstream to the atonic portion of the bowel. Distention will persist until the tone of the bowel returns to normal and peristalsis resumes. It is experienced to some degree by most patients after abdominal and renal surgery.

Gas pains are caused by contractions of the unaffected portions of the bowel in an attempt to move the accumulated gas through the intestinal tract.

ASSESSMENT. Patients with abdominal distention complain of diffuse abdominal pain. High distention may cause dyspnea by pressure on the diaphragm and lead to atelectasis. Abdominal girth is increased because of the collection of gas; this can be measured with a tape measure to determine progress. Percussion produces a drumlike (tympanic) sound as compared with a dull sound occurring with ascites or obesity. Acute gastric dilation may produce signs of shock (restlessness; rapid, weak, thready pulse; hypotension) and overflow vomiting. Gas pains in the intestinal tract usually occur as peristalsis is beginning to return and can be extremely painful. Bowel sounds are usually audible on auscultation.

INTERVENTION. Ambulation is one of the most effective means for stimulation of peristalsis and expulsion of flatus. Dilation of the stomach can be relieved by aspiration of fluid or gas with a nasogastric tube.

Gas in the lower bowel may be removed by a lubricated rectal tube inserted into the rectum. This tube is inserted just past the rectal sphincter and is removed after approximately 20 minutes. If necessary it may be used every 4 hours. Heat applied to the abdomen in the form of a hot water bottle or heating pad may be used in conjunction with the use of a rectal tube. A hypertonic enema is often effective in relieving gas pains postoperatively. If this fails, small carminative enemas of milk and molasses or of glycerin, magnesium sulfate, and water sometimes are ordered to stimulate the expulsion of flatus.

If the distention progresses and the flatus is not expelled after 48 hours, a paralytic ileus is suspected. The patient is given nothing by mouth. Nasogastric suctioning is started and continued until peristalsis returns.

OUTCOME: Postoperative pain is minimized.

Pathophysiology. Pain is a common occurrence after nearly all types of surgical procedures in which there has been cutting, pulling, or manipulations of tissues and organs. It may result from stimulation of nerve endings by chemical substances released at the time of surgery or from tissue ischemia caused by interference of blood supply to the part, such as by pressure, muscle spasm, or edema. Trauma to the nerve fibers in the skin produces sharp localized pain. Extensive dissection and prolonged retraction of muscle and fascia produce deep long-lasting pain. Pain originating in a visceral organ may be referred to a distant portion of the body surface or deeply in a different area. It is usually characterized as a deep, aching pain. A hollow visceral organ such as the ureter or bile duct can develop muscle spasms characterized as cramping pain.

Following surgery other factors can add to the pain sensation. These include pressure from tissue edema, infections, distention, muscle spasms surrounding the incisional area, and tight dressings or casts. Postoperative pain usually lasts 24 to 48 hours but may continue longer depending on the extent of the surgery, the pain threshold of the patient, and response to pain (p. 377). The presence of pain can prolong convalescence, since it may interfere with return to activity.

Assessment. When the patient complains of pain in the postoperative period, one must not assume that the pain is incisional in nature. It is important to try to ascertain the possible cause of the pain. Subjective data include origin, area involved, nature of the pain, and possible cause from the patient's viewpoint. Objective data include observation of facial expressions, body position, activity, muscle rigidity, and pulse rate.

Pain with fever may be due to wound infection. Pain with vomiting and abdominal distention is a result of gas collecting in the intestinal tract. Pain with fullness about the symphysis pubis is caused by a full bladder. Pain with coldness, paraesthesia, or numbness of a part is a result of decreased circulation from a tight bandage or cast or venous stasis. If the patient is experiencing severe pain, the assessment should be made gently and quickly but thoroughly.

Intervention. It is often impossible to prevent the occurrence of postoperative pain, but it can be minimized so that the patient is relatively comfortable. Patients who have had adequate preoperative instructions and who have confidence in the surgeon, in the nurse, and in the outcome of the surgery usually have less postoperative pain than the apprehensive patient because they have less tension. Measures to reduce anxiety and apprehension will also help reduce any pain that is present.

If the cause of pain is determined to be other than incisional, measures are taken to relieve the cause. Emptying a full bladder can relieve what was thought to be pain from a lower abdominal incision. Elevation of a part may relieve venous stasis. Loosening of a tight bandage if permissible will relieve ischemic pain.

Incisional pain can be relieved by nursing measures and by analgesics. Spasms and pain from surrounding muscles being continually contracted contributes to incisional pain. Many patients find a position that is tolerable and then hesitate to move for fear of increased pain. Muscles used to hold this position and guard the incision become strained. If the patient understands what is occurring and is helped and encouraged to move frequently, pain will be decreased. Patients with surgery

of the trunk should avoid twisting the body; they may be more comfortable if the trunk is moved as one unit. Side rails are helpful for the patient to hold onto when turning over. A limb that has been operated on should be supported. If hands are used for supporting a limb, the broad palms rather than fingers, which dig into painful tissue, are more comfortable for the patient. Pillows serve as useful "splints" during movement of a limb. Autogenic techniques for control of pain, such as the "relaxation response" technique (p. 174), may be helpful for some patients.

MEDICATIONS. In addition to making the patient as comfortable as possible, it is usually necessary during the first 12 to 48 hours after major surgery to administer a narcotic. The goal is to keep the patient fairly comfortable without overmedication. Analgesics have greater effect if they are administered *before* pain becomes severe. If severe pain is expected, medication should be offered to the patient within the prescribed limits before it is requested.

Addiction to narcotics is *not* a probability when given during the first few postoperative days for severe pain. Although certain narcotics, such as morphine, depress the respiratory center, the patient in pain may be breathing shallowly or splinting the chest and not moving about in bed adequately. Relief of pain may encourage the patient to move and breathe more deeply, thus preventing postoperative complications. During early ambulation patients receiving meperidine hydrochloride (Demerol) may develop orthostatic hypotension.

After the first 48 to 72 hours, pain usually decreases in severity and may be controlled with a less potent analgesic. Because of the variability in perception and reaction to pain, each patient must be assessed individually. It is the custom in some hospitals for physicians to write prn orders for different analgesics, thus permitting the nurse to select the one that best meets the immediate needs. If this is the practice, careful patient assessment and monitoring to prevent overlapping of drugs given are important. Some communities do not permit this practice, considering it to be prescription of drugs and therefore not under the legal jurisdiction of nursing.

Activity needs

OUTCOME: Maximal activity is carried out within established limits.

Pathophysiology. Early ambulation has been a significant factor in hastening postoperative recovery and preventing postoperative complications. Numerous benefits accrue from the exercise of getting in and out of bed and walking during the early postoperative period (Fig. 24-21). Increases in rate and depth of breathing improve ventilation, helping to prevent atelectasis

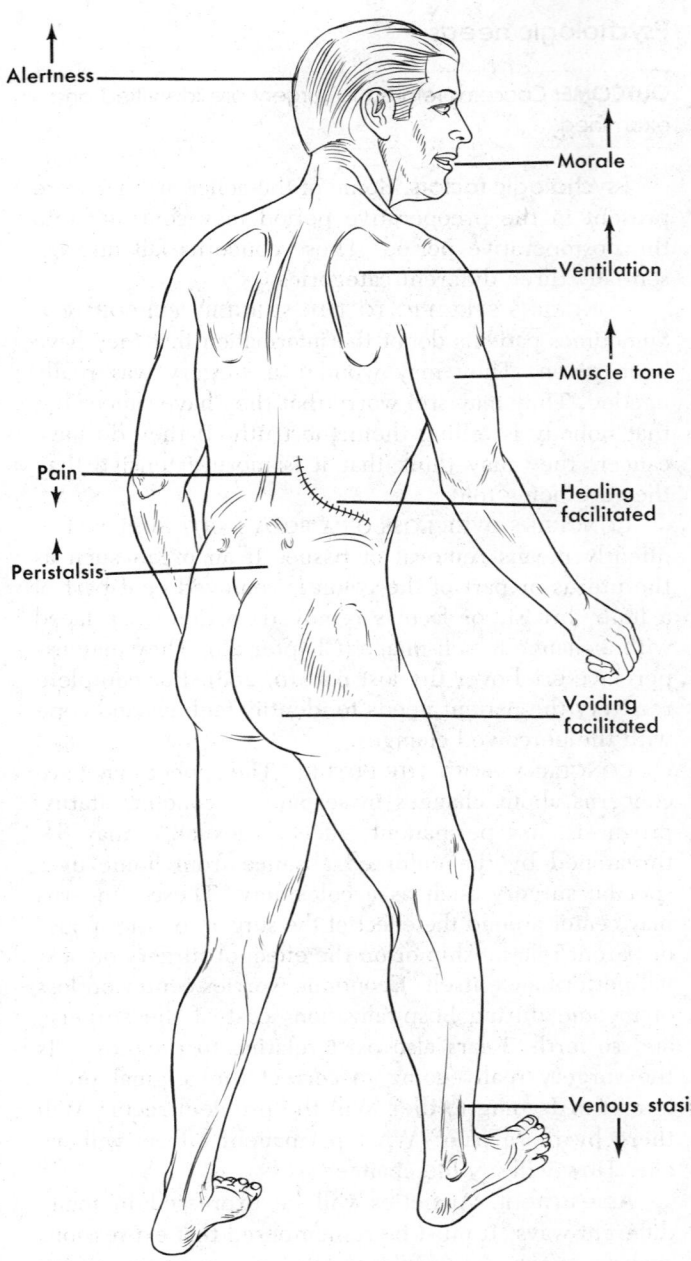

Alertness

Morale

Ventilation

Muscle tone

Pain

Healing
facilitated

Peristalsis

Voiding
facilitated

Venous stasis

Fig. 24-21. Benefits from early postoperative ambulation.

and hypostatic pneumonia. Oxygen intake increases and with the increased circulation more oxygen reaches the brain, increasing mental alertness. Cardiac output increases; more blood flows through the capillaries, providing the wound with substances needed for healing; and venous return is enhanced, decreasing venous stasis. Kidney function is increased because of the increased circulation. Activity also promotes micturition.

Metabolism increases as muscles are stimulated, preventing loss of muscle tone. Nitrogen loss is decreased, thus helping to restore nitrogen balance. Ac-

tivity stimulates peristalsis in the gastrointestinal tract, promoting passage of fluids and gas and thus helping to prevent abdominal distention, gas pains, and constipation. Pain is decreased over time as the chemical stimuli are removed through increased circulation and strained muscles around the incision, neck, back, and legs relax. Morale is also affected as the patient sees fuction returning. Ambulation is usually contraindicated when there is a severe infection or thrombophlebitis.

Exercises in bed facilitate strengthening of muscle tone (Fig. 24-3). Moving around in bed, if carried out actively by the patient with minimal help, will offer some of the same benefits but to a much less extent. Moving to different positions also helps prevent tissue ischemia from pressure.

Assessment. A postoperative patient who is to get out of bed needs to be alert enough to follow directions. Asking the patient simple questions or to follow simple commands will help to determine the level of alertness.

Assessment of the patient's cardiovascular status includes obtaining baseline pulse and respiratory rate and rhythm. A change in position from supine to sitting or standing may produce orthostatic hypotension. Pulse and respiratory rates will increase as the result of sympathetic stimulation. The patient's face may become pale and the patient may complain of dizziness. Ambulation should not be attempted until the pulse and respirations stabilize at close to their baseline level.

Assessment of motor status includes muscle strength (p. 441) and sitting ability. Sitting ability will give an indication of the patient's ability to maintain balance while ambulating. This is assessed by asking the patient to maintain an erect position while he or she is gently pushed sideways while sitting on the side of the bed.

It is also important to know of any limitations to ambulation that the patient had preoperatively. The patient with arthritis or arteriosclerosis may take longer to move and to adjust to standing and walking. The patient who used a walker preoperatively will need assistance for a longer time before progressing to using the walker again.

Intervention. Muscle strengthening exercises should be carried out by patients who are not permitted to or cannot ambulate for a period of time. Exercises of the lower extremities will also prevent venous stasis. The patient is taught to bend the knees, to lower them, and to push the backs of the knees hard against the bed. The nurse's hand can be slipped under the popliteal area while the patient pushes hard against it. The same thing can be accomplished by having the patient alternately contract and relax the calf and thigh muscles. This should be done at least 10 times, and a brief period of rest should follow each contraction and relaxation. The cycle is *contract, relax,* and *rest.* Bed exercises should be carried out several times a day. If the patient is unable to do active exercises, passive range-of-motion exercises should be carried out.

When patients are permitted out of bed, they are assisted to sit up on the side of the bed and dangle the legs over the side to become accustomed to an upright position. Orthostatic hypotension may occur at this time. After the pulse has stabilized and the patient is ready to move, assistance is given to stand and walk a few steps. Each time the patient is encouraged to increase the distance walked. There should be ample space available for walking. A very weak patient may need two helpers, one to assist the patient and the other to manage the intravenous fluid pole or other equipment. The patient is assisted and supervised in getting out of bed and walking until able to do this without difficulty or danger of injury. Small goals can be set each day to give the patient something to work for and a sense of achievement.

Children usually recover quickly from the effects of surgery and often sit up and walk around in their cribs without urging. Older children occasionally are fearful of injuring the operative site and must be encouraged to leave the bed and move about freely.

Treatments need not interfere with helping the patient out of bed. If the patient is receiving an infusion, the bottle of infusion fluid can be hung on a movable pole that can be wheeled by the nurse as the patient walks. Permission is usually given by the physician to clamp off nasogastric tubes for a short period of time. Urethral catheters should remain attached to the closed drainage system. Plastic drainage bags make ambulation for these patients possible.

The word *ambulate* means to move from place to place, to walk. Sitting in a chair is not considered ambulation. After ambulating, the patient may sit in a chair if permitted but should be advised to stand and walk at intervals and to elevate the legs while sitting to prevent venous pooling in the extremities. Sitting in a chair for long periods is to be avoided.

OUTCOME: The person returns to optimal functioning in activities of daily living.

Encouraging the patient to carry out activities of daily living (washing, combing hair, dressing) promotes activity and helps move the patient from a dependent to an independent level. Pain and tiredness are useful criteria in determining when to step in and take over for the patient. Priorities must be set between the need for activity and the need for rest. Family education is important; if the family members do not understand the basis for encouraging patient self-care, the family member may become upset or step in and do for the patient. This may prolong hospitalization and the recovery period.

Psychologic needs

OUTCOME: Concerns related to surgery are identified and examined.

Psychologic factors. Some of the concerns that were present in the preoperative period may continue into the postoperative period. These concerns fall into essentially three different categories.

CONCERNS SPECIFIC TO THE SURGERY PERFORMED. Sometimes patients doubt the information that they have been given. They may wonder if surgery was really needed. They may still worry that they have cancer but that nobody is telling them the truth. If they do have cancer, they may think that it is more extensive than they are being told.

CONCERNS OVER LOSS OF A BODY PART. Surgery frequently means removal of tissue. If an organ such as the uterus or part of the colon is removed or if part of a limb, breast, or face is removed, patients are faced with a change in self-image (Chapter 28). They may experience grief over the lost part (p. 253). For complete recovery the patient needs to identify feelings and cope with the perceived changes.

CONCERNS ABOUT THE FUTURE. The patient may have concerns about changes in sexuality, economic status, prognosis, or permanent effects. Sexuality may be threatened by the enforced absence from home or a specific surgery such as a colostomy. These concerns may center around the effect of the surgery on the spouse or parent relationship or on the effect of surgery on sexual performance itself. Economic worries center on loss of income during hospitalization, cost of the surgery, and so forth. Fears also exist relating to prognosis. Is the surgery really going to correct the original problem? Am I going to die? Will the problem recur? Will there by more pain? What permanent effects will occur? How will my life change?

Assessment. Anxieties will be expressed in many different ways. It must be remembered that expressions such as anger, resentfulness, crying, excessive joking, inappropriate laughter, or withdrawal may all be signs of anxiety and are often seen in the postoperative period. Some of these feelings may be projected against the surgeon, nurse, housekeeping aide, food, and so forth.

Intervention. Sitting down and talking with surgical patients about their concerns is as important a nursing action in many instances as any of the physical activities. Time must be planned for this. If a specific concern is expected, such as sexual functioning after a perineal prostatectomy, the topic may have to be introduced by the nurse who has established rapport with the patient in order to let the patient know that it is permissible to talk about this topic.

Some patients will talk freely about the cancer or

the heart operation but never really face their feelings about the surgery. No patient is forced to do so, but the alert nurse will watch for cues that the patient is beginning to move from a cognitive thinking level to a feeling level and may need some support while identifying and learning to cope with these feelings.

Discharge planning

Discharge planning is an important part of nursing care postoperatively. Plans for the patient's discharge may have been discussed and begun preoperatively, but most of the teaching, arrangements, and preparations are done after surgery. The patient, the family, and the members of the health team responsible for the care of the patient during hospitalization should participate in the long-range planning. Outcome criteria for the patient at discharge are listed below at right.

As a result of early resumption of ambulation and a nutritious diet, most patients regain their strength rapidly, and the average hospital stay following surgery is 5 to 8 days. During this time the patient and family should be prepared for any care that must be given at home, and any necessary arrangements for convalescent care should be completed several days before discharge. Patients are helped to become as self-sufficient as possible before being discharged so that they do not have to depend any more than necessary on the assistance of relatives and friends.

After surgery the nurse consults with the physician regarding the anticipated discharge plans for the patient. The nurse assesses the patient's ability to participate in the care to be given at home, the interest and the desire of the family to help, and the home situation and its facilities. Whenever possible both the patient and a member of the family are taught all treatments and exercises that must be done at home. Sometimes arrangements should be made for a member of the family to come to the hospital to observe and perhaps practice procedures, to talk to the dietitian, to consult with the physician, to discuss problems with the social worker, and to plan with the nurse about home care. The patient and family should have ample opportunity to ask questions.

The nurse should try to anticipate any problems that might arise and help the patient and family plan for them. For example, if a colostomy irrigation must be given and there are no private bathroom facilities, extra equipment will be necessary so that it can be done in the room available. If the patient is reluctant or unable to give himself an injection, some member of the family must be taught how to give injections or arrangements must be made for a community health nurse to give them. If the patient does not understand English, an interpreter may be needed to explain diets, medica-

tions, or treatments. If dressings are needed the patient should be given a 48-hour supply to take home unless a family member has already obtained them from the hospital. The patient and family must know where in the community they can get dressings and other needed materials. If treatment of almost any kind is to be done at home, it is advisable for the nurse to discuss with the surgeon and with the patient the advisability of having a community health nurse visit the patient at home soon after leaving the hospital. A written referral should be made, and the report returned by the community health nurse helps the nurse in the hospital learn how effective the teaching of the patient has been.

On discharge the patient is given an appointment for a follow-up examination in the surgeon's office or hospital clinic. This appointment is usually for 1 to 2 weeks after discharge. The nurse should make sure that the patient understands the importance of returning for the medical examination.

With modern surgical techniques the wound is usually healing well by the time of discharge from the hospital. Therefore the convalescent period usually is relatively short, and most patients may return to their usual activities and occupation within 2 to 4 weeks postoperatively. Normal activities should be resumed gradually. Driving is usually permitted after 2 weeks, but the patient should avoid any heavy lifting, pushing, or pulling for at least 6 weeks.

Outcome criteria for the person who has had surgery

1. No injury has occurred during hospitalization.
2. The incision heals normally without infection.
3. No avoidable complications (atelectasis, pneumonia, thrombophlebitis) have occurred.
4. Elimination patterns are reestablished.
5. The person carries out activities of daily living at his optimal level of functioning; the person may still tire easily.
6. The person has had an opportunity to explore individual concerns.
7. The person or significant others can explain and carry out any treatments to be carried out at home or medication program resulting from the surgery.
8. The person or significant others can explain any dietary changes required by the surgery after discharge.
9. The person or significant others can explain activity limits incurred by the surgery and any exercise programs to be followed at home.
10. The person or significant others can explain

health maintenance or therapeutic follow-up programs; they know where and when to see the surgeon.

11. The person or significant others can explain how to obtain any needed professional or community resources.

REFERENCES AND SELECTED READINGS
Contemporary

1. *Aldrete, J.A.: Assessment of recovery from anesthesia, Curr. Rev. Recovery Room Nurses 1:161-168, 1980.
2. Alexander, J.W., editor: Symposium on surgical infections, Surg. Clin. North Am. 60:1-240, 1980.
3. Allen. P.: Applying standards to practice, A.O.R.N. J. 31:805-813, 1980.
4. American College of Surgeons: Manual of surgical intensive care, Philadelphia, 1977, W.B. Saunders Co.
5. Andrews, I.C.: Criteria for discharge from the recovery room. I, Curr. Rev. Recovery Room Nurses 2:49-56, 1980.
6. Andrews, I.C.: Criteria for discharge from the recovery room. II, Current Reviews for Recovery Room Nurses 2:57-64, 1980.
7. Atkinson, L.J., and Kohn, M.L.: Berry and Kohn's introduction to operating room technique, New York, 1979, McGraw-Hill Book Co.
8. Association of Operating Room Nurses, Inc.: Standards of nursing practice: recovery room, Denver, 1980, The Association.
9. *Auld, M., Craven, R., and West, J.: Wound healing, Nurs. '72 2(10):36-40, 1972.
10. *Baker, P.J.: Postoperative atelectasis, Nurs. Dig. 5:42-47, 1977.
11. Bakow, E.D.: Sustained maximal inspiration: a rationale for its use, R.C. 22:379-382, 1977.
12. Bakutis, A.,: Anesthetic reactions, Nurs. '72 2(9):16-19, 1972.
13. *Barnett, L.A.: Preparing your patient for the operating room, A.O.R.N. J. 18:534-539, 1973.
14. Bastasaraswathi, K. and El-Etr, A.A.: Preoperative evaluation of drug history, A.O.R.N. J. 23:616-620, 1976.
15. Belleville, J., et al.: Influence of age on pain relief from analgesics, J.A.M.A. 217:1835-1841, 1971.
16. Bernstein, A.H.: Current status of the law of consent to treatment, Hospitals 53(3):83-85, 1979.
17. Besst, J.A., and Wallace, H.L.: Wound healing: intraoperative factors, Nurs. Clin. North Am. 14:701-712, 1979.
18. *Blackwell, A., and Blackwell, W.: Relieving gas pain, Am. J. Nurs. 75:1474-1475, 1975.
19. Bryant, W.M.: Wound healing, Clin. Symp. 29:2-36, 1977.
20. Bushong, M.E.: Principles of postanesthetic management: criteria for patient discharge, Curr. Rev. Recovery Room Nurses 1:73-80, 1979.
21. Cahill, C.A.: Yawn maneuver to prevent atelectasis, A.O.R.N. J. 27:1000-1004, 1978.
22. Caranasos, G.J.: Drug reactions and interactions in the patient undergoing surgery, Med. Clin. North Am. 63:1245-1256, 1979.
23. *Castillo. P.: Care of the patient under local anesthesia, A.O.R.N. J. 18:283-285, 1973.
24. *Castle, M.: Wound care, Nurs. '75 5(8):40-44, 1975.
25. Codd. J., and Grohar, M.: Postoperative pulmonary complications, Nurs. Clin. North Am. 10:5-15, 1975.
26. Cooper, D.M., and Schumann, D.: Postsurgical nursing as an adjunct to wound healing, Nurs. Clin. North Am. 14:713-726, 1979.
27. Copeland, W.M.: Informed consent and the OR nurse, A.O.R.N. J. 29:928-944, 1979.
28. *Croushore, T.M.: Postoperative assessment: the key to avoiding the most common nursing mistakes, Nurs. '79 9(4):46, 1979.
29. Cruse, P.J. and Ford, R.: The epidemiology of wound infection, Surg. Clin. North Am. 60:27-40, 1980.
30. Cullen, D.J.: Recovery room complications, A.O.R.N. J. 26:746-763, 1977.
31. Cullen D.J., et al.: Postanesthetic complications, Surg. Clin. North Am. 55:987-998, 1975.
32. Cullen, S., and Larson, C.P.: Essentials of anesthetic practice, Chicago, 1974, Year Book Medical Publishers, Inc.
33. Daly, B.J.: Intensive care nursing, Garden City, N.Y., 1980, Medical Examination Publishing Co., Inc.
34. *Damsteegt, D.: Pastoral roles in presurgical visits, Am. J. Nurs. 75:1336-1337, 1975.
35. Denny, J., and Denson J.: Risk of surgery in patients over 90, Geriatrics 27:115-118, 1972.
36. *Dew, T.A., Bushong, M.E., and Crumrine, R.S.: Parents in pediatric R.R., A.O.R.N. J. 26:266-272, 1977.
37. Drain, C.B., and Shipley, S.B.: The recovery room, Philadelphia, 1979, W.B. Saunders Co.
38. Dripps, R.D., Eckenhoff, J.E., and Vandam, L.D.: Introduction to anesthesia, ed. 5, Philadelphia, 1977, W.B. Saunders Co.
39. Dunphy, J.E., and Way, L.W.: Current surgical diagnosis and treatment, ed. 4, Los Altos, Calif., 1979, Lange Medical Publications.
40. Durand, O.: Respiratory care of surgical patients, Resp. Ther. 7:62-64, 1977.
41. *Dziurbejko, M.M., and Larkin, J.C.: Including the family in preoperative teaching, Am. J. Nurs. 78:1892-1894, 1978.
42. Eisele, J.H.: Recognizing and treating respiratory problems in the surgical patient, A.O.R.N. J. 17:80-87, 1973.
43. Fay, M.R.: Introduction to recovery room nursing, Denver, 1977, Association of Operating Room Nurses, Inc.
44. Feigal, D.W., and Blaisdell, F.W.: The estimation of surgical risks, Med. Clin. North Am. 63:1131-1143, 1979.
45. Felton, G., et al.: Preoperative nursing intervention with the patient for surgery: outcomes of three alternative approaches, Int. J. Nurs. Stud. 13:83-96, 1976.
46. *Field, L.W.: Identifying the psychological aspects of the surgical patient, A.O.R.N. J. 17:86-90, 1973.
47. Fitzmaurice, J.B., and Sashara, A.A.: Current concepts of pulmonary embolism: implications for nursing practice, Heart Lung 3:209-218, 1974.
48. Flaherty, G.C., and Fitzpatrick, J.J.: Relaxation technique to increase comfort level of postoperative patients, Nurs. Res. 27:352-355, 1978.
49. Flynn, N.M., and Lawrence, R.L.: Antimicrobial prophylaxis, Med. Clin. North Am. 63:1225-1244, 1979.
50. Fochtman, D., and Raffensperger, J.G.: Principles of nursing care for the pediatric surgery patient, ed. 2, Boston, 1976, Little, Brown & Co.
51. Fortin, F., and Kirovac, S.: A randomized controlled trial of preoperative patient education, Int. J. Nurs. Stud. 13:11-24, 1976.
52. Friedman, J.: Ventilatory function in the recovery room, Curr. Rev. Recovery Room Nurses 1:57-64, 1979.
53. *Garrett, J.: Oliguria in postoperative patients, Nurs. Clin. North Am. 10:59-67, 1975.
54. Gelman, S.: The recovery room care of the patient with spinal, epidural and other regional blocks, Curr. Rev. Recovery Room Nurses 2:81-88, 1980.
55. Goodman, L.S., and Gillman, A.: The pharmacological basis of therapeutics, ed. 6, New York, 1980, Macmillan Publishing Co., Inc.

*References preceded by an asterisk are particularly well suited for student reading.

56. *Gordon, M.: Assessing activity tolerance, Am. J. Nurs. **76:**72-76, 1976.

57. Goth, A.: Medical pharmacology: principles and concepts, ed. 10, St Louis, 1982, The C.V. Mosby Co.

58. Greenfield, L.J.: Surgery in the aged, Philadelphia, 1975, W.B. Saunders Co.

59. *Gruendemann, B.: The impact of surgery on body image, Nurs. Clin. North Am. **10:**635-643, 1975.

60. *Gruendemann, B.J., and Meeker, M.H.: Alexander's care of the patient in surgery, ed. 7, St. Louis, 1983, The C.V. Mosby Co.

61. Guerra, F., and Aldrete, J.A., editors: Emotional and psychological responses to anesthesia and surgery, New York, 1980, Grune & Stratton, Inc.

62. Guyton, A.: Textbook of medical physiology, ed. 6, Philadelphia, 1981, W.B. Saunders Co.

63. Hahn, A.B., Barkin, R.L., and Oestreich, S.J.K.: Pharmacology in nursing, ed. 15, St. Louis, 1982, The C.V. Mosby Co.

64. Harman, E., and Lillington, G.: Pulmonary risk factors in surgery, Med. Clin. North Am. **63:**1289-1298, 1979.

65. Harrington, J.D., editor: Intensive care of the surgical patient, Nurs. Clin. North Am. **10:**1-144, 1975.

66. Hercules, P.R.: Nursing in the postoperative care unit: a review, A.O.R.N. J. **28:**1042-1052, 1978.

67. Hoopes, N.M., et al.: An approach to preoperative visits, A.O.R.N. J. **26:**1048-1091, 1977.

68. Howard, R.B.: More on informed consent, Postgrad. Med. **65:**25-28, 1979.

69. Johnson, J.E., et al.: Sensory information, instruction in a coping strategy, and recovery from surgery, Res. Nurs. Health **1:**4-17, 1978.

70. Johnson, J.F., Dabbs, J.M., Jr., and Leventhal, H.: Psychosocial factors in the welfare of surgical patients, Nurs. Res. **19:**18-29, 1970.

71. *Johnston, M.: Outcome criteria to evaluate postoperative respiratory status, Am. J. Nurs. **75:**1474-1475, 1975.

72. *Knudsen, K.: Play therapy: preparing the young child for surgery, Nurs. Clin. North Am. **10:**679-686, 1975.

73. Laird, M.: Techniques for teaching pre- and postoperative patients, Am. J. Nurs. **75:**1338-1340, 1975.

74. Le Maitre, G., and Finnigan, J.A.: The patient in surgery, ed. 4, Philadelphia, 1980, W.B. Saunders Co.

75. *Libman, R.H.: Relieving airway obstruction in the recovery room, Am. J. Nurs. **75:**603-625, 1975.

76. Lindeman, C.A., and Van Aerman, B.H.: Nursing intervention with the presurgical patient: the effects of structured and unstructured preoperative teaching, Nurs. Res. **20:**319-332, 1971.

77. *Lipman, M.: Informed consent and the nurse's role, R.N. **35:**50, 1972.

78. *Luciano, K.: The who, when, where, what and how of preparing children for surgery, Nurs. '74 4(11):64-65, 1974.

79. *Lyons, M.L.: What priority do you give preop teaching? Nurs. '77 7(1):12-14, 1977.

80. *Marcinek, M.B.: Stress in the surgical patient, Am. J. Nurs. **77:**1809-1811, 1977.

81. Mason, J.H.: General surgery. In Steinberg, F.U., editor: Cowdry's the care of the geriatric patient, ed. 6, St. Louis, 1983, The C.V. Mosby Co.

82. *McConnell, E.A.: Meeting the special needs of diabetics facing surgery, Nurs. '76 6(6):30-37, June 1976.

83. *McConnell, E.A.: After surgery, Nurs. '77 7(3):32-39, 1977.

84. McConnell, E.A.: Applying recovery room standards, A.O.R.N. J. **31:**796-798, 1980.

85. McConnell, E.A.: Use of the nursing process in the recovery room, Curr. Rev. Recovery Room Nurses **2:**73-80, 1980.

86. *McConnell, E.A.: Toward complication-free recoveries for your surgical patient. I, R.N. 43(6):30-33, 1980.

87. McConnell, E.A.: Toward complication-free recoveries for your surgical patient. II, R.N. 43(7):34-38, 1980.

88. McCredie, J.A., editor: Basic surgery, New York, 1977, Macmillan Publishing Co., Inc.

89. *Meng, A.L.: Parents' and childrens' reactions to impending hospitalization for surgery, Matern. Child Nurs. J. **9:**83-98, 1980.

90. *Metheny, N.: Water and electrolyte balance in the postoperative patient, Nurs. Clin. North Am. **10:**49-57, 1975.

91. *Metheny, N., and Snively, W.D., Jr.: Perioperative fluids and electrolytes, Am. J. Nurs. **78:**840-845, 1978.

92. *Mitchell, J.A., and Cragin, C.L.: Informed consent: a doctor's dilemma, A.O.R.N. J. **18:**810-826, 1973.

93. Mitchell, M.A.: An RR experience: as nurse and patient saw it, R.N. **38:**46-47, 1975.

94. Morgan, D.: Prepared patients make faster surgical recovery. Can. Hosp. **50:**45-49, 1973.

95. *Nielson, M.A.: Intra-arterial monitoring of blood pressure, Am. J. Nurs. **74:**48-53, 1974.

96. *Nursing care of the patient in the O.R., Somerville, N.J., 1972, Ethicon Co.

97. O'Byrne, C.: Clinical detection and management of postoperative wound sepsis, Nurs. Clin. North Am. **14:**727-742, 1979.

98. *Parsons, M.C., and Stephens, G.: Postoperative complications: assessment and intervention, Am. J. Nurs. **74:**240-244, 1974.

99. *Patrick H.: Electrical hazards in the operating room, A.O.R.N. J. **18:**1127-1130, 1973.

100. Peacock, E.E., and Van Winkle, W.: Wound repair, ed. 2, Philadelphia, 1976, W.B. Saunders Co.

101. Phippin, M.L.: Intraoperative nursing assessment, A.O.R.N. J. **28:**160-166, 1978.

102. Powell, M.: An environment for wound healing, Am. J. Nurs. **72:**1862-1865, 1972.

103. Robbins, J.A., and Mushlin, A.I.: Preoperative evaluation of the healthy patient, Med. Clin. North Am. **63:**1145-1156, 1979.

104. *Robusto, N.: Advising patients on sex after surgery, A.O.R.N. J. **32:**55-61, 1980.

105. Rockwell, D.A., and Pepitone-Rockwell, F.: The emotional impact of surgery and the value of informed consent, Med. Clin. North Am. **63:**1341-1351, 1979.

106. Rose, S.D.: Prophylaxis of thromboembolic disease, Med. Clin. North Am. **63:**1205-1224, 1979.

107. Rose, S.D., Lourdes, C.C., and Mason, D.T.: Cardiac risk factors in patients undergoing non-cardiac surgery, Med. Clin. North Am. **63:**1270-1288, 1979.

108. Sabiston, D.C., editor: Davis-Christopher's textbook of surgery, ed. 11, Philadelphia, 1977, W.B. Saunders Co.

109. Saylor, D.: Understanding presurgical anxiety, A.O.R.N. J. **22:**624-636, 1975.

110. Schmitt, F.E., and Woolridge, P.J.: Psychological preparation of surgical patients, Nurs. Res. **22:**108-116, 1973.

111. Schumann, D.: Preoperative measures to promote wound healing, Nurs. Clin. North Am. **14:**683-699, 1979.

112. *Schumann, D.: How to help wound healing in your abdominal surgery patient, Nurs. '80 10(4):34-40, 1980.

113. *Schwab, S.M.: Caring for the aged, Am. J. Nurs. **73:**2049-2053, 1973.

114. Schwartz, S., et al.: Principles of surgery, ed. 3, New York, 1979, McGraw-Hill Book Co.

115. Silva, M.C.: Preoperative teaching for spouses, A.O.R.N. J. **27:**1081-1086, 1978.

116. *Smith, B.J.: Safeguarding your patient after anesthesia, Nurs. '78 8(10):53-56, 1978.

117. *Smith, R.B., Petruscak, J., and Solosko, D.: In a recovery room, Am. J. Nurs. **73:**70-73, 1973.

118. Smith, R.M.: Anesthesia for infants and children, ed. 4, St. Louis, 1980, The C.V. Mosby Co.

119. Starving children before operation, Br. Med. J. **3:**213-216, 1974.

120. *Strauss, R.J., et al.: Operative risks of obese patients: nursing care, A.O.R.N. J. **25**:1053-1057, 1977.

121. *Symposium on perspectives in operating room nursing, Nurs. Clin. North Am. **10**:613-686, 1975.

122. *Symposium on postoperative nursing care, Nurs. Clin. North Am. **10**:1-67, 1975.

123. Thomas, D.: Hypoglycemia in children before operation: its incidence and prevention, Br. J. Anesth. **46**:66-68, 1974.

124. Travelbee, J.: Interpersonal aspects of nursing, ed. 2, Philadelphia, 1971, F.A. Davis Co.

125. Vain, E.: Obesity in surgery, A.O.R.N. J. **16**:85-88, 1972.

126. Ward, R.J., et al.: An evaluation of postoperative respiratory maneuvers, Surg. Gynecol. Obstet. **123**:51-59, 1976.

127. Weaver, T.E.: New Life for lungs . . . through incentive spirometers, Nurs. '81 **11**(2):54-58, 1981.

128. *Webb, G.E.: Hyper and hypotension in the recovery room, A.O.R.N. J. **26**:546-574, 1977.

129. White, M.J., et al.: Memory loss following halothane anesthesia, A.O.R.N. J. **26**:1053-1064, 1977.

130. *William, J., et al.: The psychological control of preoperative anxiety, Psychophysiology **12**:50-54, 1975.

131. Williams, S.R.: Nutrition and diet therapy, ed. 4, St. Louis, 1981, The C.V. Mosby Co.

132. Wilson, W.: Routine shaving and wound infection, A.O.R.N. J. **28**:762-770, 1978.

133. *Winslow, E., and Fuhs, M.: Preoperative assessment for postoperative evaluation, Am. J. Nurs. **73**:1372-1374, 1973.

134. Wolfe, B.M., Phillips, G.J., and Hodges, R.E.: Evaluation and management of nutritional status before surgery, Med. Clin. North Am. **63**:1257-1269, 1979.

135. *Wolfer, J.A., and Davis, C.E.: Assessment of surgical patients' preoperative emotional condition and postoperative welfare, Nurs. Res. **19**:402-414, 1970.

136. Wolfer, J.A., and Visintainer, M.: Pediatric surgical patients' and parents' stress responses and adjustments, Nurs. Res. **24**:244-245, 1975.

137. Wound care, Postgrad. Med. **55**:171-177, 1974.

138. Wyatt, S., and Cullop, M.E.: Problems with patient visits by RR nurses, A.O.R.N. J. **27**:1087-1091, 1978.

139. Wylie, W.D., and Churchill-Davidson, H.C.: A practice of anesthesia, ed. 3, Chicago, 1972, Year Book Medical Publishers, Inc.

Classic

140. *Ross, R.: Wound healing, Sci. Am. **220**:40-50, 1969.

CHAPTER 25

NEOPLASIA

ROSEMARIE HOGAN
DEANNA MELTON XISTRIS

Cancer was recognized in ancient times by skilled observers who gave it the name "cancer" (L., *cancri,* crab) because it stretched out in many directions like the legs of a crab. The term is somewhat general and is used interchangeably with malignant tumor and malignant neoplasm. It denotes a tumor caused by cell growth. Forms of cancer are found in plants and in humans and other animals. It would be good if the image of the crab, suggested by Hippocrates for superficial cancer in the advanced stages, could be dropped because it helps maintain a legend of incurability.[19]

Few diseases cause greater feelings of anxiety and apprehension than cancer. Its physiologic and psychologic impact on patients and their families results in profound changes in their life-styles. Cancer may spell death to some and mutilation to others. The legends surrounding malignant disease, often focusing on incurability, help foster feelings of hopelessness and dread. Yet much progress has been made in prevention, early detection, and treatment of cancer, and research continues in these areas.

Nurses too may have the same negative attitudes that exist in society. For this reason it is extremely important that all nurses examine their own feelings about cancer and try to work them through, both by increasing their knowledge of the disease and its treatment and by discussing feelings openly with members of the health team. Nurses who have worked through their feelings are more able to be of assistance to patients and their families than nurses who have not done so.

The nurse's role in helping cancer patients is broad in scope and areas of influence. The nurse must have correct knowledge of prevention, control, and treatment of cancer and be able to apply this information in a variety of settings. Teaching about cancer is not limited to the hospital or clinic setting but takes place in industry, at PTA meetings, and at other public forums. In addition to teaching about prevention, the nurse has an active role in treatment and control programs in all settings in which clients are found. Clients and their families look to the nurse for assistance and guidance in all phases of illness from detection to terminal care.

To be effective as a helping person the nurse must be aware of the emotional impact that the diagnosis of cancer has on the patient and family because this emotional response affects every aspect of nursing care. Cancer nursing is a challenge to the creativity, skill, and commitment of the nurse.

Epidemiology

Cancer is a disease that is universal in scope. It has existed since the beginning of history and affects humans wherever they live and whatever their race, color, level of culture, and material progress.[2]

Cancer ranks second to heart disease as the cause of death in the United States, but significant progress has been made in prevention and treatment. Twenty-five years ago, one in four patients with cancer survived 5 years. Today one in three will be saved, a gain of 67,000 lives each year. Success can be attributed to (1) the diagnosis of more cancers in the early localized stage, (2) the treatment of more patients within 4 months of diagnosis, and (3) the development of new diagnostic and treatment modalities, especially chemotherapy.

Despite these advances, in 1980 an estimated 134,000 persons died of cancer who might have been cured by early detection followed by prompt treatment.[1] Although in general cancer shows no respect for economic

TABLE 25-1. Reference chart: leading cancer sites, 1982*†

Site	Estimated new cases 1982	Estimated deaths 1982	Warning signals: (if you have one see your doctor)	Safeguards	Comment
Breast	112,900	37,300	Lump or thickening in breast or unusual discharge from nipple	Regular checkup, monthly breast self-examination	Leading cause of cancer death in women
Colon and rectum	123,000	57,100	Change in bowel habits, bleeding	Regular checkup including proctoscopy, especially for those over 40 yr	Considered a highly curable disease when digital and proctoscopic examinations are included in routine checkups
Lung	129,000	111,000	Persistent cough or lingering respiratory ailment	80% of lung cancers would be prevented if no one smoked cigarettes	Leading cause of cancer death among men and rising mortality among women
Oral (including pharynx)	26,800	9150	Sore that does not heal, difficulty in swallowing	Regular checkup	Many more lives should be saved because the mouth is easily accessible to visual examination by physicians and dentists
Skin	14,800‡	6900	Sore that does not heal or change in wart or mole	Regular checkup, avoidance of overexposure to sun	Skin cancer readily detected by observation and diagnosed by simple biopsy
Uterus	55,000§	10,100	Unusual bleeding or discharge	Regular checkup including pelvic examination with Papanicolaou test	Uterine cancer mortality has declined 70% during the last 40 yr with wider application of Papanicolaou test; postmenopausal women with abnormal bleeding should be checked
Kidney and bladder	55,200	18,900	Urinary difficulty, bleeding, in which case consult physician at once	Regular checkup with urinalysis	Protective measures for workers in high-risk industries are helping to eliminate one of the important causes of these cancers
Larynx	10,900	3700	Hoarseness, difficulty in swallowing	Regular checkup including laryngoscopy	Readily curable if caught early
Prostate gland	73,000	23,300	Urinary difficulty	Regular checkup including palpation	Occurs mainly in men over 60 yr; disease can be detected by palpation at regular checkup
Stomach	24,200	13,800	Indigestion	Regular checkup	63% decline in mortality in 25 years for reasons yet unknown
Leukemia	23,500	15,900	Leukemia is a cancer of blood-forming tissues and is characterized by the abnormal production of immature white blood cells. Acute lymphocytic leukemia strikes mainly children and is treated by drugs that have extended life from a few months to as much as 10 years. Chronic leukemia strikes usually after age 25 and progresses less rapidly.		
Lymphomas	30,000	14,200	These cancers arise in the lymph system and include Hodgkin's disease and lymphosarcoma. Some patients with lymphatic cancers can lead normal lives for many years. Five-year survival rate for Hodgkin's disease increased from 25% to 54% in 20 years.		

*From American Cancer Society: 1982 Cancer facts and figures, New York, 1982, The Society.
†All figures rounded to nearest 1000. Incidence estimates based on rates from NCI SEER Program (Surveillance, Epidemiology, and End Results), 1973 to 1977.
‡Estimated new cases of nonmelanoma skin cancer about 400,000.
§If carcinoma in situ is included, cases total over 92,000.

or social status, there are some variables with regard to sex, site, age, race, and geographic location.

Sex and site

The average incidence of cancer is similar in both sexes. The overall incidence (excluding carcinoma in situ of the uterine cervix and nonmelanoma skin cancer) has decreased slightly during the past 25 years. Cancers of the stomach, esophagus, rectum, uterus, ovary, and bladder (female) have declined while cancers of the lung, pancreas, colon (male), prostrate gland, and bladder (male) have increased (Table 25-1).

Overall survival rates for some cancers have increased, such as those for cervical cancer, whereas rates for most other cancers have leveled off in the past 25 years. Dramatic increases in survival have occurred for cancers of the prostrate gland, uterine corpus, thyroid gland, kidney, bladder, and larynx, and for melanoma of the skin, Hodgkin's disease, and chronic leukemia.

The average cancer mortality in developed countries is higher for men than for women. During the past 40 years there has been a decrease of 13% in mortality from cancer among American women because of a sharp reduction in mortality from uterine cancer. Among men a 40% mortality increase has resulted from a 1400% increase in lung cancer.[1] It is revealing to note that there

has been an increase in the incidence of lung cancer in women and it may surpass breast cancer as the number one killer of women! This appears to be related to increased cigarette smoking by American women.

The death rate from cancer involving the female genital tract has dropped from between one third to one half the rate of 25 years ago, and there is ample evidence that the increased use of the Papanicolaou test to detect lesions of the cervix before symptoms develop has resulted in early treatment and a higher rate of cure (Fig. 25-1).

Age

Although more than half of the deaths from cancer occur in persons over 65 years of age, cancer is the leading cause of death in women between 30 and 54 years of age and more school-aged children die of it than of any other disease.

In children, cancer death rates have declined from 8.4 per 100,000 population under 15 years of age in 1950 to 4.9 in 1977. The actual number of deaths, as well as the rate, has also decreased during the period.[1] Although no age group is totally exempt from cancer, the death rate shows a rapid increase with aging, and some researchers believe that if one lives long enough, he will eventually develop cancer[2] (Table 25-2).

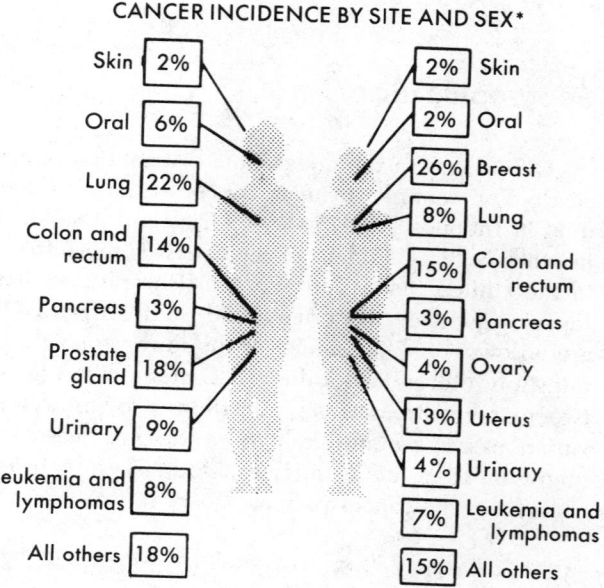

CANCER INCIDENCE BY SITE AND SEX*

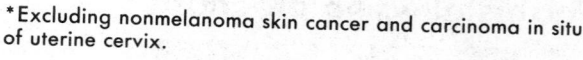
*Excluding nonmelanoma skin cancer and carcinoma in situ of uterine cervix.

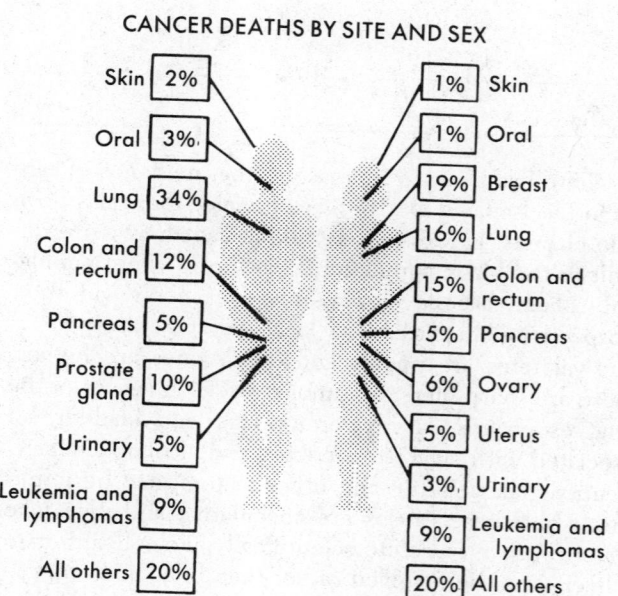

CANCER DEATHS BY SITE AND SEX

Fig. 25-1. Comparison of cancer incidence and deaths by site and sex (1982 estimates). (From American Cancer Society: 1982 Cancer facts and figures, New York, 1982, The Society.)

TABLE 25-2. Mortality for the five leading cancer sites in major age groups by sex (United States, 1978)

Age (yr)	Males		Females	
Under 15	Leukemia	550	Leukemia	411
	Brain and central nervous system	344	Brain and central nervous system	275
	Bone	47	Bone	45
	Connective tissue	43	Kidney	44
	Kidney	39	Connective tissue	43
15-34	Leukemia	827	Breast	585
	Brain and central nervous system	467	Leukemia	493
	Hodgkin's disease	335	Brain and central nervous system	347
	Testis	329	Uterus	295
	Melanoma (skin)	261	Hodgkin's disease	223
35-54	Lung	10,124	Breast	8205
	Colon and rectum	2462	Lung	4679
	Pancreas	1262	Colon and rectum	2210
	Brain and central nervous system	1282	Uterus	2111
	Leukemia	1065	Ovary	2029
55-74	Lung	46,049	Breast	17,403
	Colon and rectum	13,717	Lung	14,463
	Prostate	9047	Colon and rectum	12,551
	Pancreas	6490	Ovary	5992
	Stomach	4558	Uterus	5480
75+	Lung	14,646	Colon and rectum	12,626
	Prostate	12,298	Breast	8129
	Colon, rectum	9325	Lung	4819
	Pancreas	3208	Pancreas	3939
	Bladder	3172	Uterus	2954

Race

There has been an increase in the incidence of cancer in black males, but in black females there has been little change. However, controlling cancer is more difficult in the black population than in the white population. Blacks are developing more cancers, and their prospects for diagnosis in a localized stage are poorer. Survival rates are poorer and death rates are higher. There are sharp increases among blacks in cancer of the lung, esophagus, larynx, oral cavity, and bladder, all associated with cigarette smoking and alcohol. Dietary, occupational, genetic, and other factors may be implicated, but these causes are speculative and may take years to prove or refute scientifically. Poor health care delivery may be involved rather than biologic factors so that better education, detection, and treatment of cancer may drastically change the incidence of cancer in both black males and females.[36] Most differences in the cancer rates of black and white populations are attributed to environmental and social factors rather than to inherent biologic characteristics.[1]

Geographic factors

Differences in the geographic distribution of cancer occur. For example, primary cancer of the liver is common in Indonesia and parts of Africa and Asia but rare in other regions. Cancer of the breast is more frequent in the United States and Western Europe than it is in Japan. Ugandans, Nigerians, and South African blacks are at lowest risk for cancer of the lung, stomach, large intestine, uterus, and kidney.[99] Genetic differences between populations may contribute to international variations but are not likely to be the only reason since migration from one country to another results in major changes in the cancer pattern.[2]

Factors affecting prognosis

Trends are being evaluated to determine why the incidence of certain cancers has decreased, increased, or remained the same. There is reason to believe that the cure rate and the prognosis of cancer would improve substantially with earlier recognition and more complete reporting of early signs. Success in treating many cancers awaits better and more sensitive diagnostic aids to detect lesions in their early stages. In some parts of the body such as the skin and cervix, early recognition and prompt treatment often result in cure.

The prognosis is also affected by the intrinsic characteristics of the tumor such as histologic type and grade, size, and rate of growth. Another important factor is the general condition of the patient. The presence of debilitating conditions such as infection, diabetes, or malnutrition may adversely affect the outcome.[19]

Cancer is not only a threat to life, but its cost in loss of income and disruption of the lives of families cannot be estimated. Nurses must be in the forefront of the thousands of health professionals who are working to eradicate the disease.

Pathophysiology

Characteristics of normal cells

Normal tissue contains large numbers of mature cells of uniform size and shape, each containing a nucleus of uniform size. Within each nucleus are the chromosomes, a specific number for the species, and within each chromosome is *deoxyribonucleic acid* (DNA). DNA is a giant molecule whose chemical composition controls the characteristics of *ribonucleic acid* (RNA), which is found both in the *nucleoli* of cells and in the cytoplasm of the cell itself and which regulates cell growth and function. When ovum and sperm unite, the DNA and RNA within the chromosomes of each will govern the differentiation and future course of the trillions of cells that finally develop to form the adult organism. In the development of various organs and parts of the body, cells undergo differentiation in size, appearance, and arrangement; thus the histologist or the pathologist can look at a piece of prepared tissue through a microscope and know the portion of the body from which it came.

Mitosis

Mitosis refers to the splitting of one cell into two cells. In the normal cell, multiplication takes place by an orderly process. Reproduction begins in the nucleus by duplication (replication) of the 23 pairs (46) of the chromosomes, as well as the genes within the chromosomes. This duplication is followed by the division of the two sets of chromosomes into two separate nuclei and finally the splitting of the cell to form two daughter cells. Mitosis, which is preceded by a phase called in-

CELL REPLICATION: INTERPHASE AND MITOSIS

Interphase	Two centrioles (small cell structures) begin to move apart. Microtubules grow radially away from centrioles, some penetrating cell nucleus, some connecting the centrioles forming a spindle. Within nucleus each chromosome splits to form two new chromosomes.
Mitosis	
Prophase	Nuclear envelope dissolves and some of the microtubules become attached to the chromosomes.
Metaphase	The two centrioles are pushed further apart by the growing spindle, pulling the chromosomes to center of cell.
Anaphase	Each pair of chromosomes breaks apart; 46 daughter chromosomes are pulled toward one mitotic spindle and the other 46 chromosomes to the other spindle.
Telophase	The two sets of chromosomes are pulled completely apart and are enveloped by new nuclear membranes. The cell then separates into two cells with a nucleus in each cell.

terphase, consists of four phases; prophase, metaphase, anaphase, and telophase (see box above and Fig. 25-2).

Cell cycle time

The concept of cell cycle time is pertinent to understanding normal cell replication and has implications for drug use in cancer therapy (p. 498). Cell cycle time may be described as the interval from mitosis of a cell to its mitosis into daughter cells. Initially, there is a stationary period (G_0) of apparent rest after mitosis takes place. The cells are not in the cycle but are viable and capable of undergoing mitosis if necessary. The cell cycle is divided into four phases (Fig. 25-2): (1) a quiescent phase consisting of G_1 (G denotes a gap) in which RNA and protein synthesis begin; (2) S_1, a period of DNA synthesis; (3) G_2, further RNA and protein synthesis and the development of the mitotic spindle; and (4) mitosis (M). These processes of normal cell multiplication take place in response to a need and then stop.

Differentiation

Another characteristic of normal cell growth and cell division is cell differentiation. Changes in physical and functional properties of cells occur in the embryo to form different organs and tissues. Differentiation of cells,

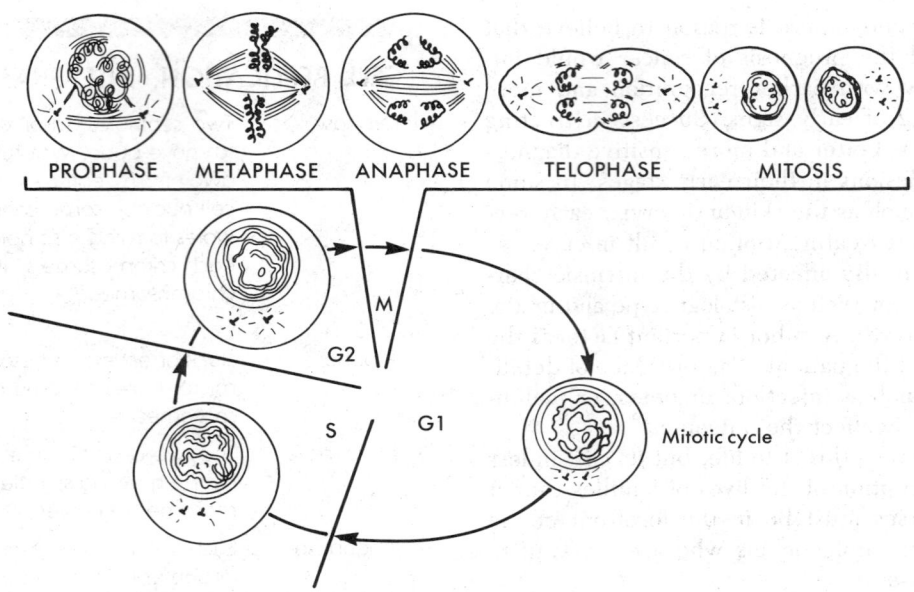

Fig. 25-2. Cell cycle. *G1,* RNA/protein synthesis; *S,* DNA synthesis; *G2,* RNA/protein synthesis and interphase; and *M,* mitosis. (Adapted from Krakoff, I.: Cancer chemotherapeutic agents: American Cancer Society professional education publication, New York, 1977, American Cancer Society.)

consequently, refers to the extent to which the cells resemble their normal forebears and thus have fully mature, specialized function and morphology. For example, all kidney cells are similar but are different from muscle cells, and each type has its specialized function. In malignant cells, changes in differentiation take place.

The method by which differentiation takes place is unknown. One current thought is that all cells carry the same genetic material but that selective repression of different genetic characteristics occurs because of buildup of different repressor substances in the cytoplasm. Different cells repress different genetic characteristics.

Normal alterations in cell growth

Some abnormal changes in cell growth are malignant growths (neoplasias). Other types of cellular growths are benign. *Hyperplasia* is an increase in cell number, whereas *hypertrophy* is an increase in cell size but not in number. Although many neoplasms are characterized by hyperplasia, many normal tissues may also undergo increase in cell number. Wound healing, callus formation, and growth of embryonic tissue are all normal forms of hyperplasia.[88]

Metaplasia is a reversible process in which one adult cell type in an organ is replaced by another adult cell type. The new cell type usually is not one normally seen in the area in which metaplasia occurs. The most common type of epithelial metaplasia is the change of columnar or pseudostratified columnar epithelium of the respiratory tract to squamous epithelium or squamous

metaplasia. *Dysplasia* is an alteration in adult cells characterized by changes in their size, shape, and organization (Table 25-3).

Benign tumors

Benign (nonmalignant) tumors involve cellular proliferation of adult or mature cells growing slowly in an orderly manner in a capsule. These tumors do not invade surrounding tissue but may cause harm through pressure on vital structures within an enclosed structure such as the skull. Benign tumors remain localized, do not metastasize (spread), and do not recur once they are completely removed (see box, p. 469).

Characteristics of malignant cells

A malignant cell is one in which the basic structure and activity have become deranged in a manner that is unknown and from a cause or causes that are still poorly understood. It is believed, however, that the basic process involves a disturbance in the regulatory functions of DNA. It is known that the DNA molecule is affected by radiation in certain instances, and it is speculated that it may be affected by other factors as well.

In the neoplastic cell, normal restraints on growth are defective. It is believed that malignant neoplasms occur as the result of faulty mechanisms inside the cell nucleus.[11]

DNA, the permanent genetic material in nuclear

TABLE 25-3. Terms denoting cellular changes

Type of cellular change	Definition	Example
Mitosis	Formation of new cell by cell division	Normal cell growth
Hyperplasia	Increase in cell number	Breast epithelium in pregnancy
Hypertrophy	Increase in cell size	Increase in muscle cell size with exercise
Atrophy	Decrease in cell size	Disuse of muscles
Metaplasia	Replacement of one adult cell type by a different adult cell type	Replacement of columnar epithelium of respiratory tract by squamous epithelium
Dysplasia	Changes in cell size, shape, and organization	Changes in cervical epithelium in long-standing cervicitis
Anaplasia	Reverse cellular development to a more primitive cell type	Irreversible change accompanying cancer
Neoplasia	Abnormal cellular changes and growth of new tissues	Malignancies

DIFFERENCES BETWEEN BENIGN AND MALIGNANT NEOPLASMS

Benign	Malignant
Limited growth potential	May proliferate rapidly or grow slowly
Localized	Spreads (metastasizes) throughout the body
Fibrous capsule	No enclosing capsule
Rarely recurs after removal	May recur even after treatment
Usually regular in shape	Irregular shape with poorly defined border
Cells similar to cell of parent tissue (well differentiated)	Cells much different from parent cells (poorly differentiated)
Expansive growth	Infiltrative growth

CHARACTERISTICS OF NEOPLASTIC CELLS[11,115]

1. Nuclei are larger and irregular in shape.
2. DNA is coarsely distributed and tends to appear near nuclear membrane.
3. Nucleoli are large, usually increased in number, and contain more chromatin than usual.
4. Mitosis is increased and atypical in appearance.
5. Abnormal multipolar mitoses and multinucleated cells may appear.
6. Cytoplasm is comparatively scanty and stains more deeply than normal cytoplasm, indicating greater RNA concentration.
7. Cells vary in size from normal cells.

chromosomes, contains information necessary for cell replication, the chemical code for cell growth and development. To convey this information, RNA serves as a messenger. Any small change in DNA (mutation) causes a distortion of biologic information, which results in the affected cells running wild. Malignant neoplasm is the result.[11] The malignant cells lose the normal specialized function of the normal cell or may take on new characteristics and functions.

A characteristic of malignant cells that can be observed through a microscope is a loss of differentiation, or a likeness to the original cell (parent tissue) from which the tumor growth originated. This loss of differentiation is called *anaplasia*, and its extent is a determining factor in the degree of malignancy of the tumor.

Anaplasia is characterized by alterations in intracel-

lular macromolecular synthesis and intercellular relationships and associations. Two types of anaplasia have been identified. In positional or organizational anaplasia, the usual distinct histologic patterns in tissues are altered. In cytologic anaplasia there is increased or altered nucleic acid synthesis in growing tissues.[88] Anaplasia is one of the most reliable indicators of malignancy. It is seen only in cancers and does not appear in benign neoplasms.

Other characteristics of malignant cells that can be seen through a microscope are the presence of nuclei of various sizes, many of which contain unusually large amounts of chromatin (hyperchromatic cells), and the presence of mitotic figures (cells in the process of division), which denotes rapid and disorderly division of cells (see box above at right for characteristics of malignant cells).

Tumor cells show less contact inhibition in vitro and therefore "pile up" in cultures, suggesting that surface properties of cancer cells are different from normal cells. In addition, the proportion of cancer cells actively proliferating in malignant tumors is generally greater than that of normal cells in benign tumors.[88]

Malignant tumors have no enclosing capsule; thus they invade adjacent or surrounding tissue, including lymph and blood vessels, through which they may spread to distant parts of the body to set up new tumors (*metastases*). Unless completely removed or destroyed, they tend to recur after treatment, and their continued presence causes death by replacing normal cells and by other means not fully understood.

Growth of neoplasms

The term *neoplasm* has been defined as a relatively autonomous growth of tissues, the term *autonomy* meaning that a malignant tumor is not subject to the "rules and regulations" that govern cells and cell interaction of the healthy individual. This autonomy is relative in that the tumor is not completely independent of the tissue from which it arose.

There are considerable differences in the rate of growth of malignant tumors. Occasionally, one grows so slowly that it can be removed completely after a long period of time. This characteristic probably accounts for the good results obtained in a few circumstances even when treatment has been delayed. No physician, however, ever relies on this possibility to justify delay in treatment. Occasionally, a malignant tumor grows slowly for a long time and then undergoes change, and the rate of growth increases enormously.

Factors causing tumor growth. The first overt cellular change in the development of cancer is transformation. Transformed cells are morphologically different from the cells that gave rise to them. Whether the cells become a tumor depends on a number of factors, many of which are host mediated (p. 472). Replication of transformed cells may be prevented if the immune system recognizes the tumor as foreign and destroys the cells, a hypothetical concept known as "immune surveillance." This ability decreases with age, since it depends on the physiologic state of the individual (p. 475).

Several factors may be involved in failure of immune surveillance: (1) a deficiency in T cells and B cells (see Chapter 19), (2) the presence of "blocking factor," which binds tumor cells and prevents their destruction by sensitized lymphocytes, and (3) the presence and extent of "recognition factor" (RF). RF appears to combine with tumor cells before they are attacked by macrophages. Healthy persons and many persons with nonmalignant diseases have large amounts of RF in their serum. It has been found that persons with terminal cancer have less RF than do those with less advanced disease. Failure of the recognition mechanism may play a role in growth of tumors.

Factors inhibiting tumor growth. Some tumor growth may be checked by lack of vascularization. One researcher has shown that some tumors produce an angiogenesis factor that attracts capillaries to the tumor. Tumors will not grow over a diameter of 3 to 4 mm unless this vascularization occurs.[88]

Growth of tumors that arise in tissues regulated by sex hormones may be affected in positive or negative ways. For example, breast cancers that occur during pregnancy often grow rapidly but tend to grow less rapidly after delivery.

There are also a number of growth-inhibiting factors called chalones. For example, epithelial cells produce a glycoprotein chalone that interacts with adrenaline to inhibit proliferation. Some experimental tumors have been inhibited by a tissue-specific chalone from which the tumor arose.

Although it is rare, tumors have regressed spontaneously, in some cases as a result of maturation and differentiation of tumor cells. This happens most frequently in neuroblastoma, a tumor of embryonic neuroblasts. The cause and physiologic action of spontaneous maturation are not known.

Factors affecting rate of tumor growth. Most tumors continue to grow and evolve, and when a large number of rapidly growing cells are present, additional mutation and arrangement of chromosomes may occur. Stem cells, a subpopulation of tumor cells with an extreme ability to proliferate, develop and may eventually be the predominant tumor cells. Different stem lines have marker chromosomes, large chromosomes with unusual morphologies. The ability to metastasize may be the result of the production of a stem cell line with greater invasive properties.[88]

The rate of growth of a tumor is expressed in terms of volume doubling time. Human tumors generally have a long doubling time, from 1 week to more than 1 year with a median time of about 60 days. Since tumors contain many different types of cells, the length of the cell cycle time (median generation time) varies and is 2 to 3 days among the various cells.

Three factors affect *rate* of tumor growth: (1) the rate of replication of proliferating cells (cell cycle time; p. 467); (2) the proportion of total cell population that is actively proliferating (growth fraction); and (3) the rate of cell loss from the tumor, which depends on the type and age of the tumor. Cell cycle time is relatively constant in tumors of similar histology, but there is considerable difference between normal and tumor tissue. Tumor doubling time is influenced by the cell cycle time. Although early tumor growth is exponential, this soon stops and the required time for doubling increases with tumor age. For a given cycle time, a tumor with a high growth fraction will double faster than a tumor with a low growth fraction.

Cell loss may be caused by cell death as a result of senescence and differentiation, nutrient deficiency (including oxygen deprivation), and destruction of stem cells by host defense mechanisms. Cells also may be lost by their moving out of the tumor through exfoliation and metastasis. Knowledge of cell population kinetics is important since the sensitivity of the cell to chemotherapy and radiotherapy depends heavily on the proliferative state of the cell at a specific time. In addition, study of cell cycle kinetics will help increase understanding of tumor growth and regulation, laying the foundation for better methods of controlling tumor cells.

Tumor size may also be increased by hemorrhage,

by accumulation of a secretion such as mucin, or by some degenerative process. Escape of these secretions into the body may produce profound local or general symptoms such as endocrine disturbances and neurologic degeneration.

Metastasis

Types of metastases. The rate of growth of a tumor determines its capacity to metastasize (spread). Cancer spreads in several different ways (Fig. 25-3).

Local spread involves infiltration into surrounding

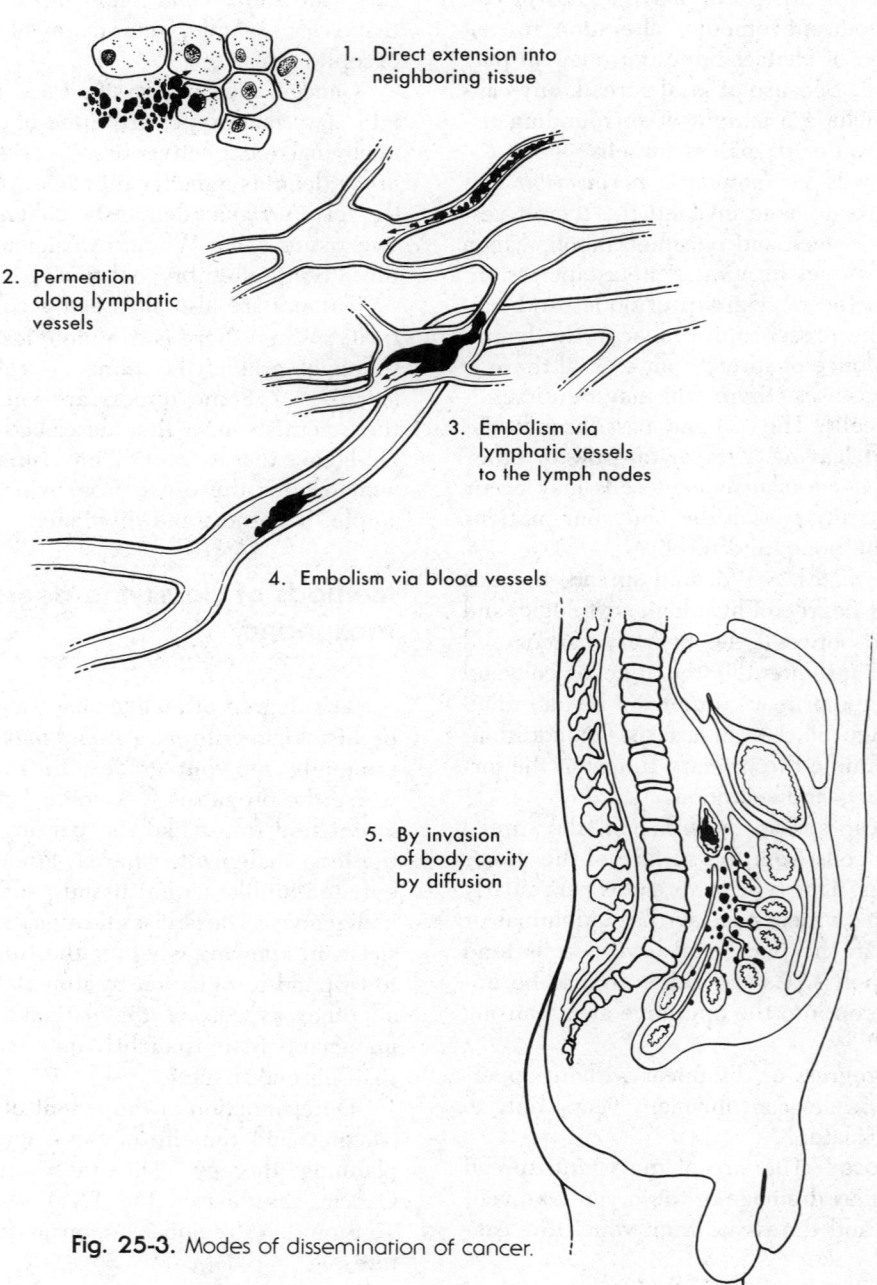

CANCER SPREADS IN MANY WAYS:

1. Direct extension into neighboring tissue

2. Permeation along lymphatic vessels

3. Embolism via lymphatic vessels to the lymph nodes

4. Embolism via blood vessels

5. By invasion of body cavity by diffusion

Fig. 25-3. Modes of dissemination of cancer.

tissues and may involve hemorrhage, necrosis, ulceration, and fibrous replacement of the involved tissues. This produces the typical local effects of ulcerating, bulky, hemorrhagic masses or indurative, fibrosing lesions with tissue fixation, distortion of the structure, and the pitting of the skin that may be seen in some cancer of the breast. Infection may accompany this local infiltration. The cancer cells tend to spread along the path of least resistance, in tissue clefts, along blood vessels or the perineural spaces. The fibrous capsule that covers some organs may limit growth from either side. For example, primary tumors of the kidney, liver, or testes may increase the size of the organ without destroying the capsule. Local spread is not an orderly process, but stages of penetration can be identified, serving as a method of classifying extent of spread (pp. 472-473). Loss of cell cohesiveness, ameboid movements, alteration in cell membranes, and loss of contact inhibition may all play a role in local spread. Because of local spread, any cancer excision must include a margin of surrounding tissues to ensure removal of all malignant cells.

Cancer also spreads by *lymphatic permeation* and *embolization*. Once cells have invaded the lymph vessels, they then may detach and become emboli, which lodge in the lymph node, forming a metastatic lesion. Spread continues to the next group of nodes and into the other organs. The presence of cancer in the lymph nodes is certain evidence of spread, but even if there is no lymph node metastases, there still may be dissemination of malignant cells. The cell may pass through the lymph node without leaving a trace, to grow in other areas. *Vascular embolism* of malignant cells may occur through the veins to any part of the body but particularly to the lungs, the bone, and the liver.[2]

In *disseminative metastasis* (distant spread) there is almost always a high degree of histologic, cytologic, and functional similarity between the primary cancer and these metastases. Consequently, the type of cell and the probable site of the primary tumor can be identified from the morphology of the metastasis. In addition, metastases usually mimic the primary tumor in the formation of cell products and secretions.

Finally, cancer can spread by *diffusion*, the spread of clumps of cancer cells from the surface of the tumor by mechanical means. This type of spread is particularly prevalent in serous cavities such as the abdominal or the pleural cavity. In the peritoneal cavity, cells tend to gravitate to the pelvis. Cancer cells can also be implanted by the surgeon into the operative area, causing metastatic lesions.[11,19]

Metastasis may regress or disappear without apparent cause and may be dormant for many years, only to resume growth years later.

Sites of metastases. The site of metastatic spread depends on the venous drainage of the organ involved, the type of cancer, and the tissue from which the cancer arises.[2] Cancer of an organ that ordinarily drains into systemic veins usually metastasizes to the lungs. Various body tissues seem to have different attraction for metastases, common sites being, in order, the liver, lungs, bone marrow, brain, and adrenal glands. Spleen, muscle, and skin are rarely involved.[19]

Classifying and naming neoplasms

Tumors derive their names from the types of tissue involved (Table 25-4), but classification of malignant tumors is difficult, since many contain several types of cells and may have benign tissue incorporated within them as well. In general, the names of benign tumors carry the suffix *-oma* following the name of the parent tissue, for example, neuroma or fibroma; there are some exceptions.

Cancers may be classified according to cell type origin. Two main types are those of epithelial and of mesenchymal (connective tissue) origin. The term *carcinoma* denotes a malignant tumor of epithelial cells, and the term *sarcoma* denotes a malignant tumor of connective tissue cells. When a malignant tumor contains all three types of embryonal tissue, it is called a *teratoma*.

Tumors are also classified according to cellular maturity. When there is complete loss of identity with the tissue of origin, the tumor is called *undifferentiated* (anaplastic). Some tumors are known by the names of the scientists who first described them, for example, Hodgkin's disease and Wilms' tumor. Other tumors are named after the organ from which they arise, for example, hepatoma and thymoma.

Methods of classifying degree of malignancy

The degree of malignancy (stage) may be estimated by histologic criteria. Tumors may be graded by roman numerals into four grades; the higher the grade, the worse the prognosis.[19] A grade 1 tumor is the most differentiated (most like the parent tissue) and therefore the least malignant, whereas grade 4 is the least differentiated (unlike parent tissues) and has a high degree of malignancy. These classifications are useful to the physician in knowing whether the tumor may be expected to respond to radiation treatment as well as in planning all other aspects of the patient's treatment. Usually, malignant tissue is slightly more sensitive to irradiation than normal tissue.

Determination of the extent of the spread of cancer (staging) and the site of the original tumor is vital for planning therapy. The International Union Against Cancer has devised the TNM system of classification: *T*, tumor; *N*, regional lymph nodes; *M*, distant metastases.

TABLE 25-4. Classification of neoplasms

Parent tissue	Benign tumor	Malignant tumor
Epithelium		
Skin and mucous membrane	Papilloma Polyp	Squamous cell carcinoma Basal cell carcinoma Transitional cell carcinoma
Glands	Adenoma Cystadenoma	Adenocarcinoma
Endothelium		Endothelioma
Blood vessels	Hemangioma	Hemangioendothelioma Angiosarcoma
Lymph vessels	Lymphangioma	Lymphangiosarcoma Lymphangioendothelioma
Bone marrow		Multiple myeloma Ewing's sarcoma Leukemia Lymphosarcoma
Lymphoid tissue		Reticulum cell sarcoma (difficult to classify because of cell embryology) Lymphatic leukemia
Connective tissues		
Embryonic fibrous tissue	Myxoma	Myxosarcoma
Fibrous tissue	Fibroma	Fibrosarcoma
Adipose tissue	Lipoma	Liposarcoma
Cartilage	Chondroma	Chondrosarcoma
Bone	Osteoma	Osteogenic sarcoma
Synovial membrane	Synovioma	Synovial sarcoma
Muscle tissue		
Smooth muscle	Leiomyoma	Leiomyosarcoma
Striated muscle	Rhabdomyoma	Rhabdomyosarcoma
Nerve tissue		
Nerve fibers and sheaths	Neuroma Neurinoma (neurilemoma)	Neurogenic sarcoma
	Neurofibroma	Neurofibrosarcoma
Ganglion cells	Ganglioneuroma	Neuroblastoma
Glia cells	Glioma	Glioblastoma Spongioblastoma
Meninges	Meningioma	
Pigmented neoplasms		
Melanoblasts	Pigmented nevus	Malignant melanoma Melanocarcinoma
Miscellaneous		
Placenta	Hydatidiform mole	Chorion-epithelioma (choriocarcinoma)
	Dermoid cyst	Embryonal carcinoma Embryonal sarcoma Teratocarcinoma

Adding a number to the letters (e.g., T1, T2, N1, N2) indicates the extent of the malignancy[19] (see box in next column). This system provides a type of "shorthand" notation to describe the particular tumor. The

TNM STAGING CLASSIFICATION SYSTEM

Tumor

T0	No evidence of primary tumor
TIS	Carcinoma in situ
T1, T2, T3, T4	Ascending degrees of tumor size and involvement

Nodes

N0	No regional nodes demonstrably abnormal
N1a, N2a	Demonstrable regional lymph nodes, metastasis not suspected
N1b, N2b, N3	Demonstrable regional lymph nodes; metastasis suspected
Nx	Regional nodes cannot be assessed clinically

Metastasis

M0	No evidence of distant metastasis
M1, M2, M3	Ascending degrees of metastatic involvement of the host including distant nodes

purpose of the TNM system is to define categories for all cases and also to allow subsequent and more detailed information to be added. A TNM classification has been identified for major cancer sites, and the choice of treatment depends on the clinical TNM stage, both for the primary tumor and the lymph nodes.

Nurse's responsibility regarding pathophysiology

As individuals take more responsibility for their own health care and as their knowledge of disease processes grows, they want more explanations of and information about their illness. Physicians may give adequate explanation about cancer and its treatment, but the patient may not understand because of anxiety or misinterpretation of vocabulary. The nurse can clarify information for both patient and family, using appropriate but understandable terms and illustrations. If there is any question of the patient's or the family's understanding of the information given by the physician, the nurse clarifies with the physician what the patient and family have been told. The nurse may also interpret to the physician the patient's or family's readiness for more information.

Etiology: carcinogenesis

The factors that contribute to the development of cancer are many and at the present time are not fully understood; however, certain health practices are known to decrease the possibility that cancer may occur. Factors involved in carcinogenesis include host susceptibility, environmental carcinogens, habits and customs, and viruses.

Host susceptibility

Genetic factors

Certain conditions and predispositions of the individual seem to contribute to the development of cancer. Studies of genetic factors have focused on specific cancer sites and the disease in general. Chromosomes have been studied to find evidence of the genetic origin of cancer. Human carriers seem to have an abnormal number of chromosomes, usually approximate multiples of the diploid state. The question is whether these changes are the cause or the effect of cancer. Abnormalities in chromosome numbers 7 and 17 have been found in cells with malignant characteristics. These experiments, however, involved studying simian viruses, not human chromosomal changes.

A second indication of genetic origin is that cancer cells are a population of cells descendant from a single cell of origin (clones). Future generations of cancer cells are always malignant; they inherit and pass on the trait.

Finally, there is the possibility that cancer arises from an innate genetic inability, possibly a defect in mitotic regulation. Theoretically, in normal cells mitosis is either inhibited or induced by diffusible substances. The repressor substances are called chalones. Cancer cells may fail to be regulated by the chalones either because the chalones may not be secreted, or if they are, they fail to respond.[30]

Hereditary cancer has certain general characteristics: (1) an early age of onset, occurring 20 or more years earlier than in the general population; (2) a marked incidence of bilateral cancer in paired organs, e.g., breasts, kidneys, thyroid glands; (3) multiple primary or multicentered cancers with greater frequency than expected; and (4) well-established autosomal recessive sex-linked and cytogenic cancer and precancerous disorders. In addition, in many cases there is evidence of vertical transmission in consecutive generations with autosomal dominant inheritance.[69]

Familial polyposis of the colon, a precursor of cancer, is indisputably hereditary. There is also a high incidence of breast cancer in a vertical line of descent, such as from mother to daughter.[2] Risk of breast cancer in the first-degree relatives of a patient is five times that of the general population. Heredity in some way seems to be connected with bronchogenic cancer. It seems to interact with cigarette smoking to cause a synergistic effect.[61]

Cancer family syndrome (CFS) is characterized by adenocarcinoma involving the colon and endometrium and less frequently the stomach, breasts, and ovaries. The tumor incidence is transmitted vertically, and there is an autosomal dominant mode of inheritance. Familial atypical multiple mole-melanoma (FAMMM) syndrome is a familial disease in about 3% to 10% of occurrences and it is believed that primary genetic factors may predispose individuals to the disease. Three types of multiple endocrine adenomatosis (MEA) involving various endocrine glands are also familial diseases.[69]

Other autosomal dominant disorders include retinoblastoma, hemochromatosis, and multiple exostosis. Autosomal recessive diseases are gonadal dysgenesis and skin cancer precursors: xeroderma pigmentosum and disseminated superficial actinic porokeratosis.

In general, inherited cancers are a direct expression of an inherited defect, but these syndromes are rare and account for only a small percentage of familial cancer.[72] Studies have shown that the pattern of inheritance is not usually that of a single mendelian gene, and it is still not known whether the incidences of many specific cancers are a result of a combination of genetic or environmental factors.[83]

Hormonal factors

Some evidence suggests that hormones may in some way be connected with the development of certain cancers. In addition, some metabolites of cancers may also act as antihormones or have new physiologic effects. Hormones do not appear to be primary carcinogens, but rather they seem to influence carcinogenesis in three ways: (1) by a preparative action on the target tissues making them susceptible to the carcinogenic agent, (2) by a "permissive" influence on carcinogenesis allowing the process to progress, and (3) by a conditioning effect on the tumor. Hormones are capable of restraining or enhancing growth of tumors that have developed.[83] Hormone therapy (p. 504) and some surgical therapies (hypophysectomy and oophorectomy) are based on this fact.

There is evidence that tissues that are endocrine responsive (e.g., breasts, endometrium, and prostate) do not develop cancer unless they are stimulated by their growth-promoting hormones. Estrogens have been associated with cancers such as adenocarcinoma of the vagina, hepatic tumors, breast tumors, and uterine cancer.[67]

In addition to tissue stimulation by the hormone,

carcinogenesis may be determined by the length of time of the hormonal effect. The longer the preparative influence of the hormone, the greater is the chance of cancer development.

Precancerous lesions

Certain benign lesions and tumors have a tendency toward malignant change. These cancers are preventable if minor precursor conditions are treated carefully. These precancerous conditions include polyps of the colon and rectum, certain pigmented moles, dysplasias of the cervical epithelium, Paget's disease of the bone, and radiodermatitis and senile keratosis.[2]

Senile (solar) keratoses are thickened patches on the skin of the face and hands of those who are exposed to sunlight. Xeroderma pigmentosum, a rare congenital hypersensitivity to light, results in warty precancerous elevations of the skin in childhood. Epidermal carcinoma or malignant melanoma frequently develops. Leukoplakia, precancerous white thickened patches, may occur on the mucous membranes of the lips, mouth, tongue, vulva, and cervix.

Precancerous lesions are a large and heterogeneous group; in some, cancer is inevitable, whereas in others the risk is so low that medical management disregards the cancer risk. For example, the risk of cancer is high in xeroderma pigmentosum but low in leukoplakia of mucous membranes, especially of the oral cavity, larynx, and vulva.[93]

Chronic irritation

It is also known that cancer may follow chronic irritation of any part of the body. There are many ways to prevent irritation that may lead to cancer. Effort is being made in industry to protect workers from coal-tar products known to contain carcinogens. Masks and gloves are recommended in some instances, and workers are urged to wash their hands and arms thoroughly to remove all irritating substances at the end of the day's work. Industrial nurses participate in intensive educational programs to help workers understand the need for carrying out company rules that may help prevent cancer.

Prolonged exposure to wind, dirt, and sun may also lead to skin cancer. Skin cancer of the face and hands is particularly frequent among farmers and cattle ranchers who have fair complexions and who do not protect themselves from exposure.

Any kind of chronic irritation to the skin should be avoided, and moles that are in locations where they may be irritated by clothing should be removed. Shoelaces, shoetops, girdles, brassieres, and shirt collars are examples of clothing that may be a source of chronic irritation. Glasses, earrings, dental plates, and pipes that are in repeated contact with skin and mucous membrane may contribute to cancer. Chewing food thoroughly is recommended to lessen irritation in the throat and stomach. Cancer of the mouth is sometimes associated with rough jagged teeth and the constant irritation of tobacco smoke. The habit of drinking scalding hot or freezing cold liquids is also thought to be irritating to the mouth and to the esophagus. Indiscriminate use of laxatives is believed to have possible carcinogenic effects on the large bowel.

Immunologic factors

Immunologists have been increasingly aware of the role of the immune system in the natural history of malignant disease. It may be possible that failure of the normal immune mechanism may predispose to certain cancers.[78] The change from normal to malignant cells is relatively common. These new cells are antigenically different and are recognized as such by the body's immune system. If the immune response is initiated, the malignant cell will be destroyed. That a kind of immune surveillance system may exist is suggested by the following evidence: (1) The two peaks of high incidence of tumors in humans are in early childhood and old age, periods when the immune system is weak. (2) Individuals with rare immunodeficiency diseases in which there is a defect in cellular immunity have increased evidence of tumor development. (3) Individuals receiving immunosuppressive drugs to prevent organ transplant rejection have an increased evidence of neoplasia.[47]

The question arises, if a surveillance system exists, why do initial tumor cells progress to clinical cancer? There are no clear-cut answers but some are suggested. Some tumors arise in areas that are poorly served by the immune system, areas such as the central nervous system or the retrobulbar aspect of the eye. Some tumors do not stimulate antibody formation because they are so similar to normal cells. The normally occurring system, called suppressor lymphocytes, which check the immune response, may become overly active and overwhelm the immune system. The problem may reside in individuals who do not have the same genetic ability for immune response as others have, just as not all have the same physical strength. A problem of time also exists, since the immune system can handle only about 10 million cells. A 1 cm tumor mass contains over 1 billion cells, therefore it is not controlled by normal immunologic response. Consequently, a tumor that develops faster than the immune system can respond to it will escape destruction.[47]

Cancer itself appears to suppress the immune response early in the disease as well as late in its progression. It has not been definitely established that cancer develops because of failure in immune surveillance and at the present time there is not enough data to make a strong case, but investigations continue.[73] (The role of the immune system and cancer therapy is discussed later in this chapter and in detail in Chapter 19.)

Environmental factors

Many years ago it was observed that skin cancers developed more often in men who were employed as chimney sweeps in English homes in which coal was burned in fireplaces. It was then learned that when the suspected substance (methylcholanthrene) contained in the sweepings was repeatedly painted on the ears of experimental animals, cancer developed.

It has been estimated that 70% to 90% of human cancers result from environmental factors and that we have the knowledge to prevent 30% to 40% of cancers in the United States. One to five percent of human cancer is caused by occupational exposure, and the Environmental Protection Agency indicates that as many as 50,000 chemical substances, *excluding* pharmaceuticals and food additives in common use, are carcinogenic.[99]

The Occupational Safety and Health Act of 1970 authorized the Occupational Safety and Health Administration to enforce maximal allowable concentrations of exposure to carcinogens (threshhold limit values [TLVs]). The National Institute for Occupational Health and Safety at present believes that it is not possible to show precise tolerance levels of chemical carcinogens and consequently stresses that exposure to any known or suggested carcinogens must be reduced to the least possible level by any means available.[99]

There are several types of chemical and physical carcinogens (cancer-producing substances). Various carcinogens may have an additive or enhancing effect on one another, and even small amounts of these substances in the environment may constitute a hazard. Carcinogens act on different organs depending on the portal of entry and the distribution in the body.[1]

Ionizing radiation

Radiographs and radium may cure cancer, but in other cases they cause it. Ionizing radiation consists of electromagnetic waves or material particles that have sufficient energy to ionize atoms or molecules (i.e., remove electrons from them) and thereby alter their chemical behavior. In adequate amounts it destroys the cells.

Every living thing from the beginning of time has been exposed to small amounts of radiation from the sun and from certain natural elements in the earth, such as uranium, that emit gamma-rays (γ-rays) in the process of their decay. This is called natural background radiation. No problem regarding radiation existed until after 1895, when the roentgen-ray (x-ray) machine was developed and became widely used in diagnosis of disease. The development of this machine was followed by the discovery of radium and the use of both radium and radiographs for treatment of diseases such as cancer. With developments in the field of nuclear energy, it has been possible to produce radioactive isotopes of a number of the elements, although only a few of them, such as gold, iodine, cobalt, and phosphorus, have medical application at the present time. The problem of overexposure and possible harm to patients and to personnel caring for them has increased greatly with the increased use of radiographs in diagnosis and treatment and the more recent use of radioisotopes in diagnosis and treatment. Also, radiation in the environment resulting from atomic testing has become a widely feared and much debated subject in many parts of the world.

No one really knows how much exposure to radiation is safe for persons working with patients and for patients having repeated radiographs taken for various purposes. Relatively small amounts of exposure have produced serious damage in experimental animals, but humankind has not lived through enough generations of relatively high exposure for conclusive evidence of safe levels to be obtained. It is reasonable to assume that the less exposure one has the better. This does not mean that a patient receiving radiation treatment should not receive adequate nursing care. There are ways to protect persons from exposure, and hospitals are required to have protective procedures and guidelines for persons who care for patients receiving radiation therapy. All nurses should be familiar with the procedures used in the institution in which they are employed.

The ionizing effect of radiation on the body cells remains, so that exposure is cumulative throughout life. Exposure of the entire body enormously increases the amount of radiation received. For this reason all of the body except the part being treated is protected from exposure when relatively high doses are given for therapeutic purposes.

The National Academy of Science's Advisory Committee on Radiation has recommended that the exposure limit for the population be set at 170 mrem per year per person. It has been calculated that an exposure of 500 mrem per year could be allowed for an occasional individual. At this level it was felt that there might be some increase in mutation rate but not sufficient to cause a significant increase in genetic disease. Scientists no longer assume nor can they prove that there is a threshold below which there is no radiation damage. There are certain effects of radiation that do show a threshold but scientists suspect that some irreparable residual damage exists at even the smallest dose. They postulate that a damaged cell might ultimately become cancerous. There is no assumption that any level of radiation is completely safe, but present arguments focus on how large a risk arises in the dose of natural background radiation.[109]

The U.S. government's Interagency Task Force on Ionizing Radiation has recommended that physicians be more cautious in the use of radiographs both in the number of exposures and in the amount of radiation per exposure.

The amount of exposure the patient receives from a series of radiographs taken for diagnostic purposes depends on the machine used and the technical skill involved. Usually, the fluoroscopic examination entails more exposure than radiography. To prevent excessive exposure with fluoroscopy, the physician allows time for his or her own eyes to accommodate to the darkened room so that the patient can be observed with a lower intensity of the machine. The exposure of the average nurse working in a hospital and occasionally assisting a patient while a radiograph is taken is almost negligible.

Radiation effects. Systemic reactions to excessive radiation exposure are leukopenia, leukemia, and sterility or damage to the reproductive cells. Leukemia and skin cancer are occupational diseases among radiologists.[109] Because of the increased risk, badges are worn by persons whose daily work exposes them to radiation. The badge, which contains photographic film capable of absorbing radiation, is developed each month. A darkening or blackening of the film indicates excessive exposure. Personnel who are becoming overexposed are removed, at least temporarily, from direct contact with radiation.

Because of the possible danger to the fetus, particularly between the second and sixth weeks of life, radiographs are seldom taken of pregnant women. If they must be taken, the lower abdomen is carefully protected. Also, pregnant women usually are not employed in radiology departments or in caring for patients receiving radioactive materials internally.

Nurses who work where they are exposed to x-rays repeatedly or who care for patients receiving radioactive substances must take responsibility for learning how to protect themselves from too much exposure.

Effects of the sun. Our society at times seems sun addicted and a tanned skin is eagerly sought by many, yet sunlight is the most universal carcinogen.[24] Skin cancer occurs mostly in people who work in the open air, such as sailors and farmers, and on areas of the body most exposed to sunlight. Light-complected individuals are the most cancer susceptible.[19]

Chemical pollutants

Air pollution has been blamed for the rising cancer incidence in the twentieth century. Ten polycyclic aromatic hydrocarbons have been recognized as carcinogenic.[19]

In addition to the high incidence of epithelioma of the scrotum among the chimney sweeps mentioned earlier, tar and pitch and their derivatives as well as mineral oils containing aromatic hydrocarbons were discovered to be carcinogenic many years ago.

Skin cancers caused by arsenic have been found among farmers and vineyard workers who handle arsenicals. Bladder cancer from aromatic amines is an occupational disease of workers in the rubber industry. The risk of contacting lung cancer is 15 to 30 times greater among those exposed to the chromium compounds. Other common occupational cancers are respiratory cancers from asbestos and leukemia resulting from long-term inhalation of benzol.[19]

Many nitrosamines cause a variety of cancers in different species. Nitrates are commonly used as food additives, while nicotine may be a source of amines. A new liver carcinogen, aflatoxin 13, has been isolated from a common mold that grows on peanuts, soybeans, fruit, some meats, and mild and cheddar cheese. The most recently indicated carcinogenic agents are chloromethyl methyl ether and vinyl chloride (a basic precursor of polyvinyl plastics). A rare form of vaginal cancer in young women has been linked to the ingestion by their mothers of diethylstilbestrol (DES) prescribed to prevent spontaneous abortion.[53]

Various red dyes used in the coloring of food products have been banned because they may be potentially carcinogenic. In late 1969 cyclamates, which were widely used as sugar substitutes, were banned when experimental studies revealed that in high doses they could produce cancer of the bladder in mice. Saccharin has also been identified as being carcinogenic in a study of rats, and the Food and Drug Administration (FDA) has recommended that it not be used as an artificial sweetener. In 1977 the United States Congress approved an 18-month moratorium on the proposed ban to allow for further scientific study of the effects of saccharin because of questions raised about the validity of applying the results of the study to humans. Cancer has been implicated in the use of some hair dyes.

Health practices

Smoking

There is now no question that cigarette smoking is linked with the increased incidence of lung cancer. More and more reports are appearing that incriminate moderate and heavy cigarette smoking as a predisposing factor in the development of lung cancer, which now causes 14 times as many deaths each year as it did 30 years ago. In 1981 lung cancer killed approximately 105,000 persons in the United States (77,000 men and 28,000 women).[1] Although the rate of lung cancer in men has been alarming, separate and independent studies have noted a rise in the rate of lung cancer in women. The rise appears to parallel an increase in women smokers, particularly teenage girls, over the last 5 years. In 1968 the number of girls between the ages of 12 and 18 who smoked was about half the number of teenage boys who smoked. By 1972 there was only a 2.4% difference, and by 1980 the difference had dropped to less than 0.5%. The rise in the number of women smokers has captured the attention of cigarette manufacturers, who have increased their advertising efforts in this direction to the point of designing cigarettes expressly for women. An enormous amount of effort is being put forth by both private and public agencies concerned with the health of the public to alert everyone, smokers as well as nonsmokers, to the dangers of cigarette smoking.

It has also been demonstrated that there is a correlation between cancer mortality and the number of cigarettes smoked daily, number of years an individual has smoked, and the age at which he or she began to smoke cigarettes.[19] Smoking has also been connected with esophageal cancer and possibly bladder cancer.[19,116] If smoking is discontinued even after a habit of 30 years, there is a decrease in the evidence of lung cancer.[118]

After the release of the Surgeon General's Report on Smoking and Health in 1964, the National Interagency Council on Smoking and Health was formed. This group, composed of 27 public and private health, educational, and youth organizations, has as its major objective combating smoking as a health hazard. Several of these participating organizations have produced films and other educational materials that are available to schools, organizations, and individuals. Assistance in securing films and other materials can be obtained from the Library, National Clearinghouse for Smoking and Health, Public Health Service.* One of the main concerns of the Interagency Council is how to convince young people not to start smoking. A new film, *Breathing Easy,* was produced by the American Lung Association† especially for the preteen group. The American Cancer Society is designing smoking cessation clinics for places of employment and for schools. Antismoking education drives in schools are conducted through school courses, assemblies, and exhibits.

Since January 2, 1971, no cigarette advertising has been permitted on either television or radio. On the same date the warning on packages was changed from "Caution: cigarette smoking may be hazardous to your health" to "Warning: the Surgeon General has determined that cigarette smoking is dangerous to your health." While the campaign to convince people to stop smoking has been slow and arduous, there has been change noted in smoking patterns. There is a trend toward increased use of filter cigarettes and pipes among smokers. The two thirds of the population who are nonsmokers have been active and in some instances successful in getting smokers to refrain from smoking in public places such as specified sections of airplanes and public buildings. In 1972 the Surgeon General of the

United States declared that smoking in the presence of a nonsmoker might be considered an act of aggression. Experiments have shown that cigarette smokers in a crowded, ill-ventilated room or automobile can raise the level of carbon dioxide to the point that all within the area can experience trouble discriminating time intervals and visual and sound cues as well as difficulty with eye-hand coordination. Action in the form of bills, ordinances, and restrictions on smoking and the sale of tobacco in places of public assembly are being instituted at all government levels on a nationwide basis.

Nurses have a responsibility, both as well-informed citizens and as professional persons, to be aware of the most recent antismoking programs and to interpret them to the public. One of the best ways for nurses to do this would be to stop smoking themselves. Although there are no figures available on the number of nurses who have stopped smoking, the American Cancer Society estimates that 50,000 physicians have done so.

Nutrition

Nutritional habits are increasingly being investigated and implicated in the cause of cancer. A high incidence of cancer of the colon occurs in populations whose diet is high in refined food and low in nonabsorbable cellulose "roughage" or fiber. Evidence indicates that there is a low incidence of colonic carcinoma among persons who eat a largely vegetarian diet that has relatively few animal products[48,102] and is especially low in fats.[118] Breast cancer appears to be associated with a diet high in animal fat, but the precise relationship has not been identified.[67]

Other factors in the daily diet may be responsible for cancer. These are not only specific carcinogenic agents but also certain nutritional deficiencies. Breast and colon cancers have also been correlated with nutritional deficits, especially with vitamins A, B (riboflavin), and C, although these may play an indirect role.[29] Ingestion of smoked foods, which contain benzopyrene, has been correlated with an increased incidence of stomach cancer. Some epidemiologic and experimental evidence suggests that high caloric intake may lead to cancer and calorie deprivation may prevent it. Obesity may increase the risk of endometrial cancer.[67]

Some foods may protect against cancer. The food additives BHA (butylated hydroxyanisole) and BHT (butylated hydroxytoluene) seem to inhibit cancer. Although reports are conflicting, some investigators believe vitamins A, B, and C actually have anticancer effects. The *Lactobacillus bulgaris* and *Streptococcus thermophilus* microorganisms found in yogurt have been found to inhibit tumor cell proliferation.[29]

Many food substances contain additives, contaminants, and naturally appearing substances such as aflatoxin, which may be carcinogenic. Food additives being studied include food dyes, flavoring agents, and antimicrobial preservatives such as sodium and potassium ni-

---

*5401 Westbord Ave., Bethesda, MD 20016
†1740 Broadway, New York, NY 10019

trite and nitrate. Although some potential carcinogens are present in the diet, the time trends do not indicate that additives now in use are significant in the etiology of cancer. The present government policy is to keep the levels of potential carcinogenic agents in food as low as feasible, recognizing that it is almost impossible to state with absolute certainty that any ingested chemical is safe.[48]

The U.S. Delaney amendment to the Federal Food, Drug and Cosmetic Act requires that no substance producing tumors in experimental animals should be permitted in food for human beings. The problem is that effects from ingesting carcinogenic agents may not be seen for decades because of the long latency periods. Childhood exposure, particularly, may provide the time for cancer to appear.[29]

Alcohol

There is a significant association between high alcohol intake and cancer of the mouth, pharynx, larynx, and esophagus. However, alcoholism is often associated with smoking and with vitamin and dietary deficiencies, whose roles in the etiology of cancer are not known. It is speculated that alcohol and nutritional deficiencies enhance carcinogenesis by increasing the metabolic activities of specific tobacco carcinogens.[29] Tumors of the involved sites occur with greater frequency in men, blacks, lower socioeconomic groups, increasingly urbanized societies, and the elderly.[98]

Sexual practices

Carcinoma of the uterine cervix is less common in virgins than in married women. It is higher in those who have first coitus at an early age, who have an early first marriage, and who have had multiple sex partners. Cervical cancer is more frequent in women who have had multiple pregnancies, but this factor decreases in importance when the groups of women compared started their sex life at the same age. The development of cancer seems to be connected with coitus rather than pregnancy.

Carcinoma of the penis is virtually unknown among circumcised men. The means by which circumcision provides protection is not clear, but it is probably related to better hygiene. There is also a lower incidence of cancer of the uterine cervix in women whose sexual partner has been circumcised and in cultures in which the men, even though not circumcised, have a high standard of genital hygiene.[19]

The correlation with sexual experience and breast cancer is the reverse of that for the uterine cervix. Breast cancer patients have usually been married and become pregnant later in life. Lactation may provide some protection against breast cancer, since women who have breast-fed their infants show a lower incidence of breast malignancy. Cancer of the breast is reported to be unknown among Eskimo women and to be relatively rare among Japanese women; both cultures practice breast-feeding.

Viruses

Studies in animals have established that there is a viral role in carcinogenesis, but proof that humans are affected has not been definitely established.[2,103,115] Viruses have been isolated and identified as the cause of cancer in mice, rabbits, and frogs.

Cervical cancer may result from a virus introduced into the cervix during sexual intercourse. This virus may be a member of the herpes group, *herpesvirus hominis* (HV-2). Carriers of HV-2 in the population are generally uncircumcised males with poor personal hygiene.[115]

Herpeslike viruses have been visualized by electron microscopy in Burkitt's tumor and Hodgkin's disease cells. Investigators, however, have been unable to demonstrate human oncogenic viruses from human tumors. This may be a technical problem, since the ideal laboratory conditions for the isolation of tumor viruses have not been found. In addition, the long latency period in humans makes study of viruses difficult.

The viruses found in animal tumors indicate that viruses may act individually or as co-carcinogens in causing malignancy in humans.[115] The question is no longer, however, whether viruses have a role in the cause of cancer but when they will be definitely implicated and whether one or many will be involved.[103]

Psychosocial factors

Stressors such as life changes, loss of a significant other, and personality variables have been suggested as etiologic factors in the development of cancer. Some researchers believe that stress alters the body's immune system, making a person more susceptible to cancer. Depression has also been linked to cancer deaths by causing changes in immune mechanisms.

Social support in the form of institutions, family, and friends also may be an important variable. The individual with low social support and high need may be at a higher risk for developing cancer. In addition, lack of social support may adversely affect coping responses to therapy and to the illness. At the present time, however, how one defines the nature of social support and the degree to which it is present or lacking is unclear.[82]

Conclusions

Carcinogenesis is a dynamic process that is influenced by many independent and poorly defined variables. The initial molecular changes are irreversible, but they may not be expressed when cooperative conditions are absent. Changes in these conditions may alter the carcinogenic process, resulting in either acceleration, inhibition, or even reversal of the process.[53] Etiologic agents may be co-carcinogens. A genetic predisposition for a "weak" immune system along with a viral infection may lead to cancer, or oncogenic viruses may act as suppressants of the immune system. Chemical carcinogens may activate latent viral genes or inhibit the immune system's effectiveness in destroying cancer cells. Fig. 25-4 illustrates the relationship between various carcinogenic factors in the etiology of cancer.

Nurses have a vital role to play in communicating to the public the factors involved in carcinogenesis. They can clarify misconceptions as well as do health teaching so that known carcinogenic practices may be eliminated. They can also set an example of good health practices for the general public, perhaps a more difficult role. As knowledgeable and concerned citizens, nurses must be initiators and supporters of efforts to have carcinogens removed from the environment.

Prevention and health education

Health teaching

The American public is more widely read and informed about health problems than ever before. Health-seeking behavior and a desire to be more knowledgeable about health problems are indicated by the frequency of articles about topics such as cancer in the lay press. The topic of cancer is also discussed more openly than ever before. Nurses have a major responsibility in the prevention of cancer. Because of their knowledge about the disease and their opportunity for contact with the public in the inpatient and outpatient setting, nurses have the opportunity to teach about cancer and to help motivate patients to seek treatment.

Case finding is a responsibility of all nurses. The nurse must be able to (1) counsel and direct patients to the proper sources of help, (2) have information about

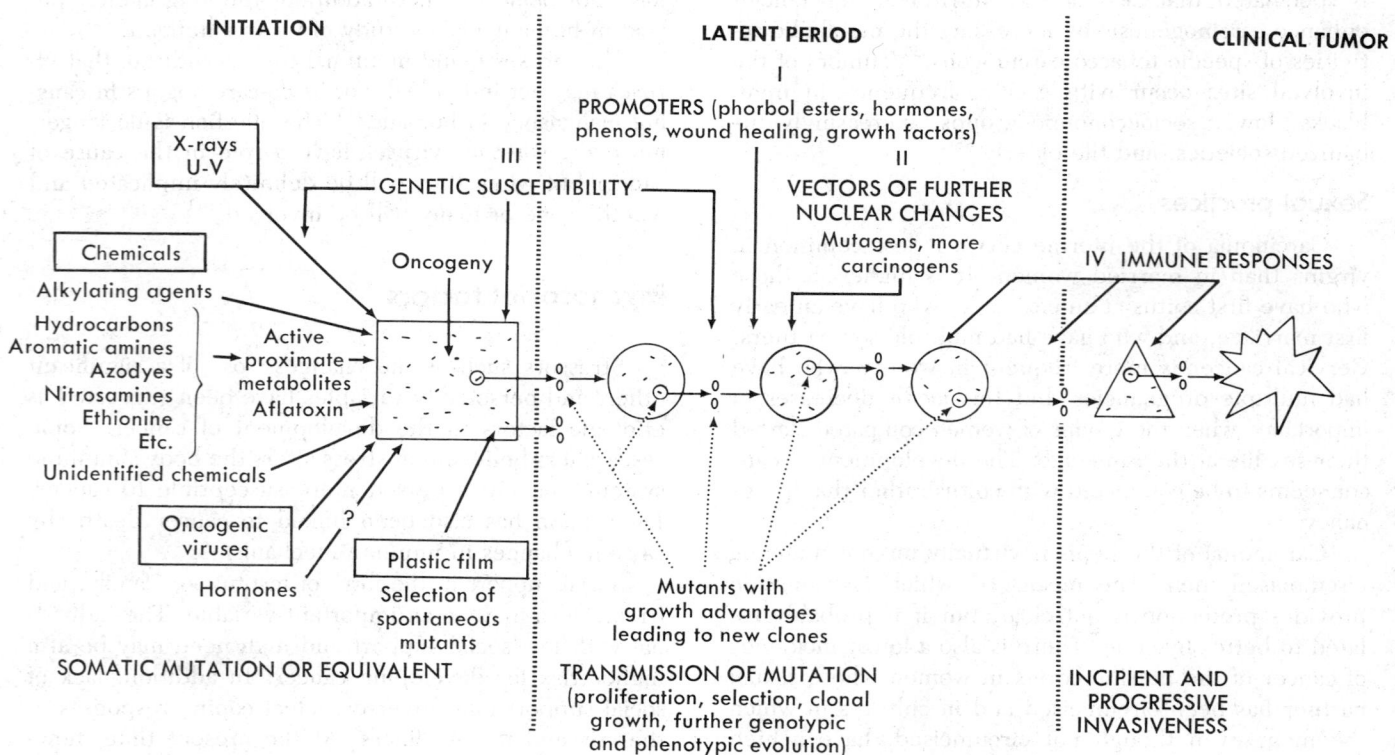

Fig. 25-4. Physical, chemical, and viral carcinogens may cause damage in cells of target organs *(dots in square)*. Changes are transmitted by cell division resulting in clones of modified cells *(small circles)*. These cells undergo further genotypic and phenotypic changes as a result of exposure to same or different carcinogens. Promoters of proliferation, whether chemical, hormonal, or viral, enhance carcinogenic process. Successive selection of new clones *(large circles)* leads to premalignant state. From complex interplay of host and tumor, affected by genetic, endocrine, immunologic, and other environmental factors, populations of cells characteristic of clinical tumors arise. (From Ryser, H.J.: CA **24:**358-359, 1974.)

those conditions that are known to predispose individuals to the development of the disease, and (3) educate the public about these factors. In addition, the nurse must be sensitive to the needs of patients who may be afraid and embarrassed when confronted with the possibility of cancer.

Since prevention of cancer is a primary goal of health professionals, the nurse must be aware of and able to communicate to others the importance of good health habits and the importance of avoiding conditions that predispose to cancer.

Early detection and treatment

The approach to early detection of cancer is worldwide. General criteria for cancer screening and testing programs have been drawn up by the epidemiology section of the American Public Health Association, and these criteria have been adapted by the World Health Organization. Multiphasic screening and a periodic health examination are being accepted by the public. In some cases diagnosis can be made months before the development of symptoms causes the person to seek care.[96]

Cancer detection is expensive. Education of the public often includes convincing them that a periodic health examination is a sound investment. Some cities have cancer detection centers where a complete physical examination including chest radiograph, Papanicolaou smear, breast examination, proctoscopy, urinalysis, and blood count are performed for a moderate fee. Nurses should be aware of clinics in their area where persons needing such resources may be referred.

The American Cancer Society has revised its guidelines for cancer-related checkups to provide essentially the same benefits with greatly reduced cost, risk, and inconvenience. Protocols for the early detection of cancer in asymptomatic persons are listed in Table 25-5. In general, persons over 20 years of age should have a cancer-related health checkup every 3 years, and those over 40 years old should have one every year. These checkups should also involve health counseling including information about personal cancer risk factors.[43] Women should request that the Pap test (Papanicolaou stain) be done if it was inadvertently overlooked by the health care provider. If the test is done early, cancer may be diagnosed before metastasis occurs (see Chapter 63).

Early detection of cancer can decrease mortality. The nurse must know and be able to explain the significance of the seven warning signs of cancer, stressing that any of these signs should be reported immediately to a physician. These warning signs as listed by the American Cancer Society are:

1. **C**hange in bowel and bladder habits
2. **A** sore that does not heal
3. **U**nusual bleeding or discharge
4. **T**hickening or a lump in the breast or elsewhere
5. **I**ndigestion or difficulty in swallowing
6. **O**bvious change in a wart or mole
7. **N**agging cough or hoarseness

It should be emphasized that any of these signs should be investigated medically (Table 25-1), but their occurrence does not necessarily mean that the person has cancer.

All persons should know the most common sites of cancer. In women these are the breast, uterus (cervix), and gastrointestinal tract (Fig. 25-1). Women should be taught to examine their breasts each month immediately after the menstrual period or, if postmenopausal, on a designated day each month. Such self-examination (p. 1742) is a much better method of detecting early breast cancer than an annual physical examination.

TABLE 25-5. Guidelines for cancer related checkups*

Test or examination	Sex	Age (yr)	Recommendation
Papanicolaou test	Female	Over 20; under 20 if sexually active	q 3 yr after two initial negative tests 1 yr apart
Pelvic examination	Female	20-40	q 3 yr
		Over 40 or at menopause	Yearly
Endometrial tissue sample	Female	At menopause if high risk	High risk: history of infertility, obesity, failure of ovulation, abnormal uterine bleeding, estrogen therapy
Breast self-examination	Female	Over 20	Monthly
Breast physical examination	Female	20-40	q 3 yr
		Over 40	Yearly
Mammogram	Female	35-40	One baseline mammogram
		Over 50	Yearly
Stool guaiac slide test	Male and female	Over 50	Yearly
Digital rectal examination	Male and female	Over 40	Yearly
Sigmoidoscopic examination	Male and female	Over 50	q 3-5 yrs after two initial negative examinations 1 yr apart

*American Cancer Society recommendations.

Women of all ages should know the importance of reporting any abnormal vaginal bleeding or other discharge occurring between menstrual periods or after menopause (see p. 1698 for details of early symptoms of cancer of the female reproductive system). (Further information about cancer of specific organs can be found in appropriate chapters in Part Three of this book.)

Two common misconceptions that lead the person to ignore symptoms should be corrected. The first is a belief that a disease as serious as cancer must be accompanied by weight loss. Weight loss is usually a late symptom of cancer, yet the person often remarks, "I wasn't losing weight so I thought nothing serious could be wrong." Another reason for neglect of cancer is that it may not cause pain, and again the person believes the absence of pain means that the indisposition is minor. It must be repeatedly emphasized to the public that pain is not an early sign of cancer and that cancer often is far advanced before pain occurs.

Nurses also have a role in prevention and early detection of genetic cancer. They systematically obtain family cancer histories, teach about health maintenance, and do genetic counseling.[72] They may be involved in centralized familial cancer registries analogous to the monitoring of communicable diseases by health departments. Familial cancer registries would be helpful in pooling data on suspected cancer-prone families, as well as in disseminating current methods of surveillance and management of the conditions.[69]

In addition to being knowledgeable about measures for prevention and early detection of cancer, nurses must be aware of current therapeutic modalities and their rationales. Because of lack of information, misinformation, or fear of the effects of treatment, persons may put off seeking help. Clearly presented information about therapy will help to allay anxiety and confusion.

Factors that interfere with health-seeking behavior

Even though there is more widespread knowledge of cancer, a more positive attitude toward the disease is essential if individuals are to follow good health practices and seek help when warning signs of cancer are noted. The public underestimates the incidence of cancer although they are aware of and concerned about it. This suggests that defense mechanisms are at work. The public does not view the conventional types of therapy as optimal, although they have a high level of awareness of cancer's warning signals. Less-educated people and men in general are less likely to have physical examinations.[90] These are all factors that may interfere with health-seeking behaviors.

Unfortunately, anxiety and fear may immobilize the individual. Despite all the public announcements that have been made in the last few decades, there are still people who think of cancer as a disgraceful disease that must be hidden from others. Cancer is talked about in whispers by some people who look on it as a punishment for past sins, a shameful disease, or a disgrace to the family. This attitude stems partly from the fact that cancer in its terminal stages may be a painful and demoralizing disease that is sometimes accompanied by body odor and other signs of physical debility that are deeply etched on the consciousness of friends and relatives. Actually, there is no characteristic odor of cancer, although diseased tissue that breaks down and becomes infected with odor-producing organisms will be as unpleasant as any other infected wound. The essential point—so often missed by the public—is that this tragic situation is by and large an unusual one.

Some people fear cancer and shun persons who have the disease because they believe it is contagious. Scientific speculation on the possibility that a virus may be the cause has added to this fear. At this time, there is no conclusive evidence that cancer can be spread among humans in a way similar to the spread of infectious diseases, and absolute proof of the specific role of viruses in human malignancy is still not available.

The positive aspects of cancer care should be emphasized. It is estimated that approximately one third of the persons for whom a diagnosis is made are cured by medical treatment. Another one third could perhaps be cured by medical treatment if the cancer is diagnosed early enough. Only a third have cancer occurring in locations in which the disease advanced beyond permanent medical aid before sufficient signs appear to warn the patient of trouble. In spite of these facts, some persons think it is useless to report symptoms early, since they believe that if they do have cancer they cannot be cured. It can only be hoped that the recent publicity given to well-known persons who have been treated for cancer will help overcome some of these beliefs. If nothing else, the open discussion of the diagnosis and treatment in all types of media should result in a better informed public than ever before.

Cancer quackery

Fatal delay in seeking medical care may occur because of the patient's reliance on a "quick, painless cure." Despite public education and efforts of the medical profession to control extravagant claims of a few unethical practitioners, cancer quackery still exists, feeding on the ignorance and fear of the cancer patient and family.[2,108]

Quacks rely on testimonials of people they have "cured." Books and testimonials in magazines may be so appealingly written that the reader gets the impression that the content is factual and accurate. Electronic gadgets, dietary regimens, and various drugs and enzymes have all been purported to cure cancer.

Two drugs still available mostly outside the United States are krebiozen and Laetrile, a substance derived from apricot kernels. Use of Laetrile for cancer therapy has been outlawed by the FDA, whose regulations prohibit the transportation of Laetrile across state lines. In response to active lobbying by various groups, however, 11 states in 1977 passed legislation legalizing use of Laetrile within their borders. The American Cancer Society and the American Medical Association do not recommend use of Laetrile or krebiozen, since neither drug has been scientifically demonstrated to result in objective benefit to the person or show evidence that metastatic growth has been controlled.

In 1979 the National Cancer Institute (NCI) announced that it would sponsor human testing of Laetrile. In 1981 investigators reported that the drug was a failure as a cancer treatment based on a study of 156 patients at four medical centers. These patients had advanced cancer, usually of the lung, breast, colon, and rectum, that could not be treated by standard methods. In addition to intravenous and oral administration of the drug, the patients received the metabolic program prescribed: vitamins, pancreatic enzymes, and a diet containing fresh fruits, vegetables, and whole grains. Within 1 month cancer had progressed in 50% of the patients and cancer had progressed in 3 months in 90%. Only one fifth were alive after 8 months, findings comparable to no therapy at all.

Laetrile advocates state that the drug used was not pure Laetrile and charge that the study was designed to discredit Laetrile. However, NCI stated that the drug was structurally the same as that used in Mexico's Laetrile clinics. The tragedy in the use of these drugs is the false security the treatment gives to patients. The security results in delay in seeking medical care until it is too late.[54]

Federal legislation is aimed at controlling quackery. The nurse must teach the danger of unproved methods of treatment in contacts with individuals and families.

Cancer research

Cancer research is multifaceted. Investigations are ongoing into the cause, prevention, and treatment of cancer. Research on the cause of cancer has explored the effect of several factors acting together to stimulate aberrant cell growth, the role of chemicals and other environmental pollutants, genetic factors, and the role of viruses in the development of cancer.

Many investigators are focusing their interest on subcellular components. There is increasing interest in changes in the chromosome and in the nucleic acids, essential cell constituents, DNA, and RNA. In addition, investigations using animals yield much useful information. For example, a strain of mice has been developed in which all the mice develop breast cancer. Evidence obtained through animal experimentation, however, does not necessarily prove that human beings react in the same way, but it raises the possibility that they may do so.

Immunologists in cancer research have become increasingly aware of the role of the immune system in both the natural history and the therapy of malignant disease. They suggest that it is possible to strengthen the body's natural responses so that the body would be able to destroy malignant cells when they first appear. The discovery that human neoplasms contain tumor-specific antigens not found in normal cells has opened up new avenues of therapy in controlling the progression and in inducing the regression of human neoplasms.

Around the world many research centers are developing better treatment modalities. Use of a combination of surgery, radiation, and chemotherapy has shown that there may be significant prolongation of life and in some instances complete cure of children with Wilms' tumor, an extremely malignant embryonal tumor of the kidney. Continued study of the use of chemotherapeutic drugs has resulted in effective new combination therapies for many types of cancer.

Future research against cancer will probably be directed toward developing and screening new drugs that can act alone or with other drugs; applying new forms of radiation such as laser beams that spare normal tissue and are not carcinogenic themselves; developing new regimens for the use of bacille Calmette-Guérin (BCG) vaccine and other forms of immunotherapy, both alone and in combination; developing new combinations of known effective drugs; and combining treatment modalities such as surgery, irradiation, chemotherapy, and immunotherapy.[103]

Research in cancer nursing is increasing; nurses, individually or working with others in clinical centers specializing in cancer, are studying the effects of cancer on client and family.

Too often effective nursing care practices have been passed on by word of mouth rather than being validated by careful investigation. There are many topics that if diligently and imaginatively studied might result in increased comfort to patients and their families. The psychologic response of patients and families, innovative approaches to care, and attitudes of care givers are just a few of the topics that might be investigated. Nurses are now looking systematically at priorities in cancer nursing research. New treatment regimens force nurses to look at their old assumptions about patient's needs and to identify where nursing research efforts should be focused.[86]

Organizations involved in cancer education, detection, and rehabilitation

Federal organizations

Federal recognition of the need to give intensive assistance to educational programs in cancer began in 1926 when Congress proclaimed April of each year as National Cancer Control Month. In 1937 the National Cancer Institute was created within the National Institutes of Health. This institute, with generous support from the federal government, conducts an extensive program of research in the field of cancer.

Cancer patients may also obtain help from both Medicare and Medicaid. The Community Services Administration provides services through state agencies such as Welfare and Aging or by direct grants. The Rehabilitation Services Administration will arrange and pay for services that help the cancer patient return to productive living.[2] With the passage of the National Cancer Act of 1971, impetus was given for the development of Cancer Clinical Research Centers. The goal was to translate research results into medical practice so that no one will be denied professional advice and care because of lack of facilities and knowledge. These centers combine research capability, demonstration of recent techniques and therapy, and community outreach programs.[110]

Nurses can be articulate speakers for the cause of cancer care and cure, since they are intimately aware of the effects of cancer in threat to life and cost in dollars, disrupted lives, and human suffering. Nurses must assertively express to their representatives in government the importance of a combined effort to eradicate cancer.

American Cancer Society

The American Cancer Society, Inc. (ACS), a large national voluntary organization, has branches in all states and in 11 major cities. It was organized in 1913 as the National Society for the Control of Cancer with the major objective of combating the fear, shame, and ignorance that were outstanding obstacles in the early treatment of the disease. This huge organization, which is supported by voluntary gifts, has expanded its functions and now has three main objectives: research, education, and services to cancer patients.

Research is a major focus, and the Society finances studies that seek the cause of cancer and the development of better methods of treatment. As part of its education efforts, ACS publishes booklets and pamphlets for the use of health care providers and it stimulates better preparation of professional persons in the care of patients with cancer by sponsoring institutes and other programs for these special groups. Information about available teaching materials may be obtained from the main office of the Society or from state or lcoal offices.*

In addition, the American Cancer Society strives constantly to educate the public. It works intensively through magazines, radio, television, women's clubs, insurance companies, state departments of health, and medical and nursing organizations in an effort to reach all the population with the educational message of how cancer may be prevented and controlled. A large amount of literature for the laity is prepared and distributed annually. Also, many excellent films for use in public education may be borrowed from the Society.

The Society also performs services for patients and their families. Branches in most communities provide assistance for cancer patients who cannot afford to pay for adequate care and for those who, although they can presently afford to pay, will eventually leave their families with too great a financial burden. Depending on how much community support is given to the society, the services may include dressings, transportation to and from clinics and physicians' offices, special drugs such as expensive hormones, blood, prostheses, and the loan of equipment such as hospital beds. In some communities homemaking, visiting nurse, and rehabilitation services are also provided. Of the money collected, 60% remains with the local chapter for the community's use. The remaining 40% supports the activities of the national office. Patients and their families should know about these services before their own resources are depleted, and local citizens should be urged to support the Society.

Other voluntary organizations

In addition to the American Cancer Society, some large cities have other voluntary organizations that serve only cancer patients. For example, Cancer Care, a large voluntary organization in New York City, confines its activities solely to the tremendous needs of patients with advanced cancer and to the needs of their families. The nurse who works in a small community or a rural area may learn of the resources available to cancer patients through local or state health departments.

Lists of available films for both professional and lay use can be obtained from the American Cancer Society and from state and local health departments. Some insurance companies, such as the Metropolitan Life Insurance Company and the John Hancock Insurance Company, prepare very useful pamphlets on control of cancer and the care of persons who have the disease. These pamphlets are useful to nurses in conducting health education programs and in teaching relatives of a patient with cancer how to care for him.

Cancer patients' groups

Patient groups have been organized to help others with the same disability. Lost Chord Clubs (laryngectomy patients), Encore and Reach to Recovery (both for mastectomy patients), and ostomy clubs have been formed in many cities. Individuals share what they have learned about coping with the problems resulting from therapy for their conditions. They visit patients either in the hospital or at home and hold regular group meetings.

*Headquarters: 777 Third Ave., New York, NY 10017.

Public health agencies

Many other agencies may be needed for the rehabilitation of the cancer patient. Community health nurses have a vital role in helping patients and families adjust after the cancer patient returns from the hospital. It is by the coordinated effort of hospital and community nurses that the patient and family can return to a satisfying and self-fulfilling life.

Assessment

Subjective data

The physician obtains a careful medical history inquiring into family history to determine those with a familial tendency for cancer, social history, marital and sex history, habits, occupation, and past medical history, since all may provide valuable clues to identify the presence of cancer.

It is especially important that the nurse obtain baseline data in relation to the cancer patient's health and health habits, since the treatment of cancer often involves complex changes in the patient's ability to meet psychologic, physiologic, and sociologic health needs. By careful collection of data the nurse can plan and carry out the complex nursing care that may be needed by the patient with cancer.

Knowledge of diagnosis

Some initial data are needed to plan care. The first important question to be answered is whether the patient knows the diagnosis. This information should be recorded on the nursing care plan and discussed with other health team members. This will ensure that the person does not receive different answers to the same questions from the health care providers. Some hospitals have partially overcome this problem by having regular meetings of all the members of the professional staff at which the information given to each patient is reviewed. If meetings of this type are not being held, nurses should take the initiative in planning such a meeting.

The nurse should also elicit from both the patient and the physician what the patient has been told. Because of anxiety and the need for denial to protect the ego, the patient may have only heard part of the information given by the physician or may have misinterpreted the information. The nurse can identify any discrepancies in order to plan the care on the basis of the patient's perceptions of the illness.

Members of the medical profession differ in their opinions as to whether the patient with cancer should be told the diagnosis. The decision is usually made by the physician after consultation with the patient's family. The present trend is toward telling patients they have cancer. When patients are not informed, the reasons seem to be related much more to the physician's own attitudes and emotional reactions than to concern about patients' reactions. The nurse may help by discussing with the physician the reactions of the patient and the feelings expressed. It is the nurse's responsibility and sometimes a challenge to work effectively for the ultimate benefit of the patient within the seeming limitation it may impose.

Many spiritual advisers recommend telling the truth. Some persons, however, may not want to know the diagnosis and may ask and then answer their own questions negatively. Some do not ask for the diagnosis because they do not wish to have confirmed what they already suspect. Some insist on knowing the diagnosis and are preoccupied with every detail of their progress and treatment in a detached but completely abnormal fashion. Finally, there are some who wish to know the facts and who can accept them in a realistic way when given an opportunity to discuss their feelings with others. Some physicians prepare the patient over a period of time and tell the complete truth when they feel the patient is ready to accept it.

It is also important to determine how long the patient has known the diagnosis. The patient who has just been told may be going through the initial grief reactions. The person who has known for many years may have made a realistic adaptation and may see cancer as a chronic disease and not as a death sentence. The nurse should ascertain from the physician whether the cancer has already metastasized and, if so, whether the patient is aware of this fact. Responses of the patient with metastatic cancer will be different from those of the patient who can be more hopeful of a cure.

Coping skills

Coping skills should be identified, for in no other disease are the person's inner resources and those of friends and families tested to a greater degree. Some persons cope by directly verbalizing fears and seeking support from others, while other persons are less direct. Some deal with problems with a problem-solving approach, while others try to avoid dealing with the problem.

The patient's and family's interpersonal, physical, and financial resources must be determined. What kind of support can be expected from the family? (See Chapter 3 for discussion of family.) The financial burden the patient anticipates because of the therapy may affect the reaction to the disease.

Psychologic response to cancer

Once the diagnosis of cancer has been made, the patient and family may be overwhelmed and immobilized. As one patient stated, "I cried all day Saturday, Sunday, and Monday. My daughter and my husband wanted to help but they didn't know what to do or say. I know my daughter was scared that she'd get cancer, too." Not all patients can openly express their feelings. Consequently, the nurse may have difficulty gathering data in order to assess and plan intervention. Some individuals are stoic, feeling it is a sign of weakness to display their psychologic devastation in public. The nurse must be alert for subtle cues that may indicate that intervention is needed.

Grief. The general psychologic responses to a diagnosis of cancer are those accompanying the grieving process (see Chapter 17). The patient and family may go through a period of denial, during which there may be a delay in beginning therapy. Anxiety, depression, regressive behavior, and anger may all be manifested (see Chapter 14).

To many the diagnosis of cancer signifies the end of life itself, the ultimate loss. Nurses must be careful that they do not communicate any negative reactions to cancer. Beginning practitioners must look at their own attitudes toward the disease.

Guilt. Guilt is also a frequent psychologic response. Cancer patients may feel that the disease is punishment for actions of their past life. They may also feel guilty if they have delayed seeking treatment (see Chapter 14).

Sense of isolation. Perhaps one of the most prevalent reactions described by patients with cancer is a sense of isolation, of being cut off from those persons and things that are important to them. Patients with cancer may report that there is a gradual break in relationships. In some cases the isolation is patient initiated,[59] in others it may result from actions of significant others because of their negative attitude toward the disease. Perhaps the most profound isolation is psychologic isolation, an inability to relate to and derive comfort from others, the feeling of being alone in a crowd.

Sexual disequilibrium. Nurses must be comfortable with their own sexuality and sensitive to the patients' responses, which may indicate that sexual tension is present.

Cancer is particularly destructive to the sexual relationship. It may so occupy the patient's life that all energy is directed to the illness. Sexual roles change. There may be fear that sexual activity may either cause the cancer to spread or that the well partner may "catch" it. Treatment modalities that affect the genital organs may cause sexual dysfunction, and the psychologic responses of anxiety, anger, depression, and body image disturbance may do violence to the sexual relationship[50] (see Chapter 67).

Fantasies of death and dying. Some patients report that they are overwhelmed with fantasies of death and dying. Most patients are more concerned about the process of dying, fearing pain, mutilation, and deterioration in both their physiologic and psychologic status, than with death itself. Patients may be open about their fantasizing, but they are more apt to communicate this in less obvious ways. Patients may focus their attention and discussion on the suffering and pain of others. They may express concern about the future of their families and may speculate what will happen to their loved ones. The nurse must be alert to these signs that patients need to talk about their view of their future (see Chapter 17).

Objective data

Local effects

Benign tumors cause serious problems if they obstruct the lumen of tubular structures such as the ureter, trachea, or intestinal tract. Intraspinal and intracranial tumors cause problems because of the pressure they exert in a closed space. Tumors may also degenerate or by the pressure they exert cause atrophy and ulceration of overlying epithelium.

Malignant tumors may produce the same problems as benign tumors. In addition, because of their size and ability to infiltrate and destroy surrounding tissue, there is danger of obstruction, hemorrhage, ulceration, and secondary infection.

Systemic effects

The term *paraneoplastic syndrome* is used to describe the systemic effects of cancer. These can be divided into the following categories: (1) hematologic, immunologic, and vascular abnormalities, (2) hormonal and endocrine effects, (3) neuromyopathies; (4) skin and connective tissue disorders; (5) gastrointestinal disorders; and (6) general and metabolic disorders.[88]

Anemia, leukopenia, and platelet deficiency may result from replacement of bone marrow by cancer cells. Patients with cancer of the gastrointestinal tract often develop anemia secondary to chronic blood loss and malabsorption. Tumors of the endocrine glands usually cause an increase in secretion from the glands, resulting in various syndromes such as Cushing's disease or hyperthyroidism. In addition, some malignant tumors of the lung secrete trophic hormones, which can result in conditions resembling Cushing's syndrome.[20]

When there is a metastatic implant in the peritoneal or pleural cavity, this causes an increased production of serous fluid, and the patient develops either pleural effusion or ascites (peritoneal).

Degenerative changes can occur in the central nervous system of patients with advanced cancer, even in the absence of metastases to the area. The patient may show signs of cerebellar disease and peripheral neuritis. There may be severe muscle weakness or dermatomyositis, and hemorrhage may occur if blood vessels are eroded by the growing tumor.

There is destruction of muscle protein, impaired cellular respiration (often a complication of anemia), and neuromyopathies followed by failure of important muscle masses, such as intercostal and abdominal muscle. This results in poor pulmonary ventilation, stasis of secretions, and pneumonia. Smooth muscle failure in the urinary bladder wall and the intestinal tract results in urinary tract infection or constipation.

Cachexia is almost universal in malignant disease at some point in its development and is usually a sign of advanced cancer. It is characterized by anorexia, hypermetabolism, excess of energy consumption over nutritional supply, and wasting as a result of negative protein and fat balance in the body. Weight loss may be gradual or rapid.

Four factors are involved in the etiology of cachexia:

1. It is possibly caused by inhibition of the hypothalamic appetite center. Appetite may fail to increase in the face of the increased nutrient needs of the tumor.
2. There is altered gastrointestinal function, malabsorption of nutrients, especially in the small intestine, and exudation of protein and electrolytes.
3. There is increased utilization of nutrients by some tumors that require more amino acids and vitamins than do normal tissues. There may also be insufficient utilization of available nutrients.
4. There is increased excretion of nutrients such as urinary excretion of electolytes and metabolic products.[88]

In addition, other factors that may be implicated include immobilization, drugs, and reactive depression that may accompany metastatic cancer. Along with this may be insomnia and a feeling of hopelessness,[11] which also may contribute to anorexia and cachexia.[97] There is an increased susceptibility to infection.

Therapy for the cachectic state is rarely successful unless the underlying cancer is treated. Glucose plus insulin, or androgens for males, may stimulate anabolism.[52]

Pain does not always occur with cancer; when it does occur, it is usually a late sign. Cancer pain is described later in the chapter (p. 512).

Diagnostic studies

The nurse needs to be able to give a simple description of various diagnostic procedures to patients and families. The tests may involve the use of complex equipment as well as the injection or ingestion of various substances. The patient's anxiety may be high, and the nurse's ability to give factual information often will help decrease anxiety. Several of the most widely used tests are discussed below.

X-ray, isotope, and scanning procedures

X-ray and isotope studies are usually ordered. Chest radiography is absolutely necessary if the patient is a smoker. Gastrointestinal series, intravenous pyelogram, and mammography may be done depending on areas where lesions are expected to be present.

Lymphangiography is a newer development in radiology. It is useful in diagnosing lymphoma and metastatic cancer. A mixture of vital blue stain and Novocain is injected in the skin of the web between the first and second toes to show lymphatic drainage of the lower extremities. If the upper extremity is to be investigated, the injection is made in the web between the index and second finger.

Five to ten minutes after the injection of the dye, the skin of the dorsum of the foot or hand is prepared. An incision is made and the lymphatics that can be visualized are dissected. Ethyl ester iodinated poppyseed oil (Ethiodol) is injected. Normal lymphatics appear as thin beaded vessels. Lymphomatous nodes are usually enlarged and sometimes have a "foamy" or "lacy" architecture. "Moth eaten" is the term used to describe the appearance of metastatic nodes.[19] Skin discoloration from the dye may persist for a week after the procedure.

Xeroradiography, taking of an x-ray picture on a plate of selenium-coated metal, results in a detailed picture of soft tissue. Another examination used to visualize soft tissue is *tomography,* an x-ray technique with ability to penetrate dense shadows.[2] *Thermography* is a method of constructing photographic images of surface temperature; localized skin temperature elevations that occur over inflammatory or malignant lesions are sharply delineated.

Computed tomography (CT) of the brain is a method for diagnosing intracranial lesions by the use of an x-ray beam in conjunction with a computer. It produces a detailed study of the brain without patient discomfort (p. 739).

Radioisotope studies

Various scanning procedures that involve the introduction of a radioactive substance into the body are used to detect primary or metastatic cancer. The radioisotope either concentrates in the tumor and shows up as a "hot spot" in the scan of the organ, or the tumor does not concentrate the isotope and a "cold spot" surrounded by normal tissue that did concentrate the isotope is found.

Radioactive iodine is a commonly used isotope employed in the diagnosis of thyroid gland disease. Researchers are also experimenting with it in other diagnostic tests. Radioactive iodine-tagged albumin has proved useful in locating tumors in the brain, and it is frequently used to determine blood volume.

In diagnostic procedures a tracer dose of the radioactive iodine either is taken by mouth or is injected intravenously as radioactive iodine-tagged albumin. The test is dependent on either the percentage of the dose picked up (blood volume) or on the rate of excretion (hyperthyroid studies). This is only one example of the advances that have occurred in the diagnostic use of radioactive isotopes. The scanning technique, which permits the mapping of organs by the detection and measurement of radioactive substances, plays an important part in the evaluation of the patient with cancer (see Fig. 30-11).

Ultrasound

Ultrasound probing, or *echography*, is done by an electronic instrument that detects and records echoes of sound when they are reflected at the junction of tissues with different densities. The procedure is helpful in differentiating between cystic and solid tumors.

Endoscopy

Hollow metal tubes equipped with a light are used to illuminate various body cavities and to permit visual inspection of the interior of the cavity being examined. These instruments are commonly referred to as scopes and are named for the organs they are to visualize. Thus a bronchoscope is used to examine the bronchus, a gastroscope is used to visualize the stomach, and a proctoscope to visualize the anus and sigmoid colon. A biopsy of tissue or secretions is usually obtained during these endoscopic procedures. A local anesthetic that diminishes the gag reflex is used before bronchoscopy or gastroscopy. Usually, no anesthetic is necessary for sigmoidoscopy. Peritonoscopy, which is employed to examine the peritoneal cavity, is particularly helpful in visualizing peritoneal metastasis. A local anesthetic is used with this procedure.

Cytology

In 1942 Dr. George Papanicolaou demonstrated that the diagnosis of cancer can be made from the study of cells that have sloughed or exfoliated from a tumor. These cells are found in body secretions such as cervical discharges, sputum, gastric washings, pleural fluid, and urinary washings. The secretion is spread on a slide, stained, and examined by a pathologist. The main use of the Pap smear, as it is often called, is to diagnose cancer in an asymptomatic person and to identify precancerous lesions or noninvasive cancer. If suspect cells are found, a biopsy must be performed to diagnose cancer.[1,19] The Pap smear is most widely used in routine examination of the cervical washings.

Biopsy

Biopsy is the only definitive way that cancer can be diagnosed. *Incisional biopsy* is the surgical removal of a section of the neoplasm. If the tumor is small, the entire growth may be removed, a procedure called an *excisional biopsy*. When possible, an *aspiration biopsy*, removing a small plug of tumor by use of a needle or syringe, is used to avoid the larger incisional or excisional biopsy.

The biopsy specimen is examined under a microscope to obtain a histologic diagnosis as to the type of cancer. In some cases it may be possible to determine the degree of malignancy.

Contrary to a belief sometimes expressed by patients, a biopsy, properly taken, adds little or no risk of causing the spread of cancer. Nurses must be careful to dispel the idea that biopsy should be avoided.

General laboratory tests

The patient's general health status must be determined in addition to determining the presence of cancer. Routine blood and urine studies are done. In addition, tests that are especially valuable in cancer detection are employed. Measurement of an enzyme, acid phosphatase, which is produced almost entirely by the prostate gland, gives evidence of the extent of prostatic disease. Another enzyme, alkaline phosphatase, is elevated in individuals with bone metastases and sometimes in those with liver metastases. Blood in the stool, identified by the guaiac test, may be a sign of gastrointestinal cancer.

Nursing intervention during assessment phase

The emotional climate produced during the period of diagnostic examination and initial treatment is very important in determining whether patients will continue diagnostic examination, treatment, or repeated follow-up care after discharge. The care they receive in the hospital may shape their attitudes toward the disease and may determine whether they can return home and either care for themselves or be cared for by the family. An important nursing function in the care of patients with cancer is building up faith in the physician and in the clinic or the medical center where care is received. The patient needs to feel certain that everything possible is being done and that new measures will be tried if there is any promise whatsoever of their being helpful.

Many patients must undergo extensive diagnostic examinations and surgery in large medical centers a long distance from their homes. Some patients have reported that, although they were confident that they were in "good medical hands," such confidence did not make up for the feelings that they were not always known as individuals. They needed desperately to feel that at least one person knew and understood them. Some patients experience near panic at the thought of their loved ones coming to visit and being unable to locate them. The nurse who works with the patient in the community, in the small hospital, or in the physician's office can help patients by preparing them for what they may experience in the large medical center. In most instances it is best for the patient to be accompanied by a relative or a close friend. It should also be recognized that even a patient in familiar surroundings may feel very much alone when awaiting diagnostic tests or surgical treatment for known or suspected cancer.

The patient needs something to help pass the time while awaiting completion of diagnostic tests and treatment and between steps of treatment such as surgery or x-ray therapy.

The family also needs to keep busy while awaiting the results of diagnostic tests and the outcome of surgery or other treatment. One woman, on learning that her husband had far advanced carcinoma, went home immediately and made his favorite cake, even though he was in the hospital and unable to enjoy it. Psychologic relief may sometimes come from keeping occupied with usual daily activities. Anxious relatives also receive satisfaction from doing things that the patient would do if possible, thus preserving parts of cherished routines. Taking the dog for his daily walk is an example. Members of the family often need direction in their activity when they have just learned that a loved one has cancer. They may need to talk over immediate and long-term plans with someone not close to the family situation. The nurse can sometimes be this listening person. At other times the family can best be served by a social caseworker, who will help them talk through and think through a course of action (see Chapter 14).

Intervention

Planning care

A sound personal philosophy and an objective, positive attitude toward the disease based on knowledge will help the nurse who is caring for the patient with cancer. The nurse should be able to give support and hope to the patient and family or friends.

Four principles should be considered by the nurse when planning nursing interventions that are patient or client centered: (1) persons have a right to be part of the treatment team; (2) persons have the right to choose the desired degree of privacy or communication; (3) the nurse must respect the coping mechanisms of patients who are trying to maintain themselves through a difficult illness; and (4) the nurse must remember not to give the appearance of hurrying, thus blocking communications and "turning the patients off."

Meeting psychologic needs

Cancer nursing demands not only caring *for* the patient but also caring *about* the patient, who may be angry, depressed, and perhaps physically unattractive because of the effects of the disease or its treatment. Communication is vital in meeting the needs of the cancer patient and the family. Validating assumptions and assisting patients to describe, clarify, and identify reasons for feelings are important to promote communications. In addition, the nurse must try to make explanations clear and uncomplicated. Getting feedback from the patient is one way to ensure that the message has been received.

Nursing interventions to help the patient cope

Since the threat to life and the potential for other losses are great for patients with cancer, they need especially to have their existing coping mechanisms supported or to receive support if coping mechanisms are inadequate to meet their needs.

Each patient's reaction to cancer is unique, so there can be no easy formula for care. The nurse must be able to work with and accept patient's behavior and coping style. Avoidance of false reassurance and pat answers that block communication will contribute to patient comfort. Openness, honesty, and creativity of the nurse are essential. The nurse reinforces patients' hope but is careful to avoid giving false hope, which can be more devastating than none at all. At times patients may need to deny their illness, while at other times they may want to talk about it.

Trusting patients' resilience and their will to try and helping them live as fully as possible are all appropriate interventions. When patients complain, perhaps the best response is, "Tell me how you feel. Perhaps we can do something about it." Self-esteem is maintained by fostering patients' independence, even if this only involves taking part in decision making about the care to be given.

Persons working with these patients must have confidence in themselves and the ability to suspend their own concerns, needs, and desires in order to concentrate on patients' problems. In order to do this one must be able to tolerate a high level of anxiety and to look at problems on both a feeling (affective) and a thinking (cognitive) level.

Listening carefully and attentively to concerns of patients helps to calm fears. In addition, nurses who are knowledgeable about cancer, who can answer questions and clear up misconceptions, help promote the patient's psychologic well-being.

Nursing interventions to help the family cope

The interventions that help the patient cope are also important in helping the family cope. The nurse must get to know them and their reactions. They may feel guilty, helpless, and angry just as the patient does. Letting them know that their feelings are normal may increase their comfort. Families should not be pushed into responsibilities that they cannot handle. Some want to participate in care, others are overwhelmed by the disease and are afraid to or may not want to help. Their feelings need to be respected.

Teaching the family is a major responsibility. They should be reminded not to cut the patient off from family activities and concerns. If possible, the patient should be included in family decision making and planning. In their desire to help their loved ones, families may unintentionally contribute to the patient's sense of isolation by shielding him or her from family concerns.

Interdisciplinary approach to care

The skills of many members of the health team may be required to meet the needs of the cancer patient. Clear, concise communication of ideas about care and the planned interventions is essential for coordination, continuity, and integration of care. Team conferences are helpful in promoting the sharing of expertise.[101] The social worker, occupational therapist, minister, and psychologist may all be needed to contribute to the patient's well-being. The nurse, who spends the most time with the patient, may be the first to recognize that the patient and family could benefit from the services of other health team members.

Rehabilitation of the cancer patient to an optimal level of functioning through the efforts of many health team members results in a more satisfying life for the patient and the family. Often the community health nurse is called on to give care, teach, counsel, and support the patient and family after discharge.

Therapeutic regimens

Often several physicians are involved in determining the appropriate treatment for cancer. The medical team decides on the choice of treatment on the basis of the biologic characteristics of the tumor, its clinical stage (p. 473), and the condition of the patient.[19] The histologic type of tumor is particularly important in determining the treatment to be used.

Therapy may be curative (removal of all traces of the disease from the body) or palliative (directed only toward relieving symptoms). At the present time there are four major forms of treatment: surgery, radiotherapy, chemotherapy, and immunotherapy. The latter is the newest form of treatment for cancer. Combinations of the four treatment modalities are often employed to achieve the best result for each patient.

Surgical intervention

Surgery, the oldest method of treating cancer, may be either curative or palliative. The best treatment for cancer at the present time is complete surgical removal of all malignant tissues before metastasis occurs. Surgery must often be extensive and may require adjustments beyond that needed in many other conditions. There may not be time to accustom oneself gradually to the idea of surgery and the effect it can have on one's body and on one's life-style. The individual often faces the prospect of mutilating surgery with only the hope that it will cure the cancer and be lifesaving. Concern about what will happen to the family may be utmost in the patient's mind. Obviously, the individual and family need empathy and understanding as they attempt to accept the recommendation for immediate surgery.

The operative procedures used to treat various types of cancer are discussed in Part Three of this book under the particular systems.

Radiotherapy

Radiotherapy, or the use of radiation in the treatment of disease, has been used in the treatment of cancer for about 80 years. The principal radiation agents are: (1) x-ray, which consists of electromagnetic radiation produced by waves of electrical energy traveling at a very high speed; (2) radium, which is a radioactive isotope occurring freely in nature; and (3) the artificially induced radioactive isotopes produced by bombarding the isotopes of elements with highly energized particles in a cyclotron. The most common sources of radiation for external beam therapy are the linear accelerator, the cobalt-60 teletherapy machines, and the betatron. These machines produce radiation of varying types of energy, which control the depth of penetration of the x-rays into tissues.[112]

Radiotherapy is effective in curing cancer in some instances; in other instances it controls the growth of cancer cells for a time. Because it may deter the growth of cancer cells, it may relieve pain even when extension of the disease is such that cure is impossible.

Principle underlying radiotherapy

Radiotherapy is based on the fact that rapidly reproducing malignant cells are more sensitive to radiation than are normal cells. Therapeutic doses of radiotherapy are calculated to destroy or delay the growth of malignant cells without destroying normal tissue. Rotation of either the target site in the patient or the radiation beam makes it possible to deliver a high total dose to the tumor while at the same time only part of the dose reaches the noncancerous tissue surrounding it.

The radiation used medically consists of alpha- (α-),

Fig. 25-5. Relative penetrating power of three types of radiation. (From Bouchard-Kurtz, R., and Speese-Owens, N.: Nursing care of the cancer patient, ed. 4, St. Louis, 1981, The C.V. Mosby Co.)

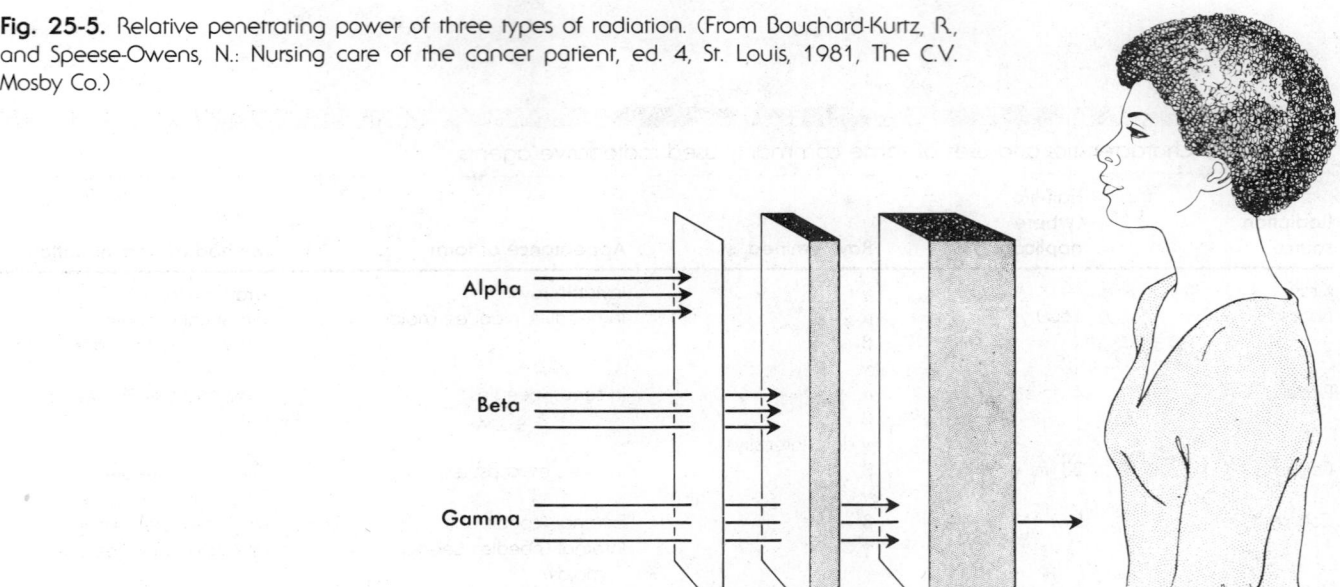

beta- (β-), and gamma- (γ-) rays (Fig. 25-5). α- and β-Rays cannot pass through the skin. γ-Rays, however, have been found to penetrate several inches of lead, although lead shielding offers a considerable degree of protection. X-rays, which are similar to γ-rays, require lead protection.

Radiation can be delivered to the patient *externally* by exposure to rays, such as from an x-ray machine or from cobalt 60, or *internally*, either by placing radioactive material such as radium within the tissues or body cavity (sealed internal radiation) or by administering the materials intravenously or orally so that they are distributed throughout the body (unsealed internal radiation).

Protection of health workers from radiation hazards

Radiation delivered externally (including x-rays) can do harm to persons working with the patient *only during* the time that the patient is being treated. This is true also of the radiation from some radioactive substances used for other methods of treatment (p. 476). Patients with internal radiation who emit γ-rays, however, may expose other persons to radiation for varying periods of time, and the time one can be exposed safely to the patient is important in planning care. The time interval required for the radioactive substance to be half dissipated is called its *half-life* (Table 25-6). This period varies extremely widely, but as the end of the half-life is reached, danger from exposure decreases.

There are three ways by which exposure to radiation can be controlled: *time, distance,* and *shielding.* All emanations are subject to the physical law of inverse-square. For example, a person who stands 2 m away from the source of radiation receives only one fourth as much exposure as when standing only 1 m away. At 4 m only one sixteenth of the exposure will be received. Therefore increasing the distance from the emanations decreases the exposure (Fig. 25-6). When a patient such as an infant must be held for x-ray treatment, the nurse or person who holds the patient must be careful to keep at arm's length or as far away as possible and to avoid having any body part in the direct path of the rays. *Lead-lined gloves and a lead apron, which act as a shield to reduce exposure, should be worn by anyone who attends patients during x-ray treatment or during examination by fluoroscopy.*

When the nurse knows the kind of substance used, the kind and amount of rays it emits, its half-life, and its exact location in the patient and considers these facts in relation to control of exposure, safe and adequate care for the patient can be planned.

Nurses wishing to know about radioactive substances can obtain information from the Division of Radiological Health of the Public Health Service or from their state health department. Several drug companies also publish pamphlets that contain helpful information. In cities with large medical facilities a radiation physicist may be consulted.

External radiotherapy

Preparation of the patient. Teaching the patient and family is an important aspect of care. Orientation programs, information booklets, and weekly group sessions for patients and families are useful methods of communicating information. In group meetings, topics such as scheduling, whom to see for assistance with special problems, or care of the skin are discussed. There is an

TABLE 25-6. Characteristics and uses of some commonly used radioactive agents

Radiation source	Half-life (where applicable)	Rays emitted	Appearance or form	Method of administration
X-ray	—	γ	Invisible rays	X-ray machine
Radium	1600 yr	α β γ	In needles, plaques, molds	Interstitial (needles) Intracavitary (plaques, mold)
Radon	4 days	α β γ (low intensity)	In seeds, needles	Interstitial (seeds, needles)
Cesium (^{137}Cs)	33 yrs	β γ	In needles, capsules	Interstitial (needles) Intracavitary (capsules)
Cobalt (^{60}Co)	5 yr	β γ	External (cobalt unit) Internal (needles, seeds, molds)	Machine (teletherapy) Interstitial (needles, seeds)
Iodine (^{131}I)	8 days	β γ (low intensity)	Clear liquid	By mouth
Phosphorus (^{32}P)	14 days	β	Clear liquid	By mouth, intracavitary, intravenous
Gold (^{198}Au)	3 days	β γ	Purple liquid	Intracavitary
Iridium (^{192}Ir)	74 days	β γ (low intensity)	In needles, wires, seeds	Interstitial
Yttrium (^{90}Y)	3 days	β	Beads, needles	Interstitial

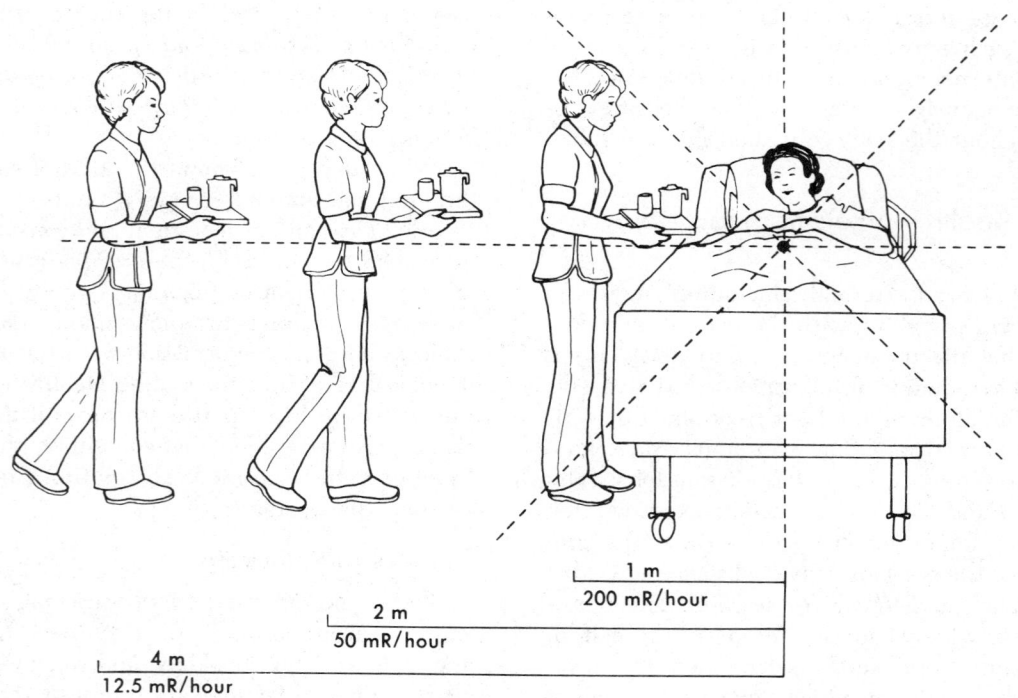

1 m
200 mR/hour

2 m
50 mR/hour

4 m
12.5 mR/hour

Fig. 25-6. Nurse nearest source of radioactivity (patient) is exposed to more radioactivity. (Adapted from Bouchard-Kurtz, R., and Speese-Owens, N.: Nursing care of the cancer patient, ed. 4, St. Louis, 1981, The C.V. Mosby Co.)

opportunity to discuss fears and misconceptions about radiation and cancer. Both inpatients and outpatients can attend.[112]

Patients who are to receive radiation therapy should know that they will be attended by radiotherapists who will be stationed outside the treatment room and who will observe the treatment and be in communication at all times. The patient must often lie absolutely still for a period of time, a very tiring experience. There is no pain associated with radiation therapy.

Procedure. In giving treatment, rays can be directed at the tumor from several different angles so that normal tissue receives a minimum of exposure. The areas through which rays pass are known as *ports*. Different ports may be used on different days, or the position may be changed at intervals during a daily treatment so that only a certain amount is given through each of several ports. The patient may be placed on a rotating device such as a rotating chair so that although the tumor mass receives the full dose of radiation, skin areas receive less exposure.

In medical centers where hyperbaric oxygen chambers are available, patients may receive radiation therapy while receiving hyperbaric oxygen. The rationale for this combined therapy is that malignant cells, in which the oxygen tension is increased, are more susceptible to the effects of radiation. At the same time the sensitivity of normal cells to the radiation effects is not increased.[49,52]

Early reaction. When radiation therapy is used some degree of radiation reaction may occur. Early reactions include blanching or erythema of the skin and mucous membranes, possibly progressing to dry or moist desquamation. If the mucosa of the mouth, pharynx, bladder, or rectum is affected, there may be pain, inhibition of the normal secretions, and impairment of functions.

When treatment is directed toward abdominal organs or any deep tissues there is almost always some skin reaction. There may be itching, tingling, burning, oozing, or sloughing of the skin. The term *burn* should never be used in referring to this reaction, since it implies incorrect dosage. Reddening may occur on or about the tenth day, and the skin may turn a dark plum color after about 3 weeks. The skin may also become dry and inelastic and may crack easily.

Gastrointestinal reactions to radiation therapy are more common when treatment includes some part of the gastrointestinal tract or when the ports lie over this system. The patient may have nausea, vomiting, anorexia, malaise, and diarrhea. This difficulty is usually not discussed with the patient before treatment is started because it is thought that the power of suggestion may contribute to symptoms. Almost all patients who receive moderate or large doses of radiation, however, have these symptoms in varying degrees.

Radiation therapy also causes depression of the he-matopoietic system and in turn a low white blood cell count, predisposing the patient to infection. Sloughing of tissue and subsequent hemorrhages are complications that must be considered when radiation is used in any form. Hemorrhage is not mentioned to the patient, but ambulatory patients are told that they should call the physician at once should any sloughing of tissue occur.

Late reaction. Effects of radiation may be apparent months or years after therapy. Genital tissue, muscles, and kidneys may be affected, resulting in painful radionecrosis.[19] Radiation causes destruction of fine vasculature, and the skin may show signs of atrophy (thinning and blanching), pigmentation, and telangiectasis. If there is severe vascular damage or if there are other complications that require further surgery, the irradiated tissues may fail to heal.[19]

Nursing intervention for patients receiving external radiation

PREVENTING SKIN BREAKDOWN. Skin preparation for external radiation therapy includes removal of any ointment and dressing and thorough cleansing of the skin. This procedure usually is followed by an alcohol rub. After this preparation nothing should be used on the skin. The area to be treated is usually outlined by the radiologist at the time of the first treatment. Occasionally, a small tattoo mark is used instead of the conspicuous skin markings when treatment is given to exposed parts of the body. Marks must not be washed off until the treatment is completed because they are important guides to the radiologist (Fig. 25-7). Sponge bathing of other parts of the body must replace showers and tub

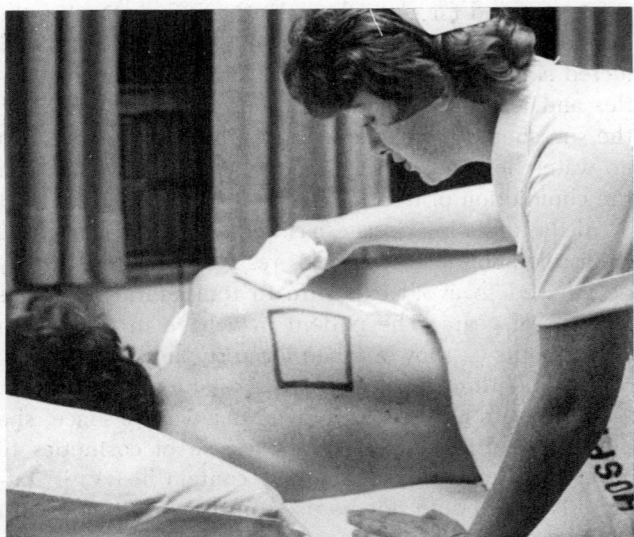

Fig. 25-7. When bath is given, care must be taken not to remove skin markings used to guide radiologist in giving x-ray treatments.

baths. A vegetable fat or oil may be ordered to protect the affected skin.

Medicated solutions or ointments and even powders that may contain heavy metals such as zinc are not permitted on the skin until the series of treatments is completed because they may increase the radiation dosage. Cornstarch may be used instead of powder.

The radiologist is consulted about skin care when a local radiation reaction occurs. The area may be cleansed gently with sterile mineral oil, but crusts should not be removed. Lanolin or petroleum jelly may be used to protect the area, and healing ointments containing vitamins A and D and healing oils such as cod-liver oil may be used if breakdown of superficial tissues occurs. Saline soaks, antibiotic ointments, or steroid creams may be used if moist desquamation occurs.[57] Healing usually starts approximately in the fifth week of treatment and should be completed about a month later.

Ointments are best applied by spreading them on a piece of sterile gauze and fastening the gauze to the patient's clothing. If this procedure is not possible, dressings may be bandaged loosely or anchored to healthy skin outside and beyond the treatment ports. If tape must be used instead of a bandage, a nonirritating tape is used. In removing dressings the greatest care must be taken to pull toward the middle of the area and thus avoid any pull on affected skin. Dressings should be loose to permit circulation of air and to avoid pressure on the skin.

Because the skin exposed to radiation treatment may become irritated and break down easily, it should be protected from constricting clothing or friction of any kind. For example, the patient receiving treatment to the trunk should not wear a girdle, tight panty hose, or a constricting trouser or skirt belt during the period of treatment and for several weeks thereafter. During the period of treatment, excesses of heat and cold to affected skin surfaces should be avoided. Hot water bottles and ice caps should not be used, and exposure to the sun should be avoided. Some physicians advise that no water be used on the skin for at least 2 weeks after the completion of treatment.

If the radiation dosage has been high and blanching or discoloration of the skin has resulted, the patient may be advised to avoid exposure to temperature changes for several years. The patient may have to take much cooler baths or showers than formerly and may have to avoid sunbathing or any other extreme of temperature. If x-ray treatment has been given to a woman's face, she must be cautioned regarding the use of cosmetics to cover discolored skin. They may contain heavy, irritating oils and should not be used until consultation with the physician.

When treatment must be given to any part of the head, women may ask about the danger of loss of scalp hair and men about loss of beard. Whether hair will return after falling out depends on the amount of radiation received. Attractive scarves and wigs are useful for patients with alopecia or when returning hair is too thin.

DECREASING GASTROINTESTINAL TRACT UPSET. Many patients find that resting just before meals and lying down immediately after eating help to control nausea and vomiting. Frequent small meals instead of the usual three a day may be more helpful. Some patients find that it helps to avoid food for 2 to 3 hours before and about 2 hours after each treatment. Sour beverages and effervescent liquids may also relieve nausea. Usually breakfast is the meal best tolerated; therefore it should be substantial, and the patient should be encouraged to eat as much as possible. One author has suggested that nausea and vomiting can be prevented by a high-protein, high-carbohydrate, fat-free, low-residue diet.[100] Problems related to radiation therapy in specific body locations are discussed in the appropriate sections of this book.

Intravenous solutions of glucose in physiologic solution of sodium chloride are used for nausea, anorexia, and dehydration. Pyridoxine (vitamin B_6), dimenhydrinate (Dramamine), chlorpromazine (Thorazine), and trimethobenzamide hydrochloride (Tigan) relieve nausea in some patients. Camphorated tincture of opium (paregoric), kaolin and pectin (Kaopectate), or diphenoxylate hydrochloride (Lomotil) may be used to control diarrhea, but drugs such as bismuth subcarbonate are not given because they contain a heavy metal that will increase radiation dosage. Low-roughage diets are recommended by some authors to prevent diarrhea. When it occurs, a diet with increased calories and fluids, low residue, and low roughage is suggested.[100]

PREVENTING INFECTION. As previously mentioned, radiation therapy depresses the hematopoietic system, thus reducing the white blood count and making the patient more vulnerable to infection. Clients receiving treatment on an ambulatory basis are cautioned to avoid persons with upper respiratory tract or other infections. In the hospital the patient should never be in the same room with patients who have an infection, and a private room and even protective isolation may be required if the white blood cell count is very low. Antibiotic drugs may be ordered to be given prophylactically both during and following a course of treatment.

Internal radiotherapy

Internal radiation may be delivered by sealed or unsealed methods. In either type special precautions may be necessary, depending on the amount of radioactive material used, its location, and the kind of rays being emitted (Table 25-5). Special precautions may be taken if more than a tracer diagnostic dose has been given. Hospitals in which therapeutic doses of radioactive isotopes are administered are required to have a radiation safety officer. Quite often this person is a physicist. The radiation safety officer determines the precautions to be observed in each situation. Most hospitals have printed instruction sheets stating the precautions to be followed for each substance used. Personnel should be fully acquainted with all precautions and should be supervised in carrying them out. Generally, the patient will be placed in a single room or in a double room with another patient who is also receiving radiation therapy. A radiation precaution sign should be placed on the door to the patient's room, and visitors should be restricted.

Sealed internal radiotherapy. Brachytherapy is used to deliver a concentrated dose of radiation directly to the malignant lesion or tumor area. Usually this involves insertion of radioactive substances within hollow cavities or within tissues. The radioactive isotopes commonly used are cobalt 60, iridium 192, iodine 125, phosphorus 32, cesium 137, gold 198, and radium 226.[112] These radioactive substances may be used in the form of molds, plaques, needles, wires, special applicators, or ribbons that are carefully placed and left in position for a specified length of time (Fig. 25-8). Emanations from the radioactive substances may also be sealed in

tiny gold tubes (seeds) and left indefinitely within the tissues into which they are inserted (Fig. 25-9). The half-life of the seeds is much less than that of the substances from which their emanations come.

A fairly common site for the implantation of seeds is the mouth. Plaques and molds also are used for lesions in the mouth. Sealed internal radiation also is used widely in treatment of cancer of the cervix.

PREVENTION OF RADIATION HAZARD: SEALED RADIOTHERAPY. Safe practice for the nurse caring for a patient receiving sealed internal radiotherapy depends on the principles of time, distance, and shielding (p. 490). Radioactive materials for sealed internal therapy usually are kept in a lead-lined container in the radiology department and are inserted into the patient in the operating room. They should never be touched with bare hands. A pair of forceps should be kept in the patient's room for handling in case the radioactive implant becomes dislodged.

Sealed radioactive material is often reused. On removal from a patient the radioactive material should be cleansed using the precautions just described and returned to the radiology department in a lead-lined container at once so that it may be safe from accidental handling or loss. Even if it is not to be reused, it is returned in a lead-lined container. To prevent accidental loss in cleansing, radioactive material is cleansed in a basin of water instead of in an open sink. If a brush must be used, it must be grasped with forceps so that close contact with the material is avoided.

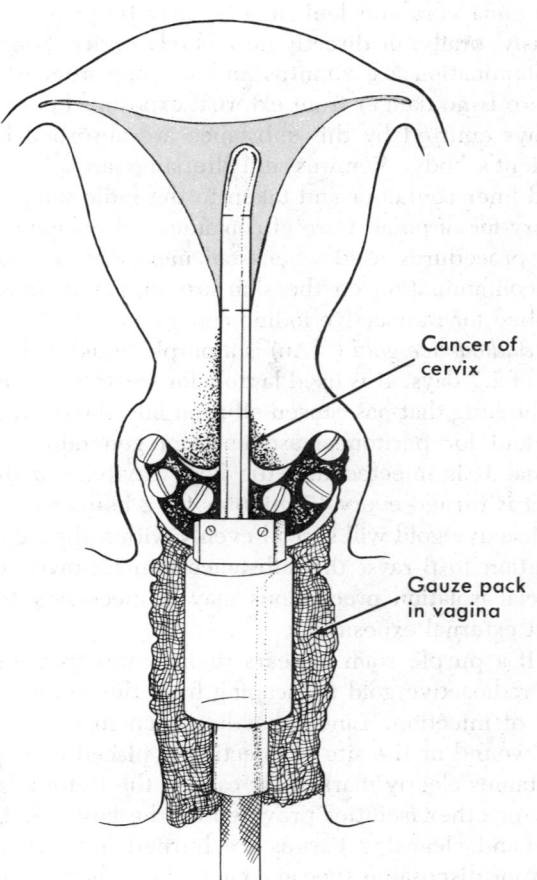

Fig. 25-8. Ernst applicator in place for treatment of cancer of cervix. Note gauze packing in vagina to help maintain applicator in position.

Cancer of cervix

Gauze pack in vagina

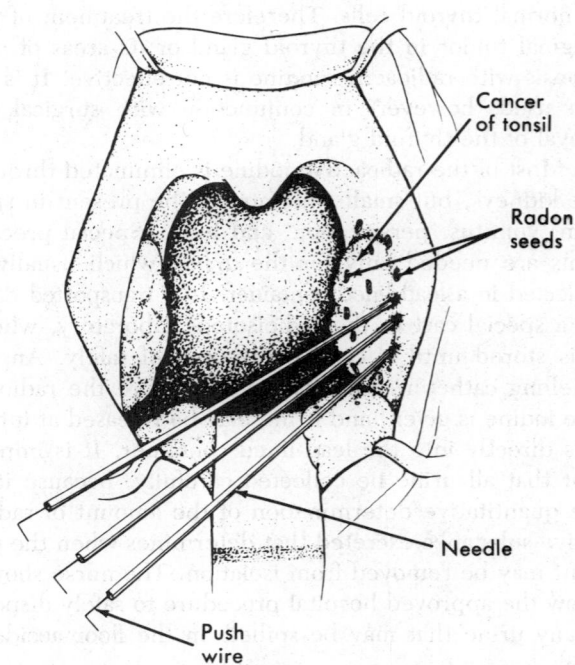

Fig. 25-9. Radium emanations may be sealed in tiny gold tubes (radon seeds) and left indefinitely within tissue into which they are inserted. Schema shows insertion into tonsil.

Cancer of tonsil

Radon seeds

Needle

Push wire

Exposure is sometimes termed *external* in that it can occur only by direct exposure to the encased radioactive substance. It cannot result from contact with linen, vomitus, or urine or from touching the patient. Knowing where the radioactive material is implanted helps the nurse to plan activities of care. If, for example, the substance is in the patient's mouth, there is less exposure if one stands toward the foot of the bed. If it is in the uterus or bladder, standing at the head of the bed is safer.

Unsealed internal radiotherapy. Unsealed internal radiation is delivered to the patient by mouth as an "atomic cocktail" or as a liquid instilled into a body cavity. Exposure for persons caring for the patient can result from direct contact with emanations from the substance in the patient (external exposure) or from contact with the patient's discharges that contain the radioactive substances (internal exposure). It may be inhaled, ingested, or absorbed through the skin. The exposure varies with each of the substances used, and safety for the nurse and for other persons caring for the patient depends on a thorough knowledge of the substance used and its action within the body. If only tracer doses (very small amounts) of radioactive substances are used, as for diagnostic purposes, no precautions are necessary.

PREVENTION OF RADIATION HAZARDS: UNSEALED RADIOTHERAPY. *Radioactive iodine* (^{131}I) is a clear liquid with a half-life of 8.1 days. Originally, it was hoped that it might destroy malignant cells in the thyroid gland, but results of its use have been disappointing because malignant thyroid cells do not concentrate iodine as well as normal thyroid cells. Therefore the treatment of the original tumor in the thyroid gland or its areas of metastasis with radioactive iodine is not effective. It is often used, however, in conjunction with surgical removal of the thyroid gland.

Most of the radioactive iodine is eliminated through the kidneys, but small amounts will be present in sputum, vomitus, perspiration, and feces. Special precautions are needed only for the *urine*, which usually is collected in a lead-lined container. It is transported daily on a special cart to the radioisotope laboratory, where it is stored until it can be disposed of safely. An indwelling catheter may be inserted before the radioactive iodine is given, and urine may be released at intervals directly into the lead-lined container. It is important that all urine be collected carefully, because it is the quantitative determination of the amount of radioactive substance excreted that determines when the patient may be removed from isolation. The nurse should know the approved hospital procedure to safely dispose of any urine that may be spilled on the floor accidentally.

No linen or equipment should be removed from the room until it is monitored with a Geiger-Muller counter for contamination. If the isolation gown and linen show

contamination, they are placed in a special container labeled "Radioactive" and stored in lead containers in the isotope laboratory, or they are burned. Paper dishes are used and then burned. If the nurse's skin should become contaminated, it should be washed thoroughly with soap and water and then monitored. If contamination remains, washing should be continued until monitoring shows that additional cleansing is not necessary. Because washing is essential to prevent or to lessen contamination, the patient must be in a room that has running water. Nurses may be required to wear rubber gloves when handling linen to lessen the possibility of contamination.[40]

When the patient is removed from isolation, all equipment is monitored and carefully scrubbed by attendants who have been instructed in safe methods by persons who are in charge of the administration of the radioactive substance. It is then remonitored. The room is aired until monitoring shows that radioactivity is negligible and that the room is safe for any other patient. Airing takes at least 24 hours.

Radioactive phosphorus (^{32}P) is a clear liquid with a half-life of 14 days. It is used in the treatment of polycythemia vera and leukemia. It may be given intravenously, orally, or directly into a body cavity. Sources of contamination are vomitus and seepage from wounds. There is no danger from external exposure because the β-rays emitted by this substance are absorbed by the patient's body. Vomitus and dressings are placed in a lead-liner container and taken to the radioisotope laboratory for disposal. Care of contaminated equipment and the procedures used when staff members are exposed by contamination on the skin are similar to those described for radioactive iodine contamination.

Radioactive gold (^{198}Au) is a purple liquid with a half-life of 2.7 days. It is used largely for treatment of cancer of the lung that has caused effusion into the pleural cavity and for peritoneal ascites from generalized carcinoma. It is injected into the body cavity, and the patient is turned every 15 minutes for 2 hours so that the radioactive gold will spread evenly within the cavity. In addition to β-rays, the substance emits x-rays, so that special isolation precautions may be necessary to prevent external exposure.

If a purple stain appears, it indicates that some of the radioactive gold is escaping from the wound or the site of injection. Linen that has been in contact with the wound or the site of injection is placed in a special container clearly marked for care in the isotope laboratory or other facilities provided by the hospital. Dressings and cleansing tissues are burned immediately or sent for disposal in special containers to the isotope laboratory.

The patient who receives radioactive gold is usually terminally ill. If he dies soon after receiving ^{198}Au, a notation that the patient was receiving radioactive gold immediately before death is made on a tag, and the tag should be conspicuously placed on the body for the protection of the coroner and the mortician. If the nurse has any questions about precautions that should be taken, the radiation safety officer is consulted.

Nursing intervention for patients receiving internal radiotherapy

TEACHING THE PATIENT. It is important to explain the routine to the patient and the reason for the precautions that are to be taken. The patient should know that isolation is temporary, that the restrictions will be removed on a certain day, and that members of the nursing staff will be available but that they will work quickly and will remain in the room only long enough to carry out essential activities. The patient can assist in notifying significant others about the restriction on visitors and how long it will last. The patient should know how the radioactive substance is eliminated lest he or she fear indefinite danger to other people and become concerned about social isolation or about the possibility of harming others after returning home.

DECREASING PATIENT ISOLATION. A radio or television will help the patient keep in contact with outside happenings. The patient needs to see the nursing staff, and if treatment permits they should interact from the open doorway.

Trips made in haste into the patient's room are disturbing psychologically because they imply that the patient is not acceptable to others. The nurse who plans thoughtfully might deliver a letter, a telephone message, fresh water, and the newspaper and make pertinent observations in much less time than the one who plans less well and must make several trips into the patient's room.

PROMOTING COMFORT. Before treatment requiring a period of precaution or isolation is started, the patient should have a complete bath, since bathing will not be permitted for a few days. The bed is made with clean linen, and all personal linen should be fresh. If the patient is very ill and requires help in turning and moving, a turning sheet may be placed so that the nursing staff can turn and raise the patient in bed in the shortest possible time and with little close contact. If treatment requires lying still in a specified position, measures for comfort should be anticipated. For example, if the patient is receiving treatment to the cervix and must lie on her back, a small pillow should be provided for use against the curve of the back before fatigue and discomfort become a major problem.

Outcome criteria for the person receiving radiotherapy

1. The person is free from infection on discharge from the hospital.
2. The person or significant others can:
   a. Describe measures to prevent skin breakdown.
   b. Describe the measures to decrease nausea and vomiting and increase food and fluid intake.
   c. List the components of an adequate diet.
   d. Describe measures to prevent infection.

Chemotherapy

Advances in knowledge of cancer growth and chemotherapeutic agents have led to concomitant advances in cancer treatment. Improvement in overall survival and longer disease-free intervals can be directly ascribed to the use of chemotherapeutic agents, particularly in combination chemotherapy regimens and as adjuvant therapy.

Benefits of chemotherapy

Chemotherapy is potentially curative in gestational choriocarcinoma, acute lymphocytic leukemia (ALL), Ewing's sarcoma, advanced Hodgkin's disease, diffuse histiocytic lymphoma, Burkitt's lymphoma, testicular cancer, and ovarian cancer. Prolonged disease-free or controlled intervals may be achieved by chemotherapy in the treatment of several non-Hodgkin's lymphomas, multiple myeloma, breast cancer and oat cell carcinoma of the lung. In other advanced malignancies, such as colorectal carcinoma, chemotherapy rarely produces a complete response and only a few such patients experience an increased survival time. In the treatment of chronic myelogenous leukemia (CML) and chronic lymphocytic leukemia (CLL), although the duration of life may not be prolonged, the quality of life may be enhanced by chemotherapy because of control of symptoms. Patients and families may be told that incurable does not mean untreatable or uncontrollable.

In the care of an individual patient with cancer, the expected benefit of chemotherapy (cure, control, or palliation) should be known by the physician, nurse, and patient. This allows for realistic goal setting by the care givers, patients, and family. Such background also provides a perspective from which to view side effects. The potential for cure, prolonged disease-free survival, or reduction of symptoms is a benefit that most often outweighs the risk and discomfort of short-term toxicity and side effects. Conditions in which risk may outweigh benefits include overt or occult infections, bleeding dyscrasias, bone marrow depression, severe metabolic disturbances, renal or liver dysfunction, and pregnancy.

Adjuvant chemotherapy refers to chemotherapy administered after surgical removal of all known cancer present in the body. It is aimed at the destruction of micrometastases thought likely to be present but too small to be detected by current diagnostic techniques. Left untreated, the micrometastases have a high potential for tumor growth and cancer recurrence. With the use of chemotherapy at a time when the malignant cell population is small and likely to be susceptible, complete tumor cell eradication is possible. The goal is cure.

Adjuvant chemotherapy is now generally considered to be indicated after mastectomy in all women with involved axillary lymph nodes at the time of surgery and it has demonstrated a significant decrease in recurrence rates and prolonged disease-free intervals. Adjuvant chemotherapy also appears to be beneficial in osteogenic sarcoma and Wilms' tumor. Evidence is currently equivocal regarding its benefit in other malignancies, such as colon cancer and malignant melanoma. The precise role of adjuvant chemotherapy will be more clearly delineated during the next decade, but it is already established as one of the major recent developments in health care.

A feeling of well-being and knowledge that all diagnostic tests are negative for cancer understandably may cause the patient to question the need for adjuvant therapy. This is emphasized when side effects are experienced. A sensitivity to these feelings, coupled with the knowledge of the expected benefit of therapy, is the basis for both patient teaching and the supportive encouragement often needed for continued therapy.

Despite an intellectual understanding of the benefits of chemotherapy, it is sometimes difficult for a nurse to maintain an appropriately optimistic and realistic outlook if all one sees are those patients who did not respond to or are no longer responsive to therapy, manifest severe toxicity, or are dying. The practitioner must take into account the setting in which patients are seen. Hospital-based nurses tend to see patients at the time of diagnosis, when they are critically ill, or during the final days of life. The public health nurse may see the patient at comparable points of illness while providing nursing care in the home. Discussion between the nurse and primary physician, contact with the outpatient clinic, and readmission to the same nursing unit are useful ways of acquiring a more complete picture of an individual's response to treatment. Such positive experiences are a means of nurturing one's own beliefs in therapy so that a realistic and at times very optimistic approach to caring for, supporting, and teaching the chemotherapy patient exists.

Clinical trials

The general public and, at times, health professionals outside of oncology view chemotherapy with some mystique and feelings of it being experimental. The patient may ask, "Am I a guinea pig?" For this reason it is helpful for the nurse to be able to explain that chemotherapeutic drugs are carefully tested before being identified as an acceptable mode of treatment. Chemotherapeutic drugs reach a phase of clinical trial in humans according to a drug-screening process established by the National Cancer Institute. This screening process identifies compounds with antitumor activity,

TABLE 25-7. Phases of clinical trials for chemotherapeutic drugs

Phase	Action
I	Identify toxic reactions; determine optimal dose within safe limits and set schedule
II	Determine extent of antineoplastic activity
III	Compare action of new drug with standard antineoplastic drugs
IV	Determine effect on advanced cancer, effect of combined therapy with other antineoplastic drugs, and effect with adjuvant therapy

demonstrates the activity in animals, studies and determines all of the pharmacologic aspects of the drug (kinetics, absorption, dose, metabolism, and excretion), and defines toxicity. The drugs next go through the four phases of clinical trial outlined in Table 25-7. The effectiveness of the new agent is then compared with standard therapy to determine if the new drug is equal to or better than drugs currently used.

Pathophysiologic principles of chemotherapy

Normal and malignant cells progress through various phases in the cell cycle as they replicate (Fig. 25-2) (p. 468). Cancer chemotherapy is based on the actions of certain drugs, creating changes in the cell cycle phases. Fig. 25-10 summarizes how some of the commonly used chemotherapeutic agents interrupt cell growth and replication. Drugs such as antimetabolites and vinca alkaloids that are effective during a particular point of the cell cycle are said to be *phase-specific drugs*. Drugs that are active throughout the cell cycle (*phase nonspecific*) include the alkylating agents, antibiotics, nitrosoureas, procarbazine, and dacarbazine (Dtic-Dome). Combinations of cycle-specific and cycle-nonspecific drugs have proved useful in constructing treatment regimens. One major factor that influences the response of a cancer to chemotherapy is the fraction of tumor cells in replication at a given time, a percentage that varies among different tumors, among individual patients, and at different times in the same patient. It is at this point that malignant cells are most vulnerable to drug therapy.

Combination chemotherapy. Increased knowledge of how specific cytotoxic drugs exert their effect and of the potential for the emergence of tumor cells resistant to a specific therapy, similar to antibiotic resistance, has led to the use of combination chemotherapy. Combination chemotherapy demonstrates a therapeutic effect superior to a single agent therapy for many cancers. Drugs considered for combination chemotherapy are those that (1) are active when used alone, (2) have different mechanisms of action, (3) have a biochemical ba-

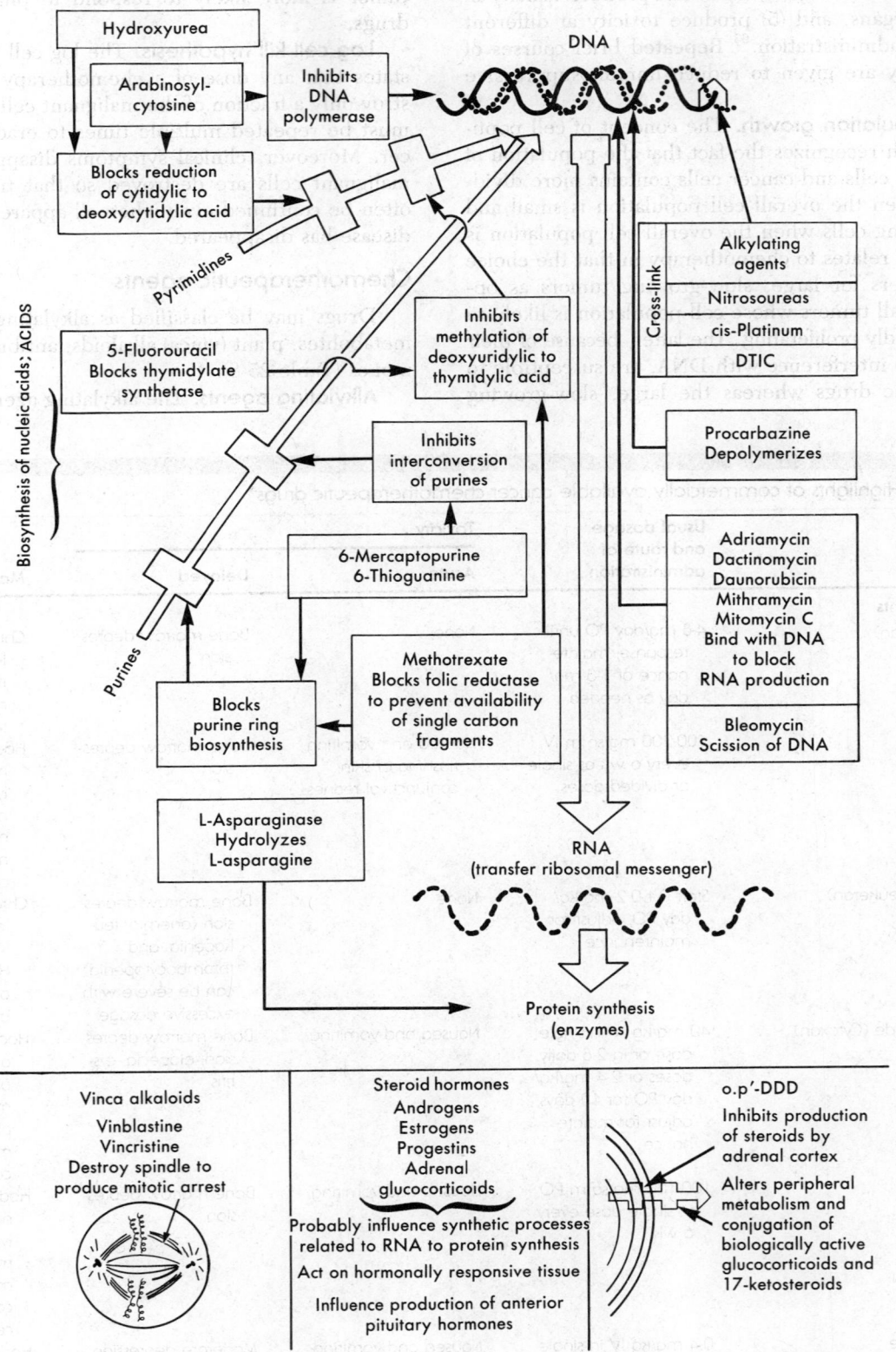

Fig. 25-10. Summary of chemotherapy drug interference with cell replication. (Adapted from Krakoff, I.: Cancer chemotherapeutic agents: American Cancer Society professional education publication, New York, 1977, American Cancer Society.)

sis for possible synergism, (4) do not produce toxicity in the same organs, and (5) produce toxicity at different times after administration.[63] Repeated brief courses of drug therapy are given to reduce immunosuppressive effects.

Cell population growth. The concept of cell population growth recognizes the fact that the population of both normal cells and cancer cells contains more dividing cells when the overall cell population is small and fewer dividing cells when the overall cell population is large.[44] This relates to chemotherapy in that the choice of drug differs for large, slow-growing tumors as opposed to small tumors whose cell population is likely to be more rapidly proliferating. The latter, because of their sensitivity to interference with DNA, are susceptible to phase-specific drugs whereas the large, slow-growing tumor is more likely to respond to phase-nonspecific drugs.

Log cell kill hypothesis. The log cell kill hypothesis states that any dose of a chemotherapy drug will destroy only a fraction of the malignant cells.[44] Treatment must be repeated multiple times to eradicate the cancer. Moreover, clinical symptoms disappear before all malignant cells are destroyed so that treatment must often be continued even when all apparent evidence of disease has disappeared.

Chemotherapeutic agents

Drugs may be classified as alkylating agents, antimetabolites, plant (vinca) alkaloids, antibiotics, and hormones (Table 25-8).

Alkylating agents. The alkylating agents are cell cy-

TABLE 25-8. Highlights of commercially available cancer chemotherapeutic drugs*

Drug	Usual dosage and route of administration	Toxicity Acute	Delayed	Major indications
Alkylating agents				
Busulfan (Myleran)	4-8 mg/day PO until response; maintenance of 1-3 mg/day as needed	None	Bone marrow depression	Chronic granulocytic leukemia; polycythemia vera; primary thrombocytosis
Carmustine (BCNU)	100-200 mg/sq m IV every 6 wk as single or divided doses	Nausea and vomiting; flushing of skin; conjunctival redness	Bone marrow depression	Hodgkin's disease; non-Hodgkin's lymphomas; primary brain tumors; malignant melanoma; renal cell myeloma
Chlorambucil (Leukeran)	Start 0.1-0.2 mg/kg/day PO; adjust for maintenance	None	Bone marrow depression (anemia, leukopenia, and thrombocytopenia) can be severe with excessive dosage	Chronic lymphocytic leukemia; Hodgkin's disease; non-Hodgkin's lymphoma; trophoblastic neoplasms
Cyclophosphamide (Cytoxan)	40 mg/kg IV in single dose or in 2-8 daily doses or 2-4 mg/kg/day PO for 10 days; adjust for maintenance	Nausea and vomiting	Bone marrow depression; alopecia; cystitis	Hodgkin's disease and other lymphomas; multiple myeloma; lymphocytic leukemia; many solid cancers
Lomustine (CCNU)	100-130 mg/sq m PO in single dose every 6 wk	Nausea and vomiting	Bone marrow depression	Hodgkin's disease, non-Hodgkin's lymphomas, primary brain tumors; renal cell, colon, and oat cell carcinoma
Mechlorethamine (nitrogen mustard; HN_2; Mustargen)	0.4 mg/kg IV in single or divided doses	Nausea and vomiting; vesicant	Moderate depression of peripheral blood count	Hodgkin's disease and other lymphomas; bronchogenic carcinoma

*Adapted from Carter, S.K., and Kershner, L.M.: Resident Staff Physician, pp. 55-56, Jan. 1976.

TABLE 25-8. Highlights of commercially available cancer chemotherapeutic drugs—cont'd

Drug	Usual dosage and route of administration	Toxicity Acute	Delayed	Major indications
Melphalan (1-phenylalanine mustard; Alkeran)	0.25 mg/kg/day for 4 days PO; 2-4 mg/day as maintenance or 0.1-0.15 mg/kg/day for 2 wk	None	Bone marrow depression	Multiple myeloma; malignant melanoma; ovarian carcinoma; testicular seminoma
Thio-TEPA (triethylene-thiophosphoramide)	0.2 mg/kg IV for 5 days	None	Bone marrow depression	Hodgkin's disease; bronchogenic and breast carcinomas
Uracil mustard	1-2 mg/day PO until response; then 1 mg/day for 3-4 wk	None	Moderate depression of peripheral blood count	Chronic lymphocytic leukemia; non-Hodgkin's lymphomas; Hodgkin's disease; ovarian primary thrombocytosis
Antimetabolites				
Cytarabine hydrochloride (arabinosyl cytosine; Cytosar; Ara-C)	2-3 mg/kg/day IV until response or toxicity or 1-3 mg/kg IV over 24 hr for up to 10 days	Nausea and vomiting	Bone marrow depression; megaloblastosis	Acute leukemia
Fluorouracil (5-FU, FU)	12.5 mg/kg/day IV for 3-5 days or 15 mg/kg/wk for 6 wk	Nausea	Oral and gastrointestinal ulceration; stomatitis and diarrhea; bone marrow depression	Breast, large bowel, and ovarian carcinomas
Mercaptopurine (6-MP; Purinethol)	2.5 mg/kg/day PO	Occasional nausea and vomiting; usually well tolerated	Bone marrow depression; occasional hepatic damage	Acute lymphocytic and granulocytic leukemia; chronic granulocytic leukemia
Methotrexate (amethopterin; MTX)	2.5-5.0 mg/day PO; 0.4 mg/kg rapid IV daily 4-5 days (not over 25 mg) or 0.4 mg/kg rapid IV twice weekly	Occasional diarrhea; hepatic necrosis	Oral and gastrointestinal ulceration; bone marrow depression (anemia, leukopenia, thrombocytopenia); cirrhosis	Acute lymphocytic leukemia; choriocarcinoma; carcinoma of cervix and head and neck area; mycosis fungoides; solid cancers
Thioguanine (6-TG)	2 mg/kg/day PO	Occasional nausea and vomiting; usually well tolerated	Bone marrow depression	Acute leukemia
Plant alkaloids				
Vinblastine sulfate (Velban)	0.1-0.2 mg/kg/wk IV or every 2 wk	Nausea and vomiting; local irritant	Alopecia; stomatitis; bone marrow depression; loss of reflexes	Hodgkin's disease and other lymphomas; solid cancers
Vincristine sulfate (Oncovin)	0.01-0.03 mg/kg/wk IV	Local irritant	Areflexia; peripheral neuritis; paralytic ileus; mild bone marrow depression	Acute lymphocytic leukemia; Hodgkin's disease and other lymphomas; solid cancers

Continued.

TABLE 25-8. Highlights of commercially available cancer chemotherapeutic drugs—cont'd

Drug	Usual dosage and route of administration	Toxicity Acute	Delayed	Major indications
Antibiotics				
Doxorubicin (Adriamycin)	60-90 mg/sq m IV, single dose or over 3 days; repeat every 3 wk to total dose of 550 mg/sq m	Nausea; red urine (not hematuria); vesicant	Bone marrow depression; cardiotoxicity; alopecia; stomatitis	Soft tissue, osteogenic, and miscellaneous sarcomas; Hodgkin's disease; non-Hodgkin's lymphoma; bronchogenic and breast carcinoma; thyroid cancer
Bleomycin (Blenoxane)	10-15 mg/sq m/wk or twice/wk IV or IM to total dose 300-400 mg	Nausea and vomiting; fever; very toxic	Edema of hands; pulmonary fibrosis; stomatitis; alopecia	Hodgkin's disease; non-Hodgkin's lymphoma; squamous cell carcinoma (head and neck); testicular carcinoma
Dactinomycin (actinomycin D; Cosmegen)	0.015-0.05 mg/kg/wk (1-2.5 mg) 3-5 wk IV; wait for marrow recovery (3-4 wk), then repeat course	Nausea and vomiting; local irritant; vesicant	Stomatitis; oral ulcers; diarrhea; alopecia; mental depression; bone marrow depression	Testicular carcinoma; Wilm's tumor; rhabdomyosarcoma; Ewing's and osteogenic sarcoma; other solid tumors
Mithramycin (Mithracin)	0.025-0.050 mg/kg IV every 2 days for up to 8 doses	Nausea and vomiting; hepatotoxicity	Bone marrow depression (thrombocytopenia); hypocalcemia	Testicular carcinoma; trophoblastic neoplasms
Mitomycin C (Mutamycin)	0.05 mg/kg/day IV for 5 days	Nausea and vomiting; flulike syndrome	Bone marrow depression; skin toxicity; pulmonary, renal, and CNS effects	Squamous cell carcinoma of head and neck, lungs, and cervix; adenocarcinoma of the stomach, pancreas, colon, and rectum; adenocarcinoma and duct cell carcinoma of breast
Other synthetic agents				
Dacarbazine (DTIC-Dome; DIC)	4.5 mg/kg/day IV for 10 days; repeated every 28 days	Nausea and vomiting; flulike syndrome	Bone marrow depression (rare)	Metastatic malignant melanoma
Hydroxyurea (Hydrea)	80 mg/kg PO single dose every 3 days or 20-30 mg/kg/day PO	Mild nausea and vomiting	Bone marrow depression	Chronic granulocytic leukemia
Mitotane (ortho-para-DDD, o-p-DDD; Lysodren)	6-15 mg/kg/day PO	Nausea and vomiting	Dermatitis; diarrhea; mental depression	Adrenocortical carcinoma
Procarbazine hydrochloride (methylhydrazine; ibenzmethyzin; Matulane)	Start 1-2 mg/kg/day PO; increase over 1 wk to 3 mg/kg; maintain for 3 wk, then reduce to 2 mg/kg/day until toxic	Nausea and vomiting	Bone marrow depression; CNS depression	Hodgkin's disease; non-Hodgkin's lymphoma; bronchogenic carcinoma

TABLE 25-8. Highlights of commercially available cancer chemotherapeutic drugs—cont'd

Drug	Usual dosage and route of administration	Toxicity Acute	Delayed	Major indications
Hormones				
Diethylstilbestrol (DES)	15 mg/day PO (1 mg in prostate gland cancer)	None	Fluid retention; hypercalcemia; feminization; uterine bleeding; during pregnancy may cause vaginal carcinoma in offspring	Breast and prostate gland carcinomas
Ethinyl estradiol	3 mg/day PO	None	Fluid retention; hypercalcemia; feminization; uterine bleeding	Breast and prostate gland carcinomas
Fluoxymesterone	10-20 mg/day PO	None	Fluid retention; masculinization; cholestatic jaundice	Breast carcinoma
Medroxyprogesterone acetate	100-200 mg/day PO; 200-600 mg twice weekly	None	None	Endometrial carcinoma; renal cell and breast carcinomas
Prednisone	10-100 mg/day PO	None	Hyperadrenocorticism	Acute and chronic lymphocytic leukemia; Hodgkin's disease; non-Hodgkin's lymphomas
Testolactone (Teslac)	100 mg IM three times weekly	None	Fluid retention; masculinization	Breast carcinoma
Testosterone propionate	50-100 mg IM three times weekly	None	Fluid retention; masculinization	Breast carcinoma

cle nonspecific and act against already formed nucleic acids by cross-linking DNA strands, thereby preventing DNA replication and the transcription of RNA.

Antimetabolites. The antimetabolites act by interfering with the synthesis of chromosomal nucleic acid. Antimetabolites are analogues of normal metabolites and block the enzyme necessary for synthesis of essential factors or are incorporated into the DNA or RNA and thus prevent replication. Most antimetabolites are pyrimidine analogues, purine analogues, or folic acid antagonists and are, in general, cycle specific.

Vinca alkaloids. Vincristine sulfate and vinblastine sulfate are plant alkaloids that act as mitotic inhibitors. These agents exert their cytotoxic effect by binding to proteins within the cells causing metaphase arrest. The vinca alkaloids are cell cycle specific. Although these two agents are similar in composition, mechanism of action, and metabolism, their antitumor spectrum, dose, and clinical toxicity differ.

Antibiotics. Those antibiotics that demonstrate antitumor activity appear to effect either the function or synthesis of the nucleic acids. In addition, antimitotic

and cell surface effects may be caused by these agents. The cytotoxic antibiotics are cell cycle nonspecific agents.

Steroids. The corticosteroids are produced by the adrenal cortex and include mineralocorticoids and glucocorticoids. It is the glucocorticoids that, in addition to their use in numerous nonmalignant diseases, are effective in the treatment of many neoplastic disorders. In some malignancies (e. g., lymphomas, breast cancer, multiple myeloma, acute lymphocytic leukemia, and chronic lymphocytic leukemia) steroids exert a direct antitumor effect. Steroids are also able to reduce edema and inflammation around a tumor and therefore are useful for symptom relief. There are many side effects associated with long-term steroid use, most notably a compromised immunologic response to infection, osteoporosis, and a cushingoid syndrome.[60] Steroids in cancer treatment regimens are often given intermittently and for short periods of time and are not often associated with the debilitating side effects associated with chronic, long-term use. Patients often describe an improved sense of well-being and an increased appetite while on prednisone. With completion of a prescribed course of therapy, a brief period of fatigue, malaise, and emotional liability may be experienced.

Hormones. Hormonal alteration may be a desired therapeutic goal when tumor growth is directly influenced by certain hormones. The mechanism whereby the steroid hormones stimulate or inhibit cellular growth is not clear; an important mechanism may be interference or alteration at the cell membrane.

Estrogen receptor assays are now routinely done at the time of mastectomy for breast cancer. This technique has made it possible to evaluate the ability of a breast tumor to bind estrogen and thus project the probable sensitivity of the tumor to hormonal therapy.

Dose calculations

The dosage range for a particular drug is determined at the time of clinical trial and regimen development. Given these guidelines, the dosage for a specific individual must be calculated before starting therapy. Although some regimens may still prescribe milligrams per kilogram, drug doses are usually stated in terms of body surface area, and therefore, the doses are given in milligrams per square meter (sqm).[60] An individual's height and weight are used to determine body surface, therefore it is very important that height and weight are measured *accurately*.

Methods of administration of chemotherapeutic agents

The route of administration is based on the metabolism and absorption of a given drug. The route of choice is that which will deliver the optimal amount of drug to the tumor. Chemotherapeutic agents are given orally, intravenously, intramuscularly, intraarterially, and by local instillation (i.e., intrapleurally and intrathecally). If tumor cells are in an area that drugs cannot reach, cancer cells will survive with a consequent increase in disease recurrence. An example is the sanctuary effect afforded leukemic cells by the meninges in patients with acute lymphocytic leukemia. For this reason, local instillation of chemotherapy via an Ommaya cerebrospinal reservoir or intrathecally (directly into the spinal fluid by lumbar puncture) is used to treat tumor cells present in the CNS.

Before administering a cytotoxic drug, the clinician consults a reference for usual dosage, acceptable routes of administration, and any precautions that should be taken for that particular drug. Since protocols may deviate from drug manufacturers' guidelines, discussion with the prescribing physician may also be indicated.

Oral administration. Many cytotoxic drugs are given in pill form. Since these may be prescribed on a daily basis to be taken at home, careful instructions need to

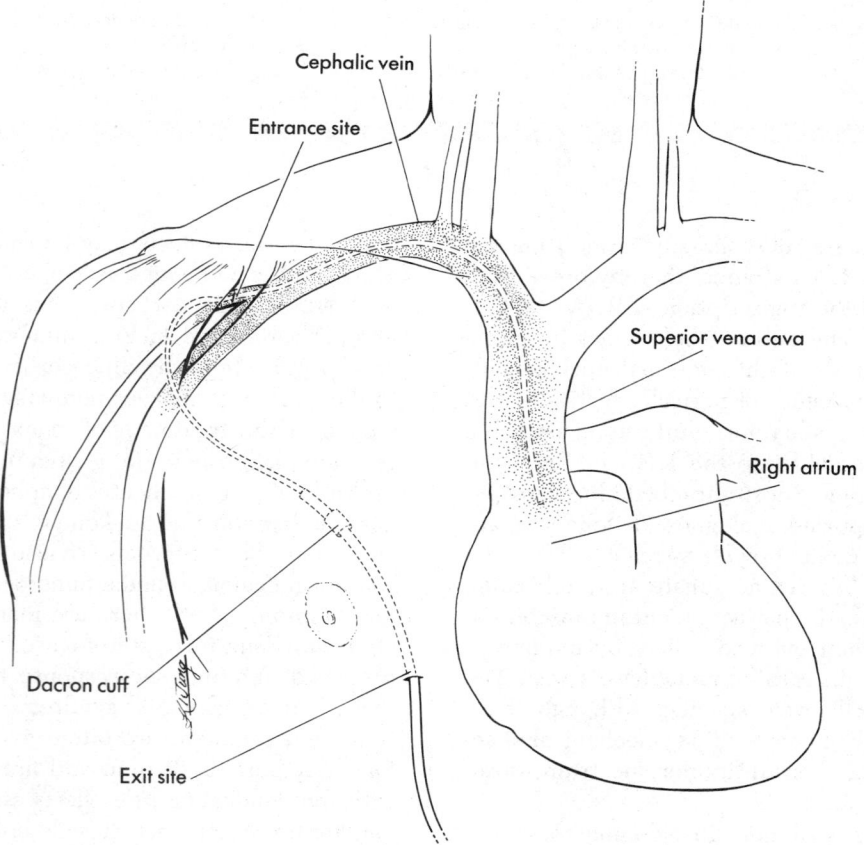

Fig. 25-11. Placement of a Hickman catheter through chest incision between right nipple and sternum through cephalic vein into superior vena cava at entrance to right atrium.

be given to patients. Areas to be discussed include the importance of taking the drug as prescribed, the relationship to meals, fluid intake, and the use of an antiemetic.

Intravenous administration. The clinician must know specific properties for each drug to be administered. Of particular importance is the identification of those drugs that are vesicant (produce blisters). If infiltration and extravasation occur, extensive tissue damage and necrosis may result. Nitrogen mustard, doxorubicin (Adriamycin), vincristine, and vinblastine are the principal vesicant drugs. The intravenous site is evaluated before

the administration of these drugs. If *any* suspicion of an infiltration or leak exists, the site is changed. Most often, vesicant drugs are given via the side arm of a running IV. If extravasation occurs, immediate action is taken to minimize damage. Guidelines vary but may include the administration of methylprednisolone (Solu-Medrol) or sodium bicarbonate to the area of infiltration and the intermittent application of ice for a 24-hour period.

For patients with poor venous access, an indwelling Hickman catheter (Fig. 25-11) may be used for chemotherapy administration.[8,22] Aside from the daily care of dressing changes to the insertion site and the flushing

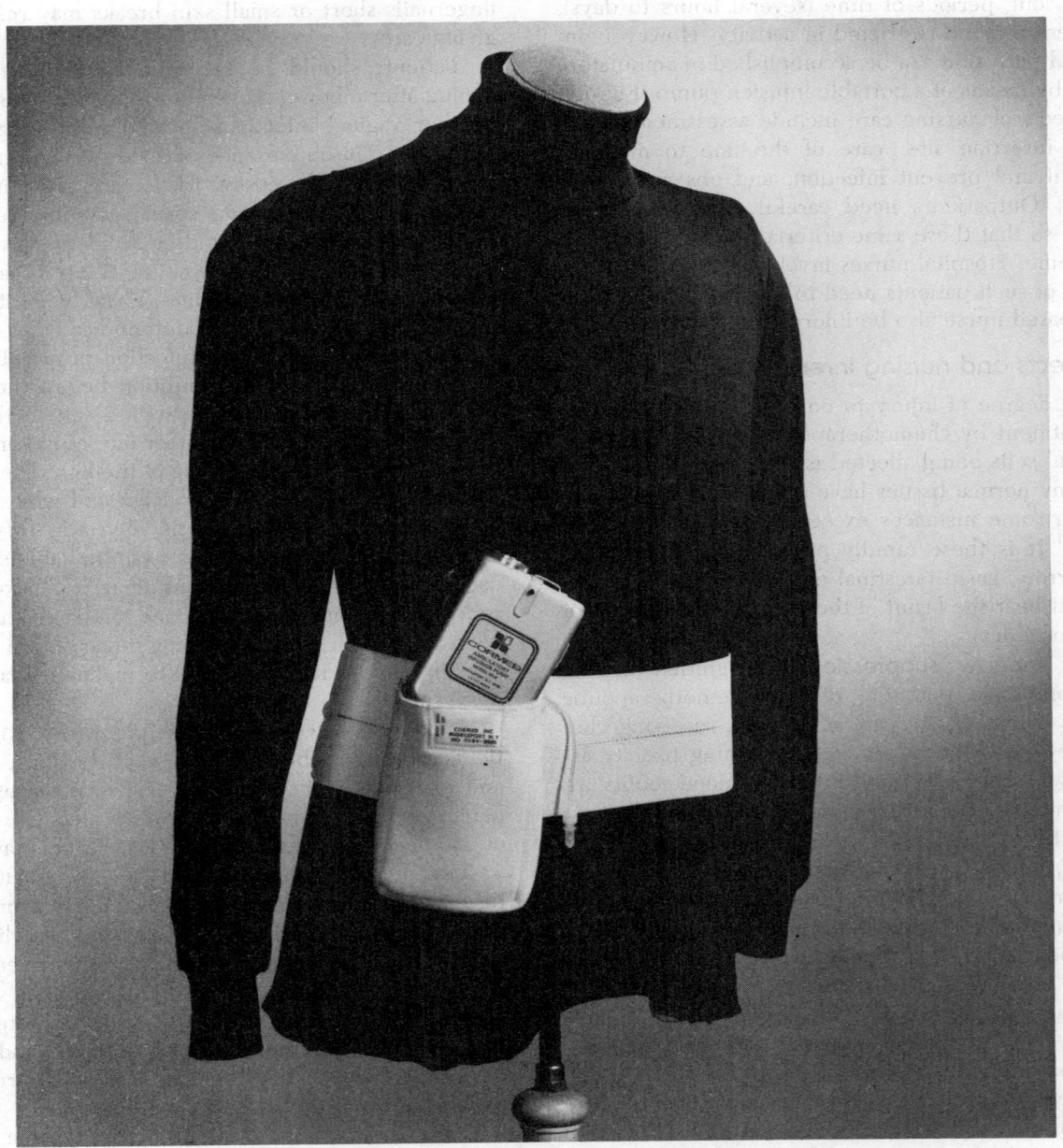

Fig. 25-12. Lightweight, battery-operated infusion pump for ambulatory patient. Flow rate is adjustable. Power pack operates for 7 days before needing recharging. (Courtesy CORMED, Inc., Middleport, N.Y.)

of the line with a heparin solution, the presence of the catheter requires little attention by the patient.

Perfusion. Regional and isolation perfusion is a means of delivering a high dosage of a drug directly to a tumor. This is accomplished by the placement of a catheter into an artery that provides the blood supply to the area being treated.[32] By this method, a high percentage of the drug is delivered because it is not diluted in the general circulation.

Intraarterial perfusion is used occasionally for cancers of the head and neck and of the liver, and as adjuvant chemotherapy with radiotherapy for advanced cancer of the cervix. Because infusions may be continuous for long periods of time (several hours to days), the patient may be restricted in activity. However, intraarterial perfusion can be accomplished in ambulatory patients by means of a portable infusion pump (Fig. 25-12). Aspects of nursing care include assessment of the catheter insertion site, care of the line to maintain placement and prevent infection, and observation for bleeding. Outpatients need careful and detailed instruction so that these same criteria can be maintained in the home. Hospital nurses involved in the discharge planning of such patients need to ensure that the community-based nurse also be informed of these details.

Side effects and nursing intervention

Some degree of injury to normal cells often occurs with treatment by chemotherapeutic agents. The basis for normal cells being affected is their rate of proliferation. Many normal tissues have a high proliferation capacity, in some instances exceeding that of malignant disease.[39] It is these rapidly proliferating tissues (the bone marrow, gastrointestinal epithelium, and hair follicles) that bear the brunt of the toxic effects of many of the cytotoxic drugs.

Bone marrow suppression. Recognition of the myelosuppressive potential of the chemotherapeutic agents is critical to the care of patients receiving chemotherapy. It is the major life-threatening toxicity associated with chemotherapy. Frequent blood counts are done to monitor this toxicity and astute attention must be given to the results of the white blood count, platelet count, and hemoglobin with appropriate modification of drug dosage. Patients who have received previous chemotherapy or radiation therapy, particularly to areas of bone marrow reserve (sternum, hips, or pelvis) may have an increased sensitivity to myelosuppression. Blood counts are done before the administration of chemotherapy and at regular intervals to assess the predictable nadir effect, which varies with the drugs used. Nursing care of patients with neutropenia, thrombocytopenia, and anemia is discussed in Chapter 47.

Infection. The prevention of infection is of utmost importance in the care and teaching of the cancer patient. Body areas with high potential for infection should be inspected daily. The skin and mucous membranes, especially the mouth, axillae, and perineal areas, are infection prone. Assessment of the respiratory tract is also important to identify early signs of respiratory infection. In preventing all types of infection, good medical asepsis and especially careful hand washing by the medical and nursing staff are important.

MAINTAINING INTACT SKIN AND MUCOUS MEMBRANES. Nursing intervention includes teaching the patient to avoid bumping and breaking the skin. Injections are usually avoided. Aseptic technique must be scrupulously maintained during intravenous infusions and dressing changes. It is important that the nurse keep fingernails short or small skin breaks may result while giving care.

Patients should be taught the proper method of wiping after a bowel movement to help prevent urinary tract or vaginal infections. Sexual counseling may be necessary. The importance of good perineal hygiene is stressed. Avoiding excessive friction and providing proper vaginal lubrication during sexual activity are emphasized. Anal intercourse should be avoided, since the area is very prone to abscess formation if any breaks in the tissue occur. The use of enemas, rectal medications, and rectal thermometers is also contraindicated.

The mouth is also very infection prone. Teeth and gums should be in good condition before therapy begins. Fastidious oral hygiene with a soft toothbrush is essential. Petroleum jelly or other lubricants can be used to prevent drying and cracking of the lips. The patient's mouth is inspected daily for ulcers and white patches, which may indicate moniliasis. Nystatin (Mycostatin) mouthwash may be used, or nystatin tablets, usually used for intravaginal infections, may be sucked. Antiseptic sprays, mouthwashes, and oral irrigations help keep the mouth clean. Irrigating devices such as a Water Pik may be recommended to maintain oral cleanliness.

MAINTAINING OPTIMAL RESPIRATORY FUNCTION. Patients are susceptible to middle-ear infections, sinusitis, and pharyngitis. Pneumonia is especially prevalent in patients with leukemia and in elderly persons. Families of patients are instructed not to visit if they have colds.

USE OF PATIENT ISOLATION. Reverse isolation may be ordered, but it is not usually effective unless life islands or laminar airflow units are used. The life island consists of a special large plastic canopy placed around and over the patient's bed. All equipment is sterilized and the air is filtered to remove airborne bacteria. Objects are passed in and out through locks irradiated by ultraviolet light. Patient contact is through arm-length gloves built into the side of the canopy.

Laminar airflow units are rooms that have a constant flow of purified air flowing across the width and breadth of the room (Fig. 25-13). Anyone in the room remains downstream from the patient. If the patient must be

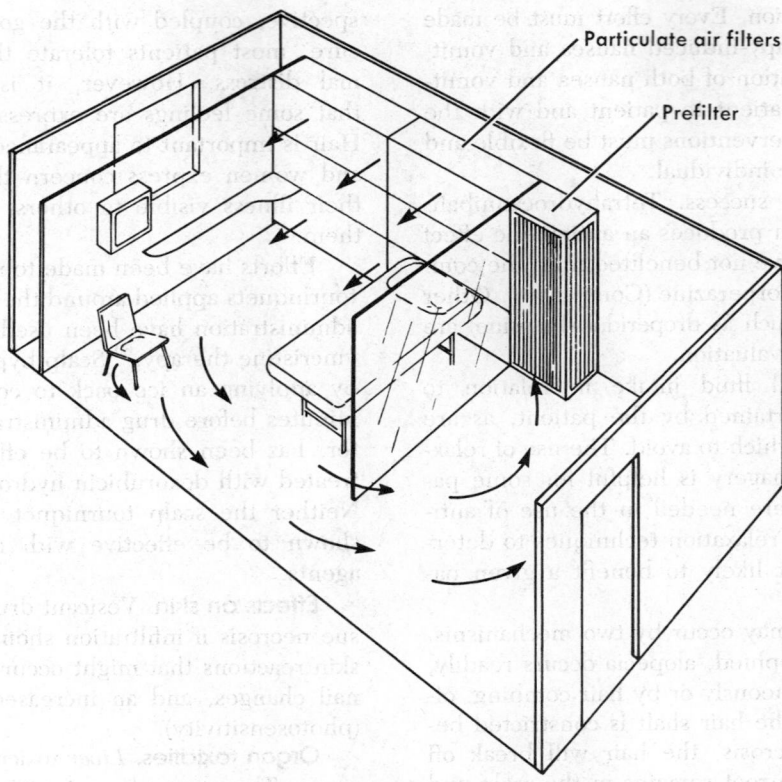

Fig. 25-13. In laminar airflow units constant flow of purified air flows across width and breadth of room. (From American Cancer Society: Proceedings of the National Conference on Cancer Nursing, New York, 1973, The Society.)

touched a mask, cap, and gown are worn. The advantage of the laminar airflow room is that it is large and allows more freedom of movement than the life island.

One danger of any type of isolation is that the patient may experience psychotic episodes because of sensory deprivation. In addition, patients may react adversely when allowed out of the unit. They may feel unsafe, vulnerable, and angry because they are removed from the protected environment.

Gastrointestinal effects. Changes in bowel habits commonly occur but usually do not require intervention. If diarrhea becomes marked or persists, an antidiarrheal medication such as diphenoxylate with atropine (Lomotil) may be prescribed. Alertness to the possibility of other gastrointestinal pathologic conditions such as bleeding or ulceration must be part of the assessment in interpreting symptoms of diarrhea and cramping. Since vincristine may cause paralytic ileus, patients receiving this drug are specifically evaluated for and instructed to report constipation. Patients receiving narcotic-based pain medications may have constipation as a result and a daily bowel regimen program may be indicated.

STOMATITIS. Stomatitis, an inflammation of the mucous membranes of the oral cavity, may range from an erythema of the oral mucosa to mild or severe ulcera-

tion. Methotrexate, 5-fluorouracil, doxorubicin, dactinomycin, and bleomycin are the chemotherapeutic drugs most frequently associated with stomatitis. Patients may also develop a superimposed *Candida* infection of the mouth and esophagus.

Oral nystatin is usually prescribed and is effective in alleviating infection and associated discomfort. A useful regimen for stomatitis includes the use of a rinse and lidocaine (Xylocaine Viscous) before meals (provides lubrication and some analgesic effect so that meals can be taken more easily).[23] After meals, the mouth is again rinsed as a cleansing, either with plain water or a dilute hydrogen peroxide mixture. If necessary, nystatin is then used.

NAUSEA AND VOMITING. Oncology nurses and patients often identify nausea and vomiting as one of the most uncomfortable and distressing side effects of chemotherapy.[58] For the ambulatory patient, nausea may interfere with the ability to continue daily work. Persistent vomiting may result in fluid and electrolyte imbalance, general weakness, and weight loss. Decline of nutritional status renders the patient more susceptible to infection and perhaps less able to tolerate therapy. Such physiologic symptoms can accompany or precipitate psychologic responses that might include depression, withdrawal, and humiliation. Every effort must be made to minimize chemotherapy-induced nausea and vomiting. The onset and duration of both nausea and vomiting vary greatly from patient to patient and with the drugs given. Nursing interventions must be flexible and addressed to the specific individual.

Antiemetics vary in success. Tetrahydrocannibalis (THC) taken in pill form produces an antiemetic effect in some patients who have not benefited from the commonly prescribed prochlorperazine (Compazine). Other antinausea medications such as droperidol (Inapsine) are currently under active evaluation.

Timing of food and fluid intake in relation to treatment is often ascertained by the patient, as are which foods to eat and which to avoid. The use of relaxation techniques and imagery is helpful for some patients. Further studies are needed in the use of antiemetics and the various relaxation techniques to determine the methods most likely to benefit a given patient.

Alopecia. Alopecia may occur by two mechanisms. If the hair roots are atrophied, alopecia occurs readily, either falling out spontaneously or by hair combing, often in large clumps. If the hair shaft is constricted because of atrophy or necrosis, the hair will break off very near the scalp. The root remains in the scalp and a patchy thinning pattern of hair loss occurs.[60] In addition to scalp hair, body hair, pubic hair, and chest hair may also be affected. Loss of leg, arm, and facial hair is seen less often although loss of eyebrows and eyelashes may occur. The pattern and extent of hair loss cannot be accurately predicted for a given patient. However, when treatment is given with a drug known to cause alopecia (see boxes below), the patient needs to be told that severe hair loss can begin within a few days or weeks of treatment and that partial or complete baldness can quickly ensue. Drug-induced alopecia is never permanent. Occasionally, hair growth may return while chemotherapy treatment continues. Given this per-

spective, coupled with the goal of disease control or cure, most patients tolerate the hair loss with minimal distress. However, it is common and normal that some feelings are expressed about the hair loss. Hair is important to appearance. Moreover, many men and women express concern that the hair loss makes their illness visible to others, which is distressing to them.

Efforts have been made to minimize hair loss. Scalp tourniquets applied around the scalp at the time of drug administration have been used with some benefit with vincristine therapy.[60] Scalp hypothermia, accomplished by applying an ice pack to cover the entire head 10 minutes before drug administration and 30 minutes after, has been shown to be effective in those patients treated with doxorubicin hydrochloride (Adriamycin).[68] Neither the scalp tourniquet nor the pack has been shown to be effective with other chemotherapeutic agents.

Effects on skin. Vesicant drugs may cause severe tissue necrosis if infiltration should occur (p. 505). Other skin reactions that might occur are hyperpigmentation, nail changes, and an increased sensitivity to the sun (photosensitivity).

Organ toxicities. *Liver* toxicity is uncommon but may occur. There may be a transient increase in liver enzymes. Alteration in liver function has been associated with Ara-C, methotrexate, and 6-mercaptopurine. *Cardiac* status is carefully monitored in patients receiving doxorubicin. A baseline echocardiogram is usually done before beginning treatment and at regular intervals while therapy continues. Two forms of cardiac damage may occur : arrhythmias, most commonly associated with a

---

DRUGS COMMONLY CAUSING ALOPECIA*

Bleomycin	ICRF-159
Cyclophosphamide	Hydroxyurea
Dactinomycin	Methotrexate
Daunomycin hydrochloride	Mitomycin
Doxorubicin hydrochloride	VP-16-213
5-Fluorouracil	Vincristine

*From Knopf, M., et al.: Cancer chemotherapy treatment and care, New Haven, Conn., 1979, Yale Comprehensive Cancer Center.

DRUGS NOT CAUSING ALOPECIA*

5-Azacytidine	Melphalan
Busulfan	Mercaptopurine
Carmustine	Mithramycin
Chlorambucil	Nitrogen mustard
Cis-platinum	Procarbazine
Cytarabine	Semustine
Dacarbazine	Streptozotocin
Estramustine phosphate	Triazinate
Frorafur	Vinblastine
Hexamethylmelamine	Zinostatin
Lomustine	

*From Knopf, M., et al.: Cancer chemotherapy treatment and care, New Haven, Conn., 1979, Yale Comprehensive Cancer Center.

preexisting cardiac disease, and a delayed moderate to severe congestive heart failure.[44] Other drugs associated with some potential for cardiac toxicity are daunorubicin (Daunomycin) and high-dose cyclophosphamide (Cytoxan). *Pulmonary* toxicity may occur with methotrexate and some of the alkylating agents. The most common cause of chemotherapy-induced pulmonary toxicity is bleomycin. Pulmonary fibrosis can occur and may be irreversible. Each time bleomycin is administered, the pulmonary status of the patient is assessed by auscultation and questioning regarding the presence of cough or shortness of breath.

Urinary effects. Hemorrhagic cystitis occurs in about 10% of patients being treated with cyclophosphamide but rarely occurs with other agents.[38] Patients receiving cyclophosphamide are encouraged to drink a large amount of fluid to minimize this effect. Taking the cyclophosphamide early in the day may also be of some benefit. Renal toxicity is associated with several drugs, but most notably with cis-platinum and Streptozotocin. Before the administration of each dose of these drugs renal function is evaluated by either a serum creatinine or a 24-hour urine collection for creatinine clearance.

Sterility. Cancer chemotherapy reaches the reproductive organs at dose levels similar to those achieved at the site of the target tumor. The potential exists for a disruptive effect on genetic and fetal development.[56] It is recognized that chemotherapy, particularly some of the alkylating agents, may cause transient or permanent sterility. Patients on chemotherapy need to be informed of the known and possible effects on fertility. Birth control and reproductive counseling need to be factors included in patient teaching. If a nurse does not feel comfortable or qualified to discuss the topic, resources useful to the patient and spouse should be identified. Sperm banking before the initiation of therapy offers male patients the option of future conception. Following completion of chemotherapy, conception and the birth of normal, healthy children are possibilities for couples. It is customary to recommend that procreation be avoided until at least 18 months after completion of treatment.

Outcome criteria for the person receiving chemotherapy

The person or significant others can:
1. State the names of chemotherapeutic drugs and any special instructions related to each.
2. State the importance of close medical follow-up, especially for blood studies.
3. Describe interventions for anticipated side effects of prescribed drugs.
4. State who to call if side effects persist or new symptoms occur.
5. Describe how to contact support groups for chemotherapy patients.

Immunotherapy

The role of immunotherapy in the prevention and treatment of cancer is being studied. Many scientists believe cancer occurs in the body more frequently than once in a lifetime; however, in most cases clinical evidence of the disease is not apparent. It is postulated that there is a natural immunity against the development of the disease and that cancer cells are destroyed almost as fast as they develop.[104] Clinical malignancy may occur as a result of failure in the immunologic surveillance system of the body (see p. 475).

Studies of cancer in lower animals and in humans show that when the normal cell becomes malignant it often undergoes biochemical changes resulting in formation of new cellular antigens that cause an immune response.

This response has two major components. The first, or *cellular immune response* (see chapter 19), produces lymphocytes capable of destroying tumor cells on contact. These lymphocytes (T cells) undergo division and are released into the bloodstream when stimulated by an antigen. In addition to destroying cancer cells on contact, T cells may release cytotoxins, which cause holes in the cell membrane, eventually resulting in lysis or death of the malignant cell.

Another important cell, which collaborates with the T cell, is the macrophage. The macrophage, which is attracted to the immune lymphocyte, is immobilized in its vicinity and then activated by the lymphocyte. It is a relatively nonspecific cell that seems to have the ability to kill selectively malignant cells with which it comes in contact.

The second component of the immune response is *antibody production* resulting from activation of lymphocytes (B cells). When stimulated by antigen, B cells proliferate and differentiate into plasma cells, which are the major source of antibody production.

In addition to B cells and T cells, a third immunologic component, natural killer (NK) cells, has been discovered in animals having a natural resistance to tumors.

The cells involved in the immune response interact and seem to exchange signals at both cellular and humoral levels.[75] Antigenic human tumors such as carcinomas of the skin, colon, lung, stomach, esophagus, breast, and thyroid and parathyroid glands have been identified. Some leukemias, sarcomas, and melanomas have been responsive to immunotherapy.

Approaches used in immunotherapy

There are three major approaches to immunotherapy. The first, *nonspecific immunotherapy,* uses substances such as BCG (bacille Calmette-Guérin) vaccine and *Corynebacterium parvum,* which appear to in-

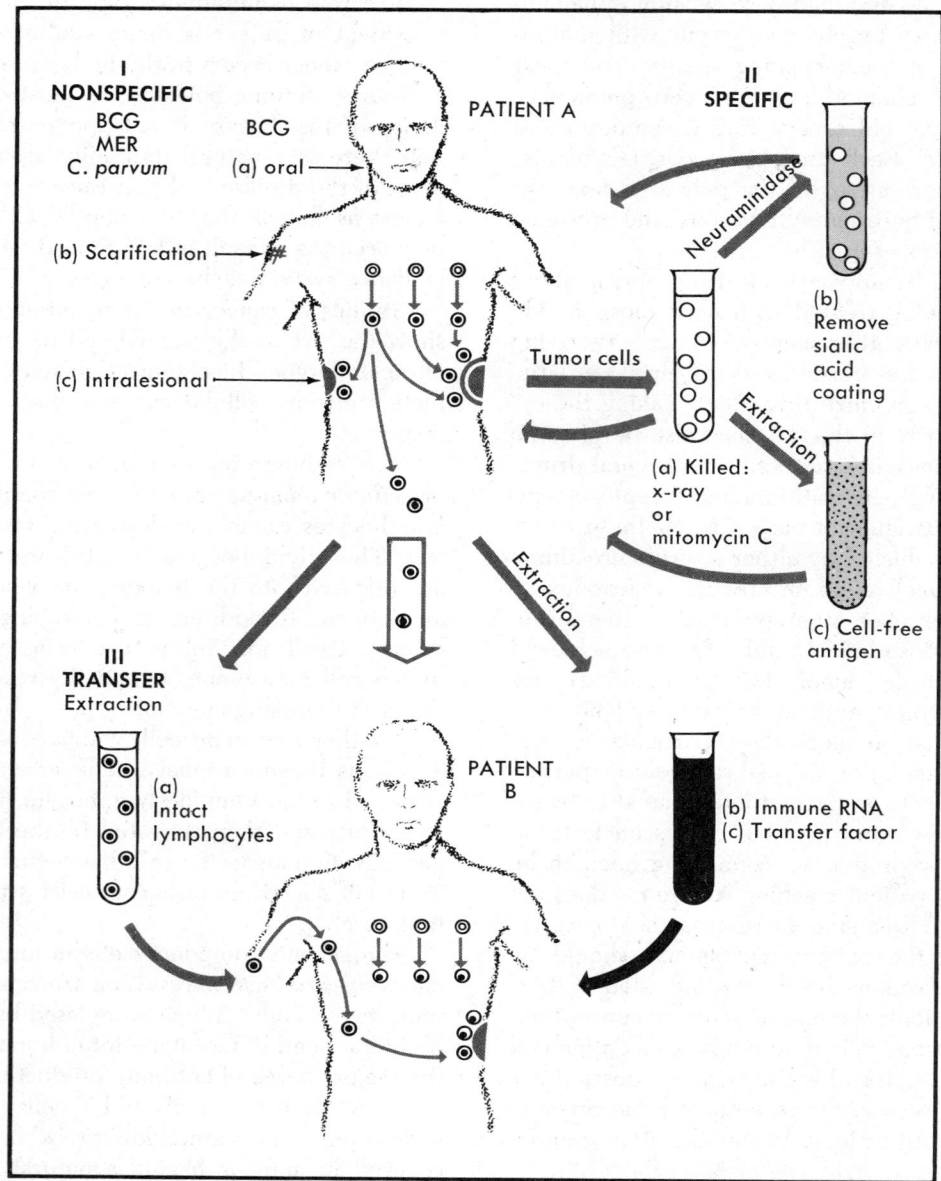

Fig. 25-14. Three major approaches to immunotherapy are active nonspecific immunization, active specific immunization, and transfer of immunity. In each case nonimmune lymphoid cells (⊙) are converted to specifically or nonspecifically sensitized cells (⊙), which
are then capable of attacking tumor. Specific immunotherapy requires inactivating or killing
tumor cells and then returning killed cells to host in multiple injections. Cells may be altered
with such materials as neuraminidase, which removes surface coating of sialic acid, thus
increasing immunogenicity, or cell-free antigen extracts made from tumor cells. Nonspecific
immunization and specific immunization are carried out in original tumor-bearing individual,
while transfer of immunity delivers specific immune capacity to another individual with similar
tumor by intact lymphoid cells or with extracts of immune RNA or transfer factor made from
such cells. (From McKhann, C.F., and Yarlott, M.A.: CA **25:**196, 1975.)

crease the general immune capacity of the patient. Experimentally, these agents prevent tumor growth and halt the growth of small tumors. BCG vaccine has been used against acute leukemia, malignant melanoma, and soft-tissue sarcoma.

Specific immunotherapy, the second type of immunotherapy, uses substances that are antigenically related to the tumor or its products. These substances may be (1) killed tumor cells from the same patient or from another patient with an antigenically similar tumor; (2) tumor cells that have been altered in vitro, making them more immunogenic; or (3) antigen substance extracted from tumor cells.

The third type of immunotherapy is accomplished by *transfer of tumor immunity*, either by transfering lymphocytes from one tumor patient to another or more recently by transferring tumor immunity at the informational level. Two sources of informational molecules recovered from lymphoid cells are immune RNA and transfer factor. Their advantage is that, unlike intact lymphoid cells, they are nonimmunogenic and therefore do not produce a host immune response[75] (Fig. 25-14).

The ultimate goal of immunotherapy is to immunize patients effectively against their own tumors. A perhaps more utopian goal is prophylactic immunization. When more is known about the cause of some tumors, use of attenuated virus or tumor antigen may be a real possibility.[74]

At the present time the immune response can handle only a limited number of tumor cells, up to 10 million. After a growth to 100 million cells the immune response is not capable of preventing further growth. Once the cancer is large, it cannot be totally controlled by the immune system, so immunotherapy cannot be the primary mode of cancer therapy at the present time. It is used after surgery, radiotherapy, and chemotherapy have removed the bulk of the tumor.[104]

Much is yet to be learned about the immunology of cancers. The number of cancers once thought to be immunogenic and responsive to immunotherapy is less than originally supposed. If cancer vaccines are developed, they will be effective in tumors caused by viruses and these are probably limited in number. Even if a cancer-carrying virus is isolated, it must be attenuated so that it can be given safely.

Research is attempting to define cancer detection techniques in the undiagnosed high-risk individual so that knowledge of the immune system can be directed toward those who can benefit from therapy. Although there have been some disappointments and problems because factors that can be controlled and altered in vitro and in animals cannot be controlled in humans, research continues.[73] Much knowledge is needed of the complex host-tumor relationship before specific immunotherapy for cancer can be a reality.

Complications of immunotherapy

Some complications of immunotherapy may occur. Intratumor injection of BCG vaccine has resulted in fever, chills, localized abscesses, and draining sinuses. Regional lymphadenitis, systemic infections, anaphylactic reactions, malaise, and influenza-like reactions may also occur. Fewer problems (mild fever, malaise) have arisen with the intradermal multiple-tine technique of administration. There has been some evidence of liver dysfunction, although the incidence is low.[81] Immunotherapy holds promise for the future prevention as well as treatment of cancers.

Interferons

The newest and one of the most exciting forms of cancer therapy is the use of interferons, a family of secretory glycoproteins produced by leukocytes in response to viral infections or to other stimuli. Interferons induce cellular resistance to a broad spectrum of viruses and are a first line of defense against viral infections. In addition, they may protect against intracellular parasites, neoplastic changes in cells, and the tumor growth itself. They appear to have an inhibitory effect on DNA synthesis and cell growth and may suppress the tumor directly.[73] Interferons were discovered in 1957 and a number of different forms have been identified over time.[65]

All nucleated cells are capable of interferon production, which can be induced by many natural and synthetic agents. Exogenous interferon is interferon induced in cells that are either propagated or maintained in cultures, secreted into the culture medium, concentrated, and purified to give a preparation that can be injected. The cost of large-scale production of interferon has hampered its use for therapy. Dr. Kari Cantell of Finland has developed a process that enables human white blood cells to be used as sources of a considerable amount of interferon.[65] More important, however, is the manufacture of biologically active synthetic interferon by gene-cloning technique, which may reduce the present high cost of about $30,000 to treat one patient.[3]

Interferon's antitumor effect develops from its ability to augment NK cell activity, which is the spontaneous killing of tumor cells by lymphocytes from an animal or person not previously sensitized by tumor cells. Interferon appears to convert inactive lymphocytes into cytotoxic NK cells. Second, it enhances cytotoxicity of monocytes and of antibody-related mechanisms. In addition, human cancer patients have decreased amounts of NK activity, and in most patients this is enhanced for a short time by administration of BCG, which stimulates interferon production.[3] Antitumor effects in humans include marked regression of benign and malignant tumors.

Leukocyte interferon given systemically results in little or no toxicity. Some patients who have responded were resistant to other therapy. The number of patients treated is small and the length of therapeutic response cannot be assessed because of the scarcity of interferon and the lack of definition of an optimal regimen, especially in regard to length of treatment.[66]

At the present time interferon is being used in treatment of melanoma, multiple myeloma, breast carcinoma, prostatic cancer, laryngeal papilloma, and osteogenic sarcoma.

The American Cancer Society has invested almost 6 million dollars in interferon research. Controlled clinical testing with interferon supplied by the Society is in progress at 10 American medical centers. Since research is in the early stages, data about final tumor response and possible long-term side effects are unknown. Precise doses, dose timing, immune effects, and coordination with other types of treatment must be identified before interferon's role in cancer therapy can be delineated.

Nursing assessment of the patient receiving interferon therapy includes knowledge about the patient's emotional status, family and community support systems, previous therapy, and general condition. Side effects include fever to 39° C (103° F), local discomfort at the injection site, and minimal nausea and vomiting. Acetaminophen (Tylenol) is given for fever and antiemetics for nausea and vomiting. At some centers nurses teach the patients to give their own intravenous injections.[71] Nurses must be careful not to raise false hopes in clients who may view interferon as a last resort therapy.

Cancer pain

Pain is one of the most feared effects of cancer, although, contrary to popular belief, it is frequently the last symptom to appear. Even in terminal stages, 60% of persons with cancer will experience mild or no pain. The etiology of cancer pain is complex since it has physical, psychologic, social, and spiritual aspects.[105]

Stages of cancer pain

Three stages of cancer pain have been described: early, intermediate, and late. Early pain usually occurs after initial surgery for diagnosis or treatment and usually subsides after the third day; thus this pain is an acute episode, that is, short term and temporary.

Intermediate-stage pain results from postoperative contraction of scars and nerve entrapment or from cancer recurrence or metastasis. This pain may subside or may be controlled by palliative therapy such as radiation, chemotherapy, neurosurgery, and analgesics. Therapy itself may initiate the pain.[91]

Late-stage pain occurs in terminal cancer when therapy no longer controls the disease. This pain is chronic, may slowly increase in intensity, and at times may be intractable. Severe chronic pain occurs in only about 20% of patients who die from cancer.[64]

Pathophysiology

Malignant neoplasms cause pain by five physiologic changes: bone destruction, obstruction of lumens (viscera or vessels), peripheral nerve involvement, pressure of growing tumors causing ischemia or distention, and inflammation, infection, or necrosis of the tissue.

Bone destruction with infraction (fractures without displacement) is the most frequent cause of pain, usually resulting from metastatic lesions. Bone destruction may cause increased sensitivity over the area or sharp, continuous pain.

Obstruction of a viscus, such as in the gastrointestinal or genitourinary tract, causes severe, colicky, crampy-type pain. Visceral pain is dull, diffuse, and poorly localized. Obstruction of an artery, vein, or lymphatic vessel may initiate arterial ischemia, venous engorgement, or edema. This pain is dull, diffuse, and aching.[91]

Infiltration or compression of peripheral nerves or nerve plexuses causes continuous, sharp or stabbing pain sometimes accompanied by hyperesthesia or paresthesia.

Infiltration or distention of the integument, fascia, or tissue initiates a severe localized pain that is dull and aching, increasing in intensity as tumor size increases. An example of this is the pain resulting from distention of the abdomen by ascites or the stretching of the skin by carcinoma of the neck.

Finally, inflammation, infection, and necrosis of the tissue itself may cause pain by producing either pressure or ischemia. Chemical mediators of pain are present during inflammation and necrosis.

Psychosocial aspects

The psychologic component of cancer pain is associated with the patient's perception of the threat and stress of cancer and varies from individual to individual. Three categories of stressors have been identified: injury or threat of injury as a result of the cancer, loss or threat of loss (body part or death), and frustration of drives as a result of disabilities from the cancer per se or from the effect of therapies. Patients may respond with depression, decreased self-esteem, hostility, and irritability.

The sociologic effects include decreased interaction and participation in activities of daily living. There is decreased productivity characterized by absenteeism from work, economic problems, and deterioration in family relationships. The spiritual effects of pain are evidenced by loss of hope and trust and an overwhelming feeling of despair, rejection, and sense of isolation.

Side effects of cancer pain include fatigue, sleeplessness, anorexia, and decreased movement followed by the complications of immobility, namely, muscle weakness, decubiti, contractures, and respiratory dysfunction.

Intervention

Medical therapy in early-stage pain focuses on therapy directed at the cancer per se. Late-stage pain is treated symptomatically by analgesia, neurosurgery, and nerve blocks. Surgical procedures to relieve the pain include simple intercostal nerve block where feasible, surgical section of posterior sensory roots adjacent to the spinal cord, and spinothalamic tractotomy (interruption of pain- and temperature-conducting tracts).[12] Dorsal column stimulators and transcutaneous electrical stimulators (p. 390) may be helpful in selected cases.

Cancer pain, as with other types of severe pain, may occupy the patient's entire attention and, unless treated vigorously, may demoralize the patient and interfere with eating, resting, or sleeping. Interventions are directed toward helping the patient live as normal a life as possible and cope with the pain. Pain tolerance is increased when the patient's energy is preserved for enjoyable activities. General comfort measures to promote rest and sleep, good body positioning, and nutrition may do much to increase the patient's pain tolerance. Teaching patients conscious muscle relaxation (p. 174) during which they systematically contract and relax muscle groups throughout the body may decrease pain resulting from muscle tenseness as well as anxiety associated with the pain.

Diversionary activities help decrease the patient's perception of the pain by distraction. These activities may be physical (work, walking, rocking, swimming, etc.), social, or mental (watching television, reading, crafts, etc.). Some patients find imagery (waking-imagined analgesia) helpful. Others may try to separate the pain from their bodies thereby "quieting the mind by letting the body drop away."[91]

Medications. Drugs may be the one significant method that alleviates the pain of cancer. Aspirin is the most effective single analgesic for mild to moderate pain.[64] There is an additive and perhaps synergistic effect between aspirin and codeine; therefore combinations of these drugs are useful in moderate acute pain and in chronic aching pain.

In severe chronic cancer pain the narcotics, with the exception of codeine and oxycodone, are the most effective. Although there are no significant differences among the various drugs in potency or side effects, there are significant differences in the duration of action. Those with long duration of action are preferred for relief of chronic cancer pain. Tolerance and dependence in these drugs are less common with cancer pain than when the narcotics are used for acute pain.[64]

There are three important principles in administra-

tion of narcotics. The first is that the optimal dose must be determined, and initial pain control may require seemingly large doses of the narcotics. The second principle is to start with a dose that is too high rather than one that is too low since the person may become anxious if there is no analgesia despite analgesic administration. This anxiety may exacerbate the pain. The third and most important principle is that the narcotic must be *administered regularly,* not prn. Each dose must be given before the previous dose loses effect. Prevention of pain recurrence usually requires less analgesia than treatment of pain after it has recurred.

Oral administration is preferred. Parenteral therapy produces higher initial serum and tissue levels of the narcotic, but the oral doses are as effective as parenteral doses in maintaining drug levels in the body. Intramuscular and subcutaneous injections are more difficult to administer and are painful to patients with marked muscle wasting. In addition, parenteral administration may make the patient dependent on others for drug administration.[64]

Analgesic drug "cocktails," such as Brompton's cocktail mixture, have become more widely used. This liquid commonly contains morphine, cocaine, alcohol, syrup, and chloroform water. In countries where it is legal heroin may be substituted for morphine, although a controlled double blind study has shown morphine to be as effective as heroin. More recently, at St. Christopher's Hospice in London, directed by Dr. Cicely Saunders, simple aqueous solutions of morphine are being used as the primary analgesic. Dr. Saunders, a pioneer in symptomatic care of patients with advanced cancer, no longer advocates use of heroin or Brompton's cocktail over simple narcotic analgesics that are available in the United States.[64]

Phenothiazines are the principal adjunct drug given to control severe chronic cancer pain. They are effective as antiemetics and also have an antianxiety effect.

Nurses provide the psychologic and social support necessary to help the cancer patient cope with severe pain. Administration of analgesics over the 24-hour period and explanations of the physiologic and pharmacologic effects of the drugs can be very helpful to patients and their families (see Chapter 23).

Supportive care of the patient with advanced cancer

Planning care

When all possible surgery and maximal radiation therapy have failed to control the spread of cancer, the patient and family have many special problems. They need encouragement and help in living as normally as possible, in planning for the late stages of the patient's illness, and in adjusting to death and its implications for the family.

Before nurses can help the patient and family, they must have developed a mature philosophy that allows acceptance of death as an eventual reality for everyone. This philosophy is not acquired overnight. The nurse needs the opportunity to discuss feelings about caring for the patient whose death is imminent, since the nurse's attitude toward death and suffering will affect the ability to plan and give care to the patient with advanced cancer. (See Chapter 17 for discussion of death and dying.)

No one can say with certainty when death will come. The patient may ask about the length of time remaining, but no absolute answer can be given. Physicians may have made a statement to the patient about life expectancy. The nursing staff should know what the patient has been told, since the patient's willingness to participate in self-care and attitude toward the illness may be influenced by perception of life expectancy.

Planning, doing, and achieving are the best way to prevent the hopelessness and despair that may overwhelm the patient. Every effort must be put forth to meet the patient's physiologic needs so that higher order psychologic needs may be expressed. The patient who is in pain or feels "dirty" will have difficulty expressing concerns and fears.

Other factors to consider in planning care are the personality of the patient, feelings about death and illness, and the reactions of those significant others whose opinion the patient values. The goal of nursing care should be to relieve physical, mental, and spiritual distress.

Planning for home care

At least half of all deaths from cancer occur in the patients' homes. Planning for home care of the patient without completely disrupting the rest of the family takes the concerted efforts of many people. Patients must always be consulted, and their wishes should be respected in the early stages of the disease. In the final stages they may be too ill to be bothered or concerned with making decisions. The physician, the social worker, and the nurse must work together with the local community agencies, such as the American Cancer Society, to ensure continuity of care from the hospital to the home. The principles governing suitability for home care are similar to those for any patient receiving home care, although the patient with cancer may not live as long as many others with chronic long-term illnesses. Medical and nursing supervision must be available; it must be possible for required care to be given; both patient and family must want the patient home; and home facilities must be suitable. Rehabilitation teams may also be sent into the home to help the patient and family.

The growth of the *hospice* concept, a place where

patients may come for short or long periods for nursing care and then return to their homes as their condition warrants, is exciting. The hospice tries to maintain a homelike setting while relieving the family of the emotional and physical burden of constant care.[35] Hospice programs provide medical, social, and psychologic support for patients and their families so that dying can be truly dignified.

The hospice concept may also be implemented by home care for the patient with the inpatient facility as a backup for home care. If a family wishes to go away on a trip, for example, the patient may request to stay in the hospice. The ultimate goal of the hospice is for the family to develop its ability to give care; thus the relationship of the hospice to the family becomes primarily one of consultation and referral. The family is aided in remaining the patient's primary support system.

Hospice staff are multidisciplinary and are employed and evaluated based on their interests and abilities to care for the terminally ill person. The focus of activities is care rather than cure, with an emphasis on symptom control. Actions are identified to help the patient and family deal with their chief concerns.

Nursing intervention to meet psychologic needs of patients with advanced stages of cancer

Avoiding false hope. Occasionally, there is a mistake in diagnosis or the disease is in some way arrested for a long time. If the patient assumes that one of these occurrences may take place, the nurse should not suggest facing probable reality. The nurse must, however, avoid encouraging false hopes. Many patients accept their prognosis philosophically, with the hope that a cure for cancer will be found before their disease is far advanced. Some patients are better able to accept the situation if their religious faith can be strengthened. Some patients and their families find it helpful to live each day as fully as possible without looking too far ahead. Sometimes patients with cancer have few symptoms and are able to carry on quite well until shortly before death.

Nurses also must be careful that they do not experience false hope. The inability to fulfill the hope to sustain life may make it more difficult for nurses to accept the patient's death and they may see themselves as having failed.[27]

Encouraging social and vocational activities. Patients with advanced cancer should resume their regular work if they can possibly do so, for work makes them feel as though they are still an active part of their group and worthy of the approval of others. It was said many centuries ago that employment is a person's best physician, and this concept applies particularly to persons whose existence is seriously threatened by cancer. Social activities and all experiences associated with normal family life should be continued whenever possible. There is probably no greater service the nurse can give to patients with uncontrollable cancer than to help them continue their everyday lives in any way possible. Family members often need guidance in seeing the patient's need to live as normally as possible. Sometimes the patient appears almost unduly concerned with the details of some aspect of the immediate treatment and almost oblivious to the entire problem. Such a patient senses that success with the immediate treatment is the only way to remain up and about or to carry on at that time.

Decreasing fear of helplessness. Patients may be haunted by fear of brain involvement, loss of mental faculties, and the possibility that they may become completely helpless and dependent on others.[26] By these fears they express a basic human wish: the wish to leave the world with as much dignity as possible. The nurse should urge the patient and family to discuss such fears with the physician. The patient may feel that the physician is too busy and that questions are too trivial to justify the use of the physician's time. Some questions, however, are not trivial at all, and a satisfactory answer to them adds tremendously to the patient's peace of mind. Metastasis to the brain in persons who have other metastases is somewhat rare, and some patients suffer more from fear of damage to the brain than is justified. The patient should know that good general hygiene, good nutrition, being up and about for part of each day, and doing deep-breathing exercises with attention to posture all help to prevent helplessness. A positive approach to all problems certainly shortens the time of helplessness and makes the patient more content.

Nursing interventions to meet physiologic needs of patients with advanced stages of cancer

Increasing comfort. Giving good nursing care to the patient with advanced cancer is challenging. Promoting the patient's comfort should be high on the list of goals. Nursing measures that increase rest and sleep and reduce pain will help maintain the patient's physical and psychologic well-being.

Maintaining nutrition. Cachexia is a frequent problem. Anorexia may accompany therapy, and the increased protein needs of the body resulting from tumor growth may be difficult to meet. Mealtimes should be incorporated with family visiting, or patients can eat together if possible. A high-protein diet enhances the response from therapy, and an adequate intake of calories spares protein for cell building. Because chewing may be difficult, food should be cut in small pieces and creamed or combined with cooked vegetables, rice, or noodles. Meat may also be ground or used as a base for soup or stews. Fish, cottage cheese, and eggs are also good sources of protein.[85]

Intravenous hyperalimentation (total parenteral nutrition [TPN]) may be used as an adjunct to therapy. Studies have found that this did not stimulate tumor growth and that it often resulted in a return of immune system competence, a decrease in sepsis, wound healing, and an increase in response to chemotherapy.[20]

Maintaining elimination. Diarrhea may be a problem, but constipation is more likely. If the patient is receiving narcotics, especially opium derivatives, peristalsis is decreased. Patients receiving the plant alkaloid vincristine (Oncovin) may develop neurotoxicity, causing a high fecal impaction.[26] Increasing the intake of roughage and fluids in the diet, maintaining activity, and using stool softeners may be helpful. Enemas and laxatives may be necessary.

Maintaining personal hygiene. Careful and meticulous hygiene is essential. Careful bathing and attention to skin, hair, and clothing will all promote self-esteem in the patient. Odors from body exudates, draining wounds, and incontinence may occur. Soiled dressings and bed linen are changed immediately. Judicious use of deodorizers is helpful, but deodorizers do not take the place of good hygiene.

Preventing the effects of immobility. Pressure sores may be a severe problem. The combination of inactivity, poor nutrition, and incontinence seen in patients with advanced cancer predisposes them to skin breakdown. Maintaining the patient's activity by getting him or her out of bed as much as possible will prevent pressure and also promote the patient's joint mobility and muscle strength.

Teaching the patient and family. The nurse is involved in teaching during most interactions with the patient and family. Careful explanations about care and sensitivity to what the patient thinks and feels about the disease contribute to the nurse's effectiveness in promoting change in the patient's behavior. When possible, self-care activities should be emphasized. Maintaining the patient's independence whenever possible should be the goal while recognizing that the time may come when dependence is necessary.

Outcome criteria for the person with advanced cancer

The following outcomes occur to the extent that is physically and emotionally possible:
1. The person makes his or her own decisions as long as desired.
2. Skin does not break down.
3. Pain is minimized.
4. Hope is maintained.

REFERENCES AND SELECTED READINGS
Contemporary
1. American Cancer Society: 1981 Cancer facts and figures, New York, 1981, The Society.
2. American Cancer Society: A cancer source book for nurses, New York, 1975, The Society.

3. At year's end: what's new with interferon, J.A.M.A. **242**:2829-2830, 1979.

4. Austin, D.F., et al.: Cancer symptoms and survival rates, Am. J. Public Health **70**:474-475, 1980.

5. Ayers, R., Baker, V., and Padilla, G.: Research in cancer nursing. In Proceedings of the National Conference on Cancer Nursing, New York, 1974, American Cancer Society.

6. *Baird, S.B.: Economic realities in the treatment and care of the cancer patient, Top. Clin. Nurs. **2**:67-80, 1981.

7. *Barlock, A., Howser, D., and Hubbard, S.: Nursing management of adriamycin extravasation, Am. J. Nurs. **79**:94-96, 1979.

8. *Bjeletich, J., and Hickman, R.: The Hickman indwelling catheter, Am. J. Nurs. **80**:62-65, 1980.

9. Bloomer, W.D., and Hillman, S.: Normal tissue responses to radiation therapy, N. Engl. J. Med. **293**:80-83, 1975.

10. Blumberg, F., Flaherty, M., and Lewis, J.: Cancer in the adult. In Coping with cancer, Bethesda, Md., 1980, National Cancer Institute.

11. Bouchard-Kurtz, R.E., and Speese-Owens, N.F.: Nursing care of the cancer patient, ed. 4, St. Louis, 1981, The C.V. Mosby Co.

12. Bourke, R.S.: Metastases and disseminated cancer, New York, 1979, American Cancer Society.

13. *Bullough, B.: Nurses are teachers and support persons for breast cancer patients, Ca. Nurs. **4**:221-225, 1982.

14. *Buehler, J.A.: What contributes to hope in the cancer patient, Am. J. Nurs. **75**:1353-1356, 1975.

15. Carter, S.K., and Kershner, L.M.: Cancer chemotherapy: what drugs are available, Resident Staff Physician **22**:56-65, 1976.

16. Cassileth, B., et al.: Information and participation preferences among cancer patients, Ann. Intern. Med. **92**:832-836, 1980.

17. Cline, M.J.: Cancer chemotherapy, ed. 2, Philadelphia, 1975, W.B. Saunders Co.

18. Cobb, A.B.: Medical and psychological problems in the rehabilitation of the cancer patient. In Hardy, R.E., and Cull, J.G.: Counseling and rehabilitating the cancer patient, Springfield, Ill., 1975, Charles C Thomas, Publisher.

19. Committee on Professional Education of International Union Against Cancer, editors: Clinical oncology: a manual for students and doctors, New York, 1973, Springer-Verlag New York Inc.

20. Copeland, E.M., Van Eys, J., and Shils, M.: Nutrition and cancer, New York, 1978, American Cancer Society.

21. Crowley, M., and Baker, M.: Preparing nurses for Hickman catheter care: a self-learning module, Oncol. Nurs. Forum **7**(4):17-19, 1980.

22. *Daeffler, R.: Oral hygiene measures for patients with cancer, Ca. Nurs. **3**:347-355, 1980.

23. Daniels, F.J.: Sunlight. In Schottenfeld, D.: Cancer epidemiology and prevention, Springfield, Ill., 1975, Charles C Thomas, Publisher.

24. Devita.: Cancer treatment: medicine for the layman. NIH pub. no. 80-1807, Washington, D.C., May 1980, National Institute of Health.

25. Donovan, M.I., and Pierce, S.G.: Cancer care nursing, New York, 1976, Appleton-Century Crofts.

26. Drugs and dosages; interferon, Occup. Health Nurs. **8**(5):47-51, 1980.

27. *Duncan, S., and Rodney, P.: Hope: a negative force, Can. Nurse **74**(11):22-23, 1978.

28. Enstrom, J.E.: Cancer mortality among low-risk populations, Ca: A Cancer Journal for Clinicians **29**:352-360, 1979.

29. Fagin, C., and Dubin, L.: Causes of cancer, Ca. Nurs. **2**:435-441, 1979.

30. Fisher, B., et al.: Ten year follow-up of patients with carcinoma of the breast in a cooperative clinical trial evaluating surgical adjuvant therapy, Surg. Gynecol. Obstet. **140**:528-534, 1975.

31. Fortner, J., and Pahnke, L.: A new method for long-term intrahepatic chemotherapy, Surg. Gynecol. Obstet. **143**:979-980, 1976.

32. Freihofer, P., and Felton, G.: Nursing behaviors in bereavement, Nurs. Res. **25**:332-337, 1976.

33. Frytak, S., Sallon, S., and Cronin, C.: Is THC an effective antiemetic for cancer patients? New York, 1981, American Cancer Society.

34. Gahart, B.L.: Intravenous medications: a handbook for nurses and other allied health personnel, ed. 3, St. Louis, 1981, The C.V. Mosby Co.

35. Galton, V. Cancer nursing at St. Christopher's Hospice. In Proceedings of the National Conference on Cancer Nursing, New York, 1974, American Cancer Society.

36. Garfinkel, L., et al.: Cancer in black Americans, Ca: A Cancer Journal for Clinicians **30**:39-44, 1980.

37. George, M.M.: Long-term care of the patient with cancer, Nurs. Clin. North Am. **8**:623-631, 1973.

38. Golden, S., et al.: Chemotherapy and you, a guide to self-help during treatment, NIH pub. No. 80-1136, Washington, D.C., Aug. 1978, Natiional Institute of Health.

39. Goodman, L., and Gilman, A.: Goodman and Gilman's pharmacological basis of therapeutics, ed. 6, New York, 1980, Macmillan Publishing Co., Inc.

40. Greenfield, L.D., and Herman, M.W.: Radiation safety precautions with ^{131}iodine therapy, Ca. Nurs. **1**:379-384, 1978.

41. *Greenwald, E.S.: Cancer chemotherapy, ed. 2, Flushing, N.Y., 1973, Medical Examination Publishing Co., Inc.

42. Greenwald, E.S.: Cancer chemotherapy, N.Y. State J. Med. **72**:2541-2556, 1972.

43. Guidelines for the cancer-related check-up, Ca: A Cancer Journal for Clinicians **30**:195-196, 1980.

44. Haskell, C.: Cancer treatment, Philadelphia, 1980, W.B. Saunders Co.

45. Helping cancer patients effectively, Horsham, Pa., 1977, Nursing '77 Books.

46. Hensinkveld, K.: Cues to communication with the terminal cancer patient, Nurs. Forum **11**:105-113, 1972.

47. Herrman, C.S.: Immunology, the method to our madness, Ca. Nurs. **2**:359-363, 1979.

48. Higginson, J., Terracini, B., and Agthe, C. Nutrition and cancer: ingestion of foodborne carcinogens. In Schottenfeld, D.: Cancer epidemiology and prevention, Springfield, Ill., 1975, Charles C Thomas, Publisher.

49. Hoffman, E.: "Don't give up on me!" Am. J. Nurs. **71**:60, 1971.

50. Hogan, R.: Human sexuality, a nursing perspective, New York, 1980, Appleton-Century-Crofts.

51. Holland, J.: Understanding the cancer patient, Ca: A Cancer Journal for Clinicians **30**:135-139, 1980.

52. Horton, J., and Hill, G.J.: Clinical oncology, Philadelphia, 1977, W.B. Saunders Co.

53. Hughes, J., and Ryser, P.: Chemical carcinogenesis, CA **24**:351-360, 1974.

54. Isler, C.: Cancer quackery, R.N. **37**:55-59, 1974.

55. Isler, C.: The cancer nurses: how the specialists are doing it, R.N. **35**:28-34, 1972.

56. Kaempfle, S.: The effects of cancer chemotherapy on reproduction: a review of the literature, Oncol. Nurs. Forum **8**:11-18, 1981.

57. *Kelly, P.P., and Tinsley, C.: Planning care for the patient receiving external radiation, Am. J. Nurs. **81**:338-342, 1981.

58. Kennedy, M., et al.: Chemotherapy related nausea and vomiting: a survey to identify problems and interventions, Oncol. Nurs. Forum **8**:19-22, 1981.

*References preceded by an asterisk are particularly well suited for student reading.

59. *Klagsbrun, N.C.: Communications in the treatment of cancer, Am. J. Nurs. **71**:944-948, 1971.

60. Knopf, M., et al.: Cancer chemotherapy treatment and care, New Haven, Conn., 1979, Yale Comprehensive Cancer Center.

61. Knudson, A.G.: Genetic differences in human tumors. In Becker, F.F.: Cancer: a comprehensive treatise, New York, 1975, Plenum Publishing Corp.

62. *Koons, S.B.: The future of cancer nursing, R.N. **39**:23, 1976.

63. Krakoff, I.: Cancer chemotherapeutic agents, New York, 1977, American Cancer Society.

64. Kipman, A.G.: Drug therapy and cancer pain, Ca. Nurs. **3**:39-46, 1980.

65. Krim, M.: Toward tumor therapy with interferons. I. Interferon's production and properties, Blood **55**:711-721, 1980.

66. Krim, M.: Toward tumor therapy with interferons. II. Interferon's in vivo effects, Blood **56**:875-882, 1980.

67. Lippsett, M.B.: Interaction of drugs, hormones, and nutrition in the causes of cancer. In Proceedings of the American Cancer Society and National Cancer Institue's National Conference on Nutrition in Cancer, New York, 1979, American Cancer Society.

68. *Lovejoy, N.: Preventing hair loss during adriamycin therapy, Ca. Nurs. **2**:117-120, 1979.

69. Lynch, H.T., et al.: Hereditary cancer: ascertainment and management, Ca: A Cancer Journal for Clinicians **29**:216, 1979.

70. Marinao, E.B., and LeBlanc, D.: Cancer chemotherapy, Nurs. '75 **5**(11):22-32, 1975.

71. *McAdams, C.W.: Interferon: the penicillin of the future, Am. J. Nurs. **80**:714-718, 1980.

72. McGuire, D.B.: Familial cancer and the role of the nurse, Ca. Nurs. **2**:443-451, 1979.

73. McKhann, C.: Cancer immunotherapy: a realististic appraisal, Ca: A Cancer Journal for Clinicians **30**:286-293, 1980.

74. McKhann, C.F.: Immunotherapy of cancer. In Gottlieg, A.A., Plescia, P.J., and Bishop, D.H.: Fundamental aspects of neoplasia, New York, 1975, Springer-Verlag New York Inc.

75. McKhann, C.F. and Yarlott, M.A.: Tumor immunology, CA **25**:187-197, 1975.

76. Modell, W., editor: Drugs of choice 1980-1981, St. Louis, 1980, The C.V. Mosby Co.

77. Miller, F.N.: Perry and Miller's pathology, Boston, 1978, Little, Brown, & Co.

78. Miller, S.: Nursing actions in chemotherapy administration, Oncol. Nurs. Forum **7**(4):8-16, 1980.

79. Morrin, B.M.: Meeting the immunological challenge: cancer immunology, Heart Lung **9**:686-689, 1980.

80. Morton, D.L., et al.: Response to active immunotherapy of malignant melanomas. In Gottlieb, A.A., Plescia, O.J., and Bishop, D.H.: Fundamental aspects of neoplasia, New York, 1975, Springer-Verlag New York Inc.

81. Mudinger, M.: Nursing diagnosis for cancer patients, Ca. Nurs. **1**:3-9, 1978.

82. Murawski, B.J., Penman, D., and Schmitt, M.: Social support in health and illness, Ca. Nurs. **1**:365-371, 1978.

83. Newell, G.R.: Prologue: the national cancer plan and its relationship to basic research. In Gottlieb, A.A., Plescia, O.J., and Bishop, D.H.: Fundamental aspects of neoplasia, New York, 1975, Springer-Verlag New York Inc.

84. Niles, A.G., and Paulen, A.E.: A humanistic approach to nursing care, Superv. Nurse **4**:42-44, 1973.

85. Nutrition for patient receiving chemotherapy and radiation treatment, New York, 1978, American Cancer Society.

86. Oberst, M.T.: Priorities in cancer nursing research, Ca. Nurs. **1**:281-290, 1978.

87. Paulen, A.E.: Patient and family teaching in the hospital. In Proceedings of the National Conference on Cancer Nursing, New York, 1974, American Cancer Society.

88. Pitot, H.C.: Fundamentals of oncology, New York, 1978, Marcel Dekker, Inc.

89. Prosnitz, L.R.: Radiation therapy: treatment for malignant disease, R.N. **34**:42-47, 1971.

90. Public attitudes toward cancer and cancer tests, New York, 1980, American Cancer Society.

91. Rankin, M.: The progressive pain of cancer, Top. Clin. Nurs. **2**:59-73, 1980.

92. Rodman, M.J., and Smith, D.W.: Clinical pharmacology in nursing, Philadelphia, 1980, J.B. Lippincott Co.

93. Rosai, J., and Ackerman, L.V.: The pathology of tumors. I. Precancerous and pseudomalignant lesions, CA **28**:331-342, 1978.

94. *Rumerfield, P.S., and Rumerfield, M.J.: What you should know about radiation hazards, Am. J. Nurs. **70**:780-786, 1970.

95. Ryser, H.J.: Special report: chemical carcinogenesis, CA **24**:351-360, 1974.

96. Sackett, D.: Periodic examination of patients at rest. In Schottenfeld, D.: Cancer epidemiology and prevention, Springfield, Ill., 1975, Charles C Thomas, Publisher.

97. Schmale, A.H.: Psychologic aspects of anorexia. In Proceedings of the American Society and National Cancer Institute's National Conference on Nutrition in Cancer, New York, 1978, American Cancer Society.

98. Schottenfeld, D.: Alcohol as a co-factor in the etiology of cancer. In Proceedings of the American Cancer Society and National Cancer Institute's National Conference on Nutrition in Cancer, New York, 1978, American Cancer Society.

99. Schottenfeld, D., and Haas, J.F.: Carcinogens in the workplace, Ca: A Cancer Journal for Clinicians **29**:144, 1979.

100. Schreier, A.M., and Lavenia, J.: The nurse's role in nutritional management of radiotherapy patients, Nurs. Clin. North Am. **12**:173-183, 1977.

101. Shepardson, J.: Team approach to the patient with cancer, Am. J. Nurs. **72**:488-491, 1972.

102. Shills, M.E.: Nutrition and cancer: dietary deficiency and modifications. In Schottenfeld, D.: Cancer epidemiology and prevention, Springfield, Ill., 1975, Charles C Thomas, Publisher.

103. Shinkin, M.B.: Reporting on cancer research, CA **25**:105-106, 1975.

104. Silverstein, M.J., and Morton, D.L.: Cancer immunotherapy, Am. J. Nurs. **73**:1178-1181, 1973.

105. Steel, J.F.: Nursing looks at pain. In Proceedings of the Second National Conference on Cancer Nursing, New York, 1977, American Cancer Society.

106. *Teitelbaum, A.C.: Intra-arterial drug therapy, Am. J. Nurs. **72**:1634-1637, 1972.

107. Theologides, A.: Cancer cachexia. In Proceedings of the American Cancer Society and National Cancer Institute's National Conference On Nutrition in Cancer, New York, 1979, American Cancer Society.

108. Unproven methods of cancer management: cancer quackery, CA **25**:66-71, 1975.

109. Upton, A.C.: Low level radiation, New York, 1979, American Cancer Society.

110. U.S. Department of Health, Education and Welfare: The cancer Centers Program, Nov. 1973, Division of Cancer Research Resources and Centers, National Cancer Institute.

111. Van Scoy-Masher, M.: Chemotherapy: a manual for patients and families, Ca. Nurs. **1**:234-240, 1978.

112. *Varricchio, C.G.: The patient on radiation therapy, Am. J. Nurs. **81**:334-337, 1981.

113. Warren, B.: Adjuvant chemotherapy for breast disease: the nurse's role, Ca. Nurs. **2**:32-37, 1979.

114. Welch, D.A.: Assessment of nausea and vomiting in cancer patients undergoing external beam radiotherapy, Ca. Nurs. **3**:365-371, 1980.

115. Winters, W.D., and Morton, D.L.: Immunobiology. In Schottenfeld, D.: Cancer epidemology and prevention, Springfield, Ill., 1975, Charles C Thomas, Publisher.

116. Wintrobe, M.M., et al.: Harrison's textbook of medicine, ed. 8, New York, 1977, McGraw-Hill Book Co.

117. Wynder, E.L.: Dietary habits and cancer epidemiology. In Proceedings of the American Cancer Society and National Cancer Institute's National Conference on Nutrition in Cancer, New York, 1979, American Cancer Society.

118. Wynder, E.L., and Mabuch, K.: Tobacco and cancer epidemiology and prevention. In Schottenfeld, D.: Cancer epidemiology and prevention, Springfield, Ill., 1975, Charles C Thomas, Publisher.

Classic

119. *Boeker, E.H., editor: Symposium on radiation uses and hazards, Nurs. Clin. North Am. 2:1-113, 1967.

120. Warren, W.: Ionizing radiation and medicine, Sci. Am. 201:154-176, 1959. (Entire issue devoted to radiation, including articles on what it is, its circulation in the body, and how it affects the cell, evolution, and the whole animal.)

AUDIOVISUAL RESOURCES

Cancer: Series 1 (kit), Concept Media, 1971, Costa Mesa, Calif. 1. The malignant cell: physiology of disordered function; 2. The malignant cell: etiology of disordered function, 3. The malignant neoplasm: growth, invision metastasis, 4. The malignant neoplasm: interactions with the host, 5. Diagnostic procedures.)

Cancer: Series 2: Focusing of feelings, Concept Media, 1971, Costa Mesa, Calif. (Four filmstrips and four cassettes. 1 and 2. Viewpoint: the nurse; 3 and 4. Viewpoint: the cancer patient.)

Highlights of the National Conference on Cancer Nursing, Chicago, 1973, American Cancer Society. (Two cassette-audiotapes.)

CHAPTER 26

SENSORY OVERLOAD AND SENSORY DEPRIVATION

MARIANN DiMINNO

Individuals as open systems are continuously interacting with the environment. Their boundaries, as unique systems, have been developmentally defined through their sensory apparatus. It is through their senses that individuals learn to differentiate themselves as separate entities.

Infants initially respond to the environment almost exclusively through their skin, since the first nerve endings to be myelinated are those of touch, temperature, and pain.[32] Eventually, as the sensory apparatus develops and refines, children perceive their boundaries as separate from the environment and learn to use their senses to expand their knowledge of the world. It is this very process of receiving and responding to environmental cues that an individual uses throughout the life cycle to form the basis for adaptive responses.

Since our sensations are such an integral part of our ability to perceive and interact with our environment, it follows that any alteration of this process will result in system disequilibrium. As open systems, individuals constantly receive inputs or cues from the environment. If these inputs were suddenly altered, either diminished or overloaded in some way, the normal method of receiving environmental cues would be affected, and the individual would have to adapt to this sudden change. As anyone knows who has played childhood games involving patching of the eyes, the immediate response on the part of the patched individual is to place the arms in a frontal position to obtain from the environment through touch those cues no longer available through vision. This illustrates one way in which the organism adapts to a loss of sensation from one modality by obtaining data through another modality.

Clients in health care settings may also experience system disequilibrium. The mechanized hospital environment may result in altered sensory input and may be compounded further by the physiologic alterations of illness, which add further stress to the client system.

The purpose of this chapter is to explore sensory alteration and its resultant disequilibrium for both theoretical and clinical perspectives.

Interest in the area of sensory alteration began in the 1950s. Early experiments manipulated the environment in an attempt to seek some answers to the phenomena of brainwashing and the effects of monotony on an individual's performance.[43] The findings indicated that by manipulating the amount of sensory-perceptual inputs, behavioral changes could be elicited from experimental subjects. When exposed to sensory and perceptual deprivation, subjects experienced hallucinations, difficulty in cognitive tasks, disorientation, anxiety, and somatic complaints.

Since these first studies, interest in sensory deprivation has grown considerably. Nurses have also evidenced particular interest in what happens to clients experiencing sensory deprivation and, to some extent, sensory overload. Although the nursing profession requires additional rigorous clinical research to substantiate some of the nursing interventions proposed for clients with a sensory alteration, it is useful to consider a model of sensory overload and underload for intervening with clients whose behavior often seems confusing and perplexing to the nurse. In viewing this model of sensory overload and underload from a systems perspective, it enables the nurse to use a systematic approach for processing inputs that could be possible system stressors and to intervene to assist the client in making adaptive responses.

Sensory process

Sensory perception

Humans orient themselves to their environment through their ability to receive and organize sensory stimuli. This *reception* and *organization of stimuli* is collectively known as *sensory perception*. The process of sensory perception is dependent on several factors: a stimulus, adequate sensory receptors, intact neural pathways, and adequate processing by the brain to interpret the stimulus input.

A stimulus is received by a sensory receptor, which then synapses with a cranial, peripheral, or autonomic nerve. The nerve then either synapses with sensory nerve tracts in the spinal cord or with areas of the brain. The exact mechanism by which the brain interprets sensory input is not known, but there is evidence that the *reticular activating system* (RAS) plays an integral role in processing sensory input. The RAS is composed of a network of neurons, called the reticular formation, which forms a central core extending from the medulla of the lower brain to the thalamus in the diencephalon.[42] The RAS can be stimulated by two major sources: cortical impulses and sensory stimulation from visual, auditory, olfactory, somatic, and visceral sources.[42] It controls general central nervous system activity and selectivity of attention (arousal) to the environment. It serves a monitoring function for both inputs and outputs to the human system.

It is believed that the RAS in conjunction with the thalamus and hypothalamus collects and combines sensory input. *Perception* takes place when the sensory input is received, decoded (synthesized), and interpreted by the cortex. When interpretation occurs, a conscious awareness of sensation begins. Perception provides the individual with an awareness of reality, which then serves as a basis for determining if an adaptive or maintenance action is required. To clarify this further, consider the following example: if the cortex interprets an auditory stimulus to be loud, unpleasant, and painful, the individual becomes consciously aware of the discomfort and may adapt by covering the ears or moving to a quieter environment. If the cortex interprets an auditory stimulus to be pleasant, the client becomes consciously aware of this sensation and may utilize a maintenance action of remaining stationary in the pleasant environment.

It is important to note that without the function of the ascending reticular activating system, perception does not occur. Lindsley[40] gives the example of an individual who is under barbiturate anesthesia: the sensory pathways can conduct their messages to the primary receiving areas, but discrimination and perception do not occur. Thus it is seen that the RAS not only plays an im-

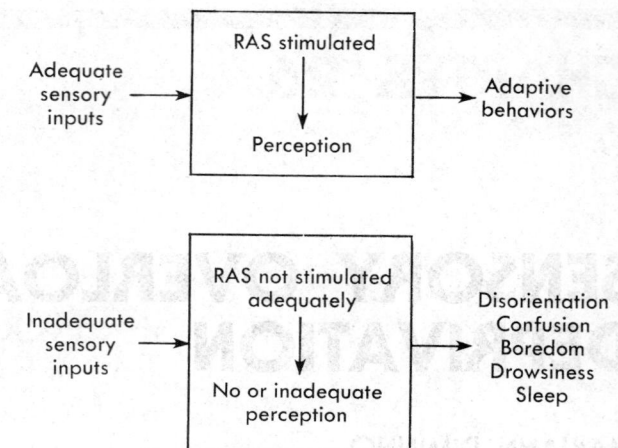

Fig. 26-1. Relationship between sensory inputs, arousal, and outcome.

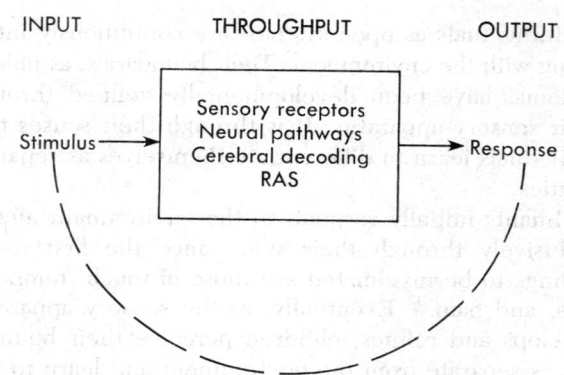

Fig. 26-2. Sensory process from a systems perspective.

portant role in providing a mechanism for general arousal and alerting of the individual, but it must also be stimulated for perception to take place.

If sensory inputs are adequate, the RAS is stimulated and an alert aroused state is created in the individual—a state that allows perception and adaptive responses to occur. If there is inadequate stimulation of the RAS, disorientation, confusion, boredom, drowsiness, and sleep may occur (Fig. 26-1).

In viewing the sensory process from a systems perspective, the input would be the stimulus; the sensory receptors, neural pathways, and cerebral decoding necessary for processing (the RAS) would be throughput; and the resulting adaptive response or behavior of the individual would be output (Fig. 26-2).

Sensory apparatus and modalities

The sensory apparatus provides stimulus inputs into the system; the eyes, ears, nose, skin, tongue, muscles, and visceral organs all provide information relevant to system functioning. It is not hard to imagine what would happen if one of the sense organs was no longer providing cues about the environment. It is easy to see, then, the relevance of this function to everyday life situations.

Sensory *modalities* can be broadly classified as either originating internally or externally (Table 26-1). The internal sources of stimuli are *kinesthetic,* such as those arising from muscles and specialized neural tissue, or *visceral,* originating from hollow organs. These internal sensations provide information about our placement and position in space, that is, where parts of the body are in relation to one another. These internal sensations are primarily involved with the sensations of pain and with the regulatory mechanisms of the internal environment of the body.

The external sources of stimulation arise from the eyes, ears, nose, and skin, while the tongue provides both internal and external inputs of stimulation.

It is important to emphasize that sensation has both internal and external components, since both sources contribute to the overall sensory information processed by the brain. An alteration in the amount of stimulation received from either an internal or external source will affect the amount of sensory input to the brain and may necessitate an adaptive response. The importance of this will be more evident in the discussion of the clinical applications of sensory alteration.

Sensoristasis

Schultz[42] has defined *sensoristasis* as a drive state of cortical arousal that propels the awake individual to seek an optimal level of sensory variation. In other words, each individual has a drive or need for a constant range of varied sensory input. This varied input is required for the organism to function optimally. Schultz compares sensoristasis as being similar to the homeostasis concept of Cannon[29]—a dynamic changing condition that adapts to subject and task variables but that also has a relatively constant pattern. The RAS appears to play a monitoring function by its mediation of system inputs and outputs in maintaining the sensoristatic equilibrium. This equilibrium, however, can be disturbed under conditions of sensory restriction or overload, and the organism must then use adaptive behaviors to restore the balance. For example, if sensory stimulation is below the optimal level, the organism will adapt to seek alternative stimuli or become more sensitized to existing stimuli. If stimulation is greater than the optimal level, the organism will adapt by attempting to decrease system inputs.

Schultz[42] lists four major corollaries of his sensoristatic model:

TABLE 26-1. Sources of sensory inputs, modalities, and their functions

Source and function of stimulus inputs	Sense organs	Modality
Internal: provide internal environmental cues	Muscle and specialized neural tissue	Kinesthetic
	Hollow organs	Visceral
External: provide external environmental cues	Eyes	Visual
	Ear	Auditory
	Nose	Olfactory
	Skin	Tactile
Internal and external: provide internal and external environmental cues	Tongue	Gustatory

1. The drive or need mechanism implemented in the sensoristasic concept is equivalent with arousal as mediated by the RAS.
2. An optimal range of external stimulation exists that influences cortical arousal. Only when this optimal level is maintained can the organism function adaptively with its environment. If there is alteration of stimulation, there is a disruption of learned responses and prevention of new learning.
3. An organism behaves in a way that will maintain this optimal arousal level.
4. The optimal range of sensory stimulation can alter depending on several factors: the task to be performed, the present status of the organism, and the preceding level of stimulation. Also, there may be individual differences in need for sensory inputs and differences over time within the same individual.

There seems to be general agreement that there is an optimal level of arousal required to maintain perceptual and adaptive functions; however, it is still unclear what the exact limits of normal sensory stimulation are. What is considered optimal seems to vary widely among individual subjects.

Deprivation and overload

Definitions

The term *sensory deprivation* has been used synonymously in the literature with many different terms, ranging from social deprivation to restricted stimulation

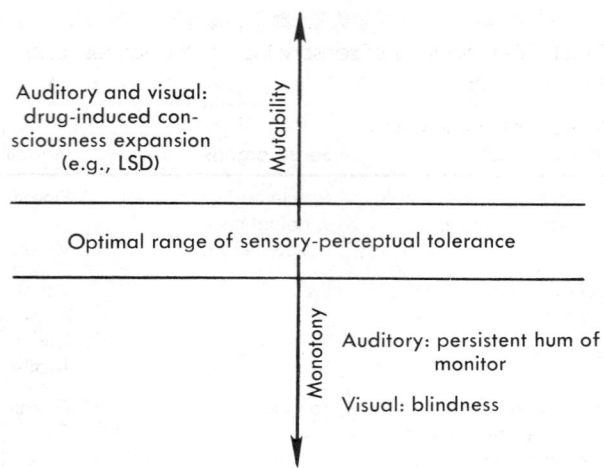

Fig. 26-3. Sensory-perceptual deprivation. Change in patterning of sensory input may create mutability or monotony.

and solitude. For the purposes of this discussion, *sensory deprivation* is defined as a state of being in which the amount or intensity of sensory inputs is below the individual's range of tolerance. Tolerance is the unique range each person has for tolerating every type of sensation and that enables each person to function well and comfortably. The state of being in which the sensory inputs exceed the optimal range of tolerance is termed *overload*.

Deprivation refers to the general concept of decreasing sensory inputs, but in the specific case of a reduction in the pattern of meaningfulness of stimuli, the term *perceptual deprivation* is employed. This occurred in experimental studies when subjects wore translucent goggles or translucent halved Ping-Pong balls as eye shields to produce diffused, unpatterned light. The subject saw light, but the form and pattern did not alter. Another example is the consistent hum of a monitor in the intensive care unit (ICU). The state of being in which the patterning of sensory input is below the individual's optimal range of tolerance is defined as *monotony;* that which is above the optimal range is termed *mutability* (Fig. 26-3). It should be emphasized that both sensory and perceptual deprivation refer to a reduction of stimulation from a previous condition and not the total absence of all stimulation, which is logistically impossible.

Effect of early alteration on growth and development

Deprivation or overload of system inputs will affect an individual's capacity for adaptive responses. Experimental literature indicates that there are effects on adult behavior from alteration of sensory stimulation early in life.[41,45] The normal growth and maintenance of neural structures depend on adequate stimulation at an early level of development.[21,41] Experimental work with cats, monkeys, and chimpanzees demonstrated that organisms reared in restricted sensory environments show perceptual visual deficits, which may never be eliminated.[5,41] The primates also reacted violently to a marked increase in stimulation.

From these studies it appears that the adaptive capacity and neurologic structures of an organism can be severely affected when there is early sensory deprivation. Although deprivation can limit sensory development, it can also lead to physiologic adaptation. The findings of Freeman and Bradley[9] on monocularly deprived humans suggest that although the affected eye has an irreversible deficit (decreased ability to activate cortical neurons) the unaffected eye has increased visual sensitivity in alignment discrimination.

Studies of institutionalized children reveal that early childhood deprivation results in behavioral changes and developmental problems. When children who spent their first 3 years in an institution before being placed in a foster home were compared with children raised continuously in a foster home, the children who were institutionalized experienced less intellectual and emotional capacity.[34] The institutionalized children demonstrated aimlessness, poor concentration, poor impulse control, and a decreased capacity for abstract thinking as compared with the control group. Thus it is evident that a decrease in critical inputs from a consistent source, such as a mother, adversely influenced the emotional and intellectual development of these children.

Another study compared the developmental patterns of institutionalized children with children raised in their own homes for the first year of life. Children were observed in two different institutions. The first was a foundling home where children had only minimal brief contacts with a nurse. The other institution was a nursery located in a penal institution for delinquent girls, where the children had consistent, frequent contacts with their own mothers.[44] The children raised in a foundling home began at a normal developmental level but did not maintain it and eventually fell behind the other children in social, perceptual, and motor development. Both of these studies indicate the critical nature of early sensory inputs from a consistent source and the importance of perceptual and social stimulation to normal human development.

Others investigated the effects of increased sensory inputs on infants. They found that infants who had experienced increased handling and exposure to objects within their visual field demonstrated "visually directed reaching" and "visual attentiveness" earlier than infants who had not been exposed to such stimuli.[25,47]

Early environmental inputs also affect the infant's ability for self-soothing, first as a child and later as an

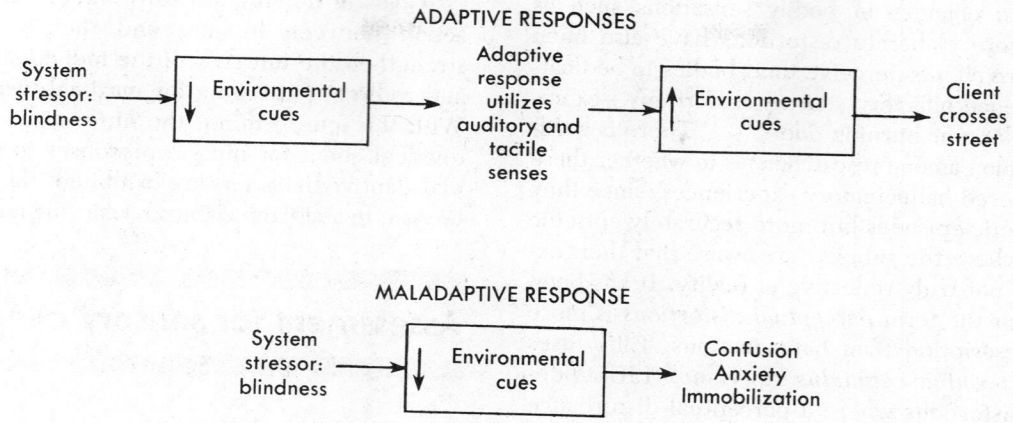

Fig. 26-4. Adaptive vs. maladaptive responses to blindness.

adult. For example, the sensory stimulation of a mother soothing a child through holding and rocking becomes an internalized structure, which the adult draws on later in times of distress. It has been hypothesized that the self-soothing psychic structure of the adult is linked to early repetition of infant satisfaction from the environment in meeting basic biologic needs and the supportive sensory inputs provided by a parent. Deficits in this early process adversely affect the adult's ability for psychic self-soothing.

It has been suggested that early levels of stimulation influence the optimal level of sensory variation in the adult. The child's level of stimulus variation will influence the arousal of the RAS for adaptive behavior as an adult. Thus adaptation levels may be determined by the amount of variety of early sensory input. This may explain individual differences in the optimal level of stimulation within which the organism can function effectively.[42]

The fact that early sensory input is critical to the normal growth and development of children has definite implications for nurses, who may be called on to assess the amount of stimulation available to an infant in the home environment.

The same assessment process is called for when children are hospitalized. Nurses are entrusted with the care of hospitalized children whose needs include a stimulating sensory environment to enhance normal development. Contact with families, other children, play therapy and various sensory stimulators such as mobiles, toys, colors and patterns on walls, curtains, and furniture all contribute to adequate sensory inputs.

Adaptive and maladaptive responses

When system inputs either exceed or fall short of the optimal range for the organism, the overload or deprivation state is considered a system stressor. Any

conditions that alter sensory inputs would also be considered stressors. These can be environmental, social, physical, psychologic, or developmental factors. For example, anxiety, immobilization, paralysis, flotation mattresses, body casts, isolation, and neurologic deficits alter sensory inputs and can be categorized as system stressors. The degree to which each individual tolerates system stressors differs, and this influences how a client will respond—whether in an adaptive or maladaptive manner. Roy[20] defines adaptation as a human's positive response to a changing environment. An adaptive response maintains client integrity, whereas a maladaptive response does not and is disruptive to the individual.

Mitchell[17] cites examples of adaptive behaviors by newly blinded individuals who can no longer perceive traffic lights through their visual apparatus. These individuals can adapt and obtain environmental cues through other sensory modalities, such as their auditory sense by listening to traffic patterns to determine if traffic has stopped, or through their sense of touch by becoming aware of the motion against their person as the crowd begins to move across the street. A maladaptive response to the same situation would occur if this individual became anxious, confused, and immobilized on the street corner and unable to utilize alternative environmental cues (Fig. 26-4).

Stressors that exceed the optimal tolerance level of the client will result in maladaptive responses, which can be cognitive, perceptual, motor, or affective disturbances.

Cognitive changes experienced by subjects range from poor concentration, altered sequencing of thoughts, or unusual ideas to bizarre or primary process thinking—defined as the instinctual thought patterns experienced in dreams. There is also alteration in ability to perform unstructured cognitive tasks.[42]

Perceptual changes include visual and auditory distortions, perceived movement of stable objects, warping and curvature of surfaces and lines, changes in color and form, and changes in bodily sensations such as numbness. More elaborate distortions have also been reported where clients perceive their bodies to be floating or experience olfactory sensory distortions—exemplified by cooking or burning odors.[5,7,14] There is a difference of opinion among researchers as to whether these can be considered hallucinatory experiences, since they are not psychotic episodes but more accurately episodic occurrences where the subjects are aware that their experiences are not truly reflective of reality. It has been contended that the term *perceptual distortions* is more accurate a description than hallucinations. Ellis[7] uses the term *indeterminate stimulus experience* (ISE) to describe such distortions where a perceptual disturbance occurs for which there is no known stimulus. This can occur without disorientation to time, place, or person.

The experimental literature supports the contention that sensory and perceptual alteration will produce changes in *motor* coordination. Dexterity, other measures of eye-hand coordination, balance, and body coordination have been found to be negatively affected by deprivation conditions.[46,52]

Affective disturbances noted by researchers include anxiety, fear, mood swings, irritability, depression, exaggerated emotional responses, and anger.[42] The intensity of the disturbances varies from mild discomfort to panic.

Additional responses include somatic complaints and noncompliant behavior. Noncompliant behavior would include actions clients display that are contrary to the instructions of health care providers and detrimental to the client. A study of postoperative eye surgery patients identified behaviors such as removing eye patches and getting out of bed as noncompliant.[49]

It should be emphasized that clients may not openly or easily share with staff some of these disturbances, such as perceptual distortions, because of the anxiety or embarrassment that may accompany such experiences. The nurse must be alert for maladaptive responses and investigate further, seeking additional data from the client if the situation warrants intervention.

It is also important for the nurse to be aware that clients in a hospital setting can display maladaptive behaviors in response to an altered sensory environment. It is not unlikely that the nurse may be in a situation where an apparently "normal" client is exhibiting psychotic-like behavior such as confusion, noncompliance, disorientation, anxiety, mood swings, or perceptual distortions. This does not mean the client has suddenly become psychotic, toxic, or senile but may be responding to an altered sensory environment. However, in applying research findings to the clinical situation, certain limitations must be noted. Although it is hypothesized that responses are correlated with alterations in sensory inputs, this hypothesis needs further testing. It is not a ready explanation but a framework to use in attempting to assess and understand client behavior.

Goals of nursing are to promote harmonious interaction between humans and their environment, to strengthen the integrity of the individual, and to direct and redirect patterning for maximal health potential.[20] With this aim in mind, the nurse must assess each individual client for unique responses to stressors and if maladaptive behaviors are exhibited, the nurse must intervene to assist the client in achieving an adaptive state.

Assessment for sensory alterations

In assessing for altered sensory inputs, the nurse includes both individual and environmental variables, since both contribute to the total amount of sensory input. Data can be collected either by direct questioning or by observation of the client.

Individual factors

Following are individual factors to be considered:

1. *Sensory status of visual, auditory, olfactory, gustatory, and tactile modalities:* Does the client have normal visual and auditory functions? Are there any impairments,[10,13] defects, or corrective devices required such as glasses or a hearing aid? Can the clients discriminate between odors and various taste sensations? Can they perceive changes in temperature, feel pain, and discriminate between various forms of touch such as sharp and light? Do they have the ability to define placement or position in space?

2. *Neurologic status:* What is the client's level of consciousness? (See Chapter 27.) Are the normal pathways and processing functions intact? Are there any neurologic deficits that would affect sensory inputs, such as spinal cord injuries, stroke conditions, or hyperirritability of neural tracts, that would cause excessive stimulation?

3. *Motor status:* Is the client capable of independent movement? Is there any alteration as a result of illness, such as paralysis, casts, or immobilization?

4. *Cognitive status:* Can the client perceive, process information, and respond appropriately to the environment? Can the person read or write and follow simple commands?

5. *Communication status:* Is the ability to communicate within normal range? Can the client understand and initiate speech and respond to verbal communications? Is there any impairment of speech organs or neural pathways necessary for verbal communications?

6. *Age and developmental level:* What is appropriate for the client in terms of age and developmental level?

7. *Psychologic status:* Is the client an independent, self-reliant person? What coping mechanisms are used?

Does the person appear anxious, irritable, angry? Oriented to time, place, person?

8. *Utilization of drugs:* Has the client been exposed to central nervous system depressants, such as alcohol or narcotics, which decrease awareness of the environment? Have stimulants, such as amphetamines, or consciousness expanding drugs, such as LSD, been used that would alter perception?

9. *Presence of maladaptive behaviors:* Are there any cognitive, perceptual-motor, or affective disturbances noted?

10. *Presence of specific stressors:* Are there any additional specific stressors to which the client is exposed that would further alter sensory input? This could include pain, drug toxicity, immobilization, isolation, or specific system disorders such as alterations in gas exchange or regulatory mechanisms.

Environmental factors

Two variables are considered when assessing the effect of environment on sensory input: (1) the amount and intensity of environmental inputs and (2) the increase or reduction of pattern or meaningfulness of sensory inputs from the environment. It is important to assess whether these two variables are sufficient to maintain an arousal state in the individual that permits adaptive responses to occur.

Much of the clinical literature concerns itself with two alterations that can occur in the environment of the client. The environment can be analyzed on the basis of being either a therapeutically restricted environment or a socially restricted environment.

Therapeutically restricted environment

Because of particular health care needs, clients may be placed in a therapeutic environment that is at the same time restrictive. The following clinical situations provide some examples.[6,17]

1. Clients who are kept isolated in sterile environments to protect themselves or others from pathogenic organisms constitute one major category of clients. Their environments are generally unchanging, and contacts with staff are minimal and often directed through gowns and masks.

2. Clients with orthopedic or neurologic injuries are often placed in traction, casts, or in Stryker or Foster frames, which limit their mobility and commonly confine them to bed. They are not only restricted in movement but can also be restricted visually, since their position may not afford them a changing environment. They may be positioned, for example, on their backs, with the major visual field being the ceiling.

3. Clients placed in intensive care units (ICUs) or coronary care units (CCUs) make up another category of individuals with a restricted environment. These clients are removed from their familiar world often under an acute crisis situation that did not allow time for client preparation or a transitional period. They are exposed to unfamiliar repetitious sounds, constant light, constant activity, immobilization, and strange equipment and commonly are stressed further by the alterations of illness, pain, sleep, and anxiety. This restricted environment may also be one that predisposes to sensory overload.

Socially restricted environment

Living circumstances that lead to social deprivation are also restrictive to clients. Several variations of this condition have been cited[15,17]:

1. Infants raised in nonstimulating institutions with minimal contact with care givers or infants raised by families who do not provide an adequately stimulating environment

2. Institutionalized individuals of any age whose living situation is devoid of adequate social or perceptual inputs

3. The depressed or psychotic client, the elderly, and the chronically ill individual (these persons constitute another group who may live in their own homes but are physically, socially, or emotionally unable to venture out or whose home environment is restricted or monotonous.)

4. Persons isolated by disfigurement (these persons may also have restricted interaction with their environment. Persons with cancer of the head and neck, for example, contend not only with the physical impact of the disease but also with the psychologic trauma and social effects inflicted on them.[15])

In summary, all factors considered, both individual and environmental variables should be assessed as possible contributory factors to sensory alteration.

Clients predisposed to sensory alteration

It appears that many clinical situations contain elements of sensory deprivation or overload. It also appears that certain clients are prone to developing cognitive and behavioral impairments. There is no research to support specific predictions of exactly who will experience the effects of sensory alteration, but there is evidence to suggest the categories of clients that might be considered as possible risks.

Clients experiencing *eye surgery* are in the most common situations discussed in the literature; the majority of these persons have had cataract surgery.[35] These clients were relatively immobilized postoperatively and wore eye patches, a combination that greatly reduced sensory input. They experienced anxiety, perceptual and thought disturbances, and confusion and exhibited noncompliance behavior such as getting out of bed and removing their bandages.[35,36] Nursing interventions that were reported to be most useful in these situations were reassurance, reality orientation, and providing information to the client.

Immobilized clients also experienced sensory impairments. The hallucinatory behavior of clients with bulbar poliomyelitis confined to tank-type respirators has been described as exemplifying the possible effects of sensory alteration[39] It has been suggested that immobility with the reduction of kinesthetic input produces perceptual and motor abnormalities. Downs[5] investigated the effects of bed rest on young, healthy adults. The subjects, who were relatively immobile for a fixed period of time, experienced difficulty in concentration, disorientation in time and place, olfactory distortions, and "indeterminate stimulus experiences" (ISEs). Similar effects may also be seen in orthopedic clients immobilized for long periods of time.

The third category discussed in the literature are those clients placed in *intensive care units* (ICUs). The environment of the ICU has received attention as a possible stressor. Clients interviewed stated that they felt restricted by the monitoring equipment and experienced a feeling of being trapped—that they could not escape.[33] Researchers have also found that noise levels of the ICU and recovery room environment have potential for both sensory overload to the client and as a possible stressor for the staff's own work environment.[8,26] The psychotic-like symptoms exhibited by open heart surgery clients have prompted researchers to analyze the ICU for psychologic hazards.[15] It has been found that approximately 10% to 20% of persons experiencing open heart surgery develop ICU syndrome. This is a form of acute organic brain syndrome that is manifested by decreased intellectual functioning, decreased orientation and memory, agitation, and confusion. It ranges from mild disorientation to psychotic episodes and can last from 2 to 14 days. Generally, the condition resolves with sufficient sleep and a return to a more normal routine.[6]

It has been suggested that critical care areas be designed to promote the client's sense of well-being and to promote appropriate adaptive response. Health care providers should influence decisions regarding architectural details, such as isolating utility areas from client areas, providing adequate privacy for individual clients, and utilizing carpeting and drapes to absorb sound. Interventions can also be initiated by staff to promote client adaptation. Preparing the client for the ICU environment when appropriate (prescheduled surgery, for example), freeing the client from restrictive equipment as soon as possible or placing equipment in such a way to diminish noise levels, limiting conversation to that which is essential, and speaking in a normal tone are all appropriate interventions (see Chapter 75).

The three conditions of eye surgery, immobiliza-

tion, and exposure to the ICU environment are the primary alterations considered in the clinical literature for client predisposition to sensory alteration. However, in considering the experimental literature, we can hypothesize that the research results are also applicable to other clients. This would encompass clients with a sudden alteration in one or more sensory modalities such as clients with acute blindness, neurologic impairments, spinal cord injuries, strokes, cancer,[4] surgical clients who may be experiencing multiple stressors, clients in drug-induced states that alter perception of the environment, and clients experiencing social isolation.

Intervention

There are no clear-cut differences between clinical manifestations of sensory deprivation or overload. The nurse may be in a position where an individual client's unique situation must be assessed and the nurse must utilize professional judgment in making a decision to either increase or decrease sensory inputs as an intervention measure. It may be a trial-and-error approach until the client responds adaptively.

In managing manifestations of sensory alteration, the logical first step in the process is to perform an assessment including both individual and environmental variables, as discussed previously in this chapter. In addition, the nurse would consider the temporal variable. Is it an *acute* manifestation or is it indicative of a *chronic* condition, such as social restrictions that can occur with institutionalization?

Consider the following clinical example: M.H. is an 84-year-old woman recovering from abdominal surgery, which was performed yesterday. She is in a private room. Although she was alert on admission, the staff has noted that since surgery she has become disoriented—she does not recognize her visitors and calls staff by her granddaughter's name. She appears confused and has been combative with staff when they approach to check her dressing. She has pulled out both her intravenous line and her Foley catheter. She is complaining of pain and is presently receiving medication for both pain and sedation. Restraints have been applied.

In assessing M.H. the following data were gathered:

1. This is her first hospital admission. She is unfamiliar with this environment and was not prepared for hospitalization because of the emergency nature of her illness. She requires glasses to visualize the environment clearly and has diminished hearing.

2. This client, whose sensory input is generally altered because of the aging process, has suddenly been placed in a strange environment where familiar orienting clues are not available. Sensory inputs have been

further altered by the presence of pain, sedatives and pain medication, immobility as a result of restraints, and the physiologic stressors of illness. The problem has been further compounded by her being placed in a private room where social contacts are minimal.

3. The sudden manifestation of the behavior plus the supporting assessment data are indicative of an acute reaction to sensory alteration. This can occur after exposure to a restricted environment and generally occurs more frequently with an older client, although it can occur regardless of age or diagnostic factors.

4. This condition can clear spontaneously or, in the specific situation of M.H., nursing intervention can be initiated by staff, such as increasing sensory inputs in the form of environmental stimulations—night light, a radio, increased social contacts with family members and staff, and frequent orientation to reality.

Specific client problems

Perceptual disturbances

Clients experiencing hallucinations or perceptual disturbances are often frightened and anxious, even when the client has an awareness that the experience is not based in reality. The nurse should not indulge or appease the client in an attempt to allay anxiety. A more useful intervention is to encourage the client to describe the experience and to allow opportunities to ventilate feelings. It may also be helpful to the client for the nurse to clarify possible environmental stimuli that were misinterpreted, such as an intercom message, and for the nurse to remain in the room with the client to provide reassurance.

Delusional thinking

Clients may articulate beliefs that are contrary to reality, such as that the staff is persecuting or mistreating them. This generally is an episodic occurrence that passes when the client becomes reoriented. The client should not be ridiculed, dismissed, or strongly confronted when such beliefs are expressed. Instead, it would be more helpful to allow the client to verbalize thoughts and, when appropriate, be presented with the nurse's perception of the facts.

Confused, combative clients

When the client's behavior indicates confusion or combativeness, attempts should be made to reorient the client repeatedly to time, place, and person. Explanations should also be provided regarding identification of staff, tasks to be performed, and environmental stimuli to which the client is exposed. If the client is combative and requires restraints, the rationale for the restraints should be given and reassurance provided that the client is not being punished. Restraints that allow the most freedom in movement (body vs. limb restraints) should be utilized, and safety measures should be taken regarding careful supervision and protection of the client. *Restraints should not be utilized indiscriminately, but only when the client's condition absolutely necessitates it.*

Decreased sensory inputs

As stated throughout this chapter, nurses have many options at their disposal to increase sensory inputs when conditions necessitate such interventions. In summary, the nurse can intervene with both individual and environmental variables. Visual inputs can be increased through the utilization of mobiles, pictures, greeting cards, flowers, color, or something as simple as providing the client with glasses to see the environment clearly. Auditory inputs can be increased through the use of radio, TV, and increased verbal interaction with staff, family, or other clients. Tactile stimulation can be provided by administering back rubs or allowing the client to explore objects in the environment through the sense of touch. Social contacts can be initiated through group activities. Group sessions with the chronically ill have been described as one way to increase social interactions.[31] Also, utilizing natural meeting places in the hospital environment for staff and patients, such as a solarium or day room, appears to increase social stimulation and client satisfaction. Clarifying and providing meaning to the environment through the use of calendars, clocks, and other measures to provide reality orientation are additional sources of increasing sensory inputs.

Increased sensory inputs

If inputs are above the client's range of tolerance, the nurse can intervene to reduce the amount and intensity of stimuli by reducing noise, light, or social contacts. The pattern of stimuli may also require a change. It appears that this is most problematic in critical care areas where the client's condition often necessitates constant monitoring.

REFERENCES AND SELECTED READINGS
Contemporary

1. Bellak, L.: Overload, New York, 1975, Human Sciences Press.
2. *Chodil, J., and Williams, B.: The concept of sensory deprivation, Nurs. Clin. North Am. 5:453-459, 1970.
3. *Cullinan, J.: Quality of life is the challenge—not quantity, Nurs. Times 76:1604-1605, Sept. 11, 1980.
4. Daw, N.W., and Ariel, M.: Properties of monocular and directional deprivation, J. Neurophysiol. 44:280-293, 1980.
5. *Downs, F.: Bed rest and sensory deprivation, Am. J. Nurs. 74:434-438, 1974.

*References preceded by an asterisk are particularly well suited for student reading.

6. *Eisendrath, S.J.: ICU syndromes: their detection, prevention and treatment, Crit. Care Update **7:**5-8, 1980.

7. *Ellis, R.: Sensory and thought disturbances after cardiac surgery, Am. J. Nurs. **72:**2021-2025, 1972.

8. *Falk, S.A., and Woods, N.F.: Hospital noise: levels of potential health hazards, N. Engl. J. Med. **289:**274-281, 1973.

9. Freeman, R.D., and Bradley, A.: Monocularly deprived humans: nondeprived eye has supernormal Vernier acuity, J. Neurophysiol. **43:**1645-1653, 1980.

10. Goldberg, H.: Hearing impairment: a family crisis, Soc. Work Health Care **5:**33-40, Fall 1979.

11. *Haslam, P.: Noise in hospitals: its effect on the patient, Nurs. Clin. North Am. **5:**715-724, 1970.

12. *Hearth, K.: Beyond the curtain of silence, Am. J. Nurs. **74:**1060-1061, 1974.

13. Heppen, C.J., and Petersen, S.B.: Visual impairment: facing possible blindness, Soc. Work Health Care **5:**41-49, 1979.

14. *Jackson, C.W., and Ellis, R.: Sensory deprivation as a field of study, Nurs. Res. **20:**49, 1971.

15. Kaplan, B.E., and Hurley, F.L.: Head and neck cancer: a threat to life and social functioning, Soc. Work Health Care **5:**51-58, Fall 1979.

16. Lipowski, Z.J.: Sensory overloads, information overloads and behavior, Comp. Psychiatry **16:**199-220, 1975.

17. Mitchell, P.H.: Concepts basic to nursing, ed. 3, New York, 1981, McGraw-Hill Book Co.

18. *Perron, D.: Deprived of sound, Am. J. Nurs. **74:**1057-1059, 1974.

19. Rogers, M.: An introduction to the theoretical basis of nursing, Philadelphia, 1970, F.A. Davis Co.

20. Roy, C.: Introduction to nursing: an adaptation model, Englewood Cliffs, N.J., 1975, Prentice-Hall, Inc.

21. Sackett, G.: Innate mechanisms, rearing condition, and a theory of early experience effects in primates. In Jones, M.: Miami Symposium on the Prediction of Behavior, Coral Gables, Fla., 1970, University of Miami Press.

22. Suedfeld, P.: The benefits of boredom: sensory deprivation reconsidered, Am. Sci. **63:**60-69, 1975.

23. *Thompson, L.R.: Sensory deprivation: a personal experience, Am. J. Nurs. **73:**266-268, 1973.

24. Tolpin, M.: On the beginnings of a cohesive self, Psychoanal. Study Child **26:**316-352, 1971.

25. White, B.L.: Human infants: experience and psychological development, Englewood Cliffs, N.J., 1971, Prentice Hall, Inc.

26. *Woods, N.F., and Falk, S.A.: Noise stimuli in the acute care area, Nurs. Res. **23:**144-150, 1974.

Classic

27. Berrien, K.F.: General and social systems, New Brunswick, N.J., 1968, Rutgers University Press.

28. Brownfield, C.A.: Isolation: clinical and experimental approaches, New York, 1965, Random House, Inc.

29. Cannon, W.: The wisdom of the body, New York, 1932, W.W. Norton & Co., Inc.

30. *Carlson, S.: Selected sensory input and life satisfaction of immobilized geriatric female patients. In ANA clinical sessions, New York, 1968, Appleton-Century-Crofts, Inc.

31. Cockburn, K.: Sensory stimulation in the nursing care of chronic schizophrenic patients. In ANA regional clinical conference, New York, 1967, Appleton-Century Crofts, Inc.

32. Cohen, S.: Contact deprivation in infants, Psychosomatics **7:**85-88, 1966.

33. DeMeyer, J.: The environment of the intensive care unit, Nurs. Forum **6:**262-272, 1967.

34. Goldfarb, W.: Emotional and intellectual consequences of psychological deprivation in infancy: a reevaluation: psychopathology of childhood. In Proceedings of The American Psychopathological Association, New York, 1955, Grune & Stratton, Inc.

35. Jackson, C.W.: Clinical sensory deprivation: a review of hospitalized eye-surgery patients. In Zubek, J.P.: Sensory deprivation: 15 years of research, New York, 1969, Appleton-Century-Crofts, Inc.

36. Jackson, C.W., and O'Neil, M.: Experiences associated with sensory deprivation reported for patients having eye surgery. In Jeffries, J.E., editor: Disturbances in sensory input in nursing practice and research, Columbus, Ohio, 1966, Ross Laboratories.

37. *Kornfeld, D., Maxwell, T., and Momrow, D.: Psychological hazards of the intensive care unit, Nurs. Clin. North Am. **3:**41-51, 1968.

38. Kornfeld, D., Zimberg, S., and Malm, J.: Psychiatric complications of open-heart surgery, N. Engl. J. Med. **273:**287-292, 1965.

39. Leiderman, H., et al.: Sensory deprivation: clinical aspects, Arch. Med. **101:**389-396, 1958.

40. Lindsley, D.: Common factors in sensory deprivation, sensory distortion and sensory overload. In Somomon, P., et al.: Sensory deprivations, Cambridge, Mass., 1961, Harvard University Press.

41. Riesen, A.: Excessive arousal effects of stimulation after early sensory deprivation. In Solomon, P., et al.: Sensory deprivation, Cambridge, Mass., 1961, Harvard University Press.

42. Shultz, D.: Sensory restriction, New York, 1965, Academic Press, Inc.

43. Solomon, P., et al.: Sensory deprivation, Cambridge, Mass., 1958, Harvard University Press.

44. Spitz, R.: Hospitalism: an inquiry into the genesis of psychiatric conditions in early childhood, Psychoanal. Study Child **1:**53-74, 1945.

45. Thompson, W.R., and Schaefer, T.: Early environmental stimulation. In Fiske, D.W., and Maddi, S.R., editors: Functions of varied experience, Stonewood, Ill., 1961, Dorsey Press.

46. Vernon, J., et al.: The effect of human isolation upon some perceptual and motor skills. In Solomon, P., et al.: Sensory deprivations, Cambridge, Mass., 1961, Harvard University Press.

47. White, B.L.: An experimental approach to the effects of experience in early human behavior, Minn. Symp. Child Psychol. **1:**201-226, 1967.

48. Winnicott, D.W.: The maturational processes and the facilitating environment, New York, 1965, International Universities Press, Inc.

49. Ziskind, E.: A second look at sensory deprivation, J. Nerv. Ment. Dis. **64:**223-230, 1964.

50. Ziskind, E., et al.: Observations on mental symptoms in eye patched patients: hypnogogic symptoms in sensory deprivation, Am. J. Psychiatry **116:**893-900, 1960.

51. Zubek, J., editor: Sensory deprivation: 15 years of research, New York, 1696, Appleton-Century-Crofts, Inc.

52. Zubek, J.P., Sansom, W., and Prysiaznuik, A.: Intellectual changes during prolonged perceptual isolation, Can. J. Psychol. **14:**233-243, 1960.

CHAPTER 27

ALTERED LEVELS OF CONSCIOUSNESS

JUANITA LEE LONG

Caring for a client with an altered consciousness is one of the most demanding situations in nursing practice. Any alteration in consciousness decreases the reliability of information received from the patient and increases the potential that the patient will need assistive care. The unconscious patient is totally dependent on the skill and good judgment of the nurse. There is no way to get subjective cues from the unconscious patient, so all care is based on continuing assessment of objective data and the conclusions that can be drawn from that data. It is the purpose of this chapter to explore altered states of consciousness, their causes, assessment, and care.

Definitions of levels of consciousness

Consciousness is an ongoing process of awareness of the self and the environment and the mental ability to evoke feelings and provide meaning to that awareness based on previous experiences. One can only infer awareness in others by observed behaviors. There may, however, be occasions when full consciousness is present without the caretaker being able to verify it, as in the case of a patient with severe polyneuritis. Such a patient may be able to see, hear, and think yet seem unaware because of lack of motor ability to indicate that awareness.

One should distinguish between the level of consciousness (LOC) and the content of consciousness. Plum and Posner[36] refer to the two aspects of consciousness as *arousal* and *content*. Arousal is a physiologic function associated with wakefulness. One level of arousal is a simple response to environmental stimuli, such as withdrawal from a painful stimulus. Another level is based

on reflective conscious awareness, for example, avoiding contact with a hot stove. Content is the sum of all cognitive and affective functions. When the content is disturbed, the person is said to be *confused*. The problems of caring for the patient experiencing confusion will be discussed later in the chapter, apart from the problems of altered LOC. Use of word *level* implies a graded phenomenon, a continuum from greatest to least awareness.

The *conscious* person is able to respond to sensory stimuli, has subjective experiences, exercises will, and is capable of thought and reasoning. Consciousness may also be defined as self-awareness, being able to function mentally and physically in a manner appropriate to the level of one's normal ability and to experience life to the fullest degree. All body activities are controlled and coordinated by the nervous system. The cerebrum plays the central role in the higher functions. Rather than experiencing sensory inputs individually and discretely, they are integrated into a single consciousness, a perception; for example, one can identify items by touch that one has seen but not touched before.[10] Guyton[24] proposes that each instant of awareness can be defined as a thought, and the awareness itself as consciousness.

In contrast, to be *unconscious* implies that there is no response to sensory stimuli—no thinking and no feelings or emotions. The conscious person is aware of what is going on in the environment. To differentiate between these two ends of the continuum are many levels of awareness and mental ability not so easily defined or precisely described.

While it is not known precisely what the neural mechanisms are that make awareness possible, it is known that many different parts of the nervous system work together to determine the nature of one's awareness. To date, knowledge of brain mechanisms is insufficient to explain the functioning of the mind as we experience it. No unified representation of one's environment exists in any single cortical area. Necessary conditions for consciousness, such as perception, memory, and language, depend on cortical functions. The presence of consciousness depends on a normally functioning interplay between certain neurons, the brain, and the reticular activating system (RAS).[25] The RAS, or deep central core of gray matter beginning in the brain stem, extends into the hypothalamus and thalamus either directly or indirectly, transmitting stimuli to the cerebral cortex and influencing arousal or wakefulness (p. 520). Conscious behavior is dependent on an intact functioning cerebrum. The organization of the reticular network is vague; however, it does contain some distinct nuclei with long overlapping fibers and dendrites. Anatomic and physiologic details of brain stem nuclei are not yet fully understood.[36] (For an in-depth review of the anatomy and physiology of the consciousness system, the reader is referred to Plum and Posner.[36]) Impulses from the RAS keep us active and serve as an alerting system. When the effects of an insult impinge on the RAS, the state of consciousness can be altered. As the severity of the insult or dysfunction increases, the client experiences an increasing impairment of responsiveness to events in the internal and external environment. If the dysfunction is great enough, unconsciousness or coma will result. Any impairment, reduction, or absence of consciousness indicates a serious dysfunction of the brain.

Consider a continuum with awareness and consciousness at one extreme and unawareness and coma at the other. Inasmuch as consciousness is a complex expression of the mind, and not just a single function, there will be a wide spectrum of levels of consciousness between the two ends of the continuum: consciousness and coma. To set these levels into neatly defined patterns is impossible. The use of such common terms as "alert," "confused," "obtunded," "stuporous," "light coma," and "deep coma" is likely to lead to misunderstanding on the part of the health team providing care, since there is overlap in behaviors from one term to another.

Since the nomenclature used to describe the various levels of consciousness is vague and ill defined, communication between health care providers is often tentative when labels are used. One therefore avoids the use of labels and clearly states the behavior observed. Clear descriptions of things the patient can do and say will be much more likely to indicate the changing status of the patient and will afford the best opportunity for prompt, high-quality care.

While it is better that one should not use labels, it is still incumbent on the nurse to have an understanding of them in order to have some idea of what is being said when they are encountered. The term *obtunded* implies a reduction in alertness and a decreased interest in the surroundings. *Stupor* has been described as unresponsiveness from which the subject can be aroused only by vigorous and repeated stimuli, whereas *coma* is unarousable responsiveness.[36] Different clinical pictures of coma have been described. The most common one is a sleeplike condition with eyes closed; the closed eyes are not seen in the chronic state. Second is a hypersomnia state very much like normal sleep since patients can be aroused, but they return to sleep immediately. The third state is one in which the individual's eyes are open, but no movement or speech can be elicited.[37]

The chronically brain-damaged comatose patient may have periods when the eyes are open alternating with closed eye periods and may seem to be making some response to environmental stimuli. This is referred to as *vegetative* state.[37] Brain stem function may be intact and respirations remain normal, yet forebrain damage is too extensive to permit any awareness.

The *locked-in* state refers to those persons who may be awake and alert, completely able to think and reason, yet who because of a metabolic or structural disease in the nervous system are unable to realize any motor expression of the cerebral function. Some of these patients have the ability to move their eyes in an up-and-down direction. Most commonly this state is caused by lesions in the brain stem.[5,17,37] There are three categories of events that may do this: (1) supratentorial masses or lesions that secondarily compress or damage both cerebral hemispheres; (2) subtentorial lesions or masses damaging the RAS, which normally activates the cerebral hemispheres; and (3) metabolic disorders that interrupt function of supratentorial and subtentorial brain structures. The tentorium cerebelli is an extension of the dura mater that separates the cerebellum from the occipital lobe of the cerebrum.

Table 27-1 places the commonly utilized terms for altered levels of consciousness into an organizational framework to help provide an understanding of how each level relates to the others. It also describes some of the behaviors often observed for each of the levels cited.

Etiology of altered levels of consciousness

Impaired consciousness may be the result of two general types of pathologic processes: first, conditions that widely and directly depress the function of the cerebral hemispheres, and second, conditions that depress or destroy the brain stem activating mechanisms that lie in or near the central core of the gray matter of the diencephalon, midbrain, and rostral pons.[36]

A single factor, then, is not the cause of an altered LOC.[17,36] Indeed, an altered LOC may be the end result of any one of a number of causes typified by the

TABLE 27-1. Commonly used states of awareness and associated behaviors,

State	Conscious-aware		Semiconscious-semicomatose		Unconscious-comatose	
Level	Alert	Confused	Obtunded, drowsy	Stupor	Light coma	Deep coma
Behaviors	Normal activity Aware; mentally functional	Poor coordination Delirium Hallucinations Restlessness Excitable May be combative Short attention span Inappropriate actions and judgments Decreased awareness Disorientation	Sleepy Very short attention span Can respond appropriately if aroused	Apathetic Slow moving Blank expression Drooping head Staring Aroused only by vigorous stimuli	Not oriented to time, place, or person Aroused only by painful stimuli Response is only to grunt, grimace, or withdraw limb from pain	No response except decerebrate or decorticate reflexes

two types of processes. Following are possible causes of alterations in LOC:

1. Vascular lesions: epidural hematomas; subdural hematomas; subarachnoid hematomas; thrombosis, embolism
2. Pressure: tumors (malignant or benign) that compete for limited space within the cranium; hydrocephalus; brain edema
3. Trauma: contusions of the brain; concussion (this is more likely to cause confusion); ruptured aneurysm
4. Toxins: barbiturates; narcotics; alcohol; anesthetics; gases, malfunctioning kidneys or liver causing excess of usually normal substances
5. Deficits: decreased oxygen as in respiratory diseases or with overexertion; decreased blood flow in arteriosclerotic conditions; fluid and electrolyte imbalance causing reduced amounts of normal substances
6. Infections: bacterial or viral infiltration of the meninges and brain tissue; cerebral edema, very high temperatures
7. Epilepsy: grand mal or petit mal seizures
8. Shock: diabetic; electrical; hematogenic; sunstroke; emotional stress
9. Nonorganic diseases: mental illness

As can be seen, causes for altered levels of consciousness are many, and nursing care will need to be individualized according to the cause and the symptoms manifested. The brain must be protected against serious damage, which would occur through loss of oxygen or glucose needed to meet cerebral metabolic needs.[36] However, the fact that the patient has a decreased ability to think and plan leads to certain general guidelines for nursing care regardless of the cause of the altered LOC.

Pathophysiology

Cerebral function is most commonly affected by lack of oxygen or glucose. The brain is extremely sensitive to hypoxia, and only a few seconds of anoxia can lead to loss of consciousness. The amount of oxygen available to cells of the cerebral cortex depends on adequacy of blood flow, blood oxygen tension, hemoglobin concentration, and serum pH. Delirium usually results with a Po_2 level below 55 mm Hg and coma when the level falls below 25 mm Hg.

Glucose is the major energy source for cerebral metabolism, although other substances may be utilized for a short period of time during periods of decreased glucose availability. Confusion usually results when the blood sugar level is less than 30 mg/100 ml and coma when the level falls below 15 mg/100 ml.

Cerebral cells are also affected by the same conditions that affect cellular metabolism elsewhere in the body. Thus altered levels of consciousness can result from conditions such as fluid and electrolyte imbalances or toxins that interfere with metabolism of cerebral cells.

Intervention for the patient with an altered level of consciousness

Following are general guidelines for caring for the patient with an altered level of consciousness.

1. *Provide for alert and knowledgeable assessment.*

Technology is valuable for monitoring individual aspects of the patient's response. Machinery gives objective data, but nurses make judgments that may be lifesaving. Assessment will vary according to the patient's changing level of consciousness and whether it is an initial or subsequent assessment.

2. *Prevent complications resulting from altered biopsychosocial functioning.* The nurse asks, "Will the patient be safe? What precautions should be taken? Will the patient move frequently enough? Will he eat properly? What will happen if he does not eat, move, etc.?"

3. *Support normal physiologic functioning wherever there is a need.* The nurse thinks beyond the evident, asking such questions as "What will this patient be unable to do because of the deficit in reasoning? What are the routine requests from any rational patient, and which of those requests might this patient be unable to make? Are all essential body functions taking place?"

4. *Support and participate in the medical therapy directed at eliminating the cause of the problem.* This will be dictated by the cause and the prescribed therapy.

Assessment of the patient manifesting decreasing consciousness

When a patient begins manifesting a decreased LOC, an initial baseline of information is gathered against which later assessments may be compared. This baseline includes a measurement of history, vital signs, and LOC. (See Chapter 34 for further information on the neurologic assessment.)

Elicit the *history* from the patient (recognizing that the sensorium is impaired and the data may not be accurate) *and* any other person (family member, friend, another client) with such knowledge. Since changes in the sensorium emanate from so many sources, what the nurse will monitor may be varied according to clues found in the assessment.

Vital signs include blood pressure, temperature, pulse and respiration, as well as a pupil check. The anatomic proximity of brain stem areas controlling consciousness to areas controlling the pupils makes *pupillary changes* a valuable guide to the presence and location of pathological conditions causing coma[15,36] (p. 1884). Also, the size and reaction of the pupils to light provide a reliable indication of the status of the brain stem; for example, impending herniation or brain stem lesions. One should be aware of drugs that confuse the assessment of pupillary reactions. Atropine and scopolamine (in large amounts) result in fully dilated and fixed pupils and may cause confusion and a decreased awareness. Since these

GLASGOW COMA SCALE SCORING*

Eyes open

4—Spontaneously

3—On request

2—To pain stimuli (supraorbital or digital)

1—No opening

Best verbal response

5—Oriented to time, place, person

4—Engages in conversation, confused in content

3—Words spoken but conversation not sustained

2—Groans evoked by pain

1—No response

Best motor response

5—Obeys a command ("Hold out three fingers.")

4—Localizes a painful stimulus

3—Flexes either arm

2—Extends arm to painful stimulus

1—No response

*Adapted from Teasdale, G.: Nurs. Times **71**(24):914-917, 1975.

drugs are often given in cardiac arrest resuscitation attempts, the comatose patient may have fixed pupils after cardiac arrest. If the fixed pupils are caused by anoxia one drop of pilocarpine eye drops will cause an immediate pupillary constriction. Heroin and morphine may result in pinpoint pupils. In an unconscious patient without serious neurologic injury, pupils are in the midposition. If the pupils do not react at the same rate, it is of no concern as long as the pupils are equal in size initially and following their reaction to light.

Another aspect of the assessment is to establish the *level of consciousness*, the best indicator of the function of the entire brain.[15] The ability of the nurse to note changes in the LOC and interpret them could mean the difference between life and death. The nurse is sensitive to where the patient is on the continuum between awareness and coma and knows how long the patient has been at that level, the direction in which change is taking place, and how fast the change is occurring. If the patient is unconscious, the nurse needs to know how long the condition has existed, for the length of unconsciousness and speed of change will give valuable clues to the severity of the problem.

Accuracy is best attained when a systematic approach is used by all persons involved in the continuing assessments. Although some efforts have been made to

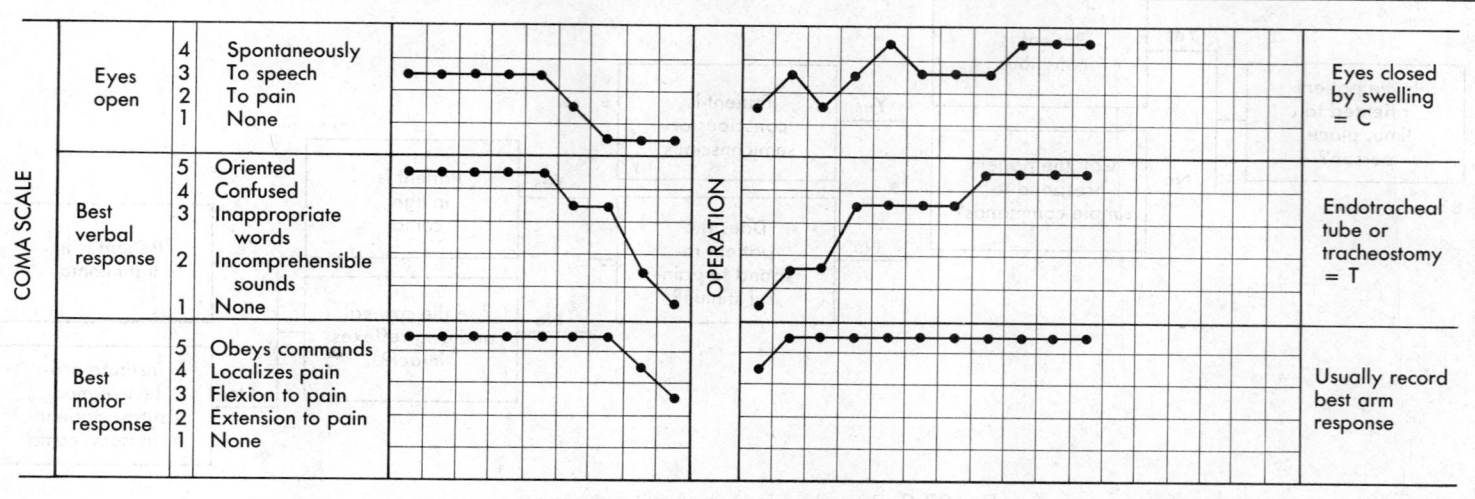

Fig. 27-1. Glasgow Coma Scale.

develop scales to measure LOC, there is a paucity of tools. What is vital is that all persons in a facility consistently use a single technique. The clues or evidence that might lead to the use of a descriptive term are recorded or reported as opposed to the descriptive term itself.

A promising objective measure to describe LOC is the Glasgow Coma Scale (GCS), which has been shown to be reproducible by professional and other health personnel.[4,27,40] The scale is simple, based on the patient's response in three areas: eye opening, motor response, and verbal response. Numbers are assigned to the best performance in each of the three areas (see box, p. 532) and the total score gives a view of the patient's LOC. When a sequence of the numbers for each of the three categories is plotted on a graph over time, a visual picture of the direction of progress evolves (Fig. 27-1). It may show stability, or it may indicate deterioration or improvement in the condition. While the GCS does not take the place of a comprehensive neurologic check, it is extremely useful in conjunction with motor and brain stem assessment in rapidly changing situations to detect deterioration in the patient's status. Scores of seven or less (but not scores of nine or more) represent coma.

When the onset of unconsciousness is *not* immediate, as it is with fainting or extreme shock or trauma, there is usually a consistent pattern of deterioration, although each patient is unique and may depart somewhat from the usual pattern. In the early stages of a deteriorating LOC the changes are so subtle they may not be noted. The behavior may appear to be a normal mood change. For instance, there may be less interest in the surroundings or in events taking place; the client may seem bored or drowsy, inattentive or irritable, and

restless. If these behaviors are noted and if there is any history that could lead one to suspect altered brain function, further exploration is necessary (p. 726).

When checking the LOC, the nurse explains to the patient the content and purpose of the examination. With a small child, verbal assessment is unlikely to be valid; therefore a check of motor ability should be used (p. 734). With the adult patient, however, there is a sequence of questions and examinations to be used in assessing awareness.

Another procedure for assessing level of consciousness is outlined in Fig. 27-2. One begins by determining the patient's orientation by means of several questions regarding time, place, and person. The month and year are more readily recalled than days and dates. One can be satisfied if patients know they are in a hospital even if they cannot recall the name of the institution. Persons can be asked their name and occupation.

Next the person is requested to respond to simple commands such as blinking the eyes or touching the nose or ear with the fingers. Lack of symmetry can be noted by testing both sides of the body. This is important in localizing some lesions. The person can be asked to squeeze your hand with first the right and then the left hand or to lift both feet simultaneously. If the person cannot perform in response to these commands, then proceed to assess the response to pain.

There are several techniques for checking response to pain that do not cause trauma to the patient. Pinching and pricking may damage tissues and are avoided when possible. Other ways to test for pain include use of supraorbital pressure, pressure on the fingertips, and on the trapezius muscle. To perform the supraorbital pain maneuver, put the thumb on the upper edge of the bony groove of the eye socket about one third the

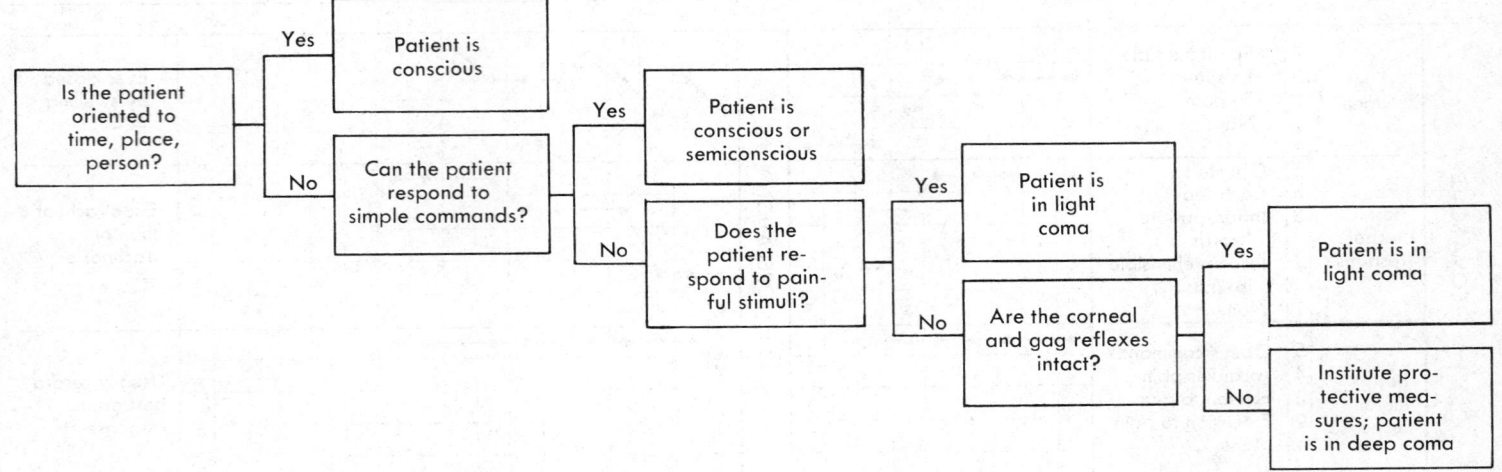

Fig. 27-2. Procedure for assessing level of consciousness.

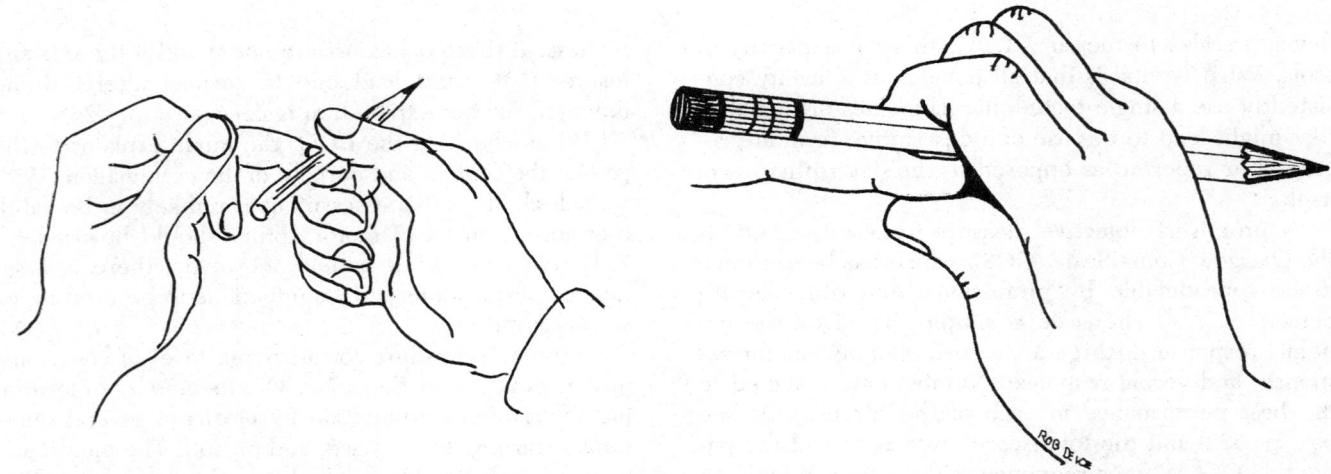

Fig. 27-3. Fingertip pressure stimulation.

distance from the inner aspect of the orbit and press. Probably the best check and the one with the least potential for harm is shown in Fig. 27-3.[36] One can apply pressure to the nail bed using a pencil held between the examiner's thumb and the patient's finger. One can also apply pressure to the trapezius by pinching it between the patient's neck and the shoulder. (Practice on yourself to see how much pressure is necessary.) The response showing the highest level of consciousness is for the patient to withdraw from the stimulus or try to push it away. If the response is by grimaces or by moving or thrashing around but in a nonpurposeful manner, the level of awareness is lower. Finally, with very deep coma there may be no response at all. Regardless of the response, be sure to record the type of stimulus and the response behavior.

If none of the pain stimuli lead to responses, the final check is of reflexes, since they will be the last responses to be lost. To check the corneal reflex, hold the eyelid open and gently stroke the eye with a thin wisp of cotton. A positive reflex is indicated by immediate blinking. Checking the cornea more than once or twice a day is avoided, since the cornea is quite sensitive and may easily be irritated. The gag reflex is checked by touching the posterior of the pharynx with a cotton swab or tongue depressor.

As the status changes, dependency needs become either greater or lesser, based on the direction of change. Assessments may need to be made every 15 minutes—more frequently if the level of consciousness is decreasing or less frequently if the level is maintained over time or is improving. The nurse independently institutes more frequent observations when the patient's status so indicates.

Care of the comatose patient

The nurse who cares for an already unconscious patient is constantly aware of the *patient's total dependency* on others. For the nurse the word *coma* is equated with helplessness. The unconscious patient cannot approve or disapprove of what is being done and cannot participate or select the person providing the care. Aside from involuntary motor activities such as cardiac, respiratory, and gastrointestinal actions, the patient is unresponsive. It then becomes paramount for others to provide for additional life-sustaining requirements including nourishment, elimination, and protection of tissues.

Such a comatose state may lull the nurse into thinking that nothing is taking place in the patient's social world. We can only speculate about receptiveness. Myco and McGilloway[34] propose that *meaningful stimuli can be introduced* into the comatose patient's environment. To do this, the nurse must first learn as much of the patient's life-style as possible: social activities, work, friends, family. Key factors in the patient's former 24-hour routine are then selected, and the care should concur closely with previous habits. As an example, tube feedings should be scheduled about the same time of day as the patient was accustomed to eating, so that stomach distention is closely related to former habits. If the patient worked in a noisy factory, provide sound during the former working hours. Record familiar sounds and play them at appropriate times, for example, table talk when the family has dinner. For the long-term unconscious patient, this approach appears to have merit in keeping the focus of care from becoming too oriented to body functions to the exclusion of social factors.

Since *hearing is probably the last sense to be lost,* the monitoring of what is said in the presence of the unconscious person is vitally important. At present there is no sure device to assess when patients are no longer able to hear; therefore, even when patients appear incapable of receiving messages, they may still understand what is said. Grave prognoses or flippant comments are best kept outside a patient's range of hearing. In fact, positive and hopeful comments made in the patient's presence may give the patient motivation to struggle back to consciousness. Thus the nurse speaks to the patient and explains what is being done as if the patient were fully aware.

The fourth factor to consider is the *therapeutic effect of touch*. The patient is spoken to before being touched and is handled with gentleness. Because there is no pain response to remind care providers when stress is increased, the tendency is to move the unconscious patient without consideration of soft tissue. Touch is one of the first sensations experienced by the human organism, and without proper touch, normal development would not take place.[33] Touch is a medium for communication. Holding and cuddling infants seems to make them more tranquil and content. Research has shown positive results from the use of touch with disoriented and some mentally ill persons. It is highly possible that some of the same positive responses can be elicited in the unconscious patient. Using a firm hand grasp while talking to the patient about the day or the environment, smoothing the hair away from the face with the full palmar surface of the hand, or tucking the bed covers snuggly around the patient may stimulate the feeling of being cared for or encompassed.

A fifth concern relates to the environment. The *environment should be low key*, with loud noises kept to a minimum. Soft music may be beneficial, but unnecessary sounds should be eliminated. The unconscious person with improving awareness often has an overly excitable nervous system response and is unable to attend to multiple stimuli. To facilitate the patient's ability to focus on any stimulus, eliminate all but necessary noises.

Assessment of the comatose patient

The assessment of the patient who is comatose for an extended period of time is similar to the assessment of a patient with a changing level of consciousness but is broader in scope, focusing on needs for health maintenance. Following is a guideline for assessment of the comatose patient:

1. General impressions
   a. Skin
      (1) Color and consistency of color
      (2) Temperature
   b. Olfactory cues
      (1) Odor of breath
      (2) Other odors (e.g., incontinence)
   c. Activity level
      (1) Presence of movement
      (2) Character and symmetry of movement
2. Specific aspects of assessment
   a. Pupillary response
      (1) Size and equality
      (2) Reaction to light
      (3) Consensual movement of eyes
   b. Respiratory status
      (1) Breath sounds
      (2) Excursion of chest, abdomen
      (3) Respiratory rate
   c. Muscular status
      (1) Tonus

(2) Symmetry of paralysis
(3) Posturing—decorticate or decerebrate
   d. Elimination
     (1) Presence of incontinence
     (2) Skin irritation
     (3) Palpation of abdomen for impaction
   e. Cardiovascular status
     (1) Pulse rate
     (2) Rhythm

One begins with a general inspection of the patient's body. *Skin color* and *consistency of color* are noted. A bluish area or swelling may indicate trauma in the comatose patient and be significant in determining the cause of unconsciousness. Redness may indicate beginning skin breakdown.

A significant change from normal *skin temperature* prompts the nurse to take the body temperature. A gradual increase in temperature may indicate that an infection is beginning. Infections may develop in wounds but are equally prone to develop in the urinary tract (especially in the presence of an indwelling catheter) or lungs (because of decreased movement of secretions caused by immobility and the inability to cough voluntarily). Dehydration may cause an elevated temperature. Rarely, the temperature-regulating center in the hypothalamus is disturbed by pressure or trauma, and there will be significant increase or decrease in temperature.

The *olfactory sense* may provide cues. A sweet acidotic breath may indicate hyperglycemia. An objectionable odor may signify the need for better mouth care, signal bleeding gums, or indicate incontinence.

Next note the *activity level*. Watch the patient from a short distance. Is the patient motionless or moving? Are the movements purposeful or jerky and erratic? Convulsive movements may indicate increasing intracranial pressure. Movement on one side and not the other may indicate hemiplegia. Observe fingers, eyelids, and lips for tremors, as these may be a prelude to a seizure. Report any changes to the physician to allow for preventive intervention or further evaluation. General restlessness may indicate increasing cerebral pressure, discomfort from a distended bladder, a tight bandage, or poor positioning. Restlessness may also be a positive sign indicative of an increasing awareness.

Next one determines if the *pupils* are equal in size and reaction. Their size is recorded in millimeters, and the reaction to light is noted for symmetry and speed. Sluggish responses are reported. Findings are compared with the patient's "normal" or predetermined standard. Being unaware that the patient has an artificial eye or pupil that does not respond to light as readily as the other may lead to erroneous inferences. The unconscious patient will usually stare straight ahead without eye movements, but from time to time the eyes will move. When this happens the eyes should move consensually. If there is deviation of either eye from the midline (disconjugate), toward the midline (strabismus), or back and forth oscillation (nystagmus), this is significant to report.

Next one listens to *breath sounds* and observes the *rise and fall of the chest or abdomen*. The pattern and rate of breathing and character of respiration (easy or labored, fast or slow, regular or irregular, deep or shallow) are noted. Many different parts of the brain influence respirations. Trauma to the brain or reactions to drugs and toxins may cause abnormal and inadequate breathing.

Next the *muscle tone* is noted. Are the muscles tight? Flaccid? Each arm and leg is put through passive range of motion, comparing one side to the other side and upper extremities with lower extremities. Changes or asymmetry give clues about the location of the problem and are reported. When the arms are lifted and allowed to fall, the paralyzed arm will fall faster than the unaffected arm. When the patient's heels are placed on the bed and the legs flexed and released, the paralyzed leg will fall outward.

Unusual movements such as decorticate or decerebrate rigidity are observed. *Decorticate* rigidity is characterized by stiff, extended legs, with arms flexed on the chest, and is caused by damage to the pyramidal motor tract above the brain stem. Upper brain stem damage may cause the *decerebrate* position, with all limbs extended and arms hyperpronated. This indicates a grave condition.

Finally, the patient is inspected for *incontinence*. Continued contact of the skin with either feces or urine exposes the patient to skin problems such as rashes or decubitus ulcers and should be avoided stringently. A consistent check will enable quick care to prevent skin breakdown or to plan intervention when there has been no elimination over a period of time. The abdomen is palpated daily to check for fecal buildup and impaction.

Palpation may also be used to check the *pulse* for rate and rhythm. A slow pulse may indicate increasing intracranial pressure or overreaction to medication. The significance of pulse in relation to electrolyte imbalance may be found in Chapter 21.

Intervention for the comatose patient

Intervention begins even as assessment and goal setting are being accomplished. There are two functions of intervention on behalf of the patient experiencing a diminished level of consciousness—maintenance and prevention. As consciousness begins to improve, intervention may include rehabilitative measures also.

Maintenance

While there is often overlap in the maintenance and prevention functions, maintenance may be thought of as that care essential to the support of life. It is often described as those activities carried out when a person is suddenly rendered unconscious, before the body has returned to a state of dynamic equilibrium. An example of maintenance would be to provide sufficient oxygen to maintain life processes. This would require the nurse to clear the air passages, loosen clothing, position the patient in such a way that breathing and circulation are facilitated, and, if necessary, turn the patient on the side to facilitate drainage from the oral cavity. (See Chapter 73 for an in-depth discussion of other emergency measures.) Maintenance intervention for the patient experiencing coma of long duration includes provision of adequate nutrition, promotion of regular elimination, promotion of adequate circulation, and control of body temperature.

Nutrition. When a patient is experiencing rapidly decreasing awareness, nutrition is not a primary concern; however, if the patient becomes comatose and remains so for an extended period of time, nutritional support becomes a major concern. For the first few days of unconsciousness the patient will probably be maintained on intravenous fluids, as prescribed by the physician. Close observation of the needle site for inflammation or infiltration, as well as attention to flow rate to prevent excessive fluid intake, are essential. After 2 or 3 days a nasogastric tube may be inserted into the stomach through which nourishment will be supplied in liquid form (p. 1373). Feedings are usually prescribed every 2 to 3 hours in small amounts to decrease the possibility of regurgitation and aspiration. The tube should be changed every 5 to 7 days unless it becomes clogged sooner, but the naris through which the tube is placed should be cleaned daily with warm water and lubricated with a water soluble lubricant to decrease the formation of crusts.

The presence of a tube in the nostril is irritating and may cause tissue damage, so if coma lasts for an extended period of time, there may be a need for a gastrostomy tube to provide a means for feeding. The gastrostomy tube is inserted through the abdominal wall into the stomach. A catheter with an inflatable tip (to prevent the tube from slipping out of the stomach) is then sutured in place. This tube remains clamped or plugged except during feedings, and the area around the tube is cleaned daily and covered with a dry dressing (p. 1396).

Elimination. Measures must be taken to assist in elimination and maintain the tone of the bowel muscles. Without intervention, the tendency is for the comatose patient to become constipated and possibly impacted. Routinely palpate the abdomen to determine when a fecal mass is present. This palpation may also serve to stimulate peristalsis and induce a bowel movement. If possible, determine the patient's normal elimination schedule and place the patient on a bedpan at that hour. If a suppository is needed, administer it about 30 minutes before the regular elimination schedule.

Bisacodyl (Dulcolax) is an effective suppository to use for bowel training. When laxatives are needed, a mild one such of milk of magnesia is often used and can be administered via the nasogastric tube.

Sometimes it becomes necessary to give a cleansing enema. Usual techniques for administering an enema are used; however, it may be necessary to hold the patient's buttocks together to prevent expulsion of the solution before the enema is ready to be expelled. The enema may also be administered through a Foley catheter placed in the rectum. The balloon is inflated before the fluid is introduced, thus preventing the expulsion of the fluid until the desired amount has been administered. The balloon is deflated (before removing the catheter) to allow expulsion of the enema. When placing the patient on the bedpan, care is taken to align the body correctly and to protect the skin. Gentle massage of the abdomen along the path of the transverse and descending colon will assist in the expulsion of the fecal mass. Stool softeners such as dioctyl sodium sulfosuccinate (Colace) administered via the nasogastric tube will also help facilitate elimination. Assuring an adequate liquid intake helps keep the fecal mass soft, and juices that have a laxative effect, such as prune juice, may be included in the diet. In the event that an impaction does occur, a retention enema is administered. If this is unsuccessful, the impaction may require manual removal; that is, using a gloved, lubricated finger to remove small pieces of the fecal material until the mass is eliminated.

The need for communication between health care providers is especially great with reference to bowel function. Only when bowel movements are carefully recorded as to time, amount, and consistency can the nurse make competent judgments about laxatives and enemas.

Circulation. Circulation can be assisted in several ways. Conscientiously turning the patient from side to side at least every 2 hours will enhance circulation, for muscle movement stimulates circulation. Careful attention to positioning so that there are no constricted areas, as would be caused by twisted clothing, tight bedclothes, or a misplaced limb, will allow for maximum circulation. Joints bent at sharp angles slow circulation and should be avoided. Passive range-of-motion exercises planned into the nursing care regimen at least every 8 hours will increase blood flow. Padding of dependent bony prominences when they are being laid upon decreases pressure and helps to maintain good circulation. Back massage with application of increasing pressures toward the level of the heart and decreasing pressure away from the heart is thought to increase circulation to the skin. A commonly overlooked area is the ear. If it is folded over, circulation to the outer area is occluded and tissue necrosis occurs quickly. Always check the lower ear after turning the patient. Frequent monitoring of infusions to prevent overloading the circulatory system will also enhance good circulation. The use of elastic stockings or wraps from toe to thigh on the lower extremities decreases the potential for stasis. These should be removed every 8 hours and the skin observed. They can be replaced after 30 minutes. When putting them on, raise the leg above the heart level to assist in having the volume of blood as near normal as possible before putting on the wrap.

Temperature. A normal body temperature is generally considered to range from 36° C (97° F) to 37.2° C (99° F). Since the comatose patient is unable to express being too cold or too warm, it becomes the nurse's responsibility to monitor the body temperature at least every 4 hours and more frequently if a problem arises. If the heat center in the hypothalamus is disturbed, as it often is by trauma or by certain medical problems, the temperature may change rapidly. When the temperature is excessively elevated, it is called *hyperthermia*. An elevated temperature may also be indicative of an infection or dehydration. When a patient is experiencing hyperthermia, the nurse can assist in maintaining the temperature within a normal range by removal of bedclothes and lowering the room temperature. If necessary, remove all of the patient's clothes except enough to protect modesty and the family's sense of propriety. Antipyretics may be given via the nasogastric or gastrostomy tube or by suppository. Ice bags covered with protective wraps to prevent tissue damage may be placed on the groin and axilla where there is a large blood supply. This helps to hasten body cooling. Sponging the body with a water and alcohol solution causes evaporation and subsequent cooling. The use of a fan to blow over the patient while the patient is being sponged further enhances cooling. Electrically controlled hypothermia blankets are now available and are often used to reduce fever when a patient suffers from hyperthermia. The patient should not be allowed to get chilled and shiver, since shivering increases body metabolism and produces heat, thus raising the temperature. Continued hyperthermia will result in brain damage and ultimately death, so the temperature is kept as near normal as possible. On the other end of the continuum, a subnormal temperature (hypothermia) may be experienced. Additional clothing and covers and increased room temperature will help. Warmed blankets may help to elevate temperature in the hypothermic patient.

Prevention

Preventive interventions include safety measures and those actions aimed at avoiding damage to the eyes, ears, nose, mouth, and hair, as well as to the musculoskeletal, gastrointestinal, integumentary, urinary, and cardiovascular systems.

Safety. Numerous activities of the nurse are geared toward providing a safe environment for the comatose patient experiencing a changing level of consciousness. Side rails are kept up at all times for the unconscious patient unless the nurse is present. When the patient is restless and likely to be thrashing about, the railing should be padded. Equipment is placed far enough from the bed that a confused patient would be unlikely to interfere in its operation. Any prosthetic device such as false teeth, an artificial eye, or contact lenses should be removed and carefully stored in a safe place until the patient is lucid enough to use them appropriately. Restraint should be avoided unless the patient is agitated enough to do harm. When any type of restraint is used, caution should be taken that it is put on properly and is not too tight. Periodic checks should be made for tissue damage.

Musculoskeletal positioning. To protect musculoskeletal integrity, there are numerous possible interventions and aids. Perhaps the most crucial is positioning. Improper positioning can lead to contractures, foot drop, wrist drop, and other deformities (p. 948). The preferred position of the comatose patient is in the *side-lying position*.

The comatose patient is at risk of pulmonary complications. Therefore frequent changes of position are essential. Turning the patient from side-to-side at frequent intervals prevents pooling of pulmonary secretions. In some instances, tracheal suctioning may be necessitated by the patient's inability to cough. Unless neurologic complications contraindicate it, postural drainage may be initiated.

Patients who are comatose may be placed in a prone or supine position; however, care must be taken to ensure a patent airway. The reader is referred to a text on fundamentals of nursing for information about turning and positioning patients.

Exercise. Passive range-of-motion exercise is done a minimum of twice daily and ideally several times a day (p. 924). One way to accomplish this is to put the upper side through complete range-of-motion each time the patient is turned. Doing it systematically helps assure that it is not postponed and subsequently overlooked. This too will increase circulation and decrease the likelihood of thrombi.

When the physical condition is stable enough and consciousness returns, the patient should sit in a chair at least once and preferably twice a day. The upright posture fosters weight-bearing on the long bones, thus limiting calcium loss, and enhances pulmonary expansion, circulation, and digestive motility. Unless the patient is small enough for two people to manage, use a mechanical lift. Position the patient so that he or she is seated squarely on the buttocks with the spine straight and feet flat on the floor or footrest. Support the arms and head with pillows. Use a chest harness support tied behind the chair or secure the patient's torso by wrapping a sheet around the torso and the chair.

Skin care. The integument of the comatose patient is prone to many assaults: being pulled across bed linens, lying too long on bony prominences, dryness or moisture, and increased bacteria from incontinence of urine and feces. A warm water bath daily is recommended. While tub baths are not always feasible, the patient can be placed in a tub or shower when consciousness returns if there are an adequate number of people present to prevent injury. Until such time, a daily bed bath should include a brisk rub (except when the skin is fragile) with sparing use of soap and a thorough rinse. Soap residue causes dryness and skin irritation, and moisture increases the potential for skin breakdown.

To prevent dryness, place a lotion (such as Alpha-Keri oil or Jeri-Bath) in the bath water. If this is not sufficient, rub the body with a lanolin preparation or other cream. The family may suggest a lotion the patient has used routinely.

The skin of the feet is especially prone to drying, and the nails harden with decreased circulation. Rub the feet daily with a lubricant such as Vaseline. Never use alcohol unless specially indicated, for it makes the skin extremely dry. Comatose patients perspire just as alert patients do. If talcum powder is used, it tends to hold this perspiration. Since moist skin is more prone to necrosis, avoid using talcum.

Linens are kept dry and crumb free. Keep them pulled taut so there will be no wrinkles underneath the patient that might cause decubitus ulcers. Protect the patient's skin from the shearing effect of sliding on the sheets by positioning the head of the bed at not more than a 10 degree angle so that the patient will not constantly be sliding down in bed. Additional ways to prevent decubitus ulcers include the use of lamb's wool under pressure areas. A water or air mattress to equalize pressure can be used, although if the patient is turned carefully, this is not needed. Be sure never to use a doughnut or rubber ring, as it simply causes a circle of pressure and cuts down on the blood supply to the area within that circle, making skin breakdown more likely.

Incontinence. A condom catheter connected to a urinary elimination bag may be placed on the male patient. The condom is unrolled on the penis and secured by an elasticized piece of tape around the penis. Care should be taken that the tape is not placed on the skin, but on the condom, and is wrapped around the penis snuggly enough to prevent the condom from slipping, but not so tight as to interfere with circulation. Tactile stimulation may cause a temporary engorgement of the penis. When the size of the penis diminishes, the condom may slip off unless it has been securely wrapped. The condom is removed and the penis cleansed with soap and water daily.

An indwelling catheter with closed drainage may be needed for the female patient. While the catheter remains in, continual observation for signs of infection, chills, or fever is required. Accurately monitor intake in relation to output. Irrigation of the bladder through an indwelling catheter increases the possibility of introducing organisms; therefore irrigate only when absolutely necessary. When irrigation must be done, observe scrupulous sterile technique. Infections from prolonged use of an indwelling catheter cause the urine to become alkaline. This, in turn, causes inorganic materials such as phosphorus and calcium to settle out, and as a result, bladder stones may form. A fluid intake of at least 3000 ml/day will keep the urine dilute enough to lessen the risk of bladder stones.

The catheter should be changed before mineral deposits plug the lumen or tip of the catheter. If no manufacturer's information is available regarding how frequently the catheter must be changed, a safe estimate is every 10 days.

Hair. Shampoos are indicated every 1 or 2 weeks, unless contraindicated by the patient's underlying problems, for the scalp of the comatose patient continues to secrete oils and perspiration; the hair becomes sour-smelling and difficult to manage when not properly cleansed. Comb hair daily, and braid or arrange long hair to prevent matting. Take care that there are no lumps of hair on the part of the head where the patient lies.

Hair care for black persons differs from that recommended for white persons. For the black person, cleansing the hair with a warm solution of one part alcohol with four parts of mineral oil is followed by an application of warm olive oil, baby oil, or Vaseline oil to the scalp and hair.[23] Excess oil may be removed with a towel. Long hair can be braided; very short hair can be left loose after combing. Afro combs make combing less uncomfortable.

Hair care is important to the patient's sense of well-being and comforting for the family because a well-groomed patient conveys that he or she is "cared about" as well as "cared for."

Mouth and teeth. The unconscious patient is often a mouth breather and therefore has a dry mouth. Regardless of how he or she breathes, the patient experiencing a decreased level of consciousness will require mouth care. When not cleansed, the mouth becomes inflamed and prone to other infections. Mucus and bacteria form plaque. Plaque, tartar, and food debris collect in gingival crevices around the teeth and cause mechanical and bacterial irritation. The tissue becomes swollen and inflamed. In time, gingival tissue will separate from the teeth and form pockets where still more debris can accumulate.[38] Teeth may be lost and bone may become involved. Elderly persons have thinner oral membranes and less flow of salivary juices to help wash the mouth, so their problem is compounded. Refer to Chapter 56 for oral care guidelines.

Nose. The nares are cleansed daily to help keep them patent. Inspect for secretions and note the type. If crusts are forming, gently remove with a moist applicator unless the patient's condition contraindicates. A thin application of a water-soluble lubricant helps decrease accumulation of debris. This is especially important when a nasogastric tube is in place, for it causes some trauma to the tissues, and inflammation may ensue if the naris is not kept cleaned.

Ears. The folds of the ears are cleansed and dried carefully. The area behind the ear is easily over-looked when drying, but is prone to skin irritation when soap or moisture is not removed. Check the ears for wax while bathing the patient. Over a period of time large amounts of wax may accumulate, but are easily removed with a small wire loop. When head trauma is the basis of coma, be very cautious about introducing anything into the ear until it has been ascertained that there is no damage within the ear.

Eyes. When a person becomes unconscious, one of the first interventions is to remove contact lenses (p. 864). When properly done, there is little likelihood of causing damage. The cornea receives its oxygen supply primarily through exchange of gases in the atmosphere. When eyes are closed during sleep, the metabolic rate of the cornea goes down and the oxygen supply from the blood system is adequate to maintain health. When contact lenses are worn, however, the metabolic rate of the cornea increases. If the eyes are closed for a long time with the contact lenses in place, the cornea cannot remain healthy. The damage will be directly related to the time the lenses have been in place and the extent of interference with metabolic rate of the tissue.[21] The contact lenses, having been removed, should be stored either in saline solution or distilled water, keeping the right and left lens separated and labeled.

Since the eyes are very precious and cannot be replaced, special caution should always be given to prevent any damage occurring to them. Pull the lid back and check the eyes several times a day. Make sure they do not become dried out. Cleanse them with clear water or one of the commercial lubricants. Keep the eyelids closed. If there is any problem with keeping the eyelid closed, shield the eye to prevent irritation from scratching or from dryness.

Support of significant others

The unconscious patient has no awareness of the severity of the situation, but the alert family does. This awareness creates great anxiety and stress. During the initial phase of injury or onset of disease when consciousness is being affected, the family has many decisions to make about the patient's care. If the outcome of those decisions is not positive, family members may feel guilty for having made those decisions. Addition-

ally, they will experience feelings of loss and grief. As time passes, the family members remain in limbo, unable to complete the grieving process, yet equally unable to sustain the high pitch of grief initially experienced. Guilt feelings may be expressed in anger and hostility toward those who are providing care.[30] It is difficult for family members to understand what is going on, and it is very frightening to stand by feeling inadequate and unable to help. The family then becomes part of the responsibility of the nurse. From the beginning, they need special understanding and special consideration. For them the patient's condition may precipitate a crisis. They can be helped to cope by becoming involved in the patient's care.

A good way of involving the family in the care of the patient is by asking for help with positioning the patient. They are usually quite capable of doing an excellent job of monitoring and maintaining position and are often with the patient extended periods of time when the nurse cannot be. The involvement not only ensures more consistent care for the patient, but it is very beneficial to the family, giving them a sense of accomplishment and purpose. The hours of waiting are lessened for significant others when they feel they are needed and involved. For this reason, carefully explain what is to be done and the principles underlying the actions; then allow them to help you, not only with positioning but in other aspects of care as they desire. The value of their contributions is acknowledged.

Family members often will wish to stay at the bedside. If they do, share with them that their talking is providing sensory stimulation to the patient. The assumption is made that some of this talking may be filtering through to the awareness of the patient even though the patient is unable to respond to it.

The nurse conveys to the family a willingness to listen, to be involved, and to help them explore their thoughts. Keeping the family informed of what is being done, what is planned, and the changing condition is very crucial. Provide the family with a comfortable environment. An expression of a willingness to help is frequently all that is required.

When a patient begins to recover, the first response often is to a familiar voice or face, and this may be in the form of a verbal comment. The patient will need the security of knowing that family, friends, and staff are concerned and will need much support and encouragement, as well as explanation.

Outcome criteria for the person who has been comatose

The person will:
1. Demonstrate no further signs of brain damage attributable to lack of oxygen or glucose.
2. Exhibit minimal loss of body weight.

3. Be free of fecal impaction, urinary tract infection, decubitus ulcers, thrombi, effects of pulmonary infiltrates, corneal abrasions, hyperthermia, joint contractures, and oral and dental problems resulting from inability to provide self-care.
4. Be free of bodily injury from falls or other accidents.

Confused or disoriented patient

When one has a disturbed consciousness, rather than a decrease in the level of consciousness, one is said to be experiencing a confused or disoriented state. It is the *content* of consciousness that is altered. The disoriented person may experience hallucinations or have illusions or delusions. With *disorientation* the patient is awake, but perceives phenomena incorrectly. Thinking and reasoning are inappropriate, and remembering is difficult.

A *hallucination* is an impression on any of the senses in the absence of a stimulus. The patient believes he or she sees, hears, tastes, feels, or smells something, but the source of this occurrence is within the patient's thinking rather than in reality. Confusion and hallucinations may be caused by injury, drugs, psychologic problems, or organic problems. Organic causes may be acute infections with high fever, drug toxicity from alcohol or psychedelic drugs, withdrawal from drugs, brain tumors, senility, or exhaustion.

It is well to consider the causes of confusion in the *elderly* apart from the other confused states. It is probable that much of the confusion of the elderly may be the result not of insult, but of normal physiologic aging of tissues and organs. In the aged person the lungs do not expand as well as in the younger person, thereby decreasing the ability to cough and deep breathe. Cardiovascular changes in the myocardium of the older person prohibit the heart from responding quickly to stress with a resulting decrease in blood flow throughout the body. This decreased oxygen supply to the brain tissue may bring about a lowering in sensory perception, making contact with reality more difficult. A new environment such as a hospital or nursing home increases the likelihood of misperceptions. This is especially true in the elderly. When drugs that are eliminated through the kidney are given to the elderly, unless there are fully functioning nephrons, there may be accumulations of the drug. In increased amounts, many drugs have the capacity to cause confusion. The nurse is advised to be aware of the changed physiology in older persons and mediate the care given accordingly. Disorientation in the elderly commonly manifests itself during the evening and night hours.

An *illusion* is a sensory experience based on fact, but misinterpreted. This may happen when one of the senses is faulty or when environmental conditions prohibit a true interpretation of what is sensed. For example, the older person who has failing vision may think there is someone present in the room when a shadow moves.

Assessment and intervention

The care of the *confused* patient begins with a thorough assessment to determine the cause and needs. There may be some metabolic imbalance or deficit in circulation or respiration, or the client may be experiencing pain. Try to determine if the patient has been eating and eliminating. The patient's reply to such inquiries may not be reliable if confusion is present, hence it is extremely important for all staff to be accurate in recording all objective data. Check on other possibilities: Is the client positioned in poor body alignment? Is there an elevated temperature? Is the client experiencing an overload or deficit that might create a confused state? When causes are found, one makes adjustments, trying to eliminate the cause.

Establish communication with the patient. A good way to get the patient's attention is through touch. Once the contact is made, use a calm, quiet, unhurried voice. To keep the patient oriented, explain in advance what you will do. Include the patient in planning and discussions. See that the room is well lighted. Keep a calendar in view. Introduce yourself each time you care for the patient. Talk slowly and distinctly and use short statements. Face the patient and stay within a conversational distance of 4 ft. When speaking to the patient, eliminate extra stimuli such as the radio and television, which would tend to clutter the sensory field and might prevent a clear communication between the nurse and patient. When it is possible, provide consistency by having the same staff members care for the patient every day. It is advisable to keep decision making at a minimum for the confused person.

Help family members or significant others to understand what is happening and what such behavior might imply. Let them know that their presence provides a familiar stabilizing force. Let them make plans for the patient's care in the hospital and at home. Support them as much as possible in whatever they decide.

Delirium is a response often encountered in an intensive care unit.[2] It is characterized by progressive disorientation first to time, then place, then person. Illusions, hallucinations, and delusions also commonly occur. Patients become agitated and combative or secretive and withdrawn. Sleep deprivation is implicated as a causative factor when it is impossible for the patient to get even one complete sleep cycle because of frequently interrupted sleep. Either too much stimulation (constant pain) or too little stimulation (eye patches) can initiate delirum. Microemboli in the postcardiotomy patient have been suggested as a possible cause. Analgesic and antipsychotic agents, metabolic imbalance, and shock are all contributory factors. High fevers, drug overdose, alcoholism, and strong fears can also lead to delirium.

The nurse can minimize effects of confusion by recognizing environmental areas likely to precipitate delirium and teaching the patient what to expect before placement there. When emergency placement is required, discussion and explanation should take place as soon as possible after the crisis situation. Emphasize that physical and environmental factors are contributing to the confusion, fears, and memory loss; reassure the patient that the state will eventually pass. Other interventions include keeping the environment simplified and well organized. Place noisy machines as far from the head as possible. Change lighting to facilitate sleep. Organize care to provide the longest possible rest periods. Place familiar personal objects within view. Use touch judiciously. Treatment directed at known causes such as fever, shock, and drug overdose will result in decreasingly confused responses.

Regardless of the specific treatments, the nurse provides safety for the patient and protection from self-injury. This may include keeping the environment quiet and nonstimulating or using side rails if the patient is to be left alone. If side rails disturb the patient by their presence, as they sometimes do, a judgment must be made whether to use them and risk increased agitation or not use them and risk a fall. Occasionally it becomes necessary to restrain the patient.

One also monitors the physiologic processes, ensures the adequate intake of fluid and food, and monitors and supports elimination. Speak slowly and clearly. This facilitates communication with the person who experiences delirium. Recognizing that the patient cannot control behavior fosters acceptance and patience.

Outcome criteria for the person who has been confused or disoriented

The person will:
1. Be free of bodily injury, either self-inflicted or from falls.
2. Be free of physiologic effects attributable to inability to perform self-care tasks related to nutrition, elimination, and mobility.

REFERENCES AND SELECTED READINGS

1. *Adam, N.R.: Prolonged coma: your care makes all the difference, Nurs. '77 **7**(8):21-27, 1977.
2. *Adams, M., et al: The confused patient: phychological responses in critical care units, Am. J. Nurs. **78**:1505-1512, 1978.
3. *Alexander, M., and Brown, M.: Physical examination: neurological examination, Nurs. '76 **6**(6):38-43, 1976.
4. *Allen, N.: Prognostic indicators in coma, Heart Lung **8**:1075-1082, 1979.
5. *Baxter, S.: Psychological problems of intensive care, Nurs. Times **71**:22-23, 1975.
6. Burnside, I.M., and Moehrlin, B.A.: Health care of the confused elderly at home, Nurs. Clin. North Am. **15**:385-401, 1980.
7. *Burton, G.: Families in crisis, Nurs. '75 **5**(12):36-43, 1975.
8. *Cahall, J., and Smith, D.: Considerate care of the elderly, Nurs. '75 **5**(9):38-39, 1975.
9. *Canning, M.: Care of the unconscious patient, Nurs. Mirror **139**:61-62, 1974.
10. Carlson, N.R.: Physiology of behavior, Boston, 1977, Allyn and Bacon, Inc.
11. Conway, B.: Carini and Owens' neurological and neurosurgical nursing, ed. 8, St. Louis, 1982, The C.V. Mosby Co.
12. Creutzfeldt, O.D.: Neurophysiological mechanisms and consciousness, brain and mind: Ciba Foundation Symposium 69, Elsevier, Holland, 1979, Exerpta Medica.
13. Darmody, W.R.: Current concepts in emergency medicine, vol. 1, Management of the unconscious patient, St. Louis, 1976, The C.V. Mosby Co.
14. Downie, P.: Physiotherapy and the care of the progressively ill patient: the unconscious and bedridden patient, Nurs. Times **69**:922-923, 1973.
15. Erickson, R.: Cranial check: a basic neurological assessment, Nurs. '74 **4**(8):67-72, 1974.
16. *Field, W., and Ruelke, W.: Hallucinations and how to deal with them, Am. J. Nurs. **73**:638-640, 1973.
17. *Finklestein, S., and Ropper, A.: The diagnosis of coma: its pitfalls and limitations, Heart Lung **8**:1059-1064, 1979.
18. Fuerst, E., Wolff, L., and Weitzel, M.: Fundamentals of nursing, ed. 6, Philadelphia, 1979, J.B. Lippincott Co.
19. Gifford, R., and Plant, M.: Abnormal respiratory patterns in the comatose patient caused by intracranial dysfunction, J. Neurosurg. Nurs. **7**(7):57-61, 1975.
20. *Glass, S.J.: Nursing care of the neurosurgical patient: head injuries, J. Neurosurg. Nurs. **5**(12):49-55, 1973.
21. *Gould, H.: How to remove contact lenses from comatose patients, Am. J. Nurs. **76**:1483-1485, 1976.
22. *Grant, M., and Kubo, W.: Assessing a patient's hydration status, Am. J. Nurs. **75**:1306-1311, 1975.
23. *Grier, M.: Hair care for the black patient, Am. J. Nurs. **76**:1781, 1976.
24. Guyton, A.C.: Human physiology and mechanisms of disease, ed. 3, Philadelphia, 1981, W.B. Saunders Co.
25. Hafey, L., and Keane, B.: Patients with acute insult to the central nervous system: an observation tool, Nurs. Clin. North Am. **8**:743-749, 1973.
26. Hunt, P.: Confusion in the elderly, Nurs. Times **73**:1928-1929, 1977.
27. *Jones, C.: Glasgow Coma Scale, Am. J. Nurs. **79**:1551-1553, 1979.
28. Kroner, K.: Dealing with the confused patient, Nurs. '79 **9**(11):71-78, 1979.

*References preceded by an asterisk are particularly well suited for student reading.

29. *Kunkel, J., and Wiley, J.K.: Acute head injury: what to do when, and why, Nurs. '79 9(3):23-33, 1979.
30. Loen, M., and Snyder, M.: Psychosocial aspects of care of the long-term comatose patient, J. Neurosurg. Nurs. 11:235-237, 1979.
31. Meyd, C.J.: Acute brain trauma, Am. J. Nurs. 78:40-44, 1978.
32. Mitchell, P.H., and Lousteau, A.: Concepts basic to nursing, ed. 3, New York, 1981, McGraw-Hill Book Co.
33. Montague, M.F.A.: Touching: the human significance of the skin, ed. 2, New York, 1978, Harper & Row, Publishers.
34. *Myco, F., and McGilloway, F.A.: Care of the unconscious patient: a complementary perspective, J. Adv. Nurs. 5:273-283, 1980.
35. *Norsworthy, E.: Nursing rehabilitation after severe head trauma, Am. J. Nurs. 74:1246-1250, 1974.
36. Plum, F., and Posner, J.: The diagnosis of stupor and coma, ed. 3, Philadelphia, 1980, F.A. Davis Co.
37. *Posner, J.B.: Coma and other states of consciousness: the differential diagnosis of brain death, Ann. N.Y. Acad. Sci. 315:215-227, 1978.
38. Reitz, M., and Pope, W.: Mouth care, Am. J. Nurs. 73:1728-1730, 1973.
39. Rimel, R.W., Jane, J.A., and Edlich, R.F.: Assessment of recovery following head trauma, Crit. Care Q./Neurol. Injuries 2:97-104, 1979.
40. *Rimel, R.W., Jane, J.A., and Edlich, R.F.: Care of CNS trauma at the site of injury, Crit. Care Q./Neurol. Injur. 2:1-6, 1979.
41. *Rudy, E.: Early omens of cerebral disaster, Nurs. '77 7(2):59-62, 1977.
42. Scarbrough, D.: Reality orientation: a new approach to an old problem, Nurs. '74 4(11):12-13, 1974.
43. Schwab, M.: Caring for the aged, Am. J. Nurs. 73:2049-2053, 1973.
44. Swift, N.: Head injury: essentials of excellent care, Nurs. '74 4(9):26-33, 1974.
45. Teasdale, G. and Jennett, B.: Assessment of coma and impaired consciousness: a practical scale, Lancet 2:81-84, 1974.
46. *Trockman, G.: Caring for the confused or delirious patient, Am. J. Nurs. 78:1495-1499, 1978.
47. *Tyson, G.W., et al.: Acute care of the head injured patient, Crit. Care Q./Neurol. Injur. 2:23-44, 1979.
48. *Wahe, S.: Only a concussion, Nurs. '76 6(8):44-45, 1976.
49. *Wallhagen, M.P.: The split brain, Am. J. Nurs. 79:2118-2125, 1979.
50. *Wilkinson, O.: The confused patient: out of touch with reality, Am. J. Nurs. 78:1492-1494, 1978.

CHAPTER 28

ALTERED BODY IMAGE

DOROTHY J. BRUNDAGE
DEBRA C. BROADWELL

Body image is the mental idea a person has of his or her body at any moment and is based on past as well as present perceptions. This mental picture of one's body develops over time and is derived from internal sensations, postural changes, contact with outside objects and people, emotional experiences, and fantasies.[36] Body image is formed by the interaction between the perceptual pool and the experiential pool.[15,32] The perceptual pool consists of all present and past sensory experiences, while the experiential pool consists of all experiences, affects, and memories.

Body image is influenced by cognitive growth as well as by changes in the body that give rise to physical stimuli.[27] These stimuli may be internal or external to the body and include stimuli from the social and physical environment.

Three levels of body experiences play a role in the development of body image: somatic, behavioral, and topologic.[32] Somatic stimuli include neurologic, metabolic, endocrine, and hormonal sensations. This sensory level of experience is observed in infants as they respond to internal stimuli. As a toddler becomes aware of separateness from the environment, behavioral aspects of the development of body image, involving perceptual, cognitive, motor, and personality variables, become evident. During adolescence topologic stimuli, (e.g., superficial sensations and physical characteristics of the body surface) become influential. Modification of one's body image occurs with new percepts and new experiences.[31] Throughout all stages of growth and development and with changes in health stage, body image is continually being altered.

Body image makes up one aspect of the individual's self-concept. The importance of body image within the self-concept will vary mainly according to the nature and intensity of values and emotions invested in it.[35] Self is what a person is, whereas self-image is what a person thinks of self. An essential factor in the development of self-image is body image. Body image is an interpersonal experience of the body, including one's attitudes and feelings. One's body image becomes a standard that influences performance and the way one thinks of oneself.

Many societal and cultural standards influence the development of body image.[32] The attitudes of society, parents, and peers will be reflected in the way persons view their bodies. There has been much discussion of the emphasis on youth, wholeness, and beauty seen in the American culture. Body image includes both reality and ideality[12]; thus body image does not always coincide with objective body.[2] Components of a person's ideal body image may be youth, slenderness, or beauty. Individuals may incorporate so much ideal into their body image that when confronted by the reality of a videotape or a mirror they are genuinely shocked. They do not feel older, and the face in the mirror does not seem to belong.[12]

Since body image is a dynamic, constantly changing perception, change in the structure, function, or appearance of the body requires modification of the image an individual has. The idea of body image disturbances arises from observations that persons with altered structure, function, or appearance may fail to perceive the changes and to adapt to the body as it exists.[56]

Current clinical literature related to persons with altered structure, function, or appearance includes studies of patients following amputation,[16,26] heart attacks,[40] and facial disfiguration.[2,59] Such studies frequently have direct application to patient assessment and intervention by a variety of the health professions involved in rehabilitation of the physically disabled.

A major assumption underlying this chapter is that physical disability or a change in body structure that results in altered function or appearance or both are accompanied by an alteration in the person's body image. Interventions by the health team to help the patient manage the results of the physical change must include help in the pyschosocial areas of life also affected. Much of the effort made in this latter area is focused on helping the patient recognize, accept, and live with the change in self-concept, which includes both body image and self-esteem. These conditions occur not only in the young but also in the older person.

Alteration in body function or appearance usually is not an isolated problem. People are often faced with high hospital costs and long-term use of medications and prosthetic devices. The chronicity of the problem may affect the entire family. Change in body image often creates anxiety, distortion of self, self-depreciation, and mourning for a loss.[24]

This chapter will focus on (1) physical causes of alterations in body image; (2) reactions to such alterations; (3) responses to physical disability by the patient, family, health team, and community; and (4) nursing interventions and desired patient outcomes when changed body image occurs. The content of this chapter will be limited to acquired physical alterations. Please refer to pediatric texts for information about congenital problems.

Physical disability and change in body image

The nature of the change causing altered body image may include (1) altered appearance; (2) altered patterns of eating, breathing, communicating, and elimination; (3) action and motion limitation; (4) deformity; (5) discomfort; (6) stigma; (7) social isolation; and (8) vocational threat.

Altered structure: change in function and appearance

Physical disability is often associated first with a change in body image. Physical changes in body structure may be temporary or permanent. An example of a temporary change is a temporary colostomy, which may be done for a variety of reasons (e.g., diverticulitis, gunshot injuries.) Many patients tolerate the change because it is of a temporary nature. Problems in management of the physical care can develop, however, when

a patient refuses to participate in self-care because the colostomy is temporary. Additional problems may develop if the temporary change becomes permanent. The major problems requiring body image alteration are the result of permanent changes in structure. These alterations may be readily visible, as in an amputation of an extremity or facial disfigurement, or invisible, as in impaired cardiac function after myocardial infarction.

Physical disability can cause loss of function or change in appearance or both. Loss of function occurs in paraplegia, hemiplegia, and chronic renal failure. Partial loss of function occurs in chronic respiratory insufficiency and chronic cardiac disease. Renal, respiratory, and cardiac problems show relatively few visible signs of their presence until the problems are far advanced. Appearance is modified in paraplegia as the muscles of the legs atrophy and contractures occur. Facial muscles may droop and the hands may appear flaccid or spastic on the affected side of a patient with hemiplegia. Change in appearance without loss of function occurs with a traumatic injury to the external ear that leaves hearing unimpaired and with facial scarring after multiple lacerations received in an automobile accident. Enucleation of the eye and amputation of an extremity cause marked changes in both function and appearance.

While some physical changes are immediately visible, some must be disclosed during the activities required to replace the functional loss or to improve appearance. A patient with chronic renal failure who requires hemodialysis two or three times a week cannot hide this fact except from strangers. The person with an artificial eye, ear, or nose may under some circumstances (e.g., hospitalization) be forced to share this information.

While health care professionals often discuss and initiate intervention for body image alteration following traumatic injuries, cancer surgeries (mastectomies, laryngectomies, colostomies), and paralysis, it is important to remember that obesity, pregnancy, and aging also result in body image alteration. Nathan[30] found that obese subjects failed to develop an organized, differentiated, and inner sense of self and of integrity. Wagner and Bye[43] found that patients with chemotherapy-induced alopecia refocused on spiritual values and inner worth as opposed to physical appearance.

Causes of body image alteration

Major causes of conditions that result in physical disability and altered body image are (1) injuries from accidents and war, (2) diseases of the sensorimotor systems, and (3) changes in body structure from toxic or metabolic disorders (box, p. 546). Body image changes related to these conditions may also include the need to incorporate prosthetic devices or a donated body part.

SELECTED CAUSES OF BODY IMAGE ALTERATIONS

Injuries from accidents or war

 Amputation

 Burns: scars and contractures

 Lacerations: scars

Sensorimotor system disease

 Paralysis: paraplegia, hemiplegia

 Blindness, deafness

 Parkinsonism, muscular dystrophy, multiple sclerosis

Change in body structure

 Cardiac, renal, respiratory disease

 Cushing's syndrome

 Rheumatoid arthritis

 Cancer: colostomy, ileostomy, laryngectomy

Excessive overweight or underweight

Reactions and responses to body image changes and losses

Individuals are disturbed when serious threats to or actual deficits in the structure, function, or appearance of the body occur. They must revise long-accepted assumptions about their bodies. Life patterns may need to be changed. The patient faces problems regarding work, social activities, and family. Sexual activities may require modification. Patients may believe that goodness is lost, the ability to accomplish is lost, and that valued skills and talents are impaired. They may feel they are receiving "deserved punishment." One reaction that may interfere with recovery is expectation of rejection and separation. The individual also may feel vulnerable, resigned, rebellious, defiant, rejected, dependent, avoided, resentful, timid, self-conscious, unhappy, humiliated, stigmatized, inferior, and hypersensitive. Indecision, decreased self-respect, bitterness, and cynicism also occur. The hostility of a disabled person toward the healthy may interfere with communication. The attitudes of disabled persons toward themselves are more important than the nature of their disabilities.

Important determinants of reactions

Regardless of the body image alteration, the response of the person will depend on (1) the personal meaning and the significance of the change, (2) the responses of significant others, (3) the availability of help for the person and the family, (4) previous coping behaviors, and (5) the availability of positive role models. The outcome of the alteration in body image is also influenced by the physiologic status of the person; that is, the amount of pain present, the extent of the change or disability, and the realistic expectations of therapy. The physiologic status is relatively fixed for the specific disability; therefore this section will explore the broader psychosocial factors that are amenable to intervention by health professionals.

Meaning of the change

The value the individual assigns to what was lost, the meaning the part or the function has, and the intensity of the person's feelings about the loss all influence how the individual will respond. A person may attribute the successes in life to specific body features. When there is an overvaluation and reliance on security through body beauty or activity, alteration in the body image is likely to cause severe emotional disturbances. Women appear to be less disturbed by threats to the body than men.[14] Women are often concerned about cosmetic effects.[38]

The self-concept is closely linked to sexuality and perception of body image. The response to mastectomy in part is a response to the culture's preoccupation with the breast as a symbol of femininity. This represents the integration of the ideal into the body image. Thus the loss of a breast is often followed by lowered self-esteem, postoperative depression, and concerns of psychosexual role and sexual functioning. The ability of a woman to integrate the trauma of loss of her breast into her life depends on her reactions, real, perceived, or anticipated, and the acceptance of her partner.[25] Her response reflects the value she assigns to the loss, rehabilitation and reinforcement from health professionals, and positive role models.

Men are often concerned about their ability to work and their earning capacity. The loss of earning power and the resultant loss of self-esteem are important determinants of family relationships. Dyk and Sutherland[47] reported that after ostomy surgery, the reduction in housework seemed to be more acceptable to wives than the reduction in gainful employment was to husbands. Most men expressed fears of dependence on spouse or children. The thought of getting old and being ill can be disabling; however, when fears of ostomy spillage and other problems are added, the older person with a stoma may view the burden as insurmountable. Work is important to a sense of achievement, and many persons express who they are in terms of their work.

Social interactions are also affected. Dropkin[11] reported that social interactions decreased after head and neck surgery as the deformity became more pronounced. To varying degrees everyone has a need to feel that the presentation of one's body is acceptable to others. The person who has sustained facial alterations may feel isolated, excluded, stigmatized, helpless, or ashamed. Physical unattractiveness is often associated with social devaluation, denied opportunities, inaccurate judgments of worth, and low self-esteem. The individual with a low need for social approval does not rely as heavily on others to maintain body image, but a low need for social approval does not preclude fear of social rejection. This individual, however, may show earlier signs of integration through early efforts toward self-care.[11]

The meaning of the threat is also influenced by the expected duration of the change and its permanency. A body image alteration resulting from a diagnosis of cancer involves the fear of recurrence or death. The alteration in the body function or structure may be of lesser significance if the person equates the change with an extension or saving of life.

The rapidity of onset is another variable and a sudden unexpected change may be devastating. A traumatic injury that results in sudden loss of mobility may completely alter a person's life goals; for example, a football player with a spinal cord injury must find a new career in addition to coping with everything else. A slow, progressive change, as in rheumatoid arthritis or chronic ulcerative colitis, may allow time for anticipatory mourning.

The source of the change, its type, and the opinions of others are important. Hirschfield and Behan[53] describe acceptable and unacceptable disability following accidents. Changes resulting from heroic sacrifice are viewed differently from changes resulting from socially unacceptable activities. The loss of a leg saving a comrade in battle is viewed quite differently from loss of a leg in a motorcycle accident during a high-speed chase from the scene of a crime. Sterility following venereal disease may be viewed as deserved punishment, while sterility caused by exposure to prescribed radiation therapy carries no stigma. The cause of the disability (active combat injury vs. the sequelae of venereal disease), the type of disability (paralysis vs. weakness or anxiety), and the opinion of others (sympathy vs. scorn) make a difference in the meaning of the disability.

Responses of significant others

Satisfactory social adaptation to a body change depends to a great extent on family relationships and cultural attitudes toward the body structure involved. The sociocultural milieu plays an important role in the acceptance of the change.

What are the attitudes of others, including parents, siblings, and peers, toward physical disability? Satisfactory social adaptation to a body defect depends to a great extent upon family relationships and cultural attitudes

toward the body structures involved. The sociocultural milieu is important. What are the specific body values of the subculture of the patient? What prejudices are there related to wholeness, independence, and attractiveness?

Does stigma accompany the change? A stigma is an attribute that is deeply discrediting. Goffman[51] discusses the idea of being discredited (having a disability fairly readily noted) and being discreditable (having a disability that may be discovered).

Myths and misconceptions abound regarding one whose body is scarred or misshapen by disease or is distorted during movement. There is an overabundance of largely unfounded opinion and folklore regarding physical disability. A strange belief exists that suffering and misfortune somehow make one "a better person." It is also believed that the disabled person mysteriously develops untapped assets and achieves a new depth of understanding and sensitivity.

Help available to patient and family

How a client deals with the loss may well depend on the kind of help available. The help available from the health team and specifically the nurse's role in helping clients with altered body image is discussed later in this chapter. Much of the outcome will depend on whether the client can and does make use of the help offered.

The rehabilitation program generally has as its goal the recovery of physical function. Psychosocial diagnoses and psychosocial therapy are often secondary. Kutner and Abramson[21] speak strongly for considering the person needing rehabilitation as a complete person with a partial disability.[22] They believe that attempts should be made to strengthen the individual's inner resources and the relationship between the individual and the immediate family. A family assessment should be made and family therapy instituted, if necessary.

The family needs help from health care providers to be supportive during this time of change. The reactions of patients discussed earlier also apply to the family. Their reaction will depend on the meaning of the threat, their coping patterns, available resources, and positive role models. They also are frightened by the altered appearance of the patient or the loss of function. They wonder and speculate about the significance of the change on their lives. Since their response plays a significant role for the patient in the integration of the body image alteration and rehabilitation, the family needs cannot be ignored.

Patient care conferences that involve physicians, nurses, social workers, and the family are extremely beneficial in delineating the reality of the situation and the available resources. Rehabilitation centers often use these conferences appropriately when the patient is admitted. More acute care centers are holding patient care conferences throughout the patient's hospitalization.

Involvement of the patient and family is encouraged.

Coping behaviors

Health problems have different meanings at different stages in the life cycle; however, the same problem may be perceived quite differently by persons of the same age. By 4 years of age body image is becoming stabilized and can be affected by body changes. Special care must be taken to assess children's perceptions of their body image because it influences personality organization and ego strength. The level of psychosocial development, the quality of the child's relationship with the parents, and previous adjustment are important. In adolescence the body image undergoes a massive upheaval. Physical changes in the body as a result of accident or illness place an enormous strain on the coping abilities of the young person. Surgical intervention for congenital craniofacial lesions *before* school age is more likely to allow for normal development of body image.[27]

The young adult needs independence. The nurse who "does for" the young adult rather than permitting self-care may precipitate conflicts. Young war veterans with disabling injuries experienced at a time of high physical abilities find adjustment very difficult, and aggressive behavior is common. Concern for sexual identity is prominent. Older persons face the changes of aging: physical and social losses and death. Esberger[12] describes a phenomenon known as "body monitoring" found most often in older persons because the body at this time requires more care in order to maintain adequate performance. Because older persons have more health problems, they often require daily medications, more frequent contacts with health care agencies, special diets, and prosthetic aids. It often becomes more difficult for the older person to maintain activities and hobbies that contribute to a positive self-concept.

All persons as a result of their life history have a well-developed and predictable pattern of coping with threats, real or perceived. Some people immediately begin to problem solve, looking for alternatives; others are immobilized and require help to return to a balance.[41]

Positive role models

The use of positive role models in the rehabilitation plan following body image alteration has increased significantly. Trained visitation programs sponsored by the American Cancer Society have resulted in Reach to Recovery, Ostomy Visitors, and Laryngectomy Visitors. The value of visitors and self-help groups is readily apparent in the growth of these services around the country.

Patients gain from talking with someone who has been through a similar situation and has coped and adapted well. One important aspect is the timing of the visit. The nurse needs to assess each person carefully and offer the choice of a visitor, preoperatively or postoperatively. The visitor should be close to the patient's age and have had a similar diagnosis and surgery. Most important, the visitor should have reached a successful level of rehabilitation, know how to talk with others, and be prepared for a mixed reaction from the patient.

Adaptive responses

Those responses in which the patient works through and accepts the loss are considered adaptive. Any situation perceived by a person as resulting in a major body change and profoundly affecting body image may precipitate a crisis. Most commonly the period of crisis is followed by unrealistic defenses, gradual acceptance, and then reduction of the problem to manageable proportions. Responses depend on the number and intensity of the stresses in comparison to the degree of emotional support and the strength of personal attributes. Patients are helped to meet the challenge of disability if they are mature and secure from the start. An acute sense of proportion helps them recognize reality. A sense of humor helps them live with reality. The urge to fight back and pick up the pieces of an interrupted life may motivate the patient. Hunt[54] has edited a series of essays written by persons with disabilities that provide profound insights into their perceptions of living with a disability.

Several authors note that the loss of a valued body part or function is followed by a period of reaction and adjustment that can be compared to the grief and mourning process that follows the death of a loved one* (see also Chapter 17). Grief is the subjective state of one who has sustained the loss of a valued object, in this instance, physical function or body appearance or both. Mourning is the psychologic process by which one works through to acceptance (ideally) of the loss. The subjective reactions to grief include helplessness, loneliness, hopelessness, sadness, guilt, and anger. Mourning usually leads to relinquishing that which was lost. Eventually the person looks at the past realistically and comfortably.

Rubin[60] describes the losses associated with body image change as the loss of the *capacity for functioning* and the loss of the capacity for *control of functioning* in time and place. A sense of shame accompanies such losses. This reaction reflects a private judgment of failure. The intensity of the emotional response seems to be related to the intensity of the struggle to maintain control.

An individual facing a real or threatened change or loss may experience several stages of grieving, including (1) shock and panic, (2) defensive retreat, (3) acknowledgment, and (4) adaptation.[44] During the first stage the person may be unable to understand or com-

---

*References 8, 17, 22, 38, 62.

prehend the event, its meanings, and its implications. During defensive retreat the person acknowledges the event but is unable to cope with the meaning and implications. The retreat provides time and distance and may appear as denial. Acknowledgment is the recognition of the reality of the situation, its meaning, and its significance. Adaptation is the integration of the change or loss in a way that is supportive of functional living. The person is realistic about the event, its meaning, and its significance.

The reactions of individuals are different throughout the grief process. Some people may lack initiative during shock, have high energy levels during panic, and demonstrate goal-directed behavior later. Other people may feel helpless, angry, guilty, or lost.

Maladaptive responses

When a person is unable to accept the reality of the situation, the response is maladaptive. Patients may deny the change in appearance or the loss of function. They may completely deny the change, may appear withdrawn, aloof, joke and laugh, or present a pseudo–self-confidence. They may use a variety of defense mechanisms such as denial, projection, repression, or regression (see Chapter 15).

The loss may be acknowledged but its significance denied and the situation intellectualized. The person may project concern onto others: "My wife is very upset about my having to change jobs." Tasks may be avoided. Overcompensation for the loss may occur. Patients may project hostile feelings that interfere with acceptance. The resumption of a social, sexual, and emotional life may be impossible. Some may reject others out of a fear of being rejected themselves.[20]

Some persons may try to hide the disability to forget it, and they often pay a high price for such a futile endeavor. Exaggerated independence, overdependence, and pseudocooperation are responses that interfere with the necessary acceptance of help from the family and health team.

Occasionally, the disability may be used as a crutch and if the defect is then corrected, problems may occur. For example, a person may attribute failures in life to an external facial feature; when this feature is changed by plastic surgery, the person may be forced to examine the realities. A similar situation may exist after changes resulting from illness and injury, and in both cases extreme emotional upsets are possible.

Another strategy is to focus attention on a healthy part in order to deny or shut out the damaged part. Idealizing normal standards commits the disabled person to repeated feelings of inferiority. On the other hand, overidentification with the disabled may occur and limit efforts toward achievable levels of rehabilitation. The patient may use the disability as the excuse for early retirement. A return to work can thus be avoided. Another defensive response is the illusion of restoration of the part (phantom).[14] A complete rejection of reality is a psychotic response and may require intense therapy.

The effects of the disability may spread beyond the specific structure, function, or change in appearance to other areas of life and activity and increase the patient's limitations. Perceptions of being incompetent, unlovable, insecure, and unworthy reflect low self-esteem. The person's perception of the situation, the responses received from others, and previous experience with losses determine the level of self-esteem and affect coping mechanisms.

The initial response of the family to the loss depends on many factors already discussed. The *rapidity of onset*, the *specific loss*, and *its meaning* are especially important. The patient is the center of attention, and the family is unified by dread, numbness, a sense of unreality, and the shared threat of loss. During the time the patient is denying the situation, the family may also be denying it. Fear and anger may be directed at the staff. The family may lose interest and patience. They may urge the patient to make a more rapid recovery.

The *degree and quality of support* are important. Sometimes families deal well with the immediate threat but have difficulty with the long-term kinds of help needed. The family must acknowledge the change in the patient, their way of life, and the patient's reactions. Family conflicts over the prescribed regimen occur. Families may use the patient's changed state to keep the patient dependent. Rejection by the family complicates the life of a disabled person. They may attempt to conceal the defect by avoiding and isolating the patient. They may be angry, blaming, and rejecting or indifferent. Ambivalence is not uncommon.

The family must acknowledge the change in the patient and deal with changes in the interpersonal reactions within the family. Constructive, supportive attitudes in the family increase the possibilities for successful adaptation for compensatory development without personality disorder. As patients move to reorganize their lives, their families reexamine interactions, modify living arrangements, encourage social activities, and try to improve family relationships.

Community responses

Society values youth and beauty, good looks in facial features, physical wholeness, and activeness. Social discrimination against those who are different is common. Physical disability, its thought and reality, provoke stereotyped responses in the general public. The type of deformity rather than its severity evokes the stereotypic response. Subtle and overt negative reactions occur. Repulsion, revulsion, rejection, contempt, ridicule, taunts, discrimination, patronizing aversion, tactless curiosity, staring, questioning, and devaluing pity are frequent.

Goffman[51] describes two sets of sympathetic others: those who share stigma and the "wise" who are normal but are acquainted intimately with the secret life of the stigmatized. The latter includes family members and professional persons involved in the patient's care.

Reactions to one who is physically disabled may range from overly sympathetic to unsympathetic. One takes on the attitude of others toward one's body. Negative feelings already present about one's body thus may be reinforced by society.

Visible handicaps alter social and psychologic functioning in important ways. Confronting a damaged face disrupts one's sense of inner security. The thought of disfigurement or scarring causes fear of public reaction in most people, and not withouse cause. Social ostracism is a real possibility. Physical disability is accompanied by a fear of being unable to perform one's regular routines, the fear of loss of control of oneself. If the disability is not visible, it may not be considered to be important by others.

The part of the body that is lost or nonfunctioning will also influence the reactions of others. People are usually very uncomfortable discussing ostomies or the wearing of a pouch. Loss of sexual function is not usually easily accepted. Others will often respond with comments such as "he should be thankful he's alive," showing a lack of concern for the values of the individual.

Some disabilities are more acceptable than others. Breast cancer and mastectomies have received recent national television coverage. Several movies have been made about recoveries following spinal cord injuries. Recovery from drug abuse has made headlines as television stars seek help for drug and alcohol problems. Yet there are many other disabilities that are poorly understood by the general public.

Attitudes toward body structures affect responses to those with physical disabilities. The attitudes of well people affect the social adaptation of those with body defects. Disapproval may be present when those persons with disability appear not to be helping themselves. Generalized indifference rejects the reality of the person facing real threats. Studies show that women are more accepting than men, while adolescents are less accepting than those of college age of persons with disability.[27] No significant difference in attitude was found according to socioeconomic status.

Health team responses

Members of the health team are not immune to negative attitudes toward the disabled. They may subscribe to certain stereotypes, especially with regard to sexual functioning in persons with disabilities. Conde-

scension, resentment, insensitiveness, and aloofness can be found in those "dedicated to help." The health team may expect a passive, compliant, dependent patient. They may feel protective or they may react with superiority. Examples of negative attitudes are reflected in the use of such labels as "unmotivated" as justification for closing a case. The use of stereotype labels—"CPs," "CVAs," "quads"—reflects obvious disregard for the individuality of the patient. The reactions of health professionals may include embarrassment, undefined anxiety, relief if the patient is cheerful, abandonment by disregarding stress signals, and maintenance of a superficial atmosphere to being thoughtful, understanding, and helpful. Anger at being unable to help is a recurring phenomenon.

Health professionals can contribute to a patient's lowered self-esteem when they express openly or covertly negative reactions to the change in structure, function, or appearance. A patient's loss of control threatens the health professional's control. Sarcasm covered with saccharine sweetness and teasing may be signs of displaced anger. People reject what they cannot cope with, and they may withdraw from the situation. Health professionals should honestly explore their feelings toward the patient with body changes.

Little investigation of health team attitudes has been done. This is unfortunate, for the health team probably is more important in shaping the patient's response than any other group.[58] Persons who work with the disabled should try to be as sensitive and perceptive as possible about their own responses to disability and the disabled and about the patient's emotional reactions to the problems. Recently, group experiences have been made possible so that health care providers can explore their feelings and be better able to facilitate rehabilitation. Specialization in certain areas has occurred within nursing as people identify those patients with whom they are best capable of working. Values clarification is one method of helping nurses identify their values and the effect of personal values on the care provided.

Reactions to physical disability and rehabilitation

Rehabilitation attempts to enable disabled persons to live within the limits of their disabilities but to the full extent of their capacity. How do reactions to physical disability affect the rehabilitation of the physically disabled?

Rehabilitation will be impeded if the person with the disability feels inferior, self-conscious, frustrated, preoccupied with the deformity, hypersensitive, anxious, hostile, or paranoid. One measure of the capacity to adapt is the person's willingness to participate in a program of restoration or rehabilitation.[38]

Disability may be perceived by some as deserved punishment or by others as a source of pride: the person is specially selected by God to suffer. Dependency in disability may be hard to accept or be welcomed, temporary or permanent. The exemptions and privileges of illness may be tempting, and some patients find it to their advantage to be disabled.[14] Such a person gains the satisfaction of security and other pyschosocial needs without stigma or shame attached to the role change.

There are many successfully rehabilitated persons who have experienced body image alteration. The level of rehabilitation is often directly reflective of the therapeutic intervention supplied throughout the hospitalization and posthospitalization period.

Intervention for persons with altered body image

Persons with changes in structure, function, and appearance face problems related to (1) physical limitations and failures; (2) discomfort from appliances, abnormal sensations, and fatigue; (3) visual or auditory changes in appearance; (4) vocational and economic limitations; and (5) social interaction limitations.

Assessment

Bernstein and Cope[2] have delineated six axes for adjustment to disability: (1) active coping—passive surrender; (2) leading and comanaging treatment—resisting treatment; (3) loving exchange—rage; (4) denial—overawareness; (5) adaptive defenses—maladaptive defenses; and (6) mental (activity) mode—physical (activity) mode. Along each axis are important variables. Complex interwoven patterns form within a matrix of factors including money, education, family support, religious help, and rehabilitation services. Bernstein and Cope have found this framework helpful in looking at the catastrophe of burn disfigurement.

The patient's perception of the situation and his usual pattern of adapting must be considered in planning nursing intervention. How does the patient deal with stress? What threats are seen as dangerous? What are the patient's goals? Consider the patient's personality, values, needs, and readiness for learning.

Does the patient cry? If not, consider the following possibilities. The patient cannot cry or does not want to cry or perhaps the loss will not be missed. Usually, however, there is ambivalence with feelings of guilt and shame.

Recognize the energy used to handle the enforced awareness of the disability. Be aware of how far the patient has come and the distance yet to go.

Appraise the response of family members and significant others. Identify the patient's support systems—those people and resources that may assist during the period of adaptation. Consider the importance of the patient's peers.

Transitional points of entry and termination are critical points of emotional adjustment—they reflect periods of change. The move from rehabilitation center to home for a patient with paraplegia or the first hemodialysis treatment at home for a patient with chronic renal failure are examples of such points.

The nurse's ability to assess accurately the patient's response and adaptation to loss requires an understanding of (1) the visibility of the loss, (2) the loss of function, and (3) the patient's emotional investment in the part affected.[10] This information is useful in predicting (1) the patient's and the family's coping abilities, (2) the nature of assistance needed for adaptation, and (3) the identification of those persons who can provide the assistance.

Intervention

Nursing care is important during the *acute, convalescent,* and *rehabilitative* phases following disability. During the acute phase the nursing focus is on activities such as lifesaving techniques, assisting with diagnosis, and preoperative and postoperative care. Most frequently the patient is hospitalized. The goal is to save life, halt illness, and to prevent helplessness and deformity.

During the convalescent phase nursing activities include assisting the patient to adjust to change, maintaining physical abilities through occupational therapy and physical therapy, and home planning with the family, community health nurse, and social worker. During this phase patients may still be hospitalized but some individuals may be at home. The goal is to prepare for the rehabilitative phase. Patient education plays an important role in the rehabilitation of persons with altered body image. They need the information necessary for self-care to recognize signs and symptoms of potential problems and to identify who to see for additional supportive services.

Rehabilitation includes the coordination of a number of specialized services. Rehabilitation should focus on physical social, emotional, and sexual aspects of the person's life. The patient's response and needs will vary in each stage of adaptation (see box, p. 552). Assist the patient to identify reasonable goals and objectives; then carefully plan ways of implementing a sequence of events that will enable the person to complete the goals successfully.

ADAPTATION PROCESS*

I. Shock and panic (message: "Oh!")
  A. Shock
   1. Critical issue: The mind is communicating an inability to integrate the critical event, its meaning, and its implications.
   2. Thought process: Immobilized, devoid of problem-solving ability, decision making difficult.
   3. Physical behavior: Immobilized, responsive primarily to external suggestions. May have difficulty caring for self. (At times, the individual may appear to be functional in problem solving and self-care because "automatic" survival response occurs.)
   4. Affect: Blunted or devoid of affect.
   5. Intervention: Dependent on an accurate assessment of the individual's mental, physical, and affectual status. Individuals in shock respond to directive intervention and support that provides for very basic physical and psychosocial needs.
  B. Panic
   1. Critical issue: The mind is communicating an inability to integrate the event, its meaning, and its implications.
   2. Thought process: Scattered thoughts, often tangential in nature. They may also be in the form of "racing thoughts," numerous, constant, repetitive questioning with limited or no ability to integrate answers or data in response to questioning.
   3. Physical behavior: Extensive energy release through nondirected or non-goal-oriented behavior; high-level motor activity.
   4. Affect: Obviously anxious.
   5. Intervention: Allow opportunity for physical release and expression of energy and anxiety. Provide very calm, accepting environment. Provide appropriate intervention for client safety.

II. Defensive retreat (message: "No")
  A. Critical issue: The mind is communicating an acknowledgment of the critical event or situation and an inability to integrate or cope with the affectual meaning and implications of the event. The retreat acts as a time and distance maneuver, allowing the individual the space and opportunity to integrate the psychosocial impact of the critical event.
  B. Thought process: Denial is an unconscious process that protects the individual from further intrusion of fearful or threatening implications related to the critical event. Specific information related to the critical situation or the event itself may be negated as nonexistent. In rationalization/intellectualization the critical event and related information are treated with seeming objectivity and distance. Request for information is seemingly appropriate to resolution of the "problem."

  C. Physical behavior: Appears goal-directed, reasonable, and logical excepting those areas of information that may be negated as non-existent with denial.
  D. Affect: May appear to be minimal or at least cautiously covered. Affectual responses of fear or anxiety minimally acknowledged.
  E. Intervention: Acknowledge to yourself as therapist that significant affect is being defended against, not that information has not been received. Do not challenge the areas of information being denied or negated. This will only precipitate the strengthening of this defense. Acknowledge to the individual the normalcy of his difficulty integrating this "confusing and upsetting" information and your willingness to be available to discuss feelings. Provide open-ended opportunities for feeling expression without being intrusive. Use feeling words that are nonspecific and nondiagnostic in encouraging feeling expression (e.g., "You seem a bit confused or upset by all this information" rather than "You seem to be denying very important aspects of your diagnosis and treatment"). It is imperative that the therapist keep in mind that effective feeling expression will diminish the need for defensive retreat mechanisms. Often time and distance (if realistic to the critical nature of the situation) will be themselves give the individual the opportunity to integrate the meaning and implications of the critical situation.

III. Acknowledgment (message: "Yes, but I don't want it!")
  A. Critical issue: The mind has integrated the critical event, its meaning, and its implications in a way that is supportive of functional living.
  B. Thought process: Equilibrium has returned, effective problem solving is in process, learning of new information related to the integration of the situation is more possible.
  C. Physical behavior: Returned to prevent function with the integration of necessary alterations related to critical change or loss.
  D. Affect: Hopeful and realistic. Life is now worth living. Feelings of sadness and anger may be experienced from time to time, but the individual is not immobilized or ruled by his feelings.
  E. Intervention: Effective teaching and learning may now occur. Anticipate with the individual the possibility of emotional upset in the future, which is normal rather than regressive. Be available over time (4 to 6 months at least) for further follow-up and exploration of the adjustment process.

---

*From Sultenfuss, S.: Psychosocial issues and therapeutic intervention. In Broadwell, D.C., and Jackson, B.S.: Principles of ostomy care, St. Louis, 1982, The C.V. Mosby Co.

The person with a disability needs understanding. Assume that such patients are coping with an overwhelming experience, support the self-esteem necessary for them to reorganize the body image, and permit crying in such a manner that patients still have a sense of self-respect and worthiness. Give patients time, and help them confront the problem in manageable steps. Acknowledge appropriate feelings, recognize assets and strengths, and provide support to the extent needed, that is, the degree mutually agreed upon.

Let the patient ventilate, helping clarify misconceptions. Promote a sense of trust, respect, security, and comfort. It is essential for the patient to come to terms with the change. Reassurance that "you'll be as good as new" delays adjustment and raises false hopes. Do not encourage the patient to blame others; rather, assist the patient to accept help with everyday tasks. Counteract the effects of deprivation and immobilization by helping the patient understand what is occurring and maintaining the remaining body integrity. The focus of care is on what is left—not what is lost.

Be accepting within appropriate limits. Assure the patient that grief is normal. The patient must also accept the fact that permanently unattainable goals exist. Privacy and a safe environment are necessary for the patient to achieve control of a lost or altered body function. Avoid overprotection and unnecessary restrictions. Explore realistic alternatives rather than being overly optimistic or pessimistic. Help the patient find the facts, as speculating can be worse than the truth. Help the patient develop compensatory personality traits.

Predict the occurrence of body image problems, prevent them where possible, and be ready to intervene to help solve them when necessary. Anticipatory guidance and preventive intervention help to promote the capacity of individuals to cope with life crises. Prepare patients before surgery or before receiving drugs that alter body image. Consider various influencing factors. Recognize the need for grief and mourning. Help the patient strengthen both coping mechanisms and problem-solving skills.

Health team

All the health team members must work through their feelings regarding loss, disability, and disfigurement, and examine their behaviors used in coping with such threats. If this conscious self-examination is omitted, feelings and behaviors may interfere with the patient's rehabilitation and may result in the professional's leaving this field of service. Staff responses to persons with disability should be honest, patient, consistent, realistic, and firm, but not hostile. Often they must accept the patient despite his hostility and rejection toward them. Every effort must be made to avoid rein-

forcing the person's low self-esteem. Special preparation is needed for open, honest discussion of the patient's problems with sexuality.[48] Consistent support promotes the trust vital to learning to cope with altered structure, function, and appearance.

Evaluation

Positive attitudes of the patient toward rehabilitation, the staff, and program of help are desirable. Acceptance and use of prosthetic devices are expected. Desired patient outcomes include self-assurance, confident behavior, self-reliance, stable motivation, self-acceptance, and adequate social interactions. It is generally accepted that a person is happier if involved in productive activities.

Siller[39] suggests that one outcome measure of the acceptance of the loss is the degree that the reconstituted self is oriented toward self-approval and is responsive to reality.

Some dependency may be legitimate, and some physical help may be needed. Retirement from gainful employment may be required, or reduced household responsibilities and a sharp curtailment of social activities may be unavoidable.

Litman's[57] study of family disruption because of disability shows no significant relationship between the degree of family solidarity and rehabilitation response. However, family support during rehabilitation has a significant effect on the patient's response to the program. The family consequently reexamines and probably reorients interpersonal relationships and readjusts living arrangements.

Employment, school attendance, or home responsibilities are insufficient measures of outcomes for many patients. Areas to be considered include cognition, activities of daily living, home activities, activities outside the home, and social interaction. Evaluation is best accomplished after the patient is discharged. Many tools have been designed to assist in measuring body image, but there is no one tool that adequately measures the whole of body image.[13] Most tools measure body perception or body attitude. Body perception is the mental experience of the body's physical appearance. Body attitude reflects feelings, attitudes, and emotional reaction toward the body. Since patients are not regularly tested, behavioral responses are usually used to evaluate the effectiveness of the integration of a change in body image. A therapeutic relationship established early in the rehabilitative phase is often beneficial in evaluating change.

The change in body image does not occur quickly. Adaptation to a change may take a year or longer, but that does not signify maladaptation. The integration of a new mental image takes time and a reorganization of thoughts and images.

REFERENCES AND SELECTED READINGS
Contemporary

1. Abramson, A.S., and Kutner, B.: A bill of rights for the disabled. In Meislin, J.: Rehabilitation medicine and psychiatry, Springfield, Ill., 1976, Charles C Thomas, Publisher.
2. Bernstein, N.R., and Cope, O.: Emotional care of the facially burned and disfigured, Boston, 1976, Little, Brown & Co.
3. *Blaesing, S., and Brockhaus, J.: The development of body image in the child, Nurs. Clin. North Am. 7:597-607, 1972.
4. *Blues, K.: A framework for nurses providing care to laryngectomy patients, Ca. Nurs. 1(6):441-446, 1978.
5. *Brown, M.S.: Distortions in body image in illness and disease. In Bower, F.L., editor: Wiley nursing concept modules, New York, 1977, John Wiley & Sons, Inc.
6. *Brown, M.A.: Normal development of body image. In Bower, F.L., editor: Wiley nursing concept modules, New York, 1977, John Wiley & Sons, Inc.
7. Brundage, D.J.: Assessing rehabilitation in home dialysis patients. Paper presented at Thelma Ingles Scholarly Paper Presentation, Sigma Theta Tau, Beta Epsilon, Durham, N.C., 1976.
8. Compton, C.Y.: War injury: identity crisis for young men, Nurs. Clin. North Am. 8:53-66, 1973.
9. Dempsey, M.O.: The development of body image in the adolescent, Nurs. Clin. North Am. 7:609-615, 1972.
10. *Donovan, M.I., and Pierce, S.G.: Cancer care nursing, New York, 1976, Appleton-Century-Crofts.
11. Dropkin, N.J.: Compliance in postoperative head and neck patients, Ca. Nurs. 2(5):379-384, 1979.
12. Esberger, K.: Body image, J. Gerontol. Nurs. 4(4):35-38, 1978.
13. Fawcett, J., and Frye, S.: An exploratory study of body image dimensionally, Nurs. Res. 29:324-327, 1980.
14. Fisher, S.: Body experience in fantasy and behavior, New York, 1970, Appleton-Century-Crofts.
15. Fujita, M.T.: The impact of illness or surgery on the body image of the child, Nurs. Clin. North Am. 7:641-649, 1972.
16. Garrett, J.F., and Levine, E.S.: Rehabilitation practices with the physically disabled, New York, 1973, Columbia University Press.
17. Gruendemann, B.J.: Problems of physical self: loss. In Roy, S.C.: Introduction to nursing: an adaptation model, Englewood Cliffs, N.J., 1976, Prentice-Hall, Inc.
18. *Gruendemann, B.J.: The impact of surgery on body image, Nurs. Clin. North Am. 10:635-643, 1975.
19. Harris, R.: Cultural differences in body perception during pregnancy, Br. J. Med. Psychol. 52:347-352, 1970.
20. Kaplan, S.: Some psychological and social factors present in the condition of obesity, J. Rehabil. 45(3):52-54, 1979.
21. Kutner, B., and Abramson, A.S.: Rehabilitation goals: myth or reality. In Meislin, J.: Rehabilitation medicine and psychiatry, Springfield, Ill., 1976, Charles C Thomas, Publisher.
22. *Lee, J.M.: Emotional reactions to trauma, Nurs. Clin. North Am. 5:557-587, 1970.
23. *Leonard, B.J.: Body image changes in chronic illness, Nurs. Clin. North Am. 7:687-695, 1972.
24. Liss, J.L.: Psychiatric issues in ostomy management. In Broadwell, D.C. and Jackson, B.S.: Principles of ostomy care, St. Louis, 1982, The C.V. Mosby Co.
25. May, H.J.: Psychosexual sequelae to mastectomy: implications for therapeutic and rehabilitative intervention, J. Rehabil. 46:(1):29-31, 1970.
26. Mital, M.A., and Peirce, D.S.: Amputees and their prostheses, Boston, 1971, Little, Brown & Co.
27. Murray, J., et al.: Twenty year experience in maxillocraniofacial surgery, Ann. Surg. 190:320-331, 1979.
28. *Murray, R.L.E.: Body image development in adulthood, Nurs. Clin. North Am. 7:617-630, 1972.
29. *Murray, R.L.E.: Principles of nursing intervention for the adult patient with body image changes, Nurs. Clin. North Am. 7:697-707, 1972.
30. Nathan, S.: Body image in chronically obese children as reflected in figure drawings, J. Pers. Assess. 37:456-463, 1973.
31. Norris, C.M.: The professional nurse and body image. In Carlson, C.E.: Behavioral concepts and nursing intervention, ed. 2, Philadelphia, 1979, J.B. Lippincott Co.
32. *O'Brien, J.: Mirror, mirror, why me? Nurs. Mirror 150(17):36-37, 1980.
33. Riddle, I.: Nursing interventions to promote body image integrity in children, Nurs. Clin. North Am. 7:651-661, 1972.
34. Rosillo, R.H., Welty, MJ., and Graham, W.P.: The patient with maxillofacial cancer. II. Psychologic aspects, Nurs. Clin. North Am. 8:153-158, 1973.
35. Safilios-Rothschild, C.: The sociology and social psychology of disability and rehabilitation, New York, 1975, Random House, Inc.
36. Salkin, J.: Body ego technique, Springfield, Ill., 1973, Charles C Thomas, Publisher.
37. Sarno, J.E., Sarno, M.T., and Levita, E.: The functional life scale, Arch. Phys. Med. Rehabil. 54:216-220, 1973.
38. Schoenburg, B., et al., editors: Loss and grief: psychological management in medical practice, New York, 1970, Columbia University Press.
39. Siller, J.: Psychosocial aspects of physical disability. In Mesilin, J.: Rehabilitation medicine and psychiatry, Springfield, Ill., 1976, Charles C Thomas, Publisher.
40. Smith, C.: Body image changes after myocardial infarction, Nurs. Clin. North Am. 7:663-688, 1972.
41. Sultenfuss, S.: Psychosocial issues and therapeutic intervention. In Broadwell, D.C., and Jackson, B.S.: Principles of ostomy care, St. Louis, 1982, The C.V. Mosby Co.
42. Tourkow, L.P.: Psychic consequences of loss and replacement of body parts, J. Am. Psychoanal. Assoc. 22:170-181, 1974.
43. Wagner, L., and Bye, M.G.: Body image and patients experiencing alopecia as a result of cancer chemotherapy, Ca. Nurs. 2(5):365-369, 1979.
44. Wineman, N.M.: Obesity, Nurs. Res. 29:231-237, 1970.
45. *Woods, N.F.: Human sexuality in health and illness, St. Louis, 1979, The C.V. Mosby Co.
46. Woods, N.F.: Altered levels of sexual function. In Boroch, R.M.: Elements of rehabilitation in nursing, St. Louis, 1976, The C.V. Mosby Co.

Classic

47. Dyk, R.B., and Sutherland, A.: Adaptation of the spouse and other family members to the colostomy patient, CA 9:123-125, 1956.
48. Engel, G.L.: Grief and grieving, Am. J. Nurs. 64:93-98, 1964.
49. Engel, G.L.: Psychological development in health and disease, Philadelphia, 1962, W.B. Saunders Co.
50. Fisher, S., and Cleveland, S.E.: Personality, body perception and body image boundary. In Wapner, S., and Werner, H., editors: The body percept, New York, 1965, Random House, Inc.
51. Goffman, E.: Stigma: notes on the management of spoiled identity, Englewood Cliffs, N.J., 1963, Prentice-Hall, Inc.
52. Gorman, W.: Body image and the image of the brain, St. Louis, 1969, Warren H. Green, Inc.
53. Hirschfield, A.H., and Behan, R.C.: The accident process: disability, acceptable and unacceptable, J.A.M.A. 197:85-89, 1966.

*References preceded by an asterisk are particularly well suited for student reading.

54. Hunt, P., editor: Stigma: the experience of disability, London, 1966, Geoffrey Chapman Publishers.
55. Kaplan, L.: Foundations of human behavior, New York, 1965, Harper & Row, Publishers.
56. Kolb, L.C.: Disturbances of the body-image. In Arieta, S.: American handbook of psychiatry, vol. 1, New York, 1959, Basic Books, Inc.
57. Litman, T.J.: The family and physical rehabilitation, J. Chronic Dis. 19:211-217, 1966.
58. McDaniel, J.W.: Physical disability and human behavior, New York, 1969, Pergamon Press, Inc.

59. MacGregor, F.C.: Psychosocial approach to patients with facial disfigurement. In Wood-Smith, D., and Porowski, P.C., editors: Nursing care of the plastic surgery patient, St. Louis, 1967, The C.V. Mosby Co.
60. Rubin, R.: Body image and self esteem, Nurs. Outlook 16:20-23, 1968.
61. Shontz, F.C.: Perceptual and cognitive aspects of body experience, New York, 1969, Academic Press, Inc.
62. Wright, B.A.: Physical disability: a pyschological approach, New York, 1960, Harper & Row, Publishers.

CHAPTER 29

CHRONIC ILLNESS

ELEANOR E. BAUWENS
SANDRA VANDAM ANDERSON
PATRICIA BUERGIN

Prevention and control of chronic disease constitute one of the major health problems in the United States today. In the past the impact of chronic diseases on individuals, families, and communities has been overlooked. Recently, there has been an increasing awareness in the United States of great pockets of unmet needs among people with long-term health problems. These individuals have needs that extend beyond the strictly medical. Their problems demand the use of multiple sources of help and care. In many cases the coping capacities of chronically ill individuals are reduced because of advancing age, serious functional impairment and disability, and limited personal, social, and financial resources.

Chronic disease is not an entity in itself but an umbrella term that encompasses long-lasting diseases, which are often associated with some degree of disability. Each chronic illness is unique and has a different impact on the individual, family, and community. Nevertheless, common problems and complications that accompany the various chronic health problems can be studied in general to help the nurse understand and care for individuals with specific long-term illnesses.

The incidence and prevalence of chronic diseases have increased since the beginning of the twentieth century. This increase has been brought about by a number of developments including decreased mortality from infectious diseases, improved sanitation, and the development of effective vaccines and mass immunizations. Today only 1% of people who die before age 75 in the United States die from infectious diseases. Although the mortality from infectious diseases declined between 1900 and 1970, the proportions of deaths from major chronic diseases such as heart disease, cancer, and stroke have increased more than 250%.[32] According to the surgeon general's report, 80% of the over-65 population has one or more chronic illnesses.[32] Since the late 1960s, declining mortality from heart disease (particularly ischemic heart disease) and the cerebrovascular diseases has contributed to increased longevity. In fact, 1977 was the first year in which cardiovascular causes were responsible for less than 50% of all deaths in the United States.[31] Longevity of the total U.S. population has increased by 3.1 years since 1970, compared with a gain of 0.8 year in the sixties. This gain in longevity is undoubtedly due to measures by individuals to help themselves.

Differences between acute and chronic illness

An *acute illness* is one caused by a disease that produces symptoms and signs soon after exposure to the cause, that runs a short course, and from which there is usually a full recovery or an abrupt termination in death. Acute illness may become chronic. For example, a common cold may develop into chronic sinusitis. A *chronic illness* is one caused by disease that produces symptoms and signs within a variable period of time, that runs a long course, and from which there is only partial recovery. The Commission on Chronic Illness in 1949 defined chronic illness as any impairment or deviation from normal that has one or more of the following characteristics: it is permanent; leaves residual disability; is caused by nonreversible pathologic alteration; requires special training of the patient for rehabilitation; or may be expected to require a long period of supervision, observation, or care. This definition is still in use.

The symptoms and general reactions caused by chronic disease may subside with proper treatment and care. The period during which the disease is controlled and symptoms are not obvious is known as a *remission*. However, at a future time the disease may become active again with recurrence of pronounced symptoms. This is known as an *exacerbation* of the disease.

Acute exacerbations of chronic disease often cause the patient to seek medical attention and may lead to hospitalization. The needs of a patient who has an acute illness may be very different from those of the patient with an acute exacerbation of a chronic disease. For example, a young person may enter the hospital with complaints of fever, chest pain, shortness of breath, fatigue, and a productive cough. If the diagnosis is pneumonia, the patient usually can be assured of recovery after a period of rest and a course of antibiotic treatment. However, if the diagnosis is rheumatic heart disease and if the patient is being admitted to the hospital for the third, fourth, or fifth time, the reassurance needed will not be so definite, clear-cut, or easy to give. In such a case it is necessary to begin planning care that will extend beyond the period of hospitalization, taking into consideration many aspects of the patient's total life situation. The concerns of the patient who has repeated attacks of illness will be very different from the concerns of the one who has a short-term illness.

Further, the needs of patients who are admitted to the hospital with an acute illness but who also have an underlying chronic condition must not be overlooked. For example, elderly patients who enter the general hospital with pneumonia may receive treatment for the pneumonia and recover from their illness. However, they may still be hampered by the arteriosclerotic heart disease and arthritis that they have had for years. Also, these two chronic conditions may have been aggravated by the acute infection, or the return to former activity may be hindered by joint stiffness resulting from the enforced bed rest and inactivity. Consideration of a patient's several diagnoses can help in preventing new problems associated with the chronic illness.

Neither completely well nor acutely ill, the individual with chronic disease must make daily adjustments in living. Strauss[27] has listed some problems surrounding chronic illness: (1) preventing and managing medical crises as they occur, (2) controlling symptoms, (3) following a prescribed regimen and managing attendant problems, (4) normalizing interactions with others, (5) adjusting to recurrent patterns in the disease course, and (6) arranging payment for treatment. Emotional,

social, and economic implications of chronic illness will be discussed later in this chapter.

Chronic illness as a force in society

Extent and effects of chronic illness

According to the National Health Survey, 80 million people have one or more chronic conditions. The National Health Survey list of chronic diseases includes asthma, allergy, tuberculosis, bronchitis, emphysema, sinusitis, rheumatic fever, arteriosclerosis, hypertension, heart disease, cerebral vascular accident and other vascular conditions, hemorrhoids, gallbladder or liver disease, diabetes mellitus, thyroid disease, epilepsy or convulsions, spinal disease, cancer, chronic dermatosis, and hernia.

Many of these specific illnesses cause a limitation of activity, which affects the life-style of the chronically ill. Data on limitation of activity can be obtained from the National Center for Health Statistics. One of the trends that has been documented is that the impact of acute illness has seemed to diminish, whereas the burden of chronic health problems and related disability has increased. Limitation of activity is a measure of long-term disability resulting from chronic health problems or impairment and is defined as the inability to carry on the major activity for one's age group, such as cooking, keeping house, going to school, or going to work.[21] Approximately 15% of the population experience some limitations in their activities, whereas almost half of the persons over 65 years of age are limited in their activities by one or more chronic conditions. Some activity limitations are associated with mental disabilities, but most are the result of physical handicaps caused by heart conditions and arthritis. Since chronic disability increases in direct proportion to age, persons over 65 years of age are most prone to severe chronic disability.[13]

The inability to work or to move about influences greatly the kind of medical treatment and health supervision needed by persons who have a chronic illness. Some persons only need periodic medical examination and perhaps continuing treatment with medications; others may require complete physical care. Some have a disease that progresses very slowly without remissions, while others may have episodes of acute illness and then seem comparatively well for a time. Each person requires a thorough assessment to determine the stage of the illness, the course the illness is likely to take, the type of care needed, and the method by which that care will be delivered if the individual is to be helped appropriately.

Factors that influence chronic illness

Age

Different age groups have different kinds of experience with acute and chronic diseases. The young are more likely to experience short, intense, acute conditions that are quickly over. The elderly are more likely to have long, drawn-out chronic diseases; nevertheless, it is true that anyone can have either an acute or a chronic disease at any age. Chronic illness and disability may date from birth (e.g., spina bifida with neurologic damage), or it may originate in childhood, adolescence, or early adult life (e.g., multiple sclerosis, rheumatoid arthritis). Table 29-1 depicts the prevalence of selected chronic conditions by age groups for selected years from 1970 to 1977.

Because of strides made in pediatric medicine, children who 30 years ago would have died for lack of knowledge and treatment of diseases such as cystic fibrosis are now living longer with those chronic diseases. The reduction in death rates among the younger age groups has allowed a higher percentage of the population to reach the age of greatest risk from chronic diseases. Cancer develops far more frequently in older people. Because the average age of our population continues to rise, one out of four people now alive will eventually contract cancer.[3]

Much remains to be learned about interactions of the normal, pathologic, and physiologic changes of aging with various diseases. A common question that is asked is "When does aging end and illness begin?" Differences found in age groups or changes found in individuals as they age represent normal aging; that is, a universal, intrinsic process of growth and development that is inevitable, irreversible, unpreventable, but ulti-

mately detrimental. Even though aging, a normal process, is distinct from chronic disease, a pathologic process, chronic illness is often concomitant with aging. The problems of aging and chronic disease are influenced in major ways by each other; for example, the social problems confronting the aged are strongly influenced by the presence and severity of chronic disabilities. Remissions and exacerbations are possibilities with chronic illness; they are not with aging.

Cultural values

Health is a major value in Western culture; thus few people are interested in personalized, prolonged contact with the ill. Because Western culture tends to be cure oriented, health care for acute conditions is often more valued than is health care for the chronically ill. In contrast to the exciting aspects of sophisticated and mechanical technology, caring for chronically ill persons is often considered boring. The continual struggle to cope with day-to-day living soon becomes tedious for ill persons, their families, and health professionals. The rewards of treating chronic illness cannot be measured by a cure but by the prevention of complications and by helping individuals function at their optimal level.

The cultural context has many symbolic meanings, beliefs, and values that health professionals need to understand to meet individual's health needs (see Chapter 3). Some individuals may view their chronic disease as a form of punishment from God. Thus they may experience a sense of guilt. Individuals who view their chronic disease as a "leper phenomenon" may experience a sense of social rejection. Others may see their chronic illness as a destructive force without meaning or simply as a physical response of their body. Appreciation of the person's beliefs and behavior in the context of his or her cultural heritage rather than denial of the cultural influ-

TABLE 29-1. Prevalence of selected chronic conditions, 1970 to 1977*

Condition	17 to 44 years		45 to 64 years		65 years and older		All ages	
	A†	B‡	A	B	A	B	A	B
Arthritis (1976)	45.5	13.1	255.8	18.3	436.6	25.5	116.7	20.3
Asthma (1970)	26.0	17.0	33.0	19.0	36.0	27.0	30.0	17.0
Cerebrovascular diseases (1972)	NA§	NA	12.0	NA	48.0	NA	8.0	22.0
Diabetes (1975)	9.4	23.5	50.3	30.3	83.0	34.4	22.9	30.6
Emphysema (1970)	NA	NA	14.0	NA	32.0	NA	7.0	45.0
Heart conditions (1972)	25.0	22.0	89.0	46.0	199.0	52.0	50.0	42.0
Major extremity missing (1977)	0.8	56.3	3.1	61.9	6.2	73.2	1.7	65.9
Vision impairment, severe (1977)	1.2	42.7	6.0	36.4	44.5	35.5	6.6	37.0

*From National Center for Health Statistics, Division of Health Interview Statistics; data from the Health Interview Survey.
†Per 1000 persons.
‡Percent resulting in limitation of activity.
§NA-Not available.

ence will increase understanding between the health professional and the chronically ill person. Differences need not imply deviance. It is possible to introduce health practices in a manner congruent with the individual's cultural values.

Race and ethnicity

Race or ethnic group membership is a factor that influences chronic health problems. Race-specific rates measure the association between disease occurrence and race. Data on specific conditions indicate not only that some problems are more prevalent among nonwhites (blacks, American Indians, and Asiatics), but also that nonwhites fail to receive necessary care. For example, nonwhites are more than three times more likely to die of hypertension than whites of the same age group.[16] They are also more likely to die from other conditions resulting from untreated hypertension. For example, nonwhites face a 60% higher risk of dying of cerebrovascular disease than do whites and are almost four times as likely to die of hypertensive heart disease. They are also twice as likely as whites to die from diabetes and four times as likely to die of chronic kidney disease.

Ethnic and racial factors can help identify individuals at risk for various chronic diseases. For example, after 45 years of age nonwhite women in the United States have an incidence of diabetes about twice that of whites. Pima Indians in Arizona have a 50% incidence of diabetes among those 35 years of age and older. This is 10 times higher than the incidence of diabetes for the same age group in the United States.[16]

Cost of disability

For the individual and family the costs of disability are temporal, emotional, and financial. The goal of maintaining the patient in the best possible condition relative to the illness must be the primary concern, since a good program of maintenance is the best way to help the patient avoid excessive financial drain caused by unnecessary or preventable complications. Meeting the goal, however, can require that extensive periods of time be spent on treatments, maintenance regimens, and follow-up appointments. Further, each chronically ill person and family are subjected to great personal and emotional losses that must be dealt with—loss of self-esteem, loss of status within the family, loss of independence, feelings of rejection, and feelings of helplessness are only a few. These can be more devastating than economic deprivation.

The economic cost to the patient and family is considerable. The cost of hospitalization rises yearly. Frequent or extended hospitalization and medical expenses can be ruinous if the patient is inadequately insured or if he or she is unable to qualify for insurance programs.

Many are forced to seek public assistance merely to survive. Placement in quality nursing homes is frequently financially impossible for patients or their families to manage. The cost of medications to control or maintain a patient's health status may require a major portion of the family budget. Additional expenses may include special diets and equipment, home modifications (e.g., ramps or widening of doors for wheelchairs), transportation, and support services provided by homemakers, day or live-in attendants, or nurses.

The ability of the individual family to pay its own way is determined in part by which member of the family becomes disabled. Studies show that if the wife is disabled, the family suffers less economic deprivation than if the husband is disabled. However, three fourths of the chronically ill persons unable to carry on their major activity are men.[24]

Some financial assistance is provided by Medicare. This federally administrated program provides hospital and medical insurance protection for individuals 65 years of age and over as well as for people under 65 who are disabled and eligible for Social Security benefits. The Social Security Administration in 1972 was mandated by Congress to finance treatment for individuals with chronic kidney disease. An original estimate for the program was an annual cost of approximately $250 million; however, at the end of 4 years, the cost was double that amount. The estimated cost of the program by 1983, approximately 10 years after the start of the program, is $2.7 billion per year.[25]

In considering the cost of disability to the community, it must be realized that most individuals who are unable to work must be supported by others, either from private or from public funds. There are 3 million adults between the ages of 18 and 64 years who are unable to work because of chronic disabilities. There are an additional 9.4 million who are partially limited in their ability to work.[24]

Chronically ill persons and their families

The effects of chronic illness on individuals and their families are numerous and varied. The first impact of the disability may nearly immobilize them. Time must be provided them to talk through their concerns and fears before they can be expected to begin coping with their new situation.

Marked changes often take place, and are often required to take place, in family living as a result of chronic illness. Some families may find themselves drawn closer together. Other families may drift apart, the individual members being incapable of helping one another. At times, chronic illness may threaten an individual's basic emotional stability, and the whole situation may be unbearable to others. Sometimes the individual's emotional needs may not have been apparent to the family early in the illness, but when such needs grow obvious, relatives feel inadequate to cope with the situation. The length of illness, periodic hospitalizations, and increased financial, emotional, and social burdens are stressors that threaten the family's integrity.

Families with chronically ill children must face many difficulties. Among these difficulties are marital stresses. Sultz et al.[29] reported that 9% of the mothers in their study group felt that the ill child was a disruptive factor to their marriages. Problems contributing to weakening of the marriage included avoidance of sex for fear of having another sick child or of being unable to cope with another child along with the ill one, too little time left for each other after caring for the ill child and other children, and anxiety over finances. Disagreement between parents over what to expect from the sick child can also pose a problem. Indications are that suicide and divorce rates are higher in families with chronically ill children than in the general population. A divorce rate of nearly 50% was seen in one group of parents with children with meningomyelocele.[14]

Jealousy, insecurity, and resentment may be problems for the siblings of a chronically ill child. Since most children equate love with attention, it is perfectly normal for them to resent the child who receives more attention from the parents because of a chronic illness that requires treatments, special diets, and hospitalization. Furthermore, many parents feel their chronically ill child cannot be held to usual standards of behavior.[15] Again, if healthy siblings see differential treatment given to their ill sibling, they often interpret it as preferential. During angry outbursts at the ill child, siblings often wish the other child dead. If the child is then hospitalized or dies, they experience guilt.

Lastly, chronic illness can cause significant and permanent interference with the physical and emotional growth and development of the ill child and with the development of healthy family functioning. A large number of chronically ill children have psychologic and social handicaps secondary to their conditions. They exhibit more behavioral deviation and have significantly more problems with eating, bedtime activities, speech, temper, nervous tics, and body management than healthy children.[15]

Many persons struggle on their own to assume the full financial burden of the illness and consequently expose other members of the family to lower standards of nutrition, housing, and care. Many times relatives move in with one another, arguments develop, and family ties are strained or broken. Public assistance may be acceptable to some families, whereas others find it impossible to accept.

Chronic illness imposes additional problems of learning how to cope with restrictions on activities of daily living, how to prevent or identify medical crises that occur, and how to carry out treatment regimens as delineated by the health care provider. Family members also need to learn about the restrictions, not only to be of assistance to the chronically ill person, but also because their own activity patterns may be disrupted by the person's activities.

Since chronic illness may have periods of exacerbation when symptoms become more acute and medical crises may occur, patients and family members need to know which symptoms must be reported to the health care provider as well as the time interval for reporting these symptoms. They also need to know how to contact the provider and what measures to take if a medical crisis occurs. For example, the person who has a history of myocardial infarction as well as family members must know what to do if the person experiences severe chest pain. Should the person be taken immediately to a hospital emergency room or should the physician be contacted first? Patient and family should plan in advance the sequence of actions to take during a medical crisis, depending on the nature and extent of the presenting symptoms.

Persons with chronic illness are often labeled as "compliant" or "noncompliant" in carrying out regimens prescribed for them. There are many factors that influence the person's ability or motivation to carry out the prescribed regimen. If the person does not carry out the regimen (noncompliant), it does not necessarily mean that the individual is refusing to do so deliberately, although this may sometimes occur. One reason for noncompliance may be lack of knowledge of the importance of doing what is required because learning the appropriate regimen never occurred. The person may have been "told" the reason for the regimen, but he or she may not have perceived it or have internalized it. In many situations, however, there are other more influential factors for noncompliance: (1) time-consuming activities, (2) difficult techniques to learn or carry out, (3) presence of side effects, (4) expense, (5) visibility to others, (6) inefficient as perceived by clients, or (7) social isolation.[27] Social and cultural patterns will also affect compliance. (For further information on sociocultural effects, see Chapter 3.) Conflicts occur within the family structure when one family member recognizes the importance of carrying out the prescribed regimen but another does not. For example, a wife may see the need for continuing checkups and medication for her husband's hypertension, whereas he may perceive this as a needless expense since he feels well and has no symptoms. Persons vary from time to time in the extent of compliance. Individuals who are not hospitalized are their own health care agents and they (or their significant others) determine the actions that are taken.

Coping mechanisms that have been developed should not be tampered with unless, based on a thorough understanding of the situation, viable and more appropriate alternatives can be proposed. If the goal of maintaining the chronically ill person in the optimal state of health is being interfered with by the individual's or the family's attitudes or capacities, a change in those attitudes or capacities is necessary, but it must be a change that is mutually acceptable.

Epidemiology

Epidemiology examines the distribution of chronic disease as well as the measurement of health status in the general population. It is both a body of knowledge and a method for obtaining knowledge (see Chapter 5). As a methodology, epidemiology can be used to assist in explaining the multifactorial causal patterns of chronic diseases.

Problems in investigation of causality of chronic diseases

Some of the factors that contribute to the difficulty of studying the etiology of chronic disease are the following:

1. *Multifactorial nature of etiology.* The operation of multiple factors is particularly important in chronic diseases. The interaction of factors may be purely additive or it may be synergetic; that is, the combined potential for harm of many risk factors is more than the sum of the individual potentials. They interact, reinforce, and even multiply each other. Asbestos workers, for example, have increased lung cancer risk. Asbestos workers who smoke have 30 times more risk than coworkers who do not smoke and 90 times more risk than people who neither smoke nor work with asbestos.[32]

2. *Absence of a known agent.* Since there is no specific diagnostic test for many chronic diseases, the distinction between diseased and nondiseased persons may be more difficult to establish than in most infectious diseases.

3. *Long latent period.* Many chronic diseases have a long latent period, which is the equivalent of the incubation period in infectious disease except that it is generally longer. Because of the extended length of latency, it is often difficult to link antecedent events with outcomes. However, evidence is increasing that onset of ill health is strongly linked to influences of physical, social, economic, and family environments. It is easy to identify the common exposure to chickenpox in a school setting, but it is much more difficult to identify the impact of drastic alterations in family circumstances and resulting mental disorders or slow-onset physical illnesses.

4. *Indefinite onset.* The problem of pinpointing the initial occurrence of the disease exists with many chronic conditions such as degenerative diseases and mental illnesses. Because of the vague onset of chronic illnesses, it is difficult to collect statistics on the number of new cases in any given year.

5. *Differential effect of factors on incidence and course of disease.* Factors in the socioeconomic environment that affect health include income level, housing, and employment status. Another factor to consider is culture; for example, Mormons who abstain from smoking and alcohol have lower cancer rates than the general population as a whole.

6. *Disease-specific mortality rates.* These rates are difficult to determine with chronic illness because the cause of death may be due to factors other than the chronic disease itself.

One approach for studying chronic illness from an epidemiologic viewpoint is to emphasize that interrelated factors determine illness; that is, disease is a process that results from the breakdown of a multiplicity of factors: biologic, cultural, economic, emotional, and social. The multiple interactions involving the *host*, the *environment*, and the *agent* are sometimes described as the "web of causation." With this approach an attempt is made to identify the multiple related factors that lead to the disease process. Until a disease can be understood as a "web of causation," it is difficult to make rational decisions regarding therapeutic interventions, and it is even more difficult to identify early preventive actions. To develop a chain of causation, one must identify first the natural history of disease by systematic studies of groups of people.

Natural history of disease

All diseases have a natural history. For example, chronic diseases extend over time and develop through a sequence of stages. When people speak of the epidemiology of a disease, they are referring to its natural history. That is, the outcomes of a particular disease are observed over a period of time and the numbers of the affected persons developing each outcome are measured. This information is used to predict an individual's possible future health. Knowledge of the natural history of disease allows us to intervene to prevent or limit the effects of diseases. The stages involved in the natural history include the following:

1. *Stage of susceptibility.* The disease has not yet developed, but the groundwork has been laid by the presence of factors that favor its occurrence. These factors may be referred to as "risk factors." The need to

identify such factors is becoming more apparent as awareness grows that chronic diseases present our major health challenge. Some major risk factors are environmental and behavioral and therefore are amenable to change; for example, smokers can be persuaded to give up smoking.

2. *Stage of presymptomatic disease.* There is no manifestation of disease, but pathologic changes have begun. An example of presymptomatic disease is atherosclerotic changes in coronary vessels before any overt signs or symptoms of illness appear.

3. *Stage of clinical disease.* By this stage sufficient anatomic or functional changes have occurred so that there are recognizable signs of disease. At present there is incomplete understanding of the natural history of many diseases. For example, it is not known why some individuals with several risk factors do not progress to clinical disease while others with fewer risk factors do develop disease.

4. *Stage of disability.* Disability, which can result from an acute or chronic condition, reduces a person's activity. The extent of protracted disability resulting from chronic disease is of great significance to the person and to society because of the person's reduced income, the impact on psychosocial role, and the burden on community resources.

The subtlety of the natural history of chronic diseases often leaves the person unaware of a disease process for an extended period. Recently, predisposing characteristics or habits that help identify the person at risk to develop a particular chronic disease have been studied extensively. By altering habits of eating, rest, activity, or smoking, the course of certain chronic illnesses such as emphysema, hypertension, or heart disease may be changed. Unfortunately, many chronic conditions begin without the individual's awareness of significant physiologic changes. An important step in prevention is early detection of these changes.

Prevention

Because chronic disease evolves over time and pathologic changes may become irreversible, the goal is to detect risk factors as early as possible. Although the degenerative diseases differ from their infectious disease predecessors in having more complex causes, it is now clear that many are preventable.

Generally, prevention means inhibiting the development of a disease before it occurs. More specifically, the term includes several levels of prevention to interrupt or slow the progression of disease: (1) primary prevention, (2) secondary prevention, and (3) tertiary prevention. Primary prevention, appropriate in the stage of susceptibility, is concerned with health promotion and specific protection against diseases. Secondary preven-

tion, applied in presymptomatic and clinical disease, includes early detection and prompt intervention to halt the progression of the disease. Tertiary prevention, appropriate in the stage of disability, uses rehabilitation activities to prevent further complications and to restore optimal functioning as much as possible.[7]

Another way of looking at prevention has been identified by Albee.[1] He has developed a "prevention equation" for preventing dysfunction:

$$\text{Incidence of dysfunction} = \frac{\text{Stress + Constitutional vulnerabilities}}{\text{Social supports + Coping skills + Competence}}$$

The two major strategies for preventing dysfunction are decreasing the values in the numerator (i.e., decreasing stress or constitutional vulnerabilities) and increasing the values in the denominator (i.e., increasing social supports, coping skills, and competence). It is more difficult to have an impact on the numerator of the prevention equation since stress in our lives cannot always be controlled, but creative ways to decrease individual and societal stress must continually be sought. It is easier to affect the denominator by strengthening social supports, coping skills, and competence.[1]

One valuable tool that has been developed to assist clients to identify their own risk factors and hopefully help them change their life-styles is the health hazard appraisal (HHA).[6] The HHA is a screening process that includes a comprehensive questionnaire and the taking of certain physical measurements. Based on probability tables, a risk assessment is then calculated from each client's profile along with goals that would result in risk reduction. Counseling and follow-up are provided to reinforce the data.

Assessment

Before a plan of care can be devised for the chronically ill person, a thorough assessment of needs and capabilities must be carried out. Included in such an assessment are the individual's physical, psychologic, social, and financial status.

Physical status

Since medical diagnoses do not accurately reflect the physical status and functioning of the chronically ill person, the use of a profile system or assessment tool may be instituted as a guide for those working with the patient. One such tool[40] provides a guide for grading the patient in six different categories: (1) physical condition including cardiovascular, pulmonary, gastrointestinal, genitourinary, endocrine, or cerebrovascular disorders; (2) upper extremities, structure and function, including the shoulder girdle and cervical and upper dorsal spine; (3) lower extremities, structure and function, including the pelvis and lower dorsal and lumbar sacral spine; (4) sensory components relating to speech, vision, and hearing; (5) excretory function, including the bowels and bladder; and (6) mental and emotional status. The ability of the person to carry out activities of daily living (e.g., dressing, feeding, bathing, brushing teeth, combing hair, toileting, and moving from place to place) specifically need to be assessed. The completed assessment should indicate in what areas the patient has difficulty and the extent of that difficulty. Such a guide can be used in planning care, both immediate and long term, and will be useful in assisting the individual and the family to make realistic plans for care. Since a chronic condition is not static, reassessment should be carried out at regular intervals whether there is improvement or regression.

Psychologic status

Assessment of the individual's psychologic needs and capabilities includes determining attitudes and stage of adaptation to the illness, feelings concerning how illness affects the family or significant others, and the person's own goals in regard to living with an illness.[35] For example, individuals who are almost totally helpless as a result of an accidental spinal cord injury may seem to have no interest in learning ways to help themselves. Their families may react in the same manner and be of little help to them. Both the individuals and their families need interest and support from professional persons as they learn to cope with the change in their life situations.

Feelings of anxiety, frustration, irritability, bitterness, and guilt may be expressed by some chronically ill persons who face unending pain and loss of economic and social security. Some persons become hypochondriacal, obsessed with their health problems, and spend much of each day thinking about what will happen and what to do. Guilt may result from being unable to work and support oneself or from the belief, as a result of a search for some purpose or reason for the affliction, that one must deserve the suffering.

Social and financial status

Social and financial status must be considered, as they relate specifically to the kind of support and resources available to the individuals in meeting their goals. It would be unrealistic, for example, to plan for a hydraulic bathtub chair if the patient could not afford it, family members were unavailable to help operate it, or

the patient's apartment manager would not permit it to be installed. Alternative methods of helping the patient to take a tub bath would have to be explored.

The social assessment includes living arrangements, family roles, support of significant others, cultural and social group memberships, education, and vocational and avocational activities. The data collected through the performance of this kind of thorough assessment should make it possible to devise a plan of care directed toward the accomplishment of attainable goals that are mutually acceptable to the patient, the family, and the care givers.

Intervention

Chronically ill persons and their families require long-term care. The nursing profession has been concerned with chronic health problems and the challenge involved in providing long-term nursing care to chronically ill individuals and their families.

The American Academy of Nursing has made a statement regarding long-term care:

Long-term care is the provision of that range of services—physical, psychological, spiritual, and social, including socioeconomic—needed to help people attain, maintain, or regain their optimal level of functioning. It includes health maintenance throughout the life span as well as care during acute and protracted illness and disability. Such care is the legitimate province of nurses who now are making social contributions through health teaching and promotion, prevention of illness, and rehabilitation.[2]

In the past nursing has followed the general pattern of providing health services by placing the emphasis on acute and episodic care rather than on health promotion and health maintenance. However, there is an emerging consensus among the health community that the health strategy must be changed dramatically to emphasize the prevention of disease. In the same vein, the American Academy of Nursing has proposed that "nursing assume major responsibility for health promotion, maintenance, and teaching within the context of its definition of long-term care."[2]

Physical considerations

The first focus in intervention for the chronically ill person is on prevention and reduction of disability and on enabling the person to remain a socially functioning individual in every respect. Some of the disability seen among the chronically ill might have been prevented if prompt, aggressive, suitable medical and nursing care had been available at the onset of the illness. Many of the difficulties that limit the chronically ill may not have been caused by the disease itself but may have developed because of immobility during the acute phase of the illness.

Keeping the person's body in good alignment, maintaining joint range and strength, and preventing decubitus ulcers are physical measures that must constantly be borne in mind. (For further information see Chapter 41.) A careful plan of rest and activity helps preserve physical resources and makes the day purposeful. If assistance is needed, it should be given until the persons can manage the activity by themselves or until an alternative method of management can be taught.

Second, recognizing what is meaningful to the individual is a primary step toward helping develop self-care. Physical needs become of paramount importance to chronically ill persons. Meeting these physical needs provides a way to convey to such individuals an interest in their progress and welfare. Helping them to take their own baths, to attend to toilet needs, and to groom themselves can give some sense of accomplishment and help them maintain their self-respect. Helping them to be dressed appropriately promotes a sense of wellness. Success in performing portions of their own self-care may be stimulating enough to strengthen the persons' motivation so that they and their families may make amazing strides in thinking through and working out future problems themselves. In order for their planning to be realistic and ultimately functional, all health care personnel must teach chronically ill persons the total physiologic ramifications of their disability as well as methods of coping with those ramifications.

Persons who are in their homes or in substitute homes should be encouraged to dress in regular, comfortable street clothing rather than in pajamas or gowns. Visitors coming into the home and members of the family who constantly see such individuals dressed in bedclothes think of them as sick and are reminded of their illness. Seeing them dressed as they ordinarily would be helps to maintain normal attitudes, relationships, and expectations.

Psychosocial considerations

The care of chronically ill persons requires alertness of feeling, seeing, and hearing. Continued warmth and interest are necessary to the well-being of any chronically ill person. Very often it is a relationship based on an understanding of these requirements that helps the individual to become highly motivated. It may be taxing to listen to the same questions and to say the same things day after day, but the nature of chronic illness may require this attention, and the manner in which responses are given will convey warmth and interest. The world of chronically ill persons, whether they are

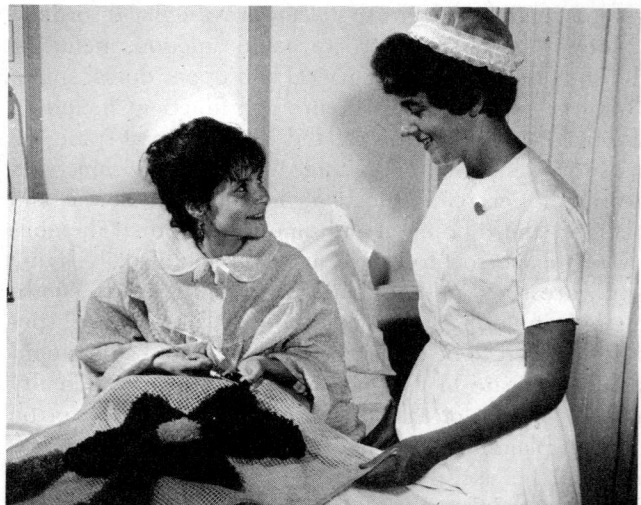

Fig. 29-1. Occupational therapy provides patient with purposeful activity. Interest shown by nurse encourages patient to complete project.

in the hospital or elsewhere, becomes narrowed and circumscribed. They treasure and are interested in those things and those people who are close to them. Their conversations may be largely about themselves, their immediate environment, a few close objects, and the persons who are close to them. Although they may be confined to bed and to their room, others can keep them up-to-date on outside news. Depending on their level of adaptation to their illness, they may welcome hearing about outside events, or they may not be able to think beyond themselves. When they reach the stage of being able to look beyond themselves, newspapers, magazines, radio, television, or creating something with their own hands (Fig. 29-1) may help to keep up their interest in others and in outside events.

Coping skills may be challenged by persistent, ongoing problems such as chronic pain, recurring medical expenses, or continuing difficulties in carrying out activities of daily living. Usual coping methods may become impossible; for example, a person who usually copes by expending energy in physical activity may become unable to do so. The person who usually copes by discussing problems with family members will need to find an alternative method if family communication patterns break down. The person can be helped to identify usual coping methods and to explore alternative approaches when necessary (see Chapter 12).

It is important to recognize that chronically ill persons or their families may suffer from unresolved sadness known as chronic grief. Chronic grief may be defined as accumulated or prolonged grief. Chronic grief extends over long periods of time with permanent characteristics in a large number of sufferers. It carries with it a potential for decreased functioning. The causes are varied, and new waves of grief are constantly triggered. One example is that of the mother of the retarded child who has accepted her situation and is coping well, but over and over is faced with unattainable goals, repeated frustrations, and an uncertain future. Another example is grief caused by the losses associated with aging: youth, dreams, jobs, hair, friends, family, health, visual acuity, social role, money, body parts, and mobility. Each loss is accompanied by grief, which builds on previous grief like bricks placed by the mason creating a wall. In chronic grief the patient may be faced with repeated acute episodes. These episodes may coincide with exacerbation of the condition, facing a new limitation, or meeting new indignities. Each new episode requires a renewed struggle back and forth through the various stages of grief.[27]

The nurse can assist by listening and helping the person explore feelings and the content related to these feelings. Since the grief is ongoing, family members can also be helped to identify their feelings and to strengthen the communication patterns within the family structure for mutual support of its members.

Those who work with chronically ill persons need to be able to distinguish between their own values, standards, and goals and those of the patient. In day-to-day contact with individuals who are making little or no progress, it is tempting to make plans for their future because of a sincere interest in helping them. This is particularly true when the patient's age is similar to one's own. There may be a feeling that something must be done to speed progress. One may become frustrated by the feeling of wanting to do something or wanting to see some marked change. However, it must be recognized that management of chronically ill persons requires a slow-moving, persistent pace with possibly little or no change for a long time. The person's physical and mental condition must be maintained at its present level or improved, and effort must be made to further progress and to encourage the family's adaptation to the patient's condition. Eagerness and readiness to progress will be determining factors for the future. The "doing" in the care of the chronically ill person is not always an active, physical "doing" with the hands. Many times the maintenance of a positive approach and attitude and a demonstration of real interest are the greatest help to the patient. Teaching patients to perform activities related to their own care independently rather than performing those activities for them may also lead to progress.

Health care personnel must also be prepared to provide care for those patients whose disease will follow a course of inexorably progressive disability, for example, multiple sclerosis or rheumatoid arthritis. In these instances, goals of care must be modified to retard the downhill progression of disability rather than to achieve maintenance or improvement of physical status. Help-

ing the patient and family cope with progressive deterioration and, in some cases, eventual death is a demanding task. Those who wish additional information relating to this aspect of care are referred to the literature treating this subject.[27,35]

Community activities

There has been an increasing interest in providing programs for the chronically ill and in assisting chronically ill or disabled persons to assume a more active role in their communities. Volunteer workers may act as readers both in hospitals and in homes (Fig. 29-2). Institutions receiving federal funds are required to make aids such as ramps available to individuals who are unable to climb stairs or who are in wheelchairs. With the development of structural changes that facilitate mobility, some persons with physical limitations are becoming more actively involved in local activities and associations. Nurses can assist by supporting the further development of these structural changes in all community buildings and by encouraging the participation of chronically ill persons in community activities of interest. Various kinds of information may be obtained from national organizations involved with chronic illness and disability. Many of these agencies have services available in the community (see box, pp. 566 to 568). Programs, facilities, and legislation of this nature reflect an increasing awareness on the part of the public of the difficulties that are faced by the chronically ill or disabled.

Rehabilitation

Rehabilitation is the process of assisting the individual with a handicap to realize his or her particular goals, physically, mentally, socially, and economically. As such, "rehabilitation" is an active concept and must be clearly differentiated from the concept of "maintenance" care. Following a thorough assessment of patients' disabilities and capabilities, assumptions can be made regarding the potential for improving their condition. If improvement can be made, patients are candidates for rehabilitation. If improvement cannot be made, care is directed toward maintaining the current condition, that is, preventing further disability. The process of rehabilitation can be viewed more appropriately as patient education rather than patient "care." It must be remembered, however, that the rehabilitation of every patient will reach an end point; that is, a point at which no further progress is possible. At that point, the focus of care reverts to that of maintenance.

The purpose or extent of rehabilitation ranges from employment or reemployment for the handicapped

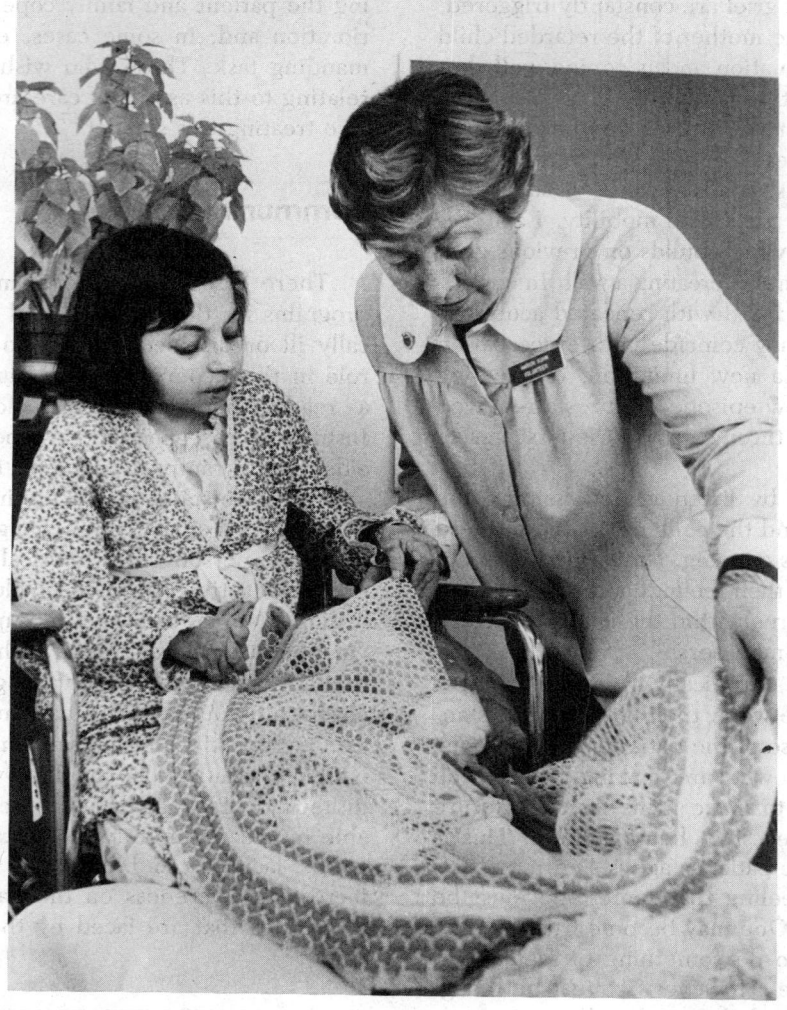

Fig. 29-2. Volunteer helping patient who has a chronic illness with some handwork.

COMMUNITY RESOURCES INVOLVED IN CHRONIC HEALTH PROBLEMS

Various kinds of information may be obtained by writing these national organizations. In addition, services of the various agencies are usually available at the local level.

General

American Association of Diabetes Education
3553 W. Peterson Ave.
Chicago, IL 60659

American Association or Retired Persons
1909 K St., N.W.
Washington, DC 20006

American Cancer Society
777 3rd Ave.
New York, NY 10017

American Diabetes Association
1 W. 48th St.
New York, NY 10020

American Heart Association
44 E. 23rd St.
New York, NY 10010

American Lung Association
1740 Broadway
New York, NY 10019

American Parkinson Disease Association
147 E. 50th St.
New York, NY 10022

COMMUNITY RESOURCES INVOLVED IN CHRONIC HEALTH PROBLEMS—CONT'D

Arthritis Foundation
221 Park Ave. S.
New York, NY 10003

Easter Seal Society for Crippled Children and Adults
2023 W. Ogden Ave.
Chicago, IL 60612

Juvenile Diabetes Foundation
23 E. 26th St.
New York, NY 10010

Leukemia Society of America, Inc.
211 E. 43rd St.
New York, NY 10017

Mental Health Materials Center
419 Park Ave. S.
New York, NY 10016

Muscular Dystrophy Association, Inc.
810 7th Ave.
New York, NY 10019

National Aid to Retarded Citizens (formerly N.A.R. Children)
2709 E. St.
Arlington, TX 76011

National Association for Down's Syndrome
628 Ashland Ave.
River Forest, IL 60305

National Association for Mental Health, Inc.
1800 N. Kent St.
Rosslyn Station
Arlington, VA 22209

National Association for Sickle Cell Disease, Inc.
945 S. Western Ave., Suite 206
Los Angeles, CA 90006

National Association for Visually Handicapped
305 E. 24th St.
New York, NY 10010

National Asthma Center
875 Avenue of the Americas
New York, NY 10001

National Council on the Aging
1828 L. St. NW
Washington, DC 20036

National Cystic Fibrosis Research Foundation
3379 Peachtree Rd. N.E.
Atlanta, GA 30326

National Epilepsy League
6 N. Michigan Ave.
Chicago, IL 60602

National Foundation—March of Dimes
1275 Mamaroneck Ave.
White Plains, NY 10605

National Genetics Foundation
250 W. 57th St.
New York, NY 10019

National Hemophilia Foundation
Room 903
25 W. 39th St.
New York, NY 10018

National Kidney Foundation
116 E. 27th St.
New York, NY 10016

National Multiple Sclerosis Society
205 E. 42nd St.
New York, NY 10017

Nutrition Foundation, Inc.
489 5th Ave.
New York, NY 10017

Parents of Down's Syndrome Children
11507 Yates St.
Silver Spring, MD 20902

Shriners Hospital for Crippled Children
323 N. Michigan Ave.
Chicago, IL 60601

Stroke Clubs of America
805 12th St.
Galveston, TX 77550

United Cerebral Palsy Association, Inc.
66 E. 34th St.
New York, NY 10066

United Ostomy Association
1111 Wilshire Blvd.
Los Angeles, CA 90017

Rehabilitation

American Coalition of Citizens with Disabilities
1346 Connecticut Ave. N.W., Rm. 817
Washington, DC 20036

Architectural and Transportation Barriers Compliance Board
330 C St. W.W., Rm. 1010
Washington, DC 20201

Closer Look, National Information Center for the Handicapped
Box 1492
Washington, DC 20013

Mainstream, Inc.
1200 15th St., N.W., Rm. 403
Washington, DC 20005

National Center for a Barrier-free Environment
8401 Connecticut Ave.
Washington, DC 20015

National Center for Law and the Handicapped
1235 N. Eddy St.
South Bend, IN 46617

Continued.

COMMUNITY RESOURCES INVOLVED IN CHRONIC HEALTH PROBLEMS—CONT'D

National Congress of Organizations of the Physically
  Handicapped
7611 Oakland Ave.
Minneapolis, MN 55432

National Paraplegia Foundation
333 N. Michigan Ave.
Chicago, IL 60601

Paralyzed Veterans of America
7315 Wisconsin Ave. N.W.
Washington, DC 20014

President's Committee on Employment of the Handicapped
111 20th St., N.W., Rm. 636
Washington, DC 20210

Prevention/wellness

American Association of Fitness Directors in Business and
  Industry
President's Council on Physical Fitness and Sports
Room 3030
400 Sixth Ave. S.W.
Washington, DC 20201

Bureau of Health Education
Centers for Disease Control
Atlanta, GA 30333

Center for Health Promotion
American Hospital Association
840 N. Lake Shore Dr.
Chicago, IL 60611

Know Your Body Project
American Health Foundation
320 East 43rd St.
New York, NY 10017

Society of Prospective Medicine
Department of Family Medicine
University of South Florida
12901 North 30th St.
Tampa, FL 33612

Well Aware About Health
University of Arizona Health Sciences Center
P. O. Box 43338
Tucson, AZ 85733

Wellness Associates
42 Miller Ave.
Mill Valley, CA 94941

Wholistic Health Center
137 S. Garfield Ave.
Hinsdale, IL 60521

---

person to the more limited achievement of developing the ability to give his or her own daily care. This latter accomplishment can be just as important to the individual as earning money and may represent that person's greatest life achievement. This might be true, for example, for a person who was born with a severe physical handicap such as cerebral palsy.

Considerations for ongoing care

Success in learning to adjust to living with a disability will depend on the person's premorbid personality, total life experience, and premorbid family relationships, as well as the current behavior and motivation the person presents. Certainly, some rehabilitation can occur in any health agency; nevertheless, the greater the number of rehabilitation disciplines that can be made available as needed to individuals, the greater is their chance of achieving their highest potential. The rehabilitative process, as with any form of education, is involved as deeply in the motives and purposes of the teacher as in those of the learner.[44]

Persons with a disability, whether it is obvious to others or unrecognizable, should not be viewed from the standpoint of their disability alone. Usually the greatest need is for comprehensive health services and continuing care. Comprehensive care is that which is provided to patients according to their needs in an appropriate, continuous, and dynamic pattern. Accommodating the plan of care to the needs and goals of individual patients rather than to those of the providers of care is the essence of comprehensive care.

Teamwork and special services in rehabilitation

The number of professional people required to assist the patient and family with rehabilitation will vary. Most often the patient, the family, the physician, and the nurse can work out a practical plan. If a patient's problems are complex, other members may be added to the team. Typically, such a team consists of a physician, nurse, medical social worker, vocational counselor, psychologist, speech pathologist, occupational and physical therapists, and a caseworker from the patient's social agency. Teamwork requires that members of the team be able to use their special knowledge and skill and understand the value of their contribution to the patient's care. In addition, team members need some understanding of each other's professional functions and contributions. One of the cooperative efforts of the involved team members

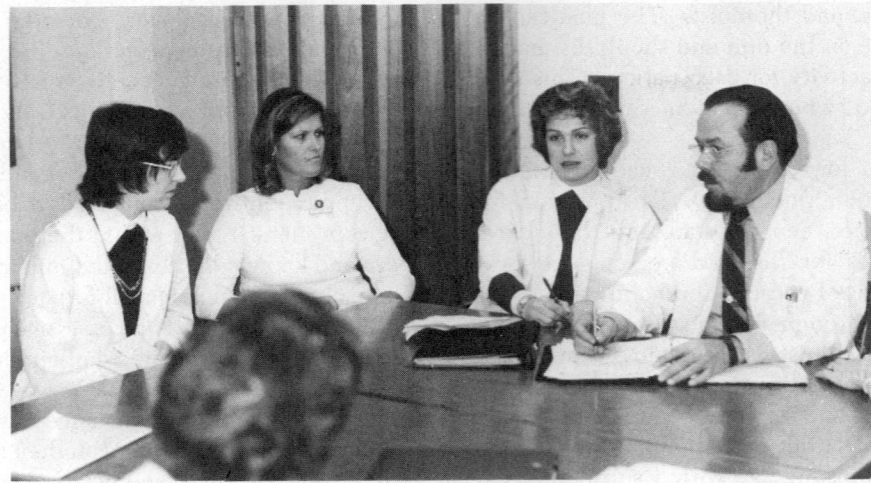

Fig. 29-3. Team approach to rehabilitation is essential. Here, physician, nurse, physical therapist, social worker, and occupational therapist review a patient's program and progress.

is to meet regularly to thoroughly evaluate patients and their abilities. Based on this assessment, each patient and the team devise a plan to foster readjustment, compensation, and the learning of new ways of managing self-care and living. In Fig. 29-3 some of the members of a team review a patient's rehabilitation program.

Persons with very complex problems of rehabilitation may need to receive care at specialized centers for rehabilitation or they may receive care at home combined with visits to day rehabilitation centers. The variety of specialized centers includes teaching and research centers (centers located in and operated by hospitals and medical schools), community centers with facilities for inpatients, community out-patient centers, insurance centers, and vocational rehabilitation centers. In addition to centers that provide multiple services for the physically disabled, there are specialized centers for rehabilitation of the blind, deaf, mentally ill, and mentally retarded. Most centers offer a wide range of services that usually fall into three areas:

Physical area

Physical, nursing, and medical evaluation
Physical therapy
Occupational therapy
Speech therapy
Medical and nursing supervision of appropriate activities

Psychosocial area

Evaluation
Personal counseling
Social service
Psychometrics
Psychiatric service
Recreational therapy

Vocational area

Work evaluation
Vocational counseling
Prevocational experience
Industrial fitness of programs
Trial employment in sheltered workshops
Vocational training
Terminal employment in sheltered workshops
Placement

There are several advantages for patients participating in organized programs for rehabilitation. They have an opportunity to see and be with others who have similar or more extensive disabilities. Often they progress more rapidly when they realize that others have similar difficulties and are overcoming them. Group therapy often arouses a competitive spirit, and a formerly reluctant person may become willing and diligent. On the other hand, all personnel need to be alert to those patients who have had the opposite reaction. Patients who see others advance in activity while they either do not improve or progress very slowly may become so discouraged that they give up trying.

On a rehabilitation unit activities are scaled so that individuals can see their own progress in comparison with their beginning abilities. Patients may take an active interest in keeping their own scores. After a program of therapy has been planned and is scheduled as to time of day, patients can help to keep themselves on the schedule by having a copy of it at the bedside. Individuals can then be helped to gradually assume more and more responsibility for getting themselves ready for scheduled activities. In addition, a master plan of activities for all patients on the unit can be a useful device for nurses, physicians, and therapists. The plan can be kept in a central place on the unit and should list name, activity, and time of activity for each patient. This type of plan is helpful, too, when a patient's progress is to be reevaluated.

A public program for vocational rehabilitation has been serving the nation since 1920. The program involves a partnership between the state and the federal governments. Services for disabled persons are provided by state divisions of vocational rehabilitation. The federal government, through the Social and Rehabilitation Service (SRS), administers grants-in-aid and provides technical assistance and national leadership for the program. Opportunities and services are available in each of the 50 states, the District of Columbia, and Puerto Rico. All persons of working age with a substantial job handicap resulting from either physical or mental impairment are eligible for help or assistance. The purpose of this service is to preserve, develop, or restore the ability of disabled persons to earn their own livings. The individual services offered are medical care, counseling and guidance, training, and job finding. All 50 states have separate rehabilitation programs for the blind. Application for such services can be made to the SRS or to the agency in the state for serving the blind.

Nurse's role in rehabilitation

The concepts of comprehensive nursing care and rehabilitation can be considered synonymous. Helping the patient and the family to help themselves is an integral part of nursing care. Nurses who work with patients who have disabilities have two major responsibilities: (1) to see that disability from disease is limited as much as possible and (2) to see that a rehabilitation program is planned and implemented. Limitation of disability requires attention to the prevention of complications, to the early recognition of symptoms of exacerbations or complications, and to the prevention of deformity. For patients with chronic illnesses, the onset of exacerbations or complications is frequently subtle, marked by minute changes in functional ability or general performance or attitude. Nurses, working closely with such patients and understanding the pathophysiology of their diseases, are frequently the first to recognize initial signs of difficulty and to make provision for appropriate intervention.

The second responsibility, planning and implementing a program of rehabilitation in accordance with the patient's goals, is a process in which nurses are intimately involved. Nursing personnel are likely to be in contact with a patient and the family for a greater period of time each day than are members of any other single discipline on the rehabilitation team. Both in the hospital and in the home, nurses are in an excellent position to plan a reasonable care program with the patient, as well as to teach the patient, the family, and, if necessary, the employer about the patient's limitations and rehabilitative expectations.

Much of the nursing activity in the rehabilitation process is no different from the nursing care given to all patients. Measures such as appropriate bowel and bladder programs, providing proper diet and fluid requirements, and implementing new methods of bathing and maintaining skin integrity fall within the domain of nursing concern and knowledge. Initially, nursing personnel may assume almost total responsibility for performing these activities for the patient. After assessing patient needs in these areas, nurses formulate, implement, and evaluate a teaching plan in much the same way as do therapists from other disciplines. The assistance nurses can give the patient and family will depend on their ability to understand self, personal feelings, and personal behavior as well as the behavior of the patient, family, and other professional team members.

One of the most important aspects of giving continuing care to a patient with a disability is the nurse's own attitude, perseverance, and expectations. Improvement may be slow, and patients may reach a "plateau" in their progress. Such a time can be critical for patients because they may become discouraged and not wish to continue with their program of care. Realistic encouragement can often sustain patients so that they will not regress until some improvement is noted.

Patients in a rehabilitation program must often learn and practice special physical techniques to strengthen muscles and to improve mobility. Such measures as physical exercise to improve walking, activities to improve self-care abilities, and the use of prostheses require the special knowledge and skills of physical and occupational therapists. To be effective in the rehabilitation process, nurses must have an understanding of the techniques used by the various therapists so that they can plan and work cooperatively with them in caring for the patient. This knowledge is also used to help the patient employ appropriate techniques in carrying out activities of daily living (ADL).

Patient's role in rehabilitation

The most important contributions to patients' rehabilitation are made by the patients themselves. The patient, the nurse, the physician, the social worker, the occupational therapist (Fig. 29-4), and sometimes others planning together can arrive at the best plans for the future, but the patient's attitudes, acceptance, and direction of motivation are the most important considerations. If the patient cannot adjust to the disability, whatever it may be and however extensive it may be, attempts at rehabilitation usually are hindered. Patients are the persons who really make the decisions, and they change at their own pace. If they are agreeable to suggestions but make little or no effort to try them, one should question if they really have accepted them.

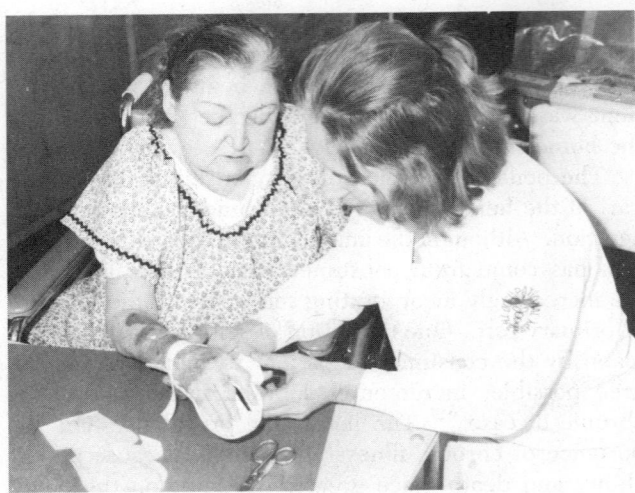

Fig. 29-4. Occupational therapist makes resting splint for patient whose hands are severely deformed by rheumatoid arthritis. Splint will be worn by patient in effort to prevent further deformity.

Self-care is encouraged within existing limitations. The patient's behavior from day to day can be the first indication of the direction of positive motivation. For example, if the patient makes every effort to resume normal daily activities such as feeding, bathing, and dressing, one can be quite certain that this is a person with a sincere desire to be independent. As patients become ready for more advanced activities such as ambulation and work in the occupational therapy shop, they need continuing genuine interest and support (Figs. 29-5 and 29-6). As obstacles present themselves, patients may be able to accept them and eventually overcome them. Patients who are truly motivated toward helping themselves never seem to give up, finding ways of accomplishing activities that professional personnel might believe impossible. Each person working with the chronically ill has seen that many times life has meaning for the individual even though it may not be readily apparent to others. However, there are some patients

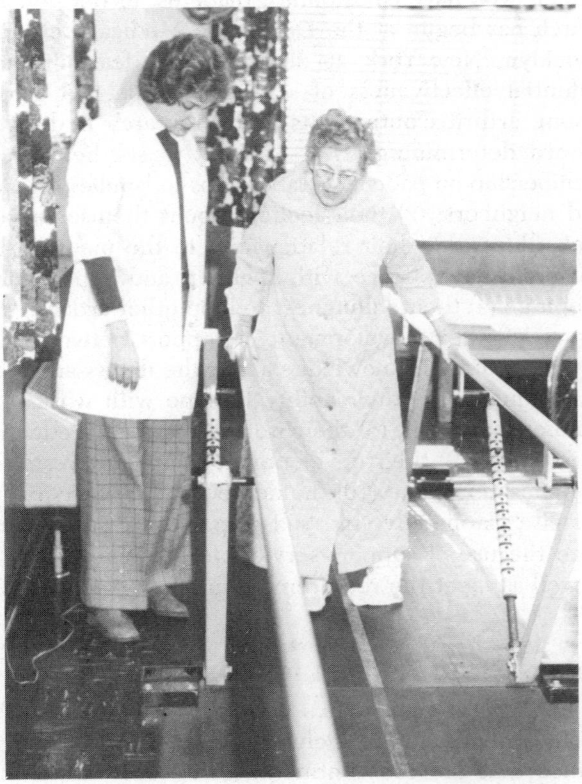

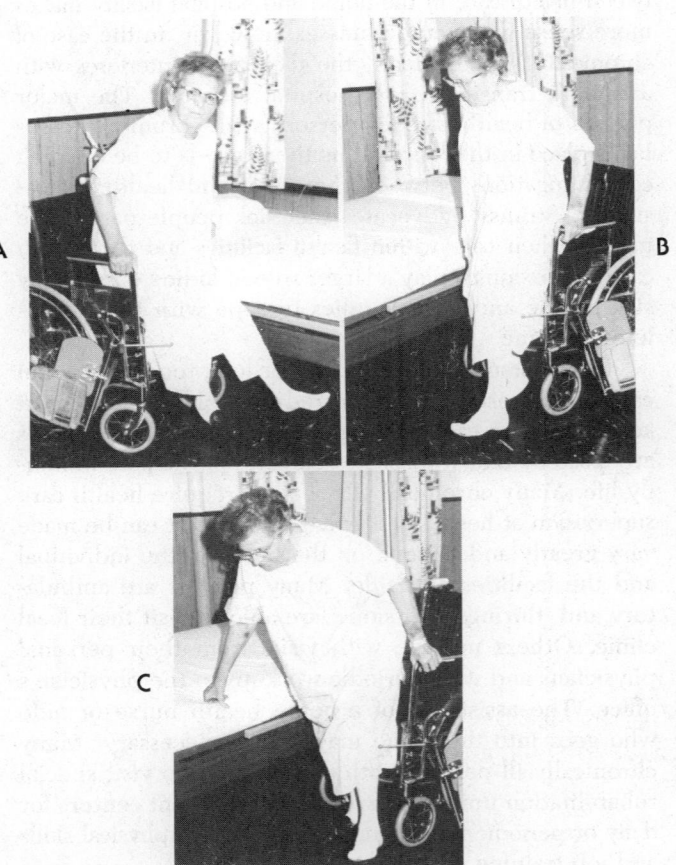

Fig. 29-6. A, Patient executes transfer from bed to chair. She is not bearing weight on her left leg; thus she moves toward her right, or strong side. **B,** Here, patient moves back into bed from wheelchair, again leading with her right, or strong side. She pushes up from chair, using arms of chair for support. **C,** Patient places her right hand on the bed for support, pivots on her right foot, and sits down.

Fig. 29-5. Physical therapist begins patient's ambulation training by teaching her to walk with support of parallel bars. Patient's left foot is wrapped in a towel to remind her not to bear weight on it.

who, when faced with an added burden, cannot accept it and give up trying. Guidance and support for the families of such patients become tremendously important. Health care personnel who understand these attitudes and behaviors can help make life more satisfying for the chronically ill person and can positively influence the behaviors of the family, professional co-workers, and the public.

Continuing care

Considerations for continuing care

Traditionally, health care professionals have assumed responsibility for the patient's well-being within the hospital and little to no responsibility for the client and family in the home setting. This dichotomy between health care in the home and hospital facility makes more sense with acute illnesses; however, in the case of chronically ill individuals, the dichotomy interferes with a smooth transition from hospital to home. The major portion of health care for persons with chronic illnesses takes place in the home; thus there needs to be ongoing communications between the client and health professionals. Strauss[27] advocates that sick people participate more in their care within health facilities and that health care professionals play a larger role in aiding chronically sick people and their families to cope with their problems at home.

Most persons with a chronic or long-term illness can care for themselves or be cared for at home, and most actually prefer to be at home, where family and friends are close by and where they can still participate in family life. Many chronically ill persons require health care supervision at home. The arrangements that can be made vary greatly and depend on the needs of the individual and the facilities available. Many persons are ambulatory and, during remissions, are able to visit their local clinic. Others manage with visits from their personal physicians and with periodic workups in the physician's office. The assistance of a home health nurse or aide who goes into the home may also be necessary. Many chronically ill persons with disabilities also visit special rehabilitation units of hospitals or outpatient centers for daily or periodic instruction and practice in physical skills and job training.

Nurses from voluntary and official health agencies help the chronically ill in their homes. Nurses who visit the home to assist the individual or family members to accomplish daily care will need to understand the patient. Chronically ill persons are very often misjudged by even the closest members of the family because of blinding emotional ties or lack of knowledge and under-

standing. Families need to be helped to understand the limitations and necessary restrictions on the patients. Hopefully this process will have begun while the patient was hospitalized, but it will need to continue in the home setting.

The benefits and the necessity of self-care as a valid part of the health care system are undergoing new recognition. Although the main impetus for this recognition has come from consumers, health care providers are increasingly incorporating self-care into the delivery of primary care. One definition of self-care is "an action taken by the consumer or patient to reduce to the degree possible, incremental debilitation resulting from chronic disease."[17] The increasing prevalence and importance of chronic illness as a principal cause of disability and death place greater demands on the client and family for involvement in self-care.

Self-help groups are associated with self-care. These groups may or may not include the guidance of health care providers. They provide social support to their members through the creation of a caring community, and they increase members' coping skills through the sharing of information, experiences, and problem solutions. Examples of self-help groups include those for women who have had mastectomies and those for individuals who have colostomies, diabetes, or obesity. Research has begun at the Downstate Medical Center in Brooklyn, New York, to determine the feasibility and potential effectiveness of self-help mutual aid groups among arthritis outpatients.[1] The research is directed toward determining (1) the impact of self-help group membership on patients' relationships to families, friends, and neighbors; (2) their feelings about themselves and their illness; (3) their relationships to the medical staff (including compliance with regimen and appointment keeping); (4) their willingness to help other arthritis sufferers; (5) their development of support networks and hotlines; (6) their knowledge about the illness and ways of treating it; (7) their ability to cope with work, life, families, and pain; (8) their isolation and any reduction in isolation; (9) their development of new interests and compensations; and (10) the degree of their activity and exercise. Hopefully, the self-help modality will maximize the use of support services for the chronically ill as well as meet the requirement for cost effectiveness.

Patterns and facilities for continuing care

It is impossible to include here all of the many facilities that provide continuing care. Only those programs that have been developed or emphasized recently will be covered. It must also be noted that each of the programs that will be mentioned has its own criteria for acceptance of patients for the services it renders. Before application for service is made, a determination of the individual patient's eligibility for that service must be carried out.

Ambulatory care

The term *ambulatory care* is used interchangeably with *outpatient care* and refers to first contact health care services as well as to continuing contact services in settings that do not require overnight stays. There has been a marked increase in the use of ambulatory care facilities because of the increase of chronic illness and the increase in cost of inpatient services. A good ambulatory care service constitutes one of the most important elements of the hospital's contribution to community health. There is a trend toward development of ambulatory care facilities in neighborhood health centers to assist the disabled, the aged, or the disadvantaged person obtain needed health care. An ambulatory care center usually provides long-term follow-up care needed by the person with a chronic illness, in addition to preventive health care, diagnostic workups, and treatment of acute illnesses for which hospitalization is unnecessary.

Home care

Before the 1940s the home was the place where medical treatment was given. Well-to-do persons rarely thought of going into a hospital, and they received the services of a private physician in their own home. The family was responsible for the day-to-day care. Poor families were among the first persons to use hospitals. The philosophy of home care can be traced as far back as 1796, when the Boston Dispensary provided medical care to the sick poor in their homes. One of the first institutions to study and demonstrate the advantages of continuous medical care for patients at home was University Hospital in Syracuse, New York, in 1940. By 1950, 16 New York City hospitals were offering this service. In 1959 the Commission on Chronic Illness defined care of the aged and disabled as one of the foremost national health problems and recommended the development of home nursing care as an alternative to institutionalization.

One of the most obvious reasons for the development of home care programs was to provide care to patients with long-term illnesses who did not need the around-the-clock services of an institution and yet who were too ill to go to an outpatient center. Caring for patients at home is what the individual and the family often want, and it also releases hospital beds for use by acutely ill patients.

Frequently the issue arises as to who should pay for home health services and who should be reimbursed for health care provided. The American Nurses Association's (ANA's) position is that reimbursement systems should foster care of individuals in their homes based on the following premises[4]:

1. Home care is humane and respectful of the dignity and integrity of the individual.
2. Home care or care within the community can be less costly than institutional care.
3. Nursing care is the primary element in home care.
4. Payment systems for home care should recognize nurses as the major providers of home care, and as such their services should be reimbursed on their own authority.

Home care is not the solution for all patients. For those living in smaller dwellings, adequate space for the patient and other members of the family may be at a premium. The choice of home care, independent living center, or institutional care will depend largely on the desires of the patient and the family. Despite many inconveniences some families wish to have the patient with them. The family's understanding of the patient and their ability to assist one another will make a great difference in choosing between home care or other living arrangements. Not only may space be inadequate, but many times it is impossible to have a member of the family in attendance with the patient during the day. Members of the family who work cannot afford to sacrifice jobs to stay with the patient. However, many families find it easier financially to have the patient at home and are able to make satisfactory arrangements even though the facilities are limited.

Many communities now provide portable meals (Meals-on-Wheels) for homebound persons. Most programs provide one hot meal daily and unheated food for at least one other meal. The cost differs widely and depends on the services offered, such as special diets, and on the sponsorship of the plan. Volunteer groups frequently act as delivery messengers. The local public health nursing service usually participates actively in the plan by selecting suitable patients and by being a resource for the workers who encounter health problems on their "rounds." This service alone often makes it possible for a chronically ill or aged person to remain at home.

Home health aide services

Home health aide services have developed with the increased use of home care plans and particularly since Medicare plans came into existence. The greater number of persons eligible for home health aide services under Medicare has spurred the growth of such services, not because the services were not needed before, but because the cost of such services would have been prohibitive for most of the persons who needed them. Home health aides, who provide actual physical care to the patient, are being trained in many states and are assigned to home care through a central office that coordinates plans of care, often in collaboration with community health nursing agencies. The community health nurse assists by evaluating the home situation and the patient's need for physical personal care. Consequently, the community health nurse supervises the home health aide in the provision of continuing care.

Homemaker services

Homemaker services also have developed with the increased use of home care plans. These services are increasingly in demand in many communities and may be sponsored by a public or voluntary health or welfare agency. Homemakers provide service to families with children and to the person who is convalescing, aged, or acutely or chronically ill. Homemakers are trained to assist in homes where the responsible family manager is temporarily unable to perform his or her usual responsibilities because of illness or absence.

Day care centers

In a number of communities some nursing homes are expanding their facilities and services to include day care centers. There are a great number of chronically ill persons who are able to live with their families, but who require 24-hour attendance. Often the caretaker in the family has to work 8 hours a day. Homemaker or home health aide services are generally not available 8 hours a day, 5 days a week. Day care centers fill this gap in care by providing a place where the chronically ill person can be looked after on a daily basis. Nursing services, physical and occupational therapy, recreational facilities, meals, and in some instances, transportation to and from the center are provided. This kind of service may allow a person to remain at home with the family rather than have to resort to fulltime institutional care.

Independent living centers

Some persons with chronic illnesses may be unable to cope with the demands of maintaining a home but wish to live as independently as possible. There are a variety of options available in some communities that range from living units where persons cook their own meals but are provided with maintenance of the living unit to assisted living units where persons can have their own physical living area but are assisted with activities of daily living, as necessary. Living units in such centers are designed with such features as hand rails for support in ambulation or wide doors to facilitate passage of wheelchairs.

Institutional resources

Many patients and families have to resort to institutional care for the patient because their own facilities are not suitable, no member of the family can be in attendance during the day, community alternatives are not available, or the kind of care needed by the patient requires close professional supervision. A large or a limited selection of outside facilities may be available,

depending on the community. These include chronic disease hospitals, skilled care facilities, convalescent homes, rest homes, homes for the aged, and nursing homes. The patient's potential for rehabilitation, need for maintenance care, or the level of physical disability are factors that will determine eligibility for placement in any of these facilities.

Foster homes

Care in foster homes is a relatively new service that is now being widely used in many communities. Carefully selected families volunteer to take chronically ill persons into their own homes and provide the nonprofessional care that is needed. The family is paid either by the patient or the patient's family, from public funds, or by some social agency. The plan is primarily for those patients who have no family and cannot live alone, but who neither desire nor need institutional care.

Nurse's role in continuing health care

A nurse may be involved in continuing health care in a number of ways: (1) as an independent nurse practitioner assisting the person with chronic illness to cope with problems incurred by the illness; (2) as a public health nurse or visiting nurse involved in a primary rehabilitative program in the home; (3) as a supervisor of home health aides; or (4) as a nurse in a hospital concerned about the care patients will be receiving after they leave the hospital, particularly in situations where the patient's rehabilitation program is not completed or where rehabilitation is not possible. Any of these nurses may also be involved in research pertaining to chronic illness. Some concepts that need further study in the area of chronic disease include social stigmatization, effects of isolation, and effects of chronic illness on the family, marriage, and domestic and occupational roles. Research will make a major contribution to clarification of these general concepts by identifying their relationship to chronic health problems.

Nurses must know the community resources available to patients in order to interpret to them and their families what resources they may be able to obtain, the types of service from which they may benefit, and what kinds of referrals they need for obtaining those services (see list of community resources). When care is to be continued beyond the hospital setting, the hospital nurse should clearly communicate to the continuing care agency data pertinent to the care of the patient in order to provide continuity in the transfer of services. Teamwork and continuity are the keys to successful rehabilitation and management services for patients, and they must be practiced at all stages of care if patients are to realize their fullest potential.

Outcome criteria for the person with a chronic illness

Discharge outcomes for specific chronic diseases are discussed in the chapters dealing with those diseases. However, it may be stated on a general basis that on discharge from the hospital patients with a chronic disease or their family members should be able to:

1. Demonstrate or explain those measures that must be taken to avoid further preventable disability.
2. Demonstrate or explain those self-care activities of which they are capable.
3. Identify those activities for which help is needed.
4. Explain who will be available to help them with those activities and on what basis that help will be available.
5. Explain what community resources are available to them for help and how they may obtain that help.
6. Discuss in reasonable detail their plans for follow-up care and reevaluation.

Focus on the future

Five measurable and achievable national goals for public health action have been identified in the 1979 surgeon general's report.[32] These goals include one major goal for each major age group in our society. The time frame for the achievement of these goals is between now and 1990. The goals are concerned with the major health problems and the preventable risks for diseases throughout the life span. These goals and their relationship to chronic health problems follow:

1. *To continue to improve infant health and, by 1990, to reduce infant mortality by at least 35%, to fewer than 9 deaths per 1000 live births.* The two principal threats to infant survival and good health are low birth weight and congenital disorders, including birth defects. Low birth weight may be associated with long-term health problems such as mental retardation, cerebral palsy, and other conditions that impede growth and development. Many birth defects that include congenital disorders, mental retardation, and genetic diseases are immediate serious hazards to infants. Many others, if not diagnosed and treated immediately after birth or during the first year of life, can affect health and well-being in the later years.

2. *To improve child health, foster optimal childhood development, and, by 1990, to reduce deaths among people aged 1 to 14 years by at least 20%, to fewer than 34 per 100,000.* The major cause of death among children is accidents, followed by cancer, birth defects, influenza and pneumonia, and homicide. But not all health problems are reflected in mortality figures. Habits and attitudes developed during childhood can lead to adult disease and disability. As many as 40% of school children ages 11 to 14 are estimated to already have one or more of the risk factors associated with heart disease: overweight, high blood pressure, high blood cholesterol, cigarette smoking, poor physical fitness, or diabetes.

3. *To improve the health and health habits of adolescents and young adults and, by 1990, to reduce deaths among people aged 15 to 24 by at least 20%, to fewer than 9.3 per 100,000.* Despite improvements in health over the past 75 years, death rates for adolescents and young adults are increasing. The principal health problems of this age group include violent death and injury, sexually transmitted diseases, alcohol, drug abuse, and emotional problems. Young men are at particular risk, since their death rate is almost three times that of young women. Although chronic diseases are not among the major causes of death at this period of life, the life-styles and behavioral patterns that are shaped during these years may determine later susceptibility to chronic diseases.

4. *To improve the health of adults and, by 1990, to reduce deaths among people aged 25 to 64 by at least 25%, to fewer than 400 per 100,000.* The leading causes of death in this age group are heart disease, cancer, stroke, and cirrhosis of the liver. Accidents are a prominent problem for the younger members of this group, but overall the chronic diseases predominate. In addition to causes of death, disability from mental illness presents a major health problem. More than one third of all deaths in this group are due to cardiovascular diseases, principally coronary artery disease and stroke. However, such deaths have declined in recent years and account for most of the recent decreases in mortality.

5. *To improve the health and quality of life for older adults and, by 1990, to reduce the average annual number of days of restricted activity due to acute and chronic conditions by 20%, to fewer than 30 days per year for people aged 65 and over.* Today there are 24 million people aged 65 years and over in the United States, accounting for 11% of the population. This group is the fastest growing segment of the population. By the year 2030 there will be more than 50 million Americans in the over-65 group, and they will represent nearly 17% of the population. The leading causes of death for this age group are heart disease, cancer, stroke, influenza, and pneumonia. The long-term goal of a health-promotion and disease-prevention strategy for older people must be not only to achieve further increases in longevity but also to allow such individuals to seek in-

dependent and rewarding lives in older age, unlimited by the many health problems that are within their capacity to control.

Even though it is possible to identify health goals for a nation, it is far more difficult to carry them out so that the effect is noticeable to the individual seeking health care.

The challenge of providing health care to all people includes the challenge to promote the full participation of individuals with physical and mental disabilities. The United Nations proclaimed 1981 as the International Year of Disabled Persons (IYDP). The United States Council for the IYDP has worked to strengthen public understanding of the needs and contributions of 35 million people. The council has defined the following long-term national goals of and for the disabled:

1. Expanded educational opportunities
2. Improved access to housing, buildings, and transportation
3. Greater opportunity for employment
4. Broader recreational, social, and cultural activities
5. Expanded and strengthened rehabilitation programs and facilities
6. Increased biomedical research aimed at conquering major disabling conditions
7. Reduced incidence of disability through accident and disease prevention
8. Increased application of technology on behalf of persons with disabilities
9. Expanded international exchange of information and experience to benefit the disabled everywhere

The commitment of health care providers must be not only to find ways to help the disabled and other chronically ill individuals cope with chronic health problems but also to educate individuals in the prevention of disease and the promotion of health.

REFERENCES AND SELECTED READINGS
Contemporary

1. Albee, G.: In Curtis, N., editor: Self help reporter, vol. 3, no. 4, Sept.-Oct. 1977.
2. American Academy of Nursing: Long-term care: some issues for nursing, Kansas City, Mo., 1976, American Nurses Association.
3. American Cancer Society: 1980 Cancer facts and figures, New York, 1981, The Society.
4. American Nurses Association: A national policy for health care: principles and positions, 1977, The Assocation.
5. Anderson, H.C.: Newton's geriatric nursing, ed. 5, St. Louis, 1971, The C.V. Mosby Co.
6. *Anderson, S.V., and Bauwens, E.E.: Chronic health problems: concepts and application, St. Louis, 1981, C.V. Mosby Co.
7. Archer, S.E., and Fleshman, R.P.: Community health nursing, ed. 21, North Scituate, Mass., 1970, Duxbury Press.
8. Boroch, R.M.: Elements of rehabilitation in nursing, St. Louis, 1976, The C.V. Mosby Co.
9. Cowdry, E.V., and Sternberg, F.U., editors: The care of the geriatric patient, ed. 5, St.. Louis, 1976, The C.V. Mosby Co.
10. Expectation of life in the United States at a new high, Statistical Bull. **61**(4):13-15, 1980.
11. Ford, A.B., et al.: Results of long-term home nursing: the influence of disability, J. Chronic Dis. **24**:591-596, 1971.
12. Hirschberg, G.G., Lewis, L., and Vaughn, P.: Rehabilitation: a manual for the care of the physically disabled and elderly, ed. 2, Philadelphia, 1976, J.B. Lippincott Co.
13. Kalisch, P.A., and Kalisch, B.J.: Nursing involvement in the health planning process. DHEW pub. no. (HRA) 78-25, Hyattsville, Md., 1977, U.S. Department of Health, Education and Welfare.
14. Kalin, I.S., et al.: Studies of the school-age child with meningomyelocele: social and emotional adaptation, J. Pediatr. **78**:1013-1019, 1971.
15. Lawson, B.A.: Chronic illness in the school aged child: effects on the total family. In Anderson, S.V., and Bauwens, E.E.: Chronic health problems: concepts and application, St. Louis, 1981, The C.V. Mosby Co.
16. Lefkowitz, B.: Health differentials between white and non-white Americans, Washington, D.C., 1977, U.S. Government Printing Office.
17. Martin, N., King, R., and Suchinski, J.: The nurse therapist in the rehabilitation setting, Am. J. Nurs. **70**:1694-1697, 1970.
18. Martinelli, R.P., and Dell Orto, A.E.: The pyschological and social impact of physical disability, New York, 1977, Springer Publishing Co., Inc.
19. McCaffery, M.: Patients in pain, Nurs. '73 3(6):41-50, 1973.
20. Morris, R., editor: Allocating health resources for the aged and disabled, Lexington, Mass., 1981, Lexington Books.
21. National Center for Health Statistics: State estimates of disability and utilization of medical services: United States, 1974-76, DHEW pub. no. (PHS) 78-1241, Washington, D.C., 1978, U.S. Government Printing Office.
22. *Palmer, I.S., editor: Nursing in long-term illness, Nurs. Clin. North Am. **5**:1-84, 1970.
23. Public Health Service: Vital and health statistics—current estimates from the Health Interview Survey (1974). U.S. Department of Health, Education and Welfare, series 10, no. 100, Rockville, Md., Sept. 1975.
24. Public Health Service: Vital and health statistics—health characteristics of persons with chronic activity limitations (1978), U.S. Department of Health and Human Services, series 10, no. 112, Rockville, Md., Oct. 1980.
25. Rettig, R.A.: End-stage renal disease and the cost of medical technology. In Altman, S.H., and Blendon, R.J., editors.; Medical technology: the culprit behind health care costs? DHEW pub. no. PHS-79-3216, Washington, D.C., 1979, U.S. Government Printing Office.
26. *Rifle, K.L., editor: The patient with long-term illness, Nurs. Clin. North Am. **8**:571-681, 1973.
27. Strauss, A.L.: Chronic illness and the quality of life, St. Louis, 1975., The C.V. Mosby Co.
28. Stryker, R.: Rehabilitative aspects of acute and chronic nursing care, Philadelphia, 1972, W.B. Saunders Co.
29. Sultz, H.A., et al.: Long-term childhood illness, Pittsburgh, 1972, University of Pittsburgh Press.
30. U.S. Congress, House Committee on Interstate and Foreign Commerce: National Health Promotion and Disease Prevention Act, 1976.
31. U.S. Department of Health, Education and Welfare: Final mortality statistics, 1977. Doc. PHS-79-1120, Washington, D.C., 1979, U.S. Government Printing Office.

*References preceded by an asterisk are particularly well suited for student reading.

32. U.S. Department of Health, education and Welfare: Healthy people. Surgeon general's report on health promotion and disease prevention, Washington, D.C., 1979, U.S. Government Printing Office.
33. Williams, S.R.: Nutrition and diet therapy, ed. 4, St. Louis, 1981, The C.V. Mosby Co.

Classic

34. Christopherson, V.A.: Role modifications of the disabled male, Am. J. Nurs. **68**:290-293, 1968.
35. Crate, M.: Nursing functions in adaptation to chronic illness, Am. J. Nurs. **65**:72-76, 1965.
36. Garrett, J.F., and Levine, E.S.: Psychological practices with the physically disabled, New York, 1962, Columbia University Press.
37. Guidelines for the practice of nursing on the rehabilitation team, New York, 1965, American Nurses Association.
38. Katz, S., et al.: Studies of illness in the aged. The index of ADL: a standardized measure of biological and psychosocial function, J.A.M.A. **185**:914-919, 1963.
39. Litman, T.J.: An analysis of the sociological factors affecting the rehabilitation of physically handicapped patients, Arch. Phys. Med. Rehabil. **45**:9-16, 1964.
40. Moskowitz, E., and McCann, C.B.: Classification of disability in the chronically ill and aging, J. Chronic Dis. **5**:342-346, 1957.
41. Myers, J.S.: An orientation to chronic disease and disability, New York, 1965, Macmillan Publishing Co., Inc.
42. Olson, E.V., editor: The hazards of immobility, Am. J. Nurs. **67**:780-797, 1967.
43. *Sorensen, K., and Amis, D.B.: Understanding the world of the chronically ill, Am. J. Nurs. **67**:811-817, 1967.
44. Talbot, H.S.: A concept of rehabilitation, Rehabil. Lit. **22**:358-359, 1961.

PART THREE

CLINICAL INTERVENTIONS

FOR PERSONS WITH MEDICAL-SURGICAL PROBLEMS

FAILURE OF INTEGRATIVE MECHANISMS: REGULATORY PROBLEMS

The effect of stress on the human body and the response of individuals to stressors are greatly affected by the status of the regulatory mechanisms of the body. Nurses assist persons to cope with deficiencies in regulatory mechanisms, to promote optimal functioning possible when deficiencies exist, and to decrease external stressors when the regulatory mechanisms are not at the optimal functioning level.

The neuroendocrine integrating mechanisms were discussed in Chapter 18. The endocrine system and the liver are the focus of this unit for their role in regulating body functions. Chapter 30 identifies the parameters of *assessment of regulatory mechanisms*. Chapter 31 discusses interventions for persons during an acute phase of a *disturbance in some regulatory function* or during long-term care when learning to care for oneself. Specific problems and special nursing interventions for *dysfunctions of the endocrine system* and the *liver* are discussed in Chapters 32 and 33.

CHAPTER 30

ASSESSMENT OF REGULATORY MECHANISMS

VIRGINIA L. CASSMEYER

The regulation of body mechanisms is controlled by the endocrine and hepatic systems. The hepatic system consists of the liver and gallbladder. Although the endocrine system consists of eight special glands—pituitary, thyroid, parathyroid, adrenals, pancreas, gonads, pineal, and thymus—only the first five will be considered in this chapter. The gonads are discussed in Chapter 63. The endocrine functions of the pineal and thymus glands are as yet poorly understood.

Anatomy and physiology

Endocrine system

Development and location

The various endocrine glands are located throughout the body (Fig. 30-1). The *pituitary gland* is approximately 1 cm in size and weighs approximately 500 mg. It is composed of two functionally distinguishable components: the adenohypophysis (anterior pituitary) and the neurohypophysis (posterior pituitary). The adenohypophysis develops from an outpouching of ectodermal cells (Rathke's pouch). It is connected to the hypothalamus by the hypothalamic hypophyseal portal vascular system. The neurohypophysis and neural stalk (infundibulum) arise embryonically from ectodermal cells of the floor of the third ventricle. The nerve fibers of the neurohypophysis traveling through the neural stalk are connected to various nuclei in the hypothalamus. The pituitary gland lies in the pituitary fossa of the sella turcica of the middle cranial fossa.

The *thyroid gland* is located in the anterior aspect of the neck just below the larynx. It consists of two lobes connected by the isthmus that lies on the upper part of the trachea. The thyroid gland originates from downward growth of endodermal cells from the floor of the pharynx and appears as a discrete organ at approximately the twelfth week of embryonic development. The thyroid gland consists of two cell types, the follicular cells concerned with iodine and thyroid hormone metabolism and the parafollicular cells (C cells), which arise during embryonic development from the ultimobranchial body and are concerned with calcitonin metabolism. The *parathyroid gland* consists of four minute glands, two of which are located on the posterior aspect of each thyroid lobe. It originates from endodermal cells of the third and fourth pharyngeal pouch.

The *adrenal gland* is a retroperitoneal abdominal organ capping the upper pole of each kidney. It consists of two glands that have different embryonic origins: the *adrenal cortex,* which arises from mesodermal cells, and the *adrenal medulla,* which arises from ectodermal cells. The adrenal cortex consists of three zones: the zona glomerulosa, the zona fasciculata, and the zona reticularis. The products of the adrenal medulla are associated with the neuroendocrine integrating functions described in Chapter 13.

The *pancreas* is both an exocrine and endocrine gland. It lies retroperitoneally behind the stomach, with its head and neck in the curve of the duodenum, its body extending horizontally across the posterior abdominal wall, and its tail touching the spleen. The pancreas embryonically arises from an outpouching of the primitive gut that arises from the endodermal cells. The *islets of Langerhans* are the cells that serve the endo-

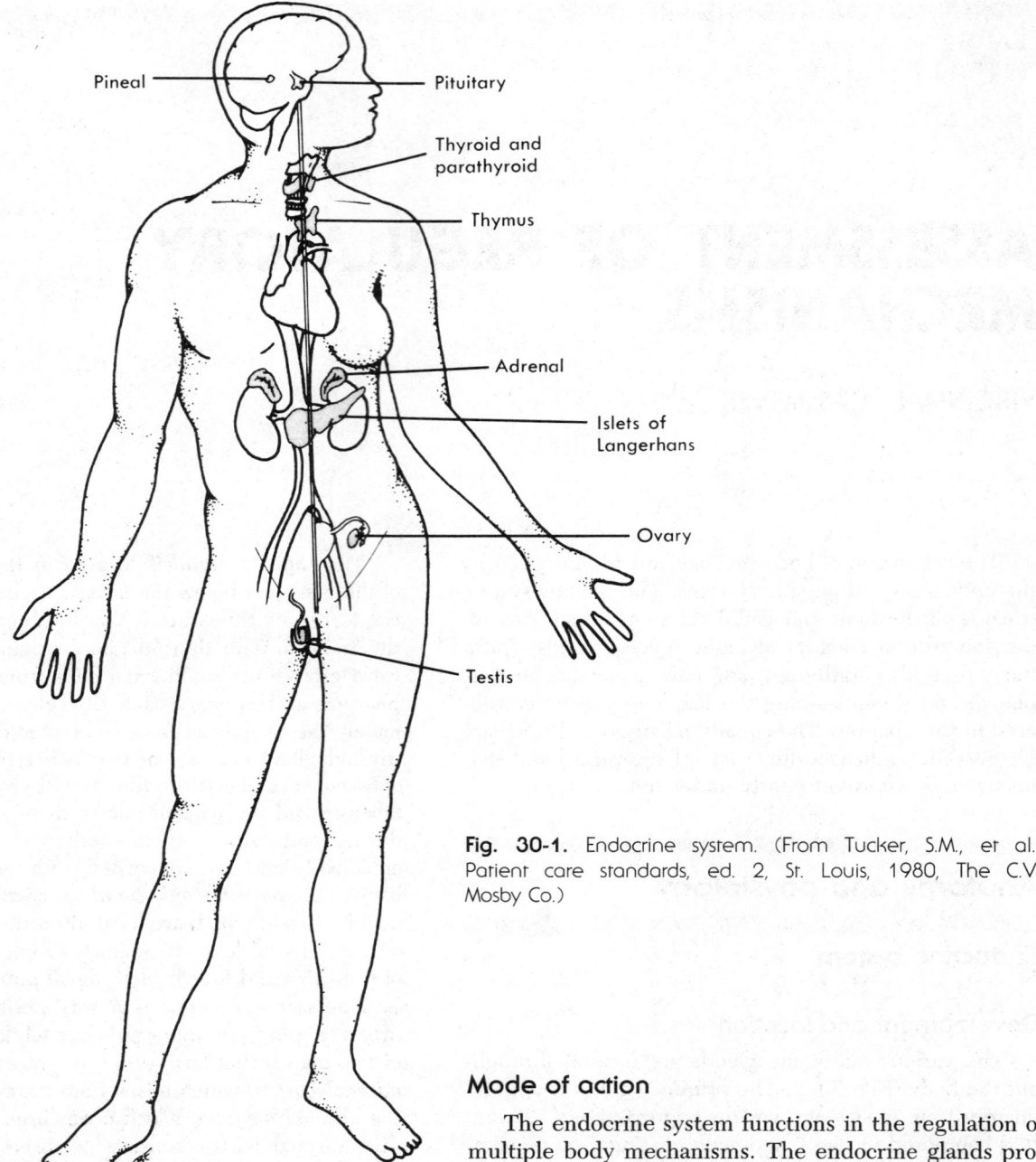

Pineal
Pituitary
Thyroid and parathyroid
Thymus
Adrenal
Islets of Langerhans
Ovary
Testis

S.E. BEEBE

Fig. 30-1. Endocrine system. (From Tucker, S.M., et al.: Patient care standards, ed. 2, St. Louis, 1980, The C.V. Mosby Co.)

Mode of action

The endocrine system functions in the regulation of multiple body mechanisms. The endocrine glands produce specific chemical compounds *(hormones)* that are synthesized in the glands under genetic control and then secreted into the blood. Hormones are continually lost either by excretion or metabolic inactivation.

The secretion of hormones varies. No hormone is secreted at a uniform rate; some seem to have rhythmic patterns (daily or periodic), such as adrenal cortisone or the female reproductive hormones. Others, such as insulin, glucagon, and aldosterone, are secreted in response to blood levels of specific substances. How hormonal production is stimulated or how the hormones act in the cell is not fully understood. No hormone is believed to initiate reactions in the cell de novo. The biochemical machinery of the cell responds to the pres-

crine function. There are over 1,000,000 islet cells, and they make up 1% to 2% of the pancreatic mass. The islet cells are located throughout the entire organ. The islets of Langerhans consist of three cell types: (1) *alpha (α) cells,* which make up 20% of the islet cells and *secrete glucagon,* (2) *beta (β) cells,* which make up 75% of islet cells and *secrete insulin;* and (3) *delta (δ) cells,* which make up 5% of the islet cells and *secrete gastrin and somatostatin.*

ence of the hormone by increasing or decreasing the rate at which a reaction takes place, but all the equipment for the reaction is present in the cell.

It is hypothesized that hormones initiate cellular activity in one of two ways. The two models of hormone activity are the mobile receptor model and the fixed receptor model. In the *mobile receptor model* the hormones are believed to cross the plasma cell membrane and combine with receptors in the cytoplasm of the cell. The combination of the hormone and receptor changes the receptor in some way so that it can cross the nuclear membrane and react with particular acidic proteins in the chromatin of the nucleus or bind with DNA and initiate transcription of DNA. In general, steroid hormones such as adrenal steroids, androgens, active derivatives of vitamin D, estrogen, and progesterone act in this manner. Thyroid hormone is believed to act in this way, but the data to support this belief are not conclusive.

In the *fixed receptor model* the hormone combines with a receptor on the plasma membrane of the cell and initiates a sequence of events coordinated by a second messenger. Cyclic adenosine monophosphate (AMP) has been found to be the second messenger for many hormones. The idea behind this model is that the combination of the hormone with the receptor activates adenylcyclase, which causes the formation of 3',5'-cyclic AMP from ATP (adenosine triphosphate). Once cyclic AMP is generated, it activates protein kinase. Activated protein kinase phosphorylates the specific proteins in the stimulated cell. The phosphorylation causes the cell to initiate whatever activity it is equipped to do. It is believed that adrenocorticotropic hormone (ACTH), prolactin, thyroid stimulating hormone (TSH), glucagon, thyroid releasing factor (TRF), luteinizing hormone releasing factor (LHRF), parathyroid hormone, and catecholamines initiate cellular activity in this manner. Insulin seems to function by a fixed receptor model, but cyclic AMP is not the second messenger in this case.

Relationship between the hypothalamus and the endocrine glands

The anterior pituitary gland, often called the "master gland" because of its regulation of the production of other hormones, is under the control of the hypothalamus. The hypothalamus regulates anterior pituitary gland secretion by the release of *neurosecretory releasing* and *neurosecretory inhibitory factors*. The number and type of releasing and inhibitory factors are unknown. It has been stated that for every pituitary hormone, there are two companion hypothalamic factors, a stimulating factor and an inhibitory factor. Only three of the hypothalamic factors have been isolated. They are TRF, LHRF, and growth hormone inhibitory factor (somatostatin). Other factors for which there is some data to support their presence are follicle stimulating hormone releas-

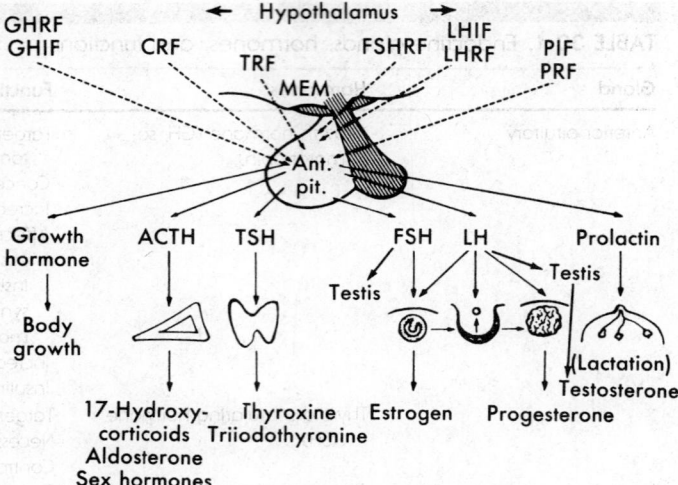

Fig. 30-2. Releasing factors that control output of hormones from anterior lobe of pituitary gland and ultimate hormone release from peripheral glands. *GHRF,* Growth hormone releasing factor; *GHIF,* growth hormone inhibitory factor; *CRF,* corticotropin releasing factor; *TRF,* thyrotropin releasing factor or hormone; *FSHRF,* follicle stimulating hormone releasing factor; *LHRF,* luteinizing hormone releasing factor; *LHIF,* luteinizing hormone inhibitory factor; *PIF,* prolactin inhibitory factor; *PRF,* prolactin inhibitory factor; *MEM,* median eminence. Note that combination of FSH and LH produced maturation of follicle, ovulation, and corpus luteum formation in female. In male, FSH regulates spermatogenesis and LH regulates testosterone production. (Modified from Mountcastle, V.B., editor; Medical physiology, vol. 1, ed. 14, St. Louis, 1979, The C.V. Mosby Co.)

ing factor (FSHRF), luteinizing hormone inhibitory factor (LHIF), growth hormone releasing factor (GRF), prolactin releasing factor (PRF), prolactin inhibitory factor, (PIF) and corticotropin releasing factor (CRF). These factors are produced by cells scattered throughout the hypothalamus.

Stimulation of the hypothalamus leads to the liberation of selected factors into the hypothalamic hypophyseal portal blood system, which carries them to the anterior pituitary gland to stimulate the release of appropriate hormones. The relationship between the hypothalamus, anterior pituitary gland, and target organs is summarized in Fig. 30-2.

The hypothalamus also produces two other hormones, which are stored and released from the posterior pituitary gland. These hormones are produced in two discrete nuclei of the hypothalamus, the paraventricular and supraoptic nuclei, and they are carried down neurons by axonal transport to the posterior pituitary.

The various endocrine glands, hormones, and the major known functions of the individual hormones are summarized in Table 30-1.

TABLE 30-1. Endocrine glands, hormones, and functions

Gland	Hormones	Functions
Anterior pituitary	Growth hormone (GH; somatotropin)	Target organ: whole body, possibly works on all tissues through action of somatomedin or other compounds Concerned with growth of cells, bones, muscles, and soft tissue Increases mitosis Affects carbohydrate, protein, and fat metabolism: decreases utilization of glucose, amino acid catabolism, and plasma levels of amino acids; increases insulin sensitivity, pancreatic activity, amino acid transport, RNA and protein synthesis, fat mobilization, and free fatty acid levels; inhibits lipogenesis; promotes ketosis Increases electrolyte retention and extracellular fluid volume Insulin antagonist
	Thyroid stimulating hormone (TSH)	Target organ: thyroid Necessary for growth and function of thyroid gland Controls release of thyroid hormones
	Adrenocorticotropic hormone (ACTH)	Target organ: adrenal cortex Necessary for growth of zona fasciculata and the zona reticularis of the adrenal cortex Controls release of glucocorticoids and adrenal androgens Has minor role in release of aldosterone
	Gonadotropins Follicle stimulating hormone (FSH) Luteinizing hormone (LH; also referred to as interstitial cell stimulating hormone [ICSH] in males)	Target organs: sexual organs Necessary for development of primary and secondary sex characteristics
	Luteotropic hormone (LTH; prolactin)	Target organ: breast Necessary for development and lactation
Posterior pituitary	Antidiuretic hormone (ADH)	Target organ: kidney (distal convoluted tubules and collecting ducts) Necessary for maintenance of body fluid osmolarity by controlling water reabsorption in kidneys; may stimulate the pumping of sodium in loop of Henle and rate of blood perfusion to different parts of kidney
	Oxytocin	Target organs: breast and possibly uterus Causes milk "let-down" in lactating breast Exogenous oxytocin causes contraction of pregnant uterus Role of endogenous oxytocin in onset of labor is uncertain
Thyroid	Thyroxine (T_4) and triiodothyronine (T_3)	Regulates protein, fat, and carbohydrate catabolism in all cells Regulates metabolic rate of all cells Regulates body heat production Insulin antagonist Maintains growth hormone secretion, skeletal maturation Affects CNS development Necessary for muscle tone and vigor Maintains cardiac rate, force, and output Maintains secretion of gastrointestinal tract Affects respiratory rate and oxygen utilization Maintains calcium mobilization Affects RBC production Stimulates lipid turnover, free fatty acid release, and cholesterol synthesis
	Thyrocalcitonin	Lowers serum calcium and phosphorus levels by inhibiting osteoclastic activity Decreases calcium and phosphorus absorption in gastrointestinal tract
Adrenal medulla	Epinephrine and norepinephrine	Necessary for maintenance of neuroendocrine integrating functions of body Elevates blood pressure, increases heart rate, and causes vasoconstriction Stimulates conversion of glycogen to glucose for emergency fuel Stimulates gluconeogenesis Increases lipolysis

TABLE 30-1. Endocrine glands, hormones, and functions—cont'd

Gland	Hormones	Functions
Adrenal cortex	Glucocorticoids (cortisol)	Overall effect is to maintain blood glucose level by increasing gluconeogenesis; decrease rate of glucose utilization by cells
		Increases protein catabolism
		Promotes lipolysis
		Promotes sodium and water retention
		Antiinflammatory
		Degrades collagen
		Decreases T-lymphocyte participation in cellular-mediated immunity by decreasing circulating level of T-lymphocytes
		Increases neutrophils by increasing release and decreasing destruction
		Decreases new antibody release
		Decreases eosinophils, basophils, and monocytes
		Decreases scar tissue formation
		Increases RBC formation and possibly increases platelet formation
		Increases gastric acid and pepsin production
		Maintains emotional stability
	Mineralocorticoids (aldosterone)	Major stimulus is renin-angiotensin system
		Primarily responsible for maintenance of normovolemic state by increasing sodium and water retention in distal tubules
		Cause potassium excretion
		Cause increased excretion of ammonium and magnesium ions
	Androgens	Same functions as gonadal sex hormones
Parathyroid	Parathyroid hormone (PTH)	Increases serum calcium levels and decreases serum phosphorus levels by (1) increasing bone resorption, (2) increasing calcium absorption from gastrointestinal tract (needs vitamin D), (3) decreasing urinary excretion of calcium, and (4) increasing urinary excretion of phosphorus
		Inhibits H+ secretion, decreases bicarbonate reabsorption, and decreases sodium reabsorption in proximal tubules
		Increases renal threshold for glucose
Pancreas: islets of Langerhans		
β-Cells	Insulin	Overall, decreases blood glucose level
		Increases uptake and utilization of glucose by adipose and muscle cells
		Increases phosphorylation of glucose by liver
		Increases glycogenesis
		Increases lipogenesis
		Increases amino acid incorporation into protein
α-Cells	Glucagon	Actions contrary to insulin
		Increases blood glucose level by increasing glycogenolysis and gluconeogenesis
		Increases serum lipid level

Control mechanisms

In a state of health the level of any one hormone is kept within very definite limits. The endocrine glands are regulated by a number of control mechanisms. The *closed-looped negative feedback system* is illustrated in Fig. 30-3. Gland A produces hormone X, which stimulates organ B. In turn, organ B produces substance Y,

Fig. 30-3. Closed-loop negative feedback system. A principle of control that is applicable to all endocrine glands. (Redrawn from Harvey, A.M., et al.: The principles and practice of medicine, ed. 18, Englewood Cliffs, N.J., 1972, Prentice-Hall, Inc.)

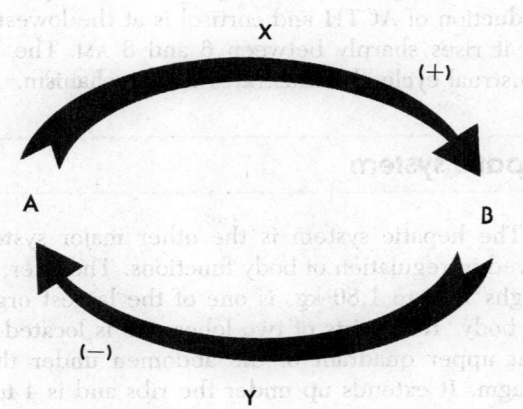

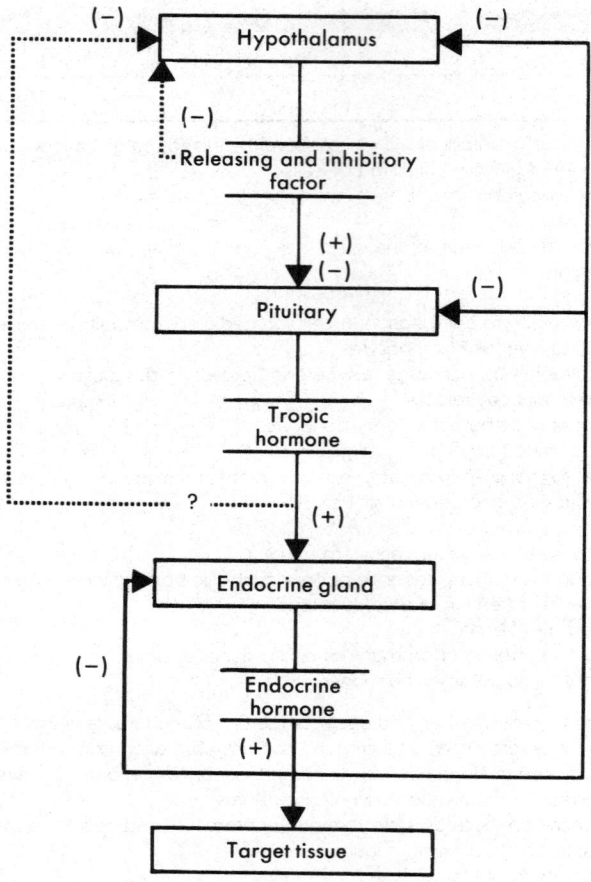

Fig. 30-4. Complex negative feedback loop system between hypothalamus, pituitary, other endocrine glands, and target tissue. (Redrawn from Harvey, A.M., et al.: The principles and practice of medicine, ed. 18, Englewood Cliffs, N.J., 1972, Prentice-Hall, Inc.)

which then inhibits secretion of gland A. An extensive feedback loop exists between the hypothalamus, pituitary gland, other endocrine glands, and target organs. Fig. 30-4 identifies the negative- and positive-feedback loops. A third regulating phenomenon is *internal rhythm*. The diurnal variations of ACTH and cortisol production provide examples. While a person is asleep at 2 AM, production of ACTH and cortisol is at the lowest level, but it rises sharply between 6 and 8 AM. The human menstrual cycle also illustrates this mechanism.

Hepatic system

The hepatic system is the other major system involved in regulation of body functions. The liver, which weighs 1.35 to 1.80 kg, is one of the largest organs of the body. It consists of two lobes and is located in the right upper quadrant of the abdomen under the diaphragm. It extends up under the ribs and is 4 to 8 cm

in height in the midsternal line and 6 to 12 cm in height in the midclavicular line. The gallbladder lies under the inferior surface of the liver (Fig. 30-5).

The liver is made up of small liver lobules (Fig. 30-6) composed of hepatic cellular plates. Each hepatic cellular plate is usually two cells thick, and between these cells run bile canaliculi. Hepatic sinusoids, which receive blood from the portal vein and hepatic artery, lie on the opposite sides of the hepatic cells. After flowing through the hepatic sinusoids, the blood is emptied into the central vein and from there flows into the hepatic vein. The hepatic sinusoids are lined with Kupffer's cells. Kupffer's cells are reticuloendothelial cells that phagocytize bacteria and other foreign products.

The liver, as can be seen from this description, is ideally structured to receive large supplies of blood to carry out multiple functions. The major functions of the liver are (1) participation in various parts of fat, carbohydrate, and protein metabolism; (2) metabolism of bilirubin and production of bile; and (3) detoxification of endogenous and exogenous substances. The liver cells contain many enzymes to carry out these functions.

Fat, carbohydrate, and protein metabolism

The liver plays a major role in the metabolism of fats, carbohydrates, and proteins. Through various enzymatic activities the liver can oxidize fats, carbohydrates, and proteins for energy; use fat, carbohydrate, and protein products to produce compounds that can be stored for future use; or use fat, carbohydrate, and protein products to manufacture needed compounds. In fat metabolism the liver is responsible for the production of phospholipids, lipoproteins, and cholesterol. It functions in protein metabolism by synthesizing essential proteins such as albumin, which is necessary for the maintenance of osmotic pressure, some globulin, blood-clotting factors such as fibrinogen and prothrombin, and converting the ammonia produced from the deamination of proteins to urea. In carbohydrate metabolism it is responsible for the production and storage of glycogen for glycogenolysis and gluconeogenesis and is primarily responsible for the metabolism of galactose.

Bilirubin metabolism

Bilirubin is a by-product of the heme portion of red blood cells and is released when red blood cells are destroyed. The bilirubin released from the red blood cell is non-water-soluble (unconjugated) and is carried in the blood attached to protein. The liver is responsible for picking up this unconjugated bilirubin, combining it with glucuronide into a conjugated water soluble form, and secreting conjugated bilirubin into the bile. The bilirubin in bile is secreted into the duodenum and is broken down by bacteria into urobilinogen. Some of the urobilinogen is excreted with the feces, becoming stercobi-

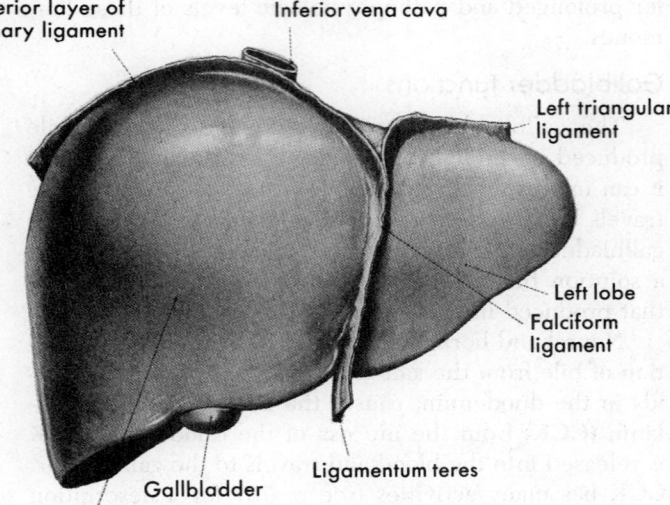

Fig. 30-5. Anterior view of liver. (From Hamilton, W.J., editor: Textbook of human anatomy, ed. 2, St. Louis, 1976, The C.V. Mosby Co. By permission of Macmillan, London & Basingstoke.)

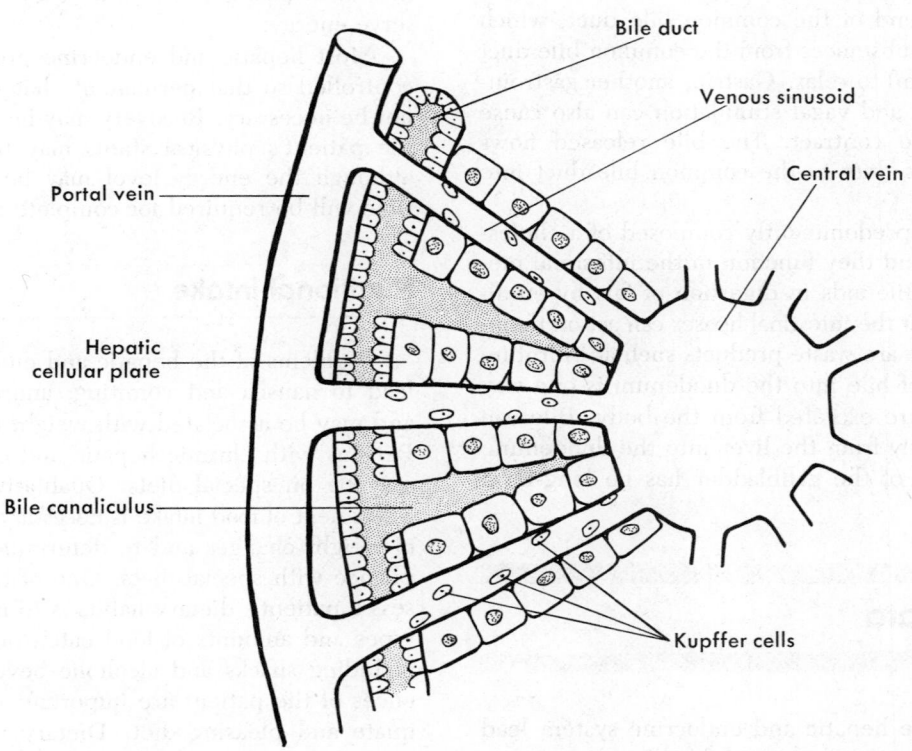

Fig. 30-6. Diagram of liver lobule. (Adapted from Guyton, A.: Textbook of medical physiology, ed. 4, Philadelphia, 1971, W.B. Saunders Co.)

lin and giving the stool its brown color. Some is eliminated in the urine, and the remainder returns to the liver and is reconverted to bilirubin.

Detoxification

The liver has a prime role in detoxification of both exogenous and endogenous substances. It also has a major role in the detoxification of many drugs. All barbiturates (except phenobarbital and barbital) and many other sedatives are inactivated by the liver. The status of the liver plays an important role in the effectiveness or toxicity of these and other drugs. The liver also detoxifies corticosteroids, aldosterone, and estrogen. The inability of the liver to inactivate these hormones may account for prolonged and pathophysiologic levels of these hormones.

Gallbladder functions

The gallbladder serves as a storage place for bile produced in the liver. Its capacity is usually 50 ml, but it can increase in size under normal conditions. The bile travels by a system of ductules from the liver to the gallbladder. In the gallbladder, bile is concentrated to a solution that is five to ten times as concentrated as that produced in the liver.

Neural and hormonal mechanisms control the secretion of bile from the gallbladder. Food, particularly lipids in the duodenum, causes the release of cholecystokinin (CCK) from the mucosa of the duodenum. CCK is released into the blood and travels to the gallbladder. CCK has many activities (see p. 707 for a description of its other actions), one of which is to stimulate the gallbladder musculature to contract. At the same time CCK causes the muscle of the sphincter of Oddi (the sphincter at the end of the common bile duct, which controls entry of substances from the common bile duct into the duodenum) to relax. Gastrin, another gastrointestinal hormone, and vagal stimulation can also cause the gallbladder to contract. The bile released flows through the cystic duct to the common bile duct into the duodenum.

Bile acids are predominantly composed of a cholesterol derivative, and they function in the intestinal metabolism of fats. Bile aids in digestion of fats by emulsifying them so that the intestinal lipases can act on them. Mixed in with bile are waste products such as bilirubin; thus the release of bile into the duodenum is one way in which wastes are excreted from the body. Bile can be released directly from the liver into the duodenum; thus the removal of the gallbladder has no long-term consequences.

Subjective data

Diseases of the hepatic and endocrine system lead to varied manifestations because of inadequate energy production, insufficient metabolism of nutrients and other products, water and electrolyte imbalance, abnormal growth and development, altered reproductive processes, and inadequate removal of toxic and waste products. Because of these varied manifestations, systematic assessment of numerous parameters is necessary to define the patient's total problems and needs. Since their anatomic locations for the most part preclude direct examination of the health of the various organs, assessment of the status of the regulatory mechanisms requires a thorough history from the patient or significant others. Special attention should be paid to the patient's *energy level, nutritional intake, elimination patterns, subjective perception of changes in body characteristics,* and *tolerance to stress.*

Energy level

Since the liver and the endocrine system are directly involved in the metabolism of nutrients for energy and the production of elements necessary for the formation of red blood cells to carry oxygen, diseases of these systems will change the patient's energy level. Many patients will complain of "not being able to do their normal things." It is important to assess the person's energy level and to use this as a guide for helping plan activities of daily living. Some patients need help in adjusting their activities to allow for rest periods; they may need assistance in eliminating activities or in changing the ways they do activities to conserve energy.

Most hepatic and endocrine problems can be well controlled so that permanent changes in life style will not be necessary. Recovery may be slow, however, and the patient's physical status may be so damaged that although the energy level may be normal, additional time will be required for complete recovery.

Nutritional intake

Problems of the hepatic and endocrine systems can lead to nausea and vomiting, anorexia, or polyphagia and may be associated with weight loss or weight gain. Persons with chronic hepatic and endocrine problems may be on special diets. Qualitative and quantitative assessment of food intake is necessary to decide the cause of weight changes and to determine the level of compliance with special diets. One of the best ways to assess a patient's dietary habits is to have the patient list types and amounts of food eaten on the previous day, including snacks and alcoholic beverages. The preferences of the patient are important in planning an adequate and pleasing diet. Dietary restrictions may be necessary for some conditions, and providing adequate dietary intake in cases of anorexia, nausea and vomiting, and dietary restrictions is a tremendous challenge. In some instances the restriction will be necessary for life, so it is very important to show the patient that the diet can be pleasing as well as therapeutic.

Elimination pattern

Both the hepatic and endocrine systems are involved in maintenance of water and electrolyte balance.

The history should include information on the frequency, approximate amount, and color of urinary elimination. The presence of nocturia or dysuria is also solicited. In liver disease a history of decreased output with a relative increase in weight may be elicited. In endocrine disease, depending on the cause, the client may give a history of increased output and increased thirst, or decreased output and increased weight. Some patients may be on diuretics, and their compliance with the therapy should be assessed. The frequency and color of bowel movements is also determined. Constipation or other changes in bowel habits that may be caused by changes in water balance, dietary intake, or sluggishness of the bowel may be elicited. Treatment of disease states may include changes in diet and fluid intake; the patient's previous pattern of intake will assist the nurse in teaching the patient about needed changes.

Body characteristics

Changes in hair distribution, body proportions, voice, skin pigmentation, and facial appearance may accompany problems of the regulatory mechanisms. A description of changes by patients or their significant others is very important because the characteristics of persons vary so greatly, and changes may not be so great that observation alone will pick them up.

The collection of information regarding changes in body characteristics is not only important in helping to define the physiologic problem but also is very important in identifying potential or present emotional or psychologic problems. Some of the changes that occur with endocrine and hepatic problems are irreversible even when the physiologic problem is controlled. Body characteristics are part of the identity of the person, and the patient may have problems dealing with the changes. (See Chapter 28 for a detailed discussion of body image.)

Tolerance to stressors

The regulatory mechanisms help to maintain the body's ability to respond to all types of physical and psychologic stressors. The patient or significant others should be questioned in relation to the patient's ability (or change in ability) to tolerate stressors. Such things as intolerance to heat and cold, increased frequency of infections, increased irritation, euphoria, depression, increased crying, or increased anger may be elicited. Depending on the patient's ability to handle stressors, special environmental controls to decrease the chance of infection and to maintain an even physical and emotional environment may be necessary.

Objective data

The collection of objective data about the endocrine and hepatic system requires a thorough inspection and the use of the techniques of palpation and percussion. Most of the information that can be collected by physical examination is gathered by inspection.

Inspection

Inspection should be used to assess the patient's body growth and developmental status. Such things as height, weight, body proportions, amount and distribution of muscle mass, fat distribution, skin pigmentation, and hair distribution should be assessed. A great variation in these parameters exists in the general population, and often the changes will not be obvious. Inspection of family members for like characteristics will provide information as to whether the characteristics seen in the patient are caused by hereditary or pathophysiologic alterations. The patient's alertness and speech patterns can be assessed when the history is being collected.

The regulatory mechanisms play a major role in growth and development, metabolism of food products, and regulation of sex hormones. All of these functions, if affected, cause changes in body characteristics. Some examples of specific changes are (1) dwarfism caused by thyroid and pituitary problems, (2) jaundice caused by liver abnormalities (best seen in the sclera in dark-skinned persons), (3) changes in fat distribution, producing "buffalo hump" and "thickened girdle," from adrenal cortical excess, (4) presence of purplish striae instead of white striae because of adrenocortical excess, (5) muscle wasting with a wide variety of regulatory problems, and (6) change in sexual characteristics because of abnormalities of hormonal levels or hepatic problems. All of these changes can be identified during inspection.

Inspection along with palpation is used to check skin turgor, mucous membrane moisture, and the presence of edema. Abdominal girth should be measured. All of this data will give information about the fluid and electrolyte status of the patient.

Following are changes that may be found: The finger should slide over the mucous membrane easily. In states of fluid depletion the mucous membranes are sticky. Edema can be graded from 1+ to 4+ (see Chapter 21). Skin turgor can be checked on the forearm, forehead, or over the sternum (p. 1783).

Palpation and percussion

Of all the organs discussed, only the thyroid and liver will be routinely examined by use of palpation and percussion. In disease states, sometimes the pancreas and parathyroid gland can be palpated.

Examination of thyroid gland

The thyroid gland is usually examined along with examination of the head and neck. Palpation of the thyroid provides information about the size, shape, and symmetry of the gland, and the presence of nodules or tenderness.

The first step in the examination is to inspect the neck for any visible thyroid tissue. Normally no tissue is visible. Palpation of the thyroid gland can be done from either in front of or from behind the patient. Frequently the normal thyroid gland is not palpable and, if felt, is a layer of tissue that moves with swallowing. Normally, each lobe is approximately 5 cm long and 2 cm thick. The right lobe is slightly larger than the left. A light rotary motion is used to delineate nodules and irregularities. Each step in the following description should be done before and while the patient swallows. Sips of water will assist the person to swallow.

Palpation from behind. Seat the person in a chair and stand behind him or her. Have the person lower the chin, place your thumbs on the back of the neck, and curve fingers anteriorly over the thyroid. Feel for the thyroid isthmus and anterior surface of the lobes. Next, have the patient flex the neck slightly forward and to the right. Displace the thyroid cartilage to the right with the fingers of your left hand. Palpate with your right hand, placing the right thumb behind the sternocleidomastoid and the index and middle finger in front of it. Reverse the procedure for the left side (Fig. 30-7).

Palpation from the front. Stand in front of the patient. With the second and third fingers, feel below the cricoid cartilage for the thyroid isthmus. Then move your fingers laterally and deep to the borders of the sternocleidomastoid muscle. Feel for each lateral lobe. Lastly, have the client flex the neck forward and to the right. Place your right thumb on the lower portion of the patient's thyroid cartilage and displace it to the client's right. Hook the tips of the second and third fingers of your left hand behind the sternocleidomastoid muscle while feeling in front of the muscle with your thumb. Reverse the procedure for the left side (Fig. 30-8).

Occasionally, the thyroid gland is more easily palpated if the neck is extended. The procedures de-

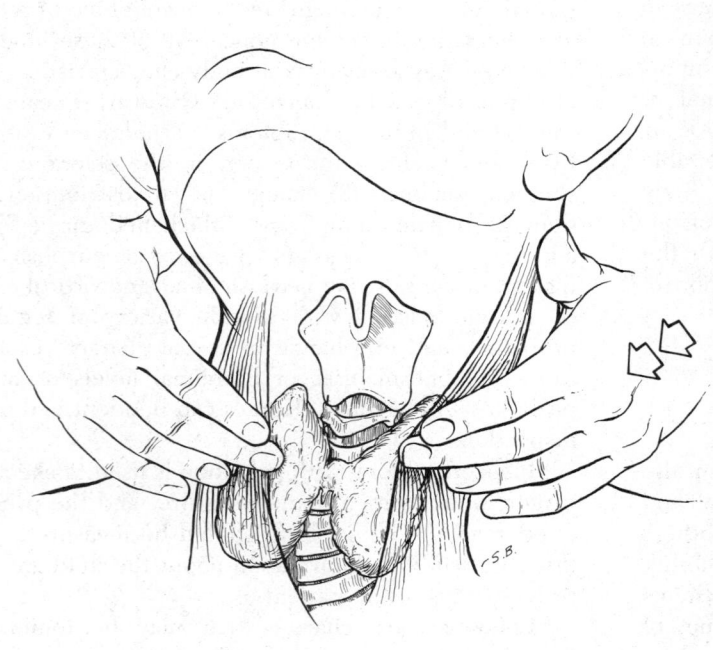
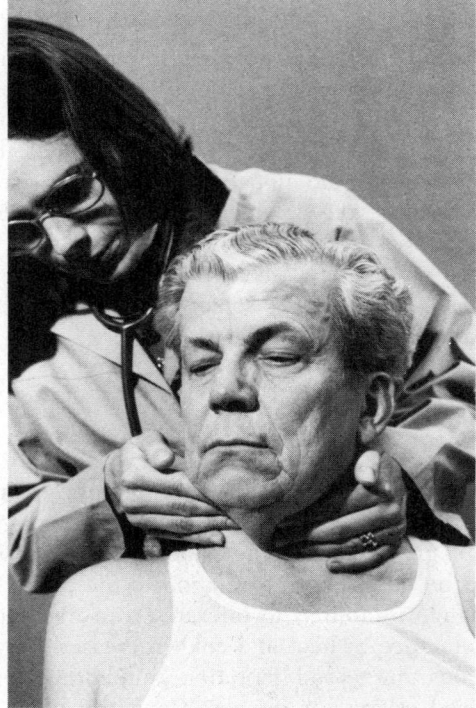

Fig. 30-7. Posterior approach to thyroid examination. In order to examine right lobe of thyroid gland, examiner displaces trachea slightly to right with fingers of left hand and palpates for right thyroid robe with fingers of right hand. (From Malasanos, L., et al.: Health assessment, ed. 2, St. Louis, 1981, The C.V. Mosby Co.)

scribed above can be repeated with the neck extended. If an enlarged thyroid is felt, the thyroid should be auscultated for the presence of *bruits*. The increased vascular flow that occurs with hypertrophy of the gland can cause bruits.

Examination of the liver

Examination of the liver is done while examining the abdomen. The examination begins with inspection of the abdomen for striae, which may be caused by ascites; engorged veins, which may be caused by obstruction of portal flow; and abdominal distention, which also may be caused by ascites. When auscultation of the abdomen is desired, it must be done before palpation and percussion of the abdomen.

Percussion. The technique of percussion is used to examine the liver. In percussion the fingers of one hand are placed over the organ to be examined. The fingers of the other hand are flexed and used to tap the fingers of the other hand (Fig. 8-4).

To percuss the liver, start at an area below the umbilicus in the midclavicular line and percuss upward until dullness is heard. Then start at about the third or fourth intercostal space, midclavicular line, and percuss downward until dullness is heard. Measure the vertical span of liver dullness. It should be approximately 6 to 12 cm in width. If this percussion reveals an enlarged liver, the liver can be percussed in the same manner at the midsternal line. At this point it normally is 4 to 6 cm in width (Fig. 30-9). Lung consolidation or right pleural effusion can obscure the upper border dullness, while gas in the colon can obscure the lower border dullness.

Percussion is also used to examine for the presence of ascites. Ascites causes bulging of flanks and dullness when the patient is supine. If the patient is turned to the side, the bulging is shifted to the dependent side, and the dullness is localized to that side.

Fluid wave. While the patient is lying supine, the abdomen can be examined for presence of a fluid wave. In performing this test, the left hand of the examiner is on the patient's right flank, and the ulnar edge of the hand of an assistant or the patient is placed over the upper middle abdomen as the examiner's right hand sharply strikes the left flank of the patient. A sharp wave will be felt by the examiner's left hand in the presence of a significantly large amount of fluid (ascites).

Palpation. Gently work the fingertips of the right hand deep into the right upper quadrant and place the left hand under the patient's back at the eleventh and twelfth rib to palpate the liver (Fig. 30-10). Instruct the patient to take a deep breath. The liver edge, if palpable, presents a firm, sharp, regular ridge with a smooth surface. When felt more than 1 cm below the costal margin, it is considered abnormal.

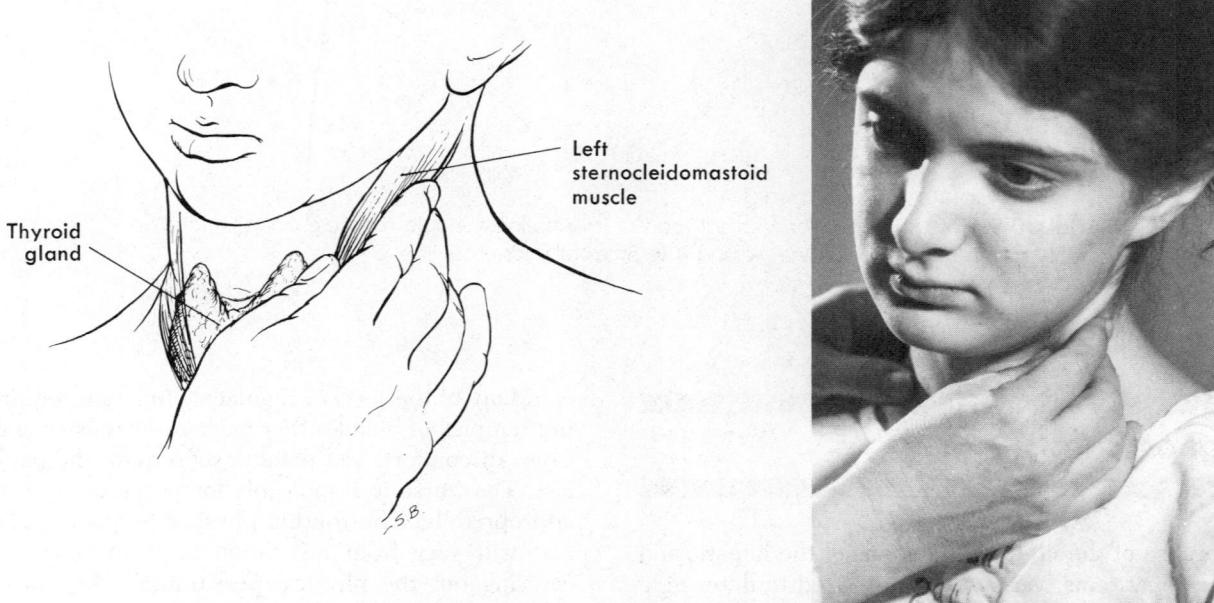

Fig. 30-8. Anterior approach to thyroid examination. Examiner grasps around left sternocleidomastoid muscle with right hand to palpate for enlarged left thyroid lobe. (From Malasanos, L., et al.: Health assessment, ed. 2, St. Louis, 1981, The C.V. Mosby Co.)

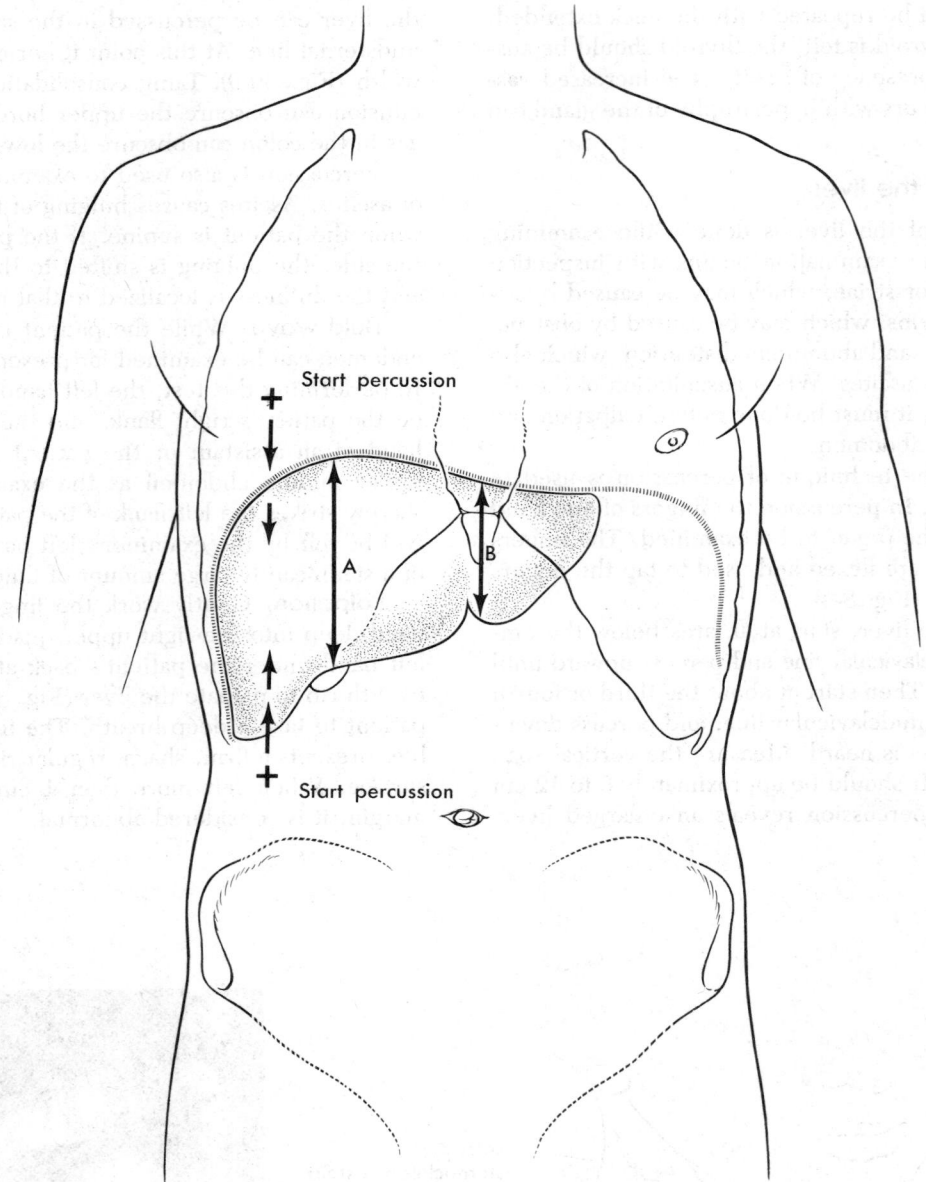

Start percussion

A

B

Start percussion

Fig. 30-9. Percussion of liver. Vertical span of liver dullness should measure approximately 6 to 12 cm at midclavicular line, *A*, and 4 to 8 cm at midsternal line, *B*.

Diagnostic tests

Because of the multiple functions of the hepatic and endocrine systems, various tests are used to determine whether disease of these regulatory systems is present and, if so, to identify the cause of the patient's symptoms.

Many of the tests of regulatory function require taking samples of blood; other tests are extensive and may cause discomfort, and many tests require the patient to fast. The nurse is responsible for preparing the patient appropriately. The routine physical preparation for any test will vary from institution to institution. Besides carrying out the physical preparation, the nurse prepares the patient for the test by explaining the purpose of the test, what can be expected prior to and during the test, and special care required after the test.

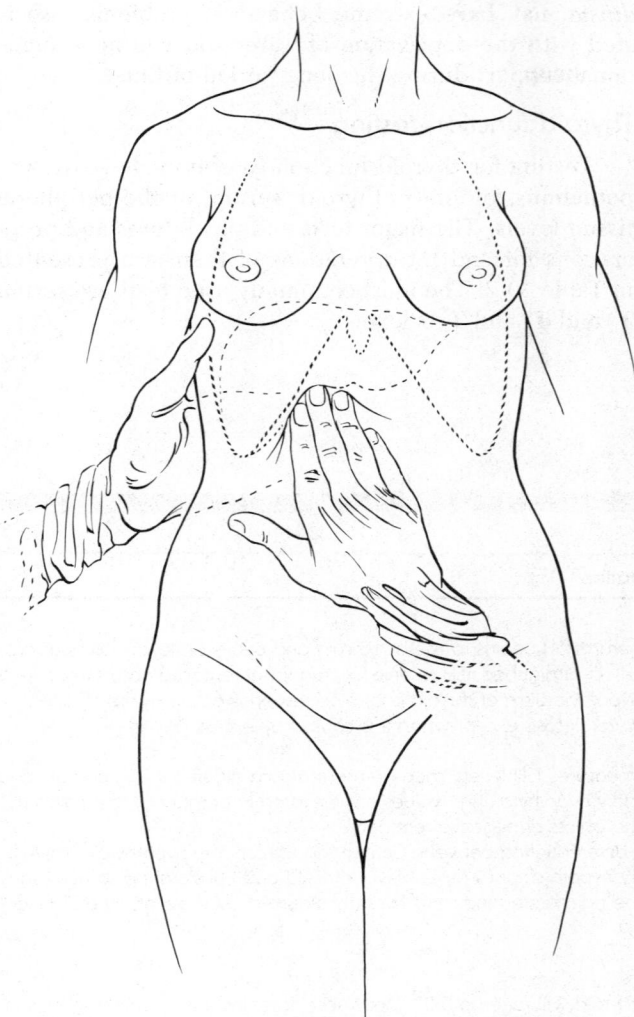

Fig. 30-10. Correct placement of hands for palpating liver.

Endocrine function testing

The suspicion that an endocrine disorder exists can be derived from information gained from the patient's history and physical examination. Since the endocrine system affects multiple body functions, all persons with suspected malfunction will have evaluations of the levels of normal blood constitutents. In this section specific diagnostic tests of endocrine function will be described. These tests are divided into two categories: direct measurement of various hormones or their by-products and measurements of specialized body functions or particular blood and urine constituents known to be controlled by the hormone. The specific diagnostic tests will be discussed separately in relation to each gland.

Pituitary function testing

Pituitary gland malfunction can lead to a wide variety of symptoms, depending on which hormone is in excess or in deficit. The pituitary gland, as described previously, is interrelated with functions of the thyroid, the adrenal glands, and the gonads. The tests for the function of the pituitary with regards to TSH, ACTH, and gonadotropins will be discussed when the diagnostic tests of each gland are discussed. Pituitary malfunction may be associated with pituitary tumors, and skull roentgenograms to assess the size of the pituitary gland will be carried out. Computed tomography (CT) scanning may be used to demonstrate the presence of intrasellar masses. In some instances pneumoencephalograms may be necessary to define the size of the mass or to exclude empty sellar syndrome.

Somatotropin hormone. The absence or deficit of somatotropin (growth hormone) leads to dramatic changes in appearance. Diagnostic tests for somatotropin will include skeletal roentgenograms to assess changes in bone structure. Assay of the growth hormone is possible. Growth hormone (GH) release follows a diurnal pattern and basal levels can best be determined in the morning, but basal levels of growth hormone are usually less than 3 μg/ml. Growth hormone secretion can be stimulated by L-dopa, arginine hydrochloride, and hypoglycemia. The provocative tests are done as follows: (1) basal levels of GH are determined; (2) L-dopa (500 mg PO), arginine hydrochloride (0.5 g/kg IV over 30 minutes), or insulin (0.1 unit/kg IV) is given; and then (3) serum levels of GH are drawn at various times up to 120 minutes after the stimulation. GH usually peaks at approximately 60 minutes after provocative stimuli. In some instances patients are given L-dopa and arginine simultaneously.

Prolactin. Prolactin excess is seen in some pituitary tumors. Prolactin deficiency may result in failure of postpartum lactation. Prolactin levels can be measured by radioassay. Provocative tests for prolactin using chlorpromazine or thyroid releasing hormone (TRH) are available. The tests are done as follows: (1) basal levels of prolactin are measured; (2) chlorpromazine (0.7 mg/kg IM) or TRH (400 μg IV) is given; and then (3) serum levels of prolactin are drawn at timed intervals up to 240 minutes.

Antidiuretic hormone. Absence of ADH leads to a disease called *diabetes insipidus*. The major symptom of this problem is an output of large quantities of dilute urine (greater than 7 to 11 liters per day). Before diabetes insipidus can be conclusively diagnosed, the patient must be shown to have a deficit in ADH, and the patient's kidney must be able to respond to ADH. Exogenous sources of ADH have no effect if the patient's kidney cannot respond. Exogenous ADH will increase the osmolarity of the urine whether the dilute urine is caused by excess intake of water or by diabetes insipidus. The differentiation between these two conditions is made by demonstrating response or lack of response to osmolarity changes in the serum.

Water deprivation test. Water is withheld until 2% to 5% of body weight is lost. This may require up to 12 hours of deprivation. The patient who has no ability to produce ADH is susceptible to vascular collapse because the massive output of urine will continue unabated. Close monitoring for impending collapse during the test is required. The patient with *psychogenic poly-* *dipsia* may have extreme behavioral problems associated with the deprivation of water and will need emotional support during this long period of time.

Thyroid function testing

Testing for thyroid function can be made at the hypothalamus, pituitary, thyroid, serum, or the peripheral tissue levels. The major tests and procedures and preparations for and interpretations of them are presented in Table 30-2. The most commonly used tests are serum T_4 and T_3 and T_3U levels.

TABLE 30-2. Tests of thyroid function

Function test	Procedure and preparation	Interpretation
Hypothalamus level test TRH stimulation test	TRH is given IV and then serum TSH levels are repeatedly measured	Normal serum TSH begins to rise at 10 min and peaks at 45 min, subnormal tests reflect diminished TSH reserve; supranormal response occurs in patients with hypothyroidism of thyroid origin; no response occurs in most patients with thyrotoxicosis except when it is caused by excess TSH
Pituitary level test TSH radioimmunoassay	Blood sample, no special preparation	Directly measures TSH levels; measurement aids in differentiating primary and secondary hypothyroidism; values are elevated in primary hypothyroidism because of loss of negative feedback
Thyroid stimulating hormone (TSH) stimulation test	Baseline levels of radioactive iodine uptake (RAIU) and protein-bound iodine (PBI) are taken, TSH injection is given and repeat RAIU and PBI levels are taken	Assists in differentiating between primary and secondary hypothyroidism; in primary hypothyroidism repeat level of RAIU and PBI stays the same; if they become normal, this indicates hypothyroidism caused by too little TSH (secondary)
Thyroid level test Radioactive iodine uptake (RAIU)	A tracer dose of radioactive iodine (^{131}I) is given by mouth. At 2, 6, and 24 hr following administration, scintillation detector is placed over neck in region of thyroid and amount of accumulated radioactive iodine is measured; excess iodine in any foods, cough medicines, x-ray media, other medications, and enriched iodine foods affect test by giving low readings; diarrhea, causing decreased absorption of tracer dose, gives low readings, renal failure, causing decreased excretion, can cause elevated readings; no radiation precautions are necessary.	Normal thyroid will take up 5-35% of tracer dose; increased uptake occurs in hyperthyroidism; excess tracer dose is excreted in urine and can be measured; urine is collected for 24 hr; decreased amounts in urine indicate hyperthyroid state
Thyroid scan	Dose of ^{131}I is given and scintillation scan is done: scanner is moved over thyroid, and a picture of distribution of radioactivity is recorded; no radiation precautions necessary	Size, shape, and anatomic function of gland assessed; areas of increased or decreased uptake noted
Thyroid suppression test	RAIU test and serum T_4 levels are done, patient given thyroid hormone for 7-10 days, RAIU and serum T_4 repeated	If euthyroid (normal), repeat RAIU and serum T_4 will be low; failure of hormone therapy to suppress RAIU and serum T_4 indicates hyperthyroidism

TABLE 30-2. Tests of thyroid function—cont'd

Function test	Procedure and preparation	Interpretation
Tests related to serum levels of thyroid hormone		
Thyroxine binding globulin (TBG)	Blood sample, no special preparation	Measures levels of TBG; TBG can be elevated or depressed by other conditions unrelated to thyroid problems; helpful in determining amount of bound and active T_3 and T_4
Serum T_4 concentration	Blood sample; test determines ability of T_4 extracted from serum to displace radioactive T_4 from T_4-binding proteins; not affected by iodides and dyes that elevate PBI and depress RAIU	Measures circulating thyroxine that is bound to TBG and free T_4; normal, 3-7 μg/100 ml; increased TBG such as occurs in pregnancy, and estrogen therapy causes increased T_4 values; decreased TBG as seen with glucocorticoid therapy and hypoproteinemia caused decreased T_4 values
Serum T_3 concentrations	Radioassay of blood sample; no special preparation	Measure circulating T_3 that is bound to TBG and free T_3; normal values are 100-170 ng/100 ml and are elevated in T_3 thyrotoxicosis; variations in thyroxine-binding globulin (TBG) can influence test results as they do for serum T_4
Triiodothyronine (T_3) resin or red cell uptake	Blood sample drawn; in laboratory resin and radioactive T_3 are added to sample of blood; radioactive T_3 will bind to unoccupied sites of thyroxine-binding globulin (TBG); radioactive counts are done on blood and resins to determine amount of T_3 (radioactive) bound to resin	Normally 25-30% of radioactive T_3 will bind to resin; in hyperthyroidism, where there are increased amounts of endogenous thyroid hormone, value will be increased; in hypothyroidism T_3 resin uptake will be low; this is not a measure of the patient's endogenous T_3 level; test is affected by total amount of TBG; in wasting diseases where amount of TBG may be decreased, reading may be falsely elevated; in conditions such as pregnancy and estrogen therapy abnormal amounts of TBG may be available and a false-low T_3 may be obtained; phenytoin (Dilantin) and salicylates compete with thyroxine for TBG sites and may give false-negative T_3 resin uptake
Free T_4 and free T_3	Blood sample, special laboratory procedures	Measures unbound metabolically active T_4 or T_3; is a difficult test and is not used frequently; instead FT_4I is calculated; FT_4I varies directly with FT_4
Free T_4 index (FT_4I)	Serum T_4 and T_3U measured	Free T_4I is product of serum T_4 and T_3U; changes in TBG causes reciprocal alterations in serum T_4 and T_3U, so that FT_4I stays normal
Protein-bound iodine test (PBI)	Serum blood sample; results of test are invalidated if patient has high exogenous sources of iodine; cough syrups, x-ray media, estrogens, and enriched iodine foods may cause false-high levels and should be avoided for 1 wk before test; mercury causes abnormally low readings	Test indirectly measures circulating T_4 concentration; normal range is 4-8 μg/100 ml of serum, decreased PBI indicates hypothyroidism; increased PBI indicates hyperthyroidism; test is being used less frequently because of availability of more specific tests
Thyroid antibodies	Blood sample; in laboratory red cells are latex coated with thyroid globulin and mixed with blood	Test may differentiate cause of thyroid enlargement; if antibodies are present, agglutination occurs
Tests related to peripheral effects of thyroid hormone		
Basal metabolism rate (BMR)	Patient at rest; amount of oxygen used while at rest is calculated; patient's oxygen utilization is compared with established norms for people of same sex, age, and size; results expressed in percentage above or below normal; patient receives nothing by mouth (NPO) the night before test, should have 8 hr of sleep, and should stay in bed morning of test; no food or smoking is allowed; anxiety will increase BMR, so patient needs explanation of what to expect	Normal range is -15% to $+15\%$; in hyperthyroidism patient's BMR will be greater than $+15\%$; in hypothyroidism patient's BMR will be less than -15%; BMR is less accurate than other tests described above but may be used to observe patients on thyroid therapy
Serum cholesterol level	Blood sample; patient placed on NPO list night before	Normals vary from laboratory to laboratory; high levels found in hypothyroidism and low levels found in hyperthyroidism; data augment other tests
Achilles tendon reflex recording	Electrodes from recording drum attached to patient's ankle; while ankle tendon is tapped, recording is done	Slow, sluggish jerk indicates hypothyroidism; rapid jerk indicates hyperthyroidism

Parathyroid function testing

Since the maintenance of normal calcium and phosphorous metabolism involves multiple systems besides the parathyroid (skeletal, gastrointestinal, and urinary), when parathyroid function is being assessed, the patient will also have diagnostic tests of these other systems. This is necessary to determine whether the problem with calcium and phosphorus metabolism is caused by parathyroid metabolism or other disease states. In addition, because calcium has a very important role in the maintenance of normal neuromuscular irritability and because hypocalcemia can be lethal, when hypoparathyroidism is suspected, the patient will be assessed and continually monitored for the presence of Trousseau's and Chvostek's signs (see Chapter 21).

The specific tests of parathyroid function consist of radioimmunoassay of parathyroid hormone (PTH), serial lab determinations of serum calcium and phosphorus, urinary calcium and phosphorus, and serum alkaline phosphatase. In addition, two other commonly performed tests are the Ellsworth-Howard excretion test and the phosphate reabsorption test.

Ellsworth-Howard excretion test. This test provides for differentiation between normal parathyroid function and decreased parathyroid function. The test is done as follows: the patient fasts prior to the examination, 200 units of parathyroid extract are given intravenously, urine is collected on an hourly basis for 3 to 5 hours and examined for the amount of phosphate excreted. Normally there will be a fivefold to sixfold increase in urinary excretion of phosphate. In hypoparathyroidism there is a tenfold increase in phosphate excretion.[41]

Phosphate reabsorption test. This test is used in the diagnosis of suspected hyperparathyroidism. It consists of collecting a urine sample for 4 to 24 hours, and a blood sample is collected at the beginning or end of the test. The amount of phosphate in the urine and blood is measured, and tubular reabsorption of phosphate is calculated. The normal tubular reabsorption of phosphate is 90% or greater. In hyperparathyroidism, values are less than 85%.[41] Although this is a relatively simple test, it is only valid if renal function is proven to be normal.

Adrenal function testing

The adrenal function tests can be divided into those designed to test *medullary* function and those designed to test *cortical* function.

Adrenal cortical function test. Since the adrenal cortex affects so many physiologic functions, tests that are diagnostic for many disorders may be ordered. Analysis of blood to ascertain electrolyte balance, a glucose tolerance test to determine the ability of the patient to utilize carbohydrates, and a test of the ability of the renal tubules to concentrate and dilute urine will probably be done. In addition, roentgenograms of the kidney area may be taken to ascertain the presence of adrenal tumors.

Diagnostic tests of adrenocortical function include tests of all three types of hormonal secretions. Plasma cortisol follows a diurnal pattern and is measured at 8 AM and 4 PM. Plasma aldosterone, angiotensin II, and renin are measured to evaluate the aldosterone-angiotensinogen system. Plasma levels of aldosterone are increased by dietary potassium loading, sodium restriction, and assumption of an upright position. Aldosterone levels may be measured before and after manipulating these factors. Plasma levels of androgens are also measured to evaluate the adrenal androgen system. ACTH levels can also be measured.

Twenty-four-hour urine collections, which are analyzed for 17-ketosteroids (17-KS), 17-ketogenic steroids (17-KGS), and 17-hydroxycorticosteroids (17-OHCS) will also be measured. These compounds are metabolites of the hormones produced by the adrenal gland. These 24 urine collections require special preservatives, and the nurse should know the institution's requirements and make sure the appropriate container is available.

In addition to the above studies, other definitive tests are available to determine whether hypofunction or hyperfunction of the adrenal cortex is present and to establish whether the malfunction is caused by a primary adrenal cortical problem or whether the malfunction is secondary to pituitary malfunction. These studies are described in Table 30-3.

Adrenal medulla function test. The function of the adrenal medulla can be assessed by the assay of catecholamines and their metabolites in the urine. A 24-hour urine collection is carried out, and the end product, 3-methoxy-4-hydroxymandelic acid, also called vanillylmandelic acid (VMA) or catecholamines is assayed.

Pressor tests to establish a diagnosis of *pheochromocytoma* (adrenal-medullary tumor) employ manipulation of the blood pressure. In one test, histamine 0.01 to 0.025 mg is given intravenously. A dramatic rise in blood pressure of at least 50 mm Hg higher than an elevation provoked by the immersion of the patient's hand in cold water will be seen if the patient has pheochromocytoma. Urine collection after the test will contain increased catecholamines. The patient needs to be monitored closely for hypertensive crisis, and intravenous antihypertensive agents should be readily available.

Another test employs phentolamine (Regitine). Phentolamine will cause a drop of at least 35 mm Hg in the systolic blood pressure and at least a 25 mm Hg drop in the diastolic blood pressure if the elevated pressure is caused by excess catecholamines. The patient can have a major hypotensive crisis during this test and needs very careful monitoring.

TABLE 30-3. Tests of adrenocortical function

Function test	Procedure and preparation	Intereration
ACTH stimulation test (various tests available)	Synthetic ACTH given in 500-1000 ml of normal saline at 2 units/24 hr; then 17-OHCS and plasma cortisol levels are measured; alternative way is to infuse 25 units of ACTH over an 8-hr period on 2-3 days and measure 17-OHCS and plasma cortisol levels on these days	Normally 17-OHCS excretion increases to 25 mg/24 hr and plasma cortisol increases to 40 μg/100 ml or greater; in patients with secondary adrenal insufficiency, the 17-OHCS rate is 3-20 mg/24 hr and the cortisol level is 10-40 μg/100 ml
Screening ACTH stimulation test	ACTH, 25 units, is given IM and plasma cortisol level is measured before and 30 and 60 min after tests	Normally plasma cortisol increases 7 μg/100 ml
Cortisone suppression test	Twenty-four-hour urine specimen for 17-OHCS is collected for baseline; dexamethasone, 0.5 mg, is given every 6 hr for 2 days; 24-hr urine is collected for these 2 days	Dexamethasone suppresses pituitary secretion of ACTH but does not change steroid excretion; normally by second day of dexamethasone, 24-hr urinary level of OHCS should drop more than 50% below baseline, patients with adrenocortical excess (primary) will show decrease in 24-hr urine levels; patients with secondary adrenocortical excess will have drop, but less than 50%
Screening suppression test	Dexamethasone 1 mg, given at 12 PM, at 8 AM cortisol level is drawn	Normally cortisol should be less than 5 μg/100 ml
Mineralocorticoid suppression test (various tests are available)	IV infusion of saline 500 ml/hr for 4 hr	Normally saline infusion depresses plasma aldosterone to < 8 μg/100 ml if patient has been on a sodium-restricted diet and to < 5 μg/100 ml if the patient has been on a normal sodium diet
	Alternative: patient placed on normal sodium diet (100 mEq) or high sodium diet (200 mEq), after patient is in sodium balance, DOCA (10 mg q 12 hr) administered IM for 3-5 days	Normal persons on a sodium diet of 100 mEq/day will have a 70% decrease in aldosterone

Pancreatic endocrine function testing

The pancreas has both exocrine and endocrine capabilities. The major endocrine disorder of the pancreas is caused by disturbance in production, action, or metabolic rate of utilization of insulin. The relative lack of insulin leads to elevated blood glucose levels and the presence of glucose in the urine. The majority of diagnostic tests of pancreatic endocrine function are based on assessment of urine and blood glucose levels. The hormone, insulin, can be measured by radioimmunoassay.

Urine tests. Urine testing is familiar to most of the public. Testing of urine for sugar is part of a complete urinalysis, and the urine of patients with known or suspected diabetes mellitus is tested frequently for sugar and acetone by one of the following methods. Patients with known diabetes mellitus may be asked to do the tests themselves at regular intervals as an indication of adequate control of the blood sugar level.

Clinitest is a copper reduction method of testing the urine for sugar. It comes in a compact kit and is convenient for use because it is small and easy to carry and store. The kit contains a test tube, a medicine dropper, caustic tablets, and a color chart. Either 2 or 5 drops of urine are placed in the test tube with 10 drops of water,

and a Clinitest tablet is added. The tablet generates heat, and the color of the solution is graded by comparing it with the 2-drop or 5-drop color chart. Certain drugs can affect the accuracy of this testing product. Large amounts of vitamin C and cephalosporin preparations such as cephalothin (Keflin) can give false-positive readings.

Tes-Tape, Clinistix, and *Diastix* are strip tests for glucose. Since color charts vary for each product, caution must be exercised in interpreting results. Also, test results must be read at specified time intervals to be accurate. *Acetest* tablets may be used to test for acetone. Urine is dropped on the tablet. If acetone is present, varying shades of lavender will appear and can be compared with a color chart. *Ketostix* is a strip product that can also be used to detect the presence of ketones.

Increasingly, single specimens of urine are used to test the urine for the presence of sugar. If the physician desires to know the amount of sugar being excreted in the urine at a particular time, a *double-voided urine* is ordered. To obtain this type of specimen the patient is asked to void, then is given water to drink, and voids again in 30 minutes. The second specimen is tested by one of the methods described above. If the patients are taught to test their urine at home, usually the double-void technique is taught. *If insulin is being regulated on the basis of urine checks, double-voided specimens for testing are required.*

In some situations the physician may wish to find out what time of day the most sugar is excreted. To determine this, *fractional* or *group* urines may be collected. All the urine voided from before breakfast to just before lunch is collected, and a sample is tested for sugar. This is the first specimen; the second is collected from before lunch to just before dinner; the third, from dinner to before bedtime; and the fourth, from bedtime until the next morning.

Twenty-four–hour urine collections also may be obtained to determine the quantity of sugar excreted in a day. In this collection the first specimen of the morning is discarded. All urine excreted for the next 24 hours is collected in a gallon container and sent to the laboratory. It is important that the patient knows he must add the first urine voided the next morning to the specimen.

Blood tests. Common tests to assess blood glucose

levels are described in Table 30-4 and a more detailed explanation of them can be found on p. 647.

Liver function tests

Liver function tests include (1) blood, urine, and stool examination to determine amount and distribution of bile pigments; (2) blood tests that demonstrate the ability of the liver to carry out its metabolism functions; (3) tests that identify presence of hepatic damage; and (4) tests that determine the liver's excretory functions. Other diagnostic procedures may be employed to determine causes of biliary and hepatic malfunction. Because the liver can be affected by processes outside of the hepatic system, the tests are of great importance in determining whether signs and symptoms are caused by disease of the hepatic cells themselves (hepatocellular) or by pathologic processes outside the hepatic system.

TABLE 30-4. Diagnostic blood tests for pancreatic endocrine function

Test	Procedure and preparation	Interpretation
Fasting blood sugar (FBS)	NPO after midnight	Normal level at 80 to 120 mg/100 ml; elevated level indicates a need for further study to rule out diabetes mellitus
Two-hr postprandial blood sugar	Blood sugar measured 2 hr after heavy meal or 2 hr after receiving loading dose of 100 g of sugar	Blood sugar should be within normal limits; levels above 120 mg/100 ml should be investigated further
Glucose tolerance test (GTT)	NPO after midnight; samples of blood and urine are collected at beginning of test; patient is given mixture of glucose to drink or a meal containing 150-300 g of carbohydrate; blood and urine are collected at intervals of ½, 1, and 2 hr (2-hr GTT); samples may be collected at 3-, 4-, and 5-hr intervals (5-hr GTT); presence of gastrointestinal disorder that interferes with oral glucose absorption requires administration of intravenous glucose; test is done in same manner as for oral GTT	Interpretation of results differs according to source of blood, method of analysis, and critical levels established by various authorities; patient with diabetes mellitus or hyperfunction of adrenal cortex will have high levels initially that remain higher than normal; patients with hypoglycemia may have drop in blood sugar much below normal levels and must be monitored for signs of hypoglycemia
Cortisone-glucose tolerance test	Performed similar to GTT except that cortisone is administered at start of test	Used when GTT results are inconclusive; cortisone causes an abnormal increase in blood glucose and decreased peripheral utilization of glucose in persons predisposed to diabetes; blood glucose level of 140 mg/100 ml at end of 2 hr is considered positive test
Tolbutamide test	NPO after midnight; FBS is drawn and sodium tolbutamide, 1 g, is given intravenously, blood samples for glucose analysis are drawn at intervals of 15, 30, and 45 min and 1, 1½, 2, 2½, and 3 hr	In normal persons, FBS level will fall to at least 70% of fasting level within 3 hr; in abnormal response, FBS fails to fall; in patients with insulin-producing tumors, blood sugar may drop drastically; patient must be monitored for signs of hypoglycemia

Laboratory tests

Multiple tests may be necessary to determine the extent and seriousness of hepatic disease. Many tests require serial reading to be of benefit. The test, procedure and special preparation, and interpretation of commonly used blood, stool, and urine studies for evaluation of liver function are summarized in Table 30-5.

Various other tests to measure different aspects of liver function are available and have been used in the past, but have been abandoned as more specific tests became available. These tests may be used in rare cases. A full description of other tests and their interpretation can be found in the identified references.[12,34]

Other diagnostic tests

Roentgenologic and other diagnostic tests are used to assist in identifying the cause and site of hepatic mal-

TABLE 30-5. Laboratory tests of liver function

Function and test	Procedure and preparation	Interpretation
Fat metabolism		
Serum total cholesterol and cholesterol esters	Blood drawn; fasting may be required	Normal level is 140-220 mg/100 ml of blood; approximately 70% is cholesterol ester; in hepatocellular disease, amount of total serum cholesterol and cholesterol ester may be decreased; in obstructive biliary tract disease, total serum cholesterol is increased, but amount of esterified cholesterol is decreased; normal cholesterol levels rise with age
Serum phospholipids	Blood drawn; no special preparation	Normal level is 150-250 mg/100 ml; serum phospholipids tend to be low in severe hepatocellular disease and high in obstructive biliary tract disease
Protein metabolism		
Total serum protein	Blood drawn; no special preparation	Normal level is 6-8 g/100 ml; measures all serum protein; may be normal in hepatocellular disease because an increase in serum globulin will replace decreased serum albumin; increased globulins are seen in chronic inflammatory disease, neoplastic diseases, and biliary obstruction
Albumin	Blood drawn; no special preparation	Normal level is 3.4-5 g/100 ml; albumin made only in liver; in hepatocellular disease there may be decrease in serum albumin level
Protein electrophoresis	Blood drawn; no special preparation, protein fraction of blood will migrate in characteristic directions in electrical field; after separation of fractions, specimen is stained and densitometer used to measure amounts of various serum protein	Normal fractions in relation to total serum protein (100%) are albumin, 52-68%; α-globulins, 12-17%, β-globulins, 7-15%; and immune serum globulins (γ-globulins), 9-19%; in severe hepatocellular damage, amount of albumin may be decreased; inflammatory processes of the liver may produce increased amounts of α_1 globulins, neoplastic disease is associated with increased levels of α_2-globulins, and some patients with obstructive biliary tract disease may have high levels of β-globulins
Immunoglobulins	Blood drawn; no special preparation	Five classes of antibodies; IgA, IgG, IgM, IgE, and IgD; IgA and IgG are often increased in presence of cirrhosis; IgG is elevated in presence of chronic active hepatitis; biliary cirrhosis and hepatitis A cause an increase in IgM component
Blood urea nitrogen (BUN)	Blood drawn; no special preparation	Normal is 10-20 mg/100 ml; in severe hepatocellular disease if portal vein flow is obstructed, level may decrease; varies with dietary protein intake and fluid volume
Serum prothrombin time (PT)	Blood drawn; no special preparation; reflects activity of prothrombin, fibrinogen, and factors V, VII, and IX	Normal prothrombin time is 12-15 sec or 100%, as compared to control level; prothrombin time may be increased in hepatocellular disease because of inability of liver to produce clotting factors or in obstructive biliary tract disease because of malabsorption of vitamin K; persistence of abnormal prothrombin time after parenteral administration of vitamin K indicates hepatocellular damage
Serum partial thromboplastin time (PTT) and activated partial thromboplastin time (APTT)	Blood drawn; no special preparation; reflects activity of prothrombin, fibrinogen, and factors V, VII, IX, X, XI, and XIII	Normal level is 68-82 sec with standard technique; activated PTT levels are 32-46 sec; this test is more sensitive in detecting minimal deficiencies than prothrombin time; PTT and APTT will be increased for same reasons as those stated for prothrombin time
Blood ammonia levels	Blood drawn; may require fasting	Normal level is less than 75 μg/100 ml; may be elevated in severe hepatocellular disease because of decreased urea production or obstruction of portal blood flow
Bilirubin metabolism		
Total bilirubin Conjugated (direct) Unconjugated (indirect)	Blood drawn; no special preparation	Total serum bilirubin measures both conjugated and unconjugated bilirubin; normal values range from 0.1-1 mg/100 ml; conjugated bilirubin acts directly with diazo reagents; unconjugated bilirubin requires addition of methyl alcohol; thus the terms *direct* and *indirect*; conjugated bilirubin increased in presence of hepatocellular and obstructive biliary tract disease; unconjugated bilirubin elevated with increased hemolysis of red blood cells or with hepatocellular disease

Continued.

TABLE 30-5. Laboratory tests of liver function—cont'd

Function and test	Procedure and preparation	Interpretation
Urine bilirubin	Spot urine specimen; no special preparation	Normally no bilirubin is excreted in urine; urine with abnormal bilirubin is mahogany colored and has a yellow foam when shaken (foam test); unconjugated bilirubin not excreted in urine; conjugated serum bilirubin levels greater than 0.4 mg/100 ml will lead to conjugated bilirubin being excreted in urine—indicates hepatocellular or obstructive biliary tract disease; bilirubinuria may be present before jaundice
Urine urobilinogen	Twenty-four–hr urine collection or 2-hr afternoon collection	Normally 0.2-1.2 units found in specimen; fresh urine urobilinogen is colorless; decreased amounts of urine urobilinogen found in obstructive biliary tract disease; increased amounts found in hepatocellular disease; alterations in intestinal flora by broad-spectrum antibiotics may change test
Fecal urobilinogen	Stool specimen; no special preparation	Normally 90-280 mg/day; presence of urobilinogen gives stool brown color; absence of urobilinogen causes stools to become clay to white colored; increased amounts found in increased hemolysis of red blood cells; absence of fecal urobilinogen (stercobilinogen) indicates obstructive biliary tract disease
Serum enzymes		
Serum glutamic-oxaloacetic transaminase (SGOT)	Blood drawn; no special preparation	Normal values vary depending on measurement used; these enzymes are present in hepatic cells, and with necrosis of hepatic cells, enzymes are released and elevated serum levels will be found; GGT is found in high levels in kidney and liver; SGPT is primarily present in liver; SGOT is also present in high levels in skeletal and heart muscle; LDH is also present in heart, kidneys, skeletal muscle, and erythrocytes, but in each tissue the LDH enzyme has a characteristic composition: thus the source can be determined by isoenzyme tests; with the other three tests necrosis of other organs must be ruled out; GGT is elevated early in liver disease and elevation persists as long as cellular damage continues; GGT is routinely elevated in alcohol-induced liver disease and increased levels are often seen before other abnormal test results occur
Serum glutamic-pyruvic transaminase (SGPT)		
Lactic dehydrogenase (LDH)		
Gamma-glutamyl transpeptidase (GGT)		
Alkaline phosphatase	Blood drawn; no special preparation	Normal values vary depending on measurement used; this enzyme originates in liver, bone, intestine, and placenta; alkaline phosphatase is slightly to moderately elevated in hepatocellular disease but extremely elevated in obstructive biliary tract and bone disease
Excretory function		
Bromsulphalein (BSP) excretion	Patient is weighed and BSP, 5 mg/kg of body weight, is injected intravenously; blood sample is drawn from other arm 45 min later; patient must be fasting	Normally less than 5% of test dose is retained in serum after 45 min; abnormal retention reflects presence of hepatic cell damage and inability of liver to remove dye and excrete it; biliary tract obstruction may also cause retention; extrahepatic conditions such as shock and congestive heart failure can cause retention of BSP; BSP dye causes necrosis of tissue if it extravasates during injection; certain drugs (iopanoic acid) may cause retention; phenolsulfonphthalein test of kidney function should not be done for 24 hr after BSP test
Antigens and antibodies of hepatitis	Blood drawn; no special preparation	Normally no hepatitis antigens or antibodies should be found in serum; hepatitis A virus (HAV) found in stool and serum early in course of hepatitis A[20] and identified by immune electron microscopy; there are many serum particles associated with hepatitis B virus; complete hepatitis B virus is called the Dane particle; a core antigen (HB_cAg), a surface antigen (HB_sAg) and antibody (anti-HB_sAg), and several antigenic subtypes can be found by various serologic procedures; test for presence of HB_sAg is the only test readily available; Australian antigen is the original name for HB_sAg

function. Examination of the liver, portal system, gallbladder, and biliary duct is possible. Besides the examinations described below, the diagnostic examination of the patient with liver problems may include abdominal films, barium swallow (p. 1382), barium enema (p. 1439), and gastroscopy (p. 1382). The latter three tests assist in the detection of varices.

Cholecystography. A normal liver will remove radiopaque drugs such as iodoalphionic acid (Priodax), iopanoic acid (Telepaque), and iodipamide methylglucamine (Cholografin Meglumine) from the bloodstream and store and concentrate them in the gallbladder. Because the roentgen rays cannot penetrate the dye, the dye-filled gallbladder shows up as a dense shadow on x-ray examination (*cholecystogram, gallbladder series*). A satisfactory gallbladder shadow would indicate a functioning gallbladder. A total absence of opaque material in the gallbladder would suggest a nonfunctioning gallbladder. After ingestion of a fatty meal, a functioning gallbladder should contract and expel the radiopaque dye along with the bile through the common bile duct into the duodenum. X-ray examination at this point would outline the bile ducts. Stones, which are not radiopaque, show up as dark patches on the film. Visualization of the gallbladder depends on absorption of the dye through the intestinal tract, isolation of it by the liver, and a free passageway from the liver to the gallbladder. Therefore if the results show a nonfunctioning gallbladder, sometimes the test is repeated to be sure that failure to visualize the gallbladder by x-ray examination was not caused by insufficient dye.

On the evening before cholecystography is scheduled, the purpose of and preparation for the test is explained to the patient. The importance of following instructions regarding food restriction the morning of the test, as well as the need for the high-fat intake, which may cause nausea, should be discussed.

The average adult dose of both iodoalphionic acid and iopanoic acid is 3 g (45 grains) given orally following a low-fat evening meal, after which no food is given. The dose is calculated by body weight. An obese person would receive a larger dose than normal, and a very small person a smaller than normal dose. These drugs may cause nausea, vomiting, and diarrhea in some people. The nurse should check dosages accurately and watch carefully for toxic signs, which should be reported to the physician. If vomiting occurs soon after ingestion of the drug, the physician may ask that the tablets be repeated when nausea subsides, or the test may be delayed for several days. If the patient cannot tolerate the drug by mouth, a radiopaque substance such as iodipamide methylglucamine may be given intravenously by the physician in the radiology department. The radiopaque dyes are organic iodine compounds and may cause allergic reactions when given intravenously. Symptoms may include dyspnea, chills, diaphoresis, faintness, and tachycardia and are identical to symptoms that can occur when radiopaque substances containing iodine are injected intravenously for other tests such as pyelography or arteriography. (See discussion of intravenous pyelogram [IVP] for precaution and care.)

On the morning of the examination the patient may have only black coffee, tea, or water. One or more enemas may be given to help remove gas from the intestinal tract so that it will not interfere with a clear roentgenogram. The patient goes to the radiology department where two roentgenograms are taken during the morning. The first one is on a fasting stomach, and the second is taken after ingestion of a high-fat preparation. Ingestion of fat should stimulate flow of bile and emptying of the gallbladder. The dye is finally excreted in the urine, and some patients report slight temporary pain on urination following the test.

Cholangiography. Cholangiography is the x-ray examination of the bile ducts to demonstrate the presence of stones, strictures, or tumors. The radiopaque substance may be administered intravenously or injected directly into the common bile duct with a needle or catheter at the time of surgery. Following operations on the common bile duct, the radiopaque drug, usually iodipamide methylglucamine, may be instilled through a drainage tube such as the **T** tube to determine the patency of the duct before the tube is removed. This dye also may be injected through the skin and abdominal wall into a bile duct in the main substance of the liver (*percutaneous transhepatic cholangiography*). This technique is useful in visualizing the location and extent of a pathologic process such as obstructive jaundice and permits decompression of the liver for improved function. The procedure helps the surgeon identify the location of pathologic processes prior to surgery or may indicate that surgery is not necessary. The hazards of the examination occasionally may include bile leakage leading to bile peritonitis or bleeding caused by accidental rupture of a blood vessel.[14]

Angiography. Catheterization of the hepatic artery, portal venous system (by various routes), and the hepatic vein allows the injection of a contrast media and the visualization of the vascular supply of the hepatic system. The patency of the system and the presence of tumors, abscesses, collateral circulation, varices, and bleeding may be determined by use of angiography.

Portal and hepatic vein pressure (wedged hepatic vein pressure [WHVP]) can be measured. These readings may be done in conjunction with angiography or as a separate study. These measurements help in determining the degree of portal hypertension.

The presence of allergy to contrast media must be ascertained prior to angiography. After both angiography and pressure readings, the site of insertion is observed for bleeding, and the patient's vital signs are checked frequently.

Radioisotope scanning. The liver may be outlined by radioisotope scanning techniques. Radioisotopes such as ^{131}I rose bengal, which is taken up by the hepatocytes, colloidal technetium (^{99}Tc), which is taken up by the reticuloendothelial cells, or gallium citrate (^{67}Ga), which is concentrated in inflammatory and neoplastic cells, are given intravenously. After the injection of the radioisotope, the patient is placed supine, and a scintillation detector is passed over the abdomen in the area of the liver. The radiation coming from the isotopes immediately beneath the probe of the scanner is detected, amplified, and recorded. Scanning helps to differentiate nonfunctioning areas from normal tissue and helps to identify hepatic tumors, cysts, and abscesses (Fig. 30-11). Usually a nonfunctioning area will appear as an area of decreased activity. However, ^{67}Ga is preferentially taken up by hepatocellular carcinomas and abscesses, and these areas will appear as areas of very heavy radioactivity. Untoward reactions to these radioisotopes are unusual, and the procedure is relatively safe. Discom-

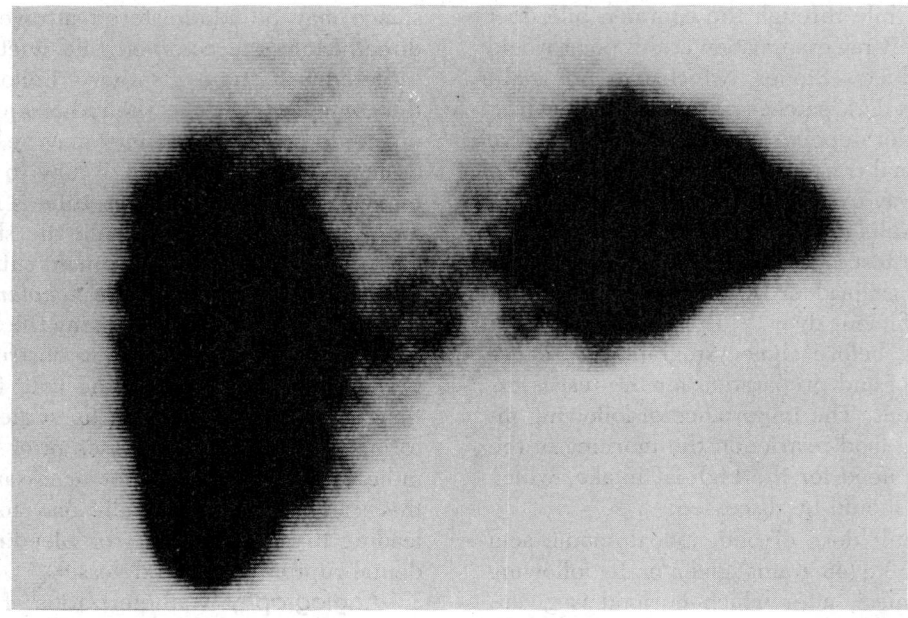

Fig. 30-11. Liver scan showing metastasis to liver (light area on right) of carcinoma of colon. (Courtesy Abbas M. Rejali, M.D., Department of Radiology, Case Western Reserve University, Cleveland.)

fort is minimal and is related to the intravenous injection and the position on the x-ray table. Only small amounts of radioactive material are given, and radiation precautions are *not* necessary. Except for ^{67}Ga scanning, no special preparation is required. Gallium citrate is excreted by the gastrointestinal tract. To avoid absorption of the radioisotope by the gastrointestinal contents, cleansing of the bowel with laxatives and enemas will be prescribed. The exact preparation will vary from institution to institution.

Ultrasound examination. In ultrasonic hepatography the liver is bombarded with sound waves and the reflected sound is recorded. The ability to portray an image is caused by the different sounds generated by solid tissue, air-filled cavities, and fluid-filled cavities. Air almost completely impedes transmission so that a 100% reflection occurs. The liver, predominantly a solid organ, provides no impedance; therefore no reflections occur. The vascular system and biliary ducts in the liver impede some transmissions, and small reflections occur from these areas. The presence of diffuse liver disease such as cirrhosis, the presence of cystic and solid tumors, and the presence of cavities cause the recording of different sound patterns.[34]

Ultrasound is a noninvasive procedure that can be used safely on most patients. Preparation for the test requires the bowel to be cleansed, since the presence of solid content in the gastrointestinal tract would cause changes in reflected sounds and distort the recording.

Endoscopy. The hepatic system and gallbladder can be examined by endoscopy. Two types of endoscopy

procedures can be done. The tube can be inserted through the peritoneum (peritoneoscopy), thus affording direct visualization of the abdominal organs and the taking of biopsies. Also the tube can be passed through the oral pharynx to the duodenum and into the biliary tract. This is known as endoscopic retrograde cholangiopancreatography (ERCP). Direct visualization is possible, dye can be injected through the scope, and biopsies can be taken.

Endoscopy is an invasive procedure that is not without risk and is used only when absolutely necessary. The patient is required to fast prior to the test and may be given a sedative before the procedure.

Biopsy of the liver. A biopsy of the liver may be used to aid in establishing the cause of liver disease. In this procedure a specially designed needle is inserted through the chest or abdominal wall into the liver, and a small piece of tissue is removed for study. This procedure is contraindicated if the patient has an infection of the right lower lobe of the lung, ascites, a blood dyscrasia, or is unable to cooperate by holding his breath. To avoid hemorrhage, vitamin K may be given parenterally for several days before and after the biopsy is taken. A biopsy may not be done if the prothrombin time is below 40%. The physician should explain the procedure to patients; for example, patients should know that they must hold their breath and remain absolutely still when the needle is introduced. Movement of the chest may cause the needle to slip and to tear the liver covering. Most hospitals require that the patient give written permission for the procedure to be done. Food and fluids may be withheld for several hours preceding the test, and a sedative usually is given about 30 minutes before the biopsy is to be taken.

The method is as follows: The patient lies supine; the skin over the area selected (usually the eighth or ninth intercostal space) is cleansed and anesthetized with procaine hydrochloride. A nick is made in the skin with a sharp scalpel blade. Then the patient is instructed to take several deep breaths and to hold his or her breath while the needle is introduced through the intercostal or subcostal tissues into the liver. The special needle assembly is rotated to separate a fragment of tissue and then is withdrawn. The specimen is placed into an appropriate container, which is then labeled and sent to the pathology laboratory. A simple dressing is placed over the wound.

The dangers of this procedure, which is done relatively "blind," are accidental penetration of blood vessels, causing hemorrhage, and accidental penetration of a biliary vessel, causing a chemical peritonitis from leakage of bile into the abdominal cavity. After the procedure the patient's pulse rate and blood pressure should be taken every 30 minutes for the first few hours and then hourly for at least 24 hours. The physician may order pressure applied to the biopsy site to help stop any bleeding. Pressure may be applied by having the patient lie on the right side with a small pillow or folded bath blanket placed under the costal margin for several hours after the biopsy. The patient remains on bed rest for 24 hours after the test.

REFERENCES AND SELECTED READINGS
Contemporary

1. Bates, B.: A guide to physical examination, ed. 2, Philadelphia, 1979, J.B. Lippincott Co.
2. *Berk, R.N.: Radiology of the gallbladder and bile ducts, Surg. Clin. North Am. 53:973-1005, 1973.
3. *Black, M.: Diagnostic methods in liver disease, Med. Clin. North Am. 59:1015-1023, 1975.
4. *Boyer, C.A., and Oehlberg, S.M.: Interpretation and clinical relevance of liver function tests, Nurs. Clin. North Am. 12:275-290, 1977.
5. Brody, D.H., and Leichter, T.: Clearance tests of liver function, Med. Clin North Am. 63:621-630, 1979.
6. *Burke, M.D.: Hepatic function testing, Postgrad. Med. 64:177-182, 185, 1978.
7. *Byrne, J.: Liver function studies. I. Introduction and bilirubin, Nurs. '77 7(7):12-14, 1977.
8. *Bryne, J.: Liver function studies. II. Conjugation and excretion tests, Nurs. '77 7(9):88-90, 1977.
9. Cryer, P.E.: Diagnostic endocrinology, ed. 2, New York, 1979, Oxford University Press.
10. DeGroot, L., et al.: Endocrinology, 3 vols., New York, 1979, Grune & Stratton, Inc.
11. Dolman, L.I.: Plasma ACTH radioimmunoassays in the diagnosis of pituitary adrenal dysfunction, Ann. N.Y. Acad. Sci. 297:205-219, 1977.
12. Dworken, H.: The alimentary tract: basic principles and case problems, Philadelphia, 1974, W.B. Saunders Co.
13. Eddy, R.L., Gilliland, P.F., and Ibarra, J.D.: Human growth hormone release. Comparison of provocative test procedures, Am. J. Med. 56:179-183, 1974.
14. Evans, J.A., and Mujahed, Z.: Percutaneous transhepatic cholangiography, Postgrad. Med. 53:182-185, 1973.
15. *Gold, E.M.: Hypothalamic-pituitary function tests, Postgrad. Med. 62:105-108, 110, 1977.
16. Gorman, C.A.: Some problems in thyroid diagnosis, Med. Clin. North Am. 56:841-847, 1972.
17. *Hallal, J.: Thyroid disorders, Am. J. Nurs. 77:418-432, 1977.
18. Harvey, A.M., et al.: The principle and practice of medicine, ed. 20, Englewood Cliffs, N.J., 1980, Prentice-Hall, Inc.
19. Huang, S.H.: Nursing assessment in planning care for diabetic patients, Nurs. Clin. North Am. 6:135-143, 1971.
20. Isselbacher, K., et al.: Harrison's principles of internal medicine, ed. 9., New York, 1980, McGraw-Hill Book Co.
21. Jubiz, W.: Endocrinology: a logical approach for clinicians, New York, 1979, McGraw-Hill Book Co.
22. Krueger, J.M., and Ray, J.C.: Endocrine problems in nursing, St. Louis, 1976, The C.V. Mosby Co.
23. *Leopold, G., and Sokoloff, J.: Ultrasonic scanning in the diagnosis of biliary disease, Surg. Clin. North Am. 53:1043-1052, 1973.
24. Loeb, P.M.: Endoscopic pancreatocholangiography in the diagnosis of biliary tract disease, Surg. Clin. North Am. 53:1007-1018, 1973.
25. Lomas, F.: Increased specificity of liver scanning with the use of ^{67}Ga citrate, N. Engl. J. Med. 286:1323-1329, 1972.
26. Malasanos, L., Barkauskas, V., Moss, M., and Stoltenberg-Allen, K.: Health assessment, ed. 2, St. Louis, 1981, The C.V. Mosby Co.
27. *May, P.: Initial evaluation and management of patients with suspected pituitary tumors, Primary Care 4:89-129, March 1977.
28. Mountcastle, V.B., editor: Medical physiology, ed 14, St. Louis, 1979, The C.V. Mosby Co.
29. Ontjes, D.A., and Ney, R.L.: Tests of anterior pituitary functions, Metabolism 21:159-165, 1972.
30. Pierce, L.: Anatomy and physiology of the liver in relation to clinical assessment, Nurs. Clin. North Am. 12:259-273, 1977.
31. Sanders, T.P.: Liver scanning, Postgrad. Med. 53:191-195, 1973.
32. Sawin, C.T., et al.: The free triiodothyronine (T_3) index, Ann. Intern. Med. 88:474-476, 1978.
33. Schein, C.J.: Influence of choledochoscopy on the choice of surgical procedure, Am. J. Surg. 130:74-77, 1975.
34. Schiff, L., editor: Diseases of the liver, ed. 4, Philadelphia, 1975, J.B. Lippincott Co.
35. Schwartz, S.I., et al.: Principles of surgery, ed. 2, New York, 1974, McGraw-Hill Book Co.
36. Shultzev, G., Bogen, Y., and Sokolova, G.: Ultrasonic diagnoses of hepatic disorders, Am. J. Gastroenterol. 65:432-436, 1976.
37. Small, D.M.: Gallstone diagnosis and treatment, Postgrad. Med. 51:187-193, 1972.
38. *Solomon, B.L.: The hypothalamus and the pituitary gland: an overview, Nurs. Clin. North Am. 15:435-452, 1980.
39. Tepperman, J.: Metabolic and endocrine physiology, ed. 3, Chicago, 1973, Year Book Medical Publishers, Inc.
40. Vennes, J.A.: Endoscopic cholangiography for biliary system diagnosis, Ann. Intern. Med. 80:61-64, 1974.
41. Widmann, F.: Goodall's clinical interpretation of laboratory tests, ed. 8, Philadelphia, 1979, F.A. Davis Co.
42. Williams, S.M.: Diabetic urine testing by hospital nursing personnel, Nurs. Res. 20:444-447, 1971.

Classic
43. Stauffer, M.H.: Needle biopsy of the liver, Surg. Clin. North Am. 47:851-860, 1967.

---

*References preceded by an asterisk are particularly well suited for student reading.

CHAPTER 31

INTERVENTION FOR PERSONS WITH IMPAIRED REGULATORY MECHANISMS

VIRGINIA L. CASSMEYER

Persons with impaired regulatory mechanisms will have some problems that are similar regardless of the particular site of pathology. This chapter will focus on the needs of these persons and measures to meet their needs. Desired patient outcomes to guide care are presented with each problem. Care of persons with specific problems is discussed in later chapters.

Persons with impaired regulatory mechanisms will have a problem maintaining physiologic stability and integrity. Physiologic functions under the control of the hepatic and endocrine systems are diverse, and dysfunction may be reflected in many parts of the body. Because these functions are vital ones, disorders of any of the regulatory mechanisms may be extremely serious. A majority of the problems arising from dysfunction of these mechanisms are chronic in nature and require the individual to learn how to keep the problems under control. Regardless of cause, nursing management of these persons is centered on three areas: *prevention of the primary problem or complications, care during the acute episode, and preparation of individuals (and significant others) to care for themselves on a long-term basis.*

Prevention

The public is becoming better informed about certain diseases of the regulatory mechanisms, such as viral hepatitis and diabetes mellitus. This in' turn may lead to better health habits in the future. At the same time many persons have friends or relatives who have died or have been handicapped by disease of the regulatory mechanisms; and this may cause fear and lead them to be hesitant in seeking help.

Certain diseases of the hepatic system can be prevented. For example, the spread of viral hepatitis can be halted if the public is taught to use good hygienic practices and proper sterilization techniques. Some degenerative diseases of the liver also can be prevented if the public is informed about precautions in the use of substances such as alcohol and carbon tetrachloride. Serious damage to the hepatic system can be avoided if early symptoms such as jaundice, light-colored stools, or dark-colored urine are recognized and the patient referred appropriately.

Some endocrine diseases can also be prevented. Simple goiter can occur because of a lack of iodine in the diet. Nurses also can do primary prevention of endocrine problems by working with the public on weight control. Obesity can lead to many health problems, including diabetes mellitus. Control of obesity is needed with all age groups, and nurses can be involved in teaching nutrition, weight control, and exercise regimens that assist in reduction of weight and maintenance of ideal weight. Nurses need to be able to identify persons who are at high risk of developing diabetes and work with them to ensure that they are checked for diabetes periodically and, if diabetes is diagnosed, that appropriate follow-up care is received.

As mentioned above, many of the diseases of the regulatory mechanisms are chronic in nature. The progression of many of them can be halted or slowed if the patient knows what he or she can do to control the disease process. Adequate control is dependent on knowledge and motivation to follow prescribed regimens.

Nurses carry a major responsibility for teaching these patients and for supporting them in following the prescribed therapy.

Intervention

Nursing care for all types of regulatory problems is directed toward returning the body to a state of physiologic stability and maintaining that stability. There are common outcomes and interventions that are needed by many patients with diseases of the regulatory mechanisms and these are discussed next.

Care during acute phase

The care of the patient during the acute phase is guided by five desired outcomes.

OUTCOME: The person will have improvement in presenting signs and symptoms.

The most obvious signs and symptoms are the presence of fluid and electrolyte imbalance, lack of adequate nutrition for cell repair and growth, and lack of ability to handle waste products.

Fluid and electrolytes will return to normal. The liver and the hormones of the endocrine system play a major role in maintaining adequate fluid and electrolyte balance. Depending on the abnormality, excessive amounts of fluid and electrolytes may be lost or retained. The patient may enter the hospital with any of a number of fluid and electrolyte problems. Specific therapy will depend on the fluid and electrolyte status, which is determined by history, physical examination, and diagnostic tests (see Chapter 21). In most instances the identification of the particular pathologic condition will provide data on which fluid and electrolyte problems will be present. Chapters 32 and 33 describe the problems that the nurse should anticipate when a particular problem is present. Replacement therapy for fluid or electrolyte deficits, or restriction of intake and therapy to rid the body of excess fluids or electrolytes, will be instituted as appropriate. In all instances the nurse needs to know the goals of medical therapy. The nurse functions in meeting this outcome by instituting the ordered therapy, adequately maintaining intake and output records, and recording losses by abnormal routes such as perspiration, vomiting, and diarrhea. Monitoring the patient's weight by careful weighing and recording is extremely important, since weight is used to determine adjustments in therapy. Weights should be taken on the same scale at the same time daily. The patient should wear the same amount of clothing each day and should void before being weighed. The patient with problems of regulatory mechanisms can easily and quickly move from a state of deficit to a state of excess or from a state of excess to a state of deficit, so that the importance of careful monitoring cannot be overemphasized.

In addition, in all instances, whether there is a deficit or an excess, the status of the cardiovascular system needs to be assessed and monitored until fluid and electrolyte state is stable. The patient's cardiac reserve may be so limited that modifications in activities and independence need to be made. With the addition of each new activity or increase in independence, monitoring of tolerance to these measures is necessary.

Nutrition level will return to normal. Disturbances of regulatory mechanisms cause a deficit in nutrients for cell growth. The lack of nutrients may be caused by the inability of the cells to utilize the nutrients present, inadequate dietary intake of nutrients because of anorexia, nausea and vomiting, or abnormal loss of nutrients through vomiting and diarrhea. Early in the treatment the patient may have anorexia, nausea, and vomiting. In addition, some patients may require various food restrictions as part of the treatment of their underlying disease. All of this makes the food that the patient is allowed seem unappealing and unappetizing. Some foods may not be well tolerated, and the patient may be apprehensive about eating.

In recent years a great deal of attention has been given to diet and its relation to chronic degenerative disease of the liver. It is suspected that the liver's ability to excrete toxins and carry on its many other functions is seriously hampered by inadequate intake of protein and of vitamin B. If liver damage has occurred, the organ's ability to store glycogen and vitamins A, B complex, C, and D may also be decreased, and the patient may be in much greater need of regular intake of complete foods than before the illness. In the absence of bile salts, a major component of bile, the digestion and absorption of fats and the absorption of vitamin K and other fat-soluble vitamins are seriously hampered.

A diet high in calories, protein, and vitamins, fairly high in carbohydrates (unless weight reduction is desired), and with moderate amounts of fat is often ordered for patients with diseases of the liver. Many physicians believe that the patient who has liver damage should have 100 to 300 g of protein per day, but it is exceedingly difficult to have the patient eat this amount. Lean beef (broiled steak if it can be afforded), broiled chicken, and fish are some of the best high-protein foods. Egg white, gelatin, and cottage cheese provide large amounts of protein and can be prepared in a variety of ways. Yeast is particularly high in protein and in vitamin B. Dried skim milk is very useful for fortifying drinks taken between meals and can be added to muffins, sauces, and many other foods.

Diet therapy for persons with endocrine diseases may be directed toward increasing or decreasing calories and other nutrients. It is often exceedingly difficult to get patients to take the amount and type of food necessary.

Persons with anorexia need considerable support to eat some essential nutrients, and those who are nauseated require a carefully controlled environment conducive to retaining the food they ingest. (See Chapter 53 for more information.)

Waste products will be eliminated. Drug therapy may be used to facilitate elimination of excess fluid, electrolytes, and waste products. The nurse assists in these functions by carrying out appropriate medical therapy and by monitoring for effectiveness of therapy and for side effects. Most important from the nurse's point of view is that restriction of certain products will be necessary to supplement the patient's inability to handle certain solutes. In addition, excess waste products from endogenous protein must be prevented from accumulating. Stressors increases caloric needs and can lead to the breakdown of proteins for energy, thus adding more nitrogenous waste products. Also, the proteins in the diet will be used for caloric needs rather than to repair tissue, since catabolism is increased when the neuroendocrine response is triggered. Care to decrease stressors in the environment and to prevent infection and other complications of bed rest that can initiate the neuroendocrine response is of primary importance and is a major responsibility of the nurse.

OUTCOME: The person will have energy to carry out activities that are necessary for well-being.

The person will need constant monitoring, have many physical and preventive care needs, and may need to undergo many diagnostic tests. Careful planning and scheduling of activities are necessary to provide adequate rest and prevent fatigue. The nurse must set priorities on a day-to-day basis. Consultation with the physician in arranging diagnostic tests so that the patient does not receive unnecessary repeat preparation is very important. Not all hygiene needs may be met each day. The most important thing the nurse does to meet this second outcome is to make a total care plan so that important needs will not be missed.

OUTCOME: The person will be free of avoidable stressors.

The environment must be free of physiologic and psychologic stressors. Providing an environment that is restful and as anxiety free as possible may be one of the greatest challenges for the nurse. The emotional responses to hepatic and endocrine disease are often severe and require much support and understanding on the part of the nurse. Often these diseases are chronic,

and permanent changes in the individual's life-style are usually required. Involving the patient and the significant others in developing a suitable plan of care for the hospital and at home will help reduce fear and anxiety and will also provide an opportunity for the nurse to explore fears about the disease with the patient and to determine where teaching emphasis needs to be placed.

The patient may be lethargic or extremely restless. It is important that family and friends be told that the change in behavior is caused by the disease. Otherwise, they may become upset and add to the problem. Unexpected events and disturbing news usually are not well tolerated, and the patient must be spared from these. The effects of visitors on the patient must be assessed, and in some instances visitors may need to be restricted if they are upsetting the patient. In other instances, visitors are comforting to the patient and should be encouraged to visit often.

Planning with patients the activities they find restful and relaxing, modifying routines they find upsetting, avoiding controversial topics, and remaining calm are important points in care.

OUTCOME: The person remains free of complications.

The major complications of impaired regulatory mechanisms are infection, hemorrhage, and those arising from immobility secondary to bed rest.

Free of infection. The person with a pathologic regulatory mechanism is a prime candidate for infection. This may be because of decreased phagocytosis, decreased ability to produce white blood cells and antibodies, masking of signs of infection, or a generalized decrease in resistance. Infections are acquired easily and may be difficult to cure. They increase catabolism and add stress. The patient needs to be protected from any kind of infection. This is accomplished by placing the person who is seriously ill in a private room, ensuring that no one (staff or visitors) with an upper respiratory infection has contact with the patient, and observing strict technique in care of intravenous lines and drainage tubes and in changing dressings. Skin care, respiratory hygiene measures, and frequent oral hygiene should be part of the patient's routine care. Careful ongoing monitoring for early signs of infection is essential. The most common sites of infection are the respiratory, genitourinary, and gastrointestinal tracts and the skin.

Free of skin and foot problems. Because patients with problems of the regulatory mechanisms are more susceptible to infection and generally heal more slowly than other persons, special attention is given to skin care. A daily bath or shower is desirable. If this is not possible, emphasis is given to daily bathing of areas most likely to become infected. The back of the neck, the axillae, and the groin are prime sites for carbuncles to develop, and these areas should be bathed daily. Women who are obese need to give special care to areas under the breasts, since any place where two skin surfaces meet is a likely place for infection to develop. To prevent dry, cracked skin, a skin lubricant is helpful after bathing or showering. Areas between the toes are dried carefully after bathing since warm, moist areas are conducive to bacterial growth. The patient should wear clean socks and well-fitting shoes to prevent injuries while ambulating.

Free of hemorrhage. Hemorrhage may be a major problem in diseases of the hepatic system. Because the jaundiced person may have a low prothrombin level, the prothrombin and coagulation time of the blood may be prolonged and the person may bleed easily. For this reason the person is a poor surgical risk and may bleed profusely from minor procedures such as a venipuncture or an intramuscular injection. Normal production of prothrombin is dependent on four things: (1) *ingestion of foods that can undergo synthesis in the intestine;* (2) *presence of bile in the intestine, thus enabling the intestine to produce vitamin K from food constituents;* (3) *absorption through the intestinal wall of the vitamin K produced; and* (4) *use of the vitamin K by the liver in the formation of prothrombin.*

Since vitamin K depends on the presence of bile salts for its manufacture in and absorption from the intestine, bile salts are often given by mouth to patients who are jaundiced. Vitamin K may be given both orally and parenterally in the hope that it will enable the liver to form more prothrombin. If vitamin K, which is not water soluble, is given by mouth, bile salts must be given as well. However, menadione sodium bisulfite (Hykinone), a water-soluble preparation of vitamin K, usually is ordered. The usual dose is 0.5 to 2 mg daily, given parenterally. If the jaundice is caused by obstruction in the biliary tract and not by liver disease, it can be treated satisfactorily. If the liver is severely diseased and unable to make use of the vitamin K provided, the prothrombin level will remain low despite the administration of bile salts and vitamin K. Fresh blood then may have to be given to provide the prothrombin essential for clotting.

Since the jaundiced person may bleed more than usual from such minor procedures as drawing blood from a vein, plans should be made for samples of blood to be taken at the same time for several tests. If an infusion is ordered, it should be started at the time blood is drawn. After venipunctures, pressure should be applied for 5 minutes or longer if necessary. When giving intramuscular and hypodermic injections, the nurse selects the smallest needle that can be used safely and is particularly careful that the needle is sharp and that, following an injection, firm pressure is exerted for longer than is normally necessary. The patient should be instructed to take special care when brushing the teeth. If the prothrombin level is very low, a toothbrush is not used, but mouthwash or cotton swabs may be used instead to prevent bleeding gums. Urine and stools are checked for either old or fresh blood, and if bleeding is suspected, specimens are saved. Steady oozing of blood from hemorrhoids is not unusual in severe jaundice. Incisions heal more slowly when jaundice is present, and the nurse should inspect dressings frequently for bleeding. The patient's activity may be restricted until wounds have healed completely.

Free of injury. Persons with regulatory problems frequently have changes in sensorium secondary to an increase in toxic products, to a decrease in blood volume, or to inadequate brain perfusion. Precautions to prevent injury are necessary, and significant others require careful explanation of the reasons for the precautions.

Free of complications from bed rest. Because these persons may be treated with bed rest, have decreased nutrient levels for adequate cellular nutrition, may be dehydrated or have edema, leading to decreased perfusion to the periphery, and have decreased resistance to infection, they require care directed toward preventing skin breakdown, thrombophlebitis, and pneumonia. Frequent turning and good back care, range of motion exercises, and respiratory care must be part of the nursing care plan.

OUTCOME: The person will be free of avoidable discomforts.

One of the major discomforts associated with disease of the hepatic system is pruritus caused by jaundice.

Jaundice. Jaundice is a symptom complex caused by a disturbance of the physiology of bile pigment and is present in many diseases of the hepatic and biliary system. There is an excess of bile pigment in the blood, which eventually is distributed to the skin, mucous membranes, and other body fluids and body tissues, giving them a yellow discoloration. Jaundice, caused by faulty liver function as a result of disease of the hepatic cells, is described as *hepatocellular.* When jaundice results from intrahepatic or extrahepatic obstruction that interferes with the flow of bile, it is described as *obstructive. Hemolytic* jaundice presumably is caused by destruction of great numbers of blood cells, which results in the production of excessive amounts of bilirubin and the inability of the liver to excrete the bilirubin as rapidly as it is formed. In any of these conditions the plasma concentration of bilirubin rises, the amount of conjugated bilirubin excreted in the urine increases, the amount of bilirubin that gets to the intestines is altered (increased or decreased), and the amount of urobilinogen excreted in the urine is altered. The results of interference with bile flow or bilirubin production are summarized in Table 31-1.

TABLE 31-1. Bile pigment metabolism: jaundice

Types of liver cell dysfunction	Serum bilirubin (conjugated)	Serum bilirubin (unconjugated)	Total serum bilirubin (conjugated and unconjugated)	Urine urobilinogen	Urine bilirubin	Stool	Jaundice (icterus)
Normal	<0.2 mg/100 ml	<0.2 mg/100 ml	+	±	0	Brown	0
Hemolytic	<0.2 mg/100 ml	>0.2 mg/100 ml	+ +	+ + + +	0	Dark brown	Light reddish yellow
Familial	<0.2 mg/100 ml	>0.2 mg/100 ml	+ +	±	0	Brown (normal)	Reddish yellow
Hepatitis	+	>0.2 mg/100 ml	+ +	+ + +	+ +	Light brown	Deep reddish yellow
Cirrhosis	+	>0.2 mg/100 ml	+ +	+ + +	+ +	Light brown	Deep reddish yellow
Incomplete biliary obstruction	+ +	>0.2 mg/100 ml	+ + +	Variable and fluctuating	+ + +	Light	Light to deep greenish yellow
Complete biliary obstruction	+ + +	>0.2 mg/100 ml	+ + + +	0	+ + +	Clay colored	Deep greenish

Pruritus. The presence of bile pigment in the skin causes pruritus (itching) in about 20% to 25% of the patients who have jaundice. Pruritus was defined centuries ago as a disagreeable sensation that stimulates the urge to scratch. Actually, very little is known about the physiologic mechanism that causes pruritus. It is believed to be closely associated with the nerve mechanism that causes pain. The sensation arises in the nerve endings in the skin; it is unknown in lesions in which skin layers have been destroyed. Pruritus is known to be aggravated by dilation of capillaries, tissue anoxia such as occurs in venous stasis, and the presence of abnormal constituents such as bile pigment in the skin.

Pruritus can be exhausting and demoralizing. It is impossible for most people not to scratch the skin even when told not to do so. Giving the person a soft cloth with which to rub the skin may help.

Medications such as an antihistamine or a tranquilizer may be prescribed to reduce the itching or to reduce the patient's response to the itching. Whenever possible, bed linens should be old and soft, since these will increase the patient's comfort. The patient's fingernails are kept short and hands are kept clean so that scratching is less likely to excoriate skin lesions that can become readily infected.

Cool, light, nonrestrictive clothing and bedclothes are desirable, and contact with wool is avoided, since it makes many persons itch. Because pruritus worsens when body temperature is increased, every attempt is made to keep the patient quiet and to avoid activities that increase metabolic needs.

Women with diabetes may develop pruritus vulvae, which will require special attention. They are taught to sponge the area after voiding and to pat the area dry. Some women find applying cornstarch to the vulvae is helpful. It is cheaper than talcum powder and is free of perfumes and other agents that may increase itching.

In general, a warm, not hot, tub bath is more soothing than a shower and may relieve a great deal of discomfort. Colloidal baths using oatmeal or starch may be ordered. Medicated ointments or lotion to reduce itching also may be prescribed. Diversional activities may be helpful in reducing the patient's perception of pruritus.

A summary of the outcomes for the acute phase follows.

Outcome criteria for the person with impaired regulatory mechanisms during the acute phase

The person will:
1. Have improvement in signs and symptoms.
   a. Fluid and electrolytes will return to normal.
   b. Nutrition level will return to normal.
   c. Waste products will be eliminated normally.
2. Have sufficient energy to carry out activities that are necessary for well-being.
3. Be free of avoidable stressors.
4. Be free of complications such as infection, hemorrhage, injury, or complications from bed rest.
5. Be free of avoidable discomfort.

Preparation for discharge

Since many of the problems of regulatory mechanisms are chronic and often require the patient to take daily medications, adhere to a diet and learn measures to conserve energy, and prevent stressors and infections; both children and adults are taught early to take care of these particular needs for themselves unless this is not possible for some reason. Children as young as 6 or 7 years of age can begin to learn to take care of their own needs. Patient outcomes should provide guidelines to meet these long-term needs. Family members should be included in the teaching even though they may not take an active part in carrying out procedures. Including them helps them to understand what is required of the patient. They can then encourage the patient to carry out instructions and can take over the care if this becomes necessary.

The teaching should be planned so that the patient is not rushed and has enough time for sufficient self-practice. If a significant other is to learn the care, arrangements must be made for this person to be taught in a similar manner.

Group teaching, in addition to individual teaching, is often desirable. Both the patient and significant others derive support and consolation from contact with persons with similar problems. In all of the teaching, emphasis is on the fact that the condition can be controlled and that the required restriction will help promote the physiologic and pyschologic stability necessary to allow the patient to have energy to do the things he or she enjoys. Filmstrips, booklets, and other teaching aids are available from the U.S. Department of Health and Human Services, pharmaceutical companies, and voluntary agencies such as the American Diabetes Association. These materials should be reviewed before using them to assess their appropriateness for the individual or group being taught.

OUTCOME: The person or significant others can explain the replacement therapy planned for after discharge.

Persons with problems of the endocrine system may be on hormonal replacement therapy. Hormonal replacement therapy presents important implications for patients whose prognosis depends on acceptance of drug therapy. They need to learn the name, amount, and time of drug therapy, signs and symptoms indicating that the therapy is not effective, what to do if the therapy is not effective, and times when the amount of drug may need to be increased. Although hormonal replacement treatment may seem to restrict an individual's life, the person who has been helped to accept limitations and live within them is able to have a relatively normal life and is far less restricted than is a person with an uncontrollable problem. It is important for the individual to have the support of family members and for the family to understand the therapy and be willing to assume responsibility for it should this become necessary.

The patient must know that the treatment cannot be discontinued for a single day without specific direction from the physician and that the therapy does not usually provide for the excessive hormonal demands produced by unusually stressful physical or emotional situations. Because of this fact, stress-producing situations should be recognized and avoided. Sudden bouts of unaccustomed exercise, fasting, extremes of temperature, and fatigue are examples of stressors. If any infection, no matter how minor, or any illness occurs, the person should seek medical advice. Because sudden, unexpected, stressful situations such as accidents or incapacitating illness may occur, the person on hormonal therapy should carry an identification card on which is noted the physician's name, address, and telephone number, the prescribed hormone being taken, and the dosage to be used in event of an emergency.

Even in the absence of stressful situations, the normal person has changing needs for hormones. In replacement therapy, however, a specified amount of hormone must be given. It is not unusual therefore for the patient to develop symptoms of hypofunction or hyperfunction of the gland for which the hormone is being given. Both the patient and the family should be able to recognize signs and symptoms of dysfunction of the gland and know what to do about them. If there is a means of compensating for too much or too little of the hormone, such as taking some form of sugar for insulin reaction, the method should be taught. If this is not possible and the symptoms are acute, the patient must be taken at once to the physician or the emergency department of a hospital. Many times, if medical advice is sought at the first sign of even minor symptoms of dysfunction, the dosage of the hormone can be adjusted and further problems avoided.

A 2-month supply of the special drugs and equipment should be on hand so that an emergency does not interfere with obtaining supplies. As new supplies are bought, they should be kept in reserve and the old ones used. Continuous hormonal therapy is expensive, and the patient may require assistance from an appropriate social agency in the community. If the hormonal replacement therapy must be given by injection, the patient must be taught how to give the injection and how to maintain the necessary equipment (see p. 655).

Temporary replacement. The patient requiring only temporary replacement of hormones may be at home while taking them and, if so, must be taught the importance of taking the prescribed dosage regularly. Usually, the dosage is reduced gradually and finally discontinued. While therapy is being tapered off, the person should be observed for symptoms of hypofunction of the gland that produces the hormone that has been given. The individual and the family should know the signs and symptoms of hormonal deficiency and should understand the need to seek immediate medical attention if these signs and symptoms occur. They also should know that signs and symptoms of hypofunction of the gland may occur even after the therapy has been discontinued. Regular medical follow-up should be continued until the physician determines that it is no longer needed.

OUTCOME: The person or significant others can explain dietary requirements.

Persons with problems of the regulatory mechanisms will often require dietary modifications to assist in control of the problem. They and their significant others must be able to explain the type and amount of food needed and when needed, foods to be avoided or limited, how to measure foods, and foods that can be substituted for each other.

The nurse has an important role in helping the patient and his or her significant others understand dietary modifications. In all instances the patient's age, weight, activity level, medical problem, and nutritional state are considered when planning the dietary modification. Social and economic background and cultural preference should be accommodated, if possible. Dietary modifications may have to be adjusted for work, increased exercise, and other stressors.

The diet is part of the total treatment program and must be taken as ordered each day. In some cases, such as with diabetes mellitus, the diet is adjusted with the medications so that it becomes even more important that meals are not omitted or that unapproved changes are not made in meals. Sometimes patients may think that if they do not feel well, they can omit the meals and decrease the medications. This is not allowed. Clear liquids and full liquids in appropriate amounts can provide the essential amounts of nutrients for a short time. Directions on how to adjust the diet and how to prepare these foods should be given to patients and their families.

The restrictions in diet may require the elimination of certain foods or may require the measurement of food with kitchen equipment or with a scale. If the persons are required to weigh food, they should learn how to estimate usual weighed amounts so that they can make adjustments when they eat out. The diet, whatever the restrictions, should be well balanced in selection of foods.

A clinical dietitian, if one is available, may initiate or participate in the diet teaching program. The nurse, however, often must give the diet instructions. If the dietitian does the teaching, the nurse and dietitian need to work closely together to ensure adequate follow-up. A good time for teaching about diet is during mealtimes.

In planning the diet, written material on the type of diet being taught should be available. The material should explain foods that can be substituted for each other, foods that must be avoided, and foods that must be calculated. Sugar and salt substitutes can be purchased in most grocery stores.

If the nurse can help with menu planning on a weekly basis, patients can learn through demonstration how the diet can be varied and how they can have the food that they like even though restrictions are necessary. Most patients find it helpful to *see* food portions, especially such "unmeasurable" things as a small potato, an ounce of meat, or a slice of cheese. When possible, foods are measured using standard household measures such as an 8-oz. measuring cup, a teaspoon, or a tablespoon. All measurements are level, and cooked foods are measured after cooking. Persons on special diets do not need to buy special foods but can select their diet from the same foods purchased for the rest of the family. Fruits may be fresh, dried, cooked, canned, or frozen as long as no ingredients that are restricted are added. Vegetables can be prepared with those for the rest of the family except that the patient's portion should be removed before ingredients that are restricted are added. Meats should be baked, broiled, or boiled. Any fat used must be accounted for in the measurements for the meal. Special cookbooks with recipes that can be used for patients as well as for other members of the family are available. They may help patients make meals more varied and appetizing. Special diet foods are expensive, and the patient should be reminded that they usually are not free of restricted items and must be counted in the daily dietary allowance.

OUTCOME: The person will have the energy necessary to carry out activities of daily living and social activities.

Conservation of energy. The regulatory mechanisms have a major role in the production of adequate energy. Most patients with problems of the regulatory mechanisms will complain of fatigue and weakness. Nursing measures designed to assist them with this problem during the acute phase were presented earlier in this chapter. Some persons may continue to lack energy even after the problem is under control.

Achieving this outcome requires that the nurse know the patient's normal schedule and evaluate the things that the patient must do, things other persons can do, and the things the patient enjoys doing. The patient and nurse can plan how the significant others can be of most assistance without infringing on the patient's independence.

Activities of daily living can be spaced to allow rest periods. Some activities such as shaving or ironing can be carried out from a sitting rather than a standing position. Especially fatiguing activities are best scheduled at times of the day when there will be more opportunity to rest after completion of the activity. Rearranging the household might be indicated, since it can assist in preventing excess use of energy in walking stairs or reaching objects on high shelves. Significant others need to understand the patient's need for increased rest and their role in providing an environment that allows rest.

Patients are often guided by how they feel and can use their feeling of well-being as a measure of what activities can be tolerated.

OUTCOME: The person or significant others can identify stressors in the environment, explain ways to cope with or limit stressors, and explain changes required in therapy when a stressor is encountered.

Stressors are an everday part of life but are increased at times. Each individual has unique ways of dealing with stressors. Stressors are often associated in peoples' minds with sad or depressing events, but they also may occur with happy or exciting events. The stressors in each person's life are different. The regulatory mechanisms play a role in how persons deal physiologically and psychologically with stressors. With dysfunction of the regulatory mechanisms, the person does not always have the ability to cope with additional stressors.

Reaching the above outcome requires that the nurse have good rapport with patients so that they will feel free to discuss their stressors. Some stressors may concern very personal matters such as marital relationships and financial problems. The patient may need help from others in identifying ways to cope with identified stressors. If the patient is receiving hormonal replacement therapy, increased amounts may be necessary, since the daily therapy is only designed to meet normal requirements.

OUTCOME: The person or significant others can explain the recommended program for preventing infections.

The person with diseases of regulatory mechanisms has decreased ability to handle the stress of infection and has decreased resistance to infection.

To attain this outcome there must be appropriate ongoing monitoring for the presence of infection. Infections can cause serious problems, and the patient should know the signs and symptoms of common infections such as those of the respiratory tract and urinary tract. Patients also should be able to explain ways to decrease the chance of infections. They should recognize the need to avoid crowded places, areas with poor ventilation, and persons with upper respiratory infections. Because young children have frequent upper respiratory infections, contact with children may need to be limited.

In addition, patients with diabetes mellitus are especially prone to infections of the feet. All patients with this particular regulatory problem should know how to care for their feet properly and should see a podiatrist regularly. The care of the feet is similar to that for clients with diminished peripheral circulation described on p. 1149. Two pamphlets that are helpful in teaching clients are *Foot Care for the Diabetic Patient** and *Feet First.** Patients need to understand that the incidence of neuropathy is increased among diabetics and that neuropathy produces insensitivity to pain. As a result, blisters or cuts can become infected before they are noticed.

Finally, the patient and his or her significant others should be able to explain what to do if signs and symptoms of infection occur. Too frequently patients are taught signs and symptoms to monitor but are not told what to do should they occur. Since patients with problems of the regulatory mechanism have very poor resistance to infections, they must report any manifestations immediately. They also need to understand that infection is a stressor and may lead to a need for an increase in their replacement therapy.

The outcomes for care in the discharge phase are summarized below.

Outcome criteria for the person with impaired regulatory mechanisms during the discharge phase

1. The person will have the energy necessary to carry out activities of daily living and social activities.
2. The person or significant others can:
   a. Explain replacement therapy to be maintained after discharge:
      (1) Name, amount, and time of therapy.
      (2) Signs and symptoms indicating when therapy is ineffective.
      (3) What to do if therapy is ineffective.
      (4) Times when therapy may need to be increased.
      (5) What do do if unable to take therapy.
   b. Explain dietary requirements:
      (1) Type and amount of food needed and when needed.
      (2) Foods to be avoided or limited.
      (3) Ways of measuring foods.
      (4) Foods that can be substituted for each other.
   c. Identify stressors in the environment, explain ways to deal with or limit stressors, and explain changes in therapy when a stress situation is encountered.
   d. Explain the recommended program for preventing and treating infection:
      (1) Avoid crowds.
      (2) Avoid persons with upper respiratory infection.

---

*Published by the Department of Health and Human Services; available from the Superintendent of Documents, U.S. Government Printing Office, Washington, DC 20402.

(3) Notify the physician at the first sign of any infection, even a cold.

(4) Follow prescribed therapy for infection.

REFERENCES AND SELECTED READINGS
Contemporary

1. *Backsheider, J.E.: Self-care requirements, self-care capabilities and nursing systems in the diabetic nurse management clinic, Am. J. Public Health 64:1138-1146, 1974.
2. *Blout, M., and Kinney, A.B.: Chronic steroid therapy, Am. J. Nurs. 74:1626-1632, 1974.
3. Burke, E.L.: Insulin injection: the site and the technique, Am. J. Nurs. 72:2194-2196, 1972.
4. DeGroot, L., et al.: Endocrinology, vol. 3, New York, 1979, Grune & Stratton, Inc.
5. *Dolan, P., and Greene, H.: Conquering cirrhosis of the liver, Nurs. (Jenkintown) 6(11):44-53, 1976.
6. *Garber, R.: The use of a standardized teaching program in diabetes education, Nurs. Clin. North Am. 12:375-391, 1977.
7. Gotch, P.: Teaching patients about adrenal corticosteroids, Am. J. Nurs. 81:78-81, 1981.
8. Greenberger, N.: Gastrointestinal disorders, ed. 2, Chicago, 1981, Year Book Medical Publishers, Inc.
9. Hahn, A.B., Barkin, R.L., and Oestreich, S.J.K.: Pharmacology in nursing, ed. 15, St. Louis, 1979, The C.V. Mosby Co.
10. *Hallal, J.C.: Thyroid disease, Am. J. Nurs. 77:417-433, 1977.
11. Hirsham, J.: Endocrine pathophysiology: a patient-oriented approach, Philadelphia, 1977, Lea & Febiger.
12. Isselbacher, K., et al., editors: Harrison's principles of internal medicine, ed. 9, New York, 1980, McGraw-Hill Book Co.
13. Jubiz, W.: Endocrinology: a logical approach for clinicians, New York, 1979, McGraw-Hill Book Co.
14. Kappas, A., and Alvares, A.: How the liver metabolizes foreign substances, Sci. Am. 232:22-31, 1975.
15. *Laugharne, E.: The role of the nurse in education of the diabetic, Diabetes Educator 1:9-10, 1975.
16. Meltzer, L.E., Abdellah, F.G., and Kitchell, J.R.: Concepts and practices of intensive care for nurse specialists, ed. 2, Philadelphia, 1975, The Charles Press Publishers.
17. Mountcastle, V.B.: Medical physiology, ed. 14, St. Louis, 1980, The C.V. Mosby Co.
18. Nickerson, D.: Teaching the hospitalized diabetic, Am. J. Nurs. 72:935-938, 1972.
19. Nursing skill book: managing diabetics properly. Nursing 77 books, Horsham, Pa., 1977, Intermed Communications.
20. Porter, A.L., McDonald, A., and Levine, M.E.: Giving diabetics control of their own lives, Nurs. (Jenkintown) 3(9):44-49, 1973.
21. Redman, B.K.: The process of patient teaching in nursing, ed. 4, St. Louis, 1980, The C.V. Mosby Co.
22. Rodman, M.J.: Controlling chronic liver disease II, R.N. 39:75-79, 1976.
23. *Salzer, J.E.: Classes to improve diabetic self-care, Am. J. Nurs. 75:1324-1326, 1975.
24. Schmed, R.: Bilirubin metabolism: state of the art, Gastroenterology 74:1307-1312, 1978.
25. Sherar, L.: Ascites: pathogenesis and treatment, Postgrad. Med. 53:165-170, 1973.
26. Small, D.: A patient education program, Am. J. Nurs. 78:889-890, 1978.
27. Solomon, B.: The hypothalamus and the pituitary gland: an overview, Nurs. Clin. North Am. 15:435-451, 1980.
28. Strauss, A., and Glaser, B.: Chronic illness and the quality of life, St. Louis, 1975, The C.V. Mosby Co.
29. *Suren, J.: Education of the culturally and educationally deprived diabetic, Nurs. Clin. North Am. 12:427-437, 1977.
30. U.S. Department of Health, Education and Welfare: Healthy people: the surgeon general's reports on health promotion and disease prevention, Public Health Service pub. no. 79-55071, Washington, D.C., 1979.
31. Williams, R.: Textbook of endocrinology, ed. 5, Philadelphia, 1974, W.B. Saunders Co.
32. Williams, S.R.: Essentials of nutrition and diet therapy, ed. 2, St. Louis, 1978, The C.V. Mosby Co.

Classic

33. Gartner, L.M., and Arias, I.: Formation, transport, metabolism and excretion of bilirubin, N. Engl. J. Med. 280:1339-1345, 1969.
34. U.S. Department of Health, Education and Welfare: Diabetes source book, Washington, D.C., 1969, U.S. Government Printing Office.

*References preceded by an asterisk are particularly well suited for student reading.

CHAPTER 32

PROBLEMS OF THE ENDOCRINE SYSTEM

VIRGINIA L. CASSMEYER
CAROL J. MITTEN
WILMA J. PHIPPS

Etiology

Because of the diverse physiologic functions under hormonal control, alteration in function of the endocrine glands usually results in a wide variety of signs and symptoms that may be reflected in many parts of the body. Since many of the functions controlled by the endocrine system are vital, dysfunction is very serious and can even be fatal.

Disturbances in the functioning of an endocrine gland have vast effects on many activities of the body. Endocrinopathies can result from a variety of problems and can result in a decreased or increased secretion or activity of hormones. The following is a summary of common causes of alterations in hormonal level or activity.

1. Increased or decreased secretion and activity of hormones resulting from primary problems of specific endocrine glands
2. Increased or decreased secretion and activity of hormones resulting from secondary failure of a target gland as a result of problems in the pituitary gland or hypothalamus
3. Increased hormonal levels and activity resulting from secretion of hormones by nonglandular tissue, such as increased antidiuretic hormone (ADH) or adrenocorticotropic hormone (ACTH) associated with carcinoma of the lung
4. Alterations in hormonal level and activity caused by alterations in the metabolism or degradation of hormones, such as increased estrogen and the resultant feminization seen in males with liver failure

5. Alteration in hormonal activity because of a change in the peripheral tissue's sensitivity to hormones
6. Loss of cyclic patterns

Primary and secondary dysfunction can result from tumors (benign and malignant growths), abnormal embryonic development, alteration in blood supply to glands, destruction of glands by infection or autoimmune diseases, overstimulation or overgrowth of glands, or decreased amounts of functioning tissue.

Pathophysiology

Overstimulation results in a proliferation of active secreting cells and the size of the gland increases. This is called *hyperplasia*. In *hypertrophy* there is an increase in size of the gland caused by the increase in functional demands. Hypertrophy may or may not be accompanied by hyperplasia. *Hypoplasia* is a decrease in the amount of functioning tissue, and thus there is a decrease in the amount of hormone produced. It is caused by anything that inhibits tissue growth. *Atrophy* is a decrease in the size of the gland and is caused by a decrease in functional demands. The decrease in functional demands may be caused by glandular failure or it may result from an exogenous intake of hormones that makes the endogenous production of the hormone unnecessary.

In this chapter only the more common diseases of the endocrine system will be discussed. For those occurring less frequently, the reader should consult specialized texts.

• • • •

A number of diseases can interfere with the functioning of the pituitary gland, causing hypersecretion or hyposecretion of one or more hormones. Because the anterior pituitary trophic hormones influence other endocrine glands, alterations in anterior pituitary function may cause signs and symptoms of hypersecretion or hyposecretion of those target glands. Dysfunctions of the pituitary that result in hypersecretion or hyposecretion of hormones from specific target glands will be discussed in the sections that discuss alterations of those target glands.

Anterior pituitary problems

Hyperpituitarism

Etiology and pathophysiology

Hyperpituitarism is the oversecretion of one or more of the hormones secreted by the pituitary gland and usually refers to anterior pituitary hormones. *The most common cause of hyperpituitarism is pituitary adenomas.*

Pituitary adenomas account for 5% to 10% of all intracranial tumors, and they most frequently arise in the anterior pituitary lobe. The factors responsible for the development of pituitary adenomas are unknown. Two hypotheses have been proposed. They are (1) that the tumors develop because of chronic hyperstimulation of normal pituitary cells by an altered hypothalamus and (2) that there is an autonomous growth of pituitary cells that have become independent of factors that normally limit their proliferation.

Anterior pituitary adenomas have been classified according to the staining qualities of the cells of the tumor; namely, *chromophobic, acidophilic,* or *basophilic.* Approximately 75% of all anterior pituitary adenomas are of the chromophobic type. In the past chromophobes were thought to be nonfunctioning; that is it was believed that they did not secrete any hormones. With finer diagnostic tests, however, it has been found that many of the chromophobic tumors do secrete hormones. *Prolactin* is the most common hormone secreted by chromophobic tumors, although *growth hormone* (GH) or *adrenocorticotrophic hormone* (ACTH) may also be secreted by chromophobes. *Acidophilic tumors* are the next most frequently occurring type of adenomas. These adenomas secrete prolactin, GH, or both. ACTH and rarely thyroid stimulating hormone (TSH) are secreted by basophilic tumors, the least frequently occurring adenomas. Pituitary adenomas almost never secrete follicle stimulating hormone (FSH) or luteinizing hormone (LH).

As can be seen, the classification of adenomas by the staining qualities of the tumor cells does not help in identifying the type of endocrine dysfunction associated with the adenoma. Therefore tumors are frequently identified by the type of hormone secreted; for example, prolactin secreting adenomas, GH secreting adenomas, ACTH secreting adenomas, and so on. The reader should be familiar with both classification systems, since both are used in clinical practice and in the literature.

Clinical picture

Pituitary tumors cause two clinical problems depending on the size, location, and secreting capacity of the tumor. These are (1) hypersecretion of one or more anterior pituitary hormones and (2) neurologic alterations resulting from pressure on surrounding nervous system structures.

Neurologic alterations. Since the pituitary lies in the cranial vault, abnormal growth will cause neurologic signs and symptoms. The major neurologic alteration is caused by pressure on the optic chiasm and optic nerves. Patients experience progressive loss of vision and, if untreated, permanent blindness results. Most adenomas cause midline pressure and damage the fibers subserving vision in the upper temporal fields, causing a *bitemporal hemianopsia.* Often the visual defect is asymmetric. Visual acuity is commonly spared, and nasal field defects are rare.

Other symptoms include headache that is characteristically bitemporal and bifrontal and that results from pressure on the diaphragma sella.[19] Confusion and impaired memory may occur but are rare. As compared with other types of suprasellar tumors, pituitary adenomas rarely cause signs and symptoms of increased intracranial pressure, such as hydrocephalus or papilledema.

Endocrine alterations. The clinical picture seen may be the result of excessive secretion of prolactin, GH, ACTH, or TSH. The signs and symptoms of increased secretion of ACTH and TSH are discussed in the sections in this chapter on adrenal problems and thyroid problems respectively.

PROLACTIN EXCESS. Prolactin excess is almost always caused by pituitary adenomas, usually microadenomas that have only been recognized during the last decade. Women usually seek help for endocrine dysfunction before neurologic signs and symptoms are present. They may complain of amenorrhea and galactorrhea (amenorrhea-galactorrhea syndrome) but may have one without the other. They often will complain of depressed libido. Men frequently will seek help for neurologic complaints. They may give a history of depressed libido, infertility, or impotence. Other signs and symptoms of hypogonadism, such as changes in secondary sex characteristics, may be present.

GROWTH HORMONE EXCESS. An excess of GH is almost always caused by a secreting pituitary tumor, although occasionally there is no distinct tumor.[19] Hypersecretion of growth hormone that occurs in children before fusion of the epiphyses results in *gigantism*. Such children reach enormous proportions because of the massive growth in both the length and width of bones. Soft tissue enlarges along with the skeleton.

Hypersecretion of GH that occurs after the fusion of the epiphyses results in *acromegaly*. This disorder affects men and women equally and most frequently begins between the second and fourth decade. The changes are slow and progressive and frequently go unrecognized for some time.

Enlargement in acromegaly is most apparent in the extremities (hands, feet) and the nose and mandible (Fig. 32-1). The patient may note an increase in ring, shoe, glove, and hat size. The hands become spadelike in appearance. The enlargement of the mandible causes prognathism, with an underbite and increased spacing of the lower teeth. The forehead and orbital ridges become prominent. Widening of spaces between joints occurs with increased cartilage growth. This leads to osteoarthritis with pain and limitation of joint motion. Changes in the spine may cause nerve root and cord compression.

Soft tissue enlargement also occurs. This causes coarsening of facial features with increased size of nose, lips, and cheeks. The tongue enlarges. Visceral enlargement may occur and result in *hepatomegaly, splenomegaly, cardiomegaly,* and *enlarged kidneys*. Prominent muscular development is present. At first, the

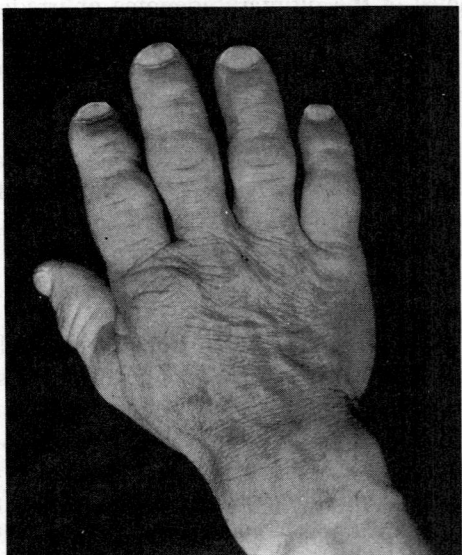

Fig. 32-1. Hand showing characteristics of acromegalic condition. (From Schottelius, B.A., and Schottelius, D.D.: Textbook of physiology, ed. 18, St. Louis, 1978, The C.V. Mosby Co.)

person experiences increased muscle strength, followed by myopathy and weakness. Another change noted is development of a husky voice.

Increased metabolic rate occurs, and the person complains of increased sweating and sebaceous gland activity. The skin is warm, moist, and coarse. Hypertension occurs in approximately 25% of these patients and congestive heart failure (CHF) may result from the cardiomegaly and hypertension.

GH excess precipitates other endocrine abnormalities. Glucose intolerance is present in approximately 50% of these persons as a result of the insulin-resistant state produced by the GH. Physiologically, most of these individuals tolerate the glucose intolerance, but some will develop overt diabetes mellitus. The adrenal cortex may secrete increased quantities of cortisol, but this is metabolized and excreted in the urine so that the plasma cortisol level stays normal. Individuals with pituitary adenomas have a higher incidence of parathyroid and pancreatic islet cell tumors than the general population.[19]

Almost all patients with GH excess will eventually develop the neurologic alterations described previously. Frequently, help is not sought until the neurologic symptoms occur.

Diagnostic tests

All patients with suspected pituitary tumors will have blood drawn to determine hormonal levels. Basal levels and levels stimulated by provocative tests will be taken (p. 595). Radiographic studies of the sella turcica will be obtained. Computed tomography (CT) and sometimes pneumoencephalography are used to identify presence of tumor growth. All persons with suspected pituitary tumors should have visual field checks and a complete ophthalmologic examination. Patients with signs and symptoms of GH excess will also have x-ray studies of the feet and hands.

Intervention

The medical interventions are directed toward decreasing abnormal hormonal levels and removing the adenoma. In some instances drug therapy to lower the excess growth hormone or prolactin may be prescribed. Estrogen, medroxyprogesterone, and chlorpromazine have been used to decrease GH levels but have shown limited success.[99] Dopamine receptor agonists such as bromocriptine methylyslate (Parlodel) have been used with good success in cases of *hyperprolactinemia*, but symptoms will recur when therapy is stopped.[99] Bromocriptine methylyslate has also been used to suppress GH secretion.

In most instances removal or destruction of the adenoma by surgery or irradiation is the intervention of choice. Surgery is the most frequently used therapy since hormonal levels return to normal immediately, whereas with irradiation it may take several years for hormonal levels to return to normal.

Care of the patient undergoing surgical removal of a pituitary adenoma. Pituitary adenomas may be removed either through a transfrontal open craniotomy or via a transsphenoidal approach. The transfrontal approach is used when there is extensive suprasellar spread.[19] (See p. 773 for a discussion of care of the patient having a craniotomy.)

Transsphenoidal surgery is being used increasingly. In this surgery the sella turcica is entered from below through the sphenoid sinus and the tumor is removed with the aid of a surgical microscope. There is no external incision, since the incision is made between the gums and the upper lip. Because the postoperative needs of these patients differ somewhat from those of patients who have had open craniotomies, transsphenoidal patients will be discussed first, before a discussion of care applicable to all patients treated with surgery or irradiation.

The opening made in the dura mater on entering the sella turcica is frequently patched with a piece of fascia taken from the leg; thus the patient must be prepared for the leg incision. The patch is to prevent cerebrospinal fluid (CSF) leak. Leaking of CSF may occur for a few days postoperatively but should then stop. The nose is packed and a gauze sling is worn under the nose to absorb drainage. The patient can be out of bed immediately after anesthesia effects have worn off; however, activities such as bending over and straining are forbidden because they cause increased intracranial pressure, which increases pressure on the graft site. Coughing, sneezing, and blowing the nose also can put pressure on the graft site and increase intracranial pressure and thus they too are prohibited.

The patient should be monitored for the presence of a CSF leak. Complaints of postnasal drip and constant swallowing may alert the nurse to the presence of such a leak. CSF itself is clear and when mixed with serous fluid on the gauze sling will form a "halo ring." To differentiate CSF fluid from the nasal secretions, a check for glucose is made. Nasal drainage will be free of glucose unless serous drainage is mixed with the nasal drainage, whereas CSF contains glucose. If glucose is found, a specimen of drainage is sent to the laboratory for positive identification. If a persistent leak is present, bed rest with the head elevated to decrease pressure on the graft site is prescribed. Occasionally, repair of the graft site will be necessary to close a leak, but most leaks heal spontaneously.

The patient often receives oxygen and humidity by face mask. This helps to keep nasal and oral mucous membranes moist and reduce the dryness associated with mouth breathing. Oral hygiene consists of rinsing the mouth with saline or mouth wash and cleansing the teeth with a toothette or cotton swab. Brushing the teeth is forbidden, since it can disrupt the suture line.

Oral fluids and a clear liquid diet may be started as soon as the patient is alert and no longer nauseated from the anesthetic. Diet is increased as tolerated. While the nasal packing is in place, the patient may loose the sense of smell. This often inhibits the appetite as well as being very frightening. The patient should be told the reason for the loss of smell and that it is only temporary.

Headache may be present and is treated with nonnarcotic analgesics or codeine. Persistent headache may indicate the presence of meningitis and should be reported immediately. Because of the risk of infection, prophylactic antibiotics may be ordered preoperatively or postoperatively.

Care of the patient with a pituitary tumor during the pretreatment and posttreatment period. *Irradiation therapy* or *cranial surgery* is very frightening to most patients and their significant others and they need time to share concerns, fears, and questions with the nurse. All questions should be answered as honestly and completely as possible.

The patient needs to be aware that the surgery or irradiation will remove excess hormone levels. Some of the coarsening of features may disappear because soft tissue swelling will decrease, glucose intolerance will disappear, and visceral enlargement may decrease; but most of the physical changes associated with excessive growth hormone are irreversible.

Usually with transsphenoidal surgery and irradiation only the adenoma is removed or destroyed and normal pituitary tissue is not disturbed. However, tumor removal requiring a transfrontal approach usually involves such large invasive tumors that a total *hypophysectomy* is done; thus *panhypopituitarism* results. Even though panhypopituitarism is not expected after transsphenoidal removal of the pituitary adenoma or irradiation, it can occur as a complication and all patients should be monitored for hormonal deficiencies, which may be temporary or permanent.

ACTH deficiency and thus glucocorticoid deficiency will occur immediately if the total pituitary has been removed, and they may occur as temporary deficits after removal of an adenoma. The following signs and symptoms are seen if an ACTH deficiency is not treated. Patients will frequently have vague symptoms such as nausea, vomiting, and prolonged lethargy. They may be more tired than expected, and their recovery does not proceed at the usual rate. Hypotension, at first mild, will occur. As the deficiency continues, fluid and electrolyte imbalances (dehydration, low sodium, increased potassium) will become apparent. Hypoglycemia may occur. If untreated, *addisonian crisis* can occur (p. 639). Therefore all patients should be on hourly vital sign checks until all vital signs are stable and then patients' vital signs should be checked every 4 hours. Intake and output are tabulated every shift; daily weights and daily electrolyte determinations are made so that complications will be identified early if they occur.

When the total pituitary is removed, an intramuscular or intravenous cortisone preparation will be given preoperatively and immediately postoperatively. Oral replacement therapy using cortisone acetate, prednisone, or another of the synthetic preparations will be started as soon as oral intake can be tolerated. Replacement therapy will be necessary for life, and the patient will need the same care as the patient with *adrenocortical insufficiency* (see p. 637). If a temporary deficit occurs, the patient is treated with replacement therapy as long as necessary. Plasma levels of cortisol will be checked before discharge to make sure they are normal and that the deficit has been corrected.

Temporary *diabetes insipidus* occurs very frequently in patients following transspenoidal or transfrontal surgical removal of a pituitary adenoma or following irradiation. It is usually not permanent, even if all of the pituitary gland has been removed, because ADH is produced in the hypothalamus and adequate amounts can be released from there. All patients should have their intake and output tabulated every 8 hours, and specific gravity should be determined on each urine specimen. Polyuria and continuously dilute urine (specific gravity of 1.000 to 1.005) are signs of diabetes insipidus. No treatment will be instituted if the deficit is mild and the patient is able to take enough fluid to maintain sufficient fluid volume. If the deficit is more severe or if fluid intake is inadequate, vasopressin (Pitressin) will be given. When diabetes inspidus occurs, thirst is a frequent complaint. It can usually be managed by providing ice chips and adequate water intake.

Deficiency of thyroid stimulating hormone (TSH) and of thyroid hormones usually does not occur on a temporary basis, and it is not seen immediately even after the total pituitary has been removed, since the thyroid gland stores enough hormone to last for several weeks. If the total pituitary has been removed, the patient will eventually require thyroid replacement similar to the patient with *hypothyroidism* (p. 624).

Gonadotropin deficiency requires lifetime therapy. If the total pituitary has been removed, replacement of sex hormones will be necessary. To maintain libido, secondary sexual characteristics, and well-being, men will be given testosterone and women will receive estrogen-progesterone preparations. If childbearing is desired, the gonadotropins (luteinizing hormone [LH] and FSH) must be replaced in both the male and female partner.

Total removal of the pituitary (hypophysectomy) has been used to treat *mammary carcinoma* and *diabetic retinopathy*. In these instances a transsphenoidal or transfrontal approach will be used. Care of the patient is the same as that described above. These patients will need lifetime replacement therapy of glucocorticoids and thyroid hormones. Gonadal hormones or gonadotropins will be replaced in the patient having a hypophysec-

tomy for diabetic retinopathy. They will not be given to the patient who undergoes a hypophysectomy for treatment of mammary cancer, since the purpose of the surgery is to remove these hormones because they stimulate mammary tumor growth.

Outcome criteria for the person who has had removal of a pituitary adenoma with or without removal of the total pituitary

The person or significant others can:
1. Describe the treatment and the expected effects of treatment.
2. Describe the mouth-care regimen to be used after discharge.
3. State plans for regular follow-up care.

If a total hypophysectomy is done, the following additional outcome criteria need to be met:
1. Explain the prescribed medication program.
   a. State awareness of need for lifelong replacement therapy.
   b. State name, dosage, and frequency of prescribed medications.
   c. Describe desired effects and side effects of drug therapy.
   d. State the side effects, if undertreatment or overtreatment occurs that indicate the need for immediate medical care.
2. Explain the effects of stressors on the need for glucocorticoids, identify stressors in own life and ways to control them, and state awareness of the need for additional medication in times of severe stress.
3. Show the Medic Alert bracelet or necklace or personal identification card stating drugs, dosages, and physician's name and telephone number.
4. State plans for regular follow-up care.

Hypopituitarism

Etiology and pathophysiology

A number of diseases can interfere with the function of the anterior pituitary and cause hyposecretion of one or more hormones. *Hypopituitarism* can result from vascular lesions (e.g., hemorrhage or aneurysm), infections, granulomatous lesions, genetic and developmental disorders, trauma, surgery, nonsecreting pituitary adenomas, or tumors arising from surrounding structures whose growth compresses the pituitary.

Panhypopituitarism (deficiency of all anterior pituitary hormones) may be present or there may be isolated deficiency of one hormone. If panhypopituitarism occurs, the deficiencies usually do not appear simultaneously. Deficits of growth hormone and gonadotropins usually occur first, followed by deficits of TSH and then ACTH.[19]

Clinical picture

The clinical picture will vary greatly depending on the hormonal deficit or deficits present and the cause of the deficit. If a tumor is present, the patient will have neurologic alterations similar to those seen with secreting pituitary adenomas (p. 616). If the tumor arises from regions surrounding the pituitary, such at Rathke's pouch (craniopharyngiomas), the hypothalamus, or the region of the third ventricle; the neurologic signs and symptoms may be more severe. Signs and symptoms of increased intracranial pressure, such as *hydrocephalus* and *papilledema* are usually present.

Deficiency of growth hormone in the adult is usually not significant. Congenital deficiency of growth hormone in the child results in short stature (dwarfism). *Dwarfism* is a rare disorder and is characterized by short stature that is apparent at about 4 years of age (Fig. 32-2). In addition to short stature, the child typically appears immature and has increased truncal fat. Bone age and height age are usually approximate, and as the child matures, the body proportions approach those of an adult. Sexual development although delayed is normal. Deficiency of the gonadotropins in the adult results in infer-

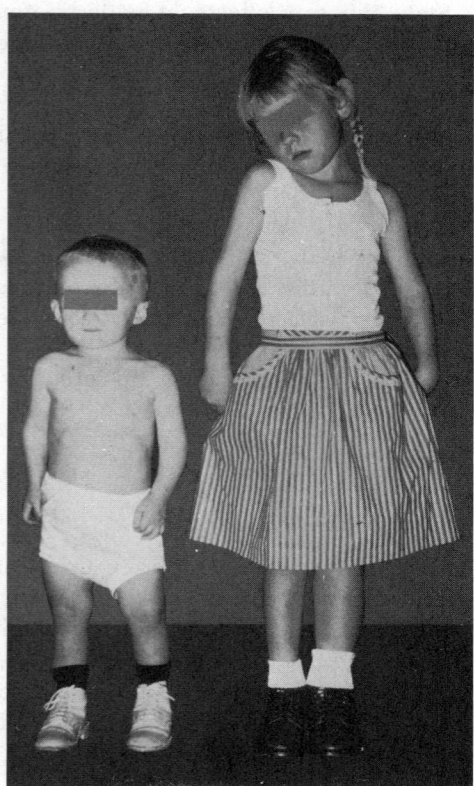

Fig. 32-2. Hypopituitary dwarfism in a 4-year-old boy whose height is 25 in. Girl is also 4 years old and has a normal height of 39 in. Dwarf has a normal face, as well as head, trunk, and limbs of approximately normal proportions. (From Brashear, H.R., and Raney, R.B.: Shand's handbook of orthopaedic surgery, ed. 9, St. Louis, 1978, The C.V. Mosby Co.)

tility, amenorrhea in females, impotency in males, and change in secondary sexual characteristics. Deficiency in the child will result in signs and symptoms of impaired sexual development (see p. 1770 for a discussion of hypogonadism). Deficiency of TSH results in signs and symptoms of hypothyroidism (see p. 624 for a discussion of hypothyroidism). Deficiency of ACTH secretion results in signs and symptoms of adrenal insufficiency (see p. 637).

If *panhypopituitarism* is present, the patient will have signs and symptoms of hypogonadism, hypothyroidism, adrenal insufficiency, and growth hormone deficits (in children only).

Diagnosis is based on history, physical assessment, and diagnostic tests. Basal hormonal levels and hormonal levels following stimulatory or inhibitory tests will be done. Radiographic examinations, CT scans, and pneumoencephalograms will be used to evaluate the pituitary gland and identify the presence of a tumor.

Intervention

If a tumor is present it will be removed via the transfrontal or transsphenoidal approach or destroyed by irradiation. The care is the same as that described for patients having removal of a pituitary adenoma (see p. 618).

Hormonal deficiencies will be replaced as described on p. 619 for the patient experiencing panhypopituitarism after a total hypopysectomy. Human growth hormone replacement is not necessary in adults. Its use in children has been limited because of its scarcity. If children are treated, they are usually treated only until they attain a height of 5 ft. A new development, the production of biologically active human growth hormone (HGH) by recombinant DNA technology, may make more treatment and longer treatment available. Research is ongoing in this area.[187]

Outcome criteria for the person with hypopituitarism

The person or significant others can:
1. Describe the hormonal deficit or deficits and relate them to the signs and symptoms.
2. Explain the planned treatment measures and effects of treatment.
3. Explain the prescribed medication program.
   a. State awareness of the need for lifelong replacement therapy.
   b. Describe drugs, dosage, and frequency of therapy.
   c. Explain desired effects and side effects of therapy and what to do when signs and symptoms of undertreatment or overtreatment occur.
4. Describe the times when extra hormonal therapy is necessary.

5. Show the Medic Alert bracelet or necklace or personal identification card stating drugs, dosages, and physician's name and telephone number.
6. State plans for regular follow-up care.

Posterior pituitary problems

Syndrome of inappropriate antidiuretic hormone

Etiology and pathophysiology

In the syndrome of inappropriate antidiuretic hormone (SIADH) there is a continual release of ADH unrelated to plasma osmolality. The patient is unable to dilute the urine appropriately and therefore retains water. The extracellular fluid volume is expanded, and *dilutional hyponatremia* occurs.

This syndrome is associated with a wide variety of problems. Most frequently, it is seen in the presence of *small cell* or *oat cell carcinoma* of the lung. These cells are capable of secreting ADH. Diseased pulmonary tissue such as that affected by pneumonia or abscesses may also produce inappropriate amounts of ADH. Diseases of the central nervous system (CNS), such as skull fractures, subdural hematoma, cerebrovascular thrombosis, and subarachnoid hemorrhage, may also cause SIADH. Stressors, both physical and emotional, pain, and positive pressure breathing can also cause a sudden release of ADH resulting in SIADH.

Clinical picture

The patient may have weight gain because of water retention. Edema is rarely present. Weakness, lethargy, and CNS changes such as confusion or convulsions may occur. These result from the *dilutional hyponatremia*. The serum sodium level is usually less than 130 mEq/L and the plasma osmolality is less than 275 mosmols/kg. Urine is hypertonic as compared to plasma.

Intervention

Intervention is directed toward treatment of the etiologic factors. Water retention is treated with water restriction of 800 to 1000 ml/day. Hyponatremia is not treated unless the patient is experiencing signs of convulsions and then hypertonic saline is given. In most instances SIADH will disappear as appropriate treatment of the underlying etiology is instituted. SIADH associated with stressors and pain is self-limiting.

Intake and output and daily weight are monitored for improvement of the problem. Thirst will be a major complaint during water restriction. The nurse must work with the patient to space fluids throughout the 24-hour period. Ice chips instead of water will allow the patient to have more frequent relief of thirst without excess intake of fluid. Frequent mouth care will also help relieve the thirst. Nursing measures directed toward the problems caused by the etiologic factors must also be part of the care plan.

Outcome criteria for the person with SIADH

The person or significant others can:
1. Explain the syndrome and purpose of treatment.
2. Describe the amount of fluid restrictions prescribed and ways to space fluids over 24 hours.
3. State that thirst is controlled.
4. Explain plans for follow-up care.

Diabetes insipidus

Etiology and pathophysiology

Diabetes insipidus is a disease caused by failure of the *posterior* lobe of the pituitary gland to secrete ADH (p. 595). Primary diabetes insipidus is a rare disease, but its symptoms are seen fairly frequently, since they may occur when a tumor develops in the gland, following head trauma, or following hypophysectomy or irradiation of the pituitary gland.

Clinical picture

ADH increases reabsorption of water from the renal tubules, and in its absence a very large amount of urine is excreted—as much as 15 L may be excreted daily. This causes fluid and electrolyte imbalance. Persons with diabetes insipidus also have insatiable thirst (polydipsia), anorexia, weight loss, and weakness.

The thirst (polydipsia) results from the polyuria. The patient usually prefers ice water, although the reason for this is unknown. The urine is dilute and has a specific gravity of 1.000 to 1.005. The serum osmolality is slightly elevated as a result of the urine loss. *Dehydration* and *hypernatremia* seldom develop because the thirst prompts the patient to drink. If something occurs to prevent replacement of water, dehydration, sodium imbalance, and vascular collapse will occur. The diagnosis is based on the dehydration test (p. 596).

Intervention

The goal of therapy is to provide adequate replacement of posterior pituitary hormone and correct the underlying pathologic condition if possible. Surgical removal of a primary or secondary tumor may be necessary.

Vasopressin tannate (Pitressin Tannate) in oil, given intramuscularly, is usually recommended for immediate treatment for 24 to 48 hours to reduce urinary volume. Administration is easier if the vial is warmed first. Vigorous shaking of the vial is necessary for administration, since the active ingredient tends to precipitate out.

A synthetic lysine-vasopressin solution (Lypressin) can be used every 3 to 6 hours as a nasal spray or drops for ongoing therapy. Patients should watch for symptoms of rhinopharyngitis. They are taught to use the medication whenever they notice polyuria or polydipsia. In severe cases, Lypressin may be used as adjunct therapy between injections. Patients should carry an identification card that explains their condition and treatment program or should wear a Medic Alert bracelet in case an accident or injury should occur.

Outcome criteria for the person with diabetes insipidus

The person or significant others can:
1. State dosage and side effects of prescribed medication.
2. Demonstrate how to use prescribed medication (nasal spray or drops).
3. State signs and symptoms that indicate the need to take prescribed medication (polyuria, polydipsia).
4. State when immediate medical follow-up is required (worsening of symptoms or symptoms not relieved by prescribed medication).
5. State plan for regular follow-up care.
6. Show the identification card or Medic Alert bracelet or necklace that the person will carry at all times.

Thyroid problems

Alterations in the thyroid gland may be associated with hyperthyroid, hypothyroid, or euthyroid metabolic states.

Simple goiter

Etiology

Any enlargement of the thyroid gland is spoken of as a goiter. A *goiter* may be caused by various disorders that prevent the synthesis of normal quantities of thyroid hormones. If the impairment is severe enough, the goiter may be associated with hypothyroidism.

Pathophysiology

Goiter occurs because of an impairment in hormonal synthesis associated with a reduction of serum triiodothyronine (T_3) and thyroxine (T_4) levels. This reduction prevents the normal feedback inhibition of TSH. The TSH level is increased, which in turn causes an increase in thyroid mass. The thyroid enlargement may be sufficient enough to allow for adequate hormonal synthesis. Simple goiter may result from *iodide deficiency*; the incidence of simple goiter in the United States is greatest in the Great Lakes Basin, Minnesota, the Dakotas, the Pacific Northwest, and the Upper Mississippi Valley because of the limited amount of iodine in the water and food supply of those regions. Iodine normally is found in seafood, and small amounts of iodine are found in green leafy vegetables that have been grown where iodine is present in the water and soil. Simple goiter may also occur because of congenital metabolic defects that prevent the synthesis of thyroid hormones. It can result from the blocking of hormone synthesis by chemical agents such as L-5-vinyl-2-thio-oxazolidone (a naturally occurring substance in cabbage, turnips, and soybeans) and drugs such as thiocarbamides, sulfonylureas, and lithium. Simple goiter is frequently seen in girls, appearing at puberty, when the metabolic rate is highest and the body's need for thyroid hormone is greatest. It may disappear spontaneously after the age of 25 years. Chronic thyroiditis may also be associated with simple goiter.

Prevention

The nurse can help to prevent simple goiter by teaching the importance of eating foods that contain iodine. The patient should be asked about the quantity of leafy vegetables and seafoods eaten and the kind of table salt used. Encouraging uses of iodized salt is important in parts of the country where there is a known deficiency of iodine in the natural water.

Clinical picture

Changes in the contour of the neck may give a clue to thyroid enlargement. Palpation may identify an enlarged thyroid (see Figs. 30-7 and 30-8). A simple goiter may go unnoticed, or the person may ignore it unless it becomes nodular or symptomatic. Difficulty in breathing may occur as a result of pressure on the trachea.

Intervention

Large goiters may have to be removed surgically to relieve symptoms of pressure or for cosmetic improvement. More conservative methods include medication and diet therapy.

If the goiter is a result of iodine deficiency, iodine replacement therapy will be given. One drop of saturated solution of potassium iodide (SSKI) each week usually provides enough additional iodine for the thyroid gland to produce adequate thyroid hormones, and the hyperplasia will gradually decrease. Using iodized table salt is an easy and inexpensive way of ensuring sufficient iodine intake, since the average adult can obtain more than twice the daily iodine requirement from the amount of salt normally used.

If the goiter is caused by goitrogens, these should be eliminated.

Most commonly, no known specific etiologic factor for a goiter can be identified, and then suppressive therapy is used. For this therapy, sodium L-thyroxine (levothyroxine) in a dose of 150 to 200 μg daily is given. This amount of exogenous thyroid will elevate the serum T_3 and T_4 levels and inhibit TSH secretion. Early goiters will disappear in 3 to 6 months. The therapy is continued until the goiter is reduced. At times, the goiter will return when suppression therapy is withdrawn; in these instances it is necessary for therapy to be reinstituted.

Patients need adequate teaching about the therapy prescribed. They should understand the need to continue therapy until it is discontinued by the physician.

Outcome criteria for the person with simple goiter

The person or significant others can:
1. Explain the medication program (effects, desired dosage, frequency, and side effects).
2. Explain the dietary changes required (use of iodized salt).
3. State plans for follow-up care.

Cancer of the thyroid

Epidemiology

Cancer of the thyroid gland is less prevalent than other forms of cancer, and only a small percentage of thyroid lumps are found to be malignant. Encouraging persons to have yearly physical examinations can be very helpful in early detection.

This cancer appears in all age groups and especially in those with a past history of irradiation to the neck structures. Recently, there has been a concerted search in the United States for young adults who received irradiation of the thymus gland as children. These individuals are urged to seek medical attention so that they can be watched closely for the development of thyroid cancer. Chronic TSH stimulation has also been identified with the formation of thyroid carcinoma.[9] The cell type determines the rapidity with which the malignancy will advance and therefore influences the type of therapy required and the prognosis. Carcinomas that are well differentiated and encapsulated and can be completely surgically removed carry a good prognosis.

Clinical picture

Cancer of the thyroid is usually suspected from a painless nodule or by palpable lymph nodes along with thyroid enlargement. Surgical exploration may be necessary to confirm the diagnosis. Thyroid function tests are usually normal.

Intervention

Surgical removal of the lesion is the treatment of choice. Whether a subtotal or total thyroidectomy will be necessary depends on the findings at the time of surgery. In all cases, doses of thyroid hormone large enough to suppress endogenous TSH are given before and after surgery because many of the tumors are TSH dependent. The parathyroid glands are preserved and may be transplanted if necessary.

Radioactive iodine (^{131}I) is used following surgery for patients with metastases or lymph node involvement. Thyroid hormone is discontinued while the radioactive iodine is being administered. Certain types of cancer of the thyroid (medullary) are treated by surgery and then by x-ray therapy of the neck because this tumor usually does not concentrate ^{131}I.

Presently, bleomycin and doxorubicin (Adriamycin) are being used to treat thyroid cancer unresponsive to surgery, radioactive iodine, or x-ray therapy.[9]

Outcome criteria for the person with cancer of the thyroid

The person or significant others can:
1. Explain the necessary follow-up therapy (x-ray, radioactive iodine, or chemotherapy).
2. List signs and symptoms requiring immediate medical attention.
3. Describe suppressive drug therapy dosage, frequency, desired effects, and side effects.
4. State plans for follow-up care.

Thyroiditis

There are three types of thyroiditis; acute, subacute, and chronic. *Chronic thyroiditis* occurs in two forms, one is a lymphocytic thyroiditis, also known as *Hashimoto's struma*. The other is *Riedel's struma* or ligneous thyroiditis, which is a rare disease that causes slowly progressive fibrosis of the thyroid.

Acute thyroiditis occurs when there is an infection of the thyroid gland. It is not common and is treated symptomatically. *Subacute thyroiditis* may last weeks or months, but the majority of persons become asymptomatic and return to normal thyroid function in time.

Hashimoto's struma

Epidemiology. The incidence of Hashimoto's struma has tripled in the last 3 decades. It is 20 times more common in women than in men. It can occur in children but is most common in adults between 30 and 50 years old.[9]

Etiology and pathophysiology. In Hashimoto's struma the thyroid is infiltrated with lymphocytes and plasma cells. Since 1956, when antibodies were identified, it has been believed to be an autoimmune disease.

Positive titers have been found to thyroglobulin and thyroid cell cytoplasm, and in some individuals both titers are positive. The mechanisms for the autoimmunity are not understood, although there appears to be a strong hereditary link that is a dominant trait. Hashimoto's struma is associated with other possible autoimmune diseases such as pernicious anemia, rheumatoid arthritis, lupoid hepatitis, disseminated lupus erythematosus, and idiopathic adrenal insufficiency.

Some experts believe that hyperthyroidism (Graves' disease), Hashimoto's struma, and myxedema are variants of a common process.[9] It is not unusual to find family members with one of the three diseases.

Clinical picture. There may be diffuse thyroid enlargement, and some persons complain of difficulty in swallowing or choking. Signs and symptoms of hypothyroidism or hyperthyroidism may also be present. Early in the disease, during exacerbations of chronic thyroiditis, when functioning thyroid tissue is still present, excessive thyroid hormone may be released resulting in signs and symptoms of hyperthyroidism. As the disease progresses, the thyroid gland may be destroyed, and signs and symptoms of hypothyroidism may be present.

The diagnosis is not always easy to establish, and several tests may be necessary to confirm the diagnosis. Early in the disease antibody levels are determined, and protein-bound iodine, radioactive iodine uptake tests, and serum T_4 and T_3 levels will also be used. When the diagnosis is still inconclusive, a needle biopsy of the thyroid is indicated.

Intervention. The treatment depends on the clinical findings. Signs and symptoms of hyperthyroidism are not usually treated. Persons with signs of hypothyroidism are treated with thyroid hormone. The hormone is also used to treat some persons with an enlarged thyroid gland; others may receive no therapy unless they develop symptoms of hypothyroidism later on.

Hypothyroidism

Hypothyroidism is a metabolic state resulting from deficient thyroid hormones. It may occur at any age. Congenital hypothyroidism results in a condition known as *cretinism*. *Myxedema* is a term used to refer to a severe form of hypothyroidism accompanied by an accumulation of *hydrophilic mucopolysaccharides* in the ground substance of the dermis as well as in other tissue.

Etiology and pathophysiology

Hypothyroidism can result from primary deficits of the thyroid hormones. Congenital developmental or genetic defects, idiopathic thyroid dysfunction, iodine deficiency, chronic thyroiditis, and thyrotoxic drugs such as lithium, antithyroid drugs, or iodide can all cause thyroid deficiency. *The most common cause of hypothy-*

roidism results from destruction of the thyroid gland by surgery or radioiodine therapy.

Hypothyroidism may be secondary to pituitary failure and is then called *pituitary hypothyroidism*. Hypothalamic hypothyroidism (tertiary hypothyroidism) results from hypothalamic disease that causes a deficiency of thyroid releasing hormone.

Regardless of the cause, the clinical findings are the same. The signs and symptoms result from a deficiency of T_3 and T_4, leading to a decrease in the normal metabolic functions that are under the control of T_3 and T_4. (See p. 586 for an outline of the functions of T_3 and T_4.)

Clinical picture

The picture presented by the person with hypothyroidism will vary with the age of onset and the severity of the deficiency. Manifestations of *cretinism* may be present at birth but usually are not noticeable for several months (Fig. 32-3). Abnormally persistent physiologic jaundice, hoarse crying, somnolence, feeding problems, and constipation are common early symptoms of cretinism. In later months physical and mental retardation will appear. The characteristic cretin appearance includes a broad flat nose, protruding tongue, widely set lips, protuberant abdomen, dry skin, and short stature. The child will not reach the normal mental and sexual developmental milestones. If hypothyroidism starts in childhood, physical, mental, and sexual development stops.

In adults early signs and symptoms are vague and of insidious onset. Early complaints may consist of sluggishness, weight gain, or sleepiness. Intolerance to cold and constipation are usually present. Menorrhagia in younger women may be severe. Slowing of intellectual functioning and slurred speech may occur as the disease progresses. The person may complain of dry skin and changes in hair (hair is sparse and dry). Complaints of stiff, aching muscles and joints may also be given. About 12% of persons with hypothyroidism have pernicious anemia.

Other possible findings include slow pulse rate, an elevation of diastolic blood pressure, and possibly pericardial effusion. Pleural effusion also may be present, and some individuals have ascites. The heart is enlarged. All body functions are slowed. Deep tendon reflexes are diminished, and there may be joint effusion and arthritis or bursitis. Despite these marked changes, some individuals do not seem to be aware of the changes in their physical functioning, appearance, or behavior.

The individual may or may not have an enlarged thyroid, depending on the cause of hypothyroidism. Enlargement (goiter) occurs in hypothyroidism caused by genetic defects, iodine deficiency, thyroiditis, and chemical agents. Goiter is present because in these states there is an increase in TSH as a result of the lack of feedback, and the TSH acts on the thyroid tissue to produce hyperplasia. In hypothyroidism caused by a congenital developmental defect or destruction of the gland by radiation or surgery, there is no tissue for TSH to act on. In hypothyroidism resulting from pituitary or hypothalamic problems, TSH is depressed and no hyperplasia occurs.

The severest form of hypothyroidism in adults is called *myxedema* (Fig. 32-4). When this form is present, the patient has a dull, expressionless face, periorbital puffiness, nonpitting edema of the feet and hands, and a large tongue. The skin feels rough and doughy and is pale and cool. The puffiness of the periorbital area, the nonpitting edema, and the changes in the skin are caused by an accumulation of mucopolysaccharides.

Myxedema coma. Myxedema coma occurs as the myxedema worsens. The individual becomes less responsive and may be difficult to arouse or go into a coma. Sometimes an infection such as pneumonia, cellulitis, or pyelonephritis precipitates the coma. There is decreased blood flow to the brain. Hypotension, hypoglycemia, bradycardia, hypothermia, and carbon dioxide retention resulting from hypoventilation may result from the decrease in metabolic function.

Despite improvement in therapy, which is directed toward gradual reversal of the signs and symptoms, the mortality is still between 50% and 90%.[9]

Intervention

Treatment of hypothyroidism is by the administration of the deficient thyroid hormone. The drugs used

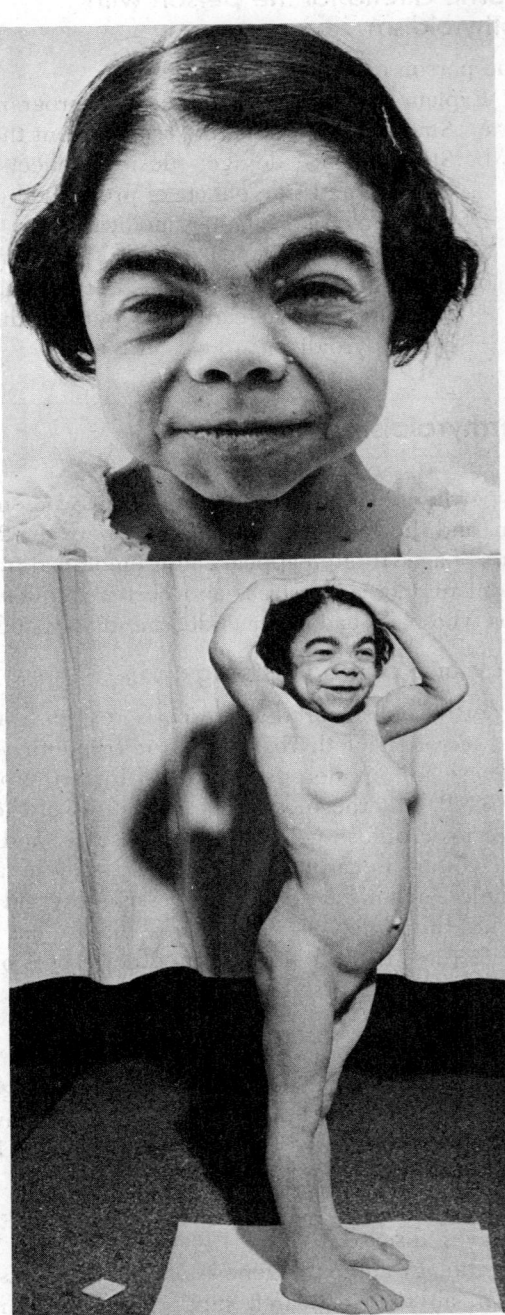

Fig. 32-3. Adult cretin (33 years old, untreated). Note characteristic cretinoid features, dwarfism (height of 44 in.), absent axillary and scant pubic hair, poorly developed breasts, potbelly, and small umbilical hernia. Patient has primary amenorrhea (protein-bound iodine [PBI] 5.9, butanol-extractable iodine [BEI] 0, radioactive iodine uptake [RAIU] 0, thyroid stimulating hormone [TSH] response 0). Increased PBI/BEI ratio suggests that this patient was a goitrous cretin in early life and goiter regressed. (From Schneeburg, N.G.: Essentials of clinical endocrinology, St. Louis, 1970, The C.V. Mosby Co.)

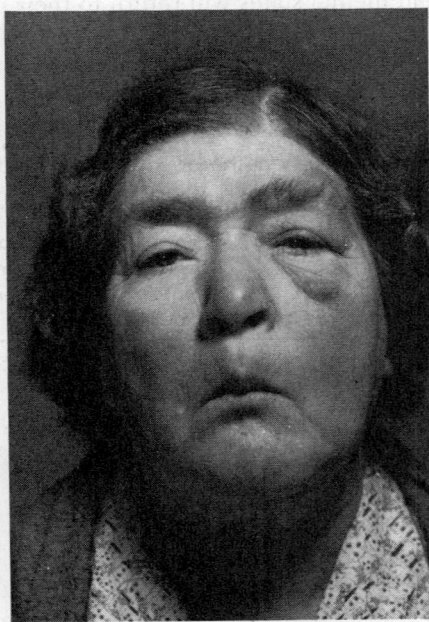

Fig. 32-4. Person with myxedema. (From Schottelius, B.A., and Schottelius, D.A.: Textbook of physiology, ed. 18, St. Louis, 1978, The C.V. Mosby Co.)

to treat hypothyroidism are listed in Table 32-1. It is important that dosages be increased gradually because a sudden increase in metabolic rate can cause death from cardiac failure. The daily maintenance dose of thyroid hormones varies widely. The correct dose is determined by a remission in the symptoms of hypofunction. Adults with hypothyroidism respond quickly to the administration of thryoid hormones. Changes in appearance and physical symptoms occur within 2 to 3 days. Treatment must be continued throughout life, and the individual must be taught that failure to take the prescribed medication will result in an exacerbation of the disease. Medication dosage may need periodic adjustments to avoid symptoms of hyperthyroidism or hypothyroidism. A diet fairly high in protein and low in calories is often prescribed until weight returns to normal as a result of therapy.

In addition to administering replacement therapy and monitoring the patient for effectiveness of the therapy and for side effects, the nurse will need to provide appropriate physical and emotional care.

Some patients will require complete care at first, and constipation is a frequent problem. Environmental stressors should be kept at a minimum, since the patient lacks the ability to respond to them.

Cardiovascular and respiratory support may be required. The patient's slowed mental functioning requires understanding and patience on the part of caregivers. A thorough explanation of the cause of the changes in the patient's physical and mental responses should be given to the patient's significant others. As the thyroid hormone levels return to normal, the patient's physical and mental states will return to their preillness levels.

TABLE 32-1. Replacement therapy in hypothyroidism: approximate equivalents

Thyroid: combination of T_4 and T_3	Levothyroxine sodium: synthetic L-thyroxine*	Liothyronine sodium: synthetic triiodothyronine†	Liotrix: synthetic combination of T_4 and T_3‡
30 mg	0.05 mg	12.5 μg	0.5
65 mg	0.1 mg	25 μg	1
130 mg	0.2 mg	50 μg	2
200 mg	0.3 mg	75 μg	3

*Trade names are Synthroid, Letter, and Levoid.
†Trade names are Cytomel and Trionine.
‡Trade names are Euthroid and Thyrolar.

It is imperative that newborns, infants, and children receive replacement therapy immediately to avoid physical and mental retardation. It is estimated that 1 of every 5000 children born has hypothyroidism. Every

newborn should undergo screening for hypothyroidism because of the seriousness of nontreatment.[99]

Outcome criteria for the person with hypothyroidism

The person or significant others can:
1. Explain the prescribed medication program.
   a. State reason for lifelong replacement therapy.
   b. State name, dosage, desired effects, frequency, and side effects of prescribed drugs.
2. Describe need for ongoing medical follow-up.
   a. State plans for regular medical follow-up.
   b. Describe signs or symptoms necessitating immediate medical care of hypothyroidism or hyperthyroidism.

Hyperthyroidism

Hyperthyroidism is more common in women than in men, and there is a higher incidence between 20 and 40 years of age. It often appears after emotional trauma, infection, or increased stress and occurs frequently in persons who have had other endocrine disturbances.

Etiology and pathophysiology

Hyperthyroidism or thyrotoxicosis results from excessive secretion of thyroxine (T_4) or triiodothyronine (T_3). There are numerous causes of hyperthyroidism (Table 32-2), but the most common causes of the disease are toxic diffuse goiter (Graves' disease) and toxic nodular goiter. Regardless of the cause, the metabolic and clinical manifestations of excessive thyroid hormones are the same. Because Graves' disease has some unique features that are not seen in other causes of thyrotoxicosis, it is discussed separately below.

Graves' disease

Graves' disease is characterized by a *triad* of *goiter*, *hyperthyroidism*, and *exophthalmos*, although any one or two signs may appear without the other signs being present. The three signs may occur in any order. Pretibial myxedema occurs in a small percentage of persons with Graves' disease.

The etiology and pathogenesis of Graves' disease are unknown, although research supports an autoimmune basis for the disease. What is known is that in the disease the homeostatic mechanisms that normally adjust hormone secretions are disrupted, and hyperthyroidism and the goiter develop.

In 1965 a thyroid stimulator distinct from TSH was discovered. This stimulator has a maximal stimulating effect at 9 to 12 hours after injection, whereas TSH's maximal stimulating effect is 2 to 3 hours after injection; thus it was named long-acting thyroid stimulator (LATS). Because LATS was found in only approximately one half of the patients with Graves' disease, its role in the

TABLE 32-2. Causes and definitions of types of hyperthyroidism

Cause	Definition	Cause	Definition
Toxic diffuse goiter (Graves' disease)	See discussion in text	Pituitary hyperthyroidism	Hyperthyroidism becuase of secretion of excess TSH by pituitary adenomas, rare cause of hyperthyroidism but can occur; treatment involves removal of pituitary tumor
Toxic nodular goiter	Multiple aggregates of follicular cells that function autonomously; cause unknown, although can occur as consequence of long-standing simple goiter	Chorionic hyperthyroidism	Chorionic gonadotropin has weak thyrotropin activity; tumors such as choriocarcinoma, embryonal cell carcinoma, and hydatidiform mole have high concentrations of chorionic gonadotropins that can stimulate T_4 and T_3 secretion; hyperthyroidison disappears with treatment of tumor
Thyroiditis	Early in thyroiditis, before gland is destroyed by the inflammatory process, acute inflammation of gland can cause release of increased amounts of T_4 and T_3; self-limiting and usually requires no treatment; hyperthyroid state followed by euthyroid state and then over time by hypothyroidism	Struma ovarii	Ovarian dermoid tumor made up of thyroid tissue that secretes thyroid hormones
T_3 thyrotoxicosis	T_3 elevated but cause unknown; T_4 normal or low; T_3 thyrotoxicosis should be suspected in patients who have normal T_4 but have signs and symptoms of thyrotoxicosis	Factitious hyperthyroidism	Hyperthyroidism that results from ingestion of exogenous thyroid extracts; may result when thyroid hormone is used in weight reduction
Hyperthyroidism caused by metastatic thyroid cancer	Thyroid cancer does not usually concentrate iodine efficiently and thus rarely causes hyperthyroidism; occasionally, large metastatic follicular carcinomas produce hyperthyroidism		

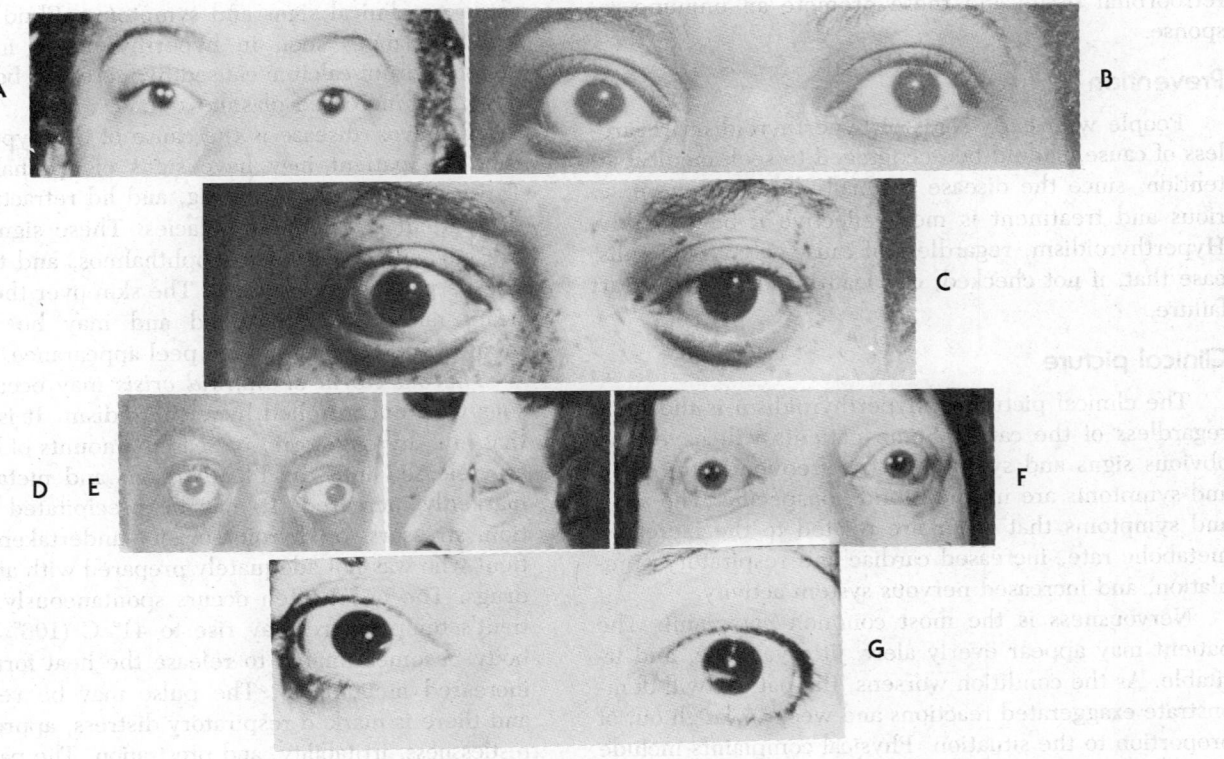

Fig. 32-5. Ophthalmopathy in Graves' disease. **A,** Minimal retraction of lower lids, no exophthalmos. **B,** Lid retraction with mild exophthalmos (18 to 19 mm). **C,** Asymmetric exophthalmos (OD 24 mm, OS 18 mm). **D,** Ophthalmoplegia (partial paralysis, left lateral gaze, OD). **E** and **F,** Infiltrative ophthalmopathy with severe exophthalmos. **G,** Residual corneal scar in left eye after unilateral malignant exophthalmos. (From Schneeburg, N.C.: Essentials of clinical endocrinology, St. Louis, 1970, The C.V. Mosby Co.)

pathogenesis of the disease was at first questioned. However, more recent research has demonstrated that the failure to detect LATS in many patients was a result of problems with assay technology. The thyroid stimulating activity of sera in patients with Graves' disease is the result of a *polyclonal immunoglobulin* that causes various responses directed against some component of the thyroid. The various responses caused by this immunoglobulin G and the corresponding factors have been given various names. Because the use of various names has been confusing, it is recommended that the term *thyroid stimulating immunoglobulins* (TSI) be used to refer to all the immunoglobin G that stimulate thyroid activity in sera of patients with Graves' disease.[19]

The cause of this abnormal development of immunoglobulins is unknown. It has been proposed that a heritable abnormality in immune surveillance allows a particular clone of lymphocytes to survive and secrete immunoglobulins to a precipitating factor.[19] Another hypothesis is that because of heredity, the TSH receptor is altered and evokes the production of antibodies.

The pathogenesis of the exophthalmos is even less clearly understood (Fig. 32-5). One hypothesis is that fragments of TSH bind with immunoglobulins and cause the retroorbital edema. A second hypothesis proposes that the lymphatic system transports thyroglobulins to retroorbital tissue and these promote an immune response.

Prevention

People with early signs of hyperthyroidism regardless of cause, should be encouraged to seek medical attention, since the disease gradually becomes more serious and treatment is more effective if begun early. Hyperthyroidism, regardless of cause, is a serious disease that, if not checked, can lead to death from heart failure.

Clinical picture

The clinical picture in hyperthyroidism is the same regardless of the cause. Some patients will have very obvious signs and symptoms, but frequently the signs and symptoms are insidious and nonspecific. The signs and symptoms that occur are related to the increased metabolic rate, increased cardiac and respiratory stimulation, and increased nervous system activity.

Nervousness is the most common complaint. The patient may appear overly alert, jittery, tense, and irritable. As the condition worsens, the patient will demonstrate exaggerated reactions and weep or laugh out of proportion to the situation. Physical complaints include increased sweating, intolerance to heat, palpitations, and sometimes tachycardia, fatigue, and weakness, weight loss with an increased appetite, and dyspnea. Some patients will complain of increased frequency of bowel movements or diarrhea.

Physical examination will reveal a goiter in almost all instances of hyperthyroidism, and a *thyroid bruit* is usually present. The cardiovascular system is very seriously affected by hyperthyroidism because of the increased metabolic rate and the direct effects of thyroid hormones on the heart. Changes include increased blood volume, increased cardiac output, and increased blood pressure. The patient usually has tachycardia. *Angina, arrhythmias,* and *congestive heart failure* may be present. The physical status of the patient with underlying cardiac disease can be severely threatened by hyperthyroidism. Cardiovascular abnormalities may be the presenting signs and symptoms of hyperthyroidism.

Typically, the skin is warm, moist, and reddened. These changes are caused by increased blood flow to the skin. The hair is fine and some alopecia may occur. The neuromuscular examination will reveal fine tremors in almost all patients. Hyperactivity is usually present. Muscle weakness and muscle atrophy are common.

Abnormalities in menstruation are common. Oligomenorrhea and sometimes amenorrhea are present. In males there may be a decrease in libido.

Hyperthyroidism may cause signs and symptoms of other metabolic abnormalities such as glucose intolerance, which results from decreased insulin release.[19] There may be abnormalities in growth hormone secretion and changes in corticosteroid metabolism, but these cause no clinical signs and symptoms. Fluid and electrolyte changes seen in hyperthyroidism include increased serum calcium caused by increased bone breakdown and increased plasma volume.

If Graves' disease is the cause of the hyperthyroidism, the patient may have signs of ophthalmopathy. These include a stare, lid lag, and lid retraction giving the patient a "frightened" facies. These signs may be present with or without exophthalmos, and there may also be pretibial myxedema. The skin over the tibia appears raised and thickened and may be hyperpigmented and have an orange peel appearance.

Thyroid storm or *thyroid crisis* may occur in persons with uncontrolled hyperthyroidism. It is believed that in a thyroid storm, increased amounts of hormones are released into the bloodstream, and metabolism is markedly increased. It may be precipitated by infection, stressors, or thyroid surgery undertaken on a patient who was not adequately prepared with antithyroid drugs. The onset often occurs spontaneously. The patient's temperature may rise to 41° C (106° F) as the body becomes unable to release the heat formed with increased metabolism. The pulse may be very rapid, and there is marked respiratory distress, apprehension, restlessness, irritability, and prostration. The patient may become delirious and finally comatose, with death resulting from heart failure.

Diagnostic studies to identify hyperactivity of the thyroid gland are described in Table 30-3. The expected results for hyperthyroidism are also described.

Intervention

Therapy is directed toward reducing the output of thyroid hormone and treating other signs and symptoms. There are two approaches that may be used to reduce the output of thyroid hormone: (1) the use of antithyroid drugs or (2) ablation of thyroid tissue by surgery or radioactive iodine. Usually a trial of antithyroid therapy is used. Ablation therapy is used when there is a relapse during drug therapy, drug toxicity, failure of the patient to follow the regimen, or a large goiter. Subtotal thyroidectomy is the procedure of choice for persons under 40 years of age; radioactive iodine is usually used with older patients.

Drug therapy. *Propylthiouracil* and *methimazole* (Tapazole) are the most commonly used antithyroid drugs. The action of these drugs is slow, and it usually takes 2 to 4 weeks before improvement is noticeable. This is because these drugs block thyroid hormone synthesis and not the secretion of the hormone and the supply stored in the gland must be reduced before improvement is seen. This takes from 2 to 4 weeks. The patient usually is started on a relatively large dose of an antithyroid drug, and then the dosage is gradually reduced to a level sufficient to maintain the euthyroid state. When antithyroid drugs are used as the primary therapy, they commonly are continued for 6 to 18 months or longer. Some patients will stay in remission without further therapy. Others will require longer drug therapy, additional therapy, or lifelong therapy. The patient should see the physician at regular intervals after drugs are discontinued so that early signs of recurrence will be noticed. It is important to give the drugs at regularly spaced intervals, since their blood levels are reduced in about 8 hours.

Patients are instructed to look for toxic signs of the drugs, such as fever, sore throat, and skin eruptions and to call their physician if these signs appear. If toxic reaction occurs, blood counts may show leukopenia. Continued use of antithyroid drugs may not be tolerated by some persons.

Preparations of iodine, such as *Lugol's solution*, also are used in the treatment of hyperthyroidism. These preparations can reduce the metabolic rate rapidly because they block the synthesis and release of thyroid hormone. However, their action is less sustained. They reduce glandular vascularity and help to prevent postoperative hemorrhage when a partial thyroidectomy is necessary. Lugol's solution is often prescribed after a course of propylthiouracil to prepare the patient for surgery. When Lugol's solution is ordered, it is more palatable given in milk or fruit juice. It should be taken through a straw because it may stain the teeth. A brassy taste in the mouth and sore teeth and gums are signs of toxicity, but these complications rarely occurs.

There are some disadvantages to the use of iodides, including (1) the patient cannot be treated for some time with radioactive iodine (RAI) because the thyroid gland is saturated with iodide and the RAI will not be taken up; (2) some persons develop an exacerbation of their disease when RAI is given following iodide treatment; and (3) if iodide is given before treatment with other antithyroid drugs, this also may result in an exacerbation of hyperthyroidism.[84]

The beta-adrenergic (β-adrenergic) blocking drugs, such as propranolol (*Inderal*), are used to treat tachycardia, arrhythmias, and angina present in the hyperthyroid patient. These drugs also improve tremors, restlessness, anxiety, and sometimes myopathy. Propranolol is used in all patients with thyroid storm.

Lithium has been found to block hormone secretion. However, it has not been used as frequently as other drugs and is saved for times when the patient develops toxicity to other drugs or as an adjunct to other therapy during thyrotoxic crisis.

Radioactive iodine therapy. Radiation can decrease thyroid activity. The most effective way is by the use of ^{131}I, a radioactive isotope of iodine. The isotope is given by mouth, is absorbed rapidly in the stomach, and becomes concentrated in the thyroid. Usually, a single dose is given in a radioactive "cocktail." If an unusually large dose of radioactive iodine is given, hospitalization for several days may be necessary. Patients receiving usual amounts of the isotope may go directly home, and no special precautions are advised. It takes about 3 weeks for the symptoms of hyperthyroidism to subside, and over 2 months for thyroid function to become normal. Occasionally, remission is not achieved with one dose, and the treatment is repeated after an interval of several months.

Radioactive iodine is not used in pregnant women because of the potential effect on the fetus since the placenta transports iodine easily. Some physicians do not use it in persons in the childbearing years because of the potential for destruction of the gonads.

Patients who receive radioactive iodine for hyperthyroidism need to have the treatment explained to them with special care, and they usually need repeated reassurance that the radioactive properties are quickly dissipated. Since they may be more emotional than other persons, they sometimes think they are experiencing reactions to the drug long after this is possible. Permanent hypothyroidism is a potential complication of radioactive iodine therapy.

Care of the eyes. Persons with exophthalmos need to have their eyes protected from irritation. Dark glasses will afford some protection from wind, sun, and dust, while soothing eye drops, such as methylcellulose, 0.5% to 1%, may provide comfort. For more severe protrusion shields, tarsorrhaphy (suturing the eyelids together), or surgery for orbital decompression may be necessary.

Rest. Since the advent of the antithyroid drugs and the trend toward early treatment, most persons with hyperthyroidism can be cared for at home. Although those allowed to stay at home usually are not particularly hyperactive, they are likely to be very nervous and irritable. It is important that family and friends understand that extreme sensitivity and excessive irritability are part of the disease; otherwise, they may become upset with the individual and aggravate the situation. Plans for maintaining a quiet environment should be made with the individual and the family. Assisting the individual to obtain sufficient rest is a real challenge. Quiet activities, such as handicrafts that require gross motor movements (e.g., weaving) or reading, may provide rest. Family members should try to remain calm and avoid discussion of controversial subjects.

When individuals are nervous, they may drop articles or be clumsy in handling them. This usually is upsetting and may become a source of real frustration. It may be necessary, therefore, to do small things for these persons that they may seem physically able to do for themselves, and they need to understand why they are being helped.

Diet. There is usually an increased need for food because of the increased metabolism. A high-caloric, high-protein diet with snacks between meals may be needed to maintain weight and meet energy requirements. Decaffeinated drinks are encouraged.

Complications. Therapy may be ineffective, causing thyroid crisis (p. 628), or may decrease thyroid activity to a point of hypothyroidism (p. 624). The goals of treatment and nursing care for thyroid crisis are to control the release of thyroid hormones and maintain vital functions. Treatment includes antithyroid drugs, oxygen, hypothermia blankets to reduce fever, intravenous fluids, steroids, sedatives, and cardiac drugs as indicated. Emotional and physical care is needed to decrease metabolic needs. Cardiovascular monitoring is necessary, because severe cardiovascular complications can occur.

Hypothyroidism may occur as a result of any of the prescribed treatment programs; however, it occurs more frequently after surgery or radiation. Significant decrease in pulse rate, rapid weight gain, mental dullness, or a change in tolerance to cold are some of the possible indications of hypothyroidism.

Relapse may occur in a number of patients treated for hyperthyroidism; therefore patients must be alert to return of former signs and symptoms and seek medical advice should they occur.

Outcome criteria for the person with hyperthyroidism on antithyroid drugs

The person or significant others can:
1. Explain the medication program (desired effects, dosage, frequency, toxic effects).
2. Describe plans for a quiet, restful environment.
3. Plan meals to meet energy requirements.

4. State plans for follow-up care.
   a. State symptoms necessitating immediate follow-up (signs of remission, thyroid crisis, hypothyroidism).
   b. State plans for regular medical appointments.
5. Describe eye care if exophthalmos is present.

Surgery of the thyroid

Before thyroid surgery is undertaken, a *euthyroid* state is produced by drug therapy. The patient is ready for surgery when signs and symptoms of hyperthyroidism are absent and weight gain is normal. An ECG is made before surgery in order to detect evidence of heart damage. Patients with heart damage are preferably treated with radioactive iodine.

Part or all of the thyroid gland may be removed surgically, depending on the purpose for which the operation is done. In the case of a malignancy the gland may be removed completely *(total thyroidectomy),* and the patient must then take thyroid hormones regularly for the remainder of his life. When antithyroid drugs do not correct the hyperthyroidism and treatment with radioactive iodine is contraindicated, hyperthyroidism may be treated surgically by removing approximately five-sixths of the gland *(subtotal thyroidectomy).* In most cases this operation permanently alleviates symptoms, while the remaining thyroid tissue provides enough hormones for normal function. The remaining tissue can hypertrophy, however, and hyperthyroidism can recur.

Preoperative care

Because the patient who has a thyroidectomy must protect the suture line from strain while raising secretions and while repositioning in bed or ambulating, preoperative teaching includes this information. The patient is taught to support the neck by placing both hands behind the head; this action avoids flexion and hyperextension during moving or coughing.

Postoperative care

The *complications* following thyroid operations are extremely serious, and if they are not recognized and treated at once, they can result in death. Complications that the nurse should be alert for are recurrent laryngeal nerve injury, hemorrhage, tetany, and respiratory obstruction. Since the thyroid gland partially surrounds the larynx and trachea, there is danger of respiratory obstruction from a variety of causes, and a tracheostomy set should be kept readily available.

The dressing is observed for signs of *hemorrhage* for the first 12 to 24 hours postoperatively. Since blood may drain back under the patient's neck and shoulders, the nurse's hand should be slipped gently under the neck and shoulders each time the patient is observed to be certain that any bleeding will be detected early. A choking sensation, difficulty in coughing and swallowing, or tightening of the dressing usually means there is bleeding into the surrounding tissues, causing pressure on the trachea and epiglottis. If these symptoms occur, the dressing should be loosened at once and the surgeon notified. If loosening the dressing does not relieve the *respiratory difficulty* and medical assistance will not be immediately available, the surgeon may instruct the nurse to remove the clips or sutures from the wound to relieve pressure on the trachea. The procedure to follow until the surgeon arrives should be ascertained whenever the nurse is caring for a patient having a thyroidectomy. The surgeon may need to perform an emergency tracheostomy, and the patient often must be taken to the operating room for retying of the blood vessels and resuturing of the wound.

Although slight hoarseness is normal, the nurse observes the patient for any increase in it and for any respiratory difficulty accompanying it, since these conditions may be caused by injury to the recurrent laryngeal nerves, hemorrhage, or excessive edema about the vocal cords and larynx. The most common condition to suspect when the patient has difficulty in speaking or breathing is edema, but if the recurrent *laryngeal nerves* have been *injured* during an operation on the thyroid gland, the patient may have vocal cord spasm. If the nerve to one vocal cord only is injured, hoarseness may develop. If the nerves on both sides are injured, the vocal cords will become tight and close off the larynx, causing the patient to shows signs of respiratory obstruction. As the patient attempts to pull air in through tightened vocal cords, a crowing sound is made and the tissues around the neck are retracted. To recognize early symptoms of recurrent laryngeal nerve injury, the patient is asked to speak as soon as he or she has reacted from anesthesia and at intervals of 30 to 60 minutes.

When thyroid surgery was first used, the parathyroid glands were sometimes removed by mistake. Although this is uncommon today, injury to the parathyroids can occur during surgery or inflammation may block the normal release of parathyroid hormone. When such an injury or blockage occurs, symptoms of calcium deficiency, *tetany,* may develop (p. 341). This complication may appear from 1 to 7 days postoperatively. If not treated promptly, it can cause contraction of the glottis, respiratory obstruction, and death. Serum calcium levels are usually monitored, and hypocalcemia is treated by replacement of calcium intravenously.

Calcium gluconate is given intravenously as immediate treatment. Daily oral doses of calcium chloride are then given until normal function returns. If not all the glands were destroyed by injury, the remaining glands hypertrophy, so that hypoparathyroidism is only temporary. If all were destroyed, the patient must have lifetime replacement therapy.

Diet. High-carbohydrate fluids by mouth and a soft diet are given as soon as tolerated. The throat is usually sore for several days, and this may make swallowing difficult. Analgesic throat lozenges or a narcotic may be ordered to be given as necessary. When possible, they are given about 30 minutes before meals to make swallowing easier. A humidifier may be used to decrease discomfort and to thin secretions, making them easier to raise.

Activity. Following surgery, any activity that does not put tension on the suture line is permitted. When the suture line has healed sufficiently, the patient begins gradually to practice full range of neck motion to prevent permanent limitation of head movements.

Outcome criteria for the person who has had a thyroidectomy

The person or significant others can:
1. Demonstrate neck exercises to be done at home.
2. State plans for follow-up care.

Parathyroid problems

Primary hyperparathyroidism

Etiology and epidemiology

The most frequent causes of primary hyperfunction of the parathyroid glands are benign neoplasms, although malignant tumors and hyperplasia may occur. In about 80% of the cases there is a single adenoma.

The disease most frequently occurs in adults between the third and fifth decades.

Pathophysiology and clinical picture

Parathyroid hormone regulates the level of calcium and phosphate ions in the body fluids (see Table 30-1); therefore hypersecretions cause a disturbance in these ions. The serum calcium becomes elevated (hypercalcemia), and the phophorus level is decreased (hypophosphatemia). There is increased urinary excretion of both calcium and phosphorus, and renal calculi frequently develop.

The increased parathyroid hormone can cause bone destruction. *Osteopenia* and rarely *osteitis fibrosa cystica* occur. Although serious bone destruction is not a frequent problem, all patients should be monitored for it, since they all have the potential for developing pathologic fractures resulting from weight bearing or pressure. Other symptoms related to the calcium imbalance are anorexia, nausea, vomiting, weakness, fatigue, bone pain, polyuria, polydipsia, constipation, and proximal muscle weakness and myopathy. Some patients may develop duodenal ulcers or acute pancreatitis, and gastrointestinal complaints may be the first clue to the diagnosis.

Mental changes are found in one half of the persons with primary hyperparathyroidism. They may vary from behavior disorders, confusion, and depression to personality changes, psychosis, and stupor. Relatively small elevations of calcium may cause major mental changes. This must be kept in mind, particularly when working with elderly persons.

Laboratory changes that may occur, in addition to elevated serum calcium, decreased serum phosphorus, and elevated urinary calcium and phosphorus, include hyperchloremic acidosis, hyperglycemia, hyperuricemia, and hypomagnesemia. Serum alkaline phosphatase is always elevated when there is significant bone involvement.

Intervention

Before definitive therapy for the hyperparathyroidism is undertaken, the altered electrolytes must be normalized. This involves rehydration. After this is achieved, an infusion of isotonic sodium chloride, 4 to 5 L daily, and a potent diuretic, such as furosemide (Lasix), are given. This regimen allows for the excretion of several grams of calcium per day, but the therapy can only be used in patients with adequate renal function. Intake and output must be monitored closely in all patients receiving this treatment.

Intravenous phosphate is effective in lowering calcium levels, but it is associated with the danger of widespread calcification. In some instances, mithramycin (Mithracin), 25 to 50 μg/kg of body weight, is used to lower calcium levels. This is used if the sodium chloride–furosemide regimen is contraindicated.

Surgery (partial parathyroidectomy) is usually the treatment of choice in primary hyperparathyroidism. The usual surgery involves removing three glands totally and part of the fourth gland. An alternative approach involves removing all four glands and implanting some of the removed tissue into the muscle of the forearm. Implantation avoids vascular failure and death of residual parathyroid tissue left in the neck.[99] If no glandular abnormality is found at the time of surgery, extensive exploration of the neck and surrounding areas for additional glands that could be the source of the symptoms is necessary.

The serum calcium level will decrease within 24 hours after successful surgery. The patient must be monitored carefully for signs of tetany (p. 341). Parathyroid function usually returns to normal in 5 to 7 days. By this time the remaining parathyroid tissue resumes normal secretion. If mild hypocalcemia occurs, oral calcium is given. If hypocalemia is severe, calcium gluconate or calcium chloride at a concentration of 1 mg/ml in 5% dextrose will be given intravenously. Calcium replacement will be continued until serum calcium is returned to normal. This usually takes a few days. If signs and symptoms of hypocalcemia continue to be present, calcium and/or vitamin D replacement therapy in the same amount as that used to treat hypoparathyroidism will be necessary. While patients are on replacement therapy, they must be monitored carefully for signs and symptoms of hypercalcemia.

The other electrolytes must also be monitored. Magnesium deficiency may also precipitate tetany and will need to be treated if present.

If parathyroid cancer is found during surgery, wide excision with total parathyroidectomy will be necessary. These patients will develop hypoparathyroidism and will need the same treatment as any other patient with hypoparathyroidism (p. 633).

Outcome criteria for the person with primary hyperparathyroidism and postoperative partial parathyroidectomy

The person or significant others can:
1. Explain the expected results of surgery.
2. List signs and symptoms of hypocalcemia and hypercalcemia and describe action necessary if they occur.
3. Explain planned medication regimen if appropriate (drugs, dosage, frequency, expected effects, and side effects).
4. Describe plans for follow-up care.

Secondary and tertiary hyperparathyroidism

Secondary hyperparathyroidism is a disease characterized by excessive production of parathyroid hormone resulting from chronic hypocalcemia. Malabsorption and chronic renal failure are two common causes of secondary hyperparathyroidism. In these conditions the calcium level is chronically low. The low calcium level is a chronic stimulus to the parathyroid glands and results in hyperplasia of the parathyroid glands. The hyperplasia and excessive production of parathyroid hormone may be enough to keep the calcium level normal, but at the expense of bone destruction. The bone lesions are characterized by *osteomalacia, osteosclerosis,* and *osteitis fibrosa cystica*.

Treatment involves correction of the calcium level with a calcium supplement and vitamin D in persons with malabsorption problems and a calcium supplement, vitamin D, and a phosphorus depleting agent such as aluminum hydroxide in persons with chronic renal failure (see p. 1577 for a discussion of calcium problems in chronic renal failure). If medical therapy does not bring the calcium level to normal and halt the chronic stimulation of the parathyroid gland, a subtotal parathyroidectomy may be necessary to stop the severe bone destruction.

Tertiary hyperparathyroidism is the result of long-standing secondary hyperparathyroidism and is characterized by the development of autonomous parathyroid function that no longer functions under normal homeostatic control mechanisms. When tertiary hyperparathyroidism occurs, the patient with chronic renal failure or malabsorption syndrome will develop hypercalcemia as the underlying calcium alteration is reversed. In most instances the reversal of the original alteration removes the chronic stimulus and the hyperplasia will regress. The only treatment for tertiary hyperparathyroidism is to prevent complications of hypercalcemia until the gland returns to normal. In some patients the glandular hyperplasia does not regress and a partial parathyroidectomy is necessary.

The care for patients who undergo partial parathyroidectomies for secondary or tertiary hyperparathyroidism is the same as for patients who have partial parathyroidectomies for primary hyperparathyroidism. Nurses play a major role in helping patients with malabsorption syndrome or chronic renal failure to follow prescribed regimens so that secondary or tertiary hyperparathyroidism is prevented.

Hypoparathyroidism

Etiology

Hypoparathyroidism is a metabolic disorder that results in hypocalcemia. It most commonly results from a deficiency in parathyroid hormone resulting from excision of the parathyroid glands or damage to them during thyroid surgery, surgery for hyperparathyroidism, or radical neck surgery. It may also be idiopathic with no known cause.

Pathophysiology and clinical picture

In acute hypofunction of the parathyroid gland, there is a diminished level of parathyroid hormone and increased bone resorption, and the serum calcium level falls. Since parathyroid hormone is involved in the renal clearance of phosphate, serum phosphate levels increase. The decreased level of serum calcium results in neuromuscular irritability. The individual may complain of numbness and tingling in the extremities and around the mouth. These complaints suggest tetany. Chvostek's and Trousseau's signs are present. (See Chapter 21 for a description of these signs.) Carpal spasm, marked anxiety and apprehension, laryngeal stridor, dyspnea, and cyanosis may be present. The increased neural activity may also result in seizures, and abnormal EEG changes may be present. ECG changes and arrhythmias are frequently present. Prolongation of the Q-T interval is frequently seen. The ECG changes result from the fact that calcium is needed for proper electrical conduction in the myocardium. Nausea, vomiting, and abdominal pain may also be present, and this is thought to be caused by the effect of decreased calcium on the sympathetic ganglia in the gastrointestinal tract.

Even though the serum calcium is low, some persons will develop calcification in various organs. Neurologic defects as a result of calcification of various parts of the nervous system develop. Cataracts also occur. Calcification is most frequently seen in chronic hypocalcemic states, and persons with chronic hypoparathyroid function may demonstrate personality changes and lethargy secondary to neurologic calcification among their early symptoms.

The symptoms of hypoparathyroidism are more severe in persons with alkalosis because alkalosis causes more of the dissolved calcium to bind to serum albumin. The reader needs to remember that only the ionized calcium is metabolically active in maintaining normal neuromuscular and cardiovascular function.

Hyperphosphatemia may cause soft tissue calcification. The nurse must always be aware when assessing the laboratory results of serum calcium that the serum protein level must also be assessed. (See Chapter 18 for a discussion of effects of serum protein on serum calcium.)

Intervention

Care of the patient with tetany includes careful observation of beginning symptoms so that prompt treatment can be given and severe reactions such as convulsions can be prevented. Calcium gluconate, 10 to 30 ml of 10% solution in saline, is given intravenously for immediate replacement. Large daily doses (50,000 to 100,000 units) of vitamin D taken orally are also given. Calcium salts are started orally as soon as possible.

Maintenance doses of calcium salts and dihydrotachysterol (Hytakerol) or calciferol (vitamin D_2) will be prescribed. Vitamin D appears to be the principal regulator of the level of calcium ions in the body and therefore increases the absorption of calcium. A diet high in vitamin D will need to be followed. The amount of calcium and vitamin D is gradually adjusted until serum calcium level is normal. During reduction, recognition of early symptoms of hypoparathyroidism, such as numbness or tingling of fingers or toes, is important so that adjustment in dosage can be instituted. Hypercalcemia is a continuous hazard during therapy, and serum and urinary calcium levels are evaluated at regular intervals (every 6 to 12 months).

Outcome criteria for the person with hypoparathyroidism

The person or significant others can:

1. Explain the prescribed drug therapy.

a. State name, desired effect, dosage, frequency, and side effects of prescribed calcium salts and vitamin D.

b. State reasons for lifelong calcium and vitamin D therapy if total parathyroid function is lost.

2. Plan a diet high in vitamin D.

3. Describe measures to prevent complications (renal calculi, fractures).

4. Describe need for medical follow-up.

a. List symptoms of tetany or hypercalcemia that necessitate immediate attention.

b. State plans for ongoing follow-up care.

Adrenal problems

The *adrenal cortex* is essential to life. Without its hormones, cortisol and aldosterone, the body's metabolic processes respond inadequately to even minimal physical and emotional stressors, such as changes in temperature, exercise, or excitement. Severe stressors, such as those caused by serious infections or extreme anxiety, may result in shock and death.

The *adrenal medulla* is not essential to life because the sympathetic nervous system produces similar although slower responses. Dysfunction of the adrenal gland can be manifested as an increased or decreased function of the cortex or increased function of the medulla (Fig. 32-6).

Hyperfunction of the adrenal gland: cortisol excess

Etiology and pathophysiology

Cortisol excess was first described in 1932 by Harvey Cushing.[99] There are three causes of the increased secretion of cortisol: (1) adrenocortical hyperplasia resulting from excessive production of ACTH by pituitary microadenomas or from pituitary-hypothalamic dysfunction (also called Cushing's disease or pituitary Cushing's syndrome); (2) adrenocortical hyperplasia resulting from secretion of ACTH by a nonpituitary neoplasm, such as bronchial carcinoid or undifferentiated small cell carcinoma of the lung (also called ectopic Cushing's syndrome); or (3) primary adrenocortical hyperplasia resulting from adrenal adenomas or carcinomas or nodular hyperplasia (also called Cushing's syndrome). Manifestations of Cushing's syndrome are also seen in patients being treated with corticosteroids for their antiinflammatory effects (also called iatrogenic Cushing's syndrome).

The most common cause of increased cortisol is bilateral adrenal hyperplasia resulting from oversecretion of ACTH by the pituitary or by nonendocrine tumors. Approximately 25% of patients with Cushing's syndrome have excessive cortisol production secondary to adrenal neoplasms.

Clinical picture

Excessive cortisol, regardless of the cause, has widespread effects. Manifestations result from an increase in all the known actions of glucocorticoids (see Chapter 30). Because of increased protein catabolism, muscle wasting, weakness, fatigability, osteoporosis, and purple cutaneous striae occur. The muscle wasting is most obvious in the extremities, resulting in very thin arms and legs. The striae result from weakening of collagenous fibers so that subcutaneous tissues are exposed. Because of the lack of support, there is easy bruisability and ecchymosis formation at sites of trauma.

Increased cortisol results in alteration in adipose deposition. Characteristically, the adipose tissue is deposited in the face, resulting in "moon facies," in the interscapular area resulting in "buffalo hump," and in the abdomen resulting in "truncal obesity." The cause of this adipose distribution is unknown.[99]

Increased gluconeogenesis and decreased rate of glucose utilization result in impaired glucose tolerance. Some patients will have diabetes mellitus, with all the characteristic signs and symptoms.

Increased sodium and water retention results in hypertension and edema. The antiinflammatory action of

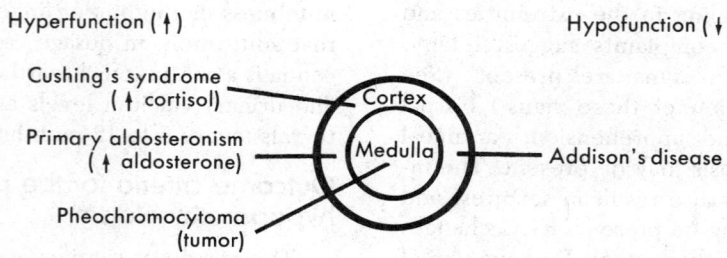

Fig. 32-6. Adrenal gland dysfunctions.

the cortisol results in decreased resistance to infections. Cortisol excess can also cause emotional changes. The patient may be irritable, demonstrate emotional lability, be depressed, or in some cases, develop frank psychosis. Emotional changes may also be the result of changes in appearance and the resulting change in self-concept.

Frequently, excessive adrenal androgen secretion occurs simultaneously with excessive cortisol. In females this results in changes in sexual characteristics. Acne, hirsutism, and oligomenorrhea or amenorrhea are frequently present. Excessive androgens in young males result in precocious sexual development. Characteristic laboratory changes are usually found. Increased plasma cortisol levels and increased urinary 17-hydroxycorticoid levels are present. Lymphopenia, increased eosinophils, and neutrophilic leukocytosis are present. With severe excess hypokalemia, hypochloremia and metabolic alkalosis occur. Serum sodium is usually normal because of isotonic sodium and water retention.

Intervention

Treatment of cortisol excess depends on the cause. Before definitive therapy for the underlying cause of excessive cortisol production can be instituted, the patient will undergo various blood and urinary studies to determine the cause of cortisol excess (see Chapter 30). Radiologic studies will be used to identify the presence of adrenal or pituitary tumors. Other tests necessary to identify ectopic ACTH secreting tumors will also be carried out. If a tumor of the adrenal cortex is found, the tumor may be surgically resected. When there is a tumor of one of the adrenal glands, the increase in corticosteroids produced by that gland will cause suppression of ACTH (by negative feedback) and subsequent atrophy of the unaffected gland. In this situation the treatment of choice is the removal of the affected gland with replacement therapy given until the atrophic gland resumes normal functioning. If there is hyperplasia of both glands, then a bilateral total adrenalectomy is usually done. In this case the patient must be on *lifetime replacement therapy*. In nonpituitary neoplasms (ectopic Cushing's syndrome), surgical removal of the neoplasm is the treatment of choice. However, it is often not possible to remove the tumor surgically.

When this happens, the patient may be treated with drugs that block cortisol synthesis. There are three drugs currently being used. These are mitotane (o-p'-DDD), aminoglutethimide, and metyrapone. Mitotane is capable of destroying the adrenal gland and can precipitate adrenal insufficiency. Aminoglutethimide blocks cortisol production by preventing the conversion of cholesterol to pregnenolone, and thus adrenocortical replacement therapy is necessary. Metyrapone only partially blocks steroid synthesis and thus can not be used alone. It is recommended that metyrapone be used in conjunction with aminoglutethimide so that the dose of both can be decreased and thus side effects can also be decreased. In some instances, when the site of ectopic ACTH secretion cannot be found, bilateral adrenalectomy may be performed.

In pituitary Cushing's syndrome the pituitary tumor may be ablated by irradiation. The results are not apparent for 1 to 4 months, and the patient may be treated with mitotane, aminoglutethimide, or metyrapone until irradiation is successful. The pituitary gland may be removed surgically by transsphenoidal microdissection, or radioactive gold or yttrium may be implanted. (See p. 618 for discussion of care of persons undergoing transsphenoidal surgery.)

The patient with excessive secretion of cortisol needs very skilled nursing care. The patient is usually very ill and the changes in metabolic homeostasis, the hypertension, the fluid and electrolyte imbalances, and the decreased resistance to infection all make the patient very prone to physiologic complications. The patient needs to be monitored on a continual basis. Intake and output calculated every 8 hours, daily weights, and observation of laboratory data are used to monitor fluid and electrolyte status. Vital signs are taken every 4 hours or more frequently to monitor the hypertension. Increases in blood pressure should be reported immediately. Serum glucose and urinary glucose or urinary ketones are checked at least four times per day to monitor the abnormal glucose state. Patients must not be exposed to infections, and they should be isolated from other patients with infections. Staff members who have *any* signs and symptoms of infections should not care for these patients. Nutritional support is a primary need. The patient may be on a low-sodium, low-calorie, and high-protein diet.

The patient needs considerable support to deal with the changes in body image and resulting changes in self-concept. Some of the body changes are reversible with successful treatment. Patients should be encouraged to accentuate positive physical attributes, and as they recover they should be helped to see their self-worth. Emotional lability and the inability to handle emotional stressors should be anticipated. Stressors should be decreased as much as possible. One way to do this is to include the patient and family in developing the plan of care, so that all needs can be met and the activities scheduled for the day are known to the patient. As much as possible a consistent routine is maintained.

Education of the patient and significant others is a major need. The patient needs to learn about the diagnostic tests, the treatment planned, and the potential complications of treatment (adrenocortical insufficiency).

Many nurses may never see a patient with excess cortisol secretion from one of the causes described above. However, most nurses come in contact with patients with iatrogenic Cushing's syndrome (*Cushing's syndrome medicamentous*). In this situation the patient is receiving large enough doses of the glucocorticosteroids to develop iatrogenic Cushing's syndrome. In these instances, it is necessary for the patient to remain on the steroids and the side effects will be treated. The patient may need to be on limited fluid intake and a salt-restricted diet. Occasionally, diuretics will be used to control sodium and water retention. The nurse must remember that most diuretics promote hypokalemia. The patient may need potassium supplements and should eat foods high in potassium. Hypertension will be treated with antihypertensive drugs. Diabetes mellitus, if it occurs, is treated as described in the section on diabetes mellitus. If weight gain is a problem, caloric restriction is necessary. These patients must learn how to protect themselves from infections and must understand the need to report any signs and symptoms of infection immediately. They also need to know that they must take their medications (steroids) daily and that sudden withdrawal can precipitate *adrenal insufficiency*.

Outcome criteria for the person with excessive cortisol secretion

The person or significant others can:
1. Explain the cause of the disease and how the signs and symptoms are related to the disease.
2. Describe the treatment and the expected effects.
3. Describe replacement therapy or other medication prescribed, if appropriate (drug, dosage, frequency, side effects, and expected effects).
4. Describe plans for follow-up care.
5. State need for Medic Alert bracelet or necklace or identification card if on replacement therapy.

For the person who has iatrogenic Cushing's syndrome, the person or significant others can:
1. Describe diet for restricted calories and sodium.
2. Describe fluids allowed and how the fluids will be distributed throughout the day.
3. Describe any therapeutic regimens prescribed for hypertension or diabetes mellitus, if appropriate.
4. Explain ways to avoid infections and describe what to do if infections occur.
5. Describe plans for follow-up care.
6. State need for Medic Alert bracelet or necklace or identification card stating name of drug, dosage, frequency, and physician's name and phone number.

Primary aldosteronism

Etiology

Primary aldosteronism is a rare disorder that is usually caused by an aldosterone-secreting adenoma (Conn's syndrome). It also can result from adrenal hyperplasia.

Females are reported to have the condition twice as often as males.

Pathophysiology and clinical picture

Hypersecretion of aldosterone increases the renal tubule exchange of sodium for potassium and hydrogen ions; hypernatremia, hypokalemia, and hypertension result. Metabolic alkalosis may be present. The hypertension is related to the increased sodium reabsorption, whereas severe muscle weakness and ECG abnormalities are the result of potassium depletion. Headache is a common complaint. The most definitive diagnostic tools are an abnormally high aldosterone secretion rate and abnormally low plasma renin activity.[9] Laboratory findings include hypokalemia and sometimes hypernatremia. The bicarbonate level may be elevated because of a loss of hydrogen ions.

Intervention

The desired treatment is *surgical excision* of tumors or resection of hyperplastic glands. Successful surgery reverses the hypertension in about two thirds of the patients. Early diagnosis and treatment are the goals, since patients who are untreated will in time develop the sequelae of hypertensive cardiovascular disease and renal insufficiency. In preparation for surgery, spironolactone, an aldosterone antagonist, is given daily in doses of 200 to 400 mg.

There is considerable controversy about the incidence of primary aldosteronism. Some experts believe that as many as 7% of the patients who appear to have essential hypertension may in fact have primary aldosteronism.[9] Persons who cannot be treated surgically are given spironolactone, 100 to 400 mg daily, for life.

Pheochromocytoma

Etiology

Pheochromocytoma is a catecholamine-producing tumor, usually benign, of the sympatheticoadrenal system, which causes hypertension. Although pheochromocytomas account for less than 1% of cases of hypertension, it is important that they be diagnosed, since they can be cured.

A single benign adrenal tumor is the most common pathologic finding. *Pheochromocytomas* are most frequently found between the fourth and fifth decades of life. The tumors are most frequently found in the abdomen around or in the adrenal medulla, but they can be found anywhere along the sympathetic nervous system trunk.

Clinical picture

The prominent sign is hypertension, which may be labile, depending on blood levels of the catecholamines, or may stay persistently elevated. Most persons have an elevated blood pressure reading at least 50% of the time.[9] Along with hypertension there is usually a history of headache, excessive sweating, and palpatations. The headache is abrupt, severe, throbbing, and generalized. It usually has a short duration. Sweating may be continuous or paroxysmal. Along with palpitations, tachycardia may be present. Other symptoms include nervousness, tremors, apprehension, and pallor followed by flushing and heat intolerance. The patient usually gives a history of weight loss and is thin. During paroxsymal attacks pupillary dilation will be present. If hypertension is long standing, the patient may have hypertensive retinopathy.

Frequently there is a history of paroxysmal attacks that are precipitated by multiple factors. Postural changes (especially flexion or bending of the body), sneezing, abdominal pressure, sexual activity, eating, urination, the Valsalva maneuver, exercise, pain, and changes in environmental or body temperature are some of the major precipitating factors.

The diagnosis is confirmed by assays of catecholamines and their metabolites in the urine. In pheochromocytoma the levels of these compounds are increased.

Intervention

Immediate treatment may be directed toward control of hypertensive crisis. This involves use of phentolamine or nitroprusside (Nipride). Propranolol (Inderal) will be used to control tachycardia. The patient should be in an intensive care unit during the hypertensive crisis phase. Cardiac monitoring and frequent monitoring of vital signs are necessary. During nitroprusside or phentolamine therapy, the blood pressure is taken every 15 minutes. These drugs are given by a controlled infusion pump at a rate that keeps the blood pressure at a prescribed level. When the blood pressure is at the desired level, the drugs will be gradually decreased. The blood pressure is closely monitored during this time.

Surgical excision of the pheochromocytoma is the usual treatment and is successful in 90% of the cases. Removal of the tumor results in complete remission of the symptoms unless there is metastasis to another site. During surgery there may be excessive production of catecholamines as the tumor is manipulated. This causes very high blood pressure levels and cardiac arrhythmias. Administration of the α-adrenergic blockers (trimethaphan camsylate and phentolamine) is common. Trimethaphan camsylate is given daily for 7 to 10 days prior to surgery and may be used to control preoperative hypertension and reduce these complications of surgery. Propranolol (Inderal), a β-sympathetic blocker, may be used when there are catecholamine-induced arrhythmias and tachycardia. It is given either by mouth or intravenously. The drug is used with caution, and

patients receiving it must be carefully monitored.

Hypotension occurs as soon as the tumor is removed. This is best treated with plasma or a plasma substitute, preferably 5% albumin in normal saline. Volume expanders administered appropriately usually control the hypotension, and vasopressors are not necessary.[9]

On the first postoperative day, hypertensive episodes are common and are caused by the response to pain and the hypervolemia resulting from the treatment of hypotension following surgery. At this time the most effective therapy is with a rapidly acting diuretic such as furosemide (Lasix) or ethacrynic acid (Edecrin).

Persons with pheochromocytoma who cannot be treated surgically or who are not cured by surgery are treated with adrenergic blocking agents or α-methyl p-tyrosine,[9] a research drug that reduces the production of norepinephrine by about 75%.

Outcome criteria for the person with pheochromocytoma

The person or significant others can:
1. Explain the relationship between the disease and the patient's signs and symptoms.
2. Explain the treatment and the expected results.
3. Explain signs and symptoms (recurrence of signs of pheochromocytoma or hypotension) that should be reported.
4. If appropriate, explain medication regimen ordered (drugs), dosage, frequency, expected effects, and side effects.
5. Explain plans for follow-up care.

Hypofunction of the adrenal gland: adrenocortical insufficiency

Etiology

Adrenocortical hypofunction results when there is a decrease in adrenocortical secretions. This decrease may be caused by (1) primary insufficiency of the adrenal cortex resulting from infection, hemorrhage, surgical removal, congenital hypoplasia, destruction by chemicals such as mitotane (o-p'-DDD), or idiopathic atrophy; or (2) secondary failure resulting from pituitary insufficiency or suppression of the hypothalamic-pituitary adrenal axis as a result of the use of exogenous steroids. Primary insufficiency is also called *Addison's disease*. The adrenocortical hormones are essential for life, and the person with insufficiency will die unless treated.

In primary adrenal insufficiency, as a result of the destruction of the adrenal cortex, there is a deficiency of glucocorticoids and mineralocorticoids. The deficiency in glucocorticoids leads to an impairment of metabolism, which in turn leads to an inability to maintain a normal glucose level. The loss of mineralocorticoids reduces the person's ability to retain sodium and water, and various fluid and electrolyte problems result. In secondary insufficiency, the level of mineralocorticoids is normal, and there will be less severe problems with fluid and electrolyte balance. (For further information see Chapter 30.)

Clinical picture

The symptoms of adrenocortical insufficiency have a gradual onset, and the person's initial complaints are often vague. The major early complaints are asthenia, anorexia, nausea and vomiting, abdominal pain, and diarrhea. There may be a history of frequent hypoglycemic reactions with nervousness, headache, trembling, and diaphoresis. Weight loss is common. *Asthenia* (weakness) is a cardinal complaint and usually is more severe at times of stress. It eventually may require the person to stay in bed. However, often the gastrointestinal complaints are the reason that the person initially seeks help.

Hyperpigmentation with *bronzelike coloration* of skin and mucous membranes is a common sign in primary adrenal insufficiency. This is caused by increased levels of melanocyte stimulating hormone (MSH). In normal persons, cortisol causes negative-feedback inhibition. The lack of cortisol in adrenal insufficiency allows the MSH level to increase. Persons with secondary insufficiency do not usually have hyperpigmentation because their levels of ACTH and MSH are low.

Hypotension, hyponatremia and *hyperkalemia* are characteristically seen in primary adrenocortical insufficiency because of a lack of mineralocorticoids. In secondary insufficiency mineralocorticoids are not deficient because they are under the control of the renin-angiotensin system (see Chapter 20). Therefore hypotension is usually not as severe. Hyponatremia and hyperkalemia do not usually occur.

Diagnosis is based on hormonal levels. Cortisol is low in all cases of adrenal cortex insufficiency. In primary adrenal insufficiency the mineralocorticoid level is also low and the level of ACTH is high.

Intervention

The treatment of adrenal insufficiency consists of administration of hormones. In primary insufficiency a *glucocorticoid*, usually cortisone or hydrocortisone, and a *mineralocorticoid*, usually 9-alpha-fluorohydrocortisone (fludrocortisone) are prescribed. The usual dosage of cortisone is 37.5 mg daily, with 25 mg given on awakening and 12.5 mg given before 4 PM. Since cortisone is ulcerogenic, it should always be given after meals or with milk. Antacids may also be prescribed. The dose of fludrocortisone is 0.1 to 0.2 mg daily. Other forms of these drugs may be prescribed. If a different adrenocortical derivative with glucocorticoid properties, such as prednisone, is prescribed, the dosage will be equivalent to the antiinflammatory potency of hydrocortisone. For example, the dosage of predisone will be approximately 10 mg/day. Table 32-3 compares the antiinflammatory potency of the adrenocortical steroids relative to the glucocorticoid potency of hydrocortisone and the mineralocorticoid potency of desoxycorticosterone acetate (Doca). In secondary insufficiency only glucocortical replacement is necessary.

Patients with adrenocortical insufficiency should understand the serious nature of the disease and the importance of taking prescribed replacement therapy (Fig. 32-7). They should also know that they should never omit a dose of the drug and if they are unable to take the drug or retain it for any reason, the physician should be notified at once. Since the prescribed replacement therapy is planned to meet normal requirements of daily living, patients will require additional glucocorticoids and mineralocorticoids if subjected to stressors such as infection, trauma, surgery, or emotional upset. For this reason, persons with adrenocortical insufficiency should wear an identification bracelet and carry an identification card at all times. It is recommended that the card

TABLE 32-3. Comparison of antiinflammatory and mineralocorticoid potency of derivatives of adrenocorticosteroids

Drug	Antiinflammatory potency *	Mineralocorticoid potency †
Hydrocortisone (cortisol)	Potency = 1	Potency 0.03 times that of Doca
Cortisone acetate	Potency 0.8 times that of hydrocortisone	Potency 0.03 times that of Doca
Prednisone	Potency 4 times that of hydrocortisone	Potency 0.04 times that of Doca
Methylprednisolone	Potency 6 times that of hydrocortisone	Potency 0.02 times that of Doca
Triamcinolone	Potency 5 times that of hydrocortisone	No mineralocorticoid activity
Dexamethasone	Potency 30 times that of hydrocortisone	Only mild natriuretic effect
Desoxycorticosterone (DOC)	Zero antiinflammatory effect	Potency = 1
Fludrocortisone	Potency 10 times that of hydrocortisone	Potency 4.2 times that of Doca

*Potency relative to hydrocortisone, whose potency = 1.
†Potency relative to Doca, whose potency = 1.

state which of the adrenocortical hormones is to be given in case of illness or injury and the name and phone number of the patient's physician. In addition, it is recommended that persons with little or no function of the adrenal glands carry an emergency supply of cortisone, hydrocortisone, or desoxycorticosterone at all times with directions as to when and how they should be administered. One expert recommends that persons with Addison's disease carry a kit containing 100 mg of hydrocortisone in a sterile syringe ready for injection with directions to inject it under the skin if the patient is injured, vomiting, or loses consciousness.[9]

The person with adrenocortical insufficiency who is on adequate replacement therapy can live a normal, productive life as long as undue stress is avoided.

Adrenal crisis (addisonian crisis)

Adrenal, or addisonian, crisis is a severe exacerbation of adrenal insufficiency. It is a very serious condition in which there is severe hypotension, shock, coma, and vasomotor collapse, and it quickly leads to death unless treated promptly. It may occur in any person with an insufficient amount of adrenocortical hormones, regardless of the cause, and may be precipitated by strenuous activity, by infection or other stressful situations, or by failure to take prescribed steroids. (The latter is one of the most frequent causes of adrenal crisis.) It often is a complication of surgery or other treatment of the pituitary or adrenal glands. The signs of impending crisis are those of the disease in exaggerated form.

When adrenal crisis occurs, a large dose of hydrocortisone phosphate is given immediately by the intravenous route. A continuous and rapid infusion of normal saline solution is started immediately. Cortisone may be given intramuscularly also. These patients must do *absolutely nothing* for themselves. If they are conscious, they are cautioned not to attempt to turn or otherwise help themselves.

The patient is *not moved* unless absolutely necessary and then only with physician consultation. It is essential that all forms of stimuli such as loud noises and bright lights be eliminated. Vital signs usually are taken every 15 minutes and temperature every hour. If hypotension is severe, a vasopressor drug may be given. Whole blood and concentrated serum albumin are given if hypotension persists, since the protein in these fluids tends to hold fluid in the vascular compartment. The patient often complains of severe headache; an ice bag may be used to relieve it. The patient has an extremely low resistance to infection, and reverse isolation (p. 374) usually is used to protect the patient from exposure to infection. The patient must be protected from anyone, including members of the family and hospital personnel, who has a cold or other infection. If the adrenal crisis was precipitated by an infection, appropriate antimicrobial therapy will be instituted.

Surgery of the adrenal glands

A bilateral adrenalectomy (surgical excision of the adrenal glands) is sometimes done for persons with cancer of the breast with metastasis, and occasionally for persons with cancer of the prostate gland with metastasis. Adrenalectomy is also performed for the treatment of hypersecretion of either the medullary or cortical portion of the adrenal gland.

Preoperative care

When any surgery on the adrenal glands is planned, hormonal blood levels should be normal. If antihypertensive drugs are being used, they are discontinued, since the surgery may cause a rather severe drop in blood pressure. Sedation may be given at this time.

Postoperative care

The immediate postoperative care for patients having any type of adrenocortical surgery is quite similar. Adrenocortical function is very labile when part of the

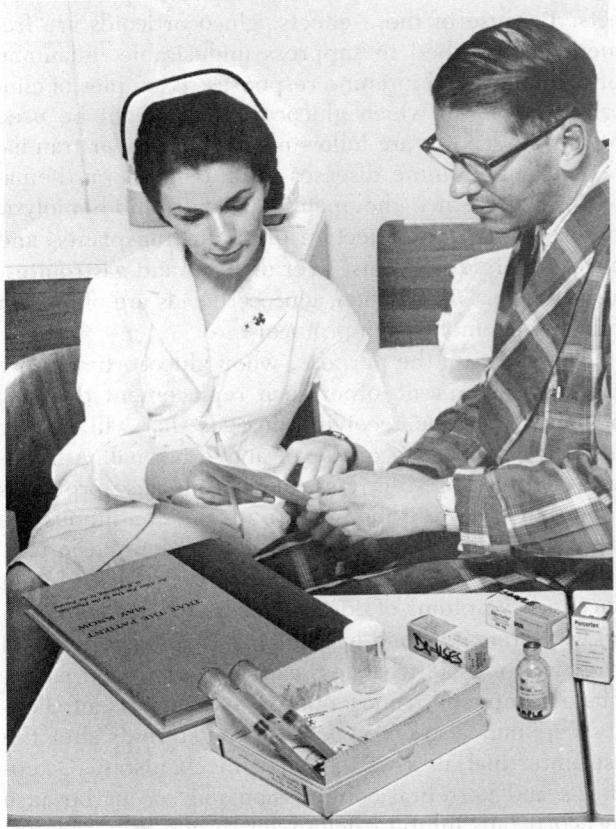

Fig. 32-7. Patients with adrenocortical insufficiency should be taught about the disease, about hormones they must take, and how they can live safely with the disease. (Reprinted with permission from Shea, K.M., et al.: Am. J. Nurs. **65:**80-85, 1965.)

adrenocortical tissue is removed, and, of course, it is labile when all the tissue is removed, since maintenance of the hormonal level then must be controlled completely by replacement therapy. The patient's special needs center around maintaining appropriate amounts of adrenocortical hormones in the blood.

Hormonal control and monitoring. Immediately after surgery, replacement of corticosteroids is started. Hydrocortisone is given continuously by intravenous drip, and dosage is adjusted at intervals according to the clinical findings. Since hormonal replacement is delicately regulated on the basis of continuous observations of electrolyte balance, blood sugar, and blood pressure determinations, the patient needs to be given constant nursing attention until hormonal stability is regained or a maintenance regimen established. Vasopressors may need to be given. Frequent blood pressure readings will be necessary to determine medication dosage needs.

The nurse should also observe the patient carefully for signs of *hypoglycemia*. This condition is most likely to occur if the patient had diabetes mellitus as a symptom, but it can occur in any patient who has adrenal gland surgery. Intravenous solutions containing glucose are usually ordered. If the patient is able to eat, the nurse should check to see that all food on the tray is eaten. Hypoglycemic reactions are most likely to occur in the early morning, and they may follow any unusual physical activity or any emotional upset. The nurse also should be alert for symptoms of *adrenal crisis* (p. 639), which requires immediate treatment. *Markedly increased* urinary output may indicate the need for vasopressin (Pitressin) to control excessive diuresis.

Hypotension. Because of the instability of the vascular system following adrenalectomy, patients must be monitored closely for signs of hypotension. Blood pressure is taken every 15 minutes when the patient is first ambulated. If the blood pressure drops, the patient is assisted back to bed and the physician is consulted before ambulation is attempted again. Elastic stockings applied prior to ambulation may help to prevent hypotension.

Replacement therapy. The treatment for persons who have a bilateral adrenalectomy is the same as for patients with adrenocortical insufficiency disease. They must be on replacement therapy for life and must understand the need to take their medication daily. They also need to know what to do when they are vomiting and cannot take the drug.

It is not unheard of for patients to be admitted in adrenal crisis because they did not understand the seriousness of not taking their medication as ordered.

Outcome criteria for the person with adrenocortical insufficiency

The person or significant others can:
1. State why medications must be taken daily as prescribed.

2. Describe the effect of stressors on the disease and measures to be taken to reduce them.
3. Explain the home medication program.
   a. State name, dosage, frequency, and side effects of prescribed medications.
   b. State need for continued treatment if replacement therapy is necessary.
   c. State situations that will require an increase in the dose of medication.
4. Describe medical follow-up program.
   a. State symptoms indicating adrenal crisis and need for immediate medical attention.
   b. State need for continued medical follow-up.
   c. Show the card that the patient will carry at all times. The card will give the patient's name, address, and phone number; the name of the drug and its dose; and the physician's name and phone number.

Care of persons on glucocorticoids for their antiinflammatory effects

As described in Chapter 30, the glucocorticoids have profound antiinflammatory and immunosuppresive effects. Because of these effects, glucocorticoids are frequently prescribed to suppress undesirable inflammatory reactions and immune responses. Examples of clinical situations in which glucocorticoids might be used for these purposes are following eye surgery or trauma; to treat autoimmune diseases such as lupus erythematosus, scleroderma, rheumatoid arthritis, and hemolytic anemia; to prevent rejection of organ transplants, and to treat allergic reactions, liver disease, and gastrointestinal problems. In addition, glucocorticoids are often part of cancer chemotherapy protocols.

Regardless of the purpose, when glucocorticoids are given for any reason other than replacement therapy, the person will be receiving dosages that will elevate the serum glucocorticoid level above normal. Adrenocorticosteroids used in this manner can cause problems when they are prescribed for long-term, continuous use and when they are withdrawn following long-term use.

Prolonged use (longer than 2 weeks) will result in signs and symptoms of cortisol excess (p. 634). Sodium and water retention and hypokalemia, hyperglycemia and glycosuria, muscle weakness and wasting, moon facies, buffalo hump, and truncal obesity may be present. Peptic ulcers may also occur because the steroids alter the gastrointestinal mucosal defense mechanisms. Osteoporosis and vertebral compression may occur because glucocorticoids inhibit calcium absorption from the gastrointestinal tract and osteoblast activity, which are necessary for bone formation. Persons receiving glucocorticoids are very susceptible to cataract formation. Behavorial disturbances are also frequently seen and may take various forms such as manic behavior, depression, or insomnia. Therapy in children results in stunted growth. Because steroids are prescribed for their antiinflammatory effects, resistance to all types of antigens is suppressed, and there is increased susceptibility to infection by all types of organisms (bacterial, viral, and fungus).

When steroids are given for a prolonged period, they must be withdrawn slowly. The reason for this is that the high blood levels of exogenous glucocorticoids cause negative feedback to the hypothalamus and anterior pituitary gland, and the production of corticotropin releasing factor (CRF) and ACTH is suppressed. The lack of ACTH results in adrenal atrophy. Thus, if glucocorticoids are stopped suddenly, the person develops signs and symptoms of adrenal insufficiency (p. 637) because of an inability to produce the steroids internally. It has been found that it may take as long as 9 months for return of normal hypothalamic-pituitary-adrenal function.[75] In some instances, the person may be able to produce enough steroids to meet body needs in nonstressful times but may need additional steroids during times of increased stress.

Intervention

The side effects discussed cannot be completely avoided, but they can in some instances be minimized. To prevent fluid retention, the patient will often be placed on a sodium-restricted diet. The person should be weighed frequently and the extremities should be observed for signs of edema, and changes should be reported as soon as possible, since diuretic therapy may be necessary. To prevent hypokalemia the person should be on a diet high in potassium, and a potassium replacement may be prescribed unless there is some underlying condition that results in potassium retention.

Urinary glucose and acetone should be monitored as described on p. 599. If the person is a diabetic, the diabetic regimen may need to be adjusted. Some patients may develop type IV diabetes (p. 643). Most persons receiving steroids experience an increase in appetite. If weight gain is a problem, a calorie-restricted diet may be necessary.

The changes in body structure (moon facies, buffalo hump, and truncal obesity) may not be avoidable. Patients should be aware of these side effects and be supported as they deal with a change in their self-concept. To prevent the gastrointestinal problems, steroids should always be taken with food. Antacids may also be ordered. Stool guaiac should be checked regularly to monitor for early signs of ulcerations and gastrointestinal bleeding secondary to ulceration of the gastrointestinal tract. The person and significant others must be aware of the potential changes in behavior that may occur. Usually the person will adjust to the therapy, but at times the psychiatric disturbance may lead to suicidal tendencies.[75]

The person on prolonged steroid therapy must avoid anyone with an infection. Since young children frequently have upper respiratory infections, close contact with them may have to be limited. Crowded, poorly ventilated environments should also be avoided. The patient should be monitored constantly for signs of infection, and the patient's primary health care provider should be notified immediately if any signs of infection occur. All persons placed on prolonged steroid therapy should have a tuberculin skin test, unless they have a history of a positive test. Persons who have a positive test should have isoniazid (INH) therapy (p. 1302) for the duration of their steroid therapy. A positive tuberculin test implies that the person has been exposed to tuberculosis and has tubercle bacilli in the body. The organisms are kept under control in the body by being encapsulated in fibrous tissue. The steroids, however, can cause fibrous tissue to be broken down, liberating live tubercle bacilli, and an active tuberculosis can occur.

To prevent adrenal insufficiency secondary to sudden withdrawal, persons on steroids for a prolonged time must have the steroids withdrawn gradually to allow the hypothalamic-pituitary-adrenal axis to recover. During the time the drug is being withdrawn, these persons should be monitored for signs and symptoms of adrenal insufficiency. If symptoms occur, withdrawal is slowed. To prevent sudden withdrawal in emergency situations, the person should wear an identification bracelet or carry an identification card that states the name and dosage of the prescribed steroid. If the person is ill or injured and requires emergency care, those treating the patient will be able to determine if more steroids will be needed because of the increase in stressors; additional steroids can be given intravenously if they cannot be tolerated by mouth.

To prevent depression of the hypothalamic-pituitary-adrenal axis, some physicians prescribe every-other-day steroid therapy. In these instances *double the patient's daily dose is given at 8 AM every other day*. The benefit of this schedule is that it allows the serum glucocorticoid level to drop low enough every other day to prevent the negative inhibition of the hypothalamus and the pituitary gland. Thus every other day the person will have a normal secretion of endogenous CRF and ACTH and normal stimulation of the adrenal cortex. Thus atrophy of the adrenal gland does not occur. Even though the glucocorticoid level drops low enough to prevent negative feedback, the antiinflammatory effect is not reduced. Even though every-other-day therapy should prevent hypothalamic-pituitary-adrenal axis depression, the dose of glucocorticoids is still tapered off when they are withdrawn.

Persons on prolonged steroid therapy need considerable teaching to be able to monitor themselves for side effects of the steroids. They must understand all the potential side effects discussed above and must be able to manage any additional therapy that is prescribed for treatment of side effects. Because it may take 1 to 2 years for the adrenal cortex to recover sufficiently to be able to respond to stressors, nurses caring for persons who have a disease that may have been treated with steroids should ask, as a part of the initial interview and assessment, if the person has ever received steroid therapy. If the patient has a history of steroid therapy, he or she should be monitored for early signs of insufficiency.

Although most of the emphasis in this section has been on the care of persons on oral therapy, the information applies equally to persons receiving steroids intravenously. In addition, the nurse should be aware that steroids are commonly found in ointments prescribed for the treatment of dermatologic conditions. Steroids applied topically are absorbed through the skin and can have systemic effects. The systemic effects that occur depend on the frequency of the topical application and the amount of body surface covered with the ointment. Therefore persons treated with topical steroids may develop the same complications and need the same care as described above for others receiving steroid therapy.

Pancreatic endocrine problems

Diabetes mellitus

Diabetes mellitus is a complex, chronic metabolic disease involving disorders in carbohydrate, protein, and fat metabolism and the development of microvascular and macrovascular complications and neuropathies. Disturbances in the production or utilization of insulin, a hormone secreted by the islets of Langerhans in the pancreas, is one hormonal abnormality involved in the disease.

Epidemiology

Diabetes mellitus is one of the most common diseases affecting humans. According to the National Diabetes Commission, there are 6 million known diabetics in the United States and an additional 4 million with undiagnosed diabetes. Diabetes mellitus is found most frequently in persons over the age of 40, although it does occur in children and young adults. The incidence increases steadily until the seventh decade of life. It is more common in females. The increased incidence of diabetes can be attributed to a longer life span, better detection, and the decreased mortality in younger people.

Etiology

The etiology of diabetes mellitus is unknown. Diabetes mellitus is probably not a single entity but a heterogeneous group of diseases with diverse etiologies.[66] Various factors have been implicated in the develop-

ment of diabetes. Each of these factors will be discussed briefly.

Genetic factors have long been thought to be a causative factor, but the results of studies of monozygotic twins, offsprings of conjugal diabetics, and siblings and parents of diabetics show no proven mode of inheritance. Genetic factors are most frequently implicated in the etiology of non-insulin-dependent diabetes (type II).

The relationship between *histocompatibility antigens* (HLA antigens) and diabetes mellitus has been explored as more information has been gained about these antigens and the role they play in resistance or susceptibility to infection. Research studies designed to discover the association between the major histocompatibility complex (MHC) antigens and specific diseases have been done. These studies show that persons with HLA-B8, HLA-Bw15, HLA-Dw3, and HLA-Dw4 are at increased risk of developing insulin-dependent diabetes (type I).[148,211] No specific HLA complexes have been associated with non-insulin-dependent diabetes (type II).[65]

Certain viruses, particularly those of mumps, rubella, and Coxsackie virus B have been associated with the development of severe insulin-dependent diabetes (type I). It has been hypothesized that HLA antigens may be involved in an interaction between these viral agents and the beta cells (β-cells) of the pancreas to produce diabetes mellitus.[66]

The endocrine glands have long been known to be affected by autoimmune disease. Diabetes mellitus is often found in persons with other clinically diagnosed autoimmune diseases, and autoimmunity may be a factor in the development of diabetes mellitus.

Ethnic and socioeconomic factors also seem to be causative factors. The prevalence of diabetes mellitus increases from country to country as affluence, improved nutritional factors, and urbanization occur.[66] It has been noted that as the weight of the population of a country increases, the prevalence of diabetes also increases.[21] But the role of obesity in causation is unknown. Not all obese persons develop diabetes although obesity is frequently seen in diabetics between the ages of 30 and 69.

None of the above factors alone can account for all cases of diabetes mellitus or account for diabetes mellitus in any one person. Diabetes mellitus may indeed result from the interaction of environmental, viral, and socioeconomic factors with pancreatic endocrine cells that are less stable because of genetic factors or HLA type.[14]

Classification

Diabetes mellitus has long been classified according to the age of onset as *juvenile-onset diabetes* and *maturity-onset diabetes*, but a type of maturity-onset diabetes does occur in the young. Given this fact and the

TABLE 32-4. Classification of diabetes mellitus and descriptive characteristics for each type

Class	Clinical and associated factors and former terminology
Type I: insulin-dependent diabetes mellitus (IDDM)	Persons dependent on insulin to prevent ketosis; onset usually in youth but may occur in adults; associated with certain HLA types, islet cell antibodies are frequently present; formerly called juvenile-onset diabetes, ketosis-prone diabetes, brittle diabetes
Type II: non-insulin-dependent diabetes mellitus (NIDDM)	Persons not dependent on insulin to preserve life, although they may be treated with insulin (even if treated with insulin, they are still classified as NIDDM); ketosis resistant except in very special circumstances such as presence of infection; not HLA related; onset usually after age 40 but may occur in youth; serum insulin levels may be depressed, normal, or elevated; 60% to 90% of diabetics in this class are obese; formerly called maturity-onset diabetes, adult-onset diabetes, ketosis-resistant diabetes, and stable diabetes; class may be subdivided into two classes: (1) obese type II, and (2) nonobese type II
Type III: gestational diabetes mellitus (GDM)	Glucose intolerance occurs during pregnancy; group does not include known diabetics who become pregnant; after delivery, glucose intolerance may remain but not be serious enough to be treated or the person may have characteristics of type I or type II diabetes, or glucose intolerance may disappear; patient is reclassified after delivery; formerly called gestational diabetes
Type IV: other types, includes diabetes mellitus associated with pancreatic disease, other hormonal abnormalities, drugs, etc.	Persons in this class must have diabetes mellitus and one of the other diseases, syndromes, or causal factors; formerly called secondary diabetes

results of studies on etiologic factors, a new classification system that divides persons with overt diabetes into four types has been proposed by an international work group sponsored by the National Diabetes Data Group of the National Institute of Health.[147] *This new classification system is based on etiologic factors, insulin dependency,* and *other chemical findings.* There are probably subcategories within each of the first two types, but further research is necessary before these subcategories can be identified. See Table 32-4 for the classifications of diabetes mellitus and for descriptive characteristics of each class.

In the past, terms like prediabetes, subclinical diabetes, chemical diabetes, and latent diabetes were used to describe certain groups of persons. These terms are no longer helpful, and the National Diabetes Data Group recommends that they not be used. Instead, they recommend the following classification: (1) persons who were classified as *prediabetics* because they had a potentially higher risk of developing diabetes should be termed as having a *potential abnormality* of *glucose tolerance;* (2) persons who were classified by terms such as latent diabetics because they had transient glycosuria or hyperglycemia but who now have no abnormalities should be termed as having a *previous abnormality* of *glucose tolerance;* (3) persons who have glucose levels intermediate between normal and those considered to be diabetic and who were previously classified using terms such as chemical, latent, borderline, or subclinical diabetics be termed as having *impaired glucose tolerance.*

Use of a consistent pattern of classification for diabetes mellitus and for states of impaired glucose tolerance will allow for better comparison of research studies and case studies reported in the literature. In this chapter, when the information applies to all classes of diabetics, the term diabetes mellitus without a designation of type will be used. If the information is specific for one particular class, that class will be identified. It is important that the reader be familiar with the old terminology such as juvenile-onset diabetics, maturity-onset diabetics, latent, subclinical, and chemical diabetes, and secondary diabetes since these terms are still used clinically and by some authors writing for current literature.

Pathophysiology

To understand the pathophysiology of diabetes, the normal functions of insulin and other selected hormones must be understood. These functions will be reviewed briefly before pathophysiologic changes are discussed.

Normally, insulin, acting by a fixed receptor model, has a major role in controlling the metabolism of carbohydrates, fats, and proteins. Although insulin acts by activating a "second messenger" (see Chapter 30) in the affected cells, as many peptide hormones do, the second messenger is not cyclic AMP. Insulin suppresses cyclic AMP production. The second messenger is probably cyclic guanosine 3,5-monophosphate (CGMP).[22] The primary target tissues for insulin are muscle, fat, and liver cells. Insulin also exerts effects on the heart and some smooth muscles, but it has no effect on intestinal mucosa, renal tubule cells, nervous tissue, erythrocytes, or leukocytes.

Insulin is secreted in response to various factors. Although glucose is probably the major stimulus for insulin secretion in humans, amino acids, fatty acids, and ketones also stimulate insulin secretion. Glucose is a more potent stimulator when given orally than when given intravenously. This suggests the presence of an anticipatory signal from the gastrointestinal tract to the pancreas that may be important for the effective utilization of all foods. It is know that the gastrointestinal hormones (gastrin, secretin, pancreozymin-cholecystokinin, gut glucagon, and a glucagon-like polypeptide termed *gastric inhibitory polypeptide*)[24,165] all stimulate insulin secretion. Glucose stimulates insulin release from the pancreas by reacting with glucose receptors on the surface of the beta cells or through the intracellular metabolism of glucose. There are two phases of insulin secretion in response to glucose stimulation. There is an initial rapid secretory burst beginning within 1 minute of glycemic stimulation. This burst reaches a peak within 2 minutes and then declines over the next 5 minutes. A second phase, characterized by a more gradual increase in insulin, commences in approximately 10 minutes and continues over an hour.

Insulin secretion can be directly or indirectly affected by other hormones and neurotransmitters. ACTH, thyrotropin, and glucagon directly stimulate insulin secretion. Growth hormone and glucocorticoids cause increased insulin secretion by increasing glucose production. β-Adrenergic stimulation increases insulin secretion, whereas α-adrenergic stimulation suppresses insulin secretion. Somatostatin suppresses insulin secretion.

Insulin's effects are anticatabolic and anabolic in nature. In Chapter 30 the overall effects are described, but the specific effects on muscle, liver, and fat cells will be briefly reviewed here.

Liver cells. Glucose enters liver cells freely, but insulin is needed to activate the hormone glucokinase. This enzyme is needed to promote phosphorylation of glucose. Phosphorylation of glucose is the first step in the metabolism of glucose by the anaerobic glycolytic pathway or in the synthesis of glycogen. Insulin is also necessary to activate the hormone glycogen synthetase, which is necessary for glycogen formation. It inhibits glycogenolysis by inactivating the enzyme phosphorylase. Gluconeogenesis is inhibited because insulin inhibits enzymes necessary for this activity. Also lipogenesis and protein synthesis are stimulated, and lipolysis and protein catabolism are depressed by insulin.

Muscle cells. In the *resting* muscle insulin is needed for the transport of glucose across the cell membrane. Glucose can enter *active* muscle cells without insulin. In active muscles glucose is oxidized to carbon dioxide and water for energy production. In resting muscles insulin increases glycogen synthesis by activating the enzyme glycogen synthetase and inactivating the enzyme phosphorylase. Amino acid uptake, protein synthesis, and prevention of protein catabolism all are facilitated by insulin.

Adipose tissue. Insulin is necessary for transport of glucose across the cell membrane. It promotes glucose metabolism and the production of α-glycerolphosphate (a product from the anaerobic metabolism of glucose). Insulin promotes fatty acid synthesis and if adequate α-glycerolphosphate is available, it will combine with the fatty acids produced in the liver and in fat cells to form triglycerides. Insulin decreases lipolysis. Table 32-5 summarizes these metabolic effects.

In diabetes mellitus there is an absolute or relative lack of insulin or ineffective utilization of insulin. In *insulin-dependent diabetes* there is usually an absolute deficiency of insulin. In *non-insulin-dependent diabetes* there is often a normal or near normal serum insulin level and in some instances an above normal level. In non-insulin-dependent diabetes with normal or above normal insulin levels, it is felt that ineffective utilization of insulin is caused by a decreased number of insulin receptors on body cells, impaired binding of insulin to body cells because of a receptor defect, or the presence

TABLE 32-5. Metabolic effects of insulin on liver, muscle, and fat cells

| Cell type | Substrate metabolism | | |
	Carbohydrate	Protein	Fat
Liver cell	↑ Phosphorylation of glucose ↑ Glycogen formation ↓ Gluconeogenesis ↓ Glycogenolysis	↑ Protein synthesis ↓ Protein catabolism	↑ Lipogenesis ↓ Lipolysis ↓ β-Oxidation
Muscle cell	↑ Transport of glucose ↑ Glucose oxidation (active muscle) ↑ Glycogenesis (resting muscle) ↓ Glycogenolysis	↑ AA uptake ↑ Protein synthesis ↓ Protein catabolism	
Fat cell	↑ Transport of glucose ↑ Formation of α-glycerolphosphate		↑ FFA synthesis ↑ Triglyceride formation ↓ Lipolysis

of circulating antibodies against insulin or insulin receptors that inhibit binding.[5] It has been shown that obese non-insulin-dependent diabetics often have decreased insulin receptors.[5]

The physiologic alterations in metabolism seen with a lack, deficiency, or underutilization of insulin are (1) hyperglycemia from overproduction of glucose because of increased gluconeogenesis and glycogenolysis and from decreased peripheral utilization of glucose; (2) protein catabolism and loss of amino acids from muscles; and (3) impaired triglyceride synthesis, increased release of free fatty acids from adipose tissue, and increased beta oxidation of fats. The hyperglycemia causes the serum glucose level to exceed the renal threshold and glycosuria results. The β-oxidation of fats can proceed faster than their utilization resulting in increased serum ketone levels and *ketonuria*. The protein loss can be so severe that it results in muscle wasting and stunted growth.

The serum glucose level is influenced by four other hormones besides insulin: *epinephrine, growth hormone, glucocorticoids*, and *glucagon*. Because hyperglycemia is the primary symptom in diabetes mellitus, the role of these hormones in the pathophysiology of diabetes mellitus is important.

Epinephrine opposes the action of insulin and is released in response to physical and emotional stressors, exercise, and pain. It may play a role in enhancing the severity of diabetes mellitus but does not seem to be a causative factor. *Growth hormone* has both insulin-mimicking and anti-insulin effects. Persons with increased levels of growth hormone often have diabetes mellitus, and it may be an etiologic factor in some cases of type IV diabetes (see Table 32-4). *Glucocorticoids* increase blood glucose levels by preventing the uptake of glucose by tissues, by facilitating protein breakdown, and by promoting gluconeogenesis. Some persons on long-term glucocorticoid therapy may develop type IV diabetes mellitus.

Glucagon has been studied intensively in relation to its role in the pathophysiology of diabetes mellitus.[216] Studies suggest that diabetes mellitus may not simply be the result of a deficiency, lack, or underutilization of insulin, but may also involve a disturbance in the level of glucagon. In normal persons glucagon prevents hypoglycemia. It has many metabolic effects, most of which are opposite to those of insulin. Glucagon activation of phosphorylase promotes glycogenolysis and glucose production in the liver. After the liver glycogen is depleted, it stimulates gluconeogenesis by increasing the transportation of amino acids to the liver, increasing proteolysis in muscle tissue, thereby increasing amino acids levels, and increasing lipolysis in adipose tissue, thereby providing α-glycerolphosphate for gluconeogenesis and free fatty acids for energy production. Glucagon stimulates β-oxidation of fats by the liver. It also stimulates the release of epinephrine and norepinephrine, which then cause glycogenolysis of muscle glycogen to lactate and pyruvate, providing more substrates for gluconeogenesis in the liver. Epinephrine and norepinephrine also assist in the mobilization of fat from adipose tissue.

Recent research suggests that glucagon contributes to the pathophysiology of diabetes mellitus only when there is a deficiency, lack, or underutilization of insulin.[186] Glucagon may indeed be responsible for the severity of hyperglycemia and hyperketonemia in diabetes mellitus, but it can cause these problems only if there is a deficiency, lack, or underutilization of insulin. Normally glucagon and insulin are kept in a fine ratio. Research to explore whether a change in the ratio of glucagon to insulin may be a causative factor in the altered physiology seen in diabetes mellitus is ongoing. Table 32-6 summarizes the metabolic alterations seen in diabetes mellitus.

Preventive health care and health education

Preventive health care and health education about diabetes focuses on two levels: (1) measures directed towards the prevention of the primary disease and (2) measures directed towards the prevention of complications of the disease. Because the etiology of diabetes mellitus is unknown, primary preventive measures are limited. A major focus in primary prevention is the prevention or correction of obesity, since obesity is related to the occur-

TABLE 32-6. Metabolic alterations seen in diabetes mellitus

| Cell type | Substrate metabolism | | |
	Carbohydrate	Protein	Fat
Liver cell	↑ Glycogenolysis ↑ Gluconeogenesis	↑ Protein breakdown	↑ β-Oxidation of fats
Muscle cell	↑ Glycogenolysis liberating lactate and pyruvate ↓ Glucose uptake	↑ Protein catabolism ↑ Liberation of amino acids ↓ Amino acid uptake	
Fat cell	↓ Glucose uptake		↑ Lipolysis ↓ Lipogenesis

rence of non-insulin-dependent diabetes mellitus. Nurses in all settings who are aware of the dangers of obesity can support appropriate health practices.

Secondary prevention is focused on (1) detection of diabetes, follow-up of suspected cases to confirm diagnosis, and the institution of effective treatment and (2) keeping persons with diabetes mellitus under appropriate health supervision and their diabetes under control. It is estimated that there are 4 million persons with undiagnosed diabetes mellitus in the United States. If these persons are to be identified, education programs designed to promote an understanding of diabetes mellitus and programs to screen persons for diabetes mellitus must be carried out. Currently, some form of education and mass screening is being carried out in many states. These programs vary in scope, methods, and goals. Educational and case-finding programs can be carried out in health departments, neighborhood clinics, hospital outpatient clinics, physicians' offices, industry, or in the community at health fairs or by mobile health units offering screening programs for diabetes and other health problems. Follow-up of all positive findings is essential for a screening program to be successful.

Community health nurses can help by making home visits if diabetes is definitely established, if retesting needs to be done, if individuals have indicated that they have no physician or are under no medical supervision, or if persons being tested request home visits by a nurse at the time of the first testing. Through the nurse's visits, misunderstandings about retesting can be clarified. Family reactions to the possibility of diabetes can be determined, and appropriate education and promotion of self-care in the treatment of diabetes mellitus can be instituted for those persons with confirmed diagnoses.

To improve the efficiency of educational and screening programs, efforts of such projects should be concentrated on high-risk groups. These groups include obese persons, persons with a family history of diabetes mellitus, and the elderly. Another high-risk group includes women who have given birth to large babies. Statistics show that diabetes mellitus develops later in life in 17% of mothers whose babies weighed over 9 lb and in 80% to 90% of those whose babies weighed over 13 lb. A summary of persons at risk for diabetes mellitus appears in the box below.

PERSONS AT RISK FOR DEVELOPING DIABETES MELLITUS

1. Obese persons
2. Persons with a family history of diabetes
3. The elderly
4. Women who give birth to babies weighing more than 9 lb

Another area of emphasis for preventive health care is working with pregnant women who are known diabetics. Studies of women with diabetes have shown that there is a high fetal and neonatal death rate, a high proportion of large babies with a high mortality rate, and a great tendency toward other abnormalities in pregnancy. Thus there is now greater emphasis on preventive intensive prenatal care. With improved monitoring devices available to determine placental function and fetal maturity, the pregnant women with diabetes may be subjected to less risk to herself and the fetus.

In some sections of the country there are high-risk perinatal networks set up to provide specialized care to pregnant women with conditions such as diabetes, which put them and their fetus at risk. It has also been discovered that women who have repeated spontaneous abortions, although showing no signs of carbohydrate intolerance by a regular glucose tolerance test, often show evidence of a decreased insulin reserve when cortisone is given prior to the glucose tolerance test. A significantly large number of relatives of persons with diabetes also respond in this manner. Therefore it is suspected that these people may need close medical supervision during stress situations such as pregnancy, extensive surgery, or serious illness to determine a need for insulin or oral hypoglycemic agents. The nurse should look at the medical history of patients and watch those with family histories of diabetes mellitus closely for symptoms of the disease.

Increased awareness of diabetes mellitus as a major health problem, promotion of research and professional and lay education, and promotion of detection efforts have been facilitated by national legislation and organizations. The passing of the National Diabetes Mellitus Research and Education Act in 1974 provided recognition of diabetes as a major health problem. In addition, the National Diabetes Advisory Board was created in 1976 to facilitate coordination of funds to provide several new diabetes research and training centers throughout the country.

The American Diabetes Association, Inc., furthers patient education, professional education, diabetes detection, public education, and research. It publishes both a professional journal, *Diabetes*,* that helps to keep health professionals informed and a bimonthly magazine, *Forecast** for persons with diabetes. Each year a National Diabetes Week is sponsored by the Association to stimulate early case finding in persons who do not know that they have diabetes and to educate the public about the disease. The Association has 50 local groups that work in their own areas. They sponsor camps for diabetic children and cooperate on nationwide projects.

The Juvenile Diabetes Foundation has also gained

*American Diabetes Association, Inc., 18 East 48 St., New York, NY 10017.

national prominence. This relatively new organization raises funds for research but also provides public education and counseling for Type I diabetics and their families.

Clinical picture

The clinical picture will vary depending on the type of diabetes mellitus. Insulin-dependent diabetes mellitus is characterized by a sudden onset with symptoms such as increased appetite *(polyphagia)*, increased thirst *(polydipsia)*, increased urine volume *(polyuria)*, and loss of weight and strength. These signs and symptoms are directly related to the altered metabolism of carbohydrates, proteins, and fats resulting from a deficiency or underutilization of insulin and possibly other hormonal changes.

The inability to metabolize carbohydrates properly causes *hyperglycemia* and *glycosuria*. The glycosuria promotes polyuria because glucose acts as an osmotic diuretic. This eventually leads to dehydration and stimulates thirst, causing polydipsia. Although the blood glucose level is high, most cells in the body are subjected to starvation conditions. The appetite is increased, so the person eats constantly. The cellular starvation, insulin changes, and other hormonal changes lead to mobilization of fats and proteins with resultant loss of body weight and strength.

If fat mobilization increases greatly, the metabolic intermediaries of fatty acid metabolism *(ketone bodies)* may increase in the blood and be excreted in the urine *(ketonuria)*. Urinary excretion of ketones causes loss of sodium, water, and other electrolytes. This can intensify the dehydration and electrolyte imbalance caused by hyperglycemia. The loss of sodium and the increase in ketones can disturb the acid-base balance, and metabolic acidosis can result. The diabetic with ketosis and acidosis commonly complains of nausea, vomiting, and abdominal pain. The person with undiagnosed diabetes may seek medical help because of symptoms suggestive of acute appendicitis. If metabolic acidosis is severe, the person may show typical signs and symptoms of *diabetic ketoacidosis*, although this is a rare initial complaint. In many instances the initial symptoms of the person with *insulin-dependent diabetes mellitus* are the metabolic abnormalities described above, which have been precipitated by an infection or other stressor. Occasionally, persons with insulin-dependent diabetes present a clinical picture more insidious in nature. Their major complaints are weakness, lethargy, and weight loss. Vaginitis in females may also be an early complaint.

The patient with *non-insulin-dependent diabetes* may shown initially the classic signs and symptoms of metabolic imbalance: *polyuria, polydipsia,* and *polyphagia*. Weight gain rather than weight loss is usually present. Patients with non-insulin-dependent diabetes mellitus are ketosis-resistant, but can have diabetic coma not as-sociated with ketoacidosis. This type of coma is called *hyperglycemic, hyperosmolar, nonketotic coma (HHNC)* (see p. 665). In the instances where HHNC is the initial problem, the usual precipitating factor is an infection or another stressor. Frequently, persons with non-insulin dependent diabetes mellitus are not diagnosed until they seek medical help for signs and symptoms secondary to the complications of diabetes. These complications include *macrovascular disease* affecting *cerebral, coronary,* or *peripheral vessels, microangiopathy* affecting *vision* or *renal* function, or *peripheral neuropathy*. The initial complaint may also be a history of recurrent infections such as infections of the feet, candidal infections and vulvovaginitis, or pyogenic dermatitis. Thus it can be seen that the clinical picture may vary greatly, and thus diabetes mellitus should be suspected in persons with a wide variety of complaints.

A fasting blood sugar (FBS) test for glucose level is used to diagnose diabetes. Because fasting blood sugar test results may be misleading, a 2-hour postprandial test is used in diagnosis of some cases of diabetes. These tests and the other blood tests useful in the diagnosis of diabetes mellitus are described in Table 30-5.

There has been some controversy over what fasting blood glucose level is diagnostic for diabetes mellitus. The following criteria are recommended by the National Diabetes Data Group.[147] For nonpregnant adults the diagnosis of diabetes mellitus is made in those persons with (1) classic symptoms of diabetes and unequivocal hyperglycemia, (2) a fasting venous plasma glucose concentration greater than 140 mg/100 ml, or (3) a venous plasma glucose concentration during an oral glucose tolerance test greater than or equal to 200 mg/100 ml at 2 hours and also at some other time between 0 and 2 hours. For children the diagnosis is made in those persons with (1) classic symptoms of diabetes and a random plasma glucose greater than 200 mg/100 ml or (2) fasting plasma glucose concentration greater than 140 mg/100 ml and a 2-hour plasma glucose concentration during an oral glucose tolerance test greater than or equal to 200 mg/100 ml and at another time between 0 and 2 hours.

For pregnant women the diagnosis of diabetes requires a 3-hour glucose test.[173] *Normal results* are (1) fasting venous plasma glucose less than 105 mg/100 ml, (2) 1-hour results less than 190 mg/100 ml; (3) 2-hour results less than 165 mg/100 ml; and (4) 3-hour results less than 145 mg/100 ml. The pregnant female is considered diabetic if laboratory results demonstrate two or more values above normal. All pregnant women should be screened for diabetes, and if diabetes is discovered they should be followed by a health team that includes an endocrinologist as well as an obstetrician.

Intervention

Diabetes can be controlled in most instances. The controversy continues regarding the relationship between the degree of control and long-term complications. Some authorities believe that long-term problems are caused by an inherited defect and are not related to reduction of the blood sugar to close to normal levels; others feel that long-term complications are directly related to increased blood sugar levels and can be prevented by proper control. Recent findings support the effectiveness of control of hyperglycemia in preventing long-term complications. Criteria for control vary, but it is felt that the patient is in good to excellent control if (1) the fasting blood glucose is normal, (2) the blood glucose 1 hour after meals is no greater than 200 mg/100 ml in diabetics on insulin and 180 mg/100 ml in diabetics controlled by diet alone or by diet and oral hypoglycemic agents, (3) the 2-hour postprandial glucose is no greater than 120 mg to 140 mg/100 ml, (4) the urine glucose and acetone are negative, (5) the 24-hour urinary glucose is less than 5% to 10% of daily carbohydrate intake, (6) the patient maintains optimal weight, and (7) the hemoglobin A_{1C} (Hb A_{1C}) is no greater than 1.5 times normal.

Long-term control of diabetes mellitus is being monitored by Hb A_{1C}. Hb A_{1C} is a minor hemoglobin that results from the glycosylation of normal hemoglobin A, when normal hemoglobin A is exposed to a high glucose environment. The glycosylated hemoglobin accumulates during the 120-day life span of red blood cells. The level of Hb A_{1C} concentration reflects the average glucose level over several preceding weeks. In normal persons the level of Hb A_{1C} is 3% to 6%. The goal of therapy is to have the person with diabetes mellitus maintain Hb A_{1C} no greater than 1.5 times normal. Since Hb A_{1C}, is formed during the total life span of the red blood cells, it reflects the blood glucose level over previous weeks and cannot be used to make decisions about insulin, diet, or fluid needs in the acute situation.

The degree of control should be the optimal level that can be reasonably maintained considering the lifestyle of the person with diabetes. The degree to which the individual participates in control of the disease depends on how well he or she has adapted emotionally to having diabetes and on his or her knowledge of the disease and motivation to pursue control measures.

The emotional response to a diagnosis of diabetes is often severe and is not easily dealt with. Part of this may result from fear of disability and eventual death. Since diabetes is so widespread, many people know of relatives and friends who have had the disease and who have eventually had an amputation or have become blind. Perhaps an even greater cause of emotional reaction is that diabetes affects the life pattern in regard to food. Food and eating have meaning beyond the actual meeting of nutritional needs, and changes in eating habits are extremely difficult for some persons to accept. Adolescents, perhaps more than any other age group, may find restrictions almost intolerable and need much un-

derstanding in their adjustment to the disease.

Initiating a suitable plan of care for diabetes will often make a great difference in how the person continues with care. It can help the person and significant others avoid undue stressors and concerns that may make it difficult to control the diabetes. Since most persons with diabetes are now treated in a physician's office or a hospital clinic, the community health nurse very frequently needs to help them with the initial adjustment.

The majority of nursing interventions for persons with diabetes mellitus involve assisting them to learn about their condition, promoting self-care, and teaching measures for control of the disease and prevention of complications. Various teaching aids on diabetes are available from many sources, such as the American Diabetes Association.

Many diabetics are hospitalized for conditions other than their diabetes. In these situations the nurse identifies during the initial interview the diabetic regimen being followed at home. Whenever possible, patients should continue this regimen in the hospital. This includes administering insulin, monitoring their status, and making personal food selections. Continuing to carry out their own regimen allows patients independence and promotes self-care. Sometimes, however, the patient cannot be independent, and the nurse makes judgments as to when and how much self-care should be assumed by the patient.

Diet. Nutritional management is a primary part of the treatment for all persons with diabetes mellitus. The person with diabetes has the same nutritional needs as anyone else but needs some restrictions to control the metabolic abnormalities. The type of restrictions recommended have varied over the years. At present, the most highly recommended diet consists of sufficient calories to promote normal growth and activity in the child and to maintain normal weight and activity in the non-obese adult with diabetes mellitus. Calorie restriction to promote weight reduction is needed in a large percentage of non-insulin-dependent diabetics.

Traditionally proteins have formed a large part of the diet for persons with diabetes mellitus, since restriction of carbohydrates is a priority. The current recommendation is that proteins should provide from 10% to 20% of the total calories in the diet. The goal is to provide the recommended RDA levels plus 0.5 g/kg of body weight.[149]

Carbohydrates (CHO) have traditionally been restricted, but research has demonstrated improved glucose tolerance with increased carbohydrates.[2] A usual recommendation is that 45% of the total calories be from carbohydrate foods. Ten to fifteen percent of the CHO calories should come from sugar in milk, fruit, and vegetables and 30% to 35% of the CHO calories should come from starches. There should be sharp limitations on refined sugars.[149]

The proportion of fat in the diabetic diet has traditionally been high, but the current recommendation is to reduce the fat to 35% of total calories. The amount of saturated fat should be 10% or less and the remainder should be monounsaturated and polyunsaturated fats.

The person with diabetes needs the normal amount of vitamins and minerals. Meal size and frequency are adjusted to the individual's life-style and to the medications the person is taking. Consistency in timing and the distribution of calories, carbohydrates, fats, and proteins for each meal is most important. This is particularly true when the person is on insulin. Typically the diet prescribed consists of three meals and one or more snacks a day, but adjustments must be made so that the diet is satisfactory to the patient.

A new dietary approach that is being recommended is a high-fiber, high-CHO diet. High-fiber, high-CHO diets have been shown to decrease insulin requirements, fasting and postprandial glucose levels, and cholesterol levels. Anderson[2] recommends a diet of 55% to 60% CHO, 20% proteins, 20% to 25% fats, and 25 g to 30 g of plant fiber per 1000 kilocalories.

The exact dietary restrictions prescribed will vary. Some persons will be on calorie restriction only; others will be required to control calories and carbohydrates; and others will be required to regulate calories, carbohydrates, fats, and proteins. Once the goal of nutritional therapy has been established, the specific diet will be prescribed. Individuals may then be taught one of several methods to assist them in calculating and maintaining their dietary intake on a daily basis.

The most frequent method taught to and used by those with diabetes mellitus to calculate their diets is use of the exchange list. The exchange list is divided into seven food groups. Foods are grouped according to the amount of carbohydrate and fat they contain. The first six groups consist of foods that must be measured: *milk* and *milk products, vegetables, fruits, breads* and *starchy vegetables, meats,* and *fats*. The meat group is subdivided into three groups: lean meat sources, meats with moderate fat content, and meats with high fat content. The seventh group consists of foods with negligible calories that do not need to be measured. Examples are coffee, tea, bouillon, plain gelatin, mustard, lemon, rhubarb, spices, and vinegar. Everything added to food (cream, sugar) is counted as part of the meal's exchange.

The total number of exchanges for each day is determined by the prescribed calorie, carbohydrate, fat, and protein restrictions. The number of exchanges is then divided into a meal/snack pattern that takes into account the life-style and the medication-taking pattern of the individual. The person selects food from the appropriate groups on the exchange list according to the distribution of the exchanges in the prescribed meal/snack pattern. The advantage of this method is that it is widely used throughout the country. A disadvantage is that the list does not include mixed dishes, but the list does include the staple food items that can be combined for mixed dishes. Exchange list values for items sold at popular fast food chains have been published and there are cookbooks available which provide recipes and exchange list equivalents. Booklets that simplify the exchange list have been developed by the Greater Cleveland Diabetes Association. Table 32-7 gives examples of meal plans using exchange lists.

Another method that can be used by those with diabetes mellitus to assist them in calculating and maintaining their dietary intake is the point system. Foods are categorized according to calorie, carbohydrate, protein, and fat content. The total daily food allowance is written as number of calories and carbohydrate points. The person is then instructed to select foods according to a point distribution. Meat, milk, and fats are included at each meal. Other methods that may be taught are the *percent of carbohydrate system* and the *calculation of dietary intake* from tables of food values. See reference 149 for a discussion of these systems.

Some individuals who have difficulty with the systems described above will be given a rigid menu plan that tells them the amount and type of food to eat or drink for each meal and snack (e.g., 4 oz of apple juice, 8 oz of milk, 3 oz of baked chicken). They will use this menu plan until they are ready to use the exchange list or some other system.

The described systems require that all food be measured or weighed. This should be done until the person becomes familiar with the amounts of food in one serving. They can then estimate portions. If problems develop, measurements as well as other aspects of the diet must be reviewed. Some physicians will prescribe unmeasured diets for some individuals, particularly young diabetics. The number and time of meals and snacks, however, are prescribed. Those individuals on unmeasured diets are told to eat sufficient food from all categories of food to satisfy their appetite. Some sweets may be included or all sweets may be restricted on the unmeasured diet.

The diabetic diet does not require the use of special or dietetic foods. Persons with diabetes mellitus must be warned about being misled by the word *dietetic*. Dietetic may refer to low-sodium content rather than to low-sugar content. Dietetic candies also must be used with care. They are not necessarily low in calories. Sugar substitutes can be used and still are available despite the controversy about the possible carcinogenic effects of saccharin.

Some persons who develop diabetes are accustomed to having an alcoholic beverage daily. With approval of the physician, the diabetic may have small amounts of alcohol. Since alcohol is a high-caloric food, it must be exchanged for the fat calories in the diet.

TABLE 32-7. Sample of two menu plans using the exchange list*

Exchanges	Menu I	Menu II
	Breakfast	**Breakfast**
1 Fruit	½ Glass orange juice	¼ cantaloupe
1 Milk (low-fat)	1 Glass skim milk	1 Glass skim milk
1 Meat	1 Egg, poached	1 Scrambled egg
3 Bread	2 Toast, ½ C oatmeal	1 English muffin, ½ C bran flakes
2 Fat	1½ tsp Margarine	1½ tsp Margarine
	Lunch	**Lunch**
1 Fruit	1 Peach	½ Banana
1 Milk (low-fat)	1 Glass skim milk	1 Glass skim milk
2 Meat	Tuna salad sandwich (¼ C tuna, with	1 MacDonald's cheeseburger (2 bread, 2 meat, 1 fat)
2 Bread	celery, 2 slices of bread, 3 tsp mayon-	1 Lettuce salad with 2 tbsp French dressing
	naise and lettuce)	
	Afternoon snack	**Afternoon snack**
1 Bread	6 Thin round crackers	Pretzels
1 Fruit	1 Apple	Grapes
	Dinner	**Dinner**
1 Fruit	¾ C strawberries	½ C pineapple
2 Vegetable B	1 C green beans	Sliced tomatoes
4 Meat	4 oz Round steak	4 oz Ham (boiled)
1 Milk (low-fat)	1 Glass skim milk	1 Glass skim milk
2 Bread	1 Small baked potato	2 Slices bread
	1 Roll	
3 Fats	1 tbsp Sour cream/2½ tsp Butter	1 tsp Mayonnaise
	Evening snack	**Evening snack**
1 Bread	3 Rye wafers	6 Salt crackers
1 Meat	1 oz Low-fat cheese	¼ C low-fat cottage cheese

*Diet distributed over three meals and two snacks. Diet based on 2000 calories with 45% CHO (225 g); 35% fats (78 g); and 20% proteins (100 g).

No matter what type of diet the individual is on or what method is used to calculate daily intake, instructions on how to meet dietary needs when ill must be given. All individuals have days when they cannot eat solid foods. Persons with diabetes must know how to replace normal foods with liquids. They also must know that they should consult the physician or nurse who is providing their follow-up care if they are unable to take any food.

The nutritional therapy used to treat diabetes must be matched to the drug activity for persons on insulin or oral hypoglycemics. In addition, the exercise level of all such persons must be considered. Exercise facilitates the movement of glucose into muscle cells without requiring insulin. Therefore, when individuals with diabetes mellitus increase their activity level with work, sports, and other physical activity, they will have to know how to increase their calories or decrease their insulin or they may become hypoglycemic. Persons with diabetes should not limit their activities as long as there are no other medical reasons for the limitation.

Although the diet is prescribed by the physician and

the use of the exchange list or other method of calculating and maintaining the diet is usually taught by a dietitian or nutritionist, every nurse needs to know what method is being used, how to use the particular method, and how to teach others to use it. Often individuals do not know what they do not understand about the method of calculation until they begin using it on their own. Reinstruction and follow-up are consistently needed. Whenever a nurse encounters patients with diabetes, their level of knowledge about their prescribed diet should be assessed and reinstruction given as necessary.

Medications: insulin. Insulin is used in the treatment of all persons with *insulin-dependent diabetes mellitus* and in the treatment of some patients with non-insulin-dependent diabetes whose metabolic status is not controlled by diet alone or by diet and oral hypoglycemic agents. It must be kept in mind that even though insulin may be used with the latter group, the patient is still classified as having non-insulin-dependent diabetes mellitus.

TYPES OF INSULIN. There are eight insulin prepara-

TABLE 32-8. Action of insulin preparations

Type of insulin	Time of onset (hr)	Peak of action (hr)	Duration of action (hr)	Insulin appearance
Rapid acting				
Regular	<1	2-4	4-6	Clear
Crystalline zinc	<1	2-4	5-8	Clear
Semilente	<1	4-7	12-16	Cloudy
Intermediate acting				
NPH	1-2	8-12	18-24	Cloudy
Globin zinc	2-4	6-10	12-18	Clear
Lente	1-4	8-12	18-24	Cloudy
Slow acting				
Protamine zinc	4-8	16-18	36+	Cloudy
Ultralente	4-8	16-18	36+	Cloudy

tions on the market. The insulin preparation most commonly used is a combination of beef and pork insulin. Pure beef or pure pork insulins are also available. Recombinant insulin (bacterially produced human insulin) has been tested on healthy volunteers in the United States, Great Britain, Greece, and West Germany and was found to be free of toxic effects. It is now being tested on diabetic patients at several centers in the United States.[28] In the past insulin preparations contained significant amounts of pro-insulin and other antigenic components. Procedures that allow the preparation of more pure preparations of insulin are now available. Two such preparations are single-peak insulin (70% to 75% insulin and 25% to 30% desamino insulin) and single-component insulin (99% pure insulin).[171] Most insulin in the United States is now of the single-peak variety.[75] Single-component insulin is available but is very expensive, and its use is restricted to those patients with problems such as persistent allergy.[75]

Insulins are classified as to their time of action as rapid, intermediate, and slow acting. *Regular insulin* is a *rapid-acting* form of insulin that is prepared by precipitation of insulin from solution in a noncrystalline form and then prepared for subcutaneous injection by mixing it with water of neutral or acidic pH. *Crystalline zinc insulin* is also *rapid acting* and is produced by precipitation of the hormone in the presence of zinc crystals. It has a slightly longer duration of action than regular insulin.

In the search to find an insulin that had a longer duration of action, insulin has been modified in various ways. The first such modification was made by reacting insulin and zinc with the protein protamine to form *protamine zinc insulin (PZI)*. PZI is a *long-acting* insulin. *Isophane insulin,* also known as NPH insulin, is a modified protamine zinc insulin preparation with an *intermediate onset* and *duration of action*. *Globin zinc insulin* is an *intermediate-acting insulin* that is made by reacting insulin with zinc and the protein globulin. Be-

cause it does not provide coverage for 24 hours, it is rarely used at this time.

Research has also revealed that the absorption of insulin can be modified by changing the size of the crystal, the zinc content, and the nature of the buffer.[75] Extended insulin zinc suspension *(ultralente insulin)* is prepared by dissolving large crystals of insulin with high zinc content in a solution of sodium acetate. It is a long-acting insulin. Prompt insulin zinc suspension *(semilente insulin)* is a microcrystalline high pH preparation that has a rapid onset and short duration of action. Insulin zinc suspension *(lente insulin)* is an intermediate-acting insulin made from 7 parts of ultralente and 3 parts semilente.

All insulin preparations are usually given by the subcutaneous route. *Only regular and crystalline insulin can be given intravenously*. Various preparations of insulin can be mixed together. Regular and crystalline insulin can be mixed with all other insulin preparations. Semilente can be mixed with lente and ultralente insulin. Table 32-8 summarizes the properties of various insulin preparations.

It is important that nurses know the time of onset of action as well as the peak action and duration of action so that food intake is coordinated with the insulin. Food must be taken within one hour after the injection of rapid-acting insulin to prevent a hypoglycemic reaction, while intermediate or slow-acting insulin require a supplementary feeding in the midafternoon or a bedtime feeding or both. The between-meal snacks are timed to meet the peak action of the insulin being used. Most important to coordination of insulin and nutrition therapy is consistency in timing and the amount and type of food intake.

FACTORS INFLUENCING ABSORPTION OF INSULIN. Other important factors that nurses must be aware of are factors that influence absorption and excretion of insulin. Sachs[171] identifies the following four factors that can influence absorption.

1. The rate of absorption following subcutaneous administration of modified insulin decreases as volume increases, whereas the absorption rate of regular insulin increases as volume increases.

2. The greater the amount of adipose tissue present at the injection site, the slower the absorption.

3. Subcutaneous injections given in the arms are usually absorbed more rapidly than injections given into the thighs; but leg exercises can increase absorption following injections into the thighs and can precipitate a hypoglycemic reaction.

4. Hypertrophy of injection sites can occur with repeated injections and can delay absorption.

The kidneys play a major role in the metabolism of insulin and thus the activity of insulin. The metabolism and excretion of insulin decrease in the presence of renal damage; thus diabetics on insulin may require less insulin if renal damage occurs.

FACTORS IMPORTANT TO SAFE ADMINISTRATION OF INSULIN. Insulin dosage is measured in units and is available in three concentrations: U-40, U-80, and U-100. U-40 insulin has 40 units/ml, U-80 has 80 units/ml, and U-100 has 100 units/ml. U-100 insulin was introduced in 1973, and it is hoped that it will become the standard preparation in use. All types of insulin presently come in all three concentrations.

Insulin should be administered only in an insulin syringe. For each concentration of insulin there is an insulin syringe with a maximal volume of 1 ml that is calibrated in the appropriate unit scale (Fig. 32-8). Therefore U-40 insulin should only be administered in U-40 syringes, U-80 insulin should only be administered in U-80 syringes, and U-100 insulin should only be administered in U-100 syringes. If syringes and insulin concentration are mismatched, errors leading to hypoglycemia or uncontrolled diabetes will occur. There is also a U-50 insulin syringe to use with U-100 insulin. This syringe holds a maximum of 0.5 ml (50 units) and allows for more accurate calibration of small insulin doses.

In the past dual-scaled glass syringes to be used for either U-40 or U-80 insulin were available. These syringes can easily lead to errors, and persons with diabetes mellitus should be encouraged to purchase single-scale insulin syringes. These older types of syringes have not been on the market for some time, but some individuals may still be using glass syringes of this type. Persons with diabetes also need to be instructed to make sure that the concentration of insulin matches the scale on the insulin syringe each time they purchase insulin or new syringes. Reusable glass or plastic disposable syringes for all strengths of insulin are available at most pharmacies.

Errors in dosage can occur even if the person has the appropriate syringe and the correct type of insulin. These errors can occur if the technique for drawing up insulin varies on a day-to-day basis. Normally, with

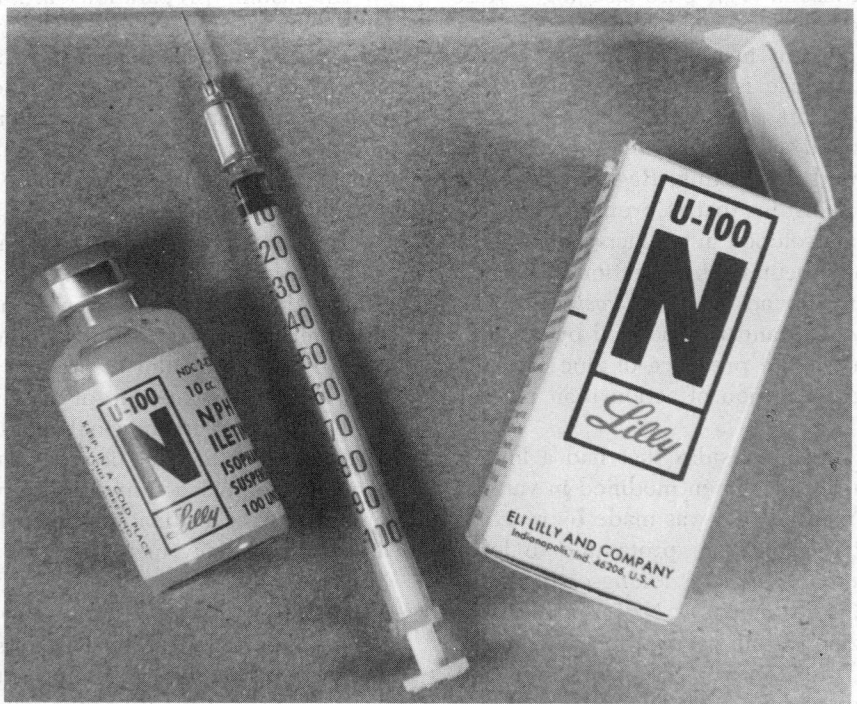

Fig. 32-8. U-100 insulin and disposable U-100 insulin syringe.

subcutaneous injections, an air bubble is not added to the syringe to clear the needle of solution. Therefore, a certain amount of insulin is retained in the needle's dead space after each injection. The needle may contain as much as 0.1 ml (10 units of U-100 insulin) dead space. If the technique is not correct and at times an air bubble is kept in the syringe, it will clear the dead space and a significant increase in dosage may be administered. If the person makes sure that all air bubbles are eliminated from the syringe, this error in dosage can be avoided.

When individuals are mixing two insulins in the same syringe, it is important that they use the same sequence for drawing up the two insulins each time or the amount of both insulins will vary. The dead space skews the dosage because an extra amount of insulin equal to the dead space is drawn up with the first insulin. This insulin is then included in the measurement of the second insulin withdrawn. Therefore, the person actually gets too much of the first insulin and less than prescribed amount of the second insulin. If the insulins are mixed in the same sequence, the person will always be getting the same dosage and probably will have no problems. Some producers of syringes claim that their syringes have no dead space. Since the amount of dead space in syringes varies, patients should use the same brand of syringe at all times. To prevent dead-space effects, insulin can be premixed in a vial. Some practitioners recommend that if a fast-acting insulin and an intermediate or long-acting insulin are being mixed in the same syringe, the fast-acting insulin be drawn up first. The reason for this is that there is always a chance that some of the first insulin withdrawn will be inadvertently injected into the second bottle of insulin. Adding a small amount of fast-acting insulin to a vial of intermediate or long-acting insulin will not affect the activity of the intermediate or long-acting insulin.

METHODS FOR PROVIDING DAILY INSULIN. Each individual has his or her own insulin needs. Today the majority of persons with diabetes are treated with NPH and regular or crystalline insulin. The long-acting insulins are seldom used. Some persons will be treated with one injection per day. This injection may be NPH or lente insulin or a combination of regular or crystalline and NPH or lente insulin. For many individuals one injection per day does not provide adequate control. In these instances two injections per day may be given. One injection is given before breakfast and the other before the evening meal. Each injection may be a combination of regular and NPH or lente insulin or a single type of insulin. If the person is on a two-injection schedule, usually two thirds of the daily insulin requirement is given in the morning and the remainder is given before the evening meal.

In recent years research has led to a better understanding of normal insulin levels in humans, and differ-

ent techniques of insulin administration are now being used. It is now known that nondiabetics have a continuous basal level of insulin which rapidly increases with food intake (p. 643). Health care providers are trying to mimic this normal pattern when treating insulin-dependent diabetics. This is being accomplished in several different ways. For some diabetics this can be achieved with two injections per day using a combination of regular or crystalline and NPH or lente insulin in each injection. With this schedule, the morning dose of regular or crystalline insulin provides the peak needed at breakfast, the morning dose of NPH or lente provides the peak needed at lunch, and the overlap of their duration of activity provides the basal insulin level needed during the day.[84] The evening dose of regular or crystalline insulin provides the peak needed for the evening meal. The NPH or lente insulin given before the evening meal provides the peak needed for the bedtime snack and the basal level needed during the night.[83] This schedule of injections does not control all insulin-dependent diabetics and if the person is late in eating a meal, hypoglycemic reactions will occur. Therefore some insulin-dependent diabetics are being treated with multiple injections with the person taking a prescribed dose of *regular* insulin 30 minutes before each meal and possibly before each snack.[83,173] This method mimics the normal burst of insulin that is seen in nondiabetics when food is eaten and provides the basal level needed during the day. To provide the basal level of insulin needed during sleep, the person takes a small dose of NPH or lente insulin at bedtime or a small dose of long-acting insulin at the time of the evening meal. Because of the difference in the time of peak and duration of action, NPH or lente insulin, if used, must be given at bedtime. With the latter schedule the individual patient must take four or five injections per day and some may find this impossible.

One of the major goals of diabetic research has been to develop an implantable artificial pancreas. To achieve this requires the following components:

1. A sensor that continually monitors glucose levels and transmits this information to a computer
2. A computer that can analyze the information, calculate based on preprogramming the amount of insulin needed, and then activate a delivery system
3. A delivery system that would deliver the proper amount of insulin

This is an example of a *closed-loop system* and most closely resembles the system in the human body. A number of these devices, which can control glucose concentrations in insulin-dependent diabetics, are available. However, at this time the glucose sensors that have the reliability desired are bulky and not implantable. They are being used in research centers and in some university hospitals.

An *open-loop system* consists of a device that provides a variable insulin delivery system. It does not have the ability to monitor glucose or calculate insulin needs. With this system the patient's daily insulin dosage is determined, the dose necessary for each meal and snack, and the dose necessary to maintain an adequate basal level are calculated, and the insulin is delivered by a battery-powered pump. There are multiple types of pumps available, and each varies in some minor way, but the general description that follows applies to all pumps.

The pump is loaded with a syringe that contains the total 24-hour insulin dose in the form of regular insulin. The syringe in the pump is attached by a loop of tubing to a subcutaneous needle. The needle is inserted into subcutaneous tissue, usually in the abdomen, using the same technique as is used for any subcutaneous injection, and it is then taped in place. The pump is worn on a belt at the waist or in a pocket (Fig. 32-9). It is about the size of a pocket calculator. The pump has two settings, one for delivery of a basal rate and one for the delivery of a bolus dosage. The pump setting is set so that a continuous basal infusion is delivered and then at meal times, the person changes the setting to deliver a bolus infusion. Usually, all that is required to deliver the bolus is to change the setting and press a button. The setting then is either manually or automatically switched back to the basal infusion rate. Each pump has alarms that inform the patient if the battery is low, if there is an occlusion in the line, or if the insulin is in-

fusing too fast. The injection can also be given intravenously into a Broviac catheter or some other intravenous site.

The insulin dose is altered based on home monitoring of blood glucose, and the subcutaneous injection site is changed every 48 hours. The tubing, needle, and syringes are also changed at this time. The individual is instructed not to allow the pump or injection site to become wet. The advantage of this system is that it does not require multiple injections daily. The disadvantages are the expense of the pump, the need to wear the pump at all times, and the restrictions the pump places on some activities.

There are many methods for initiating therapy in the newly diagnosed insulin-dependent diabetic or the non-insulin-dependent diabetic who is going to be treated with insulin to achieve better metabolic control. Regardless of the method used, once therapy has been initiated, adjustments are made based on the individual's response until the desired level of control is obtained.

PRINCIPLES FOR MEETING INSULIN NEEDS WHEN ILL. Regardless of what type of insulin or what administration routine is used, all persons with diabetes mellitus must be taught what to do when they are ill. Many persons will skip their insulin when they are ill and are unable to eat their regular diet. *They should be taught that usually in times of illness their insulin needs are greater. Optimally, the goal is for them to continue to*

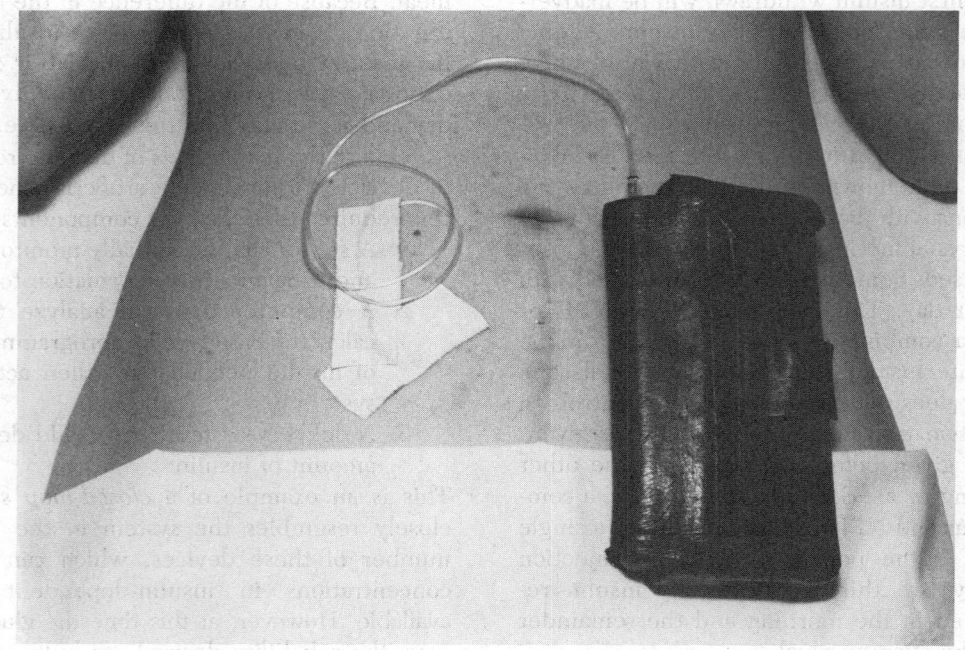

Fig. 32-9. Insulin infusion pump in place. (Courtesy Dr. Ralph Weiland, Case Western Reserve University, Cleveland.)

take their insulin and prescribed calories and carbohydrates in some manner. Physicians will vary on what they desire the diabetic to do when the person is ill. Most important is that the individual with diabetes know what to do.

TEACHING THE PATIENT TO ADMINISTER INSULIN. The major goals of a teaching program are to help the patient (1) understand the basic characteristics of insulin so that it is stored and mixed appropriately, (2) learn how to prepare the injection site and know the importance of rotating sites, (3) gain the ability to withdraw the appropriate amount of insulin and administer it with aseptic technique, and (4) learn how to care for the equipment (Fig. 32-10).

Typical trays for the injection at home can be set up for use in demonstrations and for patients to use in practice. The nurse can discuss boxes or trays that can be set up at home to keep all equipment together. The equipment should be stored on a shelf or closet out of reach of children, out of sight, and in a cool place. Equipment needed for insulin injections and preparation of the skin includes insulin syringes, subcutaneous needles, cotton (box of rolled or balls), alcohol, and, if using a pump, the pump and tubing. It is now known that insulin does not need to be stored in the refrigerator since all insulins (except regular and crystalline) are stable for 24 months at room temperature, while regular and crystalline insulins are stable for 12 months at 37° C.

The patient must know that all forms of lente insulin, NPH, and protamine zinc insulin separate into layers on standing. To obtain an accurate dose of the active ingredient, *the solution must be mixed by rotating the bottle between the palms of the hands and inverting the vial from end to end several times. Vigorous shaking should be avoided.*

The site of injection must be rotated to assure proper absorption of insulin. Lipodystrophy or atrophy can occur with repeated injections and can cause poor absorption of the medication. The major areas for injection of insulin are the arms, legs, buttocks, and abdomen. Each of these areas has multiple sites. See Fig. 32-11 for a diagram of these major areas and sites. Injections should not be given in any one spot more often than every 2 weeks. A diagram of the possible sites can be made as a guide and the sites numbered so that they can be rotated according to the plan.

The patient can choose one of two different methods to sterilize nondisposable equipment. The syringe and needle can be stored immersed in 70% alcohol between injections and boiled weekly for 10 minutes or they can be boiled daily for 10 minutes. A strainer placed in a saucepan makes it easier for the patient to drain and handle the boiled equipment.

Because there are many things the patient and family must learn, this particular skill may be delayed until the patient feels more comfortable with other skills. Disposable equipment may be used at first, and then reusable equipment employed when the skill has been learned. The nurse may need to teach the patient how to *mix two insulins* in the same syringe so that they may be given in one injection. A simple way of mixing insulins in the same syringe is to inject the correct amount of air into the second insulin bottle first. Then the correct amount of air is injected into the first insulin bottle and the insulin withdrawn. As a final step, the correct dose is withdrawn from the second insulin bottle. Reg-

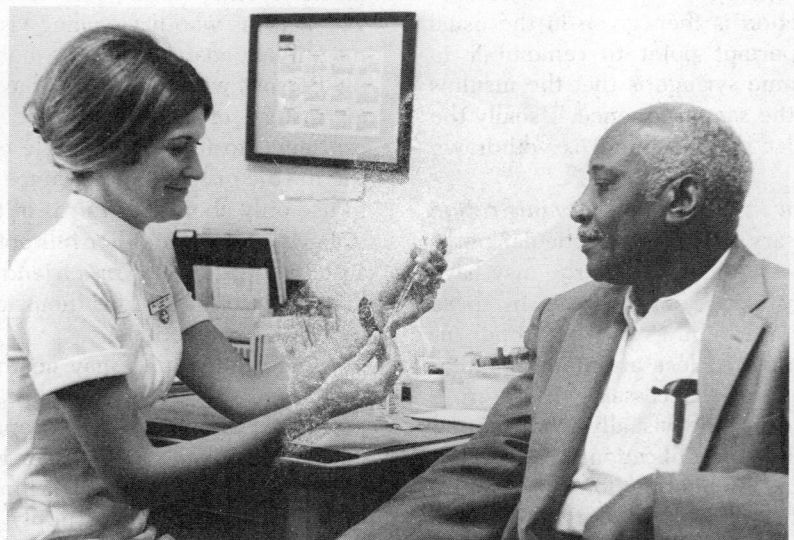

Fig. 32-10. Clinic nurse begins instruction in insulin administration by demonstrating procedure to patient.

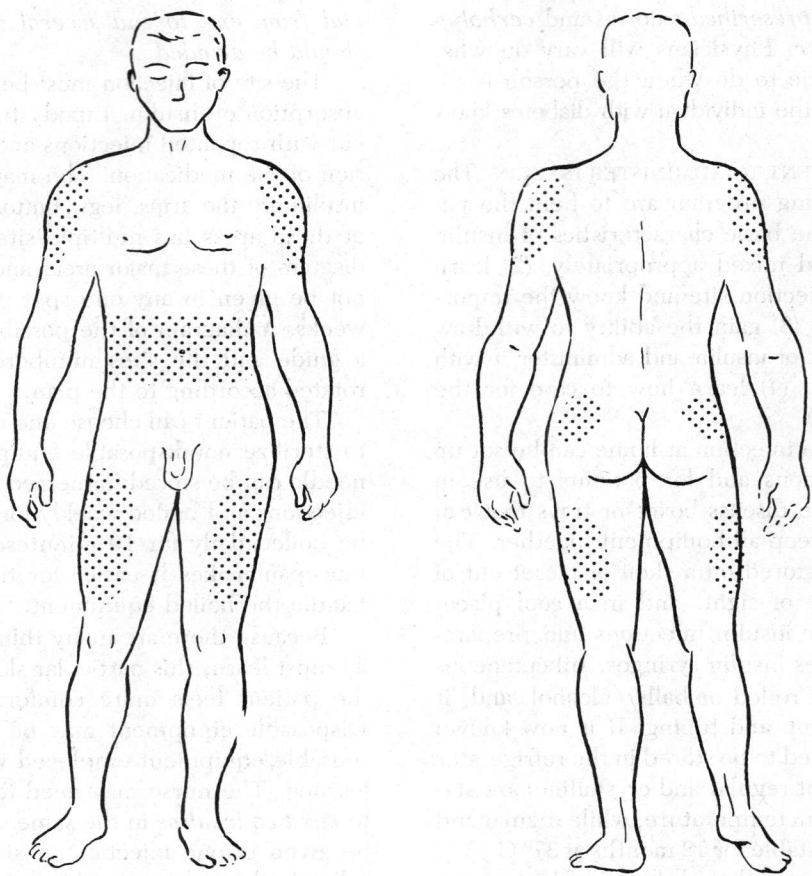

Fig. 32-11. Arms, legs, buttocks, and abdomen can be used for insulin injection. A different site (indicated by each dot) should be used for each injection.

ular insulin can be mixed with any other type of insulin. The lente insulins can also be mixed together. The syringe should be rotated gently to obtain a well-distributed solution. The injection is then given in the usual manner. The most important point to remember in mixing insulins in the same syringe is that the insulins are always drawn up in the same sequence. Usually the fast-acting insulin (regular or crystalline) is withdrawn first (p. 653).

At times *modification in methods of administration of insulin* may be necessary because of particular problems; for example, the person may be elderly, may have unsteady hands, or may have failing vision. In these instances, measurement of insulin as well as proper injection technique will require close attention. Adaptation of equipment may also be necessary. There are a number of aids available for the visually handicapped that are advertised in diabetic publications or are available from the American Foundation for the Blind.* Special syringes with plunger locks and attachable de-

---

*American Foundation for the Blind, Inc., 15 West Sixteenth St., New York, NY 10011.

vices for locking the plunger can be purchased, as well as attachable needle guides and insulin bottle guides to facilitate entry of the needle into the bottle (Fig. 32-12). Persons who have failing vision may also use a small magnifying adapter that can be clipped to a syringe.

Persons with poor vision have the danger of drawing air instead of insulin into the syringe. They must be cautioned to invert the bottle completely and to insert the needle only a short distance. Often they are advised to use only about two-thirds of the bottle of insulin and to have on hand another full bottle. Some persons have a public health nurse or a friend withdraw the last doses in a bottle of insulin for them, or they go to a clinic for the last few injections.

Some individuals may not be able to prepare their own insulin dose accurately because of motor or sensory problems, but they may be capable of giving their own injections. A family member or neighbor could be taught to prepare the correct dose of insulin, or a public health nurse could fill a week's supply of syringes. The syringe would need to be rotated gently before use to mix the insulin. In some instances a member of the family may have to give the insulin. A family member should al-

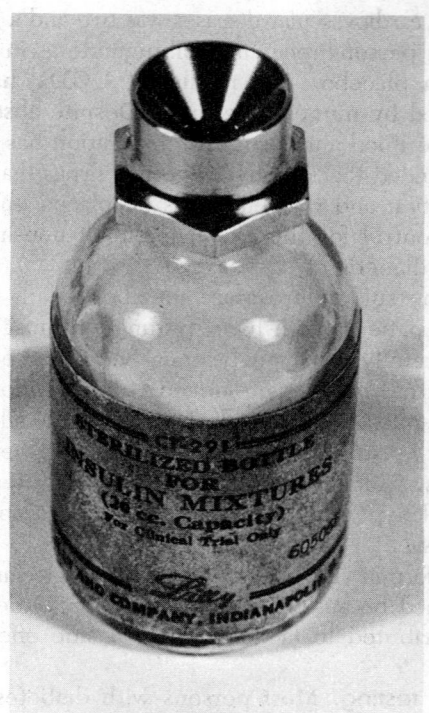

Fig. 32-12. Insulin needle guide that fits over top of insulin vial. Patient cleans stopper and guide with alcohol before placing guide on vial. Needle is laid in **V** of guide and vial is pushed toward it. (Courtesy American Foundation for the Blind, Inc., New York, N.Y.)

ways know how to do this in case impending coma or other illness makes it impossible for the individual to administer his or her own insulin. If the patient is using an insulin pump, the same material as described above would have to be taught. In addition, the patient would need to learn about the pump and its care.

COMPLICATIONS OF INSULIN USE. The major complications that the nurse must be aware of will be briefly described. *Hypoglycemia* is one of the major complications. However, it occurs in many persons with diabetes even though they are not on insulin; it is discussed on p. 660 along with the other metabolic complications of diabetes mellitus.

Lipodystrophies. Two forms of lipodystrophy can occur: hypertrophy and atrophy. *Hypertrophy* is a thickening of an injection site because of the development of fibrous scar tissue that results from repeated injections in the same site. A hypertrophic area is usually devoid of nerve endings, and the patient likes to reuse it because injections given in this area are painless. Absorption from this area is slow and erratic. Teaching the patient the importance of rotating injection sites and supporting their doing so helps prevent hypertrophy.

Atrophy is a loss of subcutaneous fat. The cause is unknown. It is felt to be the result of repeated injections in the same site, faulty injection technique resulting in injection into fat tissue, or impurities in the insulin. Again, a major nursing role is to ensure that the patient rotates the sites and gives injections deep enough to bypass fat tissue. Some researchers,[75,82] believing the cause of atrophy was impurities in the insulin and that insulin was naturally lipohypertrophic, have successfully treated atrophy by injecting purified insulin into atrophic areas.

Insulin hypersensitivity. Insulin hypersensitivity occurs in some patients. Most reactions are local, consisting of wheals at the site of injection, but systemic symptoms and anaphylactic reactions can occur. The hypersensitivity may be the result of several factors. These include improper injection technique, sensitivity to the alcohol used to prepare the skin, sensitivity to the modifying proteins in the insulin, or sensitivity to the species source.

Treatment varies depending on the cause. Improper technique or hypersensitivity to the alcohol is ruled out first. Proper injection technique is ensured, and then a more purified form of alcohol or a different antiseptic agent is used to prepare the skin and sterilize the equipment. If the modifying protein is thought to be the causative factor, the patient may be switched from NPH to lente insulin. If the species source is thought to be the cause, the patient is switched to porcine (pork) insulin, which is thought to be less antigenic than other forms. Single-component insulin may also be used. If the hypersensitivity is severe, an antihistamine may be given to treat the symptoms until the allergic response disappears. Corticosteroids may be used for severe reactions. If the patient is found to be allergic to all types of insulin, desensitization may be necessary.

Insulin resistance. Insulin resistance occurs in some patients. It is defined as an insulin requirement greater than 200 units a day for a period longer than 2 days in the absence of infection or other factors that would increase insulin need. The etiology of insulin resistance is unknown, but is thought to be a result of the development of antibodies which render insulin inactive. All patients who have been on insulin for 6 weeks to 3 months develop some antibodies to insulin. Usually these antibodies are not sufficient to interfere with the response to insulin and the control of diabetes.

Insulin resistance may be treated by porcine insulin or by single-peak and single-component insulin. In some instances, ACTH or adrenal glucocorticoids may be used for short-term treatment.[171] In most instances insulin resistance is self-limiting. For this reason, some physicians do not use adjunctive therapy such as the steroids. Instead they treat the patient during the period of resistance with higher doses of insulin. When high doses of insulin are used to treat insulin resistance, the patient must be monitored carefully for hypoglycemia since the dose will need to be decreased when the resistance period passes.

Medications: oral hypoglycemic agents. Several oral agents are available for use in controlling blood sugar levels in persons with diabetes mellitus. These agents have proved effective in the treatment of many adults whose diabetes is stable. These drugs are not hormones, and it is a misnomer to refer to them as oral insulins.

As a result of a study conducted in the 1970s by the University Group Diabetes Program (UGDP), the Food and Drug Administration recommends that oral hypoglycemic agents be limited to persons with symptomatic adult onset nonketotic diabetes mellitus that cannot be adequately controlled by diet or weight loss alone, and in whom the addition of insulin is impractical or unacceptable. The oral hypoglycemic agents are most effective in the treatment of elderly persons; they are not used to treat insulin-dependent diabetes or pregnant diabetics. They are useless in treating diabetic ketoacidosis.

Persons taking oral hypoglycemic medication instead of insulin need to be as careful about taking the prescribed dosage of the drug, following the prescribed diet, maintaining the usual amount of exercise, testing their urine for sugar, and taking general health precautions as do persons taking insulin.

The sulfonylurea compounds, which include acetohexamide (Dymelor), chlorpropamide (Diabinese), tolazamide (Tolinase), and tolbutamide (Orinase), are the oral agents prescribed. Micronase (Glyburide) is a new oral hypoglycemic agent of the sulfonylurea class that has been used in European countries for some time. It is now being used in research studies in the United States which are comparing it to presently available drugs for effectiveness and side effects. The sulfonylurea compounds are thought to act primarily by increasing the ability of the islet cells of the pancreas to secrete insulin, although other methods of action are being studied.

The dosages for the commonly used agents are presented in Table 32-9. In the UGDP study, tolbutamide was the oral hypoglycemic agent investigated. The death rate from cardiovascular diseases was two and a half times higher in persons receiving tolbutamide as in those receiving a placebo. The results of UGDP have been challenged by numerous groups. Despite absolute evidence the Food and Drug Administration has therefore recommended that oral hypoglycemic drugs may be used with caution and that emphasis be placed on diet and weight control for the management of non-insulin-dependent diabetics.

All the sulfonylureas are metabolized in the liver. Diabetic patients with liver dysfunction must be monitored carefully for hypoglycemia because the action of sulfonylureas may be prolonged. Complications of oral hypoglycemic agents include hypoglycemia, allergic skin reactions, gastrointestinal complaints, and hematologic disorders. Chlorpropamide causes water retention and dilutional hyponatremia in addition to the above complications.

Phenformin (DBI), another oral hypoglycemic agent, was banned because a significant number of deaths have been attributed to lactic acidosis, a side effect of this drug.

Urine testing. Most persons with diabetes mellitus must know how to test their urine for sugar and acetone in order to monitor their control. The urine testing equipment used will depend on the stability of the disease, the degree of glycosuria anticipated, the life-style of the person, visual acuity, and the person's physical limitations. Different urine testing products can give 0.5%, 2%, or 5% maximum readings of glycosuria. Some require accurate timing or an ability to measure drops of urine. The individual may be able to distinguish shades of color more accurately on one specific color chart. (See p. 599 for urine testing techniques.)

What the person *does* if the test is abnormal depends entirely on the individual and the instructions that have been given. Instructions should be in writing. The physician may, for example, instruct the patient to do nothing except repeat the test again during the same day and to keep a careful record of urine reactions, or instruct the patient to increase or decrease insulin or oral drug dosage, increase or decrease food intake, or get in touch with the physician at once. Some physicians may want certain patients to show a trace or even 1% sugar in their urine once daily as evidence that the blood sugar is not going too low, whereas for other individuals this would not be considered good control. The age of the individual and the stability of the disease affect the physician's decision in advising a course of action. The nurse can assist the person in interpreting the urine test results and in understanding the rationale for the specific regimen.

Home blood glucose monitoring. Increasingly persons with diabetes mellitus are using home blood glucose monitoring to monitor their metabolic status on a day-to-day basis rather than testing urine for glucose.

TABLE 32-9. Oral hypoglycemic agents

Classification	Proprietary name	Usual daily dose	Divided dose per day
Sulfonylureas			
Acetohexamide	Dymelor	250 mg-1.5 g	1-2
Chlorpropamide	Diabinese	100-500 mg	1
Tolazamide	Tolinase	100 mg-1 g	1-2
Tolbutamide	Orinase	0.5-2 g	2-3 after meals

Blood or serum glucose monitoring has always been the test used to monitor patients in the hospital, and the development of glucose oxidase sticks and reflectance meters now allows the use of blood glucose monitoring at home (Fig. 32-13). There are various types of tests for home blood glucose monitoring, and all have been shown to give results that correlate well with laboratory measurement of blood glucose.[31,164,185,233] Most of the tests require the use of a reflectance meter for valid interpretation of results. This adds to the cost and inconvenience of monitoring. Chemstrips bG is a test strip that eliminates the need for a reflectance meter; in preliminary tests it seems to be as accurate as strips used with a meter as long as the patient can detect color differences.[31,164,185]

Numerous articles report that home monitoring of blood glucose is a means of optimizing glycemic control.[31,158,199,224] Home monitoring has been found to facilitate the attainment of glycemic control in type I insulin-dependent diabetics and pregnant diabetics.* It is always used for those on multiple injection schedules or infusion pumps. Because the main emphasis with home monitoring has been on adjustment of insulin dosage on a daily basis, it has not been used with persons with other types of diabetes at this time. Home monitoring has other advantages in that it can be used to validate subjective symptoms of hypoglycemia or hypergly-

*References 39, 96, 101, 159, 178, 193, 199.

cemia, and it allows more immediate feedback to the individual about the effects of nonadherence with the prescribed therapeutic regimen. Some experts feel home glucose monitoring will replace urine testing in all diabetics within the next few years.[103]

Glucose monitoring is done before meals and at bedtime and at other times to document symptoms of hypoglycemia. At times, more frequent testing may be recommended if medicines are being changed. To do the testing the person does a finger stick and applies a drop of blood to a commercially prepared glucose oxidase stick. The timing for the reading and the preparation of the specimen are very important in obtaining accurate results. As stated, most strips require the use of a reflectance meter for valid interpretation of results.

Home blood glucose monitoring is expensive and not all insurance companies reimburse for this expense. As more data are collected showing the improved benefits that can be achieved with home blood glucose monitoring, it is expected that more health insurance carriers will reimburse for this expense. Nurses in some university centers will increasingly be involved in research studies about the benefits and limitations of this type of monitoring.

As is true regarding urine testing, the person with diabetes must know what to do with the results of home monitoring of blood glucose. When the person is on an insulin pump, he or she is advised to call the primary health care provider daily to report that day's results. The insulin for the next day is then adjusted as appro-

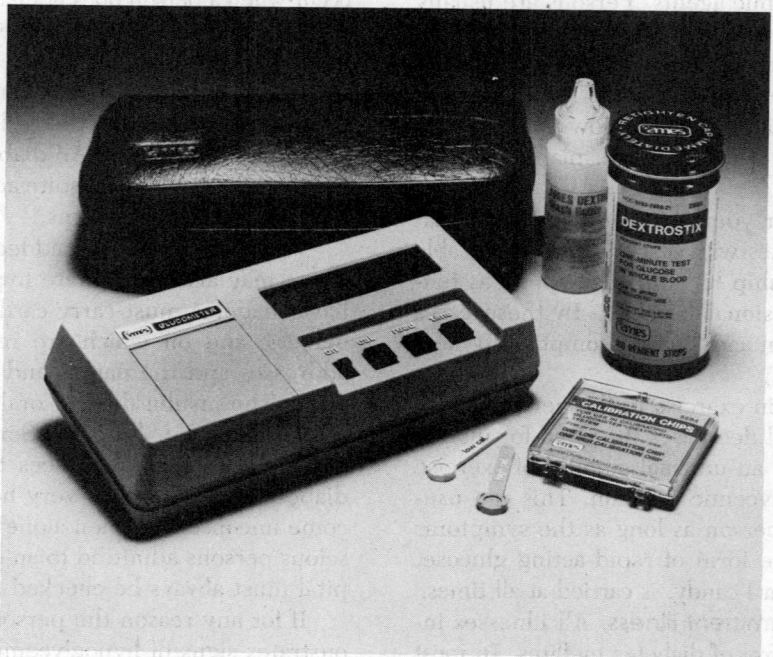

Fig. 32-13. Glucometer to measure blood glucose levels at home. Reflectance photometer to the left, calibration chips, wash bottle, Dextrosticks, and leatherette case. (Courtesy Ames Division, Miles Laboratories, Elkhart, Ind.)

priate. Over time the person is taught how to increase or decrease the insulin dose independently.

Prevention of infection. Persons with diabetes are more susceptible to infection. The effectiveness of the skin as a first line of defense is diminished. Uncontrolled diabetes leads to loss of fat deposits under the skin, loss of glycogen, and catabolism of body proteins. Protein loss can hamper the inflammatory response and wound healing. In addition, leukocyte function, migration of leukocytes to the site of infection, phagocytosis, and bacterial killing, all of which are involved in the ability of the body to combat infection, are impaired. Decreased circulation to the part can also delay healing. The skin must be kept supple and as free of pathogenic organisms as possible. This is especially true in warm moist areas that encourage growth of the organisms (i.e., between the toes, under the breasts, and in the axillae and groin). It is therefore very important that persons with diabetes carry out hygienic measures for prevention of infection, with special emphasis on good foot care (p. 1149). They should also avoid persons with upper respiratory tract infections. These persons must be taught to seek medical attention immediately if an infection occurs.

Exercise. All persons with diabetes need regular exercise, and this should be discussed with them as part of the overall treatment plan. Those receiving insulin or oral hypoglycemic agents should understand that the amount of medication as well as diet prescribed by the physician is planned around their usual exercise pattern. An increase in activity will decrease the need for insulin or the hypoglycemic agents. Persons are usually taught to increase their dietary intake by eating a quick-acting form of glucose just before starting activities that are more strenuous than usual. In some instances physicians will teach those taking insulin how they may reduce their insulin dose when they are planning more exercise than usual.

It may be helpful for young diabetics to know that several well-known athletes with diabetes have been able to perform at championship level in such sports as tennis, hockey, and professional baseball. In these cases they adjusted their insulin and food consumption to meet their athletic schedule.

Because an increase in exercise in the person whose diabetes is under control decreases the need for insulin or hypoglycemic agents, an unusual amount of exercise can precipitate a hypoglycemic reaction. This can usually be handled by the person as long as the symptoms are recognized and some form of rapid-acting glucose, such as sugar cubes or hard candy, is carried at all times.

Care during an intermittent illness. All illnesses influence the status of control of diabetes mellitus. In most instances the person with diabetes needs increased insulin in the presence of a concurrent illness, especially an infection. Yet many mistakenly believe that if they cannot eat, they do not need to take the prescribed insulin or oral hypoglycemic agent. Optimally, the individual should take calories and CHO in a liquid form such as soups, broths, or soft drinks and take the normal dose of insulin. The diet should be advanced toward the normally prescribed diet as soon as possible. The person should also institute urine or blood glucose monitoring on a more frequent basis. For example, at least every 4 hours urine testing for ketones should be carried out. The result of these tests will help the person make decisions about alterations needed in the diabetic regimen.

The person should know when the primary health care provider should be called. Each person will receive individual instructions, but in general the primary health care provider should be called if any of the following occur: (1) a full day's urine glucose results are at maximal readings or blood glucose levels are consistently elevated beyond a specified level, (2) ketones are present in the urine, (3) the person is not able to take *any* food or fluids, (4) the person has been unable to eat normally for longer than 4 hours, or (5) the person has a fever.

Metabolic complications of diabetes

Hypoglycemic reactions. Hypoglycemia is a major metabolic complication that can occur in any person with diabetes who is treated with insulin or oral hypoglycemic agents. Severe reactions are usually caused by too little food or too large a dose of insulin or of an oral hypoglycemic agent or a combination of these two events. Hypoglycemia can occur when a person does not eat all the prescribed food or skips between meal or bedtime feedings. Sometimes the individual increases the dosage of insulin to cover excessive eating, and the amount of insulin taken may be greater than needed. At other times the cause of hypoglycemia cannot be ascertained. All diabetics may experience hypoglycemic reactions despite adherence to diet, medication, and exercise regimens.

Vomiting, diarrhea, added exercise, or emotional stress may also precipitate hypoglycemia. Persons who have diabetes must carry cards that state that they are diabetic and on which are recorded their names and addresses and the names and addresses of their physicians. The insulin dose or oral antidiabetic drug dosage is also listed on the card. Some diabetics wear Medic Alert bracelets or necklaces that alert others to their diabetic status. This is very helpful if they faint or become unconscious when alone in a public place. Unconscious persons admitted to an emergency room of a hospital must always be checked for such identification.

If for any reason the person who is a diabetic demonstrates signs of hypoglycemia, additional food should be given or taken. Many persons with diabetes carry lump sugar or hard candies to be eaten in such emergencies. If the person is at home, a glass of orange juice, other fruit juice, ginger ale, or any other readily available source of glucose may be taken. Sometimes hypoglycemia comes on suddenly, and the person may not sense early signs. In such an instance a family member may have to give the orange juice or some other sweet fluid. One of the safest ways to administer sugar to a groggy person is to place a teaspoonful of corn syrup or honey in the person's mouth. This will be rapidly absorbed by the mucous membrane of the oral mucosa, and the person will usually arouse sufficiently to be able to drink a glass of juice or sweetened coffee or tea.

The signs and symptoms of hypoglycemia can be related to two factors: increased sympathetic activity and the effects of low blood glucose levels on the central nervous system. The signs and symptoms are listed in the box at right. The signs and symptoms seen in any particular person will vary with the individual and with the type of insulin, if insulin is being used. In slow-developing hypoglycemia, such as might result when intermediate or long-acting insulin is used, the central nervous system signs and symptoms predominate. Although the type of signs and symptoms seen may vary, the pattern in a given person is usually the same and the person can generally tell when hypoglycemia is occurring. Hypoglycemia can occur during sleep, particularly in patients on intermediate and long-acting insulin; and the only symptoms may be nightmares, sweating, and headache upon arising. Nighttime hypoglycemia may be part of the *Somogyi phenomenon* (p. 662).

Symptoms similar to those seen in hypoglycemia may occur when the blood glucose level is elevated and drops raipdly to a level that is still within the elevated range. The sudden rapid drop in blood sugar, regardless of the final level reached or the levels at which this occurs, is a stimulus for the neuroendocrine integrating mechanisms (see Chapter 18) to come into play. Thus, a patient whose glucose level goes from 500 mg/100 ml to 300 mg/100 ml very rapidly may demonstrate the same signs and symptoms as a patient whose glucose drops to 30 mg/100 ml. Frequently patients with uncontrolled diabetes may complain of feeling hypoglycemic, even though their plasma glucose levels are high. The patient is often labeled as a "malingerer" or "uncooperative" because the health team may believe that the patient is trying to obtain more food. The nurse who is aware of the above phenomena may be able to help others understand the patient's complaints and help avoid such labeling.

The treatment for hypoglycemia is carbohydrates. If a question exists concerning the validity of the diabetic's feeling about an impending insulin reaction, blood should be drawn immediately for a blood sugar test and *sugar given at once*. The nurse should understand that when in doubt, it is always safer to give sugar than to risk nervous system damage from hypoglycemia. Usually 20 to 25 g of carbohydrate will be sufficient to over-

SIGNS AND SYMPTOMS OF HYPOGLYCEMIA

Sympathetic nervous system activity

Pallor

Perspiration

Piloerection

Tachycardia

Palpitation

Nervousness

Irritability

Weakness

Trembling

Hunger

Central nervous system activity

Headache

Blurred vision

Diplopia

Incoherent speech

Emotional changes

Fatigue

Numbness of lips, tongue

Mental confusion

Convulsions

Coma

come hypoglycemia. This can be obtained from 8 oz of fruit juice or sweetened soft drinks, 4 teaspoons of sugar, 2 tablespoons of syrup, or 4 pieces of hard candy. If the individual is already unconscious, 50% glucose will usually be given intravenously. When the person's symptoms have passed, a snack consisting of complex carbohydrates and proteins such as cheese or peanut butter and crackers should be given. If the next meal is due soon, it should be eaten instead of the snack.

Glucagon, a pancreatic hormone that acts primarily by mobilizing hepatic glycogen, may be given to treat insulin reactions. The effects of this glycogen conversion last about 1½ hours, and therefore treatment with sugar, complex carbohydrates, and proteins will also be required to prevent a recurrence of the hypoglycemia. Glucagon is given intramuscularly, and some physicians instruct their patients to take it when an insulin reaction occurs. If the patient is unconscious, the family administers the drug and then seeks medical assistance.

The reason hypoglycemia is so serious is that hypoglycemia interferes with the oxygen consumption of nervous tissue. Repeated or prolonged attacks can cause irreparable brain damage.

Somogyi phenomenon. The Somogyi phenomenon is a reaction characterized by alternating hypoglycemic reactions and periods of hyperglycemia. This phenomenon is most frequently seen during initial periods of blood glucose regulation. The person being treated with intermediate or long-acting insulin may experience hypoglycemia at peak times of insulin activity. As is true with healthy nondiabetic persons, hypoglycemia stimulates the production of counterregulatory hormones (glucagon, ACTH, glucocorticoids, growth hormone, and catecholamines). These hormones promote glycogenolysis and gluconeogenesis. In normal persons the blood glucose level is brought only to the normal range because, as it is elevated, insulin secretion would be stimulated and the blood glucose level lowered. In persons with diabetes, the blood glucose goes to abnormally high levels because insulin secretion does not respond in the normal way. Very frequently the signs and symptoms of the hypoglycemia are not obvious enough to be detected. In many instances the hypoglycemia occurs at night and is undetected. The hyperglycemia is recognized in the early morning and the assumption is made that the patient needs higher doses of insulin, but this treatment just worsens the problem.

The signs and symptoms of the *Somogyi phemonenon* can be those normally seen with hypoglycemia, but frequently they consist only of nighttime sweats, nightmares, and a headache on arising. There may be weight gain in the presence of glycosuria, negative urine glucose with positive ketones (remember that counter-regulatory hormones stimulate lipolysis and β-oxidation of fats), and wide fluctuations in blood and urine glucose unrelated to meals.

Treatment consists of decreasing the insulin dosage. A primary nursing role is to document complaints of hypoglycemia, glucose intake, and laboratory results, and in particular to look for complaints of night sweats, nightmares, and early morning headaches. The nurse should also correlate these complaints and laboratory results with the time of meals. Such data will help to identify the phenomenon. Continual monitoring of the person's response to treatment is important.

Diabetic ketoacidosis. Diabetic ketoacidosis is one of the major metabolic complications of diabetes mellitus. It is most frequently seen in persons with insulin-dependent diabetes mellitus. Although unusual, it can occur in persons with non-insulin-dependent diabetes. It also can occur in gestational diabetes mellitus and diabetes associated with other problems.

ETIOLOGY. Acute insulin insufficiency is the cause of diabetic ketoacidosis. It is usually precipitated in the known diabetic by stressors that increase insulin needs, although it may occur when diabetes is out of control because of noncompliance with prescribed therapy. The most frequent precipitating factor is an infection, such as those of the urinary or respiratory tracts. Other major stressors that can precipitate diabetic ketoacidosis are surgery, trauma, major illnesses, therapy with steroids, and emotional upset. Occasionally, diabetic ketoacidosis will be the presenting problem in persons with undiagnosed diabetes.

PATHOPHYSIOLOGY. Diabetic ketoacidosis occurs when there is insufficient insulin for appropriate metabolism of glucose, fats, and proteins. When this happens (as explained on p. 644), glucose is not utilized appropriately, resulting in hyperglycemia. In addition, gluconeogenesis and glycogenolysis also occur and add to the hyperglycemia. Glycosuria results when the glucose threshhold is exceeded. The glycosuria results in osmotic diuresis with the excretion of large amounts of water and electrolytes, and dehydration. The loss of sodium prevents the formation of sodium bicarbonate and the alkali reserve is decreased. Proteins are broken down for the gluconeogenesis, causing liberation of potassium and an increase in urea nitrogen. Fats are broken down for energy in the absence of insulin. This process occurs faster than complete metabolism can occur and ketone bodies accumulate. The increase in acid sources calls on the alkali reserve to combat acidosis, thus furthering loss of water and electrolytes as the kidneys try to maintain acid-base balance. When the alkali reserve is depleted, the pH of the blood decreases. The decreased pH stimulates the compensatory mechanisms (p. 353). The kidneys attempt to excrete even more acids, worsening the dehydration and electrolyte balance. The lungs compensate by excreting hydrogen ions in the form of carbon dioxide. Since the acid products (ketones) continue to be formed, compensation can usually not completely correct the acidosis, and the pH remains low. The end result of the water loss is hemoconcentration and hyperosmolality. This can cause tissue hypoxia. In the presence of hypoxia, increased lactic acid is produced, worsening the acidosis. If the process is not interrupted, the patient will lapse into coma, since hypoxia, dehydration, and acidosis interfere with the function of the central nervous system. Although the precipitating event in this metabolic crisis is acute insulin insufficiency, as mentioned in the preceding column, glucagon excess may add to the severity of the hyperglycemia and ketone buildup. See Fig. 32-14 for a summary of the pathophysiology involved.

CLINICAL PICTURE. The signs and symptoms of diabetic ketoacidosis can be directly linked to the acidosis, severe dehydration, and electrolyte imbalance. The acidosis and its compensatory mechanisms cause hyperpnea (Kussmaul's breathing), and the elimination of ketones through the respiratory tract accounts for the fruity breath odor that may be noticeable in some persons. Acidosis can induce nausea and vomiting. The person

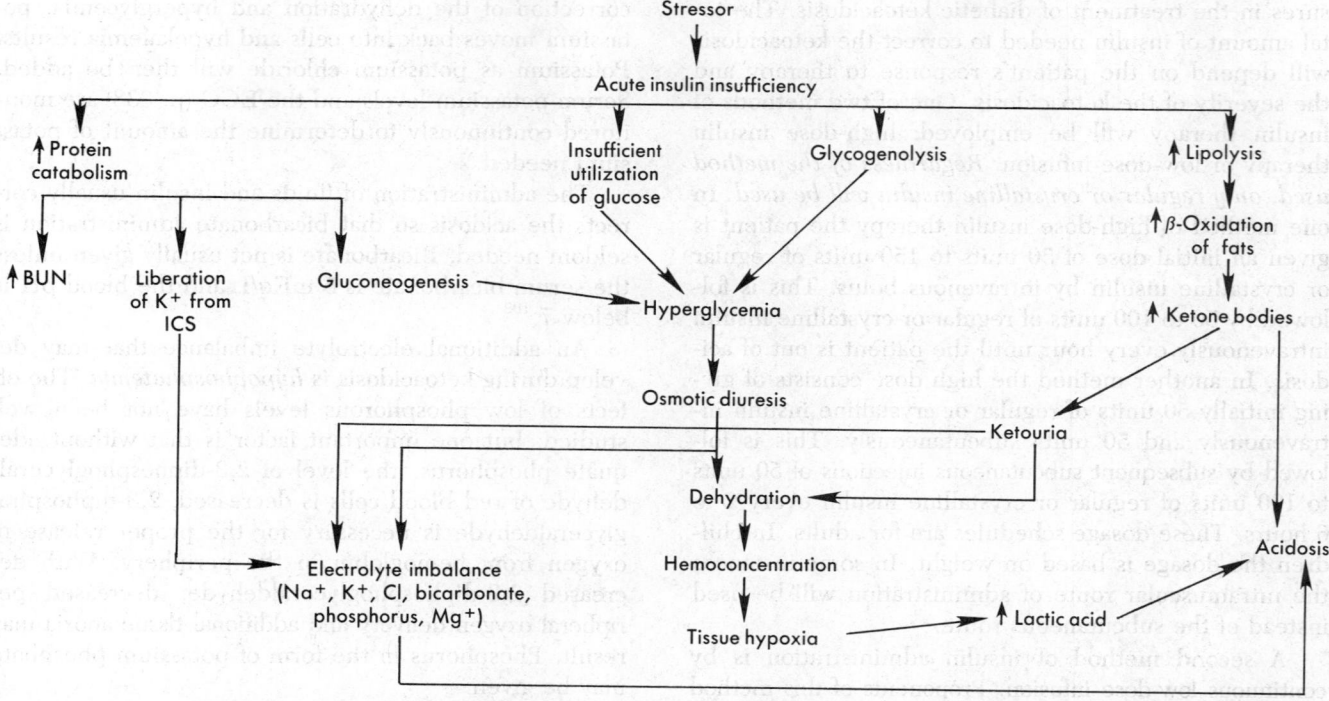

Fig. 32-14. Summary of metabolic alterations and relationship to clinical problems seen in diabetic ketoacidosis.

may come to the hospital with signs and symptoms of an acute abdomen, but this is usually a result of the nausea, vomiting, and electrolyte imbalances. Dehydration causes the following characteristic changes: dry mucous membranes, loss of skin turgor, increased thirst (in conscious patients), red, parched lips and tongue, and soft or sunken eyeballs. Hypovolemic shock, which can result from the dehydration, is common. The systolic blood pressure may be as low as 60 to 70 mm Hg. The patient, if not treated, will become anuric, and circulatory collapse can occur. Other signs and symptoms that result from a combination of dehydration, acidosis, and electrolyte imbalance are weakness, fatigue, general malaise, headache, and flushed face. Body temperature is usually elevated but will decrease with treatment.

The diagnosis and severity of the patient's condition are determined by laboratory tests. The serum glucose level usually exceeds 500 mg/100 ml, but may be lower. The urine glucose value, if renal threshold is not altered, will be 5%. Urine tests for ketones will be strongly positive and the blood ketone level will also be positive. Blood is tested for ketonemia as follows: first, the patient's blood, undiluted, is tested for a 4 + ketone reading. Then the patients' plasma is diluted to determine the extent of the ketonemia. The greater the number of dilutions in which ketones remain 4 +, the more severe the ketoacidosis. Most patients' serum ketones are elevated to 3 or more dilutions of the serum. These dilu-

tions are converted to an approximation of the acetone values per 100 ml of blood. Values over 50 mg/100 ml are considered severe ketosis, while those 80 mg or over are considered to be evidence of clinical coma.

Serum electrolytes at initial diagnosis do not usually depict the true body levels because hemoconcentration masks the loss. The initial serum potassium level is usually elevated, although the total body potassium level is low. As osmotic diuresis occurs, potassium is liberated from the intracellular space and extracellular potassium levels will appear elevated. With correction of dehydration and hyperglycemia, the potassium level will return to normal. Serum sodium levels are often normal initially because of hemoconcentration, but there is a total sodium deficit because of the osmotic diuresis. The serum chloride and bicarbonate levels are also low because of the acidosis. The anion gap (p. 352) is usually greater than 20 mEq/L. The blood urea nitrogen level is usually increased because of the protein breakdown, dehydration, and decreased filtration. The patient will usually have increased triglyceride levels and hyperlipidemia. Tissue enzymes may be elevated.

INTERVENTION. Diabetic ketoacidosis is a medical emergency that requires intensive nursing care. Therapy is directed towards correction of the hyperglycemia, dehydration, electrolyte imbalances, acidosis, and other precipitating factors. All of these interventions will be carried out simultaneously.

Insulin therapy is one of the main therapeutic measures in the treatment of diabetic ketoacidosis. The total amount of insulin needed to correct the ketoacidosis will depend on the patient's response to therapy and the severity of the ketoacidosis. One of two methods of insulin therapy will be employed: high-dose insulin therapy or low-dose infusion. *Regardless of the method used, only regular or crystalline insulin will be used*. In one method of high-dose insulin therapy the patient is given an initial dose of 50 units to 150 units of regular or crystalline insulin by intravenous bolus. This is followed by 50 to 100 units of regular or crystalline insulin intravenously every hour until the patient is out of acidosis. In another method the high dose consists of giving initially 50 units of regular or crystalline insulin intravenously and 50 units subcutaneously. This is followed by subsequent subcutaneous injections of 50 units to 100 units of regular or crystalline insulin every 2 to 6 hours. These dosage schedules are for adults. In children the dosage is based on weight. In some instances the intramuscular route of administration will be used instead of the subcutaneous route.

A second method of insulin administration is by continuous low-dose infusion. Proponents of this method feel that it allows the delivery of insulin at rates that maintain serum levels closely approximating those of normal persons, avoids peaks and valleys in the insulin levels, and allows for a constant, predictable rate of decrease in blood glucose so that hypoglycemia can be avoided. With this method regular or crystalline insulin is added to intravenous fluids and infused at a rate of 4 to 12 units per hour. The initial infusion is usually preceded by an intravenous bolus of 10 units of regular or crystalline insulin.

The high-dose or low-dose insulin therapy is continued until the acidosis is corrected and the serum glucose level is 200 to 300 mg/100 ml. When these two conditions are met, the patient is given small doses of rapid-acting insulin to maintain control. Once the patient is stable, a normal regimen of diet, exercise, and insulin, if necessary, will be started. Serum and urinary glucose levels are continuously monitored.

To correct the dehydration and sodium deficit normal saline or 0.45% saline (half-strength normal saline) solution is given intravenously. Initially, the saline is infused rapidly and may be started at a rate of 1 L/hr in adults without cardiac or renal failure. When the urine output is 1 to 2 ml/min[120] and the blood pressure is stable, the rate is reduced to 1 L in 2 to 4 hours. The usual fluid deficit is 3 to 5 L. When the blood glucose level falls to 300 mg/100 ml, 5% glucose solutions (D_5NS, $D_5\frac{1}{2}NS$, etc.) are used. The patient must be monitored very carefully for signs and symptoms of fluid overload and hypoglycemia.

Potassium is not initially added to the intravenous fluids because the patient's potassium serum level is usually elevated at the beginning of therapy. With the correction of the dehydration and hyperglycemia, potassium moves back into cells and hypokalemia results. Potassium as potassium chloride will then be added. Serum potassium levels and the ECG (p. 338) are monitored continuously to determine the amount of potassium needed.

The administration of fluids and insulin usually corrects the acidosis so that bicarbonate administration is seldom needed. Bicarbonate is not usually given unless the serum bicarbonate is 5 mEq/L and the blood pH is below 7.[102]

An additional electrolyte imbalance that may develop during ketoacidosis is *hypophosphatemia*. The effects of low phosphorous levels have not been well studied, but one important factor is that without adequate phosphorus, the level of 2,3-diphosphoglyceraldehyde of red blood cells is decreased; 2,3-diphosphoglyceraldehyde is necessary for the proper release of oxygen from hemoglobin in the periphery. With decreased 2,3-diphosphoglyceraldehyde, decreased peripheral oxygen delivery and additional tissue anoxia may result. Phosphorus in the form of potassium phosphate may be given.

The nursing interventions planned for the patient depend on the severity of the ketoacidosis and the prescribed therapy. One thing all patients require is careful, frequent monitoring of vital signs, level of consciousness, and intake and output. In addition, the patient should be monitored for resolution of other signs and symptoms of dehydration and acidosis and for signs and symptoms of fluid overload. Urine and blood specimens are obtained frequently and checked for glucose and ketones. Other blood specimens will need to be obtained to check for electrolytes and pH levels. The nurse must make sure that the specimens are collected as ordered and that the appropriate tests are done. It is important that the nurse monitor the results of the tests. The assessments made by the nurse and the results of laboratory tests will be used to make appropriate adjustments in therapy. A flow sheet with all pertinent laboratory and assessment data should be instituted so that all changes in the patient's status are displayed in a readily comprehensible manner.

As the patient's condition improves, the serum ketone levels will decrease and the blood glucose level will return to normal. At this time the patient must be monitored closely for signs and symptoms of hypoglycemia. It should be remembered that blood levels of ketone and sugar will return to normal before urinary levels will. When the patient is able to take fluids by mouth, fruit juices, broth, cooked cereal, and milk will be given. Solid foods are added as soon as possible to improve gastric tone and prevent further ileus.

As the patient recovers, the cause of the acidosis should be reviewed so that the patient understands how to avoid a recurrence.

The patient or the family should contact the physician at once if any signs or symptoms of acidosis occur. Carrying a card stating that the person has diabetes helps to ensure prompt treatment in the event that coma develops while the person is away from home. Such a card also helps prevent this condition from being mistaken for head injury, cerebrovascular accident, or drunkenness.

Hyperglycemic, hyperosmolar, nonketotic coma. Another major metabolic complication is hyperglycemic, hyperosmolar, nonketotic coma (HHNC). This complication is approximately one sixth as frequent as diabetic ketoacidosis.[72] Most patients admitted with HHNC are elderly persons with a history of non-insulin-dependent diabetes, but a number of such patients have no prior history of diabetes.[72] The mortality for HHNC is very high (40% to 60%).

ETIOLOGY. In most instances HHNC is associated with another major illness. The most common associated illnesses are gram-negative infections such as pneumonia and pyelonephritis, uremia, lactic acidosis, myocardial infarction, gastrointestinal hemorrhage, subdural hematoma, pancreatitis, and arterial thrombosis.[196] HHNC has also been associated with various medications and therapeutic interventions such as diuretics, glucocorticoids, peritoneal dialysis, and tube feedings.

PATHOPHYSIOLOGY. HHNC is a syndrome of profound hyperglycemia and dehydration without ketosis and ketoacidosis. The cause of the hyperglycemia is the same as that of diabetic ketoacidosis, but in this instance the hyperglycemia is more severe (often greater than 1000 mg/100 ml) and causes osmotic diuresis and depletion of extracellular fluid volume and hyperosmolality. In addition, the fluid depletion and hyperosmolality are worsened because the patient, as a result of associated illnesses, is unable to replace any of the excess fluid loss with oral intake. The hyperosmolality results in a fluid shift, pulling fluid from the intracellular space, and intracellular dehydration occurs. The reasons for the lack of ketoacid formation are unknown. It was originally believed that patients with HHNC secreted enough insulin to prevent lipolysis, but research has shown that there is no difference in the basal insulin levels of patients with HHNC and those with ketoacidosis. Another hypothesis is that patients with HHNC have lower levels of free fatty acids, limiting substrate availability. A third hypothesis is that patients with HHNC, although they do not have higher insulin levels, have higher portal venous concentrations of insulin, thus preventing activation of the enzymatic machinery necessary for ketone formation.

CLINICAL PICTURE. Clinically, the patient has blood glucose levels of 1000 mg/100 ml or higher, a urine glucose of 5%, and a serum osmolality of 370 to 380 mosmols/L. Signs and symptoms of dehydration, similar to those seen in ketoacidosis (p. 662), are present. Vascular collapse may be present. One of the major characteristics of HHNC is the accompanying neurologic signs and symptoms. The most common neurologic signs and symptoms are hemisensory and motor deficits and focal seizures. The patient's level of consciousness varies from states of lethargy and confusion to coma. Many other neurologic deficits such as aphasia, nystagmus, hyperthermia, hyperreflexia, and nuchal rigidity, may be present. The most common laboratory changes, in addition to those described earlier are normal to high serum sodium, normal to high chloride, elevated potassium, and an elevated blood urea nitrogen (BUN) level greater than 60 mg/100 ml. The BUN level is higher than that seen in ketoacidosis because of the more severe gluconeogenesis and dehydration. In addition, the patient frequently has some underlying renal insufficiency. Although ketoacidosis is not present, most patients will have a slightly depressed pH (approximately 7.25). The acidosis can be a result of starvation, uremia, bicarbonate loss from the gastrointestinal tract or from diuretic therapy, or lactate buildup.

INTERVENTION. The patient with HHNC is critically ill and requires a very high level of care. Fluid therapy is the cornerstone of therapy. The patient with HHNC may have a fluid deficit of 8 to 12 L.[3] As much as 2 to 3 L of fluid may be required over the first 1 to 2 hours, and the patient often receives 5 to 6 L within the first 12 hours.[136] Usually half-strength normal saline solution will be used for the initial therapy, but if the patient shows signs and symptoms of vascular collapse, normal saline will be used initially. Subsequent laboratory values will determine the type of fluids used. As the glucose level nears normal, dextrose solutions will be given. As the dehydration, hyperosmolality, and hyperglycemia are treated, potassium deficits will appear and potassium will be added to the intravenous fluids. A phosphorus deficit may also be present, and replacement similar to that used in diabetic ketoacidosis is necessary.

Insulin will be used to treat the hyperglycemia, but in most instances these patients are very sensitive to insulin and require only very small amounts of it. Regular or crystalline insulin given by the subcutaneous, intramuscular, or intravenous route will be used. In most instances the total insulin dose will be 25 to 50 units. Most patients are given an initial dose of 5 to 15 units and some require no additional insulin. As soon as possible the patient is started on oral food and fluids.

The nursing care required for these patients is the same as that described for the patient with diabetic ketoacidosis (p. 662). Additional care appropriate to the underlying illness will be required. On recovery the patient has teaching needs similar to those for any patient with diabetes. See Table 32-10 for a summary of

TABLE 32-10. Summary of differences between hypoglycemia, diabetic ketoacidosis, and HHNC

Factors	Hypoglycemia	Diabetic ketoacidosis	HHNC
Onset	Rapid	Slow	Slow
Precipitating factors			
Food	Insufficient	Excessive	Excessive
Complications	None	Infection	Infection
Insulin	Excess	Too little	Too little or normal
Exercise	↑	Too little	Nonsignificant factor
Symptoms			
Thirst	Absent	↑	↑
Vomiting	Absent	Frequent	Frequent
Hunger	Frequent	Absent	Absent
Abdominal pain	Absent	Frequent	Not a major complaint
Vision	Double	Dim	Dim
Signs			
Temperature	Normal or ↓	↑	↑
Respirations	Normal	Hyperpnea (Kussmaul's breathing, acetone odor to breath)	Depressed
Blood pressure	Normal or ↑	Lowered, may be in hypovolemic shock	Lowered, may be in hypovolemic shock
Skin	Moist and pale	Hot, dry flushed	Hot, dry
Dehydration	None	Loss of skin turgor, sunken eyeballs	Loss of skin turgor, sunken eyeballs
Neurologic signs	Tremors frequent, syncope → coma	Lethargy → coma	Multiple, major signs
Laboratory findings			
Urine			
Glycosuria	Negative	5%	5%
Ketonuria	Negative	Highly positive	Usually negative
Blood sugar	↓	↑ above 200 mg/100 ml	↑ >1000 mg/100 ml
Ketones	Normal	↑	Usually negative
Electrolytes	Normal	↓ except serum K+, which will ↑ as treatment begins and ↓ later with treatment	↑ Cl+, Na+ because of loss of ECF K+ normal to ↑; as H_2O replaced, Na^+ and Cl^- return to normal
Treatment	Glucose supplement	↑ Insulin, fluids, electrolytes	↑ Insulin, fluids, electrolytes

the differences between hypoglycemia, DKA, and HHNC.

Long-term complications

The person with diabetes is susceptible to a number of long-term complications resulting from macrovascular changes, microvascular changes, and neuropathy. The resulting effects of these changes include cardiovascular disease, renal failure, blindness, and diabetic gangrene. These three types of changes will be described briefly and then the major systemic effects of the pathologies will be discussed.

Macrovascular changes. Diabetics develop macrovascular changes caused by atherosclerosis that are the same as those seen in nondiabetics. However, it is well known that diabetics are prone to develop atherosclerosis at an earlier age and that the disease progresses faster and is more severe and extensive in diabetics than in nondiabetics. The exact mechanism underlying the formation of atheromatous lesions is unknown, but probably involves the interaction of many factors. It has been hypothesized that the initial event involves endothelial injury, which is followed by the proliferation of smooth muscle cells with an accumulation of intracellular matrix. Endothelial lesions can result from mechanical and chemical factors such as hypertensive lipid disorders, tissue hypoxia, and possibly hyperglycemia. The smooth muscle cell proliferation, lipid accumulation, and extracellular matrix formation which follow are accelerated by various factors such as presence of abnormal lipids, tissue hypoxia, platelet changes, and hormonal changes. Diabetes is associated with various of these atherogenic factors in addition to the hyperglycemia and hormonal changes.

Insulin plays a major role in the metabolism of fats and lipids. Lipid disorders are frequently found in persons with diabetes mellitus. The hyperlipoproteinemia seen in diabetes is usually identified as type IV or type V and is often the result of an excess of very low density lipoproteins (p. 643).[15] In addition, diabetes is considered to be a contributing factor in the development of hypertension. The patient with diabetes mellitus needs teaching not only with regards to control of the diabetes but also with regards to control of the risk factors for complications.

Microvascular changes. In addition to the macrovascular changes previously discussed, microvascular changes characterized by thickening and damage to the basement membrane of the capillaries may occur. These changes do not occur in nondiabetics. The causes of these changes are unknown but are felt to be related to uncontrolled diabetes.[83] Various factors such as the role of protein fractions, glycoproteins, lipids, and lipoproteins have been studied, but no conclusive evidence is yet available about the relationship between these factors and the microvascular changes seen in persons with diabetes.

Neuropathy. All persons with type I and type II diabetes have one or more alterations that affect peripheral nerves, the autonomic nervous system, the spinal cord, or the central nervous system. The neuropathies seen in diabetics result from two different processes. Neuropathies unique to diabetics may result from increased metabolism via the polyol pathway that results in an accumulation of sorbitol in nerve cells and in hyperosmolality, fluid shifts with swelling, and consequent rupture and destruction of the cell.[38,234] In addition, other factors such as decreased nerve myoinositol and altered myelin synthesis may be involved. Diabetics as well as nondiabetics may develop neuropathies as a result of vitamin deficiencies and electrolyte disturbances.[38] In the neuropathies, found in diabetic patients sensory fibers are usually affected first, then motor fibers. Most diabetics have mixed (sensory and motor) polyneuropathy of the lower extremities.

Cardiovascular changes. The macrovascular changes result in cerebrovascular disease and coronary artery disease. Approximately three fourths of all cerebrovascular accidents are related to diabetes; myocardial infarction is the most common cause of death among older diabetics.[16] Microvascular changes can cause cardiomyopathy. The signs and symptoms, problems, complications, and medical and nursing interventions for diabetics with these problems are the same as they are for nondiabetics. The nurse must keep in mind that the underlying diabetes must be controlled for the best recovery from the cardiovascular complications. Likewise the cardiovascular complications will make the diabetes more difficult to control.

Renal changes. One of the major results of the microvascular changes is alterations in renal structure and function. Renal failure frequently results from these changes in structure and function. Four types of lesions can occur: (1) *pyelonephritis*, (2) *glomerular lesions*, (3) *arteriosclerosis of the renal arteries* and *afferent and efferent arterioles*, and (4) *tubular lesions*. The pyelonephritis seen in diabetics is similar to that seen in nondiabetics and is treated in the same way.

Three types of glomerular lesions can occur. *Diffuse glomerulosclerosis* resulting in severe proteinuria and renal failure is one type of glomerular lesion. A second type is *nodular glomerulosclerosis (Kimmelstiel-Wilson syndrome)*, which involves nodular masses of laminated hyaline material that occur randomly throughout the kidney and result in a *nephrotic syndrome* with *proteinuria, edema,* and *hypertension*. This lesion is found only in diabetics and occurs in 10% to 35% of all persons with diabetes. A third type of glomerular lesion is an exudative one in which *eosinophilic fibrinoid deposits* are found in Bowman's capsule or over the outer surface of glomerular capillary loops. These glomerular lesions along with arteriosclerosis obliterate vascular channels and glomeruli and lead to *renal failure*. Tubular lesions result from deposits of glycogen, fat, and mucopolysaccharides within the epithelial cells of the distal tubules and the descending loop of Henle.

The progression of renal disease varies from individual to individual. An early sign of a glomerular lesion is *proteinuria* which gradually increases in severity. As renal insufficiency develops the serum creatinine and urea levels increase and other signs and symptoms of renal insufficiency (see p. 1570) appear. The treatment and nursing care for the renal insufficiency seen in diabetes are the same as for nondiabetics. It is important to remember that as renal insufficiency occurs, the patient on insulin may require less insulin because insulin will be excreted more slowly.

Vision changes. Blindness is a frequent complication of diabetes; diabetes is the leading cause of blindness in persons between the ages of 20 and 65. The blindness can result from *cataracts* or *retinopathy*. The cataracts may be caused by prolonged hyperglycemia, resulting in polyol increased metabolism via the polyol pathway with increased sorbital formation and intralens hyperosmolality, swelling, and opacity formation. Cataracts are treated the same in diabetics as in nondiabetics (p. 892).

Retinopathy causes the greatest amount of visual impairment in the diabetic. The primary lesion is the formation of microaneurysms in the retinal vessels. The microaneurysms are followed by hemorrhage and exudate formation. These early retinal changes may progress to a more serious stage—*proliferative retinopathy*. In proliferative retinopathy there is the formation of new blood vessels on the retina. These new vessels bleed causing vitreous hemorrhage and retinal detachment. The bleeding is usually repetitive and causes permanent loss of vision.

There are no symptoms of early retinal changes, and patients with diabetes should be encouraged to have yearly eye examinations or eye examinations at all outpatient visits.

The treatment for retinopathy has included various measures. Procedures such as adrenalectomy and hypophysectomy have been used in the past in an attempt to interfere with the process. *Photocoagulation,* the use of thermal energy, is the treatment most frequently employed now to control retinopathy. Photocoagulation results in protein denaturation and a therapeutic burn, which seals capillary leaks and destroys new vessels. This treatment is very frequently performed on an outpatient basis.

Vitrectomy, the removal of vitreous humor that has been infiltrated by hemorrhage, is another treatment for retinopathy. The vitreous humor removed is replaced by saline. Improved vision is seen in 50% to 75% of the patients who have vitrectomies.[19]

All nurses working with persons with diabetes should continually monitor them for visual changes. In addition to making appropriate referrals, the nurse working with the diabetic experiencing visual loss must help the person make adaptations in self-care routines.

Lower extremity changes. The macrovascular changes, microvascular changes, and neuropathies all cause changes in the lower extremities. Diabetics develop gangrene five times more frequently than nondiabetics. The anesthesia resulting from loss of sensory nerve function contributes to minor trauma and infections that can go undetected and result in gangrene. The infections start in cracks in hypertrophied skin, ingrown toenails, corns, and calluses as well as in traumatized areas. Healing is retarded because of the vascular changes.

The gangrene that results may be dry or wet. *Dry gangrene* occurs when tissue death is not associated with inflammatory changes. Autoamputation of toes affected with dry gangrene is the treatment of choice. The area is kept dry during the process. Close monitoring for signs of infection or extension of the gangrene is necessary.

Wet gangrene is gangrene coupled with inflammation. *Septicemia* and *septic shock* may occur. Bed rest, antibiotic therapy, appropriate cleansing and debridement, and continuous monitoring for signs of extension are the preliminary treatment. Various diagnostic tests to determine the extent of the lesion, status of the circulation, and presence of bone involvement are done. Very frequently amputation will be required. (See Chapter 46 for care of the patient experiencing an amputation.)

Prevention of ulcers, trauma, and infections of the lower extremities is the key to prevention of these complications. Ulcers, injured areas, and infections heal very slowly. The following measures will help to prevent these problems: (1) Persons with diabetes should wear well-fitting shoes and clean stockings at all times when ambulating and should never walk barefooted. (2) They should bathe their feet daily and dry them well, paying particular attention to areas between the toes. (3) Patients should not self-treat calluses, corns, or ingrown

toe nails; a podiatrist should be consulted if these are present. (4) Bath water should be 85° to 90° F and should be tested with a bath thermometer or the elbow before immersing the feet. (5) Heating pads and hot water bottles should not be used. (6) Measures that help increase circulation to the lower extremities should be instituted. These include not smoking, not sitting with legs crossed, appropriate protection of extremities when exposed to cold, not immersing the feet in cold water, not using elastic stockings, socks with elastic tops, or panty girdles that constrict circulation to the lower extremities, and the institution of a regimen of exercises (see Chapter 46, p. 1147). (7) Patients should be instructed to visually inspect their feet at least once per week. If they are unable to do this, someone else must do it. Any cuts, cracks, redness, blisters, or other signs of trauma should be reported immediately so that early treatment can be instituted and hopefully prevent more serious damage.

Other changes. The diabetic may develop neuropathies that affect the autonomic nervous system and result in gastric motility changes that lead to unpredictable and irregular absorption of food and bowel incontinence. (See Chapter 58 for a discussion of care of the patient who has bowel incontinence.) *Urinary incontinence* may also result from changes in the autonomic nervous system. Prompt recognition and treatment for this is essential to prevent urinary tract infections. See Chapter 61 for a discussion of the care of patients with urinary incontinence. *Impotence* resulting from destruction of autonomic fibers is often a complaint. Diabetics very frequently will not share this complaint with the nurse because of embarrassment. Careful, frank questioning by the nurse will often allow the individual to express concern about this problem so that appropriate rehabilitation can be instituted. See Chapter 67 for a discussion on sexual counseling.

Although all late complications have specific treatment measures as discussed, a primary nursing role is to help the person with diabetes mellitus maintain normal weight and euglycemia (normal blood glucose). These persons also need to be taught the need for regular follow-up care so that *early* signs and symptoms of complications will be recognized and treated and more severe complications avoided. This will help prevent hospitalization and time lost from work and may allow such persons to use their energy doing things they enjoy.

Outcome criteria for the person with diabetes mellitus

The person or significant others can:
1. Explain the metabolic alterations that occur in diabetes mellitus.
2. Explain signs and symptoms of hyperglycemia and hypoglycemia and what to do when these occur.

3. Explain the daily plan of care at home.
4. State dietary regimen prescribed and demonstrate the use of an appropriate method (exchange list, point system, etc.) in calculating daily dietary intake.
5. Describe medications being used and how to take them (if on medications).
6. If on insulin, state the dosage and demonstrate the appropriate technique for drawing up and administering insulin.
7. If on insulin, state the dosage and describe where it is stored, the sites used for administration, and the need to rotate sites.
8. Test urine or blood accurately.
9. Describe what to do if abnormal glucose is present.
10. Demonstrate proper foot care.
11. Show the Medic Alert bracelet, or necklace or identification card the patient will wear or carry at all times.
12. State the plan for regular follow-up care.
13. Describe situations requiring immediate medical care.

Summary of the teaching needs of the person with diabetes mellitus

The many teaching needs of the person with diabetes mellitus have been discussed in various parts of this section. The nurse is usually responsible for seeing that the person with diabetes mellitus gains the information, skills, and attitudes necessary for accurate self-care. Teaching is usually begun at the time the diagnosis is made, but the nurse working with the person at this time must be aware that the person cannot learn everything during the first visit. Priorities need to be set and the person should be given the skills necessary to meet their needs for a 24- to 48-hour period. The person should then be referred to a visiting nurse, community health nurse, or outpatient diabetic teaching program for continued teaching. The ability of persons to handle such information varies, depending in part on what the diagnosis of diabetes mellitus means to the person. There are multiple reports on various types of diabetic education programs in the nursing literature. All programs present similar content, but they vary in the methodology used. Research is needed to evaluate the effectiveness of these various types of programs.

The box at right presents a summary of some of the knowledge and skills that the person with diabetes must eventually master for effective self-care. Attitudes that show an appreciation and value for these self-care measures and knowledge must also be attained. Each time the nurse has contact with the person with diabetes mellitus the person's self-care habits should be assessed and reteaching given as necessary.

SUMMARY OF THE KNOWLEDGE AND SKILLS THE PERSON WITH DIABETES MELLITUS MUST LEARN FOR ADEQUATE SELF-CARE

Basic understanding of diabetes mellitus and how metabolism is changed by it

Therapeutic regimen prescribed and how it works to keep the blood sugar normal

Diet (calories, carbohydrates, etc.) ordered, how to calculate diet for each meal, ability to incorporate personal preferences

If on insulin, type, amount, time to be administered, method of administration, ability to give the insulin accurately, and ability to care for equipment properly

If on oral hypoglycemia agents, type, dosage, time schedule, and potential side effects and what to do if new or unexpected symptoms occur

Self-monitoring routine for monitoring glucose status (urine or serum glucose monitoring); how to do the tests accurately; what to do if results show hyperglycemia, ketonuria, or hypoglycemia; and how to care for equipment and supplies

Exercise and its effect on caloric and insulin needs; how to manage if exercise level is increased above usual

Signs and symptoms of hypoglycemia, how to treat them, and what to do if they occur frequently

Signs and symptoms of hyperglycemia and what to do when they occur

How to manage diabetes mellitus on days when usual diet cannot be eaten because of illness

Measures to take to prevent lower extremity trauma or injury

Type of follow-up care necessary

Who to contact with questions

Management of the person with diabetes mellitus undergoing surgery

Surgery is a physical and psychologic stressor for anyone. For the person with diabetes mellitus there are additional risks from surgery as compared with the risks to nondiabetic persons. The stressors of surgery can result in disruption of metabolic control. Persons with diabetes mellitus have an additional risk of infection because of their decreased resistance to infection and slower wound healing. Many persons with diabetes mellitus are elderly and that also increases the risks associated with surgery. If the person has already developed some of the macrovascular and microvascular complications of diabetes mellitus, those changes further increase the risks associated with surgery.

The person with diabetes mellitus faces the risk of developing hypoglycemia or hyperglycemia during the perioperative period. To understand this, a brief review of factors that change insulin needs follows. During the perioperative period, persons usually are not given anything by mouth and are given intravenous fluids. This decreases total calorie intake and may also decrease insulin needs. However, the effects of surgery on contrainsulin hormonal changes may increase the need for additional insulin, and this is the case in most persons with diabetes mellitus. The stressors of surgery cause the release of ACTH, glucocorticoids, and catecholamines, all of which elevate serum glucose.

There are many methods used to manage the person with diabetes during periods of fasting. To minimize the disruption in metabolic control, the person should be thoroughly regulated before surgery. In addition, the surgery should be scheduled for the early morning since this results in the least amount of variation from normal control measures. Diabetics are kept on their normal food and fluids and medication routine until the night before surgery.

Management of glucose in the diabetic on insulin. For the diabetic who is on insulin, one of the most commonly used perioperative protocols is to start an intravenous infusion of glucose the morning of surgery and to give one half the usual insulin dosage subcutaneously. The glucose in the intravenous infusion will usually be sufficient to cover insulin needs during the intraoperative period and prevent hypoglycemia. If the surgery is long, blood sugar levels may be checked during the surgery so that insulin or extra glucose can be given as needed.

During the postoperative period, the person is maintained by intravenous glucose infusion until food can be taken orally. Insulin is given either by dividing the normal dose equally over the 24-hour period and giving it subcutaneously or by adding regular or crystalline insulin directly to the intravenous fluids. In addition, if the person is on a standard dose of insulin, extra insulin may be administered based on urine or blood glucose checks. These checks must be carried out on an every 4-hour or every 6-hour schedule. Some patients may receive no daily insulin dose and instead will be given insulin based on the amount of glucose found in urine and blood checks.

Management of glucose in the diabetic who is not normally on insulin. Diabetics who are not normally managed with insulin will receive an intravenous infusion of glucose on the morning of surgery after being NPO during the night. Such patients may be able to meet all their usual insulin needs with their internal insulin supply, but in times of stress they may require exogenous insulin. Following surgery, blood and urine glucose and acetone levels are checked every 4 to 6 hours, and if glycosuria or hyperglycemia are present, exogenous insulin may need to be given.

All diabetics, regardless of whether they are treated with insulin or not, should receive 125 to 250 g of carbohydrates per day until their normal diet is resumed. Fewer carbohydrates than this may result in starvation ketosis. The patient's normal regimen should be reinstituted as soon as possible. Monitoring of urine and blood glucose and acetone levels should be continued on a routine basis even after the patient's usual diet is resumed since the increase in catabolism because of the surgery will continue for some time and additional insulin may still be needed. By the time patients are discharged, they should be back on their normal regimen. Other postoperative care measures are similar to those necessary for all surgery patients (see Chapter 24). Initiation of the above measures should prevent complications.

Hypoglycemic states

Hypoglycemia is that condition in which the plasma or blood glucose concentration falls to levels below normal. This can occur in diabetes mellitus as described on p. 660.

Etiology

Hypoglycemia may also result from other conditions that cause an underproduction of glucose. Hormonal deficiences (hypopituitarism, adrenal insufficiency, catecholamine deficiency, glucagon deficiency), enzyme defects, acquired liver disease, and drugs such as alcohol, propranolol and salicylates (which decrease glucose production) are conditions that cause underproduction of glucose. Hypoglycemia may also result from conditions that promote overutilization of glucose, such as insulinoma and extrapancreatic tumors that secrete an insulin-like material. Autoimmune diseases with production of antibodies against insulin may also cause hypoglycemia. The mechanism causing hypoglycemia in this instance is believed to be the sudden release of insulin from the antibodies.[18] Reactive or functional hypoglycemia is a condition in which the person has a normal fasting blood glucose concentration, but becomes mildly hypoglycemic within 2 to 4 hours after a carbohydrate meal. This state can be induced by any stimulus that stimulates insulin, such as a glucose tolerance test. In most instances the cause of reactive hypoglycemia is unknown.

Clinical picture

The clinical picture seen in hypoglycemia is the same despite the etiology and is the same as that described for hypoglycemia seen in diabetes mellitus (p. 660). The diagnosis is based on history, plasma insulin and plasma glucose levels, and the identification of one of the etiologic factors discussed previously. The patient may be admitted for fasting to see if hypoglycemia develops, for glucose tolerance tests to stimulate hypoglycemia, or for other diagnostic tests necessary to rule out other etiologic factors.

Intervention

Treatment is directed toward removal of the underlying etiology; for example, correction of other hormonal deficiencies, discontinuance of hypoglycemia-inducing drugs, control of liver disease, or removal of *insulinoma* or *extrapancreatic tumors*. If the underlying etiology cannot be corrected, management is directed toward maintaining a normal blood glucose level. In reactive or functional hypoglycemia this involves avoidance of fasting and avoidance of a high-carbohydrate diet that would stimulate insulin production. The patient is treated with a high-protein, low-carbohydrate diet. Protein is metabolized more slowly than carbohydrate, so the blood sugar remains more stable from meal to meal. It is important that meals be evenly spaced.

These patients may be advised to carry lump sugar or candy with them at all times for immediate use if faintness occurs. Candy with nuts is best, since the nuts are a source of protein. However, the person should not rely on these sugars as a substitute for regularly spaced meals, since functional hypoglycemia is provoked by glucose stimulation, and more frequent attacks of hypoglycemia may occur.

REFERENCES AND SELECTED READINGS
Contemporary

1. Alexander, N.B., and Cotanch, P.H.: The endocrine basis of infertility in women, Nurs. Clin. North Am. 15:511-524, 1980.
2. Anderson, J.W.: Newer approaches to diabetes diet: high-fiber diet, Med. Times 1108:41-44, 1980.
3. Arieff, A.: Nonketotic hyperosmolar coma with hyperglycemia, Medicine 51:73-94, 1972.
4. Asplen, C., et al.: Detection of unrecognised noctural hypoglycaemia in insulin-treated diabetes, Br. Med. J. 280:357-360, 1980.
5. Bar, R., and Roth, J.: Insulin receptor status in disease states of man, Arch. Intern. Med. 137:474-481, 1977.
6. Baxter, J.: Recombinant DNA and medical progress, Hosp. Pract. 15(2):57-67, 1980.
7. Beahrs, O.H.: Operative management of hyperparathyroidism, Milit. Med. 146:98-99, 1981.
8. Beahrs, O.H.: Operative surgical management of thyroid nodules and carcinoma, Milit. Med. 146:100-102, 1981.
9. Beeson, P.B., and McDermott, W., editors: Textbook of medicine, ed. 15, Philadelphia, 1981, W.B. Saunders Co.
10. Beland, I.L., Rice, V.H., and Power, L.: Metabolic crises. In Meltzer, L.E., Abdellah, F.G., and Kitchell, J.R.: Concepts and practices of intensive care for nurse specialists, ed. 2, Philadelphia, 1976, The Charles Press Publishers.
11. Bernstein, R.K.: Role of glycosylated hemoglobin in diabetic vascular disease, Arch. Intern. Med. 140:442, 1980.
12. Bernstein, R.K.: Virtually continuous euglycemia for 5 years in a labile juvenile-onset diabetic patient under noninvasive closed-loop control, Diabetes Care 3:140-143, 1980.
13. Birch, K., et al.: Self-monitoring of blood glucose without a meter, Diabetes Care 4:414-416, 1981.
14. *Blevins, D., editor: The diabetic and nursing care, New York, 1979, McGraw-Hill Book Co.
15. Blevins, D.R., and Breckbill, V.: The diabetic with vascular complications. In Blevins, D.: The diabetic and nursing care, New York, 1979, McGraw-Hill Book Co.
16. *Bodhan, S.T., and Jans, K.: A new diabetic with complications, Nurs. Clin. North Am. 12:393-406, 1977.
17. *Boden, G., et al.: Monitoring metabolic control in diabetic outpatients with glycosylated hemoglobin, Ann. Intern. Med. 92:357-360, 1980.
18. *Bolinger, R.E.: Hypoglycemia, Crit. Care Q. 2:99-109, 1980.
19. Bondy, P., and Rosenberg, L.: Metabolic control and disease, Philadelphia, 1980, W.B. Saunders Co.
20. *Boyles, V.A.: Injection aids for blind diabetic patients, Am. J. Nurs.' 77:1456-1458, 1977.
21. Bray, G.: New developments in diabetes: obesity and insulin resistance, Calif. Med. 119:22-25, 1973.
22. Breckbill, V.: Physiological alterations in diabetes. In Blevins, D.: The diabetic and nursing care, New York, 1979, McGraw-Hill Book Co.
23. Brown, J., et al.: Thyroid physiology in health and disease, Ann. Intern. Med. 81:68-81, 1974.
24. Brown, J.C., and Otte, S.C.: Gastrointestinal hormones and the control of insulin secretion, Diabetes 27:782-787, 1978.
25. *Burke, E.L.: Insulin injection: the site and the technique, Am. J. Nurs. 72:2194-2196, 1972.
26. *Cahill, G., and McDevitt, H.: Insulin-dependent diabetes mellitus: the initial lesion, N. Engl. J. Med. 304:1444-1464, 1981.
27. *Cataland, S.: Hypoglycemia: a spectrum of problems, Heart Lung 7:459-462, 1978.
28. *Check, W.A.: Bacterially produced human insulin given therapeutically, J.A.M.A. 4:322-323, 1981.
29. *Clancey, J., and Abruzzi, L.: Pituitary tumors, growth disease. Nurses intervention of patients with pituitary tumor, J. Neurosurg. Nurs. 10:24-28, 1978.
30. Clements, R.S.: What's new for neuropathic syndromes, Med. Times 5:45-53, 1980.
31. Clements, R.S., et al.: Comparison of various methods for rapid glucose estimate, Diabetes Care 4:392-395, 1981.
32. *Cooperman, D., and Malarkey, W.B.: Pituitary apoplexy, Heart Lung 7:450-454, 1978.
33. Costen, G.: Endocrine disorders associated with tumors of the pituitary and hypothalamus, Pediatr. Clin. North Am. 26:15-31, 1979.
34. *Cranley, M.S., and Frazier, S.A.: Preventive intensive care of the diabetic mother and fetus, Nurs. Clin. North Am. 8:489-499, 1973.
35. *Cryer, P.E.: Diagnostic endocrinology, ed. 2, New York, 1979, Oxford University Press.
36. Cryer, P.E., et al.: Diagnosis and therapy of acromegaly, Arch. Intern. Med. 135:338-343, 1975.
37. Danowski, T.S., and Sunder, J.: Jet injection of insulin during self-monitoring of blood glucose, Diabetes Care 1:27-33, 1978.
38. *Danowski, T.S., et al.: Diabetic complications and their prevention or reversal, Diabetes Care 3:94-99, 1980.
39. Danowski, T.S., et al.: Parameters of good control in diabetes mellitus, Diabetes Care 3:88-93, 1980.
40. David, D.S.: Calcium metabolism in renal failure, Am. J. Med. 58:48-56, 1975.
41. Davidson, J.K.: Newer approaches to diet management of diabetes: calorie control, Med. Times 5:35-40, 1980.
42. deBoer, M.J., et al.: Glycosylated haemoglobin in renal failure, Diabetologia 18:437-440, 1980.
43. Deckert, T., and Larsen, M.: The prognosis of insulin-depen-

---

*References preceded by an asterisk are particularly well suited for student reading.

dent diabetes mellitus and the importance of supervision, Advances Exp. Med. Biol. **119:**21-27, 1979.

44. DeGroot, L., et al.: Endocrinology, 3 vols, New York, 1979, Grune & Stratton.

45. DeLuca, H.T.: Vitamin D endocrinology, Ann. Intern. Med. **85:**367-377, 1976.

46. Drash, A.: The control of diabetes mellitus: Is it achievable? Is it desirable? J. Pediatr. **88:**1074-1076, 1976.

47. *Dudley, J.D.: The diabetes educator's role in teaching the diabetic patient, Diabetes Care **3:**127-133, 1980.

48. *Dupuis, A.: Assessment of the psychological factors and responses in self-managed patients, Diabetes Care **3:**117-120, 1980.

49. Editorial: Endocrine aspects of aging, Ann. Intern. Med. **92:**429-431, 1980.

50. *Elliott, D.D.: A self-instruction unit: adrenocortical insufficiency, Am. J. Nurs. **74:**1115-1130, 1974.

51. Etzwiler, D.D.: Teaching allied health professionals about self-management, Diabetes Care **3:**121-123, 1980.

52. Evered, D.: Diseases of the thyroid gland, Clin. Endocrinol. Metab. **3:**425-450, 1974.

53. *Fairchild, R.S.: Diabetes insipidus: a review, Crit. Care Q. **2:**111-118, 1980.

54. Fass, B.: Glucocorticoid therapy for nonendocrine disorders: withdrawals and "coverage," Pediatr. Clin. North Am. **26:**251-256, 1979.

55. *Fauci, A., et al.: Glucocorticosteroid therapy. Mechanisms of action and clinical considerations, Ann. Intern. Med. **84:**304-315, 1976.

56. Felig, P., et al.: Amino acid and protein metabolism in diabetes mellitus, Arch. Intern. Med. **137:**507-513, 1977.

57. *Fletcher, H.P.: The oral antidiabetic drugs: pro and con, Am. J. Nurs. **76:**596-599, 1976.

58. Frasier, S.D.: Growth disorders in children, Pediatr. Clin. North Am. **26:**1-14, 1979.

59. *Friedland, G.M.: Learning behaviors of a preadolescent with diabetes, Am. J. Nurs. **76:**59-60, 1976.

60. Frohlich, E.D., editor: Pathophysiology, ed. 2, Philadelphia, 1976, W.B. Saunders Co.

61. Frohman, L.: Neurotransmitters as regulators of endocrine function, Hosp. Pract. **10**(4):54-57, 1975.

62. Frohman, L., and Stachura, M.: Neuropharmacologic control of neuroendocrine function in man, Metabolism **24:**211-234, 1975.

63. *Fulton, M., et al.: Vision, Am. J. Nurs. **74:**54-57, 1974.

64. Galloway, J.A.: When the patient is resistant or allergic to insulin, Med. Times **5:**91-101, 1980.

65. Ganda, O.P.: Pathogenesis of macrovascular disease in the human diabetic, Diabetes **29:**931-942, 1980.

66. *Ganda, O.P., and Soeldner, S.S.: Genetic, acquired, and related factors in the etiology of diabetes mellitus, Arch. Intern. Med. **137:**461-469, 1977.

67. *Garber, R.: The use of a standardized teaching program in diabetes education, Nurs. Clin. North Am. **12:**372-391, 1977.

68. *Garofano, C.: Travel tips for the peripatetic diabetic, Nurs. '77 **7**(4):44-46, 1977.

69. Garofano, C.: Deliver facts to help diabetics plan parenthood, Nurs. '77 **7**(4):13-16, 1977.

70. Geola, F., and Chopra, I.: Hyperthyroidism and hypothyroidism, Med. Times **108:**64-69, 73-74, 1980.

71. Gerich, J.E., et al.: Characterization of the glucagon response to hypoglycemia in man, J. Clin. Endocrinol. Metab. **1:**77-82, 1974.

72. *Gerich, J.E., et al.: Clinical and metabolic characteristics of hyperosmolar nonketotic coma, Diabetes **20:**228-238, 1971.

73. Gill, G.N.: Mechanism of ACTH action, Metabolism **21:**571-588, 1972.

74. *Gillies, D.A., and Alyn, I.B.: Caring for parients with thryoid disorders: how good are your skills? Nurs. '77 **7**(10):71-80, 1977.

75. Gilman, A.G., Goodman, L.S., and Gilman, A.: Goodman and Gilman's the pharmacological basis of therapeutics, ed. 6, New York, 1980, MacMillan Publishing Co., Inc.

76. Gonen, B., and Rubenstein, A.H.: Haemoglobin A and diabetes mellitus, Diabetologia **15:**1-8, 1978.

77. *Gotch, P.M.: Teaching patients about adrenal corticosteroids, Am. J. Nursing **81:**78-85, 1981.

78. Graf, R.J., et al.: Nerve conduction abnormalities in untreated maturity-onset diabetes: relation to levels of fasting plasma glucose and glycosylated hemoglobin, Ann. Intern. Med. **90:**298-303, 1979.

79. *Gribbons, C.A., and Aliapoulios, M.A.: Treatment for advanced breast carcinoma, Am. J. Nurs. **72:**678-682, 1972.

80. *Guthrie, D.W.: Exercise, diets and insulin for children with diabetes, Nurs.' 77 **7**(2):48-54, 1977.

81. *Guthrie, D.W., and Guthrie, R.A.: DKA: breaking a vicious cycle, Nurs. '78 **8**(6):54-57, 61, 1978.

82. *Guthrie, D.W., and Guthrie, R.A.: Nursing management of diabetes mellitus, ed. 2, St. Louis, 1982, The C.V. Mosby Co.

83. Guthrie, R.A.: What's happening with the young, Talk presented at conference on What's new in diabetes for health professionals. Sponsored by University of Kansas College of Health Sciences and Hospital and University of Missouri-Kansas City at Kansas City, Kan., April 13-14, 1981.

84. Hahn, A.B., Barkin, R.L., and Oestreich, S.J.K.: Pharmacology in nursing, ed. 15, St. Louis, 1982, The C.V. Mosby Co.

85. *Hallal, J.: Thyroid disorders, Am. J. Nurs. **77:**418, 1977.

86. Hamburger, S., and Rush, D.: Syndrome of inappropriate secretion of antidiuretic hormone, Crit. Care. Q. **2:**119-129, 1980.

87. Harvey, A.A., et al.: The principles and practice of medicine, ed. 20, Englewood Cliffs, N.J., 1980, Prentice-Hall, Inc.

88. Hays, R. and Levine, S.: Antidiuretic hormone, N. Engl. J. Med. **295:**659-665, 1976.

89. *Hayter, J.: Fine points in diabetic care, Am. J. Nurs. **76:**594-599, 1976.

90. Hellman, R.: The evaluation and management of hyperthyroid crises, Crit. Care. Q. **2:**77-92, 1980.

91. Hershman, J.: Clinical application of thyrotropin-releasing hormone, N. Engl. J. Med. **290:**886-889, 1974.

92. Hoffman, J.T.: Syndromes of ectopic hormone production in cancer, Nurs. Clin. North Am. **15:**499-509, 1980.

93. Hoffmann, J.T., and Newby, T.B.: Hypercalcemia in primary hyperparathyroidism, Nurs. Clin. North Am. **15:**469-480, 1980.

94. Horton, R.: Aldosterone: Review of its physiology and diagnostic aspects of primary aldosteronism, Metabolism **22:**1535-1545, 1973.

95. *Hurwitz, L.S.: Nursing implications of selected pediatric endocrine problem, Nurs. Clin. North Am. **15:**525-534, 1980.

96. Ibeda, Y., et al.: Pilot study of self-measurement of blood glucose using the Dextrostix-Eyetone system for juvenile onset diabetes, Diabetologia **15:**91-93, 1978.

97. Inada, M., et al.: Clinical evaluation of measuring glycosylated hemoglobin levels for assessing the long-term blood glucose control in diabetics, Endocrinologia Japanica **27:**411-415, 1980.

98. *Isaf, J.J., and Alogna, M.T.: Better use of resources equals better health for diabetics, Am. J. Nurs. **77:**1792-1795, 1977.

99. Isselbacher, K., et al., editors: Harrison's principles of internal medicine, ed. 9, New York, 1980, McGraw Hill Book Co.

100. Jeanrenaud, B.: Insulin and obesity, Diabetologia **17:**133-138, 1979.

101. Jovanovic, L., and Peterson, C.M.: Management of the pregnant insulin-dependent diabetic woman, Diabetic Care **3:**63-68, 1980.

102. Jubiz, Wm.: Endocrinology: A logical approach for clinicians, New York, 1979, McGraw-Hill Book Co.

103. *Judd, S., and Sonksen, P.H.: Teaching diabetic patients about self-management, Diabetes Care **3:**134-139, 1980.

104. Kaplan, S.: Disorders of the adrenal cortex. I, Pediatr. Clin. North Am. **26**:77-89, 1979.

105. Kaplan, S.: Disorders of the adrenal cortex. II, Pediatr. Clin North Am. **26**:77-89, 1979.

106. *Kaufman, S.J.: In diabetic diets, realism gets results, Nurs. '76 **6**(11):75-77, 1976.

107. *Keyes, M.: The somogyi phenomenon in insulin-dependent diabetes, Nurs. Clin. North Am. **12**:439-445, 1977.

108. Kilo, C., Miller, J.P., and Williamson, J.R.: The crux of the UGDP. Spurious results and biologically inappropriate data analysis, Diabetologia **18**:179-185, 1980.

109. Kilo, C.: The use of oral hypoglycemic agents, Hosp. Pract. **14**(3):103-110, 1979.

110. Kjaergaard, J.J., et al.: Vitreous fluorophotometry and hemoglobin A^{IC} in non-proliferative diabetic retinopathy, Endocrinologica **238**(suppl.): 75-76, 1980.

111. Kuivisto, V.A., and Sherwin, R.S.: Exercise in diabetes: therapeutic implications, Postgrad. Med. **66**:87-91, 94-96, 1979.

112. Kolata, G.B.: Blood sugar and the complications of diabetes, Science **203**:1098-1099, 1979.

113. *Koppers, L.E.: Pheochromocytoma—critical care, Crit. Care Q. **2**:93-97, 1980.

114. Krieger, D.T., and Hughes, J.C., editors: Neuroendocrinology, Sunderland, Mass., 1980 Sinauer Associates Inc.

115. *Krosnick, A.: Self-management, patient compliance, and the physician, Diabetes Care **3**:124-126, 1980.

116. Krueger, J., and Ray, J.: Endocrine problems in nursing, St. Louis, 1976, The C.V. Mosby Co.

117. Kubilis, P., et al.: Comparison of blood glucose testing using reagent strips with and without a meter (Chemstrip bG and Dextrostix/Dextrometer), Diabetes Care **4**:417-419, 1981.

118. Kubilis, P., et al.: Stability of reacted reagent strips (Chemstrips) for blood glucose determinaties, Diabetes Care **4**:412-413, 1981.

119. *Kubo, W.M., and Grant, M.: The syndrome of inappropriate antidiuretic hormone, Heart Lung **7**:469, 1978.

120. *Kyner, J.L.: Diabetic ketoacidosis, Crit. Care Q. **2**:65-75, 1980.

121. Labru, F., et al.: Mode of action of hypothalamic regularity hormones in the adenophypophysis. In Martini, L., and Ganong, W.: Frontiers in neuroendocrinology, vol. 4, New York, 1976, Raven Press.

122. LaFranchi, S.: Hypothyroidism, Pediatr. Clin. North Am. **26**:33-51, 1979.

123. Lee, W.N.: Thyroiditis, hyperthryroidism, and tumors, Pediatr. Clin. North Am. **26**:53-64, 1979.

124. Levin, M.E.: Saving the diabetic foot, Med. Times **5**:56-62, 1980.

125. Lukert, B.P.: Hypercalcemia, Crit. Care Q. **2**:11-18, 1980.

126. MacLead, R.: Regulation of prolactin secretion. In Martini, L., and Ganong, W., Frontiers in neuroendocrinology, vol. 4, New York, 1976, Raven Press.

127. Malarkey, W.B.: Recently discovered hypothalamic-pituitary hormones, Clin. Chem. **22**:5-15, 1976.

128. Malone, J.I., et al.: Good diabetic control—a study in mass delusion, J. Pediatr. **88**:943-947, 1976.

129. Manfreidi, C., Cassidy, V., and Moffitt, D.: Developing a teaching program for diabetic patients, J. Contin. Educ. Nurs. **6**:46-52, 1977.

130. *Mannix, H., et al.: Hyperparathyroidism in the elderly, Am. J. Surg. **139**:581-585, 1980.

131. Martin, J.: Brain regulation of growth hormone secretion, In Martini, L., and Ganong, W.: Frontiers in neuroendocrinology, vol. 4, New York, 1976, Raven Press.

132. Maugh, T.: Diabetes therapy: can new techniques halt complications, Science **190**:1281-1284, 1975.

133. Maurer, A.: The therapy of diabetes, Am. Sci. **67**:422-431, 1979.

134. May, P.B.: Initial evaluation and management of patients with suspected pituitary tumors, Primary Care **4**:89-125, 1977.

135. *McConnell, E.A.: Meeting the special needs of diabetics facing surgery, Nurs. '76 **6**(6):30-37, 1976.

136. McCurdy, D.: Hyperosmolar hyperglycemic nonketotic diabetic coma, Med. Clin. North Am. **54**:683-698, 1970.

137. McDonald, J.M., and Davis, J.E.: Glycosylated hemoglobins and diabetes mellitus, Hum. Pathol. **10**:279-291, 1979.

138. McGarry, J., and Foster, D.: Hormonal control of ketogenesis, Arch. Intern. Med. **137**:495-501, 1977.

139. McKenna, T.J.: Acute adrenal insufficiency, Hosp. Med. **12**(6):77-79, 81, 83, 1976.

140. Meek, J.C.: Myxedema coma, Crit. Care Q. **2**:131-137, 1980.

141. Melnick, D.E.: Future management of diabetes mellitus, Postgrad. Med. **5**:101-105, 108-110, 113, 1979.

142. Michelis, M., and Murdaugh, H.: Selective hypoaldosteronism, Am. J. Med. **59**:1-4, 1975.

143. Moffitt, P.S.: Interpretation of glycosuria in the teenage diabetic patient, Diabetes Care **3**:112-116, 1980.

144. Molnar, G.D., et al.: Methods of assessing diabetic control, Diabetologia **17**:5-16, 1979.

145. Morris, M.L.: Why patient education? I. A. look at the patient with diabetes mellitus, Occup. Health Nurs. **12**:7-11, 1979.

146. Mountcastle, V.B., editor: Medical physiology, ed. 14, St. Louis, 1980, The C.V. Mosby Co.

147. National Diabetes Data Group: Classification and diagnosis of diabetes mellitus and other categories of glucose intolerance, Diabetes **28**:1039-1057, 1979.

148. Nerup, J., et al.: HLA antigens and diabetes mellitus, Lancet **2**:864-866, 1974.

149. Neville, J.: Management by nutrition. In Blevens, D.: The diabetic and nursing care, New York, 1979, McGraw Hill Book Co.

150. Nicholls, M.G., et al.: Primary aldosteronism, Am. J. Med. **59**:334-342, 1975.

151. *Nursing Skillbook: Managing diabetics properly. Nursing '77 Books, Horsham, Pa., 1977, Intermed Communications.

152. *O'Dorisio, L.M.: Hypercalcemic crisis, Heart Lung **7**:425-434, 1978.

153. Oparil, S., and Haber, E.: The renin-angiotensin system, N. Engl. J. Med. **291**:389-401, 446, 457, 1974.

154. Paisey, R.B., et al.: Home blood glucose concentrations in maturity-onset diabetes, Br. Med. J. **280**:596-598, 1980.

155. Paisey, R.B., et al.: The relationship between blood glycosylated haemoglobin and home capillary blood glucose levels in diabetics, Diabetologia **19**:31-34, 1980.

156. *Patient panel, Diabetes Care **3**:144-147, 1980.

157. Perrin, E.D.: Laser therapy for diabetic retinopathy, Am. J. Nurs. **80**:664-665, 1980.

158. Petersen, C.M., et al.: Self-management: an approach to patients with insulin-dependent diabetes mellitus, Diabetes Care **3**:82-87, 1980.

159. Peterson, C.M., et al.: Feasibility of improved blood glucose control in patients with insulin-dependent diabetes mellitus, Diabetes Care **2**:235-239, 1979.

160. *Petrokas, J.: Common sense guidelines for controlling diabetes during illness, Nurs. '77 **7**(12):36-37, 1977.

161. Podolsky, S.: Hyperosmolar nonketotic coma: death can be prevented, Geriatrics **34**:29-33, 36-37, 41-42, 1979.

162. *Powers, D., et al.: Nursing management of diabetic ketoacidosis, Crit. Care Q. **2**:139-143, 1980.

163. *Read, S.: Clinical care in hypophysectomy, Nurs. Clin. North Am. **9**:647-654, 1974.

164. Reeves, M.L., et al.: Comparison of methods for blood glucose monitoring, Diabetes Care **4**:404-406, 1981.

165. Renold, A.E., et al.: Diabetes mellitus. In Stanbury, J.B., et al.: Metabolic basis of inherited disease, ed. 4, New York, 1978, McGraw-Hill Book Co.

166. Richmond, I.: Pituitary adenomas in childhood and adolescence, J. Neurosurg. **49**:163-168, 1978.

167. Roth, J.: Insulin receptors in diabetes, Hosp. Pract. **15**(5):98-103, 1980.

168. Rude, R., et al.: Functional hypoparathyroidism and parathyroid hormone end-organ resistance in human magnesium deficiency, Clin. Endocrinol. **5**:209-224, 1976.

169. Rush, D.R., and Hamburger, S.C.: Drugs used in endocrine metabolic emergencies, Crit. Care Q. **2**:1-9, 1980.

170. Russell, P.N., and Rix-Trott, H.M.: An exploration study of some behavioural consequences of insulin induced hypoglycaemia, NZ Med. J. **81**:337-340, 1975.

171. Sachs, M.: Management of diabetes by pharmacological agents. In Blevins, D.: The diabetic and nursing care, New York, 1979, McGraw-Hill Book Co.

172. Sanford, S.J.: Dysfunction of the adrenal gland: physiologic considerations and nursing problems, Nurs. Clin. North Am. **15**:481-498, 1980.

173. Santiago, V.: Insulin pump and transplants (methods of near normalization of blood glucose of persons with insulin dependent diabetes), Talk presented at conference on What's new in diabetes for health professionals. Sponsored by University of Kansas College of Health Sciences and Hospital and University of Missouri-Kansas City at Kansas City, Kan., April 13-14, 1981.

174. Savage, P.J., Bennion, L.J., and Bennett, P.H.: Normalization of insulin and glucagon secretion in ketosis-resistant diabetes mellitus with prolonged diet therapy, J. Clin. Endocrinol. Metab. **49**:830-833, 1979.

175. Schimke, R.N.: Adrenal insufficiency, Crit. Care Q. **2**:19-27, 1980.

176. Schneeberg, N.G.: Hyperparathyroidism: early diagnosis now possible, Consultant **19**:58, 1979.

177. Schneider, A.B., and Sherwood, L.M.: Pathogenesis and management of hypoparathyroidism and other hypocalemic disorders, Metabolism **24**:871-897, 1975.

178. Schneider, J.M, et al.: Pregnancy complicating ambulatory patient management of diabetes, Diabetes Care **3**:77-81, 1980.

179. *Schulz, J.M., and Williams, M.: Encouragement breeds independence in the blind diabetic, Nurs. '76 **6**(12):19-20, 1976.

180. *Schumann, D.: Assessing the diabetic, Nurs. '76 **6**(3):62-67, 1976.

181. *Schumann, D.: Tips for improving urine testing techniques, Nurs. '76 **6**(2):23-27, 1976.

182. *Schumann, D.: Coping with the complex, dangerous, elusive problems of those insulin-induced hypoglycemic reactions, Nurs. '74 **4**(4):56-60, 1974.

183. Scott, F.B., Fishman, I.J., and Light, J.K.: An inflatable penile prosthesis for treatment of diabetic impotence, Ann. Intern. Med. **92**:340-342, 1980.

184. Service, F.J., and Nelson, R.L.: Characteristics of glycemic stability, Diabetes Care **3**:58-62, 1980.

185. Shapiro, B., et al.: A comparison of accuracy and estimated cost of methods for home blood glucose monitoring, Diabetes Care **4**:396-403, 1981.

186. Sherwin, R., et al.: Hyperglucagonemia and blood glucose regulation in normal, obese, and diabetic subjects, N. Engl. J. Med. **294**:455-461, 1976.

187. Shiner, G.: Human growth hormone: potentials for treatment are broadened. Res. Resources Reporter **12**:1-5, 1980.

188. Shuman, C.R.: When-and-how to use an oral agent, Med. Times **5**:77-86, 1980.

189. Silva, F.E., and Larsen, R.P.: Pituitary nuclear 3,5,3'-triiodothyronine and thyrotropin secretion: an explanation for the effect of thyroxine, Science **198**:617-619, 1977.

190. Siperstein, M.D., et al.: Control of blood glucose and diabetic vascular disease, N. Engl. J. Med. **296**:1060-1063, 1977.

191. Skillman, T.G.: More than one insulin injection per day improves control, Med. Times **108**:104-118, 1980.

192. Skillman, T.G.: Diabetic ketoacidosis, Heart Lung **7**:594-602, 1978.

193. Skyler, J.S., et al.: Blood glucose control during pregnancy, Diabetes Care **3**:69-76, 1980.

194. Skyler, J.S., et al.: Home blood glucose monitoring as an aid in diabetes management, Diabetes Care **1**:150-157, 1978.

195. *Slater, N.: Insulin reactions vs. ketoacidosis: guidelines for diagnosis and interventions, Am. J. Nurs. **78**:875-877, 1978.

196. *Sneid, D.S.: Hyperosmolar hyperglycemic nonketotic coma, Crit. Care Q. **2**:29-43, 1980.

197. Solomon, B.L.: The hypothalamus and the pituitary gland: an overview, Nurs. Clin. North Am. **15**:435-451, 1980.

198. Sönksen, P.H., et al.: Home monitoring of blood glucose: new approach to management of insulin-dependent diabetic patients in Great Britain, Diabetes Care **3**:100-107, 1980.

199. Sönksen, P.H., et al.: Home monitoring of blood glucose, Lancet **1**:729-732, 1978.

200. *Sowers, D.K., and Sowers, J.R.: Pituitary emergencies, Crit. Care Q. **2**:45-54, 1980.

201. Sperling, M.A.: Diabetes mellitus, Pediatr. Clin. North Am. **26**:149-169, 1979.

202. Spiro, R.G., and Spiro, M.J.: Effect of diabetes on the biosynthesis of the renal glomerular basement membrane, Diabetes **20**:641-648, 1971.

203. Stein, J.: Hormones and the kidney, Hosp. Pract. **14**(7):91-105, 1979.

204. *Stowe, S.M.: Hypophysectomy for diabetic retinopathy, Am. J. Nurs. **73**:632-637, 1973.

205. Sulway, M., et al.: New techniques for changing compliance in diabetes, Diabetes Care **3**:108-111, 1980.

206. *Suren, J.V.: Education of the culturally and educationally deprived, Nurs. Clin. North Am. **12**:427-437, 1977.

207. Sussman, K.E., and Metz, R.J.S.: Diabetes mellitus, ed. 4, New York, 1976, American Diabetes Association, Inc.

208. Svendsen, P.A., et al.: Rapid changes in chromatographically determined haemoglobin A$_{IC}$ induced by short-term changes in glucose concentration, Diabetologia **19**:130-136, 1980.

209. Tchobroutsky, G., et al.: Diabetic control in 102 insulin-treated out-patients, Diabetologia **18**:447-452, 1980.

210. Tepperman, J.: Metabolic and endocrine physiology, ed. 3, Chicago, 1973, Year Book Medical Publishers, Inc.

211. Thomsen, M., et al.: MHC typing in juvenile diabetes mellitus and idiopathic Addison's disease, Transplant Rev. **22**:125-147, 1975.

212. Tolis, G.: Prolactin: physiology and pathology, Hosp. Pract. **15**(2):85-95, 1980.

213. *Tribble, N.M., and Hollenberg, E.E.: The import of a quality assurance program on diabetic education, Nurs. Clin. North Am. **12**:365-373, 1977.

214. *Tzagournis, M.: Acute adrenal insufficiency, Heart Lung **7**:603-609, 1978.

215. Unger, R.H., and Orci, L.: Role of glucagon in diabetes, Arch. Intern. Med. **137**:482-491, 1977.

216. Unger, R.H., and Orci, L.: The essential role of glucagon in the pathogenesis of diabetes mellitus, Lancet **1**(7897):14-16, 1975.

217. Urbanic, R.C., and Mazzaferri, E.L.: Thyrotoxic crisis and myxedema coma, Heart Lung **7**:435-447, 1978.

218. VanLoon, G.: New drugs in the treatment of pituitary disorders, Primary Care **4**:721-737, 1977.

219. Voorhess, M.: Disorders of the adrenal medulla and multiple endocrine adenomatosis, Pediatr. Clin. North Am. **26**:209-222, 1979.

220. *Ventura, E.: Foot care for diabetics, Am. J. Nurs. **78**:886-888, 1978.

221. Vranic, M., and Berger, M.: Exercise and diabetes mellitus, Diabetes **28**:147-163, 1979.

222. Wake, M.M., and Brensinger, J.F.: The nurse's role in hypothyroidism, Nurs. Clin. North Am. **15**:453-467, 1980.

223. *Walesky, M.E.: Diabetic ketoacidosis, Am. J. Nurs. **78**:872-874, 1978.

224. Walford, S., et al.: Self-monitoring of blood-glucose. Improvement of diabetic control, Lancet **1**:723-735, 1978.

225. Walter, R.M., and Warsaw, T.: Diabetic ketoacidosis—a treatment appraisal, Heart Lung **10**:112-113, 1981.

226. White, V., and Kumagai, L.: Preoperative endocrine and metabolic considerations, Med. Clin. North Am. **63**:1321-1334, 1979.

227. Whitehouse, F.W., et al.: Teaching the person with diabetes: experience with a follow-up session, Diabetes Care **2**:35-38, 1979.

228. Williams, R.A., et al.: The treatment of acromegaly with special reference to trans-sphenoidal hypophysectomy, Q. J. Med. **44**:79-98, 1975.

229. Williams, R., editor: Textbook of endocrinology, Philadelphia, 1974, W.B. Saunders Co.

230 *Williams, S.R.: Nutrition and diet therapy, ed. 4, St. Louis, 1981, The C.V. Mosby Co.

231. Winter, C.C., and Morel, A.: Nursing care of patients with urologic diseases, ed. 4, St. Louis, 1977, The C.V. Mosby Co.

232. *Wolfe, L.: Insulin: paving the way to a new life, Nurs. '77 **7**(11):38-41, 1977.

233. Worth, R.C., et al.: A comparative study of blood glucose test strips, Diabetes Care **4**:407-411, 1981.

Classic

234. Gabbay, K., and O'Sullivan, J.: The sorbitol pathway. Enzyme localization and content in normal and diabetic nerve and cord, Diabetes **17**:239-243, 1968.

235. Pyke, D., and Pease, J.: Diabetic ketosis and coma, J. Clin. Pathol. **22**:57-61, 1969.

CHAPTER 33

PROBLEMS OF THE LIVER AND RELATED STRUCTURES

VIRGINIA L. CASSMEYER
JUDITH L. GREIG

The liver, the biliary system, and the pancreas are affected by a variety of pathologic processes that may present many nursing care challenges. Many of the pathologic processes are chronic in nature and require that the patient make changes in life-style to keep the problem under control. These patients need nursing support in adapting to their chronic health problem and in learning the necessary self-management skills.

Disorders that are encountered include not only those caused by infectious organisms but also abnormalities from changes in structure and function that are essential to digestion and normal metabolic processes. In this chapter nursing care specific to general problems commonly seen in patients with hepatic, biliary, and pancreatic diseases is discussed.

Focal parenchymal disorders of the liver

A variety of pathological states can affect the liver. Diseases of the liver may be classified in several ways. In this chapter disorders secondary to focal parenchymal damage and disorders secondary to diffuse parenchymal damage will be discussed. The major emphasis is given to the most common disorders, with a brief discussion of those that are less frequently seen.

Regardless of the specific pathologic condition, disorders secondary to diffuse parenchymal damage present the patient with many problems. Inadequate nutrition and metabolism are common, as are fluid and electrolyte imbalances, coagulation problems, decreased resistance to infection, and inability to detoxify substances normally detoxified in the liver. Disorders secondary to focal parenchymal damage do not cause as many problems, but all focal disorders require effective management to prevent more diffuse liver damage or death.

In many instances of diffuse parenchymal damage no specific curative therapy is available, and the treatment and care focus on providing physiologic and psychologic support until the liver heals itself. Emphasis is on assisting the individual to conserve energy and on health teaching related to preventing further liver damage.

Liver function studies, radiographic diagnostic procedures, liver biopsy, and other invasive procedures may be necessary to determine the exact disease process that is present and the extent of liver damage. Tests more frequently used are discussed in Chapter 30 along with a review of the normal physiologic mechanisms carried out by the hepatic system.

Focal parenchymal disorders can result from (1) abscess formation, (2) trauma, (3) tumors, (4) cysts, and (5) granulomatous processes. The first three disorders will be discussed next.

Liver abscess formation

Etiology and physiology

Liver abscesses may result from a variety of etiologic processes and are caused by a variety of organisms. A common etiologic process is the spread of infection from an infected biliary tract obstructed by gallstones, tumors, or strictures. Abscesses may also result from direct spread from contiguous viscera, from infections of the intestinal tract that spread via the portal vein, from seeding of the liver in septicemia, or from infection following traumatic injury.

The most common pyogenic organisms causing liver abscess are *Escherichia coli* and *Staphylococcus aureus*. *Entamoeba histolytica* is also an important worldwide cause of amebic liver abscess and dysentery. In amebic infections the vegetative form of the organism moves from the gut to the small portal caliculi in the liver, where it becomes activated, releasing enzymes that cause local tissue destruction. Multiple abscesses occur. In pyogenic abscesses the bacteria cause pus formation and a pus-filled cavity occurs.

Clinical picture

The clinical manifestations of liver abscesses are often nonspecific. The patient may complain of malaise, vague abdominal discomfort, nausea and vomiting, chills, and diaphoresis. A history of weight loss also may be present. Physical examination will usually reveal jaundice, an enlarged, tender liver, and a low-grade fever.

Laboratory tests usually reveal leukocytosis, moderate elevation of serum alkaline phosphatase, and minimal elevation of serum glutamic oxaloacetic transaminase (SGOT). A highly specific and sensitive indirect hemagglutination test provides over 95% accuracy in the diagnosis of amebic liver abscesses. Hepatic scintiscan and ultrasonography are often used for diagnosis and for follow-up evaluation.

Intervention

Treatment usually consists of surgical incision and drainage of the abscess or abscesses and treatment with broad-spectrum antibiotics for pyogenic abscesses and with emetine hydrochloride and chloroquine or mitranidiazole for amebic abscesses. The prescribed medications may have to be taken for long periods of time and the patient must realize that the abscess can rupture and cause the infection to spread. The patient is instructed about the importance of reporting any new signs and symptoms of infection. Portal hypertension can occur from scarring of the liver as part of the healing process. This is a rare complication, but patients must be instructed to report any worsening of liver function immediately.

These patients require close follow-up after discharge from the hospital.

Outcome criteria for the person with a liver abscess

The person or significant others can:
1. Explain the pathophysiology of the disorder.
2. Explain medication regimen (e.g., drugs, dosage, frequency, expected effects, and side effects).
3. Describe problems that need to be reported immediately (e.g., signs and symptoms of spread of infection and signs and symptoms of worsening of liver function).
4. Explain plans for follow-up care.

Trauma to the liver

Because of its location and size, the liver is frequently subjected to trauma, which may be either penetrating (stab wounds) or blunt (automobile accidents or falls). If the injury is severe, rupture of the liver may occur with severe internal hemorrhage.

Pathophysiology

Small lacerations or ruptures, except for temporary peritoneal irritations from blood oozing into the peritoneal cavity, usually heal leaving a subcapsular scar. In some instances the hematoma may become infected and abscess formation complicates the healing process. Hepatic cysts may also develop. Rare complications include arterial aneurysms or portal vein thrombosis. Trauma that causes severe contusions may result in subsequent degeneration of the injured hepatic cells. The prognosis depends on the amount of tissue damaged, and the final outcome for the patient may not be known for many years after the initial injury.

Severe lacerations or rupture of the liver has a mortality estimated to be between 27% and 30%. Death that occurs shortly after the injury is caused by uncontrollable hepatic hemorrhage. This happens in part because the walls of the hepatic veins are thin, the liver is very vascular, and the bile mixing with the blood interferes with clotting. Deaths occurring later after injury may be caused by biliary peritonitis, shock, or infections.

Clinical picture

If the injury has not penetrated the abdomen, there may be no external evidence of injury. If conscious, the patient may complain of pain. Symptoms of shock (pallor, tachycardia, and hypotension) may develop depending on the rapidity of the bleeding. Needle aspiration of the abdominal cavity may show the presence of blood.

Intervention

All patients with abdominal wounds should be monitored carefully for signs and symptoms of internal hemorrhage. This includes vital signs; neurologic checks for alertness and responsiveness; physical examination of skin for color, temperature, and dryness; and abdominal checks for signs of peritonitis every hour until danger has passed. Intake and output of fluids should be monitored at least every 8 hours.

If trauma to the liver has occurred, blood volume replacement is usually required. Emergency surgery may be needed to suture the ruptured liver and apply local pressure to stop the bleeding. Removal of necrotic tissue may also be indicated as well as drainage of any bile that may be leaking from the liver surface. The patient may require long-term follow-up to monitor for signs and symptoms of residual liver damage. Nursing care in the acute period is the same as for any patient requiring abdominal surgery as a result of trauma. The type of monitoring required will depend on the extent of the patient's injuries.

Tumors of the liver

Tumors of the liver may be either malignant or benign. Benign lesions include hemangiomas, cysts, and rarely adenomas. These benign tumors occasionally enlarge enough to become symptomatic and present problems in differentiation from a malignant tumor. If the latter occurs, surgical intervention may be required.

Epidemiology and etiology

Malignant tumors may be metastatic or primary. Metastatic tumors are common. They occur 20 times more frequently than primary tumors and rank second to cirrhosis as a cause of fatal liver disease.[29] The liver most commonly receives metastatic cells from the gastrointestinal tract, the lung, the breast, the kidney, and melanomas of the skin, although virtually any neoplasm can metastasize to the liver.[29]

Primary hepatic carcinomas may arise within the liver cell (hepatocellular) or the bile duct cell (cholangiocellular) or may be of mixed origin. Hepatocellular tumors are the most common. Primary liver cancer accounts for only 1% to 2% of malignant tumors found at death in the United States. They are more common in men than in women and usually occur in the fifth and sixth decades of life. Chronic liver disease from hepatitis, hemochromatosis, or any other cause appears to predispose individuals to the development of primary liver cancer.

Pathophysiology

Primary tumors may arise from either liver cells or bile ducts or from both. The lesions may be multiple or singular, diffuse or nodular, and may spread to only a lobe or to the entire liver. The cancerous cells appear to compress the surrounding normal liver cells and to spread quickly by invading the portal vein branches. Some cells infiltrate the gallbladder, mesentery, peritoneum, and diaphragm by direct extension.

Primary cancers also tend to cause hemorrhage and necrosis. The most common site for metastasis of the primary liver lesion is the lung, but it may also metastasize to the adrenal glands, spleen, vertebrae, kidney, ovary, or pancreas. Primary lesions tend to grow rapidly, sometimes without signs or symptoms, and the patient may live only a short time after their onset.

Metastatic carcinoma of the liver varies from a few small nodules to large nodes. Adjacent nodes may eventually grow together and compress the surrounding liver tissue. Usually different parts of the liver are uniformly involved so that liver biopsy may be a useful diagnostic aid.

Clinical picture

In the early stages, the signs and symptoms of primary malignant tumors may be absent, acute, or referred to other areas if metastasis has occurred. Metastases make it difficult to differentiate the tumor from cirrhosis. In a patient with early metastatic lesions of the liver, the only signs and symptoms may be those referable to the primary tumor. The liver involvement is found only during evaluation. Metastatic hepatic involvement should be suspected when a patient with a history of carcinoma develops anorexia, weakness, weight loss, secondary anemia, pain in the right upper quadrant, and general ill health.

Jaundice and ascites are signs that the metastatic or primary process is quite far advanced, and the patient may live only a short time after their onset. Unexplained temperature elevations accompany about 15% of primary or metastatic carcinomas of the liver. Extreme weakness is also usually an outstanding symptom. The major physical sign is an enlarged liver. Ascites occurs secondary to compression of the portal vein. Gastrointestinal bleeding may also be present and may confuse the diagnosis.

Diagnostic tests include blood studies and invasive procedures. Liver biopsy is necessary for definitive diagnosis. Laboratory data usually indicate abnormal liver function. Abnormal data such as an increased sedimentation rate, anemia, decreased blood sugar levels, and elevated alkaline phosphatase, SGOT, and serum glutamic pyruvic transaminase (SGPT) levels are usually present (p. 602).

A special blood test that may be used to help diagnose primary liver carcinoma is serum concentrations of alpha-fetoprotein (α-fetoprotein; AFP). AFP in concentrations of 500 ng/ml to 5 mg/ml is found in up to 70% of the patients with hepatocellular cancer. It is also found in a small percentage of patients with metastatic carcinoma or viral hepatitis but rarely is the level elevated as high as it is with hepatocellular carcinoma. High levels that occur in any adult without obvious gastrointestinal tract tumors strongly suggest the presence of primary liver cancer.[29]

Intervention

In most instances there is no medical or surgical treatment for metastatic or primary carcinoma of the liver because the disease is too far advanced when first diagnosed. Patients are usually alert at this time and will know the prognosis. The nurse and other health team members must work together to assist the patient and significant others to live with the prognosis and to do the things that they wish to do in the time remaining for the patient. This requires very skilled nursing care (see Chapter 17). Various interventions will be needed to manage physical changes that occur as liver failure progresses. These interventions will be similar to those needed in patients with cirrhosis.

Chemotherapy may be used in an effort to induce regression of tumor growth. Methotrexate, 5-fluorouracil, or doxorubicin (Adriamycin) has been used. In many instances the chemotherapy is given by perfusion into the hepatic artery. The results with chemotherapy are still poor. The patient will need assistance to deal with the side effects of chemotherapy (see Chapter 25). In a few patients with primary tumors, surgery may be possible. If the tumor is limited to a single lobe and there is no evidence of metastases elsewhere, a *hepatic lobectomy* may be done to remove metastatic as well as primary carcinoma. The remarkable regenerative capacity of the liver permits resection of 70% to 80% of the organ. *Preoperatively*, the patient may be given massive doses of vitamin K for prothrombin defects, blood volume is ascertained and necessary blood given, and preparation of the bowel is done as for intestinal surgery. The surgery usually involves a thoracoabdominal incision, and postoperative care includes care given to patients with chest surgery (p. 1252) and abdominal surgery (p. 1399) plus the general care needed by any patient with dysfunction of the liver. A nasogastric tube usually is inserted and attached to suction. Nothing is given by mouth for several days. Cortisone may be given to prevent fibrosis and enhance liver regeneration.

The patient is acutely ill following surgery and must be attended constantly. Continuous monitoring for potential complications such as hemorrhage (the most feared), infections (wound and subdiaphragmatic abscesses), pulmonary dysfunction (atelectasis and pneumonia), and decreased liver function (hypoglycemia, coagulation problems, fluid and electrolyte imbalance, and hepatic coma) must be instituted. Appropriate measures to help prevent these complications are necessary.

Following surgery of the liver the patient may be out of bed by the third postoperative day but must be attended constantly, and pulse, blood pressure, and respiratory rate are monitored before, during, and after any exertion, since complications such as hemorrhage may occur. Food will be taken by the fifth postoperative day and the patient must be monitored for ability to handle protein nitrogen waste products. Liver function tests are done frequently to check progress.

Homotransplantation of the liver is possible, but the survival rate is poor. The liver must be transplanted rapidly because of difficulty with preserving the organ. Death occurs as a result of rejection or infection secondary to depression of immune response by immunosuppressive therapy.

Diffuse parenchymal disorders of the liver

Hepatitis

Hepatitis may be defined as any acute inflammatory disease of the liver. Although the term *hepatitis* is most commonly used in conjunction with viral hepatitis, the disease can be caused by viruses, bacteria, or toxic injury to the liver. Hepatotoxins include drugs (chlorpromazine, isoniazid, tetracycline, thiazide diuretics, thiouracils, and others), agents such as phosphorus, organic solvents (carbon tetrachloride and methylenedianiline [MDA][37]), plant poisons, and alcohol.

Although there are some differences in the pathologic and clinical phenomena of viral, bacterial, and toxic hepatitis, the clinical management of the person with hepatitis is quite similar. The particular aspects of care for toxic and viral hepatitis are discussed next. It should be pointed out that any form of hepatitis can result in postnecrotic cirrhosis unless the hepatitis responds to treatment.

Toxic hepatitis

Pathophysiology

The morphologic changes in the liver will depend on the toxic agent. For example, necrosis and fatty infiltrates are present when the causative agent is carbon tetrachloride, whereas cholestasis with portal inflammation is seen when the toxic agent is chlorpromazine.[29] Microscopic examination of liver tissue obtained by biopsy helps to differentiate the causative agent. Two types of chemical hepatotoxicity occur: direct toxic and idiosyncratic. In *direct toxic* hepatitis the agent causes toxicity with predictable regularity. The occurrence of this form of hepatitis is dose dependent and usually occurs several hours to 2 days after exposure.[29]

The occurrence of *idiosyncratic toxic* hepatitis is infrequent and unpredictable, and the response is not dose dependent. Hepatitis may occur anytime, from during exposure to shortly after exposure to the toxic substance. Most cases of drug-induced toxic hepatitis are idiosyncratic reactions. It is thought that these idiosyncratic reactions may be caused by unique host susceptibility or may be immunologically mediated, although immune-mediated hypersensitivity has not been proved.[29]

Prevention

The nurse can assist in the prevention of toxic hepatitis by teaching the danger of injudicious use of materials that are known to be injurious to the liver and by emphasizing the need for a diet that is protective to the liver.

Since cleaning agents, solvents, and related substances sometimes contain products that are harmful to the liver, the public should read instructions on labels and should follow them explicitly. Dry-cleaning fluids may contain carbon tetrachloride, which can cause liver injury if warnings to avoid inhalation of the fumes and to keep windows open are not heeded. If people must use these agents inside the home, a good practice is to open the windows wide, use the cleaning materials as quickly as possible, and then vacate the room, the apartment, or the house for several hours, leaving the windows open.

Many solvents used to remove paint and plastic material and to stain and finish woodwork contain injurious substances and should be used outdoors and not in the basement, since dangerous fumes may spread throughout the house. Cleaning agents and finishes for cars should be applied outdoors or in the garage with the door open. Nurses in industry have a responsibility to teach the importance of observing regulations to avoid industrial hazards. Nitrobenzene, tetrachloroethane, carbon disulfide, and dinitrotoluol are examples of injurious compounds used in industry.

Some drugs that are known to cause mild damage to the liver must be used therapeutically. However, the nurse should warn the public regarding the use of preparations that are available without prescription that may be injurious. Many drugs reach the market before dangers of their extensive use have been conclusively ruled out; for example, chlorpromazine, which was being widely used as a tranquilizer, is known to cause stasis in the canaliculi of the liver, which may lead to serious hepatic damage. A safe rule to follow is to avoid taking any medication except that specifically prescribed by a physician for a specific ailment.

Clinical picture

The symptoms of toxic hepatitis resemble those of viral hepatitis (p. 685). Liver function tests including serum transaminase levels are valuable in evaluating the severity of injury to liver cells (see Chapter 30).

Intervention

If the liver damage is from toxic agents, the treatment consists of identifying the toxic agent and removing or eliminating it. Gastric lavage and cleansing of the bowel may be indicated to remove the hepatotoxin from the intestinal tract. Antidotes such as dimercaprol (BAL) have been used with some degree of success in binding the agent for possible excretion by the kidneys. Patients with toxic hepatitis are placed on bed rest. Nursing measures include those for patients with any hepatic disease (see Chapter 31).

Viral hepatitis

Viral hepatitis is by far the most important infection attacking the liver. Although the disease is not new, it assumed serious proportions during World War II when 50,000 men developed jaundice after receiving yellow fever vaccine containing human serum. Since that time it has become a major health problem in the United States as well as in many other countries and has been studied intensively.

There are at least three types of viral hepatitis—type A (HAV), type B (HBV), and type non-A, non-B. Research supports the fact that more than one virus may be responsible for non-A, non-B hepatitis. When more data are available, non-A, non-B hepatitis will probably be reclassified according to distinct viruses.

Epidemiology

Viral hepatitis is a reportable disease in all states. Centers for Disease Control (CDC) statistics indicate that viral hepatitis is one of the four most frequently reported infectious diseases in the United States. Although there has been a decline in the number of reported cases each year since 1971 when there were 69,000 reported cases of hepatitis in the United States, the total number of cases reported for 1980 was higher than in 1978 and 1979. In 1980 the total number of cases was 59,996. There were 29,087 cases of hepatitis A, 19,105 cases of hepatitis B, and 11,894 cases were unspecified as to type.[62] It is well accepted that the figures for any given year may be grossly underestimated, since carriers with subclinical manifestations are often not reported as having active disease. There are geographic differences in the number of cases of hepatitis, with the highest number of cases being reported in the Pacific area (Washington, Oregon, California, Alaska, and Hawaii) and the lowest in the north central area (Minnesota, Iowa, Missouri, North Dakota, South Dakota, Nebraska, and Kansas).[62]

Hepatitis B accounts for 50% of the hepatitis cases that are seen clinically with type A and type non-A, non-B being about equally responsible for the other 50% of the cases.[25] Hepatitis A seems to have a distinct pattern of occurrence. It is more common during the fall and winter. Epidemic waves have been recorded every

5 to 20 years as new segments of nonimmune population appear.

As with other infections, hepatitis seems to be more prevalent in low-income areas where there is overcrowding and among residents and staff of long-term care institutions. In 1980, persons 15 to 39 years of age were the group most affected by all types of hepatitis.[62] Patients and staff in hemodialysis units and physicians, nurses, dentists, and personnel of clinical and pathology laboratories have a higher risk for hepatitis B because of the increased exposure to equipment contaminated with blood. Homosexuals, perhaps because of the fact that many have numerous sexual partners, and drug abusers, because of the sharing of unsterile equipment, also have a higher incidence of hepatitis B. Persons who receive blood transfusions are at risk of acquiring hepatitis B or hepatitis non-A, non-B, but 90% of all cases of posttransfusion hepatitis are type non-A, non-B.

Great advances have been made in the understanding of the epidemiology of hepatitis in the last 2 decades. It has only been since the early 1940s that the true infectious nature of viral hepatitis was recognized. One problem that has constantly thwarted researchers investigating viral hepatitis was the lack of a suitable experimental animal host system for the transmission of the viral agents. Only recently has human viral hepatitis been transmitted to animals in the laboratory.

Etiology

The most significant breakthrough in the elucidation of the etiology of viral hepatitis came in 1965 when an antigen was demonstrated in the blood of an Australian aborigine and was shown to have some relationship to hepatitis. The antigen, initially called *Australian antigen,* was shown to be transiently but consistently present in the blood of several patients suffering from hepatitis type B infections. This antigen was first thought to be the hepatitis B virus (HBV), but researchers had no success in transmitting disease or growing the Australian antigen in tissue culture. In 1970, however, Dane and his co-workers discovered a larger, more complex structure in the serum from infected individuals, which is known as the *Dane particle*. The Dane particle seems to be the free virus (HBV) in the serum. The Australian antigen represents an excess of viral coats free in the serum and is now referred to as hepatitis B surface antigen (HB_sAg). HB_sAg is visible by electron microscopy in the following three forms: (1) as a sphere, (2) as the outer coat of the Dane particle, and (3) as an elongated tubular form.[25] Since these discoveries other distinct antigens and antibodies have been found. A second antigen of the Dane particle is called the hepatitis B core antigen (HB_cAg). An e antigen (HB_eAg) is found only in patients with type B infections and correlates with DNA polymerase activity, continued infectivity, and active disease. Antibodies to HB_sAg (anti-HB_s, HB_sAb) and to HB_cAg (anti-HB_c, HB_cAb) have also been identified. Currently, only the tests to detect HB_sAg are readily available and used in clinical practice.

In 1973, a virus similar to the HBV was found by immune electron microscopy in the stool specimens from individuals with hepatitis type A. Patients with type A hepatitis demonstrate a serologic response to this antigen and their sera show increased titers of hepatitis antibodies (HA Ab). The HA Ab peaks and persists after 2 to 3 months. The hepatitis A antigen (HA Ag) is cleared rapidly from the stool and sera, and thus tests for clinical detection are not feasible.

Less is known about the viruses involved in non-A, non-B hepatitis. It is felt that there are at least two viruses and the non-A, non-B hepatitis antigen is detectable 2 to 4 weeks before liver enzymes increase.[25] The antigen has been demonstrated in the liver, and its characteristics as seen by electron microscopy are similar to those of the hepatitis B virus.[25]

Data on the physiochemical and biologic characteristics of the viruses are accumulating slowly. The hepatitis viruses are extremely resistant to such antimicrobial measures as drying, chlorination, disinfectants, heat, ultraviolet light, radiation, and freezing. The viruses are especially refractive to such measures when protected by the presence of serum proteins. At boiling temperatures the viruses can survive for about 20 to 30 minutes. Autoclaving is the best method to ensure destruction of the viruses on contaminated articles.

Transmission

Hepatitis viruses are similar in some respects, but they vary in their incubation period and possibly in their mode of transmission. The older terms used to refer to the types of hepatitis reflect these differences.

Type A viral infections are still sometimes called *infectious hepatitis, epidemic hepatitis*, and *short-incubation hepatitis*. The incubation period for hepatitis A is usually about 30 days, with a range of 10 to 40 days from the time of exposure to appearance of the initial prejaundice symptoms. The source of the virus is human feces and human blood. The disease is most often spread by the fecal-oral route. Fecally contaminated food, water, milk, shellfish, and inanimate objects can serve as sources of infection. If common sources such as communal wells, streams, or food supplies are contaminated with the virus caused by a breakdown in sanitation, small or large epidemics can occur. Often secondary epidemics may result from close contact with infected persons, this is especially true of transmission to members of the household of an infected individual or to other persons in an institution. In addition to the fecal-oral route, parenteral introduction of HAV through blood products or contaminated parenteral equipment can occur, since the virus is found in the blood (viremia) during the latter half of the incubation period and the early acute phase of the infection. However, parenteral transmission is thought to be of only limited significance in the spread of HAV. The implication of a respiratory route of transmission has been suggested, but there is little experimental or epidemiologic data to support this as an important mechanism of transmission.

Type B infections are still sometimes referred to as *serum hepatitis, homologous serum jaundice,* and *long-incubation hepatitis.* The incubation period of HBV ranges from 45 to 180 days, with 90 days being about average. It is often difficult to assess the true length of the incubation period, because by the time the symptoms appear the circumstances attendant to the exposure have been forgotten. The principal source of the virus is the blood of persons who have the virus or who are carriers of the virus. HB$_s$Ag has been detected in urine, saliva, nasopharyngeal washings, pleural fluid, feces, and semen.

The virus is transmitted parenterally through blood, serum, or plasma, or through equipment used for venipuncture or pricking the skin. The virus can also be spread by contact of mucous membranes of the mouth and respiratory tract or an open cut in the skin with contaminated blood. Those caring for or closely associating with the infected individual are highly vulnerable to infection. The disease can be transmitted from infected patients to medical, nursing, and other hospital personnel by accidental pricking of the skin with a needle contaminated by the patient's blood. The virus can also pass the placental barrier and infect the fetus. Since HBV can be transmitted by nonparenteral routes, other sources of spread have been identified but occur with much less frequency. HB$_s$Ag has been found to stay persistently elevated in some patients.

Non-A, non-B hepatitis was for a very short time referred to as type C hepatitis. This term was dropped when evidence that more than one virus may be responsible for non-A, non-B hepatitis became available. Non-A, non-B hepatitis has an incubation period of 14 to 150 days, with 50 days being about average. The source of the virus is blood of persons who have the virus. It is transmitted parenterally through blood, serum, or plasma. Non-A, non-B hepatitis is primarily seen after transfusions but is also seen (1) in persons receiving hemodialysis, (2) among family members, (3) and among residents of institutions. A summary of the differences between type A, type B, and type non-A, non-B hepatitis is outlined in Table 33-1.

TABLE 33-1. Characteristics of hepatitis A, hepatitis B, and hepatitis non-A, non-B infections

Features	Hepatitis A	Hepatitis B	Hepatitis non-A, non-B
Sources	Contaminated food, water, needles, or surgical instruments	Contaminated needles, surgical instruments, or blood products, asymptomatic carriers	Contaminated blood, needles, or surgical instruments
Route of infection	Fecal-oral, parenteral, or direct contact	Parenteral, oral, direct, or sexual contact	Parenteral
Incubation period	Short (10-40 days), 30 days average	Long (45-180 days), 90 days average	Variable (14-150 days), 50 days average
Onset of disease	Abrupt, often febrile	Insidious, seldom febrile	Insidious, often anicteric
Viral antigens	Fecal antigens, liver antigens, but not used clinically	HB$_s$Ag in serum during incubation and acute phases and tested for clinically	Non-A, non-B antigen detectable 2-4 wk before enzyme increase; also demonstrable in liver but not tested for clinically
Diagnostic tests	Liver function tests, liver biopsy	Liver function tests, liver biopsy	Liver function tests, liver biopsy
Mortality	Less than 0.5%	1-5%	1-3%
Age group affected	Children, young adults, elderly persons	All age groups	All age groups but higher in adults because of blood transfusions
Immunity	Recovery provides immunity to HAV but not to HBV or non-A, non-B	Recovery provides partial immunity to HBV but not to HAV or non-A, non-B	Recovery provides immunity to non-A, non-B virus but not to HBV or HAV
Immune globulin protection	Effective	If immune globulin has a high titer of HB$_s$Ab it is effective	Questionably effective
Subsequent chronic disease	Virtually absent	Higher than HAV; about 10% develop this complication	Approximately 20-25% develop this complication

Pathophysiology

Viral hepatitis causes diffuse inflammatory infiltration of hepatic tissue with mononuclear cells and local, spotty, or single cell necrosis. The liver cells may be very swollen. With typical viral hepatitis there is no collapse of lobules, no loss of lobular architecture, and minimal or no fibrosis. Inflammation, degeneration, and regeneration may occur simultaneously, distorting the normal lobular pattern and possibly creating pressure within and about the portal vein areas. These changes may be associated with elevated serum transaminase levels, prolonged prothrombin time, and slightly elevated serum alkaline phosphatase level. Because the pathologic process is usually distributed evenly throughout the liver, biopsy has been particularly useful in studying and diagnosing the disease. In most instances of nonfatal viral hepatitis, regeneration begins almost with the onset of the disease. The damaged cells and their contents eventually are removed by phagocytosis and enzymatic reaction, and the liver returns to normal. The outcome of viral hepatitis may be affected by such factors as the virulence of the virus, the amount of hepatic damage sustained before exposure to the virus, the natural barriers to damage and disease of the liver, and the supportive care the patient receives when symptoms appear. The majority of patients recover normal liver function, but the disease may take several courses, and different terms describe each of them.

Submassive hepatic necrosis refers to destruction of substantial groups of adjacent cells without destruction of the greater part of the lobule. The liver function tests remain abnormal for a long period of time and signs of liver failure may occur. *Massive hepatic necrosis* refers to destruction of the whole lobule. In both instances chronic active liver disease with or without cirrhosis, or fulminant hepatic failure can occur.

Fulminant hepatic failure or *fulminant viral hepatitis* is used to designate sudden and severe degeneration and atrophy of the liver. This condition most often is associated with an overwhelming infection with the hepatitis virus that progresses rapidly to cause death unless corticosteroids are successful in arresting the process. The liver may shrink in size to as little as 600 g, in contrast to a weight of 1500 g in a normal adult.

Subacute fatal viral hepatitis causes acute massive necrosis, which, even though it is not evenly distributed throughout the organ, finally destroys enough of the liver to cause death. This form of the disease may vary in duration from several weeks to several months, with apparent short remissions followed by exacerbations. In its late stages subacute fatal viral hepatitis is almost impossible to distinguish from cirrhosis of the liver by clinical manifestations and by liver function tests. However, history of exposure to viral hepatitis and symptoms of acute infection aid in diagnosis.

Chronic forms of the disease can occur with all types of hepatitis but are virtually absent with hepatitis A. Chronic hepatitis occurs in 10% of patients with hepatitis B and in 25% of patients with non-A, non-B hepatitis. *Chronic active liver disease,* also called *chronic active hepatitis* and *chronic aggressive hepatitis,* is characterized by signs and symptoms of liver disease or abnormal liver function tests for periods greater than 6 months. During this time there is extension of the necrosis with loss of normal structure and function. Very frequently the disease progresses to cirrhosis. If left untreated, most patients will die within 4 to 5 years. About 75% of the patients respond well to corticosteroid treatment.

The second form of chronic disease is *chronic persistent hepatitis.* Liver function tests may be abnormal for greater than 6 months and fatigue and hepatomegaly are common, but there is no necrosis, normal liver structure is maintained, and there is no increase in mortality.

Prevention

It is in the area of prevention that the nurse can make the greatest contribution to the control of viral hepatitis. Since there is no specific treatment for the disease and no adequate immunization for type A or type non-A, non-B at this time, it is only by making use of what is known about the viruses that control can be accomplished.

Methods of destroying the viruses of hepatitis are limited. There is the possibility that undiagnosed hepatitis may be most infectious; therefore particular emphasis should be placed on *thorough washing of hands* with soap and running water after possible exposure. Hospital workers must regard all feces, blood, and other body fluids as potentially infectious and not just those of patients with hepatitis or jaundice. The patient should be taught how to wash his or her hands thoroughly and should know why this is necessary, particularly after a bowel movement. Thorough washing of all equipment that might be contaminated lessens the danger to persons who must handle it and may help protect the next patient for whom the equipment is used. Since hepatitis A can be transmitted by infected stools and contaminated food and water, food handlers should be encouraged to pay careful attention to hand-washing regulations.

At the present time dry heat and steam heat under pressure (autoclaving) are the only safe ways to sterilize needles and other equipment used to penetrate the skin. The adequate boiling time is still undetermined, and for this reason most hospitals use autoclave sterilization and sterile, disposable syringes and needles almost entirely. When boiling is the only available way to sterilize needles and other equipment, the nurse should see that everything placed in the water sterilizer is *covered completely and boiled for at least 30 minutes.*[21]

Hepatitis A, hepatitis B, and non-A, non-B hepatitis can be transmitted from one patient to another when multiple doses of a drug are put into one syringe and only the needle is changed between patients. This practice is inexcusable. Regardless of the extra expense involved and the extra time and work entailed in preparation of materials for each injection, separate or disposable syringes and needles should be used. School immunization programs and practices in large outpatient clinics such as allergy clinics have been affected by recommendations in this regard. The nurse often must help explain the need for the extra cost to administrative personnel. The use of jet-spray guns to administer injections is safe, and they are especially helpful when immunizing a large number of persons.

Since individuals may be carriers of type B viruses, all needles and other equipment that have penetrated the skin of any patient should be handled with the greatest care. Type B hepatitis occurs quite frequently among hospital personnel. This is not surprising considering how often nurses, laboratory workers, or other members of the hospital staff may unwittingly prick themselves with needles that have been used for a wide variety of parenteral treatments. The safest way to handle any needle that is to be sterilized and reused is to rinse it carefully in cold water after use and place it in a puncture-resistant rigid container. Syringes and needles should be placed in a double bag and returned to central supply for decontamination and sterilization. Needles from infusion sets should be removed from the tubing immediately after an infusion is discontinued so that persons cleaning the equipment will not accidentally prick themselves. Special precautions should be used when throwing away disposable syringes and needles, both to protect refuse handlers from accidental infection and to keep them out of the hands of drug abusers. Used needles are not to be recapped or purposely bent; they are placed in a prominently labeled, impervious, puncture-resistant container designated for that purpose. Some hospitals use bright red cardboard containers labeled "Contaminated" for this purpose. Syringes are placed in an impervious bag. Both of these containers are incinerated or autoclaved before discarding.[61]

Because it is impossible on clinical grounds alone to determine which type of hepatitis is present, persons with hepatitis-like symptoms are considered to have any of the three types of hepatitis until otherwise proved.

It is recommended that patients with hepatitis be placed on *enteric* and *blood precautions*. Children should be in a private room. Responsible adults need not be in a private room if all precautions are observed. The reasons for the precautions and how the patient can assist with them should be carefully explained to the patient and family. The greatest care should be taken in handling fecal matter and urine and in performing treatments that involve contamination of the hands. Bedpans should be isolated and should be autoclaved following the patient's discharge from the hospital. Rubber gloves are often advised when handling urinals, bedpans, and commodes. In most localities feces and urine need not be treated if proper sewage disposal is available. If there is any doubt, the local health department should be consulted.

To prevent spread of hepatitis viruses it is suggested that individual toilet paper packages, rather than rolls, be used in any public bathroom and that toilets be cleaned with 1% aqueous iodine. The use of disposable seatcovers and foot pedals for flushing the toilet would help to reduce the chances of spread of the infection.

All patients should have individual thermometers, and the thermometer used for a patient with hepatitis should be disposed of after discharge. Since there is no really safe and satisfactory method of sterilizing a thermometer, discarding it is the only way to be certain that the disease is not spread by it. The cost of a thermometer is relatively small.

During hospitalization the thermometer is kept in 70% to 90% alcohol with 2% iodine. The solution is changed every 3 days. For the protection of the nursing personnel, the patient's temperature should be taken orally whenever possible. When small children must have their temperature taken rectally, rubber gloves should be worn. Poor technique in carrying out temperature-taking procedures has been suspected as a cause of widespread infection from the hepatitis viruses in foundling homes and similar sheltered-care facilities for children.

Because both type A and type B viruses may be transmitted by the oral route from contaminated hands and food, special care should be taken in handling nose and mouth secretions. The patient should be instructed to use tissues, which are then placed in an impervious paper or plastic bag and burned. Disposable dishes are preferred. Food waste should be burned and dishes boiled for 30 minutes or (ideally) autoclaved. If feasible, utensils may be washed in the patient's room, placed in an impervious plastic bag, labeled "Contaminated" or "Isolation,"[61] and autoclaved after discharge. Rooms should be cleaned well and aired when the patient leaves the hospital. Utmost care must be given to syringes, needles, and other instruments that are contaminated with the patient's serum. They should be autoclaved at 121° C (15 lb pressure) for 15 minutes or dry-heat sterilized at 170° C for 2 hours. Use of disposable syringes and needles is highly recommended. Known or suspected carriers should not be blood donors. Patients should also be placed on stool precautions because of possible transmission by the fecal-oral route. If any doubt exists as to which of the hepatitis viruses is involved, it is safest to take the precautions necessary in the care of patients with type A hepatitis.

Anyone who has been exposed to viral hepatitis should be urged to report this fact to the physician. This is especially important for a woman in the second or third trimester of pregnancy. Although the role of transplacentally transmitted viral hepatitis in causing injury to the liver in newborn infants has not been determined, the disease is believed to increase the likelihood of abortion, stillbirth, and congenital abnormalities. Immune serum globulin (ISG) offers some protection against type A hepatitis, but it does not protect against type B hepatitis. The routine use of ISG for hospital contacts of a patient with hepatitis is not recommended. It is given to some persons with known exposure to hepatitis A.[61] It is also recommended that persons planning to travel to areas where hepatitis A is endemic receive immune serum globulin. The dose for an adult is approximately 2 ml (0.01 ml/lb body weight) intramuscularly.[23]

Immune serum globulin with a high titer of HB_sAb has been shown to modify the clinical course of hepatitis B and is used when there is a high likelihood that a person has been contaminated with blood or serum from a patient with hepatitis B. Preliminary data suggest there is some protection provided by ISG against the non-A, non-B hepatitis virus.

An important step in prevention of hepatitis has been the mandatory screening of blood donors for HB_sAg. This has greatly reduced the incidence of type B hepatitis, but type B hepatitis can occur if the donor's level of HB_sAg is below detectable levels. There is no screening test for the non-A, non-B virus.

Another step in prevention was the development of a vaccine for hepatitis B. The vaccine was developed from HB Ag purified from plasma of carriers with no apparent signs of active disease.[44] The vaccine was tested in animals and humans and early in 1982 received FDA approval for general use. Vaccination consists of three injections at specified intervals. Because it is quite expensive, the vaccine is only recommended for use in high-risk populations such as male homosexuals, dentists, and surgeons.

A simple test for bilirubinuria, the *Icotest*, has been developed. Since bilirubin is present in the urine of the person who has viral hepatitis before clinical signs appear, it has been suggested that as part of a disease detection program this test be done on anyone exposed to hepatitis, all schoolchildren, hospital patients and employees, blood donors, employees in public institutions and industrial plants, and food handlers. Early recognition of the disease would make control of its spread easier. The test is done by placing 5 drops of urine on the Icotest reagent tablet.

Clinical picture

Collection of subjective and objective data through systematic assessment should be carried out paying par-

ticular attention to those parameters previously discussed (see Chapter 30). In addition, the nurse should obtain information with regard to any recent exposure to possible hepatotoxic agents or persons who were jaundiced or with regard to any recent blood transfusions or injections. The clinical symptoms of viral hepatitis vary. Patients may be asymptomatic and show minimal laboratory evidence of liver disturbance. Some patients may have many symptoms of the disease but no jaundice. A few may have fulminating necrosis of the liver and die. In most instances, however, viral hepatitis is a mild disease, and complete recovery is the rule.

Symptoms of the various types of hepatitis are not clinically distinctive from each other except that acute symptoms may be more severe in hepatitis A. Symptoms usually appear from 4 to 7 days before jaundice is apparent. Observations that the nurse may make to assist in determining a diagnosis include the presence of *headache, elevated temperature, chills, nausea* and *vomiting, dyspepsia, anorexia, general malaise, arthralgia,* and *tenderness over the liver.* Bleeding into the skin and mucous membranes may also occur because of a prolonged prothrombin time. *Anorexia is one of the most frequent symptoms,* and often the patient who smokes is repulsed by tobacco taste and smoke and other strong odors. This *preicteric stage* lasts for approximately 1 week and then subsides as jaundice occurs.

The *icteric stage* usually reaches its intensity in 2 weeks and may last from 4 to 6 weeks. Jaundice occurs when damaged liver cells are prevented from metabolizing bilirubin, resulting in large amounts diffusing into the tissues. The patient may then be observed to have yellow sclera and skin. In addition, excess conjugated bilirubin may be excreted by the kidneys, producing dark amber urine. Clay-colored stools will result if the hepatitis prevents bilirubin from entering the gastrointestinal tract. (For additional details about jaundice refer to p. 609.) Gastrointestinal tract symptoms may increase during the icteric stage, with the temperature elevation subsiding after the onset of jaundice. The liver frequently becomes more tender and swollen as a result of necrosis of the parenchymal cells.

The *posticteric* or *convalescent stage* begins with the disappearance of jaundice and may last from a few weeks to several months. Complete recovery is usually expected in 6 months. The disease may relapse during this stage, with recurrence of previous symptoms but to a milder degree. Children usually have a milder, nonicteric form of infectious hepatitis A with symptoms predominantly those of an intestinal or respiratory tract illness.

Laboratory tests will reveal hyperbilirubinemia and bilirubinuria and elevated serum enzyme levels. In *submassive* and *massive hepatic necrosis,* blood test results may demonstrate impaired synthetic liver functions such as decreased serum albumin levels and prolonged prothrombin time and partial thromboplastin time.

Intervention

There is no specific medical treatment for viral hepatitis; therefore treatment is primarily aimed at providing sufficient rest and nutrition to allow the patient's body to tolerate the insult of the infection and to gradually return to a state of physiologic stability.

Acute phase

REST. Physical activity should be restricted and the patient usually is placed on bed rest. The amount of bed rest required will depend on the individual patient, but it will be longer in patients with severe disease and in elderly persons. Extremely elevated serum enzyme levels may be indicative of hepatic cell necrosis and thus indicate the need for restricted activity. It is believed that activity and maintaining an upright position decrease hepatic blood flow, thus preventing optimal circulation to the already compromised liver cells.[48] Continued monitoring of these laboratory values can serve as an indicator for determining the amount of increased activity that the patient can tolerate. Relapses are frequently attributed to premature increases in activity.

During the first few days after the onset of symptoms the patient feels ill, and maintaining bed rest may not be difficult. However, bed rest should not be an irritating, uncomfortable experience. Changing the patient's position frequently along with the use of pillows for comfort may aid in promoting rest. A quiet environment is maintained, and necessary activities are carried out at one time so that the patient's rest is not interrupted. The nurse may also need to intervene if the patient is having prolonged visits or frequent visitors who interfere with adequate rest.

DIET. Fluids are encouraged by mouth if nausea is not a problem. The desirable fluid intake usually is considered to be at least 3000 ml/day. If the patient's temperature is high and nausea and vomiting are severe, infusions containing glucose are given, and occasionally solutions containing other electrolytes and protein hydrolysates are ordered. Intake and output are monitored because some patients with severe viral hepatitis cannot excrete a normal amount of fluid. Occasionally, a record of daily weight is instituted to assist in monitoring for fluid retention. If diarrhea occurs, the color, consistency, frequency, and amount of stool are carefully noted. Constipation is common.

Even if nauseated the patient can usually tolerate some food by mouth. Fruit juices, carbonated beverages, and hard candy can sometimes be retained and are encouraged during the periods of anorexia. Antiemetics may be ordered one-half hour before meals and should be conscientiously administered if found to be of value in preventing nausea. No special diet is re-

quired, but usually one high in protein, calories, and carbohydrates is ordered. Fats may be poorly tolerated because of the lack of bile entering the gastrointestinal tract. General care, including attention to good oral hygiene, skin care, and elimination, is necessary. Special attention should be paid to protecting the patient from intercurrent infection.

MEDICATIONS. Therapy may include the administration of vitamin K if the prothrombin time is prolonged. Vitamins B complex and C may be ordered as a dietary supplement. Corticosteroid therapy may be used for the fulminating types of the disease. If jaundice continues to increase after 3 weeks and nausea and vomiting remain uncontrolled, steroid therapy may be initiated. The nurse should observe for signs of sodium retention and potassium loss following steroid administration.

Convalescent phase.

During the convalescent stage nursing care may become an even greater challenge. As jaundice disappears and patients begin to feel better, it is often difficult for them to accept the need to curb their activities until their liver function tests return closer to normal levels. Enforced inactivity often makes patients irritable, and it is not unusual for them to complain about their daily routines and hospital food. Because these complaints often continue after patients go home, the patients' families need to be prepared for this eventuality.

Boredom can be reduced if patients can take part in occupational therapy activities at the bedside or be taken in their beds to an area where they can view television or converse with others.

There is a trend toward earlier ambulation of patients with viral hepatitis. When acute symptoms subside and the jaundice begins to recede, patients may be permitted to walk about their rooms. Activities are increased gradually, and if there are no adverse effects they may be permitted to convalesce at home under close medical supervision. Recurrence of anorexia, enlargement or tenderness of the liver, or lack of progress as shown by studies of hepatic function indicates a need to return to bed rest. Some patients are cared for at home from the onset of symptoms to complete recovery. With the assistance of a community health nurse, many families are able to care for the patient safely and adequately.

Appropriate isolation measures have to be instituted. These include no direct contact (sexual or oral) between the patient and others, use of disposable dishes, use of separate bathroom or cleansing of toilet seat after each use, separate washing of personal articles and linens, and use of separate razors, tissues, and toothbrushes.

Whether treated at home or in the hospital, patients will have weekly liver function tests until the abnormal test results show a downward trend toward normal levels. When this occurs, the tests will be done every other week until the results are within the normal range. If the tests remain abnormal for more than 3 months, more invasive procedures will be used to determine the reason for the abnormal values.

The nurse who cares for the patient in the home should observe carefully for changes in the color of urine and stool and for jaundice and should report any changes to the physician.

Outcome criteria for the person with viral hepatitis

The person or significant others can:
1. Explain the disease and the need for isolation.
2. Describe the diet and activity schedule allowed.
3. Explain times when immediate medical care should be sought (recurrence of signs and symptoms).
4. Explain plans for follow-up care.
5. If the person is treated at home during the acute phase, the following criterion is applicable: explain isolation precautions and describe how these will be carried out at home.

Cirrhosis of the liver

Etiology

Cirrhosis of the liver is a term applied by pathologists to several diseases that are characterized by diffuse inflammation and fibrosis of the liver resulting in drastic structural changes and significant loss of liver function. The basic processes leading to cirrhosis are liver cell death with scar tissue formation and regeneration of cell mass that causes distortion of the structure with a resultant change in circulation.

There are various types of cirrhosis. Table 33-2 lists the four major types of cirrhosis, the cause of each type, and a brief description of the pathologic changes that occur. *Postnecrotic cirrhosis* is the most common type on a worldwide basis. *Laennec's cirrhosis* is the most common type in North America.

Epidemiology

In European and American studies of persons with Laennec's cirrhosis, chronic alcoholism was present from 50% to 80% of the time.[48] However, chronic alcoholism is not the only cause of Laennec's cirrhosis. Malnutrition associated with other diseases such as pancreatitis, diabetes mellitus, and ulcerative colitis has been associated with Laennec's cirrhosis. Alcoholics who develop liver disease first develop fatty degeneration of the liver. The fatty changes are usually reversible if appropriate treatment is instituted. If the degenerative process continues, acute inflammation (alcoholic hepatitis) and then cirrhosis follow. Alcohol alone may cause cirrhosis, but another major contributing cause of Laennec's cirrhosis in alcoholics is malnutrition, which is frequently found to exist simultaneously with chronic alcoholism, and the combined insult is particularly damaging to liver cells.

Rare and nonspecific types of cirrhosis account for about 10% of deaths resulting from cirrhosis.[29] Nonspecific types of cirrhosis are associated with metabolic problems, infectious diseases, infiltrative disease, and gastrointestinal tract disorders. In the United States the number of deaths from cirrhosis continues to increase, and the incidence appears to parallel increases in alcohol ingestion. Cirrhosis as a cause of death in the United States now ranks fifth in persons between the ages of 45 and 64 years of age, with more men than women and more nonwhites than whites succumbing to the disease.

TABLE 33-2. Types, causes, and description of cirrhosis

Type	Causes	Description
Biliary cirrhosis	Intrahepatic cholestasis, blockage of common bile duct	Chronic impairment of bile excretion exists; liver destruction occurs around intrahepatic bile duct; at first liver is enlarged and greenish yellow in color but evolves into smaller, firmer, nodular organ as disease progresses
Postnecrotic cirrhosis, (toxic or multilobular cirrhosis)	Massive necrosis from hepatotoxins, *usually viral hepatitis*	Liver is decreased in size with many nodules separated by fibrous tissue
Cardiac cirrhosis	Right-sided congestive heart failure (CHF)	Liver is swollen and hepatic sinusoids are dilated and engorged; changes are reversible if CHF treated effectively; long-standing CHF results in fibrosis around central vein, which extends outward
Laennec's cirrhosis (nutritional, fatty, alcoholic, or portal cirrhosis)	Alcoholism, nutritional deficiencies	Massive collagen formation appears in periportal and pericentral areas; collagen fibers destroy normal lobular structure; in fatty stage, liver is large, yellow, greasy, and firm; in late stages liver is small and nodular

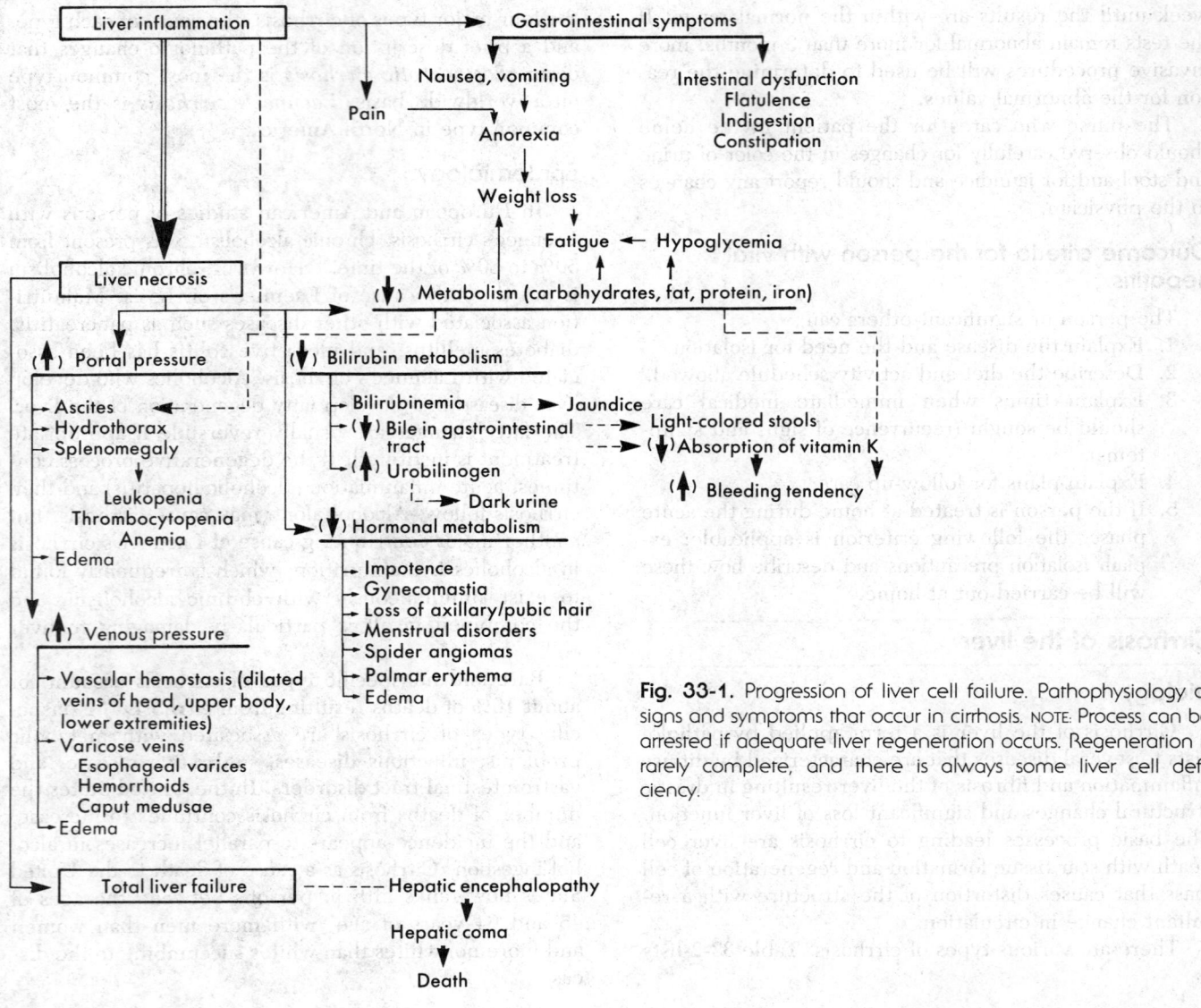

Fig. 33-1. Progression of liver cell failure. Pathophysiology of signs and symptoms that occur in cirrhosis. NOTE: Process can be arrested if adequate liver regeneration occurs. Regeneration is rarely complete, and there is always some liver cell deficiency.

Pathophysiology

The morphologic changes in the liver will vary depending on the type of cirrhosis (Table 33-2).

The signs and symptoms seen in cirrhosis are similar regardless of the cause of the cirrhosis. The signs and symptoms are caused by the progressive destruction of hepatic cells resulting in loss of the normal metabolic functions of the liver. In addition, the regeneration and proliferation of fibrous tissue cause obstruction of the portal vein. The body attempts to circumvent the obstruction to portal vein flow by establishing collateral circulation (Fig. 33-1).

Ascites, or fluid in the peritoneal cavity, usually follows obstruction of the portal vein and occasionally is one of the first signs of cirrhosis, although it usually does not occur until the disease is quite far advanced and jaundice has become marked.

Once the disease is established, it usually advances slowly to cause death. Many people, however, can be helped to live for years if they follow instructions. The liver has remarkable powers of regeneration. Sometimes sufficient collateral circulation can be established and sufficient repair of hepatic tissue can be accomplished so that symptoms subside for long periods. At other times the person appears to be doing fairly well when he or she suddenly goes into coma and may die within a few days.

Prevention

In the United States programs aimed at the prevention of cirrhosis are designed primarily to control the ingestion of alcohol. The loss of time from work related to alcoholism is estimated to cost billions of dollars annually. Many large corporations have or are organizing

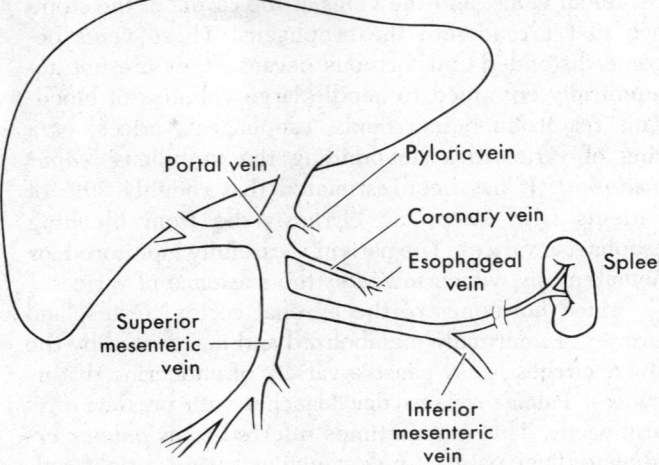

Fig. 33-2. Splanchnic veins. Venous drainage of splanchnic organs. When portal hypertension develops, other vessels can become engorged, leading to stasis and hypoxia of respective organs. (From Groër, M.E., and Shekleton, M.E.: Basic pathophysiology: a conceptual approach, ed. 2, St. Louis, 1983, The C.V. Mosby Co.)

programs to assist employees in controlling their alcoholic intake.

Clinical picture

Liver biopsy is believed to be essential for a definitive diagnosis. Assessment and eventual diagnosis of cirrhosis involve a thorough analysis of history and physical examinations, liver function tests, and radiographic examination (see Chapter 30). The patient with cirrhosis may have a long history of failing health with vague symptoms typical of many gastrointestinal disorders. Initial complaints may include weight loss, anorexia, indigestion, nausea, vomiting, flatulence, and abnormal bowel function. These symptoms are probably caused by metabolic dysfunctions of the damaged liver or venous congestion of the gastrointestinal mucosa. Abdominal pain is variable in character and may be dull, mild, sharp, steady, or wavelike. Pain may be confined to the liver or referred to the lower abdomen and is attributed to several factors: spasm of the biliary ducts, intermittent vascular spasm, swelling of the liver capsule, and inflammation of the peritoneum.

Later symptoms, which occur gradually, include jaundice, ascites, and edema. Jaundice may range from being barely visible in the sclera of the eyes to deep yellowing of the skin. The severity is usually proportional to the amount of liver damage. Peripheral edema may occur before ascites or the two may develop concomitantly. Hydrothorax may also be present in patients with ascites and is usually found in the right pleural space. Venules on the head and upper body become markedly distended. As circulation in the portal system becomes impaired because of structural changes in the liver, portal hypertension occurs (Fig. 33-2), producing splenomegaly and increasing edema of the lower extremities. As pressure increases in the portal veins, a back flow of blood into the veins emptying into the portal veins occurs. These veins in turn develop collateral channels of circulation. Collateral channels are most likely to occur in the paraumbilicus veins (Fig. 33-3), the hem-

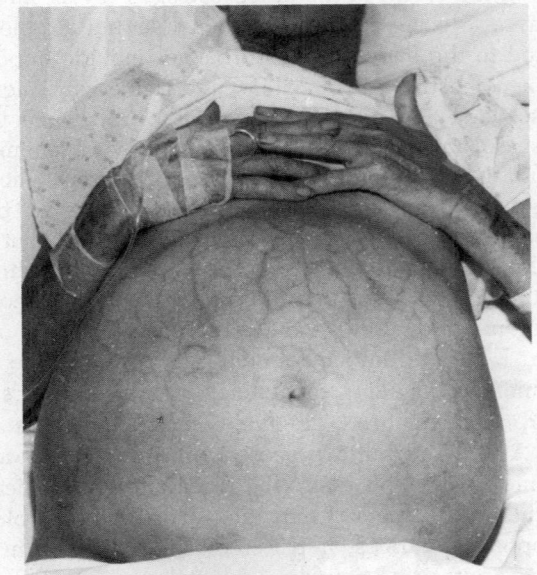

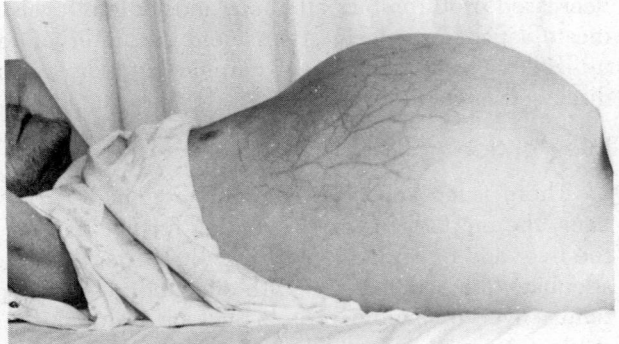

Fig. 33-3. Massive ascites. Note bulging flanks, dilated upper abdominal veins, and everted umbilicus. (From Prior, J.A., Silberstein, J.S., and Stang, J.M.: Physical diagnosis: the history and examination of the patient, ed. 6, St. Louis, 1981, The C.V. Mosby Co.)

orrhoidal veins, and the veins at the cardia of the stomach that extend into the esophagus. These veins become distended and tortuous because they are not anatomically equipped to handle large volumes of blood. This results in hemorrhoids, esophageal varices, or a ring of varicosities surrounding the umbilicus (*caput medusae*). It has been estimated that roughly 30% of patients with Laennec's cirrhosis die from bleeding esophageal varices. The patient is carefully monitored for hematemesis, which indicates the presence of varices.

Since hormones of the adrenal cortex, testes, and ovaries are normally metabolized and inactivated by the liver, cirrhosis may cause a variety of endocrine disturbances. Palmar redness that blanches with pressure may also occur. This is sometimes referred to as *palmar erythema* (liver palm). *Spider angiomas* (tiny, bright red, pulsating arterioles that disappear on pressure) frequently appear. The cause of spider angiomas and palmar redness is not fully understood, but they are thought to be the result of increased estrogen levels since they may also occur during pregnancy. Other problems related to the endocrine disturbances include impotence, gynecomastia, loss of axillary and pubic hair, menstrual disorders, and fluid and electrolyte imbalance. As the disease advances, typical signs of severe anemia, including malaise and memory loss, may occur. Increased erythrocyte destruction may also occur within the enlarged spleen. Other hematologic changes that occur include coagulation defects, leukopenia, and thrombocytopenia. Coagulation defects (caused by decreased protein production) and decreased absorption of vitamin K and thrombocytopenia may result in the development of bleeding tendencies with symptoms such as purpura, hematuria, gingival bleeding, and epistaxis.

As the cirrhotic process continues, the patient is prone to develop many life-threatening complications. Death may occur from total liver failure, bleeding esophageal varices, hepatic coma, or renal failure. Severe ascites and jaundice, neurologic symptoms, and decreased prothrombin, albumin, and sodium levels indicate a poor prognosis. Assessment and interventions utilized to treat sequelae of chronic liver disease are discussed next.

Intervention

There is no specific treatment for cirrhosis of the liver; the emphasis is on preventing further damage to the liver and on supportive care of the patient. Thus an adequate diet compatible with the ability of the patient's liver to handle protein will be ordered. Rest, moderate exercise, avoidance of exposure to infections, and protection from toxic agents of any kind are emphasized. Alcohol is forbidden. The patient is often disinterested in food and needs constant encouragement to eat the prescribed diet. As the disease progresses, increasing effort must be made to compensate for the fail-

ure of the functions of the liver. Vitamins may be given to compensate for the organ's lost ability to store vitamins A, B complex, D, and K. Bile salts are usually given if the patient is jaundiced to facilitate absorption of fat-soluble vitamin A and synthesis of vitamin K. Pruritus from the jaundice may need to be treated and is discussed on p. 610.

Because alcohol is thought to interfere with the hepatic conversion of folic acid to its active metabolites, many persons with cirrhosis have a folic acid deficiency anemia that usually responds well to treatment with oral doses of folic acid.[3]

To achieve a remission of threatened hepatic failure in cirrhosis may take a long time. There may be setbacks and periods when there is no improvement. The person and his or her family often become discouraged and require support from the physician and nurse. After discharge from the hospital, visits from the community health nurse may be requested to give whatever care, supervision, and support seem necessary. The person must be taught to avoid substances potentially toxic to the liver such as alcohol and drugs that require detoxification in the liver (p. 589).

Sequelae of cirrhosis or chronic liver disease

Any person with liver disease must be monitored for the presence of fluid and electrolyte changes, bleeding tendencies, portal hypertension, esophageal varices, and hepatic encephalopathy. Although the liver disease may be minimal, there is the possibility that any or all of these alterations may occur. Most often severe alterations will occur only when liver disease is long-standing, chronic in nature, and subject to progressive worsening such as occurs with cirrhosis.

Fluid and electrolyte changes

Pathophysiology

Retention of sodium and water by persons with liver disease is attributable to both local and systemic factors. The sequence of these mechanisms and how they interact to intensify ascites is not well established. The factors that are believed to contribute to the development of ascites include (1) decreased hepatic synthesis of albumin necessary for adequate plasma osmotic pressure, (2) increased portal vein pressure creating transudation of albumin and fluid from the intestines and mesentery into the peritoneal space, (3) increased serum aldosterone level caused by impaired degradation by the liver, and (4) transudation of fluid and albumin from the liver caused by obstruction of hepatic lymph outflow. Fig. 33-1 summarizes the changes that occur. The diminished serum albumin level, which is osmotically the most potent fraction, reduces the colloidal osmotic pressure in the blood. This leads to an increase in filtration through the capillary wall, while the reabsorption of the escaped fluid is impaired. In addition, the increased portal vein pressure facilitates the escape of fluid and albumin. A vicious cycle is established as the albumin lost into the peritoneal cavity further decreases the patient's serum albumin level.

Hydrothorax and ankle and presacral edema may accompany the ascites. The patient with cirrhosis frequently retains abnormal amounts of water and sodium. The sodium retention appears to be related to excessive aldosterone activity. It has been postulated that water is retained by excessive secretion of antidiuretic hormone, possibly caused by the liver dysfunction.

Renal function is also believed to affect fluid and electrolyte balance in patients with liver disease. Alterations in renal function may occur because of decreased blood volume secondary to vasodilation and portal hypertension. Thus the renal function of patients with liver disease is monitored for signs of increased urea and creatinine. Patients are also monitored for hypokalemia, which can result from diuretic therapy, diarrhea, vomiting, and sodium retention.

Intervention

Ascites is treated in several ways. Restriction of sodium aids greatly in limiting the formation of ascitic fluid. The amount of dietary restriction necessary to reduce sodium and water retention may initially be based on a 24-hour urine collection to determine sodium loss. Sodium is generally restricted to not more than 1 g daily. The sodium restriction along with bedrest may be enough to clear the ascites and edema.

The lack of salt in food makes it less palatable, and the patient may not consume adequate protein and total calories (see Chapter 21). The nurse should report the patient's food intake to the physician and dietitian, since adjustments may need to be made in the sodium restriction. Salt substitutes such as potassium gluconate may be permitted.

If edema and ascites do not clear with sodium restriction and bedrest, a second intervention that may be used is fluid restriction. Fluids may be restricted to as little as 500 ml/day and will usually not exceed 1500 ml/day. The fluid restriction may affect the patient's food intake. The nurse must work with the patient to provide fluids the patient tolerates best and to spread the allotted fluid throughout the total 24 hours.

Failure of bed rest and sodium and fluid restriction to improve ascites requires a pharmacologic approach. Furosemide (Lasix), 50 mg/day, is often prescribed. The dosage may be increased by 40 mg/day every 5 to 7 days until diuresis is achieved. The maximal dosage usually prescribed is 160 mg/day. Because furosemide results in loss of potassium along with sodium and wa-

ter, the patient will be monitored for hypokalemia. If hypokalemia occurs it will be treated with a potassium supplement. Patients who do not respond to the treatment with furosemide often require aldosterone inhibition with spironolactone A (Aldactone A), which inhibits the reabsorption of sodium in the distal tubules and promotes potassium retention. The usual dosage is 100 mg/day for 5 days and the dosage may be increased by 100 mg every 5 days until a maximal dosage of 400 mg daily is attained. The furosemide dose is maintained along with the spironolactone therapy.[45] Other combinations of diuretics, such as chlorothiazide (Diuril), which inhibits the reabsorption of sodium in the proximal tubules, and spironolactone A, may be used. Occasionally, one of the glucocorticoids, such as prednisone, may be given to aid in fluid loss.

Removal of fluid through the kidneys has the advantage of usually not removing essential body protein, which is contained in fluid removed from the abdominal cavity. However, diuretic therapy may cause serious side effects for the patient with cirrhosis and the patient must be monitored very carefully. Fluid and electrolyte levels must be carefully monitored during the initial administration of diuretic therapy. An extremely rapid diuresis can precipitate oliguria and uremia caused by the rapidly diminished blood volume. According to one expert, ascites cannot be mobilized at rates greater than 900 ml/day or approximately 2 lb/kg.[45] Unless the patient has peripheral edema, which could contribute to a fluid loss greater than 900 ml/day, nonascitic extracellular fluid is being lost.[45] Infusions of albumin in 25-g units to promote retention of an adequate vascular volume may be given to avert azotemia and encephalopathy and to promote diuresis. The administration of salt-poor albumin may expand the blood volume rapidly, and during and following administration, the patient is monitored carefully for signs of pulmonary edema.

In order to evaluate further the effectiveness of therapy, daily weights are required. Measurements of abdominal girth will also assist in determining the gross amount of abdominal swelling. Patients need to be taught the importance of monitoring and reporting weight gain or rapid increase in abdominal girth after discharge.

Patients with ascites may also experience dyspnea resulting from pressure being exerted upward on the diaphragm. A high Fowler's position may assist respiratory efforts. Skin care may present another problem since these patients are often emaciated despite edema.

The patient confined to bed is turned frequently to help prevent pressure areas from developing over the sacrum leading to skin breakdown. The use of alternating pressure mattresses and flotation pads may be helpful. When edema is severe, the skin may "weep" as the accumulation of fluid seeps through the pores. Frequent change of bed linen will be necessary.

When ascites is intractable to all the therapies described above, a LeVeen peritoneojugular shunt (PJS) (Fig. 33-4) may be used. The LeVeen PJS allows for the continuous reinfusion of ascitic fluid back into the venous system through a silicone catheter with a one-way pressure-sensitive valve. One end of the catheter is implanted in the peritoneal cavity, and the tube is channeled through subcutaneous tissue to the superior vena cava where the other end is implanted. The valve opens when there is a pressure differential greater than 3 mm of water between the abdominal cavity and the thoracic vein, allowing fluid to move from the peritoneal cavity into the superior vena cava. Persons treated with the LeVeen PJS may still receive furosemide ther-

apy and the two together have been successful in relieving ascites in some patients. Patients who have a LeVeen PJS may still have severe problems including disseminated intravascular coagulation (p. 1201), bleeding varices, and congestive heart failure.[45]

Although once a standard therapy, paracentesis is used with caution and usually only as a last resort in patients with severe and chronic liver disease, since it may precipitate hepatic coma. If the abdomen is tight with fluid and is producing dyspnea and anorexia, paracentesis may be necessary. In general, only small amounts of fluid are removed; this decreases the risk of rapid fluid shifts and additional protein loss. Dangers of

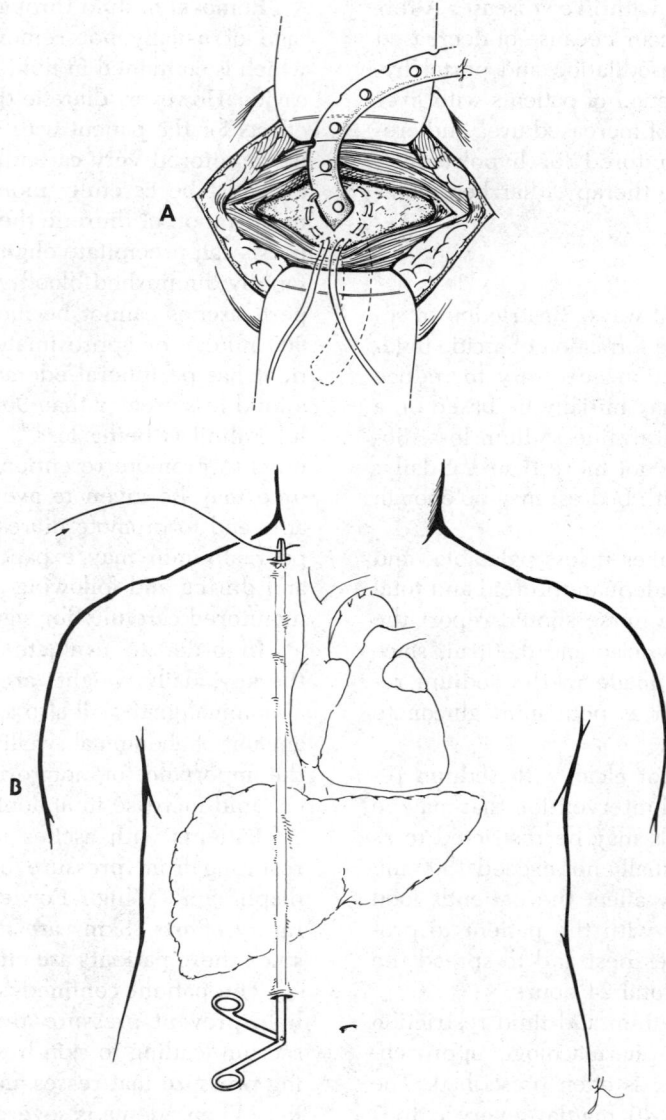

Fig. 33-4. LeVeen-Pertoneo-Vendus shunt. **A,** Peritoneal collecting tube is inserted into peritoneal cavity. Purse-string sutures are snugged around valve stem to prevent leakage of peritoneal fluid. **B,** Long alligator forceps is pushed from abdominal wound into neck.

paracentesis include shock and hypovolemia, which occur as the fluid from the general circulation shifts to the peritoneal cavity as the ascitic fluid is withdrawn. One liter of ascitic fluid contains as much protein as 200 ml of whole blood. Salt-poor human blood albumin may be administered following this procedure to counteract the loss of fluid and protein. (For details of paracentesis and the nursing care involved, see texts on fundamentals of nursing.)

Bleeding tendencies, anemia, and infection

Pathophysiology

Bleeding tendencies, anemia, and infections are common complications of liver disease. Bleeding tendencies may occur in persons with advanced hepatitis, cirrhosis, and biliary duct obstruction. These tendencies are a result of deficiencies in the formation of clotting factors, leukopenia, thrombocytopenia, and a deficiency of erythrocytes. Normally, vitamin K is utilized by the liver cells in synthesizing various clotting factors. In patients with obstructive jaundice and liver disease, this synthesis is impaired. If the patient's bile duct is obstructed, absorption of fat and fat-soluble vitamins (vitamin K) is reduced. On the other hand, even if vitamin K is absorbed, severely damaged liver cells cannot synthesize adequate amounts of these factors, especially prothrombin.

The patient with liver disease may also develop an enlarged spleen caused by portal hypertension. This is believed to be responsible for the resulting thrombocytopenia. In advanced liver cell destruction it has been suggested that a toxic effect on the bone marrow may take place causing hematologic changes in thrombocytes, leukocytes, and erythrocytes.

Vitamin deficiencies resulting from inadequate intake, decreased absorption of fat-soluble vitamins, and the inability to store vitamins also occur. The person with cirrhosis will be deficient in vitamins A, B complex, D, and K.

Anemia is a common problem. Various factors contribute to the anemia, including increased blood loss from gastrointestinal bleeding, decreased red blood cell production secondary to folic acid deficiency and poor protein intake, and increased destruction of red blood cells from hypersplenism. In addition, alcohol has a direct toxic effect on bone marrow.

Infections of various sites may occur because of decreased resistance to infection. Barriers to pathogenic organisms from loss of skin and mucous membrane integrity may be lost. The loss of the activity of the phagocytic cells of the liver and the shunting of blood around the portal circulation prevents the normal removal of pathogenic agents from the blood. Another

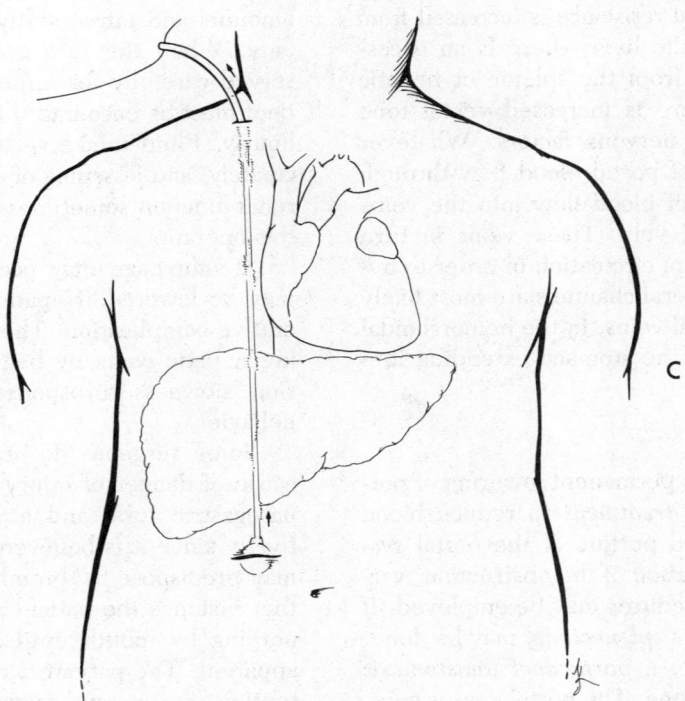

Fig. 33-4, cont'd. C, Tip of venous tubing is secured to this suture and is railroaded into neck by traction.

major factor that contributes to increased risk of infection is leukopenia resulting from hypersplenism and bone marrow destruction.

Intervention

Therapy for bleeding tendencies is aimed at the restoration of clotting factors. If a decreased prothrombin level is identified, vitamin K will be given parenterally. This will not help if liver cell damage is the cause of the reduced prothrombin formation. If this is the case, whole blood or plasma may be given to replace clotting factors at least temporarily. If the patient has a reduced platelet level, platelet transfusions may be given. Vitamin supplements of B complex, particularly thiamine, will be given. In addition, bile salts to assist in the absorption of fat-soluble vitamins may be prescribed. Anemia is treated by measures that control blood loss, a high-caloric, high-protein diet (if ammonium can be handled by the liver), and avoidance of alcohol. Anemia usually responds well to these measures. Infection is prevented by using aseptic techniques with all invasive procedures; isolating patients from staff, other patients, and visitors who have an infection; and providing good respiratory, skin, and oral hygiene.

Portal hypertension

Pathophysiology

A rise in portal venous pressure (portal hypertension) occurs when peripheral resistance is increased from damage of vessels within the liver, there is an excessive flow of arterial blood from the splenic or hepatic artery to the liver, or there is increased vessel tone caused by hormonal and nervous factors. Whatever the cause, an obstruction of portal blood flow through the liver causes a backup of blood flow into the veins that empty into the portal vein. These veins in turn develop collateral channels of circulation in order to bypass the obstruction. Collateral channels are most likely to occur in the paraumbilical veins, in the hemorrhoidal veins, and at the cardia of the stomach extending into the esophagus.

Intervention

The only way to achieve permanent lowering of portal pressure is by *surgical treatment* to reduce blood flow through the obstructed portion of the portal system. Depending on the location of the obstruction, various elective operative procedures may be employed. If the splenic vein is blocked, a *splenectomy* may be done. If the block is intrahepatic, a *portacaval anastomosis* (portacaval shunt) may be done. The portal vein is anastomosed to the inferior vena cava so that the blood from the portal system bypasses the liver (Fig. 33-7). This may be achieved by an end-to-side or side-to-side anas-

tomosis. For more effective portal decompression the end-to-side anastomosis is preferred and is considered to be technically easier to perform. With the side-to-side shunt the total portal blood flow to the liver is not diverted. When the portal vein is blocked, the splenic vein is anastomosed to the left renal vein. This procedure is called a *splenorenal shunt* and relieves pressure on the portal vein, since approximately 30% of the blood in the portal vein comes from the splenic vein.[47] If there is no portal hypertension, the varicosed vessels may be ligated through a thoracotomy incision.

Careful *preoperative* preparation is necessary, since it must be remembered that the patient with liver damage severe enough to cause bleeding esophageal varices is not a good operative risk (p. 403). Preoperative criteria for a portacaval shunt include at least one hemorrhage from esophageal varices, absence of ascites and hepatic coma, a bilirubin level below 1.5 mg, and an albumin level above 3 g/100 ml. It is generally felt that a *prophylactic* shunt is not usually justified. The patient is usually apprehensive about the recommended operation, yet in *selected* cases it is known that the operative risk is much less than the risk from recurring hemorrhage. Vitamin K, antibiotics, and transfusions are usually given preoperatively.

Postoperatively, the patient needs close observation and constant nursing attention. Narcotics should be given for severe pain, but sedative drugs usually are avoided because of their toxic effects on the diseased liver. Generally, narcotics are given in guarded amounts and infrequently in the presence of liver disease. When they are given, the patient must be observed carefully for impending hepatic coma. The patient must be encouraged to breathe deeply and to cough hourly. Fluid intake and output must be recorded accurately, and lessening of output must be reported, since renal function sometimes decreases for a time following this operation.

Hemorrhage may occur, since prothrombin levels may be lowered. Hepatic coma may also be a postoperative complication. The nurse can recognize impending hepatic coma by beginning signs of mental confusion, slowness in response, and generally inappropriate behavior.

Some surgeons do not pass a nasogastric tube because of danger of injury to the varices. Others pass a nasogastric tube and attach it to suction .postoperatively, since it is believed that postoperative distention may predispose to thrombosis of the portal vein. In either instance the patient is fed intravenously and given nothing by mouth until signs of active peristalsis are apparent. The patient is observed closely for pain, distention, fever, and nausea, which may be signs of thrombosis at the site of anastomosis. *Regional heparinization* may be employed to prevent thrombus formation at surgery. A fine polyethylene catheter is inserted into the right gastroepiploic vein, brought out through the wound, and attached to a continuous drip of heparin and saline solution. The surgeon determines the rate of flow. The catheter may be left for 5 to 7 days and during this time the nurse must see that it is not obstructed or subjected to tension in any way. During heparinization the patient remains in bed or sits by the bedside. Particular attention should be paid, therefore, to exercising the lower extremities in an attempt to prevent development of thrombi.

Some surgeons prefer to keep the patient flat in bed for several days until the anastomosis is healed. Others want their patients to get out of bed on the day after the operation. Leg and arm exercises are begun on the day after surgery. The lower extremities must be observed carefully for signs of edema, which may follow the sudden increase of blood flow into the inferior vena cava. Elevation of the lower extremities may be ordered, and the length of time the patient spends standing and walking should be medically prescribed.

After some shunting procedures none of the venous blood passes through the liver, and protein end products are not completely detoxified. For this reason the patient is usually placed on a low-protein diet. Neomycin or chlortetracycline (Aureomycin), both of which destroy the bacteria in the intestine, may be given so that fewer bacteria remain in the bowel to break down protein and increase the production of ammonia.

Bleeding esophageal varices

Pathophysiology

Bleeding esophageal varices (Fig. 33-5) occur in approximately 30% of all patients with cirrhosis of the liver.[47] The branches of the azygos and vena cava veins become distended where they join the smaller vessels of the esophagus. This occurs because of the greater volume of blood, which is under higher pressure as a result of portal hypertension. These small vessels become tortuous and fragile and may be affected by mechanical trauma from ingestion of coarse food and acid pepsin erosion, which may result in bleeding.[55] Bleeding may also occur as a result of coughing, vomiting, sneezing, straining at stool (Valsalva's maneuver), or any physical exertion that increases abdominal venous pressure. Bleeding is frequently abrupt and without pain. Severe hematemesis and resultant shock may follow, requiring emergency treatment.

Clinical picture

Along with routine liver function tests, esophagoscopy most clearly determines the diagnosis. There is danger of initiating hemorrhage while carrying out this procedure, however, and the risks should be carefully weighed depending on the patient's situation. Portal vein

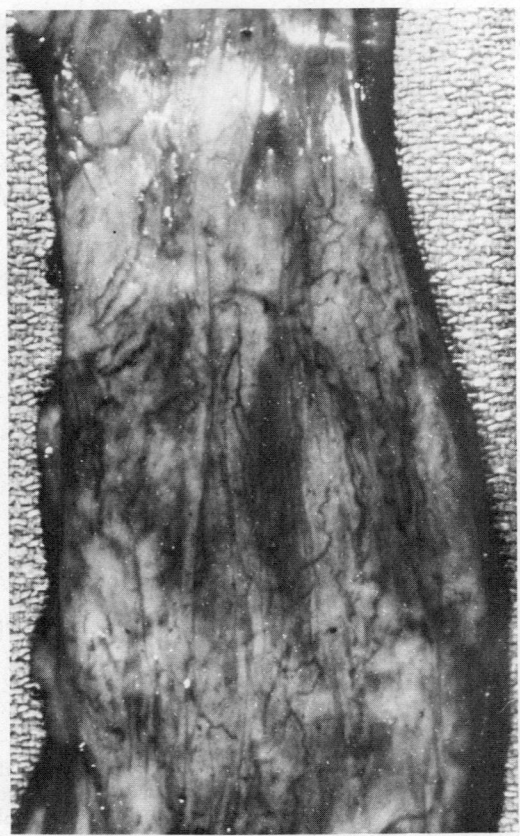

Fig. 33-5. Esophageal varices. Swollen varices and extensive collateral circulation are evident in segment of esophagus from patient with Laennec's cirrhosis. (From Groër, M.E., and Shekleton, M.E.: Basic pathophysiology: a conceptual approach, ed. 2, St. Louis, 1983, The C.V. Mosby Co. Courtesy Department of Pathology, University of Tennessee, Knoxville.)

pressure readings may also be carried out as well as other specialized radiographic procedures. Hemorrhaging is a true medical emergency and requires prompt medical and nursing action.

Intervention

Control of bleeding. Management of bleeding esophageal varices consists of restoring blood volume and controlling the bleeding. Measures that may *control the hemorrhage* include gastric lavage with ice water, local gastric hypothermia using an esophagogastric balloon, or intravenous injection of vasopressin (Pitressin), which reduces portal pressure and blood flow by constricting the splanchnic arterioles. Since vasopressin also decreases the blood supply to the liver, it should be used with caution. If the hemorrhage is considered to be *minor*, introduction of a nasogastric tube and administration of magaldrate (Riopan) may be sufficient to control the hemorrhage. Esophagogastric tamponade (with a Blakemore-Sengstaken tube) is the most widely used therapy for massive hemorrhage.

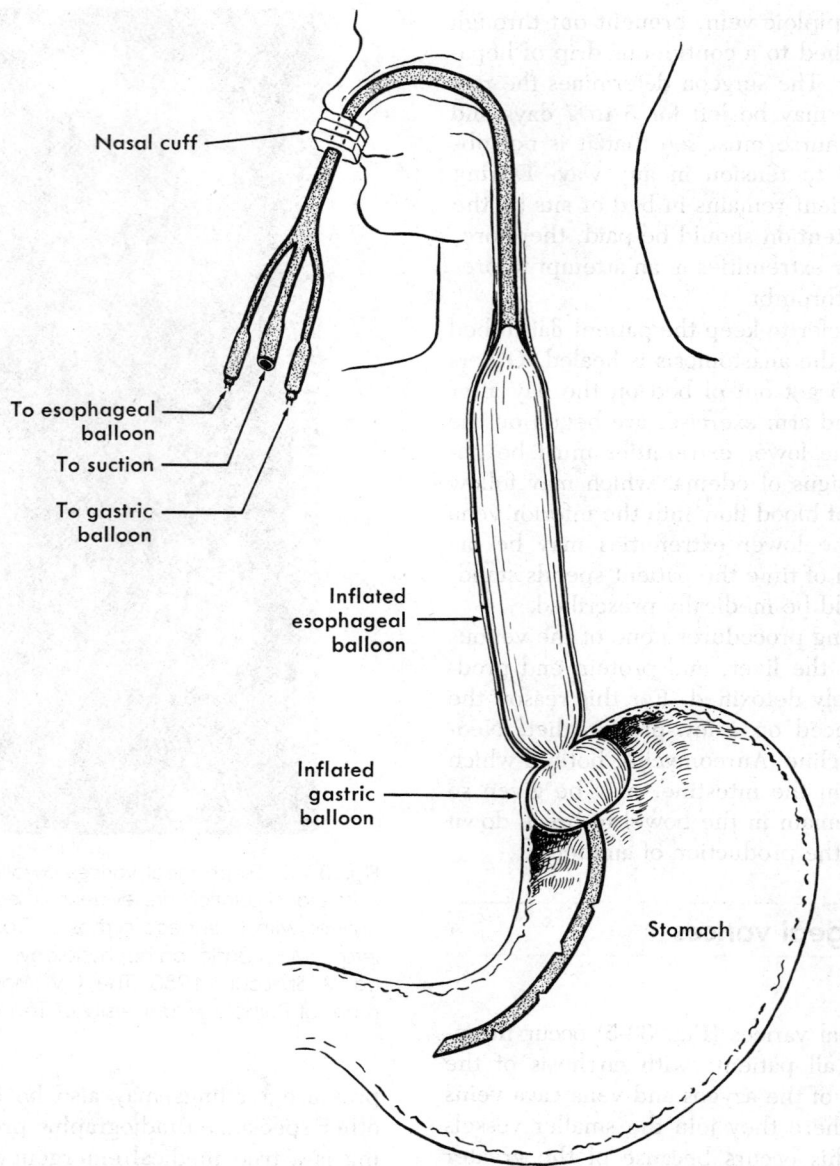

Nasal cuff

To esophageal
balloon

To suction

To gastric
balloon

Inflated
esophageal
balloon

Inflated
gastric
balloon

Stomach

Fig. 33-6. Blakemore-Sengstaken tube with esophageal and gastric balloons inflated. (Redrawn from Rubber appliances in surgery and therapeutics, Providence, R.I., Davol, Inc.)

The esophagogastric tube (Blakemore-Sengstaken) is a three-lumen tube with two balloon attachments. One lumen serves as a nasogastric suction tube, the second is used to inflate the gastric balloon, and the third is used to inflate the esophageal balloon (Fig. 33-6). The tube is passed through the nose into the stomach with the balloons deflated. When the tube is in the stomach, the gastric balloon is inflated with 100 to 300 ml of air and the lumen is clamped; the tube is then pulled out slowly so that the balloon is held tightly against the cardioesophageal junction. A cube of foam rubber called a nasal cuff is placed between the tube and the nares, and the tube is secured to the face with pressure-sensitive tape. The cube of foam rubber absorbs excess nasal se-

cretions and reduces trauma to the nostril. It also provides traction, which maintains the tube in the proper position. If after the gastric balloon is inflated there is further hematemesis or if bloody fluid is returned on aspiration, one can assume that the bleeding is from the esophagus, and the esophageal balloon should be inflated (Fig. 33-6). The esophageal lumen is connected by a Y tube to a manometer and the balloon is inflated with 20 to 45 mm Hg and clamped. In order to stop bleeding, the pressure must be greater than the patient's portal venous pressure. If bleeding is from esophageal varices, blood will no longer be aspirated from the stomach. If there is still blood present, the stomach may be lavaged with a small amount of ice water or a solution of iced alcohol and water may be circulated through the balloon to provide vasoconstriction as well as pressure. The nasogastric lumen is usually connected to intermittent gastric suction, which permits easy appraisal of whether bleeding has ceased and also serves to keep the stomach empty. It is important to remove all blood from the stomach because the presence of it may precipitate hepatic coma.

Persons who are being treated for esophageal varices are very ill and may be disoriented. They require constant attention, and if there is any chance they will pull on the tube, their arms should be restrained. The nurse must be constantly alert to the pressure in the balloons. If the gastric balloon should collapse or rupture, the entire tube may move up and obstruct the airway. Should the gastric balloon rupture, the esophageal balloon is deflated at once and the entire tube is removed.

The esophageal balloon can be left inflated up to 48 hours without tissue damage or severe discomfort for the patient. The fully inflated gastric balloon with traction exerted on it, however, compresses the stomach wall between the balloon and the diaphragm, causing ulceration of the gastric mucosa, and is severely uncomfortable for the patient. To offset the possibility of necrosis, the physician may release the traction and balloon pressures periodically. If the pressure in the gastric balloon is temporarily released to relieve pressure and the esophageal balloon is left inflated, the patient must be attended continuously to make sure the tube does not move up the esophagus.

A second tube should be in the patient unit ready for immediate use in case of damage to the one being used (the tubes are not reused). Before the tube is inserted, the balloon should be tested. The tubes have the date of manufacture stamped on them, and those over a year old should be discarded because of deterioration of the rubber. Before removal of the tube, the balloons are deflated gradually, and the tube is gently withdrawn by the physician. The patient then is observed closely for any indications of renewed bleeding.

Shock. As soon as the balloons are in place and bleeding has been controlled, transfusions of *fresh* whole blood are given to combat hypovolemic shock. Fresh blood is used for several reasons: (1) hepatic coma can be precipitated by blood that is only 3 to 4 days old because whole blood develops as increasing concentration of ammonia from hydrolysis of cells; (2) the damaged liver may be unable to metabolize citrate from the sodium citrate used to preserve stored blood, and citric intoxication can result; (3) patients with cirrhosis excrete sodium poorly; and (4) refrigerated blood is virtually devoid of prothrombin and coagulation factors essential for clotting.

Oxygen is usually administered to increase the oxygen available to the blood. A saline cathartic such as magnesium sulfate may be given through the nasogastric tube to hasten the expulsion of blood that has passed from the stomach to the intestine, and enemas may also be given in an effort to lessen bacterial action on the blood in the intestinal tract. This action produces ammonia, which passes to the bloodstream and in turn puts a burden on the liver, which must detoxify it to form urea. An antibiotic that destroys intestinal bacteria, such as neomycin, also may be given to lessen their activity in the decomposition of protein in the intestine. Antacids are commonly prescribed to reduce stomach acidity and to prevent a reflux of acid into the esophagus. They are given through the nasogastric lumen of the tube.

Emotional support. The patient with bleeding esophageal varices is acutely ill and extremely apprehensive. Discomfort from the tamponade tube and the potential onset of encephalopathy must be considered when evaluating the patient's behavior. The patient must be attended constantly, given reassurance, and kept absolutely quiet. All procedures and the patient's part in them should be quietly and calmly explained and carried out with the minimum of activity. The family generally is very frightened and should be given as much information as necessary to relieve their concern. Some member of the family should be permitted to see the patient or to stay at the bedside for a short time.

Monitoring. The nurse is responsible for checking the vital signs, which may be taken as often as every 15 minutes until the hemorrhage is controlled. The blood pressure cuff is left on the arm deflated, and care is taken to inflate it only a few degrees above the anticipated level. In this way many patients may sleep through the taking of blood pressures. Care also is taken to see that the transfusion and the infusions are running at an appropriate rate. The patient in shock may feel cold and must be kept warm but not perspiring. If iced solutions are used in the balloons, chills may occur. They should be reported to the physician, who may order a warming blanket.

When an esophagogastric tube is in place, the nurse must also check the manometer attached to the tube. If the pressure rises or falls below the prescribed level, the amount of air or solution in the balloon must be adjusted. Often this adjustment is made by the physician, but it may be made by the nurse if there are orders to that effect.

Mouth care. Because the inflated esophageal balloon occludes the esophagus, the patient cannot take anything by mouth or even swallow saliva. The patient should be provided with cleansing tissues and an emesis basin. Frequent mouth care is required and all blood in the mouth should be removed. If the patient is very weak or if movement is not allowed, gentle suctioning of the mouth and throat may be needed to prevent aspiration of saliva. The nostrils are kept clean, lubricated, and protected so that tissues do not sustain injury because of pressure from the tube. Care must be taken not to disturb the tube, and the physician is consulted as to how much movement the patient is permitted. Passive moving of extremities usually is allowed.

Operative management

If the measures already described do not control bleeding, a surgical *portal-systemic decompression* procedure may be considered in a good-risk patient. Patients with advanced hepatic failure are not good surgical candidates because the mortality in these patients is so high. The most commonly used *portal-systemic*

decompression procedures (shunts) are *end-to-side portacaval anastomosis* and *end-to-side splenorenal anastomosis*. Since postshunt encephalopathy and hepatic failure are not uncommon, surgeons are interested in modifying these operations to preserve hepatic blood flow while providing for decompression of the gastroesophageal veins. The *distal splenorenal shunt*, which preserves superior mesenteric flow to the liver while allowing for variceal decompression through the short gastric and splenic veins, may be such a procedure (Fig. 33-7). The preoperative and postoperative care is the same as that described on p. 679.

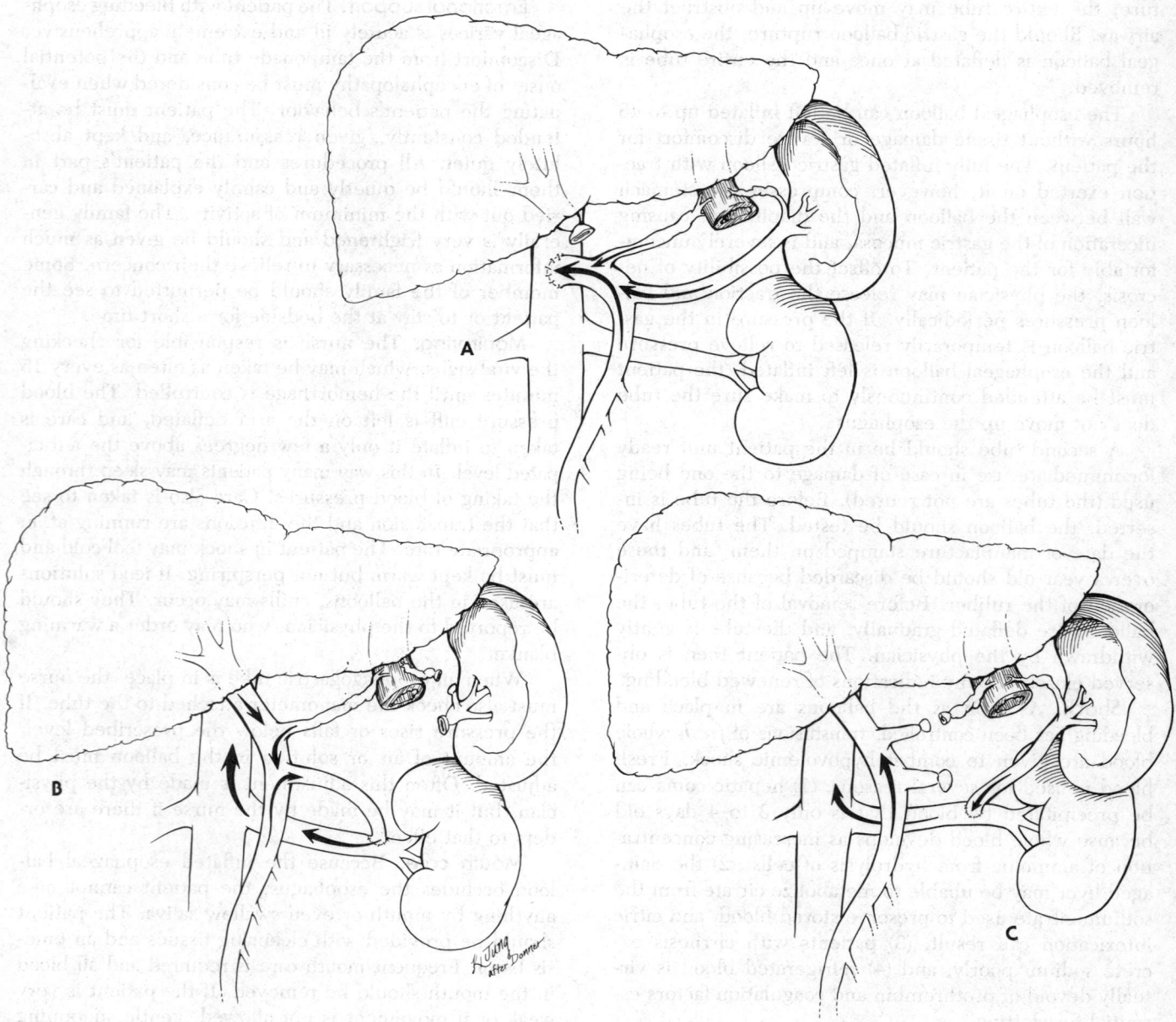

Fig. 33-7. Decompression operations for portal hypertension. **A,** End-to-side portacaval shunt. **B,** Splenorenal shunt. **C,** Distal splenorenal shunt.

Hepatic coma

Pathophysiology

Hepatic coma (hepatic encephalopathy) is metabolic encephalopathy of the brain associated with liver failure. Dysfunctions of the central nervous system are thought to be precipitated by elevated ammonia concentrations, hypoxia, changes in electrolyte concentrations with disturbances of acid-base balance, infections, and depressant drugs. Many patients with hepatic coma have an increase in blood ammonia concentration. Normally, ammonia, which is formed in the intestines from the breakdown of protein by intestinal bacteria, is converted to urea through the Krebs-Henseleit cycle in the liver. When liver failure occurs, ammonia is not converted into urea and ammonia concentration in the circulating blood is increased. The factors that may cause depression of liver function or an increase in the level of ammonia in the blood and thus may precipitate hepatic coma are summarized in the box below.

Clinical picture

The manifestations of hepatic coma vary and may occur quickly or gradually over the course of a few days. At least daily observation and interviewing of the patient are carried out and recorded in order to ascertain subtle personality and behavioral changes indicative of impending coma. Early signs may be missed if someone does not know the patient well or if a detailed assessment was not obtained initially. Manifestations may include impaired attention span, poor ability to concentrate, delayed rate of response, yawning, twitching, irritability, apathy, insomnia and restlessness, and loss of interest in the environment. Speech patterns and the ability to write should be evaluated for change. As the condition worsens, speech usually becomes slurred, confusion is more apparent, and the level of consciousness is gradually depressed. A characteristic flapping tremor (*asterixis*, or liver flap) may be elicited when the patient is asked to dorsiflex the hand while the rest of the arm is extended resting on the bed. A peculiar sweetish odor can frequently be detected on the breath (*fetor hepaticus*). Soon the patient cannot be aroused except by painful stimuli, and as the coma deepens there may be no response to pain and reflexes may be completely absent. At this point the patient's temperature may rise markedly and there may be alterations in pulse and respiratory rate.

The patient's consciousness level commonly fluctuates, and if possible the same nurse should be assigned to the patient over time in order to document accurately changes in mental functioning. Early detection of symptoms allows for more rapid treatment and consequently improves the patient's chance of recovery. Progress notes should describe actual behavioral observations as opposed to generalizations that are vague

---

FACTORS COMMONLY PRECIPITATING HEPATIC COMA

Factors depressing liver function

Hypoxia

    Secondary to hemorrhage and hypovolemic shock

    Secondary to morphine and other sedatives

Intercurrent infection

Exercise

    In patients with chronic liver disease who are in impending coma

    In patients with acute hepatitis

Acute hepatitis during pregnancy, especially during last trimester

Abdominal paracentesis

    Secondary to reduction of plasma volume

    Patients may also have hyponatremia, especially if natriuretic diuretics were being administered before paracentesis

Factors increasing level of ammonia

Gastrointestinal ammonia (old blood in bowel from gastrointestinal hemorrhage)

High-protein intake

Transfusions, especially with stored blood

Thiazide diuretics and acetazolamide (Diamox)

Hypokalemia

    Secondary to thiazide diuretics

    Secondary to potassium loss from the bowel

Shunting of blood into systemic circulation without passing through hepatic sinusoids

    Natural collateral bypass of liver

    Surgical bypass of liver

Alkalosis secondary to hyperventilation and hypokalemia

Hyperbilirubinemia (serum bilirubin level greater than 35 mg/100 ml)

and allow for various interpretations. In the assessment of the patient's ongoing clinical state, the nurse monitors for any changes in the rate or depth of respiration, the development of cardiac arrhythmias (cardiac monitors are usually used), evidence of rapid changes in peripheral edema or ascites, and neurologic changes.

Intervention

Treatment of hepatic coma centers around finding and treating the precipitating cause, general supportive measures, and avoidance of additional trauma to the liver. This is accomplished by completely eliminating protein from the diet for several days, giving carbohydrates by mouth or nasogastric feedings, and administering antibiotics such as neomycin that destroy bacteria in the intestine and subsequently reduce the amount of ammonia formed. Enemas and carthartics such as magnesium sulfate may be given to empty the bowel and prevent further ammonia formation. Some physicians prefer to rely on cathartics and cation exchange resins to help remove toxic substances from the bowel rather than to give antibiotics. Antibiotics destroy bacteria, which are active in the manufacture of vitamin K, and the absence of bacteria causes diarrhea and other symptoms which may worsen the patient's condition.

Lactulose is being used in an attempt to decrease the production of ammonia. Lactulose, which is given orally, is a synthetic disaccharide that cannot be utilized in the small intestine. It produces diarrhea, lowers the pH level, and alters the bacterial flora of the colon, thereby decreasing the production of nitrogenous substances.

In some patients large doses of the adrenocortical steroids are effective in reversing hepatic coma, providing that hepatic cell destruction has not been overwhelming. Other methods used to reverse encephalopathy include the following: (1) attempts to increase the low levels of branched-chain amino acids by administration of either the amino acid or its keto-analogues; (2) administration of levodopa, since it was felt that in coma there may be a deficiency of neurotransmitters; (3) use of hemodialysis or peritoneal dialysis to remove ammonia; and (4) exchange transfusion to remove toxins.

In selected patients a colon-bypass operation may be performed to stop function of the colon and prevent absorption of material from the intestines. Attempts have been made to replace nonfunctioning livers with those of recent cadavers. To date these transplants have not been successful because immunosuppressive therapy is inadequate and the transplanted organs have been rejected by the recipient's body.

Many patients in hepatic coma die of renal failure secondary to an inadequate circulating blood volume (hypovolemia). In some patients renal function progressively deteriorates without any apparent cause. The treatment of hepatic coma requires a careful balancing of fluid administration to maintain adequate perfusion of the kidney without creating an excessive load on the cardiovascular system. Therefore when intravenous solutions are being administered, the desired flow rate is monitored very closely and the patient is observed for signs of cardiovascular overload. In order to adequately monitor renal function, an indwelling catheter is often inserted, especially if the patient is being maintained on intravenous fluids. Central venous pressure (CVP) monitoring (p. 1055) is also commonly used. The nurse is alert to changes in the CVP readings suggestive of either hypervolemia or hypovolemia. The supportive nursing care required by any patient with hepatic disease as well as by any unconscious patient should be given.

Tracheostomy may be performed as a prophylactic measure. Intermittent positive pressure breathing with oxygen may also be used to improve oxygenation (pp. 1231 and 1243). Since most narcotics and sedatives must be detoxified by the liver, they are contraindicated in patients with impaired liver function. If a sedative must be used, drugs such as chlordiazepoxide (Librium), barbital, or phenobarbital, which are excreted by the kidney, are prescribed.

The patient in hepatic coma is very ill and is vulnerable to any increase in stress. The meticulous nursing care required for any patient who is unconscious is necessary. Particular care should be taken to protect the patient from infection. If the patient survives, long-term care as discussed for the patient with cirrhosis of the liver should be planned. The patient who has had definite or threatened hepatic coma may be kept indefinitely on a low-protein diet. When protein is added to the diet, it is added gradually and often does not exceed 40 g/day (average intake in the United States is 70 to 80 g/day). In addition, the patient may receive neomycin, 2 to 3 g/day, or lactalose daily. Patients with chronic liver disease may go in and out of coma; therefore they are monitored for any change in behavior that would indicate early coma. The patient and the family should also be taught to be alert to subtle changes in the patient's behavior and to seek medical assistance when this occurs.

Outcome criteria for the person with chronic liver disease

The person or significant others can:
1. Explain the dietary plan to be followed after discharge:
   a. List daily food and fluid requirements (e.g., amount of protein allowed).
   b. List foods and fluids not allowed in diet (e.g., sodium restriction, elimination of alcohol).
   c. Explain plans for meeting nutritional needs.
2. Explain medications to be taken at home and precautions related to them:

a. State name, dosage, expected effects, and side effects for each medication.

b. State the untoward effects of medication that need to be reported to the health care provider at once.

c. State reason for not using over-the-counter drugs.

3. Explain program to prevent complications:
   a. Explain the basic health problem.
   b. State how the prescribed treatment is helping.
   c. List daily schedule including rest periods.
   d. List ways to avoid bleeding episodes (such as using soft toothbrush, blowing nose gently, taking antacids as ordered).
   e. List ways to avoid infections.
   f. Explain plans for follow-up care.

4. Describe possible complications of illness and state what to do if they occur:
   a. State health care monitoring to be done daily (weight, abdominal girth, temperature, checking for bleeding).
   b. List signs and symptoms requiring immediate medical attention (e.g., weight gain, increase in abdominal girth, elevated temperature, bleeding from any orifice, frank blood in urine or stool, tar-colored stools, changes in behavior or memory).
   c. State name and phone number of health care provider to be called in case of emergency.
   d. State plans for follow-up care.

Disorders of the biliary system

The biliary system consists of the gallbladder and its associated ductal system. The ductal system provides a pathway for the bile that is formed in the liver to reach the intestine and also functions to regulate bile flow. The liver produces up to 1 L of bile per day. As it is formed, bile is excreted into the hepatic duct where it passes into the cystic duct to be stored in the gallbladder. After reaching the gallbladder, bile is altered to a concentrated form. When bile is needed, the gallbladder releases it into the cystic duct where it goes into the common bile duct and then into the duodenum. On reaching the intestine, bile functions to emulsify undigested fat, facilitate the absorption of fat-soluble vitamins, iron, and calcium, and activate the release of pancreatic and intestinal enzymes. (See Chapter 30 for a discussion of laboratory and diagnostic tests used to assist in identifying the cause and site of biliary malfunction.)

There are no specific means to prevent disease of the biliary system. However, since disease of this system occurs much more often in obese persons, it is reasonable to suppose that control of obesity may contribute to its prevention. Women are more often affected than men, and the description "fair, fat, and forty" is fairly accurate. In all health education the nurse stresses the importance of avoiding excess weight. Patients with biliary tract disease are usually advised to keep fat intake to a fairly low level for the remainder of their lives, although no rigid dietary regulations are needed. Patients who tend to form stones in the ducts are usually advised to be careful of their fat intake and to drink generous amounts of fluids.

Most of the problems of the gallbladder are treated surgically. The following section describes the common problems and presents surgical care and management.

Cholecystitis

Etiology and epidemiology

Cholecystitis is inflammation of the gallbladder. The condition may be acute or chronic and usually is associated with gallstones or other obstructions of bile passage.

A large variety of organisms may contribute to acute disease of the gallbladder. Colon bacilli, staphylococci, streptococci, salmonellae, typhoid bacilli, and many other organisms have been found. Infection may reach the gallbladder through the bloodstream, the lymph system, or the bile ducts. Cholecystitis is more common in women than in men, the ratio being 2.5:1. Sedentary, obese persons are affected most often, and the incidence is highest in the fifth and sixth decades of life. The incidence of cholecystitis and mortality are high in the elderly.

Pathophysiology

In acute cholecystitis the gallbladder is usually very enlarged, resembling a distended sac. Inflammation occurs and the wall of the gallbladder becomes thickened and edematous. The inflammation may be confined to the mucous membrane lining, or it may involve the entire wall of the gallbladder. In prolonged edema a cellular reaction is imposed on the already inflamed gallbladder. This cellular reaction is caused by the bile that acts as an irritant. This irritation, plus impaired circulation, edema, and distention, produce ischemia, which can proceed to anoxia and necrosis, and gangrene may result. The gallbladder may become adherent to surrounding structures.

Chronic cholecystitis may produce a variety of structural changes whether or not stones are present. This is not the result of an infectious process but is related to a diseased gallbladder wall with inefficient emptying. It is believed that chronic cholecystitis is caused by chemical or mechanical irritation from stones causing pressure on the mucosa or biliary stasis. The gallbladder walls are usually thickened, fibrosis may be present, and the gallbladder may be shrunken or distended. Eventually, because of destruction of the mucosa, outpouchings of the epithelium may form. Bacteria and other irritants may become trapped in them, which may help maintain a chronic inflammatory process.

Clinical picture

Persons experiencing an acute attack of cholecystitis may be very ill. Acute cholecystitis is usually abrupt in onset; however, the individual often has a history of intolerance of fatty foods and general indigestion. Nausea and vomiting usually occur, and there is severe pain in the right upper quadrant of the abdomen. The pulse rate and respiratory rate are increased, and the temperature and white blood count are elevated. This acute phase may subside with medical treatment, or it may require emergency surgery.

The chronic form of the disease is usually preceded by several acute attacks of moderate severity, and the individual gives a history of having learned to avoid fried foods and certain other foods such as nuts that are high in fat. Pain is usually located in the right upper quadrant but may be referred to the back. Nausea and vomiting and flatulence may also occur. Persons with chronic cholecystitis may not be as ill as those with acute disease and therefore may not seek medical attention until they experience pain from a biliary obstruction or develop jaundice.

Intervention

The treatment of choice for most patients with cholecystitis is surgery. The decision as to when to operate depends largely on the age and condition of the patient and the response to treatment. Although some surgeons favor conservative treatment until the acute infection has subsided, others believe that the danger of rupture and subsequent peritonitis is so great that immediate surgery to drain the gallbladder (cholecystostomy) is advisable. All recommend removing the gallbladder (cholecystectomy) when the acute condition has subsided. Infection may spread to the hepatic duct and liver, causing inflammation of the ducts (cholangitis) with subsequent strictures that may cause obstruction of bile flow and are exceedingly difficult to correct surgically.

When medical treatment is prescribed it includes the administration of antibiotics and infusions of glucose and appropriate electrolytes. Food is withheld until acute symptoms subside. If vomiting persists, a nasogastric tube is passed and attached to suction. Meperidine hydrochloride (Demerol) may be given for pain and is preferred because its spasmogenic effect on the biliary tract is less than that which occurs with opiates, although it is thought by some authorities to increase spasm of the biliary sphincter. The inhalation of amyl nitrite may diminish intestinal and biliary spasms. When infection is present, antibiotics are prescribed.

When food is tolerated, a reducing diet and careful avoidance of too much fat usually are recommended. Persons who have had acute attacks are more strongly motivated to follow dietary instructions, and the nurse may be of real help to them in planning attractive meals that are low in fat and total calories.

Cholelithiasis

Epidemiology and etiology

Cholelithiasis is the presence of stones in the biliary tract. *The stones are composed largely of cholesterol, bile pigment, and calcium.* Cholelithiasis may occur in either sex at any age, but it is more common in middle-aged women. The incidence increases gradually thereafter, and one out of every three persons who reach the age of 75 years will have gallstones.[47] It is not known why stones form in the gallbladder and in the hepatic duct. They may be present for years and cause no inflammation. Sometimes they appear to be preceded or followed by chronic cholecystitis. Chronic cholelithiasis is aggravated by pregnancy, perhaps because of the increased pressure in the abdomen.

Pathophysiology

Three specific factors appear to contribute to the formation of gallstones: metabolic factors, stasis, and inflammation. An increased concentration of one of the three substances present in bile (bile acids, bile pigments, and cholesterol) may result in their subsequent precipitation giving rise to the formation of stones. An increased serum cholesterol level is a *metabolic* disorder occurring in obesity, pregnancy, diabetes, and hypothyroidism. About 90% of gallstones in Western cultures are cholesterol stones. The remaining 10% consist of bilirubin pigment stones in persons with hemolytic disease.[3] Cholesterol stones are firm and radiolucent, but pure ones are uncommon. Bilirubin stones are small and soft and are found mostly in the ducts. Calcium salts usually contribute to the composition of both types of stones and make them radiopaque.

Biliary *stasis* leading to stagnation of bile in the gallbladder leads to excessive absorption of water. This allows the salts to precipitate easily and leads to the formation of mixed stones. These stones may be quite variable in size and are sometimes small enough to have a gravel-like appearance on gallbladder radiographs.

The third contributing factor to stone formation is *inflammation* of the biliary system. This condition causes the bile constituents to become altered, and the inflamed gallbladder mucosa absorbs more of the bile acids with a resultant reduction of the solubility of cholesterol.

Stones may lodge anywhere along the biliary tract where they may cause an obstruction which, if unrelieved, leads to jaundice, or they may cause pressure and subsequent necrosis and infection of the walls of the biliary ducts (Fig. 33-8). Occasionally, a stone, because of its location, blocks the entrance of pancreatic fluid and bile into the duodenum at the ampulla of Vater. This condition is difficult to differentiate from obstruction caused by malignancy.

Clinical picture

There may be no signs of cholelithiasis until a stone becomes lodged in a biliary duct, although a history of indigestion after consuming rich, fatty foods, occasional discomfort in the right upper quadrant of the abdomen, and more trouble than the normal person with gaseous eructations after eating is common. Gaseous eructations in cholelithiasis characteristically occur almost immediately following meals, in contrast to those associated with gastric ulcer, which occur when the stomach is empty (usually several hours after a meal).

Gallstone colic, or *biliary colic*, can cause what is probably the most severe pain that can be experienced. The pain may come on suddenly and is probably caused by spasm of the ducts as they attempt to dislodge the stone. There is severe pain in the right upper quadrant of the abdomen, and it radiates through to the back

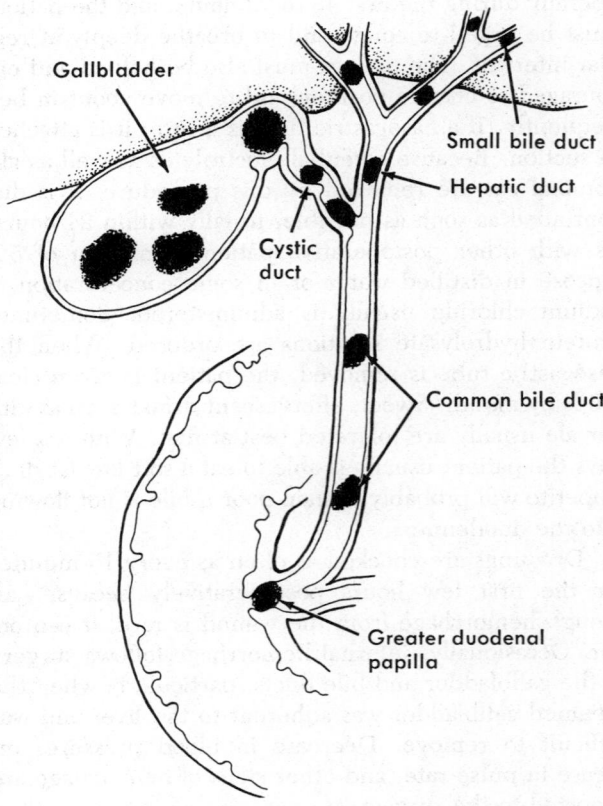

Fig. 33-8. Common sites of gallstones.

Gallbladder

Small bile duct

Hepatic duct

Cystic duct

Common bile duct

Greater duodenal papilla

under the scapula and to the right shoulder. Pain may be so severe that the patient writhes in agony despite large doses of analgesic drugs. Meperidine hydrochloride (Demerol) is used because it is thought to be less spasmogenic than morphine sulfate. Nitroglycerin or inhalations of amyl nitrite are sometimes helpful, and papaverine hydrochloride, atropine, and calcium gluconate often are given to help produce relaxation of the biliary ducts. The patient usually has nausea and vomiting, profuse diaphoresis, tachycardia, and occasionally complete prostration. A nasogastric tube attached to suction often helps to relieve distention in the upper gastrointestinal tract and thereby lessens the pain. Occasionally, following an acute attack of biliary colic the stools are saved to determine whether a stone has passed into the intestines. The stools may be sent to the laboratory, or they may be strained for examination on the patient unit.

Intervention

Because there is no suitable method at present to dissolve stones, the treatment of cholelithiasis is surgical removal of the gallbladder and exploration of the common bile duct. The physician must decide whether to treat the patient medically and wait until the acute attack has subsided or to carry out the surgery immediately. Supportive medical treatment includes relief of pain and control of nausea and vomiting. If the patient becomes dehydrated, intravenous therapy may be necessary along with the replacement of fat-soluble vitamins, which are not absorbed because of absence of bile. If surgery is further delayed, the patient is placed on a low-fat diet and given antispasmodics and anticholinergics to prevent smooth-muscle contraction. Surgery is carried out when the patient's condition has stabilized and after correction of any decrease in prothrombin level.

Carcinoma of the biliary system

Carcinoma can occur anywhere in the biliary system, and unfortunately at present there is no way of diagnosing early carcinoma in the abdominal viscera. Jaundice may be the first sign and indicates that the lesion has developed sufficiently to obstruct bile passage at some point. Carcinoma rarely develops in a normal gallbladder. Associated stones are present in a very high percentage of these patients, which suggests the need to remove all gallbladders with stones.

The treatment for carcinoma of the biliary system is surgical, and an operation is performed as soon as the patient's condition warrants it in the hope that complete surgical removal of the lesion is possible. Patients often benefit from surgery even when cure of the carcinoma is impossible, since various operations that help to restore the flow of bile into the gastrointestinal tract produce remarkable relief of symptoms, and the patient may feel relatively well for a time.

Biliary atresia

Biliary atresia is a condition in which there is a congenital absence or obliteration of the bile ducts. There is no known cause. Jaundice appears about 2 to 3 weeks after birth and progresses until the infant is a greenish bronze color. Tears and saliva may be pigmented, the urine is dark, and the stools are white or clay colored. The child may not be alert and may move slowly but usually has a good appetite. The treatment consists of an operation to establish a pathway for bile into the intestines. As surgery is possible for only a small percentage of these infants, the prognosis is poor.

Surgical management of the patient with biliary disease

The terminology used to indicate specific biliary tract surgery sounds somewhat complicated but actually is self-explanatory once common terms are understood. *Cholecyst* refers to the gallbladder, *docho* refers to the common bile duct, and *litho* refers to a stone.

Cholecystectomy is the removal of the gallbladder, whereas *cholecystostomy* refers to the creation of an opening into the gallbladder for decompression and drainage. *Choledochotomy* is a surgical incision into the common bile duct, usually for removal of a stone *(choledocholithotomy)*. When carcinoma has been found or when strictures in the ducts make other methods of treatment unsatisfactory, *choledochoduodenostomy* and *choledochojejunostomy*, which refer to anastomoses between the bile duct and the duodenum and between the bile duct and the jejunum, respectively, also may be done. *Cholecystogastrostomy* is the surgical formation of an anastomosis between the gallbladder and the stomach.

Preoperative management

A general medical examination is done before biliary surgery, including a radiograph of the chest, x-ray study of the gallbladder, and examination of the urine and stools. Usually an electrocardiogram is ordered. Various tests of hepatic function may be made if disease of the liver is suspected, and if the patient is jaundiced, tests are done to determine the cause. The prothrombin level usually is determined.

If there is jaundice, the prothrombin level usually is low, and vitamin K preparations such as phytonadione (vitamin K_1, Mephyton) may be given preoperatively. Occasionally, when the prothrombin level is very low,

yet surgery is imperative, transfusions of whole blood may be given immediately preoperatively to provide prothrombin, which is essential for blood clotting. If the patient is taking food by mouth poorly, infusions containing glucose and protein hydrolysates may be given in an effort to protect the liver from potential damage and to ensure wound healing. Signs of upper respiratory tract disease should be reported at once, since upper respiratory tract infections can lead to serious complications following surgery of the upper abdomen. A nasogastric tube may be inserted before the patient is taken to the operating room.

Preoperative preparation of the patient with biliary disease is the same as that carried out for any patient having abdominal surgery (see Chapter 24). Emphasis is placed on teaching the patient how to deep breathe and cough postoperatively. This is particularly important because of the high abdominal incision, which makes these activities very painful. An explanation of the types of drainage tubes that may be in place postoperatively may also be helpful.

Postoperative management

Immediate care. On recovery from anesthesia the patient is usually placed in a low Fowler's position. Because breathing is painful the patient may take shallow breaths in order to splint the incision and lessen pain. Analgesic medications for pain should be given fairly liberally during the first 48 to 72 hours, and the patient must be urged to cough and to breathe deeply at regular intervals. The patient must also be helped and encouraged to change position and to move about in bed frequently. If a nasogastric tube is in use, it is attached to suction. Because essential electrolytes as well as abdominal gas are removed by this procedure, it is discontinued as soon as possible, usually within 24 hours. As with other postoperative patients, infusion of 5% glucose in distilled water or in some concentration of sodium chloride usually is administered. Sometimes protein hydrolysate solutions are ordered. When the nasogastric tube is removed, the patient is given clear fluids by mouth. Sweet, effervescent drinks such as ginger ale usually are tolerated best at first. Within a few days the patient usually is able to eat a soft low-fat diet. Appetite will probably remain poor if bile is not flowing into the duodenum.

Dressings are checked as often as every 15 minutes for the first few hours postoperatively because, although hemorrhage from the wound is rare, it can occur. Occasionally, internal hemorrhage follows surgery of the gallbladder and bile ducts, particularly when the inflamed gallbladder was adherent to the liver and was difficult to remove. Decrease in blood pressure, increase in pulse rate, and other signs of hemorrhage are reported to the surgeon at once.

Wound care. If the gallbladder is removed, the cystic duct is ligated and a drain usually is inserted near its stump and brought out through a stab wound on the abdomen. This tube drains bile and small amounts of blood and other serous fluid or exudates onto the dressings. It usually is removed within 5 to 6 days when drainage has largely subsided.

If a cholecystostomy has been performed, a self-retaining catheter is inserted through an opening in the gallbladder and is attached to straight drainage. Bile will drain out through this tube until it is removed, usually between 6 weeks and 6 months.

If exploration of the common duct has been done, a T tube, with the short ends placed into the common duct, will probably be used (Fig. 33-9). The long end of this soft rubber tube is brought through the wound and sutured to the skin. The section of the T tube emerging from the stab wound may be placed over a roll of gauze anchored to the skin with adhesive tape to prevent it from occluding (Fig. 33-10). The T tube is inserted to preserve patency of the common duct and to ensure drainage of bile out of the body until edema in the common duct has subsided enough for bile to drain into the duodenum normally. If the T tube was clamped while the patient was being transported from the recovery room, it must be released *immediately* on arrival in his room. The nurse should check the operative sheet carefully and seek clarification if directions are not clear. The tube usually is connected to closed gravity drainage similar to that used to drain the urinary bladder. Sufficient tubing should be attached so that the patient can move without restriction. The purpose of the tube should be explained, and the patient should be told why it must not be kinked, clamped, or pulled. The drainage should be checked for color and amount at least every 2 hours on the operative day. The tube may drain some blood and blood-stained fluid during the first few hours, but drainage of more than a small amount of blood should be reported to the physician. After this the amount is measured and recorded each day. At first the entire output of bile (normally 500 to 1000 ml/day) may flow through the tube, but within 10 days most of the bile should be flowing into the duodenum.

Usually the T tube is removed in 10 days to 2 weeks. Before this is done the patency of the common bile duct must be assessed. The tube is clamped for variable intervals and the patient monitored for sign of distress. If distress occurs the tube is unclamped immediately and the physician informed. Otherwise a *burette test*, similar to that performed before removing a nephrostomy tube, is done to determine the patency of the biliary system (Fig. 33-9). If the common bile duct is patent the pressure readings will fluctuate very little from the initial reading unless the patient is moving, coughing, talking, or laughing just before the reading. If the com-

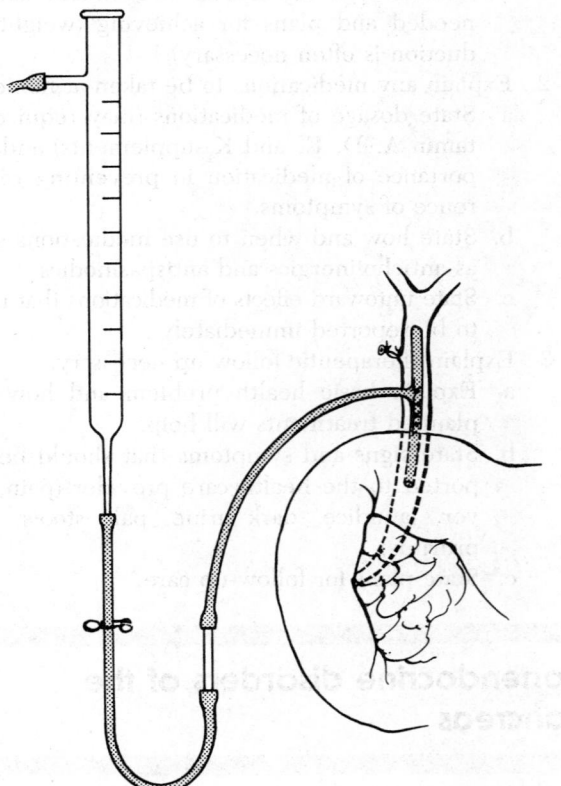

Fig. 33-9. T tube placed in common bile duct and attached to manometer for burette test. Common bile duct has been brought from its normal position for better visualization of T tube.

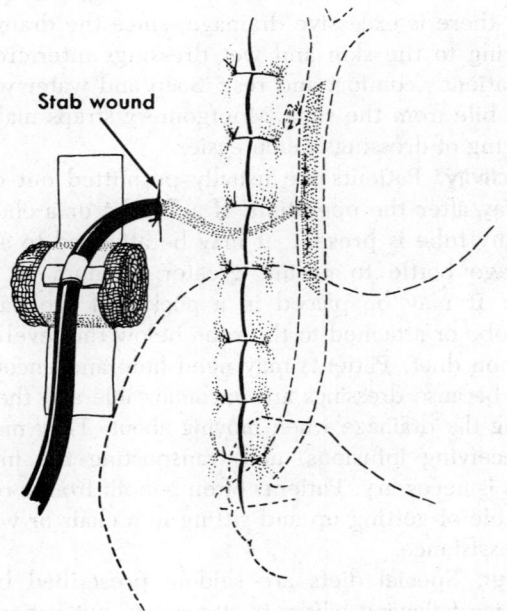

Stab wound

Fig. 33-10. Section of T tube emerging from stab wound may be placed over roll of gauze anchored to skin with adhesive tape to prevent its lumen from being occluded by pressure.

mon bile duct is still obstructed, the level of bile will rise in the burette beyond the set point, usually 15 cm above the level of the common bile duct. If this happens, the physician should be notified. A cholangiogram usually is done to confirm the patency of the duct before the tube is removed (p. 603). Following the removal of the T tube the patient may have chills and fever, but they usually subside within 24 hours. They are caused by edema and a local reaction to the bile. Occasionally, flow of bile into the abdominal cavity causes peritonitis, and therefore any abdominal pain should be reported at once.

Postoperatively, the bile should either drain out through the drainage tubes or flow into the intestine. If it does not do so, it can be assumed that the flow of bile is obstructed and that bile is being forced back into the liver and into the bloodstream. The nurse should observe the patient closely for jaundice, particularly in the sclerae. Urine should be examined for the brown color that is indicative of bile pigment. A specimen should be saved for the physician's inspection when bile pigment is observed in the urine. The nurse may observe the patient's progress by noting the stools: a light color is usual if all the bile is flowing out through the drainage tubes (unless bile salts are being given by mouth), but the normal brown color should gradually reappear as drainage diminishes and finally disappears.

Patients should be told about any drainage tubes that have been used. They should know if much bile is expected on the dressings so that they will not become alarmed by soiling of dressings, gowns, or bedclothes. Outer dressings usually should be changed frequently when there is excessive drainage, since the drainage is irritating to the skin and wet dressings interfere with the patient's comfort and rest. Soap and water will remove bile from the skin. Montgomery straps make the changing of dressings much easier.

Activity. Patients are usually permitted out of bed the day after the operation. If a T tube or a cholecystostomy tube is present, it may be attached to a small drainage bottle to permit greater freedom of movement. It may be placed in a pocket of the patient's bathrobe or attached to the robe below the level of the common duct. Patients may need help and encouragement because dressings are uncomfortable and they fear spilling the drainage when moving about. They may still be receiving infusions, and transporting the infusion bottle is necessary. Patients often benefit from a regular schedule of getting up and sitting in a chair or walking with assistance.

Diet. Special diets are seldom prescribed by the physician following biliary tract surgery, but patients are advised to avoid excessive fats. The nurse should help to teach patients the essentials of good nutrition, with emphasis on foods that are low in fat.

Occasionally, if excessive drainage through the T tube or cholecystostomy tube continues for a long time, the the bile collected in the drainage bottle is administered to the patient through a nasogastric tube to improve digestion. If this is done the funnel or Asepto syringe should be covered and the bile should be in a receptacle so that the patient does not see it. Sometimes the bile may be diluted with grape or other juices to disguise its appearance. Patients generally are not told that they are receiving bile.

Usually from 10 days to 2 weeks of hospitalization are required following biliary tract surgery. If complications occur longer hospitalization is necessary. The length of convalescence depends on the individual patient, but usually at least a month is needed before normal activites can be resumed safely. The nurse should emphasize to the patient the importance of keeping medical appointments as scheduled.

Outcome criteria for the person with chronic biliary disease

The person or significant others can:
1. Explain dietary changes required:
   a. List foods to be avoided or limited (patient is frequently placed on low-fat diet, if treated medically).
   b. Discuss type and amount of food and calories needed and plans for achieving (weight reduction is often necessary).
2. Explain any medications to be taken at home:
   a. State dosage of medications (may require vitamin A, D, E, and K supplements) and importance of medication in preventing recurrence of symptoms.
   b. State how and when to use medications such as anticholinergics and antispasmodics.
   c. State untoward effects of medications that need to be reported immediately.
3. Explain therapeutic follow-up necessary:
   a. Explain basic health problem and how the planned treatments will help.
   b. State signs and symptoms that should be reported to the health care provider (pain, fever, jaundice, dark urine, pale stools, and pruritus).
   c. State plans for follow-up care.

Nonendocrine disorders of the pancreas

The pancreas has both endocrine and exocrine functions. The endocrine functions along with diagnostic tests used to evaluate them are discussed in Chapter 30. The location of the pancreas and developmental facts about it are described on p. 583. The exocrine functions of the pancreas are carried out by acinar cells, which release their secretions into ducts that converge to form the main pancreatic duct (duct of Weesung). In most persons, the pancreatic duct merges from the common bile duct at its entry into the duodenum, but in some persons the common bile duct and pancreatic duct do not merge. The secretions from the pancreas are emptied into the duodenum through the ampulla of Vater.

The acinar cells of the pancreas secrete two substances: one is an isoosmolar solution with a high concentration of bicarbonate, and the other contains multiple digestive enzymes. The pancreatic enzymes include proteolytic (trypsinogen, chymotrypsinogen, and procarboxypeptidase), and amylolytic (amylase), lipolytic (lipases), and nucleolytic (ribonuclease and deoxyribonuclease) enzymes.

The proteolytic enzymes are secreted as inactive precursors. After entering the duodenum, trypsinogen is converted by enterokinase to trypsin. Once some trypsin is formed it can activate more trypsinogen, as well as chymotrypsinogen and procarboxypeptidase.

The pancreatic exocrine secretions are released under the influence of the vagus nerve and secretin, cholecystokinin-pancreozymin, and gastrin. The vagus nerve is involved in increased pancreatic secretion during the cephalic phase of digestion. Gastrin is released during the gastric phase and stimulates the release of the bicarbonate rich solution. The entry of chyme and acids into the small intestines stimulates the release of secretin and cholecystokinin-pancreozymin. Secretin stimulates further secretion of the pancreatic bicarbonate-rich solution, and cholecystokinin-pancreozymin stimulates the release of the pancreatic enzyme-rich solution.

The pancreatic juices complete the digestion of proteins, carbohydrates, and fats so that absorption can take place.

Pancreatitis

Pancreatitis is an inflammatory disease of the pancreas. It can be classified as follows: (1) acute pancreatitis, (2) relapsing acute pancreatitis, (3) chronic pancreatitis, and (4) chronic relapsing pancreatitis. In *acute* and *relapsing acute pancreatitis* restoration of normal function occurs. In the *chronic* forms permanent damage occurs. Common laboratory tests used for evaluating all classes of pancreatitis are described in Table 33-3.

Acute pancreatitis

Etiology and epidemiology

The three most important causes of acute forms of pancreatitis are gallstones, alcohol, and "idiopathic" processes. Other causes are carcinoma, adenomas, infections, trauma, and connective tissue disorders, or it may be induced by drugs or metabolic problems.

The amount of pancreatitis caused by biliary tract disease ranges from 10% to 95%. The percentage depends on the amount of alcoholism present in the population being studied. The association between biliary disease and pancreatitis is obscure.[3] For the reasons stated above, the percentage of persons with pancreatitis related to alcoholism ranges from 8% to 75%, depending on the socioeconomic status of the population served. The relationship between alcoholism and pan-

TABLE 33-3. Laboratory tests used for evaluating pancreatic disease

Test	Sample	Interpretation
Amylase	Serum or whole blood	Normal = 80-150 Somogyi units; in acute pancreatic damage level usually is elevated in 24-48 hr; in very acute damage level may rise to 600 Somogyi units within 4 hr of onset reaching levels up to 2000 units in short time; decrease also occurs rapidly, and values may return to normal within 48-72 hr; chronic pancreatitis produces variable elevations that are less marked, and carcinoma of pancreas does not usually affect amylase levels
	Urine (single specimen)	Normal = 2-50 Wohlgemuth units/ml
	Urine (24-hr specimen)	Normal = 6-30 Wohlgemuth units/ml and up to 5000 Somogyi units/24 hr; since amylase is excreted in urine, elevation level is dependent on serum level; if level has already declined, urine level may be diagnostically useful since it may remain elevated up to 7 days after acute attack
Lipase	Serum	Normal = 0-1.5 units; in acute pancreatitis, lipase levels usually parallel serum amylase levels; level rises somewhat slower (peaks in 72-96 hr) but may remain elevated for 5-7 days
Calcium	Serum	Normal = 4.5-5.75 mEq/L (9.0-11.5 mg/100 ml); in severe cases of pancreatitis and steatorrhea, level may be low because calcium soaps are formed from sequestration of calcium by fat necrosis
Proteins (total)	Serum	Normal = 6-8 g/100 ml; may be decreased in acute pancreatitis caused by vascular colloid loss
Glucose	Whole blood	Normal = 90-120 mg/100 ml; in severe, acute, or chronic pancreatic disease level may be elevated as a result of beta (β-) cell destruction causing decreased insulin production

NOTE: Serum bilirubin and alkaline phosphatase levels may be elevated as a result of biliary tract or liver involvement.

creatitis is not well understood, although several mechanisms have been postulated.

Pathophysiology

How the etiologic factors listed above induce pancreatitis is unknown. Autodigestion is the most popular theory. This theory proposes that proteolytic enzymes are activated within the pancreas. The activated proteolytic enzymes digest pancreatic and surrounding tissues and activate other enzymes that can digest cellular membranes. This autodigestion results in edema, hemorrhage, vascular damage, coagulation necrosis, and fat necrosis. The edema is further worsened by release of bradykinin.

The way in which the enzymes become activated within the pancreas is not understood. It has been suggested that factors such as endotoxins and exotoxins, ischemia, anoxia, and trauma may initiate the activation. Another theory proposed is that a reflux of duodenal contents through a patent sphincter of Oddi (entrance to the duodenum from the pancreatic duct) may initiate activation of pancreatic enzymes. However, research studies do not completely support the theory that reflux does occur. An old theory that is no longer accepted is that obstruction of the duct by duodenitis and hypersecretion against the obstructed duct caused pancreatitis. It is now felt that obstruction may result in pancreatic edema but not in pancreatitis. Another theory that is no longer accepted is the "common channel theory." In this theory it was proposed that obstruction of the sphincter of Oddi blocked bile and pancreatic enzymes. The bile refluxed into the pancreatic duct and activated the enzymes. Contradictions to this theory are that many persons do not have a common duct, and even in those with a common duct, reflux could not be found.

The role of alcohol in the pathogenesis of pancreatitis has been investigated and still is unknown. Several effects of alcohol on the pancreas have been proposed. It has been postulated that alcohol induces pancreatitis by an intense stimulation of pancreatic secretions, by causing atony and edema of the sphincter of Oddi allowing reflux of duodenal contents into the pancreas, by increasing intraductal pressure, by a direct toxic effect, or through dietary deficiencies usually associated with pancreatitis that hamper normal tissue repair.

Regardless of the cause or the pathogenic mechanism, the patient with *acute pancreatitis* or *acute relapsing pancreatitis* may have a spectrum of pathologic changes. Various terms are used to describe the spectrum. The patient may have *edematous pancreatitis*, which is usually a mild, self-limiting disease. *Necrotizing pancreatitis* refers to a rapid necrotic destruction of the pancreas. *Hemorrhagic pancreatitis* refers to the presence of interstitial hemorrhage within the pancreas.

Clinical picture

The signs and symptoms presented by the patient with the acute forms of pancreatitis vary greatly. Major symptoms include pain, nausea and vomiting, abdominal tenderness, and temperature elevation. Signs and symptoms of fluid and electrolyte imbalances are usually present, and shock may occur. Signs and symptoms of metabolic complications or malabsorption are usually not present, and if present they are usually mild.

Acute attacks of pancreatitis usually occur suddenly, and pain is the major complaint. The pain is severe, widespread, and constant. The pain may be experienced in the epigastrium and other parts of the abdomen and may radiate to the back, flanks, and substernal area. The pain may be more intense when the person is lying supine. Pain is caused by the distension of the capsule, obstruction of bile flow, and peritonitis. Difficulty in breathing and cyanosis may accompany the pain. The patient usually gives a history of nausea and vomiting. Vomiting at first relieves the pain, but continuing vomiting worsens the pain.

Signs and symptoms of dehydration or shock may be present. These result from the nausea and vomiting, exudation of fluid into the peritoneal space, or hemorrhage into the pancreas. In mild cases of pancreatitis only signs and symptoms of dehydration are present, such as poor skin turgor, dry mucous membranes, tachycardia, weight loss, and elevated temperature. If shock is present, signs and symptoms such as hypotension, thready pulse, cool clammy skin, subnormal temperature, poor urinary output, and altered sensorium may be present. Shock can proceed to the irreversible stage rapidly.

Physical examination reveals abdominal tenderness and muscle rigidity, jaundice, and diminished bowel sounds. Some patients, approximately 10% to 20%,[29] have signs of respiratory involvement. These include decreased breath sounds, which may be the result of atelectasis and pleural effusion. Rales may also be present. Metabolic dysfunction may cause transient hyperglycemia. Hypocalcemia may also be present.

Diagnostic tests of the greatest value in establishing a diagnosis are enzyme levels. A *serum amylase* level of greater than 300 Somogyi units in the presence of the symptoms outlined above usually establishes the diagnosis of acute pancreatitis. *Serum amylase* levels usually become elevated within 24 to 48 hours and may range from 300 to 800 units. Some clinicians have reported levels as high as 12,000 units.[3] There is no apparent relationship between the severity of the disease and the height of the enzyme levels.

Serum lipase also rises in pancreatitis and reaches its peak in 72 to 96 hours. When elevations in SGOT, alkaline phosphatase, and leucine aminopeptides occur there is usually obstruction of the common bile duct or liver disease.

Urinary amylase levels may also be used to diagnose acute pancreatitis in the absence of kidney failure. Other abnormal laboratory values include leukocytosis, elevated serum bilirubin levels, and elevated serum alkaline phosphatase levels. Laboratory findings consistent with dehydration may be present. In very severe cases serum glucose levels may be elevated and serum calcium and protein levels may be decreased.

Advances in fiberoptic techniques have made it possible to visualize the pancreatic duct by cannulation of the ampulla of Vater. It is possible to use this technique to determine an accurate diagnosis of obstructive biliary tract disease or chronic vs. acute pancreatitis. This is a highly specialized test and at present is only carried out by very experienced endoscopists.[4]

Intervention

Control of pain. Meperidine hydrochloride (Demerol), 75 to 100 mg every 4 to 6 hours, may be necessary to reduce pain. Morphine and codeine are not used because of their spasmogenic effects. Some patients find that the pain is decreased if they assume a sitting position with the trunk flexed, or with their knees drawn up to the abdomen in a side-lying knee-chest position. Sympathetic nerve blocks and epidural anesthesia can be used if pain is persistent and not relieved by meperidine.[3]

Treatment of fluid and electrolyte deficit or shock. The patient's blood volume deficit is determined, and fluids, blood, albumin, or plasma is given as appropriate. Ongoing monitoring includes vital signs, central venous pressure, and intake and output every hour and serum electrolytes frequently. Appropriate electrolytes are replaced. If shock is severe, vasopressors and other measures discussed in Chapter 21 may be necessary.

Inhibition of pancreatic activity. Several measures are taken to rest the injured pancreas. These include absence of oral intake, continuous nasogastric suction, and use of drugs such as propantheline bromide (Pro-Banthine) or methantheline bromide (Banthine) to inhibit pancreatic secretion. These drugs are contraindicated in the presence of paralytic ileus and shock, and there is some question as to their efficacy in treating pancreatitis. Antacids may be prescribed to neutralize hydrochloric acid.

Other measures. If paralytic ileus is present, a long intestinal tube such as a *Miller-Abbott* tube may be inserted. *Peritoneal* dialysis may be used for patients who are unresponsive to other therapy and whose condition is deteriorating.

Respiratory care to prevent respiratory tract infection is necessary. Monitoring for signs and symptoms of metabolic complications such as hyperglycemia and hypocalcemia is also necessary. Urinary glucose and acetone checks every 4 to 6 hours and daily calcium and observation for Chvostek's and Trousseau's signs should

be incorporated into the plan of care. All patients with *acute pancreatitis* or *acute relapsing pancreatitis* have the potential for developing chronic pancreatitis and should be monitored for signs and symptoms of malabsorption.

An exploratory laparotomy may be performed in acute pancreatitis when a diagnosis cannot be established and the possibility of general peritonitis, perforation of an organ, or a bowel obstruction cannot be excluded. If cholecystitis or cholelithiasis is present, an operation may be performed when the patient can tolerate surgery. An operation also is sometimes done in an attempt to divert or increase bile flow at the sphincter of Oddi and thereby reduce regurgitation of bile into the pancreatic duct.

After an acute attack, management is aimed at preventing further attacks. As soon as the acute attack passes, oral fluids and foods are restarted. Patients are placed on a low-fat, bland diet, distributed over five to six small feedings per day. When refeeding starts, the patient must be observed carefully for pain, nausea, and vomiting, all of which indicate continuing inflammation. If these occur the methods described above for inhibition of pancreatic activity will be reinstituted. Following discharge from the hospital, patients are advised to avoid alcohol and other gastric stimulants and to remain on the same low-fat, bland diet with several small feedings per day. Rich foods must sometimes be avoided to keep pancreatic secretions at a minimum. The dietitian may need to work with the patient to help plan an appropriate diet.

Long-term management focuses on prevention of further attacks. The patient may be given vitamin supplements to help with maintenance of an adequate nutritional status. Antacids may be continued to help maintain a decrease in pancreatic stimulation. The patient must also know what signs and symptoms need to be reported immediately.

Chronic pancreatitis

Chronic pancreatitis may take one of two forms: (1) chronic pancreatitis, in which there is permanent residual deficit; and (2) chronic relapsing pancreatitis, in which there are episodes of acute inflammation superimposed on previously injured areas. The causes and pathophysiology of chronic pancreatitis are the same as those of acute pancreatitis.

Clinical picture

The patient with *chronic* or *chronic relapsing pancreatitis* may have a clinical picture similar to the patient with acute pancreatitis, but pain is often harder to manage and the disease may progress to the point where pain is constantly present. The pain often lasts for days at a time. Between attacks the pain may disappear or be only a vague discomfort. Nausea and vomiting usually occur during the attack. Jaundice with dark urine is usually present. Fluid and electrolyte problems are not as severe as in acute pancreatitis, and shock does not occur. Temperature elevation is present.

Pancreatic exocrine and endocrine insufficiency usually occur. The exocrine insufficiency leads to diarrhea, steatorrhea, weight loss, and malnutrition. Endocrine insufficiency may result in diabetes mellitus. Calcification of the pancreas worsens.

Laboratory findings include leukocytosis, increased serum bilirubin, increased alkaline phosphatase, and elevated levels of amylase and lipase. The enzymes may not be as greatly elevated as with acute pancreatitis because acinar cells have been replaced by fibrous tissue.

Intervention

Treatment during the acute phase of chronic pancreatitis is the same as for patients with acute pancreatitis. The dietary prescription for long-term management of the patient is also the same as for the patient with acute pancreatitis. Antacids are usually continued. Calories and protein should be increased to help the patient regain weight. The exocrine insufficiency may be treated with pancreatin (Viokase) or pancrelipase (Cotazym). These substances contain amylase, lipase, and trypsin. They are taken at mealtimes to aid digestion and facilitate the absorption of fat-soluble vitamins. The patient should observe stools for the presence of steatorrhea and report this immediately to the physician.

If diabetes mellitus is present it is treated as described in Chapter 32. The patient needs to understand the relationship between pancreatitis and diabetes and needs to monitor for signs and symptoms on a continual basis. If signs and symptoms occur, they must be reported immediately.

Pain control between acute exacerbations is a major nursing challenge. The dietary restrictions, if followed, will help to control pain. If appropriate and the patient is interested, behavioral control methods such as relaxation therapy may be taught. The patient will need to be taught why narcotics should be avoided.

Outcome criteria for the person with chronic pancreatic disease

The person or significant others can:
1. Explain necessary dietary changes required after discharge:
   a. Explain the relationship of attacks to ingestion of foods.
   b. List specific foods to be avoided (e.g., alcoholic beverages, excessive use of coffee, spicy or rich foods, and heavy meals).
2. Explain medications to be taken at home and their relationship to the condition present:
   a. Explain dosage and expected effects of medications (e.g., pancreatic enzyme replacements, oral hypoglycemics or insulin, bile salts, and vitamin supplements).
   b. Explain any untoward effects of medications that need to be reported to the health care provider.
   c. Explain how and when to use medications (e.g., antacids, anticholinergics, and analgesics).
3. Explain health maintenance necessary to assist in preventing further attacks or indicate need for therapeutic follow-up:
   a. Explain the need to avoid irritants and infectious agents and identify sources of these in the environment. (These may differ slightly depending on the precipitating cause of the illness.)
   b. List signs and symptoms indicative of an attack (e.g., pain, nausea, vomiting, distention, and low-grade fever).
   c. Explain what steatorrhea is, how to monitor for it, and what it means.
   d. State whom to contact if the above signs and symptoms occur.
   e. Explain signs of diabetes (e.g., polydipsia, polyuria, polyphagia, weakness, or weight loss) and know that these must be reported to the health care provider immediately.
4. Explain need to identify, limit, and learn to cope with emotional stressors in the environment.
5. Explain how to obtain community resources if necessary:
   a. If alcoholic, is aware of available assistance programs in the community (Alcoholics Anonymous and other groups).
6. Explain plans for follow-up care.

Tumors of the pancreas

Epidemiology

Tumors of the pancreas may be malignant or benign. Benign tumors include islet cell tumors, cystadenomas, and duct cell adenomas. Malignant tumors occur more frequently and are most often found in the head of the pancreas. Men are affected far more often than women, and tumors usually occur after middle age. Cancer of the pancreas is the sixth most common cause of cancer mortality in men. Sarcomas of the pancreas may be found in infants and young adults but are very rare.

Pathophysiology

Most malignant tumors of the pancreas appear to begin in the ductal areas, causing eventual blockage and resulting in chronic pancreatitis. Direct extension of the lesion may cause its spread to the posterior wall of the stomach, the duodenal wall, the colon, and the common bile duct. The tumor may be diffusely spread over the entire gland, or it may be a well-defined growth. It commonly grows in a rapid manner, is highly invasive and vascular, lymphatic, and perineural metastases frequently occur. Many patients live only 3 to 6 months after diagnosis is confirmed.

Clinical picture

Symptoms of pancreatic malignancies are not usually detectable until late in the course of the disease. Pain occurs in about 85% of the patients. This may be preceded by vague anorexia, nausea, and weight loss over a period of months. Jaundice frequently occurs because of common duct obstruction but is seldom a primary sign. Changes in stools may occur if the pancreatic ducts are obstructed. Pain may be colicky or intermittent and often radiates to the back, abdomen, and chest.

Definitive diagnosis before surgery is difficult. Diagnostic studies include duodenal cytology, pancreatic scans, and arteriography. About half of these patients develop diabetes mellitus.

Intervention

Surgical treatment is most effective, although the prognosis is usually poor. If the tumor is operable, a pancreaticoduodenal resection (Whipple's procedure), which includes removal of the head of the pancreas, the lower end of the common bile duct, the duodenum, and the distal portion of the stomach, may be done. The common bile duct and the remaining portions of the pancreas and stomach are then anastomosed to the jejunum. If the tumor is not resectable, a palliative operation such as a cholecystojejunostomy, a choledochojejunostomy, or a palliative gastrojejunostomy may be done to help restore temporarily a normal flow of bile and some pancreatic enzyme to the intestinal tract. The type of procedure performed depends on the involvement found at operation. Palliation of the symptoms also may be achieved by the administration of chemotherapeutic agents.

In addition to routine postoperative care following abdominal surgery, the patient who has had pancreatic surgery must be watched for signs of peritonitis, gastrointestinal obstruction, and jaundice until sufficient time for healing has elapsed and until it is determined that all the anastomoses are secure and patent.

Hypotension is a common occurrence after pancreatic surgery, and good baseline data should be obtained preoperatively. The patient may require the administration of vasopressor drugs for 24 to 48 hours postoperatively. Patients with extensive pancreatic resections may not be ambulated as soon as other patients with abdominal surgery and may be prone to develop pulmonary complications if excellent pulmonary hygiene is not encouraged and persistently carried out.

Stools should be observed, and frothy, light-colored stools containing conspicuously undigested fat are reported. If most of the pancreas was removed, the patient may have to take pancreatic enzymes in tablet form by mouth to aid the digestion of fat. The patient is watched for signs and symptoms of diabetes mellitus following this procedure, although it rarely occurs unless the entire pancreas has been removed. If hypoinsulinism occurs, treatment with insulin will be necessary for the remainder of the patient's life (p. 650). The average duration of life after Whipple's procedure is about a year.

REFERENCES AND SELECTED READINGS
Contemporary

1. Aach, R.: Viral hepatites A to E, Med. Clin. North Am. **62:**59-69, 1978.
2. Are liver function tests outmoded? (editorial), Br. Med. J. **2:**75-76, 1977.
3. Beeson, P.B., and McDermott, W., editors: Textbook of medicine, ed. 15, Philadelphia, 1981, W.B. Saunders Co.
4. Belinsky, S.: Visualizing the pancreatic and biliary ducts, Am. J. Nurs. **76:**936-937, 1976.
5. Bell, J.: Just another patient with gallstones? Don't you believe it, Nurs.' 79 **9:**26-33, Oct. 1979.
6. Bossone, M.C.M.: The liver: a pharmacologic perspective, Nurs. Clin. North Am. **12:**291-303, 1977.
7. Boyer, C.A., and Oehlberg, S.M.: Interpretation and clinical relevance of liver function tests, Nurs. Clin. North Am. **12:**275-290, 1977.
8. Boyer, J.L.: Chronic hepatitis: a perspective on classification and determinants of prognosis, Gastroenterology **70:**1161-1171, 1976.
9. Butler, M.: Variceal hemorrhage, Milit. Med. **145:**766-770, 1980.
10. Byrne, J.: Liver function studies. I. Introduction and bilirubin, Nurs. '77 **7:**12-14, July 1977.
11. Byrne, J.: Liver function studies. II. Conjugation and excretion tests, Nurs. '77 **7:**88-90, Sept. 1977.
12. Byrne, J.: Liver function studies. V. Using enzyme levels to assess liver function, Nurs. '78 **8:**50-52, Jan. 1978.
13. Carey, L.C., editor: The pancreas, St. Louis, 1973, The C.V. Mosby Co.
14. Cohn, H.O.: Diuresis of ascites: fraught with or free from hazard (editorial), Gastroenterology **73:**619-621, 1977.
15. Collin, J.: Pancreatic transplantation, Nurs. Mirror **143:**51-53, 1976.
16. Dane, D.S., Cameron, C.H., and Briggs, M.: Virus-like particles in serum of patients with Australia-antigen-associated hepatitis, Lancet **1:**695-698, 1970.
17. Daniel, E.: Chronic problems in rehabilitation of patients with Laennec's cirrhosis, Nurs. Clin. North Am. **12:**345-356, 1977.
18. Dawson, J.: Cholecystitis and cholecystectomy, Clin. Gastroenterol. **6:**129-137, 1977.
19. Dolan, P., and Greene, H.: Conquering cirrhosis of the liver, Nurs. '76 **6**(11):44-53, 1976.
20. Fortner, J.G.: Technique of liver transplantation, RN **5:**OR1-OR4, 1976.
21. Fuerst, E.V., and Wolff, L.V.: Fundamentals of nursing, ed. 5, Philadelphia, 1974, J.B. Lippincott Co.
22. Given, G., and Simmons, S.: Gastroenterology in clinical nursing, ed. 3, St. Louis, 1979, The C.V. Mosby Co.

23. Gocke, D.J.: New faces of viral hepatitis, Disease a Month 1:1-32, Jan. 1973.

24. Graham, D.: Enzyme replacement therapy of exocrine pancreatic insufficiency in man, N. Engl. J. Med. **23:**1314-1317, 1977.

25. Greenberger, N.J.: Gastrointestinal disorders: a pathophysiologic approach, ed. 2, Chicago, 1981, Year Book Medical Publishers, Inc.

26. Hahn, A.B., Barkin, R.L. and Oestreich, J.K.: Pharmacology in nursing, ed. 15, St. Louis, 1982, The C.V. Mosby Co.

27. Harvey, A., et al.: The principles and practice of medicine, ed. 20, New York, 1980, Appleton-Century-Crofts.

28. Hoyumpa, A.M. Jr., et al.: Hepatic encephalopathy, Gastroenterology **76:**184-195, 1979.

29. Isselbacher, K., et al.: Harrison's principles of internal medicine, ed. 9, New York, 1980, McGraw-Hill Book Co.

30. Kalser, M.H.: Chronic pancreatitis, Compr. Ther. **2:**43-46, 1980.

31. Leery, C., and Kanagasundaram, N.: Alcoholic hepatitis, Hosp. Pract. **13:**115-123, Oct. 1978.

32. Levin, D.M., and Boyer, J.L.: Principles of therapy in cirrhosis, Primary Care **2:**311-329, 1976.

33. Mahood, W.H., Dill, J.E., and Dill, R.P.: Hepatic failure. In Meltzer, L.E., Abdellah, F.G., and Kitchell, J.R.: Concepts and practices of intensive care for nurse specialists, ed. 2, Bowie, Md., 1976, The Charles Press.

34. Marks, J.N., and Bank, S.: Chronic pancreatitis: classification, chemical aspects, diagnosis and management, Curr. Concepts Gastroenterol. **3:**5-12, 1977.

35. Mazzola, P.: Nursing care of the liver-transplant patient, RN **5:**34-37, 1976.

36. McElroy, D.B.: Nursing care of patients with viral hepatitis, Nurs. Clin. North Am. **12:**305-315, 1977.

37. McGill, D.B., and Motto, J.D.: An industrial outbreak of toxic hepatitis due to methylenedianiline, N. Engl. J. Med. **291:**278-282, 1974.

38. Mitchell, J.R., and Lauterburg, B.H.: Drug-induced liver injury, Hosp. Pract. **13:**95-106, Sept. 1978.

39. Nadkarni, S.V.: Amebic abscess of the liver, Int. Surg. **58:**112-115, 1973.

40. Nelson, W.E., Vaughn, V.C., and McKay, R.J.: Textbook of pediatrics, ed. 10, Philadelphia, 1975, W.B. Saunders Co.

41. Peterson, A.: Acute viral hepatitis, Nurse Pract. **13:**9-11, July-Aug. 1979.

42. Pierce, L.: Anatomy and physiology of the liver in relation to clinical assessment, Nurs. Clin. North Am. **12:**259-273, 1977.

43. Popper, H., and Schaffner, F., editors: Progress in liver diseases, vol. 3, New York, 1970, Grune & Stratton, Inc.

44. Purcell, R.: The viral hepatitis, Hosp. Pract. 51-62, July 1978.

45. Resnick, R.H.: Cirrhosis. In Conn, H.F., et al., editors: Current therapy 1982, Philadelphia, 1982, W.B. Saunders Co.

46. Rutherdale, J.A., et al.: Hepatitis in drug users, Am. J. Gastroenterol. **58:**275-287, 1972.

47. Sabiston, D.C., editor: Davis-Christopher textbook of surgery, ed. 11, Philadelphia, 1977, W.B. Saunders Co.

48. Schiff, L.: Diseases of the liver, ed. 4, Philadelphia, 1975, J.B. Lippincott Co.

49. Schweitzer, I.L., et al.: Viral hepatitis B in neonates and infants, Am. J. Med. **55:**762-771, 1973.

50. Seybert, P., Gardon, K.M., and Jackson, B.S.: The Leveen shunt: new hope for ascites patients, Nurs. '79 **9:**24-31, Jan. 1979.

51. Shahinpour, N.: The adult patient with bleeding esophageal varices, Nurs. Clin. North Am. **12:**331-343, 1977.

52. Sherar, L.: Ascites: pathogenesis and treatment, Postgrad. Med. **53:**165-170, 1973.

53. Sherlock, S.: Diseases of the liver and the biliary system, ed. 5, Philadelphia, 1975, F.A. Davis Co.

54. Sherwood, S.: Chronic hepatitis, Curr. Concepts Gastroenterol. **1:**21-27, 1978.

55. *Simmons, S., and Givens, B.: Acute pancreatitis, Am. J. Nurs. **71:**934-939, 1971.

56. Small, D.M.: Gallstones: diagnosis and treatment, Postgrad. Med. **51:**187-193, 1972.

57. Statement on hepatitis B antigen carriers, Hospitals **48:**95-98, 1974.

58. Syndman, D.R., Bryan, J.A., and Dixon, R.E.: Prevention of nosocomial viral hepatitis, type B (hepatitis B), Ann. Intern. Med. **83:**838-845, 1975.

59. Thorpe, C., and Caprini, R.: Gallbladder disease: current trends and treatment, Am. J. Nurs. **80:**2181-2185, 1980.

60. U.S. Department of Health, Education and Welfare, Public Health Service, Center for Disease Control: Immune globulins for protection against viral hepatitis, vol. 26, no. 52, 1977.

61. U.S. Department of Health, Education and Welfare, Public Health Service, Center for Disease Control: Isolation techniques for use in hospitals, ed. 2, 1975.

62. U.S. Department of Health, and Human Services, Public Health Service, Centers for Disease Control: Reported morbidity and mortality in the United States Sept. 1981, vol. 29, no. 54, 1980.

63. Warshaw, A.L.: A guide to pancreatitis, Compr. Ther. **5:**49-55, 1980.

64. Waterson, A.: The viruses of hepatitis, Clin. Gastroenterol. **2:**241-254, 1974.

65. Wenzel, R.P., Adams, J.F., and Smith, E.P.: Patterns of illicit drug use in viral hepatitis patients, Milit. Med. **138:**345-350, 1973.

66. Williams, S.R.: Essentials of nutrition and diet therapy, ed. 3, St. Louis, 1982, The C.V. Mosby Co.

Classical

67. Netter, F.: The Ciba collection of medical illustrations, Part III. Digestive system, vol. 3, Summit, N.J., 1964, Ciba Pharmaceutical Co.

---

*References preceded by an asterisk are particularly well suited for reading.

SENSORIMOTOR PROBLEMS

Survival through the ages has depended on the ability to sense dangers in the environment and to be ready for flight or fight. The senses are used in many ways: for protection from injury, for aid in activities of daily living, and for enjoyment of the arts and music. The senses are part of the neurologic system that also has motor function. Nerves transmit messages to and from the muscles that permit a person to move about, to carry out daily activities, to work, and to play. Thus activity, which is one of the basic physiologic needs, depends on an intact nervous system and an intact musculoskeletal system. Problems with either of these systems will affect a person's ability to function in the environment and may require coping with permanent changes in life-style.

Because both the neurologic and musculoskeletal systems are involved in the ability to be active, they have been grouped together in this unit. Three major topics are considered: *the neurologic system* itself, the *special senses (eye and ear)*, and the *musculoskeletal system*. Each section consists of a chapter on assessment, a chapter that reviews general management of persons experiencing problems with the system, and a chapter that examines specific problems. The special senses have been dealt with separate from the overall neurologic system because of the specific needs of persons who have impairment of sight and hearing.

CHAPTER 34

ASSESSMENT OF THE NERVOUS SYSTEM

ELIZABETH STRAUSS NOSSE
MARJORIE KINNEY

Persons with neurologic deficits require skilled assessment by both physician and nurse. Neurologic assessment may be performed by generalists and specialists in both fields, and data collected will be used both collaboratively and independently to permit these professionals to provide their distinct services to the individual.

For example, the physician generalist's primary purpose is to screen for neurologic symptoms. Because many systemic diseases have neurologic manifestations, individuals may have their first neurologic assessments performed during a routine physical examination. Thus the physician generalist is often the first medical professional to document the neurologic problems. However, on referral to a physician specialist (neurologist), the individual will undergo a more detailed assessment to localize the particular lesion and to identify its pathophysiology. To enable the specialist to determine the specific diagnosis, the neurologist's examination will be more detailed, exact, and comprehensive than that of the generalist.

Role of the nurse in neurologic assessment

Professional nurses are involved in initial and ongoing assessments of a patient's neurologic status. The nurse's role is that of an independent professional as well as that of a collaborator.

The nurse generalist may become involved in baseline and continuing assessments early in the patient's course of therapy. Although data collected will also be useful to the physician, its primary purpose is to enable the nurse to identify the degree to which the patient is able to perform self-care activities and to assess how such activities are limited by the identified deficits in sensory, motor, affective, or intellectual capacities. With these problem areas identified, the nurse then is able to select appropriate strategies to maximize the patient's capabilities.

The neurologic nurse specialist, because of additional experience and preparation in the speciality, has developed skills beyond those of the generalist. Like the physician specialist, the neurologic nurse's assessments are more comprehensive and detailed in nature and, as such, they are more likely to overlap with those of the neurologist.

Again, although this data will be useful to the neurologist, its primary purpose is to enable the neurologic nurse specialist to formulate more comprehensive analyses of patient conditions. Problems identified may provide more thorough descriptions of deficits observed, patient responses to these deficits, and the effects of such deficits on the patient's family and lifestyle. This thorough analysis will lead to more comprehensive plans of care extending from the acute phase through rehabilitation. Also, the neurologic nurse specialist serves as a consultant to nurse generalists caring for patients with neurologic problems.

The purposes of this chapter are to review selected neuroanatomy and physiology, to discuss aspects of history taking, to present the components and methods of and the observations to be made during the neurologic examination, and to discuss selected tests and procedures used to assist in the diagnosis of neurologic problems.

Anatomy and physiology

Neurologic assessment is dependent on the examiner's knowledge of normal neurophysiology and neuroanatomy and ability to interpret the degree of change in status from what is considered to be normal. The attainment of a logical diagnosis (nursing or medical) begins with a recognition of abnormality followed by grouping of the data, analysis of data, and conclusions about what the data mean in terms of a diagnosis.

The complexity of the nervous system limits what can be presented here. Only selected concepts relevant to neurologic assessment are included. The reader is referred to current texts for a more detailed and comprehensive coverage.[4,25] Emphasis is placed on key concepts including the *neuron, synapse, conduction, motor system pathways, sensory system pathways,* and *effector organs*.

Functionally, the nervous system, like an electrical conductance system, coordinates and controls all activities of the body. Broadly, the nervous system carries out four general kinds of functions as related to informational processes:

1. Receives stimuli or information from the internal and external environments over varied afferent or sensory pathways
2. Communicates information between distant parts of the body (periphery) to the central nervous system
3. Computes or processes the information received at various *reflex* (spinal cord) and *conscious* (higher brain) levels to determine responses appropriate to existing situations
4. Transmits information rapidly over varied efferent or motor pathways to effector organs for body action control or modifications

Neuron

The single *neuron* is the basic structural and functional unit of the nervous system. It shares all of the basic biologic and biochemical properties of other body cells. It is also a highly specialized and differentiated cell. The single neuron acts as a miniature nervous system and has properties specialized for its electrical function.

Microscopically, the neuron consists of a cell body, or *soma*, with two extensions that project from it: a *dendritic tree* and an elongated *cylindric axon*. A *cell membrane* encloses the outer boundary of the soma, dendrites, and axon, thus separating the inside from the outside of the cell. The presence of a large surface area of cell membrane makes it suitable to receive a large number of synaptic contacts at one time (Fig. 34-1). The *axon* is specialized for the transmission of information along its extension *away from* the cell body to adjacent neurons; the *dendrite* or *dendrites* are specialized for receiving information from axon terminals at special sites called *synapses*. (It should be noted that the word *axon* is used in various ways. It may be used to describe the extension of one cell or the extension of several cells making up a nerve.)

Many of the most important *functional* properties of the neuron lie within the *cell membrane* itself. Structurally, the membrane is made up of lipids and proteins and has the property of translocating materials across itself. The membrane exhibits *differential permeability* in that it is permeable to oxygen, carbon dioxide, and certain inorganic ions while it is impermeable to organic compounds (proteins) and other inorganic ions. This differential permeability results in a characteristic ionic distribution. The inside of the neuron contains a high concentration of proteins (which are impermeable) and potassium ($K+$), whereas the outside of the cell is high in sodium ($Na+$). This unequal distribution, or gradient, of $K+$ and $Na+$ results across the membrane in part from differential permeability and from the presence of an active *sodium-potassium pump* within the membrane. The pump requires metabolic energy for rapid movement of sodium and potassium across the membrane, and this produces an electrical potential difference, or charge, between the inside and the outside of the cell. The magnitude of the potential difference is a function of the ratio of charged particles on opposite sides of the membrane and is called the *resting membrane potential* (resting potential). All cells exhibit this property of resting potential, which essentially remains constant over time. Thus in the resting state all neurons possess a potential for action and are said to be *polarized* (a difference in voltage charge between inner and outer cell membrane or surface). This resting potential is quite small, -60 mV, with the inside of the cell being electronically negative compared to the outside of the cell.[25]

Additionally, the neuron exhibits the property of "excitability" as do muscles and certain glands. "Excitability" means that the resting potential of neurons is unstable under certain conditions; for example, as when a neuronal membrane is subjected to stimulation, application of chemicals, or mechanical damage. This instability gives rise to the generation of *action potentials*. The generation of an action potential is a capacity unique to excitable cells, and it is the basic phenomenon underlying all nervous system functions. It is by means of action potentials that information is conducted within the nervous system.

An action potential occurs in the following manner: when a neuron is stimulated, membrane permeability to $Na+$ significantly increases, and there is a sudden

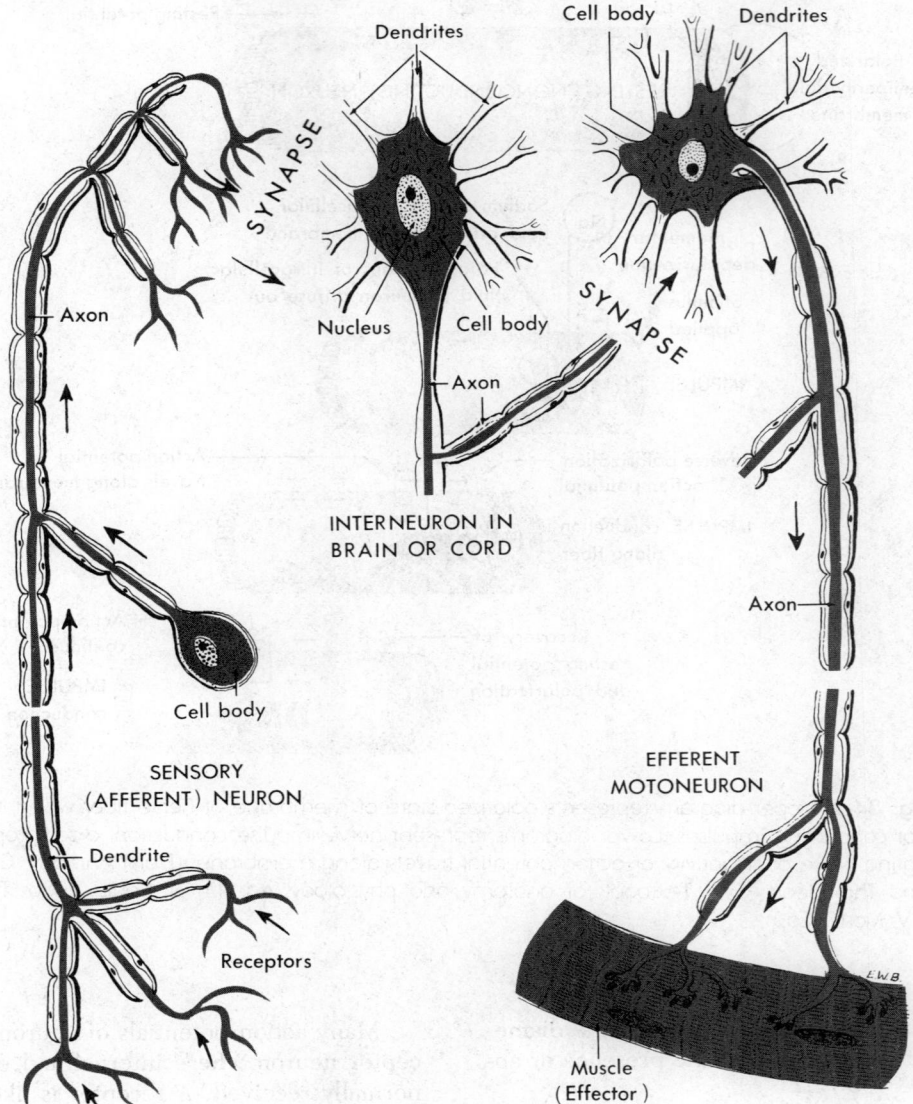

Dendrites

Cell body   Dendrites

SYNAPSE

Axon

Nucleus   Cell body

Axon

SYNAPSE

INTERNEURON IN
BRAIN OR CORD

Cell body

Axon

SENSORY
(AFFERENT) NEURON

EFFERENT
MOTONEURON

Dendrite

Receptors

Muscle
(Effector)

Fig. 34-1. Diagram of structure of three kinds of neurons. Note that each neuron has three parts: a cell body and two types of extensions, dendrite(s) and an axon. Arrows indicate direction of impulse conduction. (From Anthony, C.P., and Thibodeau, G.A.: Textbook of anatomy and physiology, ed. 10, St. Louis, 1979, The C.V. Mosby Co.)

movement of Na+ to the inside of the membrane. These ions carry a sufficiently large positive charge, which causes the disappearance of the normal resting potential. In fact, a *positive state* develops within the cell, and *depolarization* occurs.

Almost instantaneously the membrane pores return to the state of being virtually impermeable to Na+ while K+ moves to the outside of the cell. The K+ movement also quickly returns to normal, and active transport brings Na+ and K+ movement back to the original state. These mechanisms result in the disappearance of the internal positive state and a return to the

normal resting potential. This phase is called *repolarization*. These two phases together form the *action potential*. An entire AP occurs within 1 to 2 msec (Fig. 34-2).

When an action potential is generated it proceeds *automatically to completion* independent of the property of the stimulus that initiated the depolarization; that is, a strong stimulus does not give rise to a larger action potential but does cause it to proceed to completion in an "all-or-none" fashion. The action potential is also spread, or propagated, over the entire membrane without a decrease in its velocity. The propagation velocity

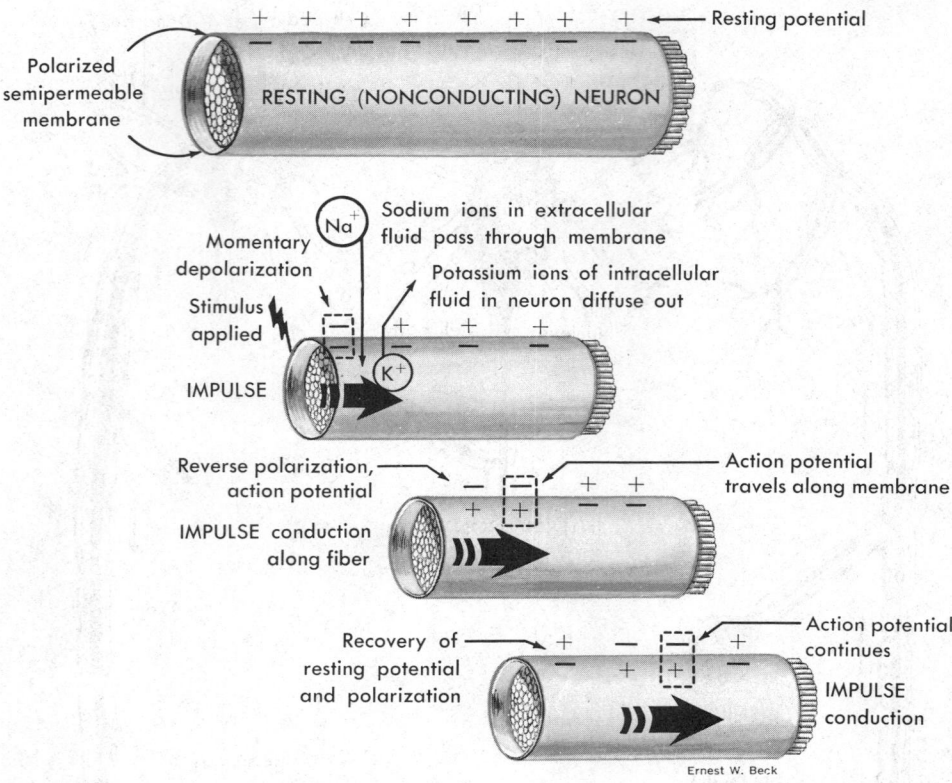

Fig. 34-2. Upper diagram represents polarized state of membrane of nerve fiber when it is not conducting impulses. Lower diagrams represent nerve impulse conduction: a self-propagating wave of negativity or action potential travels along membrane. (From Anthony, C.P., and Thibodeau, G.A.: Textbook of anatomy and physiology, ed. 11, St. Louis, 1983, The C.V. Mosby Co.)

is related to the size of the axon (the larger the diameter, the higher the velocity) and to the presence or absence of myelin.

Myelin is an excellent insulator of axons. The myelin sheath is deposited around the axons by Schwann's cells, and this layer may be as thick as the axon itself. Myelin prevents almost all ion flow across the axon and its membrane. However, at distances approximately 1 mm apart the sheath is interrupted by nodes of Ranvier. At these small, uninsulated areas, ions can flow easily between the extracellular fluid and the axon. In fact, at these nodes the axonal membrane is 500 times more permeable than the membranes of some nonmyelinated fibers.[10] Thus impulses are conducted from node to node.

The presence of myelin causes such fibers to be called *large* fibers; those without myelin are called *small* fibers. Large fibers have a greater conduction velocity because (1) the jumping effect allows depolarization to proceed quickly and (2) energy is conserved since only the nodes depolarize. Large fibers appear white because of the myelin; the "white matter" of the nervous system is made up of myelinated fibers.

Many action potentials of neurons originate in a receptor neuron where internal and external stimuli are normally received. A receptor is like a transducer and can change one form of energy into another form. A receptor, however, responds or depolarizes to *only one* type of stimulus. For example, the retina of the eye responds only to the stimulus of light, which is converted to electrical energy and travels over the optic nerves to the visual cortices for perception. In this way the receptor neuron may initiate the depolarization. It does, however, limit what the neuron responds to, although the receptor neuron does obey the all-or-none theory; a strong stimulus does make the receptor neuron fire more action potentials *per unit of time* within its time limitations than does a weak stimulus.

Neurons make functional contact with one another at specialized sites called *synapses*. Whenever an action potential is generated in one neuron that invades a synapse site, a sequence of processes results in the action potential affecting the second neuron. Transmission across a synapse is essentially a *chemical process*. The end of the axon contains a chemical substance located within its vesicles. When an action potential reaches the vesicle, it releases a transmitter substance, which then diffuses across the synapse to the adjacent neuronal cell membrane. *Synaptic transmission* is both *excitatory* and *inhibitory* in nature. Inhibition means that the dendritic membrane becomes hyperpolarized because of the release of the specific neurotransmitter. The membrane potential shifts toward K+ equilibrium, thus stabilizing the membrane and taking the potential further from threshold. Each neuron only acts when its membrane is *depolarized to threshold*. Thus whether a neuron fires depends on the sum of excitatory and inhibitory inputs. Chemicals allowing excitatory transmission are acetylcholine, norepinephrine, dopamine, and serotonin. Those that inhibit transmission include gamma aminobutyric acid (GABA) in brain tissue and glycine in the spinal cord.

In summary, the single neuron has all the structural and functional building elements of an electrical conductance system that also makes interconnections with adjacent neurons at synapses. Collectively, neurons are in turn organized into larger and larger units of function that serve to coordinate all body activities. All neurons function basically in the same way. There is, however, a major difference in the functions carried out by the sensory and motor neurons.

In neurologic assessment it should be appreciated by the examiner that any disruption in the conductance system results in dysfunction distal to the break. The degree of change in status of a particular function or functions depends on the location and nature of the stressor or lesion causing the disruption.

Divisions of the nervous system

Macroscopically, the nervous system is divided into two major divisions: the central nervous system and the peripheral nervous system.

Central nervous system

The central nervous system (CNS) is made up of collections of neurons and their connections organized into the brain and spinal cord areas. All of the basic informational processes as summarized on p. 714 occur within the CNS. Areas of the brain and spinal cord are distinguished where cell bodies are concentrated into *nuclei* and groups of axons running in *tracts* that interconnect the parts. Collections of neurons are connected in complex ways. The *connections* determine what each collection of neurons is capable of doing. The neurons are organized into circuits, some of which are simple and made up of relatively few neurons and others that are very complex. A single neuron may be a component of a number of different neuronal circuits and thus play a role in different functions.

Structurally, the brain and spinal cord are continu-

ous. They are protectively housed within the skull and vertebral column, respectively. When injured, centrally located neurons are unable to reproduce themselves because most cell bodies are located centrally and nerve cell bodies cannot reproduce. However, nerve endings can regenerate because of the presence of neurilemma. Neurilemma covers all peripheral nerves; it is theorized that the living neurilemma contains openings through which axonal growth occurs proximally to distally. This growth seems to occur at a rate of 1 to 4 mm/day. Rarely, however, is there 100% regrowth.

The brain (encephalon) is grossly divided rostrally to caudally into three main areas: the *cerebrum, brain stem* (diencephalon, midbrain, pons, and medulla), and *cerebellum*. Each circuit or area carries out unique functions. The *cerebrum* of each hemisphere (right and left) is further organized into four major lobes (frontal, parietal, temporal, and occipital). The cortex of the cerebrum, which is approximately ¼ in. thick and contains over 14 billion neurons, receives and analyzes all impulses, controls voluntary movements, and stores knowledge of all impulses received. Each cerebral lobe is named from overlying cranial bones and carries out one or more of the following functions: general sensation perception (pain, touch, temperature, and pressure), special senses perception (hearing, vision, smell, taste), and speech. Very generally, the *frontal cortex* is responsible for conceptualization, abstraction, and judgment formation. It also contains the premotor and motor areas, which govern motor activity. The *parietal cortex* is the highest integrative and coordinating center for perception and interpretation of sensory information. A lesion in this area, especially on the nondominant side, leads to inability to recognize body parts and to disturbances in body image. The *temporal cortex* is responsible for memory storage and auditory integration. The *occipital cortex* houses the visual center.

Also important to note is that speech is a function of the *dominant hemisphere*, which for all right-handed people and most left-handed people is the left side. The two identified speech centers are *Broca's area* and *Wernicke's area*. Broca's area is located in the lateral inferior portion of the frontal lobe adjacent to the motor cortex and its projections. This area appears to control verbal, expressive speech. Wernicke's area is located in the posterior part of the superior temporal convolution and may extend to adjacent portions of the parietal lobe. This area is responsible for the reception and understanding of language. Other areas of the brain that are also involved in speech include an area in the frontal lobe, which governs the ability to write words, and an area in the occipital lobe, which governs the ability to understand written material (see Fig. 34-3 for important cortical areas).

Finally, deep within the cerebrum are structures called the *basal ganglia*. These are masses of gray mat-

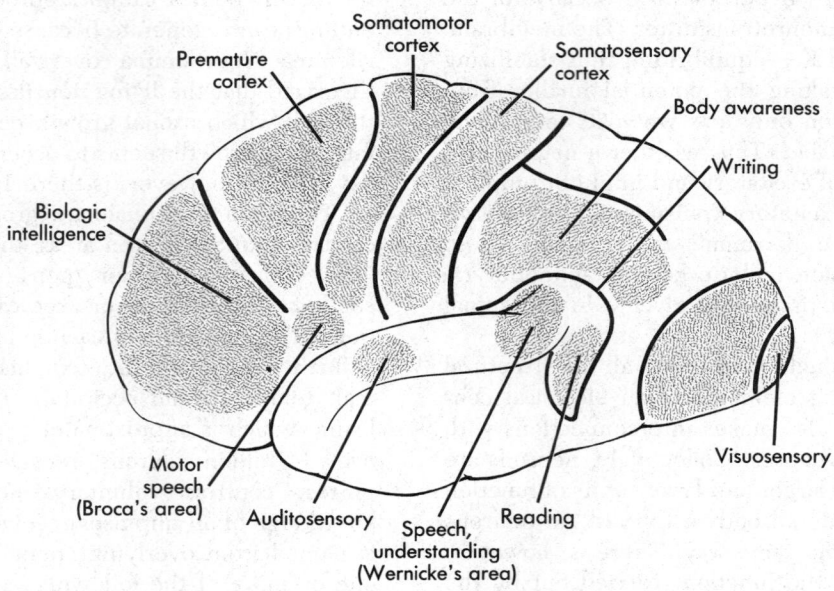

Fig. 34-3. Lateral view of cerebral cortex with identification of major cortical areas.

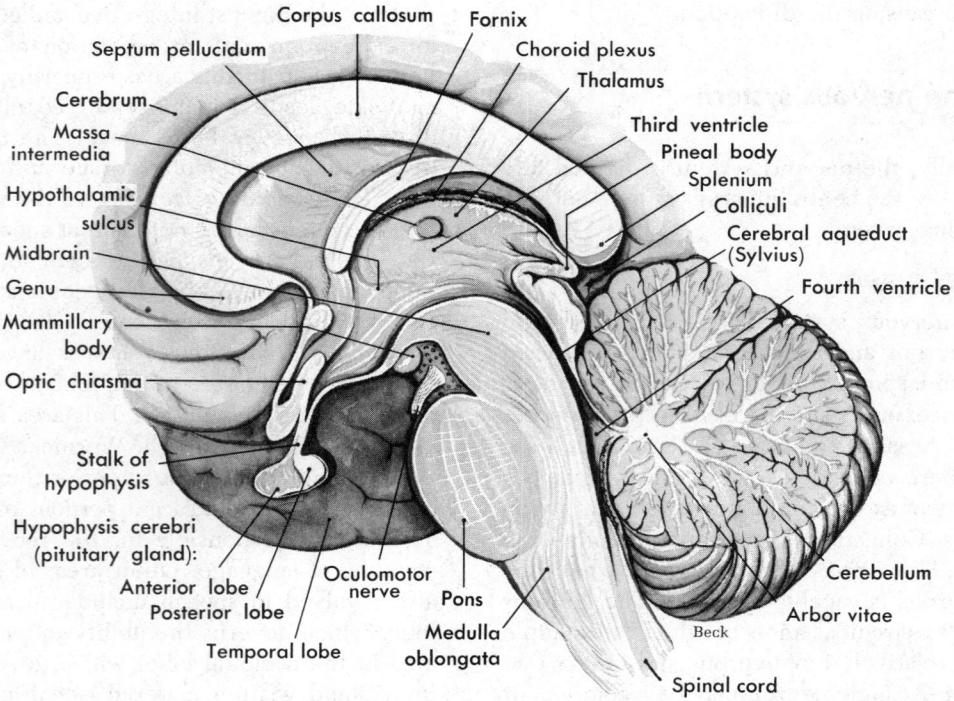

Fig. 34-4. Sagittal section through midline of brain showing continuity of brain and spinal cord. (From Anthony, C.P., and Thibodeau, G.A.: Textbook of anatomy and physiology, ed. 11, St. Louis, 1983, The C.V. Mosby Co.)

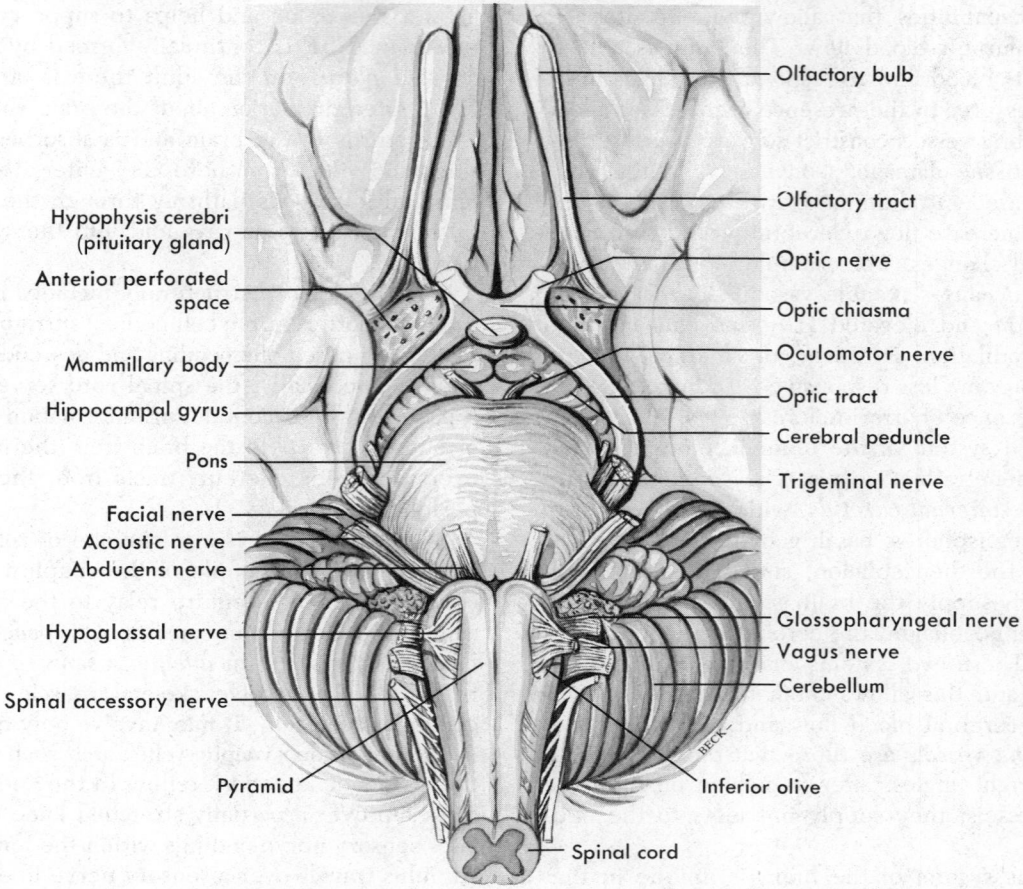

Olfactory bulb

Olfactory tract

Optic nerve

Optic chiasma

Oculomotor nerve

Optic tract

Cerebral peduncle

Trigeminal nerve

Glossopharyngeal nerve

Vagus nerve

Cerebellum

Inferior olive

Spinal cord

Hypophysis cerebri (pituitary gland)

Anterior perforated space

Mammillary body

Hippocampal gyrus

Pons

Facial nerve

Acoustic nerve

Abducens nerve

Hypoglossal nerve

Spinal accessory nerve

Pyramid

Fig. 34-5. Ventral surface of brain showing structures around third ventricle and individual cranial nerves arising from midbrain. (From Anthony, C.P., and Thibodeau, G.A.: Textbook of anatomy and physiology, ed. 11, St. Louis, 1983, The C.V. Mosby Co.)

ter (cell bodies) and include such structures as the *caudate nucleus, putamen,* and *globus pallidus.* In general, the basal ganglia function as part of the *extrapyramidal* system and are responsible for postural adjustments and gross volitional movements.

The brain stem is placed deeply in the center of the hemispheres and is not visible when viewing the intact brain. It includes a series of parts making connections with the spinal cord at the level of the medulla (Fig. 34-4), and it carries all nerve fibers passing between the hemispheres and the cord. All cranial nerves except the olfactory nerve (I) arise from it (Fig. 34-5). General functions of the brain stem's several structures are as follows: The *thalamus* serves as the end station for all sensory impulses (except for those from cranial nerve I). All sensory fibers synapse here for final relay to the appropriate portion of the sensory cortex. General sensation is perceived in the thalamus, but its meaning and locality are imparted by the cortex. The thalamus is thought to house the "pain threshold." Beneath the thalamus is the *hypothalamus,* which contains the cell

bodies mediating most autonomic functions, endocrine functions, and also emotional responses. The *medulla* houses the primitive respiratory and cardiovascular control centers.

Of special importance is the core of tissue extending throughout the entire brain stem. This is called the *reticular formation.* This interconnected network of cells has important integrating centers for respiration, cardiovascular function, afferent and motor systems, and states of consciousness. Increased stimulation leads to wakefulness, and decreased stimulation (as in anoxia caused by increased intracranial pressure) results in sleepiness.

The *cerebellum* is attached to the lower portion of the brain stem. It generally aids in coordination of voluntary muscle movements.

Circulation in the brain possesses special characteristics. For example, systemic circulation favors the central nervous system over all other body parts. This helps provide a constant supply of nutrients (glucose and oxygen) to nervous tissue. The brain's vessels themselves also possess capabilities that allow them to assist in achieving a constant blood flow. The brain is able to autoregulate its blood flow to respond to changes in intraluminal pressure. In the presence of increased blood pressure, cerebral vessels constrict so as to decrease flow and possible tissue damage. Conversely, in the presence of decreased intraluminal pressure, cerebral vessels dilate to increase flow. Cerebral vessels also react to biochemical changes. For example, *elevated carbon dioxide content* causes notable vasodilation of cerebral vessels; *hypoxia* and elevated H+s ion concentration also cause vasodilation. However, these autoregulatory mechanisms become less responsive with increasing age and in the presence of arteriosclerosis.

The arterial system of the brain includes the conducting and penetrating vessels. The *conducting* arteries are (1) the *internal carotids,* which supply most of the cerebral hemispheres, basal, ganglia, and the upper two thirds of the diencephalon, and (2) the *vertebral* arteries, which supply the brain stem, the lower one third of the diencephalon, the cerebellum, and the occipital lobes. These two systems anastomose at the *circle of Willis,* and this allows them to compensate for alterations in cerebral blood flow and blood pressure. The *penetrating* vessels are those that enter the brain substance at right angles, after branching off from the conducting vessels; they supply nutrients to the neurons.

The venous system of the brain is unique in that cerebral veins have no valves. Also, all veins of the brain terminate in dural sinuses, which eventually empty into the superior vena cava by means of the jugular veins.

Another fluid present in the nervous system is *cerebrospinal fluid (CSF).* CSF is found in the ventricles of the brain, in the central canal of the spinal cord, and in the subarachnoid space. It serves as a fluid cushion

for nervous tissue and helps to support the weight of the brain. CSF is continually formed by vessels of the *choroid plexus.* In the adult there is 90 to 150 ml of CSF. After circulation about the brain and spinal cord, CSF returns to the brain and is absorbed through the arachnoid villi. From here CSF enters the venous system and follows its pathway through the jugular veins to the superior vena cava and into the systemic circulation.

The *spinal cord* structurally includes H-shaped central gray matter (nerve cell bodies) surrounded by white matter composed of ascending and descending tracts (Fig. 34-6). Functionally, the spinal cord serves primarily as a passageway for conducting information over sensory, or afferent, tracts to the brain from the periphery, and over motor, or efferent, tracts from the brain to the periphery.

The spinal cord is also the site of reflex pathways. Reflexes are an example of the simplest neuronal circuit. They *do not* require relay to the brain level for action. A reflex action consists of a *specific stereotyped motor response to an adequate sensory stimulus.* The response may involve skeletal muscle movement or glandular secretion. It may involve only two neurons as in a simple monosynaptic reflex arch such as occurs with the myotactic knee jerk reflex. In the knee jerk reflex a brisk tap over a partially stretched knee tendon stimulates sensory nerve endings within the tendons, and the stimulus travels over a sensory nerve fiber within a peripheral nerve toward the spinal cord where it synapses with a central motor neuron (anterior horn cell). Following this, the impulse is transmitted down the motor nerve (over anterior nerve root of the spinal nerve or peripheral nerve) and across the neuromuscular junction to stimulate the muscle to contract. Fig. 34-7 shows the reflex arc. In summary, a reflex arc is dependent

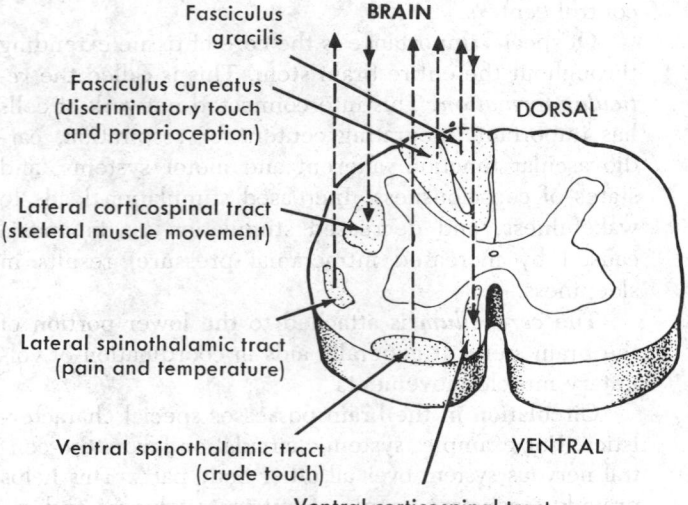

Fasciculus gracilis
BRAIN
Fasciculus cuneatus (discriminatory touch and proprioception)
DORSAL
Lateral corticospinal tract (skeletal muscle movement)
Lateral spinothalamic tract (pain and temperature)
Ventral spinothalamic tract (crude touch)
VENTRAL
Ventral corticospinal tract (skeletal muscle movement)

Fig. 34-6. Some nerve pathways between spinal cord and brain that arise from white matter of cord. Note H-shaped gray matter of cord.

on an intact sensory nerve, a functional synapse with a central neuron within the spinal cord, an intact motor nerve fiber and neuromuscular junction, and a competent muscle. A reflex may involve only one spinal cord level, as in the knee jerk reflex, or it may involve one or a few spinal cord levels (*segmental reflexes*), or it may involve structures in the brain that influence the spinal cord (*supraspinal* reflexes).

Finally, a word must be said about the *meninges*, the coverings of the nervous tissue in the brain and spinal cord. These fibrous coverings help support, protect, and nourish the brain and spinal cord. Outermost is the *dura mater*, a very tough membrane consisting of two layers. This meningeal layer is significant in that it sends four processes deep into the cranium and these processes form fibrous compartments for portions of the brain. The

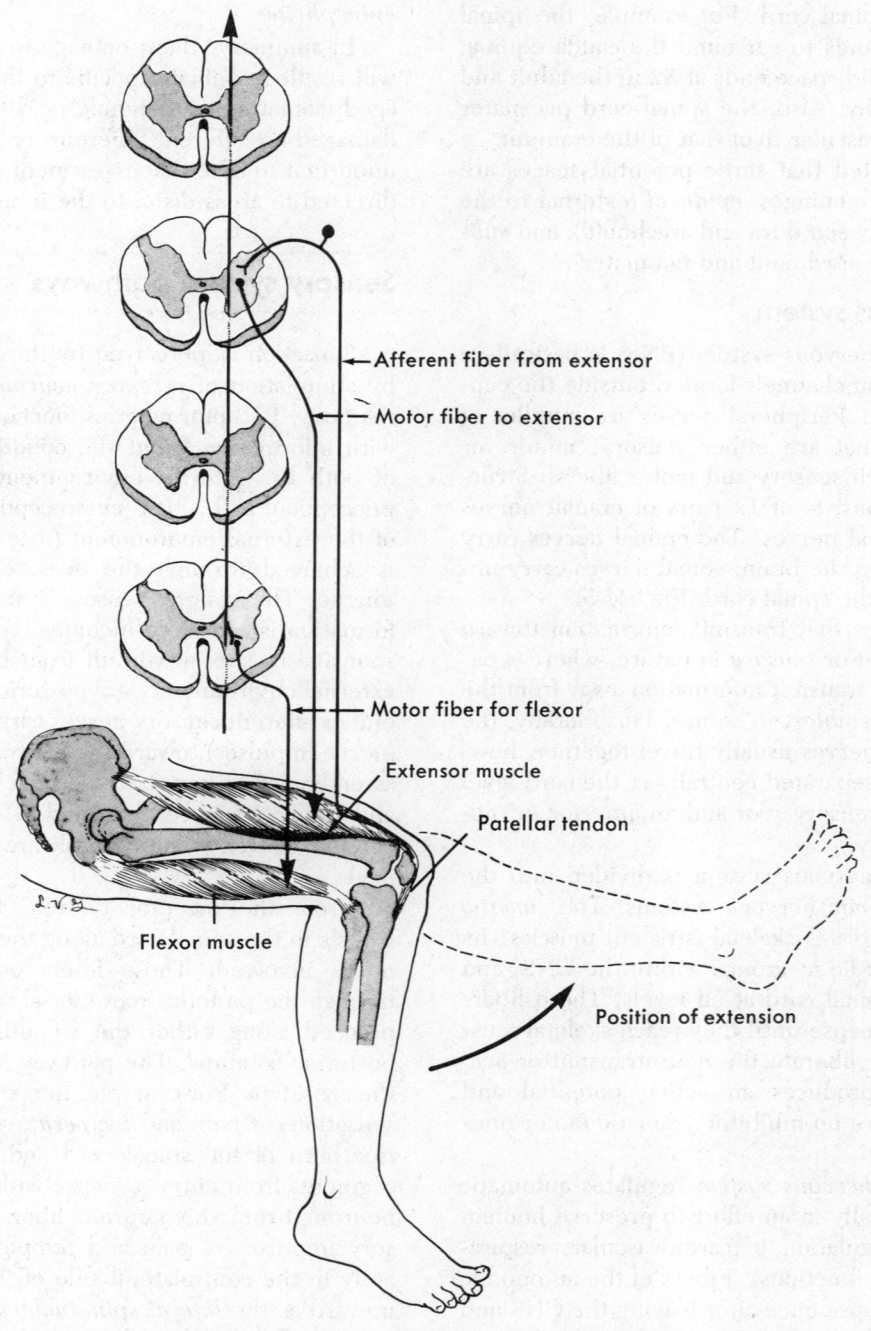

Afferent fiber from extensor

Motor fiber to extensor

Motor fiber for flexor

Extensor muscle

Patellar tendon

Flexor muscle

Position of extension

Fig. 34-7. Deep tendon reflex (knee jerk or patellar tendon reflex) representative of reflex arc. Note that patellar tendon of extensor muscle is attached to tibia below knee. (From Schottelius, B.A., and Schottelius, D.D.: Textbook of physiology, ed. 18, St. Louis, 1978, The C.V. Mosby Co.)

arachnoid, which is the delicate membrane lying beneath the dura, covers the brain more loosely. Projections extend into the overlying dura and these are called the *arachnoid villi.* The *pia mater,* innermost of the meninges, is a vascular membrane having many minute plexuses of blood vessels. The pia mater follows the course of the penetrating blood vessels as they dip into the substance of the brain.

These three coverings with only minor variations are also found in the spinal cord. For example, the spinal cord arachnoid expands to surround the cauda equina; thus the subarachnoid space ends at S2 in the adult and is most wide caudally. Also, the spinal cord pia mater is thicker and less vascular than that of the cranium.

It should be noted that three potential spaces are associated with the meninges: *epidural* (external to the dura); *subdural* (between dura and arachnoid); and *subarachnoid* (between arachnoid and pia mater).

Peripheral nervous system

The peripheral nervous system (PNS) is basically a set of communication channels located outside the central nervous system. Peripheral nerves are bundles of individual nerves that are either sensory, motor, or "mixed" (having both sensory and motor fibers). Structurally, the PNS consists of 12 pairs of cranial nerves and 31 pairs of spinal nerves. The cranial nerves carry impulses to and from the brain; spinal nerves carry impulses to and from the spinal cord (Fig. 34-5).

Peripheral nerves that transmit information toward the CNS are *afferent* or *sensory* in nature, whereas peripheral nerves that transmit information away from the CNS are *efferent,* or *motor,* in nature. Peripherally, the sensory and motor nerves usually travel together; however, they become separated centrally at the cord level into a *posterior* or sensory *root* and an *anterior* or motor *root,* respectively.

The peripheral nervous system is divided into the somatic and *autonomic* nervous systems. The *somatic nervous system* innervates skeletal (striated) muscles. Its neuronal cell bodies lie in groups within the CNS, and its axons exit the spinal cord at all levels. These fibers continue without synapse until they reach skeletal muscle cells. Here they liberate the neurotransmitter *acetylcholine,* which produces an action potential and movement. There are no inhibitory somatic motor neurons.

The *autonomic nervous system* regulates automatic body functions, usually in an effort to preserve homeostasis (e.g., the regulation of cardiovascular, respiratory, and endocrine functions). Fibers of the autonomic nervous system synapse once after leaving the CNS and before arriving at the neuroeffector junction. The site of this synapse is called a *ganglion* and its neurotransmitter is acetylcholine. The autonomic nervous system is further divided into the sympathetic nervous system,

which functions to maintain homeostasis and to provide defense against stressors (see Chapter 13) and the parasympathetic nervous system, which is responsible for conservative and restorative vegetative functions. Fibers leaving the ganglia finally synapse at the effector organ. The neurotransmitter for the postganglionic synapse of the parasympathetic nervous system is *acetylcholine,* and for the sympathetic nervous system the neurotransmitter for the postganglionic synapse is *norepinephrine.*

In summary, then, damage to any peripheral nerve will result in deficits specific to the type of nerve damaged (somatic or autonomic) and to whether the fibers damaged are afferent, efferent, or mixed in nature. It is important to note that assessment of dysfunction will be directed to areas *distal* to the injury.

Sensory system pathways

Sensation as perceived by the individual is initiated by stimulation of *receptor neurons* located throughout the body. Receptor neurons function to provide the brain with information about the condition and composition of both the internal environment (e.g., position proprioception) and action (enteroception of body parts) and of the external environment (exteroception). The latter is achieved through the eyes, ears, nose, skin, and tongue. The general sensory system by which this information is conveyed includes (1) receptor neurons responsive to special stimuli from both the internal and external environments, (2) posterior roots of the peripheral or afferent sensory nerves carrying action potentials (nerve impulses) toward the central nervous system, (3) ascending or sensory tracts located within the spinal cord and upper brain centers, and (4) sensory areas of the cerebral cortex where stimuli are perceived and localized.

From the receptor neuron, the sensory impulse travels to the spinal cord along the afferent fibers of the nerve involved. These fibers enter the spinal cord through the posterior root (dorsal root ganglion) and may proceed along either the spinothalamic tracts or the posterior columns. The pathway followed is specific to the sensation. For example, nerve fibers conducting the sensations of *pain* and *temperature* pass into the posterior horn of the spinal cord and, within a few spinal segments from entry, synapse with a secondary sensory neuron. From this neuron, fibers conducting the sensory impulses of pain and temperature cross immediately to the contralateral side of the cord and continue upward as the *lateral spinothalamic tract.* These fibers arrive at the thalamus, where they synapse with a third sensory neuron. Fibers from this neuron terminate in the appropriate area of the sensory cortex (Fig. 34-8).

Sensations for crude touch follow a very similar

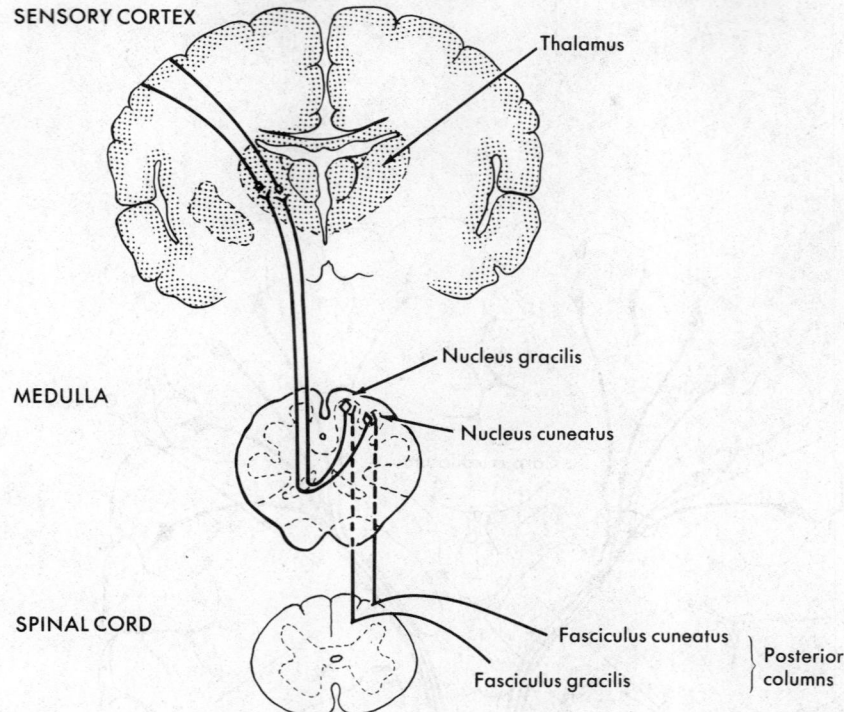

SENSORY CORTEX

Thalamus

MEDULLA

Nucleus gracilis

Nucleus cuneatus

SPINAL CORD

Fasciculus cuneatus

Fasciculus gracilis

Posterior columns

Fig. 34-8. Pathways for fine touch, deep touch and pressure, vibration, and proprioception. Note how stimuli entering through dorsal root (posterior) travel on same side as posterior columns to medulla where they cross to opposite side, ascend to thalamus, and end in somesthetic area where perception occurs.

pathway to that for pain and temperature. Nerve fibers conducting the impulses pass into the posterior horn of the spinal cord and synapse with a secondary sensory neuron. The fibers from the secondary neuron cross to the contralateral side of the cord and continue upward as the *ventral spinothalamic* tract. These travel to the thalamus where they synapse with a third sensory neuron. Fibers from this neuron terminate in the appropriate area of the sensory cortex. Sensation of fine touch, deep touch/pressure, vibration, and proprioception, on the other hand, arriving at the spinal cord are conducted directly by the *posterior columns (fasciculus gracilis* or *fasciculus cuneatus)* to the level of the medulla before synapsing with a second neuron. These fibers then cross over to the contralateral side, where they continue to the thalamus. Here they also synapse with a third sensory neuron that terminates at the appropriate area of the sensory cortex (Fig. 34-8).

Motor system pathways

After the brain perceives the state of the body's internal and external environments, it may initiate corrective actions. These impulses are conveyed by the *de-*

scending motor pathways—including the *corticospinal* (pyramidal) tracts, the extrapyramidal system, and the cerebellar system. The corticospinal system is primarily concerned with skilled voluntary skeletal muscle movements of the distal extremities and, in particular, with the alpha (α-) and gamma (γ-) motor neurons. Fibers that combine to form the corticospinal *tracts* arise from the *upper motor neurons*. Their cell bodies are located in the primary motor area of the cerebral cortex in the precentral gyrus of the frontal lobe, and in the premotor cortex in the frontal lobe.

After fibers leave the cerebral cortex, they descend through the posterior limb of the internal capsule, middle of the cerebral cerebri, break up into bundles in the basilar portion of the pons, and then collect into discrete bundles within the pyramids of the medulla. In the medulla the majority of the fibers cross over, or *decussate*, to the opposite side of the medulla and become the *lateral* corticospinal tract, which then passes to all spinal cord levels in the lateral funiculus and terminally synapse in the lateral aspect of laminae IV through VIII (Fig. 34-9). The remaining fibers descend directly from the medulla (do not decussate) and synapse directly with α- and γ-neurons in lamina IX of the spinal cord. The latter is known as the *anterior corti-*

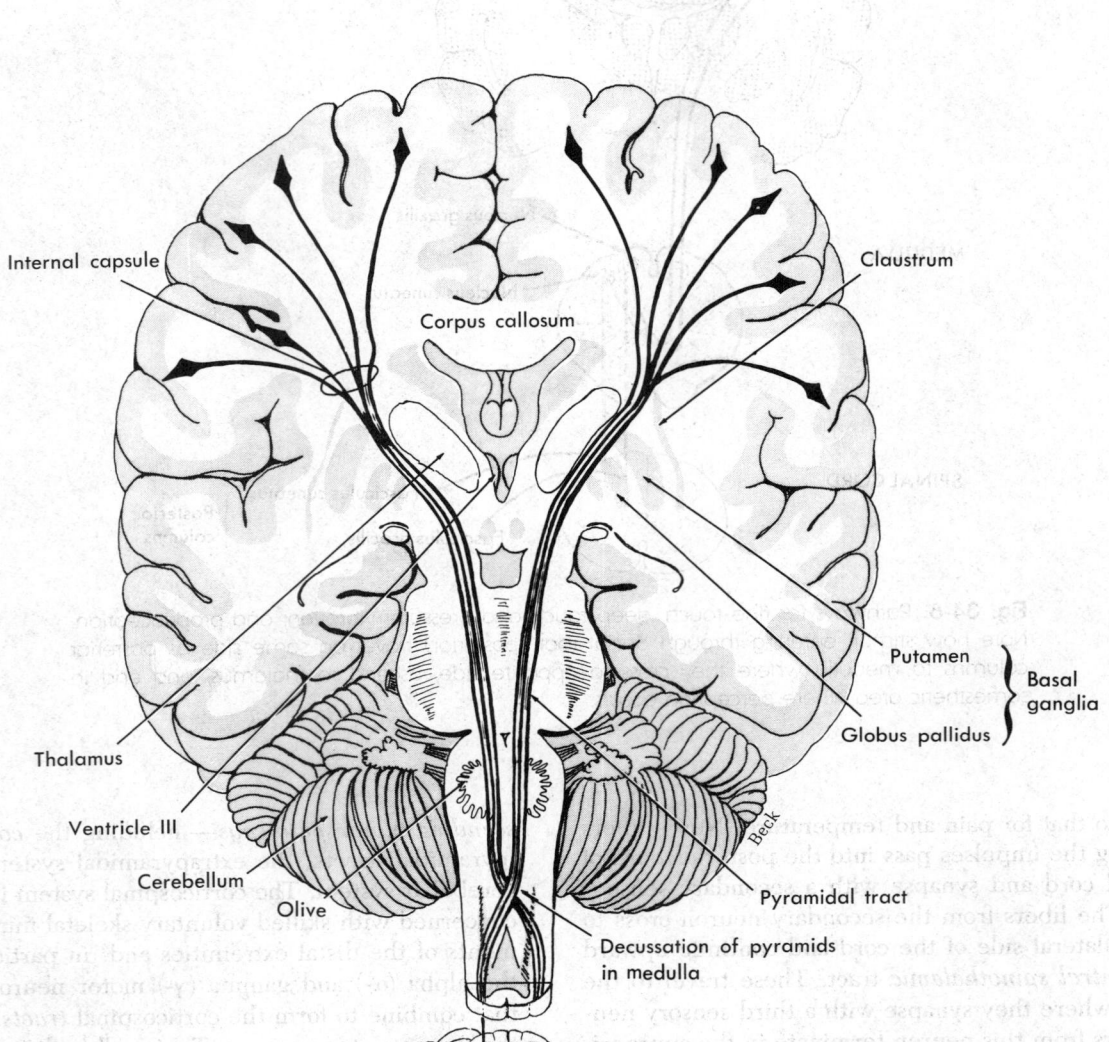

Internal capsule

Corpus callosum

Claustrum

Thalamus

Ventricle III

Cerebellum

Olive

Putamen

Globus pallidus

} Basal ganglia

Pyramidal tract

Decussation of pyramids in medulla

Spinal cord

Beck

Fig. 34-9. Crossed corticospinal (pyramidal) tracts. Axons that compose pyramidal tracts (corticospinal) come from neuron cell bodies in cerebral cortex. After they descend through internal capsule of cerebrum and white matter of brain stem, about three fourths of fibers decussate (cross over from one side to the other) in medulla, as shown. Then they continue downward in lateral corticospinal tract on opposite side of cord. Each crossed corticospinal tract therefore conducts motor impulses from one side of brain to interneurons or anterior horn motoneurons on opposite side of cord. Therefore impulses from one side of cerebrum cause movements of opposite side of body. (From Anthony, C.P., and Thibodeau, G.A.: Textbook of anatomy and physiology, ed. 11, St. Louis, 1983, The C.V. Mosby Co.)

cospinal tract. The left cerebral motor strip of the primary motor area controls the muscular movement of the right side of the body.

Eventually, these fibers synapse with large anterior horn cells located in the spinal cord as well as in the motor cranial nuclei in the brain stem. These cells are called the lower motor neurons and are responsible for providing the final direct link or final common pathway with muscles via the myoneural (neuromuscular) junction at the motor end-plates. Thus skeletal muscle activity is the result of the net influence of upper motor neurons on the α- and γ-motor neurons through the anterior horn cells (lower motor neurons) in the spinal cord and motor cranial nuclei.

The extrapyramidal tracts are complex and provide separate pathways between the cortex, the basal ganglia, the brain stem, and the cord. In general, these include all descending motor pathways other than the corticospinal tract (indicating that they do not pass through the pyramids of the medulla). In general, these tracts are named from point of origin to termination. The extrapyramidal tracts collectively assist in maintaining muscle tonus and the control of gross automatic skeletal muscle movements. Some tracts tend to facilitate extensor activity and inhibit flexor activity (lateral vestibulospinal tract and pontine reticulospinal tract), while others facilitate flexor activity and inhibit extensor activity (lateral corticospinal tract and rubrospinal tract). It should be noted that some clinicians include as upper motor neurons the extrapyramidal descending fiber systems since such neurons also influence the lower motor neurons and help to modulate skeletal muscle tone and reflex activity.

The cerebellar system is responsible for muscle synergy throughout the body. The cerebellum coordinates the action of muscle groups and controls their contractions so that movements are performed smoothly and accurately. Voluntary movements can proceed without the cerebellum, but movements would be clumsy and incoordinated (asynergia and cerebellar ataxia). The cerebellum receives both sensory and motor inputs. There are feedback circuits with all the descending motor pathways. In addition, all sensory modalities, including tactile, auditory, and visual, also feed impulses to the cerebellum. The general scheme of cerebellar operation allows nerve impulses to be returned to or fed back to the same region from which they originated. These circuits can be compared with modern automatic control devices, or servomechanisms. The cerebellar cortex, similar to a computer, can detect any errors in muscle synergy and return the proper messages to adjust muscular control within the body.

Visceral efferent motor pathways from the spinal cord mediate the action of involuntary, or smooth, muscles located within walls of tubes, hollow organs, the heart, and the glands. Most viscera are supplied by both excitatory and inhibitory fibers.

Effectors

Effectors may be thought of as the cells of the body that "do something." They in turn interact with the internal and external environments in some way and carry out the commands of the nervous system. The two classes of effectors are muscles and glands. They are both transducers and are capable of converting one form of energy into another. Effectors, like nerve tissue, are excitable tissues and are able to generate action potentials. The nervous system controls muscles and glands by directly turning them on or by altering their level of spontaneous activity through a neuron-to-effector chemical communication system.

Neurologic assessment

Complete neurologic assessment is usually done in phases and is dependent on the condition of the person and the urgency in collecting the necessary data. It includes a history, neurologic examination, and special neurodiagnostic procedures. A discussion directed primarily to a description of the components of the neurologic examination follows.

History

As in other specialties, a careful history precedes physical examination of the nervous system. In the course of the history taking, the person's chief complaints are elicited through an interview. The person is asked to give a timewise account of the illness. The onset and progression of the condition as well as the nature of symptoms should be determined. As the person describes the onset of symptoms, note particularly the speed of onset, frequency of remissions (if any), and any diurnal patterns of intensity changes in symptoms. Symptoms often reported with vagueness and thus requiring sophisticated analyses are complaints of pain, headache, seizures, vertigo, numbness, visual changes, and weakness. Identification of specific patterns of these common neurologic manifestations may provide pertinent diagnostic information regarding the pathologic process and the person's perception of limitations. Ongoing collection of psycho-sociocultural data is of special importance. Information is collected about family members and their relationships and interactions, ethnic background, housing, recreational interests, occupation, education, coping mechanisms, dependence-independence characteristics, and how usual activities of daily living are correctly managed by the person. Particular attention should be paid to reports of any recent changes in the person's usual behaviors; for example, increased irritability, memory loss, or complaints of increasing job-related pressure or tension. A family health history and developmental history are also included. During the course of the neurologic or physical examination, some of the observations made during the history may be confirmed. A skillfully taken history with accurate analysis and interpretation of the collected data often holds the key to diagnosis. Some observations made during the history that are validated during the examination will require further study through special neurodiagnostic procedures.

Neurologic examination

Neurologic examination of the conscious adult includes physical examination of the following components: *mental status* (level of consciousness, orientation, mood and behavior, knowledge, vocabulary, memory), *cranial nerves, language and speech, meninges, sensory status* (touch, pain, temperature, proprioception), and *motor status* (gait and stance, muscle strength, muscle tonus, coordination, involuntary movements, muscle stretch reflexes). The ongoing sequential discussion of each of these components provides the nurse with a framework for the kind of information that should be collected in order to make decisions about nursing care and to assist the physician in making a medical diagnosis.

The sequence in performing the neurologic examination varies with the examiner, but it should be one that ensures completeness and thoroughness without exhausting the person being examined. Throughout the examination the examiner attempts to localize the site of any abnormality. Using knowledge of normal neuroanatomy and neurophysiology, combined with a series of tests, the abnormal findings with reference to their *distribution* and *symmetry* of both sides of the body are noted by the examiner.

The examination depends largely on inspection and palpation and only occasionally on percussion. Auscultation may be used to detect related vascular abnormalities. Varied instruments are utilized. Initially, functions may be tested grossly, followed by definitive testing should an abnormality be identified.

Equipment required to perform a neurologic examination (in addition to materials used for a general physical examination) is often assembled for convenience on a neurologic tray (see box in next column).

EQUIPMENT NEEDED TO PERFORM A NEUROLOGIC EXAMINATION

Compass

Cotton applicators

Diagram of dermatomes

Dynamometer

Flashlight

Miscellaneous items of varied shapes and sizes (coin, key, marble)

Ophthalmoscope

Oroscope

Colored pencil

Pins with sharp and blunt ends

Printed page

Reflex hammer

Tape measure

Tongue depressors

Tuning fork

Snellen chart

Stroppered vials containing:
1. Peppermint, oil of cloves, coffee, soap (smell)
2. Sugar, salt, vinegar, quinine (taste)
3. Cold and hot water (temperature)

Watch with second hand

Mental status

Specific abnormalities of higher cerebral function are particularly significant in determining the presence of organic brain disease; therefore clinical observation of mental function is important.

A determination of the examinee's *level of consciousness* (awareness of self and environment) is necessary (see Chapter 27 for a more detailed discussion). Although many metabolic and toxic states produce changes in consciousness, destructive lesions of the brain do so directly. With destructive lesions that affect the reticular system, there also may be elevation of consciousness as evidenced by insomnia, agitation, mania, and delirium.

The patient is also tested for *orientation* to time (day, month, week), place, and person. Disorientation to place and person indicates a more profound cerebral disorder. It is helpful to remember that orientation depends on the ongoing sensory impressions and involves the cerebral cortex.

TABLE 34-1. Cranial nerves*

Nerve	Function	Assessments
Olfactory (I)	Sensory—smell	Identification of odors
Optic (II)	Sensory—vision	Visual acuity; inspection of fundi; determination of visual fields
Oculomotor (III)	Motor—pupil constriction, elevation of upper eyelid, extraocular movements	Tested together for extraocular movements (Fig. 34-15); also pupil reflex for CNIII
Trochlear (IV)	Motor—downward/inward eye movements	
Abducens (V)	Motor—lateral eye movements	
Trigeminal (VI)	Motor—jaw movement; Sensory facial sensation	Jaw strength; facial sensation; corneal reflex
Facial (VII)	Motor—facial muscles; Sensory taste on anterior two thirds of tongue	Facial movements; identification of tastes
Acoustic (VIII)	Hearing—cochlear division; Balance—vestibular division	Whisper; caloric test
Glossopharyngeal (IX)	Sensory—pharynx and posterior tongue, with taste; Motor—pharynx	Identification of tastes
Vagus (X)	Sensory—pharynx and larynx; Motor—palate, pharynx, and larynx	Gag reflex; uvula motion; soft palate movement; hoarseness
Spinal accessory (XI)	Motor—sternocleidomastoid, upper part of trapezius	Shoulder and neck motion
Hypoglossal (XII)	Motor—tongue	Tongue motion

*Adapted from Bates, B.: A guide to physical examination, ed. 2, Philadelphia, 1979, J.B. Lippincott Co.

The identification of mood and behavior is also included in a mental examination, since a particular mood may be associated with a specific disease. For example, emotional lability is often seen in bilateral (diffuse) brain disease, where the mood shifts easily and quickly from one extreme to the other. Euphoria is a superficial elevation of mood accompanied by unconcern even in the presence of threatening events. It needs to be determined if the person's mood is appropriate to the topic of conversation. Personality changes with the appearance of violent temper and aggressive behavior may occur with destructive lesions of the inferior frontal parts of the limbic system. Such behaviors can be validated by family and friends.

The individual's knowledge and vocabulary are tested in reference to common knowledge of current events. The ability to think abstractly may be tested by asking the person to explain the meaning of a proverb. Calculation is tested by examining the ability to subtract serially 7 from 100. *Dyscalculia* is the inability to solve simple problems. Recent memory loss is more common in brain disease than is remote memory loss. The findings of these gross tests may indicate the need for more definitive tests of mental function. Thus, it can be seen that much data concerning mental status can be collected through a careful and thoughtful patient history.

Cranial nerve examination

A general description of cranial nerve testing is included at this point. It is helpful to recall from anatomy the number of the nerve (the sequence of the nerve along the rostrocaudal axis of the brain) and the name (explains the function or distribution) and to be able to express in a few words the function or functions of each cranial nerve so that it has practical meaning. Knowledge of the brain stem anatomy assists in relating the cranial nerve locations (Fig. 34-5).

The 12 cranial nerves may be tested in numbered sequence as presented on the following pages. Some nurses prefer to test at the same time those cranial nerves that have similarity of function, such as voluntary motor function and visceral motor function and special sensory and general sensory functions. It should be recalled, however, that some cranial nerves have both motor and sensory functions, while others are purely motor or sensory. It also should be recognized by the examiner that data collected from sensory testing is subjective. To counteract this, the person should be retested several times and in a random order to avoid memorization by the examinee (Table 34-1).

Cranial nerve I (olfactory). The function of cranial nerve I is purely *sensory*, namely, smell. Special receptors located within the superior or uppermost part of each nasal chamber, when stimulated by odors, transmit neural impulses over the olfactory bulbs to the olfactory nerves terminating in the area of the central cortex concerned with olfaction. This nerve is tested with the examinee's eyes closed or blindfolded at all times. A nonpungent, familiar substance is held under each nostril while blocking the other nostril. Each nostril is tested separately and with multiple substances, such as coffee, soap, tobacco, and peppermint, in a random pattern. The substance may be placed on an applicator or the person may be asked to sniff the substance from an open vial. First, it is determined if an odor is perceived. If so, then identification of the specific odor is requested by name. Data is collected in relation to the ability to perceive odor and identify substances by their odor. The ability to be aware of an odor must be differentiated from the ability to name a specific substance. *Anosmia* (absence of smell) or *hyposmia* (decreased sensitivity of

the sense of smell) is often associated with complaints of lack of *taste*, even though tests may demonstrate that sense to be intact. Anosmia is caused by varied lesions involving any part of the olfactory pathways. Neoplasia at the base of the frontal lobe and trauma are the common causes of neurogenic anosmia. Intranasal disease affecting the epithelium containing the receptors should be excluded before a diagnosis is made.

Cranial nerve II (optic). The function of cranial nerve II is purely *sensory,* namely, sight, or vision. Rods and cones, the special receptors sensitive to light, are located within the retina of the eye. When the retina is stimulated, nerve impulses are transmitted over the optic nerves (extending from the optic disk to the chiasm), over the optic tracts with the radiations terminating in the visual cortex of the occipital lobes. It should be noted, as shown in Fig. 34-10, that the medial (nasal) fibers of each optic nerve cross at the chiasm to the opposite

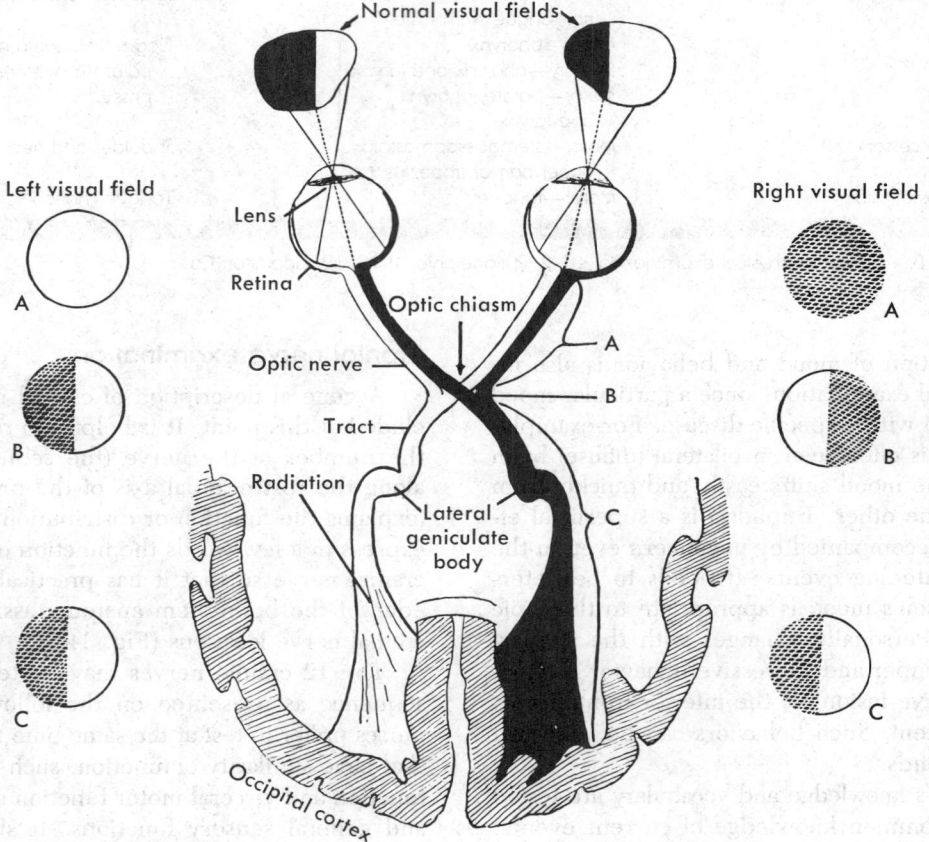

Fig. 34-10. Visual pathways showing partial decussation at optic chiasm and their radiation to end station of occipital cortex. Normal visual fields show reversal of light rays, through action of lens, from nasal and temporal sides to receptors in retina. Pathologic visual fields are illustrated. **A,** Loss of vision in right field resulting from complete lesion of right optic nerve; left field is normal. **B,** Loss of vision in temporal half of right and left fields caused by lesion involving optic chiasm (bitemporal hemianopia). **C,** Loss of vision in nasal field of right eye and in temporal field of left eye caused by lesion of right optic tract or radiation (homonymous hemianopia). Pathologic fields are lettered corresponding to sites of causative lesions. (From Conway, B.L.: Carini and Owens' neurological and neurosurgical nursing, ed. 7, St. Louis, 1978, The C.V. Mosby Co.)

side of the brain, while the lateral (temporal) fibers remain uncrossed. Thus fibers of the *left optic tract* contain only fibers from the left half of each retina and carry impulses to the left occipital lobe; fibers of the right optic tract contain only fibers from the right half of each retina and carry impulses to the right occipital lobe. Vision is dependent on the intactness of the visual pathways described above. Optic nerve function is assessed in relation to visual acuity, visual fields, and the appearance of the fundus (inner eye posterior to the lens). Each eye is tested separately.

VISUAL ACUITY. Visual acuity is mediated by the *cones* of the retina. Central vision is grossly tested by reading fine newspaper print. Distant visual acuity is assessed through the use of the Snellen chart (p. 841). Individuals with vision less than 20/20 are tested to determine light perception (LP), hand movement (HM), and finger count (FC).

VISUAL FIELDS. Field of vision is defined as that portion of space in which objects are visible during the fixation of vision in *one* direction. The field of vision thus relates to peripheral vision, or indirect vision. As in visual acuity, normality depends on the intactness of all parts of the visual pathway of the eye. The receptors for peripheral fields are the *rod* neurons of the retina. These are efficient for detection of form and movement but are poor for vision and color. Visual acuity and color are functions of the central field. The visual fields are tested grossly by *confrontation techniques*. As the name implies, the examiner faces or confronts the person directly from a distance of 2 to 3 ft. Various methods are used; only one is discussed here. The individual is instructed to cover one eye and to focus steadily at a point directly ahead. Initially, a small object, such as a pencil or the examiner's finger, is placed peripherally beyond the person's field of vision and then advanced centripetally until the examinee first indicates that the object is seen. The object should be held equidistant between examiner and examinee. Normally, the individual should see about 60 degrees nasalward, 50 degrees upward, 90 degrees temporally, and 70 degrees downward. The eye should be tested in equally spaced meridians including the upper and lower nasal and temporal quadrants of each eye. If deficits are detected, a sketch of them should be made and placed in the examinee's record. Additional visual field testing may be warranted at this point. This is often conducted by a neuroophthalmologist, who may employ perimetry using an arch marked in 90 degree sectors. In this manner specific deficits can be mapped with great precision.

Visual fields may be altered in a variety of central nervous system diseases, such as neoplasia and vascular disease. Ocular disease such as glaucoma is a major cause. Damage to one optic nerve anterior to the chiasm affects only the field of the involved eye. Lesions at the chiasm or posterior to it produce bilateral visual field defects of a wide variety. For example, a pituitary gland tumor compressing the optic chiasm damages the crossing fibers from the nasal retina and classically causes bitemporal hemianopia, or the loss of vision in the temporal halves of each eye. Loss of vision in the corresponding halves of both visual fields produces *homonymous hemianopia* and can be further designated as right or left. For example, patients with *right* cerebrovascular accidents often experience hemianopia with left visual field loss.

OCULAR FUNDUS. The fundus is examined through the use of an instrument called an *ophthalmoscope*. The ocular fundus is defined as that portion of the interior of the eyeball that lies posterior to the lens. It includes the optic disk, blood vessels, retina, and macula.

The electric ophthalmoscope permits the examiner to see into the pupil through a lens and with a light along the viewer's line of sight. The latter is achieved by the light projected through a prism, which bends the light rays at a 90 degree angle. A number of different lenses arranged on a wheel can be dialed by a number on the instrument. A lens labeled with a red numeral assists in focusing farther away; a lens labeled with a black numeral assists in focusing nearer. The shape and color of the light beam can also be adjusted by the examiner; the light must always enter the pupil. Errors of refraction in the eyes of the examiner or examinee can be corrected by the use of lenses in the ophthalmoscope; as a rule glasses need not be worn by the examinee unless there is a high degree of astigmatism. The room is darkened so that the pupil dilates. Adequate funduscopic examination requires the use of mydriatic drugs such as phenylephrine (10%) to produce dilation of the pupil.

Examination, although painless in the normal eye, does require cooperation from the person being examined, who is asked to keep both eyes open and to focus on a distant object or on an imaginary point straight ahead. Care is taken that the person does *not focus* on the light from the instrument. Each eye is examined separately. The examiner stands or sits directly in front of the examinee. To avoid misalignment the instrument rests firmly against the nose or cheek of the examiner so that the lens of the instrument is directly in front of the pupil of the eye being examined. The right hand and right eye are used to examine the person's right eye, the left hand and left eye to examine the left eye. The examiner's index finger rests on the lens dial to facilitate interchange of dials during examination. The examiner does not usually change the position of the instrument when attempting to view the inner eye structures. Instead, the examiner's head or body is repositioned to achieve clear visualization. Initially, the lens focus is directly on the pupil; *a red glow or reflex* may be noted as directed.

When the fundus is examined, the examiner is positioned at a 15 degree angle temporal to the person's line of vision. The lens focus is then adjusted. The entire fundus is not visualized at one time. The examiner *systematically* scans the fundus, examining each part in *detail* beginning with the optic disk. The blood vessels, periphery, and macula are then examined in sequence. The neurologist's primary interest in ophthalmoscopy is in determining whether neurologically related abnormalities of the optic disk and retina or vascular system are present. Discussion here is limited to these aspects. The reader is referred to Chapter 37 for further discussion of ophthalmoscopy as related to diagnosing other diseases involving the eye.

EXAMINATION AND INTERPRETATION OF OPHTHAL-MOSCOPIC FINDINGS. The optic disk (papilla) is normally the most prominent structure visible; *it is the center of observation from which the funduscopic* examination proceeds. It is the area where the blood vessels and nerve fibers enter and exit from the eyeball (Fig. 34-11). The normal characteristics of the optic disk are presented in the box at right.

The disk is examined in detail as to normality of size, shape, margins, and color. There can be excessive pallor or redness. Swelling of the optic disk, or *papilledema*, may be caused by active inflammation or passive congestion. Papilledema because of passive congestion and edema from increased intracranial pressure is called *choked* disk (see Chapter 37). The neurologist is most interested in differentiating between early and late papilledema. *Optic atrophy* indicates partial or complete destruction of the optic nerve. It is associated with decreased visual acuity and with a change in the color of

the disk to a lighter pink or gray. The recognition of advanced papilledema is relatively easy, but differentiation of physiologic variations is difficult.

The largest blood vessels just visible in the fundus, the central retinal artery and central retinal vein, branch throughout the retina. Each vessel is carefully examined along its length from the disk to the periphery. The arterioles of the retina diverge from the disk, and the veins converge toward the disk. The retina is the only site in the human body where microcirculation can be viewed directly. In examination of the blood vessels the arteries normally appear lighter in color and narrower than the veins, and they intertwine. Veins pulsate. Examination is made relative to size, color, or fullness. Normally, arteries do not indent or displace veins. *Periphery* is the area adjacent to the disk, outside the disk and between the large vessels.

The macula is situated temporal to the optic disk. It is 1 DD (disk diameter) in size and is vascular. A glis-

NORMAL CHARACTERISTICS OF THE OPTIC DISK

Size	1.5 mm
Shape	Flat round or vertically oval
Margins	Sharply defined
Color	Creamy red with a small whitish depression in the center (physiologic cup)

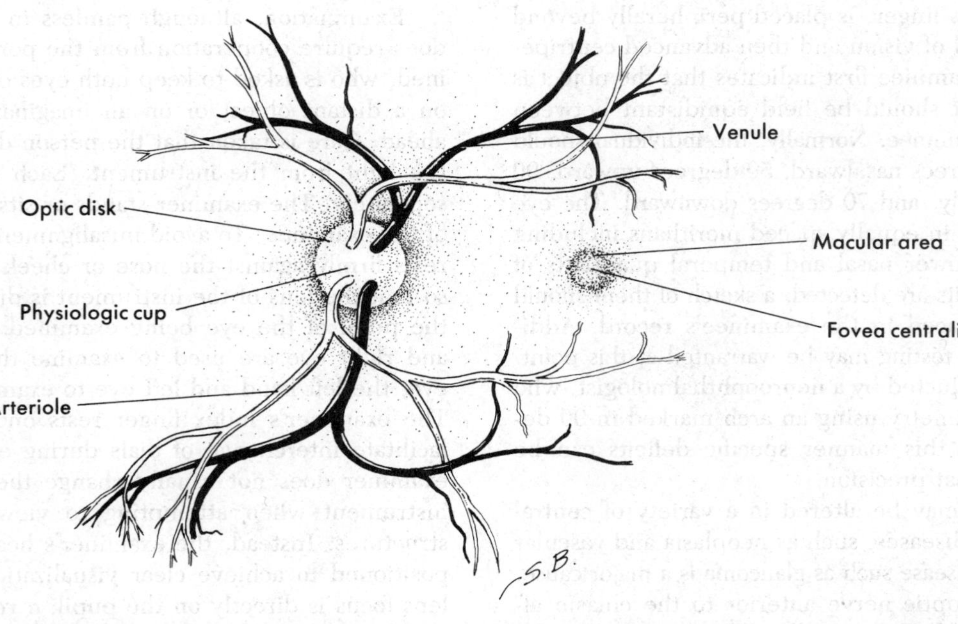

Fig. 34-11. Funduscopic structures of left eye. (From Malasanos, L., et al.: Health assessment, ed. 2, St. Louis, 1981, The C.V. Mosby Co.)

Labels: Venule; Optic disk; Physiologic cup; Arteriole; Macular area; Fovea centralis

tening spot of reflected light seen in the macula represents a pinpoint depression and is the *fovea centralis* (region of retina with highest visual acuity). For this reason a small macular lesion may be more disabling than a considerably larger peripheral lesion and results in a greater decrease in visual acuity. Last, the direction of light beam is adjusted to view the extreme periphery (examinee's eyes follow the light beam).

Cranial nerve III (oculomotor), cranial nerve IV (trochlear), and cranial nerve VI (abducens). Cranial nerves III, IV, and VI are *motor nerves* that arise from the brain stem and innervate the six *extraocular muscles* attached to the eyeball. These muscles function as a group in the coordinated movement of each eyeball in the six cardinal fields of gaze (straight, up, and down on both nasal and temporal sides). The motor nerves control the ocular muscles so that the eyes remain parallel throughout all ranges of motion and thus maintain *binocular* (stereoscopic) vision. The oculomotor nerves, in addition, send parasympathetic autonomic fibers to the constrictor muscles of the iris and to the levator palpebrae muscles of the upper eyelids.

EXTRAOCULAR MOVEMENTS. Individual eye movements are tested by covering one eye and following the examiner's finger in all fields of gaze with the uncovered eye while keeping the head stationary. Limitations of movement in all directions are observed as well as actual paralysis (*ophthalmoplegia*). If one of the extraocular muscles is paralyzed by damage to the nerve, the eye is unable to deviate fully into the corresponding field of gaze.

Conjugate movements of the eyes are also tested by asking the person to look with both eyes as far possible to either side then up and down. The examiner observes for parallel movements of the eyes in each direction or any deviation from normal (Fig. 34-12).

Double vision (*diplopia*), squint (*strabismus*), and involuntary rhythmic movements of the eyeballs (*nystagmus*) may indicate weakness of some of the extraocular muscles because of deficits of the motor nerves. These nerves may be involved singly or in unison in some neurologic diseases. *Ptosis,* or dropping of the upper eyelid over the globe, may be caused by damage to the oculomotor nerve. Normally, the upper lid minimally overlaps the iris as the examinee moves the eyes downward. The person with ptosis is unable to raise the lid voluntarily.

PUPILS. Each pupil should be inspected first as to

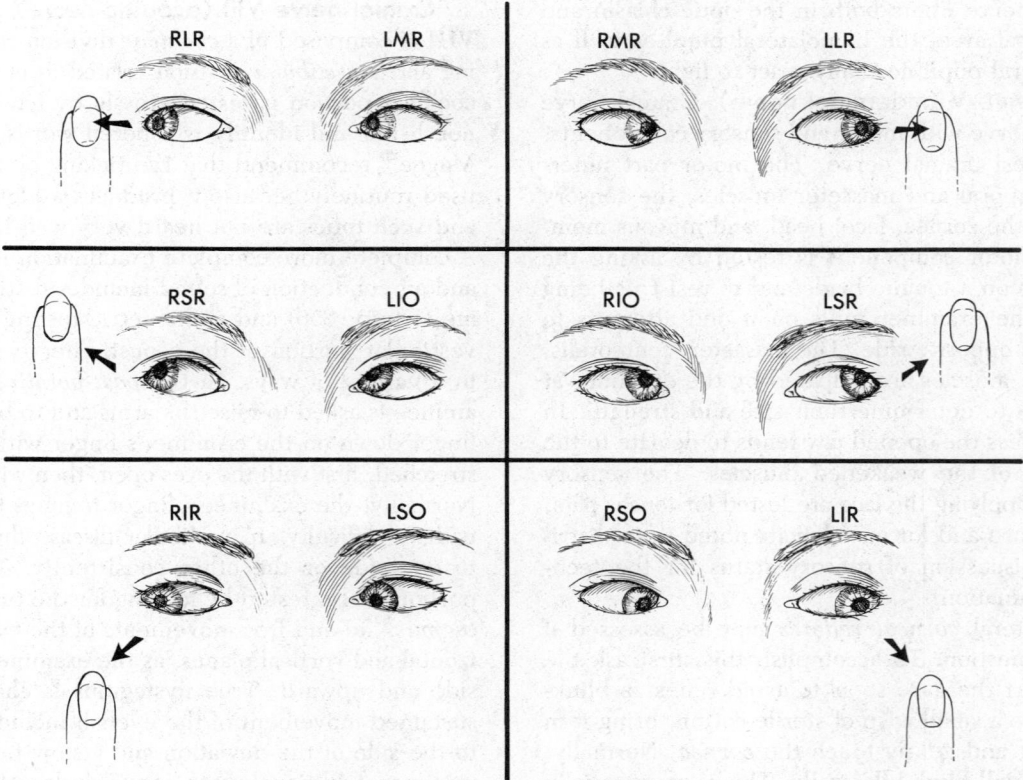

Fig. 34-12. Examination of extraocular muscles. Note that two muscles are involved in each cardinal direction. R = right; L = left; LR = lateral rectus; MR = medial rectus; SR = superior rectus; IO = inferior oblique; IR = inferior rectus; SO = superior oblique.

size and then as to shape and equality. *Argyll Robertson* pupils, for example, are constricted and do not react to light, although they react to accommodation for near objects (p. 811). Pupil inequality, or *anisocoria,* may assist in diagnosis of some neurologic diseases. The pupil is normally round, centrally placed, regular in outline, and equal in size to the other pupil. However, unequal pupils are found in approximately 25% of the normal population. Thus it is more significant to assess briskness of the pupillary response.

PUPILLARY REFLEX. The examiner darkens the room before examination. A small beam of light is focused directly into each eye in turn. The examiner avoids shining the light into both eyes simultaneously and instructs the person not to focus on the light beam, thus producing an accommodation reaction. Normally, the pupil constricts quickly when a light is focused on the homolateral retina. Constriction is reported by Simpson and Magee[26] to be especially brisk in young people and those with blue eyes. After a head injury, for example, a *dilated, fixed* pupil may be observed on the side of the cranial injury. A slow or sluggish pupil occurs as the pupil contracts slowly or imperfectly and relaxes immediately.

CONSENSUAL LIGHT REFLEX. Observations include inspection for constriction of the pupil *opposite* to the one directly stimulated. As a result of the decussation (crossing) of nerve fibers both in the optic chiasm and in the pretectal area, the homolateral pupil as well as the contralateral pupil normally react to light.

Cranial nerve V (trigeminal nerve). Cranial nerve V is a *mixed* nerve with motor and sensory components. It is the largest cranial nerve. The motor part innervates the temporal and masseter muscles; the sensory part supplies the cornea, face, head, and mucous membrane. The motor component is tested by asking the person to bite on a tongue blade and to resist its being removed as the examiner pulls on it and attempts to push it to the opposite side. The masseter, temporalis, and pterygoid muscles are palpated by the examiner at the same time to determine their size and strength. In muscle weakness the opened jaw tends to deviate to the opposite side of the weakened muscles. The sensory components supplying the face are tested for touch, pain, and temperature and for any deficits noted as to distribution (see discussion of sensory status for the technique of examination).

Next, bilateral *corneal reflexes* may be assessed if they are in question. To accomplish this, first ask the person to avert the gaze so as to avoid reflexive blinking. Next, take a small wisp of sterile cotton, bring it in from the side, and gently touch the *cornea*. Normally, the examinee will blink bilaterally. This is an especially important reflex to assess in persons with *decreased levels of consciousness* because corneal damage may result in its absence.

Cranial nerve VII (facial nerve). Cranial nerve VII is a *mixed nerve* that is concerned with facial movement and the sensation of taste. The motor part is tested by asking the person to perform specific facial movements while the examiner observes for muscle weakness. The inability to smile, close both eyes tightly, look upward and wrinkle the forehead, show the teeth, purse the lips, and blow out the cheeks constitutes weakness or paralysis of facial muscles innervated by this nerve. Distinction must be made between central and peripheral neurologic involvement. Special attention in examination is given to asymmetry. Peripheral involvement as in *Bell's palsy* is caused by compression of this cranial nerve and is a common *lower motor neuron* type of facial paralysis. (This means the lesion affects the facial nerve or its nucleus.) Lesions affecting the facial nerve produce paralysis of half of the entire face including the eyelids, forehead, and lips. Forehead function, by contrast, remains intact in *central* or *upper motor neuron* lesions. This suggests that the lesion lies somewhere on the path from the contralateral cerebral cortex to the nucleus of the facial nerve. The sensation of taste is tested by placing, in turn, salty, sweet, bitter, and sour substances on the side of the protruded tongue for identification. A loss of taste over the anterior two thirds of the tongue is present when the nerve is diseased, as in mastoid canal lesions.

Cranial nerve VIII (acoustic nerve). Cranial nerve VIII is composed of a *cochlear* division related to hearing and a *vestibular* division related to equilibrium. The cochlear portion is tested grossly by having the examinee listen and identify whispered words. Simpson and Magee[26] recommend that the ticking of a watch not be used routinely because it produces a high-pitched tone and such tones are not heard very well by the elderly. A complete more complete examination including bone and air conduction of sound includes testing with a tuning fork (p. 856) and audiometric testing (p. 853). The vestibular portion of the acoustic nerve may be tested in a variety of ways. In the *past-pointing test,* the examinee is asked to raise the arms and to bring the index finger down on the examiner's finger with the arm outstretched, first with the eyes open, then with eyes closed. Normally, the examinee's finger touches the examiner's without difficulty. In vestibular disease the finger points to one side or the other consistently. The vestibular portion is also tested by looking for the presence of *nystagmus,* "to-and-fro" movements of the eyeballs on horizontal and vertical planes, as the examinee looks to one side and upward. True nystagmus is characterized by sustained movement of the eyeball including a fast jerk to the side of the deviation and a slow jerk back to the midline. Additional tests can include caloric tests and electronystagmography (p. 856). Nerve deafness is usually the result of disease of the peripheral nerve but may also occur from central lesions involving acoustic nerves and nerve pathways in the brain stem and their termination within the temporal lobe. The vestibular portion is frequently affected in diseases of the central nervous system, and the most prominent symptom is vertigo.

Disease of the *cochlea* is characterized by nerve deafness (perception deafness). There is loss or impairment of hearing. Nerve deafness is usually the result of disease of the peripheral nerve. It may also occur from central lesions involving *acoustic nerves and nerve pathways* in the brain stem and their *termination within the temporal lobe*.

Cranial nerve IX (glossopharyngeal) and cranial nerve X (vagus). Cranial nerves IX and X are tested together. The chief function of cranial nerve IX is *sensory* to the pharynx and taste to the posterior third of the tongue. Both nerves supply the posterior pharyngeal wall, and normally when the wall is touched there is prompt contraction of these muscles on both sides, with or without gagging. This test is thus unreliable in regard to either nerve alone. Since cranial nerve X is the chief *motor nerve* to the soft palatal, pharyngeal, and laryngeal muscles, the detection of abnormalities is made through testing of voice sounds and cough sounds. In unilateral involvement of the motor portion of the vagus nerve there is harshness and nasality of the voice. When the person says "ah" the soft palate does not stay in the midline but deviates to the intact side. Bilateral involvement produces more severe effects in speech; there is also difficulty in swallowing (*dysphagia*), and fluids regurgitate through the nose because of palatal and pharyngeal involvement. Sensory function is not usually tested in the vagus nerve.

Cranial nerve XI (spinal accessory nerve). Cranial nerve XI is a motor nerve, that supplies the sternocleidomastoid muscle and upper part of the trapezius muscles. It is tested by having the person rotate the head against resistance while any weakness of the sternocleidomastoid muscle on the opposite side is observed and palpated by the examiner. The ability to shrug the shoulders while the examiner attempts to push against them is also tested. Weakness or paralysis of these muscles constitutes abnormality of this nerve.

Cranial nerve XII (hypoglossal nerve). Cranial nerve XII is a purely *motor* nerve. To begin, the examinee's tongue should first be inspected at rest in the mouth. Any asymmetry, unilaterality, decreased bulk, deviations, or fasciculations (fine twitching) should be noted. Next, the examiner should have the person stick out the tongue and move it from side to side. When this nerve is involved, there is deviation of the tongue toward the side of the lesion. Atrophy of the tongue is shown through wrinkling and loss of substance on the affected side. In an upper motor neuron lesion there is involvement of the tongue on the side opposite (contralateral) the lesion.

Language and speech

In assessing language and speech, one must first distinguish between *aphasia* and *dysarthria*. Aphasia is the general term for impairment of language function; it is a disorder of symbolic language. Dysarthria, on the other hand, is an indistinctness in word articulation or enunciation resulting from interference with the *peripheral* speech mechanisms (e.g., the muscles of the tongue, palate, pharynx, or lips).

Gross assessment of speech and language is made while the examinee's history is being taken. To further assess language, one must recall that language ability is concentrated in a cortical field that includes parts of the temporal lobe, the temporoparietal-occipital junction, the frontal lobe of the dominant (usually the left) hemisphere, and the occipital lobes. Lesions in any of the above areas will produce some impairment of language ability.

Four types of aphasia have been identified: (1) expressive (motor), (2) receptive (sensory), (3) expressive-receptive (global), and (4) amnesic (nominal). Although one type usually predominates, often one or more of the other type will be detected to some degree. *Expressive* aphasia occurs when the lesion is located in Broca's area. With this type of aphasia, the individual has difficulty finding the correct words although he or she understands part or most of what is being said. The individual may also have difficulty writing. The person with *receptive* aphasia has a lesion in Wernicke's area. This person has difficulty comprehending the spoken and often the written word (auditory-receptive and visual-receptive deficits, respectively), although hearing remains intact. With *global* aphasia there is severe loss of both sensory and motor language ability. Often such persons have extensive, destructive brain lesions. In *amnesic* aphasia the person is unable to recall the correct names for objects, conditions, or qualities. for example, the person may be able to repeat the series of days of the week but be unable to identify what day it is. This deficit is caused by a lesion located in the posterior and superior portions of the temporal lobe.

Aphasic problems can be detected by assessing spontaneous speech and by asking the examinee to follow simple commands, written and oral, to read and interpret newspaper stories, or to write down thoughts. Once a problem is identified, referral may be made to a speech pathologist for a definitive diagnosis and suggestions for treatment.

The ability to produce speech is tested through the detection of weakness or incoordination of muscles used in articulating speech. Limitations are observed during cranial nerve testing and particularly in reference to cranial nerves V, VII, IX, X, and XII. As previously discussed, involvement of the motor component of these nerves may produce alterations in phonation, resonance, and articulation. The examiner asks the individual to produce different speech sounds in order to localize the problem.

Dysarthrias are usually noticed during ordinary conversation or by having the examinee repeat a difficult phrase such as "Methodist Episcopal" or "third riding artillery brigade." Dysarthrias may be manifested by a single alteration or a variety of alterations. There are characteristic changes in particular diseases. For example, in cerebellar disease speech is often thick and explosive with a prolongation of speech sounds occurring at intervals (scanning). In parkinsonism speech is referred to as being hyperkinetic and is characterized by a decrease in loudness and in vocal emphasis patterns that makes sounds seem monotonous to the listener.

Apractic speech is a rare, yet interesting, disorder in which there is difficulty in the production of speech volitionally in the absence of motor programing through cortical integration. (Apraxia is a general term that also relates to motor acts other than speech.)

Meninges

To test for meningeal irritation, or stiff neck, the head is passively flexed sharply toward the chest while the person is in a recumbent position. In the presence of meningeal irritation there is marked resistance to flexion, accompanied by rigidity of the neck (nuchal), spasm, and pain. There is also resistance to extension and rotary movements of the neck. *Brudzinski's sign,* indicating meningeal irritation, is also elicited by passive neck flexion. When the neck is flexed, the hips and legs flex involuntarily. *Kernig's sign* is a classic test used in the diagnosis of meningitis. In this test the examiner flexes one of the patient's thighs to a right angle and then attempts to extend the leg on the thigh (there are many variations of this test). A positive Kernig's sign is present when there is spasm of the hamstring muscles with resistance to extension of the leg and with neck and head pain.

Sensory status

Accurate assessment of sensory function depends on the person's cooperation, alertness, and responsiveness. The examinee should be relaxed and have the eyes closed during all portions of the sensory examination to avoid receiving visual clues. Also, sensation should be tested side to side, and distally to proximally.

General sensory function of the trunk and extremities is tested for both superficial and deep sensations. Areas of sensory loss or abnormality are mapped out on a body diagram with a red pencil according to the distribution of the *spinal dermatomes* and peripheral nerves (Fig. 34-13). A dermatome, or skin segment, may be thought of as the area of skin supplied by one dorsal root of a cutaneous nerve. An area in which sensation is absent *(anesthesia)* is differentiated from areas in which

a sensation is intensified *(hyperesthesia)* or lessened *(hypesthesia)*. *Paresthesia* is an abnormal sensation that is perceived as burning, prickly, or itching.

Pain, temperature, and touch. *Superficial pain* perception is assessed by stimulating a suspected area by pinprick and asking the examinee to report discomfort felt. One can alternate sharp with dull objects for increased discrimination. *Deep pain* may be assessed by multiple means, some of which have the potential of causing tissue injury. It is only necessary to assess deep pain when the person being examined has a decreased level of consciousness. The method used should be chosen carefully, and the reader is directed to utilize the expertise of a nurse specialist to learn the correct techniques.

Crude touch may be assessed by touching a suspected area with cotton and requesting that the examinee indicate when the touch is felt. Temperature is tested by touching particular areas with warm to hot and cool to cold objects and asking the person to state the sensations felt. Since pain and temperature have the same nerve pathway, testing for temperature can be eliminated in the routine examination if the tests for pain perception are normal.

Motion and position. Proprioceptive fibers transmit sensory impulses from muscles, tendons, ligaments, and joints. This results in an awareness of the position of one's limbs in space (kinesthetic sense). *Proprioception* is tested by the examiner's grasping the sides of the examinee's distal phalanx and moving it up and down without assistance from the examinee. If proprioception is intact, the examinee will report correctly the direction in which the joint is being moved. (One can also assess proprioceptive abilities by the Romberg test, p. 735.)

Vibration is tested by placing a low-frequency tuning fork on a bony prominence of each extremity and assessing the examinee's ability to feel it.

Cortical sensory perception. All sensation is integrated and interpreted in the sensory cortex. The special ability to recognize objects through any of the special senses is known as *gnosia*. Lesions involving a specific association area of the cortex produce a specific type of *agnosia* (absence of this ability). One type of ability often tested is *stereognosis,* the ability to perceive an object's nature and form by touch. This is assessed by asking the examinee to identify familiar objects placed in the hand one at a time.

Motor status

Function of the motor system is assessed as to gait and stance, muscle strength, muscle tonus, coordination, involuntary movements, and muscle stretch reflexes.

Gait and stance should be recognized as complex activities that require muscle strength, coordination,

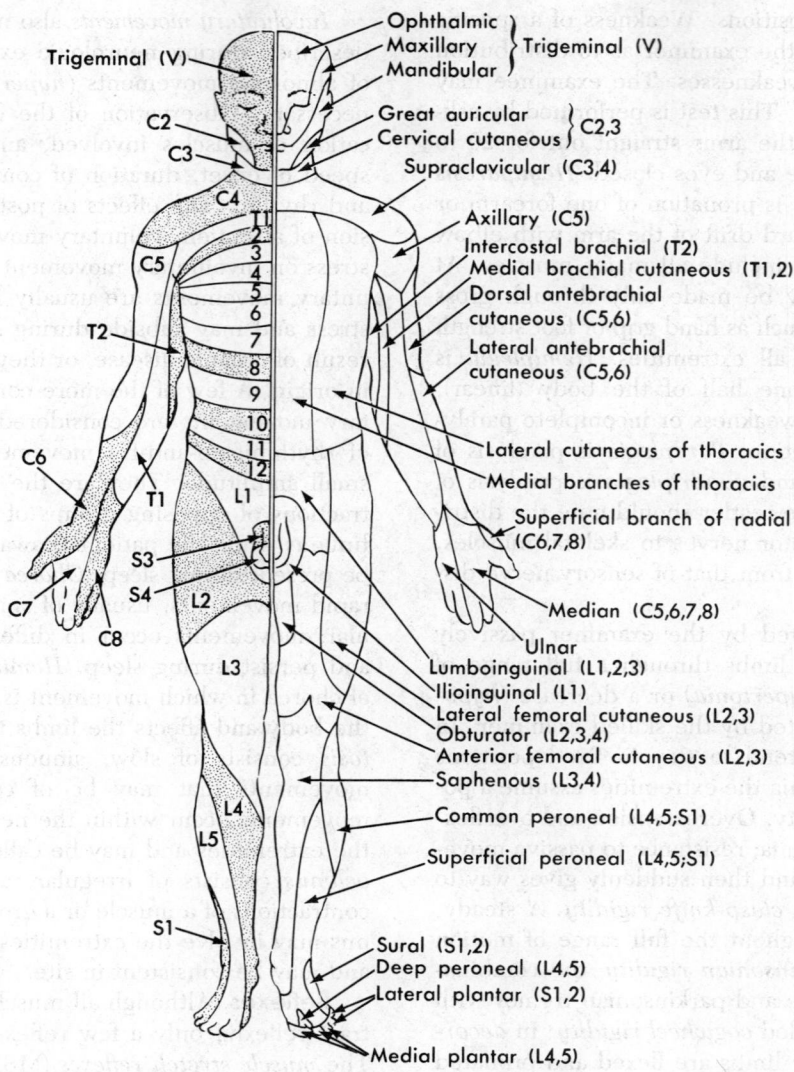

Fig. 34-13. Peripheral distribution of sensory nerve fibers. Anterior view. *Right,* distribution of cutaneous nerves. *Left,* dermatomes *(shaded)* or segmental distribution of cutaneous nerves. (Redrawn from House, E.L.: Neuroanatomy, ed. 2, New York, 1967, McGraw-Hill Book Co.)

balance, proprioception, and vision. Gait, or walking, and associated movements give considerable information about motor status. Changes in gait may be characteristic of a specific neurologic disease. *Ataxia* is a general term meaning lack of coordination in performing a planned, purposeful motion such as walking. It can be caused by disturbance of position sense or by cerebellar or other diseases. In evaluation of gait the person is asked to walk freely and naturally. A request may be made to walk *heel to toe* in a straight line, since this exaggerates any abnormalities. To evaluate stance, the person may perform the *Romberg test.* In this test the individual stands with feet close together, first with eyes open and then with eyes closed. Patients with problems of proprioception have difficulty maintaining balance with their eyes closed; patients with cerebellar

disease have difficulty even with their eyes open.

The *hemiparetic gait* seen in upper motor neuron disease is characterized by circumduction of the affected leg and inversion of the foot. Persons with Parkinson's disease walk with a slow, shuffling gait, and as they start walking there is an increase in rapidity until they are almost running *(propulsive).* They also have difficulty stopping, and deviation in the center of gravity causes retropulsion or lateropulsion. In addition, there is loss of associated movements of the arms in walking. Persons with cerebellar disease, on the other hand, walk with a wide-based, *staggering gait.*

Muscle strength, or power, is assessed systematically, including trunk and extremity muscles. During manual testing of each muscle group the examinee attempts to resist the examiner in moving his muscles when placed in fixed positions. Weakness of a specific muscle is identified by the examiner as to distribution and degree of muscle weaknesses. The examinee may also be tested for "drift." This test is performed by asking the person to hold the arms straight out for 20 to 30 seconds palms supine and eyes closed. *Hemiparesis* is suggested when there is pronation of one forearm or when there is a downward drift of the arm with elbow flexion. Evaluation may include all major muscles. At other times testing may be made only through gross tests of the extremities, such as hand grip or foot strength or the ability to move all extremities. *Hemiplegia* is complete paralysis of one half of the body (linear), whereas *hemiparesis* is weakness or incomplete paralysis in the same distribution. *Paraplegia* is paralysis of the lower extremities, and *quadriplegia* is paralysis of the four extremities. The reader should note the distribution of peripheral motor nerves to skeletal muscles. (The distribution varies from that of sensory nerve distributions.)

Muscle tonus is tested by the examiner passively moving the examinee's limbs through a full range of motion. An increase *(hypertonia)* or a decrease *(hypotonia)* can be differentiated by the skilled examiner. In hypertonia extremities tend to stay in fixed positions and feel firm; in hypotonia the extremities assume a position governed by gravity. Overextension and overflexion are found in hypertonia; resistance to passive movement increases rapidly and then suddenly gives way to *pyramidal spasticity*, or *clasp-knife rigidity*. A steady, passive resistance throughout the full range of motion is characteristic of *parkinsonian rigidity;* the combination of passive resistance and parkinsonian tremor with small regular jerks is called *cogwheel rigidity*. In *decorticate rigidity* the upper limbs are flexed and pronated and the lower limbs are extended. In *decerebrate rigidity,* on the other hand, the upper limbs are extended.

Coordination of muscle movements, or the ability to perform skilled motor acts, may be impaired at any level of the motor system. However, the cerebellum is primarily responsible for control, so that movements take place in a smooth and precise manner. Disturbance in cerebellar function may result in ataxia (as discussed relative to gait), difficulty in controlling the range of muscular movement *(dysmetria),* and an inability to alternate rapid opposite and successive movements *(adiadochokinesia)*. Simple motor activities are evaluated on command of the examiner to perform rapid and rhythmic movements. For example, the nose-finger-nose test requires the individual to alternately touch the nose and the tip of the examiner's finger with variation in rate and level. Other tests include the knee pat (pronation-supination) and heel-knee or shin test, during which the examinee slides his heel over the shin toward the dorsum of the foot. There are many such tests, often modified by the examiner.

Involuntary movements also need to be observed and described during neurologic examination. Description of abnormal movements *(hyperkinesia)* is difficult but necessary. Observation of the following is helpful: location of muscles involved, amplitude of movement, speed of onset, duration of contraction and relaxation, and rhythm. The effects of posture, rest, sleep, diversion of attention, voluntary movements, and emotional stress on involuntary movement are determined. Involuntary movements are usually increased by emotional stress and may subside during sleep. They can be the result of organic disease, or they may be psychosomatic in origin. A few of the more common types of involuntary movements are considered next. *Tremor* consists of rhythmic to-and-fro movements that are usually of small amplitude. They are the result of alternate contractions of opposing groups of muscles; they are continuous while the patient is awake and may or may not be present during sleep. *Chorea* consists of short, sharp, rapid movements, usually of small excursion and irregular; movements occur in different parts of the body and persist during sleep. *Hemiballismus* is a variation of chorea in which movement is confined to one side of the body and affects the limbs to a great extent. *Athetosis* consists of slow, sinuous, and more sustained movements that may be of considerable amplitude; movements occur within the neck and trunk as well as the extremities and may be called *torsion spasms*. *Myoclonus* consists of irregular, abrupt, and arrhythmic contractions of a muscle or a group of muscles. Myoclonus may involve the extremities, the trunk, or the face and may be consistent in site.

Reflexes. Although all muscles can be made to contract reflexly, only a few reflexes are tested clinically. The *muscle stretch reflexes* (MSRs) (also called myotactic and deep tendon reflexes) that are tested more routinely include the biceps, triceps, brachioradialis, quadriceps, and gastrocnemius and soleus muscles. (Superficial reflexes are omitted in this discussion.) Since the muscle reflexes are simply monosynaptic reflexes, they may be diminished in normal response *(hyporeflexia)* or lost completely *(areflexia)* because of interruption of afferent sensory fiber transmission or extensive destruction of efferent motor fibers of the anterior horn cells (lower motor neurons). On the other hand, release of the monosynaptic reflex from the influence of suprasegmental fibers (pyramidal and supplementary motor systems) (upper motor neuron influence) produces an increased muscular response *(hyperreflexia)*. The general method for testing muscle stretch reflexes is through mechanical stimulation of the muscle spindles through stretching and by tapping a tendon or a bone or by depressing the distal phalanx and allowing it to flip up sharply (Hoffmann's sign). The degree of response, above or below normal, is noted and graded on a scale. The most important feature of any reflex pattern is not the

TABLE 34-2. Grading of muscle stretch reflexes (MSR)

Scale	Interpretation
0	Areflexia
±	Hyporeflexia
1+ to 3+	Normal
3+ to 4+	Hyperreflexia

absolute value on the scale but the difference between one side of the body and the other (asymmetry). Stick figures are commonly used to record the bilateral values (scale may range from 0 to 4+). See Table 34-2 for one example of how reflexes are graded on a scale. Since the threshold for muscle stretch reflexes has a normal range of variability, some individuals with generalized hyporeflexia or hyperreflexia will not have pathologic conditions but will rank at the end of the normal range. On the other hand, areflexia is usually a pathologic condition.

One *pathologic reflex* often referred to clinically is the *plantar reflex*. This reflex when present in adults results in extension of the great toe (moves toward dorsum) with fanning (abduction) of the other toes when pressure is applied to the plantar surface of the foot laterally from the heel toward the toes. This response is known as *Babinski's sign* and is associated with upper motor neuron disease. Other reflexes may also be classified as pathologic. These are reflexes that are present in infancy for variable periods. They are thought to be released in adults by acquired diseases of the cerebrum. Examples include the sucking, pouting, and grasp reflexes.

A reflex when present may assist in localizing a lesion, as does the presence of a unilateral Babinski's sign. Reflex findings, however, are only used in relation to total assessment data and are not used alone. (Refer to neurology tests for techniques on eliciting specific reflexes.) Variations of grading-scale values used should be noted. It also should be recognized that grading is somewhat objective.

Special neurodiagnostic tests and procedures

Special neurodiagnostic procedures of the nervous system include examination of the cerebrospinal fluid by lumbar puncture, radioisotope brain scans, neuroradiologic studies of the spinal cord, and brain and electrodiagnostic studies to measure the electrical activity of the brain and muscles. Each is discussed generally as to use, methodology, data determined by the test, and nursing management. Some studies are invasive and carry a certain risk; they also are uncomfortable. Other studies are noninvasive and involve little risk. The reader is alerted to the fact that neurology tests give a variability of norms when interpreting laboratory findings. Tests related to specific neurologic problems are discussed in Chapter 36.

Lumbar puncture

Use

Lumbar puncture is used to obtain cerebrospinal fluid (CSF) for examination and to detect spinal subarachnoid block. The cerebrospinal fluid is examined for an increase or decrease of its normal constituents; it is also examined for foreign substances such as pathogenic organisms and blood. Cerebrospinal fluid normally is a clear fluid, since it is formed in the lateral ventricles of the brain.

Interpretation

Spinal fluid normally is under slight positive pressure; 80 to 180 mm of water is considered normal. It is measured on a manometer when a spinal puncture is done. When a brain tumor or other space-occupying lesion is within the cranium, the spinal fluid pressure usually is greatly increased. For this reason a lumbar puncture is *not* performed in the presence of signs of increased intracranial pressure or when a brain tumor is suspected, lest the quick reduction in pressure produced by removal of spinal fluid cause the brain structures to herniate into the foramen magnum, which would put pressure on vital centers in the medulla and might cause sudden death. The neurologist often writes "No spinal tap" on the patient's chart to be certain that no other medical staff member attempts this procedure.

Normally, each milliliter of spinal fluid contains up to eight lymphocytes. An increase in the number of cells may indicate an infection. Tuberculosis and viral infections may cause an increase in lymphocytes, while pyogenic infections may cause an increase in polymorphonuclear leukocytes, which may be in large enough numbers to make the fluid cloudy. Bacterial infections such as tuberculous meningitis often lower the blood sugar levels. They may also reduce the chloride level. In the presence of degenerative diseases and when a brain tumor is present, the spinal fluid protein is usually increased. (See box on p. 738 for normal values in spinal fluid.) The colloidal gold test is particularly helpful in diagnosing neurosyphilis or multiple sclerosis. Study of the spinal fluid may occasionally reveal the actual or-

NORMAL VALUES OF CEREBROSPINAL FLUID (CSF)

Pressure	75 to 180 mm H_2O
Glucose	50 to 80 mg/100 ml
Chloride	118 to 132 mEq/L
Protein	20 to 50 mg/100 ml
Gamma (γ-) globulin	3% to 9%
Lymphocytes	0 to 8/ml

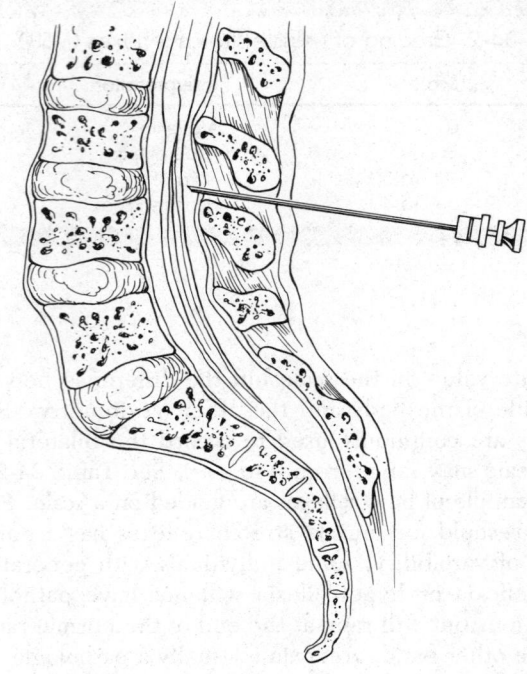

Fig. 34-14. Position and angle of needle when lumbar puncture is performed. Note that needle is in fourth lumbar interspace below level of spinal cord.

ganism causing disease. Results of the serologic test for syphilis may be positive in spinal fluid even when the blood serologic test result is negative.

Blood in the spinal fluid indicates hemorrhage from somewhere into the ventricular system. It may be caused by a fracture at the base of the skull that has torn blood vessels, or it may be caused by the rupture of a blood vessel, which may occur, for example, with a congenital aneurysm. Occasionally, the first specimen of spinal fluid contains blood from slight bleeding at the point of the puncture. For this reason the specimens of fluid are numbered, and the first one is not used to determine the cell count.

Method

Strict aseptic technique is mandatory in all procedures in which the cerebrospinal fluid system is entered. Details of the *lumbar (spinal) puncture procedure* and a list of the equipment needed are given in texts on fundamentals of nursing. An operative permit may or may not be required.

The physician or nurse will explain to the patient that the needle is inserted below the level of the spinal cord (L4-L5 or L5-S1 interspace) (Fig. 34-14) so that there is little danger of injury. The patient will be positioned on the side with both knees and head flexed at an acute angle so that there is a maximal lumbar flexion and separation of interspinous spaces. Constant nursing attention during the procedure is required. Even when a local anesthetic is used (usually procaine, 1%), the patient should be prepared to feel slight pain and pressure as the dura mater is entered. The patient should be reminded not to move suddenly and may be told that a sharp shooting pain down one leg may be experienced. This pain is caused by the needle's coming close to a nerve and is similar to hitting one's "funny bone"; however, the nerve actually is floating in fluid and is safe from injury.

The nurse prepares the patient and the equipment, assists the physician, ensures sterility, monitors the patient during and immediately following the procedure, and arranges for suitable labeling and disposition of specimens. The nurse may also assist during dynamic examination of cerebrospinal fluid as detected through manometer readings. The level of the fluid column within the manometer is measured after the needle is entered into the subarachnoid space and stabilized. The manometer is held by the nurse or another assistant above the point where the physician's hands contact the instrument. When a subarachnoid block is suspected, *Queckenstedt's* test is performed. The nurse or another assistant compresses the patient's jugular veins for 10 seconds, first on one side, then on the other side, and finally on both sides simultaneously. Pressure is exerted with the fingers flat against the patient's neck, avoiding the trachea, and the change in spinal fluid pressure during compression of the jugular veins is noted.

Headache is fairly common following a lumbar puncture. Although its exact cause is unknown, it is thought to be caused by the loss of spinal fluid through the dura mater. It is currently believed that the smaller the needle used, the less likely that there will be fluid leak and headache. The sharpness and size of the needle used, the skill of the physician, and the emotional state of the patient are probably the determining factors in whether a headache will develop. If one does develop, it is treated with bed rest, an ice cap to the head, and an analgesic. Forcing fluids is also considered to be

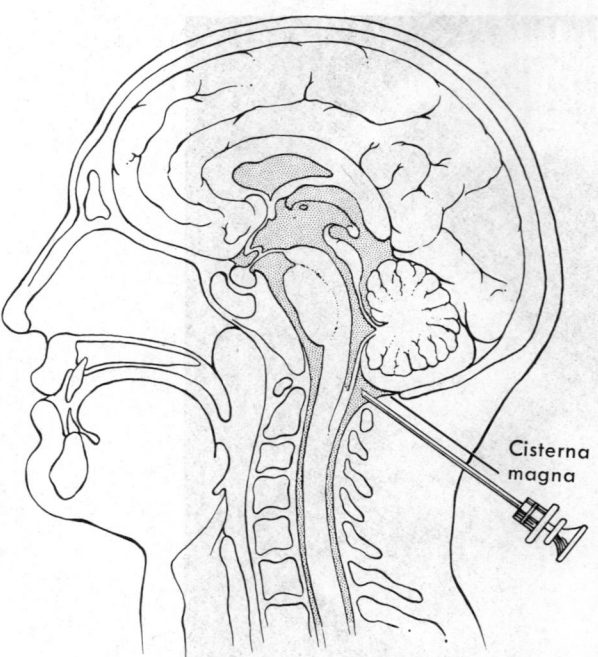

Fig. 34-15. Position of needle when cisternal puncture is performed. Note needle length and short bevel.

beneficial. Most headaches from this cause disappear within 24 hours.

Lumbar punctures are often performed on patients who are ambulatory and who go home immediately after the procedure is completed. It has been found that they suffer no more from headaches than do those who are treated more conservatively with bed rest and no elevation of the head.

In a *cisternal puncture* the cerebrospinal fluid is tapped by inserting a short-beveled needle immediately below the occipital bone into the cisterna magna (Fig. 34-15). This procedure may be more frightening to the patient than a lumbar puncture, since the approach is closer to the brain. A detailed explanation is given by the physician before the head is prepared or the patient placed in the required position. Usually a permit for surgery is required. The back of the patient's neck may be shaved. The procedure is performed in the patient's bed or in the treatment room with the patient in a side-lying position at the edge of the bed or treatment table; the head is bent forward and held by the nurse or another assistant so that it does not rotate. The patient is observed immediately following the procedure for dyspnea, apnea, and cyanosis, but these complications seldom occur. A cisternal puncture is often performed on children. In some outpatient departments it is more commonly performed than a lumbar puncture because it is less likely to be followed by headache.

Radioisotope brain scan

Radioactive isotopes are used with a scanner to detect brain lesions. This procedure is particularly successful in the detection of cerebral neoplasia and infarcts. A positive brain scan does not, however, provide histologic information about the kind of lesion, but it does provide information similar to that provided by other screening procedures such as electroencephalography. It is used adjunctively with neurologic examinations and radiologic studies.

It is known that abnormal brain tissue selectively concentrates radioactive isotopes to a greater extent than does the normal brain tissue that is peripheral to a lesion. The procedure for the brain scan is a relatively simple one and consists of no physical preparation other than the intravenous administration of a radioactive isotope indicator such as mercury. This is followed by scanning of the patient's scalp with a special sensing device to pick up the concentrated areas of uptake. Serial scans and the structural features of the isotope uptake may suggest a particular pattern that is indicative of a specific lesion, but this is not reliable for a differential diagnosis. When mercury is used as the isotope indicator, a mercurial diuretic, meralluride (Mercuhydrin), is administered several hours before the procedure. This permits a greater concentration of radioactive mercury to be circulated to the brain tissue, since meralluride minimizes the uptake of mercury by the kidneys. Areas of concentration show up as very dark areas (Fig. 34-16). Sodium pertechnetate Tc 99m (^{99m}Tc) is also becoming widely used for brain scans.

Neuroradiologic studies

There are multiple radiologic procedures of the brain and spinal cord that are best carried out and interpreted by a neuroradiologist. These include plain radiographs, special contrast studies of the ventricular system (including the cisternal and subarachnoid space) and the cerebral vessels, and computed tomography.

Routine or plain radiographs

Routine or plain radiographs of the brain and spinal cord are usually taken first, using varied projections to detect any developmental, traumatic, or degenerative bone abnormalities.

Computed tomography (CT scan)

One of the most significant technologic advances in radiographic equipment is the EMI scanner, which is capable of providing up to 100% more information than conventional radiographic techniques. The EMI scanner is also referred to as CAT, CT scan, computerized tomography, computed tomography, and computerized

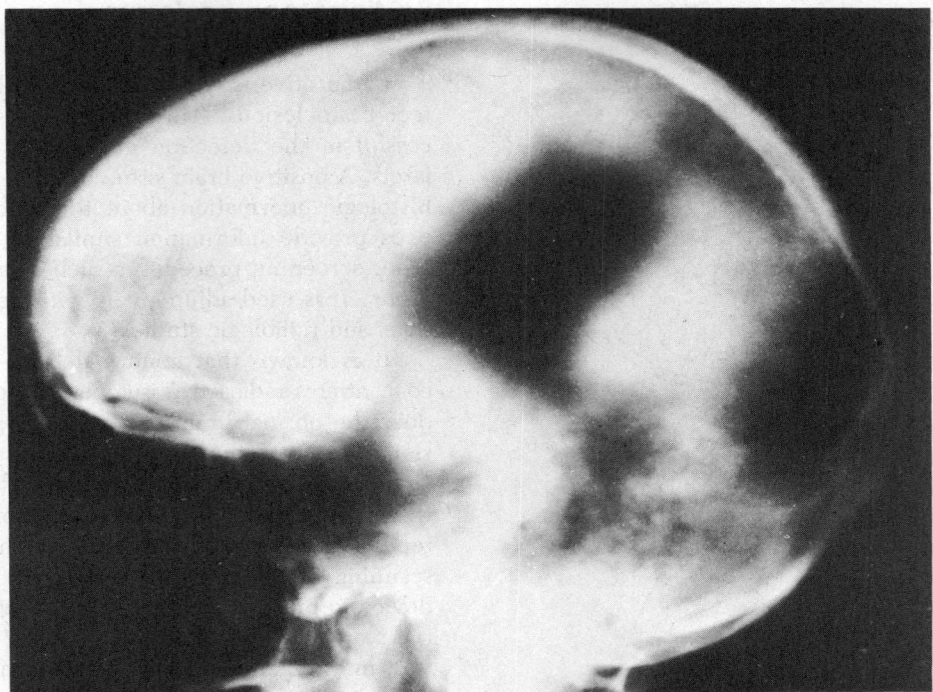

Fig. 34-16. Radioisotope brain scan. Intracranial mass (brain tumor) is seen in two dark areas (parietal and occipital) of scan where abnormal uptake of ^{197}Hg-tagged chlormerodrin accumulated. (Courtesy Abbas M. Rejali, M.D., Department of Radiology, Case Western Reserve University, Cleveland.)

assisted tomography. This technique offers increased versatility, efficiency, and enhanced image detail. It is commonly available in the United States, but is still limited by expense to larger hospitals and university medical centers. The EMI scanner is based on a technique of scanning the brain without isotopes in which series of images using the principles of tomography are x-rayed and each of the images is derived from a specific layer of brain tissue. The brain is thus scanned in successive layers by a very narrow beam of x-rays. The total system includes a scanning unit that houses the x-ray tube, two scintillation detectors, an x-ray control unit, a computer and magnetic disk unit, viewing unit, a line printer, and a teletyper. Data are thus collected in x-ray form and printout form, and information is also stored for future use.[23]

For this procedure the person lies supine with the head positioned within a rubber bag head-holder to prevent an air gap between the machine and the scalp. The cap does not cause any discomfort and ensures more accuracy, since patient movement during scanning produces blurred images resulting in a poor examination. As the patient's head is scanned in two planes simultaneously and at various angles, the computer calculates tissue absorption in contiguous tissues and displays on a printout the numerical values and a visualization of the tissue density. By comparing the tissue densities

with norms, abnormalities can be detected. Tumor masses, infarctions, displacement of bone, and ventricles can be accurately detected. The CT scan is particularly efficient in the detection of brain neoplasia and cerebrovascular lesions.

A routine CT scan is noninvasive and, as such, does not carry the risk and discomfort of other procedures, such as air contrast studies and cerebral angiography. However, occasionally a physician may choose to order a "contrast" study. What follows is two series of scan pictures, the first without contrast media and the second with contrast media. The dye used most frequently is iodine based and is similar to that used for intravenous pyleography. When a contrast study is ordered, the nurse must carefully evaluate the patient for any history of iodine allergy (seafood, etc.) Although rare, reactions range from hives to anaphylaxis and may cause local irritation, resulting in increased intracranial pressure. Before dye infusion the patient may be asked to sign a permission form.

In general, the nurse should stress the following points in preparing persons for a CT scan:

1. It is noninvasive and requires no special preparation.
2. It is painless. The only discomfort is caused by the need to lie still.
3. The person must maintain a motionless position

until the scan is completed—approximately 20 to 30 minutes for a routine scan, with an additional 30 minutes for a contrast study.

4. The scanner rotating about the head may feel like the head is in a washing machine (some persons complain of claustrophobia).

Pneumoencephalography

Pneumoencephalography (air encephalography) is a special contrast study of the ventricular and cisternal systems that permits accurate localization of brain lesions. It is known to provide greater visualization of the posterior fossa than ventriculography. This technically difficult and uncomfortable procedure combines a spinal or a cisternal puncture with an x-ray examination. Air or oxygen, used as a contrast medium, is injected (25 to 30 ml) and rises to the ventricles where its presence can be noted on x-ray examination. Abnormal shape, size, or position of the ventricles or failure of the ventricles to fill with the gas is diagnostically significant. See Fig. 34-17 for examples of normal and abnormal findings. The procedure usually is performed with the patient under local anesthesia, but a general inhalation, rectal, or intravenous anesthetic may be used for nervous or unstable patients. Headache is usually severe during and following encephalography. Nausea and vomiting are not uncommon. A nurse must be in constant attendance to observe the patient while a second person assists the physician.

The patient who is to have a pneumoencephalogram may be prepared as for surgery: no foods or fluids by mouth for 6 hours before the procedure and a sedative the evening before and ½ hour before the procedure. A permit must be signed and dentures removed.

The procedure may be started in the patient's room or in the treatment room. The patient is then taken to a special room in the x-ray department or operating room. The equipment needed is the same as that for a spinal puncture with the addition of a three-way stopcock, a 20-ml syringe with which to withdraw spinal fluid and inject air, a calibrated glass to measure any fluid that is removed, and an ampule of caffeine and sodium benzoate and an ampule of epinephrine (Adrenalin) for use in case of respiratory distress. Emergency oxygen equipment is also often requested.

The pressure of the spinal fluid is taken as soon as the needle is inserted into the lumbar spine arachnoid space. As the procedure is carried out, the patient is watched carefully for headache, nausea, and vomiting and the vital signs and color are noted and recorded. The head of the bed or table is gradually raised, and some physicians prefer to have the patient's head gently rotated after the air has been injected in the belief that this gives better filling of the lateral ventricles.

On return from the x-ray department or the operating room, the patient is placed in bed with the head flat. Usually the patient is more comfortable without a pillow. If a general anesthetic has been administered, a side-lying position with the head flat is safest. Constant attention is needed until the patient is awake and alert. Vital signs are taken every 15 minutes for the first hour, then every ½ hour, and every hour for several hours or until they become stabilized. They are then taken every 4 hours. The level of consciousness is also noted. Any changes should be reported at once. The patient usually has a severe headache and may benefit from an ice cap applied to the head. Acetylsalicylic acid (aspirin), dextropropoxyphene hydrochloride (Darvon), or other nonnarcotic analgesics are given for severe headache. If the patient complains of noises in the head assurance should be given that they are temporary, since they are caused by gas in the ventricles and will disappear when the gas is absorbed. If the patient has a history of convulsions or unpredictable behavior, side rails should be up and convulsion precautions taken. An emergency tracheostomy set may be kept on the unit for 48 hours following this procedure.

Infrequently, reactions to pneumoencephalography are severe and include continued vomiting, convulsions, shock, and signs of increased intracranial pressure with respiratory difficulty. A severe, prolonged headache may also follow this diagnostic procedure, although the headache usually disappears in 24 to 48 hours. For the first 24 to 48 hours the patient remains quiet in bed. After 48 hours the patient may be out of bed gradually. If headache and nausea increase when the upright position is assumed, they will be relieved by lying flat until the symptoms gradually subside.

Pneumoencephalography is not done as frequently as formerly because of the availability of the CT scanner in major medical centers. It is contraindicated when there is increased intracranial pressure because of the danger of herniation of the temporal uncus and cerebellar tonsils resulting in compression of the brain stem and death.

Craniotomy should be performed promptly when a tumor is detected during the procedure to prevent brain stem compression.

Ventriculography

Ventriculography is similar to pneumoencephalography except that air is introduced directly into the lateral ventricles through trephine openings (burr holes) into the skull. This procedure is always performed in the operating room. It may be used when the suspected diagnosis is such that a spinal or lumbar puncture is contraindicated because of the extreme pressure within the skull or because the spinal canal is blocked. The preparation is similar to that for encephalography except that the top or the back of the head must be partially shaved, depending on the physician's orders. An intravenous or general anesthetic is commonly used, and the patient may go directly from the x-ray department

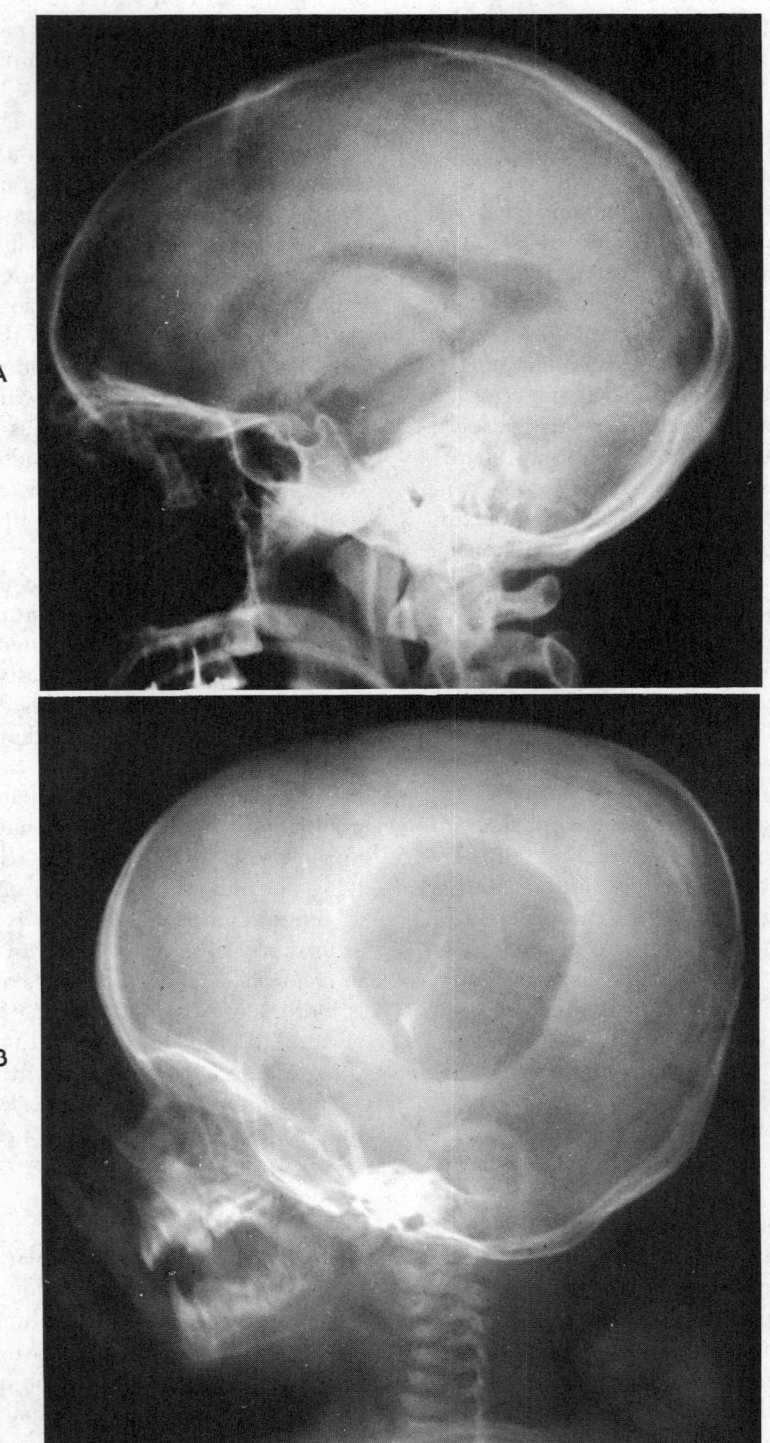

Fig. 34-17. Pneumoencephalogram. **A,** Lateral view showing outline of normal ventricle. **B,** Lateral view showing marked distention of ventricle with cerebrospinal fluid because of hydrocephalus.

to the operating room for attempted removal of a tumor or for other brain surgery. If the radiograph is normal, the patient is cared for in a manner similar to that following encephalography. Tissue and skin over the burr holes are sutured and the wounds covered with a collodion dressing.

Myelography

In myelography either gas or a radiopaque liquid is injected into the spinal subarachnoid space by way of a lumbar or cisternal puncture, and radiographs are taken. It is useful in the identification of lesions in the intradural or extradural compartments of the spinal canal. Observation of the flow of the radiopaque dye fluoroscopically through the subarachnoid space provides valuable information. Lesions in the spinal cord or in the subarachnoid space produce a blocking at some point (Fig. 34-18).

The blockage may be complete or incomplete. The exact configuration of the defect causing the block may be helpful in determining whether the lesion is intramedullary or extramedullary. Turning the patient in varied positions throughout the examination assists in securing a more complete visualization.

This procedure is thus similar to that for a spinal puncture except that after the air or the radiopaque substance is injected, the head is elevated on two pillows and the patient is taken to the x-ray department. After the fluoroscopic examination and radiographs are completed, the dye is removed by lumbar puncture because it can cause serious irritation to the meninges. If some of it remains, care is taken to keep the patient's head elevated, and repeated attempts to remove the dye are made under fluoroscopy. One disadvantage of this test is the irritating quality of the available dyes. Therefore the test is not performed when relatively certain diagnosis can be made by other means, and air is often used in preference to the dye. A new contrast material, metrizamide, is now available for use in myelograms. However, it may precipitate seizure activity

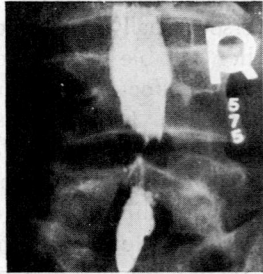

Fig. 34-18. Myelogram showing almost complete block of interspace between fourth and fifth lumbar vertebrae. (From Moseley, H.F., editor: Textbook of surgery, ed. 3, St. Louis, 1959, The C.V. Mosby Co.)

after the procedure, and special precautions must be taken. Before the myelogram the patient is encouraged to remain well hydrated for at least 12 hours and to avoid medications that lower the seizure threshold. Some examples of drugs to be avoided are phenothiazides, tricyclic antidepressants, CNS stimulants, and amphetamines. A cleansing enema may also be ordered. After the myelogram, the patient's head and thorax must remain elevated 30 to 50 degrees for at least 8 hours, and bed rest may be maintained for as long as 24 hours. The patient's head is kept elevated at 30 degrees for 24 hours. Fluids are encouraged during this period, and the drugs listed above are avoided for 24 hours.

Side effects of metrizamide are nausea, vomiting, and seizures and are most likely to occur 4 to 8 hours after the myelogram. However, the advantages of a metrizamide myelogram may outweigh its risks. Major advantages are that metrizamide is water soluble, and thus the dye does not need to be removed. Also, metrizamide is less viscous than the iodine-based dye and therefore permits better visualization of small areas.

Cerebral arteriography

Cerebral arteriography is a method of radiologic visualization of the cerebral arterial system during the injection of radiopaque material. The carotid or vertebral vessels in the neck are used directly. A four-vessel study in which a catheter is introduced percutaneously into the femoral artery and then directed into the innominate, carotid, and vertebral vessels under fluoroscopic control may be done. Each vessel is then injected with the contrast dye as serial radiographs are taken. The selection of needle puncture site is determined by the clinical problem under study. Although the indirect method is less traumatic, the carotids or axillaries may also be used. Arteriography allows detection of arterial aneurysms, vessel anomalies, ruptured vessels, and displacements by mass lesions. The large vessels of the circle of Willis and the large penetrating vessels can also often be visualized via arteriography (Fig. 34-19).

Before the test is performed, a permit is signed by the patient or a responsible relative. The patient should be prepared for the procedure and the close monitoring that will follow it. A careful history must be taken to detect allergy to iodine. Immediately before the procedure, baseline vital signs and a neurologic check should be taken and recorded. If the femoral approach is to be used, it is helpful to assess and mark the locations of the bilateral pedal pulses. If the carotid artery will be the approach used, the patient's neck circumference should be measured as part of the baseline data. Usually a sedative is given the night before, and scopolamine, atropine sulfate and sodium phenobarbital, or meperidine (Demerol) is given ½ hour before the procedure is performed. Occasionally, when the patient is confused or extremely restless, a general anesthetic is

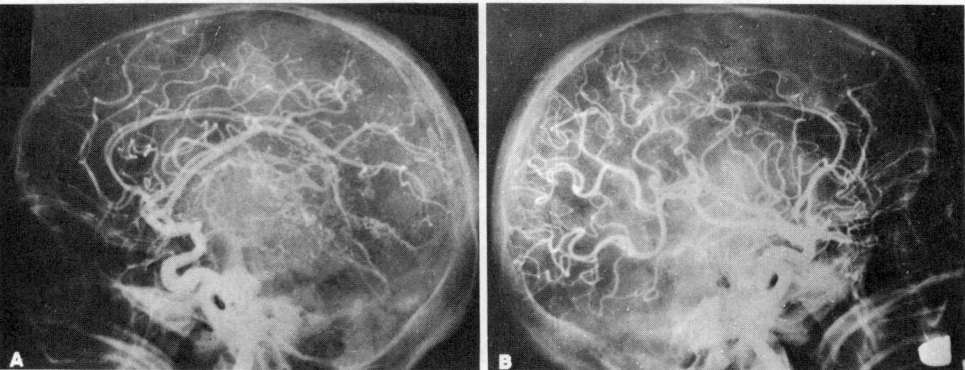

Fig. 34-19. A, Cerebral arteriogram showing elevation of middle cerebral arteries by glioblastoma multiforme containing abnormal vascular network. **B,** Arteriogram showing opposite normal side for comparison. (From Moseley, H.F., editor: Textbook of surgery, ed. 3, St. Louis, 1959, The C.V. Mosby Co.)

given. If this is necessary, the procedure is usually performed in the operating room. If the dye can be injected directly into the carotid vessel without surgical exposure of the artery and if general anesthesia is not necessary, the procedure is usually performed in the x-ray department.

Following this procedure, the patient's vital signs will be taken frequently, usually every 15 minutes for an hour, every 60 minutes for a variable period of time, and then every 4 hours for 24 hours. If a femoral approach was used, a sandbag may be placed over the puncture site. The site must be assessed frequently for hematoma formation, and pulses distal to it are checked frequently for evidence of arterial occlusion. If a direct carotid approach was used, an ice collar may be applied and frequent measurement of the neck circumference will be made. Swelling in this area could seriously compromise breathing. Also, there may be more pain associated with the carotid approach. In all cases, bed rest is usually prescribed for several hours.

Occasionally, neurologic deficits result or intensify following this procedure. Decreased hand grip on plantar pressure and facial weakness on the side opposite the injection site are significant. Convulsive seizures or aphasia may occur. Occasionally, a delayed allergic reaction to the dye occurs, and this reaction may be serious (p. 740). Usually, however, the patient experiences little, if any, discomfort.

Electrodiagnostic examination

The electrodiagnostic examinations include electroencephalography and electromyography.

Electroencephalography

An *electroencephalograph* measures the electrical impulses of the brain; the *electroencephalogram* (EEG) is a pictured recording of the electrical activity of the brain amplified many times and recorded in a manner similar to that of the electrocardiogram. The recording represents the synthesis of collective neurons. Certain characteristic patterns in the record are normal, and by study of the recordings of brain action, areas of abnormal action can sometimes be detected. This test is nonspecific and is only an adjunct to other diagnostic tests, but it may be helpful in locating the site of a lesion. Before the examination the patient should be quiet, and the procedure should be explained in advance so that no undue excitement occurs. The scalp should be clean but no other local preparation is necessary. The hair need not be cut, which is often reassuring to the patient. The procedure involves the application of electrodes to the scalp to record cortical electrical activity. Sixteen or more tiny electrodes are fixed to the scalp with collodion. They are placed in a set pattern to cover all scalp areas (frontal, parietal, temporal, and occipital). Occasionally, the electrodes used are tiny pins that are stuck into the scalp. The patient should know that this procedure will not be painful because there are very few nerve endings in the scalp. The examination is done in a special room where outside electrical activity is eliminated. The person usually sits in a comfortable chair or lies on a stretcher or table with the eyes closed. The basic resting rhythm is affected by opening the eyes or by alteration in attention. Cutaneous sensory stimulation or the induction of motor activity does not alter the scalp record. The test may last for 1 hour or more. Recordings may be made during sleep or during sleep deprivation and provide valuable information. Anticonvulsive drugs may be discontinued in patients with known convulsive disorders before the EEG. In general, the EEG is used to provide evidence of focal or diffuse disturbances of increased brain function produced by organic lesions. The EEG has been particularly helpful in the diagnosis of epilepsy, in the differential diagnosis of convulsive disorders, and in locating lesions of the cerebrum.

Electromyography

The *electromyograph* measures the electrical activity of muscles; the *electromyogram* (EMG) is a recording of the variations of electric potentials (voltage) detected by a needle electrode inserted into skeletal muscle. The electrical activity can be heard over a loudspeaker and viewed on an oscilloscope and on a graph at the same time. No electrical activity can be detected in normal muscles at rest, but during volitional movement action potentials can be detected. However, in motor disease electrical activity of various types and abnormal patterns appear in resting muscles. An EMG provides direct evidence of motor dysfunction and can be used to some extent to detect a dysfunction located in the motor neuron, the neuromuscular junction, or muscle fibers. Thus it is particularly helpful in the diagnosis of lower motor neuron disease, primary muscle disease, and defects in the transmission of electrical impulses at the neuromuscular junction, such as in myasthenia gravis. There is no special preparation for this procedure. However, some patients may be fearful, and they should be assured that there is no danger from the electrode needles. Also, the patient may be told that there may be some discomfort when the electrodes are inserted. Although there are no major after effects from the procedure, the patient's muscles may ache slightly for a short time, and persons with sensory neuropathies may experience more intense discomfort during electrode insertion. Premedication and sedation are usually avoided to ensure that the patient is better able to cooperate. A pertinent history should elicit whether the patient is on anticoagulant therapy or has an extensive skin infection. These are both contraindications to the procedure. (See p. 938 for a discussion of EMG related to primary muscle problems.)

Echoencephalography

Echoencephalography is a rapid and simple diagnostic procedure that has become popular. Information provided is supplementary to an EEG and complementary to radiologic studies as to the nature and location of brain lesions.

Ultrasonic pulses (capable of reflection or refraction at cerebrospinal fluid and brain tissue surfaces) are delivered to the head in such a way that the beam intersects the site under study at a perpendicular angle, traverses the area, and is then reflected back. The returning echoes are then converted back to electrical impulses and recorded on a screen. For example, when a transducer is placed on the right temporal bone and directed toward the opposite temporal bone, the sound beam traverses the third ventricle area (which has two parallel walls) and is reflected back. This procedure provides a right, left, and lower trace, or picture, that gives reliable information as to the position of the midline of the brain. Shifts from the midline, as caused by right or left hemispheric brain masses, can be inferred. Estimation of ventricular size can also be made from the traces.

Evoked potentials

As a group, "evoked potentials" are electrical measurements of physiologic maturation of the human nervous system. Used diagnostically, they can provide information regarding the maturational development of all the primary sensory areas of the cortex. Most commonly used are *auditory evoked potentials* and *visual evoked potentials*. The reader is directed to the literature for a further discussion of these measurements.

REFERENCES AND SELECTED READINGS

1. Alpers, B.J., and Mancall, E.L.: Essentials of the neurological examination, Philadelphia, 1971, F.A. Davis Co.
2. *Bates, B.: A guide to physical examination, ed. 2, Philadelphia, 1979, J.B. Lippincott Co.
3. *Carlson, C.E.: Psychosocial aspects of neurologic disability, Nurs. Clin. North Am. 15:309-320, 1980.
4. Chusid, J.C.: Correlative neuroanatomy and functional neurology, ed. 17, Los Altos, Calif., 1979, Lange Medical Publications.
5. Conway, B.L.: Carini and Owens' neurological and neurosurgical nursing, ed. 7, St. Louis, 1978, The C.V. Mosby Co.
6. DeMyer, W.: Technique of the neurologic examination ed. 2, New York, 1974, McGraw-Hill Book Co.
7. Donohoe, K.M., et al: Cerebral circulation and cerebral angiography, Nurs. Clin North Am. 9:623-631, 1974.
8. Eliasson, S.G., et al., editors: Neurological pathophysiology, ed. 2, New York, 1978, Oxford University Press, Inc.
9. Francis, G.M., and Munjas, B.A.: Manual of social psychologic assessment, New York, 1976, Appleton-Century-Crofts.
10. *Guyton, A.C.: Textbook of medical physiology, ed. 6, Philadelphia, 1980, W.B. Saunders Co.
11. *Johnson, J.H., and Cryan, M.: Homonymous hemianopsia: assessment and nursing management, Am. J. Nurs. 79:2131-2134, 1979.
12. Judge, R.D., and Zuidema, G.D.: Methods of clinical examination: a physiologic approach, ed. 3, Boston, 1974, Little, Brown & Co.
13. *Kolb, D.: Understanding aphasia and the aphasic, J. Neurosurg. Nurs. 9:15-18, 1977.
14. *Mahoney, E.K.: Alterations in cognitive functioning in the brain-damaged patient, Nurs. Clin. North Am. 15:283-292, 1980.
15. *Malasanos, L., et al.: Health assessment, ed. 2, St. Louis, 1981, The C.V. Mosby Co.
16. Mayo Clinic and Mayo Foundation: Clinical examination in neurology, Philadelphia, 1976, W.B. Saunders Co.
17. *Mitchell, P.H., and Irvin, N.J.: Neurological examination: nursing assessment for nursing purposes, J. Neurosurg. Nurs. 9:23-28, 1977.

*References preceded by an asterisk are particularly well suited for student reading.

18. *Norman, S., and Baratz, R.: Understanding aphasia, Am. J. Nurs. 79:2135-2138, 1979.
19. O'Reilly, A.J.: Preparing the patient for computerized tomography, J. Neurosurg. Nurs. 11:41-43, 1979.
20. *Patient assessment: neurological examination. I, Am. J. Nurs. 75:1511-1535, 1975.
21. *Patient assessment: neurological examination. II, Am. J. Nurs. 75:2037-2057, 1975.
22. *Patient assessment: neurological examination. III, Am. J. Nurs. 76:609-633, 1976.
23. *Patient assessment: examination of the eye, Am. J. Nurs. 74:2039-2059, 1974.
24. Ross, A.J., et al.: Neuromuscular diagnostic procedures, Nurs. Clin. North Am. 14:107-121, 1979.
25. Selkurt, E.E.: Basic physiology for the health sciences, Boston, 1975, Little, Brown & Co.
26. *Simpson, J.F., and Magee, K.R.: Clinical evaluation of the nervous system, Boston, 1973, Little, Brown & Co.

CHAPTER 35

INTERVENTIONS FOR THE PERSON WITH COMMON NEUROLOGIC MANIFESTATIONS

ELIZABETH SCHENK
ELIZABETH STRAUSS NOSSE
MARJORIE KINNEY

Neurology as a field of nursing practice and study is concerned with problems of the nervous system that have an organic and physical cause. Many persons with neurologic conditions have serious emotional and even psychiatric disturbances that can be related in part to the organic nature of the problem. In addition, the chronicity of many neurologic diseases as well as the multiple adjustments persons have to make in their life-styles may precipitate functional pathologic conditions. Because of this, neurology and psychiatry are often confused as fields of practice and require differentiation. Psychiatry is concerned with functional disorders of the mind, or psyche, where no organic cause can be demonstrated. It should be recognized that much about the physical basis of the psyche is unknown and that it is difficult to demonstrate the organic nature of psychologic manifestations in many instances. For this reason the nurse practicing in neurology should have knowledge that the psyche and soma (body) are one in the *person* and that often there can be no clear-cut distinction. A person must be viewed as an open system where many different subsystems interplay. (See the discussion of open systems in Chapter 2.)

The nervous system as the coordinator and regulator of all body activities collects sensory information from the internal and external environments, communicates it from distant parts of the body, processes it centrally to determine appropriate response patterns, and then generates control signals to the effector muscles and glands for action. Because of the nature of the anatomy and physiology of the nervous system, organic lesions or trauma results in clinical manifestations related to the site affected regardless of the underlying pathologic findings. When disease or injury affects a part of the nervous system, some neurons are destroyed and will not regenerate; some are partially damaged and may later recover; some are irritated into abnormal activity; others are undamaged. Manifestations reflect a complete loss or an alteration in normal function or body activity as a consequence of the degree of damage to the neurons at a particular site. Normal function and activities may thus be ablated, decreased, or increased.

Other clinical manifestations are an expression not of the damaged site itself but of other parts of the nervous system affected by the damaged site, for example, as a result of lack of control or regulation of the part. Other manifestations are caused by pathologic findings of nonneuronal tissues such as cerebral blood vessels, muscles, and other supporting tissues within the nervous system. When manifestations are long standing and the pathologic condition and its consequences are irreversible and progressive, the person is required to make necessary changes in life-style. These changes can cause social and psychologic problems for the person.

This chapter will discuss the nursing management of the person with clinical manifestations resulting from alterations in neurologic function and structure common to many types of pathologic conditions. Discussion focuses on selected manifestations and their related pathophysiology and nursing management including prevention, intervention, and expected client outcomes.

Headache (cephalgia)

Headache, or head pain, is a common symptom experienced by many persons. As a symptom of an underlying disease, it varies in degree of severity from that of relative unimportance and transience to that of very serious prognosis. It is clear that this symptom may have its source in many different pathologic processes. *The source of recurring headache should be determined through careful physical examination and neurologic testing.* Persons have been known to self-treat headache for months in the belief that it was the result of a sinus infection, only to learn later that it was caused by a more serious problem such as a brain tumor or hypertension. Because of the sites of some tumors in the brain, headache may be the only overt symptom for many months.

Headache from a neurologic perspective may be caused by an expanding cranial mass such as a neoplasm, by intracranial bleeding as in an aneurysm, by inflammation of the meninges as in meningitis and other cerebral infections, or by head trauma, cerebral hypoxia, or dilation of cerebral blood vessels. It is also important to recognize that psychologic factors may be involved in the cause of headache. Head pain is also commonly caused by systemic disease or by eye, ear, and sinus problems. Headache may be described by the person in terms of location (either diffuse or local) or in terms of the quality or nature of the pain.

The pathophysiology of head pain is not fully known. The skull and brain tissues from a neurophysiologic standpoint are not capable of sensing pain. Rather, the pain arises from the scalp and its blood vessels and muscles, from the dura mater and its venous sinuses, and from the blood vessels at the base of the brain. All of these structures have pain receptors. Pain most commonly originates in muscles (face, neck, head), blood vessels, and the dura mater. The blood vessels dilate and become congested with blood extracranially and intracranially. The pain is also thought to be the result of tension in or stretching of these tissues. For these reasons, headaches can be divided into three categories:

TABLE 35-1. Comparison of migraine, cluster, and tension headaches

Type	Onset	Frequency	Duration	Nature	Prodromal symptoms	Associated symptoms	Miscellaneous comments
Migraine headaches	Occur at any age	Episodic; tend to occur with stress or life crisis	Hours to days	Occur slowly; pain becomes severe, with one side of head affected more than other	Visual field defects; confusion; paresthesias	Nausea; vomiting; chills; fatigue; irritability; sweating; edema	Strongly hereditary; more common in women than men
Cluster headaches	Early adulthood; precipitated by alcohol or nitrates	Episodes clustered together in quick succession for few days or weeks with relatively long remissions that last for months	Few minutes to few hours	Pain intense; throbbing, deep; often unilateral; begin in infraorbital region and spread to head and neck	Uncommon	Flushing; tearing of eyes; nasal stuffiness; sweating and swelling of temporal vessels	More common in older men
Tension headaches (muscle contraction)	Often in adolescence; related to tension or anxiety	Episodic; vary with stress	Variable; can be constant	Dull, constant, uncommon aggravating pain; vary in intensity; usually bilateral and involve neck and shoulders; pain may be poorly defined	Uncommon	Sustained contraction of head and neck muscles	No family history

vascular, muscular contraction (tension), or a combination of the two.[13]

Discussion here is limited to migraine, cluster, and tension headaches and their treatment (Table 35-1).

Migraine headache

Etiology and pathophysiology

Broadly defined, migraine is a recurring vascular headache. Exactly what causes an attack is not known, and there may be multiple causes. Chemical changes in and around the cranial blood vessel walls appear to play a role in causation. It is believed that the symptoms are produced by spasm of vessels inside the skull and dilation of vessels outside the skull; the latter is related to the head pain. Hereditary incidence is high, and migraine is more common in women than in men. In the majority of cases migraine headaches begin before the age of 40, often between 16 and 30. It has also been found that the majority of persons suffering from headaches are individuals with perfectionist personalities.

Clinical picture

Prodromal signs and symptoms (aura) occurring before the acute *attack* may include *visual field defects, confusion, paresthesia,* and even *paralysis*. The usual *signs and symptoms occurring at the time of the attack* may include *nausea, vomiting, chilliness, fatigue, irritability, sweating, edema,* and *other autonomic signs*. Temporary paralysis or paresis as well as aphasia may even occur with a severe attack.

The acute symptoms are severe and vary in intensity and duration. The pain is usually severe and starts gradually. The *headache is often present on awakening,* and *one side* of the *head is usually more affected than the other*. Pain may be most severe over the temporal area but may occur anywhere in the head including the face. The associated symptoms may also be severe. The person is often forced to seek isolation in a dark room. The acute attack may last from several hours to many days. It concludes with a feeling of relaxation and need for sleep. Dull head and neck pain (probably caused by tension during the attack) may persist for sometime.

Intervention

Specific treatment for migraine includes treatment of the attack and prevention of recurrences of attacks. Acetylsalicylic acid (aspirin) is seldom effective for classic or common migraine but may be helpful after the headache has developed. Ergotamine tartrate preparations taken early in the attack may prevent the headache from developing. These drugs are the treatment of choice in migraine, and their efficacy in relieving the headache is often considered diagnostic of migraine. Ergotamine tartrate preparations act by constricting ce-

rebral blood vessel walls, thus reducing cerebral blood flow. Ergotamine tartrate may be administered orally, sublingually, or rectally in 2- to 4-mg dosages. It is also available for injection in 0.25- to 0.5-mg dosages. Ergot preparations are also available in combination with other drugs such as caffeine, phenobarbital, and belladonna. Pregnant women cannot take ergot preparations because they stimulate uterine smooth muscles, and other medications need to be substituted. Ergot preparations have the side effects of nausea, vomiting, numbness and tingling, muscle pain, and changes in heart rate and may not be tolerated by some persons. Other drugs that may be substituted include nonnarcotic analgesics, such as phenacetin, acetaminophen, or propoxyphene (Darvon), as well as narcotics such as codeine. Propranolol hydrochloride (Inderal) has been used to prevent migraine attacks with limited success. Its mode of action in relieving the headache is unclear, but it has been hypothesized that it acts similarly to the ergot derivatives.

Other treatment includes cold packs applied to the forehead or the base of the brain; this may either relieve or aggravate the condition. Pressure applied to the temporal and carotid arteries may or may not be helpful. Psychotherapy may be helpful depending on the precipitating cause. Treatment between attacks includes efforts to reduce the frequency and severity of the headaches and in establishing definitive causes for the headache if unknown. Although in many instances no obvious precipitating cause can be found for the migraine attack, in other instances specific factors have been identified. These include mental and emotional stress, fatigue, and certain foods, especially chocolate, nuts, and onions. In women migraine headaches often occur along with menstruation. It is particularly important to teach the person to initiate treatment early in the onset of headache.

Cluster headache

The onset of cluster headaches is usually in early adulthood. They occur most frequently in middle-aged men, and they are sometimes precipitated by ingestion of alcohol. In this type of vascular headache pain episodes are clustered or spaced together in quick succession for a few days or weeks and with relatively long remissions that last for months. The frequency of the attacks is a unique characteristic. The duration of the pain is usually for a few minutes to a few hours. The pain is very intense, throbbing, and deep. It is abrupt in onset and also stops abruptly. *Prodromal signs are uncommon. Associated signs may include flushing, lacrimation (tearing), nasal stuffiness, sweating, and swelling of temporal vessels.*

The pain, which is severe and unilateral, most often

begins in the face, usually in the infraorbital region, and spreads to the head and neck as it increases. The pain usually reaches its peak in 1 to 3 hours. Nausea and vomiting are seldom associated with the attack. Applications of cold may relieve the headache pain, while heat usually aggravates it. Potent pain medications may be necessary to relieve pain during the acute attack. After the pain disappears, the person usually feels perfectly well.

Tension headache (muscle contraction)

Tension headache is a common type of headache associated with tension or anxiety and resulting from sustained contraction of extracranial skeletal muscles around the face, scalp, neck, and cervical areas. The headaches vary in frequency and duration and are related to stress and fatigue. There is no aura. The pain is usually constant and bandlike; it is usually bilateral and involves the occipital region, neck, and shoulders. The headache may be intermittent and transitory or it may persist for days, weeks, or months. It may spread to all parts of the head and may be poorly defined. Treatment usually consists of analgesics and muscle relaxants. Amitriptyline HCl (Elavil) has been used by some to relieve long-standing headaches. Modification of the environment with the reduction of sensory stimulation may be helpful. Psychotherapy may be indicated depending on the underlying stressors. Biofeedback and meditation have been used with varying amounts of success to reduce tension and pain. See p. 832 for a discussion of headache as a symptom of brain tumor.

Assessment

Information collected by the nurse about the nature of the headache is extremely important in helping to define the type of headache and in determining the treatment. The history begins with a subjective description of the type of headache and the length of time the headache has been a problem. Data about the onset of headache is also important (see box in next column). For instance, organic disease usually produces a headache that has existed for a relatively short period but is progressive in nature. Vascular headaches have their onset most often between childhood and the fourth decade of life. After the fifth or sixth decade, a new type of headache often has a psychogenic cause.

It is important to determine by questioning whether the headache occurs in a focal, localized area or is generalized. A localized type of pain is usually associated with migraine headaches or organic disorders. A generalized type of headache pain, on the other hand, is usually related to psychogenic causes or to the presence of generalized increased intracranial pressure. It is also helpful to question whether the headache occurs in the

---

INTERVIEW QUESTIONS FOR PATIENTS WITH A HISTORY OF HEADACHE

1. When did the headache begin?
2. Does the headache occur on one side or part of the head or does it affect the whole head?
3. Does the headache recur in the same place each time?
4. At what time of the day does headache occur?
5. What are the intervals between head pains?
6. What is the nature of the head pain?
7. Do other symptoms (prodromal symptoms) occur before the headache starts?
8. Are there concurrent symptoms?
9. What precipitates the headaches?
10. Is there a family history of headaches?
11. What helps relieve the headache (including any medications)?
12. What makes the headache worse?

---

same place each time or whether the side or location of the pain changes. Typically, migraine headaches may switch from one side of the head to the other.

It is also important to find out about the intervals between head pains and the time of occurrence. Headaches that occur with increased intracranial pressure usually are present on awakening and may awaken the person from sleep. Sinus headaches typically occur in the early morning and increase in intensity as the day progresses. Some headaches, especially migraines, occur in an intermittent pattern and are often related to stress. For instance, the migraine type of headache usually does not occur during relaxed, happy times, and psychogenic headaches (like tension headaches) become worse during holidays or when depression occurs.

It is important to describe the nature of the headache pain. Pain described as dull, nagging, aggravating, and ever present often occurs with psychogenic headaches. Organically caused pain tends to be constant and progressive in nature, whereas intense intermittent pain is characteristic of vascular headaches. Headache pain is sometimes preceded by an aura, such as visual disturbances. These prodromal symptoms occur most frequently with migraine headaches but may also precede headaches caused by organic problems.

Many events may lead to headaches. For example, stressful situations may lead to headaches, and the onset of menstruation may be associated with migraine. Headaches may also be precipitated by eating foods ·containing monosodium glutamate or sodium nitrate or by drinking alcohol. Sleeping too long, fasting, or the inhalation of toxic fumes in work situations with inadequate ventilation may cause headache. Psychosocial problems may also be related to headaches. Familial history of headache is also important. Migraine headaches often occur in families.

Finally, it is important to assess the factors that make the headache worse and those that make it better. The assessment includes regular use of medications, such as oral contraceptives (which may make migraines worse), including those medications taken in an attempt to relieve the pain. Other measures used to relieve the pain, such as lying down in a darkened room, applying an ice bag, or taking an antihistamine, may give important clues as to the type of headache.

Identification of the triggering factors of severe recurring headaches will need to be made through ongoing assessment of personality, habits, and activities of daily living. The nurse seeks to determine what purpose if any the headache serves for the person. Internal conflicts lead to anxiety, and this may be manifested by headache. The headache may hide a serious emotional disorder or serve purposes of secondary gain, such as allowing the person to withdraw from unpleasant situations or to gain attention. Clues may be obtained from seeking information about goals and aspirations of the person, work habits, family relationships, coping mechanisms, and relaxation patterns. The person may be asked to keep a diary of activities of daily living and the occurrence of the headaches as well as their nature and treatment. Triggering factors may include fatigue, alcohol, stress, climatic changes, hunger, and menstruation. The nurse may be involved in assisting with special tests to determine the underlying cause of severe recurring headaches. These may include brain scans and an arteriogram to detect cerebral lesions. In some instances no triggering factors may be identified.

Ongoing assessment by the nurse of patient responses to diagnostic tests and treatment is important. It is necessary to record pain descriptors in the person's own words, recognizing that headache is subjective. Any interferences made should be carefully validated with the person.

Intervention

Treatment varies depending on the type of headache. In addition to the specific treatments already mentioned, there are certain broad measures that apply to the general treatment of headaches. Teaching is carried out concerning the treatment methods prescribed for the person. The person should learn about dosage, action, and side effects of prescribed medications. The dangers of over-the-counter drugs including aspirin should be explained. In teaching it is important to stress that persistent headache should be treated adequately and early. Persistent headaches (in which organic causes

have been ruled out) indicate a need for individuals to examine their life-style and make necessary adjustments. The nurse can sometimes be supportive to individuals who are trying to sort out possible causes of their headaches. Relaxation techniques including biofeedback can be demonstrated and supervised until the individual has mastered them.

Prevention of headache may be possible once the specific cause has been determined or the triggering factors have been isolated by the health professional or by the individual. Health teaching includes removal of the cause if known (and possible), the avoidance of triggering factors, and the importance of early treatment if *not* preventable. Early treatment lessens the more acute, prolonged, and incapacitating attacks such as occur in migraine.

Outcome criteria for the person with headache

The person or significant others can:
1. Explain prescribed medications.
   a. List and explain each prescribed medication as to dosage, action, side effects, and frequency.
   b. Explain how to use drugs as needed when headache recurs.
   c. Explain the reason for adequate and early treatment with prescribed drugs.
2. Explain the dangers of continued use of unprescribed drugs for chronic recurring headache.
3. Explain the importance of continued medical supervision for chronic recurring headache, whether the cause is known or unknown.
   a. State plans for follow-up care.
   b. Explain the dangers of undiagnosed headache.
   c. Recognize headache as a serious symptom.
4. Demonstrate prescribed relaxation techniques.
   a. Demonstrate the relaxation technique to the nurse.
   b. Explain in own words the values of adjustment of life-style to lessen stress.
5. Identify factors that trigger the onset of headache.
   a. Discuss the factors that trigger the headache.
   b. State plan to avoid these factors.

Neurologic pain

Pain other than headache is one of the most common symptoms seen in neurology. It is sometimes difficult to distinguish between pain produced by lesions within the nervous system that cause objective sensory abnormalities and peripherally produced somatic pain in a distant organ. The nurse working with the patient in pain must appreciate the individuality of the pain experience and understand the multiple factors that influence the patient's perception and expression of pain. Although in practice pain may be viewed from the standpoint of neural transmission, the transmission of pain impulses is not fully understood. (See Chapter 23 for a detailed discussion of pain.) However, the factors that are known about the neuroanatomy of pain transmission can serve to explain sources of neurologic pain and some of the interventions used. Neurologic pain may arise from lesions involving peripheral cutaneous nerves, the sensory nerve roots (posterior), the thalamus, and the central pain tract (spinothalamic) at some level (see sensory pathways, Fig. 34-8). It is known that pain receptors, unlike those for touch or temperature, are not adaptable. The pain impulses continue at the same rate as long as the stimulus is present. These receptors are considered specific for pain only and are present in layers of the skin, the periosteum, and the adrenal walls, as well as in the falx and tentorium of the dura. Pain receptors can be activated by (1) cellular damage, (2) certain chemicals such as histamine, (3) heat, (4) ischemia, and (5) muscle spasms. They are also triggered when sensations of heat, cold, and itching go beyond a specific intensity level.

Assessment

As in other types of pain, the quality of pain and its distribution are important for the nurse to assess. The quality of neurologic pain or *paresthesia* (abnormal sensation) may vary from mild to excruciating. The sensation of pain may be increased (*hyperalgesia*), decreased (*hypalgesia*), or blocked (*analgesia*). Pain may also be caused by a stimulus that normally would not be painful (*dysesthesia*). The nurse may find that in some types of pain it is difficult for the person to describe the pain accurately. It is perceived variously as "burning," "pins and needles," or "numbness." The constancy of the pain makes it difficult for the person to bear.

Peripheral cutaneous nerves are particularly vulnerable to trauma and vascular effects. The pain resulting from peripheral nerve lesions is usually limited to the anatomic area supplied by the affected nerve or nerves. This has been called local pain and occurs as a result of direct stimulation of the pain receptors. Thus the location or distribution may be compared with charts showing the distribution of peripheral sensory fibers (see Fig. 34-13). For example, a lesion involving the lateral femoral cutaneous nerve of the thigh produces pain limited to the area of the skin supplied by this nerve. Pain of this type is often described as a burning sensation, but it can also be described as sharp or dull and aching. The pain may be constant or periodic and is described as being severe.

It should be recalled that all peripheral nerves are mixed nerves (sensory and motor). Each nerve has a definite area of skin from which to carry sensation and a definite muscle or muscle group to supply. Damage to a nerve at its periphery results in both loss of sensation and muscle function. An occasional sequela of peripheral nerve injury is *causalgia,* that is, intense and continuous burning type of pain. An attack may arise spontaneously, or in response to touch, or even as a result of emotions and stress. The quantity and quality of pain are disproportionate to sensory intake.

Root pain, or *radicular pain,* is limited to the dermatomes supplied by the affected sensory nerve roots (see Fig. 34-13). However, pain from lesions arising from deep somatic and visceral structures may radiate beyond the dermatomes. When assessing root pain, the nurse should understand that it is often aggravated by anything that causes direct or indirect movement of the spinal cord, leading to increased spinal pressure. Such actions as sneezing, coughing, or straining increase intrathoracic and intraabdominal pressure and indirectly produce distention of veins in the epidural space, thus affecting the dura mater surrounding the nerve roots. Pain occurring with the above events is of diagnostic value. It should be remembered that sensory (posterior) nerve roots are fixed directly to the cord, and lesions in this area may extend to include the motor (anterior) nerve roots and, in addition, cause motor signs and symptoms. Because of this anatomic fact, the person with this type of pain should not lie in a horizontal plane for long periods as this causes tension or traction on the thoracic and sacral nerve roots. Sitting up may help to relieve tension on the nerve roots. When moving a person with root pain, sharp flexion of the neck and leg extension should be avoided as much as possible, since this intensifies the pain causing more direct movement of the meninges and roots.

Pain resulting from *central lesions within the thalamus* is confined to the contralateral side of the body, since the thalamus receives sensory pain impulses from the opposite side of the body. In massive thalamic lesions only contiguous portions of the body may be affected. This type of pain is described by patients as "burning," "pulling," and "swelling." It is often aggravated by emotional stress and fatigue and is influenced by cutaneous stimulations. The nurse may find it difficult to care for the person, both physically and emotionally. It is most important that the nurse understand the physiologic basis of this kind of discomfort, the factors that aggravate it, and why the person has persistent complaints.

Lesions involving the *central spinothalamic tracts* (see Fig. 34-6) produce pain sensation distributed to the level of the tract involved. Hemisection of the spinal cord involving the spinothalamic tract usually produces loss of pain and temperature perception on the contralateral side at a level one or two segments below the injury. Tract pain is similar to thalamic pain but may be less distressing.

Pain may also be called referred—that is, it occurs in a site other than its origin. This often occurs with visceral pain. Perhaps the most common example is chest pain that is referred to the left arm, the shoulder, neck, or jaw (see Fig. 23-7).

Intervention

Providing relief from discomfort and pain from lesions arising from within the nervous system is challenging. It requires the ability to try varied methods to find the one that provides the most relief. Ongoing assessment includes the location, distribution, and site of origin of the pain. Observation of associated symptoms such as muscle weakness, vasomotor response, and the presence of abnormal sensations is equally important. The emotional and cultural aspects of pain and how it is perceived by the person are necessary data for planning care (see Chapter 23). Since environmental stimuli often initiate or intensify pain, these are significant data in planning specific interventions. Analgesics are prescribed to obtain the most effective relief of pain; alternate drugs are usually tried until the one providing the best result is determined.

Intractable pain. Unbearable pain that does not respond to definitive treatment of the causative lesion is classified as intractable. The pain is chronic and often disabling. The individual's degree of disability and suffering (despite the physiologic basis for the pain) must also be related to psychologic and personality factors. It is difficult to evaluate objectively a patient's complaints of pain. The chronic complainer of pain is often stereotyped by the nurse as a difficult patient. It is usually possible to alleviate intractable pain surgically through deafferentation at varied sites by *nerve block, neurectomy, rhizotomy,* and *cordotomy*. Electrical stimulation may also be used. These techniques and the care required when instituted are described in Chapter 23.

Outcome criteria for the person with neurologic pain

The person or significant others can:
1. Explain methods to control discomfort and pain.
   a. Explain the prescribed analgesics or alternates as to action, side effects, and dosage schedules.
   b. Demonstrate physical measures that can be safely used for pain control.
   c. Explain the advantages and disadvantages of available surgical interventions used to control intractable pain.
   d. Describe positioning methods and their relationships to the occurrence of pain.
2. Explain general health practices.
   a. Explain how to maintain sleep and rest patterns.

b. Explain the relationship between pain and emotional upsets.
c. State plans for follow-up care.

Increased intracranial pressure

Etiology and pathophysiology

Increased intracranial pressure (ICP) is a complex manifestation that is the consequence of multiple neurologic conditions and often requires surgical intervention.

The cranial contents, including the brain tissues, vascular tissues, and cerebrospinal fluid (CSF), are contained within a bony vault for protection. Any increase in the volume of any of the cranial contents, singly or in combination, results in increased ICP, since the cranial vault is rigid, closed, and nonexpandable. Several neurologic lesions, either by their nature or by inciting cerebral edema, increase the volume of tissue within the cranium. Any lesion that increases tissue volume is known as a space-occupying lesion. Common examples include cerebral contusions, hematomas, infarcts, abscesses, and other inflammations of brain tissues. Intracranial tumors arising from all types of brain tissues increase cell mass and as a consequence increase ICP. An increase in the production of cerebrospinal fluid, blockage of the ventricular system, or a decreased absorption of cerebrospinal fluid can likewise increase tissue fluid volume. Activities such as coughing, sneezing, or straining at the stool or other Valsalva's maneuver type of activities also increase ICP for a short time. After the activity ceases, the pressure then returns to its baseline. It is also important to note that the contrast dye used with cerebral angiography and computed tomography (CT) scans may result in irritation to cerebral blood vessels with resulting cerebral edema and increased ICP. Patients who have had either of these tests should be observed carefully for deterioration in neurologic status.

According to the *box theory of the brain,* an increase in any one of the contents of the cranium is usually accompanied by a *reciprocal change* in the volume of one of the others. Brain tissue cannot expand without serious effects on the flow and amount of CSF and cerebral circulation. Space occupying lesions must of necessity displace and distort the brain and vascular tissues as pressure increases. Pressure may build up slowly (days or months) or rapidly (minutes or hours), depending on the cause. At first one hemisphere will be more involved, depending on the lesion site, but eventually both hemispheres may become involved if the pressure continues to increase.

As pressure increases within the cranial cavity, it is

at first compensated through venous compression and CSF displacement. Although the brain has autoregulatory mechanisms to maintain a normal cerebral blood flow in the presence of some increase in ICP (up to levels of 450 mm H_2O),[45] as the pressure continues to rise, the cerebral blood flow decreases and inadequate perfusion occurs. The inadequate perfusion initiates a vicious cycle causing the Pco_2 to increase and the Po_2 and pH to decrease. These changes cause vasodilation and cerebral edema. The edema further increases ICP, causing increased compression of neural tissue and an even greater increase in ICP.

When the pressure within the cavity exceeds the compensatory mechanisms in the adult, the only escape for the brain hemisphere is to be displaced caudally or by downward herniation. The falx cerebri oppose medial shift of the hemispheres and the tentorium cerebelli oppose downward shift to some extent. Structures that allow internal herniation are the cingulate gyrus, which permits medial subfalcial herniation (under the falx); the uncus, which permits downward transtentorial herniation (across free edge of tentorium); and the cerebellar tonsil, which permits transforaminal herniation (through the foramen magnum) (see Fig. 35-1 for identification of these structures with internal herniations and shifting of the hemisphere). As a consequence of the herniation, the brain stem is compressed at variable levels, which in turn compresses the vasomotor center, posterior cerebral artery, oculomotor nerve, corticospinal nerve pathways, and fibers of the *ascending reticular activating system* (ARAS). Internal herniation in this way represents the critical state of decompensation. The

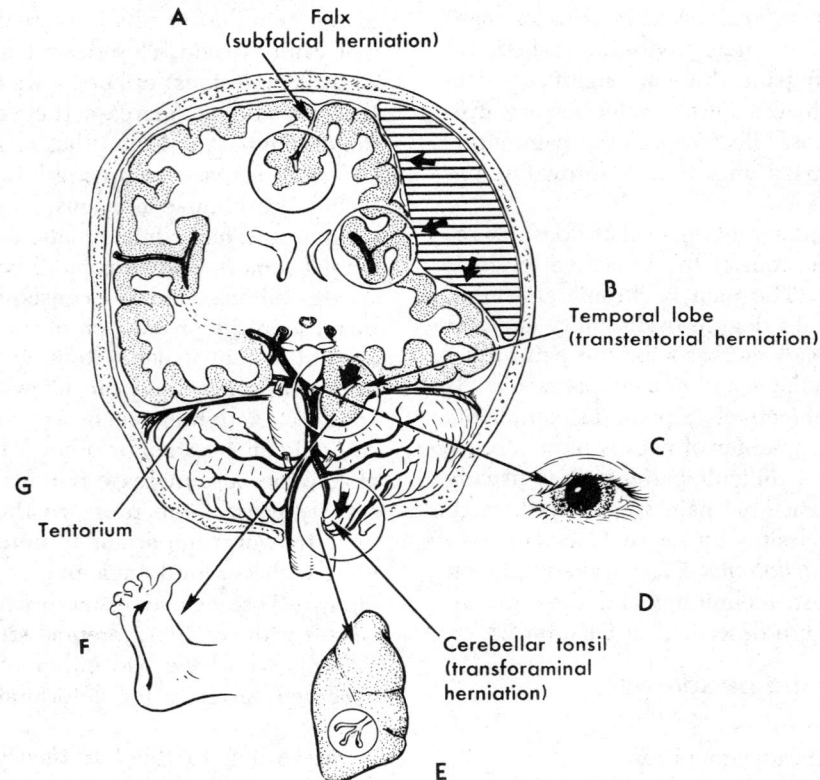

Fig. 35-1. Consequences of increased intracranial pressure. Expanding temporoparietal epidural hematoma with medial and downward pressure has produced subfalcial, transtentorial, and transforaminal internal herniations. Note distortion of falx, **A,** bulging of medial temporal lobe at tentorial edge, **B,** and herniation of cerebellar tonsil with descending pressure on brain stem, **D.** Also note how major blood vessels are collapsed in encircled areas. Some consequential effects of continuing or expanding pressure on neural structures with alterations in body functions are detailed. **C,** Homolateral dilation and fixation of pupil with ptosis of eyelid. **E,** Life-threatening respiratory centers in brain stem. **F,** Contralateral Babinski's sign showing extension of great toe and fanning of other toes following plantar stimulation. Coronal view of head, ventral view of brain stem. **G,** Intact tentorium. Herniation occurs downward with herniation across free edge. (Modified from original painting by Frank H. Netter, M.D.; from Clinical Symposia, Copyright by Ciba Pharmaceutical Co., Division of Ciba-Geigy Corp. All rights reserved.)

life-sustaining mechanisms for consciousness, blood pressure, pulse, respiration, and temperature regulation fail.

Assessment

The detection of increased ICP must occur *early*, when it is reversible and before the stage of decompensation. *The ability to make accurate observations, to interpret observations intelligently, and to record observations carefully is without question the most important part of nursing care of patients with increased intracranial pressure.* The nurse must know when to notify the physician regarding changes in the patient's condition. The nurse must be capable of implementing nursing, medical, and surgical measures appropriately. Because of the need to understand the neurophysiologic basis of observations, selected signs relative to increased ICP are discussed from a nursing standpoint.

Level of consciousness (LOC). The mesencephalon and diencephalon, which act as way stations to the ascending reticular activating system (ARAS), become compressed following herniation of the brain stem. Nerve impulses are interrupted throughout the ARAS, which is considered to be the seat of consciousness. There is hypoxia of tissue cells of the ARAS, and the increased pressure decreases transmission of sensory input through the ARAS, causing a decrease in wakefulness. A decreasing level of consciousness is an early sign of internal herniation. *Any change in the level of consciousness is one of the most important observations for the nurse to make, report, and record.* Level of consciousness is one of the earliest and most sensitive indicators of increased cranial pressure.

Although discussed in Chapter 27, the level of consciousness will be reviewed briefly here. The level of consciousness can be divided into five levels of cerebral functions:

1. Loss of ability to abstract (inattentiveness, slowed thinking, difficulty in arousal)
2. Confusion (disorientation, inability to follow simple commands)
3. Stupor (responds to vocal commands with moaning or groaning, if at all)
4. Semicomatose (loss of ability to cooperate; responds only to pain—response may range from purposeful to decerebrate)
5. Comatose (loss of ability to respond to any external stimuli loss of all basic reflexes)[8]

In describing a person's level of consciousness, it is important to describe the patient's behavior and not just label it.

The Glasgow coma scale is a tool that was developed in 1974 at the University of Gasgow to standardize observations of the level of consciousness in patients with head injuries. Its use is becoming more widespread, especially because tests of its reliability have shown it to be quick, accurate, and simple to use. The scale consists of three parts: (1) assessment of eye opening; (2) verbal response; and (3) best motor response. Each part gives information about an aspect of central nervous system functioning. As central nervous system deterioration occurs, stronger stimuli are required to obtain a response. The stronger the response needed, the lower the score (Table 35-2). The three parameters are often checked hourly and then graphed so that changes can be readily detected. The number value assigned to each parameter is added to the others to yield a score that is an objective measurement of the level of consciousness. The score for normal persons is 14. The lowest possible score is 3 with a score of 7 or less being commonly accepted as a definition of coma.[34]

Pupillary signs. Pupillary responses are controlled by the oculomotor nerve (cranial nerve III), which carries sensory, motor, and parasympathetic fibers as well as sympathetic fibers. The oculomotor nerve is compressed by the herniating tissue and specifically by the downward displaced posterior cerebral artery. The pupilloconstrictor fibers of the oculomotor nerve run in a group in the top part of this nerve and are the first to be compressed. As a consequence, the ipsilateral pupil (when the lesion is in one hemisphere) remains dilated and is incapable of constricting. The pupil appears larger than in the other eye and does not react to light. Eventually as cerebral pressure increases and both hemispheres are affected, there is bilateral pupil dilation and fixation. Inequality of the pupils may appear earlier than fixation when the nerve is only stretched. The pupil may respond to light slowly rather than with the usual brisk normal response. In examining the pupils the nurse should note the size and equality first and then test the reaction of each pupil to light in a darkened room. Di-

TABLE 35-2. Glasgow coma scale

	Stimuli	Score
Eyes open	Spontaneously	4
	To speech	3
	To pain	2
	None	1
Best verbal response	Oriented	5
	Confused	4
	Inappropriate words	3
	Incomprehensible sounds	2
	None	1
Best motor response	Obey commands	5
	Localized pain	4
	Flexes to pain	2
	None	1

lating pupils are a sign of impending tentorial herniation. When pupils dilate or changes in their ability to react are noted, the physician should be notified immediately. A pupil that is fixed and dilated is sometimes referred to as a "blown pupil."

Blood pressure and pulse. The effect of cerebral pressure on blood pressure and pulse is variable. Compensatory changes occur in the cerebral vasculature relative to hypoxia or diminished blood flow. But when the compensatory changes are no longer effective, compression of the brain stem occurs, and ischemia in the vasomotor center will be present. This excites the vasoconstrictor fibers, causing an increase in systolic blood pressure. If the ICP continues to increase; the ability of the vasomotor center to stimulate the vasoconstrictor fibers decreases and the blood pressure may fall. What is often seen in practice is an increased systolic blood pressure with a widening pulse pressure followed by a sharp drop in blood pressure as the patient's condition deteriorates.

Pressure on the vasomotor center also increases the transmission of parasympathetic impulses via the vagus to the heart and the pulse rate is slowed. As the intracranial pressure continues to rise, however, the heart rate may sharply increase. *Slowing of the pulse rate in conjunction with a rising systolic blood pressure is a significant observation to be made and reported.* For consistency blood pressure readings should be taken in the same arm and the pulse should be taken for a full minute in the same location each time.

Respiration. Herniation produces respiratory dysrhythmias that are variable and are related to the level of brain stem compression or failure. The breathing pattern may be deep and stertorous, or Cheyne-Stokes (periodic); terminally there is respiratory paralysis. The beginning of periodic episodes of apnea is significant. The usual picture is one of slowing of respiration, along with a slow pulse and a rising systolic blood pressure. The nurse should learn to look for variability in vital signs and detect trends as they occur. It is important to remember that the patient with a decreasing level of consciousness will require assistance in keeping the airway clear. Consequently respiratory difficulty is further aggravated by this problem. Hypoxia also causes increased ICP. Persons who are experiencing ICP require supplemental oxygen.

Temperature regulation. Failure of the thermoregulatory center because of compression occurs later and gives rise to high uncontrolled temperatures. It is important to understand that hyperthermia needs to be controlled, since it increases the metabolic needs of the brain tissues. Temperatures are taken rectally unless otherwise ordered.

Focal motor and sensory signs. Compression of upper motor neuron pathways (corticospinal tract) interrupts the transmission of impulses to lower motor neu-

rons, and progressive muscle weakness results. For example, a contralateral weakened hand grasp may progress to hemiparesis and hemiplegia; a weak hand, however, is not always a good indicator of motor weakness. More accurate is the observation and testing for drift, which requires the patient to close the eyes and extend the arms straight out in front for 30 seconds. If one arm is weakened, it will drift downward without the patient being aware of it. This can be tested in patients with increased ICP as long as they are capable of cooperating. Testing of the lower extremities includes the patient's ability to do straight leg raises as well as to push and pull against the examiner. Ability to do plantar and dorsiflexion of the feet can also be evaluated.

When the patient is comatose, the response to tactile or painful stimuli is important. It should be noted whether the person responds appropriately to pain or touch or whether the response is decorticate or decerebrate posturing.

The presence of the Babinski's signs, hyperreflexia, and rigidity are additional motor signs that provide evidence of decreasing motor function from upper motor neuron involvement. Transtentorial herniation of the upper or rostral part of the brain stem produces decerebrate rigidity. The motor inhibitory fibers are blocked, and the person involuntarily assumes a fixed posture with arms, legs, and trunk extended and with flexion of the palmar and plantar joints; seizures may also be present. Decorticate rigidity may also occur. This consists of a fixed posture with flexion of the arm, wrist, and fingers, with adduction of the arms and extension and internal rotation of the legs. Decorticate and decerebrate posturing may both be seen in the patient with herniation. The nurse should use gross tests or more definitive tests to determine motor changes. *The worsening in existing motor deficits is significant.*

Visual acuity and papilledema. The blind spot of the retina measures the size and shape of the optic papilla, or optic disk. As venous congestion and intracranial pressure increase, the resulting pressure is transmitted to the eyes through the cerebrospinal fluid and to the optic disk (choked disk). Since the meninges of the brain reflect out around the eyeball, they permit the direct transmission of pressure along the subarachnoid space through the cerebrospinal fluid. As the optic disk swells, the retina adjacent to it is also compressed. The damaged retina cannot detect light rays. As the size of the blind spot enlarges, visual acuity is lessened. The ability of the nurse to detect papilledema is dependent on skill in examination of the fundi.

Many nurses will not have learned to observe for papilledema and must rely on other means to assess intracranial pressure. Decreasing visual acuity can be detected through the confrontation technique (p. 729). Papilledema occurs most often when the increased ICP develops slowly. A rapid rise in the pressure may not be reflected by papilledema.

Headache. Headache may occur as an early symptom. It is thought to result from venous congestion and the tension on the intracranial blood vessels as the cerebral pressure rises. The onset of the headache should be noted along with its location and duration. It increases in intensity with cough, straining, and stooping.

Vomiting. The occurrence of vomiting that is projectile is often associated with increased intracranial pressure. Its frequency and character should be noted. The significance of vomiting and headache needs to be associated with other clinical signs such as papilledema and vital signs.

Observation

The frequency of "neurologic checks" of the patient is often ordered by the physician. However, with significant deteriorating changes in the aforementioned signs, the nurse should decide when more frequent assessments and recordings are indicated. Based on the results obtained from observations and the medical history of the patient, the nurse will need to make a decision as to frequency of monitoring. Tools for assessing the neurologic condition of a patient may vary from institution to institution. The important point is that the patient's condition is regularly compared with an established baseline through continuous monitoring.

Various methods for measurement of ICP have been devised. One of the most frequent methods requires placement of a hollow screw through the skull into the subarachnoid space. The screw is attached to a Luer-Lok, which is connected to a transducer and oscilloscope for continued monitoring.[15] The transducer is fastened to the head of the bed and must be level with the screw for accurate monitoring. The screw may be attached to a manometer for intermittent readings. Directions for the use of this measurement device can be found in the literature.[15]

With more experience with the use of continous internal intracranial monitoring, it has become evident that the traditional clinical signs of increased pressure do not always correlate with the actual pressure changes as seen on the monitor. It has been found that many of the classic signs of increased pressure do not appear until the pressure has reached extremely high levels and the opportunity to reverse the rising pressure and prevent permanent brain damage has already passed.

With internal intracranial monitoring the nurse is responsible for reading the monitor and responding to significant changes as they occur.

Intervention

The *prevention* of increased ICP may not be possible, but prevention of *further rise* of ICP and resulting damage to brain tissues is crucial. The detection of *early signs* is important to prevent irreversible effects.

The medical treatment of patients with increased ICP depends on the underlying cause for the pressure increase. For example, if it is caused by an intracranial tumor, the tumor is removed surgically. When surgery is not possible (or indicated), efforts made to reduce the pressure through the use of drug therapy or direct physical measures.

Rapidly rising intracranial pressure must be relieved directly by mechanical decompression. This may be accomplished by a variety of procedures including (1) ventricular puncture with the withdrawal of CSF by needle or cannula, (2) continuous ventricular drainage with a special device that maintains the pressure at a set rate and level, and (3) removal of a piece of skull (craniotomy) to provide room for the cranial contents to expand. Each of these measures requires careful monitoring by the nurse for signs of increased ICP and the maintenance of asepsis at the entrance site into the skull.

Medications commonly ordered to promote rapid osmotic diuresis and the reduction of brain volume include the intravenous administration of urea (Urevert), mannitol, and hypertonic solutions of glucose (25% to 50%). Corticosteroids such as dexamethasone (Decadron) may also be ordered to lessen cerebral edema. The corticosteroids act more slowly, but their effect is more sustained. All these drugs cause dehydration and promote the movement of excess fluid from the brain tissues into the blood so that it can be eliminated. Narcotics and other drugs that cause respiratory depression are avoided. Phenytoin sodium (Dilantin) may be prescribed to prevent seizures.

Conservative measures to reduce venous volume may be implemented. The person is positioned to promote venous drainage; the head of the bed is elevated 15 to 30 degrees so that the head is higher than the heart level and there is no neck flexure. Proper positioning to avoid extreme flexion of neck or hips is important. The patient should not be prone, since this increases ICP. Rotation of the head, especially to the right, was found to increase ICP, whereas passive range of motion exercises did not, unless they occurred in association with multiple activities within a short period of time. In addition, any closely spaced activity has been found to have a cumulative effect on increasing intracranial pressure.[24,26] This has important ramifications for the nurse caring for the neurologically compromised patient. Spacing of nursing activities has been found to be important in maintaining ICP as low as possible.

Fluid intake may also be restricted so that there is a less total intake than is normally desired. Urine output with the administration of osmotic diuretics must be monitored carefully through an indwelling catheter and a urimeter. The patient's use of Valsalva's maneuver is eliminated to the extent possible, since it causes increased intrathoracic pressure that indirectly increases ICP. This includes not allowing the patient to become constipated or to strain during defecation. Suctioning should be avoided because it causes coughing and gagging, which increase ICP. If suctioning becomes necessary, it should be performed gently with the patient well preoxygenated (p. 1232). It should not be performed at the same time as other procedures that cause increased ICP.

Oxygen therapy via mask or cannula is administered if the arterial blood gases reveal a decrease in Po_2 and a normal Pco_2. However, if a rise in Pco_2 occurs, controlled ventilation including endotracheal intubation or tracheostomy may be necessary. With the use of controlled ventilation, the Pco_2 can be lowered to below normal, which causes a slightly alkalotic pH. The decrease in the Pco_2 and increase in the pH to alkalotic will decrease vasodilation and ICP.

During the treatment phases the nurse makes ongoing, systematic assessment of neurologic status to detect *even slight changes in status*. In summary, nursing and medical interventions are directed toward achievement of the following treatment goals:

1. Reduction of cerebral edema and CSF excess
2. Prevention of cerebral hypoxia by maintaining a clear airway and reducing cerebral pressure
3. Reduction of activities that increase ICP
4. Limitation of fluid intake
5. Monitoring of intake and output so that the results of therapy can be evaluated.

Outcome criteria for the person with increased intracranial pressure

The person or significant others can:

1. State signs or symptoms that indicate need for immediate medical assistance.
2. Explain the action, side effects, toxic effects, and dosage schedule of medications ordered to decrease ICP.
3. State plans for follow-up care.

Alterations in muscle tone and motor function

Disturbances of motor function probably surpass all other clinical neurologic symptoms in frequency and in importance. Since the nervous system is designed primarily for movement of the body in space and of the various parts in relation to each other, damages to it often cause serious problems in mobility. The term *paralysis* refers to a loss of function, either motor or sensory. When applied to motor function as below, it means loss of voluntary movement because of interruption of

the descending efferent motor pathways. A lesser degree of paralysis is called *paresis*. Damage to sensory pathways that are intimately concerned with motor function may occur concomitantly with the loss of motor function. Loss of sensory function is discussed on p. 770.

Assessment

Injury or disease of motor neurons and their extensions at any level results in alterations of muscle strength, tone, and reflex activity. The specific clinical manifestations differ according to whether the lesion involves an *upper motor neuron* or a *lower motor neuron*. In addition, extension of lesions to the *extrapyramidal* and *cerebellar tracts* further alters normal motor activity. Diseases associated with disturbances in motor function are classified in Fig. 35-2.

An important concept in neurologic examination and diagnosis by the neurologist rests on identifying the abnormalities of motor function that result from disease or injury to upper and lower motor neurons. The ability to differentiate between upper and lower motor neuron lesions is the first step in the localization of the site of a neural lesion that manifests itself by disturbances in normal motor function. When the site of the neural lesion has been decided, the neurologist can then consider the cause.

Lower motor neuron signs. It is necessary to recall that *lower motor neurons* (LMNs) consist of the large anterior horn cells located in the anterior gray matter of the spinal cord. They are also located in the motor cranial nuclei of the brain stem. Each anterior horn cell has a long axon that exits the cord via the anterior (ventral) spinal root and extends out the peripheral nerve, eventually synapsing at the motor end-plate of the neuromuscular junction. These structures together form a *motor unit* which effects skeletal muscle activity—both voluntary and reflex (Figs. 35-3 and 35-4). When a lesion selectively involves some part (cell body, motor root, isolated peripheral nerve) of the LMN, it characteristically results in flaccid muscle weakness or paralysis, loss of reflex activity, loss of muscle tone, and atrophy confined to the involved muscle or muscles.

The *degree* of muscle weakness occurring in the involved muscle or muscles in a LMN lesion bears a direct relationship to the extent and severity of the lesion. Since each anterior horn cell innervates several separate muscle fibers and since several anterior horn cell columns exist at each spinal level, a lesion confined to *one* spinal segment may not damage all the anterior horn cells innervating an entire muscle. Thus such a lesion will cause muscle *weakness* (paresis) rather than paralysis of the entire muscle. Complete paralysis occurs in LMN lesions only when the lesion involves the column or anterior horn cells in several spinal segments that innervate an entire muscle or the ventral roots

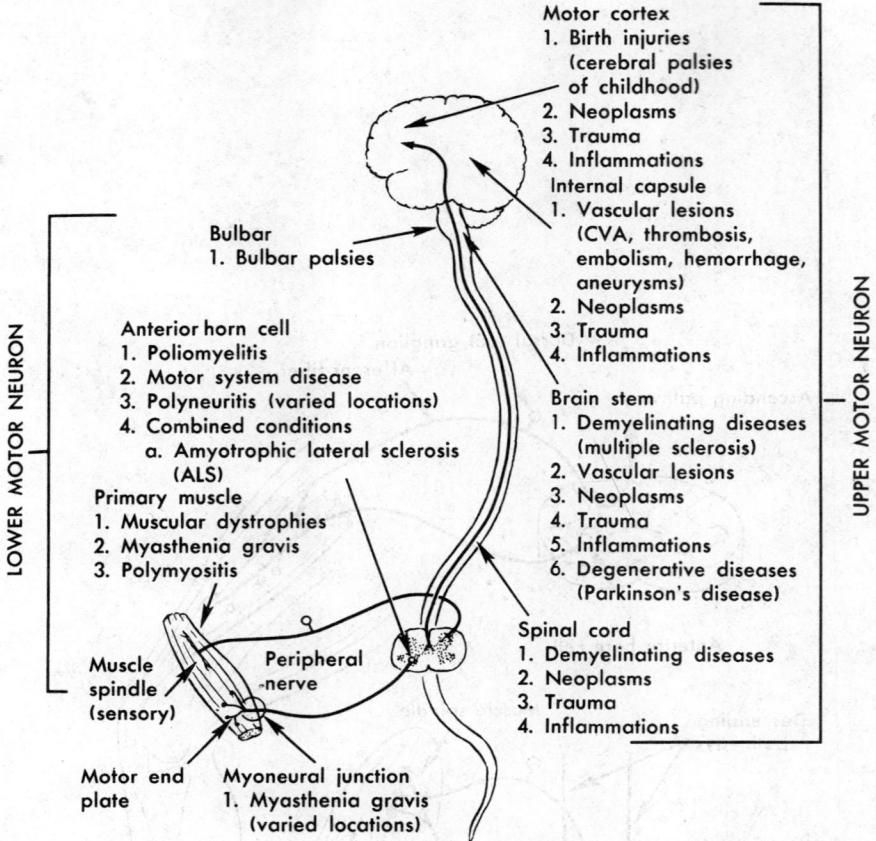

Fig. 35-2. Disturbances in motor function are classified pathologically along upper and lower motor neuron structures. It should be noted that the same pathologic condition occurs at more than one site in upper motor neuron shown on right. A few pathologic conditions involve both upper and lower motor neuron structures, as in amyotrophic lateral sclerosis, for example. Other lesion sites include myoneural junction and primary muscle, making it possible to classify conditions as neuromuscular and muscular, respectively. (Modified from Chusid, J.G.: Correlative neuroanatomy and functional neurology, ed. 15, Los Altos, Calif., 1970, Lange Medical Publications.)

arising from these cells. A lesion in a single motor nerve root will cause varying degrees of muscle weakness in several muscles. If *all* or practically all peripheral motor fibers supplying a muscle are destroyed, all voluntary postural and reflex movements are lost. The entire muscle becomes lax and soft, a condition known as *flaccidity*.

Muscle weakness itself cannot be classified as either lower or upper motor neuron, since it is common to both. It is the *distribution* of the muscle weakness that is important to distinguish. In summary, a LMN lesion weakens individual muscles or sets of muscles in the spinal root or peripheral nerve distribution.

The involved muscle or muscles become *flaccid* because the motor unit has been damaged and normal reflex activity has been interrupted. This flaccidity is further evidenced by *hypotonia* and by reduced or absent muscle stretch reflexes (*hyporeflexia* and *areflexia*, re-

spectively). This interruption of the primary motor unit results in localized muscle atrophy, or wasting, corresponding to the spinal segmental distribution of the anterior horn cells involved.

Atrophy also increases with nonuse of the muscle. In some LMN lesions the affected muscle bundle or unit exhibits small localized, spontaneous, and involuntary contractions known as *fasciculations*. These are visible through the skin and should not be confused with fibrillation. The fasciculations are thought to represent the discharge of isolated muscle fibers arising from a single-functioning lower motor neuron unit. They are coarse in large motor units but may be fine in smaller motor units, as in the hands.

The criteria for an LMN lesion site or disease includes segmental or localized muscle weakness and atrophy in the same distribution, with absent or decreased muscle stretch reflexes in the affected muscles.

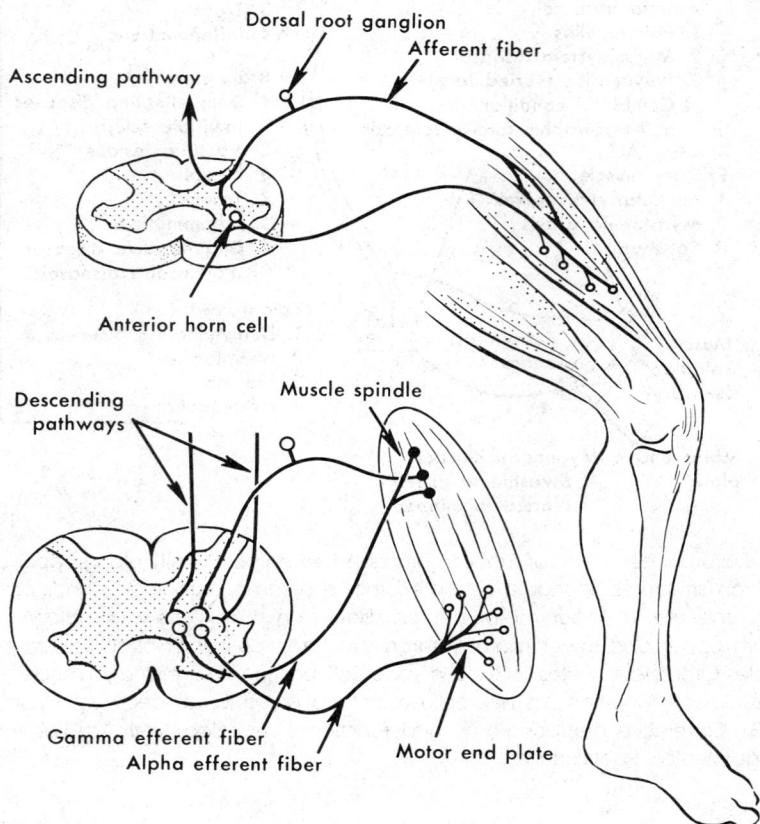

Fig. 35-3. Structures making up lower motor neuron including motor (efferent) and sensory (afferent) elements. Shown on right is anterior horn cell in anterior gray column of spinal cord and its axon terminating in motor end-plate as it innervates extrafusal muscle fibers in quadriceps muscle. Detailed in enlargement on left are sensory and motor elements of γ-loop system. γ-Efferent fiber is shown innervating polar or end region of muscle spindle (sensory receptor of skeletal muscle). Contraction of muscle spindle fibers stretch central portion of spindle and cause afferent spindle fiber to transmit impulse centrally to cord. Muscle spindle afferent fibers in turn synapse on anterior horn cell and are transmitted by way of α-efferent fibers to skeletal (extrafusal) muscle, causing it to contract. Muscle spindle discharge is interrupted by active contraction of extrafusal muscle fibers. (Adapted from Truex, R.C., and Carpenter, M.B.: Human neuroanatomy, ed. 6, Baltimore, 1969, The Williams & Wilkins Co.)

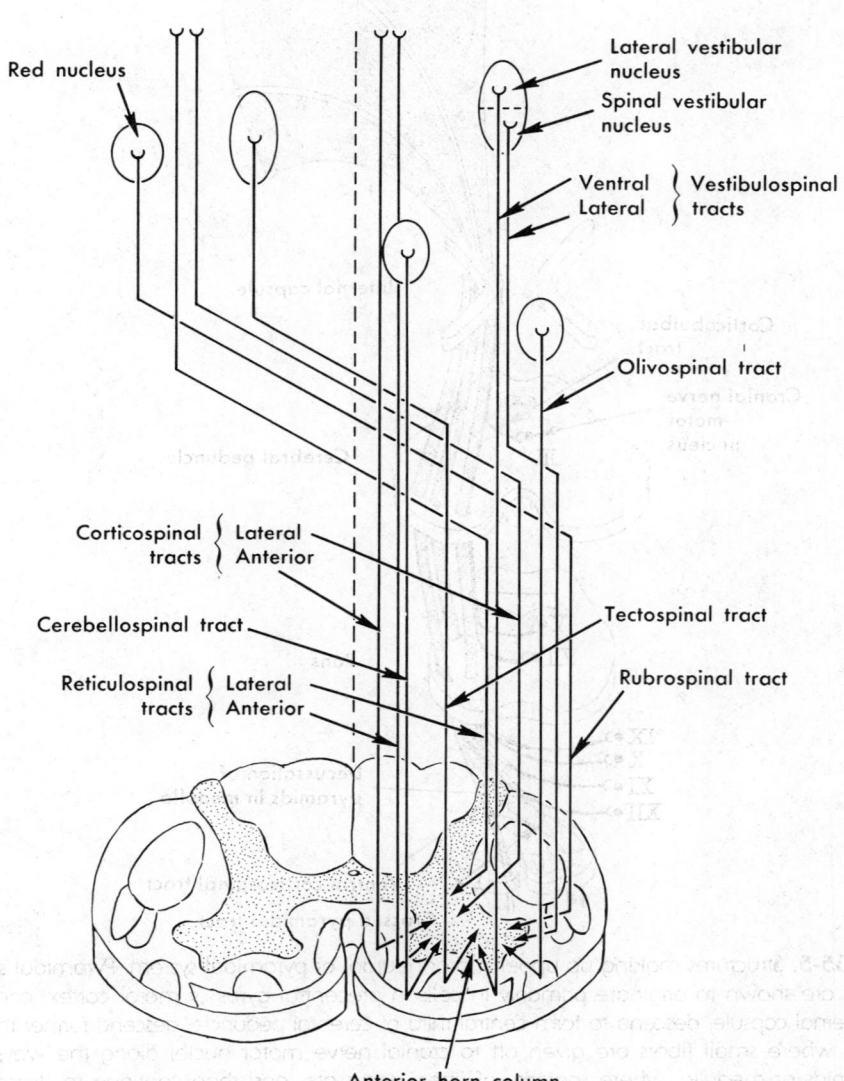

Red nucleus

Lateral vestibular nucleus

Spinal vestibular nucleus

Ventral } Vestibulospinal
Lateral } tracts

Olivospinal tract

Corticospinal { Lateral
tracts { Anterior

Tectospinal tract

Cerebellospinal tract

Reticulospinal { Lateral
tracts { Anterior

Rubrospinal tract

Anterior horn column

Fig. 35-4. Principle of final common pathway. Numerous nuclei and their respective pathways of tracts are shown descending and terminating around lower motor neuron of ventral column of spinal cord, where they exert combined influence on motor activity. (Redrawn from House, E.L., and Pansky, R.: A functional approach to neuroanatomy, ed. 2, New York, 1967, McGraw-Hill Book Co.)

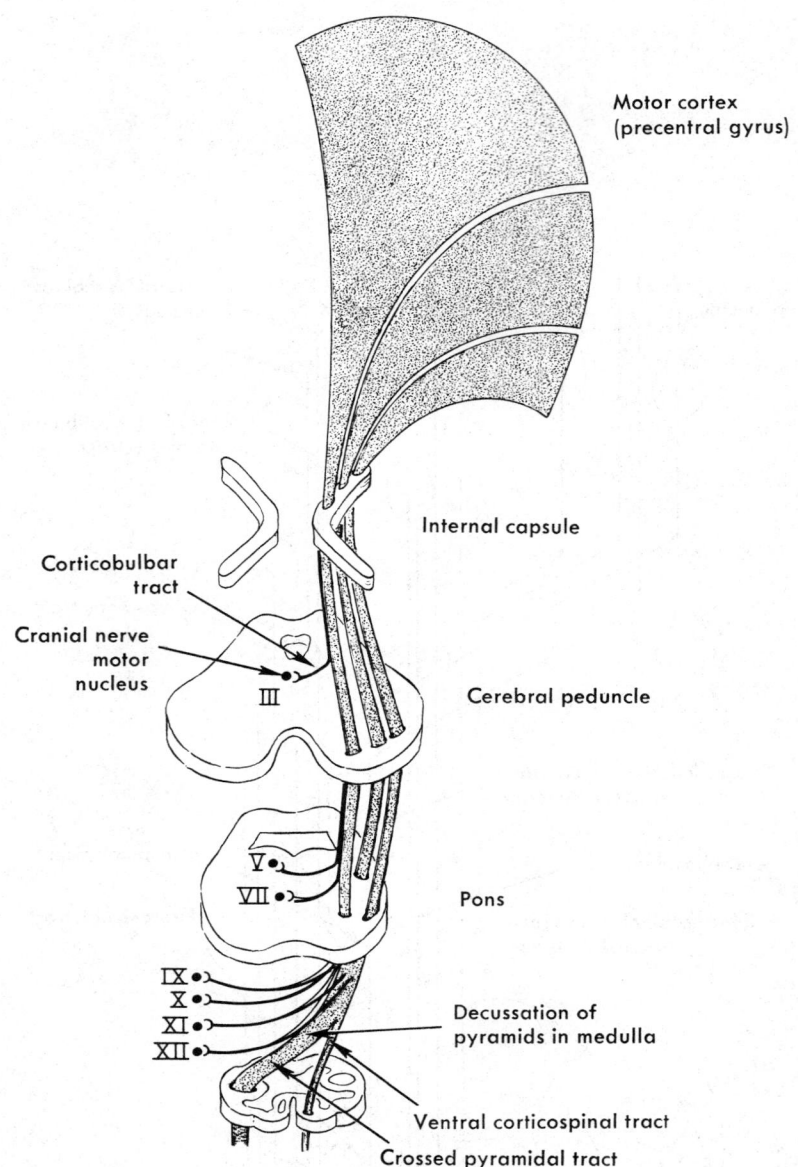

Fig. 35-5. Structures making up upper motor neuron, or pyramidal system. Pyramidal system fibers are shown to originate primarily in cells in precentral gyrus of motor cortex; converge at internal capsule; descend to form central third of cerebral peduncle; descend further through pons, where small fibers are given off to cranial nerve motor nuclei along the way; form pyramids at medulla, where majority of fibers decussate; and then continue to descend in lateral column of white matter of spinal cord, where they synapse with anterior horn cells at all segments of cord. A few fibers descend without crossing at medulla level. (Adapted from original painting by Frank H. Netter, M.D.; from Ciba Collection of Medical Illustrations. Copyright by Ciba Pharmaceutical Co., Division of Ciba-Geigy Corp. All rights reserved.)

Upper motor neuron signs. Recall that *upper motor neurons* (UMNs) originate in the motor strip of the cerebral cortex and in multiple brain stem nuclei. From the cortex these axons pass through the internal capsule and brain stem, cross over (decussate) in the medulla, and continue descending in the spinal cord via the cor-

ticospinal tracts. These fibers eventually synapse with LMNs in the spinal cord (Fig. 35-5).

It is believed that the corticospinal tracts are primarily responsible for the execution of precise, fine, voluntary muscle movements. However, together with the extrapyramidal tracts descending to the LMNs, they assist in modulating muscle tone and reflex activity to some degree. Thus all descending systems collectively combine their influences on the LMNs so that efferent neural impulses are modified, and this results in fine, orderly, and smooth muscle movements.

Any lesion, then, that destroys UMNs or interferes with their influences over LMNs is called an UMN lesion. When an UMN lesion is *rostral* to the medulla, as in a cerebrovascular accident (CVA), deficits will be contralateral to the lesion and will be demonstrated as a hemiplegia. The distribution or degree of paralysis is not always equal or the same within the hemiplegic distribution. For example, the face and arm may be weak or the weakness may involve the leg alone, depending on the part of the motor cortex involved. The following may be considered *UMN signs* following CVA: weakness of the mouth muscle associated with eye muscle weakness (forehead muscle is intact), weakness of forearm and wrist extensors, and weakness of the hip flexors and foot dorsiflexors. These muscle weaknesses result in the characteristic gait and appearance of the patient with a stroke. There is circumduction of the affected leg with inversion of the foot that drags. The arm is held semiflexed at the elbow and wrist. The facial muscles around the eye and mouth droop.

Initially and for a variable period of time the muscles affected by the lesion are flaccid (hypotonic) and hyporeflexic. Gradually the flaccidity recedes, and the reflex arcs become increasingly hyperreactive in the absence of UMN modulation. What is eventually demonstrated is paresis or paralysis of voluntary muscle movement, with increased muscle tone and spasticity. The spasticity is characterized by increased resistance to passive movement, hyperreflexia, clasp-knife phenomenon, and *clonus*. The latter is related to the hyperreflexia, in which the contraction of one muscle group is sufficient to stretch the antagonistic muscles and perpetuate the contractions. A unilateral Babinski sign is present on the hemiparetic side. Atrophy of the muscle results from disuse and occurs late and to a lesser extent than in LMN disease.

UMN lesions within the brain stem also produce the characteristic motor manifestations as just described and, in addition cause involvement of the cranial nerve nuclei and sensory pathways that are near the midbrain lesion site. The problem of localizing the site of an UMN brain stem lesion is made more difficult by the close proximity of the descending fiber systems and cranial motor nuclei in the brain stem area.

UMN lesions that are caudal to the medulla (as in spinal cord trauma) produce deficits ipsilateral to the lesion. If the cord is transected or the lesion extends into both halves of the spinal cord, deficits will be demonstrated as a quadriplegia or paraplegia. A complete transection of the spinal cord immediately produces loss of motor function, muscle tone, and reflex activity as

TABLE 35-3. Clinical syndromes of upper motor neuron (UMN) and lower motor neuron (LMN) lesions

Motor component	UMN characteristics	LMN characteristics
Reflex	Hyperreflexia, extensor toe sign (Babinski's sign)	Hyporeflexia or areflexia
Muscle tonus	Hypertonia, clasp-knife spasticity, clonus	Hypotonia, flaccidity
Muscle movement	Paralysis or paresis of movements in hemiplegic distribution, etc.	Paralysis or paresis of individual muscles in peripheral nerve distribution
Muscle wasting	Late atrophy from disuse	Early atrophy or denervation
Muscle fasciculations	Not present	Present

well as somatic and visceral sensations below the level of the injury. Usually, when examined after a year, voluntary motor losses remain but there is increased spasticity of extensor muscles and hyperreflexia of *all* cord reflexes (muscle stretch, autonomic, and nociceptive). Thus any stretch on the spastic muscles may result in marked contraction. Likewise, contact with a noxious stimulus may cause flexion withdrawal of the limb along with variations of autonomic activity. Occasionally, all three types of reflex activity may occur simultaneously as a response to a single stimulus. (For example, a full bladder or decubitus irritation may cause flexion of the lower extremities, reflex bladder or bowel emptying, and altered vasomotor response to that area.) A bilateral, positive Babinski sign is also present. Table 35-3 summarizes and compares the characteristic clinical syndromes seen in UMN and LMN lesions.

Intervention

An ongoing assessment of basic needs and the ability of the paralyzed person to independently carry out movements in bed, range of motion, and activities of daily living provides the nurse with data necessary to plan the care of the paralyzed person. Successful intervention lies in prevention of joint contractures and decubitus ulcers and in development of the person's optimal level of functioning.

Safety needs. Patients who are paralyzed need to be protected from falling. The person with hemiplegia needs to have the side rail raised on the affected side when unattended. If permitted up in a chair, a chair restraint is used.

The *eye on the affected side* should be protected if the lid remains open and there is no blink reflex. Otherwise damage to the cornea can lead to corneal ulcers and blindness. Irrigations with physiologic solution of sodium chloride, followed by drops of sterile mineral oil, sterile castor oil, sterile petroleum jelly, or artificial tears solution (methylcellulose), are sometimes used. After the lid is gently closed, an eye pad may be taped over the affected eye. If a pad is used, it must be changed daily and the eye cleansed and carefully examined for signs of inflammation or drying of the cornea. Eye shields are preferable to pads because they lessen the danger of lint entering the eye.

The *skin* over bony prominences needs to be inspected regularly for pressure signs (p. 941). Paralyzed persons are at risk for decubitus formation. Several factors account for this. First, muscles are not being used. Second, interference with the autonomic reflexes, which monitor and maintain vasomotor tone, may result in altered circulation to the paralyzed areas. Third, accompanying sensory loss may prevent the individual from perceiving pain and pressure—the warning symptoms of tissue injury. In monoplegic, hemiplegic, and quadriplegic distributions there are successively larger surfaces of skin to be protected (see p. 943 for interventions to prevent decubiti). Persons with a lesser degree of paralysis are taught to turn themselves in bed and to reposition themselves independently, if possible. Persons with paraplegia who are confined to wheelchairs are taught to change position every 15 minutes by elevating themselves with their strong upper extremities. No external heat such as that from a hot-water bottle should be used if the person has loss of sensation, since the heat will not be felt and a burn could result. Care should also be taken to be sure that bathwater is not too hot, and paralyzed areas should be inspected daily for any signs of skin irritation. Patients must be taught to use mirrors and other devices to assist in this assessment activity.

Activity needs. The limbs of a person with acute hemiplegia, as with the person with paraplegia, are often flaccid at first. Spasticity with a tendency to muscle contracture develops gradually. The joints then become flexed or extended and fixed in useless positions with deformity *unless preventive measures are taken by the nurse*. There is a shortening of joint capsules and ligaments around the immobile joint, and the limb may be drawn into flexure or extensor contracture with or without muscle spasm.

Through assessment the nurse determines the specific joints that are vulnerable to contracture and deformity formation as related to the existing degree and type of paralysis. For example, there will be a greater contracture vulnerability with quadriplegia than with paraplegia or hemiplegia, since the amount of muscle and joint involvement is greater. Assessment includes free range of motion (ROM) to determine the level of motion in all joints (p. 924). Based on assessment, the nurse carefully positions the limbs in normal anatomic posi-

tions in order to prevent deformity. By having knowledge of the distribution patterns of paralysis in UMN or LMN lesions, *counterpositioning* can also be initiated. In hemiplegia, for example, the neglected upper limb is pulled inward at the shoulder joint and the wrist drops; in the lower limb the knee flexes and the foot drops. In counterpositioning the nurse plans for the shoulder and upper arm to be in abduction, the elbow slightly flexed, the wrist in dorsiflexion, the knee in neutral position, and the foot in dorsiflexion. If the person is supine, a pillow can be placed between the upper arm and body to hold the arm in abduction. A roll made of one or two washcloths or a styrofoam cup, serves as a good support to prevent flexion of the fingers, and a splint made from a padded tongue blade may be used to ensure straightening of the thumb or other fingers for periods during the day. Dayhoff[9] questions the common use of soft devices to prevent hand deformity and believes that there should be experimentation with hard devices to improve hand functioning following an UMN lesion such as a CVA.

A firm box at the foot of the bed holds the feet at right angles and prevents contractures in the drop-foot position. Some physical therapists believe that footboards used in the prevention of foot drop contribute to increased spasticity and that their use should *not* be a routine practice for persons with UMN lesions. One author reports effective use of high-top tennis shoes as a measure to prevent footdrop.

Positioning is equally important as related to paraplegic and quadriplegic distributions. Knee flexion and foot drop are severe complications that must be prevented. The development of a flexion contracture at the knee joint interferes with the ability of the person to bear weight later in an upright position and to transfer unaided from one place to another. As a consequence, the level of self-care and independence of the person may be greatly diminished when a joint deformity occurs. Subluxation of a shoulder joint in a person with hemiplegia, related to inadequate support of the joint when in an upright position, causes pain and limits therapy of the limb. In addition, keeping the paralyzed person in a semiupright position for long periods, whether in or out of bed, results in hip deformities. Positioning in the prone position helps to counteract the formation of this type of deformity. In summary, most joint deformities in a paralyzed person are *preventable* with early and continuing nursing interventions.

In addition to positioning, interventions for the person with paralysis include range of motion (ROM) exercises to all joints (p. 923). Passive ROM is indicated at least *twice daily* for all joints that the person cannot voluntarily move. Frequent active ROM of the unaffected joints must be carried out by the individual. The regularity of ROM is most important so that limitations do not develop. The muscles of an unaffected leg need to remain strong in the person with hemiplegia as this leg must bear the person's weight when ambulation is begun. Quadriceps drills and isometric exercises are begun with the unaffected leg as soon as possible (p. 413).

During the rehabilitative phase persons with paralysis are taught how to carry out activities of daily living to the extent of capabilities. A variety of self-help devices are available (Fig. 35-6). Diversional activity should be started to keep the person constructively occupied, and an occupational therapist can help in selecting appropriate activities. The person may do any light handiwork that is enjoyable, feasible, and within physical capabilities. A radio, television, and reading material may help to pass the time. If the patient's neck is hy-

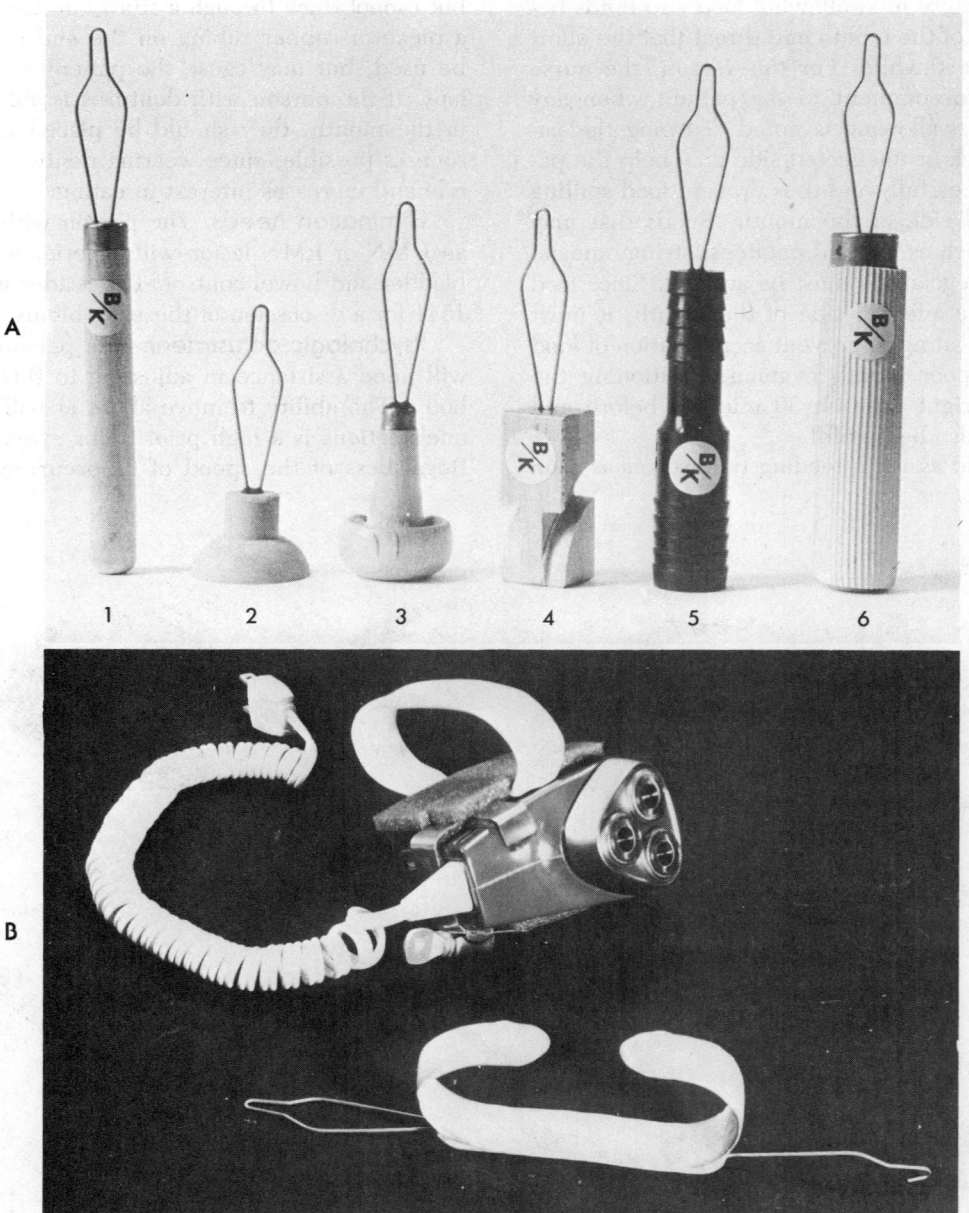

Fig. 35-6. Self-help or assistive devices. **A,** Variety of button hooks are available. Hooks are designed to meet needs of patients with *1,* hemiplegia or quadriplegia; *2,* hemiplegia (especially CVA) or upper extremity amputation; *3,* hemiplegia; *4,* upper extremity amputation and hook prosthesis (note handle is cut to be gripped by hook); *5* and *6,* hemiplegia or quadriplegia. **B,** Electric razor with universal cuff and combination button hook and zipper pull. These are designed to be used by quadriplegic patient. (Courtesy Fred Sammons, O.T.R., Chicago.)

perextended, books that can be projected on the ceiling are useful if they do not cause eyestrain or prism glasses may be obtained. Volunteers are very helpful in reading to patients.

Nutritional needs. Patience and persistence are necessary in giving food and fluids to the hemiplegic person. The nurse must make patients feel that the problem is not discouraging and that time taken to assist them in eating is well spent. Patients may encounter so much difficulty in swallowing food and fluids because of paralysis of the mouth and throat that the effort may not seem worthwhile. For this reason, the nurse should be sure to comment to the patient when any improvement in swallowing is noted. Turning the patient onto the back or unaffected side may help the patient swallow successfully and thus prevent food spilling from the affected side of the mouth. Foods that may cause choking, such as mashed potatoes, stringy meats, and semicooked vegetables, must be avoided. Since food may collect in the affected side of the mouth, it must be irrigated after eating to prevent accumulation of food and subsequent poor mouth hygiene. Positioning the patient in an upright position 30 minutes before and after meals may also be helpful.

Patients should assist in feeding themselves as soon as possible, since the helplessness of having to be fed by others is detrimental to emotional health. Self-help devices are available (Figs. 35-7 and 35-8). Food such as meats must be cut up. A covered plastic cup is available with a small center opening through which a straw can be introduced, or one can be improvised by using a straw and a covered plastic food container. This cup is useful for persons who can draw through a straw but whose hands are unsteady. If the person can swallow but cannot draw through a straw, an Asepto syringe with a piece of rubber tubing on the end or a pitcher may be used, but may cause the patient to feel like an infant. If the person with dentures is able to keep them in the mouth, they should be placed in the mouth as soon as possible, since wearing dentures improves morale and increases interest in eating.

Elimination needs. The person with paralysis from an UMN or LMN lesion will experience problems with bladder and bowel control. The reader is referred to p. 1541 for a discussion of these problems.

Psychologic adjustment. The person with paralysis will need assistance in adjusting to this change in the body. The ability to move about at will and to control one's actions is a high priority for every human being. Regardless of the speed of its occurrence, the loss of

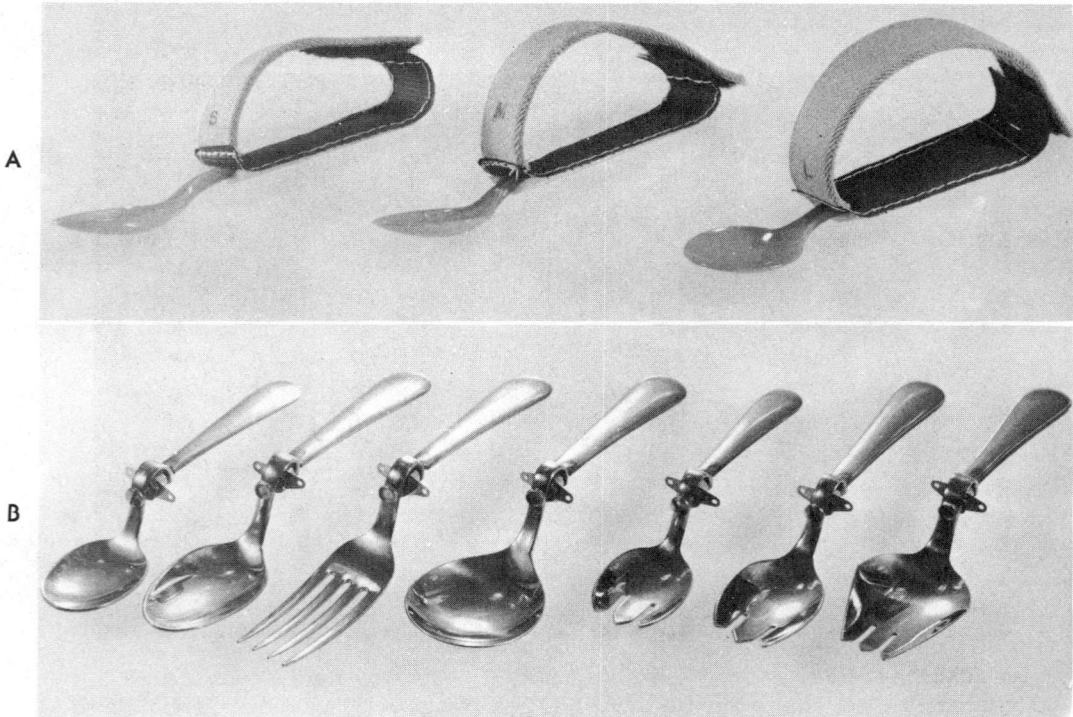

Fig. 35-7. Self-help devices for quadriplegic. **A,** Spoons with small, medium and large universal cuff attachments that fit over hand. **B,** Swivel spoons, forks, and sporks (combination spoon and fork, last three on right), which are used with universal cuff. (Courtesy Fred Sammons, O.T.R., Chicago.)

ability to function independently when paralyzed is psychologically traumatizing. There may also be fears of rejection by loved ones, concerns about the future, and loss of self-esteem. Persons faced with such a major loss of body function also experience a grief reaction much like that experienced by one mourning the loss of a love object. In addition, the person's self-image undergoes change. At times, persons may relate to the paralyzed portion of the body as though it were unrelated to them. It must be reiterated here that victims of a cerebrovascular accident with parietal lesions have an additional physiologic basis for their body image disturbances. This physiologic disturbance must be accounted for in caring for them. Interventions to assist the person to cope with losses and changes in body image are discussed in Chapter 28.

Medications. Patients experiencing ongoing problems with spasticity may be placed on one or more skeletal muscle relaxants to decrease tone and involuntary movements and to help relieve anxiety and tension. In general, the centrally acting preparations also depress the central nervous system while specifically affecting the spinal polysynaptic reflexes. Common side effects include drowsiness and dizziness; these become intensified if the drugs are used in combination with alcohol, barbiturates, sedatives, hypnotics, or tranquilizers. Because depressant effects are potentiated by such combinations, they must be avoided. Some commonly prescribed preparations are the following:

1. *Baclofen (Lioresal)*, a derivative of GABA (an inhibitory neurotransmitter). This drug acts in the spinal cord and is considered by one expert to be the most effective agent presently available to control spasticity resulting from spinal cord lesions.[6]
2. *Dantrolene sodium (Dantrium)*, which acts directly on skeletal muscle. This drug must be taken for 1 week before its effects are apparent. It is a hydantoin preparation and can cause the additional side effects of muscle weakness, slurred speech, drooling, and anuresis. It acts by impairing $Ca++$ release from the sarcoplasmic reticulum.
3. *Diazepam (Valium)*, which is a centrally acting muscle relaxant and antianxiety agent.

Outcome criteria for the person recovering from paralysis

The person or significant others can:
1. Describe dosage, function, side effects, and toxic effects of prescribed medications.
2. Demonstrate measures to prevent muscle or joint deformities.
3. Describe measures to prevent decubitus ulcers.
4. List signs of skin breakdown requiring professional intervention.
5. Demonstrate activities of daily living that can be done alone and those that require assistance.
6. Discuss plans for bowel and bladder control.
7. State plans for follow-up care.

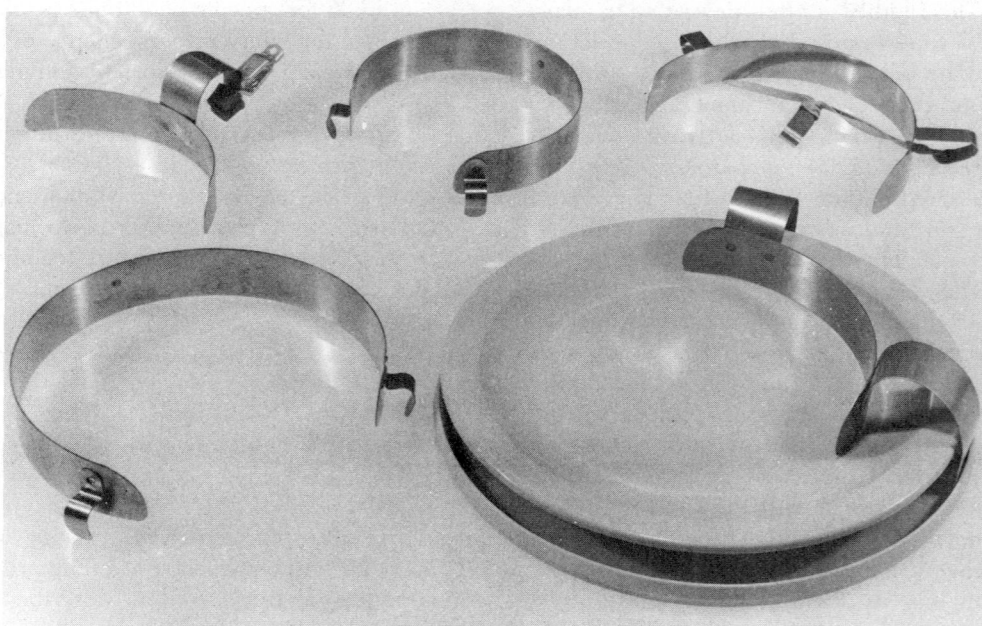

Fig. 35-8. Variety of food guards. Lower right-hand corner, food guard attached to plate. Food is pushed against guard to help get it onto utensil and to prevent it from being pushed off plate. (Courtesy Fred Sammons, O.T.R., Chicago.)

Alterations in movement and posture

Various neurologic lesions of the extrapyramidal motor system result in alterations of movement and posture. Clinically, this is seen most commonly in paralysis agitans, or parkinsonism. In this condition there is degeneration of various parts of the basal ganglia. The nuclear masses making up the basal ganglia lie deep in the center of the cerebral hemispheres to either side of the midline and are a part of the extrapyramidal system. The motor pathways between the basal ganglia interconnect with both the cerebral motor strip and the cerebellum and affect LMN activity as related to the mediations of posture and coordination of movement.

Assessment

In contrast to UMN syndrome with the loss of volitional movement and spasticity, in extrapyramidal lesions there is characteristic muscle rigidity, involuntary movements, and bradykinesia without loss of voluntary movement. Muscle rigidity, or *hypertonus*, is present in all muscle groups, both flexor and extensor, but appears to be more prominent in those muscles that maintain a flexed posture. The smaller muscles of the face, tongue, and even the larynx become involved with consequent difficulty in chewing, swallowing, and speech. The muscles remain continuously or intermittently firm and tense. Hypertonus is present even when the person is relaxed. There is an even or uniform quality to the hypertonus throughout the range of passive movement of a limb. The rigidity is often described as plastic. In addition, a superimposed rhythmic contraction of the muscle may be felt as the joint is moved through its range of motion. This is termed *cogwheel rigidity*.

Strength of muscle is not significantly decreased in bradykinesia. *Bradykinesia*, or *hypokinesia*, refers to slowness of movement rather than lack of movement (*akinesia*); the actual time in carrying out a movement is longer than normal. There is also an extreme poverty of movement. The semiautomatic or habitual movements observed in the normal state such as putting the hands to the face, folding the arms, or crossing the legs are absent or greatly reduced. In looking to the side the eyes move but not the head. In arising from a chair the necessary adjustments such as putting the feet back and the hands on the arm of the chair are not made, although the person can do it with effort or will. The muscle is not paralyzed or apraxic. There are a variety of involuntary movements such as static tremor or pill rolling of the fingers, as seen in parkinsonism; rest tremors that decrease when the limb is used; and chorea, athetosis, and deptonia. In all basal ganglia disorders, stress and nervous tension worsen motor performance; relaxation improves it.

Intervention

Muscle rigidity may be relieved by physical therapy. It is important that the person remain physically active in order to prevent the complications of immobility (p. 941). It requires much patience and understanding on the part of the family not to take over physical activities that the person can perform even though they will be performed slowly and with much effort. Nursing interventions are planned to assist with feeding problems related to swallowing, ambulation, and speech. Often the person with parkinsonism is viewed as unintelligent because of dysarthria produced by the rigid and bradykinesic muscles of articulation and phonation. Education of the patient and family is a nursing priority. They need to understand the need to reduce stress and nervous tension in order to improve rigidity.

Outcome criteria for the person with basal ganglia or extrapyramidal problems

The person or significant others can:
1. Demonstrate how activities will be carried out at home.
   a. Explain the need to remain physically active despite difficulty and slowness in performance of activities.
   b. Demonstrate prescribed treatments (exercise, speech).
   c. Explain the need to prevent the complications of immobility (joint contractures, decubiti).
   d. Explain the dosage, side effects, and toxic effects of prescribed medications. (See Chapter 36 for specific conditions.)
2. Plan for safety in performance of activities.
   a. Relate safety factors in ambulation related to gait.
   b. Demonstrate techniques in eating to prevent aspiration of food.
3. Explain the need for relaxation and freedom from stress to improve motor performance.
   a. Demonstrate relaxation techniques.
4. State plans for follow-up care.

Aphasia and dysphasia

Etiology and pathophysiology

To recall, *aphasia* is a disorder of language caused by damage to the speech-controlling areas of the brain, it is a general term used to describe organic disturbances in language. It includes all areas of language, including speech, reading, writing, and understanding.

Cerebral hemorrhage and cerebral thrombosis are the most common causes of cortical damage, but tumors, multiple sclerosis, and trauma may also lead to aphasia. Aphasia caused by cerebral edema following trauma is usually temporary. Occasionally, a person cannot speak following a cerebrovascular accident because motor function of the vocal cords is affected, not because of damage to cortical speech centers. Defective innervation of the muscles of speech articulation such as vocal cords, tongue, cheeks, and palate results in *dysarthria*.

As discussed previously, a variety of abnormalities in communication can occur. The patient may be unable to comprehend the spoken word *(sensory aphasia)* or may comprehend and yet be unable to use the symbols of speech *(motor aphasia)*. The patient may have both disorders at the same time *(global aphasia)*. Writing may be possible even though speaking is not. Some patients may be able to speak but the wrong words may be used, or there may be a selective loss of words, or the patient may be able to read but be unable to speak or to write.

Assessment

A history of the person's background pertaining to language, including education and languages spoken, should be secured from significant others. Assessment of sensory problems of vision and hearing is made as well as assessment of problems in speech articulation. Assessment of an individual's communication efforts, however, is only possible by listening to and observing that person directly.

As described in Chapter 34, gross tests must be performed to determine what specific language abilities have been lost. Simple tests may be conducted as follows. Spread several familiar objects such as keys, a pencil, a book of matches, a penny, and scissors before the patient: (1) ask the patient to name each object; (2) as you name each object, ask the patient to point to it; (3) ask the patient to write the name of each object as you point to it; (4) ask the patient to write the name of each object as you say the word; (5) show the patient a card containing the printed name of each object and ask the patient to read the word orally and point to the object. It may be too fatiguing for the patient to take all the tests at one time, and they can be phased in gradually.

Intervention

Each person reacts to language problems differently. Most persons with aphasia become tense and anxious. They may be irritable and emotionally upset because they are unable to evoke the words they need, and they become discouraged easily in their efforts to speak. Some may quickly refuse to attempt to communicate; others feel ashamed and withdraw from people, including their family and close friends. Yet desire to communicate and persistence in efforts to do so are the essential ingredients in speech rehabilitation.

Care is taken to reduce tension so that patients with aphasia can make satisfactory adjustments to their loss. The environment should be relatively free of excess stimuli. These patients are not deaf, and they should be spoken to in a normal voice. Procedures are explained to them in the same manner as that used with other patients. Recreational activities should be soothing and nonstimulating. Music is often relaxing, and some patients will enjoy listening to the radio. If the patient is able to read and comprehend written captions on television, watching television may be gratifying. Some patients do not enjoy listening to the radio or watching television when they cannot follow what is going on. Being alert to patients' facial expressions often gives clues as to the activities that are most satisfying.

The patient should be helped to understand that speech may be relearned. In the interim, gestures, pointing to objects, pointing to pictures or words on communication boards, or writing may be used to improve communication. After the most effective approach to communication is decided upon, this approach is shared with all who interact with the patient, including the family and other members of the health team.

Specific interventions are based on whether the patient's aphasia is primarily one of *comprehension* or *expression*. Some approaches for patients with *comprehension* deficits are (1) to keep distractions to a minimum (clear the patient's visual field of extraneous stimuli before initiating conversation), (2) to face the patient when speaking and speak simply and slowly, and (3) if the patient miscomprehends the message, to slow down the rate of speech and reword the message, using gestures to emphasize points. If the message is still not comprehended, go on to another topic after supplying the correct response.

When the patient has an *expressive* problem, try to anticipate the patient's words and ideas. Avoid interrupting or rushing the patient's attempts to speak. Discuss topics that are important to the patient, such as the family or other interests. Allow time for the patient to repeat what you have said or written and encourage the patient to utilize other means of communication. This latter suggestion is also appropriate for the patient with aphasia that involves comprehension. Calmness and patience on the part of the nurse are essential to the patient's acceptance of the difficult program of practicing relearned words and patterns of speech.

Although the nurse does not initiate the formal speech therapy program with the patient, the nurse's cooperation is needed to reinforce the program. As the nurse cares for the patient, common objects should be named and the patient encouraged to handle them, to speak their names, and to write or copy their names. The family can supply these words and others that are particularly important for the patient. Speech retraining should be done for short periods of time because it is exceedingly trying, and fatigue tends to increase difficulty in speaking. Praising patients for each small improvement and encouraging them to take their mistakes good-naturedly helps to make this difficult problem more bearable. A patient's progress in language retraining will depend on the level of intelligence, the age (older patients have more difficulty), the severity of the damage, and whether the brain lesion is progressive. Complete language rehabilitation may require months of painstaking work on the part of skilled pathologists.* *A Guide to Clinical Services in Speech Pathology and Audiology†* lists clinics in the United States where speech and hearing services are available. Some of these clinics offer specialized help to persons with aphasia and dysphasia.

Outcome criteria for the person with aphasia

The person or significant others can:
1. Explain the recommended communication approach of the speech pathologist.
   a. Demonstrate the approach in communication to be used.
   b. Explain the need to provide an atmosphere conducive to communication relearning.
   c. Explain the need to practice communication regularly but not to the point of frustration.
   d. Explain how to communicate basic needs associated with activities of daily living.
2. The family or significant others shall have information about effective communication techniques and can:
   a. Explain alternate communication techniques (e.g., gesture, writing, and communication board) for the person with expressive aphasia.
   b. Explain the need to encourage the person in communication efforts.
   c. Explain the need to avoid the use of complex and long sentences in communications.
   d. Explain the need to articulate clearly in communication and not to speak loudly.
   e. Explain the need to listen carefully to what the person is communicating.
   f. Distinguish between communication and speaking.
   g. Explain the need to be realistic and honest with the person about communication efforts.
   h. Explain the need to treat the person with aphasia as a person and not to discuss the person with others in the person's presence.

   i. Explain the need to prevent isolation of the person by providing for socialization.
   j. State plans for follow-up care in relation to speech.

General sensory dysfunction

Etiology and pathophysiology

The presence of a lesion anywhere within the sensory system pathways, from the receptor to the sensory cortex, alters the transmission or perception of sensory information. The parietal lobe cortex is of major importance for interpretation of sensation with the exception of sight, hearing, smell, taste, and thermoregulation. A loss, decrease, or increase in the sensation of pain, temperature, touch, and proprioception, singly or in combination, results in difficult problems in daily living for the person. Since these sensations normally help the person to be aware of alterations in the internal and external environments, any alteration in sensibility lessens the ability to be completely and accurately protected. As a consequence, there is a need to adapt to the alteration and plan for safety and comfort.

Some specific losses deserve to be mentioned. The loss of *proprioception*, or the ability to know the position of the body and its parts without looking directly at the part, is a serious loss that requires considerable adaptation. Lack of control of body temperature, or *hyperthermia*, occurs because of a malfunction in the thermoregulatory center in the brain, such as occurs following brain surgery near the hypothalamus or from head injury, brain tumors, and other cranial conditions. Hyperthermia is believed to occur as a result of hypoxia of the center. Persons also often complain of *dysesthesia* or *paresthesia* (abnormalities of the sensation of touch). These are commonly associated with peripheral neuropathies.

Fig. 35-9 presents common patterns of sensory alteration. A cerebral lesion results in various alterations in sensation *contralateral* to the lesion. This distribution results from the fact that all sensory fibers have decussated before reaching the sensory cortex of the cerebrum. On the other hand, *transection* of the spinal cord results in total *bilateral* sensory loss distal to the lesion since *all* pathways have been severed. Note, however, the characteristic distribution of deficits with hemisection of the cord (Brown-Séquard syndrome). In this situation the person experiences *Ipsilateral* loss of proprioception and vibratory sense because the posterior columns decussate in the medulla and *Contralateral* loss of pain, temperature, and crude touch sensation because the spinothalamic tracts decussate in the cord.

---

*Some institutions that specialize in working with patients who have aphasia are ICD Rehabilitation and Research Center, New York, NY; The Institute of Logopedics, Wichita, KS; and Vanderbilt University Hospital Clinic, Nashville, TN.
†American Speech-Language-Hearing Association, 10801 Rockville Pike, Rockville, MD 20852.

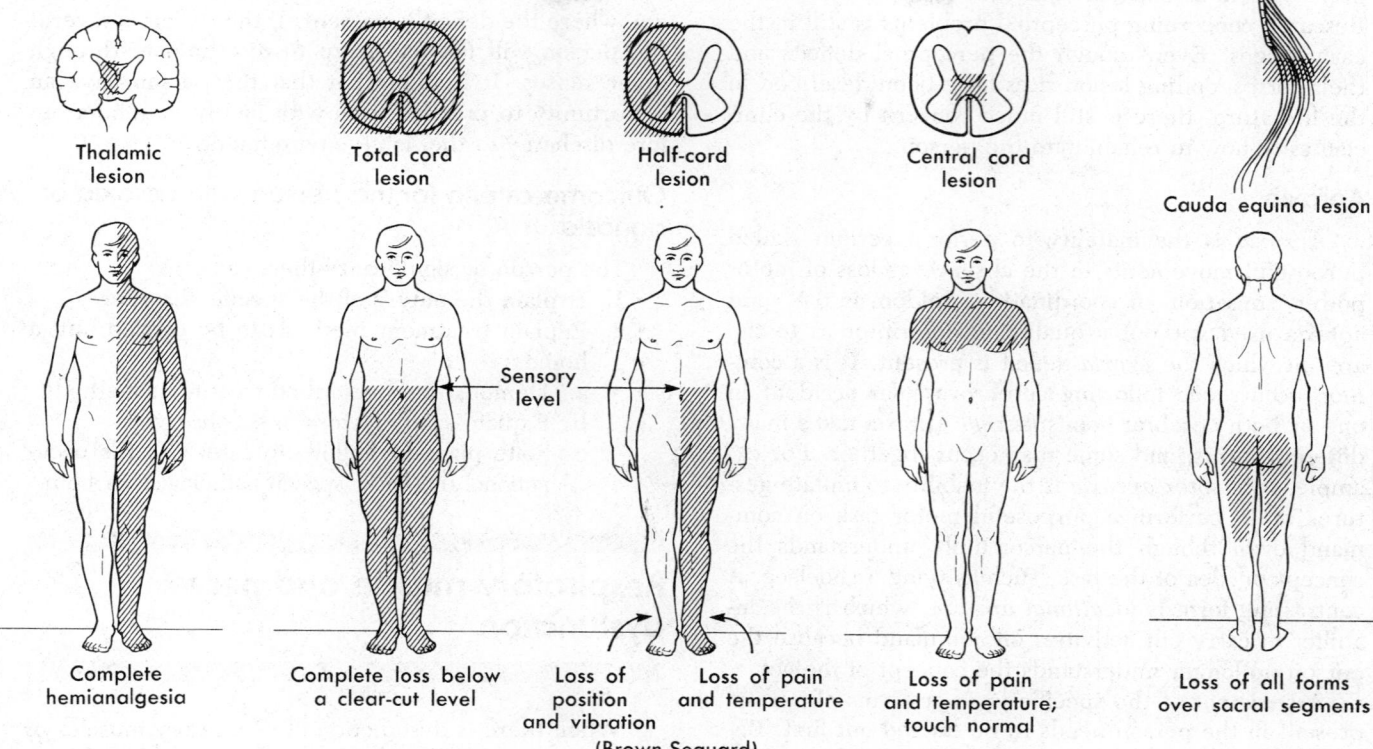

Fig. 35-9. Common patterns of sensory abnormality. Upper diagrams show site of lesion; lower diagrams show distribution of corresponding sensory loss. (Adapted from Bickerstaff, E.R.: Neurology for nurses, ed. 2, London, 1971, English Universities Press Ltd., and Hodder & Stoughton Ltd.)

Assessment

The specific sensory alterations present in the person need to be assessed as a basis for planning self-care. The nurse should recognize that sensory examination is the most difficult part of a neurologic examination. The detail in which a specific sensation is tested is determined by the clinical situation. The specific complaint of the person is thoroughly checked out by the examiner. Methods for sensory examination of each of these sensations are discussed in Chapter 34.

Intervention

The most important nursing intervention, once the alteration has been clearly identified, is teaching the person (and family) protection measures in relation to the sensory deficit or alteration. Teaching the person to utilize the noninvolved senses to an increased extent helps to avoid injuries. For example, teaching the person with hypoesthesia (lessened touch) to visually inspect involved body parts regularly will help to prevent injuries. Some nursing interventions will be more complex, such as in hyperthermia, and require lifesaving measures.

Outcome criteria for the person with alteration of one or more sensations

The person or significant others can:

1. Demonstrate how to substitute for each sensation deficit or loss.
2. Explain safety factors needed in activities of daily living to protect from injury.
   a. Demonstrate how to provide protection relative to the specific deficit.
   b. Demonstrate how to inspect the affected body parts for injury.
3. State signs or symptoms that would indicate worsening of the condition and the need to seek medical assistance immediately.
4. State plans for follow-up care.

Apraxia and agnosia

Apraxia and agnosia are both fairly common perceptual deficits that occur in neurologic conditions. They may occur in association with each other or separately. Research concerning perceptual problems is still in the early stages. Even though the perceptual deficits and their corresponding lesion sites have been described in the literature, there is still much concern by the clinician as to how to rehabilitate the person.

Apraxia

Apraxia is the inability to perform certain skilled purposeful movements in the absence or loss of motor power, sensation, or coordination. Seldom is the word apraxia used without a qualifying descriptor as to the area in which the *praxia* deficit is present. It is a common occurrence following cerebrovascular accident in one or both cerebral hemispheres. Apraxia takes many different forms, and some may occur together. For example, *ideomotor apraxia* is the inability to imitate gestures or to perform a purposeful motor task on command even though the person fully understands the concept or idea of the task, such as tying a shoelace. A contrasting form is *ideational apraxia*, which is the inability to carry out activities on command because the person no longer understands the concept of the act.

Assessment of the specific form or forms of apraxia present in the person needs to be carried out first. Because of the nature of apraxia, it is difficult to intervene in a way that assists the apraxic person to act. Some persons may be able to respond to verbal cues from the nurse and others from visual cues. Also, it is not always possible to determine if the person understands the instruction given. Collaboration with occupational therapists and speech pathologists is necessary in order that information from definitive tests and treatment administered by them be shared.

Agnosia

Agnosia is the inability to recognize familiar objects perceived by the senses. This occurs frequently in stroke patients. It may be a disturbance in one or all of the following sensory modes—visual, tactile, proprioceptive, and auditory—or it may involve additional problems in body scheme, such as somatognosia or anosognosia. The form of agnosia can be related to the perceptual site of the brain involved; that is, *visual agnosia* is caused by a disturbance in the association area of the occipital cortex. In this deficit the person is unable to recognize objects visually although pathways for visual acuity and recognition of objects by touch are intact. The person will be unable to recognize familiar persons or possessions. In other forms of visual agnosia there is difficulty in recognition of color, size of objects, and spatial relationships of objects. Tactile and auditory agnosias are common.

As in other perceptual alterations, assessment of the specific form is carried out first. Treatment measures are directed toward repeated experiences in trial rec-

ognition of objects through other senses as well as the one where the deficit is present. If the deficit is severe, the person will have to learn to discriminate through other senses. It is important that the person have an opportunity to practice tests with family members before discharge to the home environment.

Outcome criteria for the person with apraxia or agnosia

The person or significant others can:
1. Explain the nature of the specific disorder.
2. Explain treatment methods to be carried out at home.
   a. Demonstrate prescribed treatment methods.
   b. Explain safety factors to be observed.
   c. State plans for follow-up care with the occupational therapist, speech pathologist, or both.

Respiratory muscle and nerve dysfunction

When there is dysfunction of respiratory muscles or the nerves innervating these muscles, serious problems in breathing ensue. This often necessitates the use of a respirator to assist or control breathing. Although tank and chest respirators are used infrequently today, when they are used it is most often in the care of patients with neurologic conditions; therefore the nursing care needed is included here.

Etiology and pathophysiology

A few neurologic conditions produce paralysis of intercostal muscles, the diaphragm, or both, such as acute polyneuritis, poliomyelitis, toxic encephalitis, myasthenia gravis, amyotropic lateral sclerosis (ALS), and fractures of the skull. Paralysis of respiratory muscles may be accompanied by paralysis of the palate and pharynx when the brain stem is involved and create increased difficulty in respiration. There is resultant difficulty in swallowing, coughing, breathing, and speech. When this occurs, the person should be positioned so that secretions can be drained or suctioned when a tracheostomy is present.

Intervention

When patients have difficulty in swallowing, coughing, or breathing, measures to assist with these maneuvers are necessary. The patient is positioned so that secretions can be drained or suctioned if an endotracheal tube or tracheostomy is present. The side-lying postanesthesia position is commonly used to drain secretions.

For patients who cannot sustain their own respirations, a respirator that creates negative pressure outside the chest wall and causes air to enter the lungs may be necessary. A mechanical device is a poor substitute for normal respiration and is usually used only as a last resort.

There are two main types of respirators and several manufacturers of each. The *tank respirator* encases the entire body except the head. Modern tank respirators are hinged at the foot to facilitate placement of the patient and include large portholes. The *chest respirator* encloses only the chest. Chest respirators permit the patient much greater freedom and simplify nursing care. They cannot, however, be used for long periods of time, since they may not provide adequate aeration of the lungs. Several variations of equipment are available to aid breathing. Some of these respirators employ the use of a mask over the face and do not encase the body; more frequently, respirators are attached to a tracheostomy tube (p. 1228). Other aspects of acute respiratory care are discussed in Chapter 49.

Before placing the conscious patient in a respirator, the procedure and the purpose of it are explained as much as time permits. Usually the explanation includes the fact that the patient will be able to breathe easier and will be able to sleep and rest without struggling to breathe. Many patients are so exhausted from having to remain awake and consciously use their accessory muscles to breathe that they may welcome the respirator. It is not uncommon, however, for some patients to "fight" the machine. When this occurs, special measures such as sedation of the patient may be necessary. (See Chapter 49 for a detailed discussion of respirators.) Coaching and the calm presence of the nurse will help some patients adjust to the respirator, but others will continue to resist it. All patients on a respirator must be under constant nursing surveillance, and for this reason they are ideally cared for in an intensive care unit.

Altered level of consciousness related to neural causes

In the practice of neurologic nursing the clinical assessment of unresponsive and comatose patients becomes a practical necessity. Patients are frequently admitted in coma as a result of direct trauma to the head, cerebrovascular problems, epilepsy, intracranial tumors, or increased intracranial pressure. Unconsciousness occurs when there is depression of transmission of impulses between the reticular activating system and the cerebral hemispheres. Level of consciousness is a reliable indicator of neurologic status. The assessment parameters for the unconscious patient are described in detail in Chapter 27.

Alterations in cognition and personality

Cognitive behavioral changes are common in neurologic disease. Their slow development in the person may be the initial and only sign of a serious neurologic disorder. Assessment of cognition and personality should be made and reported accurately. Also, structural changes and loss of function caused by neurologic disease will affect self-concept and cause behavioral changes. Frustration resulting from restrictions and from attempts to get about, anxiety from increasing helplessness, and the feeling of powerlessness produce changes in personality. Cognition changes with resulting alteration in judgment, decision-making, memory, and attention may become so serious that restrictions on the person's freedom by family and health professionals are necessary. Such situations are extremely difficult to manage because strong emotional reactions may follow curtailment of the person's freedom. The problem is usually dealt with by the family, the physician, and the social worker. When caring for such persons, the nurse does not communicate to the patient knowledge of measures taken to prevent the consequences of errors in judgment.

Intracranial surgery

Intracranial surgery is commonly done for all types of pathologic conditions of the brain, including repair of aneurysm, evacuation of hematoma, relief of increased intracranial pressure, repair of fracture, drainage of infections, exploration of suspected pathologic conditions and brain bypass surgery.

A surgical opening through the skull is known as a craniotomy. It is a basic preparatory procedure for intracranial surgery. A series of burr holes (trephine) is made first, and then the bone between the holes is cut with a special saw (Gigli) to permit removal of the bone. Bone is then removed in such a way that it can be replaced if desired. The opening depends on the lesion site. Brain surgery may be done under hypothermia to lessen bleeding during the procedure. Drugs for hypotension may be used such as levarterenol bitartrate (Levophed). Patients may also be placed in a barbiturate coma during the surgery and for several days following it to lessen brain activity, matabolism, and oxygen needs. This may help to prevent worsening of deficits because of hypoxia.

Fluorescein sodium, a dye, may be administered intravenously 1 hour preoperatively to help localize a tumor during surgery. Tumor tissue tends to retain the dye, which can be seen under ultraviolet light. The dye will cause the skin and the scleras to appear jaundiced for several days. The nursing staff, the patient, and the family should be aware of this.

When the brain lesion is in the *supratentorium* (above the tentorium or in the cerebrum), the incision is usually made behind the hairline. When the incision is into the *infratentorium* (below the tentorium or in the brain stem and cerebellum), it is made slightly above the nape of neck. Neither of these incisions is apparent when the hair has regrown.

Following craniotomy and removal of the bone, an incision is made into the meninges and the tumor is removed or other cranial surgery performed. The removed bone is carefully saved or preserved. Following brain surgery, *the bone may be replaced immediately (as in a bone flap with muscle attachment) or when there are no evidences of infection or increased intracranial pressure*. Not infrequently the bone is left out for variable periods to prevent pressure from cerebral edema postoperatively or to permit expansion of an inoperable tumor. The preserved bone, in this instance, is used as a mold for a bone prosthesis, which is inserted with wire at a later date, or the preserved bone is reinserted. Sterile acrylic is the material presently used to make the bone prosthesis. The acrylic can be molded directly into the skull opening after covering the dura mater with a thin plastic sheet at the time of surgery, or it can be molded from the preserved bone at a later time. The removal of part of the skull without replacement is called *craniectomy*. When a tumor cannot be removed because of its location and nature, a subtemporal decompression is made by leaving an opening in the dura and skull. *Cranioplasty* is the repair of a cranial defect through use of substitute bone materials.

Limitation of some functions may necessarily follow complete removal of brain tumors occurring in cerebral hemispheres. Portions of the frontal lobe are removed in some instances with little residual damage. Patients with tumors located where they are readily accessible to removal, such as meningiomas and tumors of the outer cerebrum, have the best prognosis. Today, the decision to operate on persons with large tumors is weighed carefully by the neurosurgeon. If surgery is likely to leave the patient with a large amount of permanent disability, the decision not to operate will often be made.

Neurosurgery may also be employed to repair a cerebral aneurysm. Surgical procedures, in addition, are performed to produce destructive brain lesions in selected sites, as in the treatment of Parkinson's disease and in the control of intractable pain.

The horizons of neurosurgical care are expanding rapidly. Not only is surgery done to treat and remove brain tumors, to remove hematomas, and to repair arteriovenous malformations or aneurysms, but now some neurosurgeons are beginning to do bypass surgery. In this procedure a superficial scalp vessel, such as the superficial temporal artery, is anastomosed to the portion of the brain where blood supply has been limited. The surgery is relatively new, but good results with some regaining of functional ability are often seen.

Preoperative care

Baseline data of neurologic and physiologic status should be recorded by the nurse before surgery. Written permission for surgery on the brain must be given by the nearest relative unless the patient is able to sign the permit. Even then close relatives are usually consulted, and the neurosurgeon obtains their consent before surgery. The patient and family are usually very threatened by the prospect of brain surgery and should be encouraged to express their fears. Specific fears may be related to those of a permanent change in appearance, dependency, or death. Psychologic support of patient and family is a priority intervention. The nursing staff should provide time for this as part of essential nursing care of the patient. The patient may also wish to see a spiritual advisor before surgery.

Treatments and procedures should be explained to the patients even though they *may not* seem to understand fully. Enemas may not be given before surgery because of the danger of increasing intracranial pressure further by exertion and by the absorption of fluid. Narcotics, excepting codeine, are rarely ordered preoperatively, since they may cause further depression of cerebral function. Any order for their use should be carefully verified by the nurse. If the head is to be shaved, the procedure may be delayed until the patient is in the operating room. Hair should not be discarded but should be returned to the patient unit because the patient may wish to have it made into a wig. The availability and popularity of synthetic wigs also help in the solution of the feeling associated with the loss of hair. In many hospitals it is the practice to shave only the portion of the patient's head that must be shaved to do the surgery. Hair along the front hairline can often be left so that after the operation it can be drawn backward to cover the scar. The hair is shampooed, and the condition of the scalp is noted.

Preparation of the family

The family of the patient needs to be prepared for what they will face when they see the patient after surgery. They need to know that the patient will have a head dressing and that edema may distort facial features. They also need to know that the patient may have discolored areas about the eyes (ecchymosis). If the patient is unconscious or has a limitation such as aphasia, this should be discussed with the family before they see the patient. If the patient is alert, the family will be advised to sit quietly at the bedside since talking will tire the patient.

Postoperative care

Postanesthesia care

Whether in the patient unit or in the recovery room, the nurse should be certain that the following are readily available: side rails for the bed, suction machine or wall suction with disposable suction catheters, an airway, a padded tongue blade, a lumbar puncture set, and an emergency medication tray (cardiac and respiratory stimulants, amobarbital sodium [Amytal], anticonvulsive drugs), syringes, intravenous and hypodermic needles, and a tourniquet. An emergency tracheostomy tray should also be readily available on the unit.

The patient is *observed* regularly during the early postoperative period for signs of increased intracranial pressure (see p. 753 for a complete discussion of increased ICP). *Frequency* of making and recording specific observations *depends on the patient's condition.*

Any change in the patient's *vital signs, state of consciousness, pupillary response,* or *ability to use muscles* is reported at once. Restlessness, often secondary to tissue hypoxia, forewarnings of hemorrhage or of irritation to the brain, or other symptoms of increased ICP should be watched for and reported immediately to the surgeon. These changes are described earlier in this chapter.

Position

Immediately after surgery the patient is placed on the side to provide an adequate airway. To facilitate change of head dressings and other treatments following surgery, the patient may be placed in bed "head to foot." If a large brain tumor has been removed, the patient must not be turned on the affected side, since this position may cause displacement of brain structures by gravity. Otherwise, turning to either side is permitted. The primary objective is to eliminate pressure at the operative site. Handling of the brain tissues and surgical trauma causes cerebral edema, which contributes to increased ICP.

If there has been *supratentorial* surgery (above the cerebellum), *the head of the bed is elevated at least 45 degrees, and a large pillow is placed under the patient's head and shoulders.* This position should lessen the possibility of hemorrhage, provide for better circulation of the CSF, and promote venous return. All of these measures assist in decreasing cerebral edema and in preventing increased ICP. Internal bleeding would also contribute to a rise in ICP. If an *infratentorial* tumor has been removed, *the bed should be kept flat with only*

a small pillow under the nape of the neck and the patient turned to either side. Any *flexion* of the neck should be *avoided,* either midline or laterally. Since infratentorial incisions are made adjacent to the medulla, vital centers, and cranial nerves IX and X, there is more danger of respiratory complications and brain stem compression.

Coughing and *vomiting* are to be avoided, since these increase ICP. Suctioning, if permitted, should be done gently and cautiously to avoid initiating coughing. Suctioning through the nose is also avoided (p. 758). Deep-breathing exercises should not be followed by coughing.

Protective measures

Some patients must be protected from injuring themselves after surgery. Patients who pull at dressings or catheters or scratch or hit themselves must be attended constantly. Occasionally some kind of hand restraint such as a large mitten made of dressings, bandages, and stockinette fastened at the wrist with adhesive tape may be used. Mittens usually upset patients less than arm restraints, since with mittens they can move their arms freely. The fingers should be separated with gauze to prevent skin irritation and should be curled around a large bandage roll in the palm to prevent hyperextension of the fingers. The hand is then well covered with dressings held in place with a bandage. A piece of stockinette is closed at one end and everted so that the tied end cannot cause injury to the eye. It is then slipped over the bandaged hand and fastened securely at the wrist with adhesive tape. The wrist should be shaved and the skin protected with tincture of benzoin before adhesive is used. At least every other day the mitten must be removed, the hand washed in warm water, and passive exercise given to the fingers before the mitten is reapplied.

Ventricular drainage

Occasionally, a catheter is placed in a ventricle of the brain to drain excess spinal fluid and prevent increased ICP. The catheter is usually attached to a drainage system (Fig. 35-10). The collection bottle is frequently attached to the bed. The tubing and drainage receptacle should be sterile, and care must be taken to prevent kinking of the tubing. If drainage seems to stop, the neurosurgeon should be notified. The catheter is usually left in place for 24 to 48 hours and is then removed by the surgeon.

Head dressings

Usually the wound is covered with gauze dressings, and a special head dressing (neurosurgical roll) is then applied in a recurrent fashion from the back to the front of the head and anchored (Fig. 35-11). The head *dressing* is inspected regularly for amount and type of drain-

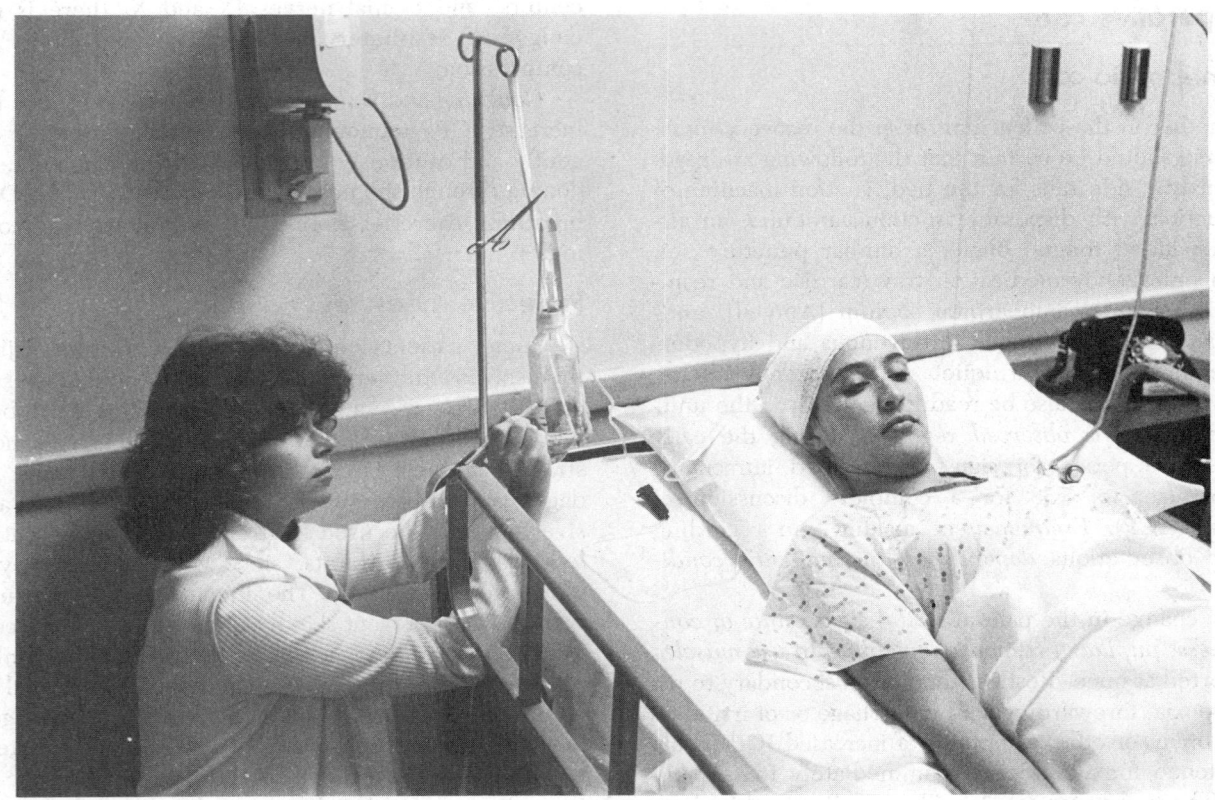

Fig. 35-10. Intraventricular drainage system. Nurse marking amount of drainage bottle. Lowering of bottle increases amount of cerebrospinal fluid removed; raising of bottle decreases amount of cerebrospinal fluid removed.

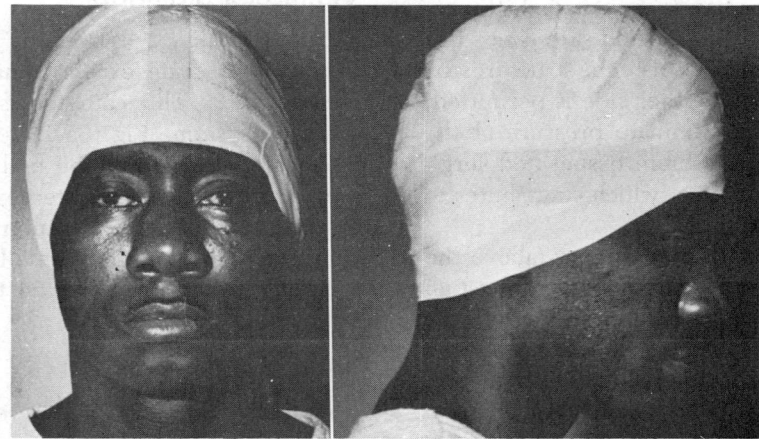

Fig. 35-11. Typical head dressing for patient who has had supratentorial craniotomy. (From Conway, B.L.: Carini and Owens' neurological and neurosurgical nursing, ed. 7, St. Louis, 1978, The C.V. Mosby Co.

age. Serosanguineous drainage on the dressings should be measured and marked, as is done with other dressings, so that it can be accurately checked for an increase in amount. Yellowish drainage should be reported immediately to the physician because it probably indicates loss of spinal fluid. If the head dressing appears to be soaked with drainage, the dressing should be reinforced. It may be necessary to apply a pressure dressing. Dressings that become wet should be removed by the neurosurgeon and replaced. It is not unusual for dressings to be removed the day after surgery and the incision left open to the air.

Fluids and food

Fluid intake and output should be accurately recorded. Fluids can be resumed when the person has good bowel sounds, is awake enough to swallow, and has a stable neurologic status. If there are no orders to the contrary, 2500 to 3000 ml of fluid should be given each day. Some neurosurgeons routinely restrict fluids to 1500 ml/day for the first 3 days after a craniotomy.

Since the gag and swallowing reflexes may be depressed or absent after *infratentorial* brain surgery, fluids by mouth are usually withheld for at least a day and intravenous fluids are substituted. They should be run very slowly to prevent increased ICP. If reflexes are present, water is carefully given by mouth. The patient should be placed in a semisitting position. Fluid should never be forced on a patient who is still neurologically depressed because of the danger of aspiration. If after several days the gag and swallowing reflexes are still absent, a nasogastric tube may be inserted. A regular diet is given to all neurosurgical patients as soon as it can be tolerated.

Elimination

Care must be taken to see that the patient voids sufficiently. Urinary output must be carefully recorded, and the specific gravity of most specimens should be measured. Sometimes an indwelling catheter may be used for a few days following surgery. A *decrease* in output must be reported, since it may indicate the onset of a metabolic disorder of central nervous system origin. Correspondingly, an increase in output with low specific gravities should also be reported for it may herald the onset of *diabetes insipidus*. Although this condition occurs most frequently after hypophysectomy for pituitary tumor, it can also occur following trauma to the head or intracranial surgery (especially involving the area near the pituitary).

Since most patients who have intracranial surgery will be on some type of steroids, it is important to test the urine for sugar and acetone. Patients who develop diabetes mellitus as a sequela of steroid treatment may require active treatment of the diabetes until the steroids are discontinued.

Laxatives or stool softeners should be used liberally to prevent constipation and straining while defecating. The patient should be instructed not to strain (p. 758). Bowel function should be monitored by the nurse to prevent fecal impaction. If an impaction does develop, enemas or manual evacuation may be necessary. Suppositories may also be used after the initial postoperative period to promote bowel regularity.

Comfort

Patients who are conscious after intracranial surgery may complain of a severe *headache* for 24 to 48 hours. Central nervous system depressants, such as opiates and sedatives, are avoided. Codeine sulfate is often prescribed and is given parenterally. Acetylsalicylic acid (aspirin) or acetaminophen (Tylenol) may be given by rectum, or by mouth if fluids can be swallowed. An ice cap may be placed on the head, and sudden movement and jarring are avoided. The patient should be protected from loud noises and bright lights. The patient may need assistance with turning and other activities of daily living.

Ambulation

The patient who has had surgery for a *supratentorial* lesion usually is allowed out of bed on the second to third postoperative day. If the surgery was extensive or complications develop, bed rest may be prescribed for longer periods. Activity is increased gradually, and the patient is watched carefully for signs of increased intracranial pressure. First the head of the bed should be elevated to high Fowler's position, and then the patient should sit on the edge of the bed with the feet dangling over the side. If this is tolerated, 4 to 6 hours later, with the help of two persons, the patient may be assisted to a chair and usually may sit up for a half hour. It is important to check the patient for postural hypotension while beginning progressive activity. Any drop in blood pressure of more than 20 points or complaints of dizziness by the patient should delay ambulation for several hours before another attempt is made. Patients then progress to normal activity as quickly as they desire and are able. The patient who has had surgery for an *infratentorial* lesion usually is not permitted up for a much longer period of time. The trend is toward getting up earlier, depending on the patient's condition. Initial progress may be slower, since patient's who have been kept flat in bed for some time may be dizzy and experience orthostatic hypotension when arising until the circulatory system readjusts to the change in position.

Head care after wound healing

When the final dressings are removed, the scalp can be gently cleansed with hydrogen peroxide to remove dried blood. Crusts can be loosened with mineral oil.

Patients are usually advised to wait 7 to 10 days after the surgery before the head is shampooed. A head covering is usually worn to protect the wound, to help remind the patient not to scratch, and for cosmetic reasons until the hair has grown back. A cap can be made by tying one end of a 10-in. piece of tubular stockinette. Head scarves or wigs are usually preferred by women, and wigs can also be worn by men. Many patients prefer to wear the disposable paper caps like those worn by the operating room staff. The patient who has had a piece of bone left out will have a depression in the scalp, and should be warned of the danger of bumping the head in this area.

Complications

Meningitis is a relatively rare complication of brain surgery; it can follow infection intraoperatively or postoperatively. Following supratentorial surgery, the nurse should watch for any clear, watery drainage from the nose. This drainage may be present if there has been a tear in the meninges, which causes subsequent loss of cerebrospinal fluid. The treatment consists of keeping the patient very quiet, avoiding suctioning the nose or blowing it, and administration of appropriate antibiotics. The leakage usually subsides spontaneously. Because of the danger of causing damage that might be followed by the drainage of cerebrospinal fluid through the nose, many surgeons request that the nose never be suctioned when supratentorial surgery has been performed. A sign with this caution may be placed at the head of the bed.

Respiratory collapse may follow infratentorial surgery. It is caused by edema of the brain stem or edema above the brain stem that causes herniation of the brain stem into the foramen magnum and pressure on the respiratory center. Any irregularity of respiration, dyspnea, or cyanosis should be reported at once. Equipment should be ready for administering oxygen, doing a ventricular tap, and inserting an endotracheal tube if one is not already present. (For details of nursing care of the patient with an endotracheal tube, see p. 1228.) Occasionally a respirator is used (p. 1244).

Convulsions are not unusual after a craniotomy, and therefore side rails should be used even if the patient is unconscious and it is believed that movement is not possible. Phenytoin sodium (Dilantin) is often ordered prophylactically to prevent convulsions. It *should not* be given intramuscularly because of its poor absorption via this route. If the patient has a history of seizures before the operation or if convulsions occurred in the postoperative period, this drug may be given for several months.

Loss of the corneal reflex may follow brain tumors or brain surgery. If the eye appears inflamed or if the patient does not seem to blink when objects approach the open eye, the neurosurgeon should be notified. Special eye care such as that given to patients who have had cerebrovascular accidents or who have had surgery for trigeminal neuralgia may be necessary (p. 829).

The patient may complain of *diplopia* after brain surgery. This condition is often temporary, and the patient should know that it will probably improve. It can be relieved by placing an opaque eye shield over one eye. The eye covered usually is alternated each day to prevent atrophy of eye muscles through disuse.

Planning with the patient's family

Few illnesses tax the entire physical and emotional resources of the patient's family as do the chronic neurologic diseases. It is imperative that the family participate in long-term plans for the patient. Members of the family may have severe emotional reactions and difficulties in adjustment that may require the assistance of specially trained persons such as a psychiatrist. Both the patient and family need time to work through their feelings. Sometimes the enormity of the significance of the diagnosis cannot be grasped for weeks or even months by either the patient or family members. Toxic polyneuritis in a young husband and father and multiple sclerosis in a young mother are examples of problems of such magnitude that long-term plans cannot be made quickly.

If the patient with neurologic disease has marked personality changes, aphasia, or convulsions, the family may even be afraid of the patient. Because the family is unaware that the patient may fully understand what is being said, they may make tactless remarks in front of the patient. When the patient is admitted to the hospital, it is often desirable to take the family aside to ascertain their insight into the situation. This interview provides an opportunity to help interpret the patient's actions and responses so that the family may better understand and be more supportive of the patient. See Chapter 29 for more information about the general care of persons with prolonged illness.

REFERENCES AND SELECTED READINGS
Contemporary

1. Adams, R.D., and Victor, M.: Principles of neurology, New York, 1977, McGraw-Hill Book Co.
2. *Belt, L.H.: Working with dysphasic patients, Am. J. Nurs. 74:1320-1322, 1974.

---

*References preceded by an asterisk are particularly well suited for student reading.

3. Benson, V.M., et al.: Traumatic cerebral edema, Arch. Neurol. **23**:179-186, 1970.
4. *Blount, M., and Kinney, A.B.: Neurological and neurosurgical nursing, Nurs. Clin. North Am. **9**:591-772, 1974.
5. Boroch, R.M.: Elements of rehabilitation in nursing: an introduction, St. Louis, 1976, The C.V. Mosby Co.
6. Bowman, W.C., and Rand, M.J.: Textbook of pharmacology, ed. 2, London, 1980, Blackwell Scientific Publications, Ltd.
7. *Conway, B.L.: Carini and Owens' neurological and neurosurgical nursing, ed. 8, St. Louis, 1982, The C.V. Mosby Co.
8. Daly, B.J.: Intensive care nursing, Garden City, N.Y., 1980, Medical Exam Publishing Co., Inc.
9. *Dayhoff, N.: Rethinking stroke: soft or hard devices to position hands, Am. J. Nurs. **75**:1142-1144, 1975.
10. *Delehanty, L., and Stravino, V.: Achieving bladder control, Am. J. Nurs. **70**:312-316, 1970.
11. Erry, M.: Spasticity: the nursing management, Aust. Nurs. J. **10**:43-44, 1981.
12. Hahn, A.B., Barkin, R.L., and Oestreich, J.K.: Pharmacology in nursing, ed. 15, St. Louis, 1982, The C.V. Mosby Co.
13. *Hoskins, L.M.: Vascular and tension headaches, Am. J. Nurs. **74**:848-851, 1974.
14. *Hughes, M.T.: Neuroradiology: a subspecialty, J. Neurosurg. Nurs. **4**:83-85, 1972.
15. *Jimm, L.R., Nursing assessment of patients for increased intracranial pressure, J. Neurosurg. Nurs. **6**(1):27-38, July 1974.
16. *Johnson, M., and Quinn, J.: The subarachnoid screw, Am. J. Nurs. **77**:448-450, 1977.
17. Jones, S.: Glasgow coma scale, Am. J. Nurs. **79**:1551-1554, 1979.
18. Loebel, S., et al.: The nurses' drug handbook, ed. 2, New York, 1980, John Wiley & Sons, Inc.
19. *Loetterle, B.C., et al.: Cerebellar stimulation: pacing the brain, Am. J. Nurs. **75**:958-969, 1975.
20. MacLeod, I.: Information processing aids for physically handicapped people, Aust. Nurs. J. **10**:46-53, 1981.
21. Maus, P., and Mitchell, P.: Increased intracranial pressure: an update, Heart Lung **5**:916-926, 1976.
22. Merritt, H.H.: A textbook of neurology, ed. 6, Philadelphia, 1979, Lea & Febiger.
23. Mitchell, P.: Intracranial hypertension: implications of research for nursing care, J. Neurosurg. Nurs. **12**:145-154, 1980.
24. Mitchell, P., and Maus, P.: Relating of patients nursing activities to intracranial pressure variation: a pilot study, Nurs. Res. **27**:4-10, 1978.
25. Mitchell, P., and Mauss, N.: Intracranial pressure: fact and fancy, Nurs. '76 **6**(6):53-57, 1976.
26. Mitchell, P., Ozwna, J., and Lipe, H.: Moving the patient in bed: effects on intracranial pressure, Nurs. Res. **30**:212-218, 1981.
27. Plum, F., and Posner, J.B.: The diagnosis of stupor and coma, ed. 3, Philadelphia, 1980, F.A. Davis Co.
28. Reinisch, E.S.: Quick assessment for hemiplegic's functioning, Am. J. Nurs. **81**:102-104, 1981.
29. Schow, R.L., et al.: Communication disorders of the aged, Baltimore, 1978, University Park Press.
30. Speers, I.: Cerebral edema, J. Neurosurg. Nurs. **13**:102-115, 1981.
31. *Stryker, R.P.: Rehabilitative aspects of acute and chronic nursing care, New York, 1977, W.B. Saunders Co.
32. Stubbins, J.: Social and psychological aspects of disability: a handbook for practitioners, Baltimore, 1977, University Park Press.
33. Swift, N., and Mabel, R.M.: Manual of neurological nursing, Boston, 1978, Little, Brown & Co.
34. Teasdale, G., et al.: Assessment of coma and impaired consciousness: a practical guide, Lancet **2**:81-84, 1974.
35. Terzian, M.: Neurosurgical intervention for the management of chronic intractable pain, Top. Clin. Nurs. **1**:75-88, 1980.
36. Vick, N., et al.: Grinker's neurology, ed. 7, Springfield, Ill., 1976, Charles C Thomas, Publisher.
37. West, B.: Understanding endorphins: our natural pain relief system, Nurs. '81 **11**(2):50-53, 1981.
38. Williams, A.: A study of factors contributing to skin breakdown, Nurs. Res. **21**:238-343, 1972.
39. Williams-Kurkland, T.E., and Berne, R.: Neurological aspects of rehabilitation. II. Spinal cord injury, Am. Rehabil. J. **8**:8-17, 1980.
40. Wing, S.: Cervical spine injuries: treatment and related nursing care, J. Neurosurg. Nurs. **9**:138-140, 1977.
41. Wintrobe, M.M., editor: Harrison's principles of internal medicine, ed. 8, New York, 1977, McGraw-Hill Book Co.
42. Young, M.S.: A bedside guide to understanding the signs of intracranial pressure, Nurs. '81 **11**:59-62, 1981.

Classic

43. Blinderman, E.E., Graf, C.J., and Fitzpatrick, T.: Basic studies in cerebral edema, J. Neurosurg. **19**:319-324, 1962.
44. Kety, S., et al.: The effects of increased intracranial pressure on cerebral circulatory functions in man, J. Clin. Invest. **27**:493-496, 1948.
45. *King, I.M., guest editor: Symposium on neurologic and neurosurgical nursing, Nurs. Clin. North Am. **4**:199-283, 1969.
46. Silverstein, A.: Arteriography of stroke, Arch. Neurol. **12**:387-389, 1965.

CHAPTER 36

PROBLEMS OF THE NERVOUS SYSTEM

MARJORIE KINNEY
ELIZABETH SCHENK

The neurologic problems selected for inclusion in this chapter are the ones most closely associated with the common clinical neurologic manifestations presented in Chapter 35. The problems are categorized for discussion both from a broad pathologic standpoint and from the standpoint of the anatomic site of the neural lesion.

Discussion of each problem includes pathophysiologic explanation and the assessment, interventive, and evaluative aspects of patient care specific to the problem.

Convulsive disorders: epilepsy

Epilepsy (convulsive disorders) is one of the oldest diseases known to humans. It was described in detail by Hippocrates, as well as being described in the Bible. It has come to be defined as "seizure" or "cetate." (For purposes of this discussion the terms *epilepsy, seizure disorder*, and *convulsive disorder* will be used interchangeably.) At one time epilepsy was thought to be of divine origin, and perhaps for this reason it has been linked in the public mind with the occult, the strange, and the unmentionable. No disease has been more carefully concealed within families, and many attitudes toward the disease have persisted from early times to the present. Attitudes may also be affected (1) by the sometimes frightening experience of seeing a person during a severe seizure, (2) by the belief that mental deterioration always occurs in epilepsy, and (3) by the fact that the tendency to develop epilepsy may be inherited.

Etiology

Epilepsy may be defined as a transitory disturbance in consciousness or in motor, sensory, or autonomic function (with or without loss of consciousness) caused by uncontrolled electrical discharges in the brain. Seizures as a sign and symptom are of particular significance in neurologic diseases. They occur in many childhood and adult illnesses. They may result from cerebral anoxia, hypoglycemia, disturbances of calcium balance, electrolyte imbalances, disturbance in hydration, injection of drugs and poisons with convulsive activity, infections that produce high temperature elevations, and numerous metabolic disturbances and disorders. In many individuals with epilepsy, a localized organic lesion serves as the focus for the abnormal neuronal discharges from the damaged brain tissues. The organic lesions include neoplasms, inflamed areas or abscesses, sclerosis, vascular formations or hematomas, congenital malformations, trauma, or other space-occupying lesions. Quite often the lesion is microscopic in size and is related to trauma at birth or scars from infantile or childhood infections. Seizures may also be caused by generalized inflammatory and degenerative brain diseases. Seizures that may be hysterical in origin are not considered true seizure disorders.

The role of heredity in the causation of epilepsy has not been completely clarified. The disease is not directly inherited, although abnormal brain waves, as shown on the EEG, are found in many relatives of persons who have seizures.[28]

Incidence

The incidence of epilepsy is probably 1 in every 200 to 300 persons. This means that more than 1 million persons in the United States are subject to seizures.

Seizures occur in all races and affect males and females equally. There seems to be no geographic distribution. Epilepsy begins at any age, but many persons have seizures before 20 years of age. The life expectancy of persons with seizures is somewhat less than that for the population as a whole because the person often dies of an accident incurred during a seizure.

Pathophysiology

Convulsions or seizures are brief cerebral storms. These are associated with sudden, excessive, disorderly electrical discharges in the neurons of the brain. The patterns or forms of seizures vary and are dependent on the area of the brain from which the seizure arises. The pattern is stereotyped in the individual, although variations may occur with progression of the cerebral lesion. Seizures can involve essentially all parts of the brain at once, as in the generalized type, or only a minute focal spot. In the former, the excessive neuronal discharges are thought to originate in the brain stem portion of the reticular activating system; these then spread throughout the central nervous system including the cortex and the deeper parts of the brain. The process may last from a few seconds to as long as 3 to 5 minutes, or it may stop immediately as in a *petit mal seizure*. It is not known what stops the seizure at a given time, but it is believed to result from fatigue of the neurons involved in precipitating the seizure or by inhibition of certain structures within the brain. Focally, the excessive neuronal discharges may result in a *tonic convulsion*, with the contraction of all muscles at once, or a *clonic convulsion*, with alternate contraction and relaxation of opposing muscle groups and characteristic jerking movements of the body. The seizure, regardless of origin or type, is always inappropriate to the immediate situation. It is followed by an inhibition of cerebral function, the length of which may last longer than the seizure itself. The inhibition of function is often incomplete and depends on the area of the brain from which the seizure arises.

Assessment

Types of seizure. There are numerous ways to classify seizures, and this causes confusion. One common way to classify seizures is the International Classification of Epileptic Seizures. In this classification, seizures are identified as partial (beginning locally), generalized (bilaterally symmetric and with no local onset), unilateral, or unclassified.[28]

Most experts find it useful to classify seizures based on the clinical features of the attack. Thus they can be classified into five large groups, depending on their severity and nature. These are (1) *grand mal* (major or generalized), (2) *petit mal*, (3) *psychomotor*, (4) *jacksonian and focal*, and (5) *miscellaneous*. This classification of seizures is not pure. Some varieties (although rare) may not fall into the above classifications.

GRAND MAL SEIZURES. The *grand mal seizure* is by far the most common and dramatic type. It is generalized and is characterized by a loss of consciousness for several minutes (variable) and tonic and clonic convulsions (motor activity). The clinical course or sequence is the *aura, cry, loss of consciousness, the fall, tonic and clonic convulsions,* and *incontinence*.

The symptoms that occur during the prodrome are called an *aura*. Prodromal symptoms occur in about 50% of all patients and usually include a change in sensation or a change in affect. The exact character of the aura varies from person to person but may include numbness, flashing lights, dizziness, tingling of the arm, smells, or spots before the eyes. The patient may find it difficult to describe the aura precisely, but it gives conclusive warning of an impending seizure. The specific warning serves a useful purpose in that it enables the individual to seek safety and privacy before the onset of the seizure. Occasionally, it occurs as much as a day before the seizure, so that the individual who works can remain at home and fellow workers may not know of the attacks. The aura really represents the "local signature" of the attack and is the result of an abnormal stimulation of the cortical area. Almost at the same time that loss of consciousness occurs there is the so-called *epileptic cry*. It is caused by spasms of the thoracic and abdominal muscles expelling air through the glottis. Another type of cry results from an inspiratory effort and sounds like the scream of a parrot. The loss of consciousness is sudden and variable in duration. It usually lasts several minutes.

The individual slumps or falls, depending on the position at the time. This is followed immediately by bilateral tonic contraction of all muscles; the legs are extended and the arms are flexed; jaws are clenched and the tongue is frequently caught between the teeth; the eyes roll upward and pupils dilate and become fixed. There is cessation of respiration, and cyanosis occurs. The tonic spasms may occasionally be so violent that a joint, such as the shoulder, hip, or temporomandibular, is dislocated. Fractures may also result. As the tonic phase ends, it is replaced by a series of clonic contractions. As the clonic movements continue, the contractions become stronger. Breathing returns and is shallow and irregular at first. There is often frothing at the mouth, which may be streaked with blood if the tongue and lips have been bitten during the convulsion. Fecal or urinary incontinence often occurs during the clonic phase or earlier. As the clonic phase subsides within a few minutes, there is relaxation of muscles. Partial consciousness is regained and color improves.

During the *postictal* (postseizure) *period* the individual appears groggy and confused. Complaints of headache or muscular pain are common. A deep sleep usually follows. During this phase the pupils may remain dilated and there may be abnormal plantar reflexes. After a variable period of time the patient awakens and is frequently unaware of the occurrence of the seizure. A dull headache and depression are common. It is possible that the depression is caused in part by knowledge that a seizure has occurred.

General fatigue may last 1 or 2 days. In addition to the injuries that may occur, the violent activity during a grand mal seizure may result in ruptures of blood vessels with the production of corneal and subconjunctival hemorrhages.

Seizures occur during sleep in some individuals. In such instances the occurrence of the seizure is known on awakening by the presence of blood on the pillow or by soiled linen from fecal or urinary incontinence.

PETIT MAL SEIZURES. Petit mal seizures are characterized by a sudden impairment in or loss of consciousness with little or no tonic-clonic movement. They usually occur without warning, and the arrest of voluntary activity is very brief, usually 10 to 20 seconds. The attacks have a tendency to appear a few hours after arising or when the person is quiet. In the classic petit mal seizure there is a sudden vacant facial expression with the eyes focused straight ahead. All motor activities cease except perhaps for a slight symmetric twitching about the eyelids or of the face and arms, or a loss of muscle tone. Consciousness returns as quickly as it left, and the individual may resume speaking at the point interrupted, unaware that the seizure occurred. The individual may learn to recognize when a few seconds of time have been lost. Petit mal seizures usually occur many times a day and have no aura, falling, or tonic and clonic phases.

This type of seizure usually occurs during childhood and adolescence, particularly at the time of puberty. The frequency of the episodes usually diminishes as the child grows older. Although petit mal seizures do not have the dramatic and frightening aspects of grand mal seizures, they are disconcerting, and the momentary loss of consciousness presents safety problems.

PSYCHOMOTOR SEIZURES. Psychomotor seizures are more complex and bizarre than either grand mal or petit mal seizures. They can occur at any age and are characterized by a sudden change in awareness or consciousness, associated with a complex distortion of feeling and thinking and partially coordinated motor activity. Any aura present is usually a complex hallucination or illusion. The length of the seizure is longer than that of petit mal. Persons with these seizures often behave as though they were partially conscious and do antisocial things such as exposing themselves or committing acts of violence. They often appear intoxicated. Talking with them during this type of seizure shows that they are out of contact with their environment. Smacking of the lips and chewing movements may take place. Visceral symptoms with autonomic complaints of chest pain, respiratory distress, tachycardia, urinary incontinence,

and gastrointestinal distress may also occur. Abnormal smell and taste sensations are common.

These persons are likely to be confused and amnesic for a period of time and often fall asleep at the end of the seizure activity. A relationship has been found between psychomotor epilepsy and lesions in the temporal lobe of the brain. Because of the crimes that may occur during this type of seizure, the diagnosis is of interest not only to physicians but to law enforcement officials, lawyers, and judges, as well.

FOCAL, OR JACKSONIAN, SEIZURES. Focal, or jacksonian, seizures are those that arise initially in the motor or sensory areas of the brain adjacent to the rolandic fissure or any localized part of the cerebral cortex. These seizures occur almost entirely in patients with structural brain disease and often occur as a symptom in persons with brain tumor, vascular malformations, scars, or infections. The clinical manifestations seen in this type of seizure are thus dependent on the site of the focus and differ from the generalized motor seizure (grand mal). If, for example, the abnormal neuronal discharge is initiated in the *precentral* or *motor region* of the cortex for the thumb, the individual will experience a tonic contracture of the thumb muscles. If the abnormal neuronal discharge spreads to adjacent parts of the motor strip, there is progressive involvement of associated musculature with a progression (march) of movements from thumb to hand, arm, face, and so forth. The discharge may or may not progress. The localized seizure that does spread progressively to other muscles following initiation is known as a *jacksonian seizure*. Focal motor seizures commonly begin in the hand, face, and foot but may arise in any part of the motor strip. The seizure may end in a shower of clonic movements, or it may end in a generalized convulsion. Consciousness is retained unless the opposite half of the body is involved. When abnormal neuronal discharges arise in the lower part of the motor strip, which controls salivation and mastication, seizures are then manifested by chewing, smacking of the lips, and swallowing movements. Salivation may be profuse. Other seizures may begin with a forced turning of the head and eyes. Such attacks are termed *adversive* and originate in the eye-turning fields of the brain; the head turns away from the side of the lesion, or focus. When the abnormal neuronal discharges arise in the *postcentral*, or *sensory, strip,* of the cortex, the seizure is initiated with complaints of disturbed sensations such as a numbness, tingling, prickling, or crawling feeling, and as in a focal motor seizure a march of sensations may or may not occur. The neuronal discharge may also spread from the sensory area to the motor area.

• • • •

The category of miscellaneous seizures includes many different types, a few of which are described here.

MYOCLONIC SEIZURES. Myoclonic seizures are characterized by the sudden involuntary contraction of a muscle group, usually in the extremities or trunk. These contractions may be very mild, or they may result in rapid, forceful movement of the part. There is no loss of consciousness. Some experts see myoclonus as a variant of petit mal seizures. The myoclonus may be found in some petit mal conditions. Myoclonus will sometimes antedate grand mal seizures by months or years.

AKINETIC SEIZURES. Akinetic seizures are characterized by a peculiar generalized tonelessness. There is rarely an aura, but the person falls in a flaccid state and is unconscious for a moment or two. Recovery comes quickly and the person is not postictal.

Status epilepticus. When recurrent generalized seizure activity occurs at such frequency that full consciousness is not regained between seizures, it is referred to as *status epilepticus*. Although this condition is relatively rare, it can lead to death from brain damage secondary to prolonged hypoxia and exhaustion. Status epilepticus is a medical emergency requiring intensive medical and nursing care.

The person with status epilepticus is often in a coma for a period of 12 to 24 hours or longer, during which time there are recurring seizures. The seizures may cease spontaneously and consciousness return, or death may result from the repeated attacks. The attack usually is related to failure to take prescribed medication. Vigorous therapy is thus directed toward arrest of the seizures. The first priority is ensuring an adequate airway, which may be compromised by the seizure and complications of certain drug therapy. Endotracheal tubes, a laryngoscope, aspirating equipment, and oxygen should be in the patient unit before administration of medications. This is important because the large drug dosages and the type of drugs used often lead to pulmonary complications. Drug therapy is given intravenously. Medications commonly used include sodium phenobarbital, diazepam (Valium), phenytoin (Dilantin), and paraldehyde. Results appear to be best from large or full (not divided) therapeutic dosages. Medications are stopped if respiratory depression occurs or mechanical ventilation is started. At times it may be necessary to give a general anesthetic. Oxygen may be used to counter the effects of cerebral anoxia. Solutions of glucose may be ordered to treat dehydration.

Constant monitoring of vital signs of respiratory depression and cardiac changes is necessary. The responsibilities pertaining to the observation and recording of seizure activity are the same as described on p. 784. It may not be possible to note the separate seizure phases because of the frequency of them. A safe, quiet, and nonstimulating environment is essential. The head of the bed should be lowered and the patient turned to a side-lying position to lessen the danger of aspiration during seizures; padded side rails should be in place.

Intervention

The treatment of persons with seizures is based on a careful study of the person to detect any remedial lesion or metabolic cause. When these have been eliminated or treated, care is then directed toward the prevention of seizures. Only rarely will the elimination of causative factors result in the complete disappearance of seizures. There is no known cure for idiopathic epilepsy, although seizures can be controlled by anticonvulsive drugs and the regulation of mental and physical hygiene. The period of treatment is years or a lifetime for the majority of patients.

The nurse has responsibilities in the diagnostic, therapeutic, and instructional programs of persons with known seizures. The community health nurse and the clinic nurse will work with selected persons with seizures for extended periods. The person and family need to learn what to do during and after a seizure, to assume responsibility for drug therapy, and to recognize the need to seek assistance when side effects and toxic effects occur.

Care during a seizure. The primary goals of the nurse and family caring for a person having a seizure are protection from injury and observation and recording of the seizure activity. The person should never be left alone. If the person is in an upright position when a generalized motor seizure begins, he or she is lowered to the floor or a bed and adjacent articles and equipment are moved away to prevent injury during uncontrolled body movements. Constricting clothing is loosened, especially about the neck. The head should be turned to the side to allow the tongue to fall forward so that it does not occlude the airway. *No effort should be made to restrain the person either manually or with restraints.* Attempting to resist body movements of a person in grand mal seizure may result in injury to bones and soft tissues. It is best to permit the person as much range of motion as possible without injury to self. Padded side rails are helpful for the person confined to bed and for individuals who have a pattern of seizures during sleep. Pillows should not be used for padding, since there is some danger from suffocation. If the person is lying on the floor or ground, all articles that can be struck during the seizure are moved. Something soft, such as a piece of clothing (sweater, jacket, etc.), should be placed under the person's head if possible. *If the jaws are not already clenched* at the time when first observed, a padded tongue blade or rubber wedge may be inserted between the back teeth to prevent injury to the tongue and mouth tissues. At the same time care must be taken to avoid pushing the tongue back and occluding the airway. In many instances the jaws and teeth are already clenched and efforts to insert a tongue blade or any nearby substitute may damage the teeth and gums. The idea that one should pry the mouth open and insert a tongue blade or other object has been overemphasized and can be dangerous. A judgment needs to be made about whether it is better to insert something, depending on the phase of the seizure and the condition of the person. It is the policy of many hospital nursing services that a padded tongue blade be kept at the patient's bedside when seizures are anticipated. It is less disturbing to the patient if the tongue blade is placed in the drawer of the bedside cabinet rather than being taped to the bed. A single oral airway may also be kept at the bedside along with other emergency equipment if the severity of seizures and the condition of the patient warrant it.

Accurate observation of the seizure (see box at right) from the beginning, when possible, is important because it provides needed information that may assist the physician in locating the site or focus of a cerebral lesion. It is more important to describe the seizure activity, sequence, and where it started than it is to name or classify the seizure.

When a person with known seizure activity is admitted to the hospital for diagnosis or reevaluation, it is important for the nurse to obtain a history of the pattern of seizure activity, the frequency and time of day, whether an aura is present, any precipitating factors, and any seizure characteristics. In this way nursing interventions can be planned more specifically. Admission of a person with known seizures who is undergoing treatment provides the nurse an opportunity to evaluate the person's understanding of the cause of the seizures and the prescribed therapy.

Mental health. From the standpoint of mental health, the individual with seizures should use all resources to cope with feelings of self-consciousness and inferiority resulting from attacks. Adults should be encouraged to lead normal productive lives. Children should be kept in school unless the frequency of attacks disturbs the activities of the classroom. Family members need to be assisted to discuss their attitudes and feelings about the individual's illness. Excessive attention to the overprotection of the person with seizures is to be avoided. The family needs understand the problems resulting from seizures and the prescribed therapy but should not make a chronic invalid of the person.

Activities of daily living. Since most persons with seizures are without symptoms between attacks and a majority of seizures can be controlled by medication, the person with seizures should be encouraged to lead as normal a life as possible. The person should not be made to feel that he or she is a chronic invalid. With treatment the person can live a useful, normal, and happy life. Until seizures are controlled the person should avoid dangerous activities such as driving a car, working on or about machinery, or swimming. Once the seizures are controlled with medications and the person has learned the importance of taking the medication regularly and avoiding alcoholic beverages these restrictions

---

OBSERVATIONS TO BE MADE ABOUT A PERSON HAVING A SEIZURE

Aura	Presence or absence; nature if present; ability of patient to describe it (somatic, visceral, psychic)
Cry	Presence or absence
Onset	Site of initial body movements; deviation of head and eyes; chewing and salivation; posture of body; sensory changes.
Tonic and clonic phases	Movements of body as to progression; skin color and airway; pupillary changes; incontinence; duration of each phase
Relaxation (sleep)	Duration and behavior
Postictal phase	Duration; general behavior; ability to remember anything about the seizure; orientation; pupillary changes; headache; injuries present
Duration of entire seizure	
Level of consciousness	Length of unconsciousness if present

---

can be relaxed. Achieving adequate rest and nutritional intake is also important.

The issue of driving a car is one that often poses a problem. Epilsepsy is one condition that imposes driver limitations. Usually, a waiting period of 1 seizure-free year should elapse before the person is eligible to drive and then *only* if seizures are completely controlled.

No special diet is needed for persons with a seizure disorder, unless mandated by the side effects of medications. The use of alcohol should be avoided, however. The person should be taught the importance of good mouth care if on long-term phenytoin (Dilantin) therapy because gingival hyperplasia is a common side effect.

Anticonvulsant therapy. Success in the prevention of seizures in persons under treatment is to a great extent dependent on the skill of the neurologist in selecting the type of anticonvulsant medication to be used and the regulation of dosage. The choice of medications depends on the type of seizure. The person and family must understand the importance of taking the prescribed drugs on schedule and in the correct dose. Anticonvulsant medications act generally on the cerebral cortex and are not selective in acting on the part of the brain involved in abnormal neuronal discharges.

TABLE 36-1. Anticonvulsants used to prevent seizures

Drug	Use related to seizure type	Average daily dose	Toxic effects
Phenytoin sodium (Dilantin)	Grand mal, focal, psychomotor	0.4-0.6 g (divided dose)	Ataxia, vomiting, nystagmus, drowsiness, rash, fever, gum hypertrophy, lymphadenopathy
Phenobarbital (Luminal)	Grand mal, focal, psychomotor (adjunctive)	0.1-0.4 g (divided dose)	Drowsiness, rash
Primidone (Mysoline)	Grand mal, focal, psychomotor	0.5-2.0 g	Drowsiness, ataxia
Mephenytoin (Mesantoin)	Grand mal, focal, psychomotor	0.3-0.5 g	Ataxia, nystagmus, pancytopenia, rash
Ethosuximide (Zarontin)	Petit mal, psychomotor, myoclonic, akinetic	750-1500 mg	Drowsiness, nausea, agranulocytosis
Trimethadione (Tridione)	Petit mal	0.3-2.0 g (divided dose)	Rash, photophobia, agranulocytosis, nephrosis
Diazepam (Valium)	Status epilepticus, mixed	8-30 mg	Drowsiness, ataxia
Carbamazepine (Tegretol)	Grand mal, psychomotor	0.3-2.0 g	Rash, drowsiness, ataxia
Valproic acid (Depakene)	Petit mal, absence of seizures	5-35 mg/kg body weight (at least tid dosage)	Nausea, vomiting, indigestion, sedation, emotional disturbance, weakness, altered blood coagulation
Clonazepam (Clonopin)	Petit mal, akinetic, myoclonic	5-20 g	Grand mal seizures, drowsiness, ataxia, hypotension, respiratory depression

There are currently many medications that can be used to prevent the occurrence of grand mal and petit mal seizures and to a lesser extent psychomotor seizures in a high percentage of individuals. Selected commonly used anticonvulsant medications as related to seizure types are listed in Table 36-1 along with average daily dose and toxic effects. Drugs may be used singly or in combinations based on the response of the person. Highly refractory seizures may require several drugs in full therapeutic dosages. Phenytoin sodium (Dilantin) has the highest therapeutic index and is the drug of choice for grand mal seizures. When the seizure fails to respond to phenytoin sodium alone, either phenobarbital or primidone (Mysoline) or related drugs may be added; in refractory seizures all three drugs may be utilized. The same three drugs are also often used in combination with psychomotor seizures, but the seizures are not so readily controlled as are grand mal seizures. Carbamazepine (Tegretol) appears to hold some promise in controlling psychomotor seizures. Ethosuximide (Zarontin) and trimethadione (Tridione) are the drugs of choice in petit mal seizures. Valproic acid (Depakene) is a newer drug that is used to treat petit mal seizures as well as mixed seizures. The dosages of anticonvulsant drugs are difficult to establish and regulate because of the high incidence of side effects and the toxicity of the drugs. The drug of choice is introduced in average therapeutic dosage and is increased in dosage until control is reached; if toxicity is reached before control of the seizures, the dosage is decreased to the previous non-

toxic or tolerated dosage. Additional secondary drugs are usually introduced at this point and increased similarly until control is obtained. It is important that convenient dosage schedules are established for the individual; dosage may be divided, with a smaller dose taken during the day and a larger dose taken during the evening.

Corticosteroids are used occasionally to treat myoclonus. Bromides are used less frequently than in the past and have been replaced to a great extent by the anticonvulsant drugs. Occasionally, a ketogenic diet may be prescribed for patients with petit mal seizures. The diet is not easy to follow, and the effectiveness of ethosuximide (Zarontin) has led to decline in its use.

Failure to take the prescribed medication or to take an adequate dose is frequently the cause of failure in treatment. Most medical centers have facilities to determine the level of drugs in the blood. This is helpful in providing an accurate check on the therapeutic and toxic levels of the medications taken by the patient, as well as to ascertain how well the person metabolizes the drug. Unfortunately, most medications that help to control seizures produce toxic effects. It should be recognized that effects on the kidneys and bone marrow can be serious. The individual must remain under medical supervision in order to regulate the medications and to make changes as necessary. Persons with seizures often engage in wishful thinking once control is reached and believe that they have outgrown their disease. They often think that they can omit the prescribed medication, since they have gone for some time without a seizure.[39]

Surgical treatment. Surgical treatment of seizures is becoming less frequent but may still be used in some cases when medical therapy is not effective. *Cortical resection* is one surgical approach. It involves removal of the brain tissue where the focus of electrical discharge is located. The localization of tissue must occur in a part of the brain that is easily accessible to surgery and that can be removed without leaving the person with a serious disability.

Another surgical approach involves *stereotactic procedures* using electrical stimulation. This technique is used in an attempt to interrupt the pathways of seizure activity, to destroy the foci, or to alter the actions of the cortical nerve cells.

Home care of the person with a convulsive disorder. Members of the family must learn to care for the person during and following a convulsion. They should be alert for accident hazards. One of the most important things for the family to learn is the need to be calm and accepting of the family member's seizures. They should attempt to prevent the person from engaging in activity that may be dangerous and keep him or her from exposure to curious persons during convulsions, but they should not contribute to the person's feelings that he or she is different from others.

Public attitudes. One of the most important aspects in epilepsy therapy is changing the public's attitude toward the disease. The individual subject to seizures and the public must view seizures not as bizarre catastrophies but as relatively normal events that can be dealt with rationally. Many persons with epilepsy lead normal productive lives. Indeed, many outstanding figures in world history had seizures (Julius Caesar, Lord Byron, and Napoleon). Studies do not bear out the popular assumption that mental deterioration occurs with epilepsy. Cognitive abilities vary among persons with epilepsy as with the population generally. Nor is there any evidence that personality changes are the result of pathologic processes; when they occur they are probably the result of society's attitude toward the person with epilepsy. For example, some people who are found to have epilepsy are immediately suspended from their work even when they are not dangerous to themselves or others. Some employers refuse to hire a person with known epilepsy, yet at least 80% of all persons with epilepsy are employable.

The Epilepsy Foundation of America has been active in trying to improve state laws regarding employment of persons with epilepsy. Children with epilepsy have been segregated to separate schools, and only recently have some major cities passed laws ensuring children with epilepsy the right to attend the public schools if they are under adequate medical care. In many schools children are barred from the classroom according to the inclination of the teacher. Limitation of environment and of education opportunity often limits the child's knowledge, but this does not mean that learning capacity is poor.

Interest in epilepsy and in the problems of the epileptic person has been increased by various organizations such as the National Association to Control Epilepsy, Inc.,* National Epilepsy League, Inc.,† Epilepsy Foundation of America,‡ and United Epilepsy Association.§

Outcome criteria for the person with known epilepsy or other convulsive disorders

The person or significant others can:
1. Explain any medications to be taken or treatment program to be carried out at home.
   a. Explain the action, side effects, toxic effects, and dosage schedule of each anticonvulsant drug prescribed.
   b. Explain the importance of taking the prescribed anticonvulsants regularly according to schedule even though seizures are controlled.
   c. Explain the need to seek medical assistance when side effects or toxic effects occur.
   d. Explain the incompatibility of anticonvulsant drugs with alcohol and drugs that counteract the anticonvulsants.
2. Explain activities of daily living to be followed.
   a. Explain the need to structure a balance between rest and activity.
   b. Explain the need to avoid excessive exercise, fatigue, and stress.
   c. Explain the importance of continuing usual activities within the above limitations when seizures are under control.
3. Explain how to secure professional and community resources necessary to structure a satisfactory home and work environment.
   a. List agencies that can be contacted.
   b. Explain how to secure legal counsel relative to state laws.
   c. State plans for follow-up care.

The significant others can:
1. Demonstrate seizure precautions to be followed during and after an attack or seizure.
   a. Demonstrate how to maintain an open airway so that aspiration and blockage of the airway by the tongue are prevented.
   b. Explain the importance of staying with the person during the attack for protection and to make observations.

---

*Headquarters: 22 East 67th St., New York, NY 10021.
†Headquarters: 203 Wabash St., Chicago, IL 60604.
‡Headquarters: 1828 L St., N.W., Washington, DC 20036.
§Headquarters: 113 West 57th St., New York, NY 10019.

c. Demonstrate how to loosen clothing around the neck and waist.

d. Explain the need to provide rest and to make observations after a seizure.

Degenerative diseases

The phrase *degenerative diseases* as used here refers to those neurologic diseases in which there is a premature senescence of nerve cells, there is a known or suspected metabolic disturbance, or the cause is unknown (see Table 36-2) for a comparison of these degenerative neurologic diseases).

Multiple sclerosis (disseminated sclerosis)

Epidemiology

Multiple sclerosis is a common neurologic disease in northern climates. The exact prevalence of this disease is not known, since in many instances the diagnosis is not made, but probably at least 500,000 persons in the United States are known to have multiple sclerosis. The onset of symptoms usually occurs between 20 and 40 years of age. The course of the disease estimated to be 12 to 25 years. Multiple sclerosis has serious implications for family life, since it affects both men and women equally in the active productive years when their responsibilities are greatest. Several studies have demonstrated that there seems to be an increased incidence of multiple sclerosis among siblings and even distant relatives. There has been no evidence found to suggest a conjugal relationship.

Etiology

During the past decade there have been major advances in the knowledge of the etiology, pathology, diagnosis, and treatment of multiple sclerosis. The etiology, however, remains unknown despite new findings and the numerous hypotheses that have been advanced as to cause. Mineral deficiency, toxic substances, disturbance of blood-clotting mechanism, viruses, and autoimmunity are a few of the causes studied. The latter two are currently the most favored. Experimental allergic encephalomyelitis has been produced in animals by the injection of the basic protein from a homologous neuron sheath.[71] Despite the resemblance to multiple sclerosis, it is not yet clear to what extent this disease represents a human model for multiple sclerosis. The recent discovery of slow viruses (those with a long latent period) in association with the frequent findings of an increase of gamma (γ-) globulin and immunoglobulin (IgG) in the spinal fluid of patients with multiple sclerosis gives support to these theories. What constitutes an elevation of γ-globulin or of IgG is not clear. Whether the γ-globulin and IgG get into the spinal fluid by transudation or by increased permeability of the blood-brain barrier is still controversial.

Pathophysiology

Multiple foci of demyelination are distributed randomly in the white matter of the brain stem, spinal cord, optic nerves, and cerebrum. During the demyelination process (primary degeneration) the myelin sheath and the sheath cells are destroyed, but there is early sparing of the axon cylinder. The outer myelin sheath in the

TABLE 36-2. Comparison of neurologic degenerative diseases

Disease	Pathologic signs	Effect
Multiple sclerosis	Multiple foci (patches) of nerve degeneration throughout brain and spinal cord	Demyelination causes nerve impulse to be interrupted (blocked) or distorted (slowed)
Myasthenia gravis	Decreased secretion of acetylcholine or an increase of cholinesterase enzyme at myoneural junction	Interference of nerve impulse across myoneural junction
Amyotrophic lateral sclerosis	Destruction of myelin sheath of motor neurons of lateral tracts of spinal cord and brain	Demyelination causes nerve impulse to be interrupted (blocked) or distorted (slowed)
Parkinsonism	Destruction of nerve cells of basal ganglia of brain	Decreased dopamine (neurotransmitter substance with anticholinergic effect)
Syringomyelia	Destruction of gray and then white matter of spinal cord by development of "syrinx" (cysts filled with CSF)	Destruction of nerve pathways in spinal cord—interruption of nerve impulses
Muscular dystrophy	*Not a neurologic disease*; atrophy of voluntary muscles	Effect is a wasting away of the voluntary muscles—no nerve effect
Alzheimer's disease	Degeneration of neurofibrils and presence of plaques in brain	Destruction of neurons leading to impairment in intellectual functioning

spinal cord neuronal pathways is often compared to the insulation on an electric wire. Its destruction causes interruption or distortion of the impulse so that it is, *slowed or blocked*. This type of demyelination differs from that of *wallerian degeneration* (p. 828) in that damage is always primary to the myelin sheath or sheath cells. There is evidence of partial healing in areas of degeneration, which accounts for the transitory nature of early symptoms. In late stages the degeneration may extend to gray areas of the cord and limit healing.

Because of the wide distribution of areas of degeneration, *there is a greater variety of signs and symptoms in multiple sclerosis than in other neurologic diseases*. The scarring that occurs at the degenerative lesions as well as the increasing sites provides the name "disseminated sclerosis."

Multiple sclerosis is a *chronic, remitting*, and *relapsing disease*. The majority of people recover from their early episodes. Usually there are acute exacerbations and remissions that may last for a year or more, although eventually exacerbations will recur. There is no record of any patients having recovered from the disease, although many have lived for 20 years or more and have died from other causes. Exacerbations may be aggravated or precipitated by fatigue, chilling, and emotional disturbances. In some cases the disease may terminate in death within a few months of onset. This so-called "malignant" multiple sclerosis is rare.

Clinical picture

Early symptoms are usually transitory and may include double vision (*diplopia*), spots before the eyes (*scotomas*), *blindness, tremor, weakness* or *numbness of a part of the body such as the hand, fatigue, susceptibility to upper respiratory infections, emotional instability* or *problems with the bowel or bladder*. Many persons with early multiple sclerosis may be considered neurotic by their associates and sometimes by their physicians because of the wide variety and temporary nature of symptoms and because of their emotional instability. As the disease progresses, symptoms may include *nystagmus, disorders of speech (scanning), urinary frequency and urgency, constipation*, and *changes in muscular coordination and gait*. Late symptoms may include urinary incontinence, difficulty in swallowing, severe muscle spasm and contractures, and spastic ataxic gait.

A sense of optimism and well-being (euphoria) also seems to be characteristic of persons with multiple sclerosis, especially during remissions. It is suspected that this reaction is due largely to patients' attempts to reassure themselves that their condition is not so serious as is supposed. This response is helpful to patients in many ways, but sometimes it may lead them to overdo, and thus increase symptoms. This euphoria may also be an indicator of involvement of selected areas of the brain.

Motor signs have upper motor neuron characteristics. Pain is not a common symptom of multiple sclerosis except when there is severe muscle spasm. Death generally is caused by infection, usually developing in the respiratory or genitourinary system.

In the hospital the nurse may care for patients for short periods when they are admitted for diagnosis or for some other condition or when they are terminally ill with advanced disease. Many patients are never hospitalized and will be cared for in their homes by their families with the support and assistance of community health nurses.

The fact that multiple sclerosis involves multiple parts of the nervous system, is often characterized by exacerbations and remissions, and frequently includes transient and bizarre signs and symptoms makes it difficult to diagnose with certainty. Because there is *no specific diagnostic test*, diagnosis is often a clinical judgment. The determination of cerebrospinal fluid γ-globulin by chemical or electrophoretic methods or of cerebrospinal fluid IgG by electroimmunodiffusion, when used with the history and neurologic examination, appears to be the most valuable single laboratory test. Testing of visual evoked potentials is now being performed to assess optic nerve integrity. Evidence of early damage has been closely linked with the diagnosis of multiple sclerosis.

Intervention

Drug therapy. At the present time there is no specific treatment for multiple sclerosis. Many physicians get favorable results from symptomatic treatments and the judicious use of adrenocorticotropic hormone (ACTH) and the corticosteroids, psychotherapy, social rehabilitation, physical therapy, patient education, and a great deal of compassion. Although ACTH and the steroids are widely used, their efficacy remains controversial. These drugs have been shown to prevent experimental allergic encephalomyelitis. Currently, some clinicians prefer oral prednisone; others prefer intramuscular ACTH; still others prefer intravenous ACTH. Dexamethasone (Decadron), administered intramuscularly or orally, has become popular. Its demonstrated antiedema effect may explain the favorable results in acute attacks of multiple sclerosis. the effects of ACTH and the steroids on the demyelinating activity per se are not known. It is known from testing that (1) there is nothing to be gained from long-term treatment with either steroids or ACTH and (2) there is possibly some gain from taking high doses of steroids at the start of a fresh episode, since the episode tends to resolve itself more rapidly if patients are treated with intensive courses of these drugs. The mood-elevating drugs are used to relieve depression, which is often present in multiple sclerosis.

The judicious use of passive and active exercises, when the person is not in an acute exacerbation, can be helpful. The use of drugs such as diazepam (Valium) and dantrolene sodium (Dantrium) as well as baclofen (Lioresal) has been found useful in relieving spasticity.

Activity and rest. Persons with multiple sclerosis should have a daily routine for rest and activity. Rest must be balanced with adequate exercise. They are usually advised to exercise regularly but never to the point of extreme fatigue, Because persons with multiple sclerosis almost always feel tired, they must look for some special sign that tells them that they have exercised enough. If they do more, they may suffer ill effects. For example, a tight feeling in the chest may indicate that the person must rest or else have severe discomfort. During the acute exacerbation, many physicians keep the patient as quiet as possible, limit all activities, and place the patient on bed rest. After an exacerbation, it may be difficult to resume exercises, but it is usually best that an established schedule be returned to as soon as possible. There is a need to conserve energy for priority activities.

One side of the body is usually affected more than the other, and the person may learn to stabilize gait by leaning toward the uninvolved side. The annoyance of having the foot slap forward in taking a step may sometimes be overcome by putting the heel down in a pronounced fashion and rolling the weight forward on the side of the foot.

Effort is made to maintain activity and work for as long as possible, and many persons have worked for 5 to 10 years and even longer after the onset of the first symptoms. Women at home can be helped to plan their shopping, housework, and other duties so that they may continue to function as wives and mothers even when the disease is advanced.

Comfort. Diplopia can be relieved by an eye patch. Peripheral neurectomies, rhizotomies, and cordotomies (p. 753) are often used for the relief of spasticity, pain, and paresthesias. Relief from severe spasticity is often obtained from intrathecal injections of phenol. In more severe cases of spasticity when contractures have developed, release of tendons may be necessary, followed by casting for a period of time.

Skin care. Many persons with multiple sclerosis have motor involvement that prevents them from moving about easily and from changing position easily. Also, they may experience sensory disturbances that affect how they sense pressure. As a result, these patients are especially prone to develop decubiti. They must be taught the importance of turning at least every 2 to 3 hours. Air mattresses or other devices may be used to help prevent pressure, but it is important to note that there is no substitute for turning.

Elimination. Urinary frequency and urgency, often the source of social disability, may respond to timed doses of propantheline bromide (Pro-Banthine). Prevention of urinary tract infection remains a problem, and such infections are a major cause of death. Cholin-

ergic drugs such as bethanechol (Urecholine) may be of help in the patient with an atonic bladder. Oxybutynin chloride (Ditropan) is a newer drug used to treat neurogenic bladder. It acts by exerting a direct antispasmodic effect on smooth muscles. Some patients are placed on prophylactic doses of medications such as trimethoprim and sulfamethoxazole (Bactrim/Septra) or nitrofurantoin (Macrodantin) indefinitely. Cystometrographic study is important to detect the specific bladder problem.

Teaching needs. Good general health and hygiene are necessary for the person with multiple sclerosis. Hot baths should be avoided because the heat can increase weakness in the person with multiple sclerosis. (In some centers, patients have been treated with ice water baths.) Traveling in hot weather should be carefully planned to prevent travel during the warmest part of the day. It is essential that the person and the family understand the importance of checking the skin routinely and take measures to relieve tissue pressure.

Since association with others is good for physical and mental health, the individual with multiple sclerosis must be encouraged and helped to remain an active, participating member of the family and the community for as long as possible. Personal cleanliness adds to a feeling of acceptance and well-being; consequently, these persons should be encouraged to pay careful attention to personal appearance and hygiene even though they may sometimes feel too tired to put forth the effort. They also should be encouraged to develop interests and hobbies that will help make up for things they cannot do, such as driving a vehicle, and that will help to fill the time when physical activity becomes more difficult. Music, writing, reading, and question games are good hobbies to develop. Interest in politics and in world affairs, which may be followed on the radio if sight is lost, may stand the person in good stead.

The National Multiple Sclerosis Society* is a national voluntary, nonprofit organization founded in 1946. Its functions are to encourage and finance research, to gather statistics, and to act as an information center for patients and for the public. A recent development is the Multiple Sclerosis Home Care course planned by the Society in conjunction with the American Red Cross on a national basis to teach relatives and friends of MS patients how to provide better care at home. Some local chapters also supply equipment to patients. Membership is open to health and welfare workers and to patients and their families. Local organizations can be found in many large cities.

A well-balanced diet with plenty of high-vitamin foods and fluids is important. Obesity must be avoided because it is more difficult for the obese person to maneuver, and this makes it more difficult to meet daily needs.

---

*257 Park Ave. South, New York, NY 10010.

Fresh air and sunshine are helpful, and overheating must be avoided because it may aggravate symptoms or bring on exacerbations. A good night's sleep is important, and a rest period after lunch is recommended. A good fluid intake should be stressed. Many persons are taught to include several glasses of cranberry juice in their diet each day to help decrease the possibility of urinary tract infections.

Adaptation. The decision as to whether the patient is told the diagnosis is controversial. There is not full agreement among physicians as to the proper course of action. Usually the decision is made on an individual basis and depends on the person's emotional makeup and on the family's ability to cope with the economic, social, and emotional problems that a condition of this kind presents.

Persons with multiple sclerosis need a peaceful, relaxed environment. They should never be hurried and should not be expected to respond quickly either physically or mentally. They may have slowness in speech and slowness in ability to respond, and this difficulty should be ignored by persons around them. Members of the family and friends need help in understanding this problem and in meeting it calmly. The person may have sudden explosive emotional outbursts of crying or laughing brought on by such simple acts as putting something hot into the mouth. Close members of the family must protect both the patient and visitors from the embarrassment of prolonged emotional outbursts. Reminding the patient of something sad may stop him from laughing, and holding the mouth open will sometimes stop the crying.

Outcome criteria for the person with multiple sclerosis

The person or significant others can:
1. Explain the prevention of urinary bladder infection and discomfort.
   a. Explain need for adequate or increased fluid intake during the day.
   b. Relate the need for a well-balanced diet for the prevention of infection generally.
   c. Explain home medications (actions and effects on the urinary system, dosage, and side effects of urinary antiinfective drugs).
   d. Explain need to consult physician when there are urinary problems.
   e. State methods to keep the urine acid.
   f. Explain the need and method of perineal cleanliness.
2. Explain general health maintenance practices.
   a. Make a plan to balance rest and work activities at home.
   b. State how to conserve energy for priority activities.
   c. Explain plan for a balanced diet.

   d. Explain the need to avoid hurry in the performance of activities.
   e. Plan for inclusion of hobbies and interests as related to mental health.
   f. Explain the occurrence of euphoria and other reactions to multiple sclerosis.
3. Explain safety factors related to the condition
   a. Explain the relationship of gait patterns to the need for safety.
   b. Explain the relationship of sensory deficits to safety.
   c. State where to secure safety equipment.
4. Explain exercise program to be followed at home.
   a. Demonstrate physical and occupational therapy exercises prescribed for continuing care.
   b. Explain the need for exercise for the preservation of muscle strength.
5. Explain how to secure human and material resources.
   a. Explain how to contact community health nurses.
   b. Explain the availability of ambulatory clinics.
   c. Explain the services that are obtained from the local multiple sclerosis chapter.
   d. List the visual and adaptive equipment available and where purchase or loan can be made.
6. State plans for follow-up care.

Paralysis agitans (Parkinson's disease, parkinsonism)

Epidemiology

Parkinson's disease is one of the more common diseases of the nervous system. It was first described in 1817 by James Parkinson. It affects both men and women in their middle and late years (50 to 60 years old). It affects all races and classes of persons. It is estimated to affect 100 to 150 persons per 100,000 population.

Etiology

The cause is not known, but the cluster of symptoms was seen in many patients following the 1916-1917 epidemic of encephalitis.

The characteristic symptoms of Parkinson's disease are sometimes found in arteriosclerotic patients, leading some researchers to believe that arteriosclerosis may be a causative factor. Viral infections have also been suggested as a cause. Drug-induced parkinsonian syndromes are linked with phenothiazines, reserpine (Serpasil), and butyrophenones (e.g., Haloperidol).

Pathophysiology

The pathologic process that occurs with Parkinson's disease is basically a depigmentation of the substantia nigra of the basal ganglia. The loss of neurons in the substantia is severe. Also with Parkinson's disease, selective depletion of dopamine occurs and can be correlated with the degree of striated degeneration. Dopamine is a neurotransmitter necessary for proper muscle movement. Without dopamine there is a loss of inhibitory influence and excitatory mechanisms (acetylcholine) are unopposed.

Clinical picture

Parkinson's disease begins with a faint tremor and progresses so slowly that the person is seldom able to recall its onset. There is not true paralysis and no loss of sensation. Tremor (pill rolling of the fingers or resting tremor) is the outstanding sign of the disease. Two other frequent signs of the disease are muscular weakness (with rigidity) and loss of postural reflexes. Parkinson's disease has some characteristics of upper motor neuron involvement (p. 762). It is essentially a problem in motion. Muscle rigidity prevents normal response in commonly performed acts and leads to characteristic changes that make the diagnosis almost unmistakable to persons who have observed patients with the disease. There is a masklike appearance to the face and slowed, monotonous speech. Drooling may occur because of the difficulty of swallowing saliva. This may cause skin irritation that is best prevented or treated by frequent sponging followed by protecting the skin with an emollient such as cold cream. There is a characteristic shuffling gait in which patients tend to walk on their toes. The trunk is bent forward, and the arms fall rigidly to the sides and do not swing as in normal rhythmic gait. Neuromuscular control may be altered so that the patient is unable to stop this propulsive gait until an obstruction is met. The patient usually as a moist, oily skin. Defects in judgment and emotional instability may occur, but intelligence is not impaired. The appetite may be increased, and there is heat intolerance. A decrease in blinking is seen. Fatigue is a common complaint, and pain in the arms or shoulders may be present. All signs and symptoms increase with fatigue, excitement, and frustration. As the disease progresses, the severity of symptoms increases. More and more symptoms develop. Patients with Parkinson's disease usually die from other causes, most commonly pulmonary or renal disease.

Intervention

Drug therapy. Treatment for Parkinson's disease is palliative and symptomatic and depends on the pharmacologic manipulation of the pathophysiologic state. The severity of symptoms and presence of associated disease processes determine the drugs to be used. Anticholinergic alkaloids such as scopolamine hydrobromide and related drugs (hyoscyamine) have been used for more than a century. They act against cholinergic excitatory effects and are more effective in lessening muscle rigidity than in controlling tremor. Many synthetic anticholinergic drugs of varied chemical structure are also available. There is little to recommend one over the other, aside from personal preference, but each has some degree of central nervous system anticholinergic action. However, they are incapable of restoring striatal balance. The preferred anticholinergic agents are trihexyphenidyl (Artane), benztropine mesylate (Cogentin), procyclidine (Kemadrin), and biperiden (Akineton).[70] These drugs have some selectivity of action in that they have greater central than peripheral anticholinergic activity. Optimal results from these drugs depend on a dosage that provides a compromise between the limited symptomatic improvement given by these drugs and the disagreeable symptoms of central and peripheral cholinergic blockade (blurring of vision, dryness of mouth and throat, constipation, urinary urgency or retention, ataxia, dysarthria, mental disturbances). Antihistaminic drugs such as diphenhydramine (Benadryl), which are not primarily anticholinergic, exert mild central anticholinergic properties when used alone or in combination with other drugs.

Some patients with severe Parkinson's disease have experienced dramatic benefits from levodopa not experienced from anticholinergic drugs. Levodopa assists in restoring striatal dopamine deficiency, since it is a precursor of dopamine. This drug does not affect the underlying process of parkinsonism.[16] In this way, levodopa is more like a replacement drug than a cure. Once benefits are obtained from levodopa, they are likely to be sustained. After prolonged periods of treatment there may be an increased appearance of side effects as well as a decrease in the effectiveness of the medication. The drug is usually increased gradually but cannot be increased indefinitely. It has been found helpful to admit some patients into the hospital for a drug holiday during which all medications are withdrawn for a period of 7 to 10 days. The medications are then restarted and often much smaller doses are able to produce favorable results. This type of drug holiday must take place within the hospital setting, however, because of the danger of aspiration pneumonia or other complications that can occur since the immobility, rigidity, and other signs and symptoms will return when the drugs are withdrawn. Usually patients remain on anticholinergic drugs or they may be added as an adjunct. Most individuals experience side effects from levodopa, such as nausea and vomiting, orthostatic hypotension, insomnia, agitation, and mental confusion, but these lessen with continued medication and dosage modification.

There have been some cases of kidney and liver damage from levodopa. Candidates for levodopa should be selected carefully.[16] Amantadine hydrochloride (Symmetrel), an antiviral agent, is known to have antiparkinsonian activity. It acts by blocking the reuptake and storage of catecholamines and allowing the accumulation of dopamine in extracellular or synaptic sites. This drug may not sustain its effectiveness for more than 3 months in some patients. Side effects, although infrequent, include mental confusion, visual disturbances, and seizures.

Carbidopa-levodopa (Sinemet) is a drug that is more recently utilized in neurologic practice. It is a combination of levodopa with an inhibitor of the enzyme dopa decarboxylase, which limits the metabolism of levodopa peripherally and provides more levodopa for the brain. The reduction in peripheral metabolism and the reduction in dose of levodopa that can occur reduces some of the side effects seen when levodopa is used alone.

Surgery. A surgical procedure has been used with some success in the treatment of selected patients with Parkinson's disease. Descriptions of successful operations in popular magazines have led some patients and their families to believe that a cure for all patients has been found. Many patients cannot be treated surgically. Results seem to be best in younger patients who have unilateral involvement following other diseases and who have marked tremor and rigidity. Treatment consists of destroying portions of the globus pallidus (relieves rigidity) or the thalamus (relieves tremor) in the brain by sterotactic methods through the use of cautery, removal, or injection of alcohol. Operative techniques involving cooling or freezing with liquid nitrogen (cryogenic surgery) have been attempted with good results in selected cases and with fewer complications than when cautery or alcohol was used. Medications used to control rigidity and tremor are discontinued several days preoperatively so that patients' symptoms will be at their maximum during the operation.[77] Nursing care *preoperatively* includes seeing that nutrition is adequate as well as other general preoperative care.

Postoperative care includes the most careful attention to the vital signs, use of side rails to prevent accidents in the event of convulsions, disorientation, or temporary hemiplegia, and frequent turning and moving to prevent respiratory and circulatory complications. Excessive salivation and difficulty in blinking the eye on the operated side may be problems requiring nursing attention.

Activity. Special attention should be paid to *posture*. Lying on a firm bed without a pillow during rest periods may help to prevent the spine from bending forward, and lying in the prone position also helps. Holding the hands folded behind the back when walking may help to keep the spine erect and prevent the annoyance of the arms falling stiffly at the sides. The tremor often is less apparent when persons are sitting in an armchair, since they can grip the arms of the chair and partially control the tremor in their hands and arms. The reader is referred to Chapter 35 for a discussion of alterations of movement and posture.

Feeding the patient becomes a real problem when the disease is far advanced because of the danger of choking in attempts to swallow; eventually, aspiration pneumonia may terminate the patient's life. Unless the patient is well controlled by medication, drooling can be a real problem and increases with general excitement. A bib can be used to protect the clothing during napping hours. When patients are dressed, garments with generous pockets well supplied with soft tissues will help them be less conspicuous and more comfortable.

The patient with Parkinson's disease should continue to work as long as possible. Most physicians advise this unless the occupation is such that continued work is dangerous.

Teaching needs. The progress of Parkinson's disease, a condition that often last for years, may be slowed by good nutrition, sufficient rest, moderate exercise in fresh air, and other measures that improve general health. Patient and family education is a primary nursing intervention. Instruction should include general health maintenance practices, prevention of the complications of poor posture and immobility, and drug therapy. The nurse needs to assist the patient and family in communication techniques. Speech exercises directed toward relaxation of speech muscles and improvement of voice volume have assisted some persons.[23]

Relatives need complete understanding of the circumstances so that they may intelligently assist in the adjustments that will eventually be necessary. Such problems as accidents, personality changes, and progressive helplessness must be anticipated. While drooling and difficulty in swallowing often limit the important social outlet of eating at group gatherings, the patient should have meals at home with the family as long as possible.

Outcome criteria for the person with Parkinson's disease

The person or significant others can:
1. Explain each home medication prescribed for the relief of parkinsonism.
   a. Explain use, action, dosage, frequency, and side effects of each medication.
   b. Explain that dosage may require modification until side effects are stabilized.
   c. Explain how to take medications for best results in the relief of signs and symptoms and side effects.
   d. Explain the value of taking medications regularly.
2. Explain the importance of adherence to general health practices.
   a. Make a plan of activities of daily living that is balanced as to rest, physical activities, and socialization.

b. Recognize emotional responses to illness and the effects of fatigue and stress.

3. Describe potential safety factors related to parkinsonism.

   a. Respiratory infection related to rigidity of respiratory muscles.

   b. Aspiration of food caused by difficulty in swallowing.

   c. Social isolation related to embarrassment about speech and physical appearance.

   d. Accidents related to difficulty in gait.

4. State plans for follow-up care.

Myasthenia gravis

Epidemiology

Myasthenia gravis is a relatively rare disease of unknown cause. It usually occurs in young adults and is thought to have a link with autoimmune reactions. It affects about 1 in 20,000 persons. In young persons, women are more commonly affected than men; in older persons the distribution among the sexes is about equal. Occurrence among families is rare; however, infants of affected mothers may have symptoms at birth, but these symptoms usually disappear within several weeks.

Pathophysiology

With myasthenia gravis there is no observable structural change in the muscle or nerve. Nerve impulses fail to pass to muscles at the myoneural junction. It is not known specifically why the motor nerve impulses fail to pass to the muscle and cause it not to contract. It is believed variously to be caused by the inability of the motor end-plate to secrete adequate acetylcholine, by excessive quantities of the cholinesterase enzyme at the nerve ending, or by a nonresponse of the muscle fibers to acetylcholine. Relative to the third theory, myasthenia gravis may be considered a primary muscle disease; relative to the first two theories it is a neuromuscular disease with lower motor neuron characteristics. About 25% of patients with myasthenia gravis have been found to have thymoma, and nearly 80% have changes in the cellular structure of the thymus gland.[64] Myasthenia gravis is considered a grave disorder, since the respiratory muscles and the bulbar cranial nerves may be involved. During periods of exacerbation or lack of drug control, the patient may have to be cared for in a respiratory intensive care unit.

Clinical picture

The outstanding symptoms of myasthenia gravis are muscle weakness and severe generalized fatigue that come on quickly, are usually more evident in the evening, and, in the early stages of the disease, disappear quickly with rest. Weakness of arm and hand muscles may be first noticed when shaving or combing the hair. Facial muscles innervated by the cranial nerves are often affected, and it may not be possible for the person to hold the eyelids open (ptosis), to keep the mouth closed, or to chew or swallow. Diplopia (double vision) is also common. As the disease progresses, the trunk and lower limbs are affected, leading to difficulty with walking and sustained sitting. Usually the distal muscles are not as affected as the proximal muscles. Muscle weakness may become so severe that the person cannot breathe without assistance. Exacerbations of the disease may be initiated by upper respiratory infections, emotional tension, and menstruation.

Because of the slow and insidious onset and the occurrence of symptoms with stress, myasthenia gravis is sometimes misdiagnosed as hysteria or neurosis. Actual diagnosis can be made partly on the basis of electromyography (EMG). A specific diagnostic test is the edrophonium chloride (Tensilon) test. In this test, Tensilon (a very short-acting anticholinesterase drug) is injected intravenously. When increased strength in a predetermined muscle group is seen, the test is considered positive. To obtain true results, it is important that the patient not know when the medication is being given.

The *Eaton-Lambert syndrome* is a condition associated with cancer that has many of the same symptoms as myasthenia gravis. It is important to differentiate between the two diseases. The Eaton-Lambert syndrome is a special form of myasthenia that is found almost invariably in persons with oat cell carcinoma of the lung. In this syndrome the muscles of the trunk as well as those of the pelvic and shoulder girdles are the ones most frequently involved by weakness, fatigue, and atrophy. Visual symptoms are less frequent. Increasing weakness occurs after exertion, but there may be a temporary increase in muscle power at first.

The onset of the Eaton-Lambert syndrome is usually insidious and the course progressive. Because the myasthenia may precede discovery of the lung tumor by months or years it is important that there be a thorough check for malignancy at regular intervals. In addition to oat cell carcinoma of the lung, the syndrome has occurred with carcinoma of the rectum, stomach, prostate, and breast.

Intervention

There is no known cure for myasthenia gravis. There is, however, a very marked improvement following the use of neostigmine (Prostigmin) or pyridostigmine (Mestinon). These drugs block the action of cholinesterase at the myoneural junction and allow acetylcholine, a chemical necessary for transmission of impulses to the muscles, to act. Acetylcholine is the neurotransmitter between postganglionic parasympathetic fibers and receptor organs. Atropine or some other anticholinergic agent that blocks these *muscarinic effects* of acetylcholine may be used to treat the side effects of neostigmine and pyridostigmine. Treatment is planned so that the patient may continue to receive the amount of drug that can be tolerated without side effects and yet carry out activities essential for normal living. Usually the patient is permitted to adjust the dosage. *The nurse should teach the importance of taking medications at the time prescribed.* If the drug is delayed, dyspnea may result, followed by severe respiratory distress, which if untreated can cause death.

It is important also to teach that (1) dosage is individually determined and related to the activity of the person; (2) dosage needs to be adjusted to maintain muscle strength; and (3) the effects of drugs need to be monitored. The nurse and family must understand that it is often difficult to distinguish between myasthenic crisis (too little drug) and cholinergic crisis (too much drug), since both conditions cause severe muscle weakness. Tensilon administered intravenously is used to differentiate between the two conditions. A positive test (increase in strength) usually indicates underdosage of medication. An increase in weakness when Tensilon is administered may be a sign of overdosage. Drugs to be avoided are muscle relaxants, morphine, barbiturates, tranquilizers, and neomycin, since they can potentiate the weakness associated with myasthenia gravis because of their effects on the myoneural junction.

Patients with myasthenia gravis should take particular care of their health. Upper respiratory tract infections may be serious because the person may not have the energy to cough effectively and may develop pneumonia or airway obstruction. Because of weakness in swallowing, food may be aspirated. The patient who is living at home may feel more secure if there is a tracheal suction apparatus and other airway and ventilatory equipment available and if a member of the family knows how to use it if an emergency arises.

During acute episodes of the disease a tracheostomy set is kept in the patient's room ready for immediate use. Changes in the respiratory status may occur rapidly. Serial determinations of vital capacity and/or tidal volume and minute volume are extremely helpful in monitoring respiratory status. Often is is necessary to suction the patient's airway before meals. If swallowing is too dangerous, a nasogastric tube is used, and great care must be taken to be certain that the tube is in the stomach before fluid is introduced, since the patient cannot cough to indicate presence of fluid in the trachea. When caring for patients with severe symptoms of myasthenia gravis, the nurse should remember that they may be too weak to do anything for themselves. Therefore the patient may not be able to take a drug or turn over in bed.

Persons with myasthenia gravis may have to change daily patterns of activity. The nurse can help the patient and family plan so that a minimum of energy is used in activities that are essential to remaining relatively self-sufficient and yet allow energy for activities the patient wishes to take part in.

Outcome criteria for the person with myasthenia gravis

The person or significant others can:
1. Explain each prescribed anticholinesterase or cholinergic drug or other drugs prescribed.
   a. Explain the action, effects, side effects, and toxic effects.
   b. Explain the reason for taking the medication at the exact time scheduled.
   c. Explain the need to monitor the effects of the medication, particularly on respiration, swallowing, and general muscle strength.
   d. List the drugs that act on the neuromuscular junction and that are contraindicated.
2. Describe measures to prevent respiratory tract infection.
3. Demonstrate use of airway and ventilatory equipment.
4. Explain the need to avoid overexertion and emotional tension.

Amyotrophic lateral sclerosis

Amyotrophic lateral sclerosis (ALS) is a motor neuron disease that affects upper or lower motor neurons lying within the brain or spinal cord or a combination of the two.

Epidemiology and etiology

ALS is sometimes called Lou Gehrig's disease since the famous New York Yankee ballplayer died of the disease. It affects men more than women. It usually occurs in middle age but may occur in younger persons. There is some thought that there is a familial or genetic component to ALS. The cause is unknown, but a slow viral infection has been suggested to be the causative agent.

Pathophysiology

Myelin sheaths are destroyed and are replaced by scar tissue. There is direct involvement of the lateral tracts of the spinal cord with possible eventual involvement of the medulla and the ventral tracts. The nerve impulses are distorted or blocked. Symptoms depend on which motor neurons are affected.[9]

Clinical picture

Early symptoms include fatigue and awkwardness of fine finger movements and muscle wasting. Dysphagia may be the first symptom in many persons. There is *progressive muscle weakness, atrophy,* and *fascicula-*

tions. Spasticity of flexor muscles is commonly present. With involvement of the brain stem and medulla there is dysphagia, dysarthria, jaw clonus, tongue fasciculations, and respiratory difficulty. As the diseases progresses, there is disability relative to both upper and lower limbs, and one side of the body becomes more involved than the other. The person remains alert. There is no sensory loss with the disease. Death occurs usually within 5 to 10 years, generally from respiratory or bulbar paralysis.

Intervention

Treatment is directed toward relieving the symptoms of the disease. Nursing interventions include assistance with activities of daily living as limb deficits increase. Prostheses are often applied to support the weakened muscles. As the disease progresses, respirations are affected. At this time constant nursing attention is required. Providing adequate nutrition to the patient can be a real challenge. As swallowing becomes more difficult a nasogastric or gastrostomy tube may be necessary. Attention to prevention of skin breakdown and contractures is important.

Emotional support is extremely important. Patients and families should be involved in making decisions about the types of interventions that will be used as the disease progresses. Some patients will decide to use ventilators at home as respiratory muscles become involved, whereas other patients will decide not to use any supportive devices. Patients and families need help and support in making decisions about how they are going to live their lives from the time the diagnosis is made until the disease causes complete dependency of the patient on others. Whatever decisions the patient and family make must be supported by the health team. Because the patient remains alert until the end, nurses should not forget they are dealing with a person who is probably very afraid of what lies ahead. Patients should be helped to retain some control over their treatment as long as possible.

Outcome criteria for the person with ALS

The person with ALS is evaluated based on the outcome criteria described relative to upper and lower motor neuron paralysis (p. 767) and bulbar respiratory failure (p. 767).

Syringomyelia

Etiology

Syringomyelia is a chronic, slowly progressive, and rare condition. It involves the spinal cord or the lower brain stem (syringobulbia). There is some tendency for it to occur in families. The causes for the development of the initial syrinx are variable, including glioma and failure of the ventricular system to circulate cerebrospinal fluid properly within its normal channels.

Pathophysiology

Syringomyelia is the name given because of small tubelike cavities or cysts called *syrinxes* that form and progressively destroy the cord from the inside out, involving first the gray matter near the central canal and then the white matter. The syrinxes become inflated with CSF and communicate with each other and with ventricular fluid pathways, causing distention. The widest parts of the cord (cervical and lumbar) become inflated with fluid first, and early symptoms can be related to cord damage at the cervical or upper arm level. There is blockage of nerve impulse transmission. At first there is involvement of the spinothalamic sensory pathway and later involvement of motor neuron pathways. As the cord inflates with fluid, the spinothalamic pathway becomes *vulnerable to destruction first because the nerve cell fibers from the cell bodies in the gray matter cross the cord to the opposite side* and then travel to the brain in the spinothalamic tract. The cell bodies lie within the posterior horn, and the fibers run across the cord.

Clinical picture

The precise clinical picture depends on the cross-sectional and vertical extent of cord destruction, but there are certain clinical signs and symptoms. An early finding is segmental loss of pain and temperature sense and preservation of the sense of touch with losses over the arms, shoulders, and neck areas in a capelike distribution. The dissociated sensory loss is explained by the cervical cord involvement and distention as discussed above. There is also weakness and atrophy of the hands and arms and loss of tendon reflexes. As the lesions continue to extend within the cord, the anterior horn cells of the gray matter become affected, producing lower motor neuron paralysis with flaccidity and loss of reflexes. Later, as cavitation of the cord widens, the corticospinal tracts become compressed with upper motor neuron involvement (spasticity and hyperreflexia). If lesions extend upward, the upper end of the cord or bulb then becomes involved. In the latter there is numbness of the face, wasting of the tongue, and difficulty in swallowing, coughing, or breathing as a result of involvement of the nerve supply to these structures. The early analgesia and thermoanesthesia account for the painless infections, skin ulceration, injuries, and burns seen in patients with this condition. Lumbar puncture, myelography, and air encephalography are the diagnostic procedures most helpful.

Intervention

There is no specific treatment for syringomyelia. Surgical treatment is attempted in carefully selected cases, depending on the cause. Decompression of a distended syrinx may temporarily relieve symptoms of local compression of ascending and descending spinal tracts. Unroofing the spinal cord by removing the posterior rim of the foramen magnum and the cerebellar tonsils has relieved neurologic symptoms in some persons. Shunt operations to relieve blocked cerebrospinal fluid and to provide a different drainage system have been successfully attempted. Nursing interventions are directed toward prevention of injury caused by sensory losses. When the brain stem is affected, respiratory care takes priority, as does the utilization of feeding techniques to prevent aspiration.

Outcome criteria for the person with syringomyelia

The person with syringomyelia is evaluated by the same outcome criteria as for the person with general sensory dysfunction (p. 771), upper and lower motor paralysis (p. 767), and respiratory failure (p. 1331), as these entities relate to the presenting clinical symptoms and signs.

Alzheimer's disease

Epidemiology

Alzheimer's disease is a degenerative disorder that affects the cells of the brain and causes impairment of intellectual functioning. It affects 500,000 to 1.5 million American adults and is recognized as the most common cause of dementia in the older adult. It affects men and women equally. Most newly diagnosed persons are in late middle age, but the disease has been documented in some persons as young as 40 years old.

Etiology

The cause of Alzheimer's disease is not known. There is some thought that perhaps it is an autoimmune disease. A slight hereditary disposition is suggested since family members of patients with Alzheimer's disease are slightly more likely to develop the disease.

Pathophysiology

The changes in the brains of patients with Alzheimer's disease are visible in the cerebral cortex. The first change is the presence of microscopic "plaques" found in brain tissue. These plaques consist of a core surrounded by strands of fiberlike material. In addition, there is degeneration of some of the small fibers (neurofibrils) that run through the body of the nerve cells. These changes were first discovered in 1907 by the German neurologist Alzheimer.

The diagnosis of Alzheimer's disease is usually made after ruling out other conditions in which there is memory loss. These conditions include pernicious anemia, drug reactions, hormonal imbalances, depression, drug or alcohol abuse, brain tumor, chronic meningitis, head trauma, Pick's disease, or Parkinson's disease with dementia.

Clinical picture

The patient with Alzheimer's disease goes through three rather distinct stages. The first stage is characterized by rather mild mental impairment, including forgetfulness, impairment in judgment, lessening of initiative, and lack of spontaneity. Gradually, the person becomes more forgetful, particularly about recent events. The second stage includes confusion, agitation, irritability, and extreme restlessness. Incontinence of urine and stool occurs, along with the need for constant supervision. In the third stage the Alzheimer's patient is totally unable to perform self-care, is totally incontinent, and may not be able to communicate with others.

Although the signs and symptoms of Alzheimer's disease occur progressively, the rate at which they occur varies from person to person. In a few cases, there may be a very rapid decline, but in most cases many months pass with little change. As persons become more and more affected, they are more likely to develop pneumonia or other illnesses that may cause death.

Intervention

At present there is no available treatment that can cure, reverse, or stop the progression of Alzheimer's disease. Nursing care is directed toward maintaining nutrition, continence, hydration, and safety. Emotional support to both the patient and family is very important. Appropriate drugs can sometimes be used to lessen agitation, anxiety, and unpredictable behavior.

Families can be advised of the national headquarters of the Alzheimer's Disease and Related Disorders Association,* which has chapters in many cities.

Vascular disease: cerebrovascular accident

Cerebrovascular accident (CVA) is the most common disease of the nervous system and is the third highest cause of death in the United States. Five hundred thousand Americans each year have an acute CVA.

In this chapter the term *cerebrovascular accident* will be discussed as a general term. It should be recognized, however, that most neurologists and neurosurgeons more specifically refer to the disturbance in ce-

---

*292 Madison Ave., New York, NY 10017.

rebral circulation as either a thrombus, embolus, hemorrhage, or transient ischemic attack. The nursing and medical care may differ depending on the specific cause. These differences will be discussed in each relevant section. *Hemiplegia* and *stroke* are also terms used when referring to CVA. Clinically, stroke refers to the sudden and dramatic development of focal neurologic deficits, and hemiplegia is one neurologic deficit that is commonly seen.

Etiology

The major causes of CVA are a thrombus, an embolus, or a hemorrhage, which can be precipitated by many underlying factors (see box at right) frequently associated with other chronic diseases that cause vascular problems. These include heart disease, kidney disease, peripheral vascular disease, hypertension, and diabetes mellitus.

Pathophysiology

The brain is very dependent on oxygen and has no reserve oxygen supply. Thus, when anoxia occurs, cerebral metabolism is promptly altered and cell death and permanent damage can occur within 3 to 10 minutes. Any condition that alters cerebral perfusion will cause hypoxia or anoxia. Hypoxia first leads to cerebral ischemia. Short-term ischemia (less than 10 to 15 minutes) causes temporary deficits but no permanent deficits. Long-term ischemia causes permanent cell death and results in a cerebral infarction. Cerebral edema accompanies the infarction and worsens the neurologic deficits seen in the patient.

The permanent focal deficits may be unknown when the patient is first seen because generalized cerebral dysfunction (coma) may be present. The generalized dysfunction may be a result of generalized ischemia affecting larger areas of the brain than the area of infarction and cerebral edema alone.

The type of permanent focal deficits will depend on the area of the brain that has been affected. The area of the brain affected depends on which cerebral vessels are involved. Table 36-3 lists the major vessels of the brain, the major areas of the brain perfused by each vessel, and the resultant deficits that will occur when blood flow is disrupted.

The vessel most frequently affected is the middle cerebral artery. The second most frequently affected vessel is the internal carotid artery. Other vessels are more rarely affected.

Since there are major differences in the clinical picture and care of the patient who suffers a CVA caused by hemorrhage, this will be discussed in a separate section. The onset, pathologic process, and incidence of CVA from thrombosis and embolism are different, and thus each will be described before discussing care of the patient.

CONDITIONS CAUSING CVA

Thrombus
Atherosclerosis in intracranial and extracranial arteries

Adjacency to intracerebral hemorrhage

Arteritis caused by collagen (autoimmune) disease or bacterial arteritis

Hypercoagulability such as in polycythemia

Cerebral venous thromboses

Emboli
Valves damaged by rheumatic heart disease (RHD)

Myocardial infarction

Atrial fibrillation (this arrhythmia causes variable emptying of left ventricle, blood pools and small clots form and then at times the ventricle will be emptied completely with release of small emboli)

Bacterial endocarditis and nonbacterial endocarditis causing clots to form on endocardium

Hemorrhage
Hypertensive intracerebral hemorrhage

Subarachnoid hemorrhage

Rupture of aneurysm

Arteriovenous malformation

Hypocoagulation (as in patients with blood dyscrasias)

Generalized hypoxia
Severe hypotension, cardiopulmonary arrest, or severe depression in cardiac output caused by arrhythmias

Localized hypoxia
Cerebral artery spasms associated with subarachnoid hemorrhage

Cerebral artery vasoconstriction associated with migraine headaches

Cerebral thrombosis

Thrombosis is the most frequent cause of a CVA and in one study of nonhemorrhagic causes of CVA it accounted for 92% of all CVAs.[4] The most frequent cause of cerebral thrombosis is atherosclerosis. CVA secondary to thrombosis is seen most frequently in the 60-to 90-year age group, and many of these persons have a history of hypertension or diabetes mellitus. The atherosclerosis is similar to that described on p. 1154 and leads to occlusion of cerebral vessels.

It is important for nurses to be aware of the relationship between CVA and (1) atherosclerosis, (2) hy-

TABLE 36-3. Deficits resulting from disruption of blood flow in the brain

Artery	Areas of brain supplied*	Defects with disruption of flow

Internal carotid artery	Retina by its branch to retinal artery; lateral and medial surfaces of cerebral hemispheres by its branches to middle cerebral artery and anterior cerebral artery; portions of hypothalamus	Occasionally asymptomatic if good collateral circulation
		Most frequently find the following:
		  Intermittent ipsilateral visual impairment or blindness caused by retinal artery insufficiency
		  Impairment similar to that seen with disruption of flow through middle cerebral artery
		  Impairment caused by disruption of flow in anterior cerebral artery not frequently seen since both anterior cerebral arteries can be fed by one internal carotid artery
		  Ipsilateral Horner's syndrome (ptosis, miosis, and absence of sweating on same side of face) from hypothalamic damage

Anterior cerebral artery	Medial and superior surfaces of cerebral hemispheres; contains motor and sensory cortex for foot and leg and supplementary motor cortex; feeds large portion of frontal lobe	Contralateral hemiparesis or hemiplegia and contralateral sensory loss of lower extremities Upper extremities and face usually spared Confusion, dementia, and personality changes
Middle cerebral artery	Lateral portion of cerebral hemispheres, which contain motor and sensory areas for face and upper extremities and speech areas	Contralateral paralysis or paresis Contralateral sensory loss Sensory and motor loss are most noticeable in face, neck, and upper extremities Dysphasia or aphasia, may be global aphasia or only difficulty with expression without loss of comprehension; aphasia or dysphasia occurs if dominant hemisphere affected (left hemisphere in right-handed persons and most left-handed persons) Spatial perceptual problems (inability to judge distances, rate of movement, form and relationship of body parts); changes in judgment and behavior; neglect of paralyzed side; and inability to recognize paralyzed extremity as own (anosognosia) if nondominant hemisphere affected Contralateral homonymous hemianopia
Posterior cerebral artery	Posterior lateral and posterior medial surface of cerebral cortex, which contains primary visual receptive areas and internal structures; multiple branches that feed parts of optic pathway and diencephalic structure (thalamus and midbrain)	Paralysis usually absent Homonymous hemianopic field defects If dominant side, difficulty with visual learning, visual recognition, and visual spatial orientation If branch to midbrain affected, can have ipsilateral oculomotor palsy and contralateral hemiparesis (Weber's syndrome) because of affect on cerebral peduncle; may have ataxia and choreoathetosis If bilateral occlusion to midbrain, will have quadriparesis (since all tracts pass through midbrain as they leave cortex); impaired consciousness; divergent gaze; and dilated unresponsive pupils Patients in coma have unusual appearance in that they seem to be awake but do not communicate and do not respond; this has been termed *akinetic mutism* If thalamus affected, may have major sensory disturbances such as abnormal pain and dysesthesia, which are increased with emotional distress and the patient also may have emotional lability (crying, laughing without motivation); these symptoms are sometimes called *thalamic syndrome*

*Only major areas identified.

TABLE 36-3. Deficits resulting from disruption of blood flow in the brain—cont'd

Artery	Areas of brain supplied*	Defects with disruption of flow
Vertebral-basilar arteries	Multiple branches supply medulla oblongata, pons, midbrain, cerebellum; no one structure receives all its blood supply from one branch; blood supply to ventral paramedian, ventrolateral, and dorsal brain stem structures all originate from different groups of arteries	Many different signs and symptoms depending on area of brain stem affected (pons, midbrain, or medulla) and what part of that area affected Because motor and sensory tracts pass through this area, paresis and sensory deficits affecting one to all four extremities may occur All cranial nerve nuclei are in this area so disruption of their function may be present as visual impairment, facial paralysis, loss of sensory innervation to face, difficulty in swallowing, dysarthria, deafness, etc. Interference with cerebellar function can occur, causing ataxia, tremors, choreoathetosis, etc. Interference with reticular activating system causes alteration in consciousness Partial or complete Horner's syndrome caused by hypothalamic problem (ptosis of eyelid, constriction of pupil, and absence of sweating on same side of face) Respiratory difficulty, syncope, nausea, vomiting caused by dysfunction of major vital centers in brain stem

pertension, and (3) diabetes mellitus so that they can be involved in appropriate preventive care. The preventive care measures discussed on p. 1154 for atherosclerosis, p. 1176 for hypertension, and p. 645 for diabetes mellitus should be used by nurses to teach individuals and to plan community educational programs directed at decreasing the incidence of CV.

The onset of symptoms of CVA secondary to thrombosis tends to occur during sleep or soon after arising. This may be related to the fact that elderly persons have decreased sympathetic activity and recumbency causes a lowering of blood pressure, which can lead to ischemia of the brain. In addition, these persons frequently have postural hypotension and poor reflex response to changes in position, which can cause hypotension on arising. Neurologic signs and symptoms very frequently deteriorate or worsen for the first 48 hours.

Cerebral arteriosclerosis may also lead to deterioration of brain tissue, even though CVAs do not occur. This condition, which usually is associated with high blood pressure, may occur in persons in their 50s, although it is usually considered a disease of old age.

Multiple small thrombi may occur in persons whose blood pressure is normal or even below normal if atheromatous changes have occurred in the lining of arteries. This condition causes frequent small and barely perceptible strokes. Both cerebral arteriosclerosis and multiple small strokes from thrombi may produce personality changes. The person who has arteriosclerosis is likely to have a more consistent downward course, whereas the one suffering from multiple small thrombi may have periods of apparently normal physical and mental response between episodes of confusion.

Both cerebral arteriosclerosis and multiple small thrombi cause slowly progressive changes that are particularly distressing to members of the person's family. Complete brain deterioration may occur. The person may feel irritable and unhappy with apparently little cause, and no amount of reassurance can make him or her feel better. The family must be prepared for gradual deterioration of the person's condition and should make provision for the person's safety and for the results of poor judgment, for example, the person may forget to dress appropriately, may give away family possessions, and may enter into unwise business dealings. The family needs help in learning how to treat the patient as an adult and yet deal with his or her limitations. The physician, the social caseworker, and the nurse can help family members care for the patient in such a way that their own lives are not completely disrupted and yet that they are not plagued by guilt feelings when the patient dies. Institutional care is sometimes necessary, and the family needs encouragement and help in arriving at joint decisions that serve the best interests of all its members.

Cerebral embolism

Embolism is the second most common cause of CVA. Patients who have CVAs secondary to embolism are usually younger and most commonly the emboli originate from a thrombus in the heart. The myocardial thrombus is most frequently caused by rheumatic heart disease with mitral stenosis and atrial fibrillation. Therefore nurses can help to decrease the incidence of CVA from emboli by instituting the preventive care measures for persons with rheumatic heart disease described on p. 1103. In addition, since cerebral embolism can originate from emboli in infarcted myocardium another set of preventive measures that nurses should be practicing are those described on p. 1112 for the prevention of myocardial infarctions. Symptoms may occur at any time and progress rapidly. Emboli that originate from infected material can produce abcesses or other types of infections.

Transient ischemic attacks

In the preceding discussion CVA has been discussed in relation to the causative agent or the vessel involved. CVA can also be described according to the temporal character of the total clinical episode. Three profiles have been defined: transient ischemic attacks, stroke in evolution (progressive stroke), or completed stroke.

The term *transient ischemic attacks* (TIA) refers to transient cerebral ischemia with temporary episodes of neurologic dysfunction. The neurologic dysfunction can be profound with complete loss of consciousness and loss of all sensory and motor function, or there may only be focal deficits of some sensory and motor functions. Focal deficits that occur depend on the area of the brain that is involved. The most common deficit is contralateral weakness of the lower face, fingers, hands, arms and legs, transient dysphasia, and some sensory impairment. Ischemic attacks may occur many times over days, weeks, months, or years. The neurologic deficit resolves, and between attacks the neurologic examination is normal.

TIA may be caused by any of the conditions listed for CVA but most commonly precedes cerebral thrombosis.

Stroke in evolution refers to development of a neurologic deficit over several hours to days. The clinical picture is the same as for a completed stroke—only the time course is different. *Completed stroke* refers to a permanent neurologic deficit.

The major importance of TIAs is that they warn the patient and health care provider of the existence of an underlying pathologic condition. At least one third of the patients who have TIAs will have a CVA within 2 to 5 years. Some patients will be treated with vasodilators, anticoagulant therapy, or drugs that inhibit platelet aggregation after they experience a TIA. The use of anticoagulants decreases the number of attacks. Aspirin (which prevents platelet aggregation) has also been shown to decrease subsequent attacks. The dose is 0.3 g four times per day. If an isolated, extracranial arterial lesion is found, surgical correction is possible.

The nurse's major role in working with the person who has experienced a TIA is to help the patient (1) understand treatment measures instituted; (2) learn and practice health habits that can help control chronic disease such as atherosclerosis, hypertension, and diabetes mellitus; (3) learn what signs and symptoms indicate another attack is occurring and what to do about it; and (4) understand the need for follow-up care.

Clinical picture

The exact clinical picture will vary depending on the area of the brain affected. The most common focal neurologic signs and symptoms are those caused by disruption of flow through the midcerebral artery (Table 36-3).

Frequently, the patient is unconscious and may experience convulsions. Both unconsciousness and convulsions result from generalized ischemia and the brain's response to abrupt hypoxia.

Depending on the amount of cerebral edema present the patient may have increased intracranial pressure (see Chapter 35 for a description of signs and symptoms of this condition).

A lumbar puncture is usually done and may reveal elevated spinal fluid pressure. If hemorrhage has occurred, there will be blood in the spinal fluid. In almost all instances a computed tomography (CT) scan will be used to visualize the infarcted areas. If the patient is in a coma and it is uncertain how severe the increase in pressure is, computed tomography may be used before the lumbar puncture. Lumbar puncture can precipitate tentorial or foraminal herniation when there is an expanding intracranial mass.

Intervention

Emergency care. A CVA may occur when the person is at work or elsewhere outside the home and may be confused with convulsize seizures, diabetic coma, or drunkenness. Emergency care at the scene of the episode consists of turning the person carefully on to the affected side (determined by the puffiness of the cheek on this side) and elevating the head without tilting the neck forward, since tilting may constrict blood vessels and in turn cause congestion of blood within the cerebrum. Turning to the affected side permits saliva to drain out of the mouth and lessens the danger of aspiration into the lungs. Elevation of the head may help to prevent edema of the brain. Clothing should be loosened about the throat to further aid in preventing engorgement of blood vessels in the head, which may lead to cerebral edema. The person should be kept quiet, moved as little as possible, and protected from chilling. Medical assistance is sought at once.

Care in initial phase. Nursing intervention during the initial phase does not differ whether the person is in the hospital or at home, although oxygen is more likely to be given in the hospital. In an attempt to prevent further thrombosis or emboli, bishydroxycoumarin (Dicumarol) and heparin may be given in the hospital if it is certain that the cause is cerebral thrombosis or emboli and not cerebral hemorrhage. The use of anticoagulants is controversial. Some patients may be treated with various types of vasodilating agents although the effectiveness of this type of therapy is not well established.

Goals are directed toward survival needs and preventing further brain damage. Care by the nurse is directed toward the unconscious state if present (see Chapter 27). Neurologic assessment is done at regular intervals to detect changes in status and complications. The vital signs should be carefully checked, and the nurse should observe for such things as a rise in temperature within the first day or two, slowing of pulse and respiration, and deepening of the coma, all of which indicate pressure on the vital centers and a poor prognosis. Drugs to reduce intracranial pressure, such as dexamethasone (Decadron), may be given.

Care in acute phase. After the patient is stabilized physically as described in the section on initial phase, the nurse has the greatest influence, of all health care givers, on the patient's recovery. Goals for care in the acute phase are directed toward preventing complications from the original CVA, from the immobility and dependency it causes, and from the loss of function caused by focal deficit.

MOTOR FUNCTION. Since the CVA frequently results in some paralysis, the reader is referred to p. 767 for a discussion of the care of the person with loss of motor function.

FOOD AND FLUIDS. Fluids may be restricted for the first few days after a CVA in an effort to prevent edema of the brain. The patients will be fed intravenous fluids, or the physician may insert a nasogastric tube and order tube feedings. When patients are no longer comatose, small amounts of fluid, 5 to 10 ml, can be given several times daily to determine patient's ability to swallow and to help them regain this function. Returning as soon as possible to a regular diet and a normal fluid intake is desirable.

ACTIVITY. Rest and quiet are important even if the CVA has not been serious enough to cause complete loss of consciousness. Some neurologists may prescribe that the head of the bed be kept flat for several days. This is believed to assist cerebral perfusion. No attempt should be made to rouse the patient from coma, although respiratory and circulatory stimulants may be prescribed by the physician if depression of these systems is present.

The length of time the patient remains in bed depends entirely on the type of CVA suffered and the judgment of the physician in regard to early mobilization. Some physicians prescribe fairly long periods of rest after CVAs, whereas others believe that early mobilization of the patient with cerebral thrombosis, and mobilization sometimes begins a day or two after the accident has occured.

Prevention of joint deformity (p. 945) is initiated during the acute stage. This includes positioning of affected limbs in anatomic position and range of motion exercises. There should be a regular schedule for turning the patient to avoid the danger of circulatory stasis, hypostatic pneumonia, and decubitus ulcer.

ELIMINATION. Urinary output should be noted carefully and recorded for several days after a cerebrovascular accident. Retention of urine may occur, but it is more likely that the patient will be incontinent. If urinary incontinence occurs, the patient who is not comatose may be told that control of excretory function probably will improve day by day. Offering a bedpan or a urinal immediately after meals and at other regular intervals helps to overcome incontinence. A retention catheter may be used for the first few days for women patients.

Fecal incontinence is fairly common following a CVA, and again the patient must be reassured that as general improvement occurs, this condition will be overcome. Some patients develop constipation, and impactions develop readily. Elimination must be noted carefully, since diarrhea may develop in the presence of an impaction, thus causing it to go unnoticed for several days. Suppositories such as bisacodyl (Dulcolax) are generally prescribed to be given daily or every other day. However, some physicians order stool softeners, laxatives, or enemas. Warm oil-retention enemas are sometimes given in an attempt to prevent impactions and when impactions occur. Milk of magnesia by mouth is often given, since straining in the act of defecation must be avoided. The patient must be cautioned not to strain and must be assured that the suppositories can easily be repeated if no results are obtained. The patient usually needs assistance in getting on and off the bedpan. Side rails that can be held onto while turning or a trapeze that be reached with the unaffected arm and hand will help the patient to move independently and to get on and off the bedpan if this actively is allowed.

EMOTIONAL SUPPORT. If the patient survives the first few days, consciousness may begin to return, and some of the paralysis may disappear. It is then that the greatest understanding is needed by persons attending the patient. The patient will become aware of the aphasia, drooling, paralysis, and unsteadiness and will be very upset by this awareness. It is at this point that the nurse's active part in rehabilitation begins. By quiet assurance a nurse can help the patient feel that progress toward recovery and self-sufficiency has begun and will continue.

The nurse can help by explaining what is going to be done even though the person may not be able to respond by speaking. If the patient has aphasia and also is unable to use the dominant hand, an additional problem of trying to write with the nondominant hand occurs. The nurse should try to anticipate patients' needs and should make every effort to understand indistinct speech, since repeated attempts to make themselves understood only augment themselves misery and frustration. Usually, if partial speech is present at the time of return to consciousness, there is likelihood that speech will improve, and the patient is heartened by the knowledge of this fact. Speech may also be affected because of involvement of the tongue, mouth, and throat muscles.

The patient who has sustained a CVA may be overly emotional, and this reaction, combined with the fear and frustration on becoming aware of his or her condition, is upsetting to the family. Crying is common, and sometimes family members believe that they are responsible for this sadness when this is usually not true. Family, staff, and other patients need reassurance that they are not the cause of the reaction.

Following a stroke, persons may have difficulty relating to themselves and to their environment. After the acute stage a multibed environment is advocated, since the sensory input from others is helpful. In the initial stage, bringing familiar articles into the patient's environment can be a very helpful stimulus. Examples are a clock, watch, family picture, or a Bible. *Hemianopsia,* or decreased visual field, occurs rather commonly. Approaching patients from the side of intact vision and teaching them to scan will not only make them more aware of stimuli but can help prevent injury. Diminished awareness or denial of the affected side (anosognosia) can occur and could be a safety hazard. This possibility should be considered when the patient runs into objects with the wheelchair or allows the affected arm or leg to drag behind when transferring from chair to bed.[27]

The nurse's observations regarding the mental status of the patient are important. The patient may be disoriented and have decreased judgment or poor memory. A constant environment and routine are quite helpful in improving orientation and the ability to function. Poor judgment and impulsiveness can be major safety hazards. Such behavior is brought to the attention of the physician. The family also will have to be aware of this if they are to care for the patient at home.

Care in rehabilitation phase. The greatest challenge for the nurse in care of the patient who has had a CVA comes after the patient is past the point of danger, for then the long, slow process of learning to use whatever abilities remain or can be relearned must be faced and adjustments to limitations must be made if the patient and family are going to have fulfilling lives.

As a member of the rehabilitation team, the nurse must be capable of exercising initiative and judgment in making a nursing diagnosis and in planning and implementing care to meet rehabilitation goals. Three basic goals are (1) prevention of further impairment, (2) maintenance of existing abilities, and (3) restoration of as much function as possible. Knowledge of the physical arrangements of the setting where the patient will go after discharge should be a priority in planning and implementing care. Return of the function of the lower extremity often occurs before the return of arm function because the vessel most commonly affected is the midcerebral artery (Table 36-3).

Return of motor impulses and subsequent return of function are evidenced by a tightening and spasticity of the affected part. This may appear from the second day to the second week after the CVA. Return of motor impulses is significant for the future use of the affected part but presents new problems for the patient, nurse, and all others who may be involved in care. Muscles that draw the limbs toward the midline become very active, and the arm may be held tightly adducted against the body. The affected lower limb may be held inward and adducted to, or even beyond, the midline. Muscles that draw the limbs into flexion are also stimulated, with the result that the heel is lifted off the ground, the heel cord shortens, and the knee becomes bent. In the upper limb, flexor muscles draw the elbow into the bent position, the wrist is flexed, and fingers are curled in palmar flexion. This is often seen following a CVA because the adductor and flexor muscles are stronger than opposing muscles.

Persistent nursing efforts must be directed toward prevention of further impairment and keeping any part of the body from remaining in a position of flexion long enough for the occurrence of muscle shortening and joint changes that might interfere with free joint action. If a physical therapist is not available, the total responsibility for preventive measures may rest with the nurse. *Every minute counts in prevention, and the nurse must not miss one opportunity to move the patient's adducted or flexed limbs back to the correct position. Passive exercise* stimulates circulation and may help to reestablish neuromuscular pathways. No difficulty is encountered with these procedures until tightening of the muscles begins to appear, then other physical measures are needed, and at this point, if not earlier, a physical therapist should be involved in the patient's treatment.

Active exercise of the affected side also may be started early. In the hospital it may be directed by the physical therapist or nurse. In consultation with the physical therapist the nurse plans the exercises while the patient is in the hospital, and the nurse or the physical therapist may teach the exercises to the family in preparation for the patient's return home.

Since the patient will depend a good deal on the unaffected arm and leg when moving about, the unaffected part of the body needs attention to prevent contractures and preserve muscle strength. Even while in bed, the patient should exercise the unaffected arm and use it in all normal positions. The unaffected leg should be in a position of slight *internal rotation* most of the time while the patient is in bed, and the knee should be bent several times each day. Exercise to strengthen the quadriceps muscle should be done because the quadriceps is the most important muscle in providing stability to the knee joint needed for walking (p. 413).

Early *ambulation* facilitates vasomotor tone and has positive psychologic effects on the patient and family members. Ambulation is usually started by the physical therapist by having the person walk between parallel bars. Transfer techniques are also taught to the patient and family members (p. 930).

When the patients begin to move about and to try to help themselves, they may have several problems that can alter their ability to proceed. They may have loss of position sense, so that it is awkward for them to handle their bodies normally even when they have the muscular coordination to do so. They may have dizziness, spatial-perceptual deficits, diplopia, and alteration of skin sensation. They may also have to work harder than other persons to receive a normal amount of air on inhalation, since the involved side of the chest does not expand easily. This difficulty may lead to excessive fatigue unless those caring for the patient plan activities so that the patient's effort is not wasted.

Before standing or walking, patients may practice raising themselves up in bed and may sit on the side of the bed while holding firmly to an overbed table or to a strap with their good hand and pressing their feet on a chair or stool. The patient benefits from wearing shoes, since it is good for morale and keeps the paralyzed foot in good position.

If preparation for walking has been adequate, the patient usually only needs one crutch when walking begins and then a cane will be used as walking progresses. When walking first begins, the nurse must remain close to allay the fear of falling. Balancing may be practiced by standing between parallel bars or by leaning on the backs of two chairs (provided the chairs are heavy enough to support weight safely). Good walking patterns must be established early because incorrect patterns are difficult and sometimes impossible to change. A sideward shuffle should be watched for and avoided. The patient should begin by leaning rather heavily on the crutch or cane and lifting the body sufficiently to bring the leg and foot forward so that the toes point straight ahead and not inward. The cane or single crutch is held in the hand opposite the paralyzed or weakened side of the body. Pivot transfers may be the easiest way to transfer the patient from bed to chair and vice versa. When a pivot transfer is used, the chair is always placed so that the unaffected side leads the transfer.

The patient is evaluated on ability to carry out the usual *activities of daily living* and is assisted by the occupational therapist or nurse in becoming independent in each activity to the extent possible. Rehabilitation in this way is essentially a teaching-learning process in which the patient is actively involved. Motivation is absolutely essential to rehabilitation but unfortunately is not found to the same degree in all patients. Some patients devote all their energies to their rehabilitation, whereas others just seem to "give up." *If there is return of hand function in 2 to 3 weeks, fecal incontinence has disappeared, and no contractures, decubiti, or other complications have developed, there is reason to believe that the patient can be independent in care.*

Patients need preparation for each new step in learning to move and care for themselves. Each new activity must be demonstrated by the nurse and then practiced by patients; supervision and encouragement must be given by the nurse. Careful and detailed instruction on how to hold and support the body will save patients much embarrassment, discomfort, and confusion. By using the unaffected hand, the patient may, for example, straighten out the flexed fingers on the affected side and move the affected arm to a position where, with the weight of gravity, the elbow will be straightened. Most patients can relearn to do activities of daily living such as those pertaining to personal hygiene and dressing.

Long-range plans. General care and the pattern of living that should be followed after a CVA vary for each patient and are determined by the circumstances, the amount of recovery, and the guidance given in the early stages of the illness. Despite all effort, the patient may, for example, never be able to negotiate stairs. The social worker and the community health nurse are indispensable in helping to arrange the patient's home so that the greatest possible degree of self-sufficiency and independence is possible. Members of the family often need help in assisting the person to accept limitations, both physical and emotional. The family must also make adjustments to actual circumstances. Almost all persons who have CVAs need health supervision for the rest of their lives. Whether the patient will be able to return home or must go to a nursing home will depend a great deal on the family's understanding and acceptance of the patient and his or her limitations when maximal rehabilitation has been achieved.

While it is not uncommon for CVAs to recur, the person may go for years with no further difficulty and eventually die of some other cause. The physician usually explains the prognosis to the person and to the family. The nurse should know what explanation has been given by the physician and must sometimes help in interpreting it to the family.

The person who has sustained a CVA and who has high blood pressure is usually advised to take prescribed antihypertensive medications religiously, to get sufficient rest, and to avoid strain and excitement. Persons involved in strenuous work may be advised to reduce their work schedule and take more frequent vacations. Those who are overweight are advised to bring their weight within normal limits, and those who smoke are advised of the hazards of vasoconstriction caused by nicotine in tobacco. Activities of daily living may be modified; sitting while shaving or doing other similar activities helps conserve enery.

Before discharge to the home or to another health care setting, certain outcomes should be achieved. The major emphasis is on maintaining structural and body integrity consistent with pathologic involvement. The parameters involved in achieving this are an intact skin, normal range of joint motion with no contractures, loss of muscle tone confined to that which is consistent with the pathologic condition, and maintenance of bladder and bowel function. When these outcomes are achieved at the highest degree possible, the person is ready for discharge. Obviously, some persons' conditions will limit their ability to become completely sufficient in activities of daily living and some persons will benefit from long-term rehabilitation either by hospitalization in a rehabilitation hospital or through outpatient follow-up care on a regular basis.

Surgery. After the patient's condition is stable, or after the acute or rehabilitation phase, surgery may be used for selected patients. If the CVA is associated with a distinct atherosclerotic lesion in the extracranial system (internal carotid artery or common carotid artery) a carotid endarterectomy may be performed.

A *carotid endarterectomy* involves the reaming out of the diseased vessel under either local or general anesthesia. Postoperative care includes close attention to neurologic signs (changes in strength, mentation, speech, and level of consciousness), as well as observation of the incision for bleeding. The patient should be observed for swelling of the neck or complaints of dysphagia. Severe respiratory distress can occur, and an endotracheal tube or tracheostomy set should be readily available.

Revascularization procedures are now possible with the use of stereoscopic microscopes. Commonly, the superficial temporal artery is anastomosed to a superficial cortical artery, but other vessels can be used. The purpose is to provide for blood flow. The surgery usually does not resolve any permanent deficits but may prevent more deficits from occurring. The care of the patient preoperatively and postoperatively is similar to that for any patient with cranial surgery (p. 773).

Outcome criteria for the person with a CVA

1. The person shall have made progress toward independence in activities of daily living consistent with neurologic deficits and can:
   a. Feed self independently with or without adaptive equipment.
   b. Bathe self independently with or without adaptive equipment.
   c. Groom self independently with or without adaptive equipment.
   d. Dress self independently with or without adaptive clothing or devices.
   e. Toilet self independently with or without adaptive equipment.
   f. Ambulate independently with or without adaptive equipment (cane, crutch, brace, walker).
   g. Transfer independently from one surface to another (bed to chair, toilet, car, and so on).
   h. Safely compensate for visual field cuts, perceptual, motor, and sensory losses.
2. The person or significant others can:
   a. Explain each prescribed therapy to be followed at home.
   b. Accurately demonstrate each exercise to pysical therapist, occupational therapist, or nurse.
   c. Explain method, rationale, and daily schedule for each exercise.
   d. Explain schedule for return visits to evaluate progress.
   e. Relate need for daily, regular therapy.
3. The person or significant others can explain long-term goals set mutually and with the rehabilitation team and can state need to be independent in activities of daily living despite effort and time involved in doing so.
4. The person and significant others are able to communicate with each other within pathologic limits and can:
   a. Demonstrate the ability to communicate utilizing verbal, written, and or gestural approaches.
   b. Explain the methods to be followed as recommended by the speech pathologist.
5. The person or significant others know about professional and community resources necessary to achieve long-term goals and can:
   a. State how to contact agencies (vocational counselor, rehabilitation counselor, community health nurse).
   b. State how to secure equipment.
   c. State plans for follow-up care.

Intracranial hemorrhage

Intracranial hemorrhages include bleeding into the subarachnoid space or into the brain tissue itself. Unlike cerebral thrombosis or cerebral embolism, intracranial hemorrhages cause damage to the brain by destroying and replacing neighboring brain tissue. Nursing and medical treatment of patients with aneurysms and intracranial hemorrhage can be significantly different from that of patients with CVAs caused by embolism or thrombosis. Because of this intracranial hemorrhages are considered separately.

Epidemiology

Intracranial hemorrhages are the third most frequent cause of CVAs. Bleeding may be from a vessel on the surface of the brain, and the bleeding may be limited to the subarachnoid space. This is called a *subarachnoid hemorrhage with intracerebral hemorrhage*. Bleeding from a vessel in the brain substance is called an *intracerebral hemorrhage* and may form a cerebral hematoma. Intracerebral hemorrhages may extend through the brain tissue to the ventricles and the subarachnoid space.

Etiology

The most common causes of cerebral hemorrhage are listed in Table 36-3. *Berry aneurysms* can result from congenital deficits. *Fusiform aneurysms* can develop from atherosclerosis. *Mycotic aneurysms* are caused by necrotic *vasculitis* occurring in the vessel at a site where septic emboli have lodged. The necrosis causes thinning of the vessel wall and aneurysm formation.

Hypertension causes thickening and degeneration of cerebral arterioles making the small arteries vunerable to rupture. Arteriovenous (A-V) anomalies are tangled, interconnected vessels that allow blood to pass directly from the artery to the vein without passing through capillaries. These vessels may be fed by one or several normal cerebral arteries and are usually malformed. Arterial pressure distends and eventually ruptures these vessels.

Pathophysiology

Any of the above problems (i.e., aneurysms, hypertensive vascular disease, and A-V malformation) can result in a subarachnoid hemorrhage, intracerebral hemorrhage, or a combination of the two. The most common site for berry aneurysms is the anterior portion of the circle of Willis at the junction between the internal carotid and posterior communicating artery. Other common sites are the middle cerebral artery or the anterior communicating artery. A small number of intracranial hemorrhages occur in the vertebral-basilar artery system. Multiple aneurysms are found in many persons. The rupture of a vessel causes disruption of the blood flow to a selected area and causes focal ischemic changes and infarction of brain tissue. In addition, the sudden release of blood acts like a concussion and unconsciousness results.[4] It also causes a rapid rise in cerebrospinal fluid (CSF) pressure with displacement of the brain. Bleeding into brain tissue itself can cause

brain damage by dissecting the brain along the fiber tracts. The blood itself is a noxious agent, and as it is hemolyzed it irritates the blood vessels, the meninges, and the brain. The blood and the release of vasoactive substances promote arterial spasms, which can further decrease cerebral perfusion.

Clinical picture

Symptoms of an intracranial hemorrhage include sudden explosive headache, photophobia, and neck rigidity (if subarachnoid), nausea and vomiting, loss of consciousness (usually), convulsions, signs and symptoms of increased intracranial pressure, respiratory distress, and shock.

The following system of grading has been developed to classify the clinical state of the patient with an intracranial bleed by level of consciousness and neurologic deficit.

grade I Minimal bleeding, alert, no neurologic deficit.
grade II Mild bleeding, alert, minimal neurologic deficit such as third nerve palsy and stiff neck.
grade III Moderate bleeding, drowsy or confused, stiff neck with or without neurologic deficit.
grade IV Moderate or severe bleeding, semicoma with or without neurologic deficit.
grade V Severe bleeding, coma, decerebrate movement.

Additional grades are also added for patients over 50 years of age and those with major heart, lung, kidney, and liver conditions that increase risk for procedures.[72]

Laboratory findings include an abnormal CT scan, increased CSF pressure, and blood and white blood cells in the CSF. Lumbar puncture may not be performed if there is evidence of extensive brain damage for fear of precipitating tentorial herniation. An arteriogram will be used to identify the exact cause of the problem.

Intervention

The immediate treatment for *intracranial hemorrhage* is to keep the person absolutely quiet to prevent additional bleeding. Many of these patients are unconscious and require care as described on p. 531. In addition, since the bleeding causes an elevation in the intracranial pressure they need care for increased intracranial pressure as discussed on p. 757. An antifibrinolytic agent (Amicar) may be used to seal the clot. The person should be very gently moved to bed. Patients are kept flat in bed in a darkened room and attended constantly to be sure that they do not raise their heads. Blood pressure may be taken as often as every 15 minutes. This procedure is best accomplished and is less disturbing to the patient if the cuff is left (deflated) about the arm. If patients are conscious, they are given small amounts of water by mouth, but the water must be given through a straw so that the head is not elevated. Intravenous fluids may be given by slow drip so that blood pressure and intracranial pressure are not increased, and often an indwelling catheter is inserted to avoid the exertion of voiding.

Bowel elimination is usually ignored for several days, and then oil-retention enemas or small doses of bulk laxatives may be given. Under no circumstances should patients be permitted to strain, cough, sneeze, or otherwise exert themselves because these activities increase intracranial pressure. Visitors must be carefully prepared so that they will not upset the patient, and it may be necessary to restrict visitors to the immediate family. No mail should be given the patient unless it is certain that it contains no disturbing information. Hypothermia may be used to lessen the need of the brain for oxygen and thereby decrease the danger of damage to vital brain tissues (p. 756).

About 50% of patients with rupture of an aneurysm recover from the initial episode, but at least 50% of these persons will have recurrences of hemorrhage if untreated. Recurrence may occur within 2 weeks, and the danger of death increases with each recurrence. If the aneurysm is not obliterated by surgery, the patient may die eventually from recurrent hemorrhage. Activities will be restricted for all patients on admission. Thus these patients are kept on bed rest until surgery is performed. Rebleeding from a ruptured A-V anomaly or hypertensive vascular disease is not as likely as from an aneurysm, so these patients are allowed up as soon as they are stable. Surgery is not usually performed to repair A-V anomalies or hypertensive vascular disease. Therefore as soon as the patient is stable, appropriate rehabilitative measures should be instituted (p. 802).

If the aneurysm cannot be successfully treated, however, the family needs to be aware that there is always the danger of sudden death. The patient must be protected from strenuous activity and excitement. The patient is kept on bed rest for approximately 6 weeks and then activities are resumed gradually. Rehabilitation for residual neurologic deficits may be necessary.

Surgery. The only satisfactory treatment for congenital aneurysm is surgery. If an intracerebral hematoma has formed, it may be evacuated after the patient is stable. Before surgery can be performed, however, the location of the aneurysm must be determined by arteriography (angiography), as described on p. 743. The time after the acute rupture when arteriograms are taken and when surgery is performed varies with the person, age, the intensity and kind of symptoms present, and the judgment of the surgeon. Since angiography may increase symptoms, it may be followed by immediate surgery.

Before surgical treatment of an aneurysm is attempted, the surgeon usually explains the hope for cure and the risks involved to the patient's family. The nurse must appreciate how distressing the situation is for the family and should realize that the time spent waiting to know whether the outcome will be favorable seems in-terminable to them. The nursing care the patient will receive postoperatively should be explained to them if they are to be with the patient. For example, it is important that both the patient and the family know that blood pressure, pulse rate, respiratory rate, and other pertinent observations will be taken frequently, since these procedures can be most upsetting if their purpose and the need to check them so frequently is not understood. Some patients may spend the initial postoperative period in the intensive care unit. The family should be prepared for this possibility.

Surgery consists of a *craniotomy* and *location of the aneurysm*. When found, the aneurysm may be obliterated by ligation at its neck with the application of a silver clip. If the base of the aneurysm is too large for ligation to be practical, it may be coated with a liquid, adherent, plastic substance that hardens to form a firm support about the weakened vessel wall and thereby prevents rupture. If the aneurysm has not ruptured but has produced symptoms, attempts may be made to produce thrombosis within the aneurysm by use of an electric current and other means.[58] Both before and after surgery the nurse should observe for signs of increased intracranial pressure (p. 755).

If the surgery is successful, patients will be cured, although usually they will be advised to avoid strenuous exercise and emotional stress of the rest of their lives. Occasionally, they may have a severe physical or mental handicap resulting from damage to brain tissue during surgery. If so, they need the same type of care as discussed for patients with a CVA.

Other procedures. Not all aneurysms can be treated surgically at the site of the lesion. If surgery is not feasible, to reduce the chances of hemorrhage the common carotid artery in the neck may be completely or partially obliterated to lessen the flow of blood to the site of the aneurysm, *provided* enough blood can be supplied from collateral vessels to preserve vital brain function. The procedure usually is done in stages of several days. A clamp (Silverstone or Salibi clamp) that has a detachable screw stem and can be tightened gradually is used.[58] Usually the surgeon adjusts it each day, and the nurse who attends the patient watches closely and is instructed to release the clamp at once if there is evidence of inadequate blood supply. Neurologic checks are done regularly by the nurse relative to placement of the clamp in the dominant or nondominant hemisphere. Any signs of muscle weakness in the face or in either extremity on the side opposite the incision or any changes in the level of consciousness, vital signs, or sensory or muscular coordination or control should be reported to the neurosurgeon at once. Immediate removal of the clamps may prevent irreversible complications such as hemiplegia, aphasia, and loss of consciousness. If symptoms of inadequate blood supply appear, further surgical treatment cannot be done safely, although the clamp may be left indefinitely to partially obliterate the vessel. If complete occlusion can be tolerated, the vessel may be permanently ligated. Serial embolizations of blood vessels that "feed" the aneurysm may also be done via the femoral or axillary route. The procedure is similar to a cerebral angiogram, and the postoperative care is the same. Thrombus formation with resultant cerebral embolism may complicate the patient's postoperative course following any surgery for a cerebral aneurysm. It is a feared and often fatal complication.

Outcome criteria for the person with an intracranial hemorrhage

1. The person does not develop any undetected changes in mental function or physical status (increased intracranial pressure, seizures, rebleeding).
2. The person does not develop any complications from the immobility (decubiti, contractions, urinary tract infection).
3. The person or significant others can explain surgery planned, risk of surgery, preoperative and postoperative care needs (if applicable).
4. Other outcome criteria are the same as for CVA (p. 804).
5. The person and significant others can explain any restriction in activities that might be necessary.
6. The person and significant others can describe the stressors in their lives and ways to decrease them.

Infections

Epidemiology and etiology

The nervous system may be attacked by a variety of organisms and viruses and may suffer from toxic reactions to bacterial and viral disease. Sometimes the infection becomes walled off and causes an abscess; sometimes the meninges, or coverings of the brain and spinal cord, are involved; and sometimes the brain itself is affected most. Organisms and viruses may reach the nervous system by a variety of routes. Untreated chronic otitis media and mastoiditis, chronic sinusitis, and fracture in any bone adjacent to the meninges may be the source of infection. Some organisms such as the tubercle bacillus and probably the pneumococcus reach the nervous system by means of the blood or the lymph system. Meningitis can also occur as a complication of invasive procedures such as lumbar puncture or procedures involving the use of contrast media. The exact route by which some infective agents, such as the meningococcus in epidemic meningitis and the viruses that

cause encephalitis, reach the central nervous system is not known.

Meningococcal meningitis (epidemic) and poliomyelitis are reportable communicable diseases. Because they are becoming less common and because they are discussed in specialized texts, they will be mentioned only briefly here.

Meningitis

Etiology

Meningitis is an acute infection of the meninges usually caused by pneumococci, meningococci (epidemic), staphylococci, streptococci, *Haemophilus influenzae*, or aseptic agents (usually viral). Any other pathogenic organism, such as the tubercle bacillus, that gains access to the subarachnoid spaces can also cause meningitis. Mild forms of the disease do occur and may be referred to as *meningism*. They may be caused by viruses. A common form of the disease is lymphocytic meningitis, believed in many instances to be associated with a virus.

Epidemiology

The incidence of bacterial meningitis is higher in fall and winter when upper respiratory tract infections are common. Children are more often affected than adults because of frequent colds and ear infections. Disease caused by the enteroviruses is more common in the summer and early fall than in other seasons of the year.

Pathophysiology

As previously stated, organisms and viruses reach the nervous system by many routes. Once organisms reach the brain the CSF in the subarachnoid spaces and in the pia arachnoid membrane becomes infected. The infection then spreads rapidly throughout the meninges and eventually invades the ventricles. Pathologic alterations include hyperemia of the meningeal vessels, edema of brain tissue, increased intracranial pressure, and a generalized inflammatory reaction with exudation of white blood cells into the subarachnoid spaces. An associated hydrocephalus may be caused by exudate blocking the small passages between the ventricles.

Clinical picture

Meningitis can be a medical emergency. The onset (except when caused by tubercle bacilli) is usually sudden and characterized by severe headache, stiffness of the neck, irritability, malaise, and restlessness. Nausea, vomiting, delirium, and complete disorientation may develop quickly. *Kernig's sign* (the inability of the patient to extend the legs completely without extreme pain) is usually present with meningitis. When the neck of the patient with meningitis is flexed, the hip and knee also flex. This is known as *Brudzinski's sign*. Temperature, pulse rate, and respirations are increased. The diagnosis is usually confirmed by examination of spinal fluid obtained from a lumbar puncture. Usually the offending organism can be isolated from the spinal fluid, and if a pyogenic organism is the cause, the fluid is cloudy. The CSF pressure is usually elevated, the protein level is elevated, and there is a decrease in the sugar content.

Intervention

Treatment consists of massive doses of the antibiotic specific for the causative organism. Culture and sensitivity studies determine the most effective antibiotic. Usually a course of at least 10 days of parenteral administration is needed. The antibiotic may be given directly into the spinal canal (intrathecally). The use of hyperosmolar agents or steroids may also be necessary to decrease cerebral edema. Anticonvulsants may be administered to prevent seizures.

Respiratory isolation is required until the pathogen can no longer be cultured from the nasopharynx. This is usually accomplished after 24 hours of effective antimicrobial therapy. Therapy is continued until the patient has been afebrile for 5 days or after 7 days of therapy (whichever is longer).

Nursing care for the patient with meningitis includes the general care given a critically ill patient who may be irritable, confused, and unable to take fluids and yet who is dehydrated because of elevation of temperature. The room is kept darkened, noise is kept at a minimum, and care is taken not to jar the bed, since any increase in sensory stimulation can cause a seizure. The patient must be observed very carefully and must be constantly attended if disorientation is present. Padded side rails should be placed on the bed. The patient should be observed for symptoms of inappropriate secretion of antidiuretic hormone (p. 304), which can occur readily in patients with meningitis.

Residual damage from meningitis includes deafness, blindness, paralysis, and mental retardation. These complications are usually the result of chronic arachnoiditis or subdural effusion. Hydrocephalus may also develop, requiring a shunting procedure. However, these complications are now less common because the infection is effectively treated with antibiotics before permanent damage to the nervous system occurs.

Encephalitis

Epidemiology and etiology

Encephalitis is inflammation of the brain tissues and its coverings. Occasionally, the meninges of the spinal cord are also involved. Encephalitis can have a variety of causes. A generalized inflammation of the brain can be caused by syphilis, and encephalitis can follow exogenous poisoning such as that which follows the ingestion or lead or arsenic or the inhalation of carbon monoxide. It can be caused by reaction to toxins produced by infections such as typhoid fever, measles, and chickenpox, and occasionally it follows vaccination.

Encephalitis caused by a virus and occurring in epidemic form was first described by von Economo in Austria, and the name Von Economo's disease is still used to identify the widespread epidemic in the United States that followed the influenza epidemic in 1918. This form of the disease has not recurred since 1926. Von Economo's disease was also called encephalitis lethargica and sleeping sickness, a term still used by lay persons. The demonstration that viruses can affect the central nervous system after a prolonged incubation period has resulted in considerable search for viral agents in many chronic neurologic diseases.

The death rate from encephalitis varies with epidemics but is generally fairly high. The most common sequela for patients who do recover from the acute disease is *paralysis agitans*, which may come on suddenly or develop slowly. Other residual neurologic symptoms may also occur and occasionally incapacitate the patient completely.

Acute viral encephalitis

Viral encephalitis appears to be caused by a number of viruses, some of which may be interrelated. Acute viral encephalitis can be classified as epidemic and sporadic forms. The primary causes of acute epidemic encephalitis are members of the *arbovirus* (those transferred by a biting arthropod to humans) or *togavirus* group (named after properties of the virus). There are about 80 viruses of the arbovirus group that cause disease in humans. Six of the viruses cause infections of the central nervous system (Table 36-4).

Clinical picture. Clinical features of *acute epidemic encephalitis*, caused by the arboviruses that infect humans, are similar. The eastern equine form is more severe than the western form. The onset is abrupt, with a *high fever, headache, meningeal signs, nuchal rigidity, and vomiting. Drowsiness or coma and focal or generalized convulsions develop within 24 to 48 hours after onset.* Focal neurologic signs develop, such as hemiplegia and cranial nerve palsies. There are typical findings in the CSF. Fatality rates may be as high as 60%. Those who survive usually have no sequelae.[4]

Intervention. Nursing care consists mainly of symptomatic or supportive care and careful observation. Any change in appearance or behavior must be reported at once, since the progress of this disease sometimes is extremely rapid. The patient is kept in bed, and side rails are used if disorientation develops. The patient must be constantly attended to prevent injury. During the

TABLE 36-4. Arbovirus infections of the central nervous system occurring in the western hemisphere*

Disease	Causal agent	Location	Incubation period (days)	Clinical manifestation
California encephalitis	Arbovirus of California virus (mosquito-borne)	United States, Canada, Alaska, the Yukon, and the northwest territories	5-15	Aseptic meningitis, encephalitis
Eastern equine encephalitis	Eastern equine encephaencephalitis virus (mosquito-borne)	Eastern seaboard and Gulf states, Caribbean	5-15	Severe encephalitis (usually infants and children)
Powassan encephalitis	Powassan virus (tick-borne)	Canada, northeastern and north-central United States	4-8	Encephalitis
St. Louis encephalitis	St. Louis encephalitis virus (mosquito-borne)	Central, southern, northwestern, western, and central United States; southern Ontario; Caribbean	4-21	Encephalitis, aseptic meningitis
Venezuelan equine encephalomyelitis	Venezuelan equine encephalomyelitis virus (mosquito-borne)	Texas, Florida, Mexico, Central and South America	2-5	Fever, headache, myalgia, malaise, cough, encephalitis
Western equine encephalomyelitis	Western equine encephalomyelitis virus (mosquito-borne)	Central and western United States and Canada, Central and South America	5-10	Encephalitis (infants), fever, aseptic meningitis

*Adapted from Report of the Committee on Infectious Diseases, American Academy of Pediatrics, 1977.

period when the temperature is high, sponging or other hypothermia measures may be ordered. Frequent changes of linen may be necessary if perspiration is excessive. There is no specific medical treatment for this disease. No isolation is necessary, since encephalitis is not transmitted from person to person. Prevention of arboviral infections consists of eradication of the mosquito or tick vector, including destruction of larvae and elimination of breeding places. Control is by avoiding bites of the mosquito or tick vectors.

Acute encephalitis (nonepidemic)

Acute encephalitis occurs sporadically and is caused by the herpes simplex virus (HSV). It occurs at any age, but over half of the cases are in persons at least 15 years of age. Upper respiratory complaints often precede the onset of neurologic symptoms by at least 24 hours or longer. Headache and focal or major convulsions are the common early signs of cerebral involvement. A persistent high fever and coma are common. Spinal fluid proteins may be moderately elevated, and red blood cells are often present when spinal fluid is examined. Herpetic skin lesions are not common. Treatment is supportive with anticonvulsant drugs and steroids to reduce cerebral edema. Adenine arabinoside (ARa-A) may be given parenterally.

Brain abscess

Epidemiology and etiology

A brain abscess is almost always secondary to a foci of infection somewhere else in the body. Common sites include the ear, sinus or mastoid, lung, heart, pelvic organs, teeth, or skin. The three most common organisms involved are streptococci, staphylococci, and pneumococci. Brain abscesses are most common in older children and young adults but may be seen at any age. At times no organism is found and the abcess is called a "sterile abscess."

Pathophysiology

In the first stage of brain abcess there is a localized inflammation of the brain with formation of exudate. Septic thrombosis of some vessels occurs, and the surrounding brain tissue becomes edematous and necrotic. After a period of time (days to weeks) the inflammatory reaction decreases as the area is walled off. It is not uncommon for "satellite" abscesses to occur and for the abscesses to rupture into the ventricles. Brain abscesses are most commonly found in the temporal lobe and the cerebellum.

Clinical picture

There may be a history of infection although the person may not recall an infection. The most common symptom is a constant or intermittent headache that is not relieved by medication and that is increased by straining. There may be drowsiness, confusion, and mental slowness. Focal or generalized seizures may occur. Fever with bradycardia is often present. There may be signs and symptoms of increased intracranial pressure (p. 755). The evolution of symptoms is variable. In some patients there may be a rapid progression of symptoms ending in death, whereas in others the course is more benign. Generally, however, the mortality is high with brain abscess and residual disability often results. Brain abscess may recur.

The diagnosis of brain abscess is made primarily on the basis of the history and examination of the CSF. EEG changes are present, and there will be areas of increased uptake of dye on the CT scan.

Intervention

Treatment consists of administering the appropriate antibiotics often for extended periods of time. Because it may take some time to isolate the causative organism, broad-spectrum antibiotics or combined antibiotic therapy may be used. Appropriate agents to reduce intracranial pressure may be necessary. Nursing care is supportive and directed toward ongoing assessment for signs and symptoms of increased intracranial pressure, seizures, and spread of the infection. Measures to prevent permanent damage from neurologic deficits that might be present should be instituted. The long hospitalization, length of treatment, neurologic deficits, and chance for recurrence all are major sources of stress, and the nurse must be prepared to spend time with the patient and significant others to help them cope with these stressors.

Poliomyelitis

Poliomyelitis is an acute febrile disease caused by poliovirus types 1,2, and 3; paralysis is more common with type 1. With discovery of the Salk vaccine, its wide use since 1956, and the availability of a safe "live virus" vaccine (Sabin vaccine), this disease, which had been a serious crippler of children and young adults, has become quite rare.

The incubation period for poliomyelitis is from 7 to 21 days. The virus attacks the anterior horn cells of the spinal cord where the motor pathways are located and may cause motor paralysis. Sensory perception is not affected since posterior horn cells are not attacked. Poliomyelitis sometimes takes a somewhat different form and attacks primarily the medulla and basal structures of the brain, including the cranial nerves; the term *bul-*

bar poliomyelitis is used for this form. Management usually includes bedrest, supportive therapy, and respiratory assistance if needed.

An important responsibility of the nurse is to help prevent poliomyelitis by encouraging immunization. In the United States there is a concerted effort to have all children immunized, since the number of immunizations have decreased in recent years.

Guillain-Barré-Strohl syndrome (polyneuritis)

Epidemiology and etiology

Guillain-Barré-Strohl syndrome, known also as acute inflammatory polyradiculoneuropathy and postinfectious polyneuritis, is often serious because of the extent to which the nervous system may be affected. This condition has become better known to the public since it was identified as a sequela of swine flu immunization. The disease is most common in persons 30 to 50 years of age and is seen equally in men and women. The cause is unknown, but two thoughts are emerging: (1) that it is caused by a viral agent or (2) that it is an autoimmune reaction.

Pathophysiology

There is patchy demyelination in the peripheral nerves, nerve roots, and root ganglia and spinal cord. For this reason it may be classified as a neuritis. Axons are generally spared so that recovery may occur early; in severe forms, *wallerian degeneration* (p. 828) occurs with involvement of the axons, making recovery slow. In the severe form there is an elevation of protein in the CSF.

If the seventh, ninth, and tenth cranial nerves are involved, the patient may have varying degrees of difficulty in swallowing, speaking, and breathing. The vital centers in the medulla oblongata may be affected, and the patient may die of respiratory failure. Patients with less severe involvement may recover fully, although a year or more may transpire before the patient is completely well.

Clinical picture

There is symmetric muscle weakness and lower motor paralysis characteristics (flaccidity). The paralysis usually starts in the lower extremities, and it ascends upward to include the thorax, upper extremities, and face. Selected cranial nerves may also be affected, as previously mentioned. Other symptoms that may be assessed clinically are paresthesias and sensory alteration as the sensory roots and nerves may also become involved. Respiratory failure may occur as intercostal muscles are affected, and without mechanical ventilation there is a 10% to 20% mortality.[4] The bowel and bladder are rarely affected. Autonomic symptoms, such as a fluctuating blood pressure, are not uncommon.

There may be variations in the pattern of onset of weakness, as well as in the rate of progression of symptoms. The progression may stop at any point.

Intervention

A priority goal for nurse and patient is the maintenance of respiratory function. Close observation of respiratory function is necessary. This should include serial measurements of the patient's vital capacity, tidal volume, and minute volume. Urinary retention occurs in about 5% of patients. Patients who develop respiratory failure require mechanical ventilation and are usually placed in an intensive care unit. Nursing care of patients with respiratory failure is discussed on p. 772. Adrenocortical steroids are used empirically to treat symptoms. Convalescence may require several months. Attention to the prevention of iatrogenic complications such as contracture, decubitus ulcers, muscle atrophy, and loss of range of motion is imperative. Recovery is usually complete.

Neurosyphilis

In the late or chronic stage of syphilis, infection may involve the brain and spinal cord. The oculomotor nerves may be involved, causing inability of the pupil to react to light (Argyll Robertson pupil). *Tabes dorsalis* is the name given to the involvement of the posterior columns of the spinal cord and the posterior nerve roots. Since the sensory nerves are primarily involved, sensory symptoms predominate. The patient may have severe paroxysmal pain anywhere in the body, although perhaps the most common location is in the stomach. This condition, known as *gastric crisis,* may be confused with ruptured peptic ulcer or other acute conditions of the stomach or gallbladder. There may be areas of severe paresthesia. A common finding in tabes dorsalis is loss of position sense in the feet and legs. The patient is unable to sense where the feet are placed, and as a result there is a slapping gait that is highly characteristic of the disease. There is increased difficulty walking in the dark because the person relies on vision in placing the feet. Visual loss or even total blindness also occurs. Tabes dorsalis can cause trophic changes in the limbs and changes in the joints so that stability is lost (Charcot's joint).

General paresis is the term used to designate another late manifestation of syphilis in which there is degeneration of the brain and deterioration of mental function and varying evidences of other neurologic disease. More specific information can be found in neurology texts.

With the success of penicillin in the treatment of syphilis the incidence of neurosyphilis has decreased. However, the recent rise in the overall incidence of syphilis among the young may indicate problems in the future.

• • •

Outcome criteria for the person with an infection of the nervous system

The person or significant others can:
1. Explain the nature of the infection, infectious agent, and method of transmission.
2. Explain any neurologic deficits resulting from the infection.
3. Explain how to prevent further infection.
4. State plans for follow-up care.

Traumatic lesions

Parts of the nervous system commonly subjected to trauma include the craniocerebrum, the spinal cord, and the peripheral nerves. With the exception of the peripheral nerves, each is protected by a bony covering. The phrase *traumatic lesions,* as used here, includes lesions resulting from direct physical force and injuries that result from sustained compression. Attention is directed primarily to the former in the following discussion.

Craniocerebral trauma

Epidemiology

Craniocerebral trauma, or head injury, causes death and serious disability in people of all ages. In the United States, head injuries result in about 80,000 deaths yearly. Primary traumatic lesions result from industrial, motor vehicle, and military accidents. Head injury is the second most common cause of major neurologic deficits, and the major cause of death between ages 1 and 35.[4] It is estimated that 70% of motor accidents result in head injury. Brain injury causes more deaths than does injury to any other organ. In some states the repeal of laws requiring motorcyclists to wear helmets has resulted in an estimated threefold increase in death and injury resulting from damage to the brain sustained in motorcycle accidents.

Etiology and pathophysiology

Craniocerebral trauma may result in injury to the scalp, skull, and brain tissues, either singly or collectively. Some of the variables that may modify the extent of the injury to the head include the location and direction of the impact, rate of the energy transfer, the surface area of energy transfer, and the status of the head at the time of the impact. Injuries vary from minor scalp wounds to concussions and open fractures of the skull with severe damage to the brain. The amount of obvious damage is not indicative of the seriousness of the trouble.

Contusions, abrasions, and lacerations of the scalp may occur. Lacerations of the scalp bleed profusely because of its large blood supply. Most bleeding is minor and controlled readily. An internal hematoma of the scalp may form as a result of the bleeding and resemble a depressed fracture. Infection of the scalp may result from the prescence of foreign debris. It should be stressed that the absence of external scalp injury does not preclude serious craniocerebral damage.

The skull indents and deforms when a physical impact occurs. Fractures commonly result, and they are classified as in other parts of the body (p. 1017). Skull x-ray films may detect the fractures; a negative x-ray film does not exclude the presence of a fracture such as a hairline fracture. Fractures can occur distal to the point of impact. A compound and depressed fracture causes serious complications. *The presence of a skull fracture does not necessarily indicate that brain injury has occurred.* There is often a reverse correlation between skull damage and brain damage. Complications of skull damage may include injury to cranial nerves, epidural hemorrhage, and brain contusion.

Types of lesions

Damage to the brain tissues per se may include concussion, contusion, or laceration. Each is discussed briefly to differentiate them as to degree of damage and significance. The dura may remain intact in brain damage and is thought of as a *closed injury,* or the dura may be opened from a direct blow or from penetrating objects such as bone fragments or knives and is then classified as an *open injury.* A *concussion* is characterized by immediate and transitory impairment of neurologic function caused by the mechanical force. There is no demonstrable structural alteration. There may be loss of consciousness that is instant or delayed and is usually recovered. The effect of a blow on the cranium to the soft brain tissues contained within the closed cavity is one of sudden movement. This effect can be likened to what happens as one stops suddenly when moving quickly with an open dish of fluid—some of the fluid spills. The only difference is that instead of spilling in the closed cavity, the brain tissues strike the bony coverings forcibly. The sustained damage is variable in degree. There may be damage to the brain stem centers and cerebral hemispheres. There can be loss of consciousness, the cause of which is not clearly understood. Any person exhibiting an alteration in consciousness following a blow on the head should be under constant observation for a period of time, since damage is not always immediately apparent.

A *contusion* is a structural alteration characterized by extravasation of blood cells. It can be likened to bruising without tearing of the tissues. The contusion may be at the site of the impact or on the opposite side. A concussion or contusion site may be classified as a *coup* (at the site), *contrecoup* (opposite the site), or *intermediate.* Contusions often damage the cortex. *Laceration* of the brain tissues and blood vessels is a tearing of the tissues that may be caused by a sharp fragment or object or a shearing force. It is obvious that hemorrhage may be a serious complication.

In summary, when the head receives a direct blow or injury, the brain moves in the skull and suffers varying degrees of damage not always at the site of the injury. In addition, the brain swells to a great extent, and the capacity of the brain to swell may exceed the capacity of the closed cranial cavity to expand. Most deaths from head injury are from the brain swelling rather than from the actual primary destruction of vital centers. Brain edema is thus a major cause of increased intracranial pressure and its consequences (as previously discussed on p. 753). Along with the swelling, local and systemic disturbances in circulation occur with resulting anoxia. The brain damage may be minor or severe. There is often a great disparity between functional neurologic derangement and structural damage that can be demonstrated.

Assessment of head injury

Most patients with head injuries will be examined in the emergency department where beginning treatment is instituted. The airway is assessed first. It is important to maintain an open airway and ensure adequate oxygenation. Anoxia with a buildup of carbon dioxide can produce cerebral hypoxia and subsequent cerebral edema, which can result in irreparable damage. It is important to assess the ability to clear the airway. Blood or mucus from injuries may block the airway, or the patient may have vomited and suctioning may be necessary. Inability to clear the airway can lead to airway obstruction as well as aspiration pneumonia. Oxygen should be given to the patient with a head injury and if the patient cannot clear the airway an endotracheal tube should be inserted.

A careful neurologic examination is done. The patient's responsiveness is determined and is described in terms of behavior. Pupils are checked for inequality as well as for reaction to light. If an enlarged pupil is present unilaterally, this is indication for immediate surgery. It is important to assess the extremities for ability to move them as well as for quality of movement. The ability to speak is also assessed, as is the presence of headache, double vision, nausea, or vomiting. Measurement of blood pressure, pulse, and respiration is also important since these become baseline data for comparison with later findings. Changes in these parameters may indicate neurologic decline. Blood is drawn for baseline tests.

Since many persons with head injury, especially those involved in automobile accidents, have sustained other injuries, the intrathoracic and intraabdominal areas are checked carefully and the limbs are examined for fractures or injury to nerves or arteries. It is important to determine what caused the injury, as well as the direction and force of the blow. A history of any bleeding from the eyes, ears, nose, or mouth is recorded. Inability to move the extremities is also noted. Baseline nursing assessment of the patient with a head injury is included in the box at right.

Diagnostic procedures are performed as necessary and most commonly include CT scan, skull roentgenograms, and possibly cerebral angiography. When a hematoma is suspected, a trephine of the skull (burr holes) may be performed. It is important to remember that the contrast media used during the CT scan and angiography will in and of itself increase intracranial pressure.

While the patient's emergency needs are being met, a history is obtained from family members or other witnesses. Details are collected about the accident and especially about the duration of unconsciousness, since this is a rough index of the severity of the injury.[4]

Neurologic examination is repeated at frequent intervals to determine changes in consciousness, respiration, pupils, motor strength, speech, and vision. Changes in any of these may indicate an expanding intracranial mass. Vital signs are also checked frequently, and intracranial pressure may be monitored continuously by a ventricular catheter.

Lumbar puncture is usually not performed in the presence of head injury because the sudden withdrawal of fluid can precipitate transtentorial or foramen magnum herniation when there is cerebral edema or an intracranial clot.

Hemorrhage resulting from craniocerebral trauma may occur at the following sites: scalp, epidural, subdural, subarachnoid, intracerebral, and intraventricular. Epidural and subdural hematomas are discussed because of the need for careful and continuing observations by the nurse. An *epidural hematoma* forms as blood collects between the dura and the skull. Since bleeding in this area is commonly caused by laceration of the middle meningeal artery, it is capable of producing rapid clot formation. *If lethargy or unconsciousness develops after the patient regains consciousness*, an epidural hematoma may be suspected. Bleeding needs to be controlled promptly and the blood evacuated. Common sites for bleeding include basal and temporal skull fractures. The nurse should be alert for potential epidural hematomas when it is known that fractures exist in these sites. A *subdural hematoma* forms as venous blood collects below the dural surface. Since the bleeding is under venous pressure, the hematoma formation

---

BASELINE NURSING ASSESSMENT OF THE PATIENT WITH A HEAD INJURY

1. Respiratory status
   a. Patent airway
   b. Need for suctioning
   c. Need for intubation and/or mechanical ventilation
2. Level of alertness and consciousness
3. Orientation
4. Pupil size, equality, and reactivity
5. Motor strengths
6. Temperature, blood pressure, pulse
7. Bleeding from ear, nose, eyes, or mouth
8. Presence of headache, visual changes (diplopia), nausea, or vomiting

---

is relatively slow. However, the clot formation will cause pressure on the brain surface and may eventually displace brain tissue. If this expanding clot is not evacuated, it can contribute to a rise in intracranial pressure and its sequelae. Thus a subdural hematoma can become serious because of its location and compression of vital areas. If a patient who has been conscious for several weeks or months after a head injury becomes unconscious and develops neurologic symptoms, a subdural hematoma should be suspected. *Nurses need to be aware of the delayed signs of head injury as well as the immediate and more obvious ones. The focal neurologic signs from clot formation can be related to the site of the clot.*

Fractures of the *base of the skull*, are usually serious because of their site. When one is sustained, *vital centers, cranial nerves, and nerve pathways may be permanently damaged.* Trauma and the resulting edema may obstruct CSF flow directly or indirectly with resultant increased intracranial pressure. If the injury has caused a direct communication between the cranial cavity and the middle ear or the sinuses, meningitis or a brain abscess may develop. Bleeding from the nose and the ears suggests a basal fracture. Serosanguineous drainage from these orifices may contain CSF and should be noted. Intracranial bleeding as a result of trauma may cause the same signs and symptoms as nontraumatic hemorrhage (p. 804). Interventions are the same as discussed on p. 805.

Intervention

The immediate care is directed toward lifesaving measures and the maintenance of normal body functions until the time when recovery is assured. With appropriate continuing care and rehabilitation, even the severely injured may regain consciousness, recover to some extent, and return to an active life.

The patient who has a skull fracture or other serious head injury must be attended constantly. The major aims of medical and nursing management are (1) to be constantly alert for changes in the patient's condition, especially changes that indicate any increase in intracranial pressure; (2) to sustain patients' vital functions until they have recovered sufficiently to resume them on their own; and (3) to minimize complications that will be life threatening or interefere with full recovery. (See p. 753 for a discussion of the components of increased intracranial pressure.)

Many neurosurgeons feel that alert and intelligent nursing care is often the decisive factor in determining the outcome of the patient. Side rails should always be on the bed, and a padded tongue blade or an airway to protect the tongue should be kept at the bedside, since restlessness may come on suddenly and convulsions may occur. Usually the bed is kept flat, although some neurosurgeons believe that the danger of edema to the brain may be reduced by slight elevation of the head of the bed.[79]

Rest and control of convulsions. The patient should be kept as quiet as possible. No vigorous effort should be made to "clean the patient up" during the first few hours after an accident. Rest and constant observation are much more important. Sudden noises, flashes of light, and the clatter of equipment can increase the patient's restlessness and should be avoided. Portable equipment should be used to take roentgenograms. Nurses must remain in the room with patients to help them move and to protect them from exertion. Restlessness may be caused by the need for a slight change of position, the relaxation of a limb, or the need to empty the bladder. If nursing measures fail to allay extreme restlessness, the physician may order sodium amytal intramuscularly or paraldehyde. Morphine is not given to relieve pain because it will depress the patient's responsiveness and cause pupillary constriction, thus interfering with the necessary observation of pupillary change. Codeine or other mild analgesics may be necessary, however.

Twitching or convulsive movement of a body part is recorded in detail and reported at once. In some medical centers, anticonvulsants are given prophylactically when seizures are anticipated; they are always given once seizures occur.

Vital signs and temperature control. Usually the blood pressure, pulse, and respiratory rate are taken and recorded every 15 minutes until they become stabilized and remain within safe limits. Leaving the deflated blood pressure cuff on the arm helps to prevent disturbing the patient unduly when the pressure must be taken often. Developing the habit of not forcing the mercury column much above the expected reading also sometimes enables the nurse to take the blood pressure and yet barely disturb the patient. The eyes are observed for inequality of the pupils and the lips and fingernails for cyanosis. A sudden sharp rise in temperature, which may go to 42° C (106° F) or higher, and a sudden drop in blood pressure indicate that the regulatory mechanisms have lost control and the prognosis is poor. When there is elevation in temperature, measures will need to be instituted to reduce the temperature, to normal. Although hypothermia has been used in the treatment of patients with severe brain contusions, it is being used less often because of some of the undesirable side effects. Instead, the nursing measures usually employed to reduce temperature, such as the administration of aspirin, tepid sponges, ice bags to the groin and axillae, and reduction of the temperature in the patient's room, are used. Electrically controlled cooling mattresses are also frequently used (Fig. 36-1).

Respiratory insufficiency. One of the most common complications of severe head injury is respiratory insufficiency. Cerebral anoxia, which is a sequela of respiratory insufficiency, is a leading cause of death in these patients. The patient who has respiratory insufficiency may have hypoxia, hypercarbia, hypotension, and dyspnea. Most generally these patients will be intubated and will receive respiratory assistance with one of the mechanical respirators (p. 773). Arterial blood gas levels and pH are checked frequently to determine whether respiratory exchange is adequate. The patient will have to be suctioned as necessary to maintain a patent airway. (See p. 1231 for further nursing care of the intubated patient.)

Drainage from ears and nose. The patient's ears and nose are observed carefully for signs of blood and for serous drainage, which may indicate that the meninges have been torn (common in basal skull fractures) and that spinal fluid is escaping. No attempt should be made to clean out these orifices. Loose sterile cotton may be placed in the outer openings only. This procedure must be done with caution so that the cotton does not in any way act as a plug to interfere with free flow of fluid. The cotton should be changed as soon as it becomes moistened. Usually the flow of fluid subsides spontaneously. Antibiotics usually are given when a basal fracture has been sustained. Suction is never used to remove nasal secretions in any patient who has a head injury or who has undergone brain surgery because of the danger of causing further damage. *Meningitis is a possible complication when communication with the nose and ears occurs.* If there is evidence of drainage of spinal fluid from the nose, the patient should not cough, sneeze, or blow the nose. These activities may, in addition to contributing to the development of meningitis, enable air to enter the cranial cavity, where it may increase

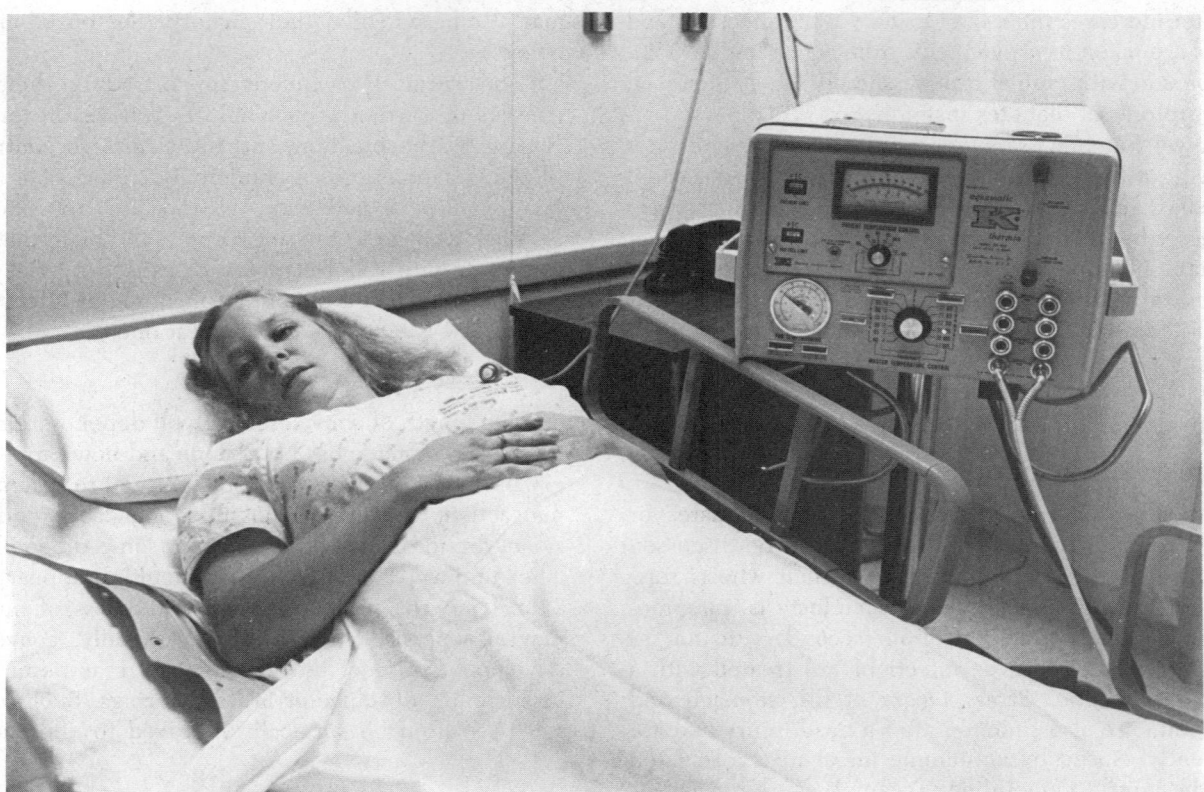

Fig. 36-1. Patient lying on cooling mattress connected to hypothermia machine.

symptoms of intracranial pressure. Sometimes it is difficult to determine whether drainage from the nose is mucus or CSF. A Tes-Tape will give a positive sugar reaction to spinal fluid and a negative reaction to mucus.[5]

Control of cerebral edema. Cerebral edema and increased intracranial pressure are common problems in patients with head injuries. Osmotic diuretics that penetrate the brain slowly, such as 30% solution of urea in 10% invert sugar or 20% mannitol, may be given intravenously for several days.[4] When the patient's condition is deteriorating because of cerebral edema, dexamethasone is usually administered intravenously. The usual dose is 10 mg initially, followed by 4 mg intramuscularly or intravenously every 4 hours thereafter. The steroids are also useful in combating shock associated with head injury. Usually they are employed only during the acute phase because of their side effects (p. 757).

Electrolyte balance. Careful monitoring of electrolytes is necessary. Several types of sodium imbalance are known to occur in head injury. *Natriuresis,* or increased urinary excretion of sodium, is common. More recently this has been attributed to the inappropriate ADH syndrome (with an increased plasma level of ADH, serum hyponatremia, and hypotonicity). This aggra-

vates cerebral edema. Hypernatremia, or cerebral sodium retention, may also occur. No specific variations in potassium or chlorides have been noted. Plasma cortisol levels are also elevated in acute head injury. Plasma, BUN, pH, electrolytes, and urinary electrolyte levels are checked frequently.

Elimination. The patient's intake and output should be carefully measured and recorded. The specific gravity of the urine is also measured and recorded. These measures may be performed hourly when the patient's condition is acute.

Fluid intake may be restricted to 1500 to 2500 ml daily, and it is the nurse's responsibility to see that this is spread over the 24-hour period. Fluids may be given parenterally, by nasogastric tube, or by mouth, depending on the condition of the patient. The nurse must use caution in administering fluids orally, since the patient may have difficulty with vomiting and aspiration. The urinary output should be approximately 0.6 to 1 ml/kg of body weight per hour. This means that a person weighing 175 lb (79 kg) should eliminate between 45 and 80 ml/hour, and if osmotic diuretics have been given, this amount may be greater. An indwelling catheter is essential when giving mannitol because of the large amounts of urine produced and the need to measure output exactly. The presence of an indwelling catheter increases the risk of urinary tract infection, and efforts are taken to prevent this from occurring (p. 372). The person with cranial trauma should also be assessed for symptoms of diabetes insipidus (p. 777).

Bowel function is not encouraged for several days following a head injury. Mild bulk laxatives, bisacodyl (Dulcolax) suppositories, and oil-retention enemas may be prescribed. The patient is cautioned repeatedly not to strain in an effort to defecate, since straining increases intracranial pressure. When the patient is receiving steroids, it is important to check stool guaiac frequently to determine the presence of occult blood. Some patients develop diarrhea secondary to antibiotic therapy.

Complications of head injury

Patients with severe head injuries are candidates for several complications, some of which will be discussed in this section. As with any other patient who is seriously ill, the patient may develop atelectasis, pneumonia, or a urinary tract infection (secondary to an indwelling catheter). These infections are treated with a suitable antibiotic. *Stress ulcers* of the stomach and duodenum are also common after a head injury and are apparently caused by autonomic imbalances associated with the injury. Cimetidine (Tagamet) can be given intravenously and acts to decrease the acid production of the stomach. Antacids can be given when the patient is able to take oral fluids. Antacids are especially important if the patient is on steroids such as prednisone, which is ulcerogenic.

Prolonged unconsciousness. General nursing care as described in Chapter 27 is necessary for the patient with a head injury who remains unconscious for some time. Patients may be unconscious for long periods of time and yet make a satisfactory recovery, provided good supportive care has been given.

Extradural hematoma. Because of the danger of extradural hematoma, as discussed previously, many physicians believe that any patient who has sustained any injury to the head with loss of consciousness should be hospitalized for at least 24 hours. If patients are asleep during this time, they should be awakened hourly to determine their state of consciousness. Some physicians believe that fluids should be restricted to 1000 to 1500 ml for the first day or two and that an osmotic diuretic should be given. If patients do remain at home, the families should be told to watch them closely for signs of increased intracranial pressure, to awaken them hourly during the night after injury, and to bring them to a hospital at once if drowsiness, stupor, paralysis, convulsions, or inequality of the pupil size occur. Written handouts with appropriate instructions about head injury can be extremely helpful to families of patients who are sent home instead of being hospitalized. It not only alerts them about what to observe the patient for but

may also help to allay their anxiety. (See boxed material below.)

The surgical treatment for extradural hematoma consists of making a burr hole to relieve the pressure caused by the bleeding and to attempt to control the bleeding. Sometimes a craniotomy, removal of a large bony window, is necessary. Occasionally, the patient has so much damage to the soft tissue of the brain that death occurs despite relief of pressure caused by the bleeding. Usually such a patient is unconscious after the accident and is taken to a hospital at once.

Convalescence

The length of convalescence will depend entirely on how much damage has been done and how rapid recovery has been. Patients are usually urged to resume normal activity as soon as possible. Headache and occasional dizziness may be present for some time following a head injury. These difficulties should disappear within 3 to 4 months. Loss of memory and loss of initiative may also persist for a time. Occasionally, convulsions develop because of the formation of scar tissue in injured brain substance or in its coverings. Such scar tissue may often be surgically removed to effect a com-

---

INSTRUCTIONS FOR PATIENTS WITH A HEAD INJURY

Patient should be awakened periodically through the first 24 hours to be sure he or she can wake up easily.

Also, for the first 24 to 48 hours, the family should watch carefully for the following warning signs:

1. Vomiting (throwing up)—often with force behind it
2. Unusual sleepiness, dizziness and loss of balance, or falling
3. Complaint of seeing two of everything or blurry objects; jerking movements of the eyes
4. Bleeding or discharge from nose or ears
5. A slight headache may be expected; however, if it gets worse and the patient complains of feeling even worse when moving about, it should be reported
6. Convulsions (fits): any twitching or movements of arms or legs that the patient is not able to stop
7. Any behavior or symptom that is not normal for the individual

Call a doctor at once if any of these signs are observed by the family. Call either your personal physician or the emergency services.

Courtesy Department of Nursing, University Hospitals of Cleveland.

plete cure. Loss of hearing and strabismus (cross-eye) sometimes complicate basal skull fractures and require a long period of rehabilitation. Sometimes corrective surgery can be performed for the strabismus.

Some persons require intensive rehabilitation in a rehabilitation center. Recovery from head injury is most likely in those under age 20. Persons between the ages of 20 and 50 who remain in a coma longer than 2 weeks rarely recover.[4]

Spinal cord trauma

Spinal cord injury from accidents is a frequent and increasing cause of serious disability and death in the United States. It has been estimated that there are more than 100,000 individuals with serious spinal cord injury in the United States today and approximately 6000 to 8000 new cases occur annually.

Violent accidents are occurring more frequently, and because of medical advances the patients are living longer. Automobile, diving and other athletic accidents, and gunshot wounds are major causes of spinal cord injuries.

Neuroanatomy

There are important variations in the neuroanatomy of the vertebral column at the cervical, thoracic, and lumbar areas as well as important segmental variations in the spinal cord itself. In the cervical area the vertebrae are unstable (to permit movement of the neck), and the cord at this level houses the most important neural structures in a copious dural tube. The anterior horn cells innervating the diaphragm (above C4) and the upper extremities are located in the cervical cord segments as well as the long motor tracts to the remainder of the body. In the thoracic area, by contrast, there is a stable bony column supported by the rib structures. The thoracic spinal cord fills the subarachnoid space almost completely, and injuries in this area produce bony malalignments and are often associated with serious neurologic deficits. Finally, in the lumbar area the vertebrae are heavier and are supported by massive lumbar paraspinal muscles. The lumbar vertebrae thus have more stability than the cervical vertebrae but less than the thoracic vertebrae. The lumbar spine is more apt to be injured at the junction between the thoracic and lumbar area. The cauda equina, rather than the spinal cord, is housed below L1. The tip of the spinal cord, or the conus, houses the micturition center.

Pathophysiology of spinal cord lesions

The spinal cord may be damaged by lesions arising outside the cord or by intramedullary lesions. The latter is a less common cause and is usually the result of intramedullary tumors (p. 834). Variable types of lesions arising *outside* the cord eventually cause damage within it. (The word *lesion* as used here includes both disease and injury.) For example, there may be direct extension of an extramedullary vertebral tumor to the cord, the protrusion of a ruptured intervertebral disk into the spinal canal (p. 993), or a fracture of the spine from direct trauma with resultant tearing of the spinal cord (Fig. 36-2). All such lesions may produce compression of the cord. The anatomy and size of the spinal cord subject the cord to compression with even minimal inward encroachment by extramedullary lesions. Edema then forms and contributes even more to cord compression. With damage to any part of the vertebral column, the cord itself becomes more vulnerable to damage. Recognition of the function of the spinal cord as the only conducting system of nerve impulses to and from the brain makes one realize the seriousness of spinal cord damage from any cause.

Severe traumatic lesions of the spinal cord, as from accident, may result in total *transection* of the spinal cord or a tearing of the cord from side to side at a particular level. This represents the most serious damage to the cord, with a complete loss of spinal cord functions. This total transection of injury is also referred to as a "complete cord injury." With the complete injury there is a loss of all voluntary movement below the level of the lesions and loss of all sensations below the level of the lesion. A partial transection or "incomplete injury" involves a partial transection or injury of the cord. The symptoms of incomplete injuries can vary depend-

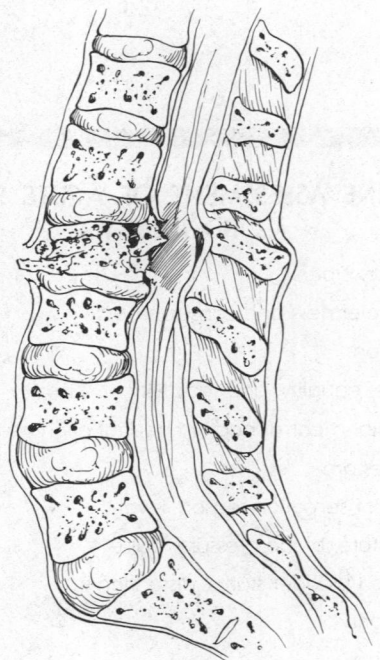

Fig. 36-2. Damage to spinal cord and distortion of adjacent structures that may occur in traumatic injuries to spine.

ing on the nature of the injury and the resultant syndrome. Possibilities include the anterior cord syndrome, central cord syndrome, Brown-Séquard syndrome, conus medullaris syndrome, and cauda equina syndrome.[7] (See a neurologic text for further descriptions of these syndromes and the respective symptoms.)

Initially, in most spinal cord injuries there is a period of flaccid paralysis and a complete (or almost complete) loss of all reflexes. This is called spinal or neural shock, or areflexia, and is a transitory event. Following the injury, afferent impulses are unable to ascend from below the injured site to the brain, and efferent impulses are unable to descend to points below the site. Because transection represents an acute form of spinal cord damage, it is used as an example to relate and discuss the symptoms of spinal cord damage. *There is considerable variability in the extent to which signs and symptoms are manifest in the individual patient.* The baseline assessment of the person with acute spinal cord injury should include the data listed in the box below.

Clinical picture

The signs and symptoms of cord transection and of lesser cord lesions depend on the level at which the lesion occurs and the degree of the damage (Table 36-5). In the *immediate stage* of a *transection* there is a complete loss or deficit of motor and sensory functions as well as somatic and visceral sensations below the level of the tear (areflexia). The individual has flaccid paralysis, areflexia, and hypotonia caused by the disruption of nerve impulses as related to the injured level. During

this period persons may require temporary respiratory assistance until the body begins to recover.

Within hours, days, or weeks the involved muscles gradually become spastic and *hyperreflexic* with the characteristic signs of an upper motor neuron lesion. These changes are thought to represent the release of the muscle stretch reflexes from the inhibitory influence of the damaged pyramidal tract, resulting in hyperactive responses. Another theory is that damage of the extrapyramidal descending fibers, in close proximity to the pyramidal fibers, permits unmodified excitatory impulses to reach the lower motor neurons via the muscle spindles. There is thus an increased sensitivity of the lower motor neurons to afferent stimulation from the muscle spindles. Nurses need to be able to explain spinal cord damage to patients and their families so that involuntary movements are not confused with voluntary movements.

Damage at the cervical cord level is the most critical level for an injury to occur. It causes paralysis of all four extremities and the trunk (*quadriplegia*). The sparing of any one muscle movement of the shoulder, arms, and fingers is dependent on the specific cervical level of the injury. At the C5 level, for example, there would remain scapular elevation movements only. All other muscle movements in the arms, chest, trunk, and legs are lost. In the immediate stage, muscles of internal organs such as the bladder and bowel are atonic. Perspiration is diminished, as is touch sensation. Since the diaphragm and intercostal muscles are affected, respiratory failure and death may result unless the patient receives adequate respiratory assistance. Respiratory

---

BASELINE ASSESSMENT OF ACUTE SPINAL CORD INJURY

1. Respiratory status
2. Level of alertness and consciousness
3. Orientation
4. Pupil size, equality, and reactivity
5. Proper alignment of body in neutral alignment
6. Motor strength
7. Absence of sensation-sensory level
8. Temperature, blood pressure, pulse
9. Bowel and bladder status; distention
10. Skin integrity
11. Pain control

TABLE 36-5. Muscle function after spinal cord injury

Spinal cord injury	Muscle function remaining	Muscle function lost
Cervical		
Above C4	None	All, including respiration
C5	Neck Scapular elevation	Arms Chest All below chest
C6-C7	Neck Some chest movement Some arm movement	Some arm, fingers Some chest All below chest
Thoracic	Neck Arms (full) Some chest	Trunk All below chest
Lumbosacral	Neck Arms Chest Trunk	Legs

assistance is sometimes necessary during transportation of the patient to the hospital. Pain is not usually an early problem.

At the thoracic level, injury results in chest, trunk, bowel, bladder, and lower extremity muscle losses. The amount of remaining function varies in this area relative to the specific level. Fortunately, the individual has use of the upper extremities; the lower extremities are not functional *(paraplegia)*.

Injury at the lumbar and sacral levels results in paralysis of the lower extremities. The center for micturition is located in the conus medullaris (S2 to S4) and is linked to the detrusor muscle of the bladder by parasympathetic sensory and motor fibers that run in the pelvic nerves; together they form the reflex arc. Sympathetic motor fibers (T11 and L2) control the trigone of the bladder. Somatic lower motor neuron fibers travel through the pudendal nerves to the external urethral sphincter and external anal sphincter and the perineal muscles. Impulses descend via the pyramidal system and synapse with the anterior horn cells at the sacral level and thus provide central control over micturition. *Lesions above the conus result in a bladder that is capable of emptying itself reflexly or involuntarily after the spinal shock phase. The bladder is hypertonic, and it is variously known as an "upper motor neuron bladder" and "automatic bladder."* The emptying occurs spontaneously or automatically. The patient has no control over the act of micturition. Voiding may occur at intervals of 3 to 4 hours; there may be frequency, urgency, and incontinence. The reflex arc of micturition is intact in this type of bladder. *When the cord lesion is at, or below, the micturition center, there is destruction of the center or the sacral nerve roots; the reflex arc is no longer intact. This type of bladder is known as a "lower motor neuron bladder" or an "autonomous bladder."* Any contractions of the bladder muscle are the result of impulses transmitted through an intrinsic nervous mechanism that is within the bladder wall. The contractions, however, are not of sufficient strength or duration to empty the bladder. This can be done only by abdominal straining or by manual compression. Since the bladder musculature is hypotonic or flaccid, retention of urine and infection are common complications.

When injury occurs in the lower sacral area and the cauda equina nerve roots, away from the cord, the signs are variable and less severe. Often there is paraparesis and scattered lower motor neuron signs.

In the past several years, nursing literature has placed increased emphasis on the problems and care of the paraplegic and quadraplegic with decreased sexual functioning.[20,34,70]

In most instances men experience impotence, decreased sensation, or difficulties with ejaculation. Impairment of fertility is common. The act of erection is under the control of sensory and parasympathetic fibers. Ejaculation requires sympathetic and parasympathetic innervation. Lesions above S2 leave the parasympathetic reflex arc intact, and patients may be able to have an erection. But, since sympathetic innervation is impaired, ejaculation is not usually possible. Lesions in the S2 to S4 area usually prevent an erection and ejaculation. The higher the level of the lesion, the more likely a man with complete cord injury will be able to attain and maintain an erection. The experience of orgasm as commonly understood will not be experienced. While the woman with spinal cord injury is able to continue to perform sexually, there is interference with the perception of sexual pleasure. Some suggestions for assisting the spinal cord injury patient to adjust to changes in sexual function are discussed later in this chapter (p. 826).

Diagnosis of spinal cord injury or compression from accidents

Diagnosis is made from the history of the trauma, neurologic examination, and selected studies. It is most important to first detect if there has been any cervical vertebra fracture or displacement and concomitant spinal cord damage. Roentgenograms are always taken to detect fracture-dislocations of the vertebrae or their parts. Roentgenograms are often taken while the injured patient is still on the stretcher in the emergency room, before the person is moved. This lessens movement of the spinal column at a critical period. A myelogram may be done to detect subarachnoid blockage. Myelography can be carried out with ease and without moving the patient when contrast material is introduced through a lateral puncture at the junction between the first cervical vertebra and the base of the skull. In this way the contrast material flows downward across the site of a cervical fracture-dislocation to demonstrate the presence or absence of subarachnoid block. Further diagnostic measures are often delayed until there has been correction of any cervical fractures as established by roentgenograms. There is a need to determine the presence of spinal compression in the thoracic, lumbar, and sacral spine areas, but the need for treatment is not as compelling as with a cervical injury. Both the lumbar and cervical spines are prone to flexion and extension movements that result from severe trauma.

Intervention

The therapeutic and rehabilitative measures are discussed briefly relative to the *immediate, intermediate,* and *late stages of care.* It should be made clear that a tremendous variation in therapy is required for the individual patient, as related to variations in levels of injuries and in combinations of injuries to the spine and the cord.

Immediate stage. During the stage immediately

following the injury the cervical area is given priority in treatment because of the neuroanatomic and physiologic features of the *cervical* vertebrae and cord. Therapy is directed first to realignment of the cervical bony column in the presence of demonstrated fractures, dislocations, or other cervical lesions. Any concomitant damage sustained by the cervical cord (or other levels) can be worsened *by continuing bony instability*. Therapeutic measures necessary to protect the cervical cord may include simple mobilization, skeletal traction, or surgery for spinal decompression through varied operative techniques. Stabilization of cervical vertebrae is usually accomplished by skeletal traction through the application of Crutchfield tongs (p. 1015) or Vinke tongs.

Patients are often placed on a Stryker or Foster frame with traction attachments. A circoelectric bed is sometimes used but is often less desirable than a Stryker or Foster frame.

Once skeletal traction for the bony cervical abnormality has been established, further diagnostic and therapeutic measures are considered. The neurologist or neurosurgeon is also guided by the presenting neurologic deficits and through continued monitoring of neurologic or spinal cord function.

Often surgical decompression is not performed until after a period of skeletal traction. This allows the patient's condition to stabilize and some initial swelling of the cord to subside. The beginning spontaneous healing of the fracture site provides more stability.

Sometimes, despite skeletal traction, extruded cervical disk materials produce continued compression of the cord. With the introduction of the anterior surgical approach to the cervical spinal column, surgical intervention is safer and can be attempted earlier in the hospitalization. The primary advantage of the anterior surgical approach (or anterior diskectomy or laminectomy) is that it provides immediate stabilization of the spinal column by techniques of interbody cervical fusion and the direct removal of any extruded disk materials. If evidences of spinal cord compression are demonstrated early, surgery may be warranted by the anterior approach.

Intubation and respiratory assistance with a ventilator may be required in the immediate stage following upper cervical cord injury. In the conscious quadriplegic patient with a spinal cord lesion below C5, respiratory function generally is not compromised unless it is associated with acute blunt trauma to the chest. A lesion at the C5 level produces paralysis of the intercostal muscles, leaving only the diaphragm to function for respiration. The nerve roots C3, C4, and C5 innervate the diaphragm and make up the phrenic nerves. C4 supplies roots mainly to the phrenic nerves. Any patient, therefore, who has a cord lesion at C4 level with quadriplegia probably will demand permanent ventilatory support.

Careful monitoring of blood gases and regular pulmonary toilet are essential. For this reason the patient may be admitted to a pulmonary intensive care unit.

Less immediate attention to *thoracic* fracture immobilization is necessary for the patient *with limited neurologic* deficits. The patient is often treated later with simple bed rest, hyperextension, and bracing (p. 823). Diagnosis is necessary, however, to determine the presence or absence of spinal cord compression at this level. Patients who show subarachnoid blockage and have associated neurologic deficits are treated through early surgical decompression. The onset of instantaneous paraplegia following direct thoracic trauma is often reversible through spinal cord decompression.

An early to an intermediate laminectomy may be performed in the presence of even severe *lumbar* neurologic deficits. Stabilization of the spine is done at the time of the primary surgical intervention or delayed until later in the posttraumatic period. Long delays in lumbar laminectomies or exploration in patients who show early partial recovery is reported to be beneficial for recovery of some neurologic function.

Also threatening to the life of the individual are the extent and effects of paralysis. Immediately, during the areflexic period, medical attention is directed toward the prevention of complications that occur as a result of the loss of motor function. In addition to the more obvious effects apparent in the involved skeletal muscles, there may be loss of vasomotor tone, bladder tone, and bowel peristalsis. Bladder and bowel distention must be avoided, since they may result in mass reflex or autonomic hyperreflexia (p. 822).

There has been increased interest in the early treatment of spinal cord injury. This interest was stimulated by demonstrations that experimentally produced cord injuries in animals are reversible if treated early. Some forms of early treatment such as localized spinal cord cooling and myelotomy are undergoing experimentation in some university centers.[73] It is too early to assess their value at this time. *Continued research in the immediate care at the time of injury is crucial to progress in treatment*. It is essential to also educate rescue squads and emergency medical technicians in the proper transportation of patients with suspected spinal cord injury. More than one person with a fractured spine has suffered paralysis because of the way they were removed from the scene of the accident.

The use of adrenal corticosteroids for the prevention and alleviation of spinal cord edema has gained acceptance. The efficacy of steroids in the reestablishment of membrane stability and in the control of central nervous tissue edema has been documented clinically. Methylprednisolone (Solu-Medrol) at a dosage level of 60 to 80 mg/day (or equivalent dosage of other corticosteroids) may be utilized for the first week or longer following injury.

Throughout all stages of hospitalization of the spinal cord–injured person, nursing and medical interventions are directed toward restoration of structural or body integrity consistent with the pathologic condition present. This means that all efforts are taken to ensure that the skin is intact, that contractures do not develop, that range of motion is maintained to the greatest degree possible, that muscle tone is consistent with pathologic condition, and that bladder and bowel functions are maintained. The following section discusses specific interventions to achieve these outcomes.

POSITION AND MOVEMENT. Before moving a patient with acute spinal cord injury onto a bed from the stretcher, the physician should be consulted about the type of bed desired. The selection will depend on the physician's preference, the type of injury, the size of the patient, and the equipment available. If a regular bed is to be used, a full-length fracture board should be placed on top of the bedspring under the mattress. This board prevents sagging of the mattress and motion of the spine. If the bed is to be gatched, the board must be hinged, or two or more boards with correctly placed breaks can be used. Mattresses containing springs should not be used. Instead of springs and one mattress, some physicians prefer two air mattresses placed on top of the fracture board. Some use the knee gatch to provide hyperextension to the spine in selected thoracic and lumbar fractures; the bed must then be made up "head to foot." Sponge rubber mattresses are widely recommended and, when available, are commonly used when there is the possibility that for some time the patient will be moved very little and with extreme difficulty. If available, an alternating air-pressure mattress often is used. Since the patient has loss of sensation and paralysis of part of the body, pressure areas develop easily. The mattress and entire bed foundation must be well protected with plastic sheeting so that incontinence will not cause damage.

To prevent injury when moving the patient, the bed foundation should be completely adjusted, with gatches raised as ordered, bolsters placed in the desired positions, and a turning sheet available so that a minimum of motion will be necessary. Three to five people are needed to move the patient from the stretcher to the bed, depending on the patient's size and the location of the spinal injury. The physician may supervise moving the patient and actually support the head and neck during the transfer. The body should be supported in proper alignment, and if necessary, a manual hyperextension should be applied to the spine as the patient is moved (p. 1904).

OBSERVATIONS. The nurse must carefully observe the patient with a spinal fracture, a cord tumor, or a ruptured intervertebral disk for signs of cord compression. The motion, strength, and sensation in the extremities should be tested at least every few hours for the first 24 to 36 hours and then at least four times a day. Any change in motion or sensation should be reported at once as related to level, since immediate surgery may be needed to relieve pressure on the cord. Some of the laminae may be removed to prevent pressure from edema.

MAINTENANCE OF FUNCTION. If cord damage has occurred, nursing care will depend on the level of the injury. Patients with cervical lesions, for instance, will be unable to do anything for themselves. Meticulous skin care, maintenance of correct body alignment, preservation of range of joint motion, and attempts to preserve muscle tone are imperative nursing measures as in the care of any paralyzed person. (See Chapter 35, p. 763, for a discussion of the care of the person with paralysis.)

ELIMINATION. The patient may have urinary retention because of injury to lumbar and sacral spinal nerves. Since there may be no sensation of needing to void, *the nurse should check carefully for voiding and for distention of the bladder*. A Foley catheter may be inserted into the bladder, or a cystostomy may be performed.

Most persons with spinal cord injuries have a reflex (autonomic or spastic) bladder, which occurs when the spinal cord reflexes are still present but the inhibiting influences from the higher cortical centers are lost. Reflex bladder is seen in persons with spinal cord injury or disease above the level of the sacral cord after the initial spinal shock phase. Because the pathways for motor and sensory impulses to the cord are still present, the reflex arc functions. Any stimulation from the bladder wall leads to contraction of the detrusor muscle and relaxation of the internal and external sphincters, resulting in involuntary bladder emptying. The spastic bladder often responds to even minor stimulus such as touching or stroking the genitalia, thighs, or lower abdomen. Small frequent voidings are common and demonstrate that the bladder empties long before it has reached normal capacity.

Some patients can be taught to recognize the stimulation for voiding and use it to induce voiding. Male patients often need to wear an external catheter for incontinence. Females unfortunately may have to wear pads and waterproof pants. One important measure that will help decrease the spasticity is the prevention of urinary tract infections.

Damage to the sacral cord or the peripheral nerves produces an atonic or areflexic bladder. Patients with spinal shock also have an atonic bladder. Any contraction from the bladder wall fails to stimulate the motor neurons in the cord. Because the reflex arc is disrupted, no sensations reach the brain. There is no awareness of the need to void, and there is no voluntary control. Because the reflex arc and voluntary control are both absent, the bladder becomes increasingly distended. Overflow incontinence occurs and if the bladder is not emptied, dribbling may occur almost continuously. The constant stretching of the bladder wall predisposes to infection and there may be reflux of urine. Depending on personal desire and residual functioning, the patient may be taught to use intermittent catheterization or the Credé maneuver or a combination of both. These procedures must routinely be done four times a day at intervals, at first by the nursing staff and then by the patient, if able. It may be necessary to continue intermittent catherization for several months before the patient is able to stimulate voiding with the Credé maneuver alone.

The presence of an indwelling catheter makes the patient highly susceptible to urinary infection. The best means of preventing infection is maintenance of fluid intake (3 to 4 L daily) and meticulous aseptic technique in changing and irrigating catheters. The patient *must* know the signs of infection and *must* have a genitourinary checkup once a year or more frequently. Following an acute injury to the spinal cord, the patient often has abdominal distention. A rectal tube may be used, and neostigmine may be administered hypodermically to stimulate peristalsis. A nasogastric tube or a Miller-Abbott or Cantor tube attached to suction may be tried.

Stool softeners, adequate fluids, prune juice, and suppositories are recommended to obtain bowel function. Long-term use of laxatives and enemas is discouraged, although they may be necessary during spinal shock. If it is necessary to give an enema, 200 ml should be sufficient; no more than 500 ml should be used. There may be fecal incontinence caused by loss of sphincter control until the patient is regulated on a suppository regimen (see p. 1448 for care of the incontinent person).

PAIN. Patients with spinal injuries often have a great deal of pain at the level of the injury that radiates along the spinal nerves. A thoracic injury causes chest or back pain, whereas a lumbar injury causes pain in the legs. Analgesics such as acetylsalicylic acid (aspirin) or other nonnarcotic analgesics are ordered. Narcotics may be given for a short time but are contraindicated for long-term use because the patient's problem may be chronic and addiction is possible. Psychologic assistance is often recommended to help the patient learn to cope with pain. If the patient has a high cervical injury, no narcotics should be administered because respirations may be further depressed. Sometimes the paravertebral nerves are injected with 95% alcohol to relieve thoracic pain. This measure may provide relief for several weeks or even months.

COMPLICATIONS. *Autonomic hyperreflexia* or autonomic dysreflexia (mass reflex) occurs in patients with cord lesions above the sixth thoracic vertebra; most commonly it occurs in cervical injuries. The clinical signs are bradycardia, paroxysmal hypertension, sweating,

"goose flesh," and severe headache (Fig. 36-3). Patients tend to develop individual symptoms of this condition. They soon are able to recognize this complication when it occurs. For instance, some patients feel flushed but never develop a headache. The wise nurse learns to listen to what the patient says is happening to him or her.

The most common causes are visceral distention (distended bladder, impacted rectum). If the patient complains of these symptoms, the patency of the catheter should be checked for kinking and a new catheter inserted *immediately* if the catheter is plugged. The patient should be placed in a sitting position to decrease blood pressure. The rectum should be checked for impaction. If it is necessary to remove stool, dibucaine (Nupercainal Ointment) should be instilled in the rectum for its anesthetic effect. At times urinary infections can lead to symptoms of autonomic dysreflexia. If no other obvious cause is found, a urine specimen is sent for culture.

Autonomic dysreflexia is a medical emergency (Fig. 36-3). The hypertension can lead to CVA, blindness, or even death. If conservative measures are not effective, a ganglionic blocking agent such as hexamethonium chloride or a vasodilator such as nitroprusside (Nipride) is given intravenously.

The major focus is to prevent such attacks. Before any bladder and bowel procedure such as cystoscopy or proctoscopy the patient is given a local anesthetic. If autonomic dysreflexia is a continual problem, the patient may need long-term therapy to block sympathetic impulses.

Respiratory complications are common following injury of the spinal cord. Any patient with a cord injury level at C4 or above can be expected to need assistance to maintain respiration, often on a long-term or permanent basis. In addition, patients with lower cervical fractures often have temporary respiratory difficulties until the spinal shock phase subsides.

Respiratory assistance may include intubation with ventilator assistance. Long-term ventilator assistance will require a tracheotomy. After the initial period these patients need continued respiratory support including postdural drainage and clapping. Deep breathing and coughing, if medically approved, are essential. At times the rocking bed, a bed that rocks on a central axis, is utilized by alternately elevating the head and foot. The bed assists in inspiration and expiration. Inspiration occurs as the diaphragm moves down as the head of the bed tilts up. With the reverse movement the patient exhales as the head is tilted down and the abdominal contents push upward against the diaphragm. If the patient is able to maintain respiration for periods of time, the bed may be turned off for eating and nursing care.

Persons who have injury at the cervical level may need respiratory assistance to prevent respiratory ar-

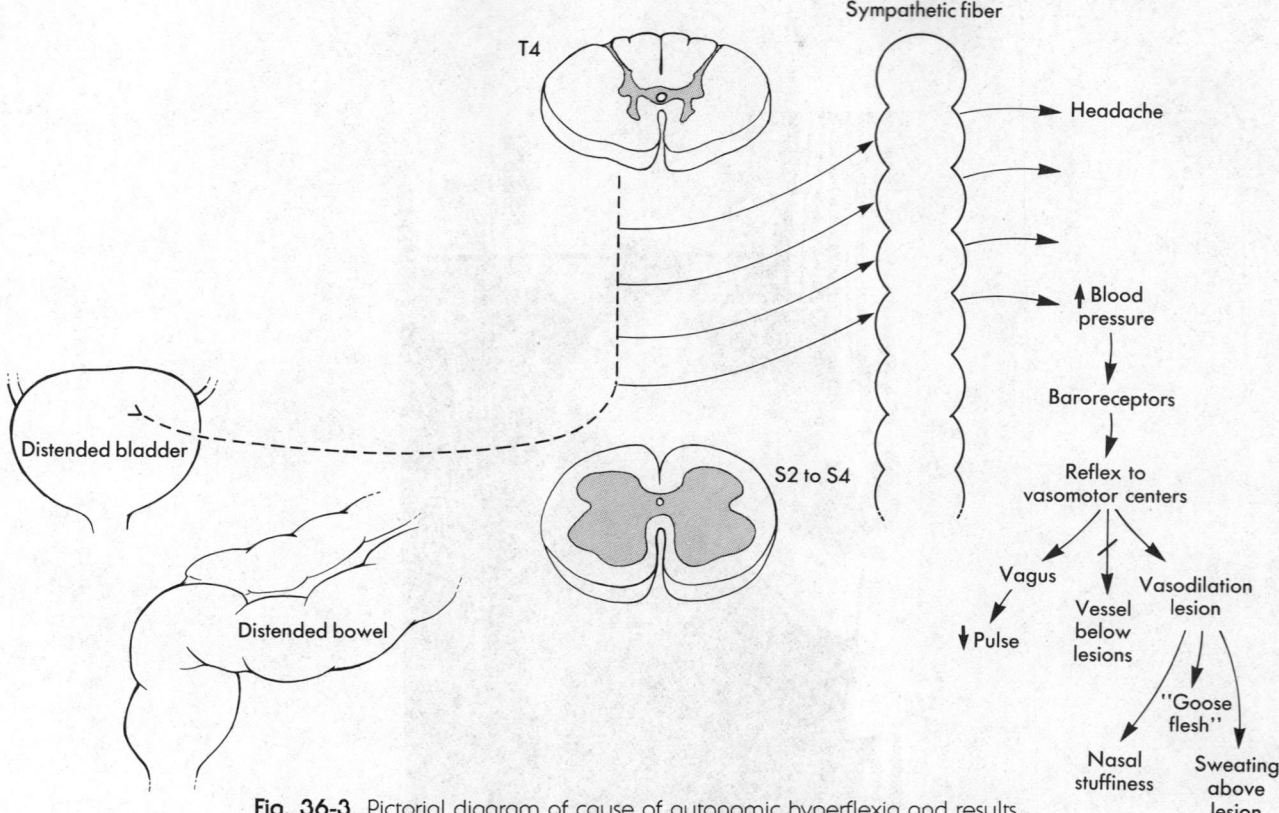

Fig. 36-3. Pictorial diagram of cause of autonomic hyperflexia and results.

rest. Those who have injury at the thoracic level tend to splint their chests and have shallow breathing; therefore measures to facilitate deep breathing and aeration of the alveoli are carried out (see Chapter 49). Since coughing can increase spinal pressure, the physician should be consulted before urging the patient to cough. Good nursing assessment of respiratory status in the patient with spinal cord injury is essential to prevent respiratory complications.

Intermediate stage. During the intermediate stage of treatment, rehabilitation and nursing care measures are focused on mobilization and patient-family education. Quadriplegics and paraplegics need to learn to live with the sequelae of paralysis. The two goals of rehabilitation are to minimize the disability and to assist the patient toward independence to the extent possible. Rehabilitation depends on the extent and level of the cord injury, the emotional reactions of the patient, his or her age, and other factors.

Early mobilization of the patient is important regardless of the level of injury. At first, mobilization includes active or passive turning movements and range of motion exercises to prevent pressure sores and contractures and to develop independence in bed activities. Later, mobilization is usually progressively effected through wheelchair activities. Most patients with spinal cord injury find it impractical to walk because of the energy required. Patients with very low injuries may

be able to ambulate with braces. If ambulation is not possible, the patient may still use the braces to stand at intervals throughout the day. This helps to decrease Ca^{++} mobilization. Mat exercises and resistive exercises are initiated to increase muscle strength and endurance in remaining muscles.

When patients, especially quadriplegics, begin to sit up, it may be necessary to wrap their legs with Ace wraps to encourage venous return. Slowly increasing the angle of sitting is essential to prevent hypotension. For this reason the new quadriplegic should use a recliner wheelchair until he or she is able to sit at 90 degrees for several hours.

The patient with paraplegia and the family are taught proper methods of transfer from bed to wheelchair or commode (Figs. 36-4 and 36-5). Physical therapy activities facilitate learning to transfer. The patient also learns how to do weight shifts if able. Even patients who are not able physically to do weight shifts can take responsibility in getting others to help.

Before the patient is permitted to be up following a spinal injury, a brace may be prescribed. All braces and corsets must be custom made and are quite expensive. The cost of a back brace varies according to the materials used in construction. The brace or corset should be applied before the patient gets out of bed. Help is needed in getting into it. The patient should wear a thin, knitted undershirt next to the skin to keep the

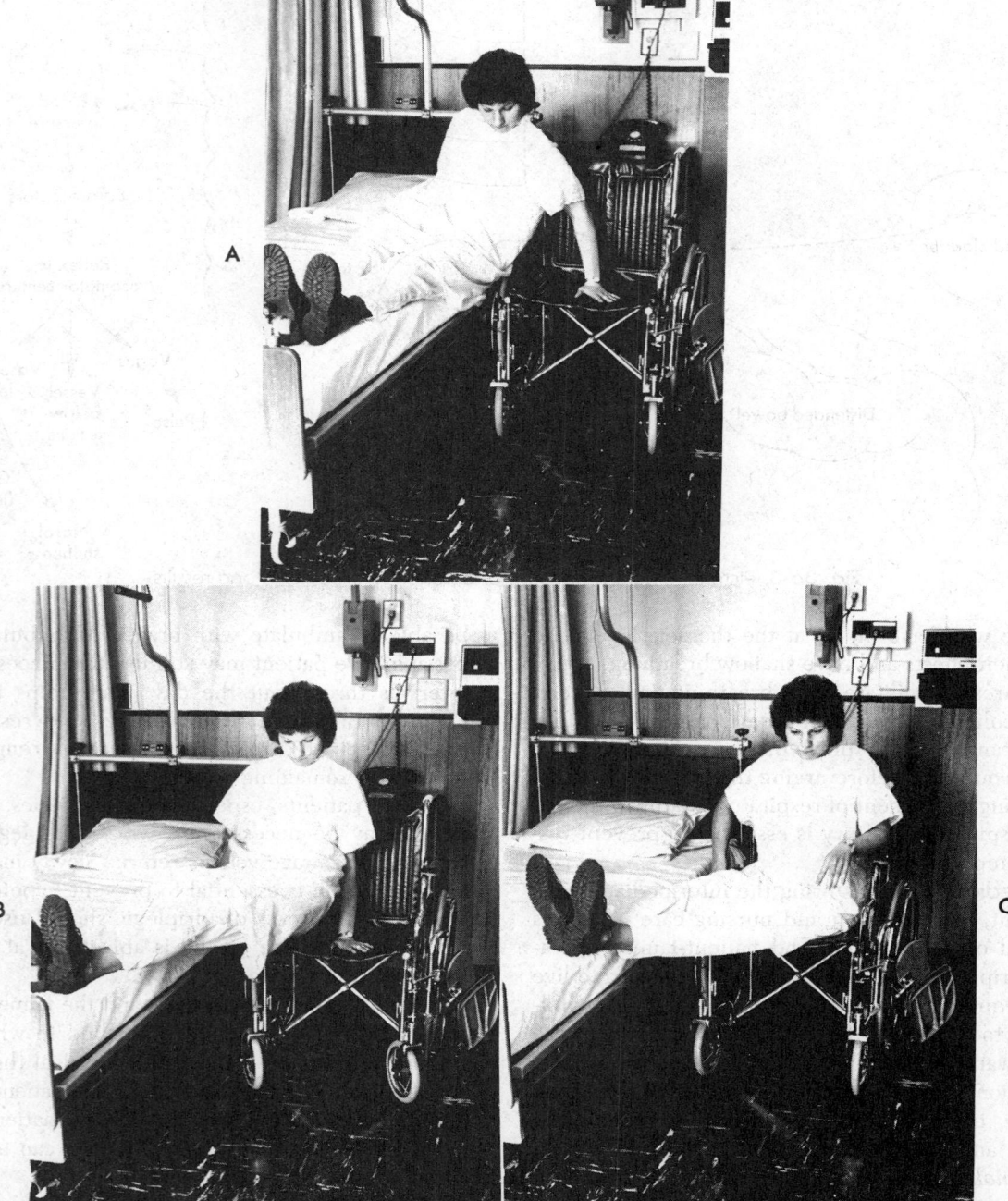

Fig. 36-4. Two methods for patient with paraplegia and strong upper extremities to transfer from bed to chair. With one method, **A,** patient moves sideways (note wheelchair, with right armrest removed, placed next to bed); **B,** Then patient uses her arms to lift trunk into chair seat. **C,** Next, patient settles her hips comfortably into chair. She will then swing footrests into place and lift her legs from bed. **D,** Second method involves patient pushing backward off bed into chair.

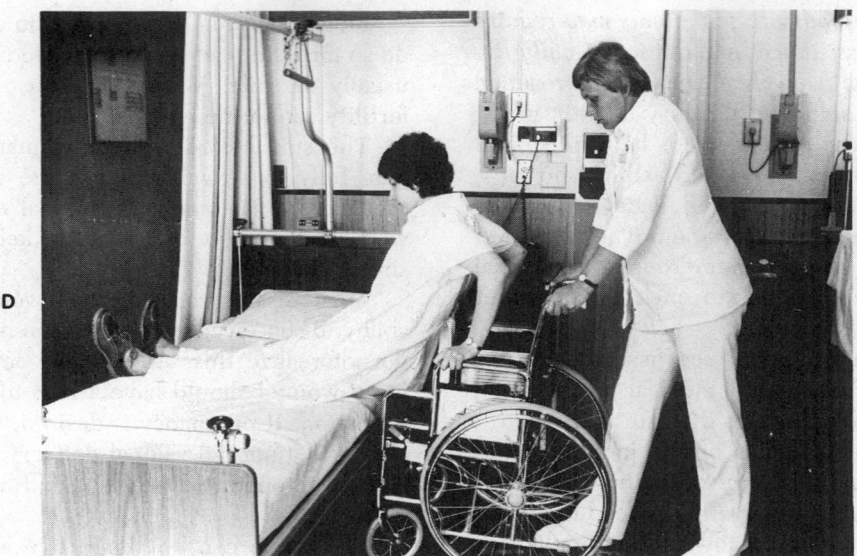

Fig. 36-4, cont'd. For legend see opposite page.

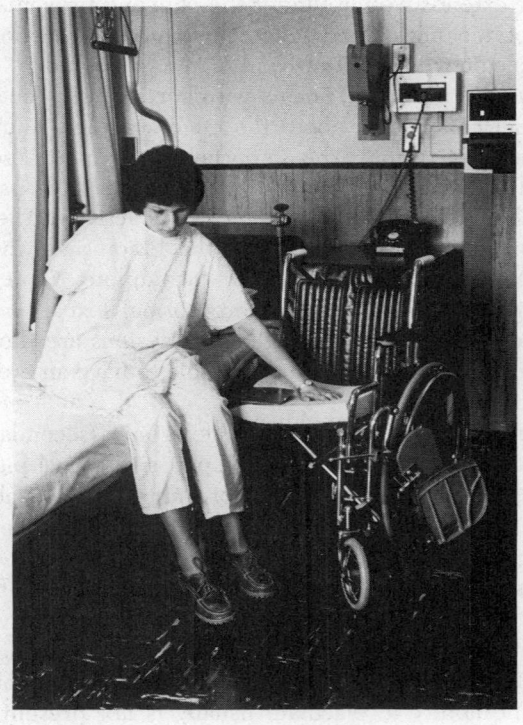

Fig. 36-5. Paraplegic whose upper extremity strength is not yet developed can use a sliding board to transfer from bed to chair. Board provides a firm surface on which to move, and trunk is supported by board through the move.

brace clean and to protect the skin. Correct use so that the brace fits contours of the buttocks and chest as designed makes a great deal of difference in the patient's comfort. The patient's emotional reaction to wearing a brace or a corset is important, since it vitally affects ultimate rehabilitation. Attention to small details that help in initial acceptance of this somewhat uncomfortable and unfamiliar piece of "clothing" is important. The patient should practice putting the brace on while in the hospital if it must be worn for some time. A close member of the family may visit the hospital and learn to assist the patient. Patients who live alone and who are unable to care for their braces themselves may need to have a community health nurse help them in the home or teach someone else to assist.

In addition to instruction about mobilization techniques, the patient is trained to be *functional in activities of daily living*, with or without equipment and as related to his or her life-style. The patient needs to know how to obtain bowel and bladder automaticity (p. 1544) and how to prevent bladder infection. It is essential to understand how to prevent decubitus ulcers when one sits in a wheelchair most of the day, and it is important to know how to manage the wheelchair itself. *The patient's family or significant others are included in in-*

struction, since many quadriplegic patients may require some supervision or assistance in activities of daily living following discharge from the hospital. The reaction of family members to spinal cord injury is often great. The family as well as the patient needs help in coping. In addition to medical and physical rehabilitation measures, there is equal need for psychologic, emotional, sociologic, and vocational rehabilitation. The trauma of spinal cord injury may result in numerous interpersonal problems and make adjustment to one's environment difficult.

Late stage. Education, continued psychologic support for patient and family, and medical and surgical follow-up are continued through the late stage as related to the rehabilitation goals of the individual patient. There may be need for surgical treatment of spasticity or mass reflex, with denervation procedures.

Orthotics, or the application of external appliances to support a paralyzed muscle or to promote a specific motion required in activities of daily living, may require further follow-up care. Patients who have a ruptured cervical disk may need to use a neck brace. The brace extends well up under the chin and prevents flexion of the neck. Leg braces may be ordered for the paraplegic who is able to ambulate or to stand.

SEXUAL NEEDS. Persons with cord injuries need assistance in learning about the effects of their injury on sexual functioning. The important thought to keep in mind is that most patients with a cooperative partner are able to engage in satisfying sexual activity. The limitation depends on the site of the lesion and whether the cord injury is complete or incomplete. Generally, the higher the lesion, the more normal sexual function is likely to be. Patients with sacral lesions are the only spinal cord injured who are not able to have an erection and to ejaculate.

In men, erections are reflexogenic (secondary to stimulation) or psychogenic (response to sexual picture, etc.). Most men with spinal cord injury are not able to have psychogenic erections but are capable of reflexogenic erections. These occur not only as a result of direct stimulation of the genitalia but may also result from stroking the inner thigh, stimulating the rectum with a finger, or manipulating the catheter. The nursing staff can help point out these "trigger" points to the patient.

The ability to ejaculate usually is not present with complete injuries. With incomplete injuries ejaculation may be possible. Even when patients have lost sensation, many report that there is increased intensity of feeling in other body parts, such as the breasts. Orgasms may be experienced, with release of tension.

Male patients with indwelling catheters can either remove the catheter just before sexual activity or turn it back on the penis where it provides extra support. The bowels should be emptied before intercourse; otherwise, bowel incontinence is common.

Since many male patients who are able to ejaculate do so into the bladder (retrograde ejaculation), they are usually infertile. Without sperm counts, however, infertility cannot be guaranteed.

The spinal cord–injured woman is able to participate fully in sexual activity. She may not experience orgasm but can enjoy the sexual experience. Women who have a Foley catheter can keep it in place if desired.

Most spinal cord–injured women maintain their ability to conceive; for some reason many of these women do not realize this. All sexually active spinal cord–injured women should have access to family planning information. If pregnancy is desired, the woman can usually have a normal vaginal delivery. She is at increased risk for autonomic dysreflexia and hydronephritis, however.

The nurse can be supportive and helpful to cord-injured patients by making it comfortable for them to discuss sexual matters. Nurses not prepared to do sexual counseling need to be aware of resources available in the community to help the spinal cord-injured person. Some general suggestions that may be helpful to any cord-injured persons are (1) sex has many meanings, and for persons with no genital function, alternate ways of expression are available; (2) it will take time for the partner to adjust to the situation; openness in communication is helpful; and (3) it is sometimes difficult for a partner who routinely provides bladder and bowel care to view the person as sexually desirable; it may be helpful in this situation if this care can be provided by a community nurse or part-time attendant.[21]

Research

Research data on spinal cord injuries contine to be gathered. It is of interest that electrostimulation of muscles of the bladder through remote control to regain micturition control in the paraplegic patient has been tested clinically. Success of this electronic spinal neuroprosthesis will assist in preventing urinary complications that are often a cause of death. Functional intramuscular electrostimulation of paralyzed upper extremities muscles is also currently being tested.[52] Since there is little or no external splinting required in the latter orthosis, it will be cosmetically appealing to the quadriplegic if successful.

In summary, although most of the complications of paralysis are now preventable, it is regrettable that complications do occur during and after hospitalization. Under optimal conditions a spinal cord–injured person would be evacuated by a knowledgeable first-aid team from the site of the accident to a regional spinal cord center. At the center a team of specialists would supervise treatment while planning a long-term rehabilitation program. Rehabilitation begun in the center eventually would be carried out consistently until patient discharge. Thereafter the center would provide a continuity in management throughout the residual stages.

Outcome criteria for the person with spinal cord injury (paraplegia, quadriplegia)

1. The person shall have made progress toward functional independence in activities of daily living, consistent with level of cord injury, in the following areas:
   a. Feeding self with or without adaptive equipment.
   b. Bathing self with or without adaptive equipment.
   c. Grooming.
   d. Toileting.
   e. Dressing.
   f. Transferring.
   g. Mobility.
   h. Utilizing communication aids.
2. The person or significant others can explain skin care measures and can:
   a. Inspect skin through use of mirror.
   b. List areas of skin vulnerable to breakdown.
   c. Demonstrate how to relieve pressure on skin surfaces when in bed or wheelchair.
   d. Explain how to avoid irritation and abrasion to skin surfaces during transfer activities.
3. The person or significant others can explain bowel training program to be followed at home and can:
   a. Demonstrate recommended method.
   b. Explain alternate methods for bowel evacuation.
   c. Relate diet and fluid intake to bowel activity.
   d. Demonstrate digital stimulation.
   e. Relate bowel incontinence to skin breakdown.
4. The person or significant others can explain bladder training program and can:
   a. Demonstrate recommended method to be followed at home.
   b. Explain alternate methods for emptying bladder.
   c. State the amount and type of fluids to be taken daily to prevent bladder infection.
   d. Demonstrate how to perform intermittent catheterization using clean technique.
   e. Relate bladder incontinence to skin breakdown.
   f. Explain the need to regularly observe amount and color of urine.
5. The person or significant others can explain prescribed therapies to be followed at home and can:
   a. Accurately demonstrate each prescribed therapy to physical therapist, occupational therapist, speech therapist, or nurse.
   b. Explain method, rationale, and daily schedule for each therapy.
   c. Explain time of scheduled return visit to outpatient therapy for reevaluation.
   d. Relate need for regular daily therapy.
6. The person can effectively utilize the wheelchair in activities of daily living and can:
   a. Explain the parts of the wheelchair and how to maintain it.
   b. Explain the importance of safety checks.
7. The person or significant others can explain how to obtain professional and community resources and can:
   a. State how to contact agencies.
   b. State how to secure equipment.
   c. State how to join social clubs for paraplegics and quadriplegics.
   d. State financial resources available to the disabled.
8. The person or significant others can:
   a. Explain long-term goals.
   b. Relate need to be independent in activities of daily living despite time and effort required.
   c. Explain motor and sensory status in relation to goal setting.
   d. State signs or symptoms that require immediate attention.
   e. State plans for follow-up care.

Peripheral nerve trauma

Etiology

The peripheral nerves that lie outside the brain and spinal cord include the cranial and spinal nerves and their branches and plexuses. The disorders involving the peripheral nerves are similar to those that affect the central nervous system and are the result of traumatic, degenerative, vascular, inflammatory, neoplastic, and metabolic causes. *Neuropathies*, noninflammatory disorders, may involve one peripheral nerve (mononeuropathy) or multiple nerves (polyneuropathies). *Neuritis* refers to an inflammatory disorder, while *neuralgia* means a painful nerve disorder. Although discussion in this section is limited to neuropathies caused by trauma, it should be clear that regardless of cause, the resulting nerve dysfunction will be similar and will be related to the site of the lesion. Some of the more common neuropathies (other than trauma) include nutritional, alcoholic, diabetic, lead, arsenic, hereditary, and infectious.

Traumatic causes of peripheral nerve injury commonly include gunshot and knife wounds, fragmented fracture wounds, and surgical transections, as in denervation surgery and amputations. They variously result in stretching, laceration, and compression of the peripheral nerve; there also is much variation in the degree of injury. Fortunately, the axons of peripheral nerves are capable of regeneration under favorable conditions.

Pathophysiology

Following trauma (or disease), the axon undergoes *secondary* or *wallerian degeneration* distal to the lesion (i.e., distal to the cells of origin) and for several segments proximal. The axon and the myelin sheath (secondary) degenerate and immediately undergo fragmentation; the fragmented particles are completely ingested within several weeks; the axis cylinder remains. Schwann's cells and fibroblasts begin to proliferate along the degenerated fibers. (Myelin in *peripheral fibers* is formed by Schwann's cells.) During the regenerative phase, new axoplasm forms at the proximal edge of the injury and the regenerating fibers now grow distally and enter the empty neurolemmal sheath, which has in the meantime proliferated. Myelin then forms around the regenerated axon. When a nerve has been severely damaged and fibrous tissue is abdundant, regeneration is interfered with by a tangled mass known as a *traumatic neuroma;* this may have to be removed surgically.

Clinical picture

The clinical signs and symptoms resulting from peripheral nerve lesions depend on the exact location of the lesion and the specific function of the involved nerve or nerves. Since peripheral nerves contain both sensory and motor components, there may be deficits in both components distal to the site. There will be alterations in pain, touch, temperature, proprioception, and stereognosis. Motor alterations include lower motor neuron signs such as flaccid paralysis and muscle wasting in those muscles innervated by the affected nerves.

Intervention

Nursing care is specific to the areas of the body affected by the sensory and motor deficits. Plans for care are based on the nurse's understanding of the distribution and function of the involved peripheral nerves. The flaccid muscles demand attention to prevent deformities. Because of the atonia or hypotonia of the paralyzed muscles, they will be pulled excessively by the muscles that normally oppose them into abnormal or contracted positions. When associated tendons shorten, the contracture is permanent. Positioning of extremities in neutral or counter positions will help in preventing joint deformities. Those areas of the body in which there is a loss of sensation need to be protected from injury. These patients need to be taught *protective measures* such as not staying in one position too long, since they cannot sense that damage is occurring in an area served by a damaged nerve. When positional sense is lost, there is also need to teach patients to protect themselves when walking and in other activities. Pain is usually localized, and there may be more paresthesia than pain. The painful areas need to be protected from external stimulation when present. Following surgical intervention, careful positioning of the operative area, as prescribed, is important. Finally, the promotion of good health measures assists in the creation of conditions favorable to nerve regeneration.

Trigeminal neuralgia

Clinical picture

Trigeminal neuralgia (tic douloureux) is characterized by excruciating, burning pain that radiates along one or more of the three divisions of the fifth cranial nerve (Fig. 36-6). The pain typically extends only to the midline of the face and head, since this is the extent of the tissue supplied by the offending nerve. There are areas along the course of the nerve known as *trigger points,* and the slightest stimulation of these areas may initiate pain. Persons with trigeminal neuralgia try desperately to avoid "triggering" the pain. It is not unusual to see them lying in bed with the covers over their heads in an effort to avoid drafts. They frequently have been unable to eat properly for some time, since chewing causes pain. They may therefore be undernourished and dehydrated. They may have slept poorly and have not washed, shaved, or combed their hair for some time. Oral hygiene may often be neglected because of pain.

Intervention

The person is usually treated medically first before attempting surgery. In caring for the person with trigeminal neuralgia *preoperatively* or in caring for the patient who is being treated medically, it is important that members of the nursing staff be sympathetic toward the person's behavior. Every effect should be made to avoid placing the bed in a draft and to avoid walking swiftly to the bed, because the slight motion of air may be enough to cause pain. The bed should not be jarred or the bedclothes fanned. It is unwise to urge the person to wash or shave the affected area or to comb the hair, since this may set off another siege of pain. The person will probably prefer to avoid self-care that involves touching the face. Some will do their own mouth care if applicators and a lukewarm mouthwash are provided. Often pureed foods or lukewarm fluids taken through a straw are the only diet that can be tolerated.

Carbamazepine (Tegretol) currently is the drug of choice for the treatment of the pain (also used for convulsions). The inhalation of trichloroethylene (10 to 15 drops on cotton) has been tried with variable success for relieving pain. Drugs such as nicotinic acid, thiamine chloride, cobra venom, and analgesics have all been tried, but usually they offer the person little if any relief. Sedatives may be given for sleep.

The peripheral branches of the trigeminal nerve may be injected with absolute alcohol. This provides relief for weeks or months, and the procedure may be repeated as necessary. Permanent relief can only be ob-

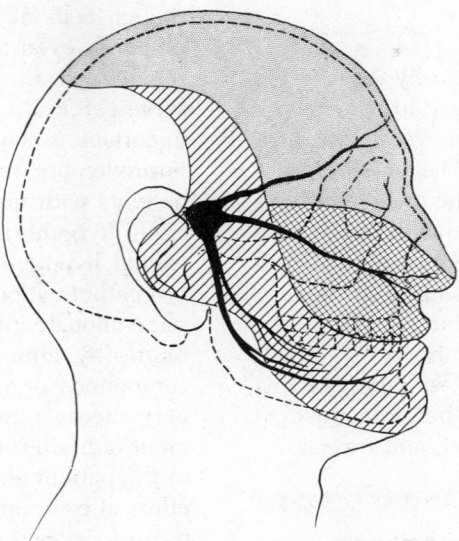

Fig. 36-6. Pathway of trigeminal nerve and facial areas innervated by each of three main divisions of this nerve.

tained by surgery that consists of dividing the sensory root of the trigeminal nerve, but this is not always successful.

Postoperatively, it is important to know what branches of the nerve have been cut in order to provide the necessary protection. If the *upper branch* is completely severed, the corneal reflex on that side will be lost. Usually an attempt is made to preserve a few of the fibers of the first division of the fifth nerve, since even a few intact fibers seem to preserve this vital function. Until the physician has tested the corneal reflex and verified its presence, an eye shield is used to prevent dust or lint from getting onto the cornea and causing injury.

The patient is instructed not to touch or rub the eye but to blink it often, since blinking helps to lubricate the eye. If the reflex is completely absent, each eye should be bathed at least every 4 hours and more often if necessary. The best solution for bathing the eye is normal saline solution. A solution of methylcellulose ("artificial tears"), 0.5% to 2%, may be prescribed to help keep the cornea moist. The lids should not be dried, since any material such as cotton, gauze, tissue, or toweling may leave lint. The patient should be taught eye care before discharge. Any contact with the eye should be carefully avoided when washing the face. The eye is inspected several times a day, and medical attention should be sought if it becomes inflamed. Persons are safer outdoors if they wear glasses, which will protect the eyes from dust and other flying particles. Contact lenses should never be worn, because the lenses are too irritating.

When the *lower branch* of the fifth cranial nerve is interrupted, hot foods will need to be avoided, since the person will not be aware if the mucous membrane is burned. There may be difficulty chewing and swallowing at first, and the person is instructed to place the food in the unaffected side of the mouth. Since food may be retained in the mouth on the affected side, mouth care should be given immediately following meals. Dental caries on the affected side will not cause pain; therefore there is need for a routine dental check every 6 months. The dentist should be informed that the person has had a fifth-nerve resection so that trauma is avoided. Care must be taken in shaving to avoid nicking the insensitive skin.

Within 24 hours after a fifth nerve resection, many patients develop herpes simplex (cold sores) about the lips. Phenol and camphor (Campho-Phenique) applied frequently seems to give more relief than any other treatment. Usually the lesions heal in about a week.

An operating microscope is used during surgery on the trigeminal nerve. Microsurgery permits greater precision in selective cutting of fibers; also, the sensation of touch and the corneal reflex are preserved.[12] A new method to sever the nerve inside the skull is presently being utilized. A thin electrode needle is inserted through the cheek and into the nerve. This avoids a surgical procedure and may provide permanent relief of pain.[8]

Outcome criteria for the person with trigeminal neuralgia

The outcome criteria are the same as for the person with neurologic pain (p. 753).

Other cranial nerve surgery

Other cranial nerves may be surgically interrupted as necessary. It is sometimes necessary to resect both the fifth and the ninth nerves to relieve severe pain caused by carcinoma of the sinuses. The nursing problems in each instance are related to the areas that have been desensitized and the resulting handicaps. Often there is temporary and sometimes permanent loss or a change of facial expression after resection of these nerves, which may cause severe psychic problems. When any nerve is resected, whether it is peripheral or cranial, the patient must understand that all sensation in this area is lost and that he or she will therefore need to avoid injury, especially from heat, cold, and trauma.

Neoplasms of the central nervous system

Neoplasms of the central nervous system include those arising from cells of structures within the cranium as well as those arising within or outside the spinal cord. In general, they occur in great variety; produce neurologic symptoms because of size, location, and invasive qualities; usually destroy the tissues in which they are situated and displace those around them; and are a frequent cause of increased intracranial pressure.

Intracranial tumors

Primary *intracranial* tumors, or *neoplasms,* arise from the intrinsic cells of brain tissues and the pituitary and pineal glands. *Secondary* or *metastatic* tumors are also a frequent contributing type of intracranial tumor. Intracranial tumors are only one example of intracranial lesions. Variable intracranial lesions occur, such as hemorrhage, abscess, and trauma, and cause similar signs and symptoms as a neoplasm, depending on the site of the lesion.

With the development of newer diagnostic techniques, modern surgical and roentgenologic methods, chemotherapeutic agents, and an increased understanding of functional anatomy of the cerebrum, the prognosis for patients with intracranial tumors is more favorable today than in the past. The prognosis, however, is dependent on early diagnosis and treatment, since as the tumor grows within the cranial cavity, it exerts lethal pressure on vital brain centers and causes irreparable brain damage and death. Although approximately one half of all primary brain tumors are benign, they also may cause death by exerting pressure on vital centers of the brain. It is important to remember that al-though cells of the central nervous system can regain function, even after cerebral edema, dead cells cannot regenerate. Early treatment is thus necessary to preserve cerebral functions. Early treatment also becomes important as newer techniques have been developed that improve operative risks and postoperative prospects for patients with intracranial tumors. These techniques include hypothermia (p. 815), the establishment of controlled hypotensive states during surgery by means of sympathetic blocking agents such as trimethaphan camphorsulfonate (Arfonad), and dehydration of cerebral tissues by administering osmotic diuretics such as urea compounds or mannitol before, during, and after surgery. Because the attitude of the nurse about the treatment of brain tumors cannot help but be communicated to the patient and the family, the nurse should make an effort to communicate a hopeful attitude while stressing the importance of early diagnosis and treatment of intracranial tumors.

Types of tumors

Brain tumors are named for the tissues from which they arise. The more frequently encountered ones include gliomas, meningiomas, pituitary adenomas, and acoustic neuromas; the brain, in addition, is a frequent site for secondary tumors from other organs.

Gliomas account for about one half of all brain tumors. They arise in any part of the brain connective tissue. As a rule, in adults they infiltrate primarily the cerebral hemisphere tissues and are not so well outlined that they can be completely excised surgically. They grow rapidly, and most persons do not live longer than a year after diagnosis.[4] The less malignant gliomas are the *astrocytomas* and the *oligodendrogliomas*. *Ependymomas* arise from the walls of the ventricular system. They cause death in about 3 years.[4] The most malignant and rapid growing forms are the *glioblastoma multiforme* and *medulloblastoma*. Gliomas not infrequently start as one type and develop into more malignant forms if untreated.

The *meningiomas*, which account for 13% to 18% of all primary tumors in the intracranial cavity, arise from the meningeal coverings of the brain. They occur most frequently in the meninges over the cerebral hemispheres in the parasagittal region along the ridge of the sphenoid bone and in the anterior fossa in relation to the olfactory groove or the sella turcica. When located in the posterior fossa, they arise from the cerebellopontine angle, from the tentorium, or rarely in the region of the foramen magnum. Meningiomas vary widely as to size and histologic findings. They are usually benign but many undergo malignant changes. The neurologic signs and symptoms produced by meningiomas relative to these sites may include anosmia, optic atrophy, extraocular palsies, visual defects, papilledema, pituitary disturbances, and cerebellar dysfunction. Meningiomas frequently cause seizures and involvement of the limbs as related to their presence in the convexity of a cerebral hemisphere.

Acoustic neuromas constitute about 8% of all primary intracranial tumors. Neuromas may arise from any cranial nerve. The tumor affecting the acoustic nerve generally arises from its sheath but usually extends to affect the nerve fibers. The signs and symptoms resulting from these slow-growing tumors are related to compression of adjacent cranial nerves (trigeminal and facial), cerebellum, and the brain stem. Pituitary tumors are another intracranial tumor. They are discussed on p. 617.

Metastatic tumors that arise primarily in the lung, kidney, breast, colon, and other organs account for about one fifth of all intracranial tumors. Primary brain tumors, conversely, rarely metastasize to other organs.

Pathophysiology

The symptoms of intracranial tumors result from both local and general effects of the tumor. Locally, the effects are from infiltration, invasion, and destruction of brain tissues at a particular site. There is also direct pressure on nerve structures, causing degeneration and interference with local circulation. Local edema develops, and if it is long standing, it is often sufficient to interfere with the function of nerve tissues. A brain tumor of any type situated anywhere in the cranial cavity

may cause an increase in intracranial pressure. The increased intracranial pressure is then transmitted throughout the brain and the ventricular system. Eventually, the ventricular system is distorted and displaced sufficiently to cause partial ventricular obstruction at some site, even though the tumor is some distance from the ventricular system. A tumor may directly obstruct a particular ventricle early when it grows adjacent to the ventricle. A tumor of the cerebrum can distort the lateral ventricles (Fig. 36-7). A tumor pressing on the third ventricle, the aqueduct of Sylvius, or the fourth ventricle can result in obstruction of cerebrospinal fluid flow into the central canal of the spinal cord. Cerebral edema forms even at some distance from the tumor and generally adds to the increasing pressure. As the edema increases, the blood supply to the brain is compromised and carbon dioxide is retained. The vessels dilate in an effort to increase blood oxygen supply. Unfortunately, this also increases edema and the situation can deteriorate rapidly. *Papilledema* results from the general effects of the increased intracranial pressure and is often a relatively late sign. Death is usually from brain stem compression resulting from herniation. The mechanism for the occasional acute focal symptoms that occur is thought to be caused by rapidly increasing cerebral edema or by functional decompensation of edematous tissues.

Common clinical circumstances in which intracra-

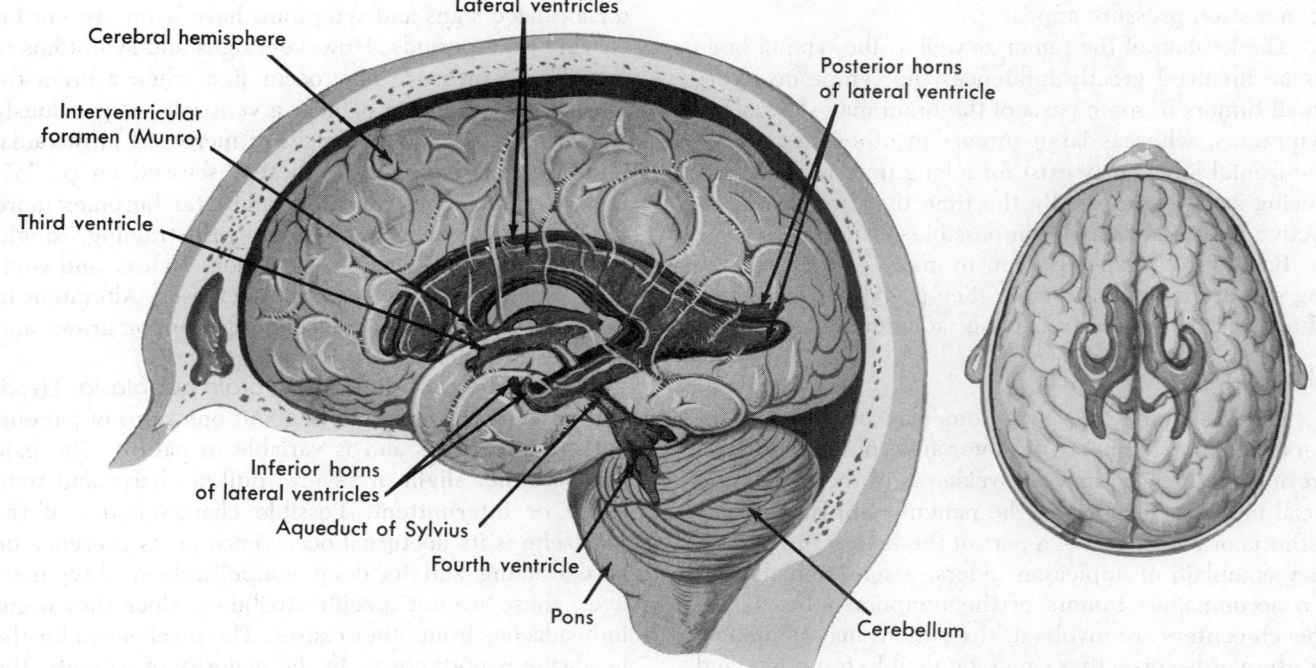

Fig. 36-7. Cerebral ventricles projected on lateral surface of cerebrum. Smaller drawing shows ventricles from above. (From Anthony, C.P., and Thibodeau, G.A.: Textbook of anatomy and physiology, ed. 11, St. Louis, 1983, The C.V. Mosby Co.)

Lateral ventricles

Cerebral hemisphere

Posterior horns of lateral ventricle

Interventricular foramen (Munro)

Third ventricle

Inferior horns of lateral ventricles

Aqueduct of Sylvius

Fourth ventricle

Pons

Cerebellum

nial tumors present, or are likely to be found, include those persons with (1) general impairment of cerebral function or a seizure, (2) evidence of increased intracranial pressure, and (3) specific or focal intracranial tumor syndrome.

Assessment

Every nurse should recognize the early and progressive symptoms of intracranial tumors. The onset of symptoms begins either with evidences of neurologic dysfunction, which can be generalized or focal, or with symptoms of increased intracranial pressure. Progressive involvement of the brain occurs in either a stepwise or linear manner regardless of the type of onset. Subsequently, both types of symptoms are present if the tumor is untreated.

Focal and generalized signs and symptoms of neurologic dysfunction as a rule are referable to a specific area of the brain. Occassionally, the concomitant occurrence of focalizing signs and symptoms and the symptoms of increased intracranial pressure produces false focalizing signs that are difficult for the neurologist to interpret. Localizing signs usually appear slowly and increase in severity over time. Such signs are rarely abrupt in appearance, but their appearance may vary from a few weeks with highly malignant tumors to years with a benign tumor. Some benign tumors may, however, produce acute signs. In many instances, especially if the tumor is infiltrating brain tissue, an alert observer may recognize subtle changes that may suggest the need for neurologic examination before the signs and symptoms of increased pressure appear.

The location of the tumor as well as the type of brain tissue involved greatly influences the symptoms. Very small tumors in some parts of the brain may show acute symptoms, whereas large tumors in other areas (e.g., the frontal lobes) may exist for a long time without producing any symptoms. By the time they are found, effective treatment may be impossible.

Radiation therapy is given to many patients following surgery for brain tumors. (See p. 493 for discussion of nursing the patient receiving radiation.)

Clinical picture

The first noticeable symptom may be a change in personality or judgment. If motor areas of the cerebrum are involved, there may be weakness of the eyelid and facial muscles. Sometimes the patient complains of paresthesia or anesthesia of a part of the body. The patient may complain of unpleasant odors, a sensation that often accompanies tumors of the temporal lobe. If the speech centers are involved, the patient may be unable to use words correctly or may be unable to understand the written or spoken word. The patient may complain of loss of visual acuity or of double vision. These signs indicate pressure on the optic nerve or on one or both

abducent nerves. Unexplained loss of hearing in one ear is suggestive of a brain tumor, although there are other causes to be ruled out. Other localized signs may include a staggering, wide-based gait that is suggestive of a cerebellar tumor. Seizures occurring for the first time after middle age are very suggestive of a brain tumor in the cerebrum or its coverings.

Intracranial tumors occurring within the cerebral lobes present disturbances that can be related to the different lobes (Fig. 36-8). A person with a tumor of the *frontal* lobe may demonstrate personality disturbances that range from subtle personality changes to frank psychotic behavior. There may be indifference to bodily functions such as urinary elimination and inappropriate affect with lack of concern.[69] Persons with tumors in the area of the *precentral gyrus* may develop convulsive seizures of the jacksonian type (involuntary clonic movements with retention of consciousness). Tumors of the *occiptal* lobe result in visual disturbances preceding convulsions. Persons with tumors in the *temporal* lobe may have olfactory, visual, or gustatory hallucinations or psychomotor seizures during which automatic behavioral patterns are carried out.[69] Lastly, symptoms of tumors in the parietal area may include the inability to replicate pictures and loss of right-left discrimination. Observations of such disturbances by the nurse assist in location of brain tumors. The signs and symptoms often develop gradually, although at times the onset may be sudden.

Signs and symptoms of increased intracranial pressure resulting from intracranial tumors usually occur after localized signs and symptoms have been present for varying time periods. However, signs and symptoms of intracranial pressure may occur first when a brain tumor is located within or near a ventricle, as previously shown in Fig. 36-7. The signs of increased intracranial pressure are the same as those discussed on p. 755. Headache at first is transitory and later becomes more constant; it increases in intensity with straining, coughing, stooping, and change of position. Nausea and vomiting usually occur as headache increases. Alteration in mental responses also occurs as the tumor grows and the pressure increases.

Headache associated with brain neoplasia. Headache is an early symptom in about one third of patients with brain tumors and is variable in nature. The pain can be either slight or severe, dull or sharp, and transitory or intermittent. Possible characteristics of the headache is its nocturnal occurrence or its presence on first awaking and its deep nonpulsatile quality; however, these are not specific attributes, since they occur in headaches from other causes. The mechanism for the headache is not known. In the majority of patients, the intracranial pressure is normal for the first weeks when headache is present. The headache may be caused by local swelling of tissues and distortion of blood vessels

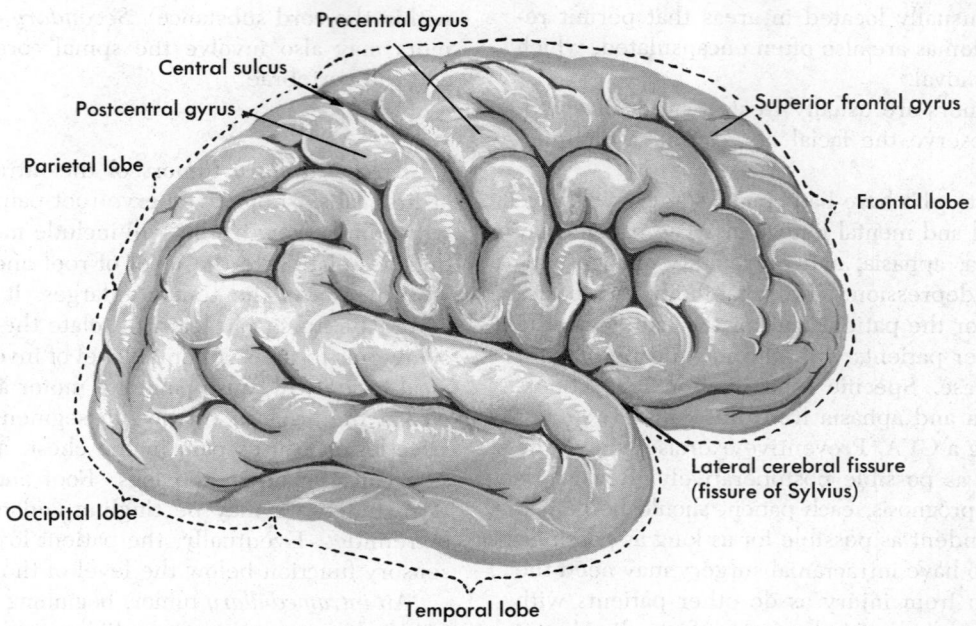

Fig. 36-8. Right hemisphere of cerebrum, lateral surface. Note location of each lobe. (From Anthony, C.P., and Thibodeau, G.A.: Textbook of anatomy and physiology, ed. 11, St. Louis, 1983, The C.V. Mosby Co.)

in and around the tumor. Later, headache seems to be related to increased intracranial pressure. Tumors above the tentorium cause headache on the side and in the vicinity of the tumor; those on the posterior fossae usually cause ipsilateral, retroauricular, or occipital headache. With elevated intracranial pressure, the headache becomes bilateral regardless of location.[1]

Diagnostic tests

No one procedure is entirely diagnostic in brain tumors, but the CT scan certainly has revolutionized the ease of diagnosis with minimal danger and discomfort to the patient. If the patient's condition is stable, electroencephalography, brain scan, or echoencephalography may be used to help determine the exact site and nature of the tumor. Patients with increased intracranial pressure but with no evidences of specific neurologic deficits are evaluated as rapidly as possible. In emergency situations, arteriography or ventriculography may be used to locate the tumor.

A lumbar puncture may be helpful in assessment of patients with potential brain tumors; as mentioned previously, it is not carried out in patients with symptoms of increased intracranial pressure except in special circumstances because of the danger of herniation (p. 753).

Brain scans are particularly useful in screening patients for suspected brain tumors by demonstrating the size and site of the tumor. A negative brain scan does not, however, exclude a tumor, since a small tumor may not be visualized. Conversely, a positive scan may be caused by a cranial lesion other than a tumor. Electro-

encephalography is particularly useful in the detection of abnormal brain waves, generally or focally, within the cerebral hemispheres or their coverings. The echoencephalogram is helpful in identifying displacement of the ventricular system and the pineal gland from their normal midline positions. Displacement to the right of the midline or to the left may be indicative of a tumor within the respective hemisphere. This so-called displacement is also referred to as a *brain shift* and is a relatively late stage of increased intracranial pressure. Radiographic studies of the skull are carried out initially and may reveal increased intracranial pressure and abnormal calcifications.

Intervention

The general methods of treatment for intracranial tumors include *surgical removal* when feasible, *radiotherapy* and *chemotherapy*. Therapy choice is related to the tumor type and specific sites of the tumor. A combination of methods is often necessary.

When gliomas are located in areas that are not critical to vital function, they are usually removed surgically. However, because gliomas infiltrate and some forms are malignant, they are difficult to completely excise and treat. Surgery is often combined with radiotherapy and chemotherapy. When the tumor is located in a more critical area, a biopsy of the tumor is done, "debrided" if possible, and the patient is treated with radiotherapy or chemotherapy (with nitrosureas).

Meningiomas are commonly treated by complete excision of the tumor (and overlying bone if infiltrated), since they are usually located in areas that permit removal. Meningiomas are also often encapsulated, which aids in their removal.

Acoustic tumors are usually treated surgically, with an effort to preserve the facial nerves and their functions.

Some patients who have had cranial surgery will have residual physical and mental limitations. The patient may have hemiplegia, aphasia, and personality changes, including severe depression. The rehabilitative care and planning both for the patient and for the family are the same as for other patients with chronic and permanent neurologic disease. Specific rehabilitation for patients with hemiplegia and aphasia from this cause is similar to that following a CVA. Preventive exercises should be started as soon as possible postoperatively. Regardless of the eventual prognosis, each patient should be helped to be as independent as possible for as long as possible.

Patients who have intracranial surgery may need the same protection from injury as do other patients with neurologic disease when judgment defect, disorientation, or locomotor difficulties make it unsafe for them to move about without assistance. (The immediate care of these patients is similar to that for any patient with intracranial surgery. See Chapter 35.)

Outcome criteria for the person with an intracranial neoplasm

The person or significant others can:
1. Explain the outcome of therapy or therapies implemented.
   a. Explain each therapy implemented and the desired outcome.
   b. State symptoms to be observed and reported (intracranial pressure).
   c. Explain neurologic deficits.
2. Explain any home medication or treatment program.
   a. State name, dosage, expected action, and side effects of each prescribed medication
   b. Explain when to use medications ordered on a prn basis (analgesics, steroids).
   c. Explain exercise program if any.
   d. Explain care of the skin in relation to radiation and surgical incision.
3. Explain the person's follow-up program.
   a. State symptoms that require immediate medical attention.
   b. State plans for ongoing care.

Intravertebral (intraspinal) tumors

Etiology

Primary intravertebral tumors, or neoplasms, occur either as extramedullary (involving tissues outside the cord substance) or intramedullary (involving tissue cells within the cord substance). *Secondary* or metastatic tumors may also involve the spinal cord, its coverings, and the vertebrae.

Clinical picture

Extramedullary tumors of the intradural type may at first cause subjective nerve root pain. Subsequently, with tumor growth, this will include motor and sensory deficits relating to the level of root and spinal cord involvement. As the tumor enlarges, it compresses the cord. The nurse can learn to relate the initial signs and symptoms to the segmental level of involvement. A cervical lesion will cause pain and motor and sensory deficits in the arms in relation to segmental level. A thoracic lesion causes pain in the chest, and a lumbar lesion causes pain in the legs. Foot and hand pain are rare, but there may be tingling and numbness in the extremities. Eventually, the patient loses all motor and sensory function below the level of the tumor.

An *intramedullary* tumor, beginning within the spinal cord substance, presents a different clinical picture. A central cord syndrome includes segmental loss of pain and temperature function. In addition, there is often loss of anterior horn cell function, especially in the hands. Most of the central long tracts next to the gray matter become dysfunctional. There is a gradual, progressive, and descending loss of pain and temperature sensations and motor weakness that is pronounced in the arms when the tumor begins in the cervical area. Caudal motor and sensory functions are the last to be lost, including loss of bowel and bladder control.

In summary, intravertebral tumors, depending on the site, can produce both upper and lower motor neuron signs as well as sensory deficits. This is also true of other intravertebral lesions such as disk herniation and syringomyelia (cavitation of the spinal medulla) and ependymoma (growths involving the central canal of the cord and ventricles).

Intervention

It is obvious that tumors involving the meninges are more likely to be removed successfully than other types. Even when complete removal is not considered possible, surgery is often performed to remove part of the tumor or to remove part of the bone surrounding the spinal column and thus reduce the obstruction for a time; this is called *spinal decompression*. It can be done at any level of the vertebral column and may include several vertebrae. The operation is sometimes palliative for malignant and nonremovable tumors. Radiation therapy is helpful in the treatment of inoperable intramedullary tumors.

Nursing care for a patient with a tumor of the spinal cord is the same as that for a spinal cord injury. The care given after a decompression operation is similar to that given the patient who has had excision of a ruptured nucleus pulposus, except that recovery is much slower (p. 993). The patient who has severe pain requires narcotics.

Convalescent care and rehabilitation depend entirely on the type of tumor and whether it has been successfully removed. Even if it cannot be removed, the decompression operation may give relief of symptoms for months and sometimes for years. If the tumor is a slow-growing one, radiation therapy may be given while the patient is recovering in the hospital and continued after discharge. The family often needs help in caring for the patient and in meeting the continuing problems. The patient often knows or guesses the prognosis (if little can be done medically) because the mental dulling that so often accompanies brain tumors is not present.

Outcome criteria for the person with an intravertebral tumor

The outcome criteria for the person with an intravertebral tumor is the same as that for the person having intravertebral surgery (p. 1016).

REFERENCES AND SELECTED READINGS
Contemporary

1. Adams, R.D., and Victor, M.: Principles of neurology, New York, 1977, McGraw-Hill Book Co.
2. Allwood, A.C., et al.: Cerebral artery bypass surgery, Am. J. Nurs. **80**:1284-1287, 1980.
3. Bartel, M.A.: Dialogue with Dementia: nonverbal communication in patients with Alzheimer's disease, J. Gerontol. Nurs. **5**:21-31, 1979.
4. Beeson, P.B., McDermott, W., and Wyngaarden, J.B.: Textbook of Medicine, ed. 15, Philadelphia, 1979, W.B. Saunders Co.
5. *Bell, M., Karb, V.B., and Nulsen, F.E.: Head injuries and craniotomies. In Meltzer, L.E., Abdellah, F.G., and Kitchell, J.R., editors: Concepts and practices of intensive care for nurse specialists, ed. 2, Bowie, Md., 1976, The Charles Press.
6. Benenson, A.S.: Control of communicable diseases in man, ed. 12, Washington, D.C., 1975, The American Public Health Association.
7. Blount, M., et al.: Management of the patient with amyotrophic, lateral sclerosis, Nurs. Clin. North Am. **14**:157-171, 1979.
8. Boroch, R.M.: Elements of rehabilitation in nursing: an introduction, St. Louis, 1976, The C.V. Mosby Co.
9. *Boyle, ·M.A., and Cluca, R.L.: Amyotrophic lateral sclerosis, Am. J. Nurs. **76**:66-68, 1976.
10. Brunnstrom, S.: Movement therapy in hemiplegia, New York, 1970, Harper & Row, Publishers.
11. Bruya, M., and Bolin, R.: Epilepsy: a controllable disease, Am. J. Nurs. **76**:388-398, 1976.
12. Burch, G.E., and DePasquale, N.P.: Axioms on cerebrovascular disease, Hosp. Med. **11**:8-10, 1975.
13. Burnside, J.: Alzheimer's disease: an overview, J. Gerontol. Nurs. **5**:14-20, 1979.
14. Center for Disease Control: Reported morbidity and mortality in the United States: 1976, Atlanta, 1977, U.S. Department of Health, Education and Welfare.
15. Cobb, B.A., and Williams, D.D.: Test your neurology nursing skills, Nurs. '80 **10**(1):40-43, 1980.
16. Cotzias, G.C., and McDowell, F.H., editors: Developments in the treatment for Parkinson's disease, New York, 1973, Medam Press.
17. *Dayhoff, N.: Rethinking stroke: soft or hard devices to position hands, Am. J. Nurs. **75**:1142-1144, 1975.
18. *Delehanty, L., and Stravino, V.: Achieving bladder control, Am. J. Nurs. **70**:312-316, 1970.
19. Donahue, R.: Symposium on care of the patient with neuromuscular disease: an overview of neuromuscular disease, Nurs. Clin. North Am. **14**:95-106, 1979.
20. Doolittle, N.: Arteriovenous malformation: the physiology, symptomatology and nursing care, J. Neurosurg. Nurs. **11**:221-226, 1979.
21. Eisenberg, M.G., and Rustard, L.C.: Sex and the spinal cord injured: some questions and answers, ed. 2, Washington, D.C., 1975, U.S. Government Printing Office.
22. Epilepsy Foundation of America: The legal rights of persons with epilepsy, ed. 4, Washington D.C., 1976, The Foundation.
23. *Erb, E.: Improving speech in Parkinson's disease, Am. J. Nurs. **73**:1910-1911, 1973.
24. Fedun, P.: Preoperative evaluation of patients undergoing microanastomosis for brain ischemia, J. Neurosurg. Nurs. **12**:46-53, 1980.
25. Felder, L.: Neurogenic bladder dysfunction, J. Neurosurg. Nurs. **11**:91-104, 1979.
26. *Feldman, J.L., and Schultz, M.: Rehabilitation after stroke, Nurs. Digest 4:63-66, 1976.
27. *Fowler, R.S., and Fordyce, W.J.: Adapting care for the brain damaged patient, Am. J. Nurs. **72**:1832-1835, 2056-2059, 1972.
28. Gastaut, H.: Clinical Electroencephalographical classification of epileptic seizures, Epilepsia **11**:102-113, 1970.
29. Gruendemann, B.J., and Meeker, M.H.: Alexander's care of the patient in surgery, ed. 7, St. Louis, 1983, The C.V. Mosby Co.
30. Hardy, A.G., and Elson, R.: Practical management of spinal injuries, ed. 2, Edinburgh, 1976, Churchill Livingstone.
31. Harkness, L.: Bringing epilepsy out of the closet, Am. J. Nurs. **74**:875-876, 1974.
32. *Hinkhouse, A.: Craniocerebral trauma, Am. J. Nurs. **73**:1719-1722, 1973.
33. Hohmann, G.W.: Consideration in the management of psychosexual adjustment in the cord injured male, Rehabil. Psychol. **19**:50-59, 1972.
34. Hunter, C.: Nursing problems of patients undergoing amino acid treatment for subarachnoid hemorrhage due to aneurysm, J. Neurosurg. Nurs. **11**:160-165, 1979.
35. *Jackson, R.: Sexual rehabilitation after cord injury, Paraplegia **10**:50-55, 1972.
36. *Jacobansky, A.M.: Stroke, Am. J. Nurs. **72**:1260-1263, 1972.
37. Jimm, L.: Nursing assessment of patients for increased intracranial pressure, Nurs. Digest 3:5-8, 1976.
38. *Kelly, R.: Management of MS, Nurs. Mirror 143(6):48-49, 1976.
39. King, R.B., et al.: Symposium on rehabilitative nursing: Rehabilitation of the patient with spinal cord injury, Nurs. Clin. North Am. **15**:225-243, 1980.
40. Kunkel, J., and Wiley, J.K.: Acute head injury: what to do when and why, Nurs. '79 9(3):22-33, 1979.
41. Kursh, E., et al.: Complications of autonomic dysreflexia, J. Urol. **118**:70-72, 1977.
42. *Larrabee, J.H.: The person with a spinal cord injury: physical care during early recovery, Am. J. Nurs. **77**:1320-1329, 1977.
43. Levitt, R.: Understanding sexuality and spinal cord injury, J. Neurosurg. Nurs. **12**:88-89, 1980.
44. Loetterle, B.C., et al.: Cerebellar stimulation: pacing the brain, Am. J. Nurs. **75**:958-960, 1975.

*References preceded by an asterisk are particularly well suited for student reading.

45. Maddox, M.: Subarachnoid hemorrhage, Am. J. Nurs. **74:**2199-2201, 1974.

46. Martin, N., et al.: Comprehensive rehabilitative nursing, New York, 1981, McGraw-Hill Book Co.

47. Melnick, J.L.: Classification and nomenclature of viruses, Prog. Med. Virol. **14:**321-332, 1972.

48. Merritt, H.H.: A textbook of neurology, ed. 4, Philadelphia, 1979, Lea & Febiger.

49. National Multiple Sclerosis Society: 1976 annual report, New York, 1976, The Society.

50. *Norsworthy, E.: Nursing rehabilitation after severe head trauma, Am. J. Nurs. **74:**1246-1250, 1974.

51. Ozuna, J.: Compliance with therapeutic regimens: issues answers and, research questions, J. Neurosurg. Nurs. **13:**1-6, 1981.

52. Peckham, P.H., et al.: Intramuscular stimulation: applications to upper extremity orthotics. In Proceedings of the Fourth Annual Meeting of the Biomedical Engineering Society, Los Angeles, 1973.

53. *Pepper, G.A.: The person with spinal cord injury: psychological care, Am. J. Nurs. **77:**1330-1335, 1977.

54. *The person with spinal cord injury: self-study program, Am. J. Nurs. **77:**1319-1342, 1977.

55. *Pfaudler, M.: Motor skill rehabilitation for hemiplegic patients, Am. J. Nurs. **73:**1892-1896, 1973.

56. Plank, N.: Multiple sclerosis: an update and review, J. Neurosurg. Nurs. **11:**44-47, 1979.

57. *Robinson, M.B.: Levodopa and parkinsonism, Am. J. Nurs. **74:**656-661, 1974.

58. *Rocklin, R.: The Guillain-Barre syndrome and multiple sclerosis, N. Engl. J. Med. **284:**803-808, 1971.

59. Romana, M.: Sexuality and the disabled female, Accent on Living, pp. 26-34, Winter 1973.

60. Rose, A.J., et al.: Neuromuscular diagnostic procedures, Nurs. Clin. North Am. **14:**107-121, 1979.

61. Sabiston, D.E., editor: Davis-Christopher textbook of surgery, ed. 11, Philadelphia, 1977, W.B. Saunders Co.

62. Schontz, F.C.: The psychological aspects of physical illness and disability, New York, 1975, MacMillan Publishing Co., Inc.

63. *Skelly, M.: Rethinking stroke: aphasic patients talk back, Am. J. Nurs. **75:**1140-1142, 1975.

64. *Stackhouse, J.: Myasthenia gravis, Am. J. Nurs. **73:**1544-1547, 1973.

65. Stryker, R.P.: Rehabilitation aspects of acute and chronic nursing care, ed. 2, Philadelphia, 1977, W.B. Saunders Co.

66. Taylor, J., and Bellenger, S.: Neurological dysfunctions and nursing interventions, New York, 1980, McGraw-Hill Book Co.

67. *Taylor, J.W.: Measuring the outcomes of nursing care, Nurs. Clin. North Am. **9:**337-340, 1974.

68. Webb, P.: Neurological deficit after carotid endarderectomies, Am. J. Nurs. **79:**654-658, 1979.

69. *Wheeler, P.: Care of the patient with a cerebellar tumor, Am. J. Nurs. **77:**263-266, 1977.

70. *Woods, N.F.: Human sexuality in health and illness, ed. 2, St. Louis, 1979, The C.V. Mosby Co.

71. Yahr, M.D., editor: Symposium on clinical neurology, Med. Clin. North Am. **56:**1225-1418, 1972.

72. Yase, Y.: Amyotrophic lateral sclerosis, Arch. Neurol. **27:**118-128, 1972.

73. *Young, J.F., and Reid, M.: Care in the surgical management of intracranial aneurysms, J. Neurosurg. Nurs. **4:**21-31, 1972.

74. *Zankel, H.T.: Stroke rehabilitation, Springfield, Ill., 1971, Charles C Thomas, Publisher.

Classic

75. Albin, M.S., et al.: Effects of localized cooling on spinal cord trauma, J. Trauma **9:**1000-1008, 1969.

76. *Hurd, G.G.: Teaching the hemiplegic self-care, Am. J. Nurs. **65:**64-68, 1965.

77. Olson, C.K., and Tollefsrud, V.E.: Chemosurgery for parkinsonism and when the patient has chemosurgery, Am. J. Nurs. **59:**1411-1416, 1959.

78. Olson, E.V., et al.: The hazards of immobility, Am. J. Nurs. **67:**779-797, 1967.

79. Ruge, D., editor: Spinal cord injuries, Springfield, Ill., 1969, Charles C Thomas, Publisher.

80. Taren, J.A., and Martin, M.A.: Cerebral aneurysm and care of the patient with a cerebral aneurysm, Am. J. Nurs. **65:**90-95, 1965.

81. *Ullman, M.: Disorders of body image after stroke, Am. J. Nurs. **64:**89-91, 1964.

AUDIOVISUAL RESOURCES

Bowel and bladder techniques, Urbana-Champaign, Ill., 1974, Rehabilitation Education Center, University of Illinois. (Films.)
The purpose of this program is to present some of the methods that may be utilized by the quadriplegic patient in the management of bowel and bladder functions.

Dressing, Urbana-Champaign, Ill., Rehabilitation-Education Center, University of Illinois. (Film.)
The purpose of this presentation is to demonstrate functional skills and techniques used in dressing, which the quadriplegic has developed through rehabilitation training to achieve independence.

Driving, Urbana-Champaign, Ill., Rehabilitation-Education Center, University of Illinois, produced by Motion Picture Production Center, 1974. (Films.)
The purpose of this program is to demonstrate functional skills necessary and equipment available to assist the quadriplegic patient in driving a car. Several types of vans are demonstrated to illustrate equipment that is available to the quadriplegic.

Human sexuality and nursing process, 1975, Concept Media in cooperation with Department of Medical Education, Memorial Hospital of Long Beach, Costa Mesa, Calif. (Filmstrips.)
This presentation describes the import of medical issues on human sexuality. It concentrates on the feelings of nursing staff with the goal of helping them to accept sexual questions and behavior as well as to answer patient's questions. Filmstrips on medical conditions, disabling conditions, and surgical conditions are especially helpful.

Initial parallel bar exercises for the paraplegic patient, Institute of Rehabilitation Medicine, New York University Medical Center, produced by Public Health Service Audiovisual Facility. (Film.)
The purpose of this presentation is to describe and demonstrate the initial parallel bar exercises the paraplegic patient must master to begin crutch walking.

Introduction to seizures, Garden Grove, Calif., 1971, Trainex. (Filmstrip.)
The purpose of this presentation is to discuss the patient who has a seizure disorder. Necessary observations are discussed.

Mobilization of the stroke patient, Ann Arbor, Mich., 1975, University of Michigan Medical Center, (Slides.)
This program describes and demonstrates useful therapeutic approaches in the mobilization of the stroke patient. This objective is achieved with the aid of clinical subjects, hospital personnel, drawings, and diagrams.

Moving in and out of your wheelchair, Minneapolis, 1969, American Rehabilitation Foundation. (Film.)
The purpose of this patient education program is to demonstrate the independent transfer of a paraplegic patient into and out of a wheelchair.

A new approach to physical therapy in parkinsonism, Norwich, N.Y., 1971, Eaton. (Film.)

The purpose of this program is to demonstrate the use of group physical therapy in parkinsonism.

Position to prevent contractures, Garden Grove, Calif., 1970, Trainex. (Filmstrip.)

This filmstrip discusses and demonstrates proper positioning to prevent the development of contractures.

Showering and grooming, Urbana-Champaign, Ill., Rehabilitation-Education Center, University of Illinois, produced by Motion Picture Production Center, 1974. (Films.)

The purpose of this presentation is to describe and demonstrate several techniques developed by quadriplegic patients for showering and grooming.

Techniques in ADL for the adult disabled, Davis, Calif., 1976, NCME, Department of Family Practice, University of California at Davis Affiliate Hospital. (Video cassette.)

This presentation presents a variety of techniques in the areas of bathing, dressing, grooming and eating. It shows time-saving as well as energy-saving techniques.

CHAPTER 37

ASSESSMENT OF SPECIAL SENSES: EYE AND EAR

LYNN CHENOWETH
LINDA ANNE BROSEMAN

Sensations in general orient people to themselves and their environment. We learn about our world and about ourselves through sensations. Sensations contribute meaning and pleasure to the human experience. A world without the sounds and sights of children playing or the esthetic pleasure of museums and symphonies may be bleak indeed. Besides pleasures, sensations provide necessary data for our safety and well-being. A fire alarm or a flashing red light provides clues to danger in our environment. We learn as infants to distinguish between what is "us" and what is the world by our senses. Our sensations directly contribute to our self-concept and feelings of personal worth and well-being.

Sensory impairment is often not the initial problem or major diagnosis but is often present in patients for whom the nurse is providing care for other medical or surgical conditions. Health workers need to be able to assess all patients in relation to sensory capabilities and plan their care accordingly.

Nursing assessment is focused on the degree to which the sensory loss affects the person's ability to carry out activities of daily living, the support systems available, and the coping skills that have been successfully utilized in the past. Nursing interventions are designed to help people meet their basic needs as they are affected by hospitalization or illness, to strengthen existing support systems, and to encourage the use of successful coping mechanisms.

Two major senses, vision and hearing, are considered in the next three chapters. Further information on other sensory alterations can be found in the discussion of management of neurologic manifestations (see Chapter 35).

Many aspects of assessment of the eyes, including visual acuity, and the ears, including hearing, may be carried out by different professionals or trained auxiliary personnel, as described in the text. The extent of the nurse's activities in assessment of the eye and ear depends on the level of preparation and place of employment.

Anatomy and physiology of the eye

Anatomy of the eye

The eyeball is composed of three coats or layers of tissue, the sclera, the choroid, and the retina (Fig. 37-1). The tough outer coat, or *sclera*, is opaque (white) but becomes transparent anteriorly over the iris and pupil to form the *cornea*. The middle layer, the *choroid*, contains blood vessels and is modified anteriorly into the ciliary body, which is attached to the suspensory ligament and to the iris. The pupil is the space in the center of the doughnut-shaped iris.

The inner coat, the *retina*, which does not have an anterior portion, contains the photoreceptors (rods and cones). These photoreceptors synapse in the retina with bipolar neurons and then with ganglion neurons, and these become the fibers of the optic nerve. The cones, which are less numerous than the rods, occur mostly near the center of the retina and are considered to be the receptors for bright daylight and color vision. The rods, which are found mostly in the periphery of the retina, are receptors for dim or night vision. Rods contain rhodopsin, a photosensitive protein that becomes

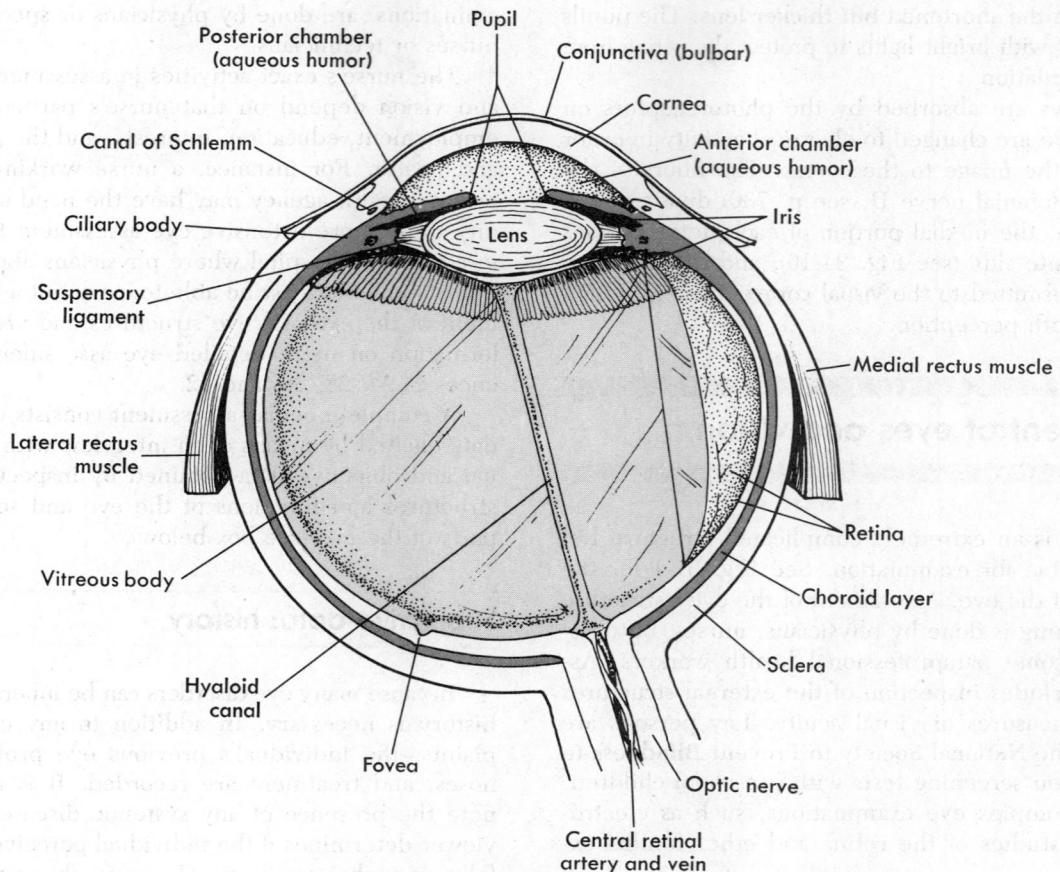

Posterior chamber
(aqueous humor)

Pupil

Conjunctiva (bulbar)

Cornea

Anterior chamber
(aqueous humor)

Canal of Schlemm

Iris

Ciliary body

Lens

Suspensory
ligament

Medial rectus muscle

Lateral rectus
muscle

Retina

Choroid layer

Vitreous body

Sclera

Hyaloid
canal

Optic nerve

Fovea

Central retinal
artery and vein

Fig. 37-1. Horizontal section through left eyeball.

rapidly depleted in bright light. The slow regeneration of rhodopsin, which is dependent on the presence of vitamin A, explains the time needed to adjust from a bright to a dim light. Vitamin A deficiency affects night vision.

The interior of the eyeball is divided into two cavities, the anterior and the posterior. The anterior cavity, which is in front of the lens, is further subdivided into an anterior chamber (between the cornea and the iris) and a posterior chamber (between the iris and the lens). The anterior cavity is filled with a clear liquid called aqueous humor, which is produced in the ciliary body, drains into the posterior chamber, passes through the pupil into the anterior chamber, and drains out the canal of Schlemm at the junction of the iris and cornea (anterior chamber angle). Obstruction of this drainage leads to glaucoma (p. 895). The posterior cavity of the eye is filled with a clear gelatinous substance called vitreous humor, which helps maintain eye body. If vitreous humor is removed, the eye collapses.

Eye muscles consist of two types, extrinsic and intrinsic. The extrinsic voluntary muscles outside the eyeball control extraocular movement. The intrinsic involuntary muscles within the eye are the ciliary body,

which controls the shape of the lens, and the iris, which controls pupil size.

Physiology of vision

Light rays entering the eye bend (*refraction*) as they pass over the curved surfaces of the cornea and through various structures of the eye (cornea, aqueous humor, lens, vitreous humor), which have different densities, to focus on the retina.

The eye can adjust (*accommodation*) to seeing objects at various distances by the flattening or thickening of the lens. Near vision requires contraction of the ciliary body, which decreases the distance between the edges of the ciliary body, thus relaxing the suspensory ligament attached to the lens. The lens then bulges to bend the light ray more acutely so that the rays will focus on the retina. Continual close vision may produce eyestrain through constant contraction of the ciliary muscle; this can be relieved by frequent shifting of the eyes to distant objects. Accommodation is also facilitated by changing the size of the pupil. With near vision the iris constricts the pupil to force light rays to pass through the shortened but thicker lens. The pupils also constrict with bright lights to protect the retina from intense stimulation.

Light rays are absorbed by the photoreceptors on the retina and are changed to electrical activity in order to transmit the image to the cortex. The fibers of the optic nerve (cranial nerve II, see p. 730) divide at the optic chiasm, the medial portion of each nerve crosses to the opposite side (see Fig. 34-10), and the impulses are then transmitted to the visual cortex. Bilateral vision provides depth perception.

Assessment of eyes and vision

The eye is an extremely complicated structure but very accessible for examination. See Fig. 37-1 for the landmarks of the eye. Assessment of the eye's structure and functioning is done by physicians, nurses, optometrists, and some paraprofessional health workers. Assessment includes inspection of the external structures and gross measures of visual acuity. Lay persons are trained by the National Society to Prevent Blindness to conduct vision screening tests with preschool children. The more complex eye examinations, such as electrophysiologic studies of the retina and other fundus ex-

aminations, are done by physicians or specially trained nurses or technicians.

The nurse's exact activities in assessment of the eye and vision depend on that nurse's particular place of employment, education, interests, and the patient's age and health. For instance, a nurse working in a community health agency may have the need and opportunity to do more extensive eye assessment than a nurse in a teaching hospital where physicians abound. Every nurse should at least be able to carry out a basic assessment of the external eye structures and vision. For information on more detailed eye assessment see references 2, 24, 28, 30, and 42.

A complete ocular assessment consists of subjective data elicited by means of an interview with the individual and objective data obtained by inspecting external structures and functions of the eye and some internal parts of the eye (see box below).

Subjective data: history

Because many eye disorders can be inherited, a family history is necessary. In addition to any current complaints, the individual's previous eye problems, diagnoses, and treatment are recorded. It is important to note the presence of any systemic disease. The interviewer determines if the individual perceives any of the following: changes in visual acuity; abnormal signs and symptoms such as burning, tearing, or blurred vision; and events surrounding onset of symptoms, duration of symptoms, and sources of relief.[42]

Objective data

Pathophysiology

When light passes through the eye, the bending of the light rays and the location of the image depend on

BASIC ASSESSMENT OF THE EYE AND VISION

Facial and ocular expression	Prominence of eyes, alert or dull expression
Eyelids	Symmetry, presence of edema, ptosis, itching, redness, discharges, blinking equality
Iris and pupils	Irregularities in color, shape, size
Pupillary reflex	Constriction of pupil in response to light in that eye (direct light reaction), equal amount of constriction in other eye (consensual light reaction)
Lens	Transparent or opaque
Peripheral vision	Ability to see movements and objects well on both sides of field of vision
Acuity with and without glasses	Ability to read newsprint, clocks on wall, and name pins, to recognize faces at bedside and at door
Supportive aids	Glasses, contact lenses, false eye

OCULAR ASSESSMENT

Recording of history

Assessment of visual acuity

Assessment of ocular movement

Assessment of pupillary reflexes

Assessment of visual fields

Inspection of external structures

Inspection of internal structures

Estimation of intraocular pressure

the shape and condition of ocular structures (see box below). The eye has the ability to adjust to near or far objects (*accommodation*) by means of the ciliary muscles, which contract or relax, causing the lens to flatten or thicken as the need arises. If the anteroposterior dimension of the eye is abnormally long, the light rays will focus in front of the retina (*myopia*). Conversely, if the anteroposterior dimension is abnormally short, the rays will focus behind the retina (*hyperopia*). When the lens becomes less elastic and responds less to the need for accommodation, as occurs in persons past the age of 40, blurring of near objects (*presbyopia*) results. The curvature of the cornea may also be asymmetric or irregular so that rays in the horizontal and vertical planes do not focus at the same point (*astigmatism*).

Measurement of visual acuity

Ocular *refraction* is a procedure that reveals the degree to which the various light-transmitting portions of the eye bring light rays into correct focus on the retina. When the image is not clearly focused on the retina, *refractive error* is present. Refractive errors account for the largest number of impairments of good vision. The refractive error is tested by means of trial lenses and the Snellen chart. (Fig. 37-2, *A*). Suitable corrective lenses are prescribed if needed. If refractive errors involving both distant and close vision are present, bifocal or trifocal lenses or separate glasses will be required. In situations where formal acuity testing equipment is not available, estimates of refractive error can be made. For instance, the person can be asked to read print or identify pictures at varying distances. The person's visual acuity can be compared with that of the examiner's.

Before refraction is done, a cycloplegic drug is in-

TERMS DESCRIBING VISUAL ACUITY

Accommodation	Ability to adjust between far and near objects
Emmetropia	Normal eye; light rays focus on retina
Ametropia	Refractive error; light rays do not focus on retina
Myopia	Nearsightedness; light rays focus in front of retina
Hyperopia	Farsightedness; light rays focus behind retina
Presbyopia	Hyperopia from loss of lens elasticity because of age
Astigmatism	Irregular curvature of cornea; light rays do not focus at same point

---

stilled into the eyes to dilate the pupils and temporarily paralyze the ciliary muscles. Cyclopentolate (Cyclogyl), 1% or 2%, is usually used, since it is effective in 30 minutes and the effect generally wears off completely by the end of 6 hours. The duration of effect will vary, however, lasting longer than 6 hours in persons with a light blue iris. A blue-eyed person's iris will dilate more rapidly and remain dilated longer than that of a brown-eyed person because more of the drug is absorbed into the iris with less pigmentation.

When the appointment is made for an eye examination with the use of a cycloplegic drug, the person is told that blurred vision will be present after the examination. It should be explained that driving or reading will not be possible until the effect of the drug subsides. In some cases a miotic drug, pilocarpine, is instilled after the examination to constrict the pupil and reduce the uncomfortable glare from lights. Homatropine occasionally is used for adults and atropine for children to dilate the pupils for refraction, but both of these drugs require longer to take effect, and their effects persist longer. Atropine must be instilled at intervals for 3 days before examination and persists in its action for at least 10 days with some residual effect for up to 3 to 4 weeks.

Distance vision is usually determined by use of a *Snellen chart* (Fig. 37-2, *A*). Examination is done with the person standing 20 ft from the chart. The chart consists of rows of letters, numbers, or other characters arranged with the large ones at the top and the small ones at the bottom. The upper-most letter on the chart is scaled so that it can be read by the normal eye at 200 ft, and the successive rows are scaled so that they can be read at 100, 70, 50, 40, 30, 20, 15, and 10 ft, respectively. Visual acuity is expressed as a fraction, and a reading of 20/20 is considered normal. The upper figure refers to the distance of the person from the chart, and the lower figure indicates the distance at which a normal eye can read the line. For example, the person who is able to read at 20 ft only the line that should be readable at 70 ft has 20/70 vision in that eye. A score of 20/30 means that the person is 20 ft from the chart and can read the line that a normal eye should see at 30 ft.[43] The distance from the chart to where the individual stands must be carefully measured. The examiner usually stands beside the chart and points to the line to be read so that no mistake occurs. Each eye is tested separately, and its performance is carefully recorded. The person is tested with and without distance lenses. When testing vision a piece of stiff paper or a plastic occluder is placed over one eye while the other eye is tested.

For preschool children and others unable to read the English alphabet, a modified Snellen chart is used (Fig. 37-2, *B*). In this chart a block **E** is shown in varying positions and the individual is asked to indicate in

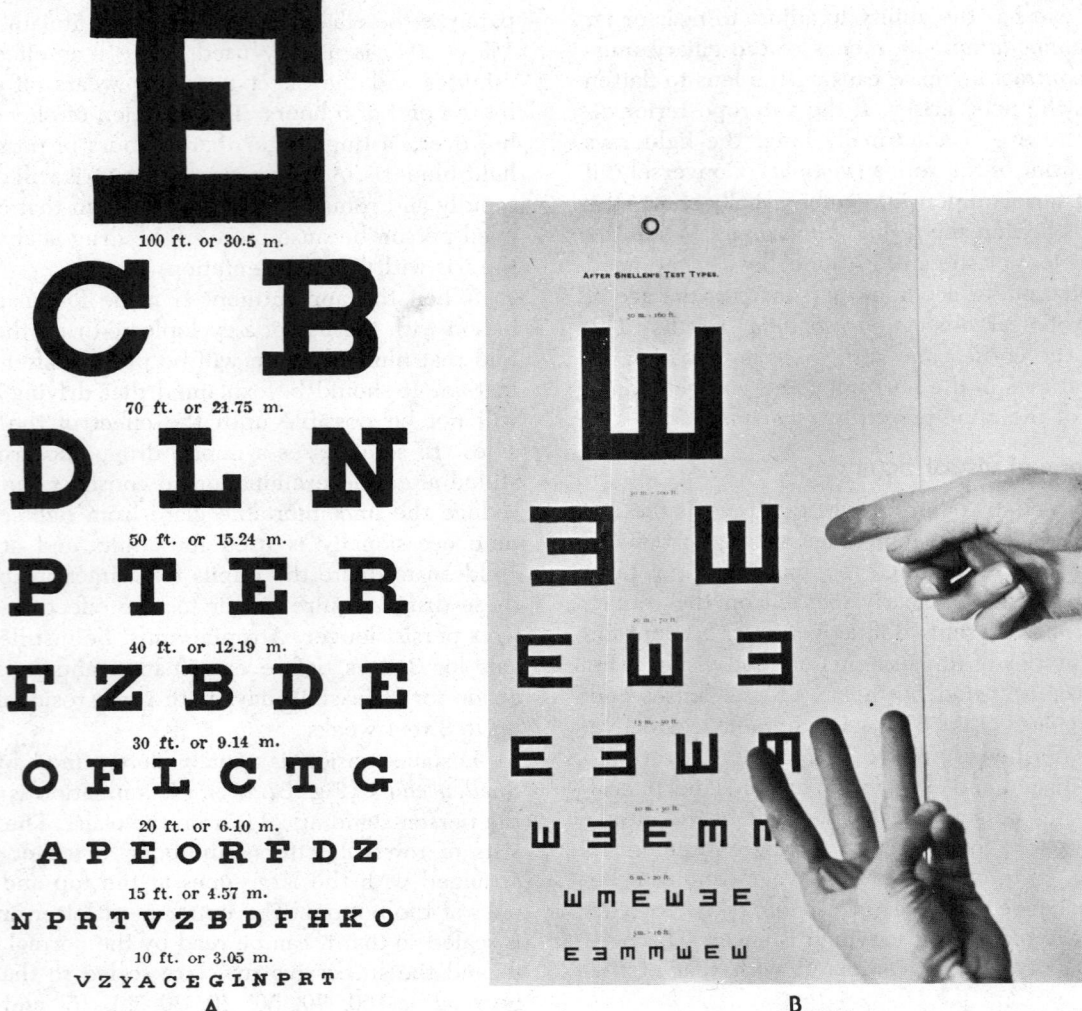

Fig. 37-2. A, Snellen chart used in testing vision. **B,** Modified Snellen chart, called "E" game, for testing vision of small children and persons unfamiliar with English alphabet.

which direction the "legs" or "fingers" of the E point.

Near vision can be tested with use of a Jaeger chart or newsprint. The Jaeger chart is a card containing varying size print, which is held 35 cm (14 in.) from the eye. The score attained can be expressed in Snellen, metric, and percentage figures.[43]

Any person with vision less than 20/30 OD (right eye) or OS (left eye) or with a two-line difference between eyes should be referred to an ophthalmologist for further testing and treatment. The Snellen, block E, or Jaeger chart examinations provide only basic screening test data. Additional detailed procedures must be done to test for nearsightedness, astigmatism, color blindness, and many other abnormalities. The nurse who works in a clinic, in an ophthalmologists's office, or in schools must know how to do vision screening tests and how to teach others to do them.

Assessment of ocular movements

Ocular movements are evaluated to determine whether the eyes are moving together in a synchronous manner. Muscle imbalances and cranial nerve damage also can be detected.

To test ocular muscles the examiner and person being tested are seated facing each other. While the person looks straight ahead at a target, a penlight is shined on the cornea. The corneal light reflex should be in exactly the same position on each pupil. The examiner then covers one of the person's eyes while the person looks at the light. When the cover is quickly removed, the examiner notes whether that eye moves to regain fixation on the light. Movement may indicate a drift of the eye behind the cover, which can indicate muscle imbalances.[24]

To evaluate possible weaknesses of individual extraocular muscles, muscle balance testing can be done in eight positions of gaze as well as straight ahead. The reader is referred to texts on physical appraisal for more detailed information about assessment of ocular movements.[2,24,28,42]

Inspection of external structures

The general appearance of the face and eyes is observed for the type of expression (dull or alert) and prominence of the eyes. When there is an abnormal protrusion or bulging of an eye, the condition is called *exophthalmia* or *exophthalmos*.

The appearance of the *eyelids* is noted in relation to color, texture, mobility, and position. The lids should be able to close completely to prevent drying of the conjunctiva and cornea. Any swelling, redness, or discharge is noted. If one upper lid seems to be in a position lower than the other, or "droops," the condition may be *ptosis* of the eyelid. When there is ptosis in both eyes, the upper lids will be observed to be in an abnormally low position covering the upper portion or more of the iris. Ptosis of the upper lids may be the result of extreme debility or neuromuscular disease.[24] Extreme ptosis can interfere with vision by covering the pupil.

The *conjunctiva* is a transparent membrane that lines the inside of the eyelids and covers the exposed portion of the eyeball except for the cornea. The conjunctiva of the lower lid is examined by pulling downward on the lid as the individual looks upward. In order to examine the conjunctiva of the upper lid, the lid must be everted. To evert the eyelid the individual looks down; the examiner grasps the eyelashes and pulls gently down and forward while pushing down on the upper lid border with an applicator or tongue blade. When the lid is everted, it is held in position by the fingers holding the lashes to the brow.

Small blood vessels are normally visible in the conjunctiva. The *sclera*, or white covering of the eye, shows through the conjunctiva and has a shiny porcelain-like appearance. Dilation of blood vessels of the conjunctiva may indicate disease of the cornea or disease within the eye. Spontaneous small hemorrhages may occur beneath the conjunctiva in the normal eye. A yellow discoloration of the sclera indicates jaundice. The *lacrimal gland* may be observed in the inner canthus of the eye and may be palpated for patency of the lacrimal puncta.

The *cornea*, which is normally invisible except for surface reflections, must be smooth and transparent for good vision. It should look shiny and bright when examined with a penlight. Moving the light and directing it from the side, the examiner looks for abrasions and opacities.

The *iris* of each eye is compared for color, pattern, and shape. When looking through the pupillary open-ing, the examiner is also inspecting the *lens,* which is normally transparent. An opaque lens is termed a *cataract*.

Pupillary reflexes

While approaching from the side, the examiner quickly shines a light into one eye causing constriction of the pupil in that eye (direct light reaction). The pupil of the other eye should also constrict the same amount (consensual light reaction, p. 732). The other eye is then tested in the same manner.

A light shined into a blind eye will not produce a pupillary response; however, a light shined into a normal eye will produce a pupillary response in the blind eye by consensual reaction if the oculomotor nerve is intact.[2]

Another test of pupillary reflex is to have the person focus on an object that is moved directly toward the nose. When focusing on the near object, the pupils of both eyes should constrict (near reaction, reaction in accommodation). The examiner looks for the presence of a response and whether the response is equal in both eyes. Loss of pupillary reflexes when sight is present is caused by neurologic disease (p. 732).

Visual fields

The visual field for an individual is that portion of the world that the eye can perceive. Lesions of the retina, optic pathways, and central nervous system affect sections of the field of vision (p. 731). The location of visual field loss indicates the location of the lesion. For instance, glaucoma decreases peripheral vision, indicating damage to the optic nerve at its head or the optic disk. A rough measurement of the visual fields can be made by using the confrontation test (p. 731). If there appears to be any abnormality in the field of vision, more precise testing should be done with precision instruments by an ophthalmologist or a specially trained technician. One precise method by which the person's peripheral vision can be plotted is the perimeter, a curved semicircular instrument measured in degrees. Another method is the tangent screen in which peripheral vision is plotted as a test object is moved against a black screen.

Evaluation of ocular fundus

The fundus, or back portion of the interior of the eye, is examined with an ophthalmoscope. The ophthalmoscope magnifies the view of the back of the eye so that the optic nerve, retina, blood vessels, and nerves can be seen through the pupil. The examiner may use either the direct (Fig. 37-3) or the indirect (Fig. 37-4) method of ophthalmoscopic examination. When examined with the indirect ophthalmoscope, the person may experience a great deal of light sensitivity. The direct method is the more commonly used approach. The en-

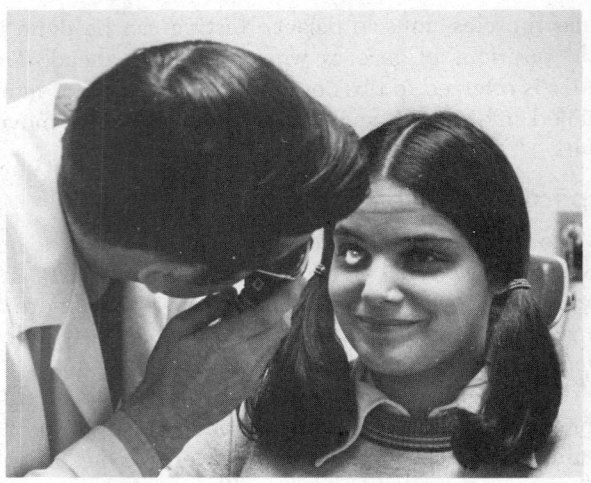

Fig. 37-3. Direct method of ophthalmoscopic examination. Ophthalmoscope is used to examine optic disk, blood vessels, macula lutea, and fovea centralis of retina.

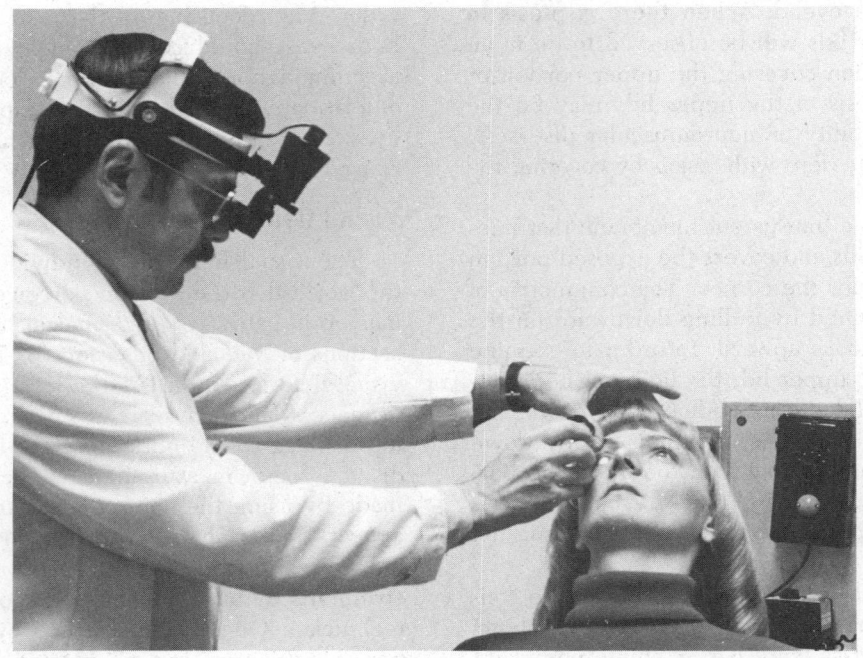

Fig. 37-4. Indirect method of ophthalmoscopic examination. Indirect ophthalmoscope provides binocular view of fundus and allows excellent observation of extreme periphery of retina.

tire retina is not visualized at one time, so the examiner moves the ophthalmoscope until the entire fundus is visualized. (For further discussion on the use of the ophthalmoscope, see p. 731.)

Difficulty in perceiving the fundus may be caused by interference with the light penetrating the eye as a result of intraocular inflammation, corneal scarring, or cataract. Data obtained from visualization of the fundus may indicate eye disease (cupping of the disk in glaucoma) or systemic disease (arteriosclerosis, hyperten-

sion). Hemorrhages in deep retinal layers occur in advanced hypertension, severe renal disease, certain collagen diseases, advanced diabetes, and blood dyscrasias.

The interior of the eye can also be examined by the ophthalmologist using a slit lamp microscope in a darkened room. By adjusting the lens, the examiner can test the person's eye for such changes as corneal ulcerations, lens changes, foreign bodies in the vitreous, or retinal changes.

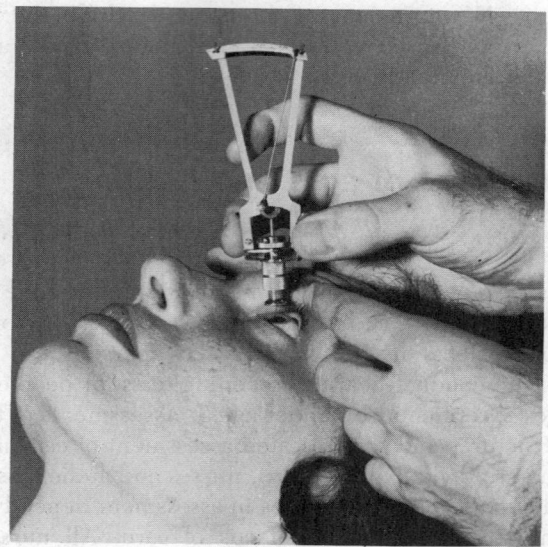

Fig. 37-5. Measurement of intraocular pressure with Schiøtz tonometer. (From Saunders, W.H., et al.: Nursing care in eye, ear, nose, and throat disorders, ed. 4, St. Louis, 1979, The C.V. Mosby Co.)

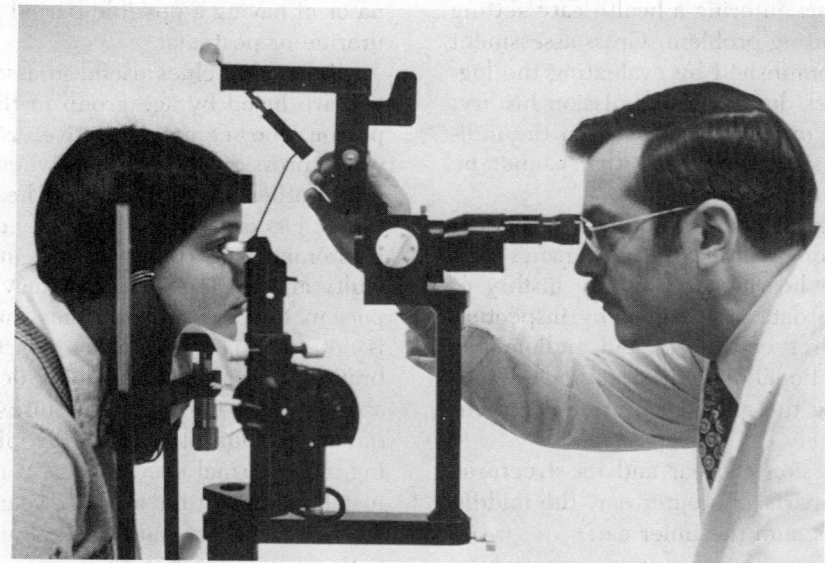

Fig. 37-6. Measurement of ocular tension with Goldmann applanation tonometer.

Estimation of intraocular pressure

An instrument known as a *tonometer* is used to measure ocular tension and is helpful in detecting early glaucoma. Some ophthalmologists suggest that tonometric readings be taken by the medical internist or the family physician as part of a regular annual physical examination. The most common indentation tonometer in clinical use is that of Schiøtz. The procedure is performed with the individual lying down and looking upward at some fixed point. The eye may be anesthetized with one or two drops of proparacaine hydrochloride (Ophthaine), 0.5%, after which the tonometer is placed on the cornea (Fig. 37-5). While the weight of the to-

nometer is supported by the cornea, the amount of indentation that the plunger of the instrument makes in the cornea is measured on the attached scale. This reading is used to determine the pressure within the eye. Readings over 24 mm Hg (Schiøtz) may suggest glaucoma, but tests usually are repeated because temporary increases sometimes may be caused by such things as emotional stress. The applanation tonometer (Goldmann) is more accurate in estimating intraocular pressure (Fig. 37-6). The applanation tonometer is attached to the slit lamp. Instead of indenting the eye, a small area of the cornea is flattened to counterbalance a spring-loaded measuring device, and the pressure is measured directly. Newer means of tonometry include the air tonometer, the scleral and air indentation types, and the electronic tonometer.

Assessment of ears and hearing*

Assessment of the ear and its functioning is done by physicians, nurses, audiologists, and occasionally by some paraprofessional health workers. Lay persons can be trained to conduct hearing screening tests for people of all ages except children under age 3. Assessments of the ear structures and sophisticated assessment of ear functioning are done by physicians, nurses and audiologists.

The nurse's exact activities in assessment depend on the nurse's education and focus of care. All nurses, however, should be prepared to carry out an inspection of the outer ear and at least a gross assessment of hearing ability for all persons entering a health care setting regardless of the presenting problem. Gross assessment of hearing may be accomplished by evaluating the logical sequences of replies during the admission history. One method is to turn one's head away from the individual when asking a simple question that cannot be answered by a yes or no response.

A complete hearing assessment consists of subjective data from the history relating to the person's perceived difficulties with hearing or a family history of hearing loss. Objective data is obtained by inspection of the external structures of the ear and audiometric testing of hearing. Additional objective data include behavioral signs indicating the need for a more complete hearing assessment.

For clarity of discussion the ear and its structures are presented in three parts: the outer ear, the middle ear and mastoid process, and the inner ear.

Early identification of hearing loss

The detection of persons with hearing impairment is an important nursing responsibility. Often the nurse is the first member of the health team to be approached by persons seeking help regarding hearing problems. Community screening programs for detecting children with possible hearing losses are helpful in limiting the handicap by getting the child under medical care.

Every school system in the United States is mandated by federal and state law (P.L. 94-142) to identify and evaluate all suspected handicapped children from birth to 21 years of age. Parents of any child with a

suspected or proven hearing loss can contact the pupil personnel director of their local school district, who must assist in directing the child into appropriate educational and diagnostic programs.

When working with children, an especially important aspect of the hearing assessment history is the identification of those children who have a high risk of having hearing loss. Highly suspect are children with any of the following risk factors[4]:

1. A birth weight of less than 1500 g
2. Neonatal hypoxia
3. Meningitis
4. Familial history of hearing loss
5. Nonbacterial intrauterine fetal infections (rubella, herpes, syphilis, cytomegalovirus, toxoplasmosis)
6. Associated congenital anomalies of the skull or face
7. Hyperbilirubinemia

All of these except heredity have the common denominator of having a possible period of anoxia, either intrauterine or postnatal.

Behavioral clues useful in assessing hearing difficulties are listed by age group in the box on p. 847. The person who seems inattentive or who has a strained facial expression, particularly when conversing or listening to others, may be hard of hearing. An early indication of loss of hearing is difficulty communicating in noisy environments as compared with quiet ones. Persons with faulty articulation in speech may be deaf. In order for persons to speak properly they must hear properly. This is not a simple hearing function but is tied to complex brain patterns. A congenitally deaf child will never be able to talk "normally" because there is no brain sequence of sound to speech. People who lose their hearing after normal speech has been learned will be able to talk normally for about 7 years after total deafness. Then for lack of auditory stimulus, the brain-speech patterns will deteriorate.

Persons who habitually fail to respond when spoken to or who make mistakes in carrying out directions should be encouraged to have their hearing tested. The repetition of, "What did you say?" or "Uh huh" with a quizzical expression is often a symptom of hearing loss. Persons who exhibit any of these behavioral clues should have their ears examined by an otolaryngologist who will obtain a hearing test. In this way a complete evaluation of the hearing problem can be made to determine the extent of the loss, possible correction, and whether the hearing loss is caused by more serious disease.

The nurse can help find and direct the person with a hearing loss and the family to the appropriate agencies for assistance (p. 881). There may be ways of improving hearing through medical or surgical therapy. If the loss is irreversible, aural rehabilitation may make it

*The author acknowledges contributions to this section by William J. Witt, M.D.

BEHAVIORAL CLUES INDICATING DIFFICULTY IN HEARING

Infant

A newborn who:

Does not startle when someone claps sharply within 3 to 6 ft

A 3-month-old who:

Does not turn the head toward sound sources

A 6- to 12-month-old who:

Does not pass routine pneumo-otoscopic and tympanometric screening test for serous otitis media

An 8- to 12-month-old who:

Does not turn toward a whispered voice or the sound of a rattle or a spoon stirring in a cup when the sound originates within 3 ft behind him or her

Any age infant who has:

Decreased or absent babbling

Failure to produce syllables with distinct consonants (e.g., mama, dada)

Decreased response to speech, musical toys, noisemakers

Any age infant who is:

Difficult to awaken without touching

Comforted only when held

Toddler, preschooler

A 2-year-old who:

Cannot identify some objects when their names are spoken

Cannot repeat a word with a single stimulus

Cannot repeat a phrase

Does not use some short phrases while talking

Any toddler who:

Communicates wants through gesturing

Is emotionally immature, demanding, fearful

Responds to vibration and touch more than speech or noise

Ignores telephone and doorbell

Child

Any age child who:

Is not awakened or disturbed by loud sounds

Does not respond when called

Pays no attention to ordinary crib noises

Uses gestures almost exclusively instead of verbalization to establish needs

Watches parents' faces intently when spoken to

Has a history of upper respiratory tract infections associated with chronic middle ear difficulties or a history of recurrent middle ear infections

Any school child who:

Has scholastic performance below level of apparent ability

Has truancy problem

May be labeled as slow learner or behavioral problem

Asks to have things repeated

Shows inattention, daydreaming

Gives irrelevant answers

Hears better when watching speaker's face

Is withdrawn, bored, or disinterested in activities involving conversation

Has deviations in speech, mispronounces or omits some sounds

Has monotonous voice tone

Interrupts without being aware of it

Hears better in a noisy environment where people shout

Shows undue tension and fatigue with normal activities

Seems to hear better at some times than others

Fails to follow directions or does so incorrectly

Turns up volume and sits close to television

Has earaches with subsequent changes in behavior

Adult

Any adult who:

Is irritable, hostile, hypersensitive in interpersonal relations

Has difficulty in hearing upper frequency consonants

Complains about people mumbling

Turns up volume on television

Asks for frequent repetition and answers questions inappropriately

Loses sense of humor, becomes grim

Leans forward to hear better, face serious and strained

Shuns large- and small-group audience situations

May appear aloof and "stuck up"

Complains of ringing in the ears

Has an unusually soft or loud voice

possible for the person with a hearing loss to understand and communicate with others. Rehabilitation is more difficult if loss of vision is present in addition to loss of hearing.

Assessment of external ear

Anatomy and physiology

The external ear has two parts: the *auricle*, or pinna, and the *ear canal* (Fig. 37-7). The auricle is generally made up of cartilage and skin with little subcutaneous fat except for the lobule. The blood and lymphatic supply to the auricle are excellent. The nerve supply to the external ear is chiefly from the trigeminal (fifth cranial) nerve and a branch of the vagus (tenth cranial) nerve going to the posterior part of the ear canal, and from the cervical nerves. The external ear and auditory canal provide a channel along which sound travels to the tympanic membrane. The outer third of the canal is lined with skin containing wax and sweat glands. The inner part of the canal is lined with squamous epithelium.

Physical assessment

The assessment of the external ear begins with inspection of the auricle and surrounding tissues for de-
formities, lumps, or skin lesions. The normal auricle varies considerably from person to person. Observations include the placement of the ears on the head; the normal ear is set so that the upper tip of the pinna is on a line with the corner of the eye and occipital protuberance at the back of the head. Shape, size, and degree of protrusion of the ears from the head are noted in addition to redness or scratches, particularly in the crevices behind the ear.

For inspection of the ear canal the adult is instructed to tip the head slightly to the opposite side while the examiner gently pulls the auricle up, back, and out. The auricle of an infant or small child is held down and out. A penlight may be used for inspection, although a good practice in assessing the ear canal is to use an adjustable light such as a standing gooseneck lamp that does not need to be held. The ear canal is examined for the presence of wax, discharge, tissue obstruction, or foreign bodies and for redness or swelling.

The use of an otoscope may be necessary to dilate and straighten the ear canal for easier examination (Fig. 37-8). The largest speculum that the ear will accommodate is used. The speculum is inserted slightly down and forward. The ear canal often has to be cleansed for cerumen (wax), desquamated epithelium, and other accumulations. Obstructing debris can be removed with a cerumen spoon or "loop" aspiration or by irrigation

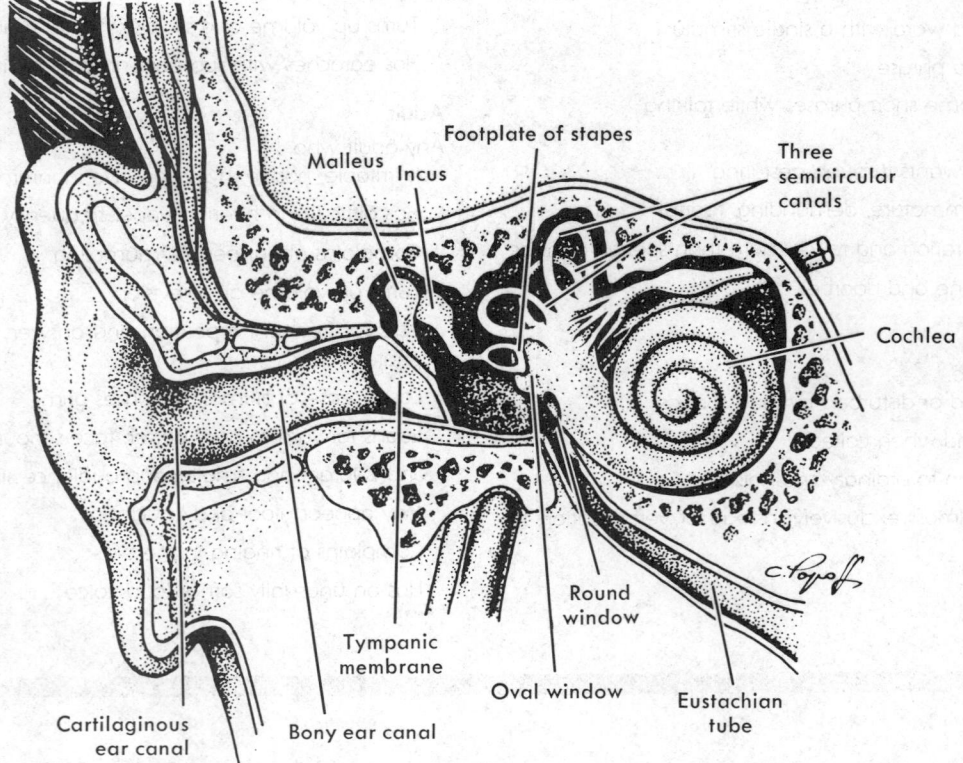

Fig. 37-7. External auditory canal, middle ear, and inner ear. (From Malasanos, L., et al.: Health assessment, ed. 2, St. Louis, 1981, The C.V. Mosby Co.)

with water at body temperature. Great care and training are needed before cleansing the canal is attempted or serious injury may result to the ear canal, eardrum, or middle ear contents. When irrigating water is used, it should be close to body temperature (37° C) or the patient may become violently dizzy because a caloric response is induced (p. 857). Irrigation should never be performed on a person with a history of tympanic membrane perforation or mastoid surgery because severe infections can be precipitated. Cotton applicators should only be used to clean the most superficial debris since they can push the debris into the depths of the canal.

Pathophysiology

Abnormalities in the height of the ear can indicate the presence of some congenital defects such as Down's syndrome as well as renal abnormalities. Normally, the ear is attached vertically to the head; attachments with deviation more than 10 degrees from vertical are abnormal and should be referred to an otolaryngologist.[2]

Redness or scratches, particularly in the crevices behind the ear, are noted because they may lead to future infection if not properly cared for. Some common nodules found in and around the ear include furuncles, palpable lymph nodes anterior to the tragus or overlying the mastoid process, sebaceous cysts especially behind the ear, tophi (deposits of uric acid crystals characteristic of gout), and chondrodermatitis helicis (a small, chronic, painful, tender nodule in the superior helix. Persons with any masses in or about the ear should be referred to an otolaryngologist since these masses may represent primary or metastatic malignant disease.

If ear pain, discharge, or inflammation is present, the ear is checked for tenderness by moving the auricle and pressing on the tragus and mastoid process. Pain on movement of the auricle and tragus is a symptom of acute external otitis (p. 903). Tenderness of the mastoid process suggests mastoiditis (p. 906).

Assessment of middle ear

Anatomy and physiology

The external ear is separated from the middle ear by the tympanic membrane (eardrum) (Fig. 37-7). It is a fairly tough membrane that serves to protect the middle ear and also vibrates with incoming sound waves for hearing. The middle ear, which lies directly behind the eardrum, is a small air-filled space in the tympanic portion of the temporal bone. It contains the three small bones (ossicles): *malleus, incus,* and *stapes.* The footplate of the stapes fits into the oval window, which is a small opening in the wall between the middle ear and the inner ear. The ossicles amplify sound waves received by the tympanic membrane and transmit them through the membrane in the oval window to the fluid in the inner ear.

Also communicating with the middle ear is the *eustachian tube,* a channel that extends into the nasopharynx. The eustachian tube allows air into the middle ear, thus equalizing pressure on both sides of the eardrum. The middle ear communicates posteriorly with mastoid air cells. A portion of the facial nerve (controlling movement of the face) and also the chorda tympani

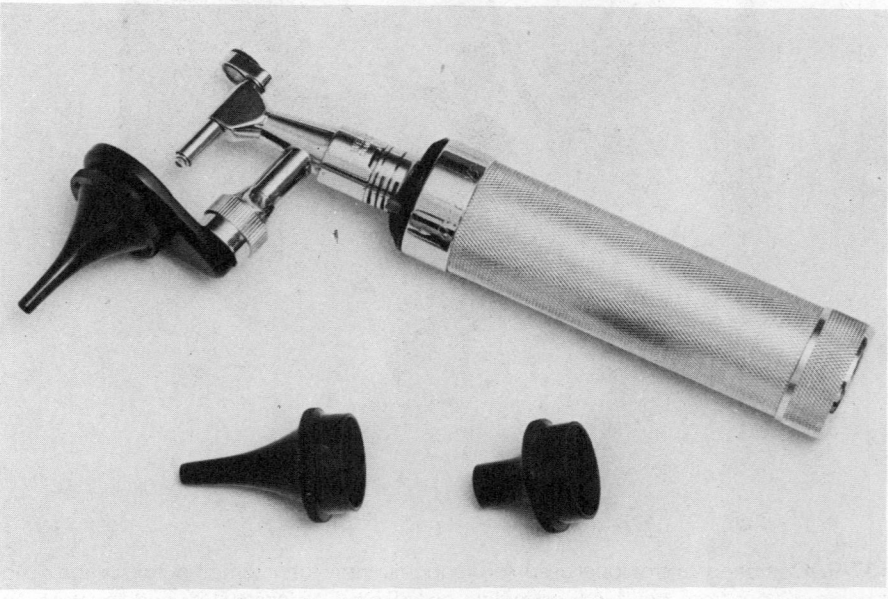

Fig. 37-8. Otoscope.

nerve (a branch of the facial nerve supplying taste to the anterior two thirds of the tongue) are located in the middle ear.

Physical assessment

The tympanic membrane is inspected by using the otoscope with the largest speculum that the ear will accommodate (Fig. 37-8). The tympanic membrane is positioned at a slant with the upper edge nearer the front; therefore care is needed when inserting the speculum so as not to push against the membrane. In addition, the skin of the ear canal becomes paper thin as it approaches the tympanic membrane; thus careless placement of the speculum too deeply in the canal may cause a laceration of that skin. Young children who have difficulty remaining still may have to be restrained for examination of the eardrum. An otoscope with a magnifying lens commonly is used to examine the ear. The ear may require examination under a binocular microscope, which provides depth perception as well as increased magnification (Fig. 37-9). Sometimes the view of the tympanic membrane may be obstructed by cerumen, which must be removed, and an ear irrigation (p. 874) may be necessary. *Pneumatic otoscopy*, in which air is compressed into the ear canal, exerting pressure against the drumhead, may be performed (Fig. 37-10). It is particularly useful in determining if the eardrum has normal mobility. Tympanic membrane retractions or perforations can also be evaluated by pneumatic pressure.

The eardrum is important in physical assessment of the middle ear because it serves as a translucent window through which disease processes in the middle ear may be inferred. The normal tympanic membrane has a wide range of colored hues, the most common being a pearly gray. Located in the membrane or seen through it are certain landmarks (Fig. 37-11). For descriptive purposes, the eardrum can be viewed as the face of a clock. Since the head divides the two ears, they must be pictured as mirror images; the right tympanic membrane will be oriented so that 3 o'clock is anterior (toward the nose) and 9 o'clock is posterior.

The *malleus* (the first of the ossicles) stands out like a tiny knot. The malleus is attached to the eardrum, with its direction going in a superior-inferior direction. It can be seen at about the 12 o'clock position and extends toward the 6 o'clock position. This inferior end of the malleus is called the *umbo*. For the right ear the portion of the drum between 12 and 9 o'clock (the posterior-superior quadrant) will have beneath it the *incus*, *stapes*, and *chorda tympani nerve*. Because the eardrum is translucent, these structures can often be seen if a brightly lighted otoscope is used. They will appear as shadows.

Under the portion of the drum between 9 and 6 o'clock (the posterior-inferior quadrant) is the *round window*, an opening into the inner ear that must be covered by an intact eardrum in order for normal hearing to occur. The portion between 12 and 6 o'clock usu-

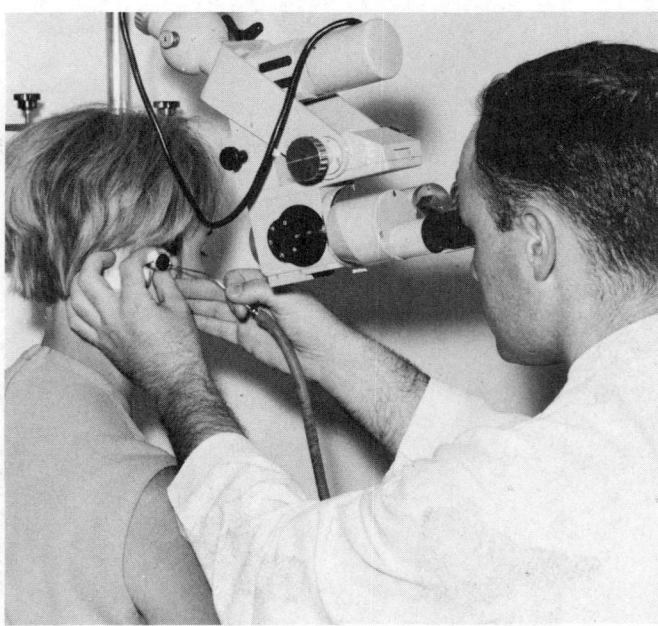

Fig. 37-9. Operating microscope used as diagnostic instrument. Small aural suction tip aspirates serum or pus from ear canal or middle ear. (From DeWeese, D.D., and Saunders, W.H.: Textbook of otolaryngology, ed. 6, St. Louis, 1982, The C.V. Mosby Co.)

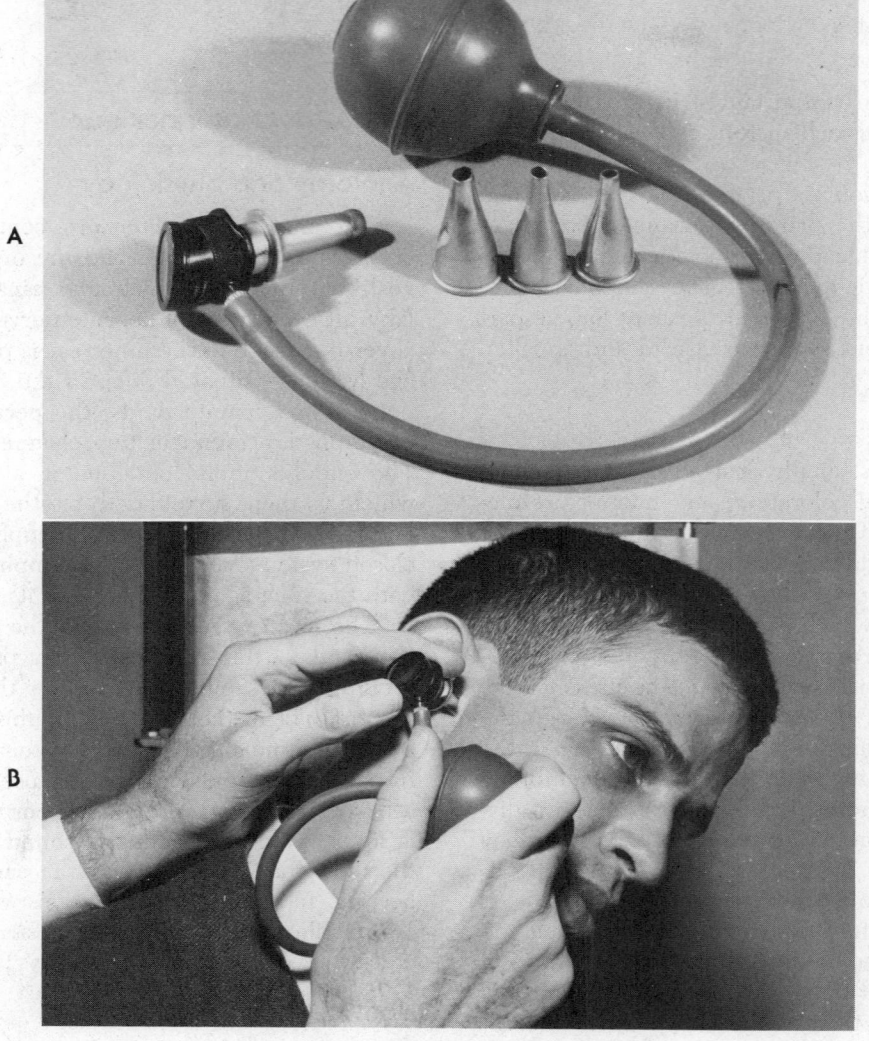

Fig. 37-10. A, Siegle pneumatic otoscope. Speculum that fits otoscope is attached. Magnifying lens also may be used with usual type of speculum if magnification only is desired. **B,** Pneumatic otoscope in use. (From DeWeese, D.D., and Saunders, W.H.: Textbook of otolaryngology, ed. 5, St. Louis, 1977, The C.V. Mosby Co.)

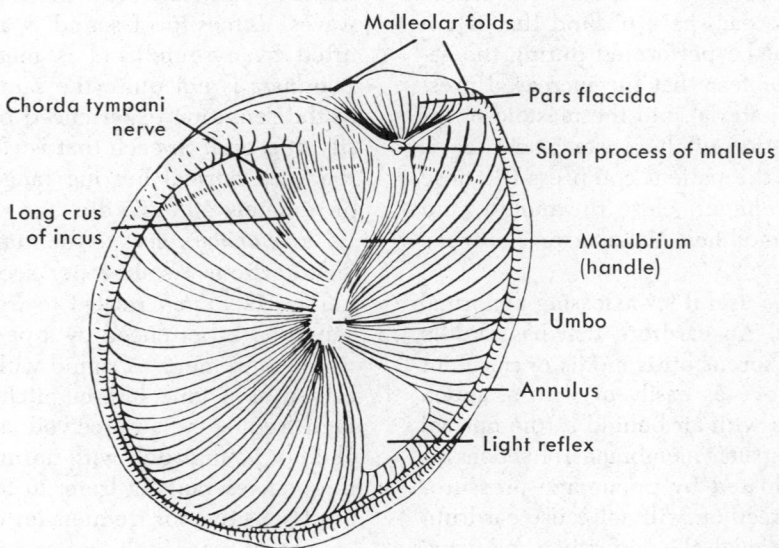

Fig. 37-11. Right tympanic membrane. (From Prior, J.A., and Silberstein, J.S.: Physical diagnosis: the history and examination of the patient, ed. 5, St. Louis, 1977, The C.V. Mosby Co.)

ally does not cover any important structures, although the opening to the eustachian tube is located between 1 and 2 o'clock.

The tympanic membrane is shaped like a cone and thus reflects light in the shape of a triangle. The triangular reflection is called the *light reflex* and is located in the anterior inferior quadrant. The tympanic membrane is stretched tight *(pars tensa)* except for the part superior to the malleus, which is flaccid and is called the *pars flaccida*.

Pathophysiology

Abnormal findings on physical assessment include inflammation, unusual coloration, and bulging, retraction, or perforation of the tympanic membrane. If the structures of the middle ear are seen very clearly when the eardrum is examined, (they usually look much like objects seen through waxed paper), this indicates an abnormality of the eardrum such as a retraction or perforation. Purulent material, such as might be present from acute otitis media (p. 904), may be seen through the thin membrane and may be white or amber. When the eardrum perforates, the fluid behind the membrane bursts out into the auditory canal and results in a discharge, which is examined for odor and color and may be cultured.

Mastoiditis may be a complication of otitis media. If the skin over the mastoid is edematous or inflamed and tender, mastoiditis should be suspected. Sensations of pressure, blockage, or pain with associated diminished hearing are signs of otitis media. Crackling in the ear may also be associated with otitis media, probably as the result of fluid in the middle ear. Insufflation of the eustachian tubes may or may not be performed during physical assessment of the middle ear. Insufflation of the middle ear space to test the patency of the eustachian tubes or to mechanically force them open can be used to clear the middle ear space of fluid that is not infected. This should not be performed during the active phase of infection for fear that the increased pressure will force infected material into the mastoid or intracranial space. Insufflation of the eustachian tube is accomplished by having the patient compress the nose with the thumb and forefinger, close the mouth, and blow both cheeks out (modified Valsalva or Politzer's maneuver).

Pneumatic otoscopy is useful for assessing abnormal mobility of the eardrum. An eardrum that has middle ear fluid behind it (as in serous otitis media or purulent otitis media) will not move as easily or with as much excursion as does a drum with air behind it (the normal condition). Similarly, tympanic membrane retractions or perforations can be evaluated by pneumatic pressure, the latter because the forced air will not cause eardrum movement as it escapes through the perforation and down the eustachian tube.

Assessment of inner ear

Anatomy and physiology

The inner ear, or *labyrinth*, contains both the organ of hearing, the cochlea, and the organ of balance, the vestibule and the semicircular canals (Fig. 37-7). The labyrinth, made up of delicate nerve tissue, will not recover if damaged. The inner ear is protected from damage by being situated deep in the head in the petrous bone. Two separate fluids, the perilymph and the endolymph, are found in tiny channels in the labyrinth. The endolymph is contained in a membranous tube, which is then surrounded by the perilymph, which cushions the tube. The endolymph is in a contained closed system, while the perilymphatic spaces connect with the subarachnoid space and its cerebrospinal fluid.

The end organ for hearing, the organ of Corti, has thousands of tiny "hair cells" that project from its neuroepithelium. Sound waves enter the cochlea and mechanically bend the hair cells. At this time sound, which had been a mechanical force, is converted into an electrochemical impulse. The impulse travels along the acoustic nerve to the temporal cortex of the brain and is interpreted as meaningful sound. The hair cells are the most fragile elements in the ear and are crucial to hearing. In some instances persons with normal hair cells are unable to hear because of destruction of the eighth cranial nerve by a tumor.

Normal hearing process

Functional examination of the inner ear may be better understood by a short review of the normal hearing process (Fig. 37-12). Sound is a form of energy generated by a vibrating source. Pure tones such as those generated by a tuning fork are simple sound waves. The human voice, however, produces more complex sound waves. *Intensity* of sound is actually the pressure exerted by a sound and is measured in decibels (db). *Loudness* is not quite the same as intensity but refers to the sensation experienced by a person to the intensity of sound. Speech that is comfortably loud to a person with normal hearing ranges in intensity from approximately 40 to 65 db.

Frequency refers to the number of sound waves emanating from a source per second and is expressed in hertz (Hz). *Pitch* relates to frequency and describes a sensation experienced by a person rather than a physical measurement. A sound with a low frequency is perceived as a tone low in pitch, whereas a sound with high frequency is perceived as a high-pitched tone. A child or young adult with normal hearing can often hear frequencies ranging from 20 to 20,000 Hz. Hearing is most sensitive for frequencies of 500 to 4000 Hz.

Sound reaches the inner ear by one of two ways: air conduction or bone conduction. Air conduction is the

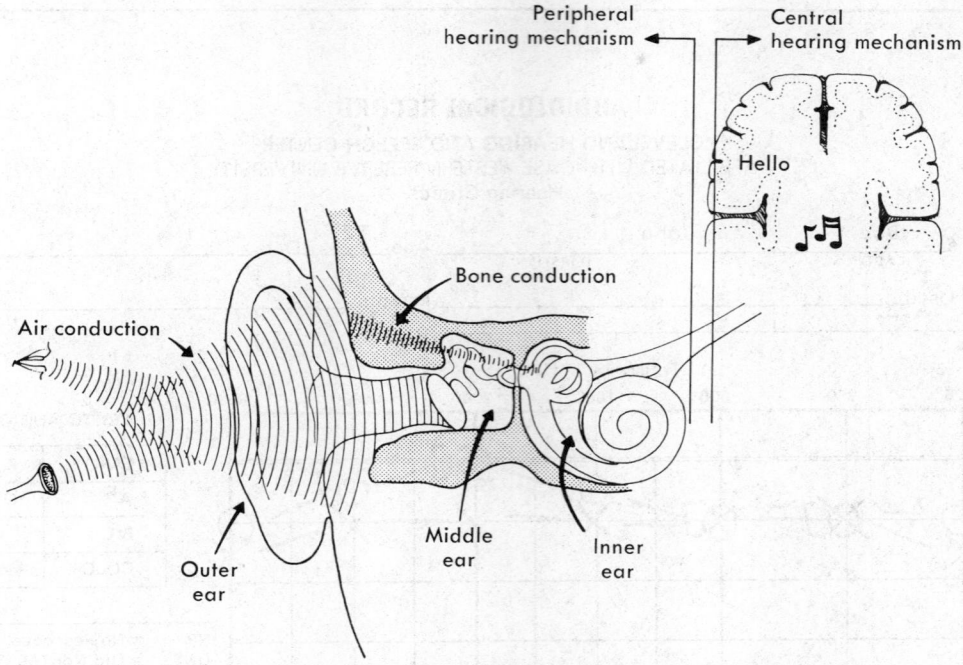

Fig. 37-12. Schema depicting functions of hearing mechanism as it translates sound waves into meaningful sensations. (From Saunders, W.H., et al.: Nursing care in eye, ear, nose, and throat disorders, ed. 4, St. Louis, 1979, The C.V. Mosby Co.)

more sensitive. In air conduction sound waves pass through the ear canal to the ossicular chain to the inner ear. In bone conduction hearing is caused by sound being transmitted through the bones of the skull to the inner ear. Sound energy is transformed in the inner ear into neural energy and is then "decoded" and interpreted by the brain as sound.

Testing

The inner ear cannot be examined visually. Functional examination is done by testing hearing by audiometry and by testing function of the semicircular canals by the caloric examination (p. 857) or electronystagmography (p. 856). Complete examination of the ear must include a hearing examination.

A child's acquisition of speech is critically dependent on proper hearing. It is imperative that if a hearing loss is suspected by the parent or health professional, the child be referred to an otologist for a medical examination and to an audiologist for proper testing. Until the child is 4 to 5 years of age, the child may be difficult to test by conventional methods. The cribogram, impedance audiometry, and brain stem evoked response audiometry can test infants for hearing potential.[1,11,14,22] In young children special testing procedures utilize rewards for correct responses and aid in conditioning the child to behave in an expected manner if the sound is heard. Audiology is presently at a very

sophisticated level and yields much information as to the child's hearing status, although definitive statements about hearing often cannot be made. All statements referring to hearing capabilities of very young children should be guarded and interpreted with care.[19] It should be remembered, however, that given the proper testing facilities and setting, it is possible for the audiologist to make a gross assessment of the hearing of a child or infant of any age. Proper management and counseling can only be initiated once hearing loss is suspected and the child is properly evaluated.

Audiometry. Functional examination for sensitivity (ability to hear sounds) and for speech discrimination (ability to distinguish different speech sounds) is done by audiometry. The graph of the hearing levels of both of these is called an audiogram (Fig. 37-13). *Hearing threshold* is defined as the lowest intensity of sound at which an auditory stimulus can be heard. Speech considered comfortably loud to a person with normal hearing ranges from 40 to 65 db. Fig. 37-14 lists the decibel level of various environmental sounds and situations.

In recent years audiologists (specialists in administering hearing tests) have developed audiometric tests to determine not only whether a hearing loss is present but also the frequency of the loss, how well the person can understand speech, and whether the problem site is in the middle ear (conductive loss), inner ear, or auditory nerve system (sensorineural loss). (See pp. 872

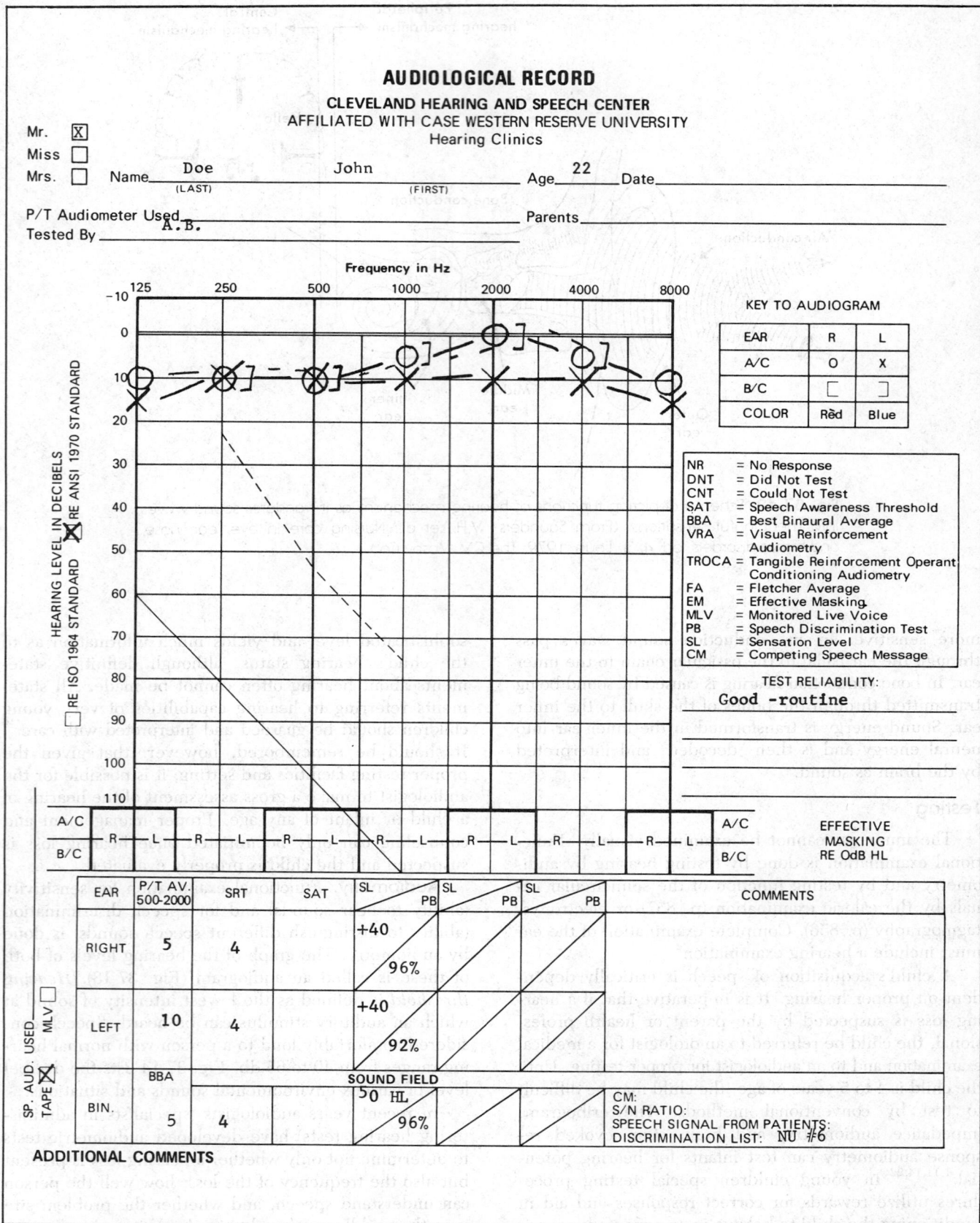

Fig. 37-13. Normal audiogram. (Courtesy Cleveland Hearing and Speech Center, Cleveland, Ohio.)

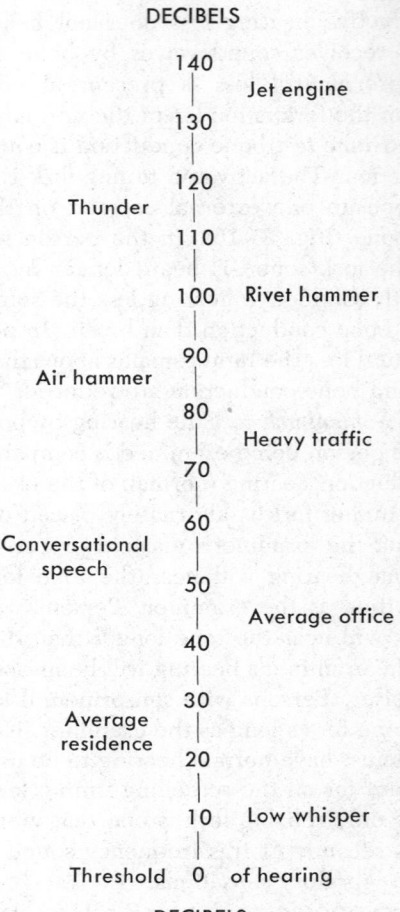

DECIBELS

140	Jet engine
130	
120	
	Thunder
110	
100	Rivet hammer
90	
	Air hammer
80	
	Heavy traffic
70	
60	
	Conversational speech
50	
	Average office
40	
30	
	Average residence
20	
10	Low whisper
Threshold 0 of hearing	

DECIBELS

Fig. 37-14. Intensity range of human hearing. Intensity levels of various environmental sounds and situations. (From Saunders, W.H., et al.: Nursing care in eye, ear, nose, and throat disorders, ed. 4, St. Louis, 1979, The C.V. Mosby Co.)

and 873 for further discussion of the types of hearing loss.) Pure tone audiometry must be performed in a specially constructed soundproof booth for best results. Group screening examinations such as are done in schools are only helpful in detecting children who need individual examinations.

To test the sound intensity by air conduction, persons wear earphones and are instructed to signal (usually with a finger) when they first hear the tone and when they no longer hear it. The middle frequencies are tested first, and the operator alternately increases and decreases the intensity of sound until the dial setting is found at which the person being tested can just perceive sound (threshold). In audiometric testing the frequencies 125, 250, 500, 1000, 2000, 4000 and 8000 Hz are commonly employed to assess the hearing sensitivity of an individual.

Hearing loss is identified as the number of decibels reached before the person hears the sound for each

specific frequency. Zero loudness is calibrated for that sound barely heard by a person with normal hearing. A range of 0- to 20-db loss for a tested frequency is considered to be within the normal range. Mild hearing loss ranges between 20 and 50 db; moderate loss, 50 to 69 db; severe loss, 70 to 89 db; and profound hearing loss, above 90 db. While the above decibel ranges for degree of deafness are generally accepted, in a practical way they are misleading. For instance, an individual with a hearing loss of 30 db, while considered to have a mild hearing loss, will have considerable difficulty in ordinary conversation and would be a candidate for a hearing aid.

Impedance audiometry is a technique that was developed because of the limitation of pure tone audiometry.[35] It provides a rapid and reliable means of assessing the presence or absence of abnormality of the conductive mechanism of the middle ear. It is an objective test in that it does not require a response from the individual and is therefore very valuable in assessing a child's hearing. The examinee sits with a headset on, and a mushroom-shaped plastic eartip is placed on a probe. This probe is inserted into the ear canal, an airtight seal is secured, and middle ear pressure measurements are obtained. The data consist of muscle reflex measurements in response to sound.

Speech audiometry is used to determine how well the person can hear and understand speech. There are two primary tests included in speech audiometry: the speech reception threshold (SRT) test and a speech discrimination test. The SRT is simply the lowest intensity level in decibels at which the person can correctly repeat specially selected bisyllabic words 50% of the time. Usually the SRT closely corresponds to the air conduction thresholds between the frequencies of 500 to 2000 cycles per second, the frequencies in which most human speech occurs. Speech discrimination tests require the person to repeat 50 monosyllabic words common to the English language. These words are usually presented at an intensity level easily heard by the person (25 to 40 db above the SRT). The number of correctly repeated words is converted to a percentage score. Individuals with normal hearing generally score 90% to 100% on this test.

Electrocochleography evoked response audiometry are also tests to assess hearing. EEG-type leads are attached, and clicks are played to the ear. Subsequent changes on the EEG recording are noted. In this way it can be determined if the central (brain) portion of hearing is intact or where the lesion interfering with the transmission of sound is anatomically located.

Tests for hearing acuity. Gross examination of hearing acuity may be made by assessing the person's ability to hear a whispered or spoken voice or to hear a ticking watch. The ticking of a watch normally produces high-pitched tones and may be useful in testing persons for high-frequency sounds. Since hearing loss is often insidious in onset, all adults entering the health care system should have at least a gross examination of hearing.

Tuning fork tests are useful in testing hearing acuity and especially for discriminating conductive and sensorineural hearing losses. In the *Weber test* a tuning fork is placed in the center of the forehead or on the maxillary incisors (Fig. 37-15). Normally the sound is heard equally in both ears. If a person has a *conductive* (middle ear) hearing loss, the hearing is *better* in the *affected* ear. This happens because the ordinary room noise tends to mask hearing in the normal ear; the ear

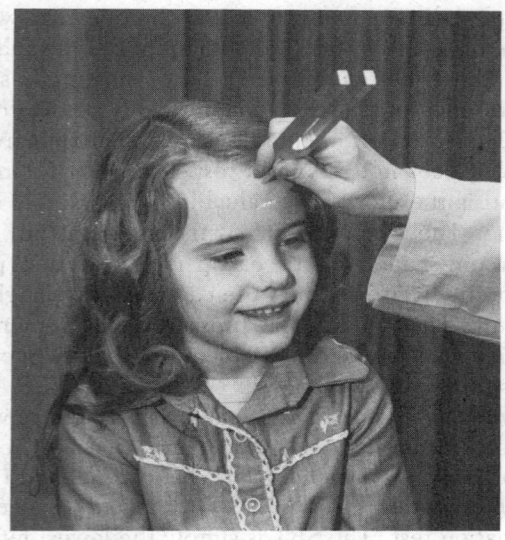

Fig. 37-15. Weber test. (From Malasanos, L., et al.: Health assessment, ed. 2, St. Louis, 1981, The C.V. Mosby Co.)

with conductive hearing loss does not hear the room noise but receives sound waves by bone conduction. When *sensorineural* loss is present in one ear, the sound from the fork is louder in the *normal* ear.[43,44]

In the *Rinne test* bone conduction is compared with air conduction. The activated tuning fork is alternately placed opposite one external ear and on the adjacent mastoid bone (Fig. 37-16). In the person with normal hearing the fork sound is heard longer by air than by bone. With conductive hearing loss the sound is heard longer by bone conduction than by air. In persons with sensorineural loss the ratio remains about the same, but both air and bone conduction are reduced.[43]

In the *Schwabach test* the hearing by bone conduction of the person being examined is compared with the bone conduction hearing (normal) of the examiner. The activated tuning fork is alternately placed on the individual's and the examiner's mastoid processes. Persons with normal hearing will hear the tone for the same length of time as the examiner. Persons with conductive losses will hear the tone longer than the examiner because the examiner's hearing will be masked by background noises. Persons with sensorineural loss will not hear the tone for as long as the examiner. Naturally the examiner must have normal hearing to be used as a reference point for all the screening tuning fork examinations. The only reliable fork is one that vibrates at 512 cycles per second. At this frequency sound is not confused with vibratory sensations.

Electronystagmography. Electronystagmography (ENG) is a test used to measure nystagmus, an abnormal rhythmic jerking of the eyes often associated with inner ear dysfunction and vertigo. ENG records the po-

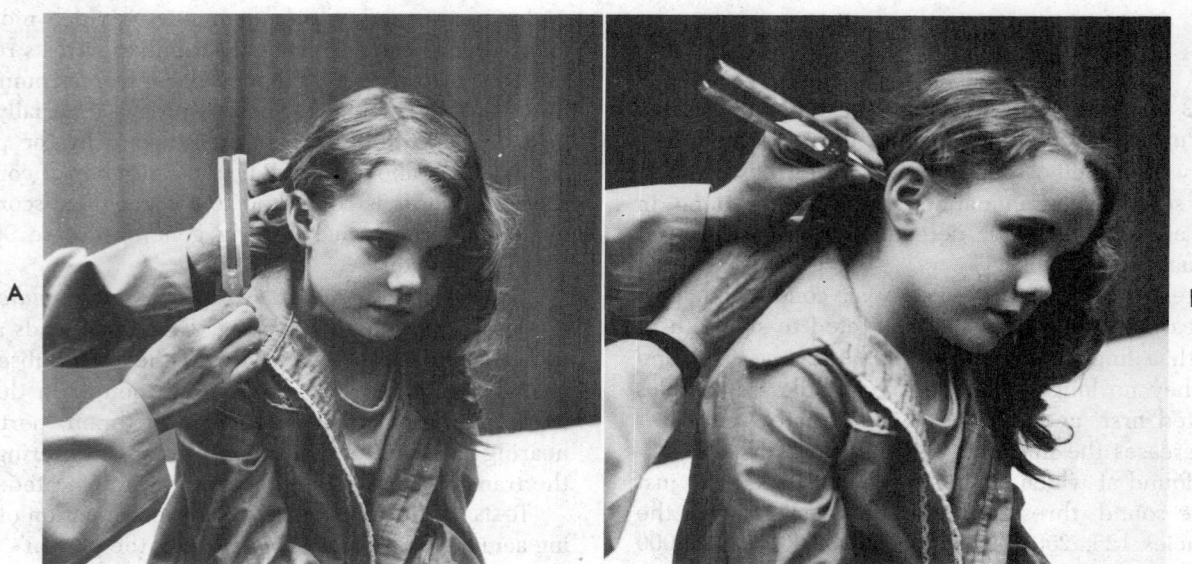

Fig. 37-16. Rinne test. **A,** Air conduction. **B,** Bone conduction. (From Malasanos, L., et al.: Health assessment, ed. 2, St. Louis, 1981, The C.V. Mosby Co.)

sition and movement of the eyeball by recording the changes in the electrical field around the eye when there is a change in position of the eye (Fig. 37-17). A graph can be made of the amplitude, direction, and speed of nystagmus. ENG is useful in diagnosing vestibular disease and is an important test in evaluating persons with symptoms of vertigo, hearing loss, or tinnitus.

Both spontaneous nystagmus and induced nystagmus can be tested. Nystagmus occurs in normal persons after stimulation of the active vestibular labyrinth with cold or warm water (caloric test). In the caloric examination cold or warm water or air is irrigated into the external auditory canal. As the labyrinth is stimulated, the person starts to become dizzy and an induced nystagmus occurs. If stimulation is excessive, some persons may vomit. To lessen the likelihood of this unpleasant sequela, the length of exposure to the thermal stimulation is designed to provide the diagnostic nystagmus without vomiting. Usually a water irrigation of 25 seconds, an air irrigation of 1 minute, or an irrigating temperature of only a few degrees above or below body temperature will accomplish this. With water the temperatures of 30° C and 44° C are used. In cases of no response, ice water irrigations may be used to determine if any labyrinthine function is present.

Diseases of the vestibular system can usually be detected by abnormal caloric responses, that is, hyperactivity or no reaction at all.[3,34,41] Different head positions can also cause dizziness, and the type of nystagmus that occurs during these measures may give an indication as to whether the disease process is occurring in the inner ear or in the brain.

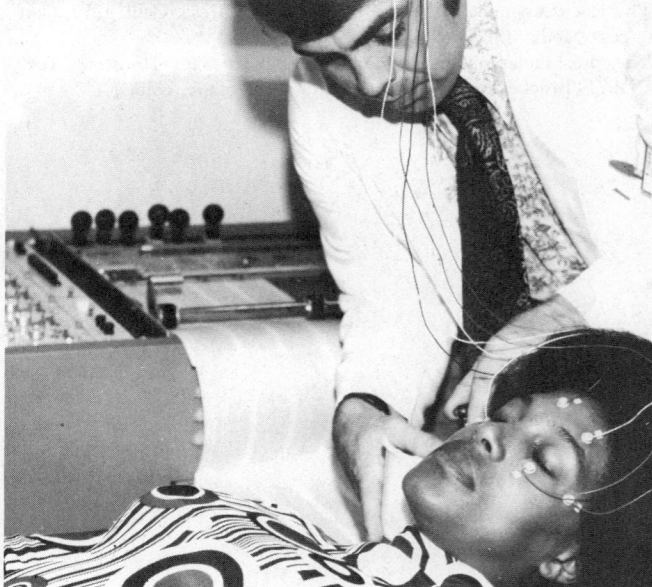

Fig. 37-17. Electronystagmography. Patient undergoing caloric stimulation as nystagmus is recorded on graph. (From Saunders, W.H., et al.: Nursing Care of eye, ear, nose, and throat disorders, ed. 4, St. Louis, 1979, The C.V. Mosby Co.)

REFERENCES AND SELECTED READINGS

1. Adams, R.M.: The ultimate hearing test: evoked response audiometry, J. Sch. Health **49:**536-537, 1979.
2. *Bates, B.: A guide to physical examination, ed. 2, Philadelphia, 1979, J.B. Lippincott Co.
3. Belal, A., Jr., and Linthicum, F.H. Jr.: Pathologic correlates of electronystagmographic tracings, Am. J. Otolaryngol. **1:**213-223, 1980.
4. Bergstrom, L., et al.: A high risk registry to find congenital deafness, Otolaryngol. Clin. North Am. **4:**369-379, 1971.
5. *Boyd, M.H.: Examining the external eye. I, Nurs. '80 **10**(5):58-63, 1980.
6. *Boyd, M.H.: Examining the external eye. II, Nurs. '80 **10**(6):58-63, 1980.
7. *Boyd, M.H.: Screening for glaucoma, Nurs. '79 **9**(8):42-25, 1979.
8. Buckingham, R.A., et al.: Correlation between micro-otoscopy, micropneumatoscopy and otoadmittance tympanometry, Laryngoscope **90:**1297-1304, 1980.
9. Cass, R.: Middle ear disease and learning problems: a school system's approach to early detection, J. Sch. Health **49:**557-560, 1979.
10. Cooper, J.C.: The audiovestibular test battery for vertigo, Ear Nose Throat J. **59**(9):347-353, 1980.
11. Dieroff, H.G.: Efficiency of subjective audiometry in children up to the third year of age, Audiology **19:**94-100, 1980.
12. Egan, J.J.: Audiology: defining hearing impairment, Ear Nose Throat J. **59**(3):6-7, 1980.
13. Finitzo-Hieber, T., et al.: A sound effects recognition test for the pediatric audiological evaluation, Ear Hear. **1**(5):271-276, 1980.
14. Galambos, R., and Despland, P.A.: The auditory brainstem response (ABR) evaluates risk factors for hearing loss in the newborn, Pediatr. Res. **14**(2):159-163, 1980.
15. Galloway, N.R.: Ophthalmic electrodiagnosis, Philadelphia, 1975, W.B. Saunders Co.
16. *Hammond, E.A., and Besley, P.K.: Screening for glaucoma: a comparison of ophthalmoscopy and tonometry, Nurs. Res. **28**(6):371-372, 1979.
17. Hatfield, E.M.: Methods and standards for screening preschool children, Sight Sav. Rev. **49:**71-83, 1979.
18. *Heinlein, D.: The nurse's role in helping to assess learning disabilities in the school setting, Sight Sav. Rev. **50:**25-29, 1980.
19. Hersch, L.B., and Amon, C.: A child has a hearing loss: reporting the diagnosis of handicaps in children and its impact on parents, Am. Ann. Deaf **120:**568-571, 1975.
20. *How to test your patient's hearing acuity, Nurs. '80 **10**(7):60-61, 1980.
21. Jerger, J.: Modern developments in audiology, New York, 1975, Academic Press, Inc.
22. Jerger, J., Hayes, D., and Jordan, C.: Clinical experience with auditory brainstem response audiometry in pediatric assessment, Ear Hear. **1:**19-25, 1980.
23. Jones, M., et al.: Assessment of the red eye, Nurse Pract. **5:**10-12, 1980.
24. Judge, R.D., and Zuidema, G.D.: Methods of clinical examination: a physiologic approach, Boston, 1974, Little, Brown & Co.

*References preceded by an asterisk are particularly well suited for student reading.

25. Kimmelman, C., and Potsic, W.P.: Electric response audiometry in pediatric otolaryngology, Trans. Pa. Acad. Ophthalmol. Otolaryngol. **33:**194-199, 1980.

26. Latham, A.D.: A pilot study to detect hearing impairment in the young, Midwife Health Visit Community Nurse **16:**370-374, 1980.

27. *Lum, S.B., et al.: Reappraising newborn eye care, Am. J. Nurs. **80:**1602-1603, 1980.

28. *Malasanos, L., et al.: Health assessment, ed. 2, St. Louis, 1981, The C.V. Mosby Co.

29. McNeer, K.W., et al.: Pediatric ophthalmology: detecting visual problems in children, Pediat. Nurs **5**(suppl.):B-G, 1979.

30. *Mechner, F., and Saffiati, L.J.: Patient assessment: examination of the eye, Am. J. Nurs. **74:**2039-2068, 1974.

31. Moller, A.: Basic mechanisms in hearing, New York, 1973, Academic Press, Inc.

32. Musiek, F.E., and Geurkink, N.A.: Auditory perceptual problems in children: considerations for the otolaryngologist and audiologist, Laryngoscope **90:**962-971, 1980.

33. Newell, F.: Ophthalmology: principles and concepts, ed. 5, St. Louis, 1982, The C.V. Mosby Co.

34. Norris, T.W.: Electronystagmography, New York, 1974, Medcom Press.

35. Northern, J.L.: Impedance screening, an integral part of hearing screening, Ann. Otol. Rhinol. Laryngol. **89:**233-235, 1980.

36. Osterhammel, K.: High-frequency audiometry and noise-induced hearing loss, Scand. Audiol. **8**(2):85-90, 1979.

37. Poland, R.M., Well, D.H., and Ferlauto, J.J.: Methods for detecting hearing impairment in infancy, Pediatr. Ann. **9:**31-32, 1980.

38. Programmed instruction: Patient assessment: examination of the ear, Am. J. Nurs. **75:**457-476, 1975.

39. Programmed instruction: Patient assessment: examination of the eye, II, Am. J. Nurs. **75:**105-129, 1975.

40. Programmed instruction: Patient assessment: examination of the eye. I, Am. J. Nurs. **74:**2038-2062, 1974.

41. Rubin, W.: Electronystagmography and its value in the diagnosis of vertigo. In Wolfson, R.J., editor: The otolaryngologic clinics of North America. Symposium on vertigo, Philadelphia, 1973, W.B. Saunders Co.

42. *Sana, J.M., and Jedge, R.D.: Physical appraisal methods in nursing practice, Boston, 1975, Little, Brown & Co.

43. Saunders, W.H., et al.: Nursing care in eye, ear, nose, and throat disorders, ed. 4, St. Louis, 1979, The C.V. Mosby Co.

44. Stankeiwicz, J.A., and Mowry, H.J.: Clinical accuracy of tuning fork tests, Laryngoscope **89:**1956-1963, 1979.

45. Symposium on sensorineural hearing loss in children: early detection and intervention, Otolaryngol. Clin. North Am. **8**(1):1-249, 1975.

46. Tos, M., and Poulsen, G.: Screening typanometry in infants and two-year old children, Ann. Otol. Rhinol. Laryngol. **89:**217-222, 1980.

47. Vargo, S.W.: Auditory screening in the schools: failure or success? J. Sch. Health **50:**32-34, 1980.

48. Weinstock, F.J.: Tonometry screening, Am. J. Nurs. **73:**656-657, 1973.

49. *Wolfsberger, J.: Precious eyesight, Nurs. Times **77**(4):158-161, 1981.

50. Younger, J.: Pediatric ophthalmology: detecting visual problems in children, Pediat. Nurs. **5**(6):E-G, 1979.

AUDIOVISUAL RESOURCES

Anatomy of the human eye series, 1972, Teaching Films. (Super 8 mm film, 15 min each, sound, color.)

Child development: testing hearing in the preschool child, Washington, D.C., 1970, National Medical Audiovisual Center. (Film, 16 mm, color.)

The ear, San Antonio, Tex., 1971, Department of Anatomy, University of Texas Medical School. (Videotape, 20 min, color.)

The ears, Washington, D.C., 1970, National Medical Audiovisual Center. (Film, 16 mm, color.)

Ear and hearing examination, Ann Arbor, Mich., 1976, University of Michigan School of Nursing, Medical Center Media Library. (Videotape, 14 min.)

Ears, Spring Valley, N.Y., 1973, Department of Nursing, Herbert Lehman College, City University of New York, Blue Hill Educational Systems. (Videorecording, 60 min.)

Impedance audiometry in otologic evaluation, Rochester, Minn., 1976, American Academy of Ophthalmology and Otolaryngology. (Videocassette, 57 min.)

Physical assessment of the eye and ear, Costa Mesa, Calif, 1977, Concept Media. (Slide-tape.)

The otorhinolaryngologic examination, Fort Sam Houston, Tex., 1971, Brooke Army Medical Center. (Videotape, color.)

CHAPTER 38

INTERVENTIONS FOR THE PERSON WITH SPECIAL SENSORY PROBLEMS: EYE AND EAR

LYNN CHENOWETH
LINDA ANNE BROSEMAN

The general public and some health professionals may feel frustrated in their attempts to interact with persons having severe vision or hearing problems. Persons with sensory impairments are often viewed as being difficult to deal with, socially unacceptable, and generally to be avoided. Reactions of persons with normal vision and hearing to persons with sensory impairments can include embarrassment, helplessness, hostility, and general discomfort. Nurses can help co-workers and the general public become more informed about the nature of vision and hearing problems and can demonstrate ways in which to relate to persons with sensory disabilities.

Impact of sensory loss

The loss of a sense, whether it is hearing or sight, should be viewed in terms of a multiple handicap. In general, a loss or a severe impairment of a sense can cause disequilibrium in a person's feelings of psychologic security. There may be a decrease in self-confidence, self-concept, or feelings of well-being. The physical integrity of the person has been breached, and confidence in the adequacy of the remaining senses may diminish. Some environmental stimuli are no longer perceived or are perceived differently.

Communication with others is also affected. If one cannot hear conversation or see others with whom one interacts, the desire or ability to retain contacts with others is impaired and the person may experience a feeling of isolation. Depending on the age at which the handicap occurs, written or spoken communication can be severely compromised. As mentioned previously, esthetic enjoyment of that which is pleasurable or beautiful is diminished and the ability to share the human experience is decreased.

Loss or impairment of one of the senses may affect a person's activity. Mobility or ability to carry out activities of daily living may be restricted or at least modified. The ability or opportunity to carry out usual sexual roles or activities may also be affected. Career options, job opportunities, and financial security may be decreased. A sensory loss may influence the person's ability to remain independent, to feel socially adequate, or to feel that one is an esteemed contributing member of society.

Coping with sensory loss

Persons with sensory handicaps experience varying degrees of stress, isolation, and behavioral changes depending on the extent and duration of the handicap, the age at which the handicap occurs, and how the person has successfully coped with stressors in the past. Other factors that influence the ability to cope include the support systems available to the person and the extent to which the handicap affects financial security and the ability to meet societal and familial role expectations.

Over a period of time persons with sensory losses appear to be able to compensate for their deficits by an increase in sensitivity in the other senses. For example, some people who are blind compensate for their deficit by increasing auditory acuity, tactile acuity, sense of smell, or kinesthetic awareness. People who are deaf tend to become keen observers.

Intervention for the person with impaired vision and eye problems

Vision, one of a person's most priceless possessions, is essential to most employment and necessary in countless experiences that make life enjoyable and meaningful. Yet in the United States there are an estimated 1 million legally blind persons. Approximately 1.5 million Americans are so visually handicapped that they cannot read ordinary newsprint even with the aid of corrective lenses. In underdeveloped countries of the world there is a high incidence of blindness from preventable causes such as malnutrition and eye infections. Although there has been a reduction of blindness in the United States from infections and certain diseases and injuries, there has been an increase in blindness resulting from diseases that occur most frequently among older persons. These include diabetic retinopathy, glaucoma, cataract, and retinal degeneration (see Chapter 39). It is likely that the incidence of blindness will increase in the future because of the steady growth in the number of persons aged 65 and older.

Implications of impaired vision

Vision enables persons to experience pleasure and safety in the world about them. Of all the senses, the capacity to see is the most highly developed, critically needed, and cherished. In an opinion poll, Americans indicated that they fear blindness more than any other physical problem with the exception of cancer.

Persons with severe vision impairment or blindness have difficulty meeting basic human needs such as security, self-esteem, safety, nutrition, and activity. Impaired vision interferes with learning, communication, mobility, and enjoyment of the environment.

Definition of impaired vision

Vision impairment ranges from refractive errors correctable with lenses to total blindness in which the per-

son may not even be able to perceive light. For legal purposes blindness is defined very precisely in order to determine eligibility for assistance of various kinds. Although many nonseeing persons now prefer to be called *visually handicapped,* the term *blindness* is still in common usage. See box below for the legal criteria of blindness.

Adjusting to impaired vision

The physician who is certain that blindness will occur or is irreversible will usually consider it best to be completely honest with the person and family. When a person has been told that blindness will result, there is a normal reaction described by psychiatrists as a period of mourning for the "dead" eyes. Grief and mourning over the loss of vision cause emotional reactions such as denial, anger, guilt, resentment, loneliness, and depression. These strong emotional feelings interfere with the blind person's ability to plan for new ways of living. It is the responsibility of the nurse working with other members of the health team to help the individual and family adjust to the condition of blindness or severe vision impairment.

Nurses can listen to the person talk of what blindness means to him or her; they can observe exaggerated reactions that might indicate thoughts of self-destruction; they can direct the person's thinking gradually along positive, constructive lines; and they can help to make available the resources that will be needed.

Children who have never known sight adjust well and are happy provided that they are treated as normal and are neither overprotected nor rejected. It is chiefly the parents who must adjust to and accept the child's handicap and be willing to use the resources available in the community to enable the child to develop independence and to face problems of living. Both the parents and the child need special consultation and training in order to achieve this end.

It is important for the health worker to provide ex-

LEGAL CRITERIA OF BLINDNESS*

A person is considered legally blind when either of the following conditions exists:

1. Visual field no greater than 20 degrees.

2. Central distance vision in better eye is 20/200 or worse with use of corrective lenses. This means the person can see at 20 ft what the person with normal vision can see at 200 ft.

*Report of the National Advisory Eye Council, U.S. Department of Health, Education and Welfare, no. (NIH) 75-664, 1975.

planations and support to family members also, so that the family can provide the help and acceptance needed by the blind person.

Prevention

Because nurses have contact with persons in all age groups and stages of development, they have the opportunity to be involved in many aspects of health care for the eye. These aspects include health education, care of the healthy eye, safety measures, and eye examination.

Health education in care of eyes

The nurse can explain the complex structure of the eye, teach people to care for their eyesight, and direct them to the proper specialist. A nurse also should recognize signs suggestive of eye disease and teach them to others (Table 38-1). Knowledge of ophthalmic drugs, first aid for eye trauma, corrective lenses, eye patching, surgical procedures, and other modalities of assessment and treatment should be understood by the nurse. Nursing activities regarding protection of sight are outlined as follows and are described in succeeding paragraphs:

1. Protection of sight from impairment or further impairment:
    a. Teaching and providing safety measures and first aid
    b. Promoting regular eye examination by an eye specialist
    c. Detecting evidence of disease or impaired acuity

TABLE 38-1. Symptoms suggestive of eye disease

Symptom	Eye disease
Conjunctival redness	Conjunctivitis, blepharitis, sty
Crusting discharge	Conjunctivitis, blepharitis, sty
Ocular pain	Foreign body, sty, acute lid infection, glaucoma, keratitis, uveitis
Foreign body sensation	Foreign body, corneal erosion, blepharitis, chronic conjunctivitis
Blepharospasm	Keratitis, corneal ulcer
Multiple spots ("floaters")	Retinal detachment, intraocular hemorrhage, diabetic retinopathy
Photophobia	Uveitis, keratitis, glaucoma, corneal abrasions
Vision changes	
Blurred vision	Refractive error, cataract, glaucoma, uveitis, retinal detachment
Double vision	Strabismus
Halos around lights	Glaucoma
Blind spots	Hemorrhage, choroiditis
Sudden vision loss	Central retinal artery or vein occlusion

d. Explaining and administering treatments used to improve sight or prevent further loss (e.g., medications, surgery, and eye patching)

2. Adjustment of the individual to impaired vision
    a. Identifying basic human needs that have been affected
    b. Understanding the effects on adaptation of different degrees of impairment (e.g., whether one or both eyes affected, partial or complete loss, and acquired or congenital loss)
    c. Assisting the newly blinded person through stages of psychologic adaptation to blindness
    d. Assisting persons to cope with unmet needs for physical and emotional security, socialization, enhancement of self-esteem, and role identification
    e. Using available community resources to help persons with impaired vision to cope more successfully (e.g., hospital, Lion's Club, school facilities, and National Society for the Prevention of Blindness)

Care of healthy eyes

Normal healthy eyes do not need special local treatment. The secretions of the conjunctiva are protective and should not be removed by frequent bathing with unprescribed solutions. Boric acid solution and numerous trade preparations recommended to cleanse the eyes are usually unnecessary. Although these preparations are generally harmless, some proprietary solutions contain substances that may cause allergic reactions in sensitive persons.

People frequently treat eye ailments with proprietary remedies or with eyedrops and other medication that they or others have used at some time in the past. Self-treatment of the eyes is not only dangerous but may also lead to loss of much valuable time for treatment. There are many disorders that can affect the eyes for which many different drugs are used, each of which has a specific purpose. Two drugs may have completely opposite effects. Since liquids evaporate and drugs deteriorate or become contaminated with bacteria or fungus, use of preparations that a person or friends have on hand can contribute to actual damage.

Boric acid solution, like other ophthalmic solutions, may present the problem of drug crystals precipitating on the tip of the dropper and then irritating the eye. Preparations containing phenylephrine hydrochloride, 0.8%, have been reported to produce sufficient mydriasis (dilation of pupil) to cause an attack of narrow-angle glaucoma in susceptible persons.[97] Contamination of ophthalmic solutions may also be a problem. It is best to *discard* any ophthalmic solution that is cloudy, is discolored, has been opened for 3 months, or contains particles.

Many people believe erroneously that eyestrain causes permanent eye damage. Eyestrain actually refers to strain of the ciliary muscles when there is difficulty in accommodation. It causes a sense of fatigue but does not produce serious damage to the eyes. To avoid eyestrain, a good light should be used when reading and doing work that requires careful visual focus, and extremely fine work should not be done for long periods of time without giving the eye muscles periodic rest. Looking at distant objects for a few minutes helps to rest the eyes after close work.

Care should be taken not to irritate the eyes or introduce bacteria into the eyes by rubbing them. Rubbing the eyes may be a natural response of many persons who are nervous, are fatigued, or wear contact lenses. It also may be the result of eczematous scaling, infection of the lids, or occasionally loose attachment on the lashes. The cause of severe or chronic irritation should be investigated.

While adequate nutrition is as important for eye health as it is for maintaining other body functions, persons with nutritionally caused eye disorders are rarely found in the United States. Vitamin deficiencies can cause night blindness (vitamin A), corneal damage (vitamin A), optic neuritis (vitamin B), and other disorders. Although a sufficient vitamin intake is necessary, an excessive amount is wasted and may actually do more harm than good. For example, too much vitamin A can damage the optic nerve.[41] Some elderly persons and teenagers eat a diet consisting mainly of carbohydrates, which does not supply the protein, vitamins, and minerals needed for body growth and cell replacement. When assessing a person's nutritional status the nurse can learn if the person needs some assistance in meeting the need for adequate quantity and quality of nutrients (p. 1345).

Safety measures

Prevention of accidental injury to the eyes should be stressed in child and parent education. Slingshots, BB guns, and even seemingly harmless rubber bands and paper wads can be dangerous. The nurse can help physical education teachers and others to be alert to hazards to the eyes in gymnasiums and on playgrounds.

Protective goggles and break-resistant corrective lenses are available for persons engaging in very active physical exertion such as sports and selected occupations (see section on lenses, p. 863). The eyes should be protected by goggles or special dark glasses from prolonged exposure to very bright light such as sunlight over snow. They also need special protection from sudden flashes of light and heat that occur in some industrial occupations. There is no evidence that prolonged watching of television will damage eyesight.

First aid measures necessary in the event of eye injury should be known by everyone; these measures can be taught in schools and in industry (p. 886). The sight of many persons could be saved each year if everyone

understood the need for immediate copious flushing of the eye with water when an acid, alkali, or other irritating substance has been accidentally introduced. Much damage is done by the layperson's well-intentioned efforts to remove foreign bodies from the eye and by not obeying the important rule of always washing the hands before attempting to examine the eye or to remove a foreign object.

It is essential to know that a person who has a foreign object lodged on the cornea must be referred to a physician; the layperson should never attempt to remove it. The eye should be closed to prevent further irritation and the lids loosely covered with a dressing or patch anchored with a piece of transparent or adhesive tape. The person is advised not to squeeze the eye and is taken to an ophthalmologist at once.

Regular eye examinations

The eyes should be examined by an ophthalmologist at regular intervals throughout life. Many authorities believe children should have their eyes examined at birth, at age 3 or 4 years, at approximately age 10, and in early adolescence. The young adult should consult an ophthalmologist at least every 5 years. After the age of 40 years, the lens become firmer and less resilient (presbyopia). Because presbyopia causes blurring of close vision, the individual holds printed material farther away. As presbyopia progresses, it becomes increasingly difficult to perform fine work or read small print without the aid of corrective lenses. Medical specialists recommend an eye examination every 2 years after the age of 35.

Since the eyes are often profoundly affected by conditions within the rest of the body, they cannot be considered alone. In fact, nearly all diseases cause some eye changes that are diagnostically important. The nurse who is teaching eye health must be aware of *total health*. When apparently minor disease or abnormality of the eyes occurs, the nurse must be particularly alert for other signs of illness. Many serious medical conditions, such as diabetes, renal disease, neurologic disease, and generalized arteriosclerosis, may be diagnosed through early recognition of eye symptoms and examination of the eyes by an ophthalmologist.

There is widespread confusion and misunderstanding on the part of the public as to the proper specialist to consult about visual problems (see box, p. 863). People who demand the best care when other medical and surgical problems arise may fail to seek help from an ophthalmologist when they have eye difficulties. The optometrist does not treat eye diseases but assesses vision and prescribes corrective lenses or exercises. The ophthalmologist is a physician and surgeon who can diagnose and treat diseases of the eye.

In their search for help some people may purchase glasses from stores or use glasses originally prescribed

PERSONS WHO SPECIALIZE IN EYE PROBLEMS OR IN VISUAL PROSTHESES

Ophthalmologist	Physician who specializes in the diagnosis and treatment of eye diseases; may also prescribe lenses
Oculist	Same as ophthalmologist
Optometrist	Professional person with special preparation in assessment of vision and in treatment of visual problems (e.g., prescribes lenses, visual training, or orthoptic exercises); is not a physician and does not treat eye diseases
Optician	Person who grinds and fits lenses according to prescriptions written by ophthalmologist or optometrist

for friends or relatives. Nurses can explain that eye conditions cannot always be remedied simply by the purchase of a pair of glasses or a change of lenses. A serious disease process, such as glaucoma or cataract formation could be the cause of the problem.

Lenses

Eyeglasses. Acceptance of glasses seems to be influenced by the improvement in vision that they afford, the personality of the wearer, and the current fashion trends. To some persons, however, glasses may appear as a cosmetic blemish. Because there may be some stigma attached to wearing glasses, the young child will have a period of adjustment after receiving glasses. Acceptance of glasses increases when children start school and realize that the glasses are needed for seeing the blackboard. The vogue for attractive frames makes the wearing of glasses more acceptable to teenagers and adults. All persons should be encouraged to wear their glasses as prescribed and to have periodic examination of their eyes by an ophthalmologist or an optometrist. Instructions for persons who wear glasses include how to clean their glasses, how to protect them from being scratched or broken, and how to care for them when they are removed.

Federal law now requires that all prescription glasses be made with impact-resistant lenses. Each finished lens must pass an impact test before it is dispensed. *Plastic* lenses weigh less than half of equivalent glass lenses but cost more and scratch more easily. They are useful for persons who wear thick lenses that are heavy when made of glass and for those who are active in sports. *Hardened* lenses have been exposed to a tempering process that makes them extremely hard and resistant to impact and breakage. *Safety* lenses are similar to hardened

lenses but are 1 mm thicker. They are used in goggles worn by workers whose eyes may be injured by such articles as chips of metal or glass.

Bifocal lenses consists of an upper portion of one focus used for distance and a lower part of another focus used for reading and close work. They make constant changing from distance to reading glasses unnecessary. *Trifocal* lenses are divided into three focuses to give correction for distance, intermediate, and near vision. *Sunglasses* should be carefully ground, large enough to exclude bright light around their edges, and dark enough to excluse about 30% of the light. The amount of light filtered can be varied according to the needs of the person.

Contact lenses. Contact lenses are thin shells of transparent, ground plastic designed to be worn over the cornea (microlenses) or the cornea and sclera (scleral type) to replace eyeglasses. Although expensive, they may be used by persons who engage in sports because they do not fog or break easily, or they may be worn for cosmetic reasons. They are sometimes prescribed for persons who have a cone-shaped deformity of the cornea (keratoconus), which may prevent satisfactory fitting with conventional glasses. Elderly persons who have lenses removed because of cataracts achieve better vision through wearing contact lenses than with the use of glasses. Some industrial occupations prohibit the use of contact lenses because of irritation of the cornea from dirt or dust, which can become trapped under the lens.

Persons interested in wearing contact lenses are encouraged to consult an ophthalmologist who will make recommendations regarding their use. The person who dispenses the contact lenses may be an ophthalmologist, optometrist, or technician supervised by the former. Hard, or hydrophobic, lenses are usually tinted, cover the cornea, and are the most frequently used type of contact lens. Soft, or hydrophilic, lenses are flexible when in contact with the cornea and have been used successfully by many persons who cannot tolerate hard lenses. Soft lenses must constantly be kept wet to prevent irreparable damage. The disadvantages of soft lenses include a higher initial cost and need for more frequent replacement. They also are more difficult to clean and maintain. Newer types of lenses that have the optical qualities of the hard lens and the comfort of the soft lens are being explored. Scleral lenses are much larger than the other types and are less frequently used.

Contact lenses are inserted after being cleaned thoroughly and immersed in a wetting agent such as methylcellulose. Conjunctival secretions provide the lubrication needed for the lenses to be worn in comfort. The lenses are held in place by capillary attraction and by the upper lid. Although some people wear the lenses continuously, a few can never physiologically or psychologically tolerate the presence of a foreign object in the eye, even for a short time. Contact lenses should not remain in the eyes for long periods of time, because the epithelium of the cornea can be damaged through lack of oxygen.[34]

If the patient is badly injured or unconscious, the nurse removes the contact lenses (see box below). The lenses are stored separately in suitable containers such as capped test tubes filled with sterile normal saline.

REMOVAL OF CONTACT LENSES

Hard lens
Method 1:
   a. Place finger at outer canthus of eye.
   b. Pull skin obliquely upward, then straight down.
   c. Lens will appear on lower lashes as the upper lid moves downward.
   d. If lens moves off center, reposition it by gentle pressure on lid or lens itself.

Method 2:
   a. Place finger or thumb of each hand at base of eyelashes (upper and lower).
   b. Bring eyelids together, trapping the lens (the lens will eject).
   c. If lens moves off center, reposition it by gentle pressure on lid or lens itself.

Method 3:
   a. Using eye irrigation set, gently flush eye with sterile normal saline.
   b. Retrieve lens in curved basin.

Method 4:
   a. Use small suction device shaped like a miniature "plumber's helper."
   b. Place over center of lens and pull lens off gently.

Soft lens
   a. Pull up upper lid with one thumb.
   b. Be sure lens is in place before attempting removal.
   c. Move lens over conjunctiva before grasping it, if possible. If lens does not move freely, put several drops of sterile saline in eye, close lid, and wait 1 min before trying again.
   d. Grasp lens with thumb and forefinger of other hand and lift.

Scleral lens
   a. Spread eyelids with both thumbs.
   b. Exert slight downward pressure on upper lid (the lower edge of the lens will lift above the lid margin).
   c. Slide thumbs to outer canthus to eject lens.

Soft contact lenses must be kept wet at all times; drying causes the soft lens to deteriorate. If a soft lens does dry, add sterile saline to soften it before handling. Label the lens storage containers with the patient's name and whether it is the right or left lens. Place the containers in a safe location and record this in the appropriate record.

Environment

People who have loss of vision in both eyes depend on sound and tactile sensation to maintain a feeling of security and kinship with those around them. They must be spoken to frequently in a quiet and reassuring voice. This is particularly important when they are in a strange hospital environment and awaiting diagnostic procedures and perhaps surgery. It is upsetting for the person who cannot see to be touched without first being addressed; such an occurrence can be irritating and humiliating, as well as actually dangerous. The nurse teaches all persons who attend the patient the importance of making their nearness known before touching. They should introduce themselves and explain why they are there. On leaving the room they should inform the person to prevent the embarrassment of talking to someone who is not there. A small bell often is given to patients with visual loss instead of a call signal. It gives the patients who can hear the assurance that their request has been made. The person who is also deaf presents another problem. If one cannot direct conversation into an ear and have it heard, there is no alternative but to touch the person gently to make one's presence known. If contact with the environment is to be retained, frequent physical contact must be made. Elderly persons who use hearing aids are urged to bring them to the hospital.

Most persons with eye conditions are more comfortable when the lighting is dimmed. Screens or curtains can be arranged so that bright light does not enter the room. Bright artificial lighting should be shaded. The patient in the hospital is usually happiest in a room with other patients, especially if both eyes are covered or if vision is lost. The sound of voices and normal activity tends to relieve the feeling of isolation that the blind person experiences. Some patients may prefer to be alone. Radios help the patient to keep up with everyday events. Recordings of entire books are also available.

Accidents present a real hazard when eye disease occurs, especially if an eye is covered or there is loss of vision. It is estimated that 20% of the field of vision is lost if one eye is covered or removed. If the onset of visual loss is slow, the person and his or her family may have sufficient time to alter common household hazards such as adding banisters to stairs. The partially blinded person who receives care on an ambulatory basis is taught to have someone accompany him to the physician's office or clinic because additional help may be needed for a short time after certain treatments. In the hospital, special measures to prevent accidents are necessary. Side rails may be used, but low beds are safer, particularly for older patients who may forget that they are in a hospital bed. Particular effort should be made to have the space around the patient's bed and chair uncluttered. Furniture should be firmly anchored with casters locked. Rails along hallways and in bathrooms are also helpful.

Life for the person who has both eyes covered should be made as normal as possible. Smoking may be permitted, although someone must be in attendance to prevent a fire. Visitors sometimes need assistance in learning how to conduct themselves when they are with the patient who cannot see. They should be as natural as possible. For example, they should not make a conspicuous attempt to avoid such common phrases in speech as "see what I mean." Common sense dictates that gifts should appeal to other senses than vision. Scented colognes and soaps or a small bouquet of highly scented favorite flowers may be brought if the patient is not allergic to these items.

Interventions

Medications

Accuracy in the administration of medications and treatments is essential. Irreparable damage can follow instillation of unprescribed or deteriorated preparations into the eyes. All medication bottles must be checked frequently for smearing or obliteration of labels. Solutions that have changed in color, that are cloudy, that contain sediment, or whose expiration date has passed are never used. Eye medications in the home are discarded when the course of the treatment is completed. The nurse must know the usual dosage and strength of medications being used as well as signs of toxicity. For example, osmotic agents that reduce intraocular pressure by increasing plasma osmolarity are contraindicated in patients with poor kidney function. Steroids may cause an exacerbation of an already existing herpes corneal ulcer or increase the intraocular pressure.[111] Children and elderly persons are particularly susceptible to side effects of medications.

Ophthalmic drugs. A large variety of drugs are used for treatment of eye diseases (Tables 38-2 and 38-3). Most of the drugs are applied as drops, irrigations, or ointments.

Mydriatics are drugs that dilate the pupil. Mydriasis is necessary for thorough examination of the back of the interior of the eye (fundus). An example is phenylephrine (Neo-Synephrine).

Cycloplegics are drugs that not only dilate the pupil but also block accommodation by paralyzing the ciliary muscles. These drugs are used to keep the pupil dilated as part of the treatment for diseases of the cornea and for inflammatory diseases of the iris and ciliary body, after certain operations, and for eye examination. Commonly used cycloplegics are cyclopentolate (Cyclogyl), tropicamide (Mydriacyl), and atropine. Cycloplegic and mydriatic drugs should not be instilled in the eyes of a person with glaucoma, because this prevents drainage of the aqueous humor, thus increasing intraocular pressure to levels where eye damage can occur.

Miotics are drugs that contract the pupil, permitting the aqueous humor to flow out more readily and thus reduce intraocular pressure. Miotics such as pilocarpine are the drugs most often used in the treatment of glaucoma. *Osmotic agents* may also be used to reduce intraocular pressure. These drugs, for example, urea and mannitol, are given intravenously in the treatment of acute glaucoma or to reduce intraocular pressure during eye surgery.

Secretory inhibitors decrease intraocular pressure by reducing aqueous humor production. Drugs in this classification inactivate the enzyme carbonic anhydrase, which is necessary for the production of aqueous humor. These drugs are given orally and include acetazolamide (Diamox).

Local *topical anesthetics* such as tetracaine (Pontocaine) are used frequently for treatments and operations on the eye. Epinephrine (Adrenalin), 1:50,000 or 1:100,000, may be used in combination with local anesthetics to prolong the duration of anesthetics by constricting blood vessels so that the drug remains longer in the injected area and its absorption is delayed. Hyaluronidase (Wydase), which makes cell membranes more permeable, often is mixed with local anesthetic solutions to increase the diffusion of the anesthetic through the tissues.

Ophthalmologists may employ uncommonly used *antibiotics* such as bacitracin, polymyxin B, gentamicin, and neomycin for ocular instillation because bacteria are less likely to be resistant to them. Because penicillin causes ocular allergy in about 5% of adult patients, it is not often used.[19]

If the patient is being treated for an active infection, individual medicine bottles, droppers, tubes of ointment, and other equipment are mandatory. This precaution is also necessary when an infected eye is being treated with an antibacterial drug such as bacitracin and the same medication is ordered prophylactically for the other eye.

A *lubricant* such as methylcellulose may be used for dryness of the cornea and conjunctiva caused by deficiency in production of tears or faulty lid closure as a result of nerve involvement or unconsciousness.

Antiinflammatory drugs such as prednisone, cortisone, and hydrocortisone as drops and in ointment, 0.1% to 2.5%, are used to control inflammatory and allergic reactions postoperatively as well as for a variety of con-

TABLE 38-2. Mydriatic and cycloplegic drugs

Drug	Form and concentrations	Duration of effect
Mydriatic action		
Phenylephrine (Neo-synephrine)	Eyedrops, 1-10%	12 hr
Epinephrine (Epitrate)	Eyedrops, 1-2%	12 hr
Cycloplegic and mydriatic action		
Atropine sulfate (Atropisol, Isopto-Atropine)	Eyedrops, 0.5-1%	2-4 wk
	Ointment 1%	
Cyclopentolate (Cyclogyl)	Eyedrops, 0.5-2%	24 hr (cycloplegic)
		2-3 days (mydriasis)
Homatropine (Isopto-Homatropine)	Eyedrops, 0.5-5%	1-2 days
Scopolamine hydrobromide	Eyedrops, 0.25-0.5%	1-2 days
Tropicamide (Mydriacyl)	Eyedrops, 0.5-1%	2-8 hr

TABLE 38-3. Other ophthalmic drugs

Drug	Form	Dose
Antibiotics and antiviral drugs		
Polymyxin B, bacitracin (Polysporin)	Ointment or eyedrops, 0.1-0.5%	As directed
Polymyxin B, neomycin, bacitracin (Neosporin)	Ointment	As directed
Bacitracin	Ointment, 500-1000 units/g	200-400 units/kg
Idoxuridine (IDU)	Eyedrops, 0.1% solution	As directed
	Ointment, 0.5%	
Gentamicin sulfate (Garamycin)	Eyedrops, 3% solution	2-4 drops q 6 hr
Chloramphenicol (Chloromycetin, Chloroptic)	Oral, IV, subconjunctival	50 mg/kg
Steroids		
Prednisone	Topical, 0.25-0.5% suspension	As directed
	Oral, 5-15 mg	1 tablet q 6 hr
Prednisolone	Topical ointment, 0.1-0.25%	As directed
	Oral, 5-15 mg	1 tablet q 6 hr
Methylprednisolone (Depo-Medrol)	Subconjunctival, 0.5 mg	q 2-4 wk
Triamcinolone (Aristocort)	Solution or ointment, 1%, subconjunctival	Lasts 4-6 wk
Dexamethasone (Decadron)	Solution, 0.1%	As directed
	Injection, 20 mg	
Fluorometholone	Eyedrops, 0.1% solution	As directed
Anesthetics		
Proparacaine (Ophthaine, Ophthetic, Alcaine)	Eyedrops, 0.5% solution	1 drop
Lidocaine (Xylocaine)	Local infiltration, 2-4% solution	4 ml
Lubricants and tear substitutes		
Methylcellulose, gonioscopic	Eyedrops, 1% solution	As needed
Methylcellulose	Eyedrops, 0.1% solution	As needed

ditions involving the eyelids, the conjunctiva, and the cornea. Steroids also may be given systemically for the treatment of acute or subacute infections such as those of the iris and choroid.

Astringents such as zinc sulfate preparations are often useful in treating chronic conjunctivitis. The *dye* fluorescein is used to stain and thereby outline superficial injuries and infections of the external globe of the eye, to check for proper fit of contact lenses, and for applanation tonometry. Strips of filter paper impregnated with the dry dye are used in place of prepared solutions because the solution is easily contaminated by *Pseudomona aeruginosa*.[35]

Systemic effects. Drugs applied topically to the eye can be absorbed and may cause systemic side effects. Systemic reactions may occur when anticholinergic drugs are instilled into the eye to produce mydriasis. Atropine is the anticholinergic drug that most frequently causes systemic reactions. Signs and symptoms of systemic atropine toxicity include flushing, dryness of mouth and skin, fever, rash, tachycardia, and confusion, but rarely progression to coma and death.

Topically instilled miotic drugs can also cause unwanted systemic effects, most frequently with the long-acting anticholinesterase drugs such as echothiophate. Signs and symptoms include hypersalivation, sweating, gastrointestinal tract disturbances, decrease in heart rate and blood pressure, and bronchoconstriction. These drugs should be used with caution in patients with intestinal obstruction or bronchial asthma.

To avoid undesired systemic reactions, care should be taken with topically applied medications to give exactly what is ordered and no more. It may also be helpful to apply pressure at the inner canthus after instillation to minimize drainage into the nose and throat.

Instillation of medications. *Solutions* such as eyedrops are the most commonly used preparations in the local treatment of eye disease. Advantages of solutions are that they (1) are easily instilled, (2) do not interfere with vision, (3) cause few skin reactions, and (4) do not interfere with the mitosis of the corneal epithelium. The major disadvantage of eyedrops is that they do not remain in contact with the eye very long.

Approximately 90% of aqueous solutions are eliminated from the eye within the first minute of application. It is sometimes necessary therefore to instill the solution at frequent intervals to achieve therapeutic results.

Eyedrops and eyedroppers must be sterile. Each patient should have his or her own bottle of medication. If the bottle is small, it may be warmed slightly by holding it in the hands for a few moments. Blunt-edged eyedroppers are available and may be used for children. The dropper is held downward so that medication does not flow into the rubber bulb, since foreign material from the bulb can contaminate the solution. Most eyedrops are packaged in small plastic bottles with a dropper attached.

If crusting or discharge is present, the eye is cleaned before instillation of medication. When eyedrops are instilled, the patient is asked to tilt the head back and look toward the ceiling. The lower lid is pulled gently outward, and the dropper should approach the patient's eye from the side and not directly from the front (Fig. 38-1, *A*). Drops are placed on the lower conjunctiva. Care must be taken not to touch the eyelids, the con-

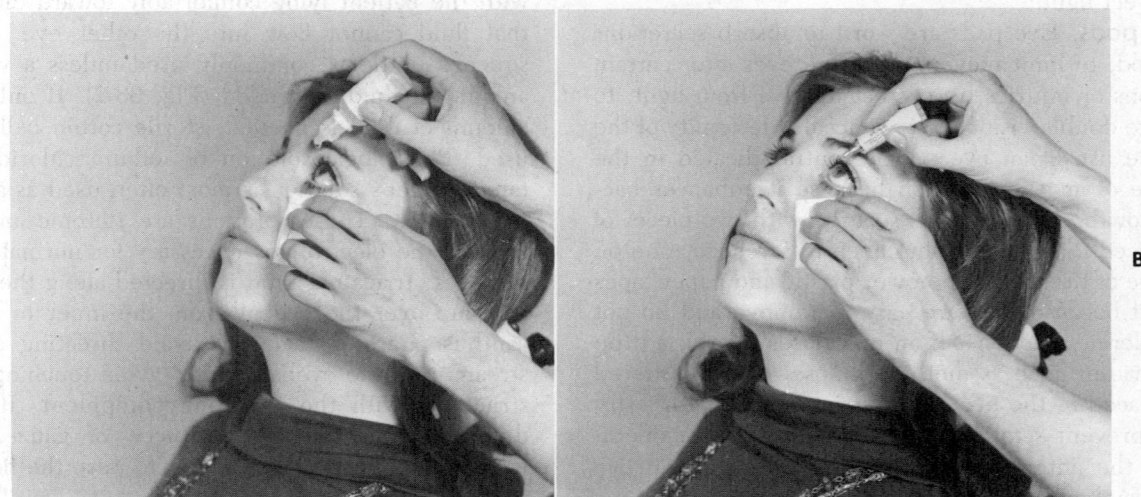

Fig. 38-1. To instill ophthalmic solution **(A)** or ointment **(B)** tilt patient's head backward supported by chairback or headrest. Use absorbent tissue pad under forefinger to depress lower lid to form conjunctival sac. Introduce medication into sac, never directly at or into eye. (Courtesy Eye and Ear Infirmary, University of Illinois Hospitals, Chicago.)

junctiva, or the eyeball with the dropper. The eyelids should then be closed. The person should be reminded not to squeeze the eye shut since this causes the medication to escape. Absorbent tissue or cotton held against the cheek will prevent the drops from running down the cheek.

Ointments remain in contact with the eye much longer, providing a prolonged effect. They usually do not cause discomfort when instilled. There is less absorption into lacrimal passages than with eyedrops. Ointments, particularly those containing antibiotics, are more stable than solutions. Disadvantages of ointments are that they (1) produce a film in front of the eye, which may obstruct vision, (2) cause contact dermatitis reaction more frequently, and (3) may inhibit mitosis of the corneal epithelial cells.

To instill ointment, the nurse asks the person to tilt the head back and to look toward the ceiling. The lower lid is gently pulled down, and the ointment is expressed directly onto the exposed conjunctiva from a small, individual tube (Fig. 38-1, *B*). Care is taken not to touch the tissues with the tube.

Treatments

Gentleness is extremely important in performing all treatments. The natural sensitivity of the eye and the reluctance of normal persons to have anything done to their eyes are increased by pain, discomfort, and fear. Nature's powers of repair may be retarded by trauma resulting from pressure on the irritated or inflamed tissues. *Hands must be washed thoroughly before giving any eye treatment*, and all materials placed in the eyes must be sterile.

Good lighting is necessary when giving treatments, but care must be taken to protect the patient's eyes from direct light.

Eye pads. Eye pads are worn to absorb secretions and blood, to limit movement of the eyes after certain operations or injuries, to protect the eye from light, to eliminate double vision, or to conceal a deformity of the eye. The use of an eye pad is contraindicated in the presence of an eye infection because it enhances bacterial growth. An eye pad is secured with two pieces of tape placed diagonally from cheek to forehead, one on each side of the pad. The newer plastic and paper tapes are used because they are easy to remove and do not cause allergic reactions. If an eye closes poorly, a drop of a lubricant such as methylcellulose may be ordered to be placed in the eye before it is covered with a dry pad to prevent scratching the cornea. After an operation on the anterior portion of the eye, a metal eye shield may be worn over the dressing to protect the eye from injury until it heals.

Compresses. Warm moist compresses are used in the treatment of surface infections of the cornea, conjunctiva, or eyelid and after many types of eye surgery

to help relieve pain, promote healing, and help cleanse the eye, which is normally cleansed by tears. Compresses may be sterile or unsterile, depending on the eye condition, and should be large enough to cover the entire orbit. If both eyes are involved and the condition is infectious, separate trays must be prepared and the hands carefully washed between treatment of each eye. The temperature of the solution used for compresses should not be over 49° C (120° F), and the treatment usually lasts for 10 to 20 minutes and is repeated hourly or several times a day. Great care must be taken not to exert pressure on the eyeball when applying compresses. If there is evidence of irritation of the skin about the eyes from the hot water, a small amount of sterile petrolatum can be used, but it should not be allowed to enter the eyes. Moist heat may be applied to the eye by using a clean washcloth soaked in hot water and squeezed free of excess moisture. When the cloth cools, the process is repeated.

Cold moist saline compresses may be ordered to help control bleeding immediately following eye injury, to prevent or control edema in allergic conditions, and to control severe itching. A small basin of sterile solution may be placed in a bowl of chipped ice at the bedside. Sterile forceps are used to wring out and apply the compress. If the compress does not need to be sterile, a washcloth or compress may be placed on pieces of ice in a basin at the patient's bedside. A rubber glove or small plastic bag packed with finely chipped ice may be applied to the eye and necessitates fewer changes of compresses. A piece of plastic material loosely filled and secured with a rubber band is effective also.

Eye irrigations. Eye irrigations are used to remove secretions, foreign bodies, and chemical irritants and to cleanse the eye preoperatively. Irrigations are done with the patient lying comfortably toward one side so that fluid cannot flow into the other eye. A plastic squeeze bottle is commonly used unless a very large amount of fluid is needed (Fig. 38-2). If only a small amount of fluid is needed, sterile cotton balls may be used. Physiologic solution of sodium chloride or lactated Ringer's solution is most often used as an irrigating solution. These solutions are isotonic and do not remove the electrolytes necessary for normal action of the eyes. Irrigating fluid is directed along the conjunctiva and over the eyeball from the inner to the outer canthus. Care is taken to avoid directing a forceful stream onto the eyeball and to avoid touching any eye structures with the irrigating equipment. If there is drainage from the eye, a piece of gauze may be wrapped about the index finger to raise the lid and ensure thorough cleansing.

Surgical management

Preoperative care. Routines for preoperative treatment and care vary with the institution and the eye

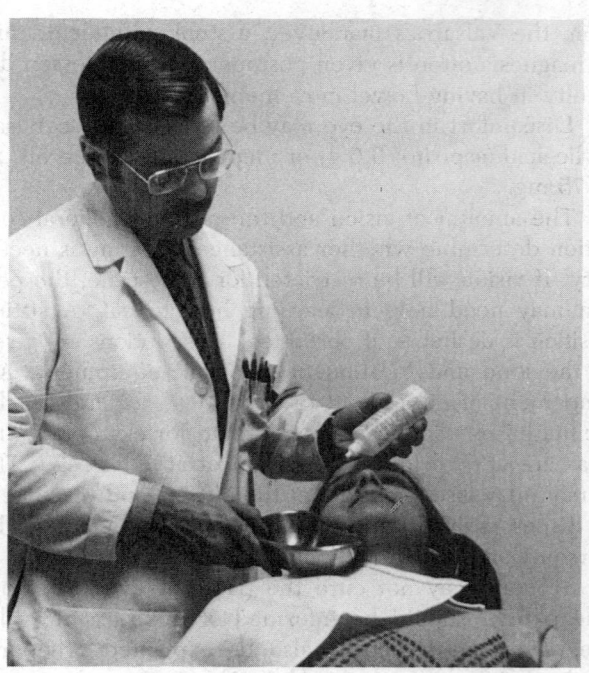

Fig. 38-2. When irrigating eye, ophthalmologist directs fluid along conjunctiva and over eyeball from inner to outer canthus.

surgeon. The patient's general condition and reaction to the anticipated surgery are assessed on hospital admission. If both eyes are to be patched following surgery, patients are introduced to all persons who will be interacting with them postoperatively. While it is unusual for both eyes to be covered at once, patients need to be prepared if this is to occur, and orientation to the immediate surroundings is necessary. Children should practice having their eyes covered so that they will not be too frightened or restless postoperatively. If possible, a parent should be permitted to remain with the child both day and night.

The preparation of the eye on the day of surgery may include the instillation of a combination of drugs such as atropine sulfate, 1%, cyclopentolate (Cyclogyl), 1%, and phenylephrine (Neo-Synephrine), 10%, into the eye at various intervals to dilate the pupil. The medications *must* be given at the prescribed times so that the eye is prepared at the time of surgery. If anesthetizing drops are instilled before the patient goes to the operating room, the patient is asked to close the eye, and a pad is applied to protect the insensitive eye from injury caused by rubbing, dryness, or dirt and dust. If only one eye is to be operated on, a mark may be placed on the forehead over that eye so that it can be identified easily in the operating room. It is vital to carefully check the patient's record so that the surgeon knows which eye is to be operated on.

If a local anesthetic is to be used, chloral hydrate,

pentobarbital sodium (Nembutal), or meperidine hydrochloride (Demerol) may be given preoperatively. Atropine sulfate may be included if a general anesthetic is to be administered. When possible, general anesthesia is avoided because the patient may be restless on reacting and disturb the eye dressing. The strain of vomiting after general anesthesia may cause tension on the suture line. Children, however, require general anesthesia and must be supervised closely until they have recovered fully from its effects.

If the eyelashes are cut, the surgeon uses straight, sharp scissors with fairly short blades that have been lubricated with petrolatum to help prevent the cut lashes from entering the eye. If local anesthesia is being used, additional anesthetic drugs such as lidocaine (Xylocaine), 2%, may be injected into the operative area.

Postoperative care. Specific routines for postoperative care following eye surgery vary and change rapidly as new techniques are developed. However, general goals of postoperative care are to *prevent* (1) increased intraocular pressure, (2) stress on the suture line, (3) hemorrhage into the anterior chamber, and (4) infection. A few general principles of postoperative care are included here.

Immediately after the operation, the patient must keep the head still and try to avoid coughing, vomiting, sneezing, or moving suddenly. The patient is positioned on the unoperated side to prevent pressure on the operated eye and to prevent possible contamination of the dressing with vomitus. The patient may turn from the back to the unoperated side but may not lie on the stomach or on the operated side.

Postoperative confusion is a problem, particularly in elderly persons and in persons who have had both eyes covered. If confusion does occur, the surgeon may decide that the danger of activity caused by confusion is worse than activity resulting from having one eye uncovered. For this reason few surgeons cover the unoperated eye.

Side rails are placed on the bed immediately postoperatively and are kept on while both eyes are covered, if the patient cannot see, or as long as necessary for protection. If both eyes are covered, it is *essential* that the call light be easily available to the patient. The bedside table is placed on the side of the *unoperated* eye to prevent turning to the operated side.

Care should be taken that the *dressing* is not loosened or removed. An unreliable patient needs constant attention. Restraints may occasionally need to be applied if the patient does not understand or cannot cooperate and if it is not possible to have constant attention. If the dressings are removed, they are replaced and the surgeon is notified. It is usual for some bleeding and serous drainage to occur, but these should be minimal. The lid is edematous, but this condition subsides with 3 or 4 days. Mild pain and pressure can be normal in the postoperative course. However, sensation of pressure within the eye may suggest hemorrhage; sharp pain may suggest infection or hemorrhage. These symptoms are quickly reported to the surgeon.

Postoperative *ambulation* depends on the type of operation, the general condition of the patient, and the surgeon's preference. The patient may be up on the first postoperative day or may be in bed 5 or 6 days after surgery. Whatever the regimen, supervision and assistance are given by the nurse to be sure that the patient is able to walk without sustaining injury. Patients who have both eyes covered should be assisted to their destinations (Fig. 38-3). They should be informed of obstacles in their path, alerted when to turn before the turn appears, and told when to move to *their* right or left. To avoid falls, the patient should not sit down until locating both arms of the chair with the hands. Bending, stooping, or lifting objects should be avoided for several weeks after the operation to prevent increasing intraocular pressure that might nullify the surgery. Slippers or shoes that do not need tying or buckling are preferable during this time.

Because increased intraocular pressure may result

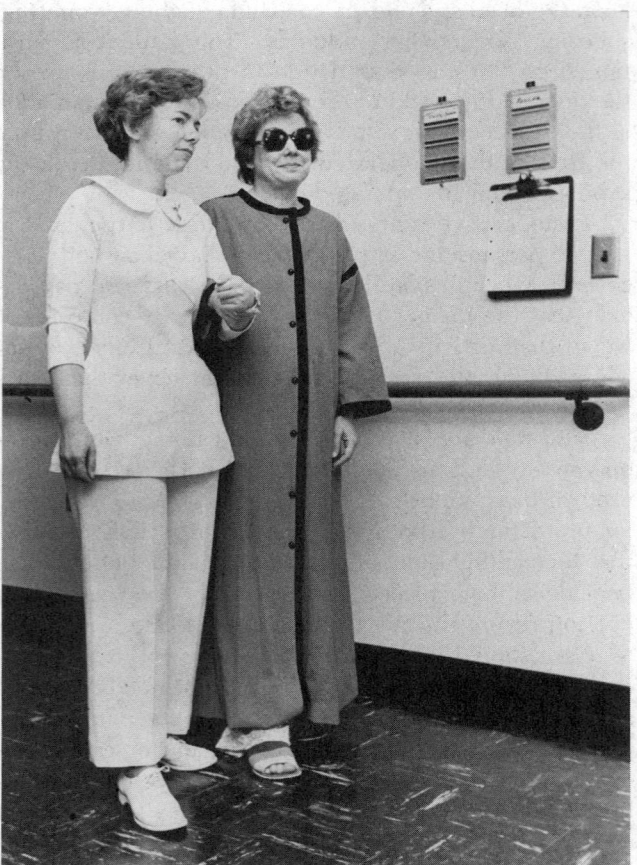

Fig. 38-3. Ambulation of patient who cannot see. Note that patient holds nurse's arm and is led without being held.

from the Valsalva's maneuver, a stool softener or milk of magnesia often is given postoperatively to lessen difficulty in having bowel movements.

Discomfort in the eye may be relieved by acetylsalicylic acid (aspirin), 0.6 g, or meperidine (Demerol), 25 to 75 mg.

The amount of vision and the person's general condition determine whether assistance in eating is necessary. If vision will be restricted for some time, the person may need help in learning how to eat. A sitting position is desirable, if permitted. Descriptions are given of the kind and location of food and equipment. Arrangement of equipment or of food on a plate can be facilitated by using the clock format; for example, "The peas are at 7 o'clock, and the meat at 1 o'clock." The person may also wish to feel the outline and placement of dishes. Privacy during eating is provided until the person learns to handle food in a normal way.

Surgery may not cure the patient's eye condition. The patient should be informed of this possibility by the physician. It should also be explained preoperatively that it may take weeks and even months to become accustomed to the type of glasses to be worn after surgery.

Outcome criteria for the person having eye surgery

1. The person does not sustain injury to eye or self during hospitalization.
2. The person is as independent as possible in activities of daily living.
3. The person or significant others can:
   a. State precautions necessary after surgery.
   b. State the dosage, method of administration, and side effects of medications to be taken at home.
   c. State how to use special lenses or eyeglasses as prescribed.
   d. Describe the rationale for and demonstrate actions that prevent increased intraocular pressure.
   e. Describe symptoms requiring medical attention and the need for medical follow-up.

Community services

Many federal, state, and local agencies provide services to persons with severe visual impairment. The health professional can refer these persons and their families to a social worker who is familiar with services and facilities available in their home area. Community health nurses often have this information readily available. Services to visually impaired persons include mobility training, personal counseling, vocational rehabilitation, relearning independent self-care, special education, and financial compensation in some instances.

National voluntary organizations

Two national voluntary health agencies concerned with blindness and the prevention of blindness are the American Foundation for the Blind* and the National Society for the Prevention of Blindness, Inc.† Both organizations have literature that is available to nurses and patients on request. The American Foundation for the Blind distributes a free catalog, *Aids and Appliances* (also available in braille, free of charge to blind persons), which contains a list of devices for the visually handicapped. The catalog includes sewing and kitchen utensils as well as various kinds of tools and instruments (Fig. 38-4). Medical appliances such as special syringes and aids for persons who must give themselves insulin or other parenteral medication can also be obtained. Founded in 1908, the National Society for the Prevention of Blindness, Inc., is engaged in the prevention of blindness through a comprehensive program of community services, public and professional education, and research. Publications, films, lecture, charts, and advisory service are available on request. The quarterly publication of this voluntary organization, *The Sight-Saving Review*, covers many aspects of sight conservation and eye health.

Recording for the Blind, Inc.‡ is a national, nonprofit voluntary organization that provides recorded educational books free on loan to anyone who cannot read normal printed material because of visual or physical handicaps. "Talking" books produced by this organization are fundamental aids to high school and college students and persons who require educational or specialized material in the pursuit of their occupations. These

---

*15 W. 16th St., New York, NY 10011.
†79 Madison Ave., New York, NY 10016.
‡215 E. 58th St., New York, NY 10022.

recordings also may be obtained from many local and state libraries. Talking-book machines are loaned free to persons who are legally blind. Information can be obtained from public libraries or organizations for blind persons.

Government assistance

Legal blindness entitles a person to certain federal assistance. A 1952 amendment to the Social Security Act made provision for assistance to blind persons, and now all 50 states and all territories have approved plans for such aid. Assistance through this program is based on need. The Internal Revenue Act of 1948 permits blind persons an extra personal deduction in reporting income. In 1943 the federal government established a counseling and placement service for the blind in the Vocational Rehabilitation Administration. This agency is now called the Social and Rehabilitation Service (SRS). It shares rehabilitation costs with the states. The Veterans Administration provides a substantial pension for the veteran who has enucleation of both eyes.

Schools

Progress has been made in improving educational opportunities for blind persons. It is believed now that the blind child, the same as any other handicapped child, does best when accepted and in as normal an environment as possible. Blind children of school age are being educated in regular public or parochial schools, where special provisions for their individual needs are being met, or they attend special residential schools. Schools emphasize the use of auditory instruction and the development of reading skills through touch perception by the braille system. The child needs to encounter as much of the environment as is practical in order to de-

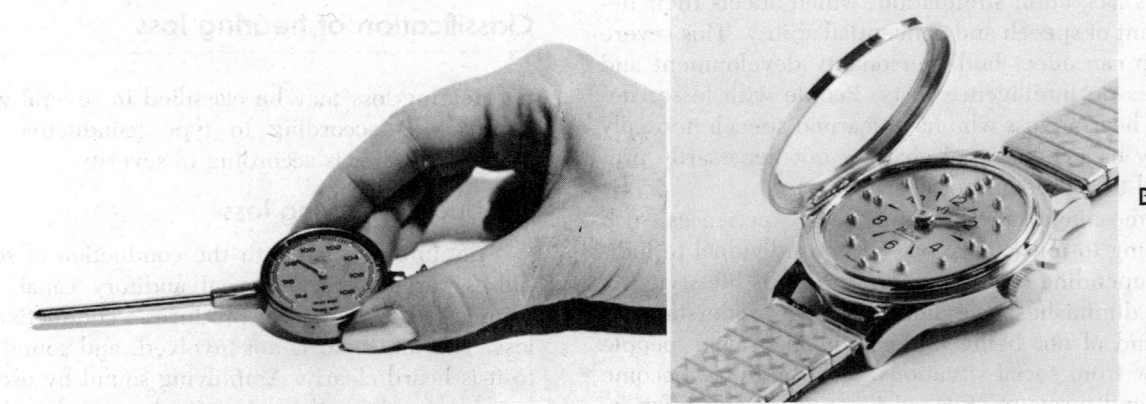

Fig. 38-4. A, Dial-type clinical thermometer with unbreakable stem. Braille (raised) dots mark scale, one dot at odd numbers and two at even numbers. Raised line is at 98.6° F. Button is pushed to register temperature, which remains set until button is released. Needle then returns to zero. **B,** One of many models of watches available in both braille and ink print. (Courtesy American Foundation for the Blind, New York.)

velop concepts that other children acquire by sight. Many states have legislated funds to provide higher education for blind persons and to provide readers for them, and many blind students go to college and compete successfully with their sighted peers.

Intervention for the person with impaired hearing and ear problems

Implications of impaired hearing

More than 13 million people in the United States have some kind of hearing impairment. Of these persons, 6 million are seriously handicapped, and more than 1.7 million are totally deaf.[28,88]

Hearing is as important as speech in our daily lives. Sound helps keep us in touch with reality and our environment; it adds esthetic pleasure as well as warnings of danger to our world. People with normal hearing are perceiving sound both consciously and unconsciously. One hears background noises, a clock ticking, or family conversations without concentrating on them; these sounds help us to be alert to our world. Other sounds, such as fire alarms or a child crying, signal us so that we consciously hear them and take action depending on our interpretation of the sound. This preconscious level of hearing is not perceived by persons who are hard of hearing and causes them to perceive the world as being "dead" about them. The sense of hearing is critical to normal development and maintenance of speech. Infants learn to speak by emulating sounds from others. They listen to the sounds they make in relationship to the sounds of others, a skill necessary in the formulation of adequate speaking skills. Congenitally deaf individuals lack aural stimulation, which affects their development of speech and conceptual ability. This severe handicap can affect both personality development and responses on intelligence tests. People with lesser degrees of hearing loss who have learned speech normally also may have behavioral changes not necessarily proportional to the degree of hearing loss.[24]

The meaning of the loss of esthetic experiences, such as listening to music, may vary from individual to individual depending on the person's previous life-style. As hearing diminishes, the impact of not understanding others and of not being understood may make people withdraw from social situations, and they may become anxious and insecure. Fear of inadequacy and inferiority may make them suspicious and depressed. When hearing is completely gone, they may find the silent world almost intolerable. Loneliness and isolation eventually may lead to disorientation or the lack of desire to live.

People who are hard of hearing or deaf are not easily recognized by others; they appear quite normal. When they fail to respond or respond inappropriately to oral communication, their actions are interpreted as slow or odd, and the speaker may withdraw. This withdrawal response of others may be perceived as rejection by the aurally handicapped person and may further increase isolation and withdrawal. The person who is hard of hearing or deaf may experience varying degrees of stress depending on personality, the extent and type of loss, the age of onset of loss, and his or her support system's (family and friends) reaction to loss.

Nursing activities regarding protection of the ears and prevention of hearing loss are outlined as follows and are described in succeeding paragraphs:
1. Protection of the ears from impairment or further impairment
   a. Teaching proper care of the ear
   b. Preventing hearing impairment from environmental forces including infection, noise pollution, and injury
   c. Working with people who evidence ear disease or impaired hearing
   d. Explaining and administering treatment to improve or prevent further hearing loss
2. Adjustment of the individual to impaired hearing
   a. Identifying those basic needs that have been affected by loss of hearing
   b. Understanding the effects on adaptation related to the different degrees and types of hearing loss
   c. Assisting the individual to cope with unmet needs of security (physiologic and psychologic), self-esteem, and love and belonging
   d. Directing individuals in using available community resources

Classification of hearing loss

Hearing loss may be classified in several ways; one approach is according to type (conductive, sensorineural), another is according to severity.

Conductive hearing loss

Any interference with the conduction of sound impulses through the external auditory canal, the eardrum, or the middle ear produces a conductive hearing loss. The inner ear is not involved, and sound directed to it is heard clearly. Amplifying sound by use of hearing aids or raising the voice may be useful so that sound will reach the inner ear. Conductive hearing loss may be caused by impacted cerumen or a foreign body in the external auditory canal; a thickening, retracting, scarring, or perforation of the eardrum; pathologic changes in the middle ear that prevent movement of one or more of the ossicles; or fixing of the stapes from otosclerosis. At the present time the conductive type of hearing loss is more effectively treated by surgery than the sensorineural type (p. 908).

Sensorineural hearing loss

Sensorineural hearing loss results from disease or trauma of the inner ear or its neural pathways. Some of the causes include arteriosclerosis; infectious diseases such as mumps, measles, and meningitis; ototoxic drugs (see box below); neuromas of the eighth cranial nerve; blows to the head or the ears; or degeneration of the organ of Corti caused by exposure to noise of high intensity, or most commonly by age (presbycusis). Treatment usually is not effective for sensorineural loss because the damage has been done by the time the individual sees the physician, and the process is irreversible. Some surgical procedures have been developed to aid in restoring this type of loss (p. 911). Amplifying sounds by shouting causes distortion of the sound and may increase the hearing problem.

SELECTED OTOTOXIC DRUGS

These drugs may affect the cochlea, vestibule of the ear, or the eighth cranial nerve.

Antibiotics	Streptomycin
	Dihydrostreptomycin
	Neomycin
	Kanamycin
	Viomycin
	Vancomycin
	Polymyxin B/Colistin
	Chloramphenicol (Chloromycetin)
	Capreomycin
Diuretics	Ethacrynic acid (Edecrin)
	Furosemide (Lasix)
	Acetazolamide (Diamox)
Salicylates	Acetylsalicylic acid (aspirin)
Other drugs	Quinine
	Chloroquine
	Nitrogen mustard
	Bleomycin
	Quinidine

Severity

Hearing loss is also classified according to severity, that is, slight loss or severe loss. Persons who have only slight hearing loss often are unaware of it or try to minimize it. Listening becomes a strain; difficulties arise in communication causing embarrassment or irritation. Exhaustion can occur, and social contacts are avoided. The recognition of the defect in hearing by the individual is necessary before corrective or rehabilitative steps can be taken.

Persons with *slight to moderate* hearing loss are found often in the aged population. Their hearing loss is most often sensorineural loss compounded at times by conductive loss. Typically, these persons have decreased ability to hear or discern higher-pitched sounds; increasing the loudness of the voice only increases the distortion of sound and compounds hearing problems.

Persons with *severe* hearing loss usually seek help because of the problems they have in functioning. Because they no longer hear themselves speak, their speech may become slurred or too loud. Severe hearing loss is exemplified by the congenitally deaf who may be severely limited in their psychologic and mental development. Deafness alters the individual's awareness of self. Early case finding of congenitally deaf children is necessary so that corrective measures can be taken early to facilitate their learning.

Prevention

Hearing difficulties may begin at any age. Understanding the many causes of hearing loss is important for all health team members in all settings. Because nurses occupy a unique position in the health care system, they have the opportunity to be involved in many aspects of health care of the ear.

Care of healthy ears

The ear should be cleaned only with a wet washcloth over the tip of a finger. Nothing should be inserted into the ear beyond the extent of vision. A certain amount of cerumen (ear wax) in the ear canal is normal, and persons who have no wax have itching and scaling in the ear canal. Usually it is not necessary to clean the ears to remove wax. Occasionally, when the cerumen becomes impacted and causes pain or temporary deafness, it must be removed by the physician, nurse, or member of the person's family who has been instructed in the procedure. The person is usually asked to instill several drops of a warm sweet oil (mineral oil or glycerin) or hydrogen peroxide or peroxide in glyceryl (Debrox) into the auditory canal for several days to soften the wax. Directions for instillation of ear drops are as follows:

1. Wash hands before and after the procedure.

2. Check the eardropper if glass or plastic to make sure it is not rough.

3. Warm the solution to body temperature (no more than 38° C [100° F]; vertigo may result from high or low temperatures. The bottle of solution may be warmed by holding it in the hand for a few minutes.

4. Have patient tilt the head so that the ear to be treated is uppermost.

5. Cleanse the external ear with a clean washcloth.

6. Straighten ear canal by pulling up and back in adults, down and back in children.

7. Instill the drops so that they run along the wall of the canal and do not entrap air.

8. Have the patient hold the head position for 5 to 10 minutes.

9. Gently insert a piece of cotton moistened with the eardrop solution into the external auditory canal to keep the drops from running out of the ear.

10. Dry the external ear thoroughly to prevent skin irritation.

To *irrigate* the ear canal, a solution of tap water or normal saline with hydrogen peroxide added to help dislodge the wax is used. The person sits with the head inclined slightly forward and toward the affected side (Fig. 38-5). Clothes are protected and a basin placed below the ear to catch excess solution. The auricle is pulled upward and backward and the solution directed along the upper wall of the meatus. If irrigation does not remove the wax easily, removal with a cerumen spoon by the physician may be necessary. It is usually necessary to dry the ear canal gently with a cotton wick. Teaching the individual or a member of the family to irrigate the ear should include the above steps in addition to the following guidelines:

1. The procedure should not be undertaken with-

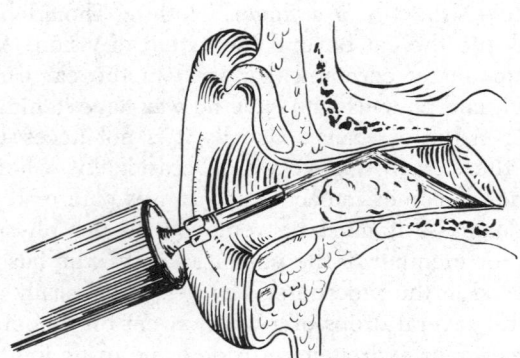

Fig. 38-5. Irrigation of external auditory canal with warm tap water. (From Saunders, W.H., et al.: Nursing care in eye, ear, nose, and throat disorders, ed. 4, St. Louis, 1979, The C.V. Mosby Co.)

out the approval of a qualified member of the health team.

2. Wash hands before and after the procedure.

3. Always warm the solution to be used to body temperature to prevent vestibular stimulation and consequent vertigo.

4. Never try to irrigate the ear canal to remove foreign objects of vegetable material; the moisture will cause the objects to swell.

5. Irrigations are not used if the eardrum is punctured, since this can cause further infection.

6. Use a steady stream of solution against the roof of the auditory canal; if directed downward, the plugging material will be forced further into the canal.

7. Do not use excessive force, and make sure the syringe used has no rough edges.

8. Air should be expelled from the bulb syringe before instilling solution, and the tip of the syringe should be directed either toward the roof or toward the floor of the canal but not straight inward.

9. The canal should not be completely obstructed by the syringe, since this will keep solution from flowing back and will cause pressure against the eardrum.

10. The person should lie on the affected side for several minutes to assure complete drainage of irrigation fluid.

11. The external ear should then be dried thoroughly to prevent excoriation of the skin.

Early adequate treatment of childhood diseases

Prevention of hearing loss involves teaching persons the necessity for adequate treatment of childhood diseases. Since viral diseases (especially measles) can cause a hearing impairment in the fetus, immunization programs and treatment of the pregnant woman who contracts the disease can prevent hearing loss in the child. Other high-risk infants who may develop hearing impairments are those who are premature or who have experienced anoxia postnatally. Good prenatal care can help prevent hearing loss in high-risk infants.

Hearing loss may also begin later in childhood. Before the advent of antibiotics, hearing loss was a frequent sequela of middle ear and mastoid process infections. Adequate treatment of upper respiratory tract and particularly of ear infections can prevent this loss. Persons need to be taught to blow the nose gently with both nostrils open (not sniffing) to avoid contamination of the eustachian tubes with mucus, especially during an upper respiratory tract infection. Individuals with upper respiratory tract infections should be encouraged to seek medical attention if they experience (1) increasing pain in the ear or increasing headache even after application of heat, (2) any reddish fluid oozing from the ear (this may indicate rupture of the eardrum), (3) temperature higher than 39° C (102° F), (4) any convulsive twitching of the facial muscles, or (5) dizziness. Medical attention should be sought if a child less than 3 years of age has any symptoms related to the ear.

Prevention of trauma

Children should be taught to avoid inserting hard articles deep into the ear canal, obstructing the ear canal with any objects, inserting unclean articles or solutions into the ear, or swimming in stagnant water or in water identified as being polluted. These practices can lead to damage of the tympanic membrane or to ear infections. Adults often insert hard articles into the outer ear in an attempt to remove cerumen.

Monitoring side effects of ototoxic drugs

Persons taking ototoxic drugs (see box on p. 873) need to know the signs and symptoms of side effects of these drugs in order to prevent loss of hearing from developing. If these symptoms (dizziness, decreased hearing acuity, tinnitus) occur, the next dose of the drug is omitted and the physician is consulted. Audiometric testing may be necessary.

Monitoring noise pollution

Hearing loss caused by loud noise is the most common type of occupational hearing loss. Exposure to industrial noise levels greater than 85 to 90 decibels (db) for months or years causes cochlear damage. Health team members in industry can help prevent deafness caused by noise of high intensity by teaching employees why they should wear earplugs. The nurse in industry faces a task calling for special knowledge and training. Industrial noise and occupational or noise-induced hearing loss are primary causes of hearing loss in our society. Some 9 million workers are exposed daily to noise levels on the job that are potentially hazardous to hearing.[29,72,100] This occupational hearing loss is preventable, and the nurse must be familiar with both the causes and the possible means of prevention of such loss. Courses are available to familiarize nurses with industrial hearing conservation requirements.

Concern with noise pollution as well as with other occupational hazards prompted the passage of the *Williams-Steiger Occupational Safety and Health Act* (OSHA) in 1970. The provisions regarding noise protection are too complex to include in detail, but in general, exposure to noise levels in excess of 90 db over an 8-hour day are considered excessive and should be avoided (Table 38-4). The requirement means that no worker should be exposed *unprotected* for over 8 hours to levels of 90 dbA or higher. The term *dbA* relates to one of three possible scales or networks found on most sound-level meters. These scales essentially respond differ-

ently to different frequencies or wavelengths in noise. The A network, like the human ear, is not responsive to (does not measure) low-frequency sound and thus is used in many situations such as the OSHA regulation or in specifying the annoyance of humans to noise. The B network is used for certain engineering applications, and the C scale measures the entire spectrum. A copy of the Occupational Safety and Health Act may be obtained from local offices or OSHA, which is part of the U.S. Department of Labor.

Other causes of noise-induced hearing loss include firearms and high-intensity music such as rock music. With an M-16 rifle or sports rifle, hearing loss tends to be greater in the ear opposite the dominant hand (i.e., left ear hearing loss in a right-handed person). With revolvers, hearing loss is equal in both ears. A person firing guns who notices tinnitus, sensation of fullness in the ear, or temporary hearing loss should stop firing guns or a least wear suitable ear protectors. Sound in front of a rock band can reach up to 120 db, and hearing losses up to 50 db have been measured in some members of rock bands. In the early stage, there is loss of hearing *at* or *near* frequencies of 4000 hertz (Hz). Later the damage extends to both higher and lower tones, with the lower tones affected least. If proximity to the high noise level cannot be avoided, ear protectors or earplugs should be worn. The earplugs are inserted into the external auditory canal and can reduce the noise reaching the middle ear by 10 to 30 db. Usually standard plugs are effective, but custom-made plugs molded to the individual's ear canal may be obtained. If the noise level is extremely high (sound levels may reach 140 db or higher), individuals are not adequately protected with earplugs alone and must wear muffs over their ears, and at times a shield must be worn over the entire head.

TABLE 38-4. Permissible noise exposures*

Duration per day (hr)	Sound level (dbA, slow)
8	90
6	92
4	95
3	97
2	100
1½	102
1	105
½	110
¼	115

*From U.S. Department of Labor, Occupational Safety and Health Administration: Noise: the environmental problem, a guide to OSHA standards, Washington, D.C., 1979, U.S. Government Printing Office.

Intervention

Local treatment of ear problems

Often treatment of external ear infections includes local application of medicated ointments or powders, hot compresses to soften crusts, or cool applications to lessen inflammation and relieve discomfort.

To apply *ointment* to the ear canal, an applicator with a tufted end is used (Fig. 38-6); a Q-Tip or other commercially prepared cotton applicator is usually too thick.[58] The tufted end of the applicator is inserted deep into the canal, and ointment is applied to the outer surface of the eardrum as well as to the ear canal. Care must be taken to prevent damage to the eardrum. A new applicator is used each time the canal is entered. The person is cautioned not to move the head during the procedure.

When *compresses* are used, the pillow is protected and a loose gauze plug is placed in the outer ear canal. This plug can be moistened with solution if the outer ear canal is also involved or may be used dry to prevent spread of the infection to the inner part of the canal. Compresses of single-thickness gauze fit the contours of the outer ear best. They should be moist but not dripping. Since ice bags are too heavy to use on the sensitive external ear, a cold application can be made by placing about 2 cupfuls of crushed ice in a small sealed plastic bag or glove. In caring for patients with infections of the external ear, it is important to avoid further infection; thus handwashing is important and all equipment and material used must be sterile.

Earwicks or *drains* may be used to encourage passage of exudate from the ear canal. Sterile wicks may be made by twisting a single layer of sterile gauze that has been picked up at its center. The wick is inserted gently only as far as the eye can see with the loose end extending outside the ear canal. Wicks must be changed often and never allowed to become hardened with exudate, because this interferes with the flow of drainage. Commercially prepared earwicks, such as the Pope earwick (Xomed Co.) or Merocel earwick (Codman Co.), are essentially expanding cellulose sponges that are harder than a gauze wick, but they serve as excellent vehicles for medicating the ear canal. A wick saturated with a medicated solution may be used both as a drain and as a local compress. A wick also may be inserted after eardrops have been given to distribute the medication and help retain it in the ear canal.

Nursing intervention for the person having ear surgery

Most persons having ear surgery have short hospitalizations. The different types of ear surgery are described in detail in Chapter 39. With any operative procedure on the middle ear, patients may experience *vertigo* for a few days postoperatively, which is probably related to the stimulation of the inner ear. Patients usually require assistance or supervision when ambulating for the first 1 or 2 days to protect them from falling. Some persons who are quite dizzy will also exhibit nystagmus resulting from labyrinthine stimulation. Keeping the patient from moving the head may help lessen vertigo. Nausea can accompany vertigo, and often both may be relieved by antimotion drugs such as dimenhydrinate (Dramamine), diazepam (Valium), or promethazine (Phenergan).

Fluids may be tolerated orally if given in small amounts with the patient keeping the head still. Pain is not usually a major problem for patients with ear surgery but may be present, and if so, it may be relieved by analgesics.

Small amounts of serosanguinous drainage on ear dressings is expected, but signs of bright blood on outer dressing are reported to the physician. Signs of facial paralysis, such as inability to smile or to wrinkle the forehead, are assessed immediately postoperatively in the recovery room and again when the patient returns to the clinical unit. Patients are cautioned not to blow their noses for a period of time postoperatively so as not to increase air pressure in the eustachian tube.

Careful hand washing before and after contact with the patient is an effective way to prevent infection. Handling contaminated dressings appropriately also helps to prevent infection. Often antibiotics are given prophylactically. Patients often are cautioned against swimming, washing their hair, or getting the affected ear wet in any way for a limited amount of time (about 2 weeks). When healing is complete, most persons may resume all normal activities. Since persons often are concerned about apparent lack of immediate improvement in hearing, especially following stapedectomy (p. 908), careful explanations about hearing restoration are necessary.

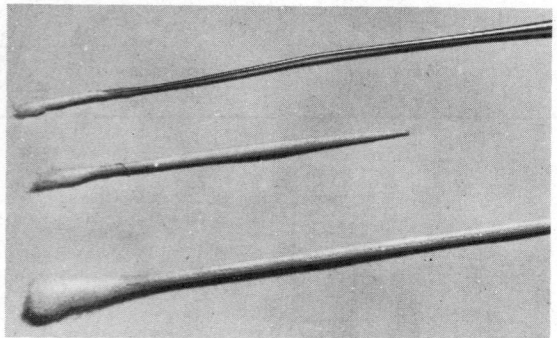

Fig. 38-6. *Top:* Physician's cotton applicator; note tuft at end. *Middle:* Toothpick with cotton. *Bottom:* Usual commercial applicator (too thick). (From Saunders, W.H., et al.: Nursing care in eye, ear, nose, and throat disorders, ed. 4, St. Louis, 1979, The C.V. Mosby Co.)

Outcome criteria for the person having ear surgery. The person or significant others can:

1. State the rationale and desired outcome of the procedure.
2. Describe the rationale for the following safety precautions:
   a. Side rails or assistance during early ambulation.
   b. No nose blowing postoperatively.
   c. Keeping the ear dry postoperatively.
   d. Hand-washing and dressing procedures.
3. State the symptoms requiring medical attention and need for follow-up care.

Aural rehabilitation

If hearing loss is irreversible and not amenable to surgical intervention, aural rehabilitation may make it possible for the individual to understand and communicate with others again. The purpose of aural rehabilitation is to maximize the hearing-impaired person's communication skills. Because the auditory sense is our primary mode of communication, it is imperative that hearing-impaired individuals be given the opportunity to utilize their hearing for this purpose. When a person exhibits irreversible hearing loss, the ability to hear conversational speech may be improved through the use of an appropriate hearing aid.

The hearing-impaired person must be helped to understand the implications of hearing loss for communication purposes. There are potential social and psychologic implications of hearing impairment,[24] and it is most helpful for the individual to gain insight into the specific communication problems. This can be accomplished through discussions pertaining to daily communicative interactions at home, at work, or at play. The presence of a family member in such discussions is often most helpful in determining how the individual's hearing impairment may have affected others. These insights are extremely important in planning appropriate rehabilitative strategies.

Formal aural rehabilitative training may be necessary to improve an individual's communication skills. Many hearing-impaired persons do not utilize their residual hearing. *Auditory training* is a process by which the person is helped to make maximum use of residual hearing. *Speech reading* is taught to supplement the hearing function and includes lipreading and the study of facial expressions, gestures, and body movements used in communication. *Speech therapy* is given to develop, conserve, or correct speech.

The person's acceptance of the fact of having a hearing impairment, desire to seek help, and use of the facilities available, coupled with motivation, perseverance and patience, contribute to the success of aural rehabilitation. Rehabilitation is affected by age and severity of impairment. Infants and children with hearing disorders require assistance from specialists to help them learn and communicate. For people who, although hard of hearing, have normally acquired communication skill, efforts are geared toward correcting, restoring, complementing, and maintaining those skills. For deaf persons who have not developed communication skills, efforts are made to teach language and speech skills by special methods.

Hearing aids

Hearing aids (Fig. 38-7) are commonly used by both hard-of-hearing individuals and deaf persons. Hearing aids are instruments through which sounds are amplified in a controlled manner. Generally an aid consists of a microphone to receive and convert speech and other sounds into electric signals, an amplifier to increase the strength of the sound, a receiver to convert electric signals back to sound, and a battery to supply the electric power. Hearing aids are used to increase the intensity of the sound reaching the ear of the person with hearing loss. *Hearing aids do not improve the ability to hear, but they make the sound louder.* They are usually recommended when the person has difficulty in understanding speech in everyday conversations.

When the person has difficulty with speech discrimination, benefits from an aid are more restricted. Persons with a conductive hearing loss benefit most from wearing a hearing aid because their ability to understand speech is usually not impaired if the speech is loud enough. They will not hear as well as they did with normal hearing, but they will be able to hear speech in the frequencies at which most ordinary conversations occur. Persons with sensorineural hearing losses often exhibit problems with amplification such as an intolerance for loud speech and noise and difficulty understanding speech even if loud enough. It should be noted, however, that this is the most common type of hearing loss and affects the majority of individuals successfully wearing hearing aids. Appropriate aural rehabilitation will ensure a successful adjustment to amplification in most instances.

Elderly persons often have difficulty adjusting to the use of a hearing aid, partially because their hearing loss usually is of sensorineural origin. Their problems also may be the result of a lack of patience, concentration, or mental energy needed to learn to use a hearing aid. Small children with a hearing loss should be fitted with a hearing aid as soon as a hearing deficit is diagnosed, usually at several months of age, because reinforcement from auditory feedback is paramount for appropriate linguistic development.

A person whose hearing problem indicates need for a hearing aid should be seen both by an otologist and an audiologist. The audiologist can perform various tests

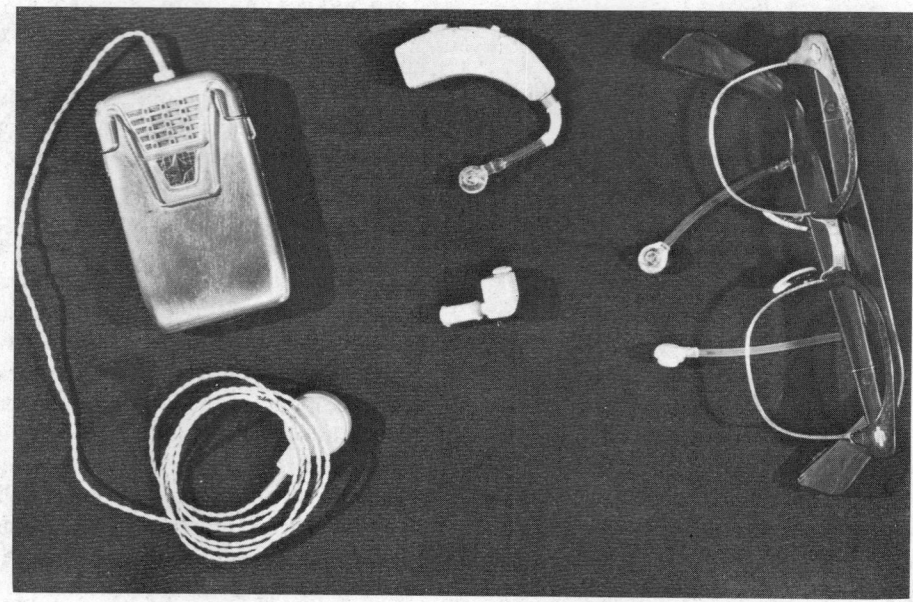

Fig. 38-7. Body and head borne hearing aids. *Left:* Body-type aid; button receiver is coupled to ear with insert, and component housing is either clipped to clothing or worn on body in harnessed cloth pouch. *Top center:* Behind-ear aid. *Center:* In-ear aid. *Right:* Eyeglass aid. (From Saunders, W.H., et al.: Nursing care in eye, ear, nose, and throat disorders, ed. 4, St. Louis, 1979, The C.V. Mosby Co.)

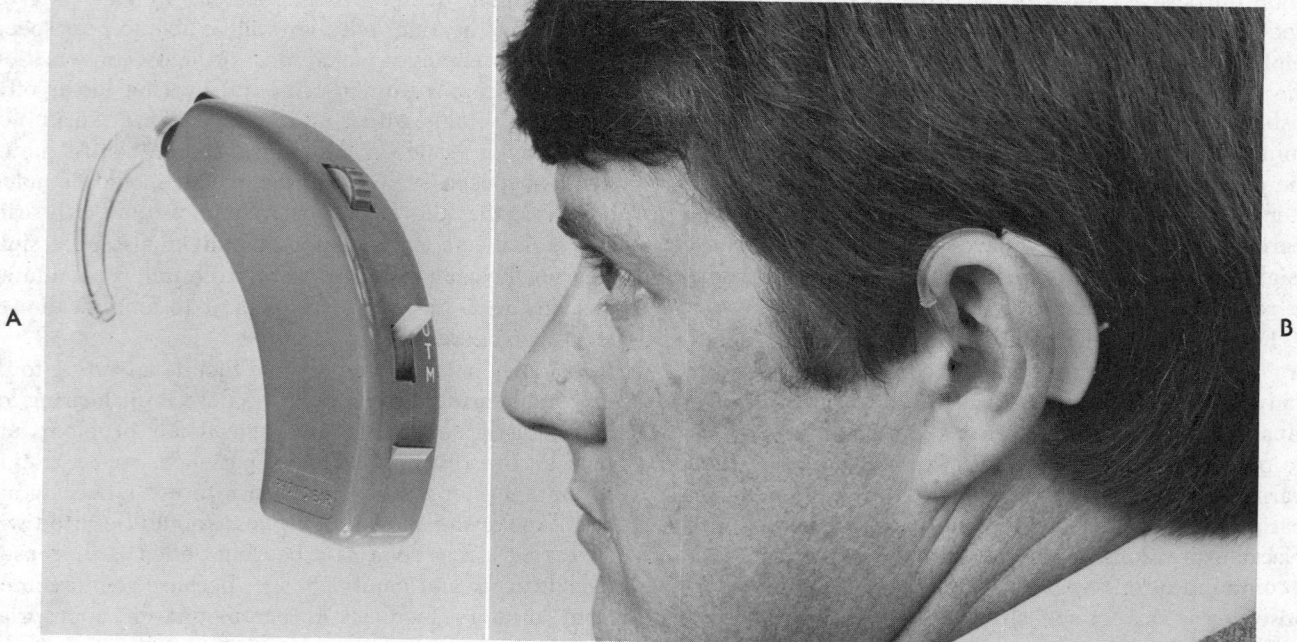

Fig. 38-8. A, Hearing aid. **B,** Hearing aid in place. (Courtesy HC Electronics, Inc. [Phonic Ear], Mill Valley, Calif.)

and help determine if a hearing aid will benefit the person and what specific type of hearing will be best. The otologist can determine the medical nature of the problem and decide whether there is any medical reason why a hearing aid cannot be worn. Food and Drug Administration (FDA) regulations[28] restrict the sale of hearing aids to those individuals who have received a medical evaluation, with the provision that any person over 18 years of age, or any parent or guardian, can be permitted to waive the medical evaluation requirement, provided they do not have any one of the following seven designated otologic conditions: (1) a visible congenital or traumatic deformity of the ear, (2) a history of active drainage from the ear within the last 90 days, (3) a history of sudden progressive hearing loss within the last 90 days, (4) a history of acute or chronic dizziness, (5) unilateral hearing loss of sudden or recent onset, (6) an audiometric air-bone gap equal to or greater than 15 db at 500, 1000, and 2000 Hz, or (7) visible evidence of cerumen or a foreign body in the ear canal. The waiver privilege has been allowed in those instances in which it would be very inconvenient to have a medical evaluation (e.g., in rural areas), and for those instances where religious beliefs forbid medical evaluation but do not forbid the wearing of hearing aids.

Over 1200 different models of hearing aids are available. They may be worn on the body, built into the temple bow of eyeglasses, or worn as individual units behind the ear (Fig. 38-8) or in the ear canal. Aids worn on the body are the most powerful and are generally fitted to persons with moderate to severe hearing losses. Aids worn in eyeglasses or behind the ear are generally equivalent to each other in amplifying power.

Implanting of hearing aids is under consideration, although it has not been demonstrated, as yet, that speech discrimination is superior with implantation than with conventional aids.

The person should be instructed in the care of the hearing aid. The ear mold or plug may be washed daily in mild soap and water using a pipe cleaner to cleanse the cannula. It should be thoroughly dried before being reconnected to the receiver. If a hearing aid is worn on the body, the microphone should face the speaker and should not be covered by heavy clothing. Men often wear the transmitter in their shirt or upper pocket. Women may fit it into a special pocket sewn on the outside of their underclothing. Children often wear it on a fabric harness placed over their undergarments. The person who uses a hearing aid should carry an extra battery and cord at all times.

Hearing aids have adjustable tone and volume controls, and several adjustments may have to be made before the aid is correctly set for the individual's needs. Since a hearing aid is not selective when amplifying sounds, often the amplified background sounds can be annoying to the individual. Persons who wear hearing aids should know what to do if the aid fails to work:

1. Check the on-off switch.
2. Inspect cleanliness of earmold.
3. Examine battery for tightness or leaks
4. Examine cord plug for tightness of insertion.
5. Examine cord plug for breaks.
6. Replace battery, cord, or both.
7. Take hearing aid to local service agency if above steps fail to correct problem.

Persons who are reluctant to wear their hearing aids (usually for cosmetic reasons) need counseling about the benefits of wearing the aid and the improvements in their ability to communicate. The aid may also serve to notify others to speak more distinctly. When a person with a hearing aid is hospitalized, it is important to encourage use of the aid during the hospitalization and its safe storage when not in use.

Outcome criteria for the person with a hearing aid. The person or significant others can:

1. Explain the rationale for using the hearing aid.
2. Demonstrate the proper care of the aid.
3. Explain what to do if the aid does not work.
4. Explain what the aid can and cannot do.

Auditory training

Auditory training is used to encourage those who are hard of hearing to use their residual hearing more effectively. The training consists of helping the affected individual to develop listening skills. It helps the hard of hearing person to (1) establish attitudes of critical listening, (2) develop an awareness of the kinds of listening errors that are most likely to be made in view of the nature of the hearing impairment, (3) compensate for these errors by using other special clues that are still heard correctly, and (4) improve listening habits and skills in general.

Speech-reading

Speech-reading (commonly known as lipreading) is taught to supplement the hearing function. It includes lipreading, the study of facial expressions, and the study of gestures and body movements used in speech. It also uses environmental clues that help supplement the hearing function in communication.

Speech training

Speech training is given to conserve speech skills, to prevent deterioration of skills, or to develop speech skills. Hearing is necessary not only for the development of speech but also for the monitoring of loudness, clearness, pitch, quality, and rate. Hearing loss reduces the reliability of the monitoring system, which may cause the speech to deteriorate.

Special interventions for the congenitally deaf child

Development of speech and language skills requires special attention for those born deaf or who become deaf in early childhood, because these persons do not develop language and speech normally. Not only is it medically important to detect deafness or hearing impairment in the young child, but also, for an educational standpoint, it is imperative that remedial measures be taken during the early years (between the ages of 2 and 5 years) when language and speech skills are most easily acquired (Fig. 38-9). Children who have never heard speech are unable to imitate it. They are educable, but their education requires more time than that for children with normal hearing. Since a period of about 3 years is required for children to learn sufficient language to begin the first grade, they should start receiving formal training as soon as a hearing loss is detected. They may then attend classes with children who have normal hearing or go to a public or private school for the deaf. The John Tracy Clinic (see box, p. 881) provides information and has correspondence classes for parents who have preschool children with severe hearing impairment or deafness.

Recent research has indicated that deaf children's learning abilities can be greatly enhanced by employing the language of signs. In these cases it appears that the *total communication* approach that includes speech reading, auditory training, and sign language is most advantageous. There is a great need for programs that focus on finding these individuals and providing services to help them learn the necessary skills for developing a sense of self-worth.

Communicating with the hearing impaired person

The following are some specific points to facilitate speech-reading or hearing for persons with impaired hearing:

1. Get the person's attention by raising an arm or hand.
2. Start with the light on your face; this will help the person speech read.
3. Talk directly to the person, facing him or her.
4. Speak clearly, but do not overaccentuate words.
5. Speak in a normal tone; do not shout. Shouting overemploys normal speaking movements and may cause distortion and be too loud for the

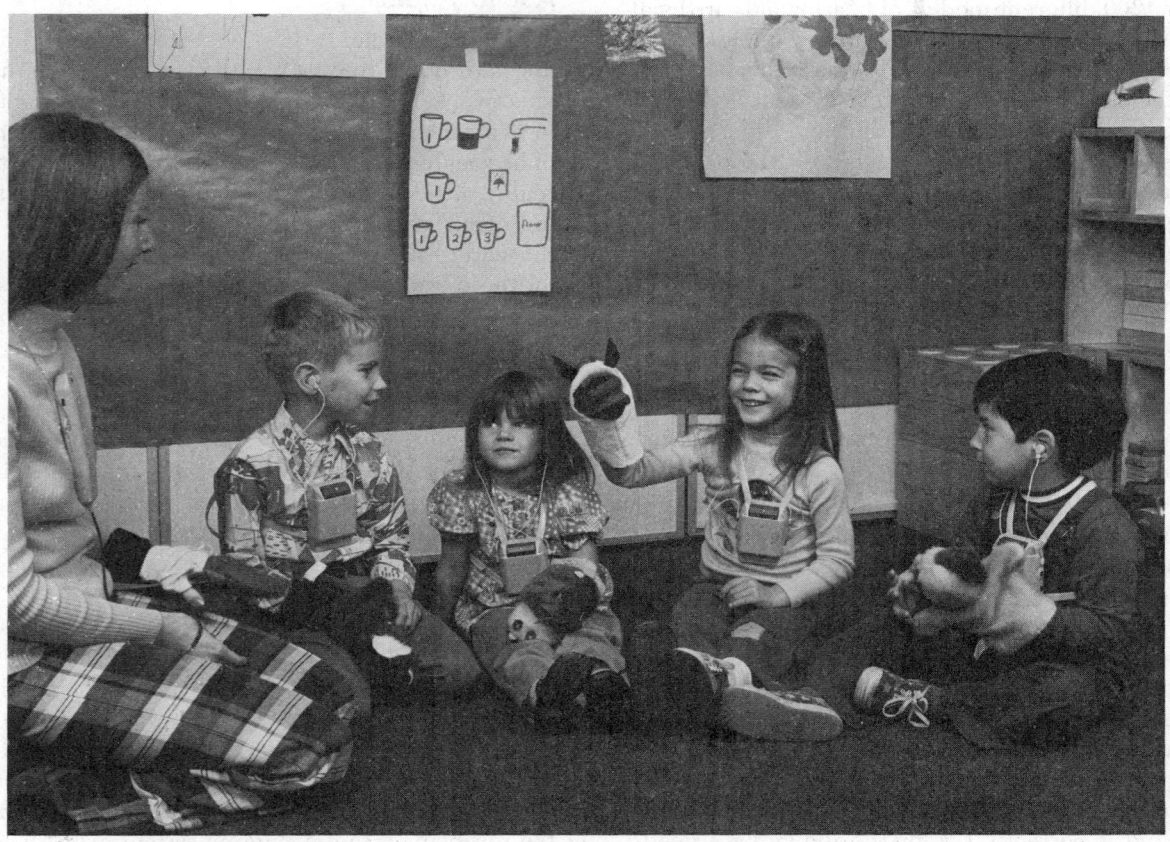

Fig. 38-9. Preschool children with hearing difficulties attend special classes to develop communication skills. (Courtesy HC Electronics, Inc. [Phonic Ear], Mill Valley, Calif.)

person with sensorineural damage. If the person has conductive loss only, sometimes making the voice louder without shouting is helpful.

6. If the person does not seem to understand what is said, express it differently. Some words are difficult to "see" in speech reading, such as white and red.

7. Move closer to the person and toward the better ear if he does not hear you.

8. Write out proper names or any statement that you are not sure was understood.

9. Do not smile, chew gum, or cover the mouth when talking to a person with limited hearing.

10. Inattention may indicate tiredness or lack of understanding.

11. Use phrases to convey meaning rather than one-word answers. State the major topic of the discussion first and then give details.

12. Do not show annoyance by careless facial expression. Persons who are hard of hearing depend more on visual clues for acceptance.

13. Encourage the use of a hearing aid if the person has one; allow him or her to adjust it before speaking.

14. If in a group, repeat important statements and avoid asides to others in the group.

15. Avoid the use of the intercommunication system as this may distort sound and cause poor communication.

16. Do not avoid conversation with a person who has hearing loss. It has been said that to live in a silent world is much more devastating than to live in darkness, and persons with hearing loss appear, by and large, to have more emotional difficulties than those who are blind.*

Hospital settings require identification of patients with difficulty with hearing. If a deaf or hard of hearing person is hospitalized, the new environment and unfamiliar faces may accentuate loneliness and isolation, and anxiety may reduce hearing even further.[14]

Persons who are hard of hearing depend on their other senses to provide information about changes in their environment. Patients are helped to use visual clues by placing them in a bed where they can observe activity and anticipate others approaching them. They will be easily startled if people suddenly enter the unit if vision is obscured. Many patients feel less isolated if the nurse touches them lightly on the arm to gain their attention and wakes them by touching them on the arm. Because hearing-impaired persons are often sensitive to light changes, they can easily be awakened by turning on a light. Special effort must be made to communicate information about the hospital routine to the deaf or

hard of hearing patients and to prepare them for special tests.

Acupuncture

Recently there has been a resurgence of interest in acupuncture for the treatment of hearing loss. Audiometric testing of large groups of persons with hearing loss who underwent acupuncture demonstrate that hearing loss is not improved.[96,102] For more information on acupuncture, see p. 394.

Community services

Selected agencies exist for helping the hearing impaired person. The telephone company can provide information with regard to special amplifiers or flashing lights that can be placed on doorbells or telephones. Services for persons with a hearing loss are offered by audiology clinics sponsored by universities, hospitals, community programs, local or state departments of health and education, or the Veterans Administration. National organizations are available to give information and counseling (see box below).

For the person whose vision and hearing both are

AGENCIES THAT PROVIDE ASSISTANCE FOR THE HEARING IMPAIRED

American Annals of the Deaf, 5034 Wisconsin Ave., N.W., Washington, DC 20016. The April issue every year lists a directory of programs and services for the deaf available by state, including information about the type of facilities.

American Federation of the Physically Handicapped, Inc., 1370 National Press Building, Washington, DC 20004. Provides counseling and information.

American Speech and Hearing Association, 10801 Rockville Pike, Rockville, MD 20852. Membership is composed of professional persons who teach individuals who have hearing and speech problems.

Gallauder College, 7th and Florida Ave., Washington, DC 20002. The only liberal arts college in the world for the deaf.

The John Tracy Clinic, 806 West Adams Blvd., Los Angeles, CA 90007. Provides information and correspondence classes for parents with deaf children.

National Association of Hearing and Speech Agencies, 919 18th St. N.W., Washington, DC 20006. Provides counseling and information.

State Office of Vocational Rehabilitation (in each state). Provides vocational training and placement services.

Veterans Administration. Provides audiology clinics and rehabilitative services for veterans.

Speech and hearing centers are found locally in many cities.

---

*Adapted from Conover, M., and Cober, J.: Nurs. Clin. North Am. **5:**497, 1970.

severely impaired, a catalog distributed by the American Foundation for the Blind includes a vibrator attachment to be used with a timer or clock. The vibrator is placed under the mattress, and its vibrations act as an alarm to wake the occupant. (For further information about the catalog, see p. 871.)

REFERENCES AND SELECTED READINGS
Contemporary

1. American Foundation for the Blind: Directory of agencies serving the visually handicapped in the United States, ed. 20, New York, 1978, The William Byrd Press.
2. American Medical Association drug evaluation, ed. 4, Acton, Mass., 1980, Publishing Sciences Group, Inc.
3. Ballenger, J.: Diseases of the nose, throat, and ear, ed. 12, Philadelphia, 1977, Lea & Febiger.
4. Becker, G., and Nadler, G.: The aged deaf: integration of a disabled group into an agency serving elderly people, Gerontologist 20:214-221, 1980.
5. Beeson, P.B., and McDermott, W., editors: Textbook of medicine, ed. 15, Philadelphia, 1979, W.B. Saunders Co.
6. *Berger, E.H.: Single number measures of hearing protector noise reduction, Occup. Health Nurs. 27(12):32-34, 1979.
7. Bitonte, J.L., and Keates, R.H., editors: Symposium on the flexible lens, St. Louis, 1972, The C.V. Mosby Co.
8. Boyles, V.A.: Injection aids for blind diabetic patients, Am. J. Nurs. 77:1456-1458, 1977.
9. Brenny, A.A.: A hearing conservation program: general considerations for the occupational health nurse, Occup. Health Nurs. 27(12):16-20, 1979.
10. *Brown, M.S.: The Gordons needed all the help they could get, Nurs. '77 7(10):40-43, 1977.
11. Bumbold, J., and Siedel, M.: Identifying and serving a multiplying handicapped population, Nurs. Clin. North Am. 10:341-352, 1975.
12. Chial, M.R.: Hearing aid evaluation methods, J. Speech Hear. Disord. 39:270-279, 1974.
13. Chung, D.Y., and Gannon, R.P.: Hearing loss due to noise trauma, J. Laryngol. Otol. 94:419-423, 1980.
14. *Clark, C.: Communicating with hearing impaired elderly adults, J. Gerontol. Nurs. 4(3):40-44, 1979.
15. Conklin, J.M., and Subtelny, J.D.: Effect of speech training upon speechreading in hearing-impaired adults, Am. Ann. Deaf 125:442-448, 1980.
16. Connolly, P.: Growing up with deafness, Commun. Outlook 9:290-293, 1980.
17. *Conover, M., and Cober, J.: Understanding and caring for the hearing impaired, Nurs. Clin. North Am. 5:497-506, 1970.
18. Craig, W.N., and Craig, H.B.: Director of programs and services for the deaf in the United States, Am. Ann. Deaf, April 1981. (New updating published every year in the April issue.)
19. *Cullin, I.C.: Techniques for teaching patients with sensory defects, Nurs. Clin. North Am. 5:527-538, 1970.
20. Downs, M.P.: The deafness management quotient, Hearing Speech News 42:8, 1974.
21. Downs, M.P.: Audiological evaluation of the congenitally deaf infant, Otolaryngol. Clin. North Am. 4:347-357, 1971.
22. Downs, M.P.: Overview of the management of the congenitally deaf child, Otolaryngol. Clin. North Am. 4:223-226, 1971.
23. *Dupont, J.: EENT emergencies, Nurs. '79 9(11):65, 1979.
24. Edsall, J.: Relationship between loss of auditory and visual acuity and social disengagement in an aged population, Nurs. Res. 27(5):296-298, 1978.
25. Egan, J.J.: Services for the hearing impaired: the case for audiologic intervention, Ear Nose Throat J. 58(8):326-327, 1979.
26. Ellis, P.E.: Ocular therapeutics and pharmacology, ed. 6, St. Louis, 1981, The C.V. Mosby Co.
27. The eye in nursing literature 1968-1973: a bibliography, A.O.R.N. J. 18:1013-1014, 1973.
28. Facts about hearing and hearing aids, HEW publ. no. (FDA) 79-4016, Washington, D.C., 1979, U.S. Government Printing Office.
29. Fox, M.S.: Workmen's compensation hearing loss claims, Laryngoscope 90:1077-1081, 1980.
30. Furth, H.: Teaching manual language to deaf children, Am. Ann. Deaf 125:3-4, 1980.
31. Gellis, S.S., and Kagan, B.M.: Current pediatric therapy, ed. 9, Philadelphia, 1980, W.B. Saunders Co.
32. Goetzinger, C.P.: The psychology of hearing impairment. In Katz, J. editor: Handbook of clinical audiology, ed. 2, Baltimore, 1978, The Williams & Wilkins Co.
33. Goldstein, B.A.: Early identification of hearing impaired infants: Public Law 94-142 falls short, Int. J. Pediatr. Otorhinolaryngol. 1:181-191, 1979.
34. *Gould, H.: How to remove contact lenses from comatose patients, Am. J. Nurs. 76:1483-1485, 1976.
35. Hahu, A.B., Barkin, R.L., and Oestreich, S.J.K.: Pharmacology in nursing, ed. 15, St. Louis, 1982, The C.V. Mosby Co.
36. Hanson, DR., and Fearn, R.W.: Hearing acuity in young people exposed to pop music and other noise, Lancet 2:203-205, 1975.
37. Hardy, B.P.: Assessment and instruction: don't push the hard-of-hearing child into the pit! Am. Ann. Deaf 120:555-557, 1975.
38. Harford, E.R.: Guidelines for hearing problems: substituting management for myth, Geriatrics 34(12):69-72, 1979.
39. Hatfield, E.M.: Why are they blind? Sight Sav. Rev. 45:3-22, 1975.
40. Hatfield, E.M.: Estimates of blindness in the United States, Sight Sav. Rev. 43:69-80, 1973.
41. Havener, W.H.: Ocular pharmacology, ed. 4, St. Louis, 1978, The C.V. Mosby Co.
42. Havighurst, R.: Optometry: education for the profession, Report of the National Study of the Optometric Education, Washington, D.C., 1973, National Commission on Accrediting.
43. Hearing aids and the older American, hearing before the Subcommittee on Consumer Interests, Washington, D.C., 1974, U.S. Government Printing Office.
44. Hemingway, W.G., and Bergstrom, L.: Symposium on congenital deafness, Otolaryngol. Clin. North Am. 4(2):369-399, 1971.
45. Hersch, L.B., and Amon, C.: A child has a hearing loss: reporting the diagnosis of handicaps in children and its impact on parents, Am. Ann. Deaf 120:568-571, 1975.
46. *Holm, C.: Deafness: common misunderstandings, Am. J. Nurs. 78:1910-1912, 1978.
47. Ivarsson, A., and Nilsson, P.: Advances in measurement of noise and hearing, Acta Otolaryngol. 366:1-67, 1980.
48. Jain, I., et al.: Cataractogenous effect of hair dyes, Ann. Ophthalmol. 11:1681-1685, 1979.
49. Jeffers, J., and Bailey, M.: Speechreading, Springfield, Ill., 1971, Charles C Thomas, Publisher.
50. Jensema, C.K.: A review of communication systems used by deaf-blind people, Am. Ann. Deaf 125:9-10, 1980.
51. *Jensen, D.: The silent minority, Nurs. '76 6(10):15-16, 1976.
52. *Johnson, J.H., and Cryan, M.: Homonymous hemianopsia: assessment and nursing management, Am. J. Nurs. 79:2131-2134, 1979.

---

*References preceded by an asterisk are particularly well suited for student reading.

53. Jones, M., and Tippett, T.: Assessment of the red eye, Nurse Pract. **5:**10-12, 1980.

54. Kabins, S.A.: Interactions among antibiotics and other drugs, J.A.M.A. **219:**206-212, 1972.

55. Katz, J.: Handbook of clinical audiology, ed. 2, Baltimore, 1978, The Williams & Wilkins Co.

56. Kiukaanniemi, H.: Speech discrimination of patients with high frequency hearing loss, Acta Otolaryngol. **89:**419-423, 1980.

57. Kornzweig, A.L.: The eye in old age, Am. J. Ophthalmol. **60:**835-843, 1965.

58. Kravitz, H., et al.: The cotton-tipped swab: a major cause of ear injury and hearing loss, Clin. Ped. Phil. **13:**965-970, 1974.

59. Kurtland, L.T., et al.: Epidemiology of neurologic and sense organ disorders, Cambridge, Mass., 1973, Harvard University Press.

60. Linnell, C., and Long, V., Sr.: The hearing-impaired infant: diagnosis and rehabilitation, Nurs. Clin. North Am. **5:**507-515, 1970.

61. Loveland, B.M.: The blind child in the hospital, A.O.R.N. J. **31:**256-259, 1980.

62. Lucente, F.E.: Psychological problems in otolaryngology, Laryngoscope **83:**1684-1689, 1973.

63. *Mamaril, A.P.: Sudden deafness, Am. J. Nurs. **76:**1992-1994, 1976.

64. Marlow, D.R.: Textbook of pediatric nursing, ed. 5, Philadelphia, 1977, W.B. Saunders Co.

65. Mattox, D.E.: Medical management of sudden hearing loss, Otolaryngol. Head Neck Surg. **88:**111-113, 1980.

66. Mausolf, F.A.: The eye and systemic disease, ed. 2, St. Louis, 1980, The C.V. Mosby Co.

67. McCrone, W.P.: Responding to classroom behavior problems among deaf children, Am. Ann. Deaf **125:**902-905, 1980.

68. Meyerhoff, W.L.: The management of sudden deafness, Laryngoscope **89:**1867-1868, 1979.

69. Morrison, A.: Management of sensorineural deafness, Reading, Mass., 1975, Butterworth Publishers, Inc.

70. Newell, F.: Ophthalmology: principles and concepts, ed. 5, St. Louis, 1982, The C.V. Mosby Co.

71. Northern, J.: Hearing disorders, Boston, 1976, Little, Brown & Co.

72. Northern, J., and Downs, M.: Hearing in children, ed. 2, Baltimore, 1978, The Williams & Wilkins Co.

73. Occupational Safety and Health Administration, U.S. Department of Labor: Williams-Steiger Occupational Safety and Health Act of 1970, Fed. Reg. **36:**105, March 1979 (revised).

74. Ohno, M.I.: The eye-patched patient, Am. J. Nurs. **71:**271-274, 1971.

75. Paparella, M.M., and Shumrick, D.A., editors: Otolaryngology, ed. 2, Philadelphia, 1980, W.B. Saunders Co.

76. Peck, A.F., et al.: Beliefs about public attitudes toward the blind, J. Rehabil. **46:**36-39, 1980.

77. Peyman, G.A., et al.: Principles and practices of ophthalmology, Philadelphia, 1980, W.B. Saunders Co.

78. Physicians Desk Reference, Oradel, N.J., 1981, Medical Economics Co.

79. Registry of interpreters for the deaf, 814 Thayer Ave., Silver Spring, MD 20910.

80. Research to Prevent Blindness, Inc.: Annual Report, New York, 1981, Research To Prevent Blindness, Inc.

81. *Reynolds, B.J.: Suddenly blind at 80, Nurs. '79 **9**(7):47-49, 1979.

82. Rose, M.: Coping behavior of physically handicapped children, Nurs. Clin. North Am. **10:**329-339, 1975.

83. Rubin, M.: Meeting the needs of hearing-impaired infants, Pediatr. Ann. **9:**46-50, 1980.

84. Ruben, M.: Contact lens practice, Baltimore, 1975, The Williams & Wilkins Co.

85. *Ruben, M.: Contact lenses, shells and prosthetics, Nurs. Times **68:**133-136, 1972.

86. *Sabatino, L.: Do's and dont's of deaf patient care, RN **39:**64-48, 1976.

87. Sahata, R.: Speech and hearing therapy, J. School Health **48:**534-537, 1978.

88. Sataloff, J.: Hearing loss, Philadelphia, 1980, J.B. Lippincott Co.

89. Sataloff, R.T.: Pediatric hearing loss, Pediatr. Nurs. **6**(5):16-18, 1980.

90. Saunders, W.H., et al.: Nursing care in eye, ear, nose, and throat disorders, ed. 4, St. Louis, 1979, The C.V. Mosby Co.

91. Schow, R.L., and Nerbonne, M.A.: Hearing levels among elderly nursing home residents, J. Speech Hear. Disord. **45:**124-132, 1980.

92. Schrader, E.S.: Perioperative nurses reassure ophthalmic patients, A.O.R.N. J. **30:**1066-1077, 1979.

93. *Shadick, M.H.: "I feel I'll be able to serve my patients more effectively because of my blindness," Occup. Health Nurs. **29**(2):16-18, 1981.

94. Sherman, F.S.: Pediatric management problems (inclusion blennorrhea), Pediatr. Nurs. **6:**18, 1980.

95. Simmons, F.B.: Diagnosis and rehabilitation of deaf newborns, A.S.H.A. **22:**475-479, 1980.

96. Simmons, F.B.: Acupuncture and hearing loss. In Northern, J.: Hearing disorders, ed. 2, Boston, 1978, Little, Brown & Co.

97. Smith, M.B.: Handbook of ocular toxicity, Acton, Mass., 1976, Publication Sciences Group, Inc.

98. Spar, H.G.: The deaf-blind. In Garrett, J.F., and Levine, E.S., editors: Rehabilitation practices with the physically disabled, ed. 2, New York, 1973, Columbia University Press.

99. *Stern, E.J.: Helping the person with low vision, Am. J. Nurs. **80:**1788-1790, 1980.

100. Sulkowski, W.J.: Industrial noise pollution and hearing impairment: problems of prevention, diagnosis, and certification criteria, Washington, D.C., 1980, Foreign Scientific Publications Department, U.S. National Center for Scientific, Technical, and Economic Information.

101. Support for vision research: interim report of the National Advisory Eye Council, U.S. Department of Health, Education and Welfare, no. (NIH) 76-1098, 1976.

102. Taub, H.: Acupuncture and sensorineural hearing loss, J. Speech Hear. Disord. **40:**427-433, 1975.

103. Taylor, I.G., et al.: A study of the causes of hearing loss in a population of deaf children with special references to genetic factors, J. Laryngol. Otol. **89:**899-914, 1975.

104. Vargo, S.: Auditory screening in the schools, J. School Health **50:**32-41, 1980.

105. Vision research program planning, U.S. Department of Health, Education and Welfare, no. (NIH) 75-664, vol. 1, 1975.

106. Ward, R.R.: Treatment of elderly adults with impaired hearing: resources, outcome, and efficiency, J. Epidemiol. Community Health **34:**65-58, 1980.

107. Wong, D., and Shah, C.P.: Identification of impaired hearing in early childhood, Can. Med. Assoc. J. **121:**529-532, 1979.

108. Wong, E.K., et al.: How ophthalmic drugs can fool you, RN **43:**36-44, 1980.

Classic

109. Carroll, F.J.: Blindness, Boston, 1961, Little, Brown & Co.

110. Gordon, R.D.: Experience with a visually disabled mother, Am. J. Nurs. **68:**1943-1945, 1968.

111. *Haddad, H.M.: Drugs for ophthalmologic use, Am. J. Nurs. **6:**324-327, 1968.

112. Kannapill, B.M., Hamilton, L.B., and Bornstein, H.: Signs for instructional purposes, Washington, D.C., 1969, Gallaudet College Press.

AUDIOVISUAL RESOURCES

Diseases causing inner-ear vertigo, Cincinnati, 1972, Video Digest, Inc. (Film, 30 min.)

Nursing techniques for the care of patients with impaired vision, Columbus, Ohio, Ohio State University. (Series of eight films.)

Churchill Films, producer: Silent world, muffled world, Washington, D.C., 1966, Deafness Research Foundation, National Audiovisual Center. (Film, 16 mm black and white, 28 min.)

Surgical management of chronic ear diseases, Cincinnati, 1970, Video Digest, Inc. (Film, 16 mm color, audiocassette or super 8 mm sound cartridge.)

Vestibular function in the dizzy patient, Rochester, Minn., 1976, American Academy of Ophthalmology and Otolaryngology. (Videotape, 43 min.)

CHAPTER 39

PROBLEMS OF SPECIAL SENSES: EYE AND EAR

LYNN CHENOWETH
LINDA ANNE BROSEMAN

Problems of the eye

The major disorders of the eye that can affect vision are trauma and infection in persons of all ages; strabismus in children; and cataract, glaucoma, retinal detachment and diabetic retinopathy in adults, primarily older adults. Information on assessment of the eye, prevention of visual impairment, general therapeutic intervention, and services for visually impaired persons is given in Chapters 37 and 38.

In order to decrease the problem of vision impairment, health workers need to focus on prevention of eye disease and injury, early detection of disease and injury, and adequate treatment. As participants in planning, providing, and evaluating health care, the nurse assumes responsibilities in all these areas.

Eye manifestations of systemic diseases

Diseases and infections that affect other parts of the body also affect the eye. The eye has been described as the most important square inch of body surface, both diagnostically and functionally.[37] By examining the back portion of the interior of the eyeball (fundus) with an ophthalmoscope, the practitioner can recognize many major diseases. Some of the diseases and pathologic states that can be identified through their typical fundus picture and other eye assessment include metabolic diseases, vascular and hematologic disorders, neurologic problems, and nutritional deficiencies. Assessment of the eye often will indicate the severity of the disease.

Metabolic diseases

Of the metabolic diseases affecting the eye, diabetes is the most common. Diabetes may affect any of the structures of the eye. Senile cataracts occur earlier in persons who have diabetes and progress more rapidly than in most elderly people. Diabetic retinopathy produces characteristic changes in the retina that can cause severe visual damage and eventually result in blindness. Diabetes also causes the growth of new blood vessels on the surface of the retina and optic disc that later extend into the vitreous humor (retinitis proliferans).

This condition often causes blindness due to recurrent vitreous hemorrhages and retinal detachment (p. 900, diabetic retinopathy).

Vascular and hematologic disorders

Vascular disorders, such as persistent systemic hypertension, will eventually produce changes in the retina (hemorrhage, edema, and exudates), which may result in the loss of sight. If the cause of the elevated blood pressure is eclampsia of pregnancy and is of short duration, the retinopathy (any disorder of the retina) usually subsides when the pregnancy is terminated. Retinopathy caused by hypertension resulting from renal arteriosclerosis or diffuse glomerulonephritis is usually progressive and irreversible. The severity of the hypertension causes narrowing of the retinal arteries, and the blood flow through the retina and choroid is diminished resulting in degenerative changes in the retina and loss of vision.

Visual loss may follow vascular accidents to vessels anywhere in the eye or in the main blood vessels outside the eye. A cerebrovascular accident may cause hemianopia (blindness for one half of the field of vision in one or both eyes) or total blindness, depending on its location. Arteriosclerosis and atheromatosis, particularly involving the carotid and cranial arteries, may release emboli that lead to occlusion of the retinal vessels.

Hematologic disorders cause characteristic retinal hemorrhages or neovascularization as in the case of sickle cell disease.

Neurologic problems

Neurologic disorders include a wide range of problems. Eye examination aids in evaluation of seven of the 12 cranial nerves (II through VIII) and provides information about the sympathetic and parasympathetic pathways (see Chapter 34). Demyelinating disorders (e.g., multiple sclerosis) and infections (e.g., syphilis) cause typical nerve damage to the eye. Increased intracranial pressure causes swelling of the optic disc (papilledema). Through eye examination (perimetry studies) lesions of the brain can be attributed to a specific lobe in the brain (temporal, parietal, or occipital). Unilateral dilation of the pupil helps diagnose severity and location of head injury.

Nutritional deficiencies

Nutritional deficiencies can cause pathologic changes in the eye. There seems to be direct relationship between good nutrition and eye health. A lack of vitamins A and B in the diet can cause changes in the conjunctiva, corneal epithelium, and retina. The lack of vitamins available for body use may also be caused by interference with absorptive, storage, or transport capacities. Tears are reduced, and eyes and lid margins become reddened and inflamed. Sensitivity to light is often present, and some loss of visual acuity is noticed at night. Significant difficulty is called night blindness (*nyctalopia*). If nutritionally caused, night blindness may respond favorably to ingestion of a nutritious diet and vitamin A. On the other hand, *excessive* amounts of vitamin A can damage the retina. Vitamin B deficiency may cause bilateral optic neuritis, especially in individuals who drink large quantities of alcohol. When damage to the optic nerve has been severe and prolonged, a diet high in vitamin B and other essential nutrients can accomplish only partial recovery. Fortunately, eye problems from nutritional deficiency are rarely found in the developed countries.

Trauma

Prevention

Although the eye is vulnerable to trauma, natural protective mechanisms can prevent or minimize injury (Table 39-1).

TABLE 39-1. Protective mechanisms of the eye

Protective feature	Function
Bony orbital rim	Prevents many mechanical injuries
Orbital fluids and tissues	Cushion direct blows
Eyelashes and eyelids	Quickly close reflexly from visual or mechanical stimuli
Bell phenomenon	Eyes reflexly rotate upward with lid closing to protect cornea
Lacrimal secretions	Can flush away chemicals or foreign bodies

TABLE 39-2. First aid for eye injuries

Injury	Interventions
Burns: chemical, flame	Flush eye immediately for 15 min with cool water or any available nontoxic liquid; seek medical assistance
Loose substance on conjunctiva: dirt, insects	Lift upper lid over lower lid to dislodge substance, produce tearing; irrigate eye with water if necessary; do not rub eye; obtain medical assistance if above interventions fail
Contact injury: contusion, ecchymosis, laceration	Apply cold compresses if no laceration present; cover eye if laceration present; seek medical assistance
Penetrating objects	Do not remove object; place protective shield over eye (e.g., paper cup); cover uninjured eye to prevent excess movement of injured eye; seek medical assistance.

In addition to the body's natural defenses against injury, *protective equipment* such as goggles, shields, and shatterproof safety lenses are advised for certain occupations and sports activities. Knowledge of safety precautions and first-aid techniques are valuable in preventing serious damage from trauma.

Prompt and appropriate care of the injured eye may prevent serious vision impairment or loss of the eye. (Table 39-2). The two major categories of trauma are *burns* and *contact* (mechanical) *trauma*.

Burns

Chemical burns, such as those caused by acid or alkali, must be treated immediately to prevent the possibility of permanent visual impairment from damage to the cornea. For chemical trauma of any nature, prompt immediate irrigation is the essential action that may result in salvaging an otherwise irrevocably lost eye. Irrigation after chemical trauma should be performed immediately after the injury and carried on for a prolonged period of time, a minimum of 15 minutes. While cool tap water is excellent for irrigation, any nontoxic solution can be used. After irrigation, and *only* after irrigation, is the patient transported to a physician.

Ultraviolet burns of the cornea may occur from exposure under a sunlamp. The individual becomes aware of painful eyes several hours after exposure. Treatment consists of cold compresses, analgesics (e.g., aspirin or codeine), and topical ophthalmic anesthetics. Topical antibiotics may also be used to prevent infection. Most patients are comfortable within 24 hours after treatment begins. Rarely is the cornea scarred permanently.[85] Ultraviolet burns may also occur from the use of germicidal lamps, electric flashes, and arc welding.

Thermal burns of the eyelids can cause lid contracture. Skin grafting may be necessary to prevent severe contractures and exposure of the eye. Full-thickness grafts can be taken from the uninjured eyelid, the inner aspect of the forearm, or behind the ear.[85]

Contact trauma

Lacerations of eyelid. Lacerations of the eyelid require treatment by an eye specialist because there is danger of scar formation as healing occurs. Although lid lacerations may bleed freely, pressure against the lid to stop bleeding can cause damage to the eye beneath. Cuts or tears in the eyelid may need to be sutured after the bleeding is controlled and any foreign material is removed. Antitetanus serum usually is given to all patients who sustain eye wounds.

Injuries to ciliary body, sclera, and orbit. Injuries to the ciliary body and sclera and injuries involving the orbit are critical because adjacent tissues usually are injured also and there may be escape of contents of the eyeball and possible infection of the interior of the eye. If these injuries result in wounds that are small and clean, treatment consists of bed rest, antibiotics given systemically and topically, suturing the wound, instilling atropine to put the iris and the ciliary body at rest, and a firm dressing. If the injury is extensive and if sight is lost, enucleation (removal of the eyeball) may be necessary.

Ecchymosis. Persons with ecchymosis of the eyelid and surrounding tissues (black eye) should be examined to rule out coexisting skull fractures and intraocular bleeding or other eye damage. Initially, cold compresses will help to control the bleeding. Subsequent warm compresses after 48 hours will speed up the reabsorption of blood from the tissues. The discoloration, which will last about 2 weeks, can be covered to some extent with cosmetics.

Penetrating injury. Penetrating injury of the eye requires medical care as soon as possible. The most important goal is to prevent further damage before reaching the ophthalmologist. It is easy to convert a minor corneal laceration without iris prolapse into the loss of an eye when applying even gentle pressure on the eye during transportation of the patient. To protect the eye against pressure, a shield can be used. A cardboard cone or a paper cup can be taped securely over the patient's eye to prevent anyone or anything from touching it. Tears, blood, and other discharges cannot be wiped away without risking dangerous pressure changes. Also, covering the *uninjured* eye will prevent excessive movement of the *injured* eye. While the patient may walk or be transported sitting up in an automobile, unnecessary exertion, such as bending over or carrying heavy objects, should be avoided. These activities could increase the intraocular pressure and cause more damage to the eye.

Corneal injuries. Corneal injuries are serious, because resistance to infection is low in the cornea, and scarring can impair vision. It has been estimated that foreign bodies on the surface of the cornea constitute about 25% of ocular injuries.[68] Tearing, photophobia, and a sensation of "something in the eye" warn a person that a foreign body is present if neuromuscular networks are functioning properly. If an abrasion of the cornea occurs, there may be considerable pain. For those persons with impaired sensorimotor function, the nurse must observe for damage to the cornea.

Sympathetic ophthalmia. Sympathetic ophthalmia is a serious inflammation of the uveal tract (ciliary body, iris, and choroid) in the *uninjured* eye that follows a penetrating injury to the other eye. While the cause of this condition is unknown, it may be caused by an allergic reaction to the uveal pigment that is set free in the bloodstream at the time of the injury. Children are especially susceptible; however, it may occur at any age. The uninjured eye becomes inflamed; photophobia, lacrimation, dimness of vision, and pain in the eye may be experienced. Sympathetic ophthalmia may appear 3 to 8 weeks after the eye injury or months or years later. The injured eye may be removed soon after the injury in an attempt to prevent the development of sympathetic ophthalmia. Because of increased medical skill in treating perforating wounds and the administration of cortisone at the earliest suggestion of inflammation, sympathetic ophthalmia has become a rare disease in recent years.

Infections and inflammation

Infections and inflammation can occur in any of the eye structures and may be caused by microorganisms, mechanical irritation, or sensitivity to some substance. Inflammation of the eye accounts for more than one half of the total incidence of acute disease conditions, with more than 1 million cases per year. Conjunctivitis represents about two thirds of the total.[92]

Styes

Styes (hordeola) are relatively mild but extremely common infections of the follicle of an eyelash or the small lubricating glands of the lid margins. Staphylococci are often the infecting organisms. These infections tend to occur in crops because the infecting organism spreads from one hair follicle to another. Poor hygiene and excessive use of cosmetics may be contributing causes. Patients should be taught not to squeeze styes because the infection may spread and cause cellulitis of the lids. If warm moist compresses are used, styes usually open and drain without surgery. A topical ophthalmic antibiotic may hasten healing.

Chalazion

A chalazion is a cyst caused by an obstruction in the ducts of the sebaceous glands (meibomian glands) located in the connective tissue in the free edges of the eyelids. The cysts present a hard, shiny, lumpy appearance as viewed from the inner side of the lid. They may cause pressure on the cornea. Small chalazions may disappear after massage, hot compresses, and topical antibiotics. If they are large or become infected, they usually require surgical incision and curettage. Chalazions usually are removed in the physician's office or in the clinic with the patient under local anesthesia. An antibacterial ointment (e.g., neomycin sulfate) may be applied to the conjunctiva, and an eyepad is worn for a few days.

Conjunctivitis and blepharitis

Etiology. Conjunctivitis (inflammation of conjunctiva) and blepharitis (inflammation of the eyelids) are common infections that can occur from a variety of causes. They may result from mechanical trauma, such as that caused by sunburn; or from infection with organisms, such as staphylococci, viruses, streptococci, or gonococci. Inflammation is often caused by allergic reactions within the body or outside irritants (e.g., poison ivy or cosmetics). Two of the viral agents that cause conjunctivitis are trachoma and herpes simplex.

Acute bacterial conjunctivitis. Acute bacterial conjunctivitis is often called "pinkeye." Common in school children, pinkeye is highly infectious. Conjunctival redness and crusting discharge deposited on the lashes and corners of the eye are the characteristic findings. Treatment includes cleansing of the lids and lashes, use of topical antibiotics, and precautions to prevent the spread to others. Firm adherent crusts may be softened by use of hot moist compresses. Because the material is infectious it should be disposed of in a sanitary way. Fortunately acute bacterial conjunctivitis is usually self-limited, leaving no permanent scars.

Seborrheic blepharitis. Seborrheic blepharitis often occurs in children and involves both upper and lower lids. The lid margins are reddened with scales attached to the base of the lashes. Some degree of conjunctivitis is present. Application of local antibiotics and local steroids is helpful. The condition can be kept under control if treated effectively before any serious eye involvement (e.g., keratitis) develops.

Trachoma. Trachoma (a form of conjunctivitis), although rare in the United States, is endemic in low-income persons living in the dry, hot Mediterranean countries and the Far East and is a major cause of blindness in these areas. It is caused by a strain of the virus *Chlamydia trachomatis*, and the disease is highly contagious in the early conjunctivitis stage and is spread by direct contact with the ocular discharge. Following the acute conjunctivitis stage, the eyelids become scarred, and granulations form on the inner surface on the lids and invade the cornea. The entire cornea may eventually become involved with subsequent loss of vision. Secondary bacterial infection is common.

Trachoma can be arrested in the early stages with topical and oral tetracycline. Eyelid granules may be removed surgically.

Conjunctivitis neonatorum. Newborn infants may develop conjunctivitis from bacteria and viruses acquired during the birth passage. The causative organism is often gonococcus but staphylococci, streptococci, and pneumonocci, as well as other bacteria and viruses, may also cause infection. Routine prophylaxis with 2 drops of 1% silver nitrate solution in each eye after birth has greatly reduced the incidence. Prognosis is good with topical antimicrobial treatment.

Keratitis

Etiology. Inflammation of the cornea is called keratitis. It may be acute or chronic and superficial or deep (interstitial). Acute epithelial keratitis commonly occurs in association with bacterial conjunctivitis caused by *Staphylococcus aureus, Streptococcus pneumoniae, Moraxella,* and *Pseudomonas aeruginosa*. Viruses such as herpes simplex may also cause a type of keratitis. Keratitis may be associated with a corneal ulcer or be caused by diseases such as tuberculosis and syphilis. Allergic reactions, vitamin A deficiency, or viral diseases (e.g., mumps, measles, and herpes simplex) may contribute to its development in children.

Clinical picture. Keratitis causes severe pain in the eye, photophobia (sensitivity to light), tearing, and blepharospasm (spasm of the eyelids). Uncontrolled keratitis can result in loss of vision caused by impairment of corneal transparency or destruction of the eye by corneal perforation.

Intervention. If possible, the systemic cause is found and treated. Cortisone may be used cautiously to control the inflammation. Except for herpes simplex, topical antibiotics are given to treat the infection. Atropine sulfate, which blurs visions for at least 1 week, will keep the iris and ciliary body at rest; hot compresses will help promote healing. Idoxuridine (IDU) applied locally is effective in helping to clear keratitis caused by herpes simplex in 80% of cases. The eyes may be covered to limit eye movements, and bed rest may be prescribed.

CORNEAL TRANSPLANTATION. When the cornea is so damaged that severe vision impairment occurs, *corneal grafting (keratoplasty)* may be done. Loss of vision caused by an opaque or destroyed cornea may be restored by replacing the damaged layers with a corresponding corneal graft obtained from a new cadaver or from an eye freshly removed by operation. For best results the donor cornea must be removed within 6 hours of death and ideally should be used within 24 hours. Transplants preserved for longer periods may be used for lamellar grafts. The present practice is to keep a waiting list of persons who need grafts, since eye banks are not able to keep up with the demand. Eye Bank for Sight Restoration, Inc.,* is a nonprofit organization that collects and distributes donated eyes throughout the country. Donors or their relatives usually make arrangements before death for donating the eyes.

Corneal transplantation cannot be done if there is any infection. The kind of corneal graft used depends on the depth and size of the damaged part that must be replaced (Fig. 39-1). Corneal transplants, or grafts, may involve the entire thickness of the cornea (total penetrating), only part of the depth of the cornea (lamellar), or a combination of these, in which a small part of the graft involves the entire thickness of the cornea (partial penetrating). Obviously, the penetrating graft is the more difficult to establish and requires the more definitive care postoperatively. For the penetrating graft, the eye surgeon seldom uses a donor eye that is over 48 hours old.

Because a large amount of tissue is removed and replaced, the patient who has had a penetrating graft transplant usually remains in bed with both eyes bandaged for 1 to 2 days so as not to disturb the graft. The patient who has had a mixed or partial penetrating graft usually has both eyes bandaged and is kept very quiet for at least 24 hours, whereas the patient who has had a lamellar graft only may not have the unaffected eye covered at all and may be out of bed and able to feed himself on the day of the operation. Corneal grafts heal very slowly because of the lack of blood vessels in the cornea and require from 3 weeks to 6 months to heal firmly. The patient is advised to avoid sudden, quick movement, jarring, bending, or lifting during this period in order to avoid disturbing the healing process. Success also depends on the basic disease process.

*210 E. 64th St., New York, NY 10021.

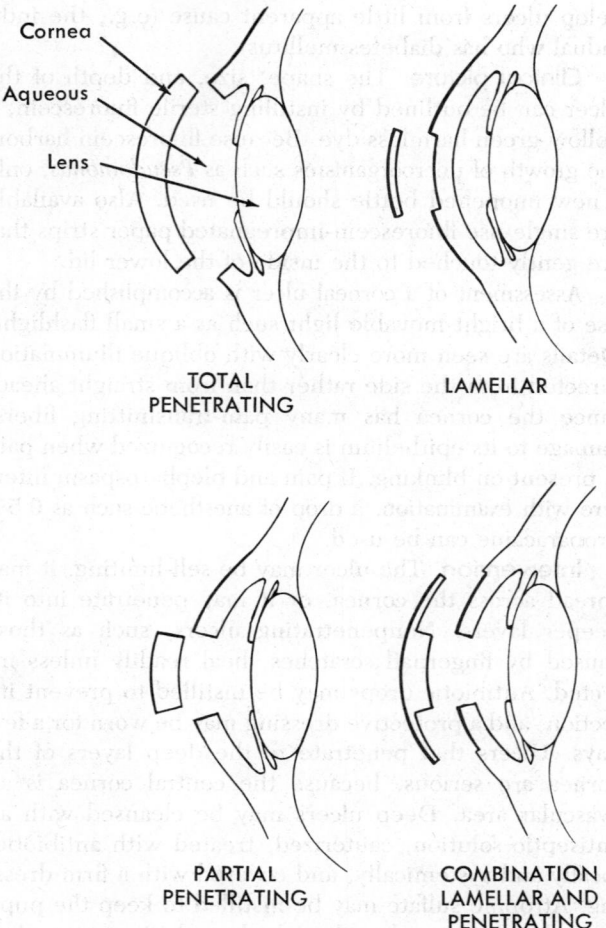

Fig. 39-1. Types of corneal grafts now being used. Note that in lamellar graft, defect does not penetrate entire thickness of cornea.

Complications of corneal transplant operations include blood vessels that grow into the new cornea (compensatory neovascularization), so that clarity may be lost, or clouding of the new cornea for no apparent reason. While the operation can usually be repeated, performing a second operation depends on the condition of the patient's eye.

Corneal ulcer

Etiology. Because of its location, the cornea is vulnerable to trauma and contamination with microorganisms. Infections of the cornea are not common occurrences. When present, however, they can lead to scarring, perforation, extensive intraocular infection, and loss of the eye. The ulcer may be caused by trauma, by contact lenses, or by infections of the conjunctiva that have spread to the cornea. Prompt treatment of ocular injuries can usually prevent the complication of infection. Persons with a low resistance to infection may develop ulcers from little apparent cause (e.g., the individual who has diabetes mellitus).

Clinical picture. The shape, size, and depth of the ulcer can be outlined by instilling sterile fluorescein, a yellow-green harmless dye. Because fluorescein harbors the growth of microorganisms such as *Pseudomonas,* only a new unopened bottle should be used. Also available are single-use fluorescein-impregnated paper strips that are gently touched to the inside of the lower lid.

Assessment of a corneal ulcer is accomplished by the use of a bright movable light such as a small flashlight. Details are seen more clearly with oblique illumination directed from the side rather than from straight ahead. Since the cornea has many pain-transmitting fibers, damage to its epithelium is easily recognized when pain is present on blinking. If pain and blepharospasm interfere with examination, a drop of anesthetic such as 0.5% proparacaine can be used.

Intervention. The ulcer may be self-limiting, it may spread across the cornea, or it may penetrate into its deeper layers. Nonpenetrating ulcers, such as those caused by fingernail scratches, heal readily unless infected. Antibiotic drops may be instilled to prevent infection, and a protective dressing may be worn for a few days. Ulcers that penetrate to the deep layers of the cornea are serious, because the central cornea is an avascular area. Deep ulcers may be cleansed with an antiseptic solution, cauterized, treated with antibiotics locally and systemically, and covered with a firm dressing. Atropine sulfate may be instilled to keep the pupil dilated and to put the ciliary body and iris at rest, thus reducing pain. Hot compresses may be applied to help clear the infection, and cortisone may be administered cautiously to control the inflammation. When the corneal ulcer causes impaired vision, corneal transplant may be done (p. 889).

Uveitis

The uvea or uveal tract is a vascular and pigmented layer of the eye that includes the choroid, the ciliary body, and the iris. Inflammation of the area is referred to as uveitis.

Etiology. Inflammatory lesions of the uvea are caused by a wide variety of factors and infectious agents, which may involve one portion or all three simultaneously. Etiologic classification includes infection, allergy, trauma, toxic agents, noninfective systemic diseases (e.g., diabetes), and unknown factors. The specific cause of most cases of uveitis cannot be diagnosed.[85]

Clinical picture. Uveitis produces pain in the eyeball radiating to the forehead and temple, photophobia (sensitivity to light), lacrimation, and interference with vision. There is edema of the upper lid, the iris is swollen because of congestion and exudation of cells and fibrin, and the pupil is contracted and irregular as a result of the formation of adhesions.

Intervention. The instillation of 0.3% scopolamine into the eye puts the iris and ciliary body at rest, relieves pain and photophobia, and diminishes congestion. By keeping the pupil dilated, a cycloplegic drug prevents adhesions from forming between the anterior capsule of the lens and the iris and tends to cause those already formed to regress. Moist, warm compresses may be applied several times each day to help diminish pain and inflammation. The eyes usually are covered, and in the convalescent period dark glasses are ordered to be worn. The patient is on bed rest during the acute stages. Although acetylsalicylic acid (aspirin) may be helpful for relieving pain, sometimes morphine sulfate is necessary. Cortisone preparations are of great value in controlling the inflammation in many patients, but the inflammation in other patients resists almost all forms of treatment. If a systemic cause cannot be found and treated, the injection of a foreign protein (fever therapy) such as the typhoid H antigen into the body to stimulate its defense mechanism may be used. Complications of these infections of the uvea include the formation of adhesions, keratitis, secondary glaucoma, and the loss of vision.

Outcome criteria for the person with inflammation of the eye

The person or significant others can:
1. State name, dosage, and frequency of eye medication to be taken and the need to destroy unused ophthalmic antibiotics after therapy.
2. Describe method and frequency of eye compresses to be used.
3. Describe measures to prevent spread of infection to the uninvolved eye.
4. Describe the activity and movements that are to be avoided after corneal grafting.
5. Describe measures to prevent spread of eye infection to others in the household.

Strabismus

Strabismus (squint, cross-eye, and walleye) is characterized by misalignment of the visual axes. Normally, when both eyes look at the same object, the image of the object is fused by the brain into a single picture (fusion). When there is fusion of the two images perceived by the eyes, binocular vision is present, providing stereoscopic (three-dimensional) vision for the individual.

Etiology

Strabismus may be paralytic or nonparalytic. *Paralytic* strabismus (inability to move the eye) is caused by loss of function of the ocular muscles resulting from damage to the muscles or the cranial nerves (III, IV, or

VI) by tumor, infection, or brain or eye injuries. Its main symptom, in addition to the strabismus, is double vision (diplopia).

Nonparalytic strabismus affects 1% of the population. The child may look straight with either the right eye or the left eye but not with both simultaneously. Alternating strabismus consists of fixing (looking straight ahead) with one eye and then with the other eye. Monocular strabismus is the constant use of one eye (the preferred eye) to the exclusion of the other eye.

Prevention

Any child who does not have straight eyes at birth or shortly after should be considered to have strabismus and be examined promptly. Although loss of sight from strabismus is *preventable*, it is the most common cause of partial blindness in one eye in children. It usually can be treated successfully before the child is 6 years of age. The younger the child, the easier is the treatment. The public health nurse and the school nurse should be particularly alert to children who show signs of strabismus and should direct them to medical care. The establishment of free preschool vision screening programs for children in the 3- to 5-year-old age group has been extremely helpful in getting the child with strabismus referred for treatment early enough to be treated satisfac-

torily. A health teaching packet, including an attractive story booklet designed by two nurses, has been developed to encourage mothers to seek eye testing for their children.* There is no cheaper, easier, or more rewarding way to restore vision to an otherwise legally blind eye than by simply patching the eye of a young child with strabismus. It is extremely important that these children be identified, referred, and properly treated.

Clinical picture

Evaluation of strabismus includes physical examination to rule out major cerebral and ocular disease, refraction with use of a cycloplegic drug to discover errors of refraction, and orthoptic evaluation to measure the angle of strabismus. During examination, when the child with strabismus looks straight ahead with one eye, the other deviates. A light source directed straight into normal eyes forms a reflected spot image symmetrically located in each pupil; in strabismus, the image is off center in one eye compared with its location in the other eye. The crossing may be slight or noticeable. If the eye is turned inward toward the nose, it is called convergent strabismus *(esotropia)*. If the eye is turned outward, it is called divergent strabismus *(exotropia)* (Fig. 39-2). If the child never uses the crossed eye, impaired vision may result. This type of defective vision is called *amblyopia*.

*Lazy Eye, Ltd., P.O. Box 161, Eau Claire, WI 54701.

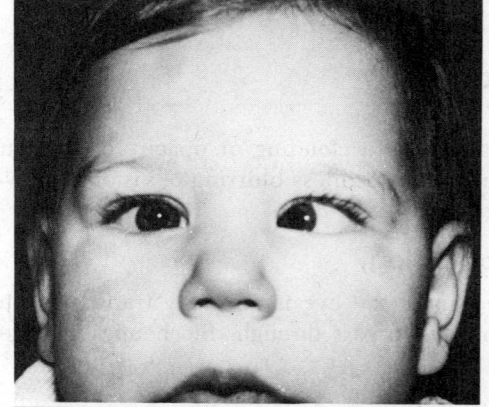

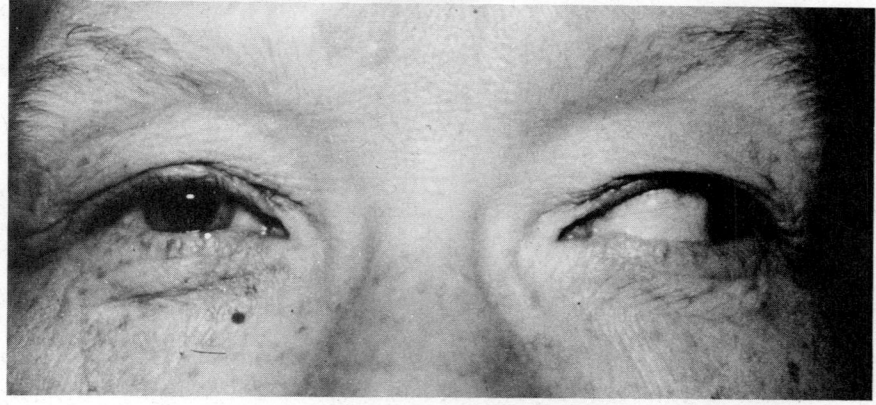

Fig. 39-2. A, Esotropia with right eye fixing and left eye deviating. There is slight epicanthus bilaterally. **B,** Comitant exotropia. (From Newell, F.W.: Ophthalmology: principles and concepts, ed. 5, St. Louis, 1982, The C.V. Mosby Co.)

Pathophysiology

When the two eyes are not coordinated and send two different mental images to the brain, fusion cannot occur. Inability to obtain fusion causes diplopia or suppression. *Diplopia* is referred to as double vision. It is possible for normal healthy persons to experience transient diplopia when they are tired or have ingested too much alcohol. These are cases of temporary failure of fusion mechanisms in the brain. In *suppression,* the mental image from one eye is ignored. Suppression of the image from one eye occurs as a normal cerebral phenomenon when a monocular microscope is used. With both eyes open, the viewer is able to see the magnified field and to disregard the picture of the table top perceived by the other eye. In strabismus, however, suppression of vision in one eye may lead to irreversible vision impairment called *suppression* (strabismic) *amblyopia.*

In amblyopia, vision is reduced in an eye that appears normal on examination. Suppression amblyopia refers to cerebral blocking of vision in an eye that either is deviated (crossed, strabismic) or has a refractive error more marked than that of the "good" eye.

Intervention

Early medical attention is important in strabismus, both to save vision and to prevent the emotional trauma that is always associated with crossed eyes. Treatment should begin as soon as the diagnosis is made. During early childhood, *occlusion* is used to improve vision. The "good" eye is covered with a patch, bandage, or attachment to the glasses, forcing the child to use the weaker eye. The length of time necessary for occlusion might be as short as 1 or 2 days in a 6-month-old child, 1 or 2 months in a 6-year-old child, and 1 or 2 years in an 8-year-old child. *Orthoptics* is nonsurgical treatment of strabismus in which prisms, glasses, and exercises are used to train the child to use the two eyes together. Orthoptics is used as an adjunct to other methods of treating strabismus.

Strabismus in children who are farsighted and who accommodate excessively may be corrected by constantly wearing glasses. Glasses with harness frames can be safely worn by children 5 to 6 months of age. As children become more independent, it is sometimes difficult to get them to wear glasses consistently. When the glasses are removed, the eyes tend to cross. Long-acting miotics such as isoflurophate (DFP) instilled daily potentiates constriction of the ciliary muscle and helps to diminish the esotropia. Sometimes the use of glasses and the use of drugs are combined.

Surgery to correct strabismus may be performed early (by 6 months of age) in an attempt to prevent the loss of fusion potential (binocularity). In most patients, particularly esotropic patients, the younger the child when surgery is performed, the more the likelihood of restoring binocular vision. After the age of 6 years, surgery may achieve only cosmetic improvement and may not restore fusion, particularly in esotropic patients. Surgery consists of shortening or lengthening the muscle to straighten the eye. The child may wear a dressing over the eye for a few days and is permitted to move about freely. Surgery may be followed by the prescription of corrective glasses and eye exercises, depending on the individual patient. The child's family should understand that the operation may need to be repeated. Parents should be encouraged to continue with medical treatment for as long as recommended. If they believe that the condition is completely cured and neglect medical attention until a conspicuous squint again appears, damage to vision may have occurred.

Cataract

A cataract is a clouding or opacity of the lens that leads to gradual painless blurring of vision and eventual loss of sight (Fig. 39-3).

Pathophysiology

The lens of the eye is normally transparent to permit light rays to pass through. Biochemical changes may

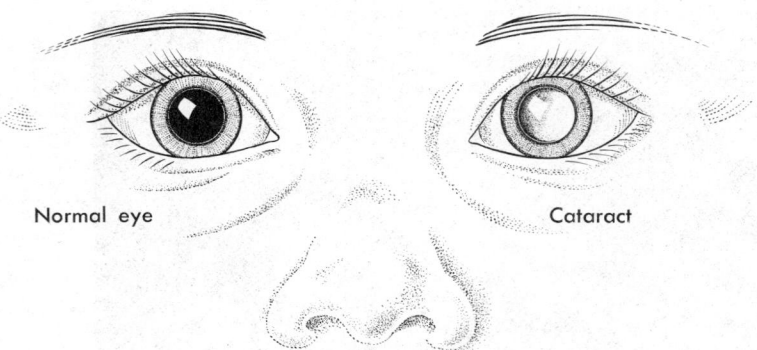

Normal eye   Cataract

Fig. 39-3. Cataract visible in left eye as white opacity of lens seen through pupil.

occur within the lens; or trauma may cause fiber changes that cause the lens to become cloudy and finally opaque, thus blocking the light rays from reaching the retina. The term *mature cataract* refers to a developed cataract that separates easily from the lens capsule. It was previously thought that a cataract had to become mature or "ripe" before it could be extracted. Now cataracts are removed whenever the decreased vision interfers with the person's activities of daily living (ADL). If both eyes develop cataracts, these usually develop at different rates.

Etiology

In general, cataracts are classified as *senile,* those associated with aging; *traumatic,* those associated with injury; *congenital,* those that occur at birth; or *secondary,* those that occur following other eye diseases.

Cataracts occur so often in the elderly that the term *senile cataract* is used. At 80 years of age, about 85% of all persons have some clouding of the lens. Senile cataracts are listed as the most common cause of blindness in older persons, yet the response of the condition to surgery often is excellent.

After aging, the next most common cause of cataract is injury to the eye.[37] The transparency of the lens may be destroyed by either a penetrating wound or a contusion. Cataracts may result from the ingestion of injurious substances such as dinitrophenol or naphthalene. Some researchers report that cataracts may result from systemic absorption of hair dyes.

While most cataracts occurring at birth (congenital) are hereditary, they may be caused by virus infections such as German measles that the mother had during the first trimester of pregnancy. Cataracts account for 11.5% of blindness in preschool children.[39] When assessing a child's eyes, the cataract may be obvious and appear as a white pupil. Cataracts also may be present in a child with strabismus, decreased visual acuity, family history of the disease, and other ocular or systemic defects. Treatment of cataracts in children depends on the degree of visual impairment and associated anomalies.

Cataracts may also occur secondary to eye diseases, such as uveitis or eye trauma; or with systemic diseases, such as diabetes mellitus, galactosemia, or sarcoidosis.

Clinical picture

Acquired cataracts resulting from aging or disease usually develop gradually. Blurring of vision may occur immediately following trauma. The predominant symptom is progressive loss of vision; the degree of loss depends on the location and extent of the opacity. Persons with an opacity in the center portion of the lens can generally see better in dim light when the pupil is dilated. The person with presbyopia may find that reading without glasses is possible in the early stages because of resulting myopia. The ophthalmoscope and the slit lamp are used to examine the lens through a dilated pupil.

Intervention

Operative treatment is the only method for treating cataracts. Unlike most other damaging diseases of the eye, vision loss from cataract can be restored by surgical removal of the cataract. Even patients who are in their 90s can often be operated on with good results. From 90% to 95% of all cataract operations are successful.[92] The decision as to when to remove the cataract depends largely on the general health of the patient and the use made of the eyes. Surgery is advised when the cataract interferes with a person's visual needs or when the cataract may lead to other eye complications such as glaucoma.

Because surgery is usually indicated only for advanced cataracts, elderly persons may believe they should wait until vision loss is far advanced before seeing an ophthalmologist. Delaying medical examination of the eye can lead to permanent vision loss if the problem is glaucoma or a combination of glaucoma and cataracts.

It is the nurses's responsibility to explain the disease, refer the person with a suspected cataract to an ophthalmologist, and encourage acceptance of treatment as recommended. Informational material designed to educate patients about cataracts is available.[37]

Cataracts usually are removed with the patient under local anesthesia. Removal has been simplified in many cases by the use of the enzyme alpha-chymotrypsin (α-chymotrypsin), which weakens the zonular fibers that hold the lens in position. Cataracts may be removed within their capsule (*intracapsular technique*), or an opening may be made in the capsule and the lens lifted out without disturbing the membrane (*extracapsular technique*).

To remove the lens and its capsule, instruments such as a forceps or vacuum cup are used. Another method is *cryoextraction*. In this case, the cataract is lifted from the eye by a small probe (cooled to a temperature below zero) that adheres to the wet surface of the cataract. All these procedures usually are preceded by an iridectomy, performed to create an opening for the flow of aqueous humor, which may become blocked postoperatively when the vitreous humor moves forward.

Congenital cataracts are never removed intracapsularly, because the capsule is adherent to the vitreous face. The method used to remove a congenital cataract depends on the size of the eye and the size of the pupil. Children may be operated on for cataract removal as early as 6 months of age.

A newer method of cataract removal is called *phacoemulsification*. This procedure breaks up the lens and flushes it out in tiny pieces. The phacoemulsification method requires an incision just large enough to insert a needle probe that vibrates 40,000 times per second to break up the lens. As the lens is broken up, the area is flushed with fluid, and pieces of the lens are carried from the eye by a tiny suction unit. Only one stitch is needed to close the incision. Healing and convalescence are considerably quicker than for patients who have had cryosurgical removal previously described. The size and shape of the eye are factors in determining if this method is suitable for a particular patient.

Postoperative care. For general care after eye surgery, see p. 869. Following any cataract operation, a dressing is applied to the eye and covered with a metal shield to protect it from injury. During the hospital stay of 1 to 3 days, the surgeon changes the dressing daily; at home the patient or family also may change the dressing daily. After 7 to 10 days, all dressings are removed. During the first month, protection of the operated eye with a metal shield at night is important. Eyedrops and moist warm compresses also may be ordered. Postoperative resumption of normal activities is much more rapid than in earlier years because of advancements in techniques of lens extraction and suturing.

If vision in the unoperated eye is not good, the patient will need considerable assistance and supervision to meet safety needs. Temporary glasses may be prescribed 1 to 4 weeks after surgery, depending on the rate of healing and the amount of vision in the other eye. Usually after 6 to 12 weeks, healing has been sufficient for the fitting of permanent glasses or contact lenses. Soft contact lenses, made from a porous flexible plastic, are now often used in place of the older hard lenses (p. 863).

The elderly person sometimes finds it difficult to adjust to removal of a cataract. The little remaining ability to accommodate the eye is lost when the lens is removed, and the patient must wear corrective lenses at all times.

Cataract glasses. While cataract glasses do restore sight, there are some problems inherent in strong glasses that cannot be avoided. The health care worker needs to be familiar with the characteristics of cataract glasses so that the patient can be helped to adjust[84]:

1. *Cataract lenses magnify.* Everything appears about one fourth closer than it is. For example, the patient may reach for a coffee cup but grasp in front of it and knock it over. This distortion of distance also causes problems in climbing stairs and many other activities.
2. *Cataract lenses distort peripheral images.* Because clear vision is only possible through the center of the lens, the wearer must learn to turn the head farther and more frequently to ensure safety.
3. *Thick lenses are heavy.* Pressure sores on the nose and ears can be troublesome. Lighter weight plastic lenses are now being made, which are much more comfortable than the glass lenses and create less peripheral distortion.
4. *Colors may be distorted.* The colors of objects seen with the eye from which the lens has been removed are slightly different.
5. *Inaccurate positioning causes distortion.* Accurate positioning of cataract glasses is important to prevent distortion. If the glasses are dropped or bumped, they should be readjusted so that they are at the correct angle and distance from the eye.

Contact lenses. Younger persons and some older persons prefer to use contact lenses after cataract surgery. On the other hand, some elderly persons may have difficulty inserting the lenses or may reject the idea without trying them. The advantages of contact lenses include improved visual correction and better cosmetic appearance. Use of contact lenses is especially recommended when only one lens is removed. Unilateral removal of a lens causes a difference in the size of the optical images perceived by the brain. This causes difficulty with binocular vision, and the person can effectively use only one eye at a time.

Lens implant. An alternative to cataract glasses and contact lenses is an artificial lens implant (intraocular lens). The lens, which is made of polymethylmethacrylate, is implanted at the time of cataract extraction. It may be held in position either by a suture to the iris (iris fixation) or by implanting it into the capsular sac. Advantages of the implanted lens include better binocular vision. When the lens is implanted without sutures, miotic agents (pilocarpine) are needed to prevent the iris from dilating too widely and causing the lens to slip.[46] Cataract glasses produce about 24% larger images on the retina than the normal eye, contact lenses produce 8%, and the implanted lens produces only 2%.[71]

Now becoming more widespread in the United States, implantation of intraocular lenses was first used in England in 1953. Several patients who underwent the procedure in 1953 have retained highly satisfactory results. Currently, the implantation procedure is generally restricted to physically handicapped and elderly persons, (those not likely to succeed with a contact lens) and is restricted to one eye. The surgeon must be skilled and well trained in this procedure. Studies are currently being conducted to establish additional guidelines for selection of likely patients and for improved surgical techniques that will keep complications at a minimum.

Outcome criteria for the person with cataract extraction

The person or significant others can:
1. Demonstrate method of changing the eye dressing.

2. State name, dosage, and frequency of any eye-drops to be given.
3. Describe extent of activity to be permitted.
   a. Avoidance of bending over.
   b. Avoidance of Valsalva's maneuver.
4. Describe expected changes in vision with and without lenses.
5. State need for follow-up by ophthalmologist.

Glaucoma

Epidemiology

The term *glaucoma* designates eye disease characterized by increased intraocular pressure associated with progressive loss of peripheral visual fields. Glaucoma is responsible for 12% to 15% of all blindness in the United States today.[37,85] About 2% of persons over the age of 40 years have glaucoma. It has been estimated that nearly 1 million persons in the United States have glaucoma that has not been diagnosed. The incidence of glaucoma is increasing as the number of older persons in our population rises. While it is seldom seen in persons under 35 years of age, it does occur in infancy. Glaucoma is the greatest threat to vision in older persons. It is important to detect and treat this disease because the permanent vision loss it causes is preventable.

In either chronic or acute glaucoma, early diagnosis and treatment are mandatory to prevent destruction of nerve fibers on the optic disk from increased intraocular pressure. Mass screening programs are important in detecting possible glaucoma in persons who do not have periodic medical eye examinations.

Pathophysiology

The anterior cavity of the eye in front of and to the sides of the lens is filled with aqueous humor, a free-flowing clear liquid similar to lymph. Aqueous humor is constantly being formed in the ciliary body located posterior to the iris, and it flow through the pupil into the anterior chamber (Fig. 39-4). The aqueous humor drains through Schlemm's canal, which encircles the eye and is located in the trabecular meshwork at the angle of the anterior chamber where the peripheral iris and cornea meet. Schlemm's canal is a thin-walled vein that permits the passage of particles as large as protein molecules to prevent increase in osmotic pressure.

Normally, there is a balance between the production and drainage of aqueous humor permitting the intraocular pressure to remain relatively constant. The normal range of intraocular pressure is 10 to 21 mm Hg, with a mean value of 16 mm Hg. The pressure may vary up to 5 mm Hg as a result of diurnal changes.[4]

Glaucoma results when the intraocular pressure is increased sufficiently to produce damage to the optic nerve. In most cases, the increased pressure results from obstruction to drainage of the aqueous humor from degenerative changes (chronic simple glaucoma). The

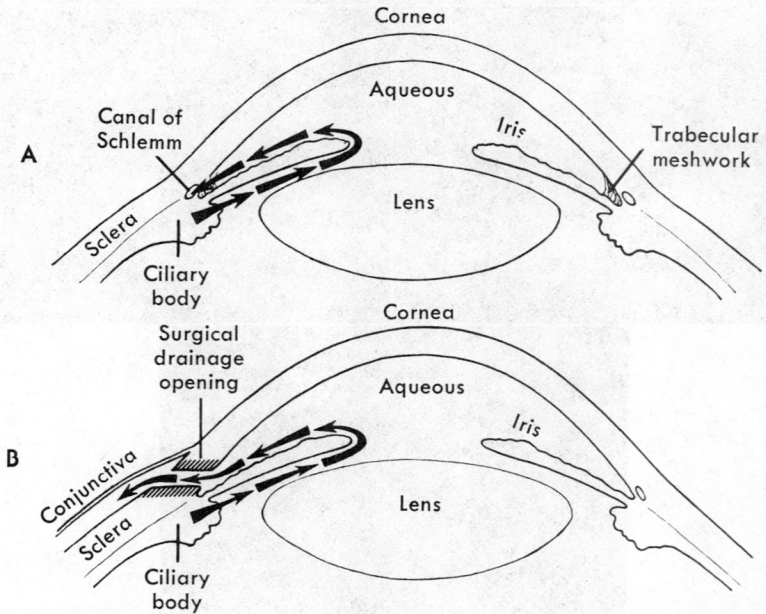

Fig. 39-4. A, Originating from ciliary processes, aqueous flows through pupil into anterior chamber and normally leaves eye by way of canal of Schlemm. **B,** In glaucoma, normal aqueous outflow is blocked. Purpose of glaucoma surgery is to create new channel through which aqueous can leave eye. (From Havener, W.H.: Synopsis of ophthalmology, ed. 5, St. Louis, 1979, The C.V. Mosby Co.)

blockage may also be secondary to infection or trauma. Most rarely, glaucoma results from abnormal placement of the iris against the angle of the anterior chamber, thus blocking the outflow of aqueous humor (acute angle closure glaucoma).

Chronic simple glaucoma

Clinical picture. The most common type of glaucoma is chronic simple glaucoma, also known as *wide-angle* or *open-angle* glaucoma. At first symptoms may be absent. Progression of the disease is slow and insidious. Permanent vision loss may occur before the individual is aware of having the disease.

Chronic glaucoma gives one characteristic sign that is important: before central vision becomes affected, the peripheral visual fields are impaired so that objects to the side are not seen (Fig. 39-5). Limitation of vision may not be so apparent as in other eye diseases, and

much damage can occur before medical assistance is sought. Patients may bump into other persons in the street or fail to see passing vehicles, yet not realize that the fault lies in their own vision. A diminished field of vision may cause the driver of an automobile to have an accident. The loss of peripheral vision ("tunnel vision") can progress until legal blindness is reached, yet the person may be able to see well straight ahead. The community nurse who recognizes this difficulty may be most helpful in early case finding and in promptly referring patients to an ophthalmologist. Because vision loss caused by glaucoma is irreversible, early diagnosis is mandatory.

Chronic glaucoma usually begins in one eye, although if it is left untreated, both eyes often become affected. Symptoms are most apparent in the morning, when a persistent dull eye pain may develop. Frequent changes of glasses, difficulty in adjusting to darkness,

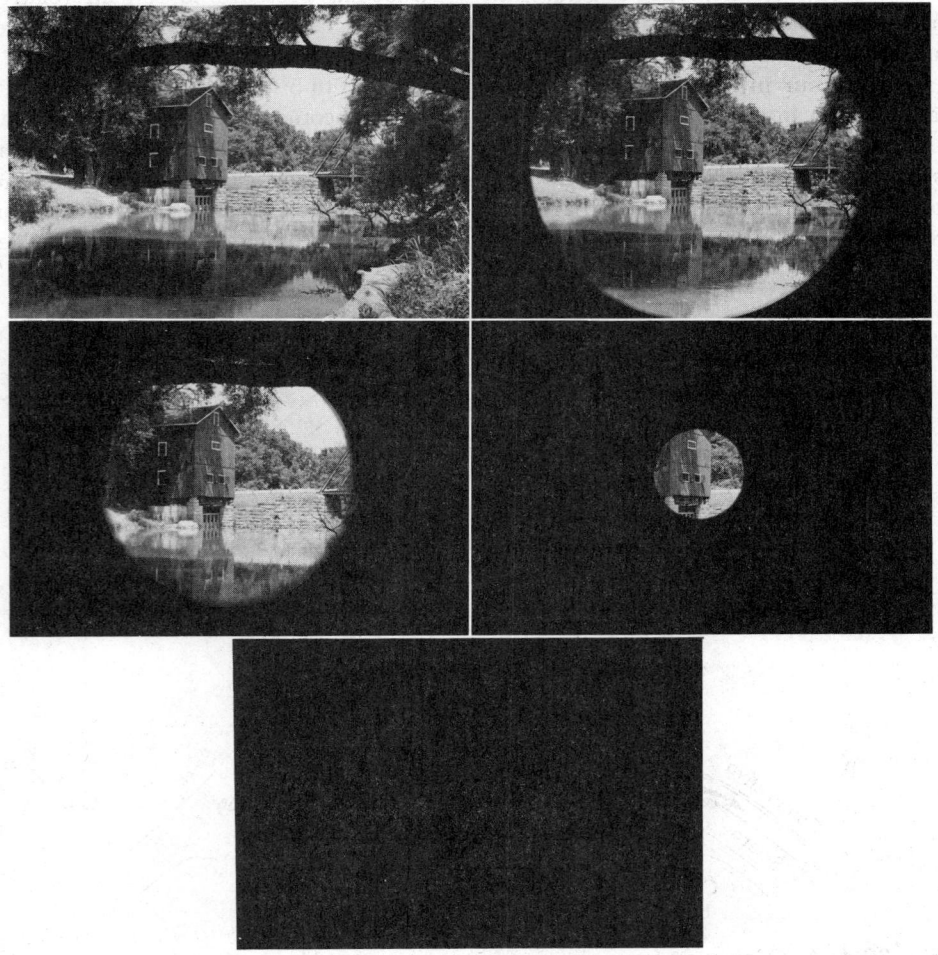

Fig. 39-5. Gradual loss of sight from glaucoma so insidiously destroys vision that person is unaware of impending blindness until extensive and irreversible damage is already present. (From Saunders, W.H., et al.: Nursing care in eye, ear, nose, and throat disorders, ed. 4, St. Louis, 1979, The C.V. Mosby Co.)

failure to accurately detect changes in color, and slight blurring of vision are fairly early signs of open-angle glaucoma. This is followed by a steamy appearance of the cornea and further blurring of vision. Tearing, misty vision, blurred appearance of the iris (which becomes fixed and dilated), headache, pain behind the eyeball, nausea, and vomiting can then occur. Halos, resembling streetlights seen through a steamy windshield, may be seen around lights.

Intervention. Treatment of chronic simple glaucoma is designed to reduce intraocular pressure and keep it at a safe level. Miotics such as pilocarpine are used to constrict the pupil and to draw the smooth muscle of the iris away from Schlemm's canal to permit aqueous humor to drain out at this point. Acetazolamide (Diamox), a drug that tends to reduce the formation of aqueous humor, is used successfully in some types of chronic glaucoma.

Surgery may be performed to produce a permanent filtration pathway for aqueous fluid. Filtering procedures, such as *trabeculectomy, sclerotomy, iridencleisis,* and *trephine* operations, provide a permanent fistula from the anterior chamber to the subconjunctival space. In selected cases, the production of aqueous fluid may be decreased by destroying part of the ciliary body. This may be accomplished by diathermy or cryosurgery. Following surgery, the patient usually is allowed out of bed at once, although one or both eyes may be bandaged for several days. Postoperative management of patients having eye surgery is discussed on p. 869.

Acute-angle closure glaucoma (narrow-angle glaucoma)

Clinical picture. Acute glaucoma has been described as one of the most dramatic and rapidly destructive diseases of the eye.[37] Characteristically, there is severe eye pain, which may radiate to any part of the head. Because nausea, vomiting, and abdominal pain also commonly occur, the primary problem is sometimes thought to be abdominal. Additional signs and symptoms include blurred vision, colored halos around lights, dilated pupil, reddened appearance of the eye, and increased intraocular pressure. Since a marked increase in intraocular pressure for 24 to 36 hours may lead to complete and permanent blindness, immediate treatment is necessary.

A relatively rare disease, acute glaucoma occurs when the iris blocks the outflow of aqueous humor. In an eye with a narrowed peripheral angle of the anterior chamber, dilation of the pupil caused by darkness, excitement, or a mydriatic drug may cause blockage of the outflow mechanism.

Intervention. Treatment consists of lowering intraocular pressure by increasing the outflow of aqueous humor and by decreasing the rate of its production. Miotics are given to constrict the pupil. Carbonic an-

hydrase inhibitors (Diamox) may be given orally or intravenously to reduce the production of aqueous humor. Osmotic agents such as glycerol also act to reduce the pressure of acute glaucoma. When the pressure is reduced and the eye is less inflamed, a portion of the peripheral iris is surgically excised (iridectomy). (See Table 39-3 for drugs used in glaucoma.) Prophylactic surgery on the fellow eye may be performed.

Other types of glaucoma

Congenital glaucoma, which is rare, may be present at birth or may develop in the first few months of life. Surgery is necessary to correct the abnormal development of the filtration angle and allow normal aqueous flow.

Secondary glaucoma occurs when the rise in intraocular pressure is caused by some other eye condition, such as uveitis, trauma, or a postoperative complication.

Absolute glaucoma is the end result of uncontrolled glaucoma. The eye is hard, sightless, and may be painful. Enucleation is often recommended to relieve the discomfort.

Long-term care

The person with glaucoma needs assistance in understanding and learning to live with the disease. Despite explanations from the physician, the person frequently hopes that an operation will cure the condition, that no further treatment will be necessary, and perhaps that the lost sight will be restored. It should be explained that the lost vision cannot be restored but that further loss can usually be prevented and life can be quite normal if the person continues under medical care. There usually is no restriction on the use of the eyes. Fluid intake generally is not curtailed, and exercise is permitted. Bright lights or darkness are not harmful to the eyes of the patient with glaucoma. There is apparently no relationship between vascular hypertension and ocular hypertension.[37]

The person with glaucoma should be under medical care for the rest of life, receiving either drug or surgical therapy, or both. One operation does not necessarily mean that drainage will be continued. Any obstruction or closing of the artificial pathway will result in reappearance of symptoms and further visual damage. The patient and family should know specifically what to do if essential eyedrops are accidentally spilled; for example, they should know which local drugstore is open at night and on holidays. The patient often is advised to have an extra bottle of medication in the home and to carry one, if working away from home. It is advisable also for the patient to carry a card or other information to identify having glaucoma in case an accident occurs.

Nurses and other health care workers must determine whether their patient has been treated for glau-

TABLE 39-3. Drugs used in treatment of glaucoma

Drug	Form	Dose
Cholinergic drugs (miotics)		
Pilocarpine	0.5-3% solution (Ocusert)	1 drop q 6 hr
		20-40 µg/hr for 1 wk
Carbachol (Carbacel)	0.25-3% solution	1 drop q 6-8 hr
Cholinesterase inhibitors (miotics)		
Physostigmine (Eserine)	0.25-1% solution or ointment	1 drop q 6-8 hr
Isoflurophate (DFP) (Floropryl)	0.01-0.1% solution	1 drop q 24-48 hr
Demecarium bromide (Humorsol)	0.125-0.25% solution	1 drop q 12-24 hr
Echothiophate iodide (Phospholine iodide)	0.06-0.125% solution	1 drop q 12-24 hr
Adrenergic agents		
Epinephryl borate (Eppy)	0.5-1% solution	1 drop q 12 hr, often used
Epinephrine hydrochloride (Glaucon)	0.5-2% solution	with miotic such as cholines-
Epinephrine bitartrate (Epitrate)		terase inhibitor
	2% solution	
Carbonic anhydrase inhibitors		
Acetazolamide (Diamox)	125-250 mg tablets	1 tablet q 6 hr
	500 mg capsules, sequential	1 capsule q 12 hr
	500 mg vials for IM or IV use	IM or IV if patient vomiting
Ethoxzolamide (Cardrase)	125-250 mg tablets	1 tablet q 6-12 hr
Dichlorphenamide (Daranide)	25-50 mg tablets	1 tablet q 6-12 hr
Methazolamide (Neptazane)	25-50 mg tablets	1 tablet q 6-12 hr
Osmotic agents		
Glycerin (glycerin, Osmoglyn, Ophthal-gan)	Mix with equal amount of orange juice (oral)	1-1.5 ml/kg body wt
Mannitol (Osmitrol)	10-20% solution for IV use	1-1.5 g/kg body wt
Urea (Ureaphil, Urevert)	30% solution for IV use	1-1.5 g/kg body wt
Beta-adrenergic blocker		
Timolol maleate (Timoptic)	0.25-0.5% solution	1 drop q 12 hr

coma so that mydriatics are not administered, and prescribed glaucoma medications are not omitted.

Outcome criteria for the person with glaucoma

The person or significant others can:
1. Describe effects of surgery or medication on visual acuity.
2. State name, dosage, frequency, and side effects of eye medications.
3. State recognition of lifetime need to continue use of eye medications.
4. Describe preventive measures.
   a. Have reserve bottle of eyedrops at home.
   b. Carry eyedrops when away from home.
   c. Carry card identifying glaucoma and the eyedrop solution prescribed.
5. List signs indicating need to report immediately to the ophthalmologist.
6. Describe purpose of regular lifetime medical follow-up.

Detachment of the retina

Pathophysiology

The retina is the part of the eye that perceives light; it coordinates and transmits impulses from receptor nerve cells to the optic nerve. There are two primitive retinal layers: the outer pigment epithelium and an inner sensory layer. Retinal detachment occurs when the two retinal layers separate as a result of accumulation of fluid or traction produced by contraction of the vitreous body (Fig. 39-6). As the detachment extends and becomes complete, blindness results. Myopic degeneration, trauma, and aphakia (absence of the crystalline lens) are the most frequent causes of retinal detachment in children and adults. It may also result from hemorrhage, tumor, or exudates that occur in front of or behind the retina. Detachment of the retina may follow sudden severe physical exertion, especially in persons who are debilitated. Most often, however, there is no apparent cause.

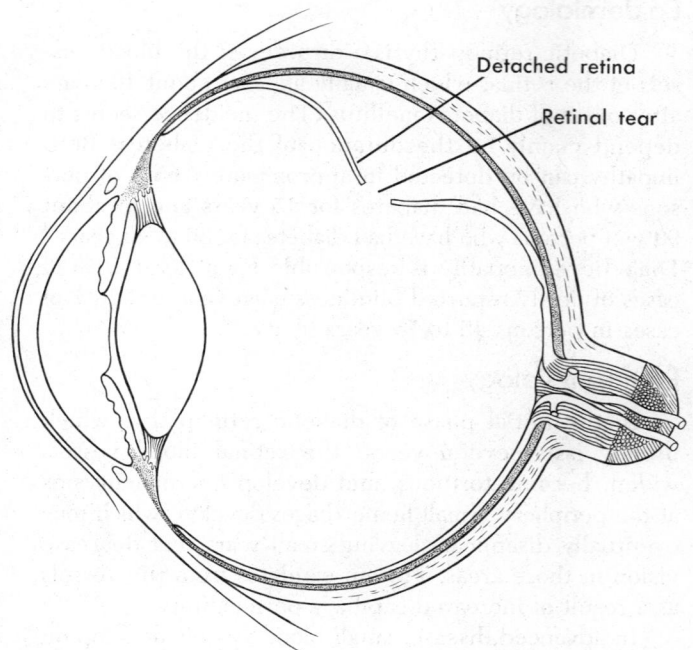

Fig. 39-6. Retinal detachment.

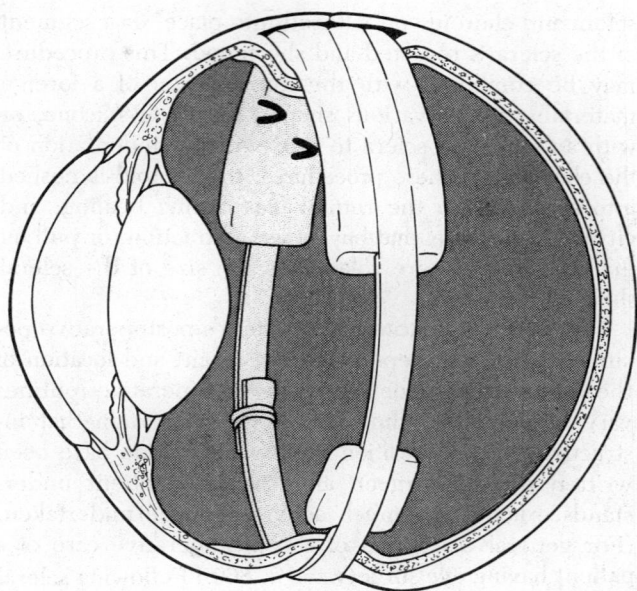

Fig. 39-7. Scleral buckle.

Clinical picture

Retinal detachment may occur suddenly or may develop slowly. Symptoms include floating spots or opacities before the eyes, flashes of light, and progressive constriction of vision in one area. The floating spots are blood and retinal cells that are freed at the time of the tear and cast shadows on the retina as they seem to drift about the eye. The diagnosis of retinal separation is based on the ophthalmoscopic appearance of the retina. The area of visual loss depends entirely on the location of the detachment. Usually there is a superior retinal detachment with inferior visual loss. When the detachment is extensive and occurs quickly, the patient may have the sensation that a curtain has been drawn before the eyes.

Intervention

Immediate care for detachment of the retina includes keeping the patient quiet in bed with the eyes covered to try to prevent further detachment. The head is positioned so that the retinal hole is in the lowest part of the eye. Because extended conservative treatment for detachment of the retina has not been successful, early surgery is now the approved method of treatment.

Surgical procedure. The surgery may be performed under either local or general anesthesia. Cyclopentolate or phenylephrine is used to keep the pupils widely dilated so that tears in the retina may be identified during the operation. The surgical procedure may include

draining the fluid from the subretinal space so that the retina returns to its normal position, thereby closing the opening in the retina. To drain the fluid from the subretinal space, the sclera and choroid are perforated at the time of the operation.

The retinal breaks are sealed off by various methods that produce an inflammatory reaction (*chorioretinitis*) in the area of the tear so that adhesions will form between the edges of the break and the underlying choroid to obliterate the opening. When the tears are small or of recent origin, diathermy may be applied through the sclera with needlepoint electrodes to produce the inflammatory process. An intense beam of visible light directed to the area by means of an elaborate ophthalmoscope may be used to close retinal tears when the retina is not elevated (*photocoagulation*). The *laser beam* is used by some surgeons as a source of intense energy to produce chorioretinitis. Subfreezing temperatures ($-40°$ to $-60°$ C) may be applied to the surface of the sclera in the area of the hole to produce the inflammatory reaction (*retinal cryopexy*). Nitrous oxide or carbon dioxide under pressure, flowing through a tube attached to a delicate instrument, is used to produce these low temperatures.

For most retinal detachments, including those previously considered inoperable, *scleral buckling* procedures are used. A scleral buckle serves as a splint to hold the retina and choroid together until the choroidal scar can form to permanently seal the hole or tear. The retinal break or tear is closed by the following procedure. The area overlying the treated tear is indented, or "buckled," inward toward the vitreous cavity (Fig. 39-7). To create the buckle, a fold is taken in the treated sclera and choroid and sutured into place, or a segment of the sclera is resected and shortened. This procedure may be combined with the implantation of a foreign material, such as various shaped pieces of silicone, or with an eye-bank sclera to cause further indentation of the choroid. By these procedures, the choroid is pushed into contact with the retinal tear during healing, and vitreous adhesions that have exerted traction, or pull on the retinal break are relaxed as the size of the scleral shell is decreased.

Postoperative care. The patient's postoperative position in bed will depend on the extent and location of the retinal detachment. Because postoperative routines vary a great deal, the nurse must be certain that instructions for bed position and for ambulation have been written by the surgeon and that the patient understands exactly how much activity may be undertaken. (For general discussion of the postoperative care of a patient having eye surgery see p. 869.) Following scleral buckle surgery, the retina is examined daily to determine if satisfactory flattening of the retina has occurred. If a redetachment occurs, a repeat operation may be done as early as the second or third postoperative day.[15]

Hemorrhage is a common complication of an operation for detachment of the retina. It may result from cryosurgery, diathermy, or puncture of the choroid to obtain release of subretinal fluids at the time of operation.

Resumption of sedentary duties may be permitted 3 weeks after surgery, while activities or occupations requiring heavy physical exertion may not be permitted for 6 weeks or more. Restoration of sight will depend on the extent and duration of the detachment before surgery, as well as the degree of success of the treatment. Some ophthalmologists advise their patients to avoid contact sports for the rest of their lives.

Outcome criteria for the person with retinal detachment

The person or significant others can:
1. State signs and symptoms indicating further retinal detachment.
2. State need for medical follow-up should further symptoms occur.
3. Describe the extent of limitations on activity.

Diabetic retinopathy

The quality of health and life expectancy of the person with diabetes have improved due to the use of insulin and regulated exercise and diet. Because of the longer life span, however, some of the complications associated with diabetes such as pathologic conditions of the retina have increased.

Epidemiology

Diabetic retinopathy is a disorder of the blood vessels of the retina, which usually appears about 10 years after onset of diabetes mellitus. The incidence seems to depend mainly on the duration of the diabetes. Retinopathy can be detected in approximately 65% of persons who have had diabetes for 15 years and in about 90% of persons who have had diabetes for 30 to 40 years.[4] Diabetic retinopathy is responsible for at least 10% of cases of newly reported blindness each year and 20% of cases in persons 45 to 75 years of age.[93]

Pathophysiology

In the initial phase of diabetic retinopathy, which usually lasts several years, the retinal blood vessels widen, become tortuous, and develop microaneurysms at the periphery. Small hemorrhages develop, which may eventually disappear, leaving small scars that decrease vision in those areas. Protein exudates from the vessels as a result of increased capillary permeability.

In advanced disease, small blood vessels develop on the retina and grow out into the vitreous. These vessels frequently rupture causing decreased vision. Some of the blood may reabsorb with some increase in vision until the next hemorrhage, but the continuing hemorrhagic process eventually leads to marked vision loss. Resolving of the hemorrhagic products may create a pull on the retina leading to tearing and detachment of the retina. Legal blindness in the affected eye usually results within 4 to 6 years from the beginning of the vessel proliferation phase.[4]

Clinical picture

The initial signs of diabetic retinopathy, tortuous vessels, small dots (microaneurysms), and "fluffy wool" exudates on the retina, can only be identified by examining the retina through ophthalmoscopy. In advanced disease, the person describes progressive loss of vision and seeing multiple spots (floaters). The floaters are minute hemorrhagic products in the vitreous humor.

Intervention

Several methods of treatment are currently being used and studied for effectiveness.

One method is photocoagulation of the retina by xenon arc or argon laser. In this therapy an intense beam of light is directed into the eye and focused on a small spot on the retina. The light energy is transformed into heat energy, coagulating the new vessels and preventing hemorrhage into the vitreous.

After severe hemorrhage into the vitreous has occurred from proliferative diabetic retinopathy, the vitreous can become permanently opaque, and vision is lost. The vitreous is the clear, gel-like fluid that fills the center of the eye. Bleeding into the vitreous blocks the transmission of light and can damage the retina. During the last 5 years, researchers have developed new instruments for surgically removing the diseased vitreous (a very difficult procedure). Removal of the vitreous (*vitrectomy*) is now being intensively studied in 14 medical centers across the United States.

Hypophysectomy (surgical removal of the pituitary gland) is another surgical procedure that has been performed in the past to treat diabetic retinopathy. The procedure was of benefit to some persons, but it is now rarely performed as a treatment for diabetic retinopathy. The effect was thought to be caused by the decreased growth hormone.[4]

Because of the limitations of surgical methods to preserve vision in diabetic retinopathy, efforts are continually being made to find medical means of preventing the condition from developing.

Retrolental fibroplasia

Etiology and pathophysiology

Retrolental fibroplasia, or retinopathy of prematurity, is a disease of premature infants in which a dense, opaque, fibrous membrane forms in the anterior vitreous behind the lens, causing blindness. An abnormality involving both eyes, retrolental fibroplasia is caused by high oxygen levels administered to premature infants in the hospital. In premature infants with incomplete vascularization of the eye, high oxygen levels cause vasoconstriction and destruction of blood vessels that supply the retina. While the excess use of oxygen has been responsible for a majority of cases, other factors such as pH changes may be involved in the response of the immature vessels to hyperoxia.[27] Incomplete retrolental fibroplasia may lead to gradual deterioration of the eye in adolescence.

Intervention

Prevention is the primary approach to retrolental fibroplasia. Premature infants suffering from respiratory distress syndrome require high oxygen levels to raise the arterial oxygen partial pressure (PO_2) to that of a normal infant. The lowest oxygen concentration required for maintenance of oxygenation should be used. These children need careful monitoring of arterial blood gas levels and of the retinal blood vessels. Ophthalmoscopic examinations are indicated at yearly intervals through life for persons with a history of retrolental fibroplasia.

Tumors

Both benign and malignant tumors may occur in the eye or related structures, such as the eyelid. Neoplasms may originate in the retina or the uveal tract or metastasize to the eye from a primary site. Orbital neoplasms include benign hemangiomas, pseudotumors, lymphomas, mucoceles from the sinuses, malignant melanomas, retinoblastomas, and others. If tumors are malignant, both vision and life are endangered. Tumors within the eyeball are often silent except for a bloodshot appearance of the eye. As in all malignant tumors, the prognosis depends on early diagnosis and prompt treatment.

Types of tumors

Tumors of the eyelids. The eyelids are subject to the usual tumors of the skin such as nevi and verrucae (warts). Carcinoma of the lids is a common type of ocular malignancy. Any warty growth in the eyelids should be removed for histologic examination. Treatment consists of surgical excision of the growth.

Retinoblastoma. Retinoblastoma is an inherited, highly malignant congenital neoplasm that arises from the retina. The most frequent ocular malignancy in childhood, it occurs in one of every 23,000 to 34,000 births.[85] The diagnosis is made in 90% of patients by the age of 4 years. Signs and symptoms may include decreased vision, strabismus, retinal detachment, white pupillary reflex, and secondary glaucoma. In about one third of the patients, the tumors invade both eyes. Retinoblastomas grow rapidly and spread backward along the optic nerve to invade the brain. Retinoblastomas can also metastasize to distant sites by way of the bloodstream and lymphatics.

Treatment of retinoblastoma consists of enucleation, with removal of as much of the optic nerve as possible. Frequent examination of the remaining eye is recommended. When the tumor is bilateral, the most involved eye is removed. An attempt is made to save the other eye by using radiation, chemotherapy, or both. If the tumor is very advanced, removal of both eyes may be necessary to save the child's life. When the tumor is unilateral and diagnosed and treated early, there is a 90% survival rate.

When normal parents have one child with retinoblastoma, there is a likelihood of less than 4% that a subsequent child will have such a tumor. There is a 50% chance that children of the individual who has survived a proved hereditary retinoblastoma will also be so affected. Persons who survive the tumors should receive genetic counseling to alert them to the danger of transmission to their offspring.

Malignant melanomas. Malignant melanomas are neoplasms that occur in the choroid and iris of adults. They grow slowly, but because of the vascularity of the choroid, they metastasize early to the liver and lungs.

Intervention

Medical treatment of tumors of the eye may include enucleation, radiation treatment, use of chemotherapeutic agents, and plastic surgery.

The emotional response to a tumor of the eye is perhaps even greater than to malignancies elsewhere. The surgeon may advise immediate enucleation of the eye in the hope of saving life. Both the patient and family need to be encouraged to talk about their feelings and concerns and helped to readjust their lives when confronted by this serious situation.

Removal of an eye

Surgical procedure

An eye, with or without its supportive structures, may be removed for four reasons: (1) in an attempt to save a life when a malignant tumor has developed, (2) to save sight in the other eye when sympathetic ophthalmia is feared or threatens, (3) to control pain in an eye blinded by disease such as chronic glaucoma or chronic infection, or (4) for cosmetic reasons following blindness from trauma or disease.

Three types of surgery may be performed. *Enucleation* is surgical removal of the entire eye including the sclera. *Evisceration* is removal of the contents of the eye with retention of the sclera. *Exenteration* involves removal of the entire eye and all other soft tissues in the bony orbit.

If feasible, the eyeball alone is removed, leaving the surrounding layers of fascia (Tenon's capsule) and the muscle attachments. A silicone, plastic, or tantalum implant is inserted into the eye socket, the cut ends of the muscle attachments are overlapped and sutured around it, and the Tenon's capsule and the conjunctiva are closed. This procedure provides a stump that supplies both support and motion for an artificial eye and therefore gives the patient whose eye has been removed a more normal appearance. The ball-shaped implant is left in place permanently.

Postoperative care

Hemorrhage, thrombosis of blood vessels, and infection are possible complications following enucleation, exenteration, or evisceration of an eye. Pressure dressings are used for 1 or 2 days to help control possible hemorrhage. Headaches or pain in the side of the head operated on should be reported at once, since meningitis occasionally occurs as a complication following thrombosis of adjacent veins. The patient is usually allowed out of bed the day following surgery.

When a person has lost one eye, the preservation of sight in the other eye becomes crucial. Wearing impact-resistant glasses provides some protection from injury. Because binocular vision is gone when there is only one functioning eye, depth perception is affected. The individual needs to be taught about the adjustments necessary in learning to carry out normal activities with one eye and of the potential safety hazards. Driving a car, for example, is dangerous for the person who suddenly must use only one eye and is not accustomed to the alteration in depth perception. With patience and practice, however, almost all normal activities are possible; surgeons who have had an eye removed have been able to operate successfully.

Artificial eye

An artificial eye can be used as soon as healing is complete and edema has disappeared, usually 6 to 8 weeks after surgery, although many patients begin to wear an artificial eye after only 3 weeks. Artificial eyes are made of glass or plastic materials. Glass eyes last longer if not broken, but they are heavier. Plastic ones are more expensive and may need to be replaced in a few years because they become more easily scratched or roughened around the edges, causing irritation to the conjunctiva. Plastic prostheses are more popular than those made of glass.

There are two kinds of artificial eyes: the shell-shaped and the hollow artificial eye. The choice of the individual patient depends on which operation has been done. Artificial eyes may be bought in shades that closely match the normal eye or they may be specially made. Most artificial eyes are plastic shells fitted and then painted by an artist. With good care, the life expectancy of the prosthesis is as great as 5 years. Despite care taken to match shape and color, the pupil of the artificial eye remains fixed, which is apparent to close observers.

Even young children can be taught to care for their own artificial eyes. A well-fitting prosthesis may not need to be removed for 30 days. When removed, however, the prosthesis should be cleansed immediately. Care should be taken not to scratch its surface. The artificial eye is removed by gently pressing upward on the lower lid, being certain that the cupped hand is held against the cheek so that the eye does not fall to the floor and break or become lost. It is inserted by gently everting the lower lid, being certain that the narrower end of the eye is placed next to the inner angle of the orifice. Then, by grasping the upper lashes and gently raising the upper lid, the eye is easily slipped into place.

Problems of the ear

Disorders of hearing and vestibular function are common and can occur at any age. Prevention, detection, and treatment of these disorders are highly diversified. Professional nursing has the responsibility of teaching preventive methods to help persons avoid damage to ear structure, including noise-induced damage, encouraging persons with aural disorders to seek appropriate medical care, caring for patients hospitalized with hearing disorders, and case finding and rehabilitation of persons with hearing disorders. The possible serious complications following infections of the ear and related structure make prompt appropriate medical care important.

For clarity in presentation, discussion of the ear and its structures is divided into three parts: (1) the outer ear, (2) the middle ear and mastoid process, and (3) the inner ear. Specific prevention and management are considered separately for each part in this chapter. Assessment of the ear, general management of hearing disorders, and general care of the person with ear problems are discussed in Chapters 37 and 38.

External ear

External otitis

Infections of the external ear are generally called *external otitis*. They are usually more common in the summer than in the winter. The external ear may be affected by acute and chronic forms of such conditions as eczematous dermatitis, diffuse dermatitis, and fungal and bacterial infections. These conditions may be associated with systemic diseases; with diseases of the skin of the adjacent face, neck, and scalp; or with diseases of the middle ear. They may be caused by trauma or may be the result of a primary invasion by organisms.

Clinical picture. Pain is the chief symptom of acute external otitis and increases with movement of the auricle and tragus. Pain or symptoms of redness, scaling, itching, swelling, watery discharge, or crusting should be referred to the otolaryngologist. If these infections are not treated, chronic changes may result causing thickening of the skin and stenosis of the external canal. There may be partial hearing loss and a blocked sensation in the affected ear. In chronic external otitis the chief symptom usually is itching.

Intervention. As described in Chapter 38, local treatment of both chronic and acute external otitis may include application of medicated ointments, drops, or powders.[24] If the ear canal is swollen secondary to the infection, a gauze or cotton wick may have to be inserted in the ear to allow a path for the topical medication to enter the canal and relieve discomfort. Systemic antibiotics may have to be included in the therapeutic regimen, and analgesics must be frequently prescribed to relieve the severe pain.

The topical medications administered generally fall into the following three categories: astringents (e.g., aluminum acetate [Burow's solution]), acidifers (e.g., acetic acid), and antibiotics (e.g., neomycin or polymyxin). These preparations usually have a "drying out" vehicle included in the solution and may contain a corticosteroid to reduce inflammation.

Recurrence is common, and steps to prevent recurrence include careful handwashing techniques by the treatment giver and use of sterile equipment and material. The patient should protect the ear canals with cotton during showering and avoid swimming, since moisture may precipitate a recurrence.

Foreign bodies in the ear canal

Children and mentally disturbed adults occasionally insert foreign bodies such as beans, peas, paper, erasers, crayons, chalk, or buttons in their ears. Depending on how loosely the foreign body fits the ear canal, removal may be by irrigation (p. 874), forceps, or cerumen loop. Irrigation should be avoided with any foreign bodies of vegetable matter, because they may increase in size if moistened and become impacted. Insects occasionally lodge in the ear canal; their movements cause pain and noise. A few drops of mineral oil, alcohol, or olive oil instilled into the ear canal will suffocate or immobilize the insect, and it may then be removed with forceps or irrigation. Nursing responsibilities include teaching parents or guardians of children or mentally disturbed adults never to poke in the ears with small or sharp objects such as cotton-tipped applicators, hairpins, matchsticks, or toothpicks. The ear should be cleaned only with a wet washcloth over the tip of a finger. *Nothing should be inserted into the ear beyond the point of vision.*

Congenital defects and deformities

Absence of the auricle is unusual; more common is a partial deformity of the ear. Often the latter is associated with absence of the external auditory meatus and at times with deformity of the middle ear and consequent deafness. Attempts have been made to surgically reconstruct the auricle with limited success. The external ear can also be deformed by trauma (cauliflower ear), which may be amenable to reconstruction surgery. Sometimes having the person wear the hair covering the area is the best solution.[84] An artificial prosthesis may also be designed.

Furunculosis of the external auditory canal

Furuncles, or boils, usually are confined to the external auditory meatus and most often are caused by *Staphylococcus aureus*. They cause severe pain because there is little expansile tissue in the area, and as they enlarge, the skin becomes taut and is under great pressure. The swelling may occlude the auditory canal, causing temporary deafness. Treatment may include the administration of systemic antibiotics, ear canal wicks impregnated with antibiotics, and incision and drainage.

Malignancies of the external ear

Cancer of the external ear is usually either a basal cell or squamous cell carcinoma.[18,74] It is not uncommon, and it usually appears as an ulcer on the auricle that fails to heal. Treatment is usually by surgical excision. Squamous cell carcinomas may metastasize to the neck or other parts of the body, although they usually remain localized for a long time. Basal cell carcinomas usually do not metastasize. The cure rate is reasonably good except when the osseous portion of the canal is invaded. Once this happens, temporal bone resection and deep irradiation therapy are employed.

Outcome criteria for the person with problems of the external ear

The person or significant others can:
1. Describe safety precautions related to the ear.
   a. Handwashing techniques in the presence of ear infection.
   b. Dangers of foreign bodies in the ear.
   c. Methods for cleaning the ear.
2. Demonstrate correct technique in the application of compresses, eardrops, ointment, or ear irrigations.
3. State symptoms requiring medical attention.

Middle ear

Serous otitis media

Etiology and pathophysiology. Serous (catarrhal) otitis media is a condition in which sterile serum is present in the middle ear, which interferes with hearing.[53,88] Normally, the nasopharyngeal end of the eustachian tubes opens periodically to permit the passage of air up into the middle ear as swallowing or yawning occurs. This air helps to maintain the pressure within the middle ear equal to that of the external ear. When the opening of the eustachian tube is blocked by nasopharyngeal infections or enlarged adenoids, or when its lumen is swollen by allergic reactions, air cannot enter. The remaining air in the middle ear space eventually is absorbed by its mucous membrane lining, and negative pressure is created, which draws fluid from the surrounding tissues into the middle ear (Fig. 39-8). A sudden change in atmospheric pressure, such as that which

occurs in flying, can also produce this condition. Ascending from a high atmospheric pressure to a low atmospheric pressure moves air from the middle ear out through the eustachian tube, but as the person descends, air may be unable to pass through the eustachian tube back into the middle ear. Chewing gum or swallowing helps to open the tube, thus permitting air to enter the middle ear.

Clinical picture. Serous otitis media may be acute or chronic. It may last for a few days or persist for years. The person may complain of a sense of fullness or blockage in the ear, hearing loss, a low-pitched tinnitus, and an earache. The eardrum may have a yellowish hue in acute cases from the amber-colored serous fluid. In long-standing cases, the eardrum may look remarkably normal or be retracted.

Intervention. Serous otitis media resolves as the cause of the eustachian obstruction is removed. Gentle inflation of the eustachian tube may bring relief. Aspiration of the fluid with a needle or through a myringotomy incision may be necessary in some instances. Polyethylene, Teflon, or stainless steel ventilation tubes can be inserted through an opening in the eardrum to equalize pressure and to prevent fluid from reforming.[34] The use of these tubes seemingly has reduced the incidence of serous otitis media, especially in children. Treatment in children may be aided by adenoidectomy (p. 1276).

Early and adequate treatment of nasopharyngeal infections and allergic conditions can often prevent chronic serous otitis media from developing. Since this disease is a cause of conduction deafness in children, the nurse should urge mothers of children who have hearing problems to seek medical advice. Any person who complains of tinnitus or who has otalgia should be advised to seek medical attention promptly.

Acute purulent otitis media

Etiology. Most of the diseases that affect the middle ear and mastoid process are caused by infection.[74] Acute purulent otitis media is an acute inflammatory process in the middle ear (Fig. 39-8). It is common in infants because their eustachian tubes are short and straight,

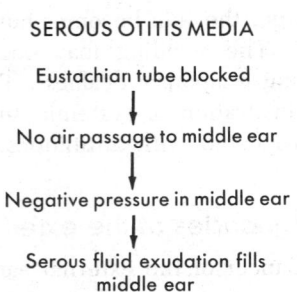

SEROUS OTITIS MEDIA

Eustachian tube blocked

↓

No air passage to middle ear

↓

Negative pressure in middle ear

↓

Serous fluid exudation fills middle ear

PURULENT OTITIS MEDIA

Bacteria enters middle ear through eustachian tube

↓

Inflammation of middle ear with pus formation

↓

Pus fills middle ear

Fig. 39-8. Pathogenesis of otitis media.

and thus almost any infection in the nasopharynx has direct access to the middle ear. This disease most often follows the common cold, but it may be a complication of measles or scarlet fever. It may also be caused by the forcing of contaminated water into the middle ear through the eustachian tube while swimming or by forcefully blowing the nose. People should be urged to avoid swimming in uninspected pools and in stagnant water, and they should be taught to blow the nose gently, lest infected material be forced into the middle ear. The offending organisms usually are pneumococci, streptococci, or staphylococci, which reach the middle ear by way of the eustachian tube. In children under 6 years of age, however, a common offending organism is *Haemophilus influenzae*.

Pathophysiology. The infection usually begins with local engorgement of the blood vessels, which causes swelling of the mucous membrane lining of the eustachian tubes and middle ear. The exudate becomes serosanguineous and later mucopurulent. The pressure of the exudate may cause the eardrum to rupture.

Clinical picture. In the early stages, the child may complain of a sensation of fullness in the ear. As infection progresses, the eardrum tenses, and pain becomes severe and throbbing. The pain may cause the child to tug on the ear, or the infant may roll the head from side to side, cry constantly, and refuse to eat. There may be decreased hearing in the affected ear, tinnitus, and fever, which in a child may range as high as 40° to 41° C (104° to 106° F).

Intervention. When otitis media develops, antibiotics are given at once, and the infection usually subsides before the eardrum ruptures.[79,88] Treatment also may include bed rest, administration of acetylsalicylic acid or codeine for pain, administration of nasal vasoconstrictors to open blocked eustachian tubes, and application of dry heat such as hot-water bottle. Eardrops (e.g., Auralgan) are contraindicated if the eardrum is perforated, because they cause a brisk mucositis of the middle ear and can damage the middle ear. Instead, antibiotic steroid drops (e.g., Cortisporin, Colymycin, Pyocidin, or VoSol) are prescribed.

A *myringotomy* (incision into the tympanic membrane) may be performed to relieve pressure and remove pus in the middle ear during acute otitis media. An older procedure, it is still performed, although less frequently since the advent of antibiotic therapy.[84] Once a purulent process is established, despite antibiotic treatment, a myringotomy is performed to prevent spontaneous rupture of the eardrum, since scar tissue that may impair hearing can develop if the membrane is allowed to rupture spontaneously. A popular misconception regarding myringotomy is that by incising the eardrum, hearing is lost. This is not true; usually a myringotomy heals rapidly with only slight scarring and does not affect hearing. The procedure is usually performed in an ambulatory setting. The physician requires a surgical microscope or a good light and a head mirror, aural speculum, and a very sharp myringotomy knife. If necessary, a short-acting anesthetic (e.g., nitrous oxide) or an injected anesthetic (e.g., lidocaine) may be used. A single incision is made, usually anteriorly and inferiorly in the eardrum to avoid injuring the ossicles (Fig. 39-9). A suction tip may be used to remove fluids from the middle ear after the incision is made, and cultures may be taken.

Free drainage must be maintained so that no pressure is put on the mastoid cells. Cotton may be placed loosely (not stuffed) in the outer ear to collect drainage. Sometimes eardrops may be ordered. The external ear is kept clean and dry. The cotton is replaced when it becomes moist to minimize the possibility of secondary infection from the draining pus. Dry wipes may be used to remove excess drainage. Petrolatum may be placed around the outer ear to prevent it from becoming excoriated from the drainage. It is important to prevent secondary infection through contamination of the wound; therefore parents and patients should know that the discharge may be infectious and that the hands should be washed before and after changing cotton plugs or cleaning the ear. Elbow restraints may be necessary to keep the young child from touching the ear and the drainage. Antibiotics are continued for several days after the discharge has stopped. If the patient has a rise in temperature, complains of headache, or becomes drowsy, irritable, or disoriented, the physician must be notified at once. These signs may indicate that the eardrum needs to be reopened, that mastoid cells are involved, or that a brain abscess or meningitis is developing.

Usually otitis media is treated on an ambulatory basis, and parents of the infant or young child need careful instruction in care of the ear. In order to prevent the complications of otitis media, all parents should be taught to seek medical attention for a child with an ear-

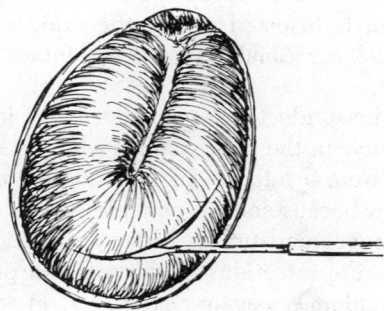

Fig. 39-9. Myringotomy incision made through anteroinferior part of eardrum to release pus in acute otitis media. (From Saunders, W.H., et al.: Nursing care in eye, ear, nose, and throat disorders, ed. 4, St. Louis, 1979, The C.V. Mosby Co.)

ache. The importance of taking prescribed antibiotics for the number of days ordered, even though symptoms have subsided, is stressed.

Acute mastoiditis

Etiology and pathophysiology. An acute infection of the middle ear usually is accompanied by some inflammatory reaction in the mucosa of the adjacent mastoid process. If the middle-ear infection is not treated early or adequately, or if the infection is particularly virulent, or if the person is very debilitated, acute mastoiditis may occur. Streptococci, pneumococci, staphylococci, or *Haemophilus influenzae* may be the causative organisms. The inflammatory reaction proceeds from edema of the tissues to the formation of exudate and pus that fills the mastoid cells. Pressure on the blood supply causes necrosis to develop and an abscess to form. There may be pain in the ear, mastoid tenderness, fever, headache, and a profuse discharge from the affected ear.

Intervention. Acute mastoiditis may be a life-threatening problem. Initially, intervention is directed toward preventing the mastoiditis from causing mastoid bone necrosis, pus under pressure, and destruction of the mastoid bone. If detected in the early stages, hospitalization with high doses of intravenous antibiotics may cause a resolution of the infection. If, however, progression has occurred to the stages as mentioned, surgical intervention is needed. The symptoms of this progression include increased ear pain, rising temperature, and vertigo. Signs include a bulging of the postauricular or ear canal areas with a forward displacement of the earlobe, tenderness of the postauricular area, and an obviously sick patient.

SIMPLE MASTOIDECTOMY. The treatment for this type of mastoiditis, which is called *surgical* (coalescent) *mastoiditis*, is a simple mastoidectomy. "Simple" does not imply that the operation is easy, but it describes the anatomic portion of the mastoid bone that is to be removed. In a simple mastoidectomy, an incision is made in front of or behind the ear (Fig. 39-10) and the air cells of the mastoid bone are removed. A small rubber drain is inserted. Since the middle ear space, eardrum, and ear canal wall are left intact, hearing is not affected.

Simple mastoidectomy was developed in the nineteenth century. In the past, patients who developed acute mastoiditis from a middle-ear infection were in danger of their lives because of the possible spread of infection to the meninges and brain. Today antibiotics are used to control acute infections of the mastoid process, and surgery is seldom necessary. However, in some underdeveloped countries, acute mastoiditis is common, and in the presence of complications, surgery may still be necessary. Preoperative preparation for a simple mastoidectomy is similar to that for any operative procedure.

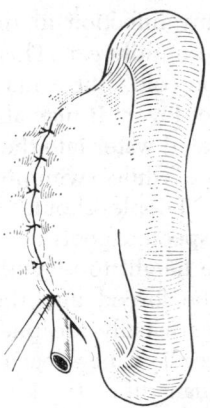

Fig. 39-10. Postauricular incision is sutured, and one Penrose drain is brought out of lower part of wound. Such incision now is commonly used for any type of mastoidectomy and often for tympanoplasty. (From Saunders, W.H., et al.: Nursing care in eye, ear, nose, and throat disorders, ed. 4, St. Louis, 1979, The C.V. Mosby Co.)

Postoperatively a bulky dressing is applied to provide some hemostasis and to absorb drainage (Fig. 39-11). The dressing may be reinforced as necessary, but it is not changed by the nurse; the surgeon usually changes it every other day. There may be a small amount of serosanguineous drainage apparent on the dressing, but signs of bright blood on the outer dressing should be reported at once. If a drain has been inserted, it is usually removed in 72 hours. Sutures are removed on the fifth or sixth postoperative day. As with any ear surgery, any signs of facial paralysis such as inability to smile or to wrinkle the forehead should be reported. Headache, fluctuating temperatures, temperature spikes, vomiting, stiff neck, dizziness, irritability, or disorientation may be forewarnings of a septic thrombosis of the lateral sinus in the brain, or meningitis, or a brain abscess. The patient is monitored for these symptoms including vital signs at least every 4 hours for the first 36 hours following surgery. Intravenous fluids and antibiotics are given for a similar length of time. Ambulation is usually permitted within 12 to 24 hours.

RADICAL MASTOIDECTOMY. Radical mastoidectomy consists of a simple mastoidectomy plus removal of the ossicles, remnants of the eardrum, the boney ear canal wall, and all of the middle ear mucosa. The middle ear and mastoid process become one large cavity. The radical mastoid cavity may be left to gradually reline with epithelium, or skin or muscle graft may be performed (musculoplasty). Sterile packing is placed in the wound to keep the graft in position, to hold the external meatus open, and to provide hemostasis. The packing is removed gradually through the external ear. The ungrafted radical mastoid cavity usually is healed 2 to 3 months after the operation. It is very important that sterile technique be observed at all times and that the external ear be kept scrupulously clean. Radical mas-

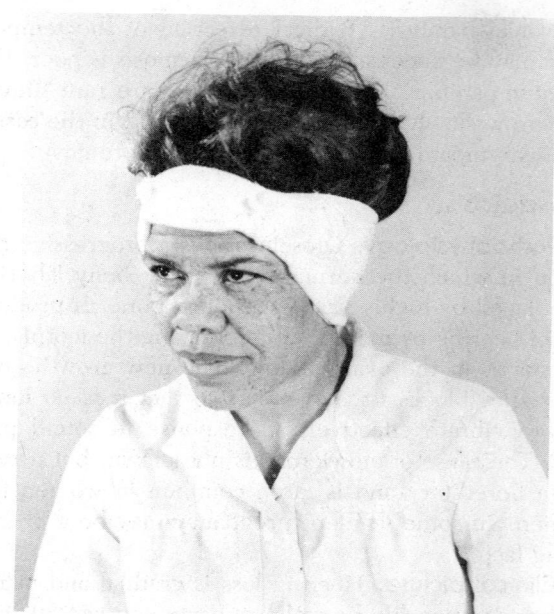

Fig. 39-11. Cling-type 3-in. roller bandage and forehead ties ensure secure and comfortable head dressing. (Courtesy Eye and Ear Infirmary, University of Illinois Hospitals, Chicago.)

toidectomy is used for the patient with chronic infection of the mastoid process. Unlike simple mastoidectomy, radical mastoidectomy *does* affect hearing. In actual practice, however, radical mastoidectomy ordinarily does not diminish hearing appreciably, because by the time the patient has the operation, hearing has already been affected.

A *modified radical mastoidectomy* is a more commonly used procedure, because it preserves as much of the eardrum and ossicles as possible. Hearing is better following the modified radical mastoidectomy than the radical mastoidectomy. Nursing care for the patient with a radical mastoidectomy is similar to that given the patient with a simple mastoidectomy.

Chronic otitis media

Chronic purulent otitis media is characterized by chronic purulent discharge from the middle ear. It is a sequela of acute otitis media and involves both the middle ear and the mastoid cells. The mastoid bone cells become thickened, and polyps may develop from the mucous membrane of the middle ear.

Clinical picture. The patient's main complaint may be deafness, occasional pain, or dizziness. If chronic purulent otitis media is permitted to progress unchecked, labyrinthitis, meningitis, brain abscess, or facial paralysis may eventually occur, because the infection gradually erodes the surrounding bone. Usually more than one bacterial organism is found on culture; streptococci, staphylococci, *Proteus,* and *Pseudomonas* organisms are most common.

Another complication of chronic purulent otitis me-

dia is cholesteatoma (cystic mass).[50,84] It often occurs when the eardrum has been ruptured and the ear has drained for some time. Skin cells from the ear canal grow into the middle ear (excrescence), where they form a mass that becomes firm and erodes the tissue surrounding it. This mass must be removed surgically.

Intervention. The best treatment for chronic purulent otitis media is prevention by early treatment of the acute disease. If the chronic condition does occur, it should be treated as soon as it is recognized. Because the infection is walled off, systemic antibiotics alone are not effective. They may be effective, however, following meticulous local debridement with suctioning and application of topical antibiotics. When this treatment is not indicated or is not effective, a radical mastoidectomy or modified radical mastoidectomy is performed. An effort is made to reconstruct the sound-conducting mechanism by tympanoplasty. Persons who have chronic otitis media should not swim or allow water to enter the ear. When showering they must keep their ears covered.

Perforation of the eardrum

The eardrum may be perforated as the result of infection (acute or chronic purulent otitis media) or trauma (skull fracture, puncture). Usually accidental perforations heal spontaneously. Often the patient is given prophylactic antibiotics. Patients with perforated eardrums should not dive, swim, or allow water to enter the ear while showering because of the danger of infection. Eardrops are avoided if the eardrum is perforated. (For further discussion on eardrops see p. 873.) Because of the increased possibility of infection with a perforated eardrum and the possibility of conductive hearing loss, surgical repair often is necessary.

Tympanoplasty is a general name given to a group of operative procedures designed to restore hearing in patients with middle ear or conductive hearing loss. It is used for people who have perforation of the tympanic membrane or necrosis of one of the ossicles due to a middle ear infection, stenosis, or dislocation of the incus following trauma. By reconstructing or preserving the middle ear conductive mechanism, hearing may be improved or maintained. Closing the tympanic membrane seals the middle ear and protects it from infection. The ear should preferably be free of infection before tympanoplasty is performed.

Tympanoplasty differs basically from mastoidectomy in that it seeks to correct hearing loss, while mastoidectomy seeks to correct infection even at the sacrifice of hearing. Reconstructive procedures of the ear are highly individualized for each patient and depend on the extent of mechanical derangement noted. Eustachian tube functions are necessary if reconstruction of the drum or middle ear space is contemplated. If the eustachian tube does not function properly the reconstruction procedure will fail because of a lack of a proper air-containing environment in the middle ear. Usual surgical approaches are postauricular or endaural. If the ear is not free of infection, the operation includes removal of all infected tissue to make sure that the grafts and prosthesis used do not become infected.

Myringoplasty is used to close a perforation in the eardrum causing conductive hearing loss secondary to trauma or infection. Myringoplasty is performed by surgically enlarging the opening in the eardrum and placing a piece of skin, vein, or fascia over the opening. An absorbable gelatin sponge (Gelfoam) or clotted blood may be used to fill the middle ear space to support the graft, and sterile packing is placed in the external ear to help keep the graft in position. If the graft takes, a considerable degree of tympanic function will return. Patients are typically given antibiotics to prevent infections and antihistamine medications to prevent sneezing. The patient should avoid sneezing and blowing the nose postoperatively so as not to disturb the graft. If sneezing cannot be avoided, the mouth should be opened and the nose should be left uncovered during the sneeze to prevent increased pressure in the middle ear. Eardrops are not used.

Occasionally, patients with small tympanic perforations who exhibit no signs of infection of the middle ear may be treated successfully by trichloroacetic acid microcauterization and placement of material for a graft to the area. The procedure is usually performed in an ambulatory setting and generally must be repeated many times. The postoperative precautions described above also apply to these patients. These procedures are usually not performed on children who are highly susceptible to infections because the infection would reach the middle ear by way of the eustachian tubes and infect the graft.

In addition to repairing a perforation of the eardrum, tympanoplasty may include examination and, if necessary, removal of any scar tissue that interferes with the function of the ossicles, replacement of diseases ossicles with plastic or metal prostheses or homograft ossicles, and reconstruction of the eardrum. Homograft or autograft ossicles are being used more frequently with a high rate of success. Some intact tympanic membranes with intact ossicles from cadavers are being used. One type of tympanoplasty changes the normal route of sound transmission across the middle ear. Usually the normal route has been disrupted by disease; therefore in this type of surgery the eardrum or graft is made to touch the head of the stapes so that sound will pass directly from eardrum to stapes. As with any operative procedure on the middle ear, patients with tympanoplasty may have problems with vertigo.

Tumors of the middle ear and mastoid process

Tumors in this region are rare and when present are squamous cell carcinomas.[74] Symptoms are usually aural discharge, loss of hearing, deep-seated pain, and eventual facial paralysis. Radical resection of the temporal bone may be necessary, and the prognosis is poor. Glomus tympanium and glomus jugulare are rare tumors; they grow slowly, rarely metastasize, and in the case of glomus tympanium are relatively easy to remove.

Otosclerosis

Pathophysiology. Otosclerosis is a progressive condition in which the normal bone of the bony labyrinth is replaced by highly vascular spongy bone. It produces loss of hearing by fixing or immobilizing the footplate of the stapes in the oval window. The new growth about the stapes blocks its movement so that it is no longer free to vibrate effectively in response to sound pressure. The cause of otosclerosis is not known, but it tends to be hereditary and is more common in women than in men. In some women, pregnancy may be a precipitating factor.

Clinical picture. Hearing loss is gradual and usually becomes noticeable between puberty and age 30. Usually both ears are affected, one more than the other, and tinnitus is a troublesome symptom. Hearing loss may be solely of the conductive variety caused by the fixation of the stapes or of the sensorineural variety caused by the direct effect on the inner ear. Audiometric testing (p. 853) is used to diagnose otosclerosis. A tuning fork demonstrates that bone conduction is superior to air conduction.

Intervention. The treatment for hearing loss as a result of otosclerosis is surgical, most commonly a *stapedectomy*. Surgery consists of removal of the stapes and replacing it with some type of prosthesis. Stapedectomy is performed on only one ear at a time, usually the poorer hearing ear. Local anesthetic is administered, and an incision is made deep in the ear canal close to the eardrum, without cutting the eardrum itself, so that the drum can be turned back and the middle ear exposed. Working through a microscope, the surgeon frees and removes the stapes and the attached footplate, leaving an opening in the oval window. The opening in the oval window is closed with a plug of fat, vein graft, or absorbable gelatin sponge (Gelfoam), which the body eventually replaces with mucous membrane cells. A steel wire, polyethylene prosthesis, or a Teflon piston is inserted to replace the stapes and is attached at one end to the incus and at the other to the graft or plug to transmit sound to the inner ear. As soon as the connection is made with the incus, the patient's hearing is improved.

When the eardrum is replaced, the patient hears better. Later in the operative day, blood forms in the middle ear and in the ear canal so that hearing is reduced temporarily. Postoperative edema and packing placed in the ear will also diminish hearing. The reasons for diminished hearing should be explained to the patient preoperatively to relieve worry about diminished hearing after surgery compared with the hearing regained initially in the operating room. Full effects of the operation cannot be evaluated until about one month postoperatively.

Postoperative routines differ in various centers. Some surgeons prefer that the patient lie with the operative ear uppermost to prevent displacement of the graft, while others prefer the patient to lie on the operative ear to facilitate drainage. Some physicians permit the patient to lie on the side that is most comfortable and does not cause vertigo. If postoperative pain occurs, it is usually relieved by codeine sulfate, 60 mg, or meperidine hydrochloride (Demerol), 100 mg. Postoperative trauma and edema may cause vertigo for a few days, and dimenhydrinate (Dramamine), 50 mg, may be given every 6 hours to relieve it. The patient is cautioned against rapid turning, since this may cause vertigo. To prevent falls, side rails should be raised when the patient is in bed, and the patient needs supervision and assistance when getting out of bed and walking. Antibiotics are given to help prevent postoperative infection or meningitis, and the patient is instructed not to blow the nose for a week to prevent air and organisms from being forced up the eustachian tube. Sneezing should also be avoided, but if a sneeze appears imminent, the patient is advised to open the mouth wide and to sneeze as lightly as possible. Bending over or lifting heavy objects should be avoided until such activity is approved by the surgeon.

The hospital stay is 1 to 5 days. The packing usually is removed in the surgeon's office or in the clinic about the sixth day, and most patients are allowed to return to work in 2 weeks. During the first week, the patient may be advised to wear cotton in the ear when outdoors. The cotton should be placed loosely in the meatus (not into the ear canal) and should be changed once or twice daily. The patient should avoid washing the hair for 2 weeks and should not get water into the ear for 6 weeks. Persons with colds should be avoided because of the danger of middle ear infections. Flying should be avoided for 6 months after the operation, especially if an upper respiratory tract infection is present, to prevent the prosthesis from moving out of place. With these exceptions, usual activities are permitted when the ear has healed.[57,90] After stapedectomy, hearing improves permanently in the majority of cases. Completely normal hearing may be restored, but occasionally hearing may become worse.

Fenestration is a surgical procedure for the treatment of otosclerosis in which the fixed stapes is bypassed and a new window is created in the inner ear. Sound then enters the new window, and hearing is partially restored. Fenestration is rarely performed. Some persons have developed reduced hearing 6 to 12 months postoperatively when sterile labyrinthitis developed, closing the new window with fibrous or bony growth. Postoperatively, patients are usually placed on their back or operative side to facilitate drainage. Severe vertigo is often present, as well as nausea and pain on moving the jaws.

Stapes mobilization, like fenestration, is a surgical procedure that was once popular but is now used less often. The stapes is broken loose and the middle ear left as normal as possible. Unfortunately, in about one half of the successful cases, refixation of the stapes developed, either by healing of the fractured footplate or by new otosclerotic growth. Stapes mobilization is performed with the patient under local anesthesia; it requires briefer hospitalization than fenestration and little postoperative care. It may produce immediate dramatic hearing improvement.

Outcome criteria for the person who has had surgery of the middle ear

The person or significant others can:
1. Describe measures to prevent infections of the middle ear until the incision is healed.
   a. Blow nose with both nostrils open.
   b. Open mouth when sneezing.
   c. Avoid getting water in the affected ear when showering or bathing.
   d. Avoid exposure to persons with upper respiratory tract infection.
   e. Avoid flying for 6 months.
2. State plans for medical follow-up until the incision is healed.

Outcome criteria for the person with problems of the middle ear not requiring surgery

The person or significant others can:
1. State preventive measures.
   a. Adequate and early treatment of upper respiratory tract infections and allergic conditions.
   b. Adequate treatment of acute purulent otitis media if necessary.
   c. Prevention of complications following a perforated eardrum, such as not swimming in contaminated water.
   d. Adequate antibiotic therapy continued for prescribed number of days even when symptoms disappear.
2. Describe symptons indicating need for medical attention (persistent earache, tinnitus, loss of hearing).

Inner ear

Presbycusis

Presbycusis is the term used to describe hearing loss associated with the aging process. Some of the degenerative change probably is the result of atrophy of the ganglion cells in the cochlea. Presbycusis is characterized by bilateral gradual loss of hearing beginning with a loss of high-frequency tones. It typically cannot be completely improved with hearing aids or surgery.

Meniere's disease

Etiology. Meniere's disease is a disorder of the inner ear that most typically occurs in women 50 to 60 years of age. The cause is unknown. Usually, there are several attacks during each year, and an emotional crisis often may precipitate an attack. The attacks may disappear without treatment, or they may continue until the person is completely deaf in the affected ear.

Pathophysiology. The membranous labyrinth of the inner ear is a closed system filled with endolymph (p. 852). In Meniere's disease, there is an increase of endolymphatic fluid circulation in the cochlea as a result of either increased production or decreased absorption of the endolymph. Pressure from the increased fluid may affect the hair cells; the acoustic nerve is not involved.

Clinical picture. Meniere's disease is characterized by recurrent episodes of vertigo accompanied by progressive deafness and tinnitus in the affected ear. The vertigo comes in attacks at irregular intervals of days, months, or years. The onset of the attack is sudden and without warning. During an attack, any sudden motion of the head or eyes tends to precipitate nausea and vomiting. There may be profuse perspiration and nystagmus. Vertigo may be so severe that persons with Meniere's disease are unable to cross a room without falling. They describe their surroundings as whirling wildly about them. Usually they must sit down to keep from falling and must hold their head very still. Persons with Meniere's disease remain vertiginous for several hours or all day, but they do not have vertigo between attacks.

Hearing loss is also present and is of the sensorineural type. Usually (in about 90% of the cases), the hearing loss is unilateral, although a lesser degree of hearing loss in the opposite ear is not uncommon. Patients with Meniere's disease often complain of a sensation of fullness in the ear.

Tinnitus or ringing is present in one ear most of the time. Like the hearing loss, it may worsen. Meniere's disease is a chronic disease; while temporary or complete remissions of the attacks of vertigo may occur, the tinnitus and hearing loss are usually permanent.

Diagnosis is made chiefly from the patient's history, which will reveal recurrent episodes of vertigo, hearing loss, and tinnitus. Initially, between attacks, the hearing and tinnitus may return to the predisease state. As attacks become more frequent, there is a tendency for the hearing loss to become permanent and progressive. Initially, audiometry reveals low-tone sensorineural loss. The caloric test (p. 857) is still performed, although it is now considered to be of limited value in establishing the diagnosis. Electronystagmography (ENG) is becoming more widely used (p. 856).

If the patient has syncope or significant pain, a neurologic consultation is usually obtained to rule out neurologic disease. Other systemic diseases (e.g., syphilis) and lipid disorders may mimic Meniere's symptomatology and need to be investigated.

Intervention. No medical treatment for Meniere's disease has proved entirely successful. In order to reduce endolymphatic hypertension, the patient's fluid intake may be restricted and a salt-free or low-sodium diet may be recommended. Diuretics, such as chlorothiazide (Diuril) or acetazolamide (Diamox), may be ordered. Other medications that may be used between attacks include histamine subcutaneously (in desensitizing doses) and antivertiginous medications such as dimenhydrinate (Dramamine), nicotinyl alcoholtrimenthobenzamide hydrochloride (Tigacol), meclizine nicotinic acid (Antivert), and nicotinic acid. Medications are changed if relief is not rapid. If a patient suffers a severe attack, diphenhydramine (Benadryl) or dimenhydrinate (Dramamine) is given parenterally. Also an attack may be relieved in 15 to 20 minutes with a high dose of atropine sulfate, 0.06 mg, subcutaneously, intramuscularly, or intravenously. Atropine acts by abolishing impulses from the autonomic system that may have precipitated the attack. Mild sedatives and tranquilizers may be prescribed. Emotional support and reassurance are important. Some patients are advised to discontinue smoking to avoid vasospasm and vasoconstriction.

About 10% of patients with Meniere's disease require surgery if medical therapy does not adequately control the vertiginous episodes. There are several surgical procedures. The initial procedure is usually one to conserve hearing, such as endolymphatic sac decompression. If the patient's hearing level is very poor or if this conservative procedure fails, a more destructive procedure may be employed. Labyrinthectomy destroys the membranous labyrinth and sacrifices the balance and hearing end organs. Relief from vertigo may not occur for several weeks in some cases. Ultrasonic labyrinthectomy is also used, especially for patients who have symptoms of vertigo but still have worthwhile hearing that should be preserved. A pencil-sized probe of the ultrasonic generator is applied directly to the bone of the horizontal canal through a mastoidectomy incision, and energy is directed into the labyrinth. Cryosurgical labyrinthectomy is also used for some patients. It is performed similarly to the ultrasonic surgery, except that it is done through the ear canal without mastoidectomy.

Caring for the patient hospitalized with Meniere's disease requires understanding of the frustrating, incapacitating, and uncomfortable acute attacks the patient suffers.[41,84] Because sudden movement or jarring aggravates vertigo, self-care and self-determination of rate of movement are often desirable. Less dizziness will be experienced if the person talking to the patient stands directly in front so that the head does not have to be turned. Although movement increases the symptoms, the patient should be encouraged to move about in bed occasionally and to permit gentle back care to preserve good skin tone. Lying quietly on the unaffected side with eyes turned toward the direction of the affected ear sometimes is recommended to relieve an acute attack. The patient should not try to read, and bright, glaring lights are avoided. Side rails should be on the bed at all times, and the patient should not attempt to get up and walk without assistance. Because it is usually difficult to get the patient with Meniere's disease to take food or fluids, efforts should be made to obtain something that the patient will eat or drink. Patients should be encouraged to call the nurse at the first indication of an attack so that medication may be given.

Labyrinthitis

Labyrinthitis is an infection of the inner ear of unknown cause, although it often follows a head cold and occasionally a middle ear infection. If labyrinthitis progresses to a suppurative stage, hearing loss will be profound and permanent. Damage to the vestibular system is compensated for by central mechanisms, and the dizziness subsides. Meningitis may develop from labyrinthitis, as well as the reverse, in which case the labyrinthitis is usually bilateral. A special form of localized labyrinthitis tends to follow infection and involves the balance mechanisms only. Since the inner ear also helps maintain equilibrium, problems there produce loss of hearing and disturb the function of the semicircular canals.

Clinical picture. Typical symptoms include severe sudden vertigo, nausea, vomiting, sudden disturbances of equilibrium, and nystagmus. The patient usually is photophobic, has a headache, has an ataxic gait, and refuses food.

Intervention. No specific treatment exists. Antibiotics are usually given in high doses. To relieve vertigo, the patient may be given dimenhydrinate (Dramamine) or promethazine. If vomiting persists, fluids must be given parenterally. However, fluids given orally are usually retained if taken in small amounts with the patient keeping the head perfectly still. Because of the severe vertigo, side rails should be kept up, and the patient is assisted when walking. If the patient prefers, the room may be kept darkened at all times. Generally after a period of several days or weeks, vertigo diminishes. If the source of infection is a surgical mastoiditis or cholesteatoma, an emergent type of mastoid operation is performed to prevent intracranial complications (p. 906). Nursing care for the person with labyrinthitis is similar to that for Meniere's disease.

Outcome criteria for persons with Meniere's disease or labyrinthitis

The person or significant others can:
1. Describe circumstances that may precipitate an attack and what to do when an attack occurs.
2. Describe symptoms requiring medical intervention.
3. State rationale for safety precautions (e.g., walking with assistance and use of side rails) during a vertiginous attack.
4. Describe dosage and side effects of prescribed medications.

Fluctuant hearing loss

Etiology. Fluctuant hearing loss is a form of sensorineural hearing loss that is now thought to be more common than Meniere's disease.[66,89]

Clinical picture. Fluctuant hearing loss is characterized by a triad of symptoms that includes fullness, roaring tinnitus, and fluctuating hearing loss. Vertigo may or may not be present. Hearing may return to normal, and the fullness and roaring may disappear after the first attack, but this is unusual. Recovery is usually not complete and becomes worse after each attack. It is thought to be caused by excessive production of endolymph or a reduction in the absorption of endolymph. Some conditions that contribute to the occurrence of fluctuant hearing loss include poor circulation, diabetes mellitus, hyperlipoproteinemia, high salt intake, allergies, smoking, and syphilis. Results of electronystagmography are positive about 20% of the time.

Intervention. Treatment is similar to the treatment for Meniere's disease; a low-sodium diet and diuretics are often helpful. Patients are usually told to refrain from tobacco. Often antihistamines are administered either intravenously or orally. Diazepam (Valium) is sometimes prescribed for both its tranquilizing and antivestibular effects. Treatment of any contributing medical condition such as diabetes mellitus is indicated.

Cochlear implantation or stimulation

Cochlear implantation or stimulation are operations designed to benefit persons who have severe sensorineural hearing loss and who do not benefit from hearing aids.[9,16,43,60] Through the procedures, an attempt is made to replace a function of the cochlea, that is, the function of transducing the mechanical energy of sound vibrations to electrical energy, which directly stimulates the auditory nerve. An electrode with a single wire of either platinum, iridium, or titanium is placed in the scala tympani (the central portion of the cochlear cavity). The wire is connected with a ground wire in the area of the temporal muscle. The leads are connected to an induction cord containing a small-amplitude modulation radio, which is imbedded in the bone of the mastoid process. The radio receiver is driven by an external antenna placed over it. Externally applied sound waves generate an audioelectrical field within the cochlea. Presently with this technique, speech discrimination is still not possible, but some hearing does take place such as hearing thunder. Cochlear stimulation also imparts a rhythm to speech, which is helpful in speech-reading. Cochlear stimulation may be helpful for at least two thirds of persons with sensorineural loss. Research and experimentation are being carried out on brain stem and cortical stimulation, which may prove helpful for sensorineural deafness.

REFERENCES AND SELECTED READINGS

1. Allen, J.H.: May's manual of the diseases of the eye, ed. 24, Baltimore, 1972, The Williams & Wilkins Co.
2. *Ammon, L.L.: Surviving enucleation, Am. J. Nurs. **72**:1817-1821, 1972.
3. *Antibiotic treatment of otitis media, J. Nurs. Care **13**:26-27, 1980.
4. Beeson, P.B., McDermott, W., and Wyngaarden, J.B., editors: Textbook of medicine, ed. 15, Philadelphia, 1979, W.B. Saunders Co.
5. Booth, J.B.: Meniere's disease: the selection and assessment of patients for surgery using electrocochleography, Ann. R. Coll. Surg. Engl. **62**:415-425, 1980.
6. *Boyd-Monk, H.: Screening for glaucoma, Nurs. '79 **9**(8):42-44, 1979.
7. *Boyd-Monk, H.: Helping the corneal transplant patient to see again, Nurs. '78 **8**(2):47-51, 1978.
8. Brackman, D., and Anderson, R.G.: Meniere's disease: treatment with the endolymphatic subarachnoid shunt, a review of 125 cases, Otolaryngol. Head Neck Surg. **88**:174-182, 1980.
9. Brackman, D., and House, W.: Direct stimulation of the auditory nerve in hearing disorders. In Northern, J.: Hearing disorders, Boston, 1976, Little, Brown & Co.
10. Bull, T., and Cook, J.: Speech therapy and ENT surgery, Oxford, London, 1976, Blackwell Scientific Publications.
11. Caruso, V.G.: When the patient has otitis externa, Geriatrics **35**(5):35-42, 1980.
12. Chadwick, D.L.: Treatment of ENT conditions, Nurs. Times **70**:424-425, 1974.
13. Chadwick, D.L.: Advances in the treatment of diseases of the ear, nose and throat, Practitioner **209**:460-473, 1972.
14. Chenoweth, R.G.: Retinal detachment. In Fraunfelder, F.T., and Roy, F.H.: Current ocular therapy, Philadelphia, 1980, W.B. Saunders Co.
15. Chignell, A.H.: Retinal detachment surgery, New York, 1980, Springer-Verlag New York, Inc.
16. Chouard, C.H.: The surgical rehabilitation of total deafness with the multichannel cochlear implant: indications and results, Audiology **19**:137-145, 1980.
17. Condl, E.D., et al.: Ophthalmic nursing, Nurs. Clin. North Am. **5**:449-496, 1970.
18. DeWeese, D.D., and Saunders, W.H.: Textook of otolaryngology, ed. 5, St. Louis, 1977, The C.V. Mosby Co.
19. Duberstein, L.E.: Myringotomy without bleeding, Otolaryngol. Head Neck Surg. **87**:237-238, 1979.
20. *Elkington, A.R.: Intraocular foreign bodies, Nurs. Times **69**:1638-1639, 1973.
21. *Elkington, A.R.: Non-perforating wounds, Nurs. Times **69**:1562-1563, 1973.
22. *Elkington, A.R.: Perforating wounds, Nurs. Times **69**:1597-1598, 1973.
23. English, G.M., Northern, J.G., and Fria, T.J.: Chronic otitis media as a cause of sensorineural hearing loss, Arch. Otolaryngol. **98**:17-20, 1973.
24. Farmer, H.S.: A guide for the treatment of external otitis, Am. Fam. Physician **21**(6):96-101, 1980.
25. *Fersberger, W.: Early diagnosis of acute angle-closure glaucoma, Am. J. Nurs. **75**:1154-1155, 1975.
26. *Fletcher, D.: Intraocular lenses: an unexpected discovery, Nurs. Mirror **150**:34-35, 1980.
27. Fraunfelder, F.T., and Roy, F.H.: Current ocular therapy, Philadelphia, 1980, W.B. Saunders Co.
28. Freeman, J.: Otosclerosis and vestibular dysfunction, Laryngoscope **90**:1481-1487, 1980.
29. *Fulton, M.K., et al.: Helping diabetics adapt to failing vision, Am. J. Nurs. **74**:54-57, 1974.
30. Gates, G.A.: Vertigo in children, Ear Nose Throat J. **59**:358-365, 1980.
31. Gellis, S.S., and Kagan, B.M.: Current pediatric therapy, ed. 9, Philadelphia, 1980, W.B. Saunders Co.
32. Girard, L.J.: Ultrasonic aspiration-irrigation of cataracts and the vitreous. In Emery, J.M., and Paton, D.: Current concepts in cataract surgery: selected proceedings of the fourth biennial cataract surgical congress, St. Louis, 1976, The C.V. Mosby Co.
33. Goldberg, I., et al.: Marijuana as a treatment for glaucoma, Sight Sav. Rev. **48**:147-155, 1978-79.
34. Gottschalk, G.H.: Nonsurgical management of otitis media with effusion, Ann. Otol. Rhinol. Laryngol. **89**(suppl.):301-302, 1980.
35. Hall, I.S., and Colman, B.: Diseases of the nose, throat, and ear, New York, 1975, Churchill Livingstone, Inc.
36. Hammond, V.: A symposium on the surgery of deafness: stapedectomy, Nurs. Mirror **140**:45-48, 1975.
37. Havener, W.H.: Synopsis of ophthalmology, ed. 5, St. Louis, 1979, The C.V. Mosby Co.
38. *Hiles, D.A.: Strabismus, Am. J. Nurs. **74**:1082-1089, 1974.
39. Hiles, D.A.: Results of the first year's experience with phacoemulsification, Am. J. Ophthalmol. **75**:474-477, 1973.
40. Hornblass, A.: Tumors of the ocular adnexa and orbit, St. Louis, 1979, The C.V. Mosby Co.
41. House, W.F.: Meniere's disease: management and theory, Otolaryngol. Clin. North Am. **8**:515-535, 1975.
42. House, W.F., and Belal, M.: Translabyrinthine surgery: anatomy and pathology, Am. J. Otol. **1**:189-198, 1980.
43. House, W.F., and Urban, J.: Long term results of electrode implantation and electronic stimulation of the cochlea in man, Ann. Otol. Rhinol. Laryngol. **82**:504-517, 1973.
44. *Huber, H.L.: Draining the "fluid ear" with myringotomy and tube insertion, Nurs. '78 **8**(7):28-30, 1978.
45. Jaffe, N.S.: Cataract surgery and its complications, ed. 3, St. Louis, 1981, The C.V. Mosby Co.
46. *Jennings, B.: Intraocular lens for cataracts, A.O.R.N. J. **23**:664-672, 1976.
47. Johnson, E.W., and House, J.: Meniere's disease: clinical course, auditory findings, and hearing aid fitting, J. Am. Aud. Soc. **5**(2):76-83, 1979.
48. Kelman, C.D.: Symposium: phacoemulsification and aspiration of senile cataracts, Trans. Am. Acad. Ophthalmol. Otolaryngol. **78**:7-9, 1974.
49. Kinney, S.E.: Middle ear reconstruction using cartilage and TORP and PORP, Laryngoscope **89**:2004-2007, 1979.
50. *Lancaster, V.: Cholesteatoma, Nurs. Mirror **145**(13):13-15, 1977.
51. Levenson, L., and Levenson, J.: Corneal transplantation, Am. J. Nurs. **77**:1160-1163, 1977.
52. Liana, J.C.: and Goldberg, M.F.: Treatment of diabetic retinopathy, Diabetes, **29**:841-851, 1980.
53. Ludman, H.: Discharge from the ear: chronic suppurative otitis media, Br. Med. J. **282**:48-49, 1981.
54. Ludman, H.: Discharge from the ear: otitis externa and acute otitis media, Br. Med. J. **281**:1616-1617, 1980.
55. Marlow, D.R.: Textbook of pediatric nursing, ed. 5, Philadelphia, 1977, W.B. Saunders Co.

---

*References preceded by an asterisk are particularly well suited for student reading.

56. Mausolf, F.A.: The eye and systemic disease, ed. 2, St. Louis, 1980, The C.V. Mosby Co.

57. Mawson, S.R.: Management of complications of stapedectomy, J. Laryngol. Otol. **89**:145-149, 1975.

58. McKenzie, W.: Vertigo, Nurs. Mirror **139**:56-57, 1974.

59. Meyerhoff, W.L., and Shrewsbury, D.: Rational approaches to tinnitus, Geriatrics **35**(10):90-93, 1980.

60. Miller, J.M., and Sutton, D.: Cochlear prosthesis: morphological considerations, J. Laryngol. Otol. **94**:359-366, 1980.

61. Mizuno, K., and Mitsui, Y.: Ophthalmology update, Amsterdam, 1980, Excerpta Medica.

62. Moody, E.: Amblyopia. In Harley, R.: Pediatric ophthalmology, Philadelphia, 1975, W.B. Saunders Co.

63. Moore, J.C.: Establishment of an outpatient ENT clinic, A.O.R.N. J. **31**:620-626, 1980.

64. Morrison, A.W., Moffat, D.A., & O'Connor, A.F.: Clinical usefulness of electrocochleography in Meniere's disease: an analysis of dehydrating agents, Otolaryngol. Clin. North Am. **13**:703-721, 1980.

65. Moses, R.A.: Adler's physiology of the eye: clinical application, ed. 7, St. Louis, 1981, The C.V. Mosby Co.

66. Naftalin, L.: The medical treatment of fluctuant hearing loss, Otolaryngol. Clin. North Am. **8**:475-482, 1975.

67. Nelson, W.E.: Textbook of pediatrics, ed. 11, Philadelphia, 1979, W.B. Saunders Co.

68. Newell, F.W.: Ophthalmology: principles and concepts, ed. 5, St. Louis, 1982, The C.V. Mosby Co.

69. Newell, F.W.: Strabismus and amblyopia, Acton, Mass., 1975, Publishing Sciences Group, Inc.

70. Nordlohne, M.E.: The intraocular implant lens development and results, with special reference to the Binkhorst lens, ed. 2, Baltimore, 1975, The Williams & Wilkins co.

71. Norton, E.: Symposium: intraocular lenses, Trans. Am. Acad. Ophthalmol. Otolaryngol. **81**:64-137, 1976.

72. Oosterveld, W.J.: Meniere's disease, signs and symptoms, J. Laryngol. Otol. **94**:885-892, 1980.

73. Pagon, R.A.: The role of genetic counseling in the prevention of blindness, Sight Sav. Rev. **49**:157-165, 1980.

74. Paparella, M.M., and Shumick, D.A., editors: Otolaryngology, ed. 2, Philadelphia, 1980, W.B. Saunders Co.

75. Pereira, P.: Screening for glaucoma, Nurs. Times **68**:771-774, 1972.

76. *Perrin, E.D.: Laser therapy for diabetic retinopathy, Am. J. Nurs. **80**:664-665, 1980.

77. Peyman, G.A., et al.: Principles and practice of ophthalmology, Philadelphia, 1980, W.B. Saunders Co.

78. *Pilgrim, M., and Sigler, B.: Phacoemulsification of cataracts, Am. J. Nurs. **75**:976-977, 1975.

79. Qvarnberg, Y., and Palva, T.: Active and conservative treatment of acute otitis media, prospective studies, Ann. Otol. Rhinol. Laryngol. **89**:269-270, 1980.

80. Reinecke, R.D., Stein, H.A., and Slatt, B.J.: Introductory manual for the ophthalmic assistant: a programmed text, St. Louis, 1972, The C.V. Mosby Co.

81. Roper-Hall, M.J.: Stallard's eye surgery, ed. 6, Philadelphia, 1980, J.B. Lippincott Co.

82. Rowe, D.S.: Acute suppurative otitis media, Pediatrics **56**:285-294, 1975.

83. Sabiston, D.C., editor: Davis-Christopher's textbook of surgery, ed. 11, Philadelphia, 1977, W.B. Saunders Co.

84. Saunders, W.H., et al.: Nursing care in eye, ear, nose, and throat disorders, ed. 4, St. Louis, 1979, The C.V. Mosby Co.

85. Scheie, H.G., and Albert, D.M.: Adler's textbook of ophthalmology, ed. 9, Philadelphia, 1977, W.B. Saunders Co.

86. *Schultz, J.M., and Williams, M.: The blind diabetic, Nurs. '76 **6**(12):19-20, 1976.

87. Schwartz, R.H.: Myringotomy: a neglected office procedure, Am. Fam. Physician **20**(6):102-108, 1979.

88. Schwartz R.H., and Schwartz, D.M.: Acute otitis media: diagnosis and drug therapy, Drugs **19**:107-118, 1980.

89. Shea, J.: Fluctuant hearing loss, Otolaryngol. Clin. North Am. **8**:263-267, 1975.

90. Shuknecht, H.F.: Stapedectomy, Boston, 1971, Little, Brown & Co.

91. Smith, J.F., and Machazel, D.P.: Retinal detachment, Am. J. Nurs. **73**:1530-1535, 1973.

92. U.S. Department of Health, Education and Welfare: Support for vision research: interim report of the National Advisory Eye Council, no. (NIH) 76-1098, 1976.

93. U.S. Department of Health, Education and Welfare: Diabetic retinopathy, no. (NIH) 75-406, National Eye Institute, 1975.

94. Walloch, R.A., and Cowden, D.A.: Placement of electrodes for the excitation of the eighth nerve, Arch. Otolaryngol. **100**:19-23, 1974.

95. Waltman, S.R., and Krupin, T.: Complications in ophthalmic surgery, Philadelphia, 1980, J.B. Lippincott Co.

96. *Weinstock, F.J.: Emergency treatment of eye injuries, Am. J. Nurs. **71**:1929-1931, 1971.

97. White, N.: OR nursing in otomicrosurgery, A.O.R.N. J. **22**:889-897, 1975.

98. Williams, S.R.: Mowry's basic nutrition and diet therapy, ed. 6, St. Louis, 1980, The C.V. Mosby Co.

99. Zweng, H.C., Little, H.L., and Peabody, R.R.: Argon laser photocoagulation of diabetic retinopathy, Arch. Ophthalmol. **86**:395-400, 1971.

AUDIOVISUAL RESOURCES

Churchill Films, producer: Silent world, muffled world, Washington, D.C., Deafness Research Foundation, National Audiovisual Center. (Film, 16 mm black and white, 28 min.)

The ear and noise, Los Angeles, 1973, Los Angeles Foundation of Otology. (Videotape, 50 min.)

Ears to hear, New York, 1975, Canadian Broadcasting Corp. Filmmakers Library. (Videotape, 28 min.)

Emergency eye care, Garden Grove, Calif, 1971, Trainex Corp. (Filmstrip.)

The function of the ear in health and disease New York, 1969, Ayerst Laboratories. (Film, 35 min.)

Nursing process with hearing disorders, La Crosse, Wis., 1977, Medical Electronic Educational Services, Western Wisconsin Technical Institute, (Filmstrip, 42 min.)

Pediatric ophthalmology, Part 1 and Part 2, New York, 1972, MEDCOM. (Slides [105, 2 × 2], color.)

Sensorineural hearing impairment, Los Angeles, 1978, Ear Research Institute. (Videotape, 56 min.)

Where old age begins, Evanston, Ill., 1970, Video Nursing, American Journal of Nursing Co. (Film, 30 min.)

CHAPTER 40

ASSESSMENT OF THE MUSCULOSKELETAL SYSTEM

PATRICIA BUERGIN

The eagle that cannot fly will starve to death. The deer that cannot run becomes the easy prey of its enemies. And if humans had to rely solely on themselves for their food, shelter, and protection, without the ability to move, they too would surely die. This is the importance of the musculoskeletal system. Yet there are many illnesses and disorders that deprive individuals of their ability to move about freely.

In order to plan appropriate interventions for individuals who have locomotor disabilities, the disabilities and the individual's reaction to them require careful assessment. Such assessment is based on knowledge and understanding of the anatomy and physiology of the musculoskeletal system, and understanding of the laboratory studies involved and what the results of these studies mean. In this chapter the anatomy and physiology of the musculoskeletal system, methods for obtaining subjective and objective data about the patients and their disabilities, and the pertinence of selected laboratory studies are discussed.

Anatomy and physiology

Bones

If you can imagine a human body without bones, you can define the three mechanical functions of bones: (1) *support* as provided by the skeletal framework itself; (2) *protection,* as in the example of the bony casing of the skull that protects the brain; and (3) *movement,* in which muscles contract, pulling on bones that act as levers to provide motion for the body. Bone also has a physiologic function as a storehouse of calcium.

Bones are composed of both living cells and nonliving intracellular material. They are derived from embryonic hyaline cartilage that undergoes a process known as *osteogenesis,* or *endochondral ossification,* to become bone. This process is accomplished through the synthesis of mucopolysaccharides and collagen by cells called *osteoblasts.* These two substances make up the material known as *bone matrix.* Calcium salts are deposited in the bone matrix, giving it the "hard" quality by which bone is characterized.

There are four types of bones according to their shape: long (femur, humerus), short (carpals), flat (skull), and irregular (vertebrae). Each bone is composed of *cancellous* (spongy) and *compact* (dense) bone. In the long bones the cancellous portions are found in the ends of the bones, and the compact bone is located in the shaft. The short and irregular bones have an inner core of cancellous bone with an outer layer of compact bone. The flat bones have two outer plates of compact bone with an inner layer of cancellous bone.

Cancellous bone and compact bone are differentiated from one another by the arrangement of the *lamellae* within them. Lamellae are concentric cylindric layers of calcified matrix. At the center of this arrangement of concentric rings is a canal, called the *haversian canal.* This canal contains a capillary. Some canals may also contain a small arteriole, venule, and lymphatics. Small spaces between the rings of the lamellae, called *lacunae,* are occupied by bone cells *(osteocytes).* Lacunae are connected with the haversian canal, and therefore the nutrient supply, by very small canals called *canaliculi.* The lamella with its haversian canal, la-

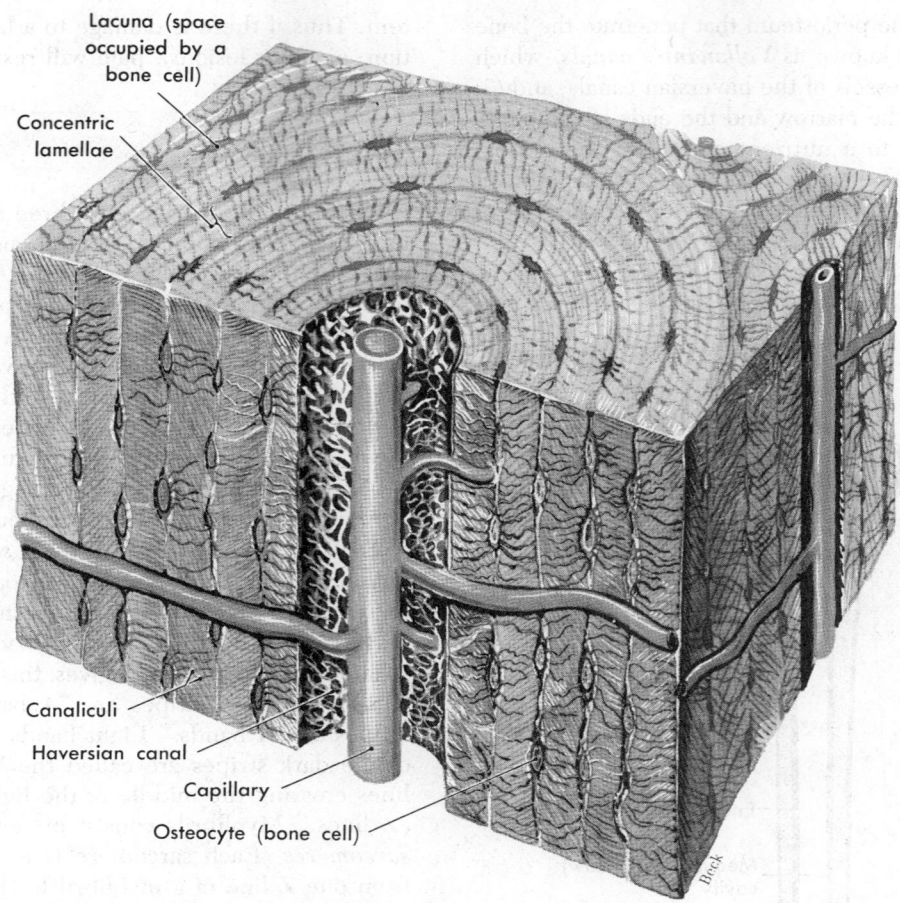

Lacuna (space occupied by a bone cell)

Concentric lamellae

Canaliculi

Haversian canal

Capillary

Osteocyte (bone cell)

Fig. 40-1. Section of compact bone showing details of haversian system. (From Anthony, C.P., and Kolthoff, N.J.: Textbook of anatomy and physiology, ed. 9, St. Louis, 1975, The C.V. Mosby Co.)

cunae, and canaliculi is called a haversian unit (Fig. 40-1). Haversian units fit closely together in compact bone. In cancellous bone, however, there are many open spaces between thin interconnecting processes of bone called trabeculae. This arrangement of fine threads of bone resembles the fine filigree work of the jeweler. Such an arrangement provides strength to the bone while reducing its weight.

A typical long bone is covered, except on its articular surfaces, by a white, fibrous membrane called the *periosteum*. The articular surfaces are covered with resilient *hyaline cartilage*. The periosteum provides a place for muscle fibers to attach, and its inner layers contain osteoblasts. Because of the presence of osteoblasts, the periosteum is considered an organ of growth and repair. The ends of the bone are called *epiphyses*, and the shaft is known as the *diaphysis*. The membranous *endosteum* lines the marrow-filled *medullary cavity* and the haversian canals (Fig. 40-2). The endosteum contains some osteoblasts.

Longitudinal growth of the long bones emanates from the epiphyseal cartilage, located between the diaphyseal and epiphyseal centers of ossification. This epiphyseal cartilage thickens because of rapid proliferation of the cartilage cells, and this additional cartilage undergoes ossification. Growth in the diameter of the bone is accomplished as osteoclasts (bone-destroying cells) enlarge the medullary cavity while osteoblasts in the periosteum produce new bone at the outside of the bone (membranous ossification). In older people or in people who are quite inactive, degeneration and reabsorption of bone occur more rapidly than growth of new bone. This leads to a condition called *osteoporosis*. In this condition bone becomes porous and fragile. Bone will reshape itself in response to alterations of its mechanical function. Such a response is in accordance with *Wolff's law:* "Every change in the form and function of bones or their function alone is followed by certain definite changes in their external configuration in accordance with mathematical laws."[11]

Blood is supplied to the bone by three routes: (1) through the arterioles in the haversian canals; (2) through vessels located in the periosteum that penetrate the bone through structures known as *Volkmann's canals*, which connect with the vessels of the haversian canals; and (3) through vessels in the marrow and the ends of the bone. Therefore damage to a nutrient artery, to the periosteum, or to the bone itself, resulting in separation of the broken ends of the bone, causes an interruption of the blood supply to the bone.

Further, bones are supplied with a network of sensory nerves that connect with the central nervous system. Thus if there is damage to a bone (fracture, infection, or other lesions), pain will result.

Muscles

Muscles are divided into three major groups: skeletal (striated, voluntary), visceral (smooth, involuntary), and cardiac. Visceral muscle, as in the stomach and intestines, is innervated by the autonomic nervous system and therefore is not under the control of the will. Skeletal muscle, however, is innervated by nerve fibers from the cerebrospinal system and is under control of the will. Skeletal muscle provides controlled movement, maintains posture, and produces heat.

Skeletal muscle cells are long and narrow. This structure causes them to be called *fibers* rather than cells. They are composed of a *sarcolemma*, or cell membrane, and *sarcoplasm*, or cytoplasm. Small, closely packed fibers within the sarcoplasm, called *myofibrils*, that alternate light and dark horizontal stripes, give the striated appearance that gives this type of muscle its name. The dark stripes are "A bands," and the light stripes are "I bands." Light bands crossing the middle of the dark stripes are called the "H zone," and dark lines crossing the middle of the light stripes are called "Z lines." Myofibrils consist of several sections called *sarcomeres*. Each sarcomere is a section that extends from one Z line of a myofibril to the next (Fig. 40-3).[1] Bundles of muscle fibers (cells) make up the muscle itself.

It is the function of muscles to contract. This is accomplished by a complex process triggered by nerve impulses arriving at the muscle fiber. Calcium ions are released when the impulse is received and bind to troponin (an inhibitor of the molecular myosin-actin interaction). Once troponin is bound, the myosin-actin interaction takes place and the sarcomeres of the myofibrils contract. The energy for muscle contraction is supplied by the breakdown of adenosine triphosphate (ATP), which the muscle cells produce by combining adenosine diphosphate (ADP) with creatine phosphate. Re-

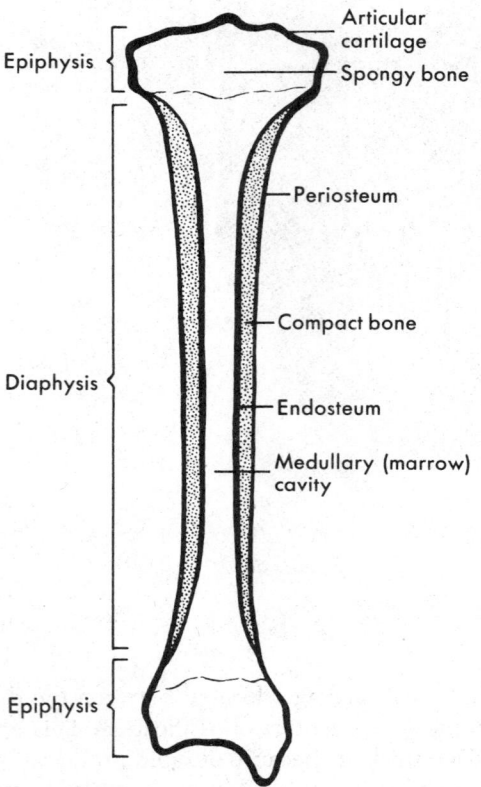

Fig. 40-2. Structure of long bone as seen in longitudinal section. (From Anthony, C.P., and Thibodeau, G.A.: Textbook of anatomy and physiology, ed. 11, St. Louis, 1983, The C.V. Mosby Co.)

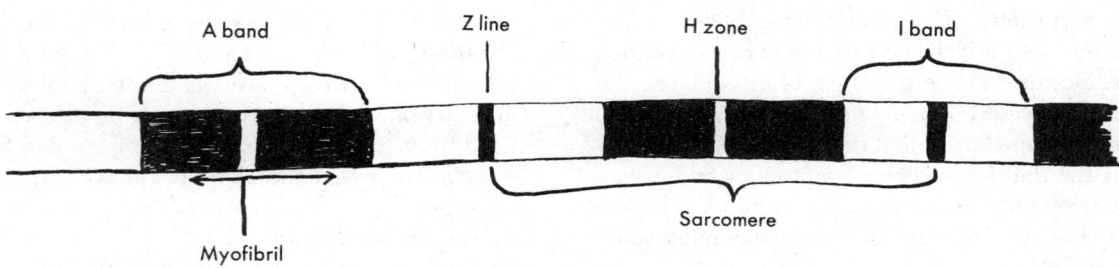

Fig. 40-3. Schematic drawing of structure of a myofibril.

laxation of the muscle occurs when the calcium separates from the troponin[1] (Fig. 40-4). Muscle cells obey the "all-or-none" law; that is, they contract fully or not at all. This does *not* mean that the entire muscle contracts fully. Just those individual cells that have received the nerve impulse contract. Muscle fibers that are adequately oxygenated will contract more forcefully than those not adequately oxygenated.

Skeletal muscles are organs; they vary in size and shape from long and thin to broad and flat, or they may form bulky masses. The arrangement of the fibers within the muscle determines the capacity of the forceful contraction of the muscle. Skeletal muscles contract only if they are stimulated. There are several types of contractions: (1) *tonic*, or a continual partial contraction that is vital in the maintenance of posture; (2) *isotonic*, where the tension within the muscle is unchanged but the length of the muscle changes (shortens); (3) *isometric*,

where the tension increases but the muscle does not shorten; (4) the *twitch* or jerky reaction to a single stimulus; (5) *tetanic*, a more sustained contraction than the twitch and produced by a series of stimuli in rapid succession; (6) *treppe*, stronger twitch contractions in response to regularly repeated constant strength stimuli; (7) *fibrillation*, asynchronous contraction of individual fibers; and (8) *convulsion*, or abnormal uncoordinated tetanic contractions occurring in varying groups of muscles.[1]

Movements of the body are produced by muscles pulling on bones, with bones serving as levers, and joints serving as fulcrums for the levers. Most movements depend on several muscles acting in a coordinated manner. *Prime movers* produce the movement; *antagonists* relax while the prime movers contract, thereby permitting movement; and *synergists* contract at the same time as the prime movers to produce movement or to stabi-

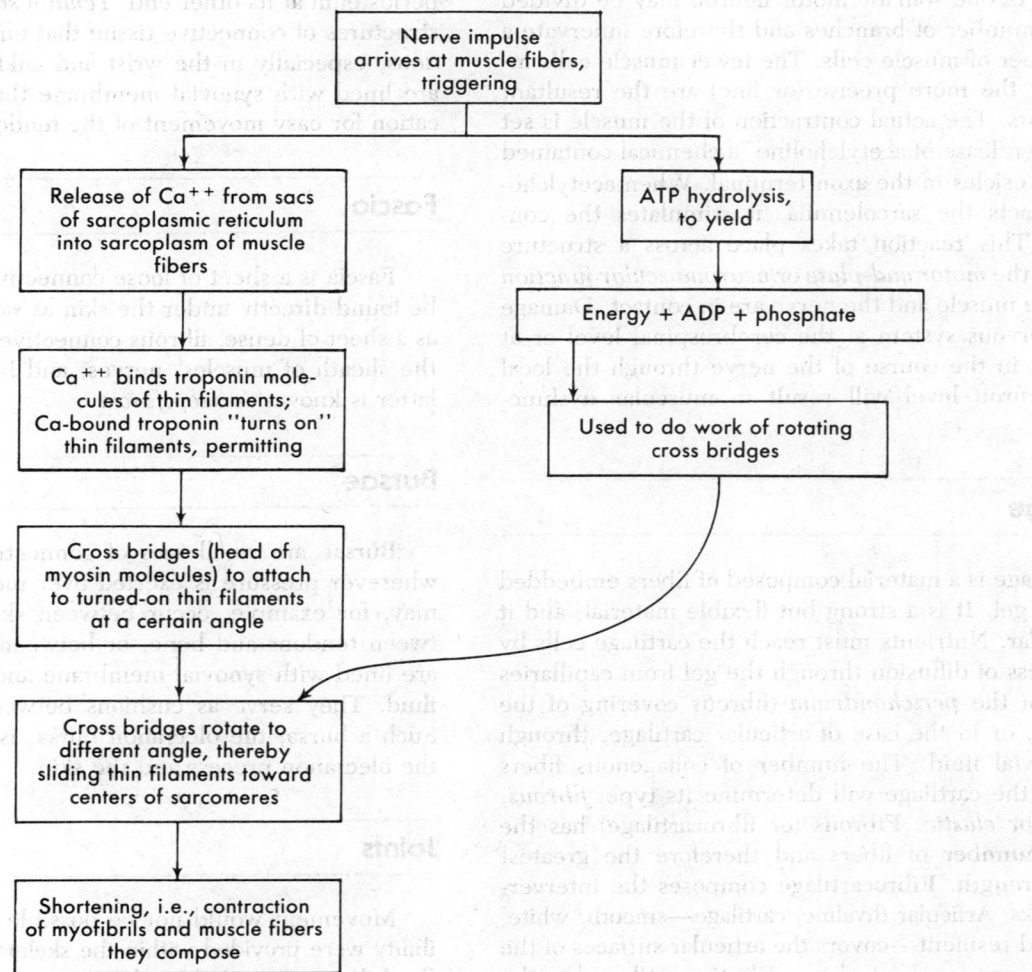

Fig. 40-4. Mechanism of skeletal muscle contraction. (From Anthony, C.P., and Thibodeau, G.A.: Textbook of anatomy and physiology, ed. 11, St. Louis, 1983, The C.V. Mosby Co.)

lize a part so the contraction of the prime movers is more efficient.[1]

Skeletal muscle is highly vascular. Waste products resulting from the chemical changes that occur during muscle contraction must be transported to the liver to be resynthesized, and oxygen must be transported to the muscle fibers if those fibers are to perform their work. Muscle fatigue and pain result when waste products cannot be adequately carried off. Conditions such as anemia, in which the amount of hemoglobin available to carry oxygen is reduced, or trauma, which interrupts circulation to the muscle fibers, will result in poor muscle work, since contractions depend on an adequate oxygen supply.

Adequate muscle contractions also depend on effective innervation. The cerebellum is primarily responsible for control of muscle movements (see Chapter 34). Every muscle cell is supplied with the axon of a nerve cell. Nerve cells that transmit impulses to skeletal muscles are known as *somatic motor neurons*. The neuron and the muscle cells it activates are called a *motor unit*. The axon of one somatic motor neuron may be divided into any number of branches and therefore innervate a like number of muscle cells. The fewer muscle cells innervated, the more precise (or fine) are the resultant movements. The actual contraction of the muscle is set off by the release of acetylcholine, a chemical contained in small vesicles in the axon terminal. When acetylcholine contacts the sarcolemma, it stimulates the contraction. This reaction takes place across a structure known as the *motor end-plate* or *neuromuscular junction* where the muscle and the nerve are in contact. Damage to the nervous system at the cerebrospinal level or at any point in the course of the nerve through the local motor neuron level will result in muscular dysfunction.

Cartilage

Cartilage is a material composed of fibers embedded in a firm gel. It is a strong but flexible material, and it is avascular. Nutrients must reach the cartilage cells by the process of diffusion through the gel from capillaries located in the *perichondrium* (fibrous covering of the cartilage), or in the case of articular cartilage, through the synovial fluid. The number of collagenous fibers found in the cartilage will determine its type: *fibrous, hyaline,* or *elastic*. Fibrous (or fibrocartilage) has the greatest number of fibers and therefore the greatest tensile strength. Fibrocartilage composes the intervertebral disks. Articular (hyaline) cartilage—smooth, white, shiny, and resilient—covers the articular surfaces of the bone and serves as a cushion. Elastic cartilage has the fewest fibers and may be found in areas such as the external ear.

Ligaments

Ligaments are bands of dense fibrous connective tissue that are flexible and tough. They connect the articular ends of bones and provide stability. Examples are the medial and lateral collateral ligaments of the knee that provide mediolateral stability to the knee joint, and the anterior and posterior cruciate ligaments within the joint capsule of the knee that provide anteroposterior stability. Ligaments may also attach to soft tissue to suspend structures. An example of this is the suspensory ligament of the ovary that passes from the tubal end of the ovary to the peritoneum.

Tendons

Tendons are bands of dense fibrous tissue that form the termination of a muscle and serve to attach it to a bone. The tendon is an extension of the fibrous sheath that envelops each muscle and is continuous with the periosteum at its other end. *Tendon sheaths* are tubular structures of connective tissue that enclose certain tendons, especially in the wrist and ankle. These sheaths are lined with synovial membrane that provides lubrication for easy movement of the tendon.

Fascia

Fascia is a sheet of loose connective tissue that may be found directly under the skin as *superficial fascia* or as a sheet of dense, fibrous connective tissue making up the sheath of muscles, nerves, and blood vessels. The latter is known as *deep fascia*.

Bursae

Bursae are small sacs of connective tissue located wherever pressure is exerted over moving parts. They may, for example, occur between skin and bone, between tendons and bone, or between muscles. Bursae are lined with synovial membrane and contain synovial fluid. They serve as cushions between moving parts. Such a bursa, the olecranon bursa, is located between the olecranon process and the skin.

Joints

Movement would not be possible unless some flexibility were provided within the skeletal framework. This flexibility is provided by the joints, or places where the bones come together. The shape of the joint will determine the amount and type of movement that are pos-

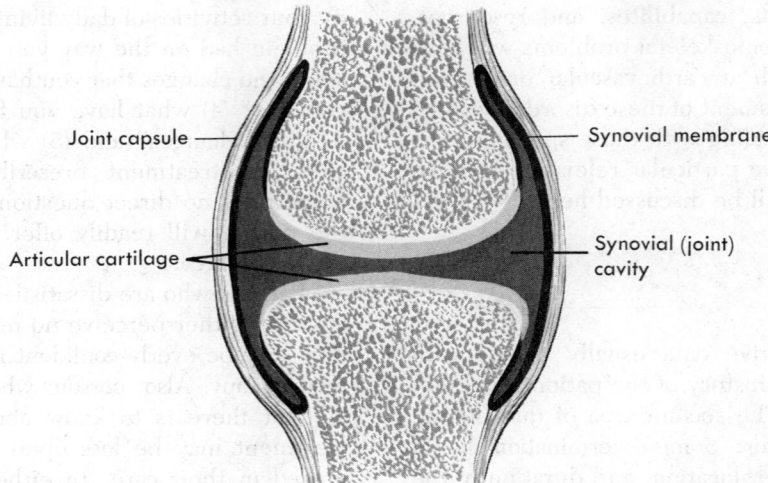

Fig. 40-5. Structure of diarthrotic joint. (From Anthony, C.P., and Thibodeau, G.A.: Textbook of anatomy and physiology, ed. 11, St. Louis, 1983, The C.V. Mosby Co.)

sible, and the classification of joints is based on the amount of movement they allow.

Classification

There are three major classifications of joints: (1) *synarthroses* (or fibrous joints), such as the sutures of the skull that do not allow movement; (2) *amphiarthroses* (or cartilaginous joints), such as the intervertebral joints that allow little movement (the synarthroses and the amphiarthroses may be classified together as synarthroses, designating that they have no joint cavity but rather tissue [fibrous, cartilage, or bone] growing between their articular surfaces); and (3) *diarthroses* or *synovial joints,* which allow free movement. Diarthroses include the hip, knee, shoulder, and elbow. Since diarthrodial joints are the joints that permit movement, they are discussed in the most detail.

Each diarthrodial joint contains a small space or *joint cavity* between the articulating surfaces of the bones that make up the joint. Articular hyaline cartilage covers the articulating surfaces of both bones. Additionally, a *joint capsule,* or sleeve of fibrous tissue, encases the joint. This capsule is lined with synovial membrane that secretes *synovial fluid,* which serves to lubricate the joint (Fig. 40-5). Additionally, ligaments may be present between the bones (as with the cruciate ligaments of the knee) to provide internal stability to the joint. Small pieces of dense cartilage may also be interposed between the articulating surfaces. These are crescent-shaped or half-moon–shaped structures that provide additional cushioning for the joint. Examples are the semilunar cartilages, or *menisci,* of the knee joint.

Diarthrodial joints are further classified by the shape of their surfaces and the type of movement they permit. Specialized texts should be consulted for discussion of

these subtypes. However, it may be generally stated that the diarthrodial joints permit one or more of the following movements: flexion, extension, adduction, abduction, rotation, circumduction, supination, pronation, inversion, eversion, protraction, or retraction. The latter six movements are considered special movements (Figs. 40-12 and 40-13).

Pathologic conditions in the musculoskeletal system

As discussed in the anatomy and physiology of the musculoskeletal system, the musculoskeletal and nervous systems are interrelated. The muscles, bones, joints, supportive structures, and sensory and motor nerves all work together to provide controlled movement. However, any problem that causes interference or disturbance at any level—innervation, contractility, articulation, or support—of this well-integrated system results in musculoskeletal dysfunction. Problems can occur when there is interruption of blood supply to the involved structures; disease affecting the contour of bones or joints; disease affecting the nerves that innervate the musculoskeletal system; or trauma, of whatever origin, that interrupts the integrity of any of the involved structures.

Assessment of the person

As for a person with any other type of illness, plans for care and eventual discharge are based on a systematic assessment of needs, capabilites, and resources. Many persons with musculoskeletal problems will have additional problems such as cardiovascular or respiratory disorders, and assessment of these disorders can be found in the chapters dealing with those specific disorders. Only data that have particular relevance to musculoskeletal problems will be discussed here.

Subjective data

Collection of subjective data usually begins with questions related to the history of the patient's present illness or dysfunction. The second area of questioning relates to pain or discomfort. Some determination should be made as to the nature, location, and duration of the patient's pain or discomfort; what measures the patient has taken to relieve it; and whether these measures were effective. A list of the patient's current medications is obtained, along with a list of any allergies, particularly drug allergies. The third area, and one of major importance, relates to questions about activities of daily living (ADL), since dysfunction of the musculoskeletal system often leads to a loss of independence in ADL. The major functions included in *personal* ADL are feeding, bathing, toileting, dressing, transfer, ambulation, and sleep. Pertinent questions include: Is assistance needed from other people to perform any of these functions? Are assistive devices used to help perform these functions independently? Do pain or other symptoms interfere with sleep? *Social* ADL functions include household activities, work activities, recreational activities, and sexual activities. Have these activities been curtailed or modified because of symptoms? How successful have the modifications been?

If the person needs assistance to perform any activities, who provides the assistance? Is that person able to provide adequate assistance? What modifications have been made in the home environment? How well do these modifications work?

Some individuals with musculoskeletal disorders are highly imaginative, inventive, or well informed regarding the variety of assistive devices that are available. These individuals are often able to determine methods of dealing with their dysfunctions in clever ways, often managing to maintain their independence despite a significant degree of pathology. Others, not so creative or so well informed and with less pathology, may find themselves markedly handicapped because they are not aware of alterations that could be made in ADL or the environment to enhance their functional ability.

Person's perception of the problem

As part of the nursing interview, specific questions may be helpful in determining the person's perception of the problem. These include (1) have you had to mod-ify your activities of daily living? (2) what effect has your problem had on the way you live? (3) how do you feel about the changes that you have had to make in the way you live? (4) what have you found helpful in adapting to these changes? and (5) what do you do to comply with the treatment prescribed by your physician? Sometimes no direct questions will be necessary since the person will readily offer comments about each of the above areas.

Persons who are dissatisfied with their current therapy may either perceive no need for further therapy or they may be overly confident in their expectations about new therapy. Also, persons who perceive that they know all that there is to know about their disease and its treatment may be less open to teaching by those involved in their care. In either of these situations the better the nurse understands the patient, the better the plans developed for the patient's care can be.

Family's perception of the patient's problem

An individual's illness generally has some effect on the other people who are intimately associated with that individual. Therefore it is important to determine the effects of the person's illness on the family or significant others. Individuals may see themselves as burdens, embarrassments, or as objects of pity. On the other hand, if the significant others are supportive, the individual may feel well accepted, respected, and loved, even though the role relationships with others have been altered.

Frequently, when a person has a disabling chronic musculoskeletal illness, family roles are changed. Not infrequently, these changes in roles and status are resented, not only by the family, but by the person who may feel worthless or inadequate. When these conditions prevail, some intervention by health personnel (physician, nurse, social worker, or psychiatrist) may be necessary in an attempt to assist the person and the family to work through these feelings and to provide support.

Listening to what the person and the family have to say about the illness, the treatment, the long-term outcomes of the illness, and their feelings about the changes the illness has necessitated in their lives will give clues for interventions that might be tried to alleviate existing problems.

Objective data

Behavior

Assessment of the person's behavior includes making observations about mental status; orientation to time, place, and person; ability to understand directions; capacity to retain information; and span of attention. (See Chapter 34 for more information.) The person's *ability*

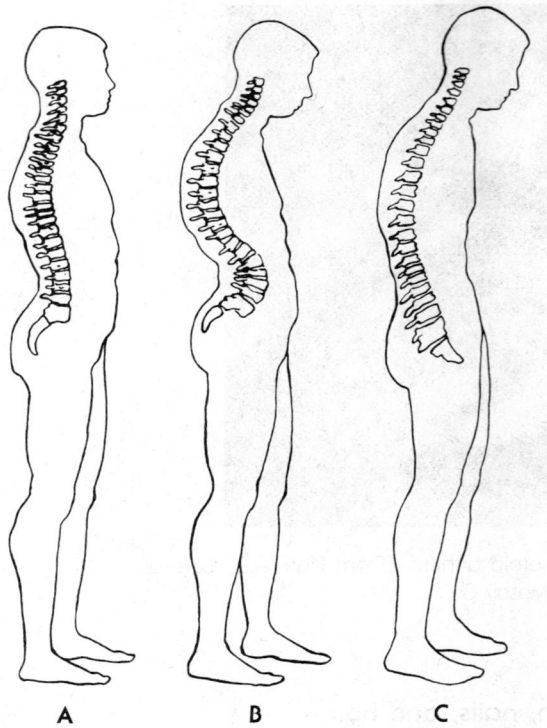

Fig. 40-6. A, Curves of spine in good posture. **B,** Curves of spine in slump posture. **C,** Obliteration of spinal curves as in early spondylitis. (From Larson, C.B., and Gould, M.: Orthopedic nursing, ed. 9, St. Louis, 1978, The C.V. Mosby Co.)

to relate to others—being withdrawn, quiet, talkative, tense, nervous, guarded, hostile—as determined from responses, affect, and behavior must also be considered. Interventions, if they are to be successful, must be based on the person's ability to understand and willingness to accept those interventions.

General appearance

General appearance is a second area to be assessed. The person's *age* and *sex* may bear a relationship to the specific disorder and can well affect the attitude toward the disorder. *Posture* can sometimes give clues to the nature of the problem, such as the severe kyphotic posture in ankylosing spondylitis (Fig. 40-6). The person may be stooped and unable to straighten up or may hold the body in a tense attitude to guard against pain from a severe whiplash.

Nutritional status—well nourished, overweight, or underweight—is also important. Obesity may be the result of general lack of activity in persons who have musculoskeletal disorders, since they do not perform enough activity to utilize the calories taken in. Extra pounds will tax a diseased musculoskeletal system, making it more difficult for the person to perform ADL. Severe underweight may be an indication of the individual's inability to secure and prepare nutritional meals

or to carry out feeding activities adequately, or it may be related to a specific systemic condition that causes nausea and vomiting or malabsorption of food. The person can usually give an accurate account of reasons for overweight or underweight.

Deformity

Many musculoskeletal problems are marked by deformity of one or more extremities or joints. Deformities should be specifically noted and described and some evaluation made of the extent to which the deformity curtails normal function. For example, the person who has severe "swan-neck" deformities of the fingers, ulnar deviation of the hand, and subluxation (incomplete dislocation) of the wrist may well be restricted in both fine and gross motor function of the hand. Deformity can be thought of as a change in size, shape, or position of a body part. Following are some of the more common deformities as related to position:

1. *Swan-neck deformity* is a flexion contracture of the metacarpophalangeal joint, hyperextension of the proximal interphalangeal joint, and flexion of the distal interphalangeal joint (Fig. 40-7).

2. In *ulnar deviation*, or drift, the fingers deviate at the metacarpophalangeal joints toward the ulnar aspect of the hand.

3. *Valgus* deformities (distal arm of the angle of the joint points away from the midline of the body) may be present in a number of joints. In *hallux valgus* the great toe turns toward the other toes. In *genu valgum* (Fig. 40-8) the knees are "knock-kneed." In *talipes valgus* the foot is everted.

4. *Varus* deformities (distal arm of the angle of the joint points toward the midline of the body) may also be present in a number of joints. *Genu varum* (Fig. 42-11) denotes a bowing of the knees, and *talipes varus* denotes inversion of the foot.

5. *Scoliosis* is a lateral curvature of the spine.

6. *Kyphosis* is also a curvature of the spine, but the convexity of the curve is posterior, usually in the thoracic area.

7. *Atrophy* (reduction in size of an organ) may lead to a difference in the appearance of an extremity or other body part. Atrophy of muscles is characterized by a wasting of the muscles so that in appearance they lack the bulk of normal muscle. This can result from disuse or from disease process such as polymyositis. Atrophied muscle will be weaker than normal muscle.

8. *Hypertrophy* is abnormal enlargement of an organ. In reference to the musculoskeletal system, hypertrophy is generally used to describe enlargement of muscle caused by a disease process. In pseudohypertrophic muscular dystrophy, for example, there is enlargement of the muscles of the calf of the leg. There is limitation of function associated with this enlargement.

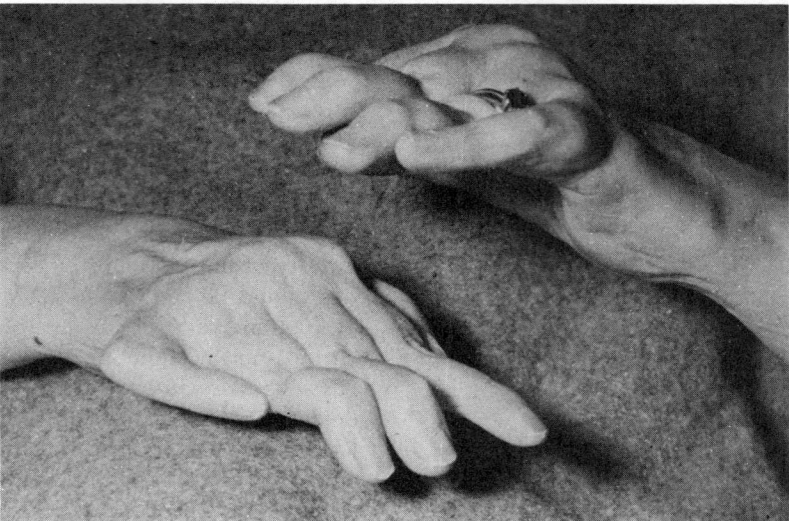

Fig. 40-7. Swan-neck deformities of fingers in rheumatoid arthritis. (From Flatt, A.E.: Care of the rheumatoid hand, ed. 3, St. Louis, 1974, The C.V. Mosby Co.)

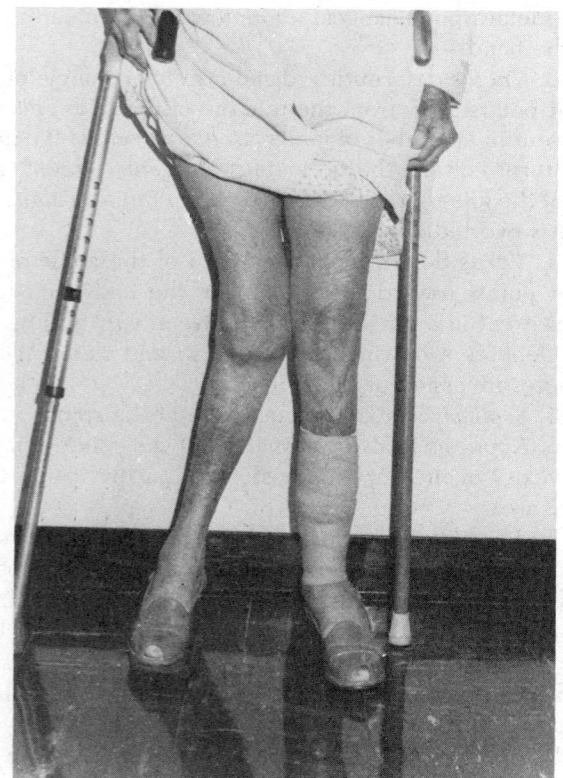

Fig. 40-8. Valgus deformity of knee.

Skin, nails, and hair

A third area of assessment is the condition of the skin and nails. The first areas to be assessed are *turgor* (fullness) and *texture* (feel). Many individuals, particularly those who are in late middle age and who have been taking steroid preparations for a prolonged period of time, will have a wasted appearance to their skin. It is dry and papery, almost having a transparent quality to it. This type of skin is easily broken. Individuals with scleroderma, on the other hand, will have patches of hard, nonelastic, leathery skin, often over the forearms, hands, chest, and face. This type of skin restricts movement of the structures underlying it.

The *integrity* of the skin must also be considered. Are there breaks in the skin, ulcerations, or reddened areas? Individuals with limited mobility are subject to skin breakdown. Pressure being exerted over skin areas and interfering with circulation to these areas may cause necrosis and breakdown of the skin, resulting in what are commonly known as pressure sores, or *decubitus ulcers* (p. 941). In addition, individuals who do not move well are subject to greater shearing forces against sheets, chair surfaces, bedpans, and other objects over which they move or are moved. Such shearing can irritate, abrade, or tear the skin. The complications that may arise from skin breakdown can last months or years longer than the acute process that brought the person to the hospital initially. Accurate assessment (which includes a determination of the status of circulation in the extremities) of potential for skin breakdown is vital in planning care that will help to prevent breakdown.

Assessing the *temperature* of the skin over painful joints (by palpating the skin) can help determine the

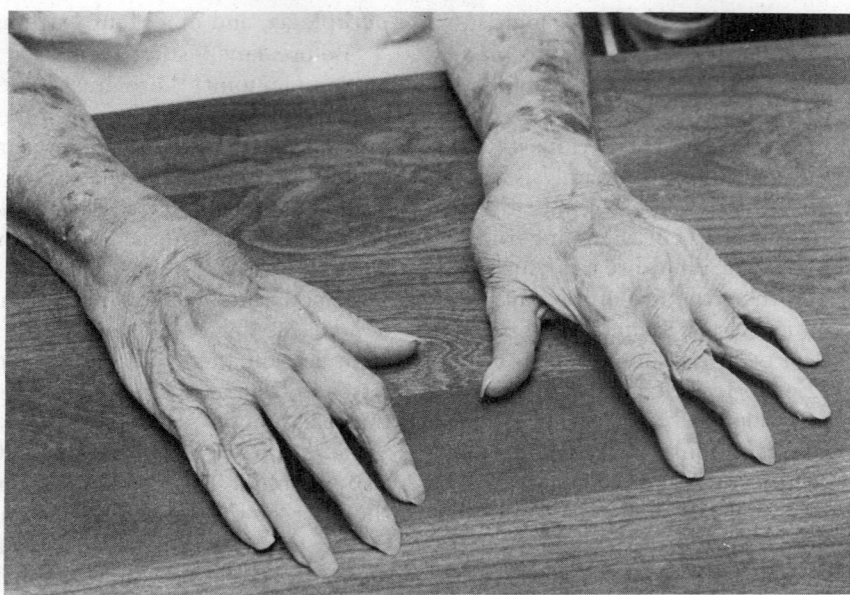

Fig. 40-9. Hands and forearms of woman with advanced rheumatoid arthritis. Note areas of bruising on forearms. Such ecchymoses are not uncommon in individuals who have rheumatoid arthritis and who take steroids in treatment. Handling of such individuals must be extremely gentle, both to avoid bruising and potential sloughing of these areas.

presence and degree of an inflammatory or an infectious process within the joint. *Erythema* of the skin may be present over acutely inflamed joints. Increased warmth is a positive indication of the presence of inflammation and the need to keep the joint at rest.

Skin *rash* may be present in psoriasis, scleroderma, rheumatic fever, dermatomyositis, and a number of other musculoskeletal disorders. A description of the nature (smooth, scaly, red, dusky) and location (over limbs, joints, face, trunk) of the rash provides a useful baseline in later determining the effectiveness of treatment.

A number of individuals with connective tissue diseases may demonstrate *color changes* in the skin of their fingers when they are exposed to cold. The characteristic color change is from white (resulting from arteriolar spasm) to blue (cyanosis caused by stagnation of blood) to red (caused by warming and reactive vasodilation).[16] These changes are known as *Raynaud's phenomenon,* the presence of which requires specific management consideration (p. 1157).

Bruising (ecchymosis) of the skin often occurs in individuals with connective tissue disease, particularly when they have had long-term treatment with corticosteroids (Fig. 40-9). Such areas of bruising may slough, become ulcerated, and at times become infected. Bruising will also be present in the soft tissue adjacent to and overlying areas that have been traumatized, as in persons who have suffered fractures or crushing injuries. The presence of bruising and skin fragility should be noted during the examination in order to plan for

precautions in the management and physical handling of the patient.

Areas of *swelling,* either of the extremities or of specific joints, must also be noted and the degree of swelling described. Peripheral edema may be present because of the prolonged dependent position of the extremity, lack of activity, circulatory disturbances, or renal involvement. Joints may be swollen as part of the inflammatory process (p. 280). The presence of serous, purulent, or bloody fluid in the joint capsule is termed *effusion* and is visible as a marked swelling of the joint. Inflamed synovium feels boggy and full on palpation. *Bony enlargements,* such as Heberden's nodes in osteoarthritis (Fig. 42-2), may be felt as hard, irregular swellings over the distal interphalangeal joints of the hands. *Subcutaneous nodules,* found in rheumatoid arthritis, are hard, most often mobile swellings found commonly in the subolecranon area. *Bursal swelling* is noted as a soft, palpable swelling over the bursa. Swelling may also be noted in the presence of a *synovial cyst,* such as Baker's cyst, which is characterized by swelling in the popliteal area, often extending into the calf. *Tophaceous deposits,* indicative of gout, are hard, translucent swellings that may be noted in cartilage such as that of the ear.

Tenderness may be elicited by direct pressure to a joint and may be grossly graded by the amount of pressure required to produce discomfort. Sometimes joints are not tender to palpation but are painful on active or passive range of motion. The degree of tenderness is usually in direct proportion to the severity of joint inflammation. Following trauma, tenderness is also present in the injured soft tissue and overlying areas of fractures.

Nails and hair are often a problem. Individuals with severe joint involvement, weakness, or paralysis may literally not be able to reach their toes or the top of their head or have the strength to cut their fingernails or toenails or comb their hair. Some diseases, such as psoriasis, cause changes in the structure of the nails (p. 1784) and a scaling condition of the scalp. Poorly cared for or diseased toenails can even prevent a person from wearing shoes or walking well. In individuals with some connective tissue diseases, alopecia (loss of hair) may occur. In most instances plans must be made for the proper care of fingernails, toenails, and hair.

Finally, during the examination of the skin there is opportunity to assess the person's *hygiene* status. Individuals with musculoskeletal disorders sometimes cannot tend to their own hygiene needs effectively, but they may not want to admit it. If evidence is found that hygiene needs are not being adequately met, plans can be made to introduce self-help devices or to assist the person in ways that will not cause embarrassment.

Strength and range of motion

Assessments of strength and range of motion are, in effect, measurements of the person's functional capacity. In discussing this area, there must first be some definition of terms:

Strength can be simply defined as the capacity to perform work.

Range of motion is the normal arc of movement provided for by the structure of a joint.

Active range of motion is the movement of a joint that can be accomplished without assistance.

Passive range of motion is the movement of a joint through its normal range by someone else.

Active assisted range of motion is active range of motion by the person with assistance to perform that motion. Active assisted range of motion can be employed, for example, with the person having polymyositis who has the strength to move the joint through only part of its normal range and needs assistance to complete the movement.

Dexterity refers to the coordination and agility with which movements are performed.

An extremity may be *flaccid*, having defective or absent muscle tone; *paralyzed*, having loss of function, especially loss of sensation or voluntary motion; or *paretic*, having incomplete loss of muscle power or partial paralysis. The suffix *-plegia* is used to describe paralysis. Involvement of one extremity is referred to as a *mono*plegia or monoparesis; of both extremities on one side of the body, *hemi*plegia; of both lower extremities,

*para*plegia; and of all four extremities, *quadri*plegia.

Before any testing of muscle strength or range of motion of a joint, there must be some assessment of the *position* of the person's extremities. Positions that vary from normal and that have an acute onset may be indications of fractures, dislocations, or ruptures of supporting structures. Typical of this kind of sudden change is the marked external rotation and shortening of the leg following a hip fracture; the inability to extend a "dropped" finger following rupture of an extensor tendon in the hand; or the postoperative "drop foot," a complication that may occur following surgical procedures to the back, hip, or knee because of stretching of the sciatic nerve.

Subluxation, or partial dislocation of a joint, should also be noted. This is often a chronic problem, as in the shoulder of the hemiplegic or in the wrist of the arthritic; but its presence is usually accompanied by some loss of function or need for support. Subluxation of the shoulder may be detected by feeling a space between the head of the humerus and the glenoid cavity of the scapula.

Loss of strength or limitation of joint motion will result in some degree of loss of function. Loss of strength or joint range of motion may be the result of a neurologic, skeletal, muscular, or traumatic disorder. Detailed tests of strength and joint range of motion require instruments such as the *dynamometer*, which measures grip strength in the hand, and the *goniometer* (an instrument resembling a protractor), which is useful in measuring joint motion (Fig. 40-10).

Gross testing of strength, however, may be done very simply. To test the upper extremities, apply moderate pressure with your hand against the person's upper arm to resist movement; then have the person (1) flex, extend, and abduct the shoulder; (2) with resistance at the forearm, flex and extend the elbow; and (3) at the wrist, flex and extend the hand. Hand grip strength may be tested by having the person squeeze your hand as hard as possible. The same maneuvers can be performed with the lower extremities. Applying moderate pressure with your hand against the person's foot to resist movement, ask the person to (1) invert and evert the foot and dorsiflex and plantar flex the ankle; (2) with resistance at the lower leg, flex and extend the knee; and (3) with resistance at the thigh, raise and lower the leg. In all these instances the area proximal to the joint being moved is stabilized by one of the examiner's hands, while moderate resistance to movement distal to the joint being moved is provided by the other hand. Trunk strength may be tested by having the person attempt to sit up from the supine position.

Gross muscle testing will provide very useful data for determining the amount of assistance the person needs. More specific testing done by a physical thera-

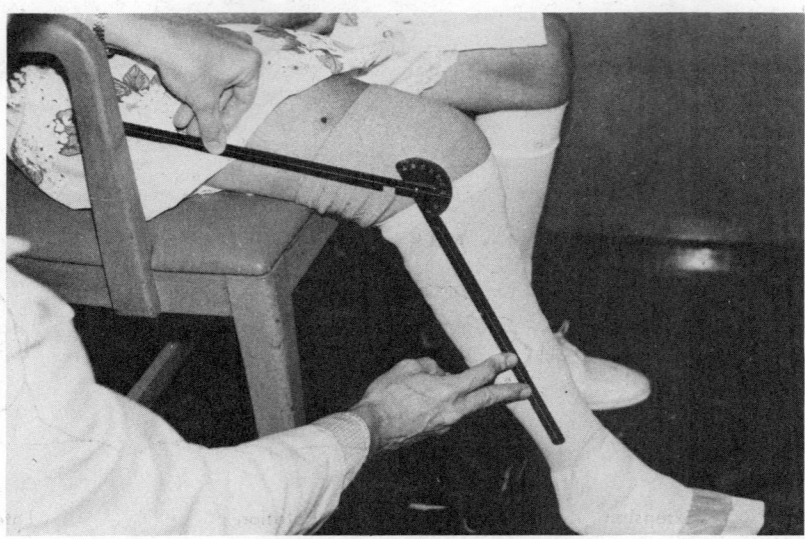

Fig. 40-10. Use of goniometer in measuring joint range.

pist is useful to the physician in diagnosis and to the therapist in planning a program of muscle-strengthening exercises (p. 938).

Coordination of the upper extremities can be tested by having the person extend an arm, touch one of the examiner's fingers with a finger, then touch his or her own nose, then the examiner's finger, and so on. The ability to pick up small objects, such as a coin or a pen, from a smooth, hard surface will provide some indication of the person's manual dexterity.

Range of motion is tested by having the person *actively* perform with each joint those motions that joint is capable of performing (Figs. 40-11 to 40-13). In some instances where the person cannot actively move a joint, as with the person in whom paralysis has previously been diagnosed, the joint may be passively moved. (Refer to Chapter 41 for discussion of passive range of motion and joint instability.) When passive range of motion is being performed, support must be given proximal to the joint moved (Fig. 40-14). Comparing the limitation of movement or instability that is present in one joint with its similar opposite joint is helpful in differentiating normal from abnormal findings.

If a joint cannot be moved beyond a certain point in its range (for example, a knee that does not extend beyond 30 degrees of flexion), it is said that the joint is contracted or that a *contracture* is present. Contractures may exist because of soft-tissue limitation (following a fracture with immobilization) or because of bony limitation (Fig. 40-15). The location and nature of contractures can be a significant indication of functional limitation. For example, a person with only 15 degrees of knee flexion in one knee will be able to climb steps only one at a time.

Crepitus, or a crunching or grating sound when the joint is actively or passively moved, is a significant indicator of the presence of a pathologic condition within the joint. This sound will also be heard if the two broken ends of a bone move against one another. *In the presence of a possible fracture, no attempt should be made to elicit crepitus*. At times, grating within a joint may be felt, rather than heard, by placing a hand over the joint as it moves.

The foregoing tests of strength, dexterity, and range of motion are simple to perform; however, it must be noted that the person's ability to perform the movements described may be limited by *pain* rather than weakness, lack of coordination, or joint limitation. It is often difficult to differentiate these factors, and while quantitatively the effect of the pain is the same as the effect of the weakness or limitation—that is, diminished function—qualitatively it makes a difference, since treatment measures will be geared to relief of pain rather than to muscle strengthening. To further confuse the situation, the person with pain may have actual concomitant muscle weakness on the basis of long-standing pain and consequent disuse of muscles. It must be remembered that in performing this kind of testing the person *must not be moved beyond the point of pain*. Pain is an indication that something is wrong. Injudicious testing techniques can produce untoward results; for example, the fracture of an osteoporotic bone. The desired result of such testing is the establishment of a baseline of strength, motion, and dexterity from which interventions to assist the person to gain strength, regain lost motion, and increase functional capacity may be planned and evaluated.

Text continued on p. 930.

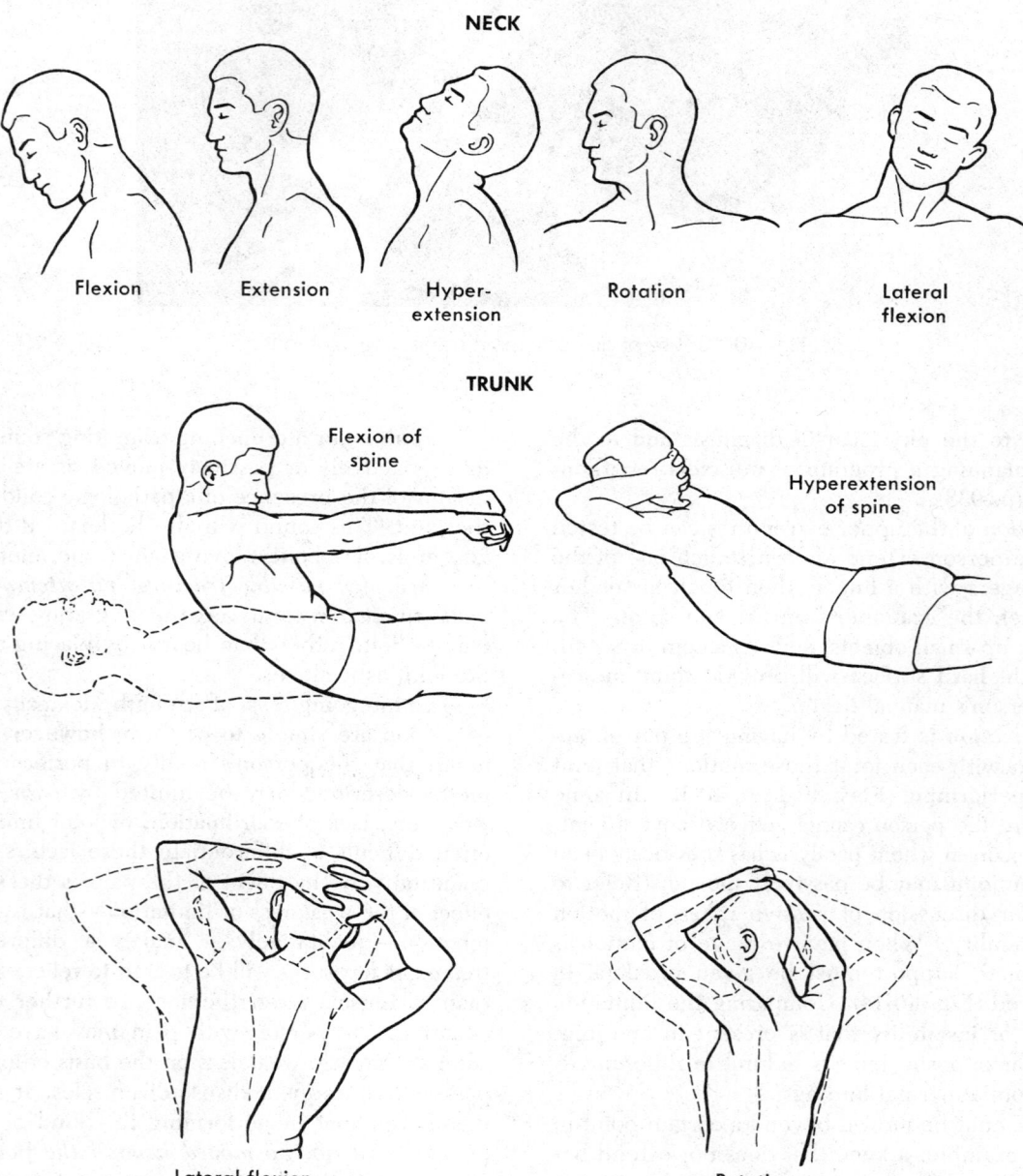

NECK

Flexion   Extension   Hyper-extension   Rotation   Lateral flexion

TRUNK

Flexion of spine

Hyperextension of spine

Lateral flexion

Rotation

Fig. 40-11. Range of joint motion for neck and trunk.

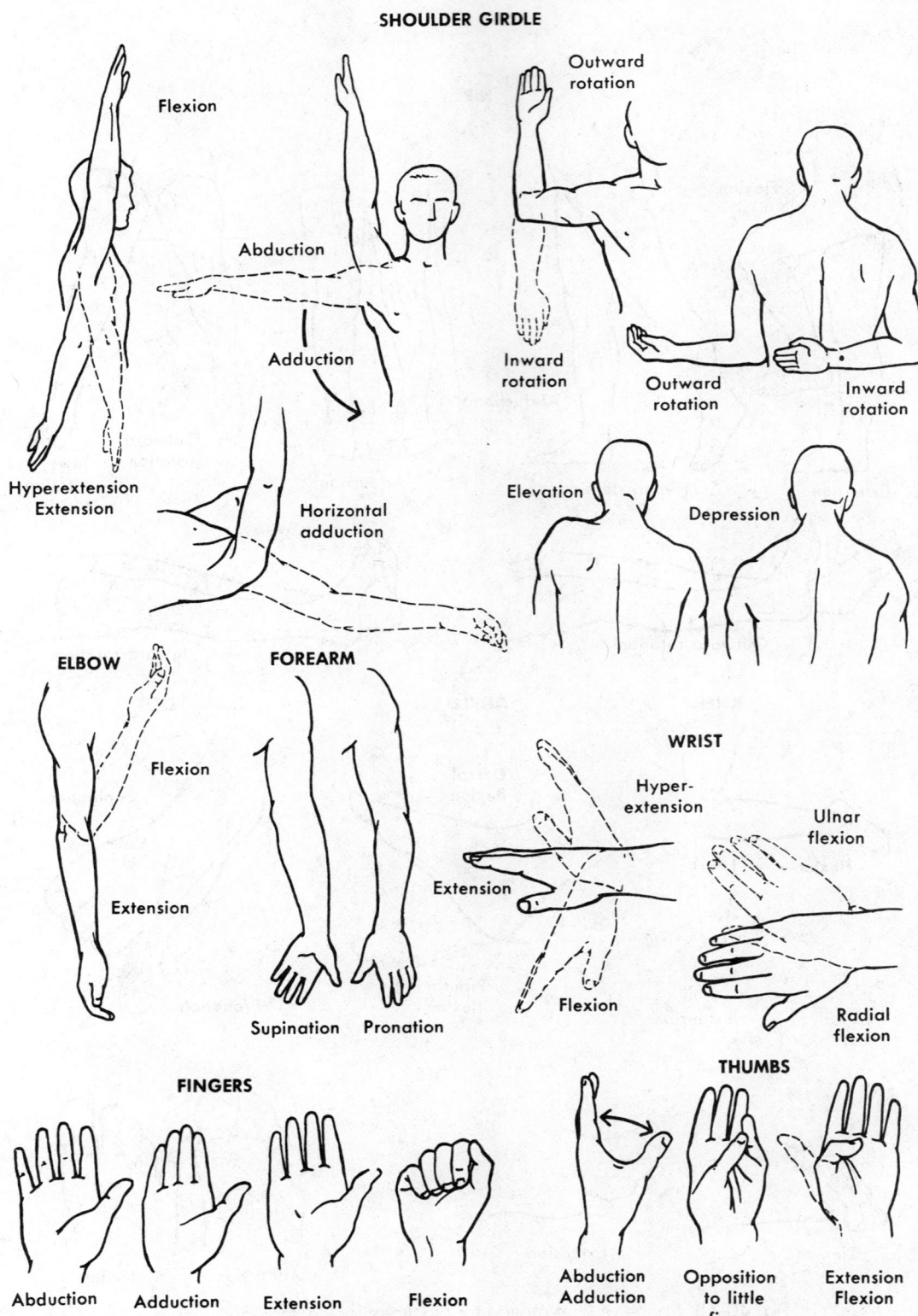

Fig. 40-12. Range of joint motion for shoulder and shoulder girdle, elbow, forearm, wrist, and hand.

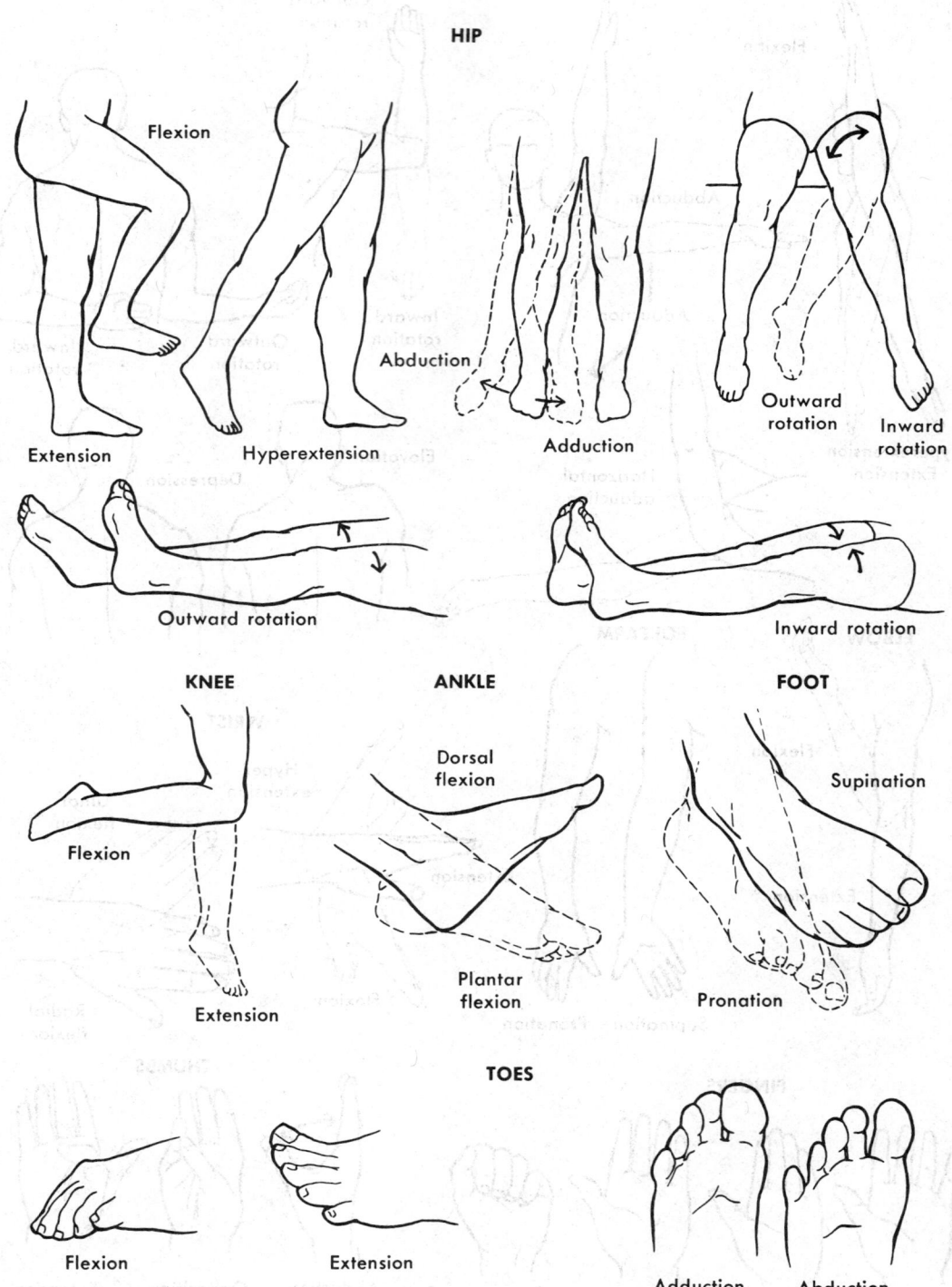

Fig. 40-13. Range of joint motion for hip, knee, ankle, foot, and toes.

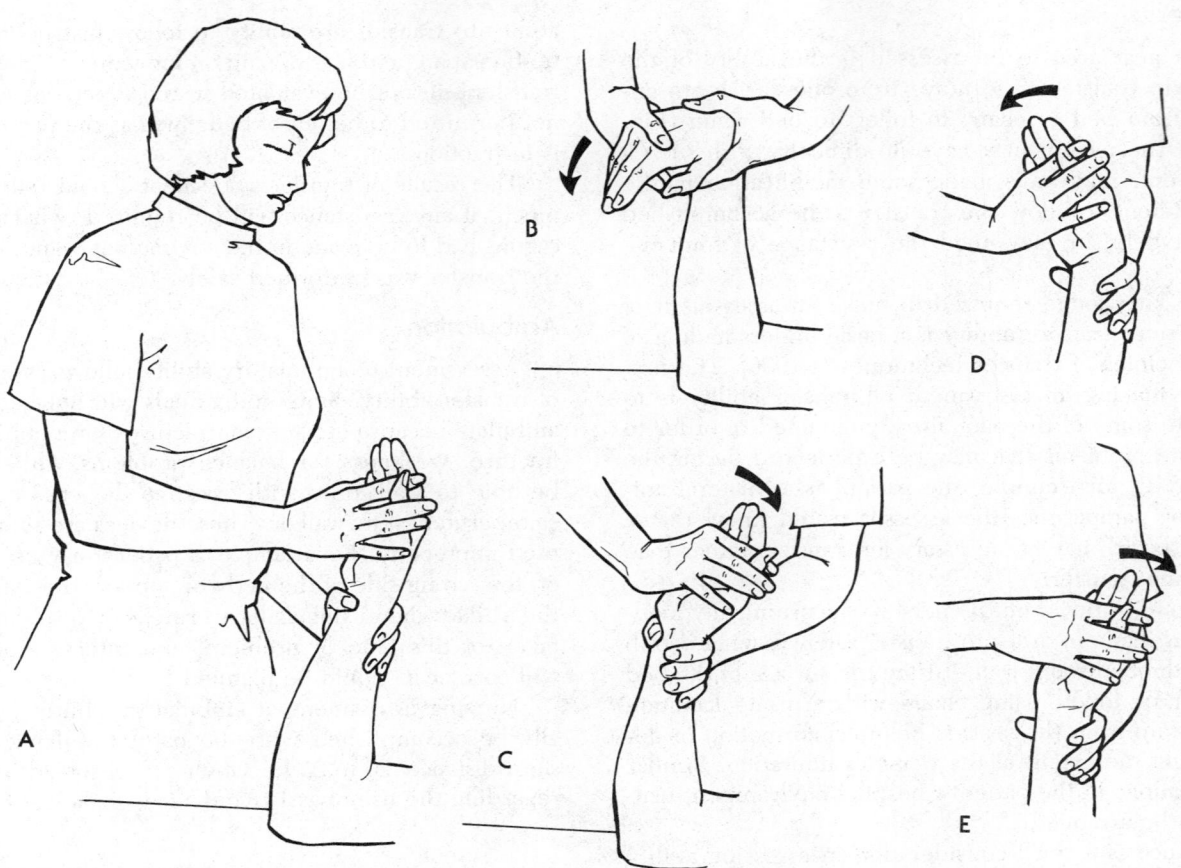

Fig. 40-14. Techniques of passive range of motion. With patient in supine position, upper arm is supported on bed. **A,** Forearm is supported with nurse's hand; hand is supported with nurse's other hand. **B,** Wrist is then flexed forward. **C,** Extended. **D,** Moved to ulnar side. **E,** Moved to radial side. (Modified from Larson, C.B., and Gould, M.: Orthopedic nursing, ed. 8, St. Louis, 1974, The C.V. Mosby Co.)

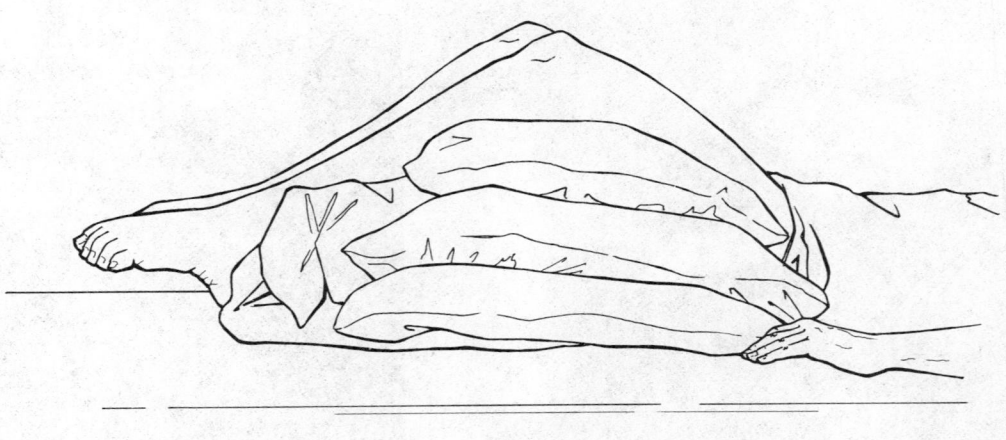

Fig. 40-15. Contractures of hips and knees in patient with rheumatoid arthritis caused by continuous use of pillows to support knees in flexed position. (Modified from Larson, C.B., and Gould, M.: Orthopedic nursing, ed. 8, St. Louis, 1974, The C.V. Mosby Co.)

Transfer

The next area to be assessed is the ability of the person to transfer or to move from one surface to another: from bed to chair, to toilet, to bed again (Fig. 40-16). The person may have no difficulty with such a movement, may have made some modification in the environment to allow the transfer to be accomplished without help, or may need the assistance of someone else.

The knowledge required to make an assessment of the person's transfer ability is a basic understanding of the principles of transfer techniques (p. 956). The first step in making an assessment of transfer ability is to correlate some of the data already obtained in order to anticipate problems that may be experienced during the transfer. If, for example, the patient is a bilateral amputee or paraparetic, the assessor would know that a transfer board may be necessary for transfers rather than a standing transfer.

Second, input from the person concerning any modifications made in order to transfer safely (having a grab bar on the bathroom wall, raising the surface of the bed or chair or toilet, using chairs with arms to facilitate pushing up from the seat) is helpful information in determining the extent of the person's limitation. Similar modifications in the patient's hospital environment usually can be arranged.

Balance is a third consideration in assessing ability to transfer. Inability to maintain balance, a problem seen in a variety of conditions, may severely limit transfer ability. Balance can be easily tested by having the person sit on the side of the bed without using the hands for support after attaining a sitting position.

Other considerations that will influence the person's ability to transfer are ability to follow instructions, attention span, and fear of pain on movement. Obviously, transfer will not be evaluated in those persons who are not permitted to be out of bed, such as the patient who is in traction.

The results of transfer assessment should reflect how much, if any, assistance will be required, what modifications had to be made in the environment, and whether the transfer was performed safely.

Ambulation

Assessment of ambulatory ability follows assessment of transfer ability. Some individuals will not be able to ambulate because of pain, contractures, immobilization, fracture, weakness, or balance problems. Others may be able to walk only with assistive devices such as a cane, crutches, or walker. These devices are sometimes used improperly. For example, a patient may use a cane on the wrong side of the body or support the weight on the axillae when using axillary crutches. Note should be taken of this kind of problem, and interventions that will correct it should be planned.

Nursing assessment of ambulatory ability can usually be accomplished with the patient walking only a short distance (20 to 25 ft). Observations should be made regarding the use of assistive devices, balance, and gait

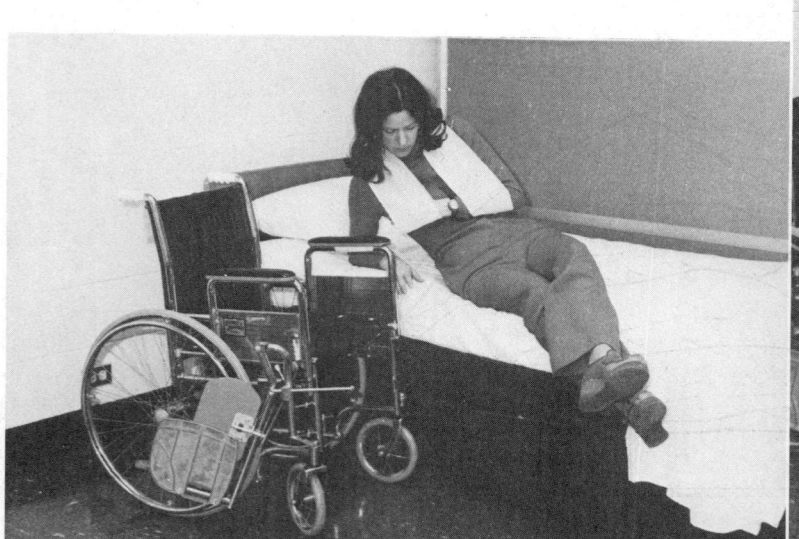
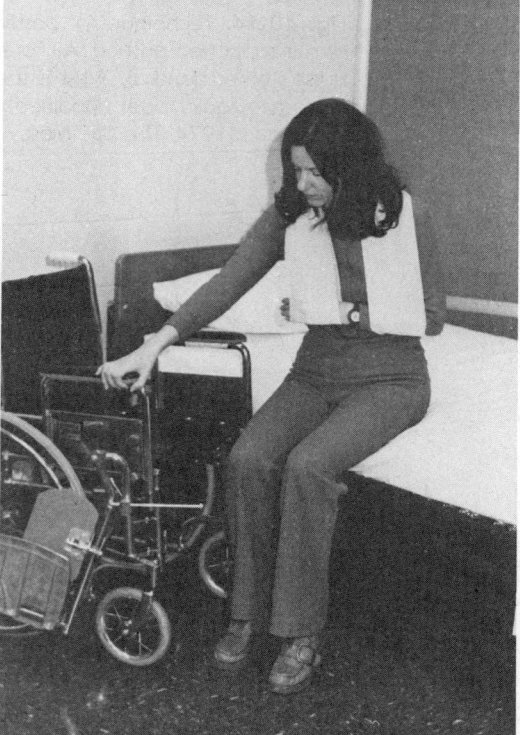

Fig. 40-16. Independent transfer from bed to chair. The chair is placed within reach of patient's uninvolved side. Movements are made leading with uninvolved, or stronger, side. Position of chair is reversed for return to bed.

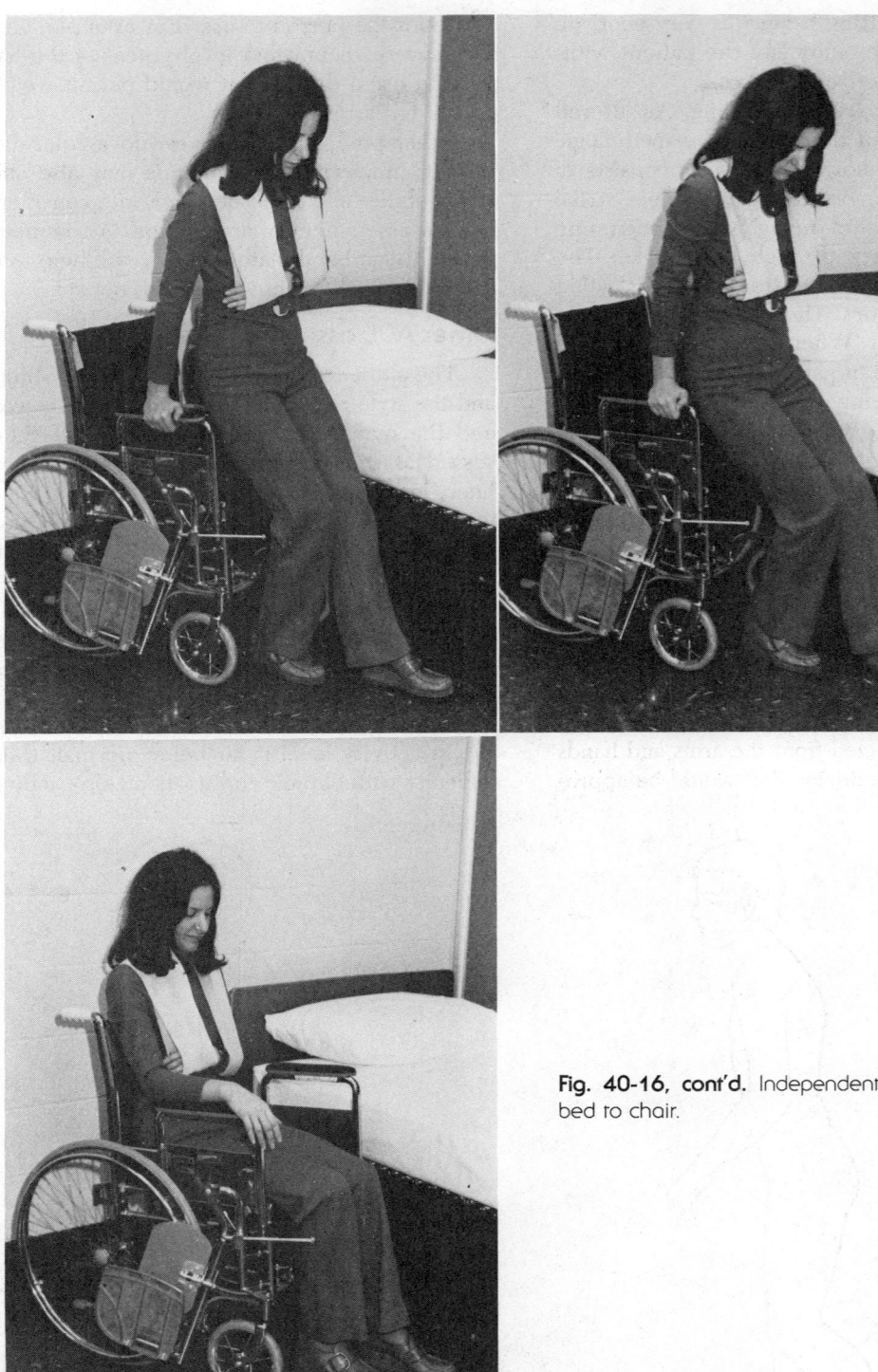

Fig. 40-16, cont'd. Independent transfer from bed to chair.

pattern. If unsupported sitting balance is very poor, no attempt should be made to ambulate the patient without assistance of another person.

Gait is the manner or style of walking. An altered *gait pattern* is indicative of the presence of pathologic process (Fig. 40-17). The normal *gait cycle* consists of two phases: *stance phase*, beginning with heel strike and ending with toe off, and *swing phase*, beginning with toe off and continuing through heel strike. The brief period when both feet are on the ground is called the period of *double support*. These phases are usually rhythmic and symmetric. When they are markedly asymmetric, the alteration in gait is called a *limp*.

While ambulation is being observed, note should be taken of the presence and type of limp displayed, the joints in which there is complaint of pain, the degree to which there is reliance on assistance for weight bearing (either on devices or on a person), balance, and the degree of deformity in the lower extremities. Deformity of the lower extremities (genu valgum, genu varum, talipes varus, and so on) may not be as apparent when the joint is examined at rest as when weight-bearing forces are exerted across the joint. Further, in persons who have significant upper extremity involvement, some consideration must be given both to the amount of weight bearing that might be expected from the arms and hands and to the type of assistive device that would be appro-

priate for the person to use. For example, an individual with severe rheumatoid involvement of the hands might have to use a device that would permit weight bearing on the forearms.

Other problems such as cardiovascular disease, respiratory impairment, or anemia may also affect ambulatory ability and must be taken into consideration during the assessment of ambulation. Assessment of transfer ability and ambulatory ability will help to determine a suitable level of activity for the person.

Other ADL assessment

The ability to dress and undress, the ability to bathe and the style of bathing employed (tub, shower, sponge), and the management of toileting needs should be assessed as soon as possible. If a physical problem has been long standing, the individual may have devised ways of managing these activities despite physical limitations that may appear prohibitive. On the other hand, if the problem is one of acute onset, methods of dealing with these activities may need to be taught. In the hospitalized patient, assessment and evaluation of ADL abilities is an ongoing process throughout the hospital stay.

Further mention must be made of toileting needs. When activity level is far below normal, there may be difficulty with chronic constipation. Also, individuals with

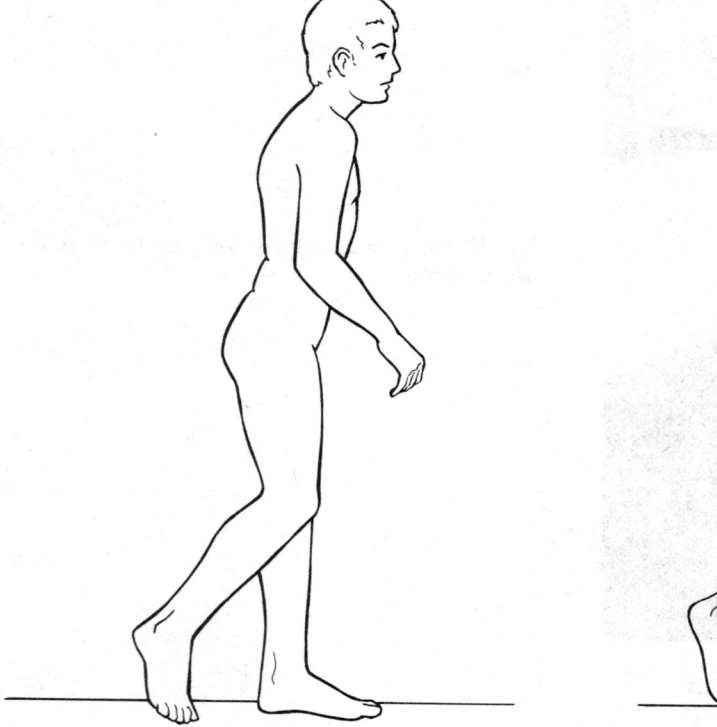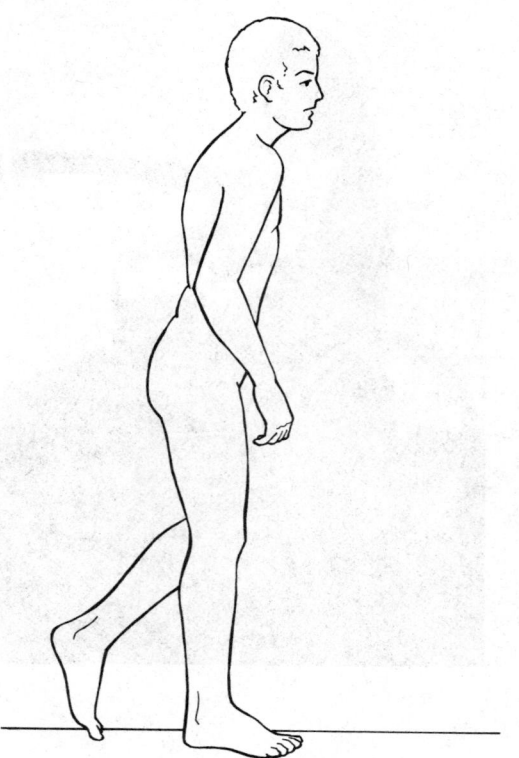

Fig. 40-17. Altered gait pattern caused by bilateral stiff hips. Angle of flexion at hips is constant, requiring that knees and ankles control leg length adjustment and propulsion. (Modified from Larson, C.B., and Gould, M.: Orthopedic nursing, ed. 8, St. Louis, 1974, The C.V. Mosby Co.)

profound muscle weakness or neurologic problems such as stroke may have lost control of bowel and bladder functions. The presence of these problems must be known and intervention programs established as soon as possible (p. 1544). The person who experiences great difficulty in getting to a bathroom may limit fluid intake to avoid making trips to the bathroom. Such individuals often have chronic bladder infections. Plans must be made to make toileting facilities easily available to the patient, and fluid intake should be encouraged.

Pain or the lack of ability to move freely often interferes with sleep. Observations regarding the person's comfort and ability to rest and sleep should be made. If problems exist in these areas, appropriate interventions must be planned.

Observations of the interactions of the patient with hospital staff, family, and friends will often verify what the patient and the patient's family have said about reaction to and acceptance of the problem and the significance the problem has in their relationships. Assessment of these interactions should take place throughout the patient's hospital stay. The data gathered will be helpful in planning with the patient and the family for the patient's eventual discharge and in devising teaching approaches for both the patient and the family.

Diagnostic tests

As with other illnesses, diagnostic tests are employed to provide information to assist in diagnosing a patient's illness and to aid in devising a treatment program for the patient. Elements of the patient's care may be dependent on the outcomes of diagnostic studies. Some of the principal studies that may be performed on the person who has a musculoskeletal problem are discussed below.

Roentgenologic examinations

Bones and joints

Roentgenologic examination of bones and joints is imperative in the identification and treatment of fractures. Roentgenograms are also most helpful in determining not only the presence of disease, such as rheumatoid arthritis, spondylitis, avascular necrosis, and tumors, but also the progress and effects of treatment of these disorders (Fig. 40-18). Specialized texts should be consulted for reference to the variety of views that are

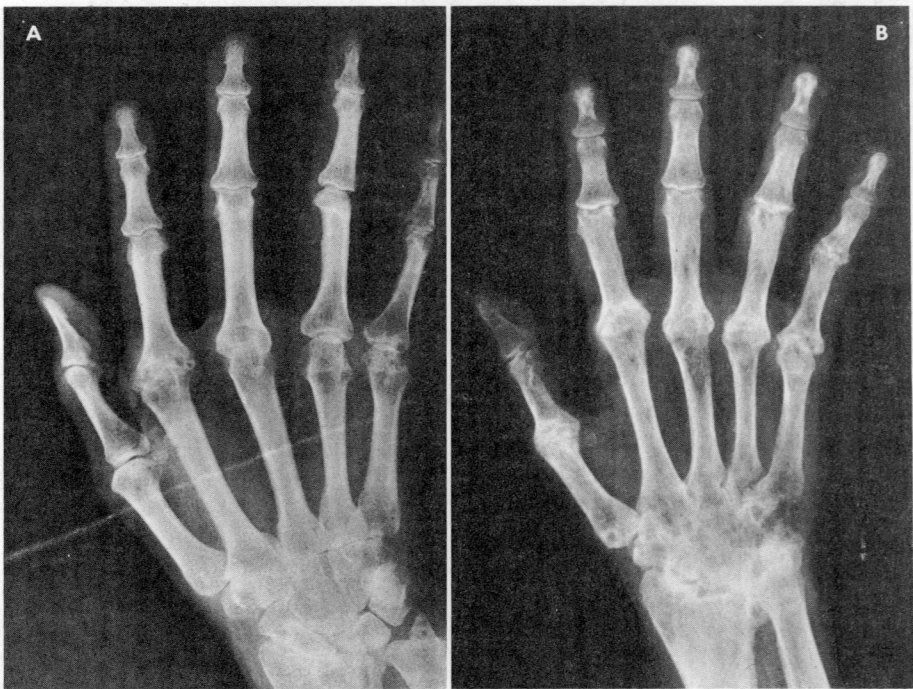

Fig. 40-18. Roentgenograms of rheumatoid arthritis in hand and wrist. **A,** Moderate changes ranging from atrophic bone areas and narrowed cartilage spaces to subluxation of second and third metacarpophalangeal joints. **B,** More advanced case with severe destructive changes including multiple subluxations in digits and ankyloses in carpus. (From Raney, R., and Brashear, H.: Shand's handbook of orthopaedic surgery, ed. 8, St. Louis, 1971, The C.V. Mosby Co.)

obtained in such examinations as well as for the specific findings that are present in the various disorders. However, it is important to remember that many patients are not able to lie on x-ray tables for long periods of time. Persons with arthritis, in particular, develop joint stiffness and pain if their ability to move about is restricted. Since roentgenologic examinations for individuals with rheumatic diseases are often quite extensive, careful thought should be given to the scheduling of these examinations. Very few of these patients can tolerate having all the required views of all the involved joints taken at one session. A day or even 2 days of rest between sessions may be required by patients with severe joint involvement. Analgesics or local heat applications for relief of joint pain may be necessary for some patients following their return from the radiology department.

Systemic roentgenologic studies

Systemic roentgenologic studies such as the barium enema, upper gastrointestinal series, esophagogram, and intravenous pyelogram are helpful in determining the extent of involvement of various internal organs (bowel, kidneys) when the patient has a systemic rheumatic disease. Discussion of these examinations will be found on pp. 1382 and 1516.

Myelography

As discussed in Chapter 34, myelography is useful in identifying lesions, such as a herniated nucleus pulposus, that are blocking the subarachnoid space. Discussion of this procedure and the precautions that must be exercised in caring for the patient after the procedure are discussed on p. 743.

Arthrography

Arthrography permits visualization of structures within the joint that are not normally seen on routine x-ray films. The joint cavity is injected with radiopaque dye, air, or both. The latter is called *a double-contrast arthrogram*. The dye or air serves as a contrast medium against which the outlines of soft tissue components of the joint may be seen. Tears of the menisci, internal derangements of the joint, and synovial cysts may be diagnosed with the aid of arthrograms. Before the study, it must be determined whether the patient has a history of an allergy to the radiopaque dye. No other special preparation is required.

Radioisotope scans

Radioisotope *bone scans* are performed primarily to demonstrate the presence of metastatic disease. Intravenously injected sodium pertechnetate Tc 99m is the isotope most frequently used in this study. The ^{99m}Tc will concentrate in areas of osteoblastic activity involved in the exchange of calcium. In malignancies this activity is accelerated. Lesions may be visualized on bone scans as early as 6 months before there is evidence of the lesions on routine roentgenograms.[10]

Technetium Tc 99m scans are also of some use in determining the degree of *parotid gland* involvement in Sjögren's syndrome. The uptake, concentration, and excretion of the isotope by the major salivary glands are measured by a technique called sequential scintiphotography.[16]

Persons being prepared for these procedures should know that the procedures will not cause them pain, that the isotopes will not harm them, but that they may have to remain in one position quietly for up to 1 hour or more.

Serologic tests

Serum muscle enzymes

The serum muscle enzymes, serum glutamic-oxaloacetic transaminase (SGOT), aldolase, and creatine phosphokinase (CPK), are elevated in the presence of primary myopathic (muscle) diseases. The SGOT is the least sensitive indicator of muscle involvement and the CPK the most sensitive. The SGOT is also elevated in patients who have myocardial or hepatic disease. The CPK is elevated in myocardial conditions or in the patient who has had frequent intramuscular injections. Elevated serum levels of these enzymes may occur as a result of the degeneration of muscle fibers or may result from diffusion of the enzymes through a muscle membrane that has increased permeability. The levels of these enzymes may be checked as an index of both the progress of the myopathic disorder and the effectiveness of treatment. If treatment is adequate, the serum enzyme levels will decrease. In patients in whom these enzyme levels are being monitored, intramuscular injections should be avoided.[16]

STS and FTA-ABS

The serologic test for syphilis (STS) is of some value in the diagnosis of connective tissue disease since 10% to 15% of persons with these diseases will have a *false-positive* STS result. In these persons the presence of syphilis may be excluded by the more sensitive fluorescent treponemal antibody absorption test (FTA-ABS).

Rheumatoid factor (latex fixation)

Abnormal proteins classified as antibodies are found in the sera of individuals with rheumatoid arthritis. These antibodies are called rheumatoid factors, and they will react with IgG (7S) gamma (γ-) globulin. The test to determine the presence of these factors is called *a latex fixation test*. Latex particles are coated with denatured IgG. The serum from the patient is heated and then added to the suspension of coated latex particles.

If the serum contains the rheumatoid factor, the rheumatoid factor will react with the IgG and cause the latex particles to agglutinate. Titrated solutions of latex particles are used, and the rheumatoid factor is considered to be present if the particles agglutinate in dilutions of 1:40 or higher. It should be noted, however, that rheumatoid factor is present in a significant number of other conditions in addition to rheumatoid arthritis: aging, scleroderma, acute pulmonary tuberculosis, parenteral narcotic addiction, systemic lupus erythematosus, and others.

Antinuclear antibodies and LE cell reaction

Circulating antibodies (protein material) that react with nuclei and various individual constituents of nuclei are known as *antinuclear antibodies*. These antibodies can be identified by fluorescent techniques utilizing antihuman γ-globulin labeled with fluorescein. Test serum from a patient is applied to a section of tissue that contains nucleated cells. Antinuclear antibodies, if they are present in the serum, bind to the nuclei of the cells. When the antihuman γ-globulin is applied to these cells, it reacts with the antinuclear antibodies and the nuclei become fluorescent when examined under ultraviolet light. Tests for antinuclear antibodies are helpful in diagnosing Sjögren's syndrome, scleroderma, and systemic lupus erythematosus. The pattern of nuclear staining varies with the different diseases.[16]

The test for LE cells is based on the interaction of antinuclear antibodies, nuclear material, and phagocytic white blood cells. The *LE cell factor* (an antinuclear antibody) reacts with nuclear material from damaged white blood cells. This interaction results in an alteration of the nuclear material. The nuclear material is then called a *hematoxylin body*. The hematoxylin body typically stains red-purple with Wright's stain and has the appearance of "ground glass." The hematoxylin body attracts polymorphonuclear leukocytes. These leukocytes surround the hematoxylin body in the form of rosettes. When one of the leukocytes ingests the nuclear material (hematoxylin body), the nuclear material is then known as an *inclusion body* (Fig. 40-19).[16]

The cell with the inclusion body is known as an *LE cell*. LE cells are seen in 80% to 85% of patients with systemic lupus erythematosus during acute disease activity.[16]

Complement

The complement studies relate to a system of protein substances (at least nine) that are found in the serum and in synovial fluid. These proteins are related both to the immune and the inflammatory mechanisms. Low serum and synovial complement levels often occur in systemic lupus erythematosus and rheumatoid arthritis.

Erythrocyte sedimentation rate

The erythrocyte sedimentation rate (ESR) is the most important index of the *presence of inflammation*. The test is a measurement of the rate of settling of erythrocytes, with an increased rate of settling indicating the presence of inflammation.[15] There are two major methods of determining the ESR: the Westergren method

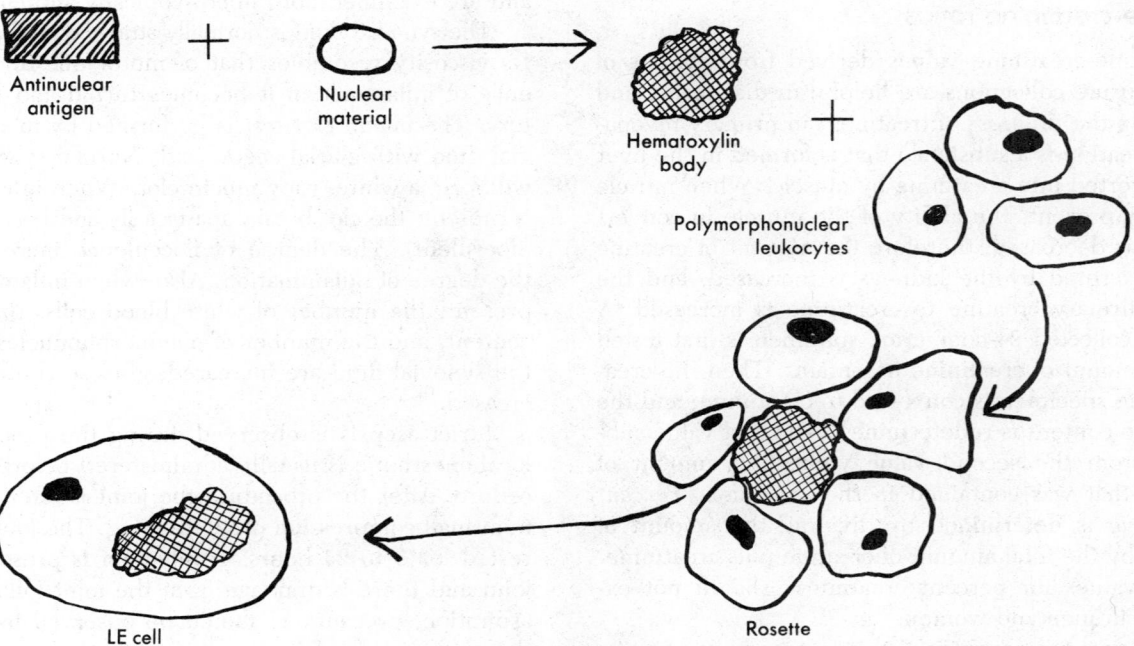

Antinuclear antigen + Nuclear material → Hematoxylin body + Polymorphonuclear leukocytes

LE cell ← Rosette

Fig. 40-19. Schematic drawing of the formation of an LE cell.

and the Wintrobe method. The Westergren method is considered by some experts to be the most dependable. Normal values for men are a fall of 1 to 3 mm per hour; for women, 4 to 7 mm per hour.[15]

Hematocrit

The hematocrit is a measure of the size, capacity, and number of cells present in a person's blood. A blood sample is centrifuged to separate the cells from the plasma. The results of the test are expressed as cubic mililiters of packed cells per deciliter of blood or in volumes per deciliter of blood. The normal range for men is 45 to 50 vol/dl; for women, 40 to 45 vol/dl. Individuals who have hematrocits *below* normal levels are considered to be *anemic*.[10]

Patients with systemic connective tissue diseases or notable rheumatoid arthritis are very often anemic. The red blood cells in this particular form of anemia are normal (normocytic) and carry a normal amount of iron (normochromic), and the anemia exists in the absence of any abnormal bleeding. In contrast, individuals who suffer trauma with subsequent blood loss or who undergo major surgery with intraoperative and postoperative bleeding will have an acute drop in hematocrit. When the hematocrit drops rapidly, symptoms of anemia—extreme tiredness, fatigue, and weakness—are more likely to be experienced. A chronically low hematocrit that develops gradually allows a person to become used to functioning at lower hematocrit levels, and there may be no acute symptoms.

Urinary tests

Creatine-creatinine ratios

Creatine-creatinine values derived from studies of 24-hour urine collections are helpful in diagnosing and evaluating the progress of treatment in primary myopathies. Creatine is a substance that is formed in the liver and converted into creatinine by muscle. When muscle disease is present, the ability of the muscle to convert creatine is decreased; therefore the amount of creatine that is excreted by the kidneys is increased, and the ratio of urinary creatine to creatinine is increased. A carefully collected 24-hour urine specimen is first tested for the amount of creatinine it contains. Then the creatine in the specimen is converted to creatinine, and the creatinine content is redetermined. The first value subtracted from the second value yields the amount of creatine that was contained in the specimen. *Percent creatinuria* is determined by dividing the amount of creatine by the total amount of creatine plus creatinine. Normal values for percent creatinuria should not exceed 6% in men and women.[16]

To ensure the accuracy of this test, two consecutive

24-hour urine specimens are obtained. If there is a variance of more than 10% in the two values obtained, the urine collections are considered inadequate and must be repeated. The person needs to be carefully taught how to collect these urine specimens.

Urinary uric acid levels

Not all individuals who have gout overexcrete uric acid. However, urinary uric acid levels, determined from 24-hour urine collections, can be helpful in establishing a diagnosis of gout. Daily uric acid excretion for individuals on a normal diet should not exceed 900 mg. Individuals with higher levels of urinary uric acid who also have only slightly elevated or high normal serum uric acid levels probably have gout.[16] Treatment decisions as to whether to give uricosuric agents that increase urinary uric acid output and therefore increase the hazard of kidney stone formation may be guided by determination of the amount of uric acid excretion. The accuracy of the collection is important in establishing the diagnosis and in determining an appropriate treatment program.

Joint aspiration

Joint aspiration is performed to obtain samples of synovial fluid from within the joint cavity. This procedure (performed by introducing a needle into the joint cavity and withdrawing fluid) will aid in determining the presence of an aseptic inflammatory process, such as rheumatoid arthritis, or a septic process, such as bacterial arthritis. Samples of synovial fluid are cultured and are examined both microscopically and chemically.

The synovial fluid is normally straw colored and clear. Its viscosity resembles that of motor oil. In the presence of inflammation it becomes turbid and more watery. The *mucin clot test* is performed by mixing synovial fluid with glacial acetic acid. Normal synovial fluid will form a white, ropy mucin clot. When inflammation is present, the clot breaks apart easily and becomes flaky (flocculent). The degree of flocculence increases with the degree of inflammation. Also, when inflammation is present, the number of white blood cells, the protein content, and the number of polymorphonuclear cells in the synovial fluid are increased; glucose content is decreased.[16]

Strict asepsis is observed during the procedure. A local anesthetic is usually administered before the procedure. After the procedure the joint is often wrapped in a small compression (Ace) dressing. The joint may be rested for 8 to 24 hours. If infection is present in the joint and there is drainage from the joint following the aspiration, precautions should be observed in dressing the wound and in handling the contaminated dressings.

Arthroscopy

Arthroscopy is a procedure performed in the operating room. A specially designed endoscope (arthroscope) is inserted through a small incision into the joint cavity, enabling the physician to visualize the structure and contents of the joint. The usefulness of this procedure is limited chiefly to the knee.[12] The procedure permits biopsy of the synovium or cartilage, is useful in the diagnosis of torn meniscus, and in some instances permits the removal of loose bodies from the joint space. The patient is treated in much the same manner as following a synovial biopsy; however, the period of time that the joint is rested is determined by the extent of the procedure. The surgeon should be consulted on how long the patient's activity is to be restricted.

Biopsy

Skin biopsy

Skin biopsy may be performed to aid in the diagnosis of such rheumatic diseases as scleroderma, systemic lupus erythematosus, or psoriatic arthritis. Generally a small "punch" biopsy is taken with a punch biopsy needle at a site where a clinical rash is evident. This skin specimen may be studied for histopathologic evidence of disease, or it may be subjected to *immunofluorescent staining*. This is done by washing the specimen, which has been placed on a glass slide, with a solution of fluorescein-labeled antihuman γ-globulin antibody. A positive reaction, indicating the presence of disease, is the appearance of a band of immunofluorescence at the epidermal-dermal junction.[16]

The biopsy site will appear as a punched-out lesion approximately 0.625 cm in diameter on the patient's skin. This area should be kept clean and may be covered with a small adhesive bandage until an eschar develops. Hydrogen peroxide (3%) may be used to cleanse the open area if necessary, particularly when healing takes more than 3 to 4 days. Generally, only very mild discomfort is experienced after this procedure.

Muscle biopsy

Muscle biopsy is performed to aid in the diagnosis of specific myopathic disorders. The muscle on which the biopsy is to be performed is determined by prior gross muscle testing by the physical therapist and by electromyography studies. In early disease a muscle that is found to be "weak" is most likely to provide histopathologic evidence of disease. Histochemical staining of muscle tissue may reveal features of lower motor neuron disease (e.g., atrophy of groups of fibers innervated by single motor units), or it may reveal degeneration, inflammatory reactions, or involvement of specific fibers that would indicate primary myopathic disease.

A muscle biopsy is an operative procedure usually performed by the general surgeon. The patient may be given either a local or a general anesthetic. Following the procedure, the patient will experience minor to moderate discomfort, depending on the location of the muscle on which the biopsy was done. The discomfort may be in the form of stiffness or pain at or around the operative site. In most instances, if the muscle is in the lower extremity (one of the gluteals or quadriceps), the patient is encouraged to resume ambulation within 24 hours of the procedure to avoid undue stiffness.

Synovial biopsy

Synovial biopsy is helpful in differentiating various forms of arthritis. It may be performed as a closed biopsy with a special synovial biopsy needle (e.g., the Parker-Pearson) or as an open biopsy. The latter is performed in the operating room. If a closed biopsy is being performed, the patient is given a local anesthetic. The specimen of synovium obtained is examined histologically for evidence of inflammation; and a specimen of synovial fluid, obtained at the same time, is sent for culture and other studies.

A closed biopsy of the synovium is performed with strict attention to aseptic technique to avoid introducing infectious agents into the joint. A small compression dressing, usually an Ace wrap, is placed around the joint involved, and the patient is generally asked to rest the joint for 24 hours to prevent hemorrhage or effusion.

Buccal biopsy

Biopsy of the buccal mucosa is performed to aid in defining the presence of Sjögren's syndrome. A small punch biopsy is taken from the lower lip, and the tissue is examined for evidence of lymphoid involvement of the minor salivary glands located in that area. The procedure causes minor discomfort, and the mucosa heals quickly. However, the diet may have to be altered slightly until healing takes place, since rough foods or hot fluids may irritate the biopsy site.

Temporal artery biopsy

Temporal artery biopsy is an operative procedure performed to definitely establish the presence of temporal arteritis (inflammation of the temporal arteries with tenderness and swelling over the temples, headaches, and visual disturbances). Histologic examination reveals stenosis and dilatation of segments of the artery in the presence of the disease. Generally, there is only minor discomfort at the biopsy site. A small compression dressing is applied over the area and should be checked frequently during the first 24 hours for evidence of bleeding.

Electromyography

Electromyography measures the electrical activity of muscles; and an *electromyogram* (EMG) is a recording of the variations of electrical potentials (voltage) detected by a needle electrode inserted into skeletal muscle. The electrical activity can be heard over a loudspeaker and viewed on an oscilloscope and on a graph at the same time. No electrical activity can be detected in normal muscles at rest, but during volitional movement, action potentials can be detected. In both primary myopathic and neuropathic disorders there are specific variations in the size of individual motor unit potentials. In neurogenic atrophy there may be fibrillations in the resting muscle. An EMG provides direct evidence of motor dysfunction and can be used to some extent to detect a dysfunction located in the motor neuron, the neuromuscular junction, or the muscle fibers. Thus it is particularly helpful in the diagnosis of lower motor neuron disease, primary muscle disease, and defects in the transmission of electrical impulses at the neuromuscular junction, such as myasthenia gravis. However, electromyography cannot be used to differentiate *specific* disease entities in either the myopathic or neuropathic categories. There is no special preparation for this procedure. The patient may be fearful that electrode needles will cause an electric shock and should be assured that there is no danger.

Manual muscle test

Manual muscle tests are used in an attempt to determine the degree of muscular weakness resulting from disease, injury, or disuse. The muscle test rates the strength of muscles by their performance in relation to gravity and manually applied resistance and is usually performed by a physical therapist. Factors such as gravity, stabilization of the tested part, proper positioning, amounts of resistance, range of the joint, pain, and abnormal muscle tone must be considered in the performance of this test and can influence the test's objectivity. There are several grading systems used, such as 0 to 5 and the percentage system. The Lovett scale is probably the system most frequently used by physical therapists. This scale employs a grading system that allows muscle strength to be rated on a scale from "zero" (no contraction seen or felt) through "trace," "poor," "fair," and "good" to "normal" (the muscle contracts to overcome greater resistance than a "good" muscle).[7]

Muscle testing is particularly helpful in determining on which muscle a biopsy should be done when confirmation of diagnosis of myopathic disorders is required. Further, the initial test is used as a baseline examination against which later test results can be compared to demonstrate progress or lack of progress in the treatment of myopathic and other musculoskeletal diseases. When muscle-strengthening exercises are indicated, the test will indicate the group of muscles that requires the most therapy.

Schirmer test

The Schirmer test is a simple test used to determine the presence of lacrimal gland involvement in suspected Sjögren's syndrome. A strip of filter paper is folded and placed in the lower conjunctival sac of both eyes for 5 minutes. In the normal individual, the portion of the paper that becomes moistened measures 15 mm or greater; in the individual with Sjögren's syndrome the moistened area measures 5 mm or less.[16] This test is painless, and no special preparation is necessary.

REFERENCES AND SELECTED READINGS
Contemporary

1. *Anthony, C.P., and Thibodeau, G.A.: Textbook of anatomy and physiology, ed. 11, St. Louis, 1983, The C.V. Mosby Co.
2. *Arthritis Foundation: Primer on the rheumatic diseases, ed. 7, New York, 1973, The Foundation. (Prepared by a committee of the American Rheumatism Association Section of the Arthritis Foundation. Reprinted from J.A.M.A. **224**(suppl.), April 30, 1973.)
3. Bluestone, R., editor: Rheumatology, Boston, 1980, Houghton Mifflin Professional Publishers.
4. *Brunner, N.A.: Orthopedic nursing: a programmed approach, ed. 3, St. Louis, 1979, The C.V. Mosby Co.
5. *Cohen, S., and Viellion, G.: Patient assessment: examining joints of the upper and lower extremities, Am. J. Nurs. **81**:763-786, 1981.
6. Committee on Trauma, American College of Surgeons: Early care of the injured patient, ed. 2, Philadelphia, 1976, W.B. Saunders Co.
7. Daniels, L., et al.: Muscle testing, ed. 3, Philadelphia, 1972, W.B. Saunders Co.
8. *Farrell, J.: Illustrated guide to orthopedic nursing, Philadelphia, 1977, J.B. Lippincott Co.
9. Flatt, A.E.: The care of the rheumatoid hand, ed. 3, St. Louis, 1974, The C.V. Mosby Co.
10. *French, R.M.: Guide to diagnostic procedures, ed. 5, New York, 1980, McGraw-Hill Book Co.
11. *Gartland, J.J.: Fundamentals of orthopedics, ed. 3, Philadelphia, 1979, W.B. Saunders Co.
12. Helfet, A.: Disorders of the knee, Philadelphia, 1974, J.B. Lippincott Co.
13. *Larson, C.B., and Gould, M.: Orthopedic nursing, ed. 9, St. Louis, 1978, The C.V. Mosby Co.
14. Malasanos, L., et al.: Health assessment, ed. 2, St. Louis, 1981, The C.V. Mosby Co.
15. McCarty, D.J., editor: Arthritis and allied conditions: a textbook of rheumatology, ed. 9, Philadelphia, 1979, Lea & Febiger.
16. *Moskowitz, R.W.: Clinical rheumatology, Philadelphia, 1975, Lea & Febiger.

*References preceded by an asterisk are particularly well suited for student reading.

17. *Mourad, L.: Nursing care of adults with orthopedic conditions, New York, 1980, John Wiley & Sons, Inc.
18. *Salter, R.B.: Textbook of disorders and injuries of the musculoskeletal system: an introduction to orthopaedics, rheumatology, metabolic bone disease, rehabilitation and fracture, Baltimore, 1970, The Williams & Wilkins Co.
19. *Stryker, R.P.: Rehabilitative aspects of acute and chronic nursing care, Philadelphia, 1972, W.B. Saunders Co.

20. Swinson, D.R., and Swinburn, W.R.: Rheumatology, New York, 1980, John Wiley & Sons, Inc.

Classic

21. Beetham, W.P., et al.: Physical examination of the joints, Philadelphia, 1965, W.B. Saunders Co.

CHAPTER 41

INTERVENTIONS FOR THE PERSON WITH MOTOR PROBLEMS

PATRICIA BUERGIN

The essence of nursing individuals with musculoskeletal problems lies in assisting individuals to make the physiologic and psychosocial adaptations necessary to minimize their temporary or permanent disability. It is the purpose of this chapter to define some of the common problems (both physiologic and psychosocial) experienced by individuals with motor disabilities, and to discuss specific methods that may be employed in managing these problems.

Physiologic disabilities

Six major problems must be considered in the area of physiologic disability: pain, stiffness, loss of strength, loss of dexterity, loss of locomotor ability, and complications common to immobility. Most patients with a motor disability will have one or more of these problems.

Pain

Pain is a problem common to many musculoskeletal disorders. When it exists, it ranks as the priority problem that must be dealt with in planning care. Regardless of its intensity, unrelieved pain can become so all consuming a concern that the individual's entire attention is focused on relieving it. Pain prevents activity, predisposes the patient to the complications of immobility, and dulls receptiveness to care and to teaching. In the extreme, it can affect the individual's attitude toward life. Therefore pain must be relieved to the greatest extent possible before other needed interventions can be implemented.

Stiffness

Stiffness (decreased flexibility) can be a result of pain or of disuse (as in the case of persons who are immobilized), or it can be a result of pathophysiologic changes (as in scleroderma or degenerative joint disease). Stiffness cannot be defined as pain; however, pain may well result as an attempt is made to use an extremity that is stiff. Stiffness may discourage activity, thereby affecting the person in much the same manner as pain.

Decrease in muscle strength

Decrease in muscle strength is sometimes a primary problem, as with some myopathic and neuropathic disorders; or it can result from prolonged bed rest or immobility. Interventions designed to improve strength (e.g., increasing mobility or exercises) can be implemented when some progress is made with treatment of the primary problem.

When it is not possible for the person to regain muscle strength, some means of modifying activities in order to maintain function must be provided.

Loss of dexterity

Loss of dexterity (skillful use of the hands or body) is a problem again encountered either as a result of a primary pathophysiologic process (e.g., rheumatoid arthritis or ataxic neurologic disorders) or as a result of pain, stiffness, or enforced immobility. And again the primary problem must be treated before measures to improve dexterity can be implemented. If the primary problem cannot be controlled, measures can be taken to provide alternative methods of performing activities so that function can be maintained. Examples of such interventions would include specially built utensils and other assisting devices as discussed on p. 950.

Loss of locomotor ability

Perhaps the most threatening component of many musculoskeletal disorders is the temporary or complete loss (or potential for loss) of the ability to move freely from one place to another. Consider what it must be like not to be able to reach for a glass of water, not have the means to escape a potentially threatening situation such as a fire, or having to be dependent on others for all of one's personal requirements. While some problems present only short-term immobility, others, such as spinal cord damage, can cause lifelong disability.

Various groups of handicapped persons throughout the United States have in the past several years been active socially and politically to inform the general public of the architectural barriers encountered by individuals with limited mobility. It is now a federal requirement that public facilities be equipped to accommodate the handicapped individual. All new public buildings must have wheelchair ramps, special toilet facilities, and easy-access parking spaces.

The concern of those caring for hospitalized persons with activity or motor restrictions is directed toward preventing complications, such as contractures, that would further restrict mobility; helping them work through their feelings about restricted mobility; assisting them to adapt to having mobility restricted (regardless of whether this is a short-term or a long-term problem); when possible, providing the patients with and teaching them how to use alternative means for moving about (wheelchair, crutches) or extending themselves (long-handled reachers); and helping them plan for adaptations that they will have to make in their home environments and life-styles.

Complications of immobility

Immobility may be accompanied by a number of complications that can involve any or all of the major systems of the body. It is of the utmost importance that those caring for the patient whose mobility is impaired be aware of these potential complications and be skilled in interventions designed to help prevent them. Perhaps the most effective method of reviewing these com-

plications is to consider them system by system in terms of the person who is most severely immobilized—the patient on bed rest.

Cardiovascular system

The three major problems associated with the cardiovascular system in the patient who is on bed rest are (1) a decreased ability to adapt to an erect posture, (2) an increased incidence of deep vein thrombosis and pulmonary embolus, and (3) an increased work load on the heart. Failure of the vessels in the legs to assume or maintain a state of vasoconstriction results in the pooling of venous blood, decreased venous return, and a diminished cardiac output. This may result in postural hypotension on assuming an erect position. While the heart beats more slowly when the patient is first placed on bed rest, the rate gradually increases. This results in decreased tolerance to exercise or activity when activity is begun.

Intervention. Active or passive range of motion, isometric exercises of the legs, frequent turning, and slow mobilization all may help offset or prevent these complications. Following trauma, both prothrombin time and platelet adhesiveness are increased, thereby increasing clotting potential. Improper positioning, with pressure being exerted over major vessels, may enhance the possibility of thrombus formations.

Respiratory system

When patients are on bed rest, decreased movement, decreased stimulus to cough, and decreased depth of ventilation all contribute to the pooling of secretions in the bronchi and bronchioles. Unabated, this will lead to hypostatic pneumonia.

Intervention. Turning, active range of motion, deep breathing and coughing and encouraging patients to move as much as they are able will help to prevent this problem.

Skin integrity

Loss of skin integrity (abrasions, decubitus ulcers) is caused by friction, pressure, or shearing forces (two or more tissue layers sliding on each other).[23] Pressure exerted over an area for a period of time will restrict the circulation of blood to that area and result in tissue destruction by the process of ischemic necrosis. Infection, trauma, obesity, sweating, increased age, and a poor nutritional state tend to hasten this process. Body weight and infections, other than genitourinary, have been found to have the highest correlation with decubitus formation.[50] Moisture from any cause, as from urinary and fecal incontinence, leads to skin breakdown and infection.

Prevention. The prevention of skin breakdown is vital in the care of all patients and especially in those with limited mobility. Persons in traction are forced to lie supine for a period of time; persons with a neurologic problem producing immobility, such as quadriplegia (p. 818), are unable to move themselves. In extreme situations, such as severely debilitated persons with diabetes or quadriplegia, large areas of ulceration can be life threatening. Measures must be taken by others to prevent decubitus formation. Nurses play a major role in preventing skin breakdown.

The skin is inspected regularly for pressure signs (erythema, induration). Areas of the skin where bone is more superficial, such as the sacrum, elbows, and heels, are most vulnerable to breakdown and require careful inspection. The frequency of inspection depends on the presence of risk factors but should be carried out at least once every 8 hours.

As noted on p. 922, turning the patient (changing points of pressure) at frequent intervals is one of the most effective methods of preventing the development of skin breakdown. Turning the patient with a turning sheet can help in preventing trauma to the skin by pressure and shearing forces (Fig. 41-1). When persons who cannot move themselves are moved to another sur-

face, such as to a cart, pull sheets or roller boards (Fig. 41-2) should be used to avoid friction against the surface of the bed or cart. Rolling patients to their sides or lifting them when placing them on bedpans will prevent friction against the surface of the pan.

Some patients cannot be fully turned because of traction apparatus or other limiting factors. For these persons especially, other methods such as air pressure mattresses, foam mattresses, sheepskin pads, flotation pads, elbow and heel pads, and elevation of the heels may be helpful in preventing circulatory compromise to a skin area. Flotation pads distribute pressure equally over large skin areas, thereby decreasing pressure on any one site. Air pressure mattresses alternate pressures on the skin. Sheepskin decreases friction, distributes pressure, and reduces moisture but must be changed if dampness occurs.

Special beds may be used to turn the immobile patient from supine to prone positions. The Stryker or Foster frame permits movement in a horizontal direction to only two positions: supine and prone. The CircOlectric bed (Fig. 41-3) permits many more posi-

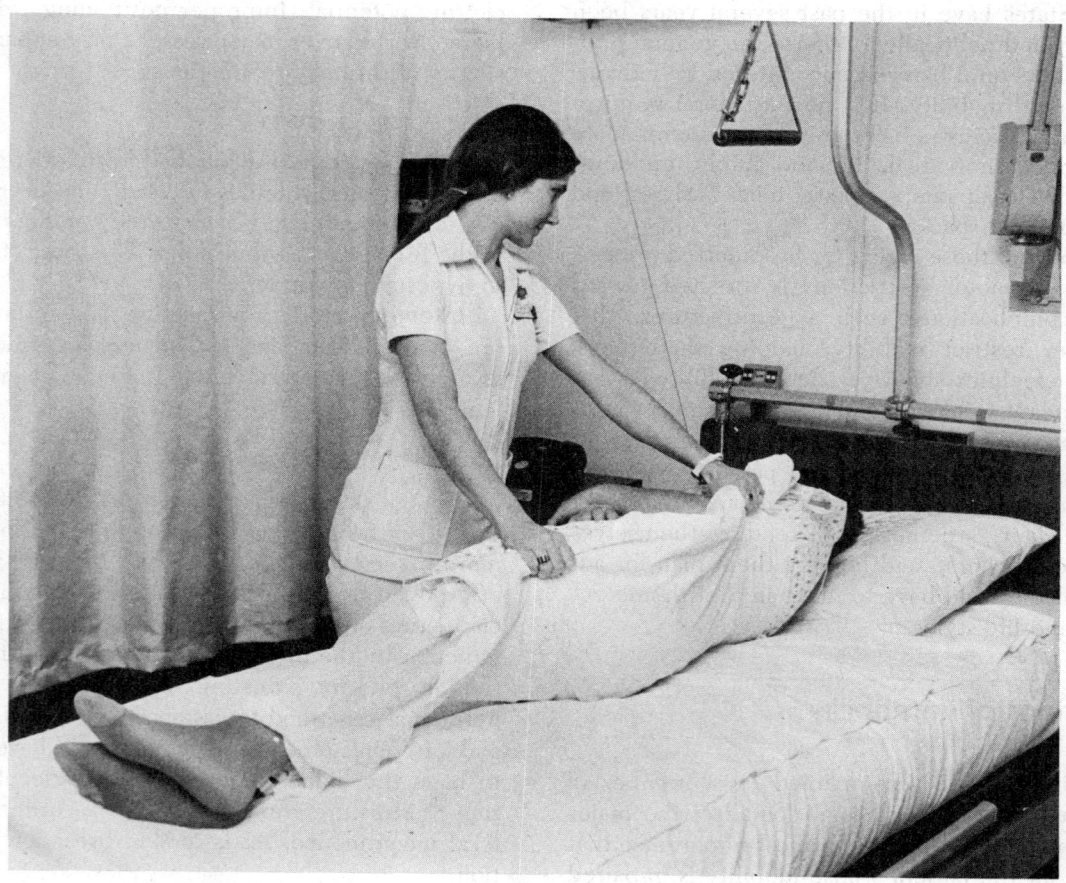

Fig. 41-1. Use of turning sheet. Sheet is held taut with one hand at level of patient's shoulder and other hand below patient's buttocks, thus providing patient with a sense of support and control.

tion changes; movement is vertical and can be stopped at any angle while good body alignment is being maintained.

Intervention for decubitus ulcers. If a decubitus ulcer does develop, treatment consists of prevention of further extension of the ulcer through vigorous application of the preventive measures listed above and in the promotion of wound healing (p. 443). The ulcer must be kept clean if healing is to occur. There are numerous topical agents that have been used over the years; the large numbers attest to the fact that no one best method has yet been found. However, when a method of treatment is decided on, it should be consistently carried out for several days. Failure to be consistent with treatment is one reason why there is little data available as to whether one method may be more efficacious than another.

The ulcer can be debrided mechanically or by the use of fibrinolytic enzyme. If the enzyme is used, the wound is cleaned first with water, peroxide, or saline and dried gently before the enzyme is applied. The ulcer is covered by a nonadhering dressing. This procedure is repeated two to three times daily. If skin erosion only is present, positioning to relieve pressure and application of heat may encourage healing. With very large deep ulcers, packing and irrigations are necessary, and excision and reconstructive surgery may be indicated. To reiterate, the most effective intervention for skin breakdown is *prevention*.

Gastrointestinal system

Constipation is perhaps the most frequent complication of immobility. The change in normal dietary habits and fluid intake, lack of activity, and having to use a bedpan are contributing factors.

Intervention. Turning, movement, elevation of the head of the bed, increased fluid intake, good dietary intake, use of stool-softening agents, laxatives, or suppositories to which the person is accustomed, and use of a commode, if possible, will help to alleviate this problem. (See Chapter 55 for further information.)

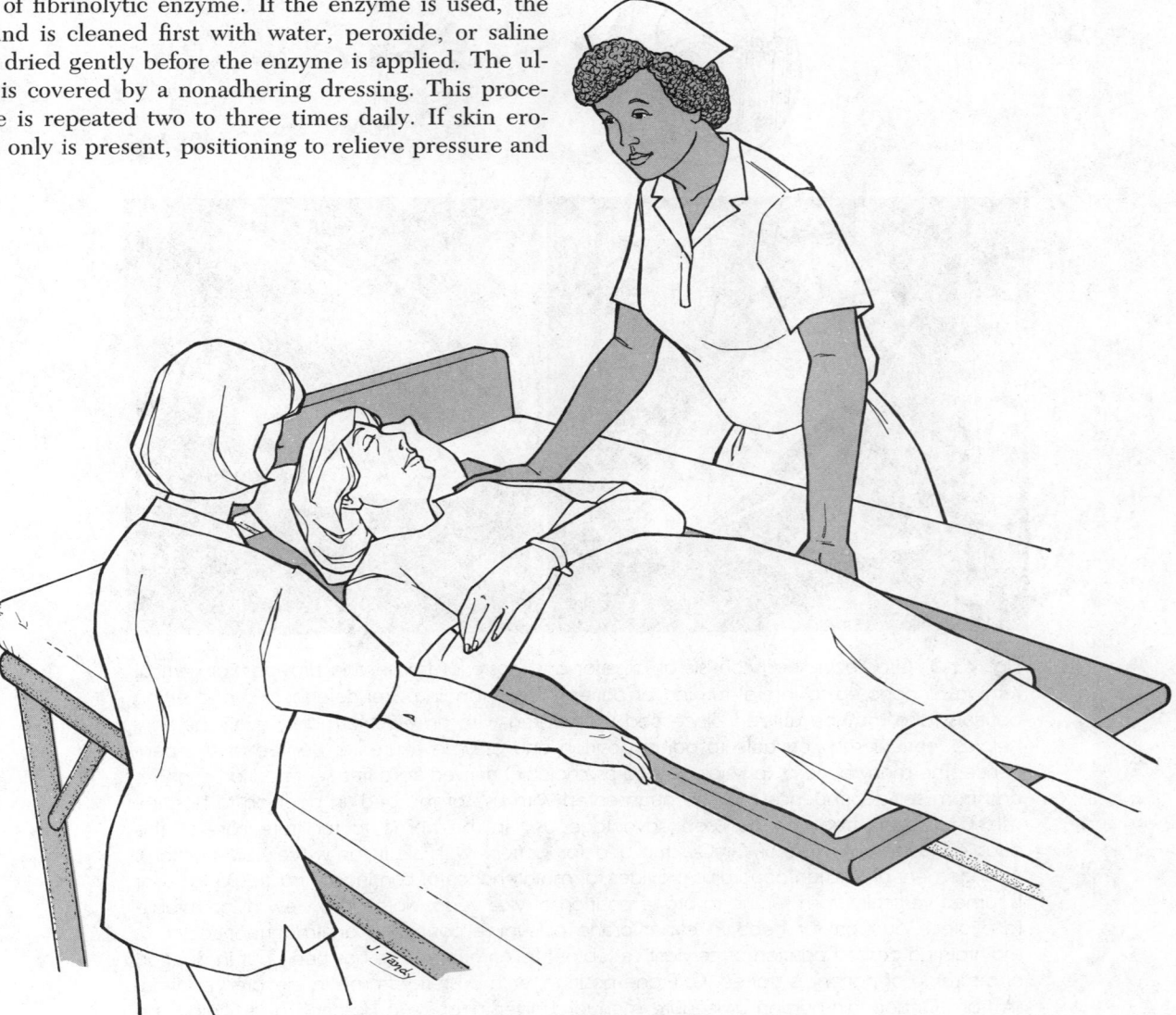

Fig. 41-2. Nurses using a roller board to move patient from bed to cart.

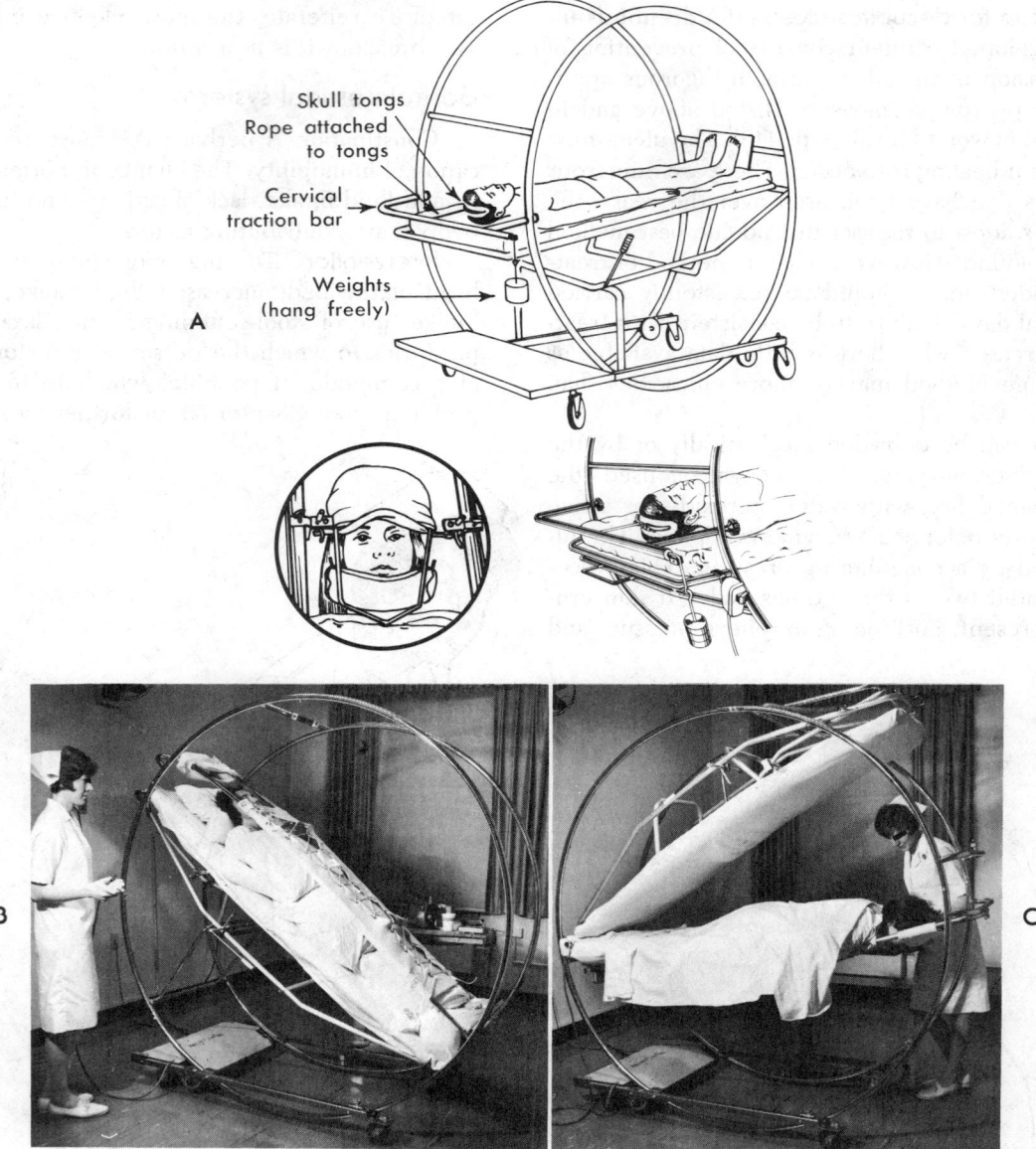

Fig. 41-3. CircOlectric bed consists of anterior and posterior frame and provides for vertical turning as opposed to lateral turning of patient. Thus standing, Trendelenburg's, and sitting positions also may be utilized. Since bed is operated with an electric motor, even the very helpless patient may be able to adjust position and assume a greater degree of independence. The many benefits (physiologic and psychologic) derived from frequent position changes and from self-dependence may be augmented with use of this bed. In addition to hospital use, CircOlectric bed can be used advantageously in the home to facilitate care of the disabled person. **A,** Use of CircOlectric bed for patient with skull tongs (cervical traction). Arrangement of traction apparatus provides for maintenance of continuous traction as patient is turned vertically from supine to prone position or vice versa. Note close view of adjustable face piece. Support for head in either prone or supine position is an important factor in maintaining desired position of cervical vertebrae. **B,** Anterior frame has been put in position and turning of patient is started. **C,** Prone position, with posterior frame in elevated position. (**A** from Orthopedic nursing procedure manual, University of Iowa Hospitals and Clinics, The University of Iowa, Iowa City, Iowa; **B** and **C** from Larson, C.B., and Gould, M.: Orthopedic nursing, ed. 9, St. Louis, 1978, The C.V. Mosby Co.)

Muscular system

Through disuse, atrophy and weakness affect the muscles within a relatively short period of time.

Intervention. Efforts made to actively exercise the muscles within the restrictions imposed by the cause of the immobility can help reduce the effects of atrophy and weakness.

Joints

Contractures secondary to muscle shortening, fibrosis, or bony ankylosis around the joints can develop quickly and take months to correct.

Intervention. Use of active and passive range of motion, isometric exercises, encouraging persons to perform all activities not restricted by the cause of their immobility, and attention to positioning can help prevent loss of joint motion.

Skeletal system

Immobility disrupts the balance of *osteoblastic* (bone growth) and osteoclastic (bone destruction) activity. Osteoclastic (destructive) activity takes precedence with the result that bone matrix is destroyed and calcium is released. The end result is *osteoporosis*.

Intervention. Exercises (active, to whatever extent possible, and isometric) may be helpful in reducing the effects of this complication.

Urinary system

Increased calcium from bone destruction, increased urinary pH (alkaline), increased citric acid (which causes the precipitation of calcium salts), stasis of urine in the bladder, and infection can all cause urinary problems.

Intervention. An increased fluid intake, decreased calcium intake (milk), and use of the commode (instead of the bedpan), whenever possible, are recommended to help reduce the potential for bladder infection and the formation of renal stones.

Neurologic system

Prolonged bed rest deprives a person of usual intellectual and social mobility. The older person in particular may respond to loss of stimuli by becoming disoriented or incapable of retaining information.

Intervention. Frequent contact by staff, provision of diversionary material such as magazines, radio, or television, and orienting mechanisms such as clocks or calendars can help to offset these complications.

In summary, those caring for the patient must understand the reason for the patient's immobility, how that immobility must be maintained to obtain maximal healing benefits, and what systems or organs are to be rested and to what extent. Organs or systems that need not be immobilized must be identified, and provision must be made for their continued use and development within the prescribed limits of rest.

Psychosocial problems

Reaction to disfigurement or disability

A major problem faced by many individuals who have problems that lead to motor impairment is that the disease itself can be disfiguring. Not only must they adapt to functional disability, but they may have to adapt to "looking different" than other people. Severe deformities such as occur with rheumatoid arthritis (see Fig. 42-1) or amputation, or uncontrolled movements that occur with Huntington's chorea are problems that affect the person's self-image. (For further information on body image see Chapter 28.) For some individuals the problem may not be so much with disfigurement but rather with loss or alteration of function (e.g., ambulatory ability), or the need to use an assistive device or prosthesis. In such situations persons view themselves as different from others.

Depending on the nature and pressures of family, social, or work situation or the individual's self-image, there may be an attempt to cover up the disability so as not to lose support and esteem of friends. Some persons even fear the loss of their jobs. If the disability cannot be covered up, some persons may withdraw and limit their contact with others. An example would be the middle-aged woman with hip disease who, although in pain, will not use a cane to assist her in walking for fear of being thought of as "old." As walking becomes more and more difficult, she limits her social contacts and even necessary functions such as shopping to avoid being seen by others.

It takes a great deal of patience and time to help individuals affected in this manner to accept that hiding their disability is not a reasonable method of dealing with it. Treatment that can restore function may be available (medical therapy or corrective surgery). If not, the hospital staff can often, by their understanding and accepting attitude, help patients adapt to their altered appearance or function. Encouraging patients to participate in activities, referring to their disabilities or disfigurements in a very matter-of-fact manner, helping them to be neatly groomed, or encouraging them when they try new activities or demonstrate an improvement in abilities can often improve their motivation and sense of self-worth.

Dependence, independence, and interdependence

Most people want to be able to live their lives independently. In the sense of this discussion, independence would mean freedom from having to make demands on others for personal and social activities of daily living. However, individuals with musculoskeletal problems may be unable to manage one or more activities of daily living for themselves. If help from another person is needed to perform certain functions, such as buttoning buttons, the individual is dependent in that area. If an assistive device (button hook, Velcro closures) can be made available and the use of it can be mastered, the individual can again be independent in that function.

The *major objectives in caring for individuals* who have motor impairment are to allow them to do what they can for themselves, to devise ways to help them achieve independent function in impaired areas, and to assist them to the extent necessary in areas where independent function cannot be achieved. If patients are not allowed to perform the functions that they can perform, they can quickly become angry and discouraged and lose motivation. Loss of the desire to be independent, subjecting oneself to a state of dependence, can be the most destructive element of a musculoskeletal disorder.

Interdependence is the third area for consideration. Very few people live truly independent lives. As a society, we depend on the farmer to grow our food, the lawyer to attend to our legal affairs, the mechanic to repair our automobile. Families also are structured around interdependent functions. Persons with motor disability may at some time be faced with losing their interdependent role; that is, they may no longer believe that they are useful or needed by anyone else. Counseling, by members of the health team, of patients and their families concerning the nature of the disability and discussing the patient's areas of independence and dependence may be helpful in assisting patients and their families to define new roles for themselves—roles in which patients can have an active part in their families' lives and concerns.

Outcomes of care in relation to these entities (dependence and independence and interdependence) are to (1) assist patients to maintain or achieve a state of independence consistent with their physical capabilities, (2) define and share with their families or significant others the areas in which they are dependent, and (3) return persons to their living situations able to resume interdependent roles with their families.

Adaptation to assistive, supportive, and corrective devices

Walkers, canes, crutches, splints, braces, and feeding aids often have negative connotations in our society. A major problem in caring for patients with motor disabilities can be that of helping them to overcome their aversion to such devices and to accept these devices as a means for maintaining their independence and safe functioning.

On the more optimistic side, many patients are quite happy to learn that there are aids that can improve or extend their abilities. Sometimes, all that is necessary is to demonstrate the effectiveness of the device in alleviating pain or eliminating dependence in a certain area of functioning. However, some patients may need constant encouragement before they will accept the device; some may never accept it. Family members or significant others may be enlisted to provide encouragement, and it is often their support that will produce the desired result.

Socioeconomic impact

Many disorders that affect motor function occur at an age when wage earning, child rearing, and other functions can be seriously impaired. Loss of income and self-esteem, the inability to maintain one's standard of living, and increased stress on the family can all result. There are agencies available to help with employment problems (bureaus of vocational guidance, vocational guidance and rehabilitation centers, sheltered workshops). Often there is an opportunity for hospital staff to advise the patient of the availability of such services and to make the appropriate referrals.

The older patient. By no means, however, is motor impairment less of a problem for the older patient. Living alone or on a fixed income and faced with the possibility of not being able to maintain independence, the patient can become very frightened, depressed, or withdrawn. Nursing homes are costly, as are persons who are hired to help in the home, if they are even available in a community. The idea of giving up one's home and way of life can be very threatening and demoralizing.

It is important, then, to identify the socioeconomic problems facing any patient with motor impairment. Often patients can be helped to work through some of their physical limitations with modifications that will not cost a great deal of money and that will allow them to continue living in their present circumstances. For example, applying a levering device to a garage door could help the individual with limited lifting ability and would be less expensive than an automatic garage door opener. For those who cannot sit in a bathtub, bathing while sitting on a chair in the tub and using a shower hose extension on the faucet would be a less expensive arrangement than purchasing a hydraulic tub seat and would be more satisfying than a sponge bath. Referrals to community resources such as the Visiting Nurse Association or arranging for Meals on Wheels can sometimes be all the support that is needed to keep an individual in his or her own home and out of a dependent setting.

In working with individuals who have motor impairment, one must be inventive and innovative and should possess a working knowledge of community resources available to help them maintain satisfactory functioning in settings that they can afford.

Family relationships

Reference has already been made to the fact that family roles and relationships (social and economic) may be changed, owing to a patient's restricted motor function and areas of dependency. It is important that those caring for the patient recognize when those relationships are destructive and help the patient and family obtain appropriate guidance. Sometimes, psychiatric counseling is necessary. Whenever it is possible, support should be given to "healthy," caring relationships that are identified in the situation.

Prevention

Factors affecting the alteration

Whatever the nature of the musculoskeletal disability, there are factors of prevention and teaching that must be considered.

Nonpreventable factors

Many of the diseases that affect the musculoskeletal system have at this time an unknown cause. Rheumatoid arthritis and the systemic connective tissue diseases are but a few examples. While these diseases are not now preventable, there are complications of the diseases that are preventable—contractures, atrophy, skin breakdown, and others. In these instances, prevention depends on teaching the patient to understand the disease process and to employ preventive measures (pp. 984 and 985).

Preventable factors

Polio vaccine, screening of school-aged children for scoliosis, and screening tests for streptococcal infections with early treatment of the infection to prevent rheumatic fever are examples of preventive measures that can be employed on a community-wide basis in combating illnesses that cause musculoskeletal disability. Early attention to posture; good dietary habits; genetic counseling for individuals with sickle cell anemia and hemophilia; teaching of good body mechanics for individuals whose jobs entail lifting or carrying heavy objects;

and concern and attention to the recommendations of the National Safety Council to help avoid accidents at home, on the job, and on the road are all examples of preventive measures that may be employed to decrease musculoskeletal disability within the general population.

Promotion of safety

For those individuals who have limitations of motion or mobility, there are a variety of precautions and protective or safety devices that can be employed in the hospital or the home. Examples would be grab bars that can be mounted on a wall near a tub or toilet, safety arms that fit around a toilet, and rails that fasten onto the side of a bathtub. These devices provide the patient with both a stable place to hold onto and a point of leverage for assuming a standing or a sitting position. Throw rugs and obstacles should be removed from areas used by individuals with ambulatory difficulties, and floors should not be highly waxed. Wheelchairs should have adequate locking devices, and patients who must use wheelchairs should be taught how to lock and unlock the chair.

While some of these measures may seem to be common knowledge, patients are frequently not aware of them or their need for them. One of the most important functions nurses can perform—and because of their 24-hour contact with the patient they are in a unique position to do so—is to assess the safety requirements of their patients and then teach the patient or family what steps are necessary to ensure safety. It is helpful if nurses know where in the community needed equipment can be obtained. Often the hospital social worker or physical therapist provides this information and assists the patient or family in obtaining the equipment. By the time of discharge from the hospital, arrangements should be made for the patient to have the equipment and instruction required for safe functioning at home.

Prevention of muscle and joint complications

Maintenance of joint mobility

For the individual with limited motion or mobility, range of motion exercises should be carried out to prevent joint stiffness or contractures from disuse. (Techniques of range of motion are discussed in Chapter 40.) Whenever it is possible, except in conditions where there is acute joint inflammation, range of motion should be performed several times a day. *Active range of motion* is most beneficial for the patient. Encouraging patients to do as much of their own care as they are able to do within the restrictions of their disability will often satisfy active range of motion requirements.

Several precautions should be mentioned. *Passive range of motion* should not be performed past the point of the complaint of pain. Particularly in individuals with skeletal pathologic conditions (gross deformity, osteoporosis), fractures can result if a joint is forced through "normal" range of motion. Also, acutely inflamed, painful, or septic joints should be rested, since harm can be done by moving the joint before inflammation has subsided. The person who has pain is also likely to resist movement in order to avoid further pain.

Maintenance of posture

Although maintenance of good posture is important for all persons, it is especially important for the patient with chronic arthritic disease. Poor posture exerts further strain on already damaged joints and not only may cause pain and fatigue but predisposes to increased deformity.

The patient who must remain in bed for a long period of time in traction or in a cast should be in a bed with a firm mattress, and a bed board should be placed under the mattress. A firm bed lessens pain by preventing motion and consequent pull on painful joints and helps to keep the spine in good alignment. Boards should be long enough and wide enough to rest firmly on the main side and end rails of the bed, not on the bedsprings. The person with arthritis should either use no pillow or should use one small pillow that fits well down under the shoulders so that forward flexion of the cervical spine is not encouraged. Knees should not be flexed on pillows, and all patients who must be confined to bed most of the day should lie prone with a pillow under the abdomen for a part of each day to relieve supine pressure areas (inferior scapular areas and the ischial tuberosities) (Fig. 41-4).

Careful positioning with trochanter rolls (rolled towels or bath blankets to brace an extremity in the desired position), supportive pillows, attention to avoiding extreme flexion of joints, and care to avoid compressing nerves or arteries (the result of which can be neurologic or circulatory compromise) are all important considerations for both skin care and general maintenance of the patient.

The unaffected foot (or feet) should rest against a footboard at least part of the day. This helps to maintain the foot in a neutral position for a more normal walking position, prevents the weight of bedclothes from contributing to footdrop, and provides a firm surface against which the person can do resistive foot exercises. Patients should be taught to check the position of their lower limbs when at rest. If their problem is nonneurologic, they should "toe in" to prevent external rotation contracture of the hip and pronation of the foot. These complications cause serious difficulty when walking is resumed.

For the general public, it should be remembered that poor posture throughout life may contribute to hypertrophic arthritis. The child should be taught to stand correctly so that strain caused by prolonged hyperextension does not occur in points such as the knee joints. Molding the pelvis correctly with a posterior pelvic tilt will help prevent increased curvature of the lower back with its resultant strain on muscles and joints. Holding the head up with the chin in takes a great deal of strain from the joints of the upper spine. It is surprising how many older persons can benefit from posture improvement even though damage may date from childhood.[26]

Attention should also be paid to correct mechanical use of the body. Techniques such as stooping with knees and hips flexed (see Fig. 42-6), rather than bending over, prevent muscle strain that may pull a joint out of alignment just enough for osteoarthritic changes to develop or to cause symptoms. Techniques for lifting, using the strong muscles of the legs rather than the weak back

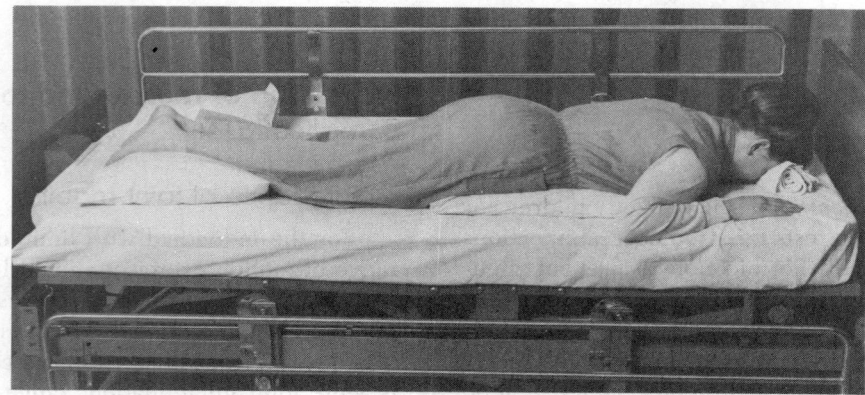

Fig. 41-4. Good body alignment in prone position. Lower legs are elevated off bed to avoid forcing feet into plantar flexed position. (From Rantz, M., and Courtial, D.: Lifting, moving and transferring patients, St. Louis, 1977, The C.V. Mosby Co.)

muscles, should be taught particularly to individuals whose work involves heavy lifting and to hospitalized patients who have suffered back injuries. Nurses are frequently in an excellent position to teach patients good body mechanics because of the work they do, and it is important that they serve as positive role models by exhibiting good body mechanics in their work.

In regard to sitting posture, furniture should be such that good posture can be maintained during working and recreational hours with a minimum of drain on vital energy resources. There are *five criteria for a good chair*: (1) the seat should be deep enough to support the thighs but not so deep that circulation in the popliteal spaces is hampered; (2) the seat should be high enough so that the feet rest firmly on the floor and do not dangle, placing increased pressure on the posterior thighs; (3) the seat should be level or tilted slightly forward so that flexion of the knees and hips is at a minimum and not at more than a right angle; (4) the chair should have arms so that arm and shoulder muscles can provide leverage to help in moving from the chair, the arms of the chair being at a level such that with the patient's arms at right angles, the shoulders are neither too high nor too low; and (5) the rungs must be such that one foot can be placed partially under the chair in preparation

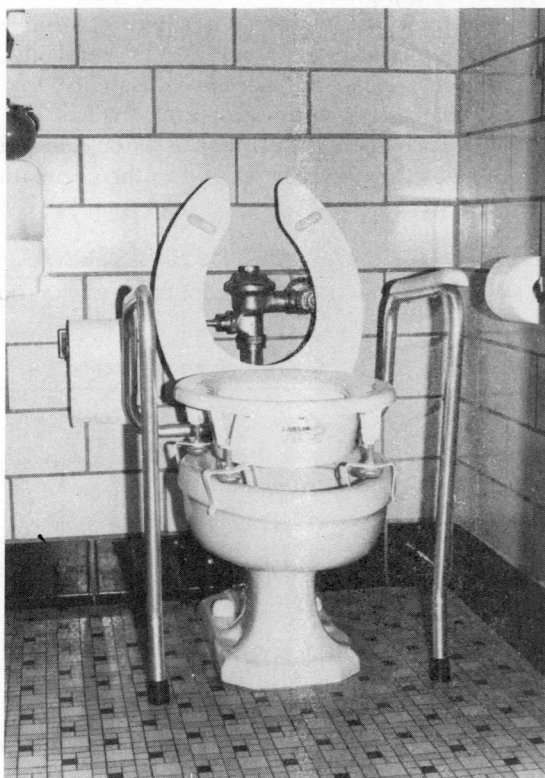

Fig. 41-5. Removable raised toilet seat and safety arms around toilet.

for rising so that the person is better able to stabilize his or her center of gravity as an erect position is assumed. Chairs with seats a little higher than is usually considered comfortable provide better leverage when rising. Sometimes, adding an inch or two to the height of the person's favorite chair will increase comfort while sitting and make rising from it easier. This is particularly true for persons with hip girdle weakness or hip or knee joint involvement. If the patient is advised to spend time with the feet elevated, a small stool on which to comfortably rest the feet should be available. Occasionally, it is also necessary to build up a toilet seat. Devices to be placed over the seat to provide height can be improvised, or they can be purchased from hospital supply stores (Fig. 41-5). A rail beside the toilet seat is necessary if support is needed in rising from the seat safely.

Intervention

Conservative intervention

The interventions that will be discussed in this section are those that are used primarily for individuals with joint and muscle diseases. They can be restorative, preventive, or analgesic in nature.

Activity

Because motor problems are essentially problems of activity limitation, many of the appropriate interventions are directed toward improving activity.

Rest, activity, and joint protection. Rest is a therapeutic measure employed in many inflammatory and in some traumatic conditions, such as back injuries. However, it cannot be overemphasized that too much rest can at times be as detrimental as too much activity. Absolute rest of a particular limb, joint, or the entire body in acute inflammatory conditions helps to prevent further tissue destruction and pain. Resting a joint of the lower extremity may mean placing that joint on a non-weight-bearing status by having the person "unload" it through the use of crutches or a walker. The usefulness of resting splints in controlling muscle spasm is discussed on p. 954. As symptoms subside, activity will be gradually increased to the limits that can be tolerated without pain or fatigue. The patient must strike a balance of rest and activity to maintain function and to prevent further disability.

The physician is usually the one to determine when activity is to begin, but the nurse can be very instrumental in helping the patient recognize when activity should be stopped in favor of rest. Clues include increase in pain, tiredness, and progressive loss of dexterity in the use of the involved part. As the condition that requires rest improves, the patient should be assisted to develop a plan for daily activites that provides for both a gradual increase in activity and adequate periods of rest. Patients are encouraged to do as much as they are able without becoming overtired.

Patients who have chronic conditions that will continue to require rest periods should try, while in the hospital, to work out a schedule for themselves approximating the activity schedule that meets their rest and activity requirements at home or work. This is often difficult to do. Many times persons will have to be helped to work through their feelings about not being able to attend to all the activities they believe are necessary or desired. They need support from both the hospital staff and their families to come to terms with their limitations.

Patients with joint involvement must be made aware of techniques they can use to protect their joints from overuse, misuse and stress. Joint protection techniques should be implemented in all possible activities of daily living (ADL) situations, and improper uses of joints should be pointed out to patients as they are observed. Learning to function in different but still effective ways is difficult for most people, but the most frequent indicator that they have overused or misused their joints is an increase in pain or fatigue. Individuals need to learn to recognize these symptoms and need to be assisted to take steps to modify the offending activity.

Splinting and bracing to protect joints are discussed on p. 954. Another form of joint protection is modification of activities that can stress or harm joints. Joint protection techniques are particularly beneficial in chronic inflammatory joint diseases such as rheumatoid arthritis. These techniques involve patients' learning to find easier ways of accomplishing what *needs* to be done. These techniques can be broken down into several categories.

The first category is *energy conservation techniques*. Examples are sliding rather than lifting objects and moving dishes, utensils, or equipment from one room to another on a wheeled cart rather than carrying them.

The second category is *avoiding positions of possible deformity*. Flexor muscles are generally stronger than extensor muscles, and joints tend to become deformed in a position of flexion. External pressures that put stress on joints in the wrong direction and internal pressures from muscles forces can produce deformities in joints that have been affected by chronic inflammatory processes. Sitting for long periods, keeping the knees or elbows bent to avoid pain, and twisting motions such as turning a doorknob or removing a jar lid are examples of stressful or harmful activities that can result in joint deformity or contracture. Performing active range of motion, varying sitting and standing activities at frequent intervals, turning sideways to a doorknob, and

using wrist motion rather than finger motion to turn it are examples of how harmful positions can be avoided.

The third approach is *learning to avoid holding muscles or joints in one position for a long time*. Varying activities as mentioned above and learning to stop activity before it becomes painful will help prevent fatigue and possible joint damage.

The fourth technique is *learning to use the strongest joints for all activities*. A good example of this is using the knees, not the back, when lifting objects, or pushing a door open with the shoulder, not the hand. Joints should be used in their best position. This means using good standing and sitting posture, working at a comfortable height, and not reaching or bending when another approach would do as well.

For patients to learn these techniques they must be introduced to them and be afforded the opportunity to practice them. The occupational therapist is instrumental in this teaching, but in areas where occupational therapists are not available, nurses are often the resource persons for teaching joint protection. Nurses are also in a position to observe the patients' follow-through on the techniques they have been taught, and nurses can provide encouragement and reminding as necessary.[30]

Assistive, supportive, and safety devices. There are many assistive devices available for persons who have impairment of upper and lower extremity function; some examples of these devices are described in Table 41-1. Although the occupational therapist is generally the person who evaluates the patient's disability, recommends specific assistive devices, and teaches the patient how to use them, the nurse is often the person who recognizes the need for referral to the occupational

TABLE 41-1. Some assistive devices for persons with motor impairments

Assistive device	Patient limitation
Utensil with built-up handle (Fig. 41-6)	Cannot adequately close hand
Utensil with cuffed handle (see Fig. 35-7)	Loss of opposition of thumb
Combination knife-fork (Fig. 41-7)	Use of only one hand
Mug with special handle (Fig. 41-8)	Unable to grasp regular cup handle
Long-handle shoehorn (Fig. 41-9)	Unable to bend to reach feet
Long-handle reacher (to reach for or pick up objects) (Fig. 41-10)	Unable to stoop or reach
Long-handle comb, fork, spoon (Figs. 41-11 and 41-12)	Limited shoulder or elbow motion
Stocking guide (Fig. 41-13)	Inability to reach feet

therapist. Nurses need to be aware of what self-help devices the person has, and should encourage the use of them in activities in the hospital or in the home. For example, it is nontherapeutic and time consuming to feed persons who can feed themselves independently with aids that can be provided.

Supportive devices or ambulatory aids (walkers, canes, crutches) are usually recommended for persons who cannot bear weight on one or more joints of the lower extremities. These devices permit part of the person's ambulatory weight to be transferred to the upper extremities. Some other indications for their use are instability, poor balance, or pain on weight bearing.

The physical therapist evaluates the patient to determine the specific device that will match the patient's needs and abilities. Axillary crutches require that the person be fairly dexterous and have a good sense of balance, especially if no weight bearing is permitted on one leg; however, crutches permit faster ambulation and can be used on stairs as well as on level surfaces (Fig. 46-10). Walkers provide more solid support than crutches and in most instances are more useful for individuals

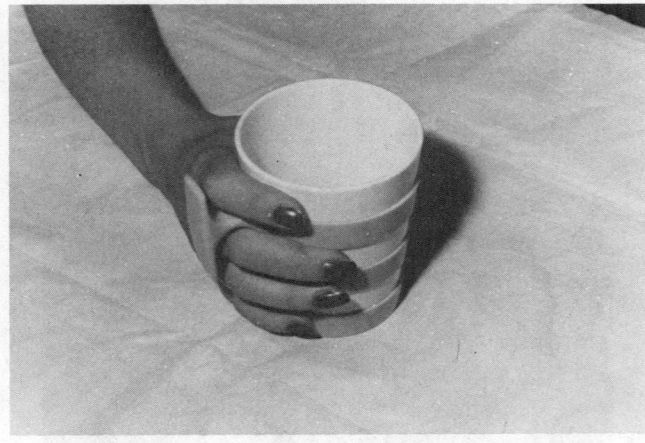

Fig. 41-8. Mug with special handle.

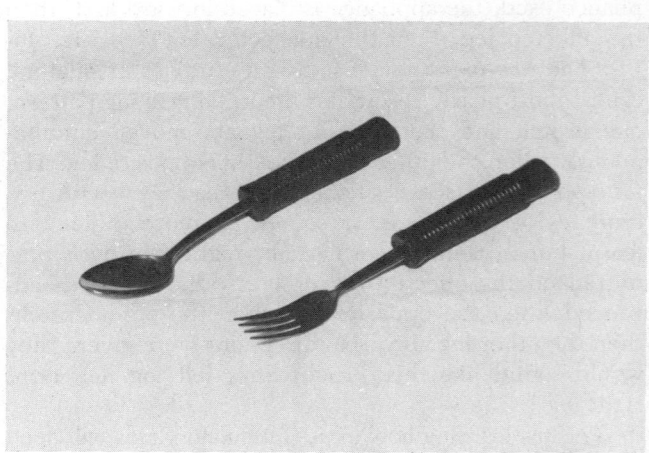

Fig. 41-6. Utensils with built-up handles.

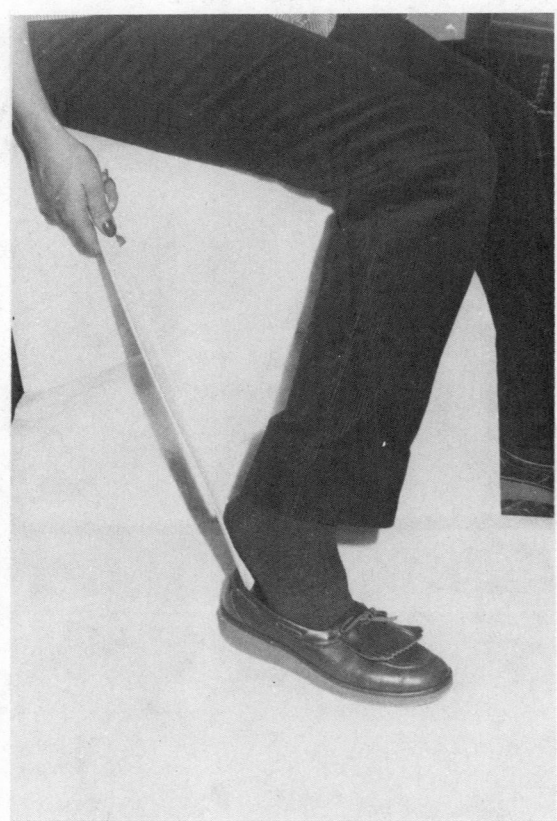

Fig. 41-9. Long-handled shoehorn.

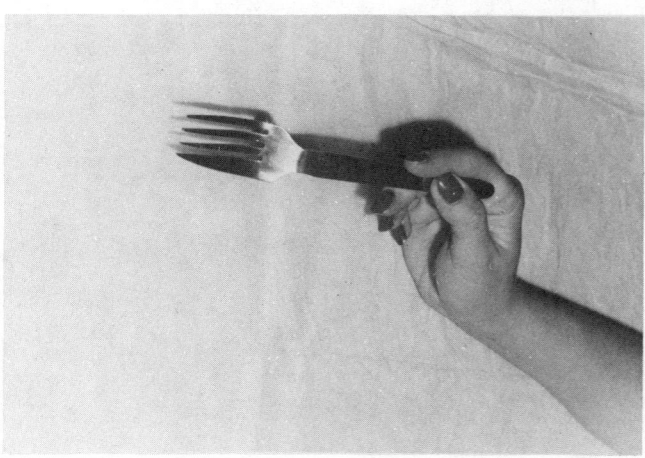

Fig. 41-7. Combination knife-fork.

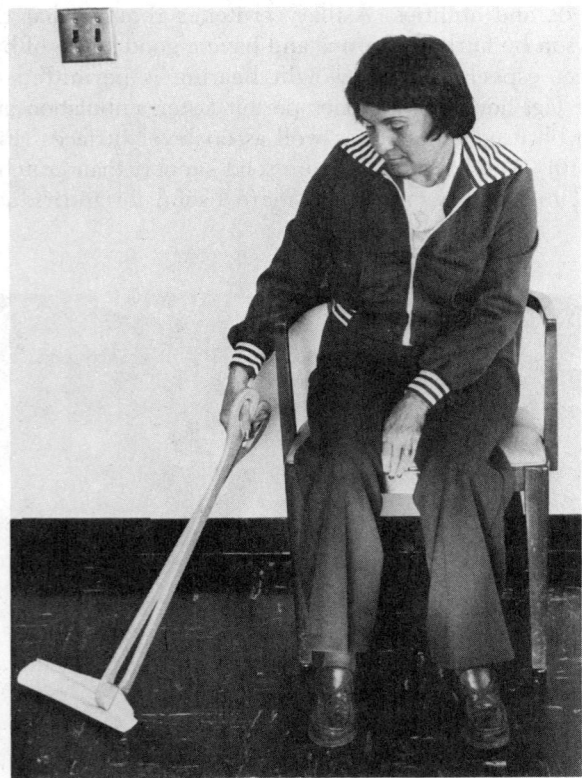

Fig. 41-10. Long-handled reachers are handy for picking things up off floor if person is not to bend or stoop.

with problems of balance and dexterity. Ambulation with a standard walker is slower than with crutches, and it is hazardous on stairs and uneven ground outdoors. Canes allow the person greater mobility and are less cumbersome than either crutches or walkers, but with a single cane the person cannot unload his weight from the affected limb as effectively as he could with a walker or crutches. A number of variations of the three basic ambulatory devices are available, depending on the person's special needs (special handles on canes, forearm supports on crutches, reciprocal walkers, elevated walkers, and others).

Physical therapists generally select and teach the person how to use ambulatory devices. However, nurses may at times be called on to do this teaching, and they must, in any case, know how to supervise the person who uses ambulatory aids. The most common gait pattern is the *three-point gait*. This pattern may be used with a walker, cane, or crutches. Regardless of the appliance used, the appliance is placed forward first, then the affected leg, then the unaffected leg (see Fig. 46-11). The *two-point gait,* used with crutches or bilateral canes, most nearly resembles a normal walking pattern: one crutch and the opposite leg are moved simultaneously, then the other crutch and its opposite leg. The *four-point gait* (see Fig. 46-12, A), also used with two crutches or two canes, is somewhat more difficult to learn, but is useful when partial weight bearing is permitted on the affected leg or legs. One crutch is advanced, then the opposite leg, then the other crutch, then the other leg. If verbal directions were given, they would sound like this: "Right arm, left leg, left arm, right leg."

Persons learning how to use ambulatory aids will need close supervision or assistance until they feel steady and confident. The person doing the supervision should walk along with the patient on the patient's *affected* side, slightly to the patient's rear and about one-half step be-

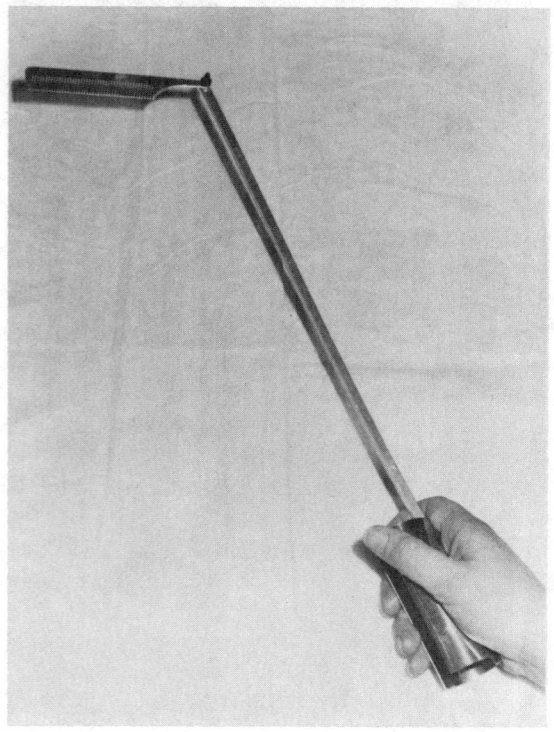

Fig. 41-11. Long-handled comb.

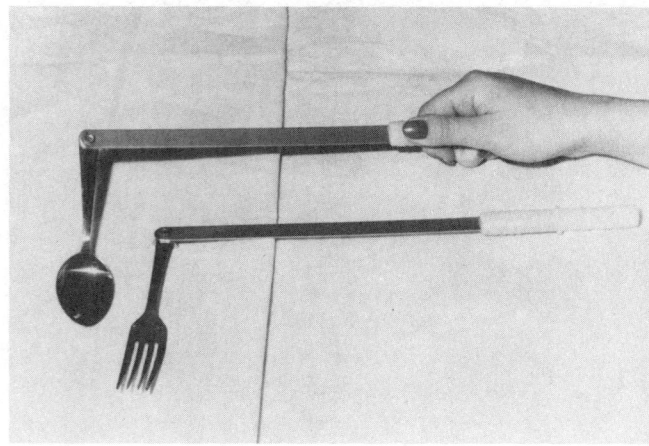

Fig. 41-12. Long-handled fork and spoon.

hind the patient, keeping in step with the patient so that both the patient and person supervising have the same balance point at any given time. The hand closest to the patient should be positioned at the patient's unaffected hip, and the hand farthest from the patient should be positioned to hold the patient's shoulder on the affected side. In this fashion the patient can be prevented from falling forward, backward, or to either side. Likewise, the person assisting will not obstruct the patient's movement of the ambulatory aid. As the patient develops more skill, assistance and supervision are gradually withdrawn.

Persons using ambulatory aids should have instruction by the physical therapist. When possible, they should practice with the device before discharge from the hospital. Proper instruction and adjustment of and practice with the device may prevent accidents after discharge.

Points of safety have already been discussed on p. 947. Examples of *safety devices* commonly employed are grab bars around toilets, tubs, or showers; elevated toilet seats; skidproof mats or adhesive strips on tub

floors; hand rails along staircases; and nonskid wax applied to floors. Areas in which the patient is unsafe or potentially unsafe can only be identified through careful observation of the patient and through testing the patient in a variety of ADL situations. Only those devices that are appropriate for a particular patient should be recommended. This requires some familiarity with the various aids available. That familiarity can be easily obtained by examining a catalogue from an orthopedic supply house.

Heat and cold. Heat and cold have a variety of uses for individuals with musculoskeletal problems. Heat, particularly moist heat, is often used for relaxation of muscles and for its sedative and analgesic effects. It is particularly useful in relieving stiffness. Heat treatments early in the morning may make it possible for an individual to move into the day more comfortably and more quickly than would be possible without treatment. Cold is often used to reduce or prevent swelling after trauma and some patients find that it reduces pain and stiffness better than heat.

One of the most effective means of delivering moist

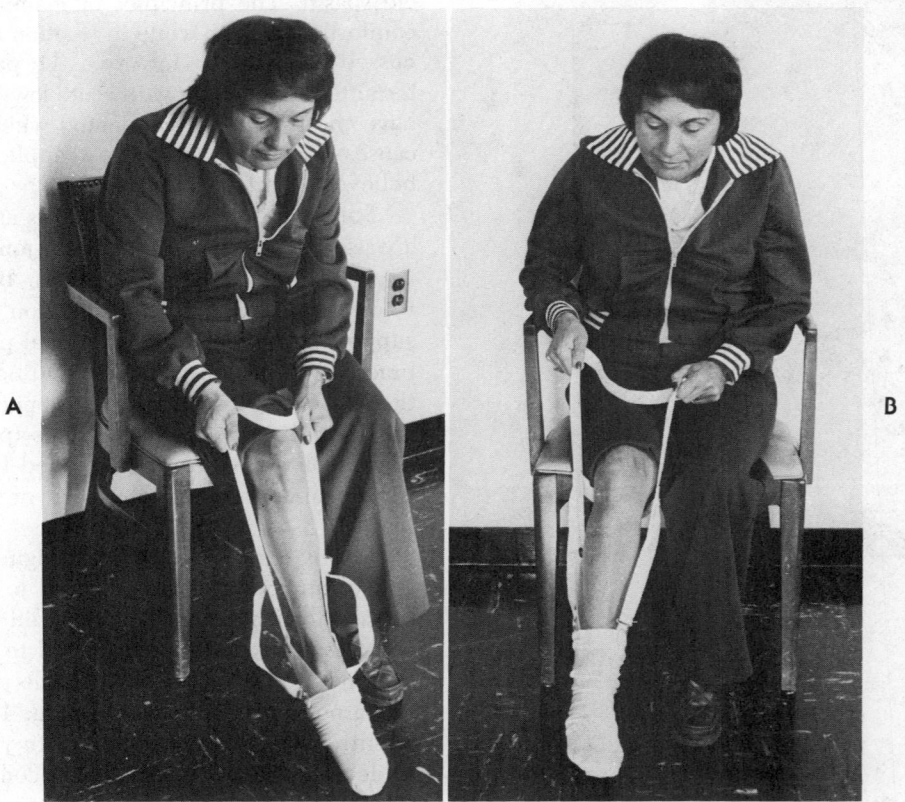

Fig. 41-13. A, Using stocking aid. Stocking has been placed over plastic guide; garter clips at ends of strap have been attached to top of stocking. Woman then places her foot into stocking. **B,** Straps are used to pull stocking over foot and up leg; when top of stocking is at knee, patient can release garters. This apparatus is useful for persons who cannot bend over to reach feet.

heat is through warm, moist compresses or hot (Hydrocollator) packs. These packs contain a chemical filler that expands in hot water and retains heat. They are heated to 80° C (174° F) in water-filled machines and are then wrapped in toweling before application. At least six to eight layers of thick toweling should separate the pack from the patient's skin (Fig. 41-14). Other forms of heating devices (Aqua-K pads and electric heating pads) provide a dry or less conductive heat to the affected part. When any form of heat application is being used, the patient's skin is checked for evidence of burning a few minutes after application. If the application is too hot, it should either be removed or additional protective toweling applied.

Moist compresses should be left on (if not contraindicated) from 15 to 20 minutes to achieve maximal ef-

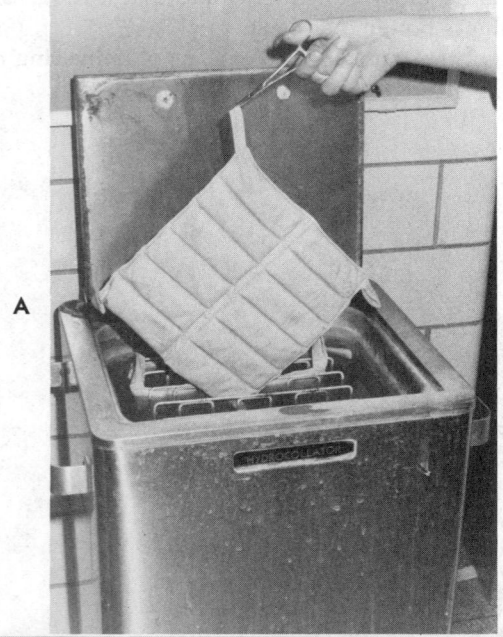

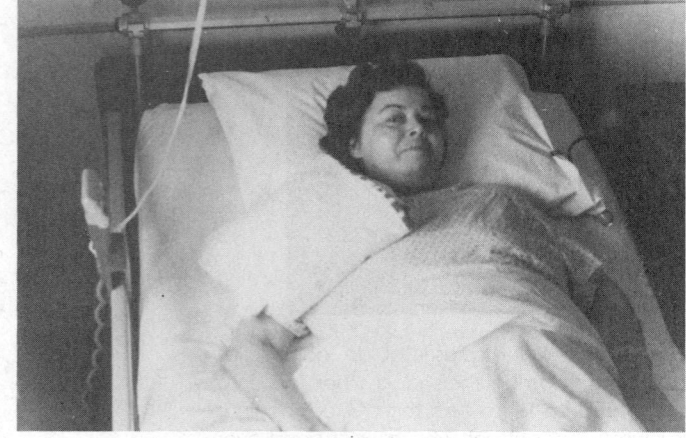

Fig. 41-14. A, Hydrocollator pack being removed from its heating machine. **B,** Patient using Hydrocollator pack.

fect. Dry heat can be left on considerably longer if there is a control device to regulate the heat at a low level. It should be noted, however, that heat is not to be used on *joints* that are or may be *infected* (p. 1002).

Ice packs must also be wrapped in toweling before application to the skin, since cold "burns" can result if the skin is unprotected. Continuous applications of ice may be required to reduce swelling following trauma to a body part; however, the skin should be checked frequently to determine if there are any signs of tissue damage.

Any person with decreased sensation must have heat or cold applied with caution, since that person will not be able to determine if damage is occurring. If heat or cold treatments are to be used at home, the patient should be taught what safety precautions to observe as well as the best methods for obtaining the desired results. For individuals with sensory deficits, this often means that someone else must be taught how to perform the treatment for them.

Traction. In addition to the use of traction in acute trauma and postoperative orthopedic situations (p. 968), *intermittent* traction can be used to assist in reducing contractures or to relieve pain in the presence of muscle spasm. The principles of maintaining the patient's comfort and safety while in traction are the same as discussed on p. 970. However, the patient who is in intermittent traction (as with acute low back injuries) should have the traction disconnected when the traction itself causes discomfort. It can be reapplied when the patient believes he or she can tolerate it.

Splinting and bracing. Splints and braces (orthoses) are used to stabilize or support a joint to protect it from improper use or external trauma. Braces are also used to mechanically correct dysfunction such as footdrop by supporting a joint in its functional position. Splints and braces are used in arthritic conditions (rheumatoid arthritis, Charcot's joints), orthopedic situations (scoliosis), and neurologic conditions (peripheral nerve lesions such as footdrop). The need for splints or braces is determined by the physician or the physical therapist.

Spring-loaded braces are designed to oppose the action of unparalyzed muscles and to act as partial functional substitutes for the paralyzed muscles[36] (Fig. 41-15). *Resting splints* are designed to maintain a limb or joint in a functional position while permitting the muscles around the joint to relax (Fig. 41-16). They are frequently used for the patient with rheumatoid arthritis to decrease muscle spasms that contribute to joint deformity. *Functional splints* maintain the joint or limb in a usable position. For example, if the patient has a drop wrist, a splint will support the wrist in a "cock-up" position so that the hand can be used for feeding or other functions.[36]

Splints and braces are designed to be as lightweight and cosmetically acceptable as possible. Advances have

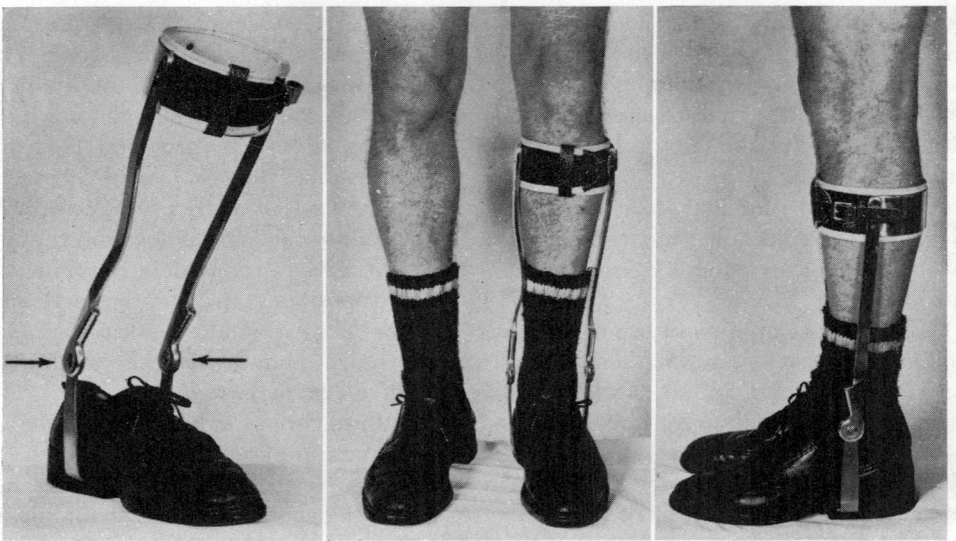

Fig. 41-15. Spring foordrop brace. When weak dorsiflexor muscles are overbalanced by stronger plantar flexors, adjustable spring at ankle hinge of each upright (Klenzak joint, Pope Foundation, Inc.) is used to supply passive dorsiflexion and thus prevent foordrop and an equinus limp. (From Brashear, H., and Raney, R.: Shand's handbook of orthopaedic surgery, ed. 9, St. Louis, 1978, The C.V. Mosby Co.)

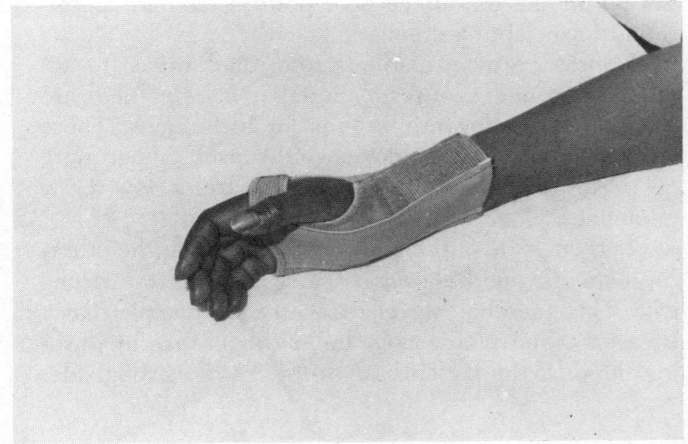

Fig. 41-16. Commercially available resting splint for wrist.

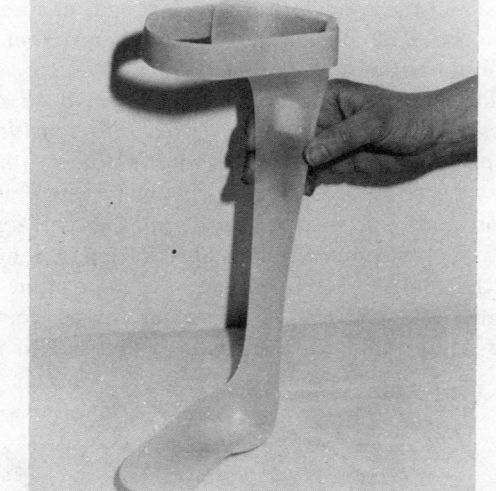

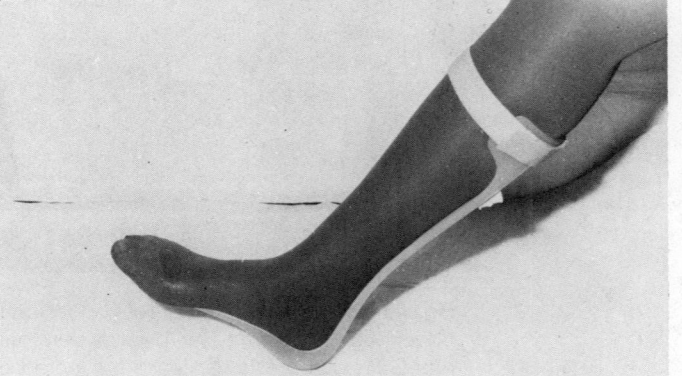

Fig. 41-17. A, Molded foordrop brace. **B,** Brace in place on foot.

been made in this area by *orthotists* (brace makers) who have developed plastic molded braces made out of lightweight materials that are custom fitted to the patient (Fig. 41-17). In some instances these have replaced the cumbersome metal and leather braces that are often obvious, even though worn under loose-fitting clothing.

Shoes may be modified, or the physician may prescribe corrective shoes to provide special support for the feet. For reasons of safety as well as support, sturdy, preferably lacing shoes of an oxford type rather than soft bedroom slippers should be worn by patients for ambulation.

Observations of the patient's skin should be made after an orthosis has been worn for a short period of time (several hours) to make certain that it has caused no skin irritation. The skin must be checked for areas of redness or abrasion. If the patient complains of discomfort or has evidence of skin irritation after wearing the brace, it will need to be checked and perhaps readjusted by the orthotist.

Nurses are frequently instrumental in helping the patient make the psychologic adjustment to wearing such appliances, as well as helping the patient learn to apply and care for them.

Patients are taught how to apply and remove their own braces or splints and how to care for them. Metal braces should be stored upright. Splints fabricated of molded materials should be stored away from sources of heat. Leather materials should be treated occasionally with Neatsfoot Compound or another leather preservative to prevent their drying and cracking. Additionally, if the patient gains or loses weight after the orthosis is made, it may no longer fit. The patient should understand this problem and the need to have the brace adjusted if there is a change in his weight.

Positioning. Principles of positioning (Fig. 41-18) can be found in most fundamental nursing texts. Special considerations for positioning of patients with specific musculoskeletal problems are discussed in Chapter 42. Posture and the specifications for a "good" chair are discussed on p. 949. Wheelchairs are another kind of device that should be mentioned briefly.

Pain. *Because pain accompanies nearly all musculoskeletal diseases, it must be taken into consideration when positioning the patient.* Pain may be exquisite in acute stages of diseases such as rheumatic fever, atrophic arthritis, gout, and diseases of the muscles and tendons. These patients require the greatest care and gentleness when they must be moved. Fear of pain often causes irritability and can lead to muscular resistance, which increases the pain. Care must be taken not to jar the

bed. Heavy bedclothes may cause added pain. If cradles are used, caution must be taken not to accidentally bump an involved part of the body when adjusting or removing the cradle. Footboards help to relieve the pressure of covers, provided the patient can be kept warm enough during their use. Sometimes a very painful joint such as a wrist, elbow, or ankle can be placed on a pillow, and the pillow and the limb can be moved together when the patient must turn over or otherwise adjust position. Frequently, patients prefer to *move themselves* rather than risk pain from having someone else move them. When that is the patient's preference, *it should be permitted*.

Wheelchairs. Wheelchairs come in a great variety of shapes and sizes and may be equipped with custom features. If patients are to use a wheelchair as their mode of moving about, the chair should fit the individual. Familiarity with the equipment available will aid in making the decision as to what chair the patient should use. *No wheelchair should be purchased for permanent use by a patient unless someone knowledgeable about wheelchairs, preferably a physical therapist, has evaluated the patient and determined what special equipment is needed.* Chairs poorly fitted to the patient's needs can be unsafe, encourage poor posture, and are an unsound financial investment.

Transfer. Moving patients from one surface to another is termed *transfer*. A number of references are available regarding proper transfer techniques. Those wishing specific information should consult one or more of those references.[28,35] Following are a few basic guidelines:

1. If one side of the body is stronger than the other, *the patient should always be moved toward the strong side*. This guideline correlates with the principle that it is easier to move objects by pulling them than by pushing them. If the patient moves toward the strong side,

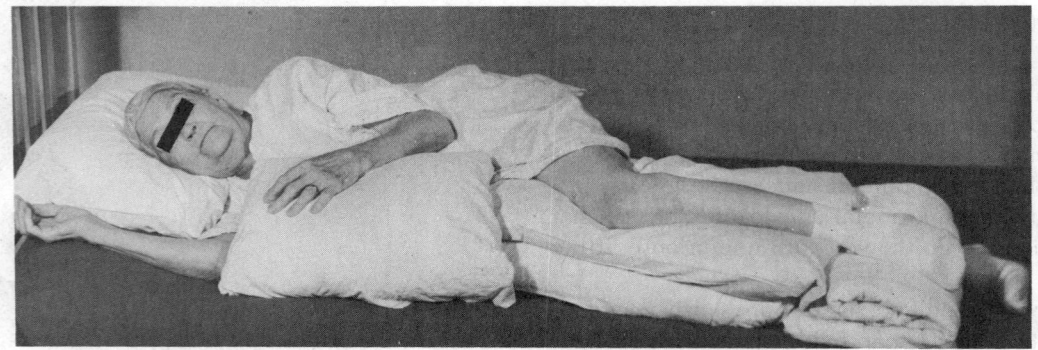

Fig. 41-18. Good side-lying position for patient who has had internal fixation of hip fracture. Upper leg is supported with pillows its entire length, maintaining hip and knee in same plane. Pressure on lower leg is prevented by bringing upper leg forward with flexion at hip and knee. (From Larson, C.B., and Gould, M.: Orthopedic nursing, ed. 8, St. Louis, 1974, The C.V. Mosby Co.)

the strong side is being used to pull the weak side through the required movement. The person assisting with the move should *support the strong side* to make it more effective.

2. If there is any question regarding the patient's ability to cooperate with the transfer, a second person should be standing by for assistance if needed.

3. If the person helping with the transfer has any doubt about his or her ability to accomplish the transfer safely, help should be obtained before attempting it.

4. The transfer should be accomplished using the strong muscles of the legs rather than the weak muscles of the back.

5. If lifting is required, there should be adequate help available. If adequate help is not available, the transfer should not be attempted at that time.

6. Whenever possible, pull sheets should be used to move the patient rather than trying to slide the patient (e.g., from bed to cart).

Therapeutic exercise. Exercise is a prescribed form of activity designed most often to preserve joint mobility or to strengthen specific muscle groups. These can be simple maintenance exercises (passive range of motion or isometric), or they can be active or resistive exercises (performed against resistance provided by another person or weights). Heat is frequently used to relax muscles and adjoining tissue before exercise; however, some individuals respond well to cold applications. *Exercise is contraindicated in the presence of acute joint or muscle inflammation* until the inflammatory process subsides.

The exercise program should be tailored to each patient's specific needs and capabilities. The physician or physical therapist generally outlines the program of exercise to be performed and instructs the patient; however, nurses should be aware of the specific exercise program the patient is following in order to give support in performing it or to provide assistance that may be needed. They should also be prepared to refer problems to the physician or the physical therapist if further instruction or closer follow-up is necessary. Whatever exercises are prescribed, the patient should be instructed about the purpose, technique, frequency, and duration of performing them and should be supervised in the performance of the exercise program until it can be done independently.

Job retraining. As soon as it becomes apparent to the health team that the patient will be unable to return to the same job as previously, the situation should be discussed with the patient and various options in jobs explored. Not infrequently, employers are responsive to the individual's need for a different job, will assist in finding an appropriate job within the same company, and will undertake any necessary retraining themselves. Sometimes, all that is needed is to change from a job with considerable walking to a desk job. Unfortu-

nately, other persons will have to seek a new job. Referrals to vocational guidance and rehabilitation services and job retraining centers (p. 569) are appropriate at this time. Social workers should be made available to such patients for discussion of these services when their use is indicated.

Medications

Although a number of medications are utilized in the treatment of various musculoskeletal problems, the emphasis here will be on those used in the treatment of the various rheumatic diseases.

Salicylates. Salicylates are specific in their antiinflammatory and analgesic effect and are generally considered the *drug of choice* in the treatment of rheumatoid and other forms of arthritis. Because aspirin is a "common" drug, many patients find it difficult to believe that it will be effective in a serious problem such as arthritis. Considerable teaching may be necessary to assure the patient that aspirin, taken as ordered, will help relieve pain, and further, by reducing inflammation, will help to prevent joint deformities and other sequelae of acute joint inflammation.

It is not unusual for as many as 12 to 16 tablets (gr v or 320 mg per tablet) of acetylsalicylic acid per day, given in divided doses, to be prescribed for the treatment of arthritic conditions. Blood salicylate levels of 20% to 30% are recommended for the drug to be clinically effective in rheumatoid arthritis.[31] Large doses of acetylsalicylic acid may cause local irritation to the stomach mucosa (gastritis). Consequently, unbuffered aspirin is nearly always given with milk or with meals or is followed in 1 hour by antacids. Enteric-coated aspirin may be prescribed to help offset the problem of gastritis and the development of ulcers. Other forms of salicylates, such as liquid choline salicylate or salicylsalicylic acid, do not seem to have this pronounced effect and may be prescribed instead of acetylsalicylic acid if the patient demonstrates gastric intolerance.[31]

The signs of salicylate poisoning—ringing in the ears (tinnitus), nausea, vomiting, tachycardia, and hepatic abnormalities—should be watched for, although aspirin usually can be taken over a long period of time without the occurrence of toxicity or the acquisition of tolerance. If tinnitus occurs, the drug is usually discontinued until the symptoms subside, and then restarted at a lower dosage level. Aspirin is also known to prolong bleeding time. This is thought to be related to its effect on platelet adhesiveness. For this reason, acetylsalicylic acid is sometimes discontinued 2 weeks before elective surgery.

Persons with rheumatoid arthritis who are taking aspirin tend to perspire a great deal. When they are on bed rest, they will require frequent bathing and frequent linen changes for comfort and skin protection.

Other nonnarcotic, antiinflammatory, and analgesic agents. Other antiinflammatory and analgesic agents may be used in the treatment of various rheumatic diseases. Indomethacin (Indocin), an antiinflammatory agent, may be effective for patients who do not respond to aspirin, but side effects (severe headaches, dizziness, confusion, and gastrointestinal disturbances) are common. Phenylbutazone (Butazolidin), a potent antiinflammatory agent, is very effective in the treatment of acute inflammatory episodes; but because of its potential to produce gastric irritation and bone marrow depression, it is generally confined to short-term use (7 to 10 days).[31] Acetaminophen (Tylenol) may be used as a helpful analgesic adjunct to acetylsalicylic acid therapy, as may propoxyphene hydrochloride (Darvon); however, they are not antiinflammatory.

Some relatively new nonsteroidal antiinflammatory agents have been receiving wide attention. They include ibuprofen (Motrin), tolmetin sodium (Tolectin), fenoprofen calcium (Nalfon), naproxen (Naprosyn), sulindac (Clinoril), and piroxicam (Feldene). While these drugs have not been demonstrated to be more efficacious than acetylsalicylic acid, they are believed to be less irritating to the gastrointestinal tract. Two of them, naproxen and sulindac, have a longer half-life than acetylsalicylic acid and need be administered only twice daily, while piroxicam needs to be taken only once a day. All of them are, however, chemically related to indomethacin, so they may produce the same side effects as indomethacin, notably drowsiness. Patients using these drugs should be thoroughly instructed in their administration and side effects.

Antimalarials. Antimalarial drugs, hydroxychloroquine (Plaquenil) and chloroquine (Aralen), are used to help control inflammatory joint disease when salicylate therapy alone is insufficient. Because response is slow, hydroxychloroquine is given on a trial basis in doses of 200 mg twice a day for a period of 3 to 6 months. If improvement occurs, the dose is adjusted to 200 mg once daily. If there is no favorable response, the drug is discontinued.[31] Toxic reactions include gastrointestinal upset, rash, headaches, and retinal changes. The latter problem is of the most concern. Persons who are given hydroxychloroquine therapy should have baseline eye examinations when treatment is begun and every 6 months thereafter. If retinal changes are detected early, they are reversible, providing the drug is discontinued. If not detected until later, changes resulting in visual loss may not be reversible. Persons who are begun on hydroxychloroquine therapy should be advised of this toxic effect and be encouraged to have regular eye examinations.

Quinacrine (Atabrine), used in the treatment of arthritis and the skin rash of systemic lupus erythematosus, will cause yellowing of the skin. This yellowing can be controlled if the drug is periodically discontinued.[31]

Patients are generally advised of this side effect before treatment is begun.

Corticosteroids. The corticosteroid drugs have a potent antiinflammatory effect. They are used in chronic connective tissue diseases (rheumatoid arthritis, systemic lupus erythematosus, progressive systemic sclerosis, polymyositis, and the various forms of necrotizing vasculitis) to control inflammation and reduce pain. They also inhibit other effects of inflammation such as the overgrowth of fibrous tissue. *In most instances, steroid drugs are not used if other, less toxic forms of treatment will be effective.* A major objective in treating patients with corticosteroids is to control symptoms at dosage levels that will cause the fewest side effects and complications. Depending on the severity of the disease being treated, the dosage may range anywhere from the equivalent of 1 mg of prednisone (Deltasone) to 200 mg of prednisone per day.[31] The latter dose, equivalent to 800 mg of hydrocortisone, is not considered excessive in the treatment of such problems as severe lupus vasculitis. Steroids may be administered orally, intramuscularly, intraarticularly (to treat inflammation in a particular joint), intravenously, or topically (in the form of creams and ointments to treat skin rashes or lesions).

Side effects and toxic effects are dose related; the higher the dose, the more likely complications are to occur. Side effects include an increased susceptibility to infection and decreased healing potential caused by suppression of the inflammatory responses; osteoporosis; psychologic disturbances (euphoria, depression, manic-depressive psychoses), particularly when dosages *per day* reach or exceed the equivalent of 40 mg of prednisone; gastrointestinal irritation and ulceration; diabetes mellitus; myopathy; hypokalemia; and hypertension. These problems are generally reversible if steroid therapy is discontinued. If treatment of the disease demands that steroid therapy be continued, some of these problems are amenable to treatment; for example, diabetes may be treated with insulin, and hypertension with sodium restriction and antihypertensive drugs.[3]

Another major problem to be considered in the management of persons who are being treated with steroids is that *prolonged steroid therapy suppresses adrenocortical activity;* therefore the body is incapable of mounting its own response in times of severe stress. If the steroids are suddenly withdrawn, or if the person is subjected to physical trauma such as accident or surgery, adrenocortical insufficiency may result. (For further information on adrenal insufficiency, see p. 637.) Persons taking steroid drugs for musculoskeletal problems should observe the same precautions as carried out by persons taking steroids as a hormonal replacement (p. 638).

Gold therapy. Treatment with gold salts is effective in inducing partial or complete remission in many patients with rheumatoid arthritis and in some patients with psoriatic arthritis.[31] Aurothioglucose (Solganal) and gold sodium thiomalate (Myochrysine) are the two forms of gold most frequently used. The usual dose is 10 mg given intramuscularly as a test dose. If no ill effects such as *nitritoid vasomotor reaction* (flushing, lightheadedness, syncope) or other evidences of clinical or laboratory toxicity are encountered, a second dose of 25 mg is given. Then 50 mg is administered at weekly intervals until the patient has received a total of 750 to 1000 mg. A maintenance dose of 25 to 50 mg is then given every 3 to 4 weeks to maintain remission. Steroids, dimercaprol (BAL), or penicillamine (Cuprimine) may be needed to treat untoward reactions.[31]

While gold salts control the symptoms of rheumatoid arthritis in some patients, they may cause serious reactions. Gold toxicity may cause severe renal and hepatic damage, and gold may be deposited in the cornea of the eye. Dermatitis is a common side effect. Before gold is administered, the patient is checked for sore mouth, a metallic taste in the mouth, skin rash or itching of the skin, and diarrhea. Blood and urinary studies are done before each of the first 15 to 20 injections and every second or third injection thereafter. Evidence of toxicity includes a decreased platelet count, leukopenia, eosinophilia, or proteinuria.[31] Mild toxicity is treated by stopping the gold therapy, while more severe reactions may be treated with corticosteroids.[31]

Penicillamine. Another agent that is proving effective in reducing inflammation in rheumatic conditions that do not respond well to other forms of therapy is pencillamine (Cuprimine). Like the antimalarials and the gold salts, it has a delayed response time. The usual beginning dosage is 250 mg/day, given on an empty stomach. Since the drug is derived from pencillin, patients who have penicillin allergies should be watched carefully for signs of allergic reaction. Albuminuria and alterations of the white blood cell count may also occur. Patients taking this drug are checked with frequent urinalyses and blood counts.

Immunosuppressive agents. Immunosuppressive agents—azathioprine (Imuran), cyclophosphamide (Cytoxan), and chlorambucil (Leukeran)—have been used on an *investigational basis* for patients with severe diseases, such as lupus vasculitis and "malignant" rheumatoid arthritis, that do not respond to treatment, or for patients who have toxic reactions to other forms of therapy.[31] *They are used only with great care because of their severe side effects and the attendant risks of the development of neoplasms.*

Narcotic analgesics. The use of narcotic analgesics (morphine sulphate, codeine phosphate, meperidine [Demerol]) is generally discouraged in patients with chronic arthritic conditions, since their effect is only temporary, they are not antiinflammatory, and the patient can develop a tolerance to them. Narcotic agents do have their place in the treatment of acute injuries to the musculoskeletal system and are a vital adjunct to the management of the patient following orthopedic surgery. They should, however, be withdrawn in favor of nonnarcotic agents when the patient's pain level permits.

Diet

The essentials of good nutrition, including fruits, vegetables, proteins, and vitamins, are as important for individuals with musculoskeletal problems as for anyone else. Special diets are usually not recommended except in instances where the patient is overweight or has some metabolic problem such as gout (p. 1002).

Patients should be urged to eat regular meals and should be given plenty of time to eat. Even if patients have marked limitation of movement, they should be urged to feed themselves (Fig. 41-19). This may require that food be prepared beforehand, for example, cut up, or that special feeding utensils be provided (p. 950).

Patients who have restricted mobility may have difficulty with constipation. Foods high in roughage or fiber should be available to help relieve this problem. The diet for a patient who has had a fracture needs to be high in protein, iron, and vitamins if bone repair is to progress normally.

During immobility, catabolic activity is accelerated, producing a rapid breakdown of cellular materials. This leads to protein deficiency and negative nitrogen balance. Decalcification and demineralization of bone take place *during immobility* regardless of the quantity of calcium intake. Increasing calcium in the diet above normal requirements is *not* recommended for the immobile patient because it cannot be used. A diet high in protein is indicated, however, in order to overcome protein deficiency and return the body to a state of *positive nitrogen balance*. At times 150 to 300 g of protein is required daily to achieve this.

Weight gain should be avoided if at all possible. Added weight increases the patient's energy consumption and causes weight-bearing joints to be abnormally stressed. For the individual who has joint problems such as degenerative joint disease or rheumatoid arthritis, every movement can be made a task because of excessive weight. For many individuals with mobility problems, the problem of weight and movement becomes a vicious circle. Mobility is impaired, therefore activity is limited, calories are not used in activity, more weight is added, and further immobility results as the individual finds it harder to move the weight he or she must carry. Weight restricts mobility, and weight gain may be inevitable if mobility is decreased. The cycle must be broken, and it must be broken by weight loss.

Psychologic and social support

The importance of family support for patients with musculoskeletal problems, especially chronic problems, is discussed in Chapter 40. When problems are serious enough to require changes in the patient's life-style and limitation of activities, family members must be given

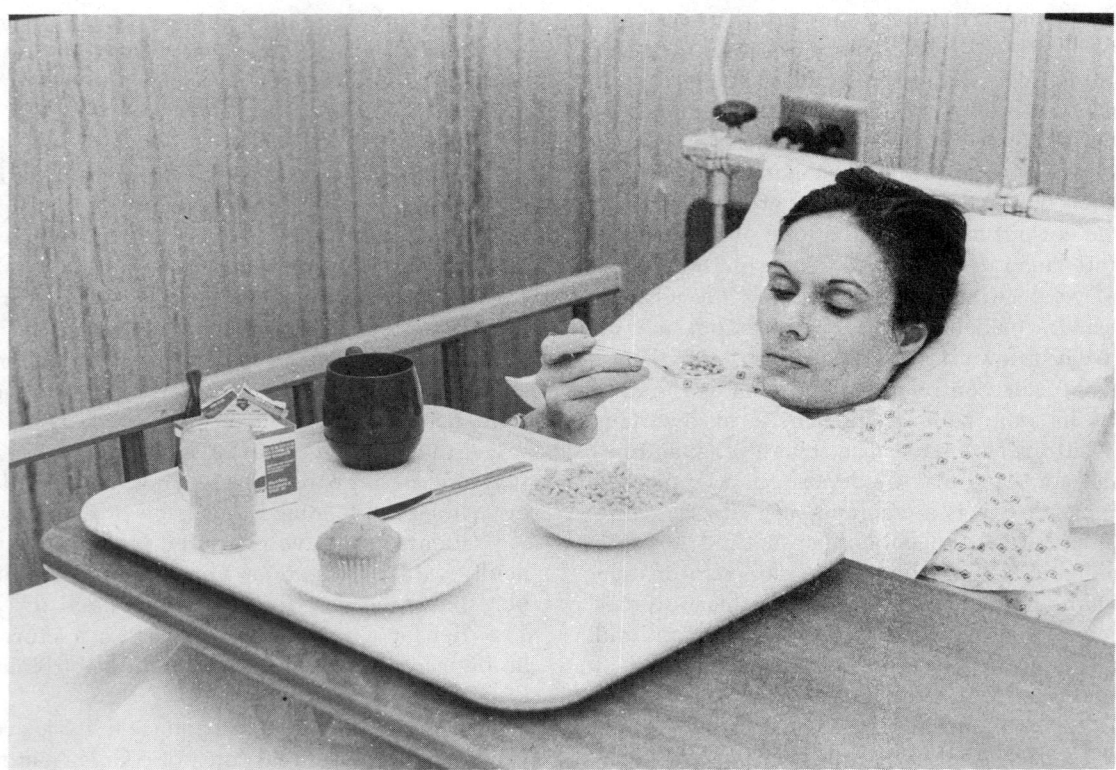

Fig. 41-19. Patient who can neither sit up nor lie on one side to eat meals can still be made comfortable with some elevation of head and shoulders on pillows. Additional means of elevating patient to a more upright position is to put frame of bed in reverse. Trendelenburg's position.

the same opportunity to cope as the patient. Social workers and other members of the health team are very often instrumental in assisting the patient and family to define new roles and responsibilities that each can assume with the least disruption in family continuity.

The idea of trying to help the patient "accept" a disability is generally not workable. Most musculoskeletal disabilities have a visible form, and patients know that they look, walk, use their hands, or sometimes even talk differently than "normal" people. They know that they are physically limited and that they cannot do all the things they would like or even need to do. As the physical problems become more pronounced and more limiting, it can be expected that the patient will go through a period of depression and grieving for these lost abilities. Sometimes psychiatric counseling is necessary before individuals can adapt to their losses. *Adaptation* is a more functional term than *acceptance* since many persons may never *accept* their condition but they may *adapt* to it very well through changes in life-style and level of activity.

It is the process of adaptation and the individual's capacity to make adaptations that must be tapped by those working with persons with musculoskeletal problems. Helping them to learn (1) new ways of doing things

in spite of limitations in motor ability, (2) that they can lead an active life in spite of activity limitation, and (3) that there are measures that can be taken toward pain relief and preservation of remaining function is appropriate and necessary in the care of these patients.

Outcome criteria for the person with motor problems requiring conservative intervention

The person or significant others can:
1. Explain the ADL program.
   a. Demonstrate competence and independence in all ADL that are within physical capabilities.
   b. Explain in what areas, if any, help is necessary.
   c. Explain what provisions have been made for obtaining that help.
   d. Explain limitations of ADL that must be observed and for what period of time.
2. Explain medication regimen.
   a. Explain the expected effect, dosage, administration times, side effects, and toxic effects of each of the prescribed medications.
   b. Demonstrate safe, competent practice in administering each medication.

c. Explain what is to be done if toxic effects occur.

d. Explain the nature and rationale for any special precautions that must be taken in relation to the prescribed drugs (e.g., taking analgesics with antacids, regular eye examination, special laboratory studies).

3. Explain measures for pain relief.
   a. Explain the use of pain-relieving agents.
   b. Explain and demonstrate the value of moderating activity and rest.
   c. Explain and demonstrate various positioning techniques that will relieve pain.
   d. Demonstrate the safe use of heat and cold applications to relieve pain and stiffness.
   e. Demonstrate the application, use, removal, and proper care of various splinting or bracing devices.

4. Explain exercise program.
   a. Explain the rationale for and demonstrate correct performance of prescribed exercise program.

5. Explain use of assistive and supportive devices.
   a. Demonstrate correct use of feeding, bathing, and dressing utensils.
   b. Demonstrate safe and proper use of prescribed ambulatory or locomotor device on level surfaces (and when appropriate, stairs).
   c. Explain weight-bearing limitations.

6. Explain safety precautions.
   a. Describe the safety devices to be obtained for use at home and how and where they will be obtained.
   b. Describe and demonstrate how these safety devices and precautions will be used at home.
   c. Describe what alterations must be made in the home environment to render it safe.

7. Explain preventive measures or techniques.
   a. Demonstrate proper positioning techniques in the prevention of contractures and atrophy.
   b. Demonstrate joint-protection techniques to prevent stress or damage to joints.
   c. Demonstrate proper body mechanics in ADL.
   d. Explain the use of bracing or splinting techniques in preventive damage to the extremities.
   e. Explain the value of maintaining an "ideal" weight to prevent joint stress and fatigue.

8. Explain diet.
   a. Explain the importance of maintaining an "ideal" weight.
   b. Demonstrate knowledge of prescribed dietary restrictions through ability to select foods that are within the dietary restrictions.

9. Explain follow-up care.
   a. Explain plans for follow-up care.

b. Explain what to do if one runs short of medication or experiences some complication.

Surgical intervention

Persons admitted to hospitals for orthopedic procedures usually fall into one of two categories: those who have suffered trauma such as a fracture, or those who require an elective orthopedic procedure for the correction of deformity, relief of pain, or the restoration of musculoskeletal function. There are four *major objectives of orthopedic treatment: (1) restoration or maintenance of function of a body part, (2) prevention of deformity, (3) correction of deformity* if it already exists, and (4) *development of the patient's powers of compensation and adaptation* if loss of function or permanent deformity is not preventable.[36]

Before performing surgery, the orthopedist considers what procedure is best suited to achieve the objectives for the individual patient. There will usually be a discussion with the patient or the patient's family concerning the outcomes that may be expected following the recommended procedure. It is important that those caring for the patient in both the preoperative and postoperative periods know and understand what the expected outcomes are so that care may be adapted to achieving them. To illustrate, the expected outcomes following a total knee replacement will not be the same for a 75-year-old woman with multiple joint involvement from rheumatoid arthritis as they would be for a 50-year-old man with degenerative joint disease in only one knee. *Orthopedic care is highly individualized to the patient being treated, and those who work with orthopedic patients must not lose sight of the practical aspects of the treatment rationale.*

Surgery for trauma: fractures

Initial care. Patients who are admitted to orthopedic units following trauma are usually seen because of fractures. Management of patients with fractures will be discussed next.

Treatment of the acute fracture is usually carried out in the hospital's emergency room or in the operating room before the patient's admission to the general hospital unit. Patients will have had little or no opportunity to become oriented to the hospital or to the care that they will be receiving. Additionally, they will most likely be frightened or overwhelmed by what has happened to them, groggy from pain medications or anesthesia, and in pain. They will need careful and often repeated explanation and direction regarding positioning, skin care routines, the need for them to perform adequate deep breathing and coughing, and measures for pain relief. Direction, explanation, and physical handling must be accomplished gently but efficiently during the initial stages of hospitalization. Patients must be given time to adjust to the situation before they can begin to understand how they can cooperate in care.

During the initial 24- to 48-hour period there are many observations that must be carried out. Circulation and sensation in the involved extremity must be checked on an hourly basis. Evidence of impaired circulation (coolness, cyanosis, poor capillary refill) or impaired sensation (diminished sensation, paresthesias, intense pain) must be reported to the physician immediately, since these signs can indicate damage to arteries or nerves. Some swelling of an injured extremity may be expected and is most often well controlled by elevating the extremity. However, unrelieved swelling of an extremity that is in a cast or a compression dressing can result in tissue damage and neurologic impairment. Unusual swelling, and the pain that usually accompanies it, must also be quickly reported to the physician so that measures may be taken to relieve pressure and reduce the swelling.

Fractures of the hip and spine may be complicated by paralytic ileus (p. 1492), and pulmonary embolus or fat embolus (pp. 1019 and 1320) is not an infrequent complication of fractures of the extremities. The patient must be observed carefully for signs and symptoms of these complications.

As with any postanesthesia patient, the patient who has been operatively treated for a fracture should have supervised pulmonary toileting, frequent turning, and leg exercises (p. 413). Positioning of the patient must be carried out with careful attention to avoid altering the alignment of the fracture, changing the direction of the pull of the traction, compromising the integrity of the cast, or placing undue stress on the internal fixation device. It is of the utmost importance that, before any changes in position are undertaken, there be an understanding of where the fracture is, the nature of the fracture, the method used to reduce the fracture, and the tolerances of that particular method. This information, as well as any special precautions that are to be observed, should be obtained from the orthopedist.

Skin care, with attention to turning, petalling rough edges of casts (p. 967), proper cleansing of pin sites (p. 976), and maintenance of good hygiene, must be conscientiously carried out, particularly when treatment of a fracture demands that the patient be confined to bed for a period of time.

Objectives in the treatment and care of fractures include reduction of the fracture, maintenance of the fragments in the correct position while healing takes place, and prevention of excessive loss of joint mobility and muscle tone. Care must also be taken to prevent complications and maintain good general health so that after healing takes place the patient can continue activity as before the accident or injury.

Reduction of fractures. *Reduction* is the term used for the return of bone fragments to their normal position. This may be accomplished by closed manipulation, traction, or surgery.

CLOSED MANIPULATION. When closed manipulation is used to reduce a fracture, the patient is often given a general anesthetic. They physician reduces the fracture by pulling on the distal fragment (manual traction) while countertraction is applied to the proximal fragment until the bone fragments engage or fall into their normal alignment. The physician may also apply direct pressure over the site of the fracture to correct angulation or lateral displacement of a fragment. Usually when this type of reduction is performed, a cast is applied to hold the fragments in the desired position while healing occurs.

TRACTION. Continuous traction (pull on the affected extremity) for a period of days or even weeks may be necessary to reduce fractures of the femur or humerus because the related large muscles draw the bone fragments out of normal alignment, making immediate reduction by manual traction impossible. Continuous traction may also be used to reduce fractures when there is very extensive tissue damage and when the physical condition of the patient is such that anesthesia cannot be safely given. Thus traction may be used (1) for reducing a fracture, (2) for maintaining correct position of fragments during bone healing, and (3) for immobilizing the limb while soft-tissue healing takes place.

OPEN REDUCTION. Open reduction may be necessary if closed manipulation or traction is unsuccessful. Open reduction has the advantage of allowing visualization of the fracture and surrounding tissues. The bone fragments can be arranged and held by internal fixation if necessary. This method is indicated when there is soft tissue caught between bone fragments or when there is known damage to nerves or blood vessels. The disadvantages of open reduction are the need for anesthesia and the possibility of introducing organisms into the fracture site at the time of surgery. In certain fractures, open reduction is the treatment of choice. Even then it may not be used if closed reduction or traction will suffice.

HEALING OF THE FRACTURES. Healing of the fracture (see Chapter 42) following reduction occurs over a period of time, depending on the location and severity of the fracture, blood supply to the body part, and the age and general physical condition of the patient. Evidence of callus formation (p. 1020) on x-ray films indicates that healing has begun. Eventually, callus is replaced by true bone that grows from beneath the periosteum of each fragment to meet and fuse across the defect. *Delayed healing* or *delayed union* is said to occur when the fracture has not healed within the usual time for the particular bone involved. Delayed healing will occur if the space between the two bones is such that neither the callus nor bone cells can bridge the gap, if the callus is broken or torn apart by too much activity, if muscle or fascia is caught between the fragments, if an infection develops, or if there is poor blood supply to the part or marked dietary deficiency. Occasionally, delayed union occurs with no obvious cause. Open reduction and more complete immobilization may be necessary.

Nonunion is the term used when healing does not take place even in much longer time than is usually required. Congenital conditions and obscure medical diseases occasionally account for this, and nonunion may occur in the aged. When it occurs, the patient may have to wear a brace to support the limb. If the fracture is in the lower extremity, crutches may have to be used indefinitely. Surgery may be performed and an attempt made to unite the fragments with a bone graft. Nonunion occurs most often in the middle of the humerus, the neck of the femur in older people, the lower third of the tibia, and the carpal bones of the wrist.

It should be noted that *impacted fractures* do not need to be reduced. However, some form of immobilization, such as a sling in the case of an impacted fracture of the humerus, may be used to prevent movement or use of the affected extremity that could lead to displacement of the bone fragments.

Immobilization of the reduced fracture. The purpose of immobilization is to hold the bone fragments in contact with each other until healing takes place. All activity of the part that might cause separation of the fragments is restricted, and the fractured bone can be kept in position by externally immobilizing the entire limb. Usually external immobilization includes the joints immediately proximal to and distal to the fractured bone. Devices for external immobilization include bandages, adhesive tape, casts, splints, braces, cast-braces, and traction. Internal immobilization (or internal fixation) may be accomplished by such devices as metal pins, screws, plates, and nails. These devices, made of inert metal alloys such as vitallium, are used to hold the bone fragments together when an open reduction is done. A cast may be used to provide extra protection in instances when a comminuted fracture has occurred.

PLASTER CASTS. Materials used for casts include plaster-of-Paris, fiberglass, and plastic. All three of these materials are available in the form of rolled bandages. Both fiberglass (light-cured) casts and plastic (thermolabile) casts are lighter in weight and faster drying than plaster. They maintain immobility as well as plaster; they do not lose their strength when subjected to water as plaster does. Plastic casts can be reheated and remolded as necessary; revisions in plaster casts usually require removal and reapplication.

However, both fiberglass and plastic are more expensive materials than plaster, and fiberglass requires drying under special ultraviolet lights. Persons wearing fiberglass or plastic casts may suffer maceration of the skin underlying the cast following immersion of the cast in water if they fail to thoroughly dry the skin with a warm air dryer. Because of these disadvantages, plaster-of-Paris remains the most widely employed cast material.[32]

Unless a cast has been applied to the entire trunk and legs, the person who is treated with a cast can usually move about and carry on most activities of daily living (Fig. 41-20). Often the person may return to school or to work and participate in many activities without damage to the site of injury. Use of casts shortens hospitalization, and many persons with simple fractures can be treated in a physician's office, the emergency room, or the outpatient department of a hospital. After a short period of observation, they can be discharged and treatment continued under close medical or nursing supervision.

Plaster-of-Paris casts can, however, restrict some activities because of their weight and their inflexibility. A cast can cause complications because of interference with normal physiologic functions and can cause actual physical injury if incorrectly applied and improperly cared for. A cast applied to the arm or shoulder may limit the kind of clothing worn and may interfere with eating, writing, or other uses of the arm. If applied to the leg, a cast may change body alignment, putting strain on the opposite leg, and limit locomotion.

Those caring for the person not only must know how

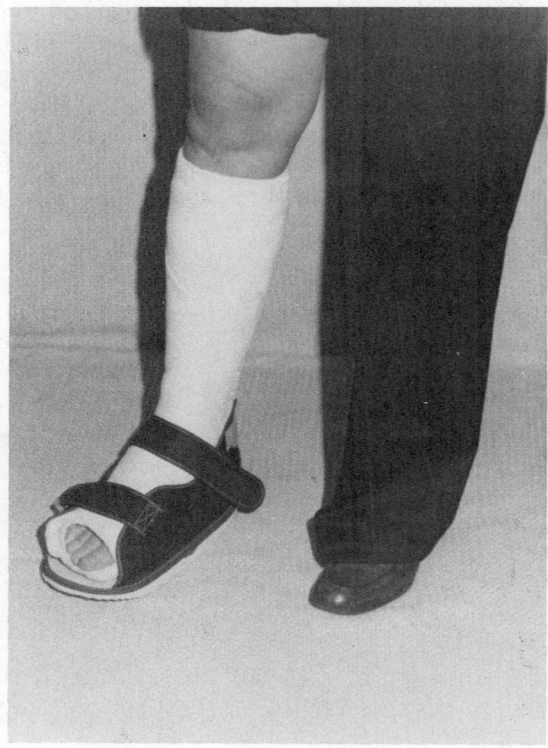

Fig. 41-20. Short leg walking cast with cast shoe.

to maintain the integrity of the cast, but also must understand how the person is affected by it. The person must be helped to be as independent as possible. Care is designed to help prevent complications, and the patient is monitored for early signs of complications. Developing complications are reported to the physician promptly.

Preparing the patient for cast application. In preparing the patient for application of the cast, skin surfaces that will lie under the cast should be thoroughly inspected for cuts, abrasions, and bruises. Note should be made of such areas so subsequent complaints of pain or tenderness under the cast can be properly evaluated. The skin must be thoroughly cleansed and then thoroughly dried with a towel.[17]

Patients undergoing cast application are likely to experience both pain and apprehension. Pain can be decreased by the judicious use of analgesia. Explanation concerning the heaviness of the cast and the fact that the cast will give off heat for a short time as it dries will reduce apprehension. Since tensing of the muscles while the cast is being applied may affect the fit of the cast, the nurse should offer reassurance and attempt to promote relaxation as the cast is applied.

Application of the cast. Most hospitals have a specially equipped cast room where casts are applied. Some hospitals also have a cart equipped with plaster and other cast material that can be taken to the bedside.

Plaster-of-Paris bandages come in various widths (5 to 20 cm). Each roll is wrapped in waxed paper to prevent sifting of the plaster from the bandage and to prevent deterioration from exposure to moisture. The bandage itself is made of crinoline into which plaster-of-Paris (gypsum or calcium sulfate dihydrate) has been rubbed (Fig. 41-21). When water is added, the gypsum assumes its crystalline state and the wet plaster bandage can be molded to fit the shape of a body part or wrapped about a limb. When the water evaporates, the cast becomes firm and can withstand considerable stress and strain. The number of layers of plaster used determines the strength of the cast.

After reduction of the fracture has been accomplished and before the cast is applied, the skin is usually protected with sheet wadding (a thick, nonabsorbent cotton web covered with starch to hold it together), and felt or sponge rubber is used over bony prominences to protect them from pressure. Tubular stockinette, from 5 to 45 cm wide, is used as lining for the cast and is applied so that it will extend over the edge to cover the round edges of the plaster. The excess stockinette and sheet wadding are usually folded back over the cast after it has been applied and bound down with a final roll of plaster.

If the cast is applied elsewhere than in a special plaster room, the floor and table should be protected from wet plaster. When the person who will apply the cast is ready, the bandage is placed in a bucket of water at 21° to 24° C (70° to 75° F) for 5 seconds. The bandage should be carefully removed from the water so that none of the plaster is lost. It should be held horizontally with an end in the palm of each hand and gently compressed to remove excess water. It should then be quickly handed to the person applying the cast so that it can be used before it begins to set. Only a few bandages should be placed in the water at a time. The bucket containing the water should be lined with a cloth or paper to collect waste plaster. When the procedure has been completed, the cloth or paper containing waste plaster can be removed and discarded into a garbage can. The water from the bucket, if it contains no loose plaster, can be emptied into the plaster sink. Plaster-of-Paris will clog ordinary plumbing and should never be emptied into ordinary drains.

Care of the cast. Plaster bandages are fast setting (3 to 7 minutes). Thin casts may dry completely in several hours, but thick casts may require several days to dry completely. The cast can be cracked or broken by inadequate support or by unwise handling before it is dry. A wrinkle in the plaster and indentations caused by the fingertips can alter the inner shape of the cast and cause pressure on the body part encased in the plaster. Wet casts should always be handled with the flat of the hand, not with the fingers.

A firm mattress and, if necessary, a bed board should be used to prevent uneven weight on the fresh plaster cast. To protect the new cast and ensure its efficiency, the patient is carefully transferred from the stretcher to the bed. The patient who is conscious can be moved onto the bed with the assistance of one nurse, while another person supports the wet cast at the areas of greatest strain—usually at the joints. If the patient is asleep or is in a body cast, three or four people will be required to lift the patient onto the bed. The entire cast

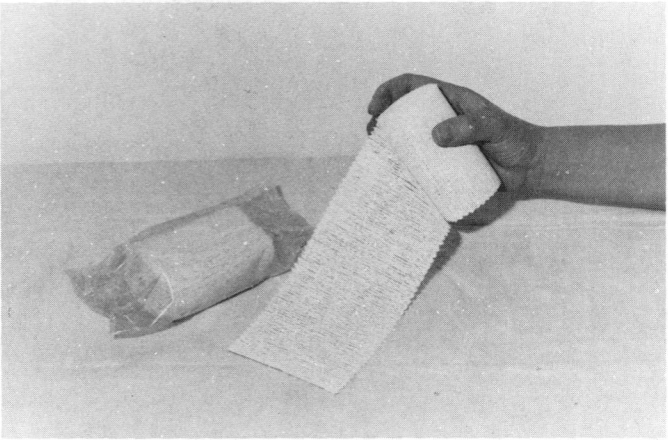

Fig. 41-21. Rolls of plaster-of-Paris bandage.

as well as the patient's head and extremities must be fully supported.

The wet cast should not lie unsupported on the hard bed because it may become flattened over bony prominences and weight-bearing areas such as the back of the heel, buttocks, and shoulders. This can cause pressure. The wet cast should always be fully supported on a pillow or pillows that are protected from waterproof material to prevent their becoming damp. Although the pillows must be protected with a waterproof material, they should also be covered with cloth so that the waterproof material is not directly in contact with the cast. Some heat is given off as the cast hardens. If the cast is completely surrounded with a waterproof material, not only will it not dry but a burn may result. The patient should be in proper body alignment, and there should not be any break in the support provided by the pillows to cause weakening of the cast. If the cast is on the leg, the foot should extend over the edge of the pillow or the bed to avoid pressure on the heel.

In order for the cast to dry, there must be provision for evaporation by exposure to circulating air. A hair dryer or cast dryer can be used to provide warm (*not hot*) moving air; this is particularly helpful when wet, humid weather delays drying. Heat from radiant lamps is not advocated because it can cause severe burns beneath the cast. Cradles equipped with electric bulbs are not recommended unless there is also provision for free circulation of air; moisture-laden air becomes trapped under the cradle and delays the drying process. The cast should not be covered with bed linen until it is dry. Therefore the bed must be made in such a way that the cast is exposed but the patient kept warm and free from drafts. Blankets may be used to protect body parts not encased in plaster.

The patient in a body cast should be turned every 2 hours to ensure uniform drying of the cast, to prevent continuous pressure on any one area while the cast is drying, and to aid in comfort. Sufficient personnel should be used in turning to ensure support of the patient and the cast. Patients are usually more comfortable turned toward the uninjured side. Whether the patient in a cast may be turned toward the affected side depends on the type of injury sustained.

To protect body and long leg casts from becoming soiled or wet, waterproof material should be applied around the perineal area. Continuous dampening will soften the cast and impair its effectiveness, and a soiled cast lining will irritate the patient's skin and cause an offensive odor. The area can be covered with plastic material, oiled silk, or waxed paper. These materials can be anchored with adhesive or cellophane tape and changed as necessary.

If the cast becomes soiled, scouring powder on a damp cloth will usually remove surface stains. The area must be allowed to thoroughly dry again. Baking soda rubbed onto the surface of the cast will help to reduce odors emanating from soiled areas. However, there is no way to clean a badly soiled cast, therefore it is essential that preventive measures be used to keep it clean.

People often like to decorate their casts; however, casts should never be covered with paint, varnish, or shellac. Plaster-of-Paris is porous and allows circulation of air to the skin. When the plaster cast is covered with a substance that decreases its porosity, the skin underneath the cast may become macerated.

Care of the patient in the cast. After the patient has been carefully transferred into bed and the cast is supported on pillows, the patient's general condition is checked. After fracture reduction and immobilization, observations are made for signs of delayed shock such as sudden faintness, dizziness, pallor, diaphoresis, or change in pulse rate. Drainage through a cast is a poor indicator of actual blood loss. The wet plaster acts as a wick to spread the drainage, often making it appear that the patient is losing large amounts of blood when this is not true. For this reason the time-honored practice of circling areas of drainage on casts to estimate the amount of drainage is now generally considered a useless activity. Monitoring the patient's systemic signs and symptoms, urinary output, and hematocrit levels much more accurately indicate blood loss.

Medication is given as ordered for general pain. Bone pain is one of the most severe types of pain, and medications may have to be given as often as every 3 to 4 hours in order to keep the patient comfortable.

The affected extremity is elevated on pillows to aid in preventing edema. Most swelling occurs within the first 24 to 48 hours. Complaints of pressure are often relieved either by elevation or by a change in position. *Continuous pressure, pain, or swelling that is not relieved by change in position or elevation must be reported to the physician at once since this often represents neurologic or circulatory impairment in the affected area.* Neurocirculatory impairment is usually caused by a tight cast or by edema, although it occasionally may be caused by bruising of a blood vessel or by stretching or bruising of a nerve during manipulation or surgery.

Areas of pressure are usually over bony prominences or places where bones lie in close proximity to the skin (the instep, lateral border of the foot, heel, malleoli, iliac crests, and sacrum). The skin distal to the cast is inspected frequently and routinely for signs of vascular impairment. Changes in skin color or temperature (cyanosis or coldness), swelling, and slow return of color (delayed capillary refill) after pressure has been applied to the fingers or toes below the cast indicate that pressure may be restricting circulation.

Signs and symptoms of neurologic impairment include complaints of tightness of the cast, numbness or tingling of the fingers or toes, and loss of motion at the

TABLE 41-2. Observations for signs and symptoms of neurocirculatory impairment

Observation	Interpretation
Tissue color white	Decreased arterial blood supply
Tissue color blue	Venous stasis and poorly oxygenated tissue
Color slow to return to nail bed after application of moderate pressure	Decreased arterial blood supply
Edema	Fluid accumulating in tissues; poor venous return
Tissue cold or cool to touch	Decreased arterial blood supply
Patient unable to move parts distal to cast	Pressure on nerves innervating parts distal to cast
Patient complaint of heightened or decreased sensation or paresthesia in part underlying or distal to cast	Pressure on nerves innervating parts underlying or distal to cast
Patient complaint of extreme pain unrelieved by elevation, analgesic, or repositioning	Pressure on nerve endings in parts underlying or distal to cast

NOTE: Comparison of tissue should be made with contralateral tissue to determine extent of deviation from normal.

free joints distal to the cast. These sensorimotor disturbances are indications of nerve compression. The nerve in the lower extremity most often affected is the peroneal nerve, located below the head of the fibula on the lateral aspect of the leg. Continuous pressure on this superficial nerve by a leg cast or by the patient lying with the leg in extreme external rotation may result in paralysis with a loss of the ability to dorsiflex or invert the foot or to extend the toes (footdrop). Any complaint of pressure on the lateral side of the leg, numbness or tingling of the foot, or burning pain in the area covered by, or distal to, the cast may be an indication of nerve compression (Table 41-2).

When there is evidence of neurologic or circulatory impairment, the pressure must be relieved at once. Failure to do so can result in nerve paralysis or lack of circulation to the part with resultant necrosis. The ultimate consequence of unrelieved pressure can be the loss of the extremity. Pressure is relieved by splitting the cast *and* the padding underneath it. If the cast is bivalved (cut in two) (Fig. 41-22), it can be held in place by Ace bandages or adhesive tape. This will provide adequate temporary immobilization for the part while relieving the pressure of the cast. A cast cutter should

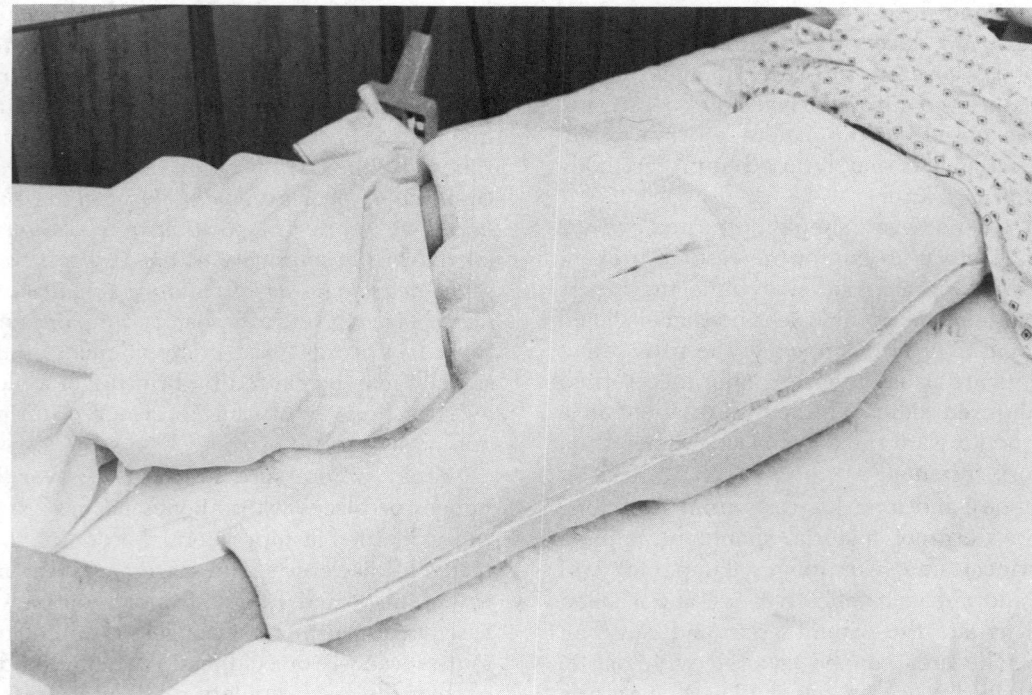

Fig. 41-22. Hip spica cast. Cast was applied to provide immobilization of left femoral fracture. Note that cast was bivalved when patient developed severe pain and swelling of left leg several hours after cast was applied. Ace bandages wrapped over cast to provide support have been removed for purposes of this picture.

be readily available, and the nurse should know how to bivalve a cast if it is necessary to do so. A new cast will be applied when the swelling is reduced.

Skin care for the patient with a cast must be thorough. Plaster on the skin should be removed with plain water. The skin around and directly under the cast edges should be washed and then massaged with alcohol to prevent skin irritation. Creams and lotions may be used with caution. They tend to soften the skin under the cast and also may cause the skin to stick against the cast lining. In addition, continuous use of excessive lotions dampens the inside of the cast. The skin should also be inspected for pressure areas and signs of irritation from rough plaster edges. Petal-shaped strips of adhesive tape or moleskin may be applied to the exterior surface of the cast, over the rough edges of the cast, and anchored smoothly to the interior surface of the cast to prevent irritation or abrasion. This process is called *petaling*. As patients remain in casts, their elbows may become irritated from bracing themselves to move about in bed. Frequent massage and protective pads will help to prevent this. An orthopedic bed frame with a trapeze will assist the patient to move about in bed.

If the patient is in a body cast or a long leg cast, the head of the bed should be elevated when a bedpan is used. This helps to keep urine or stool from running back and under the cast. If the cast is new and still damp, it is better to elevate the head of the bed on shock blocks (or use reverse Trendelenburg's position with electric beds) instead of using the gatch, since the gatch will put a strain on the cast and may cause it to crack. A pillow should be placed against the small of the back, and a cotton pad protected with plastic material may be tucked under the sacral area to protect the cast from soiling. The leg in the cast should be supported with pillows so that the patient does not feel insecure in this position. An overhanging trapeze (Fig. 41-23) permits patients to help lift themselves as the nurse places the bedpan under them. Side rails also assist patients to turn and give them protection from falling out of bed.

If abdominal distention is troublesome, a "window" or opening may be cut in the cast over the abdomen. The edges of this opening may also be petaled. Such a window is useful in checking for distention of the bladder.

For the person in a dry cast, turning from side to back to side to abdomen is seldom restricted by any consideration other than the person's discomfort. The injured part is immobilized and protected from twisting or pulling by the cast.

Many persons are discharged after the cast is dry if there is no evidence of circulatory or nerve impairment. They should be taught never to insert a sharp object (coat hanger, pencil) under the cast, since abra-

sions by such objects can easily become infected. Small objects (coins) lost in casts become sources of pressure. If a cast is applied to the arm, a sling should be worn to support the full weight of the cast, and the hand should be supported to prevent the development of wristdrop. The ends of the sling should be secured with two pins instead of being tied at the back of the neck. If the sling is to be worn for some time, sling ties may be lengthened with bandage or muslin so that they can be crossed in the back and brought around and tied in the front of the body. This helps to prevent forward and downward pull on the neck that may cause a postural defect and fatigue.

Depending on the injury, the person may or may not be permitted to bear weight on the cast. If weight bearing is permitted, a leg cast may be fitted with a rubber heel or walking iron that prevents wear on the plaster. Cast shoes having a thick, styrofoam-like, one-piece flat sole and heel, open cloth sides, and adjustable Velcro closures are also available (Fig. 41-20). (However, weight bearing on a cast is never permitted until the cast is completely dry.) If the cast is a cylinder cast that does not enclose the foot (e.g., the cast applied following a tibial osteotomy), the person's own shoes can be worn.

Cast removal. The cast is usually removed when roentgenograms show that union is sufficient to allow safe removal. This is often done in the physician's office or in the hospital cast room or emergency department. The cast is bivalved with manual or electric plaster cut-

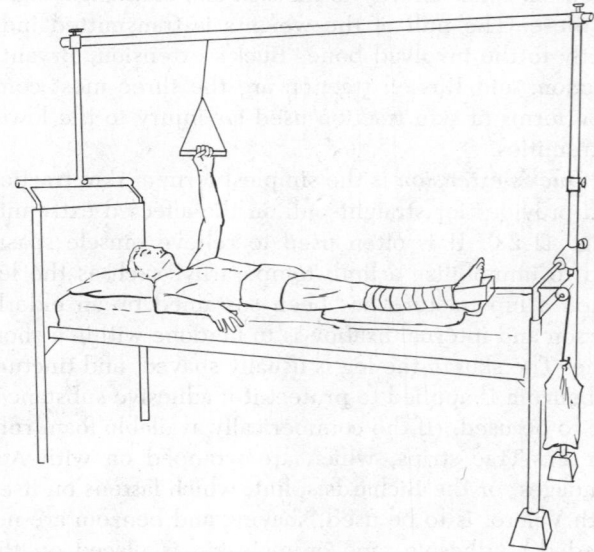

Fig. 41-23. Buck's extension. Note that limb lies parallel with bed but heel is supported off bed to prevent pressure on heel. Note also blocks to raise foot of bed to provide countertraction and to help keep patient from moving to foot of bed.

ters. While the procedure is not painful, some pressure or vibration may be felt. The skin is usually dry and scaly and is washed as soon as possible with mild soap and water and lubricated with mineral oil. Since there will usually be some stiffness of the joints, the limb should be moved very gently. The individual is usually encouraged to move the limb as much as he or she is able within limits of pain or stiffness. Exercises for the stiff joint are usually started. After a leg cast is removed, swelling and edema occur for some time when the leg is placed in the dependent position. The limb should be elevated during sleep and at intervals during the day. Elastic bandages or stockings may be prescribed to help reduce dependent edema.

Plaster jacket. A plaster jacket that extends from the shoulders to below the hips is sometimes used to immobilize the spine of the patient who has a fractured vertebra below the cervical area or another lumbodorsal disorder. Care of the patient in a plaster jacket is the same as care for the patient in a body cast except that in many instances the patient is permitted to ambulate. Once the cast is dry, transferring the patient in and out of bed should be done following the guidelines for transferring the patient who has had a laminectomy or spinal fusion (p. 1014).

TRACTION. Continuous traction, or pull, is used to reduce and immobilize fractures, to overcome muscle spasm, to stretch adhesions, and to correct certain deformities.

Skin traction. Skin traction is achieved by applying wide bands of moleskin, adhesive, or commerically available devices such as the Richards foam rubber Buck's extension splint directly to the skin and attaching weights to these. The pull of the weights is transmitted indirectly to the involved bone. Buck's extension, Bryant's traction, and Russell traction are the three most common forms of skin traction used for injury to the lower extremities.

Buck's extension is the simplest form of skin traction and provides for straight pull on the affected extremity (Fig. 41-23). It is often used to relieve muscle spasm and to immobilize a limb temporarily, such as the leg when a hip fracture has been sustained by an elderly person and internal fixation is to be done within a short time. The skin of the leg is usually shaved, and tincture of benzoin is applied to protect it if adhesive substances are to be used. (If the commerically available foam rubber Fas-Trac strips, which are wrapped on with Ace bandages, or the Richards splint, which fastens on itself with Velcro, is to be used, shaving and benzoin are not needed.) Adhesive tape or moleskin is placed on the lateral and medial aspects of the leg and secured with a circular gauze or elastic bandage. The tape should not cover the malleoli, since skin breakdown is certain to occur over these bony prominences. The tapes are attached to a spreader bar. The spreader bar should be

sufficiently wide to pull the tapes away from the malleoli. Rope is attached to the spreader, passed through a pulley on a crossbar at the foot of the bed, and suspended with weights. The maximal weight that should be applied by skin traction is 3.6 kg (8 lb). Greater amounts of weight can cause skin damage.

Not everyone will be able to be placed in Buck's extension. Contraindications include stasis dermatitis, arteriosclerosis, allergy to adhesive tape, severe varicosities or varicose ulcers, diabetic gangrene, and marked overriding of bone fragments that would require 4.5 kg (10 lb) or more of weight to reduce the deformity.

Russell traction is widely used because it permits the patient to move about in bed somewhat freely and permits bending of the knee joint (Fig. 41-24). This is skin traction in which four pulleys are used. A Balkan frame must be attached to the bed before the procedure is started. Moleskin or adhesive is then applied to the leg as in Buck's extension. The knee is suspended in a hammock or sling to which a rope is attached. This rope is directed upward to a pulley that has been placed on the Balkan frame at a point located over the tibial tubercle of the affected extremity. The rope is then passed downward through a pulley on a crossbar at the foot of the bed, back through a pulley on the footplate, back again to another pulley on the crossbar, and then suspended with weights. Because there is double pull from the crossbar to the footplate, the traction is equal to approximately double the weight used. Since there is upward pull from the hammock, skin under the popliteal space should be protected with a piece of felt or sponge rubber and should be inspected regularly. The patient's heel should just clear the bed so there is no weight or pressure on the heel. Usually a pillow is placed lengthwise under the thigh, and a second pillow is placed under the leg. This traction results in slight flexion of the hip. The angle between the thigh and the bed should be approximately 20 degrees. Usually the foot of the bed is elevated on blocks (or in Trendelenburg's position for electric beds) to provide countertraction.

Any complaints of pain or discomfort should be reported to the physician at once. Occasionally, thrombophlebitis develops from inactivity or from pressure on the popliteal vessels. Often the patient is permitted to have the head of the bed elevated slightly, but since elevation of the head of the bed does reduce the amount of the traction, the physician should be consulted about the amount of elevation permitted. Russell traction is used in the treatment of intertrochanteric fracture of the femur when surgery is contraindicated, especially in the aged. Bilateral Russell or Buck's traction may be used to treat back pain, since it immobilizes the patient and reduces muscle spasm.

Skeletal traction. Skeletal traction is traction applied directly to bone. Under general or local anesthesia a Kirschner wire or Steinmann pin is inserted distal to

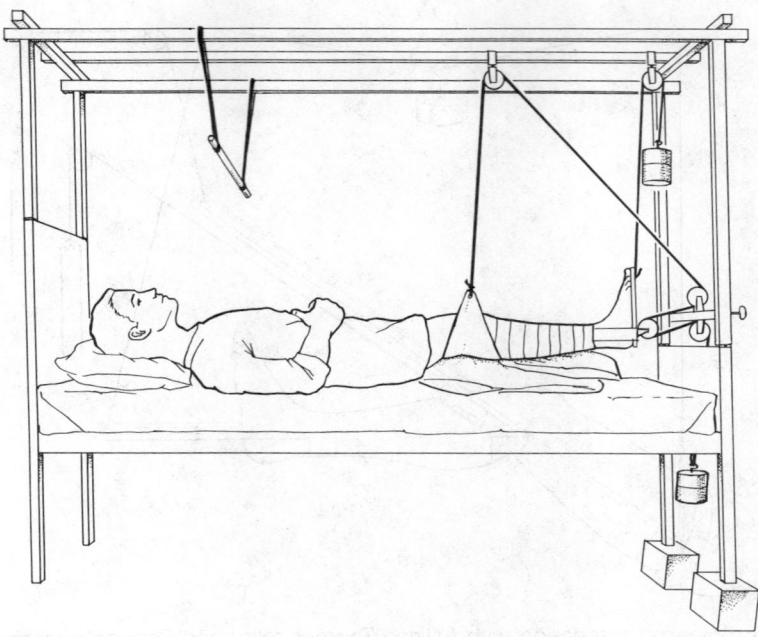

Fig. 41-24. Russell traction. Note that Balkan frame is attached to bed, that leg is supported on pillows, and that heel extends beyond pillow.

the fracture (the site of insertion varies with the type of fracture) (Fig. 41-25). For a fractured femur, the pin is often inserted through the tibia. The pin protrudes through the skin on both sides, and the ends are covered with corks or metal protectors. Small sterile dressings are usually placed over the entry and exit sites of the pin. The utmost care must be taken to guard against infection at the pin site, since infection on the surface can proceed to the bone along the pin track resulting in osteomyelitis (p. 1020). A metal U-shaped spreader or bow is attached to the pin. The rope for the traction is attached to the spreader. Skeletal traction can be used for fractures of the tibia, femur, humerus, and neck or cervical spine. Skeletal traction to the cervical spine is achieved by use of tongs applied to the skull (p. 1015).

Balanced traction. When a balanced or suspension apparatus (Fig. 41-26) is used in conjunction with skin or skeletal traction, the patient is able to move about in bed more freely without disturbing the line of traction. The extremity is balanced with countertraction, and any slack in the traction caused by the patient's movement is taken up by the suspension apparatus. The use of a balancing apparatus also facilitates nursing measures such as bathing the patient, caring for the skin, and placing the bedpan correctly.

A full or half-ring *Thomas* or *Hodgen splint* is used for balanced tractions (Fig. 41-26). (Before application, these splints should be checked to see that they are the proper size for the patients who will be using them.) Straps of canvas, muslin, or synthetic "lamb's wool" are

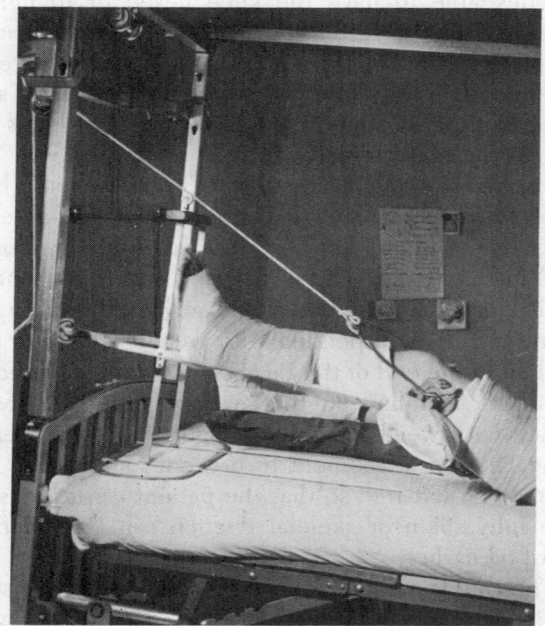

Fig. 41-25. Skeletal traction. Pin has been inserted through distal femur. Sharp ends of pin are covered with cork, and small dressing occludes pin sites. Pin and traction rope are attached to spreader. In this case, entire limb is supported by Braun-Böhler inclined plane splint. (From Larson, C.B., and Gould, M.: Orthopedic nursing, ed. 9, St. Louis, 1978, The C.V. Mosby Co.)

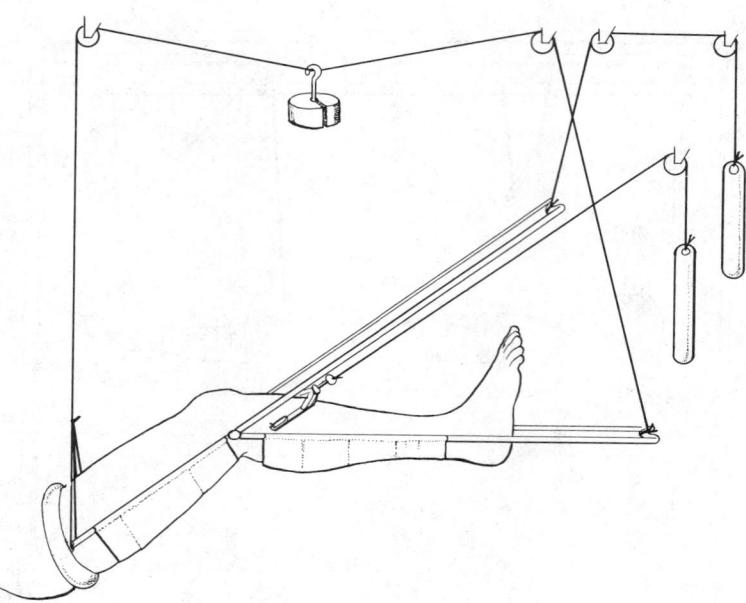

Fig. 41-26. Balanced suspension with full-ring Thomas splint and Pearson attachment used in conjunction with skeletal traction.

placed over the splint and secured to provide a support for the leg. The areas under the popliteal space and heel are left open to prevent pressure on these parts. If it is desirable to have the knee flexed or to permit movement of the lower leg, a *Pearson attachment* is clamped or fixed to the Thomas splint at the level of the knee. The attachment is also covered with a soft, strong material to support the lower leg. The leg is put through the ring and placed on the canvas support. The ring is placed firmly against the ischium. When a half-ring splint is used, the ring is placed on the anterior aspect of the thigh. Rope is attached to the ring or to the frame on either side of the ring and to the end of the Thomas splint, directed upward to pulleys on the frame, and then suspended with weights. Rope is also attached to the end of the Pearson attachment, directed upward to a pulley on the overbed frame, and suspended with weights. A foot support may be fastened to the Pearson attachment to prevent footdrop, or the foot may be left free so that the patient can exercise it more fully. Skin or skeletal traction can be added as described earlier.

The ring is made of smooth, soft, moisture-resistant plastic material or of leather. It is not necessary to wrap the ring with padding. The padding cannot be changed after it is applied, and inevitably it gets damp from perspiration, bedpan accidents, and bathing the skin. The padding holds moisture against the skin and causes skin irritation. When the patient is bathed, the skin beneath the ring must be moved back and forth so that all areas are washed, dried thoroughly, and powdered. The pa-

tient may be turned toward the leg in the splint.

Nursing intervention for the patient in traction. Before care is given to a patient in traction, the patient's problem and what is to be achieved by the use of traction must be clearly understood. For example, the patient with arthritis who is in skin traction to help release flexion contractures of the knees may be permitted to be out of traction for periods of time, whereas the patient with a recent fracture of the femur would be harmed if the traction were released.

In order for traction to be effective, patients should lie on their backs. Turning fully onto the side or sitting straight up changes body alignment, and the pull (traction) is lost or becomes less effective. However, patients in traction to the leg can usually be turned *slightly* from side to side to relieve skin pressure. The motion allowed depends on the injury and kind of traction used. Those caring for the patient must consult with the physician to determine what the limitations of motion are so that appropriate care can be planned. The patient will be extremely limited in activity. Limitations should be explained and the patient should be helped to be as comfortable as possible while remaining in the correct position. Patients who must lie flat often feel handicapped and helpless because they cannot readily see what is going on about them. Ceiling mirrors and prism glasses may be used to help them feel less isolated. Television sets are sometimes placed on high wall shelves or suspended from the ceiling so that they can be seen by those who must lie flat in bed.

Traction weight must hang free with no obstruction

to interfere with *straight, even, continuous pull*. Traction should be inspected frequently. For example, when traction is being applied to the lower limb, bedclothes must not press on the rope or against the footplate. The footplate must never push against the foot of the bed or the pulley, since this will completely negate traction. There should be no knots in the rope, since these may become caught in the pulley and interfere with traction. The rope should be long enough so that weight will not be hampered by the pulley as the patient moves up in bed, yet not long enough to rest on the floor if the patient slips down to the foot of the bed. The rope must be strong enough so that it will not break if more weights are added. The weights must be securely fastened so that they will not drop off if they are disturbed accidentally, and the equipment should be visible so that it is not jarred, is not swung inadvertently, or does not present a hazard to persons moving past the bed. If sandbags are used for weights, they are tied to the rope. When regular scale weights are used, they should be fastened with adhesive tape so that they will not slip off. Jarring the bed and swinging the weights may cause pain and upset the patient. Any extremity in traction must be checked frequently for adequate circulation. Patients in Buck's extension or Russell traction should be checked for inability to dorsiflex and invert the foot on the affected side. The inability to perform these motions would indicate peroneal nerve damage (p. 966).

An important concept in the care of patients in traction is that they should not suffer from lack of any kind of nursing care because of their immobilization. At first glance it might sometimes appear that good back care, for example, is impossible. This is not true. Patients in traction should be on a firm bed and should have an orthopedic frame or overhead attachment with trapeze bar so that they can help to lift themselves and take some weight off their backs for short periods. Usually they can be moved enough for good back care to be given and for linen to be changed. This is accomplished by having patients raise themselves straight up in bed with the help of the trapeze while care is given and the bed linen slid under them. Depending on the site and the extent of the fracture, the patient may be permitted to turn toward the side of the fracture enough for back care to be given. It is a good practice for a second nurse or an attendant to steady the traction and even increase the pull slightly as patients carefully and steadily turn or raise themselves. The same principles are followed when the bedpan is placed under the patient. A very small, flat bedpan (fracture pan) should be used, and the back above the pan should be supported by a small pillow or a bath blanket folded to the height of the pan.

The patient who is in traction needs the same attention to nutrition, elimination, exercise of noninvolved extremities, prevention of postural defects, and skin care as any other patient who is immobilized. Particular at-

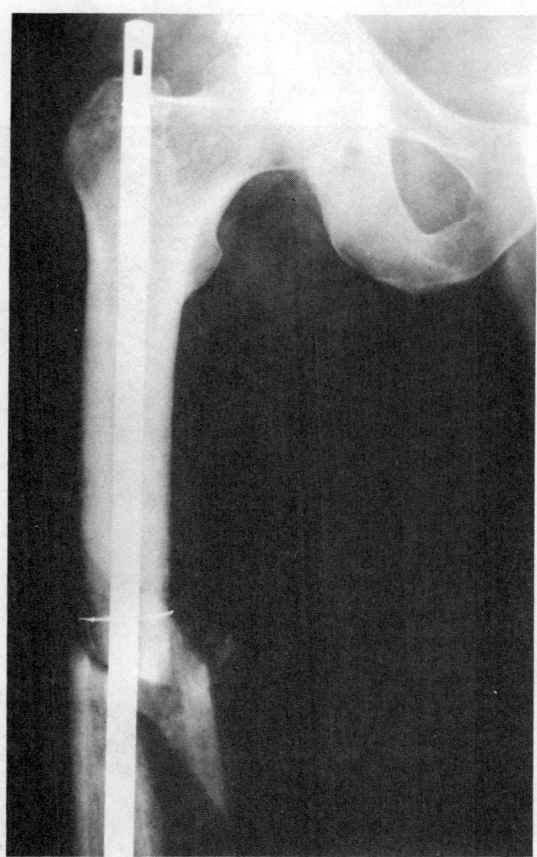

Fig. 41-27. Internal fixation of fracture of middle third of femur by means of intramedullary nail (Kirschner nail).

tention must be given to skin surfaces that come into contact with any traction apparatus. For example, the skin over the bony hip prominences may become reddened and painful if a pelvic band is being used, adhesive tape may work downward so that straps may rub against the ankle when skin traction is used on the lower limb, and a *Thomas splint* may cause injury to the skin of the groin. Skin irritation of this kind must be reported to the physician, who may alter the amount of weight used or take other action. Meanwhile, nursing measures to relieve skin irritation are initiated.

INTERNAL FIXATION. Depending on the location and type of fracture, *open reduction with internal fixation* may be necessary. Open reduction with internal fixation is used only when other methods of reduction are not suitable. Although this method allows direct visualization of the injury, it also carries the risk of infection; consequently, it is performed under the most vigorous aseptic conditions.

Internal fixation is achieved by using a metal device (Fig. 41-27). There are a wide variety of metal pins, wires, intramedullary rods, compression plates, nails, and so on available. Each has its particular advantage

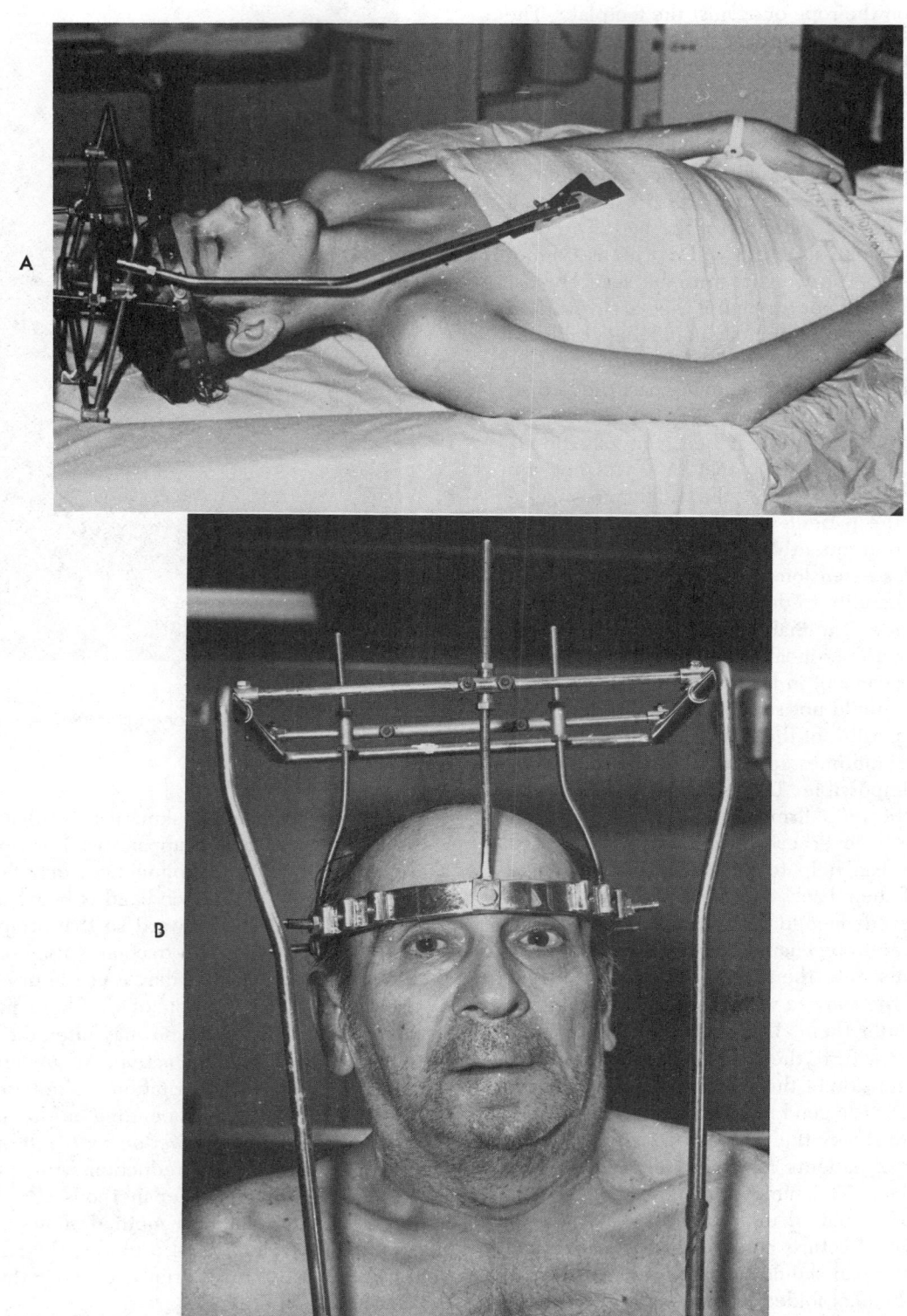

Fig. 41-28. A, Halo attached to body cast. **B,** Metal ring, or halo, that attaches to skull. (Courtesy Dr. Henry Bohlman, Cleveland.)

and indications for use. The care of the patient who has internal fixation of a fracture depends on the site of the fracture and the device used for stabilization. The major aim of care is to protect the part until healing takes place. Metal that can fatigue and break cannot be expected to substitute for intact bone. If the fixation device breaks, healing of the fracture will be disrupted. Depending on the fracture, protection may be achieved by using a cast, by limiting stressful forces on the metal by restricting positioning, or by placing the patient on limited weight bearing until healing occurs. For examples of care of patients following open reduction with internal fixation, see pp. 1021 and 1024.

CAST BRACES. The cast brace is used in the treatment of patients with femoral shaft fractures. It has three components: (1) a plaster-of-Paris cast (or thigh cuff) that encloses the patient's thigh; (2) two metal or high-density polyethylene hinges, one on either side of the knee; and (3) a short leg plaster-of-Paris walking cast that extends from just below the knee to and enclosing the foot. The proximal ends of the hinges are embedded in the plaster of the thigh cuff; the distal ends are embedded in the short leg cast. The thigh cuff compresses the thigh muscles, thus providing immobilization of the fracture fragments. The hinges allow flexion and extension of the free knee joint. The walking cast provides support for the thigh cuff and prevents the thigh cuff from slipping distally.

The advantages of using this apparatus are that the period of time required for fracture healing is shortened and the hip and knee joints can be mobilized. The cast brace is applied after the fracture has been aligned in skeletal traction for 2 to 6 weeks. The patient progresses to fairly normal ambulation with crutches and may even be permitted to return home within a week of the cast brace application.[18]

The care of the patient in a cast brace and the care of the cast are essentially the same as have been outlined on pp. 964 to 968. Particular attention must be paid to checking for neurocirculatory compromise in the affected leg *throughout the hospitalization*. Some swelling of the knee and foot may be experienced when the leg is in a dependent position during ambulation. This swelling can usually be relieved by prompt elevation of the extremity, but if it is not, the pressure of the cast must be relieved. If knee swelling is present, the knee should be carefully checked to determine if the skin is rubbing against the hinges. Friction from the hinges will quickly abrade the skin.

HALO CAST. The halo cast is another apparatus that employs both a plaster-of-Paris cast and a metal frame. It is used to immobilize the spine following cervical spinal fusion. It provides for greater stability than a neck brace and has an advantage over cervical tongs in allowing the patient to be ambulatory. A plaster cast, extending from the axillae to the iliac crests, houses a metal frame (Fig.

41-28, *A*). The struts of the frame extend to the skull at the parietal areas. These struts attach to a round metal (halolike) device. The halo itself is fixed to the skull by screws inserted in the same fashion as tongs (p. 1015). There are four screws: two located anterolaterally and two located posterolaterally (Fig. 41-28, *B*). The halo cast permits no flexion, extension, or rotational movements of the neck, thus completely immobilizing the site of the fusion to prevent displacement of the grafts.

It is helpful if patients who are to wear this apparatus have the opportunity to see it and have its function explained before it is applied. The cast and the frame are cumbersome, and the idea of having something screwed into the skull frightens most people. It is not reasonable to assure the patient that the frame will not cause discomfort, since some persons do complain of headaches. Patients in a halo cast can be taught to transfer and ambulate, but they will need help to do this in the initial postoperative period, since the weight of the cast and frame will make them feel "top-heavy."

The care of the patient in a halo cast is essentially the same as for the patient in a plaster jacket (p. 968). Additionally, the screws to the skull and the screws that hold the upper portion of the frame together must be checked several times per day *throughout the time that the patient is in the frame* to be certain that they are tight. If any part of the frame is allowed to come apart, the position of the patient's head can change and the fusion can be displaced.

STRYKER FRAME AND FOSTER BED. For patients with an injury that allows them to be placed flat in bed but who are not allowed to turn, a Stryker frame or a Foster bed may be used (Figs. 41-29 to 41-31). These devices are used for patients with some types of spinal injury. They make it possible to change a person's position from abdomen to back without altering body alignment. Usually the patient on one of these beds is turned every 2 to 4 hours. Traction, particularly cervical traction, can be used on a frame; however, the frame cannot be used for very obese patients because space between the top and bottom frames is inadequate and cannot be adjusted sufficiently.

The beds have two metal frames to which canvas covers are attached. The canvas used for the back-lying position has an opening under the buttocks to allow for use of a bedpan, and the canvas used for the prone-lying position can be cut out so that the male patient can void. When the patient is in the prone position, the canvas should extend from below the shoulders to the ankles, and a narrow head strap should be used to support the forehead. In the prone position the patient can eat, read, and do light hand activities. The canvas may be covered with thin sponge rubber mattresses cut the same size as the canvas and covered with bed linen. To turn the patient, the linen, mattress, and opposite canvas and frame are placed in that order over the patient.

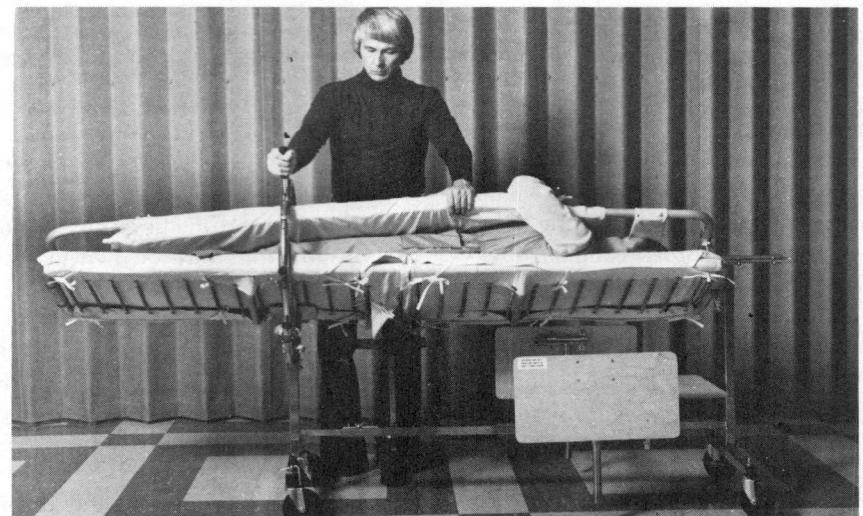

Fig. 41-29. Patient is in supine position on Foster bed. Anterior frame is fastened in place and, on other style frames, can be additionally secured by turning straps prior to turning patient. (From Rantz, M., and Courtial, D.: Lifting, moving and transferring patients, ed. 2, St. Louis, 1981, The C.V. Mosby Co.)

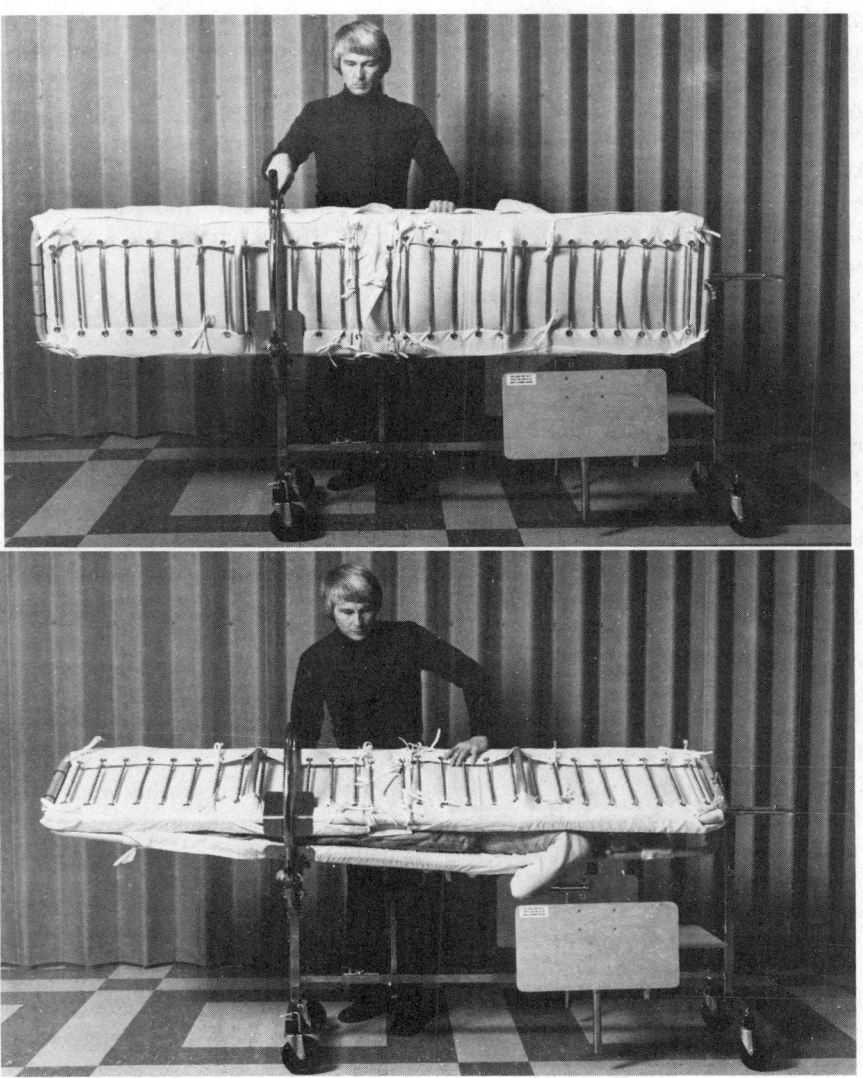

Fig. 41-30. Turning process is started. Narrow canvas strip is placed across forehead to support head when in prone position. (From Rantz, M., and Courtial, D.: Lifting, moving and transferring patients, ed. 2, St. Louis, 1981, The C.V. Mosby Co.)

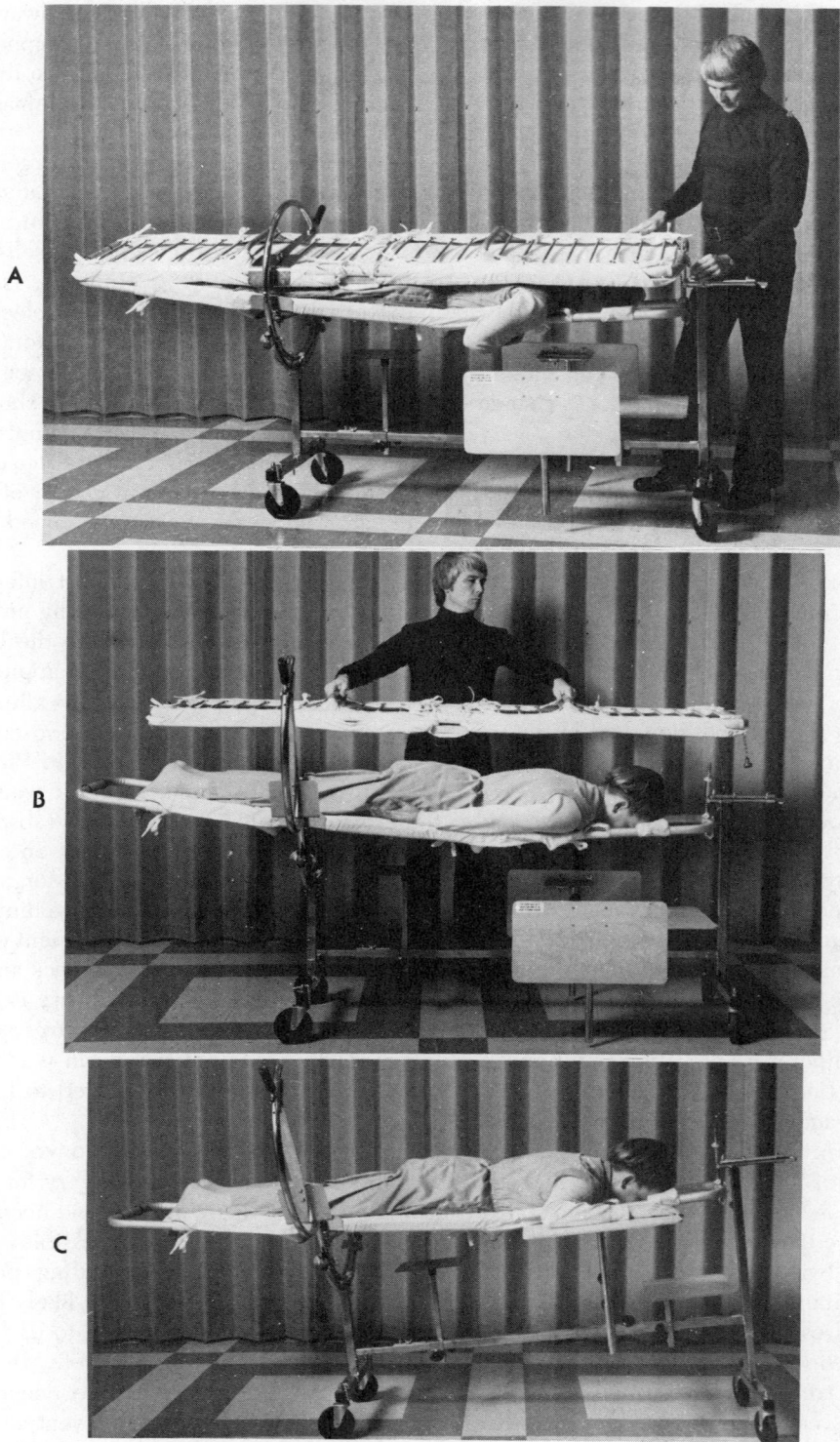

Fig. 41-31. A, Turning is complete. **B,** Posterior frame has been removed. **C,** Adjustable arm boards have been replaced for support. Lower shelf may be used to hold reading material or diet tray. (From Rantz, M., and Coutial, D.: Lifting, moving and transferring patients, ed. 2, St. Louis, 1981, The C.V. Mosby Co.)

The frame is then fastened by bolting it securely in place to the metal attachment at the head and foot. Safety straps are placed around both frames; then two people release pivot pins at either end of the frame and turn the patient on the frame. The pins are reinserted, and the upper frame, canvas, and mattress are removed. The bed has arm-board and footboard attachments to use, if desired, for permissible activity or for good alignment. Patients may be quite apprehensive about being placed on this bed, and if possible, a demonstration of turning should be given before they are moved onto it. Another advantage of these beds is that they wheel easily so that the patient may be taken to the operating room, radiology department, or to a recreational area for a change of surrounding. This type of bed is unsafe for a very restless or disoriented patient, although the safety straps may be used to give some security and protection.

Another type of turning frame, the CircOlectric bed (Fig. 41-3), also allows patients to be turned without changing their alignment. However, since this bed rotates the patients by turning them through the standing position rather than through the side-lying position, it is often not used for patients who are not permitted weight bearing. This includes patients with unresolved spinal injuries, since the standing position does load (puts weight through) the spine.[5]

Assessment and care of surgical wounds. The assessment of surgical wounds in patients who have had orthopedic surgery is often complicated by the fact that the wound is covered by a cast or other occlusive dressing, sometimes for a period of several weeks. In instances where the wound cannot be visualized, those caring for the patient may have to rely on their sense of smell to alert them to potential problems. Foul odors emanating from under occlusive material, particularly in the presence of a temperature elevation or other systemic evidence of infection, should be called to the attention of the physician and investigated. Casts and other dressings can be cut (windowed) at the site of the incision and the condition of the wound assessed. If a cast is windowed, it is necessary to replace the portion of the plaster removed—either by taping or replastering it—to prevent swelling (window edema) in the area that would no longer be contained by the cast. If necessary, irrigations, soaks, or dressing changes can be carried out by removing the window at regular intervals and replacing it when the treatment is finished. If irrigations or soaks are done, care must be taken to line the surrounding portions of the cast with moisture-resistant material to prevent the cast from becoming wet.

Initial dressings are changed as necessary to prevent drainage from coming in contact with potential sources of contamination. After the initial dressing is changed, subsequent dressings are changed as necessary using aseptic technique to keep the wound clean and dry. It has already been noted that the plaster-of-Paris cast acts as a wick to promote drainage away from the wound. Compressive-type dressings, composed of many layers of cotton wadding and wrapped on the outside with Ace bandages, will also promote drainage away from the wound.

Depending on the type of surgery and the location of the surgery, some form of wound drainage may be employed. This may be in the nature of a Penrose drain (as in surgery to the hand), a self-contained vacuum suction device such as Hemovac (see Fig. 24-12), or polyethylene tubing attached to electric suction. These types of drainage prevent hematoma formation at the operative site, and the latter two collect drainage so it can be measured accurately. It should also be noted that, because of its density, a compressive dressing can contain very large amounts of drainage before drainage becomes visible. Frequent checks of vital signs will aid in early detection of excessive blood loss by the patient who has this type dressing.

It has also been noted that infection may proceed from the surface of the skin along pin tracks (in patients who are in skeletal traction) to the bone (p. 969). Collodion dressings are sometimes applied to the entry and exit sites of pins immediately after the pins are inserted. If the wounds are not so occluded, and *if the surgeon requests care to the pin site,* drainage may be gently removed from around the wounds with hydrogen peroxide applied with cotton swabs. Dry sterile dressings may be applied to the wounds, and the wounds should be checked frequently for any signs or symptoms of infection (erythema, swelling, warmth, tenderness, unusual drainage). Movement of the pins may also carry infection along the pin track and irritate the bone the pin traverses. Therefore care is taken to avoid manipulating or putting undue stress on the pins themselves. If it is noted that a pin is moving in and out of its track, it should be reported to the surgeon as soon as possible.

Prevention of postoperative complications. Patients having orthopedic surgery for the treatment of a fracture have many of the same needs as any other surgical patient. Whenever possible, they should have preoperative teaching regarding postanesthesia care. Since these patients are very likely to be relatively immobile, they especially need to understand the importance of good pulmonary toilet. Movement of all uninvolved extremities should be encouraged in order to maintain muscle tone and prevent circulatory stasis. Full plantar flexion and dorsiflexion of the feet, isometric quadriceps-setting and gluteal-setting can be encouraged to these ends (see Fig. 24-3). Quadriceps-setting is contraindicated until specifically ordered by the surgeon for patients who have patellar or patellar tendon surgery, or when surgical drains are in the parapatellar area. These exercises are generally done five times every hour initially, and the number can be increased up to

20 times every hour as the patient can tolerate them.

Limitation on positioning, movement, and ambulation will be determined by the body part involved, the nature of the surgical procedure, the type of fixation device, or the type of immobilization device (traction, cast, and so on). This means that those caring for the patient must be familiar with the patient's problem and the method of treatment used in order to avoid giving improper care that can lead to the displacement of fracture fragments.

Because of the complex arrangement of muscle attachments and because of muscle action, the surgeon should be consulted before attempts are made to assist or encourage the patient to exercise the involved limb. A safe rule is never under any circumstances have the patient move or use the joint either immediately distal or immediately proximal to the fracture before consulting the physician. For example, if the fracture is in the radius, the wrist and elbow joints should not be moved without an order; however, the shoulder can and should be protected from muscle weakness, muscle shortening, and joint changes by regular motion and exercise. The legs, trunk, and unaffected upper limb should be checked regularly (at least daily) to be certain that the patient is doing some systematic, routine exercises. The patient is mobilized as soon as possible.

Prevention of infection is discussed under wound care. The complications of fat embolus and osteomyelitis and their treatment are discussed in Chapter 42. Other interventions relating to the prevention of complications of immobility are discussed on p. 941.

Pain relief. The person who has sustained a fracture will most often have severe pain at and around the site of the fracture. Extensive soft-tissue injury may be present adjacent to the fracture, edema is present, and there may be considerable spasm of muscles in the fracture area. In the initial stages of treatment, narcotic analgesics are effective in relieving pain and should be used as needed to help the patient obtain satisfactory relief. Continued pain and the muscle spasm accompanying it can put undue stress on the fracture fragments and retard efforts both to reduce and to maintain reduction of the fracture. Further, patients who are in severe pain will resist efforts to assist them to cough and deep breathe and other measures designed to prevent complications. If the fracture is repaired by open reduction and internal fixation, the patient will have operative pain. If muscle spasm is a continuing problem, an agent such as diazepam (Valium) can be employed to reduce the spasm. It will not, however, relieve operative pain.

As healing progresses, the strength and frequency of analgesics can be decreased. It is important, however, to try to strike a balance in the use of analgesics; that is, patients should be helped to be comfortable enough to perform required exercises and other activities, but not so heavily medicated that they are unaware of potential damage that they might do to themselves by overextending their activity. Many times, simple changes in position, within the restrictions of the prescribed treatment, are enough to relieve discomfort without having to use analgesics.

Patient education. Before leaving the hospital, patients who have been treated for a fracture must be aware of any activity restrictions or limitations that they must observe, how long they must observe them, how they are to use their ambulatory or other assistive devices (if needed), what kind of assistance they may need to perform their ADL, and who will be available to help them. If necessary, referral can be made to a community nurse or other community agency for assistance.

The easiest and most effective way to teach patients how to handle these problems is to have them function to the point of their limitations with whatever assistive aids they need while they are still in the hospital. Their functioning and abilities should be assesed and they should be helped to correct problems such as incorrect gait when using crutches while they are still in a supervised situation. Whenever possible, it is best to have patients perform all their ADL as independently as possible so that problem areas can be identified and solutions worked out so they will not be confronted with the problem when professional guidance is no longer available.

Individuals who will be returning home in a plaster cast need information related to care of the cast and the affected body part. They should be instructed to avoid damaging the integrity of the cast by wetting it or placing undue stresses on it. They should know that objects inserted between the cast and the underlying skin can cause pressure areas or skin abrasion. Unusual pain, pressure, or increased swelling in the affected part should be reported to the physician since they may be signs of developing infection or skin breakdown. Finally, the body part in the cast should be elevated when possible to ease discomfort, facilitate venous return, and prevent swelling.

Reconstructive surgery

In addition to treatment for traumatic injuries, orthopedic interventions are also carried out for patients who require correction of a deformity, relief of pain, or restoration of musculoskeletal function. These are termed *reconstructive* (or palliative) surgeries. Surgeries of this nature include osteotomies (p. 1010), arthrodeses (p. 1012), arthroplasties (p. 1005), arthrotomies (p. 1005), synovectomies (p. 1010), tendon transplants (p. 1010), and the various spinal surgeries (p. 1012). Those procedures that involve structures inside the joint capsule are termed *intraarticular* procedures; those outside the joint capsule are *extraarticular* procedures.

Patient education. One of the major advantages in

caring for the patient who is to have reconstructive surgery as opposed to the patient who has sustained a fracture is that there is more time to teach the patient preoperatively. Preoperative teaching should include information on positioning, activity limitation, exercises the patient will be required to perform, the necessity of and techniques of pulmonary toileting, and in some cases, transfer and ambulation techniques. Patients are often frightened by the propsect of surgery; and their fears are increased if they are confronted with procedures or techniques that they do not understand, or for which no rationale has been presented, or that they do not know how to perform. A few patients may be comfortable knowing as little as possible about what is going to happen to them, but most want to know as much as they can be told.

Patients who accept and understand what will be required of them in the postoperative period are more likely to follow through with exercises, activity limitation, and other requirements than patients who are poorly prepared. The least that can be said for preoperative teaching is that it involves patients in their care. If they accept and learn the information that is given, their postoperative course may be facilitated. If they do not accept information, that fact in itself provides cues for postoperative management.

Positioning. For the patient who has had an extraarticular procedure, positioning will depend on the type of immobilization device that is used. If the patient has had an intraarticular procedure, positioning will be limited both by the immobilizing device (most often a bulky compression dressing) and the tolerances of any prosthetic implant. An example of a prosthetic implant is the total hip prosthesis discussed on p. 1005. Elevation of the extremity to aid in preventing edema should be maintained for the first 24 to 48 hours following either an extraarticular or an intraarticular procedure (Figs. 41-32 and 41-33). In the lower extremities, some form of skin traction may be used in the initial postoperative period to help maintain position and to reduce muscle spasm, but it is generally removed after 2 to 5 days. The physician should be consulted to determine if there is any position that the patient should avoid, as is necessary with a total hip arthroplasty. (See also Chapter 35 for a discussion of positioning restrictions for patients having spinal surgery.) Otherwise, patients should be turned every 2 hours while in bed and should begin sitting in a chair or ambulating as soon as possible. When they are sitting (and, in the case of upper extremity surgery, standing) elevation of the operated extremity should be maintained. If the joint operated on is the knee, pillows should not be put under the knee in such a way that the knee will be allowed to flex. Full knee extension should be maintained to prevent the formation of knee flexion contracture or laxity of the knee after the immobilizing device is removed. Further, pa-

tients who have had knee surgery should not be allowed to position their legs in extreme external rotation (p. 966), thus putting pressure on the peroneal nerve.

Skin care. Care of the skin for the patient who has had reconstructive surgery is the same as for any patient who is immobilized or who is confined by a cast or traction (p. 967).

Prevention of postoperative complications. The measures pertaining to prevention of postoperative complications discussed on p. 976 are equally applicable for the patient who has had reconstructive surgery. The bulky compression dressing, usually applied following an intraarticular procedure to prevent edema and joint effusion, can contain a large amount of drainage before that drainage becomes visible; therefore systemic signs and symptoms of excessive blood loss must be frequently and carefully monitored for the first 48 hours after surgery. The compression dressing can also be as constricting as a cast if swelling does occur. Neurocirculatory checks must be carefully performed every 1 to 2 hours until the danger of excessive swelling is over. Evidence of neurocirculatory compromise should be reported to the physician immediately so that the dressing can be split and the pressure relieved.

Immobilization. Immobilization of the operated extremity is carried out by casts, bulky compression dressings, traction, braces, or bed rest. The major difference between the management of patients who are immobilized for a fracture and those immobilized following a reconstructive procedure is that the period of immobilization and non-weight-bearing is usually shorter. Immobilization following most intraarticular procedures is necessarily shorter (2 to 7 days, depending on the joint operated and the procedure performed), since prolonged immoblilzation will lead to the development of adhesions that will prevent joint motion. If adhesions develop, they often have to be broken (the joint flexed) with the patient under anesthesia.

Care of wounds. Wound care considerations are the same as discussed on p. 976. Additionally, patients who have had reconstructive surgery are often elderly, have chronic underlying diseases such as rheumatoid arthritis, or may be taking medications that will retard wound healing. If wound healing is slow, continued attention to strict asepsis in dressing techniques is required. It is also not unusual for blisters to develop adjacent to the surgical incision or, particularly with hand surgery, on the operated extremity as a result of excessive edema. Such blisters should be kept intact and allowed to resolve on their own. If they do break, however, they can be covered with a piece of sterile petrolatum gauze to size and allowed to remain on the area until healing takes place.

Mobilization. Patients who have had reconstructive procedures are mobilized as soon as possible. For example, patients who have had a knee procedure may

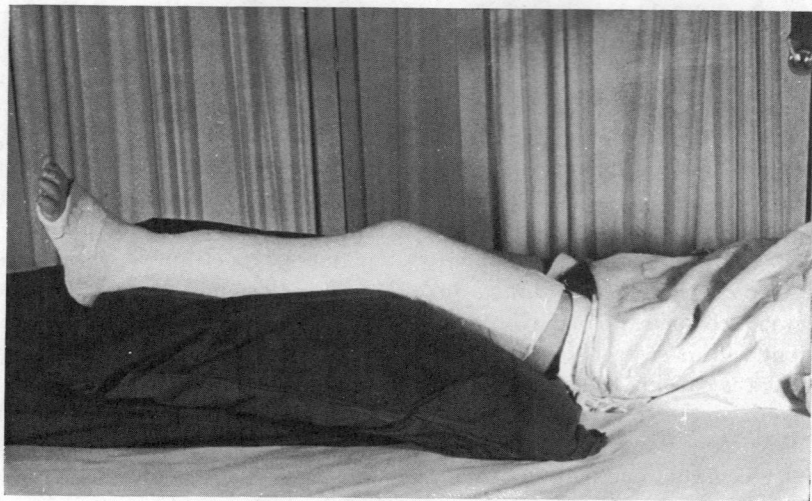

Fig. 41-32. One method of providing elevation to an extremity is to support it on pillows. Note that two pillows are wedged to provide support for entire extremity while still providing elevation for distal portion of extremity. (From Larson, C.B., and Gould, M.: Orthopedic nursing, ed. 9, St. Louis, 1978, The C.V. Mosby Co.)

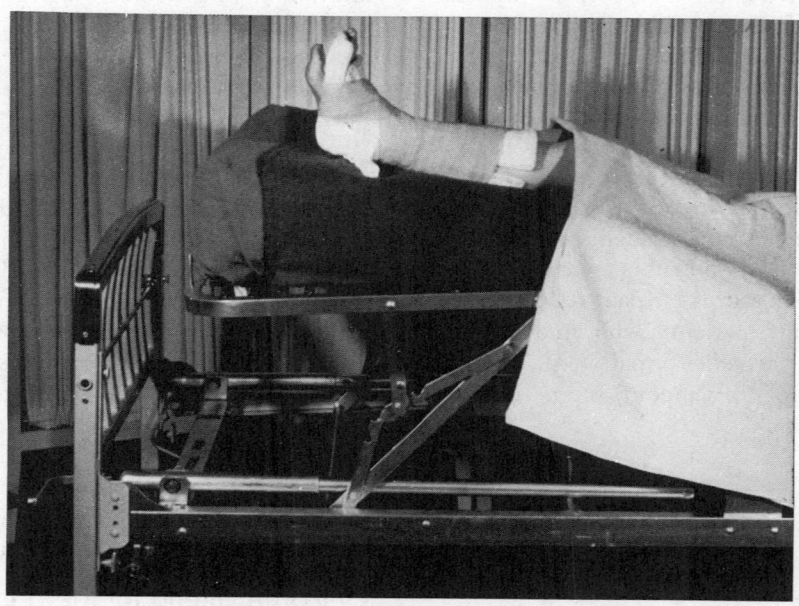

Fig. 41-33. Another method of elevating patient's foot is to gatch knee, then raise lower portion of springs. (From Larson, C.B., and Gould, M.: Orthopedic nursing, ed. 9, St. Louis, 1978, The C.V. Mosby Co.)

usually be up in a wheelchair with the leg elevated the first postoperative day. Patients who have had a wrist or hand procedure may be out of bed with the hand elevated on the operative evening, depending on their recovery from anesthesia and the type of anesthesia used. The weight-bearing status of the patient will be determined by the procedure that is performed. Some weight-bearing restrictions that will require the patient to use

ambulatory aids are generally enforced for those patients having lower extremity surgery.

In most instances, patients who have had intraarticular procedures will begin gentle *active* range of motion exercises to the involved joints as soon as the danger of joint effusion is past and the restrictive dressing is removed. These exercises will cause pain. However, if the joint is not moved, adhesions will develop. Whenever possible, pain medication should be given before the exercise period to help the patient relax to achieve the greatest range of motion possible. Local heat applied to the joint before exercising will also aid the involved muscles to relax. Application of ice following the exercise period can help retard swelling that results from exercising.

It must be stressed that these range of motion exercises must be done *actively* by the patient. *Under no circumstances should passive exercises be performed by another person*. If attempts are made to passively exercise the joint, the patient will most probably respond by resisting the exercise that is causing the pain and no movement will be achieved. If the joint is moved for the patient, and if that movement does cause pain, the patient may resist further attempts to actively move it. Most importantly, if the patient has osteoporosis, passive movement beyond the point of pain may result in pathologic fracture. Splints (or Buck's traction following knee surgery) may be used to rest the joint during periods between exercising. Balanced suspension traction or a system of slings and pulleys can be set up for the patient to perform active-assisted exercises. Special "dynamic" splints (Fig. 41-34) are fabricated by the occupational therapist to help patients exercise their fingers following arthroplasties of the metacarpophalangeal joints of the hand. With these splints, individual slings for each finger are suspended by rubber bands from a heavy wire hoop that extends over the dorsal surface of the hand. The slings hold the fingers in extension, and patients are required to flex their fingers against the gentle resistance provided by the rubber bands.

Pain relief. General measures for pain relief are discussed on p. 977. Many patients who undergo orthopedic procedures for the relief of pain (e.g., the patient who has a total hip replacement) often consider

the operative pain minor compared to the pain they experienced before the surgery. It is not unusual for these patients to require minimal analgesia postoperatively.

Adaptation to change in function. The person who has undergone a surgical procedure to correct deformity, relieve pain, or improve musculoskeletal function usually has a positive attitude toward the outcome of surgery. One problem that can be encountered is that patients expect much more of the surgery than the surgery is designed to provide. They may tend to overdo and perhaps cause themselves some damage. This is another good reason for providing preoperative instruction for the patient. Informing the patient before surgery about the limitations that must be observed may help in the adjustment to those limitations after the surgery.

A second problem that can be encountered is that the hospital staff or the patient's family can hold unrealistic expectations for the outcomes of a particular procedure on an individual patient. If it is not clearly defined before surgery that the outcomes for an individual patient will be limited by other conditions (e.g., multiple joint problems), there may be pressure on the patient to achieve the same as other patients who do not have the same limitation.

Happily, most patients do have their functional abilities extended or improved by the surgery that is performed. However, depending on how long standing was the situation that precipitated the surgery, the patient will have to be given time to adjust to these new abilities. Patterns of dependence may have to be broken down gradually as the patient discovers that "I now can do it myself." The patient's family may have to be reassured that the patient can now manage activities that formerly they carried out. These kinds of adjustments will begin in the hospital setting, and they will continue for some time after discharge. If it is anticipated that the patient will have adjustment problems at home, it may be advisable to make a referral to the Visiting Nurse Association or another community resource so the patient can have continuing support after discharge.

Outcome criteria for the persons requiring surgical management

The person or significant others can explain or demonstrate the following components of care:
1. Care of wound.
   a. Demonstrate the care of the wound, including dressing changes, that will be required until healing occurs.
   b. Explain the care of the cast (if applicable).
   c. Explain what to do if the nature or character of wound drainage changes.
   d. Explain the rationale for and use of antibiotics (if prescribed).
2. Restriction or limitation of activity.

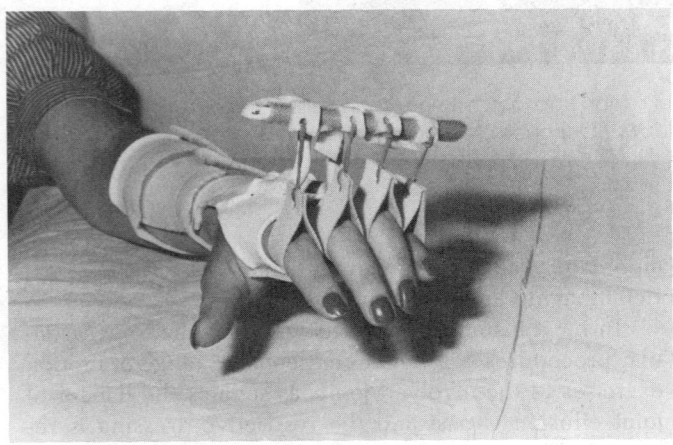

Fig. 41-34. Dynamic hand splint.

a. Explain the limitations of activity to be observed and for what length of time.

b. Explain the nature of and rationale for prescribed weight-bearing restrictions and limitations of joint movement.

c. Demonstrate the appropriate, safe use of assistive and supportive devices.

d. Demonstrate safe performance of ADL within the prescribed limitations or restrictions of activity, weight bearing, or joint movement.

3. Use of medication.
   a. State dosage of medications, when to take them, and possible side and toxic effects.

4. Safety measures.
   a. Describe the safety devices to be obtained for use at home and how and where they will be obtained.
   b. Describe and demonstrate how safety devices and precautions will be used at home.
   c. Describe what alterations must be made in the home environment to render it safe.

5. Techniques for the prevention of complications.
   a. Demonstrate the techniques appropriate to the prevention of infection, cardiorespiratory problems, skin breakdown, swelling, and neurocirculatory impairment.
   b. Demonstrate the uses, application and removal, and care of splints or braces.
   c. Demonstrate proper posture, body mechanics, and other specific joint protection techniques.

6. Infection.
   a. Demonstrate care of the wound.
   b. Explain and demonstrate the proper care of wires or pins used for fixation (if applicable).
   c. Explain what measures are to be taken if there is a change in the nature or character of drainage.

7. Follow-up care.
   a. Explain plans for follow-up care.
   b. Explain measures to take when a complication arises.

REFERENCES AND SELECTED READINGS
Contemporary

1. *Adams, J.C.: Outline of fractures, including joint injuries, ed. 6, Baltimore, 1972, The Williams & Wilkins Co.
2. *Arthritis Foundation: Primer on the rheumatic diseases, ed. 7, New York, 1973, The Foundation. (Prepared by a Committee of the American Rheumatism Association Section of the Arthritis Foundation. Reprinted from J.A.M.A. 224(suppl.), April 30, 1973.)
3. *Blount, M., and Kinney, A.: Chronic steroid therapy, Am. J. Nurs. 74:1626-1631, 1974.
4. Bluestone, R., editor: Rheumatology, Boston, 1980, Houghton Mifflin Professional Publishers.
5. Bohlman, H.: Personal communications, Dec. 1976 and Sept. 1978.
6. *Brunner, N.A.: Orthopedic nursing: a programmed approach, ed. 3, St. Louis, 1979, The C.V. Mosby Co.
7. *Buck, B.I.: Hip replacement, Superv. Nurse 3:75-78, 1972.
8. Canda, K.: The hazards of bedrest, unpublished paper, 1972. (Written in fulfillment of requirements for master's degree, Case Western Reserve University.)
9. *Ciuca, R., et al.: Active range-of-motion exercises: a handbook, Nurs. '78 8(8):45-49, 1978.
10. *Ciuca, R., et al.: Passive range-of-motion exercises: a handbook, Nurs. '78 8(7):59-65, 1978.
11. *Cohen, S., and Viellian, G.: Nursing care of a patient in traction, Am. J. Nurs. 79:1771-1798, 1979.
12. Daniels, L., and Worthingham, C.: Therapeutic exercise for body alignment and function, ed. 2, Philadelphia, 1977, W.B. Saunders Co.
13. Dequeker, J., et al.: Aging of bone: its relation to osteoporosis and osteoarthrosis in postmenopausal women, Orthopedics Dig. 4:26, 1976.
14. *Donahoo, C.A., and Dimon, J.H., III: Orthopedic nursing, Boston, 1977, Little, Brown & Co.
15. Edmonson, A.S., and Crenshaw, A.H., editors: Campbell's operative orthopaedics, ed. 6, St. Louis, 1980, The C.V. Mosby Co.
16. Ehrlich, G.E., editor: Total management of the arthritic patient, Philadelphia, 1973, J.B. Lippincott Co.
17. *Farrell, J.: Illustrated guide to orthopedic nursing, Philadelphia, 1977, J.B. Lippincott Co.
18. *Farrell, J.: Nursing care of the patient in a cast brace, Nurs. Clin. North Am. 13:717-724, 1976.
19. Gallagher, L.: When your patient has a shoulder arthroplasty, here's how to help. . ., Nurs. '80 10:46-49, 1980.
20. *Gartland, J.J.: Fundamentals of orthopedics, ed. 3, Philadelphia, 1979, W.B. Saunders Co.
21. Ghista, D.N., and Roaf, R., editors: Orthopaedic mechanics, procedures and devices, London, 1978, Academic Press, Inc.
22. *Gramse, C.A.: For control of severe pain: dorsal column stimulation, Am. J. Nurs. 78:1022-1025, 1978.
23. *Gruis, M.L., and Innes, B.: Assessment: essential to prevent pressure sores, Am. J. Nurs. 76:1762-1764, 1976.
24. *Kitching, C.: Nursing care study: subluxation of the atlanto-occipital joint, Nurs. Times 75:354-355, 1979.
25. Kuhn, R.A.: The halo in the management of cervical spine lesions, Orthop. Rev. 1:25-27, 1972.
26. *Larson, C.B., and Gould, M.L.: Orthopedic nursing, ed. 9, St. Louis, 1978, The C.V. Mosby Co.
27. Lewis, R.C., Jr.: Handbook of traction, casting and splinting techniques, Philadelphia, 1977, J.B. Lippincott Co.
28. *Long, B., and Buergin, P.: The pivot transfer, Am. J. Nurs. 77:980-982, 1977.
29. McCarthy, D.J., editor: Arthritis and allied conditions; a textbook of rheumatology, ed. 9, Philadelphia, 1979, Lea & Febiger.
30. Melvin, J.L.: Rheumatic disease: occupational therapy and rehabilitation, Philadelphia, 1977, F.A. Davis Co.
31. *Moskowitz, R.W.: Clinical rheumatology, Philadelphia, 1975, Lea & Febiger.
32. *Mourad, L.: Nursing care of adults with orthopedic conditions, New York, 1980, John Wiley & Sons, Inc.
33. Owen, B.D.: How to control that aching back, Am. J. Nurs. 80:894-897, 1980.
34. Pendleton, T., and Grossman, B.J.: Rehabilitating children with inflammatory joint disease, Am. J. Nurs. 74:2223-2226, 1974.
35. *Rantz, M.J., and Courtial, D.: Lifting, moving and transferring patients: a manual, ed. 2, St. Louis, 1981, The C.V. Mosby Co.
36. *Roaf, R., and Hodkinson, L.J.: Textbook of orthopaedic nursing,

*References preceded by an asterisk are particularly well suited for student reading.

ed. 2, Oxford, 1975, Blackwell Scientific Publications, Ltd. (Distributed by J.B. Lippincott Co., Philadelphia.)

37. *Ryan, J.: Compression in bone healing, Am. J. Nurs. **74**:1998-1999, 1974.

38. *Salter, R.B.: Textbook of disorders and injuries of the musculoskeletal system: an introduction to orthopaedics, rheumatology, metabolic bone disease, rehabilitation and fracture, Baltimore, 1970, The Williams & Wilkins Co.

39. *Schneider, F.R.: Handbook for the orthopaedic assistant, ed. 2, St. Louis, 1976, The C.V. Mosby Co.

40. *Schwaid, M.C.: Advice to arthritics: keep moving, Am. J. Nurs. **78**:1708-1709, 1978.

41. Spruck, M.: Gold therapy for rheumatoid arthritis, Am. J. Nurs. **79**:1246-1248, 1979.

42. *Sterman, L.: Clinical biofeedback, Am. J. Nurs. **75**:2006-2009, 1975.

43. *Stryker, R.P.: Rehabilitative aspects of acute and chronic nursing care, Philadelphia, 1972, W.B. Saunders Co.

44. *Swinson, D.R., and Swinburn, W.R.: Rheumatology, New York, 1980, John Wiley & Sons, Inc.

45. *Synnestvedt, N.: The do's and don't's of traction care, Nurs. '74 **3**:35-41, 1974.

46. Townley, C., and Hill, L.: Total knee replacement, Am. J. Nurs. **74**:1612-1617, 1974.

47. Turek, S.L.: Orthopaedics: principles and their application, ed. 3, Philadelphia, 1977, J.B. Lippincott Co.

48. Uhthoff, H.K., and Jaworski, Z.F.G.: Bone loss in response to long-term immobilization, J. Bone Joint Surg. [Br.] **60**:420-429, 1978.

49. *Waterson, M.: Hot and cold therapy, Nurs. '78 **8**(10):44-49, 1978.

50. Williams, A.: A study of factors contributing to skin breakdown, Nurs. Res. **21**:238-243, 1972.

51. Williams, S.R.: Nutrition and diet therapy, ed. 4, St. Louis, 1982, The C.V. Mosby Co.

52. Willkens, R.F.: The use of nonsteroidal anti-inflammatory agents, J.A.M.A. **240**:1632-1635, 1978.

53. Wilson, J.R.: Aspirin hepatotoxicity in adults with rheumatoid arthritis, Ohio State Med. J. **72**:577-579, 1976.

Classic

54. *Kirk, J.A., and Kersley, G.D.: Heat and cold in the physical treatment of rheumatoid arthritis of the knee, Ann. Phys. Med. **9**:270-274, 1968.

55. Lowman, E.W.: Clinical management of disability due to rheumatoid arthritis, Arch. Phys. Med. Rehabil. **48**:136-141, 1967.

CHAPTER 42

PROBLEMS OF THE MUSCULOSKELETAL SYSTEM

PATRICIA BUERGIN

The disorders and injuries of the musculoskeletal system are vast in scope. They range from those that cause the patient only minor discomfort and inconvenience to those that are life threatening. The purpose of this chapter is to discuss those specific musculoskeletal conditions that commonly necessitate the adult individual's hospitalization and need for specific nursing care. Included are both the rheumatic diseases and conditions that require orthopedic surgical intervention. Some clinical conditions present localized signs and symptoms, while others present systemic signs and symptoms. Assessment of the patient with musculoskeletal signs and symptoms is discussed in Chapter 40, and general management considerations for such patients are discussed in Chapter 41. The epidemiology, pathophysiology, and clinical manifestations of specific disorders will be discussed in this chapter. In instances where specific management techniques pertain, those techniques will be discussed; otherwise, the reader will be referred to the discussion in Chapter 41. This will also apply to discussion of outcome criteria.

Rheumatic diseases include a wide range of clinical conditions that cause pain and stiffness in the musculoskeletal system. The American Rheumatism Association has classified rheumatic diseases into 13 categories.[3] Diseases included in the following nine categories will be discussed in some detail:

1. Connective tissue diseases (acquired)
2. Degenerative joint disease (osteoarthritis, osteoarthrosis)
3. Traumatic or neurogenic disorders
4. Polyarthritis of unknown cause
5. Rheumatic fever
6. Nonarticular rheumatism
7. Disorders associated with known infectious agents

8. Disorders associated with known or strongly suspected biochemical or endocrine abnormalities
9. Miscellaneous rheumatic disorders

The four remaining categories are mentioned only briefly here. Information concerning the specific disorders in these categories may either be found elsewhere in this book or would repeat other information presented in this chapter if those disorders were discussed in detail.

1. Diseases with which arthritis is frequently associated. This category includes sarcoidosis (p. 1316), ulcerative colitis (p. 1484), and regional enteritis (p. 1483). Sjögren's syndrome (p. 990) is also cross referenced in this category.

2. Neoplasms. The care of patients with neoplasms is discussed in Chapter 25.

3. Allergy and drug reactions. Notable in this category are the lupuslike syndromes (p. 987) induced by procainamide and hydralazine.

4. Inherited and congenital disorders. Congenital dysplasia of the hip is the most common disorder in this category.[20,22,41]

Some commonalities are shared by many of the diseases that will be discussed; however, their differences will be emphasized. It should also be noted that many of the disorders require corrective surgical intervention at some point in their course. Synovectomy (p. 1010), osteotomy (p. 1010), arthroplasty (p. 1005), and total joint replacement (p. 1005) are vital adjuncts to the medical management of individuals with rheumatic diseases.

There are some commonalities shared by a number of these disorders; however, their differences will be emphasized. It may also be noted that many of these disorders require corrective surgical intervention at some point in their course. Surgery is more and more a vital adjunct to the management of individuals with rheumatic diseases. Nurses caring for patients with these diseases must have an appreciation for and an understanding of both the medical and the surgical approaches that will be employed in treatment.

The term *arthritis* means inflammation of a joint. Arthritis is a condition that exists in a number of specific rheumatic diseases. However, like the term *rheumatism*, it is often used by the public to apply to any pain or stiffness of the musculoskeletal system whether or not the cause is an inflammatory process. It is estimated that 20 million people in the United States are suffering from arthritis or arthritis-like conditions.[40] As such, it may be anticipated that a significant proportion of the patients with whom a nurse has contact will have some discomfort or disability caused by musculoskeletal disorders.

Rheumatic diseases

Systemic connective tissue diseases

Rheumatoid arthritis

Epidemiology and etiology. Rheumatoid arthritis is a chronic *systemic* disease. The disease process, while most prominent as a nonsuppurative inflammation in the diarthrodial joints, may also be manifested by lesions of the vasculature, nervous system, and other major organs of the body.

Rheumatoid arthritis is more prevalent in women than men by a ratio of 2:1 or 3:1. Usually it appears during the productive years of life when career and family responsibilities are greatest. While the cause of this disease is unknown, there are several theories of causation under investigation. Areas of study include (1) immune mechanisms, such as the interaction of the IgG class of immunoglobins with the rheumatoid factor that appears to play a role in perpetuating rheumatoid inflammation[3]; (2) metabolic factors; and (3) infection, with particular attention to viruses.

Pathophysiology. The disease process within the joints (intraarticular) begins as an inflammation of the synovium with edema, vascular congestion, fibrin exudate, and cellular infiltrate.[3] The amount of synovial fluid increases while the fluid itself becomes turbid and has a decreased viscosity. Continued inflammation leads to thickening of the synovium, particularly where it joins the articular cartilage. At these junctures, granulation tissue forms a *pannus*, or mantle that covers the surface of the cartilage. The pannus also invades subchondral bone. As the amount of granulation tissue from inflammation increases, it interferes with normal nutrition of the articular cartilage. The cartilage becomes necrotic. The degree of erosion of the articular cartilage will determine the amount of articular disability. If large areas

of cartilage are destroyed, adhesions form between the joint surfaces, and fibrous or bony union (ankylosis) develops between what were previously articulating surfaces. Destruction of cartilage and bone, in addition to some weakening of tendons and ligaments, may lead to subluxation or dislocation of joints. Invasion of the subchondral bone may cause eventual regional osteoporosis.

Clinical picture. The early manifestations of the disease may include fever, weight loss, fatigue, and generalized aching. Early morning stiffness lasting a few minutes to an hour or more is characteristic. The patient may describe the location of aching and stiffness in general terms, such as "in my arms," "in my hands," or "in my legs," as opposed to naming specific joints. This kind of discomfort, commonly referred to as fibrositis, is *poorly localized*. Such discomfort is often seen in rheumatoid arthritis and may be the patient's earliest complaint. This symptom picture may be present for some period of time before it is followed by more specific, or localized, problems—frank articular inflammation with joint swelling, pain, redness, warmth, and tenderness. In other patients, fibrositis and joint inflammation occur together at the onset.[40]

The proximal interphalangeal and metacarpophalangeal joints of the hands and the metatarsophalangeal joints of the feet are often affected early. As the disease progresses, the fingers develop a characteristic tapering appearance with a classic ulnar deviation of the hand. Virtually all joints can become involved—hips, knees, wrists, elbows, shoulders, and jaw. Joint involvement most often occurs in a *bilaterally symmetric* pattern with involvement of the same joints on both sides of the body. (*Asymmetric distribution* is the term used to indicate a scattered type of involvement.) Even such small structures as the cricoarytenoid joints of the larynx can be affected. Laryngeal involvement, if severe, may result in hoarseness or voice changes, dysphagia, and dyspnea on exertion.[36] Fortunately, it causes symptomatic problems in relatively few patients.

Inflammation of the tendon sheaths, particularly in the wrist, may occur. There is spasm of the muscles attached to the involved joints. Such spasm is believed to contribute to deformity of the involved joints, and since the patient will tend to guard painful joints, there may be some atrophy of muscles from disuse (Fig. 42-1). Subcutaneous nodules may develop near joints, over bony prominences, or along extensor surfaces.

The course of rheumatoid arthritis varies greatly from patient to patient. It is marked by periods of exacerbation and remission. Some individuals have been known to recover from a first attack and never suffer a recurrence. For others, particularly those in whom the rheumatoid factor is found (seropositive rheumatoid disease), the disease tends to be chronically progressive.[36] In a small number of individuals the disease may be

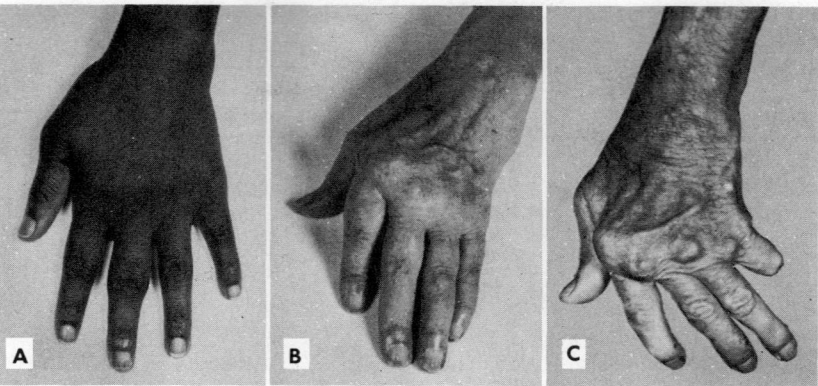

Fig. 42-1. Rheumatoid arthritis of hand. **A,** Early stage. Note fusiform swelling of proximal interphalangeal joints, especially that of middle finger. **B,** Moderate involvement. Note swelling from chronic synovitis of metacarpophalangeal joints and early ulnar drift. **C,** Advanced stage. Note marked ulnar drift and subluxation of metacarpophalangeal joints with extension of proximal interphalangeal joints and flexion of distal joints. Note also deformed position of thumb. (From Raney, R., and Brashear, H.: Shand's handbook of orthopaedic surgery, ed. 8, St. Louis, 1971, The C.V. Mosby Co.)

rapidly progressive, marked by unremitting joint destruction and diffuse vasculitis. This form of the disease is referred to as *malignant rheumatoid disease*.[3] The length of time between exacerbations varies greatly with individuals. There is some evidence that exacerbations can be triggered by mental stress such as worry or grief,[36] by overexertion, and at times by physical trauma such as surgery. The likelihood that the patient will enter a complete remission after 3 years of sustained disease activity is very slight.[36]

If it is not treated, rheumatoid arthritis has a tendency to relapse and to recur in more severe form. Continued competent medical care is of the utmost importance for anyone who has rheumatoid arthritis. Some individuals, when experiencing a remission of their symptoms, believe they are cured and discontinue their therapy, only to have a later and more severe exacerbation of the disease. Even with careful management, approximately 10% of patients with rheumatoid arthritis progress to a crippling state of complete incapacity.[36]

Laboratory findings usually include an elevated erythrocyte sedimentation rate and mild leukocytosis. A positive rheumatoid factor (latex fixation test, p. 934) is seen in 50% to 90% of patients, depending on disease duration and severity.[40] Roentgenographic examination may reveal narrowing of the joint spaces and erosion of the articular surfaces. Synovial biopsy and examination of synovial tissue can establish the presence of inflammatory changes in the synovium, and synovial fluid obtained by needle aspiration will have increased turbidity and decreased viscosity.

Intervention. The basic interventions for rheumatoid arthritis involve (1) rest, (2) relief of pain, (3) main-

tenance of joint function, (4) prevention and correction of deformities by application of orthopedic principles (p. 961), and (5) correction of other health factors. These principles, as well as the specific medications used in the treatment of rheumatoid arthritis, are discussed in Chapter 41 and in Table 42-1.

One special consideration in dealing with the rheumatoid patient requires further discussion. Depending on the disease condition, the disability may increase in spite of all efforts, including those of the patient. The patient and family often become very discouraged. The person who is discouraged and in pain is very vulnerable to promises of a "cure." Millions of dollars (estimates range as high as $400 million) are spent each year by persons who can ill afford the expense on gadgets, programs, and "medicines" that allegedly are able to "cure." While the ultimate decision to try a program rests with the individual, the health care team can provide guidance to the patient and family. Teaching patients about their care and seeing that they are referred to reputable resources for additional assistance and information is one of the most valuable services that can be rendered to them. The local chapter of the Arthritis Foundation can be of great assistance to patients and their families. The Arthritis Foundation is also keenly aware of the relative merit or lack of merit of resources available in the community.

The Arthritis Foundation* has prepared the following material, all of which is helpful to nurses working with persons who have arthritis: *Home care programs in arthritis; Arthritis and related disorders: a manual*

---

*3400 Peachtree Drive NE, Atlanta, GA 30326.

TABLE 42-1. Medications prescribed in the treatment of rheumatoid arthritis

Medication	Action	Usual dosage	Side effects/ toxic effects	Precautions
Salicylates				
Examples: acetylsali- cyclic acid, choline salicylates	Analgesic, antipyretic, an- tiinflammatory	2560-5120 mg/day in divided doses	Gastric irritation; dose-re- lated salicylism; skin rash; hypersensitivity	Take with food, milk, or antacid; space q 4-6 hr to maintain antiinflammatory ef- fect
Nonsteroidal antiinflammatory agents				
Indomethacin (Indo- cin)	Analgesic, antiinflammatory	25 mg bid or tid to maximum of 200 mg/day	Headache; dizziness; insom- nia; confusion; gastroin- testinal irritation	Take with food, milk, or antacid; discon- tinue if CNS symp- toms develop and notify physician
Ibuprofen (Motrin)	Same as indomethacin	300-400 mg tid or qid	Same as indomethacin but believed less irritating to gastrointestinal tract	Delayed absorption if taken with food
Tolmetin sodium (Tol- ectin)	Same as ibuprofen	400 mg tid to maxi- mum of 2 gm/day	Same as ibuprofen	Take with food or milk
Naproxen (Naprosyn)	Same as ibuprofen	250 mg bid to maxi- mum of 750 mg/ day	Same as ibuprofen; also drowsiness	Take with food, milk, or antacid; avoid driving until dosage effect established
Fenoprofen calcium (Nalfon)	Same as ibuprofen	600 mg qid up to 3.2 g/day	Same as naproxen	Delayed absorption if taken with food; avoid driving until dosage effect estab- lished
Sulindac (Clinoril)	Same as ibuprofen	150 mg bid to maxi- mum of 400 mg/ day	Same as ibuprofen; plus skin rash	Take with food, milk, or antacid; not to be used with acetylsali- cylic acid
Potent antiinflammatory agents				
Adrenocorticosteroids (e.g., prednisone)	Interfere with body's normal inflammatory response	Adjusted to control symptoms at lowest possible dosage per day; range: 1-40 mg/day, usually in divided doses	Fluid retention; sodium re- tention; potassium deple- tion; hypertension; de- creased healing potential; increased susceptibility to infection; gastrointestinal irritation; hirsutism, osteo- porosis, fat deposits; dia- betes mellitus; myopathy; adrenal insufficiency or adrenal crisis if abruptly withdrawn	Take with food, milk, or antacid; dosage not to be increased or decreased without physician's supervi- sion; take in morning if taken on once-a- day basis
Phenylbutazone (Bu- tazolidin)	Antiinflammatory; analgesic at subcortical site in brain	300-600 mg/day in di- vided doses for flare-ups of arthritis	Gastrointestinal irritation; hematologic toxicity; hy- pertension, impaired renal function	Used for a short term (7-10 days); take with food or milk
Slow acting antiinflammatory agents				
Antimalarials				
Hydroxychloroquine (Plaquenil)	Antiinflammatory (mecha- nism unknown); effect not expected to be noted for 6-12 mo after begin- ning therapy	Initial dosage: 400- 600 mg/day in one or two doses; main- tanance: 200-400 mg qid	Gastrointestinal disturbances; retinal edema that may result in blindness	Eye examination before beginning therapy and every 6 mo thereafter

TABLE 42-1. Medications prescribed in the treatment of rheumatoid arthritis—cont'd

Medication	Action	Usual dosage	Side effects/ toxic effects	Precautions
Chloroquine (Aralen)	Same hydroxychloroquine	Initial dosage: 250 mg bid; maintenance: 250 mg qid with evening meal	Same as hydroxychloroquine	Same as hydroxychloroquine
Quinacrine (Arabrine)	Same as hydroxychloroquine	100 mg qid	Same as hydroxychloroquine but may be better tolerated; yellow discoloration of the skin	May be stopped periodically to prevent deepening of skin discoloration
Gold salts (Myochrysine, Solganol)	Antiinflammatory	See text, p. 959; maintenance: 25-50 mg q 3-4 wk	Renal and hepatic damage; corneal deposits; dermatitis; ulcerations in mouth; hematologic changes	Urinalysis and CBC before each injection; report dermatitis, metallic taste in mouth, or lesions in mouth to physician
Penicillamine (Cuprimine)	Antiinflammatory (mechanism unclear); effect not expected to be noted until several months after beginning treatment	Initial dosage: 250 mg qid, increasing at 4-wk intervals up to 750 mg/day; maintenance: lowest possible dose to maintain clinical improvement	Fever; rash; nephrotic syndrome; hematologic changes; gastrointestinal irritation; lupuslike syndromes; allergic reactions (33% probability if allergic to penicillin); retarded wound healing	Urinalysis, CBC, differential, hemoglobin and platelet count at least weekly for 3 mo, then monthly; report skin rash, fever to physician; food interferes with absorption—take on empty stomach between meals

for nurses, physical therapists, and social workers; *Arthritis: the basic facts; Rheumatoid arthritis; Osteoarthritis;* and *Gout.* The last four of these references are written in such a way that many patients can understand and learn from them. After consulting with the physician to determine which particular books will be most appropriate for the individual patient, those planning to teach the patient will find that these books are helpful teaching aids to share with the patient.

Outcome criteria for the person with rheumatoid arthritis. The person or significant others can:

1. Explain the basic nature of rheumatoid arthritis.
2. Demonstrate the prescribed methods of joint protection.
3. Explain how medications are to be taken (dose, what times, side effects, toxic effects).
4. Demonstrate prescribed exercise program.
5. Demonstrate how to use moist heat applications to relieve pain in joints.
6. Demonstrate how to apply and explain when to use splinting devices.
7. Explain the need for plans for consistent follow-up care.

Systemic lupus erythematosus

Epidemiology. Systemic lupus erythematosus (SLE) is a chronic inflammatory disease of unknown cause. It affects women, particularly adolescents and young adults, four times more often than it affects men. The disease was named after its characteristic rash, the erosive nature of the rash being "likened to the damage wrought by a hungry wolf."[3] Once thought to be relatively rare and always fatal, better techniques for recognition of the disease have demonstrated it to be fairly common, and its course can be controlled by corticosteroids. Some patients do, however, die as a result of lesions affecting major organs or from secondary infections.

Pathophysiology. The pathologic manifestations of the disease include severe vasculitis with necrosis of the walls of the small arteries, renal involvement with thickening of the basement membrane of the glomerular tufts, and necrosis of the glomerular capillaries, lymph node necrosis, synovial involvement as a fibrous villous synovitis, lesions of the nervous system, and the development of small white spots in the retina called *cytoid bodies*. Two major areas are being investigated as possible causes of this disease. One possibility is that an aberration of the immune system causes immune complexes containing antibodies to be deposited in tissue, thereby causing tissue damage; the second possibility is the presence of a viral infection caused by or resulting from some immunologic abnormality. A third possibility is that both of these factors combine to produce the disease. Some drugs, notably procainamide (Pronestyl), isonicotinic acid hydrazide (INH, Isoniazid), and penicillin are known to induce lupuslike syndromes.

Clinical picture. The initial manifestation of SLE is often arthritis. In many instances the joint symptoms are transient and respond to treatment. Weakness, fatigue, and weight loss may be present. The patient may complain of sensitivity to the sun, developing rash and at times fever or arthritis on exposure to sunlight. Erythema, usually in a butterfly pattern, appears over the cheeks and bridge of the nose. The margins of the lesions are bright red, and the lesions may extend beyond the hairline with partial alopecia (loss of hair) above the ears. Lesions may also occur on the exposed part of the neck. The lesions spread slowly to the mucous membranes and other tissues of the body, or they may originate there. The lesions do not ulcerate, but cause degeneration and atrophy of tissues.

Depending on the organs involved, the patient may have findings of glomerulonephritis, pleuritis, pericarditis, peritonitis, neuritis, or anemia. Renal and neurologic manifestations are among the more serious manifestations of the disease.

Laboratory findings may be specific to the organs involved, as with proteinuria, abnormal cerebrospinal fluid, or roentgenographic evidence of pleural reactions. A positive lupus erythematosus (LE) cell reaction and immunofluorescent studies to identify the antibody responsible for LE cell reaction are helpful in making the diagnosis of the disease (p. 934).

Intervention. Adrenocorticosteroid therapy is used to control active manifestations of SLE. In the presence of lupus nephritis, steroids are frequently given in very high doses (60 mg or more of prednisone per day). The management considerations in caring for patients on high doses of steroids as discussed in Chapter 41 should be well understood in these instances (p. 958). Joint pains are often treated with salicylates. Antimalarial drugs may be helpful in treating the cutaneous lesions; however, the possibility of serious retinal damage with prolonged use must be carefully monitored (p. 958). If skin lesions are present or if there is exacerbation of symptoms on sun exposure, exposure to the sun is to be avoided.

Outcome criteria for the person with SLE. The person or significant others can:

1. Explain how medications are to be taken (dosage, what times, side effects, toxic effects).
2. Explain the reason for immediate medical consultation if for any reason the prescribed steroids cannot be taken.
3. Explain the reason for carrying an identification card stating name of prescribed steroid, dose, and name and phone number of physician.
4. Describe the clothing to be worn when out in the sun (all body surfaces covered, wide-brimmed hat).
5. Explain plans for follow-up care.

Polymyositis (dermatomyositis)

Epidemiology and etiology. Polymyositis (dermatomyositis) is an inflammatory disease involving striated (voluntary) muscle. Polymyositis occurs two times more frequently in women than men, and it may occur at any age. It is estimated that the disease occurs in one of every 200,000 of the population per year.[3] The cause of the disease is unknown; however, it is thought that some reaction of the autoimmune system is involved.

Pathophysiology. Pathologic findings on histologic studies of biopsied muscle are variable, but the alterations found, in order of their frequency, are the following: (1) primary degeneration of muscle fibers, either focal or extensive; (2) basophilia of some fibers with central migration of the sarcolemmal nuclei; (3) necrosis of parts or of entire groups of muscle fibers; (4) lymphocytic and plasma cell infiltrates near or surrounding blood vessels or between individual muscle fibers; (5) interstitial fibrosis varying in severity with the duration and to some extent the type of disease; (6) variation in the cross-sectional diameter of fibers.[3,36]

Clinical picture. Polymyositis, which usually runs a course of exacerbations and remissions, is usually first noted in proximal muscles, in particular the pelvic and shoulder girdles. Climbing stairs, arising from a chair, and other activities that involve lifting the body become increasingly difficult or impossible. Lifting of the arms becomes progressively more difficult. Hair combing may be impossible. Other muscles—neck flexors, the muscles of swallowing—may also become involved. Muscle pain or tenderness is present in some instances in the early stages, but not necessarily. Involvement of the skin in the form of a rash marks the disease as *dermatomyositis*. A dusky red lesion may be found in the periorbital region, along with periorbital edema. This dusky red rash may extend over the face, forehead, neck, upper shoulders, chest, and upper back. Lesions on the arms and legs commonly affect the extensor surfaces. These patches are sometimes slightly scaly.[40]

The weakness of myositis, if it persists, can lead to contractures and atrophy. Individuals with the dermatomyositis form of the disease, particularly if they are over 40 years of age, have a 40% to 50% greater chance of having evidence of a malignant neoplasm found during the first 5 years of illness than the population at large. Some physicians believe that routine yearly examinations should be performed to define or exclude the presence of neoplasms in these patients during that 5-year period.

The physical therapist is helpful in delineating which specific muscles are involved (or are weak) by performing a manual muscle test (p. 938). An electromyogram (p. 938) is useful in the diagnosis, as it can delineate a specific pattern of findings that helps to differentiate polymyositis (dermatomyositis) from other types of muscle disease. Muscle biopsy (p. 937) results may define the specific pathologic changes within the involved muscle. Serum enzymes—serum glutamic-oxaloacetic transaminase (SGOT), creatine phosphokinase (CPK), and aldolase (p. 934)—are elevated in the presence of active polymyositis or dermatomyositis. Close monitoring of these enzyme values will give indications of the progress of the disease or the effects of treatment. Twenty-four-hour urine collections for the creatine-creatinine ratio (indicating the amount of muscle disease that is present) are also obtained on a frequent basis (p. 936).

Intervention. Polymyositis (dermatomyositis) responds to corticosteroid therapy. Prednisone is often given in high (50 mg or more per day) doses. Those management principles relating to rest, positioning, assisted transfer and locomotion, prevention of skin breakdown, and care of the individual receiving high doses of corticosteroids (p. 958) are all relevant in caring for the patient who has myositis.

Outcome criteria for the person with polymyositis or dermatomyositis. The person or significant others can:

1. Describe how to balance rest and activity.
2. Demonstrate ability to safely perform activities of daily living (ADL) or explain how these needs will be met if unable to do for self.
3. Explain how medications are to be taken (dosage, what times, side effects, toxic effects).
4. Explain the reason for immediate medical consultation if for any reason the prescribed steroids cannot be taken.
5. Demonstrate prescribed program of exercises.
6. Demonstrate proper positioning in bed.
7. State symptoms that would indicate need for immediate medical assistance.
8. Explain the reason for carrying an identification card stating name of prescribed steroid, dose, and name and phone number of physician.
9. Explain plans for follow-up care.

Progressive systemic sclerosis (PSS, scleroderma)

Epidemiology and etiology. Progressive systemic sclerosis involves the connective tissue throughout the body. It affects women three times more often than men, usually in the 30- to 50-year age group. The cause of PSS is unknown. Some aberration of the immune system may be involved.

Pathophysiology. As this disease runs its course, involved tissue becomes fibrotic. These changes may be accompanied by vascular lesions, and the tissue involved may be the skin (scleroderma), synovium, esophagus, intestinal tract, heart, lungs, or kidneys. The disease may exist in a mild chronic form or, depending on the organs involved, may progress to rapid death.

Clinical picture. The word "scleroderma" means "hard skin," and that accurately describes the skin manifestations that are present. Usually local areas such as the face and fingers are affected first with gradual thickening and tightening of the skin. The skin may first appear slightly edematous, then turn pale, become steadily more firm, and finally become fixed to underlying tissue. The skin may also appear mildly pigmented. *Telangiectases* (elevated dark red spots formed by the dilatation of groups of capillaries) appear on the lips, tongue, fingers, and face. Normal skin folds are lost as the skin hardens, and as a result, the face appears "pinched."[40] This is sometimes referred to as "birdlike" facies. Articular symptoms—pain and stiffness—are present in about one third of the patients as an initial symptom. Raynaud's phenomenon (p. 923) may be pronounced. Muscle weakness (sclerodermatomyositis) may be present. In the presence of pain on joint motion, skin and muscle contractures develop to produce deformity of the joint.

As the face becomes masklike, the ability to chew food may be impaired. The patient may have difficulty swallowing. Chest expansion may be impaired by the firming of the skin so that respiratory failure threatens. If the disease progresses to its end stage, all body motion becomes so restricted that the patient has the appearance of a living mummy. Tissues of essential organs such as the heart, kidneys, and liver may be affected in a similar manner, and fatal impairment of their function may result.

Laboratory and other diagnostic tests are helpful in defining the extent of the disease. For example, a barium swallow will help to define the presence of reflux esophagitis; upper gastrointestinal studies may demonstrate decreased peristalsis in the small intestine; pulmonary function studies may indicate impaired gas exchange, decreased vital capacity, and total lung capacity (p. 1220); and antinuclear antibody studies may show a speckled pattern on nucleolar immunofluorescence (p. 935).

Intervention. There is no cure for PSS. Treatment with corticosteroids is generally limited to those patients who have evidence of myositis. Salicylates and mild analgesics are used for joint pain. Physical therapy, while only partially effective in preventing contractures, should be offered to help preserve muscle strength. Frequent small feedings and the use of antacids, along with elevation of the head of the bed, may be helpful in relieving reflux esophagitis.[3] Meticulous hygiene (including frequent mouth care), assisting the patient while eating to prevent choking, and skin care directed to the prevention of decubiti, as well as emotional support are important.

Outcome criteria for the person with PSS. The person or significant others can:

1. Demonstrate prescribed exercises.
2. Explain precautions that must be taken while

eating if experiencing difficulty chewing or swallowing. Pureeing of foods and so on may be necessary.
3. Explain skin care precautions.
4. Demonstrate a ability to safely perform ADL or explain how these needs will be met by others.
5. Explain how medications are to be taken (dosage, what times, side effects, toxic effects).
6. State symptoms that indicate need for immediate medical care.
7. Explain plans for follow-up care.

Necrotizing arteritis and other forms of vasculitis

Necrotizing arteritis and other forms of vasculitis comprise a group of syndromes in which inflammation of blood vessels is seen. This group of syndromes includes the vasculitis found in rheumatoid arthritis, systemic lupus erythematosus, progressive systemic sclerosis, and polyarteritis nodosa.

Pathophysiology. Inflammation of the arterial wall is associated with necrosis. The body's natural attempts to repair the necrosed area result in fibrosis of the arterial wall or rapid growth of the intima (inner coat of the artery). Intimal proliferation may partially or completely occlude the vessel, thus causing infarction. If only a portion of the circumference of a vessel is involved, *aneurysms* (dilatations of the wall of the artery) can develop. Such aneurysms may rupture.[3]

Clinical picture. Vessels in any part of the body—heart, lungs, kidneys, or nerves, either centrally or peripherally—may be involved. The result of such involvement can be angina, myocardial infarction, hypertension, peripheral neuropathy, or focal central nervous system involvement. *Temporal arteritis*, which usually presents with intractable headaches (p. 753), can result in blindness caused by occlusion of the central retinal artery.

Laboratory tests may reveal leukocytosis and elevated erythrocyte sedimentation rate, or may be specific to certain organs as, for example, with proteinuria in renal involvement. Angiography will often demonstrate aneurysmal dilatation of the involved vessels.

Intervention. Corticosteroids administered in high doses in the initial phases of these diseases may prompt remission. Rest is generally prescribed until there is a remission of symptoms. The sections dealing with rest (p. 949) and steroid treatment (p. 958) in Chapter 41 should be consulted for additional information.

Outcome criteria for the person with vasculitis. The person or significant others can:
1. Describe the program of rest that should be adhered to until symptoms are in remission.
2. Explain how medications are to be taken (dosage, what times, side effects, toxic effects).
3. Explain the reason for immediate medical consultation if for any reason the prescribed steroids cannot be taken.

4. Explain the reason for carrying an identification card stating name of prescribed steroid, dose, and name and phone number of physician.
5. Describe symptoms that require immediate medical attention.
6. Explain plans for follow-up care.

Sjögren's syndrome

Epidemiology. Sjögren's syndrome is a chronic inflammatory disorder affecting the lacrimal and parotid glands. The disease occurs dramatically more often in women than in men, the ratio being about 9:1. One half of the individuals who display this syndrome are people who have rheumatoid arthritis, systemic lupus erythematosus, or progressive systemic sclerosis. The syndrome presents with diminished lacrimal and salivary secretions; this is known as the *sicca complex*.

Pathophysiology. The disorder is associated with lymphocytic and plasma cell infiltration of the lacrimal and parotid glands, causing a decrease in the production and flow of tears and saliva. The parotid involvement (*xerostomia*) occurs more slowly than the lacrimal (*keratoconjunctivitis sicca*).

Clinical picture. Patients complain of a dry or gritty sensation in the eye, redness, itching, or a filmy sensation that interfers with vision. When parotid involvement is present, there may be difficulty chewing and swallowing, and some persons experience some difficulty with speech. While the symptoms of this syndrome are distressing, the complications can be even more severe. Corneal ulceration, ulcers of the tongue and lips, and dental caries may occur. In some instances the parotid glands become enlarged.

Lacrimal gland involvement can be measured by a Schirmer test (p. 938), while parotid gland function can be measured by a technetium Tc 99m uptake scan (p. 934). A biopsy of the inside lower lip, where minor salivary glands are located, may demonstrate lymphoid involvement.

Intervention. Treatment is symptomatic. It includes the use of methylcellulose eyedrops on an as needed basis to alleviate the discomfort of dry eyes. Some patients may find it necessary to use these drops as often as every hour. Fluids should be readily available to help keep the mouth moist. Some patients are able to alleviate the dry mouth by sucking on sour candy, as this stimulates the secretion of saliva. The relatively new "artificial saliva," prepared from a saline base, is dramatically effective in relieving symptoms and is safe for teeth. It is also vital to remember that the majority of patients with this syndrome have a systemic connective tissue disease as well. If they have dysfunction of their hands caused by pain, deformity, or contracture, they may not be able to administer their own eyedrops or handle a glass in order to drink fluids. Provision must be made for these complications when planning patients' care or discharge from the hospital. Mouth care is especially important; and if there is difficulty chewing, a change in the texture of the diet is indicated. Junior foods or baby foods may be helpful to some patients.

Outcome criteria for the person with Sjögren's syndrome. The person or significant others can:

1. Explain the basic nature of this syndrome.
2. Demonstrate the administration of prescribed eyedrops.
3. Demonstrate how adequate fluid intake will be maintained.
4. Explain how the texture of the diet can be changed (chopping, pureeing, junior, and baby foods).
5. Describe how to facilitate chewing and swallowing by increasing fluid intake with meals.
6. Explain plans for follow-up care.

Degenerative joint disease

Epidemiology

Degenerative joint disease, also known as osteoarthritis, hypertrophic arthritis, osteoarthrosis, or senescent arthritis, is an extremely common disease that is probably as old as civilization. Almost everyone past 40 years of age has hypertrophic changes in the joints. While symptomatic degenerative joint disease is usually noted in the 50- to 70-year age group, it has been observed as early as age 20. On the basis of one study, it is estimated that 40 million Americans have degenerative changes of the hands and feet, and estimates are that 175,000 Americans 65 years old and over have been incapacitated by degenerative joint disease of the hip.[3]

Etiology and pathophysiology

Degenerative joint disease is a disease of the articular cartilage. It is thought to accompany aging, but may develop as a result of trauma, congenital problems (e.g., hip dislocations), or childhood diseases such as Legg-Calvé-Perthes disease. The articular cartilage, normally dense, white, translucent, and smooth, becomes yellow and opaque. Areas of the cartilage may become soft and the surface becomes roughened, frayed, and cracked. Eventually this cartilage may be destroyed, and the underlying subchondral bone goes through a remodeling process (p. 915). *Osteophytes*, or spurs of new bone that appear at the joint margins and at the sites of attachment of supporting structures, may break off and appear in the joint cavity as "joint mice." While the cause of the degeneration of articular cartilage is unknown, several theories of causation include digestion of the cartilage by enzymes and alteration of the nutrition of the cartilage. Individuals affected with degenerative joint disease may be predisposed to the disease by excessive "wear and tear" of the affected joints. Obes-

ity, metabolic disturbances (e.g., acromegaly), repeated joint hemorrhages, trauma, or genetic predispositions are examples of contributing factors. Also, certain occupations such as coal mining and boxing tend to be associated with osteoarthritis.

Clinical picture

The individual with degenerative joint disease experiences pain in the movable joints, particularly on weight bearing. Inflammation is usually not present, and tenderness is mild; however, the joints may become enlarged. Crepitation may be present, and there may be changes in the alignment of the extremity. The patient may experience stiffness after periods of rest.

Characteristic changes occur in certain joints. Bony protuberances on the dorsal surface of the distal interphalangeal joints of the fingers, known as *Heberden's nodes,* may appear (Fig. 42-2). *Bouchard's nodes* on the proximal interphalangeal joints of the fingers are not uncommon. *Coxarthrosis* (degenerative joint disease of the hip) presents with pain in the hip on weight bearing and may progress to include pain in the groin and along the medial side of the knee. Range of motion of the hip becomes markedly limited. When the knee is involved, there is loss of motion, crepitus, and flexion deformity.

Serologic and synovial fluid examinations will be essentially normal. Roentgenographic examinations may reveal narrowing of the joint space, osteophyte formation, and *eburnation* (sclerosis) of subchondral bone.

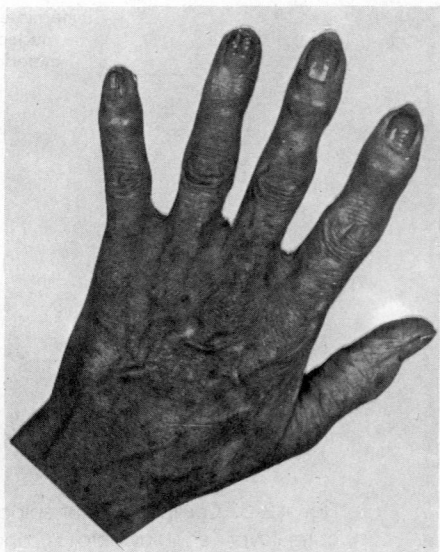

Fig. 42-2. Osteoarthritis of hand. Note enlargement of distal joints of index, middle, and little fingers (Heberden's nodes). (From Brashear, H., and Raney, R.: Shand's handbook of orthopaedic surgery, ed. 9, St. Louis, 1978, The C.V. Mosby Co.)

Intervention

The major objectives of treatment of degenerative joint disease are relief of pain, restoration of joint function, and prevention of disability or further progression of the disease. Attention to posture; loss of unnecessary weight; unloading the painful joints by using ambulatory aids such as canes, crutches, or walkers; altering activities of daily living to avoid particularly painful activities; and the use of external measures such as local heat, prescribed exercises, or traction (p. 954) can be helpful in achieving these objectives. Salicylates, used in combination with these physical measures, seem to be the most useful pharmacologic agents in the relief of the pain of degenerative joint disease. When these measures are not reasonably successful, surgery may be employed both to relieve pain and to correct deformity. Specific procedures available are (1) debridement, (2) arthrodesis, (3) arthroplasty, (4) osteotomy, and (5) total joint replacement. Principles related to the conservative management measures noted above are discussed in Chapter 41; the surgical measures are discussed on p. 1004.

Outcome criteria for the person with degenerative joint disease

The person or significant others can:
1. Explain the alterations that must be made in ADL to avoid excessive use of affected joints.

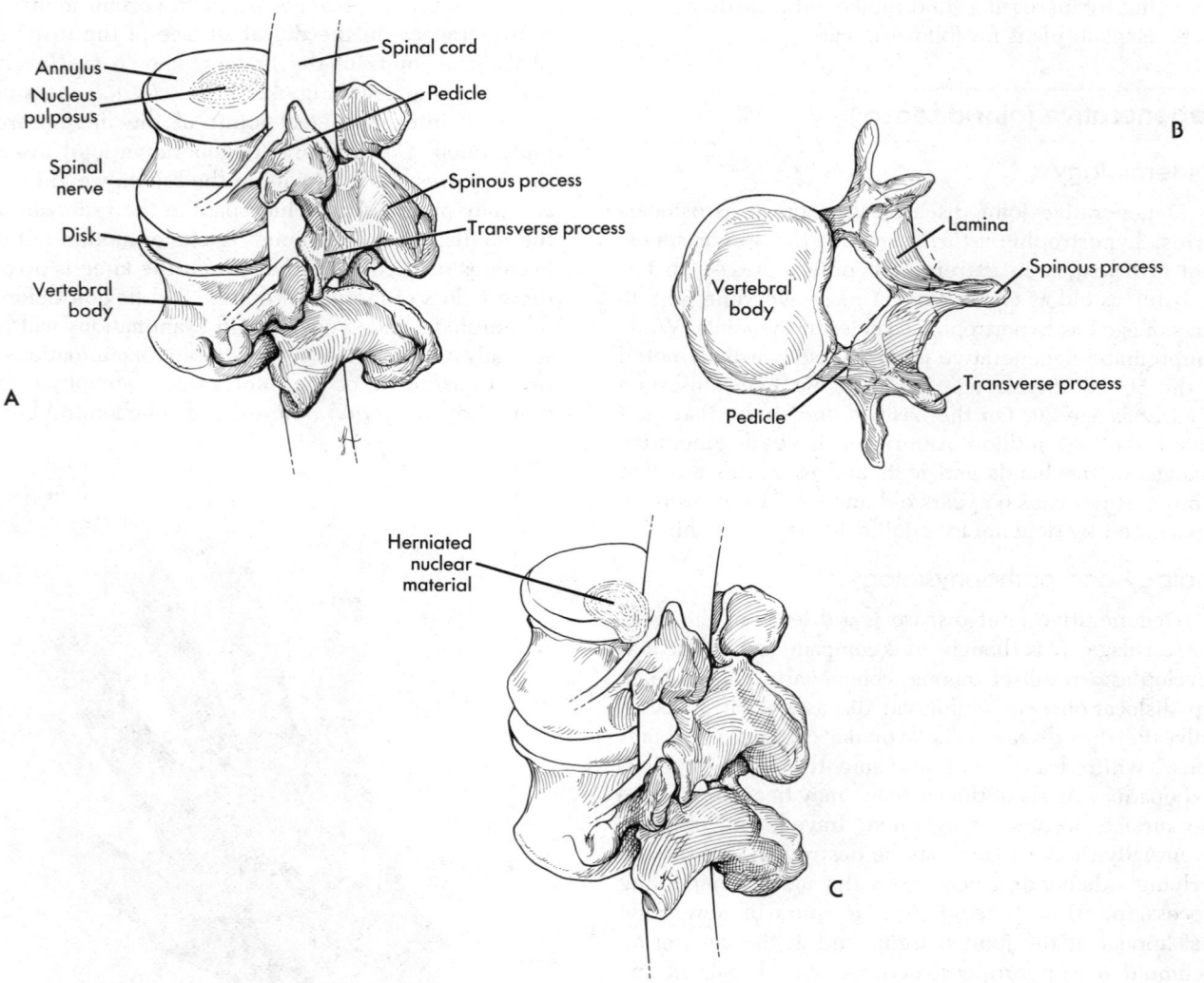

Fig. 42-3. Compression of spinal cord and nerve root. **A,** Disks, composed of cartilaginous outer layer (annulus fibrosus) and a gel-like inner layer (nucleus pulposus), lie between vertebral bodies. Spinal nerves exit the spinal cord laterally just above pedicle. **B,** Laminae compose posterior portion of vertebrae. Each pedicle joins with a lamina; the transverse and spinous processes project from laminae. (Dotted line indicates laminae). **C,** When nucleus pulposus herniates posteriorly through its fibrous covering and posterior longitudinal ligament, it may compress the spinal cord and trap the nerve root. Surgical approach to relieve this compression is through lamina, posterior to transverse process.

2. Explain the importance of losing excessive weight.
3. Review plans for reduction diet.
4. Explain the basic nature of degenerative joint disease.
5. Demonstrate safe use of ambulatory assistive devices.
6. Demonstrate ability to safely perform ADL or to explain how ADL needs will be met.
7. Demonstrate how to safely apply moist heat to painful joints.
8. Explain how medications are to be taken (dosage, what times, side effects, toxic effects).
9. Explain plans for follow-up care.

Degenerative joint disease of the spine

Pathophysiology

Degenerative joint disease of the spine is a common but difficult problem that merits special consideration. The spine has 23 intervertebral disk joints and 46 posterior facet joints, all of which are subjected to stresses and strains in holding the human body upright and moving it about. The vertebrae in the spinal column are articulated in a series of "couplets" that are able to move through an intervertebral disk joint and two posterior facet joints. The intervertebral disks are composed of an outer layer of cartilage called the *anulus fibrosus* and an inner layer of cartilage called the *nucleus pulposus*. The degeneration and dehydration of this cartilage results in a loss of elasticity. The disk normally functions as a shock absorber. As it loses its resiliency, a strong force exerted across the disk can result in herniation of the nucleus through the anulus either posteriorly or laterally. This results in compression of a spinal nerve root and subsequent pain (Fig. 42-3). The facet joints that stabilize the spine are synovial joints, and their articular surfaces are covered with articular cartilage. This means that these joints can be affected by rheumatoid arthritis as well as by degenerative joint disease (Fig. 42-4). Osteophytes developing along the vertebral column can fuse and cause a limitation of motion, usually in the lumbodorsal region. The intervertebral foramina in the cervical spine (C2-3 through C6-7) can become narrowed by spurs, thus creating pressure on the nerve roots in this area and resulting in neurologic symptoms.

Clinical picture

The diagnosis of a herniated disk is usually made on the basis of the history and physical examination. The history of low back pain that is relieved by recumbency and aggravated by flexion of the trunk, coughing, or sneezing is typical. The patient will often complain of sciatic pain radiating down the leg. Some patients, after the initial injury, will have sciatic pain but no pain in their back. Deep pressure over the interspace will usually elicit pain. Straight leg raising with the hip flexed

and the knee extended (a positive Lasègue sign) will produce the sciatic pain. Neurologic signs and symptoms help in determining the level of the disk involved. The sensory and motor changes depend on the nerve root involved.

If the back problem has been long standing, the patient may have some muscle atrophy in the affected leg. Roentgenography of the spine is performed. Myelography may be performed if necessary to confirm the physical findings before surgery or to exclude conditions such as tumors. The most common sites of lumbar herniation are L3-4, L4-5, and L5-S1.

Intervention

Unless there are major neurologic deficits indicating a need for immediate surgery, the patient is usually managed conservatively. (This course of treatment may have been attempted at home before admission.) The patient is placed on bed rest in a bed with a firm mattress and bed boards. Patients with a herniated disk are usually most comfortable when supine with their heads elevated a few degrees and their knees flexed (Fig. 42-5). Beds should be flat when patients are on their sides, and they will probably be most comfortable with pillows between their legs. The patients should be taught to turn themselves in a logrolling fashion: to cross the arms over the chest, bend the uppermost knee to the side to which they wish to turn, and then roll over. This position helps them to maintain good spinal alignment.

If there is any motor nerve loss, a footboard or splint

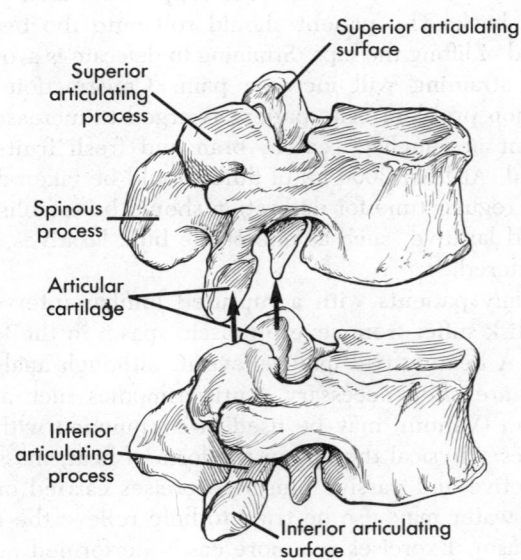

Fig. 42-4. Posterior facet joints of lumbar vertebrae. Each vertebra has four surfaces by which it articulates with its adjacent vertebrae, two on its superior aspect and two on the inferior. Superior articulating surfaces are medially located; the inferior, laterally. These joints are diarthrotic, having a joint capsule with a synovial lining.

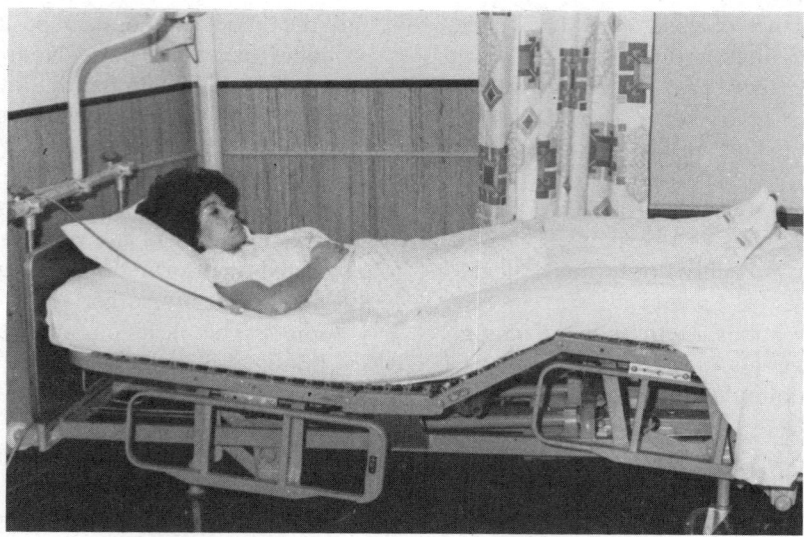

Fig. 42-5. Elevating head of bed 20 to 30 degrees and flexing knees slightly provides comfortable position for patients with acute back pain.

should be used to prevent footdrop. The patient may complain of a burning sensation in his feet because of paresthesia, and a footboard helps by keeping the bedclothes off the feet. If the patient has a sensory nerve loss, hot water bottles or heating pads should not be used on the feet or legs, and other precautions (protection from trauma, avoidance of prolonged pressure to skin surfaces, proper handling during positioning) should be taken to prevent further injury.

A small bedpan should be used with a small towel roll placed directly behind it to support the arch of the lower back. The patient should roll onto the bedpan instead of lifting the hips. Straining to defecate is avoided, since straining will increase pain. Constipation is a common problem. The patient is urged to increase the amount of roughage eaten; bran and fresh fruits are helpful. At least 3000 ml of fluid should be taken daily, and a regular time for defecation should be established. A mild laxative, such as one of the bulk laxatives, may be ordered.

Many patients with a ruptured lumbar intervertebral disk suffer from severe muscle spasm in the lower back. A heating pad may relieve it, although analgesic drugs are often necessary. Antispasmodics such as diazepam (Valium) may be used in conjunction with analgesics. Physical therapy in the form of heat, massage, and active and passive muscle exercises carried out in warm water may also be tried to help relieve the muscle spasm. Exercises are more easily performed in water, and the heat helps to relax muscles. The patient should be transferred to the physical therapy department by stretcher, and extra covers and a towel to wrap around the head if the hair becomes wet should be sent with the patient. Chilling after treatment is to be avoided.

Traction may be ordered to relieve muscle spasm. This is usually accomplished by bilateral Buck's extension (p. 968) or pelvic traction. Patients may begin with short periods in traction and gradually increase their tolerance until they remain in traction most of the time.

Patients with a ruptured disk may be discouraged by the prospects of a long period of bed rest and possible surgery. If they have motor or sensory losses, they worry that they may be unable to walk. To some people, spinal surgery is synonymous with paralysis. Worries about family relationships, finances, loss of a job, and collecting compensation if the injury was sustained at work are common. Nurses, other health care providers, and the patient's spiritual advisor may all be involved in helping to alleviate the patient's fears and anxieties.

If improvement is shown on bed rest, as occurs with 90% of the patients for whom this is the first occurrence, a brace or corset may be ordered to provide external support for the spine. This support may be needed for several months or until the patient is asymptomatic. The external supports are discarded as soon as possible, since prolonged use fosters muscle weakness, which then increases the load on the vertebral column.

The principles of body mechanics should be taught and demonstrated to the patient, since particular care will need to be taken in lifting. Some patients may have to change their type of work. Movements and positions that cause poor alignment of the spinal column and put a strain on the injured nerves should be avoided. A firm, straight chair should be used instead of an overstuffed one. (See p. 949 for a description of an ideal chair.) The knees should not be crossed or the feet or legs elevated on a footstool unless the knees are flexed. It is inadvis-

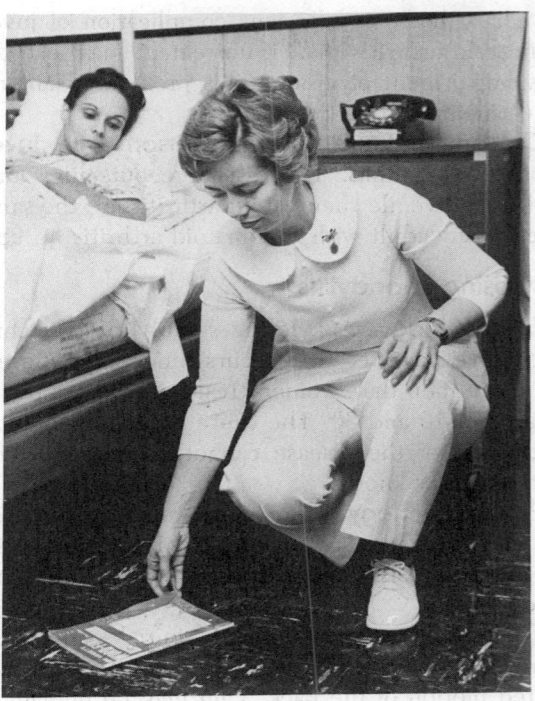

Fig. 42-6. Good body mechanics being used to pick up object from floor. Note that nurse's back is straight while her knees and hips are flexed sharply.

able for the patient to drive a car, since this activity would necessitate stretching the legs. Stairs should be climbed as infrequently as possible, and great care should be taken in walking over rough ground or in stepping off curbs to avoid sudden twisting of the back. When walking, the pelvis should be tilted forward to decrease lordosis of the lumbar spine. If a tub bath must be taken, the knees should be kept flexed. However, getting in and out of the tub may aggravate the symptoms, and showers are preferable. A warm shower before bed and on arising often helps to reduce discomfort. In picking things up off the floor, the patient should assume a squatting posture with the knees bent and the back held straight (Fig. 42-6). Anything weighing more than 2.25 kg (5 lb) should not be carried.

When the acute episode has subsided, the physician may prescribe exercises designed to strengthen the back and abdominal muscles to decrease the load carried by the vertebral column.

Outcome criteria for the person with degenerative joint disease of the spine or a herniated disk

The person or significant others can:
1. Explain the basic nature of the disorder.
2. Explain the alterations that must be made in ADL to avoid activities and positions that will cause pain or further damage to the back (bending at the waist, straight leg raising, lifting).

3. Demonstrate how to put on and take off the prescribed brace or corset.
4. Demonstrate exercise program (if prescribed).
5. Demonstrate how traction will be set up at home (if prescribed).
6. Explain how medications are to be taken (dosages, what times, side effects, toxic effects).
7. State symptoms that would indicate the need for immediate medical consultation.
8. Explain plans for follow-up care.

Traumatic or neurogenic disorders

Neuropathic arthropathy

Epidemiology. Neuropathic arthropathy (Charcot's joints) is a chronic, progressive degeneration of joints resulting from a disturbance in sensory innervation of the joints. Men over 40 years of age are most commonly affected.

Pathophysiology. The primary neurologic disorder (tabes dorsalis, diabetic neuropathy, meningomyelocele) causes loss of proprioception at the joint. As a result, the supporting structures around the joint relax and the joint becomes unstable. The patient, having lost the ability to protect the joint, overuses or misuses it while remaining relatively unaware of pain. Joints most often affected are the knees, tarsal areas, and lower vertebrae. The primary neurologic disorder will determine the specific joints that are involved.

Clinical picture. The first symptoms that may be noticed are enlargement or instability of the joint. While there may be some pain, the pain is much less than would be expected when compared to the extent of the joint effusion and destruction. Swelling, warmth, and tenderness may be present, and the joint is hypermobile. As loss of cartilage, overgrowth of bone, and formation of loose bodies in the joint progress, enlargement of the joint increases and crepitation will be present.

Intervention. Management usually includes bracing or splinting to afford support for the affected joint through immobilization. Further support and protection may be achieved by limiting weight bearing through the use of assistive ambulatory devices such as crutches. (See Chapter 41 for discussion of bracing and other forms of joint protection.)

Outcome criteria for the person with neuropathic arthropathy. The person or significant others can:
1. Explain the basic nature of the joint disorder.
2. Demonstrate appropriate joint protection techniques.
3. Demonstrate how to apply, take off, and care for the prescribed brace.
4. Explain plans for follow-up care.

Polyarthritis of unknown cause

For a discussion of rheumatoid arthritis, see p. 984.

Juvenile rheumatoid arthritis

Epidemiology. Juvenile rheumatoid arthritis is generally considered to be rheumatoid arthritis that occurs before the age of 16. As with rheumatoid arthritis, the incidence of this disease is greater among girls than boys. Onset of the disease can occur as early as 6 weeks of age, but more typically it occurs between the ages of 2 to 5 years and 9 to 12 years.[3]

Pathophysiology. Juvenile rheumatoid arthritis may be a more severe systemic disease than adult rheumatoid arthritis. An acute febrile illness and polyarthralgia (pain in many joints) may precede the onset of frank arthritis. When the presence of arthritis is preceded or accompanied by fever, hepatosplenomegaly, lymphadenopathy, a maculopapular erythematous rash, pleuritis, pericarditis, and pronounced leukocytosis, the disease is called *Still's disease*.[3] In juvenile rheumatoid arthritis, joint involvement may vary from all joints to one joint, often the knee.

Clinical picture. Premature closure of the epiphyses, failure of development of the cervical vertebrae and jaw, widening of the phalanges, and impaired development of the head of the femur and acetabulum are common manifestations of the disease. As a result, normal growth and development are also impaired. The deformities that result can be quite severe and seriously impair normal function.

Intervention. General management considerations, rest, relief of pain, and so on are the same as for adults (p. 949). Specific attention must be paid to proper positioning, splinting, an individually prescribed program of exercise, and avoidance of highly active and contact sports. Additionally, the child's family must have an understanding of the disease. Their expectations of the child to move, perform activities of daily living, and cooperate with the treatment program should be neither too great nor too small. Particularly when the child experiences pain, concerned parents may not insist on the child following the treatment regimen. Results of such lapses may be the development of contractures, loss of function in some joints, and overdependence on the parents. Such problems are difficult, if not impossible, to overcome. Therefore the family needs as much support and attention from the health care team as the patient.

Salicylates are the drug of choice in the treatment of juvenile rheumatoid arthritis. The corticosteroids are reserved for patients who have severe disease that has not responded to salicylates alone or for those patients who have evidence of systemic involvement (myocarditis or vasculitis). Iridocyclitis (inflammation of the iris and ciliary body) is a serious complication of juvenile rheumatoid arthritis that, if untreated, may lead to serious impairment of vision. This problem is amenable to treatment with corticosteroids.

Outcome criteria for the person with juvenile rheumatoid arthritis. The discharge outcomes for the child with juvenile rheumatoid arthritis are the same as those for any adult with rheumatoid arthritis (p. 987).

Ankylosing spondylitis

Epidemiology. Ankylosing spondylitis is a chronic progressive disorder that occurs nine times more frequently in men than women. It usually occurs between the ages of 10 and 30. The cause is unknown, and the progression of the disease cannot be stopped by any treatment now known.

Pathophysiology. The major joints involved are the hips and the sacroiliac joints. A chronic synovitis followed by fibrosis then ankylosis is the pattern of involvement.

Clinical picture. The patient's initial symptoms are aching and stiffness. This gives way to pain and restricted motion of the back. Pain may be intermittent. Fusion of the sacroiliac joints and spine up through the cervical vertebrae may occur over a period of 10 to 20 years; and as a result, the patient may develop either a "poker-back" deformity or a kyphosis at the cervicodorsal junction (Fig. 42-7).

Roentgenograms are most helpful in delineating this condition, since the findings are usually specific. Bony growths, called *syndesmophytes*, that bridge the adjacent vertebrae give the appearance of a "bamboo spine."

Intervention. Intervention for patients with ankylosing spondylitis includes attention to the principles of rest, proper positioning and posture, postural exercises, heat application, and in some instances external support through splinting or bracing. Spinal osteotomy or hip arthroplasty might be necessary for patients with severe symptoms. Salicylates are used to decrease inflammation, and in some instances where stronger antiinflammatory agents are needed, phenylbutazone (Butazolidin) or indomethacin (Indocin) may be tried. The objectives of treatment are to relieve pain, achieve and maintain the best possible alignment of the spine, strengthen the paraspinal muscles, and prevent interference with breathing capacity.[3] See Chapter 41 for a full discussion of these management considerations.

Outcome criteria for the person with ankylosing spondylitis. The person or significant others can:
1. Explain the basic nature of the disease.
2. Demonstrate the prescribed program of postural exercises.
3. Demonstrate how to apply heat to back and hips.
4. Explain how medications are to be taken (dosage, what times, side effects, toxic effects).

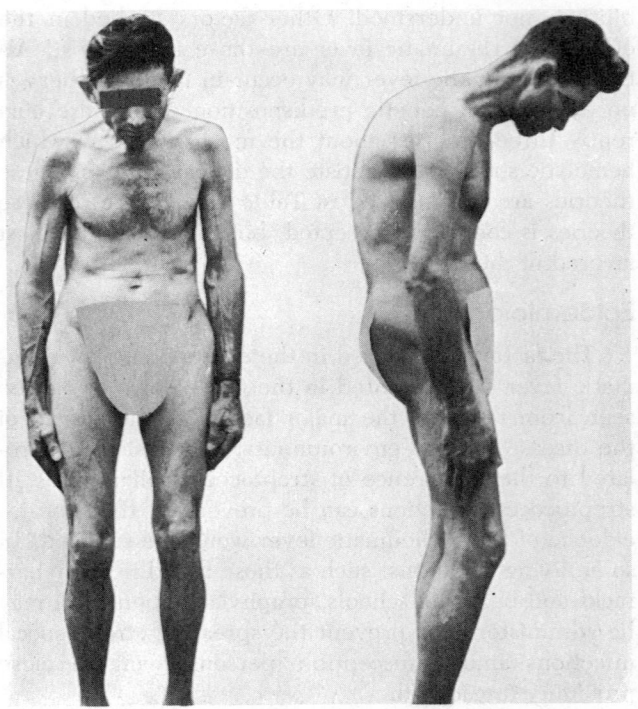

Fig. 42-7. Ankylosing spondylitis in 46-year-old man with ankylosis of entire spine in faulty position. (From Brashear, H., and Raney, R.: Shand's handbook of orthopaedic surgery, ed. 9, St. Louis, 1978, The C.V. Mosby Co.)

5. Describe signs or symptoms that would indicate need for immediate medical consultation.
6. Explain plans for follow-up care.

Psoriatic arthritis

Epidemiology. Psoriatic arthritis is a complicated problem. As many as 3% to 4% of patients with psoriasis (p. 1846) have some inflammatory joint disease. However, the epidemiology of the disease is unclear, as psoriatic arthritis can exist for a time in the absence of skin lesions.

Clinical picture. The interphalangeal and metatarsophalangeal joints of the feet and the distal interphalangeal joints of the fingers are commonly involved, usually in an asymmetric pattern, frequently only two or three joints at a time. Spine and sacroiliac joint involvement as spondylitis is common.[40] The activity of the joint disease may vary with that of the skin disease, and involvement of the nails is common. The nails become discolored, pitted, thickened, and begin to loosen from their beds. This loosening process (oncholysis) begins at the free edge of the nail and progresses gradually back to the root of the nail.[40] When other joints are involved (knee, ankle, and so on), the involvement is consistent with that of rheumatoid arthritis.

Patients with psoriatic arthritis usually can be grouped into one of several distinct categories: (1) those with asymmetric peripheral polyarthritis, usually with involvement of the distal interphalangeal joints of the fingers or the interphalangeal joints of the toes; (2) those with *arthritis mutilans;* (3) those with a pattern of involvement that cannot be distinguished from rheumatoid arthritis except that the swelling of the small joints in psoriatic arthritis appears sausage shaped; (4) those with symptoms of spondylitis; (5) those who have skin and nail changes preceding or occurring simultaneously with articular disease; and (6) those whose joint manifestations precede skin and nail changes by months or years.[40] With arthritis mutilans, areas of or whole bones (usually the phalanges) may be destroyed, causing a "telescoping" of the digit.

Intervention. Management measures for patients with psoriatic arthritis are limited generally to the physical measures available for the management of other forms of arthritis: rest, local heat, and splinting (see Chapter 41). Nonsteroidal antiinflammatory drugs such as aspirin or indomethacin (Indocin) are helpful. Antimalarials are specifically avoided as they may aggravate the psoriatic rash. The skin lesions can be treated with local applications of coal tar or steroid creams. Ultraviolet light is helpful.[40]

Outcome criteria for the person with psoriatic arthritis. The discharge outcomes for the person with psoriatic arthritis are essentially the same as for the patient with rheumatoid arthritis (p. 957). Additionally, the patient or significant others need to be able to explain the use of the various topical medications prescribed to control the psoriatic lesions.

Reiter's syndrome

Epidemiology and etiology. Reiter's syndrome mainly affects young adult men. Its cause is unknown, but its occurence usually follows exposure to venereal disease. Since it has also been associated with the occurrence of bacillary dysentery, there is some thought that it may be caused by an inflammation of the prostate or the bowel.

Clinical picture. Symptoms usually include urethritis, conjunctivitis, and arthritis. The arthritis is generally asymmetrical and mainly involves the large joints for example, the knee joints. When the sacroiliac joints are involved, a form of the spondylitis may result. A skin condition known as *keratodermia blennorrhagicum* may be present, with lesions resembling psoriatic pustules appearing chiefly over the palms of the hand and soles of the feet. Small lesions of the glans penis (circinata balanitis) may also be present.

While the disease runs its course in 6 weeks to 6 months, it recurs in about 50% of patients. Joint deformities may occur when the disease runs a recurrent course, and spondylitis may remain active for many years.

Intervention. Management techniques are designed

to provide relief of pain and inflammation in involved joints. (See Chapter 41 for specific measures.) Antiinflammatory agents such as salicylates can be used. Severe inflammation may require the use of phenylbutazone (Butazolidin), indomethacin (Indocin), or systemic corticosteroids. Local applications of steroid creams can be used to clear skin lesions.[40]

Outcome criteria for the person with Reiter's syndrome. The person or significant others can:
1. Explain the basic nature of the disease.
2. Describe the program of rest to be observed until the disease has run its course.
3. Explain the dose, side effects, and toxic effects of the prescribed medications.
4. Explain plans for follow-up care.

Rheumatic fever

Rheumatic fever is a delayed sequela of an upper respiratory tract infection (usually pharyngitis) caused by group A beta-hemolytic (β-hemolytic) streptococci. It is most common in children between the ages of 5 and 15, although it can occur at any age. The manifestations of rheumatic fever include *migratory arthritis, carditis, chorea, erythema marginatum,* and *subcutaneous nodules*. Recurrences of rheumatic fever are common following untreated streptococcal infections in persons with a previous history of the disease. Rheumatic fever can be prevented by early diagnosis and appropriate antimicrobial treatment of streptococcal pharyngitis.[4]

Etiology

There has been a dramatic decline in the incidence of rheumatic fever over the past 50 years. The usual course of the disease occurs in three phases: (1) streptococcal infection (usually pharyngitis), (2) latent period of 1 to 5 weeks, and (3) acute rheumatic fever. Rheumatic fever is believed to be a *reaction* to the streptococcal infection and not a continuation of the infectious process. During the latent period signs and symptoms are usually absent even though streptococci may be present in the throat. Despite the presence of streptococci in the throat, repeated throat cultures may be negative.[4] There are more than 70 serologic types of group A streptococci on the basis of serologically distinct M proteins (see Chapter 14). It is now known that immunity to streptococcal infections is M-type specific, and infection with one type does not confer immunity to another type. Since some children have recurrent streptococcal infections, the possibility of repeated attacks of rheumatic fever exists. Moreover, there appears to be an increased susceptibility to repeated attacks of rheumatic fever in children who have had an attack of rheumatic fever. The reason for this suscepti-

bility is not understood. Other factors studied in the etiology of rheumatic fever are those in the host. Although rheumatic fever may occur in families, there is no evidence of genetic predisposition. There are currently three theories about the mechanisms by which hemolytic streptococci initiate the disease process. These theories are summarized in Table 42-2. None of these theories is completely accepted, but the first is the most favored of the three.

Epidemiology

The factors considered in the epidemiology of rheumatic fever are presented in the box below. As can be seen from the box, the major factors in the spread of the disease are the environmental and host factors related to the occurrence of streptococcal pharyngitis. If streptococcal infections can be prevented, then the incidence of acute rheumatic fever would be reduced. In some living situations, such as those found in army barracks and boarding schools, prophylactic penicillin may be administered to prevent the spread of streptococcal infections among susceptible persons living in close proximity to each other.

Clinical picture

The attack of rheumatic fever occurs several weeks after a streptococcal infection. The latent period between the streptococcal pharyngitis and acute rheumatic fever varies from 1 to 5 weeks. It is not uncommon for the patient to have no recollection of having a sore throat. However, careful questioning of the patient, and the parents when a child is the patient, often reveals a history of a sore throat a few weeks previously. Because of the variability of the signs and symptoms of rheumatic fever, the Jones criteria are used as

TABLE 42-2. Suggested theories of etiology of rheumatic fever

Theory	Support for theory
Immunologic response or hypersensitivity reaction to streptococcal antigens, or both	Patients have exaggerated response to streptococcal antigens; most (not all) have a higher antistreptolysin O response than those with streptococcal pharyngitis who do not develop rheumatic fever
Rheumatic fever is a direct response to streptococcal toxins occurring at time of streptococcal infection	Little evidence for or against this theory
Persistence of streptococcus in body during rheumatic fever	Little bacteriologic evidence of direct infection of heart or other organs involved in rheumatic fever

a guide in establishing the diagnosis. The *Jones criteria,* which include major and minor manifestations of acute rheumatic fever, are presented in Table 42-3. One of the major criteria listed by Jones along with some of the minor criteria must be present for the diagnosis of acute rheumatic fever to be made. The onset is usually sud-

EPIDEMIOLOGY OF STREPTOCOCCAL PHARYNGITIS AND ACUTE RHEUMATIC FEVER*

Age:	5-15 yr
Peak:	6-8 yr
Sex:	No difference
Season:	Late winter and early spring with some increase after start of school in fall
Geography:	Most common in temperate zones, but increased reports of rheumatic fever from Africa, India, and Southeast Asia
Living conditions:	Overcrowding as seen in crowded tenements, army barracks, and boarding schools
Prevalence in the United States:	Estimated incidence of rheumatic fever is 50,000-100,000; disease is not reportable in all states so true figures are not known; schoolchildren—0.7-1.6 per 1000; freshmen college students and servicemen—6-9 per 1000

*From Beeson, P.B., et al.: Cecil's textbook of medicine, ed. 15, Philadelphia, 1979, W.B. Saunders Co.

TABLE 42-3. Clinical and laboratory manifestations of acute rheumatic fever (Jones criteria)

Major manifestations	Minor manifestations
1. Carditis	1. Clinical
2. Carditis	a. Previous rheumatic fever or rheumatic heart disease
2. Polyarthritis	b. Arthralgia
3. Chorea	c. Fever
4. Erythema marginatum	2. Laboratory
5. Subcutaneous nodules	a. Acute phase—elevated erythrocyte sedimentation rate, elevated C-reactive protein, leukocytosis
	b. Prolonged P-R interval
	3. Evidence of preceding streptococcal infection (increased ASO or other streptococcal antibodies, positive throat culture for group A streptococcus, recent scarlet fever)

den with the first symptoms being fever and joint pain. Some persons have a high fever, but often the fever is moderate or low grade. Other symptoms that may be present are sore throat, epistaxis, and severe abdominal pain and vomiting in children, which may be suggestive of appendicitis.

Intervention

There is no specific therapy for the treatment of acute rheumatic fever. Measures that are prescribed are those that will promote the natural healing mechanisms of the body. The management for the arthritis of rheumatic fever is the same as for other forms of arthritis and includes rest, proper positioning, and other supportive measures, which are discussed in Chapter 41. Bed rest is always instituted and continued until the acute symptoms of arthritis and carditis are under control. In mild cases without carditis the symptoms usually subside in 3 to 4 weeks. When severe arthritis and carditis are present, the natural course of the disease is 2 to 3 months.

All persons with acute rheumatic fever should be treated with penicillin to eradicate the streptococcus from the pharynx. Penicillin is the drug of choice and is used unless there is a history of allergy to it. The usual dose is 300,000 units of procaine penicillin G once daily for children and twice daily for adults for 10 days. Alternately, long-acting benzathine penicillin in a single dose of 1.2 million units may be prescribed. Oral penicillin, 200,000 units four times a day for 10 days, is also acceptable therapy if it can be ensured that the drug is taken without fail. For persons allergic to penicillin, erythromycin, 250 mg four times a day for 10 days, is given. Sulfonamides are not effective in treating acute rheumatic fever but may be prescribed for long-term prophylactic follow-up. All patients with rheumatic fever should receive prophylactic therapy to prevent recurrent streptococcal infections. Continuous prophylaxis is begun as soon as the initial 10-day course of therapy is completed. The prophylaxis for some children will continue well into adulthood. The drugs used for continuous prophylaxis are listed in Table 42-4.

Aspirin is usually effective in reducing fever and joint pain. It is given in high doses—100 mg/kg of body weight or in doses sufficient to achieve blood levels of 25 mg/ 100 ml.[40] In addition to aspirin, steroids are often prescribed, especially if carditis is present.

Observations and care considerations for patients receiving high doses of salicylates should be adhered to (p. 957). In the presence of the febrile condition, fluids are usually given in large amounts (3 to 4 L daily). Further, since these patients often become very bored and restless, especially when confined to bed for long periods of time, those caring for them may be taxed to develop diversional activities in accordance with their physical limitations. The American Heart Association

TABLE 42-4. Drugs prescribed for continuous prophylaxis for rheumatic fever

Drug*	Comments
Benzathine penicillin G, 1.2 million units every 30 days	Discomfort of monthly injection weighed against assurance that blood level is maintained; especially important for persons who cannot be relied on to take oral drugs daily
Sulfonamides daily, 1 g sulfadiazine or other sulfapyrimidine daily	Toxic reactions occur rarely; occasional failure of chemoprophylaxis; patient must be committed to take daily dose without interruption
Oral penicillin G, 200,000-250,000 units bid	Not any more effective than sulfadiazine; even twice the daily dose is no more effective than sulfadiazine; patient must be committed to taking drug daily; more expensive than sulfadiazine

*Listed in order of preference.

publishes many booklets that are helpful in understanding rheumatic fever. One of the most useful is *Home Care of the Child with Rheumatic Fever*.

Usually either aspirin or steroid therapy is withdrawn gradually over 1 to 2 weeks. Commonly, "clinical rebound" occurs after therapy is withdrawn. The most common symptoms of rebound are *fever, arthritis*, and *tachycardia*. Symptoms of rebound usually disappear in 5 to 10 days without reinstitution of therapy. If cardiac symptoms worsen, therapy will be reinstituted and continued for another 3 to 4 weeks.

Ambulation is begun after symptoms subside, and full activity, except vigorous exercise, is permitted in 3 to 4 weeks.

Prevention

In addition to prophylactic therapy, which has already been discussed, the prevention and adequate treatment of streptococcal infections are important. Populations at risk for development of streptococcal infections include military recruits, schoolchildren, schoolteachers, and medical personnel. Persons who have rheumatic heart disease should be on chemoprophylaxis for life. It also should be stressed that persons in late middle age can have a recurrence of rheumatic fever following streptococcal pharyngitis.[4]

Outcome criteria for the person with rheumatic fever

The person or significant others can:
1. Explain the program of rest to be observed until the acute symptoms have subsided.
2. Explain the importance of continuing prophylactic antibiotic therapy indefinitely.

3. Explain the doses, side effects, and toxic effects of prescribed medications.
4. Describe signs and symptoms that would indicate need for immediate medical consultation (fever, joint pain, any new symptom).
5. Explain the plans for regular follow-up care, including when and how to receive the intramuscular injection of penicillin or a supply of sulfadiazine or oral penicillin.

Nonarticular rheumatism

Nonarticular rheumatic diseases include those disorders in which the supportive structures and structures located near the joints are involved, but the joints themselves are not involved, except by the limitations imposed by the supportive structures.

Fibrositis

Fibrositis, or fibromyositis, is a common symptom complex. Its cause is unknown and its course seems self-limited. Pain and stiffness in the neck, shoulder girdle, and extremities worsen with activity and subside with rest. Occasionally there are specific areas of tenderness and ill-defined nodules. Psychogenic factors, particularly a chronic tension state, may be important to some patients.[36]

Intervention. Management is generally related to the specific symptoms. Rest, analgesics, and physical therapy may be utilized (see Chapter 41).

Outcome criteria for the person with fibrositis. The person or significant others can:
1. Explain the program of rest to be observed until acute symptoms have subsided.
2. Explain the doses, side effects, and toxic effects of prescribed medications.
3. Explain exercise program (if prescribed).
4. Explain plans for follow-up care.

Tenosynovitis

Tenosynovitis is a nonspecific inflammation of tendon sheaths. It usually involves tendon sheaths located around the wrists, ankles, or shoulders. Symptoms may vary from local tenderness to inability to move the joint because of pain. The tendon sheath may become thickened and may even prevent free motion of the joint. This disorder, the cause of which is not known, is generally idiopathic but may be found in association with rheumatoid arthritis. When it is associated with rheumatoid arthritis, granulation tissue invades the tendon as well as the tendon sheath and weakens the tendon. The tendon may rupture, requiring surgical intervention.

Intervention. Tenosynovitis tends to be self-limiting. Symptomatic relief may be obtained through rest, splinting, and antiinflammatory agents such as indomethacin (Indocin) or phenylbutazone (Butazolidin) (p. 958). Steroid injections into affected joints are very helpful in quickly relieving symptoms.

Outcome criteria for the person with tenosynovitis. The person or significant others can:

1. Explain the program of rest to be observed until the acute symptoms have subsided.
2. Demonstrate how to use prescribed splinting device.
3. Explain the doses, side effects, and toxic effects of prescribed medications.
4. Explain plans for follow-up care.

Bursitis

Bursitis, or inflammation of the bursa, may be acute or chronic. It usually is caused by trauma, strain, and overuse of the joint with which the bursa is associated. The shoulder bursa is most often affected and may be exceedingly troublesome. Severe pain can occur, especially on movement of the joint.

Intervention. Management of patients with bursitis includes rest for the involved area. Antiinflammatory agents such as salicylates, phenylbutazone, or indomethacin usually control symptoms. In some instances adrenocorticosteroids are injected into the bursa. Application of cold during the early acute phase may help to relieve discomfort. Much of the discomfort at this time is caused by the presence of additional fluid in the bursa; therefore heat is avoided as this increases the fluid exudate during the early inflammatory period. Occasionally, large calcium deposits are present, and these can be surgically removed. Care of patients receiving these forms of treatment is discussed in Chapter 41.

Outcome criteria for the person with bursitis. The person or significant others can:

1. Explain the program of rest to be observed until acute symptoms have subsided.
2. Explain modifications in ADL to avoid overuse of the joint associated with the inflamed bursa.
3. Explain the doses, side effects, and toxic effects of the prescribed medications.
4. Explain plans for follow-up care.

Carpal tunnel syndrome

Carpal tunnel syndrome is caused by pressure being exerted on the median nerve at the wrist. The median nerve passes through a tunnel bounded by the carpal bones dorsally and the transverse carpal ligament volarly (Fig. 42-8). Flexor tendons run through the tunnel parallel to the median nerve. The pressure on the nerve may derive from trauma or swelling of the tendon sheaths caused by other processes like rheumatoid arthritis. Generally the tenosynovitis is localized and not associated with any systemic disease. This condition is most common in middle-aged women.

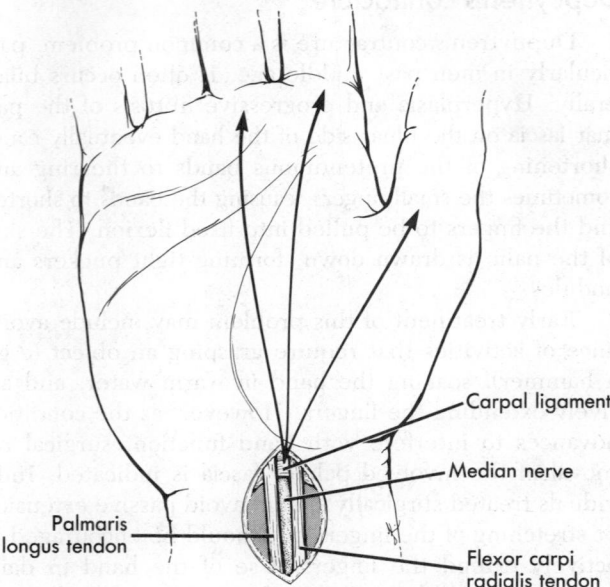

Fig. 42-8. Carpal tunnel syndrome. Volar aspect of wrist retracted to demonstrate position of median nerve. Distribution of median nerve is to thumb and first two fingers. (Adapted from Compare, E.L.: Orthopaedic surgery, Chicago, 1974, Year Book Medical Publishers, Inc.)

The patient will complain of dyesthesia, paresthesia, and hypesthesia in the middle three fingers. These complaints will usually increase when there has been forced flexion of the hand for long periods, as in knitting. The symptoms can be elicited by tapping the median nerve at the wrist (Tinel's sign). Referred pain to the upper extremity is common.[4] Atrophy of the thenar eminence (the padded area of the palm below the base of the thumb) may be present in late disease.[40]

Intervention. Rest, splinting of the wrist, local steroid injections, or, finally, surgery (release of the transverse carpal ligament to decompress the median nerve) are treatment measures that can be employed. Often the conservative measures are all that are needed. Rest, splinting, and steroid injections are discussed in Chapter 41. If surgery is performed, active use of the hand is encouraged as soon as possible following the surgery.

Outcome criteria for the person with carpal tunnel syndrome. The person or significant others can:

1. Explain the program of rest to be observed until acute symptoms subside.
2. Demonstrate how to apply and take off splint (if prescribed).
3. Demonstrate range of motion of wrist (if surgery has been performed.)
4. Demonstrate care of the surgical wound (if surgery has been performed).
5. Explain plans for follow-up care.

Dupuytren's contracture

Dupuytren's contracture is a common problem, particularly in men past middle age. It often occurs bilaterally. Hyperplasia and progressive fibrosis of the palmar fascia on the ulnar side of the hand eventually cause shortening of the pretendinous bands to the ring and sometimes the small fingers, causing the bands to shorten and the fingers to be pulled into fixed flexion. The skin of the palm is drawn down, forming tight puckers and nodules.

Early treatment of this problem may include avoidance of activities that require grasping an object (e.g., a hammer), soaking the hand in warm water, and actively extending the fingers. However, as the condition advances to interfere with hand function, surgical removal of the involved palmar fascia is indicated. Individuals treated surgically should avoid passive extension or stretching of the fingers but should be encouraged to actively extend the fingers. Use of the hand in daily activities should begin 2 to 3 days postoperatively.

Outcome criteria for the person with Dupuytren's contracture. The person or significant others can:

1. Explain what activities are to be avoided during the developmental stages of the problem.
2. Explain how hand soaks are to be done.
3. Demonstrate active extension exercises of the fingers.
4. Demonstrate care of the surgical wound (if surgery is performed).
5. Explain limitations of activity to be observed postoperatively.
6. Explain plans for follow-up care.

Rheumatic disease associated with known infectious agents: bacterial arthritis

Epidemiology

Bacterial arthritis is the result of invasion of the synovial membrane by microorganisms, most often gonococci, meningococci, staphylococci, coliforms, salmonellae, and *Haemophilus influenzae*. Factors that predispose to such infections are a high degree of susceptibility on the part of the patient, recent joint surgery or trauma, intraarticular injections, and rheumatoid arthritis.

Pathophysiology and clinical picture

The synovial tissues respond to bacterial invasion by becoming inflamed. The joint cavity may become involved, and pus will be present in the synovial membrane and the synovial fluid. If allowed to progress, the infection will cause abscesses in the synovium and subchondral bone and will destroy cartilage. Ankylosis of the joint may result. The patient will complain of pain, swelling, and tenderness of the joint.

Joint aspirations are helpful in making a diagnosis if

the presence of organisms can be demonstrated in the synovial fluid. Joint fluid white cell counts will be high, and glucose content of synovial fluid may be reduced. Roentgenograms taken days to weeks after onset of the infection may reveal loss of joint space and lytic changes in bone.

Intervention

Untreated joint infections can result in damage to contiguous bone and in osteomyelitis. Antibiotic therapy should be specific to the organism that is present. Rest or immobilization of the joint is necessary in the initial stages of the infection and may help control pain or prevent deformity. To prevent contracture the patient is urged to move the affected joint as soon as the infection subsides and motion can be tolerated. Local heat is *not* generally used in the presence of infection, as it may increase the inflammatory process.[40] Surgical drainage or a system of irrigation and drainage may be employed if the infection does not respond to antibiotic therapy or if osteomyelitis is present. Death, though rare, can result if there is dissemination of the infection. The patient is usually hospitalized until the infection is cleared, and active range of motion in the involved joint can be resumed.

Outcome criteria for the person with bacterial arthritis

The person or significant others can:
1. Demonstrate exercises (if prescribed).
2. Demonstrate how to use safely ambulatory assistive devices (if prescribed).
3. Explain the dosages and side effects of antibiotics (if prescribed).
4. State how long antibiotic therapy is to be continued (if prescribed).
5. Explain plans for follow-up care.

Rheumatic disease associated with known or strongly suspected biochemical or endocrine abnormalities: gout

Epidemiology

Gout or gouty arthritis is a metabolic disorder that affects men eight to nine times more frequently than women. It can occur at any age, the peak age of onset occurring in the fifth decade.[36] Eighty-five percent of all patients with gout have a genetic or familial tendency to develop the disease.

Pathophysiology and clinical picture

Prolonged hyperuricemia (elevated serum uric acid levels) caused by a metabolic problem in synthesizing purines or by poor renal excretion of uric acid leads to the formation of urate crystals in the synovial tissue. The inflammatory process that results is extremely rapid,

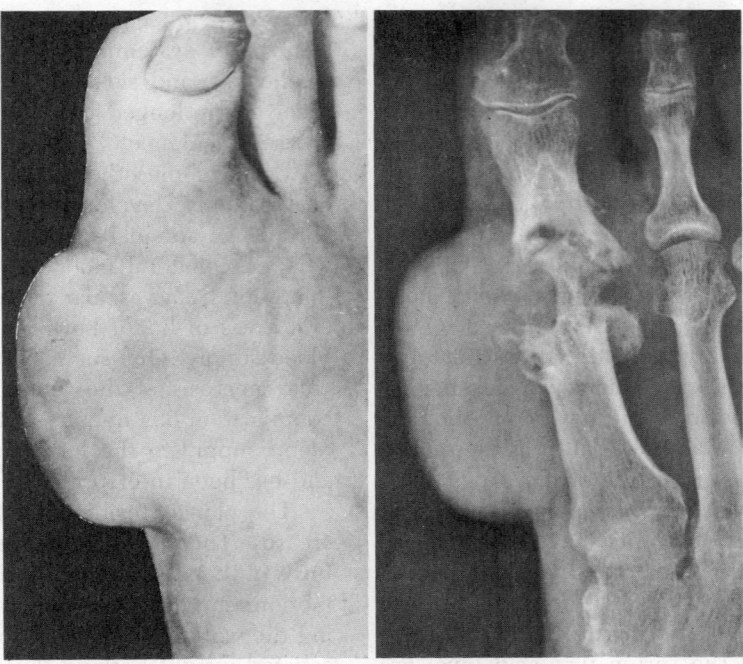

Fig. 42-9. Gout of long duration. Tophaceous mass at base of great toe, as well as destructive bone and joint changes shown in roentgenogram, are associated with extensive urate deposits. (From Brashear, H., and Raney, R.: Shand's handbook of orthopaedic surgery, ed. 9, St. Louis, 1978, The C.V. Mosby Co.)

occurring over a few hours. Gout is a chronic diathesis, but patients who have it will have acute symptoms of pain, swelling, and erythema in the involved joints. Typically the great toe is involved (the first metatarsophalangeal joint), but other joints, such as the ankles and knees, may also be affected. The pain is so severe that the patient may not tolerate even the weight of a sheet over the joint. Renal damage may occur, especially if recurrent uric acid stones have been present. Between attacks of gout, the patient may be asymptomatic, but repeated attacks can occur with gradually increased frequency if the disease is untreated. Patients with gouty symptoms may develop *tophi,* or deposits of monosodium urate in their tissues. These consist of a core of monosodium urate with a surrounding inflammatory reaction. Patients with tophaceous deposits tend to have more frequent and more severe episodes of gouty arthritis (Fig. 42-9).

Laboratory studies will indicate an elevated serum uric acid, normal or increased urinary uric acid over a 24-hour period, and the presence of monosodium urate monohydrate crystals in the synovial fluid and in the tophi.

Intervention

The management of patients is directed toward control of acute attacks and prevention of recurrent attacks and tophaceous deposits (interval therapy). In an *acute attack,* treatment consists of pain relief and rest of the affected limb. Medications such as colchicine, phenylbutazone (Butazolidin), and indomethacin (Indocin) are used to reduce pain. Colchicine is the standard drug used in the treatment of acute gout. When an acute attack of gout is imminent, the usual treatment is oral administration of 1.2 mg (2 tablets) of the drug initially followed by 0.6 mg (1 tablet) each hour until nausea, vomiting, or diarrhea develops, or until joint pain is relieved. No more than 6.0 to 8.0 mg is given for an acute attack. Colchicine may be given intravenously in doses of 1.0 to 3.0 mg in saline over a 10-minute period. This dose can be repeated in 4 to 6 hours if necessary. No more than 4.0 mg should be given within 24 hours.[4] Colchicine is not given to patients with uremia since the drug is excreted by the kidney. Camphorated tincture of opium (paregoric) is usually prescribed for the diarrhea associated with oral colchicine use.

Interval therapy to prevent the chronic manifestations of gout is directed toward reducing the body pool of urates and serum uric acid. The presence of tophi, recurrent acute gouty arthritis, or significant asymptomatic hyperuricemia (over 9 mg/100 ml) are indications for such a preventive program.[40] Because they are likely to develop renal stones, patients who overexcrete uric acid will also be treated with an interval program. The medications used in an interval program are uricosuric agents such as probenecid (Benemid) and sulfinpyrazone (Anturane), and agents that decrease uric acid formation such as allopurinol (Zyloprim). Dietary regulation in the form of a low purine diet and increased fluid intake (3 to 4 L/day) may also be helpful.[40]

The usual dosage of probenecid is an oral dose of 0.5 g daily for 1 week, then increased by 0.5 g weekly until the serum uric acid is brought into a normal range.[40] This drug may cause gastric distress and is best tolerated if taken with meals. For those patients who do not tolerate probenecid, sulfinpyrazone may be used. One hundred milligrams of sulfinpyrazone are approximately equivalent to 0.5 g of probenecid. Patients who are being treated with either probenecid or sulfinpyrazone should not use compounds that contain salicylates, as the salicylate will nullify the uricosuric action of the drugs. Allopurinol is the drug of choice for patients who have an allergy to the usual uricosuric agents, have a history of uric acid stones, have renal impairment, or who overexcrete urinary uric acid.[40] The initial dose is 100 mg twice a day, and the dose is is increased by 100 mg every 2 to 4 weeks until the serum uric acid level is normal. Sodium bicarbonate, 5 to 7.5 g daily, may be given to help prevent the formation of renal stones by making the urine more alkaline.

Patients with gout who are able to maintain normal uric acid blood levels with prescribed medication do not need to be on a restricted diet unless they have other health problems. If overweight, the patient is advised to lose weight, since excess weight will aggravate the joint symptoms. However, an alkaline-ash diet, high in fruits and vegetables with lower amounts of meat proteins, may be prescribed to increase the alkalinity of the urine, thereby decreasing the possibility of urate crystal formation. In either case, a high fluid intake is advisable to minimize uric acid precipitation. The daily urinary *output* for the patient should be 2000 to 3000 ml.

Outcome criteria for the person with gout

The person or significant others can:
1. Explain the basic nature of the disease.
2. Explain the dietary restrictions to be observed (if any).
3. Explain the dosage and side effects of the prescribed medication.
4. Explain the amount of fluid to be taken each day and the plan to achieve this.
5. Explain plans for follow-up care.

Miscellaneous rheumatic disorders: avascular necrosis of bone

Avascular necrosis of bone, or bone death caused by inadequate blood supply, is a problem resulting from a variety of conditions. It can be a complication of bone fractures, connective tissue diseases such as rheumatoid arthritis or systemic lupus erythematosus, irradiation, alcoholism, and sickle cell anemia. Patients who have received prolonged corticosteroid therapy have an increased incidence of avascular necrosis.

Unlike some other forms of connective tissue, bone has a highly developed vascular system and will die without an adequate blood supply. There is a well-developed collateral blood supply to most bones so that infarction from vascular interruption is infrequent. Several areas of bone, however, have a rather precarious blood supply. One such area is the femoral head. Avascular necrosis of the femoral head is a common late complication of a fracture of the femoral neck, since the blood supply to the head comes up through the neck and has been interrupted by the trauma.

The pain is insidious in its onset and gradually increases. There may be development of flexion contractures of the affected joint. Later, pain at rest, restricted motion, and gait disturbances are characteristic. Reducing the work of the joint through rest may help, as may assisted weight bearing through the use of ambulatory aids. Analgesics may help. However, where destruction is severe, surgery, particularly of the hip in the form of total joint replacement, is performed to alleviate pain and increase motion.

Outcome criteria for the person with avascular necrosis of bone who has undergone a conservative program of treatment

The person or significant others can:
1. Explain how to alter ADL to avoid stressing the affected joint.
2. Demonstrate how to safely use ambulatory assistive aids.
3. Explain the dosage and side effects of the prescribed medications.
4. Explain plans for follow-up care.

Surgical intervention

The goals of surgery are correction of deformity and improvement of musculoskeletal function. In some cases surgery may be the only treatment modality required; but in certain diseases it may be adjunctive to medical management. *Synovectomy* to arrest the course of rheumatoid arthritis in a particular joint is an example of adjunctive treatment. Sometimes surgery is indicated because conservative measures designed to relieve pain or prevent deformity have been ineffective. The field of orthopedic surgery has been greatly influenced and advanced by developments in other fields such as bioengineering. Techniques and devices for reconstructive surgery now make it possible to restore function effectively in patients who formerly could be offered only very limited means of treatment. The following discussion will be limited to operative orthopedic procedures commonly performed on bones and joints.

Intraarticular surgical intervention

Arthrotomy

Arthrotomy is simply the opening of a joint. This procedure is usually performed for exploration of the joint to determine the presence of a disease process, for drainage of a joint, or for removal of damaged tissue or foreign bodies within the joint. While any joint may be so opened, it is frequently the knee joint that is involved, often to remove a torn meniscus, foreign bodies, or calcium deposits.

Following an arthrotomy, the joint must be protected until healing takes place. After an arthrotomy of the knee, the patient is often placed in a modified Robert-Jones compression dressing to prevent effusion. Depending on the procedure, the surgeon may order straight leg raising exercises to be done postoperatively. Active flexion exercises may usually be started when the compression dressing is removed. Limited weight bearing will be ordered for that leg, and crutches will be utilized for a prescribed period of time.

Arthroplasty

Arthroplasty is the reconstruction of a joint that has been destroyed by injury or disease. The purpose of the procedure is to restore motion to the joint, relieve pain, and correct deformity.

Interposition arthroplasty. There are several types of arthroplasties. One type involves replacement of *part* of a joint with a *prosthesis* made of metal or other material. An example of this type of arthroplasty is the D-shaped McIntosh prosthesis designed to fit on the tibial plateau of the knee joint. This prosthesis on one or both tibial plateaus enables the surgeon to correct either genu varum or genu valgum in addition to providing a smooth articulating surface.

Another common interposition arthroplasty is the "cup" or "mold" arthroplasty of the hip joint. The usual indication for this procedure is osteoarthritis of the hip. In this procedure both the acetabulum and the femoral head are reshaped, and a Vitallium cup is interposed between the head of the femur and the acetabulum. In the immediate period following a mold arthroplasty, the patient is placed in some form of traction with an apparatus to allow the patient to begin prescribed exercises. The period of hospitalization is usually 5 to 6 weeks, during which the patient will undergo an extensive program of physical therapy. The patient will not be permitted full weight bearing for at least 6 months. Therefore crutches are necessary. An exercise program to be performed at home will be prescribed and followed for several years. The cup arthroplasty provides relief of pain, increases motion in the hip, and corrects deformity. To achieve these results, however, a patient must be highly motivated and committed to the long-term exercise program.

A second type of interposition arthroplasty involves surgical reshaping of the bones of the joint, which are then covered by *soft tissue* used as an interposition device. An example of this is an elbow fascial arthroplasty for either degenerative joint disease or rheumatoid arthritis. This surgery involves removing bone from the lower end of the humerus and the trochlear notch of the ulna, excising the head of the radius, and covering the raw bone ends with a sheet of fascia lata from the thigh. The elbow is immobilized in 90 degrees of flexion for 3 weeks; then active exercises are begun.

Replacement arthroplasty. A third type of arthroplasty is the *total joint replacement,* where both sides of the joint are replaced by metal or plastic implants. These implants are held into the bone by a cement called polymethylmethacrylate. The replacement arthroplasty is one of the most rapidly expanding areas of orthopedic surgery. The results are quickly apparent and very dramatic. Partially for these reasons this type of surgery has received wide coverage in the lay press. Many patients with diseased joints seek out an orthopedic surgeon with the expressed hope that they might benefit from joint replacement. However, not all persons with diseased joints are candidates for joint replacement. Joint replacement, still a relatively new procedure, is usually considered when there is no other operative procedure that would be effective for the individual. Although some prostheses have been in place for over 10 years, a yet unresolved problem in their use is the life expectancy of the prostheses with respect to wear. All artificial joints have a finite life; therefore they are used most frequently in older persons. However, they are considered for those individuals who have significant pain, limitation of motion, and deformity in the affected joint. The causes of these problems include osteoarthritis, rheumatoid arthritis, avascular necrosis, congenital deformities or dislocations, and numerous systemic diseases.

Replacement arthroplasties are available for the shoulder, wrist, elbow, the phalangeal joints of the fingers (in the form of silicone or Silastic implants), the hip, knee, and the ankle. The hip and knee are the most commonly replaced, and this discussion will be limited to those two joints.

TOTAL HIP REPLACEMENT. The hip prosthesis consists of an acetabular portion (cup) and a femoral component. There are numerous types of total hip replacements in use. Some prostheses (McKee-Farrar, Ring) are made entirely of metal (Vitallium or other alloys). Other prostheses (Charnley, Charnley-Müller, Trapezoidal-28) have a metal femoral component and a high-

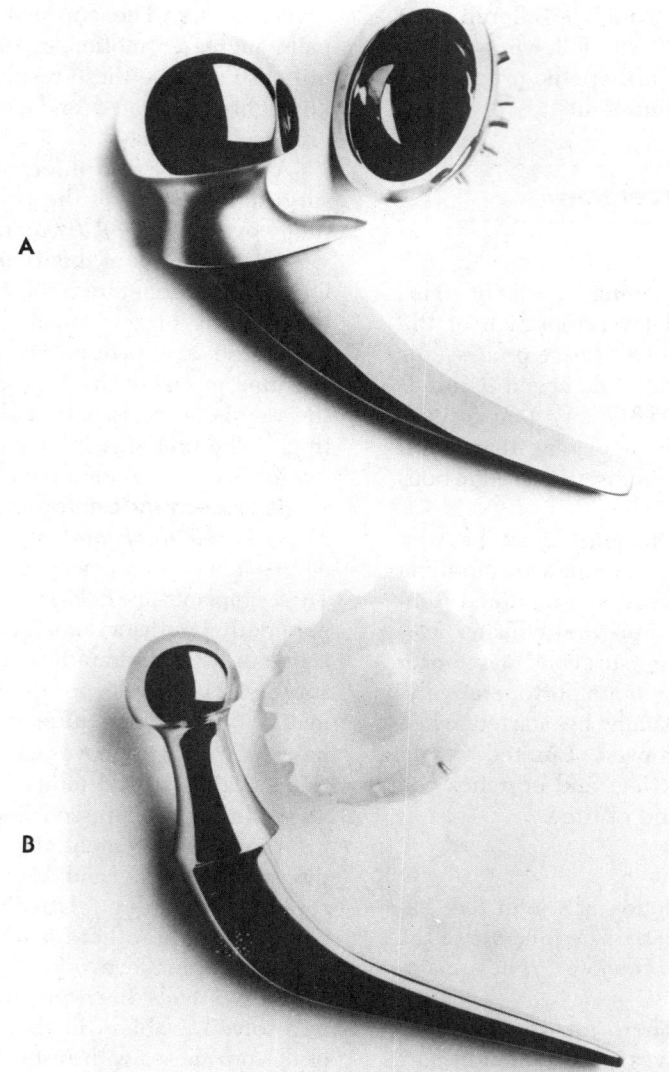

Fig. 42-10. **A,** McKee-Farrar prosthesis. **B,** Charnley prosthesis. **C,** Charnley-Müller prosthesis. **D,** Trapezoidal-28 prosthesis. (Courtesy Zimmer USA, Warsaw, Ind.)

density polyethylene acetabular component (Fig. 42-10). The metal component moving within a polyethylene cup is expected to cause less friction and therefore should wear at a slower rate. The designs of the different prostheses vary in size of the femoral head, shape and length of the femoral neck, and shape of the acetabular component. Each type of prosthesis has its own mechanical advantages and disadvantages of design, and each prosthesis is inserted by a particular operative technique. The relative merits of the design and operative techniques are discussed at great length in the orthopedic literature. As in any new and expanding field, changes are constantly being made. For this reason *it is essential that the nurse caring for a patient with a total hip replacement become familiar with the literature pertaining to the prosthesis and the procedure being used for each patient.*

Postoperative care. The postoperative positioning of the total hip patient is directly dependent on the design of the prosthesis and the method of insertion. Positioning is generally directed at keeping the patient's operative leg in *abduction* and in limiting excessive flexion of that hip. To plan care for the patient the nurse must have the following information:

1. What degree of flexion in the operative hip is permitted and for how long?
2. In what rotation is the leg to be held?
3. How much weight bearing is allowed on the operative leg?
4. What exercises, if any, are to be done?

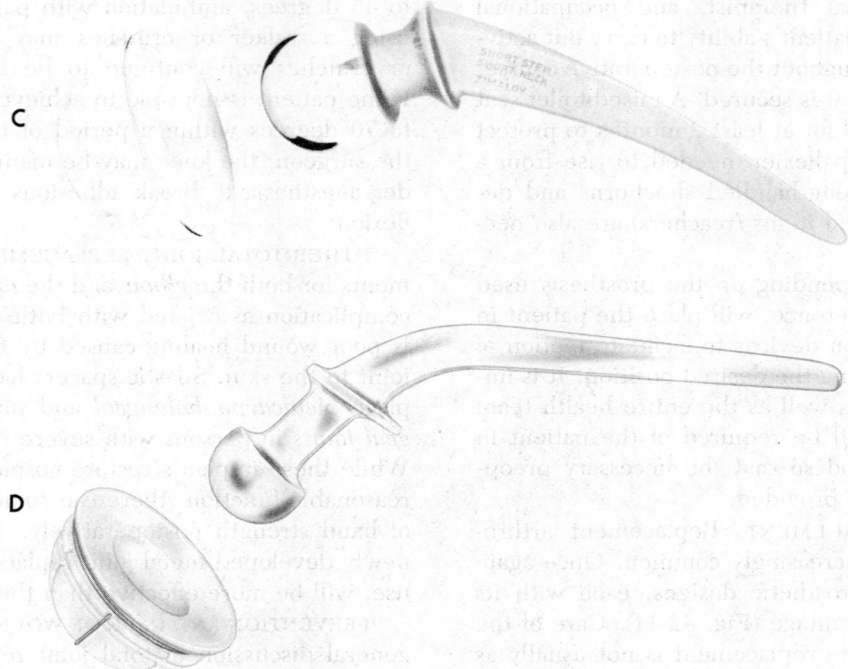

Fig. 42-10, cont'd. For legend see opposite page.

The care of the patient with a *Charnley total hip replacement* will serve as an example of a partial care plan regarding positioning and ambulating. The Charnley prosthesis has a small (22.5 mm) head that, once healing has taken place, can be flexed to 90 degrees without dislocating it. In the Charnley procedure the greater trochanter is detached with all its muscles still in place. After placement of the prosthesis, the trochanter is wired back into place. Until bony union takes place (6 to 8 weeks), pull on the abductor muscles attached to the trochanter must be avoided. However, protected weight bearing on the operative leg is permitted with the use of crutches.

During surgery, drains are placed in the wound to prevent formation of a hematoma. The drains are connected to constant suction and are usually the self-contained vacuum type such as the Hemovac (see Fig. 24-12). It is imperative that the system remain closed and that sterility be maintained. Because the drains are inserted deep in the wound, contamination of the tubing would provide a portal of entry for bacteria. The drainage is emptied as necessary to maintain an accurate record of output from the wound, and the suction device should be recompressed every few hours to maintain suction. Aseptic technique is required for these procedures.

Since patients remain in bed for at least 3 postoperative days, care is directed at keeping them as active as possible within the specified restrictions. The head of the bed may be elevated for comfort (usually about 60 degrees) for short periods of time. Patients are encouraged to spend some time flat with the operated hip in full extension. They are instructed in the use of the overbed trapeze and how to shift their weight using the unoperated leg and the trapeze. The operated leg is maintained in abduction with an abduction block, and the patient is turned only slightly side to side. Plantar flexion and dorsiflexion of the feet as well as quadriceps and gluteal-setting exercises are encouraged to promote venous return and prevent thrombi. These exercises are taught preoperatively (see Chapter 24).

Because of the increased risk of thromboembolic phenomena in hip surgery, prophylactic anticoagulant treatment is often prescribed. The various methods of treatment are debated in the literature. While there is not general agreement on which method is preferable, three types of treatment are most common: acetylsalicylic acid (aspirin), usually 600 mg two to four times a day; low molecular weight dextran, which increases microcirculation and decreases platelet cohesiveness; and small dosages of heparin. Each method has its particular advantages and hazards with which the nurse must be familiar.

Ambulation begins on the third to fourth postoperative day. Nursing personnel and the physical therapist assist the patient to stand without flexing the operative hip more than 60 degrees. The amount of walking, using a walker for support, that is permitted is variable and depends on the patient's progress. Patients are usually discharged 3 weeks after surgery. They must use crutches, avoid adduction, and limit their hip flexion to 90 degrees for 2 months.

The nurse, physical therapist, and occupational therapist evaluate the patient's ability to carry out activities of daily living throughout the postoperative course, and necessary equipment is secured. A raised toilet seat extension must be used for at least 2 months to protect against the extreme hip flexion needed to rise from a standard toilet seat. Long-handled shoehorns and devices to pick up dropped items (reachers) are also necessary.

Some surgeons, depending on the prosthesis used and their personal preference, will place the patient in various slings or traction devices to facilitate motion of the hip while maintaining the desired position. It is important for the nurse as well as the entire health team to understand what will be required of the patient in the postoperative period so that the necessary preoperative teaching can be provided.

TOTAL KNEE REPLACEMENT. Replacement arthroplasty of the knee is increasingly common. Once again there are numerous prosthetic designs, each with its distinct mechanical advantage (Fig. 42-11). Care of the patient with a total knee replacement is not usually as complex as that for a patient with a total hip replacement. The postoperative course follows that of most intraarticular procedures performed on the knee; however, there is more emphasis on active exercising. While the bulky compression dressing is still in place, usually about 5 days, the patient is strongly urged to do quadriceps-setting exercises and to attempt straight leg raising. When the dressing is removed, *active* flexion exercises are begun. These exercises may increase discomfort greatly. The patient will need considerable encouragement as well as prescribed medication and other comfort measures. Once the patient is able to do independent straight leg raising and actively flex the knee to 45 degrees, ambulation with partial weight bearing using a walker or crutches may begin. The walker or crutches will continue to be used for 2 months. If the patient is not able to achieve active knee flexion to 70 degrees within a period of time determined by the surgeon, the knee may be manipulated (flexed) under anesthesia to break adhesions that are preventing flexion.

OTHER TOTAL JOINT REPLACEMENTS. Total replacements for both the *elbow* and the *ankle* are available. A complication associated with both of these procedures is poor wound healing caused by the proximity of the joint to the skin. Silastic spacers have been used to replace *metacarpophalangeal* and *proximal interphalangeal joints* in persons with severe rheumatoid arthritis. While these implants restore cosmetic appearance and reasonable function, there can sometimes be some loss of hand strength postoperatively. It is hoped that the newly developed metal joint replacements, now in trial use, will be more effective than the Silastic spacers.

PREVENTION AND CARE OF WOUND INFECTIONS. Any general discussion of total joint replacement must include reference to the dreaded complication of *infection*. Many total prostheses are held in place by polymethylmethacrylate. This material is a filling or cement-like agent that gives off heat as it solidifies. The temperature is high enough to cause minimal local tissue necrosis. Because necrotic tissue is a good culture medium for bacterial growth and because the prosthesis is a large foreign body, there is an increased risk of infection. Although any bone infection is serious, it has especially grave consequences for a patient having a joint replacement. Infection at the site of the prosthesis results in total failure of the surgery. The prosthesis must be removed and usually cannot be replaced except un-

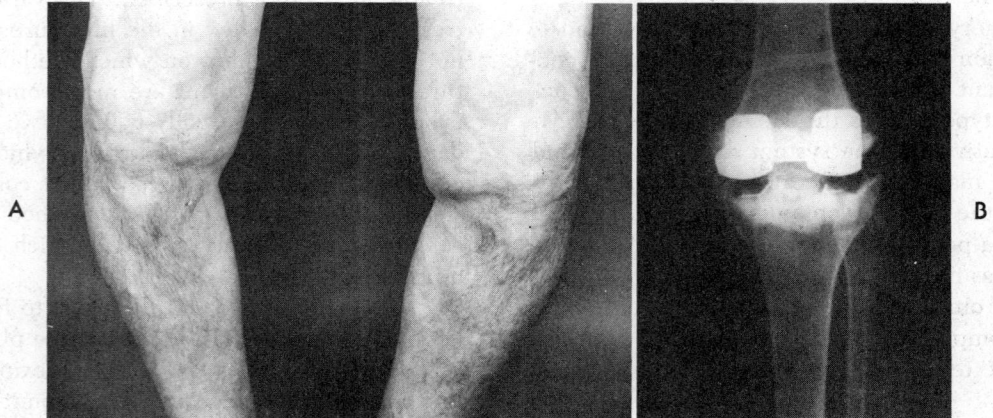

Fig. 42-11. A, Marked varus deformity in both knees. **B,** Varus deformity corrected by proper insertion and alignment of total knee replacement. Prosthesis provides joint surface for both motion and weight bearing. (From Larson, C.B., and Gould, M.L.: Orthopedic nursing, ed. 9, St. Louis, 1978, The C.V. Mosby Co.)

der unusual circumstances. When a hip prosthesis is removed, the patient is left (after healing) with a pain-free but unstable hip and must use crutches or other ambulatory aids for the rest of his or her life. If a knee joint fails, the joint can be fused. This may result in some shortening of the leg, and the patient will not be able to flex the knee; however, the knee will be stable and pain free.

Because of the possibility of infection, utmost care must be taken in preparing the operative site preoperatively. Each hospital will have its own procedure for preoperative preparation, but the goal is the same—keeping the patient and the immediate environment as free as possible from potential sources of contamination. Once the joint is replaced and the wound closed, the patient has no more risk of infection than any other surgical patient, but it must be emphasized that infection

occurring in the operated joint *at any time* will yield the same disastrous results. Precautions necessary to guard against infection should be explained before the patient is discharged from the hospital.

A system of wound irrigation offers some promise in the treatment of wound infections and may be attempted before prostheses are removed. This system involves a set-up of polyethylene tubing utilizing crisscross tubes that allow for reversal of the flow of irrigation fluid and effluent (Fig. 42-12). It is a completely closed system. The effluent is drawn off by an electric suction pump such as a Gomco or an Emerson. When an Emerson pump is used, the suction is adjustable. As the flow of irrigation fluid and effluent can be reversed, the system is self-irrigating and need not be opened. Irrigation rates are generally maintained fast enough to keep the system patent (often 200 to 300 ml per hour),

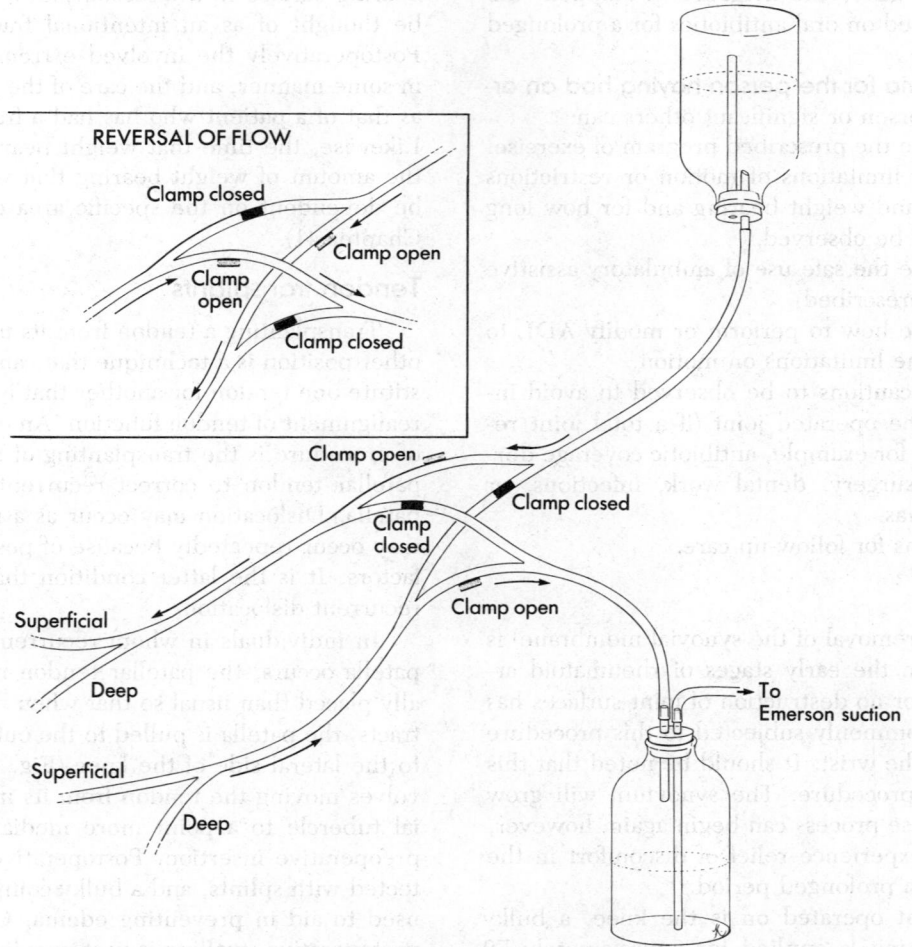

Fig. 42-12. System of closed irrigation allowing continuous irrigation of wound and reversal of flow of irrigant and effluent through tubing is made possible by opening or closing appropriate clamps. (Adapted from Compare, E.L.: Orthopaedic surgery, Chicago, 1974, Year Book Medical Publishers, Inc.)

and suction is maintained at a level that will draw off the effluent at the same rate as the flow of the irrigation fluid. Careful *running totals* of intake and output must be maintained to aid in determining if the system is patent or if fluid is being retained in the tissue surrounding the wound. Leakage of fluid out through the dressings covering the wound will indicate that the system is no longer functioning as it should. Clamping the system for longer than 60 seconds can result in loss of patency; therefore changes of irrigation fluid bottles and bottles used for the collection of the effluent must be accomplished quickly and with strict attention to asepsis. Cultures of the effluent will be obtained on a regular basis, and the irrigation will be discontinued when the surgeon is satisfied that there is no longer evidence of infection (often 2 weeks or more). The patient is maintained on appropriate intravenous antibiotics throughout the period that the irrigation apparatus is in place, and sometimes antibiotics may be added to the irrigating solution. After the irrigation is stopped, the patient is maintained on oral antibiotics for a prolonged period.

Outcome criteria for the person having had an arthroplasty. The person or significant others can:
1. Demonstrate the prescribed program of exercise.
2. Explain the limitations of motion or restrictions on activity and weight bearing and for how long these are to be observed.
3. Demonstrate the safe use of ambulatory assistive devices (if prescribed).
4. Demonstrate how to perform or modify ADL to be within the limitations on motion.
5. Explain precautions to be observed to avoid infection in the operated joint (if a total joint replacement), for example, antibiotic coverage during future surgery, dental work, infections, or major traumas.
6. Explain plans for follow-up care.

Synovectomy

Synovectomy (removal of the synovial membrane) is often performed in the early stages of rheumatoid arthritis when little or no destruction of joint surfaces has occurred. Joints commonly subjected to this procedure are the knee and the wrist. It should be noted that this is not a curative procedure. The synovium will grow back and the disease process can begin again; however, the patient does experience relief of discomfort in the operated joint for a prolonged period.

When the joint operated on is the knee, a bulky compression dressing is applied for approximately 72 hours postoperatively. While the dressing is still in place, the patient usually begins isometric quadriceps exercises prescribed by the physician. As pain decreases, the patient is encouraged to exercise more actively. Active flexion is begun after the compression dressing is

removed, usually 3 to 5 days after surgery. Ambulation is begun on the parallel bars or on a walker and progresses, as the patient is able, to crutches. Partial weight bearing on the operative leg is begun when the patient is able to demonstrate active straight leg raising and active flexion to 45 degrees (see Chapter 41).

Outcome criteria for the person having had a synovectomy. The discharge outcomes for the person having had a synovectomy are the same as those for the patient having had an arthroplasty.

Extraarticular surgical interventions
Osteotomy

An osteotomy is a frequently used orthopedic procedure that involves cutting a bone to change alignment, thereby correcting deformity in the bone or adjacent joint. This procedure may be used to correct angulation or rotational deformities, or to alter the weight-bearing surface in a diseased joint. An osteotomy may be thought of as an intentional fracture (Fig. 42-13). Postoperatively the involved extremity is immobilized in some manner, and the care of the patient is the same as that of a patient who has had a fracture in that area. Likewise, the time that weight bearing may begin and the amount of weight bearing that will be allowed will be dependent on the specific area of the surgery (see Chapter 41).

Tendon transplants

Transplanting a tendon from its usual position to another position is a technique that can be utilized to substitute one tendon for another that is not working or for realignment of tendon function. An example of this type of procedure is the transplanting of the insertion of the patellar tendon to correct recurrent dislocation of the patella. Dislocation may occur as a result of trauma or may occur repeatedly because of postural or congenital factors. It is the latter condition that is referred to as recurrent dislocation.

In individuals in whom recurrent dislocation of the patella occurs, the patellar tendon may be more laterally placed than usual so that when the quadriceps contracts, the patella is pulled to the outside and dislocates to the lateral side of the knee (Fig. 42-14). Surgery involves moving the tendon from its insertion on the tibial tubercle to a point more medial and distal to the preoperative insertion. Postoperatively, the leg is protected with splints, and a bulky compression dressing is used to aid in preventing edema. Once the danger of postoperative swelling is past, a cylinder cast is applied to immobilize the knee to permit healing; however, weight bearing is permitted. After about 6 weeks the cast may be bivalved, and active flexion exercises are begun. Postoperative management considerations are discussed in Chapter 41.

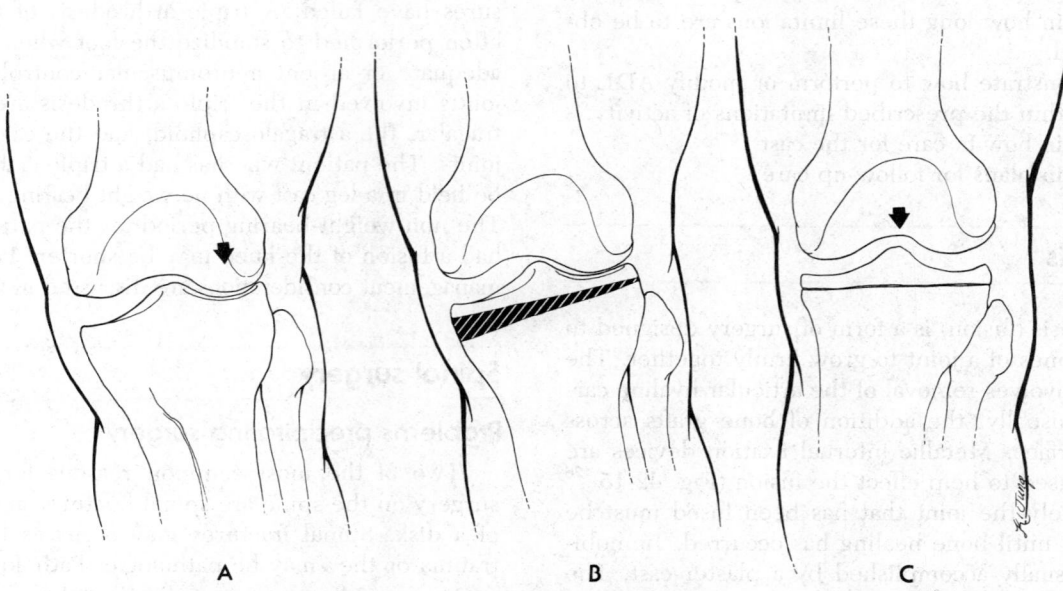

Fig. 42-13. Osteotomy of tibia. Genu valgum (anterior view of left knee). **A,** Weight-bearing force is concentrated on one compartment of knee. **B,** Wedge of bone is removed from tibia. Amount of bone removed depends on how much correction in angulation is necessary. **C,** Distal portion of tibia is swung to proximal portion. Correction of angulation obtained allows weight-bearing forces to be more evenly distributed through both compartments of knee. (Adapted from Hollander, J.L., and McCarty, D.R., Jr.: Arthritis and allied conditions, ed. 8, Philadelphia, 1972, Lea & Febiger.)

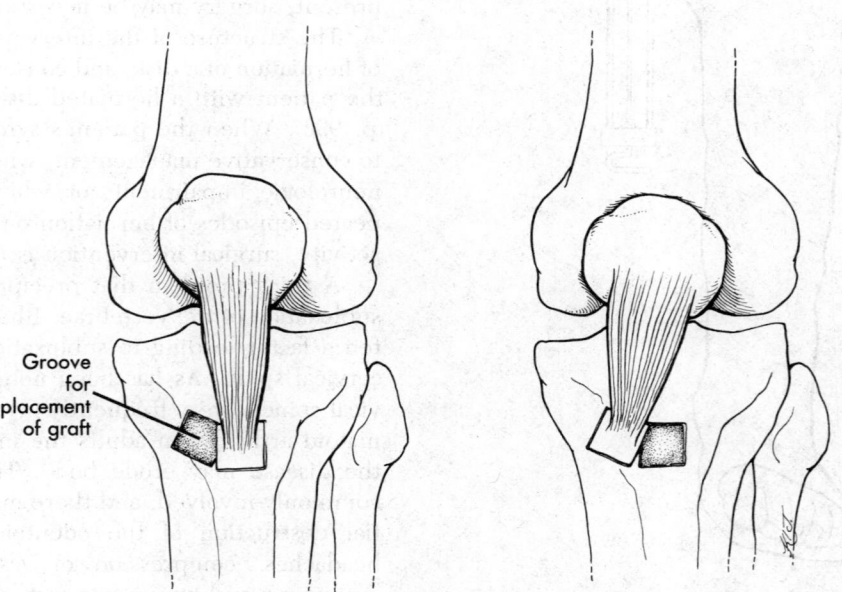

Groove for placement of graft

Fig. 42-14. Tendon transplant. Movement of patellar tendon medially by detaching it and bone it is attached to in order to correct recurrent dislocation of patella. (Adapted from Helfet, A.J.: Disorders of the knee, Philadelphia, 1974, J.B. Lippincott Co.)

Outcome criteria for the person who has had extraarticular surgery

The person or significant others can:
1. Describe the limitations of activity.
2. Explain how long these limitations are to be observed.
3. Demonstrate how to perform or modify ADL to be within the prescribed limitations of activity.
4. Explain how to care for the cast.
5. Explain plans for follow-up care.

Arthrodesis

Arthrodesis (fusion) is a form of surgery designed to cause the bones of a joint to grow firmly together. The procedure involves removal of the articular hyaline cartilage and, usually, the addition of bone grafts across the joint surface. Metallic internal fixation devices are sometimes used to help effect the fusion (Fig. 42-15).[26] Postoperatively the joint that has been fused must be immobilized until bone healing has occurred. Immobilization is usually accomplished by a plaster cast. The permanent immobilization of the joint accomplished by

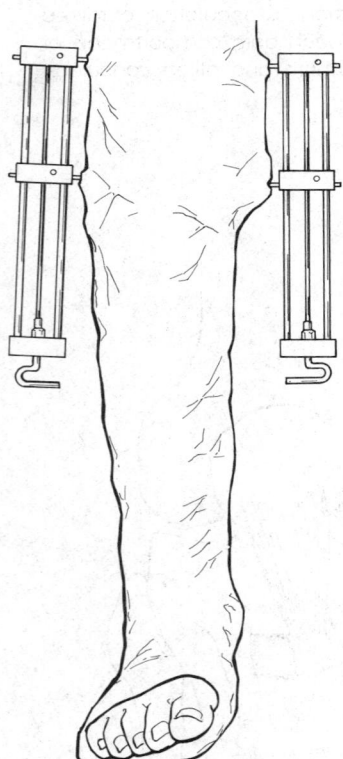

Fig. 42-15. Arthrodesis of knee with compression apparatus. Pins are placed through proximal tibia and distal femur. Compression is maintained by adjusting hand screws, bringing bone wires closer together.

this procedure provides a stiff but stable, pain-free joint.

Arthrodesis of the knee or wrist, for example, may be an end-stage procedure for rheumatoid arthritis or other destructive processes when other treatment measures have failed. A triple arthrodesis of the ankle is often performed to stabilize the foot when there is inadequate or absent neuromuscular control. The three joints involved in the triple arthrodesis are the subastragalar, the astragaloscaphoid, and the calcaneocuboid joints. The patient who has had a triple arthrodesis will be held in a leg cast with no weight bearing for 6 weeks. The non-weight-bearing period for the patient who has had a fusion of the knee may be shorter. Postoperative management considerations are discussed in Chapter 41.

Spinal surgery

Problems precipitating surgery

Two of the most common reasons for performing surgery on the spine are spinal fractures and herniation of a disk. Spinal fractures may occur as the result of trauma or they may be pathologic. Pathologic fractures occur most often as a complication of cancer, osteoporosis of the vertebrae, and other metabolic problems. Fractures in the thoracolumbar area are often compression fractures wherein the vertebral body collapses. Other types of fractures involve the transverse processes or the spinous processes of the vertebrae. Generally, these fractures are not complicated by spinal cord or nerve root compression and heal with bed rest as the only treatment. However, if there is displacement of the fracture and if spinal cord or nerve root compression is present, surgery may be necessary.

The structure of the intervertebral disk, the causes of herniation of a disk, and conservative management of the patient with a herniated disk have been discussed (p. 993). When the patient's symptoms fail to respond to conservative management, when there is progressive neurologic impairment, or when the patient has repeated episodes of herniation on attempting to resume activity, surgical intervention is usually indicated.

A third problem that precipitates spinal surgery is subluxation of the vertebrae. Rheumatoid arthritis is often a factor leading to subluxation of vertebrae in the cervical spine. As has been noted on p. 996, the cervical spine is very frequently involved in juvenile rheumatoid arthritis. In adults the inflammatory process of the disease may erode bone. The atlantoaxial area is commonly involved, and there may be complete or partial destruction of the odontoid process.[40] Occipital headaches, compression of vascular and neurologic structures, and upper extremity weakness may be present. When subluxation of vertebrae in the cervical spine is causing neurologic symptoms, surgery is generally indicated.

Types of spinal surgery

Three major types of spinal surgery will be discussed: diskectomy, laminectomy, and spinal fusion. *Diskectomy* and *laminectomy* are procedures classified as decompression procedures; that is, they are procedures designed to relieve pressure on the spinal cord or spinal nerve roots caused by herniated nuclear material. *Diskectomy* is removal of that portion of the disk that is impinging on the nerve or spinal cord, and it is most often performed through a posterior approach. A portion of the lamina may also be removed *(laminectomy)*. These procedures are generally unilateral and do not create any instability of the spine. However, removal of the disk can cause increased stress on the posterior articulations of the spine, which then may develop degenerative changes. Therefore, depending on the extent of the pathologic condition and the type of activities the patient usually engages in, the surgeon may elect to perform a *spinal fusion*. A spinal fusion may also be performed when there is an anatomic reason for instability of the spine, for unstable fractures of the spine, or to correct scoliosis. There are numerous techniques for spinal fusion, details of which may be found in orthopedic texts. Most commonly, lumbar fusion is performed through a posterior incision with the bone for the graft being taken from the iliac crest. The approach for a cervical fusion may be either anterior (through the front of the neck) or posterior (through the back of the neck). Thoracic spinal fusions may also be approached either anteriorly or posteriorly.

Postoperative care

Care of a patient who has had a *diskectomy* or *laminectomy* is similar to that required in conservative intervention (p. 993). In addition, the patient needs that care indicated for any postanesthesia patient. Patients should be told preoperatively that they may have the same pain in the *initial* postoperative period as they did before surgery. Although the pressure from the disk has been removed, there will be pressure from edema at the operative site, which causes pain.

Postoperative care must include routine checking of the patient's motion and sensation in the lower extremities along with vital signs. Prescribed analgesics should be given as necessary to control postoperative pain. Patients are encouraged to move their legs and continue plantar flexion and dorsiflexion of their feet. Bowel and bladder dysfunction may be present for several days, urinary retention and ileus being the most common complications. A Foley catheter may be used during the first few days postoperatively or until postoperative edema is sufficiently reduced to allow normal bladder function. Rectal tubes, suppositories, or enemas are used as needed to relieve abdominal distention. It is advisable to limit oral intake in the immediate postoperative period until the danger of ileus is past; however, if ileus

occurs, a nasogastric tube will probably be required. When the patient is able to take oral medications, it is very beneficial if a stool softener is prescribed.

Surgeons vary in their postoperative management of patients who have had laminectomies. Generally, the head of the bed is not raised for at least 24 hours and then the patient is allowed a position of comfort in bed. The dressing should be inspected frequently for signs of bleeding or leakage of spinal fluid. Any evidence of either is reported at once. If there is increased drainage, the patient may be placed in a supine position to put pressure on the operative site. As with any dressing, it should be kept dry to prevent contamination.

Following the surgery, the patient may be ambulated any time after the first postoperative day. Orders to ambulate depend largely on the patient's general postoperative condition and the surgeon's preference.

For the patient who has had a *lumbar fusion through a posterior approach*, the bed is kept absolutely flat. Raising the head of the bed would increase the lordosis in the lumbar spine, putting strain on and possibly dislodging the graft. The patient is usually kept flat for 10 days to 2 weeks.

Any twisting motion of the trunk must be avoided. The patient should be logrolled (Fig. 42-16) from side to side (p. 993). The technique is taught preoperatively but the patient is expected to assist with it for several days postoperatively. Patients anticipate pain with turning and tend to be very tense. Giving medication for pain before turning is beneficial. Patients are instructed to fold their arms across their chest to lessen the possibility of reaching out and twisting while being turned. A turning sheet, although not essential, makes it easier to turn the patient while keeping the trunk in good alignment. When patients are on their side, pillows between the legs are needed to maintain proper alignment, as described on p. 993. A pillow behind the back will lend support. Multiple small adjustments are usually necessary to get the patient in a position of comfort. Although for several days the patient will have a great deal of discomfort for which pain medication will be necessary, positioning is often the key factor in providing comfort. If the patient must be transferred from bed to cart, a sheet or roller board should be used along with adequate personnel to maintain proper alignment of the patient's body during transfer.

Some surgeons prefer that patients who have had posterior lumbar fusions remain flat on their backs for several hours. This is to provide additional pressure on the operative site and increase hemostasis. The patient who has had a spinal fusion is more likely to develop a hematoma than is the person who has had a laminectomy. A pressure dressing is applied and should be checked frequently for drainage. Also, the contour of the area around the dressing should be noted as the patient is turned. A change in contour may indicate that

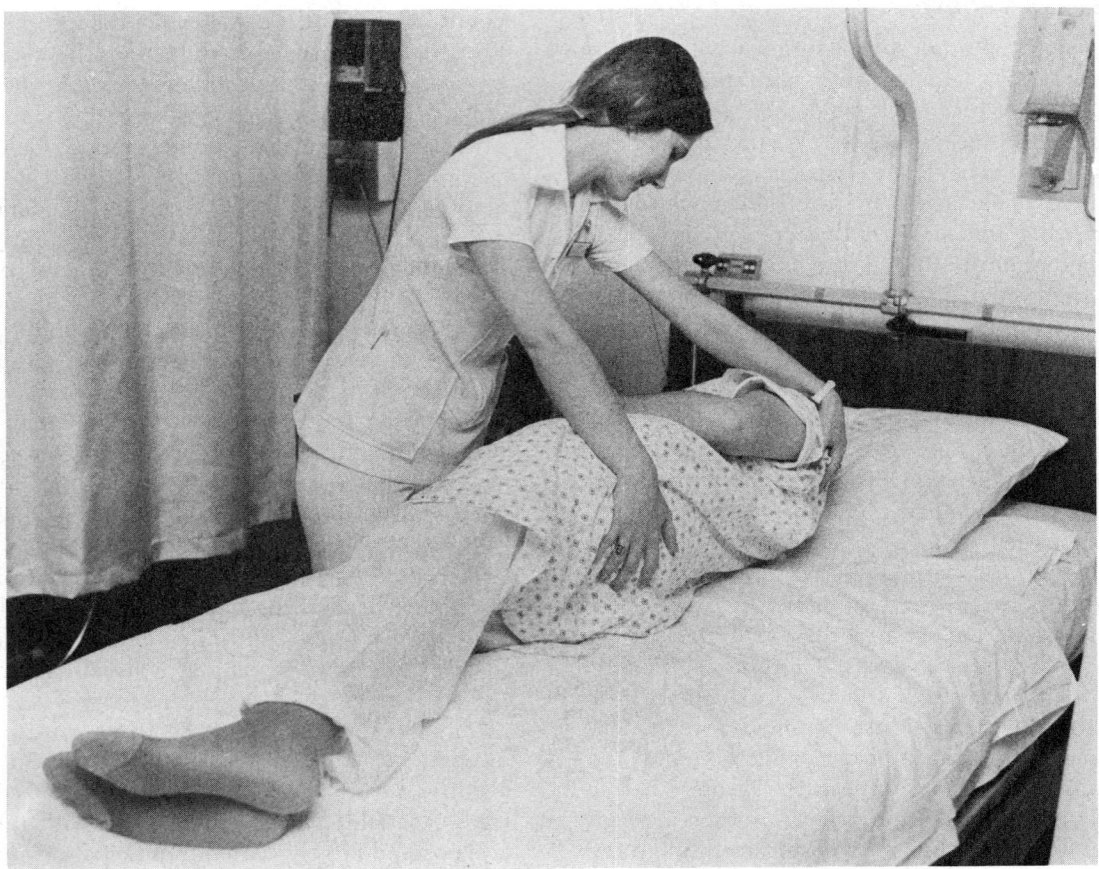

Fig. 42-16. Logrolling of patient. Patient crosses arms over chest, holds legs in extension and feet together. Nurse supports patient at level of shoulders and buttocks.

a hematoma is developing. The patient may also complain of a feeling of pressure at the site. When the bone graft is taken from the iliac crest, the patient may be very uncomfortable when positioned on that side. It is not unusual for the patient to complain of intense discomfort at the graft site.

Bowel and bladder considerations are the same as for the patient who has had a laminectomy.

Depending on the type of fusion that was done and the preference of the surgeon, the patient may have to wear a brace when ambulation is begun. If a brace is to be worn, it is obtained for use when the patient first begins getting out of bed. It is put on while the patient is lying in the bed. Transfer, which is to be accomplished without placing the patient in a sitting position, begins with the patient moving from a side-lying position in the bed. At least two people should be present the first time this is done. Patients who have been horizontal for an extended period of time may very likely have postural hypotension on assuming an upright position. They are moved to the very edge of the bed and then turned to one side. They are then instructed to push up with their lower elbow as one person lifts their

shoulders and the other person guides their legs to the floor. The weight of the lower extremities moving to the floor assists in pivoting the trunk upwards. After several days of getting out of bed in this manner, the assistance of only one person will be necessary. As postoperative pain decreases, the patient will be able to do this unassisted. A walker will be a useful source of support when ambulation is begun.

When the patient is able to ambulate without problems, bathroom privileges for bowel movements are usually allowed. A raised toilet seat results in less discomfort. The patient may not be permitted to actually sit for several weeks. When sitting is permitted, a firm, straight-backed chair with arms is provided so that sitting is bolt upright. Sitting will be the least comfortable position for the patient because of the load that this places on the lumbar spine. Although surgery may have corrected the initial disorder, the patient who has had a back problem is very vulnerable to further trauma. The teaching of good body mechanics to avoid putting unnecessary stress on the back is mandatory.

The patient who has a fusion of the *thoracic spine* is most often an individual who has sustained a fracture

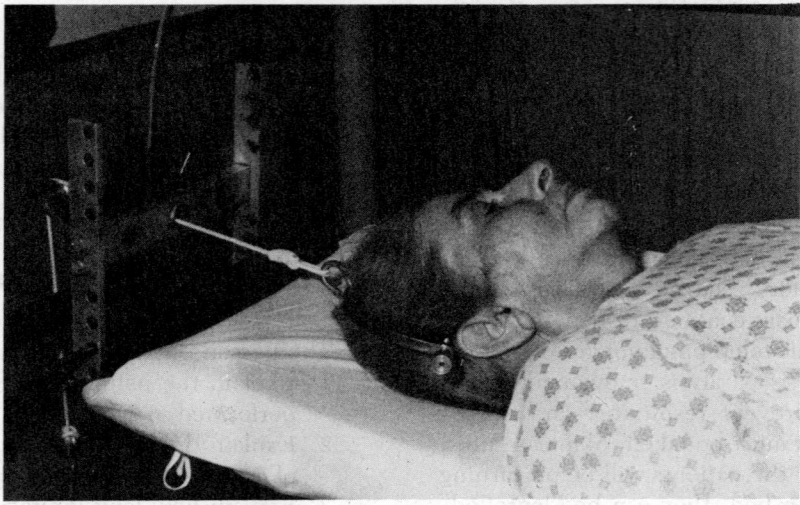

Fig. 42-17. Patient with Crutchfield tongs inserted into skull to immobilize head and neck.

with displacement of one or more of the thoracic vertebrae. If the anterior approach is used for the fusion and the pleural cavity is entered, the patient will have a chest tube postoperatively. Management of the chest tube and appropriate pulmonary toileting will be additional concerns in this patient's care (p. 1252). Because the thoracic spine is more mobile than the lumbar spine, even greater care (than with lumbar fusions) must be taken to maintain good alignment and prevent twisting motions. Bed rest may be maintained for 3 to 4 weeks or longer depending on the extent of the fusion and the degree of instability at the level of the fusion. A brace will be obtained before the patient is allowed out of bed, and the patient may be allowed to sit in a reclining chair before being allowed to stand or walk. Since weight bearing through the arms poses a threat to the integrity of the graft, pushing with the arms is usually discouraged until there is evidence of healing at the graft site. Transfer to a chair is therefore most easily accomplished by sliding the patient to a chair using a pull sheet or turning sheet.

Cervical spine involvement

Cervical spine involvement presents some different problems. Cervical disk degeneration, degenerative arthritis of the cervical spine, herniated cervical disk, trauma to the neck with subluxation of or fracture of vertebrae, or metabolic and other disease conditions leading to destruction of the vertebrae are all conditions that can require interventions designed to relieve pain, promote stability, or decompress the spinal cord or nerve roots in the cervical region. The cervical vertebrae are designed to permit more mobility than are the thoracic or lumbar vertebrae. Consequently, support and immobilization are of vital importance in situations (e.g., displaced fractures) that can result in spinal cord or nerve

root compression. Paralysis results from spinal cord or nerve root damage at the cervical level, and at the C1-2 level, respiratory failure can occur.

In non-life-threatening situations or in instances where paralysis does not threaten, symptoms of pain, muscle spasm, or mild neurologic symptoms such as tingling or paresthesias of the hands and arms can often be relieved by resting the neck. A soft cervical collar or Thomas collar worn around the neck provides a degree of immobility by preventing flexion and hyperextension movements. Cervical traction, either continuous or intermittent, may also aid in relaxing muscles. These physical measures are often used in conjunction with mild analgesic or muscle-relaxing agents. (See Chapter 41 for management of patients in splints and traction.)

For patients whose symptoms do not respond to conservative management or who are threatened with severe spinal cord or nerve root damage, surgery, usually in the form of spinal fusion, is indicated. The surgical approach for cervical fusion may be either anterior or posterior, depending on the preference of the surgeon and the location of the area to be fused.

Preoperative care. Before fusion the neck is immobilized with the spine in proper alignment. This may be done with a hard collar, brace, a halo cast (p. 973), or with traction. If traction is used, it is most often achieved with the use of tongs (usually Vinke or Crutchfield) or a halo. Small burr holes are drilled in the outer portion of the skull over each parietal region. The tongs are then inserted into the holes, the skin around the tongs is sutured, and a collodion dressing is applied. From 4.5 to 9 kg (10 to 20 lb) of weight are attached to a rope coming from the center of the tongs and extending over a pulley attached to the head of the bed (Fig. 42-17). Sandbags may be placed above the patient's shoulder's to help prevent the patient from slipping toward the head of the bed. Occasionally, the head of the bed may be elevated by placing the bed on blocks to give counter traction and to prevent the patient from slipping toward the head of the bed. However, since such counteraction increases the traction, it is not done without first consulting the physician.

Use of the *halo cast*, which is also a form of skeletal traction, or the use of the hard collar or brace permits the patient to be ambulatory. The patient who is in tong or halo traction is obviously confined to bed. Individuals so immobilized may develop pneumonia. Movement is difficult, and if there is paralysis, movement is impossible. Measures to prevent respiratory and thromboembolic complications must be taken. Skin care must be exquisite. Preferably, the patients will be on turning frames, but if they are in bed, they can be "logrolled" off their backs periodically (p. 993). In doing so, the patient's head must be held firmly and maintained in proper alignment with the body. Extreme care must be taken in feeding patients who are in cervical traction. Swallowing is difficult when lying flat, and patients cannot turn or sit up if they choke. Suction equipment should always be on hand for immediate use in case of aspiration of food into the trachea. Some attention must be given to the texture of the patient's diet to provide foods that are easy to swallow.

The patient may be immobilized in this fashion for some time, often weeks, before surgery is performed. When surgery is performed, the tongs or the halo cast remain in place to maintain alignment. If a collar has been worn, the patient may be placed in tongs in the operating room.

Postoperative care. Postoperatively the surgeon may elect to use a neck brace to maintain position rather than skeletal traction. If this is the case, the brace will have been made preoperatively and will be sent to the operating room with the patient for immediate application postoperatively. The brace will allow for early, safe mobilization of the patient. This is also true of the halo cast. Braces must be checked frequently to ensure that there is no loosening of the adjustment screws or straps. Such loosening would permit movement that could result in slippage or nonunion of the fusion.

When the anterior approach is utilized for the fusion, postoperative edema in the soft tissues of the neck makes it difficult initially for the patient to swallow and cough. Mucous secretions are thick and difficult for the patient to manage. Edema may progress to a point that the patient experiences difficulty with respirations. For these reasons, suction equipment and a tracheotomy set should be readily available until postoperative edema begins to subside. Diet should be confined to fluids until there is no longer difficulty experienced in swallowing or clearing secretions from the throat. Usually patients are allowed to sit up, and they should be assisted to do so, since often less pressure is felt over the throat in the sitting position. If a brace is in place, the patient may be mobilized as early as the evening of surgery; however, this depends on the desires of the surgeon.

Just as for lumbar fusions, bone grafts for cervical fusions are usually taken from the iliac crest. Pain over the iliac crest is to be expected, and it is often greater than the pain at the site of the fusion.

Outcome criteria for the person who has had spinal surgery

The person or significant others can:
1. Explain the nature of the surgery that has been performed.
2. Explain the limitations of motion and restrictions of activity that must be observed.
3. Explain how long limitations and restrictions are to be observed.
4. Demonstrate how to apply and remove the brace (if it may be taken off).
5. Demonstrate how to perform or modify ADL within the limitations of activity and motion to be observed.
6. Explain plans for follow-up care.

Scoliosis fusion

Lateral deviation of the spine from the midline is known as scoliosis. There are two forms of scoliosis: postural and structural. The postural form is often successfully treated and corrected by adherence to a program of exercises. The structural form of scoliosis may be congenital, idiopathic, or paralytic. Structural defects are amenable to treatment either with bracing or surgical fusion of the spine, but congenital and paralytic scoliosis nearly always require fusion.

Treatment with bracing may be approached either through the use of a Milwaukee or an Orthoplast brace, although the Orthoplast brace seems to be more comfortable. Braces are worn for periods up to 23 hours per day until skeletal maturity is reached or the spine is straightened. Braces are most effective in correcting the curvature if the curve is flexible, less than 40 degrees, and the patient is cooperative.[18]

Early fusions of the spine to correct scoliotic defects were of the in situ type, involving stripping the posterior elements of the spine of overlying muscle and periosteum and removing the outer cortex of the bone, adding bone grafts to promote bone formation, and immobilizing the patient until fusion occurred.[18] More recent techniques involve the use of internal devices such as Harrington rods or Dwyer screws and cables in conjunction with bone grafts. Surgical fusion is usually indicated for individuals whose curves exceed 40 degrees or in whom bracing has failed.

Preoperative care

Preoperatively, pulmonary function studies are obtained, since some degree of pulmonary decompensation is associated with the spinal deformity, and the need for assisted ventilation postoperatively must be predicted.[18] Additionally, since individuals with congenital scoliosis may have congenital anomalies of the genitourinary system, an intravenous pyelogram may be performed. Exercises to render the spine more flexible and correctable may be prescribed, as may Cotrell's traction, which is particularly useful with adults. Other techniques to obtain preoperative correction are Risser casts and halofemoral or halopelvic traction. Patients must be carefully prepared for application of these latter devices since they are cumbersome, confining, and very often frightening.

Surgical intervention

At surgery the spine may be approached either posteriorly or anteriorly. Harrington rod instrumentation, which involves a series of rods and hooks that apply compression to the posterior spinal elements, is accomplished through a posterior approach.[18] Dwyer instrumentation, in which tension is applied by means of titanium cables passed through the heads of titanium screws that have been embedded in each of the vertebral bodies, is accomplished through an anterior approach and may require the use of chest tubes. Bone grafts are added between the vertebral bodies in either approach.

Postoperative care

The patient is immobilized on a Stryker frame or in a cast that extends from neck to pelvis. If a frame is used, a cast will generally be applied 8 to 12 days postoperatively. The cast remains on for 6 months, although it is changed after 3 months, when radiographs are taken to determine the quality of both correction and fusion.

Individuals who have had a scoliosis fusion can be expected to have considerable postoperative pain and will require adequate analgesia. They must also be closely monitored for the first 48 to 72 hours for respiratory, bowel, and urinary problems, as well as for neurologic problems in all extremities. Nasogastric suction may be employed during the first 24 to 48 hours (or longer if necessary) to prevent the development of ileus; stool softeners may be required when bowel function is reestablished. Indwelling urethral catheters are utilized until output is stable. Skin care, as discussed in Chapter 41, is imperative as are all of the considerations related to care of the immobilized patient. Particular attention should be paid to psychologic considerations as they relate to confinement in the cast or on a frame and to alterations in body image. Adults undergoing these procedures are at higher risk for developing thromboembolic complications. Exercise programs are carried out with the assistance of the physical therapist. The therapist will also assist with mobilization once the postoperative cast is applied 8 to 12 days).

Patient education

Discharge from the hospital can be accomplished when the individual is able to walk and climb stairs without assistance. The individual and family should be instructed in cast care, skin care, shampooing, dietary intake that is high in protein and low in carbohydrates to promote healing and prevent weight gain, use of a bed board, and performance of a program of exercises.

Outcome criteria for the person who has had a scoliosis fusion

The person or significant others can:
1. Explain the nature of the surgery that has been performed.
2. Explain care of the cast.
3. Demonstrate how to perform or modify ADL within the limitations of activity and motion imposed by the cast.
4. Demonstrate the prescribed exercise program.
5. Explain the prescribed diet.
6. Demonstrate independent ambulation and stair climbing.
7. Explain how long the cast is to be on.
8. Explain plans for follow-up care.

Trauma

The patient who has suffered trauma to the musculoskeletal system has, like the postoperative patient, had an interruption in the integrity of the locomotor system. Trauma as seen in fractures—and to a lesser extent, trauma that involves tendons, ligaments, and muscles—will be considered here. When sufficient force is applied to bone, it breaks. As it breaks, the original force is dissipated through the soft tissue. Small fragments of bone may become embedded in the soft tissue such as muscle, blood vessels, and nerves. Because of the potential injury to soft tissue in an extremity that has sustained a fracture, that extremity must be carefully checked for neurocirculatory impairment.

Fractures

Definitions and terminology

A bone is said to be fractured or broken when there is an interruption in its continuity. This is usually caused by a blow or injury sustained in a fall or other accident. A fracture may also occur during normal activity or following a minimal injury when the bone is weakened by disease such as cancer or *osteoporosis*. This is called a *pathologic fracture*, a collapse of the bone. A bone may fracture when the muscles involved are unable to absorb energy as they usually do. This type of fracture, a *fatigue fracture*, has been seen in persons who have been on long foot marches and the muscles have become fatigued.

There are several types of fractures. A fracture is *complete* when there is complete separation of the bone, producing two fragments. It is *incomplete* when only part of the bone is broken. The part of the bone nearest to the body is referred to as a *proximal* fragment, whereas the one most distant from the body is called the *distal* fragment. The proximal is also called the uncontrollable fragment because its location and muscle attachments prevent it from being moved or manipulated when attempting to bring the separate fragments into correct alignment. The distal is referred to as the controllable fragment because it can usually be moved and manipulated to bring it into the correct relationship to the proximal fragment. Fractures in long bones are designated as being in the proximal, middle, or distal third of the bone.

If the skin is intact, the fracture is classified as *simple* or closed. A fracture is classified as *compound* when there is a direct communication between the skin wound and the fracture site. An open or compound fracture has a high risk of contamination, and this is an important factor in its treatment. When the two bone fragments are in good alignment with no change from the normal position despite the break in continuity of bone, the fracture is referred to as a *fracture without displacement*. If the bone fragments have separated at the point of fracture, it is referred to as a *fracture with displacement*. This may be slight, moderate, or marked.

The line of fracture as revealed by x-ray examination or fluoroscopy is usually classified as to type. It may be *greenstick*, with splintering on one side of the bone (this occurs most often in young children with soft bones); *transverse*, with a break straight across the bone; *oblique*, with the line of fracture at an oblique angle to the bone shaft; or *spiral*, with the fracture lines partially encircling the bone. The fracture may be referred to as *telescoped* if a bone fragment is forcibly pushed against and into the adjacent fragment. If there are several bone fragments, the fracture is called *comminuted* (Fig. 42-18).

Symptoms of fracture and related injury

The signs and symptoms of fracture vary according to the location and function of the involved bone, the strength of its muscle attachments, the type of fracture sustained, and the amount of related damage.

Pain is usually immediate and severe following a fracture. It may continue and is aggravated by attempted motion of any kind and by pressure at the site

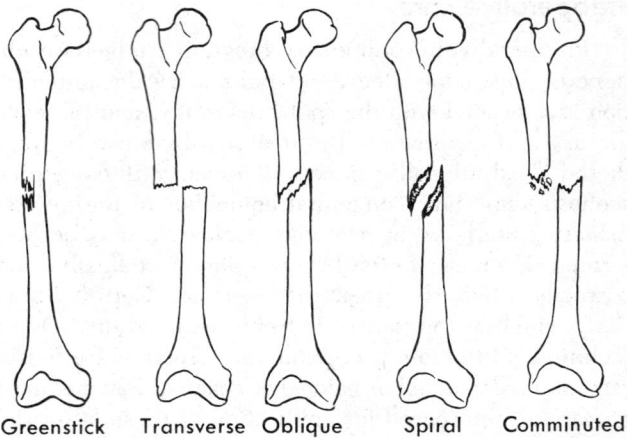

Greenstick Transverse Oblique Spiral Comminuted

Fig. 42-18. Types of fractures.

of injury. *Loss of function* is another characteristic sign, and the injured part will not be capable of movement. If there has been marked displacement of fragments, there will be obvious gross deformity, and there may be motion where motion does not usually occur. When the fractured limb is moved gently, there may be a characteristic grating sound (crepitus) as the bone fragments come in contact with each other. *No attempt should ever be made to elicit this sign when fracture is suspected, since it may cause further damage and increase pain.* It is possible, although unusual, for a fracture to occur with no displacement of fragments, little or no swelling, and pain only when direct pressure is applied to the site of fracture or on use of the limb or body part. Fractures of this kind might be missed if x-ray examinations were not routinely ordered when there was reason to suspect that a fracture may have occurred.

Since bones are firmer than their surrounding structures, any injury severe enough to cause bone fracture may also cause injury to adjacent muscles, nerves, connective tissue, and blood vessels. Bleeding, unless external, may not be fully apparent for several hours, and discoloration of the skin (ecchymosis) may not be apparent until several days after injury. Edema may follow extravasation of blood into the tissues and localization of serous fluid at the site of injury, and paralysis or other evidence of nerve injury may develop. Occasionally a large nerve becomes locked between two bone fragments, causing immediate paralysis. The patient who has a fracture usually has signs and symptoms of injury to bone and surrounding tissues and may go quickly into shock from severe tissue injury, blood loss, or intense pain.

Immediate management

Perhaps the most important basic principle in the care of any fracture is to provide some kind of splint before moving the patient. This is emphasized in the emergency care of patients at the scene of accidents (p. 1883). It is equally important to remember to preserve body alignment when caring for patients who are in traction or some other mechanical apparatus.

Since it is known that edema will occur following a fracture, the injured part usually is elevated. One or more protected pillows are used, and these can support the extremity if moving must be done. If a temporary splint has been applied, it is not removed without orders from the physician no matter how crude or soiled it may be. The limb encased in the splint can be elevated.

The injured part should be observed at frequent intervals for local changes in color, sensation, or temperature. Care should be taken that emergency splinting bandages do not cause constriction as edema develops. Tingling, numbness, or burning pain may indicate nerve injury. Coldness, blanching, or cyanosis usually indicates interference with circulation. Increased warmth and swelling may indicate infection or may relate to the body's reaction to the fracture itself. The patient should be observed for early signs of shock, especially if the injury is severe. Vital signs should be taken every 15 minutes until the patient's condition has stabilized.

It should be anticipated that the physician may order local cold applications during the first 24 hours following a fracture, since these help to reduce hemorrhage and edema and contribute to the patient's comfort. Ice bags are often used and must be covered and moved at regular intervals to prevent skin damage.

When a patient with a *compound* fracture is admitted to the hospital, the wound will be surgically cleansed to remove dirt and foreign material; surgically debrided to remove devitalized tissue and detached pieces of bone; cultured; and if the wound was extremely dirty or if there was a delay in treatment, it will be packed open. Closure of the wound will be accomplished in a few days if there is no sign of infection. Appropriate antibiotics are given intraoperatively and postoperatively. Following care to the wound, the fracture is appropriately reduced and immobilized.[26] *Osteomyelitis, tetanus,* and *gas gangrene* are *three major complications* in grossly contaminated compound fractures. The antibiotics used in conjunction with cleansing and debridement are to prevent osteomyelitis. Tetanus immunization is generally given when a compound fracture has been sustained, and the patient should be carefully observed for signs of gas bacillus infection—sudden increase in edema and pain associated with darkening of the tissues. These signs should be reported to the physician at once.

Pain is usually relieved in the first few hours by giving acetylsalicylic acid (aspirin) or narcotics. Adjustment to sudden immobilization is difficult for patients, and those caring for them must appreciate what it means to

be unable to move about freely. Even a fracture of an arm bone may make patients quite helpless at first. They may be unable to move or use the rest of their body without severe pain. Sometimes treatment of the fractured bone makes it physically impossible for them to care for some of their most basic physical needs. Patients may need a sedative such as secobarbital (Seconal) to ensure sleep during the first few nights after a fracture.

Complications

Fat embolism is a serious complication that may follow a fracture, especially a comminuted fracture of a long bone. The source of the emboli is thought to be the fat of the bone marrow. Pressure changes occurring in the interior of fractured bones force molecules of fat from the marrow into the systemic circulation. If the emboli are large, they may cause distinct problems in the respiratory and central nervous systems. The signs of a fat embolus are similar to the signs of other kinds of emboli and consist of sudden severe pain in the chest, pallor, dyspnea, prostration, and collapse. The development of these signs and symptoms constitutes a medical emergency, and the physician should be called at once. In some instances signs are less dramatic, consisting of subtle changes in the patient's behavior, for example, confusion.

Petechial hemorrhages of the skin and conjunctivae are a classic sign of systemic fat embolism. These usually appear on the second or third day after injury and are commonly found in the conjunctivae, skin of the neck, shoulders, and axillary folds.

There is no specific treatment for systemic fat embolism. Treatment is geared to supportive measures. The patient can usually breathe best in high Fowler's position and will require oxygen therapy. Blood transfusions may be necessary to relieve hypovolemic shock and maintain an adequate hemoglobin level. If heart failure occurs, the patient will be digitalized. Initially, all patients with a fracture should be kept as quiet as possible and subjected to no unnecessary movement. Some experts feel that proper immobilization and careful handling of patients with bone injuries *may* help prevent the occurrence of fat emboli.

Ischemic paralysis (contracture) is a somewhat rare complication of a fracture and develops when an artery is injured by trauma or pressure so that arterial flow is interrupted. *Volkmann's contracture* is a complication of fractures about the elbow caused by circulatory impairment because of pressure from a cast, constricting bandages, or injury to the radial artery. The muscles of the forearm atrophy, and the fingers and forearm are permanently flexed (clawhand). Signs of coldness, pallor, cyanosis, pain, and swelling of the part below the cast must be watched for and reported promptly so that pressure may be relieved by either loosening the bandage or removing the cast in order that circulation may be restored before damage can develop.

Osteomyelitis refers to an infection of bone by pyogenic bacteria. Such an infection can occur as a result of a compound fracture or as a complication of surgery. The infection involves the marrow spaces, the haversian canals, and the subperiosteal space. The bone is involved secondarily, being destroyed by proteolytic enzymes. Interference with the blood supply causes necrosis. *Acute osteomyelitis* may be caused by introduction of bacteria through a wound, but the most common route of infection is *hematogenous spread* from a preexisting focus such as a boil.

There is initially a small focus of inflammation, evidenced by hyperemia and edema. Since bone is a rigid material, this edema causes increased pressure and pain. The pus that forms further increases the pressure, which compromises local circulation and results in necrosis of the bone.

The initial treatment of *acute osteomyelitis* involves rest and large doses of appropriate antibiotics prescribed following culture and sensitivity testing. If dramatic improvement is not seen within 24 hours, the involved bone is usually opened surgically to relieve the pressure and provide for drainage. Inadequate treatment leads to *chronic osteomyelitis,* which is extremely difficult to eradicate. After a relatively long period of being symptom free, the patient may again have an acute episode. The infected dead bone separates from the living bone and becomes a *sequestrum.* The infection cannot be permanently cleared until the sequestrum is removed. This is usually done surgically, although it will sometimes happen by a natural process.

Osteomyelitis is extremely difficult to treat and often means years of recurrent episodes of disability for a patient. It can result in failure of surgical procedures such as arthroplasty. A major nursing role in osteomyelitis is in its prevention. *Aseptic technique is always indicated when caring for an open wound,* and the nurse working with the orthopedic patient must be acutely aware that this is one means by which osteomyelitis can be prevented.

Physiology of healing of fractures

Immobilization of a bone that is fractured is necessary for bone healing. Such immobilization may take place in any of three ways. The first is *physiologic splintage.* This form of splintage will occur naturally, since guarding, avoidance of use, and muscle spasm will occur as a result of pain in the affected limb. Further, there will be a desire to rest the whole body until some repair has occurred. The second method is *external orthopedic splintage* with devices such as plaster casts. The third method is *internal fixation* wherein the opposing ends of the fracture are held in place by screws, plates, or rods.

Once immobilization is accomplished, the bone heals by a process known as *callus formation* (Fig. 42-19). New growth of bone is called a *callus.* Callus formation proceeds in five general stages. First is *hematoma formation.* Since bone is highly vascular, there is bleeding at both ends of the fractured bone. More blood collects, as an increase of capillary permeability permits extravasation into the injured area. This blood collects in the periosteal sheath or adjacent tissues and fastens the broken ends together. Second, the hematoma becomes organized, as fibroblasts invade the area, forming a *fibrin meshwork.* White blood cells wall off the area, *localizing*

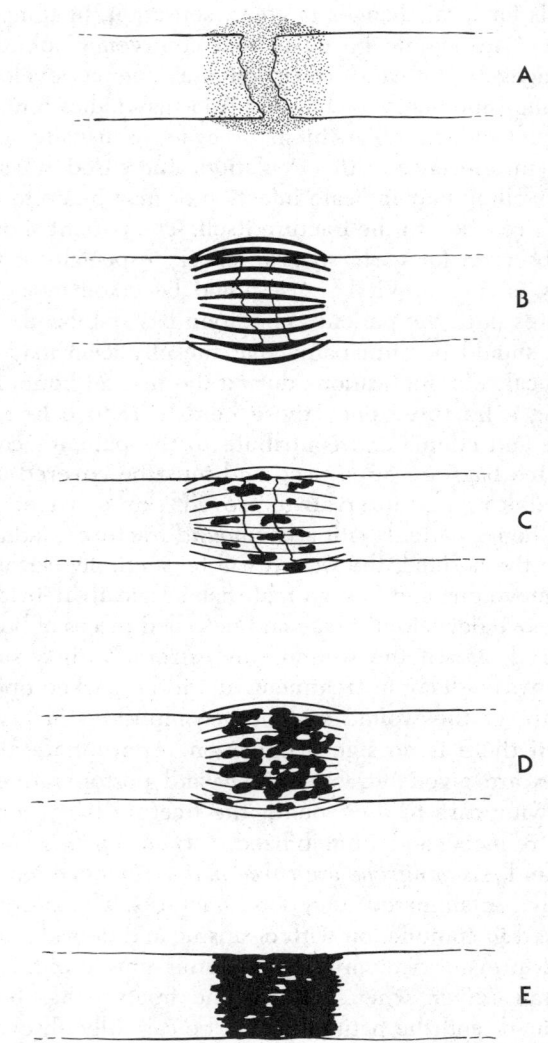

Fig. 42-19. Bone healing (schematic representation). **A,** Bleeding at broken ends of bone with subsequent hematoma formation. **B,** Organization of hematoma into fibrous network. **C,** Invasion of osteoblasts, lengthening of collagen strands, and deposition of calcium. **D,** Callus formation: new bone is built up as osteoclasts destroy dead bone. **E,** Remodeling is accomplished as excess callus is reabsorbed and trabecular bone is laid down.

the inflammation. This fibrin meshwork is not strong enough to withstand or support movement or weight-bearing forces. Third, *osteoblasts invade* the fibrous union, helping to make it firm. Blood vessels develop from capillary buds, establishing a source of supply of nutrients for building collagen. Collagen strands become longer and longer and begin to incorporate calcium deposits. The fourth stage is *callus formation*. As osteoblasts continue to lay the network for bone buildup, osteoclasts destroy dead bone and help synthesize new bone. The collagen strengthens and becomes further impregnated with calcium. *Remodeling* is the fifth step, in which excess callus is reabsorbed and trabecular bone is laid down along lines of stress in accordance with Wolff's law (p. 915).

Factors that impede good callus formation are so much edema at the fracture site that the supply of nutrients to the area is impeded; too much bone lost at the time of injury to permit sufficient bridging of the broken ends; inefficient immobilization; infection at the site of injury; bone necrosis; anemia or other systemic conditions; endocrine imbalance; poor dietary intake.[26,40] If callus formation does not occur normally and efficiently, the resulting lack of repair is termed *nonunion,* or an *ununited fracture*.

Methods of treatment

The usual methods of treatment—reduction, immobilization, traction, and internal fixation—and their management are discussed at length in Chapter 41.

Fractures of the hip

Patients with fractured hips are frequently seen in the hospital, so these fractures will be discussed in more detail. The hip joint is a ball-and-socket joint and is formed by the acetabulum, a deep round cavity in the innominate bone, and the rounded upper portion of the femur. The upper part of the femur is composed of a head, neck, greater and lesser trochanter, and shaft. The distal part of the femur ends in two condyles. The head of the femur fits into the acetabulum. The hip joint is surrounded by a capsule, ligaments, and muscles. The greater trochanter serves as a point of insertion for the abductor and short rotator muscles of the hip, whereas the lesser trochanter serves as a point of insertion for the iliopsoas muscle.

The blood supply to the femoral head is of paramount importance in fractures in or about the hip joint. The blood supply to the femoral head varies with age. The chief source of blood supply to the femoral head in adults is the posterior retinacular artery (Fig. 42-20). The nutrient and periosteal vessels of the femoral shaft extend into the trochanteric region and lower part of the neck.

Fractured hips occur more frequently in women than in men. Some factors explaining this are (1) women have a wider pelvis with a tendency to coxa vara; (2) women experience postmenopausal hormonal changes often accompanied by an increased incidence of osteoporosis; and (3) women's life expectancy is greater than that of men.

Fractures of the hip may be classified in two general categories: intracapsular and extracapsular fractures. The patient with a fractured hip will present with pain in the hip. The affected leg will be shorter and externally rotated.

Intracapsular fractures of the hip are those occurring within the hip joint and capsule. These include *subcapital, transcervical,* and *basal neck* fractures. *Extracapsular* fractures occur outside of the capsule to an area 5 cm (2 in.) below the lesser trochanter (Fig. 42-21).

Impacted intracapsular fractures may be treated by bed rest without internal fixation. *Other intracapsular fractures* of the hip may be treated by the use of nails, pins, or prosthesis. The choice of device depends on the location of the fracture and the personal preference of the surgeon. Since the blood supply to the head of the femur comes up through the neck, it is often disrupted in an intracapsular fracture (Fig. 42-20). When

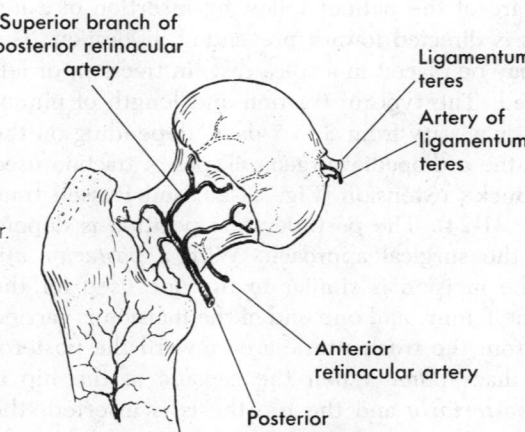

Fig. 42-20. Posterior view of blood supply to head of femur.

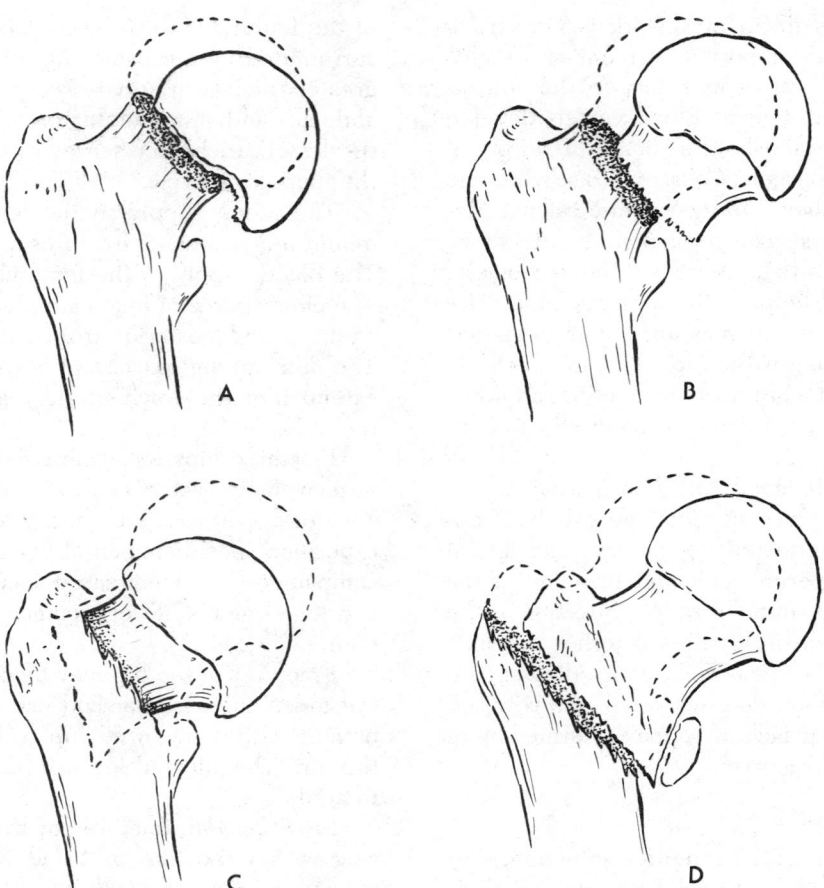

Fig. 42-21. Fractures of hip. **A,** Subcapital fracture. **B,** Transcervical fracture. **C,** Impacted fracture of base of neck. **D,** Intertrochanteric fracture.

the blood supply is interrupted, there may be eventual avascular necrosis of the femoral head (p. 1004). Since this complication occurs in a significant percentage of patients following intracapsular fracture of the hip, particularly in the elderly patient, the physician may elect to remove the head of the femur and insert a prosthesis such as the Austin-Moore prosthesis (Fig. 42-22).

The care of the patient following insertion of a hip prosthesis is directed toward preventing dislocation. The patient may be placed in a spica cast, in traction, or left free in bed. The type of traction and length of immobilization may vary from 3 to 7 days, depending on the wishes of the orthopedic surgeon. Types of traction used include Buck's extension (Fig. 41-23) and Russell traction (Fig. 41-24). The postoperative position is dependent on the surgical approach. With a *posterior approach* the incision is similar to the one used for the neck of the femur, and one end of the incision is carried upward from the trochanteric area toward the postero-superior iliac spine. When the capsule of the hip is opened *posteriorly* and the prosthesis is inserted, the leg must be placed in slight external rotation with slight

abduction. The head of the bed should not be elevated more than 45-60 degrees. Acute flexion of the hip, adduction, and internal rotation must be avoided to prevent dislocation of the hip prosthesis before complete healing has occurred. With an *anterior approach*, the upper end of the incision is carried forward to the anterior spine of the ilium. The position of the operated leg is abducted or neutral with internal rotation.

Since adduction must be avoided, if the patient does not have traction or a cast, turning to the unaffected side must be carefully executed. The nurse supports the leg in abduction while the patient turns the rest of the body (Fig. 42-23). Several pillows are placed between the thighs and staggered forward to the foot to avoid adduction. The leg must not slip off the pillows (Fig. 42-24). Sandbags may be used to help maintain this position. Careful instruction must be given to the patient.

Partial weight-bearing ambulation, assisted by a walker or crutches, may be permitted 3 to 7 days postoperatively. Sitting, being careful not to flex the operated hip more than 60 degrees, may be permitted 5 to 10 days postoperatively. In transfer, ambulation, and

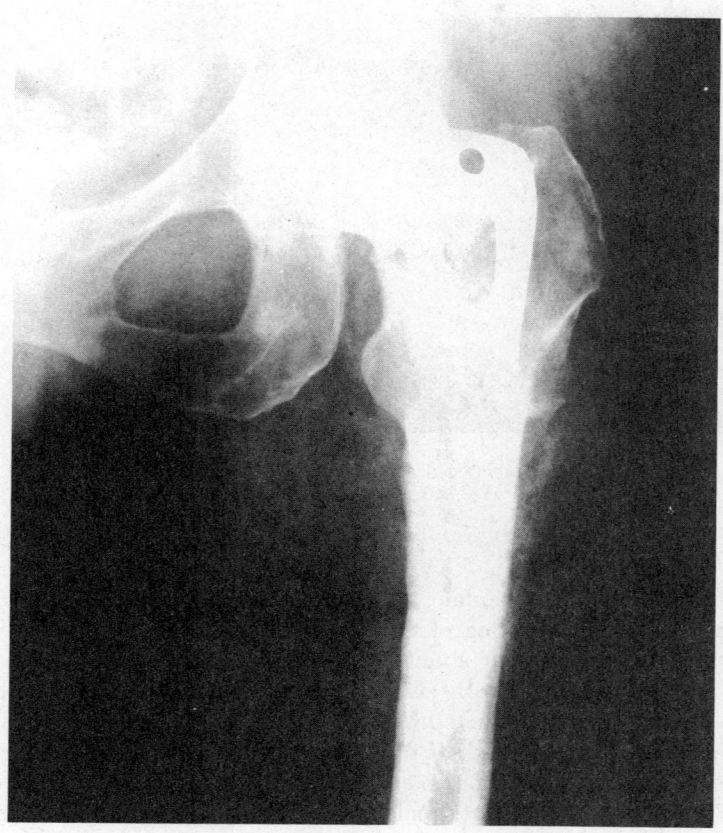

Fig. 42-22. Roentgenogram showing Austin-Moore prosthesis in place. Tracks of nails and screws of recently removed Smith-Petersen nail and plate are still visible in remaining bone. (Courtesy The University Hospitals of Cleveland, Cleveland.)

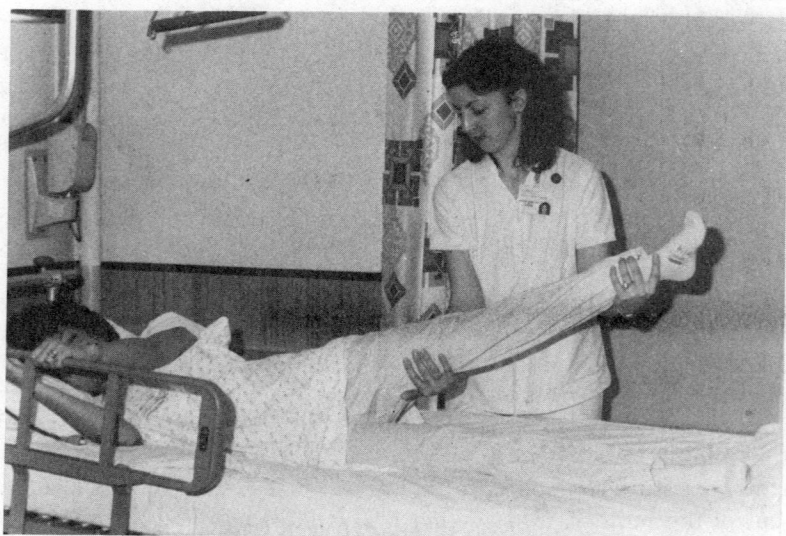

Fig. 42-23. Nurse holding patient's leg in abduction while patient turns on side.

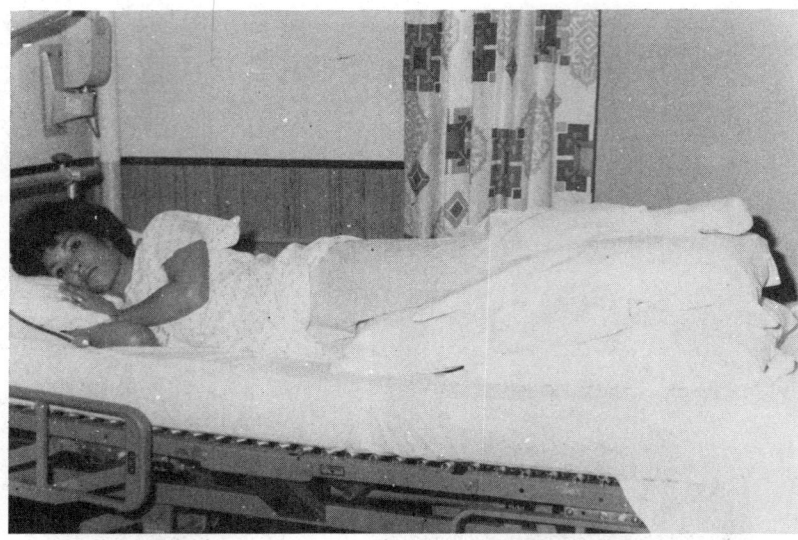

Fig. 42-24. Staggering pillows to avoid adduction of leg. Pillows must be placed so that leg does not slip off them.

sitting the patient must be reminded to maintain abduction of the operated hip. Complete healing of the capsule of the hip joint will not take place for about 2 months; until that healing is complete, the prosthesis is at risk of dislocating if the operated leg is adducted beyond the midline or if the hip is sharply flexed. If the patient's abductor muscles are weak, abduction exercises may be prescribed. When sitting, the patient should have the knees flexed and the feet on the floor, since it is easier to maintain abduction in this position than it is with the legs elevated. This position also puts less strain on the hip itself.

Extracapsular fractures are usually caused by direct violence, by a fall directly onto the trochanter, or by a twisting of the leg. The leg will be externally rotated and shortened. The shaft fragment tends to shorten, producing an acute angle between the shaft and the neck of the femur. Shortening occurs because of the fracture itself and the angulation. Such fractures may be *comminuted*. If the fracture is not treated, the leg will be externally rotated and adducted. The intertrochanteric region has a rich blood supply, and union usually occurs without difficulty, although complication can be the *varus deformity*. A varus deformity occurs when the angle of the femoral shaft to the neck is less than the normal 120 degrees.

Extracapsular fractures of the hip are reduced under general or spinal anesthesia. The objectives of treatment include (1) overcoming the shortening by traction or pull; (2) correcting the external rotation so that the leg is rotated while forward pressure is applied to lift the greater trochanter out of the buttock; (3) swinging the leg in abduction; and (4) maintaining the reduction by pinning or support. A lateral incision is made from

the greater trochanter down along the outer side of the thigh for 15 or 17.5 cm (6 to 7 in.) The incision is placed toward the posterior surface of the shaft of the femur to produce easier access to the femur's lateral surface. After reduction, the fracture may be immobilized by a *three-flanged Smith-Petersen nail*, a *Jewett nail*, a *Sarmiento nail*, *Richard's screw*, or other similar metallic device that keeps the fractured ends of the bone in good approximation (Fig. 42-25). Internal fixation permits more mobility for the patient, thereby reducing systemic complications common in the aged. Complications associated with some methods of internal fixation, in contrast to closed reduction and external immobilization, include displacement of fragments, causing deformities that may require further and more extensive surgery, including bone grafts.

Following internal fixation of an extracapsular fracture, mobilization may be started on the first postoperative day. Some of the newer fixation devices permit partial weight bearing on the operated leg; others, such as the Smith-Petersen nail, do not. The patient's weight-bearing status should be ascertained before transfer maneuvers are begun. Generally there are no restrictions on positioning in bed, and the patient may lie in a position of comfort. When sitting, the operated leg *should not be elevated* since elevation puts stress through the nail and the fracture site.

Outcome criteria for the person who has sustained a fracture

The person or significant others can:
1. Explain the nature of the injury and the treatment.
2. Explain the limitations of motion and restrictions

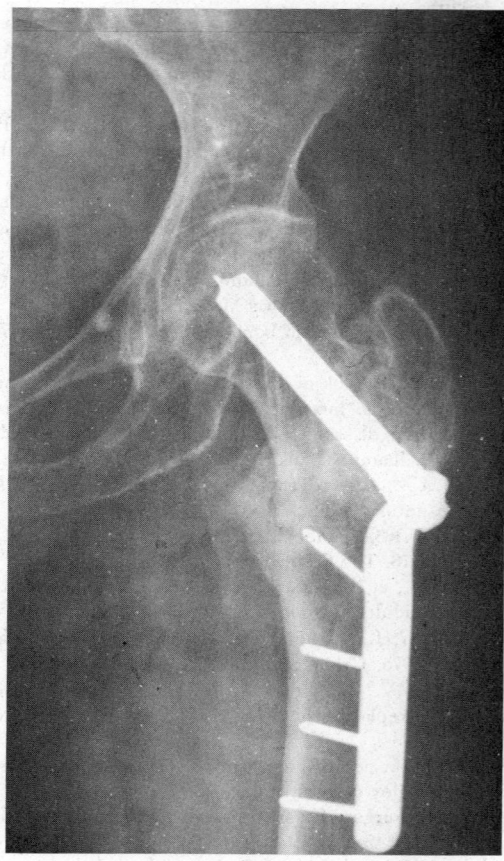

Fig. 42-25. Roentgenogram showing internal fixation of intertrochanteric fracture with McLaughlin plate and pins.

of activity to be observed and how long they must continue.

3. Demonstrate how to perform or modify ADL within the limitations of activity and motion that must be observed.
4. Explain how to care for the cast (if applied).
5. Demonstrate how to use safely an ambulatory assistive device (if necessary).
6. Explain plans for follow-up care.

Soft tissue injuries

Twisting of joints may result in damage to ligaments, muscles, or tendons. Damage to ligaments and tendons may also be secondary to degenerative changes in the tissue comprising these structures. *Sprain* usually refers to damage to ligaments, while *strain* refers to muscle damage. *All three structures—ligaments, muscles, and tendons—may rupture*. If stretching is the only damage sustained, the usual treatment is rest for the involved area. Cold applications may be used immediately to help retard swelling and ease discomfort. A soft support such as an Ace wrap may be used in less

serious injuries, whereas more severe injuries may require immobilization in a plaster cast (as with rupture of the Achilles tendon). The most severe injuries are those that involve laceration or rupture. These are treated surgically by suturing the torn ends of the structure together. Depending on the location of the surgery, immobilization of the involved part may be accomplished with a plaster cast or with an internal fixation wire (as in tendons of the finger).

Outcome criteria for the person who has sustained a sprain or strain

The person or significant others can:
1. Explain the limitations of motion and restrictions of activity that must be observed and for how long.
2. Demonstrate how to perform or modify ADL within the limitations of activity and motion that must be observed.
3. Explain how to care for the cast (if applied).
4. Explain plans for follow-up care.

REFERENCES AND SELECTED READINGS

1. *Adams, J.C.: Outline of fractures, including joint injuries, ed. 6, Baltimore, 1972, The Williams & Wilkins Co.
2. Anthony, C.P., and Thibodeau, G.A.: Textbook of anatomy and physiology, ed. 11, St. Louis, 1983, The C.V. Mosby Co.
3. *Arthritis Foundation: Primer on the rheumatic diseases, ed. 7, New York, 1973, The Foundation. (Prepared by a committee of the American Rheumatism Association Section of the Arthritis Foundation. Reprinted from J.A.M.A. **224**[suppl.], April 30, 1973.)
4. Beeson, P.B., et al.: Cecil's textbook of medicine, ed. 15, Philadelphia, 1979, W.B. Saunders Co.
5. Bennett, R.M., et al.: The arthritis of mixed connective tissue disease, Ann. Rheum. Dis. 37:397-403, 1978.
6. *Berger, M.R., and Froimson, A.I.: Hands that hurt: carpal tunnel syndrome, Am. J. Nurs. 79:264-265, 1979.
7. Bluestone, R., editor: Rheumatology, Boston, 1980, Houghton Mifflin Professional Publishers.
8. Brashear, H.R., and Raney, R.B.: Shand's handbook of orthopaedic surgery, ed. 9, St. Louis, 1978, The C.V. Mosby Co.
9. Bryan, R.S., and Lowell, F.A.P.: The quest for the replacement knee, Orthop. Clin. North Am. 2:715-728, 1971.
10. *Buck, B.I.: Hip replacement, Super. Nurse 3:75-78, 1972.
11. Carnesale, P.G.: Arthrodesis of the hip, Orthopedics Dig. 4:12-18, 1976.
12. Cautious use of anticancer drug urged for rheumatoid arthritis (Orthopedic Notes), Contemp. Surg. 9:64A, 1976.
13. Clissold, G.K.: The body's response to trauma: fractures, New York, 1973, Springer Publishing Co., Inc.
14. *Committee on Trauma, American College of Surgeons: Early care of the injured patient, ed. 2, Philadelphia, 1976, W.B. Saunders Co.
15. Compere, E.L.: Orthopaedic surgery, Chicago, 1974, Year Book Medical Publishers, Inc.
16. *Darst, B.J.: I have a new hip, Am. J. Nurs. 78:1489-1490, 1978.
17. Dee, R.: Total replacement arthroplasty of the elbow for rheumatoid arthritis, J. Bone Joint Surg. [Br.] 54:88-95, 1972.

*References preceded by an asterisk are particularly well suited for student reading.

18. *deToledo, C.H., et al.: The patient with scoliosis (series of four articles), Am. J. Nurs. **79**:1587-1612, 1979.

19. Dimon, J.H.: Complications of femoral neck fractures treated primarily by reduction and internal fixation, Orthop. Rev. **6**:47-55, 1977.

20. *Donahoo, C.A., and Dimon, J.H.: Orthopedic nursing, Boston, 1977, Little, Brown & Co.

21. Ecker, M.L., et al.: The treatment of trochanteric hip fractures using a compression screw, J. Bone Joint Surg. [Am.] **57**:23-27, 1975.

22. Edmonson, A.S., and Crenshaw, A.H., editors: Campbell's operative orthopaedics, ed. 6, St. Louis, 1980, The C.V. Mosby Co.

23. Ehrlich, G.E., editor: Total management of the arthritic patient, Philadelphia, 1973, J.B. Lippincott Co.

24. Evarts, C.M., and Kendrick, J.I.: Cup arthroplasty, Orthop. Clin. North Am. **2**:93-111, 1971.

25. *Farrell, J.: Illustrated guide to orthopedic nursing, Philadelphia, 1977, J.B. Lippincott Co.

26. *Gartland, J.J.: Fundamentals of orthopedics, ed. 3, Philadelphia, 1979, W.B. Saunders Co.

27. *Gilroy, A., and Caldwell, E.: Initial assessment of the multiply injured patient, Nurs. Clin. North Am. **13**:177-190, 1978.

28. Gurd, A.R., and Wilson, R.I.: The fat embolism syndrome, J. Bone Joint Surg. [Br.] **56**:408-416, 1974.

29. Hagemann, W.F., et al.: Arthrodesis in failed total knee replacement, J. Bone Joint Surg. (Am.) **60**:790-794, 1978.

30. Helfet, A.J.: Disorders of the knee, Philadelphia, 1974, J.B. Lippincott Co.

31. Heppenstall, R.B., editor: Fracture treatment and healing, Philadelphia, 1980, W.B. Saunders Co.

32. Hubbard, M.J.S.: One treatment of femoral shaft fractures of the elderly, J. Bone Joint Surg. (Br.) **56**:96-101, 1974.

33. *Kryshyshen, P.L., and Fischer, D.A.: External fixation for complicated fractures, Am. J. Nurs. **80**:257-259, 1980.

34. *Larson, C.B., and Gould, M.L.: Orthopedic nursing, ed. 9, St. Louis, 1978, The C.V. Mosby Co.

35. Lipscomb, P.R.: Management of preoperative and postoperative complications of rheumatoid arthritis, Orthop. Rev. **2**:11-14, 1973.

36. McCarty, D.J., editor: Arthritis and allied conditions: a textbook of rheumatology, ed. 9, Philadelphia, 1979, Lea & Febiger.

37. McKibbin, B.: The biology of fracture healing in long bones, J. Bone Joint Surg. [Br.] **60**:150-163, 1978.

38. *Meyers, M.H., McNell, D.B., and Nelson, K.: Total hip replacement—a team effort, Am. J. Nurs. **78**:1485-1488, 1978.

39. Mishler, W.G., and Mallory, T.H.: Conservative or resurfacing total hip replacement, Ohio State Med. J. **74**:636-638, 1978.

40. *Moskowitz, R.W.: Clinical rheumatology, Philadelphia, 1975, Lea & Febiger.

41. *Mourad, L.: Nursing care of adults with orthopedic conditions, New York, 1980, John Wiley & Sons, Inc.

42. Murray, D.G., and Racz, G.B.: Fat embolism, the role of respiratory failure and its treatment, J. Bone Joint Surg. [Am.] **56**:1327-1337, 1974.

43. *Nysather, J.O., Katz, A.E., and Lenth, J.L.: The immune system: its development and functions, Am. J. Nurs. **76**:1614-1618, 1978.

44. Pandey, S.: Nailing and immediate weight bearing in femoral shaft fractures, Int. Surg. **58**:712-715, 1978.

45. Polyarthritis responds to immunoglobulin treatment (Orthopedic Notes), Contemp. Surg. **9**:64, 1976.

46. *Rabb, S.: Bunion surgery, Am. J. Nurs. **74**:2185-2187, 1974.

47. Radin, E.L., et al.: Practical biomechanics for the orthopedic surgeon, New York, 1979, John Wiley & Sons, Inc.

48. *Roaf, R., and Hodkinson, L.J.: Textbook of orthopaedic nursing, ed. 2, Oxford, England, 1975, Blackwell Scientific Publications, Ltd. (Distributed by J.B. Lippincott Co., Philadelphia.)

49. Ryan, A.J.: Injections for tendon injuries: cure or cause? (editorial), The Physician and Sports Medicine **6**:39, 1978.

50. *Ryan, J.: Compression in bone healing, Am. J. Nurs. **74**:1998-1999, 1974.

51. Salter, R.B.: Textbook of disorders and injuries of the musculoskeletal system: an introduction to orthopaedics, rheumatology, metabolic bone disease, rehabilitation, and fracture, Baltimore, 1970, The Williams & Wilkins Co.

52. Savastano, A.A., editor: Total knee replacement, New York, 1980, Appleton-Century-Crofts.

53. Schneider, F.R.: Handbook for the orthopaedic assistant, ed. 2, St. Louis, 1976, The C.V. Mosby Co.

54. Steinberg, M., et al.: Nontraumatic avascular necrosis of the femoral head in adults, Orthopedics Dig. **5**:17-22, 1977.

55. Stollerman, G.H.: Rheumatic fever and streptococcal infections, New York, 1975, Grune & Stratton, Inc.

56. Swanson, S.A.V., and Freeman, M.A.R., editors: The scientific basis of joint replacement, New York, 1977, John Wiley & Sons, Inc.

57. *Swinson, D.R., and Swinburn, W.R.: Rheumatology, New York, 1980, John Wiley & Sons, Inc.

58. Testa, N.N.: Surgery for arthritis: what can and cannot be done, Consultant **18**:142-151, 1978.

59. *Torbett, M.P., and Ervin, J.C.: The patient with systemic lupus erythematosus, Am. J. Nurs. **77**:1299-1302, 1977.

60. *Townley, C., and Hill, L.: Total knee replacement, Am. J. Nurs. **74**:1612-1617, 1974.

61. Turek, S.L.: Orthopaedics: principles and their application, ed. 3, Philadelphia, 1977, J.B. Lippincott Co.

62. Vainio, K.: Orthopedic surgery in treatment of rheumatoid arthritis, Orthopedics Dig. **4**:42-43, 1976.

63. Volz, R.G., et al.: Upper extremity total joint replacement, Assoc. Operating Room Nurses J. **28**:843-847, 1978.

64. Waxman, J.: Osteoarthritis: new look, Orthopedics Dig. **4**:28, 1976.

65. Webb, K.J.: Early assessment of orthopedic injuries, Am. J. Nurs. **74**:1048-1052, 1974.

66. White, J.: Teaching patients to manage systemic lupus erythematosus, Nurs. '78 **8**(9):26-35, 1978.

67. *Wilde, A.H.: Synovectomy of the knee, Orthop. Clin. North Am. **2**:191-205, 1971.

68. Williams, S.R.: Nutrition and diet therapy, ed. 4, St. Louis, 1982, The C.V. Mosby Co.

69. Wolf, L., et al.: Classification criteria for systemic lupus erythematosus, J.A.M.A. **236**:1497-1499, 1976.

GAS TRANSPORT PROBLEMS

The ability to take in oxygen, transport the oxygen to the cells for utilization, and carry carbon dioxide and other waste products to organs of elimination is vital for survival. Failure of any part of the respiratory or cardiovascular systems to carry out these functions is incompatible with survival. The airway must be patent; gasses must be able to diffuse across the alveolar capillary membranes; the blood must have the capacity to transport the gasses; the heart must provide adequate pumping to move the blood to the tissues; and the vascular system must ensure a free passageway for the blood to reach the tissues.

Because of the interrelationship of the respiratory and cardiovascular systems to meet the body's basic need for oxygen and elimination of carbon dioxide, the care of persons experiencing problems with both systems is considered in this unit. The first portion of the unit (Chapters 43 to 47) considers the transport of oxygen and carbon dioxide to and from the cells. *Cardiovascular assessment* is followed by a discussion of *nursing considerations* of *general cardiovascular problems* (e.g., cardiac arrhythmias, sudden death) and of persons experiencing cardiovascular surgery. *Specific problems* of the *heart and major blood vessels, peripheral circulation,* and *blood and blood-forming tissues* are discussed next.

The last portion of the unit (Chapters 48 to 51) focuses on the respiratory system per se. *Respiratory assessment* is followed by *general nursing care requirements* of persons having some form of impairment obtaining oxygen or getting rid of carbon dioxide through the respiratory system. *Specific problems* of both the *upper airway* and *lower airway* complete the unit.

CHAPTER 43

ASSESSMENT OF THE CARDIOVASCULAR SYSTEM

JOAN M. KAVANAGH
MARCIA J. RIEGGER

Heart disease today remains the leading cause of death in the industrialized nations. In the United States alone, cardiovascular disease (CVD) is responsible for approximately 1 million fatalities every year. Fortunately, during the past 2 decades, cardiovascular research has drastically increased our understanding of the structure and function of the cardiovascular system in health and disease; and despite the formidable statistics regarding the prevalence of CVD, during the last 10 years a steady decline in mortality from cardiovascular disorders has been witnessed. It is hoped that the effective application of the increased knowledge regarding CVD and its risk factors will enable health care professionals to assist clients better in achieving and maintaining cardiovascular health.

Anatomy and physiology

Basic structure

The heart is a relatively small organ located in the middle of the mediastinum, where it is partially overlapped by the lungs. This pulsatile four-chambered pump beats approximately 72 times/min, pumping more than 5 L of blood each minute, or about 2000 gallons per day. It continually propels oxygenated blood into the arterial system and receives poorly oxygenated blood from the venous system. The heart muscle rests on the diaphragm and is tilted forward and to the left so that the apex of the heart is rotated anteriorly.

The heart is enclosed by the *pericardium,* which consists of two layers: the inner layer (visceral pericardium) and the outer layer (parietal pericardium). The two pericardial surfaces are separated by a pericardial space that normally contains approximately 10 to 20 ml of thin, clear pericardial fluid. This lubricating fluid moistens the contacting surfaces of the pericardial layers and serves to reduce the friction produced by the pumping action of the heart. The visceral pericardium actually encases the heart and extends several centimeters onto each of the great vessels. The parietal pericardium is attached anteriorly to the manubrium and xiphoid process of the sternum, posteriorly to the vertebral column, and inferiorly to the diaphragm.

There are three layers of cardiac tissue: *epicardium*—the outer layer of the heart, which is the same structure as the visceral pericardium; *myocardium*—the middle layer of the heart, which is composed of striated muscle fibers and is responsible for the heart's contractile force; and *endocardium*—the innermost layer of the heart, which consists of endothelial tissue. The endocardium lines the inside of the heart's chambers and covers the heart valves.

Chambers

The heart is divided into two halves by a muscular wall (septum) (Fig. 43-1). Each half has an upper collecting chamber (atrium) and a lower pumping chamber (ventricle). Oxygen-poor venous blood enters the right atrium, flows from the right atrium to the right ventricle (mainly by gravity) when the tricuspid valve is opened, and is pumped into the pulmonary artery to the lungs. Oxygen-rich blood returns from the lungs to

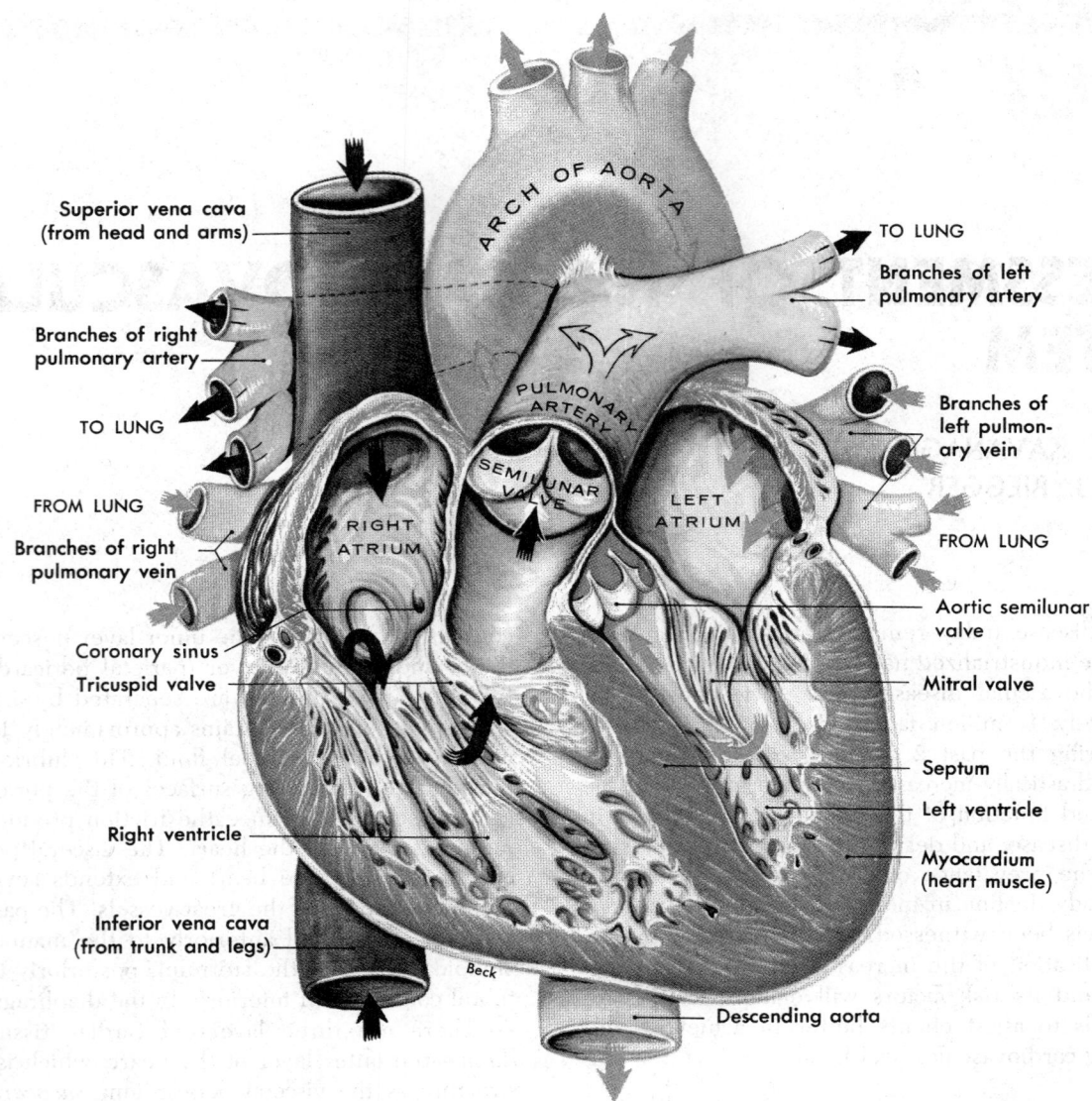

Fig. 43-1. Frontal section of heart showing four chambers, valves, openings, and major vessels. Arrows indicate direction of blood flow. Black arrows represent unoxygenated blood; gray arrows represent oxygenated blood. Two branches of right pulmonary vein extend from right lung behind heart to enter left atrium. (From Anthony, C.P., and Thibodeau, G.A.: Textbook of anatomy and physiology, ed. 11, St. Louis, 1983, The C.V. Mosby Co.)

the left atrium, enters the left ventricle when the mitral valve is opened, and is ejected into the aorta for distribution to the peripheral tissues.

The *right atrium* is a thin-walled structure that serves as a reservoir for venous blood returning to the heart. Venous blood returns to the heart via the superior and inferior vena cava and the coronary sinus, which drains venous blood from the heart muscle. Blood is temporarily stored in the right atrium during right ventricular systole (contraction). During ventricular diastole (filling), approximately 80% of the venous return to the right atrium flows by gravity into the right ventricle through the tricuspid valve. The remaining 20% of the

venous return is delivered to the ventricles during atrial systole. This additional 15% to 20% of the venous return, which is actively propelled into the ventricles, is called the "atrial kick."

The *right ventricle* is normally the most anterior structure of the heart and is situated immediately beneath the sternum. The right ventricle receives venous blood from the right atrium during ventricular diastole and then propels this blood through the pulmonic valve into the pulmonary artery and then to the lungs. Because the pulmonary system is a low-pressure system, the overall workload of the right ventricle is much lighter than that of the left ventricle. The right ventricle has a crescent-shaped chamber and a thin outer wall that is 4 to 5 mm thick. This thin structure is suitable for right ventricular systole, because the right ventricle contracts against low resistance.

The thin-walled *left atrium* receives oxygenated blood from the four pulmonary veins and serves as a reservoir during left ventricular systole. Blood flows by gravity from the left atrium into the left ventricle through the opened mitral valve during ventricular diastole. Left atrial contraction then propels the remaining 20% of the venous return and provides a significant increment of blood volume to the left ventricle. This atrial kick serves to stretch the ventricle and prime it for ventricular ejection.

The *left ventricle* receives blood from the left atrium through the opened mitral valve during ventricular diastole. Blood is then ejected through the aortic valve into the systemic arterial circulation during ventricular systole. The left ventricle must contract against a high-pressure systemic circulation in order to deliver blood flow to the peripheral tissues. Therefore the left ventricular chamber is surrounded by 8 to 15 mm of thick musculature, which is approximately 2 to 3 times the thickness of the right ventricle. The thick musculature and ellipsoidal sphere shape contribute to the powerful expulsive ability of the left ventricular chamber during systole.

Valves

The four cardiac valves are flaplike structures that function to maintain unidirectional (forward) blood flow through the heart chambers. These valves open and close in response to pressure and volume changes within the cardiac chambers. The cardiac valves can be classified into two types: the atrioventricular (AV) valves, which separate the atria from the ventricles; and the semilunar valves, which separate the pulmonary artery and the aorta from their respective ventricles.

Atrioventricular valves

The AV valves are the *tricuspid* valve, located between the right atrium and the right ventricle, and the *bicuspid* (or mitral) valve, located between the left atrium and left ventricle. The tricuspid valve contains three leaflets held in place by fibrous cords called the *chordae tendineae*, which in turn are anchored to the ventricular wall by the papillary muscles. The mitral valve on the left side of the heart is a bicuspid valve with two valve cusps or leaflets. It, too, is attached to strands of fibrous tissue called chordae tendineae, which extend to the papillary muscles. The chordae tendineae are extremely important because they support the AV valves during ventricular systole to prevent valvular prolapse into the atrium. There is a degree of leaflet overlapping

during closure of the AV valves, and this helps to prevent the backward flow of blood. Damage to the chordae tendineae or to the papillary muscles would permit valvular regurgitation of blood back into the atrium during ventricular systole. During diastole, the AV valves serve as a type of funnel as they allow blood to flow from the atria to the ventricles. The diameter of the AV cusps is almost double that of the orifice that they occlude; and in general, the AV valves are structurally much more complex than the semilunar valves.

Semilunar valves

The semilunar valves include the *aortic* and *pulmonic* valves. The structural design of the semilunar valves is quite different from the AV valves; each consists of three cuplike cusps. They lie between each ventricle and the great vessel into which it empties. These valves are open during ventricular systole (contraction) to permit blood flow into the aorta and pulmonary artery. They are closed during diastole (relaxation) to prevent retrograde flow from the aorta and pulmonary artery back into the ventricle when it is relaxed.

Coronary arteries

The coronary arteries arise from the aorta (just behind the cusps of the aortic valve) in an area known as the sinuses of Valsalva. The function of the coronary artery system is to provide an adequate blood supply to the myocardium. Despite scientific advances in the field of cardiology, coronary artery disease and its complications remain the leading cause of death in the United States (see Chapter 45).

There are two main coronary arteries—the *left* and the *right* (Fig. 43-2). The left coronary artery divides into two branches: the left anterior descending (LAD) artery and the circumflex coronary artery (CCA). The LAD branch supplies the left ventricular myocardium, the septum, anterior papillary muscle, and portions of the right ventricle. In addition, the LAD artery usually supplies the anterior apex, as well as some portion of the posterior apex. The CCA typically emerges at a sharp 90-degree angle from the left main coronary artery and is then directed toward the lateral left ventricle and apex. The CCA and its branches supply most of the left atrium, the lateral wall of the left ventricle, and part of the posterior wall of the left ventricle. Diagonal branches arise between the LAD artery and the CCA and are distributed along the free wall of the left ventricle.

There are two important external landmarks to look for when tracing coronary circulation. These anatomic landmarks are sulci or grooves, and they include the following: the *atrioventricular groove*, which encircles the heart between the atria and the ventricles; and the *interventricular groove*, which divides the right and left

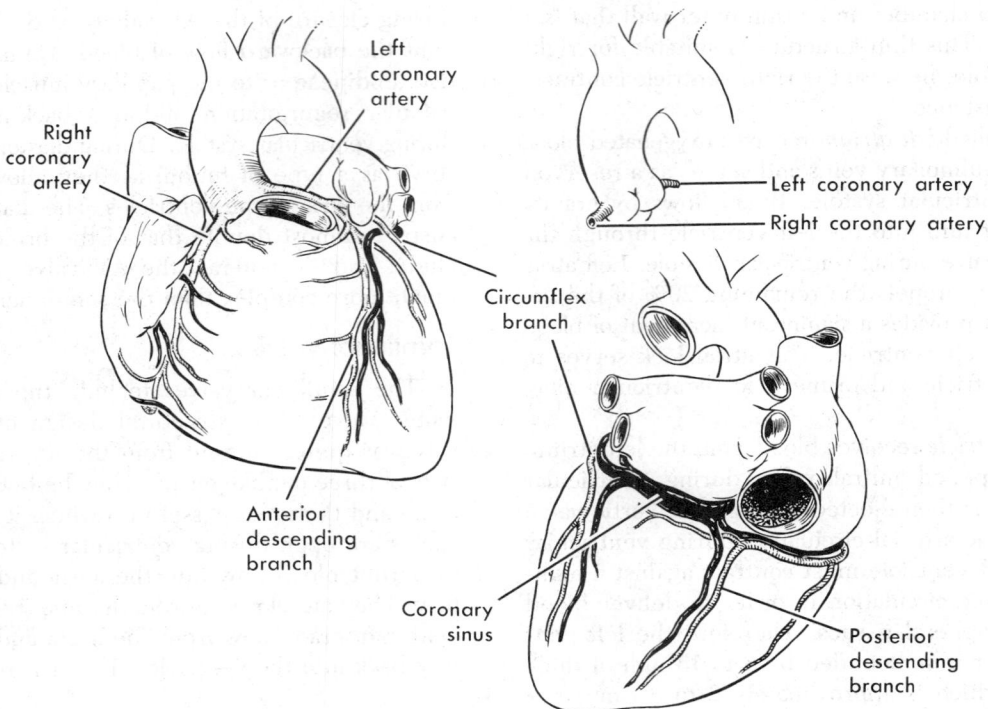

Fig. 43-2. Coronary blood vessels. (From King, O.M.: Care of the cardiac surgical patient, St. Louis, 1975, The C.V. Mosby Co.)

ventricles. The meeting of the two anatomic grooves on the posterior side of the heart is known as the crux of the heart. The location of the crux of the heart is significant, because this is the region in which the AV node is located. The phrases "dominant left" circulation and "dominant right" circulation refer to whether the right or the left coronary artery turns at the crux of the heart and supplies the posterior interventricular groove. Therefore if the CCA extends as far as the posterior interventricular groove, the circulation is considered to be dominant left. This condition occurs in only 10% to 15% of all individuals.

The right main coronary artery (RCA) arises from the right sinus of Valsalva off the aorta and courses around the right atrioventricular groove. Its branches supply the right ventricle, a portion of the septum, and in over 50% of all individuals, it supplies the SA node. In approximately 67% of all individuals, the RCA turns at the crux of the heart and descends into the posterior interventricular groove. These individuals are classified as "right dominant." The posterior descending branch of the RCA then supplies the posterior aspect of the septum and the posterior left papillary muscle before terminating in a number of branches to the left ventricular wall. There exists a great deal of variation in the branching pattern of the coronary arteries. In approximately 18% of the population, the CCA also reaches the crux of the heart with the RCA; this is the so-called

balanced coronary artery pattern. In the remaining individuals, there is no true posterior interventricular branch, but rather a large number of branches from either main coronary artery supplies the posterior septum.

Coronary artery blood flow to the myocardium occurs almost exclusively during diastole, when coronary vascular resistance is diminished. During systole, coronary vascular resistance is increased because of the increased ventricular wall tension produced by ventricular contraction. During diastole, blood enters the coronary arteries at the pressure that exists at that moment in the aortic arch. This particular pressure is termed the *aortic diastolic pressure*.

Coronary venous drainage is accomplished via three subdivisions of the venous system of the heart: the thebesian veins drain a portion of the right atrial and right ventricular myocardium; the anterior cardiac veins drain a large portion of the right ventricle; and the coronary sinus and its branches drain the left ventricle and the majority of myocardial venous return.

Conduction system

Properties of cardiac muscle

The mechanical contraction of the heart is the product of a stimulus-response process. The following prop-

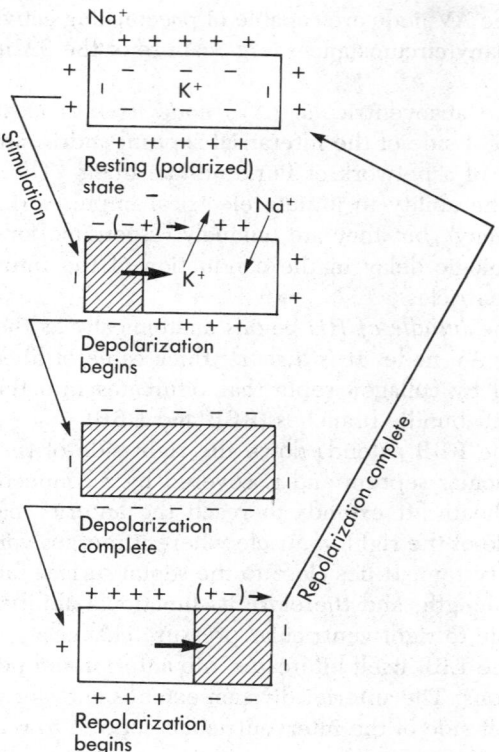

Fig. 43-3. Schematic diagram illustrating process of depolarization and repolarization.

erties are integral components of the electromechanical events in the heart.

Action potential. The resting myocardial cell has a membrane potential (i.e., an electrical charge), as a result of the relative distribution of sodium and potassium ions extracellularly and intracellularly. Whenever the cell is stimulated, the membrane potential undergoes a change. A graphic record of this change forms the basis for an electrocardiogram (ECG). The change in electrical potential in response to a stimulus is known as the action potential. The two components of the action potential are *depolarization* and *repolarization*.

In the resting state, the inside of the cell is negative with respect to the outside (Fig. 43-3). Extracellular measurements show a high sodium concentration and a low potassium concentration. Conversely, intracellular recordings reveal a high potassium and low sodium concentration. This distribution is maintained by a selectively permeable membrane, which in the resting state is more permeable to potassium than to sodium.

The initiation of a cardiac impulse begins with the process of depolarization. The term *depolarization* indicates the rapid reversal of the resting membrane potential, which results from the following sequence of events: (1) the cell membrane permeability to sodium increases spontaneously (as in pacemaking cells) or in

response to a stimulus; (2) there is a rapid influx of sodium; and (3) potassium moves out of the cell. This movement of ions across the membrane creates an electrical current. When the amount of sodium entering the cell reaches a critical level, an electrical impulse is generated. The impulse may spread as a wave of depolarization to adjacent cells.

Repolarization is the process by which the cell is returned to the resting state. The following sequence of events occurs: (1) the cell membrane permeability to sodium decreases; and (2) sodium leaves the cell and potassium returns through an active ion transport system.

Automaticity. The ability of the heart to initiate impulses regularly and spontaneously is known as automaticity or rhythmicity. Although most cardiac cells have this ability, it is the prominent property of the sinoatrial (SA) node, making it the primary pacemaker in the normal heart. Pacemaker cells are known to have lower resting membrane potentials than other myocardial cells and exhibit *spontaneous* depolarization.

Excitability. The ability of cardiac cells to respond to a stimulus by initiating a cardiac impulse is known as excitability. It should be noted that excitatory cells differ from pacemaker cells in that pacemaker cells do not require a stimulus to initiate an impulse.

Conductivity. The ability of cardiac cells to respond to a cardiac impulse by transmitting the impulse along cell membranes is referred to as conductivity. Cells, which are specialized in this function, are found in the conduction system. The arrangement of cells outside the conduction system ensures rapid conduction through intercalated disks joining adjacent cells.

Contractility. The ability of cardiac cells to respond to an impulse by contracting is known as contractility. Contractile cells compose the largest mass of the myocardium, but it should be noted that under certain circumstances, the contractile cell may become an excitable or a conducting cell and, in the case of Purkinje fibers, an automatic cell.

Refractoriness. The inability of cardiac cells to respond to successive stimuli is known as refractoriness. During the absolute refractory period, no stimulus will produce a response. This period begins with depolarization and extends through a portion of the repolarization period until the sodium ion carrier sites are again free to transport the sodium ions necessary for depolarization.

Refractoriness progressively diminishes in the relative refractory period, which occurs in the final stage of repolarization. During this interval, a stimulus of sufficient strength will produce a response. When the resting state is attained, the cell is no longer refractory. During the latter period, a mild stimulus will initiate a cardiac impulse. This is known as the supernormal period.

Anatomy of the conduction system

The pacemaking center of the normal heart is the *sinoatrial* (SA) or "sinus," node (Fig. 43-4). Located in the right atrium near the root of the superior vena cava, it is composed of two types of specialized cells within a network of dense Purkinje-like fibers. P cells in the center of the node initiate impulses at a rate of 60 to 100/min under normal conditions. T cells on the circumference transmit these impulses to surrounding atrial muscle.

Formerly, it was thought that the sinus impulse traveled to the AV node by spreading radially through the atrial musculature. More recent studies have identified that the impulse is actually conducted through tracts composed of Purkinje fibers and ordinary myocardial cells. The three tracts traveling to the AV node are designated as anterior, middle, and posterior *internodal tracts*. A fourth tract, called Bachmann's bundle, branches off the anterior nodal tract and transmits the impulse to the left atrium.

The three internodal tracts meet at the atrionodal junction. The junctional area refers to the region where atrial and ventricular tissues merge. This junction contains the AV node. The junctional cells above and below the AV node are capable of pacemaking activity under many circumstances (e.g., failure of the SA node to fire).

The atrioventricular *(AV) node* itself is located on the right side of the interatrial septum and is also composed of a network of Purkinje-like fibers. These cells lack the ability to initiate electrical impulses (i.e., automaticity), but they are uniquely responsible for a brief physiologic delay in the conduction of the impulse to the ventricles.

The *bundle of His* begins anatomically as the "tail" of the AV node. It is a short, thick cable of fibers separated by collagen septa that bifurcates into the right and left bundle branches (RBB and LBB).

The RBB extends down the right side of the interventricular septum and is covered by a connective tissue sheath. It extends to reach the anterior papillary muscle of the right ventricle where it merges with Purkinje system. It lies close to the septal surface for much of its length, and therefore its functional ability is vulnerable to right ventricular pressure changes.

The LBB itself bifurcates into anterior and posterior divisions. The anterior division extends anteriorly down the left side of the interventricular septum to reach the

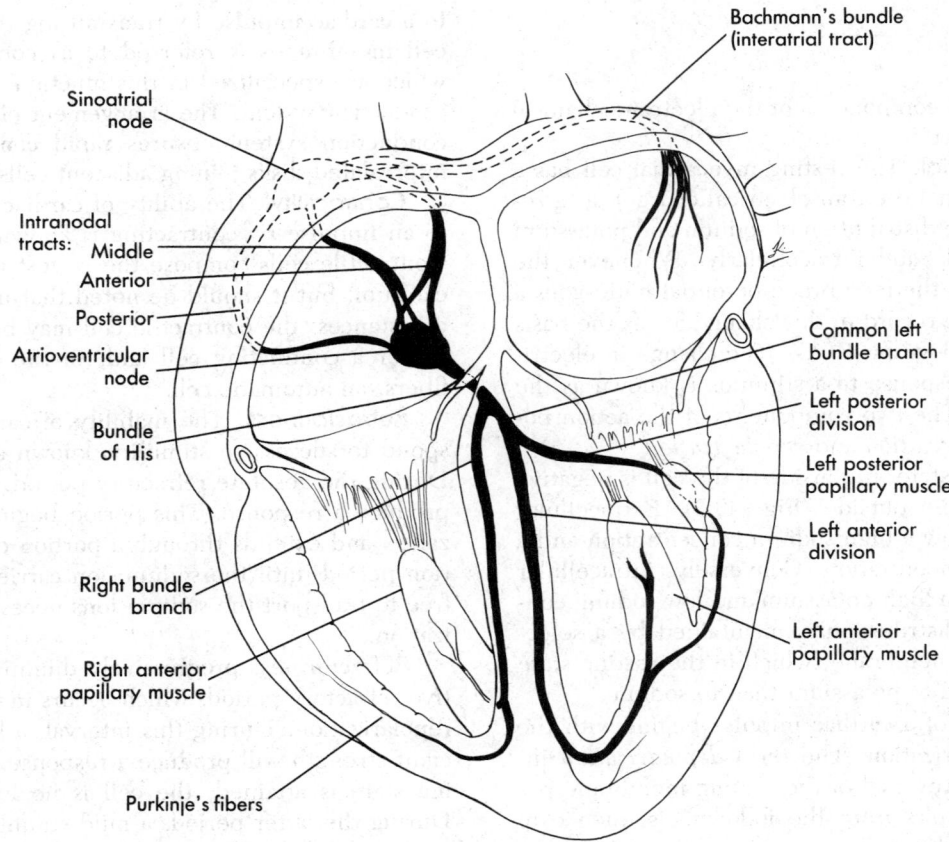

Fig. 43-4. Schematic diagram of heart illustrating the conduction system.

anterior papillary muscle. The posterior division is shorter and thicker and extends to the posterior papillary muscle of the left ventricle. Both divisions connect with Purkinje system and equally share in the spread of the impulse to the left ventricle.

Purkinje fibers lie as a network on the endocardial surface and penetrate the myocardium of both ventricles. They are responsible for the transmission of the impulse to both ventricular free walls. Purkinje cells are elongated and contain intercalated disks.

Cells outside the conduction system also play a role in the conduction of an impulse. A surface membrane, the sarcolemma, surrounds each cell and acts as a selectively permeable barrier to sodium and potassium ions. Adjacent myocardial cells are connected end-to-end by a thickened portion of the sarcolemma known as an intercalated disk. These disks act as low-resistance pathways to the transmission of an impulse between cells.

Sequence of cardiac activation

Depolarization is initiated by an impulse from the SA node. The impulse first spreads through the right atrium and then activates the left atrium. Atrial activation is normally accomplished in 0.11 second or less.

Shortly after the impulse reaches the left atrium, it also activates the junctional region and subsequently the AV node. The AV node delays the impulse about 0.1 second before the impulse enters the bundle of His.

Once reaching the bundle of His, the impulse is transmitted along the bundle branches. Within the ventricles, the first structure to be activated is the ventricular septum. The septum is activated by the impulse traveling from the left side to the right side.

The impulse then continues down the remaining length of the bundle branches and into Purkinje network, thus activating the free ventricular walls almost simultaneously. Activation of the ventricular muscle proceeds from the apex toward the base of the heart to complete the process.

Depolarization of cardiac musculature proceeds from endocardium to epicardium. Repolarization in the atria follows this same pathway. In contrast, repolarization of ventricular musculature proceeds from epicardium to endocardium. Knowledge of the sequence of activation is fundamental to analysis of the ECG.

Cardiac cycle

It is not the action potential itself that causes the myofibrils to contract. It is believed that electrical stimulation causes muscular contraction by stimulating the release of calcium ions from the cisternae of the sarcoplasmic reticulum. Once the sarcoplasmic reticulum is depolarized, the electrical excitation spreads rapidly through it, resulting in the release of large amounts of calcium. Calcium diffuses rapidly into the myofibril sarcomere, which is the basic contractile unit of the myocardial cell. Calcium ions then catalyze the chemical reaction that promotes the interdigitating and sliding of the actin and myosin filaments along each other. As these myofilaments overlap each other, they form linkages or cross-bridges, which are force-generating sites. This actin-myosin interaction produces myocardial contraction by a sliding filament mechanism, which causes a shortening of the sarcomeres. The shortening of multiple sarcomeres initiates muscle contraction. Immediately on the termination of the action potential, calcium ions are then pumped back into the sarcomere reticulum. The resultant decrease in the density of calcium ions surrounding the myofibrils is insufficient to maintain muscular contraction. Therefore a dissociation of the actin-myosin linkage occurs and the muscle relaxes.

The cardiac cycle has two phases—diastole and systole. Relaxation and filling of both atria and then both ventricles take place during diastole. Contraction and emptying of both atria and then both ventricles occur during systole.

Diastole

The diastolic phase of the cardiac cycle is subdivided into the following phases: (1) isometric ventricular relaxation, (2) rapid ventricular filling, and (3) slow ventricular filling.

The initial phase of isometric ventricular relaxation begins as soon as the aortic valve and pulmonic valve close. During this time, the myocardial muscle relaxes and ventricular pressure falls. However, the falling ventricular pressure is still higher than atrial pressure, therefore the AV valves remain closed. Because these valves remain closed, a large amount of blood collects in the atria. As ventricular pressure begins to drop more rapidly to its low diastolic level, the higher pressure in the atria pushes the AV valves open and allows blood to flow rapidly into the ventricular cavity. This second phase of diastole, the rapid filling phase, lasts for approximately the first third of diastole. Rapid ventricular filling causes intraventricular pressures to rise. As ventricular pressure increases, it impedes further rapid filling, and the resultant slowing of ventricular filling marks the third phase of diastole. This phase of slow ventricular filling is referred to as diastasis. Both the atrial and ventricular chambers are relaxed and blood entering the atria flows passively into the ventricles.

Systole

Atrial systole. Electrical depolarization spreads through the atria and pauses at the AV node for 0.10 second. The atrial musculature then contracts, propelling an additional 20% to 30% of blood into the ventricle before ventricular contraction.

Ventricular systole. The ventricular systolic phase of the cardiac cycle is subdivided into phases of isometric ventricular contraction, maximal ventricular ejection, and reduced ventricular ejection.

During the isometric ventricular contraction phase, there is an increase in myocardial tension and intraventricular pressure, while there is no change in blood volume or muscle fiber length. At this time, the aortic valve is closed, because pressure in the aortic root exceeds left ventricular pressure. The higher pressure in the aortic root is the result of a previous systole that has just ejected blood into the aorta. As this aortic blood is distributed to the periphery, aortic pressure falls slowly. At the same time, intraventricular pressure and tension are increasing. When intraventricular pressure exceeds aortic root pressure, the aortic valve opens and maximal ventricular ejection begins. Blood from the ventricles is pumped into the pulmonic and systemic circulations. As the ejection rate starts to slow, the phase of reduced ventricular ejection, or protodiastole, begins. The ventricles remain contracted, but there is little blood being ejected from the ventricle into the aorta. Ventricular pressure actually falls slightly below aortic root pressure, but some blood is still being ejected simply because of the momentum built up by the contraction. At the end of systole, ventricular relaxation begins suddenly, and there is a rapid decrease in intraventricular pressure. The higher pressure in the large arteries and in the aortic root immediately pushes blood back toward the ventricles, therefore snapping shut the semilunar valves.

Cardiac output

The amount of blood ejected from the left ventricle into the aorta per minute is called the cardiac output. Although the right ventricle ejects an equivalent amount of blood into the pulmonary artery, it is not included in the measurement of total cardiac output. Rather, cardiac output (CO) is equivalent to stroke volume (SV) (volume of blood ejected from the left ventricle with each contraction) times heart rate (HR) (number of heart beats per minute):

$$CO = SV \times HR$$

The average cardiac output is 5.6 L/min in the average man. However, during periods of strenuous exercise, the cardiac output may reach 20 to 25 L/min. Since cardiac requirements will vary according to individual body sizes, a more accurate means of assessing tissue perfusion is to compute the cardiac index. The *cardiac index* is obtained by dividing the cardiac output by the patient's total body surface area:

$$\text{Cardiac index} = \frac{\text{CO (L/min)}}{\text{body surface area (sq m)}}$$

Therefore the cardiac index represents the cardiac output in terms of liters per minute per square meter of body surface. This corrects an individual's cardiac output to match body size. The normal range for cardiac index is 2.4 to 4.0 L/min. The cardiac output is based solely on the amount of blood ejected by the left ventricle into the systemic circulation. The average 70 kg man will have an approximate cardiac index of 3 L/min.

Stroke volume

Stroke volume is the amount of blood ejected by the left ventricle into the aorta per beat. At the completion of each filling phase, or diastole, the ventricle contains approximately 120 ml of blood (end-diastolic volume [EDV]). Under normal circumstances, the heart ejects approximately two thirds of this EDV. The portion of blood that is ejected is termed the ejection fraction. The volume of residual blood in the ventricle at the end of systole is known as the end systolic volume (ESV). Therefore stroke volume can be defined as the difference between the volume of blood contained in the ventricle at the end of diastole and the volume of blood remaining at the end of systole:

$$SV = EDV - ESV$$

Control of cardiac output

Cardiac output is dependent on the relationship between two important variables—stroke volume and heart rate. Despite fluctuations in one of these two variables, cardiac output can be maintained at relatively constant levels by compensatory adjustments made in the other variable. For example, if the heart rate slows, the time for ventricular filling (diastole) is lengthened. This lengthened period allows for an increase in preload and a subsequent increase in stroke volume. Conversely, if the stroke volume falls, the heart rate can increase to compensate temporarily and to maintain cardiac output. Therefore the actual determinants of cardiac output are the mechanisms regulating stroke volume and heart rate.

Control of stroke volume. Three significant factors affecting stroke volume and thus cardiac output are preload, contractility, and afterload.

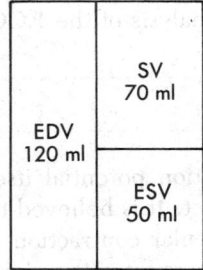

Fig. 43-5. Representation of normal ventricular function, illustrating relationship between end-diastolic volume (EDV), stroke volume (SV), and end-systolic volume (ESV).

PRELOAD. Starling's law of the heart states that myocardial fiber responds with a more forceful contraction when it is stretched. An example of this phenomenon is that of increasing the stretch of a rubber band to obtain a more forceful recoil when the rubber band is released. Myocardial fibers can be stretched by increasing the volume of blood delivered to the ventricles during diastole. The degree of myocardial stretch before contraction is expressed in terms of preload. Preload is related to the volume of blood distending the ventricles at the end of diastole. Preload is determined by the amount of venous return and the ejection fraction, which determines the amount of blood left in the ventricle at the end of systole.

According to Starling's law, increasing venous return, and thereby increasing left ventricular end-diastolic volume (preload), facilitates ventricular contraction and promotes increased ventricular function by stretching the myocardial fibers. Stretching of the sarcomeres increases the number of interaction sites for actin-myosin linkages and therefore increases ventricular contraction. Under normal conditions, the sarcomere is stretched to 2.0 mm during ventricular diastole. Maximal ventricular force is developed at a sarcomere length of 2.2 mm. It is at this length that actin and myosin are able to enjoy the greatest number of interaction sites. When myocardial stretching exceeds 2.4 mm, the myofilaments become partially disengaged and fewer contractile sites are activated. Since Starling's length-tension relationship is only functional within physiologic limits, it is important to note that prolonged, excessive stretching of the myocardial fibers will eventually lead to a decrease in cardiac output by reducing the stroke volume (as in ventricular hypertrophy).

CONTRACTILITY. Contractility is another major mechanism involved in the control of stroke volume. By definition, contractility refers only to a change in the inotropic state of the muscle without a change in myocardial fiber length or preload. Increased contractility (inotropism) is a function of the increased intensity of interaction at the actin-myosin linkages. Contractility can be increased by sympathetic stimulation or by the administration of substances such as calcium or epinephrine. Increased contractility improves ventricular emptying during systole, thereby increasing the stroke volume.

AFTERLOAD. Another factor involved in the control of stroke volume is afterload. Afterload is defined as the amount of tension the ventricle must develop during contraction in order to eject blood from the left ventricle into the aorta. The major impedance against which the left ventricle must pump is primarily determined by peripheral vascular resistance. Increase in pressure resulting from hypertension or vasoconstriction produces an increased resistance to pumping and will ne-

cessitate an increase in ventricular tension in order to eject blood. Not only is the afterload on the heart affected by the amount of aortic pressure, but it is also affected by the size of the heart. This relationship between ventricular tension, arterial pressure, and ventricular size is known as the law of Laplace:

$$\text{Ventricular tension} = \text{Arterial pressure} \times \text{Ventricular radius}$$

As this simplified version of Laplace's law indicates, both hypertension and dilation of the ventricular chamber increase ventricular tension (increase afterload). Therefore if arterial pressure increases, the ventricle must pump against higher resistance in order to empty adequately. Also, if ventricular radius increases, ventricular volume will increase. Thus at the same level of aortic pressure, the afterload against which an enlarged or dilated left ventricle must work is higher than that encountered by a normal-sized ventricle.

Excessive elevation of the afterload may impair ventricular emptying, thereby reducing stroke volume and cardiac output.

Control of heart rate. The autonomic nervous system (ANS) regulates the heart through two distinctly opposing sets of nerves—the sympathetic and the parasympathetic nervous systems. Afferent fibers accompany the efferent fibers of both these systems.

The sympathetic fibers arise from the thoracic spinal cord and reach the entire atria and ventricles as well as the SA and the AV nodes. The control of the ANS on the heart is mediated by neurotransmitters. The sympathetic nervous system neurotransmitter is norepinephrine. The sympathetic fibers have both positive chronotropic (increase rate) and inotropic (increase force) effects. Therefore with an increase in sympathetic stimulation, the neurotransmitter norepinephrine is released from the nerve endings and produces the following effects: increase in heart rate, increase in atrial and ventricular contractility, and increase in the speed of electrical conduction through the AV node.

The parasympathetic fibers originate in the medulla and have their innervation primarily in the atrial musculature and in the SA and AV nodes; however, parasympathetic stimulation has been shown to reach the ventricles. The parasympathetic fibers have a negative chronotropic effect and may exert a slightly negative inotropic effect; however, in the healthy circulatory system, this negative inotropic effect is compensated for by the increased filling that occurs as a result of a lengthened diastole. Stimulation of the parasympathetic system causes the release of the neurotransmitter acetylcholine at the vagal nerve endings and has basically the opposite effect of norepinephrine. Parasympathetic stimulation causes a decrease in the rate of discharge of the SA node, a decrease in the rate of conduction from the atria to the ventricles, and a decrease in the force of atrial contraction and probably also of ventricular contraction. The final effect of ANS control on the heart is the balance between these two opposing nervous systems at any one time. It is thought that the heart is normally under the control of vagal inhibition and maintains a resting heart rate of 65 to 75 beats/min.

The effects of the ANS can be greatly influenced by several additional factors, such as the central nervous system (CNS) and pressoreceptor reflexes. Impulses from the cerebral cortex can have a significant effect on the heart rate. Pain, fear, anger, and excitement can all cause substantial increases in the heart rate. Also, reflex changes caused by stimulation of the pressoreceptors can influence heart rate. The baroreceptor reflex, with afferent branches in the aortic arch, carotid sinus, and other pressoreceptor zones, functions as a negative feedback mechanism to regulate pressure in the arteries and regulate the resistance of vessels in the vasculature. Consequently, an episode of hypotension would cause a sudden drop of blood pressure in the aorta or carotid sinus and would stimulate the pressoreceptors less intensely. The cardiac inhibitory center would then be stimulated less, and the end result would be a reflex increase in the heart rate.

Many other important factors are involved in the control of heart rate, including body temperature, medication, catecholamines, arterial blood gas tensions, hormones other than epinephrine, and plasma electrolyte concentrations.

In summary, ventricular function and, hence, cardiac output are influenced by heart rate and stroke volume. Heart rate is primarily controlled by the ANS, and stroke volume is dependent on the three distinct variables of preload, contractility, and afterload.

Blood pressure

Blood flows out of the heart, goes through the arterial system into the capillary bed, then flows out of the tissues through the venous system and back into the heart. Blood flow depends on two variables—a *pressure gradient* (difference in pressure between two points) and *resistance* to flow. Blood flows from areas of high pressure to areas of low pressure. Arterial pressure averages approximately 100 mm Hg. This pressure falls very slightly in the larger arteries because of little resistance, but it falls rapidly in arterioles where the small size increases resistance. Blood pressure drops to about 25 mm Hg in the capillaries and is close to zero as the blood enters the right atrium.

Arterial pressure

Arterial blood pressure (P) is defined as the force exerted by the blood against the arterial wall and is *directly* related to the cardiac output (CO) (p. 1036) and peripheral vascular resistance (R):

$$P = CO \times R$$

Thus arterial blood pressure decreases when cardiac output and peripheral resistance decrease and vice versa. Factors affecting cardiac output and peripheral resistance are summarized in the box below. Peripheral resistance is *inversely* related to the size and elasticity of the blood vessel; thus peripheral resistance increases when the diameter or elasticity of the vessel is decreased.

Systolic blood pressure is the maximal pressure exerted against the arterial wall during cardiac systole (contraction phase); *diastolic blood pressure* is the maximal pressure exerted against the arterial wall during cardiac diastole (relaxation phase). In general, increases in cardiac output increase systolic pressure, whereas increases in peripheral resistance increase diastolic pressure. For example, systolic pressure increases with emotions, pain, or exercise, whereas diastolic pressure increases with atherosclerosis. The *pulse pressure* is the difference between systolic and diastolic blood pressures. For example, a pulse pressure of 40 mm Hg is present when the blood pressure is 120/80 mm Hg. A narrow pulse pressure indicates a low stroke volume, high peripheral resistance, or both.

Venous pressure

Blood flow through the veins is facilitated by pressure gradients. In the limbs the veins are surrounded by skeletal muscles that compress the veins when the muscle contracts. This rhythmic contraction of skeletal muscles propels the blood toward the heart. Forward blood flow is facilitated by valves in the veins that prevent backward or regurgitant blood flow. During inspiration, intrathoracic pressure decreases and further facilitates venous return to the heart. During ventricular systole, pressures in the atrium decrease creating a negative pressure that draws venous blood into the atrium. Dysfunction in any of these mechanisms will cause venous pressure to change.

FACTORS AFFECTING ARTERIAL BLOOD PRESSURE

Cardiac output	Stroke volume: preload (blood volume), myocardial contractility, afterload
	Heart rate: autonomic and CNS stimulation, hormones
Peripheral vessel characteristics	Diameter of vessel, elasticity of vessel

Purpose of cardiac assessment

Systematic cardiac assessment provides the nurse with baseline data useful for identifying the physiologic and psychosocial needs of the patient and for planning appropriate nursing interventions to meet these needs. The nurse is in a unique position of ongoing patient monitoring and thus is able to take immediate action when signs occur to indicate alterations of cardiac function.

Subjective data

Subjective data obtained by means of a detailed patient history are as diagnostically significant as laboratory data and ECG recordings in the assessment of the patient with suspected cardiac disease. Accurate assessment data are necessary to develop a profile of the cardiac risk factors operating in any individual situation, as well as to determine the psychodynamic family relationships that must be addressed throughout the diagnostic, treatment, and follow-up phases.

The cardinal symptoms of heart disease include *dyspnea, chest pain* or discomfort, *edema, syncope, palpitations,* and excessive *fatigue*. Cyanosis is usually a sign rather than a symptom, but it too may be an important feature of the patient's history, particularly in patients with congenital heart disease. An important principle of cardiovascular evaluation is that cardiovascular function, which may be adequate at rest, may be insufficient during exercise or exertion. Therefore careful attention should be directed to the effects of activity on the patient's symptoms.

Dyspnea

Dyspnea is one of the most common and distressing symptoms of cardiopulmonary disease. It is described as an abnormally uncomfortable awareness of breathing. The patient complains of shortness of breath. Since dyspnea is associated with a variety of diseases, as well as with anxiety, the history is a necessary tool in evaluating the etiologic factors.

There are several different types of dyspnea; therefore the history must include factors that precipitate and relieve dyspnea and data regarding the patient's body position when dyspnea occurs.

Dyspnea on exertion is a common symptom of cardiac dysfunction. In the early stages of heart failure, dyspnea is usually provoked only by effort and is relieved promptly by rest. It is important to identify the amount of exertion necessary to produce dyspnea, be-

cause the less the cardiac reserve (heart's ability to adjust and adapt to increased demands), the less effort is required to precipitate dyspnea.

Orthopnea refers to dyspnea in the recumbent position. It is usually a symptom of more advanced heart failure than is exertional dyspnea. Patients relate that they may use two or more pillows in order to sleep restfully in a semiupright position. When an individual assumes the recumbent position, gravitational forces redistribute blood from the lower extremities and splanchnic bed, increasing venous return. The augmentation of intrathoracic blood volume elevates pulmonary venous and capillary pressures, resulting in a transient pulmonary congestion. Orthopnea is usually relieved in less than 5 minutes after the patient sits upright.

Paroxysmal nocturnal dyspnea, also known as cardiac asthma, is characterized by severe attacks of shortness of breath that generally occur 2 to 5 hours after the onset of sleep. This condition is frequently associated with sweating and wheezing and wakens the patient from sleep. These frightening attacks are precipitated by an increased blood volume caused by the reabsorption of edema that was pooled in dependent portions of the body during the day. When the patient lies in a recumbent position, there is a redistribution of the increased intravascular volume with a specific rise in intrathoracic blood volume. The diseased heart is unable to compensate for this increase in blood volume, and it is not able to pump extra fluid into the circulatory system; therefore pulmonary congestion results. Paroxysmal nocturnal dyspnea is relieved by having the patient sit on the side of the bed or even get out of bed. However, unlike simple orthopnea, paroxysmal nocturnal dyspnea may require 20 minutes or more for the patient to obtain relief.

Chest pain

Although pain or discomfort in the chest is one of the cardinal symptoms of cardiac disorders, it is essential to recognize that chest pain can be precipitated by a variety of conditions. For example, chest pain may be caused by ischemic heart disease, acute dissection of the aorta, or acute pericarditis, or it may occur in pulmonary disorders (e.g., pleurisy and pulmonary embolism). The most common cause of chest pain, however, is not associated with cardiovascular disease (CVD), but rather with anxiety. Therefore to correctly evaluate chest pain, the following list of characteristic symptoms should be addressed during a thorough history.

1. Onset	When was chest pain first noticed?
2. Manner of onset	Did the pain or discomfort start suddenly or gradually?
3. Duration	How long did the pain last?
4. Precipitating factors	Ask patient to describe possible precipitating factors (e.g., exertion, food, anxiety, emotions).

5. Location — Where did the pain originate? Did it radiate? To what area?

6. Quality — Ask patient to describe how symptoms feel (e.g., sharp, dull).

7. Intensity — Ask patient to describe severity of the pain (e.g., if pain interfered with any activities).

8. Chronology and frequency — Has this pain occurred in the past? If so, how often?

9. Associated symptoms — Are there any other signs or symptoms that occur at the same time?

10. Aggravating factors — What makes pain worse?

11. Relaxing factors — What makes symptoms less intense?

Edema

Edema is defined as an accumulation of excess fluid in the interstitial spaces. The retention of considerable amounts of extracellular fluid may occur without associated edema. In fact, weight gains of up to 7 kg of water can occur before the abnormality is detected. Because early manifestations of edema may be subtle, careful comparison of daily weights is required to determine weight gains resulting from fluid retention. Normally, basal body weight varies little from day to day; therefore subtle weight gains resulting from fluid retention are readily detectable.

There are numerous causes of edema, including congestive heart failure, fluid overload, and obstruction of venous drainage. Therefore depending on the specific cause of the edema, it may be localized to one particular body part, organ, or tissue; or it may have a generalized distribution. For a more in-depth discussion of edema, see Chapter 21.

Syncope

Syncope is defined as a generalized muscle weakness with an inability to stand upright, accompanied by loss of consciousness. The most common cause of syncope is decreased perfusion to the brain. Any condition that results in a sudden reduction of cardiac output, and therefore reduced cerebral blood flow, could potentially cause a syncopal episode. In patients with cardiovascular disorders, conditions such as orthostatic hypotension, hypovolemia, or a variety of arrhythmias (e.g., heart block and severe ventricular arrhythmias) may precipitate syncope.

Palpitations

Palpitation is a common subjective phenomenon defined as an unpleasant awareness of the heartbeat. It may be precipitated by a change in cardiac rate or rhythm or by an increase in myocardial contractility. Patients may describe their heartbeat as "pounding," "racing," or "skipping." Palpitations that occur either during or after strenuous activity are considered physiologic and represent an awareness of the overactivity of the heart. Palpitations that occur during mild exertion may suggest the presence of heart failure, anemia, or thyrotoxicosis. Other noncardiac factors that may precipitate palpitations include the following: nervousness; heavy meals; lack of sleep; and a large intake of coffee, tea, alcohol, or tobacco.

Fatigue

There are numerous causes of fatigue and lassitude, and therefore these symptoms are not diagnostic of cardiovascular disorders. However, fatigue as a symptom associated with heart failure may result from such things as nocturia, insomnia, and nocturnal dyspnea. In addition, fatigue may be a direct consequence of the heart failure itself. The exact physiologic mechanism responsible for fatigue related to heart failure is not known, but it is probably a consequence of an inadequate cardiac output. Such fatigue can occur during effort or at rest and generally worsens as the day progresses. Fatigue that occurs after mild exertion may indicate a low cardiac reserve if the heart is unable to meet even small increases in metabolic demands.

Objective data

Physical assessment of cardiac function

The cardiovascular system is examined with the use of *inspection, palpation, percussion,* and *auscultation.* The following is a description of these techniques and their significance in cardiovascular assessment.

Inspection

Beginning with a cephalocaudal approach, the examiner inspects the head and neck. The color of the patient's skin and mucous membranes should be noted. A person's "normal" color depends on race, ethnic background, and life-style and is an indication of adequate cardiac output and circulation. Pallor may indicate anemia, hypoxia, or peripheral vasoconstriction. Cyanosis, a bluish discoloration of the skin, is most easily observed by examining the earlobes, oral mucosa at the base of the tongue, the lips, and the nail beds.

There are two types of cyanosis—central and peripheral. In central cyanosis the tongue is characteristically cyanotic. This form of cyanosis is caused by low arterial oxygen saturation and is generally seen in some congenital heart defects with left-to-right shunts or in pulmonary diseases that interfere with ventilation or diffusion.

Peripheral cyanosis results from low cardiac output and is generally accompanied by decreased skin tem-

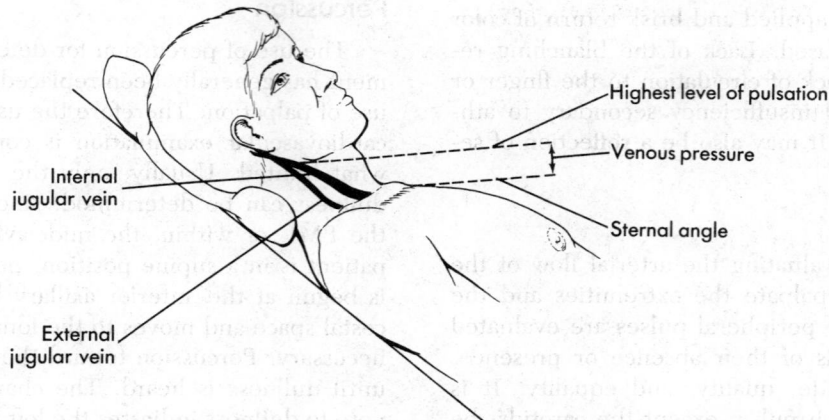

Fig. 43-6. Position of internal and external jugular veins used in measuring venous pressure.

Labels in figure:
- Internal jugular vein
- External jugular vein
- Highest level of pulsation
- Venous pressure
- Sternal angle

perature and mottling. In contrast to central cyanosis, there is no cyanosis of the tongue. (For further information on skin color, see Chapter 68.)

A general estimate of venous pressure can be obtained by observation of the neck veins (Fig. 43-6). Normally, when an individual is in a supine position, the neck veins are distended. However, when the head of the bed is elevated at a 45-degree angle, the neck veins are collapsed. To assess neck vein distention, the patient is first placed in a sitting position and the neck veins are observed. Then the patient's trunk is lowered to a 45-degree angle. The uppermost point of visible internal jugular pulsation is noted, and the height (measured in centimeters) between this level and the level of the sternal angle is recorded. The jugular veins reflect venous tone, blood volume, and right atrial pressure. Therefore distended neck veins suggest increased venous pressure, which may be caused by right-sided heart failure, circulatory volume overload, superior vena caval obstruction, or tricuspid valve regurgitation.

Next, the rate and character of the patient's respirations are assessed. Normally, an adult breathes comfortably at a rate of 12 to 20 times/min. Particular attention is paid to the ease or difficulty in breathing and noting the patient's general demeanor.

Inspection of the anterior chest is best accomplished with the patient lying in a supine position, either flat or with the head slightly elevated. Observe the precordium for the point of maximal impulse (PMI), which is a faint heaving of the chest wall caused by the forward thrusting of the ventricles during systole. The location of the PMI helps to locate the apex of the heart, which lies approximately 0.5 cm to the left of the PMI. Observation of the chest wall is best accomplished in a tangential position. The PMI is normally located in the left fifth intercostal space in the midclavicular line or 8 to 10 cm to the left of the midsternal line (p. 1043). Any pulsation noted below the third intercostal space on the

left precordium is known as the PMI; any pulsation above the third intercostal space is generally not related to the heart but rather to the great vessels. The PMI is not always visible, but it is usually palpable. Concluding the examination of the chest, the examiner observes the entire chest wall for symmetry and the presence of any abnormal pulsations.

An important indicator of cardiovascular function is the presence or absence of peripheral edema, especially in the feet, ankles, legs, and sacrum. Edema that disappears on elevation of the body part may be caused by gravity flow or by interruption of the venous return to the heart caused by constricting clothing or pressure on the veins of the lower extremities.

In contrast, pitting edema does not disappear with elevation of the extremity or body part, and it may be an indication of fluid overload or a pathologic condition (e.g., congestive heart failure) when cardiac pumping efficiency is impaired. Edema is identified by inspection and palpation. Pitting edema is present if an indentation is left in the skin after a thumb or finger has been used to apply gentle pressure (see p. 333).

Next, the nutritional state of the hair, skin, and extremities is assessed. Nutritional deficiencies caused by decreased circulation can produce dry skin, thickened nails, brittle hair, and occasional hair loss in an extremity (characteristic of peripheral vascular disease). The nails must also be assessed for clubbing and capillary refill. The exact cause of clubbing is not known at present; however, clubbing of the fingers is typical of congenital heart defects and of pulmonary arteriovenous (A-V) fistulas with right-to-left shunting. Capillary filling, commonly called blanching, is an indicator of peripheral circulation to the fingers and toes and can be tested in all nail beds. This maneuver is done by pressing the examiner's thumbnail against the edge of a patient's fingernail or toenail and then quickly releasing it. The normal response is whitening (blanching) of the area when pressure is applied and brisk return of color when pressure is released. Lack of the blanching response may indicate lack of circulation to the finger or toe because of arterial insufficiency secondary to atherosclerosis or spasm. It may also be a reflection of severe vasoconstriction.

Palpation

One method for evaluating the arterial flow of the vascular system is to palpate the extremities and the peripheral pulses. The peripheral pulses are evaluated bilaterally on the basis of their absence or presence, rate, rhythm, amplitude, quality, and equality. It is recommended that each pulse, except the carotids, be palpated on the left and right sides simultaneously in order to evaluate contralateral symmetry.

Pulses are rated on a scale of 0 to 4+ as follows:

$$0 = \text{Absent}$$
$$+ = \text{Palpable, but diminished}$$
$$+ + = \text{Normal, or average}$$
$$+ + + = \text{Full and brisk}$$
$$+ + + + = \text{Full and bounding, often visible}$$

Peripheral arterial pulses are palpated systematically using the cephalocaudal approach in the following sequence: carotid, brachial, radial, femoral, popliteal, posterior tibial, and dorsalis pedis. If any peripheral pulse is noted to be absent or unequal to the contralateral pulse, the examiner assesses the pulse proximal to that pulse to evaluate when the pulse begins to diminish. Also, the extremity is felt to assess any noticeable change of temperature.

Concentration on the precordium is the final step. Palpation of the heart should begin with the patient in a supine position. The flat of the examiner's hand is placed lightly on the patient's PMI to determine the character of the apical impulse. If the apical impulse is not palpable, the patient is turned to the left lateral position. This position will bring the heart closer to the chest wall. Locating the PMI with the patient in the lateral position is not suitable for use as an exact determinant of the location of the apex, because the heart has been displaced laterally. However, it is useful as a reference point in relocating the PMI when the patient has returned to a supine position. Normally, the apical impulse is felt as a single, light tap. The presence of anything other than a single, light tap may suggest a myocardial pathologic condition and should be reported to the physician. A thrill, or palpable murmur, indicates the presence of significant turbulent blood flow across an intracardiac shunt or a severely stenotic valve. A thrill has been described as a vibration similar to that of a cat's purr. A thrill is more readily palpated after the patient exhales forcefully. Frequently, having the patient in a left lateral position or leaning forward will accentuate the vibration.

Percussion

The use of percussion for detecting cardiac enlargement has generally been replaced by the more accurate use of palpation. Therefore the use of percussion in the cardiovascular examination is considered to be somewhat limited. Usually, only the left border of cardiac dullness can be determined, since this is located near the PMI, or within, the midclavicular line. While the patient is in a supine position, percussion on the chest is begun at the anterior axillary line in the fifth intercostal space and moves to the fourth intercostal space if necessary. Percussion toward the sternum is continued until dullness is heard. The change in the percussion note to dullness indicates the left border of cardiac dullness. Cardiac dullness noted below the fifth intercostal space, beyond the left midclavicular line, or to the right of the sternum is characteristic of cardiac hypertrophy. Unfortunately, mild to moderate degrees of cardiac hypertrophy or dilation are not usually detectable by percussion.

Auscultation

Auscultation of heart sounds enables a nurse to establish baseline data for identifying current and future cardiac problems that require nursing intervention. Cardiac auscultation also assists the nurse in evaluating a patient's progress (e.g., effect of activity on heart rate) or in monitoring responses to medications (e.g., quinidine or digitalis preparations).

Heart sounds. The first heart sound (S_1) is generally thought to be produced by the almost simultaneous closures of the mitral and tricuspid valves. Closure of the mitral valve slightly precedes clearance of the tricuspid valve, but the combined closure is usually heard as one sound. S_1 lasts approximately 0.10 second and signals the onset of ventricular systole. S_1 is generally loudest at the apex, but it can be heard over the entire precordium. S_1 is longer and lower pitched than the second heart sound (S_2), and S_1 corresponds with the beat of the carotid pulse. S_2 is mainly caused by the closure of the semilunar valves (aortic and pulmonic). Because the mechanical events in the right side of the heart are slightly slower than those in the left side of the heart, the aortic valve closes just before the pulmonic valve. S_2 is usually loudest at the base of the heart and is described as shorter, higher pitched, and "snappier" than S_1. The sounds of the cardiac cycle are depicted in Fig. 43-7.

To avoid missing abnormal auscultatory findings, cardiac auscultation should always be carried out systematically. The examiner may begin at either the apex or the base of the heart. As previously mentioned, the apex of the heart is found by palpating the left anterior part of the chest at the level of the fifth intercostal space (beginning at the left sternal border) until a pulsation is felt. The base of the heart is ap-

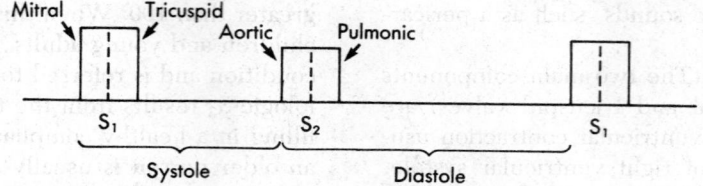

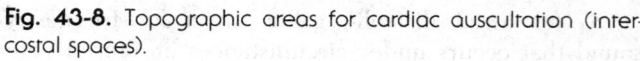

Fig. 43-7. Heart sound S_1 is the closure of mitral and tricuspid valves; S_2 is the closure of aortic and pulmonic valves. Systole is the time interval between S_1 and the start of S_2; diastole is S_2 to the start of S_1. Diastole is longer than systole.

Fig. 43-8. Topographic areas for cardiac auscultation (intercostal spaces).

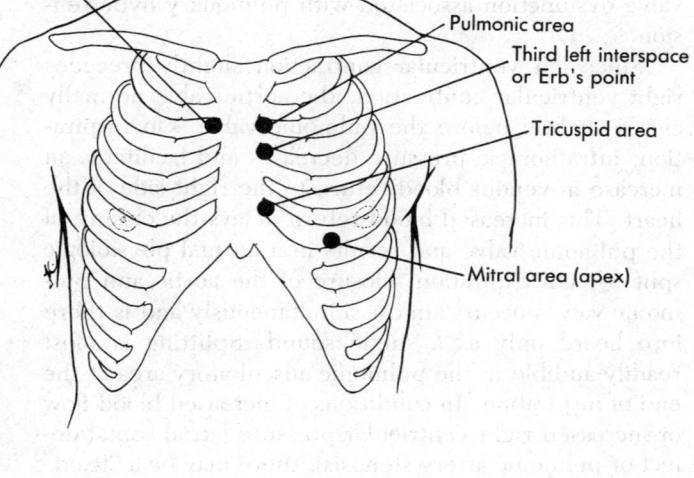

proximately in the area of the second intercostal space.

The following method is used to locate intercostal spaces. The index finger is placed at the suprasternal notch and then moved downward until a ridge is felt (angle of Louis). The finger is moved either to the right or left of the sternum. The space felt is the second intercostal space. While the index finger is still on the second intercostal space, the next finger is placed on the next space below, and so forth, ending with the little finger, which is in the fifth intercostal space.

When using the base-to-apex method of auscultation, listen in order of the following locations:

1. Aortic area (second intercostal space, just to the right of the sternum)
2. Pulmonic area (second intercostal space, just to the left of the sternum)
3. Erb's point (third intercostal space, close to the sternum)
4. Tricuspid area (fifth left intercostal space, close to the sternum)
5. Mitral area or apical area (fifth intercostal space, just medial to the midclavicular line) (Fig. 43-8)

These classic or traditional areas for auscultation are derived from the fact that the sound vibrations produced by the closure of each cardiac valve are projected in the direction of blood flow.

The auscultatory examination should not be restricted to these areas alone, but rather an "inching" method should be employed. The examiner should move the stethoscope small distances from one auscul-

tatory site toward another. This inching method will facilitate the assessment of all auscultatory sounds. Also, at each auscultatory point the examiner should use both the diaphragm and the bell of the stethoscope. The diaphragm chest piece is most useful in listening to high-pitched sounds and murmurs. These include such sounds as S_1, S_2, and ejection sounds and clicks. The diaphragm should be placed firmly on the chest wall so that when it is removed, an indentation is present on the patient's skin. The bell chest piece is most useful in detecting low-pitched sounds and murmurs. These include the third heart sound (S_3), the fourth heart sound (S_4), and mitral and tricuspid diastolic rumbles. The bell should be placed lightly on the chest wall, barely creating an airtight seal. If the bell is placed firmly on the skin, it will act as a diaphragm.

At each auscultatory site, the examiner should do the following:

1. Listen to the rate, rhythm, and intensity of the sound.
2. Listen to S_1 (corresponds with carotid pulse).
3. Listen to S_2.
4. Listen for extra sounds in systole.
5. Listen for extra sounds in diastole.
6. Note any systolic or diastolic murmurs.

7. Note any extracardiac sounds, such as a pericardial friction rub.

SPLITTING OF S_1 AND S_2. The two main components of S_1 (closure of the mitral and tricuspid valves) are asynchronous, because left ventricular contraction usually occurs slightly ahead of right ventricular systole. The dominant component of S_1 is the closure of the mitral valve; therefore a split S_1 is not easily heard. When a split S_1 is audible, the two components (mitral and tricuspid valves) are separated by more than 0.02 second. True S_1 splitting is best heard in the tricuspid area close to the xiphoid. The S_1 may be split in individuals who have right bundle branch block, left-sided mechanical defects (e.g., mitral stenosis), or tricuspid valve dysfunction associated with pulmonary hypertension.

Since left ventricular contraction slightly precedes right ventricular contraction, the aortic valve normally closes slightly before the pulmonic valve. On inspiration, intrathoracic pressure decreases and facilitates an increase in venous blood return to the right side of the heart. This increased blood return delays the closure of the pulmonic valve and results in a normal physiologic split S_2. On expiration, closure of the aortic and pulmonic valves occurs almost simultaneously and is therefore heard only as a single sound. Splitting is most readily audible in the pulmonic auscultatory area at the end of inspiration. In conditions of increased blood flow or increased right ventricular pressure (atrial septal defect or pulmonic artery stenosis), there may be a "fixed" splitting of S_2; that is, both components of S_2 are heard both in inspiration and expiration. A fixed split is considered abnormal and may occur in right bundle branch block, pulmonary hypertension, and right ventricular failure related to atrial or ventricular septal defects.

EXTRA HEART SOUNDS. Extra heart sounds include ejection sounds (systolic clicks), opening snaps, and S_3 and S_4. Of these sounds, the two that occur most frequently and will be discussed here are S_3 and S_4 (see Fig. 43-9).

Ventricular diastolic gallop, or S_3, is a faint low-pitched sound produced by rapid ventricular filling in early diastole. This occurs when the volume of early filling is increased or there is a decrease in ventricular compliance. Ventricular "gallop" describes the canter of a horse, which is frequently mimicked at heart rates

greater than 100. When this sound is present in healthy children and young adults, it is almost always a normal condition and is referred to as a physiologic S_3. A physiologic S_3 results from the transition from rapid to slow filling in a healthy compliant ventricle. An S_3 heard in an older person is usually a pathologic sign and is frequently one of the first signs of serious heart disease or cardiac decompensation as seen in congestive heart failure. An audible S_3 is associated with elevated mid-diastolic left ventricular filling pressures and left atrial and pulmonary artery pressures. Using the bell of the stethoscope barely touching the skin, S_3 is best heard at the apex and occasionally at the left lower sternal border. The presence of S_3 is common in such states as left-to-right shunts, mitral regurgitation, congestive heart failure, and constrictive pericarditis.

S_4 (or atrial diastolic gallop) is a low-frequency sound that occurs under circumstances of altered ventricular compliance, either left or right. S_4 occurs late in diastole when atrial systole ejects blood into a non-compliant ventricle. Because the presence of an audible S_4 is related to a decrease in left ventricular compliance and an increase in left ventricular end-diastolic pressure, it is often heard in hypertensive cardiovascular disease and idiopathic hypertrophic subaortic stenosis. An S_4 is frequently identified in patients with acute myocardial infarctions and in patients with coronary artery disease, especially during an attack of angina pectoris. In addition, an S_4 may be present when cardiac output and stroke volume are increased, such as in severe anemia, thyrotoxicosis, and large A-V fistulas. Although the S_4 sound occurs close to S_1, it can be easily differentiated because S_4 is lower pitched than S_1. It can be differentiated from ejection sounds because S_4 is heard only with the bell of the stethoscope, whereas S_1 and ejection sounds are readily audible using the diaphragm. S_4 is heard best at the apex and the left lower sternal border during expiration, with the patient in a left side-lying position.

Murmurs. Murmurs are audible vibrations of the heart and great vessels that occur because of turbulent blood flow. Turbulent blood flow may be produced by hemodynamic events or by structural alterations occurring in the heart or in the walls of the great vessels. In general, murmurs are heard most distinctly over the area of the valve or altered cardiac structure responsible for the vibrations. The major factors involved in the production of cardiac murmurs include the following: (1) increased velocity of blood flow through normal or abnormal valves; (2) forward flow through a stenotic or irregular valve orifice; (3) backward (regurgitant) blood flow through an incompetent valve, septal defect, or patent ductus arteriosus; and (4) turbulent blood flow produced in a dilated chamber, such as is found in a ventricular or aortic aneurysm.

Murmurs are generally characterized according to

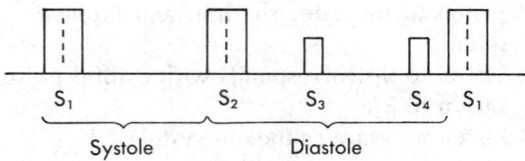

Fig. 43-9. Location of extra heart sound during cardiac cycle.

timing (position in the cardiac cycle), intensity, quality, pitch, location, and direction of radiation. These characteristics provide data concerning the location and nature of the cardiac abnormality.

TIMING. Most murmurs occur in either the systolic or diastolic phase of the cardiac cycle, hence the phrase systolic or diastolic murmurs. However, a few murmurs are heard throughout both phases of the cardiac cycle. A systolic murmur occurs between S_1 and S_2; a diastolic murmur occurs between S_2 and S_1. Systolic murmurs are also classified as early, mid, or late systolic, or holosystolic (lasting through all of systole). Diastolic murmurs are further described as early, mid, or late diastolic, or presystolic.

INTENSITY. Murmurs are traditionally graded from I to VI in terms of their loudness:

Grade I   Very faint; not usually heard during the first few seconds of listening
Grade II   Faint; but immediately recognizable
Grade III   Intermediate in intensity; but loud
Grade IV   Loud; often associated with a palpable thrill
Grade V   Very loud; associated with a thrill
Grade VI   Exceptionally loud; audible when the stethoscope is removed slightly from the chest wall

QUALITY. The quality of a murmur is described as harsh, blowing, rumbling, or musical. The characteristic shape or pattern of a murmur further describes its quality. A murmur, which progressively increases in intensity, is called a crescendo murmur. A murmur, which progressively decreases in intensity after its onset, is called a decrescendo murmur. Finally, a murmur whose intensity increases and then decreases is termed crescendo-decrescendo.

PITCH. The pitch of a murmur is in part determined by the velocity of blood flow. A high-frequency murmur composed of a large number of vibrations will be heard as being high pitched or sharp. Conversely, a low-frequency murmur will produce a sound that is interpreted as low pitched or dull.

LOCATION AND DIRECTION OF RADIATION. The location of a murmur is described in relation to the auscultatory area in which the murmur is the loudest. Not all cardiac murmurs transmit their sounds to other areas, but some murmurs radiate from the area of loudest auscultation to other areas on the precordium, or to the neck or to the axilla. Information regarding the radiating pattern of a murmur is helpful in determining the origin of the murmur. For example, certain valvular defects have typical radiation patterns, such as in mitral insufficiency, when the murmur radiates to the left axilla. The examiner may describe this murmur as a grade II/VI harsh, holosystolic murmur heard best at the apex and radiating to the left axilla.

Pericardial friction rub. A pericardial friction rub is an extra heart sound originating from the pericardial sac. This rub may be a sign of inflammation, infection, or infiltration. It occurs as the heart moves. Pericardial friction rubs may have specific subcomponents (different sounds), each associated with a particular cardiac movement. The heart moves with atrial and ventricular systole and with ventricular diastole. Each of the sound components of a pericardial friction rub corresponds to a movement of the cardiac cycle and is described as a short, high-pitched scratchy sound. The location of a pericardial friction rub may vary; however, it is usually heard best in the third interspace to the left of the sternum. The intensity of the rub may be increased by having the patient lean forward and exhale.

Vascular auscultation by sphygmomanometry

Vascular auscultation refers to measurement of the arterial blood pressure by sphygmomanometry. Blood pressure varies with the cardiac cycle, reaching a systolic high and diastolic low.

Basic principles

Although the essential procedures of obtaining blood pressure measurements are more thoroughly described in basic nursing skill books, the following overview highlights some of the salient features requisite to accurate pressure determinations.

1. A blood pressure cuff of the proper size is selected. A cuff that is too small may give a false high reading, and a cuff that is too large may give a false low reading. For the average adult, a cuff 12 to 14 cm wide and 30 cm long is appropriate. Children and thin adults will require the use of a smaller cuff. Wider cuffs (18 to 20 cm) should be used when obtaining blood pressure readings on the thigh and on large or obese persons.
2. The patient should be as comfortable and relaxed as possible. The patient's arm is positioned so that the brachial artery is approximately at heart level. Deviations of up to 10 mm Hg in both systolic and diastolic readings may occur if the arm is not positioned at heart level. The cuff is snugly secured.
3. The radial pulse is palpated and then the cuff is inflated to approximately 30 mm Hg above the level at which the radial pulse disappears. The cuff pressure is slowly lowered until the radial pulse is palpable once again. This is the palpable systolic pressure and will help the examiner to avoid missing the true systolic reading.

Initial blood pressure measurements should be taken on both arms; normally, there may be a difference in arm pressures of 5 to 10 mm Hg. However, a pressure difference greater than 10 mm Hg may suggest arterial compression or obstruction and should be reported.

All blood pressure measurements should be recorded according to Korotkoff's sounds; that is, the first, fourth, and fifth phases of sound are included in the reading (e.g., 120/80/74). The first phase of Korotkoff's sounds is a tapping sound caused by an initial spurt of blood into the collapsed artery as deflation of the cuff is begun. This sound is considered the measurement of *systolic blood pressure*. As the cuff is deflated, more blood rushes into the artery, causing a murmur that is known as the second phase of Korotkoff's sounds. The third phase occurs when the murmur changes to a tapping sound again; the fourth phase begins when the tapping of the third phase becomes muffled; and the fifth phase occurs when the sound disappears entirely. It is felt that true *diastolic pressure* is between the fourth and fifth phases. In order to identify accurately Korotkoff's sounds, the blood pressure cuff is pumped up rapidly and then slowly deflated at a rate of approximately 2 mm Hg/sec. Deviation from normal Korotkoff's sounds can indicate cardiac or vascular abnormalities. Because of this, the technique used for measuring blood pressure is very important.

Vascular auscultation also includes listening for *bruits*, especially over the carotid arteries. These sounds are murmurs caused by turbulent blood flow as a result of narrowing of the arteries.

Problems in blood pressure auscultation

Inaudible blood pressure. The most frequent cause of an inaudible blood pressure is improper positioning of the stethoscope over the brachial artery. The stethoscope should not be touching the cuff or the patient's clothing. If repeated attempts to obtain the blood pressure reading have been made on the same arm, venous engorgement may be present because of repeated cuff inflations. The patient's arm should be elevated over the head for 1 to 2 minutes, and then the procedure is repeated.

Arrhythmias. Irregular rhythms, such as frequent premature ventricular contractions (PVCs) or atrial fibrillation, may cause variations in systolic pressure. In this case, an average blood pressure should be computed from several successive readings. It should be indicated that measurements are an approximation.

Lower limb blood pressure. When a large cuff is used, the systolic pressure in the legs may be as much as 20 mm Hg higher than in the arms, but the diastolic pressure is usually identical to that in the arms. The recording of a higher diastolic pressure in the legs than in the arms may indicate that the thigh cuff is not large enough. The recording of a systolic pressure that is substantially lower in the legs than in the arms is significant and may represent aortic disease

or coarctation of the aorta and should be reported to the physician.

Abnormal pulses

A *hypokinetic* (weak) pulse signifies a narrowed pulse pressure (decreased difference between systolic and diastolic pressures) (p. 1038). It is usually produced by a low cardiac output and is associated with increased peripheral vascular resistance. This type of pulse may be palpable in such conditions as severe left ventricular failure, hypovolemia, or mitral and aortic valve stenosis.

A *hyperkinetic* (bounding) pulse represents a widened pulse pressure. It is usually associated with an increased left ventricular stroke volume and a decrease in peripheral vascular resistance. This type of pulse is frequently found in hyperkinetic circulatory states caused by exercise, fever, anemia, and hyperthyroidism.

Pulsus alternans is a condition in which the heart beats regularly, but the pulses alternate in amplitude. It is caused by an alternating left ventricular contractile force and usually indicates severe depression of myocardial function. Pulsus alternans may be detected by palpation but is more accurately assessed by auscultation of the blood pressure.

Pulsus paradoxus signifies a reduction in the amplitude of the arterial pulse during inspiration. Variations in pulse strength can be palpated, but a paradoxical pulse is most readily detected by sphygmomanometry. The procedure to test for pulsus paradoxus is as follows:

1. Have the patient breathe normally.
2. Quickly inflate the blood pressure cuff to suprasystolic levels, and then deflate the cuff slowly at a rate of 2 mm Hg per heartbeat.
3. Note the peak systolic pressure during expiration. (The systolic sound may disappear during normal quiet inspiration.)
4. Deflate the cuff more slowly and note the pressure at which Korotkoff's sounds become audible during both inspiration and expiration.

The difference between the peak systolic pressures at which sounds are audible *only* during expiration and later when sounds are audible during both inspiration and expiration is a measure of the magnitude of the paradoxical pulse. Normally, the difference between these two pressures should not exceed 8 mm Hg.

Pulsus paradoxus is an accentuation of the normal decrease in systolic arterial pressure with inspiration. This is a result of decreased left ventricular stroke volume and the transmission of negative intrathoracic pressure to the aorta. Pulsus paradoxus may occur in conditions such as cardiac tamponade and constrictive pericarditis, but it may also be found in patients with chronic obstructive airway disease who have wide swings of intrapleural pressure during respiration.

Diagnostic tests

Cardiovascular diseases are usually diagnosed by correlating laboratory test results with findings from the patient interview and the physical examination. The laboratory tests ordered most frequently in patients with heart disease or suspected heart disease include the following: blood tests, urinalysis, electrocardiography, invasive hemodynamic monitoring, sonic studies, dynamic studies, radiography, nuclear studies, and angiography.

The nurse may be directly or indirectly involved in these tests and procedures and should understand why a particular test or examination is being performed and what it will contribute to the patient's diagnosis. This information enables the nurse to prepare the patient adequately before any diagnostic procedure and to observe and record signs and symptoms while caring for the patient.

Blood tests

Blood count

A complete blood count is ordered on all patients with documented or suspected heart disease. A general analysis of the blood through hematologic studies provides useful information concerning the overall health status of the individual. The normal erythrocyte count varies from 4.7 to 6.1 million/μl for men. The erythrocyte count is almost always decreased in subacute bacterial endocarditis (SBE) with a normocytic, normochromic anemia that persists as long as inflammation is present. The blood count, therefore, provides helpful information in determining when the patient's physical activity can be increased. Erythrocytosis, or an abnormally elevated erythrocyte count, may develop as a physiologic response to inadequate tissue oxygenation. In some congenital heart defects associated with pulmonary stenosis and a right-to-left shunt, unoxygenated venous blood bypasses the pulmonary circuit and enters the systemic circulation. This partial shunting of blood may produce severe erythrocytosis.

The leukocyte count is normally 4.8 to 10.8 thousand/μl. An increase in the number of circulating white blood cells is characteristic of significant acute and chronic inflammations. For example, leukocytosis is usually present in infective diseases of the heart, such as infective bacterial endocarditis. If a myocardial infarction has occurred, producing necrotic tissue within the heart muscle, a leukocytosis will generally develop within a few hours after the onset of pain. White blood cell counts may remain elevated for 3 to 7 days and often reach levels of 12,000 to 15,000/μl. This nonspecific reaction to myocardial injury provides information about the relative size of the infarct; higher white blood cell counts are associated with larger infarcts.

Erythrocyte sedimentation rate

The erythrocyte sedimentation rate (ESR) reflects the composition of plasma and the relation of the red blood cells (RBCs) to plasma. It is a measurement of the rate at which RBCs "settle out" of anticoagulated blood in 1 hour. The rate of RBC "settling" is increased if the proportion of globulin to albumin increases or if fibrinogen levels are excessively increased. Nonspecific increases in globulin and increased fibrinogen levels occur when the body responds to injury, inflammation, or pregnancy; therefore an elevated ESR accompanies most acute inflammatory processes. Although the ESR is most useful in monitoring conditions such as rheumatoid arthritis and tuberculosis, it is also helpful in following the course of acute rheumatic fever, acute myocardial infarction, and any infectious heart disease. Because of the lack of specificity of the ESR, it may some day be replaced by more accurate, sophisticated laboratory tests.

Blood coagulation tests

Prothrombin time. A prothrombin time (PT) determination is a blood test that indicates the rapidity of blood clotting. Normal PT is 12 to 15 seconds, or 100% as compared to control level. This test is performed routinely on persons receiving anticoagulant therapy with drugs such as coumarin (Dicumarol) and warfarin sodium (Coumadin). Coumarin anticoagulants act by inhibiting hepatic synthesis of the following vitamin K–dependent factors: II, VII, IX, and X. Since the goal of anticoagulant therapy is to prevent intravascular thrombosis without inducing a dangerous bleeding tendency, careful monitoring of the PT is essential.

Partial thromboplastin time. The partial thromboplastin time (PTT) is a more sensitive test than the PT in detecting minor coagulation deficiencies, and it is used to observe patients receiving heparin therapy. The normal PTT is 30 to 45 seconds. The therapeutic range for heparin anticoagulation is a PTT that is 2 to 2.5 times the normal.

Activated partial thromboplastin time. The PTT test can be reproduced more rapidly and more reliably by standardizing a certain contact phase of the intrinsic coagulation sequence. The resultant activated partial thromboplastin time (aPTT) is just as sensitive as the

PTT in detecting minimal coagulation deficiencies and is less time consuming to perform. The aPTT is usually standardized so that the normal aPTT is 35 to 45 seconds.

Blood urea nitrogen

The blood urea nitrogen (BUN) is an extremely helpful indicator of renal function. Urea, the end product of protein metabolism (produced only in the liver), represents the primary method of nitrogen excretion. After its synthesis, urea travels through the blood and is then excreted in the urine. The normal BUN is 8 to 18 mg/100 ml. The most common cause of elevated BUN is acute or chronic renal failure. However, other prerenal factors, such as a decreased cardiac output leading to a low renal blood supply and concomitant reduction in glomerular filtration rate, will also elevate the BUN.

Serum proteins

The normal level of total serum protein is 6.0 to 8.0 g/100 ml. A decrease in the total protein level below 5 g/100 ml will undoubtedly lead to edema, because the colloid osmotic pressure is decreased and fluid shifts out of the vascular compartment into the tissues. Of the total protein composition, 68% is albumin. This fraction represents approximately 80% of the colloid oncotic pressure responsible for pulling water into the blood. Hypoproteinemia, especially a decrease in albumin, may be associated with malnutrition states.

Blood lipids

The blood (plasma) lipids are composed mainly of cholesterol, triglyceride, phospholipid, and free fatty acids, all of which are insoluble in water and require a "carrier" to transport them. The carriers for plasma lipids are the proteins to which they are bound, hence the name lipoproteins. There are four major classes of lipoproteins: chylomicrons, very low–density lipoproteins, low-density lipoproteins, and high-density lipoproteins, all of which contain varying levels of cholesterol, triglycerides, and phospholipids.

Chylomicrons are composed mainly of triglycerides and originate in the intestine following the absorption of dietary fat. Chylomicrons should not be found in the plasma after 12 to 14 hours of fasting. Studies to date have not shown elevated chylomicron levels to be associated with premature coronary artery disease.

Very low–density lipoproteins (VLDL) are composed primarily of triglycerides and are synthesized in the liver. Sustained elevations of VLDLs have sometimes been associated with atherosclerosis; however, the exact relationship of triglycerides to coronary heart disease is not yet clear.

Low-density lipoproteins (LDL) are composed of approximately 50% cholesterol and are thought to have the greatest correlation with coronary artery disease. According to the insudation theory of atherogenesis, LDL can enter the arterial intima and produce arterial endothelial injury, which can lead to progressive atherosclerotic plaque formation and eventually produce clinical manifestations, including ischemic heart disease.

High-density lipoproteins (HDL) are composed of mostly protein with a modest amount of cholesterol and a considerable amount of phospholipids. This lipoprotein appears to have the lowest atherogenic potential. In fact, recent studies have demonstrated that HDL are inversely associated with coronary heart disease. In vivo tests indicate that HDL may carry cholesterol away from tissues, including atheromatous plaques. It appears that HDL may even protect individuals against coronary heart disease.

Before blood tests are performed for the detection of elevated lipids, the patient must fast for 14 to 16 hours. No alcoholic beverages or lipid-influencing drugs (e.g., estrogens, oral contraceptives, steroids, and salicylates) may be taken, with the exception of insulin for the diabetic patient. If the patient is under stress or has any acute illness, the tests should be postponed. Since lipid levels may fluctuate markedly from day to day, repeated blood samples will be obtained before a definitive diagnosis of hyperlipidemia is assigned. Disorders of lipid metabolism are classified according to their lipoprotein pattern and are discussed in Chapter 45.

Blood cultures

Blood culture tests are crucial in the diagnosis of infective diseases of the heart such as endocarditis. Blood cultures are obtained by venipuncture, and special care should be taken not to contaminate the cultures. Meticulous skin asepsis is important; the site for venipuncture should be cleansed with tincture of iodine (not isopropyl alcohol). Usually three to six cultures taken over a 24- to 48-hour period will provide an adequate sampling. Results of these blood cultures will identify the organism responsible for the infective process and will identify the organism's sensitivity to various antibiotics. This information will aid the physician in planning an effective course of antibiotic therapy.

Enzyme studies

Enzymes, which are located in all tissues, catalyze the biochemical reactions of the body. When cell membranes are damaged, such as in myocardial infarction, enzymes leak out of the damaged myocardial cell and escape into the serum. The serum enzyme measurements that are used to detect myocardial necrosis are serum glutamic-oxaloacetic transaminase (SGOT), creatinine phosphokinase (CPK), lactic dehydrogenase (LDH), and hydroxybutyrate dehydrogenase (HBD). Since these enzymes are located in various body tissues, there are numerous conditions other than myocardial damage that may produce enzyme elevations; for example, the brain, pancreas, and liver are all rich sources of SGOT. If an individual were to develop chest pain concurrently with pancreatic or liver disease, an elevated SGOT may be mistaken for myocardial necrosis. Fortunately, two of the enzymes, CPK and LDH, have isoenzymes that are thought to be present almost exclusively in myocardial muscle.

The CPK molecule has two subunits, which have been identified as follows: M, associated with muscle; and B, associated with brain. The brain and gastrointestinal tract contain modest amounts of the BB dimer; and skeletal muscle contains large amounts of the MM form. Heart muscle contains huge quantities of MM, but it also contains the MB hybrid form of CPK. Because CPK_{MB} is not found in any other tissue, its presence in the serum is a sensitive indicator of myocardial damage.

Of the five LDH isoenzymes, LDH_1 has been found to be the most sensitive indicator of myocardial damage. Specifically, the LDH_1/LDH_2 ratio is very helpful in distinguishing myocardial infarction from other causes of chest pain or vascular instability. Normally, the LDH_1 value is less than LDH_2; however, in the presence of acute myocardial infarction, LDH_1 is not only elevated, but it also exceeds LDH_2. Further discussion of cardiac enzymes can be found in Chapter 45 (p. 1119).

Urinalysis

A routine urinalysis is done to determine the effects of cardiovascular disease on renal function and to determine the existence of concurrent renal or systemic diseases, such as glomerulonephritis, hypertension, or diabetes. Mild to moderate proteinuria (usually albuminuria), can be seen in patients with malignant hypertension and venous congestion of the kidneys secondary to congestive heart failure or constrictive pericarditis. The presence of red blood cells in the urine may indicate infective endocarditis or an embolic kidney disease.

Recently, the detection of myoglobin in the urine (myoglobinuria) has been useful in the diagnosis of myocardial infarction. At present, clinical experience with this test remains limited; however, it may prove to be a sensitive indicator of myocardial damage. Destruction of infarction of striated muscle liberates myoglobin; and because of its small size, the molecule filters through the glomerulus and is excreted in the urine.

Serologic tests

Syphilis can play an important role in the development of aortic disorders. The patient may present with aortic insufficiency, aortic aneurysms, or disease of the ostia of the coronary arteries. Because of the relationship between syphilis and heart disease, a routine VDRL (Venereal Disease Research Laboratories) test is performed on all cardiac patients.

Electrocardiogram

The electrocardiogram (ECG) is a graphic representation of the electrical forces produced within the heart. It is a necessary component in the assessment of cardiovascular status, but it is important to remember that this tool has limitations. For example, a resting ECG may be normal, even in the presence of heart disease. Conversely, abnormal variances may be seen in the ECG of a normal heart. It is therefore essential that the ECG be utilized in conjunction with data obtained from the patient history, physical assessment, and laboratory tests.

There are numerous indications for recording an ECG (see box below). In addition, since the advent of coronary care units in 1962, continuous electrocardiographic monitoring for arrhythmia detection is possible in the inpatient setting.

It is important to prepare the patient before any type of electrocardiographic procedure. For those patients who are unfamiliar with the procedure, there may be a fear of receiving a shock or of electrocution. The patient should be informed of the step-by-step procedure and assured of its safe, painless nature. Once the ECG is taken, the correct interpretation is based on knowledge of the electromechanical system of the heart as well as the significance of each portion of the ECG tracing.

The standard 12-lead electrocardiogram

The electrocardiographic tracing represents the net electrical activity or electrical potential variations of the

MOST COMMON EXAMPLES OF ECG USE

Evaluation of tachycardia, bradycardia, or arrhythmias

Sudden onset of dyspnea

Evaluation of pain occurring in the upper trunk and extremities

Evaluation of syncopal episodes

Evaluation of shock state or coma

Preoperative evaluation

Evaluation of postoperative hypotension

Evaluation of hypertension, murmurs, or cardiomegaly

Evaluation of artificial pacemaker function

atria and ventricles as each depolarizes and repolarizes. The electrical currents passing through the heart are subsequently conducted to the body surface. These currents can be detected by electrodes and then measured when they reach the surface.

Basically, the ECG machine is a galvanometer designed to measure the electrical potential difference between two locations on the body surface. The conventional 12-lead system utilizes several electrode sites to record potential differences at the body surface. A pair of electrodes, consisting of a positive and a negative terminal, constitutes an ECG lead.

The patient is first attached to the ECG machine by the examiner's placing electrode plates or suction cup electrodes on the upper and lower extremities. These are designated as right arm (RA), left arm (LA), right leg (RL), and left leg (LL). The chest (or precordial) electrode is placed and moved across the chest wall six times during the latter portion of the ECG. These 10 sites are combined in pairs through a switching network connected to the lead selector switch. The operator of the ECG machine need only select the desired lead with the selector switch.

Effective contact between the skin and the electrode is facilitated by the use of electrode jelly, which contains electrolytes and an abrasive to interrupt the waterproof layer of the skin. In addition, the position of the patient should be uniformly flat if possible. Assumption of a sitting or side-lying position severely alters the position of the heart relative to the electrodes. The discussions that follow will clarify the individual leads and their respective electrode sites (Fig. 43-10).

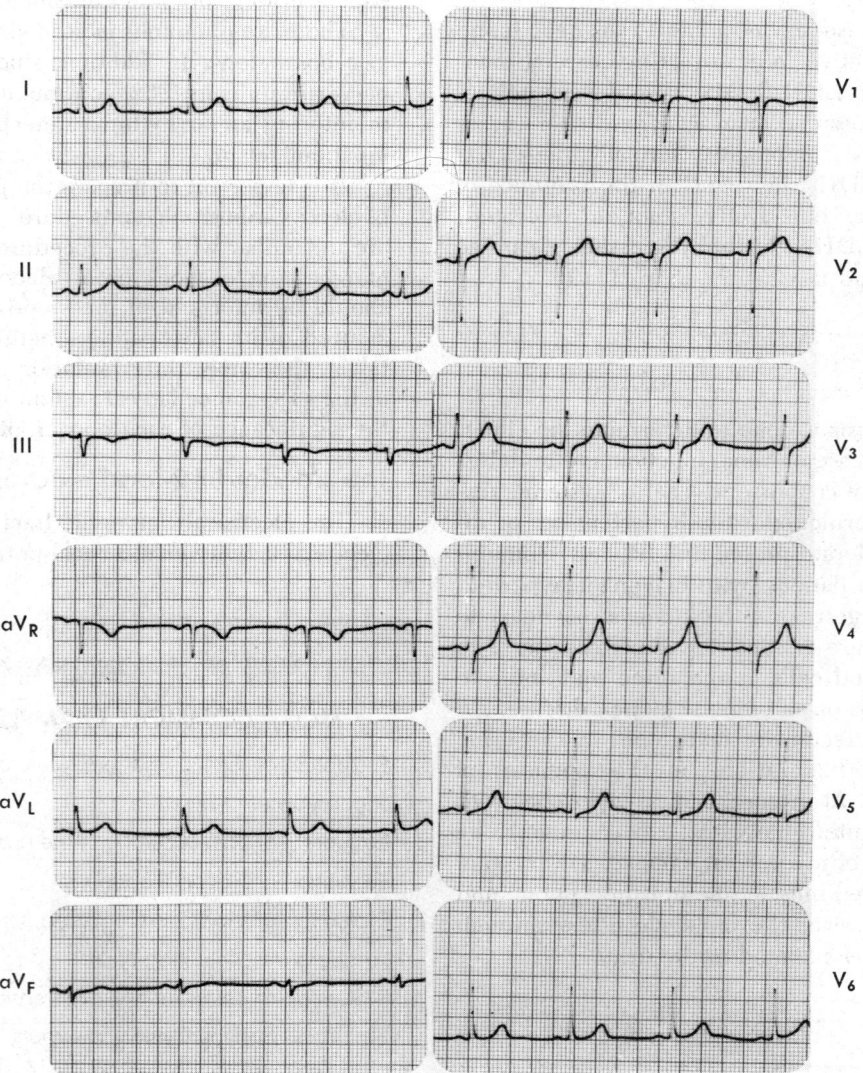

Fig. 43-10. Twelve-lead ECG showing normal sinus rhythm. (From Andreoli, K.G., et al.: Comprehensive cardiac care, ed. 5, St. Louis, 1979, The C.V. Mosby Co.)

Standard limb leads. The standard limb leads, designated by Roman numerals I, II, and III, are obtained by utilizing electrodes applied to the right arm (RA), left arm (LA) and left leg (LL) (Fig. 43-11). The right leg (RL) electrode acts only as a grounding electrode. The limb leads are termed *bipolar leads* because each registers the electrical potential difference between two anatomic sites.

Lead I records the difference between the RA and LA potentials. The LA electrode is positive. (The importance of the positive electrode will be more apparent in later discussions.)

Lead II records the difference between the RA and LL potentials. The LL electrode is positive.

Lead III records the difference between the LA and LL potentials. The LL electrode is positive.

Augmented unipolar limb leads. The augmented unipolar limb leads are designated by the abbreviated forms aV_R, aV_L, and aV_F ("a" represents augmented; "V" represents unipolar). For these leads, the right arm (R), left arm (L), and left leg (F) become the respective positive electrodes (Fig. 43-12).

The negative (central) terminal is formed by electrically joining the remaining two limb electrodes. Such a connection essentially nullifies any potential variation at the negative terminal. The electrical potential variation is only recorded by the positive electrode, thus the term *unipolar lead*. For clinical purposes, the amplitude of

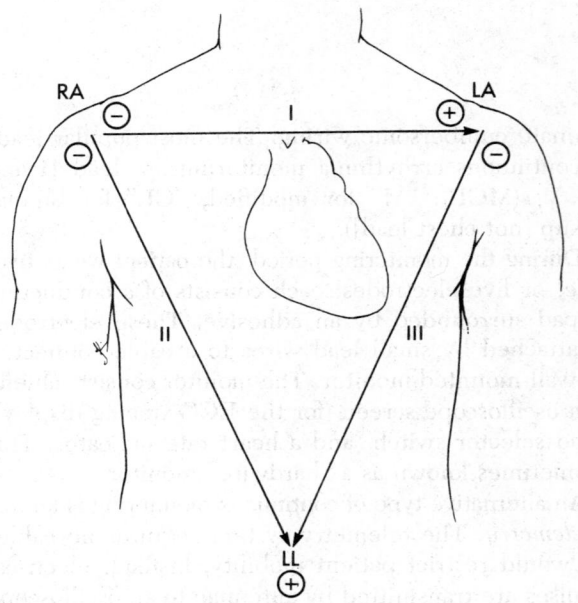
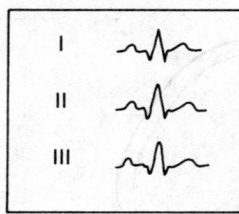

Fig. 43-11. Schematic representation of standard limb lead system.

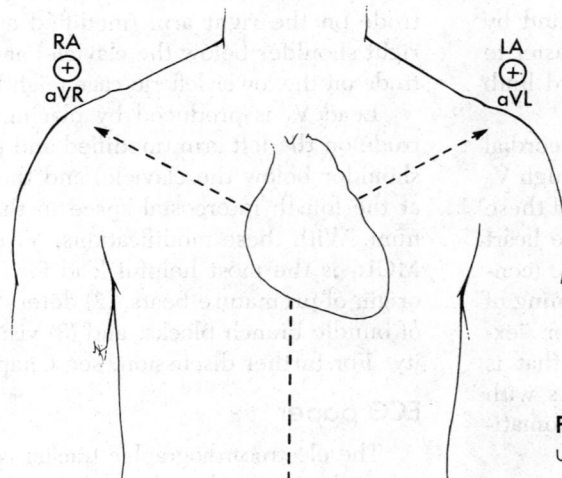
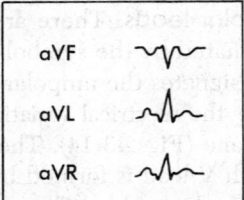

Fig. 43-12. Schematic representation of augmented unipolar limb lead system.

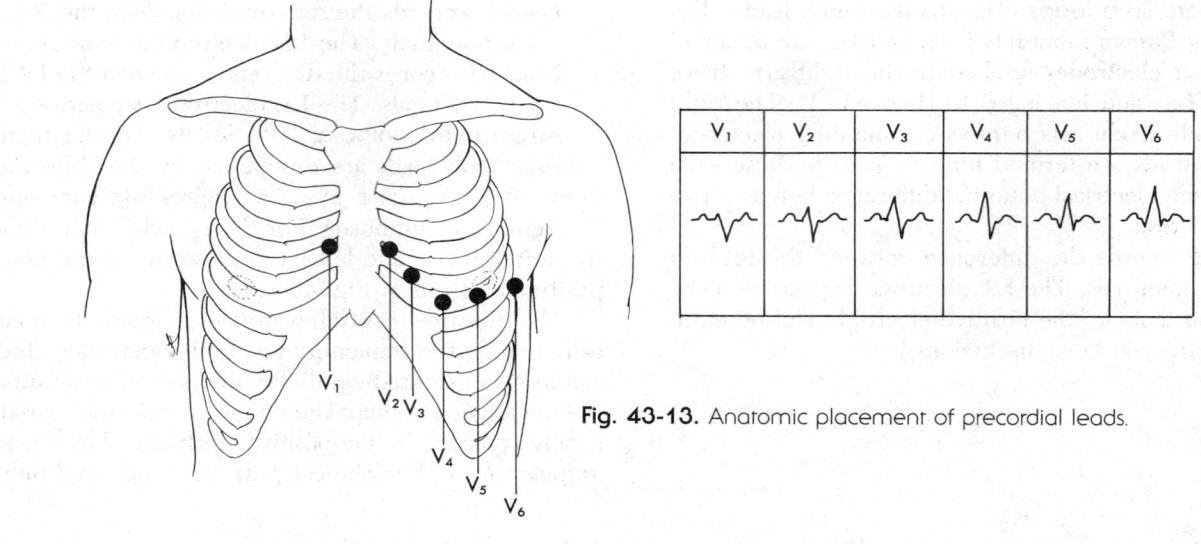

Fig. 43-13. Anatomic placement of precordial leads.

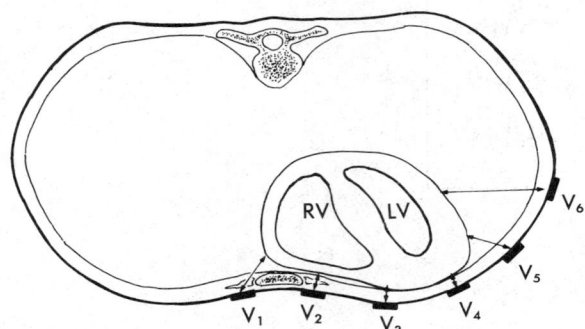

Fig. 43-14. Cross section of heart showing precordial leads V_1 through V_6 in the horizontal plane.

the recordings from these electrodes is augmented by approximately 50% to produce a tracing that is easier to interpret. Together, the augmented and standard limb leads provide the six frontal plane leads.

Precordial unipolar leads. There are six precordial or chest leads designated by the symbols V_1 through V_6 (Fig. 43-13). "V" designates the unipolar design of these leads, which register the electrical variations of the heart in the horizontal plane (Fig. 43-14). The negative (central) terminal of each V lead is formed by the joining of the three limb lead electrodes. The positive, or "exploring," electrode is a suction cup electrode that is moved to six different sites across the chest. As with the limb leads, these connections are made automatically when the lead selector is turned to "V."

Monitoring

In order to perform continuous cardiac monitoring and provide for patient mobility during hospitalization, the conventional ECG leads have been modified to

eliminate cumbersome wiring. The most popular leads for continuous arrhythmia monitoring are lead II and lead V_1 (MCL_1: "M" for modified; "CL" for bipolar hookup [not chest lead]).

During the monitoring period, the patient wears two, three, or five electrodes; each consists of a conducting gel pad surrounded by an adhesive. These electrodes are attached by small lead wires to a cable connected to a wall-mounted monitor. The monitor consists chiefly of an oscilloscope screen (for the ECG tracing display), a lead selector switch, and a heart rate indicator. This is sometimes known as a "hardwire" monitor.

An alternative type of continuous monitoring is known as *telemetry*. The telemetry system requires no cables that would restrict patient mobility; instead, electrical impulses are transmitted by antennae to an oscilloscope at the nurses' station.

Lead II is produced by placing the negative electrode on the right arm (modified and placed near the right shoulder below the clavicle) and the positive electrode on the lower left rib cage (eighth intercostal space).

Lead V_1 is produced by placing the negative electrode on the left arm (modified and placed near the left shoulder below the clavicle) and the positive electrode at the fourth intercostal space to the right of the sternum. With these modifications, V_1 is known as MCL_1. MCL_1 is the most helpful lead for (1) determining the origin of premature beats, (2) determining the presence of bundle branch blocks, and (3) visualizing atrial activity. For further discussion, see Chapter 45.

ECG paper

The electrocardiographic tracing is recorded on graph paper that passes by a heated pen at a speed of 25 mm/sec. The graph paper is divided into millimeter squares. The millimeter squares are grouped and divided into larger squares by thick lines occurring every fifth square (Fig. 43-15).

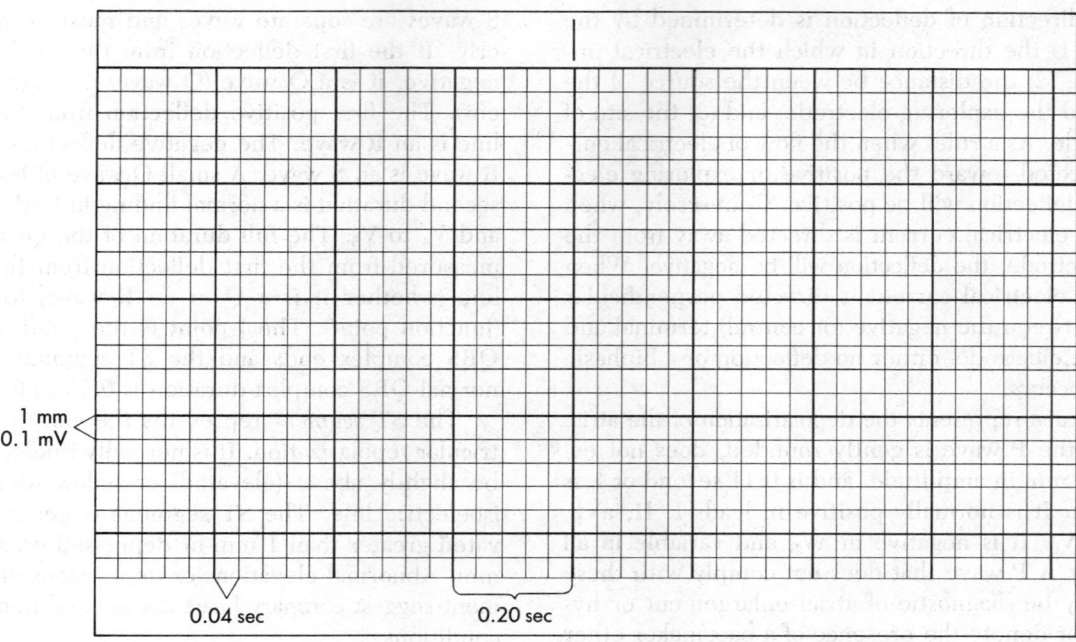

Fig. 43-15. Components of ECG paper.

Horizontally, each millimeter square represents 0.04 second of time elapsed. Each thick line denotes the passage of 0.20 second. Fifteen hundred (1500) small, or 300 large, squares represent 1 minute. With this information, one can measure the duration of any complex or interval by determining the number of small squares and multiplying by 0.04 second.

Heart rate may be measured or estimated quickly by any of the following three methods:

1. Measure the interval between consecutive complexes, determine the number of small squares, and divide 1500 by that number.
2. Measure the interval between consecutive complexes, determine the number of large squares, and divide 300 by that number.
3. Determine the number of complexes occurring between two slash marks found along the top of the ECG paper, and multiply by 20. (The time interval between two slash marks represents 3 seconds elapsed.) This is a most helpful method when the heart rate is very irregular.

Vertically, each small square is 1 mm in height and represents 0.1 mV of voltage. Thus each large square represents 5 mm or 0.5 mV. The ECG machine is standardized so that 1 mV produces a 10-mm deflection before its use.

The voltage or amplitude of a wave or complex in a given lead is indirectly indicative of the electrical activity of the muscle below the exploring or positive electrode. For example, hypertrophied myocardium will produce abnormally high voltage in some leads, while

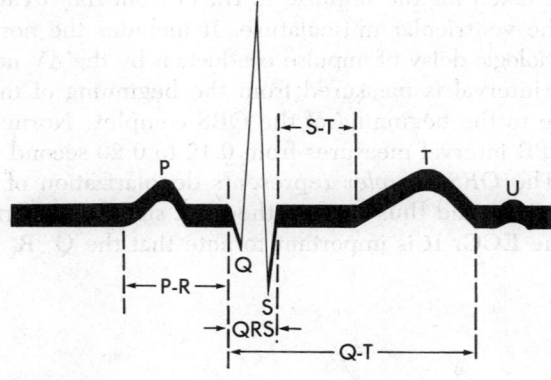

Fig. 43-16. Schematic drawing of ECG waves produced by the cardiac cycle.

infarcted myocardium could produce no voltage or low-voltage waves. The reader is referred to a coronary care text for a more detailed discussion of the significance of voltage.

Waves, complexes, and intervals

The waves recorded electrocardiographically have been arbitrarily designated by the letters P, Q, R, S, T, and U (Fig. 43-16). A discussion of each wave will be presented after the basic concept of wave generation.

The baseline of the ECG tracing is known as the isoelectric line (Fig. 43-17). Waves are deflections, either above (positive) or below (negative) the isoelectric line. The direction of deflection is determined by the following: (1) the direction in which the electrical impulse flows, (2) the distance between the source of the impulse and the exploring electrode, and (3) the site of the electrode. As a rule, when the flow of electrical current is directed toward the positive or exploring electrode, the deflection will be positive. Conversely, when the flow of electrical current is directed away from the positive electrode, the deflection will be negative. When the flow of electrical current is directed perpendicular to a line between the negative (or central) terminal and the positive electrode, either no deflection or a biphasic deflection occurs.

The *P wave* represents the depolarization of the atria. Normally, the P wave is gently rounded, does not exceed 2 to 3 mm in amplitude, and is 0.11 second or less in duration. It is normally positive in leads I, II, aV$_F$, and V$_4$ to V$_6$. It is negative in aV$_R$ and variable in all other leads. A P wave that does not comply with these criteria may be diagnostic of atrial enlargement or hypertrophy or denote the presence of a pacemaker other than the SA node. Repolarization of the atria also produces a wave, but it is generally hidden within the QRS complex.

The *PR interval* is a measurement of the amount of time taken for the impulse to travel from the SA node to the ventricular musculature. It includes the normal physiologic delay of impulse conduction by the AV node. The interval is measured from the beginning of the P wave to the beginning of the QRS complex. Normally, the PR interval measures from 0.12 to 0.20 second.

The *QRS complex* represents depolarization of the ventricles and thus is often the most significant portion of the ECG. It is important to note that the Q, R, and

S waves are separate waves and must be named properly. If the first deflection from the isoelectric line is negative, it is a Q wave (Q waves are not always present). The first positive deflection from the isoelectric line is an R wave. The negative deflection following an R wave is an S wave. A small Q wave of less than 0.04-second duration is a normal finding in leads II, III, aV$_F$, and V$_4$ to V$_6$. The full duration of the QRS complex is measured from the first deflection from the isoelectric line (whether it is a Q or an R wave) to the J-point (junction point). The J-point is the point at which the QRS complex ends and the ST segment begins. The normal QRS complex duration is 0.05 to 0.12 second.

The *ST segment* represents the early phase of ventricular repolarization. It is normally isoelectric but may be slightly above (elevated) or below (depressed) the isoelectric line. The ST segment is generally not elevated greater than 1 mm or depressed greater than 0.5 mm. Abnormal elevations or depressions of the ST segment suggest coronary heart disease and numerous other conditions.

The *T wave* represents the final phase of ventricular repolarization. It is normally rounded and slightly asymmetric. The height of the T wave should not exceed 5 mm in a limb lead or 10 mm in a precordial lead. It is normally a positive wave in leads I, II, and V$_3$ to V$_6$. The T wave is a negative deflection in aV$_R$ and variable in all other leads. Departure from these norms has the same significance as the abnormal ST segment.

The *QT interval* is measured from the beginning of the QRS complex to the end of the T wave. It represents the entire duration of ventricular systole. The normal QT value varies with age, sex, and heart rate. However, as a rule, the QT interval should be less than half the preceding R-R interval. Although difficult to measure, an abnormal QT interval may indicate a pathologic condition as well as drug and electrolyte imbalances.

The *U wave* is a small wave sometimes seen following the T wave. It always deflects in the same direction as the T wave and is best seen in V$_3$. It has been suggested that the U wave represents late repolarization of papillary muscle. The U wave is affected by numerous drugs and conditions but is best known for its prominence in hypokalemia.

Invasive hemodynamic monitoring

Invasive monitoring techniques used to evaluate the hemodynamic status of the critically ill patient have greatly increased the data base on which health professionals can plan and evaluate therapeutic modalities. There are numerous devices utilized in hemodynamic monitoring, and for a detailed description of this partic-

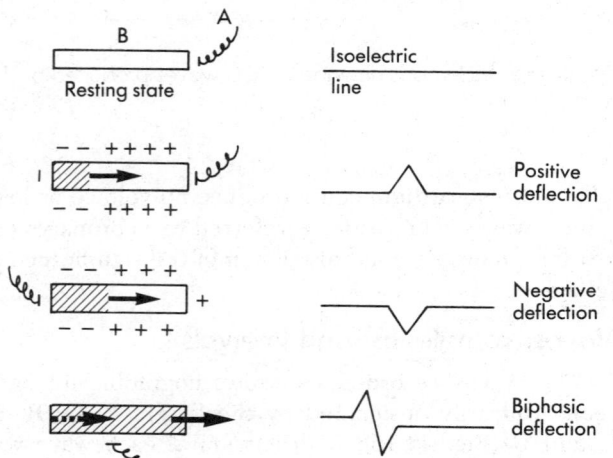

Fig. 43-17. Diagram illustrating basic changes in electrocardiographic waveform as wave of depolarization *(arrow)* moves toward or away from positive electrode *(A)*. Block B represents a group of muscle fibers in myocardium.

ular aspect of care, the reader is referred to references 12 and 33.

Central venous pressure

Central venous pressure (CVP) measurements reflect the pressures in the right atrium and provide information regarding changes in right ventricular pressure. For many years it was thought that CVP accurately reflected changes in left ventricular function. However, it has now been documented that although the CVP may provide information about left-sided heart pressures, the CVP is not as accurate as other methods in reflecting rapid changes in cardiovascular status.

The primary factors affecting CVP are the circulating blood volume, right-sided pump function, and the degree of peripheral vasoconstriction. Therefore the CVP is best utilized in monitoring blood volume and adequacy of the venous return to the heart. Since the CVP reflects the pressure in the great veins as blood returns to the right side of the heart, a low (or falling) reading may indicate an inadequate blood volume (hypovole-

mia) and fluid replacement may be necessary. A high or rising CVP is usually secondary to left-sided pump failure. This decrease in cardiac contractility may lead to congestive heart failure and pulmonary edema. Unfortunately, the patient's hemodynamic status may be severely altered before representative changes in the CVP are evident.

The normal values for CVP will vary with the use of different equipment; however, a range of 5 cm to 15 cm water is acceptable. It is important to note that a change or a trend in the CVP is more important than the actual numeric value. For example, if the CVP of a patient who has had a myocardial infarction should change from 5 cm to 10 cm in a 30-minute period, the physician should be notified. Even though both 5 cm and 10 cm are "normal" values, it is crucial to monitor the trend of a rising CVP.

To obtain an accurate CVP reading, a catheter is inserted into a major vein and threaded through the superior vena cava into the right atrium. The catheter is attached by a three-way stopcock to an intravenous infusion and a water manometer (Fig. 43-18). The intravenous solution (usually 5% glucose in water) is allowed to drip slowly into the vein to keep the vein open. When a reading is to be taken, the stopcock is opened to the manometer and the manometer is filled with the intravenous solution. The stopcock is then turned to the venous opening (the patient). The fluid level in the manometer should fluctuate with each respiration. The fluid is allowed to stabilize before a reading is taken, and the

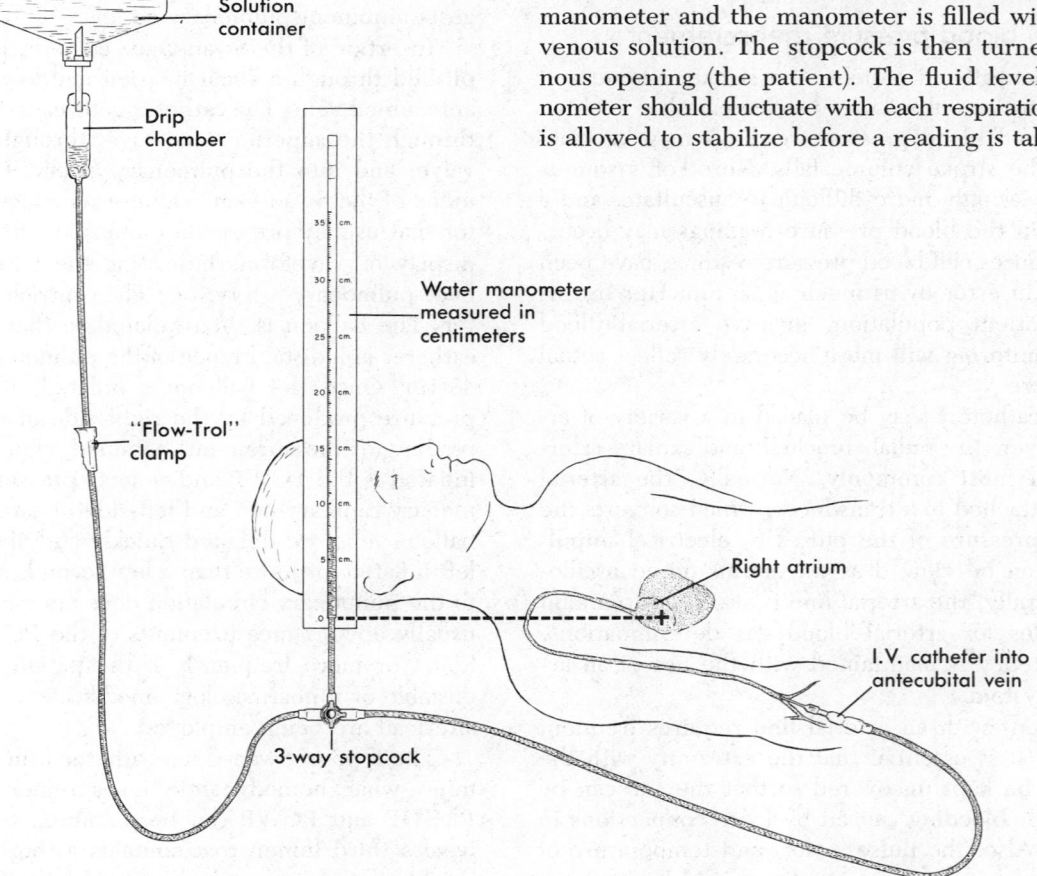

Fig. 43-18. Measurement of central venous pressure (CVP) using water manometer. Zero point on manometer is at level of midright atrium, and CVP reading is 7 cm of water.

highest level of the fluid fluctuating in the column is used for the CVP reading. As soon as the reading is taken, the stopcock is turned to the solution position, and the infusion is continued.

For the CVP reading to be accurate, the patient must be relaxed; and the zero point of the manometer must always be at the level of the right atrium, which in most people is level with the midaxillary line. If the patient cannot be flat in bed, the zero point on the manometer is adjusted to the level of the right atrium in a sitting position. Any change in the patient's position requires that the zero point be reset. The initial CVP reading and the position that the patient was in when it was taken should be recorded, because these will serve as a baseline for comparison with subsequent readings. The patient should be placed in the same position for each reading, since even a slight change in position alters the CVP.

Central venous catheters can also be used to obtain blood samples, to assess venous oxygen saturation determinations, and to administer fluids. The catheter insertion site should be kept scrupulously clean to minimize the possibility of phlebitis. Patient movement is not restricted as long as the catheter and tubing are secured adequately and intravenous flow is maintained.

Intraarterial blood pressure measurement

In the critically ill patient, the stroke volume and hence the cardiac output may be decreased to such an extent that cuff blood pressure readings may be inaccurate. As the stroke volume falls, Korotkoff's sounds become increasingly more difficult to auscultate, and a wide range in the blood pressure readings may occur. In some instances cuff blood pressure readings have been found to be in error by as much as 25 mm Hg. In this particular patient population, invasive arterial blood pressure monitoring will more accurately reflect actual blood pressure.

Arterial catheters may be placed in a variety of arteries; however, the radial, brachial, and axillary arteries are used most commonly. Normally, the arterial catheter is attached to a transducer, which converts the mechanical pressure of the pulses to electrical impulses, which can be viewed as waveforms on an oscilloscope. Generally, the arterial line is also used to obtain blood samples for arterial blood gas determinations. Catheter patency is maintained with the use of an arterial flush system.

The patient with an arterial line requires frequent observation. It is essential that the extremity with the arterial line be kept uncovered so that the site can be monitored for bleeding caused by loose connections in the system. Also, the pulse, color, and temperature of the extremity distal to the catheter should be assessed every 2 hours so that early signs of circulatory compromise or thrombosis may be detected.

Pulmonary artery and pulmonary capillary wedge pressures

To obtain essential information regarding left ventricular function, a balloon-topped catheter (Swan-Ganz catheter) may be introduced into the pulmonary artery. The Swan-Ganz catheter permits the measurement of the pulmonary artery end-diastolic pressure (PAEDP) and the pulmonary capillary wedge pressure (PCWP).

The best indicator of left ventricular function is the left ventricular end-diastolic pressure (LVEDP). Since there is a direct relationship between the PAEDP, the PCWP, and the LVEDP, an elevated PAEDP or PCWP reflects an elevated LVEDP. Elevations in LVEDP result from impaired left ventricular contractility, which does not permit adequate emptying of the ventricles.

In the healthy individual, the PAEDP and the PCWP will be similar. However, in the presence of increased peripheral vascular resistance, such as that found in pulmonary embolism, the PAEDP will rise while the PCWP remains normal. Therefore to accurately evaluate the true LVEDP, the PCWP must be monitored. The PCWP is a critical factor affecting the transudation of fluid from the vascular space to the interstitial and alveolar spaces in the lungs. Normally, the PCWP ranges from 4 to 12 mm Hg. PCWP exceeding 25 mm Hg suggests imminent pulmonary edema.

Insertion of the Swan-Ganz catheter is often accomplished through a small incision (cutdown) made in an antecubital vein. The catheter is threaded into the vein, through the superior vena cava, through the tricuspid valve, and into the pulmonary artery. One of the lumens of the Swan-Ganz catheter is attached to a monitor that usually presents a numeric reading as well as a display of waveforms indicating the location (capillary bed, pulmonary artery, or right ventricle) of the catheter. The balloon is then inflated so that it wedges the catheter in a distal branch of the pulmonary artery (Fig. 43-19). Once the balloon is inflated, it occludes the pressure produced by the right side of the heart. The reading (or measurement) obtained when the balloon is inflated is the PCWP and reflects pressures in the pulmonary capillary bed and left-sided heart function. The balloon must be deflated quickly and should never be left inflated for more than a few seconds so that damage to the pulmonary circulation does not occur. The nurse usually obtains measurements of the PCWP every few hours or more frequently if the patient's condition is unstable or if pharmacologic modifications of preload and afterload are being employed.

The type of Swan-Ganz catheter utilized will determine what hemodynamic measurements other than PAEDP and PCWP can be obtained. Some catheters have a third lumen that contains a thermistor. This is used to determine cardiac output by the thermodilution technique. A fourth (proximal) lumen ends at the level of the right atrium and is used to monitor CVP and to

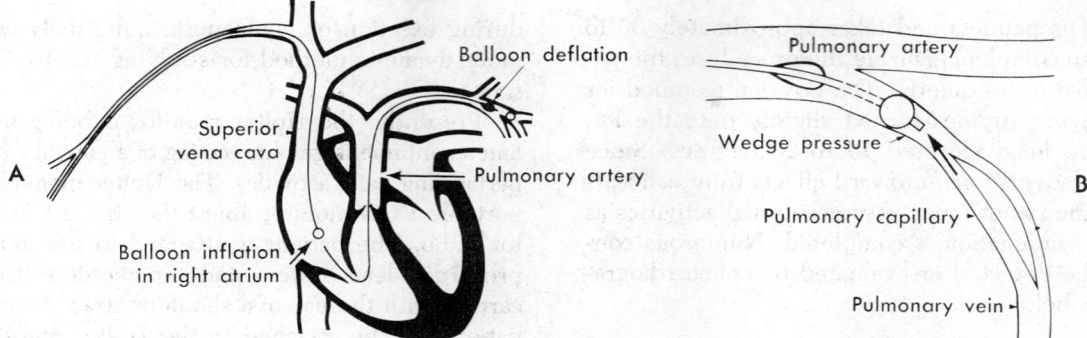

Fig. 43-19. A, Flow-directed, balloon-tipped catheter showing inflation of balloon in right atrium and consequent "floating" of catheter through right ventricle and out to distal PA branch. Balloon is deflated, advanced slightly, and reinflated slightly to obtain PCW pressure. **B,** During initial positioning of balloon-tipped catheter in pulmonary artery, balloon is deflated. Catheter is then advanced, and balloon is reinflated just enough to obtain PCW pressure. (From Schroeder, J., and Daily, L.: Techniques in bedside hemodynamic monitoring, St. Louis, 1976, The C.V. Mosby Co.)

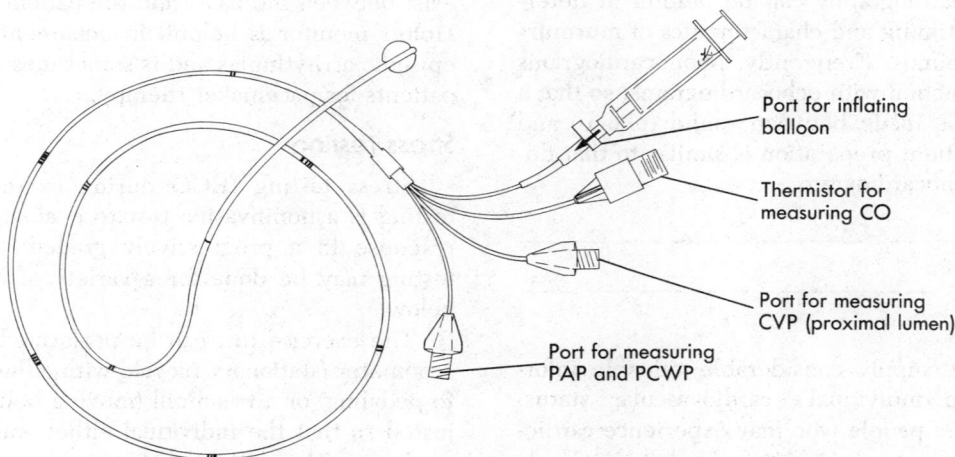

Fig. 43-20. Four-lumen thermodilution Swan-Ganz catheter for measuring cardiac output *(CO)*, central venous pressure *(CVP)*, pulmonary artery pressure *(PAP)*, and pulmonary capillary wedge pressure *(PCWP)*.

obtain blood samples. A four-lumen thermodilution catheter is illustrated in Fig. 43-20.

Sonic studies

Echocardiography

Echocardiography uses ultrasound to provide a method for assessing cardiac structure and mobility in a noninvasive manner. A small transducer is usually placed on the patient's chest at the level of the third or fourth intercostal space near the left lower sternal border. The technician then angles the transducer in varying directions to visualize specific areas of the heart. The transducer transmits high-frequency sound waves and then receives these waves back from the patient as they are reflected off different structures. The ultrasonic beam, which is reflected back from the patient's heart, produces "echoes" that are viewed as lines and spaces on an oscilloscope. These lines and spaces represent bone, cardiac chambers and valves, the septum, and muscle. A copy of the echocardiogram is recorded on paper and becomes a permanent graphic record of the findings.

Since echocardiography is a noninvasive procedure, it is safer than cardiac catheterization; thus whenever possible, echocardiography is carried out first and then followed with cardiac catheterization as necessary. There are virtually no contraindications to performing an echocardiogram. In fact, for the critically ill patient, portable echocardiography can be performed at the bedside. There is no special preparation for the test; the patient can eat and take medications as usual. Patient teaching regarding the echocardiogram should include not only the purpose of the test but also the fact that the test is painless and takes approximately 30 to 60 minutes to complete. During the procedure, the patient will have to lie quietly. The position assumed for the test is lying supine, turned slightly onto the left side with the head elevated 15 to 20 degrees. Since there are no adverse or untoward effects from echocardiography, the patient may resume normal activities as soon as the examination is completed. Numerous conditions can be detected or evaluated by echocardiography (see box below).

Phonocardiography

Phonocardiography involves the use of electrically recorded amplified cardiac sounds. Special microphones attached to the patient's chest pick up cardiac sounds produced by pressure changes in the heart and great vessels. The sounds are graphically recorded on special phonograph paper so that a permanent record is available. Phonocardiography can be helpful in determining the exact timing and characteristics of murmurs and extra heart sounds. Frequently, phonocardiograms are used in conjunction with echocardiograms, so that a comparison can be made between sound (phono) and motion (echo). Patient preparation is similar to that described for the echocardiogram.

Dynamic studies

Holter monitor

Resting ECGs supply considerable valuable information about an individual's cardiovascular status. However, for some people who may experience cardiovascular symptoms (e.g., chest pain and palpitations) only during exertion or while performing daily activities, a more dynamic method for studying the ECG is necessary.

Presently, the Holter monitor is being used to obtain a continuous graphic tracing of a patient's pulse while performing daily activities. The Holter monitor is a small portable ECG monitor about the size of a large transistor radio. The patient is attached to the monitor by a precordial lead system and the monitor itself can be carried with the use of a shoulder strap. Generally, the patient will be attached to the Holter monitor for approximately 24 hours. During this time the patient is required to keep a log or diary of daily activities. The log should include the time, present activity, any medication taken, and any unusual sensations experienced while attached to the monitor. When the monitoring period is completed, the physician compares the ECG with the patient's log to determine if any correlations exist between the ECG and the patient's activities. The Holter monitor is helpful in documenting transient or episodic arrhythmias and is sometimes used to evaluate patients for pacemaker therapy.

Stress testing

Stress testing (ECG during exercise) or exercise testing is a noninvasive test to evaluate cardiovascular response to a progressively graded workload. Stress testing may be done for a variety of reasons (see box below).

The exercise test can be performed using a bicycle ergometer (stationary bicycle with adjustable resistance to pedaling) or a treadmill (moving belt that can be adjusted so that the individual either walks or runs on a gradient). The patient's blood pressure and ECG are

---

CONDITIONS DETECTED OR EVALUATED BY ECHOCARDIOGRAPHY

Abnormal pericardial fluid

Valvular disorders, including prosthetic valves

Ventricular aneurysms

Cardiac tumors, such as atrial myxomas

Some forms of congenital heart disease, such as atrial septal defects

Cardiac chamber size

Stroke volume and cardiac output

Some myocardial abnormalities such as idiopathic hypertrophic subaortic stenosis (IHSS)

INDICATIONS FOR PERFORMING A STRESS TEST

Evaluation of the patient with symptoms suggestive of coronary artery disease

Determination of the patient's physical work capacity and aerobic capacity

Determination of the patient's functional capacity following a myocardial infarction and as an aid in planning an exercise rehabilitation program

Evaluation of exercise-induced arrhythmias

Evaluation of the asymptomatic individual over 40 years of age who is at risk for coronary artery disease

Evaluation of pharmacologic interventions for arrhythmias, angina, or ischemia

monitored closely during and after the stress test. Since the stress test is designed to progressively increase myocardial oxygen demand, some patients may experience untoward effects, and the test may need to be terminated. Conditions necessitating termination include the following: (1) ventricular tachycardia, (2) fall in peak systolic blood pressure and/or fall in heart rate, despite increased workload, (3) vertigo, (4) frequent premature ventricular beats, (5) chest pain (angina), (6) severe dyspnea, (7) severe anxiety, and (8) diagnostic ST segment depression.

The manifestations of an abnormal stress test reflect an imbalance between supply and demand for myocardial oxygen caused by myocardial ischemia. The criteria for evaluating a stress test as positive are many and may vary with individual patients. The most common criteria for evaluating a stress test are listed in Table 43-1.

Adequate preparation for stress testing is extremely important. Although the procedure is not considered painful, it can be extremely fatiguing; patients may become anxious, because they will be exercising at a level that might produce such cardiovascular symptoms as dyspnea, palpitations, and chest pain. After reviewing the purpose and method of stress testing, the patient should be advised to do the following:

1. Get adequate rest the night before the test.
2. Avoid coffee, tea, and alcohol the day of the test.
3. Avoid smoking and taking nitroglycerin during the 2-hour period immediately before the test.
4. Eat a light breakfast or lunch at least 2 hours before the test.
5. Wear comfortable, loose-fitting clothes. (Women should be advised to wear a bra for support.)
6. Wear sturdy, comfortable walking shoes.
7. Consult with the physician regarding the taking of medications before the test. (Digoxin, propranolol, and vasodilators may affect the results of the stress test.)
8. Inform the physician if any unusual sensations develop during the test (e.g., chest pain and dizziness).
9. Rest after the test. (Do *not* take a hot shower; a bath in warm water 1 to 2 hours after the test is permitted.)

Radiography

Chest radiographs

A radiograph of the chest may be taken to determine overall size and configuration of the heart, as well as individual cardiac chamber size. Most abnormalities of heart size can be detected with a standard posteroanterior and lateral view of the chest. Calcifications in the pericardium, heart muscle, valves, or large blood vessels can also be visualized in such a cardiovascular film.

Cardiac fluoroscopy

Cardiac fluoroscopy facilitates observation of the heart from varying views while the heart is in motion. Fluoroscopy can be used to detect ventricular aneurysms, which appear as a paradoxic bulging during systole. In addition, fluoroscopy is used to monitor prosthetic valve movement and to assess the position of cardiac calcifications during the cardiac cycle. Because of the increased risk of exposure to radiation during fluoroscopy, many institutions no longer use this diagnostic technique; rather, procedures such as echocardiograms and phonocardiograms are used more frequently.

Nuclear studies

The recent development of radionuclide techniques in the diagnosis of cardiovascular disorders is seen as a highly significant adjunct to the noninvasive assessment of myocardial functioning. The noninvasive nature of

TABLE 43-1. Criteria for evaluating a stress test

Assessment parameters	Possible indicators of positive stress test
ECG	ST segment depressions 1 mm or more are generally regarded as indicative of ischemia
	Arrhythmias: exercise-induced premature ventricular beats in the healthy individual are of little prognostic significance, unless they occur in conjunction with ST segment depression; individuals with both exercise-induced ventricular arrhythmias and significant ST depression, are likely to have severe coronary artery disease
Hemodynamics	An exercise-induced, sustained reduction of peak systolic blood pressure of 10 mm or more may be an inappropriate blood pressure response to stress testing and is a highly specific sign of multivessel coronary artery disease
	An inappropriate heart rate response to exercise may correlate with impaired left ventricular function
Symptoms	Typical anginal pain induced by exertion is reliable symptom of coronary artery disease
Cardiac auscultation	Development of S_3 is suggestive of advanced coronary artery disease and myocardial dysfunction
	Development of transient S_4 following stress testing may be from increased turbulence and volume of blood flow
	Development of systolic murmurs is often caused by papillary muscle dysfunction, which is suggestive of coronary artery disease

these nuclear studies allows for repetitive screening and evaluation of cardiovascular function at less cost, risk, and discomfort to the patient than traditional invasive techniques such as angiography.

Myocardial imaging

Presently, myocardial imaging is used to identify myocardial infarctions, evaluate myocardial perfusion, and assess left ventricular function. This technique can provide invaluable information in the presence of conflicting data. For example, if a patient has recently undergone coronary artery bypass surgery, the cardiac enzymes may already be elevated and may complicate the diagnosis of a new infarction. Also certain ECG abnormalities (e.g., left bundle branch block and pacer-induced beats) may complicate the usual electrocardiographic indicators of a new infarction. Unfortunately, there are also times when a patient is either unable to supply a history or presents conflicting data about a cardiovascular episode. In all of the above examples, myocardial imaging can provide a relatively safe and noninvasive technique for evaluating myocardial function.

In this procedure, a minute dose of the radioisotope technetium pyrophosphate is injected into an antecubital vein. The patient must then wait approximately 2 hours while the renal system clears the unbound technetium so that the heart can be visualized. In the healthy myocardium, there will be a homogeneous tracer distribution of the radiopharmaceutical. However, in the damaged heart there will be an increase in the uptake of the radioactive material. A gamma (γ-) scintillator camera is used to identify the area of increased uptake. This area is termed a "hot spot." This technique for identifying the extent of a myocardial infarction is best performed 1 to 3 days after the infarction. Test results obtained within the first 12 hours after infarction are not considered diagnostic. Because such a minute amount of technetium is administered during this examination, there have been no toxic or allergic reactions noted. This examination is considered radioactively safe for both the patient and the staff providing care.

Perfusion imaging

Myocardial perfusion scans enable the examiner to demonstrate regional myocardial perfusion, detect myocardial infarctions, and screen patients for coronary artery disease before arteriography.

The procedure begins with the patient undergoing a stress test. Once the patient reaches maximal activity level, a minute dose of the radioisotope thallium 201 is administered intravenously. The patient continues to exercise for approximately 1 to 2 minutes. A γ-scintillator is then used to detect the distribution of the radioisotope in the myocardium. Normally, the distribution in the heart muscle is homogeneous; however, in the presence of decreased perfusion, there is a decrease

in the uptake of the radioactive material. These areas of low radioactivity are known as "cold spots."

There are many patients with coronary artery disease who demonstrate normal perfusion scans at rest. However, during exercise, when myocardial oxygen demands outstrip the supply, perfusion deficits become apparent. If the results of the stress perfusion scan indicate decreased myocardial perfusion, a second scan (taken at rest) will be performed approximately 4 hours later. This second scan will help to differentiate between areas of transient underperfusion or ischemia and areas of scar or infarcted myocardium. Because the amount of thallium used in this procedure is small, the risk is considered to be minimal.

Gated blood pool imaging

Gated blood pool imaging is a noninvasive radionuclide method for evaluating ventricular function. ECG leads are attached to the patient, and the ECG is then synchronized to a computer and a γ-camera. A small amount of technetium 99m (attached to either human serum albumin or to autologous red blood cells) is injected intravenously. After the radioactivity reaches a state of equilibrium (approximately 3 to 5 minutes), the patient is placed in a supine position with the γ-camera positioned over the precordium. The computer then constructs an average cardiac cycle that represents the summation of several hundred heartbeats. Enough data are generated so that an outline of the left side of the heart in all phases of the cardiac cycle can be seen.

Gated pool imaging is used to evaluate regional wall motion abnormalities as well as entire left ventricular function; areas of decreased, absent, or paradoxical contractility can be identified. In addition, the effects of pharmacotherapeutics (e.g., nitroglycerin and vasodilators) on ventricular function can be evaluated, and the left ventricular ejection fraction can be calculated from the computer-reconstructed image of end-diastole and end-systole. The ejection fraction may provide an early indicator of deteriorating cardiovascular functioning in patients with congestive heart failure, with low cardiac output, or who are at risk of developing cardiotoxicity caused by high doses of doxorubicin (Adriamycin).

Stress testing ventriculography can also be performed to evaluate the ejection fraction during exercise. Some patients with coronary artery disease demonstrate a normal resting ejection value. However, under maximal stress, the ejection fraction may decrease, or an abnormality in a specific region of the heart may become apparent.

Angiography

Cardiac catheterization

Cardiac catheterization is an extremely valuable diagnostic tool for obtaining detailed information about the structure and function of the cardiac chambers, valves, and great vessels. Cardiac catheterization may include studies of the right side of the heart, the left side of the heart and coronary arteries. Studies of the coronary arteries are done to detect the presence and extent of coronary artery disease and to evaluate the

---

REASONS FOR PERFORMING A CATHETERIZATION

Confirmation of the presence of suspected heart disease, including congenital heart disease, valvular disease, and myocardial disease

Determination of the location and severity of the disease process

Preoperative assessment to determine if cardiac surgery is indicated

Evaluation of ventricular function following surgical revascularization

Evaluation of the effect of medical treatment modalities on cardiovascular function

Performing specialized cardiac techniques such as the placement of an internal pacemaker

---

effects of medical and surgical treatment of the disease. There are many indications for performing a cardiac catheterization (see box at left). Often, individuals will have undergone several other diagnostic procedures before being evaluated for catheterization.

Right heart catheterization. Right heart catheterization is performed when congenital heart disease is suspected or to evaluate certain acquired conditions, such as tricuspid stenosis or valvular incompetence. Blood samples and blood pressure readings are taken, ECG studies are done, and cineradiographs of the right chambers of the heart and the pulmonary arterial circulation are made.

To perform a catheterization of the right side of the heart, a catheter is inserted via cutdown into a large vein (e.g., the medial cubital or brachial vein). The catheter is then threaded with the use of fluoroscopy into the superior vena cava, the right atrium, the right ventricle, the pulmonary artery, and pulmonary capillaries. As the catheter is passed through the various chambers and vessels, blood samples are obtained to determine the oxygen content and saturation. In the presence of a left-to-right atrial shunt, blood samples would indicate a higher oxygen content in the right atrium than in the superior or inferior vena cava. Blood pressure measurements are also recorded (Fig. 43-21). Normal blood pressures in the heart vary among the chambers. The pressure is highest in the left ventricle

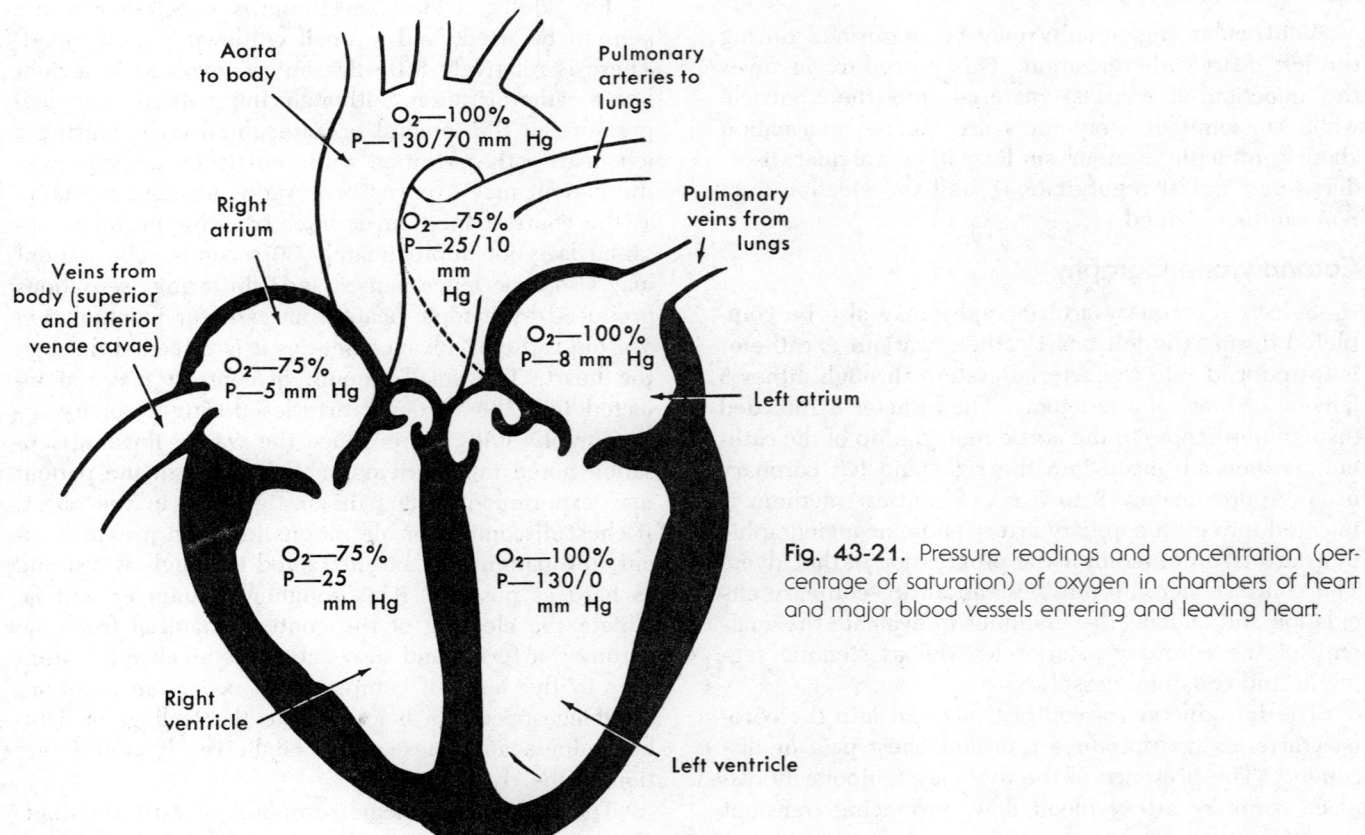

Fig. 43-21. Pressure readings and concentration (percentage of saturation) of oxygen in chambers of heart and major blood vessels entering and leaving heart.

because of the stronger ventricular contractions. Normally, the pulmonary artery pressure is approximately 25/10 mm Hg or approximately one fifth of the systemic blood pressure. Elevations in chamber pressures, such as an elevated left atrial pressure, can be indicative of mitral stenosis or insufficiency and possibly left ventricular failure.

Left heart catheterization. Left heart catheterization is performed to evaluate pressures of the left side of the heart, valvular competency, and left ventricular function. A catheter is passed into the aorta from either the brachial or femoral artery using fluoroscopic visualization. After the catheter reaches the aorta, it is manipulated around the aortic arch, down the ascending aorta, and through the aortic valve into the left ventricle. Pressure-gradient measurements are obtained to detect pressure changes across the valves. In the presence of a stenotic valve, the chamber pressure proximal to the stenosis will be significantly higher than the pressure in the distal chamber. Pressure gradients are recorded by taking continuous pressure measurements while simultaneously pulling the catheter back through a valve. Normally, a pressure gradient exists across the mitral and tricuspid valves (Fig. 43-21). Therefore a decrease in the gradient is indicative of stenosis. Conversely, no pressure gradient exists across the aortic and pulmonic valves; therefore if a gradient is present, it is of diagnostic importance.

Ventricular angiography

Ventricular angiography may be performed during the left heart catheterization. This procedure involves the injection of contrast material into the ventricle while concomitant x-ray films are taken. Information about contractility, aneurysm formation, valvular disorders (e.g., mitral regurgitation), and the ejection fraction can be obtained.

Coronary arteriography

Selective coronary arteriography may also be completed during the left heart catheterization. A catheter is introduced into the arterial system through either a femoral or brachial arteriotomy. The catheter is threaded (using fluoroscopy) to the aortic root; the tip of the catheter is then advanced into the right and left coronary ostia. Approximately 2 to 5 ml of contrast medium is injected into each coronary artery and cineangiographic films are taken to monitor the progression of the "dye." The contrast medium outlines the entire coronary circulation and enables the examiner to evaluate the anatomy of the coronary arteries as well as stenotic segments and collateral vessels.

The introduction of contrast material into the coronary arteries may produce transient chest pain or discomfort. The presence of the dye may temporarily displace coronary artery blood flow, producing transient ischemia. Sublingual nitroglycerin is frequently administered to relieve the anginal discomfort. In addition, medications such as isosorbide dinitrate (Isordil) may be given to dilate vessels so that greater visualization of the coronary arteries may be achieved. Occasionally, the injection of contrast material into the right coronary artery may suppress the SA node, producing bradyarrhythmias and intravenous atropine may be required.

Patient preparation

Preparation for cardiac catheterization is extremely important. Even after careful explanations, most patients are somewhat apprehensive. The individual may be concerned not only about the technical procedure but also about the results of the examination. Patients need to be adequately informed about the procedure as well as the more common sensations that might be experienced during the catheterization. This material should not be presented to the extent that it may increase the patient's anxiety. It should be reassuring information, so that the patient understands that various sensations that might occur during the examination are expected and not considered a complication of the procedure.

Usually, the meal before the procedure is withheld. If the procedure is scheduled for later in the day, the patient may be permitted a clear liquid breakfast. A mild sedative may be given before the procedure and an antibiotic may be ordered as a prophylactic measure.

For adults, a local anesthetic is injected over the vein to be used, and a small cutdown is performed. There is relatively little discomfort involved in a right heart catheterization, although the patient may feel pressure in the femoral or antecubital area. During a left heart catheterization with ventricular angiography, the patient may experience a warm, flushing sensation as the contrast medium is injected. This flushing sensation lasts for approximately 30 seconds. The patient may also experience nausea and "fluttering" sensations produced by ectopic beats from catheter manipulation or from catheter advancement as it is threaded through the heart. The small amount of contrast material injected into the coronary arteries during coronary arteriography does not produce the warm, flushing sensation noted in ventriculography, although the patient may experience some pain or tightness in the chest. If chest discomfort or alterations in blood pressure occur, the patient will be instructed to cough as fast and as hard as possible. This coughing maneuver will facilitate the clearing of the contrast material from the coronary arteries and also acts as a mechanical stimulus to the heart if ectopic beats occur. In addition, coughing appears to help alleviate the feelings of light-headedness and nausea that might result after injection of the dye.

The body's physiologic responses to cardiac catheterization are numerous and vary with each individual. It is therefore essential that the patient understand the importance of alerting the physician to any unexpected or unusual sensations that might arise during the catheterization.

Nursing care after catheterization

Regardless of the type of cardiac angiographic study performed, the postoperative nursing care will be the same. These procedures generally last from 1 to 3 hours and can be tiring for the patient. Following the examination, many patients like to rest or sleep, but they may resume usual activities as soon as their vital signs are stable.

The patient's pulse (on the operative side) and blood pressure (on the opposite side) are monitored every 15 minutes for 1 hour and then every 30 minutes for 3 hours. It is essential to check the pulses distal to the catheter insertion site to determine the patency of the cannulated artery. Occasionally, the amplitude of the pulse may be slightly diminished for approximately 24 hours, because of arterial spasm or edema at the site. There are occasions when thrombus formation will totally obliterate the distal pulse and surgical correction may be necessary to detect any sign of impaired circulation. The cutdown site should be closely monitored for signs of bleeding, inflammation, tenderness, or swelling. If a femoral approach was used, the patient should be kept on bed rest for 12 to 24 hours. Frequently, the patient will return from the catheterization with either a weight, sandbag, or ice applied to the femoral site. The patient should not have the head of the bed elevated more than 30 degrees and should avoid flexing the femoral area. If the brachial site is used, the patient should keep the arm straight for several hours (with the use of an armboard), but he or she can be up in the room as soon as vital signs are stable. If any bleeding occurs from the cutdown site, firm pressure is applied directly over the site and the physician is notified. For the first 24 hours after catheterization intake and output are monitored. Hypotension may develop as a result of the sometimes profound diuretic effect of the contrast material used during angiography. Complications during cardiac catheterization are infrequent; however, cardiac arrhythmias, including ventricular fibrillation, can occur. Following the procedure, the development of tachycardia or any other arrhythmia is reported to the physician immediately.

To reduce stress for the patient, many cardiac catheterization laboratories now permit patients to wear their glasses, dentures, and watches during the procedures. They may also have piped-in music or allow patients to bring a radio or favorite records with them. Children especially are enccouraged to bring a favorite toy or stuffed animal. Many times someone from the cardiac catheterization laboratory will visit the patient before and after the procedure to answer questions and offer emotional support.

REFERENCES AND SELECTED READINGS

1. Adams, N.R.: Reducing the perils of intracardiac monitoring, Nurs. '76 **6**(4):66-74, 1976.
2. Adler, J.: Patient assessment: abnormalities of the heart beat, Am. J. Nurs. **77**:647-672, 1977.
3. Andreoli, K.G., et al.: Comprehensive cardiac care: a text for nurses, physicians, and other health practitioners, ed. 4, St. Louis, 1979, The C.V. Mosby Co.
4. Bates, B.: A guide to physical examination, ed. 2, Philadelphia, 1979, J.B. Lippincott Co.
5. Benchimol, A.: Noninvasive techniques in cardiology for the nurse and technician, New York, 1978, John Wiley & Sons, Inc.
6. Berne, R.M., and Levy, M.N.: Cardiovascular physiology, ed. 3, St. Louis, 1977, The C.V. Mosby Co.
7. Boucher, C.A., et al.: Current status of radionuclide imaging in valvular heart disease, Am. J. Cardiol. **46**:1153-1163, 1980.
8. Braunwald, E.: Heart disease: a textbook of cardiovascular medicine, Philadelphia, 1980, W.B. Saunders Co.
9. Braunwald, E.: The myocardium: failure and infarction, New York, 1974, Hospital Practice Publishing Co.
10. Chung, E.K., editor: Exercise electrocardiography, Baltimore, 1979, The Williams & Wilkins Co.
11. Cogen, R.: Preventing complications during cardiac catheterization, Am. J. Nurs. **76**:401-405, 1976.
12. Daly, B.: Intensive care nursing, Flushing, N.Y., 1980, Medical Examination Publishing Co., Inc.
13. Disch, J.: Diagnostic procedures for CV disease, New York, 1979, Appleton-Century-Crofts.
14. Ellestad, M.: Stress testing, Philadelphia, 1980, F.A. Davis Co.
15. Frolich, E.: Pathophysiology: altered regulatory mechanisms in disease, ed. 2, Philadelphia, 1976, J.B. Lippincott Co.
16. Hurst, J.W.: The heart, arteries and veins, ed. 4, New York, 1978, McGraw-Hill Book Co.
17. *Lalli, S.M.: The complete Swan-Ganz, RN **41**(9):64-77, 1978.
18. Lipman, B.S., et al.: Clinical scalar electrocardiography, ed. 6, Baltimore, 1972, The Williams & Wilkins Co.
19. MacFarlane, P.: The stress test, Can. Nurse **76**:39-40, 1980.
20. Marriott, H.J.: Practical electrocardiography, ed. 6, Baltimore, 1972, The Williams & Wilkins Co.
21. McIntosh, H.D., et al.: Smoking as a risk factor, Heart Lung **7**:145-152, 1978.
22. Mechner, F.: Patient assessment: auscultation of the heart, part II (programmed instruction), Am. J. Nurs. **77**:275-298, 1977.
23. Mechner, F.: Patient assessment: examination of the heart and great vessels, part I (programmed instruction), Am. J. Nurs. **76**:1807-1830, 1976.
24. Merrill, S.A., and Froelicher, V.F.: Exercise testing, Cardiovasc. Nurs. **13**(6):23-28, 1977.
25. *Nichols, W.W., Nichols, M.A., and Barbour, H.: Complications associated with balloon-tipped, flow-directed catheters, Heart Lung **4**:74-80, 1975.
26. Noble, M.I.: The cardiac cycle, London, 1979, Blackwell Scientific Publications, Ltd.
27. Okada, R.D., et al.: Exercise radionuclide imaging approaches to coronary artery disease, Am. J. Cardiol. **46**:1188-1204, 1980.
28. Pantaleo, N., et al.: Thallium myocardial scintigraphy and its use in the assessment of coronary artery disease, Heart Lung **10**:61-71, 1981.

*References preceded by an asterisk are particularly well suited for student reading.

29. Price, S.A., and Wilson, L.: Pathophysiology: clinical concepts of disease processes, New York, 1978, McGraw-Hill Book Co.
30. Rogers-Kinney, M.: AACN clinical reference for critical-care nursing, New York, 1981, McGraw-Hill Book Co.
31. Rushmer, R.F.: Cardiovascular dynamics, ed. 4, Philadelphia, 1976, W.B. Saunders Co.
32. Scheer, E.: Enzymatic changes and myocardial infarction: a nursing update, Cardiovasc. Nurs. 14(2):5-8, 1978.
33. Schroeder, J.S., and Fitzgerald, J.W.: Indications and techniques for ambulatory electrocardiogram monitoring, Heart Lung 4:540-545, 1975.
34. Shine, KI., et al.: Noninvasive assessment of myocardial function, Ann. Intern. Med. 92:78-90, 1980.
35. Sivarajan, E., and Halpenny, C.: Exercise testing, Am. J. Nurs. 79:2163-2170, 1979.
36. *Smith, R.N.: Invasive pressure monitoring, Am. J. Nurs. 78:1514-1521, 1978.
37. Sodeman, W.A., Jr., and Sodeman, W.A.: Pathologic physiology—mechanism of disease, Philadelphia, 1974, W.B. Saunders Co.
38. Strong, A.: Caring for cardiac catheterization patients, Nurs. '77 7(11):60-64, 1977.
39. Teaching tool: a study of myocardial infarction patients receiving warfarin, Heart Lung 8:511-516, 1979.
40. Thatcher, S.K., and Lemberg, L.: Exercise stress testing in the patient with coronary artery disease. I, Heart Lung 7:1062-1065, 1978.
41. Tilkian, Am., and Conover, M.: Understanding heart sounds and murmurs, Philadelphia, 1979, W.B. Saunders Co.
42. Visich, M.A.: Knowing what you hear: a guide to assessing breath and heart sounds, Nurs. '81 11(11):64-76, 1981.
43. Widman, F.K.: Clinical interpretation of laboratory tests, Philadelphia, 1979, F.A. Davis Co.
44. Yonkman, F.F., editor: The CIBA collection of medical illustrations, vol. 5 heart, Summit, N.J., 1978, CIBA.

CHAPTER 44

INTERVENTION FOR THE PERSON WITH A CARDIOVASCULAR PROBLEM

JOAN M. KAVANAGH
MARCIA J. RIEGGER

Persons with heart disease or with conditions which can affect heart function may experience cardiac arrhythmias, which in certain situations may lead to cardiac arrest. All nurses should be certified to perform cardiopulmonary resuscitation (CPR). This chapter describes some common cardiac arrhythmias and their management and reviews the techniques of CPR. Also included are the nursing interventions for patients who have an intraaortic counterpulsation device and those patients experiencing heart surgery. Specific pathologic conditions of the heart are described in Chapter 45.

Cardiac arrhythmias

The term *arrhythmia* refers to the presence of a heart rate and rhythm other than normal sinus rhythm. There are many types of arrhythmias (Table 44-1), which are grouped in the discussion that follows according to anatomic origins. Abbreviations commonly used to name specific arrhythmias are listed in the box at right.

At present, there are a variety of pharmacologic agents, cardiac pacemakers, and electrical stimulation techniques that are useful in the control of arrhythmias. These methods and the salient features of the common arrhythmias will be presented. Since the care of persons with cardiac arrhythmias is complex, the review that follows is not sufficient for the nurse with primary responsibility for monitoring patients in an intensive

The author acknowledges the assistance of Maura A. Hopkins, RN, MSN, CCRN, in the preparation of this chapter.

ABBREVIATIONS DENOTING CARDIAC ARRHYTHMIAS

SSS	Sick sinus syndrome
PAB	Premature atrial beat
PAT	Paroxysmal atrial tachycardia
PJB	Premature junctional beat
SVT	Supraventricular tachycardia
PVB	Premature ventricular beat
VT	Ventricular tachycardia
RBBB	Right bundle branch block
LBBB	Left bundle branch block
LAH	Left anterior hemiblock
LPH	Left posterior hemiblock

care setting. For further study the reader is referred to more specialized texts.

Guide to interpretation

A heart rhythm that is benign to one person may be life threatening to another. The key lies in recognizing the many factors that may be pertinent to the occurrence of an arrhythmia. Although arrhythmias most frequently occur in persons with underlying heart disease, some are noted in the absence of disease. There are also several extracardiac factors that may precipitate arrhythmias. A careful history, physical assessment, and

TABLE 44-1. Comparison of selected cardiac arrhythmias

Arrhythmia	Description	Etiology	Symptoms/ consequences	Treatment
Sinus tachycardia	P waves present followed by QRS Rhythm regular Heart rate 100-150	Increased metabolic demands Decreased oxygen delivery, congestive heart failure, shock, hemorrhage, anemia	May produce palpitations Prolonged episodes may lead to decreased cardiac output	Treat underlying cause Occasionally sedatives
Sinus bradycardia	P waves present Rhythm regular Heart rate less than 60	Physical fitness Parasympathetic stimulation (sleep) Brain lesions Sinus dysfunction Digitalis excess	Very low rates may cause decreased cardiac output; light-headedness, faintness, chest pain	Atropine if cardiac output is decreased Pacemaker Treat underlying cause if necessary
Complete third-degree AV block	Atria and ventricles beat independently P waves have no relation to QRS Ventricular rate may be as low as 20-40/min	Digitalis toxicity Infectious disease Coronary artery disease Myocardial infarction	Very low rates may cause decreased cardiac output: light-headedness, faintness, chest pain	Pacemaker Isoproterenol to increase heart rate Epinephrine if isoproterenol is ineffective
Premature atrial beats	Early P wave QRS may or may not be normal Rhythm irregular	Stress, ischemia, atrial enlargement, caffeine, nicotine	May produce palpitations Frequent episodes may decrease cardiac output Is sign of chamber irritability	Sedation Quinidine May require no treatment
Premature ventricular beats	Early wide bizarre QRS, not associated with a P wave Rhythm irregular	Stress, acidosis, ventricular enlargement Electrolyte imbalance Myocardial infarction Digitalis toxicity Hypoxemia, hypercapnia	Same as for premature atrial beats	Procainamide Quinidine Disopyramide (Norpace) Lidocaine Oxygen Sodium bicarbonate Potassium Treat congestive heart failure
Atrial fibrillation	Rapid, irregular atrial waves (over 350/min) Ventricular rhythm irregularly irregular Ventricular rate varies, may increase to 120-150/min if untreated	Rheumatic heart disease Mitral stenosis Atrial infarction Coronary atherosclerotic heart disease Hypertensive heart disease Thyrotoxicosis	Pulse deficit Decreased cardiac output if rate is rapid Promotes thrombus formation in atria	Digitalis Quinidine Cardioversion
Ventricular fibrillation	Chaotic electrical activity No recognizable QRS complex	Myocardial infarction Electrocution Freshwater drowning Drug toxicity	No cardiac output Absent pulse or respiration Cardiac arrest	Defibrillation Epinephrine Sodium bicarbonate Bretylium CPR
Ventricular standstill	Can only be distinguished from ventricular fibrillation by ECG P waves *may* be present No QRS "Straight line"	Myocardial infarction Chronic diseases of conducting system	Same as for ventricular fibrillation	CPR Pacemaker Intracardiac epinephrine Isoproterenol

arrhythmia interpretation provide the optimal evaluation of potentially dangerous cardiac events.

A history and assessment should include (1) subjective complaints or symptoms, (2) onset of the arrhythmia (gradual vs. sudden), (3) state of hydration, (4) current medications, (5) electrolyte balance, (6) body temperature, and (7) adequacy of oxygenation.

In interpreting the ECG tracing, it is helpful to approach each tracing systematically. One suggested approach is to determine in the following order the (1) rate (atrial and ventricular), (2) rhythm (atrial and ventricular), (3) presence or absence of P waves, (4) PR interval, (5) QRS interval, (6) relationship of QRS to P wave, and (7) QT interval. A normal sinus rhythm has an atrial (P) and ventricular (QRS) rate of 60 to 100 beats/min, a regular rhythm (constant P-P and R-R intervals), and a P wave before every QRS. A review of ECG waves and normal interval and complex measurements is included in Chapter 43.

Mechanisms of arrhythmias

Arrhythmias arise from disturbances in two properties of myocardial cells: automaticity and conductivity. Enhancement or suppression of automaticity in the sinoatrial (SA) node will produce abnormalities of rate and possibly of rhythm. The same will occur if there is a change in the automaticity of a pacemaking cell outside the SA node (ectopic).

Disorders of rate and rhythm may also occur when there is a block or delay of conduction of the sinus impulse from the SA node to the ventricles. The impulse may be completely blocked, causing a pause in the rhythm. Alternatively, a conduction delay may lead to conduction via an abnormal pathway or blockage because of the arrival of the impulse during the refractory period of the ventricles.

Arrhythmias originating in the sinoatrial node

Sinus arrhythmia

Sinus arrhythmia is the most frequently noted arrhythmia. It is commonly found in young adults and the aged. The P waves are of sinus origin and have a constant morphology. The PR intervals are within normal limits and constant. The P-P or R-R intervals vary by at least 0.16 second (Fig. 44-1).

There are two forms of sinus arrhythmia, respiratory and nonphasic. In the respiratory form the cyclic pattern of changing P-P or R-R intervals correlates with the patterns of inspiration and expiration. During inspiration the intervals shorten as the heart rate increases. Conversely, the intervals lengthen during expiration. This phenomenon results from a reflex inhibition of vagal tone, an enhancement of sympathetic tone, or both. Its occurrence is favored by slower heart rates and ingestion of drugs, such as digitalis, that enhance vagal tone. The nonphasic form has no correlation to respiration. It may be caused by vagal stimulation from other vagally innervated organs.

Sinus arrhythmia is a benign rhythm that usually requires no treatment. With slower heart rates, some patients may experience palpitations or dizziness if the P-P intervals are unusually long. In such cases, exercise or medications that increase the heart rate will abolish the arrhythmia.

Sinus tachycardia

Sinus tachycardia (Fig. 44-2) is characterized by an atrial and ventricular rate of 100 beats/min or more. Generally, the upper limit with sinus tachycardia is 160/min, but the rate may increase to 200 under extreme exertion. The P waves are sinus in origin, but they may appear more peaked than usual with very high rates. Intervals and complexes are within normal limits. There is a QRS following each P wave. The onset of sinus tachycardia is gradual.

Sinus tachycardia is associated with the ingestion of alcohol, tea, coffee, or tobacco. It is a normal physiologic response to exertion, fever, fear, excitement, or any condition that requires a higher basal metabolism. Clinically, it is a short-term compensatory mechanism associated with heart failure, hypovolemia, and hypotension. It is also often seen with hyperthyroidism and may be produced by drugs such as atropine, epinephrine, and isoproterenol.

Generally, sinus tachycardia is a benign rhythm. The patient may complain of palpitations or be asymptomatic. In the patient with a compromised myocar-

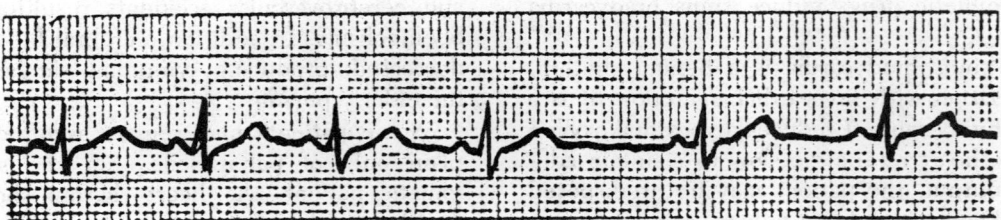

Fig. 44-1. Sinus arrhythmia. Lead II, rate (A and V) 78-58, rhythm irregular, PR 0.16 second, QRS 0.08 second.

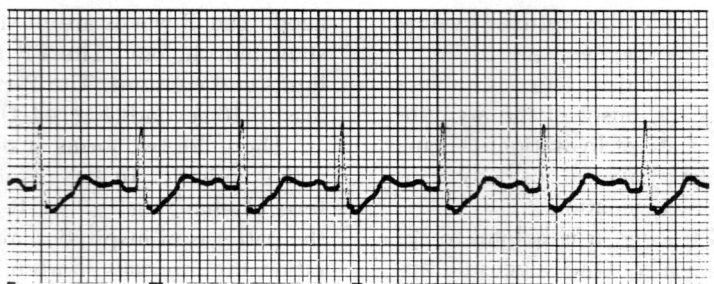

Fig. 44-2. Sinus tachycardia. Lead II showing heart rate of 115, regular rhythm, normal PR interval, and normal QRS duration.

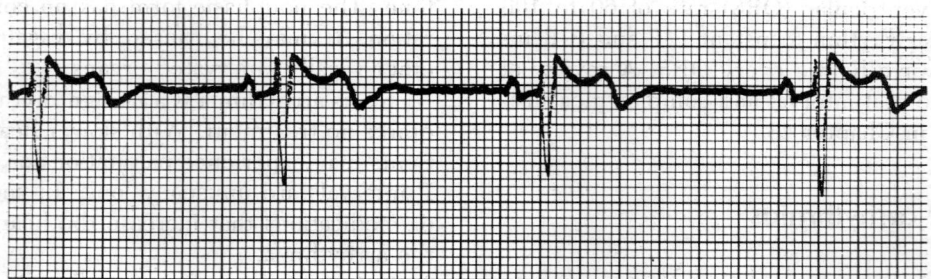

Fig. 44-3. Sinus bradycardia. Lead V₁ showing heart rate of approximately 44, regular rhythm, normal PR interval, and normal QRS duration.

dium, the tachycardia may cause a decrease in cardiac output with resultant light-headedness and heart failure. Treatment is directed toward correction of the underlying cause.

Sinus bradycardia

Sinus bradycardia (Fig. 44-3) is characterized by atrial and ventricular rates of less than 60/min. It should be noted that some researchers use a rate of 50 or below as an indication of bradycardia. In all other respects, sinus bradycardia has the normal parameters for sinus rhythm. It may develop gradually or occur suddenly for a brief period.

Bradycardia generally results from increased vagal tone or decreased sympathetic tone. It is frequently seen in the elderly and in athletes. It is associated with sleep, vomiting, eye surgery, intracranial tumors, and myocardial infarction. Carotid sinus stimulation and parasympathomimetic drugs induce sinus bradycardia in many patients.

Generally, sinus bradycardia is a benign rhythm. Often in association with myocardial infarction, it is a beneficial rhythm because it reduces myocardial oxygen demand. If the heart rate is too slow to maintain adequate cardiac output, the patient may be predisposed to syncope and congestive heart failure. Administration of atropine or isoproterenol is usually effective in in-

creasing the heart rate. The patient with refractory bradycardia that is symptomatic may require a permanent implantable pacemaker (p. 1077).

Sick sinus syndrome

Sick sinus syndrome (SSS) is a term describing a number of clinical disorders of SA node function. The SA node dysfunction is often accompanied by depressed automaticity of lower pacemakers (e.g., atrioventricular [AV] junction) as well as conduction disturbances in the atria, AV node, bundle branches, or ventricles.

The *tachycardia-bradycardia syndrome* is the most common type of SSS. Typically, it is characterized by the presence of a sinus bradycardia with intermittent episodes of atrial tachyarrhythmias. The episode of tachyarrhythmia is often followed by a long pause before returning to sinus bradycardia. Complications of this inefficient rhythm include congestive heart failure and cerebrovascular accidents resulting from thromboembolisms. In addition, cerebral blood flow may be decreased, producing symptoms similar to senility in the elderly person.

Some patients may remain asymptomatic or complain only of palpitations. For the severely symptomatic patient, the heart rhythm should be stabilized by the use of a permanent implantable pacemaker (p. 1077).

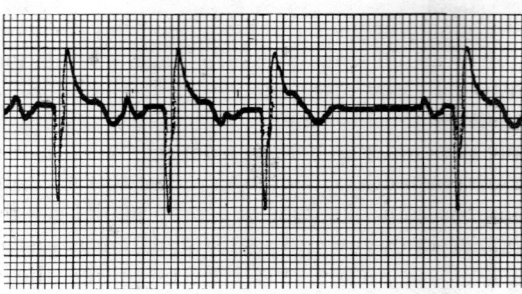

Fig. 44-4. Premature atrial beat. Lead V_1 showing third beat is premature atrial beat with abnormal, early P wave followed by normal QRS complex.

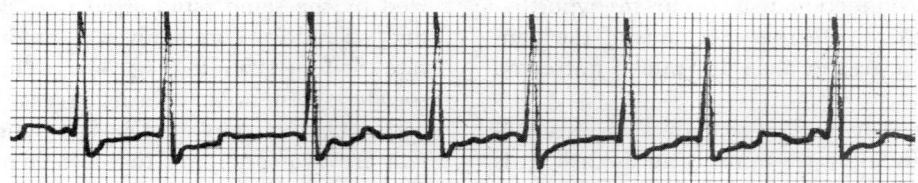

Fig. 44-5. Atrial fibrillation (lead II). Atrial rate is rapid with varying conduction to ventricles, rhythm irregular, QRS complex normal, no definite P waves visible, PR interval not measurable.

Arrhythmias originating in the atria

Premature atrial beat

The premature atrial beat is initiated by an ectopic focus in the atria (Fig. 44-4). It is characterized by a premature P wave with a contour different from that of a sinus P wave. The QRS may or may not be normal, and the premature beat is followed by a pause approximately equal to the sinus cycle (measured R to R). The atrial impulse may be nonconducted (blocked) because of refractoriness of the ventricles at the time the impulse arrives. The nonconducted atrial beat (blocked premature atrial beat) is the most common cause of irregularities in the heart rhythm.

The premature atrial beat may be associated with stress or the use of caffeine or tobacco products. It is also seen in the clinical setting with infection, inflammation, and myocardial ischemia. Frequent premature atrial beats may warn of impending atrial fibrillation or tachycardia.

In the absence of organic disease, no treatment is required. Often the omission of caffeine and tobacco will suppress the atrial focus. If symptoms are present or organic disease is known, premature atrial beats may be suppressed by digitalis, quinidine, or procainamide.

Atrial fibrillation

Atrial fibrillation (Fig. 44-5) is the most rapid of atrial arrhythmias. The atria beat chaotically at rates of 350 to 600/min. The baseline is characteristically composed of irregular undulations without definable P waves. The QRS is usually normal, but the ventricular rhythm is irregularly irregular. If untreated, the ventricular rate will generally be 100 to 180/min.

Atrial fibrillation may be paroxysmal and transient, or it may be chronic. The latter generally indicates underlying heart disease. It is commonly associated with pericarditis, thyrotoxicosis, cardiomyopathy, coronary atherosclerotic heart disease (CAHD), hypertensive heart disease, and rheumatic mitral valve disease. Its development is also related to atrial dilation, blockage of the SA node artery, and atrial infarction.

Because of ventricular rhythm irregularity and the loss of synchronous atrial contractions (*atrial kick*), cardiac output is decreased and a pulse deficit often exists. In the presence of mitral stenosis, thrombi may form in the atria and cause embolisms affecting the lungs or periphery. The goal of therapy is to prevent these complications through the control of the ventricular rate and the use of anticoagulants in certain patients.

The treatment for atrial fibrillation is dependent on the circumstances. Often, correction of the underlying condition will convert the rhythm to sinus rhythm. If the patient's condition deteriorates hemodynamically with symptoms of congestive heart failure and hypotension, immediate intervention with cardioversion (p. 1079) is highly successful. Cardioversion is contraindicated in several conditions including digitalis toxicity, AV block, and SSS. If the patient is hemodynamically stable, digitalis is the drug of choice. Propranolol may be added to the regimen. The goal is to attain a resting heart rate of 60 to 80 beats/min or restoration of sinus rhythm. The patient must be monitored for heart rate and blood pressure until stable.

Atrial flutter

The hallmark of atrial flutter is the presence of a sawtooth pattern of rapid atrial activity (Fig. 44-6). The atria depolarize at a rate of 250 to 350/min. The atrial depolarizations produce flutter (F) waves that give the baseline a sawtooth appearance. The QRS configurations are normal. There is no true PR interval because it is often difficult to determine electrocardiographically which atrial impulse is actually conducted to the ventricles. Physiologically, the AV node generally prevents conduction of each atrial impulse to the ventricles although increased conduction may occur in hyperthyroidism. Despite this protective mechanism, the ventricular rate is often greater than 150/min if untreated (2:1 conduction).

Atrial flutter is seen less commonly than atrial fibrillation but usually indicates underlying disease. It is associated most frequently with CAHD, pulmonary embolism, mitral valve disease, and thoracic surgical procedures.

The potentially rapid ventricular rate of atrial flutter may result in a decrease in cardiac output. The major goal of treatment is conversion to sinus rhythm or control of the ventricular rate. Direct current cardioversion (p. 1079) is the treatment of choice in the patient with an acute myocardial infarction to protect an already compensated myocardium from the metabolic demands of rapid contractions.

Cardioversion is highly successful in converting atrial flutter to sinus rhythm, often with 50 watt-seconds or less. If cardioversion is unsuccessful or if atrial flutter is recurrent, digitalis usually succeeds in slowing the ventricular rate by lengthening AV nodal conduction time. In some cases, the addition of quinidine, procainamide, or propranolol to digitalis therapy may result in conversion to sinus rhythm. Atrial pacing may be utilized in patients for whom pharmacologic and external cardioversion methods have been unsuccessful.

Atrial tachycardia

In atrial tachycardia the atrial rate is approximately 150 to 250/min. In contrast to atrial flutter or fibrillation, P waves are present but may be hidden in the T waves of the preceding beats when the ventricular rate is high. The QRS is generally normal, and the ventricular rate is regular.

When atrial tachycardia occurs suddenly, it is called paroxysmal atrial tachycardia (PAT). Transient episodes of PAT may occur in children and young adults in the absence of heart disease. When underlying disease is present, it is usually rheumatic heart disease.

The patient may complain of palpitations and experience anxiety during a tachycardic episode. Short, infrequent episodes require no treatment. Generally, hemodynamic changes are not severe unless the episode is persistent, the rate is greater than 200/min, or

there is underlying disease. Lengthy paroxysms may require carotid sinus pressure, vagal stimulation, or intravenous administration of edrophonium chloride (Tensilon) to slow the rate or restore sinus rhythm. Some patients may benefit from receiving instruction in the performance of Valsalva's maneuver to cause slowing of the rate. Digitalis and propranolol are the drugs of choice in the event vagal stimulation is unsuccessful. Should hypotension or CHF complicate the arrhythmia, cardioversion is indicated.

Atrial tachycardia *with block* (p. 1074) is characterized by the same rapid atrial rate. The AV nodal conduction ratio is commonly 2:1, producing a ventricular rate of 75 to 125/min (Fig. 44-7). This arrhythmia is associated with organic heart disease. Digitalis toxicity and potassium depletion in the patient receiving digitalis are two conditions that also favor its development. The treatment depends on the clinical picture and is often aimed at correcting the underlying cause.

Arrhythmias originating in the AV junction

Premature junctional beats

The premature junctional beat arises from an ectopic focus either at the junction of atrial and AV nodal tissue or at the junction of AV nodal tissue and the bundle of His. If the premature junctional beat arises from the former, the P wave will be inverted, premature, and precede the QRS complex. In the latter case, the P wave is either hidden in the QRS or is inverted and follows the QRS (Fig. 44-8). The abnormal timing and the inversion of the P wave are caused by depolarization of the atria in a retrograde fashion. The QRS is normal, but the PR or RP (when P waves follow the QRS) interval is less than 0.12 second.

Premature junctional beats may occur in the normal heart. They are also associated with congestive heart failure and digitalis toxicity. Treatment, when needed, is directed toward correcting the underlying cause. Quinidine, propranolol, and procainamide may suppress premature functional beats. Phenytoin (Dilantin) is particularly useful in the suppression of premature junctional beats secondary to digitalis toxicity.

Junctional rhythms

When the SA node fires at a rate less than 40 to 60/min, the automatic cells in the AV junction may initiate impulses (escape beats) to stabilize the rhythm. If a single junctional escape beat occurs, the cycle length is longer than the longest sinus cycle. A succession of beats from the junction is a *junctional escape rhythm*.

The P waves may occur before, during, or after the QRS. The QRS is normal, and the ventricular rhythm is regular. Junctional escape rhythm is occasionally found in the well-trained athlete with sinus bradycar-

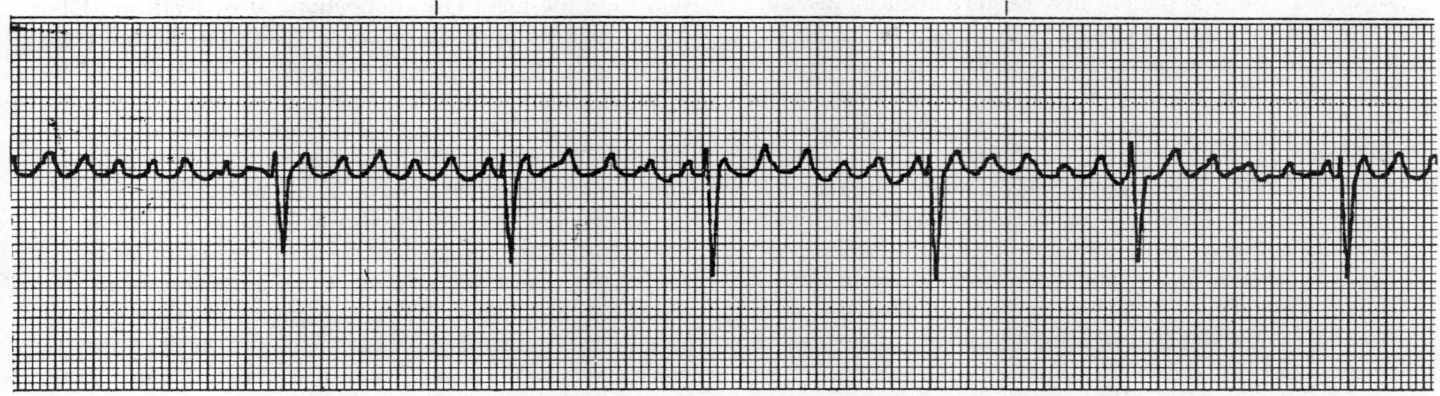

Fig. 44-6. Atrial flutter (V_1). Rate of atrial flutter waves is 300/min. Ventricular rate is 50 to 75/min.

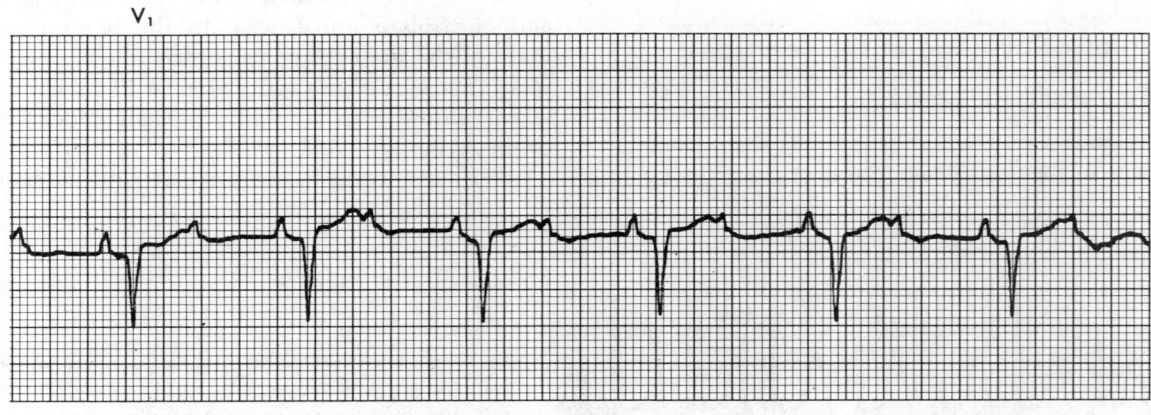

Fig. 44-7. Atrial tachycardia (130/min) with 2:1 AV conduction. (From Conover, M.H.: Cardiac arrhythmias, ed. 2, St. Louis, 1978, The C.V. Mosby Co.)

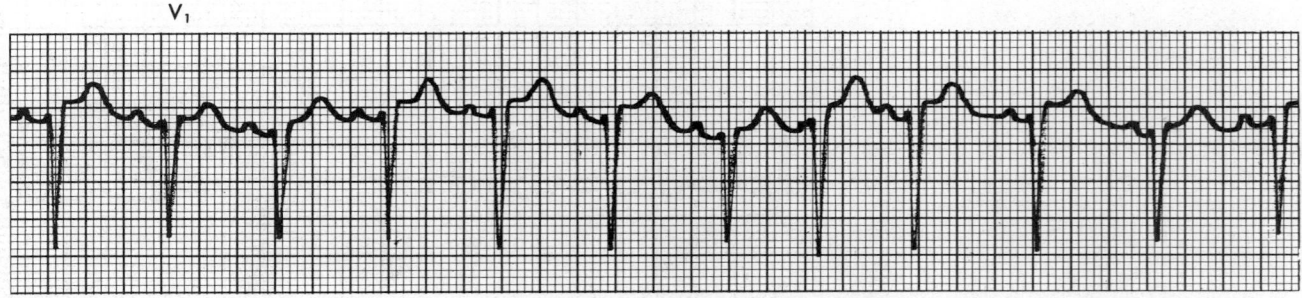

Fig. 44-8. A single premature junctional ectopic beat seen in eighth complex. (From Conover, M.H.: Cardiac arrhythmias, ed. 2, St. Louis, 1978, The C.V. Mosby Co.)

dia. It is also found when sinus bradycardia complicates an acute inferior wall myocardial infarction. Junctional escape rhythm is generally not treated unless the loss of atrial kick produces symptoms of low cardiac output. In such a case, the patient may require artificial pacing.

When the automaticity of a junctional pacemaker increases to a rate greater than 60/min, it may usurp the SA node as the pacemaker of the heart. At a rate of 60 to 100/min, the rhythm is called *accelerated* junctional rhythm.

A *junctional tachycardia* exists when the rate exceeds 100/min. Junctional tachycardia is associated with digitalis toxicity, acute inferior myocardial infarction, acute rheumatic fever, and open heart surgical procedures. Digitalis is the drug of choice to slow the ventricular rate. If digitalis toxicity is present, phenytoin or propranolol is effective.

Junctional tachycardia may occur paroxysmally. Because of the rate, it is often difficult to distinguish it from PAT. Both premature junctional tachycardia and PAT are often referred to as supraventricular tachycardia, indicating that the rhythm originates above the ventricles (Fig. 44-9).

Arrhythmias originating in the ventricles

Premature ventricular beats

The premature ventricular beat (PVB) arises from an ectopic focus in the ventricles. The characteristic wide,

bizarre QRS (usually greater than 0.12 second) makes the PVB readily identifiable on the ECG tracing (Fig. 44-10). There is no associated P wave preceding the QRS complex, and the T wave is in the opposite direction from the main QRS deflection. Most PVBs are followed by a compensatory pause such that the interval from the beat preceding to the beat following the PVB is equal to two sinus cycles.

If several PVBs of different configuration are noted in an ECG tracing, they are said to be *multifocal*, indicating the presence of more than one ectopic focus in the ventricles. PVBs may also have various degrees of prematurity. It is important to note the relationship of the PVB to the QRST waves of the preceding beat. As discussed in Chapter 43, an electrical impulse of any kind that stimulates the heart near the peak of the T wave (vulnerable period) may precipitate a more dangerous or lethal arrhythmia.

The majority of persons who experience PVBs are healthy. The incidence and frequency of occurrence are higher, however, for the population with heart disease. The patient with an acute myocardial infarction must be monitored closely for the presence of PVBs. Clinically, PVBs are also associated with CHF, digitalis toxicity, and electrolyte imbalances. In the latter cases treatment of the underlying cause may abolish the arrhythmia. Pharmacologic suppression of PVBs is most often accomplished with lidocaine, procainamide, quinidine, or disopyramide (Table 44-2).

PVBs occurring in conjunction with an acute myo-

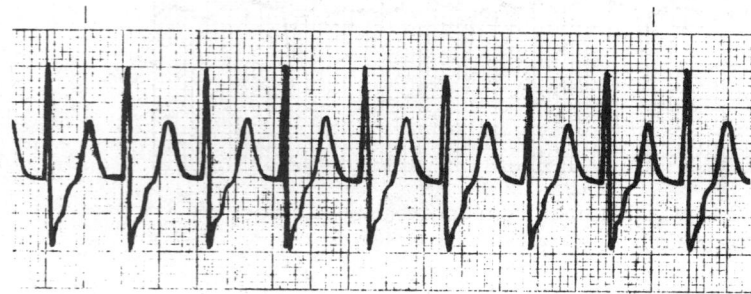

Fig. 44-9. Supraventricular tachycardia (SVT). Origin is atrial or junctional. If P waves are present, they are not visualized; they may be present in preceding T wave.

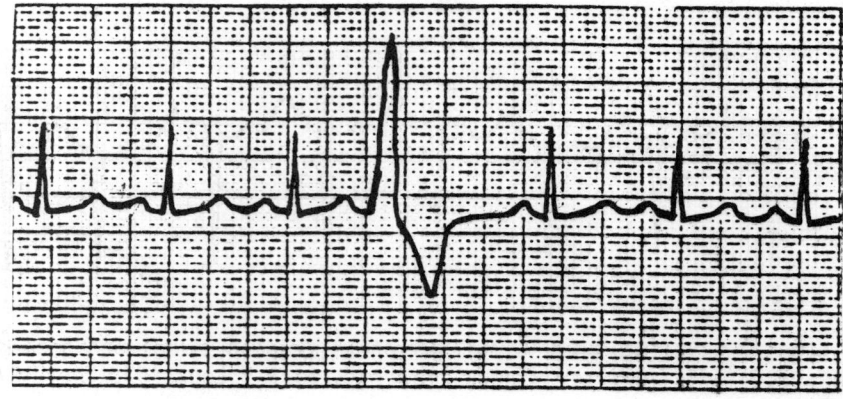

Fig. 44-10. Premature ventricular beat. Lead II showing fourth beat is a PVB with wide early QRS complex; no P wave associated with beat.

TABLE 44-2. Antiarrhythmic agents

Drug	Action	Indications	Dosage	Side effects
Procainamide (Pronestyl)	Slows conduction; prolongs the refractory period; depresses spontaneous depolarization and automaticity	Ventricular tachyarrhythmias, especially after lidocaine or cardioversion breaks tachycardia; PVB; SVT, particularly atrial fibrillation	100 mg IV q 2-4 min, not to exceed 2 g Or 2-6 mg/min by drip Or 250-500 mg PO q 4-6 hr	Nausea, vomiting, fever, leukopenia, lupus erythematosus, AV block
Quinidine	Anticholinergic effect; prolongation of refractory period of atria; same but less effect on ventricular refractory period	Conversion of atrial fibrillation or flutter to sinus rhythm; PAB, PVB; more effective in suppressing SVT than VT	200-400 mg PO q 6 hr	Thrombocytopenia purpura, nausea, vomiting, diarrhea
Propranolol (Inderal)	Inhibition of β-adrenergic stimulation; reduction of automaticity; prolongation of atrial and AV conduction times	Tachyarrhythmias, especially digitalis induced; catecholamine-induced arrhythmias (exercise, emotion, sympathetic stimulation)	1-3 mg IV, not to exceed 10 mg Or 10-30 mg PO tid or qid	Hypotension, CHF, bradycardia, nausea, vomiting, mental depression
Phenytoin (Dilantin)	Depressed automaticity of pacemaker cells; shortens refractory period and action potential duration; may improve depressed conduction	Digitalis-induced arrhythmias	125-250 mg IV slowly until arrhythmia terminates Or 200 mg PO; then 100 mg q 4 or 6 hr	Nausea, vomiting, ataxia, vertigo, gum hyperplasia
Disopyramide (Norpace)	Similar to procainamide and quinidine	Ventricular tachyarrhythmias; PVB; helpful in patients who are not helped by all of the above drugs; contraindicated in severe CHF, glaucoma, second- or third-degree AV block	200-300 mg PO, loading dose; then 100-150 mg PO q 6 hr	Dry mouth, urinary hesitancy
Verapamil	Calcium channel blocker; slows SA node discharge rate and prolongs AV conduction time; depresses myocardial contractility	Termination of paroxysmal SVT; slows ventricular rate of atrial fibrillation or flutter; coronary vasodilator	5-10 mg IV over 2 min	Headache, dizziness, nausea, constipation, bradycardia, hypotension
Lidocaine	Similar to procainamide and quinidine; depresses spontaneous depolarization and automaticity in ventricles	PVB; ventricular tachycardia; contraindicated in severe liver or renal disease	75-100 mg IV bolus (1-1.5 mg/kg), then 2-4 mg/min	Hypotension, dizziness, drowsiness, confusion
Bretylium tosylate (Bretylol)	Raises ventricular fibrillation threshold; lengthens action potential and effective refractory period of ventricles; interferes with release of norepinephrine and uptake of catecholamines by nerve endings	Ventricular tachyarrhythmias and fibrillation	5-10 mg/kg IV bolus over 10 min Or 600 mg IM; then 200 mg IM q 2 hr	Severe hypotension, nausea, vomiting

cardial infarction may lead to more serious arrhythmias and must be suppressed. Lidocaine is an intravenous preparation that is a first-line choice for immediate suppression of ventricular irritability. After initial suppression, PVBs may be controlled on a long-term basis with the oral antiarrhythmics. Most authors agree that in the face of an acute myocardial infarction, PVBs should be treated if they (1) are greater than 5/min, (2) fall in the vulnerable period (known as the R-on-T phenomenon), (3) are multifocal, (4) occur in pairs or multiples, or (5) are accompanied by a history of ventricular tachycardia or fibrillation.[2]

Ventricular rhythms and tachycardia

In the event that the SA node and AV junction fail to initiate impulses, a ventricular pacemaking cell will automatically begin to initiate impulses at an inherent rate of 20 to 40/min. This is known as *idioventricular* rhythm.

If the rate of the ventricular-initiated rhythm increases to 40 to 100/min, it is known as an *accelerated* idioventricular rhythm (commonly misnomered slow ventricular tachycardia). It may be seen in digitalis toxicity or as a complication of an acute myocardial infarction. Generally, neither of the above rhythms is treated except to correct underlying abnormalities. Suppression of the heart's dominant and perhaps only rhythm could be hazardous. If the cardiac output is low and symptoms of CHF, syncope, or hypotension develop, the patient may require temporary or permanent artificial pacing (p. 1077). Atropine may also be helpful in stimulating the return of SA node activity.

By definition three or more successive premature ventricular beats (PVBs) constitute *ventricular tachycardia* (Fig. 44-11). The ventricular rate is greater than 100/min and is usually 140 to 240. The rhythm is regular or slightly irregular. P waves may be present but are not associated with the QRS complexes. Ventricular tachycardia may complicate any form of heart disease and be a direct result of a PVB striking during the heart's vulnerable period. Conditions that favor its occurrence include hypoxemia, drug toxicity, electrolyte imbalance, and bradycardia. Some patients may tolerate ventricular tachycardia without loss of consciousness, particularly if the heart rate is closer to 100/min. If the patient remains stable, treatment may include intravenous lidocaine, procainamide, or bretylium to break the tachycardia. If pharmacologic measures are unsuccessful, the alternative is cardioversion.

Because of the high ventricular rates and the loss of atrial kick, other patients may experience severe hypotension, loss of consciousness, and respiratory arrest. CPR should be administered immediately until emergency defibrillation can be performed. Once conversion to sinus rhythm is accomplished, intravenous lidocaine is generally administered to prevent recurrence. Main-

tenance suppression is obtained with oral antiarrhythmics.

Ventricular fibrillation and standstill

In ventricular fibrillation the ventricles twitch chaotically, much like the atria in atrial fibrillation. The ECG tracing consists of a bumpy line of unidentifiable waves (Fig. 44-12). The fibrillatory waves may be coarse (as pictured) or fine (smooth).

In ventricular standstill (asystole) the ECG tracing is a flat line. There is no electrical activity noted; all pacemaking cells have failed. Clinically, ventricular fibrillation and standstill cannot be differentiated without the ECG. Both are fatal arrhythmias, requiring immediate measures. The patient has no blood pressure, pulse, or audible heart beat, and respirations quickly cease. CPR must be instituted immediately (p. 1080) and defibrillation performed within 1 minute to prevent biochemical derangements that further compromise the patient.

Coarse ventricular fibrillation is most likely to respond to defibrillation. Intracardiac administration of epinephrine or intravenous isoproterenol (Isuprel) and calcium is useful in producing a positive response to defibrillation of fine fibrillation or standstill. Unfortunately, the patient most vulnerable to these arrhythmias has suffered an acute myocardial infarction complicated by congestive heart failure. Because of these factors, resuscitation efforts are less likely to be successful.

Conduction abnormalities

Atrioventricular block

A block to conduction of an impulse may occur at any point along the conduction pathways. One common area of block is the atrioventricular (AV) junction. The severity of the block is identified by degrees; first-, second-, or third- degree AV block.

First-degree AV block is present when the PR interval is prolonged to greater than 0.20 second, indicating a conduction delay in the AV node (Fig. 44-13). It is commonly found in association with rheumatic fever, digitalis toxicity, and the degenerative changes of CAHD (p. 1118) in the conducting tissue. When a first-degree AV block occurs as an isolated defect, no treatment is necessary.

Second-degree AV block may be divided into two categories. Type I (Wenckebach or Mobitz I) is characterized by a PR interval that progressively lengthens until a P wave is not followed by a QRS (Fig. 44-14). The nonconducted beat is the result of the arrival of the impulse during the refractory period of the AV node. The ratio of P waves to QRS complexes may be 5:4, 4:3, 3:2, or 2:1. Any drug that slows AV conduction

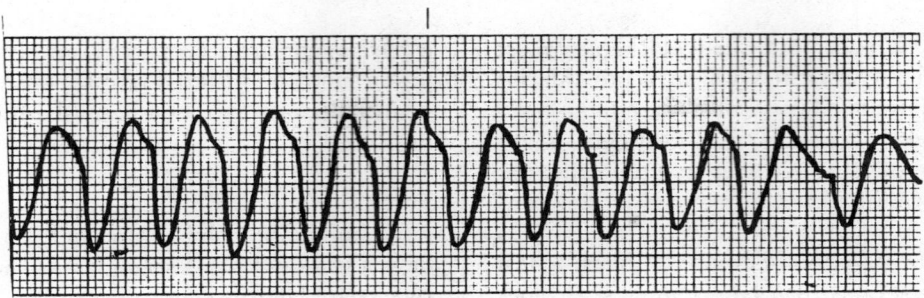

Fig. 44-11. Ventricular tachycardia at a rate of approximately 150/min; rhythm is slightly irregular.

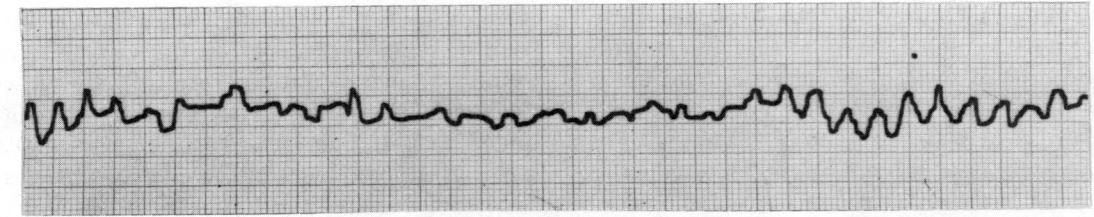

Fig. 44-12. Ventricular fibrillation (lead II). Rate is rapid, rhythm irregular, no QRS complexes, no definite P waves visible. Tracing shows electrical chaos in myocardium.

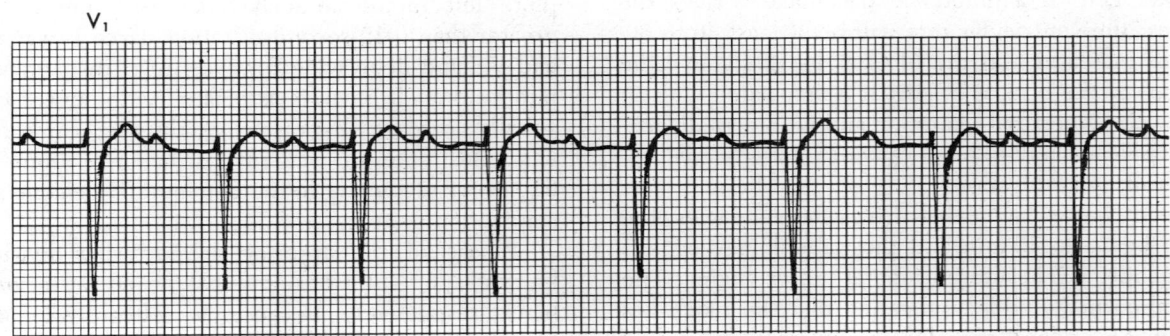

Fig. 44-13. First-degree AV block; the PR interval is 0.33 second (too long). (From Conover, M.H.: Cardiac arrhythmias, ed. 2, St. Louis, 1978, The C.V. Mosby Co.)

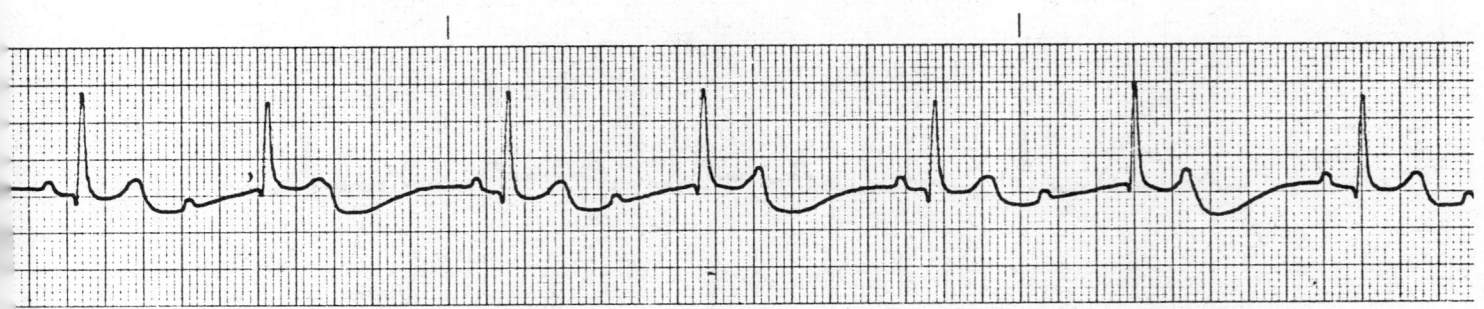

Fig. 44-14. Second-degree AV block, type I (Wenckebach). Every third P wave is hidden in preceding T wave; conduction is 3:2. Note progressive lengthening of PR interval before dropped QRS.

may cause a type I block, but such blocks are most commonly seen in the patient with an acute inferior wall myocardial infarction. Type I blocks are often transient and reversible. Generally, no treatment is required unless the patient becomes symptomatic because of the slow ventricular rate induced by 2:1 conduction.

Type II (Mobitz II) second-degree AV block is less common but more serious than type I. A type II block is characterized by nonconducted sinus impulses despite constant PR intervals. Usually the QRS complexes are widened because of a bundle branch block. The dropped beat represents a form of intermittent blockage of both bundle branches. The defect is found in either the bundle branches or the bundle of His. Type II blocks are most commonly seen in the patient with an acute anterior wall myocardial infarction and are a warning of an impending third-degree block. A temporary pacemaker is usually inserted prophylactically until the conduction stabilizes. If the block is persistent, the patient will benefit from a permanent implantable pacemaker.

In *third-degree AV block* all the sinus or atrial impulses are blocked and the atria and ventricles are forced to beat independently (Fig. 44-15). The ventricles are driven by either a junctional or a ventricular pacemaker cell. If a junctional pacemaker drives the ventricles, the ventricular rate will be at least 40 to 60/min. This indicates that the block is located above the bifurcation of the bundle of His. It is associated with an inferior wall myocardial infarction and with digitalis toxicity and is less likely to be permanent. Atropine is useful in restoring conduction.

If a ventricular pacemaker drives the ventricles, the rate will be 20 to 40/min and the patient may experience syncope, CHF, altered mentation, or angina. The QRS is abnormally wide, indicating that the block lies below the AV node. Generally, the patient will require a permanent artificial pacemaker. Epinephrine or isoproterenol administered intravenously may increase the ventricular rate temporarily until artificial pacing can be instituted.

Bundle branch block

A bundle branch block occurs as a permanent defect or as a transient block secondary to tachycardia, congestive heart failure, acute myocardial infarction, pulmonary embolus, hypoxia, or metabolic derangements. In all these cases, the electrical impulse spreads from one ventricle to the other by abnormal pathways, thus producing distinct ECG tracings.

The *right bundle branch* is the more delicate structure of the two bundles and has a longer refractory period in some individuals. In the younger patient right bundle branch block often results from right ventricular hypertrophy, while CAHD is usually the culprit in the older patient. The QRS is widened to 0.10 second or greater. Among the most classic ECG changes is the M-shaped QRS in V_1 and V_2. In the absence of other conduction defects, no intervention is necessary.

The *left bundle branch* has a main trunk that bifurcates into the left anterior and left posterior divisions. A block may occur in the main trunk or in either of the divisions. A block in the main trunk produces a complete left bundle branch block resulting in a QRS greater than 0.12-second duration, large R waves in V_5 and V_6, and deep wide S waves in V_1 through V_3. Left bundle branch block is associated with severe CAHD, valvular disease, hypertensive disease, cardiomegaly, and acute anterior wall myocardial infarction. It may also occur secondary to the degenerative changes in the conduction system.

Blocks of the anterior or posterior division are known as left anterior hemiblock or left posterior hemiblock, respectively. Because the left posterior division is the sturdier, its blockage carries a poorer prognosis.

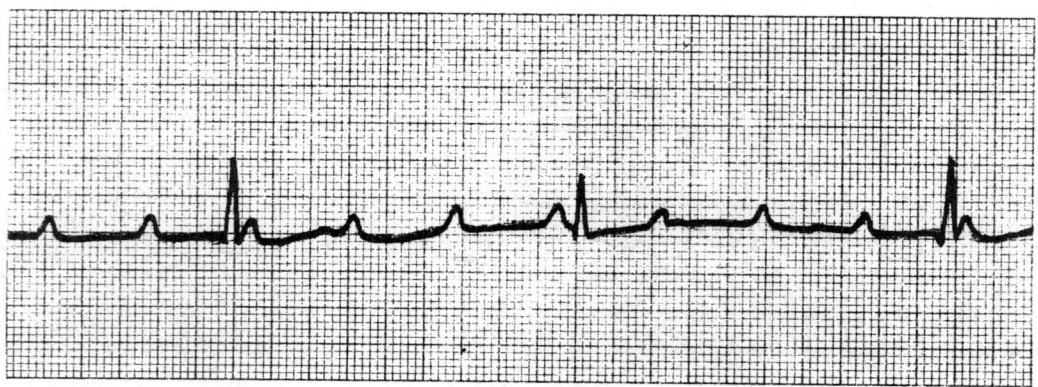

Fig. 44-15. Third-degree AV block. Atrial rate is 105/min; ventricular rate is 33/min; an idioventricular rhythm.

It is important to determine *all* blocks to conduction that may coexist. Whenever sufficient blockage is present to leave the heart dependent on one fascicle for conduction to the ventricles, the patient is a candidate for a permanent artificial pacemaker.

Treatment modalities

Pacemakers

Indications for use. As noted in previous discussions of arrhythmias and conduction defects, the artificial pacemaker has become a leading modality in the control of potentially dangerous arrhythmias. Indications for artificial pacemakers are summarized in the box at right. Some of these conditions require only temporary pacing. Permanent pacing is an option when the condition is recurrent or persistent.

Pacemaker mechanism. The artificial pacing system consists of a battery-powered generator and a pacing wire that delivers the stimulus to the heart. For temporary pacing the wire is usually passed transvenously to the right atrium or ventricle. Externally, the wire connects to a generator as seen in Fig. 44-16. The same system exists for permanent pacing except that the generator itself is more compact and may be implanted subcutaneously (Fig. 44-17). The permanent pacing generator may be implanted in the right or left subclavicular area, and the pacing wire is passed through the major veins to the right side of the heart (transvenous or endocardial). Alternatively, the generator may be implanted subcutaneously in the abdomen with the pacing wire passed upward and sutured to the left ventricle (epicardial). The generator is powered by a battery with an expected life of 4 to 6 years. Research is directed toward power sources that may function for 10 or more years.

INDICATIONS FOR ARTIFICIAL PACEMAKERS

1. Adams-Stokes attack (syncope secondary to third-degree AV block)
2. Third-degree AV block with slow ventricular rate
3. Acute myocardial infarction with Mobitz II AV block
4. Right bundle branch block plus left anterior hemiblock or left posterior hemiblock (particularly with acute myocardial infarction)
5. New left bundle branch block associated with acute myocardial infarction
6. Symptomatic sinus bradycardia unresponsive to medical therapy
7. Atrial fibrillation with slow ventricular rate in the patient who requires digitalis therapy
8. Carotid sinus syncope
9. Suppression of arrhythmias (e.g., PVBs)
10. Arrhythmias occurring during or after cardiac surgery

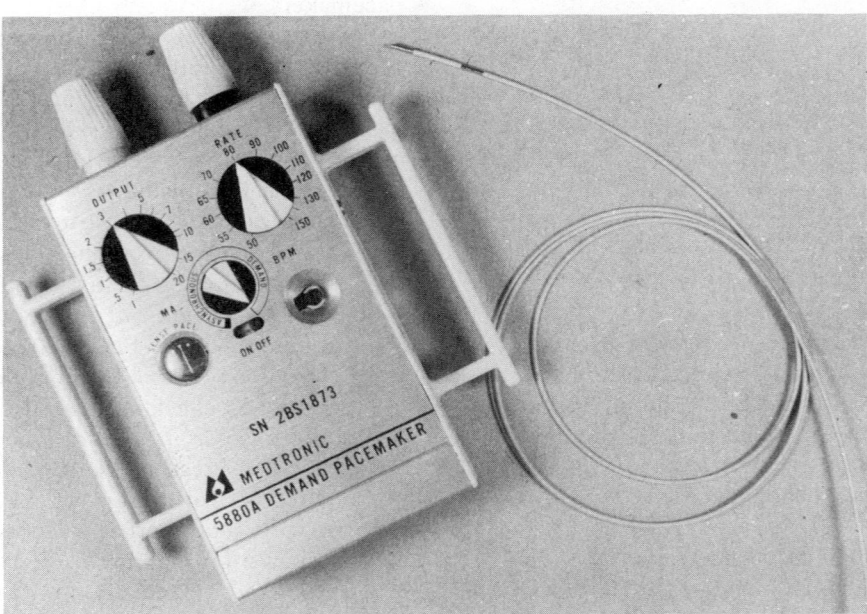

Fig. 44-16. Temporary (external) pacemaker. Pulse generator is battery powered. Electrode is passed into heart before being attached to pulse generator.

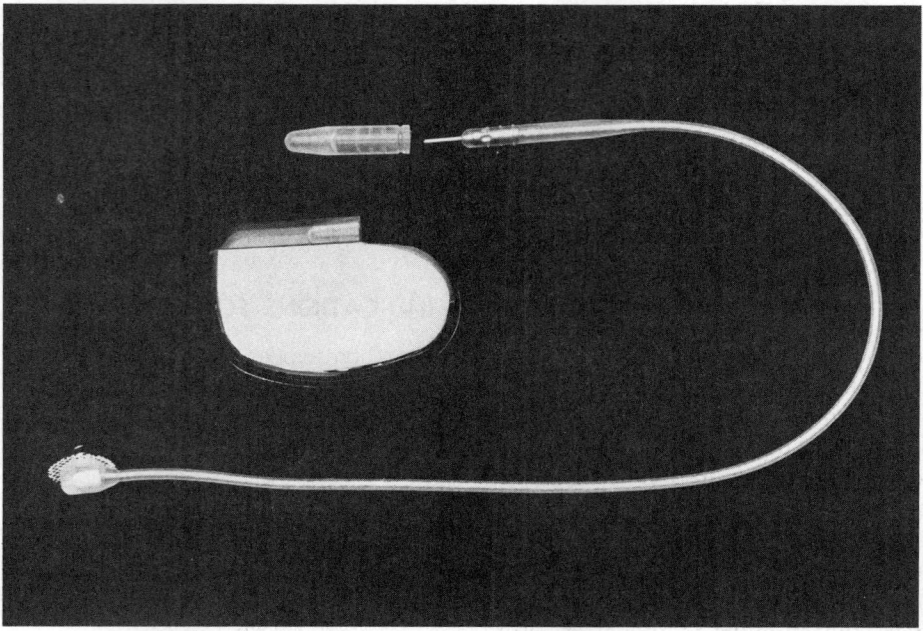

Fig. 44-17. One type of implantable pacemaker (pulse generator); usually implanted subcutaneously in right anterior chest below clavicle.

TYPES OF PACEMAKERS

1. Stimulation of ventricles only
   a. QRS inhibited (demand) pacing
   b. P wave triggered ventricular pacing (SA node still determines heart rate and atrial kick is maintained)

2. Stimulation of atria only (requires the presence of a normal conduction system below the atria)

3. Stimulation of both atria and ventricles (simulates the normal impulse formation and conduction; has artificial PR interval to maintain synchronous contraction of the cardiac chambers)

There are two basic modes of artificial pacing: fixed rate (asynchronous) or demand mode. In the fixed rate mode the pacemaker fires electrical stimuli at a preset rate regardless of the patient's inherent rhythm. Because of the hazards of a pacing stimulus falling within the vulnerable period, asynchronous pacing is rarely used today.

The most popular mode is the demand or standby mode. It is one in which an electrode at the tip of the pacing wire is able to sense the patient's own heartbeats. The pacemaker produces a stimulus only when the patient's own heart rate drops below the rate per minute that is preset on the generator by the physician. Some types of pacemakers currently available are described in the box at left.

It should be noted that the temporary pacemaker is limited to atrial or ventricular stimulation. The potential for maximizing the patient's hemodynamic status is much greater with the various types of permanent pacemakers.

ECG tracing. Fig. 44-18 shows the ECG appearance of pacemaker-stimulated heartbeats. Paced beats are readily identified by the sharp spike that precedes a paced QRS complex. The skilled practitioner is able to analyze an ECG and determine the type of pacemaker and where it is implanted.

Complications. The use of artificial pacemakers is not without potential complications. The most common causes of pacemaker failure are displacement of the pacing wire electrode and battery failure. Both of these require minor surgery to make repairs. Patients detect this failure themselves by noting drastic changes in the heart rate when checking the pulse daily.

Interference from electrical sources and infection are two other areas of concern. Infection may be a problem for any pacemaker patient, but it is a particular concern with the external temporary pacemaker. The patient should be monitored on a daily basis for signs of infection and inflammation at the insertion site. The patient with a *temporary* pacemaker must always be careful to avoid contact with any electrical machinery that is not properly grounded. A small electrical charge

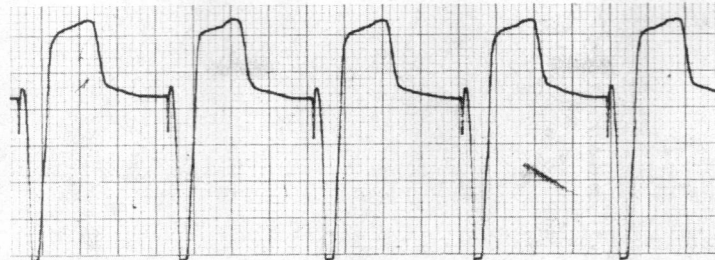

Fig. 44-18. Pacemaker ECG (lead V_1). Rate is 78, rhythm regular, QRS complex wide, no P waves visible, pacing stimulus (spike) precedes each QRS.

passing via the wire directly into the heart could initiate lethal arrhythmias.

Fortunately, current *permanently* implantable pacing generators are well shielded from outside electrical interference. The patient should, however, be instructed to use only electrical equipment that is in good working order. Persons with pacemakers need to show their pacemaker identifications to security officers at airport detector stations and to request a hand scanner in order to avoid false activation of the metal detector.

Infection may be a problem for any pacemaker patient, but it is a particular concern with the external temporary pacemaker. It is the nurse's responsibility to monitor for signs of infection and pacemaker malfunction as well as to teach the patients about their pacemaker and how to monitor themselves at home. The patient should plan for regular monitoring of the pacemaker by the physician or at a pacemaker clinic. One method of follow-up evaluation for persons who are unable to see the physician regularly is to transmit the patient's ECG by special telephone equipment.

Outcome criteria for the person with an internal pacemaker. The person or significant others can:

1. Describe the purpose and function of the pacemaker.
2. Describe plans for resuming normal life activities.
3. Describe plans to monitor pulse daily.
4. Carry an identification card with the type of pacemaker, rate, milliamperage, manufacturer, model number, and physician's telephone number.
5. Describe plans for follow-up care.
   a. State need for regular medical visits.
   b. Describe signs requiring immediate medical attention (pain or tenderness at point of insertion, fever, pulse rate below or double the preset rate).

Cardioversion and defibrillation

Cardioversion is a method of electrical countershock by which an undesirable rhythm is converted to one that is more hemodynamically stable, perferably sinus rhythm. Defibrillation is the emergency form of this method.

Electrophysiologically, the electrical countershock produces a simultaneous depolarization of all cardiac fibers, thus halting the asynchronous chaos of a fibrillation or the rapid firing of a tachycardia. The electrical stimulus must be of sufficient strength and duration to affect all cardiac fibers. In some cases, especially in elective cardioversion, the shock will be delivered more than once until the correct level of voltage is reached. Once the heart is fully depolarized, the SA node is better able to resume control of the heart.

For emergency defibrillation, the paddles from the defibrillator are placed (Fig. 44-19) at the third intercostal space to the right of the sternum and the fifth intercostal space on the left midclavicular line. Either conducting gel or saline pads (as pictured) must be applied between the paddles and the skin to ensure conductance and minimize skin irritation. The button on each paddle is depressed simultaneously to release 200 to 400 watt-seconds (joules) to the patient. Defibrillation must be performed rapidly for ventricular fibrillation and most cases of ventricular tachycardia.

When the cardioversion is elective (e.g., conversion of atrial flutter, atrial fibrillation, or PAT), the procedure differs slightly. The patient should have nothing by mouth for 8 hours in advance. In many cases the daily digitalis dose may be withheld that day or for several days in advance. Selected patients who are receiving anticoagulants should continue to receive this therapy. Oral antiarrhythmics (Table 44-2) are also frequently given in advance.

Patients should be prepared psychologically for what to expect and be reassured that they will remember none of it. The atmosphere should be quiet. The patient is generally given intravenous diazepam (until sleepy) for its amnesic effect. The defibrillator is synchronized such that when the buttons are pressed, the impulse is not initiated until the next R wave. Because of this precaution, the danger of entering the vulnerable period is eliminated. For most elective procedures, the amount of watt-seconds or joules required for con-

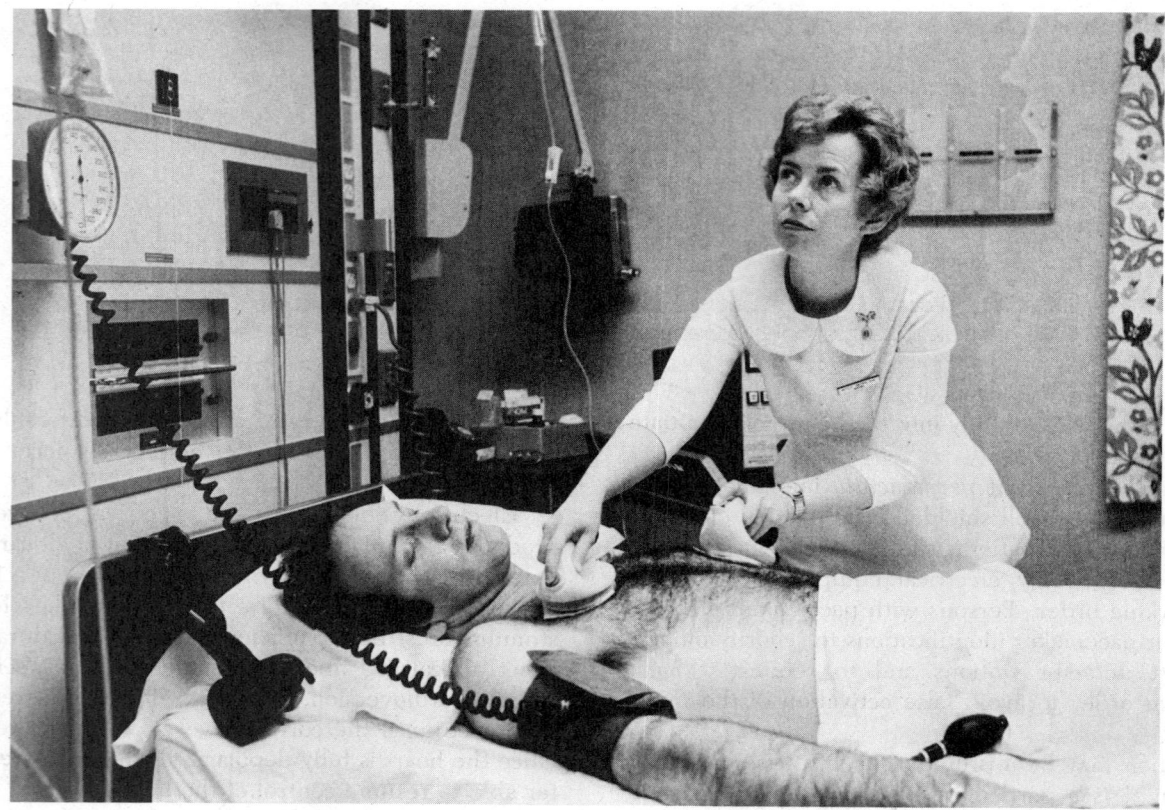

Fig. 44-19. Nurse defibrillating patient.

version is lower than that required for defibrillation. The patient is monitored after cardioversion until vital signs are stable and the gag reflex has returned.

Cardiopulmonary resuscitation

The American Heart Association estimates that each year more than 650,000 victims die of ischemic heart disease. Of these deaths 350,000 take place outside the hospital and usually occur within 2 hours after the onset of symptoms. Thus sudden death from ischemic heart disease is the gravest and most important medical emergency today. It seems reasonable to assume that a large number of these deaths might be prevented by prompt and appropriate interventions that provide either rapid entry into the emergency medical system (see Chapter 73) or cardiopulmonary support using CPR.

Cardiopulmonary arrest is recognized by the cessation of breathing and circulation and signifies a state of clinical death. Immediate and definitive action must be instituted within 4 to 6 minutes following the arrest or biologic death will occur.

Clinical picture

The person who has suffered a cardiac arrest appears clinically dead. Unresponsiveness, cessation of respirations, development of pallor and cyanosis, absence of heart sounds and blood pressure, loss of palpable pulse, and dilation of the pupils are present. (Pupillary response can be misleading in patients who are receiving drugs such as atropine or opium derivatives or in the presence of corneal pathologic conditions.) If a hospitalized patient is being monitored by means of an ECG machine or cardiac monitor, the electrocardiographic pattern of ventricular fibrillation or, less commonly, ventricular asystole will appear.

Techniques of basic life support

Basic life support is an emergency procedure that consists of recognizing an arrest and initiating proper CPR techniques to maintain life until the victim either recovers or is transported to a medical facility where advanced life support measures are available (Table 44-3).

Step I—assess level of consciousness

Persons may appear to be unconscious when in fact they are either asleep, deaf, or possibly intoxicated.

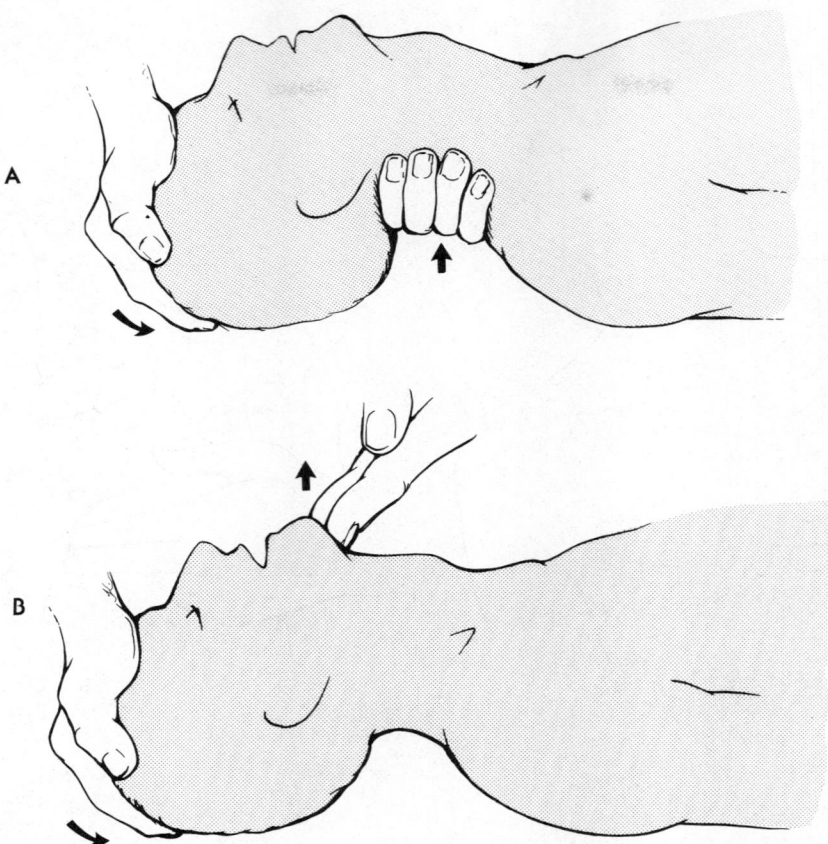

Fig. 44-20. Head tilt. **A,** Neck lift. Place one hand behind neck and other hand on forehead. Lift neck with one hand and tilt head backward by applying pressure to forehead. **B,** Chin lift. Place one hand on forehead and tips of fingers of other hand under lower jaw near chin. Bring chin forward while pressing forehead down.

TABLE 44-3. Sequence of cardiopulmonary resuscitation (CPR)

Findings	Action	ABCs of action
No response		
Absence of respirations; cyanosis; dilated pupils	Open airway	A—Open Airway
Respirations still absent	Initiate artificial ventilation	B—Restore Breathing
Carotid pulse not palpable	Initiate external cardiac compressions	C—Restore Circulation
ECG: ventricular fibrillation	Drug therapy; defibrillation	D—Provide Definitive treatment

Unconsciousness is confirmed by shaking the victim's shoulders and shouting, "Are you OK?" If the person does not respond, help is summoned and the victim is placed in the supine position on a *firm* surface.

Step II—open the airway

The tongue is the most common cause of respiratory obstruction in the unconscious person. Either the head tilt–neck lift (Fig. 44-20, *A*) or the head tilt–chin lift (Fig. 44-20, *B*) is used to open and maintain the airway. While maintaining an open airway, the rescuer should take 3 to 5 seconds to *look, listen,* and *feel* for spontaneous breathing. The rescuer places an ear over the victim's nose and mouth while looking at the victim's chest. The rescuer looks to see if the chest moves with respiration, listens for air escaping during exhalation, and feels for air movement against the face.

Step III—initiate artificial ventilation

Mouth-to-mouth ventilation. If the victim is not breathing, four quick mouth-to-mouth breaths are given. To perform mouth-to-mouth resuscitation, the head tilt–chin lift position is maintained while the victim's nostrils are gently pinched off so that no air escapes. The rescuer takes a deep breath and places the mouth around the outside of the victim's mouth form-

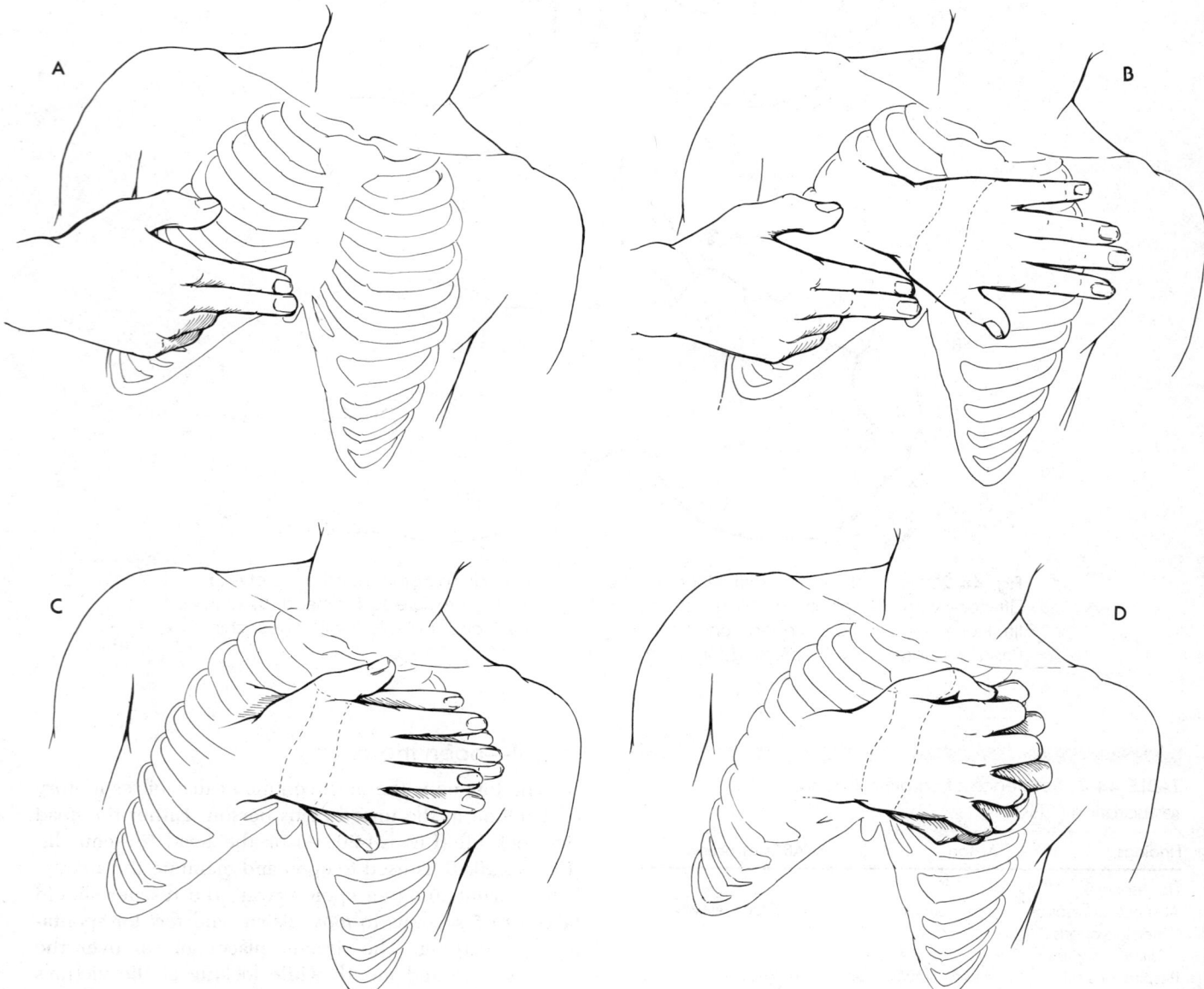

Fig. 44-21. Positioning of hands on sternum. **A,** Middle finger locates xiphoid process; index finger positioned next to middle finger. **B,** Heel of opposite hand is placed on sternum next to index finger. **C,** First hand is removed from landmark position and placed on top of other hand so heels of both hands are parallel and fingers point away. **D,** Fingers may be interlocked to avoid pressure on ribs.

ing a tight seal. Four full breaths are delivered in rapid succession, not allowing the victim to exhale completely after each ventilation. If the lungs are being adequately ventilated using mouth-to-mouth resuscitation, the rescuer should be able to (1) observe the rise and fall of the chest during respiration, (2) hear and feel air escape as the victim passively exhales, and (3) feel in the rescuer's own airway the resistance of the victim's lungs as they expand.

Mouth-to-nose ventilation. Mouth-to-nose ventilation is indicated when it is impossible to open the victim's airway, if the mouth is seriously injured, or if a tight seal cannot be established around the mouth. The rescuer places one hand on the forehead to tilt the head back and uses the other hand to lift the lower jaw and close the mouth. After taking a deep breath, the rescuer seals the mouth around the victim's nose and begins blowing until the lungs expand. Occasionally, when mouth-to-nose ventilation is used, it may become necessary to open the victim's mouth or lips to allow air to escape on exhalation because the soft palate may produce nasopharyngeal obstruction.

Mouth-to-stoma ventilation. Direct mouth-to-stoma artificial ventilation should be performed for the laryngectomy patient. For the patient with a temporary tracheostomy tube, mouth-to-tube ventilation should be initiated after the cuff is inflated.

Step IV—assess circulation

The carotid pulse is palpated rapidly to determine if cardiac compression is needed. The carotid pulse is located by finding the larynx and then sliding the fingers laterally into the groove between the trachea and the sternocleidomastoid muscle. If the carotid pulse is not palpable in 5 to 10 seconds, help is again summoned and cardiac compressions are initiated. The carotid pulse is palpated because the rescuer will already be at the victim's head and generally no clothing has to be removed to assess the pulse. In addition, the carotid arteries are central, and sometimes these pulses will persist when more peripheral pulses have diminished and are no longer palpable.

Step V—initiate external cardiac compression

External cardiac massage is the rhythmic compression of the heart between the lower half of the sternum and the thoracic vertebral column. This intermittent pressure compresses the heart, raises intrathoracic pressure, and produces an artificial pulsatile circulation. Correctly performed cardiac compressions can produce a peak systolic blood pressure of more than 100 mm Hg, but the diastolic pressure is close to zero and the mean blood pressure in the carotid arteries is approximately 40 mm Hg or one fourth to one third normal. The technique for performing external cardiac compression is outlined in the following four stages:

1. The rescuer positions himself or herself close to the victim's side. Using the middle finger of the hand closest to the victim's feet, the rescuer locates the xiphoid process (Fig. 44-21, *A*). The index finger of the same hand is then placed on the victim's sternum directly next to the middle finger. Using the index finger as a landmark, the heel of the opposite hand is placed next to the index finger on the sternum (Fig. 44-21, *B*). The first hand is then removed from the landmark position and placed on top of the hand on the sternum, so that the heels of both hands are parallel and the fingers are pointing away from the rescuer (Fig. 44-21, *C*). Fingers may be interlocked to avoid putting pressure on the patient's ribs (Fig. 44-21, *D*).

2. To perform effective external cardiac compression the rescuer must position the shoulders directly over the victim's sternum and, while keeping elbows locked in a straight position, depress the lower sternum 1½ to 2 in. (Fig. 44-22, *A*). The compressions should be regular, smooth, and uninterrupted. Following each compression the rescuer must release the pressure completely to allow the heart to refill. The rescuer's hands should not ordinarily leave the chest or change position. If hand position must be changed in order to ventilate or move the victim, proper hand position must be relocated using the technique described.

3. Artificial circulation must always be accompanied by artificial ventilation. It is hoped that two rescuers will be available to administer CPR. One rescuer positions himself or herself at the victim's side and performs external cardiac compression while the second rescuer remains at the victim's head to perform artificial ventilation. If two rescuers are available, the cardiac compression rate is 60/min with a 5:1 ratio of cardiac compression to ventilation. The rescuer who is ventilating the victim quickly delivers one breath after every five compressions without any pause or interruption in compressions (Fig. 44-22, *B*). If only one rescuer is available to perform CPR, cardiac compression is performed at a rate of 80/min with a 15:2 ratio of cardiac compression to ventilation. The rescuer delivers two quick breaths after every 15 compressions. Because a single rescuer must interrupt cardiac compression in order to ventilate the victim, a faster rate of compression is required. A rate of 80 compressions per minute is required to attain an actual compression rate of 60/min. The two breaths delivered to the victim must be in rapid succession, not allowing the victim to exhale fully.

4. After the first minute of CPR, the carotid pulse should be palpated to assess the effectiveness of CPR and to check for the return of spontaneous circulation. If there are two rescuers performing CPR, the person ventilating the victim can also assess pulses, monitor for the return of spontaneous breathing, and assess pupillary response to light. If the victim's brain is being ad-

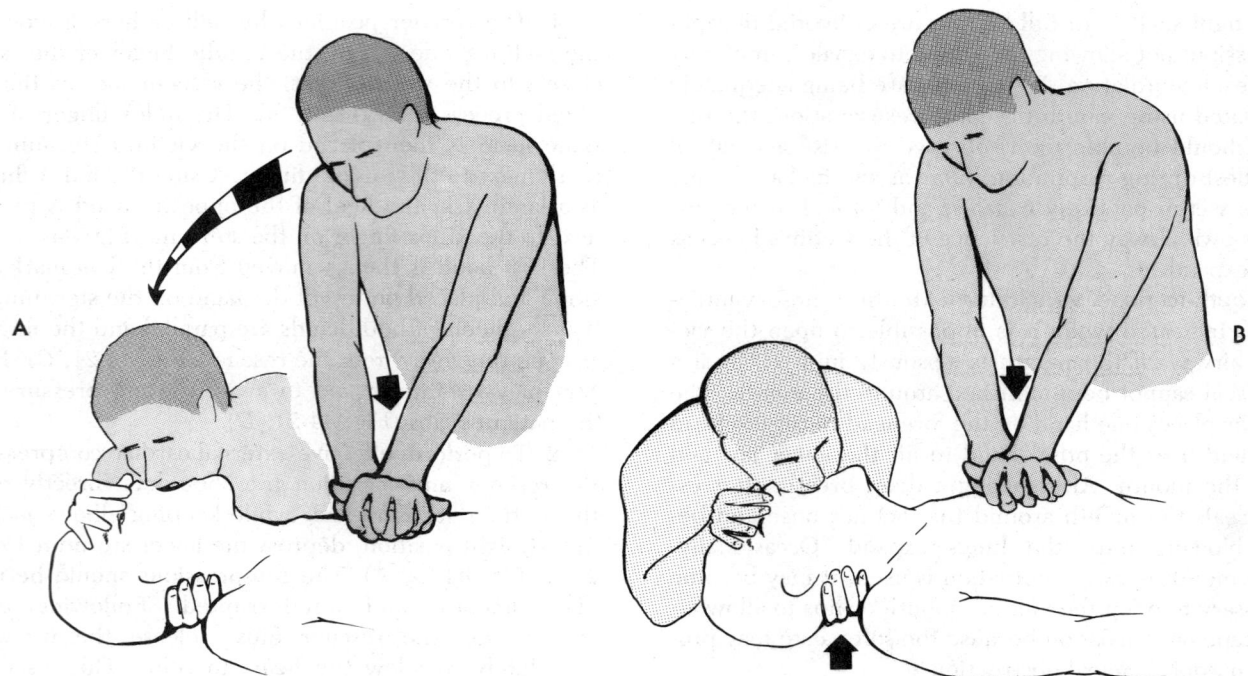

Fig. 44-22. A, One-person rescuer CPR; two rapid inflations after every 15 compressions. **B,** Two-persons rescuer CPR; one inflation after every five compressions without pause.

equately oxygenated, the pupils will constrict in response to light. If the pupils are grossly dilated and nonreactive to light, severe brain damage may be imminent or may have already occurred. CPR should be stopped for no more than 5 seconds every 4 to 5 minutes to assess the return of spontaneous pulse and respiration. Rescuers should continue CPR until one of the following takes place:

1. Spontaneous circulation and ventilation return.
2. Another rescuer takes over basic life support.
3. Victim is transported to an emergency facility where qualified personnel assume the responsibility for CPR.
4. Victim is pronounced dead by a physician.
5. Rescuer is exhausted and unable to continue.

Precordial thump

The precordial thump is a quick blow delivered to the middle portion of the sternum within 1 minute after cardiac arrest. The precordial thump has been found to be useful in cases of *witnessed* cardiac arrest and when a patient is being monitored. A precordial thump generates a small low-voltage stimulus in the heart. In a potentially reactive heart this stimulus may be effective in restoring a heartbeat in asystole caused by a block and in reversing recent-onset ventricular tachycardia and fibrillation. The precordial thump is not recommended for use on children or in the case of unwitnessed arrests. In an anoxic heart that is still beating a precordial thump could be hazardous since it may in-

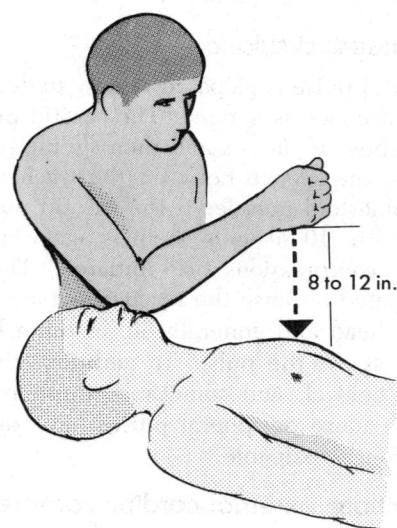

Fig. 44-23. Precordial thump. Quick sharp blow over midportion of sternum using fleshy portion of fist.

duce ventricular fibrillation. The precordial thump maneuver may be utilized at varying times during CPR, depending on the circumstances surrounding the arrest. In the case of a witnessed cardiac arrest, the precordial thump should be administered as soon as the absence of a pulse is discovered. If there is no immediate response to the thump, CPR is initiated immediately (Fig. 44-23).

In-hospital cardiac arrests

Many hospitals have prepared teams of personnel, including physicians, nurses, anesthesiologists, and technicians who can be called to give immediate and complete care in the event of a cardiac arrest. Most hospitals are equipped with a cardiac arrest tray or have access to a specially equipped cart on which all necessary emergency items are available. Equipment needed includes an ECG machine, a suction device, oxygen, defibrillator, airway and Ambu or other breathing bag, laryngoscope, a variety of endotracheal tubes, cut-down set, intravenous fluids, and tracheostomy set should this be necessary.

Medications usually administered during a cardiac arrest are generally available on the emergency cart. Some of these medications are described in Table 44-4. For a more detailed discussion of basic life support and for information on advanced life support, the reader is referred to reference 69.

Complications of cardiopulmonary resuscitation

The most common complication of external cardiac massage is fracture of the ribs. This may occur in some individuals even though the technique of external car-

TABLE 44-4. Drugs commonly used in cardiac resuscitation

Drug	Route and dosage	Actions and indications	Drug	Route and dosage	Actions and indications
Atropine sulfate	0.5 mg by IV bolus; may be repeated at 5-min intervals	Reduces vagal tone; enhances AV conduction; accelerates heart rate in cases of pronounced sinus bradycardia	Epinephrine hydrochloride (adrenalin), 1:10,000 solution	0.5-1.0 mg (6-10 ml of 1:10,000 solution) by IV bolus, intracardiac, tracheobronchial, or endotracheal route; 0.5 mg may be repeated at 5-min intervals	Positive inotropic and chronotropic action; peripheral vasoconstrictor; converts fine ventricular fibrillation to coarse ventricular fibrillation, making it more amenable to defibrillation; increases perfusion pressure of cardiac compressions
Bretylium tosylate (Bretylol)	5 mg/kg by IV bolus followed by defibrillation; may be increased to 10 mg/kg and repeated at 15- to 30-min intervals until maximal dose of 30 mg/kg has been given	For ventricular fibrillation and tachycardias that have not responded to other forms of therapy			
			Isoproterenol hydrochloride (Isuprel)	2-20 μg/min by IV bolus or intracardiac; dosage should be titrated to heart rate and blood pressure response	Positive inotropic and chronotropic effects that generally result in increased cardiac output; used in cases of asystole or cardiovascular collapse
Calcium chloride, 10% solution	5-7 mg/kg by IV bolus; may repeat at 10-min intervals	Used in ventricular standstill and all types of AV dissociation; enhances contractile state of heart (positive inotropic action) as well as conduction velocity			
			Metaraminol bitartrate (Aramine)	15-100 mg/500 ml in D5W or NS; or 2-5 mg by IV bolus every 5-10 min	Potent vasopressor; increases peripheral resistance and corrects severe hypotension and shock
Dobutamine hydrochloride (Dobutrex)	2.5-10 μg/kg/min by IV	Used to treat refractory pump failure; direct receptor stimulating agent; increases myocardial contractility			
			Levarterenol bitartrate (Levophed)	8 mg/500 ml in D5W or NS IV infusion; should be titrated to blood pressure response	Potent vasopressor and positive inotropic effects; increases peripheral resistance; used in severe hypotension with low total peripheral resistance
Dopamine hydrochloride (Intropin)	5 μg/kg/min by IV drip; may be increased up to 20-50 μg/kg/min; a range of 5-30 μg/kg/min is usually required in arrest situations	Actions depend on dosage; 2-10 μg/kg/min generally has β-receptor stimulating action on heart with resultant increase in cardiac output; greater than 10 μg/kg/min has α-receptor stimulating action with resultant peripheral vasoconstriction			
			Sodium bicarbonate (50 mEq)	1 mEq/kg by IV bolus (may be repeated in 10 min if necessary); further doses governed by arterial blood gas and pH determinations	Used to counteract metabolic acidosis
			Lidocaine hydrochloride (Xylocaine)	50-100 mg at rate of 25-50 mg/min by IV; may be repeated in 5 min if necessary	Antiarrhythmic; shortens refractory period and suppresses automaticity of ectopic foci

diac compression was performed correctly. Other complications of external cardiac compression that might occur despite correct CPR technique include fractured sternum, costochondral separation, and lung contusions. If medications were injected into the heart during the resuscitative effort, the patient is monitored carefully for signs of hemothorax, pneumothorax, or pericardial tamponade (p. 1102). Any indication of labored respiration, paradoxical pulse, muffled heart sounds, tachycardia, decreased breath sounds, or drop in blood pressure is reported to the physician immediately. Laceration of the liver may also occur as a result of compressions performed over the xiphoid process.

Internal cardiac compression

In this seldom used method of cardiac massage, a thoracotomy is performed and the heart is massaged with the hands or stimulated with an electric current. In most cases open heart compression will not succeed when proper external compressions coupled with appropriate drug therapy and ventilation have failed. There are some instances or conditions in which internal compression is necessary, such as in cardiac tamponade, in crushing or penetrating chest injuries, and in the presence of an anatomic deformity of the chest that precludes adequate and effective compression by external cardiac massage.

Intervention for the person with intraaortic balloon counterpulsation

A counterpulsation device is one that assists the circulation of blood through the body by pumping when the heart is in ventricular systole. The hemodynamic result of this action is to augment intraaortic blood pressure during diastole. The physiologic effects of counterpulsation are therefore an increase in coronary artery perfusion, a decrease in preload (the degree to which the myocardium is stretched before contracting), and a decrease in afterload (the resistance against which blood is expelled).

The two primary goals in the use of circulatory assist devices are to provide temporary assistance to the patient's circulation until the underlying pathophysiologic condition is corrected and to afford optimal conditions for repair of the heart until it can provide adequate circulation unaided. The intraaortic balloon pump (IABP) is a counterpulsation device capable of achieving these goals in selected patients.

INTRAAORTIC BALLOON COUNTERPULSATION: INDICATIONS FOR USE

Cardiogenic shock secondary to acute myocardial infarction

Other low cardiac output states

During emergency diagnostic procedures on unstable cardiac patients

In unstable cardiac patients before and during open heart surgery

Assistance in removing patients from cardiopulmonary bypass postoperatively

Drug-resistant, life-threatening arrhythmias

Unstable angina pectoris

Severe acute myocardial infarction

Indications for use

The various situations in which counterpulsation has been found useful are listed in the box above. In all cases, the timeliness of its application is essential to reduce the work load of the heart and halt the progressive deterioration of the myocardium. Individuals have been maintained on IABP assistance for periods of several hours to several months; however, the usual time is from 2 to 3 days. The IABP is not indicated for persons whose underlying pathologic condition is so severe that eventual weaning from the IABP is considered impossible, unless the individual is being seriously evaluated for a heart transplant. Absolute contraindications are few; the two primary ones are aortic valve incompetence and aortic aneurysm.

Technique

The intraaortic balloon is inserted percutaneously or by cutdown into the right or left femoral artery. It is advanced into the thoracic aorta and is sutured into place at the insertion site after the balloon tip has been correctly positioned just distal to the left subclavian artery (Fig. 44-24). The end of the balloon catheter is attached to a pump console, which alternately inflates and deflates the balloon using either helium or carbon dioxide gas.

The timing of the inflation-deflation sequence is of the utmost importance in obtaining maximal counterpulsation effect. Using the ECG to trigger the pumping mechanism and the arterial waveform to determine effectiveness of the counterpulsation, the balloon is timed to inflate just at the beginning of ventricular diastole,

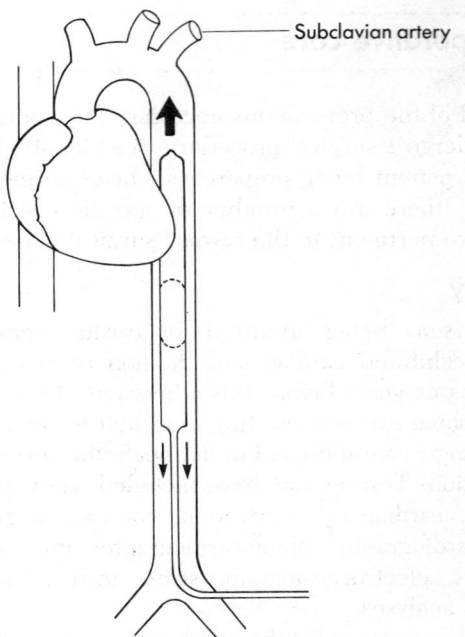

Fig. 44-24. Representation of a triple-segmented intraaortic balloon positioned just distal to left subclavian artery.

immediately after closure of the aortic valve. The balloon remains inflated during diastole and is then timed to deflate immediately before the next ventricular systolic ejection or just before the aortic valve reopens. Improper balloon timing not only defeats the purpose of counterpulsation, but also could be directly damaging to the myocardium, particularly in early inflation or late deflation in which the heart would be ejecting blood against a partially inflated balloon.

Pathophysiology

When the balloon is inflated during diastole, it causes an intraaortic pressure rise known as *diastolic augmentation*. This heightened diastolic pressure caused by balloon inflation forces blood in the aortic arch to flow in a retrograde fashion and provides increased coronary artery filling. This achieves the goal of improving oxygen delivery to the myocardium.

When the balloon deflates at the end of diastole, it reduces pressure in the aorta, causing blood in the aortic arch to move from an area of higher pressure to one of lower pressure and to fill the space previously occupied by the balloon. This decreases the pressure in the aortic arch, reducing the resistance that the left ventricle must overcome in order to eject blood during systole; hence, afterload is reduced. A sustained reduction in afterload will allow the left ventricle to eject more of

its stroke volume during each contraction, thus leaving more space for ventricular filling. This will usually result in a secondary decrease in preload as the left ventricle becomes and remains more efficient.

Nursing intervention

The patient undergoing IABP counterpulsation requires intensive nursing observation and care. All vital signs and indices of cardiac function must be observed continually and recorded; frequently the patient will be receiving vasopressor and antiarrhythmic drugs, and it will be the nurse's responsibility to titrate these for the desired effects. The patient may be intubated and be dependent on ventilatory support. All such factors require meticulous nursing intervention.

In addition, the patient with an IABP in place requires specific observation and care to prevent possible complications, such as circulatory insufficiency in the catheterized leg, aortic damage, and infection. Circulation checks of all pulses in both lower extremities are performed before insertion and hourly thereafter until the balloon is removed. No hip flexion is allowed on the catheterized side; well-padded leg restraints must be used if the patient is unable to cooperate. The head of the bed is not elevated more than 30 degrees to prevent balloon migration upward in the aorta. The patient should be tilted and carefully positioned on alternate sides every 2 hours to prevent skin breakdown and other consequences of limited mobility. The dressing on the balloon insertion site must be kept clean and dry and should be changed every 24 to 48 hours using sterile technique.

Considerable psychologic support is necessary for the patient and family during such critical therapy. Not only is the physical size and noise of the pump console very intimidating, but its presence only reinforces everyone's awareness of the frailty of the patient's heart and uncertainty about the future. Careful but simple explanations of the pump's action are necessary for those patients who are alert enough to understand; it is important that they not get the mistaken idea that the pump is working instead of their heart. Some patients with this type of misunderstanding fear that they will die if the pump stops even momentarily. Such terrific fear makes them anxious and restless and further increases the body's demand for oxygen. Continuous reassurance and repeated simple explanations are essential; some patients may benefit from mild sedation.

The IABP has become the most effective means of counterpulsation therapy, and its recent acceptance and use has spread from the medical center environment to the community hospital setting. With correct patient selection and timely application, it can be a significant lifesaving technique.

Intervention for the person requiring heart surgery

In the third decade of this century the first heart surgery procedure was performed on a human patient in England. It consisted of a closed repair of a stenosed mitral valve, or mitral commissurotomy. Since that time great progress has been made in a variety of heart surgery procedures, including valve repairs and replacements, structural defect and congenital anomaly repairs, coronary artery bypass grafting, and even total heart transplants. Currently, there is exciting research being done to develop and test prosthetic heart chambers and total prosthetic hearts. Today's surgeon has the advantage of a highly sophisticated technology to aid in performing these extremely delicate yet vital procedures; a technology advanced enough to allow many Americans to undergo heart surgery each year.

One term frequently used to describe heart surgery is also commonly misused; the term *open heart surgery* is often used in referring to any surgical procedure performed on the heart. Strictly speaking, however, open heart procedures are those in which the heart muscle itself is incised and the internal heart structures are directly visualized. A coronary artery bypass procedure is not, therefore, a true open heart procedure, and it may or may not be performed with the assistance of extracorporeal circulation (also referred to as ECC, cardiopulmonary bypass, or the heart-lung machine) (Table 44-5). True open heart procedures always involve the use of extracorporeal circulation. It is perhaps best to avoid this term entirely and instead to refer specifically to the actual procedure being performed, particularly when speaking with the patient and family. It is not uncommon to find patients scheduled for coronary artery bypass grafting who believe that their heart will be opened during the procedure.

TABLE 44-5. Types of cardiac surgery

Action	Surgical procedures	Use of extracorporeal circulation
Repair or replacement	Correction of congenital defects; valve replacements; valvuloplasty; thoracic aortic aneurysm repair	Yes
Vascular bypass	Coronary artery bypass	May or may not be used
Release of constriction	Pericardial fenestration; pericardiectomy; closed mitral commissurotomy	No

Preoperative care

All of the preparations necessary for a person about to undergo a surgical procedure (see Chapter 24) apply to the patient being prepared for heart surgery. In addition, there are a number of specific considerations that are pertinent to the cardiac surgical patient.

History

Persons being admitted for cardiac surgery may have exhibited cardiac and pulmonary symptoms for months or years before this admission. They will have undergone extensive testing to establish the underlying pathologic condition and to delineate the severity of the condition. Testing may have included chest roentgenograms, cardiac catheterization, coronary angiography, echocardiography, phonocardiography, nuclear cardiac studies, electrocardiogram, stress testing, and blood serum analyses.

It is necessary for the nurse caring for the heart surgery patient to understand each patient's pertinent medical history in order to individualize care appropriately. It is necessary to know the underlying nature of the heart condition, how long it has been diagnosed, and the particular surgical procedure chosen to correct it. The relative degree of cardiac impairment will be demonstrated in the patient's limitations in life-style. The current manifestations of the illness may range from no symptoms to intermittent pain to debilitating heart failure. It is important to be aware of past cardiopulmonary or circulatory conditions or disorders, such as myocardial infarction, bacterial endocarditis, pulmonary embolus, blood clotting abnormalities, and a history of smoking, that might place the individual at higher risk for devoping postoperative complications.

The patient's current medical regimen is very important, and medications or therapeutic measures that the patient was utilizing before admission must be noted. It may be necessary to modify some of these measures once the patient is hospitalized, and all such changes in medication, diet, activity, and other areas must be carefully explained. Without an adequate explanation, the patient or family may feel that such changes during hospitalization are an indictment of the care provided at home, rather than seeing them as necessary preoperative preparations.

Physiologic preparation

Despite the fact that the person scheduled for heart surgery may have suffered from the cardiac condition for years, it is desirable to have the person in the best physical condition possible at the time of surgery. This is one goal of patient care during the preoperative period, however short or long that may be. Efforts will have been made to help the overweight patient reach a safe body weight; to assist the patient who smokes to stop or nearly stop; to eliminate or reduce edema and establish body fluids and electrolytes in normal balance; to correct or control cardiac arrhythmias; to eliminate any signs of infection; in short, to achieve the healthiest state possible in light of the severity of the illness and the urgency of the surgery.

Therefore, along with a thorough knowledge of the patient's history, as mentioned above, it is necessary to obtain a complete data baseline to document the patient's condition just before surgery. While many of the preoperative tests and preparations may have been performed in the days or weeks before the scheduled surgery, the person is usually admitted to the hospital at least 1 or 2 days before the planned procedure. At this time, a chest x-ray film, an ECG, and full laboratory screening will be performed. For selected individuals, arterial blood gas analyses and even pulmonary function studies may be obtained to help establish a baseline of respiratory status and to plan appropriate and aggressive preoperative, intraoperative, and postoperative pulmonary care. Baseline vital signs (including apical and radial heart rates and bilateral arm blood pressures), integrity of all pulses (both proximal and distal), neurologic status, height, weight, nutritional status, elimination patterns, and psychologic status are all carefully assessed and recorded in the immediate preoperative period.

Patient education

In the past several years preoperative teaching programs for heart surgery patients have become well established. These fairly structured approaches still allow the nurse to individualize a teaching plan for any particular patient and yet ensure that all necessary topics are covered in a consistent manner for all patients.

General information. While most persons admitted for heart surgery have undergone previous hospitalizations, there will be significant differences in this particular stay, and an initial overview of general information is helpful to most patients and families. Explain that the person will first be admitted to a general patient-care division and will stay there until the day of surgery. Explain where and when the patient will move after the operation: to a postanesthesia recovery room or a cardiovascular recovery area or directly to a cardiovascular or surgical intensive care unit (ICU). Information should be given concerning visiting hours and restrictions in each of these areas, expected length of stay (usually 2 to 3 days in the ICU), and location of waiting room areas. Frequently, the family will be requested to identify one spokesperson who will be told where to meet the surgeon after the operation and who will be allowed to call the ICU nurses at any time for information. This serves to enhance the consistency and thoroughness of information given to the family while reducing the interruptions from multiple sources.

Information concerning the intensive care unit.

Many patients and family members benefit from a tour of the ICU, both to familiarize them with the equipment and to locate important areas such as waiting rooms and restrooms. Such a tour should always be conducted by ICU personnel who can accurately yet reassuringly describe the myriad of sights and sounds that assail the untrained observer. Timing of the tour must be convenient for the ICU personnel, who should greet the patient and family when they arrive, without appearing so rushed that the patient and family feel that they are imposing.

At times a tour may be omitted depending on the acuity of the ICU patients and the level of critical activity in the unit. If there is any possibility that a tour might prove distressing or unusually anxiety provoking to the patient or family, it should be replaced with a general description of the sights, sounds, and activities that the patient is likely to encounter. It is important that all discussions of the stay in the ICU center about the unique attention and in-depth care that the patient will receive from specially qualified nurses.

Description of surgery. Specific instruction must be given concerning the particular type of heart surgery that the patient will undergo. Simple diagrams or plastic heart models can be used to illustrate what type of cardiac problem the patient has and how the surgery will correct it. The type of chest incision to be made should be described: most commonly, a median sternotomy is performed for all bypasses and some valve procedures, while a left anterior axillary chest approach is used for certain selected repair procedures. In addition, the internal thigh incision for obtaining vein grafts must be described for coronary artery bypass patients.

Explanation of preoperative and postoperative procedures. It is important to describe the types of interventions and equipment that are made necessary by the intricacy of heart surgery. The patient will usually shower or bathe with special antimicrobial soap the night before surgery. In addition, a surgical shave preparation will be done either the night before or the morning of surgery; this will include a scrubbing and then a shaving of the entire chest and abdomen from neck to groin and from left midaxillary line to right. In addition, the legs will be scrubbed and shaved if the patient is to have vein segments removed for grafting.

Specific aspects of the equipment and techniques that will be of special significance to the patient are described (Table 44-6). (1) While intubated, the patient will be unable to speak, but nursing personnel will be in constant attendance and will help the patient communicate. (2) It is normal to see bloody drainage in the chest tube and bottle. (3) It is not unusual to have a sensation of needing to void while the urinary catheter is in place. (4) The tubes and lines will somewhat restrict movement, but the nurses will help the patient turn in bed and later get up. (5) Some pain will be experienced but it will not be excruciating (and will not

TABLE 44-6. Techniques and equipment commonly used after cardiac surgery

Technique/equipment	Purpose
Intubation; ventilator for 12-24 hr	Maintain open airway and ventilation
Cardiac monitoring	Identify arrhythmias
Chest tubes (one or two)	Drain blood and air from chest
Intravenous lines	Replace fluids; monitor central venous pressure (CVP)
Intraarterial lines	Monitor blood pressure; obtain arterial blood samples
Pulmonary artery line (Swan-Ganz)	Monitor pulmonary artery and capillary wedge pressure; monitor cardiac output
Indwelling urinary catheter (Foley)	Monitor urinary output for signs of impaired renal function

feel the same as the original anginal pain if this was present). (6) Frequent pain medication will be given to help relieve the pain, but the patient should always tell the nurse when pain is present.

Finally, explain that the patient will receive continuous observation in the ICU and may at times be awakened to receive necessary nursing care, such as taking vital signs, obtaining blood specimens, or x-ray films, turning, coughing, and deep breathing. Demonstrate the types of procedures in which the patient will be expected to participate actively. Have the patient practice deep breathing and coughing, using a pillow or folded bath blanket to hold across the upper abdomen for support. If a particular type of incentive spirometry or positive pressure breathing device is routinely used with postoperative heart patients, obtain the apparatus preoperatively and have the patient practice with it. Document the patient's preoperative ability to cough and use assistive breathing devices for later comparison and encouragement postoperatively.

Have the patient lie in bed and demonstrate leg exercises (p. 413), explaining their importance in maintaining circulation postoperatively. Describe the progression of patient recovery to include bed rest the first night, up in a chair the first or second postoperative day, with limited ambulation by the third day. Explain that the patient will be allowed no food or fluids until after the breathing tube is removed, but that the lips will be kept moistened.

Teaching approaches. Initial assessment of the patient's knowledge and ability to learn is essential to planning a thorough, individualized teaching plan. Continued reassessment of the patient's readiness to learn and retention ability is important throughout the preparative education period. Teaching sessions should be conducted at planned times and in a quiet area. The pace must be adapted to the patient's interest and ability to master the information presented. Opportunities should be allowed for the patient to demonstrate understanding of concepts and techniques. Adjunctive printed information should be given to all patients to reinforce what has been taught verbally.

Psychologic preparation

Patients scheduled to undergo heart surgery are usually aware that they are facing a potentially life-threatening situation; however, no two patients will manifest this awareness in the same way. A complete psychosocial evaluation is becoming a routine part of the preparative care of heart surgery patients in medical centers throughout the country. This evaluation is one part of the multidisciplinary team approach, which usually consists of the medical referral physician, cardiac surgeon, psychologist, clinical nurse specialist or practitioner, social worker, and dietitian.

The psychosocial evaluation looks at patients and significant others in relation to the presence of support mechanisms, the use of defense mechanisms (longstanding vs. situational), and established methods of adaptation. Combined with an assessment of the patient's basic levels of understanding of the experience they are about to undergo, a sound plan can be developed to enhance patients preoperative and postoperative psychologic well-being.

It has been established that a small amount of anxiety enhances learning, while too much anxiety blocks learning. The highly anxious individual may benefit from limited and carefully worded preoperative teaching, with an emphasis on a simple understanding of the surgical procedure. Highly fearful or anxious patients are most prone to serious misconceptions about their illness, the surgical procedure itself, and the anticipated outcome. It is very important to include significant others in the preoperative teaching plan when the patient is unusually worried or appears to have significant misconceptions. It is also very important to address patients' fears very seriously, no matter how unusual they might sound. Patients must be given frequent opportunity to vent their concerns to supportive, understanding staff members.

Patients who consistently reject the offer of information about their illness and impending surgery also need a supportive environment in which they feel safe. Information should not be pressed on those who truly wish not to hear it; for them, such defense mechanisms may be tremendously important. Rather, a complete psychosocial evaluation may point out ways in which staff and significant others can assist in maintaining the psychologic well-being both before and after surgery. Conversely, it may also reveal that for some patients, highly restricted visiting and family contact may be desirable for a few days postoperatively.

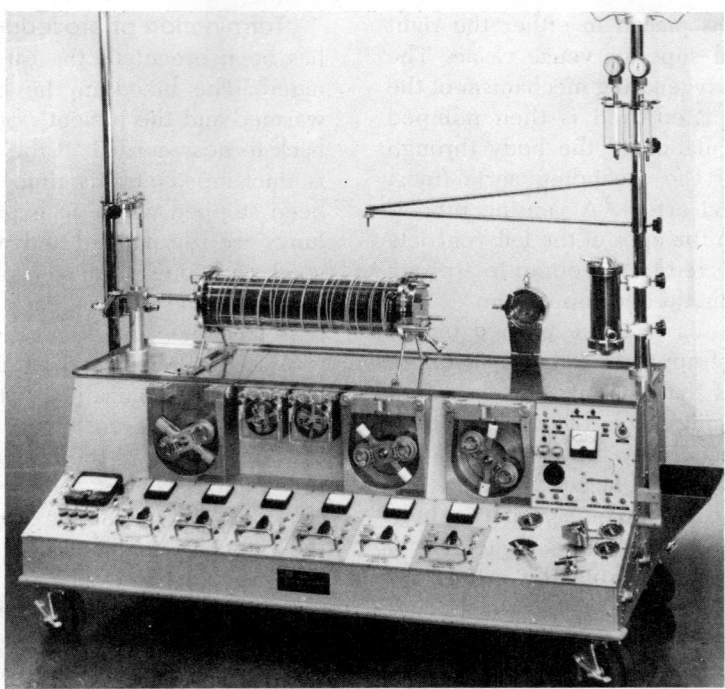

Fig. 44-25. Pump oxygenator used during open heart surgery. (Courtesy PEMCO, Inc., Cleveland.)

Finally, as more and more patients have relatives and friends who have undergone heart surgery, they may be concerned about postoperative psychologic problems that they have observed. The health professional will exercise judgment in introducing this topic in preoperative teaching, but when it appears indicated or if the topic arises, an explanation should be given of the factors that may precipitate a postoperative or ICU psychosis: sleep deprivation, stress, and sensory overload from continuous environmental stimuli. Patients who develop the psychosis may complain of depression, inability to sleep, or of having "bad dreams" when they do sleep. These symptoms usually disappear after the patient's condition will allow a few lengthy intervals of undisturbed sleep. For some patients preoperative awareness of the effects of such stressors may prevent the patients from fearing that they are "losing their minds" if such symptoms arise. A sedative may be given the night before surgery to aid the patient in maintaining a calm state and obtaining a restful night's sleep despite a normal amount of apprehension.

Intraoperative period

The preoperative medications frequently include a narcotic analgesic, a sedative, an anticholinergic agent, and sometimes an antibiotic. The patient's skin is often prepared in a specially designated area adjacent to the operating room. A light anesthetic is given first, followed by intubation, and then when fully anesthetized, the patient is placed on mechanical ventilation. Various intravenous and intraarterial lines are inserted, and the patient is placed on a cardiac monitor.

If the heart surgery to be performed is a coronary artery bypass in which autologous vein segments will be grafted, these are first "harvested." Generally, portions of the superficial saphenous vein are removed from one leg using longitudinal, interrupted incisions.

The heart is exposed through either a midline sternotomy or anterolateral thoracotomy incision, and retractors are used to hold open the chest wall.

Cardiopulmonary bypass

Some heart surgery procedures can be performed without artificial ventilation and circulation, but most procedures require either partial or total cardiopulmonary bypass. In *partial*, or left-heart, bypass, blood is drained from the left atrium and ventricle and is passed through a pulsatile pump or roller pump, which returns the blood to the common femoral artery or the descending aorta. In this type of bypass the pulmonary circulation is not interrupted.

In *total* cardiopulmonary bypass both oxygenation and circulation of the blood are performed by the bypass machine (Fig. 44-25). Venous blood is removed from the body via cannulas placed in either the right atrium or the inferior and superior venae cavae. The blood passes through the oxygenating mechanism of the bypass machine, is oxygenated, and is then pumped back into the arterial circulation of the body through cannulas placed either in the ascending aorta (most common) or in the femoral artery. A venting tube is usually introduced through the apex of the left ventricle or left atrium and is connected to the pump to aspirate intracardiac blood and maintain decompression.

The bypass pump circuits must be primed before use with a fluid volume of approximately 2500 ml. In the past a large portion of that volume was composed of cross-matched type-specific whole blood. Currently, more centers are using an entirely blood-free hemodilution primer consisting mainly of lactated Ringer's solution. The advantages of the nonblood primer include decreased viscosity, limited hemolysis, and no risk of transfusion reaction and hepatitis from the primer solution. The main concern in using a nonblood primer is maintenance of an adequate hematocrit. This can be achieved by intermittent additions of blood to the system during the cardiopulmonary bypass process.

In addition to performing blood oxygenating and circulating functions for the body, the bypass machine has two other distinct functions. It can act as a source for the direct administration of medications into the systemic circulation. It is also able to provide systemic hypothermia by cooling the perfusate to temperatures that range from mildly (30° to 34° C) to profoundly (15° C) below body temperatures. Hypothermia decreases the tissue's metabolic needs, thereby lowering the body's overall oxygen consumption. A reduced need for oxygen enhances myocardial tissue preservation during times such as when the aorta is cross-clamped.

Cold cardioplegia. Myocardial tissue preservation is of primary concern in all cardiac surgery procedures and especially in surgery for ischemic heart disease. The incidence of intraoperative or perioperative myocardial infarctions has been reported to be as high as 30%. In recent years a clearer understanding of the principles involved in myocardial tissue preservation has resulted in the widespread use of cold cardioplegia solutions.

Cold cardioplegia consists of infusing a 4° C solution with 30 mEq of potassium per liter into the aortic root. It is usually infused for a few minutes immediately after aortic cross-clamping and again after about 30 to 45 minutes or when myocardial temperatures rise above 19° C. External cardiac cooling is achieved by a continuous infusion of lactated Ringer's solution at about 4° C into the pericardium. Several variations of the cold cardioplegia technique are in use, and it appears that this development has significantly improved myocardial tissue preservation in the intraoperative phase by supercooling the myocardium and drastically reducing its oxygen requirements.

Termination of procedure. Once the surgical repair has been executed, the cardioplegia infusion is terminated. The blood in the bypass pump is slowly rewarmed and the patient's body temperature is brought back to near normal. If the aorta was cross-clamped, it is unclamped at this time and the heart, which had been stopped while on hypothermia, is restarted. The lungs are reexpanded and when the cardiac rhythm is good, weaning from the bypass machine is begun. Blood volume is given back to the patient from the bypass machine, and the patient remains on decreasing amounts of partial bypass until weaning is complete. Systemic heparinization, which was done to promote blood flow while on bypass and to prevent blood from clotting quickly in the operative field, is reversed with protamine.

Epicardial pacing wires may be attached directly to the right ventricular wall, the right atrial wall, or the internal chest wall and are then brought through the incision to the chest surface. There they may be used for temporary cardiac pacing if needed during the postoperative period. Chest tubes are inserted as indicated for blood drainage and air evacuation, if necessary. The incisions are closed and dressed, and the patient is taken to the recovery room.

Side effects of cardiopulmonary bypass. While cardiopulmonary bypass has been the most significant advance in the rapid growth of safe and effective cardiac surgery procedures, it has a number of specific, potentially deleterious side effects. Cardiopulmonary bypass creates a shocklike state, in which there is a functionally low hematocrit (produced by hemodilution), decreased systemic arterial pressures, and decreased perfusion to major organs (Fig. 44-26). During bypass there is some destruction of red blood cells because of the great turbulence of blood flow through the cannulas and the resulting trauma to the cells as they come in contact with the cannula walls and system interfaces. Any trauma to blood cells affects the blood proteins causing protein denaturation.

Despite the many potential hazards from cardiopulmonary bypass, it is clear that when scrupulous surgical technique is combined with appropriate candidate screening and thorough preoperative preparation, the potential benefits of cardiac surgery significantly outweigh the risks.

Postoperative care

After the conclusion of the heart surgery, patients are transferred to the postanesthesia recovery area or directly to a cardiovascular or surgical ICU where they will typically remain for 2 days. During this time the patient will need continuous observation and professional nursing care to promote optimal recovery and

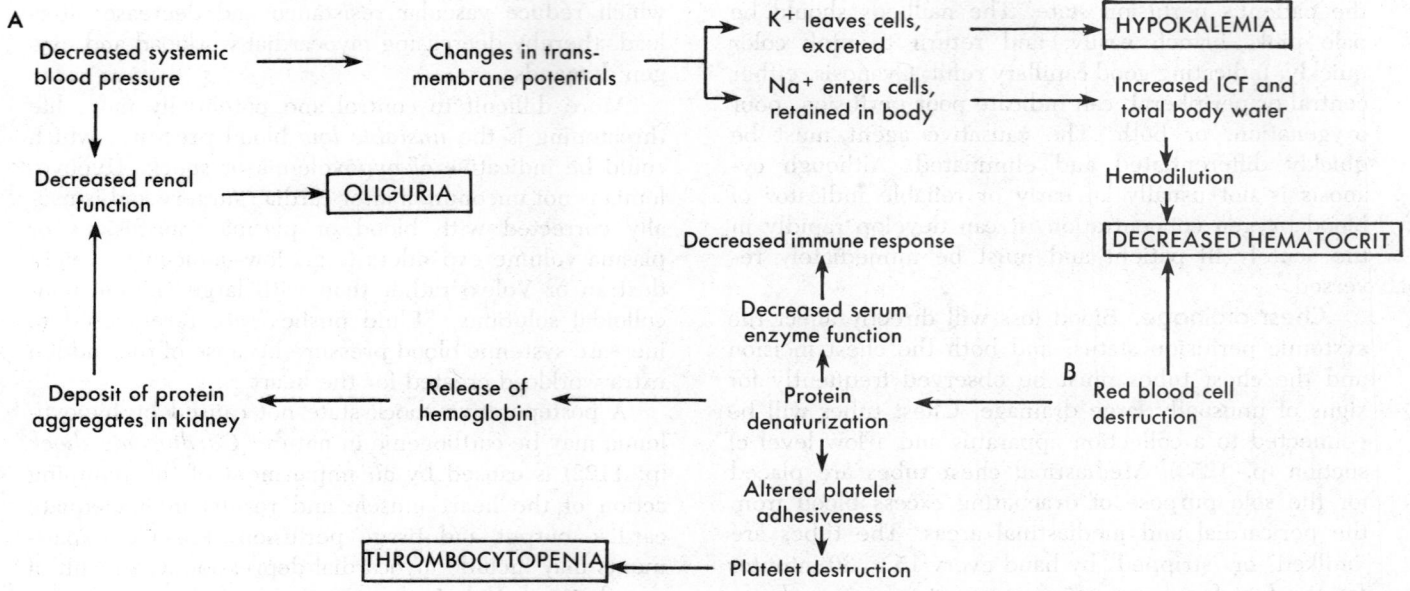

Fig. 44-26. Some effects of the shocklike state, **A,** and red blood cell destruction, **B,** that may occur with cardiopulmonary bypass. Clinical signs are indicated in boxes.

prevent complications, which are most serious in the first 48 hours after surgery.

Complete observation, thorough assessment, careful planning, and knowledgeable intervention may be organized through a systems approach to care.

Cardiovascular system

One of the major goals of patient care in the immediate postoperative period is to promote cardiovascular function, adequate tissue perfusion, and stabilization of vital signs. To evaluate cardiovascular function thoroughly, the patient will have an intraarterial line and a pulmonary artery catheter (Swan-Ganz) (p. 1056), each connected to a pressure transducer and continuous monitor; a central venous pressure (CVP) line connected to a water manometer or a pressure transducer and monitor; and a continuous electrocardiograph monitor.

Cardiac function. *Blood pressure* and *heart rate* are monitored continuously and are recorded every 15 minutes until stable, then every hour thereafter. *CVP, pulmonary artery pressure, pulmonary capillary wedge pressure,* and *cardiac output* measurements are obtained every 2 to 4 hours as indicated by changes in the patient's condition. The radial pulse is checked for rate, rhythm, and volume, with bilateral comparisons made. The apical and radial pulses are checked simultaneously for any differences (pulse deficit), which could be indicative of such complications as atrial fibrillation. Distal peripheral pulses, either posterior tibial or dorsalis pedis, are checked for strength and bilateral equality.

The *cardiac pattern* is monitored continuously for the first several days postoperatively, and the ECG pattern is compared to the preoperative baseline to detect any changes. Cardiac arrhythmias are very common in the immediate postoperative period; they may be the result of operative trauma from incision of the left ventricle, prolonged use of anesthesia, extracorporeal circulation and alterations in potassium levels, hypotension, hypovolemia, or hypoxia.

The treatment for arrhythmias depends on the cause and the type of arrhythmia produced. Treatment modalities include antiarrhythmic drugs such as lidocaine and procainamide (Pronestyl), cardiotonics such as digoxin, potassium replacement, and temporary pacing. With the increasing use of computerized monitoring systems, the nurse has a highly sophisticated adjunct to help obtain, store, and analyze ECG information when it is most vital. If the ECG status remains somewhat uncertain as recovery progresses, the patient may be transferred from the ICU to a cardiac step-down unit or telemetry unit for several days so that the ECG pattern may continue to be monitored closely.

Body temperature can be an important indication of cardiovascular function. The skin should be warm and dry, although immediately after surgery the skin may still be quite cool as a result of intraoperative hypothermia. Once the body temperature has warmed, cool or diaphoretic skin may be an indication of shock. It is not uncommon for the body temperature to rise above normal and remain elevated for the first day or two postoperatively. This is usually attributed to the time spent on cardiopulmonary bypass.

As with skin temperature, *skin color* is indicative of

the patient's perfusion state. The nailbeds should be pale pink, blanch easily, and return to pink color quickly, indicating good capillary refill. Cyanosis, either central or peripheral, can indicate poor perfusion, poor oxygenation, or both. The causative agent must be quickly differentiated and eliminated. Although cyanosis is not usually an early or reliable indicator of blood oxygen concentration, it can develop rapidly in the acutely ill patient and must be immediately reversed.

Chest drainage. Blood loss will directly affect the systemic perfusion status, and both the chest incision and the chest tubes must be observed frequently for signs of unusually large drainage. Chest tubes will be connected to a collection apparatus and a low level of suction (p. 1253). Mediastinal chest tubes are placed for the sole purpose of evacuating excess blood from the pericardial and mediastinal areas. The tubes are "milked" or "stripped" by hand every 15 to 30 minutes for the first few hours after surgery to promote drainage. Drainage should be slow and fairly consistent and does not usually exceed 50 ml/hr after the first 2 hours postoperatively. The patient is routinely turned from side to side every 2 hours to assist in proper chest drainage. The total blood drainage over the first 24 hours will usually average 500 ml.

A change in chest drainage color to a very bright red from a dark red, a sustained hemorrhage that lasts for over 1 minute, or a sudden cessation of chest drainage are all abnormal findings that must be reported immediately. Cessation of chest drainage within the first few hours postoperatively usually indicates clotting of the chest tube within the mediastinum. This could predispose the patient to *cardiac tamponade,* a life-threatening emergency. Tamponade indicates a compression of the heart caused by excessive amounts of blood or blood clots collecting between the heart and the anterior chest wall. The return of venous blood to the right atrium and the cardiac output can be significantly impaired. Other signs of cardiac tamponade, in addition to minimal or no chest tube drainage, include sudden increase in bleeding from the midline incision, restlessness, decreased blood pressure, increased CVP, and decreased urinary output. The physician must be notified at once, and cardiac decompression by needle aspiration or other methods will be undertaken.

Blood pressure. Maintenance of a stable systemic blood pressure in the postoperative period may be difficult in some patients. *High* blood pressure must be controlled so that the weakened heart muscle does not have to work excessively hard to maintain an adequate cardiac output. Excessive myocardial workload increases myocardial oxygen demands, which may not be met. Pharmacologic intervention may be necessary in the form of vasodilators, such as sodium nitroprusside, which reduce vascular resistance and decrease afterload, thereby decreasing myocardial workload and oxygen demands.

More difficult to control and potentially more life threatening is the *unstable low* blood pressure, which could be indicative of hypovolemia or shock. Hypovolemia is not uncommon after cardiac surgery and is usually corrected with blood or plasma transfusions or plasma volume expanders (e.g., low–molecular weight dextran or Volex) rather than with large volume noncolloidal solutions. "Fluid pushes" are rarely used to increase systemic blood pressure because of the sudden extra workload created for the heart.

A postoperative shock state not caused by hypovolemia may be cardiogenic in nature. *Cardiogenic shock* (p. 1122) is caused by an impairment of the pumping action of the heart muscle and results in inadequate cardiac output and tissue perfusion. Specific impairments may include myocardial depression as a result of anesthetics and hypothermia, trauma of surgery, mechanical impedance to contraction caused by an implanted prosthetic valve, decreased compliance of the ventricle because of scar tissue or hypertrophy, preexisting heart disease not corrected by surgery, or arrhythmias associated with an inadequate stroke volume.

Therapy for cardiogenic shock is directed toward improvement in myocardial contractility. Correction of any specific underlying etiology will be attempted, as in eliminating cardiac arrhythmias. Pharmacologic support may include vasoconstrictors such as dopamine hydrochloride to raise arterial pressure, although care must be taken not to increase unduly blood return to the heart and peripheral resistance unless cardiac output is increased. Sympathetic agents such as epinephrine may be used for their cardiotonic effects. Isoproterenol is a preferred catecholamine because it combines inotropic with chronotropic effects and decreases peripheral and pulmonary vascular resistance. Frequently, a combination of medications will be used to achieve the desired result of improving cardiac output with a minimum of side effects. Drug dosage administration is individually titrated to obtain desired effects. Whenever cardiac and vasopressor medications are given by continuous intravenous infusion, the patient must remain under close observation and the medications should always be administered via intravenous infusion pumps.

If pharmacologic support is inadequate in reversing or minimizing cardiogenic shock, a temporary mechanical assistive device may be employed to reduce the cardiac workload. *Intraaortic balloon counterpulsation* (p. 1086) may be used for several hours or several days and may be inserted at any time that its use is indicated in the preoperative, intraoperative, or postoperative period.

Circulatory assistance may also be obtained through the use of *left-heart assist devices,* which are becoming more sophisticated in their clinical application. They are generally indicated for profound intraoperative myocardial depression with failure to wean from the cardiopulmonary bypass. They involve a partial bypass, with diversion of some oxygenated blood from the left atrium or ventricle directly to the ascending aorta. Patients requiring this type of assistance are critically ill and must be carefully observed and cared for.

Prophylaxis. Finally, some patients may receive prophylactic medications in the postoperative period. Antibiotics may be initiated just before surgery and continued for 3 to 5 days postoperatively to help prevent infection from numerous potential sources in the perioperative period. Anticoagulants will be given, starting about the third postoperative day, to patients receiving prosthetic valve implantations. The anticoagulation is necessary to prevent embolus formation on the surface of the valves and will be continued after the patient's discharge.

Respiratory system

All patients receiving general anesthetics, especially those having undergone cardiopulmonary bypass, require meticulous attention to maintaining a clear and patent airway. Removal of excess pulmonary secretions, proper aeration of lungs and oxygenation of blood, and maintenance of chest tube patency are essential.

The rate, depth, and quality of respirations are monitored and recorded, and also the patient's breath sounds are obtained through chest auscultation. While intubated, the patient should be preoxygenated and suctioned as frequently as necessary to clear secretions. The patient is turned from side to side every 2 hours; positioning and chest percussion are used to help loosen and mobilize secretions. Arterial blood samples are obtained for blood gas analysis to document the status of the patient's systemic oxygenation. Drainage and patency of chest tubes are noted, particularly when there is a known pleural leak. Daily chest x-ray films are obtained as ordered or more frequently if a sudden change is noted. Lungs are auscultated frequently while the patient is intubated to detect any shift in endotracheal tube placement.

After extubation it is important to observe the patient for any signs of respiratory distress. The patient is helped to splint the incision and cough and deep breathe at least every 2 hours while awake. Medicating the patient before coughing may help increase the effort to cough, but some patients may require nasotracheal suctioning even after extubation. Preoperative instructions that were given regarding incentive spirometry or nebulization devices should be reinforced as the patient is assisted in utilizing them. Aggressive pulmonary hygiene must be maintained for the first week postoperatively.

Neurologic system

Following surgery the patient's neurologic status must be carefully assessed, including level of consciousness, pupil size and reaction, orientation, and movement and sensation of extremities.

Patients usually begin to awaken within 1 or 2 hours after surgery. Failure to awaken may be the result of unusually deep anesthesia or of embolization of air, calcium, fat, or thrombotic particles to the brain. A return of consciousness that seems sluggish and in which the patient does not seem to regain full alertness after a day or two may have been caused by poor cerebral perfusion or microembolization during cardiopulmonary bypass.

Pupil size, equality, and reaction to light are checked frequently in the immediate postoperative period. Pupil dilation may be caused by excessive carbon dioxide in the blood or by such cardiac medications as atropine. Constricted pupils may be caused by dopamine. Disorientation and restlessness may be signs of hypoxia or embolization to the brain in addition to being symptoms of fatigue, fear, or sensory overload. Impaired sensation or muscular control of any portion of the body postoperatively indicates a neurologic deficit that will require careful observation and complete evaluation by specialists.

Renal system

Careful observation of hourly urinary output as well as urine color, pH, and specific gravity will give essential information about renal function. Adequate urinary output is at least 20 to 30 ml/hr. It is common for the urine to demonstrate increased sugar and acetone for the first several hours after cardiopulmonary bypass. This elevation is not usually treated unless it coincides with sustained elevated serum glucose levels. Specific gravity may be elevated because of oliguria or the presence of red blood cells as a result of extracorporeal circulation.

Renal insufficiency in the patient after heart surgery is always caused by complications of extracorporeal circulation. The destruction of red blood cells can cause sludging in the kidneys. If low-perfusion states occurred during the surgical procedure, the kidneys themselves may have been damaged, resulting in acute tubular necrosis. This is marked by oliguria with increased blood urea nitrogen and serum creatinine levels. If the acute tubular necrosis is severe and prolonged, temporary peritoneal dialysis or membrane hemodialysis (p. 1589) will be initiated to sustain the patient through the acute phase. Return of kidney function after acute tubular necrosis is usually gradual but complete.

Fluid and electrolyte balance

The patient will receive necessary blood products after heart surgery to maintain a stable hematocrit. Plasma and plasma expanders such as dextran and Volex will be given to avoid hypovolemia while maintaining a normal osmotic gradient. Crystalloid intravenous solutions are given to maintain adequate circulating volume.

Extremely *accurate recording of intake and output* is essential for the first few days postoperatively. Fluids will be limited to reduce the chance of fluid overload and increased work for the heart. Daily weights are obtained, and diuretics are administered if fluid retention occurs. Intravenous fluids must be titrated very carefully, and this is usually accomplished with the aid of intravenous infusion pumps.

Serum electrolytes are obtained several times during the first 24 hours and at least daily thereafter. Initially, the serum glucose level may be grossly elevated; this is transient. Particular attention is paid to the *serum potassium level,* and supplemental intravenous potassium chloride is usually given in the immediate postoperative period, particularly in conjunction with diuretic use. Hematocrit, hemoglobin, and prothrombin time are obtained daily to assess the extent of blood loss and the effect of replacement therapy.

The patient is usually allowed sips of water 1 hour after endotracheal extubation and progresses to a clear liquid, full liquid, and then solid diet as tolerated. Solid food is usually restricted to a specific daily sodium intake while hospitalized, and the restrictions may be continued after discharge. Although few patients have much appetite initially, there is rarely any difficulty maintaining adequate nutrition within a few days.

Comfort, rest, and sleep

Alleviation of pain is very important in the postoperative period, and patients should be kept as comfortable as possible. Narcotic analgesics are administered every 3 hours for the first day and then offered to the patient as needed after that. Keeping the patient comfortable not only adds to a sense of security but reduces the stress on the heart, decreases the need for oxygen, and promotes healing. Other comfort measures are routinely employed, such as positioning in bed, controlling environmental temperature, and giving frequent oral hygiene.

The postoperative heart patient will be quite weak and will tire from activity very quickly. Activity periods should be organized so that rest periods may be frequent (even if brief) and uninterrupted. While patients are in the ICU, it is very difficult for them to obtain sufficient restful sleep. Sleep deprivation, particularly of REM sleep, is a serious problem, and significant efforts should be made to allow occasional intervals of uninterrupted sleep at least 90 minutes long.

Psychologic response

The psychologic ramifications of heart surgery, sleep deprivation, and sensory overload can be overwhelming. Some persons experience a period of depression or disorientation after surgery, whereas others may become unreasonably fearful or experience hallucinations. The disorientation may even progress to panic. The nurse should be alert to subtle behavioral changes and reassure the person and family that these reactions are common and do not mean that the patient is "losing his mind." At the same time, physiologic causes of the behavior must be ruled out.

It is very helpful to the patient and family if the nursing staff attempt to personalize the patient's experience as much as possible. It is rather easy to lose sight of the person behind the monitoring equipment in an ICU. Calling the patient by name, using frequent physical contact when orienting the patient to time and place, and including the patient in any discussions that are held at the bedside will all help to decrease the sense of isolation.

Activity

Passive arm exercises are started shortly after surgery, followed by active exercises as the person gains strength. Mobilization of the person depends on the operation and the status of the heart.

In general, persons who have had surgery of the aorta are kept flat in bed for several days to prevent unnecessary strain on the vessel (the blood pressure is lower when the patient is flat). Before getting out of bed, the person must gradually become accustomed to having the head of the bed elevated. When this procedure is first attempted, dizziness and faintness may be experienced; if this happens, the person is returned to a flat position, and elevation is attempted again later.

Persons who have had surgery for patent ductus arteriosus and mitral stenosis may be kept in Fowler's position postoperatively and are encouraged to move their arms and legs. Backache from lying flat on the back, even for short periods, is common.

The time of ambulation for each patient depends on the patient's progress and condition, but (other than the above exceptions) it usually proceeds as follows: The first day the feet are dangled over the side of the bed for 15 minutes in the morning and afternoon, and the person is allowed to sit in a chair at the side of the bed for 15 minutes in the afternoon and evening. Walking around the room is permitted by the third day. The fourth day the patient is allowed to walk around the room and to sit in the chair for gradually increasing periods of time. By the fifth day walking longer distances is encouraged. During ambulation close supervision is necessary, and activity that causes excessive fatigue, dyspnea, or an increased pulse or respiratory rate is discontinued. If any of these symptoms appear, the patient is returned to bed, and the physician is consulted before further activity is attempted.

Definite instructions must be provided regarding when the person may attempt to climb stairs. The activity should be done slowly. Only two or three steps should be attempted the first time, after which the number of steps is gradually increased. The patient should rest two or three times while climbing one flight of stairs.

Long-term care

The person and family need to be told that no marked improvement will be noticed immediately after the operation—that it will be at least 3 to 6 months before the full result of the surgery can be ascertained. It is essential that all persons be given this information so that they will not be depressed by dyspnea or pain that may still be present postoperatively.

In preparation for discharge from the hospital, the person is asked to make a list of normal daily activities. This list is discussed with the physician to determine the activities that are appropriate. Sexual intercourse is usually permitted within 3 to 4 weeks postoperatively. Patients are usually advised to start activities slowly and progress gradually to more energy-consuming tasks. The physician will want the patient to return for frequent medical follow-up examinations, at which time advice will be given regarding additional activities. The person is allowed to do anything that does not cause fatigue or pain but must be kept from attempting too much too soon.

The family should be aware of how much the person may be encouraged to do. Since the patient may have been an invalid preoperatively, the family may be as fearful as is the person about an increase in activity.

Outcome criteria for the person who has had heart surgery

The person or significant others can:
1. Describe extent of permissible activity.
   a. Describe plans for progressive return to physical activity as recommended by the physician.
   b. State awareness of when sexual activity may be resumed (3 to 4 weeks).
   c. Describe criteria to use as a guide in determining if overexertion occurs (fatigue, dyspnea, pain).

d. Describe plans to return to work if employed. Plan meals incorporating a balanced diet with any prescribed modifications (no added salt, low cholesterol).
3. State name, dosage, action, and side effects of medications ordered.
   a. How and when to use prn medications.
   b. Schedule for other medications.
4. Describe plans for follow-up health care.
   a. Explain basis of any symptoms that may persist (dyspnea, pain, night sweats).
   b. Describe signs or symptoms requiring immediate medical attention (fever, increasing dyspnea, or chest pain with minimal exertion).
   c. State plans for ongoing medical care.

REFERENCES AND SELECTED READINGS

1. American Heart Association: 1981 Heart Facts, Dallas, 1981, The Association.
2. American Heart Association: Arrhythmias in acute myocardial infarction. AHA Coronary Care Committee (James R. Margolis, director), Dallas, 1976, The Association.
3. Andreoli, K.G., et al.: Comprehensive cardiac care: a text for nurses, physicians, and other health practioners, ed. 5, St. Louis, 1979, The C.V. Mosby Co.
4. Aspinall, M.J.: Nursing the open heart surgery patient, New York, 1973, McGraw-Hill Book Co.
5. Atcheson, S., and Fred, H.L.: Complications of cardiac resuscitation, Am. Heart J. **89:**263-266, 1975.
6. Bates, B.: A guide to physical examination, ed. 2, Philadelphia, 1979, J.B. Lippincott Co.
7. Behrendt, D.: Patient care in cardiac surgery, Boston, 1976, Little, Brown & Co.
8. Berk, J.L., et al.: Handbook of critical care, Boston, 1976, Little, Brown & Co.
9. Berne, R.M., and Levy, M.N.: Cardiovascular physiology, ed. 3, St. Louis, 1977, The C.V. Mosby Co.
10. Boxonyl, S., editor: Postoperative care following coronary surgery, Heart Lung **3:**912-915, 1974.
11. Braunwald, E., editor: Heart disease: a textbook of cardiovascular medicine, Philadelphia, 1980, W.B. Saunders Co.
12. Brest, A.N.: Antiarrhythmic therapy: how to select the right method, Consultant **19:**23-26, 1979.
13. *Brzenski, T.S.: Pacemakers: pulse of life, A.O.R.N. J. **32:**967-976, 1980.
14. Calhoun, P.S., and Bozorgi, S.: Postoperative care following coronary surgery, Heart Lung **3:**912-915, 1974.
15. Carlson, R.W., and Becker, H.G.: Preventing or managing cardiopulmonary arrest, Consultant **19:**58-63, 1979.
16. *Chrzanowski, A.L.: Intra-aortic balloon pumping: concepts and patient care, Nurs. Clin. North Am. **13:**513-530, 1978.
17. Chung, E.K.: Cardiac emergency care, ed. 2, Philadelphia, 1980, Lea & Febiger.
18. *Collins, J.J., and Morgan, A.P.: Automated management of postoperative cardiac surgical care, Heart Lung **3:**929-932, 1974.
19. Committee on Emergency Cardiac Care, American Heart Association: Advanced cardiac life support, Dallas, 1975, The Association.

*References preceded by an asterisk are particularly well suited for student reading.

20. Constant, J.: Learning electrocardiography, ed. 2, Boston, 1980, Little, Brown & Co.

21. Copley, D.P., et al.: Improved outcome from prehospital cardiopulmonary collapse with resuscitation by bystanders, Circulation **56**:901-905, 1977.

22. *Cromwell, V.: Understanding the needs of your coronary bypass patient, Nurs. '80 **10**(3):34-41, 1980.

23. Daily, E.K., and Schroeder, J.S.: Techniques in bedside hemodynamic monitoring, ed. 2, St. Louis, 1981, The C.V. Mosby Co.

24. Daly, B.J., Gorenshek, N., and Mendelsohn, H.: Chest surgery. In Meltzer, L., et al., editors: Intensive care for nurse specialists, ed. 2, Bowie, Md., 1975, The Charles Press.

25. *Derrick, H.F.: How open heart surgery feels, Am. J. Nurs. **79**:276-285, 1979.

26. Dorney, E.R.: How to evaluate the implanted pacemaker, Med. Times **107**:36-42, 1979.

27. Dorney, E.R.: The indications for cardiac pacemakers, Med. Times **107**:33-35, 1979.

28. *Ellis, R.: Unusual sensory and thought disturbances after cardiac surgery, Am. J. Nurs. **72**:2021-2025, 1972.

29. Elsberry, N.L.: Psychological responses to open heart surgery, Nurs. Res. **21**:220-227, 1972.

30. Furman, S.: Recent developments in cardiac pacing, Heart Lung **7**:813-826, 1978.

31. Futral, F.E.: Postoperative management and complications of coronary artery bypass surgery, Heart Lung **6**:477-481, 1977.

32. *Giving cardiac care. Nursing Photobook Series, Springhouse, Pa., 1981, Intermed Communications, Inc.

33. Goldberger, E.: Treatment of cardiac emergencies, ed. 3, St. Louis, 1982, The C.V. Mosby Co.

34. Guyton, A.C.: Textbook of medical physiology, ed. 5, Philadelphia, 1975, W.B. Saunders Co.

35. *Hammond, C.E.: Protecting patients with temporary transvenous pacemakers, Nurs. '78 **8**(11):82-86, 1978.

36. *Hart, R.: What to do when you're number 1: a review of CPR for adults, Nurs. '79 **9**(2):54-59, 1979.

37. *Hart, R.A.: Giving artificial ventilation, Nurs. '78 **8**(6):48-53, 1978.

38. Heger, J.J., and Fisch, C.: Axions on cardiac arrhythmias, Hosp. Med. **15**:20-24, 1979.

39. Heger, J.J., et al.: New drugs for the treatment of ventricular arrhythmias, Heart Lung **10**:475-483, 1981.

40. *Hoffman, M., Donekers, S., and Hauser, M.: The effect of nursing intervention on stress factors perceived by patients in a coronary care unit, Heart Lung **7**:804-809, 1978.

41. Hurst, J.W., editor: The heart, arteries and veins, New York, 1978, McGraw-Hill Book Co.

42. Jacobson, L., and Goldschlager, N.: Cardiac pain: principles and case studies, Garden City, N.Y., 1981, Medical Examination Publishing Co.

43. Jillings, C.: Phases of recovery from open-heart surgery, Heart Lung **7**:987-994, 1978.

44. Johnson, R.A., et al.: The practice of cardiology, Boston, 1980, Little, Brown & Co.

45. Jones, P.: Cardiac pacing, New York, 1980, Appleton-Century-Crofts.

46. King, O.: Care of the cardiac surgical patient, St. Louis, 1975, The C.V. Mosby Co.

47. Kinney, M., editor: AACN's clinical reference for critical care nurses, New York, 1980, McGraw-Hill Book Co.

48. Koch-Weser, J.: Drug therapy; bretylium, N. Engl. J. Med. **300**:473-477, 1979.

49. *Kroncke, G., and Boake, W.: Practical advice for your pacemaker patients, Fam. Pract. Recertification **1**:75-76, 1979.

50. *Kroncke, G.M., et al.: What to do when your patient's pacemaker stops working, Nurs. '81 **11**(10):74-78, 1981.

51. Limberg, L., and Hamer, S.: Arrhythmias complicating acute myocardial infarction: a self-teaching program, Heart Lung **5**:576-584, 1976.

52. Lipman, B.S., Massie, E., and Kleiger, R.E.: Clinical scalar electro-cardiography, ed. 6, Chicago, 1972, Year Book Medical Publishers, Inc.

53. *Manwarning, M.: What patients need to know about pacemakers, Am. J. Nurs. **77**:825-830, 1977.

54. *Manzi, C.C.: Cardiac emergency! How to use drugs and CPR to save lives, Nurs. '78 **8**(3):30-35, 1978.

55. Marriott, H.J.L.: Practical electrocardiography, ed. 6, Baltimore, 1977, The Williams & Wilkins Co.

56. McNeal, G.J.: Tracing arrhythmias, Am. J. Nurs. **79**:98-100, 1979.

57. Meltzer, L.E., et al.: Concepts and practices of intensive care for nurse specialists, ed. 2, Bowie, Md., 1976, The Charles Press.

58. *O'Brien, J.: The nursing care of patients with cardiac pacemakers, Nurs. Times **75**:147-152, 1979.

59. Pacemaker protocol, Emerg. Med. **10**:50-53, 1978.

60. Price, S.A., and Wilson, L.M.: Pathophysiology: clinical concepts of disease processes, ed. 2, New York, 1982, McGraw-Hill Book Co.

61. *Rossel, C.L., and Alyn, I.B.: Living with a permanent cardiac pacemaker, Heart Lung **6**:273-279, 1977.

62. Scheuer, R.: Cardiopulmonary resuscitation in seven community hospitals, Heart Lung **1**:810-817, 1972.

63. Schmidt, R.M., and Margolin, S.: Harper's handbook of therapeutic pharmacology, Philadelphia, 1981, Harper & Row, Publishers.

64. Selzer, A.: Principles of clinical cardiology, Philadelphia, 1975, W.B. Saunders Co.

65. Sheldon-Czerwinski, B.: Manual of patient education for cardiopulmonary dysfunctions, St. Louis, 1980, The C.V. Mosby Co.

66. Sodeman, W.A., and Sodeman, T.A.: Pathologic physiology: mechanisms of disease, ed. 6, Philadelphia, 1979, W.B. Saunders Co.

67. Sokolow, M., and McIlroy, M.B.: Clinical cardiology, Los Altos, Calif., 1977, Lange Medical Publications.

68. Spencer, R.: Surgery of the chest, Philadelphia, 1978, W.B. Saunders Co.

69. Standards for cardiopulmonary resuscitation (CPR) and emergency cardiac care (ECC), J.A.M.A. **244**:453-508, 1980.

70. *Sweetwood, H.: Patients with pacemakers, Nurs. '77 **7**(3):44-51, 1977.

71. *Thorpe, C.J.: A nursing care plan: the adult cardiac surgery patient, Heart Lung **8**:690-697, 1979.

72. Vamiale, P., and Naclerio, E., editors: Cardiac pacing: a concise guide to clinical practice, Philadelphia, 1979, Lea & Febiger.

73. Vander, A., Sherman, J., and Luciano, D.: Human physiology, ed. 3, New York, 1980, McGraw-Hill Book Co.

74. *Van Meter, M.: Keeping cool in a code, RN **44**:29-35, 1981.

75. *Viebrock, R. and Barth, R.: The pacemaker patient; how you can spare him needless alarm, RN **43**:38-42, 1980.

76. Weiss, I.: Essentials of heart rhythm analysis, Philadelphia, 1973, F.A. Davis Co.

77. Wenger, N.K., Hurst, J.W., and McIntyre, M.C.: Cardiology for nurses, New York, 1980, McGraw-Hill Book Co.

78. *Westfall, V.E.: Electrical and mechanical events in the cardiac cycle, Am. J. Nurs. **76**:234-235, 1976.

79. Yokes, J.A., and Reed, W.A.: Heart surgery. In Meltzer, L.E., et al.: Concepts and practices of intensive care, ed. 2, Bowie, Md., 1976, The Charles Press.

CHAPTER 45

PROBLEMS OF THE HEART AND MAJOR BLOOD VESSELS

JOAN M. KAVANAGH

It is difficult to determine the exact prevalence of cardiac disorders and associated vascular conditions such as cerebrovascular and peripheral vascular disease. Unfortunately, noninvasive diagnostic techniques have not yet been perfected that can be used in mass screening for all types of cardiovascular disorders. At present, many persons are not even aware that they have heart disease until severe symptoms develop.

Epidemiology

In the United States, cardiovascular disorders cause more deaths than all other diseases combined. Over 40 million Americans are afflicted with some form of heart or blood vessel disorder, and each year over 1 million deaths are attributed to a cardiovascular disorder.[58]

Deaths caused by cardiac disorders vary with age. In the United States, congenital heart disease and closely related vascular disorders are responsible for disabling 25,000 newborns each year. Of these children, 7000 die each year. If it were possible to eliminate maternal rubella by some form of drug therapy, the incidence of congenital heart defects would be drastically reduced.[44] By far the most common cause of death from heart disease after the age of 25 years is coronary atherosclerotic heart disease (CAHD). CAHD

strikes a significant number of persons without any warning and causes prolonged suffering and disability in even larger numbers. Approximately 700,000 deaths each year are attributed to myocardial infarctions.[58]

Other cardiovascular disorders with substantial morbidity and mortality include hypertensive heart disease, rheumatic heart disease, and cerebrovascular disease. Fortunately, despite the discouraging statistics relating to the incidence of cardiovascular disorders, there has been a steady reduction in mortality from cardiovascular disease. In the United States the past decade has witnessed a tremendous expansion in cardiovascular research and much progress has been made in preventing and treating cardiovascular disease. This reduction in mortality suggests an effective application of increased knowledge regarding the causes, diagnosis, treatment, and, most significantly, the prevention of heart disease.[9]

Although the exact pathogeneses of many types of heart diseases are not yet known, extensive epidemiologic studies are in progress in an attempt to delineate further preventive measures. Observational epidemiologic studies have identified numerous risk factors for cardiovascular disease. The implication is that with pharmacologic interventions and behavior modification, especially in regard to changes in life-style, the manifestations of cardiovascular disease may be decreased, delayed, or even eliminated.[44] Further definitive research protocols are now being developed to study the validity of these implications. Presently it is felt that screening and public education can effect a significant reduction in the morbidity and mortality from cardiovascular disorders.

The author acknowledges the assistance of Noel Joyce, RN, MSN; Fred Farley, RN, MSN; and Sandy Griffiths, RN, MSN, in the preparation of this chapter.

Classification of heart disease

Heart diseases may be divided into two general groups: those that are *congenital* and those that are *acquired* after birth. Congenital heart disease follows an abnormality of structure caused by error in embryologic development of the heart. Acquired disease may affect the heart either suddenly or gradually. There may be damage to the heart from bacteria, chemical agents, or diminished blood supply. For example, inflammation may cause scarring of heart valves, muscle, or outer coverings that may impair the heart's function. Any changes in the coronary vessels supplying the heart muscle may decrease its efficiency.

Heart disease may also be classified according to a specific cause such as rheumatic fever, infective endocarditis, or hypertension. It is also classified according to anatomic change such as valvular scarring.

Despite the varied methods of classification, progression of any of these diseases may lead to cardiac failure. Varying degrees of cardiac arrhythmia and cardiac failure are the cause of many of the symptoms commonly associated with the various cardiac diseases, but with early diagnosis and treatment these complications may be prevented or controlled.

Congenital heart defects

Etiology

Congenital heart disease is discussed in detail in maternal-child nursing texts and will be only briefly discussed here. A malformation in heart structure or a *congenital heart defect* occurs during early fetal development. The incidence of congenital heart defects is estimated at approximately seven to nine per 1000 live births. The exact etiology of congenital heart defects is often unknown, but theories center around a combination of genetic and environmental influences. It is known that the more genetic defects present in one child, the greater the chances of a coexisting heart defect. Approximately 50% of children with Down's syndrome have atrial or ventricular septal defects. Prematurity has also been associated with a higher incidence of congenital heart disease in newborns.

Pathophysiology

Heart defects may be classified according to the presence or absence of cyanosis and the degree of pulmonary vascularity. The signs and symptoms of each child may be altered by the degree or severity of the defect and the presence of coexisting defects. The signs and symptoms a child presents are merely a reflection of the hemodynamic alterations of each specific defect. Some types of defects that usually cause cyanosis do not always do so, whereas lesions that usually do not produce cyanosis will do so under certain circumstances.

Acyanotic heart defects. Nine common congenital heart malformations (see box on p. 1101) represent 90% of all anomalies. Acyanotic heart disease (absence of cyanosis) is more common than cyanotic heart disease. In acyanotic heart disease, either no shunting occurs or a *left-to-right* shunt may occur where blood is diverted from the left side of the heart (oxygen enriched) to the right side (oxygen depleted); therefore only bright red oxygen-enriched blood enters the circulation. In *patent ductus arteriosus* (PDA), *atrial septal defect* (ASD), and *ventricular septal defect* (VSD) there is an increased amount of blood flow to the lungs. Children with these defects have a tendency toward frequent respiratory tract infections. PDA, normal during fetal life, is a failure of the duct between the pulmonary artery and the aorta to close at birth (Fig. 45-1, *A*). It is one of the most common congenital heart defects. Specific populations

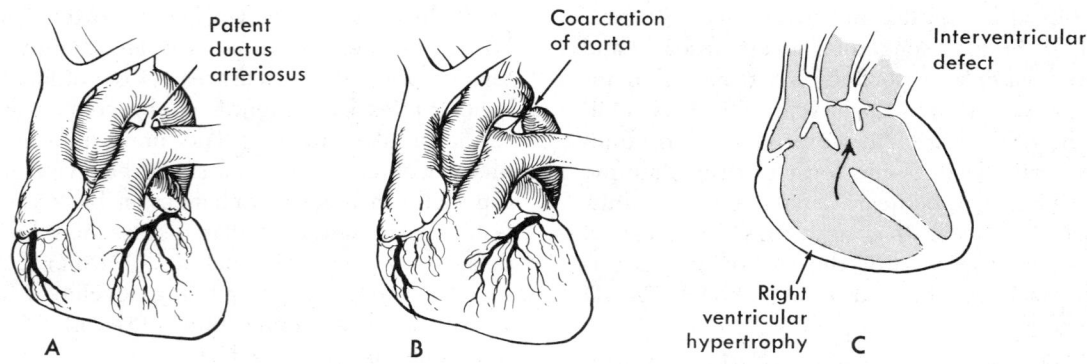

Fig. 45-1. A, Communication between aorta and pulmonary artery found in patients with patent ductus arteriosus. **B,** Abnormality found in coarctation of aorta. Note engorgement above constriction. **C,** Abnormal opening between right and left ventricles that exists when ventricular septal defect is present.

known to be at risk to have a PDA are children who were exposed to rubella in utero, premature infants, as well as infants who were hypoxic at birth. Children who have ASDs or VSDs (Fig. 45-1, *C*) have an opening in their intracardiac septum varying from one small opening to multiple openings to one large communication. Many children who have these types of defects are asymptomatic until their rate of growth exceeds cardiac tolerance. Normal pulmonary vascularity exists in *coarctation of the aorta* (narrowing of the lumen of the aorta; Fig. 45-1, *B*), and *aortic stenosis* (obstruction caused by narrowing or fusing of the valvular cusps). Decreased pulmonary vascularity is associated with *pulmonary stenosis.*

Cyanotic heart defects. The presence of cyanosis in cyanotic heart defects reflects the presence of reduced oxygen in the circulating blood as a result of *right-to-left* intracardiac shunt or a mixing of oxygenated and oxygen-depleted blood. Cyanotic heart defects are typically associated with some degree of clubbing of the fingers, slowed growth, a tendency to develop cerebral abscesses, and polycythemia. In polycythemia the tissue hypoxia related to cyanosis stimulates bone marrow to increase red blood cell production for additional oxygen-carrying ability. An increased reticulocyte count, elevated hemoglobin level, and elevated hematocrit level result. Pulmonary vascularity may be increased in children with *transposition of the great vessels* (the pulmonary artery arises from the left ventricle and the aorta originates from the right ventricle), or in *truncus arteriosus* (a VSD and a single artery supply the systemic and pulmonary circulations). Examples of cyanotic heart defects with decreased pulmonary blood flow are *tetralogy of Fallot* (VSD, overriding aorta, right ventricular hypertrophy, and pulmonary stenosis) and *tricuspid atresia* (absence or severely malformed tricuspid valve).

Clinical picture

Assessment for a child with suspected congenital heart disease begins with an inquiry about family history related to cardiovascular disorders. If relevant, the maternal childbirth history should be investigated including illnesses, complications, use of medications, and exposure to x-ray therapy or rubella. A low birth weight for gestational age, prematurity, need for respiratory assistance or cardiac resuscitation, cyanosis, or a heart murmur may indicate that the child has a congenital heart defect. After birth, signs of congestive heart failure (failure to grow, develop, and gain weight; activity intolerances such as feeding problems) as well as irritability should be evaluated carefully.

On physical examination, cyanosis, respiratory distress, upper respiratory tract infections, bounding or unequal peripheral pulses, and clubbing of the fingers may indicate a heart defect. Heart sounds are not helpful diagnostic data since the presence of a third heart sound may be heard normally in children because of the transmitted vibrations of ventricular filling. Heart murmurs, commonly benign in children (*functional* or *innocent murmurs*), are usually evaluated more closely if associated with other signs of compromised cardiac or circulatory status.

Intervention

The type of medical intervention or surgical treatment depends on the type and severity of the lesion. Children with severe heart defects may exhibit congestive heart failure (p. 1127) and are treated with a cardiac glycoside (usually digoxin) and furosemide (Lasix). Recently, indomethacin, a prostaglandin synthetase inhibitor, has been useful in producing closure of the PDA in premature infants.[64] Selective palliative surgical procedures, such as ligation of the PDA and balloon septostomies, may be done to improve oxygenation temporarily until the child grows. Total correction of the heart defect is postponed until the benefits of surgery outweigh the risks or when the child is between 3 and 5 years of age, before entry into school. Cardiopulmonary bypass is utilized, and deep hypothermia with circulatory arrest may be used with young children. Postoperatively, restoration and maintenance of maximal cardiac circulatory function are the primary goals.

Parents of children with congenital heart defects are encouraged to treat their child as they do their other children. Discipline problems are common, and sibling rivalry is seen frequently because of the attention the child receives from the parents, physicians, and nurses. Guilt feelings are experienced especially if the mother had complications during pregnancy, labor, and delivery; took medications, drugs, or alcohol; or was exposed

CONGENITAL HEART DEFECTS MOST COMMONLY ENCOUNTERED

Acyanotic heart defects

Patent ductus arteriosus

Atrial septal defect

Ventricular septal defect

Coarctation of aorta

Aortic or pulmonary stenosis

Cyanotic heart defects

Transposition of great vessels

Truncus arteriosus

Tetralogy of Fallot

Tricuspid atresia

to x-ray therapy or rubella. Early and regular contact with the health care system is stressed. Antibiotic prophylaxis is recommended before dental and surgical procedures to prevent infective endocarditis (p. 1103).

Inflammatory heart diseases

Pericarditis

Etiology

Pericarditis may occur as a result of bacterial, viral, or fungal infection, or it may occur as a complication of a systemic disease such as rheumatoid arthritis, systemic lupus erythematosus, scleroderma, uremia, or myocardial infarction.

Pathophysiology

Pericarditis is an inflammatory process of the visceral and or parietal pericardium. It can often result in compression of the heart *(cardiac tamponade)* causing a decrease in venous return to the heart and a decrease in ventricular emptying, which may lead to cardiac failure. Pericarditis can develop as a primary condition but is usually a secondary manifestation of disease such as rheumatic fever or tuberculosis, elsewhere in the body.

Pericarditis may be acute or chronic in nature and may spread from or to the myocardium. *Acute pericarditis* is further classified as fibrinous or exudative. The exudate accompanying acute pericarditis may be serous, purulent, or hemorrhagic. When fluid accumulates in the pericardial sac, cardiac tamponade may occur with impairment of ventricular filling and emptying. If not diagnosed and treated promptly, the severe reduction in cardiac output can result in shock and death. Chronic pericarditis is referred to as chronic constrictive or adhesive pericarditis. If the pericardium becomes a constrictive band surrounding the heart, it will prevent adequate filling and emptying of the ventricles, ultimately producing cardiac failure.

Acute pericarditis

Clinical picture. A predominant clinical manifestation of acute pericarditis is a pericardial friction rub along with severe precordial chest pain, which may closely resemble that of acute myocardial infarction. The patient may complain of pain over the left shoulder (left trapezial ridge), which may radiate to the neck and down the left arm; it is intensified when lying supine and is relieved by sitting. The pain may also intensify when the patient coughs, swallows, or breathes deeply.

Typically, the temperature is elevated and a leukocytosis of 10,000 to 20,000 is present. In the exudative form of acute pericarditis, the ECG may show a bradycardia with low-voltage QRS complexes caused by attenuation by the pericardial fluid or an atrial fibrillation or flutter. Occasionally, electrical alternans secondary to the heart changing position as it beats in the pericardium may be evident on the ECG.

Symptoms of cardiac tamponade may include diminished or absent point of maximal impulse (PMI) and peripheral pulses. Distended neck veins secondary to increased central venous pressure, and decreased blood pressure secondary to ineffective pumping action may be noted. A narrowing pulse pressure is a sign of cardiac tamponade. Heart sounds may be diminished and the pulse is paradoxic.

Radiographs may show a pericardial effusion, although an echocardiogram (p. 1057) is more diagnostic. If the accumulation of pericardial fluid is gradual, little pain may be noticed by the patient. As much as 1 L of clear or serosanguineous fluid may accumulate.

Intervention. If the pericardial effusion is small or absent, therapy for pericarditis is supportive with salicylates or indomethacin (Indocin) to decrease inflammation. If the effusion is large, the physician may perform a pericardiocentesis (pericardial tap). Caution is exercised to avoid puncture of the heart wall. Occasionally, after removal of the fluid the physician will instill antibiotics directly into the pericardial sac. A pericardial fenestration (pericardial window) may be performed to provide continuous drainage of pericardial fluid. Complications may include atelectasis and introduction of infectious agents. Corticosteroids may be administered to reduce inflammation.

Chronic pericarditis

Chronic constrictive pericarditis may result from fibrosing of the pericardial sac secondary to trauma or neoplastic disease. The thick fibrous pericardium tightens around the heart and decreases its efficiency as a pump.

Clinical picture. Chronic constrictive pericarditis is three times more prevalent in males. Patients may complain of dyspnea and fatigue and exhibit symptoms of congestive heart failure secondary to the diminished ability of the heart to function as a pump.

Intervention. Removal of the pericardium (pericardiectomy) may be necessary to restore cardiac function. Postoperative care is similar to that of other heart surgery (p. 1088). Other measures to restore more efficient pumping include digitalization, diuretic therapy, and a low-sodium diet.

Myocarditis

Etiology

Myocarditis is an inflammatory disease of the myocardium. Infection, drugs, chemicals, radiation, and metabolic disorders may cause myocarditis. Very often this inflammatory process develops secondary to acute endocarditis or pericarditis. Myocarditis may be classified as acute (benign or fulminant) or chronic.[48]

Infection may result in one of three ways: invasion of the myocardial tissue with organisms, production of toxins (diphtheria), or an autoimmune reaction (rheumatic fever, systemic lupus erythematosus). Worldwide, the most frequent infectious agents are rickettsiae, bacteria, protozoans, and metazoans. In North America viral causes predominate, including Coxsackie virus, echovirus, viral encephalitis, rabies, and herpes simplex.

Clinical picture

Patients may be asymptomatic or have nonspecific complaints of dyspnea on exertion, palpitations, and chest pain over the precordium. Frequently, arrhythmias such as tachycardia or premature beats occur. In some mild cases the diagnosis of myocarditis is made solely on the basis of serial electrocardiogram (ECG) tracings that demonstrate characteristic T wave abnormalities. Chest radiographs may show the heart size normal or enlarged. In the fulminant form of acute myocarditis, pulmonary rales may be auscultated.

Intervention

Persons with myocarditis often are treated with bed rest and digitalis to prevent heart failure and cardiogenic shock. Medical therapy also involves treatment of the underlying disease with antibiotics and steroids as well as management of arrhythmias.

Alcoholic cardiomyopathy

Etiology

When any form of ethanol (the chief substance in alcoholic beverages) is consumed in large quantities over a period greater than 5 years, it has a direct toxic effect on cardiac tissue. Additives in alcoholic beverages may also create their own toxic effects. Persons with alcoholic cardiomyopathy are usually well-nourished individuals; only 15% of these patients have thiamine deficiency as is seen in many alcoholics.

Clinical picture

The onset of alcoholic cardiomyopathy is usually gradual with nonspecific fatigue and dyspnea on exertion. Physical examination may reveal pulmonary rales, cardiac murmur, edema, and increasing blood pressure and central venous pressure (CVP). ECG changes may show low-voltage QRS complexes and ST segment abnormalities. Conduction defects and arrhythmias may also occur. Symptoms progress to congestive heart failure and thromboemboli, but liver enlargement is not usually present.

Electron microscopic studies of heart tissue may show fatty degeneration of myocardial cells and the heart itself may become flabby.[48] Chest radiographs show an enlarged heart with hypertrophic left ventricle and general pulmonary congestion.

Intervention

Nurses have a role in teaching the need for moderation in ethanol intake to prevent the development of alcoholic cardiomyopathy. In the early stages the disease process may be totally reversed by abstinence from alcohol. Medical treatment is primarily symptomatic. Vasodilator therapy may be helpful, and prolonged bed rest is thought by some to reduce the size of the enlarged heart.

Infective endocarditis

Infective endocarditis is an infection of the endocardium and most often of the heart valves. The disease has commonly been classified in the past on the degree of acuteness. *Acute endocarditis* occurs rapidly, often on normal heart valves, and if untreated may cause death within days to weeks. Even with treatment the mortality is high.[4] *Subacute bacterial endocarditis* (SBE) develops more gradually, usually on previously damaged heart valves, and responds well to treatment.

Etiology

The more recent method of classification of infective endocarditis is on the basis of the causative organism. The viridans streptococci are the major causative organisms, especially in the subacute form. Other major infective agents include staphylococci, such as *S. aureus* or *S. epidermidis,* and enterococci. Major causes of underlying cardiac pathologic conditions include rheumatic valvular disease, congenital heart disease, and degenerative heart disease. In some cases, endocarditis is preceded by intrusive procedures such as dental procedures, minor surgery, gynecologic examinations, and insertion of indwelling urinary catheters or renal shunts. Other persons at high risk include those who "mainline" street drugs (inject drugs directly into the veins), because of the possibility of bacteremia from contaminated needles and syringes.

Pathophysiology

The infecting organisms are carried by a turbulent blood flow and deposited on the heart valves or elsewhere on the endocardium. The turbulent blood flow occurs in areas of myocardial anomalies, such as prolapsed mitral valves or ventricular septal defects. A Venturi effect is set up around the anomalies, and the organisms bombard the heart valves, become embedded in the valve matrix, and result in vegetative growths that may scar and perforate the leaflets. One to four percent of persons who have artificial heart valve implants will develop endocarditis.

Further risk results if the vegetative growths break free of the valves, enter the bloodstream and cause emboli. If the vegetative emboli enter organs such as the spleen and kidney, abscesses may form.

Prevention

Prevention of infective endocarditis should include correction of any underlying cardiac defect, if possible, as well as utilization of measures to prevent bacteremia. For persons with underlying cardiac disease, early and vigorous treatment of infections, maintenance of oral hygiene, avoidance of intraarterial or intravenous catheters, and prophylactic use of antibiotics when undergoing dental treatment or a surgical procedure are important.

Clinical picture

The onset of SBE is gradual, and the patient reports malaise and general achiness. Low-grade fever is usually present, although a high fever usually occurs if S. aureus is the causative organism. Physical examination may reveal splenomegaly, clubbing of the fingers, the presence of Osler's nodes on fingers or toe pads, and small capillary hemorrhages (petechiae) in the conjunctiva, mouth, and extremities. On auscultation, murmurs may be audible over the cardiac valves. A normocytic, normochromic anemia is usually present.

Intervention

In infective endocarditis the affected areas have impaired cellular or humoral host defenses; therefore the major aim of therapy is to eliminate all microorganisms from the vegetative growths.[4] Antibiotic intravenous therapy is selected after several blood cultures have been drawn to identify the infecting organism. It is important that antibiotic therapy be continued *for a prolonged time*, even after symptoms abate, in order to eradicate all organisms. Abscesses may require surgical drainage. When necessary, deteriorated heart valves are surgically replaced with prostheses.

Measures are also taken to prevent further infection. Good oral hygiene is imperative, and all intrusive approaches, such as catheterization, are avoided if possible. The patients need to learn the importance of obtaining prophylactic antibiotic therapy before any dental procedures, genitourinary or gastrointestinal procedures, or surgeries are performed.

Rheumatic heart disease

Rheumatic heart disease is an acute inflammatory reaction. It may involve (1) the lining of the heart, or

endocardium, including the valves, resulting in scarring, distortion, and stenosis of the valves; (2) all muscle of the heart, or myocardium, where small areas of necrosis develop and heal, leaving scars (Aschoff bodies); or (3) the outer covering of the heart, or pericardium, where it may cause adhesions to surrounding tissues. The development of symptoms of chronic rheumatic heart disease in later life depends on the location and severity of the damage and other factors. Somewhat less than 10% of persons with rheumatic fever develop rheumatic heart disease, and about one half of those with rheumatic heart disease have mitral stenosis (p. 1105). It is possible for rheumatic fever and rheumatic heart disease with mild symptoms to go undiagnosed, or the disease may be subclinical with no noticeable symptoms. Thus the discovery of rheumatic heart disease is made years later. Careful recall of illness in childhood may include a recollection of "growing pains," confirming the likelihood that the patient had rheumatic fever during childhood. About 20% to 40% of persons who have acute rheumatic heart disease are disabled or have life shortened from this cause.

Children who have rheumatic heart disease are usually advised by the physician to lead a relatively normal, unrestricted life in which only vigorous, competitive athletics are prohibited (p. 1101). The recommendations are specific for the individual person and particular situation, and they vary a great deal. If heart damage has been severe and permanent damage is likely, the nurse should help the child's parents to direct the child's interest toward activities that can become satisfying and rewarding and yet are not strenuous.

Overprotection by parents is sometimes a serious problem. The nurse needs to be understanding and accepting of the parents' fears and concerns and provide sufficient time to allow discussion of them. The parents may also be referred to a medical social worker, if one is available, or work with the physician in seeking psychiatric consultation.

Cardiovascular syphilis

Cardiovascular syphilis usually occurs from 10 to 30 years after the primary syphilitic infection. Since the highest incidence of primary syphilis is among persons in their early 20s, persons with symptoms of cardiovascular syphilis are usually over 30 years of age.

Prevention

It is the aim of health organizations and medical personnel to treat all persons with syphilis before they develop cardiovascular disease or any of the other complications of late syphilis. Primary syphilis can be arrested; however, once syphilis has affected the aorta and the valves of the heart, little can be done except to treat the patient symptomatically.

Pathophysiology and clinical picture

In cardiovascular syphilis the spirochetes attack the aorta, the aortic valve, and the heart muscle. The portion of the aorta nearest the heart is usually affected, and the elastic wall of the aorta becomes weakened and bulges. This bulge is known as an *aneurysm*. As the aneurysm grows it may press on neighboring structures such as the intercostal nerves and cause pain. Aneurysms may also be present without symptoms. Evidence may be discovered on radiographic examination. There is a possibility that the aneurysm may rupture as it increases in size, and the person is encouraged to avoid strenuous activities that might cause a sudden increase in the pressure exerted against the bulging vessel. Surgical resection of the aneurysm sometimes is possible (p. 1139).

Syphilis may also attack the aorta more diffusely, causing *aortitis*. The aorta becomes dilated, and small plaques containing calcium are laid down. There may be complaints of substernal pain associated with exertion caused by constriction at the orifices of the coronary arteries. Thrombi may develop along the aorta, and emboli may occur, resulting in severe complications such as myocardial infarction or cerebral emboli.

Spirochetes may also attack the aortic valve, causing it to become scarred. This causes aortic insufficiency, and the person may have a bounding pulse and a high systolic blood pressure because of the extra effort demanded of the ventricles to pump blood into the systemic circulation. Heart failure eventually occurs.

Intervention

The use of penicillin in the treatment of the patient with cardiovascular syphilis is thought to possibly prolong life, since penicillin destroys any active organisms and permits healing to occur. Treatment at this stage, however, will not restore damaged aortic tissue or damaged aortic valves, and extensive scarring may occur. The person with cardiovascular syphilis should be given guidance in planning activities of daily living and in selecting work that places the least possible burden on the damaged heart and aorta. In certain cases of aortic insufficiency, surgery is possible.

Outcome criteria for the person with inflammatory heart disease

The person or significant others can:
1. Describe the rationale for the degree of rest and activity prescribed and plan activities within the established prescription.
2. Demonstrate ways to carry out activities of daily living (ADL) to conserve energy.

3. Plan a diet to include adequate nutrients and fluids and avoidance of sodium if so prescribed.
4. Describe the medication program:
   a. State name, dosage, frequency, and side effects of prescribed medications (antibiotics, analgesics, digitalis, or steroids).
   b. Describe activities (dental therapy, surgery) that require prophylactic antibiotics.
   c. State plans to follow through on prescribed antibiotic therapy even after symptoms abate.
5. State plans for regular follow-up care.

Valvular heart disease

Pathophysiology

Healthy and competent heart valves facilitate the flow of blood in the correct direction in the heart. The atrioventricular (AV) valves (mitral and tricuspid) prevent blood from flowing back into the atria from the ventricles during systole. During diastole blood flows through the AV openings and thus passively opens the AV valves. During systole, the intense ventricular contractions force the valve flaps back into a closed position. Only the simultaneous contraction of the papillary muscles and the resultant tension on the chordae tendineae prevent the valve flaps from being forced back into the atria (see Fig. 43-1). The semilunar valves (aortic and pulmonary) prevent blood from flowing back into the ventricles from the aorta and the pulmonary artery during diastole.

When the AV or semilunar valves become diseased, they may become *stenosed* and obstruct the normal flow of blood through the heart, or they may become *insufficient* and cause regurgitation or backflow of blood into the heart chamber from which the blood was previously propelled. Initially, the heart can compensate for stenosed or insufficient valves and the strain they exert on the heart through gradual hypertrophy of the myocardium. Often medical treatment can facilitate more effective compensation for the dysfunctional valve for years. If the stenosis or insufficiency worsens, however, congestive failure will eventually ensue and valve replacement is indicated.

Mitral valvular disease

Mitral stenosis

Etiology. Two thirds to three fourths of all persons with mitral stenosis are females. Mitral stenosis, the most common disease of the mitral valve, is predominantly an acquired disease. The occurrence of the congenital "parachute" mitral valve, in which all chordae tendineae insert into one papillary muscle, is rare. Rheumatic fever is most often the cause of mitral stenosis.

Pathophysiology. Rheumatic fever can cause valve thickening by calcification and fibrous tissue formation. The valve leaflets fuse together and become stiffened, resulting in a progressively narrowed and immobile valve. The chordae tendineae also shorten and thicken, and the mitral orifice can diminish in size from its normal 4 sq cm to 6 sq cm to less than 1 sq cm. Progressive stenosis of the mitral aperture causes increasingly elevated left atrial pressure as a result of the additional trapped blood in the left atrium.

Hypertrophy of the left atrium develops as the heart compensates for the increased contractile strength needed to propel the blood through the stenosed valve. The elevated left atrial pressure causes pulmonary hypertension and congestion. This pulmonary congestion impedes right ventricular function and will eventually precipitate right-sided heart failure. The left ventricle receives insufficient end diastolic blood volumes and thus the cardiac output is decreased, causing fatigue and eventual left ventricular atrophy.

To compound further the hemodynamic problems of inadequate left ventricular filling and pulmonary congestion, 50% to 80% of persons with mitral stenosis develop atrial fibrillation. When the atria fibrillate, the normal end diastolic "kick" from a unified atrial contraction is eliminated and again, less blood fills the ventricles for systole. Without an effective atrial contraction, blood may pool and stagnate in the atria, resulting in thrombus formation and arterial embolization to the brain, kidneys, spleen, and extremities.

Clinical picture. The symptoms of mitral stenosis usually develop after a latent period of about 20 years following the initial attack of rheumatic carditis. Symptoms may occur gradually or abruptly. When a person becomes acutely symptomatic, however, a rapid progression of the disease to death occurs usually between 2 to 5 years unless relieved by mitral valve replacement. Emergence of symptoms depends on the size of the orifice (see box below).

Clinical symptoms may include excessive fatigue

EFFECT OF MITRAL ORIFICE SIZE ON EMERGENCE OF SYMPTOMS*

> 2.6 sq cm	No symptoms with exertion
2.1-2.5 sq cm	Symptoms with extreme exertion
1.6-2.0 sq cm	Symptoms with moderate exertion
< 1.5 sq cm	Symptoms with minimal exertion

*From Hurst, J.W., editor: The heart, arteries and veins, ed. 4, New York, 1978, McGraw-Hill Book Co.

---

secondary to diminished cardiac output. Fatigue may be accompanied by shortness of breath, dyspnea on exertion (DOE), dry cough, bronchitis, paroxysmal nocturnal dyspnea, (PND), and orthopnea. As pulmonary hypertension and congestion progress, pulmonary edema, mild to severe hemoptysis, and peripheral and facial cyanosis may occur. Eventual right heart failure can cause hepatomegaly, jugular vein distention, pitting edema, increased venous pressure, and abdominal discomfort.

Diagnosis of mitral stenosis is established by clinical symptoms, a low-pitched, rumbling presystolic murmur and a snapping, loud, first heart sound, ECG changes that may indicate right ventricular hypertrophy, and left atrial enlargement on x-ray film. Mitral stenosis can also be diagnosed with a catheterization of the left side of the heart; however, the most sensitive and noninvasive diagnostic indicator is the echocardiogram.

Intervention

MEDICAL TREATMENT. Treatment of the disease is initially medical. Sodium restriction and oral diuretics can help to alleviate clinical symptoms caused by pulmonary congestion. In more advanced cases, bed rest or the sitting position can diminish pulmonary venous pressure and hemoptysis. Recent-onset atrial fibrillation may be cardioverted (p. 1079) to a sinus rhythm or may revert to a sinus rhythm with quinidine. Persons with atrial fibrillation of more than 1 year are treated with anticoagulant therapy to decrease the chance of thrombus formation and with digoxin to decrease ventricular response rate.

SURGICAL TREATMENT. Surgical treatment for mitral stenosis is usually indicated for persons significantly limited in activity despite appropriate medical treatment. Surgical options include either valvulotomy or replacement.

Mitral valvulotomy, also called *commissurotomy,* is the separation or incision of the stenosed valve leaflets at their borders, or commissures. Controversy exists over the two methods of performing a valvulotomy because of the risks and benefits of each. An *open* mitral commissurotomy is usually done through a sternotomy or a right anterolateral thoracotomy. A cardiopulmonary bypass pump is utilized, and after incision of the left atrium and removal of any atrial thrombi, the valve is inspected. The commissures are then opened with a scalpel under direct vision. Disadvantages of this approach include those associated with open heart surgery, that is, difficult cannulation of the heart-lung pump and clotting problems. The advantages include fewer thrombotic and embolic complications, fewer atrial tears with resultant hemorrhage, and occasionally a more complete valvulotomy.[65] If the valve disease appears to be so advanced that replacement is indicated, the heart is already open.

A *closed* commissurotomy is performed through a left posterolateral thoracotomy. The fifth rib is removed to prepare for a closed or open operation. Some closed commissurotomies are performed in the fourth and fifth interspace with transection of a rib if necessary. After the incision is made, the atrium is palpated to detect any thrombi. If a thrombus is present the procedure is converted to an open procedure to remove the clot. Otherwise, the surgeon inserts a finger through a small incision and digitally examines the atrium for thrombi and the valve for calcium particles. Some surgeons then digitally open the fused commissures. The technique of choice, however, incorporates the use of a transventricular dilator, which is inserted through the tip of the left ventricle and the mitral valve. There it is gradually opened until the stenosis is relieved. Advantages of the closed approach include a shorter operating time, greater simplicity, and less blood replacement. Systemic emboli, atrial wall tears, inadequate alleviation of the stenosis, and mitral regurgitation are all risks of this method of commissurotomy.[65]

Mitral valve replacement is considered when the valve is so stenosed and calcified that a valvulotomy would not achieve long-term relief of obstruction. The incision can be any of the three previously discussed; however, most frequently the heart is approached via a midline sternotomy. The extracorporeal bypass pump is used in an open procedure. The diseased valve leaflets are excised at the annulus, and the loose chordae are excised to avoid their becoming tangled in the new valve. The mortality with mitral valve replacement is roughly 5% to 10%, and the overall 5-year survival rate is approximately 70%. Types of valves are discussed later in this chapter (p. 1110).

Mitral regurgitation

Etiology. Rheumatic heart disease is the predominant etiologic factor in mitral regurgitation and, similar to mitral stenosis, persons with mitral regurgitation secondary to rheumatic heart disease are more commonly women than men.

Although rheumatic heart disease is the primary cause of mitral regurgitation, unlike mitral stenosis, there are many other factors, acquired and congenital, that contribute to its etiology. When these factors are considered, the incidence of mitral regurgitation is greater in men. Weakness, rupture, or fibrosis of a papillary muscle secondary to ischemic heart disease, ventricular aneurysm, or myocardial infarction can cause mitral regurgitation. Papillary muscle dysfunction allows the valve leaflets to flop in the direction of the atrium during systole and blood then flows backward. Mitral regurgitation can occur as a consequence of a congenital anomaly. A person with idiopathic hypertrophic subaortic stenosis (IHSS) can develop mitral regurgitation as a result of displacement of the anterior leaflet of the mitral valve during systole. Bacterial endocarditis is also a cause of mitral regurgitation. Abnormally long chordae tendineae can cause the floppy valve syndrome with prolapse of the valve into the atrium.

Pathophysiology. In chronic mitral insufficiency and regurgitation, a variable amount of blood from the left ventricle is shunted back through the mitral orifice to the left atrium. This causes a rise in left atrial pressure. The extra blood is returned to the ventricle during diastole, thus increasing ventricular preload (p. 1037). In response to increasing preload and increasing left atrial pressure, both the atrial myocardium and the ventricular myocardium gradually hypertrophy to compensate for the additional work load. Eventually, ventricular functioning is compromised and cardiac output falls. Concurrently, the left atrium is often fibrillating, diminishing cardiac output still more.

Clinical picture. In persons with chronic mitral regurgitation, fatigue and weakness are predominant complaints. Right-sided heart failure with its sequelae of hepatic congestion, edema, and distended neck veins may finally occur.

In acute mitral regurgitation, progressive dyspnea on exertion and frequent pulmonary edema are the primary symptoms. This different presentation of symptoms is caused by the high-pressure backflow of blood from a normal ventricle to a small left atrium. The pressure is transmitted immediately to the pulmonary veins, causing the congestive symptoms. Because the ventricle has not yet hypertrophied, cardiac output remains sufficient and fatigue is usually not a problem.

Although persons with mitral regurgitation commonly have atrial fibrillation, thrombus formation in the atria is less common than with mitral stenosis because of backflow and resultant turbulence of blood.

Diagnosis of mitral regurgitation is made by the presence of clinical symptoms and auscultation of a blowing, high-pitched systolic murmur and a third heart sound. A chest x-ray film may reveal left atrial enlargement and occasional left ventricular dilatation. The echocardiogram may identify mitral valve cusp prolapse and ruptured chordae but is not helpful in identifying the severity of the regurgitation. Definitive diagnosis is made by cardiac catheterization and left ventricular angiography in which the immediate appearance of dye in the left atrium designates a positive diagnosis.

Intervention

MEDICAL TREATMENT. Initial treatment of mitral regurgitation is again medical and similar to that of mitral stenosis. Restriction of physical activities producing fatigue and dyspnea, decreasing sodium intake, and the use of diuretics are common. Anticoagulant therapy is not usually necessary until end stages of the disease because of the turbulence of the blood in the left atrium. Because the left ventricle is more burdened in mitral insufficiency than in mitral stenosis, digitalis glycosides are important in augmenting the output of the left ventricle.

SURGICAL TREATMENT. As with mitral stenosis, when physical limitations become significant despite appropriate medical intervention, surgical intervention is implemented. The surgical treatments for mitral regurgitation are all open heart procedures. *Valve replacements* are the most common choice of treatment, and the technique, indications, and circumstances involved in replacing the mitral valve are identical to those discussed in mitral stenosis. Operative mortality ranges from 5% to 10%.

Valvuloplasty (repair) is also an indicated treatment for mitral regurgitation, especially for solitary cusp perforations seen with bacterial endocarditis and for simple mitral valve clefts. In this procedure, direct suture repair of torn leaflets or clefts is done. In patients for whom such simple repair is needed, valvuloplasty has recently been recommended as the treatment of choice over replacement.[1] Life expectancy with valvuloplasty is the same as with replacement although the reoperation rate is slightly higher. The big advantage of valvuloplasty, however, is its 0.4% thromboembolic rate per year without anticoagulation vs. a 3% to 6% rate per year with anticoagulation of xenografts and prosthetic valves.[1]

Annuloplasty (repair of the annulus) is done for a small number of patients with an enlarged valvular annulus and intact leaflets. This surgical procedure involves tightening the annulus with sutures and Teflon felt.

Aortic valvular disease

Aortic stenosis

Etiology. Aortic valvular disease is less common than mitral disease and occurs in about 25% of all persons with chronic valvular heart disease. Eighty percent of adults with aortic stenosis are men.

Aortic stenosis can be rheumatic in origin since myocarditis invades the valve, causing edema, inflammation, formation of granulation tissue, scarring, and finally, fusion of the leaflets. Rheumatic aortic stenosis is almost always concomitant with rheumatic disease of the mitral valve. Atherosclerosis in elderly persons also causes aortic stenosis and is also called idiopathic calcific aortic stenosis.

Congenital valvular disease or malformation is the predominant etiologic factor in aortic stenosis. A congenitally deformed valve may remain asymptomatic for several years; however, it is more susceptible to bacterial endocarditis, rheumatic fever, and calcification.

Pathophysiology. When the aortic valve becomes stenosed, thus obstructing left ventricular outflow during systole, left ventricular hypertrophy develops as a compensatory mechanism to continue pumping the same blood volume through the narrowed opening. As the stenosis progresses, cardiac output decreases. The left atrium cannot empty adequately, and thus the pulmonary system becomes congested. The hypertrophied left ventricle elevates myocardial oxygen needs and at the same time compresses the coronary arteries at a pressure exceeding coronary perfusion pressure. Thus myocardial oxygen needs increase and the supply decreases. This phenomenon gives rise to the myocardial ischemia and angina that are characteristic of more severe aortic stenosis. Eventually, right-sided heart failure will ensue.

Aortic stenosis rarely becomes significantly debilitating until the aortic orifice is about one third its normal size. Symptoms occur late in the disease even with severe stenosis because the hypertrophied left ventricle is able to generate pressures strong enough to maintain an adequate cardiac output and because the mitral valve prevents the high intraventricular pressures from affecting the atrium and pulmonary vasculature. When the mitral valve is also diseased, the onset of symptoms may be more rapid and may be compounded.

Clinical picture. Gradually increasing obstruction without clinical symptoms usually occurs until 40 to 50 years of age in most persons. There are three characteristic symptoms of aortic stenosis: exertional dyspnea, angina pectoris, and exertional syncope. Exertional dyspnea is secondary to diminished cardiac reserve and elevation of the pulmonary capillary pressures. Angina pectoris (p. 1115) is secondary to diminished coronary perfusion and increased myocardial oxygen needs. Exertional syncope is caused by a decline in arterial pressure secondary to vasodilatation in exercising muscles and a fixed cardiac output.

Other symptoms that also only occur in the late stages of the disease include fatigue, weakness, orthopnea, paroxysmal nocturnal dyspnea, and pulmonary edema. Symptoms of right-sided heart failure (i.e., hepatomegaly, atrial fibrillation, systemic venous hypertension) are usually end-stage symptoms.

Aortic stenosis is diagnosed by a harsh, rough, midsystolic murmur and a systolic thrill over the aortic area, by clinical symptoms, and by cardiac catheterization and angiography.

Intervention. Treatment of aortic stenosis is initially medical. Avoidance of strenuous activity is advocated as is the use of digitalis glycosides, a sodium restriction, and diuretics for the treatment of congestive heart failure. Nitroglycerin is used to treat angina.

As symptoms increase in severity, surgical treatment consisting of valve replacement is the treatment of choice and symptomatic improvement occurs. The 8-year survival rate following surgery is roughly 65%.

Valve replacement of the aortic valve is similar in technique to mitral valve replacement.

Aortic regurgitation

Etiology. Aortic regurgitation occurs less frequently than stenosis, and about 75% of those persons with aortic regurgitation are male. Etiologic factors may be congenital or acquired. The disease is rheumatic in origin in 80% of the cases. Rheumatic disease thickens, deforms, and contracts the valve leaflets. Dilation of the annulus may also occur to produce insufficiency. In persons with isolated aortic regurgitation (i.e., without associated mitral disease) rheumatic heart disease does not play such a prominent causal role.

Syphilis is a rarely seen cause of dilation of the annulus and widening of the commissures. Less than 5% of the cases of aortic insufficiency in the United States are related to syphilis. Bacterial endocarditis can cause bacterial vegetation on valve leaflets, which initiates the inflammatory response and can cause erosion of the valve.

Marfan's syndrome is another etiologic factor related to aortic regurgitation. As a generalized, systemic disease of connective tissue, it can cause necrosis of the aorta, dilation of the aortic ring, and aneurysm formation, thus causing insufficiency. Another cause is congenital malformation, which, as with aortic stenosis, renders the aortic valve more susceptible to endocarditis and rheumatic fever and can thus cause aortic insuffiency.

Pathophysiology. When the aortic valve is deformed congenitally or by infectious processes, the leaflets may not close properly and the annulus may be dilated, loose, or deformed. This allows a regurgitation of blood from the aorta back into the left ventricle during diastole. The ventricle dilates and hypertrophies with this greater volume of blood and thus compensates with a more forceful and rapid ejection.

Studies have indicated that greater than 50% of the left ventricular ejection volume must reflux into the left ventricle before a person becomes symptomatic. Because of this cardiac compensation, symptoms in uncomplicated aortic insufficiency are rare until left ventricular failure is imminent.

Clinical picture. Symptoms usually begin with an awareness of the heartbeat, which is uncomfortable and more prominent in a lying position. Sinus tachycardia may occur with exertion or stimulation, and premature ventricular beats occur. Exertional dyspnea secondary to cardiac decompensation, orthopnea, paroxysmal nocturnal dyspnea, and diaphoresis always indicates impending left heart failure. Angina may develop at rest or with exertion secondary to myocardial ischemia or pounding on the chest wall by the heart. End-stage disease is indicated by hepatomegaly, ankle edema, and ascites.

Diagnosis is determined from clinical findings of a soft, blowing aortic diastolic murmur; a widened pulse pressure; an ECG indicative of left ventricular hypertrophy with ST depressions and T wave inversions; angiocardiograms; and echocardiograms.

Intervention. As with other valve diseases, medical therapy is utilized initially with treatment to reduce congestion secondary to increasing left ventricular workload. Digitalis, a sodium-restricted diet, and diuretics are often used. Nitroglycerin, not as effective as with aortic stenosis, is still worth a try in decreasing anginal pain.

Valve replacement is usually necessary; however, surgical treatment does not always restore normal ventricular function. Valvuloplasty is rarely a viable alternative when just one valve leaflet has been torn or perforated.

Tricuspid valvular disease

Tricuspid stenosis

Etiology. Tricuspid stenosis is a more uncommon valvular disease that occurs four to five times more frequently in women than in men. This lesion is rarely isolated and usually occurs with mitral stenosis or aortic stenosis but usually not with mitral regurgitation. Rheumatic heart disease is the usual cause of tricuspid stenosis.

Pathophysiology. The fusion of the commissures and shortened and fused chordae tendineae cause the tricuspid orifice to narrow. Blood is blocked returning to the heart. The systemic pressure is increased as a result of the obstruction, and there is a reduced right ventricular output.

Clinical picture. Symptoms of right heart failure in the patient with tricuspid stenosis include hepatomegaly and jugular vein distention, as well as cardiac cirrhosis and resulting jaundice. The decrease in blood volume returned to the heart decreases cardiac output and causes fatigue, weight loss, and hypotension.

Diagnosis is made by presenting clinical symptoms, especially those of right heart failure. A chest x-ray film is a major diagnostic tool and should reveal an enlarged right atrium. Cardiac catheterization confirms the diagnosis.

Intervention. Medical treatment includes digitalis, a low-sodium diet, and diuretics. Surgical treatment may include valvuloplasty or replacement of the valve. This is usually performed simultaneously with valve repair or replacement of the mitral or aortic valve when valvular diseases occur concomitantly.

Tricuspid regurgitation

Tricuspid regurgitation is uncommon because normal valve leaflets are very small and valve closure is primarily reliant on the contraction of the valvular ring. Consequently, insufficiency caused by rheumatic, carcinoid, or bacterial destruction of the leaflets is rare. Right ventricular dilation from any cause may dilate the tricuspid ring or displace the papillary muscles and cause regurgitation. An insufficient tricuspid valve allows blood to flow back into the right atrium, causing venous engorgement and diminishing right ventricular output.

Symptoms are the same as with tricuspid stenosis. A blowing, holosystolic murmur is heard on auscultation. Atrial fibrillation often occurs. Medical and surgical treatment coincides with that of tricuspid stenosis.

Pulmonic valve disease

Lesions of the pulmonic valve are extremely rare since this valve is generally not affected by rheumatic fever and endocarditis.

Surgical treatment of valvular disease

Variables affecting the results of valve replacement are many. The patient's general clinical condition and level of myocardial functioning before surgery directly affect the prognosis. Pulmonary artery hypertension

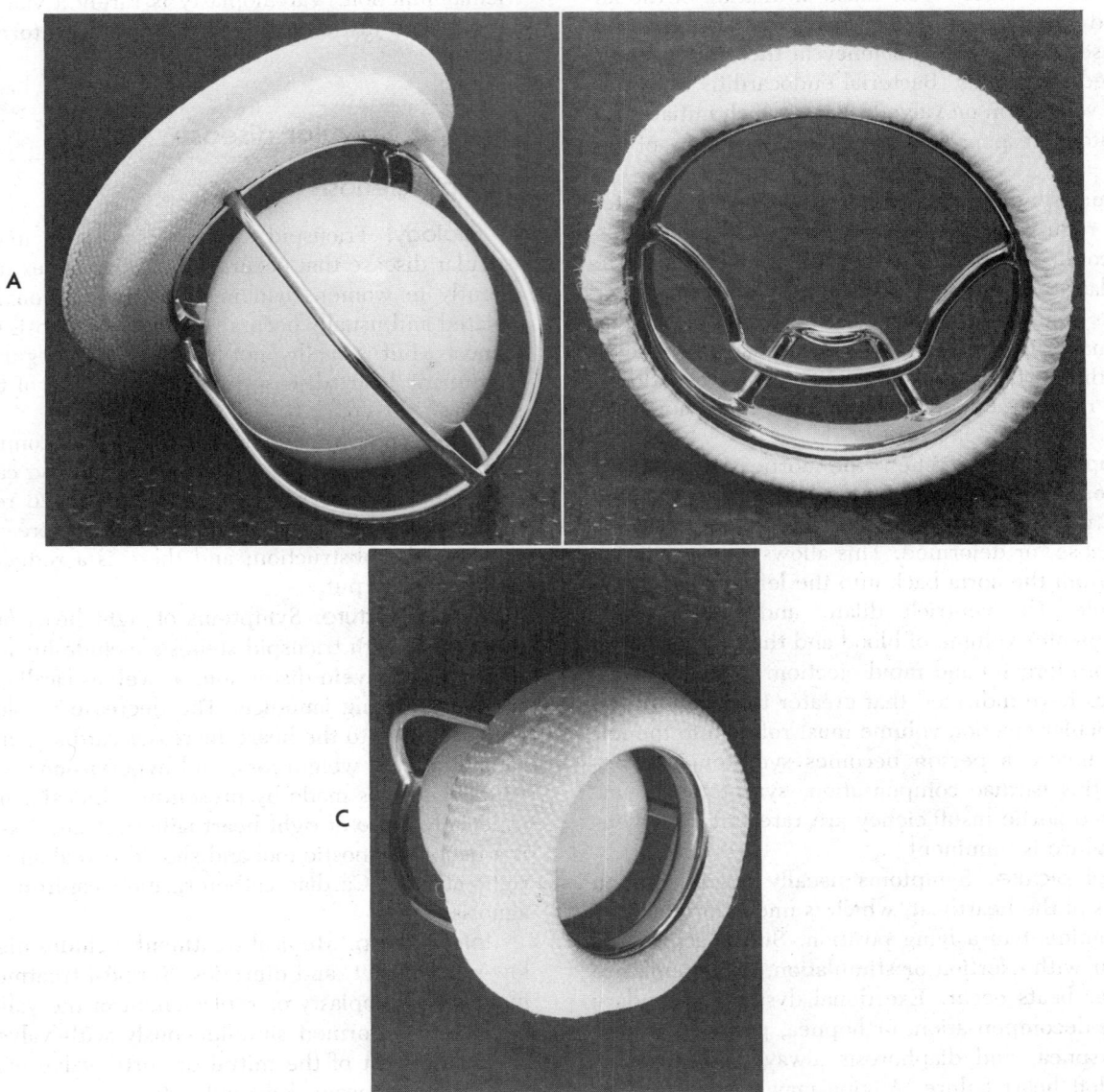

Fig. 45-2. A, Starr-Edwards mitral valve prosthesis, "ball-in-cage" mechanical valve. **B,** Bjork/Shiley mitral valve prosthesis, "tilting disk" mechanical valve. In this photo, the disk has been omitted to show metal supports that hold disk in place. **C,** Starr-Edwards aortic valve prosthesis, "ball-in-cage" valve.

greatly complicates valvular replacement. The valve used for replacement must be durable and have minimal side effects. There are a wide variety of artificial valves available.

Caged-ball prosthetic valves consist of a metal cage with a synthetic, freely moving ball inside (Fig. 45-2, *A* and *C*). The ring and struts of the cage are covered by a synthetic cloth. The cloth-covered ring is sutured carefully into the existing valve annulus. Within months, tissue covers the cloth and the incidence of a thromboembolism decreases. Starr-Edwards, Smeloff-Cutter, and Braunwald-Cutter valves are all caged-ball valves and come in varying sizes and slightly varying designs and materials.

Low-profile, caged-disk prosthetic valves occupy less space in the ventricles than other valves and require less force to move the occluding disk (Fig. 45-2, *B*). Examples of this type of valve include the Beall, Cooley-Cutter, and the Bjork-Shiley valves.

Eccentric monocusp prosthetic valves have occluders that tilt or pivot within a ring rather than balls or disks that pop back and forth. Disadvantages of this valve include the development of areas under the pivoting points where thrombi can form as a result of the stasis of blood. The advantage of this type of valve is in the nearly central blood flow through its orifice.

Stented allografts are human heart valves that are supported or "stented" by an underlying frame. The advantages of allografts include relatively normal hemodynamic characteristics with central flow, a low incidence of hemolysis, and no thromboembolic complications. Allografts are difficult to procure in quantity, however, and have had a high incidence of regurgitation.

Xenografts, or valves composed of other species

valves, are more easily available and can be obtained in all sizes. Porcine grafts (Fig. 45-3) are most frequently used. These grafts have a low rate of related thromboemboli, and graft failure has not been a problem. Their hemodynamic performance has been closely similar to human heart valves. Porcine valves are now used less often in young persons because of a higher incidence of calcification over a long time period.

Outcome criteria for the person with valvular heart disease

The person or significant others can:
1. Explain required dietary changes including any sodium restrictions.
2. State name, purpose, dosage, frequency, and side effects of any medication therapy (digitalis, diuretics).
3. Describe a work, rest, and activity program to conserve energy.
4. Describe the rationale for and the type of surgery to be performed, if surgery is indicated.
5. State plans for medical follow-up including ongoing laboratory tests, if required.

Coronary artery disease: coronary atherosclerotic heart disease

Definitions

The term *coronary artery disease* (CAD) is a generic designation for many different conditions involving the coronary arteries. Some texts still refer to coronary artery disease as coronary heart disease (CHD) and/or ischemic heart disease (IHD); however, these terms are not specific and are gradually being abandoned. Coronary atherosclerotic heart disease (CAHD) is the most common type of coronary artery disease and will be presented in this text. For a discussion of the more unusual nonatherosclerotic forms of coronary artery disease, the reader is referred to specialized texts.

Epidemiology

Coronary atherosclerosis is recognized as the leading cause of death in the industrialized Western world. In the United States, CAHD (angina, sudden death, myocardial infarction) has reached epidemic proportions. Each year approximately one-half million Americans die from the disease and another 2.5 million are

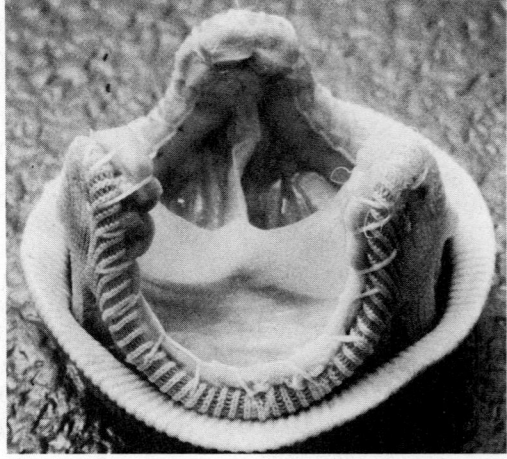

Fig. 45-3. Porcine aortic valve prosthesis; a natural-tissue valve. Note that valve leaflets are sutured to Dacron-covered fabric frame. Outer ring is sutured into heart.

disabled by it. The annual economic cost is overwhelming, averaging tens of billions of dollars.

The increased incidence of CAHD over the last 60 years has been causally linked to affluence and prosperity. There are many factors involved in this increase, however, such as increased longevity and improved recognition of the disease.

Epidemiologic studies have shown that the incidence of coronary atherosclerosis is much higher in men than in women of childbearing age, in older individuals, and in the affluent. Nutrition has become a key factor in epidemiologic studies, forming the link between affluence and an increased rate of coronary atherosclerosis. In countries such as the United States and Finland, where diets are high in calories, total fat, cholesterol, and refined carbohydrates, the incidence of coronary atherosclerosis is extremely high, whereas in a country such as Japan, where the diet is low in calories, total fat, and cholesterol, coronary atherosclerosis is infrequent or rare.

Risk factors: general considerations

Although a tremendous amount of research (both epidemiologic and experimental) is being conducted in order to learn the etiology of CAHD, the exact cause remains unknown. Certain characteristics, however, have been singled out as being common in persons who have or are at risk of developing coronary atherosclerosis (see box at right). These common characteristics or risk factors have evolved from many different types of research studies and therefore require special interpretation.

Although risk factors help to screen individuals who are at high risk for developing CAHD, the presence of a risk factor does not definitively indicate the presence or severity of coronary atherosclerosis. Conversely, the absence of risk factors for CAHD does not mean that an individual will necessarily be free from coronary atherosclerosis. At the present time there is strong evidence supporting a prudent approach to the prevention of coronary atherosclerosis. It is felt that primary prevention is both helpful and feasible.[9] Prevention requires indentification of risk factors and efforts to correct or alter those risk factors that can be modified.

Nonmodifiable risk factors

Age and sex. Clinical evidence of coronary atherosclerosis may occur in the second and third decades of life. Although women seem somewhat immune until after menopause, the disease is already a major cause of death for men aged 35 to 44 years. The mortality in CAHD rapidly increases with age, so that by age 55 to 64, 40% of all deaths among men are caused by this single disease.[44] Although there seems to be a strong and constant relationship between age and the onset of CAHD, this may simply reflect prolonged exposure to other atherogenic factors.

RISK FACTORS FOR DEVELOPING CORONARY ATHEROSCLEROTIC HEART DISEASE

Nonmodifiable risk factors

1. Age
2. Sex
3. Race
4. Family history

Modifiable risk factors

1. Major risk factors
   a. Elevated serum lipid levels (hyperlipoproteinemia)
   b. Habitual diet high in calories, total fats, cholesterol, refined carbohydrates, sodium
   c. Hypertension
   d. Obesity
   e. Glucose intolerance
   f. Cigarette smoking
2. Minor risk factors
   a. Personality type
   b. Sedentary living
   c. Psychologic stress
   d. Oral contraceptive use

Race. Before 1968, nonwhites tended to have lower mortality rates from CAHD than whites. Since that time, however, nonwhites have a higher mortality up to the age of 65. Nonwhite women also tend to have higher mortality rates than white women.

Family history. A family history of CAHD occurring in parents or siblings (before the age of 50) increases the risk of developing premature atherosclerosis. This familial disposition is thought to be related to both genetic and environmental factors. It is not clear to what extent genetic elements act in combination with environmental factors such as nutrition, socioeconomic status, and other risk factors. In addition, other mechanisms of genetic transmission are not yet known.[44]

Major modifiable risk factors

Hyperlipoproteinemia. Strong evidence indicates that an elevated cholesterol, triglyceride, or phospholipid level is a major risk factor in the development of atherosclerosis. These plasma lipids are bound to specific proteins, hence the term *lipoproteinemia*. If only one component is elevated, it is referred to as *hyperlipidemia*.

The five basic groups of lipoproteins include the chylomicrons, very low–density lipoproteins (VLDL), low-density lipoproteins (LDL), intermediate-density lipoproteins (IDL), and high-density lipoproteins (HDL) (see Chapter 43). These lipoprotein complexes transport the plasma lipids including triglycerides and cholesterol.

Cholesterol and LDL, or beta (β-) lipoproteins, have been found to have a higher associative and predictive value for CAHD than triglycerides.[44] Cholesterol in the body comes from two sources: it can be taken into the body directly in food or it can be manufactured by the liver and intestine. Approximately 0.8 g of cholesterol is manufactured by the liver each day. Cholesterol is involved in lipid transport and excreted with bile salts into the intestine to participate in the digestion and absorption of fats. The complex process by which cholesterol is manufactured, distributed, and eliminated is not not very well understood, although it is widely believed that the inherited endocrine system plays a definite part because of its effect on the metabolic processes. Studies have shown that when a large amount of saturated fat is eaten, the cholesterol level in the blood tends to rise. When the saturated fats are replaced by polyunsaturated fats, the blood cholesterol level tends to fall.

Individuals with serum cholesterol levels greater than 300 mg/100 ml have been found to have four times more risk of CAHD than those individuals with levels less than 200 mg/100 ml.[44] It would therefore appear prudent to take measures to decrease or maintain serum cholesterol levels below 200 mg/100 ml. The upper limit of normal for serum cholesterol is 220 to 240 mg/100 ml.

LDL, or β-lipoprotein, is most directly associated with CAHD. As a molecule LDL is approximately 50% cholesterol by weight. Other lipoproteins contain cholesterol, but it is in lesser amounts.

Recently, investigations have indicated a tremendous difference between HDL and LDL as predisposing factors to heart disease. Unlike LDL, HDL are inversely related to CAHD risk. In fact, HDL may serve to remove cholesterol from tissues.

The hyperlipoproteinemias have been classified on the basis of clinical and laboratory data into five types with recommendations for therapy (Table 45-1). The conditions may be primary (familial) or secondary to some other condition or process. The goal of therapy for the majority of patients is reduction of the rate of development of atherosclerosis. Many physicians are urging that blood lipid testing be done periodically and that preventive therapy begin early in childhood.

Dietary patterns. The contemporary American diet, rich in total calories, total and saturated fats, cholesterols, refined sugars, and salt, is a significant coronary risk factor. The national dietary average for fat consumption is still very high in the United States, with approximately 50% of our dietary calories being derived from fats. Studies indicate that populations that con-

TABLE 45-1. Types of hyperlipoproteinemias

Type	Abnormality	Clinical features of elevated levels
I	↑ Chylomicrons	Eruptive xanthoma, pancreatitis, organomegaly
IIa	↑ LDL	Premature atherosclerosis, corneal arcus, tendinous and tuberous xanthomas
IIb	↑ LDL and VLDL	
III	↑ IDL	Glucose intolerance, hyperuricemia, premature atherosclerosis
IV	↑ VLDL	Glucose intolerance, hyperuricemia
V	↑ VLDL and chylomicrons	Hepatosplenomegaly, eruptive xanthoma, glucose intolerance

sume low-fat diets generally have been found to have lower serum cholesterol levels than those consuming high-fat diets. In addition, populations consuming diets reduced in calories, total fats, saturated fats, and cholesterol not only have a lower cholesterol level but also have a lower incidence of and mortality from preventive CAHD.

The American Heart Association has endorsed a policy recommending some modification in diet for everyone: reducing the fat content of the diet, substituting polyunsaturated fat for saturated fat, and maintaining body weight at normal levels. Some sources of polyunsaturated fat are corn, cottonseed, soy, and safflower oils, and margarines incorporating these oils in liquid form. Oils that have been hydrogenated contain more saturated fat, as do coconut oil, butterfat, and animal fats.

Hypertension. Elevated blood pressure, either systolic or diastolic, is a significant risk factor in association with coronary atherosclerosis. However, many studies suggest that hypertension seems to accelerate atherosclerosis only in the presence of hyperlipidemia.[44]

Obesity. Although obesity has been frequently cited as a significant coronary risk factor, its independent effect in predisposing an individual to CAHD is controversial. Obese individuals are more prone to diabetes, hypertension, glucose intolerance, and hyperlipidemias. These associated factors may in fact be the link between obesity and CAHD.

Carbohydrate intolerance. Individuals with diabetes mellitus have been found to have a greater prevalence and severity of coronary atherosclerosis. However, it is difficult to isolate diabetes mellitus as a single factor since it is well established that hypertension, obesity, and hyperlipidemia are also frequent in individuals with impaired carbohydrate tolerance.[44]

Cigarette smoking. In general, the risk of death from CAHD is two to six times higher in smokers than nonsmokers, and the risk is proportional to the number of cigarettes smoked per day.[44] Fortunately, individuals who stop smoking have a lesser risk of developing CAHD than those who continue to smoke.[10] Pipe and cigar smokers have been found to have only a slightly increased risk of cardiovascular death and morbidity.

The relationship between cigarette smoking and CAHD is not totally clear, but it has been suggested that the adverse effects of cigarette smoking on the heart and blood vessels involve the effects of nicotine and carbon monoxide. Specific changes include increased myocardial oxygen demand induced by nicotine, interference with oxygen supply by carboxyhemoglobin, and adhesion of platelets. In addition, cigarette smoking has itself been associated with decreased levels of HDL as compared with levels for nonsmokers and exsmokers.[10]

Minor modifiable risk factors

At present it appears that a sedentary life-style, a particular personality type, and psychologic stress or tension are contributing factors in the development of heart disease. In the late 1950s Friedman and Rosenman described a behavior pattern they called the Type A personality. They described the Type A (coronary prone) individual as intensely competitive, aggressive, and ambitious. There is controversy over whether stress is actually atherogenic or simply precipitates the attack. However, each of the three factors may enhance proneness to premature CAHD.[44]

Pathophysiology

The exact cause of atherosclerosis (p. 1154) is still unknown. Coronary atherosclerosis involves the localized accumulation of lipid and fibrous tissue within the coronary arteries, resulting in arterial narrowing and possibly occlusion. As the atherosclerosis progresses, the narrowing of the lumen is accompanied by vascular changes that affect the functional ability of the coronary arteries to dilate. The result of this atherosclerotic process is a variable reduction of blood flow to the myocardium.

Manifestations of coronary atherosclerosis are the result of an imbalance between myocardial oxygen supply and myocardial oxygen demand. These manifestations, such as angina or coronary insufficiency, generally do not appear until the atherosclerotic process is well advanced. Despite alterations in vessel architecture and function, often greater than 75% of the coronary vessel is occluded before myocardial ischemia or dysfunction is produced. Coronary ischemia implies a relative deficit in myocardial oxygen to supply the normal aerobic metabolism of a functioning myocardium. The balance between myocardial oxygen supply and demand may be altered by a number of factors, as illustrated in Fig. 45-4.

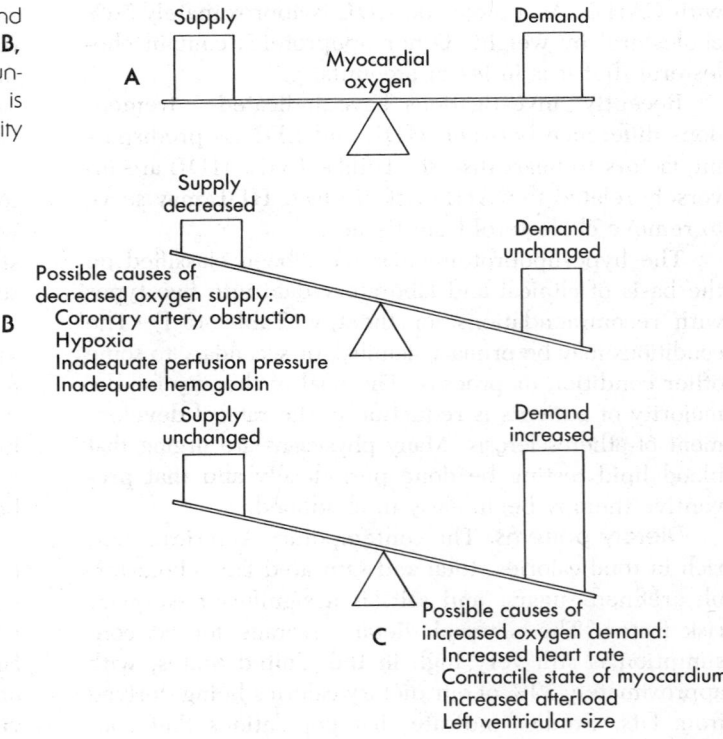

Fig. 45-4. Balance between myocardial oxygen supply and myocardial oxygen demand (mVO$_2$). **A,** Normal balance. **B,** Imbalance: supply is decreased while demand remains unchanged. **C,** Imbalance: supply unchanged but demand is increased. Atherosclerotic coronary vessels are limited in ability to increase oxygen supply.

Supply   Demand

A   Myocardial oxygen

Supply decreased

Demand unchanged

Possible causes of decreased oxygen supply:
Coronary artery obstruction
Hypoxia
Inadequate perfusion pressure
Inadequate hemoglobin

B

Supply unchanged

Demand increased

C   Possible causes of increased oxygen demand:
Increased heart rate
Contractile state of myocardium
Increased afterload
Left ventricular size

Atherosclerotic lesions usually occur near the origin and bifurcation of the main coronary vessels in the epicardial segment of the coronary artery. These lesions tend to be localized and focal; however, in advanced coronary atherosclerosis diffuse involvement of the coronary arteries can be seen.

The primary significance, therefore, of coronary atherosclerosis, is that the lesion, either alone or in conjunction with coronary occlusion, causes *myocardial ischemia*.[44] Myocardial ischemia is then responsible for producing the clinical manifestations of CAHD: (1) *angina pectoris,* (2) *acute myocardial infarction,* and (3) *sudden cardiac death*.

Angina pectoris

Etiology

Angina pectoris occurs when myocardial oxygen demand exceeds myocardial oxygen supply. Although it is usually caused by atherosclerosis of the coronary vessels, the incidence of angina pectoris is high in persons with hypertension, diabetes mellitus, thomboangiitis obliterans, polycythemia vera, periarteritis nodosa, and aortic regurgitation caused by syphilis or rheumatic heart disease.

Clinical picture

Angina pectoris is characterized by paroxysmal retrosternal or substernal pain, often radiating down the inner aspect of the left arm. The left submammary region is seldom involved. The patient frequently describes the pain as a heaviness or tightness of the chest, and at times it may be interpreted by the patient as indigestion. The pain is usually diffuse and can rarely be pinpointed at a specific site. The patient may be observed gripping the sternum with one or both hands. The pain is often associated with exertion and is relieved by rest or vasodilation by means of medication. It is believed to be caused by a *temporary* inadequacy of the blood supply in meeting the needs of the heart muscle. The location and severity of the pain vary greatly, but the same pattern recurs repeatedly in a given individual. The frequency and severity of the attacks usually increase over a period of years, and less and less exertion may cause pain. No matter how mild the attacks, they may be complicated at any time by acute myocardial infarction, cardiac standstill, or death.

Intervention

Medical therapy is aimed at reducing myocardial oxygen demand. The precipitating factors that bring on an attack of angina should be identified and avoided if possible. Risk factors that may aggravate the person's condition (e.g., hypertension, obesity) should also be corrected, if possible.

Often an exercise program is indicated as an integral component of the medical treatment for angina pectoris. Exercise training can help the heart as well as the body become trained. A trained individual experiences less of a rise in blood pressure and pulse rate on exertion. The result is a decrease in myocardial oxygen demand and an increase in the amount of exercise or work an individual can do before an imbalance occurs between myocardial oxygen supply and demand.

Medication. Nitroglycerin is presently still the drug of choice for the treatment of acute ischemic attacks. A nitroglycerin tablet placed sublingually and allowed to dissolve in the saliva will often relieve the pain of angina within 1 to 2 minutes. The nitrates dilate coronary arteries and intercoronary collateral vessels. However, their main effect is vasodilation of the peripheral vessels, especially the veins. Nitrates decrease peripheral resistance, decrease systolic blood pressure, produce venous pooling, and decrease preload (p. 1037). A reduction in preload decreases ventricular size, pressure, wall tension, heart work, and myocardial oxygen demand, thereby balancing the scale between supply and demand.

The usual dose of nitroglycerin is 0.3 to 0.4 mg ($\frac{1}{150}$ grain). If the medication has not been effective in 5 minutes, it should be repeated two or three times at 5-minute intervals. If the pain does not subside after three times, the patient should be instructed to call the physician or go to the nearest emergency department. Individuals who experience anginal pain should always carry nitroglycerin tablets with them and family members should know where the medication is stored at home. Nitroglycerin is kept in a dark brown bottle and must be stored in a dry place. Since the medication loses its potency after 6 months, patients should be instructed to check the expiration date on the bottle and make sure they always have fresh nitroglycerin. If the medication is fresh, the patient should experience a burning sensation on the tongue and may experience a throbbing sensation in the head. Some patients frequently experience flushing and headache from the vasodilation properties of nitroglycerin. Fortunately, these side effects diminish as the patient develops a tolerance for the drug. Patients taking nitroglycerin should be instructed not to stand or sit up abruptly after taking the medication since it reduces systolic blood pressure and they may become hypotensive.

Long-acting forms of nitrates are being used more commonly to diminish attacks and increase exercise capacity. Nitroglycerin ointment can be applied to any surface of the body that is not hairy. This cream is prescribed in doses of one-half to several inches and is spread on cellophane-like paper and placed on the patient's chest or another part of the body. The cream is absorbed slowly through the skin over many hours.

General skin care is necessary, and the site of application is changed daily.

β-adrenergic blocking agents including propranolol (Inderal), metoprolol (Lopressor), and nadolol (Corgard) all act to decrease myocardial oxygen demands by reducing heart rate, blood pressure, myocardial contractility, and calcium output. The use of β-blockade is contraindicated in patients with congestive heart failure, hypotension, and certain AV blocks.

NEW APPROACH IN DRUG THERAPY. A relatively new classification of drugs termed *calcium-channel blockers* (slow-channel inhibitors, calcium antagonists, or calcium inhibitors) may revolutionize cardiovascular drug therapy. In addition to myocardial ischemia, calcium-channel blockers appear to benefit persons with arrhythmias, hypertrophic cardiomyopathy, and hypertension. Only one drug, verapamil, has to date been approved by the Food and Drug Administration. Seven other drugs, (diltiazem, nifedipine, lidoflazine, flunarizine, perhexiline, prenylamine, and gallopamil) are currently under investigation. Presently, these eight drugs are thought to act at least in part as calcium-channel blockers.

The new agents appear to act in the same manner, but their cardiovascular effects are not identical. These drugs block the movement of calcium ions across cell membranes via the calcium "channel." Under normal circumstances ions cannot penetrate the lipid membrane of either heart or smooth muscle cells. However, with appropriate electrical or chemical stimulation, molecular channels are formed that permit ion passage into the cell through a gating mechanism. Unlike the rapid sodium-ion channel that permits inward depolarization, the calcium-ion channel is much slower and ionic current is much smaller, hence the term *slow* channel. The exact mechanism by which these new drugs block the calcium channel pathway is not yet clear.

The inhibition of calcium-ion transportation into the myocardial cells appears to depress inotropic and chronotropic activity, thereby decreasing the workload of the heart (p. 1035). By reducing cardiac activity a balance can be achieved between myocardial oxygen supply and demand. Decreasing the heart rate also allows for prolonged diastole, which augments perfusion of the coronary arteries. Another benefit of calcium blockaders is their potent vasodilatory effects. Exaggerated release of substances such as catecholamines and prostaglandins is known to produce vasoconstriction. Calcium-channel blockers interfere with vasoconstriction and have been shown to be effective in reducing coronary vasospasm.

Exactly where these new drugs will fit in the treatment of cardiovascular disease is still under investigation. It is felt that these new drugs will play a significant role in combination with clearly established treatment modalities and will probably be one of the major advances in the treatment of cardiac disease during the coming decade.

Activity. Most persons with angina pectoris can tolerate mild exercise such as walking and playing golf, but exertion such as running, climbing hills or stairs rapidly, and lifting heavy objects causes pain. Anginal pain is likely to be evoked more easily in cold weather, since the vessels normally constrict to conserve body heat. When persons with angina pectoris must be exposed to the cold, they should err on the side of being too warmly clothed. It is unwise to sleep in a cold room, and walking against the wind and uphill should be avoided because these activities increase the work load of the heart and cause pain.

Emotional adjustment. Since excessive emotional strain also causes vasoconstriction by releasing epinephrine into the circulation, emotional outbursts, worry, and tension should be minimized. Persons with angina may need continuing help in accepting situations as they find them. The family, the spiritual adviser, business associates, and friends can sometimes help. An optimistic outlook helps to relieve the work of the heart. Many persons who learn to live within their limitations live out their expected life span in spite of the disease. Helping a person adjust to living with this disease can be most rewarding for the individual, the family, the physician, and the nurse.

Coronary bypass surgery. Coronary arteriography is indicated for most patients with angina pectoris to confirm the diagnosis, assess any damage, estimate the prognosis, and determine the need for surgery. Coronary bypass surgery is a dramatically effective treatment for severe coronary disease. If severe narrowing of one or more branches of the coronary arteries exists, coronary artery bypass surgery may be recommended as a prophylactic measure.

The purpose of coronary artery bypass (jump graft) surgery is to increase blood flow to the myocardium (myocardial revascularization). Many persons show marked improvement after this surgery and usually do not require nitrates to maintain relief of symptoms.

The surgical technique varies somewhat among surgeons, and some surgeons routinely use extracorporeal circulation during the operation, while others do not. When the saphenous vein is used for the graft, one end is sutured to the aorta and the other end is sutured to the coronary artery distal to the occlusion (Fig. 45-5). When an internal mammary artery is used, the distal end of this vessel is freed from the anterior chest wall and sutured in place distal to the occlusion in the coronary artery (Fig. 45-6). Coronary bypass surgery is performed on the right coronary artery (RCA), the left anterior descending (LAD) artery, and the circumflex coronary artery (CCA) and their major branches. The care of the person undergoing coronary artery surgery

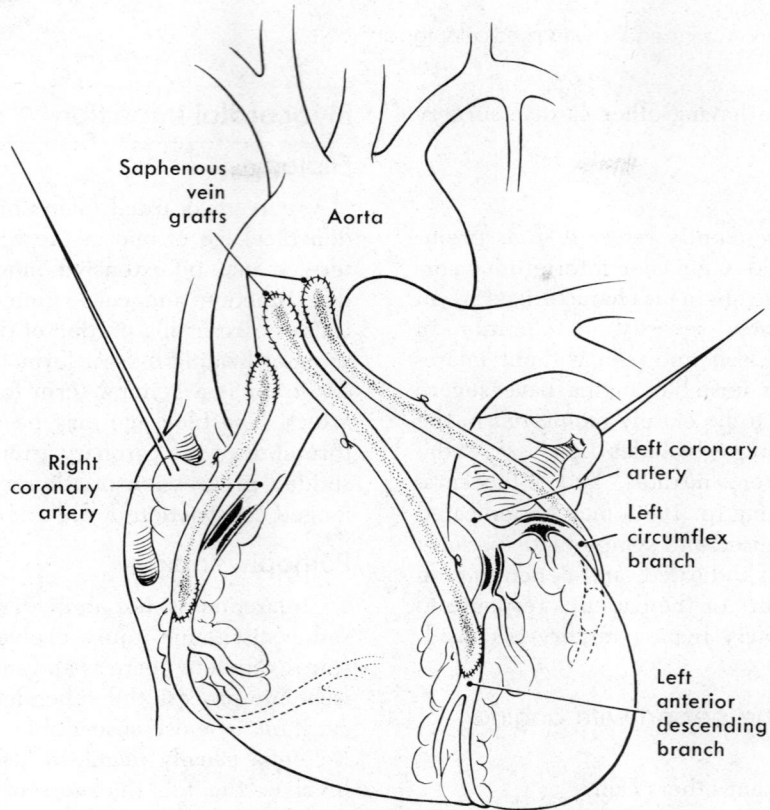

Saphenous
vein
grafts

Aorta

Right
coronary
artery

Left coronary
artery

Left
circumflex
branch

Left
anterior
descending
branch

Fig. 45-5. Triple coronary bypass in which all grafts were from saphenous veins. (Many surgeons use combination of internal mammary artery and saphenous vein grafts when performing double or triple bypass procedures.)

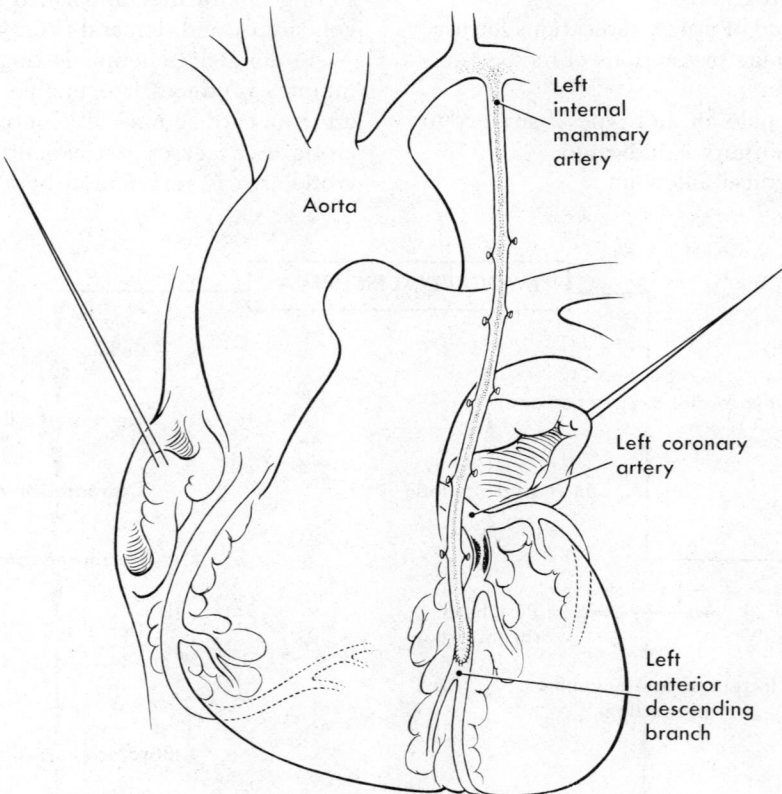

Aorta

Left
internal
mammary
artery

Left coronary
artery

Left
anterior
descending
branch

Fig. 45-6. Single coronary bypass in which left internal mammary artery has been used to bypass obstruction. Saphenous vein also may be used.

is similar to that of those having other cardiac surgery (see Chapter 44, p. 1088).

Unstable angina

Unstable angina is frequently referred to as preinfarction angina, crescendo angina, or intermittent coronary syndrome. Unstable angina is characterized by an increase in the frequency, severity, or duration of symptoms, or prolonged ischemic pain without infarction. Most patients with unstable angina have severe diffuse disease and need to be closely monitored in the coronary care unit. Therapy includes bed rest, sedation, supplemental oxygen, nitrates, and β-blockers. Intraaortic balloon pumping (p. 1086) may be indicated for the severely compromised and symptomatic patient. Coronary arteriography is indicated, and depending on the results of the procedure or the patient's response to medical treatment, coronary bypass surgery is considered.

Outcome criteria for the person with angina pectoris

The person or significant others can:
1. Describe events that may precipitate attacks (stress, exertion, overeating, exposure to cold) and plan for avoidance if possible.
2. Describe activity plans to balance myocardial oxygen demands with supply (participation in a regular exercise program).
3. State name, method of usage, indications for use, and necessary storage precautions of medications (nitrates, β-blockers).
4. Describe the rationale for and type of surgery to be performed, if surgery is indicated.
5. State plans for medical follow-up.

Myocardial infarction

Etiology

Acute myocardial infarction (MI) is caused by sudden blockage of one of the branches of a coronary artery. It may be extensive enough to interfere with cardiac function and cause immediate death, or it may cause necrosis of a portion of the myocardium with subsequent healing by scar formation or fibrosis. *Coronary occlusion* is a general term for blockage of a coronary artery. The blockage may be caused by formation of a thrombus in the coronary artery *(coronary thrombosis),* sudden progression of atherosclerotic changes, or prolonged constriction of the arteries.

Pathophysiology

Infarction is not immediately total and complete; rather, ischemic injury evolves over several hours toward complete necrosis and infarction. During an acute ischemic process the subendocardial layer of the myocardium is most susceptible to hypoxia, and cellular ischemia usually manifests itself in this area before it involves the full thickness of the ventricular myocardium. Ischemia almost immediately alters the integrity and the permeability of the cell membrane to vital electrolytes, thereby producing depressed myocardial contractility. The autonomic nervous system attempts to compensate for the depressed cardiac performance, resulting in a further imbalance between myocardial oxygen supply and demand (Fig. 45-7).

Prolonged ischemia lasting greater than 35 to 45 minutes produces irreversible cellular damage and necrosis of cardiac muscle. Contractile function in the necrotic area ceases permanently. The infarcted or necrotic area is surrounded by a zone of ischemia, made

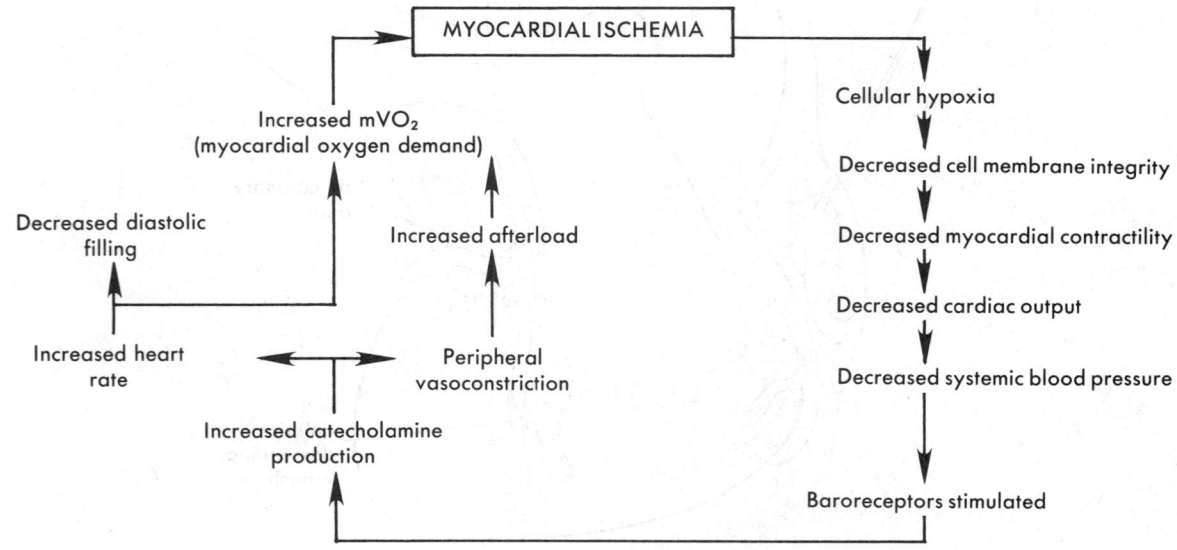

Fig. 45-7. Effects of myocardial ischemia.

up of potentially viable tissues. The final extent of the infarct size will depend on whether the marginal area in the ischemic zone succumbs to prolonged ischemia or is able to develop and maintain collateral circulation. The prognosis following an acute myocardial infarction reflects the degree of functional impairment of the heart.

The clinical features of acute myocardial infarction are determined by both the anatomic location and the extent of occlusive coronary disease. Knowledge of the anatomic location of the MI enables one to anticipate whether arrhythmias, conduction disturbances, and congestive heart failure are likely to occur. The location of the infarct is, of course, directly related to the disease in a particular region of the coronary circulation. An *anterior-wall myocardial infarction* results from lesions in the left anterior descending (LAD) branch of the left main coronary artery (p. 1031). Because the LAD branch supplies most of the left ventricle, an anterior infarct is often associated with a substantial loss of left ventricular muscle mass and can result in severe hemodynamic disturbances. An *inferior-wall myocardial infarction* is most often caused by occlusion of the right coronary artery (RCA). Since the RCA is often proximal to the origin of both the AV node and the SA node arteries, it is frequently accompanied by ischemia of the AV node, the proximal bundle of His, and the SA node as well. Abnormalities of impulse conduction and formation caused by ischemia or infarction are primary factors contributing to the development of serious arrhythmias early in the course of inferior infarction.[15] *Lateral-wall* infarcts are usually caused by occlusion of the left circumflex coronary artery and may be complicated by the hemodynamic changes similar to an anterior infarction when a large mass of myocardium is disrupted.

Clinical picture

Pain is the most frequent complaint of the patient with an MI. The individual typically complains of sudden, severe, crushing or viselike pain in the substernal region. This pain may radiate into the left and sometimes the right arm and up the sides of the neck (Fig. 45-8). At other times it may simulate indigestion or a gallbladder attack with abdominal pain. Persons often become restless and fear that they are dying. They may become short of breath and cyanotic and show signs of severe shock. The pulse is usually rapid, and it may be barely perceptible. The blood pressure usually falls, and the patient may collapse. S_1 and S_2 heart sounds are often faint; S_4 can often be heard; and at times an S_3 (gallop rhythm), which indicates left ventricular failure, may be evident. A soft systolic murmur may be heard at the apex. The symptoms of cardiogenic shock (p. 1122) occur as a result of inadequate cardiac output from decreased myocardial contractility and ineffective pumping.

Although pain is the most common initial complaint, it is not necessarily present. Approximately 15% to 20% of myocardial infarcts may be painless. The incidence of painless infarcts increases with age and in the elderly the chief complaint may be sudden shortness of breath. Other less common presenting symptoms include confusion, sudden arrhythmia, unexplained drop in blood pressure, or sudden loss of consciousness.

Diagnostic tests

Laboratory tests used in diagnosing the presence of a myocardial infarction can be divided into three categories: nonspecific indicators of tissue necrosis and inflammation, ECG, and serum enzymes. Other diagnostic procedures include myocardial scintigraphy and myocardial perfusion imaging.

Nonspecific indicators. The nonspecific reaction to myocardial injury is a *leukocytosis* that begins within a few hours after the onset of pain. This leukocytosis often reaches 12,000 to 15,000/cu mm and lasts for approximately 3 to 7 days. In general, high WBC counts are associated with larger infarcts. The *erythrocyte sedimentation rate* (ESR), another nonspecific indicator, rises during the first week after infarction and remains elevated for several weeks.

Electrocardiogram. The term *transmural myocardial infarction* denotes that the full thickness of the wall of the myocardium has been involved. If an infarct does not involve the entire thickness of the myocardium, it is termed *nontransmural* or *subendocardial*. In this situation there are no Q waves present and the characteristic ECG changes are limited to the ST segment and the T wave. It must be emphasized the ECG does not always provide definitive evidence of the ischemic process. However, pronounced Q waves, ST segment elevation, and T wave abnormalities are often evident during acute infarction. These ECG changes are apparent in the leads overlying the area of myocardial necrosis.

Serum enzymes. When cardiac muscle cells die, certain enzymes are released into the blood stream via the coronary lymphatic drainage. These enzymes include creatine phosphokinase (CPK), serum glutamic-oxaloacetic transaminase (SGOT), and lactic dehydrogenase (LDH).

A pattern of enzyme elevations following an acute MI is a valuable diagnostic indicator. However, enzyme interpretation is somewhat limited in that enzyme elevations are not solely specific to myocardial damage. For example, SGOT is found mainly in heart muscle, but it is also present in the liver and to some extent in the skeletal muscle. LDH is found in the heart, liver, kidney, brain, skeletal muscle, and erythrocytes. CPK occurs in heart, skeletal muscle, and brain cells. Because of the lack of specificity of these enzymes, coexisting processes such as cirrhosis of the liver may produce misleading enzyme elevations.

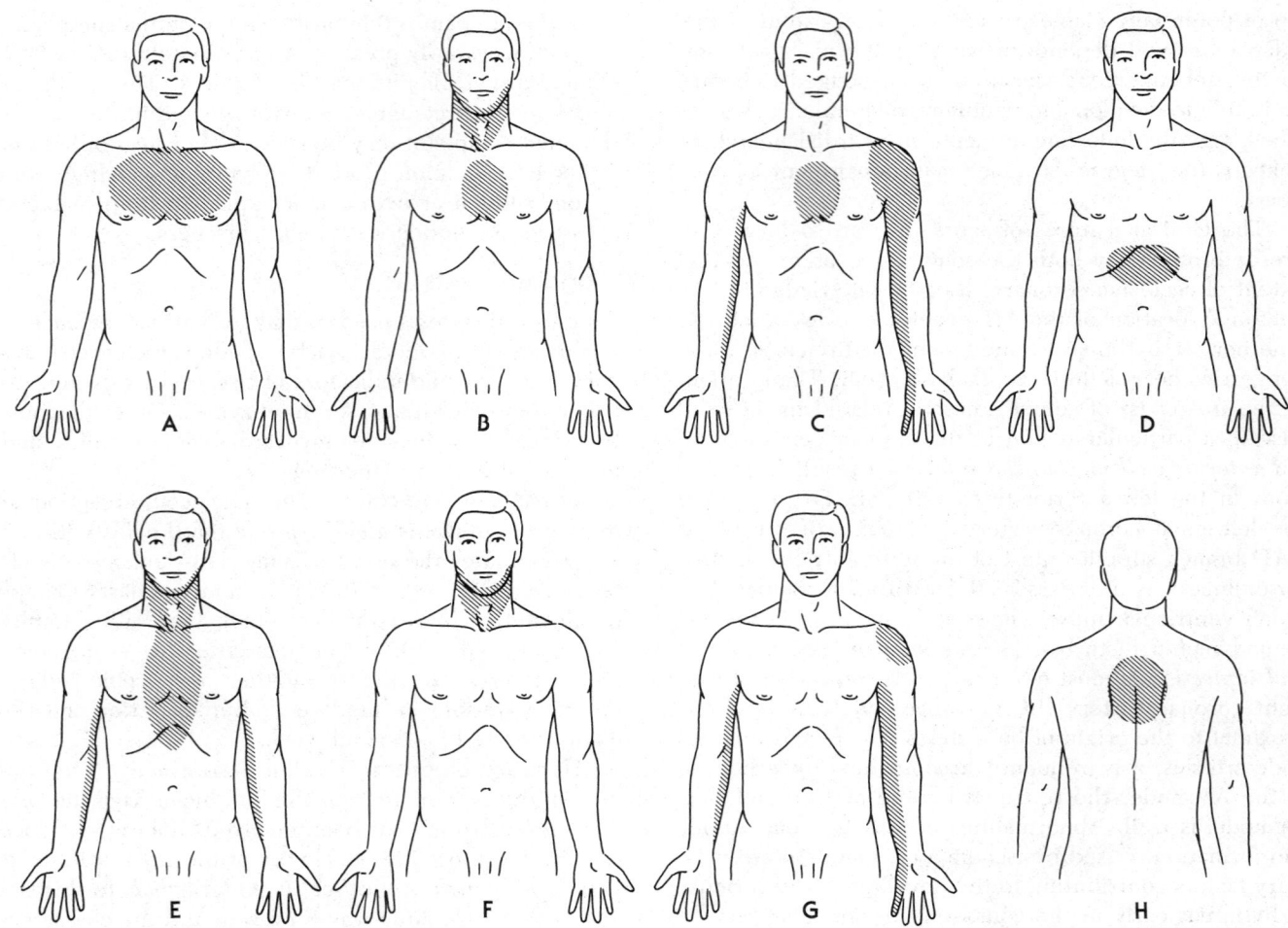

Fig. 45-8. Sites where ischemic myocardial pain may be referred. **A,** Upper chest. **B,** Beneath sternum radiating to neck and jaw. **C,** Beneath sternum radiating down left arm. **D,** Epigastric. **E,** Epigastric radiating to neck and jaw. **F,** Neck and jaw. **G,** Left shoulder, inner aspect of both arms. **H,** Intrascapular.

To increase the specificity of these enzymes, measurements of the enzyme fractions or isoenzymes are taken. Fractionating the *CPK* enzyme into isoenzymes is the most specific enzymatic indication of myocardial infarction. CPK_1 (BB) is found in brain, lungs, bladder, and bowel; CPK_2 (MB) is found almost exclusively in the myocardium; and CPK_3 (MM) is found in both skeletal and heart muscle. CPK (MB) is found in the serum of all patients for 48 hours after a transmural infarction, but it may also be elevated in the individual with crescendo, or unstable, angina, even in the absence of true infarction. The total CPK value is elevated within 3 to 6 hours after an acute myocardial infarction, peaks in 12 to 18 hours, and returns to normal in 3 to 4 days (Fig. 45-9).

The *serum LDH* level rises within 12 hours after infarction, peaks in 3 days, and returns to normal levels in 10 to 14 days. Because of the extensive tissue distribution of LDH, it can be elevated in a variety of disorders. Fractionating LDH into its five isoenzymes allows for greater specificity. Normally, LDH_2 is most prominent in the serum. The myocardium is especially rich in LDH_1, so that when an infarction occurs the serum level of LDH_1 becomes higher than LDH_2 and the LDH pattern is said to be "flipped."

The *SGOT* level rises within 4 to 6 hours following infarction, peaks in 24 to 36 hours, and returns to normal in 4 to 7 days.

Myocardial scintigraphy. The scintigram is a diagnostic tool capable of identifying the presence of myocardial infarction. A radionuclide such as technetium-tagged pyrophosphate (^{99m}Tc-PYP) is administered intravenously and a scintigram is performed 1 to 3 hours after injection (p. 1060). The procedure is not painful and takes approximately 15 minutes to perform. The scintigram identifies areas of necrosis termed *hot spots*

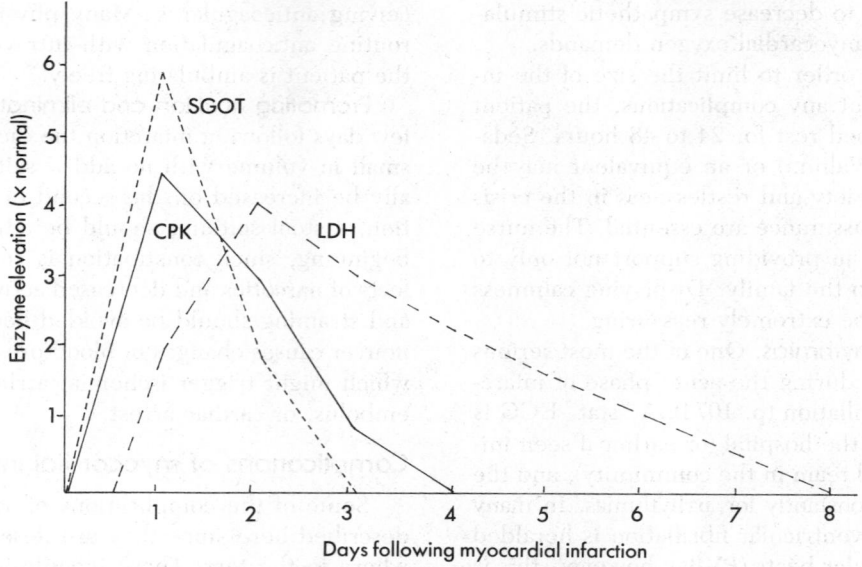

Fig. 45-9. Patterns of serum enzyme levels following myocardial infarction.

in both transmural and subendocardial infarction and is regarded as a sensitive technique for identifying myocardial necrosis.

Myocardial perfusion imaging. Thallium 201, another radioisotope, is used effectively for imaging well-perfused areas of the myocardium (p. 1060). By combining technetium-tagged pyrophosphate to pinpoint areas of irreversible damage and thallium to locate the perfused areas of the myocardium, the physician can then plan appropriate therapies.

Prognosis

The mortality for persons suffering an acute MI is high, ranging from 30% to 40%; however, a substantial number of these deaths take place before the patient reaches the hospital. Among those patients who reach the hospital, approximately 80% survive. Most in-hospital deaths from myocardial infarction take place during the first 3 or 4 days.

Intervention during acute phase

The patient is usually admitted to a coronary care unit that is equipped with special monitoring equipment and staffed by nurses with expertise in cardiovascular nursing. Medical and nursing interventions during the acute phase of myocardial infarction are aimed at reducing the workload on the heart, anticipating, preventing, and treating complications, and helping to provide psychologic support (Table 45-2).

Promoting comfort. The amount of pain and discomfort an individual will experience is highly variable. Some persons experience severe pain, and others have minimal discomfort. After an intravenous route is estab-

TABLE 45-2. Interventions for myocardial infarction in acute phase

Actions	Rationale
Morphine sulfate (IV or IM)	Relieves pain and apprehension; prevents shock
Psychologic support to patient/family	Patient: decreases oxygen demands
	Family: decreases anxiety, which can be transmitted to patient
Bed rest initially	Decreases myocardial oxygen demand
Diazepam (Valium) prn	Decreases anxiety and restlessness
Oxygen by nasal cannula	Increases myocardial oxygen supply
Monitor for arrhythmias (PVB, ventricular fibrillation)	Facilitates early recognition and treatment
Monitor vital signs	Facilitates early recognition of complications
Lidocaine (IV)	Prevents ventricular fibrillation
Heparin (IV) (may be omitted for mild cases)	Prevents thromboembolic events
Soft diet, in small amounts initially, with no added salt	Decreases oxygen demands; prevents fluid retention
Stool softener	Prevents constipation from effects of opiates and decreased mobility

lished, the patient is given morphine sulfate to relieve pain and apprehension and also to produce vasodilation. Continued episodes of chest pain may be related to the size of the infarction, the relative lack of collateral circulation, and an increased myocardial oxygen demand. Control of this pain is essential in order to provide comfort and rest and also to decrease sympathetic stimulation, which increases myocardial oxygen demands.

Providing rest. In order to limit the size of the infarction and to prevent any complications, the patient is usually placed on bed rest for 24 to 48 hours. Sedation with diazepam (Valium) or an equivalent may be ordered to relieve anxiety and restlessness in the crisis situation. Rest and reassurance are essential. The nurse plays an integral role in providing support not only to the patient but also to the family. Displaying calmness and competence can be extremely reassuring.

Monitoring for arrhythmias. One of the most serious threats to the patient during the acute phase of infarction is ventricular fibrillation (p. 1074). A "stat" ECG is obtained on arrival at the hospital (or earlier if seen initially by a paramedical team in the community), and the patient is monitored constantly for arrhythmias. In many patients the onset of ventricular fibrillation is heralded by premature ventricular beats (PVBs); however, this is not always the case. Many physicians now administer prophylactic lidocaine intravenously. Lidocaine is not effective for atrial arrhythmias, but prophylactic lidocaine in acute myocardial infarction has been shown to prevent most episodes of primary ventricular fibrillation.

Providing oxygenation. Oxygen therapy is administered to correct a decrease in arterial oxygen pressure (PO_2) caused by ventilation-perfusion abnormalities. Oxygen administered by nasal cannula should be given for the first 24 to 48 hours and longer if persistent pain, hypotension, dyspnea, or arrhythmias occur. The patient's vital signs are monitored carefully for changes indicating possible complications (Table 45-3).

Preventing thromboembolic events. Despite multiple retrospective and clinical studies over the past 30 years, anticoagulation therapy is still controversial. However, most studies show a decreased incidence of thrombophlebitis and pulmonary emboli in patients re-

ceiving anticoagulants. Many physicians now advocate routine anticoagulation with intravenous heparin until the patient is ambulating freely.

Promoting nutrition and elimination. During the first few days following infarction the diet should be soft and small in volume with no added salt. The diet can usually be increased on the second or third day. In addition, a stool softener should be administered from the beginning, since constipation is common from the effects of narcotics and decreased activity. Use of bedpans and straining should be avoided because Valsalva's maneuver causes changes in blood pressure and heart rate, which might trigger ischemia, arrhythmias, pulmonary embolus, or cardiac arrest.

Complications of myocardial infarction

Some of the complications of acute MI will not be described here since they are described in detail elsewhere in the text. These include arrhythmias, congestive heart failure, pericarditis, pulmonary embolism, systemic embolism, and interventricular septal rupture. Other complications include cardiogenic shock, ventricular aneurysm, and postmyocardial infarction syndrome.

The person who has had a myocardial infarction is at high risk for recurrent heart attacks. In the past, antithrombotic therapy has been given in attempts to prevent recurrences. More recently, β-adrenergic blocking drugs, such as alprenolol, have been found to decrease the incidence of death in the months after myocardial infarction.[4]

Cardiogenic shock. Cardiogenic shock is a shock state of primary cardiac origin. It is most frequently caused by myocardial infarction, but it may also be the result of critical aortic stenosis, intractable arrhythmias, ruptured aortic aneurysm, obstruction to flow between cardiac chambers (atrial myxoma), severe congestive heart failure, massive pulmonary embolism, or cardiac tamponade.

PATHOPHYSIOLOGY. Shock occurs in approximately 15% of all patients hospitalized with the diagnosis of acute myocardial infarction. When cardiogenic shock follows a myocardial infarction, it is the result of severe left ventricular failure. So much myocardium has been damaged (usually more than 40% of the left ventricle) that inadequate systemic perfusion occurs secondary to low cardiac output. As the shock state progresses, there is decreased coronary artery perfusion, leading to the development of extended areas of cardiac muscle ischemia and necrosis throughout both ventricles. This progressive ischemia and infarction lead to further deterioration of left ventricular function, and, if unchecked, to death. The mortality for cardiogenic shock is very high; 80% to 90% do not survive.

CLINICAL PICTURE. The severe organ hypoperfusion is characterized by metabolic acidosis (caused by anaer-

TABLE 45-3. Interpretation of changes in vital signs during an acute myocardial infarction

Vital sign	Change	Interpretation
Blood pressure	High	Increased myocardial oxygen demand
	Low (<80 mm Hg)	Decreased coronary perfusion with further myocardial ischemia
Heart rate	Increased	Possible shock
Heart rhythm	Irregular	Potential life-threatening arrhythmia
Respirations	Slow	Possible morphine toxicity
	Gurgling (rales)	Pulmonary edema

obic metabolism and lactate production), hypotension with a systolic blood pressure less than 90 mm Hg, tachycardia, urinary output less than 20 ml/hour, cold clammy skin, and mental confusion or lethargy.

INTERVENTION. Cardiogenic shock is a medical emergency that requires immediate intervention and constant attention to prevent irreversible cell damage and death. Therapy is aimed at correcting factors that contribute to decreased tissue perfusion, such as cardiac arrhythmias, hypoxemia, and pain. Lactic acidosis may be partially compensated for through use of hyperventilation and buffering agents such as sodium bicarbonate. Invasive monitoring lines that are usually placed include catheters in the pulmonary artery, systemic artery, and urinary bladder. The left ventricular end-diastolic pressure is reflected in the pulmonary capillary wedge pressure, which is used as a guide to fluid therapy. Hypovolemia must be carefully corrected without inducing a fluid overload, which could result in acute pulmonary edema.

Vasopressors and cardiotonic agents are chosen to raise the systemic arterial pressure without increasing the workload (and therefore the oxygen requirements) of the myocardium. Dopamine and norepinephrine are frequently used to raise the systemic arterial pressure and cardiac output. Nitroprusside may be added in small amounts to decrease after load and to reduce systemic vascular resistance. Every effort is made to maintain systemic arterial pressure at an absolute minimum of 60 mm Hg, preferably 90 mm Hg; total coronary artery collapse occurs at approximately 40 mm Hg.

Unless the shock state can be reversed with reinstatement of adequate cardiac output and tissue oxygenation, the patient will continue to deteriorate and death will ensue. Patients who require extensive pharmacologic support and in whom it is felt sufficient myocardium remains undamaged to allow for eventual recovery may benefit from initiation of intraaortic balloon counterpulsation (p. 1086).

Ventricular aneurysm. Aneurysms of the ventricular myocardium are predominantly a result of transmural myocardial infarctions. Traumatically induced or congenitally formed aneurysms are very rare. In 12% to 15% of the victims of myocardial infarctions, the resultant myocardial necrosis and scar formation develop a weakened ventricular wall. During systole the high pressures within the ventricle cause the weakened myocardium to bulge outward. Blood collects in the aneurysm or outpouched area and is a potential source of emboli. Cardiac output may be compromised. If symptomatic, the patient usually presents with congestive heart failure and recurring arrhythmias. Symptoms usually occur when 20% or more of the ventricle has been involved. The majority of ventricular aneurysms occur in the apex and anterior part of the heart.

Diagnosis is usually made in the presence of a ventricular gallop, persistent ST elevations following a myocardial infarction, a chest x-ray film showing an enlarged left ventricle, a paradoxic expansion of the aneurysmal sac during systole on fluoroscopy, and cardiac catheterization.

Treatment consists of a ventricular aneurysmectomy in which the aneurysm sac is excised and the ventricle sutured together. If the area excised includes part of a coronary artery, bypass surgery is done simultaneously. Operative mortality is less than 5%.

Postmyocardial infarction syndrome (Dressler's syndrome). A few patients develop a syndrome approximately 1 to 6 weeks after an acute myocardial infarction, characterized by pleural pain, joint pains, and fever. It is thought to be due to an autoimmune reaction to the myocardial necrosis. Aspirin is usually effective for the discomfort, and more severe symptoms usually respond quickly to a short intensive course of corticosteroids.

Cardiac rehabilitation

Cardiac rehabilitation is a process by which a person is restored to and maintains optimal physiologic, psychosocial, vocational, and recreational status. This process of rehabilitation involves progressive activity and exercise and education of the patient and family. Rehabilitation of the person who has suffered a myocardial infarction begins the moment the person is admitted to the hospital for emergency care and may continue for months and even years after discharge from the hospital.

Progressive activity. During the 1960s, 2 to 3 weeks of bed rest were recommended for the person who had myocardial infarction. Today the hazards of prolonged bed rest are well documented and patients with uncomplicated myocardial infarctions (no evidence of severe arrhythmias, congestive heart failure, or shock) progress rapidly through a supervised program of increased activity. Activity progression is based on METs, a term used to describe the energy expenditure for various activities. A MET is a metabolic equivalent that can be assigned to activities regardless of a person's weight. One MET represents the energy expenditure of a person at rest; it equals approximately 3.5 ml/O_2/kg of weight per minute.

A hospitalized myocardial infarction patient is usually limited to activities with low MET levels (i.e., 1 to 3 METs). For example, using a bedside commode requires 3 METs and using a bedpan requires 4 METs. Consequently, most coronary care units have changed from requiring patients to stay on strict bed rest using the bedpan to using a bedside commode. Champion athletes can perform at equal to or greater than 20 METs, while the average middle-aged man following an uncomplicated MI is capable of performing at a level of 8 to 9 METs (Table 45-4).

TABLE 45-4. Approximate metabolic cost of activities*†

	Occupational	Recreational
1½-2 METs‡ 4-7 ml O$_2$/min/kg 2-2½ kcal/min (70-kg person)	Desk work Auto driving§ Typing Electric calculating machine operation	Standing Walking (strolling 1.6 km or 1 mile/hr) Flying,§ motorcycling§ Playing cards§ Sewing, knitting
2-3 METs 7-11 ml O$_2$/min/kg 2½-4 kcal/min (70 kg person)	Auto repair Radio, television repair Janitorial work Typing, manual Bartending	Level walking (3.2 km or 2 miles/hr) Level bicycling (8.0 km or 5 miles/hr) Riding lawn mower Billiards, bowling Skeet,§ shuffleboard Woodworking (light) Powerboat driving§ Golf (power cart) Canoeing (4 km or 2½ miles/hr) Horseback riding (walk) Playing piano and many musical instruments
3-4 METs 11-14 ml O$_2$/min/kg 4-5 kcal/min (70 kg person)	Brick laying, plastering Wheelbarrow (45.4-kg or 100-lb load) Machine assembly Trailer-truck in traffic Welding (moderate load) Cleaning windows	Walking (4.8 km or 3 miles/hr) Cycling (9.7 km or 6 miles/hr) Horseshoe pitching Volleyball (6-person, noncompetitive) Golf (pulling bag cart) Archery Sailing (handling small boat) Fly-fishing (standing with waders) Horseback (sitting to trot) Badminton (social doubles) Pushing light power mower Energetic musician
4-5 METs 14-18 ml O$_2$/min/kg 5-6 kcal/min (70-kg person)	Painting, masonry Paperhanging Light carpentry	Walking (5.6 km or 3½ miles/hr) Cycling (12.9 km or 8 miles/hr) Table tennis Golf (carrying clubs) Dancing (foxtrot) Badminton (singles) Tennis (doubles) Raking leaves Hoeing Many calisthenics
5-6 METs 18-21 ml O$_2$/min/kg 6-7 kcal/min (70-kg person)	Digging garden Shoveling light earth	Walking (6.4 km or 4 miles/hr) Cycling (16.1 km or 10 miles/hr) Canoeing (6.4 km or 4 miles/hr) Horseback ("posting" to trot) Stream fishing (walking in light current in waders) Ice- or roller-skating (14.5 km or 9 miles/hr)
6-7 METs 21-25 ml O$_2$/min/kg 7-8 kcal/min (70-kg person)	Shoveling for 10 min (4.5 kg or 10 lb)	Walking (8.0 km or 5 miles/hr) Cycling (17.7 km or 11 miles/hr) Badminton (competitive) Tennis (singles) Splitting wood Snow shoveling Hand lawn mowing

*From Fox, S.M., Naughton, J.P., and Gorman, P.A.: Mod. Concepts Cardiovasc. Dis. **41**:6, June 1972. By permission of the American Heart Association, Inc.
†Includes resting metabolic needs.
‡1 MET is the energy expenditure at rest, equivalent to approximately 3.5 ml O$_2$/kg body weight/minute.
§A major excess metabolic increase may occur due to excitement, anxiety, or impatience in some of these activities, and a physician must assess his patient's psychological reactivity.

TABLE 45-4. Approximate metabolic cost of activities—cont'd

	Occupational	Recreational
		Folk (square) dancing
		Light downhill skiing
		Ski touring (4.0 km or 2½ miles/hr) (loose snow)
		Water skiing
7-8 METs	Digging ditches	Jogging (8.0 km or 5 miles/hr)
25-28 ml O₂/min/kg	Carrying 36.3 kg or 80 lb	Cycling (19.3 km or 12 miles/hr)
8-10 kcal/min (70-kg person)	Sawing hardwood	Horseback riding (gallop)
		Vigorous downhill skiing
		Basketball
		Mountain climbing
		Ice hockey
		Canoeing (8.0 km or 5 miles/hr)
		Touch football
		Paddleball
8-9 METs	Shoveling for 10 min (6.4 kg or 14 lb)	Running (8.9 km or 5½ miles/hr)
28-32 ml O₂/min/kg		Cycling (20.9 km or 13 miles/hr)
10-11 kcal/min (70-kg person)		Ski touring (6.4 km or 4 miles/hr) (loose snow)
		Squash racquets (social)
		Handball (social)
		Fencing
		Basketball (vigorous)
10+ METs	Shoveling for 10 min (7.3 kg or 16 lb)	Running: 6 mph = 10 METs
32+ ml O₂/min/kg		7 mph = 11½ METs
11+ kcal/min (70-kg person)		8 mph = 13½ METs
		9 mph = 15 METs
		10 mph = 17 METs
		Ski touring (8+ km or 5+ miles/hr) (loose snow)
		Handball (competitive)
		Squash (competitive)

Over 50% of all myocardial infarctions are uncomplicated, and these patients will be discharged from the hospital in 7 to 14 days. Since most patients will need to do 3 to 4 MET level activities when they return home, in-hospital activities should be geared toward reaching this level. In some institutions it is the physical therapist who supervises the exercise program, working closely with both the medical and nursing personnel to coordinate activities. During the first few days after an uncomplicated myocardial infarction, the patient is instructed and encouraged to perform lying or sitting exercises (arms, legs, and trunk) at low MET levels. Then exercises progress to standing and slow walking in the hall. Patients are supervised constantly during these activities, and their vital signs and heart rhythms (ECG) are constantly monitored.

Patients are taught early in the exercise program how to check their own pulses. This enables them to become familiar with the normal rate, rhythm, and response to exercise. Normally, patients can expect to have an increase in heart rate and systolic blood pressure with exercise. An exercise session is terminated if any of the following abnormal responses occur during exercise:

1. Cyanosis, cold sweat, faintness, extreme fatigue, severe dyspnea, marked pallor, ataxia, chest pain
2. Resting heart rate greater than 100 or an increase in heart rate greater than 20 over resting pulse; decrease or no change in heart rate despite exercise
3. Dysrhythmias, frequent PVBs, supraventricular tachycardia, various AV blocks, tachycardia greater than 120
4. Resting blood pressure greater than 160/95 mm Hg or an increase in systolic blood pressure of more than 40 mm Hg; decrease or no change in systolic pressure despite exercise

Progressive exercise is continued throughout the hospitalization. The nurse may be an integral member of the interdisciplinary team involved in instructing and supervising the program. Patients should exercise twice a day for approximately 20 minutes. Patients who will need to climb stairs at home gradually progress so that they can climb stairs in the supervised hospital environment. There are many psychologic as well as physiologic benefits to early and progressive activity. Most patients feel that activity is a positive sign and that they are making progress and are recovering from their infarction. Exercise also gives the patients a sense of control over their bodies and tends to decrease anxiety and depression during the convalescent period.

Home exercise program. During the posthospitalization convalescent period many patients are encouraged to begin a 2- to 12-week walking program. This is a structured program designed to have the patient walk 2 miles in less than 60 minutes by the end of the 12 weeks. Individuals are encouraged to work through this program at their own rate until they have achieved a pace just below a slow jog and their heart rate is below the prescribed rate set by the cardiologist.

After completion of the walking program, some individuals will progress on to a supervised outpatient exercise training program. Physical conditioning improves the maximal oxygen uptake (VO_2 max), which is a measure of the maximal rate at which oxygen can be delivered to the tissues. Unfortunately, not all postinfarction patients are physiologically capable of participating in a rigorous exercise program. Eventually, most patients are encouraged to participate in a maintenance (lifetime), unsupervised, home-based exercise program designed specifically for them.

Education of patient and family. Education of the patient and family enables them to assume a more active role in their own health care. A great deal of anxiety and apprehension can be allayed by providing information about the cardiac condition and its management. Although teaching methods and the amount of information presented may vary, several key concepts need to be presented. A typical education program includes a basic presentation of CAHD, risk factors, medications, and diet and stresses the importance of gradual progressive increases in activity. During the teaching sessions, patients and families are encouraged to talk about their feelings and concerns. Often in group teaching sessions a feeling of camaraderie develops as several individuals face similar problems.

During the hospitalization period many patients experience denial, depression, and anxiety. Generally, patients tend to become more anxious on the second day of hospitalization, after the immediate threat of death from the infarction has passed. Depression may begin several days later and may continue after the patient is discharged. The majority of individuals who experience a myocardial infarction adjust extremely well. Over 85% of all patients with uncomplicated myocardial infarctions are able to return to work, and this, along with resuming normal sexual functioning, aids tremendously in the adjustment process.

The patients and their partners may need teaching and reassurance regarding resuming *sexual activities*. Many feel that after an MI their sex life is over. Edu-

cation should aim at supplying information and dispelling misinformation. In general, persons should abstain from having sexual intercourse for 4 to 6 weeks following a myocardial infarction. Approximately 80% of all postcoronary patients will be able to resume sexual activity without serious risk. The other 20% need not totally abstain, but their sexual activity should be limited according to their cardiac capacity.

Once patients with an uncomplicated MI are capable of walking two flights of stairs without difficulty, they are generally able to perform sexual intercourse safely. In many hospitals, exercise stress tests are done to help the physician determine the patient's cardiac capacity and when sexual activity can be resumed.

There are five danger signs that the patient should be aware of with regard to sexual activity. These five symptoms may indicate that sexual intercourse is causing physiologic problems:
1. Dyspnea or increased heart rate that continues longer than 15 minutes after intercourse
2. Extreme fatigue the day after intercourse
3. Chest pain during intercourse
4. Palpitations lasting 15 minutes or longer after intercourse
5. Insomnia after intercourse

If any of these warning signs of possible cardiac stress should occur, the physician should be notified so that further evaluation can be performed.

Outcome criteria for the person with myocardial infarction

The person or significant others can:
1. Explain the nature of myocardial infarction and how the healing process relates to the treatment regimen.
2. Describe risk factors to be avoided and plans regarding any modifications in life-style.
3. State name, dosage, action, and side effects of prescribed medications.
4. Describe any dietary restriction, particularly those related to salt, fluids, and fats.
5. Describe exercise plans.
   a. Describe plans for progressive activity.
   b. Describe plans for a maintenance lifetime exercise program.
   c. Describe plans for resumption of sexual activity (if appropriate).
6. State plans for ongoing follow-up care.

Sudden cardiac death

It is estimated that in the United States each year at least 200,000 people are victims of sudden cardiac death. Sudden cardiac death is defined as death that occurs unexpectedly over a short period of time in a person who has been functioning adequately at the time of the event.[44]

Pathologic examinations performed on individuals who died suddenly have revealed several significant factors. It is especially common in persons with severe CAHD. Acute myocardial infarction as well as acute coronary occlusion are uncommon; however, signs of earlier infarctions are common. These observations suggest that the most predominant single cause of death in coronary arterial disease is cardiac arrhythmia. Ventricular fibrillation is thought to be the mechanism through which sudden cardiac death occurs.

Hypertensive heart disease

Hypertensive heart disease refers to changes in the heart from prolonged sustained hypertension (p. 1176), which increases afterload. The heart enlarges (as seen on radiographic examination) in an attempt to compensate for the increased cardiac workload. If the underlying hypertension is untreated, cardiac failure results.

Congestive heart failure

Heart failure (also known as congestive heart failure, cardiac decompensation, cardiac insufficiency, and cardiac incompetence) has been described clinically, physiologically, and biochemically, yet no definition has been accepted universally. One widely accepted definition of heart failure is a state in which the heart no longer is able to pump an adequate supply of blood to meet the demands of the body.

Heart failure can be classified as acute or chronic. *Acute* heart failure develops quickly and often without warning. The clinical picture may include syncope, shock, cardiac arrest, or sudden death. These outcomes are clearly the results of the myocardium failing to function adequately. Acute heart failure may result from decreased effectiveness of the heart after myocardial infarction. *Chronic* heart failure, on the other hand, develops gradually and the patient is seen initially with milder symptoms. The heart has the capability to compensate for the decreased performance, thus lessening the severity of symptoms.

Etiology

The causes of heart failure can be divided into three groups. The first group is made up of conditions that

result in direct damage to the heart and includes myocardial infarction, myocarditis, myocardial fibrosis, and ventricular aneurysm.

The second is made up of conditions that result in ventricular overload (p. 1037). Overload can be described in two subgroups:

1. *Preload.* Preload is the ventricular blood volume at end-diastole, the maximal ventricular blood volume for that beat of the heart. According to Starling's law, once the preload has reached a given limit, the effectiveness of the contraction diminishes resulting in heart failure. Increased preload can result from mitral or aortic regurgitation, atrial or ventricular septal defects, or rapid infusion of intravenous solutions.

2. *Afterload.* Afterload is the force that the ventricle must develop to eject blood into the circulatory system. This is the pressure against which the heart must work. Increased afterload may develop from aortic or pulmonary valve stenosis, systemic hypertension, or pulmonary hypertension.

The last major group of conditions that can lead to heart failure are those resulting in constriction of the ventricle, which limits ventricular filling and thus decreases stroke volume. Constriction can result from cardiac tamponade, constrictive cardiomyopathies and pericarditis.

Pathophysiology

Cardiac compensatory mechanisms

Three mechanisms of compensation that enable the weakened heart to continue to meet the metabolic demands of the body are tachycardia, ventricular dilation, and hypertrophy of the myocardium.

Tachycardia. By increasing the heart rate, cardiac output is also increased (see p. 1036 for discussion of cardiac output). As the heart rate continues to increase, however, diastole is shortened to the point where an inadequate filling of the ventricles occurs and cardiac output actually decreases.

Ventricular dilation. The myocardium has been demonstrated to function according to Starling's law of the heart. Starling's law states that within certain limits, cardiac muscle fibers contract more forcibly the more they are stretched before contraction. By increasing venous return to the heart, the fibers are stretched, which allows for a more forceful contraction, thus increasing stroke volume. This mechanism then results in increased cardiac output.

Hypertrophy of the myocardium. Hypertrophy, which is an increase in the diameter of muscle fibers, is seen as a thickening in the walls of the heart. This increase in muscle mass results in more effective contraction of the heart, further increasing cardiac output. The greatest limitation to hypertrophy as a compensatory mechanism is that the muscle mass outgrows the coronary artery supply, resulting in hypoxia and decreased effectiveness.

Homeostatic compensatory mechanisms

When cardiac compensatory mechanisms become inadequate to continue to meet the metabolic needs of the body, homeostatic compensatory mechanisms are activated. Knowledge of these physiologic responses are essential in understanding the treatment modalities for congestive heart failure.

Vascular system. As the circulating blood volume is decreased, sympathetic stimulation and release of norepinephrine result in generalized vasoconstriction. Both arterial circulation and venous circulation are affected.

Kidneys. Vasoconstriction and low cardiac output have a profound effect on renal perfusion. When cardiac output falls to one half to two thirds of normal, complete anuria can occur. As arterial pressure in the kidneys is diminished, glomerular filtration is reduced, resulting in retention of sodium and water. Aldosterone secretion by the adrenal cortex is stimulated, resulting in further reabsorption of sodium by the renal tubules. Osmotic pressure is increased by the rising sodium concentration, leading to release of antidiuretic hormone by the hypothalamus. The end result is increased tubular reabsorption of water, leading to fluid overload and edema (Fig. 45-10).

Liver. The venous volume increases to such an extent that hepatic congestion develops, resulting in decreased effectiveness of all hepatic functions. The liver normally metabolizes aldosterone and antidiuretic hor-

mone. Since the congested liver has a reduced ability to metabolize these substances, hepatic congestion serves to further compound heart failure.

Classifications of heart failure

Heart failure has been classified into three main categories. These include backward vs. forward, left vs. right, and low vs. high output heart failure.

Backward vs. forward heart failure. Backward vs. forward heart failure is perhaps the oldest method of classifying heart failure. Backward failure is said to be the result of damming up of blood in the vessels proximal to the heart. Forward heart failure, conversely, is the result of the inability of the heart to maintain cardiac output. It should be emphasized that since the heart is part of a closed system, forward failure and backward failure will always be associated with each other.

Left vs. right heart failure. The most common event would be for one ventricle to fail before the other. Since the left ventricle is most often affected by coronary atherosclerosis and hypertension, heart failure usually begins there. Left ventricular failure is usually signalled by pulmonary congestion and edema. Right ventricular failure is most often triggered by left ventricular failure. Right ventricular failure usually leads to systemic venous congestion and peripheral edema. However, when the patient usually seeks health care, signs and symptoms of both right and left heart failure are present.

Low- vs. high-output heart failure. With the development of diagnostic tools that allow for the measurement of cardiac output (cardiac catheterization), heart

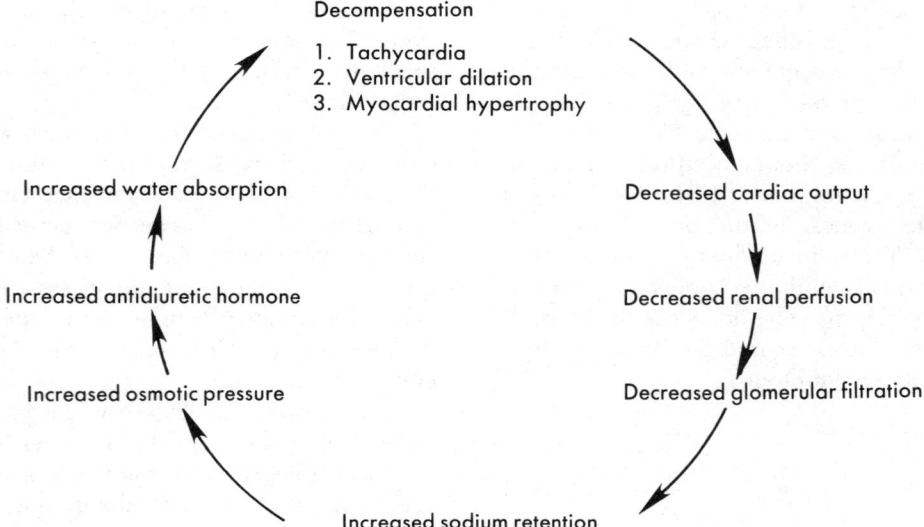

Fig. 45-10. Sequel of events compounding decompensation in chronic heart failure.

failure can be classified by the effectiveness of the heart as a pump. When cardiac output remains normal or above normal but the metabolic needs of the body are not met, the heart failure is termed *high output*. Causes of high output failure include hyperthyroidism, anemia, Paget's disease, and arteriovenous fistula. When cardiac output falls below normal, the results are termed *low-output heart failure* and can result from arteriosclerosis, hypertension, myocardial infarction, and valvular disorder.

Clinical picture

The symptoms of heart failure are the result of excessive fluid retention by the body. The congestion that results can involve either the venous system or the pulmonary system and eventually both. As the effectiveness of the heart as a pump decreases, venous stasis occurs and venous pressure increases. The result is further fluid retention by the kidneys, leading to the following clinical picture. For ease of description, the symptoms have been described individually for both right and left ventricular failure.

Right ventricular failure

The most common cause of right ventricular failure is left ventricular failure; therefore right ventricular failure is rarely seen alone. In right ventricular failure the right ventricle compensates in response to an increase in pulmonary artery pressure. The heart becomes less effective and is unable to maintain adequate output against the increased resistance. This results in blood damming back into the systemic circulation, leading to peripheral edema. This edema is of the pitting type and is nontender. It is also known as dependent edema because it occurs in dependent parts of the body such as the legs or sacrum. As the edema becomes more pronounced, it progresses up the legs into the thighs, external genitalia, and lower trunk. As the tissue becomes extremely engorged, the skin cracks and fluid may "weep" from the tissues.

The liver may also become engorged with intravascular fluid, resulting in enlargement and tenderness in the right upper quadrant of the abdomen. As the venous stasis increases, pressure within the portal system becomes so great that fluid is forced through the blood vessels into the abdominal cavity. The collection of fluid within the abdomen, known as ascites, can reach volumes of more than 10L. This great volume of fluid can displace the diaphragm, resulting in severe respiratory distress. A paracentesis (p. 690) may be required to relieve the pressure on the diaphragm. Distended neck veins as a result of the increased systemic venous pressure are usually observed when the patient is in a sitting position (see Fig. 43-6).

Left ventricular failure

In left ventricular failure, the left ventricle cannot pump oxygenated blood coming from the lungs at a volume necessary to meet the demands of the body. Symptoms are the result of congestion of the lungs with fluid that is forced from the pulmonary circulation into the pulmonary tissues, causing pulmonary edema (p. 1135) and pleural effusion. Fluid may be present in the interstitial tissues, alveoli, bronchioles, or pleural space.

Respiratory signs and symptoms. *Dyspnea*, labored breathing, is an early symptom of left ventricular failure. It is caused by interference with gas exchange as a result of the fluid in the alveoli. Dyspnea may occur or may become worse only on physical exertion, such as climbing stairs, walking up an incline, or walking against the wind, since these activities require increased amounts of oxygen.

Orthopnea, difficulty in breathing when lying flat, may be present and persons often must sleep propped up in bed or in a chair. When the person is lying flat there is decreased ventilation and the blood volume in the pulmonary vessels is increased. The orthopnea is often described by the number of pillows required for the patient to rest comfortably when in bed, for example, three-pillow orthopnea. Although orthopnea may occur immediately after lying down, it often does not occur for several hours, at which time, it causes the person to wake with severe dyspnea and coughing. This condition is known as *paroxysmal nocturnal dyspnea* and results from the accumulation of fluid in the lungs as the person is lying in bed. The patient usually experiences a feeling of suffocation and often awakens in panic.

In heart failure the patient may experience alternating periods of *apnea* and *hyperpnea* (Cheyne-Stokes respirations). Often because of respiratory insufficiency, an inadequate amount of oxygen is delivered to the brain. The decrease in oxygen makes the respiratory center in the brain insensitive to the amounts of carbon dioxide in the arterial blood, and respirations cease either until the carbon dioxide content in the arterial blood increases enough to stimulate the respiratory center or until the oxygen level in the blood drops to a level that is low enough to stimulate the respiratory center. This results in hyperpnea. These periods of overbreathing result in greater than normal decreases in carbon dioxide content of arterial blood, producing another period of apnea. Periodic overbreathing often begins as the patient goes to sleep and decreases as sleep deepens and ventilation decreases. Cheyne-Stokes respiration can often be improved by administration of morphine sulfate, which suppresses respirations. The use of morphine sulfate has the added advantage of reducing patient anxiety. High concentrations of oxygen generally are contraindicated since this would prevent the reflex stimulus to respiration caused by low oxygen content in the blood.

A persistent hacking *cough* is often a symptom of left-sided heart failure. The cough is usually productive of large quantities of frothy sputum, which is occasionally blood tinged. Coughing results from congestion of trapped fluid, which is irritating to the mucosal lining of the lungs and bronchi. On auscultation *rales* can be heard. Rales are the moist popping and crackling sounds heard most often at the end of inspiration.

Fatigue. Persons with heart failure commonly note fatigue following activities that ordinarily are not tiring. The fatigue results from impaired blood circulation to tissues as a result of the decreased cardiac output. The reduction in tissue oxygen decreases the aerobic production of adenosine triphosphate (ATP), the immediate energy source for muscle contractions. In addition, the impaired circulation decreases removal of metabolic waste products, resulting in further decreased muscle function.

Pain. Cardiac pain is *not* a typical symptom of heart failure; however, angina pectoris can occur from the decrease in cardiac output. Cardiac pain associated with congestive heart failure is most likely to occur in patients with coronary artery disease. Coronary artery disease increases the patient's sensitivity to a deficiency in the oxygen content in the circulating blood. As heart failure develops, the blood is less effectively oxygenated and angina occurs. As the fluid overload state is corrected, the chest pain resolves.

Anxiety. Most persons are aware of the importance of an effective functioning heart to maintain life and persons are acquainted with symptoms that indicate a failing heart. Anxiety usually occurs, therefore, when symptoms of heart failure are present. Anxiety can cause increased breathlessness, which is then interpreted by the patient as an increase in the severity of the heart failure, and this in turn increases the anxiety.

Intervention

At many acute care hospitals patients with acute congestive heart failure are admitted to medical or cardiac intensive care units if the institution has such a facility. Occasionally, the physician may elect to place the patient in the usual room accomodations where the environment is less stressful and where family members can visit more routinely. The decision about room placement is made on the basis of degree of failure and specific responses of the individual patient to the acute situation.

The primary goals of treatment for congestive heart failure are to restore a balance between the supply and demand for blood by body tissues and removal of excessive fluid from the circulating blood volume. The desired outcome of therapy is improvement in signs and symptoms as seen by (1) easier breathing patterns (nonlabored), (2) absence or marked reduction in edema, and (3) normal respiratory rate without the use of supplemental oxygen. These objectives are accomplished by reducing the requirements of the body for oxygen and by optimizing cardiac output.

Providing oxygenation. In heart failure the oxygen content of the bloodstream may be markedly reduced because of the less effective oxygenation of the blood as it passes through the congested lungs. The patient may be more comfortable and better able to rest when receiving oxygen, since it helps in reducing dyspnea and fatigue. Oxygen is usually administered by nasal cannula at 2 to 6 L/min. Baseline arterial blood gases are obtained at initiation of oxygen therapy and intermittently during therapy to assess effectiveness of the treatment. Breathing is often made easier by maintaining the patient in semi-Fowler's or high Fowler's position. These positions maximize oxygenation by permitting greater lung expansion.

Promoting rest and activity. Reducing the requirements of the body for oxygen can best be effected by providing the patient with the degree of activity that does not compromise myocardial function, as demonstrated by the presence of symptoms. If the degree of heart failure is mild, with only edema of the legs or minimal pulmonary congestion, the patient may be treated on an ambulatory basis with only a regimen of less strenuous activity and more rest than usual.

If the degree of heart failure is severe, a program of bed rest or limited activity may be necessary until symptoms abate. The amount of activity permitted each person is a function of the extent of symptoms such as dyspnea and fatigue. A careful assessment must be made each day to determine to what extent the person can perform ADL such as eating and bathing. Most patients prefer to maximize their independence, and this is encouraged within the limitations of their symptoms.

Sedation is used judiciously for patients with heart failure since oversedation may mask symptoms of increasing failure. In addition, immobility increases the risk of venous thrombosis and embolus. Patients with heart failure are often apprehensive and may have difficulty relaxing; thus diazepam (Valium), 2 to 10 mg three to four times a day, may be prescribed. Chloral hydrate or flurazepam hydrochloride (Dalmane) may be used if the person is unable to sleep despite nursing measures to promote rest.

The patient is often orthopneic and tends to be more comfortable sitting than lying in bed. If the patient is placed in a chair, the feet are elevated to reducing pooling of fluid in the dependent limbs. When the patient is placed on bed rest, high Fowler's position is often most comfortable. A pillow may be placed lengthwise behind the shoulders and back in such a manner

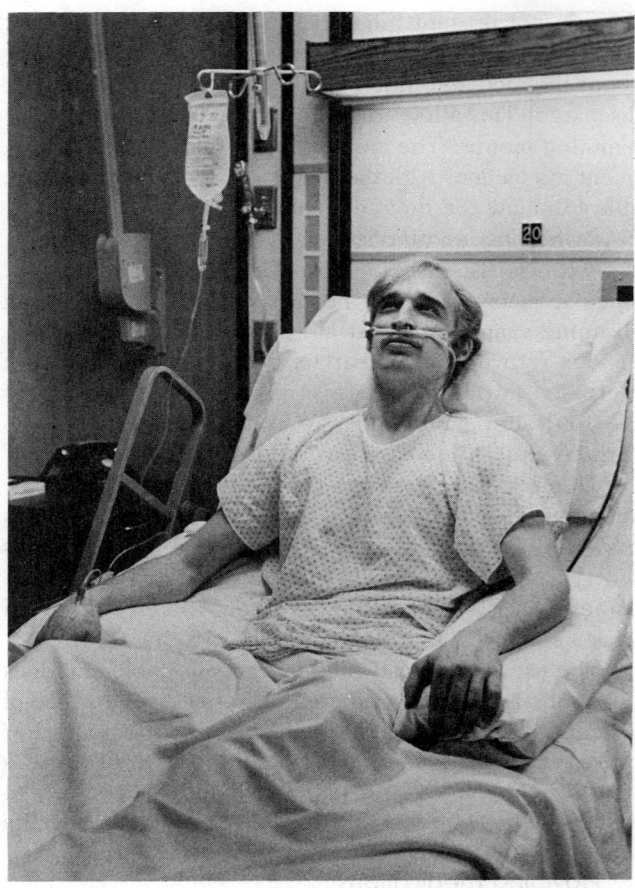

Fig. 45-11. Patient is sitting upright with pillows under head and each arm to promote chest expansion and comfort.

that full expansion of the rib cage is possible. A foot block can be used to keep the patient from slipping toward the foot of the bed. The arms may also be supported on pillows to reduce the pull on the shoulder muscles (Fig. 45-11). An over-the-bed table may be placed close to the patient to allow resting the head and arms (see Fig. 49-8).

AMBULATION. Ambulation is started slowly to avoid overloading the heart and to determine how much activity the heart can tolerate without again showing signs of failure. The regimen varies depending on individual patient response. When a patient has been on restricted bed rest, activities progress slowly through stages of dangling, sitting up in a chair, and then walking increased distances under close supervision. The patient is assessed for signs indicating that activity cannot be tolerated, including dyspnea, fatigue, and increased pulse rate that does not stabilize readily. If these signs or symptoms occur, the person is returned to bed. If dyspnea is present, the head of the bed is elevated and oxygen is administered at a low flow of 1 to 3 L/min. The physician is consulted before further ambulation is attempted.

The plan for increased activity is explained to the patient and family. They should understand that if activity tires the person excessively, it may be curtailed. Overactivity can produce physical and mental setbacks that delay ultimate recovery. In the early stages of ambulation it is important to begin stressing the importance of the rate of activity; that is, the demand on the heart is decreased when a normal activity is performed more slowly than before.

Providing emotional support. An assessment is made of the degree of the patient's anxiety and coping skills (see Chapter 14). The goal of intervention is to help break the anxiety–increased symptoms–anxiety circle by helping the patient (1) identify feelings and the content related to those feelings, (2) identify strengths that can be used for coping, and (3) learn what can be done to decrease the anxiety. Learning about measures to control heart failure and measures to reduce stress (see Chapter 13) may be helpful. Working with family members in the same manner is also helpful to decrease their anxiety so that they can be of greater support to the patient.

Monitoring daily weights. Although careful records of intake and output are kept on most patients with cardiac failure, the best method to estimate progress and response to prescribed diet, medications, and other forms of treatment is daily monitoring of the patient's weight. Weight gain indicates fluid retention; 1 kg of weight gain represents 1 L of fluid retention. The weight is carefully recorded on admission and then daily while the patient is hospitalized.

The patient with severe heart failure is weighed on a litter scale, which contains a stretcher to minimize exertion. The patient should be weighed at the same time of day with the same amount of clothing. A good practice is to weigh the patient each morning after the bladder had been emptied and before breakfast is eaten. The patient is also encouraged to continue to take his or her weight daily after being discharged to provide weight gain information for the health care provider.

Providing skin care. Edematous skin is poorly nourished and very susceptible to breakdown. Edema of the sacrum is prevalent in patients with heart failure restricted to bed rest and decubiti can develop quickly. The patient is carefully positioned and turned frequently to minimize breakdown. Measures to prevent skin breakdown (p. 941) are instituted early since prevention is more cost effective for both patient and care provider in addition to promoting patient comfort, both physical and mental. Flotation mattresses and water beds are of assistance in preventing decubiti; however, neither eliminates the need for turning the patient.

Promoting nutrition. During the acute stage of congestive heart failure the diet should be soft or liquid, and easily digested foods should be served. Anorexia is often present due to edema in the gastrointestinal tract, dyspnea, fatigue and the effect of medications. Frequent small feedings minimize exertion and reduce gastrointestinal blood requirements, which can tax the failing heart. Care must be taken in providing a diet that meets the metabolic demands of the body so that body wasting does not occur.

SODIUM INTAKE. Edema is often effectively controlled in patients with heart failure by restriction of sodium intake. The degree of restriction depends on the severity of the failure and the extent of diuretic therapy. The severely restricted sodium diet is rarely prescribed, since the diet is unpalatable and expensive, resulting in poor patient compliance.

The amount of sodium in the normal diet is 3 to 10 g/day. Sodium restriction in persons receiving diuretics may not be dropped below 3 to 5 g/day because of the dangers of hyponatremia from removal of sodium as well as water by the action of the diuretic on the kidneys. In mild cardiac failure sodium may be restricted to 1 to 2 g/day. This is known as a no-added-salt (NAS) diet and is essentially a normal diet except that no extra salt is added to prepared foods and obviously salted foods such as potato chips are omitted. For moderate or severe heart failure the amount of sodium permitted is specifically prescribed. Vitamin supplements are usually required when severely restricted sodium diets are prescribed.

Low-sodium diets can be made more appealing by adding salt substitutes to food in place of table salt. Since many salt substitutes contain potassium, the patient's need for potassium must be assessed. Often the increased intake of potassium is beneficial when the patient is on diuretic therapy. The use of herbs, such as basil, dill, bay leaves, garlic (powder not salt), and tarragon, often makes the food more appetizing.

FLUIDS. Fluid restriction is less commonly instituted than in the past as long as the person is on a sodium-controlled diet and is receiving diuretics or digitalis or both. When sodium intake is controlled, patients usually do not experience thirst and will control their own fluid intake. The kidneys will also remove water from the body to maintain proper sodium concentration. If fluids are restricted, the amount of fluid permitted is prescribed by the physician and a plan is made, in conjunction with the patient if possible, to space the fluids over the day depending on patient preferences. Usually one half of the fluids are planned for meals and the other half for between meals. If thirst does present a problem, frequent mouth care may add to patient comfort.

NUTRITION EDUCATION OF PERSON AND FAMILY. The rationale for dietary and fluid restrictions must be explained to both the patient and the family. The family must understand the necessity for these restrictions so they do not present the patient with food or fluids that are unacceptable. The patient needs to learn early about the food and fluid restrictions to be followed after discharge. This allows time for answering questions and planning menus. The ambulatory patient may need frequent interactions with the dietitian or nurse before being able to follow the diet adequately.

Promoting elimination. It is advisable for the person with cardiac disease to avoid straining at defecation, since it places an extra burden on the heart. During straining against a closed glottis (Valsalva's maneuver), venous return to the heart is decreased as a result of increased intrathoracic pressure. When this pressure is released after straining, a large amount of venous return creates an increased work load on the heart.

The feces can be kept soft by giving a mild cathartic such as milk of magnesia, a mild bulk cathartic such as psyllium (Metamucil), or a stool-softening agent such as dioctyl sodium sulfosuccinate (Colace). If an enema becomes necessary, it should be of low volume and given with a small rectal tube inserted only 3 to 4 in.

The use of a bedpan is often uncomfortable and does not facilitate bowel evacuation. The necessity for use of a bedpan often will create anxiety in the patient. For these reasons the patient is usually permitted to use a bedside commode. The patient should be assisted to and from the commode. Privacy is provided, but the patient is not left unattended.

Providing medications

DIGITALIS THERAPY. Digitalis is the major therapeutic approach in the treatment of congestive heart failure. Digitalis and its derivatives usually are effective in improving myocardial function in persons with congestive heart failure. The positive inotropic action of digitalis preparations enhances mechanical performance by strengthening the force of myocardial contraction. This leads to increased cardiac output and increased blood flow to the kidneys. Digitalis preparations also decrease heart rate (automaticity) and cardiac conduction velocity, which permits the ventricles to relax more in order to allow time for better filling of the ventricles with blood.

When acute congestive heart failure occurs, the physician usually orders an *optimal therapeutic dose* of a digitalis preparation to slow the ventricular rate and decrease symptoms. This larger dose given over a short period of time, usually 24 to 48 hours, is called a *loading*, or *digitalizing*, dose. In some instances the dose may approach the toxic level, and the person is observed carefully for signs and symptoms of toxicity (see box, p. 1133). The full effect of the digitalizing drug is realized when the heart and circulation return to normal under treatment, and the symptoms of toxicity are more evident at this time. Since digitalis preparations have a *cumulative effect* and are slowly eliminated, early recognition of toxic symptoms and discontinuance of the

SIGNS AND SYMPTOMS OF DIGITALIS TOXICITY

Cardiovascular effects
  Bradycardia

  Tachycardia

  Bigeminy

  Ectopic beats

  Pulse deficit

Gastrointestinal effects
  Anorexia

  Nausea and vomiting

  Abdominal pain

  Diarrhea

Neurologic effects
  Headache

  Double vision

  Blurred or colored vision

  Drowsiness, confusion

  Restlessness, irritability

  Muscle weakness

drug will decrease their severity. After the optimal therapeutic dose has been determined, the person is given a daily maintenance dose of digitalis.

Several factors predispose the person to digitalis toxicity. One of the most common is hypokalemia, which potentiates the effects of digitalis. When potassium is depleted in the body or myocardium, the heart becomes more excitable and arrhythmias may occur. Decrease in potassium levels below the normal range of 4.0 to 5.4 mEq/L can occur whenever excess potassium is lost from the body such as occurs in vomiting and diarrhea or induced diuresis. Most of the diuretics used to treat congestive heart failure result in the loss of potassium along with sodium and water. Therefore the nurse must be alert to changes in the patient's serum potassium blood levels. In order to replace the potassium lost through diuresis, persons are often placed on a supplemental form of potassium such as potassium chloride. Some diuretics have potassium added to them, but many physicians prefer to order the diuretics and potassium separately. In addition, foods such as orange juice or bananas, which are high in potassium and low in sodium content, should be encouraged (p. 339).

Other predisposing factors to digitalis toxicity include severe liver and kidney disease, since the liver inactivates the drug and the kidney excretes it, and primary myocardial disease, which makes the myocardium more sensitive to the drug. Increased toxicity also oc-

curs with alkalosis, hypercalcemia, hypomagnesemia, and hypothyroidism. If digitalis toxicity occurs, the medication is stopped at once and other therapy instituted as necessary. This often includes administration of procainamide and potassium chloride.

Numerous types of digitalis preparations may be used (Table 45-5). For rapid digitalization in emergency situations, deslanoside (Cedilanid-D) or G-strophanthin (Ouabain) is usually selected. Digoxin or digitoxin is most commonly used for maintenance drug therapy. Digoxin has a more rapid effect than digitoxin yet has sufficient duration for adequate maintenance therapy. If given intramuscularly, digoxin should be injected deeply and the area massaged after injection because the drug is a tissue irritant. Powdered digitalis is highly toxic and is therefore rarely used.

Before a digitalis preparation is given, the apical pulse rate is taken. If this rate is below 60, the medication should be withheld until the physician has been consulted. The pulse rate of persons with irregular rhythm should always be taken for a full minute for accuracy. Response to digitalis is evaluated on the basis of relief of symptoms, that is, decreased edema, loss of weight, fluid output greater than fluid intake, and no dyspnea or cyanosis.

DIURETIC THERAPY. Diuretic therapy is not a substitute for digitalis therapy, which has a direct action on the myocardium. Diuretics are potentially dangerous medications and their use is instituted only after symptoms of heart failure persist following digitalization and sodium restriction. The purpose of diuretic therapy is to decrease cardiac workload by reducing circulating volume and thus decrease symptoms.

Essential to proper initiation of diuretic therapy is determining how much fluid should be removed from the patient by establishing a "dry weight," or edema-free weight. This can be accomplished by gradually removing fluid by use of diuretics and assessing the patient's blood pressure. When the patient becomes hypotensive, particularly orthostatic, this signals the physician that too much fluid has been removed. The patient is then permitted to reaccumulate a small amount of fluid until hypotension no longer occurs. The weight at which this occurs is then considered the patient's dry weight. This can all be accomplished by adjusting the dose of diuretics. Adjustments in diuretic therapy can best be accomplished while the patient is hospitalized; however, changes in the patient's diet when discharged will affect the equilibrium obtained while the patient is hospitalized. The patient is instructed to seek medical attention for signs of dyspnea, rapid weight gain or weight gain in the absence of increased food intake, and edema.

Diuretics function by increasing the urinary output, which decreases blood volume, thereby reducing cardiac workload. This is accomplished primarily by inhibiting the reabsorption of sodium by the kidneys. Mer-

TABLE 45-5. Digitalis preparations

Generic name	Trade name	Digitalizing dose (time)	Maintenance dose	Route	Onset	Duration
Purple foxglove *(Digitalis purpurea)*						
Powdered digitalis	Digifortis Digiglusin	1-2 g (24-48 hr)	100-200 mg	Oral	Slow	Long
Digitoxin	Crystodigin Purodigin Digitaline Nativelle Unidigin	1.2-1.6 mg 0.05-0.6 mg (24-48 hr)	100-200 mg	IV Oral	Slow	Long
Gitalin	Gitaligin	2.5-6 mg (3-4 days)	0.5 mg	Oral	Fast	Moderate
White foxglove *(Digitalis lanata)*						
Digoxin	Lanoxin	1.0-1.5 mg 0.25-0.5 mg (12-24 hr)	0.125-0.50 mg	Oral IV IM	Fast	Moderate
Deslanoside	Cedilanid-D	0.8-1.6 mg (12 hr)	0.25-0.5 mg	IV IM	Fast	Short
Lanatoside C	Cedilanid	10 mg (4 days)	0.5 mg	Oral	Variable	Short
Acetyldigitoxin	Acylanid	1.6-2.2 mg (24 hr)	0.1-0.2 mg	Oral	Moderate	Short
Strophanthus gratus						
G-strophanthin	Ouabain	0.25-0.5 mg (12-24 hr)	—	IV	Fast	Short

TABLE 45-6. Diuretics used in the treatment of heart failure

Type	Example	Onset/peak/duration	Dose	Side effects
Thiazide	Chlorothiazide (Diuril)	2 hr/4 hr/6-12 hr	0.5-1.0 g once or twice a day	Gastrointestinal upsets (can be minimized by taking medication with meals); hypokalemia; hyperglycemia
	Hydrochlorothiazide (Esidrix, Hydrodiuril)	2 hr/4 hr/6-12 hr	25-100 mg/day	
Loop	Furosemide (Lasix)	1 hr/1-2 hr/6-8 hr	20-80 mg/day orally (may be given intravenously in doses up to 600 mg in 24 hr to treat pulmonary edema)	Similar to thiazide diurectics; also ototoxicity and blood dyscrasias
	Ethacrynic acid (Edecrin)	30 min/2 hr/6 hr	50-200 mg/day	
Potassium sparing	Spironolactone (Aldactone)	Gradual/3 days/2-3 days after therapy discontinued	25-50 mg four times a day	Gastrointestinal irritation; hyperkalemia
	Triamterene (Dyrenium)	Rapid/7-9 hr/12-16 hr	150-200 mg once a day	

curial diuretics affect the proximal tubules, furosemide and ethacrynic acid affect the ascending loop of Henle, thiazides and triamterene affect the distal tubule, while spironolactone exerts its effect on the collecting duct. Dosages and side effects of these diuretics are listed in Table 45-6.

The development of newer more potent oral diuret-

ics in the late 1950s has enhanced the success of relieving symptoms of excessive fluid retention in persons with severe congestive heart failure. Before that time, mercurial diuretics were often potentiated by the use of other drugs, such as acidifying chlorides (ammonium chloride), carbonic anhydrase inhibitors (e.g., Diamox), and aminophylline. Occasionally these treatment methods are used when current routine methods of treating heart failure are unsuccessful.

Currently, the *thiazides* are the diuretics of choice in the treatment of heart failure. The thiazides are inexpensive, easy to take, and effective when taken over a long period of time. Because these potent drugs can lead to electrolyte imbalance, serum chemistry levels should be observed closely, particularly at the onset of therapy. The major complication is hypokalemia, which can be prevented by the intake of foods high in potassium or by potassium supplements.

If thiazides are ineffective, an oral aldosterone antagonist, such as spironolactone (Aldactone) or triamterene (Dyrenium), may be given with the thiazide. These drugs work by competitive inhibition of aldosterone, resulting in retention of potassium and excretion of sodium and water.

The most potent diuretics currently available are furosemide (Lasix) and ethacrynic acid (Edecrin). These medications are reserved for severe congestive heart failure or when other forms of treatment are ineffective in relieving symptoms. These agents also increase renal blood flow and therefore may prove effective in treating heart failure when renal function is also impaired. Therapy is best initiated in the hospital setting so that electrolyte and acid-base balance may be monitored. The patient needs to be thoroughly knowledgeable about the use of these medications before being discharged from the hospital.

Complication of congestive heart failure: acute pulmonary edema

Etiology

Acute pulmonary edema is a medical emergency arising from severe left ventricular failure. It usually results from prolonged strain on a diseased heart. It may also result from inhalation of irritating gases or from too rapid administration of plasma, serum albumin, whole blood, or intravenous fluids; or it may be associated with barbiturate or opiate poisoning.

Pathophysiology

In pulmonary edema caused by heart failure, cardiac output is decreased, resulting in an increase in left atrial pressure. This results in an increase in pulmonary vein and capillary pressure. As the pulmonary capillary pressure exceeds the intravascular osmotic pressure, serous fluid is rapidly forced into the alveoli. Fluid rapidly reaches the bronchioles and bronchi, and patients literally begin to drown in their own secretions.

Clinical picture

Signs and symptoms of pulmonary edema include restlessness and vague uneasiness at the onset. As pulmonary edema progresses, the patient develops profound dyspnea, pallor, cough productive of large quantities of blood-tinged frothy sputum, audible wheezing, and cyanosis. Tachycardia is often present.

Intervention

The goals in the treatment of acute pulmonary edema include physical and mental relaxation, relief of hypoxemia, retardation of venous return, and improvement of cardiovascular function.

The patient with acute pulmonary edema is placed in bed in high Fowler's position, and the physician is summoned immediately. Treatment is usually begun by administering morphine sulfate, 10 to 15 mg intravenously. The intravenous route is preferred since vascular collapse may hinder its absorption from subcutaneous tissues. The mechanism of action of morphine in this setting is not completely understood; however, the drug reduces anxiety, slows respirations, and reduces venous return.

To relieve hypoxemia, the physician often orders oxygen at 40% to 70% to be delivered by face mask. Humidification is desirable to keep secretions moist and facilitate mobilization of these secretions. Occasionally, the patient with severe pulmonary embarrassment will require intubation to deliver adequate tidal volumes and oxygen concentration. Intubation also aids in removing secretions by suctioning. The patient is often extubated within hours of the initiation of therapy. Aminophylline may also be administered intravenously in the treatment of pulmonary edema to dilate the bronchi, increase urinary output, and increase cardiac output.

The treatments described earlier for congestive heart failure are also implemented for pulmonary edema, including rapid digitalization and institution of diuretic therapy using furosemide. Serum potassium levels are obtained immediately since these patients have large diuresis and lose large amounts of potassium.

Two more radical treatments that may be used when the preceding regimens fail include phlebotomy and rotating tourniquets. The purpose of phlebotomy is to decrease the amount of circulating blood to decrease pulmonary engorgement; however, this removes hemoglobin that may further contribute to hypoxemia.

The purpose of rotating tourniquets is to pool blood in the extremities, thus reducing cardiac overload. As much as 1 L of blood may be trapped in the extremities when tourniquets are used. The tourniquets are placed on three extremities at one time (Fig. 45-12). Every 15 minutes in clockwise or counterclockwise order, one tourniquet is placed on the extremity that has no tourniquet and one tourniquet is removed. Thus each extremity is occluded for 45 minutes. A rotating tourniquet machine uses blood pressure cuffs as tourniquets and automatically pumps and deflates the cuffs to obtain the desired effect. Since the purpose of this

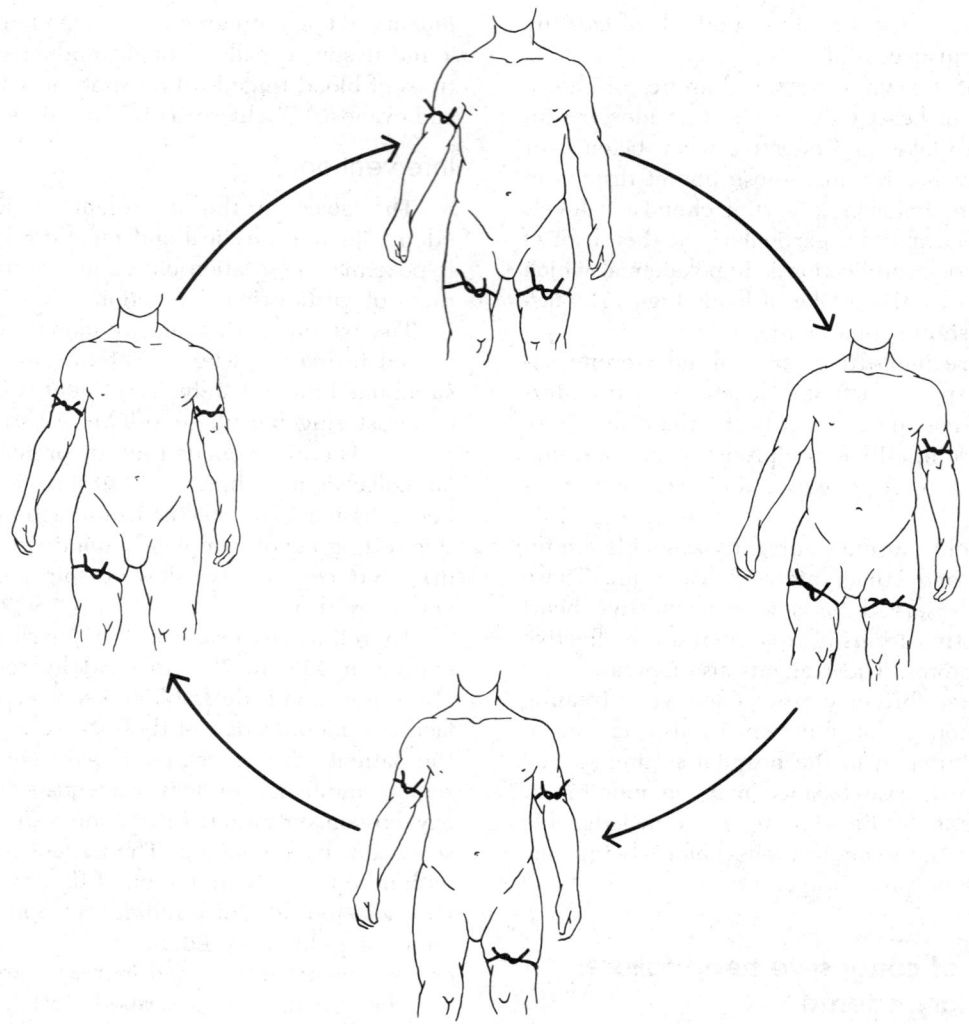

Fig. 45-12. Clockwise method of removing and applying rotating tourniquets.

therapy is to occlude venous blood, the tourniquets should not obliterate arterial pulses in the extremity. If an extremity does not return readily to normal color on release of a tourniquet, the physician is informed. When the procedure is terminated, the tourniquets are released, one every 15 minutes to prevent a sudden increase in venous return and recurrence of pulmonary edema.

Long-term care

The patient with congestive heart failure needs to know the reasons for symptoms and the rationale for the therapies, especially those that will be carried out on a long-term basis. Digitalis and diuretic medications are often prescribed for long periods of time, and it becomes difficult for the patient to remember when to take the correct medications. A method should be es-

tablished to ensure that the patient can carry out the medication regimen correctly. A medication chart listing all medications, doses, times of doses, and side effects may prove helpful. Teaching should also be directed at prevention of overexertion. If diet and/or fluid restrictions have been prescribed, the nurse assesses the patient's comprehension of these before discharge. Ongoing health management of persons who have congestive heart failure and whose condition has been stabilized is one area in which nurses are assuming a more active role.

Outcome criteria for the person with congestive heart failure

The person or significant others can:
1. Describe a plan for activity (ADL, work, recreation) that will avoid fatigue or dyspnea.

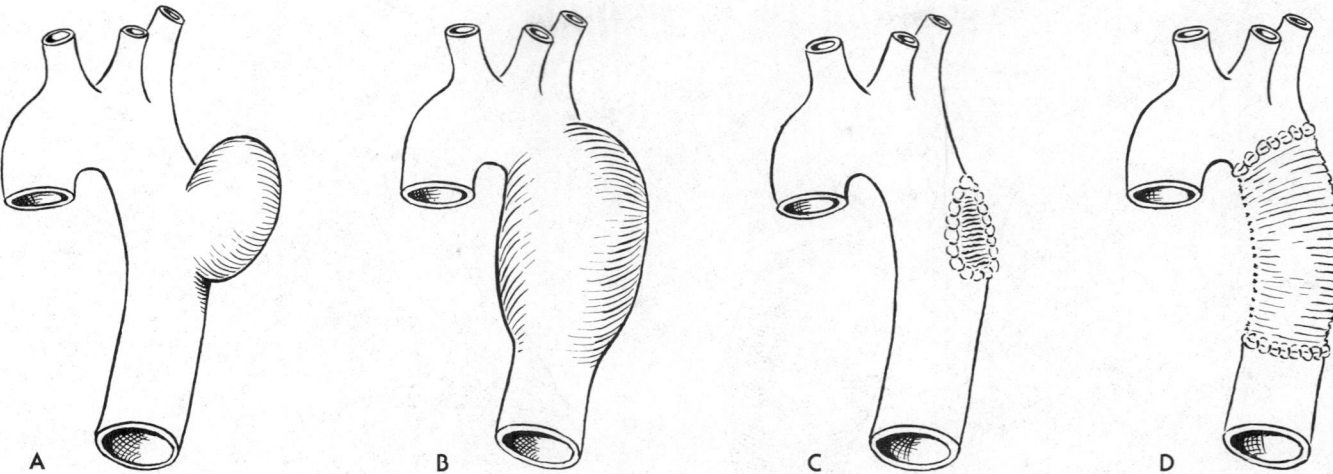

Fig. 45-13. Aneurysms of thoracic artery. **A,** Saccular aneurysm. **B,** Fusiform aneurysm. **C,** Patch-graft repair of saccular aneurysm. **D,** Replacement graft for fusiform aneurysm. (Redrawn from Bloodwell, R.D., et al.: Surg. Clin. North Am. **46:**901-911, 1966.)

2. Plan a diet incorporating any prescribed sodium or fluid restrictions.
3. Explain the medication therapy.
   a. State name, purpose, dosage, frequency, and side effects of prescribed medications (digitalis, diuretics).
   b. Describe a method for remembering to take prescribed medications as directed
   c. State what to do if a medication has been omitted.
4. State plans for follow-up care.
   a. State signs and symptoms requiring health care follow-up (dyspnea, rapid weight gain or weight gain in absence of increased food intake, edema).
   b. State plans for ongoing care with a health professional.

Aneurysms

Etiology

An aneurysm is a localized or diffuse enlargement of an artery at some point along its course. Aneurysms occur when the vessel wall becomes weakened from trauma, congenital vascular disease, infection, and atherosclerosis. Syphilitic aneurysms of the arch of the aorta still occur, but the vast majority of aneurysms, regardless of location, are caused by atherosclerosis.

Pathophysiology

Although the pathologic processes involved in the formation of an aneurysm are varied, certain factors are common to all. Once an aneurysm develops and the arterial tunica media (the middle coat composed of layers of smooth muscle and elastic tissue) is damaged, there is a tendency toward progressive dilation, degeneration, and a risk of rupture. Aneurysms may develop in any blood vessel, but the most common site is the aorta.

A *saccular* aneurysm involves only part of the circumference of the artery. It takes the form of a sac or pouchlike dilation attached to the side of the artery. A *fusiform* aneurysm is spindle shaped and involves the entire circumference of the arterial wall (Fig. 45-13). A *dissecting* aneurysm involves hemorrhage into a vessel wall, which splits and dissects the wall causing a widening of the vessel. Dissecting aneurysms are caused by a degenerative defect in the tunica media, probably as a result of the great hemodynamic stresses to which it is subjected.

Clinical picture

The most common site for the formation of an aortic aneurysm is the abdominal aorta below the renal arteries. The person may be asymptomatic and the condition evident only as a pulsatile abdominal mass, which may be found on a routine physical examination. At other times the person may have pain or tenderness in the mid or upper abdomen. Aneurysm of the abdominal aorta is a serious disease entity, and the mortality is high with rupture. A dissecting aneurysm of the aorta may develop slowly with few symptoms or may be acute with severe chest pain that may be mistaken for a myocardial infarction.

Routine chest and abdominal radiographs have proved to be very helpful in case finding and preliminary diagnosis of aortic aneurysms. Such studies frequently reveal a ring of calcification outlining the aneu-

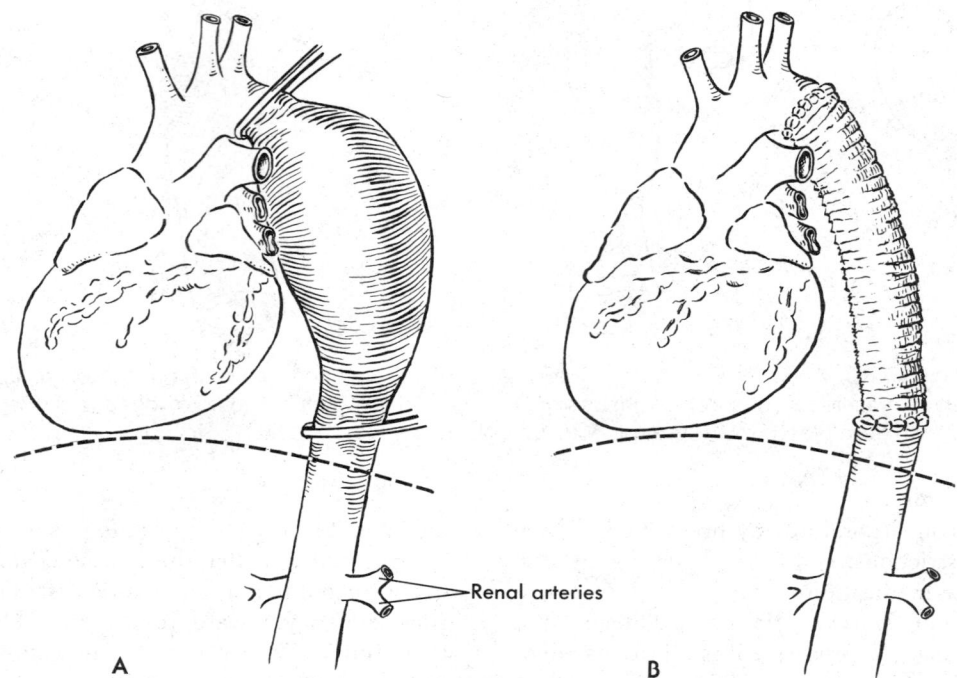

Fig. 45-14. Aneurysm of descending thoracic artery. **A,** Resection of thoracic aorta with cardiovascular clamps in place. **B,** Permanent replacement graft after resection of aneurysm. (Redrawn from Bloodwell, R.D., et al.: Surg. Clin. North Am. **46:**901-911, 1966.)

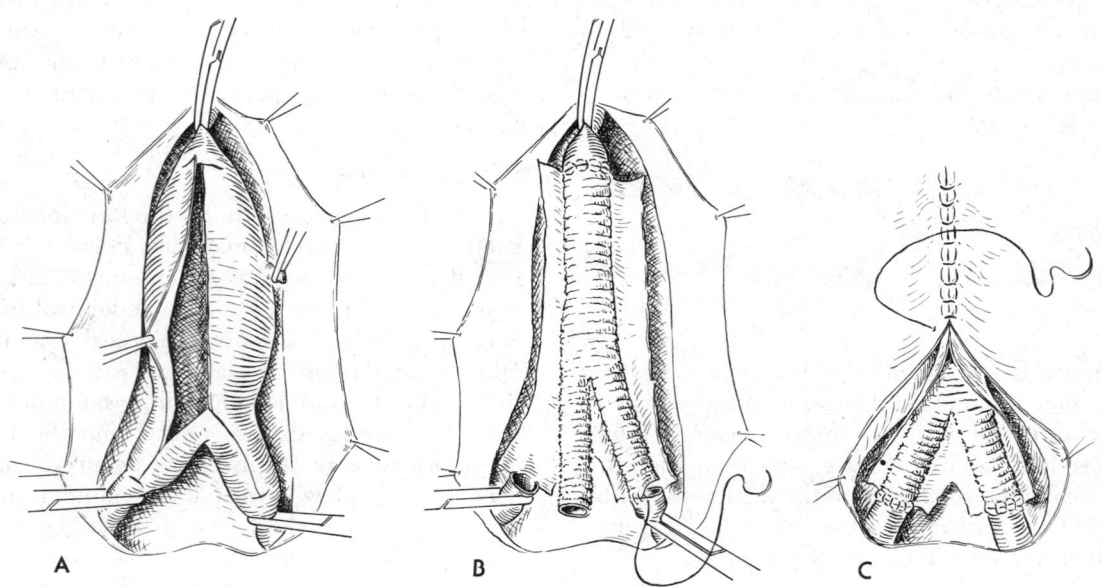

Fig. 45-15. Abdominal aneurysm. **A,** Aneurysm of aorta and iliac arteries. **B,** Bifurcation graft used to replace excised aneurysm. **C,** Closure of posterior peritoneum over graft and suture line. (Redrawn from Crawford, E.S., et al.: Surg. Clin. North Am. **46:**963-978, 1966.)

rysm and displacement of surrounding structures. Angiographic studies are usually conducted to provide the surgeon with a definite diagnosis, accurate location, and delineation of the lesion. Numerous techniques are used for these studies, and selection of the particular angiographic procedure (p. 1060) depends on a number of factors including the clinical condition of the person and the location of the lesion. Ultrasound is useful in measuring the size and position of infrarenal aortic aneurysms.

Intervention

If the aneurysm is a small chronic aneurysm with no worsening of symptoms, the person may be treated medically with antihypertensives, pain medication, and negative inotropic agents that decrease the force of muscular contractions (Inderal).

Surgery. Surgical treatment and nursing care differ depending on the location of the aneurysm.

Surgical treatment of aneurysms that involve the ascending, transverse, and descending *thoracic aorta* may involve the use of extracorporeal circulation during surgery. Operative mortality is highest in those persons who have an acute onset of symptoms and in whom a dissecting aneurysm begins in the ascending aortic arch and causes insufficiency of the aortic valve. A form of total cardiopulmonary bypass (p. 1091) is needed to maintain tissue oxygenation when the aorta is clamped. Hypothermia may be used to decrease the need of tissues for oxygen and thus decrease metabolic waste production (p. 425). After the chest is opened, the aneurysm exposed, and an extracorporeal bypass instituted to produce a satisfactory flow of oxygenated blood, cross clamps are applied proximal and distal to the lesion (Fig. 45-14). The aneurysm is then resected and replaced with a Teflon or Dacron prosthesis. (See p. 1092 for care of the person after open heart surgery.)

Treatment of an *abdominal aneurysm* is resection of the lesion and replacement with a graft. Extracorporeal perfusion (heart-lung bypass) is *not* necessary because arterial flow to the lower extremities can be interrupted safely for the time needed to complete the operation. The aneurysm is opened, the clots and debris are removed, the graft replacement is inserted, and the remaining arterial wall is closed over the graft (Fig. 45-15).

Immediate postoperative management of the person who has had an *abdominal* aortic prosthesis replacement includes constant nursing observation in the recovery room and intensive care unit. Continual reassessment and monitoring of all parameters are essential in the first 24 to 48 hours. The blood pressure, pulse (radial and apical), and respirations are taken every 15 minutes until stabilized. The central venous pressure (CVP) is also monitored to evaluate the adequacy of total blood volume. Of most concern would be a rising CVP, which would indicate overload of the venous circulation as a result of administration of too much blood or fluid replacement, inadequate cardiac function, or both (p. 1055). The pulses of the distal arterial vessels of the extremities are taken hourly, as is done with peripheral arterial bypass grafts. These include the posterior tibial and dorsalis pedis pulses. Initial spasm or trapping of air bubbles may cause these pulses to be absent on the person's return from the operating room.

If pulses continue to be absent for more than 6 to 12 hours (even less if a prosthetic failure has occurred), it generally indicates an arterial occlusion. Signs of *poor peripheral perfusion* include a drop in blood pressure and a weak and thready pulse. The person may feel cool to the touch and be perspiring. Signs of *advanced occlusion* distal to the thrombus are pain, cramping, or numbness in one or both of the extremities. The leg or legs may be blanched (white) or blue in appearance and be cool or cold to the touch. The person may appear anxious, and the elderly patient may even be disoriented. These signs and symptoms are reported to the surgeon immediately. The person who has had an abdominal aneurysm resected must be observed for complaints of back pain, which may indicate a retroperitoneal hemorrhage or a thrombus at the graft site.

Renal failure may be a complication of abdominal aortic aneurysm resection. Maintenance of adequate urinary output is essential. Accurate *hourly* intake and output records must be maintained. An indwelling (Foley) catheter is inserted for more accurate measurement. Anuria deserves immediate attention and must be reported to the physician. Oliguria (less than 30 to 50 ml/hr) may indicate poor hydration and also should be reported.

The patient usually is placed flat in bed, and sharp flexion of the hip is avoided because it causes pressure on the femoral artery. Flexion of the knee also is avoided because it causes pressure on the popliteal artery. The person is moved gently from side to side and should dorsiflex and extend the feet at regular intervals to prevent congestion of venous blood in the lower legs. Because the incision is long and pain may be pronounced, the person is able to breathe more deeply, cough productively, and move more easily if a firm abdominal binder is used and if instructions are given to support the incision while coughing or moving. The nurse often needs to help the patient. Narcotics are given fairly liberally for pain during the first few days postoperatively.

Since some handling of the viscera must occur during surgery, postoperative ileus and distention are sometimes problems. Aspiration of flatus from the stomach with a nasogastric or intestinal tube may be necessary. On about the second postoperative day the person usually is permitted out of bed for a short time. Persons having abdominal aortic surgery are at high risk of developing thrombophlebitis, and preventive measures are carried out such as the use of elastic stockings, encouragement of ambulation, and avoidance of leg massage.

REFERENCES AND SELECTED READINGS

1. Advantages of valvuloplasty over prostheses stressed, Hosp. Pract. **15:**45-51, 1980.
2. Alpert, J.S., and Francis, G.S.: Manual of coronary care, Boston, 1977, Little, Brown & Co.
3. Andreoli, K.G., et al.: Comprehensive cardiac care: a text for nurses, physicians, and other health practitioners, ed. 4, St. Louis, 1979, The C.V. Mosby Co.
4. Beeson, P., McDonald, W., and Wyngaarden, J., editors: Textbook of medicine, ed. 15, Philadelphia, 1979, W.B. Saunders Co.
5. Berk, J.L.: Handbook of critical care, Boston, 1976, Little, Brown & Co.
6. Berne, R., and Levy, M.N.: Cardiovascular physiology, ed. 3, St. Louis, 1977, The C.V. Mosby Co.
7. Berwick, D.: The evidence against cholesterol, vol. 5, Cambridge, Mass., Summer 1980, Center for the Analysis of Health Practices (Harvard School of Public Health).
8. Borgman, M.: Coronary rehabilitation: a comprehensive design, Int. J. Nurs. Studies **12:**13-21, 1975.
9. Braunwald, E.: Heart disease: a textbook of cardiovascular medicine, Philadelphia, 1980, W.B. Saunders Co.
10. Cardiac reconditioning and work evaluation unit exercise equivalents, Denver, 1976, American Heart Association.
11. *Chrzanowski, A.L.: Intra-aortic balloon pumping: concepts and patient care, Nurs. Clin. North Am. **13:**513-530, 1978.
12. Chung, E.K.: Cardiac emergency care, ed. 2, Philadelphia, 1980, Lea & Febiger.
13. Cohn, J., and Franciosa, F.A.: Selection of vasodilator, inotropic or combined therapy for the management of heart failure, Am. J. Med. **65:**181-188, 1978.
14. Cohn, J., and Franciosa, F.A.: Medical intelligence, drug therapy, vasodilator therapy of cardiac failure, N. Engl. J. Med. **297:**27-31, 254-258, 1977.
15. Conday, E., and Swan, H.J.: Myocardial infarction, Baltimore, 1973, The Williams & Wilkins Co.
16. *Cromwell, V.: Understanding the needs of your coronary bypass patient, Nurs. '80 **10:**34-37, 1980.
17. Daily, E.K., and Schroeder, J.S.: Techniques in bedside hemodynamic monitoring, ed. 2, St. Louis, 1981, The C.V. Mosby Co.
18. Daly, B.: Intensive care nursing, Garden City, N.Y., 1980, Medical Examination Publishing Co., Inc.
19. DeBusk, R.F.: The role of auscultatory monitoring in post-infarct patients, Heart Lung **4:**555-561, 1975.
20. *Dehn, M.M.: Rehabilitation of the cardiac patient: the effects of exercise, Am. J. Nurs. **80:**435-440, 1980.
21. *Devrey, A.M.: Rehabilitation of the cardiac patient: bridging the gap between inhospital and outpatient care, Am. J. Nurs. **80:**446-449, 1980.
22. *Dracup, K.: Unraveling the mysteries of cardiomyopathy, Nurs. '79 **9:**84-87, 1979.
23. Exercise testing and training of individuals with heart disease or at high risk for its development: a handbook for physicians, Denver, 1975, American Heart Association.
24. Fishman, A.: Heart failure, Washington, D.C., 1978, Hemisphere Publishing Co.
25. Fitzmaurice, J.B.: Rheumatic heart disease and mitral valve disease, New York, 1980, Appleton-Century-Crofts.
26. Forrester, J.S., et al.: Medical therapy of acute myocardial infarction by application of hemodynamic subsets. I, N. Engl. J. Med. **295:**1356-1413, 1976.
27. Forrester, J.S., and Waters, D.D.: Hospital treatment of congestive heart failure: management according to hemodynamic profile, Am. J. Med. **65:**173-180, 1978.
28. Fowler, N.: Cardiac diagnosis and treatment, ed. 3, New York, 1980, Harper & Row, Publishers.
29. Franciosa, J.A.: Nitroglycerin and nitrates in congestive heart failure, Heart Lung **9:**873-883, 1980.
30. *Futral, J.: Postoperative management and complications of coronary artery bypass surgery, Heart Lung **6:**477-481, 1977.
31. *Germain, C.P.: Exercise makes the heart grow stronger, Am. J. Nurs **72:**2169-2177, 1972.
32. *Giles, T.D.: Principles of vasodilator therapy for left ventricular congestive heart failure, Heart Lung **9:**271-276, 1980.
33. Glancy, D.L.: Medical management of adults and older children undergoing cardiac operations, Heart Lung **9:**277-283, 1980.
34. Green, A.W.: Sexual activity and the postmyocardial infarction patient, Am. Heart J. **89:**246-252, 1975.
35. Guyton, A.: Textbook of medical physiology, ed. 5, Philadelphia, 1976, W.B. Saunders Co.
36. Hahn, A.B., Backin, R.L., and Oestreich, S.J.K.: Pharmacology in nursing, ed. 15, St. Louis, 1982, The C.V. Mosby Co.
37. *Hahn, W.E., and Weber, T.M.: Rehabilitation of the cardiac patient: progressive exercise to combat the hazards of bed rest, Am. J. Nurs. **80:**440-445, 1980.
38. *Hansen, M.S., and Woods, S.L.: Nitroglycerin ointment: where and how to apply it, Am. J. Nurs. **80:**1122-1124, 1980.
39. *Hartsock, D.: Differentiation of chest pain in the emergency department, J. Emerg. Nurs. **7:**6-10, 1981.
40. *Haughey, C.W.: Alcoholic cardiomyopathy: abstinence makes the heart grow stronger, Nurs. '80 **10:**36-38, 1980.
41. Health promotion at the worksite. Public Health Report, vol. 95, no. 017-001-00424-3, Washington, D.C., March-April 1980, U.S. Government Printing Office.
42. Hellerstein, H.K., and Friedman, E.H.: Sexual activity and the post coronary patient, Arch. Intern. Med. **125:**987-999, 1970.
43. Hoepfel-Harris, J.A.: Rehabilitation of the cardiac patient: improving compliance with an exercise program, Am. J. Nurs. **80:**449-450, 1980.
44. Hurst, J.W., editor: The heart, arteries and veins, ed. 4, New York, 1978, McGraw-Hill Book Co.
45. Isselbacher, K.J., et al.: Harrison's principles of internal medicine, ed. 9, New York, 1980, McGraw-Hill Book Co.
46. Jacob, S.W., and Francone, C.A.: Structure and function in man, Philadelphia, 1974, W.B. Saunders Co.
47. Johanson, B.C., et al.: Standards for critical care, St. Louis, 1981, The C.V. Mosby Co.
48. Kaltenbach, M., et al., editors: Cardiomyopathy and myocardial biopsy, New York, 1978, Springer-Verlag New York, Inc.
49. *Kannel, W.B., Castelli, W.P., and Gordon, T.: Cholesterol in the prediction of atherosclerotic disease: new perspectives based on the Framingham study, Ann. Intern. Med. **90:**85-89, 1979.
50. Kenmer, C.V., Guzzetta, C.E., and Dassey, B.M.: Critical care nursing: body, mind, spirit, Boston, 1981, Little, Brown & Co.
51. *Lamont, L., and Reynolds, M.: Developing an individualized program for physical fitness, Occup. Health Nurs. **28:**16-19, 1980.
52. Larson, J.L., et al.: Heart rate and blood pressure responses to sexual activity and a stair-climbing test, Heart Lung **9:**1025-1030, 1980.
53. Maroko, P., and Braunwald, E.: Assessment of intervention designed to reduce myocardial ischemic damage, Circulation **53:**162-168, 1976.
54. Mason, D., et al.: Vasodilator therapy of congestive heart failure, Compr. Ther. **5**(7):6-14, 1979.
55. Miller, R.R., Awan, N.A., and Mason, D.T.: Nitroprusside ther-

apy in acute and chronic coronary heart disease, Am. J. Med. **65**:167-171, 1978.

56. Netter, F.: The CIBA collection of medical illustrations, vol. 5. The heart, Summit, N.J., 1978, CIBA.

57. Pozen, M., et al.: A nurse rehabilitation's impact on patients with myocardial infarction, Med. Care **15**:830-836, 1977.

58. Price, S.A., and Wilson, L.M.: Pathophysiology: clinical concepts of disease processes, ed. 2, New York, 1981, McGraw-Hill Book Co.

59. *Programmed instruction: new concepts in understanding congestive heart failure, Am. J. Nurs. **81**:119-142, 357-380, 1981.

60. *Purcell, J.A., and Giffin, P.: Percutaneous transluminal coronary angioplasty, Am. J. Nurs. **81**:1620-1626, 1981.

61. Reichgott, M.L.: Problems of sexual function in patients with hypertension, Cardiovasc. Med. **4**:149-156, 1979.

62. Roberts, R.: Diagnostic assessment of myocardial infarction based on lactate dehydrogenase and creatine kinase isoenzymes, Heart Lung **10**:486-506, 1981.

63. *Rodman, M.J.: Preventing post-MI thromboembolism, RN **44**:79-82, 1981.

64. Rowe, R.: Patent ductus arteriosus. In Keith, J., Rowe, R., and Vlad, R.: Heart disease in infancy and childhook, ed. 3, New York, 1978, Macmillan Publishing Co., Inc.

65. Sabiston, D.C.: The biological basis of modern surgical practice: textbook of surgery, ed. 11, Philadelphia, 1977, W.B. Saunders Co.

66. Schamroth, L., and Jaspon, J.: Variant angina pectoris: a typical Prinzmetal's angina pectoris, Heart Lung **2**:431-433, 1973.

67. Schlesinger, Z., and Barzilay, J.: Prolonged rehabilitation of patients after acute myocardial infarction and its effects on a complex of physiological variables, Heart Lung **9**:1038-1043, 1980.

68. Schneider, R.R., and Seckler, S.G.: Evaluation of acute chest pain, Med. Clin. North Am. **65**:53-65, 1981.

69. *Shor, V.: Congenital cardiac defects: assessment and case finding, Am. J. Nurs. **78**:256-261, 1978.

70. Singh, S., and Fletcher, R.D.: The site of myocardial infarction: effect on presentation and management, Pract. Cardiology **6**:35-47, 1980.

71. Sokolow, M.: Clinical cardiology, ed. 2, Los Altos, Calif., 1979, Lange Medical Publications.

72. Stiles, Q.: Myocardial revascularization: a surgical atlas, Boston, 1976, Little, Brown & Co.

73. *Stuart, E.M.: Care of the patient with a mitral commissurotomy, Am. J. Nurs. **80**:1611-1632, 1980.

74. *Thorpe, C.: A nursing care plan: the adult cardiac surgery patient, Heart Lung **8**:690-694, 1979.

75. Tilkian, S.M., Conover, M.B., and Tilkian, A.G.: Clinical implications of laboratory tests, ed. 3., St. Louis, 1983, The C.V. Mosby Co.

76. Wanamaker, L.W., and Kaplan, E.L.: Acute rheumatic fever. In Moss, A.J., et al.: Heart disease in infants, children, and adolescents, ed. 2, Baltimore, 1977, The Williams & Wilkins Co.

77. Wenger, N., and Hellerstein, H.K.: Rehabilitation of the coronary patient, New York, 1978, John Wiley & Sons, Inc.

78. Wenger, N.K., Hurst, J.W., and McIntyre, M.C.: Cardiology for nurses, New York, 1980, McGraw-Hill Book Co.

79. *Westfall, V.F.: Electrical and mechanical events in the cardiac cycle, Am. J. Nurs. **76**:231-235, 1976.

80. WHO Bulletin: Classification of hyperlipidemias and hyperlipoproteinemias, Circulation **45**:501-504, 1972.

81. *Yacone, L.A.: Is it an MI? RN **44**:53-59, 1981.

CHAPTER 46

PROBLEMS OF PERIPHERAL CIRCULATION

BARBARA J. DALY

Peripheral vascular disease refers to a number of disease entities that may affect any part of the vascular system. Diseases of the heart and coronary arteries are *not* usually included in this classification, although the pathophysiologic changes may be identical. The term peripheral vascular disease also refers to the pathologic sequelae that result from any interruption in the normal circulatory mechanics.

This chapter also discusses lower limb amputation as one of the surgical interventions for vascular disease. Techniques of treatment and management are similar to those used for the patient who has had an amputation following trauma, although rehabilitation of the latter usually is less difficult because the amputation is less likely to accompany a chronic medical disease.

Hypertension, one of the major etiologic factors in peripheral vascular disease, is discussed as a separate entity. It may exist without the presence of significant arterial or venous disease, or it may be a complicating factor.

All of the clinical conditions included under peripheral vascular disease manifest signs and symptoms in the individual because of some type of interference in normal blood supply to the tissues. The interference may be of an obstructive nature, as with the presence of a thrombus or fatty plaque on the wall of the vessel, or it may be an interruption caused by anatomic abnormalities, such as is the case with varicose veins and arteriovenous fistulas.

Etiology

Several general factors lead to the development of peripheral vascular disease. The most common of these are pathologic processes occurring in the vessels themselves, such as occur in atherosclerosis and the inflammation of lymphedema. Changes in blood hemodynamics such as hypertension, states of hypercoagulability, and stasis may be the significant factor leading to circulatory interference in some disorders. Damage to vessels caused by external agents, such as the phlebitis associated with intravenous therapy, may also be implicated in peripheral vascular disease. In addition, in some individuals an inherent weakness in the vessel may lead to the development of an abnormality such as an aneurysm.

Regardless of the specific disorder or primary cause, many factors significantly influence both the occurrence of the disease and its course once symptoms are manifested. General interventions designed to enhance those factors that promote good circulation and to eliminate or reduce factors that further inhibit circulation are appropriate for any client with known or suspected peripheral vascular disease. Common presenting signs and symptoms and diagnostic procedures are discussed under assessment before reviewing these interventions. Specific disorders, pathophysiology, and interventions are then considered.

Assessment

Because peripheral vascular disease affects so many individuals, particularly in later life, the nurse should incorporate assessment for signs and symptoms of diminished circulation in working with all patients regardless of the primary problem. Assessment of patients with known peripheral vascular disease is, of course, much more thorough.

Subjective data

A *history of pain* is of prime significance. Pain is one of the most common symptoms of diminished circulation to an extremity, and the type of pain may help differentiate between embolic phenomena and arteriosclerosis. The length of time since pain first occurred is a guide to how far the disease has progressed. Other areas to investigate include when the pain occurs, what factors initiate pain, and what relieves the pain.

The presence of *intermittent claudication* is especially significant. This is pain in the muscles caused by inadequate arterial circulation to the contracting muscles and occurs primarily in the calf. Except in rare instances it is brought on only by continuous exercise and is relieved at once by resting. Knowing the amount of exercise that can be performed before claudication occurs helps determine the severity of the condition. The presence of rest pain, or pain that occurs without any activity, is indicative of severe disease.

In advanced disease, and occasionally in early stages, the individual may notice a change in functional ability. Persistent diminished circulation will cause atrophy of muscles of the extremity, and occlusion of the aortic and femoral trunks may result in impotence. Before a change in function the individual may note a change in appearance in an extremity. Table 46-1 lists distinguishing characteristics of arterial and venous disease.

Information should also be sought about healing. Has the patient had any abrasions or cuts recently? If so, how quickly or slowly did they heal? Was treatment required or obtained?

Diet information includes the caloric intake, type of fats predominantly used, amount of carbohydrates, and general nutritional adequacy of the diet.

The patient's life-style and daily habits often significantly influence the course of the illness. If the patient smokes, the nurse determines how much is smoked and for how long. Although occupation itself has not been linked with peripheral vascular disease, knowing the patient's occupation assists in judging the level of physical activity and may also point out the need for counseling in other areas. For example, if the patient is involved in physical labor, special precautions may need to be taken to avoid trauma to the hands and feet. The same information can be partly elicited by asking about leisure-time activities.

As part of the nursing history, the nurse learns about how the patient's life-style affects the ability to comply with the prescribed therapy. For example, does the patient have to walk a long distance or climb several flights of stairs to bring groceries home? Climbing may cause severe pain in the legs because of inadequate oxygenation of the tissues. Some arrangements therefore must be made to assist the patient with this task. If the patient lives alone it should be determined whether someone in the building or neighborhood can do the necessary shopping. A thorough nursing history might reveal that the young mother with a stubborn ulcer that complicated phlebitis before delivery is so harassed with feeding the baby or with getting other children off to school that she neglects her own breakfast and lunch. The nurse may discover that the elderly man with arteriosclerosis develops intermittent claudication when he walks from his rooming house to the nearest restaurant, causing him to skip one or two meals each day. The assistance of the family or social worker may be needed to solve such problems.

TABLE 46-1. Differentiating characteristics of arterial and venous disease

	Arterial disease	Venous disease
Skin	Cool or cold; hairless, dry, shiny; pallor on elevation and rubor on dangling	Warm; tough, thickened; mottled, pigmented areas
Pain	Sharp, stabbing; worsens with activity and walking; lowering feet may relieve pain	Aching, cramping; activity and walking sometimes help; elevating feet relieves pain
Ulcers	Severely painful; pale, gray base; found on heel, lateral malleolus, toes, and dorsum of foot	Moderately painful; pink base, with irregular, pigmented skin edge; found on medial aspect of ankle
Pulses	Often absent or diminished	Usually present
Edema	Infrequent	Frequent, especially at end of day and in areas of ulceration

Objective data

The first part of the physical assessment usually involves checking all peripheral pulses for the presence or absence of pulses, their quality or strength, and also the comparison of pulses in each extremity with those of the other. The pulses that should routinely be checked with each assessment include the *radial, ulnar, posterior tibial, dorsalis pedis, popliteal,* and *femoral.*

Inspection of the skin yields valuable information about the adequacy of circulation. Poorly oxygenated skin has a pale, bluish, or mottled appearance, and the affected arm or leg will be cooler than the other extremity. There is often a loss of hair in the affected area, and the skin has a tight, shiny look to it. Nails may be thickened and black or brownish. The entire extremity should be inspected to determine how far from the tips of the fingers or toes the circulatory impairment extends.

Neurologic deficits also serve as indications of the extent of disease. Absent or diminished sensation, tingling, or reduced sense of temperature may all result from insufficient oxygen supply to the nerves.

Tests and examinations

Several specific procedures help in diagnosis of vascular disease and determine the progress in treatment. Most tests are relatively simple and require no specific preparations. The patient, however, usually is in pain and fears any procedure that may even temporarily increase pain. Nervousness sometimes causes spasm of blood vessels and sensations of chilliness that may interfere with the accuracy of a test by diminishing pulsations and altering circulation. The patient should be told that the tests are painless, and the nurse should explain what is to be done if the physician has not already done so.

The room in which the tests are done should be kept warm, and if the patient has to be transported to another area for the tests the nurse should check to see that sufficient covering to prevent chilling is provided.

Skin temperature studies

Attempts are made to record the skin temperature as a gauge of the effectiveness of the circulation to an extremity. These tests are not performed often because to be accurate they must be carried out in an environment with carefully controlled temperature and humidity. Normal skin temperature can be recorded by applying a thermocouple (a device for measuring skin temperature) to the skin. The temperature then is recorded on a potentiometer. With a humidity of 40%, the surface temperature of the skin usually varies from 24° to 35° C (73° to 93° F). Normal persons have a wide range of temperature difference in various parts of the body. For example, the forehead and the thorax are usually 5° to 8° warmer than the toes. People with arterial disease may have even greater temperature variations between the extremities and the rest of the body. Skin temperature readings are considered as only suggestive because many factors (e.g., a rise in metabolic rate) increase the temperature of the skin surface. The patient who is excited or upset by the anticipated test may have an increase in skin temperature. The test is usually scheduled several hours after a meal, since eating alters the skin temperature. Smoking also affects the accuracy of the readings.

A test for the efficiency of vasodilation in the extremities consists of immersing one of the limbs in water heated to 42° to 44° C (107.6° to 112° F) and then recording the skin temperature of the opposite limb. In the normal person with no vascular disease the temperature of the unimmersed limb will rise to a minimum of 34° C (93° F) within 35 minutes. A person with arterial disease may have little elevation in the skin temperature. An accurate bath thermometer is needed to measure the water temperature, and sufficient blankets should be used to protect the patient from chilling during and after the test.

Arterial disease can be confirmed by the *cold pressure test*. The patient's blood pressure and pulse pressure are determined under normal conditions. The patient then immerses a hand in ice water, and the blood pressure and pulse pressure are taken again. Normal subjects have an average blood pressure increase of 25 mm Hg with no change in pulse pressure; patients with internal occlusive disease have an average increase in blood pressure of 45 mm Hg with an increase in pulse pressure of 20 mm Hg.

Reactive hyperemia refers to the reaction of the skin to immersion in hot water (35° to 40° C) after emptying and occlusion of arterioles by blood pressure cuff. The normal response is for a flush to spread to the fingertips within 2 to 5 seconds and to fade within 15 seconds. Arterial occlusion delays the flush and may result in a patchy appearance. This test is sometimes combined with Doppler ultrasound (p. 1145) to measure velocity of flow. This is also done after exercise (*exercise hyperemia*).

It should be noted that skin temperature studies are never used as the sole diagnostic technique, but always in combination with other studies. They are particularly useful in comparing one extremity to another. Many experienced clinicians prefer to rely on assessing skin temperature simply by touching the skin of the patient.

Angiography

Angiography is an x-ray procedure that permits visualization of the internal anatomy of the heart and blood vessels through the intravascular injection of radiopaque contrast material. By this method calcification and other anomalies of the arteries may be demonstrated. Calcified atherosclerotic plaques at the site of an occlusion may be visualized, and calcification can sometimes be traced distally throughout the entire length of an artery and can even be seen as far away as the great toe. The information revealed by such an examination is not of itself evidence of arterial insufficiency, because some patients who have extensive calcification of the small arteries evidently have sufficient collateral circulation to permit good blood supply and thus have no symptoms of arterial insufficiency.

Radiopaque substances such as Hypaque or Renografin are injected into an artery, and serial radiographs are taken during the last few seconds of the injection and immediately thereafter. Usually this test is done in the radiology department. A cutdown on the vessel may be required in order to inject the dye. When visualization of the arteries of a lower extremity is desired, the dye is injected into the femoral artery.

The radiopaque substances used contain iodide, and the patient may have a severe allergic reaction to the dye, with dyspnea, nausea, vomiting, numbness of the extremities, diaphoresis, and trachycardia. Any signs of a reaction should be reported at once. Occasionally, a delayed reaction occurs after the patient leaves the x-ray department. Antihistaminic drugs, epinephrine, and oxygen are used to treat these hypersensitivity reactions to the dye. The site of injection of the dye must be monitored for signs of irritation or local thrombosis, which may occur if any of the irritating dye gets into the surrounding tissue. The area may have to be treated with massive warm moist packs.

The procedure is uncomfortable because even without a reaction to the dye the patient feels a flushing and burning sensation. One or more injections into deep arteries are made, and the patient must remain on the x-ray table for an hour or more. Afterward, water is given in generous amounts to hasten the excretion of the dye through the kidneys. A backrub to relieve pressure areas resulting from lying on the hard x-ray table is part of the nursing care plan.

Of utmost importance after arteriography is assessment of the involved limb. The injection site must be closely observed for excessive bleeding. The patient will return from having the arteriogram with just a small dressing over the site, and a 1- or 2-lb sandbag should be placed over the dressing for 3 to 4 hours. Peripheral pulses distal to the injection site are checked every hour for the first 4 to 8 hours after angiography.

Venography

Radioactive isotopes may be used to confirm the presence or absence of deep vein thrombosis. A substance that will become incorporated into the thrombus, such as *fibrinogen* or *urokinase*, is administered intravenously, and the area is scanned by x-ray. An increased uptake of the radioactive material indicates the presence of a thrombus.

Plethysmography

Plethysmography is also used as an aid to diagnosis. This is a graphic device that measures variations in the electrical resistance associated with changes in blood volume. It involves applying electrodes that are connected to a recorder to the extremity. Venous flow is occluded with a cuff, and changes in resistance are measured as blood pools in the extremity. Plethysmography has become one of the most commonly used tools for assessing arterial flow to the hands, feet, and calves. It is sometimes performed in combination with exercise to test for hyperemic flow and thus gain more information about functional capacity during activity. *Oculoplethysmography* refers to detection of changes in the blood volume of the eye and is used in detection of carotid lesions.

Capillary fragility test

A test for capillary fragility is sometimes ordered for patients with peripheral vascular disease. Since it is more often ordered for patients with suspected disease of the blood or blood-forming organs, it is described in Chapter 47.

Lumbar sympathetic block

Paravertebral injection of the sympathetic rami or sympathetic ganglia may be used to diagnose peripheral vascular disease. Evidence of vasodilation after the block indicates that the circulation to the limbs may be improved by subsequent injections of procaine or by sympathectomy.

With the patient in a prone or semiprone position, a needle is inserted at the level of the second or third lumbar vertebra into the sympathetic tract within the spinal canal, and 10 to 20 ml of a 1% solution of procaine hydrochloride is injected. If the procedure is successful the sympathetic tracts will be blocked, causing a definite warming and drying of the skin surface of the limb on the same side as the injection. This response may be grossly measured by touch, or skin temperature studies may be done.

The patient should be told that there will be little pain associated with the test beyond the first needle prick and that there may be a sensation of tingling and warmth in the legs for several hours following the test. The patient is observed carefully during and immediately following the procedure for signs of shock, which may result from the sudden shifting of so much blood into the peripheral circulation that the blood volume in the heart and vital vessels is depleted.

Ultrasound

Ultrasound is used to detect aneurysms and to measure flow through vessels. This technique involves directing an ultrasound beam at the involved area; the beam is reflected off red cells moving through the ves-

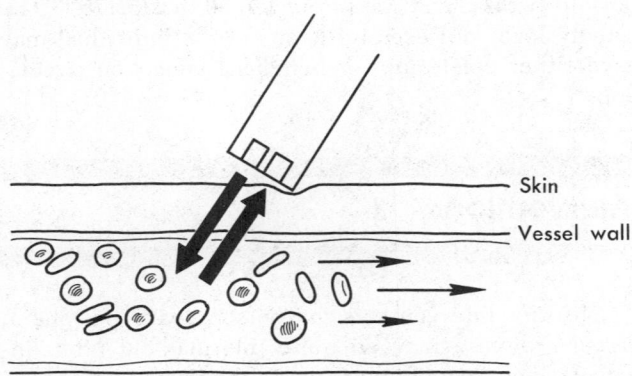

Fig. 46-1. Doppler effect showing red blood cells reflecting sound.

sel. The reflection varies according to the velocity of flow in the vessel. This change in the frequency of reflected sound according to velocity is referred to as the Doppler effect (Fig. 46-1).

Simple, portable Doppler devices are often used both to diagnose arterial disease and to ascertain the effectiveness of corrective procedures. They may also be used to measure blood pressure in low-flow states.

Prevention

Health teaching about the factors influencing peripheral vascular disease should be done by the nurse working in any clinical setting. With advancing age, arterial walls lose elasticity and undergo a thickening of the intima; this predisposes to vascular problems, and all individuals will benefit from education about this as they grow older. All hopsitalized patients with restricted activity, regardless of their primary disease, need to be taught measures to reduce the stasis associated with immobility. Intervention in areas of everyday life such as diet and activity of the nonhospitalized individual may prevent or at least slow the development of acute disease. This is one of the most important disease groups with which the nurse works and one in which the rewards of early interventions are greatest.

Clinical picture

Because of our upright posture, the danger of peripheral vascular disease is greatest in the lower extremities, where adequate circulation is most difficult to maintain. Both the arteries and veins are subject to hydrostatic change; for example, when a person rises from a lying to a standing position the pressure in the dorsalis pedis artery rises from 120/80 to 215/175.[55] The activity level and exercise habits of the individual may have either deleterious or beneficial effects on circulation.

Intervention

Nursing interventions for persons with peripheral vascular disease may be quite informal but often involve a good deal of ingenuity on the part of the nurse. In industry the nurse who helps the employees find chairs of a suitable height in order to prevent sharp knee flexion is contributing to prevention of disease.

Promoting activity

Sitting for long hours with the knees bent causes pressure on the arteries and veins of the legs, resulting in slight swelling and discomfort. The nurse may plan with supervisors in industry to provide short rest periods at frequent intervals for persons who must stand still or sit with knees bent while they work. Since walking and moving about improve circulation, such activities should be encouraged during rest periods.

The nurse making an antepartal home visit is contributing to prevention of vascular disease when questioning the woman about her posture and the kind of girdle and shoes she wears. The woman is also reminded to take regular exercise such as walking and to rest periodically with her legs elevated above heart level. A careful balance of rest and activity is essential for any person with progressive peripheral vascular disease.

Exercise improves arterial circulation by promoting alternate muscle contraction and relaxation, thereby causing blood vessels to contract and dilate. Exercise not only improves return of venous blood from the extremities to the heart but also is one of the most important stimuli for the development of collateral circulation. Too much exercise, however, increases metabolism, thereby increasing the demands placed on the circulation to take nutrients to the tissues and to remove the products of metabolism. Complete rest may be necessary in the presence of associated medical conditions, such as heart disease, thrombophlebitis, or gangrene. The nurse should plan with the physician so that proper instruction can be given regarding achieving a balance between rest and activity. In regard to posture the following is a safe guide for all persons, especially those with peripheral vascular disease: do not remain in *any* one position too long; this is particularly important for the elderly person, who often has both arterial and venous disease.

Much emphasis has been placed on *elevation of the feet,* and many persons believe that this is beneficial. However, elevation of the feet may cause damage when the patient has *arterial* insufficiency because it interferes with adequate circulation through arteries in the lower extremities. The nurse must *clearly understand* the patient's condition and the physician's orders before giving instructions in this regard. The effect of position on circulation can be best understood by relating direction of blood flow to the effects of gravity. Arteries take oxygenated blood away from the heart; elevating the extremities tends to deliver blood back to the heart; hence it tends to hamper arterial function. Long periods of standing may result in venous congestion since the effect of gravity increases the work of the veins as they return deoxygenated blood to the heart. It is safe to assume that, unless otherwise ordered, the flat position is best for circulation over an extended period.

Long periods of standing still should be avoided by

persons with either venous or arterial disease, and short periods should be alternated with exercise such as walking. Persons who have venous disease should alternate standing and walking with elevation of the affected limbs.

The importance of *posture* must be stressed in the care and teaching of patients with peripheral vascular disease. The person should sleep on a firm mattress. A soft mattress may allow enough flexion of the trunk at the hips to impede circulation to the lower extremities. It may also permit the lower limbs to be higher than the heart, which is undesirable in arterial disease. *The height of a chair should be such that the knees are not bent at more than a 90-degree angle, and the depth of the seat should permit two fingers between the chair seat and the popliteal spaces.* Both of these provisions will help to prevent pressure on the popliteal vessels, which would obstruct arterial flow to the limbs and interfere with venous return.

Furthermore, persons with peripheral vascular disease should never cross their legs at the knee because this also causes pressure on the popliteal vessels. They should develop the habit of rotating the foot at the ankle, bending the foot up and down, and straightening the knee at intervals. They should be taught to do these exercises while traveling. The importance of frequent stops if traveling by automobile or getting out of one's seat and walking in the aisle for a few moments if traveling by airplane, bus, or train should be emphasized. Attendance at movies or other sedentary diversions may be made safe and comfortable for persons with impaired circulation by the use of the above measures to improve circulation.

Specific exercises *(Buerger-Allen)* to empty blood vessels and stimulate collateral circulation are rarely used today. Instead, moderate exercise is recommended. One of the best exercises for stimulating the flow of blood to the legs is walking. Patients may be able to build up tolerance so that they can walk a mile or more a day. They should be instructed to stop and rest if pain develops and then to continue walking after it disappears. Some physicians also recommend the use of a rocking chair because rocking helps to stimulate the muscles in the legs to contract and relax.

Preventing compromise of circulation

Persons with peripheral vascular disease must not wear anything that constricts. Rolled garters, socks with thin tight bands, and girdles or pantyhose that cause constriction should be avoided. Some physicians believe that tight waistbands also should not be worn. Men may be advised to wear suspenders instead of belts. Shoelaces should be tied loosely. If edema of the feet occurs at the end of the day, the shoelaces should be loosened and relaced several times each day. Some persons who have a moderate amount of edema of the feet or ankles prefer to use elastic shoelaces. As mentioned before, any activity, posture, or position that impedes circulation is to be avoided.

It must be remembered that exposure of any part of the body to cold can cause chilling of the entire body. This in turn causes vasoconstriction and lessens circulation in a diseased extremity. In cold weather the person with peripheral vascular disease should wear warm clothing, such as thermal underwear, fleece-lined shoes or boots, hats with ear flaps or earmuffs, scarves, and warm coats, suits, or dresses. Several layers of lightweight clothing are preferable to heavy bulky garments. If chilling has been experienced, the individual should drink something hot and get to a warm room as soon as possible.

These patients should be in a warm environment whenever possible. The temperature of the room should be at least 21° C (70° F), and hospitalized patients may need even more warmth for maximal comfort. They should be able to sense that they are rather warm but should not be warm enough to perspire more than usual.

Counseling for proper diet

Diet affects the development and course of peripheral vascular disease in two ways. First, the presence of obesity places an added burden on the heart and blood vessels. Not only must the heart pump more forcefully to circulate blood effectively in the obese individual, but the excess fat tissue tends to compromise vessels and increase venous congestion. Obesity is often associated with decreased physical activity.

The second way in which diet contributes to peripheral vascular disease is related to the level of serum lipids. All lipids, or fats, in plasma are transported as constituents of lipoproteins; elevations in serum lipids are classified according to the specific lipoprotein that is elevated. Levels of *cholesterol* and *triglycerides* have been implicated for some time in the development of atherogenic disease and its sequelae such as stroke and myocardial infarction. For more detailed discussion see p. 1112.

Dietary counseling is an especially important area for nursing intervention because obesity and hyperlipidemia are contributing factors to disease and an attempt should be made to eliminate them if possible. The nurse and dietitian, in consultation with each other, may provide patients not only with the necessary teaching but also with the emotional support and encouragement required to change lifetime eating habits.

When a reduction diet has been prescribed, the nurse can be of assistance in helping to plan meals that are satisfying and yet within caloric restrictions and financial means. Because protein helps to prevent breakdown of tissues, a diet high in protein but low in saturated fats is usually advised. If a lesion such as a varicose ulcer is present, a diet high in protein should help to promote healing. The diet should include foods high in B-complex vitamins, which are important in maintaining tonicity of smooth muscle of blood vessels, and vitamin C, which is essential to healing and the prevention of both internal and external hemorrhage.

It is generally recommended that persons with peripheral vascular disease take more fluids than the normal person. As many as 15 to 20 glasses of water or equivalent fluids are often recommended. This amount may improve the quality of the limited blood supply to the limbs by increasing the elimination of waste products. It is also believed that it may decrease the viscosity of the blood and thus help to prevent the formation of thrombi. The fluid intake may, however, be restricted in the presence of other medical conditions, such as congestive heart failure.

Teaching effects of smoking

Nursing intervention to teach patients about the hazards associated with smoking and to assist them to stop smoking are essential, since smoking is one of the greatest risk factors in the development of peripheral vascular disease. Both the incidence and the mortality of myocardial infarction, cerebral infarction, aortic aneurysm, intermittent claudication, and thromboangiitis obliterans are increased in the smoker.[80] Smoking exerts an influence on circulation in two ways.

First, nicotine causes vasoconstriction and spasm of the peripheral arteries; therefore smoking is contraindicated in all vascular diseases. Damage results from inhaling smoke; there is no evidence that chewing tobacco or using snuff contributes to vasospasm. The relationship between arteriospasm and smoking is so definite that many physicians feel it is useless to try to treat patients unless they give up smoking. Smoking should be discontinued immediately in any kind of arterial vascular disease and is also contraindicated in venous disease because the arteries surrounding a thrombosed vein often develop spasms. Nicotine also increases the heart rate, causing further stress on the circulatory system.

Second, the carbon monoxide inhaled in cigarette smoke raises the carboxyhemoglobin level and reduces the oxygen carrying capacity of the blood.[80] Thus in addition to causing vasoconstriction, smoking lowers the oxygen available in the blood for tissue demands.

Although difficult for some nonsmokers to understand, the giving up of cigarettes is almost impossible for some people. In some individuals the dependency on cigarettes can be almost as strong as a dependency on narcotics. Many persons continue to smoke even after they have lost a toe or a foot as a result of vascular

disease and are informed that the incidence of amputation decreases when smoking is stopped.[34] Even if individuals have smoked for many years, stopping smoking lessens their risk. The reduction in mortality is related to the length of time that they have not smoked and the amount previously smoked.[80] The heavier the smoker, the longer it takes before there is a significant reduction in risk. Because of this and because smoking causes immediate and consistent vasoconstriction, assisting the individual to stop smoking is of highest priority for the nursing care plan.

Again, teaching the effects of smoking is the first step, coupled with support of the person's efforts to stop. Although there is no sure way to help the individual give up smoking, there are some measures that may be helpful. Chewing gum or engaging in distracting activities sometimes helps. Some persons find that cutting down to fewer and fewer cigarettes each day is easier than stopping suddenly. Constant reminders and strict discipline often do more harm than good. Patience, understanding, and reiteration of faith in the person's ability to stop smoking are more helpful than disapproval of lapses. The essential factor for success is that the person wants to stop smoking. Group support and behavior modification are other methods being used to help people try to stop smoking. The nurse needs to be aware of resources available in the community to assist persons who wish to quit smoking.

Preventing skin breakdown

Because resistance to infection is low when tissues are inadequately nourished and oxygenated, the risk of infection is high in persons with peripheral vascular disease. A great deal of teaching is required in order for patients to know which activities will help maintain skin integrity and which may contribute to skin breakdown and secondary infection.

Keeping extremities warm

Warmth is advised for most patients with peripheral vascular disease because it *causes vasodilation* and thereby *improves circulation to the affected part*. However, warmth in the form of direct heat is seldom if ever applied to the affected part because it results in an increased demand for blood in the extremity already suffering from depleted circulation. Another reason for not applying local heat is that *many patients with peripheral vascular disease* also *have peripheral nerve degeneration, which lessens sensitivity to heat, thus predisposing to burns. A safe rule to follow is never, under any circumstances, apply hot water bottles, heating pads, or other forms of local heat to the legs or feet of persons with peripheral vascular disease without a specific medical order.* Soaking the feet in hot or even very warm water is seldom advised. The temperature of the water into which the individual places his or her feet should always be tested; it should not exceed 32° C (90° F). Patients must be cautioned not to attempt to warm their feet by placing them on a warm radiator, too close to a fire in the fireplace, or in an open oven. Warmth to the extremities can be increased by placing a hot water bottle or heating pad on the abdomen. This causes reflex dilation of the blood vessels of the legs. Immersing the entire body in a warm bath also warms the extremities. Loose woolen bed socks can be worn at night.

Teaching care of feet

All persons with vascular disease need instruction in the care of their feet. A daily bath is recommended except for the elderly, for whom two or three baths a week are sufficient. The person should be advised to check the temperature of the bathwater carefully with the elbow before stepping into the tub because sensation in the feet may be diminished. This simple practice would prevent many persons from being burned. A small amount of a superfatted soap should be used. The skin should be dried by gentle patting; vigorous rubbing should be avoided.

While bathing, the person should look for any skin changes on the legs and feet. A dry scaling over the tibia may be the beginning of "bath itch," common in older people who have dry skin and who bathe often and use regular soaps. If dry scales appear, fewer baths should be taken, superfatted soap should be used, and the skin should be lubricated with lanolin or a moisturizing agent after bathing and between baths. Blueness or swelling around varicosities, and hard, reddened, or painful areas, which may indicate phlebitis, should be reported to a physician at once. Trophic changes such as dryness, cracking, hardness, thickening, and brownish discolorations of the toenails indicate impairment of blood supply and should also be called to the physician's attention.

If the individual does not bathe each day, the feet should be washed in tepid water, dried thoroughly, paying special attention to areas between the toes, and inspected for calluses, blisters, or any other abnormality. For older persons with failing vision, a member of the family or the community health nurse should inspect their feet periodically. In the daily routine care of the feet, the skin and base of the nails should be gently massaged with lubricants or moisturizing agents. Alcohol is drying to the skin and should not be used. Each toe should be gently massaged from the distal end proximally to stimulate circulation. Powder may be used between the toes, with care being taken that it does not cake and that it is thoroughly removed at the next washing. Authorities maintain that epidermophytosis (athlete's foot), which is often a precursor of infection, ulceration, and gangrene in the feet of persons with ar-

terial insufficiency, will seldom develop if the toes and feet are kept dry at all times. The individual who perspires profusely should powder between the toes more than once a day and socks should be changed at least daily. Over-the-counter preparations available in drugstores should not be used, since they are usually too strong for feet with impaired circulation. Foot powders should only be used if prescribed. Directions should always be read carefully. Small pieces of lamb's wool or cotton can be placed between the toes to absorb perspiration.

To avoid fungal infections of the feet, socks or stockings should be washed daily. If they are wool or have a tendency to shrink, they should be initially purchased one size too large or stretched before being worn.

To prevent ingrown toenails the nails should be cut carefully at regular intervals. Before the nails are cut the feet should be soaked in tepid water. The nails should be cut straight across and rounded slightly at the sides with a file. They must never be cut down to the level of the tissue. Pocketknives, razor blades, or scissors should never be used. Patients should equip themselves with a pair of toenail clippers. Nail files are usually considered safe; however, tissues can be traumatized by emery boards and files, particularly when the patient lacks normal sensation in the toes. Elderly persons with poor vision should not cut their own toenails; a member of the family or a podiatrist should do it for them.

With daily care a toenail that has a tendency to "curl under" at the side of the toe can be trained to grow more normally, but no effort should be made to "straighten" the nail by vigorous treatment. With the rounded end of an ordinary toothpick, a small wisp of cotton may be inserted gently under the edge of the nail. The cotton must be changed daily. Although it may be weeks before any improvement is seen, with patience and persistence most nails that tend to grow under can be made to grow more normally unless there is aggravation by a condition such as pressure from shoes. Nails that are thickened or deformed should not be cut or filed but should be treated by a podiatrist or physician who knows of the individual's circulatory impairment.

Medical care should be sought for blisters and for corns, calluses, and areas of thickened skin that cannot be rubbed away with a washcloth and an emery board following soaking. Soap poultices made of any soft soap such as shaving cream may be used to soften corns and calluses before rubbing is attempted. The patient with circulatory disease of any kind should seek medical advice before going to a podiatrist.

Preventing trauma and pressure

Persons with vascular diseases should be warned to avoid injury to their feet and legs and to watch carefully for infection following trauma. They should not walk barefoot. It also is dangerous for them to scratch any minor skin lesions. Many stubborn ulcers of the leg have followed the vigorous scratching of mosquito or other insect bites. Venous stasis may cause itching that can be most annoying. This itching usually follows long periods of standing and will subside if the person rests with the feet elevated for a few minutes every hour or two. The warning not to scratch the skin is hard to heed at times. Calamine lotion is sometimes suggested when pruritus is troublesome. Any minor infection of the legs or the feet should be viewed as a major one by persons with peripheral vascular disease. They should never attempt self-treatment when signs of infection are present.

These individuals should have at least two pairs of shoes and should wear them on alternate days, thus giving each pair a chance to air. If shoes become wet, they should be dried slowly on shoe trees to help preserve their shape. New shoes should be broken in gradually. Leather shoes are best because they give good support to the feet. Canvas, linen, or perforated nylon shoes provide ventilation, are comfortable in warm weather, and are safe if they have leather soles. *Rubber-soled shoes are not advised for persons who have any kind of vascular disease because they retard evaporation and thus may contribute to the development of fungal infection.* Shoes should be carefully fitted by an experienced person. They should extend about ½ in. beyond the longest toe and should be wide enough to avoid pressure anywhere on the foot and to allow fairly free movement of the toes within the shoe. The inner last of the shoe should be straight, and longitudinal arch of the shoe should support that of the foot. Shoes that afford little or no support are not recommended for persons with peripheral vascular disease, although there is no objection to women wearing pumps with moderately high heels. In fact, pumps are good because the feet can be readily slipped out of the shoes and the toes wiggled at intervals; however, the shoes should be roomy enough so that they can be put on again easily.

When sleeping, persons with peripheral vascular disease should have lightweight covers that are loose and do not cause any pressure on the toes, which often burn and are painful. They can be taught how to improvise a board at the foot of the bed to keep the weight of covers off the feet. During hospitalization the patient is provided with a padded board or box at the foot of the bed. These devices are preferable to a cradle, which may hamper freedom of movement and against which the patient may accidentally strike his or her foot. If a cradle must be used, it should be padded, and bath blankets should be placed over the cradle and tucked securely under the mattress to prevent drafts on the feet.

Treating ulceration

Despite many precautions some patients with peripheral vascular disease still develop areas of ulceration secondary to trauma or pressure. Even the smallest of cuts can rapidly develop into a deep ulcer when the tissue is inadequately nourished; the ball of the foot, the ankle, and the lower calf are the most commonly involved areas.

Ulcers occurring in any person with vascular disease require meticulous care to prevent infection or to prevent further infection with new organisms. Since local tissue resistance to infection is lessened and the rate of healing is slowed because of impaired circulation to the area, a long period of healing must be anticipated. Wet-to-dry dressings are often used for debridement. These dressings are applied wet, using sterile saline solution, allowed to dry, and then removed, taking away necrotic and sloughed tissue that adheres to the dried dressing. Foot soaks may be used, although this procedure cannot be sterile because it is impossible to cleanse the entire foot properly.

Preventing infection is one of the two most difficult problems confronting the nurse in caring for patients with ulcers. The second is providing for comfort. Although there is often diminished sensation in superficial tissue, there may be considerable pain when deep tissue layers are involved, and the patient may suffer a great deal of pain during dressing changes and wound soaks. Administering pain medication 15 to 30 minutes before wound care is of major importance.

Patients with an ulcer of the foot usually are urged to keep off their feet, although there is not complete agreement on the value of this restriction. Some physicians believe that, provided there is no direct weight bearing on the wound, the arterial circulation and healing are improved by a moderate amount of moving about and by keeping the limb in a dependent position for part of the day at least.

Cradles with lights are seldom used, but occasionally the physician may feel that dry warmth will improve healing of the ulcer. Using extreme caution, the nurse then leaves the wound exposed and places a cradle with a light in it over the ulcerated part. The bulb should never be larger than 25 W, and there should be a definite order from the physician as to how long it should be left on and how far from the limb it should be placed. Too much heat will increase the metabolic needs of the tissues and thus will be injurious.

A wide variety of agents are used in the local treatment of ulcers. These include castor oil and zinc oxide, nitrofurazone (Furacin), and scarlet red ointment. The effects of antibiotic and antibacterial topical agents such as penicillin, nitrofurazone, bacitracin, and neomycin need to be carefully monitored, since local allergic reactions are common. Streptokinase-streptodornase (Varidase) may be applied locally. Deep ulcers that do not heal properly often require skin grafting. (For special treatment of ulcers occurring in conjunction with varicose veins see p. 1163.)

Since many persons who have chronic ulcers of the legs and feet are not hospitalized, they must be taught how to bathe and otherwise care for themselves without contaminating the ulcer. Many elderly persons have lived with a chronic ulcer for so long that they become careless about their technique in changing soiled or loosened dressings. A periodic visit from a community health nurse, who can reemphasize essentials of care both to the person and to members of the family, is often beneficial.

Providing medications

Patients being treated with medications for peripheral vascular disease must have an understanding of the purpose of the medication and the way in which it is to be taken. Four general types of agents are used: anticoagulants, vasodilators, fibrinolytics, and antiplatelet agents.

Anticoagulants

Two of the commonly used anticoagulant drugs are *heparin* and *bishydroxycoumarin* (Dicumarol), although many other prothrombin depressants are now available. These drugs are used widely in the treatment of both venous and arterial thrombosis and are used prophylactically for persons with threatened thrombosis or threatened recurrence of a condition such as thrombophlebitis. They act therapeutically by prolonging the clotting time of the blood. They will not dissolve clots already formed but will prevent extension of a clot and inhibit formation of new clots.

Heparin antagonzies the activation of prothrombin to thrombin and inhibits aggregation of platelets. It can be given only parenterally because it is destroyed by the gastric secretions of the stomach. Its effect is almost immediate, but its action ceases after 3 to 4 hours. Heparin dosage is expressed in units or milligrams and is calculated individually for each patient; 5000 units (50 mg) is an average dose and is administered through an intravenous line every 3 to 4 hours. This drug is often used to lower the prothrombin time until an oral anticoagulant that acts more slowly can take effect; frequent clotting time determinations must be done.

In order to achieve uniform blood levels over a period of time, heparin is sometimes administered as a continuous intravenous drip of 10,000 to 40,000 units over 24 hours. It may be administered prophylactically in this form to patients on prolonged bed rest before overt signs and symptoms of clot formation are evident. For prophylactic purposes it may also be administered subcutaneously in dosages of 5,000 units every 12 hours.

The effect of heparin is best measured by the partial thromboplastin time, which is usually maintained at twice the normal level. Planning of nursing care must emphasize the increased tendency for bleeding to occur in these patients. Nursing responsibilities are discussed below.

Bishydroxycoumarin acts by suppressing the activity of the liver in its formation of prothrombin. It takes 12 to 24 hours to take effect, and its action persists for 24 to 72 hours after the drug is discontinued. The usual maintenance dosage is 25 to 100 mg/day administered orally.[45] Frequent determinations of the prothrombin level must be obtained and the dose regulated accordingly. Daily prothrombin levels are important while the dose is being regulated. Most physicians believe that the prothrombin level should be kept between 10% and 30% of normal. The prothrombin time should be at least 50% above the normal, or control, values.

Warfarin sodium (Coumadin, Panwarfin, Prothromadin) is also widely used. *Ethyl biscoumacetate* (Tromexan) is another synthetic drug that has an action similar to that of bishydroxycoumarin, although it acts more quickly and its effect lasts for a shorter time.

Any anticoagulant drug requires very careful regulation as to amount and continuity of dosage. If the dosage is too large, the increased tendency to bleed reaches dangerous levels, and if given in combination with other drugs predisposing to bleeding, such as acetylsalicylic acid preparations (aspirin), the problem becomes aggravated. If the dosage is too small the patient may have no relief from symptoms of thrombosis and may even have additional thrombus formation.

If bleeding results from too much heparin, protamine sulfate, a heparin antagonist, is given. Protamine acts almost immediately, and its effect persists for about 2 hours. The physician slowly injects a 1% solution intravenously. The total amount given depends on the amount of heparin that was given and on the patient's symptoms. If a patient taking bishydroxycoumarin should bleed from any body orifice, such as the nose, mouth, or urinary tract, the physician should be notified before another dose is given. Usually the drug is discontinued, and vitamin K (menadione sodium bisulfite) or vitamin K_1 (phytonadione) is given intravenously or orally. If the hemorrhage is excessive, transfusions are given. Nursing care includes reassurance of the patient and careful observation for signs of further hemorrhage.

Anticoagulant therapy has prolonged the lives of many persons and enabled them to live quite satisfactorily and productively. The person who must remain on this drug indefinitely, however, needs encouragement and supportive medical and nursing care. Unfortunately, the vein must be punctured at regular intervals to obtain blood for prothrombin determination. If large doses are needed, this procedure must be performed at least two to three times a week and sometimes daily. When smaller doses of anticoagulant are given over long periods, a prothrombin determination is done every 1 to 4 weeks. This experience is unpleasant for patients, and its continuance over weeks and months may place restraints on their activities. Vacations, for example, present problems, and even short trips must be carefully planned.

Teaching is one of the most important nursing measures in caring for patients receiving anticoagulants. Patients must be taught to recognize the signs of bleeding from any site and to report them immediately. They should carry an identification card or wear a Medic-Alert bracelet stating that they take anticoagulant drugs so that in the event of accident persons who give emergency care will have this information. The identification card should also contain the name and telephone number of the physician prescribing the drug.

Patients should also be taught not to take any other medications while taking anticoagulants without first consulting a physician. Aspirin and steroid preparations can be particularly dangerous in conjunction with heparin and warfarin (Coumadin). Other anticoagulants still being investigated are those that decrease fibrinogen levels, such as snake venom derivatives and staphylcoagulase.

Vasodilators

The second type of medications used to treat peripheral vascular diseases are vasodilators. Vasodilators are given to lessen vasospasm in the arterioles of the lower extremities when arteriosclerosis has caused narrowing of the lumen of the vessel or neighboring vessels, or when a thrombus has formed and caused partial or total obstruction. If a clot is adherent to a blood vessel, an anticoagulant drug may be given with the vasodilator to prevent further clot formation. While several drugs are useful for vasodilation, the excellent vasodilatory effects of warm baths, heat to the abdomen, and hot fluids taken orally should not be overlooked.

Papaverine, a non-habit-forming alkaloid of opium, has long been known to have a relaxing effect on the smooth muscle of the blood vessels, especially when spasm occurs. The usual dose is 300 mg orally once a day. This drug may be used in the treatment of acute arterial occlusion associated with arteriosclerosis obliterans.

Tolazoline hydrochloride (Priscoline), 25 to 50 mg (⅜ to ¾ grain), given orally three to four times a day, is an adrenergic blocking agent (sympatholytic drug). It also may be given intravenously. It prevents the transmission of impulses from the ends of the vasoconstrictor sympathetic fibers to the smooth muscle of the arterioles and thus produces vasodilation. Other drugs that have a similar effect and are prescribed for vasodilation in peripheral vascular diseases are *azapetine phosphate* (Ilidar), *dibenzyl-B-chlorethylamine* (Dibenamine), and

phenoxybenzamine hydrochloride (Dibenzyline). Toxic reactions to these drugs include palpitation, tachycardia, nausea and vomiting, pruritus and abnormal skin sensations, and drop in blood pressure. Toxic signs should be carefully watched for in any patient receiving these drugs and are reported to the physician at once. The patient who cannot tolerate one of these drugs may be able to take another without untoward effects.

Besides the adrenergic blocking agents there are other drugs that are used for their beneficial effect in peripheral vascular disease. *Isoxsuprine* (Vasodilan) and *nylidrin hydrochloride* (Arlidin) are sympathomimetic amines chemically similar to epinephrine. They possess vasodilatig effects, particularly in the vessels in skeletal muscles. Favorable results have been reported with the use of these agents in the treatment of intermittent claudication. Isoxsuprine is usually given orally (10 to 20 mg four times a day); an intramuscular form is also available. Nylidrin is administered orally (6 to 12 mg three times a day) or intramuscularly (5 mg once daily). Side effects include nervousness, palpitation, and nausea and vomiting. *Cyclandelate* (Cyclospasmol) and *nicotinyl tartrate* (Roniacol) produce direct vasodilation of the smooth muscle of the peripheral blood vessels. The usual dosage of cyclandelate is 100 to 200 mg four times daily; the dose of nicotinyl is 50 to 150 mg three times daily after meals. Both can produce dizziness, flushing, and nausea and vomiting. The latter is more likely to occur with nicotinyl because it acts like nicotinic acid.

Alcohol is a very useful drug in dilating the blood vessels. The usual dosage is 30 to 60 ml three to four times a day. The alcohol preparation often ordered is whiskey and soda, but any of the common beverages containing alcohol can be used. Some physicians order a double dose at bedtime to produce maximal effect during the hours when muscle action is not assisting the flow of blood to the legs. *Caffeine* (contained in tea and coffee) and *theobromine* (found in chocolate) also are peripheral vasodilators, but these drugs are seldom given for their vasodilating effect. However, because they have this effect there usually is no need to eliminate tea, coffee, and chocolate from the diet of the person with peripheral vascular disease.

Fibrinolytics

The third type of medication that may be ordered is a fibrinolytic drug. Unlike heparin and warfarin, these drugs will dissolve fibrinous material through direct enzyme action. They are generally available in topical forms or for systemic use.

Streptokinase-streptodornase (Varidase), purified *trypsin crystalline* (Tryptar), and *fibrinuclease* (Elase) are ointment forms that will dissolve fibrinous material and purulent accumulations. They are valuable in removing necrotic tissue for debridement. These enzymes are frequently ordered in treatment of leg ulcers, which occur as a complication of peripheral vascular disease. These enzymes used in conjunction with antibiotics seem to promote more rapid healing. They are usually applied topically in the form of wet dressings.

Streptokinase and urokinase are two fibrinolytic agents recently developed for systemic use in treating thrombosis. Streptokinase is derived from bacterial protein and converts plasminogen to plasmin. It is given as an intravenous loading dose of 25,000 units; then 100,000 units is given over 24 to 72 hours. The disadvantage of this drug is the high incidence of allergic reactions. Urokinase acts more quickly, directly activating plasminogen. It is administered in doses of 4400 units/kg of body weight, followed by 4400 units/kg of body weight over 12 to 24 hours. Although urokinase is not as antigenic as streptokinase, its high cost ($2000 for 24 hours of therapy) prevents its wide usage.[74]

Antiplatelet agents

Several pharmacologic agents have been investigated for use in preventing thrombosis through inhibition of platelet activity. The most common of these include aspirin, dipyridamole (Persantin), sulfinpyrazone (Anturane), and dextran, also referred to as a plasma expander. Dextran is administered as 500 ml of a 6% solution, and care must be taken to avoid circulatory overload during administration.

Preventing complications

The person with peripheral vascular disease has a chronic, potentially disabling process and is subject to periods of exacerbation. The single most important treatment is prevention. The person must be assisted and encouraged to become knowledgeable about all facets of the disease, particularly those that indicate a worsening condition. Prompt medical attention can often preclude complications such as infection or even amputation.

The most serious change in condition that warrants contacting a physician is an area of skin breakdown that does not heal rapidly. Once the integrity of the skin is broken, the diminished circulation often cannot supply the area with sufficient oxygen, nutrients, and leukocytes to protect against infection, and once begun, small infections readily become worse.

Persons with any vascular disease are prone to thrombosis, and any *sudden* change in circulation to an extremity must be promptly evaluated. This would include any change in sensation, color, or temperature in the extremity.

Pain that grows progressively worse over time may also indicate a worsening condition. The patient's physician must be kept aware of changes of this nature in order to evaluate therapy and make necessary alterations.

Peripheral vascular disease has no single cure, and the patient must be knowledgeable about the disease as it affects and is affected by life-style and daily habits. This same knowledge guides the nurse in providing care in the hospital setting. For example, when patients are hospitalized for treatment of a leg ulcer, they must be provided with a warm environment to prevent chills and vasoconstriction and with a diet high in protein to facilitate healing. A sheepskin or flotation pad may be needed to prevent further skin breakdown.

Persons with peripheral vascular disease often have many hospitalizations or frequent ambulatory care visits. It is essential that the patient's record reflect what teaching has been accomplished and how the patient responded to it so that subsequent teaching can build on this knowledge and level of understanding.

Providing emotional support

Emotional support of the person with peripheral vascular disease warrants special consideration because the disease is chronic, affects the person throughout his or her life, and often requires changes in lifetime habits. It may be difficult for the person to perceive how much control over the disease process he or she can exert, although this perception is essential in eliciting active involvement in the treatment program. Improvements in circulation are often slow, and the person needs constant encouragement to maintain the therapeutic regimen. What may seem like minor external changes, such as a better color of nailbeds, can be pointed to as signs of significant internal improvement in the change of the vasculature. Again, the person needs to be taught what to observe.

The pain associated with peripheral vascular disease can also be quite discouraging. The more the nurse can learn about patients' pain, how it affects them, and how they cope with it, the better the nurse will be able to plan with them measures to alleviate their discomfort. Interest in patients as individuals, recognition of the difficulty in coping with persistent pain, and willingness to listen are often the first steps in helping.

The problems that peripheral vascular disease presents often complicate the adjustments involved in the aging process. Additional physical limitation may be imposed when the individual is already attempting to cope with a less active life-style. Dependency-independency conflicts may be aggravated by the older individual's need for health care at home. For further information on assisting the individual with a chronic disease, see Chapter 29.

Outcome criteria for the person with peripheral vascular disease

The person or significant others can:

1. Explain restrictions on activity or prescribed exercise routines.
2. Explain the prescribed diet and plan appropriate meals.
3. Explain the hazards of smoking.
4. Demonstrate measures to prevent skin breakdown.
5. Explain how to avoid external factors that compromise circulation (not crossing legs, avoiding binding clothing such as garters, etc.).
6. Explain medication and treatment program.
    a. State dosage, action, frequency, and side effects of prescribed medications.
    b. If taking anticoagulants, can state precautions to be observed (attention to bleeding, prevention of bleeding, carrying an identification card or wearing a Medic-Alert tag).
    c. Describe how and when to apply any topical medication or dressings.
7. Explain health maintenance program.
    a. State symptoms that indicate the need for obtaining medical attention (bleeding, pain, skin breakdown).
    b. State plans for follow-up care.

Arterial disease

The function of the arteries is to transport blood from the heart to the tissues, utilizing the pressure pulses generated by the heart. Any disturbance in the structure of the arteries interferes with this function, resulting in diminished blood and decreased oxygen supply to the tissues. The symptoms of arterial disease are not caused by the degree of obstruction or narrowing but by the degree to which the involved body part is deprived of circulation. This in turn is affected by such factors as blood pressure and presence or absence of collateral circulation. For example, 50% occlusion of one artery may cause severe symptoms, while 50% occlusion of another artery will cause no symptoms if collateral circulation is sufficient to provide oxygenation.

The arteries are composed of three layers: the *intima*, consisting of endothelium; the *media*, containing smooth muscle cells and elastic fibers; and the *adventitia*, the outermost layer of connective tissue. The proportion of elastic tissue and muscle tissue varies with location in the body and age.

Arteriosclerosis is a general term that literally means hardening of the arteries. It primarily affects the intimal and medial layers and occurs normally as the result of changes of aging and calcification. Over time the arteries become less distensible and lose their elastic properties. The cerebral arteries and arteries of the lower extremities are the most commonly affected.

Atherosclerosis

Etiology

Atherosclerosis is generally viewed as a type of arteriosclerosis or as a part of the aging process that also results in arteriosclerosis. It has been definitely associated with several *risk factors*, including *hypercholesterolemia, cigarette smoking, stress, plasma triglycerides*, and *obesity*. Of these factors, hyperlipidemia carries the greatest risk. The increased levels of serum lipids in individuals in the United States correlates with higher mortality rates from atherosclerotic vascular diseases such as coronary artery disease and cerebrovascular accident when compared to countries such as Italy and Japan, whose inhabitants have lower rates of cholesterol intake and of degenerative heart disease.[68]

Lipoprotein levels may be elevated as a result of dietary excesses alone; may be genetically determined, as in *type II hyperlipoproteinemia;* or may be a combination of excessive intake of saturated fats in combination with inborn errors of carbohydrate metabolism, as in *type IV hyperlipoproteinemia*. Although all types are associated with an increased incidence of coronary artery disease, types II and III carry the greatest risk.

Other variables associated with atherosclerosis include diabetes, hypertension, and gender. Cornary and peripheral atherosclerosis is two to three times more prevalent in the diabetic, regardless of serum lipid levels. Hypertension is believed to accentuate the process of lesion formation, perhaps by producing mechanical stress. The incidence is also greater in men than women.

Pathophysiology

Atherosclerosis refers to the development of lesions on the intimal wall. Three types of lesions have been identified: (1) fatty streaks, which consist of smooth-muscle cells, and lipid depositions, which are present in the aorta of all individuals by age 10 years but which do not necessarily progress to produce disease; (2) fibrous plaques, which involve a thickening of the intima and are surrounded by lipids, collagen, and elastic fibers; and (3) the complicated lesion associated with disease, which is a large mass consisting of lipids and extracellular and intracellular debris, ulceration, hemorrhage, and thrombus formation.

The exact pathogenesis of atherosclerosis is not clearly understood. Endothelial cell injury, smooth-muscle cell proliferation, and lipid and cell debris accumulation are among the factors that seem to be inherent in the development of lesions. It is thought that an alteration in endothelial permeability is one of the first changes, predisposing to secondary processes. This change in permeability could result from damage by endotoxins or hypoxia, from hypertension, or from imbalances in levels of immune complexes.[118] The exact sequence of events, the mechanism for transport of lipids into the arterial wall, and the factors that promote cell proliferation are unknown.

The lesions of atherosclerosis tend to be focal rather than diffuse, increase with age, and involve primarily the larger arteries, particularly the lower portion of the aorta. Persons who develop myocardial infarctions or cerebral infarctions are usually found to have atherosclerotic involvement in many other sites.[33]

Clinical picture

The clinical picture of the individual with compromise of arterial circulation caused by atherosclerosis depends on the target organs and areas involved. The reader is referred to p. 1111 for a discussion of coronary artery disease and to p. 797 for a discussion of cerebrovascular accident. Atherosclerosis of the extremities is referred to as arteriosclerosis (or atherosclerosis obliterans).

Atherosclerosis obliterans

Etiology

Atherosclerosis obliterans is the most common form of obstructive disease after 30 years of age. The femoral artery is the most commonly involved, although the carotid artery may also be involved. The disease affects men more often than women, and the greatest incidence is between 50 and 70 years of age. It is associated with diabetes and with cigarette smoking.

Pathophysiology

Atherosclerosis obliterans is an obstructive, degenerative arterial disorder representing a late stage of atherosclerosis and involving both the medial and intimal layers. It is characterized by partial or complete occlusion of arteries by atheromas on the intima, segmental in nature, but with changes evident distal to and proximal to the stenosis. The media gradually loses elasticity as the disease progresses, and the development of thrombi is common.

As a result the artery gradually becomes unable to transport the required amount of blood to the affected part. Symptoms appear when the blood vessels can no longer provide enough blood to supply oxygen and nu-

trients to the limbs and to remove the waste products of metabolism.

Clinical picture

Early signs and symptoms of atherosclerosis obliterans may include skin temperature changes, differences in color and size of lower limbs, altered arterial pulsations, and the presence of *bruits* (sounds heard over the artery on auscultation). Intermittent claudication (p. 1143) is the most common symptom. Later the patient may complain of pain in the affected part even at rest. Pain at rest indicates that the artery cannot supply sufficient circulation to meet even minimal metabolic demands. The pain often occurs at night, and the patient may report that it subsides with movement and particularly with walking. Very elderly patients may be awakened by excruciating cramplike pains in the muscles of the calf and the thighs that are believed to be due to lack of oxygen to the tissue *(ischemia)*. Tingling and numbness of the toes may be mentioned by the patient, and a very common complaint is difficulty in keeping the feet and hands warm enough for comfort. Occasionally, the first sign of limited circulation is necrosis following mild trauma such as cutting the skin when trimming the nails; ulcers and gangrene may develop.

The disease is usually present to some extent in both limbs, although symptoms may be grossly apparent in only one. Occlusion of a fairly large artery by a thrombus will cause numbness, marked coldness, and a chalk-white appearance in the part of the limb supplied by the obstructed vessel.

Intervention

An essential nursing function when caring for patients with peripheral vascular disease is the checking of the arterial pulses.

Medical treatment for atherosclerosis obliterans includes provision for general warmth, use of drugs to produce vasodilation, carefully prescribed general exercise to maintain circulation and yet not tax the arterial system, encouragement, and instruction in avoiding injury, preventing infection, and maintaining nutrition. Pain at rest may be treated by having the patient sleep with the head of the bed elevated on blocks 7.5 to 15 cm (3 to 6 in.) in height to aid gravity in carrying arterial blood to the legs and feet. Patients should be advised not to walk about during the night unless they are warmly clothed and to avoid sitting with their legs over the side of the bed because they may become chilled and knee flexion further hampers circulation. They should not rub the extremity because of the danger of trauma and of releasing an embolus into the circulation. *Vigorous massage is always contraindicated in any patient with vascular disease*. A graduated program of exercise may be prescribed.

Nursing intervention is directed toward helping patients to live within their limitations and encouraging them to carry out medical instructions so that the disease may be held in check for an indefinite time. All nursing measures discussed earlier in this chapter under general interventions may be necessary in caring for these persons. If the condition cannot be checked, gangrene of the extremity may occur, making amputation necessary.

If the disease is rapidly progressive and the patient is in reasonably good health otherwise, surgery to correct the obstruction may be indicated. The most common procedure is a bypass of the obstructed arterial segment, using prosthetic material such as Teflon or Dacron, or autogenous (the patient's own) artery or vein, such as the saphenous vein. The bypass may involve the aorta itself, as with an aortofemoral bypass, or more distal vessels such as the femoral-popliteal (Fig. 46-2).

Procedures that may be performed either in conjunction with a bypass or by themselves include *patch grafting* (replacing a damaged segment of the arterial wall with a vein patch), *profundoplasty* (widening of the origin of the femoral artery with a vein patch), and *endarterectomy* (stripping arteriosclerotic plaques from the intima and inner media using balloon catheters or other instruments).

Carotid endarterectomy has become more frequently used as diagnostic methods have improved. Pa-

tency rate of the artery following surgery has averaged 95% with a mortality of 0.5% to 3%. Patients who have undergone carotid endarterectomy must be observed postoperatively for bleeding and for any neurologic change that could indicate inadequate cerebral circulation as a result of obstruction of the carotid artery. Vasopressors or vasodilators may be used during the first 24 postoperative hours to maintain the blood pressure at a level that will favor good flow through the operative artery. As when caring for any patient undergoing surgery for arterial obstructive disease, the nurse must keep in mind that these patients are at high risk for postoperative myocardial infarction because of their underlying disease process.

Postoperative nursing intervention for patients undergoing arterial reconstructive surgery centers around assessment of circulation to the involved extremities. The nurse needs to be aware of the preoperative condition of the extremities in order to make meaningful postoperative comparisons. The color, temperature, sensation, and quality of pulses in the extremity must be checked hourly for the first 8 hours. Initially, vasospasm may make it difficult or impossible to palpate the pedal or posterior tibial pulses, and a Doppler machine may be used (p. 1145). When adequate circulation has been restored, it will be evident from the color and temperature of the limb, which often will be warmer

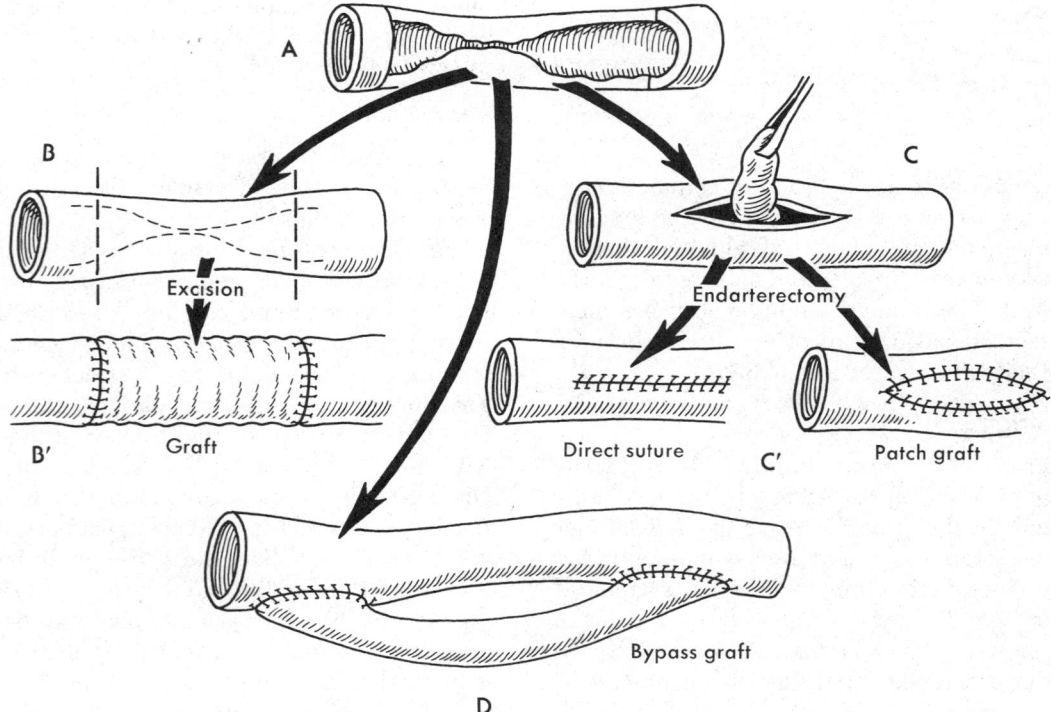

Fig. 46-2. A, Obstructed artery. Methods of restoring arterial blood flow include, **B,** excision; **B',** graft; **C,** endarterectomy; **C',** direct suture and patch graft reconstruction; and **D,** bypass graft. (Redrawn from Fairbairn, J.F., Jurgens, J.L., Spittell, J.A.: Peripheral vascular disease, Philadelphia, 1972, W.B. Saunders Co.)

than its counterpart. Obstruction is indicated by a marked coldness, sudden disappearance of a pulse that was palpable the previous hour, or a progressive whitening, later changing to cyanosis, of the toes and foot. The surgeon is notified immediately if these changes occur.

Patients are usually kept flat in bed for the first 12 to 24 hours and then are allowed out of bed but must *avoid sharp flexion in the areas of the grafts*. The success of the surgery is dependent on the general health of the patient and the size of the vessels involved. The larger the vessel, the more effective the surgery, with aortic-iliac and aortofemoral grafts having success rates of 90%.[8,59] The nurse must be alert to any sign of infection in the incisional area (redness, swelling, or purulent drainage). Infection of a prosthetic graft, although occurring rarely, invariably means failure of the graft.

Thromboangiitis obliterans

Etiology

Thromboangiitis obliterans (Buerger's disease) is an obstructive, idiopathic disease affecting small- and medium-sized arteries and veins. The exact etiology remains unknown. This disease is most common in men between 25 and 40 years of age and is slightly more prevalent in Jewish persons. It rarely occurs in females or in blacks. Tobacco may play a primary role in its development in that most patients with thromboangiitis obliterans are heavy smokers and symptoms abate when smoking is stopped. Hypercoagulability of the blood is also thought to play a role.

Pathophysiology

The primary pathophysiologic event in thromboangiitis obliterans is an inflammatory process, usually in small arterioles and sometimes in veins. The inflammation is associated with thrombosis and spasm. It occurs as a focal rather than a diffuse process, affecting the lower more often that the upper extremities. Large, central vessels, such as the aorta and carotid arteries, are not involved.

Clinical picture

The signs and symptoms of thromboangiitis obliterans are a result of peripheral ischemia. Pain is the most common complaint. This may occur as *intermittent claudication, pain at rest* or a *generalized aching. Ischemic neuropathy* may lead to numbness and tingling. *Superficial thrombophlebitis* may be evidenced by hardened, red, raised areas along the length of the affected vein. The extent of symptoms depends on the size of the area involved and the amount of collateral circulation. Ulcers and gangrene of fingers and toes are common. Arterial pulses are usually present. The involved limb may feel cooler than uninvolved areas, and

environmental cold generally causes an exacerbation of symptoms. The distal extremity exhibits dependent rubor, a dark reddish color when lowered, or cyanosis in advanced disease.

Intervention

It is often possible to arrest thromboangiitis obliterans completely and indefinitely by merely having the patient stop smoking. This restriction is considered the most important aspect of treatment. Smoking must be given up immediately, completely, and forever. Other measures prescribed to foster circulation include warmth, moderate exercise, and instruction to prevent infection and to avoid trauma and exposure to the cold. Some physicians believe that *bilateral preganglionic sympathectomy* is helpful when the lower extremities are involved because it produces permanent vasodilation of the blood vessels. Sympathetic impulses may also be blocked by paravertebral injection of alcohol. Although pain may be severe, narcotics are rarely prescribed because of the obvious danger of drug addiction in young persons with a chronic disease such as thromboangiitis obliterans. Vasodilators and anticoagulants may be tried but are generally found to be ineffective.

The nurse can often help by emphasizing the precautions that the patient should take to prevent the onset of acute symptoms including pain. The patient should be encouraged not to smoke and should be advised to wear warm gloves and footwear in cold weather. Both of these measures prevent extensive vasoconstriction. He or she should be taught to avoid any injury to the feet, especially when cutting toenails. Wounds heal slowly, and gangrene may develop.

Raynaud's phenomenon

Etiology

Raynaud's phenomenon is a condition or episode of arterial spasm of the extremities, most often the hands. When this occurs without association with another disease or vascular injury, it is termed *primary Raynaud's phenomenon,* or *Raynaud's disease*. Although the exact mechanism is unknown, abnormal sympathetic innervation, or hypersusceptibility to certain stimuli, is thought to be a possible cause. Raynaud's disease occurs almost exclusively in women and is usually diagnosed before age 40.

Secondary Raynaud's phenomenon occurs as a result of another disease process, such as scleroderma, occlusive arterial disease, or thoracic outlet syndrome, or as a result of occupational hazards. Individuals whose occupation involves subjecting their hands to repeated percussive or vibratory forces, such as operators of pneumatic hammers and chain saws or typists, may exhibit Raynaud's phenomenon.

Pathophysiology

Little is known about the actual pathophysiologic changes in vessels involved in Raynaud's phenomenon. Atrial intimal thickening occurs over time, but this may be a result of, rather than part of the cause of, vasospasm. Cold and emotional stress are the usual precipitating factors, contributing to the thought that neurogenic factors initiate the disease.

Clinical picture

The chief complaint of individuals with Raynaud's phenomenon is of cold, numbness, and tingling of one or more fingers. This always occurs as a bilateral process, affecting both hands. The involved fingers appear normal except when the spasm occurs, when they become white or mottled. When the spasm abates, they often become reddish for a few moments. In long-standing disease, small ulcerated areas may appear at the tips of the fingers.

Intervention

Patients in whom this condition is mild are advised to avoid smoking and keep the hands and feet warm. Gloves and fleece-lined boots should be worn whenever the individual is exposed to cold weather. Vasodilators, particularly reserpine, are prescribed if symptoms are incapacitating, and sympathectomy may be performed for severe disease.

Embolism

Etiology and pathophysiology

Emboli are blood clots floating in the circulating blood. These clots most commonly originate in the heart. They may be a fragment of an arteriosclerotic plaque loosened from the aorta or a thrombus released when inefficient heart pumping is suddenly corrected by digitalization. Emboli usually lodge at the bifurcations, or divisions, of the arteries because of the diminishing caliber of the vessels beyond these points. An embolus lodging at the bifurcation of any artery is called a *saddle embolus*. As soon as an embolus lodges, thrombi (propagated emboli) form in the involved vessel. The reader is referred to pp. 1154 and 1159 for a discussion of the pathophysiology of the two major underlying conditions associated with embolization—atherosclerosis and phlebitis.

Clinical picture

The signs of sudden lodging or formation of a large thrombus in an artery are dramatic and vary with the part of the arterial system and associated organ system involved. There is severe pain at the site of the thrombus formation. Fainting, nausea, vomiting, and signs of pronounced shock may appear. Almost immediately areas supplied by the vessel may become white, cold, and blotched, and they may tingle and feel numb. Cyanosis, followed by even greater darkening and gangrene, occurs if the blood supply is completely obstructed and collateral circulation is inadequate.

Intervention

Vasodilating drugs are given to improve the collateral circulation, warmth is applied to the body, and a sympathetic block of the lumbar ganglia may be performed in an attempt to produce vasodilation of other vessels. Oxygen may be administered to alleviate hypoxemia and dyspnea. Vasopressors may be necessary if shock ensues. Heparin and bishydroxycoumarin may be administered to help prevent further thrombus formation. The patient who is suspected of having or who has an acute embolic obstruction of a larger artery needs constant nursing supervision. Pain is severe, and fear is pronounced.

If the patient does not respond to the medical treatment within a few hours, surgery may be performed. Surgical procedures that may be used include opening the vessel and removing the clot (*embolectomy*), removing the clot and also removing adherent substances and part of the lining of the vessel (*endarterectomy*, or "reaming"), arterial resection with removal of the clot and the adherent diseased artery surrounding it with subsequent grafting, and bypassing the diseased portion of the vessel with a graft as is sometimes done for an aneurysm. Embolectomy is usually the treatment of choice for aortic embolus and for an embolus of the common iliac artery.

Nursing care following embolectomy is similar to that for the patient who has had surgery for an aneurysm. Blood pressure must be carefully recorded preoperatively so that suitable comparisons can be made postoperatively. It is important that the blood pressure not vary too much from what it was preoperatively because variation will predispose to thrombus formation. A complication that must be carefully watched for is hemorrhage. Small arteries that may have been useless while the embolus was in the artery may not bleed freely during surgery and may therefore be missed when bleeding vessels are tied off. They may resume normal function after the operation and cause hemorrhage.

Aneurysm of the extremity and arteriovenous fistula

Etiology

Aneurysms and arteriovenous fistulas are often considered together because of their similar clinical picture. Both may occur congenitally or may be acquired following trauma.

Pathophysiology

An *aneurysm* is an enlarged, dilated portion of an artery. Although it may follow trauma, such as an automobile accident, it is more commonly associated with arteriosclerosis. The destruction of the medial layer leads to weakening of the wall of the artery and eventual aneurysm formation. Aneurysms are particularly common in the popliteal area (Fig. 46-3).

An *arteriovenous fistula* is an abnormal communication between artery and vein. The arterial blood bypasses the capillary bed, which has a strong resistance to blood flow, and flows instead directly into the vein. Persistence of this high-pressure flow in the vein will eventually result in venous dilation and may be associated with aneurysm formation.

Clinical picture

The most common signs of both aneurysms and arteriovenous fistulas are the presence of a large, pulsating mass and a characteristic sound over the mass, a *bruit*, or soft, blowing sound heard with a stethoscope. Aneurysms are sometimes first diagnosed following the formation of a thrombus at the site of the aneurysm and the traveling of an embolus into distal portions of the artery. Pain is more common with large artery aneurysms, such as in the aorta, than in smaller arteries.

Arteriovenous fistulas usually are associated with signs

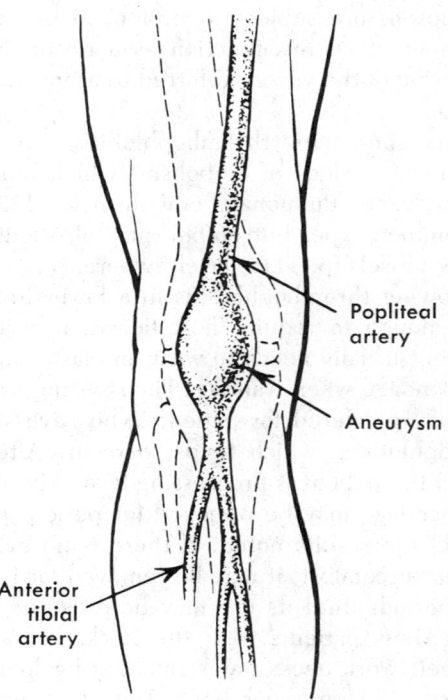

Fig. 46-3. Posterior view of knee with aneurysm of popliteal artery. (From Anderson, H.C.: Newton's geriatric nursing, ed. 5, St. Louis, 1971, The C.V. Mosby Co.)

of venous insufficiency, such as mottled, darkened skin, enlarged girth or edema of the extremity, and increased skin temperature when compared with the normal limb. In both cases, arteriogram and ultrasound studies are used as diagnostic tools.

Intervention

Closure of the fistula or removal of a portion of the aneurysm is the preferred treatment. When one of these measures is not possible, the vessel may be ligated unless ligation is incompatible with the life of tissues distal to the lesion. *Homografts* (a section of the patient's vein) or Teflon or Dacron grafts can be used in larger blood vessels of the extremities either to replace portions of the artery that contain the aneurysm or to bypass the abnormality. In addition to general postoperative care, the patient who has had this surgical procedure may be treated with any or all of the medications and other means described in this chapter to augment circulation when arterial supply is limited or when thrombosis threatens.

Venous disease

Thrombophlebitis

Etiology and pathophysiology

Thrombophlebitis, or venous thrombosis, is characterized by inflammation of a vein and by clot formation. Although much is known about some mechanisms producing inflammatory changes and thrombus production, the incidence of this condition continues to increase,[1] and the exact interrelationship of the factors is not clearly understood. In some cases the thrombosis appears to be the primary event, and in others inflammation of the vein endothelium is thought to precede the development of the thrombus.

Many factors are associated with thrombophlebitis. Venous stasis, damage to the endothelium, and hypercoagulability of the blood are all significant etiologic mechanisms. Stasis may result from relatively simple circumstances such as taking a long trip during which hours were spent sitting with the knees flexed. Pregnancy is often complicated by thrombophlebitis because of interference with venous return in the lower abdomen. Before the days of early ambulation and emphasis on exercises postoperatively, thrombophlebitis was a frequent complication of surgery. It remains a dreaded complication of any illness that requires immobilization for any length of time, and the use of low-dose heparin prophylactically is becoming more common.

Trauma to venous walls may result from the irritating effects of certain drugs or hypertonic solutions. The presence of intravenous catheters, particularly when left in place longer than 48 hours, has been associated with increased thrombosis. Damage to the veins may accompany trauma such as fractures and has been known to follow unusual physical exertion and muscle strain.

States of hypercoagulability, such as occur with hematologic diseases (e.g., polycythemia and severe anemia); also *predispose to the development of thrombophlebitis*. Thrombosis is known to occur to some degree in all types of systemic infections, and this may reflect hypercoagulability caused by endotoxins. It is believed that the use of oral contraceptives is correlated with increased intravascular clotting, but the exact mechanism responsible for this association is not yet known.

Clinical picture

Thrombophlebitis of superficial veins is readily apparent. On palpation the veins appear hard and thready and are sensitive to pressure. The entire limb may be swollen, pale, and cold, and the area along the vein may be reddened and feel warm to the touch. Deep veins in the legs may be affected, and the pain they cause when the patient dorsiflexes the foot or walks is known as *Homan's sign*. Thrombophlebitis may be accompanied by reflected pain in the entire limb. Systemic reaction to the infection, which may occur in any blood vessel when free flow of blood is interrupted, may rarely cause symptoms such as headache, malaise, and elevation of temperature. Of utmost importance in the assessment of patients is the knowledge that thrombophlebitis is a common condition, occurring in at least 5% of all surgical patients and going unrecognized in half of these. Embolization of the thrombus to lungs, heart, or brain may be a fatal complication and at the very least results in prolonged hospitalization and increased cost to the patient.

Intervention

Superficial thrombophlebitis is usually treated by rest; however, physicians differ in regard to the amount of activity that is allowed. Some believe that the clot is sufficiently adherent to the vein wall to make its release unlikely and that moving about helps to improve general circulation and to prevent further congestion of blood in the veins. Others believe that complete immobilization is necessary to prevent a part of the thrombus from breaking away and becoming an embolus. The patient who has thrombophlebitis of large and deep vessels, however, usually is kept quiet. Care must be taken that the patient is not frightened by being kept quiet; explanations from both the physician and the nurse will be helpful in reassuring the patient. Occasionally, the vein is ligated above the involvement (usually at the femoral junction) to decrease the danger of embolism, but this procedure is not possible unless there is adequate collateral circulation. The period of immobilization depends entirely on the response of the patient to treatment.

Continuous applications of warm moist heat are often used for both deep and superficial thrombophlebitis. Some physicians feel, however, that heat increases the risk that emboli will be released because it induces vasodilation, and they order ice packs for their patients, especially for those with deep vein thrombosis. When warm packs are used they are usually ordered to cover the entire extremity.[12] Heating pads permanently set on "low" may be used to keep the packs at a consistently safe temperature.

Many physicians prefer that the affected limb be elevated slightly to reduce edema and to prevent stasis distal to the thrombus. It may also relieve pain. Some physicians believe, however, that the danger of an embolus being released is greater if the limb is elevated. Therefore the nurse will need to check on the procedure to be followed in the care of each patient.

Heparin and bishydroxycoumarin are used for patients with thrombophlebitis, and sometimes patients must remain on prophylactic doses of bishydroxycoumarin for an indefinite period to prevent recurrences of the disease. Vasodilating drugs are given to combat the arterial vessel spasm that occurs at the site of a venous thrombus and to improve general circulation, thus increasing the rate of absorption of the thrombus.

Streptokinase may also be used to treat acute deep vein thrombosis and has been reported as successfully resolving the thrombus in 70% of patients.[2] However, all patients who have experienced thrombophlebitis in the lower extremities, regardless of which treatment has been chosen, are subject to prolonged or permanent impairment of venous function as a result of damage and scarring of the vessel, referred to as postthrombotic syndrome.

All persons with thrombophlebitis are observed closely for any signs of embolism, which must be reported at once. Pulmonary embolism (p. 1320) is the most common type, but emboli may also lodge in the coronary vessels (p. 1114) or elsewhere.

Following thrombophlebitis in a lower limb that is severe enough to require hospitalization or bed rest, the patient usually needs to wear an elastic stocking or elastic bandage when walking. The stocking or bandage is also often ordered for patients who have superficial thrombophlebitis, which tends to recur. After 4 to 6 weeks, if the patient is progressing favorably, the stocking or bandage may be removed for periods of ½ to 1 hour and the results noted. If there is no evidence of edema or discomfort, it may be removed for longer and longer periods until its use may be discontinued completely. Many patients wear the stockings indefinitely when their work necessitates standing for long periods or sitting with the knees bent. Two stockings or bandages are necessary for each affected limb so that they can be laundered as necessary.

The *elastic stocking*, accurately fitted to the patient's measurements, must be obtained before the patient gets out of bed for the first time. The stocking is used to compress superficial veins, increase flow through the deep veins, and prevent venous pooling. Stockings of various sizes and lengths are usually stocked by hospital supply stores, and many large department stores also carry them. The measurements that must be taken are printed on the box or can be obtained by calling the store. The most satisfactory length is 2.5 cm (1 in.) below the bend of the knee joint. The patient must be taught how to put on the stocking. It should be rolled on evenly before getting out of bed in the morning. It should be removed once during the day for a few moments and the skin very gently stroked and powdered as necessary. The stocking need not be worn during sleeping hours.

Elastic bandages may be used instead of an elastic stocking, but they are more conspicuous and are difficult to apply evenly. They may be used for short periods following surgery and are sometimes ordered for use on those occasions when the person will be lifting heavy objects or standing still for a period of time. When a bandage has been ordered for continuous use, it should be applied before the person gets out of bed in the morning. The bandage is applied with equal pressure and overlap from the foot upward. Usually the entire foot, including the heel, is wrapped. The bandage will extend either to just below the knee or to the groin, depending on the physician's orders. It should be smooth and snug but must not be so tight that it interferes with circulation.

Swimming and wading in water are among the best activities for prevention of recurrences of thrombophlebitis of the lower extremities and are highly recommended for persons with other venous diseases as well. Water, which is denser than air, exerts a smooth, even pressure on the skin, and wading is especially beneficial because the greater pressure (the deeper water) surrounds the distal portion of the extremity and helps in the return flow of venous blood.

If conservative measures such as bed rest and anticoagulation are not successful, if the thrombosis is extensive and recurrent, or if embolization is recurrent, surgical treatment may be necessary. The peripheral vein involved, such as the superficial femoral vein, may be ligated or the vena cava interrupted by ligation or placement of a vena caval umbrella or grid to impede blood flow.

Caval ligation and plication are major surgical procedures requiring general anesthesia. In addition to the usual postoperative nursing interventions, the nurse must focus on assessing all parameters of circulation. Postoperative bleeding and hematoma formation occasionally occur, especially if anticoagulants are continued. Collateral circulation should be sufficient to prevent pooling of blood in the extremities, but stasis and edema may be noted in the late postoperative period. The caval umbrella can be inserted with instruments transvenously while the patient is under local anesthesia and is much more commonly used (Fig. 46-4). Postoperative nursing

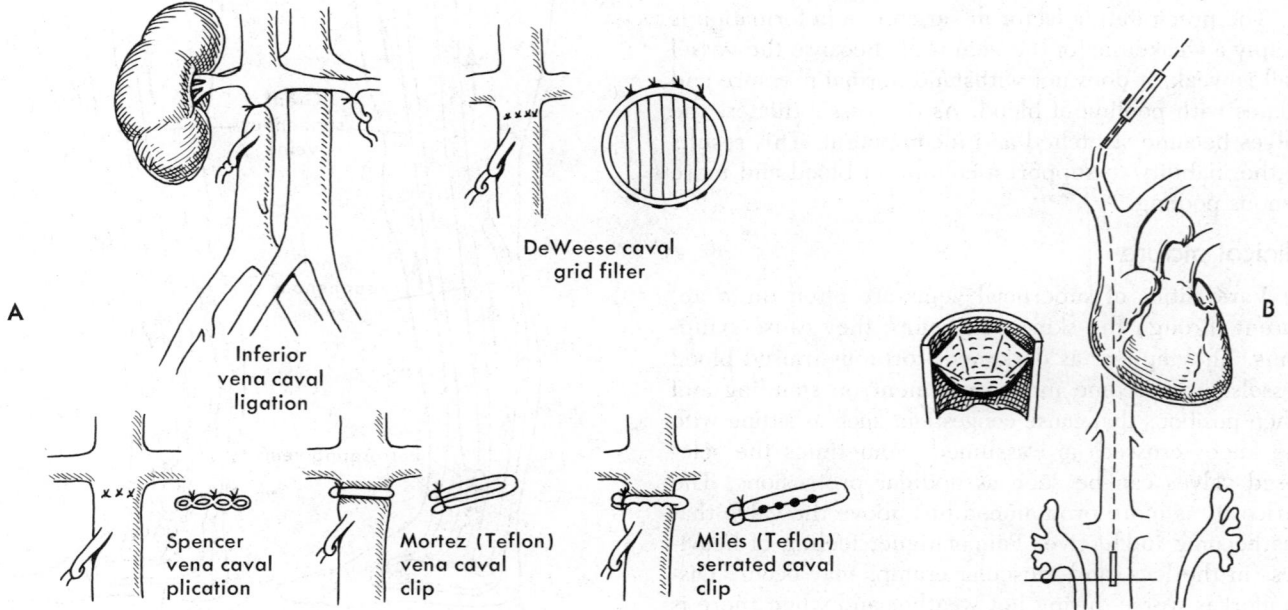

Fig. 46-4. A, Various surgical techniques for preventing embolism from pelvic and lower extremity veins. **B,** Transvenous method of vena caval interruption using caval prosthesis of umbrella design. Insert illustrates open umbrella. (Redrawn from Fairbairn, J.F., Jurgens, J.L., and Spittell, J.A.: Peripheral vascular disease, Philadelphia, 1972, W.B. Saunders Co.)

care is similar to that for the patient who has had a cardiac catheterization (p. 1060).

Varicose veins

Etiology

Varicose veins are abnormally dilated veins with incompetent valves, occurring most often in the lower extremities and the lower trunk. In the lower limbs the great and small saphenous veins are most often involved. At least 20% of the total population is affected by varicose veins. The highest incidence is in the third, fourth, and fifth decades of life. Factors that predispose a person to the development of varicosities include congenitally defective valves, hereditary weakness of the vein walls, and prolonged standing, which places strain on the valves because muscle action is not helping to return the blood. Our upright position further aggravates the problem, and poor posture with sagging of abdominal organs causes additional pressure. Pregnancy and abdominal tumors that cause pressure on the large veins of the lower abdomen and interfere with good venous drainage predispose a person to the development of varicose veins. Chronic systemic disease such as heart disease and cirrhosis of the liver may interfere with adequate return of blood to the heart and contribute to varicosities. Infections and trauma to the veins with resultant thrombophlebitis may also lead to varicose veins, since the valves are destroyed as the acute inflammation subsides.

Pathophysiology

The precipitating factor in varicose vein formation is simply a weakening of the vein wall. Because the vessel wall is weak, it does not withstand normal pressure and dilates with pooling of blood. As the vessel dilates, the valves become stretched and incompetent. This results in the inability to support a column of blood and more venous pooling.

Clinical picture

Varicosities of superficial veins are often quite apparent through the skin even before they cause symptoms. They appear as darkened, tortuous, raised blood vessels that become more prominent on standing and when positions that cause congestion, such as sitting with the knees crossed, are assumed. Sometimes the sclerosed valves can be seen as nodular protrusions. The varicosity is more pronounced just above the valve that has become ineffective. Pain, fatigue, feeling of heaviness in the legs, and muscular cramps may occur. Discomfort is worse during hot weather and when there is a change from a low to a high altitude. It is greatly increased by prolonged standing.

The simplest test for varicose veins is known as *Trendelenburg's* test. The patient lies down with the

leg raised until the vein empties completely, and a tourniquet is then applied above the knee. The patient then stands, and the vein is observed as it fills. A normal vein fills from below; a varicose vein fills from above because the valve fails to retain the blood that has drained into the portion of the vessel above (Fig. 46-5).

Intervention

Conservative management. Mild discomfort from varicose veins may be treated conservatively by advising patients to elevate their feet for a few minutes at regular 2- to 3-hour intervals throughout the day, to avoid constrictions about the legs, to avoid standing for long periods of time, and to wear an elastic stocking or elastic bandage. All of these measures help to reduce venous pooling and increase venous return. Improvement in posture sometimes helps to prevent further development of the varicosities, and the patient may be advised by the physician to lose weight.

Ligation and stripping of veins. Surgical treatment for varicosities consists of ligation of the vein above the varicosity and removal of the varicosed vein distal to the ligation, provided that the deep veins are able to return the venous blood satisfactorily (Fig. 46-5). The

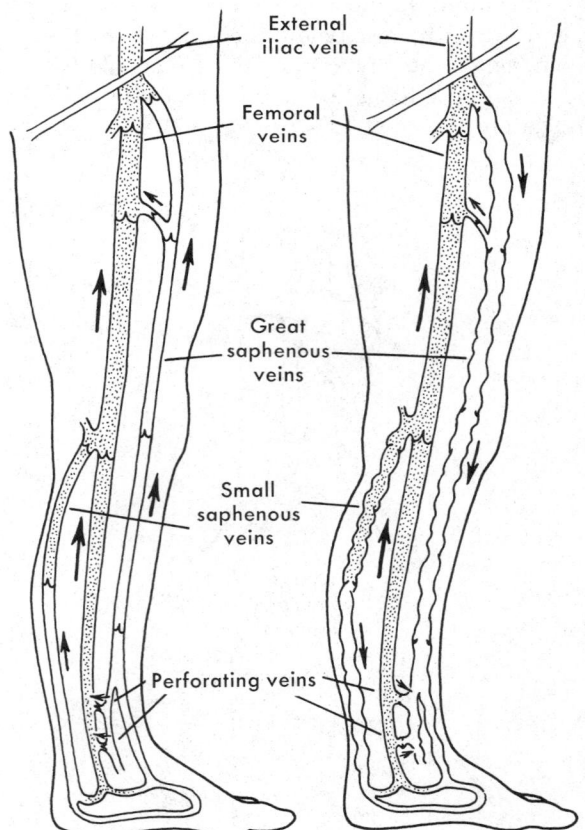

Fig. 46-5. *Left,* Venous flow in normal veins. *Right,* Venous flow in varicose veins. (Redrawn from Fairbairn, J.F., Jurgens, J.L., and Spittrell, J.A.: Peripheral vascular disease, Philadelphia, 1972, W.B. Saunders Co.)

great saphenous vein is ligated close to the femoral junction if possible, and the great and small saphenous veins are then stripped out through small incisions at the groin, above and below the knee, and at the ankle. Sterile dressings are placed over the incisions, and an elastic bandage extending from the foot to the groin is applied firmly.

General anesthesia is usual, since the procedure is very tiresome and painful. To prevent the development of thrombi in other veins, the patient usually walks about on the day of the operation and at frequent intervals during the remaining 2 to 3 days in the hospital. Unless the patient is elderly and also has arterial insufficiency, the foot of the bed is usually elevated on blocks for the first 24 hours to help in venous return of blood. Moving, walking, and bending the leg are extremely difficult for the patient, and he or she may have more pain and discomfort following this surgical procedure than following much more serious surgery. Analgesic drugs may be necessary for the first 24 to 48 hours.

Although the operation is considered a relatively minor one and the patient is out of bed at once, nursing care is important. Patients will require assistance when they walk on the first postoperative day and sometimes longer. Some patients have difficulty in walking because of the firm binding around the knees; therefore care is taken to prevent accidents. The elastic bandage and the dressings are checked several times a day because they may become loosened with walking and the incisions may become exposed. Hemorrhage may occur and should be watched for, especially on the operative day. If bleeding does occur, the leg is elevated, pressure is applied over the wound, and the surgeon is notified.

Patients who have surgery for varicose veins should know that the condition may recur, since large superficial collateral vessels may develop and in turn become varicosed. They should take the general precautions of any patient with varicosities, since the operation cures the acute symptoms but does not remove the tendency to develop varicose veins. Weight reduction, posture improvement, avoidance of pressure on blood vessels, and elevation of the lower limbs should be practiced postoperatively exactly as is recommended for the patient with mild varicosities who is receiving conservative treatment only. The booklet *Varicose Veins*, which can be obtained from the American Heart Association, is useful in teaching patients.

Treatment by sclerosis. Sclerosing solutions are occasionally used in the treatment of very small varicosities. The solutions cause an irritation within the vessel, development of a thrombus, and eventual occlusion of the lumen of the vein. This treatment is used rarely anymore because of the frequency of allergic reactions, the need for repeated treatments, and the danger of tissue sloughing if the solution touches healthy tissue. Sodium tetradecyl sulfate (Sotradecol) and monoetha-

line oleate (Monolate) are two of the solutions commonly used.

The injection of sclerosing solutions is usually performed in the clinic or the physician's office. The nurse assumes responsibility for seeing that emergency equipment for treating allergic reactions is available and for preventing accidents to patients. Many patients are elderly, and some tend to become faint while standing for the treatment. Footstools can be equipped with side attachments and handlebars on which the patient may lean for comfort and security. The site of injection is covered with a small dressing. Patients are urged not to scratch the skin over the site of injection because scratching may lead to an infected excoriation and eventual ulceration. They also should be cautioned about bruising or otherwise traumatizing the veins, which also may lead to ulceration. Patients are usually instructed to walk about immediately, and elastic stockings or bandages may be ordered.

Management of varicose ulcers. Stasis of blood in tissues around marked varicosities, particularly when deep veins are also involved, leads to changes in normal tissue. The tissue becomes pigmented and edematous as fluid and the waste products of metabolism are inadequately cleared. There is often *severe pruritus* and *discomfort*. Small arteriovenous fistulas may develop as a result of the increased pressure in the thrombosed venous system, and tissue hypoxia occurs around the capillary bed when the blood is diverted into the venous system. As a result of these changes, *stasis ulcers* develop following small bruises or scratches or may develop spontaneously.

As part of the treatment of a stasis ulcer, ligation of varicose veins may be necessary because the ulcer will not heal while marked varicosities persist in the vessels above it. In addition to the general measures already mentioned for any ulcers of vascular origin, treatment of *varicose ulcers* includes grafting of skin to cover the wound and the use of pressure bandages. Grafting may not be successful if the arterial supply is also affected because poor circulation to the fibrotic tissue surrounding the ulcer causes healing to be slow. (See p. 1802 for care of a graft.)

Medical treatment of ulcers consists of bed rest, protection of the area from trauma and infection, and promotion of healing. If the ulcerated area is small and the patient is able to remain ambulatory, a semirigid boot may be applied. The boot protects the ulcer and provides constant, even support to the area. An Unna paste boot is a commercial preparation containing gelatin, glycerin, and zinc oxide (Fig. 46-6). It is not used often because the mixture must be melted and brushed on in several coats and is somewhat inconvenient and cumbersome to apply. Instead, an elastic bandage (Elastoplast) over a layer of foam rubber and dry sterile gauze or gauze impregnated with medication may be prescribed. The boot is generally left on for 10 days to

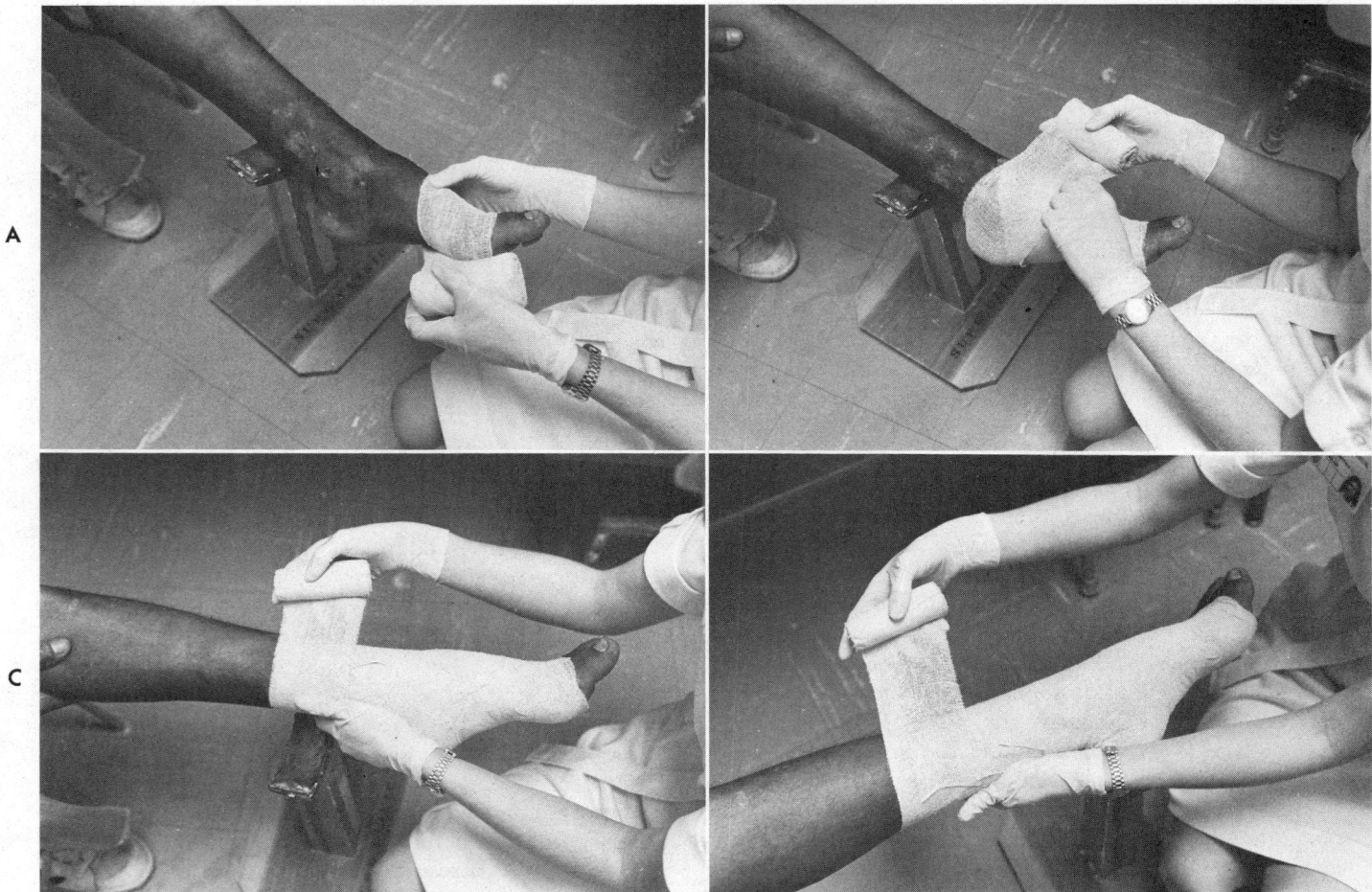

Fig. 46-6. Nurse applying Unna paste boot using specially impregnated gauze. Note ulcers on interior aspect of patient's foot.

2 weeks, although it may be changed sooner if there is copious drainage from the ulcer.

Lymphedema

Etiology

Lymphedema is a swelling of soft tissue that occurs as a result of an increase in the quantity of lymph. It may be a primary disorder or secondary to other diseases. It always involves either inflammation or obstruction of the normal lymph channels. It primarily affects females. Primary lymphedema may be congenital or may occur at puberty (lymphedema praecox) and is thought to result from hypoplastic development of lymph vessels.

Secondary lymphedema may follow mastectomy and surgical removal of lymph channels (p. 1756). It is also seen when malignant tumors cause mechanical obstruc-

tion to lymph drainage and with repeated infections and cellulitis as occurs with filiarisis and malaria. Repeated, severe attacks of lymphedema may result in eventual fibrosis and hyperplasia of lymph vessels; the progressive, severe enlargement of the extremity led to the term *elephantiasis* being used for this condition.

Pathophysiology

The pathophysiologic changes found in lymphedema vary somewhat with the type of lymphedema. Usually there is roughening of the surface of the lymphatic vessel. There may be dilation of some lymph channels, with thickening and edema of the lymphatic tissue. Fibrosis and separation of elastic fibers may be present in inflammatory states. Lymph node damage exists in many persons who have secondary lymphedema.

Clinical picture

Lymphedema of the lower extremities begins with mild swelling on the dorsum of the foot, usually at the end of the day, which gradually extends to involve the entire limb. It is aggravated by prolonged standing, pregnancy, obesity, warm weather, and the menstrual period. When the cause of the swelling is in question, lymphography, injection of radiopaque contrast medium into the lymph channel, is helpful in differentiating lymphedema from venous disease.

Intervention

There is no cure for lymphedema, although there are measures to control the progression of the disease. Treatment is conservative, and use is made of basic physiologic principles to improve the lymph drainage. Because gravity helps to drain lymph from the extremities, the person may be advised to sleep with the foot of the bed elevated 10 to 20 cm (4 to 8 in.). Very light massage in the direction of the lymph flow is recommended,[34] and the patient is advised to wear elastic stockings or an elastic sleeve and to do moderate exercise regularly. Constricting clothing must not be worn, and avoiding salty or spicy foods that increase thirst and predispose to edema may be helpful. Thiazide diuretics are often prescribed to minimize fluid accumulation. Long-term antibiotic therapy may be needed when recurrent cellulitis and infection are present. Surgery may be performed to remove hypertrophied lymph channels and hypertrophied, disfiguring tissue.

One of the greatest problems in lymphedema is the emotional reaction of patients to disfigurement. Patients often attribute difficulties encountered in working in their chosen field or social rebuffs to their disfigurement and tend to become withdrawn and depressed. The emphasis on women's legs in our culture adds to the difficulties. One leg only may be involved, accentuating the abnormality even in fairly mild cases. The patient needs help and encouragement in learning to live with this exasperating chronic condition.

Special surgical procedures

Sympathectomy

Vasospasm often accompanies arterial diseases, and a sympathectomy often is performed in an attempt to relieve it, although there is not full agreement as to its value. Occasionally, the operation, which helps dilate the blood vessels, is performed as an emergency when there is severe vasospasm from poisons such as ergot, when a limb has been frozen, or when an arterial embolism has lodged in a major vessel supplying the limb. Usually, however, before a sympathectomy is performed the ganglia are injected with procaine to determine whether the treatment will be of value for the particular patient (p. 1145).

A *lumbar sympathectomy* deprives the leg and foot of sympathetic innervation and thereby dilates the vessels in the lower extremity. It is accomplished by making a small incision in the lower lateral aspect of the abdomen. The peritoneal cavity is not opened, but the sympathetic ganglia supplying the lumbar region are removed and their fibers are cut. This operation may be unilateral or bilateral, depending on whether dilation of vessels in both legs is desired.

After a lumbar sympathectomy the patient is placed in a side-lying position. Blood pressure must be taken every 15 minutes until it is stable. *Pulse rate and respiratory rate are also checked,* and *the patient is watched closely for signs of shock, which may result from the sudden reallocation of the blood in the dilated vessels of the lower abdomen and legs.* Distention may be troublesome after a lumbar sympathectomy, and a rectal tube or rectal irrigations may be used to expel the flatus. *Hourly turning should be insisted on, and deep breathing is to be encouraged.* Following a lumbar sympathectomy the patient may notice a new feeling of warmth in the feet and legs. Very occasionally, this warmth causes a slight discomfort and a feeling of fullness, which is relieved by wearing an elastic stocking.

To relieve vasospasm in the arms and hands, the thoracic ganglia of the sympathetic chain may be resected (*cervicothoracic sympathectomy*). Because the ribs must be resected in this operation, nursing care is similar to that for any patient having chest surgery (p. 1252). The problem of postoperative shock encountered in the patient with a lumbar sympathectomy also is present. In addition, the patient may become quite dizzy on assuming an upright position. Dizziness gradually subsides as the circulation becomes readjusted, but in the meantime the patient must be assisted while he or she is up. Elastic bandages may be ordered to prevent pooling of blood in the legs and thus lessen the circulatory problem.

Amputation

Although partial or complete amputations of either the legs or the arms may be necessary as a result of sarcoma or trauma, the majority are necessitated by atherosclerosis obliterans. The presence of diabetes and superimposed infection in an extremity increases the likelihood of amputation in this condition.

It is believed that the number of amputations will increase each year because of the longer life span and consequent increase in the number of elderly people in whom peripheral vascular disease is likely to develop.

An amputation is a serious operation and usually is performed as a lifesaving measure; it may be necessary at any age. Occasionally, a deformed leg or arm is amputated because it is believed that the patient will do better with a prosthesis than with the deformed limb. Only simple amputations of the lower limb are considered. The reader is referred to selected reading pertinent to amputations of the arms.[73]

Preoperative preparation

Because of the seriousness of amputation and its impact on the patient, preoperative nursing care is of major importance. The two areas of greatest significance are the patient's emotional readiness for the amputation and physical readiness for rehabilitation.

The first goal of nursing intervention is for the patient and family to be in accord with and able to state the goals of the procedure. Throughout the hospitalization it is essential that all care be coordinated among the patient, nurse, physician, physical therapist, and prosthetist.

The initial response on learning of the need for amputation is usually distress, anger, or grief. The patient has already undergone a period of hospitalization during which conservative treatment was attempted. The failure of this treatment may generate feelings of anger and discouragement. It is not unusual for the patient to refuse the amputation initially. The patient and family need to have factual information about the consequences of the decision to amputate or not amputate, the rehabilitative program, and what to expect. The timing of the presentation of this information is important in determining whether the patient will agree to the amputation.

Loss of the power of locomotion means loss of the power of flight, which is one of the instinctive means of self-preservation. It may be for this reason that loss of a leg depresses the patient more than loss of an arm, even though the latter is a much greater handicap. Something about the loss of power to move about at will casts a shadow on the patient's spirit that can be relieved only by the most thoughtful and sensitive care. Even patients who have suffered for a long time with a chronic disease that has hampered their freedom of motion feel the anticipated loss keenly. Perhaps this is because there is such finality in an amputation. As long as the limb is there, imperfect though it may be, the patient usually retains the hope that normal or near-normal function will be restored. If amputation is necessary because of an accident, the suddenness of the change in the patient's self-image may produce real shock.

Whether the amputation is sudden or planned, it will have an impact on the individual's body image. The individual facing an amputation is confronted with the task of incorporating a major body change into his or her self-image and then dealing with the meaning of this. The feedback or information received from others concerning the impact of this body change is a major determinant of the success of the patient's efforts and resultant attitude. The nurse must therefore not only be sensitive to the patient's needs and questions but must help the family work through them so they can support the patient.

Other emotional reactions to amputation are more tangible and more easily understood. The handicap is obvious (or at least patients believe that it is), and they fear that they will be pitied. Young children, although they adjust to the physical limitations readily, may be taunted by their playmates for being different. Older children and adolescents may be handicapped in their social life and may develop serious emotional problems. To the wage earner an amputation may mean learning a new occupation. To the older person it may mean dependence on children or on the community.

Emotional reactions to an amputation have an enormous effect on the patient's rehabilitation. The reactions depend on the patient's emotional makeup and response to other life crises as well as on circumstances leading to the amputation and the support received from family and health care providers. The most perfect surgical operation and the best-fitting prosthesis are useless if patients remain invalids and a burden to themselves, their families, and the community. The nurse must think of the long-range plans for the patient from the time that it is learned that an amputation is necessary. It is at this time, when emotional reactions to the amputation and the idea of using a prosthesis are forming, that the nurse can make the greatest contribution to the patient's rehabilitation by providing appropriate support and by coordinating plans for the patient's care and rehabilitation.

The second goal of preoperative intervention focuses on exercises that will prepare the patient for the activities to be performed postoperatively. The time available before surgery may limit what can be accomplished, but the nurse can at least explain postoperative routines and demonstrate these to the patient. Patients should be told that they will be repositioned frequently and that they must be prone at intervals. Depending on the type of amputation to be performed, the patient can be shown exercises that strengthen the thigh muscles and prevent knee and hip contractures.

When time permits, the patient is assisted to do exercises to strengthen the arms. This will facilitate teaching transfer techniques postoperatively. Push-ups and weight lifting are excellent for improving muscle tone and strength in the arms and shoulders. If the patient is able to be ambulatory, instructions in crutch walking may be started. The more fully the postoperative routine can be explained, demonstrated, and practiced by the patient preoperatively, the smoother will be rehabilitation.

The amputation

The choice of anesthetic depends on the surgeon and the condition of the patient. General anesthetic (intravenous and inhalation) is the most frequently used. However, an amputation can be performed with the patient under spinal anesthesia or with only the leg being cooled (refrigeration anesthesia), but the procedure is then very distressing to the patient, since the sawing of bone can be heard despite large doses of sedation.

In amputating a limb the surgeon attempts to remove all diseased tissue yet leave a stump that permits satisfactory use of a prosthesis. Many factors determine the level of amputation. Transmetatarsal and toe amputations (phalangectomy) are performed whenever possible, since these do not usually necessitate a prosthesis.

Below-the-knee (BK) amputations make up about one third of all amputations for peripheral vascular disease.[9,89] This amputation is usually done in the middle third of the leg, leaving a stump at 12.5 to 17.5 cm (5 to 7 in.) below the knee. This type of amputation is preferable for younger persons who will remain physically active because preservation of knee function permits a more natural gait. Also, the lower the level of amputation, the less energy and balance will be required for walking.

Above-the-knee (AK) amputations are frequently necessary because of the extent of disease. The most important factor in determining the level of amputation is the adequacy of arterial blood supply, and although the BK amputation is preferred for rehabilitation, the AK procedure has been found to require reamputation less frequently, and it heals more successfully. The AK amputation is usually performed between the lower third to the middle of the thigh.

For the best function of the limb, the stump should be long enough to permit sufficient leverage to move the artificial limb but not long enough to interfere with the movement of the joint distal to the amputation. The end of the bone should be covered with skin and subcutaneous tissue and with muscle that is not adherent to the bone end. The stump should be healthy and firm without creases, folds, or flabby parts. It should be painless with no nerve endings remaining in the scar, and the scar should not fall over the weight-bearing end of the bone. The stump should have a smooth, conical contour and should be freely movable by the patient in any normal range of motion.

There are two common types of amputations. One, the *guillotine, circular,* or *open-flap amputation,* is used when there has been serious trauma, when gas bacilli are present in the wound, or when the patient cannot tolerate a long operative procedure. The disadvantage of this amputation is that a second operation is necessary. The blood vessels and nerves are ligated, but the wound is left open and a secondary closure is necessary in 3 to 7 days. Because the wound is not sutured there may be muscle and skin retraction, which makes the fitting of a prosthesis difficult or impossible unless the stump is operated on again. After final healing the resultant stump is as adequate for prosthetic fitting as in other types of amputation.

The *flap* type of amputation is by far the more satisfactory if it can be done. In this operation a long flap of full-thickness skin is loosened from the anterior portion of the limb about to be amputated. Following the amputation the end of the flap is sutured to the skin edges of the stump so that the stump is covered and the suture line is along the back of the stump. This wound usually heals completely within 2 weeks.

Postoperative care

Amputation of a lower extremity is a major surgical procedure with a 10% mortality.[1] The most common complication occurring in the postoperative period is pulmonary embolus, and the nurse must be alert to the signs and symptoms of this (p. 1320).

When the patient returns from the operating room or the recovery room, vital signs are monitored and the stump dressing observed for signs of hemorrhage. If there is bright red drainage, an outline of the stain should be marked on the outside of the dressing with pencil so that the rate of bleeding can be determined easily. The patient may have a wound catheter attached to suction.

The stump is usually elevated on a plastic-covered pillow for 12 to 24 hours immediately after surgery to lessen edema and bleeding or serous oozing from the wound. However, *the pillow must be removed after 24 hours to prevent hip and knee contracture.*

When the guillotine procedure has been used, the patient usually has traction applied to the stump to prevent retraction of skin and muscle away from the surgical incision. Wide bands of adhesive tape are placed on the skin above the wound and attached to a metal spreader bar placed below the stump. Weights are attached to provide traction (see skin traction, p. 968). Traction pulleys at the foot of the bed should be placed toward the center so that the patient can turn onto the abdomen. A Thomas splint sometimes is used for traction so that the patient can be moved more easily and can be out of bed without the traction being released (see p. 970 for care of the patient in traction).

If the amputation is below the knee, the stump may be firmly bandaged on a padded board to prevent contracture of the knee joint. The nurse must check the padding carefully because muscle spasm that results in pulling of the limb against the board may be so great that a pressure sore develops. If spasm seems severe, a piece of sponge rubber can sometimes be slipped between the bandaged stump end and the padded board for additional protection. The surgeon may remove the limb from the board for part of the day.

Immediate postsurgical fitting. Some surgeons utilize the techniques of rigid plaster dressings or immediate postsurgical fitting. This procedure is also referred to as immediate postoperative prosthesis (IPOP). After surgery, while the patient is still in the operating room, a plaster bandage is applied to the dressing over the stump. Embedded in the base of the cast is a metal socket to which a metal pylon can be attached when the patient is to bear weight (Fig. 46-7). This plaster mold or cast reduces postoperative edema, hastens desired stump shrinkage, and if a foot attachment is to be used, allows for early standing and ambulation. In fact, the plaster mold becomes the patient's first or temporary

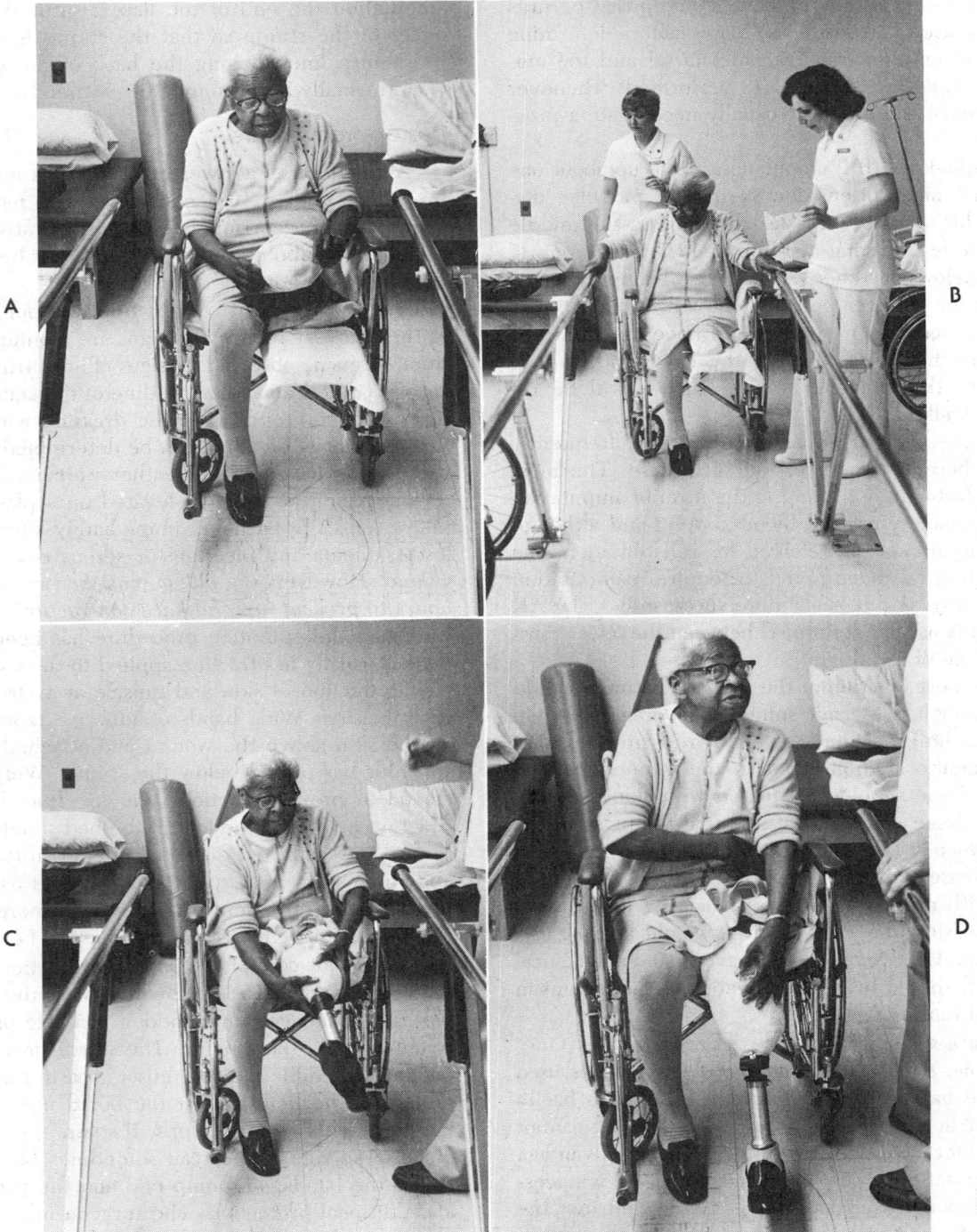

Fig. 46-7. A, Patient uses care in putting on stump sock. **B,** Patient makes sure that she is close enough to bars to have a secure grip. Note smooth fit of sock. **C,** Prosthesis is slipped over sock. **D,** Patient seeks more information about buckle on prosthesis.

prosthesis; the permanent prosthesis can usually be fitted in 3 to 4 weeks. IPOP procedures may also be used for upper extremity amputees. This technique is not used if there is significant risk of wound infection or problems in healing because the incision will not be visible for the first 2 weeks, and this limits its use in patients with vascular disease.

For the plaster mold to be effective it must remain tight and snug. If the cast slips on the stump or comes completely off, the physician and prosthetist must be

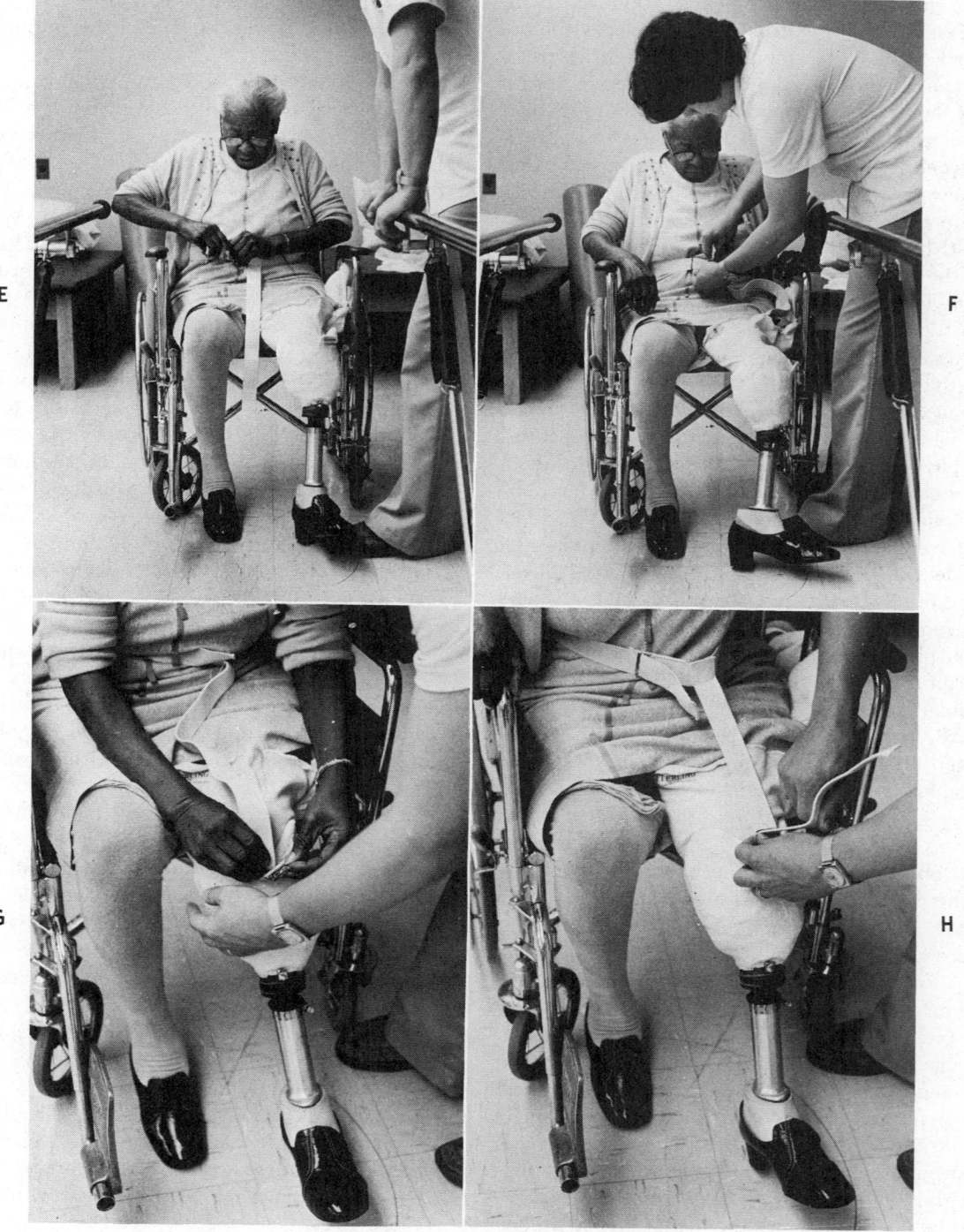

Fig. 46-7, cont'd. E, Belt is secured around waist. **F,** Fit of belt is checked. It must be secure enough to support weight of prosthesis but loose enough for comfort. **G,** Strap is buckled to prosthesis. **H,** Length of strap is adjusted.

notified immediately so that a new cast can be applied. A heavy strap, attached proximally and on the anterior surface of the cast, is fastened to a waistband to help secure the cast and prevent it from slipping. This strap is loosened to a slight degree when the patient is in bed and tightened when he or she is out of bed. The site of any drainage coming through the cast is marked (including the time) with indelible pencil. Hemovac drainage or a Penrose drain will have been inserted before the plaster is applied, so drainage should not be great. In 48 hours a window may be cut in the cast to permit removal of the drain. The opening in the plaster is then closed. This rigid dressing is kept in place for approximately 2 weeks, when it is taken off for removal of sutures. A new cast is then applied. As the stump shrinks in size, the cast becomes too large and will have to be replaced by a tighter one. Usually after the application of the third plaster cast, the cast can be removed daily for stump hygiene and inspection for pressure areas.

Usually a foot-ankle attachment with a shoe is attached to the pylon when the patient is to stand (Fig. 46-7). In this case the prosthetist will mark on the pylon the place where the attachment is to be placed. Most often the physician will be in attendance when the patient first bears weight. *No weight is to be placed on the stump until the cast is completely dry*. The exact amount of weight the patient should bear on the amputated side will be specifically ordered by the physician. Unless otherwise ordered, the prosthetic foot should always be removed when the patient is in bed because the tension produced by the twisting of the prosthesis can be harmful to remaining muscle and bone (e.g., the anterior tibial crest in the BK amputee).

In IPOP, as with any cast prohibiting full view of the involved area, the nurse must be alert to the patient's complaints of pain under the cast, elevated temperature, or foul odor coming from the cast. Such signs or symptoms are reported to the physician at once. Continued observation will be necessary to determine whether the cast is sufficiently snug.

Exercises. To *prevent flexion contracture* of the hip, unless there is a medical order to the contrary, patients who have a lower limb amputation are turned prone for a short time the day after surgery. Thereafter, they should be prone for some time at least three times daily. Even patients who have on leg in traction can turn prone with assistance. If the leg has been amputated below the knee, hyperextension of that thigh and leg can be begun while the patient is lying on the abdomen. This exercise strengthens muscles in preparation for walking. If the amputation is above the knee, a medical order should be obtained before the patient hyperextends the thigh because this exercise may cause strain on the suture line. While lying prone, the patient can practice the push-up exercises begun before surgery, thus strengthening arm and shoulder muscles in preparation for crutch walking.

While on the back the patient with a recent mid-thigh amputation should be kept flat or in low Fowler's position except for short periods such as for meals. A firm trochanter roll (a sheet or bath blanket firmly rolled) should be placed along the outer side of the affected limb to prevent its outward rotation. If permitted the patient should lie on the side of the amputation part of the time.

The patient with a BK amputation can be in mid or high Fowler's position if desired, but special care must be taken to prevent flexion contracture of the knee. Usually the physician orders the stump removed from the padded board or splint several times a day so the patient can sit on the edge of the bed. While sitting, the knee and lower limb are extended. The nurse may be asked to press slightly against the lower limb to provide resistance.

The patient with either type of amputation should practice lifting the stump and buttocks off the bed while lying flat on the back. This exercise helps develop the abdominal muscles, which are necessary for stabilizing the pelvis when the patient stoops or bends.

If the amputation involves only one limb, the nurse must not become so occupied with the affected side that the other leg and foot are neglected. Supervision of regular exercises to strengthen leg muscles and prevention of drop foot and pronation deformities are nursing responsibilities. The patient should have a firm board or block of wood at the foot of the bed against which the uninvolved leg can be pushed and thereby receive essential active exercise.

When the patient is permitted out of bed, usually on the first or second postoperative day, he or she is taught self-care activities such as rising from a chair. To preserve his or her center of gravity and balance, the patient keeps the remaining leg under him or her before shifting weight and when rising from a chair. When assisting the patient to stand, it is helpful if the nurse faces the patient and locks his or her knee against the patient's good knee as the patient rises to a standing position. This helps to stabilize the patient until a walker or crutches are in place. This same procedure is used when assisting the patient from bed to chair or from chair to bed. After locking the knee against the patient's leg, the nurse and patient pivot together and the patient is assisted into the bed or chair.

If physical therapy services are available, the physical therapist will teach exercises to the patient. It is helpful if the nurse knows which exercises were taught so that the patient can be supervised while performing the exercises.

The patient who has had an amputation because of vascular disease must be reminded to take particular care of the remaining foot and leg. Exercises and other measures to keep the arterial supply as adequate as possible must be carried out while in the hospital and after returning home.

Stump care. If a prosthesis is to be worn comfortably, a healthy stump is necessary. Teaching the patient how to care for the stump is a nursing responsibility that is carried out both in the hospital and in the patient's home. The patient may be discharged from the hospital within a few weeks but may not be fitted for a prosthesis for 6 weeks to 6 months after surgery, depending on the condition of the stump.

When the wound is completely healed, the patient is taught to wash the stump daily. Most surgeons advise their patients not to soak the stump because soaking may cause maceration of the skin. The skin should be massaged gently, directing the motion toward the suture line. The use of oils or creams should be avoided since these agents only increase the possibility of skin maceration; lanolin may be used sparingly. Usually the patient is instructed to push forcefully over the bone to toughen the limb for weight bearing. Sometimes this

process is begun by placing a pillow on a footstool, chair, or high stool (depending on the site of operation) and having the patient bear some weight on the stump while steadying himself or herself on the bed or against the wall.

There should be no tenderness, redness, or other signs of skin irritation or abrasion at the end of the stump. The skin and underlying tissue should be firm and without flabbiness and should be without tautness over the bony end of the limb (Fig. 46-8).

For 2 to 3 weeks postoperatively the stump is kept bandaged at all times in order to reduce swelling and shape the stump (Fig. 46-9). Some patients are taught to bandage the stump themselves. However, they need careful instruction and supervision. The bandage must not be so tight as to cause pain or numbness from hampered circulation, and if it is too loose it will defeat its purpose. If the patient is unable to apply a firm, even bandage, a member of the family may help with the application. The bandage should be removed and reapplied at least twice daily, and the skin should be washed, dried, powdered, and exposed to the air for a short time

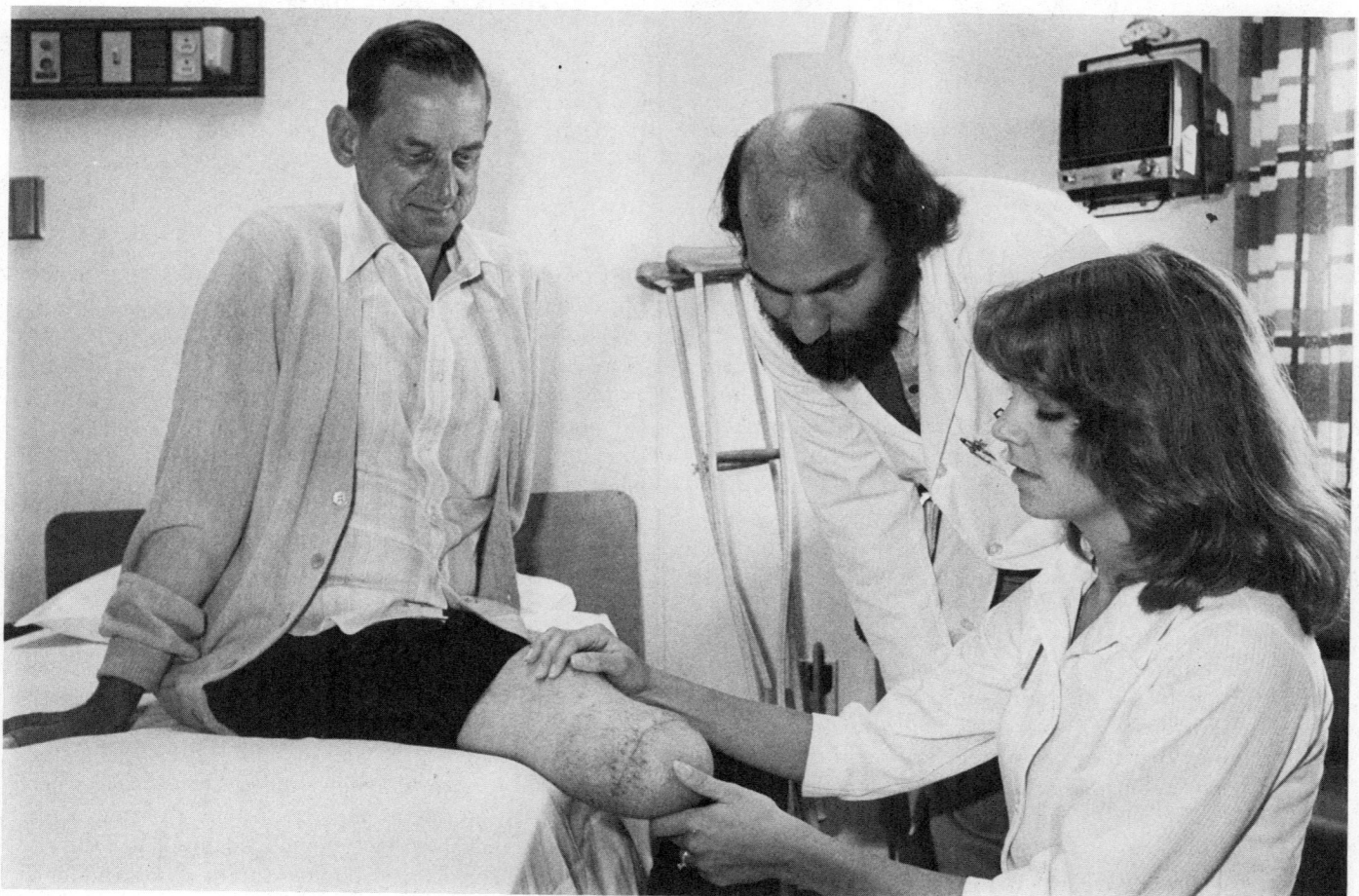

Fig. 46-8. Nurse and physician examine well-healed stump of patient with A-K amputation.

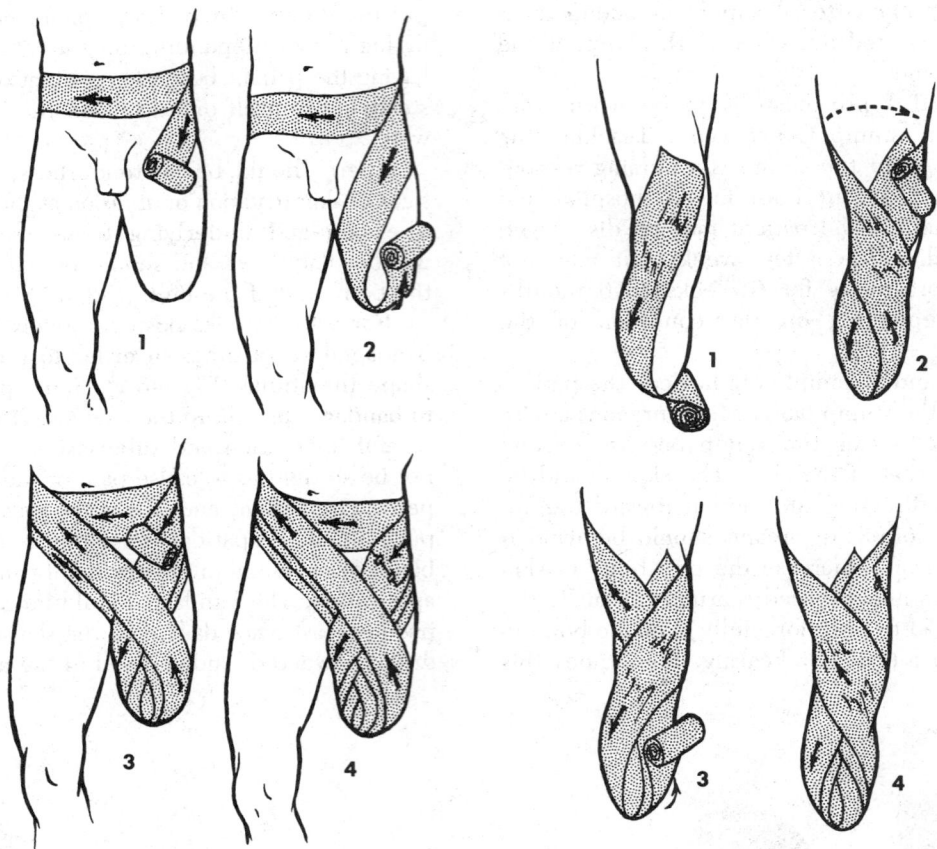

Fig. 46-9. *Left,* Correct method for bandaging midthigh amputation stump. Note that bandage must be anchored around patient's waist. *Right,* Correct method for bandaging midcalf amputation stump. Note that bandage need not be anchored about waist.

before the bandage is reapplied. The patient should have at least two bandages so that one may be washed daily; they should be laid flat to dry so as not to stretch.

When a leather prosthesis is used, the patient should have several pairs of stump socks of the right size. They should be made of cotton and wool and should be washed daily after use and dried over a mold to prevent shrinkage. Usually the patient wears out one sock a month when beginning to use a prosthesis. A worn sock should not be mended because it may cause irritation to the stump. Routine care of the stump, including bathing, massage, and inspection, should be continued. If the weather is warm and the skin perspires freely, the limb should be removed from the prothesis socket and bathed and exposed to the air more often than during cooler weather. Persons who work may take extra stump socks with them so that they can change the socks during the day in hot weather. To prevent tension on the sock as the limb is placed in the socket, a string may be attached to the end of the sock and brought through a hole that is usually left in the prosthesis below the level of the stump. The patient should be instructed to re-

port calluses or any abnormalities on the stump to the physician at once.

Phantom limb sensation. Phantom limb sensation is an unpleasant complication that sometimes follows amputation and is difficult to treat. It is a sensation that the limb is still present. The sensation may disappear if the patient looks at the stump and recalls that the limb has been amputated. *Phantom limb pain* also occurs. The patient may have the sensation, for example, that something is burning the foot or that there is pressure on it, or the pain may be identical to that experienced before surgery. The cause is not fully understood, but it is thought possibly to result from stimulation of afferent nerves severed in surgery. Phantom limb pain may disappear of its own accord, or it may lessen for a time and then recur with severity. When it is really troublesome to the patient, the nerve endings may be injected with alcohol to give temporary relief. Occasionally when pain persists, an operation is performed to remove the nerve ends that may have developed to form a tuft on the weight-bearing part of the stump. A few patients are troubled with phantom limb pain for an indefinite time following amputation, and it may interfere seriously with their rehabilitation. Reamputation is sometimes necessary, but even this procedure does not always bring relief, since the same sensations may be experienced at the end of the new stump.

Ambulation. Teaching the patient who has had an amputation to walk with crutches, with crutches and prosthesis, and then with the prosthesis alone is a complicated task that lies within the responsibility of physical medicine and nursing. In the past, teaching the patient to walk with a prosthesis often was left to the limb maker. However, learning to walk well with an artificial limb requires instruction by a skilled physical therapist (Fig. 46-7). It is the responsibility of nurses working with the surgeon, the social worker, the physical therapist, the prosthetist, and other members of the professional health team to see that the patient receives continuous care, teaching, and encouragement until the patient is able to manage independently.

Crutch walking. The nurse has the responsibility to prepare every patient for crutch walking and may have to teach the patient to use crutches, especially if a physical therapist is not available. Therefore every nurse should know the essentials about using crutches and something about the gaits that can be used. Preparation for the use of crutches should include exercises to strengthen the triceps muscles, which are used to extend the elbows and are therefore most important in the satisfactory use of crutches. These exercises can be started before the operation by teaching the patient to lie on the abdomen and to do push-up exercises (p. 1166). When lying on the back the patient can hold bags of sand or other weights on the palms and straighten the elbows. In another exercise that strengthens the triceps muscles, the patient sits on the edge of the bed with the foot in a chair and, while pressing the palms against the mattress, lifts his or her hips off the bed. This procedure provides good exercise in extension of the elbow and helps the patient become accustomed to resting the weight on the hands. Use of an overbed trapeze bar postoperatively is helpful since it enables the patient to be much more independent than would otherwise be possible. Its use, however, strengthens primarily the biceps muscles, which are less essential in crutch walking than are the triceps muscles. Further preparation includes prevention of contractures and deformities that will interfere with the use of crutches and with the use of a prosthesis. Exercises to prevent hip and knee contractures and to maintain the muscle tone and strength in the unaffected leg are described on p. 1170. Even before the stump is healed enough to permit use of a prosthesis, the patient can learn to do a good deal of self-care.

Crutches should be measured for each patient. In *method 1*, the patient lies on the back with the arms at sides. The measurement is taken from the axilla to a

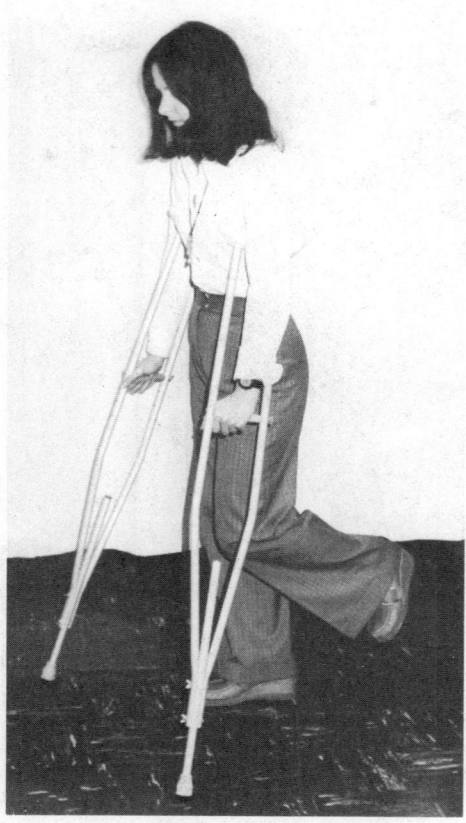

Fig. 46-10. Axillary crutches are ambulatory aids best used by young persons or persons with good motor ability, particularly if patient is non-weight-bearing on one leg. Here patient has good balance and erect posture.

point 15 cm (6 in.) out from the side of the heel. This is the length of the crutch minus 1.9 cm (¾ in.) for crutch tips. In *method 2*, the patient is measured from 5 cm (2 in.) below the level of the axilla to the base of the heel. In *method 3*, 40 cm (16 in.) is subtracted from the patient's total height. Even with careful measurement, alterations may have to be made after the crutches are used. Posture, for example, may change, altering the length needed. The crutches should not cause pressure on the axillae, and the patient is taught not to rest the weight on the axillary bars more than a few minutes at a time. Pressure on the axillae causes pressure on the brachial plexus, which can lead to severe and sometimes permanent paralysis of the arms ("crutch paralysis"). The patient is taught that weight should be borne on the palms of the hands.

Before attempting crutch walking, the patient is assisted out of bed and should stand with help to get the feel of normal balance. A walker or parallel bars may be used until the patient feels secure. At this time the patient begins to practice correct standing posture with head up, chest up, abdomen in, pelvis tilted inward, a 5-degree angle in the knee joint, and the foot straight (Fig. 46-10). Practice in front of a mirror is very helpful.

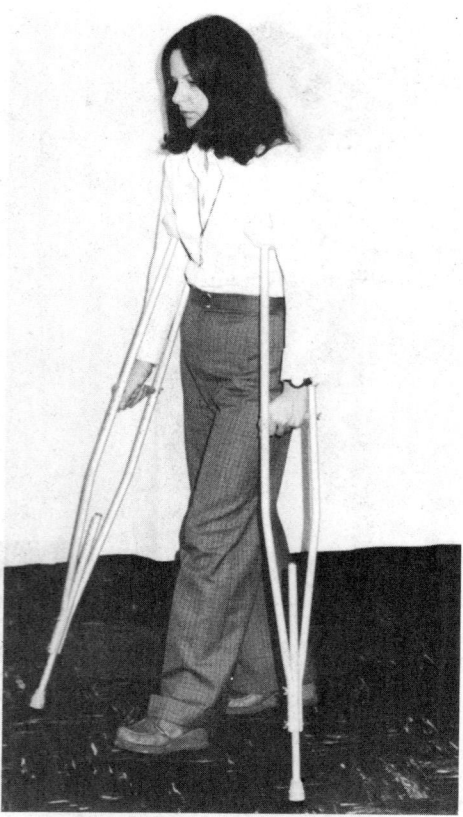

Fig. 46-11. Three-point gait is more stable crutch gait and can be used by most patients who can use walker. It provides for greater mobility than walker, so patient may also negotiate stairs.

The patient is encouraged not to look toward the foot. Next the patient should practice standing while supported by crutches to get the "feel" of them. The nurse should be sure that the patient begins at this time to bear weight on the palms and not on the axillae. Before the patient begins to try to use crutches, the proper hand and arm position and gait should be demonstrated. This will help the patient understand what is to be done. In all crutch walking the patient is taught to concentrate on a normal rhythmic gait, such as the *three-point gait* (Fig. 46-11).

The first gait that the patient will use is the *swing-through* (Fig. 46-12, *A*) or *swing-to gait* (Fig. 46-12, *B*), which require no carefully guided instruction provided the patient knows how to bear weight and has been taught to check posture, balance, and rhythm. In this gait the amputated limb and the crutches both advance either to or beyond the level of the normal limb and are followed by the normal leg. This is a simple fast gait that gives little leg exercise but is useful for rapid maneuvers such as are needed in crossing streets. The patient may use this gait when beginning to walk with one prosthesis, in which case both crutches and the prosthesis move forward, followed by the normal leg.

When the patient with double amputations has been fitted with prostheses, the *four-point gait* (Fig. 46-12, *C*) may be taught. This gait is taught to the count of four as follows: right crutch, left foot, left crutch, right foot. Some patients with bilateral amputations must always use this gait (which is also widely used by those with involved neuromuscular disabilities and poor balance). It is a safe gait because the patient always has three points of contact with the ground at any time. Most patients progress to the *two-point gait,* in which the foot and the opposite crutch move together and then the prosthesis and the opposite crutch. It is often taught to the count of two as follows: left crutch and right foot (one) and right crutch and left foot (two). The two-point gait is much faster and is easier to maintain in a rhythmic pattern than the four-point gait.

The patient with one prosthesis may progress to one crutch and then to a cane, which should be abandoned eventually. The crutch or cane should be held in the hand on the side *opposite* the prosthesis because, as the patient normally walks, the arm on the opposite side of the body alternately swings forward. Holding the cane or crutch on the same side as the prosthesis results in an awkward, unrhythmic gait.

It is important for the nurse to know which gait the physical therapist is teaching the patient so that he or she may be reminded not to revert to a previous gait. It is to be expected that the patient with a double amputation will learn to manage much more slowly than if only one limb were gone. Persons with AK amputations also take much longer to learn to walk and otherwise manage their movements than do persons with BK amputations.

The prosthesis

The physician prescribes the type of prosthesis and usually refers the patient to a limb maker. After the limb is made, the patient returns to the amputee clinic, hospital department of physical medicine, physician's office, or rehabilitation center to learn the best use of the artificial limb (Fig. 46-7). The community health nurse, particularly if also trained in physical therapy, often gives care and supervision to the person in his home.

The type of prosthesis is selected for the individual. Most prostheses are made of well-seasoned willow wood, although some are made of metal (Duralumin and aluminum) and fiber materials. Metal prostheses are lighter in weight than wooden ones, but they tend to be noisy. Usually the BK prosthesis weighs about 2.25 kg (5 lb) and the midthigh prosthesis about 2.67 kg (7½ lb), although the weight of the prosthesis is adapted to the size and weight of the individual and his or her kind of work.

The prosthesis has a socket, or "bucket," into which the limb fits. In the past the socket was usually made

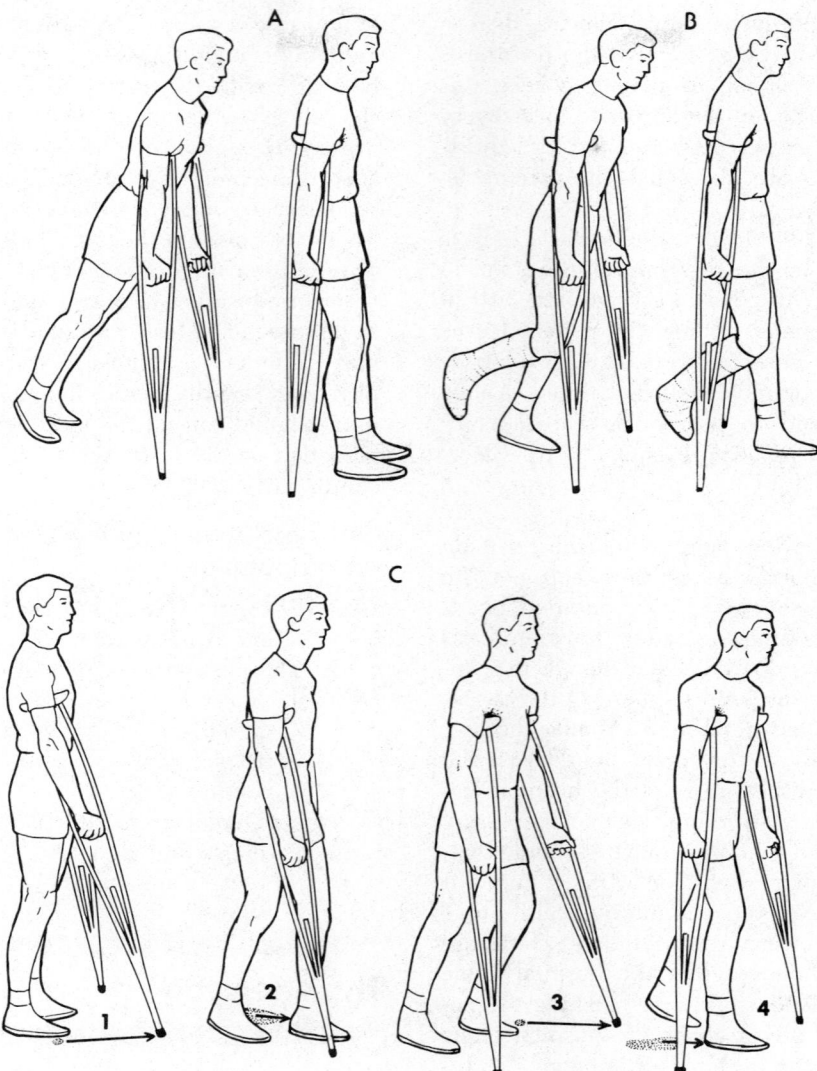

Fig. 46-12. A, Swing-through gait. **B,** Swing-to gait. **C,** Four-point gait.

of leather, but plastic materials are now widely used since they are lighter, easier to keep clean, and odorless. The socket has a one-way valve that allows air to escape but not reenter as the stump is inserted. It eliminates the need for a stump sock but does require a good fit between stump and prosthesis. Shrinkage of the stump may interfere with obtaining a good fit. It is usually greater after amputation of the foreleg than after amputation of the thigh. Suction is now quite generally used to hold the stump in the socket and obviate wearing a heavy, laced belt about the waist, although persons with high, amputations may wear a pelvic band. The patient needs constant encouragement to use the prosthesis, particularly in the beginning when he or she is adjusting to all features of the device. The prosthesis should be used as soon as stump has healed.

The nurse should determine whether the person is using the prosthesis when at home. If not, the reason should be identified and reported to the physician. Often the nurse can help make the arrangements for more instruction. It is important that there be no delay, because the longer the person puts off using the prosthesis, the less likelihood of a satisfactory adjustment to it. If crutches are used for too long or the person uses a wheelchair to get about, developing a normal rhythmic gait may be very difficult.

Care of the prosthesis should be reviewed carefully with the patient being taught to fasten the cuff above the stump from the bottom up, even though this method may seem more difficult at first (Fig. 46-7). The cuff should be snug but not uncomfortable. If the cuff is leather, care should be taken that the stump sock is long enough to protect the cuff from perspiration, and it should be rubbed with saddle soap at least weekly. The inside of the stump socket should be washed frequently to ensure cleanliness. Shoes should be kept in good repair and should have rubber heels. Broken shoelaces should be replaced at once. If the prosthesis has a joint, the person should be taught to keep this free from lint and dust, to oil the joints and locks every few weeks, and to keep screws tightened. If adjustments in the prosthesis are necessary, the patient returns to the limb maker.

The person should be told that the artificial limb is a tool and that it will be most useful when he or she has mastered its use. With good care it will last 3 to 10 years. Its value will depend on how the patient learns to balance, how much muscle strength is developed, and how smooth and rhythmic a gait is learned. Above all, its value will depend on the person's attitude toward the challenge that its use presents.

Long-term care

Most persons who have an amputation must remain under medical supervision for a long time, and it is safe to assume that any person with an amputation needs nursing care and supervision long after the wound has healed. It must be remembered that although the amputation has removed a diseased segment of the vasculature, the person still has peripheral vascular disease. If possible, a community health nurse should visit the patient's home before discharge from the hospital and help the family make any structural changes necessary for facilitating the person's ambulation. If it should happen that a person is equipped with an artificial limb but is not taught how to use it, the community health nurse should initiate steps toward rehabilitation. Occasionally, the limb maker believes that the hospital clinic personnel are taking responsibility for teaching the patient to walk, and the physician or the hospital clinic personnel believe that the limb maker is taking the responsibility. The person may become discouraged and, after months of what appears to be a good adjustment, may lay the limb aside and return to a wheelchair or crutches. Sometimes the patient reports that the prosthesis is not comfortable and is reluctant to go back to the limb maker because of costs. If so, the nurse can help to find agencies in the community that can give appropriate assistance. It may be, however, that this statement is made to conceal a much more important and deep-seated rejection of difficulties. When the nurse suspects that the patient is not accepting his or her prosthesis, consultation with the physician and other health professionals may be necessary to determine the appropriate step to be taken to assist the person.

Occasionally, a patient especially an elderly one, can use neither a prosthesis nor crutches but must be confined to a wheelchair. The nurse should give special attention to the rehabilitation of this patient in an effort to make him or her as self-sufficient as possible. Many patients can be taught to move themselves from the bed to the wheelchair, from the chair to the toilet, and even in and out of a car. The patient and family often need help in arranging facilities at home, and plans should be made with the family to let the patient do useful chores such as fixing vegetables, mending, or doing small repairs. It is often helpful if the person can be encouraged to become interested in some hobby or pastime.

There are many rehabilitation centers in the United States, but most of them are located in the larger cities. The division of vocational rehabilitation of the department of education in every state is, however, available to all patients. Most communities, counties, and states have voluntary programs that are designed to help the physically handicapped, including the amputee. The nurse should consult the local health department for information on the resources available in the person's own community.

Outcome criteria for the person who has had an amputation

1. The person achieves the established goal in relation to ambulation.
2. The person or significant others can:
   a. State the plan for obtaining a permanent prosthesis.
   b. Explain how to care for the prosthesis and stump.
   c. Demonstrate the prescribed program of exercise and activity.
   d. State plans for follow-up care.

Hypertension

As discussed earlier in this chapter, hypertension is often considered in conjunction with peripheral vascular diseases for several reasons: both are disorders of the circulation, the courses of both diseases are affected by similar factors, and hypertension is a major risk factor in atherosclerosis, the largest single cause of peripheral vascular disease.

The blood pressure level in a given individual is determined by many variables, such as age, activity, emotional state, presence of other diseases, pumping effectiveness of the heart, amount of circulating blood, and the state of the vasculature. Although 120/80 is commonly given as the "normal" level for adult blood pressure, many individuals, such as infants, most adults while sleeping, and athletes, have very adequate circulation at lower levels. Conversely, older persons, individuals under emotional stress, and obese individuals often demonstrate levels above this with no adverse consequences.

Because of these variables, statistics describing the prevalence of this disease are quite varied. When hypertension is defined as a consistent systolic level above 150 mm Hg or diastolic level above 90 mm Hg, the incidence is 15% among men in their 30s and 20% among men in their 50s. According to this common definition 20 million Americans have hypertension. It has also been estimated that of this number hypertension is undiagnosed in one half, and of those in whom the disease has been diagnosed, one half are receiving no or inadequate treatment.[109]

The incidence of hypertension varies considerably among different groups in the population. Hypertension occurs slightly more often in men than in women and is twice as prevalent among blacks as among whites. The degree of hypertension is also more severe in blacks than whites. In all groups the incidence of this disease increases with age.

Epidemiology

The effects of hypertension are numerous. The exact correlation of hypertension with other disease states and the associated mortality rates are difficult to discuss because of the varied ways in which hypertension is defined. However, there are several very definite trends that point to the importance of preventing and treating this disease.

The major complications associated with hypertension are stroke, coronary artery disease with myocardial infarction, and chronic renal failure. Hypertension is also associated with aneurysm formation and congestive heart failure. Mortality from these causes increases as blood pressure, either systolic or diastolic, increases. For example, when the diastolic pressure is over 105 mm Hg, mortality is three times greater than normal.[50] A blood pressure of 150/100 mm Hg in men at 35 years of age reduces life expectancy by 16½ years.[64] In the late 1970s hypertension and related cardiovascular diseases cost the United States over $20 billion yearly for medical and nursing care, nursing home services, and medications. Successful treatment of hypertension and lowering of blood pressure reduce the incidence of pressure-related complications, particularly stroke, aneurysm rupture, and congestive heart failure.

Etiology

Hypertension may be classified into three groups: hypertension from a known cause, essential hypertension, and malignant hypertension. In only a small percentage of cases is the cause known. Examples of these are coarctation of the aorta, which may be corrected surgically; pheochromocytoma, a catecholamine-secreting tumor; Cushing's disease and other disorders of the adrenal gland; toxemia of pregnancy; and thyrotoxicosis, which causes increased stroke volume of the heart. Chronic glomerulonephritis is the most common known cause. In the majority of cases the exact cause of hyper-

tension is unknown; this is classified as *essential hypertension*.

Malignant hypertension (accelerated hypertension) refers to hypertension that is severe and rapidly progressive, resulting in fibrinoid necrosis, especially of the heart, kidneys, brain, and eyes. The patient often has papilledema and retinal exudates and hemorrhages. The eye changes are rated according to severity from 1+ to 4+. Unless medical treatment is successful, the course is rapidly fatal and most persons do not survive longer than 2 years. Causes of death in malignant hypertension are secondary to the fibrinoid necrosis of the kidney, heart, and brain. Thus the patient may succumb to uremia, myocardial infarction, congestive failure, or a cerebral vascular accident. Malignant hypertension is seen most often in blacks, especially men under age 40 years.

Although no single causative mechanism has been identified in *essential hypertension*, several risk factors are known. As mentioned earlier, many of the factors influencing the course of other peripheral vascular diseases also influence hypertension and the likelihood of the development of pathologic sequelae. In attempts to predict the occurence of hypertension, it has been found that both a positive family history and the occurrence of episodes of elevated blood pressure in youth correlate highly with the eventual development of adult hypertension.

Because the blood pressure is the result of several interacting factors, dysfunction in any one area may result in hypertension. Research is currently focusing on clarifying the role of each of these factors. Abnormal sodium retention and corresponding water retention may be a triggering mechanism. An increased sensitivity to the renin-angiotensin system, which regulates both vasoconstriction and sodium retention, may be a primary defect. It is also thought that a deficiency of natural vasodilating substances, such as prostaglandins, may exist in hypertension.

Diet is also of significance in the course of this disease. Obesity, increased serum sodium levels, and hypercholesteremia all increase the risks of hypertension, as does smoking. In men aged 30 to 59 years, the death rate of those with hypertension is twice as high as in those without hypertension; this rate is tripled in the presence of either hypercholesteremia or smoking and is five times higher if both risk factors exist.[109] Hypertension is also thought to increase the problems of arteriosclerosis by favoring hyperplasia of connective tissue in the intima of arteries.

Pathophysiology

Blood pressure is determined by two factors: flow and resistance. Blood flow is in turn determined by cardiac output (strength, rate, rhythm of heart beat, and blood volume). The resistance to flow is primarily de-

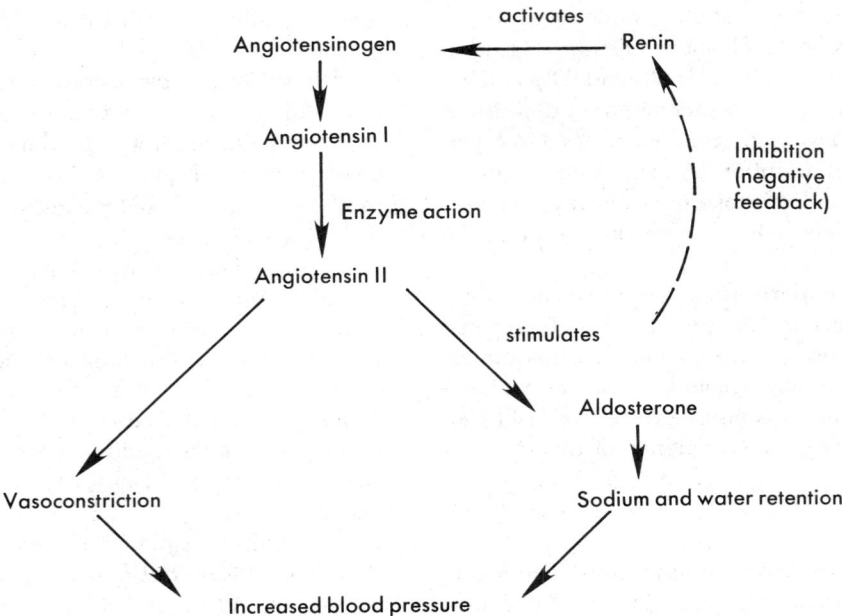

Fig. 46-13. Diagram of effect of renin-angiotensin system on blood pressure.

termined by the diameter of blood vessels and, to a lesser degree, by the viscosity of the blood. Increased peripheral resistance as a result of narrowing of the arterioles is the single most common characteristic in hypertension. Dilation and constriction of peripheral arterioles may be controlled by several mechanisms.

Renal regulation is an essential component of blood pressure control. Fig. 46-13 illustrates the normal steps in the renin-angiotensin system. Note that, as with most natural control mechanisms, this system has a negative feedback loop to prevent excessive response.

Stimulation of the sympathetic nervous system causes the release of the catecholamines epinephrine and norepinephrine. This stimulation can be the result of environmental stressors, adrenal hormones, or autonomic nervous system activity (e.g., impulses from the carotid sinus). Epinephrine is an inotropic agent that increases the force of cardiac contraction, thus increasing cardiac output; norepinephrine primarily causes vasoconstriction, which increases peripheral resistance. Stress therefore increases the force while narrowing the passageway, causing the blood pressure to increase. Parasympathetic stimulation has the opposite effect, causing relaxation of the smooth muscle of the vessels.

With prolonged hypertension the elastic tissue in arterioles is replaced by fibrous collagen tissue. The thickened arteriole wall then becomes less distensible, offering even greater resistance to the flow of blood. The left ventricle then must exert more force in order to empty completely; it becomes more distended as it fails to eject a normal stroke volume, and the muscle fibers stretch (hypertrophy) in an attempt to increase

the strength of contraction. Inadequate blood supply through the coronary arteries may cause angina pectoris, or a myocardial infarction may occur. Eventually, the hypertrophy of the left ventricle results in congestive heart failure.

Outside the heart itself, the changes in the arteriolar walls may result in permanent damage to organs. The kidney is especially susceptible, and when fibrinoid necrosis occurs in the afferent arteriole, the glomerulus is deprived of its blood supply; permanent kidney damage and possible renal failure result. Cerebral vessels are also frequently affected; neurologic changes or frank stroke may result either from hemorrhage from a leaky vessel or from thrombosis.

Prevention

Because of the alarming statistics regarding this disease, national attention has been focused on the task of detecting persons with hypertension and assuring that they receive treatment. The National Institutes of Health, part of the Department of Health and Human Services, has created and coordinated the National High Blood Pressure Education Program, including a Task Force on Nursing in High Blood Pressure Control. In addition, other organizations, such as the American Heart Association, the National Heart Institute, and the Public Health Service, have all been involved in this effort to identify and treat persons with hypertension.

One of the most problematic aspects of this disease is that it is asymptomatic until pathologic and sometimes fatal sequelae occur. Although it has been shown that proper treatment can greatly reduce the incidence

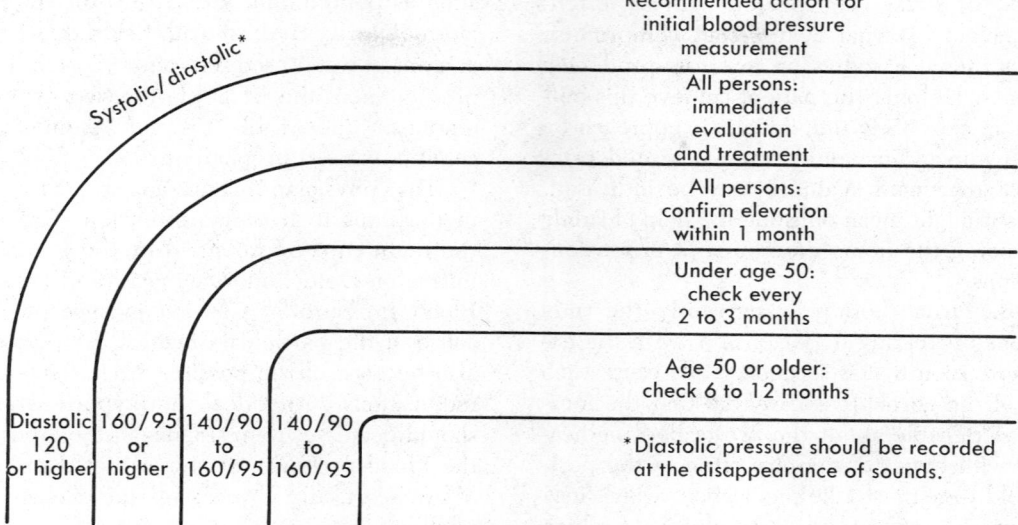

Fig. 46-14. Detection and confirmation of high blood pressure. Anyone measuring blood pressure should have resources available for confirmation and follow-up. (From U.S. National High Blood Pressure Education Programs, Recommendations of the Joint National Committee on Detection, Diagnosis, and Treatment of High Blood Pressure, Bethesda, Md., 1973, National Institutes of Health.)

of these sequelae, it has required a program of this magnitude to educate both the lay public and health professionals as to the importance of obtaining early treatment and follow-up for all persons with hypertension.

There have been three general approaches to this problem. First, efforts have been directed at public awareness, informing them and making available educational materials explaining hypertension and its treatment. Second, screening programs in schools and shopping centers have been organized in order to identify the hypertensive population. Third, there has been an attempt to develop innovative techniques to motivate hypertensive individuals to obtain and continue treatment. For example, persons have been taught to check their own blood pressure at home in order to monitor more closely their response to treatment without requiring frequent trips to the physician's office, and many insurance companies offer reduced premiums to persons with hypertension who maintain treatment regimens.

The National Task Force on Nursing in High Blood Pressure Control has confirmed that nurses are an invaluable resource in dealing with this major health problem. Industrial nurses can set up formal and informal screening programs in their work settings. Individual nurses can become involved in community screening and education programs. Community health nurses can ensure that blood pressure checks of every family member are part of every initial visit. Fig. 46-14 gives recommended steps in the screening program. In addition, the nursing profession has a unique contribution to make in the identification of methods that ensure patient compliance and research into those factors that hamper patient compliance.

Clinical picture

Unfortunately, hypertension is essentially asymptomatic in its early stages. When symptoms do occur, they generally indicate an advanced state, or very high blood pressure. Because of this, the nurse should be alert to the common complaints associated with hypertension and assess the blood pressure of anyone exhibiting these.

The most common symptom of high blood pressure is *headache*. The headache is usually *occipital* and is commonly *present in the early morning*. Sometimes the headache may be severe enough to waken the patient from sleep. *Flushing of the face* may be noted, and occasionally the *nose bleeds*. If the patient is older or has some degree of congestive heart failure, he or she may experience fatigue or shortness of breath on exertion. *Angina pectoris* may be present.

Intervention

Diet. In addition to the restrictions in caloric intake and specific prescription of the type of fat intake, a low-sodium diet is frequently ordered. Very often the nurse, together with the dietitian, can be helpful in assisting the client in determining how to stay within dietary limits without exceeding financial resources.

Modification of stress. The person with hypertension needs to avoid external factors that compromise circulation; this means a reduction in stress-producing activity or events. Helping the patient achieve this outcome requires an extremely individualistic approach on the part of the nurse. For some patients a mild tranquilizer such as diazepam (Valium) may be indicated, while for others it might mean enlisting the help of family members in freeing the home environment of tension-creating situations.

Medications. Drug therapy is currently the only successful means of treating hypertension, with the exception of hypertension that is secondary to a cause such as coarctation of the aorta. It is essential that the individual be knowledgeable about the prescribed medications. Persons with hypertension are often in the position of being told they must take medication, which may have unpleasant side effects, for a condition of which they were unaware and which is producing no symptoms! A thorough comprehensive teaching program is necessary if patient cooperation is to be enlisted (Fig. 46-15).

Medications commonly used in the treatment of hypertension fall into several categories, including sympathetic nervous system depressants, such as the alkaloids of rauwolfia; selective sympathetic nervous system inhibitors such as guanethidine (Ismelin) and methyldopa (Aldomet); drugs acting on smooth muscle to cause vasodilation such as hydralazine hydrochloride (Apresoline) and prazosin (Minipres); ganglionic blocking agents such as pentolinium tartrate (Ansolysen); and the thiazides (Diuril, Hydrodiuril, Esidrix), which reduce the amount of water, sodium, and chloride in the body and may augment the effect of other antihypertensive preparations.[10] (See Table 46-2 for a summary of the most commonly used preparations.)

The physician makes a very careful selection of medications to treat hypertension. Fig. 46-16 outlines the regimen recommended by the Joint National Committee on Detection, Diagnosis, and Treatment of High Blood Pressure.[112] Caution is necessary not only because of the particular stage of the person's illness but also because of the possible side effects of some of the medications. An ideal antihypertensive preparation should decrease the resistance of the arterioles and lower the blood pressure. It should not decrease the output of the heart, and unpleasant side effects should be minimal.

In general, there are two aspects of drug therapy on which the nurse focuses attention. First, the patient must know how and when to take the medication. Some medications that are taken only once a day can be taken at bedtime so that the patient is asleep during the peak action of the drug when side effects will be greatest. Diuretics are generally taken early in the day so the patient will not be awakened with the need to void at night.

Second, the patient must be informed of possible side effects. Many of the untoward effects, such as the depression associated with reserpine or impotence as-

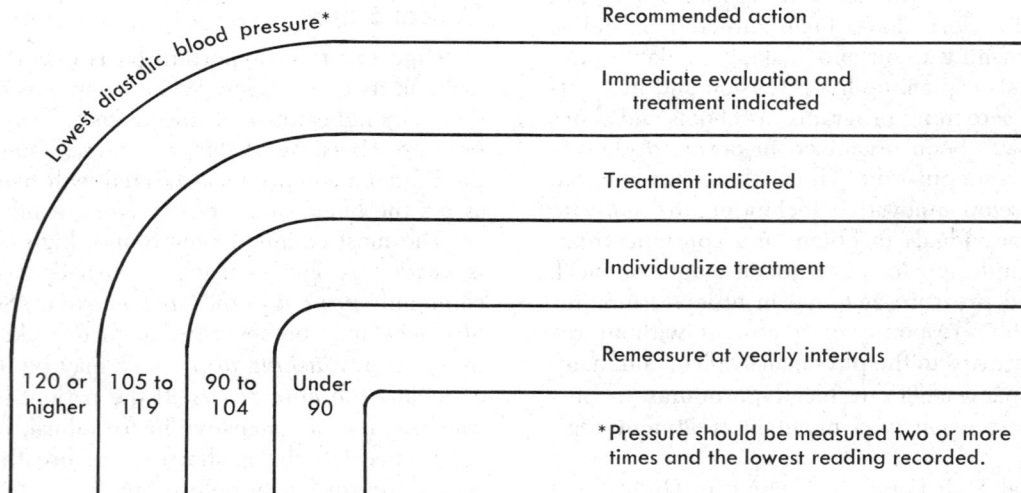

Fig. 46-15. Follow-up recommendations for persons with high blood pressure. Patient education begins when blood pressure is measured initially. Without alarming patient, person taking pressure should inform patient of blood pressure reading and carefully communicate importance of following recommended action. Patients not requiring evaluation or treatment are to be reassured and importance of annual blood pressure measurement strongly emphasized. (From U.S. National High Blood Pressure Education Programs, Recommendations of the Joint National Committee on Detection, Diagnosis, and Treatment of High Blood Pressure, Bethesda, Md., 1973, National Institutes of Health.)

TABLE 46-2. Oral drugs used in hypertension

Drug	Trade name	Dosage*	Mode of action	Side effects
Diuretics				
Thiazide derivatives				
Chlorothiazide	Diuril	500-1500	Block sodium reabsorption	↑ BUN
Hydrochlorothiazide	Hydrodiuril	50-150	in cortical portion of as-	↑ Uric acid
	Esidrix	50-150	cending tubule; water is	↓ Potassium
	Oretic	50-150	excreted with sodium,	↑ Blood glucose
Trichlormethazide	Naqua	4-8	producing decreased	↑ Calcium
	Metahydrin	4-8	blood volume	Less common: sensitivity reactions, gastrointestinal tract irritation, rashes, anemia, thrombocytopenia, purpura, pancreatitis
Methylclothiazide	Enduron	10-15		
Benzthiazide	Exna	100-150		
	Aquatag	100-150		
Polythiazide	Renese	2-8		
Cyclothiazide	Anhydron	2-6		NOTE: Thiazides are ineffective in renal failure
Furosemide	Lasix	40-160	Block sodium reabsorption	Same as for thiazides; more
Ethacrynic acid	Edecrin	50-200	in medullary portion of ascending tubule; same action as thiazides	likely to result in hypovolemia and dehydration
Chlorthalidone	Hygroton	50-100	Same action as thiazides	Same as for thiazides; more
Quinethazone	Hydromox	100-150		likely to result in hypovolemia and dehydration
Potassium sparing				
Spironolactone	Aldactone	100-400	Antagonizes the effect of aldosterone on tubular cells; sodium is excreted in exchange for potassium	Hyperkalemia, gynecomastia, hirsutism, irregular menses, rash, drowsiness, confusion
Triamterene	Dyrenium	100-300	Acts directly on sodium pump to excrete sodium in exchange for potassium	Hyperkalemia, diarrhea, nausea, vomiting, rash, photosensitivity
Combination drug				
Spironolactone-hydrochlorothiazide	Aldactaside			
Drugs acting on central nervous system				
Rauwolfia compounds				
Reserpine	Sandril	0.1-0.25	Depletion of catechol-	Drowsiness, lethargy, nasal
	Serpasil	0.1-0.25	amines in sympathetic	congestion, bradycardia,
	Reserpoid	0.1-0.25	postganglionic fibers	depression, gastric hyperacidity
Whole root	Raudixin	50-100		
Alseroxylon fraction	Rauwiloid	2-4		
Deserpidine	Harmonyl	0.25		
Guanethidine	Ismelin	10-150	Blocks norepinephrine release from adrenergic nerve endings	Orthostatic hypotension (very common), diarrhea, impotence or loss of ejaculation
				NOTE: Poor, inconsistent absorption from gastrointestinal tract
Methyldopa	Aldomet	500-2500	Metabolized into a false neurotransmitter displacing norepinephrine from its receptor sites; sympathetic activity reduced	Orthostatic hypotension, drowsiness, fever, liver damage, anemia, impotence
				NOTE: Drug of choice in presence of renal disease
Propranolol	Inderal	80-320	β-Adrenergic blocker at peripheral autonomic site	Gastrointestinal tract disturbance, thrombocytopenia, rash, congestive heart failure, aggravation of asthma, fever; increase in conduction disturbance

*In milligrams per day, except as noted.

Continued.

TABLE 46-2. Oral drugs used in hypertension—cont'd

Drug	Trade name	Dosage*	Mode of action	Side effects
Metoprolol	Lopressor	100-400	Same action as propranolol	Same as for propranolol
Nadolol	Corgard	80-320		
Timolol	Blocadren	60		
Phenoxybenzamine	Dibenzyline	20-80	α-Adrenergic blocker at peripheral autonomic site	Nasal congestion, blurred vision, tachycardia, gastrointestinal tract disturbance
Phentolamine	Regitine	200	Same action as phenoxybenzamine	Same as for phenoxybenzamine; produces direct vasodilation
Pentolinium	Ansolysen	40 to no limit	Block both parasympathetic and sympathetic nerve transmission at ganglia	Orthostatic hypotension, dry mouth, blurred vision, constipation, urinary retention
Mecamylamine	Inversine	5 to no limit		
Trimethaphan	Arfonad	40-80 μg/kg/ min, IV		Hypotension, urinary retention, angina
Clonidine	Catapres	0.1	Stimulates α-adrenergic receptor in brain; causes inhibition of sympathetic vasoconstriction	Orthostatic hypotension, dry mouth, sedation, headache, constipation, fatigue
Vasodilators				
Hydralazine	Apresoline	50-250	Direct relaxation of arteriolar smooth muscle causing vasodilation	Headache, tachycardia, nausea, weakness, angina, rash, dizziness, fever
Prazosin	Minipres	3-20		
Sodium nitroprusside	Nipride	0.5-3 μg/kg/ min, IV	Same action as hydralazine	Hypotension, gastrointestinal disturbance, tachycardia, cyanide toxicity
Diazoxide	Hyperstat	300 by rapid IV	Same action as hydralazine	Hypotension, sodium and water retention, angina, gastrointestinal disturbances

sociated with methyldopa (Aldomet) and guanethidine (Ismelin), are such that the individual does not automatically associate them with the antihypertensive medication and may be hesitant about discussing them. By informing patients when medications are started that these effects occur in a small percentage of people, that they are transient, and that they should inform their physicians if they do occur in order that the medication can be changed, there is a greater chance that patients will continue their therapy. The patient must also know the hazard of sudden cessation; for example, hypertensive crisis can follow withdrawal of clonidine (Catapres), and when this medication is withdrawn careful supervision by the physician is required. All aspects of the patient education program require careful coordination of the efforts of the nurse and physician.

All individuals with hypertension require close medical supervision. The blood pressure of some persons tends to be quite labile, and frequent adjustment in the dosage of their medications may be necessary. With certain drugs, response varies according to other variables such as the variability of guanethidine associated with shifts in extracellular fluid. Tolerance to the prescribed drug may also occur, and persons need to know what symptoms indicate the need to contact their physician.

If the blood pressure becomes very high, some symptoms may occur. The most important symptoms have been discussed previously (p. 1179). Patients should be aware that if any of these symptoms occur they should contact their physician immediately. Since the blood pressure can increase substantially without symptoms, the person should also be aware that supervision by health professionals for the rest of his or her life will probably be necessary.

Outcome criteria for the person with hypertension

The person or significant others can:
1. Explain dietary modifications including decreased sodium intake.
2. Describe how to avoid external factors, such as stress, that compromise circulation.
3. Describe the medication and treatment program.
   a. State name, dosage frequency, and side effects of prescribed medication; state how to avoid side effects such as postural hypotension.
   b. Demonstrate awareness of probable need to continue medication for the rest of his life.

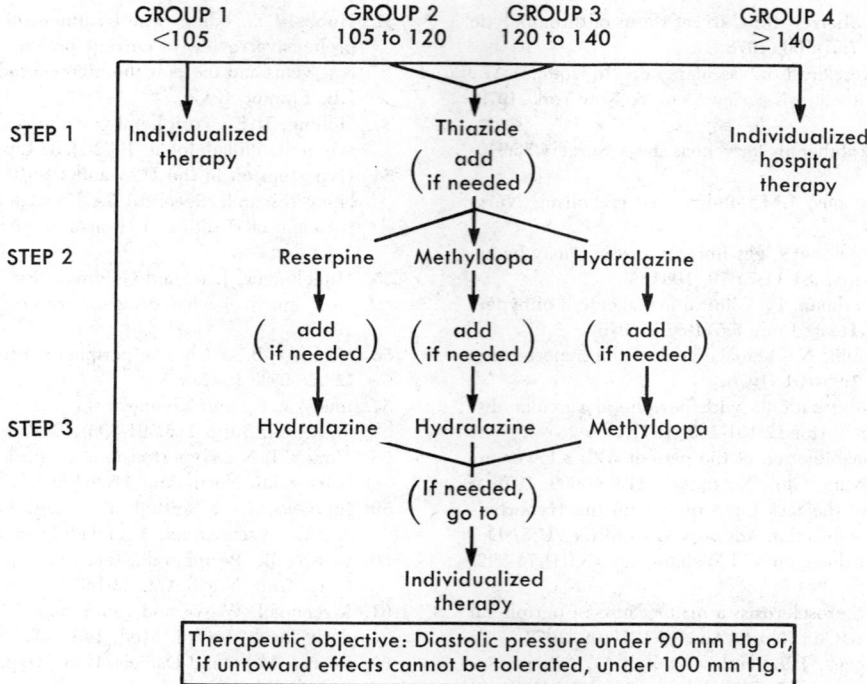

Fig. 46-16. Outline of recommended antihypertensive regimens for groups with varying degrees of severe hypertension as indicated by diastolic pressure in mm Hg. (From U.S. National High Blood Pressure Education Programs, Report of Task Force 1, Data Base, Bethesda, Md., 1973, National Institutes of Health).

c. Demonstrate ability to take blood pressure correctly (if applicable).
4. Explain health maintenance program.
  a. State symptoms that necessitate immediate medical attention.
  b. State plans for follow-up care by health professionals for the rest of his or her life.

REFERENCES AND SELECTED READINGS
Contemporary

1. Abramson, D.I.: Vascular disorders of the extremities, ed. 2, New York, 1974, Harper & Row, Publishers.
2. Albrechtson, U., et al.: Streptokinase treatment of deep venous thrombosis and the post-thrombotic syndrome, Arch. Surg. **116**:33-37, 1981.
3. Alderman, D.B.: Surgery—and schlerotherapy—for varicose veins, RN **39**:OR-1, OR-4, OR-6, 1976.
4. Alderman, M.H., editor: Hypertension: the nurse's role in ambulatory care, New York, 1977, Springer Publishing Co., Inc.
5. Alderman, M.H., and Schoenbaum, E.E.: Detection and treatment of hypertension at the work site, N. Engl. J. Med. **293**:65-68, 1975.
6. *Atchison, J.S., and Murray, J.: Post-vascular surgery, Nurs. '78 **8**:36-39, 1978.
7. Baird, R.N., and Abbott, W.M.: Vein grafts: an historical perspective, Am. J. Surg. **134**:293-296, 1977.

8. Barker, W.F.: Peripheral arterial disease, ed. 2, Philadelphia, 1975, W.B. Saunders Co.
9. Barnes, R.W., et al.: Prediction of amputation wound healing, Arch. Surg. **116**:80-83, 1981.
10. Batterman, B., Stegman, M.R., and Fitz, A.: Hypertension. I. Detection and evaluation, Cardiovasc. Nurs. **11**:35-40, 1975.
11. Batterman, B., Stegman, M.R., and Fitz, A.: Hypertension. II. Treatment and nursing responsibilities, Cardiovasc. Nurs. **11**:41-44, 1975.
12. Bergan, J.J., and DeBoer, A.: Venous thrombosis and pulmonary embolism: total care, Surg. Clin. North Am. **50**:173-192, 1970.
13. Bibliography on hypertension therapy, Postgrad. Med. **56**:95-97, 1974.
14. Borhani, N.O.: Epidemiology of hypertension as a guide to treatment and control, Heart Lung **10**:245-253, 1981.
15. *Bosanko, L.A.: Immediate postoperative prosthesis, Am. J. Nurs. **71**:280-283, 1971.
16. Buck, B., and Lee, A.D.: Amputation: two views, Nurs. Clin. North Am. **11**:641-657, 1976.
17. *Clark, A.B., and Dunn, M.: A nurse clinician's role in the management of hypertension, Arch. Intern. Med. **136**:903-904, 1976.
18. *Cobey, J.C., and Cobey, J.H.: Chronic leg ulcers, Am. J. Nurs. **74**:258-259, 1974.
19. Coffman, J.D.: Vasodilator drugs in peripheral vascular disease, J. Maine Med. Assoc. **66**:262-268, 1975.
20. Collins, G.J., et al.: Chronic abnormalities in patients with arterial, venous, and combined arterial and venous thrombosis, Arch. Surg. **112**:1347-1351, 1977.
21. *Craven, R.F., and Curry, T.D.: When the diagnosis is Raynaud's, Am. J. Nurs. **81**:1007-1009, 1981.

*References preceded by an asterisk are particularly well suited for student reading.

22. *Cudkowicz, L., and Sherrry, S.: Current status of thrombolytic therapy, Heart Lung **7:**97-100, 1978.

23. DePalma, R.G.: Atherosclerosis in vascular grafts. In Gotto, A.M., and Paoletti, R.: Atherosclerosis reviews, vol. 6, New York, 1979, Raven Press.

24. DePalma, R.G.: Surgical therapy for venous stasis, Surgery **76:**910-917, 1974.

25. *Dorsey, B., and Passons, J.M.: Pulmonary embolism, Nurs. '81 **11:**26-31, 1981.

26. *Doyle, J.E.: If your patient's legs hurt, the reason may be arterial insufficiency, Nurs. '81 **11:**74-79, 1981.

27. *Dhar, S.K., and Freedman, P.: Clinical management of hypertensive emergencies, Heart Lung **5:**571-575, 1976.

28. Draye, M.A., and Robin, N.: Management of the hypertensive patient, Nurs. Pract. **1:**98-101, 1976.

29. *Eddy, M.E.: Teaching patients with peripheral vascular disease, Nurs. Clin. North Am. **12:**151-159, 1977.

30. *Engstrand, J.L.: Rehabilitation of the patient with a lower extremity amputation, Nurs. Clin. North Am. **11:**659-669, 1976.

31. Executive summary of the task force reports to the Hypertension Information and Education Advisory Committee, U.S. Department of Health, Education and Welfare, no. (NIH) 74-592, 1973.

32. *Fagin-Dubin, L.: Atherosclerosis: a major cause of peripheral vascular disease, Nurs. Clin. North Am. **12:**101-108, 1977.

33. Fairbairn, J.F., Juergens, J.L., and Spittell, J.A., editors: Peripheral vascular disease, ed. 5, Philadelphia, 1980, W.B. Saunders Co.

34. *Falotico, J.B.: Pulmonary embolism, Crit. Care Update **8:**5-15, 1981.

35. *Fenn, J.E.: Reconstructive arterial surgery, for ischemic lower extremities, Nurs. Clin. North Am. **12:**129-142, 1977.

36. *Finnerty, F.A., Jr.: Treatment of hypertensive emergencies, Heart Lung **10:**275-284, 1981.

37. *Finnerty, F.A., Jr.: Aggressive drug therapy in accelerated hypertension, Am. J. Nurs. **74:**2176-2180, 1974.

38. Finnerty, F.A., Jr.: Hypertension as a clinical problem: the hospital based population, Prev. Med. **3:**323-327, 1974.

39. *Frank-Stromberg, M., and Stromberg, P.: Test your knowledge of managing the patient with hypertension, Nurs. '81 **11:**56-59, 1981.

40. *Freis, E.D.: Introduction to the nature and management of hypertension, Bowie, Md., 1974, Robert J. Brady Co.

41. *Gordon, T., and Kennel, W.B.: Predisposition to atherosclerosis in the head, heart, and legs: the Framingham study, J.A.M.A. **221:**661-666, 1972.

42. Greep, J.M., et al.: A combined technique for arterial embolectomy, Arch. Surg. **105:**869-874, 1972.

43. Gross, F.: Drug therapy of hypertension: what we have, what we need, what we expect, Am. J. Cardiol. **34:**471-475, 1974.

44. *Habel, M.: Plasma expanders, Crit. Care Update **8:**14-21, 1981.

45. Hahn, A.B., Barkin, R.L., and Oestreich, S.J.K.: Pharmacology in nursing, ed. 15, St. Louis, 1982, The C.V. Mosby Co.

46. Haimovici, H.: Vascular surgery: principles and techniques, ed. 2, New York, 1976, McGraw-Hill Book Co.

47. *Hartshorn, J.C.: What to do when the patient's in hypertensive crisis, Nurs. '80 **10:**36-45, 1980.

48. Haslam, P.: Hypertension: antihypertensives and how they work, Can. Nurse **75:**25-31, 1979.

49. *Haughey, C.W.: Understanding ultrasonography, Nurs. '81 **11:**100-104, 1981.

50. Helgeland, A.: Treatment of mild hypertension—the five year Oslo study, Am. J. Med. **69:**725-732, 1980.

51. *Hirschberg, G.G., et al.: Rehabilitation: a manual for the care of the elderly and disabled, ed. 2, Philadelphia, 1976, J.B. Lippincott Co.

52. Hobbs, J.T., editor: The treatment of venous disorders: a comprehensive review of current practice in the treatment of varicose veins and the post-thrombotic syndrome, Philadelphia, 1977, J.B. Lippincott Co.

53. Holling, H.E.: Peripheral vascular diseases: diagnosis and management, Philadelphia, 1972, J.B. Lippincott Co.

54. Hypertension in the USA and USSR: basic, clinical, and population research. Second USA-USSR Joint Symposium, U.S. Department of Health and Human Services, NIH pub. no. 80-2016, 1980.

55. *Ingelfinger, J.A., and Goldman, P.: Therapy for hypertension. How much of what drug for whom? J.A.M.A. **238:**1369-1370, 1977.

56. *Jackson, B.S.: Chronic peripheral arterial disease, Am. J. Nurs. **72:**928-934, 1972.

57. Jones, A.F., and Kempczinski, R.F.: Aortofemoral bypass grafting, Arch. Surg. **116:**301-305, 1981.

58. *Jones, L.N.: Hypertension: medical and nursing implications, Nurs. Clin. North Am. **11:**283-295, 1976.

59. Juergens, J.L., Spittell, J.A., and Fairbairn, J.F.: Peripheral vascular diseases, ed. 5, Philadelphia, 1980, W.B. Saunders Co.

60. Kessro, B.: Peripheral arterial insufficiency: postoperative care, Nurs. Clin. North Am. **12:**143-149, 1977.

61. Kirkendall, W.M., and Hammond, J.J.: Hypertension in the elderly, Arch. Intern. Med. **140:**1155-1161, 1980.

62. Kochar, M.S., and Daniels, L.M.: Hypertension control for nurses and other health professionals, St. Louis, 1978, The C.V. Mosby Co.

63. Larson, C.B., and Gould, M.L.: Orthopedic nursing, ed. 9, St. Louis, 1978, The C.V. Mosby Co.

64. Leonard, A.R., Igra, A., and Hawthorne, A.: Status of high blood pressure control in California, Heart Lung **10:**255-268, 1981.

65. *Long, M.L., et al.: Hypertension: what patients need to know, Am. J. Nurs. **76:**765-770, 1976.

66. *Loustau, A., and Blair, B.J.: A key to compliance, Nurs. '81 **11:**84-87, 1981.

67. *Lowther, N.B., and Carter, V.D.: How to increase compliance in hypertensives, Am. J. Nurs. **81:**963, 1981.

68. Mahley, R.W.: Dietary fat, cholesterol, and accelerated atherosclerosis. In Paoletti, R., and Gotto, A.M.: Atherosclerosis reviews, vol. 4, New York, 1979, Raven Press.

69. Malone, R.: Helping your hypertensive patient live longer, Nurs. '78 **8:**26-34, 1978.

70. Mancini, M., et al.: Role of diet in atherosclerosis. In Hegyeli, R.: Atherosclerosis reviews, vol. 7, New York, 1980, Raven Press.

71. Mannick, J.A., and Coffman, J.D.: Ischemic limbs: surgical approach and physiological principles, New York, 1973, Grune & Stratton, Inc.

72. Marshall, A.J., and Barritt, D.W.: The hypertensive patient, Baltimore, 1980, University Park Press.

73. *Martin, N.: Rehabilitation of the upper extremity amputee, Nurs. Outlook **18:**50-51, 1970.

74. *Maschak-Carey, B.J., and Moore, K.: Anticoagulation therapy, Crit. Care Update **8:**5-16, 1981.

75. *McClinton, V.S.: Nursing of the upper extremity amputee and preparation for prosthetic training, Nurs. Clin. North Am. **11:**671-677, 1976.

76. *McCulley, M.: Hypertension: questions and answers, Can. Nurse **75:**24-25, 1979.

77. *Mitchell, E.S.: Protocol for teaching hypertensive patients, Am. J. Nurs. **77:**808-809, 1977.

78. Moser, M., editor: Hypertension: a practical approach, Boston, 1975, Little, Brown & Co.

79. Murphy, B.S.: Management of hyperlipidemia, J.A.M.A. **230:**1683-1691, 1974.

80. National Heart and Lung Institute Task Force on Arterioscle-

rosis: Arteriosclerosis, vol. II, U.S. Department of Health, Education and Welfare, no. (NIH) 72-219, 1971.

81. National High Blood Pressure Education Program: Guidelines for the evaluation and management of the hypertensive patient, High Blood Pressure Information Center, National Institutes of Health, U.S. Department of Health, Education, and Welfare, no. (NIH) 76-744, 1976.

82. Nicholas, G.G., and DeMuth, W.E.: Evaluation of the use of the rigid dressing in amputation of the lower extremity, Surg. Gynecol. Obstet. **143:**398-400, 1976.

83. O'Neill, M.F.: Patients with hypertension: a study of manifest needs with self-actualization, Nurs. Res. **25:**349-351, 1976.

84. *Pasnau, R.O., and Pfefferbaum, B.: Psychologic aspects of post-amputation pain, Nurs. Clin. North Am. **11:**679-685, 1976.

85. Perloff, D., editor: Symposium on hypertension, Med. Clin. North Am. **61:**463-700, 1977.

86. Perloff, D.: Diagnostic assessment of the patient with hypertension, Geriatrics **31:**77-83, 1976.

87. Pfefferbaum, B., and Pasnau, R.O.: Post-amputation grief, Nurs. Clin. North Am. **11:**687-690, 1976.

88. *Pierce, P.F.: Gains and losses of vascular surgery patients, Nurs. Clin. North Am. **12:**119-127, 1977.

89. Porter, J.M., Baur, G.M., and Taylor, L.M.: Lower extremity amputations for ischemia, Arch. Surg. **116:**89-98, 1981.

90. Pratt, G.H.: Vascular surgery: a guide and handbook, St. Louis, 1976, Warren H. Green, Inc.

91. Proceedings of the symposium on venous surgery in the lower extremity, Walter Reed Army Medical Center, 1973, St. Louis, 1975, Warren H. Green, Inc.

92. *Ram, C.V.: Newer antihypertensive drugs, Heart Lung **6:**679-684, 1977.

93. Reis, R.L., and Hannah, H.: Management of patients with severe, coexistent coronary artery and peripheral vascular disease, J. Thorac. Cardiovasc. Surg. **73:**909-918, 1977.

94. Richardson, D.W.: Can physicians effect persistent control of blood pressure? Arch. Intern. Med. **137:**1598-1599, 1977.

95. *Robinson, A.M.: Detection and control of hypertension: challenge to all nurses, Am. J. Nurs. **76:**778-780, 1976.

96. Rodman, M.J.: Thromboembolic disorders. I. Venous thrombosis, RN **39:**81-82, 85-86, 1976.

97. Rodman, M.J.: Thromboembolic disorders. II. Arterial thrombosis and embolism, RN **39:**61-66, 1976.

98. Roon, A.J., Moore, W.S., and Goldstone, J.: Below-knee-amputation: a modern approach, Am. J. Surg. **134:**153-158, 1977.

99. *Rose, M.A.: Home care after peripheral vascular surgery, Am. J. Nurs. **74:**260-262, 1974.

100. Ross, R., and Glomset, J.: The pathogenesis of artherosclerosis. I, N. Engl. J. Med. **295:**369-377, 1976.

101. Ross, R., and Glomset, J.: The pathogenesis of atherosclerosis. II, N. Engl. J. Med. **295:**420-425, 1976.

102. Royster, T.S., Mulcare, R.J., and Marks, R.A.: Peripheral arterial disease: recognizing the need for surgery, Postgrad. Med. **62:**153-159, 1977.

103. Rutherford, R.B., editor: Vascular surgery, Philadelphia, 1977, W.B. Saunders Co.

104. Ryzewski, J.: Factors in the rehabilitation of patients with peripheral vascular disease, Nurs. Clin. North Am. **12:**161-168, 1977.

105. *Sexton, D.L.: The patient with peripheral arterial occlusive disease, Nurs. Clin. North Am. **12:**89-99, 1977.

106. *Shank, L.F., and Ludewig, J.: Hypertension, Nurs. Clin. North Am. **9:**677-692, 1974.

107. Simpson, F.O., editor: Symposium on hypertension: drugs, **11**(suppl. 1):2-5, 1976.

108. Stahl, S.M., et al.: Motivational interventions in community hypertension screening, Am. J. Publ. Health **67:**345-352, 1977.

109. Stubbins, J., editor: Social and psychological aspects of disability: a handbook for practitioners, Baltimore, 1977, University Park Press.

110. *Task Force on the Role of Nursing in High Blood Pressure Control: Nursing education in high blood pressure control: report, National Institutes of Health, U.S. Department of Health, Education and Welfare, no. (NIH) 76-1052, 1976.

111. Thompson, G.R.: Management of familial hypercholesterolemia and new approaches to the treatment of atherosclerosis. In Paoletti, R., and Gotto, A.M.: Atherosclerosis review, vol. 4, New York, 1979, Raven Press.

112. U.S. National High Blood Pressure Education Program: Directory of community high blood pressure control activities, ed. 2, National Institutes of Health, U.S. Department of Health, Education and Welfare, no. (NIH) 77-1243, 1977. (Prepared by the National High Blood Pressure Education Program with the assistance of Merck Sharp & Dohme.)

113. U.S. National High Blood Pressure Education Program: Report to the Hypertension Information and Education Advisory Committee: task force reports, Bethesda, Md., 1973, National Institutes of Health.

114. *Walter, J.: Coping with a leg amputation, Am. J. Nurs. **81:**1349-1352, 1981.

115. Warren, R.: Procedures in vascular surgery, ed. 2, Boston, 1976, Little, Brown & Co.

116. *Webb, P.H.: Neurological deficit after carotid endarterectomy, Am. J. Nurs. **79:**654-656, 1979.

117. Weber, G., Fabbrini, P., and Resi, L.: Arterial intimal changes in the early phases of experimental atherogenesis. In Paoletti, R., and Gotto, A.M.: Atherosclerosis review, vol. 4, New York, 1979, Raven Press.

118. Wilhelmsen, L., and Berglund, G.: Prevalence of primary and secondary hypertension, Am. Heart J. **94:**543-546, 1977.

Classic

119. Burgess, E., et al.: Immediate postsurgical prosthetics in the management of lower extremity amputees, Washington, D.C., 1967, Department of Medicine and Surgery, Veterans Administration.

120. *Garrett, J.F., and Levine, E.S., editors: Psychological practices with the physically disabled, New York, 1962, Columbia University Press.

121. Laughlin, E., Stanford, J., and Phelps, M.: Immediate postsurgical prosthetics fitting of a bilateral, below-elbow amputee: a report, Artif. Limbs **12:**17-19, 1968.

122. *Plaisted, L.M., and Friz, B.R.: The nurse on the amputee clinic team, Nurs. Outlook **16:**34-37, 1968.

CHAPTER 47

PROBLEMS OF THE BLOOD AND BLOOD-FORMING ORGANS

DEANNA MELTON XISTRIS

Diseases associated with the reticuloendothelial system are diverse in their underlying pathologic manifestations, disease course, and response to treatment. Most often, the symptoms manifested are the result of interference with the normal development and function of the blood components: erythrocytes (red blood cells), platelets, and leukocytes (white blood cells) (Fig. 47-1), and altered hematopoiesis (blood cell production). Normally, homeostasis is maintained through a balance between the rate of production of normal blood cells and the rate of destruction. Disorders of the blood are manifested when this balance is lost. Disturbances in the coagulation mechanism also result in blood disorders.

Discussion of the blood components and lymph system is presented in this chapter along with the related disease processes.

Assessment

A wide variety of disorders affect the hematopoietic system. In addition to primary hematologic disorders, secondary effects from disease of another body system may manifest themselves in abnormal hematologic findings. For example, the anemia associated with azotemia is the consequence of disease outside of the hematopoietic system.

The cause of any hematologic abnormality must be assiduously pursued. The importance of accurate diagnosis combined with the very diverse and frequently nonspecific signs and symptoms makes it likely that the person will become involved in an arduous diagnostic process. At the time of initial contact the patient is already experiencing the stress of sudden onset of illness or the gnawing fear or suspicion that all is not well. The explanations that are offered and the time allowed for verbalization and questions are means of providing a positive foundation for the long-term care that may follow.

Subjective data

A thorough history includes detailed information about the person's symptoms and a thorough review of systems. In the history taking of a person with suspected hematologic disease, other key points to include are family history, drug history, exposure to chemicals, and general nonspecific complaints offered by the patient.

Family history

The existence of inherited hematologic disorders necessitates a detailed family history. Questions regarding disease or presence of symptoms among relatives should include reference to parents, siblings, grandfathers, uncles, and nephews. Questions should explore instances of severe or prolonged bleeding in relation to minor trauma, dental extractions, or surgery. The occurrence of jaundice or anemia in relatives should also be ascertained.

Drugs and chemicals

Drugs may induce or potentiate hematologic disease. Most notable are the hematologic effects of the cytotoxic drugs used in cancer chemotherapy and the neutropenia associated with chloramphenicol. A thorough history of drugs ingested by a person is a crucial

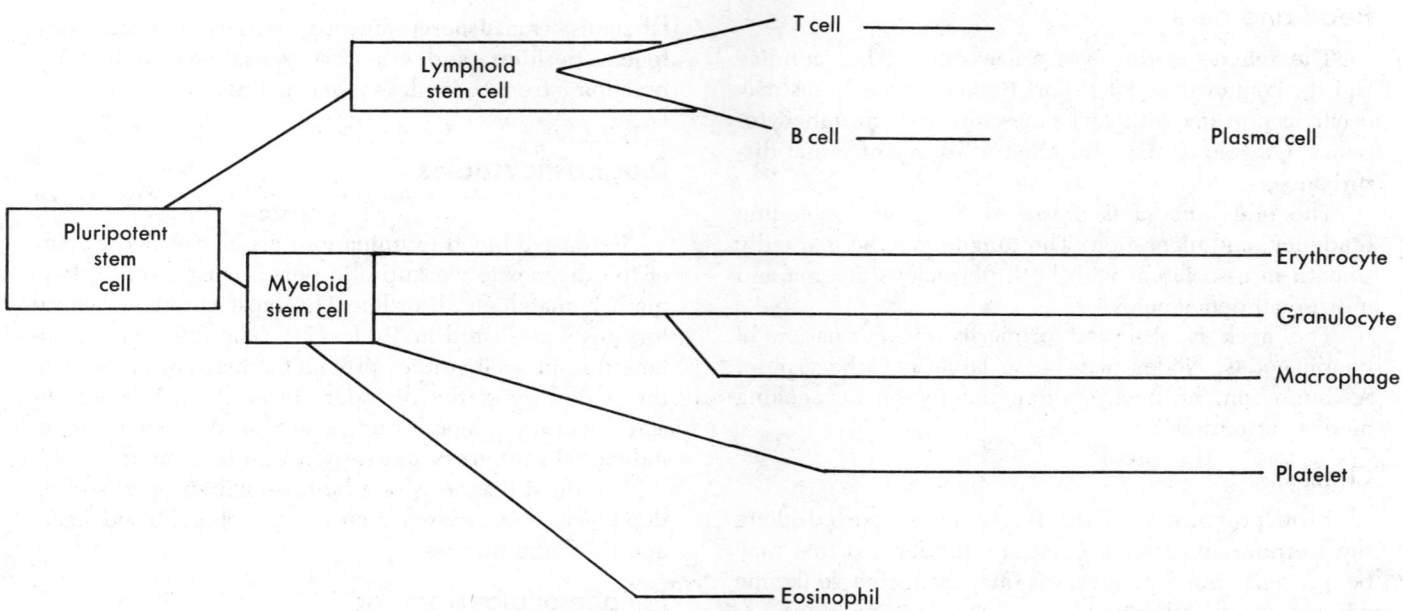

Fig. 47-1. Scheme of stem cell differentiation showing common progenitor cell for erythrocytes, granulocytes, and platelets. (Adapted from Clinc, M., and Golde, D.: Blood **53**:157-164, 1979.)

part of assessment. Many persons regularly ingest "something to help me sleep," "something to calm me down," or "just aspirin." Analgesics, tranquilizers, laxatives, and sedatives are often overlooked by persons when asked about drugs. Specific, often rephrased questioning is necessary to obtain a complete drug history.

Certain chemicals may exert a potentially harmful effect on the hematopoietic system. To obtain a history of exposure to chemicals, an occupational history is useful. In addition, such common practices as the use of hair dye should also be explored.

Fever

Fever is a common manifestation of many of the hematologic disorders and is an important question to be asked during the history. Fever is a common manifestation in lymphoma, primarily Hodgkin's disease and leukemia. Severe chills may accompany hemolytic disorders. Night sweats are frequently associated with both lymphoma and leukemia.

Fatigue and malaise

Fatigue and malaise are difficult symptoms to evaluate, since they frequently accompany many physical and emotional disorders. Information regarding the occurrence of these symptoms should be included in the history. When combined with physical and lab findings, they are of some diagnostic value. In addition, the person's subjective description of such symptoms lends some insight into perception of the illness, the extent to which

the illness is affecting daily living, and the ability to adapt.

Objective data

A thorough physical examination is performed in the assessment of a person with a hematologic disorder. It is useful to recognize target organs and alterations that may be reflective of hematologic disease.

Skin

Skin manifestations of hematologic disease are often readily visible. *Petechiae* and *ecchymoses* are associated with decreased platelets (thrombocytopenia) and other bleeding disorders. *Jaundice*, when observed, may be associated with pernicious anemia or hemolytic disease. *Pallor* is commonly associated by the lay person with disorders of the blood. Pallor as a criteria for assessment may be deceptive, since many healthy persons have pale complexions, while some severely anemic patients may have ruddy complexions.

Changes in skin texture may also be observed. Except in severe cases it will most likely be the person who observes such changes. With iron deficiency anemia the person may notice dry skin, dry hair, and brittle nails. Severe itching is commonly associated with Hodgkin's disease and may also occur with polycythemia vera, especially after bathing. In persons with leukemia and lymphoma, infiltrative lesions of the skin may be observed on any portion of the body.

Head and neck

The sclerae of the eyes are examined for jaundice and the conjunctivae for pallor. Retinal hemorrhages may occur in persons with severe anemia and thrombocytopenia. Questions may also elicit a history of visual disturbances.

The oral mucosa is observed for pallor, bleeding tendency, and ulceration. The tongue may be markedly smooth in association with both pernicious anemia and nutritional deficiencies.

The neck is observed primarily for evaluation of lymph nodes. Nodes may be so large as to be visible. A "lump" on the neck is often the reason for seeking medical attention.

Chest

Firm pressure with the fingertips is exerted along the sternum and ribs to elicit any tenderness that may be present. Such tenderness may reflect a leukemic process or multiple myeloma.

Abdomen

The abdomen is percussed and palpated with special attention to the liver and spleen. Both organs are prone to enlarge in association with hematologic disease.

Back and extremities

The skeletal system is evaluated primarily for pain, joint deformity, and arthritis. Bone pain may be associated with hematologic malignancies. In persons with hemolytic processes and some hematologic malignancies, there is increased uric acid production and a corresponding increase in the incidence of gout. Joint deformities are associated with bleeding disorders.

Lymph nodes

Lymph nodes are widely distributed in the body and are routinely examined by palpation of the body part being examined. In the healthy adult the only palpable nodes are in the inguinal region and less commonly in the axilla. With the disease the cervical and supraclavicular nodes may become palpable. Further evaluation of lymph nodes requires radiographic examination and lymphangiography. It is important to recognize that any enlarged lymph node may reflect a disease process and should be evaluated thoroughly.

Nervous system

Many neurologic abnormalities may be manifested in persons with hematologic disorders. These catastrophic complications are caused by bleeding or infection within the central nervous system. Infiltration of malignant leukemic or lymphomatous cells may produce signs and symptoms of cerebral tumor. In addition some of the lymphomas, especially Hodgkin's disease, may produce a dementia as a remote effect. Initial physical examination should therefore include assessment of mental status, cranial nerve function, sensory function (pain, touch, position, and vibratory sensation), and motor function (strength, reflexes, and plantar response).

Diagnostic studies

Extensive blood examinations are performed as part of the diagnostic workup of a person suspected of having a hematologic disorder. The most common laboratory tests are listed in Table 47-1. The information obtained from such studies provides important clues as to the pathology of the disorder. In addition to their diagnostic value, blood studies are used to monitor an individual's progress and response to treatment.

The final diagnosis of a hematologic disease is often dependent on an examination of a peripheral blood smear and the bone marrow.

Peripheral blood smear

Each blood cell possesses microscopic features that identify and set the cell apart from other cell types. Examination of the peripheral blood smear allows for the determination of the morphology of the cells (type, origin), the extent of cell maturity, and the ratio of the various cell types to each other. Often this information, when combined with the data from the history, physical examination, and other laboratory tests, determines the medical diagnosis.

Bone marrow examination

An adjunct to the peripheral blood smear is the bone marrow examination. Generally the bone marrow is examined in those instances in which the diagnosis is not clearly established from the peripheral blood smear or when further information is needed. A bone marrow specimen is obtained by bone marrow aspiration or bone marrow biopsy.

Bone marrow asipiration. Aspiration is the most common procedure for obtaining a bone marrow sample. The procedure is possible because normal bone marrow is soft and semifluid and can therefore be removed by aspiration through a needle. Bone marrow aspiration is most likely to be performed in persons with marked anemia, neutropenia (decreased number of white blood cells), acute leukemia, and thrombocytopenia (decreased number of platelets).

PROCEDURE. The skin surrounding the puncture site (Fig. 47-2) is shaved, if necessary, and cleansed with an antiseptic such as povidone-iodine complex (Betadine). Sterile towels are placed around the site. The skin and periosteum are anesthetized to avoid pain. First, the most superficial layer of the skin is infiltrated with procaine. After a few seconds the needle is further advanced until bone is touched. Procaine is then injected to anesthetize the periosteum.

The marrow aspiration needle is inserted and when

the marrow cavity is entered, the marrow stylet is removed from the needle and a sterile syringe is attached. The syringe plunger is drawn back until marrow appears in the syringe. As the plunger is drawn back the person will experience a brief, sharp pain, sometimes described as a burning sensation. The pain is caused by the suction exerted as the plunger is pulled back. At this point the nurse's hands placed gently on the person's shoulder and a calm warning coupled with a reminder to lie still serve well to prevent a sudden jerk or movement by the person.

After the needle is removed, pressure is applied

briefly over the aspiration site to arrest the scant bleeding that occurs. If the patient is thrombocytopenic, pressure is applied for 3 to 5 minutes.

Some persons may complain of tenderness at the aspiration site for a few days. Most often, no pain or discomfort is experienced following the procedure.

Bone marrow biopsy. A bone marrow biopsy is indicated when a large sample of bone marrow is needed. Persons most likely to undergo a bone marrow biopsy are those with pancytopenia (more than one altered cell type), myelofibrosis, metastatic tumor, lymphoma, and multiple myeloma. The most common site for bone

---

TABLE 47-1. Laboratory tests for hematologic assessment

Blood cell	Function	Diagnostic test
Erythrocytes (RBCs)	Mediate the exchange of oxygen and carbon dioxide between lungs and tissue	RBC, hemoglobin, hematocrit, reticulocyte count
		Blood indices: Mean corpuscular hemoglobin concentration (MCHC), mean cell volume (MCV), mean corpuscular hemoglobin (MCH)
		Red cell fragility
		Morphologic description in stained smear
Platelets	Platelet plug; promotion of thrombin production	Platelet aggregation
		Platelet count
		Bleeding time
Leukocytes (WBCs)		WBC
Granulocytes		WBC with differential
Neutrophils	Phagocytosis	
Eosinophils		
Basophils	Allergic and immunologic responses	
Lymphocytes	Formation of immunoglobulins	
Monocytes	Phagocytosis	

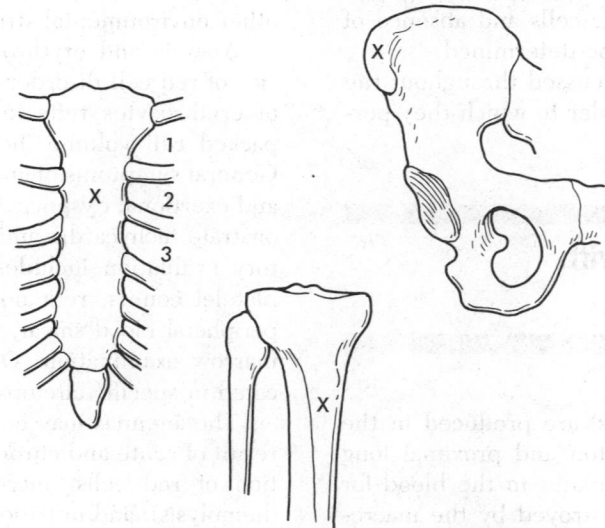

Fig. 47-2. Sites for bone marrow aspiration: sternum, iliac crest (most common), and tibia.

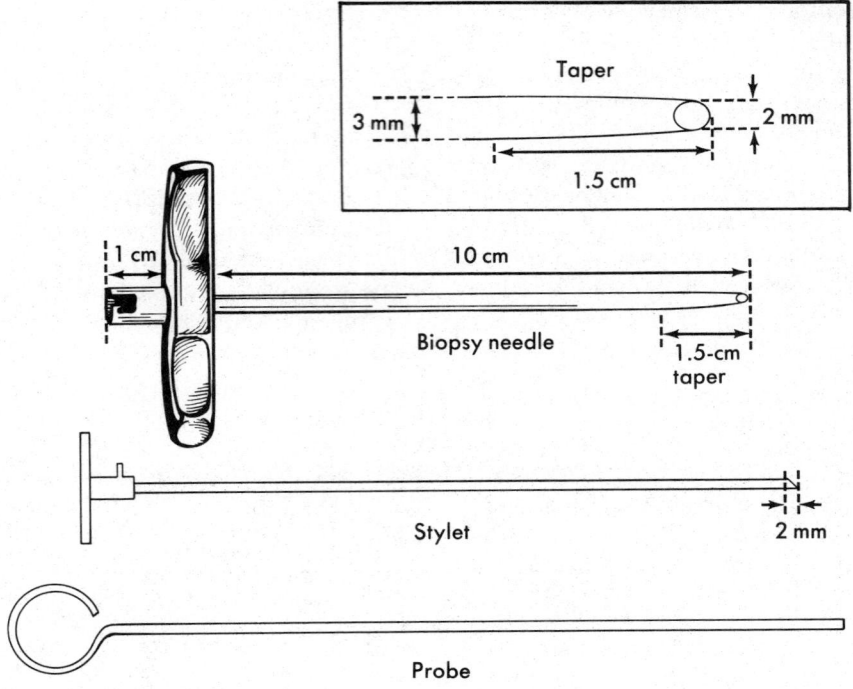

Fig. 47-3. Bone marrow biopsy needle showing shape and size.

marrow biopsy is the posterosuperior iliac spine. (The sterum is also used.) The initial steps in the biopsy procedure are similar to those outlined for bone marrow aspiration. The use of a Jamshidi needle allows for a core of marrow to be collected (Fig. 47-3).

Following a bone marrow aspirate or biopsy, patients are assessed for bleeding from the site. Some other comfort measures such as assisting the person to freshen up are often needed to help the person relax and rest comfortably.

From microscopic examination of the bone marrow, iron stores can be determined as can the morphology of the progenitor cell. Megaloblastic changes may be observed; infiltration with leukemic cells and absence of cells, as in aplastic anemia, can be determined.

Other diagnostic tests are discussed throughout the text along with the specific disorder to which they pertain.

Disorders associated with erythrocytes

Erythrocytes (red blood cells) are produced in the bone marrow of the axial skeleton and proximal long bones. The normal red cell circulates in the blood for 120 days, at which time it is destroyed by the macrophages of the reticuloendothelial system. The primary function of the red cell is the transport of oxygen to tissues. The oxygen is picked up in the lungs and binds to the principal protein constituent of red cells, *hemoglobin*. Hemoglobin is a complex molecule consisting of an iron-containing porphyrin portion (heme) and two pairs of polypeptide chains (globin). The mature red cell contains, in addition to hemoglobin, multiple enzymes involved in the metabolism of glucose. Energy is derived from the process of glycolysis in the form of high-energy phosphate bonds (adenosine triphosphate [ATP]) and is required to maintain cell membrane integrity, the relatively low sodium and high potassium content of the red cell, and as a defense against oxidation and other environmental stressors.

Anemia and erythrocytosis are the general categories of red cell disorders. *Anemia* refers to a deficiency of erythrocytes reflected in a decreased hemoglobin, packed cell volume (hematocrit), and red cell count. General symptoms of anemia include fatigue, weakness, and exertional dyspnea. Physical examination may demonstrate tachycardia and postural hypotension. Laboratory evaluation includes white blood cell (WBC) and platelet counts, reticulocyte count, examination of the peripheral blood smear, red cell indices, and often bone marrow examination. Other specialized tests are indicated in specific circumstances.

The anemias may be divided into those that are the result of acute and chronic blood loss, impaired production of red cells, increased destruction of red cells (hemolysis), and nutritional deficiency. The anemias are summarized accordingly in the box on p. 1191.

CAUSES OF ANEMIA

1. Blood loss
   a. Acute
   b. Chronic
2. Impaired production of erythrocytes
   a. Aplastic anemia
3. Increased destruction of erythrocytes (hemolysis)
   a. Congenital
      (1) Hereditary spherocytosis
      (2) Hemoglobinopathies (sickle cell anemia)
      (3) Thalassemia
      (4) Enzyme deficiency (G6PD [glucose-6-phosphate dehydrogenase] deficiency)
   b. Acquired
      (1) Autoimmune
      (2) Drug induced
4. Nutritional deficiency
   a. Iron deficiency
   b. Megaloblastic anemia
      (1) B_{12} deficiency
      (2) Folic acid deficiency

Anemia secondary to blood loss

Acute anemia

Etiology. The anemia associated with acute blood loss is the direct result of the decrease in circulating red blood cells. The adult of average build has a total blood volume of approximately 6000 ml. Usually an adult can lose 500 ml of blood without serious or lasting effects. If the loss reaches 1000 ml or more serious acute consequences may result.

Clinical picture. The patient with anemia secondary to acute blood loss has signs and symptoms of hypovolemia and hypoxemia. Weakness, stupor, irritability, and cool moist skin are all symptoms that may be observed. Vital signs will demonstrate hypotension and tachycardia. Decreased hemoglobin and hematocrit may not be evident until several hours after the blood loss has occurred. The severity of the patient's symptoms correlates with the severity of the blood loss.

Chronic anemia

Etiology and clinical picture. The body has remarkable adaptive powers and may adjust fairly well to a marked reduction in red blood cells and hemoglobin, provided the condition develops gradually. An individual may remain asymptomatic even though the total red cell count may drop to almost half of its normal figure of between 4.5 and 5 million/cu mm. Chronic, unrecognized blood loss may occur in the presence of an unsuspected gastrointestinal tract malignancy, a slowly bleeding peptic ulcer, or bleeding hemorrhoids. Chronic blood loss is the most common cause of *iron-deficiency anemia*. When blood loss is continuous and moderate in amount, the bone marrow may be able to keep up with the losses by increasing the production of red blood cells. Eventually, if the cause of chronic blood loss is not found and corrected, the bone marrow will not be able to keep pace with the loss, and symptoms of anemia appear.

Intervention for acute and chronic anemia

Treatment for anemia secondary to blood loss depends on the identification of the source of blood loss. In addition to the treatment of the underlying cause, the anemia may be corrected by the administration of iron, usually in the oral form unless there are malabsorptive problems. Bleeding depletes iron stores because the most abundant source of iron in the body is the hemoglobin of the red blood cells.

In patients with chronic anemia who are asymptomatic, transfusion is usually not indicated since it unnecessarily exposes the patients to the risks associated with transfusion. Transfusion of erythrocytes is reserved for those patients with anemia whose cardiovascular system is compromised by the anemia and in whom rapid correction by other means is not possible.

Transfusion of whole blood may be used in the treatment of anemia secondary to acute blood loss. For virtually all of the other anemias, packed red cells rather than whole blood is utilized in transfusions, since the total blood volume is generally normal and administration of whole blood may produce circulatory overload and pulmonary edema. (See care of patients receiving transfusions, p. 1868.)

Anemia secondary to impaired production of erythrocytes

Etiology

In approximately one half of the cases of aplastic anemia in the United States, no etiologic agent is identifiable. Predictable bone marrow depression occurs with antineoplastic drugs. Aplastic anemia may follow exposure to certain drugs such as chloramphenicol, sulfonamides, phenylbutazone (Butazolidin), and anticonvulsant agents such as mephenytoin (Mesantoin). Insecticides, such as DDT, and chemicals, particularly benzene, are also thought to cause aplastic anemia. The defect leading to aplastic anemia is most likely injury or destruction of a common stem cell (Fig. 47-1) affecting all subsequent cell populations. Aplastic anemia may also be congenital.

Pathophysiology

Aplastic anemia (anemia secondary to impaired erythrocyte production) is usually characterized by depression or cessation of activity of all blood-producing elements. There is a decrease in white blood cells (leukopenia), a decrease in platelets (thrombocytopenia), and a decrease in the formation of red blood cells leading to an anemia.[19]

Clinical picture

Symptoms of aplastic anemia usually develop gradually over a period of weeks and months but may appear suddenly. Pallor of the skin and mucous membranes is characteristic, in addition to fatigue and exertional dyspnea. Infections of the skin and mucous membranes occur with severe granulocytopenia; and hemorrhagic symptoms (bleeding into the skin and mucous membranes and spontaneous bleeding from the nose, gums, vagina, and rectum) occur with severe thrombocytopenia. Physical examination is often normal. The hemogram characteristically reveals a pancytopenia (a marked decrease in the numbers of all cell types). The reticulocyte count is low. Definitive diagnosis is made by bone marrow examination. Attempts at bone marrow aspiration may yield a "dry tap" because of hypocellularity and a decrease in active marrow, and bone marrow biopsy is often necessary.

Intervention

The most immediate treatment for aplastic anemia is the removal of the causative agent if it is known. Androgen therapy, aimed at stimulating hematopoiesis, may be of benefit. For those persons with marked aplasia, diligent medical care and nursing care are required. Because the levels of all of the blood cells are decreased, the individual is prone to severe and life-threatening complications, primarily infection and bleeding. (The nursing care of persons with a decreased white blood count and platelet count is discussed on p. 1202.) Intensive supportive care through transfusion of the specific components that are lacking (red blood cells, platelets, white blood cells) is frequently necessary. In recent years bone marrow transplantation has emerged as a treatment for persons with aplastic anemia, and in patients with an HLA-identical donor it is the current treatment of choice.[8,42,46]

Anemia secondary to increased destruction of erythrocytes

Pathophysiology

Hemolytic anemia (anemia secondary to increased erythrocyte destruction) results when the red cells are destroyed at such a rapid rate that the bone marrow is unable to compensate for the loss. The severity of the anemia is determined by the degree of lag between the rate of erythrocyte destruction (hemolysis) and the rate of bone marrow production of red cells (erythropoiesis). Hemolytic anemias may be congenital or acquired.

Clinical picture

The reticulocyte count is usually elevated, as is the serum bilirubin level. Bilirubin is derived from the breakdown of the hemoglobin released by the destroyed red cells. Occasionally, red cell survival time will need to be determined. This is done by labeling the cells with radioactive chromium and measuring the rate of decrease of radioactivity for 1 to 2 weeks (chromium survival). Symptoms include those commonly associated with anemia (pallor, fatigue, exertional dyspnea), jaundice from the increased serum bilirubin level, and an enlarged spleen from the increased red blood cell destruction.

Congenital hemolytic anemias

Hemolytic anemias are divided into congenital and acquired. *Congenital hemolytic anemias* include hereditary spherocytosis, the hemoglobinopathies, thalassemia, and enzyme-deficiency anemia. *Hereditary spherocytosis,* inherited as an autosomal dominant trait, is characterized by a membrane abnormality that leads to osmotic swelling of the red cell and susceptibility to destruction by the spleen. It is most commonly detected in childhood but may become manifest initially in adulthood. Diagnosis depends on observation of spherocytes on the peripheral blood smear and by demonstration of increased osmotic fragility of the red cells in the laboratory. It is almost invariably corrected by splenectomy.

Hemoglobinopathies refer to a group of diseases in which there is substitution of one or more amino acids in the globin chain of the hemoglobin molecule, leading to the formation of abnormal hemoglobins (e.g., hemoglobins S and C). Their diagnosis and differentiation are facilitated by hemoglobin electrophoresis. The most common hemoglobinopathy is hemoglobin S disease, or sickle cell anemia.

Sickle cell anemia

ETIOLOGY AND EPIDEMIOLOGY. Sickle cell anemia occurs predominantly in the black population. Approximately 8% of American blacks are heterozygous for hemoglobin S and therefore have *sickle cell trait* (Table 47-2). They produce both hemoglobin S and normal hemoglobin A. Sickle cell trait is a benign disorder, often asymptomatic, with no anemia and a normal life span. Genetic counseling and screening may be suggested to inform affected individuals that marriage to another person who is also heterozygous for hemoglobin S may lead to offspring with sickle cell disease.

Individuals who are homozygous for hemoglobin S

TABLE 47-2. Phenotypes for sickle cell

Genetic relationship	Hemoglobin alleles	Sickle cell disease
Homozygous dominant	Hemoglobin A Hemoglobin A	No disease
Heterozygous	Hemoglobin A Hemoglobin S	Sickle cell trait
Homozygous recessive	Hemoglobin S Hemoglobin S	Sickle cell anemia

can only produce the defective hemoglobin S. It is these individuals who have *sickle cell disease* and are affected with a chronic hemolytic anemia, episodes of painful "crisis," and an anticipated shortened life span.

PATHOPHYSIOLOGY. The basic abnormality lies within the globin (protein) fraction of the hemoglobin, where a single amino acid is substituted for another in one of the polypeptide chains. This single amino acid substitution profoundly alters the properties of the hemoglobin molecule. As a consequence of the intermolecular rearrangement, hemoglobin S is formed instead of normal hemoglobin A. The tendency toward sickling is dependent on both the relative quantity of hemoglobin S in the red blood cells and the levels of oxygen tension within the tissues of the body.

The clinical manifestations of the disease result from the sickling phenomenon. Sickling occurs when red cells containing hemoglobin S are deoxygenated; it is the result of the poor solubility of the hemoglobin S, which crystallizes in the red blood cells. The sickle shape represents conformity of the red cell membrane to the spindle cell aggregates of the sickle hemoglobin. Sickling is always present to some extent in the patient with sickle cell anemia.

CLINICAL PICTURE. Anemia is usually severe, but clinical signs of anemia may be absent. Pain, which is frequently experienced in the bones, joints, and back, may be localized, generalized, or migratory. Episodes of severe abdominal pain, vomiting, and fever may resemble severe abdominal disorders. Growth and sexual maturation may be delayed. Pneumococcal infections and chronic ulcers of the ankle are frequent. Hepatosplenomegaly is common in children but rarely seen in adults. The heart is usually enlarged, and murmurs are common. Sickle cell crises may occur. Symptoms, especially sickle cell crises, may be exacerbated by pregnancy, infection, surgery, trauma, and dehydration. Basically, any event that increases the body's need for oxygen or alters the transport of oxygen may lead to the exacerbation of symptoms.

INTERVENTION. Since there is no specific therapy for sickle cell anemia, treatment is symptomatic. Health teaching includes maintenance of optimal oxygenation, hydration, and good hygiene and prevention of infections. Polyvalent pneumococcal vaccine is often advised because of the high risk for pneumococcal infections. When surgery is performed, special attention should be given to maintaining adequate ventilation, oxygenation, and hydration. Long-term counseling may be needed for severe psychosocial difficulties. Support is given to help the person be as independent and productive as possible, a difficult situation when sickle cell crises are frequent.

SICKLE CELL CRISIS. The sudden exacerbation of sickling can bring about a condition known as "crisis." Sickle cell crisis may be thrombotic, aplastic, or megaloblastic. *Thrombotic crisis* is the most common type and is caused by the occlusion of blood vessels by the sickled cells. Pain is the primary symptom in thrombotic crisis; it often involves the abdomen and musculoskeletal systems and may be quite severe. Pain management regimens, often including the use of narcotics, may be necessary. Astute evaluation of the pain and its management are key nursing activities. Sickle cell patients may be labeled as malingerers because some of them demonstrate difficult behavior patterns that are influenced by their chronic illness and at times by drug abuse. Counseling and the use of support groups are to be encouraged so as to minimize behavioral dependency. In caring for this patient population it is also helpful to maintain a sense of respect and consideration for persons who experience frequent crises and yet continue to try to live as normal a life as possible.

The treatment of a *thrombotic crisis* requires adequate hydration to decrease blood viscosity. Limited exchange transfusions (replacing the person's blood with packed red cells, unit for unit, until the concentration of sickle cells is below 50% of the concentration of erythrocytes) may be used to reduce the number of circulating sickle cells.

Aplastic crisis is most often secondary to infection and a temporary decrease in erythropoiesis. Because of the shortened red cell survival, the anemia rapidly worsens. Diagnosis may be made by bone marrow examination. Treatment is by packed red cell transfusion.

Megaloblastic crisis appears in some cases to be the result of the depletion of bone marrow stores of folic acid. In such cases the crisis may be treated or prevented by administration of folic acid.

Thalassemia

ETIOLOGY AND PATHOPHYSIOLOGY. Thalassemia is an inherited disorder characterized by a decreased synthesis of one of the globin chains of hemoglobin. The beta (β-) chain is most often affected (β-thalassemia). There is, as a result, decreased synthesis of hemoglobin as well as an accumulation in the erythrocyte of the unaffected globin chain. These alterations result in decreased red cell production and a chronic hemolytic anemia.

CLINICAL PICTURE. The heterozygous state, *thalassemia minor,* is associated with a mild anemia that is usually asymptomatic; no therapy is required. The homozygous condition, *thalassemia major,* is characterized by a severe anemia. The red cells are characteristically hypochromic (low MCH) and microcytic (low MCV). Hemoglobin electrophoresis is diagnostic.

INTERVENTION. Currently, the only treatment available for thalassemia is transfusion therapy. The life span is usually significantly shortened. Transfusions may be administered either when severe symptoms occur or to maintain the hemoglobin at a near normal level continuously to allow for a more normal life-style. The latter approach incurs the risk of producing iron overload from frequent transfusions, a problem that can be ameliorated by the use of an iron-chelating agent such as desferrioxamine.

Enzyme deficiency

ETIOLOGY AND PATHOPHYSIOLOGY. Deficiency of enzymes in the pathways that metabolize glucose and generate ATP (Embden-Meyerhof and pentose phosphate shunt pathways) frequently leads to premature red cell destruction. The most common clinically significant enzyme abnormality is that of *glucose-6-phosphate dehydrogenase*. This disorder is common in a mild form among the black population in the United States.

CLINICAL PICTURE. Anemia occurs, in general, only when the patient is exposed to an oxidant drug (aspirin, sulfonamides, and antimalarial drugs), which places the cells under unusual stress with which they are unable to cope. *Acute hemolysis* results. Diagnosis is established by assay for the enzyme.

INTERVENTION. Treatment is recognition of the disorder and cessation of the offending drug. This disorder occurs in a more severe form in certain population groups in the Mediterranean area and may cause a chronic hemolytic anemia.

Acquired hemolytic anemia

Etiology and pathophysiology. Acquired hemolytic anemia is most often drug induced or is caused by an autoimmune disorder. In the latter case an antibody develops that is directed against an antigen on the individuals own erythrocytes. The antibody-coated red cells are destroyed prematurely by reticuloendothelial cells, particularly in the spleen. This autoimmune disorder may occur secondary to lymphocytic lymphomas or to chronic lymphocytic leukemia, in the course of certain connective tissue disorders, or it may occur idiopathically. Diagnosis is confirmed by demonstrating the presence of the antibody on the red cells (antiglobin or Coombs' test).

Drugs produce hemolysis in a variety of ways. Alpha methyldopa (Aldomet) is associated with production of an autoantibody and a positive Coombs' test in approximately 20% of patients and a hemolytic anemia indistinguishable from an idiopathic autoimmune hemolytic anemia in 1%. More rarely, high-dose penicillin produces hemolysis through production of an antibody that requires the presence of penicillin on the red cell membrane for its effects to occur.

Intervention. Therapy for autoimmune hemolytic anemia is with corticosteroids, which are beneficial in approximately 50% of patients, and with splenectomy in those patients not sufficiently responsive to steroids. This disorder is often fatal, in part because transfusion is often made difficult and dangerous by the fact that the autoantibody reacts not only with the patient's red cells but also with all donor cells.

Anemia secondary to nutritional deficiency

The nutritional anemias include *iron-deficiency anemia* and the *megaloblastic anemias*. The most common causes of megaloblastic anemia are vitamin B_{12} deficiency and folic acid deficiency.

Iron-deficiency anemia

Etiology and pathophysiology. Iron is a fundamental part of the hemoglobin molecule, and its deficiency leads to production of red cells with a decreased amount of hemoglobin and ultimately to a decreased number of red cells. The average adult body contains approximately 4 g of iron, 3 g of which are in hemoglobin, 500 mg to 1 g in iron stores in the liver and bone marrow, and the rest in certain tissues and enzyme systems. Average daily loss of iron by the body is approximately 1.5 mg, which is compensated for by absorption from the diet of aproximately that amount of iron daily. This tenuous balance may be compromised by chronic blood loss, which may be physiologic such as in menstruation or pathologic as in gastrointestinal or other bleeding.

Clinical picture. Gradual development of iron-deficiency anemia may permit adaptation with few clinical signs of anemia. Some persons may develop fatigue and exertional dyspnea. With severe iron-deficiency anemia, the nails become brittle and spoon shaped (concave) and they develop longitudinal ridges. The papillae of the tongue atrophy and the tongue has a smooth, shiny, bright red appearance. The corners of the mouth may crack and become red and painful (cheilosis). The anemia, which is characteristically hypochromic and microcytic, may be detected by observation of the peripheral blood smear and/or by blood cell indices. Diagnosis may be confirmed by a low serum iron and elevated serum iron-binding capacity or by low serum ferritin or absent iron stores in the bone marrow.

Intervention. The treatment of iron-deficiency anemia is to determine and correct the cause. Repletion of iron stores in the body may then be accomplished by the administration of iron. Oral iron supplement is usually given in the form of ferrous sulfate. If the person is to take the medication at home, patient instruction is necessary. Because it may be irritating to the gastrointestinal tract, ferrous sulfate should be taken after meals. The person should also be told that stools will be black and that he or she should report to the physician any symptoms of diarrhea or nausea. When the individual cannot tolerate oral preparations of iron, parenteral iron therapy is used. Parenteral therapy is also indicated when the person is unable to absorb iron properly from the gastrointestinal tract.

Poor diet is only rarely the sole cause of iron-deficiency anemia, but it may be a contributing factor. All persons with iron-deficiency anemia should be assessed for their knowledge of a well-balanaced diet and their ability and willingness to provide themselves with such a diet. When indicated, follow-up through a clinic, home visits by a dietitian, and such community resources as Meals on Wheels can be effective ways of assuring the person of a well-balanced diet.

Megaloblastic anemia

Megaloblastic anemia refers to anemias with characteristic morphologic changes. On the peripheral blood smear, macrocytic red cells and hypersegmented neutrophils (increased number of nuclei) are present. In the bone marrow, erythroid precursors that are two to three times larger than normal with nuclei that are immature relative to their cytoplasmic development are found.

Etiology and pathophysiology. Most megaloblastic anemias are caused by deficiency of either vitamin B_{12} or folic acid. Both are essential in the synthesis of DNA, and their deficiency leads to impaired nuclear development in cells throughout the body. Deficiency of either leads to anemia and often leukopenia and thrombocytopenia.

Vitamin B_{12} deficiency. Vitamin B_{12}, obtained from dietary sources, combines with intrinsic factor in the stomach and is carried to the ileum where it is absorbed and transported by a carrier protein to the tissues of the body.

CLINICAL PICTURE. Diagnosis of B_{12} deficiency is made by demonstration of a low serum vitamin B_{12} level in a patient with macrocytic anemia and megaloblastic bone marrow. In addition to the general symptoms associated with anemia, patients with B_{12} deficiency may manifest neurologic abnormalities; in particular, they may develop a peripheral neuropathy and a loss of balance resulting from an abnormality of the posterior and lateral columns of the spinal cord (subacute combined degeneration).

A deficiency of vitamin B_{12} may be the result of dietary deficiency, surgical removal of the stomach, malabsorption syndromes, or pernicious anemia. *Pernicious anemia* (PA) is caused by the absence of intrinsic factor. Dietary vitamin B_{12} therefore cannot be absorbed. Diagnosis of PA is confirmed by an abnormal Schilling test, which demonstrates the inability to absorb vitamin B_{12} unless intrinsic factor is also administered.

INTERVENTION. Treatment of vitamin B_{12} deficiency is the parenteral administration of vitamin B_{12}, usually once a month. The most common cause of relapse in persons with pernicious anemia is their reluctance to continue therapy for life. Patient teaching is a focus of nursing care and discharge planning. The individual must be assisted to understand the nature of the illness and the absolute necessity for continued treatment.

Folic acid deficiency. Folic acid–deficiency anemia may be caused by dietary deficiency, often in association with chronic alcoholism, malabsorption syndromes, and certain medications that inhibit the enzyme involved in normal absorption of folate through the intestinal wall.[50]

CLINICAL PICTURE. Signs and symptoms are those associated with the underlying disease and anemia in general. Laboratory findings include macrocytic anemia, megaloblastic changes in the bone marrow, and a low serum folate level.

INTERVENTION. Most people respond promptly to oral folic acid and a well-balanced diet. Return visits to nurse clinics and community health nurse home visits are frequently needed to assist the person in incorporating dietary modifications into daily life. Patients who drink alcohol excessively may be referred to Alcoholics Anonymous.

Outcome criteria for the person with anemia

The person or significant others can:
1. Explain the basis of the anemia.
2. Describe dietary modifications (nutritional deficiency anemias); describe components of a well-balanced diet; plan menus based on the inclusion of deficient substances (iron, B_{12}, folic acid).
3. State name, dosage, frequency, desired action, and side effects of prescribed medications.
4. State plans for receiving B_{12} injections (vitamin B_{12} deficiency) or demonstrate accurate technique for self-administration.
5. State awareness of the availability of genetic counseling services (sickle cell anemia).
6. State awareness of community resources: community health nurse, Alcoholics Anonymous, Meals on Wheels, and family counseling services.
7. State plans for follow-up care.

Erythrocytosis

Erythrocytosis refers to an abnormal increase in erythrocytes. It may be caused by hypoxia (secondary to pulmonary and cardiac disease), certain erythropoietin-producing tumors, or the disorder polycythemia vera. Principal laboratory tests to determine the nature of erythrocytosis include determination of the arterial oxygen concentration, red cell volume, and plasma volume.

Stress erythropoiesis

Elevation of the hemoglobin and hematocrit may occur when the total red cell mass volume is normal but the plasma volume is decreased, leading to a contraction of the plasma volume. This "stress erythropoiesis" occurs predominantly in males, is self-limiting, and requires no therapy.

Polycythemia vera

Pathophysiology. Polycythemia vera is characterized by erythrocytosis and usually a simultaneous leukocytosis and thrombocytosis. Hypervolemia, increased blood viscosity from the increased red cell mass, and platelet dysfunction occur.

Clinical picture. Symptoms are frequently absent in the early stages. As hypervolemia develops, symptoms include headaches, vertigo, tinnitus, and blurred vision. Thromboses with embolization may result from the increased blood viscosity, and the skin may develop a more reddened appearance. Platelet dysfunction may lead to nosebleeds, ecchymoses, and gastrointestinal bleeding.

Splenomegaly is commonly found on physical examination. Laboratory tests demonstrate an increased total red cell volume and a plasma volume that is either increased or normal. Arterial oxygen concentration is usually normal.

Intervention. Usual treatment is periodic phlebotomy aimed at maintaining the hematocrit and hemoglobin at a normal level. In some patients who need phlebotomy too frequently, other modes of therapy may be required, such as the use of radioactive phosphorus (^{32}P) or an alkylating agent such as busulfan. There is an increased incidence of other hematologic disorders arising in the course of polycythemia vera, especially acute leukemia, and this has been accentuated with the use of alkylating agents in the treatment regimen.

Outcome criteria for the person with polycythemia vera. The person or significant others can:

1. State importance of continued medical care, blood tests, and phlebotomy.
2. State name, dosage, frequency, desired action, and side effects of prescribed medications.
3. Describe signs of extremity thromboses (swelling, redness, pain) requiring immediate medical attention.
4. State plans for follow-up care.

Disorders associated with platelets

Platelets are formed in the bone marrow. In the normal adult approximately 80% of the platelets are in free circulation and 20% are stored in the spleen. It is estimated that the normal life span of platelets is approximately 10 days. The senescent platelets are removed from the circulation by the reticuloendothelial system, primarily in the spleen. The principal function of platelets is in hemostasis. Their attachment to the damaged blood vessel wall provides the first barrier against blood loss caused by trauma.

Platelet disorders may be separated into thrombocytopenias, thrombocytosis, and disorders of platelet function.

Thrombocytopenia

Thrombocytopenia is defined as a lower than normal number of circulating platelets. Laboratory values for a normal adult count range from 150,000 to 400,000/cu mm.

Etiology and pathophysiology

The most common cause of increased destruction of platelets is *idiopathic thrombocytopenia purpura* (ITP). This disorder occurs most commonly in the second and third decades of life and is caused by production of an autoantibody (IgG) directed against a platelet antigen. It is manifested by excessive bleeding, which may be reflected in purpuric lesions on the skin or by visceral bleeding.

Clinical picture

The major symptoms of thrombocytopenia observable through physical examination reflect a bleeding tendency. Petechiae and ecchymoses are hallmarks of a decreased number of platelets and are most commonly present on the arms, legs, and upper chest. The person may give a history of menorrhagia, epistaxis, and gingival bleeding. Patients should be questioned for a history of recent viral infection, since this may produce transient thrombocytopenia. A detailed history of drug and alcohol use also should be obtained. Alcohol, thiazide diuretics, and quinidine are among drugs associated with thrombocytopenia.

Diagnosis is made essentially by exclusion of other disorders that produce thrombocytopenia and by a bone marrow that is normal except for an increase in the megakaryocytes. Complete laboratory studies are done to ascertain the status of all blood components. The most commonly used tests for assessment of platelets are *platelet count, peripheral blood smear,* and the *bleeding time.* In addition, a bone marrow examination is performed to determine the presence or absence of *megakaryocytes* (precursors of platelets in the bone marrow). Their presence suggests that the thrombocytopenia is caused by peripheral platelet destruction, and their absence or decrease suggests a failure of thrombopoiesis. Examination of the bone marrow also reveals the presence or absence of primary bone marrow abnormalities such as neoplastic invasion, aplastic anemia, and fibrosis.

Intervention

Treatment for thrombocytopenia includes corticosteroids or splenectomy. Steroids appear to decrease both antibody production and phagocytosis of the antibody-coated platelets. Splenectomy removes the principal organ involved in destruction of the antibody-coated platelets.

Certain drugs may produce increased destruction of platelets and a resultant thrombocytopenia. Quinidine, a drug used in the treatment of certain cardiac arrhythmias, has been most frequently implicated, and cessation of this drug leads to improvement in platelet counts within 1 to 2 weeks.

Excessive consumption of alcohol is a relatively common cause of thrombocytopenia. Alcohol appears to both impair production and increase destruction of platelets. The platelet count generally returns to normal within 1 to 2 weeks of discontinuing alcohol intake.

Transfusion with platelet concentrates may be utilized in patients with thrombocytopenic bleeding. It is not usually helpful in thrombocytopenia caused by increased destruction because the transfused platelets are rapidly destroyed by the same mechanism as the person's own platelets and they have an extremely short survival. In conditions of impaired platelet production the platelet concentrates increase the platelet count for 1 to 3 days.

A primary concern in the nursing care of persons with decreased numbers of platelets is the concomitant bleeding tendency.[51] Bleeding associated with trauma is likely with a platelet count less than 60,000/cu mm. Spontaneous hemorrhage looms as a life-threatening possibility in individuals with a platelet count of less than 20,000/cu mm.

Ongoing nursing assessment of the patient is essential and includes alertness for increased ecchymoses, petechiae, and any change in mental status. The need for avoidance of trauma is obvious. For persons with a platelet count of 20,000/cu mm or less, bleeding precautions should be instituted. Routinely, these precautions include the following:

1. Testing of all urine and stools for blood (guaiac)
2. No rectal temperature taking
3. No intramuscular injections
4. Pressure applied to all venipuncture sites for 5 minutes
5. Pressure applied to all arterial puncture sites for 10 minutes

If the individual is to be discharged to home with glucocorticoid or steroid therapy, explicit patient education is needed. The individual must have knowledge of the importance of not omitting a dose and the danger inherent in suddenly stopping the medication.

Before discharge from the hospital, the individual should be able to describe the signs of decreased numbers of platelets (e.g., bleeding gums, petechiae, ecchymoses) and the corresponding risk of a bleeding tendency. The patient needs to be advised to continue under medical supervision and to report any signs of bleeding to the primary physician at once. The patient should be cautioned not to use aspirin or preparations containing aspirin since platelet function may be adversely affected.

Thrombocytosis

Thrombocytosis is defined as the presence of an abnormally high number of platelets in the circulating blood. It rarely occurs as a single entity (hemorrhaging thrombocythemia) and is usually seen in association with polycythemia vera, myelofibrosis, splenectomy, iron-deficiency anemia, and chronic inflammatory diseases such as tuberculosis.

The danger of thrombocytosis is that it may lead to thrombosis or abnormal bleeding. Medical and nursing care is similar to that described for persons receiving anticoagulation therapy (p. 1151).

Disorders of platelet function

Mild bleeding syndromes may be caused by quantitatively normal but functionally defective platelets. The most common cause of functional platelet abnormalities is drugs, in particular, aspirin. Aspirin inhibits the release of intrinsic platelet ADP and produces a defect in platelet aggregation. The defect remains for the life span of the platelet. A variety of familial and nonfamilial platelet disorders have also been described, and defective platelet function is common in persons with uremia. The abnormality may be detected by a test of bleeding time or, more sensitively, by platelet aggregation tests. Disorders of platelet function have clinical manifestations and patient-care needs similar to those of thrombocytopenia although the bleeding abnormality is almost invariably mild.

Outcome criteria for the person with a platelet disorder

The person or significant others can:
1. Describe signs of decreased platelets (petechiae, ecchymoses, gingival bleeding, hematuria).

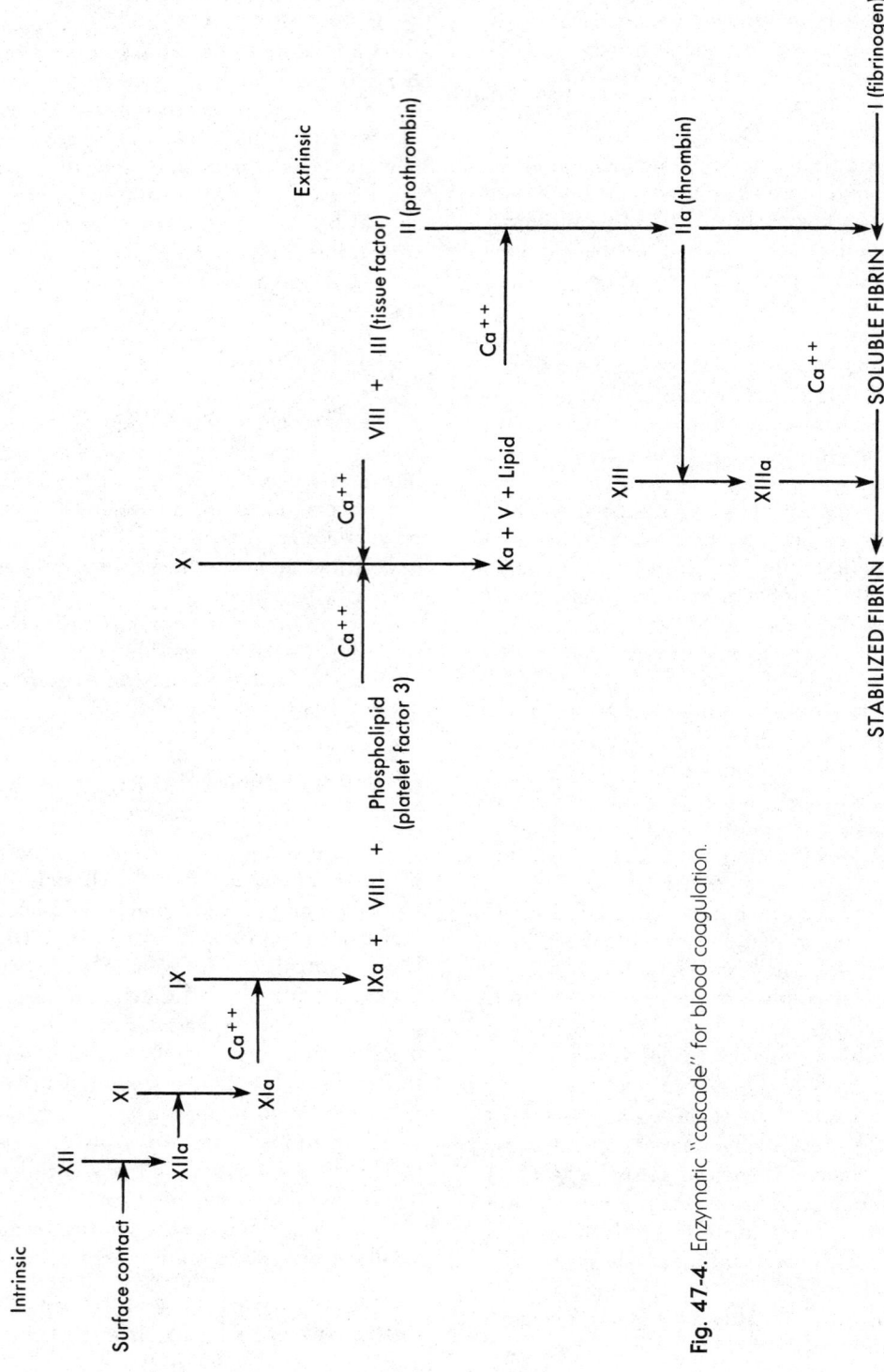

Fig. 47-4. Enzymatic "cascade" for blood coagulation.

2. State name, dosage, frequency, purpose, and side effects of prescribed medication; state awareness of the importance of not stopping steroid or glucocorticoid medications suddenly.
3. Describe signs and symptoms of phlebitis and thromboses (thrombocytosis).
4. State the importance of medical follow-up and describe plans for follow-up care.

Disorders of coagulation

Etiology and pathophysiology

Coagulation of blood results from the interaction of a number of clotting factors in a sequence of events termed *coagulation cascade* (Fig. 47-4). Coagulation disorders may occur from the depletion or absence of one or more clotting factors and may be congenital or acquired. Congenital coagulation disorders include hemophilias A, B, and C, and von Willebrand's disease. The acquired disorders include liver disease, vitamin K deficiency, and disseminated intravascular coagulation.

Hemophilias A and B are congenital disorders asso-ciated with a decrease in factors VIII and IX, respectively. In von Willebrand's disease there is a deficiency of factor VIII and defective platelet aggregation. Bleeding manifestations range from mild to severe. It may be effectively treated when bleeding occurs with cryoprecipitate.

The most common acquired disorder of coagulation is liver disease. The liver produces most of the clotting factors: II, V, VII, IX, X, and fibrinogen. Liver disease may produce impaired production of these clotting factors and an elevation of the prothrombin time. Treatment involves therapy for the underlying disease.

Hemophilia

Hemophilia is a hereditary coagulation disorder. Both hemophilia A (factor VIII deficiency) and hemophilia B (factor IX deficiency) are inherited as sex-linked recessive disorders and are therefore almost exclusively limited to males. An example of the inheritance pattern of hemophilia is shown in Fig. 47-5.

Clinical picture

The diagnosis of hemophilia may be made in infancy or early childhood. The clinical history is one of lifelong

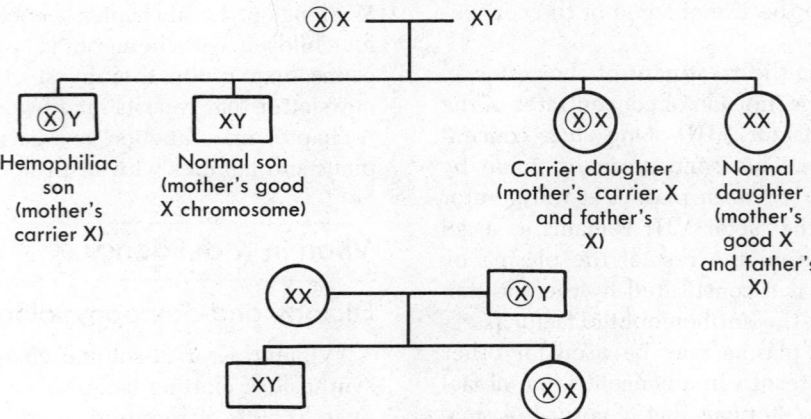

Defective gene is found on X chromosome.
When faulty X chromosome is present in a male,
the male will be a hemophiliac.

Ⓧ Y

When faulty X chromosome is present in a female,
she will be a carrier of hemophilia.

Ⓧ X

In conception between a normal male and a carrier
female, four possibilities arise:

ⒻX ——— XY

Hemophiliac son (mother's carrier X) | Normal son (mother's good X chromosome) | Carrier daughter (mother's carrier X and father's X) | Normal daughter (mother's good X and father's X)

In conception between a hemophiliac male and a normal female,
son will be normal but daughter will be carrier.

Fig. 47-5. Pattern of inheritance of hemophilia.

bleeding tendency. A history of excessive bleeding following circumcision or dental extractions is frequently obtained. Individuals with hemophilia may give a history of bleeding into any part of the body, spontaneously or following trauma.

A diagnosis of hemophilia is made by specific assays for factors VIII and IX. The partial thromboplastin time, which reflects the intrinsic pathway of coagulation, is prolonged in both hemophilia A and hemophilia B. The platelet count and prothrombin time are normal.

Complications associated with hemophilia are the direct result of the bleeding tendency. Frequently, the individual experiences repeated episodes of spontaneous bleeding into the joints resulting in several joint deformities. Bleeding that is life threatening involves retroperitoneal, intracranial, and paratracheal soft-tissue hemorrhages.

Intervention

Treatment consists of replacement of the deficient coagulation factor when bleeding episodes do not respond to local treatment (ice bags, manual pressure or dressings, immobilization, elevation, and topical coagulants such as fibrin foam and thrombin). Because the deficient factors are contained in plasma, the treatment used for many years was fresh plasma and blood or fresh frozen plasma. In major hemorrhages, adequate blood levels were difficult to maintain without overloading the person's circulation with large volumes of blood and plasma. The discovery of cryoprecipitate in 1964 led the way to the development of commercially prepared concentrated preparations such as fibrinogen, factor VIII, and a concentrate containing the four vitamin K–dependent factors (prothrombin and factors VII, IX, and X). Concentrates avoid the problem of circulatory overload and produce fewer adverse effects (e.g., urticarial or febrile reactions) in some patients. High cost and contamination with the virus of serum hepatitis are drawbacks, however, to the use of some of the concentrates.

In classic hemophilia the treatment of choice for an acute bleeding episode is infusion of concentrates of the antihemophilic factor (factor VIII). One such concentrate is cryoprecipitate. This concentrate is made by slowly thawing previously frozen plasma at refrigerator temperature. Most of the factor VIII remains as a gel and can be separated from the rest of the plasma by centrifugation. The gel is reconstituted by the addition of saline solution. After the antihemophilic factor is extracted, the remaining plasma may be used for other purposes. This process results in a concentration of factor VIII as much as 15 to 40 times that of normal plasma. It can be produced and stored in any well-equipped blood bank at a cost well below that of other concentrates. Treatment with cryoprecipitate is being given in

outpatient departments and clinics. Home infusion programs have gained interest and are seen as a way of controlling bleeding episodes more quickly, thereby decreasing the need for hospitalization and long absence from school or work.

The outlook for the person with hemophilia has been greatly improved by the availability of transfusion therapy. In the past many persons with factor VIII deficiency died in infancy or in the first 5 years of life. Today persons with moderate or mild hemophilia may live normal, productive lives.

Adults with hemophilia are generally very knowledgeable about their disease. They must be aware of the possibility of hemorrhage after dental extraction, injury, or surgery. Persons who have hemophilia should carry a card or wear a Medic-Alert tag that includes their name, blood type, physician's name, and the fact that they have hemophilia so that medical treatment will not be delayed if they should accidentally sustain injury and lose consciousness.

Pain control and the threat of spontaneous bleeding episodes are ongoing stressors the individual must confront. Those individuals who are able to meet the demands of their illness and adapt their life styles accordingly are able to live productive lives as individuals, spouses, parents, and employees. Genetic counseling, aimed at explaining the pattern of inheritance of hemophilia, may be of great value to adults contemplating parenthood. Such counseling can serve to assist potential parents to evaluate realistically their ability to raise a child afflicted with hemophilia and to anticipate ways to meet the demands placed on both them and the child.

The National Hemophilia Foundation* is an organization established for persons with hemophilia and their families. There are 51 chapters scattered across the United States. The basic function of the national organization is hemophilia research. In addition, it establishes standards for chapters, publishes literature, produces films, and promotes health care legislation in Washington. Local chapter services include special camps for children with hemophilia; parent, child, and adult counseling; group therapy sessions for parents; and a newsletter that reports on advances in hemophilic care. A chapter may function as a liaison agent between hospitals and families with insurmountable bills for blood.

Vitamin K deficiency

Etiology and pathophysiology

Vitamin K, a fat-soluble vitamin, is a cofactor in the synthesis of clotting factors II, VII, IX, and X. Approximately 50% of required vitamin K is obtained from a normal diet and 50% is produced by intestinal bacteria.

*25 West 39th St., New York, NY 10018.

Deficiencies in vitamin K can be anticipated in persons who have a decreased intake and who are given broad-spectrum antibiotics that decrease the growth of intestinal bacteria. Interference with vitamin K absorption occurs with primary intestinal disease (e.g., ulcerative colitis, Crohn's disease, cystic fibrosis), biliary disease, and malabsorption syndromes. Drugs such as coumarin derivatives and large doses of salicylates, quinine, and barbiturates interfere with vitamin K function.

Clinical picture

Symptoms are those of hypoprothrombinemia superimposed on the underlying disease. Bleeding is similar to other coagulation disorders; that is, bleeding of the mucous membranes and into the tissues. Postoperative hemorrhage may be observed. In severe cases gastrointestinal bleeding may be massive. Diagnosis of vitamin K deficiency is established by a significantly prolonged prothrombin time (p. 601).

Intervention

Treatment consists of therapy for the underlying disorder and cessation of causative drugs. For mild disorders a water-soluble vitamin K preparation (menadione) is given orally or parenterally. In severe disorders a fat-soluble vitamin K preparation (phytonadione) may be given. Fresh frozen plasma will partially correct the disorder but places the patient at risk for fluid overload.

Disseminated intravascular coagulation

Disseminated intravascular coagulation (DIC) is a recently recognized pathophysiologic response of the body's hemostatic mechanisms to disease or injury. DIC is a complicated and potentially fatal process that is characterized initially by clotting and secondarily by hemorrhage. It almost always occurs in response to a primary disease.

Etiology

DIC is essentially an imbalance between the processes of coagulation and anticoagulation. Many diseases states may alter the normal balance of clotting factors and fibrinolytic factors, which under normal conditions prevent bleeding while maintaining the fluidity of the blood. DIC may be initiated by diseases that involve the introduction of a foreign substance into the bloodstream such as endotoxins, snake venom, or placental matter from abruptio placentae. This syndrome may also be triggered by conditions associated with thrombus formation such as hypotensive states. The third group of diseases that may lead to DIC are those in which there is massive tissue damage such as blunt trauma or neoplasms.

Pathophysiology

The primary disease causes the initiation of the clotting process. This response is generalized and occurs throughout the vascular system, creating a state of *hypercoagulability*. The fibrinolytic processes, which normally operate to limit clot extension and dissolve clots, are then stimulated. As clotting factors are depleted and fibrinolysis continues, a state of *hypocoagulability* develops.

The most common sequela of DIC is hemorrhage. This paradox is caused by decreased platelets and the depletion of clotting factors II, V, VIII, fibrinogen, and the production of fibrin degradation products (FDP) through fibrinolysis. The fibrin degradation products act as anticoagulants, which increase the hemorrhagic tendency.

Clinical picture

Laboratory findings may be the only indications of the disorder in the early stages. Laboratory determinations that confirm the diagnosis of DIC are the presence of thrombocytopenia, low levels of fibrinogen, and prolonged prothrombin and partial thromboplastin times. In addition, low levels of factors V and VIII are present, and abnormal red blood cells may be found on peripheral smear. Characteristically, there is evidence of fibrinolysis, which is reflected in increased fibrin split products and prolonged thrombin time. As the disorder progresses, clinical manifestations that may become evident include bleeding of the mucous membranes and tissues (petechiae and ecchymoses). Oral, vaginal, and rectal bleeding may occur as well as bleeding following injections and venipunctures. Pain may be present with joint bleeding.

Intervention

The management of DIC must always begin with treatment of the primary disease. Once this has been initiated, the goal is to control the bleeding and restore normal levels of clotting factors. Blood products such as platelet packs, cryoprecipitate, and fresh whole blood may be administered to replace the depleted factors. Heparin has been used to inhibit the underlying thrombotic process. However, it too often promotes rather than decreases bleeding and is not commonly used. Another aspect of the management of DIC involves therapy for renal failure. Hemodialysis often becomes necessary.

Nursing intervention in the care of the patient with DIC is extremely challenging. The person who develops DIC is critically ill and frequently has numerous sites of bleeding before DIC becomes evident. The amount and nature of drainage from chest and nasogastric tubes, oozing from surgical incisions, or progressive discoloration of the skin should be noted and recorded. Continual observation for new bleeding sites and for an increase or decrease in bleeding is an integral part of the nursing plan, especially if heparin therapy is being employed. The susceptibility of these persons to bleeding presents special problems; medications should be given intravenously if at all possible and small-gauge needles used when other injections are necessary. The precautions previously described for thrombocytopenia are applicable to the patient with DIC (p. 1197).

Maintaining fluid balance assumes great importance. Persons with DIC usually lose large quantities of blood and receive frequent transfusions and other fluid replacement. In addition to carefully monitoring blood infusion rates, the nurse must be alert to signs of fluid overload such as increasing pulse rate and central venous pressure. Hourly urine output is recorded not only as another indication of cardiac function but also because of the possibility of renal thrombi formation and subsequent renal failure.

Frequently the patient is comatose, and the presence of purpura, numerous intravenous lines, and drainage tubes makes the patient's appearance especially upsetting to the family. Most of the primary conditions associated with DIC are of a sudden nature, and the family requires help in understanding this catastrophic occurrence and support during the long period of treatment.

Outcome criteria for the person with a disorder of coagulation

The person or significant others can:
1. Describe signs and symptoms requiring immediate medical intervention (excessive bleeding, hematuria, melena, pain or swelling in joints or muscles, head trauma, abdominal pain).
2. State name, dosage, frequency, purpose, and side effects of prescribed medications.
3. State awareness of genetic counseling services (hemophilia).
4. State plans to obtain Medic-Alert identification tag (bracelet or necklace).
5. State an awareness of community resources (National Hemophilia Foundation support and counseling services).
6. State plans for follow-up care.

Disorders associated with white blood cells

The white blood cell (leukocyte) system is comprised of neutrophils, lymphocytes, monocytes, baso-

phils, and eosinophils. All but the lymphocytes are derived from a common stem cell. The primary function of white blood cells (WBCs) is to provide for humoral and cellular response to infection. Neutrophils are primarily responsible for phagocytosis and the destruction of bacteria and other infectious organisms. Lymphocytes are the principal cells involved in immunity, which is responsible for the development of delayed hypersensitivity and the production of antibodies (p. 283). Any compromise in the integrity of the white blood cell system renders the individual susceptible to infection.

Neutropenia

Etiology and pathophysiology

Neutropenia is defined as a neutrophil count of less than 2000/cu mm. Neutropenia may occur as a primary hematologic disorder, but more often it is seen in association with other disorders, including malignant diseases of the bone marrow, aplastic anemia, megaloblastic anemia, use of chemotherapeutic agents, and hypersplenism. The degree of susceptibility to infection is in direct proportion to the degree of neutropenia. Individuals with marked neutropenia are at risk of contracting a life-threatening infection.

Severe neutropenia (sometimes referred to as agranulocytosis) occurs as a reaction to a variety of drugs and chemicals including sulfonamides, propylthiouracil, and chloramphenicol. Specific treatment consists of removing the offending agent.

Intervention

An individual with a compromised white blood cell system is highly susceptible to life-threatening infections. Nursing care is directed toward protecting the patient from potential sources of infection and assiduous monitoring to detect the earliest signs of infection so that prompt therapy may be instituted. Likewise, patients and families must be taught to recognize early signs of infection. Meticulous washing of the hands by medical and nursing personnel and strict asepsis are mandatory. The environment should be kept scrupulously clean and dustless, and no person with any type of infection should be allowed in contact with the patient. Family members and hospital personnel need frequent reminders of this. Mild colds and respiratory tract infections, taken for granted in daily life, are serious threats to patients with decreased numbers of WBCs.

Patients should be in private rooms. When this is not possible, cautious screening of roommates for a potential source of infection is mandatory. Occasionally, isolation technique (reverse precautions) is ordered to protect the patient from hospital personnel and visitors (p. 374). However, recent studies suggest that reverse isolation does not significantly alter the incidence of infection in this patient population.[14,34] Granulocyte transfusions may be used for the markedly neutropenic patient.[2,7,48] This is usually reserved for life-threatening situations, such as when a markedly neutropenic patient acquires an infection. (Further discussion of the nursing care of patients with neutropenia is given in Chapter 25, p. 506.)

Neutrophilia

Neutrophilia is defined as a neutrophil count greater than 10,000/cu mm. Such an increase is a normal response to infections, primarily bacterial infections. Prolonged elevation of the neutrophil count, especially in the absence of an apparent cause, is a reason for a diligent search for the underlying cause. Persistent elevated neutrophil counts are associated with leukemia, polycythemia vera, myeloid metaplasia, and a variety of systemic and inflammatory disorders.

Leukemia

Etiology and pathophysiology

Leukemias are malignant disorders of the hematopoietic system involving the bone marrow and lymph nodes; they are characterized by uncontrolled proliferation of leukocytes and their precursors. The large number of cells accumulate first at the site of origin (granulocytes in the bone marrow, lymphocytes in the lymph nodes), then spread to hematopoietic organs, leading to organ enlargement (splenomegaly, hepatomegaly). The proliferation of one type of cell often interferes with the normal production of other hematopoietic cells, leading to the development of immature cells and to cytopenias (decreased numbers). The immaturity of the white cells leads to decreased immunocompetence with increased susceptibility to infections.

The cause of leukemia is unknown. An increased incidence of leukemia in siblings has led to hypotheses of genetic predispositions or viral origins. The incidence of leukemia is high among those with Down's syndrome. Radiation and chemicals (including antineoplastic drugs) have also been implicated.

The leukemias are classified as acute or chronic and further subdivided according to cell type or maturity of the cell. Acute leukemias involve immature cells and are classified according to the predominant cell in the bone marrow, either lymphoblasts (acute lymphocytic leukemia) or myeloblasts (acute myelogenous or granulocytic leukemia). Chronic leukemias are classified according to the predominant mature white cell, either lymphocytes (chronic lymphocytic leukemia) or granulocytes (chronic granulocytic or myelogenous leukemia) (Table 47-3).

Clinical picture

Acute leukemias have a rapid onset and a short course ending in death if untreated. The immaturity of the white cells leads to numerous *infections*, such as ulcerations of the mucous membranes, pneumonias, and septice-

TABLE 47-3. Characteristic signs and common chemotherapeutic agents used in different leukemias

Leukemia	Type	Peak age (yr)	Characteristic symptoms	WBC level	Bone marrow cell predominance	Common chemotherapeutic agents
Acute lymphocytic leukemia (ALL)	Acute	2-4	Fever, infections of respiratory tract, anemia, bleeding of mucous membranes, ecchymoses, lymphadenopathy	Decreased	Lymphoblasts	Regimens with vincristine and prednisone, 6-mercaptopurine, methotrexate
Acute myelogenous leukemia (AML)	Acute	12-20, after 55	Same as ALL except less lymphadenopathy	Normal or decreased	Myeloblasts	Cytosine arabinoside, 6-thioguanine, doxorubicin (Adriamycin), daunomycin
Chronic lymphocytic leukemia (CLL)	Chronic	50-70	Weakness, fatigue, lymphadenopathy, pruritic vesicular skin lesions, thrombocytopenia, anemia, splenomegaly	Increased (20,000-100,000)	Lymphocytes	Alkylating agents (e.g., chlorambucil), glucocorticoids
Chronic myelogenous leukemia (CML)	Chronic	30-50	Weakness, fatigue, anorexia, weight loss, splenomegaly	Increased (15,000-500,000)	Granulocytes, Philadelphia chromosome	Busulfan, vincristine, prednisone

mias. Early symptoms include fever, lymphadenopathy, pallor and fatigue from anemia, and ecchymoses. WBC count may be normal or decreased.

Chronic leukemias have a more insidious onset and a median survival time (MST) of 3 to 4 years. Initially, there are fewer infections than in acute leukemias because of the maturity of the white cells in the chronic disorder, but eventually infections of the skin and pneumonias result from decreased immunocompetence. Early signs of chronic leukemias include fatigue, weakness, anorexia, and weight loss characteristic of a hypermetabolic state. An enlarged spleen and liver can usually be palpated. The WBC count is usually elevated.

Acute lymphocytic leukemia

Epidemiology. Eighty percent of persons with acute lymphocytic leukemia (ALL) are children, with a peak incidence between 2 and 4 years, and a marked decrease after the age of 10.

Pathophysiology. ALL is a malignant disorder arising from a single lymphoid stem cell (Fig. 47-1), with impaired maturation and accumulation of the malignant cells in the bone marrow. It is common to find different stages of lymphoid development in the bone marrow from very immature to almost normal cells. The degree of immaturity is a guide to the prognosis; the greater the number of immature cells, the poorer the prognosis. Leukocytes in the bloodstream are predominantly in the blast form.

Clinical picture. Signs and symptoms of ALL include respiratory infections, anemia, severe bleeding of mucous membranes and retina, and infiltration into the lymph nodes, spleen, and liver. The WBC count is often decreased (granulocytopenia), but a blood smear will show immature lymphoblasts. Diagnosis is confirmed by bone marrow biopsy.

Intervention. Perhaps more dramatically than in any other malignancy, chemotherapy has improved the prognosis of children with ALL. Untreated patients have an MST of 4 to 6 months. With current chemotherapy, MST is close to 5 years. Although late relapses can occur, approximately 50% of children with ALL can now be cured.

Complete remissions are obtained in over 90% of patients treated with chemotherapeutic regimens, most of which include vincristine and prednisone. Maintenance of remission is accomplished with a combination of drugs, usually including the antimetabolites 6-mercaptopurine and methotrexate. In most regimens vincristine and prednisone are administered intermittently during the maintenance program. Appropriate duration of therapy in patients who continue free of disease remains unsettled but in most centers is approximately 3 years.

Prognosis for patients with ALL has significantly improved; the use of "prophylactic" treatment of the central nervous system has markedly diminished recurrences in that area. Intrathecal administration of methotrexate, with or without craniospinal radiation, has proved effective.

Acute myelogenous leukemia

Epidemiology. Acute myelogenous leukemia (AML) is an acute leukemia that can occur at any age but is more common at adolescence and after age 55.

Pathophysiology and clinical picture. AML arises from a single myeloid stem cell (Fig. 47-1) and is characterized by the development of immature myeloblasts in the bone marrow. Clinical manifestations are the same as for ALL. The WBC count is usually in the low ranges of normal. Bone marrow aspiration reveals an increased number of myeloblasts.

Intervention. In the untreated patient or the patient who is nonresponsive to therapy, the MST is approximately 2 to 3 months. Current therapy includes the use of cytosine arabinoside, 6-thioguanine, and adriamycin or daunomycin. Complete remission occurs in 50% to 75% of treated patients, and there is a MST of approximately 2 to 3 years. Approximately 20% of patients are in complete remission at 5 years and are capable of prolonged disease free periods (remission). Although patients in remission clearly have an improved quality of life, induction of therapy is arduous, often requiring weeks in the hospital, with the need for intensive supportive care (blood component replacement and antibiotic therapy). Bone marrow transplantation, using HLA-identical bone marrow, has recently been used with increasing frequency and promises to have an increasing impact on this disease in the future.[35,46,47]

Chronic lymphocytic leukemia

Epidemiology. Chronic lymphocytic leukemia (CLL) occurs at any age but is found mostly between ages 50 to 70. It is three times more common in men.

Pathophysiology. CLL is characterized by a proliferation of small abnormal mature β-lymphocytes, leading to decreased synthesis of immunoglobulins and depressed antibody response. The accumulation of abnormal lymphocytes begins in the lymph nodes, then spreads to other lymphatic tissues. There is a marked increase in the number of both leukocytes and mature lymphocytes. At the time of diagnosis the bone marrow is often filled by lymphatic infiltration.

Clinical picture. The onset is insidious with weakness, fatigue, and lymphadenopathy. Symptoms include pruritic vesicular skin lesions, anemia, thrombocytopenia, and an enlarged spleen. The WBC count is elevated to a level between 20,000 and 100,000. Bone marrow biopsy shows infiltration of lymphocytes.

Intervention. The MST of persons with CLL is 4½ to 5½ years. As a general rule, persons are treated only when symptoms, particularly anemia, thrombocytopenia, or enlarged lymph nodes and spleen, appear. Chemotherapeutic agents used in the treatment of CLL are most often one of the alkylating agents, such as chlorambucil, and the glucocorticoids (p. 503).

Chronic myelogenous leukemia

Epidemiology. Chronic myelogenous leukemia (CML) occurs at any age but primarily from ages 30 to 50. The incidence is slightly higher in males.

Pathophysiology. The primary defect in CML is an abnormal stem cell leading to an uncontrolled proliferation of the granulocytic cells. As a result of this proliferation, there is a marked increase in the number of circulating granulocytes. In most cases, a characteristic chromosomal abnormality, the *Philadelphia chromosome,* is present involving deletion of a portion of one of the arms of chromosome no. 22 and its addition to chromosome no. 9.

Clinical picture. Characteristic symptoms of chronic leukemia occur: fatigue, weakness, anorexia, weight loss, and splenomegaly. Diagnosis of CML is made on the basis of an elevated WBC count (15,000 to 500,000), granulocytes on the peripheral blood smear that range in maturity from blast cells to mature neutrophils, granulocytic hyperplasia in the bone marrow, and the presence of the Philadelphia chromosome.

CML frequently changes from a chronic indolent phase into an accelerated phase that progresses rapidly into a fulminant neoplastic process sometimes indistinguishable from an acute leukemia. The accelerated phase of the disease (blastic phase) is characterized by increasing numbers of granulocytes in the peripheral blood ($\geq 30\%$). Often there is a corresponding anemia and thrombocytopenia. The patient may also develop fever and adenopathy. Fifty to sixty percent of patients with CML progress to the blastic phase.

Intervention. Although CML is less responsive to chemotherapy than acute myelogenous leukemia, agents used in the treatment of AML are occasionally effective. Some patients may respond to vincristine and prednisone. Busulfan (Myleran), an alkylating agent, is often the agent of choice.

Interventions for persons with leukemia

Leukemia, by its nature, is a diverse illness. The varied courses and response or lack of response to treatment also add to the diversity.

In acute phases of the disease and during aggressive chemotherapy, nursing care is aimed toward the prevention of complications and supportive therapy. Decreased WBC and decreased platelet counts render the individual vulnerable to severe infections and bleeding episodes. Frequent transfusions of both whole blood and component therapy (platelets, WBC) are often necessary.[47,50]

There are many foci of nursing care beyond those found in the life-threatening situations. Each individual with leukemia responds in a different way. It cannot be predicted for certain if an individual will respond to a prescribed treatment or how long a remission will last. Likewise, how the individual incorporates the illness into life is also unique to each person. Nursing has a key role in patient education. Before discharge from the hospital, the person should possess basic knowledge of the disease process and the importance of continued medical follow-up. Knowledge of specific drug therapy and anticipated side effects is also a component of the teaching plan. Of utmost importance in learning is the ability of the person to identify the body's signals that blood abnormalities exist. Petechiae, ecchymoses, and gingival bleeding are again the hallmarks to seek prompt medical attention. Bone pain, often severe, may signal blast crisis (acute proliferation of immature cells).

Individuals whose illness runs the course of several months to years often become very knowledgeable about their disease, blood components, related symptoms, and specific chemotherapeutic drugs. These persons sometimes discuss their progress in terms of changes in their blood counts. Over time many individuals become attuned to how such changes affect them. For example, they often can predict their count by how they feel. Many such persons respond well to being included in their plan of care during hospitalization and in preparation for discharge.

Time set aside for patient teaching also allows for a sharing time with the individual. This time may provide the foundation for an honest nurse-patient relationship from which emotional support may be given the person as attempts are made to adapt to the many stressors associated with leukemia.

Outcome criteria for the person with leukemia

The person or significant others can:
1. State their understanding of the disease, its treatment, and prognosis.
2. State the name, dosage, frequency, and side effects of prescribed medications. (See outcome criteria for persons receiving chemotherapy, p. 509.)
3. State the importance of and describe plans for follow-up medical care.
4. Describe symptoms requiring immediate medical attention, (fever, bleeding).
5. Describe arrangements for chemotherapy administration and periodic blood counts.
6. State resources available in the community; financial (National Leukemia Society) and local support groups.

Disorders associated with the lymph system

Assessment of lymph nodes

The normal lymph node consists of connective tissue encapsulating a fine mesh of reticular cells. The reticuloendothelial cells function chiefly in the phagocytosis of cellular debris. The chief function of lymphocytes, which are the main cells comprising the lymph nodes, is to provide an immune response to antigens presented to the node from the structure being drained by the node.

Lymph node enlargement results from an increase in the number and size of lymphoid follicles with proliferation of lymphocytes and reticuloendothelial cells. Lymphadenopathy may also occur when the node is invaded by cells normally not present (leukemic cells, cancer cells). In the lymphomas the actual nodal structure is destroyed by the malignant cells.

Normally lymph nodes are not palpable. With disease and the consequent increase in size, the nodes become palpable. In the course of a routine physical examination the lymph nodes are examined by palpation.

Lymphangiography is a radiologic technique used for evaluation of lymph nodes to detect the presence of disease. This procedure is especially valuable in the assessment of those nodes that are anatomically too deep to allow for evaluation by palpation (paraaortic). For this procedure a small incision is made on the dorsal surface of each foot so that the small lymph glands are made accessible. The glands are then cannulated, and a dye is slowly instilled over a few hours. All lymph chains and nodes fill with dye and are then visible on radiographs. Radiographs are usually done immediately after the dye is absorbed and again at intervals of 24 and 48 hours after the procedure. In addition, because the dye remains in the lymph nodes for as long as 6 months after the initial study, disease status and response to therapy can be periodically evaluated with routine abdominal x-ray films (KUB [kidney, ureter, and bladder]).

Computed tomography (CT scan) is also utilized to evaluate abdominal lymph nodes.

Hodgkin's disease

Etiology and pathophysiology

Hodgkin's disease is a malignant disorder of lymph nodes. The cause is unknown. Diagnosis requires biopsy and pathologic examination of the suspicious node. The presence of the Reed-Sternberg cell remains the pathologic hallmark of the disorder, but four pathologic

ANN ARBOR CLINICAL STAGING CLASSIFICATION OF HODGKIN'S DISEASE

Stage	Definition
I	Involvement of a single lymph node region (I) or of a single extralymphatic organ or site (I_E)
II	Involvement of two or more lymph node regions on the same side of the diaphragm (II) or localized involvement of an extralymphatic organ or site and of one or more lymph node regions on the same side of the diaphragm (II_E)
III	Involvement of lymph node regions on both sides of the diaphragm (III), which may also be accompanied by involvement of the spleen (III_S) or by localized involvement of an extralymphatic organ or site (III_E) or both (III_{SE})
IV	Diffuse or disseminated involvement of one or more extralymphatic organs or tissues, with or without associated lymph node involvement

The presence or absence of fever, night sweats, or unexplained loss of 10% or more of body weight in the 6 months preceding admission are denoted by the suffix letters B and A, respectively. Biopsy-documented involvement of stage IV sites is also denoted by letter suffixes: M, marrow; L, lung; H, liver; P, pleura; O, bone; D, skin and subcutaneous tissue.

variants of Hodgkin's disease have been recognized: *lymphocyte predominant*, *nodular sclerosis*, *mixed cellularity*, and *lymphocyte depletion*. The lymphocyte predominant and nodular sclerosis types have the best prognosis and lymphocyte depletion the worst. The most important prognostic indicator is the stage of the disease at the time of diagnosis. Accurate staging is crucial to the subsequent treatment regimen. The diagnostic workup is often arduous and difficult, and explanation of the many facets of the diagnostic procedures helps provide the emotional support so often needed during this time.

Clinical picture

Systemic symptoms that may be associated with Hodgkin's disease include fatigue, weakness, anorexia, unexplained fever, night sweats, and generalized pruritus. Physical examination may show enlargement of lymph nodes, liver, and spleen. A chest x-ray film may identify the presence of a mediastinal mass. A bone marrow biopsy is done to determine if there is marrow involvement. The liver and spleen are evaluated by radionuclide scanning or by computed tomography (CT scan). Lymphangiography is done to evaluate the retroperitoneal nodes. A "staging laparotomy" is performed in some circumstances to obtain a biopsy spec-

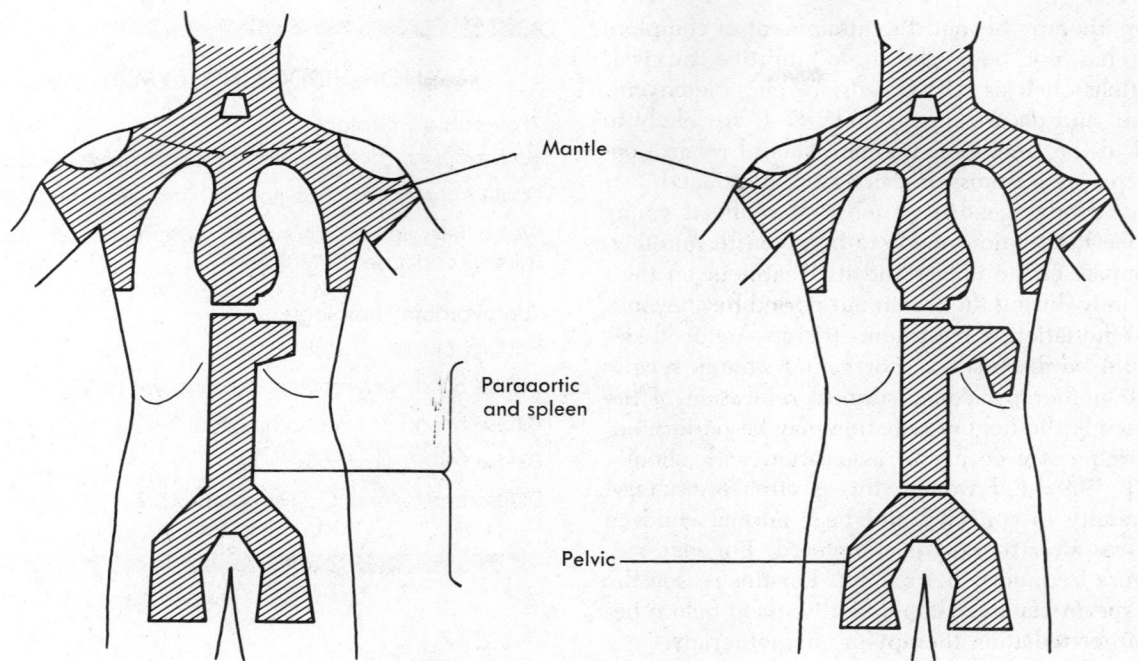

Fig. 47-6. Diagram of mantle and inverted **Y** fields used in total lymphoid radiotherapy of Hodgkin's disease. (From Rosenberg, S.A., and Kaplan, H.S.: Calif. Med. **113**:23, 1970.)

TABLE 47-4. Chemotherapeutic regimens for treatment of Hodgkin's disease

Name	Drugs	Dosage	Method	Schedule	Cycle
MOPP	Mechlorethamine (nitrogen mustard)	6 mg/sq m	IV	Days 1 and 8	4 wk
	Vincristine	1.4 mg/sq m	IV	Days 1 and 8	
	Prednisone	40 mg/sq m	Oral	Days 1-14	
	Procarbazine	100 mg/sq m	Oral	Days 1-14	
ABVD	Adriamycin	25 mg /sq m	IV	Days 1 and 15	4 wk
	Bleomycin	10 mg/sq m	IV	Days 1 and 15	
	Vinblastine (Velban)	6 mg/sq m	IV	Days 1 and 15	
	Dacarbazine (DTIC)	150 mg/sq m	IV	Days 1-5	

imen of retroperitoneal lymph nodes and of both lobes of the liver and to remove the spleen. The rationale for this procedure is that nonoperative diagnosis of involvement of the liver or spleen has proven to be unreliable.

The classification into stages allows for comparison of persons with similar disease involvement and their response to a given treatment regimen. Over time such comparisons have identified the treatment course most appropriate for a described disease. The revised Ann Arbor staging classification for Hodgkin's disease is shown in the box on p. 1206.

Intervention

Radiation therapy (Fig. 47-6) is used for stages IA, and IB, IIA, and IIB. Stage IIIA is most often treated with a combined modality regimen including radiation and chemotherapy. This treatment yields a cure rate of approximately 90% for stage I and 80% for stage II. Combination chemotherapy is the treatment of choice for stage IIIB and stage IV. The most commonly used combination is the MOPP regimen, which consists of nitrogen mustard, vincristine, procarbazine, and prednisone (Table 47-4). This regimen is administered in a 2-week course each month with prednisone added during the first and fourth course. The drugs are administered for at least 6 months or for two or three courses following the attainment of complete remission. Complete remissions are achieved in approximately 80% of these patients, and long-term, disease-free remissions and probable cures occur in half of this group. Continuing chemotherapy beyond the attainment of complete remission has not been shown to improve survival. Combinations such as ABVD (adriamycin, bleomycin, vinblastine, and dacarbazine) (Table 47-4) are likely to be added to the treatment regimen should relapse occur, and complete remission can again be attained.

Because Hodgkin's disease most often affects young adults, special attention needs to be given to minimizing the impact of the illness and its treatment on their lives, not only during the treatment period but beyond. Before the initiation of treatment, therapy-induced sterility should be discussed.[23] For young women receiving radiation therapy alone, surgical relocation of the ovaries outside the field of radiation may be performed. Sterility frequently occurs in association with chemotherapy (p. 509). For women this is often temporary, and the ability to conceive and bear normal children often returns after therapy is completed. For men sterility is more frequently permanent. For this reason the option of sperm banking should be discussed before beginning either radiation therapy or chemotherapy.

To allow for work and career development every effort should be made to schedule treatment at those times and days of the week that least interfere with work and other important events in the person's life. The nurse has a crucial role in assisting individuals to develop a realistic approach to the illness and in successfully meeting the demands and limitations imposed by the illness and its treatment.

Non-Hodgkin's lymphomas

Etiology and pathophysiology

The non-Hodgkin's lymphomas include a broad spectrum of lymphoid malignancies with different histopathologies, disease courses, and responses to therapy. The cause is unknown although viruses have been implicated. Accurate identification of the histopathology is crucial to the determination of the treatment plan. The classifications are reviewed here only briefly so that familiarity with terminology will allow the reader to review charts and treatment plans. Also, recognition of the diversity of the disease course, prognosis, and the importance of an extensive diagnostic workup is useful to the nurse for patient and family teaching.

Current classification separates the non-Hodgkin's lymphomas into *lymphocytic, histiocytic,* or *mixed cell types,* each of which may appear as nodular or diffuse on microscopic exam. (This classification replaces the previously used one that categorized the non-Hodgkin's lymphomas a lymphosarcoma, reticulum cell sarcoma, or giant follicular cell lymphoma.) Recently, these have been divided into "favorable" and "nonfavorable" histology (see box above) based on response to treatment. In general, a nodular pattern of cell structure conveys

---

NON-HODGKIN'S LYMPHOMAS

"Favorable" histology

Nodular poorly differentiated lymphocytic lymphoma (NLPD)

Nodular mixed lymphocytic and histiocytic lymphoma (NML)

Well-differentiated lymphocytic lymphomas of the nodular (NLWD) or diffuse (DLWD) type

"Unfavorable" histology

Nodular histiocytic (NHL)

Diffuse poorly differentiated lymphocytic (DPDL)

Diffuse histiocytic lymphoma (DHL)

Diffuse mixed lymphoma (DML)

Diffuse undifferentiated lymphoma (DUL)

---

a more favorable prognosis than a diffuse pattern. A lymphocytic cytology is more favorable than a histiocytic one, and a mixed cellularity-histiocytic is intermediate in its prognosis.

Clinical picture

Characteristically, patient's with non-Hodgkin's lymphoma have a median age of 50 to 60 years. Patients present to their physician most often with nontender peripheral lymphadenopathy that may appear bulky. The liver and spleen may be moderately enlarged. Other symptoms that may occur include unexplained fever, night sweats, and weight loss.

The diagnosis of non-Hodgkin's lymphoma is made by examination of pathologic lymph node tissue. Accurate histologic classification is of importance, and often slides are sent to major cancer centers for consultation regarding the classification. Once the diagnosis is made, the extent of the disease (staging) must be determined. As with Hodgkin's disease, accurate staging is a crucial factor required to determine the treatment regimen. The staging workup is similar to that previously described for Hodgkin's disease (p. 1206). Explanations of the extensive work-up and its importance in determining the treatment plan are an important focus of patient teaching during the diagnostic period.

Intervention

The complexity of the disease and the array of treatment regimens used encourages nurse-physician discussion of the treatment plan. It is especially important that the goals of therapy be shared, be they curative or only local or systemic palliation.

In general, radiotherapy is the initial treatment when the disease has a localized presentation. Local field ra-

TABLE 47-5. Chemotherapeutic regimens for treatment of non-Hodgkin's lymphomas

Name	Drugs	Dosage	Method	Schedule	Cycle
COP	Cyclophosphamide (Cytoxan)	800 mg/sq m	IV	Day 1	2 wk
	Vincristine (Oncovin)	2 mg	IV	Day 1	
	Prednisone	60 mg/sq m	Oral	Days 1-5	
CHOP	Cytoxan	750 mg/sq m	IV	Day 1	3 wk
	Adriamycin	50 mg/sq m	IV	Day 1	
	Vincristine	1.4 mg/sq m	IV	Day 1	
	Prednisone	100 mg/sq m	Oral	Days 1-5	
CHOP-Bleo	Cytoxan	750 mg/sq m	IV	Day 1	3 or 4 wk
	Adriamycin	50 mg/sq m	IV	Day 1	
	Vincristine	2 mg	IV	Days 1 and 5	
	Prednisone	100 mg	Oral	Days 1-5	
	Bleomycin	15 units	IV	Days 1 and 5	
COPP	Cytoxan	650 mg/sq m or 600 mg/sq m	IV	Days 1 and 8	2 wk with 2-wk rest period
	Vincristine	1.4 mg/sq m (max. 2 mg)	IV	Days 1 and 8	
	Procarbazine	100 mg/sq m	Oral	Days 1-10	
	Prednisone	40 mg/sq m	Oral	Days 1-14	
BACOP	Bleomycin	5 units/sq m	IV	Days 15 and 22	4 wk
	Doxorubicin (Adriamycin)	25 mg/sq m	IV	Days 1 and 8	
	Cytoxan	650 mg/sq m	IV	Days 1 and 8	
	Vincristine	1.4 mg/sq m (max. 2 mg)	IV	Days 1 and 8	
	Prednisone	60 mg/sq m	Oral	Days 15-28	

diation is used. Total nodal radiation is reserved for patients whose disease is more widespread. Chemotherapy is the mainstay of treatment of non-Hodgkin's lymphomas that are not localized (Table 47-5).

Nodular poorly differentiated lymphocytic lymphoma is the most commonly occurring non-Hodgkin's lymphoma. Treatment with a single alkylating agent, most often chlorambucil, has achieved prolonged survival periods for individuals affected by this disorder. Cyclophosphamide, Oncovin, and Prednisone (COP) make up one of several chemotherapy regimens which produce responses in 90%, and complete response in 60% to 70% of these individuals. It appears thus far that combination chemotherapy in this condition is more effective than single agents. Oral cyclophosphamide or chlorambucil produces complete remissions in 55% of patients with an approximate MST of over 5 years.

In *diffuse histiocytic lymphoma,* which includes most of the cases previously designated as reticulum cell sarcoma, combination chemotherapy has been superior to single-agent therapy. Survival is significantly prolonged in those who demonstrate a complete response, and a significant minority of this group have been disease free long enough to consider that they may be cured. COP,

COPP (COP and procarbazine), MOPP and CHOP (COP and doxorubicin [Adriamycin]), among other combinations, produce complete responses in 40% to 50% or more of patients, whose mean survival time is well over 3 years.

Data are more limited in other types of lymphomas. In *nodular histiocytic* and *nodular mixed histiolymphocytic* types, complete responses have been achieved with single agents, and 50% to 70% of those treated with COP, COPP, MOPP, and other combinations have shown a median survival of 55 months for those who attained a complete response and 13 months for those in whom only a partial response was attained.

Like persons with leukemia and Hodgkin's disease, individuals treated for non-Hodgkin's lymphomas may have periods of remission and recurrence. Such peaks and valleys are stressful and disruptive. Many patients describe subsequent courses of treatment following a recurrence as more stressful than the initial treatment. Comments include "Is it worth it? I don't have the same faith." Other patients, realistically encouraged by the initial response to treatment, are able to express an optimistic outlook, "It worked the first time. It will work again." Recognition of the stress involved in therapy requires that support systems be available to the individual. The health care team can provide some of the needed support and guidance as the individual learns to incorporate the illness into daily life.

Outcome criteria for the person with Hodgkin's disease or non-Hodgkin's lymphoma

The person or significant others can:
1. State an understanding of the disease, its treatment, and prognosis.
2. State the name, dosage, frequency, and side effects of medications. (See outcome criteria for persons receiving chemotherapy, p. 509.)
3. State the importance of and describe plans for follow-up medical care.
4. Describe symptoms requiring immediate medical attention (fever, bleeding).
5. Describe arrangements for chemotherapy treatments, radiotherapy treatments, and periodic blood counts. (See outcome criteria for patients receiving radiation therapy, p. 497.)
6. State resources available in the community: financial (American Cancer Society) and local support groups (American Cancer Society).

Infectious mononucleosis

Epidemiology and etiology

Infectious mononucleosis is an acute disease caused by a herpeslike virus, the Epstein-Barr virus. It is more common in young persons, the highest incidence occurring between 15 and 30 years of age.

Clinical picture

Signs and symptoms of infectious mononucleosis are varied. It is a benign disease with a good prognosis. Malaise is a frequent early complaint, and it is often accompanied by fever, enlargement of lymph nodes, sore throat, headache, generalized aches and pains resembling those of influenza, and moderate enlargement of the liver and spleen. Rupture of the spleen and encephalitis are rare complications. Diagnosis is established by the heterophil agglutination or Monospot blood test. This test is based on the fact that a certain substance present in the blood of a person with infectious mononucleosis causes clumping, or agglutination, of the washed erythrocytes (antigen) of another animal. The test is almost always positive at the end of 10 to 14 days of the illness. Another laboratory finding is a marked increase in the number of mononuclear leukocytes, which lends the name to the disease. At the height of the disease the WBCs may range between 10,000 and 20,000 cells/cu mm.

Intervention

Infectious mononucleosis is self-limiting and, with rest, affected individuals will usually recover spontaneously within a few weeks. Nursing care is aimed at relief of symptoms and promotion of rest and comfort.

Outcome criteria for the person with infectious mononucleosis

The person or significant others can:
1. Describe the nature of the disease and the need for avoidance of fatigue.
2. Describe a plan for rest until the temperature returns to normal.
3. Describe measures to relieve discomfort (aspirin, warm gargles).
4. Describe measures to prevent spread of infection by the oral route.
5. State plans for follow-up care.
   a. Describe symptoms requiring further medical attention (continued fever, malaise, anorexia).
   b. State plans for medical follow-up.
   c. State the continued need for adequate rest even after symptoms have resolved.

REFERENCES AND SELECTED READINGS

1. Abramowicz, M.: Blood products, Med. Lett. Drugs Ther., vol. 21, no. 3 (issue 544), Nov. 1979.
2. Barber, S.M.: Blood cell products in the supportive care of patients with acute leukemia, Nurs. Times **76:**152-154, 1980.
3. Beeson, P., McDermott, W., and Wygarden, J.: Cecil textbook of medicine, vol. II, Philadelphia, 1979, W.B. Saunders Co.
4. Beutler, E.: Iron. In Goodhart, R., and Shiels, M., editors: Modern nutrition in health and disease, Philadelphia, 1980, Lea & Febiger.
5. *Bick, R.: Disseminated intravascular coagulation and related syndromes, etiology, pathophysiology, diagnosis and management, Am. J. Hematol. **5:**265-282, 1978.
6. Brown, M.: Standards of care for the patient with "graft vs. host disease" post bone marrow transplant, Ca. Nurs. **4:**191-198, 1981.
7. *Buickus, B.A.: Blood therapy: administering blood components, Am. J. Nurs. **79:**937, 1979.
8. Card, R.T., et al.: Successful pregnancy after high dose chemotherapy and marrow transplantation treatment for aplastic anemia, Exp. Hematol. **8:**57-60, 1980.
9. Carter, S., Glatstein, E., and Livingston, R.: Principles of cancer treatment, New York, 1982, McGraw-Hill Book Co.
10. Cline, M., and Golde, D.: Controlling the production of blood cells, Blood **53:**157-164, 1979.
11. Coltman, C.: Management of the unfavorable histology non-Hodgkin's lymphomas. In Carter, S., et al, editors, Principles of cancer treatment, New York, 1982, McGraw-Hill Book Co.
12. Crosby, W.: Red cell mass: its precursors and its pertubations, Hosp. Pract. **16:**71-81, 1980.
13. *Cullins, L.: Preventing and treating transfusions reactions, Am.

*References preceded by an asterisk are particularly well suited for student reading.

J. Nurs. **79**:935-941, 1979.

14. *Curry, A.: Protective isolation study. Practice corner, Oncology Nurs. Forum **8**:42, 1981.

15. *Dietz, K.: Radiation therapy: programmed instruction, Ca. Nurs. **2**:127-138, 1979.

16. Diggs, L.W., Sturm, D., and Bell, A.: The morphology of human blood cells, ed. 4, Chicago, 1978, Abbott Laboratories.

17. Firshein, S., et al.: Prenatal diagnosis of classic hemophilia, N. Engl. J. Med. **300**:937-941, 1979.

18. *Flynn, K.T.: Iron deficiency anemia among the elderly, Nurs. Pract. **3**:20-24, 1978.

19. Goldstein, M.: Aplastic anemia, Hosp. Pract. **15**:85-96, 1980.

20. *Guy, R., and Rothenberg, S.: Sickle cell crisis, Med. Clin. North Am. **57**:1591-1598, 1973.

21. Haskell, C.: Cancer treatment, Philadelphia, 1980, W.B. Saunders Co.

22. Herbert, C.: Folic acid and vitamin B 12. In Goodhart, R., and Shiels, M., editors: Modern nutrition in health and disease, ed. 6, Philadelphia, 1980, Lea & Febiger.

23. *Kaempfle, S.: The effects of cancer chemotherapy on reproduction: a review of the literature, Oncology Nurs. Forum **8**:11-18, 1981.

24. Katz, F.: Transfusion therapy: its role in anemia, Hosp. Pract. **16**:77-81, 1980.

25. *Kenny, M.W.: Sickle cell disease, Nurs. Times **76**:1582-1584, 1980.

26. Knobf, M. et al.: Cancer chemotherapy treatment and care, Boston, 1981, G.K. Hall & Co.

27. Kozak, A.: Blood therapy. Processing blood for transfusion, Am. J. Nurs. **79**:931-934, 1979.

28. Lamberg, L.: Genetic screening: learning what you never wanted to know, Today's Health **54**:28-31, 53-54, 1976.

29. Levine, P.: Efficacy of self therapy in hemophilia, N. Eng. J. Med. **291**:1381-1384, 1974.

30. Linman, J.: Hematology, pathophysiologic and clinical principles, New York, 1975, McMillan Publishing Co., Inc.

31. Lund, D.: Eric, Philadelphia, 1974, J.B. Lippincott Co.

32. *Massie, R., and Massie, S.: Journey, New York, 1976, Warner Books, Inc.

33. *Miller, V.G.: The sickle cell anemia patient in surgery, A.O.R.N. J. **30**:1083-1090, 1979.

34. *Nausef, W.M., et al.: A study of the value of simple protective isolation in patients with granulocytopenia, N. Engl. J. Med. **304**:448-452, 1981.

35. *Owen, H., et al.: Bone marrow harvesting: nursing implications, Ca. Nurs. **4**:199-205, 1981.

36. *Parker, A.: Blood therapy, massive transfusions, Am. J. Nurs. **79**:941-948, 1979.

37. Portlock, C.: The management of favorable histology non-Hodgkin's lymphomas. In Carter, S., et al., editors: Principles of cancer treatment, New York, 1982, McGraw-Hill Book Co.

38. Refkind, R., et al.: Fundamentals of hematology, Chicago, 1976, Year Book Medical Publishers, Inc.

39. *Ruttman, R., et al.: Blood therapy. Screening donors and the phlebotomy procedure, Am. J. Nurs. **79**:926-930, 1979.

40. *Rossman, M., Slavin, R., and Taft, E.: Phoresis therapy; patient care, Am. J. Nurs. **77**:1135-1141, 1977.

41. Sherman, M.: The leukemic child. NIH pub. no. 81-863, 1981.

42. Silver, H., editor: Blood, blood components and derivatives in transfusion therapy. In a technical workshop, 1980, Washington, D.C., American Association of Blood Banks.

43. *Smith, I.E.: Hodgkin's disease—drug therapy working toward a cure for all, Nurs. Mirror **147**:37-39, 1978.

44. Spears, D.: The morbidity of sickle cell trait, a review of the literature, Am. J. Med. **64**:1021-1036, 1978.

45. *Tenczynski, J.: Leukophoresis: the process, Am. J. Nurs. **77**:1133-1134, 1974.

46. Thomas, E.D., et al.: Bone marrow transplantation—risks, successes achieved, Resident Staff Physician **22**:53-63, June 1976.

47. Thomas, E.D.: Bone marrow transplantation, N. Engl. J. Med. **292**:832-901, 1975.

48. *Thomas, S.: Transfusing granulocytes, Am. J. Nurs. **79**:942-945, 1979.

49. *Varricchio, C.: The patient on radiation therapy, Am. J. Nurs. **81**:334-342, 1981.

50. Victor, H.: The nutritional anemias, Hosp. Pract. **15**:65-89, 1980.

51. *Welch, D.: Thrombocytopenia in adult patients with leukemia, Ca. Nurs. **1**:463-466, 1978.

52. Wintrobe, M.M., et al.: Harrison's principles of internal medicine, ed. 8, New York, 1977, McGraw-Hill Book Co.

53. Wintrobe, M.M., et al.: Clinical hematology, ed. 7, Philadelphia, 1974, Lea & Febiger.

CHAPTER 48

ASSESSMENT OF THE RESPIRATORY SYSTEM

MARY A. WYPER
BARBARA J. DALY
ALICE NORMAN

Anatomy and physiology

Assessment of the lungs requires knowledge of the airways that conduct air to and from the lungs, the lungs themselves, and the surrounding structures and landmarks. A brief review of these will be provided, with emphasis on the significant characteristics and functions of each.

Structure and function of respiratory tract

The upper airway consists of the nose and nasopharynx, mouth and oropharynx, and the larynx. The lower airway comprises the trachea, main-stem bronchi, bronchioles, and alveolar ducts, which lead to the alveoli themselves (Fig. 48-1). The airway, in addition to providing a passageway for air, serves three functions: filtering, warming, and humidifying air.

Air inspired through an intact respiratory tree is cleansed of all particles larger than 2 μm in diameter before reaching the alveolus. The removal of this particulate matter, such as dust and bacteria, preserves the sterility of the alveolus. Foreign material is filtered through several mechanisms. *Goblet cells* in the epithelial layer of the airways secrete copious amounts of a thick mucopolysaccharide substance, mucus, which coats the airways and entraps particles. *Cilia*, which are found as far into the respiratory tree as the bronchi, then propel the mucus and foreign material up into the pharynx where it can be expelled by coughing or sneezing.

The warming and humidifying functions are made possible by the rich capillary blood supply in the submucosal layer of the airways. During inspiration, air is heated to body temperature, and up to 1000 ml of water is utilized per day to raise the humidity of the inspired air to at least 80%. On expiration some of this water is reabsorbed, thus conserving fluid; an average of 300 ml per day is lost in normal respiration.

The basic gas exchange unit of the respiratory system is the alveolus. Alveoli, which number over 300 million in the healthy adult, are minute sacs that arise from alveolar ducts. The ducts are composed of smooth muscle that is capable of expanding and contracting; the alveolus itself is composed of a single layer of squamous epithelium and an elastic basement membrane. These two layers, in addition to the endothelial and basement layers of the adjacent capillary, form the *alveolar-capillary* membrane or interface. It is across this membrane, a distance of less than 1 μm, that gas exchange takes place.

The lungs themselves are subdivided into lobes. The right lung has three lobes: upper, middle, and lower. The left lung has only two lobes: upper and lower. Air is conducted to each lobe through lobar bronchi that branch off the main-stem bronchus. An important difference between the right and left lungs is the size of the airways leading to them. The right bronchus is significantly wider and shorter and extends at a straighter angle from the trachea, making it the more likely lodging point of aspirated material. The left bronchus is nar-

RESPIRATORY SYSTEM

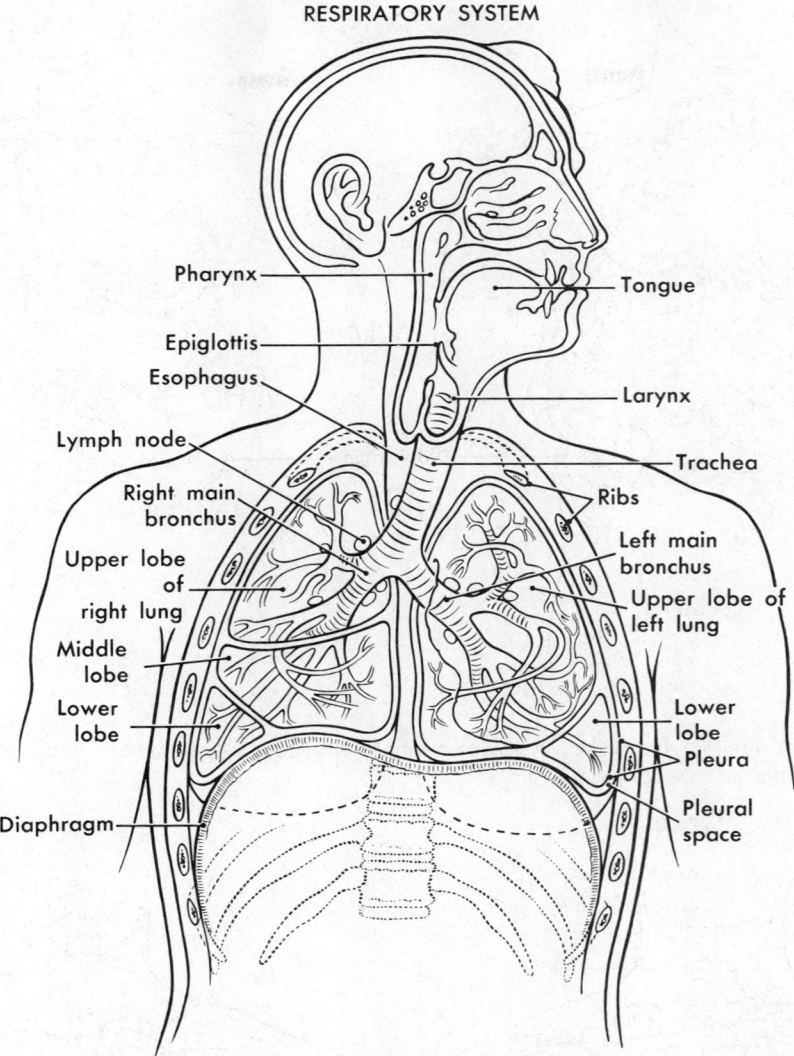

Fig. 48-1. Anatomy of thorax and lungs.

rower and extends at more of a right angle off the trachea, making it more difficult to suction secretions from the left lung.

The thoracic cavity is lined with pleura. The pleura is a continuous *serous* membrane, one surface of which lines the inside of the rib cage (parietal pleura) while the other surface (visceral pleura) covers the lungs. The space between the two surfaces is known as a *potential space*. It normally contains a few milliliters of serous fluid that prevents friction rub when the two surfaces come together.

The lungs lie in and are protected by the thoracic cavity. This bony cage is composed of the sternum and ribs anteriorly and the ribs, scapulae, and vertebral column posteriorly. On the anterior surface the apices of the lungs lie just above the clavicles and posteriorly extend to the eleventh or twelfth rib. Figs. 48-2 and 48-3

illustrate the borders of each lobe and placement of the stethoscope for auscultation.

Mechanism of pulmonary ventilation

Air moves in and out of the lungs as a result of the principle of gas flow; that is, movement is from an area of greater pressure to an area of lower pressure. At the start of inspiration the atmospheric air pressure is greater than alveolar pressure; therefore air moves through the respiratory passageway into the alveoli. When the alveolar pressure exceeds atmospheric pressure, expiration occurs and air moves out of the lungs into the atmosphere.

The pressure gradient between the alveoli and the atmosphere is established by changes in the size of the

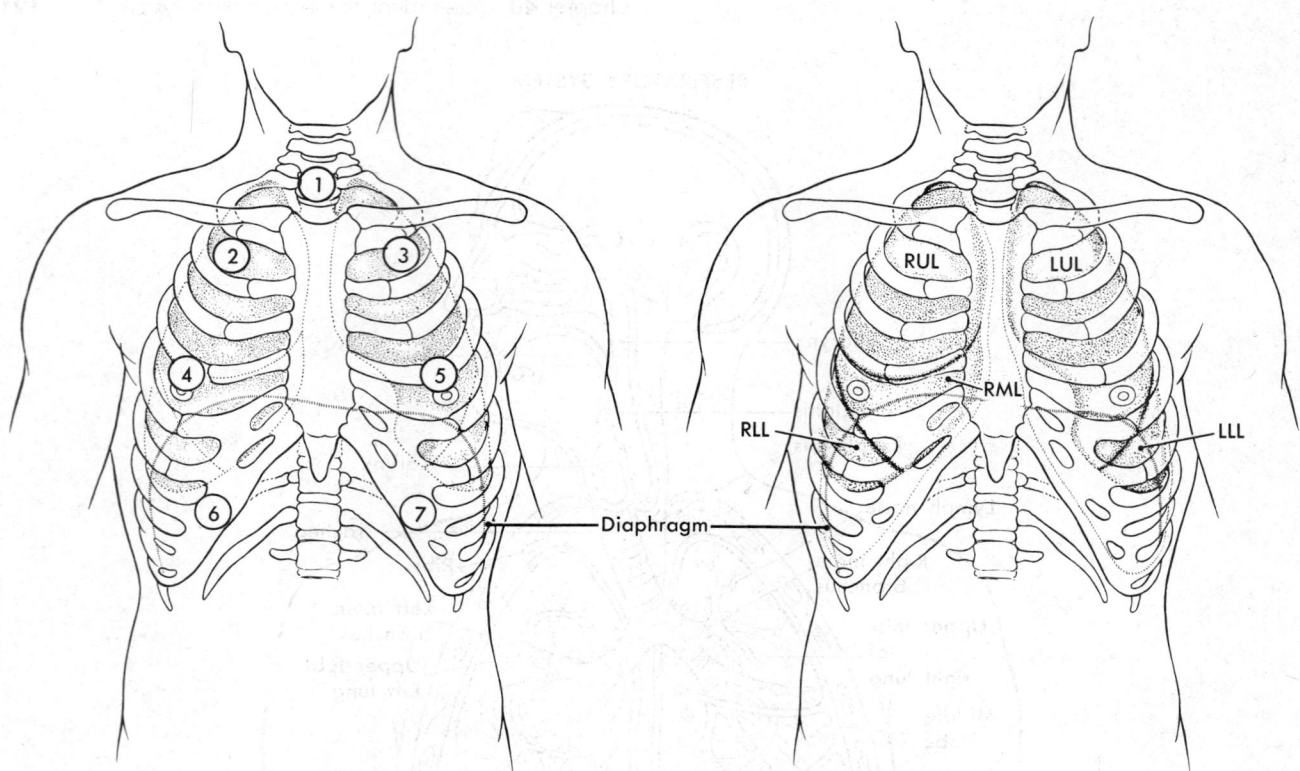

Fig. 48-2. Anterior thorax showing placement of stethoscope when listening to breath sounds and position of lobes of lungs.

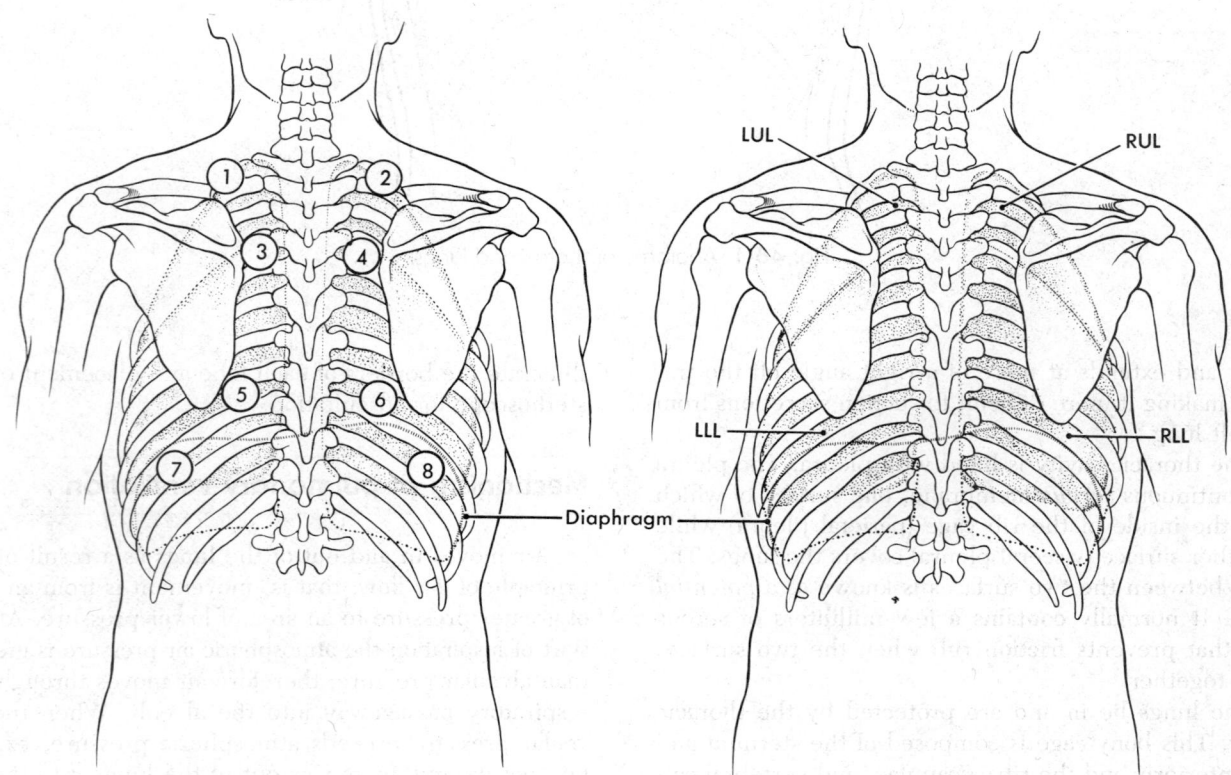

Fig. 48-3. Posterior thorax showing placement of stethoscope when listening to breath sounds and position of lobes of lungs.

thoracic cavity. As the size of the thorax increases, pressure decreases and air flows into the lung. Thoracic size is increased by contraction of the diaphragm and the external intercostal muscles. The diaphragm descends as it contracts and flattens, increasing the longitudinal diameter of the thorax. The external intercostal muscles pull the ribs up and out, elevating the sternum and increasing both anteroposterior and lateral diameters of the chest. The accessory muscles (scalene, sternocleidomastoid, trapezius, and pectoralis) are active only in labored respiration.

As the thorax expands, it pulls the lungs with it because of cohesion between the moist surfaces of the lungs and chest wall. Expiration is normally a passive process that results from the elastic recoil of the lungs and thoracic muscles. Any condition that interferes with contraction of the diaphragm or intercostal muscles will decrease pulmonary ventilation.

Control of respiration

Breathing is an automatic process but may also be controlled voluntarily; that is, we do not have to think about breathing but we can breathe slower or faster at will. Voluntary control of respiration is centered in the cerebral cortex, from which impulses are sent to innervate the muscles of respiration.

Automatic control of respiration is centered in the medulla and pons. The pons is responsible for maintaining rhythmicity of respirations. The respiratory center that is located in the medulla is controlled primarily by the carbon dioxide tension (PCO_2), oxygen tension (PO_2), and acidity (pH) of arterial blood (p. 1222). Chemoreceptors in the carotid bodies (near the carotid bifurcation) and aortic bodies (near the arch of the aorta) are stimulated by a rise in PCO_2 or by a fall in PO_2 or pH of arterial blood (more acid), leading to an increase in respiratory rate. Additional chemoreceptors near the medulla are sensitive to small changes in PCO_2. Other factors that influence respirations include emotions, pain, stretching of the anal sphincter, and stimulation of the pharynx or larynx.

Gas exchange in the lung

In the alveoli oxygen diffuses across the alveolar-capillary membrane from the alveoli into the blood because the partial pressure of oxygen (oxygen tension, PO_2) of *alveolar air* (100 mg Hg) is greater than the PO_2 of venous blood (40 mm Hg). Carbon dioxide diffuses in the opposite direction because the PCO_2 of *venous blood* (46 mm Hg) is greater than the PCO_2 of alveolar air (40 mm Hg). The pulmonary diffusion capacity for carbon dioxide is much greater than the capacity for oxygen, and thus carbon dioxide diffuses more easily. Diffusion capacity of oxygen is decreased by decreased PO_2 of atmospheric air (high altitudes), by decreased surface area in the alveoli, or by decreased alveolar ventilation volumes (amount of oxygen reaching the alveoli).

Subjective data

Before performing the physical examination, the nursing history is obtained. The nurse reviews with the individual the development of symptoms, precipitating events, and previous respiratory problems. In assessing the person's current status, the nurse specifically inquires about diet and fluid intake, activity tolerance, sputum production, use of medications (both prescription and nonprescription substances such as decongestants and allergy preparations), and exposure to known allergens.

Risk factors are particularly relevant. Smoking habits and the presence of other diseases should be established. The role that environmental pollutants have played in the patient's illness may be investigated through inquiries about the individual's occupation and knowledge of the pollution level in the geographic area at that time. Exposure to others with respiratory tract infection may also be a precipitating event.

Objective data

The methods for physical examination are described below. The techniques are used in the order listed.

Inspection

If possible, the individual should be sitting upright. The examiner first observes the person's general appearance before inspecting the thorax itself. Color of the skin is not a very reliable indicator of oxygenation but should be obtained as part of the baseline data. Central cyanosis of the tongue and mucous membranes more accurately reflects respiratory status than does peripheral cyanosis, which may be caused by vascular disease or a cold environment. The ease with which the person can talk in complete sentences without stopping to catch his or her breath often yields a clue to respiratory function. Posture and any variations from normal structure of the thorax, such as scoliosis, kyphosis, funnel or barrel chest, and pigeon breast are observed.

The quality of respirations is assessed next; this includes rate, rhythm and depth of respiratory excursions, and symmetry of chest wall expansion. Diminished chest expansion may occur with pulmonary embolus, pneumonia, pleural effusion, pneumothorax, or the pain caused by fractured ribs. The examiner compares respiratory excursion of both sides of the posterior thorax by placing the hands so that the thumbs meet at the midline as the hands extend over the chest wall. The entire thorax should move as one unit as the thumbs move away from each other; expect 7.5 cm (3 in.) expansion.

Abnormalities that may be observed in the presence of disease include the use of accessory muscles or the presence of nasal flaring, both present with labored respirations. The trachea may also be deviated from the midline. Deviation occurs in pleural effusion, pneumothorax with mediastinal shift, mediastinal shift following pneumonectomy, and atelectasis. Rapid (*tachypnea*) and slow (*bradypnea*) respiratory rates should be noted, as well as alterations in depth such as shallow respirations or *hyperpnea* (rapid, deep respirations).

Palpation

Palpation of the chest is performed with the palmar surface of the hand flat against the posterior chest to determine the presence of tactile fremitus when the patient is asked to say "ninety-nine." Normally, a vibration is felt over the exterior chest wall when the patient speaks. The examiner uses the same hand to palpate all areas of the chest. Diminished or absent fremitus may occur with pleural effusion, pneumothorax, and atelectasis. Increased tactile fremitus occurs over areas of consolidation. One may also detect areas of pain or masses of the thorax with this examining technique.

Percussion

Percussion of the chest is performed by placing the middle finger flat against the chest at an interspace and striking the distal phalanx sharply with the end of the middle finger of the other hand (p. 102). Percussion is done from apex to base with the patient in the supine position for examination of the anterior thorax and in a sitting position for examination of the posterior thorax. Normally, percussion elicits a resonant sound. The examiner compares the sound of each area with the sound of the opposite side as percussion proceeds. During percussion of the posterior bases the individual is asked to hold his or her breath at the end of inspiration and then at the end of an expiration. This maneuver allows the examiner to determine the amount of diaphragmatic descent during inspiration. Normally, the diaphragm moves downward 5 to 6 cm.

Dull or flat percussion tones are heard in the presence of atelectasis, pneumonia, pleural effusion, or a tumor mass. The same dull sound is normally heard over the heart and liver. Hyperresonance occurs when there is air trapped in the lungs or chest, as with pulmonary emphysema or pneumothorax.

Auscultation

Auscultation consists of listening to the chest to determine the presence of normal breath and voice sounds and to detect the presence of any abnormal sounds. If possible, the patient should be sitting upright. With the diaphragm of the stethoscope, the examiner begins auscultation of the anterior and posterior thorax at the position shown in Figs. 48-2 and 48-3. The patient is instructed to take slow, deep breaths through the mouth. When listening to the posterior chest, the examiner has the patient bring the shoulder forward to abduct the scapula so that a greater lung surface can be auscultated. The examiner auscultates the anterior and posterior thorax from apices to bases, comparing one side with the other.

It is particularly important when examining the patient who is on bed rest to have the patient sit up in bed or turn onto the side while you listen to the posterior aspect in order to detect pooled secretions.

Breath sounds

The three types of breath sounds are vesicular, bronchovesicular, and bronchial (Fig. 48-4).

Vesicular breath sounds are heard over most of the lung, especially the regions toward the periphery (Fig. 48-2, areas 4 through 7). These sounds are of a low pitch and have a soft rustling or swishing quality. The sound of the inspiratory phase is longer and higher in pitch than that of the expiratory phase, which is a soft, short, low-pitched, almost inaudible sound.

Bronchovesicular breath sounds may be heard over the major airways, such as at the point at which the

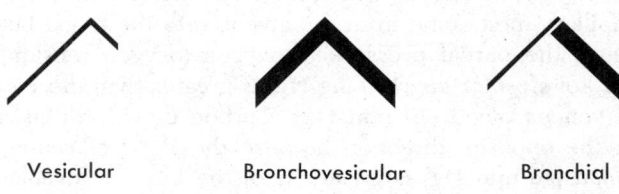

Vesicular   Bronchovesicular   Bronchial

Fig. 48-4. Schematic representation of three types of breath sounds.

trachea bifurcates into the bronchi (Figs. 48-2, areas 2 and 3, and 48-3, areas 3 and 4). Inspiration and expiration are loud and nearly equal in duration and intensity. Bronchovesicular breath sounds heard over areas of the lungs other than those indicated above are abnormal and indicate an area of partial consolidation.

Bronchial breath sounds are not heard normally over any area of lung tissue, and their presence indicates consolidation or compression of lung tissue or a pleural effusion. These breath sounds are high pitched and loud; during the expiratory phase they increase in duration, pitch, and intensity. A close approximation of bronchial breath sounds can be heard by placing the stethoscope over the trachea.

Voice sounds

Auscultation for voice sounds also aids in detecting abnormal conditions in the lung, such as atelectasis and consolidation. Whispers, normally indistinct, are well heard over these affected areas. This change is termed *whispered pectoriloquy*. Egophony is an "E" to "A" change in which the patient says "E" and the examiner hears "A" through the stethoscope. Egophony is also heard over areas of atelectasis and over areas of consolidation.

Abnormal sounds or extra sounds

Sounds that are superimposed on breath sounds are termed *adventitious* and include rales, rhonchi, wheezes, and friction rubs. *Rales* are divided into fine, medium, and coarse. Fine rales produced in the small airways, as in pneumonia or heart failure, are heard at the end of inspiration and likened to the sounds of several hairs rubbed together between the fingertips. Medium rales produced in the medium airways occur in the later stages of pneumonia, heart failure, and pulmonary edema. The medium rales have been compared to the fizzing of a carbonated drink. They are heard about midway through the inspiratory phase. Coarse rales are heard at the beginning of inspiration and produce a rough, gurgling sound; they often can be cleared with a cough, since they are produced by secretions in the larger airways. *Rhonchi* and *wheezes* are continuous sounds, although they may be more prominent in expiration. Some authors use the terms coarse rales and rhonchi synonymously. Rhonchi and wheezes are produced by air flowing through passages narrowed by secretions, mucosal swelling, tumors, or other obstructions; like coarse rales, they may be cleared with coughing. They are classified as *high-pitched, sibilant rhonchi*, which have a musical quality and originate in smaller air passages, and *low-pitched, sonorous rhonchi*, which originate in larger air passages and have a snoring sound. *Friction rubs* are crackling, grating sounds that originate in inflamed pleura. They are usually, but not always, heard on both inspiration and expiration and are not affected by coughing. Rubs are heard most easily over the anterolateral area where the greatest expansion occurs.

Diagnostic tests

Roentgenologic examination of the chest

Plain chest films

Roentgenologic examination is probably familiar to most patients and the general public. Roentgenology has had extensive use as a screening test and as a diagnostic measure. Some persons are concerned about the radiation hazards associated with x-rays and may need reassurance that the knowledge gained from the examination outweighs the risks.

When chest disease is suspected, a roentgenogram is almost always ordered to help identify the disease and to visualize the extent of the disease process. Various types of roentgenograms may be ordered. For survey purposes a minifilm may be used. If the history and physical examination or survey film indicate possible pulmonary pathologic findings, full-size chest films are obtained. These include posteroanterior and lateral views.

When the patient goes to the radiology department, the nurse should be sure that an open-backed gown is worn and that all metal objects above the waist have been or will be removed, since metal restricts passage of the x-rays and will cause a shadow on the film. Care should be taken that such articles are not misplaced or lost. If the patient is acutely ill, a portable x-ray machine is brought to the bedside, and the nurse assists the patient into correct position. The x-ray plate is covered and then placed flat on the bed. If the patient can sit up, the plate is put in place, the patient leans back on it, and the head of the bed is lowered as far as can be tolerated; or the patient may sit on the side of the bed, holding the x-ray plate against the anterior chest, resting it on a pillow. When the roentgenogram is taken, the nurse should step out of the room to avoid being exposed to unnecessary radiation. If the patient requires nursing assistance during the procedure, the nurse should wear a lead-lined apron.

Fluoroscopic examination

For certain types of information in which visualization of thoracic contents in a dynamic rather that static manner is helpful (e.g., diaphragmatic movement and size and contour of the heart), fluoroscopy is the preferred examination.

Whether fluoroscopic examination is performed in the physician's office or in the hospital, the patient must go to a room where the fluoroscope is installed. Assistance may be required in rising to a sitting or standing position or in remaining still during the examination. If the patient is in a wheelchair, a stool in front of the machine will be used to sit on. Before the examination the physician wears dark red goggles to aid adaptation to the darkened fluoroscopy room. During the examination the physician wears a protective lead apron and gloves. Fluoroscopic examination is performed with the lights off, and the machine is operated with a foot pedal. Patients need a careful explanation of the procedure and should be told that they will be in darkness and that they may be asked to hold their breath for a few seconds during the examination. They should be assured that there will be no discomfort.

Bronchography

A *bronchogram* enables the physician to visualize the bronchial tree by x-ray film after the introduction of an iodized radiopaque liquid, which coats the bronchial mucosa (Fig. 48-5). To lessen the number of bacteria introduced from the mouth into the bronchi, the patient should pay particular attention to oral hygiene on the night before and on the morning of the procedure. No food or fluids are allowed for 8 hours preceding the examination. Since, if the smaller bronchi contain secretions, the radiopaque liquid will not reach them, postural drainage may be ordered for the morning the bronchogram is made (Fig. 49-12). The patient should be asked about any loose or capped teeth or dental bridges. Dental prostheses should be removed, and loose teeth should be brought to the physician's attention. Bronchograms are *contraindicated* during acute infections and in individuals sensitive to iodine.

Approximately 1 hour before the examination the patient is given a short-acting barbiturate to minimize the stimulating effects of the anesthetic agent and for sedation. To lessen the patient's discomfort during the procedure, a local topical anesthetic agent is administered. Usually 0.5% tetracaine (Pontocaine) or cocaine is used. These drugs can cause toxic reactions in some patients. Thus the patient is observed closely for signs of central nervous system stimulation. Rapid pulse rate, excitation, headache, and palpitation are some of the signs of toxicity. When these occur, the physician is notified at once. Usually a short-acting barbiturate such as secobarbital (Seconal) is given intravenously. Oxygen may also be administered. If the patient is not treated promptly, the central nervous system can become depressed and the patient may die from respiratory failure.

The pharynx, larynx, and major bronchi are anesthetized immediately before the radiopaque substances is introduced. The patient is informed that the local anesthetic will taste bitter and that it should not be swallowed but expectorated into tissues or an emesis basin, which will be provided. When the gag reflex disappears, a metal laryngeal cannula is passed into the trachea, and then a catheter is passed through the nose into the cannula and into the trachea. The radiopaque substance is then introduced, and the patient is tilted into various positions to distribute it to the bronchi and bronchioles. These positions are the reverse of those used in postural drainage. A series of radiographs is then taken. Following this procedure, postural drainage is usually ordered to help remove the radiopaque sub-

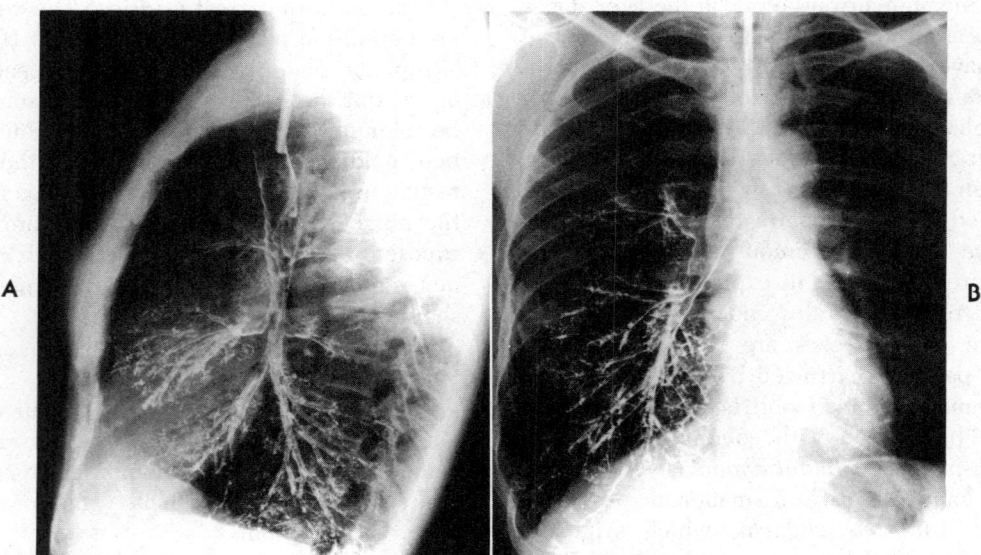

Fig. 48-5. Normal bronchogram of right lung, lateral **(A)** and anteroposterior **(B)** views. (From DeWeese, D.D., and Saunders, W.H.: Textbook of otolaryngology, ed. 6, St. Louis, 1982, The C.V. Mosby Co.)

stance from the lungs. Follow-up films may also be taken to ascertain how much dye remains in the tracheobronchial tree. No permanent damage results, however, if some of it remains for an indefinite period. Food and fluid should be withheld until the gag reflex returns, which can be tested by gently tickling the posterior pharynx with a cotton swab.

Pulmonary angiography

Pulmonary angiography is used to detect pulmonary emboli and a variety of congenital and acquired lesions of the pulmonary vessels. A radiopaque material is injected via a catheter into a systemic vein, the right chambers of the heart, or the pulmonary artery, and the distribution of this material is recorded on film. Following this procedure the nurse observes the site of insertion of the catheter and reports any adverse signs and symptoms such as inflammation, formation of a hematoma, absence of peripheral pulses, or complaint of numbness, tingling, or pain in the extremity involved.

Special roentgenologic examinations

Special views of the lungs may be obtained by placing the patient in various positions. The most common are the *right* and *left anterior oblique*, the *recumbent lateral (decubitus)*, and the *lordotic* positions. The oblique positions allow better visualization of the mediastinum and areas of the lung often hidden or obscured by normal thoracic structures in the posteroanterior position. The decubitus film is used to locate fluid in the pleural space and the lordotic to better visualize the posterior apices.

Laminography (tomography, planography) is a technique whereby a specific layer of lung tissue is visualized. It is used to study cavities, neoplasms, and densities of the lung. *Computed tomography scanning* (CT scanning) provides more accurate information than conventional tomography in some cases, but its use on thoracic structures is in the early stages of development. *Ultrasound* (echograms) of the thorax can provide information about pleural effusions or opacities.

Examination of sputum

Examinations of sputum are usually required when chest disease is suspected. The mucous membrane of the respiratory tract responds to inflammation by an increased flow of secretions that often contain causative organisms. Volume, consistency, color, and odor of the sputum are recorded. These observations are helpful both in diagnosis and evaluation of therapy. For example, thick, tenacious mucoid sputum is characteristic of asthma; green, musty-smelling sputum, *Pseudomonas* pneumonia; and rusty sputum, pneumococcal pneumonia. A *smear of sputum* gives information about the

morphology and staining characteristics of organisms. The presence of neutrophils and eosinophils is also noted. A *culture of the sputum* is also ordered. On culture the specific organism can be identified. *Sensitivity studies* done on the culture serve as a guide to the selection of antimicrobial therapy. A *cytologic* examination of the sputum is ordered if carcinoma is suspected.

Tests to be done on sputum are explained to the patient so that a suitable specimen will be obtained. The patient is instructed to collect only sputum that has come from deep in the lungs. When instructed inadequately, patients often expectorate saliva rather than sputum. They are likely to exhaust themselves unnecessarily by shallow, frequent coughing that yields no sputum suitable for study and that affords them little relief from discomfort. *The first sputum raised in the morning is usually the most productive of organisms.* During the night, secretions accumulate in the bronchi, and just a few deep coughs will bring them to the back of the throat. If patients do not know this fact, on awakening they may almost unconsciously cough, clear their throats, and swallow or expectorate before attempting to produce the specimen.

The patient should be supplied with a wide-mouthed container and instructed to expectorate directly into it. Because the sight of sputum is often objectionable to the patient and to others, the outside of a glass container is covered with paper or other suitable covering. Usually 4 ml of sputum is sufficient for necessary laboratory tests and examinations. Initial specimens for culture and sensitivity are usually collected before antibiotic therapy is started. Occasionally, however, all sputum collected over a period of 24 to 72 hours is needed. If there is any delay in sending the specimen to the laboratory, it should be placed in the refrigerator.

Sputum collection using saline inhalation

Inhalation of a heated saline solution is used to help some persons raise sputum for specimens. A 10% solution of saline in distilled water is placed in a heated nebulizer, and a fine spray is produced by attaching the nebulizer to compressed air or oxygen. When inhaled, the heated vapor condenses on the surface of the tracheobronchial mucosa and stimulates production of secretions.

Patients who have difficulty raising sputum for specimens can learn this procedure readily. The patient is taught how to deep breathe and cough before the procedure. The mouth is placed over, but not sealed around, the nebulizer before inhaling. Inhalation of the vapor is repeated for a few minutes or until coughing is stimulated. Some patients begin to cough after the first inhalation. The patient should have a supply of tissues to cover the cough and should expectorate sputum into the collection container.

It is important to encourage patients to rest for a few seconds between periods of inhaling and coughing so that they do not become overtired. If the patient complains of lightheadedness or dizziness caused by hyperventilation, sitting quietly and breathing slowly for a few minutes will normally bring relief. If nausea occurs, the inhalations should be discontinued. The patient usually feels nauseated for only a few minutes, and it may be associated with factors other than inhalation. The advantage of this method of raising sputum is that the patient can do the procedure at any time of the day and needs no special preparation.

If the patient is suspected of having tuberculosis and specimens are being collected for screening purposes, the hospital or outpatient personnel should use appropriate precautions. The room should be well ventilated so that there are frequent changes of air. If the patient is known to have sputum positive for tubercle bacilli, the extra precaution of wearing a high-filtration mask may be taken. Special ultraviolet lights may be installed to rid the rising circulating air of infectious droplets. They are installed high enough to protect the patient and the personnel from direct exposure to the light.

Gastric washings

Gastric aspiration is occasionally used to collect gastric contents, which may contain swallowed sputum. It is usually done when the diagnosis or suspected diagnosis is tuberculosis. Since most patients swallow sputum when coughing in the morning and during sleep, an examination of gastric contents may reveal causative organisms. Breakfast is withheld for gastric aspiration. (The procedure for passing the nasogastric tube is the same as that discussed on p. 1384.) Once the tube is passed, a large syringe is attached to the end, and by gentle suction a specimen of stomach contents is withdrawn. The specimen is placed in a covered bottle, and the tube is withdrawn. The specimen is examined microscopically on slides, and culture media are inoculated as is done with other sputum samples. For the patient the disadvantages of this method of sputum collection are the discomforts of going without food and the passage of the nasogastric tube.

Pulmonary function measurements and arterial blood gases

Physiologic tests of pulmonary function are performed in order to provide information regarding abnormalities in function, progression or improvement in clinical status, effects of medication, and degree of disability present. These tests cannot be used by themselves to diagnose specific diseases, but they are an integral part of the diagnostic process.

There are two general kinds of respiratory function tests. One measures the bellows action of the chest and lungs, or the ability to move air in and out of the alveoli (*ventilation*); the other measures *diffusion*, the movement of the gas across the alveolar-capillary membrane, and *perfusion*, the supply of blood to the lungs.

DEFINITIONS OF LUNG VOLUMES

Definitions of lung volumes (nonoverlapping measures)

Tidal volume (TV)	Volume of gas inspired and expired with a normal breath
Inspiratory reserve volume (IRV)	Maximal volume that can be inspired from the end of a normal inspiration
Expiratory reserve volume (ERV)	Maximal volume that can be exhaled by forced expiration after a normal expiration
Residual volume (RV)	Volume of gas left in lung after maximal expiration

Definitions of lung capacities (combinations of various volumes)

Inspiratory capacity (IC)	Maximal amount of air that can be inspired after a normal expiration (TV + IRV)
Functional residual capacity (FRC)	Amount of air left in lungs after a normal expiration (ERV + RV)
Vital capacity (VC)	Maximal amount of air that can be expired after a maximal inspiration (TV + IRV + ERV)
Forced vital capacity (FVC)	Maximal amount of air that can be expelled with a maximal effort after a maximal inspiration)
Total lung capacity (TLC)	Total amount of air in lungs after maximal inspiration (TV + IRV + ERV + RV)

Volume/time relationships

Minute volume (MV)	Volume inspired and expired in 1 min of normal breathing
Forced expiratory volume in 1 sec FEV$_1$)	Amount of air expelled in the first second of the forced vital capacity maneuver
FEV$_1$/VC ratio	Amount of air forcefully expelled in 1 sec compared to total amount forcefully expelled
Maximal voluntary ventilation (MVV) (also termed maximal breathing capacity [MBC])	Amount of air exchanged per minute with maximal rate and depth of respiration

In order for the lung to perform gas exchange efficiently, the ventilation-perfusion ratio ($\dot{V}/\dot{Q}$ ratio) must be balanced. That is, areas that receive ventilation should be well perfused with blood, and areas that receive blood flow should be capable of ventilation. Although in the normal lung with its many millions of gas exchange units some imbalance in ventilation and perfusion exists, this has little effect on overall gas exchange function. In fact, adaptive mechanisms appear to exist that divert blood flow to the best-ventilated regions of the lungs or redirect ventilation away from nonperfused areas in order to maintain a normal ratio in the range of 0.8 to 1.0. Alteration in ventilation-perfusion relationships (either overall or in circumscribed areas of lung tissue) is largely responsible for the *hypoxemia* or *hypercapnia* seen in clinical practice. The nurse should be familiar with pulmonary function tests to be able to explain them to the patient.

Measurement of pulmonary volumes and capacities

To determine the functional capacity of the lungs, basic ventilation studies are performed by using a spirometer. Some measurements, such as the *residual volume,* cannot be measured directly and are calculated mathematically. The total gas content of the lungs can be subdivided into volumes and capacities as defined in the box on p. 1220.

A spirogram giving the normal volumes and lung capacities is shown in Fig. 48-6. These volumes and capacities vary with age, sex, weight, and height. Two ventilatory studies are of particular clinical significance. They are the *forced expiratory volume* (FEV), or *timed vital capacity*, and the *maximal voluntary ventilation* (MVV), or *maximum breathing capacity* (MBC). The FEV measures the volume expired forcefully at 1, 2, and 3 seconds after a full inspiration. The FEV at *1 second* is the most useful of the three values, particularly when it is compared with the vital capacity (FEV_1/VC ratio). The MVV measures the volume of air exchanged per minute with maximal rate and depth of respiration. FEV and MVV can be affected by lung *compliance* (distensibility of the lung) because of the increased muscular effort required. FEV and MVV are decreased in obstructive lung disease and may be normal or decreased in restrictive lung disease.

The patient is usually instructed in how to participate in the tests by the physician or the technician in the testing laboratory. For all these tests the patient must breathe only through the mouth. A recording device and a spirometer are used. When the patient breathes through the mouthpiece and connecting tube, a noseclip is usually used so that the patient cannot breathe through the nose. Although a noseclip may seem like a small, harmless piece of equipment, the patient often becomes apprehensive about it. Time should be allowed for the patient to adjust to the clip. Fear of cutting off the air supply, particularly when a person has a breathing limitation, may cause anxiety. Because these tests are dependent on patient effort and can also be very exhausting to a patient with respiratory disease, rest both before and after the testing is necessary. If the patient is receiving regular bronchodilator treatments, these are withheld for 4 hours before testing if a part of the examination is to include measurements taken before and after the use of nebulized bronchodilators. Nurses can allay some of the patient's apprehension by giving clear and confident explanations.

Blood gas studies

Arterial blood gas studies have become a common tool to aid in physiologic diagnosis and therapeutic management of patients. These studies determine blood

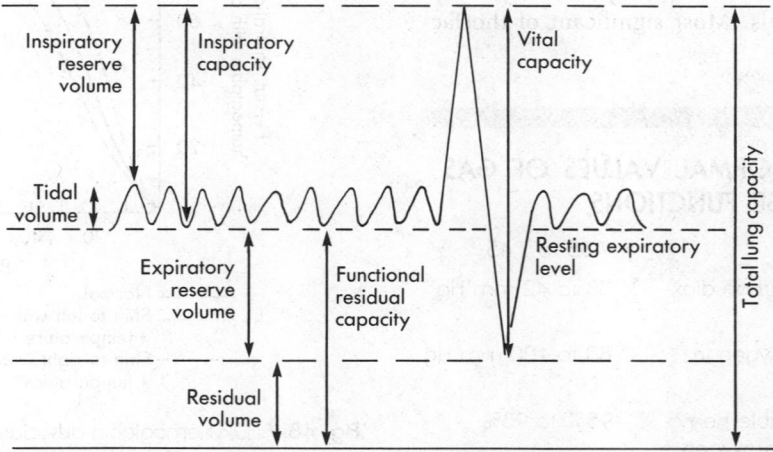

Fig. 48-6. Lung volumes and capacities illustrated by spirography tracing. (Adapted from Wade, J.F.: Respiratory nursing care, ed. 2, St. Louis, 1977, The C.V. Mosby Co.)

pH, carbon dioxide tension (Pco_2), oxygen tension (Po_2), and percent of oxyhemoglobin saturation (Sao_2). Blood gas studies are obtained to assess the adequacy of oxygenation and ventilation and to assess acid-base status. The blood sample is obtained from the radial, brachial, or femoral arteries using a preheparinized syringe to prevent clotting. The syringe is capped after obtaining the blood sample to prevent contact with air and is placed in an ice water container until analyzed. Pressure is maintained over the puncture site for at least 2 minutes after needle withdrawal to prevent bleeding.

Gas tensions refer to partial pressure, or that part of the total pressure exerted by a specific gas. For example, pressure exerted by the atmosphere at sea level is 760 mm Hg. The amount of oxygen in air at sea level is 21%; that is, 21% of the total pressure is exerted by oxygen. Since 21% of 760 is approximately 159, the Po_2 of air at sea level is 159 mm Hg. Definitions of gas exchange functions and their normal values are given in the box below.

The measurement of oxygen values includes both the Po_2 and Sao_2. The Po_2 measures oxygen dissolved in the blood; however, the amount of oxygen carried in the blood in this form is small, since most oxygen is transported in chemical combination with hemoglobin. Oxyhemoglobin saturation refers to that percentage of the hemoglobin that is combined with oxygen. More than 90% of the oxygen-carrying capacity of blood is accounted for by oxyhemoglobin, with the partial pressure of oxygen acting as the driving force for this chemical combination. Therefore both Po_2 and Sao_2 levels must be examined in order to determine the adequacy of oxygenation of the tissues.

It is particularly important to understand the relationship of the Po_2 to oxyhemoglobin saturation in order to assess adequacy of tissue oxygenation. This relationship is not directly linear; many factors affect the affinity of the heme molecule for oxygen. A sigmoid curve (Fig. 48-7) represents the saturation percentages that occur at various Po_2 levels. Most significant of the factors that affect the ability of the blood to carry oxygen is the partial pressure of the oxygen itself in the blood. As can be seen in the oxyhemoglobin dissociation curve (Fig. 48-7), in the upper portion of the curve, hemoglobin has an increased affinity for oxygen, so that large changes in Po_2 levels can be tolerated without significantly changing the saturation. For example, at a Po_2 of 100 mm Hg, hemoglobin saturation is almost total, 97%; even if the Po_2 should fall to 70 mm Hg, the saturation would only decrease to 94%. This serves as a protective mechanism that ensures adequate tissue oxygenation even when there is mild hypoxemia. It should be noted, however, that once the Po_2 level falls below 60 mm Hg, saturation begins to decrease sharply, thus reducing the ability of the hemoglobin to transport oxygen.

Other factors that influence the oxygen affinity of hemoglobin are temperature, pH, and Pco_2. At higher temperatures, increased levels of Pco_2 (hypercapnia), and acidosis, the curve shifts to the right. This means that at any given Po_2 the hemoglobin has less affinity for oxygen and lower saturations will result. The converse of this is also true; with decreased temperature, decreased Pco_2, and alkalosis, higher saturations occur with any given Po_2.

The Pco_2 is utilized as a measurement to determine the adequacy of ventilation and is dependent on the amount of carbon dioxide produced by the body and the ability of the lungs to eliminate it. *Hypoventilation* therefore is shown by an elevated Pco_2, while *hyperventilation* is indicated by a decrease in Pco_2 below normal levels.

The pH refers to the acidity of the blood and is an

DEFINITIONS AND NORMAL VALUES OF GAS EXCHANGE FUNCTIONS

pH	Acidity of blood	7.35 to 7.45
Pco_2	Partial pressure of carbon dioxide in blood	38 to 42 mm Hg
Po_2	Partial pressure of oxygen in blood	80 to 100 mm Hg
Sao_2	Percentage of available hemoglobin saturated with oxygen	95% to 98%

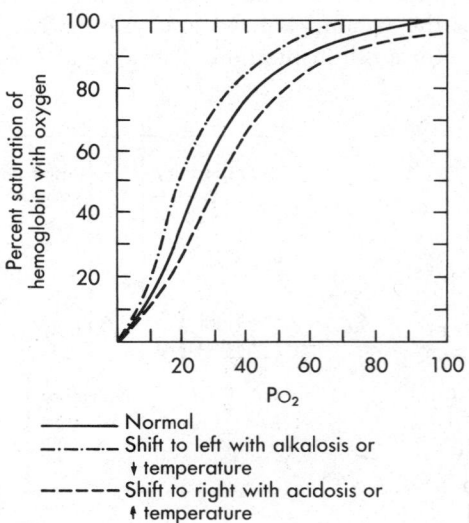

Fig. 48-7. Oxyhemoglobin dissociation curve. (Reproduced with permission from Comroe, J.H., Jr.: Physiology of respiration, ed. 2. Copyright © 1974 by Year Book Medical Publishers, Inc., Chicago.)

expression of the hydrogen ion concentration. Because pH is expressed as a negative logarithm, as hydrogen ion concentration increases and blood becomes more acid, the pH value falls. When hydrogen ion concentration decreases, the blood becomes more alkaline and the pH value rises.

The P_{CO_2} is related to the pH because of the chemical reaction of carbon dioxide and water in the blood, which results in the formation of carbonic acid. Carbonic acid, in turn, dissociates to form hydrogen and bicarbonate ions, as illustrated in the following equation:

$$CO_2 + H_2O \rightleftarrows H_2CO_3 \rightleftarrows HCO_3^- + H^+$$

The maintenance of a normal pH is dependent on a ratio of 20 bicarbonate ions to 1 hydrogen ion. It can be seen from the equation that the presence of an elevated P_{CO_2} will result in an excess of hydrogen ions. When this occurs, the pH falls and the patient is said to be in *respiratory acidosis*. Conversely, when P_{CO_2} is decreased, the pH increases and the result is termed *respiratory alkalosis* (p. 354).

Bronchospirometry

Bronchospirometry measures the ventilation and oxygen consumption of each lung separately. For this procedure a specially constructed double-lumen catheter with two balloons is used. When the catheter is in place, one balloon is inflated to seal off the contralateral lung. After measuring the ventilation of one lung, that balloon is deflated; the other balloon is inflated, and the procedure is repeated on the opposite side. This test aids the surgeon in determining whether the ventilatory capacity of the unaffected lung is sufficient to maintain the patient after pulmonary resection. This determination is most crucial before pneumonectomy.

Bronchoscopy

A *bronchoscopic examination* is performed by passing a bronchoscope into the trachea and bronchi (Fig. 48-8). Preparation of the client for a bronchoscopic examination is similar to that for bronchography except that postural drainage is less often ordered. In addition to a spray anesthetic, cocaine may be applied locally by holding small cotton pledgets soaked in solution in the posterior fossa of the pharynx. If the patient is very apprehensive or if a sponge biopsy (abrasion of the lesion with a sponge) is to be done or a tissue biopsy specimen obtained, intravenous anesthesia may be used. A bronchoscope is a long, rigid, slender, hollow instrument through which light can be reflected and visual examination of the trachea and major bronchi with their branchings can be made. In recent years the *fiberoptic*

bronchoscope, which is a flexible instrument allowing greater visualization with passage into segmental and subsegmental bronchi, has been employed with increasing frequency particularly for diagnostic examinations (Fig. 48-9). The use of this instrument is also associated with less discomfort for the patient as compared to the rigid metal bronchoscope. Bronchoscopy may be done to remove a foreign body, to facilitate free air passage by removal of mucus plugs with suction, to obtain a biopsy sample and samples of secretions for examination, and to observe the air passages for signs of disease.

Following bronchoscopy the patient is given no food or fluids until the gag reflex returns. Some physicians prefer that the patient lie flat after this procedure, while others prefer semi-Fowler's position. Unless intravenous anesthesia is used, the patient is awake and conscious, although drowsy from sedation. Lying on the side facilitates removal of secretions into disposable tissues or a small emesis basin. The patient usually produces large amounts of sputum. All sputum is saved for culture and cytologic studies because the postbronchoscopy specimens are often positive diagnostically. However, if the patient has had bronchograms, the sputum is often not helpful for cytologic examination, since the base of the dye makes fixation of the cells difficult.

The patient frequently complains of a sore throat and may have hoarseness after the procedure. Lidocaine

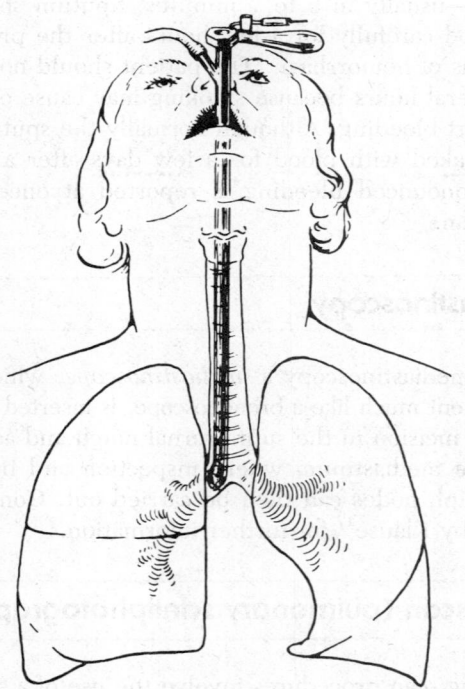

Fig. 48-8. Bronchoscope inserted through trachea into bronchus. (From DeWeese, D.D., and Saunders, W.H.: Textbook of otolaryngology, ed. 6, St. Louis, 1982, The C.V. Mosby Co.)

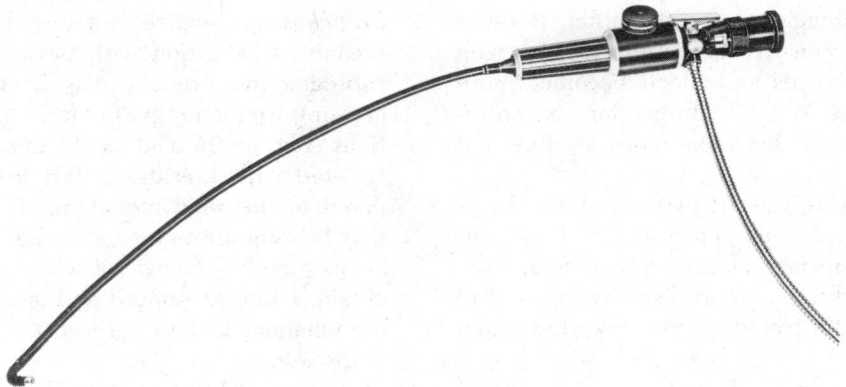

Fig. 48-9. Fiberoptic bronchoscope. Because of its flexibility, it allows better visualization of bronchi. (Courtesy American Cystoscope Makers, Inc., Pelham, N.Y.)

(Xylocaine) is often helpful in reducing discomfort. In some instances, laryngeal edema follows bronchoscopy and can cause airway obstruction. Shortness of breath and laryngeal stridor are symptoms of this complication, and if they occur the physician is notified immediately. Cool mist is often given prophylactically to prevent the development of laryngeal edema. When cocaine is used for local anesthesia, the patient is watched for the signs of central nervous system stimulation described previously (p. 1218).

If a biopsy sample is taken during bronchoscopy, the patient is kept under close surveillance until clotting occurs—usually in 5 to 7 minutes. Sputum should be observed carefully for a few hours after the procedure for signs of hemorrhage. The patient should not smoke for several hours because smoking may cause coughing and start bleeding. Although normally the sputum may be streaked with blood for a few days after a biopsy, any pronounced bleeding is reported at once to the physician.

Mediastinoscopy

In mediastinoscopy a *mediastinoscope,* which is an instrument much like a bronchoscope, is inserted through a small incision in the suprasternal notch and advanced into the mediastinum where inspection and biopsy of the lymph nodes can then be carried out. Consult the article by Klause[17] for further information.

Lung scan (pulmonary scintiphotography)

Lung scan procedures involve the use of a scanning device that records the pattern of pulmonary radioactivity after the inhalation or intravenous injection of gamma ray–emitting radionuclides, thus providing a visual image of the distribution of ventilation or blood flow in the lungs. These studies provide valuable information regarding *ventilation-perfusion patterns* and aid in the diagnosis of parenchymal lung diseases and vascular disorders such as pulmonary embolism.

Thoracentesis

Thoracentesis involves the insertion of a needle into the pleural space and aspiration of fluid for either diagnostic or therapeutic purposes. Biopsy specimens of the pleura may also be obtained by the use of needles specially constructed with a cutting edge and a mechanism for retaining the biopsy specimen. When thoracentesis is done for diagnostic purposes, the fluid may be examined for specific gravity, white blood cell count, differential cell count, red blood cell count, protein, glucose, and amylase concentrations. The fluid may also be cultured and checked for the presence of abnormal or malignant cells. The gross appearance of the fluid, the quantity obtained, and the location of the site of the thoracentesis should be recorded.

When a thoracentesis is to be done, the procedure is explained to the patient. It is necessary that the patient understand the importance of not moving when the needle is inserted to avoid damage to the lung or pleura. Usually a local anesthetic such as procaine or lidocaine is used to eliminate pain at the site of insertion of the needle. However, when the pleura is entered, a sensation of pain or pressure may occur. Whenever possible, the patient should be in an upright position, either sitting on the side of the bed with the feet supported and arms and head on a padded overbed table or straddling a chair with the arms and head resting on the back of the chair. This position with arms and shoulders raised elevates the ribs and makes it easier to carry out the procedure. Patients who cannot sit up are turned onto the unaffected side so that the side to be tapped is uppermost.

Vital signs (pulse, respiration, and blood pressure) are taken several times during the procedure, and the patient is monitored for changes in color and character of respirations and the presence of diaphoresis. The needle and syringe should be carefully checked to see that they fit snugly so that no air is permitted to enter the pleural space. Fluid may be aspirated directly into the syringe, or a three-way adaptor may be used with one end attached to tubing leading to a receptacle into which the fluid is drained. Specimens are placed in the appropriate containers and labeled according to the examinations ordered by the physician. Following a thoracentesis the patient is watched for signs of coughing or expectoration of blood, since these signs might indicate that the lung was traumatized inadvertently. (For details on the equipment needed, see texts on fundamentals of nursing.)

REFERENCES AND SELECTED REFERENCES

1. Alexander, M.M., and Brown, M.S.: Physical examination. XII. Chest and lungs, Nurs. '75 **5**(1):44-48, 1975.
2. *American Lung Association: Introduction to lung diseases, New York, 1973, The Association.
3. *Bates, B.: A guide to physical examination, ed. 2, Philadelphia, 1979, J.B. Lippincott Co.
4. Beeson, P., McDermott, W., and Wyngaarden, J., editors: Textbook of medicine, ed. 15, Philadelphia, 1979, W.B. Saunders Co.
5. *Blood-gas and acid-base concepts in respiratory care: programmed instruction, Am. J. Nurs. **76**:963-992, 1977.
6. Bouhuys, A.: The physiology of breathing, New York, 1977, Grune & Stratton, Inc.
7. *Broughton, J.: Chest physical diagnosis for nurses and respiratory therapists, Heart Lung **2**:200-206, 1972.

8. *Cohen, S.: Pulmonary function tests in patient care: programmed instruction, Am. J. Nurs. **80**:1135-1161, 1980.
9. Comroe, J.H.: Physiology of respiration, ed. 2, Chicago, 1974, Year Book Medical Publishers, Inc.
10. Delaney, M.T.: Examining the chest. I. The lungs, Nurs. '75 **5**(8):12-14, 1975.
11. Demers, R.R., and Saklad, M.: Fundamentals of blood gas interpretation, Respir. Care **18**:153-159, 1973.
12. Finch, C.M., and Lenfant, C.: Oxygen transport in man, N. Engl. J. Med. **286**:407-415, 1972.
13. *Foley, M.F.: Pulmonary function testing, Am. J. Nurs. **71**:1134-1139, 1971.
14. *Hudak, C.M., Gallo, B.M., and Lohr, R., editors: Critical care nursing, ed. 2, Philadelphia, 1977, J.B. Lippincott Co.
15. Keyes, J.L.: Blood gas analysis and the assessment of acid-base status, Heart Lung **5**:247-255, 1976.
16. Keyes, J.L.: Blood gases and blood gas transport, Heart Lung **3**:945-954, 1974.
17. Klause, M.L.: Mediastinoscopy, A.O.R.N. J. **15**:55-59, 1972.
18. Malasanos, L., et al.: Health assessment, ed. 2, St. Louis, 1981, The C.V. Mosby Co.
19. *Phipps, W.J., Barker, W.L., and Daly, B.J.: Respiratory insufficiency and failure. In Meltzer, L.E., Abdellah, R.G., and Kitchell, J.F.: Concepts and practices of intensive care for nurse specialists, ed. 2, Bowie, Md., 1976, The Charles Press.
20. Shapiro, B.A., Harrison, R.A., and Trout, C.A.: Clinical application of respiratory care, ed. 2, Bowie, Md., 1979, The Charles Press.
21. Simmons, D.H.: Evaluation of acid-base status. In American Thoracic Society: Basics of RD, New York, 1974, The Society.
22. Slonim, N.B., and Hamilton, L.H.: Respiratory physiology, ed. 4, St. Louis, 1981, The C.V. Mosby Co.
23. *Tinker, J.H.: Understanding chest x-rays, Am. J. Nurs. **76**:54-58, 1976.
24. *Thompson, J., and Bowers, A.: Clinical manual of health assessment, St. Louis, 1980, The C.V. Mosby Co.
25. Traver, G.A.: Respiratory nursing: the science and the art, New York, 1982, John Wiley & Sons, Inc.
26. *Traver, G.: The nurses' role in clinical testing of lung function, Nurs. Clin. North Am. **9**:101-110, 1974.
27. *Traver, G.: Assessment of thorax and lungs, Am. J. Nurs. **73**:466-471, 1973.
28. Wade, J.F.: Respiratory nursing care: physiology and technique, ed. 2, St. Louis, 1977, The C.V. Mosby Co.
29. Winslow, E.H.: Visual inspection of the patient with cardiopulmonary disease, Heart Lung **4**:421-429, 1975.

*References preceded by an asterisk are particularly well suited for student reading.

CHAPTER 49

INTERVENTION FOR THE PERSON WITH A RESPIRATORY PROBLEM

WILMA J. PHIPPS
BARBARA J. DALY

In order for breathing to take place normally several factors are necessary: (1) an adequate supply of oxygen in the environment, (2) a patent airway, (3) normal functioning bellows motion of the chest wall and diaphragm, (4) an adequate number of functioning alveoli and capillaries that together form a terminal respiratory unit (TRU), (5) an adequate amount of hemoglobin to carry oxygen to the cells, (6) an intact circulatory system and an effective heart pump, and (7) a functioning respiratory center. Problems in one or more of the above can result in inadequate exchange of oxygen and carbon dioxide and, if severe enough, can cause death. Table 49-1 lists some of the conditions that can lead to inadequate oxygen–carbon dioxide exchange.

Prevention

Prevention of conditions that impair oxygen–carbon dioxide exchange requires that health care providers be aware of the factors that cause problems and try to prevent their occurrence. Prevention involves teaching the public about certain hazards, such as the need to become acclimated to high altitudes before engaging in other than minimal activities, and working with parents and others who have contact with toddlers to emphasize the need to keep the environment free of small objects that could be aspirated by curious youngsters who have a tendency to put everything in their mouths.

Because of the deleterious effects of cigarette smoking on the cardiopulmonary systems, a concerted effort is indicated to teach persons about the hazards of smoking. In addition, the prevention of pulmonary infections requires that all persons understand how pulmonary infections are spread and what they can do to keep from acquiring frequent infections.

Many conditions that affect oxygen–carbon dioxide exchange may be difficult to prevent, but the nurse has a major role to play in preventing the airway of an unconscious person from becoming obstructed and in recognizing complications, such as atelectasis, congestive heart failure, pulmonary edema, and cardiac or pulmonary arrest, that require immediate intervention if adequate oxygenation is to be provided.

The interventions needed to maintain adequate tissue oxygenation are discussed in the following sections.

Interventions

Maintaining an adequate supply of oxygen in the environment

The major nursing emphasis in maintaining an adequate supply of oxygen is on prevention. One of the major interferences with oxygen in the environment is smoke inhalation. Here the emphasis must be on fire prevention and what to do if a fire occurs. In addition, the public needs to be reminded of the benefits of having smoke alarms in their homes. Some communities have local ordinances that require that all homes and apartments have smoke alarms. Since smoke alarms can now be purchased more cheaply, they should be within the means of most persons.

TABLE 49-1. Factors interfering with oxygenation and normal oxygen–carbon dioxide exchange

Necessary component	Interference
Adequate supply of oxygen	Inhalation of air containing oxygen at subnormal pressure caused by:
	Smoke inhalation
	Carbon monoxide poisoning
	High altitudes
	Dilution of inspired air with inert gases (nitrogen, helium, hydrogen, methane, or anesthetic gases such as nitrous oxide)
Patent airway	Interference with the passage of oxygen from air through tracheobronchial tree to alveolar-capillary membrane caused by mechanical obstruction such as drowning, foreign bodies in tracheobronchial tree:
	Children (aspiration of objects such as pennies, pins, jacks)
	Unconscious adults (tongue obstructing airway, aspirated vomitus, loose dentures)
	Mucus plug resulting in atelectasis
	Allergic reactions resulting in bronchoconstriction, increased mucus secretions, and increased capillary permeability
Normally functioning bellows	Trauma to chest wall with possible sequelae of paradoxical breathing, pneumothorax, mediastinal shift
	Muscle or nerve trauma or impairment (quadriplegia, paraplegia, poliomyelitis, myasthenia gravis, Guillain-Barré-Strohl syndrome, Landry ascending paralysis, muscular dystrophy)
Adequate functioning alveoli and capillaries (TRU)	Pulmonary edema
	Adult respiratory disease syndrome (interstitial edema)
	Physiologic shunts
	Damage to alveolar-capillary membrane secondary to conditions such as pulmonary emphysema
Adequate amount of hemo-globin	Severe anemia
	Carbon monoxide poisoning
	Methemoglobinemia
Intact circulatory system and pump	Congestive heart failure
	Hemorrhage
Functioning respiratory center	Depression of respiratory center by drugs (heroin, morphine, barbiturates, alcohol, or a combination of alcohol with a tranquilizer or barbiturates)
	Increased intracranial pressure (head injury or disease such as meningitis)

Carbon monoxide poisoning is a cause of both accidental death and suicide. The public needs to be reminded about the dangers of running the motor of an automobile in a closed garage. They also need to understand the danger of driving a car with a faulty exhaust system with all the car windows closed.

High altitudes do not change the composition of the air, but the oxygen pressure (PO_2) decreases.[53] Persons exposed to high altitudes, such as pilots, astronauts, mountain climbers, and those moving to high altitudes, will have various reactions depending on the rate at which hypoxia develops, the degree of oxygen requirements as determined by physical exertion, and the duration of exposure.[53]

The initial reaction to high altitudes results in the same signs and symptoms as seen in anyone experiencing oxygen lack. Headache, dizziness, breathlessness, weakness, nausea, sweating, palpitation, dimness of vision, partial deafness, and sleeplessness occur with moderate hypoxia.[53] With exertion, dyspnea and other symptoms worsen. These signs and symptoms have been referred to as *mountain sickness* since they are evident as persons drive through or take a train through higher altitudes than they have been accustomed to.

These symptoms gradually disappear over days or weeks depending on the altitude, and the person will be able to carry out more activities without becoming short of breath. This is known as *acclimatization* and is caused in part by an increased capacity for supplying oxygen to the tissues and in part by overcoming the consequences of hypocapnia produced by excessive breathing.[53]

The factors involved in acclimatization include (1) a sustained increase in alveolar ventilation, (2) adjustment in the acid-base composition of the blood and other body fluids, (3) an increase in oxygen-carrying capacity, and (4) an increase in cardiac output.[53]

Persons moving to higher climates, such as mountain climbers, are advised to allow time for their bodies to adjust to changes in various altitudes. Trained climbers, especially those ascending to very high altitudes, allow themselves weeks or even months at base camps at various altitudes in preparation for their ascent.[53]

Maintaining a patent airway

Several measures may be used to ensure a patent airway. The most basic one involves simply positioning the person in such a way as to prevent obstruction of the airway. This is most relevant in resuscitations or in caring for an unconscious person. The position of choice is supine or side-lying with the neck hyperextended. Persons who are unconscious or very lethargic may suffer airway obstruction if the tongue is allowed to fall back and cover the glottis; the side-lying position prevents this from happening (see Fig. 24-9).

When a person has a mechanical obstruction of the airway and is expected to be unconscious for some time, it may be necessary to use an artificial airway.

Types of artificial airways

An endotracheal tube is usually chosen initially as a means of providing the airway; tracheostomy is only performed if airway maintenance is necessary for a prolonged period of time or if trauma to the airway prevents the use of an endotracheal tube. Although the tracheostomy has the *disadvantage* of a higher risk of infection, it is often elected for airway management because it is much more comfortable than an endotracheal tube and allows the person to eat.

In endotracheal intubation a tube is passed through either the nose or mouth into the trachea, while in a tracheostomy an artificial opening is made in the trachea into which a tube is inserted (Fig. 49-1). These procedures are used (1) to establish and maintain a patent airway, (2) to prevent aspiration by sealing off the trachea from the digestive tract in the unconscious or paralyzed person, (3) to permit removal of tracheobronchial secretions in the person who cannot cough adequately, and (4) to treat the patient who requires positive pressure ventilation that cannot be given effectively by mask.[73] Whether an intubation or a tracheostomy is performed initially depends on the facilities available and the wishes of the physician. Most physicians now consider it safer to do an emergency endotracheal intubation and then perform a tracheostomy as a nonemergency procedure in the operating room if prolonged support of the airway is needed. In this instance the endotracheal tube is not removed until after the tracheostomy opening is made.

A tracheostomy is necessary when an endotracheal tube cannot be inserted or when it is contraindicated, as in severe burns or laryngeal obstruction caused by tumor, infection, or vocal cord paralysis.[73] Tracheostomy may also be required when a patient is conscious and cannot tolerate an endotracheal tube. Once the airway is secured either by intubation or by tracheostomy, secretions are aspirated and well-humidified oxygen is usually given. If the patient is unable to sustain respi-

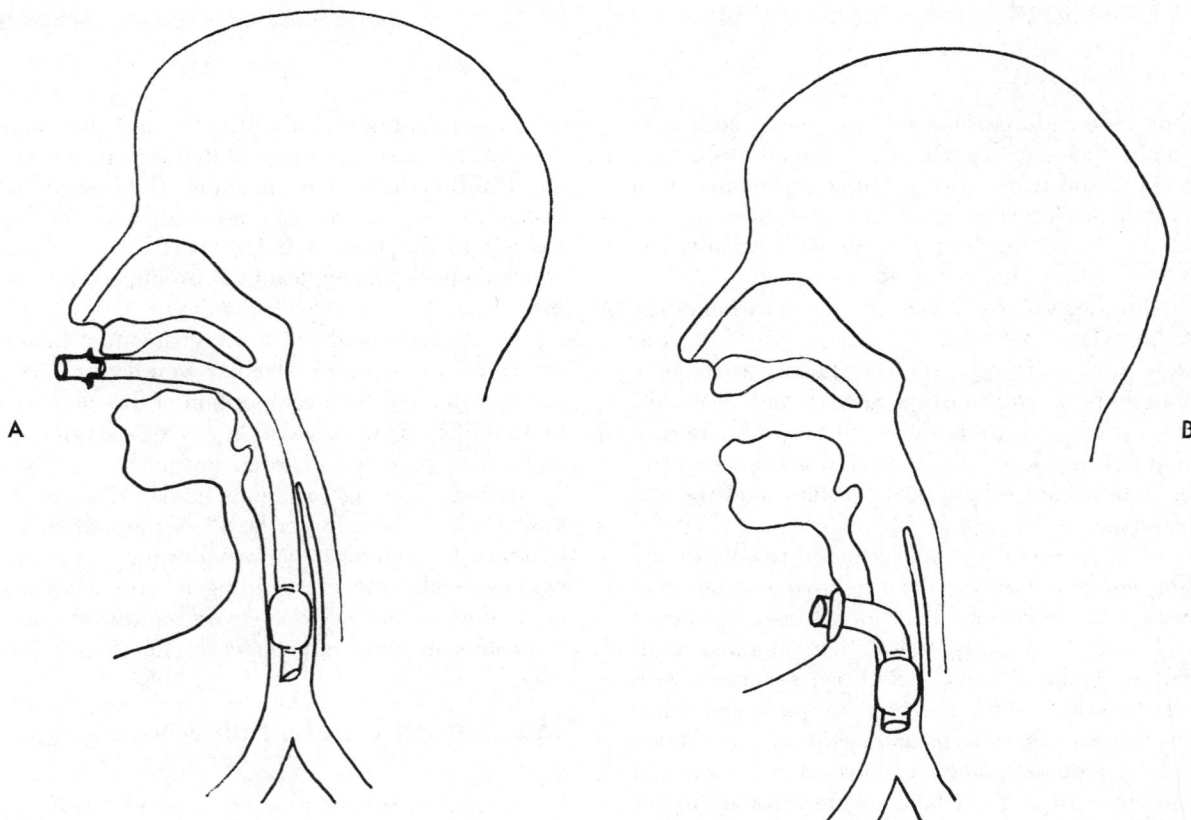

Fig. 49-1. A, Position of endotracheal tube. **B,** Position of tracheostomy tube.

ration, a mechanical ventilator (e.g., a Bennett or a Bird ventilator) is attached to either the endotracheal tube or the tracheostomy tube. When mechanical ventilation is required, a cuffed tube is used. Usually an endotracheal tube is not left in place longer than 5 to 7 days. If the patient is unable to maintain a free airway after this period of time, a tracheostomy is performed.

The endotracheal tube may be made of either plastic or rubber with an inflatable cuff so that a closed system with the ventilator may be maintained (Fig. 49-2).

The tube is inserted via the mouth or nose through the larynx into the trachea. If an oral endotracheal tube is used, a rubber airway or bite block is often necessary to prevent the patient from biting down on the tube and obstructing the airway.

The tracheostomy tube is usually made of plastic, silver, or nylon. It may be either a single-lumen or double-lumen (Jackson) type (Fig. 49-3). Both types of tubes may be cuffed, and the newer plastic tubes come with high-volume, low-pressure cuffs that are less likely

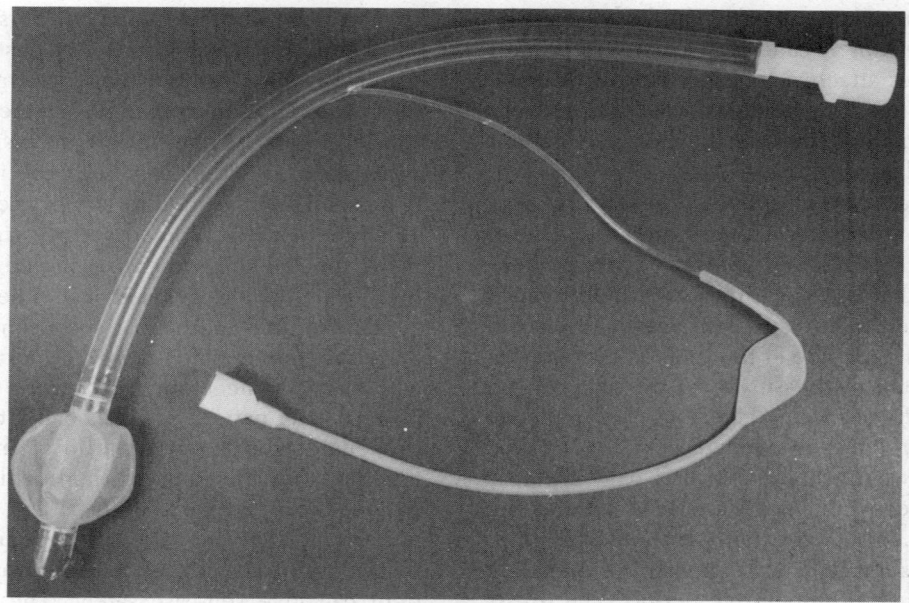

Fig. 49-2. Forregar high-volume, low-pressure cuffed endotracheal tube. Cuff shown here is not inflated. Low-pressure cuff is preferred because it is less likely to cause tracheal damage.

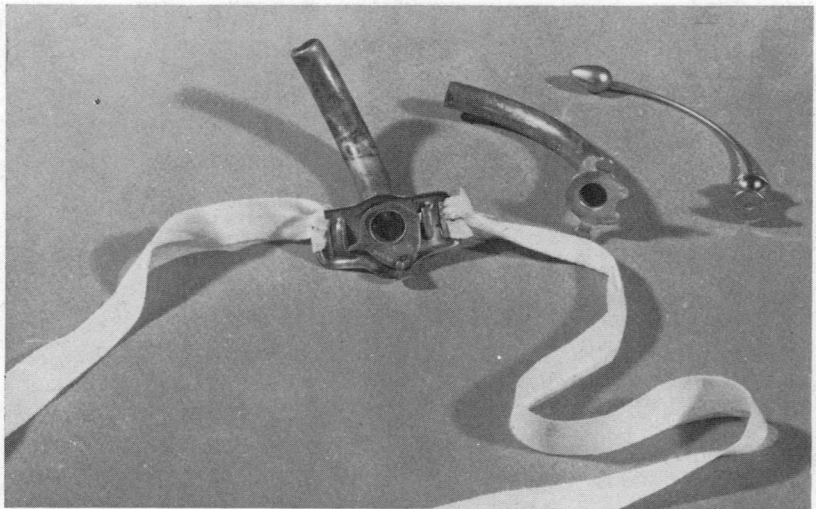

Fig. 49-3. Parts of silver tracheostomy tube: outer tube with ties attached, inner tube, and pilot. (From DeWeese, D.D., and Saunders, W.H.: Textbook of otolaryngology, ed. 6, St. Louis, 1982, The C.V. Mosby Co.)

to cause damage to the trachea (Fig. 49-4). Single-lumen tubes must be changed about every 72 hours, since they are more difficult to clean and more likely to become plugged than are double-lumen tubes.

Silver tubes are commonly available in sizes nos. 00 to 8 (no. 00 is used for the premature or newborn infant, while a no. 6 or 7 is used for most adults). The silver tracheostomy tube consists of two parts, an inner and an outer cannula. The outer cannula is removed only by the physician, while the inner cannula is removed regularly by the nurse for cleaning. The silver tracheostomy tube has a lock that must be turned in order to remove the inner cannula. The lock should be secured when the inner cannula is reinserted after cleaning. Twill tapes attached to either side of the tube (Fig. 49-3) are tied securely behind the neck to prevent the tube from becoming dislodged when the patient coughs or moves about.

Should the tube be coughed out, the opening may close and the patient will be unable to breathe. Therefore a tracheal dilator or curved hemostat is always kept at the bedside so that the opening can be held open if the tube is dislodged. Some surgeons prefer to place a retention suture on each side of the tracheostomy opening and tape the end of the suture to the skin. If the opening shows signs of closing, tension can be placed on the sutures to widen the opening.

The operative wound may be sealed with a plastic spray, or a small dressing may be placed around the tracheostomy tube. Although drainage should be minimal, the wound is inspected frequently for bleeding during the immediate postoperative period. The dressings are changed as they become soiled with drainage

of mucus. Occasionally, young children require elbow restraints to prevent them from removing the tube or putting objects into it.

Immediately after insertion of the endotracheal tube and periodically thereafter the chest is auscultated to ensure that there are breath sounds on both sides. If a cuffed tube is inserted too far, it will slip into one of the main-stem bronchi (usually the right) and occlude the opposite bronchus and lung, resulting in atelectasis on the obstructed side. Even if the tube is still in the trachea, airway obstruction will result if the end of the tube is located on the carina (area at lower end of trachea at point of bifurcation of main-stem bronchi). This will result in dry secretions that obstruct both bronchi. Although these complications are more common with the use of an endotracheal tube, they can occur with a tracheostomy tube, especially in a small person with a short neck. In either case the tube is pulled back until it is positioned below the larynx and above the carina. The tube is then fastened securely in place. A replacement tube of the same size should always be kept at the bedside in the event that it is needed.

Depending on the patient's condition, a tracheostomy can be either temporary or permanent; the person who has a laryngectomy will have a permanent tracheostomy. Any patient who has had a tracheostomy is apprehensive and is often fearful of choking. Thus when feasible, the procedure is thoroughly explained to the patient before surgery. Both patient and family need to understand that the patient will be unable to speak and that constant attendance will be provided until the patient can give self-care safely. The nurse should plan with the patient for some means of communication after

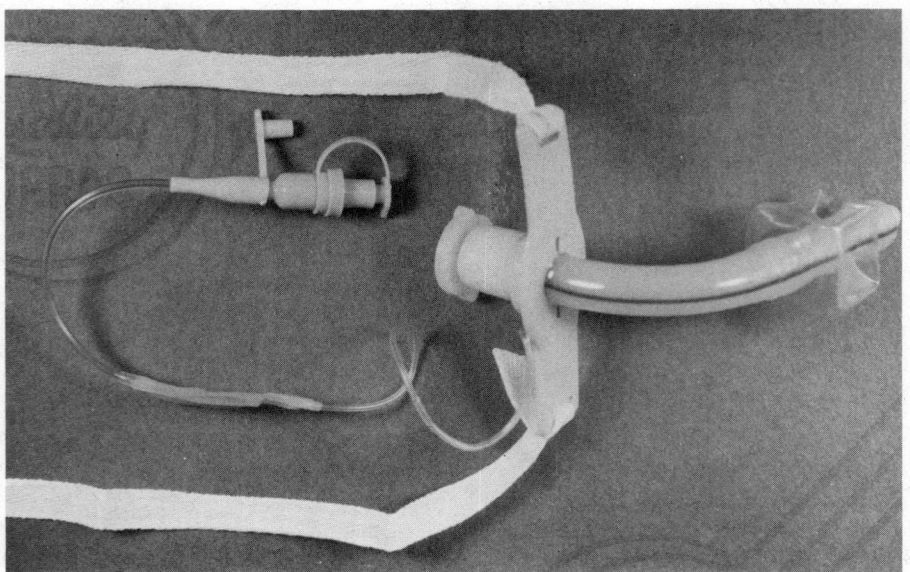

Fig. 49-4. Portex high-volume, low-pressure cuffed tracheostomy tube.

the surgery. Hand signs such as the OK sign or a raised finger might be used as a means of expressing, for example, the need to void. The patient may want to write on a pad or a Magic Slate, or a word or picture chart can be used. The patient's ideas about means of communication should be considered. Patients should have their bell cords within reach, and a tap bell is reassuring to some patients.

Care of a person with a cuffed tube. The use of a cuffed endotracheal or tracheostomy tube has several implications for nursing care. Although the advent of low-pressure cuffs has significantly lowered the incidence of tracheal erosion and necrosis from pressure on the wall of the trachea, there are still some hazards inherent in the use of artificial airways.

The cuff on the tube is used to maintain a closed system (Fig. 49-4) that will permit positive pressure ventilation. It is also used to prevent aspiration of secretions by the unconscious person. Sometimes the cuff is used to exert pressure on bleeding sites in patients who have undergone throat or neck surgery, such as a radical neck dissection. If none of these considerations apply, the cuff does not need to be inflated.

If the patient is being mechanically ventilated, the cuff should be inflated during the positive pressure phase (inspiration) of the ventilator. Two different methods may be used to inflate the cuff, depending on the patient's condition and the preference of those responsible for care. In the first method, air is injected into the cuff until a full seal is attained. At this point a pressure-cycled respirator will turn off and no air will escape around the tube or through the nose and mouth. The tubing leading to the cuff is then clamped. In the other method, air is injected until a full seal is attained, and then 0.5 ml of air is withdrawn and the tubing clamped. This latter method creates a partial leak for which the respirator can be set to compensate. The nurse should note the amount of air needed to inflate the cuff and use the smallest amount required to attain a seal. Overinflation of the cuff is extremely dangerous because it can lead to the development of tracheomalacia, tracheal stenosis, tracheoesophageal fistula, or erosion through a major blood vessel.

In the past it had been recommended that the cuff be routinely deflated for several minutes each hour in order to prevent tracheal necrosis. This is not necessary with low-pressure cuffs. It is sufficient to deflate the cuff and reinflate it once every 8 hours. This is necessary to ensure that the cuff is not overinflated and to check for tracheal dilation, indicated by the requirement of progressively larger amounts of air in order to obtain a seal.

It is important to remember that speaking is impossible with a cuffed tube in place because air does not pass directly through the larynx. The person is informed that speech will be normal when the tube is removed. Persons who are not informed of the change in function may believe that they have permanently lost their ability to speak.

Often the person with a tracheostomy tube can speak when the cuff is not fully inflated. Speech is still difficult since air must be forced around the tube and up through the larynx. For those who can tolerate it, it is often helpful to obstruct the opening of the tracheostomy tube while the cuff is deflated. This allows the person to breathe through the upper airway. See discussion of means of communication provided for the patient who cannot speak.

SUCTIONING THE TUBE. All persons with tubes require suctioning and should be suctioned as often as necessary. The frequency of suctioning is a nursing judgment. Many patients in respiratory failure have an infection and accumulation of secretions before intubation or tracheostomy is performed. Once the patient is intubated, the tube produces a natural route for introduction of bacteria into the lower airway, increasing the risk of infection. Much of the ability to produce an effective cough is lost, since it is impossible for the person to build up the pressure needed to create an expulsive cough. Because the patient has difficulty moving secretions up the tracheobronchial tree, it is important to suction as deeply as possible. The depth to which a catheter can be inserted through an *endotracheal tube* in an adult is approximately 45 to 55 cm (18 to 22 in.). Postural drainage with percussion and vibration (p. 1239) is extremely helpful in moving secretions up to a point where they can be suctioned.

If the catheter cannot be inserted as far as usual, a mucus plug may be obstructing passage of the catheter. Saline irrigation (approximately 5 to 10 ml) will often liquefy the obstructing secretions so they can be aspirated. When plastic suction catheters and plastic tubes are used, it is not uncommon for the surface of the catheter and tube to stick to each other, inhibiting passage of the catheter. Instilling 1 to 2 ml of sterile saline solution during insertion of the catheter usually prevents this problem.

Care of the person with a tracheostomy. Analgesics and sedatives are given judiciously so as not to depress the respiratory center. The patient is suctioned as often as necessary, possibly every 5 minutes during the first few postoperative hours. The need for suctioning can be determined by the sound of the air coming from the tracheostomy tube, especially after the patient takes a deep breath. When respirations are noisy and pulse and respiratory rates are increased, the patient needs to be suctioned. Patients who are conscious can usually indicate when they need to be suctioned. With any sign of respiratory distress, the tube should be suctioned. If mucus is blocking the inner cannula of a silver tube and cannot be removed by suction, the inner cannula is removed to open the airway. When the mucus is thick, the inner cannula should be cleaned and replaced at once because the outer tube may also become blocked. If, despite these measures, the patient becomes cyanotic, the physician should be summoned at once. A patient who is able to cough up secretions probably will require suctioning less frequently. The amount of mucus subsides gradually and the patient eventually may go for several hours without being suctioned. However, even when secretions are minimal, the patient is apprehensive and needs constant attendance.

Suctioning technique needs to be carefully performed in order to prevent damage to the tracheobronchial mucosa. Some of the problems associated with suctioning are discussed in more detail in various sources.[36,45,73,81] The purpose of the following section is to provide detailed guidelines about how to suction the tracheostomy tube efficiently and safely.

SUCTIONING THE TRACHEOSTOMY TUBE. The aim in suctioning is to remove all secretions that have accumulated in the tracheobronchial tree since the last suctioning. In general, suctioning techniques are the same no matter what type of tracheostomy tube is in use. However, silver tubes have both an inner and an outer cannula, while plastic tubes have only one cannula. Physicians vary in their preference as to the type of tube used. Some otolaryngologists prefer that only metal tubes with an inner cannula be used because they believe that they are safer. When a double-lumen tube is used, the inner cannula can readily be removed for suc-

tioning and cleaning, whereas tubes without an inner cannula may have to be completely removed and replaced should they become plugged with secretions. This can usually be prevented, however, by adequate humidification and frequent suctioning. The following guidelines apply to the suctioning of any type of tracheostomy tube.

1. Sterile technique is mandatory; sterile gloves or forceps and a sterile catheter are used for suctioning. In some hospitals, clean rather than sterile technique is believed to be sufficient when suctioning patients with a *permanent tracheostomy* who will be caring for their own tubes after they go home (Fig. 49-5). In the clean technique the hands are washed well with soap or pHisoHex before suctioning.

2. The catheter must be of a small enough size that it does not occlude the cannula (one half to two thirds the diameter of the tube). Commonly, when a silver-tube is suctioned, a no. 8 or 10 catheter is used for children, and a no. 14 or 16 for adults.

3. A sterile catheter is used each time the tube is suctioned.

4. Before beginning suctioning, the patient is hyperoxygenated with 100% oxygen. An Ambu bag or anesthesia bag with attached oxygen is held lightly over the face, and the patient is instructed to take five or six deep breaths. Preoxygenation with 100% oxygen is necessary since oxygen will be removed during suctioning. If the PO_2 falls in a patient with an already reduced

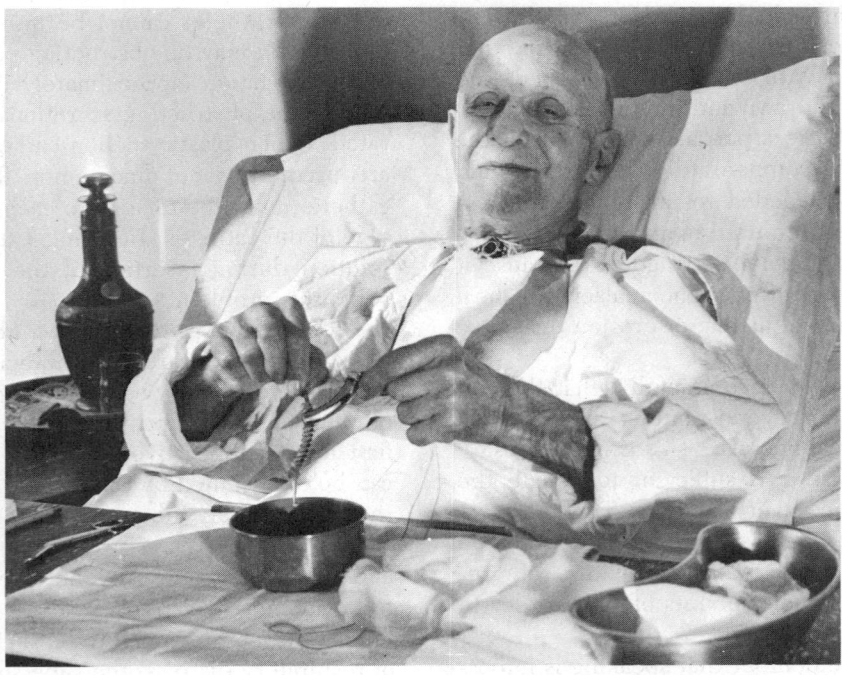

Fig. 49-5. This 82-year-old man cares for his own tracheostomy tube. He is about to clean inner tube with small tube brush. (From Anderson, H.C.: Newton's geriatric nursing, ed. 5, St. Louis, 1971, The C.V. Mosby Co.)

PO_2, cardiac arrhythmias such as ectopic beats and bradycardia may occur.

5. A fenestrated catheter with a whistle tip is attached to the suction machine. If a nonfenestrated catheter is used, it is connected to the suction machine with a Y tube. The catheter is always inserted without suction. Once the catheter is in place, suction is applied by placing the thumb over the fenestration in the catheter or over the open end of the Y tube (Fig. 49-6).

6. The suction catheter is lubricated with water or a water-soluble lubricant and is inserted deep enough into the bronchus to stimulate coughing. Unless otherwise ordered, the recommended depth through the tracheostomy tube is 20 to 30 cm (8 to 12 in.) since this permits removal of secretions lying beyond the tip of the cannula. If the patient coughs, the catheter is removed because its presence obstructs the trachea and the patient must exert extra pressure to cough around it. As coughing occurs, the nurse or the patient should have tissues ready to receive mucus, which may be ejected with force. When the patient coughs, the tracheostomy tube is held in place, since it could come out with vigorous coughing.

7. If mucus is tenacious and difficult to remove, sterile saline solution may be instilled into the tube just before suctioning. From 5 to 15 ml is commonly ordered.

8. Although some clinicians recommend that the patient's head and shoulders be turned to the right when suctioning the left bronchus and vice versa, there is no objective evidence that this technique improves suctioning the desired bronchus. In most patients the right main-stem bronchus is easier to enter anatomically and thus is suctioned more often than the left bronchus. The catheter is rotated as it is withdrawn with suction on.

9. To prevent hypoxia, the patient must *not* be suctioned longer than 10 to 15 seconds at a time, the patient should rest 3 minutes between aspirations, and 100% oxygen should be administered between suctionings. If secretions are interfering with breathing, suctioning may have to be more frequent.

10. The inner cannula of a silver tube is removed for cleaning every 2 to 8 hours, depending on the amount and consistency of secretions. If mucus collects and partially obstructs the lumen, it may be necessary to clean the inner cannula even more often than every 2 hours. Sterile water, detergent solution, pipe cleaners, and a small test-tube brush are used for cleaning. Hot water is not used because it coagulates mucus. The tube may be soaked in a solution of half-strength hydrogen peroxide to soften congealed secretions. The tube is inspected to see that all mucus has been removed. Gauze can be threaded through it to extract excess secretions and solution. Before reinserting the inner tube, the outer tube is suctioned.

AIR HUMIDIFICATION. Because the insertion of the endotracheal or tracheostomy tube bypasses the upper airway, the patient's ability to humidify and warm in-

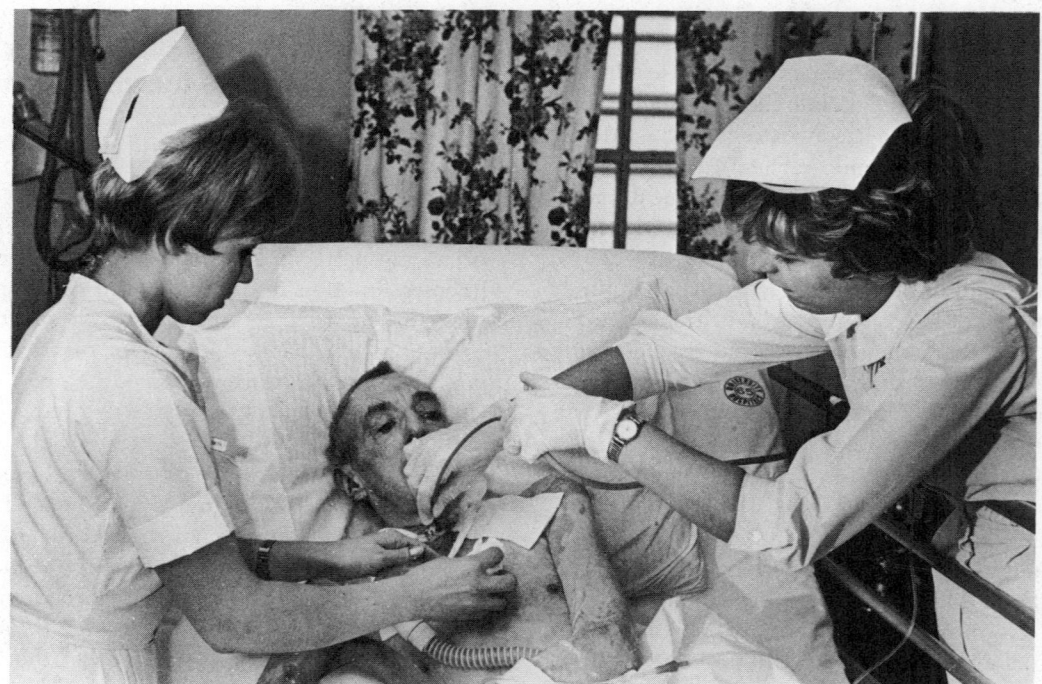

Fig. 49-6. Nurse is wearing sterile gloves and using **Y** tube attachment to suction patient's tracheostomy tube. (Courtesy Medical-World News.)

spired air is lost. Therefore whether the patient is on or off the respirator, the inspired air should be heated and humidified to prevent mucosal irritation and drying of secretions. *Large-bore* tubing is needed to provide this mist, since water particles will condense in *small-bore* tubing. A noticeable difference in the viscosity of secretions is evident in patients who do not receive mist for even as short a period as 30 minutes. Other important nursing care measures and observations vary with the route of intubation—via the larynx or from below the larynx. The patient who has an endotracheal tube in place usually has an increased volume of oropharyngeal secretions because of irritation from the tube. The patient also has great difficulty in swallowing (especially if an oral tube is used), necessitating frequent oropharyngeal suctioning.

NOURISHMENT. The patient with an endotracheal tube is allowed nothing by mouth. Nourishment will be given intravenously or by nasogastric tube feedings. The patient with a tracheostomy tube in place is usually able to swallow and have a normal oral intake. Some experts prefer that the cuff on the tracheostomy tube be inflated while the patient is eating to prevent aspiration. Others believe that the inflated cuff bulges into the esophagus and makes swallowing more difficult, and they therefore prefer the cuff to be deflated. Nursing assessment will determine which technique to use. In determining if the patient aspirates food, it is often helpful to feed the patient red gelatin. The consistency of gelatin makes it easier to swallow than water, and the red color makes it easy to detect if aspirated into the lower airway.

COMPLICATIONS. Both a tracheostomy tube and an endotracheal tube have a direct effect on the airway, but the potential damage of an endotracheal tube is more extensive than that of the tracheostomy tube. Movement with rubbing of the endotracheal tube may produce laryngeal erosion and damage to the vocal cords. There is also the danger of laryngeal edema when the tube is removed. The nurse must be alert to signs of laryngeal stridor and upper airway obstruction. If upper airway obstruction occurs, reintubation or tracheostomy is necessary. With both endotracheal and tracheostomy tubes, tracheal stenosis may result from irritation and scarring at the cuff site. Conscientious nursing care can often prevent this complication.

An additional consideration after the removal of a tracheostomy tube is assisting the patient to cough effectively. When an endotracheal tube is removed, the normal airway is restored and the patient is usually able to cough without difficulty. However, when a tracheostomy tube is removed, there is an air leak at the incision site. This air leak prevents the buildup of intrathoracic pressures high enough to produce an effective cough until the incision is healed. The patient can be taught to place two or three fingers firmly over the

dressing that covers the tracheostomy site to reduce the air leak. If this is not successful in helping to generate a cough that clears the airway, the stoma can be suctioned. Frequent use of the stoma for suctioning, however, can delay closure and healing of the tracheostomy incision.

PERSONS DISCHARGED WITH A TRACHEOSTOMY. Persons to be discharged with a tube in place are taught to care for and change the tube while in the hospital. A mirror will be necessary to do this procedure, which may be begun a few days after surgery.

Patients who go home with the tracheostomy tube still in place must be provided with necessary supplies or with instructions as to where to secure them and with knowledge of how to care for themselves. They should have suction equipment. Suction machines can be rented for home use or obtained in many communities through the local chapter of the American Cancer Society. Suction can be provided by attaching a suction hose to a water faucet. Many hardware stores carry the necessary equipment. The amount of suction is controlled by the stream of water.

Persons who have a permanent tracheostomy must take some special precautions. They must not go swimming and must be careful while bathing or taking a shower that water is not aspirated through the opening into the lungs. They are advised to wear a scarf or a shirt with a closed collar that covers the opening, yet is of porous material. This material substitutes for some functions normally assumed by nasal passages, such as the warming of air and the screening out of dust and other irritating substances.

Maintaining bellows function of the chest wall and diaphragm

Whenever there is interference with the bellows function of the chest wall, there will be changes in the breathing pattern. The major cause of disruption of the bellows function is trauma to the chest involving fractures of the ribs or penetrating chest wounds. These conditions and their sequelae of paradoxical breathing and pneumothorax are discussed below.

Chest trauma

Trauma to the chest is a major problem most often seen first in the emergency department. The injuries to the chest range from a few fractured ribs to major trauma to the chest wall, sternum, lungs, heart, and major blood vessels. Injuries to the chest are broadly classified into two groups—blunt and penetrating. *Blunt* or nonpenetrating injuries include fractures of the ribs in which there is no damage to the pleura and lung. These injuries occur most commonly as the result of automobile accidents, falls, or blast injuries. Automobile accidents in the United States kill approximately 45,000 persons each year. Of this number, 40% have a major thoracic injury.[67] The injury is most often sustained when striking the steering wheel or being hurled from the car.

Fractures of the ribs. The fourth, fifth, sixth, seventh, and eighth ribs are most commonly fractured. Fractures of the ribs are caused by blows, crushing injuries, or strain caused by severe coughing or sneezing spells. If the rib is splintered or the fracture displaced, sharp fragments may penetrate the pleura and the lung. Persons with possible rib fractures should have an x-ray examination of the chest and should be observed carefully for signs of pneumothorax or hemothorax. The person with a rib fracture complains of pain at the site of the injury that increases on inspiration. The area is very tender to the touch, and the individual splints the chest and takes shallow breaths. Unless the lung has been penetrated, the usual treatment for rib fracture is conservative and includes strapping the chest with adhesive tape from the affected side to the unaffected side

or applying a circular strapping, using an Ace bandage. A chest binder also may be used. If adhesive tape is used, the skin may be shaved and painted with tincture of benzoin to prevent blistering and other irritation. When the pain is severe and is not relieved by strapping and analgesic medications, the physician may do a regional nerve block. This procedure consists of infiltrating the intercostal spaces above and below the fractured rib with 1% procaine. If the lung has been penetrated, the person may raise bright red sputum.

PARADOXICAL BREATHING. When ribs are fractured in more than one place, the chest wall on that side becomes unstable and the result is a *flail chest*. Thus the chest wall no longer provides the rigid bony support that is necessary to maintain the bellows function required for normal ventilation. This causes paradoxical breathing. In paradoxical breathing the portion of the lung underlying the unstable chest wall moves opposite to the remainder of the lung (Fig. 49-7, *C* and *D*). On inspiration that portion of the lung sucks in while the

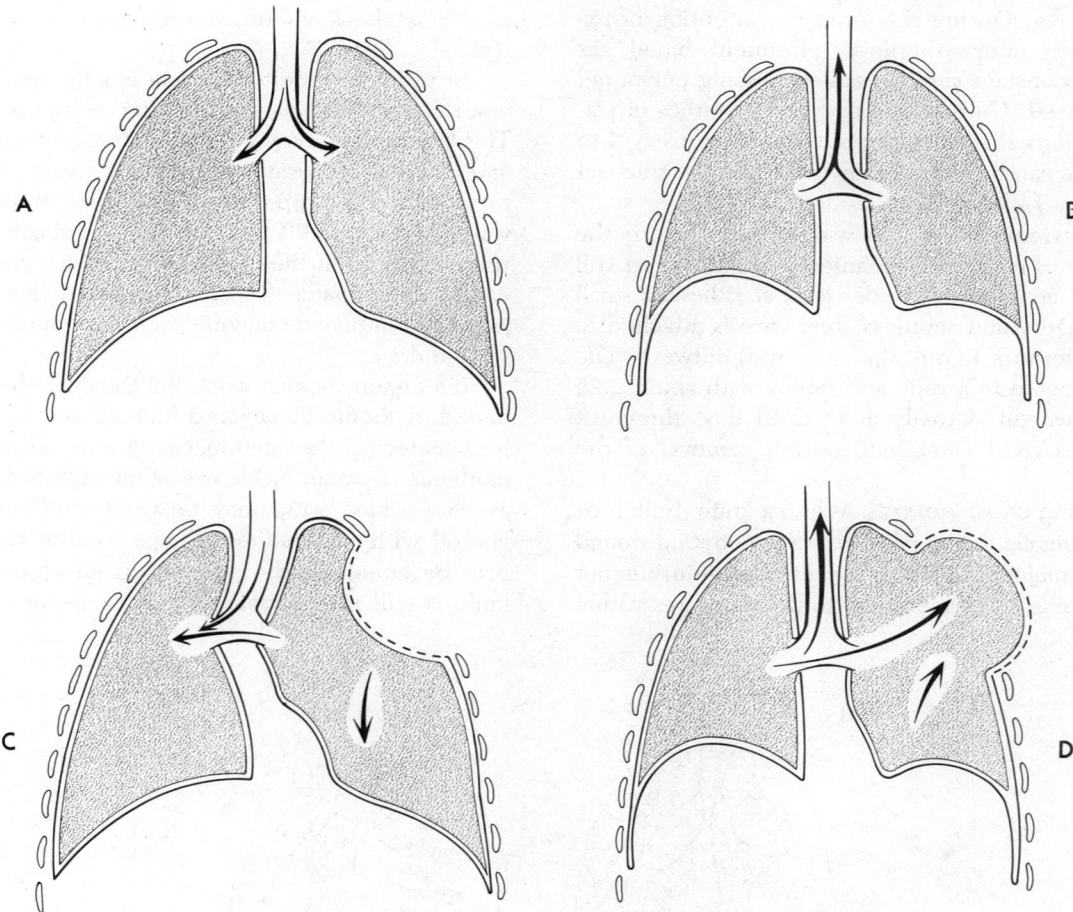

Fig. 49-7. Normal respiration: **A,** inspiration; **B,** expiration. *Paradoxical motion:* **C,** inspiration, area of lung underlying unstable chest wall sucks in on inspiration; **D,** same area balloons out on expiration. Note movement of mediastinum toward opposite lung on inspiration.

remaining lung expands (Fig. 49-7, *C*). On expiration it balloons out as the remaining lung contracts (Fig. 49-7, *D*). This results in a vicious cycle of events leading to *hypoxia*. The treatment of paradoxical motion is to *stabilize the chest wall*. The treatment may either be by internal or external stabilization of the chest wall.

Internal stabilization is the treatment of choice and is best obtained by use of a *volume-controlled* ventilator attached to a cuffed tracheostomy tube (p. 1244). The ventilator is set to automatically control the patient's respirations. The patient who is breathing against the ventilator will need to be sedated. Narcotics, sedatives, and even muscle relaxants may have to be given. When the patient also has a head injury, narcotics are contraindicated and muscle relaxants will be used until ventilatory control is achieved. Once the person is quieted down and is no longer resisting the ventilator, hyperventilation can be used to depress the respiratory center so that ventilatory control is maintained.[67] The patient will require meticulous tracheostomy care in order to maintain a clear airway and to prevent infection. The patient may have to be on the ventilator for as long as 8 to 14 days. During this time the attention of experienced respiratory therapists, frequent blood gas studies, and constant care by skilled nursing personnel will be required. Culture and sensitivity studies of tracheal aspirations should be repeated at least every 4 to 5 days. These can be obtained by collecting the tracheal aspiration in a Luken's tube.

External stabilization was widely used before the development of modern mechanical ventilators and still may be used occasionally. Under local anesthesia a small incision is made, and stainless steel wire is attached to the ribs or sternum to pull the chest wall outward. The wire is connected to a rope and pulley with about 2.25 kg (5 lb) of weight. Usually in 14 to 21 days the chest wall becomes rigid enough to permit removal of the traction.

Penetrating chest wounds. When a knife, bullet, or other flying missile enters the chest, a penetrating wound occurs. The major problem in penetrating injury is not injury to the chest wall but injury to the structures within the chest cavity. Penetration of the lung is associated with leakage of air from the lung into the pleural cavity (pneumothorax) (Fig. 49-8, *B*). Blood may also leak into the pleural cavity (hemothorax). As the air or fluid accumulates in the pleural cavity, it builds up positive pressure, which causes the lung to collapse and may even cause a mediastinal shift, thus compressing the opposite lung and interfering with cardiac action. The person then has serious difficulty in breathing and may go into shock. The pulse may become weak and rapid and the skin cold and clammy, and blood pressure falls rapidly.

Emergency treatment is directed toward sustaining oxygen exchange and correcting circulatory failure. Usually the patient is intubated with an endotracheal tube and then is checked for air or blood in the pleural cavity. An emergency thoracentesis is done, and air and fluid are removed by syringe. Usually a catheter is inserted into the pleural space and connected to water-seal drainage (p. 1254). If the lung fails to reexpand with this treatment or there is evidence of internal bleeding, surgical exploration may be necessary and will be done as soon as shock and other complications are under control.

In order to monitor the patient for hypovolemia, a central venous pressure (CVP) line is inserted (p. 1055). This line can also be used to administer intravenous fluids and blood as necessary. The CVP is a very effective way to monitor for tamponade. A pressure above 15 cm of water or a rising CVP in a patient in shock with penetrating trauma in the region of the heart often indicates cardiac tamponade.[67] If it is suspected that cardiac injury and tamponade may be present, a *pericardicentesis* will be done.

If an open sucking wound of the chest has been sustained, it should be covered immediately to prevent air from entering the pleural cavity and causing a pneumothorax. Several thicknesses of nonporous material such as plastic food wrap may be used, and these are anchored with wide adhesive tape, or the wound edges may be taped tightly together. If an object such as a knife is still in the wound, it must never be removed

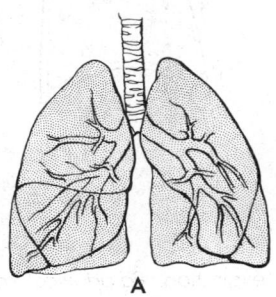
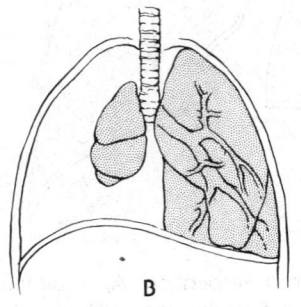

Fig. 49-8. A, Normal expanded lungs. **B,** Complete collapse of right lung caused by air in pleural cavity (pneumothorax).

until a physician arrives. Its presence may prevent the entry of air into the pleural cavity, and its removal may cause further damage. The person who has sustained a penetrating wound of the chest should be placed in an upright position and taken to the nearest emergency room.

Pneumothorax

Pneumothorax is a condition in which there is air in the pleural space between the lung and the chest wall (Fig. 49-8, *B*). It usually results from the rupture of an emphysematous bleb on the surface of the lung, but it may also follow severe bouts of coughing in persons with a chronic chest disease such as asthma. It also occurs when wounds have penetrated the chest wall and perforated the pleura. Rather frequently it occurs as a single or recurrent episode in otherwise healthy young people. As atmospheric pressure builds up in the pleural space, the lung on the affected side collapses and the heart and mediastinum shift toward the unaffected lung. If untreated, the person may die. If the cause of the condition is trauma, the immediate treatment is to seal the chest wound surgically and then to aspirate air from the pleural space.

A *spontaneous pneumothorax* occurs without warning. The person has a sudden sharp pain in the chest, accompanied by dyspnea, anxiety, increased diaphoresis, weak and rapid pulse, fall in blood pressure, and cessation of normal chest movement on the affected side. Roentgenograms are always ordered to determine the amount of collapse of the lung as well as the degree of mediastinal shift. When roentgenograms are taken, the patient needs help to prevent overexertion.

When a spontaneous pneumothorax is suspected, a physician should be summoned immediately. The patient should not be left alone and should be reassured and urged to be quiet and not move about. Oxygen and equipment for a thoracentesis should be assembled at once. Air is immediately aspirated from the affected pleural space, and the intrapleural pressure is brought to normal if possible. If air continues to flow into the pleural space, a chest tube will be inserted and connected to water-sealed drainage (p. 1254).

The person who has had a spontaneous pneumothorax is usually most comfortable in a sitting position. Physical activity is kept at a minimum for at least 24 hours. The patient is asked to remain as quiet as possible and to avoid stretching, reaching, or moving suddenly. Breathing should be normal, and the breath should not be held. Pulse rate and respirations must be checked frequently.

When air no longer is expelled from the pleural space through the underwater drainage system and a roentgenogram reveals that the lung has completely reexpanded, the chest tube is removed and the person is allowed out of bed. Strenuous exertion, which increases

rate and depth of respirations for a time, should be avoided, but relatively normal activity may be resumed rather quickly. If there are frequent recurring episodes, some physicians instill silver nitrate into the pleural space to cause adhesions between the visceral and parietal pleurae. If this procedure is unsuccessful, the portion containing the defect may be resected from the lung and the parietal pleura abraded so that it will adhere to the visceral pleura and obliterate the pleural space.

Maintaining an adequate number of terminal respiratory units

Aeration of the alveoli

The individual with pulmonary disease may have impaired ability to aerate alveoli. This impairment may be related to several factors. These include (1) inability to move adequate amounts of air in and out of the lungs, (2) interference with alveolar expansion secondary to an accumulation of secretions resulting in collapse (*atelectasis*) of portions of the lungs, and (3) restriction of lung expansion by mechanical factors such as air in the pleural space (*pneumothorax*) or fluid or blood in the pleural space (*pleural effusion* or *hemothorax*).

The person with pulmonary disease may have very slight or severe difficulty in breathing (dyspnea). There may be obstruction of the free passage of air through the bronchi, or there may be damage to lung tissue itself, or both may be present. If so, more effort is required for breathing, and the person is very conscious of breathing. This is tiring and unpleasant. With increased difficulty in breathing, most persons become apprehensive and even panicky. A nurse who understands this can be a great comfort to the patient. The presence of another person often helps to control fear and eases breathing efforts. The person with chronic obstructive pulmonary disease has often discovered ways to minimize these breathing difficulties (p. 1325). The nurse needs to assess the person's wishes about position, exercise, and so on and should utilize these in planning nursing care.

Position. The most comfortable position for more relaxed breathing is a semiupright or upright sitting position. In these positions the lungs and respiratory muscles are not cramped and thus are not working against resistance. A pillow placed lengthwise at the patient's back provides support and keeps the thorax thrust slightly forward, allowing freer use of the diaphragm, and increases the ability to breathe deeply. For those persons who must be upright to breathe, the overbed table with a pillow on top can be used as a support and a resting place for the head and arms (Fig. 49-9). If the patient has marked breathing difficulty and is not sufficiently

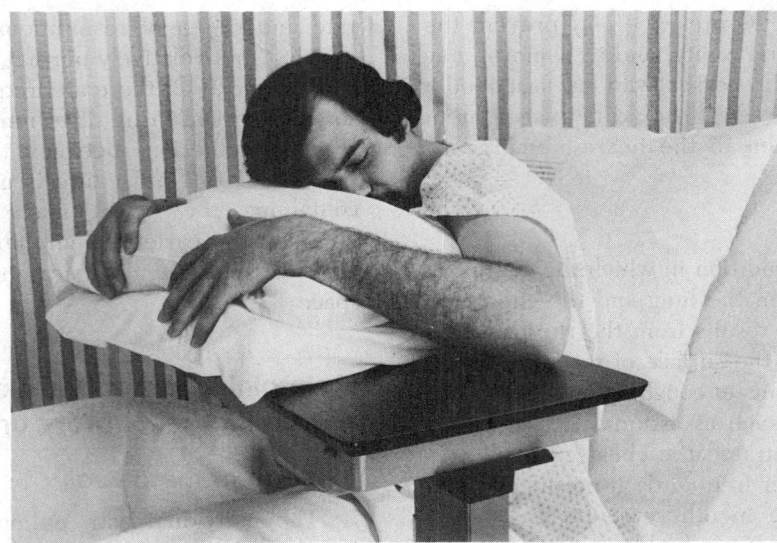

Fig. 49-9. Pillows placed on overbed table provide comfortable support for patient who must sleep in upright position.

alert or is alert and fearful, side rails can provide additional security. They also may be used to assist patients to pull themselves up into a higher sitting position. At home, some persons may prefer to sit up in a large armchair that supports them well and to lean on a smaller chair placed in front of them. This chair should be blocked to prevent it from slipping.

Since the diaphragm becomes flattened and less active in persons with chronically overinflated lungs secondary to an increase in residual volume, some patients find breathing is helped by wearing an elasticized abdominal support. The support is often made of material similar to that used in elasticized girdles. Men may need to be persuaded to wear this kind of support but, on trial, learn how much the support adds to comfort and accept it quite readily. Pressure from the girdle must be from below the umbilicus upward so that the flattened diaphragm is forced up into the thorax.

Environment. Proper ventilation, humidity, and temperature of the room will help the patient to breathe more easily. Irritants such as tobacco smoke from cigarettes, cigars, and pipes should be excluded. Patients may have preferences as to room temperature and amount of fresh air, and the nurse assesses and responds to those preferences. In general, most patients breathe more easily if the air is cool and not too humid. An air-conditioned room may make breathing easier.

Persons with nose, throat, and bronchial irritation may benefit from warm, moist air produced by a *humidifier* or *vaporizer*. A vaporizer can be used to humidify the air throughout the room, or it can be placed close so that steam is inhaled as it is released. The electrically operated vaporizers used in hospitals serve to moisten the air in the entire room. Water flowing from a gallon-sized jar is heated to form steam that is then directed out through a long, flexible spout. Inhalation of plain steam or of an aromatic medication such as tincture of benzoin or menthol is often ordered.

In recent years concern has been raised about cross-infection from room humidifiers. For this reason, the Centers for Disease Control (CDC) has issued recommendations about their use:

1. Use only a direct *heated* humidifier or nebulizer with a bacterial filter. Cold vapor or cool mist humidifiers are not recommended because they cannot withstand daily sterilization.
2. Use only sterile water in the humidifier and drain remaining water each time the humidifier is refilled, or at least every 24 hours. Tap water is not safe to use because it is frequently contaminated with *Pseudomonas, Flavobacterium, Acinetobacter,* or other organisms.
3. Establish a routine maintenance schedule.
4. Set medical guidelines to determine which patients should receive humidification and which should not. It may not be advisable to use humidifiers for immunosuppressed patients.
5. Do not send humidifying units home with patients because of the concern about transporting highly resistant hospital organisms into the community.[43]

Small electric vaporizers can be purchased at most local drugstores. However, when the person cannot afford to purchase one, the nurse can assist in improvising equipment for inhalation and for proper humidity. An empty coffee can or a shallow pie tin can be filled with water and placed on an electric plate in the person's room to increase humidity. If the inhalation is to

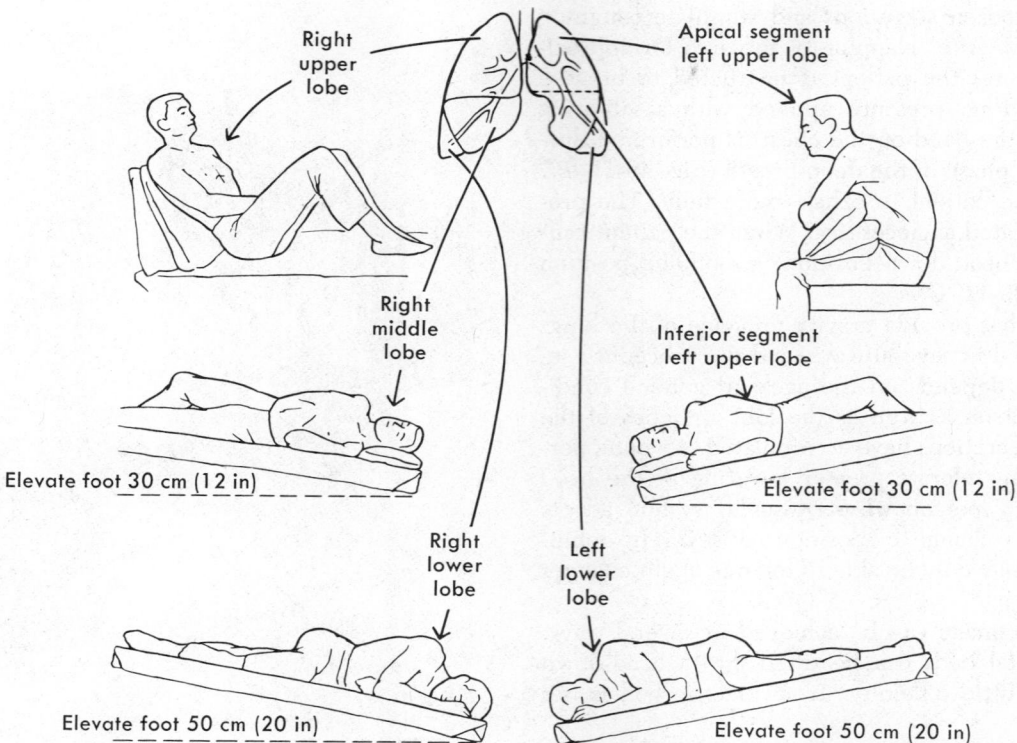

Fig. 49-10. Postural drainage requires that patient assume various positions to facilitate flow of secretions from various portions of lung into bronchi, trachea, and throat so that they can be raised and expectorated more easily. Drawing shows correct positions to drain various portions of lung.

be directed, an ordinary steam kettle or a kettle with a longer improvised paper spout may be used. The paper should be changed frequently. A few drops of menthol or oil of eucalyptus can be put into the water. Benzoin will cause corrosion in the kettle, which is exceedingly difficult to remove. The kettle and electric plate should be placed a safe distance from the face so that the medicated steam can be breathed freely, and yet the person will not be burned by accidentally tipping the kettle or by touching the hot plate. After the 25- to 30-minute treatment, equipment should be removed from the bedside.

Continued uncorrected difficulty in breathing may result in carbon dioxide being accumulated in the blood. This is the result of inadequate exchange of oxygen and carbon dioxide and is termed *carbon dioxide narcosis*. It causes flushing of the skin and a slow, deep respiratory pattern. The nurse notifies the physician at once if this occurs. (See p. 1325 for a discussion of the use of low-flow oxygen and the danger of administration in the person with chronic obstructive lung disease.)

Pulmonary physiotherapy

The person who has difficulty in breathing may be taught how to increase the efficiency of his or her breathing pattern. Breathing exercises are usually a part of pulmonary physiotherapy, which may also include *segmental postural drainage, clapping,* and *vibrating*. Although pulmonary physiotherapy activities may be performed by a physical therapist, they are often part of a nurse's responsibility. Regardless of where the primary responsibility lies, nurses must be familiar with the techniques so that they can demonstrate and reinforce them and be sure that the individual is doing them correctly. Also, the need for pulmonary physiotherapy may occur at a time when the physical therapist is not available to the patient.

Segmental postural drainage. Segmental postural drainage with clapping and vibration is a technique used to combine the force of gravity with the natural ciliary activity of the small bronchial airways to move secretions upward toward the main bronchi and the trachea. From this point the patient can cough them up, or they can be suctioned. In the treatment of chronic obstructive pulmonary disease, drainage of all segments is usually accomplished by placing patients in various postural drainage positions (Fig. 49-10). Treatment may also be directed at draining specific areas of the lung. While the patient is in each position, *clapping* with a cupped hand is done over the area being drained. This maneuver helps to loosen secretions and stimulate coughing (Fig. 49-11, *A*). After clapping of the area for approximately 1 minute, the patient is instructed to breathe deeply. *Vibrating* (pressure applied with a vibrating movement of the hand on the chest) is performed during expiratory phase of the deep breath (Fig. 49-11, *B*). This assists the patient to exhale more fully. The procedure is repeated as necessary. When the patient cannot tolerate a head-down position, a modified position is used (Fig. 49-11, *C*).

Positions that provide gravity drainage of the lungs can be achieved in several ways, and the procedure selected usually depends on the age and general condition of the person as well as the lobe or lobes of the lungs where secretions have accumulated. A young person usually can tolerate greater lowering of the head than an elderly person whose vascular system adapts less quickly to change of position. A severely debilitated patient may only be able to tolerate slight changes in position.

Postural drainage can be achieved in several ways. Electric hospital beds can be tilted into a head-down position with little difficulty. If an electric bed is not

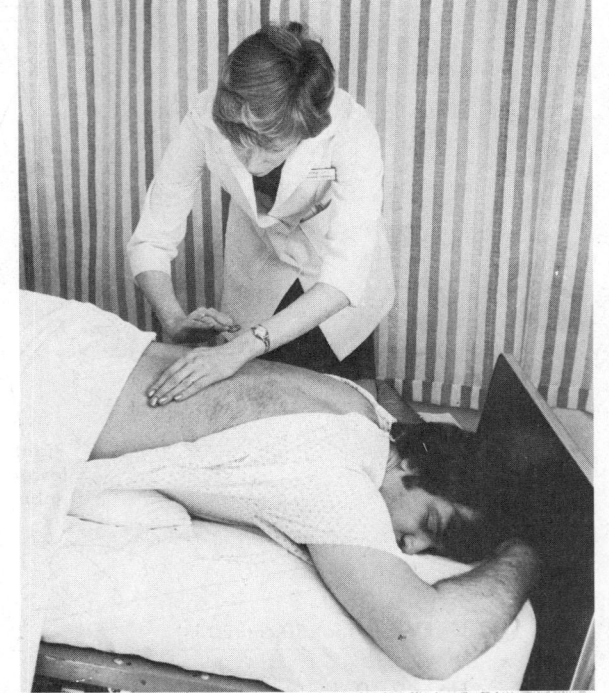

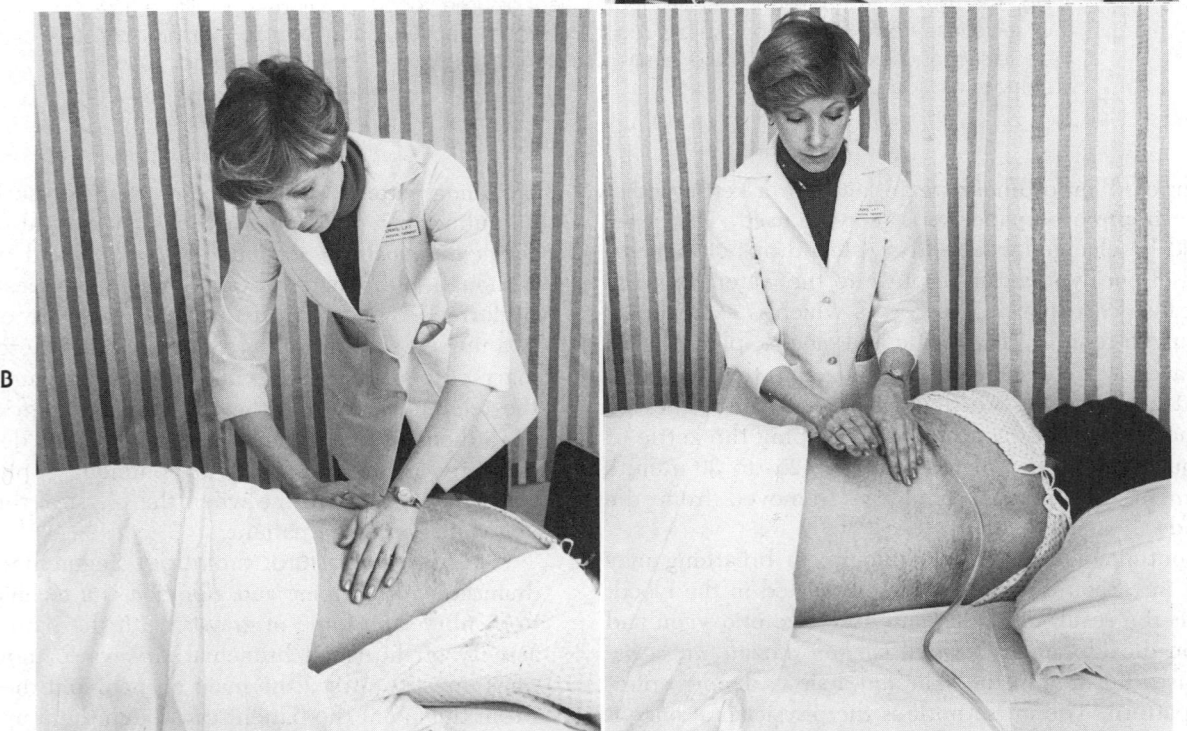

Fig. 49-11. A, Patient is in supine position with head down at 15-degree angle for postural drainage of lower lobes. Note cupped position of physical therapist's hands as she claps patient. Patient's gown is pulled aside for purposes of illustration; ordinarily clapping is never done on bare skin. **B,** Physical therapist follows clapping with vibrating, applying pressure during expiration. **C,** Even when patient cannot tolerate head-down position, such as after thoracic surgery, patient can still receive chest physiotherapy in modified positions.

available (e.g., in the home), blocks can be placed under the casters at the foot of the bed or a hydraulic lift can be used under the foot of the bed. If these are not available, the foot of the bed can be supported on the seat of a firm chair to provide a position in which the head is lowered.

The nurse needs to know the part of the lung affected and how to position the patient to drain that portion of the lung (Fig. 49-10). For example, if the right middle lobe of the lung is affected, drainage will be accomplished best by way of the right middle bronchus. The patient should lie supine with the body turned at approximately a 45-degree angle. The angle can be maintained by pillow supports placed under the right side from the shoulders to the hips. The foot of the bed is raised about 30 cm (12 in.). This position can be maintained fairly comfortably by most patients for half an hour at a time. On the other hand, if the lower posterior area of the lung is affected, the foot of the bed can be raised 45 to 50 cm (18 to 20 in.) with the patient assuming a prone position for drainage. A summary of the positions for segmental postural drainage is given in Table 49-2.

Postural drainage and percussion should be planned so as to achieve maximal benefit. The best time is generally in the morning soon after arising and at night before retiring. Frequency of treatments will depend on each person's needs, but care should be taken to avoid exhaustion, which will result in shallow ventilation and negates the positive effects of the treatment.

Patients having postural drainage of any kind are encouraged to breathe deeply and to cough forcefully to help dislodge thick sputum and exudate that is pooled in distended bronchioles, particularly after inactivity. Humidity, bronchodilators, or liquefying agents often are given 15 to 20 minutes before postural drainage is started, since they facilitate the removal of secretions. The patient may find that sputum can best be raised on resuming an upright position even though no drainage appeared while lying down with the head and chest lowered.

Since some patients complain of dizziness when assuming positions for postural drainage, the nurse stays with the patient during the first few times and reports any persistent dizziness or unusual discomfort to the physician.

Postural drainage may be contraindicated in some persons because of heart disease, hypertension, increased intracranial pressure, extreme dyspnea, or advanced age. However, most people can be taught to assume the positions for postural drainage and can proceed without help after being supervised once or twice.

Chest percussion (clapping) is contraindicated in the case of pulmonary emboli, hemorrhage, exacerbation of bronchospasms, severe pain, and over areas of resectable carcinoma. Often patients with a chronic pulmonary problem need to be taught to do postural drainage independently so that they can continue at home. The position usually is maintained for 10 minutes at first, and the period of time is gradually lengthened to 15 to 20 or even 30 minutes as the patient becomes accustomed to the position. At first, elderly persons usually are able to tolerate these positions only for a few min-

TABLE 49-2. Positions for segmental postural drainage, clapping, and vibrating

Area of lung	Position of patient	Area to be clapped or vibrated
Upper lobe		
Apical bronchus	Semi-Fowler's position, leaning to right, then left, then forward	Over area of shoulder blades with fingers extending over clavicles
Posterior bronchus	Upright at 45-degree angle, rolled forward against a pillow at 45 degrees on left and then right side	Over shoulder blade on each side
Anterior bronchus	Supine with pillow under knees	Over anterior chest just below clavicles
Middle lobe (lateral and medial bronchus)	Trendelenburg's position at 30-degree angle or with foot of bed elevated 35-40 cm (14-16 in.), turned slightly to left	Anterior and lateral right chest from axillary fold to midanterior chest
Lingula (superior and inferior bronchus)	Trendelenburg's position at 30-degree angle or with foot of bed elevated 35-40 cm (14-16 in.), turned slightly to right	Left axillary fold to midanterior chest
Lower lobes		
Apical bronchus	Prone with pillow under hips	Lower third of posterior rib cage on both sides
Medial bronchus	Trendelenburg's position at 45-degree angle or with foot of bed raised 45-50 cm (18-20 in.) on right side	Lower third on left posterior rib cage
Lateral bronchus	Trendelenburg's position at 45-degree angle or with foot of bed raised 45-50 cm (18-20 in.) on left side	Lower third of right posterior rib cage
Posterior bronchus	Prone Trendelenburg's position at 45-degree angle with pillow under hips	Lower third of posterior rib cage on both sides

utes. They need more assistance than most other patients during the procedure and immediately thereafter. They should be assisted to a normal position in bed and requested to lie flat for a few minutes before sitting up or getting out of bed. This helps to prevent dizziness and reduces the danger of accidents.

The patient may feel nauseated because of the odor and taste of sputum. Therefore the procedure should be timed so that it comes at least 1 hour before meals. A short rest period following the treatment often improves postural drainage. Aromatic mouth washes should be available for frequent use by any patient who is expectorating sputum freely.

Care of sputum. Since the causative organisms may not be known early in the respiratory disease, the nurse should use caution in the disposal of sputum and should instruct the patient how to protect others. Patients who are coughing or clearing their throats forcefully should be told to cover their mouths and noses with several thicknesses of disposable tissues to prevent possible spread of infectious organisms. Used tissue should be crumpled and placed in a paper bag or flushed directly down the toilet. If a bag is used, it is closed securely and preferably burned. Used tissues should be col-

lected from the bedfast patient at frequent intervals, and whoever handles the bags should wash his or her hands thoroughly to avoid transfer of infection to others.

Patients who have a copious amount of sputum are instructed in the use of a sputum container.

When patients cannot care for and dispose of their own sputum, assistance must be provided. Tissues may be placed in the patient's hand, and a paper bag may be placed on each side of the bed so that the patient does not have to turn to dispose of the soiled tissues. The bedfast patient should be offered soap and water for handwashing before meals.

Breathing exercises. Persons who have a restriction to chest expansion, such as those who have had thoracic surgery, and patients with chronic obstructive lung disease are taught to use an augmented abdominal breathing (diaphragmatic pattern). In teaching, exhalation is stressed rather than inspiration. The person is taught to exhale slowly and fully through *pursed lips* while contracting the abdominal muscles. Manual pressure on the upper abdomen during expiration facilitates this maneuver (Fig. 49-12). On inhalation through the nose, the abdominal muscles are relaxed. This technique will slow the respiratory rate, encourage deep breathing, and

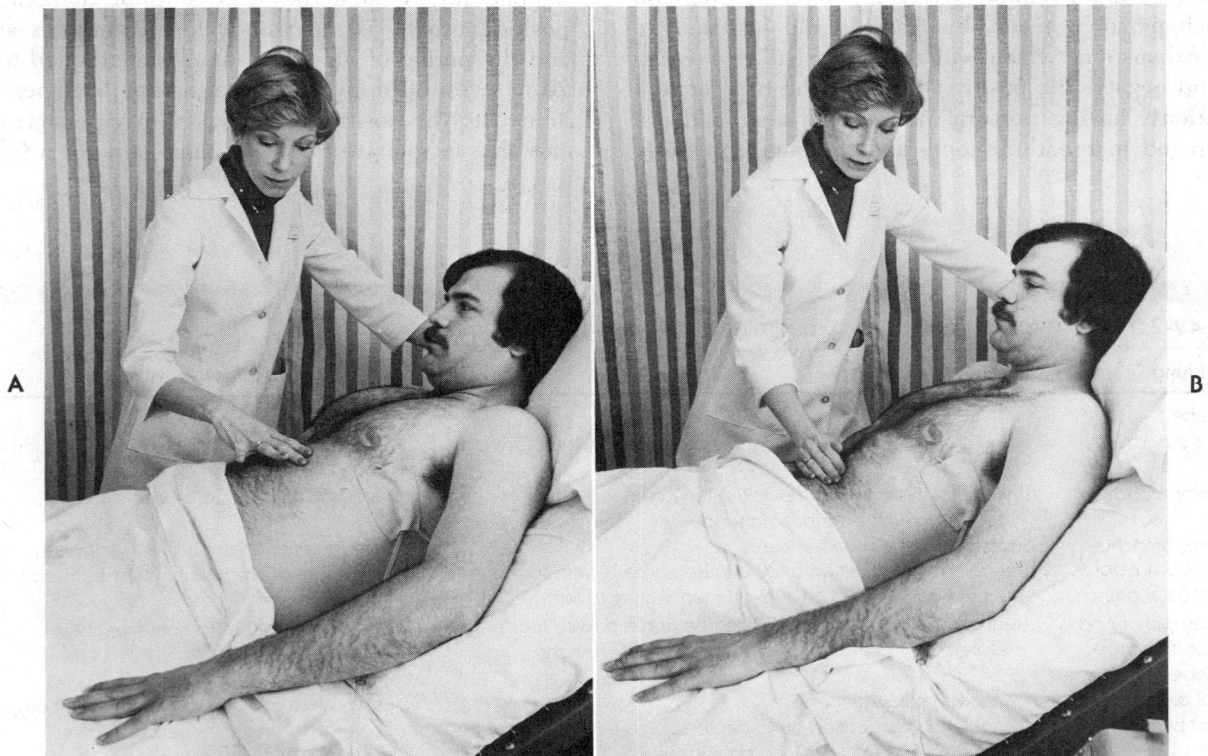

Fig. 49-12. A, Physical therapist assists patient in learning augmented abdominal breathing. Patient is instructed to inhale through nose, using abdominal muscles and concentration on moving lower ribs under therapist's hand. This exercise improves ventilation of bases of lungs. **B,** Physical therapist places hand on upper abdomen in assisting patient to exhale fully.

facilitate expiration. This "controlled" breathing pattern is to be used while performing various activities of daily living—from sitting, standing, walking, and climbing stairs to more complex activities. As this pattern becomes natural, it will be used automatically during periods of increased shortness of breath. Persons who do not know how to use controlled breathing tend to increase their respiratory rate and their work of breathing when they are short of breath. As a result, physiologic obstruction increases, oxygen requirements increase, and effective ventilation decreases. Changing a person's respiratory pattern requires a great deal of effort by both the individual and those providing care.

This same method of teaching augmented abdominal (diaphragmatic) breathing can be used to teach the patient to cough. The difference is that expiration is forced down to residual volume. This maneuver often stimulates the cough reflex. If it does not, the person is taught to actively cough at the end of full expiration. Physiologically, forced expiration simulates the effects of a cough and is therefore more effective than telling the patient to take a deep breath and then cough.

Respiratory assistive devices

A variety of devices may be used to help the patient to breathe more easily and more effectively and to assist in raising secretions. These devices may be directed at improving either the inspiratory or the expiratory phase of respiration.

Devices to assist inspiratory phase. The respiratory maneuver currently believed to be most effective in promoting alveolar gas exchange is the voluntary sustained maximal inspiration. This is accomplished by taking a deep breath, thereby inflating even small, distal alveoli, and holding the breath for at least 3 seconds to allow time for gas exchange. The device used to assist patients in performing this maneuver is the *incentive spirometer* (see Fig. 24-18). Available in several models, this device consists of one or more small plastic balls in closed chambers, which are connected to tubing and a mouthpiece. The patient is instructed to inhale slowly and steadily through the tubing, thus creating a vacuum in the chamber and raising the ball to the top. The number of times the patient can raise the ball or balls and the length of time the inspiration can be held reflects the effectiveness of the patient's efforts.

Intermittent positive pressure breathing (IPPB) was the most commonly used method in the past for improving the inspiratory phase of ventilation. The IPPB machine delivers air or oxygen under pressure until a preset pressure limit is reached. It is cycled and controlled by the patient's own respiratory rate. Specifically, it is used to (1) prevent and reverse atelectasis, (2) clear secretions, (3) deliver medications, and (4) improve gas exchange in patients with respiratory tract infections and decompensation of pulmonary status.[41] The use of IPPB remains a controversial issue. Some clinicians believe this method is no more, and possibly less, effective than other methods,[7,83] while others believe there are still some patients who can benefit from this modality.[41]

Devices to assist expiratory phase. The device most commonly used to assist expiration is the blow-bottle. Blow-bottles consist of two bottles half-filled with water and connected by tubing. The person is instructed to move the water from one bottle to another by blowing into a short tube in the first bottle, thus increasing the pressure in the bottle and displacing the water with air. In doing so the person may increase alveolar pressure through prolonged expiration against resistance.

Initially, many persons cannot move the entire contents of one bottle into the other with one breath, especially if they have had recent chest surgery. They can be encouraged to work toward increasing the amount of fluid moved with each use. If the person understands the reason for the use of blow-bottles, the therapy will be carried out more faithfully and will be treated more seriously.

Use of blow-bottles increases intrathoracic pressure, creating pressure on the vena cava similar to that in Valsalva's maneuver. Pulse rate will increase when the pressure is relieved with the surge of blood returning to the heart. Blow-bottles should therefore be used cautiously by persons with any signs of cardiac failure.

The cough is also an expiratory maneuver. While coughing is essential in raising and removing secretions, it is now believed that expiratory maneuvers are not effective in reexpanding collapsed alveoli and that forced expiration may in fact contribute to the collapse of small, distal alveoli through excessively high pleural pressures. *Consequently, devices designed to assist persons in inspiration are currently the preferred method of improving pulmonary function.*

Aerosol and mist therapy. Another category of devices designed to assist patients with respiratory problems are those that promote the humidification of gases in the respiratory tract or use humidified gases (air or oxygen) to deliver medication.

The simplest method to provide added humidity is the room humidifier, discussed on p. 1238. This is the preferred method for delivering humidity to patients who are breathing independently. The delivery of continuous bland aerosols through a mask is not recommended because most of this moisture is deposited in the nose, mouth, and upper airway, rather than the lower portion of the respiratory tract, and is thus ineffective.

If the patient is being mechanically ventilated and requires additional humidity, an ultrasonic nebulizer may be added to the respirator. Medications, such as bronchodilators, may be administered to the intubated patients through the ultrasonic nebulizer. When using this form of therapy, the nurse must be alert to the possibility of side effects from the medication and also to the likelihood of increased secretions as a result of more effective humidification.

Bronchodilators and mucolytic agents may also be administered to patients who are not intubated in aerosol form via nebulizer. Several types of nebulizers may be used. Some medications are available in commercial metered-dose nebulizers, or the medication may be diluted with saline and administered via a hand-held bulb nebulizer that looks much like a perfume atomizer. With all methods the person needs to be taught how to self-administer prescribed medications. Following are steps to be followed in teaching a person to use a hand nebulizer:

1. Exhale fully.
2. Position nebulizer in mouth *without* sealing lips around it.
3. Take a deep breath through the mouth while squeezing the bulb of the nebulizer *once*.
4. Hold breath for 3 to 4 seconds at full inspiration.
5. Exhale slowly through pursed lips.

Usually one inhalation is sufficient. Several inhalations of a bronchodilator may cause medication overdosage and result in side effects (tachycardia, palpitation, nervousness).

For the hospitalized patient who cannot use the hand-held nebulizer, a mask with attached nebulizer powered by wall oxygen or air can be used to deliver intermittent medicated aerosol therapy.

Mechanical ventilation. If, despite the use of the techniques and devices mentioned, the patient is still unable to ventilate well enough to maintain desired blood levels of oxygen and carbon dioxide, mechanical ventilation by a respirator is indicated. This requires the use of a cuffed endotracheal or tracheostomy tube (p. 1229).

Many different kinds of respirators are available. In general, there are two kinds, pressure cycled and volume cycled. The Bird and Bennett (PR series) are pressure-limited ventilators, whereas the Möerch, Emerson, Engstrom, Air Shields, Bennett MA-1, Siemen's Servo, and Ohio 560 are volume-limited machines. Both types of machines can be used intermittently or continuously to assist or to control respiration.

When a *pressure-cycled* ventilator is used, the machine is set to deliver a predetermined amount of pressure (usually 15 to 25 cm of water) with each breath. When this pressure is reached, the machine turns off and normal exhalation begins. The volume of gas delivered to the patient is not necessarily constant because it depends on the resistance of the entire system, including the patient's lungs. For this reason the expired tidal volume must be monitored frequently and adjustments made in the respirator controls as needed.

With a *volume-controlled* machine a *constant volume* of air is delivered with each breath. The volume is preset and is delivered to the patient at whatever pressure is necessary to attain that volume. A volume-cycled machine should have a pressure cutoff valve. Such a mechanism allows a pressure limit to be set. If the pressure required to deliver the set volume exceeds the pressure limit, the machine will turn off before the entire volume is delivered. The pressure limit on a volume-cycled machine usually has an audible alarm. The nurse can set the limit slightly above (approximately 5 cm of water) the pressure required to ventilate the patient. The alarm will then go off if the patient coughs, accumulates secretion, or starts to resist the machine.

Regardless of which type of ventilator is used, mechanisms for various regulations are necessary if the machine is to be adjusted to each patient. It is preferable to have a respirator that can be used to assist or control the patient's breathing. "Assist" means that the patient's own inspiratory effort triggers (turns on) the machine. Most respirators have a *sensitivity control knob* that can be adjusted to respond to weak inspiratory efforts. "Control" implies the use of automatic cycling. The patient may be apneic and the machine set at the desired rate; the patient's own respiratory rate may be too slow, and the automatic cycling can be used to force an increase in the rate; or the patient's own respiratory efforts can be ignored and an automatic rate used to ventilate the patient. (Some machines with automatic cycling do not allow for the latter adjustment.) It is also helpful to be able to regulate the flow rates at which the gas is delivered to the patient. For example, patients breathing at rapid rates and high volumes need faster flow rates than those breathing slowly and at moderate volumes. A final necessity is the ability to regulate the inspired concentration of oxygen from 20% (room air) to 100%.

All respirators used for mechanical ventilation must:

1. Provide for the heating and humidification of inspired air
2. Provide a means for measurement of expired volumes
3. Be dependable for long periods of use
4. Be easily cleaned

Any patient on continuous mechanical ventilation should be "sighed" (given a deep breath) several times an hour. Some respirators automatically "sigh" the patient, while with others the patient is "sighed" manually using a self-inflating (Ambu) or anesthesia bag. This periodic deep breathing is necessary to prevent alveolar collapse and resultant atelectasis.

A negative pressure respirator such as the tank respirator (iron lung) may also be used. This type of respirator is usually used for patients with neuromuscular problems without intrinsic lung disease. The tank respirator creates subatmospheric pressure around the chest. Since there is atmospheric pressure at the mouth and nose, air enters the lungs. This type of ventilator does not require tracheal intubation and is usually not used in patients with increased airway resistance.

WEANING FROM THE VENTILATOR. The nurse plays an important role in weaning the patient from the ventilator. Both physiologic studies (blood gases, tidal volume) and clinical status determine the patient's readiness to breathe without mechanical assistance. Before weaning, the person should have been taught breathing exercises. Removal from the respirator is very frightening to most patients. Ideally, a nurse with whom the patient has developed rapport is present when the respirator is removed. It is also helpful if the environment around the patient is calm. Much of the success of weaning is dependent on the interrelationship between the person's physiologic and psychologic responses. Those who become very anxious and take rapid, shallow breaths often will not tolerate being off the respirator. If a pattern of controlled breathing can be maintained, success is much more likely. Weaning is usually begun with short periods of breathing independently, either off the respirator completely or with intermittent mandatory ventilation (IMV). IMV is an adaptation of the ventilator that allows the patient to take independent breaths while still attached to the ventilator. The ventilator delivers several "mandatory" breaths per minute. The amount of time off the respirator or the amount of independent breaths allowed on IMV is increased according to the patient's tolerance. The nurse must carefully assess the adequacy of ventilation while the patient is being weaned. If, in the nurse's judgment, the patient cannot tolerate breathing alone because of inadequate tidal volume, cyanosis, tachycardia, diaphoresis, or restlessness, mechanical assistance should be reinstituted.

Throughout the treatment of the patient in respiratory failure, ventilation should be carefully monitored by blood gas studies and simple spirometry (tidal volume, vital capacity). Alert nursing observation of the patient can determine the adequacy of ventilation. Meticulous attention is given to maintaining a patent airway, which is the prime nursing responsibility. (See specialized material for further details.[73,92,97])

Removal of secretions

Coughing. Two of the most troublesome symptoms of respiratory disease are the increase in mucous secretions secondary to mucous membrane inflammation or allergic response and the stimulation of coughing caused by irritation of the respiratory tract. If coughing is productive, the person needs to be encouraged to cough effectively in order to keep air passages clear and allow sufficient oxygen to reach the alveoli. Periodic changes in position will help to prevent pooling of secretions in the lungs and will stimulate coughing. The patient is instructed to breathe as deeply as possible to loosen secretions and to stimulate productive coughing. For an effective cough, the patient should take a deep inspiration, force it down to residual volume, contract the diaphragm and intercostal muscles, and exhale forcefully. Any sputum raised should always be expectorated, not swallowed. When a patient cannot cough forcefully enough to raise sputum and when respirations are very shallow or sound very moist, extra fluids or a liquefying agent to thin the secretions may be given. The liquefying agent is often given as a nebulized aerosol so that it reaches deep into the tracheobronchial tree.

Many patients with obvious, noisy respirations caused by accumulated sputum hesitate to cough because coughing causes pain. To assist such a patient the nurse's hands can be placed on the front and back of the chest to give support as the patient coughs (Fig. 49-15). A towel placed around the chest and held snugly as the patient coughs may also be used.

Although coughing is a physiologic protective reflex, constant nonproductive coughing and hacking can lead to exhaustion. Medications therefore are often prescribed for problems related to cough. The type prescribed depends on the nature of the cough and the type of secretions. The purposes of various cough medications are to increase secretions, to decrease secretions, to thin secretions so that they can be raised and expectorated more easily, or to *depress* the cough reflex. Some of these medications are summmarized in Table 49-3.

Sedative expectorants increase secretions, protect irritated membranes, and lessen the amount of coughing. Increased secretions may result in a productive cough and make paroxysms of coughing less frequent. For this purpose, ammonium chloride in wild cherry or orange syrup is often ordered, and other mixtures such as iodide solutions or ipecac syrup are sometimes used. Aerosolized normal or half-normal saline solution is also effective in thinning secretions. The mucolytic enzyme pancreatic dornase (Dornavac) is useful if the secretions are purulent. Stimulating expectorants such as terpin hydrate diminish secretions and promote repair and healing of the mucous membrane.

When the main objective of treatment is to suppress coughing, drugs depressing the cough center in the medulla are ordered. Codeine is frequently used and may be added to elixir of terpin hydrate, but there is danger of addiction with its prolonged use. Some non-narcotic drugs with actions similar to codeine have been prescribed widely. Among them are dextromethorphan (Romilar) and noscapine (Nectadon).

When respiratory difficulty is severe, secretions are present, coughing is unproductive, intratracheal suctioning and occasionally bronchoscopy are necessary. By means of bronchoscopy, mucous plugs may be loosened or removed and intratracheal suctioning made more effective. Equipment for emergency bronchoscopy may be kept in the patient's room. When this procedure is ordered, the nurse must see that electrical outlets are adequate and that the necessary equipment is assembled in one place and ready for immediate use. (See p. 1223 for care of the patient during bronchoscopy.)

Fluid balance. Persons with respiratory disease often have a tenuous fluid balance. The older person, whose respiratory disease may be complicated by the existence of congestive heart failure (p. 1127) or cor pulmonale (p. 1324) may be on diuretic therapy in order to avoid overloading the vascular system. The person with chronic lung disease often has inadequate food and fluid intake because of anorexia and fatigue.

Accurate assessment of fluid balance, as indicated by daily weights, is of utmost importance. Excessive fluid administration may lead to pulmonary edema in a patient whose cardiopulmonary system is already compromised. Dehydration, on the other hand, will result in thick, tenacious secretions. The best liquefying agent is water, and it is preferable to adequately hydrate the patient rather than attempt to loosen secretions by administering mist therapy. Providing the patient does not have cardiovascular disease requiring fluid restriction, a fluid intake of 3 to 4 L/day should be provided.

Nasotracheal suctioning. If the patient is unable to clear secretions effectively by coughing, suctioning of the tracheobronchial tree may be necessary to maintain a patent airway and achieve adequate oxygenation. Suctioning is uncomfortable and is used only when the patient is too tired or weak to raise secretions through coughing. The procedure is carried out as follows:

1. The patient is prepared for suctioning by a thorough explanation of what is to be done. If coughing is painful, as with the postthoracotomy patient, for example, analgesic medication is administered 30 minutes before the procedure. Suctioning is *not* done immediately before or after meals.

2. Proper positioning of the patient will asist with suctioning. The patient should be in a sitting position, with the head of the bed elevated. A pillow under the shoulders will help hyperextend the neck, which facilitates entry of the catheter into the trachea. It may also be helpful to elevate each shoulder in turn while having the patient turn the head to the opposite side in an attempt to direct the catheter first into the right and then into left main-stem bronchi.

3. Nasotracheal suctioning is a *sterile procedure;* each piece of equipment, catheter, glove, water, lubricant, and basin are used only once. A suction source that is capable of creating a vacuum of -80 cm of water is necessary. For adults, a size 14 French catheter, 35 cm (14 in.) in length, is usually used. A water-soluble lubricant should be applied to the outside of the catheter. The sequence of steps of the procedure is as follows:

    a. Preoxygenate the patient with a few breaths of a high concentration of oxygen (80% to 100%) from an anethesia or Ambu bag. This helps prevent hypoxia during suctioning.

    b. Insert the lubricated catheter, without applying suction, through the nares. When the catheter reaches the posterior pharynx (a distance of about 10 to 12.5 cm [4 to 5 in.]), the patient is asked to cough in order to facilitate entry into the trachea. If the tongue is obstructing passage of the cateter, have the patient stick the tongue out while coughing or have another person pull the tongue forward.

    c. Continue to insert the catheter until meeting resistance. At this point suction is applied intermittently while removing the catheter, rotating the catheter 360 degrees at the same time.

    d. Administer oxygen as in *a* above.

Endotracheal suctioning. The procedure for suctioning a patient who has an endotracheal or tracheostomy tube is described on p. 1231. The principles underlying the procedure are the same; it is much easier in the patient who has an endotracheal tube, however, since the pathway to the trachea is ensured. Because

TABLE 49-3. Medications used to treat cough

Desired effect	Medications prescribed
↑ Secretions	Expectorants
	Ammonium chloride
	Ammonium carbonate
	Sodium iodide
	Potassium iodide (saturated solution; SSKI)
	Ipecac
	Terpin hydrare
↓ Secretions	Anticholinergic agents
	Atropine
Thin secretions	Mucolytic agents
	Acetylcysteine (Mucomyst)
	Desoxyribonuclease (Dornavac)
Depress cough reflex	Antitussives
	Narcotic
	Codeine
	Nonnarcotic agents
	Benzonatate (Tessalon)
	Noscapine (Nectadon)
	Dextromethorphan hydrobromide (Romilar)
	Carbetapentane citrate (Toclase)
	Levopropoxyphene napsylate (Novrad)
	Chlophedianol hydrochloride (Ulo)

the patient who has an endotracheal tube cannot clear this artificial airway by coughing, suctioning is performed routinely and the frequency of suctioning depends on the amount of secretions.

Maintaining transportation of oxygen and adequate oxygenation of tissue

In order to supply oxygen to the cells there must be (1) an adequate amount of hemoglobin available to transport oxygen and an effective heart pump and circulatory system to deliver the oxygen to the tissues. The amount of oxygen delivered to body tissues each minute equals the cardiac output in liters per minute times the number of milliliters of oxygen contained in 1 L of arterial blood. In the resting state this is about 5×200, or 1000 ml O_2/min. About one fourth of this is used by the tissues, and three fourths returns to the heart in mixed venous blood. During exercise the amount of oxygen contained in 1 L of arterial blood does not increase, but the cardiac output does increase. With cardiac output of 24 L/min, the oxygen delivered would be 24×200, or 4800 ml/min. The tissues would use three fourths of this amount, and only one fourth would be returned to the heart in mixed venous blood.[15]

An inadequate amount of hemoglobin, such as occurs in anemia, or an inadequate heart pump or a problem with the circulatory system can each have a deleterious effect on the delivery of oxygen. In these situations the basic problem is treated in an attempt to increase the amount of available hemoglobin, to strengthen the heart pump and thus increase the cardiac output,

or to improve the circulatory system. As can be seen in Table 49-1, severe anemia, carbon monoxide poisoning, methemoglobinemia, congestive heart failure, or hemorrhage are possible interferences that will need to be corrected before an optimal amount of oxygen will be avilable to the tissues.

If hypotension is present secondary to hemorrhage or a failing heart pump there may be several sequelae. These include (1) anginal pain, since the coronary vessels that normally extract almost the maximal amount of oxygen from the blood cannot significantly increase oxygen uptake to meet their needs; and (2) changes in sensorium and behavior secondary to cerebral anoxia. If this situation continues and there is inadequate oxygenation of tissues, respiratory or cardiac arrest may result. If an arrest occurs, cardiopulmonary resuscitation (CPR) must be instituted. CPR is discussed in detail on p. 1080, and the reader is referred there for details.

In any of the above situations oxygen therapy will be instituted.

Oxygen therapy

When supplemental oxygen is necessary it may be administered by nasal catheter, by nasal prongs, or by mask (Fig. 49-13). The method used will depend on the patient's condition and the concentration of oxygen required. The nurse should be familiar with the various devices used to administer oxygen, and when oxygen is in use the nurse should check the equipment frequently to be sure that it is working properly.

When the patient is having difficulty exchanging oxygen and carbon dioxide, such as occurs in pulmonary edema, oxygen may be given under positive pressure. In some situations, such as chronic obstructive pulmo-

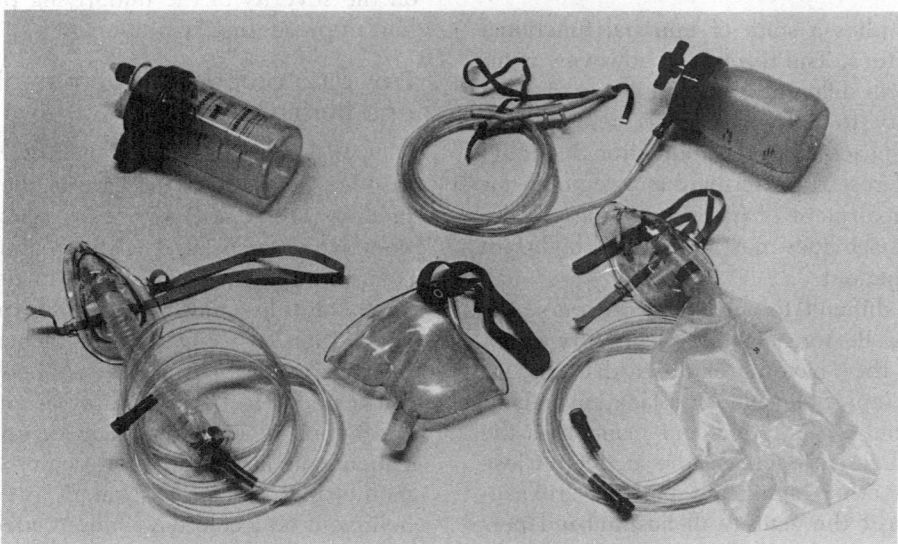

Fig. 49-13. *Top left,* Oxygen humidifying bottle. *Top right,* Nasal prongs with tubing and humidifying bottle. *Bottom,* Three types of oxygen masks.

nary disease, low-flow rates of oxygen are indicated. The use of low-flow oxygen is discussed on p. 1325. In all situations, the nurse should remember that a patient suffering from hypoxemia may not be breathless or cyanotic since cyanosis does not occur until there is 5 g or more of deoxygenated hemoglobin. In a person with anemia all the available heme is completely saturated with oxygen and thus these patients are never cyanotic even though they may be hypoxemic. For this reason an increase in the pulse rate may be the first indication that the patient is experiencing hypoxemia. When patients are receiving oxygen therapy they will be monitored by arterial blood gas studies. These studies are explained on p. 1221. The oxyhemoglobin curve and factors affecting it are discussed in Chapter 48.

Providing rest

Rest is frequently prescribed as a regimen for persons who have some impairment of tissue oxygenation. The cause may be a respiratory problem interfering with oxygen reaching the blood, a cardiac problem interfering with oxygen being pumped to the tissues, or a red blood cell (hemoglobin) deficiency interfering with the oxygen-carrying capacity of the blood. Any excess demand on the body for oxygen, resulting from increased need by the muscles during increased activity, places a severe burden on the already compromised lungs or heart. Dyspnea or hyperventilation may occur as the person attempts to increase oxygen intake, and the pulse rate increases as the heart works harder to send more oxygen to the muscles. Fatigue occurs as products of anaerobic metabolism build up in the muscles. The person with impairment of tissue oxygenation may require periods of decreased activity at regular intervals in order to provide decreased cellular demand for oxygen.

Physical rest implies a state of minimal functional and metabolic activities. The term *rest*, however, is interpreted by people in different ways and may vary from complete immobility to fairly strenuous activity that achieves a sense of peace and relaxation after the activity is completed. If rest is prescribed as a regimen for the person with impairment of tissue oxygenation, the extent of permissible activities must be clarified by health personnel and the patient.

Physical rest is difficult to achieve if the person is restless or anxious. Persons having respiratory problems or who know they have an acute cardiac disease may be extremely apprehensive. Explanations about what is occurring, and a calm, confident manner on the part of the nurse, help to decrease the anxiety. Close family members or other significant persons are usually permitted to visit the acutely ill hospitalized person, but other visitors should be restricted. Family members and significant others should be kept informed about the person's condition and therapy to decrease their anxiety and gain their cooperation. Calmness on their part will contribute to the patient's rest. Members of the family should be encouraged not to worry the person, but mention of daily problems should *not* be avoided, since the person may suspect that information is being withheld, and the worry will interfere with achieving rest.

Adequate rest is important in combating respiratory disease. During respiratory illness, however, normal sleep may be interrupted for a number of reasons. The patient may be plagued with frequent coughing, and breathing may be difficult. Airways may become blocked with secretions, and the patient may be awakened by shortness of breath.

The nurse should be alert for signs of what irritates the patient, precipitates cough, and therefore prevents rest. For example, excessive talking, smoking, or laughing or sitting in a draft or in a dry, overheated room may predispose to coughing. Cough medications given before the hour of sleep and when rest is disturbed by coughing are often helpful. However, when noisy breathing occurs and it is obvious that secretions are present in the respiratory tract, the person should be encouraged to cough deeply and to expectorate until the airway is free of obstruction before cough medication is given. A suitable position in bed and changes in position also help the patient to rest more quietly. Room temperature and ventilation should be kept at the level most comfortable for the patient.

As the person's condition improves and a greater number of activities are permitted, the person needs to guard against overexertion as evidenced by dyspnea, fatigue, or chest pain. Periods of more strenuous activity should be interspersed with periods of decreased physical activity. The amount of rest required will depend on the severity of the underlying problem and the extent of presenting symptoms.

Providing proper environmental temperature and humidity

Considerations related to environmental temperature are relevant in the care of the person with a respiratory problem in two ways. First, the vasoconstriction that is associated with breathing cold air further compromises oxygen delivery to tissues. Second, cold air contains less moisture than warm air. Consequently, in addition to using calories to heat the inspired air, moisture is taken from the tracheobronchial tree. The nurse needs to be alert to environmental temperature and humidity and its physiologic effects on the patient. Patients in air-conditioned rooms may require closer monitoring. Before discharge, precautions related to being out on a cold day without adequate covering over the face should be discussed with the patient. Many persons with chronic heart and lung problems wear some type of face mask when they must be out in cold weather.

Providing adequate nutrition

The person with hypoxia often experiences anorexia, nausea and vomiting from decreased gastrointestinal motility, fluid and electrolyte imbalances, dyspnea, or fatigue. The odor and taste in the mouth caused by frequent raising of sputum may affect appetite and impair nutrition. Provision should be made for oral hygiene before meals—washing of hands is encouraged; sputum containers should be removed before meals.

Frequently, persons with breathing difficulties cannot tolerate regular-sized meals, and smaller and more frequent feedings provide for better nutrition. Gas-forming foods should be avoided. For the person with respiratory problems who does not have a fluid restriction, taking adequate amounts of fluids helps to liquefy the secretions so that they may be coughed up more easily. If generalized edema is present as a result of inadequate pumping by the heart, sodium may be restricted in the diet.

Following is a list of the types of foods to be avoided on restricted sodium diets:

1. *No-added-salt diet* (2 to 3 g sodium). Avoid salting food at table, highly salted foods such as potato chips, luncheon meats, pickled foods, and seasonings such as catsup and mustard.
2. *Moderate low-sodium diet* (1 g sodium). Avoid (in addition to above) milk and cheese; canned fruits, vegetables, or soups; products containing baking powder or baking soda; commercial salad dressings; carbonated beverages; and antacids.

Persons may need help in planning diets to meet prescribed sodium restrictions. Special foods need not be prepared for the person on a restricted sodium diet. The simplest method is to cook the food for the entire family without salt, set aside the one portion, and then season the remainder.

Maintaining a functioning respiratory center

Hypoventilation or apnea can occur if there is depression of the respiratory center by general anesthesia, morphine, heroin, barbiturates, or alcohol. Diseases of the central nervous system, such as bulbar poliomyelitis or meningitis, also will depress the respiratory center, as will an increase in intracranial pressure. In these situations the patient's respirations will have to be supported until the patient is able to maintain his or her own breathing. Intubation with an endotracheal tube, supplemental oxygen, and artificial respiration with a ventilator may all be required. The conditions causing depression of the respiratory center will need to be identified and treated while the person's ventilation is being maintained. Details of management of patients in respiratory failure are discussed on p. 1331.

Intervention thoracic surgery the person requiring

Intelligent nursing racic surgery depends physiology of the chest, of procedures and practice of the anatomy and recover from the operatie ry performed, and thesia became possible, su st the patient to a great impetus. Before tha otracheal anes- sible, except in the rarest o est was given on the lung without causing t been pos- and death. By means of endo o operate possible to keep the unaffected d lung and functioning even when it spheric pressure. Endotracheal it is surgery involving the lungs and f c led in which the pleural space is enter

Principles of resectional surgery

In order to understand resectional purpose of chest tubes and water-seal c it is important to review a few points abo of the lung. The pleura, which lines the c covers the lung, is one continuous serous The portion that covers the lung is the *visce* and that covering the inside of the chest wall *parietal pleura*. Together they form a *potential spac* which normally contains a few milliliters of serous fluid that lubricates the surfaces and prevents friction rub during respiration. The pressure in the pleural space is subatmospheric (less than 760 mm Hg) and is referred to as being negative. This pressure is usually 756 mm Hg and goes down to about 751 mm Hg before inspiration. It is this change in pressure that allows air (atmospheric pressure) to enter and expand the lungs. The pressure within the lung itself (*intrapulmonic*) always remains near 760 (758 to 762) mm Hg.

When the pleura is entered surgically or by trauma to the chest, atmospheric pressure (positive pressure) enters the pleural space and the lung collapses. Thus after resection of the lung (except pneumonectomy) two drainage tubes are inserted into the pleural space and each tube is connected to a water-seal drainage bottle. The tubes have holes in them that allow air and fluid to be removed from the pleural space. As long as the tip of the tube in the chest bottle is 1 to 2 cm under water and all connections between it and the patient's chest tube are secure, the system is "sealed" (Fig. 49-17); that is, air and fluid can escape from the pleural space into the drainage bottles and no air (positive pressure) or fluid can reenter.

1250

In all resectional surgery ... pt pneumonectomy) the remaining portions of t... ated lung must over-expand and fill the spac... left by the removal of the resected portion. *Ins ...rimary purpose of chest tubes and water-se...is to (1) aid in the expansion of the remo... in the pleural space*. This is establish nego... fluid are removed from the accomplish... ...tions necessary to maintain the pleural s... are discussed on p. 1253. integr...

...edures

...resents the types of resectional surgery ...tions for the use of each type. A brief ...each type of resectional surgery follows.

...ry thoracotomy

...xploratory thoracotomy is an operation done to ... a suspected diagnosis of lung or chest disease. ...sual approach is by a posterolateral parascapular ...ion through the fourth, fifth, sixth, or seventh in-...costal space. Occasionally, an anterior approach is ...ed. The ribs are spread to give the best possible exposure of the lung and hemithorax. The pleura is entered and the lung examined, a biopsy usually is taken, and the chest closed. This procedure may also be used to detect bleeding in the chest or other injury following trauma to the chest. Since the pleural space was entered, a chest tube and water-seal drainage are necessary.

Pneumonectomy

A pneumonectomy, the removal of an entire lung, is most commonly done to treat bronchogenic carci-

noma (Fig. 49-14, *A*). It may also be used to treat tuberculosis. However, a pneumonectomy is only done in those instances when a lobectomy or segmental resection will not remove all the diseased tissue. A thoracotomy incision is made in either the posterior or anterior chest using the method described under exploratory thoracotomy. Before the lung can be removed, the pulmonary artery and vein are ligated and then cut. The main-stem bronchus leading to the lung is clamped, divided, and sutured, usually with black silk. To ensure an airtight closure of the bronchus, a pleural flap is placed over it and sutured into place. The phrenic nerve on the operative side is crushed, causing the diaphragm on that side to rise and reduce the size of the remaining space. Because there is no lung left to reexpand, drainage tubes are not used. Ideally, the pressure in the closed chest is slightly negative. This pressure is taken postoperatively using a pneumothorax machine, and air can be removed or added to attain the desired pressure. The fluid left in the space will consolidate in time, preventing the remaining lung and heart from shifting toward the operative side (mediastinal shift).

Lobectomy

In a lobectomy one lobe of the lung is removed (Fig. 49-14, *B*). It is used to treat bronchiectasis, bronchogenic carcinoma, emphysematous blebs or bullae, lung abscess, benign tumors, fungal infections, and tuberculosis. For a lobectomy to be successful the disease must be confined to one lobe and the remaining lung tissue must be capable of overexpanding to fill up the

TABLE 49-4. Types of resectional surgery and indications for their use

Procedure	Indications
Pneumonectomy	Bronchogenic carcinoma when lobectomy will not remove all of lesion; tuberculosis confined to one lung
Lobectomy	Bronchiectasis, bronchogenic carcinoma, emphysematous blebs or bullae; lung abscess; fungal infections; benign tumors; tuberculosis
Segmental resection (segmentectomy)	Bronchiectasis; lung abscess; lung cyst; metastatic carcinoma; hemartoma (benign developmental tumor of the lung)
Wedge resection	Well-circumscribed benign tumors; metastatic tumors) localized inflammatory disease
Decortication	Fibrinous peel on visceral pleura secondary to chronic empyema
Exploratory thoracotomy	To confirm suspected diagnosis of lung or chest disease; to obtain a biopsy specimen

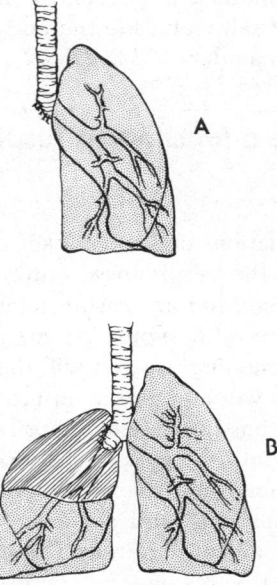

Fig. 49-14. A, Surgical absence of right lung following pneumonectomy. **B,** Surgical absence of right upper lobe following lobectomy.

space. Two chest tubes are connected to water-seal bottles for postoperative drainage.

Segmental resection (segmentectomy)

In a segmental resection one or more segments of the lung are removed. This operation is used in an attempt to preserve as much functioning lung tissue as possible. It is a very taxing operation for the surgeon, since the dissection between segments must be done very carefully and slowly, and the identification of the segmental pulmonary artery and vein and bronchus is more difficult than when a lobe is involved. Since there are ten segments in the right lung and eight segments in the left lung, only a portion of a lobe or lobes may need to be removed. The most common indication for segmentectomy is bronchiectasis. It is also used to treat the other conditions listed in Table 49-4. Chest tubes and water-seal drainage are necessary postoperatively. Because of air leaks from the segmental surface, the remaining lung tissue may take longer to reexpand.

Wedge resection

In a wedge resection a well-circumscribed diseased portion is removed without regard to the segmental planes. The area to be removed is clamped, dissected, and sutured. Chest tubes and water-sealed drainage are used postoperatively.

Decortication

In a decortication a fibrinous peel is removed from the visceral pleura, allowing the encased lung to reexpand and obliterate the pleural space. This procedure is discussed further under the treatment of empyema (p. 1309). Chest tubes and chest suction are used to facilitate the reexpansion of the lung. If the lung has been encased for a long time, it may be incapable of reexpanding following decortication. In this situation thoracoplasty may be necessary.

Thoracoplasty

A thoracoplasty is an extrapleural procedure involving the removal of ribs. By removing ribs it is possible to reduce the size of the chest cavity. Before the widespread use of resectional surgery, thoracoplasty was the basic surgical treatment for tuberculosis. Today thoracoplasty is used (infrequently) primarily to prevent or treat the complications of resectional surgery. When it is felt that a patient's lung may not be able to expand sufficiently after a resection to fill the space, a thoracoplasty is done 2 or 3 weeks before the resection. It also may be done before pneumonectomy, since this will reduce the chance of mediastinal shift after surgery. This type of thoracoplasty is often called a *preresection* or *tailoring* thoracoplasty; that is, the chest wall is tailored to reduce its size.

If the remaining portions of the lung fail to reexpand

sufficiently after resection or if another complication such as empyema occurs, a thoracoplasty is done. In general, it is employed when there is a space in the chest that cannot be olbiterated by other means. Usually no more than three ribs are removed, and therefore paradoxical motion following thoracoplasty is seldom seen anymore. Paradoxical motion is discussed under chest injuries (p. 1235).

Preoperative care

Evaluation

In addition to the screening tests that are run on all preoperative patients, special tests are usually required for persons having chest surgery. These may include chest radiography including laminography and computed tomography (CT) scan, pulmonary function tests, arterial blood gases, bronchoscopy and, in some instances, bronchography. All of these procedures are discussed in detail in Chapter 48. If the patient is being considered for a pneumonectomy, the evaluation will be even more precise since it must be determined if the uninvolved ("good") lung will be able to maintain adequate pulmonary function after surgery. In one center, patients being considered for pneumonectomy are evaluated on their forced expiratory volume in the first second (FEV_1) as follows: 1. If the FEV_1 is greater than 70% of the predicted normal level (approximately 2.5 L of flow), the patient's lung function is essentially normal and the patient should be able to tolerate a pneumonectomy as long as cardiac status and arterial blood gases are acceptable. 2. If the FEV_1 is less than 35% of the predicted normal level (less than 1.1 L of flow), there is severe ventilatory impairment, and surgical resection is not feasible. 3. If the FEV_1 is between 35% and 70% of the predicted normal level (1.2 to 2.4 L of flow), there is mild to moderate ventilatory impairment, and further studies will be necessary to determine the maximal tolerable resection.[64]

Since the tests may be done on an outpatient basis, the office nurse or clinic nurse must be sure that the patient understands what tests are to be performed and the preparation for them. The person's significant others also are kept informed.

Teaching

The operation is discussed with both the patient and family. The preoperative nursing care is similar to that discussed on p. 406. The purpose of the teaching is to prepare the patient for what he or she must do postoperatively. If the patient will go from a recovery room to an intensive care unit, this should be explained to the patient and family. In some medical centers, nurses from the operating room, recovery room, or intensive care unit make a preoperative visit and explain the routines to the patient. In other settings, the nurse caring for the patient preoperatively will be responsible for the teaching.

The patient should be told that oxygen usually by mask or nasal prongs is given postoperatively to all patients undergoing thoracic surgery. The patient also needs to know that frequent turning and coughing every 1 to 2 hours postoperatively will be necessary to maintain a clear airway and to aid in the reexpansion of the remaining portions of the lung.

The nurse teaches the patient how to cough before surgery. Patients who practice coughing preoperatively usually will cough more effectively postoperatively. Exercises to preserve symmetric body alignment, full range of motion of the shoulder, and maximal pulmonary function are usually started during the preoperative period and continued postoperatively. In some hopsitals the physical therapist instructs the patient. The nurse, however, provides follow-up instructions and is responsible for seeing that the patient carries out the instructions properly. Many times the nurse must take the responsibility for teaching the exercises. If so, the nurse should find out which exercises the surgeon believes should be used and, if possible, should obtain assistance from a physical therapist in how best to provide each specific exercise.

If chest tubes are to be used for drainage of the chest, the patient can be told that they will be used to drain fluid and air that normally accumulates after a chest operation. The patient should be told to expect to have pain for some time postoperatively because intercostal nerves are severed, but that medication will be given for this pain and that pain cannot be allowed to interfere with the need to cough as directed. The patient should also understand that it is all right to ask whether pain medication can be given. The patient should know that an intravenous infusion may be started in a vein in the arm or leg before he or she leaves for the operating room.

Postoperative care

Immediate care

Usually the patient is kept flat in bed until vital signs are stabilized. After vital signs are stable, frequent turning is instituted, with care being taken that the patient is not lying on the tubes so that drainage is occluded. Oxygen is usually administered and continued until the patient has fully reacted from anesthesia.

Vital signs are taken every 15 minutes for 2 hours and then every hour for several hours. It is not unusual for blood pressure to fluctuate during the first 24 to 36 hours, and close monitoring of the patient is essential. *Bleeding on chest dressings is unusual, and should it occur, it should be reported at once.*

When fully recovered from the anesthesia, the patient can usually breathe best in semi-Fowler's position. Patients are most comfortable if a pillow is placed under the head and neck but not under the shoulder and back. When assisting the patient to and from a sitting position, the nurse should use the arm on the patient's unoperated side. The back of the neck should also be supported. When the patient lies back down, the head and neck are supported until they are on the pillow.

Coughing

The patient should be assisted to cough as soon as conscious. If the blood pressure is stable, the patient is assisted to a sitting position and the incision is supported anteriorly and posteriorly by the nurse's hands. Firm, even pressure over the incision with the open palm of the hands is a most effective method. The nurse's head should be behind the patient for coughing (Fig. 49-15). The patient is encouraged to breathe deeply, exhale, and then cough. Sips of fluids, especially warm ones such as tea or coffee, often facilitate coughing. Coughing keeps the *airway patent, prevents atelectasis, and facilitates reexpansion of the lung*. The patient should cough every hour for the first 24 hours and then every 2 to 4 hours. The patient should cough until the chest sounds clear. Otherwise, secretions will accumulate in the tracheobronchial tree. If the patient is unable to cough effectively, tracheal suctioning may be necessary.

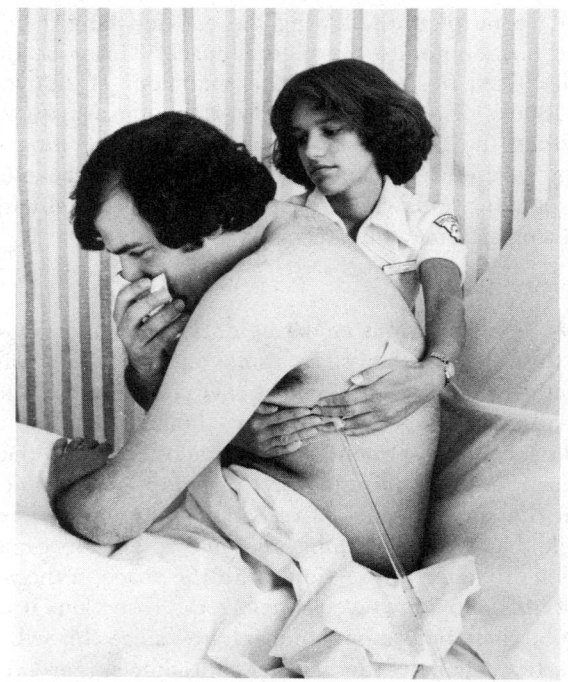

Fig. 49-15. Nurse assists patient to cough by splinting incision with firm support from hands. This lessens muscle pull and pain as patient coughs. Note that nurse keeps her head behind patient while he coughs, and patient uses tissue to cover mouth.

The patient can cough most effectively 20 to 30 minutes after receiving pain medication, and this should be capitalized on by the nursing staff.

Pain

Morphine or meperidine hydrochloride is usually ordered for pain. Medication for pain should be given as needed and may be required as often as every 3 to 4 hours during the first 48 to 72 hours. The patient is extremely uncomfortable and will not be able to cough or turn unless there is relief from pain. In some instances the dose of the narcotic is decreased so that it may be given oftener and yet not depress respirations. The tubes in the chest cause pain, and the patient may attempt rapid, shallow breathing to splint the lower chest and avoid motion of the catheters. This impairs ventilation, makes coughing ineffective, and causes secretions to be retained. Thus it is a nursing responsibility to do all that is possible to make the patient comfortable, since this facilitates deep breathing and coughing. If, despite all efforts, the patient's discomfort is interfering with adequate chest excursion, an intercostal nerve block may be performed.

Nutrition

The patient is encouraged to take fluids postoperatively and to progress to a general diet as soon as it is tolerated. Forcing fluids helps to liquefy secretions and makes them easier to expectorate. Usually fluids by mouth and mist therapy are all that are needed to thin and loosen secretions.

Exercises

Abdominal breathing exercises such as those described on p. 1242 are a valuable adjunct to the care of the patient with chest surgery because they improve ventilation without increasing pain and assist in coughing more effectively. The exercises should be taught preoperatively so that the patient has time to practice them before surgery.

Passive arm exercises are usually started the evening of surgery. The purpose in putting the patient's arm through range of motion is to prevent restriction of function. Most patients are reluctant to move the arm on the operative side, but with proper preoperative instruction and postoperative follow-through they do so readily. It is important for both the patient and nurse to understand that the longer the arm is unexercised, the stiffer it will become. The patient should put both arms through active range of motion two or three times a day within a few days. The recommended exercises are similar to those done following mastectomy (p. 1752). The exercises are best done when the patient is upright or lying on the abdomen. Exercises such as elevating the scapula and clavicle, "hunching the shoulders," bringing the scapulae as close together as possible, and

hyperextending the arm can only be done in these positions. Since lying on the abdomen may not be possible at first, these exercises are done when the patient is sitting on the edge of the bed or standing.

Chest tubes and closed drainage

As described earlier, the lungs are surrounded by the pleural space. Under normal conditions subatmospheric (negative) pressure exists within the pleural space. This vacuum keeps the lung adherent to the chest wall so that as the thorax expands with respiration, the lung also expands. When the pleural membrane is disrupted by thoracic surgery, atmospheric (positive) pressure enters the pleural space.

All patients who have resectional surgery of the lung, except those having a pneumonectomy, will require drainage of the pleural space by chest tubes connected to closed drainage. Usually two tubes are used. One catheter is inserted through a stab wound in the anterior chest wall above the resected area. This is referred to as the *anterior* or *upper tube*. It is used to remove air from the pleural space. The second tube is inserted through a stab wound in the posterior chest and is referred to as the *posterior* or *lower tube*. It is primarily for the drainage of *serosanguineous* fluid that accumulates as the result of the operative procedure. The lower tube may be of a larger diameter than the upper tube to prevent it from becoming plugged with clots. Fig. 49-16 shows the placement of tubes within the pleural space.

Initiating chest tube drainage. When initiating chest tube drainage, a 2-L clear glass bottle is usually used, although other commercial devices, such as the PleureVac system, are available. Approximately 300 ml of sterile water, or enough to fill the bottle 1 to 2 cm from the bottom, is then added. The tubing is fastened to the bed so that there are no dependent loops between the bottles and the bed (Fig. 49-17). The tip of the tube should be kept from 1 to 2 cm under water so that if the bottle accidentally tips over, the tube will remain under water. The water level in the bottle is marked by placing an adhesive strip at the waterline. The date and hour are written on the tape, which gives a ready indication as to the amount of drainage. If considerable drainage accumulates in the bottle, this will increase the amount of subatmospheric (negative) pressure in the system, and it will be more difficult for the patient to expel air and fluid. In this instance the glass rod may be pulled up so that less of it is under water or the surgeon may order that the drainage bottle be changed. In this case a sterile setup is prepared. When the bottle with sterile water and the tubing are ready, the chest tube is clamped as close to the patient's chest as possible. The chest tube is then disconnected from the drainage tubing, the new setup is connected, and the chest tube is unclamped. The drainage should be measured and may be sent to the laboratory for examination.

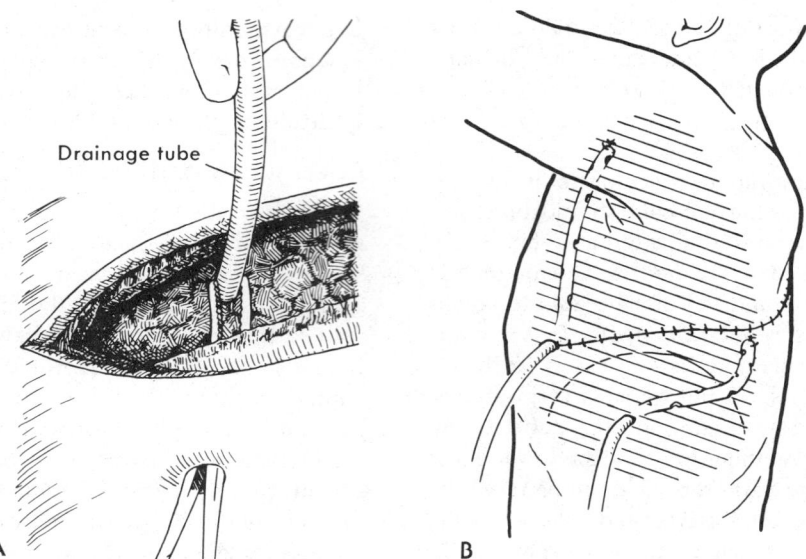

Fig. 49-16. A, Drainage tube being inserted into pleural space. **B,** Note that upper and lower tubes are placed well into pleural space. (From Johnson, J., MacVaugh, H., III, and Waldhausen, J.A.: Surgery of the chest, a handbook of operative surgery, ed. 4. Copyright © 1970 by Year Book Medical Publishers, Inc., Chicago. Used by permission.)

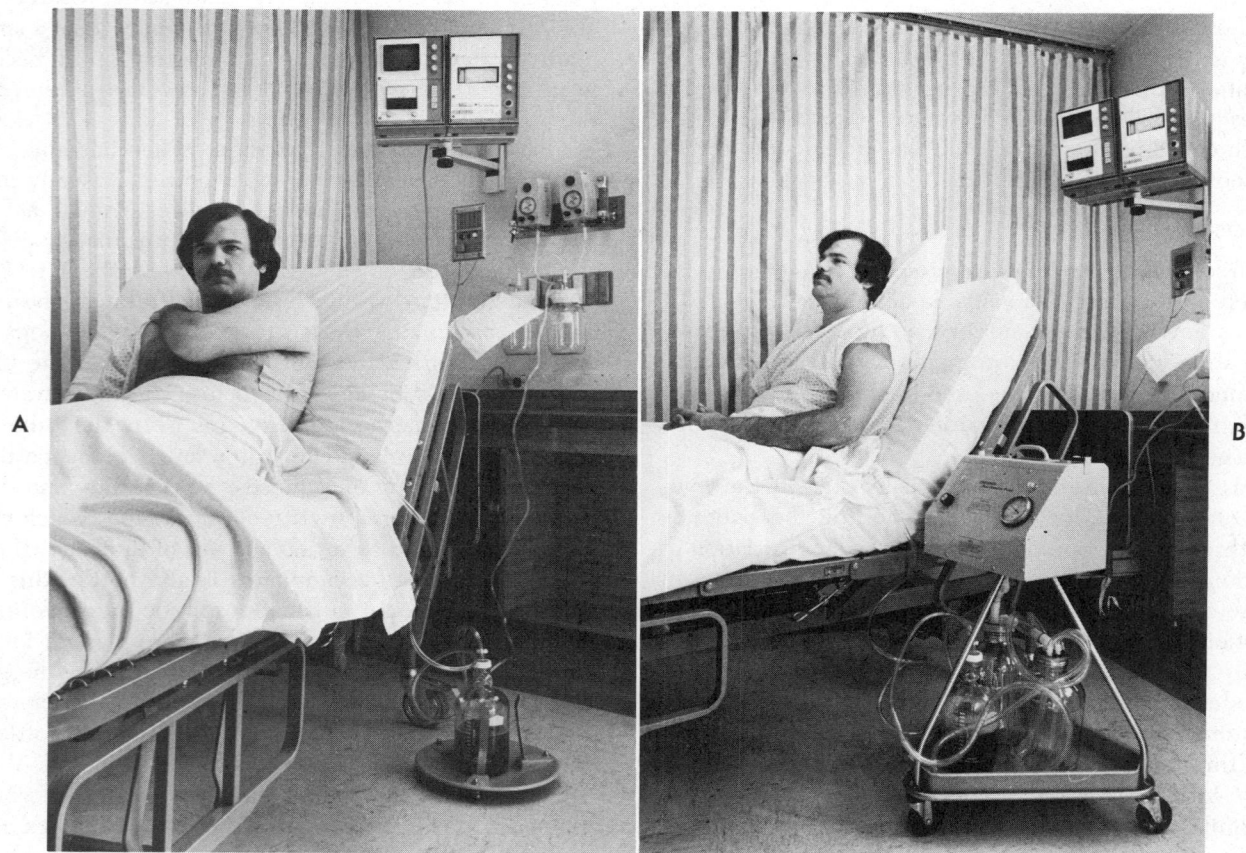

Fig. 49-17. Chest tube with water-seal suction, **A,** Wall outlet provides source of suction. Note holder used to secure bottle in upright position. **B,** Emerson suction machine as source of vacuum.

As the patient breathes, there will be movement of fluid in the glass tube that is under water. This is known as *fluctuation* or *oscillation,* and the column will move up when the patient inhales or coughs, and it will fall when the patient is exhaling. The tubes should be checked for fluctuation frequently. If the column of water is not fluctuating, the nurse should be sure that the patient is not lying on the tubes or that they are not blocked by a clot. Asking the patient to cough or to change position often restores visible fluctuation. If fluctuation still does not occur, this should be reported.

Some thoracic surgeons wish to have the chest tubes "milked" or "stripped" every hour to prevent formation of clots that could plug the tubes. Recently, questions have been raised about routinely stripping chest tubes since the practice increases the negative pressure exerted on the pleural space. A study by two nurse–clinical specialists revealed the following: (1) the pressure generated by stripping was considerably higher than the suction pressures of -15 to -20 cm of water commonly applied to chest drainage systems; (2) the amount of pressure was directly related to the length of the tubing stripped; and (3) even stripping only a few centimeters produced pressures near -100 cm of water and stripping the entire tube produced pressures exceeding -400 cm of water.[21] They also found that higher negative pressures resulted when a roller was used to strip the tubes rather than the hands.[21]

Undesirable side effects of increased levels of negative pressure reported in the literature include (1) lung entrapment in the thoracic tube eyelets and focal tissue infarction and (2) persistent pneumothorax.[88] The persistent pneumothorax occurs when the pleural surface of lung, which normally has air leaks at the close of the operative procedure, does not "seal off." Usually fibrin will seal the air leaks; however, the presence of an increased amount of negative pressure may prevent the air leaks from sealing off and may even increase the size of the air leaks. This is the reason why some thoracic surgeons do not attach additional suction to the water-sealed drainage system for the first 24 hours or so after surgery. They believe that this amount of time is sufficient in most instances to allow the pleural surface to seal off.

In view of the above findings, the nurse should consult with the thoracic surgeon about the desirability of routinely stripping chest tubes. Because the anterior (upper) tube usually evacuates mainly air there is less reason to believe that this tube will clot off. Posterior tubes, which are commonly inserted lower in the chest, usually drain more fluid and blood and are more likely to clot off. However, gentle squeezing of the tube is usually sufficient to move the bloody drainage along in the tubing. Another important factor is to ensure that there are no loops in the tubing since these impede drainage. Special caution should be used in stripping tubes of patients with a known history of fragile tissue, such as occurs in emphysema.[21]

Two hemostats should be kept at the bedside at all times (Fig. 49-18). These are to be used to clamp the tube if the water-sealed bottle is accidentally broken. For this reason the patient and all personnel should know what to do if a bottle is broken. When a bottle is broken, the chest catheter should be clamped and then reconnected to a sterile setup as soon as possible. Sterile water should be used in the bottle. As soon as the system is reconnected with the tip of the tube under water, the clamp should be removed. Except in case of an emergency, such as a broken bottle, most thoracic surgeons prefer that tubes not be clamped, and a specific order is written if clamping is desired. The reason for this is that when the tubes are clamped, air (positive pressure) may leak from the pleural surface and further collapse the lung. Therefore if the patient is being transported from one place to another, such as to the radiology department, tubes should not be clamped unless it is for a very few minutes. In general, water-sealed bottles are changed only on specific order of the physician or if the bottle is broken, which is rare. If the nurse is expected to change the bottles routinely, the procedure outlined at the beginning of this section should be employed using strict asepsis.

Water-sealed bottles should never be lifted above the level of the patient's chest, since this would allow the water in the bottle to be pulled into the pleural space. The bottle should be placed on the floor so that they will not be broken by a lowered side rail. When a Hi-Lo bed is being used, care must be taken not to lower the bed onto the bottles.

Suction. Suction is usually used to speed reexpansion of the lung after surgery, using either wall suction or an Emerson suction machine (Fig. 49-17, *B*). Most often -30 cm of suction is applied, but this varies according to the surgeon's preference. When it is particularly important to regulate the exact amount of suction used, a "breaker" bottle may be added to the system between the suction source and the patient's drainage bottle. The use of a breaker bottle provides for control of the amount of suction that is applied to the water-sealed bottle and thus to the patient's pleural space. The stopper in the control bottle has three openings. One is connected to the water-sealed bottle, one is connected to the suction source, and the third contains a glass rod that is under water and open to the outside (Fig. 49-18). The amount of suction produced will be determined by the distance between the surface of the water and the tip of this tube. When the suction source is turned on, the level of water in the open tube will sink in proportion to the amount of negative pressure in the system. Thus if there is 15 cm of water between the surface of the water and the tip of the tube, the amount of negative pressure in the system will be 15

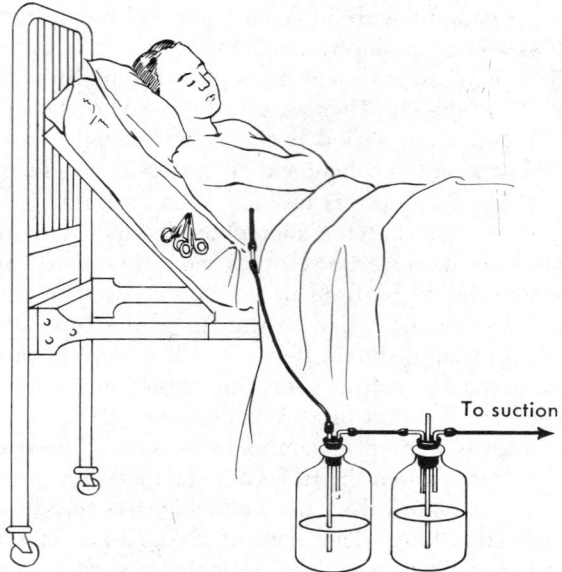

To suction

Fig. 49-18. Chest catheter in place. Chest catheter is attached to closed drainage system. Note that glass tube in drainage bottle connected to tubing of chest catheter is below level of water. Bottle to right of drainage bottle is "breaker bottle" and regulates amount of suction transmitted to drainage bottle, chest catheter, and pleural cavity. Two hemostats attached to bed are available if bottle breaks or water-seal system is otherwise interrupted.

cm of water pressure. Since the water will be at the bottom of the tube when this amount of pressure is reached, any increase in negative pressure will cause air to be drawn in from the outside, *breaking* the suction at this level. Therefore it can be expected that the water in the breaker bottle will bubble almost continuously. If it fails to bubble at all, the desired level of suction is not being attained. When the water in the breaker bottle is not bubbling, the tubing should be checked for air leaks. If there are no leaks and bubbling still does not occur, the surgeon should be notified at once since the air leak in the pleura may be so great that the amount of negative pressure is not sufficient to overcome it. In this instance water may be added to the breaker bottle to increase the distance between the surface of the water and the tip of the tube, thereby increasing the amount of negative pressure being exerted on the pleural space.

The distance the tube is placed under water in the breaker bottle is determined by the surgeon. A breaker bottle and suction may be attached to one or both tubes. Most commonly it is attached to the upper tube, since this is where air is most likely to be leaking from the pleural surface. A small empty trap bottle is usually attached by tubing between the breaker bottle and the suction source. The purpose of this bottle is to protect the suction motor from becoming wet should the breaker

bottle overflow. (Further information about other kinds of chest suction devices in common use can be found in other sources.[19,47,105,109])

Ambulation. There is no contraindication to ambulating with a chest tube in place. As long as the water-sealed bottle remains below the level of the chest, the patient may assume any position of comfort in bed or may be out of bed in a chair.

Removal of the chest tube. Chest tubes are removed when there is no fluctuation of fluid in the tubing, and when roentgenograms confirm the full reexpansion of the lung. The patient should receive medication for pain 30 minutes before removal of the tube. Physicians vary in the exact procedure used to remove the tube, but generally a sterile scissors, 4-in. × 4-in. gauze squares, and adhesive tape are required. The suture holding the tube in place is cut, the patient is asked to exhale deeply, and the tube is removed. If a purse-string suture was used, it is retied and a dry sterile dressing is placed over the site. Some physicians cover the site with a Telfa dressing instead of gauze squares to ensure an airtight dressing. The dressing is covered securely by three strips of 2-in. adhesive tape.

Complications of resectional surgery

The most common complications of resectional surgery include a persistent air space that is not filled by the remaining lung, bronchopleural fistula, and empyema. A thoracoplasty may be necessary eventually to correct any of these complications.

Special care following pneumonectomy

Chest tubes are not necessary following pneumonectomy since there is no lung tissue to reexpand. At the same time, serous drainage will accumulate in the empty space and over time will congeal to about the consistency of axle grease. The presence of this fluid in the pleural space may help prevent the remaining lung and mediastinum from shifting toward the empty space (mediastinal shift).

Generally, the patient is permitted to be only on his or her back or operated side, since some surgeons fear that the sutured bronchus may not stay closed. If it should open while the patient is lying with the operative side uppermost, fluid in the operative side would drain into the good lung and drown the patient. Although the chances of this occurring are small, this precaution is usually observed. Another reason for not allowing the patient to lie on the unoperated side is that this compresses the remaining lung and restricts lung excursion and ventilation. The patient is watched immediately postoperatively for cardiac overload, and CVP monitoring (p. 1055) is common. The patient should also be watched closely for mediastinal shift. If pressure builds up within the operative side, it can cause the mediastinum to shift toward the unoperated side. Conversely, the unoperated lung may shift toward the empty space left after a pneumonectomy. For this reason the surgeon will palpate the patient's trachea at least daily to be sure that it is in midline. If a shift occurs toward the good lung, it is treated by removing air (positive pressure) from the empty space. If the shift is toward the empty space, air may be instilled into the space to increase the pressure and cause the mediastinum to shift back. If the mediastinum persists in shifting toward the empty side, a thoracoplasty may be necessary. This will reduce the size of the space and keep the mediastinum in midline. A patient with mediastinal shift resembles the patient in congestive heart failure. Neck veins are distended, the trachea is displaced to one side, pulse and respirations are increased, and dyspnea is present.

Patients who have had a lung removed may have a lowered vital capacity, and exercise and activity should be limited to that which can be carried out without dyspnea. Before the widespread use of pulmonary function tests such as FEV_1 to determine whether the patient could tolerate a pneumonectomy safely, it was assumed that pulmonary function might improve after the body became accustomed to having only one lung. However, it is now known that pulmonary function remains relatively stable after pneumonectomy and there is no significant change with time. This is not true in lobectomy, however, where there is a gradual increase in function over time.[64] If the diagnosis is cancer, radiation therapy is usually given, and it may be started before the patient leaves the hospital. (See p. 490 for further discussion of nursing care for patients receiving radiation therapy.) The patient who has had a pneumonectomy for cancer is urged to report to the physician at once if there is hoarseness, dyspnea, pain on swallowing, or localized chest pain, since these difficulties may be signs of complications.

Special care following thoracoplasty

Since thoracoplasty is an extrapleural procedure, chest tubes are not necessary unless the pleura is inadvertently entered during surgery. Because portions of several ribs (usually three or four) have been removed, the patient may have considerable pain. Drainage on the dressings may also occur. Although paradoxical motion is rarely seen unless more than three ribs are removed, the patient's breathing pattern should be watched closely. (See p. 1235 for description of paradoxical motion.)

Since thoracoplasty is performed either before or after resectional surgery, the patient is faced with more than one surgical procedure. Therefore the patient may require additional emotional support in accepting the need for two operations.

Outcome criteria for the person undergoing thoracic surgery

The person or significant others can:
1. Explain recommended changes in activities of daily living (ADL).
   a. Which usual activities to limit and for how long.
   b. Exercise program.
2. Explain any changes required in life-style (reason and plans for changes in occupation and habits such as smoking, activity level, and so on).
3. State name, dosage, action, and side effects of medications ordered.
   a. How and when to use prn medications.
   b. Schedule for other medications and how to take them.
4. Describe professional and community resources necessary for structuring an environment compatible with convalescence.
   a. Plans for obtaining assistance of agencies such as VNA.
   b. Plans for necessary modifications of home.
5. Describe plans for follow-up care.
   a. Signs or symptoms requiring immediate medical assistance.
   b. State plans for ongoing medical care.

REFERENCES AND SELECTED READINGS
Contemporary

1. Amborn, S.A.: Clinical signs associated with the amount of tracheobronchial secretions, Nurs. Res. **25**:121-126, 1976.
2. *American Lung Association: Introduction to lung diseases, New York, 1973, The Association.
3. Baier, H., Begin, R., and Sackner, M.A.: Effect of airway diameter, suction catheters, and the bronchofiberscope on airflow in endotracheal and tracheostomy tubes, Heart Lung **5**:235-238, 1976.
4. Bartlett, R.H., Gazzaniga, A.B., and Geraghty, R.T.: Respiratory maneuvers to prevent postoperative pulmonary complications: a critical review, J.A.M.A. **224**:1017-1021, 1973.
5. Bates, D., Macklem, P.T., and Christie, R.V.: Respiratory function in disease, ed. 2, Philadelphia, 1971, W.B. Saunders Co.
6. Beeson, P.B., and McDermott, W., editors: Cecil-Loeb textbook of medicine, ed. 15, Philadelphia, 1979, W.B. Saunders Co.
7. Belinkoff, S.: Introduction to respiratory care, ed. 2, Boston, 1976, Little, Brown & Co.
8. Borman, J.B., editor: Recent trends in cardiovascular and thoracic surgery, New York, 1975, Grune & Stratton, Inc.

*References preceded by an asterisk are particularly well suited for student readings.

9. Brannin, P.: Oxygen therapy and measures of bronchial hygiene, Nurs. Clin. North Am. **9**:111-121, 1974.

10. *Broughton, J.: Chest physical diagnosis for nurses and respiratory therapists, Heart Lung **2**:200-206, 1972.

11. Butler, E.K.: Dyspnea in the patient with cardiopulmonary disease, Heart Lung **4**:599-606, 1975.

12. Centers for Disease Control: Humidifiers: tips given on trimming hazards, Atlanta, Feb. 1979 The Centers Hospital Infection Control

13. Cherniack, N.S.: Abnormal breathing patterns: their mechanisms and clinical significance, J.A.M.A. **230**:57-58, 1974.

14. *Codd, J., and Grohar, M.E.: Postoperative pulmonary complications, Nurs. Clin. North Am. **10**:5-15, 1975.

15. *Comroe, J.H.: Physiology of respiration, ed. 2, Chicago, 1974, Year Book Medical Publishers, Inc.

16. Crosby, L., and Parsons, L.C.: Measurements of lateral wall pressures exerted by tracheostomy and endotracheal tube cuffs, Heart Lung **3**:797-803, 1974.

17. *Cullen, D.J., et al.: A well-positioned endotracheal tube, RN **39**:ICU1, ICU4, 1976.

18. *Cullen, P., et al.: Ventilation for flail chest: controlled mechanical vs. intermittent mandatory, RN **39**:ICU1-2, ICU-4, 1976.

19. *Daly, B.J., Gorenshek, N., and Mendelsohn, H.: Chest surgery. In Meltzer, L., et al., editors: Intensive care for nurse specialists, ed. 2, Bowie, Md., 1975, The Charles Press.

20. Downs, J.B., Block, A.J., and Vennum, K.B.: Intermittent mandatory ventilation: a new approach to weaning patients from mechanical ventilators, Chest **64**:311-335, 1973.

21. *Duncan, C., and Erichson, R.: Pressures associated with chest tube stripping, Heart Lung **11**:166-171, 1982.

22. Effler, D.B., editor: Blades' surgical diseases of the chest, ed. 4, St. Louis, 1978, The C.V. Mosby Co.

23. Egan, D.F.: Fundamentals of respiratory therapy, ed. 3, St. Louis, 1977, The C.V. Mosby Co.

24. Finch, C., and Lenfant, C.: Oxygen transport in man, N. Engl. J. Med. **286**:407-415, 1972.

25. *Fitzgerald, L.M.: Mechanical ventilation, Heart Lung **5**:939-949, 1976.

26. *Fitzgerald, L.M., and Huber, G.L.: Weaning the patient from mechanical ventilation, Heart Lung **5**:228-234, 1976.

27. *Foley, M.F.: Pulmonary function testing, Am. J. Nurs. **71**:1134-1139, 1971.

28. *Garfinkel, L.: Cigarette smoking among physicians and other health professionals, 1959-72, CA **26**:373-375, 1976.

29. *Graas, S.: Thermometer sites and oxygen, Am. J. Nurs. **74**:1862-1863, 1974.

30. Green, G.M., et al.: Defense mechanisms of the respiratory membrane, Am. Rev. Respir. Dis. **115**:479-514, 1977.

31. Griggs, B.M., and Reinhardt, D.J.: Fundamentals of nosocomial infections associated with respiratory therapy, ed. 2, New York, 1976, Projects in Health.

32. Guenter, C.A., editor: Pulmonary medicine, Philadelphia, 1977, J.B. Lippincott Co.

33. Haberman, P.B., et al.: Determinants of successful selective tracheobronchial suctioning, N. Engl. J. Med. **289**:1060-1062, 1973.

34. Hahn, A.B., Barkin, R.L., and Oestreich, S.J.K.: Pharmacology in nursing, ed. 15, St. Louis, 1982, The C.V. Mosby Co.

35. *Hanline, D.S.: Bronchoscope's benefits, Nursing **5**:55-56, 1975.

36. Hardy, K.L.: Tracheostomy: indications, technics, and tubes: a reappraisal, Am. J. Surg. **126**:300-310, 1973.

37. Harmson, H., Fergus, S., and Cole, F.H.: Pneumonectomy: review of 351 cases, Ann. Surg. **183**:719-722, 1976.

38. *Harrington, J.D., editor: Symposium on intensive care of the surgical patient, Nurs. Clin. North Am. **10**(1):1-4, 1975.

39. Hedley-Whyte, J., et al.: Applied physiology of respiratory care, Boston, 1976, Little, Brown & Co.

40. Hirsch, E.F., et al.: The lung: responses to trauma, surgery, and sepsis, Surg. Clin. North Am. **56**:909-928, 1976.

41. *Hodgkin, J.E.: Chronic obstructive pulmonary disease, Park Ridge, Ill., 1979, American College of Chest Physicians.

42. *Humbrecht, B., and Van Parys, E.: From assessment to intervention: how to use heart and breath sounds as part of your nursing care plan, Nurs. '82 **12**:34-42, 1982.

43. *Humidifiers: tips given on trimming infection hazards, Hosp. Infect. Control **8**:24-26, 1979.

44. *Hunt, W.J., and Bespalec, D.A.: An evaluation of current methods of modifying smoking behavior, J. Clin. Psychol. **30**:431-438, 1974.

45. *Jacquette, G.: To reduce hazards of tracheal suctioning, Am. J. Nurs. **71**:2362-2364, 1971.

46. Jarvis, C.M.: Vital signs: how to take them more accurately and understand them more fully, Nursing **6**:31-37, 1976.

47. Johnson, J., et al.: Surgery of the chest, ed. 4, Chicago, 1970, Year Book Medical Publishers, Inc.

48. *Johnson, M.: Outcome criteria to evaluate postoperative respiratory status, Am. J. Nurs. **75**:1474-1475, 1975.

49. Karetzky, M.S., and Khan, A.U.: Review of current concepts in aspiration pneumonia, Heart Lung **6**:321-326, 1977.

50. *Kersten, L.: Chest tube drainage system—indications and principles of operation, Heart Lung **3**:97-101, 1974.

51. Klause, M.L.: Mediastinoscopy, A.O.R.N. J. **15**:55-59, 1972.

52. *Koss, J.A., and Christoph, C.: Oxygen therapy and other respiratory therapy in acute respiratory failure, Crit. Care Q. **1**:53-63, 1979.

53. Kryger, M., editor: Pathophysiology of respiration, New York, 1981, John Wiley & Sons, Inc.

54. Kudla, M.S.: The care of the patient with respiratory insufficiency, Nurs. Clin. North Am. **8**:183-190, 1973.

55. Lagerson, J.: Nursing care of patients with chronic pulmonary insufficiency, Nurs. Clin. North Am. **9**:165-179, 1974.

56. *Lareau, S.: The effect of positive-pressure breathing on the arterial oxygen tension in patients with chronic obstructive pulmonary disease receiving oxygen therapy, Heart Lung **5**:449-452, 1976.

57. Lee, C.A., Stroot, V.R., and Schaper, C.A.: What to do when acid-base problems hang in the balance, Nursing **5**:32-37, 1975.

58. *Lewis, E., and Browning, M., editors: Nursing in respiratory disease, New York, 1972, The American Journal of Nursing Co.

59. Lynne-Davies, P.: Influence of age on the respiratory system, Geriatrics **32**:57-60, 1977.

60. MacDonnell, K.F., and Segal, M.S., editors: Current respiratory care, Boston, 1977, Little, Brown & Co.

61. Malkus, B.: Respiratory care at home, Am. J. Nurs. **76**:1789-1791, 1976.

62. *McCormick, K.A., and Brinbaum, M.L.: Acute ventilatory failure following thoracic trauma, Nurs. Clin. North Am. **9**:181-194, 1974.

63. *Moody, L.E.: Primer for pulmonary hygiene, Am. J. Nurs. **77**:104-106, 1977.

64. Mountain, C.F.: Primary lung cancer. In Conn, H.F.: Current therapy, Philadelphia, 1982, W.B. Saunders Co.

65. *Nett, L.: The use of mechanical ventilators, Nurs. Clin. North Am. **9**:123-136, 1974.

66. *Nett, L., and Petty, T.L.: Oxygen toxicity, Am. J. Nurs. **73**:1556-1558, 1973.

67. Neville, W.E.: Care of the surgical cardiopulmonary patient, Chicago, 1971, Year Book Medical Publishers, Inc.

68. *Niewoehner, D.E., Kleinerman, J., and Rice, D.B.: Pathologic changes in peripheral airways of young cigarette smokers, N. Engl. J. Med. **291**:755-758, 1974.

69. Parfrey, P.S., et al.: Pulmonary function in the early postoperative period, Br. J. Surg. **64**:384-389, 1977.

70. *Petersen, G.M.: Application of oxygen therapy devices, Nurs. Clin. North Am. **16**:241-257, 1981.

71. *Petty, T.L.: Complications occurring during mechanical ventilation, Heart Lung **5**:112-118, 1976.

72. Petty, T.L.: Intensive and rehabilitative respiratory care, ed. 2, Philadelphia, 1974, Lea & Febiger.

73. *Phipps, W.J., Barker, W.L., and Daly, B.J.: Respiratory insufficiency and failure. In Meltzer, L.E., Abdellah, F.G., and Kitchell, J.R.: Concepts and practices of intensive care for nurse specialists, ed. 2, Bowie, Md., 1975, The Charles Press.

74. Podgorny, G.: How to insert a chest tube, RN **39**:OR1-3, OR6, 1976.

75. *Powaser, M.M.: The effectiveness of hourly cuff deflation in minimizing tracheal damage, Heart Lung **5**:744-741, 1976.

76. Ravitch, M.M.: Congenital deformities of the chest wall and their operative correction, Philadelphia, 1977, W.B. Saunders Co.

77. *Risser, N.L.: Preoperative and postoperative care to prevent pulmonary complications, Heart Lung **9**:57-67, 1980.

78. *Roediger, D.: We should have been tougher with Emma and ourselves, Nursing **7**:48-49, 1977.

79. Sabiston, D.C., and Spencer, F.C., editors: Gibbon's surgery of the chest, ed. 3, Philadelphia, 1976, W.B. Saunders Co.

80. *Sackner, M.A.: Pathogenesis and prevention of tracheobronchial damage with suction procedures, Chest **64**:284-290, 1973.

81. Sedlock, S.A.: Detection of chronic pulmonary disease, Am. J. Nurs. **72**:1407-1411, 1972.

82. *Selecky, P.A.: Tracheal damage and prolonged intubation with a cuffed endotracheal or tracheostomy tube, Heart Lung **5**:733, 1976.

83. *Selecky, P.A.: Tracheostomy: a review of present day indications, complications, and care, Heart Lung **3**:272-283, 1974.

84. *Sexton, P.: A nurse shows how to help the patient stop smoking, Am. Lung Assoc. Bull. **61**:10-11, 1975.

85. *Shapiro, B.A., Harrison, R.A., and Trout, C.A.: Clinical application of respiratory care, Chicago, 1975, Year Book Medical Publishers, Inc.

86. Simmons, D.H.: Evaluation of acid-base status. In American Thoracic Society: Basics of RD, New York, 1974, The Society.

87. Slonim, N.B., and Hamilton, L.H.: Respiratory physiology, ed. 4, St. Louis, 1981, The C.V. Mosby Co.

88. Stahly, T.L., and Tench, W.D.: Lung entrapment and infarction by chest tube suction, Radiology **122**:307, 1977.

89. *Stewart, E.: To lessen pain: relaxation and rhythmic breathing, Am. J. Nurs. **76**:958-959, 1976.

90. Stone, E.W., and Zuckerman, S.: The esophageal obturator airway, Am. J. Nurs. **75**:1148-1149, 1975.

91. Stufflet, S.K.: If you want to do patient teaching, become a pulmonary nurse specialist, Nursing **6**:94, 96-97, 1976.

92. *Traver, G., editor: Respiratory nursing: the art and the science, New York, 1982, John Wiley & Sons, Inc.

93. *Traver, G.: Assessment of thorax and lungs, Am. J. Nurs. **73**:466-471, 1973.

94. Up-to-date survey of tracheal tubes, Nursing **6**:66-72, 1976.

95. *Van Meter, M.: Chest tubes: basic techniques for better care, Nursing **4**:48-55, 1974.

96. Van Way, C.W.: Persistent pneumothorax as a complication of chest suction, Chest **77**:815, 1980.

97. *Wade, J.F.: Respiratory nursing care: physiology and technique, ed. 2, St. Louis, 1977, The C.V. Mosby Co.

98. *Wagner, M.M.: Assessment of patients with multiple injuries, Am. J. Nurs. **72**:1822-1827, 1972.

99. Warner, K.E.: The effects of the anti-smoking campaign on cigarette consumption, Am. J. Public Health **67**:645-650, 1977.

100. White, H.: Tracheostomy care with a cuffed tube, Am. J. Nurs. **72**:75-77, 1972.

101. Wood, C.: Alveolar ventilation, Nurse Pract. **2**:31-32, 38, 1976.

102. Woods, S.L.: Monitoring pulmonary artery pressures, Am. J. Nurs. **76**:1765-1771, 1976.

103. Wynder, E.L., Covey, L.S., and Mabuchi, K.: Current smoking habits by selected background variables: their effect on future disease trends, Am. J. Epidemiol. **100**:168-177, 1974.

Classic

104. Bendixen, H.H., et al.: Respiratory care, St. Louis, 1965, The C.V. Mosby Co.

105. *Enerson, D.M., and McIntyre, J.: A comparative study of the physiology and physics of pleural drainage systems, J. Thorac. Cardiovasc. Surg. **52**:40-46, 1966.

106. *Kurihara, M.: Postural drainage, clapping and vibrating, Am. J. Nurs. **65**:76-79, 1965.

107. Rie, M.W.: Physical therapy in the nursing care of respiratory disease patients, Nurs. Clin. North Am. **3**:463-478, 1968.

108. Traver, G.A.: Effect of intermittent positive pressure breathing and use of rebreathing tube upon tidal volume and cough, Nurs. Res. **17**:100-103, 1968.

109. U.S. Public Health Service: Closed drainage of the chest: a programmed course for nurses. Pub. no. 1337, Washington, D.C., 1965, U.S. Department of Health, Education and Welfare.

CHAPTER 50

PROBLEMS OF THE UPPER AIRWAY

LINDA ANNE BROSEMAN

Disorders of the upper airway are very common, and nurses in particular are often asked to give advice about these problems. To be effective, nurses need a basic understanding of the structure and function of the organs of the upper airway, as well as knowledge of the medical and nursing regimens for problems affecting these organs. For clarity, this chapter will be divided into the following three sections: problems of the nose and sinuses, problems of the upper throat (pharynx and tonsils), and problems of the lower throat (larynx and hypopharynx). For problems of the mouth and parotid gland, see Chapter 56.

Problems of the nose and sinuses

Anatomy and physiology

The nose is supported by the nasal bones, the nasal processes of the maxillary bones, the cartilaginous and bony parts of the septum, and the upper and lower nasal cartilages. Air enters the nose through the two nostrils (nares), which are separated by the septum. The septum, which is usually straight and thin in the child, is rarely straight in adults because it is subject to injury.[31]

The nasal cavities are located between the roof of the mouth and the frontal, ethmoid, and sphenoid bones. Three projections, lined with mucous membrane and called the turbinate bones, are located on the lateral walls of each nasal cavity (Fig. 50-1). Their purpose is to increase the mucous membrane surface over which air passes as it travels to the nasopharynx to allow for precipitation of inhaled particles and to warm and moisten the inhaled air.

The vestibule of the nose is the anterior part of the nose. The vestibule extends posteriorly a short distance where its lining changes from skin to mucous membrane. This mucous membrane posterior to the vestibule contains cilia that beat in a constant wavelike motion to carry mucus into the nasopharynx. Trapped in the mucus are bacteria, dust, and other foreign matter entering the nose. The olfactory epithelium is located in a small area superiorly and provides the end-organ of smell. The lateral walls of the nose contain the opening for the paranasal sinuses and the nasolacrimal ducts. These openings provide a means of aeration of and mucus drainage from the sinuses. The blood supply to the nose comes from both the external and internal carotid systems.

There are four sets of paranasal sinuses located on either side of the head (Fig. 50-2). These sinuses are air-filled spaces in the skull that serve to lighten the head. They drain into the nasal cavities through the openings behind the turbinates. The maxillary sinuses are the largest and most accessible. The sinuses are lined with mucous membrane that is continuous with that of the nose. The chief functions of the nose include providing an airway to warm and moisten air in preparation for the lungs and as the organ of smell.

Assessment

Inspection of the nose includes looking for deformities, asymmetry, and inflammation.[6] To visualize the nose, a nasal speculum or an otoscope fitted with a nasal speculum is inserted about 1 cm into the vestibule, avoiding the nasal septum (Fig. 50-3). The lower portion of the nose is inspected first by using a light source such as a penlight. The person then tilts the head back so that the upper portions of the nose can be visualized.

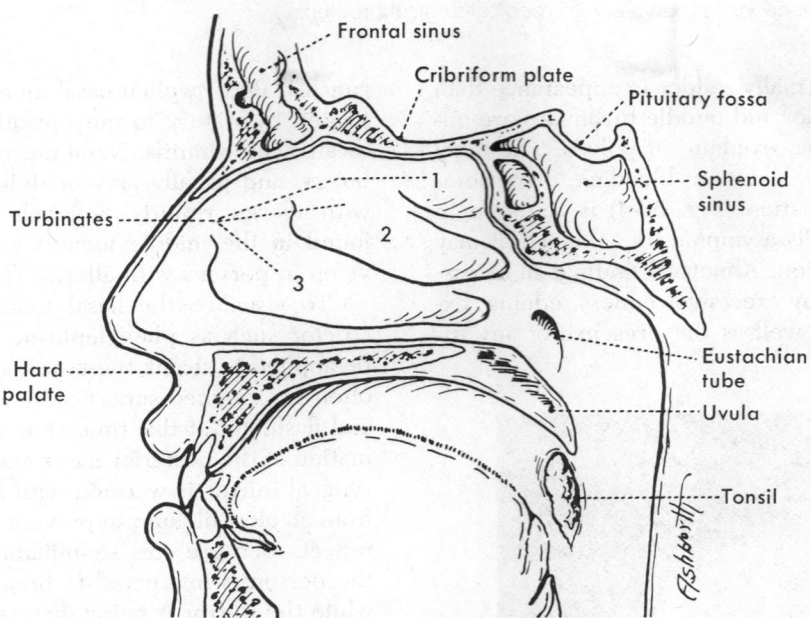

Fig. 50-1. Turbinates of nose: *1*, superior; *2*, middle; *3*, inferior. (From DeWeese, D.D., and Saunders, W.H.: Textbook of otolaryngology, ed. 6, St. Louis, 1982, The C.V. Mosby Co.)

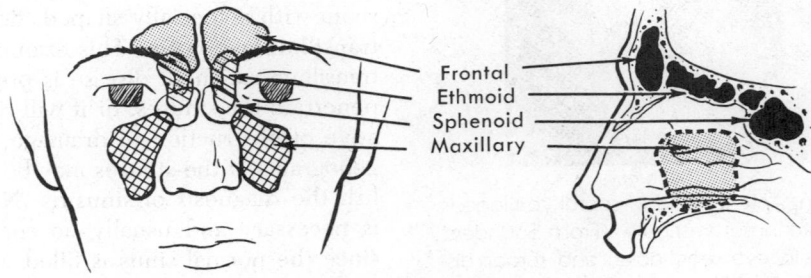

Fig. 50-2. Location of sinuses.

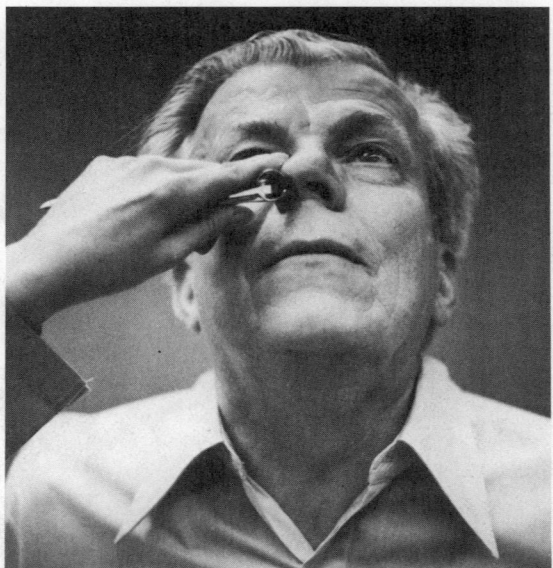

Fig. 50-3. Proper position for insertion of nasal speculum with index finger on side of nose. (From Malasanos, L., et al.: Health assessment, ed. 2, St. Louis, 1981, The C.V. Mosby Co.)

Nasal mucosa is normally redder in appearance than oral mucosa. The inferior and middle turbinates are observed for color, edema, exudate, or polyps. The nasal septum is observed for deviation, bleeding, or perforation. Some septal deviation (Fig. 50-4) is common in most adults and is usually asymptomatic, although it may produce nasal obstruction. Abnormal findings in assessing the nose include any excessive redness, edema, exudate, or bleeding, as well as the presence of any fu-

runcles. Red, swollen nasal mucous membranes accompanied by watery to mucopurulent nasal discharge indicate acute rhinitis. Nasal mucosa that is swollen, pale, boggy, and usually gray or dull red is seen in persons with allergic rhinitis. Soft pale gray mobile structures found in the middle meatus are polyps that may develop in persons with allergic rhinitis.

To visualize the nasal mucosa clearly, a vasoconstrictor such as phenylephrine (Neo-Synephrine) may be applied to shrink the mucous membrane. The throat often is examined superficially with a tongue depressor and flashlight at this time. For a more extensive examination of the posterior nares and the throat, a nasopharyngeal mirror is warmed with hot water or in a flame from an alcohol lamp to prevent fogginess and failure to reflect. Because this examination may cause gagging, the person is instructed to breathe through the mouth while the mirror is being directed toward the pharynx.

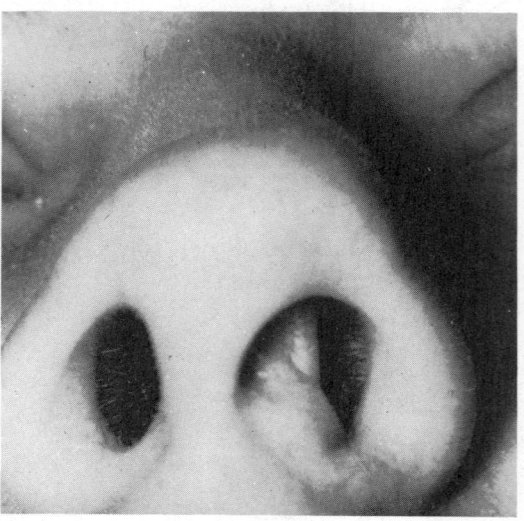

Fig. 50-4. Septal deviation. Anterior end of septal cartilage is dislocated and projects into nasal vestibule. (From Saunders, W.H., et al.: Nursing care in eye, ear, nose, and throat disorders, ed. 4, St. Louis, 1979, The C.V. Mosby Co.)

The sinuses are palpated for signs of tenderness of the frontal and maxillary areas when inspecting the nose (Fig. 50-5). The normal frontal and maxillary sinuses can be visualized by illuminating them in a dark room with a specially shaped, lighted bulb or a lighted transillumination tip. This examination is referred to as transillumination. If disease is present, the light will not penetrate the sinuses, or it will reveal fluid levels indicative of obstruction to drainage of the sinuses. Roentgenograms of the sinuses may be ordered to help establish the diagnosis of sinusitis. No physical preparation is necessary and usually no contrast medium is used since the normal sinus is filled with air, which in itself casts a shadow in contrast to surrounding structures.

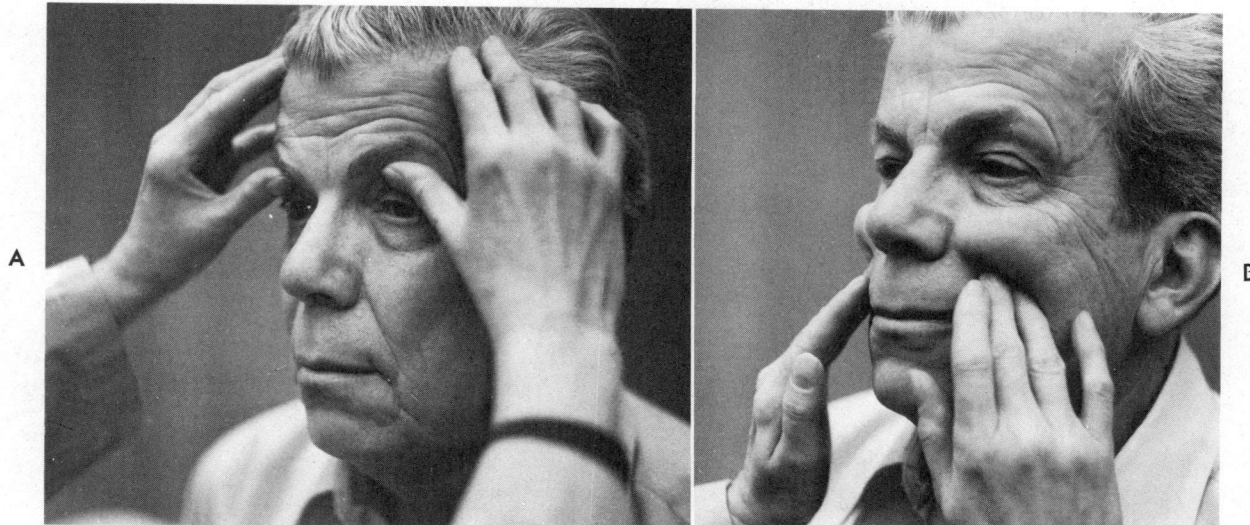

Fig. 50-5. Palpation of frontal, **A,** and maxillary, **B,** sinuses. (From Malasanos, L., et al.: Health assessment, ed. 2, St. Louis, 1981, The C.V. Mosby Co.)

Anosmia

Anosmia is the loss of the sense of smell. It may be the result of (1) nasal obstruction, which prevents air currents from reaching the olfactory epithelium; (2) skull fracture across the cribiform plate at the roof of the nose where the part of the olfactory nerve enters the nose; (3) viral infections, which affect the olfactory nerve; or (4) some meningiomas, which may form in the olfactory area. A perverted sense of smell, called *parosmia*, may also be present during sinusitis or an upper respiratory tract infection.

Infections of the nose and sinuses

Rhinitis

Rhinitis refers to inflammation of the mucous membrane of the nose. Rhinitis may be acute or chronic.

Acute rhinitis.

ETIOLOGY. Simple, acute rhinitis (coryza, common cold) is an inflammatory condition of the mucous membranes of the nose and accessory sinuses caused by a filtrable virus. It affects almost everyone at some time in life and occurs most often in the cold winter months. It is generally believed that the infecting agent is present in the nose and sinuses at all times and that fatigue and chilling are among many factors influencing susceptibility. Some of the known agents causing the common cold are more than 30 identified rhinoviruses, adenovirus, echovirus, influenza and parainfluenza viruses, and coxsackie virus. The common cold is spread by droplet nuclei from sneezing. The condition is contagious for the first 2 to 3 days.

PREVENTION. The best prevention is to avoid exposure. Since this is not possible, adequate diet, rest, and exercise presumably help to maintain resistance to a cold. Persons with colds should avoid crowded places where the cold can be easily transmitted to many others, and they should avoid infants or very young children, elderly persons, or persons with chronic lung diseases. Frequent washing of hands, covering of coughs and sneezes, and careful disposal of waste tissue are protective health measures that are advisable for everyone.

CLINICAL PICTURE. The person usually complains of dryness of the nose, eyes, and soft palate; general malaise; chilliness; and headache. These symptoms are followed in 12 to 24 hours by obstruction to nasal breathing caused by swelling of the mucous membrane and a profuse, watery nasal discharge. Sneezing, tearing of the eyes, and nasal irritation also occur, and the postnasal discharge may cause pharyngitis, laryngitis, or bronchitis, although a sore throat is not always associated with a cold. If uncomplicated, the cold is usually self-limiting and lasts for about 6 to 7 days.

INTERVENTION. Most people with colds do not go to their physician unless symptoms persist or make them very uncomfortable. Medical therapy, if sought, usually consists of rest, fluids, moist inhalations, and antihistamines and decongestants. The antihistamines do not cure the cold but are helpful in alleviating symptoms, such as sneezing and tearing of the eyes, during the initial inflammatory phase only. Since the antihistamines cause drowsiness in most persons, they should not be used when driving a car or working near moving machinery.

People with acute rhinitis are instructed not to blow their nose too hard or unnecessarily. The mouth should be open slightly when blowing the nose and both nostrils should be open to prevent any infected matter from being forced into the eustachian tube. Nose drops are sometimes recommended for infrequent use (every 4 hours for a few days) if there is some nasal obstruction. Many otolaryngologists now believe that the frequent use of nose drops results in rhinitis medicamentosa (p. 1264), an "addiction" of the nasal mucosa to their use.[18] Some physicians believe that the obstruction of the nose may be a protective device that prevents the spread of infection to other parts of the body.

When *nose drops* are ordered, the individual is taught how to use them correctly as follows:

1. Sit in a chair and tip head well backwards, *or* lie down with head extended over edge of bed, *or* lie down with a pillow placed under shoulders and head tipped backward.
2. Place no more than 3 drops of solution into each nostril at one time (unless ordered otherwise).
3. Remain in position with head tilted backwards for 5 minutes to permit solution to reach posterior nares.

If after 10 minutes following insertion of nose drops marked congestion is still present, another drop or two of solution may be administered. The mucous membrane of the anterior nares by this time should have become constricted so that the solution may reach the posterior nares more easily. Some physicians feel that the instillation of nose drops is too upsetting for children and thus order nasal decongestants such as pseudoephedrine, 30 mg every 3 to 4 hours, and steam inhalations. A rubber bulb ear syringe may be used to *aspirate* the mucous discharge from the nose of infants so that they can breathe and be able to take their feedings. Nasal decongestants may be administered by means of an atomizer or inhalator as follows:

1. Sit upright with head tilted backward.
2. Place inhalator or atomizer in nostril.
3. Occlude the opposite nostril with finger pressure to prevent entrance of air (allows medication to penetrate further).
4. Administer no more than three sprays of solution into each nostril.

Secondary invasion by bacteria may complicate the cold, causing symptoms to persist and become worse. If the nasal discharge persists for more than 7 to 10 days, or if the person develops an elevation of temperature, medical attention should be obtained. Possible *complications* include pneumonia, bronchitis, sinusitis, and otitis media. Infants and young children are particularly susceptible to colds and the complication of otitis media (p. 904). They should be isolated from persons with colds, and if they develop a cold, they should be observed carefully for symptoms suggesting otitis media. If a high temperature occurs, or if the infant becomes restless, rolls the head from side to side in bed, or pulls at the ear, medical attention should be sought.

Persons who have symptoms of *recurrent* colds should seek medical attention, because nasal deformity, such as enlarged turbinates, a deviated septum, chronic sinusitis, or allergy may cause the recurrent symptoms. Repeated attacks eventually may lead to chronic rhinitis.

Allergic rhinitis

ETIOLOGY AND CLINICAL PICTURE. Allergic rhinitis (hay fever) can be acute and seasonal when caused by the pollens of grasses and flowers, or it may be chronic and perennial when associated with numerous allergens, such as dust, animal dander, wool, and certain foods. Common symptoms include sneezing, nasal obstruction, tearing, recurrent thin watery nasal discharge, frontal headache, and itching of the eyes and nose. Typically on physical examination the turbinates are pale, edematous, and mucoid.

INTERVENTION. The best intervention for any kind of allergy is to separate the person from the sensitizing allergens. If that is not feasible, then attempts are made to desensitize the individual. For some persons a series of injections for desensitization is effective. Antihistamines are helpful in alleviating symptoms.

If nasal obstruction persists, surgery such as submucous resection or septoplasty may be performed. Often people with allergic rhinitis develop polyps, which are pale, soft edematous outpouchings of nasal or sinal mucosa. Polyps are usually bilateral and may cause obstruction of the airway. Multiple polyps may cause severe nasal obstruction as well as anosmia. Polypectomy (p. 1270) is the surgical procedure used to remove polyps.

Chronic rhinitis

ETIOLOGY. Chronic rhinitis is a chronic inflammation of the mucous membrane caused by repeated, acute infections, by an allergy, or by vasomotor rhinitis. The cause of *vasomotor rhinitis* is unclear but may result from an instability of the autonomic nervous system resulting from stress, tension, or some endocrine disorder. Often it is mistaken for nasal allergy, but the allergen cannot be identified. There is an increased formation of nasal mucus.

CLINICAL PICTURE. Regardless of the cause of chronic rhinitis, the symptoms are similar. Nasal obstruction accompanied by a feeling of stuffiness and pressure in the nose is the chief complaint. A nasal discharge is always present and may be serous, mucopurulent, or purulent, depending on the amount of secondary infection present. Polyp formation may occur, and the turbinates may enlarge as a result of the chronic irritation. Complaints of frontal headache, vertigo, and sneezing are common.

INTERVENTION. Antibiotics may be used to treat the secondary infection. If the cause is allergy related, the offending allergen is removed, or the person is desensitized to it. Antihistamines are helpful in alleviating symptoms. Polyps or hyperplastic tissues may require surgical removal.

Nasal irrigations are no longer used frequently in the treatment of chronic rhinitis. Details of this procedure are described in texts on fundamentals of nursing or in textbooks on otolaryngology.[18] Care should be taken to ensure that both nostrils are open and that the pressure in the nostrils is not excessive (the irrigating container should not be higher than 12 to 15 in. above the level of the nose). Excess pressure may force infected material into the sinuses or the middle ear. This procedure should not be performed on a child who is crying or struggling to avoid it.

Rhinitis medicamentosa.
Rhinitis medicamentosa is a common condition caused by the overuse of nose drops.[18,31] A rebound phenomenon occurs after the immediate effect of the nose drops with return to congestion. Treatment consists of stopping the use of all nose drops completely. Usually within a week or two the person can breathe through the nose again. Orally administered decongestants may often help.

Outcome criteria for the person with rhinitis.
The person or significant others can:
1. Describe ways to prevent future attacks (e.g., avoiding persons with colds, avoiding allergens to which the person is sensitive).
2. List allergens to which the person is sensitive and describe how to avoid them (e.g., environmentally controlled room [p. 1867], electrostatic filter, air conditioning, face masks).
3. Demonstrate procedure for instilling nose drops or using nasal spray.
4. State name, dosage, frequency, and side effects of medications being used; and state danger of using over-the-counter preparations.
5. Describe symptoms requiring medical intervention.
6. State plans for follow-up care.

Sinusitis

The sinuses are air-filled cavities lined with mucous membrane. Any inflammation of the mucous membranes of the sinuses is referred to as sinusitis. This is still a frequent disorder, although it is less common since the advent of antibiotics. Often persons who complain of sinusitis do not have sinus trouble but actually have other disorders. When an otolaryngologist refers to sinusitis, a bacterial invasion of the mucous membrane is implied. This can be either an acute or a chronic condition.

Acute sinusitis

ETIOLOGY. The most common cause of acute sinusitis is the obstruction of the paranasal sinuses that blocks the egress of secretions of the sinuses. These secretions become infected, giving rise to acute sinusitis. Sinusitis may follow acute or allergic rhinitis or other respiratory diseases such as pneumonia or influenza. Streptococci, staphylocci, pneumococci, or anaerobes are the infecting organisms. Abscessed teeth or tooth extraction may cause acute maxillary sinusitis, since the apices of many of the upper teeth roots are in close contact with the mucosal lining of these sinuses.

CLINICAL PICTURE. The person with acute sinusitis often complains of a constant, severe headache and of pain over the infected sinuses. Maxillary sinusitis will cause pain under the eyes, whereas frontal sinusitis often causes pain over the eyebrows. The person may have the sensation of "pain in the bone" with even slight pressure over the affected sinus.[6] Pain from the ethmoid and sphenoid sinuses usually is referred and is felt at the top of the head. Occasionally there may be noticeable swelling over the maxillary or frontal sinuses, or there may be orbital edema. The person may have nausea, purulent discharge from the nose if the duct is not closed, obstruction to nasal breathing, fever, and general malaise. Fever is proportional to the amount of obstruction present and the virulence of the infection, but usually it is a low-grade fever with the temperature rarely above 38.5° C (101° F). If the sinus is abscessed, the temperature may be as high as 40° C (104° F). The throat may be sore from irritation caused by postnasal drainage.

Medical evaluation usually consists of sinus roentgenograms, which are useful in determining the presence and extent of disease and indicate involvement of the bony walls (Fig. 50-6). When infection is present, the film appears cloudy. Complications of severe untreated sinusitis include osteomyelitis in the adjacent bone, an abscess that may involve the brain, venous sinus thrombosis, orbital cellulitis, orbital abscess, and septicemia.

INTERVENTION. Treatment is directed at relieving pain, establishing drainage of the sinuses, and controlling the infection. Broad-spectrum antibiotics such as penicillin, ampicillin, erythromycin, or the cephalosporins are given systemically for their specific action on the causative organism. Medications such as phenylephrine (Neo-Synephrine), 0.25%, and ephedrine sulfate, 0.25% to 3%, which constrict the blood vessels and thus reduce hyperemia and improve drainage, may

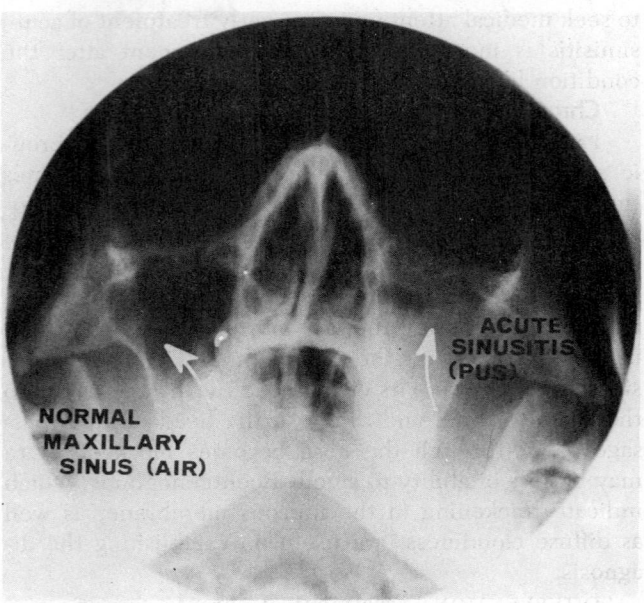

Fig. 50-6. Roentgenogram of maxillary sinus showing normal sinus on left and acute sinusitis on right. (From Saunders, W.H., et al.: Nursing care in eye, ear, nose, and throat disorders, ed. 4, St. Louis, 1979, The C.V. Mosby Co.)

be given as nose drops or by spray inhalation. Forced air pressure of the atomizer breaks the large droplets of fluid into a fine mist. If a nebulizer is used, the solution if usually forced through the apparatus by a current of oxygen or compressed air.

Pain may be relieved by the administration of various analgesics. Because aspirin may be associated with nasal polyposis, it is usually avoided as a pain medication. Acetaminophen (Tylenol) is a good substitute for the aspirin, and occasionally codeine or even morphine sulfate or meperidine may be necessary to relieve the pain. Heat over the sinuses also gives some relief from pain. Warm, wet dressings or a heat lamp may be used. Vaporizers in the room may help facilitate drainage by liquefying the secretions. The room temperature should be kept constant, since changes in room temperature aggravate sinusitis.

If conservative measures do not alleviate an acute sinus infection, the physician may irrigate the maxillary sinuses by means of an *antrum puncture*. The nasal mucosa is usually anesthetized with cocaine, and the maxillary sinus (the antrum) is perforated with a trocar and cannula. The patient is urged to breathe through the mouth during the procedure. The person's head is supported while the treatment is given, since a sensation of pressure is felt that, although not painful, may produce dizziness and nausea. Saline, rather than air, is used for irrigation, since deaths caused by air embolism have been reported.

Persons with symptoms of acute sinusitis are urged

to seek medical attention, since early treatment of acute sinusitis is more successful than treatment after the condition becomes chronic.

Chronic sinusitis

PATHOPHYSIOLOGY AND CLINICAL PICTURE. In chronic sinusitis, the mucous lining of the sinus becomes thickened from prolonged or repeated irritation and infection. The person usually has a chronic purulent nasal discharge, a chronic cough caused by a postnasal drainage, and a chronic dull sinus headache that characteristically starts during the late morning hours and gradually subsides during the evening hours. The varied positions and movements of the head during the day help the sinus to drain and diminish the headache. As passage of air through the nose becomes blocked, there may be loss of ability to smell. Roentgenograms, which indicate thickening in the mucous membrane, as well as diffuse cloudiness, are useful in establishing the diagnosis.

INTERVENTION. Treatment of chronic sinusitis may be surgical. Removal of nasal deformities, such as a deviated nasal septum, hypertrophied turbinated bones, or nasal polyps that are obstructing the sinus openings, may give relief. Sinus irrigations may ensure better drainage. If the condition is caused by an allergy, it responds to general treatment of the allergy. In general, antibiotics are not very helpful in treating chronic sinusitis.

The person with chronic sinusitis should avoid chilling and cold, damp atmospheres. Change to a warm, dry climate, though helpful to some people, is not necessarily helpful to all. The person is advised not to smoke, because smoking further irritates the damaged mucous membranes. Air conditioning often causes discomfort, particularly if the outside air is warm and moist. Persons with chronic sinusitis often sleep poorly and lack pep and vigor in their living and in their work. Persistent postnasal discharge is believed to contribute to bronchiectasis, a chronic lung disease, as the person grows older.

Outcome criteria for the person with sinusitis. The person or significant others can:

1. State factors that contribute to development of sinusitis and how to prevent future attacks.
2. Explain medication program.
   a. State name, dosage, frequency, route of administration, and side effects of prescribed medications.
   b. State rationale for full course of antibiotics even when obvious symptoms have subsided.
3. State plans for follow-up health care.
   a. Describe symptoms of secondary infections that require further medical attention.
   b. State plans for stopping smoking, if appropriate.
   c. State plans for controlling environmental temperature.

d. State plans for seeking medical attention for acute episodes.

Infections of external tissues about the nose

The skin around the external nose is easily irritated during acute attacks of rhinitis or sinusitis. Furunculosis and cellulitis (inflammation of connective tissue) occasionally develop. (See p. 1835 for discussion and treatment of furunculosis.) Infections about the nose are extremely dangerous, since the venous supply from this area drains directly into the cerebral venous sinuses. Septicemia therefore can occur easily. No pimple or lesion in the area should ever be squeezed or "picked"; hot packs may be used. If any infection in or about the nose persists or shows even the slightest tendency to spread or increase in severity, medical aid should be sought.

Nasal obstructions

Nasal obstruction is a common complaint caused by a number of conditions. Physical inspection of the nose is necessary for identification of the cause of obstruction.

Deviated septum

Deviated septum is a common cause of nasal obstruction. The septum, which is normally thin and straight, may be deviated from the midline and protrude more to one side of the nasal passage than to the other. The deviation may cause a nasal obstruction that increases when infection or allergic reaction occurs. If the obstruction is marked, noisy and difficult breathing will result. There may be a postnasal drip, or the mucosa may become dry so that crusts form. This deformity of the septum is common in older children and adults. It may be congenital but usually is the result of an injury. The person with trauma to the nose should be encouraged to seek medical attention, since a broken nose can lead to chronic sinusitis if not treated, even though it may cause no immediate problem. If the deformity causes nasal obstruction, a submucous resection or septoplasty (reconstruction of the septum) may be performed (p. 1270).

Hypertrophy of the turbinates

The inferior turbinates are sometimes the cause of considerable nasal obstruction. Hypertrophied turbinates may be medically treated by the use of aerosols containing corticosteroids such as dexamethasone (Decadron Turbinaire).[5] These aerosols are used for their antiinflammatory response and have proven to be effective for allergic and inflammatory nasal conditions as well as for treatment of nasal polyps. Although not employed as often since the advent of the corticosteroid aerosol, local surgery on the turbinates such as cryosurgery or electric fulguration may still be used to restore the airway.

Nasal polyps

Nasal polyps are grapelike growths of mucous membrane and loose connective tissue. They are usually bilateral and may be caused by irritation to mucous membranes of the nose or sinuses from an allergy or by chronic sinusitis. Nasal polyps in children may be caused by cystic fibrosis. Polyps also cause anosmia by preventing air from reaching the olfactory mucosa high in the nose. Since they may obstruct breathing or block sinus drainage, nasal polyps are removed if they do not respond to treatment (polypectomy, p. 1270). Aerosol sprays such as the ones discussed for hypertrophied turbinates have also proven effective for the treatment of nasal polyps. Since the sinus mucosa may also be involved in the polypoid process, surgery on the sinuses such as an ethmoidectomy may be necessary (p. 1271).

Foreign bodies

Foreign bodies of the nose are suspected when a child has nasal obstruction, discharge, or bleeding. It is usually necessary to use a vasoconstrictor such as ephedrine or phenylephrine (Neo-Synephrine), 1%, topically to provide shrinkage of the intranasal membranes and to make it easier for extraction of the foreign body. Usually it is necessary to restrain the arms of the child during the procedure.

Tumors

Both benign and malignant tumors can produce nasal obstruction, either unilaterally or bilaterally. Nasopharyngeal carcinomas obstruct the nose, at first on one side and then on both sides. These tumors metastasize early to the neck. Carcinomas of the maxillary or ethmoid sinuses may erode through the adjacent nasal walls and thus cause obstruction. They often bleed easily.[1,59,78,81]

Nose trauma

Fractures of the nasal bones and septum

Fractures of the nasal bones and septum commonly occur from relatively minor injuries such as falls or from more severe injuries such as automobile accidents or fights. If there is no displacement of the bone, no obstruction to the airway, nor any cosmetic deformity, treatment is not needed. When airway obstruction or bone displacement occurs (Fig. 50-7), then simple reduction is performed. Most simple nasal fractures can be reduced by applying firm pressure on the convex side of the nose. Fractures that cannot be reduced by

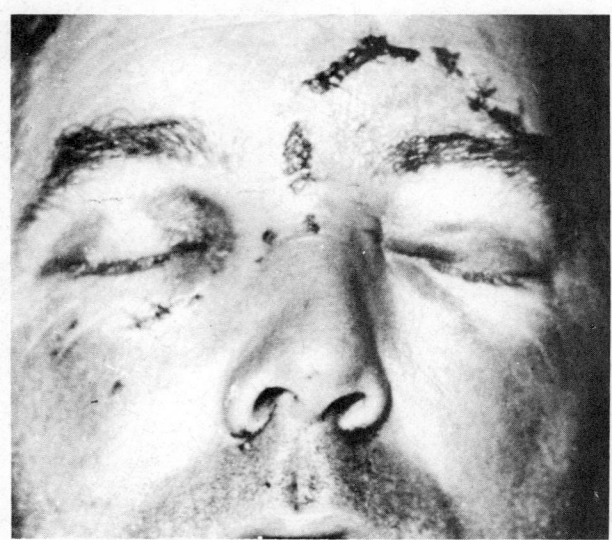

Fig. 50-7. Laterally displaced fracture of nose secondary to trauma. Pressure on convex side will restore alignment. (From Saunders, W.H., et al.: Nursing care in eye, ear, nose, and throat disorders, ed. 4, St. Louis, 1979, The C.V. Mosby Co.)

this technique are reduced surgically under local anesthesia.

Fractures of the maxillary and zygomatic bones

Fractures of the maxillary and zygomatic bones are seen after automobile accidents and fights. These fractures are generally reduced under anesthesia. Patients may also have some teeth wired together with all the attendant problems of that procedure (see p. 1410 for nursing interventions for patients with fractured jaws).

Epistaxis

ETIOLOGY. Epistaxis, or nosebleed, may be caused by local irritation of mucous membranes, chronic infection, lack of humidity in the air that is breathed, violent sneezing or nose blowing, or trauma to the nose resulting in damage to or rupture of superficial blood vessels. One of the most common causes of nosebleeds is picking of the nose. General or systemic causes may be hypertension and arterial blood vessel changes, blood dyscrasias such as leukemia, or a deficiency of vitamin K. In adulthood, nosebleeds are more common in men than in women. They are most frequent in early childhood and puberty. Persons who have frequent nosebleeds should have a complete medical examination to determine the cause.

INTERVENTION. Most nosebleeds come from the tiny blood vessels in the anterior part of the nasal septum. This bleeding usually can be controlled at least temporarily by compressing the soft tissues of the nose against the septum with a finger. Firm pressure should be

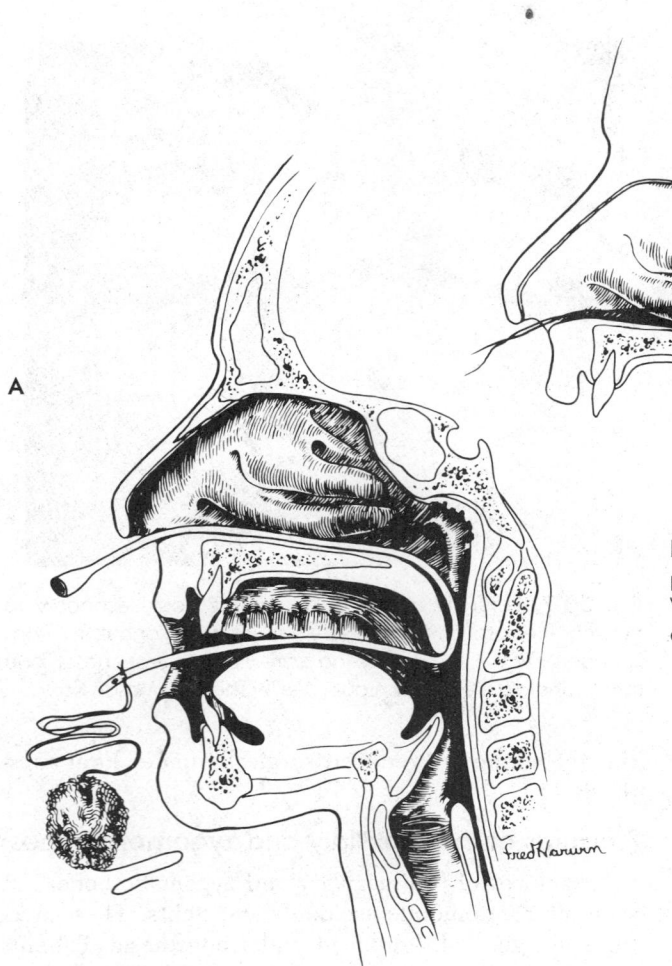

Fig. 50-8. Postnasal packing. **A,** Rubber catheter used to place packing. **B,** Anterior packing with strings attached. (From De-Weese, D.D., and Saunders, W.H.: Textbook of otolaryngology, ed. 6, St. Louis, 1982, The C.V. Mosby Co.)

maintained for at least 5 to 10 minutes, and it may be necessary for as long as 30 minutes. The person should breathe through the mouth during this time. Ice compresses may be applied over the nose; however, the primary benefit of the application of ice is that is requires the patient to remain still. Bleeding may be controlled by placing a cotton ball soaked in a topical vasoconstrictor such as phenylephrine (Neo-Synephrine) into the nose and applying pressure. Other first-aid measures include having the person sit quietly with the head up and inclined slightly *forward* to prevent blood from entering the pharynx and causing gagging or swallowing of blood. The person is instructed not to blow the nose for several hours after a nosebleed.

If the above measures do not control bleeding, the help of a physician should be sought. In order to treat a nosebleed effectively, the physician must first determine the site of the bleeding. This is done best with the person seated in a chair facing the physician. Both should wear gowns to protect their clothing. An angulated suction tip is used to suck clots from the nose. If suction is not available, the person is instructed to blow the nose to remove the clot. The physician will then use a bright light (either head mirror or lamp) to in-

spect the anterior nares. After anesthetizing the nasal mucosa with topical lidocaine (Xylocaine), the bleeding point is cauterized with a silver nitrate stick or electrode cautery.

Bleeding from the posterior part of the nasal septum is more common in elderly persons and is more likely to be severe.[40] If the bleeding point cannot be seen and treated as described above, a *postnasal pack* may be inserted (Fig. 50-8). Because this procedure is extremely painful and sometimes causes faintness, patients usually are admitted to the hospital. The pack is left in place 2 to 5 days and then removed very gently. If bleeding has been severe, a transfusion may be necessary. Severe bleeding results in a drop in blood pressure, which may cause the bleeding to stop; therefore exsanguination from the usual nosebleed is rare. Sedation may be ordered, since bleeding tends to be increased by apprehension and restlessness. To prevent recurrent hemorrhage, the person is warned not to blow the nose vigorously and to avoid dryness of the nose. This can be accomplished by using saline or nasal lubricants.

Nosebleeds can cause severe apprehension, since bleeding may be profuse, not only from the nose but also flowing into the throat. The patient is usually kept in Fowler's position and is urged not to swallow blood because it may cause nausea and vomiting. Adequate oxygenation with humidification is important with persons who have posterior packing in place. Pain medication, antibiotic therapy, and sedation may also be ordered for a person with posterior packing. The position of a postnasal pack must be checked frequently, since it may slip out of place and cause airway obstruction.[42] Nasal packs make eating and swallowing difficult. A liquid diet may be ordered. Persistent or recurrent profuse epistaxis, especially posterior epistaxis, may require surgical ligation of the external carotid artery, the ethmoid artery, or the internal maxillary artery, which supply blood to the nose.

Outcome criteria for the person with epistaxis. The person or significant others can:

1. Describe dangers inherent in picking of nose and violent nose blowing.
2. State rationale for medical examination if nosebleeds are frequent.
3. Describe simple first aid for nosebleeds.
4. Describe when simple first aid is not adequate and medical attention is required.

Carcinoma of the maxillary and ethmoid sinuses

Carcinoma of the *paranasal* sinus is relatively uncommon. Carcinoma of the *maxillary* sinus presents no early symptoms. The first complaints usually are dental in origin; either the person complains of loosening of the upper teeth, or if a denture is worn, of the upper plate no longer fitting.[1,67,81] Other symptoms may include nasal obstruction caused by the tumor eroding into the nose, nosebleeds, and displacement of the eye. Carcinoma of the *ethmoid* sinus presents no oral or dental symptoms. The tumor causes outward displacement of the eye, disturbance of the sense of smell, and nosebleeds. Often tearing of the eye or diplopia occurs. Treatment usually consists of irradiation therapy and surgery and has a grave prognosis.

Surgery of the nose and sinuses

Intervention for the person requiring nasal surgery

Most nasal surgery on adults is done under local anesthesia. The person should not be given anything orally for 6 hours preoperatively, since nausea may occur during the operation. A sedative and a narcotic are usually given preoperatively. Children require general anesthesia and may be given a medication such as atropine to reduce secretions.

The nose is usually packed with ½-in. gauze at the conclusion of the operation. Commonly used packs are petrolatum-impregnated gauze, Adaptic gauze, iodoform gauze with bacitracin, and Cortisporin-impregnated gauze. The latter is particularly effective in reducing the odor of the nasal pack. If the packing should slip back into the throat, the surgeon is notified immediately. The pack is usually removed and replaced as necessary.

Following nasal surgery, there is danger of hemor-

rhage. Blood may be evident on the external dressing that is applied under the nose, or the person may expectorate or vomit bright red blood. The back of the throat should be examined to see if blood is running down into it. The pulse may be rapid, or the patient may swallow repeatedly. Some oozing on the dressing is expected, but if it becomes pronounced or if any other symptoms appear, the surgeon is notified, and material for repacking the nose is prepared. This material consists of a hemostatic tray containing gauze packing, umbilical tape for posterior packing, a few small gauze sponges, a small rubber catheter (used for inserting a postnasal plug), a packing forceps, tongue blades, and scissors. A head mirror, a good light, epinephrine 1:1000 or some other vasoconstrictor, 4% topical lidocaine (Xylocaine) or 4% cocaine solution, applicators, a nasal speculum, suction, and metal Frazer tip aspirators should be available.

If the dressing under the nose becomes soiled, it may be changed as necessary. This is very important from an aesthetic standpoint. Sedation and encouragement are necessary because of general discomfort and apprehension caused by having the nasal passages packed and having to breathe through the mouth. Antihistamines may be administered to reduce nasal secretions.

Frequent oral care is given,[27] and fluids are given freely. Since packing blocks the passage of air through the nose, a partial vacuum is created during swallowing, and the patient may complain of a sucking action when attempting to drink. Postnasal drainage, the presence of old blood in the mouth, and the loss of the ability to smell lessen the person's appetite. Because it is difficult to eat while the nose is packed, most persons prefer a liquid diet until the packing is removed, but they can have whatever food is tolerated.

In some persons, packing may remain in the nares as long as 1 week, while in others it is removed in 48 hours. After the nasal packing has been removed, the person is asked not to blow the nose for 48 hours because blowing may start bleeding. Fever is reported to the surgeon, because it may be caused by infection. Since the person has swallowed blood, it is normal for the stools to be tarry for a day or two. Because *Valsalva's maneuver* can initiate bleeding, the person is instructed not to bear down, and milk of magnesia or prune juice is usually ordered to be given as necessary. The person is also cautioned about coughing too vigorously.

Following external nasal surgery, the person frequently has discoloration about the eyes and can be told preoperatively that this will occur. To decrease local edema, the person is kept in mid-Fowler's position. Ice compresses can be used over the nose for 24 hours to lessen discoloration, bleeding, and discomfort. If a bowl of ice and several wet 4-in. × 4-in. gauze sponges are left within easy reach at the bedside, patients can apply the ice compresses themselves.

Specific surgical procedures on the nose

Polypectomy. Polypectomy is usually performed in a hospital under local anesthesia. Polyps are removed with a small snare or biting forceps, and the nostrils are packed.[68] Packing is left in place about 24 hours. Polypectomy would give lasting relief except that nasal polyps tend to recur and often affect the sinus mucosa, thus requiring ethmoidectomy for more complete removal.

Submucous resection. Submucous resection is used for relief of nasal obstruction related to septal deformities. This surgery is usually performed under local anesthesia. An internal incision is made on one side of the nasal septum from top to bottom. The mucous membrane is elevated away from the bone, the obstructive parts of the cartilage and bone are removed, and the mucous membrane is sutured back into place. Packing is placed in both nostrils to prevent bleeding and to splint the operative area. *Nasoseptoplasty* is becoming more widely used to treat a deviated nasal septum. Plastic reconstruction (septoplasty) may be necessary if a large part of the septum must be removed.

Rhinoplasty. Reconstruction of the external nose is called rhinoplasty; it is often done for cosmetic reasons (p. 1807) and is often combined with septoplasty. Rhinoplasty is an operation that may improve nasal function and will improve appearance. The operation is usually done under local anesthesia, and the nasal bones or cartilaginous framework of the nose are altered. A protective plaster-of-Paris splint, or a dressing of adhesive tape, or a plastic mold usually is placed over the nose after a plastic procedure on the nasal bones and also after a reduction of a fractured nasal septum. When plaster of Paris is used, care must be taken to keep droplets of plaster out of the patient's eyes. If the person has a fractured nose, however, the surgeon usually removes the protective dressing daily to manually mold the broken parts. Firm healing develops about the tenth day. If a splint is used, the skin adjacent to the splint is observed for signs of pressure areas. Usually only the surgeon changes a rhinoplasty dressing. Immediately postoperatively, the patient is placed in Fowler's position to minimize oozing. Discoloration about the eyes is common. To avoid disappointment, the person should know that the cosmetic result of the operation cannot be evaluated for several weeks.

Outcome criteria for persons having nasal surgery. The person or significant others can:

1. Describe measures to prevent complications (e.g., not blowing nose for 48 hours after packing removed and avoidance of Valsalva's maneuver until healing occurs).
2. Describe comfort measures (e.g., ice packs and frequent oral care).
3. Describe signs indicating complications (e.g., fever and excessive bleeding).
4. State reasons why discoloration of eyes is present.
5. State reasons for not judging cosmetic effect of rhinoplasty until several weeks after surgery.
6. Describe plans for follow-up care.

Intervention for the person requiring sinus surgery

If the person has recurrent attacks of sinusitis, it may be necessary to provide better drainage by permanently enlarging the sinus openings or by making a new opening and removing the diseased mucous membrane.[31] Surgery usually is performed during the subacute stage of infection. Surgery on the sinuses is done under general as well as under local anesthesia.

To prevent swallowing or aspiration of bloody drainage from the nose and throat postoperatively, the patient who has had a general anesthetic is turned well to the side. On recovery from the anesthesia or following local anesthesia, the patient may be in mid-Fowler's position, which will help decrease edema at the operative site and promote drainage. Ice compresses are usually applied over the nose, or an ice bag is placed directly over the maxillary or frontal sinuses. Ice constricts blood vessels, decreasing oozing and edema, and relieves pain. The patient should be watched carefully for hemorrhage. The nasal drip pad may be changed when it becomes soiled. Excessive bleeding should be called to the surgeon's attention. Repeated swallowing by the patient who is recovering from anesthesia may indicate hemorrhage.

Gauze packing is usually inserted into the nares and usually remains there for 48 hours. Consequently, the person breathes through the mouth, and the lips and mouth become dry and need frequent care. Aromatic solutions are refreshing, and petrolatum helps to prevent dryness of the lips. Warm or cool vapor inhalations often are ordered. The person should be reminded not to blow the nose, since this procedure may cause trauma to the operative site and can cause an increase in local blood pressure and cause bleeding.

A gross check of the person's visual acuity is advisable after sinus surgery to be sure that there is no damage to the optic nerve. A check for diplopia is advisable to determine any damage to the nerves or muscles at the globe of the eye. Fever or complaints of tenderness or pain over the involved sinus is reported to the physician, since they may indicate postoperative infection or inadequate drainage. Antibiotics may be given prophylactically. For a week or two postoperatively, there may be swelling or ecchymosis of the area. Fluids should be given liberally to all patients following surgery of the sinuses. If there is an oral incision, mouth care is given before meals to improve appetite and after eating to decrease the danger of infection.

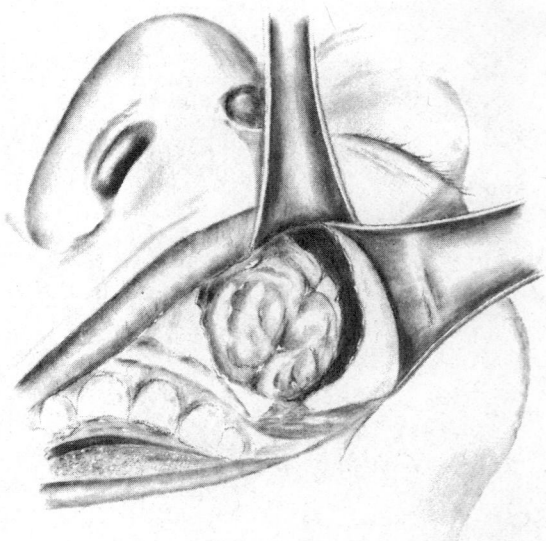

P. SAUNDERS

Fig. 50-9. Caldwell-Luc incision under upper lip to expose maxillary sinus. (From Saunders, W.H., et al.: Nursing care in eye, ear, nose, and throat disorders, ed. 4, St. Louis, 1979, The C.V. Mosby Co.)

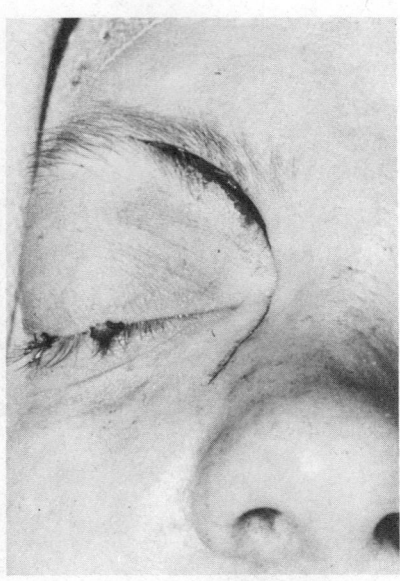

Fig. 50-10. Incision in inner half of eyebrow to expose ethmoid and frontal sinuses. Almost no visible scar results. (From DeWeese, D.D., and Saunders, W.H.: Textbook of otolaryngology, ed. 6, St. Louis, 1982, The C.V. Mosby Co.)

Specific surgical procedures on the sinuses

Caldwell-Luc surgery. The Caldwell-Luc operation is surgery of the maxillary sinus through an incision under the upper lip (Fig. 50-9) and is indicated as partial treatment for chronic sinusitis. An opening is made in the anterior wall of the sinus, and the infected contents of the sinus are stripped out. A larger opening in the nose is created to promote better aeration and drainage. The sinus is packed with petrolatum or antibiotic-impregnated gauze for about 48 hours. Numbness of the upper lip and upper teeth may be present for several months after a Caldwell-Luc operation, because some nerves to these structures pass through the site of the incision.

After Caldwell-Luc surgery, the patient usually is given only liquids for at least 24 hours and a soft diet for several days. The person should not chew on the affected side and should avoid wearing upper dentures for about 10 days, since the plate will rub on the suture line. Oral hygiene is important after Caldwell-Luc surgery, but the person must be careful not to abrade the incision about the teeth. Blowing the nose should be avoided for about 2 weeks after the packing is removed. The Caldwell-Luc operation is usually not performed on children, because they may have unerupted teeth near the site of the incision.

Ethmoidectomy. The *ethmoid* sinuses can be surgically approached either intranasally or externally through an incision made in the inner half of the eyebrow downward along the side of the nose[68] (Fig. 50-10). The latter is usually preferred, since visualization is better.

Ethmoidectomy is performed for ethmoiditis and for correction of nasal polyps, since nasal polyps frequently originate in the ethmoid cells. The *sphenoid* sinuses are approached either intranasally or externally through the eyebrow incision.

Osteoplastic flap surgery. *Frontal* sinus surgery differs from that of the other sinuses with the advent of the osteoplastic flap operation. Surgery of the other sinuses basically provides for an open, well-drained cavity, which in the past proved inadequate for the frontal sinuses, since recurrence of disease was common. The osteoplastic flap operation allows for complete removal of diseased mucosa of the frontal sinus and for obliteration of the sinus so that it is no longer functional or in continuum with the inner nose.

The osteoplastic flap procedure is performed through a "gull-wing" incision. In men, the incision extends along the eyebrows and connects along the bridge of the nose. In women, where baldness is not a problem in later life, the incision connects both temporal areas a few centimeters posterior to the hairline. Both incisions give excellent postoperative cosmesis and are extended to the periosteum of the bone overlying the frontal sinus.

The skin overlying the sinus is reflected, and a radiograph of the frontal sinus (obtained preoperatively) is used as a template for sawing the lateral and superior borders of the anterior frontal bone. The anterior bone is then reflected inferiorly, thus exposing the entire contents of the frontal sinus. The mucosa is removed under direct vision, and an operating microscope is used to ensure that all fragments of mucosa are removed. An

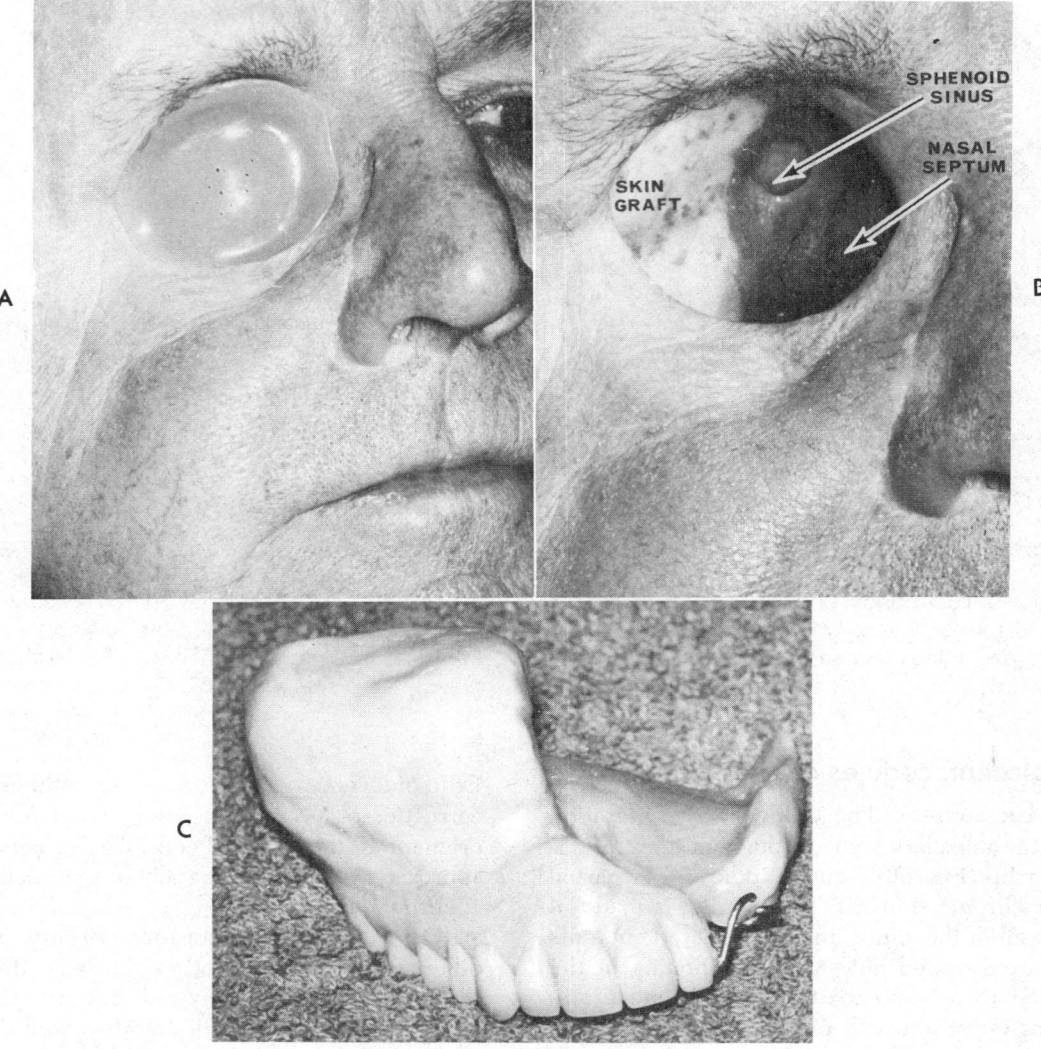

Fig. 50-11. Patient after maxillectomy and orbital exenteration. **A,** Orbital prosthesis in place. Eyeglasses worn over this further improves appearance. **B,** Defect in orbit with skin graft lining upper and lateral wall of orbital-maxillary cavity. **C,** Upper denture worn with large obturator to fill in defect created by maxillectomy. (From Saunders, W.H., et al.: Nursing care in eye, ear, nose, and throat disorders, ed. 4, St. Louis, 1979, The C.V. Mosby Co.)

incision is then made in the left-lower-abdominal quadrant and subcutaneous fat obtained for placement into the frontal sinus cavity. The bony flap and skin are then repositioned. Nasal packs are not required. Postoperatively, pain in the frontal area is not significant after 24 hours. Pain in the abdominal area, however, often lasts several days and serous drainage from this area is common after the drain is removed. Sutures are removed about the fifth postoperative day. Because nasal packs are not used, special oral hygiene care is not needed.

Outcome criteria for the person having sinus surgery. The person or significant others can:

1. Describe rationale for frequent oral care.
2. Describe rationale for not blowing the nose until healing occurs.

3. Describe signs of possible complications (fever, sinus pain).
4. State plans for follow-up care.

Surgery for carcinoma of the maxillary or ethmoid sinuses. Surgery for sinal malignancy often consists of removal of the entire upper jaw (maxillectomy) and one eye (orbital exenteration). Split-thickness skin grafts (p. 1801) are usually applied to the operative area. Postoperatively, the deformity of the jaw is managed with a dental prosthesis which closes off the defect in the mouth (Fig. 50-11). Radical surgery is required because of the danger of recurrence. Postoperatively, the patient must be watched for the complication of meningitis; usually antibiotics are given prophylactically. A nasogastric tube is usually inserted to ensure adequate liquid and caloric intake, since eating is difficult until the prosthesis is fitted. Several different prostheses may be needed before a final one fits because of shrinking of the cavity as healing progresses. All patients are uncomfortable and require analgesics following the procedure. Early ambulation is desirable. Maintenance of an airway is critical for these patients.[31,67] Often tracheostomy is performed (see p. 1231 for care of a patient with tracheostomy).

Mouth care for patients with this type of surgery is important.[27] Sometimes a gentle spray or oral irrigation using saline with hydrogen peroxide, weak sodium bicarbonate, or antibiotic solution may be used. Because the person may have difficulty swallowing, it may be necessary to aspirate the irrigating solution from the mouth; care must be taken to prevent trauma to the sutures by the suction tip. Management of saliva may also be a problem because of the swallowing difficulty (dysphagia).

Persons who undergo radical surgery of this type have a number of emotional adjustments to make.[46,58,78] The alteration in their physical appearance is readily visible; the person feels conspicuous and different. In addition to disfigurement, the person has all the normal fears of surgery and of cancer. Fear, anger, and grief are normal reactions to the situation. Fear is focused on concerns about the future, the ability to live normally, and also of being rejected. Anger and grief are common responses to the loss and the helplessness to control the loss. Oral communication also may be a problem immediately following surgery, and every effort is made to allow the person to express needs and feelings by writing if necessary. Conveying compassion and concern to the person is important.

Outcome criteria for the person having radical surgery of the sinuses. The person or significant others can:

1. State plan for achieving adequate nutritional meals.
2. Demonstrate proper care of prosthesis.
3. Demonstrate procedure to be used for maintaining oral hygiene.
4. Describe rationale for not blowing the nose until healing occurs.
5. Describe plans for socialization.
6. State plans for follow-up care.

Problems of the upper throat (pharynx and tonsils)

Anatomy and physiology

The pharynx is the space behind the oral cavity that extends from the base of the skull to the larynx. The

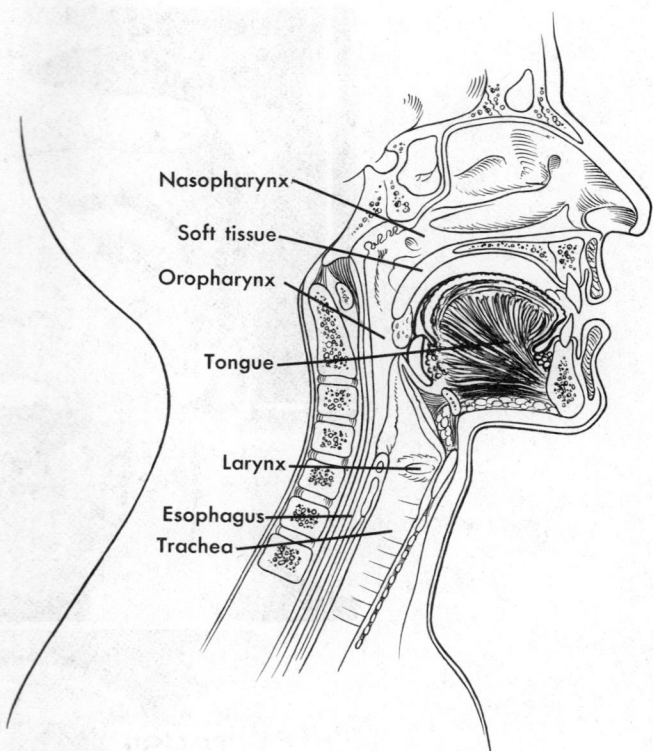

Fig. 50-12. Sagittal section of head showing pharynx and larynx.

pharynx can be considered in three parts: the nasopharynx, the oropharynx, and the hypopharynx (Fig. 50-12). It is lined with mucous membrane. The adenoids are located in the nasopharynx, the palatine tonsils in the pharynx, and the lingual tonsils in the hypopharynx; all are lymphoid tissue.

Assessment

To inspect the pharynx, the examiner asks the person to open the mouth without protruding the tongue. A tongue blade is pressed firmly down on the midpoint of the arched tongue; pressing farther back may cause gagging (Fig. 50-13). The person then says "ah" while breathing through the mouth to prevent gagging.

The oropharynx, that portion of the pharynx directly posterior to the oral cavity bounded by the nasopharynx above and laryngopharynx below, is examined with a tongue blade and a mirror. The anterior and posterior tonsillar pillars, the uvula, tonsils, and posterior pharynx are inspected for color, symmetry, evidence of exudate, edema, ulceration, and tonsillar enlargement. Redness and swelling of the tonsils, pillars, and uvula with white or yellow exudate on the tonsils may indicate streptococcal infection. Tonsils may be enlarged without being infected.

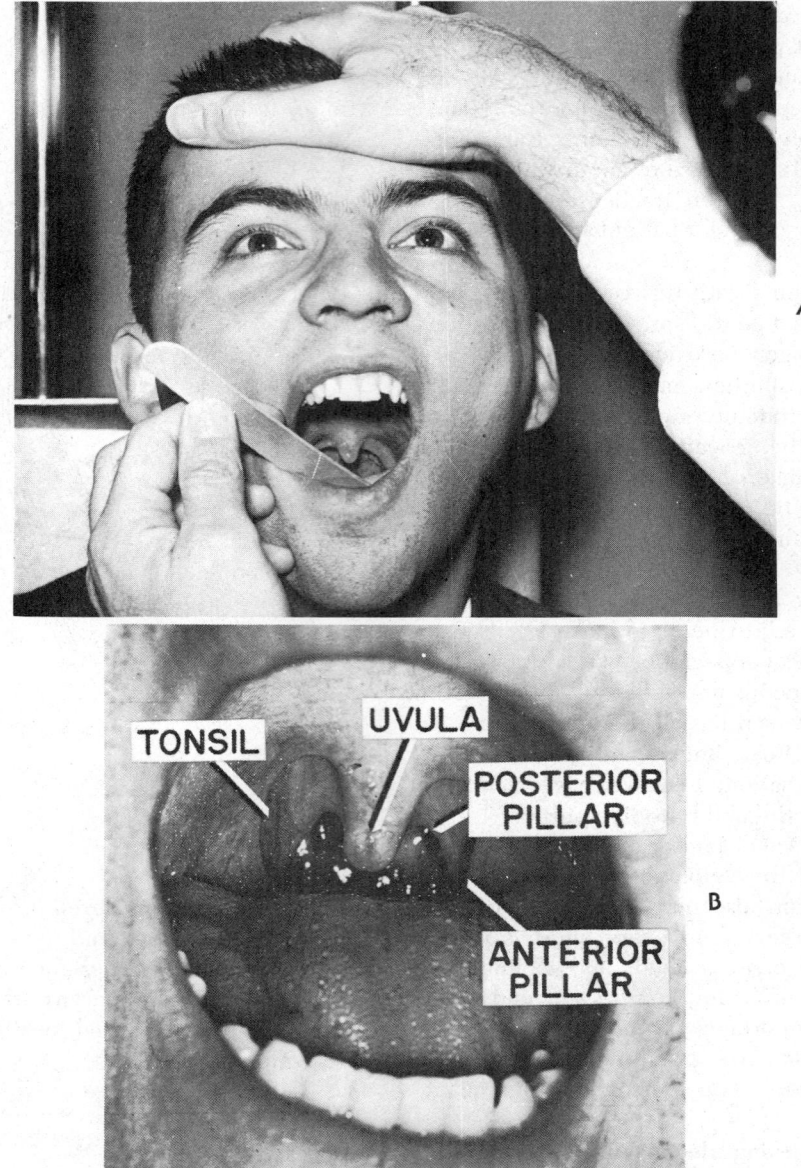

Fig. 50-13. A, Depressing of tongue. Tongue blade is held in left hand, which leaves right hand free for positioning of head and use of other instruments. Hand is braced on patient's cheek as tongue is depressed and scooped forward. **B,** Landmarks of pharynx. (**A** from Saunders, W.H.: Ears, nose, and throat. In Prior, J.A., Silberstein, J.S., Stang, J.M.: Physical diagnosis, ed. 6, St. Louis, 1981, The C.V. Mosby Co.; **B** from Saunders, W.H., et al.: Nursing care in eye, ear, nose, and throat disorders, ed. 4, St. Louis, 1979, The C.V. Mosby Co.)

Specific problems

Chronic enlargement of the tonsils and adenoids

Tonsils and adenoids are lymphoid structures located in the oropharynx and the nasopharynx. They reach their full size in childhood and begin to atrophy during puberty. When adenoids enlarge, usually as a result of chronic infections but sometimes for no known reason, they cause nasal obstruction. The person breathes through the mouth, may have a dull facial expression, and may have a reduced appetite, since the blocked nasopharynx can interfere with swallowing. In children, enlarged adenoids may block openings to the eustachian tubes in the nasopharynx, predisposing to middle ear infections and hearing impairment. Hypertrophy of the tonsils does not usually block the oropharynx but may affect speech and swallowing and cause mouth breathing. Occasionally, adenotonsillar hypertrophy in children may so restrict breathing as to precipitate pulmonary hypertension and cor pulmonale. The condition is reversed by surgical removal of the tonsils and adenoids.

Infections

Acute pharyngitis

ETIOLOGY. Acute pharyngitis is the most common throat inflammation. It may be caused by hemolytic streptococci, staphylococci, or other bacteria or filtrable viruses. There is increased evidence of gonococcal pharyngitis caused by the gram-negative diplococcus *Neisseria gonorrhoeae*. The disease is increasingly found in both men and women. When gonorrhea is suspected, a throat culture is indicated.[25] A severe form of acute pharyngitis often is referred to as *strep throat* because of the frequency of streptococci as the causative organisms.

CLINICAL PICTURE. Dryness of the throat is a common complaint. The throat appears red, and soreness may range from slight scratchiness to severe pain with difficulty in swallowing. A hacking cough may be present. Children often develop a very high fever, while adults may have only a mild elevation of temperature. Symptoms usually precede or occur simultaneously with the onset of acute rhinitis or acute sinusitis. Pharyngitis can occur after the tonsils have been removed, since the remaining mucous membrane can become infected.[51] Pharyngitis is also a common manifestation of infectious mononucleosis (p. 1210).

INTERVENTION. Acute pharyngitis usually is relieved by hot saline throat gargles. An ice collar may make the person feel more comfortable. The physician may prescribe acetylsalicylic acid administered orally as a gargle or in Aspergum. Lozenges containing a mild anesthetic may help relieve the local soreness. Moist inhalations may help relieve the dryness of the throat. A liquid diet usually is more easily tolerated, and fluids to at least 2.5 L/day are encouraged. Oral hygiene may prevent drying and cracking of the lips and usually refreshes the mouth. If the temperature is elevated, the person should remain in bed and, even if ambulatory and afebrile, should have extra rest. Occasionally, antibiotics such as penicillin or erythromycin are used to treat severe infections, or they are prescribed prophylactically to prevent superimposed infections, particularly in persons who have a history of rheumatic fever or bacterial endocarditis (see discussion of rheumatic fever, p. 998). Most pharyngitis in children is caused by viruses; therefore antibiotics should not be used for treatment, since antibiotics are not effective against viruses.

Acute follicular tonsillitis

ETIOLOGY. Acute follicular tonsillitis is an acute inflammation of the tonsils and their crypts. It is usually caused by the *Streptococcus* organism. It is more likely to occur when the person's resistance is low and is very common in children.

CLINICAL PICTURE. The onset is almost always sudden, and symptoms include sore throat, pain on swallowing, fever, chills, general muscle aching, and malaise. In children, the temperature may rise suddenly to 40.5° C (105° F). These symptoms often last for 2 or 3 days. The pharynx and the tonsils appear red, and the peritonsillar tissues are swollen. Sometimes a yellowish exudate drains from crypts in the tonsils. A throat culture usually is taken to identify the offending organism.

INTERVENTION. The person with acute tonsillitis is encouraged to rest and take generous amounts of fluids orally. Warm saline throat irrigation may be ordered, and antibiotics are given for streptococcal pharyngitis. Acetylsalicylic acid and sometimes codeine sulfate may be ordered for pain and discomfort. An ice collar may be applied to the neck.

Complications of untreated tonsillitis include heart and kidney damage, chorea, and pneumonia. Incidence of these complications is decreasing with the widespread use of penicillin and early diagnosis. Most physicians believe that persons who have recurrent attacks of tonsillitis should have a tonsillectomy. This procedure is usually performed from 4 to 6 weeks after an acute attack has subsided.

Since the person with acute tonsillitis is usually cared for at home, the nurse should help in teaching the general public the care that is needed. The office nurse, the clinic nurse, the nurse in industry, the school nurse, and the community health nurse have many opportunities to do this teaching.

Outcome criteria for the person with pharyngitis or tonsillitis. The person or significant others can:
1. Describe measures for relief of discomfort (e.g., hot gargles, ice collar, moist inhalations, and mouth care).
2. State rationale for prophylactic antibiotic therapy for pharyngitis in persons with a history of rheumatic fever or bacterial endocarditis.
3. State plans for drinking fluids, at least 2.5 L/day (adults).
4. Describe sypmtoms indicating need for medical supervision (e.g., recurrence, prolonged fever, excessive pain, presence of pus and dysphagia).
5. State plans for follow-up care, if appropriate.

Peritonsillar absecess. A peritonsillar abscess, or quinsy, is an uncommon, local complication of acute follicular tonsillitis in which infection extends from the tonsil to form an abscess in the surrounding tissues. The presence of pus behind the tonsil causes difficulty in swallowing, talking, and opening the mouth; and the person may be unable to swallow. Pain is severe and may extend to the ear on the affected side.

INTERVENTION. If antibiotics to which the offending

organism is sensitive are administered early, infection subsides. It is felt that some cases of peritonsillar abscess are caused by anaerobic organisms. In these instances, hydrogen peroxide (an oxidizing agent) in the form of a mouth wash may help relieve symptoms. Acute streptococcal or staphylococcal tonsillitis may also cause a peritonsillar abscess to form. If an abscess forms, incision and drainage are necessary. During the operation, the patient's head usually is lowered, and suction is applied as soon as the incision is made to prevent the patient from aspirating the drainage. Warm saline irrigations, an ice collar, or narcotics may relieve discomfort. If acute follicular tonsillitis is treated adequately, peritonsillar abscess is unlikely to occur.

Diphtheria. Diphtheria is a serious disease of the throat that most often affects children. It is caused by the bacillus *Corynebacterium diphtheriae*. It is highly contagious and is transmitted by droplet nuclei. There are also "carriers," that is, healthy people who carry the illness, although they are not ill. The incidence of diphtheria has rapidly decreased because of effective immunization programs. Occasional infections do occur, which increases the importance of preventive measures. Parents should be strongly encouraged to have their children immunized with the DPT (diphtheria, pertussis, tetanus) immunizations. Three separate injections are given, 1 month apart, beginning when the infant is about 2 months old.

Malignancy of the tonsils

Malignancy of the tonsils is second only to malignancy of the larynx in malignancies of the upper respiratory tract. The malignancy can be one of three types: carcinoma, lymphoepithelioma, or lymphosarcoma. Carcinomas are more common in men, possibly related to the increased incidence of smoking among men. The carcinomas spread upward into the soft palate and usually metastasize early to the neck. Local ulceration and otalgia (earache) are early symptoms. Lymphoepitheliomas often remain small and do not ulcerate, but neck metastasis occurs early. Lymphosarcomas produce large tonsils, usually without ulceration or pain, and metastasize early to the neck. Medical intervention for all tonsillar malignancies includes irradiation, which usually produces a good initial response. Extensive surgery is required if radiation therapy fails or if the carcinoma is large. Recurrence often occurs locally or with distant metastasis.[25]

Surgical procedures: tonsillectomy and adenoidectomy

The tonsils and adenoids are removed when they become enlarged and cause symptoms of obstruction, when they are chronically infected, when the person has repeated attacks of tonsillitis, or after repeated peritonsillar abscess. Chronic infections of these structures usually do not respond to antibiotics, and they may become foci of infection by spreading organisms to other parts of the body such as the heart. If a child's tonsils must be removed, the adenoids, even if they are not infected or enlarged, usually are removed also as a prophylactic measure. If possible, the removal of the tonsils is postponed until the child is about 6 years of age, but obstructing adenoids may be removed earlier. The former practice of routinely removing tonsils and adenoids for recurrent upper respiratory tract infections is no longer advocated.

Preoperative care

The patient who is to have a tonsillectomy and adenoidectomy usually is admitted to the hospital on the morning of the operation. Some physicians prefer that the child be admitted the evening before surgery to become accustomed to the hospital and have special laboratory tests. These tests would include bleeding and clotting times, a partial thromboplastin time test, and a sickle cell preparation test for black children.

In children, the operation is performed under general anesthesia; in adults, the tonsillectomy may be done under either general or local anesthesia. In the operating room, after the tonsils are removed, pressure is applied to stop superficial bleeding. Bleeding vessels are tied off with sutures, or an electrocoagulation current is used.

Postoperative care

Postoperatively, the person who has had a tonsillectomy may have a small amount of dark, bloody drainage from the operative area and may vomit blood that has been swallowed. The person is placed on the side or abdomen with a pillow under the chest until fully recovered from the anesthesia (Fig. 50-14). The patient is permitted to sit up in mid-Fowler's position when fully awake. Sometimes an ice collar is applied about the throat for comfort and to lessen the chance of hemorrhage. Young children usually resist the application of an ice collar, and therefore it is not used.

BLEEDING. Following a tonsillectomy or an adenoidectomy the patient is observed carefully for signs of hemorrhage. The person is urged not to cough or attempt to clear the throat immediately after surgery and thereafter, since these actions may initiate bleeding. Efforts are made to prevent the small child from crying lustily, and the child may be rocked if fully recovered from anesthesia. If the person swallows frequently, hemorrhage should be suspected, and the throat is inspected, since any signs of hemorrhage must be reported to the surgeon at once. Vomitus containing bright red blood is reported, and the specimen is saved for the surgeon's inspection. It is especially important

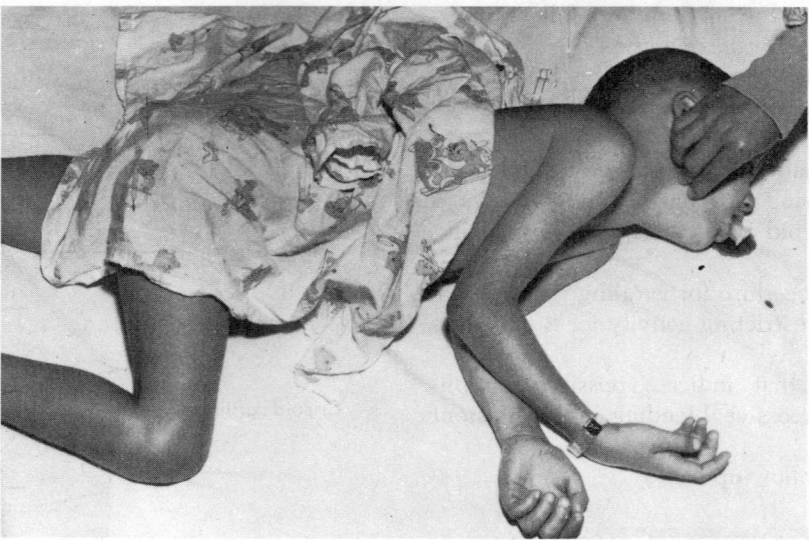

Fig. 50-14. Child is in recovery room after tonsillectomy. Note that he is propped on his side. Oral airway is in place. Nurse is supporting jaw to assist airway. (From Saunders, W.H., et al.: Nursing care in eye, ear, nose, and throat disorders, ed. 4, St. Louis, 1979, The C.V. Mosby Co.)

to observe the sleeping patient for signs of hemorrhage, since a very large amount of blood may be lost without any external evidence of bleeding.

The physician may be able to control minor postoperative bleeding by applying a sponge soaked in a solution of epinephrine to the site. The person who is bleeding excessively often is returned to the operating room for surgical treatment to stop the hemorrhage. This may be done by ligating or by cauterizing the bleeding vessel. If sutures must be used, the person will have more pain and discomfort than following a simple tonsillectomy. The patient may be unable to take solid foods for several days. Some otolaryngologists no longer prescribe acetylsalicylic acid for pain after tonsillectomy, since it increases the tendency to bleed. Acetaminophen or another aspirin substitute is usually ordered.

DIET. When vomiting has ceased, fluids and bland nourishment are offered. While the person usually will only take small amounts because of pain, he is urged to take large swallows because they hurt less, and because more fluid can thus be taken. Drinking through a straw is not advisable because of the danger of physical trauma, and because the suction on the throat may cause bleeding. Ice cold fluids are most acceptable and are given frequently. Ice cream usually is well tolerated, and ginger ale, cold milk, and cold custard often are offered next, followed by cream soups and bland juices such as pear juice. The morning after surgery, the person is usually offered foods such as refined cereal and soft-cooked or poached eggs. The patient is advised to avoid citrus fruit juices, hot fluids, rough foods (e.g., raw vegetables and crackers), and highly seasoned foods for at least 1 week because these foods irritate the operative area.

DISCHARGE TEACHING. Most persons are discharged from the hospital the day after surgery; some are permitted to return home the night of the operation, and if so, the child's parents are instructed to watch for bleeding and to report it to the physician at once. The child is usually kept indoors for 3 days. Usually the person is told to avoid vigorous exercise, coughing, sneezing, clearing of the throat, and vigorous blowing of the nose, since these actions can cause bleeding. If bleeding occurs at any time, the physician should be contacted immediately. The tough, yellow, fibrous membrane that forms over the operative site begins to break away between the fourth and eighth postoperative days, and hemorrhage may occur. The separation of the membrane accounts for the throat being more painful at this time. Pink granulation tissues soon become apparent, and by the end of the third postoperative week the area is covered with mucous membrane of normal appearance.

The person should continue to drink sufficient fluids (2 to 3 L/day) to help relieve the objectionable mouth odor common after any oral surgery. The stool may be black or dark for a few days, because blood has been swallowed during surgery.

A temperature of 37.5° to 38.5° C (99° to 101° F) may occur after tonsillectomy, but a persistent temperature elevation is reported to the physician. Discomfort in the ears may also occur and should be reported if it persists. The person usually reports to the surgeon for a follow-up examination about 1 week after the operation.

Outcome criteria for the person who has had a tonsillectomy and adenoidectomy. The person or significant others can:

1. Describe rationale for not coughing, clearing throat, and blowing nose until healing occurs.
2. State plans to avoid citrus juices and hot, rough, or spicy foods.
3. Demonstrate procedure for gargling if ordered.
4. State plans for restricting activity for 2 to 3 days after discharge.
5. Describe signs that indicate possible complications (e.g., excessive bleeding and persistent fever).
6. State plans for follow-up care.

Problems of the lower throat (larynx and hypopharynx)

Anatomy and physiology

The larynx forms the upper extremity of the trachea. The framework of the larynx is made up of several cartilages held together by muscle and ligaments (Fig. 50-15). The cartilaginous framework of the larynx protects the vocal cords and affords a stiffness that permits an airway. The thyroid cartilage, the "Adam's apple," is the largest cartilaginous element in the larynx and serves to protect the inner structures. The hyoid bone lies just above the thyroid cartilage and forms an attachment for the larynx and tongue. The cricoid cartilage lies just below the thyroid cartilage and articulates with the arytenoid cartilages, which swing in and out to open and close the vocal cords, opening and closing the glottis (the opening formed between the vocal cords). The larynx is lined with mucosa continuous with that of the hypopharynx and trachea. The vagus nerve innervates the larynx by means of the recurrent laryngeal nerve.

The chief function of the larynx is to serve as an airway between the pharynx and trachea. A leaf-shaped lid of fibrocartilage (epiglottis) protects the glottis by covering the entrance to the larynx during swallowing to prevent aspiration of food or fluids. The closing of the glottis also allows for an increase of intrathoracic pressure, which is needed, for example, in coughing or lifting. This increased pressure gives added advantage to the use of the muscles of the shoulder and thorax. In addition to these, a most important function of the larynx is *phonation*. The larynx creates sounds as a result of vocal cord vibrations that are formed into speech patterns by the movement of the pharynx, palate, tongue, teeth, and lips.

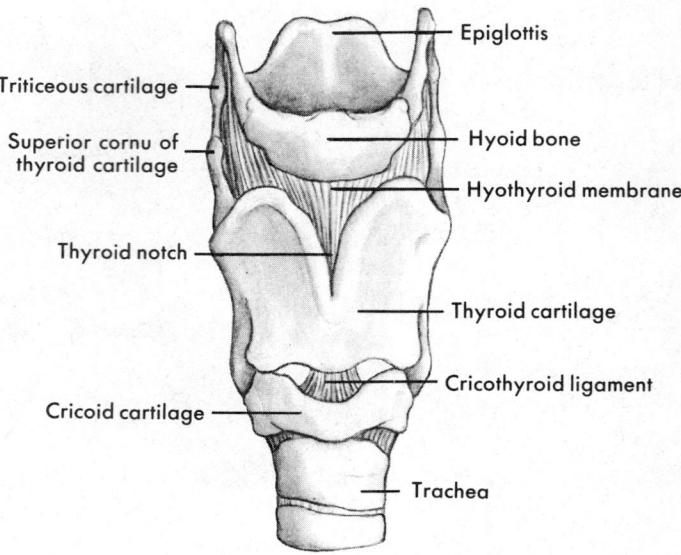

Fig. 50-15. Anterior aspect of larynx. (From Francis, C.C.: Introduction to human anatomy, ed. 6, St. Louis, 1975, The C.V. Mosby Co.)

Labels: Epiglottis; Triticeous cartilage; Hyoid bone; Superior cornu of thyroid cartilage; Hyothyroid membrane; Thyroid notch; Thyroid cartilage; Cricothyroid ligament; Cricoid cartilage; Trachea

Assessment

The larynx may be examined by an indirect laryngoscopy; the patient sits in a chair with the head tilted back and is asked to stick out the tongue. The examiner then grasps it with a gauze sponge and pulls it forward and downward. A warmed laryngeal mirror is introduced into the back of the throat until the larynx is visualized. It is examined at rest and during attempts to speak (phonation). If the gag reflex is very sensitive, the pharyngeal wall may be sprayed with a topical anesthetic such as 2% cocaine or 2% tetracaine (Pontocaine). Pontocaine is preferred by some physicians because it is less toxic than cocaine.

A direct laryngoscopy is performed on children, on adults who are unable to cooperate for an indirect examination, and on all persons with suspicious lesions of the larynx.[18] Direct laryngoscopy is usually performed under local anesthesia with 10% cocaine or under general anesthesia. A sedative (e.g., secobarbital, meperidine, or other narcotic) and atropine sulfate is given 1 hour before the examination. Atropine is essential before administering both local and general anesthesia because it reduces the volume of secretions. For direct laryngoscopy, the person is placed in a reclining position, with the head in a head holder. If no head holder is available, the person's head is extended over the edge of the table and manually supported by a physician or nurse. In some cases, a suspension device may be applied to the laryngoscope so that the physician's hands are free for instrumentation or manipulation of the fo-

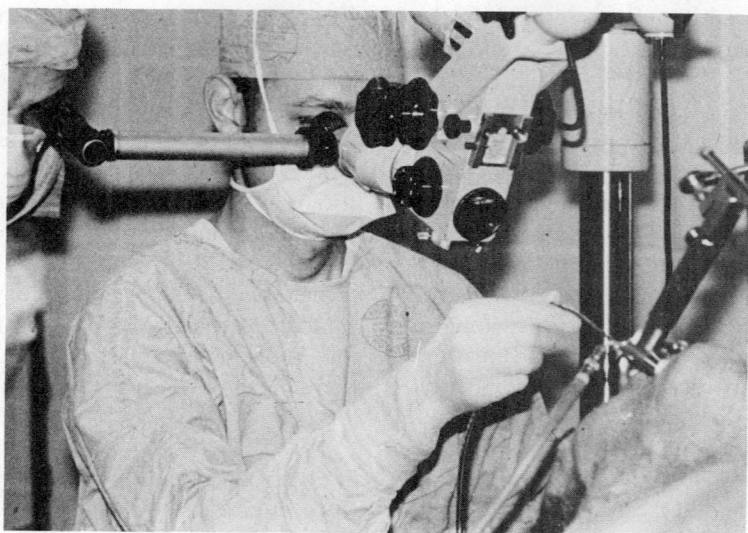

Fig. 50-16. Laryngoscopy using operating microscope to provide both illumination and magnification. Laryngoscope is self-retaining. (From DeWeese, D.D., and Saunders, W.H.: Textbook of otolaryngology, ed. 6, St. Louis, 1982, The C.V. Mosby Co.)

cus of the microscope. Microlaryngoscopy using an operating microscope is becoming more widely used (Fig. 50-16). This method provides magnification and binocular vision.

The laryngoscope, a hollow, metal tube with a handle at the proximal end and a light at the distal end, is introduced by a physician through the mouth into the hypopharynx, elevating the epiglottis, and making the interior of the larynx easily visible. Minor surgical procedures, such as a biopsy or the removal of a small benign tumor, may be performed by looking through this instrument.

After a laryngoscopy under local anesthesia, the person should not eat or drink anything until the gag reflex returns, usually within 2 hours. The gag reflex can be tested by "tickling" the throat with a tongue blade or applicator. After the gag reflex returns, the person should try first to drink water, since if it is accidentally aspirated into the trachea or lungs, it is the fluid least likely to cause aspiration pneumonia.

The interior of the larynx may also be visualized by radiographs and tomography. Radiopaque contrast material is instilled into the larynx (as in a bronchogram). These radiographs are less commonly used than laryngoscopy. Xerography is also used to evaluate the larynx.

Specific problems

Laryngitis

Simple acute laryngitis. Simple acute laryngitis is an inflammation of the mucous membrane lining the larynx accompanied by edema of the vocal cords. It may be caused by a cold, by sudden changes in temperature, or by irritating fumes. Symptoms vary from a slight huskiness to a complete loss of voice. The throat may be painful and feel scratchy, and a cough may be present.

Laryngitis usually requires only symptomatic treatment. The person is advised to remain indoors in an even temperature and to avoid talking for several days or weeks, depending on the severity of the inflammation. Steam inhalations with aromatic vapors (e.g., tincture of benzoin, oil of pine, and menthol) may be soothing. Cough syrups or home remedies for coughs provide relief to some persons. Smoking or being where others are smoking should be avoided.

Acute laryngitis may cause acute respiratory distress and prostration in children under 5 years of age. Because the larynx of the infant and young child is relatively small and is susceptible to spasm when irritated or infected, it easily becomes partially or totally obstructed. After exposure to cold air or as a result of an upper respiratory tract infection, a hoarse, barking cough may result. The child may become restless and sit up and grab the throat in an attempt to breathe. The nostrils may flare, and muscles about the clavicle may be visibly retracted. The child may be completely well before and after the attack, which may last 30 minutes to 3 hours. The usual treatment is the administration of copious amounts of vaporized cool mist. Some children's hospitals have "croup rooms" where a continuous "fog" of cool mist is generated into the room. If cool mist is not available, warm steam inhalations may be used to provide humidity and liquefy secretions. In the home, an improvised steam room can be created by running a hot shower.

Acute epiglottitis. A second and more serious form of croup syndrome, which usually occurs in young children between 2 and 12 years of age, is called *acute epiglottitis*.[63] The child rapidly develops fever, inspiratory stridor, and progressive toxicity. The symptoms are caused by inflammatory edema of the epiglottis from the *Haemophilus hemolyticus* organism.

The treatment of acute epiglottitis is directed toward preserving the airway, because a significant number of children with this disease will suffocate. In the past, tracheostomy was performed in order to ensure a patent airway. With modern pediatric intensive care units, the tracheostomy can usually be avoided, and an orotracheal intubation is done in its place. With the administration of intravenous antibiotics, usually ampicillin, cephalosporin, or chloramphenicol (Chloromycetin), the danger of respiratory obstruction usually passes within 48 hours, and the patient can be extubated and discharged in another 24 to 48 hours. Intravenous steroid therapy usually does not prevent the need for an artificial airway in acute epiglottitis but may be very beneficial in decreasing the edema in the area immediately below the vocal cords and upper trachea.

The airway must remain patent to prevent suffocation, and an artificial airway, however, may be necessary. In certain emergency situations, when endotracheal intubation or tracheostomy equipment is not available, the most expedient method of establishing an airway to avoid asphyxia and death is to perform a "mini" tracheotomy or cricothyroid stab. A large-bore intravenous needle may be inserted into the cricothyroid space. The needle is inserted slightly downward and backward. Another method of maintaining an airway during an acute attack of epiglottitis is by using a breathing bag attached to a mask and performing positive pressure ventilation. This method seems to be most helpful when the medical treatment has already been started but has not yet been effective, or when the patient must be transferred to another unit and tracheostomy is to be avoided if possible.[37]

The child with croup will be less frightened if held or if someone remains during the attack. Sedatives will not be ordered unless an artificial airway is in place and forced ventilation can be maintained, since sedatives tend to depress the person's limited respiratory effort.

Chronic laryngitis. Some people who use their voices excessively, who smoke a great deal, or who work continuously where there are irritating fumes develop a chronic laryngitis. Hoarseness usually is worse in the early morning and in the evening. There may be a dry, harsh cough and a persistent need to clear the throat. Treatment may consist of removal of irritants, voice rest, correction of faulty voice habits, steam inhalations, and

cough medications. The physician may order spraying of the throat with an astringent antiseptic solution such as hexylresorcinol (S.T. 37). To carry out this procedure properly the person must use a spray tip that turns down at the end so that the medication reaches vocal cords and is not dissipated in the posterior pharynx. The spray tip is placed in the back of the throat with the bent portion behind the tongue. The person should then take one or two deep breaths and spray the medication on inhalation. This procedure may cause temporary coughing and gagging. Many medications used as throat sprays are now sold in plastic squeeze bottles with tube and spray tip attached.

Laryngeal paralysis

Laryngeal paralysis may result from disease or injury of either the laryngeal nerves or the vagus nerve. Some causes include aortic aneurysm, mitral stenosis, bronchial carcinoma, neck injuries, and severing or stretching of the recurrent laryngeal nerve during thyroidectomy. The major diagnostic method is laryngoscopy.

Either one or both vocal cords may be paralyzed. If only one cord is affected, the airway is adequate and only the voice may be affected.[18] Efforts to improve the voice in persons with unilateral cord paralysis have been accomplished by injecting a small quantity of Teflon into the paralyzed cord. This swells the cord and pushes it toward the midline where the other cord can approximate it better during phonation.

With bilateral paralysis, the voice is weak. Bilateral paralysis causes a poor airway that results in incapacitating dyspnea and stridor on exertion. Treatment of bilateral cord paralysis is aimed at restoration of the airway, not at improvement of the voice. An arytenoidectomy may be performed, which consists of resection of one of the arytenoid cartilages, thus increasing the diameter of the posterior portion of the glottis sufficiently to improve breathing. Other procedures include external surgical approaches to lateralize (i.e., hold vocal cords open by lateral fixation) the paralyzed vocal cord. A new technique of reinnervation of the paralyzed vocal cord restores cord function in some cases. If both cords are paralyzed and the airway is inadequate, a tracheostomy will be necessary to restore the airway (p. 1231).

Laryngeal edema

Acute laryngeal edema is a potential medical emergency and may be caused by anaphylaxis, urticaria, acute laryngitis, serious inflammatory disease of the throat, and edema following intubation.[31] Acute laryngeal edema causes the airway to narrow or close and requires restoration of the airway. Treatment of acute laryngeal edema consists of administration of an adrenal corticosteroid or epinephrine. A tracheostomy or intubation may be necessary. Edema of the larynx may be chronic because of irradiation treatment of the larynx or tumors of the neck, thus requiring a tracheostomy.

Carcinoma

Squamous cell carcinoma of the larynx is increasing in frequency. It is estimated that in the United States there are over 10,000 new cases every year.[2] Cancer of the larynx limited to the true vocal cords grows slowly because of the limited lymphatic supply. Elsewhere in the larynx (e.g., the epiglottis, false vocal cords, and pyriform sinuses), lymph vessels are abundant; and cancer of these tissues often spreads rapidly and metastasizes early to the deep lymph nodes of the neck.

Cancer of the larynx is eight times more common in men than in women, and it occurs most often in persons over 60 years of age. There appears to be some relationship between cancer of the larynx and heavy smoking, alcohol, chronic laryngitis, vocal abuse, and family predisposition to cancer. Because of the increase in the number of women who are heavy smokers, the incidence of carcinoma of the larynx among this group is increasing. Any person who becomes progressively hoarse or is hoarse for longer than 2 weeks should be urged to seek medical attention at once. Hoarseness is an early symptom of cancer of the vocal cords. If treatment is given when hoarseness appears (caused by the tumor's preventing the complete approximation of the vocal cord), a cure usually is possible. Signs of metastases of cancer to other parts of the larynx include a sensation of a lump in the throat, pain in the Adam's apple that radiates to the ear, dyspnea, dysphagia, enlarged cervical nodes, and cough. The diagnosis of cancer of the larynx is made from the history, from visual examination of the larynx with indirect laryngoscopy, and from a biopsy and microscopic study of the lesion. Treatment is usually surgical.

Surgical procedures

Partial laryngectomy

If the tumor is limited to portions of the vocal cords or areas just above them, a partial laryngectomy may effect a cure. Patients suitable for partial laryngectomy have only one diseased vocal cord, and there is complete mobility of both cords.[31] The most common technique for partial laryngectomy is to make an opening into the larynx through the thyroid cartilage (laryngofissure) and remove the involved cord and tumor. As healing takes place, scar tissue fills the defect where the diseased cord was removed and becomes a vibrating surface within the larynx. This tissue permits husky but acceptable speech. A tracheostomy tube is inserted at the time of operation but is removed when edema in the surrounding tissues subsides. For 48 hours postoperatively, nutrients may be supplied intravenously or by a nasogastric tube. Fluids and soft foods may then be taken orally. Soft foods may be easier for the pharyngeal musculature to handle than fluids. Foods usually well tolerated include scrambled eggs, cottage cheese, and baked potatoes. Other care is similar to that given any patient having a tracheostomy.

A hemilaryngectomy is sometimes performed through the same operative approach as a laryngofissure. One side of the thyroid cartilage behind the true and false vocal cords is also removed. A supraglottic partial laryngectomy is performed for carcinoma of the epiglottis and adjacent structures above the level of the true vocal cords. The vocal cords are left intact, while a horizontal cut passes just above the true cords to remove the diseased tissue. The postoperative rehabilitation of persons with these two procedures is more arduous than those with a laryngofissure.

The person who has had a partial laryngectomy usually is not on absolute voice rest but is not permitted to use the voice until the surgeon gives specific approval (usually 3 days postoperatively). Then, only whispering is done until healing is complete, after which time the person usually adjusts quite readily to relatively minor limitation of speech. The main problems encountered by patients undergoing partial laryngectomy are those of swallowing and aspiration.

Total laryngectomy

When cancer of the larynx is advanced, a total laryngectomy may be performed. This includes removal of the epiglottis, thyroid cartilage, hyoid bone, cricoid cartilage, and three or four rings of the trachea. The pharyngeal opening to the trachea is closed, the anterior wall of the hypopharynx is closed, and the remaining trachea is brought out to the neck wound and sutured to the skin. It forms an opening (permanent tracheostomy) through which the patient breathes (Fig. 50-17).

The sense of smell is affected after laryngectomy. The presence of a tracheal stoma has a deleterious effect on the sense of smell, because breathing through the nose is impossible, therefore the patient does not receive olfactory sensations.

Preoperative care. The person who is to have a laryngectomy is told by the physician that breathing will occur through a special opening made in the neck and that normal speech will not be possible. This is often depressing to the patient, because it threatens economic status as well as life. In some instances, it is helpful to receive a visit from another person who has made a good recovery from laryngectomy and who has undergone rehabilitation successfully. In other instances, this visit may depress the patient further. Careful assessment must be made to determine if the person will benefit from such a visit and whether the visit should be made preoperatively, immediately after surgery, or later in the recovery period. Often no one else can give a person the reassurance that speech can be regained as well as a fellow patient. Many large cities have a "Lost Chord Club" or a "New Voice Club," and the members are willing to visit hospitalized patients. Information regarding these clubs may be obtained by writing to the International Association of Laryngectomees.* Local speech rehabilitation centers may supply instructive films and other resources. The local chapter of the American Cancer Society and the local health department also have information available. If possible, the family also should learn about the method of esophageal speech that the person will learn to use.

Postoperative care. Postoperative care of the person is essentially the same as that described for tracheostomy (p. 1231) except that these persons will have a laryngectomy tube in place—a tube that is shorter and wider in diameter than a tracheostomy tube. Some patients may not have a tube in the stoma after the operation because the stoma is a permanent one kept open initially by the sutures and because their surgeon believes that there is less tissue reaction and a better stoma if no tube is used. Most otolaryngologists believe that a laryngectomy tube is better than a tracheostomy tube,

because it is shorter. The tube will remain until the wound is healed and a permanent fistula has formed, usually in 2 or 3 weeks (Fig. 50-18). Frequent suctioning is necessary in the early postoperative period to keep the trachea free of secretions.

A nasogastric tube is usually inserted during the surgical procedure for the instillation of food and fluids at regular intervals postoperatively for about 10 days (Fig. 50-19). The use of the tube to give food is thought to minimize contamination of the pharyngeal and esophageal suture lines and to prevent fluid from leaking through the wound into the trachea before healing occurs. The nasogastric tube is removed as soon as the person can safely swallow. The person then needs careful attention in the first attempts to swallow. There may be a sensation of choking as well as severe coughing that is frightening and painful. Aspiration cannot occur because the trachea no longer communicates with the esophagus.

SPEECH REHABILITATION. Speech rehabilitation may be started as soon as the esophageal suture line is healed. In addition to the International Association of Laryngectomees and the local chapter of the American Cancer Society, information on laryngeal speech can be obtained from the American Speech and Hearing Associ-

---

*American Cancer Society, 777 Third Ave., New York, NY 10017.

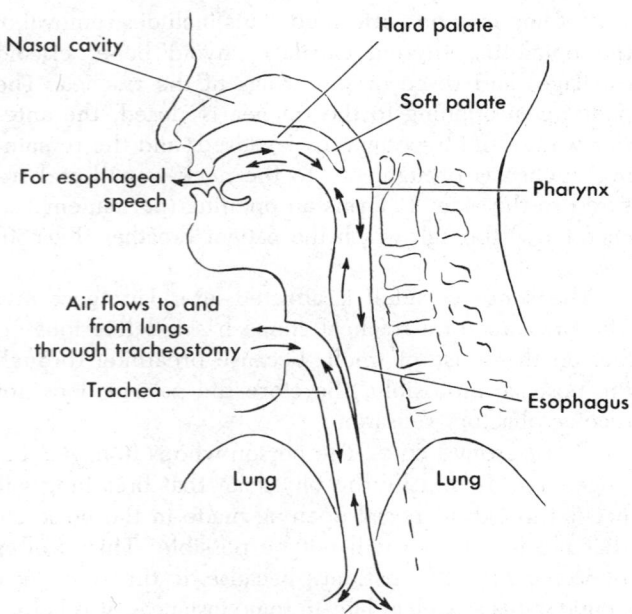

Fig. 50-17. Permanent opening in trachea following total laryngectomy. Note that nose is not used for breathing and that all air enters throuth tracheostomy opening. Air swallowed through mouth is used to produce laryngeal speech. (Redrawn from Saunders, W.H., et al.: Nursing care in eye, ear, nose, and throat disorders, ed. 4, St. Louis, 1979, The C.V. Mosby Co.)

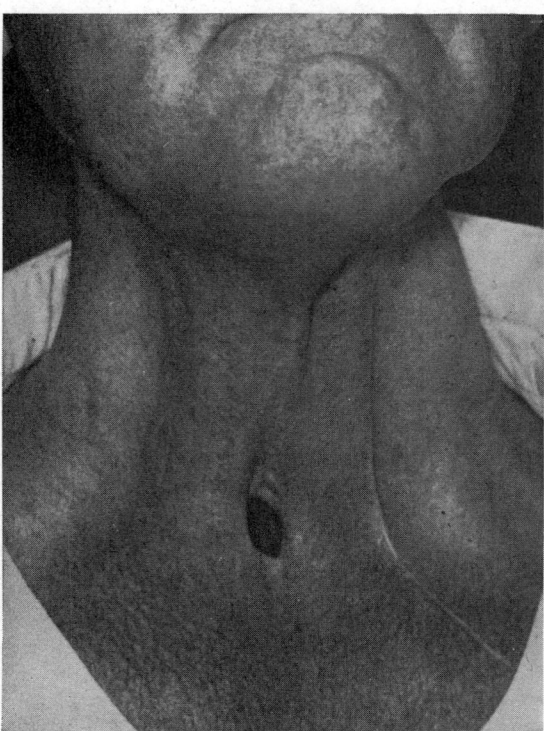

Fig. 50-18. After laryngectomy. Note scars of bilateral radical neck dissections. (From DeWeese, D.D., and Saunders, W.H.: Textbook of otolaryngology, ed. 6, St. Louis, 1982, The C.V. Mosby Co.)

ation.* Most persons learn esophageal speech best at a special clinic. Although some persons may need to go to a nearby city for this instruction, they usually must remain away from home for only 1 or 2 weeks. Motivation and persistent effort are essential in learning this

---

*10801 Rockville Pike, Rockville, MD 20852.

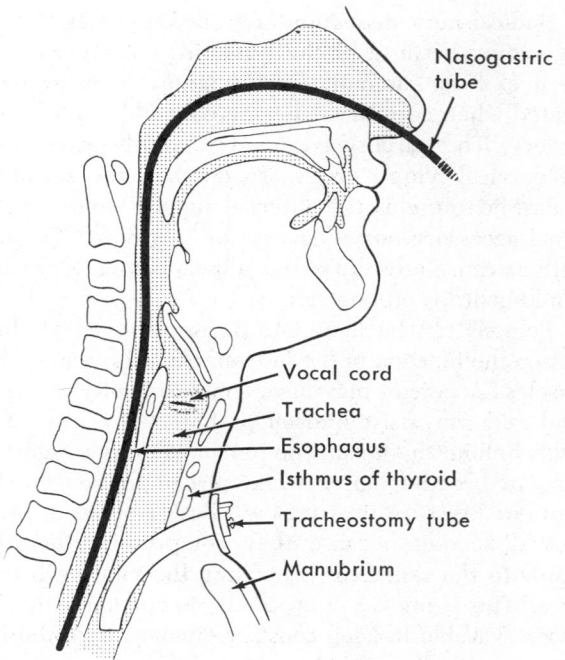

Fig. 50-19. Position of tracheostomy tube and nasogastric tube if both are used.

kind of speech; encouragement and support from the professional staff and the person's significant others are important to the person's morale. About 75% of all persons who have their larynx removed master some sort of speech, and the average person can return to work 1 or 2 months after leaving the hospital.

To learn *esophageal speech*, the person must first practice burping. This provides the moving column of air needed for sound, while folds of tissue at the opening of the esophagus act as the vibrating surface. The person must learn to coordinate articulation with esophageal vocalization made possible by aspirating air into the esophagus. The new voice sounds are natural, although somewhat hoarse. The qualities of speech provided by the use of the nasopharynx are still present, however. The client may have digestive difficulty during the time while learning to speak, caused by swallowing air during practice, by unusual strain on abdominal muscles, and by nervous tension. The individual should be told that digestive difficulty may occur but that it is not cause for alarm; it abates with proficiency in speaking.

If a person is unable to learn esophageal speech in 60 to 90 days after surgery, a speech aid such as a vibrator or an electronic artificial larynx (Fig. 50-20) may be prescribed. An individual who has a hiatal hernia may not be able to accomplish esophageal speech and will have to use another method for speech. Various mechanical devices are available, and the new ones permit a natural type of speech, providing pitch inflections and volume control. The local chapter of the American Cancer Society or the local telephone com-

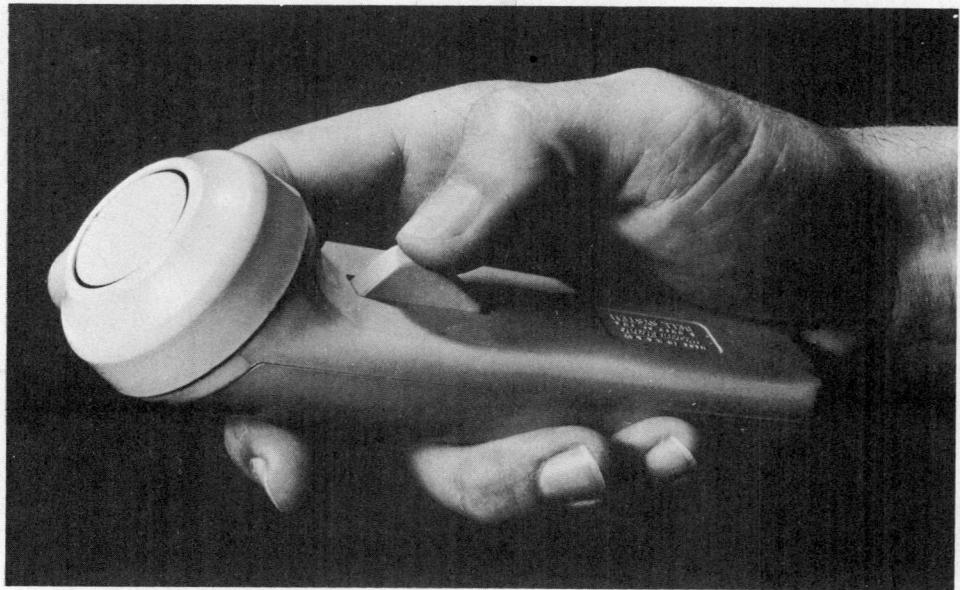

Fig. 50-20. Battery-powered electronic artificial larynx for patient who has total laryngectomy and cannot learn esophageal speech. (Courtesy Illinois Bell Telephone Co.)

pany can provide information about the purchase of these devices.

Several other surgical and prosthetic techniques are being tested. Most have not been widely used because of technical complications, and for most patients, esophageal speech is still the best method of communication. A summary of some of these procedures can be found in the literature.[23,29]

DISCHARGE TEACHING. Persons with laryngectomies must take some special precautions. They must be careful while bathing or taking a shower that water is not aspirated through the opening into the lungs. Some otolaryngologists caution their patients not to go swimming or take boat trips; others state that as long as the person is careful, these activities are permitted. A snorkle device to fit over the stoma is available to laryngectomized persons so that swimming can be permitted. Persons with laryngectomies are advised to wear a scarf or a shirt with a closed collar that covers the opening, yet is of porous material. This material substitutes for the nasal passages to warm the air and screen out dust and other irritating substances.

Usually by the time of discharge, persons with laryngectomies do not need to be suctioned but can cough up secretions. If suctioning is deemed necessary, the person or family needs to be provided with necessary supplies or with instructions as to where to secure the necessary suction equipment and of how to care for themselves. Suction equipment can be rented for home

use or obtained in many communities through the local chapter of the American Cancer Society. Suction can be provided by attaching a suction hose to a water faucet. Many hardware stores carry the necessary equipment. The amount of suction is controlled by the stream of water.

Radical neck dissection

Radical neck dissection often accompanies total laryngectomy because of the possibility of metastases to the neck from carcinoma of the larynx. It is always indicated when cervical nodes are palpable at the time of surgery. The surgery is aimed primarily at removing the cervical lymph nodes. To do that, the sternocleidomastoid muscle, the internal jugular vein, and the spinal accessory nerve have to be sacrificed. These resections cause atrophy of the trapezius muscle, and the shoulder drops on one side.

Persons can be taught to do exercises to gradually replace the function of the lost muscles with that of other muscles. A person may have some difficulty lifting the head and can assist himself or herself by placing the hands behind the head. The person is more comfortable and can breathe better when placed in mid-Fowler's position. Pressure dressings are best avoided in radical neck dissection because they compromise the blood supply to the skin flaps protecting the vital neck structures. The Hemovac (Fig. 50-21) is currently the best device available to keep constant drainage from the neck

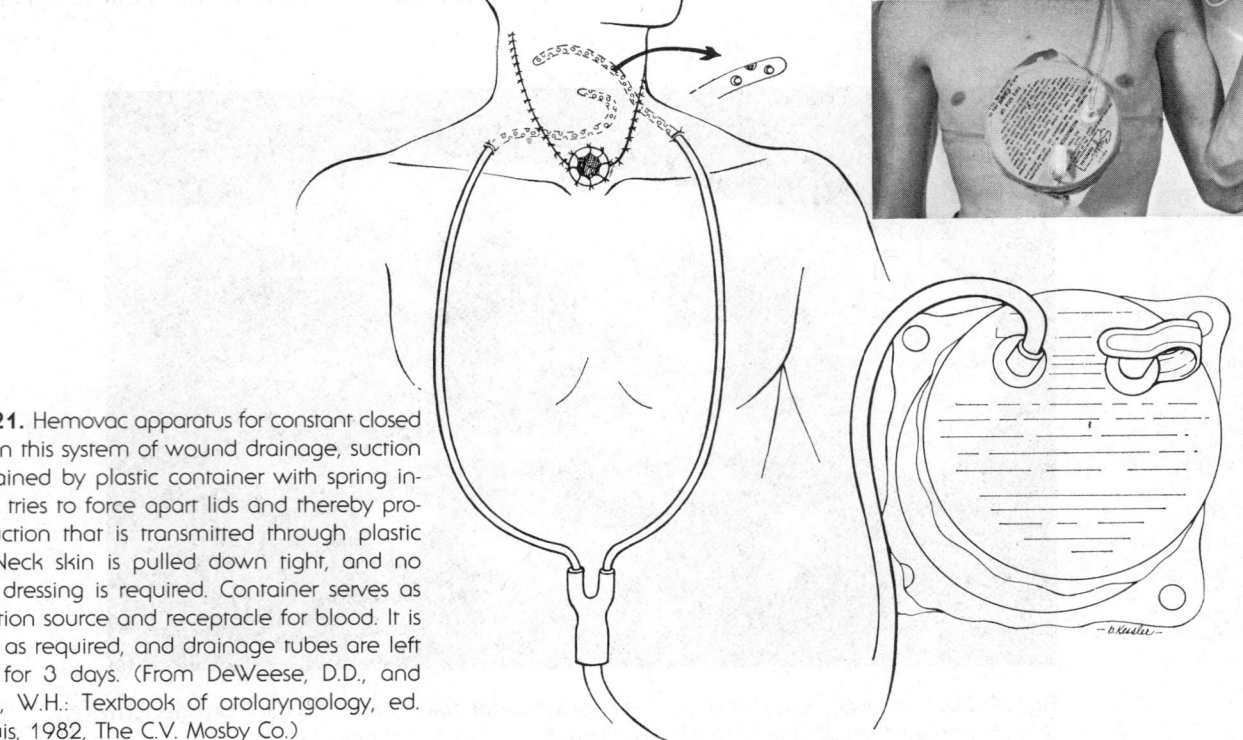

Fig. 50-21. Hemovac apparatus for constant closed suction. In this system of wound drainage, suction is maintained by plastic container with spring inside that tries to force apart lids and thereby produces suction that is transmitted through plastic tubing. Neck skin is pulled down tight, and no external dressing is required. Container serves as both suction source and receptacle for blood. It is emptied as required, and drainage tubes are left in neck for 3 days. (From DeWeese, D.D., and Saunders, W.H.: Textbook of otolaryngology, ed. 6, St. Louis, 1982, The C.V. Mosby Co.)

wound without pressure on the flaps. The Hemovac must be checked to see that it is working properly and that there is no edema, which might indicate hematoma.

There is some readily visible alteration of appearance that may cause the person to feel somewhat conspicuous. Anger, grief, or denial may be part of the person's normal response to the change in body image. (For further information on body image, refer to Chapter 28.)

Radical neck dissection can be performed without laryngectomy for persons whose primary malignant lesion is in the tongue, tonsil, lip, nasopharynx, or thyroid. Often the procedure accompanies other procedures and is termed a *composite* resection. Composite resections may include radical neck dissection in addition to either the removal of the mandible; removal of the mandible and resection of the floor of the mouth; or removal of the mandible, floor of the mouth, and the tongue. The nursing care for these patients is similar to the care given for maxillectomy and orbital exenteration (p. 1272). Emotional reactions to this type of radical surgery may be profound. Disfigurement is readily visible, and reactions to the change in body image are marked. In addition to the usual fears of surgery and cancer, the person having a composite resection may have fears of rejection and fears concerning the future.

Outcome criteria for the person having a laryngectomy or radical neck dissection. The person or significant others can:
1. Verbalize feelings about the surgery and changes in life-style.
2. Discuss plans for speech rehabilitation, including community resources available (e.g., laryngectomee clubs and American Cancer Society).
3. State reasons for wearing a scarf or other porous material over stoma.
4. Demonstrate suctioning if this is to be necessary after discharge.
5. Identify persons who can provide needed emotional support.
6. State plans for follow-up care.
   a. Time of next medical appointment.
   b. Signs or symptoms indicating need for immediate medical attention (e.g., respiratory tract infection and bleeding).

REFERENCES AND SELECTED READINGS

1. Agarwal, M.K., et al.: Fibrosarcoma of nose and paranasal sinuses, J. Surg. Oncol. **15**:53-37, 1980.
2. American Cancer Society: 1981 cancer facts and figures, New York, 1981, The Society.

3. Baker, D.C.: Intranasal steroid injections: indications, technique, results, complications, Laryngoscope **89**:998-1003, 1979.
4. Baker, D.C.: Treatment of obstructing inferior turbinates with intranasal corticosteroids, Ann. Plast. Surg. **3**:253-259, 1979.
5. Ballenger, J.: Diseases of the nose, throat, and ear, ed. 2, Philadelphia, 1977, Lea & Febiger.
6. *Bates, B.: A guide to physical examination, ed. 2, Philadelphia, 1979, J.B. Lippincott Co.
7. *Blues, K.: A framework for nurses providing care to laryngectomy patients, Ca. Nurs. **1**:441-446, 1978.
8. *Brown, M.H.: Cancer audit, nursing patient care outcome, audit criteria: laryngectomy with radical neck dissection, Ca. Nurs. **1**:331-334, 1978.
9. Brown, R.B., and Clinton, D.: Vesicular and ulcerative infections of the mouth and oropharynx, Postgrad. Med. **67**:107-116, 1980.
10. Burki, N.K.: Chronic airway obstruction, J. Fam. Pract. **11**:310-315, 1980.
11. Bye, C.E., et al.: Effects of pseudoephedrine and tripolidine, alone and in combination, on symptoms of the common cold, Br. Med. J. **281**:189-190, 1980.
12. Cachin, Y., et al.: Nodal metastasis from carcinomas of the oropharynx, Otolaryngol. Clin. North Am. **12**:145-154, 1979.
13. Carpenter, R.J., DeSanto, L.W., and Devine, K.D.: Reconstruction after total laryngopharyngectomy, Arch. Otolaryngol. **105**:417-422, 1979.
14. Clemons, J.E., and Portilla, W.: Laryngeal abscess, Otolaryngol. Head Neck Surg. **87**:339-341, 1979.
15. Conservation surgery of the larynx (clinical conference), Clin. Bull. **10**:70-75, 1980.
16. *Corkery, C.M.: Nursing care study: removal of a child's tonsils and adenoids, Nurs. Times **75**:742-743, 1979.
17. *Daly, K.M.: Oral cancer, everyday concerns, Am. J. Nurs. **79**:1415-1417, 1979.
18. DeWeese, D.D., and Saunders, W.H.: Textbook of otolaryngology, ed. 5, St. Louis, 1977, The C.V. Mosby Co.
19. Dobie, R.A., and Tobey, D.N.: Clinical features of diphtheria in the respiratory tract, J.A.M.A. **242**:2197-2210, 1979.
20. *Dropkin, M.J.: Compliant behavior and changed body image, Am. J. Nurs. **79**:1249, 1979.
21. *Dupont, J.: Ambulatory nursing, EENT emergencies, Nurs. '79 **9**(11):65-70, 1979.
22. Elman, A.J., et al.: In situ carcinoma of the vocal cords, Cancer **43**:2422-2428, 1979.
23. *Ewing, D.: Electronic larynx for aphonic patients, Am. J. Nurs. **75**:2153-2157, 1975.
24. Ferlito, A., et al.: Therapeutic prospects in cancer of the larynx, J. Laryngol. Otol. **94**:405-410, 1980.
25. Fiumara, N.J.: Pharyngeal infection with Neisseria gonorrhoeae, Sex. Transm. Dis. **6**:264-266, 1979.
26. Gann, D.S.: Emergency management of the obstructed airway, J.A.M.A. **243**:1141-1142, 1980.
27. *Gannon, E.P.: Giving your patient meticulous mouth care, Nurs. '80 **10**(3):70-75, 1980.
28. *Gardner, M.E.: Notes from a waiting room, Am. J. Nurs. **80**:86-69, 1980.
29. Glazer, D.C.: Audiologic management of head and neck carcinoma patients, J. Speech Hear. Disord. **45**:216-222, 1980.
30. Goodman, W.S.: Septo-rhinoplasty: surgery of the nasal tip by external rhinoplasty, J. Laryngol. Otol. **94**:485-494, 1980.
31. Hall, I.S., and Colman, B.: Diseases of the nose, throat, and ear, New York, 1975, Churchill Livingstone, Inc.
32. Hintz, B., et al.: Randomized study of local control and survival following radical surgery or radiation therapy in oral and laryngeal carcinomas, J. Surg. Oncol. **12**:61-74, 1979.
33. Ho, L.: Primary meningioma of the nasal cavity and paranasal sinus, Cancer **46**:1442-1447, 1980.

---

*References preceded by an asterisk are particularly well suited for student reading.

34. Howard, J.C., et al.: Effectiveness of antihistamines in the symptomatic management of the common cold, J.A.M.A. **242**:2414-2417, 1979.

35. Hutchinson, R.: The common cold primer, Nurs. '79 **9**(3):57-61, 1979.

36. Hybels, R.L.: Selected new techniques of laryngeal surgery, Surg. Clin. North Am. **60**:637-647, 1980.

37. *Isler, C.: This technique may make tracheostomy unnecessary, RN **40**:32-33, 1977.

38. Johnson, J.T., Newman, R.K., and Olson, J.E.: Persistent hoarseness: an aggressive approach for early detection of laryngeal cancer, Postgrad. Med. **67**:122-126, 1980.

39. *Kerth, C.C.: Wound management following head and neck surgery, Nurs. Clin. North Am. **14**:761-778, 1979.

40. Key, G.: Stopping nosebleeds in the elderly: pressure, cautery, or packing? Geriatrics **36**:74-80, 1981.

41. Kraus, S.J.: Incidence and therapy of gonococcal pharyngitis, Sex. Transm. Dis. **6**:143-147, 1979.

42. Lin, Y.T., and Orking, L.R.: Arterial hypoxemia in patients with anterior and posterior nasal packings, Laryngoscope **89**:140-144, 1979.

43. Linscott, M.S., and Horton, W.C.: Management of upper airway obstruction, Otolaryngol. Clin. North Am. **12**:351-373, 1979.

44. Liston, S.L., and Siegel, L.G.: Nasal and sinus disorders in the elderly: which ones are life-threatening? Geriatrics **36**:91-102, 1981.

45. Lucente, F.E.: The dying patient in otolaryngology, Laryngoscope **83**:292-298, 1973.

46. Lucente, F.E.: Psychological problems in otolaryngology, Laryngoscope **83**:1684-1689, 1973.

47. Malasanos, L., et al.: Health assessment, ed. 2, St. Louis, 1981, The C.V. Mosby Co.

48. Masterson, A.: Larynx reconstruction, Nurs. '79 **9**(3):78-80, 1979.

49. McCaffrey, T.V., and Kern, E.B.: Clinical evaluation of nasal obstruction: a study of 1000 patients, Arch. Otolaryngol. **105**:542-545, 1979.

50. *McConnell, E.A.: How to truly help the patient with radical neck dissection, Nurse. '76 **6**:58-65, 1976.

51. Merenstein, J.H., and Rogers, K.D.: Streptococcal pharyngitis: early treatment and management by nurse practitioners, J.A.M.A. **227**:1278-1282, 1974.

52. Merland, J.J., et al.: Place of embolization in the treatment of severe epistaxis, Laryngoscope **90**:1694-1704, 1980.

53. Moore, J.C.: Establishment of an outpatient ENT clinic, A.O.R.N. J. **31**:620-626, 1980.

54. Morgenstern, K.M.: Experiences in middle turbinectomy, Laryngoscope **90**:1596-1603, 1980.

55. Newmann, R.K., and Johnson, J.T.: The diagnosis and treatment of acute sinusitis, Milit. Med. **145**:638-640, 1980.

56. Newmann, R.K., and Johnson, J.T.: Nasal airway obstruction: approach to diagnosis and treatment, Postgrad. Med. **68**:184-190, 1980.

57. *Nicholson, E.: Personal notes of a laryngectomee, Am. J. Nurs. **75**:2157-2158, 1975.

58. *Oser, J.: Oral cancer: coping with the changes, Am. J. Nurs. **79**:1418-1419, 1979.

59. Pearman, K.: Malignant melanoma of the nasal mucous membrane, J. Laryngol. Otol. **93**:1003-1009, 1979.

60. Peter, G.: Streptococcal pharyngitis, Compr. Ther. **5**:51-58, 1979.

61. *Pilgrim, M.C., and Sands, D.: Reconstructive nasal surgery, Am. J. Nurs. **73**:451-456, 1973.

62. *Price, J.: Oral health care for the geriatric patient, J. Geriatr. Nurs. **5**(2):25-29, 1979.

63. *Reeves, K.R.: Acute epiglottis, Am. J. Nurs. **71**:1539-1541, 1971.

64. Redstone, P.M., Bergstrom, L., and Dans, P.E.: The diagnosis and treatment of acute maxillary sinusitus, Colo. Med. **77**:407-408, 1977.

65. Richie, M.C., et al.: The role of embolization in the treatment of severe epistaxis, J. Neuroradiol. **6**:207-220, 1979.

66. Robbins, K.T., et al.: Non-healing granulomas of the nose, J. Otolaryngol. **9**:342-347, 1980.

67. Russ, J.E.: Management of osteosarcoma of maxilla and mandible, Am. J. Surg. **14**:572-576, 1980.

68. Sabiston, D.C., editor: Davis-Christopher's textbook of surgery, ed. 11, Philadelphia, 1977, W.B. Saunders Co.

69. Saunders, W.H., et al.: Nursing care in eye, ear, nose, and throat disorders, ed. 4, St. Louis, 1979, The C.V. Mosby Co.

70. Schaefer, S.D., and Hill, G.C.: Epidermoid carcinoma of the nasal vestibule: current treatment and evaluation, Laryngoscope **90**:1631-1635, 1980.

71. *Schwartz, S.L.: Carotid catastrophe, Am. J. Nurs. **79**:1566-1567, 1979.

72. *Schweiger, J.L.: Oral assessment, Am. J. Nurs. **80**:654-657, 1980.

73. *Sheehan, M.: Reflections of a cancer nurse, Ca. Nurs. **1**:309-311, 1978.

74. Steiner, W.: Techniques of diagnostic and operative endoscopy of the head and neck, Endoscopy **11**:51-59, 1979.

75. Stone, J.W.: External rhinoplasty, Laryngoscope **90**:1626-1630, 1980.

76. *Stuart, M.: Skin flaps and grafts after head and neck surgery, Am. J. Nurs. **78**:1368-1375, 1978.

77. Symposium on reconstruction of the larynx and trachea, Otolaryngol. Clin. North Am. **12**:735-917, 1979.

78. *Tierney, E.: Accepting disfigurement when death is the alternative, Am. J. Nurs. **75**:2149-2150, 1975.

79. *Trowbridge, J.: Caring for patients with facial or intraoral reconstruction, Am. J. Nurs. **73**:1930-1935, 1973.

80. *Trowbridge, J., and Williams, C.: Oral care of the patient having head and neck irradiation, Am. J. Nurs. **75**:2146-2149, 1975.

81. *Wadsworth, P.V., MacLachlan, M., and Saxby, M.: Tumors of the nose and accessory sinuses, Nurs. Times **75**:526-529, 1979.

82. Weissbluth, M.: Diagnosis and treatment of streptococcal infections of the throat, Compr. Ther. **6**:47-52, 1980.

83. Wills, P.I., and Russell, R.D.: Percutaneous embolization to control intractable epistaxis, Laryngoscope **89**:1385-1388, 1979.

84. *Wong, R.: Sore throat, Am. J. Nurs. **77**:1796-1798, 1977.

85. Yarington, C.T., Jr.: Sinusitis as an emergency, Otolaryngol. Clin. North Am. **12**:447-454, 1979.

86. Zapka, J., and Averill, B.W.: Self-care for colds: a cost-effective alternative to upper respiratory infection management, Am. J. Public Health **69**:814-816, 1979.

AUDIOVISUAL RESOURCES

The artificial larynx handbook, New York, 1978, Grune & Stratton, Inc. (Audiocassette, 30 min.)

Cancer of the larynx, Rochester, Minn., 1975, American Academay of Ophthamology and Otolaryngology. (Two videocassettes, each 57 min.)

Cancer of the larynx and hypopharynx, New York, 1971, American Cancer Society. (Film, 22 min.)

Challenges in nursing care of patients with head and neck cancer, New York, 1976, American Cancer Society. (Film, 20 min.)

Examination of the nose, Rochester, Minn., 1975, Audiovisual Center of the Mayo Clinic. (Videocassette, 12 min).

Foreign bodies of the nose, Philadelphia, 1980, Health Education Programs, Inc., University of Pennsylvania School of Medicine. (Videocassette, 20 min.)

The larynx, Atlanta, 1976, National Library of Medicine, National Medical Audiovisual Center. (Videocassette, 38 min.)

The otorhinolaryngologic examination, Fort Sam Houston, Tex, 1971, Brooke Army Medical Center. (Videotape, 27 min.)

A second voice, New York, 1967, American Cancer Society. (Film, 13 min.)

To speak again, New York, 1968, American Cancer Society. (Film, 19 min.)

Treatment of nosebleeds, Rochester, Minn., 1968, Audiovisual Center of the Mayo Clinic. (Film, 13 min.)

PATIENT INFORMATION

Helping words for the laryngectomee, International Association of Laryngectomees, 777 Third Ave., New York, NY 10017. (Brochure, 26 pages, free.)

Looking forward: a guidebook for the laryngectomee, Schmidt Printing Inc. 1416 Valley High Dr., Rochester, MN 55901. (Brochure, 56 pages, $1.25 plus postage and handling.)

CHAPTER 51

PROBLEMS OF THE LOWER AIRWAY

WILMA J. PHIPPS
BARBARA J. DALY

There are numerous diseases that affect the respiratory system. They include both acute (short-term) and chronic (long-term) diseases. Substantial changes in the relative incidence of diseases affecting the respiratory system have occurred in the past few decades. Although chronic infectious disorders such as tuberculosis, lung abscess, and bronchiectasis have decreased, persons with chronic bronchitis and emphysema now survive longer and constitute an increasing number of persons with chronic respiratory disease, along with those with environmental lung disease. In addition, modern intercontinental travel has increased the incidence of parasitic lung infestations in the Western world, and the reduction of immunologic competence that occurs in the treatment of persons with various malignancies and following organ transplantation has resulted in an increasing incidence of opportunistic infections of the lungs with a variety of microorganisms rarely pathogenic in the past.

The most significant pulmonary diseases are those that are chronic. It is estimated that there are nearly 50 million persons in the United States who have chronic respiratory conditions such as asthma, chronic bronchitis, emphysema, and chronic sinusitis. This number can be expected to increase yearly as the number of elderly persons in our society increases. Since most diseases of the respiratory tract are not reportable, the full extent of both acute and chronic illness is difficult to estimate. However, known facts about disability from chronic pulmonary diseases indicate that they are a major health problem and that they cause tremendous losses in the nation's productivity. Disability benefits reported by the Social Security Administration show that emphysema is the fourth most frequent condition for which disability claims are made. Disability benefits for emphysema and other chronic respiratory diseases were about $500 million in the 1970s and are expected to increase in the 1980s. Whereas mortality from tuberculosis has declined, mortality from bronchitis, emphysema, and cancer of the lung has continued to rise yearly.

The objectives of health education in relation to pulmonary diseases are the same as for other diseases. Prevention, early diagnosis, prompt and often continued treatment, limitation of disability, and rehabilitation should be emphasized for all persons. Early symptoms of respiratory diseases are probably those most often ignored by the general population. Perhaps this is because, with the exception of influenza and some types of pneumonia, respiratory diseases often develop slowly and progress without the individual's awareness. Nurses should encourage individuals and families to seek proper medical attention if they have symptoms such as cough, difficulty in breathing, production of sputum, shortness of breath, and nose and throat irritation that does not subside within 2 weeks. These symptoms are suggestive of respiratory disease and should be investigated.

In recent years many organizations, but most notably the American Lung Association (ALA) and the American Cancer Society (ACS), and the federal government have launched campaigns to reduce cigarette smoking in the United States. A major emphasis has been on preventing children and teenagers from beginning to smoke. These campaigns have been somewhat successful, and it is now estimated that only one third of the population in the United States smokes. However, the number of women smokers has increased, and this is reflected in the ever rising increase in morbidity and mortality from lung disease, especially cancer of the lung and chronic obstructive pulmonary diseases, among women.

Along with the campaign to decrease smoking there has been increased emphasis on reducing pollution in the environment, which has resulted in legislation such as the Clean Air Act. Some of the measures taken to reduce pollution are presently under threat, since they are believed by some to be too costly for the benefits achieved. This issue will be at the forefront during the 1980s, and nurses as health professionals and concerned citizens will need to keep themselves informed about proposed changes and their effects on health.

Nurses seeking current information about respiratory diseases and their treatment are referred to the ALA and its local branches for information.

The American Thoracic Society, the medical section of the ALA, publishes a journal* that is an excellent source of current information on all acute and chronic respiratory diseases. The ALA also publishes the *Bulletin*, many booklets and pamphlets, and newsletters that are useful to nurses in education of the public and in teaching patients.

RESTRICTIVE LUNG DISEASES

There are several ways to classify diseases of the lung, but one of the most helpful is to divide them into those that are restrictive and those that are obstructive.

In *restrictive lung disease* there is a restriction in lung volume and a reduction in compliance. As a result there is a reduction in total lung capacity (TLC), and vital capacity (VC) is less than the predicted normal capacity.[27] Diseases that restrict lung movement and inhibit the ability to inspire properly are considered restrictive disorders. A wide variety of factors can cause a reduction in TLC and VC. These include atelectasis; fluid or air in the pleural space; changes in the bony thorax, such as kyphoscoliosis; conditions that limit thoracic mobility, such as abdominal distention (from a tumor, ascites, or ileus) or splinting of the chest because of pain from high abdominal or thoracic incisions; neuromuscular diseases such as Guillain-Barré syndrome, poliomyelitis, or myasthenia gravis; CNS depression from drugs such as heroin or morphine; fibrotic diseases such as tuberculosis, pneumonconioses, or collagen diseases; space-occupying lesions such as cancer of the lung; and the adult respiratory distress syndrome.

In *obstructive lung disease* there is an increase in airway resistance resulting in prolonged exhalation. The most prominent examples of obstructive disease are chronic in nature and include chronic bronchitis, emphysema, and asthma.

---

*American Review of Respiratory Diseases, published by the American Lung Association, 1740 Broadway, New York, NY.

In this chapter, restrictive diseases are presented first beginning with infectious diseases. Obstructive lung diseases are discussed later in the chapter.

Infectious diseases of the pulmonary tract

For an infection of the lung to occur, pathogens must be able to enter the lower respiratory tract. This means that the defense mechanisms of the lung must be overcome in some manner. There are many lung defense mechanisms including upper airway defenses, lower respiratory tract clearance mechanisms, and intrapulmonary detoxification mechanisms. These mechanisms are outlined in the box on p. 1290.

Viral infections

Many respiratory diseases are probably caused by viral infections. Presently, over 30 have been found to be directly related to viral infections, and there are probably many more. Some diseases may be caused by one virus, or different viruses may cause the same symptoms.

If specific signs are not evident, the clinical illness is termed a common cold, viral infection, fever of unknown origin, or acute respiratory illness. The most common specific respiratory diseases caused by the various viruses are epidemic pleurodynia (Bornholm's disease), acute laryngotracheobronchitis, viral pneumonia, and influenza. Most adults have developed antibodies for the more common viruses, and most viral infections are relatively mild. However, they are frequently complicated by secondary bacterial infections. When new strains of the influenza virus develop, severe epidemics may ensue, and many people may die from secondary infections such as pneumonia.

Common cold

Epidemiology. Few persons escape having a "cold." The average among the general population is three colds per person each year.[140] Respiratory diseases, primarily virus infections, are responsible for 30% to 50% of time lost from work by adults and from 60% to 80% of time lost by children from school. The frequency of their occurrence, the number of people affected, the resulting economic loss, and the possibility that a cold may lead to more serious disease are reasons why colds merit serious attention.

Since persons with colds are rarely hospitalized, nurses will encounter them at work, in public places,

LUNG DEFENSE MECHANISMS*

I. Upper airway defenses against pulmonary infection
  A. Removing particulate matter from inspired air
    1. Particles greater than 20 μm settle back on surfaces
    2. Particles 5-10 μm deposited in nose
    3. Particles 0.1-10 μm remain suspended in air for long periods and are then inhaled
    4. Particles 1-5 μm deposited in tracheobronchial tree
       a. Droplet nuclei 2-4 μm (dried particles from sneezing, coughing, talking)
       b. May contain viruses or bacteria
       c. Spread organisms from person to person
  B. Minimizing the microbial population on membranes of upper respiratory tract
    1. Mucociliary transport
       a. Posterior two thirds of nasal cavity, sinuses, and nasopharynx lined by *ciliated epithelium* covered with thin layer of mucus
       b. Dense concentration of small blood vessels present beneath ciliated epithelium and mucous layers
       c. Mucus and fluid produced = 1000 ml/24 hr in normal persons
       d. Mucus and fluid carried at rate of 5-10 mm/min back into hypopharynx by beating action of cilia
       e. Substances in secretions inhibit microbial growth and prevent organisms from sticking to mucous membranes
          (1) Immunoglobulins (secretory IgA)
          (2) Lysozyme
          (3) Complement
  C. Minimizing possibility of aspiration
    1. Motor function of upper airway
       a. Laryngeal mechanism—closes glottis when swallowing to protect larynx
          (1) Gag reflex also closes glottis
          (2) Clearing throat, spitting, clears upper airway
    2. Contamination of lower respiratory tract
       a. Impaired clearance of particles in upper airway = spread of bacteria
       b. Accumulation of debris and microbes → penetration of tissues = sinusitis, otitis media
       c. Accumulation of debris and microbes → aspiration into trachea; lung abscess caused by anaerobic bacteria secondary to severe gingival disease
       d. Intoxication or distraction → aspiration
       e. Normal sleep → minor aspiration
       f. Aspiration of pharyngeal contents → lung → bacterial pneumonia

II. Lower respiratory tract clearance mechanisms
  A. Pulmonary reflex
    1. Cough—an involuntary reflex elicited by stimulation of irritant receptors in subepithelium of hypopharynx, larynx, and tracheobronchial tree: mediated by vagus nerve
       a. Facilitator of mucociliary clearance
       b. Aids in dealing with gross contamination from above larynx
    2. Bronchoconstriction—reflex response to airway irritants
       a. Decreased size of bronchus and forced expiration and cough propel debris toward mouth
       b. Excessive bronchoconstriction (asthma) = decreased expiratory airflow, air trapped in lung, effective cough difficult
  B. Mucociliary clearance
    1. Mucus secreted by epithelial gobler cells from submucosal glands 0.10-100 ml passes up trachea into hypopharynx and is swallowed; amount and nature of mucus secreted are controlled, in part, by parasympathetic nervous system affected by neurohumoral stimulation (adrenergic or cholinergic), and by direct mucosal irritation
    2. Cilia (200 cilia/each cell surface) beat rhythmically 1200 beats/min mouthward beginning at terminal bronchioles → larynx; beating of cilia → overlying mucous layer → mouthward at rate of 0.5 mm/min in small airways to about 10 mm/min in major bronchi
    3. Clearance increased by:
       a. Bronchodilator drugs
          1. β-Adrenergic agents (ephedrine) stimulate transport of water and salt into mucus = ↓ viscosity of mucus
          2. Methylxanthines (aminophylline)— ↑ mucous production and ciliary activity

---

*Adapted from Light, B.: Respiratory infections. In Kryger, M.H., editor: Pathophysiology of respiration, New York, 1981, John Wiley and Sons, Inc.

LUNG DEFENSE MECHANISMS—cont'd

4. Ciliary function depressed by:
   a. Chronic exposure to airway irritants—cigarette smoke and other irritants
   b. Pharmacologic agents—100% O_2, anticholinergic agents, alcohol
   c. Infection such as viral bronchitis
5. Mucous production increased by:
   a. Chronic irritation of respiratory tract → increase in number of mucus-secreting goblet cells = ↑ mucus
   b. Inflammatory response to irritation→ ↑ numbers of phagocytic cells and amount of cellular debris in mucus (especially DNA) = ↑ viscosity of mucus, which is less readily moved along by ciliary action
6. Immotile cilia—congenital impairment
   a. *Kartagener's syndrome*—sinusitis, recurrent lung infection and sinusitis
   b. *Cystic fibrosis*—infection, chronic inflammatory increases in respiratory mucous volume and viscosity = impaired lung clearance and progressive lung damage

III. Intrapulmonary detoxification mechanisms
   A. Phagocytes
      1. Alveolar macrophage
         a. Phagocytosis of particles—inhaled particulate debris, bacteria, or cell constituents
         b. Kills most microbes
      2. Polymorphonuclear neutrophil present in blood (normally only small number in lung)
         a. Avid phagocyte—kills microbes
         b. Defends against established infectious processes
         c. Infection—products of inflammation attract neutrophils to site of infection (chemotoaxis)
      3. Factors interfering with phagocytosis
         a. Inhibition of alveolar macrophage function
            (1) Cigarette smoke
            (2) Other inhaled pollutants—ozone, nitrogen dioxide, oxygen
            (3) Drugs—corticosteroids, antineoplastic and antiinflammatory cytoxic agents, and ethanol (alcohol)
            (4) Metabolic derangements—uremia, hyperglycemia of diabetes mellitus
            (5) Acquired granulocytopenia—bone marrow depression from cytotoxic drugs and other drugs
   B. Immunoglobulins
      a. IgG and IgA—most important for lung defense; present in secretions of respiratory tract as well as in blood
         (a) IgA antibodies—specific for viral antigens; neutralize viruses and prevent infection
         (b) IgG predominates in terminal lung units; antigen-specific IgG contributes to local defense against bacterial infections (important in neutralizing highly pathogenic encapsulated bacteria [especially *Streptococcus pneumoniae* and *Haemophilus influenzae*], which are resistant to phagocytosis)
   C. Cell-mediated immunity (CMI)
      1. One half of lymphocytes in and around airways are thymus-derived lymphocytes, or *T cells*
         (a) Found in lymphoid aggregates adjacent to bronchi (bronchus-associated lymphoid tissues, or BALT)
         (b) T cells important in:
            (1) Resistance to some viral infections
            (2) Resistance to most fungal infections
            (3) Infections by organisms that survive and multiply inside host cells: *Mycobacterium* tuberculosis, *Brucella*, *Listeria monocytogenes*, and *Pneumocystis carinii*
      2. Impaired CMI = ↑ susceptibility to infection
         (a) Deficient T cell function (anergy) associated with:
            (1) Neoplasms—lymphoma
            (2) Cytotoxic or corticosteroid therapy
            (3) Systemic diseases—sarcoidosis, malnutrition
         (b) Some lung infections occur almost exclusively in severely impaired CMI—pneumonia caused by cytomegalovirus, herpes zoster, *Aspergillus* species, or *Pneumocystis carinii*

or in their homes. It is important to note the symptoms at the onset of the cold. Many other more serious diseases begin with a cold or with symptoms resembling those of the common cold. Because a cold is considered a minor but bothersome condition and because the person has possibly had many colds, the person, rather than a physician, makes the diagnosis. Helping persons to realize the importance of an illness that may appear slight but that may have serious consequences is an integral part of the nurse's role.

Etiology. Although the specific agent causing the common cold is unknown, it can be stated that it is a syndrome that is produced by a variety of viral infections. Viral studies do not yield the causative agent, nor is there usually any immunologic evidence of infection.

Prevention. The common cold is a communicable disease spread by droplet nuclei. The only known way to prevent spread of a cold from one individual to another is to isolate the infected person, and this is extremely difficult in our society. However, there are measures that help to prevent the development of a cold, its complications, and transfer to other persons. Good general hygiene, adequate rest, adequate diet, sufficient exercise, and fresh air presumably help maintain resistance to colds. Most persons can go through the usual course of a common cold without difficulty if they obtain enough rest.

There are several ways to minimize the spread of infection. Crowded places such as theaters should be avoided by persons with colds. The individual should particularly avoid contact with, and therefore exposing, infants and young children, persons who have chronic lung diseases such as bronchitis and emphysema, those who have recently had an anesthetic, and elderly people. Covering the nose and mouth when sneezing and coughing prevents the contamination of the air breathed by others. Frequent washing of hands, covering of coughs and sneezes, and careful disposal of waste tissues are protective health measures that are advisable for everyone, but they become increasingly important when known respiratory tract infection exists. Since the common cold is a communicable disease, the principles for protection of oneself as well as others should be practiced.

Clinical picture. Symptoms of a cold usually appear suddenly, and the infection may be full-blown within 48 hours. The acute inflammation usually begins in the pharynx, and there is a sensation of dryness or soreness of the throat. This is followed by nasal discharge and frequent sneezing. The eyes may water, the voice may become husky, breathing may be obstructed, and ability to smell and taste may diminish. Often a cough develops, and it may produce sputum.

The person with a cold may have various complaints. Lethargy and vague, aching pains in the back and limbs may be experienced. Most adults are afe-brile, but those with a tendency toward developing complications, such as persons with chronic illness and lowered resistance, may have a temperature elevation. The course of the cold is variable, but ordinarily it lasts from 7 to 14 days. It is difficult to determine when the cold ends and when complications appear. Laryngitis and tracheitis may be part of the cold, while tracheobronchitis is a complication usually caused by secondary bacterial infection. Acute sinusitis and otitis media may also follow the common cold.

Intervention. All treatment of colds is directed toward relief of symptoms and control of complications. If the person has an elevated temperature and complains of headache and muscular aching, the advice of a physician should be sought. Acetylsalicylic acid may be prescribed for mild aches and discomfort. Salicylates, however, do not influence the course of the common cold and lack specific action in this disorder.

If the patient has *nasal congestion*, the physician may recommend nose drops. Ephedrine, 0.5% to 2% aqueous solution, with isotonic sodium chloride solution, is used frequently. (See p. 1263 for method of administration.) This medication shrinks swollen nasal tissues and allows for free passage of air. Many physicians advise against the use of nose drops, maintaining that constriction of blood supply to the tissues lowers resistance. In general, oily solutions are not recommended because of the danger of inhaling oil droplets, which might cause lipid pneumonia. Nasal sprays containing antihistamine may be ordered. They should be given with the person sitting upright. The nurse should emphasize to patients and their families the importance of using only prescribed solutions and only those that are fresh, since old solutions frequently become more concentrated. Nose drops should be prescribed by a physician, and only the specified amount should be used; excessive use may aggravate symptoms. Many persons prefer a medicated nasal inhaler, since it can be carried easily in a pocket and is more pleasant to use. Benzedrex containing propylhexedrine is one that is widely used. Propylhexedrine is a volatile drug with a minimal stimulating effect on the central nervous system.[49] Soft disposable paper tissues should help to prevent dryness, redness, and irritation about the nose. Some dryness can be prevented by treating the skin early with mild, soothing creams such as cold cream.

The *dryness, cough,* and *"tickling sensation"* in the throat so often associated with a cold can be relieved in a variety of ways. There are many cough drops and lozenges on the market. Lozenges relieve irritation and are pleasant to use. Persons should be advised not to use them just before dozing off to sleep, since they may be accidentally aspirated into the trachea during sleep. A mixture of honey and lemon may be preferred to cough medications by some persons. This mixture increases mucous secretions and thereby softens exudate and facilitates its expectoration. It also relieves dryness that predisposes to coughing. Some people report that undiluted lemon or orange juice is helpful. A section of the fruit with the rind may be placed at the bedside for easy accessibility during the night. Hot fluids often relieve coughing. The person may be advised to keep a small vacuum bottle of hot water or other liquid at the bedside. If cough medication has been taken, it should not be followed by water because the effect will be dissipated. If the cough associated with a common cold persists or does not yield to the simple home remedies mentioned or to specific medication that may have been ordered, the patient should be urged to consult the physician.

Acute bronchitis

Etiology and epidemiology. Bronchitis can be acute or chronic. Acute bronchitis is an inflammation of the bronchi and sometimes the trachea (tracheobronchitis). It is often caused by an extension of an upper respiratory tract infection such as the common cold and is therefore communicable. It also may be caused by physical or chemical agents such as dust, smoke, or volatile fumes. As air pollution increases, the incidence of acute bronchitis increases.

Clinical picture. The person with acute bronchitis usually complains of chilliness, malaise, muscular aches, headaches, a dry, scratchy throat, hoarseness, and a cough. The temperature may be elevated and the person may be confined to bed at home or in the hospital. In either case, exposure to others should be kept to a minimum. Early in the disease the complaints are the dry, irritating cough and the feeling of tightness and soreness in the chest that follows coughing.

Intervention. The person may obtain relief by the same means as those described for the common cold. Cough may be relieved by cough mixtures or aerosol medications. Humidifying the air eases breathing and lessens irritation. Tincture of benzoin, menthol, or oil of eucalyptus may be ordered for the steam vaporizer for its soothing and aromatic effect. As the disease progresses, secretions usually increase. Congestion and dryness of the bronchial mucous membrane are then relieved.

Treatment of acute tracheobronchitis is usually conservative in an attempt to prevent extension of infection to the smaller bronchi, the bronchioles, and the alveoli of the lungs. Measures that maintain good drainage of tracheobronchial secretions are prescribed. (See details in discussion on chronic obstructive pulmonary disease, p. 1320.) The patient should be protected from chilling and should take from 3 to 4 L of fluid daily. A simple bland diet is usually most easily eaten. Antibiotics are commonly prescribed for an elevation in temperature.

Most persons need a period of convalescence following an attack of acute bronchitis because of weakness and fatigue. The person should not return to work without medical approval. Extra rest, a well-balanced diet, and avoiding exposure to further infection are recommended. Chronic bronchitis is discussed later in this chapter.

Bacterial infections

Pneumonia

Epidemiology. Acute pneumonias are responsible for 10% of hospital admissions in the United States.[143] Pneumonia can occur in any season but is most common during winter and early spring. Persons of any age are susceptible, but pneumonia is more common among infants and the elderly. Pneumonia is often caused by aspiration of infected materials into the distal bronchioles and alveoli. Certain individuals are especially susceptible. This includes persons whose normal respiratory defense mechanisms are damaged or altered (those with chronic obstructive pulmonary disease, influenza, and tracheostomy, and those who have recently had anesthesia); persons who have a disease affecting antibody response (those with multiple myeloma, hypogammaglobulinemia, and so on); and alcoholics in whom there is increased danger of aspiration and persons with delayed white blood cell response to infection. Increasingly, nosocomial pneumonia (acquired in the hospital) is a cause of morbidity and mortality. This is the direct result of an increase in the number of patients with impaired defenses resulting from certain types of therapy and of an increase in the number of patients whose lives are being prolonged with life support therapy.[41]

Etiology. Pneumonia is a communicable disease; the mode of transmission is dependent on the infecting organism. Pneumonia is classified according to the offending organism rather than the anatomic location (lobar or bronchial) as was the practice in the past. A recent classification of pneumonia in adults is presented in the box on p. 1294.

Typical or classic pneumonia

EPIDEMIOLOGY. Typical or classic pneumonia occurs in both males and females of any age. It is found both in persons without underlying disease and in those with diminished defense mechanisms. Commonly, there is a history of alcoholism, recent respiratory tract infection, or viral influenza.[41]

CLINICAL PICTURE. The person with typical pneumonia has the classic signs and symptoms found in the historical descriptions of pneumonia. The onset is usually sudden with a shaking chill, fever (39° to 40° C), pleuritic chest pain, and a productive cough. Sputum is greenish and purulent and may be blood tinged giving the typical "rusty" sputum.

Respirations are rapid and shallow and may be described as "grunting" because of the sound the patient

ORGANISMS CAUSING INFECTIOUS PNEUMONIA IN ADULTS*

I. Typical or classic pneumonia syndrome
A. Bacterial pneumonia
1. Common
a. *Streptococcus pneumoniae*
2. Uncommon
a. *Haemophilus influenzae*
b. *Staphylococcus aureus*

II. Atypical pneumonia syndrome
A. Common
1. *Mycoplasma pneumoniae*
B. Uncommon
1. *Legionella pneumophila*

III. Aspiration pneumonia syndrome
A. Hospitalized, debilitated, or antibiotic-treated patients
1. Mixed anaerobic/aerobic pharyngeal flora
2. *Staphylococcus aureus*
3. *Klebsiella pneumoniae*
4. *Pseudomonas aeruginosa*
5. *Serratia marcescens*
6. *Acinetobacter* species
7. Enteric gram-negative aerobes (*Eschercichia coli, Enterobacter, Proteus*)
B. Outpatients with normal pharyngeal flora
1. Mixed anerobic/aerobic pharyngeal flora

IV. Hematogenous pneumonia syndromes
A. *Staphylococcus aureus*
B. *Escherichia coli*
C. Enteric/pelvic anaerobes

*From Frame, P.T.: Basics RD **10**:1-8, 1982.

makes at the end of each breath. Close observation of the chest may show that the patient is restricting motion of the chest on the affected side in an attempt to reduce pain, which is often severe. The patient may exhibit nasal flaring, intercostal rib retraction, and use of accessory muscles. Cyanosis may be present.

Fine crackling inspiratory rales are heard early in the disease; later, as consolidation occurs in the lung, percussion elicits a dullness of sound. Bronchial breath sounds and egophony (p. 1217) are present. A chest roentgenogram showing lobar consolidation is most common with pneumococcal or *Klebsiella* infections. Multiple infiltrates are more common with *Staphylococcus* and *Haemophilus* infections.[41]

About 60% of persons with pneumococcal pneumonia have some degree of pleural effusion. Empyema may also occur in some patients with pneumonia.[41]

Other findings include a leukocyte count of usually over 15,000 bacteremia (in about 25% of patients), and hypoxia and hypocarbia.

INTERVENTION. Since the treatment and prognosis of pneumonia depend on the causative organism, sputum smears are examined and cultures obtained *before* administration of an antibiotic is started. Blood cultures may also be drawn. If antibiotic therapy is begun before cultures can be collected, it may be impossible to grow the causative organism. Diagnosis is confirmed by roentgenographic examination and by positive blood cultures.

Bacterial pneumonia is treated with antibiotics that are ordered by the physician based on the sputum or blood culture and sensitivity tests.

Table 51-1 lists the antibiotic therapy currently employed in treating pneumonia. Response to therapy usually occurs within 24 to 48 hours, the temperature decreases, and the pulse rate returns to normal. During the period of hyperthermia, the person requires rest, fluids, mouth care, and control of environmental factors similar to those of any person with a fever.

Hypoventilation results from decreased chest expansion caused by chest pain and secretions that block passage of oxygen in the airway, or exudations that fill the alveoli. The surface area available for gas exchange becomes decreased. Many patients are less dyspneic and more comfortable with supplemental oxygen. If arterial blood gas studies reveal a PO_2 less than 60 mm Hg, oxygen should be given by mask or nasal cannula.[41] Low-flow oxygen is used with caution if the pneumonia is superimposed on chronic obstructive pulmonary disease (p. 1325). Strict isolation precautions should be used for the patient with staphylococcal pneumonia. For other forms of pneumonia, isolation is not required; however, strict adherence to hand-washing techniques should be mandatory. Hand washing is the most important measure in preventing spread of pneumonia from one patient to another via the hands of hospital personnel.

Chest expansion should be encouraged to increase ventilation through deep-breathing exercises. Analgesics may be ordered for chest pain that restricts deep breathing. Narcotics inhibit the cough reflex but may be required if pain is severe; codeine is less likely to inhibit productive coughing than are stronger narcotics. The person with severe chest pain often requires help and encouragement to move about in bed and to cough productively in order to mobilize and expectorate the secretions. Measures to splint the chest (p. 1252) may be helpful. The person is encouraged to cough *deeply* to produce sputum from the lungs and not expend needless energy in raising secretions from the upper trachea and posterior pharynx only.

Atypical pneumonia

ETIOLOGY AND EPIDEMIOLOGY. The most common form of atypical pneumonia in adults is caused by *Mycoplasma pneumoniae*. *Legionella pneumophila* is an uncommon cause of atypical pneumonia. It occurs more commonly in older adults and in persons who smoke or

TABLE 51-1. Initial antibiotic therapy for pneumonia in adults*

Infective agent	Drug(s) of choice	Other effective drugs	Infective agent	Drug(s) of choice	Other effective drugs
Classic syndromes			**Atypical syndromes**		
Streptococcus pneumoniae, uncomplicated	Penicillin G procaine, 300,000 units IM q 8 hr; aqueous crystalline penicillin G, 400,000 units IV q 6 hr; penicillin V, 250 mg PO q 6 hr	Erythromycin, clindamycin, cephalosporins, other penicillins, trimethoprim with sulfamethoxazole	*Mycoplasma pneumoniae* *Legionella pneumophila*	Erythromycin, 500 mg q 6 hr Erythromycin, 500-1000 mg q 6 hr	Tetracycline Rifampin, gentamicin (?), tetracycline(?)
			Aspiration syndromes		
			Mixed anaerobic/aerobic pharyngeal flora, uncomplicated	Penicillin G, 1 million units IV q 4-6 hr	Clindamycin, cefoxitin (?)
Streptococcus pneumoniae, complicated (empyema, metastatic infection)	Penicillin G, 3-4 million units IV q 4-6 hr		Mixed anaerobic/aerobic with empyema or abscess	Penicillin G, 3-4 million units IV q 4-6 hr	
Haemophilus influenzae	Ampicillin, 1-2 g IV q 4-6 hr	Chloramphenicol, cefamandole, trimethoprim with sulfamethoxazole	Anaerobic with suspected gram-negative aerobe	Penicillin G, as above, plus gentamicin or tobramycin	Clindamycin plus gentamicin or tobramycin
Staphylococcus aureus	Nafcillin, 1.5 g IV q 4 hr	Methicillin, oxacillin, cefazolin, cephalothin, vancomycin, clindamycin	Anaerobic with *Staphylococcus aureus*	Clindamycin, 600 mg IV q 6 hr	
			Hematogenous syndromes		
			Staphylococcus aureus	Nafcillin as above	
Staphylococcus aureus (methicillin resistant)	Vancomycin, 1 g IV q 12 hr		*Escherichia coli*	Ampicillin, 1.5 g IV q 4 hr, plus gentamicin or tobramycin	
Klebsiella pneumoniae	Cefazolin, 1 g IV q 6 hr, plus gentamicin or tobramycin, 1.7 mg/kg/8 hr		Septic emboli from pelvic or enteric source	Clindamycin, 600 mg IV q 6 hr, plus gentamicin or tobramycin	

*Adapted from Frame, P.T.: Basics RD **10**:1-8, 1982.

have abnormal pulmonary defenses.[41] *Legionella pneumophila* is the agent causing Legionnaires' disease (legionellosis). It is three times more common in men than in women. A number of conditions are felt to predispose one to legionellosis. These include chronic renal disease, chronic bronchitis or emphysema, diabetes, cancer, immunosuppressive medications, and smoking. It is currently estimated that about 25,000 cases of Legionnaires' disease occur each year.[105]

Both epidemics and sporadic cases of Legionnaires' disease occur. Epidemics have been associated with common source exposures such as air-conditioning water-cooling towers, and excavation sites. *Legionella pneumophila* has been isolated from soil and fresh water and from shower heads in hospitals.[22]

CLINICAL PICTURE. The onset of atypical pneumonia is gradual (over 3 to 4 days), and malaise, headache, sore throat, and dry cough are present. Pleuritis is not common, but patients complain of chest wall soreness from coughing. Respiratory distress is not common with *Mycoplasma pneumoniae* but is common with legionellosis. Patients with *Legionella* infections may also have abdominal pain and diarrhea. Some are markedly confused. A temperature elevation of 40° C or greater is common. Shaking chills are common with legionellosis but are rare with myocoplasma infection.[41]

Fine inspiratory rales may be present, but there is no evidence of consolidation. A roentgenogram of the chest shows patchy segmental infiltrates, which may progress from unilateral to bilateral. Pleural effusion is uncommon. Patients with legionellosis may have renal failure, hyponatremia, hypophosphatemia, and an elevation of creatine phosphokinase.

INTERVENTION. The usual treatment for both *Mycoplasma pneumoniae* and *Legionella pneumophila* is erythromycin (Table 51-1). If a patient is seriously ill with Legionnaires' disease, rifampin may be added to the treatment with erythromycin. Rifampin should never be used alone because of the high likelihood of resistant organisms developing during monotherapy. Because relapses have occurred within 1 to 2 weeks of therapy, it is recommended that treatment for legionellosis be continued for 3 weeks.

The overall mortality of Legionnaires' disease is almost 15%. Most of this is attributed to respiratory failure.

When mycoplasma pneumonia is untreated, the fever and malaise generally resolve in 1 to 2 weeks. Serious systemic complications are quite rare, although hemolytic anemia, disseminated intravascular coagulation (DIC), thrombocytopenic purpura and renal failure, myocarditis and pericarditis, meningoencephalitis and other neurologic syndromes, arthritis, and hepatitis have been reported.[76] The mortality for mycoplasma pneumonia is less than 1%.[41]

Aspiration pneumonia

ETIOLOGY. The common factor in all forms of aspiration pneumonia is the aspiration of material into the airways. There are three major clinical syndromes that may follow aspiration. The first two are not infectious but are discussed here because they cause a pneumonia and they can result in a bacterial superinfection. The *first noninfectious aspiration pneumonia* is caused by aspiration of gastric acid; only a small quantity of gastric acid will cause severe respiratory distress within a few seconds of aspiration. If a bacterial superinfection occurs, it usually does not become evident for 48 to 72 hours.[41]

The *second noninfectious aspiration pneumonia* results from the aspiration of large quantities of inert substances such as water, barium, tube-feeding liquids, and nonacid gastric contents.[41] These substances cause little chemical injury, but they obstruct the airways causing respiratory distress. A secondary infection may occur in the segments of the lung that have obstructed airways.[41] In both of these noninfectious aspiration syndromes, the aspiration is either witnessed or known to have occurred because of coughing or the suctioning of foreign material from the lungs.

Bacterial aspiration pneumonia is the third syndrome. It occurs in patients who have a disorder of consciousness, such as anesthesia, coma, seizures, or excessive alcoholism.[41] It also occurs in patients with poor cough mechanisms such as those resulting from laryngeal dysfunction or respiratory muscle paralysis.[41] In these patients the mixed anerobic and aerobic flora of the upper respiratory tract is the most common cause of pneumonia.[41]

If *Streptococcus pneumoniae* or *Staphylococcus aureas* is present in the pharyngeal aspirate, classic pneumococcal or staphylococcal pneumonia may develop. If the pharynx has been colonized with any of the other organisms listed on p. 1294, then these organisms may be primary pathogens in their own right or may cause a synergistic infection with the *Streptococcus pneumoniae* or *Staphylococcus aureus*.[41]

CLINICAL PICTURE. In a mixed anaerobic aspiration pneumonia, the clinical course is mild and gradual in the early stages. There is cough and low-grade fever over several days or weeks, slowly progressing to expectoration of large amounts of foul-smelling sputum.[19] The chest film reveals pneumonitis in dependent portions of the lung. The lateral segments of the upper lobes are dependent in the lateral decubitus position, and the superior segments of the lower lobes are dependent in the supine position. Later, abscess formation occurs in these segments of the lung and empyema is not uncommon.[41]

When aspiration pneumonia is acquired in the hospital it may be insidious in onset, and the only early symptoms may be an unexplained fever and mild tachypnea. If the involved organisms are staphylococcal or gram-negative pathogens, the patient's condition can take a rapid downhill course accompanied by bacteremia and septic shock.[41]

INTERVENTION. Treatment will be symptomatic and will include the measures discussed under classic pneumonia (p. 1295). If bacterial infection is present, some of the drugs outlined in Table 51-1 will be prescribed.

Hematogenous pneumonia

ETIOLOGY. Bacterial infections of the lung can also occur when pathogenic organisms are spread to the lungs via the bloodstream. *Staphylococcus aureus* and *Escherichia coli* are the most commonly involved agents in hematogenous pneumonia. Most often the patient has an endovascular focus of infection (infected intravascular catheter, endocarditis, or intravenous drug abuse). *Escherichia coli* pneumonia is seen in patients with deep-seated *Escherichia coli* infections, such as intraabdominal abscess, pyonephrosis, or empyema of the gallbladder.[100]

CLINICAL PICTURE. The pulmonary symptoms of hematogenous pneumonia are minimal compared with the symptoms of the septicemia.[42] Nonproductive cough and pleuritic chest pain similar to that seen with pulmonary embolism are the most common complaints.[41] There may be multiple infiltrates throughout the lung, and central areas of cavitation may develop because of pulmonary infarction.

INTERVENTION. The antibiotic therapy will depend on the organism involved and the appropriate antibiotics are listed in Table 51-3. The other measures discussed under intervention for patients with classic pneumonia are also indicated for patients with this form of pneumonia.

Prevention of influenza and pneumonia. Two vaccines are now available to prevent respiratory infections: influenza vaccine and pneumococcal vaccine. *In-*

fluenza vaccine should be given yearly to all persons at high risk of developing complications of influenza (pneumonia). The vaccine is recommended for all persons with chronic heart or lung disease unless they are allergic to eggs or egg products or had a previous reaction to the vaccine. It is also recommended for all persons age 65 or older since they are at high risk of developing complications of influenza.

Pneumonia polysaccharide vaccine is recommended for the same persons who receive influenza vaccine. The vaccine should not be given more often than every 3 to 5 years.[41]

The other major preventive measure is strict adherence to hand washing as discussed previously. In addition, attention needs to be paid to reducing the likelihood of gram-negative colonization of patients. For this reason, many hospitals have instituted tighter control policies on the use of antibiotics except in situations where they are strictly necessary. A reduction in this use of antibiotics also reduces the incidence of antibiotic-resistant hospital flora, which are the source of many nosocomial infections (see Chapter 22).

Complications of pneumonia. With the advent of antibiotics and better diagnostic measures such as x-ray procedures, complications during or following pneumonia are rare in otherwise healthy persons. Atelectasis, delayed resolution, lung abscess, pleural effusion, empyema, pericarditis, meningitis, and relapse are complications that were common in the past. The fact that pneumonia and influenza rank fifth as a cause of death in the United States is an impressive reason for strict adherence to the prescribed medical treatment. Careful and accurate observation as well as sufficient time for convalescence will also help to ensure the average patient a smooth recovery. Aged persons and those with a chronic illness are likely to have a relatively long course of convalescence from pneumonia, and there is a greater possibility of their developing complications. There has been an increase in the incidence of staphylococcal pneumonia subsequent to influenza. Consolidation of lung tissue, pleural effusion, and empyema frequently occur soon after the onset of this type of pneumonia and may cause death.

Tuberculosis

Epidemiology. In 1900 tuberculosis was the leading cause of death in the United States. It remained a major cause of death until the introduction of antituberculosis drug therapy in the late 1940s and early 1050s. The most effective of these agents is isoniazid, which first became available clinically in 1952. The use of isoniazid in combination with two agents introduced earlier, streptomycin and para-aminosalicylic acid, resulted in a striking decrease in tuberculosis death rates. It also made it possible for patients with tuberculosis to be treated on an outpatient basis. However, some pa-

tients still have to be hospitalized at some time in their illness, and most nurses will care for a patient with tuberculosis at some time in their careers. At one time patients with tuberculosis were hospitalized in specialized hospitals called sanitoria. Today these sanatoria are being used for patients with other illnesses, and the patient with tuberculosis is being admitted to the general hospital. Because many persons in our society, including medical personnel, are afraid of tuberculosis, it is important that nurses learn as much as possible about the disease so that they can give effective care to the person with tuberculosis. Unfortunately, some persons still associate tuberculosis with lack of cleanliness and careless living. This may make both the individual and the family unwilling to speak openly about the disease, making treatment of the disease difficult.

Although tuberculosis is now considered a preventable and curable disease, it still is a disease requiring public health attention. In 1980 there were 27,749 cases of tuberculosis reported to the CDC. This represented an increase of 0.3% from 1979. These new cases were not evenly distributed throughout the population, however, and some differences bear mentioning.

In the past few years the greatest numbers of tuberculosis cases have been found in the counties with the largest populations, especially when the county encompasses a major city. Nearly one half of the tuberculosis cases are found in cities (Fig. 51-1), and rates are highest in the largest metropolitan areas.[123] Other regions where the case rates are higher than the average are counties close to the Mexican border and a few areas where there is a large population of American Indians. Persons of Hispanic origin accounted for about 12% of the new cases reported in 1980. Tuberculosis rates are also higher than the average in areas of the United States where there are large numbers of immigrants from countries where tuberculosis is far more prevalent than in the United States. For example, in Hawaii, which had the highest case rate in the United States in 1976, a large portion of the new cases are among persons who have lived in Hawaii for 1 year or less. Indochinese refugees accounted for approximately 7.8% of the reported cases for 1980.[25] Other places where similar situations are reported are San Francisco, Dade county, Florida, and Boston. Canada reports a similar finding. These figures point out that with a few exceptions most countries of the world have much higher tuberculosis morbidity and mortality than does the United States. In general, Latin America, Africa, Asia, and Oceania have considerably higher case rates than do the United States and the English-speaking and Western European countries. Thus Americans residing for prolonged periods of time in countries where the tuberculosis rates are very high run an increased risk of becoming infected with tubercle bacilli.

As had been true for several years the new active

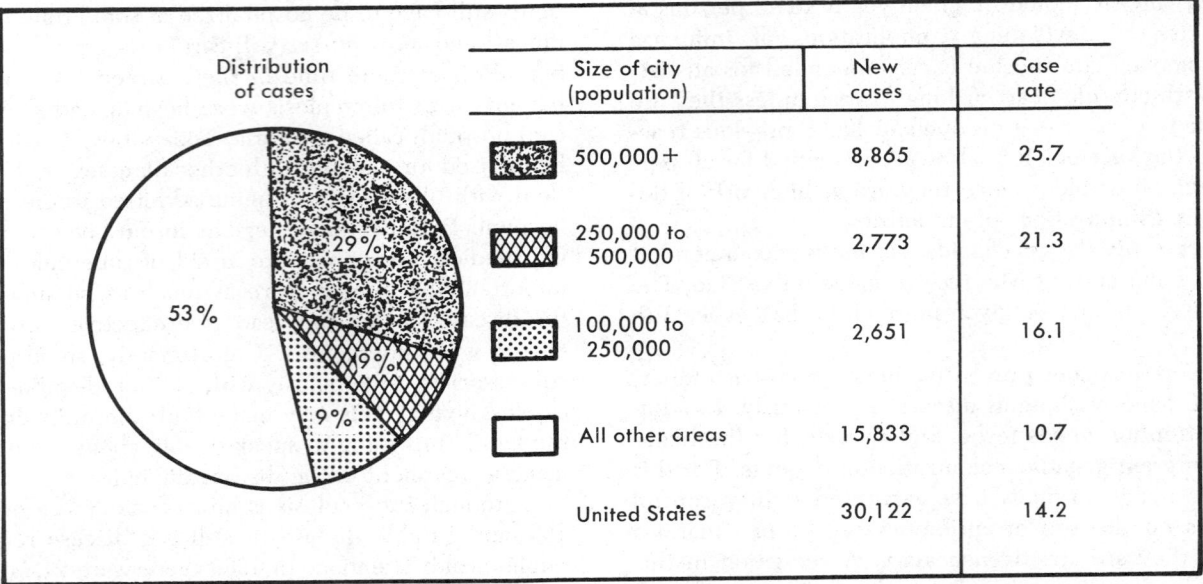

Fig. 51-1. Tuberculosis cases in large cities of United States in 1974. (From Department of Health, Education, and Welfare, Public Health Service: Tuberculosis in the United States, Atlanta, 1976, Center for Disease Control.)

case rate for men is double that for women (Fig. 51-2). Almost half of all new active cases occurred among white men. In both white men and white women the greatest number of cases are found in those age 65 and over (Fig. 51-3). In other races the greatest number of cases also occur in men age 65 and over and in women between age 25 and 44 and over age 65. The case rates for children under age 5 and those age 5 to 14 have shown a decline every year since 1964.

As was pointed out earlier, there has been a steady decline in deaths caused by tuberculosis in the United States since the introduction of effective chemotherapeutic agents. Today the tuberculosis death rate is around 2/100,000 people. However, the tuberculosis death rate for males is more than double that for females, and the death rate for nonwhites is three times that for the white population.

In an attempt to eliminate tuberculosis from the United States, concerted efforts must be made to prevent persons from becoming infected with the tubercle bacillus. Measures to do this are discussed under prevention on p. 1301.

Etiology. Tuberculosis is caused by a bacillus, the *Mycobacterium tuberculosis*, or tubercle bacillus, a gram-positive and acid-fast organism. If microscopic study of a slide prepared from the sputum of an individual reveals tubercle bacilli, the individual is said to have positive sputum, and this confirms the diagnosis of tuberculosis. Some persons with tuberculosis will not have positive sputum on smear, however, and a positive spu-

tum culture will be necessary to confirm the diagnosis. Patients who have a positive culture and negative smear are less infectious than are those with both a positive smear and culture.

When a person with tuberculosis speaks, coughs, sneezes, or sings, minute droplets fall to the ground, while the smaller ones evaporate, leaving *droplet nuclei* that remain suspended indefinitely in the air and are carried on air currents. Droplet nuclei are 1 to 10 μm in size and are small enough to be inhaled into the alveoli. Thus it is by inhalation of tubercle-laden droplet nuclei that tuberculosis is transmitted.

Pathophysiology. When an individual with no previous exposure to tuberculosis (negative tuberculin reactor) inhales a sufficient number of tubercle bacilli into the alveoli, tuberculosis *infection* occurs. The body's reaction to the tubercle bacilli depends on the susceptibility of the individual, the size of the dose, and the virulence of the organisms. Inflammation occurs within the alveoli (parenchyma) of the lungs, and natural body defenses attempt to counteract the infection. Lymph nodes in the hilar region of the lung may be involved as they filter drainage from the infected site. The inflammatory process and cellular reaction produce a small, firm, white nodule called the *primary tubercle*. The center of the nodule contains tubercle bacilli. Cells gather around the center, and usually the outer portion becomes fibrosed. Thus blood vessels are compressed, nutrition of the tubercle is interfered with, and necrosis occurs at the center. The area becomes walled off by

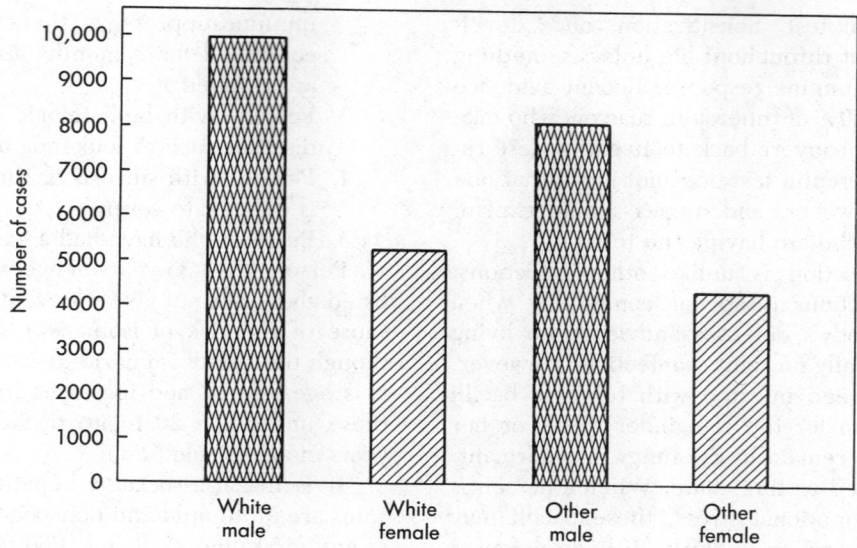

Fig. 51-2. Tuberculosis case rates by race and sex in the United States, 1980. (From Centers for Disease Control: Annual summary 1980: reported morbidity and mortality in the United States, Morbid. Mortal. Weekly Rep. **29**:54, 1981.)

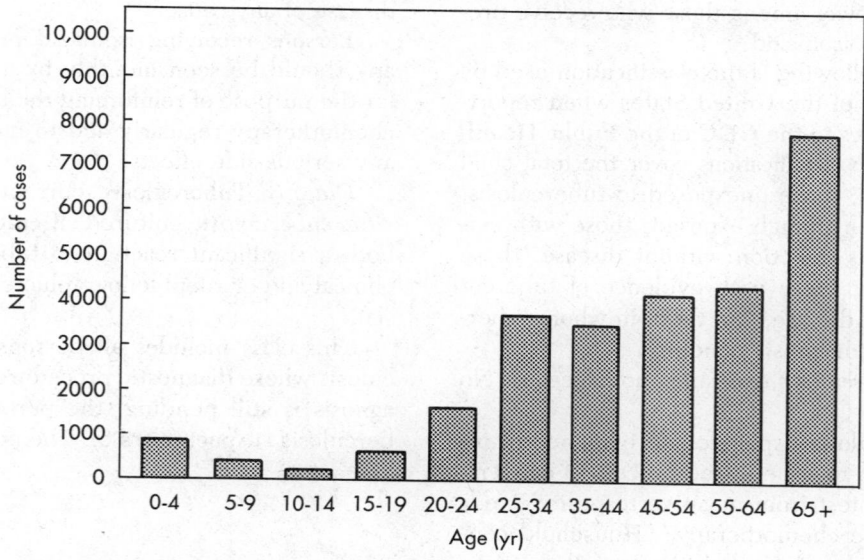

Fig. 51-3. Tuberculosis case rates by age in the United States, 1980. (From Centers for Disease Control: Annual summary 1980: reported morbidity and mortality in the United States, Morbid. Mortal. Weekly Rep. **29**:54, 1981.)

fibrotic tissue around the outside, and the center gradually becomes soft and cheesy in consistency. This latter process is known as *caseation*. This material may become calcified (calcium deposits), or it may liquefy and is known as *liquefaction necrosis*. The liquefied material may be coughed up, leaving a *cavity* or hole in the parenchyma of the lung. The cavity or cavities are visible on chest x-ray films and result in the diagnosis of *cavitary* disease. Most individuals who are ex-

posed to tuberculosis and develop a tuberculosis infection (confirmed by a positive tuberculin test) do not develop an active case of tuberculosis. The only x-ray evidence of their tuberculosis infection is a calcified nodule known as the *Ghon tubercle*. The evidence on x-ray film of enlarged hilar lymph nodes and a Ghon tubercle is sometimes referred to as the *primary complex*.

Persons who have been exposed to the tubercle bacillus become sensitized to it, and this is confirmed by a positive tuberculin test. Sensitization, once developed, usually remains throughout life unless something interferes with the immune response. Recent evidence suggests that about 50% of tuberculin reactors who take isoniazid for 1 year convert back to negative test results. A positive tuberculin test does not mean that one has tuberculosis, however, and nurses should explain this fact to persons who are having the test.

Tuberculosis infection is unlike other infections. Usually, other infections disappear completely when overcome by the body's defenses and leave no living organisms and generally no signs of infection. However, a person who has been infected with tubercle bacilli harbors the organism for the remainder of his or her life. Tubercle bacilli remain in the lungs in a dormant, walled-off, or so-called resting, state. When a person is under physical or emotional stress, these bacilli may become active and begin to multiply. If body defenses are low, active tuberculosis may develop. Most persons who have active tuberculosis developed it in this manner. However, it is generally accepted that only 1 out of 20 persons with a positive tuberculin test will ever develop active tuberculosis, and the incidence is expected to be much lower among those who receive preventive therapy with isoniazid.

Classification. Following is the classification used by states and territories of the United States when reporting morbidity statistics to the CDC of the Public Health Service. The six basic classifications cover the total child and adult population, those unexposed to tuberculosis, those uninfected even though exposed, those with evidence of tuberculosis infection without disease, those with current disease, those with evidence of tuberculosis without current disease, and those in whom tuberculosis is suspected (diagnosis pending).

Class 0: No tuberculosis exposure, not infected. No therapy necessary.

Class 1: Tuberculosis exposure, no evidence of infection. Persons who may be in the process of converting their tuberculin test from negative to positive may be given "preventive chemotherapy." Household contacts should be considered for such therapy. Preventive chemotherapy is standard for all children and most especially for those under 5 years of age. It is absolutely essential for neonates.

Class 2: Tuberculosis infection, no disease. Positive reactors under 35 years of age are considered candidates for preventive chemotherapy. The recommended chemotherapy is isoniazid (INH), 300 mg daily for 1 year. It is recommended for all persons who are at risk of developing current tuberculosis including the following groups:

1. Persons whose tuberculin test has increased by at least 6 mm in size within 24 months from less than 10 mm in diameter
2. Persons receiving prolonged corticosteroid or immunosuppressive therapy (isoniazid usually continued for 3 months after these medications are stopped)
3. Persons with hematologic or reticuloendothelial diseases such as leukemia or lymphoma
4. Persons with silicosis or those with diabetes that is difficult to control
5. Persons who have had a gastrectomy

Persons over 35 years of age without the risk factors listed above are not given preventive chemotherapy because of the risk of isoniazid-associated hepatitis. Although the risk of isoniazid-associated hepatitis is small, it is age related and increases from less than 0.2% in those under age 20 to up to 2.3% in those 50 to 64 years of age (Table 51-2).

If isoniazid-associated hepatitis occurs, the symptoms are quite mild and nonspecific and resemble those of any viral illness. (See p. 680 for a discussion of viral hepatitis.)

Contraindications to the use of isoniazid preventive therapy are (1) previous isoniazid-associated liver disease; (2) severe adverse reactions to isoniazed, including fever, chills, rash, and arthritis; and (3) *acute* liver disease of any cause.[132]

Persons receiving isoniazid preventive chemotherapy should be seen monthly by a health care provider for the purpose of reinforcing the necessity of taking the chemotherapy regularly and to monitor the patient for any serious side effects.

Class 3: Tuberculosis: current disease (*Mycobacterium tuberculosis* cultured, if culture done; otherwise, both a significant reaction to tuberculin skin test and clinical and/or roentgenographic evidence of tuberculosis).

This class includes all persons with current tuberculosis whose diagnostic procedures are complete. If diagnosis is still pending, the person is classified as tuberculosis suspect (class 5). The person remains in class

TABLE 51-2. Relationship between age and isoniazid-associated hepatitis*

Age (yr)	Occurrence of hepatitis (%)†
20 and under	0.2
35-49	0.3
50-64	2.3
64 and over	0.8

*From Weg, J.G.: Tuberculosis and other mycobacterial diseases. In Conn, H.F., editor: Curent therapy, Philadelphia, 1982, W.B. Saunders Co.

†The risk also increases in those who drink alcohol daily.

3 until treatment for the current episode is completed and the person is judged to have no clinical or roentgenographic evidence of disease.

Treatment with at least two of the first-line or primary drugs (isoniazid, ethambutol, rifampin, or streptomycin) is instituted. The most commonly prescribed drugs are isoniazid, 300 mg/kg, and ethambutol (EMB), 15 mg/kg, daily given once a day for 18 to 24 months.

If the person's organisms are resistant to the first-line drugs, second-line drugs are prescribed (Table 51-3). A person may be infected with drug-resistant bacilli inhaled from a person with drug-resistant tuberculosis. Drug resistance is more common in persons of Hispanic or Asian origin and in Americans who were infected while in Asia.[132] Primary drug resistance rates vary widely in the United States and Canada, and nurses need to know the local resistance rates for the area in which they are working. It can be postulated that resistance rates will be higher in those areas where large numbers of Hispanics and Asians are living. Resistance to isoniazid is more common than is resistance to other antituberculosis drugs.

At least two drugs and preferably three are prescribed when resistant organisms are present. The ones used will depend on the findings of sensitivity studies. All these drugs are more toxic than the first-line drugs, and viomycin, capreomycin, kanamycin, and streptomycin are usually not given together because of their toxic effect on the eighth cranial nerve and the kidneys. Some persons with resistant organisms may require more than 18 months of therapy. The most commonly prescribed drugs used to treat tuberculosis caused by resistant organisms are rifampin (RIF), 600 mg daily, and ethambutol, 15 mg/kg daily.

Class 4: Tuberculosis: no current disease. Persons in this class have (1) a history of a previous episode or episodes of tuberculosis or (2) abnormal roentgenographic findings along with no significant reaction to the tuberculin test and no clinical, laboratory, or roentgenographic evidence of current disease. Thus the person may never have had chemotherapy, may be on chemotherapy, or may have completed chemotherapy.[132]

Class 5: Tuberculosis: suspect (diagnosis pending). This classification is used until all diagnostic tests are completed and a decision is made about the person's status. No one should be in this class longer than 3 months. Preventive chemotherapy may be instituted while diagnostic studies are underway.

Each case of tuberculosis is to be reported to the local health department, using the new classification described above. It is important that all cases of tuberculosis be reported so that accurate morbidity statistics are available and control programs can be instituted as necessary. In most areas of the United States drug therapy including preventive chemotherapy is provided free of charge.

Prevention. In order to eliminate tuberculosis, the organism must be prevented from being transmitted from one person to another. Preventive measures are directed toward the recommendations described under classification. Preventive therapy emphasis is on (1) finding all persons who have tuberculosis and getting them under adequate treatment, (2) identifying persons who should be on preventive chemotherapy and getting them under treatment, and (3) locating persons who had tuberculosis in the past who did not receive adequate treatment with chemotherapy.

Following is a listing of persons who should be considered for preventive chemotherapy:

1. Persons known to be exposed to tuberculosis who may be in the process of converting their tuberculin test (recent converters under 35 years of age)
2. Household contacts of persons diagnosed as having tuberculosis, especially children under age 5
3. Positive reactors to the tuberculin test under age 35
4. Tuberculin reactors over age 35 who are at special risk
    a. Those on corticosteroid therapy
    b. Those on immunosuppressive therapy
    c. Those having a disease that impairs the immune response

VACCINATION. Efforts continue in search of a more satisfactory tuberculosis vaccine. Presently, BCG (bacillus Calmette-Guérin) vaccine is in use in many countries throughout the world. This vaccine contains attenuated tubercle bacilli that have lost their ability to produce disease. It is administered only to persons who have a negative reaction to the tuberculin test. It is not widely used in the United States because of disagreements among physicians as to its safety and effectiveness. Also, vaccination with BCG induces hypersensitivity to tuberculin in vaccinated persons. Thus the tuberculin test loses its value as a diagnostic tool for these persons, and this is one of the major objections to its use in the United States.

The vaccine should be given only by persons who have had careful instruction in the proper technique. A multiple-puncture disk is used. When there is a positive reaction to skin testing with tuberculin, when acute infectious disease is present, or when there is any skin disease, BCG vaccine is not given. Possible complications following vaccination are local ulcers, which occur in a relatively high percentage of persons vaccinated, and abscesses or suppuration of lymph nodes, which occur in a small percentage.

In countries where living conditions are such that transmission of the disease is to be expected, BCG vaccine is given early in life and then repeated after 12 to 15 years. The intradermal method is used to administer the vaccine so that a uniform controlled dose can be

TABLE 51-3. Treatment of mycobacterial disease in adults and children*

Drugs	Dosage		Most common side effects	Tests for side effects	Remarks
	Daily	Twice weekly			
First-line drugs					
Isoniazid (INH)	5-10 mg/kg up to 300-600 mg	15 mg/kg PO or IM	Peripheral neuritis, hepatitis, hypersensitivity, convulsions	SGOT/SGPT (not as a routine)	Bactericidal; pyridoxine, 10 mg, as prophylaxis for neuritis; 50-100 mg as treatment
Ethambutol (EMB)	15-25 mg/kg PO	50 mg/kg PO	Optic neuritis (reversible with discontinuation of drug; very rare at 15 mg/kg), skin rash	Red-green color discrimination and visual acuity	Use with caution with renal disease or when eye testing is not feasible
Rifampin	10-20 mg/kg up to 600 mg PO	Not recommended	Hepatitis, febrile reaction, purpura (rare)	SGOT/SGPT (not as a routine)	Bactericidal; orange urine color; negates effect of birth control pills
Streptomycin (SM)	15-20 mg/kg up to 1 g IM	25 to 30 mg/kg	Eighth cranial nerve damage, nephrotoxicity (rare)	Vestibular function, audiograms; BUN and creatinine	Use with caution in older patients or those with renal disease
Second-line drugs					
Viomycin	1 g q 12 hr/ twice weekly		Auditory toxicity, nephrotoxicity, vestibular toxicity (rare)	Vestibular function, audiograms; BUN and creatinine	Use with caution in older patients; rarely used with renal disease
Capreomycin	1 g		Eighth cranial nerve damage, nephrotoxicity	Vestibular function, audiograms; BUN and creatinine	Use with caution in older patients; rarely used with renal disease
Kanamycin	0.5-1 g		Auditory toxicity, nephrotoxicity, vestibular toxicity (rare)	Vestibular function, audiograms; BUN and creatinine	Use with caution in older patients; rarely used with renal disease
Ethionamide	750-1000 mg		Gastrointestinal disturbance, hepatotoxicity, hypersensitivity	SGOT/SGPT	Divided dose may help gastrointestinal side effects
Pyrazinamide (PZA)	15-30 mg/kg up to 2 g PO		Hyperuricemia, hepatotoxicity	Uric acid, SGOT/SGPT	Combination with an aminoglycoside is bactericidal
Para-aminosalicyclic acid (aminosalicylic acid; PAS)	150 mg/kg up to 12 g PO		Gastrointestinal disturbance, hypersensitivity, hepatotoxicity, sodium load	SGOT/SGPT	Gastrointestinal side effects very frequent, making cooperation difficult
Cycloserine	750 mg		Psychosis, personality changes, convulsions, rash	Psychologic testing	Very difficult drug to use; side effects may be blocked by pyridoxine ataractic agents, or anticonvulsant drugs

*Adapted from American Thoracic Society: Am. Rev. Respir. Dis. **115**:185-187, 1977.

given. BCG vaccine is not generally recommended for use in the United States, although some highly susceptible groups such as migrant workers may be immunized.

Diagnosis

TUBERCULIN SKIN TESTING. Tuberculin skin testing provides evidence of whether the individual tested has been infected by tubercle bacilli. It is based on the fact that a hypersensitivity reaction develops to certain products of *Mycobacterium tuberculosis*. This cell-mediated or delayed hypersensitivity reaction is manifested by induration caused by cellular infiltration at the site of the injection in persons who have been sensitized to the tubercle bacillus. Such persons are called "reactors." In the past the terms *negative* and *positive* were used to describe the results of tuberculin testing. In 1981 the American Thoracic Society (ATS), the medical section of the ALA, suggested that the terms positive and negative are not the most accurate way to describe the results of tuberculin skin testing.[11] They recommend that the number of millimeters of induration be recorded and then interpreted appropriately.

Two substances are used in tuberculin skin testing: OT (old tuberculin), which is prepared from dead tubercle bacilli and contains their related impurities; and PPD (purified protein derivative), which is a highly purified product containing protein from the tubercle bacilli.

The tuberculin test that gives the most accurate results is the *Mantoux test,* or intracutaneous injection of either PPD or OT. A tuberculin syringe and a short (½-in.), sharp, 24- to 26-gauge needle are used. With the skin (usually the inner forearm is used) held taut, the injection of 0.1 ml of PPD or OT is made into the superficial layers, and it produces a sharply raised white wheal. Weak dilutions are used first. If the reaction is negative, stronger dilutions are used. This precaution prevents severe local reactions that might occur in highly sensitive individuals if the higher dilutions were used initially. If old tuberculin is used, tests are begun with a dilution of 1:10,000, or 0.001 mg of OT. If there is no reaction, successive tests with stronger dilutions are made. The most frequently used strength of PPD is an intermediate strength of 0.0001 mg/dose, or 5 tuberculin units (5 Tu). PPD is also available in first- and second-strength dilutions. For broad-screening and case-finding purposes, a single test of intermediate strength is recommended. Interpretations of the test are made after 48 hours. A tuberculin reaction may begin after 12 to 24 hours with an area of redness and a central area of induration, but it reaches its peak in 48 hours. The area of induration (not the erythema) indicates how positive the test is. Induration should be examined in a good light and palpated gently. Tuberculin reactions should always be measured and recorded in millimeters at the largest diameter of the induration. When succes-

sive dilutions are being used, it is advisable to have tests read by the same person so that individual variation in interpretation can be prevented. If the test is negative, there may be no visible reaction or there may be only slight redness with no induration.

One of the most important steps in tuberculin testing is the accurate measurement of reaction. A reaction is considered to be significant when it is 10 mm or more in diameter. Reactions between 5 and 9 mm are considered to be doubtful reactions and are more likely to indicate infection with atypical acid-fast bacilli (p. 1307) than with *Mycobacterium tuberculosis*, except in persons who are suspects or close contacts of persons with tuberculosis. In this instance a reaction of 5 mm or more is considered significant.[11]

OTHER DIAGNOSTIC STUDIES. Results of roentgenograms and sputum examinations will either rule out the possibility or confirm a diagnosis of tuberculosis. Both tests have been described (pp. 1217 and 1219). Bacteriologic confirmation of the presence of *Mycobacterium tuberculosis* is necessary to establish the diagnosis of tuberculosis. Because it is impossible to differentiate between typical and atypical acid-fast bacilli by a sputum smear, cultures are obtained on all persons. Cultures are also used for antimicrobial susceptibility (sensitivity) studies. *Despite the introduction of improved culture media, the tubercle bacillus grows slowly on artificial media, and culture reports will not be available for 3 to 6 weeks.*

Blood-streaked sputum in the absence of pronounced coughing may be the first indication to the person that anything is wrong. Pathologic changes may have occurred in the lungs, but sputum examination may not show tubercle bacilli. However, if the nodules produced in the parenchyma of the lung become soft in the center and then caseated and liquefied, the liquefied material may break through and empty into the bronchi and be raised as sputum. Cavities in the lung may appear on x-ray film and may be present in more than one lobe of the lung.

Intervention. Once the diagnosis of "tuberculosis: infection, with disease" is made, steps are taken to prevent the patient from contaminating the air with tubercle bacilli. This is accomplished by (1) *treatment of the patient with antituberculosis drugs* and (2) *preventing contamination of air with tubercle bacilli*. Each of these measures will be discussed in detail.

PREVENTION OF TRANSMISSION: CHEMOTHERAPY. Whether the patient with tuberculosis is being treated at home or in the hospital, the same drugs are given. Isoniazid (INH), streptomycin, ethambutol, and rifampin are the drugs in common use. These four drugs are considered to be the "first-line," or *primary*, medications in the treatment of tuberculosis. If they prove to be ineffective or if the patient develops resistant tubercle bacilli, the "second-line," or secondary, drugs are used—

cycloserine (Seromycin), pyrazinoic acid amide (Pyrazinamide), viomycin (Viocin), kanamycin (Kantrex), ethionamide (Trecator), para-aminosalicylic acid (PAS), and capreomycin (Capastat). (See Table 51-5 for additional information.)

Previously untreated pulmonary tuberculosis can nearly always be controlled bacteriologically with drugs alone. Most failures of antimicrobial therapy are caused by errors in choice of drug, inadequate dosage, or failure of the patient to take the drugs regularly as prescribed. Choices of drugs are made with the objective of both effective treatment of disease and minimizing the development of drug-resistant organisms.

Susceptibility testing. Prescriptions for antituberculosis drugs are made according to the susceptibility of the organisms isolated from the patient's sputum to the primary drugs. Susceptibility testing indicates the effectiveness of a specific drug in inhibiting the growth of the organism or the organism's resistance to the drug. Until testing can be completed, the physician will start the patient on the drugs to which it is believed the bacilli are most likely to be susceptible.

Testing is done by growing cultures of the organisms in special media. The culture plate is divided into sections so that the organisms, if present in the patient's sputum, will grow on one section. Each of the other sections contains a medium plus one of the primary drugs. Thus if the organisms multiply on one section of medium but do not appear on other sections of the medium, the organisms are susceptible to those drugs that inhibit their growth. Testing usually takes about 3 weeks, about half the time formerly required to grow cultures of tubercle bacilli.

Although it is the physician's responsibility to make susceptibility tests, the nurse should understand the basis on which drugs are prescribed and help the patient understand the drugs that are prescribed.

In the last few years it has been recognized that there are naturally occurring drug-resistant tubercle bacilli. It is estimated that in every group of 100,000 bacilli there is one naturally occurring isoniazid-resistant organism, while for each group of 1 million bacilli there is one streptomycin-resistant organism.[60] Therefore antituberculosis drugs are always given in combination. Usually two of the drugs are combined, but patients with far advanced cavitary disease often receive three drugs.

Drugs frequently used. The peripheral neuritis associated with isoniazid therapy is more common in persons who are malnourished or who are receiving large doses of the drug. To prevent neuritis, the physician usually orders pyridoxine, 50 to 100 mg daily. Occasionally, isoniazid may affect memory and the ability to concentrate, and rarely it may cause psychosis.

Streptomycin is often given as part of an initial program of *triple drug therapy*. It is given intramuscularly in 1-g doses daily or twice a week for 6 to 12 weeks or more, depending on the patient's improvement. Smaller doses may be prescribed for elderly patients or for patients who have hearing impairment or renal damage. The most important untoward reaction to streptomycin is labyrinth damage with resulting vertigo and staggering. Skin rash, itching, and fever can occur. Although renal damage is uncommon, urinalyses and blood urea nitrogen determinations usually are ordered at periodic intervals.

Patients' problems with chemotherapy. It is *imperative* that the patient who has tuberculosis *take the prescribed medications regularly and without interruption*. Because patients usually must take drugs as prescribed for 18 to 24 months, some persons become discouraged and stop taking the drugs. If symptoms of intolerance to a drug such as those produced by PAS occur, the patient may simply stop taking the one drug and continue with the other. The patient may feel quite well, work regularly, yet must continue the therapy. Because most patients feel well, they may be tempted to discontinue the drugs altogether or perhaps take the one drug that bothers them the least. *All patients must be taught that the discontinuance of even one drug will allow drug-resistant organisms to flourish and will make the disease more difficult to treat.* The nurse should help all patients develop a routine for taking the drugs. For those who have difficulty remembering to take their medications, pill calendars that have each day's medications in a plastic bag stapled to a large cardboard calendar may be helpful.

Some persons stop taking drugs and then restart them. Because they may feel guilty about this interruption in therapy, they do not tell the physician or nurse, and it may not be evident until their condition fails to improve. The nurse can help by allowing time for patients to talk about themselves, their families, and their treatment. This may be done when the patient visits a health department clinic to receive a new supply of drugs, when the person comes for periodic medical examination, or when the nurse visits in the home. Patients may be asked to collect a urine specimen periodically for examination. Since the metabolic products of some of the drugs are excreted in the urine, a urinalysis will indicate whether the patient is following the therapy. The best indication, of course, is the progress of the patient. If there is improvement, therapy is effective and the medications probably have been taken as prescribed.

PREVENTING TRANSMISSION: PREVENTING CONTAMINATION OF THE AIR. As soon as the diagnosis of tuberculosis is established, the person is taught to cover the nose and mouth with disposable tissues when coughing, sneezing, or laughing. This stops the organisms at the source and prevents them from becoming droplet nuclei capable of transmitting disease (p. 1298). Soiled tissues are collected in a paper bag for subsequent burning, or they may be discarded in the toilet. The patient should wash the hands after expectorating or handling the sputum container.

The most effective way to kill the tubercle bacillus in moist sputum is by burning. All tissues and disposable receptacles for collection of sputum should be burned. Direct sunlight destroys the bacillus in 1 to 2 hours. Five minutes at boiling temperature and 30 minutes at pasteurizing temperature (61.7° C [143° F]) kill the bacillus. Autoclaving also destroys the bacillus. Disposable articles may be used if desired.

The natural movement of air in a room carries droplet nuclei containing the tubercle bacillus, and if windows are kept open or air is circulated mechanically, changes of air dilute the contaminated air below the level where infection can take place. If patients who have positive sputum have been taught to cover coughs and sneezes, air contamination in the room is even lower.

Tubercle bacilli in droplet nuclei are highly susceptible to sterilization by sunlight. *Ultraviolet light* also kills tubercle bacilli in droplet nuclei. Ultraviolet lights installed in air ducts through which room air passes or mounted high on side walls of the room are effective.

It is important that nurses understand how tubercle bacilli are transmitted through air so that they can teach the patient how to protect others and also allay fears that family members and others may have about contracting the disease. It has been well documented that patients taking antituberculosis drugs are not likely to transmit the infection even when their organisms are resistant to treatment. *Because only droplet nuclei are capable of transmitting tubercle bacilli, there is no need for those caring for the patient with active tuberculosis to wear either a mask or a gown. Droplet nuclei are so small (1 to 5 μm) that they readily pass through conventional masks or are breathed in around the edges of them.* Chemotherapeutic treatment of the patient and adequate air changes in the patient's room offer all the protection that is needed. In a situation in which the patient is unable to cover the mouth when coughing, it is more effective for the patient to wear a mask than for personnel to do so. *Newer-type high-filtration masks such as the Ultra-Filter have proved to be effective filters. If a mask is deemed necessary, this type should be used.*

Since many people with active tuberculosis are cared for in their homes, the nurse should help them and their families to understand the communicability of tuberculosis and the precautions that must be taken. Family members and friends may be frightened at the thought of contact with the patient and with articles the person has touched. On the other hand, they have often had long, intimate contact with the patient without developing the disease. Careful observation of the family will help the nurse determine how many and what kind of explanations are needed regarding spread of infection. If the family is overly cautious in handling the patient's

personal articles, the nurse may need to advise against discarding articles that are costly to replace. In contrast, if the family is too casual about spread of the disease, the nurse should urge more caution in care of sputum and in exposure to the patient's cough. If possible, the patient should occupy a room alone, but usually the patient does not need to be strictly isolated from the rest of the family. Careful planning with the family often helps ensure that the patient will not infect others yet can be part of the family. The susceptibility of infants and very young children must be emphasized in all teaching.

ACCEPTANCE OF THE DIAGNOSIS. Acceptance of a diagnosis of tuberculosis and of its many implications for the future is difficult for anyone. The patient or the patient's family should be referred to a community health nurse immediately after the diagnosis of tuberculosis is made so that initial explanations can be given and essential teaching begun. It is important that any problems that might interfere with acceptance of the disease and the need to take antituberculosis drug therapy be identified early, since the earlier efforts are made to solve them, the less difficult they may be to overcome.

Real acceptance of the disease, however, may come only after months of illness and after steady help and support from the family, the physician, the social worker, and the nurse. The acceptance of facts and realities varies according to each patient's basic personality and lifelong pattern of behavior in stress situations. The nurse should realize that for some time after the diagnosis is made, patients may deny having tuberculosis or may be very angry that it has happened to them. Some persons may become depressed and may have periods of withdrawal as they work through their feelings about the diagnosis. Many of their feelings about the diagnosis are more emotionally than intellectually determined. Even though persons having tuberculosis understand that the disease is not caused by being "unclean" or "sinful," there may still be a carry-over of these kinds of feelings from things they heard when they were a child, since these are common feelings expressed by some persons with tuberculosis.

The nurse should be aware that there is a stigma attached to persons with tuberculosis, especially in some cultural groups. The fear of stigma and being labeled as dirty, sinful, and so on may keep many patients and their families from revealing the patient's real diagnosis. In these situations family and friends are not informed that the person has tuberculosis and are left to their own conjectures about the person's illness.

There is a high incidence of alcoholism among patients with tuberculosis, probably because of the increased possibility of alcoholics coming into contact with tubercle bacilli during drinking bouts and because of their decreased resistance to infection. Some of these patients have been committed to the hospital by legal action after refusal to obtain treatment, since their disease is a threat to the health of their family and community. These patients present the dual problem of the patient with alcoholism and the patient with tuberculosis who cannot accept the disease.

Increased attention needs to be given to patients who refuse treatment and thus stand in the way of eradication of tuberculosis. The nurse often is the member of the health team called on to work with these patients. Patience and understanding as well as flexibility in trying new approaches are essential in working with them. Although the patient needs explanations as to the need for treatment and time to make decisions regarding means of obtaining it, delaying tactics should be discouraged by setting limits. Avoidance of questions that permit categorical refusal is wise. It is often helpful to discover the person for whose judgment the patient has the greatest respect and to seek his or her help in encouraging treatment. This person may be a physician, a member of the clergy, a family member, or a close friend. Persons who have completed treatment for tuberculosis and are well again often are helpful in answering specific questions the person may have and may thus relieve many of the patient's anxieties. Every effort should be made to help the person feel there is sincere concern for his or her welfare. In spite of all efforts, some patients will not consent to treatment. Sometimes, if they become suddenly worse, they may then be receptive to treatment, and the opportunity to work with them and help them at this time should not be missed.

Nurses working with patients having tuberculosis must be able to accept the diagnosis if they are to help the patient. Nurses who have a fear of tuberculosis show it in their behavior. Most patients with tuberculosis are extremely sensitive to ways in which various health workers approach them. If personnel are obvious about precautions in giving care, this may make the patient feel rejected. Nurses may be fearful of the disease for various reasons. If the nurse is aware of being fearful, talking it over with an experienced person who is unafraid of tuberculosis may prove helpful. Reassurance that tuberculosis is not highly communicable is usually very helpful to the nurse who has not previously cared for a patient with tuberculosis.

The majority of patients with tuberculosis are able to assume responsibility for their own care. The nurse's major responsibility is to help patients learn what they should do and why and to give encouragement and supervision in the simple but essential elements of good care. Group teaching often is a very productive method of instructing both patients and family members, since they often learn from each other and give each other emotional support.

ACTIVITY. Although tuberculosis previously was treated with bed rest, restriction of activity is no longer ordered except as warranted by the patient's general physical condition. Persons who are febrile are usually kept in bed until the fever subsides.

SURGICAL INTERVENTION. When medical intervention has failed to check and heal the disease process, surgical intervention for tuberculosis may be necessary. Surgical intervention for tuberculosis includes pneumonectomy, lobectomy, segmental lobe resection, and wedge resection. Usually parts of the lungs with active disease are resected, and as much unaffected lung tissue as possible is preserved. The nursing care and descriptions of operative procedures are explained on p. 1250.

Extrapulmonary tuberculosis. Tuberculosis may affect other parts of the body besides the lungs, such as the larynx, gastrointestinal tract, lymph nodes, skin, skeletal system, nervous system, and urinary and reproductive systems.

TUBERCULOUS MENINGITIS. The onset of symptoms of tuberculous meningitis usually is sudden. The patient has marked constipation, an elevation of temperature, chills, headache, convulsions, and sometimes loss of consciousness. The disease is most common in infants and young children who most often contract the disease from an adult with an undiagnosed case of pulmonary tuberculosis. If untreated, this disease causes death, but with the use of antituberculosis drugs it is usually controllable. A 12-month course of chemotherapy is essential, however, and the nurse must help the patient and family realize that it is absolutely necessary. Ethambutol, streptomycin, and isoniazid are given concurrently. Corticosteroids are usually ordered to reduce neurologic complications.[132] Nursing care is the same as that for any other type of meningitis.

SKELETAL TUBERCULOSIS. Since the advent of antituberculosis drugs, better case-finding methods, pasteurization of milk, and tuberculin testing of cattle, skeletal tuberculosis is less common. It is most common in children, but adults also are sometimes affected. Although tubercle bacilli may attack any bone or joint in the body, the spine, hips, and knees are most often involved. Deformities occur as a result of bone destruction. Tuberculosis of the spine is now rare in the United States. The "hunchback" deformity it causes can still be seen in some people, particularly in those who have come from countries where standards for pasteurization of milk and tuberculin testing of cattle were not rigid. (For nursing care of patients having tuberculosis of the spine, see specialized texts on orthopedic nuring.)

Outcome criteria for a person with tuberculosis. The person or significant others can:

1. Explain how tuberculosis is spread and those measures necessary to prevent spread (remain on chemotherapy, cover mouth and nose when coughing or sneezing).
2. Explain basic food groups and how a nutritionally adequate diet will be achieved.

3. State name, dosage, actions, and side effects of prescribed medications.
4. State why at least two chemotherapy agents must be taken uninterruptedly.
   a. Explain drug-resistant organisms and relate this to the need to take chemotherapy uninterruptedly.
   b. Explain why the health care provider should be notified immediately if for any reason (e.g., side effects) chemotherapy cannot be taken.
5. State where to receive new supply of chemotherapy and date it is to be obtained.
6. State plans for follow-up care.
   a. List signs and symptoms that indicate need for immediate medical care (increased cough, hemoptysis, unexplained weight loss, fever, night sweats).
   b. State when next sputum test or roentgenogram is to be taken and where.
   c. State plans for ongoing follow-up care.

Infection with atypical acid-fast bacilli

Pulmonary disease that is indistinguishable from tuberculosis can be produced by a number of species of mycobacteria other than *Mycobacterium tuberculosis*. These organisms are strongly acid-fast, but differ from *Mycobacterium tuberculosis* on culture. Four groups have been classified by Runyon: group I, *Mycobacterium kansasii* (photochromogens); group II, scotochromogens, which are commonly found in soil and water; group III, Battey bacilli (nonphotochromogens), which are found mainly in Georgia; and group IV, *Mycobacterium fortuitum* (rapid growers). These atypical organisms are found in various geographic locations. Group I is the most widely distributed, and many organisms have been identified in the Midwest. Group III is found more in the southeastern portion of the United States.

The pulmonary disease caused by atypical bacilli closely resembles tuberculosis. The disease often causes lung cavities, responds poorly to antituberculosis drugs, and quite often requires surgery. It occurs most commonly in persons in high socioeconomic groups—especially those residing in suburban areas of large cities. The pulmonary disease caused by these mycobacteria is more common in white males in their 30s, 40s, and 50s, especially those with chronic obstructive pulmonary disease, silicosis, or a history of arc welding.[11] Atypical bacilli are not believed to be airborne; thus isolation is not required. Because of the seriousness of the pulmonary disease caused by these organisms, patients are usually given chemotherapy for at least 2 years and should have careful medical follow-up after discharge from the hospital. It is possible for persons to be infected with both tubercle bacilli and atypical bacilli at the same time.

Lung abscess

Etiology and pathophysiology. A lung abscess is an area of localized suppuration within the lung. It usually is caused by bacteria that reach the lung through aspiration. The infected material lodges in the small bronchi and produces inflammation. Partial obstruction of the bronchus results in the retention of secretions beyond the obstruction and the eventual necrosis of tissue. The necrotic lung tissue is coughed up, and an air-filled cavity is left in the lung.

Food particles and perigingival debris, which contain both aerobic and anaerobic organisms, are the most commonly aspirated substances. Laboratory cultures of sputum or transtracheal aspirates are necessary to identify the causative organism. When only normal oropharyngeal flora is found, aerobic cultures may demonstrate the presence of fusospirochetal organisms, peptostreptococci, and members of the *Bacteroides* group. All of these organisms are commonly found in gingival infections. The most common aerobic bacteria causing lung abscess are *Staphylococcus aureus* and *Klebsiella pneumoniae*. Aerobic gram-negative organisms are found most frequently in persons with nosocomial infections or in persons who are immunosuppressed. Sputum should also be examined for tumor cells and for tuberculosis and fungal organisms. Before the advent of antibiotics and specific chemotherapy, lung abscess was a fairly frequent complication following pneumonia.

Lung abscess may follow bronchial obstruction caused by a tumor, a foreign body, or a stenosis of the bronchus. Children particularly may aspirate foreign material such as a peanut, and a lung abscess results. Metastatic spread of cancer cells to the lung parenchyma may also cause an abscess, and occasionally the infection appears to have been borne by the bloodstream. In recent years the incidence of lung abscess caused by infection has decreased, and secondary lung abscess following bronchogenic carcinoma has increased. Bronchoscopy maybe used to identify the infected segment and to obtain specimens for culture.

Clinical picture. Symptoms of lung abscess include cough, elevation of temperature, loss of appetite, and malaise. Unless the abscess is walled off so that there is no access to the bronchi, the patient usually raises sputum. There may be hemoptysis, and often the patient raises dark brown ("chocolate-colored") sputum that contains both blood and pus.

Intervention. The course of lung abscess is influenced by the cause of the abscess and by the kind of drainage that can be established. If the purulent material drains easily, the patient may respond well to segmental postural drainage, antibiotic therapy, and good general supportive care. When obstruction interferes with drainage into the bronchi, bronchoscopic procedures should be employed not only to improve drainage but to rule out obstructing foreign bodies or neoplasms.[73] Today, surgical treatment to establish drainage has become increasingly less necessary, but if after several weeks of medical treatment a cavity persists, a segmentectomy or lobectomy may be performed.

Penicillin G is the drug of choice, and 2 g is given intravenously every 6 hours until the fever is relieved and the patient's condition shows marked improvement. Penicillin G (potassium phenoxymethyl penicillin) or ampicillin in doses of 500 mg four times daily is then given orally. When the patient has a sensitivity to penicillin, clindamycin, 600 mg every 8 hours, is prescribed. For staphylococcal infections oxacillin or nafcillin, 6 to 8 g intravenously in divided doses, is often prescribed. Lung abscesses caused by gram-negative organisms are treated with appropriate antibiotics as determined by in vitro sensitivity tests.

Antibiotic therapy is continued until all signs of the illness have subsided and the chest roentgenograms show the cavity has completely disappeared or has reduced significantly in size.[107] Most cavities close within 6 weeks, but occasionally a cavity may persist for months.

If the patient does not improve with the therapy discussed above, bronchoscopy is performed to search for a possible obstruction to drainage such as carcinoma or a foreign body.[107]

Medical treatment cannot cause a walled-off abscess to disappear, and surgery may be necessary. If surgery is necessary, the portion of lung containing the abscess is removed. If the abscess is caused by carcinoma, the surgery may be much more extensive.

Bronchiectasis

Etiology and pathophysiology

Bronchiectasis is abnormal dilation of the bronchial tree. When infection attacks the bronchial lining, inflammation occurs and an exudate forms. The progressive accumulation of secretions obstructs the bronchioles. The obstructed bronchioles then break down and ciliated columnar epithelium is replaced by nonciliated cuboidal epithelium and sometimes fibrosis tissue resulting in localized areas of dilation or saccules.[140] The expulsive force of the bronchioles is diminished, and they may remain filled with exudate. Only forceful coughing and postural drainage will empty them. Bronchiectasis may involve any part of the lung parenchyma, but it usually occurs in the dependent portions or lobes. Before the widespread use of antibiotics in treating persons with respiratory tract infections, this disease began to develop in young people, with many showing symptoms in childhood or by age 20. Although the incidence of childhood bronchiectasis is decreasing, it is increasing in individuals with cystic fibrosis, immunodeficiency diseases, or atopic asthma in which repeated respiratory infections have been successfully treated with antibiotics. These persons now survive the acute episodes of bacterial infection that complicate their underlying disease but not infrequently develop bronchiectasis as a sequela.

A contributing factor in bronchiectasis may be a congenital weakness in the structure of the bronchi that results in impairment of elasticity. Bronchiectasis may occur without previous pulmonary disease, but it usually follows such diseases as bronchopneumonia, lung abscesses, tuberculosis, or asthma. A bronchogram in which radiopaque dye is instilled into the bronchial tree through a catheter shows trapping (puddling) of dye in the dilated bronchi (Fig. 48-5).

Clinical picture

The chief complaint in bronchiectasis is severe coughing (brought on by changing position) that is productive of large amounts of blood-tinged sputum and causes dyspnea. Paroxysms of coughing when arising in the morning and again when lying down are common.

Symptoms of bronchiectasis vary with the severity of the condition. Complaints of fatigue, weakness, and loss of weight are common. Appetite can be affected by the fetid sputum. The condition may develop so gradually that the person in often unable to tell when symptoms first began. Clubbing of the fingers is common, as it is in other chronic respiratory diseases.

Intervention

Treatment of bronchiectasis is not very satisfactory. Surgical removal of a portion of the lung is the only cure (p. 1250). Therefore patients who have bronchiectasis that involves both lungs are not candidates for surgery and do not have a good prognosis. The life expectancy usually is considered to be no more than 20 years. Many patients develop cardiac complications (cor pulmonale) resulting from the extra strain on the heart caused by inability of the lungs to oxygenate the blood adequately.

Postural drainage at least twice a day helps to remove secretions and thus helps to prevent coughing (p. 1239). During severe episodes of coughing the patient should not be left alone, since thick secretions may block a large bronchiole and cause severe dyspnea and cyanosis. Occasionally, a bronchoscopy may be done to remove the plug of mucus or to break adhesions that may be interfering with postural drainage by blocking passage to the main bronchi. Antibiotics may be used in the treatment of bronchiectasis. Although they do not cure the condition, they may prevent further infection and are often used before surgery. If the involvement of the the lung is widespread, oxygen may be used. Nursing care should stress good general hygiene, which may contribute to relief of symptoms. Adequate diet, rest, exercise, and diversional activity are important, and avoiding superimposed infections such as colds should be emphasized. Frequent mouth care is essential, and cleansing the mouth with an aromatic solution before meals often makes food more acceptable.

Empyema

Epidemiology and etiology

Empyema means pus within a body cavity. It usually applies to the pleural cavity. Empyema occurs as a result of, or in association with other respiratory diseases such as pneumonia, lung abscess, tuberculosis, and fungal infections of the lung and also following thoracic surgery or chest trauma. It now occurs fairly commonly as a complication of staphylococcal pneumonia.

Clinical picture

The patient with any kind of lung infection or chest injury should be observed closely for signs of empyema, which include cough, dyspnea, unilateral chest pain, elevation of temperature, malaise, poor appetite, and unequal chest expansion. The condition may develop several weeks after an apparently minor respiratory tract infection. The diagnosis can usually be made from the signs and symptoms and the medical history, but it is confirmed by a chest roentgenogram that demonstrates the presence of a pleural exudate. A thoracentesis is done to obtain a sample of the pus for culture and sensitivity studies and to relieve the patient's respiratory symptoms.

Intervention

The aim in the treatment of empyema is to drain the empyema cavity completely and thus obliterate the pleural space. This can be accomplished in several ways. Initially, the cavity may be aspirated daily and antibiotics instilled in it an an attempt to sterilize this space. If the cavity cannot be evacuated within a few days or if the lung fails to reexpand so as to obliterate the space, surgical treatment is necessary. Depending on the situation, either closed or open chest drainage may be employed. In closed chest drainage a trocar is inserted between the ribs at the base of the empyema cavity. A chest catheter is then threaded through the trocar, the trocar is removed, and the tube is connected to water-seal drainage (p. 1253). This allows the pus to drain from the cavity into the water-seal bottle. It will only be effective, however, if the pus is thin enough to drain out readily and if the visceral pleura is capable of moving out to the parietal pleura to eliminate the space. When empyema is chronic and the lung is adherent to the chest wall, rib resection with open drainage is often employed. In this procedure a portion of one or two ribs is removed. A large tube is inserted into the cavity and allowed to drain into a chest dressing. The tube is changed weekly. If this method of treatment is successful, the empyema cavity will gradually be eliminated as the space is filled in with granulation tissue. In some instances of chronic empyema a fibrinous peel forms on the visceral pleura, keeping the lung from reexpanding and filling the space left after the empyema cavity was drained. In this situation a *decortication* is performed. In decortication the fibrinous peel is removed from the lung by blunt dissection, freeing the lung so that it can expand and fill the pleural space. In order to ensure that expansion will occur, chest tubes are inserted into the pleural space and connected to water-seal drainage and suction. When there is evidence that the lung has reexpanded, the tubes are removed. (See p. 1254 for further discussion of chest drainage.) If none of these methods are successful in closing the pleural space, a thoracoplasty (removal of ribs) may be necessary. In this case the removal of ribs alters the shape of the thorax and the chest wall is brought inward to obliterate the pleural space.

Fungal infections

There are three major fungal infections of the lungs: *histoplasmosis, coccidioidomycosis,* and *blastomycosis.* They are classified as deep mycoses because there is involvement by the parasite of deeper tissues and internal organs.[142]

Histoplasmosis

Epidemiology and etiology. Histoplasmosis results from the inhalation of spores of *Histoplasma capsulatum* that are carried on air currents. *Histoplasma capsulatum* grows, multiplies, and produces spores in soil that has been contaminated with fowl excreta. The reason for this is unknown. The fowl are not infected, probably because of their higher body temperatures.[142] Bats do become infected, however, and areas where bats deposit feces, such as caves, attics, and hollow trees, can be extremely infectious because of the high concentration of spores.

The incidence of histoplasmosis is quite high in the United States, and it is especially common in certain areas of the central and eastern part of the country. Endemic areas are found in Missouri, Kentucky, Tennessee, southern Illinois, Indiana, and Ohio. It is not communicable from human to human. Organisms are transmitted to humans by inhaling spores that thrive in moist, dark, protected soil contaminated with fowl excreta.

Pathophysiology. The spores are inhaled, phagocytized by alveolar macrophages within which they germinate, form yeast cells, and multiply by budding. In persons previously uninfected there is a primary or initial infection that resembles the infection in primary tuberculosis with involvement of regional lymphatics and early dissemination via lymphatics and blood to other organs. Yeast cells spread hematogenously and are phagocytized by reticuloendothelial cells in the liver, spleen, and bone morrow. The process in the lung is similar to that seen in tuberculosis with necrosis and healing by fibrosis encapsulation. Eventually, the areas show calcification in the original parenchymal foci in the lung and in the hilar lymph nodes. This results in a *Ghon complex* similar to that found in pulmonary tuberculosis (p. 1299). Usually the initial infection is self-limiting and does not require antifungal chemotherapy. However, some persons, such as infants and adults with immunologic incompetence (lymphoma), may develop a rapidly progressive primary infection that will be fatal without antifungal therapy.

Reinfection histoplasmosis and *progressive histoplasmosis* can also occur. Reinfection with *Histoplasma* causes an illness resembling the initial infection. Since some degree of immunity to histoplasmosis is conferred by the initial infection, the extent of disease will be modified by the degree of fungal immunity.[5] Heavy inoculation may cause *pneumonitis*, which is usually self-limiting over days to weeks. The onset is acute with nonproductive cough, fever, malaise, and dyspnea. Some persons who are fully immune may develop a hypersensitivity-like pneumonitis with small discrete granulomatous foci that may give a *miliary* appearance on x-ray examination. This means that the infection is spread throughout the lung giving the appearance of the presence of small millet seeds throughout the lung.

Progressive histoplasmosis is usually chronic; chronic pulmonary histoplasmosis is the most frequently encountered symptomatic form of the disease. It develops almost exclusively in middle-aged white men who have chronic obstructive pulmonary disease. There are recurrent episodes of necrotizing segmental or lobar granulomatous pneumonitis, which have a tendency to cavity formation, contraction, fibrosis, and compensatory emphysema.

Progressive disseminated histoplasmosis usually occurs as a consequence of the initial infection in persons with very low resistance to the infection (infants, persons with immunologic imcompetence). Rarely, it can occur in adults of both sexes and all ages with no known immune disorder. These persons have fever, weakness, weight loss, hepatosplenomegaly, leukopenia, and mucous membrane ulceration involving the oropharynx, tongue, or larynx. Adrenal insufficiency occurs in about 50% of these persons.[5]

Prevention. Nurses working in areas where this disease is prevalent have an important role in helping to locate sources of infection and in teaching the public to prevent inhalation of potentially infected material. Since the disease can be fatal and children appear to be particularly susceptible, the nurse should point out potential danger to rural families when it is known that the soil is contaminated.

Clinical picture. Chest films demonstrate a nodular infiltrate. Special stains are required to see *Histoplasma capsulatum* on sputum smears. Skin tests for histoplas-

mosis are available, but if active disease is suspected, a serum complement fixation test should be obtained rather than using the skin test. Skin testing with histoplasmin is helpful in screening programs. In endemic areas, between 90% and 95% of young adults have positive test results. The signs and symptoms of histoplasmosis show a variable range from those of a slight self-limited infection to fatal disseminated disease. Severe infections are characterized by acute onset, fever, chest pain, dyspnea, prostration, weight loss, widespread pulmonary infiltrates, hepatomegaly, and splenomegaly. Some infected persons may have only a benign acute pneumonitis lasting a week or less, while others may be symptom free.

Intervention. Amphotericin B (Fungizone Intravenous) is the standard therapy for histoplasmosis. The dose and length of therapy are determined by the difficulty in eradicating the different types of *Histoplasma* infections and the likelihood of relapse.[5] The therapy may last 2 to 3 weeks or 2 to 3 months.

Amphotericin B must be given intravenously and has many toxic properties including local phlebitis, systemic reactions, renal toxicity, hypokalemia, and anemia. In rare instances anaphylaxis, bone marrow suppression, and cardiovascular and hepatic toxicity develop.

Systemic toxicity (chills, fever, aching, nausea, and vomiting) can be lessened by premedication with 600 mg of aspirin along with 25 to 50 mg of diphenhydramine (Benadryl) or promethazine (Phenergan) or 10 mg of prochlorperazine (Compazine) orally.[5] Heparin and hydrocortisone succinate (Solu-Cortef) are sometimes added to the infusions to minimize phlebitis.

A reversible azotemia occurs regularly when amphotericin B is administered. The level of azotemia is monitored by biweekly BUN or serum creatinine determinations. A BUN of greater than 40 or a creatinine nearing 3.0 indicates a need to temporarily reduce or stop the drug. Therapy is not continued until the azotemia is improved.[5] Serum potassium levels are checked biweekly, and hypokalemia is treated with oral potassium. Anemia is common, and the hematocrit usually stabilizes at 25% to 35%.[5]

Ketoconazole (Nizoral) is a newer drug, administered orally, that is effective in the treatment of systemic fungal infections. The recommended dosage is 400 mg daily for a minimum of 6 months. Toxicity appears to be minimal; pruritus, minor gastrointestinal intolerance, and liver function abnormalities have been reported. It is not known whether late relapses of histoplasmosis will occur in persons treated with ketoconazole, since the drug has been in use for only a short time.

Resectional pulmonary surgery is seldom required, and it is reserved for patients with adequate pulmonary reserve and residual cavities who are not able to tolerate amphotericin B.[5]

Nursing care of patients with histoplasmosis is determined by their symptoms and their response to therapy with amphotericin B. Because of the toxicity of the drug, the nurse is involved in monitoring the patient for all the side effects described above.

Coccidioidomycosis

Epidemiology and etiology. Coccidioidomycosis (valley fever, San Joaquin Valley fever) is a fungal infection caused by *Coccidioides immitis*. This fungus is endemic to well-defined areas in the southwestern United States, Mexico, and South America. In the United States the endemic areas are the central San Joaquin Valley and southern counties of California, southern Arizona, New Mexico, and southwestern Texas. The spores of *Coccidioides immitis* survive for many months in soil. Heavy rainfall in the desert enhances growth of the fungus and direct sunlight inhibits it.[68] Liberation of dust in the spring disperses the mature arthrospores, which are inhaled into the tracheobronchial tree.

Pathophysiology. The process following inhalation of spores is believed to be very similar to that described under histoplasmosis (p. 1309). The arthrospores reach the alveoli where they are phagocytized. If the disease becomes disseminated there is marked hilar adenopathy and fungi can be isolated from lymph nodes. A pneumonic disease with necrosis and cavitation may occur after development of delayed hypersensitivity.[142] The disease process is controlled and resolved in most persons as the result of cell immunity to infection. Thus progressive disseminated coccidioidomycosis or progressive pulmonary disease is found only in those persons whose ability to resist infection or develop immunity has been compromised in some way. Susceptibility to infection is in part genetically determined. Coccidioidomycosis is 50 times more common in Philippine men and 10 times more common in black men than it is in white men.[142] This increased susceptibility to progressive disease in these groups of men parallels their susceptibility to tuberculosis. The increased susceptibility of some races to diseases such as coccidioidomycosis and tuberculosis is believed to be the result of a genetically determined impairment of their capacity to develop cellular immunity to infection.[142]

Prevention. The only means of protection presently available is the wearing of masks by persons engaged in activities that disturb the desert dust.[68] Archeologists, argicultural workers, construction workers, and others working the the desert should be taught how to protect themselves.

An experimental vaccine is being field tested in Arizona and California. Until it is proved effective, the best protection available is a mechanical barrier such as a mask.[68]

Clinical picture. Coccidioidomycoses causes an asymptomatic upper respiratory tract infection in about 60% of those who inhale the infected dust. The remaining 40% develop symptoms ranging from a flulike illness to frank pneumonia.[68] Fewer than 10% of this latter group require therapy, and the remainder will undergo spontaneous remission of their disease.

Skin testing with coccidioidin, 1:10 or 1:100, is available to test for the disease. The test is read in 48 hours. It takes 3 to 6 weeks after exposure for the test to become positive. In severe disseminated disease the test may be negative indicating that the patient's immune system is no longer able to respond.

Roentgenograms of the chest may exhibit pneumonic infiltrate, hilar adenopathy, pleural effusion, or a cavitary lesion.[68] About 5% of persons with primary pulmonary involvement will have residual lung lesions such as cavities or nodules. Only about 0.5% of infected individuals go on to develop a severe, progressive mycosis.

Intervention. The therapy for coccidioidomycosis is the same as for histoplasmosis, namely, amphotericin B. It is used to treat individuals in whom spontaneous remission is unlikely. These include (1) persons with disseminated disease; (2) those in whom there is a high probability of dissemination (Asiatics, blacks, pregnant women, persons with severe diabetes mellitus, and immunocompromised patients); (3) persons with a severe primary infection characterized by a persistent pneumonic infiltrate lasting longer than 8 weeks, a miliary chest x-ray pattern, a necrotizing pneumonia, or a prolonged course of the disease; and (4) the very young and very old.[68]

The dose of amphotericin B and the duration of treatment are highly individualized. The patient is monitored for the side effects discussed on p. 1310.

Extrapulmonary dissemination of coccidioidomycosis can occur. One of the most frequent sites of dissemination is the meningeal surfaces of the brain. If there is any indication of involvement of the central nervous system, a lumbar puncture is performed. A positive complement fixation titer in the spinal fluid is diagnostic of meningitis.[68]

Dissemination can also occur to skin, soft tissue, and bones, and the patient is monitored by physical examination of the skin, gallium scanning of soft tissues, and bone scans. A bone scan should be performed before starting amphotericin B therapy.

Surgical intervention for localized lesions may involve either excision or drainage to facilitate healing.

Blastomycosis

Epidemiology and etiology. Blastomycosis is caused by the fungus *Blastomyces dermatitidis*. The disease is most prevalent in the United States and Canadian valley areas surrounding the Mississippi, Missouri, Ohio, and St. Lawrence rivers. It is also present in Africa, South America, and Mexico.

The source of infection with *Blastomyces dermatitidis* is not definitely known.[142] Because of the nature of the parasite, and the parallels among blastomycosis, histoplasmosis, and coccidioidomycosis, it is assumed that the microorganism lives and grows in soil, producing spores that are carried by air currents and inhaled by humans and other animals.[142] Dogs can acquire the disease, and the possibility of transmission of the disease from animals to humans cannot be excluded. However, it is most likely that both humans and lower animals are infected from the same source.[142]

Clinical picture. The outstanding clinical feature of blastomycosis is skin lesions that appear initially as small papular or pustular lesions on exposed parts of the body, such as the hands and face.[142] The lesions enlarge peripherally and may become raised. They develop slowly and do not itch.

It is now believed that the initial site of infection is the lung. During the primary infection in the lung *Blastomyces dermatitidis* is disseminated by way of the lymphatics and blood throughout the body. The cutaneous lesions represent metastic infection from the primary pulmonary disease.[142]

Acute pulmonary blastomycosis in the form of a self-limited pneumonia can occur. Otherwise, blastomycosis is a chronic progressive disease with a mortality of about 90% when untreated. For this reason it is recommended that every person in whom the diagnosis is established be treated.[91]

Intervention. The treatment for all forms of blastomycosis is the same as for histoplasmosis and coccidioidomycosis, that is, amphotericin B. The toxic effects of the drug have been discussed under the treatment of histoplasmosis on p. 1310.

Hydrocortisone succinate (Solu-Cortef) may be added to the amphotericin infusion to suppress febrile reactions. Aspirin, diphenhydramine (Benadryl), and prochlorperazine (Compazine) may be prescribed to control fever and nausea as described on p. 1310.

Usually a cumulative dose of 2 g of amphotericin B is recommended for treatment of most forms of blastomycosis.[91] About 10% of patients treated with 2 g of amphotericin will experience a relapse. The drug of choice for retreatment is amphotericin B.[91]

Occupational lung diseases

Epidemiology and etiology

There are many pulmonary diseases that are believed to be caused by substances inhaled in the work place. They are more common (1) in blue-collar workers than in white-collar workers, (2) in industrialized areas than in rural areas, and (3) in small and medium-sized businesses than in larger industrial plants.

In some instances it is debatable whether a person's lung disease is clearly occupation specific. This is especially so in cases of bronchitis, asthma, emphysema, or cancer since all of these conditions can be caused or aggravated by several factors found in many different occupations and by nonoccupational factors such as smoking and pollution of the atmosphere.[12]

Millions of Americans are believed to be suffering from job-related diseases. Since these diseases are not reportable, exact statistics do not exist. The Department of Health and Human Services (HHS) has estimated that 400,000 persons develop job-related diseases each year. They also estimate that there are 100,000 deaths each year from occupational diseases. The National Heart, Lung, and Blood Institute stated in a 1977 report that lung diseases cause more than half of these deaths.[12] Over $5 billion a year is paid out in workers' compensation for job-related illnesses and injuries.[12]

Prevention

Occupational lung diseases are preventable. However, there must be a concerted effort by the public, governmental agencies, and industry if these diseases are to be prevented.

Governmental action has been slow and has only occurred, in some instances, in response to public interest groups that have lobbied for stricter regulation of harmful substances. However, countervailing political pressures have sometimes prevented laws from being passed or have resulted in less strict laws being passed because of the costs involved in meeting the strict standards required to control certain hazards.

The ALA believes that several things need to be done to reduce the incidence of occupational-related lung diseases: (1) education of the public about the relationship between polluted air in the work place and lung diseases; (2) general commitment to reducing, eliminating, or avoiding air pollution of the work place; and (3) elimination of the most prevalent and notorious lung hazard: cigarette smoke.[12]

Education of the public includes not only employers and employees but also engineers and planners who design operations; buyers and purchasers who select ingredients, cleaning agents, and equipment; and physicians who see persons with occupational-related diseases. Many times workers who are instructed about the hazards involved in certain occupations and work places are helpful in deciding what preventive measures need to be taken to combat or minimize the effects of hazards. The commitment to reduce, eliminate, or avoid pollution of work place air requires full consideration of possible health effects whenever operations are planned and improvement of conditions whenever possible.

It is well documented that smokers get occupational lung diseases more often than nonsmokers and that smokers' lungs are more vulnerable to the effects of these diseases than are nonsmokers' lungs. The combined effects of cigarette smoke and industrial pollutants are very great. The risk of developing chronic bronchitis, emphysema, lung cancer, and heart disease is much increased when the worker smokes.[12] Some of these risks, such as lung cancer in asbestos workers who also smoke, are becoming more commonly known.

Occupational lung diseases can be divided into several categories. The major ones are (1) the pneumoconioses, including silicosis and coal miner's pneumoconiosis (black lung disease); (2) asbestos-related lung disease; (3) other pneumoconioses such as chronic berylliosis; (4) mixed-dust pneumoconioses; and (5) hypersensitivity diseases, including occupational asthma, allergic alveolitis (farmer's lung), and byssinosis (brown lung disease). Details about these diseases are presented in Table 51-4.

TABLE 51-4. Major occupational lung diseases*

Type	Etiology and epidemiology	Pathophysiology	Clinical picture and prevention
Pneumoconioses†	1 million people in United States run risk of developing silicosis		
Chronic silicosis	Inhaled silica dust; commonest form seen in miners, foundry workers, and others who inhaled relatively low concentrations of dust for 10-20 yr	Dust accumulated in tissue → tissue reaction with whorl-shaped nodules throughout lungs	Breathlessness with exercise
Complicated silicosis	20-30% of persons with chronic silicosis develop this	Progressive massive fibrosis (PMF) throughout lungs → ↓ lung function and cor pulmonale	Breathlessness, weakness, chest pain, productive cough with sputum, respiratory cripple, dies of heart failure
Acute silicosis	Rapidly progressive disease, leading to severe disability and death within 5 yr of diagnosis	Inflammatory reaction within alveoli, diffuse fibrosis	Early symptoms: difficulty in breathing, weight loss, fever, cough Prevention: dust control, wetting down of mines, and improved ventilation can reduce dust levels; sandblasters in enclosed spaces can use special suits and breathing apparatuses; some experts believe such protective measures are still inadequate
Coal worker's pneumoconiosis (CWP; "black lung disease")	150,000 coal miners in the United States at risk; amount, size, and nature of dust in air vary according to type of coal, machinery, and technique used, efficiency of ventilation, and other dust control measures; 10-30% of all coal miners develop simple form of the disease; more prevalent in miners of anthracite, or hard coal; other minerals found in miner's lung (silica, kaolin, mica, beryllium, copper, cobalt, and others); unknown whether these minerals contribute to development or progression of CWP	Simple CWP: dust accumulation in lungs visible on x-ray film; over years dust piles up and respiratory bronchioles are dilated (called focal emphysema)	Simple CWP: no symptoms, no respiratory difficulty
Complicated CWP or progressive massive fibrosis (PMF)	3% of persons with simple CWP develop complicated form; more often occurs in miners with heavy deposits of coal dust in lungs; may appear suddenly years after miner has	Fibrosis develops in some of dust-laden areas; fibrosis spreads and fibrotic areas coalesce; eventually most of lung is stiffened and useless; silica plays some role in fibrosis	PMF shortens life span; may die from respiratory failure, cor pulmonale, or superimposed infection Prevention: dust control; reduced levels of coal dust can lower simple

*From American Lung Association: Occupational lung diseases: an introduction, New York, 1979, The Association.
†Also known as "dust in the lungs."
‡Asbestos is a fire-proofing and insulating agent.

Continued.

TABLE 51-4. Major occupational lung diseases—cont'd

Type	Etiology and epidemiology	Pathophysiology	Clinical picture and prevention
Complicated CWP or progressive massive fibrosis (PMF)—cont'd	left the mines; can stop suddenly for no discernible reason; smoking seems to have no affect on development of CWP, but smoking has adverse effect on miners' health; miners who smoke have 5-6 times more lung obstruction than non-smoking miners; cigarette smoking causes chronic bronchitis and emphysema as in nonminers	but despite international research, role of silica in CWP is not understood	CWP and reduce number of miners who develop complicated CWP
Asbestos-related lung disease‡	Asbestos is one of the most dangerous occupational hazards; can cause both fibrosis and cancer in asbestos workers; also a general environmental hazard because of its extensive use before health hazards were recognized; most dangerous to those who mine the ores and process the crude material into pure form; no asbestos mines in United States, but it is processed and used in United States; federal agencies and state governments moving to tighten controls on use of asbestos; lung cancer associated with all types of asbestos; 20-25% of deaths of workers with heavy exposure are from lung cancer; cancer is related to degree of asbestosis and to cigarette smoking, which enhances carcinogenic properties of asbestos; asbestos worker who smokes is 90 times as likely to get lung cancer as smoker who never worked with asbestos	Asbestos occurs in several different forms or ores; commercially important ores are chrysolite, crocidolite, and amosite; most hazardous medically are crocidolite and amosite; fibrosis caused by asbestos is called *asbestosis*; asbestos fibers accumulate around terminal bronchioles; body surrounds fibers with iron-rich tissue = asbestos body with characteristic picture on x-ray film; more asbestos bodies as more fibers are inhaled; after 20-30 yr of exposure, fibrosis begins in lungs; if heavy exposure, fibrosis appears in 4-5 yr	After fibrosis begins, cough, sputum, weight loss, increasing breathlessness; most die within 15 yr of first symptoms
	Mesothelioma (cancer of the pleura) accounts for 7-10% of deaths of asbestos workers; inoperable and always fatal; can occur after very little exposure to crocidolite; has been reported in wives of asbestos workers and in persons living near asbestos plants; cigarette smoking not a contributing factor; only a few fine, straight crocidolite fibers are necessary; asbestos workers have a higher incidence of other cancers (esophagus, stomach, and intestines); swallowing of asbestos-contaminated sputum responsible for these cancers	Occurs in persons exposed to crocidolite fibers of a certain size; a few cases involve amosite fibers; needlelike shape of crocidolite fibers enables them to pass through lung tissue to pleura	Prevention: number of asbestos-related diseases has been increasing despite recognition of hazards and dust-control measures; much tighter controls are needed; some countries have taken such steps; there is need for massive efforts to educate general public of dangers of asbestos

Some other pneumoconioses

Type	Etiology and epidemiology	Pathophysiology	Clinical picture and prevention
Aluminum	Inhaled particles of a certain size induce disease		
Beryllium	Greatest risk of exposure in plants that extract beryllium from crude ore; beryllium is metal used in metallurgy, certain machine tools, making of ceramics, and nuclear power industry	Affects most body systems; in lung produces a severe chemical pneumonia after acute exposure; chronic form is called *berylliosis*	

TABLE 51-4. Major occupational lung diseases—cont'd

Type	Etiology and epidemiology	Pathophysiology	Clinical picture and prevention
Chronic berylliosis	Disease of hypersensitivity, unrelated to level of exposure; beryllium exposure also associated with ↑ rates of cancer of lung, liver, and gallbladder	Diffuse fibrosis over 15-20 yr → cor pulmonale	Difficulty in breathing
Talc	Inhaled by miners and millers of crude ore and soapstone and by workers in cosmetic, paint, pottery, asphalt, and rubber industries; high incidence of lung cancer; not known whether high incidence is caused by asbestos in talc or whether increased incidence in those who smoke	*Pure* talc produces a characteristic pneumoconiosis; less fibrosis than with silica inhalation; evaluation of fibrosis is difficult because most talc contains traces of asbestos and silica	
Mixed-dust pneumoconioses	Many workers exposed to a mixture of dusts; foundry, steel, and iron workers inhale dust from a variety of ores and may also inhale fumes; miners exposed to mixed dusts; some workers are exposed to one dust, then change jobs and are exposed to another dust	Individual dusts usually deposit in patterns that can be recognized on x-ray film; mixed dusts result in different patterns; patient's work history important in diagnosing occupational lung diseases	
	Not known whether mixed dusts in lungs are additive (1 + 1 = 2) or potentiating (1 + 1 = 5)	Amount of fibrosis present depends on amount of silica inhaled	
Hypersensitivity diseases	Hypersensitivity diseases fall into occupational category when antigen is found primarily in work place; lung hypersensitivity can occur in bronchi, bronchioles, or alveoli; coarse dust causes bronchial reactions; fine dust provokes small airway and alveolar reactions		
Occupational asthma	More common in the 10% of the population who are atopic (genetic tendency to develop an allergy); nonatopic persons can also become sensitized; substances with antigenic properties include detergent enzymes, platinum salts, cereals and grains, certain wood dusts, isocyanate chemicals used in polyurethane paints and other products, agents used in printing, and some pesticides	Hypersensitivity reaction mediated by histamine → bronchoconstriction and ↑ mucous production; repeated attacks if cause unrecognized and asthma is untreated may lead to permanent obstructive lung disease; asthmatic response that is well established can be provoked by other factors (house dust, cigarette smoke) and by fatigue, breathing cold air, and coughing	Wheezing is major symptom Prevention: total elimination of antigen; desensitization not successful
Allergic alveolitis (farmer's lung)	Hypersensitivity disease caused by fine organic dust inhaled into smallest airways; cause of farmer's lung is moldy hay; other dusts can cause allergic alveolitis: these include moldy sugar cane and barley, maple bark, cork, animal hair, bird feathers and droppings, mushroom compost, coffee beans, and paprika; often disease is named for cause (mushroom, worker's lung, etc.); fungus spores growing in the apparent antigen are thought in many cases to be real cause of the disease	Alveoli are inflamed, inundated by WBCs, sometimes filled with fluid; if exposure infrequent or level of dust low, symptoms are mild, and treatment not sought, chronic form develops over times; eventually, fibrosis occurs, and fibrosis may be so well established that it cannot be arrested	Symptoms begin some hours after exposure to offending dust and include fatigue, shortness of breath, dry cough, fever, and chills; symptoms may be severe enough to require emergency treatment and hospitalization; acute attacks treated with steroids; recovery may take 6 wk and patient may suffer residual lung damage; real cure is permanent separation of patient and antigen Prevention: Properly dried and stored farm products (hay, straw, sugar cane) do not cause allergic alveolitis; presumably fungi only grow in moist conditions

Continued.

TABLE 51-4. Major occupational lung diseases—cont'd

Type	Etiology and epidemiology	Pathophysiology	Clinical picture and prevention
Byssinosis (brown lung)	Occupational disease occurs in textile workers; mainly in cotton workers but also afflicts workers in flax and hemp industries; cause is found in bales of raw cotton that contain not only cotton fibers but fragments of cotton plant; something in plant matter, rather than pure cotton, is cause	Chronic bronchitis and emphysema develop in time; constriction of bronchioles in response to something in crude cotton; symptoms of asthma and allergy persist as long as there is exposure to cotton antigen	Tightness in chest on returning to work after a weekend away (Monday fever); strong relationship between amount of dust inhaled and symptoms; persistent productive tight chest with chronic bronchitis and emphysema; person leaves industry as respiratory cripple Prevention: dust control measures; pretreating bales of cotton by washing with steam and other agents may inactivate causative agent; try to detect persons who are likely to become sensitized to cotton dust and keep them out of high-risk areas

Other restrictive diseases

Sarcoidosis

Epidemiology and etiology

Sarcoidosis is a systemic granulomatous disease. Although the cause is unknown, there is evidence of an antigen-antibody reaction manifested by reticuloendothelial response in which both thymus-derived (T) cells and plasma (B) cells participate[140] (see Chapter 19 for more information). It is believed that the antigen is airborne because bilateral hilar lymphadenopathy is frequently present at the onset and bronchopulmonary macrophages are increased.[140]

Although sarcoidosis is worldwide in distribution, it is most likely to be diagnosed where the medical community is alert to the disease and diagnostic facilities are available. It is most common in adults between 20 and 40 years of age. The incidence is almost equal in men and women, but it is twice as common in women in childbearing years. In the United States, it is 10 times more common in blacks than in whites. There is some evidence that the incidence is higher in blacks than whites in other parts of the world, especially if the disease is sought out.[140]

Clinical picture

The central pathologic event involves the growth of granulomas and proliferation of lymph tissue. Sarcoidosis commonly is seen on chest x-ray films as enlarged lymph nodes in the hilar area. The patient with sarcoidosis may initially complain only of vague symptoms of malaise, fever, aching in the joints, or weakness. In addition to mediastinal lymph node enlargement, ocular manifestations, such as uveitis and conjunctivitis, and dermatologic changes, such as erythema nodosum, are commonly found.

Diagnosis of sarcoidosis is based on roentgenographic findings, organ biopsy, and positive skin test. The Kveim-Siltzback test involves the injection of sarcoid tissue; if the reaction is positive, a visible, palpable nodule develops at the site 3 to 6 weeks after the antigen is injected. A biopsy of the nodule must then be done to confirm the presence of granulomatous tissue. The Kveim-Siltzback test is not always performed as part of the diagnostic process, however, because it is difficult to obtain the active antigen and because the test is associated with frequent false-negative results. Organ biopsy yields the most conclusive evidence of sarcoidosis and is most helpful in differentiating it from Hodgkin's disease and tuberculosis.

Intervention

In most cases, sarcoidosis is a benign, self-limiting process that resolves with no residual damage within 2 years of diagnosis. However, about 10% of patients do have the chronic form of sarcoidosis. In this form, the disease proceeds to nodular granulomatous depositions in lung tissue and eventual pulmonary fibrosis. In severe cases, this will advance to pulmonary hypertension and right ventricular failure (cor pulmonale). The only treatment available at this time is the administration of corticosteroids. Nursing care is similar to that of the patient with pulmonary fibrosis and includes teaching the patient about the use of the corticosteroids.

Fibrosing alveolitis

Epidemiology and etiology

Fibrosing alveolitis (interstitial pneumonitis) is a disease of unknown etiology with a poor prognosis. It occurs mainly in persons over 40 years of age, and men and women are equally affected.

Pathophysiology

Fibrosing alveolitis is characterized by inflammation of the alveoli resulting in cellular thickening of alveolar walls with a tendency toward fibrosis. The cellular infiltrate contains lymphocytes, plasma cells, and granulocytes.[69] Serum rheumatoid factor, antinuclear factor, and circulating immune complexes are sometimes present. Fibrosing alveolitis can be associated with the collagen diseases. It is also known as interstitial fibrosis or pulmonary fibrosis.

Clinical picture

The patient becomes progressively short of breath because of the reduction in the size of the lungs and reduction in the amount of alveolar-capillary membrane available for gas exchange. Blood gas findings demonstrate hypoxemia and often hypercapnia. Clubbing of the fingers is common, and cardiac complications may develop.

Intervention

There is no cure and no specific treatment for fibrosing alveolitis since the cause is unknown. Persons who have circulating immune complexes or have abnormal cells on lung biopsy may show improvement if given adrenocorticosteroids. Patients usually must curb activities because of dyspnea, and they should be advised to guard against exposure to respiratory tract infections, since an infection could be fatal.

Cancer of the lung

Epidemiology and etiology

During the last 45 years there has been a startling increase in the incidence of cancer of the lung.

The American Cancer Society estimates 129,000 new cases in 1982 and 11,000 deaths. It is also estimated that by the mid 1980s lung cancer may well surpass breast cancer as the number one killer of women.[8] Cancer is the leading cause of death in men with the rate per 100,000 population increasing by 172% from the period of 1951 to 1953 to the period of 1976 to 1978. In that same period of time there was a 256% increase in the number of deaths from lung cancer in women. Thus it is clearly evident that the death rate is increasing at a much faster rate in women. The increase in death rates for both men and woman is directly related to cig-

TABLE 51-5. Deaths caused by lung cancer, according to smoking habits*

	Deaths per 100,000 population
Nonsmokers	3.4
10-20 cigarettes per day	54.3
20-40 (1-2 packs) per day	143.9
More than 40 (2 packs) per day	217.3

*From American Cancer Society: Cancer facts and figures, New York, 1976, The Society.

arette smoking. A history of smoking, especially for 20 years or more, is considered to be a prime risk factor. Other risk factors include exposure to certain industrial substances such as asbestos, particularly in those who smoke (p. 1314).

The mortality of persons with lung cancer is primarily dependent on the specific type of cancer and the size of the tumor when detected. Squamous cell carcinoma is the most common, followed by adenocarcinoma; undifferentiated small cell (oat cell) carcinoma is the least common and has the lowest 5-year survival rate (less than 1%). If the tumor is of the squamous cell type and is detected while still small and localized (less than 3 cm), the 5-year survival rate is as high as 40%.[58] Most people who develop the disease are over 50 years of age. Some of the factors believed to be involved in the increased incidence of cancer of the lung include an increase in smoking among women, more accurate diagnosis, and a tendency to name the lung as the primary site.

Cancer of the lung may be either metastatic or primary. Metastatic tumors may follow malignancy anywhere in the body. Metastasis from the colon and kidney is common. Metastasis to the lung may be discovered before the primary lesion is known, and sometimes the location of the primary lesion is not determined during the person's life.

Prevention

The cause of cancer of the lung is closely related to cigarette smoking. Table 51-5 shows the extreme increase in mortality from lung cancer in those persons who smoke. Prevention is the best protection against cancer of the lung because early detection of the disease if difficult, and at the present time only about 1 person in 9 (9%) is "cured" (living at the end of 5 years). From available research data it seems evident that curtailing smoking is a primary preventive measure. The nurse should be active in teaching the dangers of smoking and should set a positive health example in this regard. It is especially important that teenagers be given specific facts concerning the dangers involved in cigarette smoking, because they are not likely to be habitual smokers at that age. Recent studies indicate that the incidence of smoking among teenagers is increasing. People who are already habitual smokers should also be urged to stop smoking, although it may be difficult for them to do so. Various types of programs to assist persons to stop smoking are available. Since air pollution affects the lungs and may predispose to the development of cancer the nurse should encourage and actively support community programs to decrease the amount of air pollution.

Clinical picture

Since most new growths in the lungs arise from the bronchi, the term *bronchogenic carcinoma* is widely used. The symptoms that a patient has will depend on whether the neoplasm is located peripherally or centrally. Peripheral lesions may not cause any symptoms and be discovered only on routine chest roentgenograms. If peripheral lesions perforate into the pleural space, there will be *pleural effusion* (fluid in the pleural space), and direct invasion of the ribs and vertebral bodies may follow. If this occurs, the pain may be severe.

Centrally located lesions arise from one of the larger branches of the bronchial tree. They cause obstruction and ulceration of the bronchus with subsequent distal suppuration. Symptoms include cough, hemoptysis, dyspnea, chills, and fever. Unilateral wheezing may be heard on auscultation.

In the later stage of the disease, weight loss and debility usually indicate metastases, especially to the liver. Cancer of the lung may metastasize to nearby structures such as the prescalene lymph nodes, the walls of the esophagus, and the pericardium of the heart or to distant areas such as the brain, liver, or skeleton.

Intervention

Time is very important in the treatment of lung cancer. If cancer is detected while it is still confined to a local area, immediate surgery, with removal of all or part of a lung (pneumonectomy or lobectomy), may be successful. Unfortunately, most patients are not seen by a surgeon early enough. It is estimated that one third of the patients are inoperable when first seen, and one third are found to be inoperable on exploratory thoracotomy. Of the third who are operable, the surgical mortality is 10% for pneumonectomy and 2% to 3% for lobectomy. The nursing care of the patient following surgery of the lung is discussed on p. 1252.

Palliative treatment (irradiation, chemotherapy, or both) may be used for those persons who cannot be treated surgically, particularly when there is obstruction of an airway, obstruction of major vessels, severe pain, or recurrent pleural effusion. Presently, about one third of the patients who have surgery experience tumor spread. Radiation and chemotherapy are frequently prescribed for these patients.[8] Experimental studies with immunotherapy as an adjuvant to surgery and radiotherapy are also under way.

Efforts to detect malignant lesions of the lung early, while curative treatment may be possible, must be continued. The nurse should urge all persons over 40 years of age to have an x-ray examination of the chest periodically in addition to a yearly physical examination. As a result of various public education media, many people have become more conscious of early signs of pulmonary cancer, but there is still a great need for them to learn about diagnostic tests that are available, including x-ray examinations, bronchoscopic examinations, and cytologic studies of sputum. The nurse should know of available cancer detection clinics in the community and should assist patients to secure proper medical supervision (see Chapter 25).

Adult respiratory distress syndrome

Epidemiology and etiology

Adult respiratory distress syndrome (ARDS) was first described by T.L. Petty in 1967. ARDS is often fatal and is characterized by severe dyspnea, hypoxemia, and diffuse bilateral pulmonary infiltrations following lung injury in previously healthy persons.[94] Before 1967, what is now known as ARDS was known by several other names including pump lung, traumatic wet lung, shock lung, progressive pulmonary congestion, and Da Nang lung.

Etiologic factors that lead to ARDS include shock from any cause, multisystem trauma, overwhelming infection, overdoses of drugs, inhaled substances, and pulmonary infections including bacterial and nonbacterial pneumonia.[94] The box on p. 1319 summarizes the clinical conditions associated with ARDS.

Pathophysiology

In ARDS, several changes occur. First, there is damage to the alveolar-capillary membrane. The damage can be on either the alveolar or capillary side of the membrane. Second, as a result of damage to the alveolar-capillary membrane, there is an increase in vascular permeability, and fluid may leak into the interstitial space and into the alveoli causing pulmonary edema. Fluid and red blood cells can be found in the interstitial space and in the alveoli. Later, hyaline membranes (made up of proteins, mainly fibrinogen) that have leaked into the alveoli are seen.[94] The alveolar-capillary damage and the presence of interstitial and pulmonary edema impair gas exchange between the alveoli and the capillaries, and ventilation-perfusion abnormalities result (p. 1221). Third,

CLINICAL CONDITIONS ASSOCIATED WITH ARDS*

1. Shock
   a. Septic
   b. Hemorrhagic
   c. Cardiogenic
   d. Anaphylactic
2. Trauma
   a. Pulmonary contusion
   b. Nonpulmonary, multisystem
3. Infection
   a. Pneumonia
      (1) Viral
      (2) Bacterial (staphylococcal or streptococcal)
      (3) Legionellosis
   b. Miliary tuberculosis
4. Disseminated intravascular coagulation (DIC)
5. Fat emboli
6. Near-drowning
7. Aspiration: highly acid gastric contents (pH < 2.5)
8. Inhaled toxic agents
   a. Smoke
   b. Phosgene
   c. Oxides of nitrogen
9. Pancreatitis
10. Oxygen toxicity
11. Narcotic drug abuse
   a. Heroin
   b. Methadone
   c. Propoxyphene (Darvon)
12. Radiation pneumonitis
13. Drugs
   a. Ethchlorvynol
   b. Salicylates

*Adapted from Petty, T.L.: Adult respiratory distress syndrome. In Kryger, M.: Pathophysiology of respiration, New York, 1981, John Wiley & Sons, Inc.

surfactant is inactivated resulting in an increase in surface tension and collapse of alveoli, especially smaller ones that are more dependent on surfactant to reduce their surface tension and keep them open. As areas of the lung become atelectatic, it is more difficult to inflate them with each breath, compliance decreases, and the work of breathing increases. The atelectasis also further increases the ventilation-perfusion disparity. The end result of these processes is severe hypoxemia, which is resistant to oxygen therapy. These changes are summarized in Fig. 51-4.

There are many similarities between infantile respiratory distress syndrome (IRDS) and ARDS. For example, deficient surfactant plays a major role in IRDS. In both ARDS and IRDS there is congestive atelectasis, alveolar debris, and hyaline membrane formation. The approach to treatment is comparable in IRDS and ARDS.[94]

Clinical picture

As mentioned earlier, ARDS occurs in previously healthy persons. There is usually a latent period of 18 to 24 hours from the time of lung injury to the development of symptoms. Tachypnea, labored breathing, air hunger, and cyanosis are all present, and arterial blood gas studies confirm hypoxemia. The chest x-ray film shows diffuse, bilateral, and usually symmetric interstitial and alveolar infiltrations. These x-ray findings are commonly described as a "wet snowstorm."

Intervention

Patients with ARDS are critically ill and require mechanical ventilatory support. They are best cared for in an intensive care unit. The airway is secured with either an endotracheal tube or a tracheostomy to which a volume-cycled ventilator is attached. The tidal volume is usually set at 10 to 12 cc/kg of body weight with

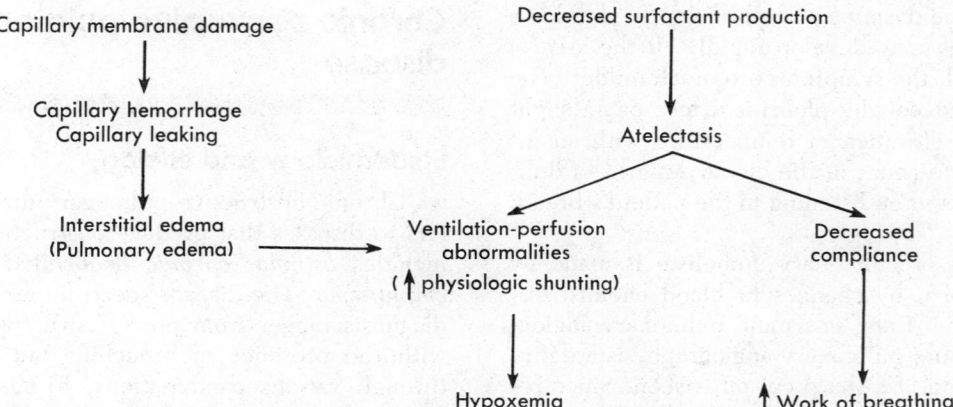

Fig. 51-4. Pathophysiologic events in adult respiratory distress syndrome.

a patient-initiated respiratory rate.[94] Positive end-expiratory pressure (PEEP) is usually used, and this and other therapeutic measures are the same as those for any patient in respiratory failure (p. 1331).

Pulmonary embolism and pulmonary infarction

Epidemiology and etiology

Pulmonary embolism is the lodgement of a clot or other foreign matter in a pulmonary arterial vessel, and pulmonary infarction is the hemorrhagic necrosis of a part of the lung parenchyma caused by interruption of its blood supply, usually as a result of embolism.

The source of the embolism may be thrombi originating in the iliac, femoral, or pelvic veins, the prostatic venous plexus; the vena cava; and the right atrium. They are common in older persons who are confined to bed. Postoperative embolism usually comes from a thrombosed vein in the pelvis or the lower extremities. It may cause symptoms before any signs of venous thrombosis appear at its place of origin.

Pathophysiology

The size of the pulmonary artery in which the clot lodges and the number of emboli determine the severity of symptoms and the prognosis. If the embolus blocks the pulmonary artery or one of its main branches, immediate death may occur, and it is often mistaken for a coronary occlusion. The actual incidence of pulmonary emboli is difficult to determine; many small emboli remain undiagnosed. Depending on the population studied, the occurrence in hospitalized patients may be as high as 14%.[141]

Clinical picture

If the embolus blocks a smaller vessel, the person may complain of sudden sharp upper abdominal or thoracic pain, become dyspneic, cough violently, and have hemoptysis; shock may develop rapidly. If the area of infarction is small, the symptoms are much milder. The patient may have cough, pleuritic chest pain, slight hemoptysis, and elevation of temperature with an increase of leukocyte count in the blood. An area of dullness can be detected on listening to the patient's breath sounds.

The diagnosis of pulmonary embolism is made by the clinical history, by changes in blood chemistries, and by chest films. Lung scans and pulmonary angiography are also done; pulmonary angiography is a definitive diagnostic tool if a sharp cut-off is seen. Since recannulization often takes place rapidly, the procedure must be done in the acute phase, or else it may be negative. The diagnosis of pulmonary embolism is often, of necessity, based on clinical criteria alone.

Intervention

If the person survives a severe pulmonary infarction, immediate medical attention is required. While awaiting the physician, the person should be kept in bed and as quiet as possible. High Fowler's position usually helps breathing. The subsequent medical and nursing care is similar to that needed by the person who has an acute myocardial infarction (p. 1118). If the infarction is a mild one, the treatment is more conservative and resembles that provided for the patient with pneumonia. In either case an immediate attempt is made to locate the original source of the embolus and to treat the thrombosis with anticoagulants. (See references 75 and 140 for a detailed discussion of therapy.)

The development of techniques to provide extracorporeal circulation (p. 1091) has made it possible to remove emboli from the pulmonary arteries—a major step forward, since pulmonary emboli cause many deaths. At present this surgery is done rarely. The nursing care following pulmonary artery surgery combines that needed after any operation on major blood vessels and the postoperative care of patients having thoracic surgery as well as the care of the patient being treated medically for pulmonary embolism.

Another optional treatment for recurrent emboli is the placement of a venacaval umbrella, which is discussed on p. 1161.

The best treatment for pulmonary embolism is prevention. Prevention of thrombophlebitis in patients undergoing surgery is discussed on p. 412. The same nursing measures should be used to prevent emboli in patients, especially when the patient is elderly and has chronic vascular or heart disease.

OBSTRUCTIVE LUNG DISEASES

Chronic obstructive pulmonary disease

Epidemiology and etiology

Chronic obstructive pulmonary disease (COPD) refers to diseases that produce obstruction of airflow and includes *asthma, chronic bronchitis,* and *pulmonary emphysema.* The disease spectrum associated with this diagnosis ranges from pure obstructive airway disease with the presence of bronchitis but no emphysema, through various combinations, to severe emphysema without bronchitis. The pathophysiologic processes that cause these changes are neither static nor are they necessarily progressive. Thus all stages are possible, from reversible abnormalities to relentlessly progressive cardiopulmonary insufficiency. There has been much confusion concerning the clinical usage of the terms chronic bronchitis, emphysema, and asthma; therefore the term *chronic obstructive pulmonary disease* is now frequently used rather than a designation of the specific disease. However, as more is being learned regarding the pathophysiologic factors involved in these diseases, the trend is once again to define each specific abnormality more precisely.[118] These diseases often begin insidiously and progress slowly. Early symptoms may be only a slight morning cough and slight shortness of breath on exertion that is not noticed, because the person has gradually reduced activities to compensate for shortness of breath. By the time medical attention is sought, pathologic changes have occurred and symptoms are often moderately severe.

The incidence of COPD has increased spectacularly in recent years. Both the prevalence of COPD and the death rate attributed to it have reached epidemic proportions according to the ALA.[10] During the 1970s, there was a sevenfold increase in the mortality attributed to COPD, and in 1980 COPD was the sixth leading cause of death following heart disease, neoplasms, strokes, accidents, and influenza-pneumonia.[10]

This increase in death rate from COPD is believed to be related to (1) the growing tendency of physicians to list it as a primary cause of death, (2) the greater use of pulmonary function testing, and (3) more emphasis in medical literature on the importance of this syndrome.[10] Despite these facts, it is believed that the mortality is even higher than reported since many persons who were reported to have died from pneumonia, asthma, or congestive heart failure probably had COPD. The major factors in this increase in mortality, in addition to improved reporting and the increased aging of the population, is an increase in cigarette smoking.[10] These diseases are more prevalent among men than women, but death rates are now showing a higher percentage rate of increase in women than in men. This is believed to be directly related to the increase in smoking among women.

Chronic bronchitis and emphysema

Chronic bronchitis and emphysema are discussed together for a number of reasons: they are difficult to differentiate clinically; they often coexist in the same individual; and many of the medical and nursing care measures are similar. In specifying the differences that do exist, however, it is helpful to examine the effect that each disease has on the individual.

Chronic bronchitis

Chronic bronchitis is defined *symptomatically* by hypersecretion of mucus and recurrent or chronic productive cough for a minimum of 3 months per year for at least 2 consecutive years in patients in whom other causes have been excluded. It is characterized *physiologically* by hypertrophy and hypersecretion of bronchial mucous glands.

Epidemiology and etiology

Chronic bronchitis is caused by the inhalation of physical or chemical irritants or by viral or bacterial infections. The most common inhaled irritant is cigarette smoke, and heavy cigarette smoking is believed to be the major etiologic factor. Occupations in which dust or other irritants are inhaled may cause bronchitis, but the evidence for this is not conclusive.[53] However, in Great Britain it has been recognized for years that the highest incidence of bronchitis occurs in large industrial cities.

Pathophysiology

Persons with chronic bronchitis are susceptible to infection because of their inability to clear their bronchial tree of excess mucus. Bacteria proliferate in the mucous secretions in the lumen of the bronchi. The most common infectious agents are *Streptococcus pneumoniae* and *Haemophilus influenzae*. As bacteria multiply, they exert a neutrophilic chemotaxis, and pus cells migrate from between bronchial epithelial cells to produce a mucopurulent exudate in the lumen, or it may progress to ulceration and destruction of the bronchial wall. When this occurs, granulation and fibrotic tissue replace the normal ciliated epithelium with flattened squamous epithelium.[53] The scarring in the airways leads to stenosis and airway obstruction. Small airways may be completely obliterated and others may become dilated. This chain of events further traps secretions and promotes multiplication of bacteria. Airway obstruction will occur first in airways that are less than 2 mm in diameter.[53] Small airway obstruction can be detected only by pulmonary function tests, and this is why symptoms alone are not sufficient to establish the diagnosis.

Clinical picture

The earliest symptom of chronic bronchitis is a productive cough, especially on awakening. This symptom is often ignored by cigarette smokers who become so accustomed to an early morning cough that they take it for granted; and some of them even refer to it as their "cigarette cough."

Often it is only when the person develops a respiratory infection that he or she seeks medical attention. As chronic bronchitis progresses in severity, there is significant physical incapacitation and breathlessness even when walking on a level surface. The patient is noticeably short of breath, uses accessory muscles of respiration, and complains of a persistent cough and sputum production. Cyanosis is common, and the person appears stout or overweight often from retained fluid. For this reason they are sometimes referred to as "blue bloaters."

Pulmonary function studies demonstrate reduced expiratory flow rates, reduced vital capacity, and increased residual volume, but the total lung capacity is frequently within normal limits. As the disease progresses, hypoventilation occurs and arterial blood gases usually show a low *resting* PO_2, and if the obstruction is severe, an *elevated* PCO_2. During exercise the PCO_2 increases and the PO_2 may also rise, perhaps because of an improvement in ventilation-perfusion relationships. Cor pulmonale (right ventricular hypertrophy, which develops as the result of increased pulmonary vascular resistance in response to hypoxemia and hypercapnia), right-sided heart failure, and respiratory failure are also frequent complications of chronic bronchitis.

Intervention

The goals of treatment for the patient with chronic bronchitis are to (1) improve the patient's symptoms, (2) improve the ability to carry out ADL, and (3) reduce the progression of the disease when the disease is detected early.[53] Specifics of therapy are presented after the discussion on emphysema since the treatment for both of these diseases is similar.

Emphysema

Emphysema is defined *pathologically* by destructive changes in alveolar walls and enlargement of air spaces distal to the terminal nonrespiratory bronchioles. It is characterized *physiologically* by increased lung compliance, decreased diffusing capacity, and increased airway resistance.

Epidemiology and etiology

The etiology of emphysema is not known; however, recent evidence suggests that proteases released by polymorphonuclear leukocytes or alveolar macrophages are involved in the destruction of the connective tissue of the lungs. Connective tissue in the lungs is composed primarily of elastin, collagen, and proteoglycan, which can be damaged and destroyed by enzymes such as proteases and elastase. It has been demonstrated that elastase (produced by alveolar macrophages) can destroy or damage the elastin in the connective tissue of the parenchyma of the lung.[53] Normally, inhibitors found in human serum, lung tissue, peripheral airways, and bronchial mucus protect the lung from the proteolytic enzymes. It is believed that some change in the en-

zyme-inhibitor balance occurs, which allows the proteolytic enzymes to attack lung tissue.

It has been known since 1965 that some persons have a deficiency of α_1-antitrypsin and that these persons develop severe, disabling emphysema early in life, usually of the bullous type. Recent studies indicate that cigarette smoke increases the amount of elastase secreted by the alveolar macrophages and neutrophils and that it impairs the inhibitor functions of α_1-antitrypsin.[53]

It is not known, however, why some smokers develop bronchitis and others develop emphysema. Differences in susceptibility and the predominant type of disease are believed to be influenced by hereditary or environmental factors or those related to the patient's history.[53] It is established, however, that there is familial tendency to α_1-antitrypsin deficiency and that relatives of persons with this type of emphysema should be screened and provided with counseling.[74,81]

Pathophysiology

The diagnosis of emphysema is inferred from pulmonary function tests that show a decrease in airflow. The type of emphysema can be determied only by descriptive morphology. There are two principal types of emphysema morphologically—*centrilobular* emphysema (CLE) and *panlobular* emphysema (PLE). In CLE, there is distention and damage of the respiratory bronchioles selectively. Openings develop in the walls of the bronchioles; they become enlarged and confluent and tend to form a single space as the walls enlarge. The disease tends to be unevenly distributed throughout the lung but usually is more severe in the upper portions.

In PLE, there is a more uniform enlargement and destruction of the alveoli in the pulmonary acinus. PLE is usually more diffuse and is more severe in the lower lung. It is found in elderly persons who have no evidence of chronic bronchitis or impairment of lung function.[10] It occurs just as commonly in women as in men, but PLE is less frequent than CLE. PLE is a characteristic finding in persons with homozygous α_1-antitrypsin deficiency.[10]

Clinical picture

Because of destruction of tissue, there is physiologic obstruction by collapse of airways on expiration. As a result, full exhalation is difficult, and air trapping ensues. Pulmonary function studies demonstrate decreased expiratory flow rates, particularly forced expiratory volume and maximal midexpiratory flow, increased total lung capacity, and increased residual volume (p. 1220). The vital capacity may be normal or only slightly reduced until late stages of the disease; thus the FEV_1/VC ratio is changed. Arterial blood gas tests of persons with emphysema usually show a normal PCO_2 and a PO_2 that is normal or only slightly low *at rest* but falls during *exercise*. Late in the course of the disease the PCO_2 is elevated, and cor pulmonale and respiratory failure may arise as complications.

Clinically, cough and sputum production *are not* striking symptoms unless there is a superimposed infection. Because of the increased total lung capacity, the diaphragm becomes relatively fixed in a flattened position. Many patients use abdominal muscles as well as other accessory muscles to aid breathing. Pursed-lip breathing is often used naturally by the patient since this aids exhalation. (Pursed-lip breathing on exhalation slows expiratory flow rates and results in less of an increase in intrathoracic pressure that "pushes in" on the airways.) Patients with emphysema are often not as cyanotic as patients with bronchitis; they are usually thin and often have a barrel chest. Because *resting* hypoxemia is absent and ventilation is high, these patients maintain a normal PCO_2 despite abnormal gas exchange function and are frequently termed "pink puffers."

Although the terms "blue bloater" and "pink puffer" have been used above, these are not pure types and represent the two extremes seen in persons with chronic airway obstruction. Rencently, it has been suggested that it is not the underlying disease alone that determines whether the person is "blue" or "pink," but it is the interaction between the lung disease and the drive to breathe. For example, the pink puffer may just fight harder to maintain a normal PCO_2, while the blue bloater settles for less work and allows the PCO_2 to rise.

Intervention

Therapy for persons with chronic airway obstruction centers around general supportive measures, medications, respiratory therapy, and physical conditioning and rehabilitation.[10]

Supportive measures. General supportive measures include the following: patient and family education, avoidance of smoking and other inhaled irritants, avoidance of infection, proper environment, adequate hydration, and proper nutrition.

PATIENT AND FAMILY EDUCATION. The patient and family need to understand the nature of the disease and how the patient can manage at home.

AVOIDANCE OF SMOKING. Encouraging the patient who smokes to stop smoking should be a goal of every health care provider. It is not easy for some people to stop smoking, and much support may be needed. Local branches of the ALA and the ACS are good sources of information regarding clinics and workshops designed to assist people to stop smoking. It may be helpful for the nurse to know that no technique for stopping smoking is superior to another, and the method needs to be tailored to the individual. Studies indicate that older persons are more likely to quit smoking than are younger persons, men have more success in quitting permanently than do women, and persons with chronic

diseases are more likely to quit smoking than are healthy persons.[53]

AVOIDANCE OF INHALED IRRITANTS. As discussed earlier, inhalation of grain dust with cigarette smoke increases the risk of developing COPD (p. 1315); smoking and working with asbestos also increase the risk of lung cancer (p. 1314). Air pollution is a common problem in modern civilization and warnings are issued regularly on television to persons with chronic lung or heart disease to avoid being outdoors when the pollution index is high. For persons with symptomatic COPD, their home and work environments should be kept as free of pollutants as possible. High-efficiency particulate air filters or electrostatic filters are effective in removing particulate matter from the air. When offending fumes and odors or gas pollutants are a problem, an activated charcoal filter can be helpful. Since electrostatic filters may produce ozone, an activated charcoal filter may need to be attached distal to the electrostatic filter to minimize the concentrations of ozone in the air.[53]

AVOIDANCE OF INFECTION. Persons with COPD need to avoid exposure to respiratory tract infections since such infections may exacerbate their symptoms and result in further irreversible damage. In some patients, a respiratory tract infection may be so severe that patients will need to be hospitalized. When respiratory tract infections are prevalent in the community, the patient should avoid crowds and minimize intimate contact with young children who are common carriers of viruses uncommon to adults. It is recommended that all persons with COPD have annual influenza immunizations unless there are contraindications to this as discussed on p. 1296.

PROPER ENVIRONMENT. Abrupt changes in the weather or hot or cold environments can increase sputum production and bronchial obstruction. For optimal mucociliary function, a humidity of 30% to 50% is ideal. This can be maintained by the use of a humidifier during the winter months when heating air reduces the humidity in the air. A humidifer is also helpful in hot, dry climates. An air conditioner may reduce dyspnea in many patients with COPD because it controls temperatures and prevents pollutants from the outside air from entering. In cold weather, the patient may be helped by wearing a scarf over the nose and mouth to warm the air. Because of the effects of high altitudes on arterial oxygen levels, persons with COPD living in such areas may be advised to move to a lower altitude or to use supplemental oxygen continuously. When air travel is planned, supplemental oxygen may be necessary, and the airline needs to be informed of this in advance.

PROPER NUTRITION. The patient with COPD should maintain normal weight as much as possible. Persons who are overweight are more likely to be tired and dyspneic. Eating is difficult for persons who are chronically short of breath, and many patients with severe COPD suffer from anorexia. Frequent small feedings of high-protein foods are desirable. Heavy meals and foods that the patient perceives cause "gas" and abdominal distention should be avoided. In some patients, milk appears to increase respiratory tract secretions and will need to be curtailed.

ADEQUATE HYDRATION. It is generally believed that an adequate fluid intake is helpful in thinning secretions; thus it is a good expectorant. However, there is little objective evidence to support this concept.[53] Nevertheless, many physicians recommend an intake of 2 to 2.5 L of fluid daily unless contraindicated. Persons with *cor pulmonale* may have fluids restricted. Some persons with COPD will develop bronchospasm or an increase in secretions when drinking very hot or cold fluids, and these will need to be avoided.

Specific therapy

MEDICATIONS. The types of medications that may be prescribed for persons with COPD include bronchodilators, expectorants, antimicrobials, corticosteroids, digitalis, diuretics, and psychopharmacologic agents.

There are two basic categories of *bronchodilators*—sympathomimetic (adrenergic) agents and xanthine compounds. These bronchodilators act at different sites and appear to work synergistically when used together.[10] Table 51-6 lists the commonly used bronchodilators and their mode of action. Adrenergic agents that work at β_2-sites located in smooth muscles of the airways have fewer cardiac side effects than do β_1-agents whose receptor sites are in the myocardium. For this reason, isoetharine, metaproterenol sulfate, and terbutaline sulfate may be prescribed for patients with hypertension and those who have excessive palpitations or tachycardia from β_1-agents.

TABLE 51-6. Bronchodilators commonly used to treat COPD

Name	Mode of action
Methylxanthines	
Aminophylline	Block action of phosphodiesterase and interfere with degradation of cyclic AMP, resulting in bronchodilation
Theophylline	
Dyphylline	
Sympathomimetics*	
β_1-receptor sites	Activate adenylcyclase leading to increased production of cyclic AMP, resulting in relaxation of smooth muscle of airway; increase in cyclic AMP also inhibits release of chemical mediators that cause bronchospasm (histamine and SRS-A)
Epinephrine (adrenaline HCl)	
Isoproterenol (Isuprel)	
β_2-receptor sites	
Terbutaline (Brethine)	
Metaproterenol (Alupent)	
Isoetharine (Bronkosol)	

*β-adrenergic drugs.

Although *expectorants* are sometimes prescribed, some experts believe they do more harm than good.[53] Water is still considered to be the best expectorant, and adequate hydration without fluid overload as mentioned above should be encouraged.

Antimicrobials are prescribed to treat respiratory tract infections in persons with COPD. The most commonly used ones are *tetracycline* or *ampicillin*, 1 to 2 g/day for 7 to 10 days. Some patients have a prescription on hand and self-administer the antimicrobial after telephone consultation with their physician. Antimicrobials should be started within 24 hours of the first sign of a respiratory infection (increased sputum production and purulence).[53] Patients who are febrile or have other signs and symptoms of infection that do not respond to the prescribed therapy should have a Gram stain and culture and sensitivity studies. When antibiotics are used inappropriately, especially in patients who are not adequately clearing their lungs of secretions, superinfection with bacteria or fungi may occur.[53]

Corticosteroids may be prescribed for patients with intermittent bronchial obstruction and blood or sputum eosinophilia whose condition is not controlled by bronchodilators.[53] Usually a short course of corticosteroids is prescribed to alleviate acute symptoms. Prednisone is often prescribed for a total of 7 to 10 days. In some patients with asthma, a longer course of prednisone may be prescribed and some patients will be on low-maintenance doses (5 to 10 mg/day) for several months or even years. Long-term corticosteroid therapy is usually not recommended for patients with chronic bronchitis or emphysema unless their disease is rapidly progressing.[53]

Persons who are on long-term steroid therapy should have a tuberculin test before initiation of therapy. Those with tuberculin reaction of 10-mm induration or more are candidates for isoniazid therapy (p. 1300). The purpose of isoniazid therapy is to prevent reactivation of tuberculosis that can occur in persons receiving prolonged steroid therapy.

Digitalis may be prescribed for patients with COPD and left ventricular failure. The patient receiving a digitalis preparation should be carefully monitored for side effects (p. 1133).

Patients with increased dyspnea secondary to pulmonary edema, or with right ventricular failure, or corticosteroid-induced fluid retention may benefit from *diuretics*. When diuretics are given, the patient should be carefully monitored for side effects (p. 1133). Those on thiazide diuretics will need to be taught about eating foods high in potassium such as bananas, oranges, prunes, and raisins.

Psychopharmacologic agents may need to be prescribed for some patients with severe emotional disturbances. The type of agent and size of dose are individually determined; but in general, the older the patient, the smaller the dose. When these agents are prescribed, a pharmacology book should be referred to for information about the side effects and precautions to be used in administering these agents.

RESPIRATORY THERAPY. Respiratory therapy for the person with COPD encompasses three modalities—aerosol therapy, oxygen therapy, and intermittent positive pressure breathing (IPPB).

Aerosol therapy. Aerosol therapy is one of the most effective ways to deliver bronchodilators. There are several ways in which aerosolization of medications can be achieved. These include a Freon-propelled, metered-dosage cartridge inhalator; hand-bulb nebulizer; compressor pump; or IPPB machine.[53] These devices have been discussed in Chapter 49, and the reader is referred there for specific details of their use. In general, metered-dosage cartridge inhalators and hand-bulb nebulizers are used more commonly than IPPB. However, IPPB is still used to deliver aerosols to persons who cannot inhale repetitively to near total lung capacity (TLC) or in those persons who are unable to use a hand-bulb nebulizer because of lack of coordination or fatigue. When administering bronchodilators, the solution should be diluted with either water or saline. Some experts recommend that the diluent be water, since saline solutions already contain a solute (NaCl) in water.[53] All bronchodilator solutions are high–molecular weight concentrated solutions and have a high solute content. When they are diluted with water, there is a maximal decrease in solute concentration; thus smaller particle size and deeper deposition of the aerosol result.[53]

Aerosol devices are excellent sites for bacterial growth, and patients using such equipment at home should be advised how to clean them appropriately.

Oxygen therapy. Oxygen therapy is required for patients with COPD who are unable to maintain a Po_2 of 50 mm Hg or more at rest and for those who cannot carry out ADL (bathing, eating, dressing, toileting) without becoming very short of breath. In these instances, 1 to 2 L of oxygen is usually given via nasal prongs. In addition, some patients only require supplemental oxygen during sleep. Patients who complain of restlessness, insomnia, or headaches may be helped to sleep more comfortably if they receive low flow oxygen during the night.[9] Because many patients with COPD have chronic carbon dioxide retention, they need to understand that the risk of high flow rates of oxygen tension to greater than 60 to 70 mm Hg may remove the hypoxic drive and put them into respiratory failure. (See section on respiratory failure later in this chapter.)

PHYSICAL CONDITIONING. Persons with COPD need carefully thought out programs to assist them to attain the highest level of functioning possible for them. Some institutions have specific programs for patients with COPD; however, most nurses work in settings where such programs are not availble. Therefore it is important to emphasize here activities in which the nurse can play a major role in assisting patients to achieve their highest possible level of functioning. These activities include relaxation exercises, breathing retraining, muscle reconditioning, and psychosocial motivation.

Relaxation exercises. Exercises that are helpful to these patients involve progressive relaxation techniques where each muscle is contracted to a count of 10 and then relaxed. An exercise that is helpful to some patients with COPD is to raise their shoulders, shrug them, and then relax. Another commonly used relaxation exercise is to make a fist of both hands, squeeze them very tightly for about 5 seconds, and then relax them completely. Exercises should be performed in a quiet room while sitting or lying in a comfortable position. Often the nurse or another person can serve as a coach to the patient by giving a command about what muscle group to tense and then giving the command to relax. Over a period of time, individuals can learn to repeat the commands to themselves and follow through as they have been taught. Some persons like to do their exercises while listening to relaxing music. There are several articles that have been written in the nursing literature regarding relaxation techniques, and the reader is referred to references 33, 144, and 145 at the end of this chapter.

Meditation. Meditation is another technique that is becoming more widely used to assist persons to relax. One technique involves sitting or lying quietly with the eyes closed and then attempting to relax all muscles by beginning with the feet and working upward. Quiet, rhythmic breathing through the nose is stressed. Patients with COPD may not be able to breathe completely through the nose, but they can breathe slowly through pursed lips. It is recommended that a person meditate for 10 to 20 minutes once or twice daily. On completion of the mediation period, the person should sit or lie quietly for several minutes. Relaxation techniques are best practiced before meals or 2 or more hours after eating, since digestion seem to interfere with the ability to relax fully.[53]

Breathing retraining. Pursed-lip breathing, leaning-forward position for exhalation, abdominal breathing techniques, inhalation-exhalation exercises, and exhalation with exertion are all part of breathing retraining.

Pursed-lip breathing is a natural response that occurs in some patients with COPD, while other patients must be taught to do it. The patient is asked to purse the lips and exhale slowly. Exhaling through pursed lips keeps the airways open longer and allows the patient to empty the lungs more fully.

Using a forward-leaning position of 30 to 40 degrees with the head tilted at a 16- to 18-degree angle is a very effective way to improve exhalation. As mentioned earlier, patients with emphysema have increased TLC and residual volume (RV) with the diaphragm in a fixed flattened position. For this reason, the diaphragm cannot assist in exhalation as it does normally. Leaning forward allows more air to be removed from the lungs on exhalation. The leaning-forward position can be achieved in either a sitting or standing position. For example, (1) the patient can sit on the edge of the bed or a chair and lean forward on two or three pillows placed on a table or overbed stand; (2) the patient can sit in a chair with the legs spread apart shoulder width (or wider, if obese) with the elbows on the knees and the arms and hands relaxed; or (3) the patient can stand with the back and hips against the wall with the feet spread apart and about 12 in. (30 cm) from the wall. The patient then relaxes and leans forward.[103] In these positions, the patient cannot use the accessory muscles of respiration, and the upward action of the diaphragm is improved.

Abdominal breathing improves the breathing efficiency of persons with COPD, because it assists the patient to elevate the diaphragm. Abdominal breathing can be taught in the sitting or lying position. In the sitting position, the patient sits on the side of the bed or in a chair and holds a small pillow or a book against the abdomen. The patient then exhales slowly while leaning forward and pressing the pillow or book against the abdomen. In the lying position, a small pillow or a book is placed on the abdomen and the patient is asked to "puff out" the abdomen and raise the pillow or book as high as possible. The patient then exhales slowly through pursed lips while pulling in on the abdominal muscles. In addition to abdominal breathing, exercises to strengthen the abdominal muscles will assist patients to use their abdominal muscles more effectively in emptying their lungs (Fig. 49-12).

Leg-raising exercises, with each leg being raised alternately as the patient exhales, is one way to strengthen abdominal muscles. Another way is to have the patient raise the head and shoulders from the bed while he or she exhales. Not all patients can do all exercises, but most can do some of them on a daily or twice daily basis. With practice and encouragement the patient can do the exercises 10 times each morning and evening after clearing the lungs as completely as possible of secretions.

Inhalation-exhalation exercises emphasize the need to prolong exhalation about four to five times longer than inhalation. Patients who are up walking can be taught to count in seconds and to concentrate on exhaling slowly and fully. While learning to *exhale with exertion*, the patient exhales during an activity such as bending over or sitting down.[103]

Muscle reconditioning refers to a variety of exercises that will tone muscles. For patients who are able to be up and about, walking, using a treadmill, or riding a stationary bicycle is helpful. The exercise period is started slowly with 10 minutes twice daily three times a week, increasing to 20 minutes twice daily three times

a week. The patient needs to be assessed for his or her ability to carry out such an exercise program, and a staff member should be present during the exercise period.

Psychosocial motivation involves reinforcing the worth of the individual. As mentioned in the literature, some of the patients feel worthless and "consigned to the junk heap."[3] Group meetings that provide mutual support are often helpful, and in some cities there are emphysema clubs sponsored by the local Christmas seal agencies, which are affiliates of the ALA. These clubs are open to persons with emphysema and their significant others.

In addition to all the measures discussed above, patients with COPD are taught how to do postural drainage. Postural drainage and clapping and vibrating are discussed in Chapter 49.

Rehabilitation. It is now recognized that patients with chronic obstructive pulmonary disease can maintain a much higher level of functioning for longer periods than was once thought possible. The patient is no longer told, "You have emphysema—there is nothing we can do to help you. Go home and don't overexert yourself."

Pulmonary rehabilitation programs stress the attainment and maintenance of optimal functioning for the individual patient. Emphasis is placed on bronchial hygiene, using all the measures described previously as well as physical retraining. Specific exercise programs vary, but all programs attempt to rebuild muscle strength so that the patient can undertake activity at a smaller oxygen cost. The psychosocial aspect of care is also stressed in these programs, which utilize a multidisciplinary approach whenever possible. Therapy is structured according to the individual's medical stability, physiologic need, stamina, personality, and life-style. Studies have shown that while overall lung function may not improve and the course of the disease is not halted, the patient and family can be helped to cope with the symptoms of disease and therefore to lead a more satisfying life.

Although it is difficult to measure the physiologic effects of these programs, hospitalization of patients who have participated in them is less frequent, and most patients state that they feel better.[2] The patient is seen regularly by the physician, and it is extremely helpful if both the hospital and community health nurses are able to be involved in the long-term care of the patient. In some centers, clinical nurse specialists follow the patients and refer them to the physician when problems requiring medical consultation arise.

Outcome criteria for the person with chronic bronchitis or pulmonary emphysema

The person or significant others can:
1. Explain dietary changes required after discharge.
   a. Explain food and fluid requirements and plan for meeting them.

b. List specific foods to be avoided.

c. Explain plan for frequent, small feedings that are soft and that do not require much chewing, and the need for increased time required for eating if indicated.

2. Explain any home medication or treatment program.

a. State name, dosage, action, and side effects of each home medication.

b. Explain how and when to use medications ordered on a prn basis (e.g., bronchodilators, antibiotics, steroids, antacids).

c. Demonstrate techniques necessary for follow-up care (e.g., segemental postural drainage, clapping and vibrating, inhalation therapy treatments [IPPB]).

3. Explain exercise program to be followed at home.

a. Demonstrate effective methods of coughing.

b. Demonstrate efficient breathing patterns with emphasis on increasing time of exhalation in relaxation to inhalation (e.g., use of diaphragm, expansion of lower thoracic cage, use of abdominal muscles, use of pursed-lip breathing).

4. Explain health maintenance or therapeutic follow-up program.

a. Explain basic pathologic condition and overall treatment for medical problem in own words.

b. Explain need to avoid respiratory irritants and infectious agents and identify sources of these in environment (e.g., tobacco smoke, industrial pollutants, allergens, persons with upper respiratory tract infections).

c. List signs or symptoms requiring institution of specific therapy or contact with physician (e.g., change in amount, color, consistency of sputum; increased cough, hemoptysis, drowsiness, changes in behavior, increasing fatigue, weight gain, increase in peripheral edema, change in color of stool).

5. Explain how to obtain professional and community resources necessary to structure a satisfactory environment at home.

a. State how to contact other agencies (e.g., vocational counselor, Visiting Nurses Association).

b. Describe how to obtain and maintain any needed equipment or supplies (e.g., oxygen, nebulizers, humidifiers, mistometers, IPPB, syringes, medications).

6. State plans for ongoing follow-up care.

Asthma

Asthma is discussed separately from bronchitis and emphysema because it results in intermittent rather than continuous airway obstruction. Its onset is sudden as opposed to the slow insidious progression of symptoms seen in bronchitis and emphysema. Asthma is characterized by increased responsiveness of the trachea and bronchi to various stimuli with difficulty in breathing caused by narrowing of the airways.[10]

Epidemiology and etiology

Asthma is divided into two basic types—immunologic and nonimmunologic. *Immunologic* or allergic asthma (formerly called extrinsic) occurs in persons who are atopic. This type of asthma usually occurs in childhood and often follows another allergic disease such as eczema. Children with allergic eczema are often highly allergic and may outgrow their eczema; however, 80% to 85% of them develop hay fever or asthma by 6 years of age. *Nonimmunologic* or nonallergic asthma (sometimes referred to as intrinsic) occurs in individuals who are not atopic, usually does not occur until adulthood, and is often associated with a history of recurrent respiratory tract infections.[53] Some persons with asthmatic conditions do not fit into either category.

In one third of asthmatic persons, no allergic component can be demonstrated, and in many individuals no obvious cause for an attack can be identified. In individuals with allergic asthma, levels of immunoglobulins (IgE) are higher than normal, although there is no direct correlation between changed serum levels and the severity of an asthmatic attack.[112] Atopic allergy is discussed more fully in Chapter 72.

In those persons whose asthma is caused by allergy, attacks are precipitated by contact with the allergen to which they are sensitive. This type of asthma is seen most often in children and young adults.

Nonimmunologic asthma usually develops in adults over 35 years of age. Attacks are most frequently triggered by an infection in the sinuses or bronchial tree. Asthma may also be classified as *mixed* asthma. In this type of asthma, attacks are initiated by viral or bacterial infections or by allergens. At different times, attacks may be precipitated by different factors.

In any type of asthma, the airway is in a state of easy provocation, and attacks may be precipitated by a variety of factors including changes in temperature and humidity, irritating fumes and smoke, strong odors, physical exertion, and emotional stress. Some allergists refer to asthma in children as the "Christmas and birthday disease," because the excitement and stress related to these special days often precipitate an asthmatic attack.

Hypoxemia, hypercapnia, and the overuse of bronchodilators may also lead to an acute asthmatic attack.[20,66,95]

Pulmonary function studies done during nonsymptomatic periods may show no significant changes, unless the previous bronchospasm was not treated adequately. In this instance, pulmonary function studies will indicate some degree of bronchospasm. During periods of airway obstruction, however, FEV_1, FEV, and MVV are decreased, while FRC is increased. Hypoxemia may be present; the degree depends on the severity of the obstruction and the resultant changes in the ventilation-perfusion $(\dot{V}/\dot{Q})$ ratio (p. 1221). Pulmonary function studies for asthmatic patients include measurements before and after the use of a bronchodilator to determine therapeutic response.

Persons who have asthmatic attacks usually seek medical care, because the attacks are both incapacitating and frightening. The individual must often make an attempt to reduce emotional stress and to control physical exertion, since these factors are less amenable to management than are specific allergens. If the underlying cause of an allergy is obscure, if it is resistant to treatment, or if the person has nonallergenic asthma, the recognition and control of secondary factors may be the main approach to treatment. *It is imperative to understand that even though psychologic factors may precipitate an attack, the response to it is physiologic and requires the same treatment as that prescribed for an attack precipitated by an allergen or any other factor.*

There is perhaps no disease in which knowing the patient well is more important than in asthma. Since sensitivity tests can be done with only a very small fraction of the substances with which the patient is on contact, the physician usually makes the diagnosis on the basis of a careful history. Knowing about the person's life-style such as the type of work, leisure-time activities, and even food preferences may give useful clues as to what precipitates the asthmatic attack. Although the allergist urges persons to report seemingly trivial and insignificant details, they often hesitate to do so, since they are accustomed to reporting only physical changes within themselves. The alert nurse can be of help in learning the cause of an allergic reaction. It is often the nurse who may learn that a relative has just visited in the home and was accompanied by a cat or a dog. This information would be of great importance because animal dander is one of the most common allergens for individuals with atopic asthma.

The nurse may make observations regarding emotional stressors that appear to aggravate the patient's condition. Careful observation of relationships between the person and his or her significant others may give clues to sources of emotional stress. Some patients remain in the hospital during an acute episode and return home relieved of serious symptoms. However, unless life circumstances can be altered, family relationships and general socioeconomic conditions that cause stress may send the patient back to the hospital with another attack.

Patients with chronic asthma may gain a sense of security while in the hospital, and they may be reluctant to return home. Asthmatic attacks can be precipitated by plans for discharge, and the patient's stay may

thus be prolonged. Patients with severe emotional problems may benefit from psychotherapy.

Pathophysiology

An asthmatic attack is the result of an antigen-antibody reaction in which chemical mediators are released. The chemical mediators, which include histamine, slow releasing substance of anaphylaxis (SRS-A), eosinophilic chemotactic factor of anaphylaxis (ECF-A) and perhaps others, cause three main reactions: (1) constriction of smooth muscles of both the large and small airways resulting in bronchospasm, (2) increased capillary permeability that contributes to mucosal edema and further narrows the airways, and (3) increased mucus gland secretions and increased mucous production. As a result, the person with an asthmatic attack struggles to breathe through a narrowed airway, which is in spasm. Because breathing is labored, the person breathes through the mouth, which dries the mucus and further occludes the airway.

Clinical picture

Asthmatic attacks often occur at night. The person awakens with a feeling of choking, since there is difficulty moving air in and out of the lungs. The bronchioles react with swelling of the mucosa, muscle spasm (bronchospasm), and increased amounts of thick secretions. The patient's breathing has a characteristic wheezing sound as air moves through the constricted and obstructed airways. Cyanosis may develop. When an attack starts, the patient should sit upright and be given something on which to learn forward such as an overbed table. During an acute attack, the patient uses the accessory muscles of respiration in an effort to get enough air, and leaning forward helps to use the muscles more effectively. During an acute attack, the person's major concern is breathing. Medication for relief of the attack should be given as soon as possible, and the patient should be constantly attended until acute symptoms subside. The attack usually ends with the patient coughing up large quantities of thick, tenacious sputum. Most attacks subside in 30 minutes to 1 hour, although repeated asthmatic attacks associated with infection may continue for days or weeks. The person is usually exhausted and should rest quietly after the attack. Diaphoresis is common because of the expenditure of energy, and linen changes may be necessary.

Persons who are severely affected with asthma and who have attacks that are difficult to control with the usual medications may develop *status asthmaticus*. In this case, the symptoms of an acute attack continue despite measures to relieve them. The patient is acutely ill. When admitted to the hospital, emergency treatment is begun. The patient is questioned as to medications already taken. Usually a bronchodilator has failed to relieve the attack, and that is why the patient is seeking medical assistance. The patient is often very anxious and may be in a near-panic state because of inability to relieve the symptoms. Aminophylline, 500 mg in an intravenous drip, is given over a 20-minute period. A prolonged attack causes exhaustion, and death from heart failure may occur. Oxygen is administered, and IPPB may be used intermittently. Blood gases are carefully monitored, and intravenous steroids are frequently given. During an acute attack, the alveoli progressively distend as in emphysema; actually, acute emphysema exists. Unless relaxation of the bronchioles can be accomplished, insufficient oxygen passes through the alveolar-capillary membrane into the bloodstream (hypoxemia), and the person becomes progressively more cyanotic. At the same time, the person is usually hyperventilating and exhaling CO_2, and for this reason PCO_2 is usually reduced. If the PCO_2 becomes elevated and the person becomes hypercapnic, this is a danger sign because it indicates that the person is tiring and ventilatory efforts are becoming inadequate. Intubation and assisted ventilation may also be necessary. The person needs constant observation and support and should have everything done for him or her. Repeated attacks of status asthmaticus may cause irreversible emphysema, resulting in a permanent decrease in total breathing capacity.

Some persons have *chronic mild asthma*. Symptoms are not noticeable when the person is at rest. However, after exertion such as laughing, singing, vigorous exercise, or emotional excitement, dyspnea and wheezing develop rapidly. These attacks are controlled with medications, and patients usually can continue their usual mode of living with a few modifications and no serious lung changes. They are not hospitalized, but they sometimes come to outpatient clinics for medical supervision.

Intervention

The management of asthma is directed toward symptomatic relief of attacks, control of specific causative factors, and general care for maintenance of optimal health. The chief aim of various medications is to afford the patient immediate and progressive bronchial relaxation. Following are some approaches to therapy*:

1. Acute asthma
    a. Moderate severity: treated safely on an outpatient basis when *no danger signs* are present
        (1) Nasal oxygen
        (2) IV aminophylline in a loading dose or subcutaneous terbutaline or both may be given simultaneously
        (3) Monitor FEV and symptoms; when they improve, begin oral therapy

*Adapted from Jenne, J.W.: Basics RD 6:1-6, Sept. 1977.

        (4) Observe carefully for 48 hours and monitor for signs of relapse
    b. Severe attack with *one or more danger signs*: vital capacity < 1.0 L, FEV_1 < 0.5 L, PO_2 under 50 mm, increase in PCO_2, exhaustion, disturbed consciousness.
        (1) Hospitalize; give supplemental oxygen; intubate if necessary
        (2) Administer IV steroids (100 mg Solu-Cortef or equivalent every 6 hours for four doses); begin prednisone, 60 to 80 mg every 24 hours until FEV_1 nears best previous value, then reduce dose over next 2 to 3 weeks; begin use of beclomethasone inhaler
        (3) IV aminophylline in a loading dose and then in maintenance dose for 48 to 72 hours; monitor aminophylline blood levels
        (4) Administer β_2-adrenergic agents subcutaneously (terbutaline or epinephrine initially); oral therapy after 24 hours
        (5) IPPB may be used to deliver adrenergic agents and to facilitate bronchodilation
2. Chronic asthma
    a. Mild to moderate, or recurring
        (1) Theophylline compounds; cromolyn sodium may be tried; adrenergic inhaler as needed
        (2) Oral β_2-adrenergic agents added in divided doses if above not effective
    b. Moderately severe: add beclomethasone inhaler to 2.a.(1) and 2.a.(2) above
    c. Severe asthma causing interferences with work; give oral steroids every other day in addition to 2.a.(1), 2.a.(2), and 2.b., above; keep steroids to minimal effective dose

In an asthmatic attack, the β_2 receptors are blocked, causing bronchoconstriction. For this reason, a β-adrenergic agent is administered to relax the bronchi. Some of the most commonly prescribed ones are epinephrine, ephedrine, isoproterenol (Isuprel), isoetharine (Bronkosol), and terbutaline (Bricanyl).

Epinephrine is usually administered during an acute attack. The usual dose is 0.3 to 0.5 ml of a 1:1000 solution. If relief is not obtained within a few minutes, a repeat dose may be ordered. *Ephedrine* is a longer-acting agent and therefore is not effective during an acute attack. It is believed that ephedrine produces bronchodilation by stimulating the production of cyclic 3,5 AMP (adenosine monophosphate), thus producing bronchodilation. The usual dose is 25 to 50 mg every 4 to 6 hours. Many persons with asthma take this medication regularly. One of its side effects is cerebral agitation, and for this reason a barbiturate such as phenobarbital, 8 to 15 mg, may also be prescribed to be taken at the same time as the ephedrine. Combined medications are also available. Most contain theophylline (aminophylline), ephedrine, and phenobarbital. Tedral and Bronkotabs are examples of agents containing all three medications.

Isoproterenol (Isuprel) and *isoetharine* (Bronkosol) are widely used inhaled bronchodilators. These medications come in metered-dose cartridges and should not be used more than two inhalations at a time and not over three times a day to avoid dependence. Sudden death during status asthmaticus has been attributed to overuse of these gas-propelled inhalants.

Terbutaline is a newer bronchodilator that works at β_2-receptors in smooth muscle (bronchi, blood vessels). A dose of 2.5 mg of terbutaline is equivalent to 25 mg ephedrine orally. Frequent side effects include increased heart rate (average 30 beats/min) and tremors. Less frequent side effects are palpitations, sweating, headache, and cramps in hands and feet. Terbutaline is almost four times as expensive as ephedrine, and since the effects of the two drugs are comparable, cost may be a factor to consider in determining which of the two drugs will be prescribed, especially for persons on chronic maintenance therapy.

Cromolyn sodium (Aarane, Intal) was first released for use in the United States in 1973. It is used to prevent asthmatic attacks and is of no benefit in the treatment of an acute attack. Cromolyn sodium is believed to stabilize the mast cells and prevent the release of the chemical mediators, histamine, SRS-A, and ECF-A, that cause the symptoms seen in an asthmatic attack.

Cromolyn sodium is available as a powder in 20-mg capsules for inhalation. The usual dose is 20 mg four times a day. It is administered through an inspiration-activated turboinhaler (Intal, Spinhaler). Cromolyn should be administered four times a day for a full month to dertermine its effectiveness in a given asthmatic patient, since its effect can be quite delayed. In the United States, its greatest use is prophylactically before exertion in exercise-induced asthma and before unavoidable exposure to a known allergen in persons with allergic asthma. Another newer drug being used in treating persons with asthma is *beclomethasone*. It is a synthetic corticosteroid closely related to prednisolone in structure. It possesses potent antiinflammatory activity (500 times that of *dexamethasone*) but very weak systemic corticoid effects. For this reason, it may be preferable to other corticosteroids in treating persons with asthma. Beclomethasone is available as an aerosol inhalant. For adults the dose is two inhalations (100 μg) three to four times a day. Sometimes a smaller dose is instituted first and then the dose is adjusted according to the response of the patient.

Beclomethasone is being prescribed as a substitute for systemic corticosteroids by some physicians. When this is done, care has to be taken to withdraw the systemic corticosteroids slowly so as not to precipitate symptoms of adrenal insufficiency. Patients should be advised to resume or increase their systemic corticosteroids during periods of increased stress, if their asthma symptoms worsen, or if symptoms of adrenal insufficiency occur.

Beclomethasone is not prescribed alone for an acute asthmatic attack because it does not work that rapidly, and in acute asthma systemic corticosteroids should be given.

Sedatives are used with caution during an asthmatic attack to avoid depressing the respiratory center. During an acute attack, the patient is usually very frightened and much reassurance is necessary—the patient is never left alone. Intubated patients who are receiving assisted ventilation may be sedated, and frequently morphine is prescribed.

If the asthmatic attack is very severe, it may be necessary to administer a neuromuscular blocking agent, such as curare (Pavulon), to cause respiratory paralysis and effectively ventilate the patient mechanically. Because the patient who receives a neuromuscular blocking agent is totally paralyzed, he or she must be cared for on a one-to-one basis and never left unattended. Since curare paralyzes muscles but does not affect consciousness, the patient requires frequent sedation with morphine or diazepam (Valium).

One of the main nursing measures is to provide frequent care to remove secretions from the airway before they become impacted. Mucous plugs are commonly a problem, and liquefying agents and humidification are indicated.

When an infection is present, appropriate antibiotic therapy is prescribed.

Outcome criteria for the person with asthma

The person or significant others can:
1. State the factors most likely to precipitate an asthmatic attack (e.g., stress, allergens, infections).
2. State the impotance of keeping a diary of symptoms and medications (time and dose) during asthma attack.
3. If the cause is allergic, state how to prepare an environmentally controlled bedroom (p. 1867).
4. Explain any home medication program.
   a. Give name, dose, action, and side effects of each medication.
   b. State conditions under which medications might be increased (e.g., infection—start or increase antibiotics; increased stress or worsening of symptoms—increase corticosteroids).
5. Demonstrate how to take inhaled medications.

6. Describe what to do when an acute attack occurs (e.g., take medication, be quiet).
7. State signs and symptoms that indicate need for immediate medical attention (e.g., asthmatic attack unrelieved by usual treatment).
8. If on corticosteroid therapy, show card to be carried at all times giving data about the drug, dose, and name of physician; alternative is to wear Medic-Alert bracelet.
9. State plans for ongoing follow-up care including plans for desensitization if appropriate.

Respiratory insufficiency and respiratory failure

Epidemiology and etiology

The term *respiratory insufficiency* is usually used to indicate that the exchange of oxygen and carbon dioxide is not adequate to meet the needs of the body during normal activities. Respiratory failure is said to occur when ventilation is not sufficient to achieve gas exchange even at rest. Many disorders can lead to or are associated with both respiratory insufficiency and failure; these are listed in Table 51-7.

The diagnosis of respiratory insufficiency or failure is based on arterial blood gas studies, pulmonary function testing, and the clinical status of the patient. The criteria in the box below, at right, are generally used in defining a state of failure. However, it cannot be overemphasized that these parameters are only *guidelines* and must be applied in light of the individual's history, age, and overall condition.

TABLE 51-7. Disorders associated with respiratory insufficiency and failure

Pulmonary disorders	Nonpulmonary disorders
Severe infection	CNS disturbance secondary to drug overdose, anesthesia, head injury
Pulmonary edema	
Pulmonary embolus	
COPD	Neuromuscular disorders (e.g., Guillain-Barré syndrome, myasthenia gravis, multiple sclerosis, poliomyelitis, muscular dystrophy, spinal cord injury)
Adult respiratory distress syndrome	
Cancer	
Chest trauma	
Severe atelectasis	
Airway compromise secondary to trauma, infection, or surgery	Postoperative reduction in ventilation following thoracic and abdominal surgery
	Prolonged mechanical ventilation

Pathophysiology and clinical picture

Regardless of the underlying condition, the resultant events or processes that occur in respiratory failure are the same. With inadequate ventilation, the arterial PO_2 falls and tissue cells become hypoxic. The PCO_2 accumulates, leading to a fall in pH, and the patient becomes acidotic. The reader must keep in mind while working with the patient with COPD who has developed respiratory failure, that this patient normally exists in a compensated state with decreased PO_2 levels and elevated PCO_2 levels. Thus the parameters in the boxed material are not applicable; the pH, however, is a useful guide in assessing the degree of insufficiency. When the pH begins to fall below 7.3, it is an indication that the patient is no longer able to compensate for the elevated PCO_2 level.

Respiratory insufficiency and failure can result from a worsening in the condition of the patient with any of the disorders already mentioned.

Intervention

Intervention for the patient who has respiratory insufficiency or failure always begins with a recognition of the underlying disease state or cause of the disturbance in ventilation. Therapy is first directed at improving the underlying condition, such as sepsis, or by removing the cause, such as fluid overload.

The goals of intervention are to improve oxygenation and ventilation in order to restore the person's normal PO_2 and PCO_2 levels. The initial medical management can often be conservative if the diagnosis is made early enough. All of the intervention measures discussed in Chapter 49 may be used.

Oxygen. Particular care is needed in working with the patient who has chronic lung disease. As mentioned earlier, individuals with COPD normally exist with elevated PCO_2 levels and have lost the usual respiratory drive, carbon dioxide stimulation. They no longer respond to increased carbon dioxide levels by increasing their rate and depth of respiration; rather, the elevated PCO_2 depresses the respiratory center. Their respiratory drive is now derived from their low PO_2 levels;

CRITERIA FOR DIAGNOSIS OF RESPIRATORY FAILURE

PO_2 < 50 mm Hg when breathing room air

PCO_2 > 50 mm Hg

Vital capacity < 15 ml/kg

Respiratory rate > 30/min or below 8/min

therefore even though these persons lack oxygen, it is extremely dangerous to raise their PO_2 to normal levels. If the arterial PO_2 is normal and there is retention of carbon dioxide (*hypercapnia*), the person will have no respiratory drive. Hypoventilation becomes more severe and PCO_2 continues to rise. This situation results in *carbon dioxide narcosis*, a markedly elevated carbon dioxide level that causes coma or semicoma. Persons with COPD are therefore treated with low flow or controlled flow oxygen; that is, inspired oxygen concentrations of 24% to 30%. These concentrations can easily be obtained by using a Venti-mask or a two-pronged nasal cannula with a 1 to 2 L oxygen flow. This amount of oxygen can significantly increase the amount of oxygen carried by hemoglobin without a significant increase in arterial PO_2; therefore the patient's blood carries much more oxygen even though hypoxemia is still present. The person continues to have respiratory drive, and the PCO_2 does not rise.

Low concentrations of oxygen are obtained by using compressed air for the driving force and adding 1 L per minute of oxygen through the nebulizer. By the use of low-flow oxygen, the amount of oxygen carried in the patient's blood can often be increased enough to maintain basic body functions without further reduction of ventilation. Persons who do not have COPD, who have a normal PCO_2, but who are hypoxic are usually able to tolerate high flow rates of oxygen (5 to 10 L/min). Oxygen is an integral part of the therapy of patients with respiratory insufficiency and failure; however, some hazards are associated with prolonged use.

Oxygen toxicity is the term used to describe the damage to lung tissue that results from prolonged exposure to high concentrations. Although the exact effects of oxygen in any one individual may be dependent on the person's underlying pathologic condition, it is believed that exposure to greater than 60% oxygen for a period of more than 36 hours, or exposure to 100% oxygen for a period of more than 6 hours, will result in atelectasis and alveolar collapse. Breathing very high concentrations of oxygen (80% to 100%) for prolonged periods (24 hours or more) is often associated with the development of ARDS.[109,129] Thus it is a firm general principle that the lowest amount of oxygen that will achieve an acceptable PO_2 is the amount that should be used.

Airway management. In addition to providing supplemental oxygen, care of the person with respiratory insufficiency usually also includes aggressive airway management and attempts to improve ventilation. Thus suctioning, IPPB, ultrasonic mist therapy, and postural drainage with clapping and vibrating are all employed in an attempt to halt the progression of insufficiency.

Rest. The patient who is subjected to many treatments can become excessively fatigued, further compromising ventilatory capacity. Frequent rest periods must be interspersed with treatments, and it is the nurse's responsibility to see that the patient is provided with a quiet environment and is not disturbed by unnecessary interruptions at rest times. Unfortunately, persons who have severe insufficiency must have frequent treatments and interventions; it is *not* appropriate, although the person may be quite tired, to allow the patient to sleep through the night and omit treatments. This will inevitably lead to a worsened status.

Although persons with respiratory insufficiency are often anxious and frightened, sedation is contraindicated because it depresses respirations. Therefore it is especially important that the nurse be supportive of the patient and be skillful in assisting the patient to breathe effectively. The patient can be extremely demanding, and the nurse must understand the fear and anxiety that is often the basis for the patient's behavior.

Monitoring. Aggressive, constant nursing care is essential for these patients. The nurse must be continually alert to clinical changes that represent changes in the patient's ventilation. Increasing confusion and behavioral changes often indicate an elevated PCO_2. The behavioral changes may range from pugnacious, combative behavior to lethargy. Other clinical signs of *hypercapnia* are flushed skin color caused by reflex vasodilation, muscle twitching, and headache. Signs commonly seen in *hypoxia* include tachycardia, increased pulse rate, cyanosis, changes in blood pressure, and changes in behavior. In *early* stages of hypoxia, the blood pressure is elevated as a result of vasoconstriction and increased peripheral resistance. In *later* stages the blood pressure falls to hypotensive levels, and circulatory arrest can occur. It is important to point out that cyanosis is not an early sign of hypoxia, since it does not occur until arterial oxygen saturation is less than 85%; thus the nurse needs to be alert to earlier signs of hypoxia.

Mechanical ventilation. If, despite all the measures discussed, the person is unable to maintain ventilation (as indicated by a rising arterial PCO_2), mechanical ventilation is necessary. The basic use of respirators, endotracheal and tracheostomy tubes, and the suctioning procedure used with an artificial airway are discussed in Chapter 49.

Positive end expiratory pressure (PEEP) is a ventilator mode that has been shown to increase the effectiveness of mechanical ventilation in certain patients. PEEP involves the maintenance of positive pressure, usually between 5 and 15 cm water pressure, at the end of expiration, rather than allowing airway pressure to return to normal (atmospheric) as usually occurs. By maintaining positive pressure, alveoli that would otherwise collapse on expiration are held open, thus increasing the opportunity for gas exchange across the alveolar-capillary membrane. This is accomplished by the increase in functional residual capacity. The result is a decrease in physiologic shunting and the ability to achieve a higher level of PO_2 with lower concentrations of delivered oxygen (F_1O_2). PEEP has its greatest use in the treatment of ARDS, but is also used in treating any patient who would otherwise require unacceptably high concentrations of oxygen.

The hazards of PEEP are related to the increase in intrathoracic pressure. Most serious of the dangers related to this technique is the increased incidence of pneumothorax, particularly in those with friable lung tissue, as seen in persons with emphysema or lung cancer. The sudden disappearance of breath sounds on one side, in conjunction with signs of respiratory distress, in the patient being ventilated with PEEP *must be taken as an indication of a pneumothorax*. This can develop into a life-threatening episode if the pneumothorax is large, and the physician must be called immediately. Another less serious consequence of PEEP may be a reduction in venous return, which is impeded by the increased intrathoracic pressure, and a subsequent fall in cardiac output. This effect seems to be particularly common in patients who are relatively dehydrated and can sometimes be avoided by careful fluid administration.

The nurse plays an important role in weaning the patient from the ventilator. Both physiologic studies (blood gases, tidal volume) and clinical status determine the patient's readiness to breathe without mechanical assistance. Before weaning, the patient should have been taught breathing exercises. When the patient is taken off the respirator, a nurse in whom the patient has confidence should be present. It is also helpful if the environment around the patient is calm. Much of the success of weaning is dependent on the interrelationship between the patient's physiologic and psychologic responses. If the patient becomes very anxious and takes rapid, shallow breaths, being off the respirator will be poorly tolerated. If a pattern of controlled breathing can be maintained, success is more likely. Weaning is usually begun with short periods off the respirator. The amount of time off the respirator is increased according to the patient's tolerance. The nurse must carefully assess the adequacy of the patient's ventilation during the time off the respirator. If, in the nurse's judgment, the patient cannot tolerate breathing on his or her own because of inadequate tidal volume, cyanosis, tachycardia, diaphoresis, or restlessness, mechanical assistance should be reinstituted.

A more recent technique of weaning is the use of *intermittent mandatory ventilation (IMV)*. This involves the addition of an oxygen reservoir with a one-way valve to the respirator circuit. The rate on the ventilator is reduced below the patient's normal rate. The ventilator then delivers the set minimum, and the patient spontaneously breathes several breaths in addition to this from the oxygen reservoir. For example, if the patient's natural respiratory rate is 16, the ventilator might be set to deliver 10 breaths per minute. The patient will then take an additional six breaths independently. In this way, the patient can gradually build up strength and gain respiratory independence without having to be taken completely off the ventilator for periods of time.

Throughout the treatment of the patient in respiratory failure, ventilation should be carefully monitored by blood gas studies and simple spirometry (tidal volume, vital capacity). Alert nursing observation of the patient can determine the adequacy of ventilation. Meticulous attention is given to maintaining a patent airway, which is the prime nursing responsibility. (See specialized material for further detail.[85,97,121,129])

REFERENCES AND SELECTED READINGS
Contemporary

1. Abraham, A.S.: The management of patients with chronic bronchitis and cor pulmonale, Heart Lung **6:**104-108, 1977.
2. Agle, D.P., and Baum, G.L.: Psychological aspects of chronic obstructive pulmonary disease, Med. Clin. North Am. **61:**749-758, 1977.
3. Agle, D.P.: et al.: Multidiscipline treatment of chronic pulmonary insufficiency. I. Psychologic aspects of rehabilitation, Psychosom. Med. **35:**41-49, 1973.
4. *Albanese, A., and Toplitz, A.: A hassle-free guide to suctioning a tracheostomy, RN **45:**24-30, 1982.
5. Alford, R.H.: Histoplasmosis. In Conn, H.F.: Current therapy 1982, Philadelphia, 1982, W.B. Saunders Co.
6. Ali, J., et al.: Consequences of postoperative alterations in respiratory mechanics, Am. J. Surg. **128:**376-382, 1974.
7. American Academy of Pediatrics: Report of the Committee on Infectious Diseases, ed. 17, Evanston, Ill., 1974, The Academy.
8. American Cancer Society: Cancer facts and figures, New York, 1982, The Society.
9. American College of Chest Physicians: A report of the Committee on Emphysema: recommendations for continuous oxygen therapy in chronic obstructive lung disease, Chest **64:**505-507, 1973.
10. *American Lung Association: Chronic obstructive pulmonary disease, New York, 1981, The Association.
11. *American Lung Association: Diagnostic standards and classification of tuberculosis, New York, 1981, The Association.
12. *American Lung Association: Occupational lung disease: an introduction, New York, 1979, The Association.
13. American Thoracic Society: Guidelines for the investigation and management of tuberculosos contacts, Am. Rev. Respir. Dis. **114:**459-563, 1976.
14. American Thoracic Society: Guidelines for long-term institutional care of tuberculosis patients, Am. Rev. Respir. Dis. **113:**253-254, 1976.
15. American Thoracic Society: Intermittent chemotherapy for adults with tuberculosos, Am. Rev. Respir. Dis. **110:**374-376, 1974.
16. American Thoracic Society: Treatment of mycobacterial disease, Am. Rev. Respir. Dis. **115:**185-187, 1977.
17. Austrian, R., editor: Pneumococcal infection and pneumococcal vaccine, N. Engl. J. Med. **297:**938-939, 1977.
18. Bartlett, J.G.: Aspiration pneumonia, Clin. Notes Respir. Dis. **4:**3-8, 1980.

*References preceded by an asterisk are particularly well-suited for student reading.

19. Bartlett, J.G., and Garbach, S.L.: The triple threat of aspiration pneumonia, Chest 68:550-556, 1980.

20. Bates, D., Macklem, P.T., and Christie, R.V.: Respiratory function in disease, ed. 2, Philadelphia, 1971, W.B. Saunders Co.

21. *Brannin, P.K.: Physical assessment of acute respiratory failure, Crit. Care. Q. 1:27-41, 1979.

22. Brenner, D.J., et al.: Classification of the legionnaires' disease bacterium: an interim report, Curr. Microbiol. 1:71-75, 1978.

23. Reference deleted in proofs.

24. Carr, D.T., and Rosenow, E.C.: Bronchogenic carcinoma, Basics RD 5:1-6, 1977.

25. Centers for Disease Control: Annual summary 1980: reported morbidity and mortality in the United States, Morbid. Mortal. Weekly Rep. 29:54, 1981.

26. *Cimprich, B., Gaydos, D., and Langan, R.: A preoperative teaching program for the thoracotomy patient, Ca. Nurs. 1:35-39, 1978.

27. Comroe, J.: Physiology of respiration, ed. 2, Chicago, 1975, Year Book Medical Publishers, Inc.

28. Cunningham, J.H., Richardson, R.H., and Smith, J.D.: Interstitial pulmonary edema, Heart Lung 6:617-623, 1977.

29. *Cushing, R.: Pulmonary infections, Heart Lung 5:611-613, 1976.

30. Danday, S., and Wiggins, K.: Current status of general hospital use for patients with tuberculosis in the United States: an update, Am. Rev. Respir. Dis. 110:442-445, 1974.

31. de Tornyay, R., Sordelett, S.S., and Jackson, B.S.: Nursing decisions: experiences in clinical problem solving, series 2, no. 5. Dan B.: a man with COPD, RN 40:61-67, 1977.

32. Donahue, F.J., and Capshaw, V.: The great smoking survey, Am. Lung. Assoc. Bull. 63:2-5, 1977.

33. Dudley, D.L., et al.: Psychosocial aspects of care in the chronic obstructive pulmonary disease patient, Heart Lung 2:389, 1973.

34. Eickhoff, T.C.: The current status of BCG immunization against tuberculosis, Ann. Rev. Med. 28:411-423, 1977.

35. *Einstein, H.E.: Coccidioidsmycosis, Basics RD 9:1-6, 1980.

36. *England, A.C., et al.: An outbreak of legionnaires' disease associated with a contaminated air-conditioning cooling tower, N. Engl. J. Med. 302:365-370, 1980.

37. Fergus, L.C., and Cordasco, E.M.: Pulmonary rehabilitation of the patient with COPD, Postgrad. Med. 62:141-144, 1977.

38. Fisher, L.: National smoking habits and attitudes, Am. Lung Assoc. Bull. 63:6-9, 1977.

39. *Fitzgerald, L.M.: Mechanical ventilation, Heart Lung 5:939-949, 1976.

40. *Fitzmaurice, J.B., and Sashara, A.A.: Current concepts of pulmonary embolism: implications for nursing practice, Heart Lung 3:209-218, 1974.

41. *Frame, P.T. Acute infectious pneumonia in the adult, Basics RD 10:3, 1982.

42. Fromm, G.: Using basic laboratory data to evaluate patients with acute respiratory failure, Crit. Care Q. 1:43-52, 1979.

43. Fuhs, M.F., and Stein, A.M..: Better ways to cope with COPD, Nurs. '76 6:28-38, 1976.

44. *Gracey, D.R.: Adult respiratory distress syndrome, Heart Lung 4:280-283, 1975.

45. *Gracey, D.R.: Home oxygen therapy for the COPD patient, Heart Lung 4:792-794, 1975.

46. *Gracey, D.R.: Radiation pneumonitis producing respiratory failure, Heart Lung 4:452-455, 1975.

47. Greenfield, L.J.: Assessing operability of lung cancer, RN 39:OR1, OR4-5, 1976.

48. *Grimes, O.F.: Neuromuscular syndromes in patients with lung cancer, Am. J. Nurs. 71:752-755, 1971.

49. Hahn, A.B., Barkin, R.L., and Oestreich, S.J.K.: Pharmacology in nursing, ed. 15, St. Louis, 1982, The C.V. Mosby Co.

50. *Hanson, R.R., and Kasik, J.E.: The pneumoconioses, Heart Lung 6:645-652, 1977.

51. Herron, S.C.: Home care of the patient with C.O.P.D., Nurs. (Jenkintown) 6:81-82, 84-86, 1976.

52. Herxheimer, H.: A guide to bronchial asthma, New York, 1975, Academic Press, Inc.

53. *Hodgkin, J.E.: Chronic obstructive pulmonary disease, Park Ridge, Ill., 1979, American College of Chest Physicians.

54. *Hudgel, D.W., and Madsen, L.A.: Acute and chronic asthma: a guide to intervention, Am. J. Nurs. 80:1791-1792, 1980.

55. Hunt, W.J., and Bespalec, D.A.: An evaluation of current methods of modifying smoking behavior, J. Clin. Psychol. 30:431-438, 1974.

56. Hunter, P.M.: Bedside monitoring of respiratory function, Nurs. Clin. North Am. 16:211-224, 1981.

57. Israel, H.L., and Atkinson, G.W.: Sarcoidosis, Basics RD 7:1-6, 1978.

58. Israel, S., and Chahinian, A.: Lung cancer—natural history, prognosis, and therapy, New York, 1976, Academic Press, Inc.

59. *James, O.: Respiratory failure after injury: a review and a plea for accuracy, Heart Lung 6:303-307, 1977.

60. Johnston, R.F., and Wildrick, K.H.: State of the art review: the impact of chemothrapy on the care of patients with tuberculosis, Am. Rev. Respir. Dis. 109:636-664, 1974.

61. Jones, R.H., and Sabiston, D.C.: Pulmonary embolism, Surg. Clin. North Am. 56: 891-907, 1976.

62. Jones, R.W., and Weill, H.: Occupational lung disease, Basics RD 6:1-6, 1978.

63. Kamholz, S.L., and Pinsker, K.L.: Bacterial pneumonia. In Conn, H.F.: Current therapy 1982, Philadelphia, 1982, W.B. Saunders Co.

64. Karetzky, M.S., and Khan, A.U.: Review of current concepts in aspiration pneumonia, Heart Lung 6:321-326, 1977.

65. Keim, L.W., Schuldt, S., and Bedell, G.N.: Tuberculosis in the intensive care unit, Heart Lung 6:624-634, 1977.

66. Kopetzky, M.: Normal and asthmatic lungs: how they work. In Essays in medicine: asthma, New York, 1972, Medcom Books, Inc.

67. Koss, J.A., and Christoph, C.: Oxygen therapy and other respiratory therapy in acute respiratory failure, Crit. Care Q. 1:53-63, 1979.

68. Kravetz, H.M.: Coccidioidomycosis. In Conn, H.F.: Current therapy 1982, Philadelphia, 1982, W.B. Saunders Co.

69. *Kryger, M. editor: Pathophysiology of respiration, New York, 1981, John Wiley & Sons, Inc.

70. *Kudla, M.S.: The care of the patient with respiratory insufficiency, Nurs. Clin. North Am. 8:183-190, 1973.

71. Lagerson, J.: Pulmonary rehabilitation, Crit. Care Q. 1:75-83, 1979.

72. Lance, E., and Sweetwood, H.: Chest trauma, Nurs. '78 8:28-33, 1978.

73. Langston, H.T., and Barker, W.S.: The adult thoracic surgical patient. In Neville, W.E., editor: Care of the surgical cardio-pulmonary patient, Chicago, 1971, Year Book Medical Publishers, Inc.

74. Larson, R.K., et al.: Generic and environmental determinants of chronic obstructive pulmonary disease, Ann. Intern. Med. 72:627-632, 1970.

75. LeQuense, D.M.: Relation between deep vein thrombosis and pulmonary embolism in surgical patients, N. Engl. J. Med. 291:1202-1204, 1974.

76. Levine, D.P., and Lerner, M.: The clinical spectrum of *Mycoplasma pneumoniae* infections, Med. Clin. North Am. 62:961-978, 1978.

77. *Linn, L.J.: Psychosocial needs of patients with acute respiratory failure, Crit. Care Q. 1:65-74, 1979.

78. *Malkus, B.L.: Respiratory care at home, Am. J. Nurs. **76**:1789-1791, 1976.

79. *Martini, N.: Lung cancer—an overview, Ca. Nurs. **1**:31-33, 1978.

80. Miller, W.C.: Chronic bronchitis, bronchiectasis, and emphysema. In Conn, H.F.: Current therapy 1982, Philadelphia, 1982, W.B. Saunders Co.

81. Mittman, C.: Chronic obstructive lung disease: the result of the interaction of genetic and environmental factors, Heart Lung **2**:222-226, 1973.

82. Moody, L.E.: Primer for pulmonary hygiene, Am. J. Nurs. **77**:104-106, 1977.

83. Moorthy, S.S., LoSasso, A.M., and Gibbs, P.S.: Respiratory failure in patients following surgery and trauma, Crit. Care. Q. **1**:15-25, 1979.

84. Moser, K.M.: Pulmonary embolism, Am. Rev. Respir. Dis. **115**:829-852, 1977.

85. Nett, L.: The use of mechanical ventilators, Nurs. Clin. North Am. **9**:123-136, 1974.

86. Nett, L., and Petty, T.L.: Oxygen toxicity, Am. J. Nurs. **73**:1556-1558, 1973.

87. *Neville, W.E.: Care of the surgical cardiopulmonary patient, Chicago, 1971, Year Book Medical Publishers, Inc.

88. Niewoehner, D.E., Kleinerman, J., and Rice, D.B.: Pathologic changes in peripheral airways of young cigarette smokers, N. Engl. J. Med. **291**:755-758, 1974.

89. On the brink of disaster. Nursing grand rounds, Nurs. (Jenkintown) **6**:27-32, 1976.

90. Pasch, S., and Jamieson, T.: Going home with COPD: is your patient ready? Can. Nurs. **71**:34-25, 1975.

91. Penn, R.L.: Blastomycosis. In Conn, H.F.: Current therapy 1982, Philadelphia, 1982, W.B. Saunders Co.

92. Pennoyer, D., and Sheffer, A.L.: Asthma in adults. In Conn, H.F.: Current therapy 1982, Philadelphia, 1982, W.B. Saunders Co.

93. Peterson, L.D., and Green, J.H.: Nurse-managed tuberculosis clinic, Am. J. Nurs. **77**:433-435, 1977.

94. Petty, T.L.: Adult respiratory distress syndrome. In Kryger, M.H., editor: Pathology of respiration, New York, 1981, John Wiley & Sons, Inc.

95. *Petty, T.L.: A chest physician's perspective on asthma, Heart Lung **1**:611-620, 1972.

96. *Petty, T.L.: Respiratory failure and the heart, Heart Lung **1**:84, 1972.

97. *Phipps, W.J., Barker, W.L., and Daly, B.J.: Respiratory insufficiency and failure. In Meltzer, L.E., et al.: Concepts and practices of intensive care for nurse specialists, ed. 2, Philadelphia, 1975, The Charles Press Publishers.

98. Pontoppidan, H., Geffin, F., and Lowenstein, E.: Acute respiratory failure in the adult, N. Engl. J. Med. **27**:690-698, 743-752, 799-806, 1972.

99. *Rassmusen, D.L.: Black lung in southern Appalachia, Am. J. Nurs. **70**:509-511, 1970.

100. Reyes, M.P.: The aerobic gram-negative bacillary pneumonias, Med. Clin. North Am. **64**:363-383, 1980.

101. Reference deleted in proofs.

102. Reference deleted in proofs.

103. *Rifas, E.M.: How you and your patient can manage dyspnea, Nurs. '80 **6**:34-41, 1980.

104. Rodman, M.J.: Drugs for acute respiratory failure, RN **38**:49-50, 52-56, 1975.

105. Rogers, B.H., et al.: Opportunistic pneumonia: a clinicopathological study of five cases caused by an unidentified acid-fact bacterium, N. Engl. J. Med. **301**:959-961, 1979.

106. *Rokosky, J.S.: Assessment of the individual with altered respiratory function, Nurs. Clin. North Am. **16**:195-209, 1981.

107. *Sachs, M.: Primary lung abscess. In Conn, H.F.: Current therapy 1982, Philadelphia, 1982, W.B. Saunders Co.

108. Saltman, J.: The patient has chronic lung disease. Then what? He needs comprehensive services. There's hope in the ALA/ATS task force plan, Am. Lung Assoc. Bull. **61**:5-12, 1975.

109. *Shapiro, B.A., Harrison, R.A., and Trout, C.A.: Clinical application of respiratory care, Chicago, 1975, Year Book Medical Publishers, Inc.

110. Silva, J., Jr.: Anaerobic infections, Heart Lung **5**:406-410, 1976.

111. Speir, W.A., Jr.: Outpatient management of chronic bronchitis and emphysema, Geriatrics **31**:77-80, 1976.

112. Stechschulte, D.J.: Asthma and immunology. In Essays in medicine, New York, 1972, Medcom Books, Inc.

113. Stephens, G.J., and Parsons, MC.: A delicate balance: managing chronic airway obstruction in a neurosurgical patient, Am. J. Nurs. **75**:1492-1497, 1975.

114. Stevens, P.M.: Positive end expiratory pressure breathing, Basics RD **5**:1-6, 1977.

115. Straus, M.J.: Lung cancer: clinical diagnosis and treatment, New York, 1977, Grune & Stratton, Inc.

116. Stroud, S.D.: What you need to know to save a shock-lung victim, RN **40**:47, 1977.

117. Taylor, C.M.: Pneumococcal pneumonia: your patient's second threat? Nurs. (Jenkintown) **6**:31-38, 1976.

118. Thurlbeck, W.M.: Chronic bronchitis and emphysema—the pathophysiology of chronic lung disease. In American Thoracic Society: Basics of RD, New York, 1974, The Society.

119. Tomashefski, J.F., editor: Chronic obstructive pulmonary disease: a perplexing and challenging spectrum: core curriculum symposium (pulmonary disease), Postgrad. Med. **62**:87-151, 1977.

120. Traver, G.A.: Living with chronic respiratory disease, Am. J. Nurs. **75**:1777-1781, 1794, 1975.

121. *Traver, G.A.: Respiratory nursing: the science and the art, New York, 1982, John Wiley & Sons, Inc.

122. Turino, G.M., et al.: Mechanisms of pulmonary injury, Am. J. Med. **57**:493-505, 1974.

123. U.S. Center for Disease Control, Tuberculosis Branch: Tuberculosis statistics: cities and states—1976, Atlanta, 1977, The Center.

124. U.S. Department of Health, Education, and Welfare: Current trends. Isoniazid-associated hepatitis: summary of the report of the tuberculosis advisory committee and special consultants to the director, U.S. Center for Disease Control, Morbid. Mortal. Weekly Rep. **23**:97-98, 1974.

125. U.S. Department of Health, Education, and Welfare: Guidelines for prevention of TB transmission in hospitals, Atlanta, 1975, U.S. Center for Disease Control.

126. U.S. Department of Health, education, and Welfare: Recommendation of the public health service advisory committee on immunization practices—BCG vaccines, U.S. Center for Disease Control, Morbid. Mortal. Weekly Rep. **24**:69-80, 1975.

127. U.S. Department of Health and Human Services/Public Health Service, Centers for Disease Control: Morbid. Mortal. Weekly Rep. **31**:10, March 19, 1982.

128. VanArsdal, P.P., Jr., and Glennon, G.H.: Drug therapy in the management of asthma, Ann. Intern. Med. **87**:68-74, 1977.

129. Wade, J.F.: Respiratory nursing care: physiology and technique, ed. 2, St. Louis, 1977, The C.V. Mosby Co.

130. *Wagner, M.M.: Assessment of patients with multiple injuries, Am. J. Nurs. **72**:1822-1827, 1972.

131. Ward, J.: Cromolyn sodium: a new approach to treatment of asthma, Heart Lung **4**:415-419, 1975.

132. *Weg, J.G.: Tuberculosis and other myocobacterial disease. In Conn, H.F.: Current therapy 1982, Philadelphia, 1982, W.B. Saunders Co.

133. Weiss, E.B., and Sega, M.S.: Bronchial asthma: mechanisms and therapeutics, Boston, 1976, Little, Brown & Co.

134. West, J.B.: Pulmonary pathophysiology—the essentials, Baltimore, 1977, The Williams & Wilkins Co.

135. West, J.B.: Respiratory physiology—the essentials, Baltimore, 1974, The Williams & Wilkins Co.

136. West, J.B.: Ventilation/ blood flow and gas exchange, ed. 3, Oxford, England, 1980, Blackwell Scientific Publications.

137. Wilson, P.: Evaluating chest films, Nurse Pract. 2:6-13, 1977.

138. *Wilson, R.F.: The diagnosis and treatment of acute respiratory failure in sepsis, Heart Lung 5:614-620, 1976.

139. *Wilson, R.F., and Sibbald, W.J.: Acute respiratory failure, Crit. Care Med. 4:79-89, 1976.

140. Wyngaarten, J.B., and Smith, L.H.: Cecil textbook of medicine, ed. 16, Philadelphia, 1982, W.B. Saunders Co.

141. *Wyper, M.A.: Pulmonary embolism: fighting the silent killer, Nurs. '75 5:31-38, 1975.

142. Youmans, G.P., Patterson, P.Y., and Sommers H.M.: The biologic and clinical basis of infectious diseases, Philadelphia, 1975, W.B. Saunders Co.

143. *Ziskind, M.M.: The acute bacterial pneumonias in the adult. In American Thoracic Society: Basics of RD, New York, 1974, The Society.

Classic

144. *Broussard, R.: Using relaxation for COPD, Am. J. Nurs. 69:1962-1963, 1969.

145. *Richter, J.M., and Sloan, R.: A relaxation technique, Am. J. Nurs. 69:1960-1964, 1969.

146. *Riley, R.L.: Air-borne infections, Am. J. Nurs. 60:1246-1248, 1960.

AUDIOVISUAL RESOURCES

Care of the patient with pulmonary emphysema, Garden Grove, Calif., 1971, Trainex. (Cassette tape, filmstrip, instructors's guide, and script.)

Chronic obstructive pulmonary disease: breathing patterns, Washington, D.C., 1974, National Medical Audiovisual Center. (Film, 16 mm.)

Chronic obstructive pulmonary disease: diaphragmatic pattern, Washington, D.C., 1975, National Medical Audiovisual Center. (Film, 16 mm.)

The pathophysiology of emphysema, Garden Grove, Calif. 1971, Trainex. (Cassette tape, filmstrip instructor's guide, and script.)

Postural drainage: patient positioning, Washington, D.C., 1976, National Medical Audiovisual Center. (Film, 16 mm.)

PROBLEMS OF NUTRITION

Without food, human beings cannot survive. A person must be able to take in food and swallow it (ingestion) and to dilute and process the food in such a manner that nutrients are available to be transmitted to cells (digestion). Problems with structure or function of the upper gastrointestinal system or with amount or quality of food being processed can affect life itself. Problems with nutrition also affect other organs of the body, rendering them more susceptible to infections or other diseases. Maintenance of health therefore requires an intact and functioning gastrointestinal system and practices leading to the ingestion of adequate amount and quality of nutrients.

This unit consists of five chapters. The first two chapters discuss *assessment of nutritional status* and *intervention* for the person with *impaired nutrition*. The last three chapters focus on the digestive system and include *assessment of upper gastrointestinal function*, general *interventions* for the person with a *digestive disorder*, and specific *problems* of the *upper gastrointestinal tract*.

CHAPTER 52

ASSESSMENT OF NUTRITIONAL STATUS

JANICE NEVILLE

Nutritional needs and nutritional care are major concerns of the general public, government agencies, and health professionals.* Malnutrition has been indicated as a major problem in hospitalized patients.[35] Nurses, physicians, and dietitians have been challenged to identify the nutritional needs of patients and to improve the quality of care.† The patient also has responsibilities,[29] whether hospitalized or at home, but should be able to expect nutritional care as an integral component of health care.

Nutrition has been identified as a national health priority.[43] In assessing relative contributions to death and disease, the surgeon general reported that as much as 50% of the U.S. mortality in 1976 was the result of unhealthy behavior or life-styles; 20% to human biologic factors; and only 10% to inadequacies in health care. Data such as these were used to determine a national strategy for improvements in health. The objectives for the nation identify 15 priority areas with specific objectives for each. Achievement of the objectives by 1990 is identified as a shared responsibility for all. Nutrition objectives include specific goals for the improvement of health status, reduction of risk factors, and improved services. For example, "by 1990, virtually all routine health contacts with health professionals should include some element of nutrition education and nutrition counseling."[43]

Objectives with nutrition implications are presented in sections on high blood pressure control, pregnancy and infant health, and fluoridation and dental health, in addition to the 17 items under nutrition. The emphasis in the national objectives is twofold—promoting health and preventing disease. Individuals with good nutritional status are less likely to get sick, and they are generally less seriously ill if sickness does occur. They are better able to withstand trauma and stress. Recovery is significantly affected, and it can be enhanced by appropriate nutrition therapy.

Many persons enter the hospital in poor nutritional status, and the nutritional status may deteriorate during hospitalization.[51,56] Studies of general populations in the United States have identified very few cases of frank deficiency disease, but a significant proportion of the population is either malnourished or at significant risk of developing nutritional problems. Obesity is a major health problem in the United States and is present in the population at all age levels. Adolescents have the highest prevalence of unsatisfactory nutritional status, and many persons over 60 years of age present evidence of poor status. People are adopting new eating styles that may increase nutritional risk,* and eating patterns have been identified as a critical public health concern.

Good nursing care has always included attention to the patient's food needs. Maintenance of good nutrition is a major nursing objective. Nutritional evaluation is an important part of total patient assessment and provides essential information for differential diagnosis and for planning appropriate interventions. An awareness of nutritional deficits, excesses, or imbalances that may exist can be of particular importance in determining management of the person. Monitoring the nutritional well-being of the person throughout hospitalization or on an ongoing basis to assure maintenance of or improvement in status is as important as the initial assessment.

---

*References 2, 13, 17, 19, 24.
†References 7, 14, 28, 32, 46.

---

*References 3, 10, 16, 18, 25, 37, 49.

Nutrition needs

Good nutritional status exists when protein, fat, carbohydrate, minerals, vitamins, and water are consumed in sufficient amounts and are used appropriately by the body to meet needs regardless of age, sex, life-style, or state of health. All persons need the same nutrients throughout life (see box, p. 1341). The amounts required vary in predictable patterns. Growth, basal metabolic needs, and physical activity are the major factors responsible for changing nutrient needs. Disease, trauma, variations in metabolism (normal and abnormal), medications, and treatments can also affect needs.

Since 1940, the Food and Nutrition Board of the National Academy of Sciences has periodically reviewed existing nutrition knowledge and research to formulate recommendations for the amounts of the different nutrients to be used as a basis for planning nutritionally adequate diets.[44] Table 52-1 illustrates the changes in amounts of nutrients recommended from infancy throughout life. Not all of the nutrients identified in the box are listed in the table, because it is assumed that when an appropriate variety and amount of ordinary foods are consumed to meet the levels of nutrients recommended, the diet will supply the other nutrients as well. The level of iron intake recommended for women during the reproductive years is high because many young women do not include iron-rich foods in their diet and their iron stores are poor.[8,53]

TABLE 52-1. Recommended daily dietary allowances, revised 1980* (Designed for the maintenance of good nutrition of practically all healthy people in the United States)

		Weight		Height			Fat-soluble vitamins		
	Age (yr)	kg	lb	cm	in.	Protein (g)	Vitamin A (µg RE)†	Vitamin D (µg)‡	Vitamin E (mg α-TE)§
Infants	0.0-0.5	6	13	60	24	kg × 2.2	420	10	3
	0.5-1.0	9	20	71	28	kg × 2.0	400	10	4
Children	1-3	13	29	90	35	23	400	10	5
	4-6	20	44	112	44	30	500	10	6
	7-10	28	62	132	52	34	700	10	7
Males	11-14	45	99	157	62	45	1000	10	8
	15-18	66	145	176	69	56	1000	10	10
	19-22	70	154	177	70	56	1000	7.5	10
	23-50	70	154	178	70	56	1000	5	10
	51 +	70	154	178	70	56	1000	5	10
Females	11-14	46	101	157	62	46	800	10	8
	15-18	55	120	163	64	46	800	10	8
	19-22	55	120	163	64	44	800	7.5	8
	23-50	55	120	163	64	44	800	5	8
	51 +	55	120	163	64	44	800	5	8
Pregnant						+30	+200	+5	+2
Lactating						+20	+400	+5	+3

*From Food and Nutrition Board, National Academy of Sciences–National Research Council: Recommended dietary allowances, 9th rev. ed., National Academy of Sciences, 1980. The allowances are intended to provide for individual variations among most normal persons as they live in the United States under usual environmental stresses. Diets should be based on a variety of common foods in order to provide other nutrients for which human requirements have been less well defined. See Table 52-8 for weights and heights by individual year of age. See Table 52-5 for suggested average energy intakes.
†Retinol equivalents. 1 retinol equivalent = 1 µg retinol or 6 µg β-carotene.
‡As cholecalciferol. 10 µg cholecalciferol = 400 IU of vitamin D.
§α-tocopherol equivalents. 1 mg d-α tocopherol = 1 α-TE.
‖1 NE (niacin equivalent) is equal to 1 mg of niacin or 60 mg of dietary tryptophan.

NUTRIENTS REQUIRED BY THE HUMAN BODY

Water

Protein

  Total nitrogen

  Isoleucine

  Leucine

  Lysine

  Methionine
  (cystine)

  Phenylalanine
  (tyrosine)

  Threonine

  Tryptophan

  Valine

  Histidine
  (infant)

Carbohydrate

  Starch, sugar,
  fiber

Fat

  Linoleate
  (arachidonate)

Minerals

  Calcium

  Chromium

Phosphorus

Copper

Fluorine

Iron

Iodine

Magnesium

Manganese

Molybdenum

Selenium

Zinc

Sodium

Potassium

Chloride

Vitamins

  Vitamin C

  Biotin

  Folacin

  Niacin

  Pantothenic acid

  Riboflavin

  Thiamin

  Vitamin B_6

  Vitamin B_{12}

Vitamin A
(carotene)

Vitamin D

Vitamin E

Vitamin K

Water-soluble vitamins							Minerals					
Vitamin C (mg)	Thiamin (mg)	Riboflavin (mg)	Niacin (mg NE)‖	Vitamin B_6 (mg)	Folacin¶ (µg)	Vitamin B_{12} (µg)	Calcium (mg)	Phosphorus (mg)	Magnesium (mg)	Iron (mg)	Zinc (mg)	Iodine (µg)
35	0.3	0.4	6	0.3	30	0.5#	360	240	50	10	3	40
35	0.5	0.6	8	0.6	45	1.5	540	360	70	15	5	50
45	0.7	0.8	9	0.9	100	2.0	800	800	150	15	10	70
45	0.9	1.0	11	1.3	200	2.5	800	800	200	10	10	90
45	1.2	1.4	16	1.6	300	3.0	800	800	250	10	10	120
50	1.4	1.6	18	1.8	400	3.0	1200	1200	350	18	15	150
60	1.4	1.7	18	2.0	400	3.0	1200	1200	400	18	15	150
60	1.5	1.7	19	2.2	400	3.0	800	800	350	10	15	150
60	1.4	1.6	18	2.2	400	3.0	800	800	350	10	15	150
60	1.2	1.4	16	2.2	400	3.0	800	800	350	10	15	150
50	1.1	1.3	15	1.8	400	3.0	1200	1200	300	18	15	150
60	1.1	1.3	14	2.0	400	3.0	1200	1200	300	18	15	150
60	1.1	1.3	14	2.0	400	3.0	800	800	300	18	15	150
60	1.0	1.2	13	2.0	400	3.0	800	800	300	18	15	150
60	1.0	1.2	13	2.0	400	3.0	800	800	300	10	15	150
+20	+0.4	+0.3	+2	+0.6	+400	+1.0	+400	+400	+150	**	+5	+25
+40	+0.5	+0.5	+5	+0.5	+100	+1.0	+400	+400	+150	**	+10	+50

¶The folacin allowances refer to dietary sources as determined by *Lactobacillus casei* assay after treatment with enzymes (conjugases) to make polyglutamyl forms of the vitamin available to the test organism.

#The recommended dietary allowance for vitamin B_{12} in infants is based on average concentration of the vitamin in human milk. The allowances after weaning are based on energy intake (as recommended by the American Academy of Pediatrics) and consideration of other factors, such as intestinal absorption.

**The increased requirements during pregnancy cannot be met by the iron content of habitual American diets nor by the existing iron stores of many women; therefore the use of 30-60 mg of supplemental iron is recommended. Iron needs during lactation are not substantially different from those of nonpregnant women, but continued supplementation of the mother for 2-3 mo after parturition is advisable in order to replenish stores depleted by pregnancy.

TABLE 52-2. Estimated safe and adequate daily dietary intakes of selected vitamins*

	Age (yr)	Vitamin K (μg)	Biotin (μg)	Pantothenic acid (mg)
Infants	0.0-0.5	12	35	2
	0.5-1.0	10-20	50	3
Children	1-3	15-30	65	3
	4-6	20-40	85	3-4
	7-10	30-60	120	4-5
Adolescents	11-18	50-100	100-200	4-7
Adults	19+	70-140	100-200	4-7

*From Food and Nutrition Board, National Academy of Sciences—National Research Council: Recommended dietary allowances, 9th rev. ed., National Academy of Sciences, 1980.

TABLE 52-3. Estimated safe and adequate daily dietary intakes of selected trace elements*

	Age (yr)	Copper (mg)	Manganese (mg)	Fluoride (mg)	Chromium (mg)	Selenium (mg)	Molybdenum (mg)
Infants	0.0-0.5	0.5-0.7	0.5-0.7	0.1-0.5	0.01-0.04	0.01-0.04	0.03-0.06
	0.5-1.0	0.7-1.0	0.7-1.0	0.2-1.0	0.02-0.06	0.02-0.06	0.04-0.08
Children	1-3	1.0-1.5	1.0-1.5	0.5-1.5	0.02-0.08	0.02-0.08	0.05-0.1
	4-6	1.5-2.0	1.5-2.0	1.0-2.5	0.03-0.12	0.03-0.12	0.06-0.15
	7-10	2.0-2.5	2.0-3.0	1.5-2.5	0.05-0.2	0.05-0.2	0.10-0.3
Adolescents	11-18	2.0-3.0	2.5-5.0	1.5-2.5	0.05-0.2	0.05-0.2	0.15-0.5
Adults	19+	2.0-3.0	2.5-5.0	1.5-4.0	0.05-0.2	0.05-0.2	0.15-0.15

*From Food and Nutrition Board, National Academy of Sciences—National Research Council: Recommended dietary allowances, 9th rev. ed., National Academy of Sciences, 1980.

TABLE 52-4. Estimated safe and adequate daily dietary intake of selected electrolytes*

	Age (yr)	Sodium (mg)	Potassium (mg)	Chloride (mg)
Infants	0.0-0.5	115-350	350-925	275-700
	0.5-1.0	250-750	425-1275	400-1200
Children	1-3	325-975	550-1650	500-1500
	4-6	450-1350	775-2325	700-2100
	7-10	600-1800	1000-3000	925-2775
Adolescents	11-18	900-2700	1525-4575	1400-4200
Adults	19+	1100-3300	1875-5625	1700-5100

*From Food and Nutrition Board, National Academy of Sciences—National Research Council: Recommended dietary allowances, 9th rev. ed., National Academy of Sciences, 1980.

Nutrient recommendations now include information about safe and adequate levels for three vitamins, six trace elements, and three electrolytes. See Table 52-3, and note that since the toxic levels for many trace elements may be only several times usual intakes, the upper levels for the trace elements should not be habitually exceeded.[43] Levels of safe intake vary from small to wide. For example, rather small but constant consumption of energy (kilocalories [kcal]) will produce excess fat. Protein and sodium are nutrients with intermediate ranges. Intakes of these nutrients twofold or threefold over recommendations produce chronic, subtle, adverse effects. The range is relatively wide for most vitamins and some trace elements where intakes of tenfold or more produce undesirable effects.[31]

All nutrients are of equal importance, although they are not required in equal amounts (Fig. 52-1). The nutrients providing energy (protein, fats, carbohydrates) and water are required in much larger quantities than vitamins that regulate body processes. The differences in the quantities of various nutrients required by an individual are much greater than the change in amounts of any one nutrient over the life cycle. Note in Table 52-1 that 0.5 μg of vitamin B_{12} are recommended for the infant and 3.0 μg for the adult; 360 to 1200 mg of calcium are recommended at different points in the life cycle. There is no overlapping of requirements. If a person consumed vitamin A in the quantities recommended for calcium or phosphorus, toxicity would result.[34,38] When food is used as the source for nutrients, such imbalances are unlikely to occur; however, nutrients are available in concentrated forms as dietary supplements, over-the-counter preparations, and prescription drugs. Should these concentrated nutrients be prescribed for the person, the nurse handles them with the same care as any other medication. There is an unsupported intuitive feeling that nutrient supplements are essential.[12,54] However, response to these supplements occurs only when persons have been relatively nutrition deficient, eating foods marginal in nutrient value, and when the supplement provides the specific nutrient or nutrients that are deficient. There is a point beyond which supplementation does not help the person and *may actually cause harm.* Continued intake of vitamins and minerals at levels from 10 to 100 times the recommended daily allowance (RDA) is associated with chronic toxicity. As a guide, recommended levels of energy intake for the public are published (Table 52-5). There can be great differences in the amount of energy needed to maintain appropriate body weight depending on the lean body mass and vigor of physical activity.

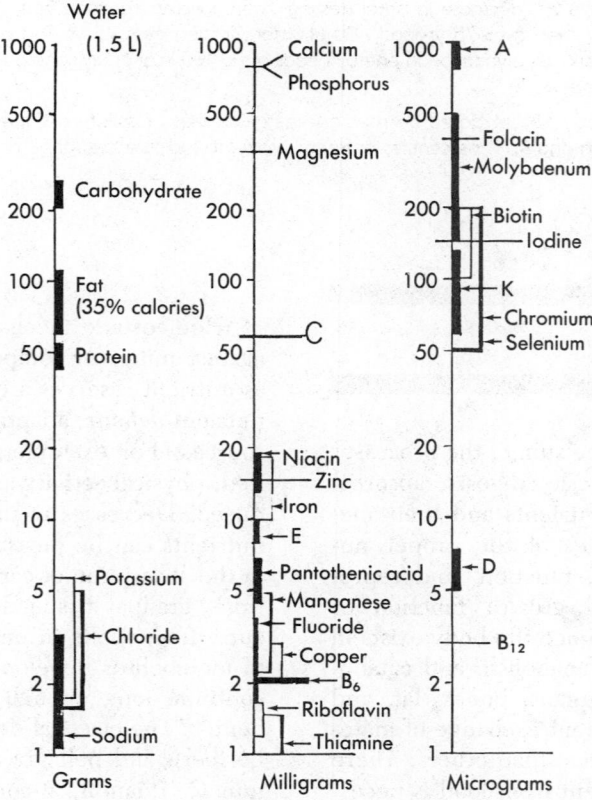

Fig. 52-1. Recommended dietary allowances (1980) from the National Research Council, National Academy of Sciences. Carbohydrate and fat vary with energy needs and are calculated from the average kilocalories for male and female adults in Table 52-3.

TABLE 52-5. Mean heights and weights and recommended energy intake*

	Age (yr)	Weight		Height		Energy needs	
		kg	lb	cm	in.	kcal	range
Infants	0.0-0.5	6	13	60	24	kg × 115	(95-145)
	0.5-1.0	9	20	71	28	kg × 105	(80-135)
Children	1-3	13	29	90	35	1300	(900-1800)
	4-6	20	44	112	44	1700	(1300-2300)
	7-10	28	62	132	52	2400	(1650-3300)
Males	11-14	45	99	157	62	2700	(2000-3700)
	15-18	66	145	176	69	2800	(2100-3900)
	19-22	70	154	177	70	2900	(2500-3300)
	23-50	70	154	178	70	2700	(2300-3100)
	51-75	70	154	178	70	2400	(2000-2800)
	76+	70	154	178	70	2050	(1650-2450)
							(1500-3000)
Females	11-14	46	101	157	62	2200	
	15-18	55	120	163	64	2100	(1200-3000)
	19-22	55	120	163	64	2100	(1700-2500)
	23-50	55	120	163	64	2000	(1600-2400)
	51-75	55	120	163	64	1800	(1400-2200)
	76+	55	120	163	64	1600	(1200-2000)
Pregnancy						+300	
Lactation						+500	

*From Food and Nutrition Board, National Academy of Sciences–National Research Council: Recommended dietary allowances, 9th rev. ed. National Academy of Sciences, 1980.

The energy allowances for young adults are for men and women doing light work; allowances for two older age groups represent mean energy needs over these age spans, allowing for a 2% decrease in basal (resting) metabolic rate/decade and a reduction in activity of 200 kcal/day for men and women 51-75 yr, 500 kcal for men over 75 yr, and 400 kcal for women over 75 yr. The customary range of daily enery output is shown in parentheses for adults and is based on a variation in energy needs of ± 400 kcal at any one age emphasizing the wide range of energy intakes appropriate for any group of people.

Energy allowances for children through age 18 are based on median energy intakes of children of these ages followed in longitudinal growth studies. The values in parentheses are 10th and 90th percentiles of enery intake, to indicate the range of energy consumption among children of these ages.

Nutrition process

Nutrition can be defined as the sum of the processes by which a living organism ingests, digests, absorbs, transports, uses, and excretes nutrients and their metabolites. With adequate supplies of the proper nutrients, the organism can grow, function, and reproduce. When supplies are limited, growth, function, or reproduction may be impaired. Since the body exists in a state of dynamic equilibrium, anabolism and catabolism are continuous. Muscles, organs, bones, fat, and the blood participate in the constant exchange of materials, with some tissues more active than others. There is some loss; therefore replacement from food is necessary throughout life. Periods of growth increase requirements for nutrients and energy.

Homeostatic mechanisms tend to protect the body against minor or temporary changes in nutrient status as nutrient reserves are mobilized to meet needs. With nutrient *deficits*, adaptations occur to conserve body resources. For example, when energy supplies are limited, physical activity and then basal metabolism are reduced. Decreases in urinary excretion levels of certain nutrients can be measured, as can increased efficiency in the absorption of certain nutrients such as iron. Over time, gradual tissue desaturation of the nutrients occurs. Reductions in enzyme activity and altered levels of metabolites develop. If this process is permitted to continue long enough, anatomic lesions become evident.[5,9] The classical deficiency diseases such as scurvy, beriberi, and pellagra are results of depletions of vitamin C, thiamin, B-complex vitamins, and niacin that are continued long enough for identifiable lesions in skin, tongue, and organs to develop as clinical signs of malnutrition. If untreated, progressive depletion results in death.

Nutrition *excesses* can also produce malnutrition.[34,36,57] Mechanisms tend to protect the body by accumulating reserves or, for some nutrients, by increasing the rate of excretion from the body or decreasing efficiency of absorption. When excesses are large or prolonged over time, increased concentrations of nutrients and alterations in enzyme activities and levels of metabolites develop. Over time, clinical signs and symptoms develop. The most common example of this type of malnutrition in the U.S. population is obesity. Consumption of energy-yielding compounds (e.g., protein, fat, carbohydrate, and alcohol) in amounts greater than needed for energy expenditure result in storage of energy as body fat. Eventually, the stores of body fat become large enough to affect body functioning, physical mobility, and health. Obese persons have greater risk of osteoarthritis, diabetes mellitus, cardiovascular disease, and hypertension.[24]

Nutritional status

In order to assess nutritional status, it is necessary to determine the nutrient supply to the body, availability for stores and metabolic processes, body size and composition, and physical signs. The basic principles are those used in general evaluation: (1) observing the person's general appearance and (2) obtaining careful medical and dietary histories, physical examination, and selected laboratory measurements. There is no one simple test of a person's nutritional state. Furthermore, long periods of time may elapse from the initial limitation of nutrient supply until malnutrition becomes clinically obvious. A person with good body stores of a nutrient as a result of consuming a nutritionally sound diet can tolerate relatively long periods of deprivation of that nutrient. The rate at which depletion progresses will be affected by the stores available and the rate of body utilization or excretion of the nutrient. The time elapsing between the insult to nutrient supply and the actual appearance of clinical signs obvious on physical examination can be as little as a week or as long as several years. For this reason, it is important to remember that dietary, laboratory, and clinical data may appear to be poorly correlated. This lack of correlation has been interpreted by some persons as demonstrating the impossibility of making an assessment and by others as evidence that one type of data is superior or more reliable than another. Actually, these data measure different points along a continuum of deprivation or excess. It is hoped that attention to the nutritional needs of the person, assessment, and appropriate interventions will protect the person and reduce the risk of impaired growth and body function. Prevention or alleviation of malnutrition requires identification of its degree and cause so that appropriate remedies may be instituted.

The nurse has the opportunity to incorporate questions and observations relevant to nutritional needs in the health assessment. Not only does this identify nutrition-related nursing diagnoses, but it also identifies persons at risk who require more extensive evaluation. As stated previously, the person's nutritional well-being is a shared responsibility and frequently requires the knowledge and skills of nurse, dietitian, physician, and others. The initial assessment is important, but nursing responsibility does not end there, since the patient's condition may improve or regress, and changes need to be identified. The earlier problems are identified, the earlier appropriate interventions can be formulated and the person protected from serious sequelae.

Assessing nutrient supply

Taking dietary history

Information about nutrient supply obtained during the initial assessment is necessarily subjective. It must be obtained from the patient or family by interview. Since both kinds and amounts of nutrients are important, intake data must be both qualitative and quantitative.[20,60] Skill in interviewing is required, since biases can be introduced or "proper" answers supplied by leading questions. The following questions should be considered, one at a time:

When did you first have something to eat or drink yesterday?

Did you eat breakfast yesterday?

Did you have orange juice for breakfast yesterday?

Notice that the first question makes no assumptions. The second question reminds one that breakfast is desirable and tempts one to provide information about breakfast, whether real or imaginary. The third question restricts freedom to answer even more and includes the interviewer's perception of an appropriate food choice. Further it implies that orange juice at breakfast is essential, in effect misinforming the patient.

Directing specific questions about food consumption to the day preceding the interview is a technique frequently used in nutrition surveys designed to assess the nutritional status of groups. It is simple and rapid and takes about 15 minutes. Although the 24-hour recall is useful as a device for continued monitoring, it should not be used for initial assessment. Food intake on a single day is a poor indicator of nutrient supply for an individual.[20,60] Not only does food intake vary over the week according to work, school, and family schedules; but intake immediately preceding hospitalization or appointments for care is often atypical.

It is more useful to ask the person to describe his or her *usual eating patterns*, including when, what, and how much foods or liquids are consumed, with gentle probing to obtain details about food preparation, use of seasonings, and so forth. Far too often the questions about diet provide a social rather than information exchange:

"Has the baby been eating well?" "Yes."
"How's your diet?" "Fine."

Unfortunately, exchanges such as these may be charted as "Nutrition no problem" or "Patient well nourished." Any problems the patient may have are unidentified and are likely to remain so.

Questioning should elicit a picture of total food consumption for the day. Designation of meals and snacks is not really necessary and may bias answers by implying value judgments. The following approach is more likely to provide useful information:

What usually is the first thing you eat or drink? When? How much? What else? You said you usually have 2 slices of toast; do you put anything on your toast? When do you eat or drink again? Let's review this now. You said you usually have a cup of soup for lunch at work; what do you have on the days when you're not working? What kind of milk do you buy?

The interviewer should make no assumptions. Some people put cream, milk, or sugar in coffee or tea, and some do not. Some people put dressing on their salads, and some do not. Find out what the person does by asking.

Portion sizes are important and are difficult to estimate without some visual reference. A hamburger can vary from 42 g (1.5 oz) to 168 g (6 oz) or more, making a significant difference in determining whether nutrient supply is adequate. The glass used at home may hold 90, 240, 300, 360, or even 480 ml (3, 8, 10, 12, or 16 oz) of fluid. Dietitians frequently use food models, measuring cups, spoons, and other aids for obtaining intake data. For the hospitalized patient, the equipment and portions on the tray can be used as a basis for comparison.

When the usual eating pattern has been determined, any *recent changes* from the pattern should be identified and described together with any explanations. Changes may be the result of illness (e.g., anorexia, nausea, vomiting and diarrhea), self-imposed dietary regimens, or emotional or physical stress. Experience with special or prescribed diets should be recorded.

Since nutrient supply is affected by use of *supplements, medications,* and *drugs*[48] the person is asked about intake of these items, whether they have been pre-

scribed by a physician or not. Whenever possible, the product, content, and size of dose should be recorded.

Food and fluid *preferences* and *dislikes* should be identified. This information is most frequently asked in order to be sure a patient is satisfied with hospital meals. It is also useful in determining fluid intake, potential inadequacies or excesses, and food intolerances. If a person reports not eating a particular food, it is important to determine if taste, intolerance, or allergy is a determinant.

Information about *financial resources* for food, *facilities* for purchasing, storing, and preparing food, as well as occupation and *daily activities* provide information about nutritional needs and the ease with which needs are met.

The person should be invited to describe any *problems with diet*. These can include problems resulting from a lack of information about a diet previously prescribed; concerns or fears about food, which may generate from the media or from ideas of others; and physical difficulties with sight, taste, chewing, movement, or pain, which may affect intake. Does the person need help with eating? What kind of help?

It is also useful to have the person describe *weight* and *nutrition status*. Does the person perceive body weight as normal, excessive, or low? Have there been major fluctuations in weight over the last year? Does the person consider diet or nutritional state a problem?

An important source of objective information about intake of the institutionalized patient is frequently ignored, that is, the choice of food the patient makes from menus and the food actually consumed from the tray, snack bar, and gifts, as well as from other modes of nutrient supply such as medications, intravenous or tube feedings, and fluids kept at the bedside. Not only can the patient be asked about these, but also direct observations can be made. Unexpected or inappropriate response to nutrition therapy may be explained by the difference between plans and implementation, if someone takes the time to observe what is happening and intervenes. For example, two women were admitted to the hospital for evaluation and treatment of heart disease. Both women had severe hypertension and were obese; both were prescribed 1000-calorie, limited-sodium diets. After 1 week, the physician noted that one patient was responding well, with significant weight loss recorded, while the other was gaining weight, both as body fat and increased edema, despite eating only half the food on the tray. The dietitian, when called, determined that the second patient was consuming a high-calorie, high-sodium diet consisting primarily of candy and other items brought daily by visitors at the patient's request.

The information gathered by the nurse about usual dietary patterns and changes provides basic data that can be evaluated rapidly to estimate adequacy of intake and to identify current and potential problems. For more complete and detailed study of intake and analysis, the dietitian can offer special expertise and assistance.

Evaluating nutrient intake

The food guides that have been developed to help people choose the kinds and amounts of food to eat for health can be used for a rapid evaluation of adequacy of the diet eaten at home or food intake in the hospital. There are many different food guides, since to be effective they must be devised for a specific country or culture and feature the foods readily available and acceptable to the people being evaluated.

A daily food guide used in the United States is shown in the box below. The guide groups staple food items rich in protein, vitamins, and minerals into four major classes according to their major nutrient contributions. Recommendations are made for the number and size of servings to be selected from each food group. One can evaluate a diet quickly by checking to see if the recommended types of food and servings are included in the usual dietary pattern.

Since foods are mixtures of nutrients, the protein, vitamin, and mineral requirements are substantially met when the daily intake includes the recommended servings from each group.[22,50] The calorie level of the basic diet is low (Table 52-6) but is approximately sufficient for adult basal metabolism. Adequacy of energy intake is best judged by evaluation of body weight. In this method of evaluation, fats, oils, and sweets are not tabulated, since they provide primarily energy.

Each food grouping contributes particular nutrients to the total diet. The absence of any one food group from the diet or particular types of food should alert the nurse that the patient has a potential nutrition problem.

Milk and milk products and foods from the *meat group* are excellent sources of high-quality protein. In contrast to the meat group milk provides calcium, phosphorus, and riboflavin abundantly as well as other minerals and vitamins. Milk is not a rich source of iron or vitamin C and should not be used as the sole protein food in the diet. There are many different types of milk: homogenized, 2%, skim milk, buttermilk, yogurt, and

---

DAILY FOOD GUIDE

Food group	Servings recommended
A Milk:	
Fluid milk—whole, skim, cultured, evaporated; milk solids may be in beverage or mixtures fortified with vitamin D	Children: 3-4 glasses Teenagers: 4 glasses Adults: 2 or more glasses Pregnant women: 4 glasses
B Vegetables and fruits:	
Vitamin A rich—dark green or deep yellow (e.g., broccoli, kale, carrots, squash, turnip, mustard greens)	1 serving (½ C) at least every other day
Vitamin C rich—citrus fruits and juices, cantaloupe, tomato, cabbage, pepper, strawberries	1 serving (½ C or usual portion)
Other fruits and vegetables	2 or more servings (½ C or usual portion; i.e., medium potato or apple)
C Meat	
Meat, fish, poultry, eggs, dried beans and peas, nuts	2 or more servings (60-75 g [2-3 oz] meat, fish, poultry, liver; 2 eggs; 1 C beans, peas, lentils; 4 tbsp peanut butter)
D Bread and cereal— whole grain or enriched	4 or more servings (1 slice bread; 30 g [1 oz] dry cereal; ½-¾ C cooked cereal, rice, macaroni, noodles, spaghetti)

Amounts recommended for a preschool child are ½ L (1 pt) milk, ½ C fruits or juices, ½ C vegetables, 75 g (3 oz) meat and eggs, and 2 servings bread and cereal.

TABLE 52-6. Protein and calorie values of basic diet selected to meet recommendations outlined in food guide for an adult

Group and food chosen	Protein (g)	Calories
Milk, ½ L (1 pint)	18	330 (180)
Whole (skim)		
Vegetable-fruit, 4 servings	6	190
Broccoli (½ C)		
Potato, 1 medium		
Lettuce, ⅙ head		
Apple, 6 cm (2½-in.) diameter		
Meat, 2 or more servings	56	341
Cheese, 30 g (1 oz)		
Beef, 75 g (2½ oz)		
Poultry, 75 g (2½ oz)		
Bread-cereal, 4 servings	8	290
Cornflakes, 30 g (1 oz)		
Bread, 3 slices		
	88	1151 (1001)

powdered, evaporated, and condensed milk. Use of milk fortified with vitamin D is desirable, especially for children, pregnant or lactating women, and persons with limited exposure to sunlight as a result of their life-style. The person should be questioned, therefore, to determine if fortified milk is used. Skim milk may be fortified with vitamin A as well as vitamin D, since that fat-soluble vitamin is removed when milkfat is removed. Cheese is included in this group because of its calcium value. When evaluating the diet, all milks and cheeses used should be considered. There is a tendency to consider only milk used as a beverage, but it is an important ingredient in soups, puddings, ice cream, and frozen desserts. Five level tablespoons of dried "skim" milk solids are equivalent to 240 ml (8 oz) of fluid milk. Two cups of cottage cheese, 40 g (1½ oz) of cheddar cheese, 1 cup of pudding, or 1¾ cups of ice cream yields calcium equivalent to 1 cup of fluid milk.

Vegetables and fruits are important primarily as sources of vitamins and minerals. They contribute some protein depending on their type, but the plant foods in the meat group and cereal grains contribute more. Fruits and vegetables are low in calories unless prepared with additional fats or sugars; they are high in nutritional value. Since vitamins A and C are not evenly distributed in all fruits and vegetables, the diet should be checked to be sure that a food rich in vitamin C is included daily and a food rich in vitamin A is included at least every other day. Foods rich in vitamin C include citrus fruits and juices, melons, berries, dark green leafy vegetables, broccoli, cabbage, green peppers, and tomatoes. Foods rich in vitamin A include dark green or deep yellow vegetables. As a general guide, foods with the deeper colors are richer sources of vitamins. Other fruits and vegetables may contribute varying amounts of vitamins C and A, but the choices described above are needed to ensure adequate intake. In addition, fruits and vegetables contribute a wide range of other vitamins including folacin (folic acid) and minerals including potassium. They are quite low in sodium unless salt is added in preparation. They also contribute fiber to the diet.

The *meat* group includes animal and plant products that are rich in protein. Meat, fish, poultry, and eggs contribute protein, fat, vitamin B complex, including B_{12}, and minerals (e.g., iron and copper). Nuts and seeds contribute protein and fat, while the legumes contribute protein and starch. The plant products also contribute vitamins and minerals except vitamin B_{12}. The meat-plant group described here is primarily important for protein content, trace minerals, thiamin, and niacin.

Bread and cereals should be whole-grain or enriched. They contribute some protein, but most of their energy value is supplied as complex carbohydrates. The whole-grain forms are important sources of fiber. These foods are important as sources of many vitamins and minerals, especially because they are inexpensive in comparison with most food items. In surveys it has been noted that these foods provide important amounts of iron in the diet for many people. They are not good sources of vitamins A and C, however, although they contribute valuable levels of thiamin, riboflavin, and niacin. Desserts (e.g., cookies, cake, and doughnuts) are grain foods of high caloric value because of added fats and sugars.

The box on p. 1349 is an assessment of a diet history. The individual is a 45-year-old woman with obesity and hypertension; her meals are eaten at home.

When using the *Daily Food Guide* for rapid screening of nutrient supply, the nurse should remember that the food group system is not a complete diet, but it is the foundation for meal planning. Additional servings from the groups, as well as fats, oils, and sweets, are used to meet energy and growth needs. Alcoholic beverages may be used by the person as well, thus increasing caloric intake with little contribution of protein, vitamins, or minerals. Levels of folacin and magnesium are likely to be low unless the diet includes green leafy vegetables. Levels of vitamin E might be low if vegetable oils are not used in food preparation or as salad dressings. The diet histories of girls and women should be checked to see if iron-rich foods are included, because menstruation and child-bearing increase iron needs. Iron-rich foods include green leafy vegetables, meat, liver, seafood, egg yolks, nuts, legumes, and whole and enriched grains and cereals.

The *Daily Food Guide* can also be used for evaluating vegetarian diets. Many people are vegetarians, and their reasons vary (e.g., religion, food cost, and philosophy[15]). The diets vary as well. Some persons eliminate only red meat such as beef, lamb, veal, and pork but do eat fish. Others eliminate all muscle meats including fish and poultry. Still others use animal products such as milk, cheese, and eggs; these persons are called lacto-ovo-vegetarians. There are some who eliminate all foods of animal origin from the diet and some who choose from a very limited list of plant products. Some eat only cereal grains, others only fruits or seeds. Generally, the lacto-ovo-vegetarian diet is nutritionally sound when a variety of foods is included.[11,39,45] Persons on more restricted vegetarian (vegan) diets should be considered at nutritional risk and candidates for more detailed study. One potential problem is vitamin B_{12} insufficiency unless fortified cereal or a dietary supplement is taken. The young adult who has changed to a vegan diet may use body stores of B_{12} for a time (a 5-year store is possible) but is at potential risk especially if intake of folacin in vegetables is high, masking the signs of megaloblastic anemia.

Other dietary guides could be used in the same manner if the population served represents a particular ethnic or cultural group with a different pattern of food

ASSESSMENT OF A DIET HISTORY

45-year-old woman with obesity and hypertension; meals eaten at home

7:00 AM
1 C cooked oatmeal
2 tsp sugar
1 C skim milk (fortified)
3 C coffee, plain

10:15 AM
2 C coffee, plain

1:00 PM
Sandwich
    2 slices white bread, enriched
    ½ tsp margarine
    ½ tsp mayonnaise
    60 g (2 oz) meatloaf or luncheon meat
4 cookies (fig bars, gingersnaps)
3 C coffee, plain

4:00 PM
7 cookies
½ C unsweetened fruit (canned, frozen, or fresh)
2 C tea, plain

10:00 PM
8 soda crackers
60 g (2 oz) American cheese
360 ml (12 oz) cola (sweet)
½ C homemade bread-and-butter pickles

Midnight
2 aspirin
1 C tea, plain

ASSESSMENT

Food group	Servings	Evaluation
Milk		Choice from milk group adequate. Fruit and vegetable intake low; choice of items rich in vitamin C or A happenstance. Meat intake low. Bread intake is 6 servings. Intake of sweets, particularly cookies, high. Use of pickles and soda crackers questionable, since patient reports that low-sodium diet was prescribed for her several years ago.
Skim milk	1	
Cheese	1	
Fruits, vegetables		
Fruit	1	
Vegetable	1	Dietitian was asked to check caloric value. Intake is 1500-1600 cal/day, which includes about 800 cal from basic food items; remainder from sweets and fat. Protein levels adequate, although source of protein could be improved.
Meat-protein		
Meatloaf	1	
Bread, cereal		
Oatmeal	2	
Bread, enriched	2	
Crackers	2	
Sweets		
Cookies	11	
Cola (360 ml [12 oz])		
Pickles, cucumber		
Fats		
Margarine		
Mayonnaise		

To the reader: Identify nutritional risks for this person; identify appropriate interventions and behavioral goals for her.

use. The pattern described here is applicable for the majority of the U.S. population. Hospital diet manuals also provide food patterns that can be used as evaluation tools. In addition to describing regular or normal diets, the manuals provide patterns for modified diets prescribed as therapeutic regimens. When these patterns are used for evaluation, they provide a mechanism for separating quickly those persons who are most likely consuming an adequate nutrient supply from those who are not. When an individual's food intake does not adhere to a recommended pattern, he or she may or may not be obtaining adequate nutrients. The evaluation of the diet must be extended, and the evaluation becomes more arduous. Tables of food composition can be used and nutrient intake estimated through calculation of the nutrient value of each food.* Referral to the dietitian is appropriate.

---

*References 1, 33, 40, 41, 52.

Assessing nutritional deficiency

At one time, a great deal of emphasis was placed on looking for specific signs of nutritional deficiency as part of the clinical examination. This was based on the observation made of populations with classic deficiency diseases. One can find lists of the signs in most nutrition textbooks. One need not to be a physician to rec-

ognize major signs of nutritional deprivation. It is hoped that nutrition problems can be identified before major signs and symptoms appear.

Signs of malnutrition may be caused by a nutrient lack or nonnutritional factors such as poor hygiene (e.g., bleeding gums and bad teeth). They may be the result of inadequate nutrient intake or a disease or condition that interferes with the body's ability to digest, absorb, or metabolize nutrients. It is important to make these differentiations.

TABLE 52-7. Physical signs indicative or suggestive of malnutrition*

Body area	Normal appearance	Signs associated with malnutrition
Hair	Shiny, firm, not easily plucked	Lack of natural shine; hair dull and dry, thin and sparse; hair fine, silky, and straight; color changes (flag sign); can be easily plucked
Face	Skin color uniform; smooth, pink, healthy appearance; not swollen	Skin color loss (depigmentation); skin dark over cheeks and under eyes (malar and supraorbital pigmentation); lumpiness or flakiness of skin of nose and mouth; swollen face; enlarged parotid glands; scaling of skin around nostrils (nasolabial seborrhea)
Eyes	Bright, clear, shiny; no sores at corners of eyelids; membranes a healthy pink and moist. No prominent blood vessels or mound of tissue or sclera	Eye membranes are pale (pale conjunctivae); redness of membranes (conjunctival injection); Bitor's spots; redness and fissuring of eyelid corners (angular palpebritis); dryness of eye membranes (conjunctival xerosis); cornea has dull appearance (corneal xerosis); cornea soft (keratomalacia); scar on cornea; ring of fine blood vessels around cornea (circumcorneal injection)
Lips	Smooth, not chapped or swollen	Redness and swelling of mouth or lips (cheilosis), especially at corners of mouth (angular fissures and scars)
Tongue	Deep red in appearance; not swollen or smooth	Swelling; scarlet and raw tongue; magenta (purplish color) tongue; smooth tongue; swollen sores; hyperemic and hypertrophic papillae; atrophic papillae
Teeth	No cavities; no pain; bright	May be missing or erupting abnormally; gray or black spots (fluorosis); cavities (caries)
Gums	Healthy; red; do not bleed; not swollen	"Spongy" and bleed easily; recession of gums
Glands	Face not swollen	Thyroid enlargement (front of neck); parotid enlargement (cheeks become swollen)
Skin	No signs of rashes, swellings, dark or light spots	Dryness of skin (xerosis); sandpaper feel of skin (follicular hyperkeratosis); flakiness of skin; skin swollen and dark; red swollen pigmentation of exposed areas (pellagrous dermatosis); excessive lightness or darkness of skin (dyspigmentation); black and blue marks from skin bleeding (petechiae); lack of fat under skin
Nails	Firm, pink	Nails are spoon shaped (koilonychia); brittle, ridged nails
Muscular and skeletal systems	Good muscle tone; some fat under skin; can walk or run without pain	Muscles have "wasted" appearance; baby's skull bones are thin and soft (craniotabes); round swelling of front and side of head (frontal and parietal bossing); swelling of ends of bones (epiphyseal enlargement); small bumps on both sides of chest wall (on ribs), beading of ribs; baby's soft spot on head does not harden at proper time (persistently open anterior fontanelle); knock-knees or bow-legs; bleeding into muscle (musculoskeletal hemorrhages); person cannot get up or walk properly
Internal systems		
Cardiovascular	Normal heart rate and rhythm; no murmurs or abnormal rhythms; normal blood pressure for age	Rapid heart rate (above 100, tachycardia); enlarged heart; abnormal rhythm; elevated blood pressure
Gastrointestinal	No palpable organs or masses (in children, however, liver edge may be palpable)	Liver enlargement; enlargement of spleen (usually indicates other associated diseases)
Nervous	Psychologic stability; normal reflexes	Mental irritability and confusion; burning and tingling of hands and feet (paresthesia); loss of position and vibratory sense; weakness and tenderness of muscles (may result in inability to walk); decrease and loss of ankle and knee reflexes

*From Christakis, G.: Am. J. Public Health **63**(suppl):1-82, 1973.

Subjective data

The patient's (or family's) description of the current illness, previous illness and surgery, pregnancy, weight, weight change, and growth, and use of prescribed and over-the-counter medications provide information, most of which can be checked by examination, measurements, and appropriate laboratory studies. The history provides data for determining likely problems and defining the priorities for testing.

Objective data

The World Health Organization (WHO) has published classifications of the physical signs most often associated with malnutrition, and these have been adapted for use in the United States.[9,59] Table 52-7 lists the signs associated with normal appearance and with malnutrition. Evaluation also includes height, weight, and growth patterns.

Height and weight

Height and weight are easily measured and are important data to obtain and use. Delayed growth and development in a child should be regarded as an important sign. This may be determined by comparing the child's measurements with normal values on growth charts. Better yet, if available, are serial measurements over time so that deviations in growth rate may be

identified for the specific child. There should be records of height and weight for children whether care is provided in office, clinic, or hospital.

Height and weight for adults is also easily measured, with weight and height compared with tables of recommended values as a guide. A useful item of historical information is the weight of the adult at age 25 and the person's perception of desirable body weight. The first provides data about a good weight for the person (if not obese at 25), and the second helps predict the person's response to attempts to change weight (Table 52-8).

For all persons, periodic recording of weight changes can provide valuable data about health status, and response to therapy and can serve as an early warning of problems. Even in hospitals where weight is measured, the data usually are not used as they should be.

The nurse should review the methods for obtaining accurate measurements of height or length. Errors of up to 5 cm have been recorded in measurements made on the commonly used type of clinical scale with a measuring rod. The most reliable measurement of weight is made in the morning after voiding and before food or drink are taken.

Interpretation of weight requires some knowledge of body fluid compartments (p. 301). Very rapid fluctuations in weight (possibly as much as 5 kg in 24 hours) are usually caused by body fluid changes and may signal difficulties with edema or dehydration. A steady downward course in weight may signal that the person is ca-

TABLE 52-8. Height and weight tables for adults; desirable weights for persons age 25 and over*

Men					Women†				
Height (with shoes, 1-in. heels)		Small frame (lb)	Medium frame (lb)	Large frame (lb)	Height (with shoes, 2-in. heels)		Small frame (lb)	Medium frame (lb)	Large frame (lb)
ft	in.				ft	in.			
5	2	112-120	118-129	126-141	4	10	92-98	96-107	104-119
5	3	115-123	121-133	129-144	4	11	94-101	98-110	106-122
5	4	118-126	124-136	132-148	5	0	96-104	101-113	109-125
5	5	121-129	127-139	135-152	5	1	99-107	104-116	112-128
5	6	124-133	130-143	138-156	5	2	102-110	107-119	115-131
5	7	128-137	134-147	142-161	5	3	105-113	110-122	118-134
5	8	132-141	138-152	147-166	5	4	108-116	113-126	121-138
5	9	136-145	142-156	151-170	5	5	111-119	116-130	125-142
5	10	140-150	146-160	155-174	5	6	114-123	120-135	129-146
5	11	144-154	150-165	159-179	5	7	118-127	124-139	133-150
5	0	148-158	154-170	164-184	5	8	122-131	128-143	137-154
6	1	152-162	158-175	168-189	5	9	126-135	132-147	141-158
6	2	156-167	162-180	173-194	5	10	130-140	136-151	145-163
6	3	160-171	167-185	178-199	5	11	134-144	140-155	149-168
6	4	164-175	172-190	182-204	6	0	138-148	144-159	153-173

*Metropolitan Life Insurance Company, New York.
†For women 18-25 yr, subtract 1 lb for each yr under 25.

tabolizing body protein or possibly body fat. For some persons this weight loss represents significant deterioration and should be stopped if possible. If loss of fat is the goal, the record represents progress. In general, loss of body fat is a slower process (about 0.5 to 1 kg/wk), since fat is a concentrated source of energy.

Body fatness can be estimated from weight for height. Generally a weight of 15% to 20% above the standard tables represents excessive body fat, although some persons can be overweight but not overfat because of muscle development. The person's general appearance gives one a rapid estimate of overweight or underweight. Fatness can be checked with the use of calipers.

Mouth and teeth

Although all of the physical signs listed in Table 52-7 should be considered, evaluation of the mouth and teeth are especially important. Persons with missing or decayed teeth or dentures that are uncomfortable may have poor nutritional status because eating is painful and unpleasant. They may have problems with appropriate oral hygiene as well. Not only may these difficulties be present at the initial contact, but further problems may develop such as increased pain, bleeding, and infection. Identification of these problems and care directed toward them are essential to the person's well-being. The mouth is checked for cleanliness, odor, evidence of irritation or lesions, soreness, paralysis, and ability to chew. Although bleeding gums usually are associated with vitamin C deficiency, they are more frequently associated with poor oral hygiene and periodontal disease in the U.S. population.

Diagnostic tests

The blood and urine analyses routinely done for patients contain data useful in the evaluation of nutritional status. There are also special tests that can be used to confirm impressions obtained from evaluation of nutrient supply and the clinical examination.*

Urinalysis routinely includes tests of pH, protein, glucose, and acetone. Urine can also be tested for creatinine, thiamin, riboflavin, N'methylnicotinamide, and pantothenic acid. If these tests are ordered, a protocol for collecting and handling the specimens should be requested from the laboratory.

Blood is frequently tested for hemoglobin, hematocrit, serum protein, and cholesterol. The values will be influenced by recent blood loss, so one should deter-

mine whether the person was a recent blood donor as well as checking for loss from bleeding. The values may also be affected by blood transfusions or intravenous solutions; therefore timing of the sample is important.

Low levels of *hemoglobin* most frequently are associated with iron or protein deficiency; however, a variety of nutritional and nonnutritional factors may be involved. About 10% of the U.S. population is estimated to have some degree of anemia related to low *iron* intake.[8] Women and children are at risk because of menstruation and growth, and often because intake of iron-rich foods is low. Hemoglobin levels are also affected by increased volume of blood in late pregnancy. Elevated hemoglobin levels are also seen with dehydration and polycythemia. Hematocrit values are indicative of anemias resulting from low intake of iron and are elevated in polycythemia. More specific evidence of iron deficiency is obtained from tests of serum iron and transferrin, which detect reduced stores before anemia develops. If these are normal, another explanation for the anemia must be sought.

Protein deficiency is uncommon in the United States but not necessarily in the hospitalized patient. The patient's appearance, muscle mass, and body weight are indicative of protein status. The serum protein level, and especially albumin in relation to globulin, falls with protein deficiency but is not considered particularly sensitive or specific for protein. Serum protein levels may be maintained for some time even with limited protein intake. Nitrogen-creatinine ratios in the urine and ratios of specific amino acids in plasma have been used but are not standard procedures as yet for determination of protein deficiency.

Other blood tests are available to test nutritional status. Some tests measure the stores of a nutrient, some measure the circulating nutrient, and others measure the activity of enzymes dependent on the nutrient for activity. These are not routine tests and may be costly to the patient in terms of laboratory fees or discomfort. The decision to request such tests is based on the evaluation of the patient's nutrient intake and physical condition and identification of the possible nutrient problem and the proper test to verify it. For many nutrients, especially the trace elements, laboratory methods have not been standardized and criteria for interpretation of results have not been developed. When the information is essential for patient care, the knowledge and skills of nurse, physician, dietitian, and laboratory personnel are needed.

Although many persons in the United States consume diets that do not provide the recommended levels of *calcium*, there is no suitable method for documenting calcium lack by means of clinical or laboratory studies. Blood levels of calcium are used to test parathyroid function, not nutrient adequacy, since they are relatively constant over wide ranges of intake. Bone

---

*References 9, 23, 26, 42.

serves as a calcium reserve for the body, but there is no standard method as yet to determine degree of mineralization. Visualization by radiograph provides some information on mineralization, particularly for children. Unfortunately by the time problems are identified by radiograph, they are far advanced. Children and postmenopausal women appear to be at highest risk, and identification of risk relies heavily on evaluation of nutrient intake, particularly of calcium and vitamin D.

Serum *copper* levels and ceruloplasmin can be measured, as can *zinc* levels.[23] Hair has been proposed as a biopsy material for determination of trace mineral nutrition, but standardization and interpretation of results remain to be firmly established.[26]

Iodine evaluation relies principally on functional tests such as protein-bound iodine and other standard clinical tests for thyroid gland function.

Tests for levels of *glucose, cholesterol,* and *triglycerides* are often part of the regular series of studies. These have implications for nutritional status and for health status, particularly as related to the development of diabetes mellitus and coronary heart disease. They are discussed in the chapters describing these diseases.

Vitamin C status can be checked by measuring the level of the vitamin in serum. The levels vary substantially with intake and thus can be interpreted to represent stores. Serum levels over 0.2 ml/100 ml are considered acceptable, providing sufficient vitamins to meet needs although the recommended levels of intake (Table 51-1) are set to provide higher serum levels. The blood sample should be a fasting sample for best results, which is true for all tests described here. If this is not possible and a casual sample is obtained, this should be recorded along with the person's food intake for at least 4 hours preceding the test.

Thiamin status can be checked by testing urine or by a funtional enzyme test. *Transketolase* is an enzyme in red blood cells that requires thiamin to function. Measurement of its activity before and after adding thiamin pyrophosphate to the sample is made. An increase in enzyme activity after the addition of cofactor in a ratio of more than 15% indicates thiamin lack. Thiamin content of the blood can be directly estimated with microbiologic assays.

Riboflavin status is most often tested by urinary excretion, with high levels of excretion denoting good intake, fasting, or protein depletion (thus dietary history is important in interpretation). Recently, functional enzyme tests have been developed using erythrocyte glutamic oxaloacetic transaminase (EGOT) or erythrocyte glutamic pyruvate transaminase (EGPT). The principle is similar to thiamin testing, with measurement of the increase in activity as a result of the addition of flavin adenine dinucleotide. Chemical and microbiologic methods are available to measure riboflavin concentration in blood as well as in urine. Since riboflavin is sensitive to ultraviolet light, handling of the sample is critical. In practice, riboflavin status is rarely checked. Riboflavin lack is rarely a problem in persons consuming the equivalent of 480 ml (1 pint) or more of milk daily.

Niacin status has been of particular interest in the United States since pellagra was a major public health problem in the Southwest in the early 1900s. It is rare now, but it occurs occasionally in chronic alcoholics or persons on severely limited diets. This in part is the result of enriched grain and bread products, but probably more to the generous protein level of most American diets. In addition to obtaining preformed niacin found from food, the body can obtain the vitamin from the amino acid tryptophane. When evaluating intake, one considers the protein content of the diet as well as the niacin content. Testing urine for end products of niacin metabolites is the most frequently used method, although microbiologic methods are available to test for circulating niacin.

Of all the vitamins, *folacin* is probably the most frequently tested in patients. This is because deficiency has been reported as common in pregnant women and in women taking estrogens. In addition, megaloblastic anemia can be identified readily in standard clinical blood examinations. The concentration of folacin in serum or red blood cells can be determined by microbiologic methods. Another test measures the excretion of formiminoglutamic acid (FIGLU) in the urine, since increased excretion of this metabolite of histidine metabolism may occur with B_{12} deficiency and other causes. Serum folacin is a more specific test.

Vitamin B_{12} status can also be checked by measuring serum levels. Since B_{12} deficiency may be caused by inadequate intake or by an inability to absorb the vitamin from food (pernicious anemia), a series of tests is used by the physician for differential diagnosis. Megaloblastic anemia is a clinical sign of folacin or B_{12} inadequacy. When folacin intake is very high in relation to B_{12} supplies in the body, megaloblastic anemia may not be apparent, and the permanent damage to the body may occur if one waits until clinical signs appear. This can happen in persons whose diet appears adequate in B_{12} but who cannot absorb it. It may occur in persons on diets inadequate in B_{12} (e.g., vegans) whose folacin intake is high because of good intakes of foods such as green leafy vegetables or, more frequently, because of folic acid supplements that may be self-chosen.

Pantothenic acid and *biotin* usually are not nutrition problems. They are widely distributed in foodstuffs, and deficiencies have been rarely documented. Although the picture may change in the future, there is little evidence that these two vitamins pose problems for many people. Identification of growth retardation or of inadequate weight for height should warn of possible nutrition problems, and an evaluation of intake for all of the vitamins would help identify the specific problem. The few cases of biotin deficiency that have been identified have been associated with intake of excessive amounts of raw egg white, with otherwise limited diet, over a long period or long-term parenteral feeding. This can be identified from the dietary history.

Assessment of *vitamin A* nutriture is important for two reasons. Repeated studies of the American population show significant numbers of people with inadequate vitamin A intake and low vitamin reserves in the liver.[8] Persons with impaired fat absorption or other absorption problems such as gluten enteropathy will have impaired absorption of fat-soluble vitamins. In addition, vitamin A is a popular dietary supplement for persons concerned about their skin or health, and they frequently take very large doses of the vitamin over long periods. Vitamin A is toxic when taken in excess and may result in either acute or chronic, hard-to-identify symptoms. Plasma levels of vitamin A and of the provitamin carotene can be measured. An individual may maintain acceptable levels (20 μg/100 ml) even with low intake, if liver stores are available for mobilization. Plasma carotene levels reflect one form of vitamin intake: that from green leafy and yellow vegetables. A low plasma carotene level would be expected in persons not including these foods, just as a high level would be expected in persons eating generous amounts. The high intake of carotenes does not pose the same hazard of toxicity as does high intake of vitamin A.

Tests for *vitamin D* nutriture are not particularly satisfactory. The signs of rickets in children can be identified radiographically, but one does not wait for this condition to develop before correcting the problem. Elevated serum alkaline phosphatase levels have been associated with vitamin D deficiency, but they are not specific. With the identification of the forms of vitamin D in body processes, tests to measure compounds such as 1,25-dihydroxycholecalciferol have been developed. These tests are difficult and expensive and are not suitable for general determination of nutritional status. For these reasons, it is useful to check on exercise or play in sunlight and the use of vitamin D fortified milks or yogurts.[38]

Vitamin E status may be checked by determining plasma vitamin E concentrations. A plasma fragility test has been used also, since red blood cell fragility increases with vitamin E. Inadequate vitamin E status is not reported frequently. It does occur in infants (especially the premature), apparently because the absorption of the vitamin is limited in the immature gastrointestinal tract. Increased hemolysis has been noted in adults consuming diets high in polyunsaturated fatty acids, although this is not usual, because the oils high in polyunsaturates are also good sources of vitamin E.

The test for *vitamin K* nutriture is the test for prothrombin time. Since vitamin K is present in many foods, including green leafy vegetables, and is synthesized by the flora of the intestinal tract, dietary deficiency is rare. One dose of the vitamin is given at birth to prevent hemorrhagic disease until the flora are established in the infant within a week or so. Vitamin K inadequacy is more often seen in patients who receive antibiotics for long periods, antibiotic enemas before surgery of the colon, or intravenous feedings without the vitamin. Since many patients are treated with anticoagulants as a component of therapy, the physician must be concerned with the relative supplies of vitamin K and the anticoagulant to maintain the prothrombin time desired for the particular patient.

The nurse, in accepting the responsibility of providing care for the person as an individual, accepts responsibility for aspects of nutritional care as well. The perceptive nurse identifies problems, seeks answers, and incorporates solutions in the nursing care plan. Identification of nutritional problems, current and potential, is the purpose of assessing nutritional status. Although medical, dietary, and laboratory personnel share responsibility, the nurse must be alert to the person's needs. Assessment should be made at the initial contact and at regular intervals to ensure the person's well-being. The nutrition assessment forms the basis for care plans and specific interventions.

REFERENCES AND SELECTED READINGS

1. Adams, C.F., and Richardson, M.: Nutritive value of foods, revised April 1981, Home and Garden Bulletin no. 72, Science and Education Administration, U.S. Department of Agriculture, Washington, D.C., 1981.
2. American Society for Clinical Nutrition, Inc., symposium: Report of the Task Force on the evidence relating six dietary factors to the nation's health, Am. J. Clin. Nutr. **32**:2621-2748, 1979.
3. Baird, P.C., and Schutz, H.G.: Life-style correlates of dietary and biochemical measures of nutrition, J. Am. Diet Assoc. **76**:228-235, 1980.
4. *Beal, V.A.: Nutrition in the life span, New York, 1980, John Wiley & Sons, Inc.
5. Beisel, W.R., et al.: Single-nutrient effects on immunologic functions, report of a workshop sponsored by the Department of Food and Nutrition and its Nutrition Advisory Group of the American Medical Association, J.A.M.A. **245**:53-58, 1981.
6. *Briggs, G.M., and Calloway, D.H.: Bogert's nutrition and physical fitness, ed. 10, Philadelphia, 1979, W.B. Saunders Co.
7. Caly, J.C.: Helping people eat for health: assessing adults' nutrition, Am. J. Nurs. **77**:1605-1609, 1977.
8. Center for Disease Control, Health Services and Mental Health Administration: Ten-state nutrition survey 1968-1970, Department of Health, Education, and Welfare DHEW (HSM) pub. nos. 72-8130, 72-8131, 72-8133, and 72-8134, Washington, D.C., 1972, U.S. Government Printing Office.
9. *Christakis, G.: Nutritional assessment in health programs, Am. J. Public Health **63**(suppl.):1-82 Nov. 1973.
10. Committee on Nutrition, American Academy of Pediatrics: Nutritional aspects of vegetarianism, health foods and fad diets, Pediatrics **59**:460-464, 1977.

*References preceded by an asterisk are particularly well suited for student reading.

11. Committee on Nutrition, American Academy of Pediatrics: Plant fiber intake in the pediatric diet, Pediatrics **67**:572-575, 1981.

12. Committee on Nutrition, American Academy of Pediatrics: Vitamin and mineral supplement needs in normal children in the United States, Pediatrics **66**:1015-1021, 1980.

13. Council on Scientific Affairs: American Medical Association's concepts of nutrition and health, J.A.M.A. **242**:2335-2338, 1979.

14. Dansky, K.H.: Helping people eat for health: assessing children's nutrition, Am. J. Nurs. **77**:1610-1611, 1977.

15. *Deutsch, R.M.: The new nuts among the berries, Palo Alto, Calif., 1977, Bull Publishing Co.

16. Dwyer, J.T., et al.: The "new" vegetarians: group affiliation and dietary structures related to attitudes and life style, J. Am. Diet Assoc. **64**:376-382, 1974.

17. Edelman, R., and Calloway, C.W., editors: Nutritional support of the patient: research directions for the 1980's, Am. J. Clin. Nutr. **24**(suppl.):1182-1259, 1981.

18. Edidin, D., et al.: Resurgence of nutritional rickets associated with breast-feeding and special dietary practices, Pediatrics **65**:232-235, 1980.

19. *Food and Nutrition Board, Division of Biological Sciences, Assembly of Life Sciences: Toward healthful diets, Washington, D.C., 1980, National Academy of Sciences–National Research Council.

20. Gersovitz, M., Madden, J.P., and Smiciklas-Wright, H.: Validity of the 24-hr. dietary recall and seven-day record for group comparison, J. Am. Diet Assoc. **73**:48-55, 1978.

21. *Goodhart, R.S., and Shils, M.E.: Modern nutrition in health and disease, ed. 6, Philadelphia, 1980, Lea & Febiger.

22. Guthrie, H.A.: Concept of a nutritious food, J. Am. Diet Assoc. **71**:14-19, 1977.

23. Hambidge, K.M., et al.: Low levels of zinc in hair, anorexia, poor growth, and hypogeusia in children, Pediatr. Res. **6**:868-874, 1972.

24. *Healthy people, the Surgeon General's report on health promotion and disease prevention, DHEW (PHS) pub. no. 79-55071, Washington, D.C., 1979, Public Health Service, U.S. Department of Health, Education, and Welfare.

25. Henderson, L.M.: Nutritional problems growing out of new patterns of food comsumption, Am. J. Public Health **62**:1194-1198, 1972.

26. Hilderbrand, D.C., and White, D.H.: Trace element analysis in hair: an evaluation, Clin. Chem. **20**:148-151, 1974.

27. *Hunt, S.M., Froff, J.L., and Holbrook, J.M.: Nutrition: principles and clinical practice, New York, 1980, John Wiley & Sons, Inc.

28. Karp, R.J., et al.: School health service as a means of entry into the inner-city family for the identification of malnourished children, Am. J. Clin. Nutr. **29**:216-218, 1976.

29. Knowles, J.H.: Responsibility for health, Science **198**:1103-1107, 1977.

30. *Krause, M.V., and Mahan, L.K.: Food, nutrition and diet therapy, ed. 6, Philadelphia, 1979, W.B. Saunders Co.

31. Mertz, W.: The new RDA's: estimated adequate and safe intake of trace elements and calculation of available iron, J. Am. Diet Assoc. **76**:128-133, 1980.

32. Michel, L., Serrano, A., and Malt, R.A.: Current concepts: nutritional support of hospitalized patients, N. Engl. J. Med. **304**:1147-1152, 1981.

33. Murphy, E.E., Willis, B.W., and Watt, B.K.: Provisional tables on the zinc content of food, J. Am. Diet Assoc. **66**:345-355, 1975.

34. *National Research Council, Committee on Food Protection, Food and Nutrition Board: Toxicants occurring naturally in foods, ed. 2, Washington, D.C., 1973, National Academy of Sciences.

35. Nehme A., and Nehme, E.: Nutritional support of the hospitalized patient: the team concept, J.A.M.A. **243**:1906-1908, 1980.

36. Nutrient toxicity, special report, Nutr. Rev. **39**:249-256, 1981.

37. Nutrition Coordinating Committee of the National Institutes of Health: Symposium on the role of dietary fiber in health, Am. J. Clin. Nutr. **31**(suppl:)291, Oct. 1978.

38. The nutritional requirements of man, a conspectus of research from the Journal of Nutrition, Washington, D.C., 1980, The Nutrition Foundation.

39. Pearson, A.M.: Some factors that may alter consumption of animal products, J. Am. Diet Assoc. **69**:522-530, 1976.

40. Pennington, J.A.T., and Church, H.N.: Bowes and Church's food values of portions commonly used, ed. 13, Philadelphia, 1980, J.B. Lippincott Co.

41. Perloff, B.P., and Butram, R.R.: Folacin in selected foods, J. Am. Diet Assoc. **70**:161-179, 1977.

42. *Prasad, A.S.: Trace elements in human health and disease, Foundation monograph series. I. Zinc and copper; II. Essential and toxic elements, New York, 1976, Academic Press, Inc.

43. Promoting health/preventing disease: Objectives for the nation, Washington, D.C., Fall 1980, Public Health Service Department of Health and Human Services.

44. Recommended dietary allowances, ed. 9, Washington, D.C., 1980, National Academy of Sciences–National Research Council.

45. Register, U.D., and Sonnenberg, L.M.: The vegetarian diet: scientific and practical considerations, J. Am. Diet Assoc. **62**:253-261, 1973.

46. Richard, K., et al.: Care of children with conditions characterized by high nutritional risks, J.A.M.A. **68**:546-549, 1976.

47. Robinson, C., and Lawler, M.: Normal and therapeutic nutrition, ed. 15, New York, 1977, Macmillan Publishing Co., Inc.

48. Roe, D.A.: Drug-induced nutritional deficiencies, Westport, Conn., 1976, Avi Publishing Co.

49. Shannon, B.M., and Parks, S.C.: Fast foods: a perspective on their nutritional impact, J. Am. Diet Assoc. **76**:242-247, 1980.

50. Smith, E.B.: A guide to good eating the vegetarian way, J. Nutr. Ed. **7**:109-112, 1975.

51. Steffee, P.: Malnutrition in hospitalized patients, J.A.M.A. **244**:2630-2635, 1980.

52. U.S. Department of Agriculture, Agricultural Research Service: Nutritive value of American foods in common units, Handbook 456, Washington, D.C., 1975, U.S. Government Printing Office.

53. U.S. Department of Health, Education, and Welfare, National Center for Health Statistics: Dietary intake findings, United States 1971-1974, data from the National Health Survey, Health and Nutrition Examination Survey, Vital and Health statistics, series 11, no. 202, DHEW pub. (HRA) no. 77-1647, Hyattsville, Md., 1977, Public Health Service, Health Resources Administration.

54. Willett, W., et al.: Vitamin supplement use among registered nurses, Am. J. Clin. Nutr. **34**:1121-1125, 1981.

55. *Williams, S.R.: Nutrition and diet therapy, ed. 4, St. Louis, 1981, The C.V. Mosby Co.

56. Winick, M.: Nutritional disorders of American women, New York, 1977, John Wiley & Sons, Inc.

57. Winter, S.L., and Boyer, J.L.: Hepatic toxicity from large doses of vitamin B_3 (nicotinamide), N. Engl. J. Med. **289**:1180-1182, 1973.

58. *Wurtman, J.J.: Eating your way through life, New York, 1979, Raven Press.

Classic

59. Jelliffe, D.B.: The assessment of the nutritional status of the community, WHO monograph no. 53, Geneva, 1966, World Health Organization.

60. Young, C.M., et al.: Comparison of dietary study methods: dietary history vs, seven-day record vs. 24-hr. recall, J. Am. Diet Assoc. **28**:218-221, 1952.

CHAPTER 53

INTERVENTIONS FOR THE PERSON WITH IMPAIRED NUTRITION

JANICE NEVILLE

Nutritional impairment can be defined in broad terms as any situation in which an inadequate, excessive, or imbalanced supply of nutrients to the body results in impairment of growth or productivity, increased susceptibility to infection or chronic disease, or impairment in functioning in the day-to-day activities of life. A child consuming a diet with marginal levels of iron and zinc may grow and function at relatively normal rates until challenged by one of the common infectious diseases of childhood. The obese person pays a price for excessive energy intake in the large deposits of adipose tissue that create increased risks of diabetes mellitus, coronary artery disease, or gallbladder disease and that interfere with functioning of organs and with ordinary activities such as walking or running or with finding attractive clothing at a reasonable price. The adolescent girl who has maintained a slim and attractive appearance by limiting caloric intake without considering the vitamin and mineral content of foods has set the stage for nutritional impairment both of herself and of the child she bears. The middle-aged woman whose diet is low in calcium and vitamin D because of diet or lack of exposure to the sun has increased risk of osteoporosis and bone fracture, conditions for which postmenopausal women are already at considerable risk. The person who takes large doses of protein or vitamin or mineral supplements can produce imbalances that may result in physical impairment, symptoms mimicking serious disease, impairment of growth (in children), or deficiencies of other nutrients.

Management of nutritional impairment requires assessment of the nutritional status of the individual (see Chapter 52) so that the nutritional needs of the person are identified and appropriate interventions to meet the needs are devised. This includes seeing that hospitalized patients receive and eat the foods they need, whether a regular or modified diet is prescribed, and that persons learn how to meet their nutritional needs at home. The nurse serves as a liaison between the patient and other professional persons in interpreting the patient's nutritional and dietary problems. Interpretation to family and friends is often needed as well.

Nutrition science has identified the nutrients required by human beings, the quantities needed for optimal growth and function, and the effects of environment, metabolism, disease, and activity on these needs. Research continues in these areas with much effort devoted to defining the relationship between diet, disease, nutrition processes, and people. Foods have been analyzed so that their nutrient composition is known. The ability of the body to absorb and utilize nutrients has been and continues to be an important area of research. Although much remains to be learned, there is a significant body of knowledge to be applied in patient care.

The nurse in accepting responsibility for patient care accepts responsibility for applying principles of nutrition. This requires knowledge of the principles and appreciation of food composition, understanding of the role of food in the person's life, and appreciation of modifications of diet and food behavior as a part of the total therapeutic regimen. The patient may be nourished by food served in the traditional manner, by tube or intravenous feedings, by nutrients supplied as medication, or by blood transfusion. The person's perceptions of food or nutrient need may differ from reality. Acceptance of proposed interventions may be affected by sociocultural factors, difficulties with appetite or taste perception, pain, weakness, depression, or a myriad of other reasons. The perceptive nurse must identify these problems, seek answers, and incorporate solutions in the nursing care plan.

Promoting adequate intake

The adequacy of the diet, in terms of quality and quantity, can be quickly estimated by comparing it with recommended patterns of food intake (see Chapter 52). A good, or balanced, diet consists of any combination of foodstuffs that yields needed nutrients in sufficient amounts to promote growth and metabolism. For most persons a good diet is one that is tasty, filling, refreshing, or desirable for some special reason important to that person. Persons may believe that a particular food or nutrient has special properties to improve or harm health.[11,14,27,50] The terms "normal," "usual," or "average" diet are ambiguous and uninformative.

Diagnoses of malnutrition are of five general types:

Quantity	Quality
Excessive	Satisfactory
Inadequate	Satisfactory
Satisfactory	Inadequate
Inadequate	Inadequate
Excessive	Inadequate

Quantity refers to volume of food intake and particularly to the energy intake. Quality relates to the protein, vitamin and mineral content.

Quantity of diet

Requirements

Energy needs can be predicted from patterns of growth and body size and from physical activity. There is a constant need for energy to maintain circulation, respiration, muscle tone, and body temperature. People of similar size have similar basal energy requirements, since the requirement is related to the amount of muscle tissue and can be predicted from body weight (excluding excess body fat, since adipose tissue is relatively inert). The total energy requirement may vary widely depending on physical activity (Table 53-1). Recommendations for caloric intake are based on the growth, activity, and life-style of most Americans (Fig. 53-1). Since this is a sedentary life pattern, the levels recommended are moderate, particularly for the adult. To emphasize the differences in energy needs associated with differences in physical activity, the range of kilocalorie needs for persons doing different types of light physical work is illustrated. The range of energy needs

TABLE 53-1. Comparison of calories used in 1 hr for different types of physical activity (exclusive of basal energy needs)

Activity	Calories expended per hour	
	Woman (121 lb)	Man (143 lb)
Lying quietly	6	7
Sitting	22	26
Standing	28	32
Ironing, dishwashing, driving car	55	65
Working in office, painting furniture	82	98
Walking, waltzing, bicycling	138	162
More active walking, skating, doing foxtrot	220	260
Running, climbing stairs, sawing wood	358	422
High-speed walking, swimming	468	552

is wide. The best method for determining the adequacy of energy intake for the person is to evaluate weight for height (and rate of growth for children) in relation to energy intake assessed from dietary information.

Problems of inadequate quantity of food often are not given the attention they deserve, possibly because Americans are so conditioned to regard obesity as a national problem that loss of weight seems benign. For many patients loss of weight impedes recovery at best and well may be life threatening. Interference with growth caused by inadequate energy intake may impose a burden on a child for his or her lifetime.

Methods of promoting adequate intake

How can the nurse ensure the patient's intake of adequate quantities of food? In the hospital setting there are some very simple and practical measures that can be taken. Make sure that the patient gets the right tray, that the food on it is acceptable to the patient, that enough food is available, that the environment is pleasant and that the patient is fed if necessary.

Regardless of the diet prescribed (regular "house diet" or a modified diet), adjustments can be made to fit the patient's likes and dislikes for particular food items. Most hospitals offer selective menus for regular and many modified diets. This system provides patients an opportunity to choose foods they like. No institutional food will match individual tastes in methods of preparation or seasoning, and the patient's taste perception can also be altered by illness or medications. Nevertheless, flexibility is built into the food service system to permit menu changes to meet patient requests. The nurse can request assistance from the dietitian if necessary. Should nothing be satisfactory to the patient except food from home, food from home should be permitted. It is nec-

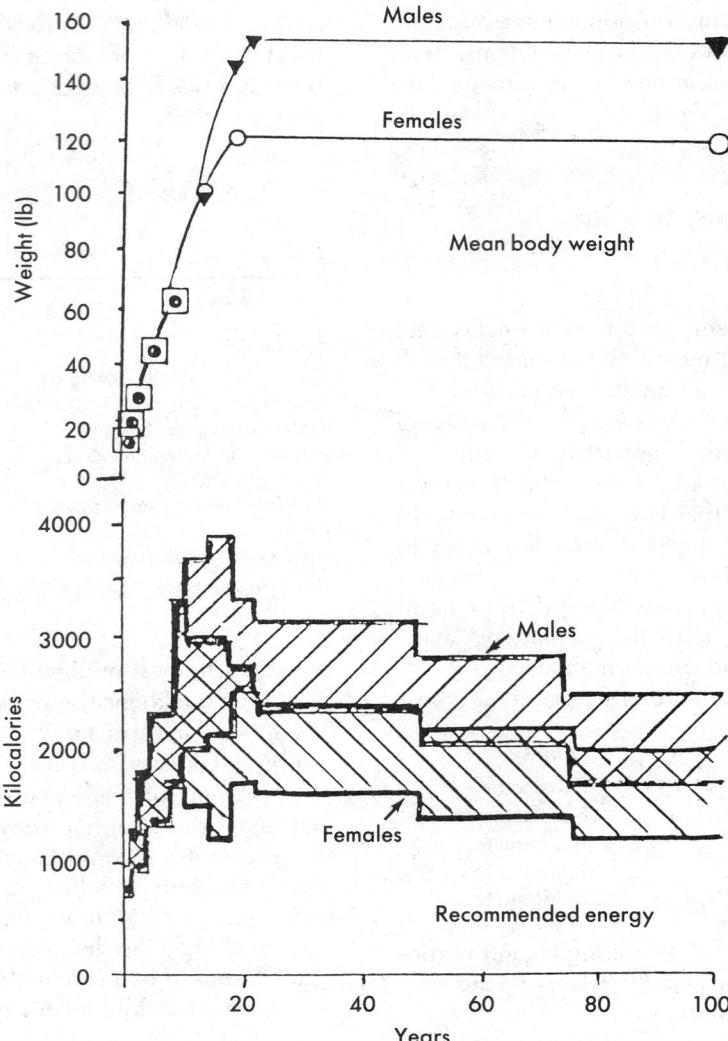

Fig. 53-1. Recommended daily dietary allowances (1980) for kilocalories over the life cycle.

essary to be sure that food provided by family and friends meets any constraints imposed by prescribed dietary modifications. Special dietary desires such as kosher foods or vegetarian meals require consultation with the dietitian.

Is the person getting enough to eat? If not, larger portions of food at regular meals may be the answer. More frequent meals of moderate size might be better, or the person might be able to handle smaller portions of food of greater caloric density.

Environment and appearance are important. The food (and tray) should be neat and attractive in appearance, and utensils should be clean. Lukewarm soup, melted ice cream, soggy toast, and tepid tea are not likely to appeal to anyone and especially not to someone who is not feeling well or who has loss of appetite. Is the room pleasant? Unpleasant smells and sights abound in hospitals and can reduce an already finicky appetite. Visi-

tors or other patients may help by providing social ease. Guest trays can be provided in most institutions.

Is the patient comfortable? A clean face and hands are refreshing. Are the patient's dentures in? Is the mouth clean and free of foul odors? Is the patient free of pain? Position is also important. Eating is most comfortable when one is sitting up. If the patient is unable to sit in a chair or sit upright on the bed with feet dangling, the bed should be adjusted and the patient assisted up in the bed to a comfortable position. If the head cannot be raised, the patient should be helped to lie on the side and the food placed for easy access. Delivery of food to the mouth is difficult for the recumbent person, and there is increased risk of choking. Fear, discomfort, embarrassment, and possibly distaste for clothing or linen spotted with food may keep a patient from eating.

Is the patient able to get the food to the mouth and

swallow it? Arranging food on the tray, opening the milk carton, or cutting meat into bite-sized pieces may be needed. Patients should be encouraged to do as much as possible for themselves, and this is determined in the nursing assessment. If patients cannot lift a spoon to their mouth, the nurse may make arrangements for someone else to feed them or may suggest that the diet be supplied as a liquid that can be drunk through a straw. Many devices are available to assist persons with physical weakness and inability to feed themselves.[25,48] These include plate guards, weighted dishes and cups, specially designed forks, knives, and spoons, and spouted cups (p. 765).

Fatigue can be a major problem for the patient or for the person feeding the patient. Rest periods before and during meals may be advisable. Often fatigue can be lessened by attention to details such as placement and height of table, tray, or chairs.[25,48]

General quantitative diet problems

Most problems of excessive quantity of food are problems of weight control. This is discussed separately. There are problems of excessive intake of vitamins and minerals that are associated with pharmaceutical products rather than food. Vitamins and minerals, alone and in various mixtures, are available to anyone who wishes to purchase them and are often prescribed for persons in and out of the hospital. The symptoms and signs of excessive intake are vague and difficult to determine. Therapeutic preparations contain concentrations far beyond daily needs and are meant to be used for a short period to meet an acute need and to replenish stores. Therapeutic levels of iron may cause severe gastrointestinal tract distress and eventually iron overload.

A person's daily energy requirements are large and measured in thousands of calories. In addition to the question of adequate but not excessive energy supply to meet patient needs is the question of the importance of the energy source. In the United States from 10% to 12% of the fuel value of the diet is obtained from protein, about 44% from fat, and about 46% from carbohydrate. These figures reflect the variety of foods available and American food preferences. The relative contributions of protein, fat, and carbohydrate to the fuel value of the diet can be varied within wide limits without harm. Up to 80% of dietary calories may be supplied by carbohydrate in persons whose major food staple is grain. This pattern is seen in some persons, although it is not typical. The usual American food pattern includes generous use of animal foods (particularly beef), fats, oils, and sugars. As much as 25% of total calories may come from protein in self-selected diets. Levels above this are rare, since the diet becomes unpalatable and expensive. Provision of 10% of required calories as protein from a variety of foods (animal and plant) is generally sufficient to meet needs for protein of good quality, that is, containing the essential amino acids and sufficient nitrogen for body needs. Some fat in the diet is needed to provide the essential fatty acids and to ensure adequate supplies and efficient absorption of fat-soluble vitamins. Dietary fats are concentrated sources of energy and are useful in providing calories for persons unable to consume large volumes of food. There is a basic requirement for some carbohydrate in the diet as starch and sugar (to prevent ketosis) and as fiber. Most foods are mixtures of protein, fat, and carbohydrate (Fig. 53-2).

It is difficult to separate consideration of calories and protein. The recommended daily dietary allowances (RDA) for protein and the growth curve for the reference woman and man are illustrated in Fig. 53-3. The curves are similar, since protein needs vary with growth and with body size. For both men and women the RDA is 0.8 g/kg of body weight. The average man needs more protein per day than the average woman because of his larger body size. The pregnant woman should be supplied with extra protein for fetal growth. The child's diet should supply more protein per unit of weight than the adult's diet to allow for growth (see Table 52-1). The recommendations exceed actual protein requirements for most persons. The protein not needed for synthesis is used as energy or converted to body fat. If energy intake is not sufficient to meet needs, protein may be used for fuel rather than for synthesis of new tissue. Scrimshaw has said:

There is no doubt that good nutrition requires a balanced complement of protein and calories, and neither can be neglected in the diets of the underprivileged and the vulnerable. To the extent that the pendulum swung too far in emphasizing protein in the 1960s, and too far in emphasizing calories in the 1970s, it must come to a more appropriate intermediate position for the 1980s and beyond.[45]

This is true when considering nutritional needs of individuals as well as needs of populations. Severe limitations in protein supply (50% or less RDA) can stunt growth and reduce body protein content. Adequate protein supplies in a diet of insufficient fuel value help set the stage for protein-calorie malnutrition. Generous supplies of protein will not result in increased body protein or muscle mass without exercise or physical activity. Body protein (and body calcium) may be lost despite adequate dietary intake in the absence of physical activity. Early ambulation of patients, bed exercises, and physical therapy may contribute to improved nutritional status.

When there is doubt that the patient is obtaining sufficient food to meet quantitative needs, the nurse should check the patient's selection of foods from the menu and inspect the patient's tray to determine how much food has been eaten. Strategies are then devised

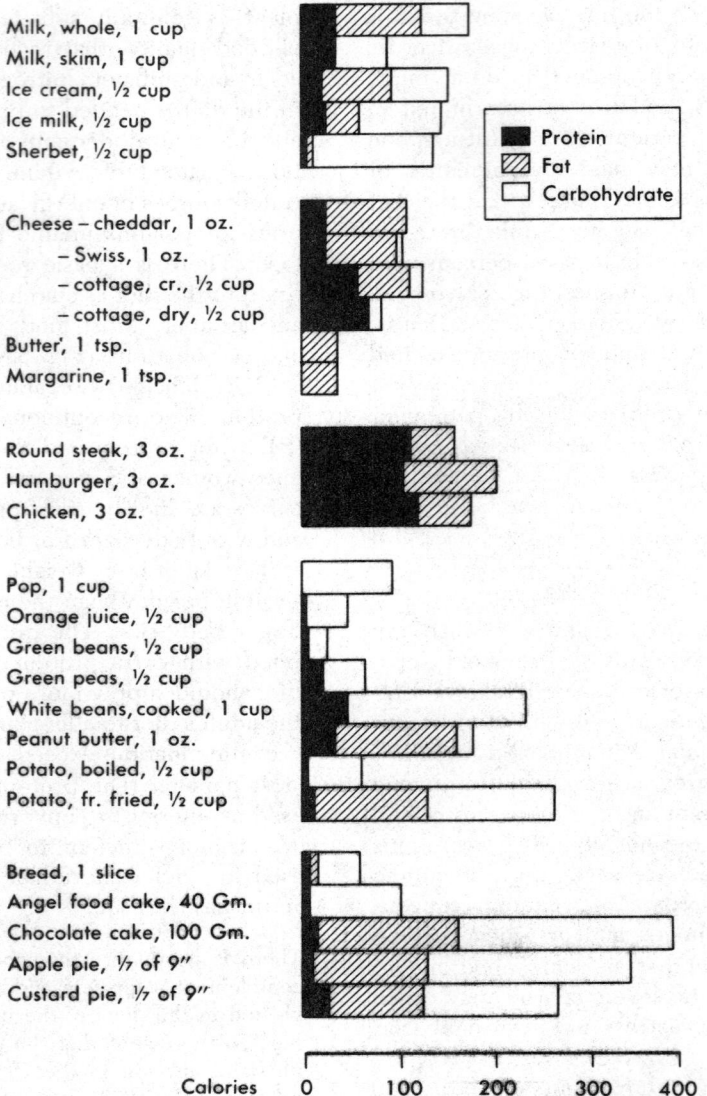

Fig. 53-2. Protein, fat, and carbohydrate concentrations in some common foods, presented as calories contributed by each and total calories in ordinary portions.

with the patient, and the dietitian if necessary, to increase intake. For some patients a combination of food by mouth and by vein may be needed for a time.

Weight control

Obesity is malnutrition resulting from the intake of foods in amounts exceeding body needs. *Underweight* and *emaciation* are malnutrition resulting from the intake of foods in amounts insufficient to meet body needs. Weight control involves evaluation of gross body size and proportions of body fat, lean body mass, and body water in assessing the person's nutritional status. The goal of therapy is to promote optimal gross body size and distribution of weight in proper proportions of muscle, bone, fat, and water throughout the life cycle.

Obesity. Obesity is the most frequently encoun-

tered type of malnutrition in the general population. In practice the person's weight is compared with a standard table of weight for height to determine degree of overweight or underweight (see Table 52-8). Skin-fold measurements give a direct estimate of fat. Therapy goals are then stated in terms of the number of pounds of body weight to be lost. This is an oversimplification. Some persons may be normal in body weight but overfat. Others may be overweight but not overfat because of muscular development. In the first group reduction of body fat but not necessarily of body weight is indicated. Obese children belong in this group, since the goal is to promote normal growth and increase of muscle while reducing the proportion of body fat. In the second group weight is not a problem.

Therapy for the obese person should have three ob-

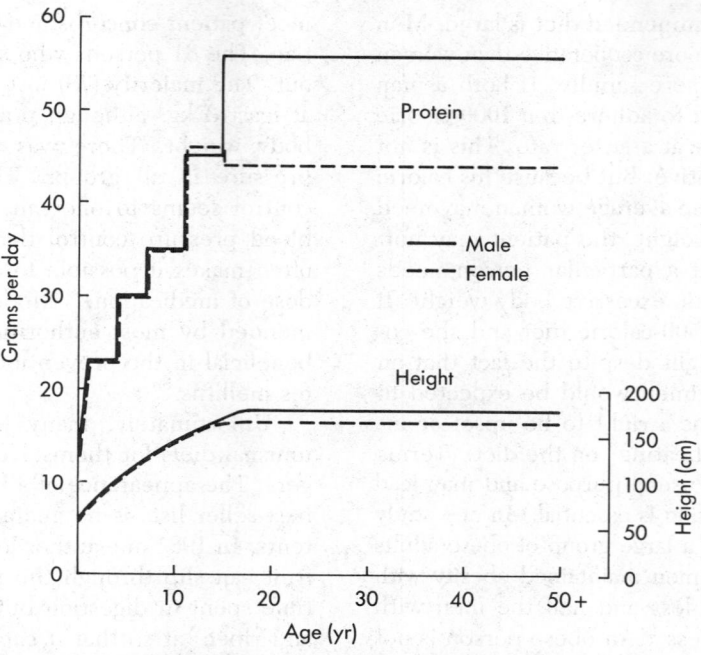

Fig. 53-3. Recommended levels of protein over the life cycle. For women an additional 30 g/day is recommended during pregnancy and 20 g/day during lactation.

jectives: (1) reduction of the body fat component, (2) reduction of total body weight when indicated, and (3) maintenance of desirable body size and composition. Far too often both patient and therapist look only at the pounds of weight lost or the rate of loss.[9,55,63] No differentiation is made as to whether the pounds represent water, muscle, or fat. Very rapid weight loss is satisfying to both patient and therapist, whether the loss is in body fat or water and whether the loss is permanent. Fasting regimens are popular because they induce rapid weight loss in a relatively easy way and are immensely satisfying to "scale watchers." Yet these regimens result in marked protein catabolism with losses of nitrogen, phosphorus, calcium, potassium, sodium, and water and may precipitate undesirable effects such as gout or orthostatic hypotension. The questions remain to be answered about the long-term effect of such losses on the health of the individual.[7,17,49,56]

Weight reduction is not achieved simply by lowering the fuel value of the person's diet. A deficit must be produced between energy expenditure and fuel intake so that body stores of fuel will be mobilized. The deficit may be achieved by increasing energy expenditures or decreasing calorie intake as illustrated in Fig. 53-4. A pound of adipose tissue has an energy potential of 3500 calories.[66] To lose 1 lb of adipose tissue per week, a calorie deficit of 500 calories/day must be induced. If a person requires only 1500 calories to maintain current weight, that person should not be expected to lose more than 1 lb of body fat per week when adhering to a 1000-calorie diet. Weight loss is more rapid

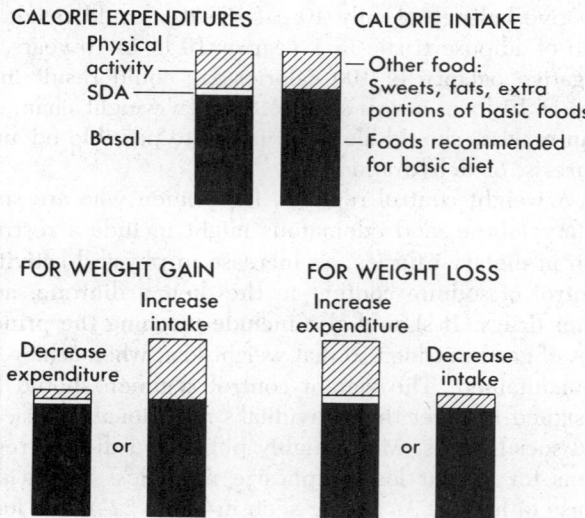

Fig. 53-4. Calorie balance in average adult.

when lean body tissue is catabolized, since lean tissue has an energy potential of about 1850 calories. If a deficit of 500 calories/day were met by catabolizing lean tissue, the rate of loss would be about 2 lb/week. Dehydration produces very rapid loss. Water has no calorie value per se, but 1 L of water weighs approximately 1 kg.

Persons consuming high levels of calories before weight reduction therapy are likely to be successful in achieving rapid weight loss because the calorie deficit between need and the recommended diet is large. Men have a reputation for being more cooperative than women because they lose weight more rapidly. If both a man and a woman are instructed to adhere to a 1000-calorie intake, the man should lose at a faster rate. This is not because he is more cooperative, but because his calorie deficit is larger. Although the average woman may need 2000 calories to maintain weight, the patient may not. It is not inconceivable that a particular person needs only 1400 calories to maintain excessive body weight. If she is told to consume a 1500-calorie diet and she cooperates, she will gain weight despite the fact that an average woman on this regimen would be expected to lose weight. This person has a right to be upset or indignant when accused of "cheating" on the diet. (Terms such as "cheating" serve no useful purpose and may lead to silence when communication is essential.) In one study evaluation of food intakes of a large group of obese adults revealed that half of the women maintained obesity with intakes of 1500 calories or less and half the men with intakes of 2200 calories or less.* An obese person is not necessarily a glutton. Obesity is not a condition that develops suddenly. Body fat may accumulate slowly over years. A positive calorie balance of 100 calories/day could, in a year's time, result in 10 lb of adipose tissue. A positive balance of only 10 calories/day could result in 1 lb of adipose tissue in 1 year or 10 lb in 10 years. A negative balance of 100 calories/day could result in a loss of 10 lb in a year's time. Sudden weight changes, gain or loss, should alert the nurse to possible edema, diuresis, or dehydration.

A weight control regimen for women who are sedentary, obese, and edematous might include a restriction in dietary calories, an increase in physical activity, control of sodium content in the diet, a diuretic, and other drugs. It should also include teaching the principles of good nutrition so that weight loss, when achieved, is maintained. The weight control regimen should be designed to meet the individual's nutritional, physical, and social needs. Many highly publicized dietary regimens for weight loss emphasize rapid loss at the expense of health. As can be seen in Table 52-4, the food guide used for evaluation provides a good pattern for weight control as well as for needed nutrients. Obese individuals have large fuel reserves but not necessarily large reserves of vitamins and minerals.

Weight control for the obese person can be effective in improving health. In a study of overweight persons with uncomplicated hypertension, one group was placed on a weight-reduction program, one group on a weight-reduction program plus antihypertensive drug therapy, and one group received antihypertensive drug therapy but no dietary program. Salt intake was not restricted. The dietary program included individual planning to meet patient concerns and regular visits with the dietitian. The 81 persons who started the diet did not drop out. The majority (73) lost more than 5 kg, and all lost at least 3 kg, although practically none achieved ideal body weight. There was a significant drop in blood pressure in all groups. The authors noted, "Weight control seems to offer an efficient, low-cost means of blood pressure control that is free of side effects and often makes it possible to avoid or to institute a lower dose of medication.[39] Modest salt restriction is recommended by most authorities.[53] Weight control is also beneficial in the prevention and management of diabetes mellitus.[59]

Unfortunately, many people prescribe bizarre or unusual diets for themselves without realizing the dangers. The appearance of a book on diet or health in the best-seller lists is no guarantee of the value of its contents. In 1981 one author focused on fruit, claiming that fruit can slip through the mouth and stomach without time spent in digestion but that the stomach does "rot and ripen" it so that it can slide through the small intestine.[31] This author presents a lurid picture; if carbohydrate hits your stomach without being in the form of maltose, it will stay in the stomach festering, fermenting, rotting, and turning into fat. Although this interpretation of physiology has *no* support in science, the public buys the books and grocery stores run special advertising on the recommended fruits. Another best-selling author blames diet volume as the cause of excess weight and offers a three-part program of a food plan, physical exercises, and mental exercises.[47] Three food plans are offered, the choice depending on the number of pounds to be lost. These diets provide a variety of foods, with protein-rich choices emphasizing chicken or fish. Calcium-rich foods are limited to low-fat milk for breakfast. A low-calorie diet can be useful when chosen from a variety of foods and when eating patterns are changed.

Despite current emphasis in both the popular press and professional journals, weight reduction is not the goal of nutrition care or diet therapy for the obese person. Weight control throughout the life span is the goal. There are times when the physician may decide rapid weight loss is essential to the patient's physical or psychologic well-being. Fasting regimens, of which there are many types, may be used. Close medical supervision is important, since risk may be high. In some instances of massive "morbid" obesity, surgical procedures may be performed consisting of gastric partitioning to reduce the amount of food ingested or intestinal bypass surgery to reduce the amount of fat absorbed (p. 1456). Gastric partitioning is the preferred method because of fewer complications.

Weight loss. Weight loss and emaciation are major malnutrition problems in the hospitalized population. Weight loss is often the first sign of ill health. Loss may

---

*From Neville, J.: Unpublished data, 1965.

be mild or severe, insignificant or serious. It may be caused by inadequate calorie intake, by problems in digestion or absorption, by abnormalities in metabolism, or by excretion of nutrients before they can be utilized. Sometimes weight loss is a result of failure to increase calorie intake when physical activity is increased. Calorie levels sufficient for inpatient activities may not be enough for outpatient activities. Management will vary depending on the basic cause of weight loss.

Missed meals, blood loss, and anorexia contribute to emaciation in many patients. In every instance, however, the goal is to restore normal body composition, not just weight. A patient will derive no advantage from becoming obese. Restoration of muscle mass occurs slowly. Providing excessive amounts of dietary protein will not hasten this process. Since growth requires energy, calorie intake should exceed calorie expenditures for basal and physical activity. There are strong physiologic arguments for preventing obesity and debilitation rather than waiting to treat it after it occurs. Every child, ill or healthy, should be provided with the essentials for attaining his growth potential. As a result, weight control is a component of the health care program for any patient and includes ensuring that the person knows the principles of weight control and food choice.

Anorexia

Lack of appetite, or anorexia, needs to be differentiated from hunger. *Hunger* is a physiologic state that occurs when the lateral nuclei of the hypothalamus are stimulated. A satiety center in the ventromedial nuclei of the hypothalamus inhibits the hunger center. "Hunger pangs" are sensations experienced in the abdomen from contractions of the empty stomach. The mechanisms that regulate the amount of food eaten and provide for a rhythmic supply of food are not clear, but a number of theories have been postulated.[51] Low serum concentration of glucose and amino acids appear to stimulate hunger. It is also thought that sensory receptors of the mouth, throat, stomach, and intestine may meter the amount of food intake.

Anorexia is a mental state, a desire not to eat, whether hunger is or is not present. It is affected by feelings about the food, either because of present factors such as the appearance of the food or because of past experiences. Offensive sights and smells or unattractive food can decrease the desire to eat. A number of people will not eat food that is new to them or that is not a regular item in their usual dietary pattern. Eating is also related to the development in childhood of love and security, and a desire not to eat may develop when love and security are threatened at a later date. Severe stress may lead either to anorexia or to excessive eating.

A number of other factors may contribute to anorexia. Poor oral hygiene decreases the sense of smell and taste and leads to dryness of the mucous membranes, all of which reduce the desire to eat. Providing good oral hygiene is important, therefore, when trying to encourage a person to eat. Increased blood temperature from hot weather or fever, or the systemic effect of the inflammatory response as seen in acute infectious diseases or allergies contribute to anorexia. Decreased tonus as seen in chronic gastritis, constipation, failure of the detoxifying function of the liver, and distention of abdominal viscera are additional contributing factors to anorexia. Drugs such as the amphetamines may act directly to reduce appetite; other drugs contribute to decreased food intake because of the side effects of nausea and vomiting.

Motivating a person with anorexia to eat can be a challenge. Interventions that can correct the cause will lead to improved appetite. Persons with inadequate nutrition stores need encouragement to eat, although forced feeding may lead to frustration or nausea and vomiting. Determining the person's likes and dislikes, providing an environment conducive to eating (p. 1358), and providing several small meals rather than three large meals a day may facilitate an adequate nutrition intake.

Anorexia nervosa. A severe form of anorexia that leads to emaciation and death is termed anorexia nervosa. One group noted that "an effective therapy for this disorder is crucial, since it is one of the few psychiatric disorders that can result in death."[21] The typical patients are young and female. Diagnostic criteria include age of onset before 25 years of age; anorexia with weight loss of at least 25% of original body weight; a distorted implacable attitude toward food, eating, or weight that overrides hunger; no known medical illness to account for the loss of appetite and weight; and no other known psychiatric disorder. Amenorrhea occurs before dieting in at least 25% of the cases and concurrently with dieting and weight loss in others. Vande Wiele suggests that the condition be named "puberal starvation-amenorrhea" because the cause is in doubt. In the series of patients reported, spontaneous recovery occurred if there was early diagnosis and a policy of benign neglect. As weight loss continued, the patients' perception of body image became more distorted and weight goals became lower. This author suggests that the distorted body image may lessen with weight gain and that weight loss is a cause rather than a result of the distortion. In the series of 42 persons studied, 32 improved, 5 were unchanged, 2 deteriorated, and 3 died.[57]

An initial treatment regimen has been suggested that emphasizes a firm and open approach with high-calorie liquid feedings dispensed as medication by the nursing staff when the specified weight gain is not achieved daily. Once weight gain is achieved so that the threat to life is reduced, the patient is discharged with psychotherapy scheduled if needed. In this approach weight gain is praised but failure to gain is not criticized. Behavior modification without drug therapy has been reported, using positive reinforcements by granting privileges tied to weight gain.[21] There is concern that behavior modification may be effective in the management of mild cases only.[6]

Quality of diet

Individuals need energy, nitrogen, essential amino acids, at least 17 mineral elements, and 13 vitamins. Foods are mixtures of these nutrients. No one food provides the full range of nutrients in proper proportions to meet needs. It is important to know whether the patient is consuming a sufficient variety of different foods

to provide the full spectrum of nutrients. The system of food grouping (p. 1347) is based on analysis of foods to determine their nutrient concentration. The recommended numbers of servings from different classes of foods are designed to provide the range of nutrients needed in amounts relative to body needs. Persons who eliminate one or more types of food from the diet are likely to have diets of poor quality.

Fig. 53-5 illustrates the vitamin contributions of different types of foods. The standard is rigorous in that one serving (e.g., 240 ml [8 oz] of milk, two eggs, ½ cup of fruit) is modest in size and judged against the amount of the vitamin recommended for total intake (RDA, Table 52-1, Fig. 52-1). The food guide suggests two servings of milk or milk products, two servings of protein-rich meats, eggs, nuts, or legumes, four serv-

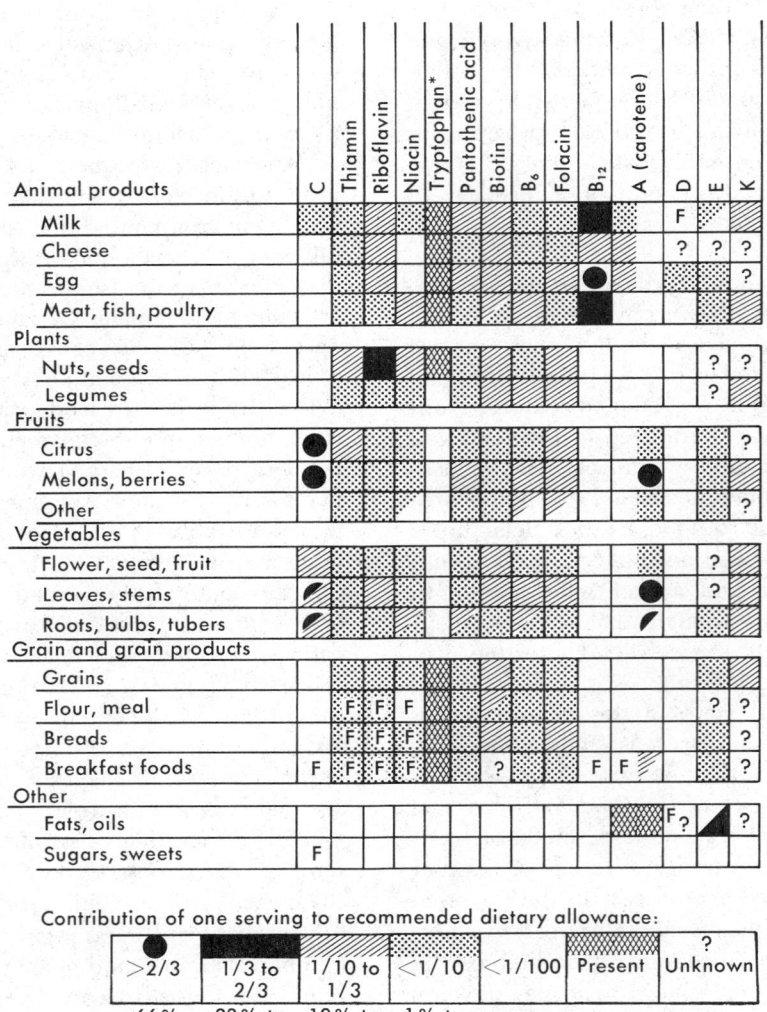

Fig. 53-5. Foods as sources of vitamins. Serving size is household portion.

ings of fruit and vegetables, and four servings of grain and grain products to make a total of at least 12 servings of food per day as a minimum. To interpret Fig. 53-5, one might judge any food that provides one tenth of the day's recommended vitamin intake as being an important source. Note that for the range of vitamins provided by each food, none provides 10% or more of each of the 13 vitamins. Milk comes closest in that all vitamins are provided. Of plant foods, vegetable leaves and stems are consistent in providing important quantities of many, but not all, vitamins. Milk also provides high-quality protein, significant calcium, and other minerals and is readily available at reasonable cost. It is a basic food in most hospital diets and is recommended in most nutrition education materials for that reason. The green leafy vegetables are superior sources of vitamins A and C and of iron as well as other minerals, thus complementing milk and improving the nutritional quality of the diet.

The vitamins are not equally distributed in foods. Note in the column for vitamin C in Fig. 53-5 that foods appear to be either rich sources of the vitamin or severely limited. This is also true for vitamin A, B$_{12}$, and D. Certain fruits or vegetables must be selected to assure adequate intake of vitamins C and A. Animal products contribute vitamins B$_{12}$ and D, although some ready-to-eat breakfast cereals and some soy-milk products may be fortified with these vitamins. Sunshine provides ad-

ditional vitamin D, and our symbiotic relationship with intestinal flora appears to provide biotin and vitamin K. Deficiencies in these nutrients are rare, as are deficiencies in vitamin E. In contrast to vitamin C, thiamin is found in most foods, but no one food is superior in content. When persons substitute sugars and sweets (including honey) or alcohol for other foods, they obtain concentrated sources of energy that yield small levels of vitamins or minerals.

A similar illustration could be presented for many of the minerals, but complete analyses of food for all the mineral elements are not yet available. Table 53-2 illustrates the contributions of calcium and iron of various foods in relation to their energy value. The contributions of calcium from milk and green leafy vegetables are obvious. Calcium and iron are not evenly distributed in foods. Meat, vegetables, breads, and cereals are important contributors.

The contributions to protein, vitamin, and mineral intake are illustrated in Fig. 53-6. Note the variation recorded in the sodium content of oatmeal. Sodium varies with the amount of salt, baking powder, and baking soda used in the preparation of foods. The variation in thiamin content illustrated for bread is based on the choice of whole-grain or enriched breads. Labels should be checked since local bakeries may not enrich their products.

A warning is needed. This discussion of diet quality

TABLE 53-2. Nutrient densities of foods: calcium and iron contributions of common foods yielding 1000 calories*

Food	Amount	Calcium (mg)	Iron (mg)
Milk (regular, whole)	190 ml (6⅓ C)	1814	0.6
Milk (fluid, skim)	340 ml (11⅓ C)	3362	1.1
Cheese	220 g (½ lb)	1701	2.3
Beef (lean, cooked)	450 g (1 lb)	54	15.9
Eggs (large)	12	324	14.4
Almonds	1¼ C	380	7.6
Kidney beans	4⅔ C	327	20.5
Orange juice	9 C	243	4.5
Lettuce	14 heads	1512	37.8
Potatoes	1.35 kg (3 lb [9 medium])	91	7.2
Bread, (white, enriched)	16 slices, standard	348	9.0
Oatmeal (cooked)	7½ C	165	10.5
Honey	1 C	17	1.7
Margarine	150 g (5 oz)	29	0
Beer	2.4 L (80 oz [6⅔ bottles])	120	Trace
Whiskey	450 ml (15 oz)	0	0
Apple pie	⅔ of pie	33	1.1
Chocolate cake with icing	⅓ of cake	216	3.1
Recommended dietary allowance for 1 day			
Man		800	10.0
Woman		800	18.0

*Based on data from United States Department of Agriculture, Agriculture Research Service: Nutritive value of American foods in common units, Agriculture handbook no. 456, Washington, D.C., 1975, U.S. Government Printing Office.

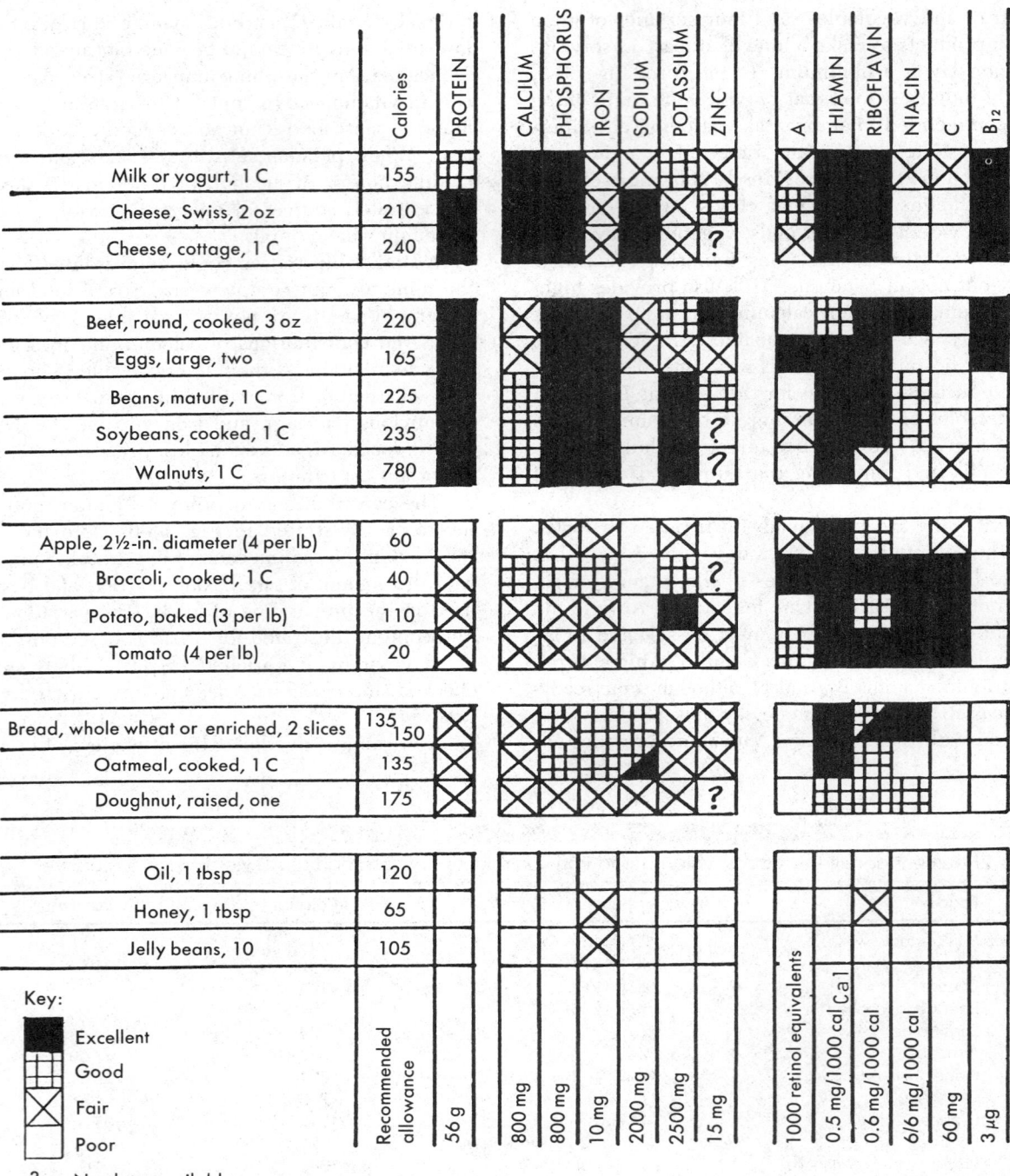

Fig. 53-6. Foods as sources of nutrients. Serving size is household portion, and recommended allowance is that for adult men.

and the importance of careful choice in kinds and amounts of food might tempt one to conclude that it is simpler to rely on vitamin and mineral supplements. These drugs, when subjected to the same rigorous examination for the range of nutrients and amounts in relation to people's needs, are no panacea. One popular brand with an advertising campaign directed primarily at women provides three times the level of iron recommended, with none of the other minerals important for hemoglobin formation, and "some" vitamins. Many over-the-counter vitamin preparations provide excess amounts of vitamins relatively inexpensive to produce and minimal quantities of others. It is not an uncommon occurrence for a person to be carefully taking a diet supplement that does not provide the nutrient really needed. The pharmacist can provide information concerning content adequacy of the dosage and potential toxicity of dietary supplements.[27]

The quality of the diet is most easily judged by determining whether the person is consuming the recommended amounts of the different types of foods. Intervention can be of two different types: (1) working with the person to include the missing items in dietary intake or (2) finding an acceptable alternate food that provides the missing nutrients.

Protein is widely distributed in foods (Fig. 53-2). When these foods are consumed in quantities sufficient to provide adequate protein, the fats and carbohydrates are also provided to meet minimum needs. Energy needs have already been discussed. The question of the quality of protein remains. As a general rule, proteins of animal origin provide the essential amino acids in appropriate quantities. Plant proteins may be limited in one or more of the essential amino acids, but few persons limit their intake to only one protein source even if they eliminate meat. The quality of dietary protein is a function of the amino acid supply provided by the combination of foods eaten at one feeding. A mixture of plant-animal protein or of plant-plant protein can provide the full range of essential amino acids. The protein status of the patient is more often at risk because total food intake is limited in quantity than because of poor quality of protein. An exception to this is the patient being maintained too long on a clear-liquid diet or intravenous saline or dextrose as the sole source of nourishment. Problems incurred from imbalances of fluid and electrolytes are discussed in Chapter 21.

Diet modifications

The modification needed by the person may be simply assistance in changing the usual food intake pattern to the normal pattern recommended for health. It may involve adjustments to meet special dietary problems imposed by disease, trauma, or metabolic abnormalities. For this reason dietary modifications must be considered before determining intervention. Therapeutic diets should not be imposed on the person without good reason. Principles basic to prescribing diets are listed in the box at right. A diet prescription is based on the determination of each patient's nutrient needs. When no constraints have been imposed by temporary or permanent alterations in nutritional processes (e.g., digestion or absorption) or body functioning by illness or trauma, the "normal" ("house") diet is prescribed. This is not considered a "modified diet," since "modified" is used to describe diets different in some way from nor-

PRINCIPLES OF THERAPEUTIC DIETS*

In deciding on the dietary management of a disease certain general principles should govern the prescription and formulation of any special diet.

1. The diet should provide all essential nutrients as generously as its special characteristics permit.

2. The special therapeutic regimen should be patterned as much as possible after a normal diet.

3. The special diet should be flexible; it should consider the patient's gustatory habits and preferences, his economic status, and any religious rules that may govern his food intake.

4. A diet should be adapted to the patient's habits with regard to work and exercise.

5. The foods that are included in the special diet must agree with the patient.

6. The diet should emphasize natural, commonly used foods that are readily available and easily prepared at home.

7. A simple and clear explanation of the purpose of the diet and reason for it should be given to the patient and to the members of his family who are responsible for the preparation of his meals.

8. Except for cases where a maintenance diet must be adhered to for life, patients should be taken off special diets as soon as possible. Practically anybody required to follow a therapeutic diet feels conspicuous and set apart; this is especially important in the case of young children, who are more impressionable and for whom a prolonged special diet may be the making of an emotional problem.

9. The diet must be absolutely justified and defensible. Hospitals, patients, and patients' families alike will benefit if the number of special diets is reduced to those that are really necessary.

10. Feeding by mouth is always the method of choice; only when the patient is incapable or will not eat and drink enough should tube feeding or, if this is contraindicated, parenteral feeding be resorted to.

*From Human nutrition, ed. 3, by Benjamin and Burton. Copyright © 1976, McGraw-Hill Book Co. Used with permission of McGraw-Hill Book Co.

mal. The nurse will find, however, that meeting the prescription for a "normal" diet does require modification of usual food behavior for persons whose food practices are poor. The diet prescription may consist of one or many modifications to be followed for varying lengths of time—from 1 day to a lifetime. The person with chronic disease is often faced with the necessity for permanent changes in food habits. In some instances dietary modification does not necessitate change in food behavior, since the person's usual diet actually meets the prescribed modification. A brief discussion of diet modifications and possible applications is included here to illustrate the scope of diet therapy. Consult this text and suggested reading lists for details.

Protein modification

Protein may be increased to levels twice those usually recommended for persons with protein losses from tissue catabolism, bleeding, and exudates. On the other hand, protein may be decreased to levels one half to one third those recommended. In chronic renal failure diet management involves providing sufficient protein to prevent tissue protein catabolism and yet avoid accumulations of urea. In hepatic coma dietary protein is adjusted to individual tolerance. In some instances control of the amino acid content of the diet may be required. Children with phenylketonuria need the same nutrients for growth as the healthy child. Their diet must be modified, however, because they cannot convert phenylalanine to tyrosine and subsequent normal metabolites. The diet should provide sufficient phenylalanine for growth but not enough to raise serum levels to those causing central nervous system damage. Phenylalanine cannot be eliminated from the diet as it is an essential amino acid. Tyrosine becomes an essential amino acid for this child as his body cannot convert phenylalanine to tyrosine as normal children do. Specific proteins may be eliminated with gluten-induced enteropathy or allergies.

Fat modification

Fat modifications include increasing or decreasing total fat intake, altering the proportion of dietary calories obtained from fat, and altering the fatty acid composition of the diet. Total fat may be increased to provide essential calories in a concentrated form. Total fat may be decreased for patients with gallbladder disease to reduce pain and contraction of the gallbladder. Alterations in the proportion of dietary calories from fat may be used for patients with primary or secondary disorders of lipid metabolism or to induce ketosis. The prescription should specify the proportions desired for the patient: 10% to 15% of total calories ("low"); 25% to 30% of total calories ("moderate"); 40% to 45% of total calories ("usual"); 60% to 80% of total calories ("ketogenic"). Modifications may also be made in the kind of fat in the diet: short-chain, medium-chain, or long-chain triglycerides or saturated, monounsaturated, and polyunsaturated fatty acids. Modifications in chain length may be prescribed for patients with disorders of digestion and absorption. Modifications in saturated and unsaturated fatty acids may be prescribed to alter serum lipid levels.

Carbohydrate modification

Carbohydrate modifications include increasing or decreasing total carbohydrate intake, altering the proportion of dietary calories obtained from carbohydrate, controlling the type of carbohydrate, and eliminating or reducing specific carbohydrate components. The dietary prescription for a patient with diabetes mellitus might include a decrease in total carbohydrates, a change in the ratio of simple to complex carbohydrates, and substitution of carbohydrate derivatives such as hexitols or dextrins for sucrose. Lactose may be eliminated from the diet of patients with lactase insufficiency and sucrose from the diet of patients with invertase insufficiency. Fructose and sucrose are excluded from the diet of persons with hereditary fructose intolerance and galactose and lactose from the diet of patients with galactosemia.

Vitamin modification

Modifications in vitamin concentrations are generally limited to increasing dosage or providing the vitamin in an alternate form to enhance absorption or utilization. Medicinal sources are frequently used. A diet low in vitamin A and carotene is prescribed for patients with vitamin A toxicity.

Mineral modification

Often the mineral content of a diet must be controlled. Sodium restriction is one of the most common dietary modifications prescribed and is frequently combined with modifications in calories, sources of carbohydrate, and other minerals. Persons with hypertension, fluid retention, or kidney disease are usually expected to control the amount of sodium they eat. The term "control" is used here deliberately, since the goal is to balance sodium intake with sodium need, with the body's ability to handle sodium, and with the physiologic effects of drugs or medications. The level of sodium recommended may vary from 250 mg to 2 g or more per day. Elimination of sodium from the diet can precipitate dehydration.

Potassium levels may be specified for patients with kidney disease and for those with disorders of electrolyte imbalance. Other mineral modifications include diets low or high in calcium and diets low in copper. Medicinal sources of minerals are frequently prescribed.

Modifications in consistency and amounts

Liquid (clear and full), *puréed,* and *soft* diets represent modifications in consistency. They may be used when the patient has difficulties in chewing or swallowing or when the patient has lesions of the gastrointestinal tract. They may be used serially for the postoperative patient. Modifications in fiber or residue content of the diet are often prescribed.

Meal size and *frequency* may be modified for treatment of appetite disorders, diabetes mellitus, dumping syndrome, hypoglycemia, peptic ulcer, and other disorders. Modifications in the *method of feeding* include tube feeding, parenteral or intravenous infusions, and sterile food service.[58]

In some cases the prescription may specify *elimination of specific foods* or beverages from the diet. This approach is used in food allergy. Food elimination may lead to rather bizarre and unusual dietary patterns that should be checked closely for adequacy. Sometimes the diet order specifies foods that may be served to the patient. This is usually a list of bland items such as gelatin, soft-cooked egg, farina, and mashed potato. The nurse may alleviate patient distress and boredom by asking the physician to change the order to "diet as tolerated."

Any diet modification, when imposed, should be justified. Theories of the appropriate nutritional therapy in some diseases vary depending on the interpretation of indirect evidence. Carefully controlled studies are needed to determine the efficacy of modifications, including some that have been used for years (e.g., the elimination of "gas-forming" or strong-flavored foods). At times it appears as though folklore rather than scientific method fathered some diet and food restrictions. In recent years there has been a trend toward liberal interpretation of dietary therapy. In part this has been the result of a recognition that many restrictions were without basis in fact and that life lived according to these restrictions was so onerous that emotional well-being was lost without a compensating increase in physical well-being.

Diet/drug modifications

Various drugs and medications that a person is taking may affect body functions in such a way that diet modification is needed. The obvious illustration of this phenomenon is the treatment regimen for persons with diabetes mellitus: diet, exercise, insulin activity, and hypoglycemic drugs. Moderate to severe elevations in blood pressure may be experienced by patients taking monoamine oxidase inhibitors when they consume large quantities of foods such as aged cheddar cheese, herring, or wines. These foods are rich in tyramine, and metabolism of tyramine is dependent on monoamine oxidase. Some persons receiving penicillamine therapy may experience a subjective loss of taste for salt and sweet. The diarrhea commonly associated with high-dosage neomycin therapy reflects an induced malabsorption syndrome. Some persons being maintained on barbiturates or anticonvulsants may develop folic acid deficiency, and some taking large doses of isoniazid may show signs of vitamin B_6 deficiency. Thiazide diuretic therapy may deplete cellular potassium. Some medications or products may yield so much sodium as to negate any benefit from a sodium-controlled diet; some products contain lactose as a filler. Since new and more powerful drugs are constantly being developed, this list is certain to grow. A diet prescription must be translated into a diet plan or food pattern that will meet the person's physical needs and yet provide enough flexibility that the patient will enjoy the food. If a modification is required for only a short time, it may not be difficult to plan. However, if the modification is one to be followed at home after discharge from the hospital, such things as cost, availability, ease of preparation, and relationship to family food requirements must be taken into account.

Considerations when making dietary modifications

An unwritten but essential part of each diet order is that the diet should provide all nutrients as generously as its special characteristics permit. If the modification is so restrictive that the food plan will not provide adequate supplies, the physician should be notified so that appropriate adjustments in diet or medication can be made. Clear-liquid diets, for example, supply important fluids, some calories, and some sodium and chloride, but they have little other nutrient value. When milk must be eliminated from the diet, it is necessary to identify and eliminate all food items containing milk and replace the calcium, phosphorus, riboflavin, and protein value of milk by incorporating other foods into the food plan. Alterations in the diet—changes in the proportions of calories from protein, fat, and carbohydrate—may in themselves change nutrient requirements. For example, increased polyunsaturated fat should be accompanied by increased dietary levels of vitamin E and increased protein accompanied by increased vitamin B_6. This is accomplished by including foods rich in the desired components in the patient's diet. For example, the polyunsaturated fat may be provided by corn oil or safflower oil which contain both the desired fat and vitamin E.

Vigorous therapeutic measures aimed at treating one condition may precipitate others when care is disease focused. For example, the traditional regimen for peptic ulcer emphasized maintaining the patient on a diet of milk, cream, and foods high in calories and fat for months or years. Gain in weight and particularly in body fat was not unusual. Ulcers are most prevalent in middle-aged men, the group most at risk from coronary artery disease.

Foods contain a variety of nutrients in varying proportions. The diet plan should guide selection of the kinds of foods in the amounts dictated by the diet prescription. Calorie, protein, fat, and carbohydrate concentrations of some common foods are shown in Fig. 53-2. Notice how many of the foods contain protein. Intake of all these foods would have to be limited if protein is restricted. Calorie needs would have to be supplied by foods consisting primarily of carbohydrate or fat.

Some dietary prescriptions can be met only by using different or unusual food items such as casein hydrolysate (low in phenylalanine or starches) made from wheat or corn or other plant sources. These cannot be handled in the same way as the foods they replace. New techniques and recipes must be developed. The final products differ in appearance, texture, and taste from those they replace. Patients whose diets require such products should have help in learning how to cook the products and use them in the diet. Since information about staple food items is the best available, food plans for diet modifications tend to emphasize staple foods and do not include many new items on the food market.

Interest in dietary fiber is high, although there is disagreement regarding the definition of fiber, conflicting data about the values of high-and low-fiber diets, and disagreements as to the relative merits of fiber from grains, vegetables, and fruits. Bran may be prescribed as an adjunct to diet together with increased use of foods containing complex carbohydrate. Sufficient fiber in the diet has been recommended for many years for proper elimination of waste products.

Dietary counseling

Assessment

The dietary history of a person serves as a useful screening device. The adequacy of the diet in terms of quality and quantity can be quickly estimated by comparing it with recommended patterns of food intake. It may also provide information about unusual or bizarre uses of food, which in turn may be a key factor in the health problem. Examples are hypokalemia associated with excessive intake of licorice or cathartics and fever associated with consumption of a gallon of coffee. These imbalances are rare. Identification of factors affecting nutrition status (e.g., faulty dietary habits, inadequate

intake, poor absorption, decreased utilization, increased excretion, increased destruction, increased requirements) permits designing an effective treatment program. Treatment may require dietary modifications, medications, and changes in living patterns.

Planning

The goals for dietary counseling are determined by the results of the nutritional assessment (see Chapter 52) and the diet prescribed while the patient is hospitalized or to be followed at home.

The definition of "good" food is very personal and is a product of all the experiences associated with food over a lifetime. The major challenge in diet therapy can be summarized as providing "good" food for the person within the limits imposed by his health and nutrient needs. One basic principle of learning is that persons learn by building on what they already know. People know about their present dietary intake and are much more likely to learn when taught about how to make changes in their current dietary pattern to meet the diet prescription. Too often diets are imposed on people as though they had no previous experience with food. Instructions for diet modifications should begin with the person's current food habits and should stress the necessary changes to be made.

The person's history of usual food intake is compared with the appropriate guide for food choice (basic food pattern or therapeutic regimen as described in the diet manuals or nutrition texts). The patient's food consumption in the hospital is observed. Good food practices that should be continued, practices that are neither particularly valuable nor harmful, and practices that need to be changed are identified. Treatment and medications are checked to determine if these affect appetite, nutrient need, meal composition, or frequency. It is determined whether the diet to be followed at home is the same as or different from the current diet.

The special services the person requires need to be coordinated so that schedule conflicts are avoided. For example, some laboratory studies require that patients fast; others require that they eat a special type of test meal. Coordination of laboratory, dietary, and nursing care schedules in such situations is essential to the accuracy of the results and to the patient's comfort. Quite often the need for consultation can be identified by the nurse early in the patient's hospital stay. The consultation can then be scheduled and provided before the day of discharge. The so-called discharge diet instruction is often omitted or rendered useless because it is left until the last minute when the patient's major interest is to get home as quickly as possible.

Intervention

The nurse serves as an interpreter to the patient by providing brief and easily understood explanations about the diet, any modifications in it, and the food selections on the tray. The nurse also serves as an interpreter by providing pertinent information about the patient to the physician, dietitian, or food service unit so that the diet prescription or food on the tray provides not only nutrients but also conforms insofar as possible to ethnic, religious, or personal preferences and provides eating pleasure.

One goal of patient education is to provide information so that the person can make informed choices. The final goal, however, is a change in behavior related to food so that the person is well nourished. Even small changes in food behavior can benefit the person. An obese person who reduces caloric intake from 3000 to 2500 calories/day has made a significant behavior change, although one cannot credit the person with complying to a dietary prescription of 1000 calories. The person with inadequate calcium intake may be willing to use milk instead of cream substitutes in coffee. The final goal of dietary adherence is more obtainable when changes are taken in small steps, one at a time. In part this is because the goal is realistic and progress can be measured. In addition, the patient has been involved in setting the goals, and the patient, not the nurse, is the one who must implement the goal.

This approach to patient teaching is more efficient for the therapist and less frustrating for the patient. It is irritating to be lectured on the importance of including milk in the diet when milk and cheese are favorite foods. It can be boring to listen to a description of the evils of salt and calories in potato chips or french-fried potatoes when one never eats them. A patient can say, "Yes, I understand" aloud and in many instances truly understand but not accept the recommendations. Consideration must be given to social, cultural, and economic factors as well as to the person's knowledge of and beliefs about nutrition.

Eating intervals. The convention of three meals a day is just that—a convention and a convenience. For many it is a fiction. Most people eat more often, while the economically deprived may eat only once a day. There may be some advantage to eating smaller meals at shorter intervals as long as total nutrient needs are met. Although physiologic evidence does not support a rigid pattern of three feedings a day, there is evidence that omitting breakfast impairs physiologic and mental efficiency. Except in special circumstances (insulin-dependent diabetes, for example), the number of feedings a day can be determined by the person's desires and life-style. If no breakfast is eaten, however, consumption of some food at the beginning of the day should be considered as a desirable goal. Since breakfast is generally the meal most enjoyed by hospitalized patients, this can be a useful mechanism for initiating breakfast as a meal at home as well. Each feeding, whether called a meal or snack, should include a mixture of nutrients.

Food costs. Cost is an important factor in family food patterns.[43] The nurse, when attempting to teach a person about diet, is frequently challenged about food cost. Vague generalities such as "use cheaper cuts of meat" are not particularly helpful. Suggestions should be specific, based on the person's diet and income. They should provide enough information to serve as a basis of action. The price of an envelope of flavored sugar used by many low-income families to make a beverage is equivalent to the price of enough dried skim milk solids for 1 L of milk. Which is the better buy? Where and how can a person get food stamps? The nurse with personal experience in managing food budgets, purchasing, cookery, and so forth, is in a position to offer practical advice. There are many useful materials available on food purchasing, storage, and preparation. The dietitian will be able to help select the materials that are best for the patient.

In most cases, money spent for food can be reduced and the nutritive value of the diet improved by (1) planning the menu at home, (2) listing kinds and amounts of food to be bought, (3) purchasing items on this list, and (4) controlling waste caused by preparing more food than is needed or from foods spoiling before use.

Food labeling. Food labels can be used as a basis for food choice. Currently many changes are being made in food-labeling practices and regulations governing the use of certain terms describing foods. These changes are designed to improve the nutrition information given on food labels and to provide meaningful information to the public. The nutrition-labeling program is voluntary for most foods; however, if a nutrient is added to any product or if a nutritional claim is made either on the label or in advertising, the product label must have full nutrition labeling. On food labels the levels of vitamins and minerals will be listed as a percentage of the US-RDA. To meet the regulations the label must include size of serving, number of servings per container, calories, protein, carbohydrate, fat, and the percentage of the US-RDA for vitamin A, vitamin C, thiamin, riboflavin, niacin, calcium, and iron. Another 12 vitamins and minerals may be listed at the option of the food producer. The US-RDA is based on the standard RDA but is condensed to four categories: infants, children under 4 years of age, adults and children over 4 years of age, and pregnant or lactating women. Consumer memos describing the regulations are available from the Food and Drug Administration. The regulation allows for a statement on the label of cholesterol, total fat, and polyunsaturated and saturated fat. This is helpful for persons on fat-modified diets.

The data in Table 53-3 were taken directly from food labels. One advantage to the system is that information on the label is based on the analysis of the specific brand so that differences in an item such as tuna packed by several different companies can be identified by com-

TABLE 53-3. Nutrition label as a guide for choosing food

	Tuna packed in oil	Chocolate bar	Skim milk	Gelatin dessert
Serving	3¼ oz	1½ oz	1 C	½ C
Servings per container	2	1	4	4*
Required				
Calories	230	230	90	80
Protein (g)	22.5	3	8	2*
Fat (g)	15	4	1	0
Carbohydrate (g)	0.5	12	11	18
US-RDA	%	%	%	%
Required listing				
Protein	100	4	20	†
Vitamin A	†	†	10	†
Vitamin C	†	†	4	†
Thiamin	2	2	6	†
Riboflavin	8	6	25	†
Niacin	120	†	†	†
Calcium	†	8	30	†
Iron	8	2	†	†
Optional listing				
Vitamin D			25	
Vitamin B₆	25		4	
Vitamin B₁₂	45		15	
Vitamin E	10			
Pantothenic acid			6	
Phosphorus			20	
Magnesium			8	
Zinc			4	

*Not a significant source of protein.
†Contains less than 2% of the U.S. Recommended Daily Allowances.

paring the labels. The labeling system may be changed, but the concept of nutrition labeling has apparently been accepted. The advantages to persons attempting to control energy intake or modifying protein, fat, or carbohydrate intake are obvious. For those concerned with cost, the attraction of getting more nutritional value for the money may provide motivation for reading labels.

Nutrition labeling does not include the listing of the ingredients. Lists of ingredients are not required on foods covered by "standards of identity" such as mayonnaise, ice cream, or peanut butter. Current regulations require that ingredients be listed in descending order by weight. This does help, although general terms such as "spices," "vegetable oil," or "starch" offer insufficient information for someone who must avoid a particular spice or choose food high in polyunsaturated fat.

Many new products are specifically designed by intent and advertising to replace staple items. Several breakfast drinks are being marketed that look and taste like orange juice and that have been enriched with ascorbic acid so that they may have as much or more ascorbic acid as orange juice. But these breakfast drinks are high in sodium and low in potassium, whereas orange juice is low in sodium and high in potassium. A wide variety of substitutes for coffee cream, sour cream, and whipped cream are on the market. They are convenient to use, easy to store, and acceptable in flavor to most people. Can they be used by persons on restricted diets? Many of these products are made from coconut oil, which is a highly saturated fat. Such products cannot be recommended as a source of polyunsaturated fat. They are excellent calorie sources, however.

Notice the difference in protein, fat, and carbohydrate in ice cream, ice milk, and sherbet in Fig. 53-2. The fat of ice cream is butterfat; that of ice milk is vegetable fat; sherbet is essentially fat free. All contain sucrose. "Diabetic" ice creams substitute other carbohydrates for sucrose and usually have a high-fat level to provide good texture. As a result the calorie content of "diabetic" ice creams is often higher than that of conventional ice cream.

Food additives. The public has become more interested in food and nutrition. The consumer movement has, among other things, focused attention on food processing and food additives.* Additives may be foods, derived from foods, or products created in the laboratory. The most widely used food additive is sucrose, ordinary table sugar. Sodium chloride, table salt, is the second. Monosodium glutamate, mustard, and black pepper are food additives used in large quantities also. Most of the current concern about food additives relates to safety. Excessive intake of sugar has been related to obesity, tooth decay, and coronary artery disease; excessive intake of salt has been related to hypertension. Questions have been raised about the safety of nonnutritive sweeteners, nitrates used in curing meats, and antioxidants such as BHT used to keep fat from becoming rancid. The food industry's use of additives is regulated by the Food and Drug Administration. In 1958 the food additives amendment to the Food, Drug, and Cosmetic Act of 1938 was passed; it requires proof of safety before a substance may be added to food. In 1960 the color additive amendment was enacted to control all color additives, natural and synthetic.

Generally recognized as safe (GRAS) substances have been classified by technical effect, and each group is being reviewed for use and safety. One such group is Technical Effect Code 16, leavening agents that include yeast and baking powder. The review for each group is published as completed.

Concern with pesticide residues (as well as food additives) has caused some people to turn to a "natural" or "organic" diet. Some believe that the body can use

*References 12, 13, 16, 20, 26, 36.

only nutrients from a natural source despite evidence to the contrary. Others want food that has been grown without the use of chemical fertilizers or pesticides and processed without additives. Foods labeled "organic" or "natural" usually cost more. The terms are not defined by law, and values are being claimed for products without evidence to support them. Current concern with food additives and pesticides has obscured other issues of food safety. It is just as important to be sure that food is free of microbiologic and insect contamination. Foods themselves contain natural substances that can be harmful. Legislation cannot protect the individual from poor food choices nor ensure good food handling practices in the home.

Enteral and parenteral nutrition

Oral feeding is the method of choice; however, when patients cannot take food by mouth, alternative methods are employed. The time period may be short or long. The same considerations governing oral nourishment apply to nourishment by tube or vein. Are all of the nutrients being supplied? For short-term care, patient stores may provide missing nutrients. For long-term care or for persons without stores (infants, debilitated persons), adequacy of all nutrients should be checked, or deficiencies may occur.[37] Providing sufficient calories without unfavorable reactions may present a problem.

Tube feeding (gavage)

The type of feeding and route are usually determined by the physician. Nasogastric tubes may be used for short-term feeding. For long-term feeding a new opening (gastrostomy) may be made in the stomach (p. 1396). The nasogastric tube is left in place for adults and older children, but for infants it usually is passed and removed for each feeding (see p. 1384 for the technique of passing the tube).

No feeding should be introduced into a nasogastric tube until it has been ascertained that the tube is in the stomach. The most accurate method is aspiration of gastric contents. A *left* side-lying position facilitates aspiration of gastric contents as the tip of the tube will move toward the greater curvature of the stomach. If gastric contents are aspirated, they are returned to the stomach to prevent loss of electrolytes. Some physicians request that the tube feeding not be given if a specified large amount of gastric contents are aspirated. Alternative methods of checking the placement of the tube are (1) inserting approximately 5 ml of air in the tube and

listening with a stethoscope over the left upper abdominal quadrant for the sound of air entering the stomach, (2) placing the end of the tube in water and observing a continual rhythmic flow of air bubbles indicating that the tip of the tube is in the upper air passages rather than the stomach, or (3) injecting 1 to 2 ml of sterile water into the tube and observing a forceful cough resulting from fluid in the upper respiratory tract.

A sitting position is best for the patient receiving a tube feeding. If this is not possible a *right* side-lying position facilitates movement of the fluid to the distal portion of the stomach and permits easier filling of the stomach.

The feeding should be nutritionally adequate, well tolerated (no vomiting, diarrhea, constipation, or distention), easily prepared, and reasonable in cost.[18,19] The tube feeding should be handled carefully with attention to sanitation. It is kept refrigerated until ready to use and may be given either at room temperature or cold depending on patient tolerance and preference.

The tube feedings used in an institution are usually described in the hospital diet manual. Three types of formulas are common: blended formulas, milk-based formulas, and elemental-diet formulas. *Blended* formulas are foods (baby food, ordinary foods from a normal diet) liquified with a high-speed blender. The formulas are similar to the usual adult diet and are generally well-tolerated and relatively inexpensive. *Milk-based* formulas may be mixtures of egg, milk, and sugar with skim milk powder and protein hydrolysates. Recipes for formulas to be made in the hospital or at home are available. Diarrhea may result from the high content of simple sugars such as lactose. *Elemental-diet* formulas are synthetic low-residue mixtures of amino acids, sugars, vitamins, and minerals that may be given orally or by the tube. They are expensive and require careful monitoring of blood glucose and electrolytes. Commercial formulas are available for tube feedings and are convenient although more costly.

The proportions of protein, carbohydrate, and fat should approximate that of the normal diet. High-protein tube feedings have been associated with severe effects.[64] The concentration is important and is usually adjusted to about 1 kcal/ml. If the patient is very young, elderly, or severely debilitated, the initial feeding should be more dilute, about 0.5 kcal/ml. Two liters every 24 hours is a customary volume. If the patient can tolerate 1000 kcal over a 24-hour period, the concentration can gradually be increased. Rapid or forced feedings of large volumes or excessively concentrated mixtures, especially with insufficient water, increase danger of dehydration. The patient should be monitored for thirst, abdominal cramping, diarrhea, and low urinary output. In patients with an inadequate swallowing reflex, vomiting should be avoided since aspiration of the vomitus may occur. Positioning of these patients to avoid aspiration is important, and suction equipment must be readily available at the bedside. A patient with a cuffed endotracheal or tracheostomy tube in place is never left alone while fluids are being given by gavage. Feedings should be given at a slow constant rate, either through a gavage drainage system or by an electric food pump. Water should be given in a small quantity before the feeding in the event that the tube is displaced and after the feeding to flush out the tube, in sufficient quantity to avoid dehydration and to permit excretion of urinary waste products.

Parenteral feeding

An alternative route for nourishing patients who cannot be fed by mouth or through the digestive tract is by intravenous infusion. The nutrients and fluid may be delivered into a peripheral vein (intravenous feeding) or into the vena cava (total parenteral nutrition [TPN]). (The reader is referred to Chapter 21 for a discussion of these two methods.) The supply of calories and amino acids that can be delivered by the intravenous route is limited. TPN has made it possible to deliver a slow, continuous infusion of hyperosmolar fluid without damage to the vein. The benefits of TPN, however, have their costs as well, such as complications related to the central venous catheter, electrolyte imbalance, metabolic disturbances, and occasionally allergic reactions following administration of protein hydrolysates. The composition of the infusate varies. Certain vitamins and minerals may be absent and others provided in concentrations high enough to produce overload if continued for long periods.[3,15,23] The ingestion of foods and fluids by way of the gastrointestinal tract is a far more efficient and effective method of meeting the body's nutrition needs.

REFERENCES AND SELECTED READINGS
Contemporary

1. American Dietetic Association: Position paper on bland diet in the treatment of chronic duodenal disease, J. Am. Diet. Assoc. **59**:244-245, 1971.
2. American Dietetic Association Statement: Infant and child nutrition: concerns regarding the developmentally disabled, J. Am. Diet. Assoc. **78**:443-452, 1981.
3. Arakawa, T., et al.: Zinc deficiency in two infants during total parenteral alimentation for diarrhea, Am. J. Clin. Nutr. **29**:197-204, 1976.
4. Beagle, W.S.: Fetal alcohol syndrome: a review, J. Am. Diet. Assoc. **79**:274-276, 1981.
5. Bradley, H., and Sundberg, C.: Keeping food safe, Garden City, N.Y., 1975, Doubleday & Co., Inc.
6. Bruch, H.: Perils of behavior modification in treatment of anorexia nervosa, J.A.M.A. **230**:1419-1422, 1974.
7. *Bruch, H.: Eating disorders: obesity, anorexia nervosa and the

8. Clayman, C.B., Jejunoileal bypass: pass it by, J.A.M.A. **246**:988, 1981.
9. Coates, T.J., and Thorensen, C.E.: Treating obesity in children and adolescents: a review, Am. J. Public Health **68**:143-151, 1978.
10. Cone, T.W.: The nursing bottle caries syndrome. Photo essay, J.A.M.A. **245**:2334, 1981.
11. Cornacchia, H.J., and Barrett, S.: Consumer health: a guide to intelligent decisions, ed. 2, St. Louis, 1980, The C.V. Mosby Co.
12. DeRitter, E.: Stability characteristics of vitamins in processed foods, Food Technol. **30**:48-54, 1976.
13. *Editors of Consumer Reports Books: Nutrition as therapy: health quackery, ch. 10, Mt. Vernon, N.Y., 1980, Consumer's Union.
14. Fineberg, S.K.: The realities of obesity and fad diets, Nutr. Today **7**(4):23-26, 1972.
15. Fleming, C.R., Hodges, R.E., and Hurley, L.S.: A prospective study of serum copper and zinc levels in patients receiving total parenteral nutrition, Am. J. Clin. Nutr. **29**:70-77, 1976.
16. Food and Drug Administration: Consumer nutrition knowledge survey, report 11, 1975, U.S. Department of Health, Education and Welfare, no. (FDA) 76-2059, 1975.
17. Genuth, S.M., Castro, J.H., and Vertes, V.: Weight reduction in obesity by outpatient starvation, J.A.M.A. **230**:987-991, 1974.
18. Gormican, A., and Liddy, E.: Nasogastric tube feedings, Postgrad. Med. **53**:71-76, 1973.
19. Gormican, A., Liddy, E., and Mrush, L.B.: Nutritional status of patients after extended tube feeding, J. Am. Diet. Assoc. **63**:247-251, 1973.
20. Hall, R.L.: Food additives, Nutr. Today **8**(4):20-28, 1973.
21. Halmi, K.A., Powers, P., and Cunningham, S: Treatment of anorexia nervosa with behavior modification effectiveness of formula feeding and isolation, Arch. Gen. Psychiatry **32**:93-96, 1975.
22. Hathcock, J.N.: Nutrition: toxicology and pharmacology, Nutr. Rev. **34**:65-70, 1976.
23. Heird, W.C., and Winters, R.W.: Parenteral nutrition: pediatrics. In Schneider, H.A., Anderson, C.E., and Coursin, D.B.: Nutritional support of medical practice, New York, 1977, Harper & Row, Publishers.
24. *Herbert, V.: Nutrition cultism: facts and fictions, Philadelphia, 1980, George F. Sickley Co.
25. Institute of Rehabilitation Medicine, New York University Medical Center: Mealtime manual for the aged and handicapped, New York, 1977, Essandess Special Editions, Simon & Schuster, Inc.
26. Johnson, P.E.: Misuse in foods of useful chemicals, Nutr. Rev. **35**:225-229, 1977.
27. Jukes, R.H.: Megavitamin therapy, J.A.M.A. **233**:550-551, 1975.
28. Kark, R.M.: Liquid formulas and chemically defined diets, J. Am. Diet. Assoc. **64**:476-480, 1974.
29. Mason, M.: Intervention in pregnancy. In Henning, D.E., editor: Costs and benefits of nutritional care. Phase I, Chicago, 1979, American Dietetic Association.
30. Maxmen, J.S., Siberfarb, P.M., and Ferrell, R.B.: Anorexia nervosa: practical initial management in a general hospital, J.A.M.A. **229**:801-803, 1974.
31. Mazel, J.: The Beverly Hills diet, New York, 1981, MacMillan Publishing Co., Inc.
32. Meng, H.C.: Parenteral nutrition: principles, nutrient requirements, techniques and clinical applications. In Schneider, H.A., Anderson, C.E., and Coursin, D.B.: Nutritional support of medical practice, New York, 1977, Harper & Row, Publishers.
33. Mock, D.M., et al.: Biotin deficiency: an unusual complication of parenteral alimentation, N. Engl. J. Med. **304**:820-822, 1981.
34. Nutritional misinformation and food faddism, Nutr. Rev. **32**(suppl.):1-73, July 1974.
35. *Ohlson, M.A.: Diet therapy in the U.S. in the past 200 years: a bicentennial study, J. Am. Diet. Assoc. **69**:400-497, 1976.
36. Packard, V.S., Jr.: Processed foods and the consumer: additives,

*References preceded by an asterisk are particularly well suited for student reading.

labeling, standards and nutrition, Minneapolis, 1976, University of Minnesota Press.

37. Paulsrud, J.R., et al.: Essential fatty acid deficiency in infants induced by fat-free intravenous feeding, Am. J. Clin. Nutr. **25**:897-904, 1972.

38. Pavry, M.: Dietetic food diarrhea, J.A.M.A. **244**:270, 1980.

39. Reisin, E., et al.: Effect of weight loss without salt restriction on the reduction of blood pressure in overweight hypertensive patients. N. Engl. J. Med. **298**:1-6, 1978.

40. Roberts, H.J.: Perspective on vitamin E therapy, J.A.M.A. **246**:129-131, 1981.

41. *Robertson, L., Flinders, C., and Godfrey, B.: Laurel's kitchen: a handbook for vegetarian cookery and nutrition, Berkeley, Calif., 1976, Nilgiri Press.

42. Safety of hydrolysates in parenteral nutrition (editorial), N. Engl. J. Med. **289**:426-427, 1973.

43. Schafer, R.B.: Factors affecting food behavior and the quality of husbands' and wives' diets, J Am. Diet. Assoc. **72**:138-143, 1978.

44. Schuman, B.M.: Tube feeding using a food pump, Am. Fam. Physician **5**:85-88, 1972.

45. Scrimshaw, N.S.: Through a glass darkly: discerning the practical implications of human dietary protein-energy interrelationships, Nutr. Rev. **35**:321-337, 1977.

46. Shuls, M.E.: A program for total parenteral nutrition at home, Am. J. Clin. Nutr. **28**:1429-1433, 1975.

47. Simmons, R.: Never-say-diet book, New York, 1980, Warner Books, Inc.

48. Smith, M.A.: Feeding the handicapped child, Memphis, 1970, Child Development Center, University of Tennessee.

49. Sours, H.E., et al.: Sudden death associated with very low calorie weight reduction programs, Am. J. Clin. Nutr. **34**:453-461, 1981.

50. Stephanson, M.: The confusing world of health foods, FDA Consumer **12**(4):18-22, 1978.

51. *Theologides, A.: Why cancer patients have anorexia, Geriatrics **34**(6):69-71, 1976.

52. Thiele, V.F.: Clinical nutrition, ed. 2, St. Louis, 1980, The C.V. Mosby Co.

53. Tobian, L.: Hypertension and obesity, N. Engl. J. Med. **298**:46-48, 1978.

54. Trowell, J.: Definition of dietary fiber and hypotheses that it is a protective factor in certain diseases, Am. J. Clin. Nutr. **29**:417-427, 1976.

55. Tullis, I.F.: Reational diet construction for mild and grand obesity, J.A.M.A. **226**:70-71, 1973.

56. Van Italie, T.B., and Kral, J.G.: The dilemma of morbid obesity, J.A.M.A. **246**:999-1003, 1981.

57. Vande Wiele, R.L.: Anorexia nervosa and the hypothalamus, Hosp. Pract. **18**:45-51, Dec. 1977.

58. Watson, P., and Bodey, G.P.: Sterile food service for patients in protected environments, J. Am. Diet. Assoc. **56**:515-520, 1970.

59. West, K.M.: Prevention and therapy of diabetes mellitus, Nutr. Rev. **33**:193-198, 1975.

60. White, M.J.: Intervention in selected problems of children, In Henning, D.E.: Costs and benefits of nutritional care, Phase I, Chicago, 1979, American Dietetic Association.

61. White, P.L., and Nagy, M.E., editors: Total parenteral nutrition, Acton, Mass., 1974, Publishing Sciences Group, Inc.

62. Wolff, R.J.: Who eats for health? Am. J. Clin. Nutr. **26**:438-445, 1973.

63. Worthington, B.S., and Taylor, B.F.: Balanced low-calories vs. high-protein-low-carbohydrate reducing diets. I. Weight loss, nutrient intake and subjective evaluation. II. Biochemical changes, J. Am. Diet. Assoc. **64**:451, 1974.

Classics

64. Gault, M.H., et al.: Hypernatremia, azotemia and dehydration due to high-protein tube feeding, Ann. Intern. Med. **68**:778-791, 1968.

65. Wilmore, D.W., and Dudrick S.: Growth and development of an infant receiving all nutrients by vein, J.A.M.A. **203**:860-864, 1968.

66. Wishnofsky, M.: Calorie equivalents of gained or lost weight, Am. J. Clin. Nutr. **6**:542-546, 1958.

AUDIOVISUAL RESOURCES

Eat right to your heart's delight, West Hollywood, Calif., 1976, International Producers Services. (Six 16-mm films or 8-mm videocasettes, color, sound, 12-15 min. each.) (For teenage and adult audiences, food demonstrations.)

Guide to good eating, Rosemont, Ill., 1977, National Dairy Council. (Full-color poster, miniature posters in English and Spanish.)

Nutritional principles of nasogastric tube feeding, Columbus, Ohio, 1975, Ross Laboratories. (Slides and audiocasettes.)

CHAPTER 54

ASSESSMENT OF UPPER GASTROINTESTINAL TRACT FUNCTION

BARBARA C. LONG

NANCY DURHAM

Maintenance of an adequate nutritional status requires a functioning upper gastrointestinal tract. Normally, food and fluids are placed in the mouth, pushed to the pharynx by the tongue, and swallowed by automatic reflex activity down the esophagus into the stomach. Digestion starts in the mouth and terminates in the small intestine, although fluids continue to be reabsorbed in the colon. Abnormalities that interfere with passage of food will interfere with nutrition; therefore assessment of nutrition requires assessment of the gastrointestinal tract. (For assessment of the lower gastrointestinal tract, see Chapter 57.)

Anatomy and physiology

The upper gastrointestinal tract consists of those structures that facilitate the ingestion and digestion of food, namely, the mouth, esophagus, stomach, and duodenum (Fig. 54-1). The subconscious or actively conscious thought of food initiates the physiologic responses of the body that are ultimately responsible for delivery of a particular nutrient to the individual cell. The hypothalamus is responsible for notifying the body that it is satiated or has received sufficient food substances to maintain proper homeostasis.

Salivation

The cortical thought regarding "food" initiates saliva production from the parotid, submaxillary, buccal, and sublingual glands. The salivary secretions are made up of *serous* secretion containing ptyalin for starch digestion (produced by the parotid and submaxillary glands) and *mucous* secretion for lubrication (produced by the buccal, sublingual, and submaxillary glands). These two secretions account for one half of the upper gastrointestinal tract secretions.

Mastication

The teeth serve the function of initial food breakdown. No other part of the gastrointestinal tract can perform this function if the teeth are missing. Enzymes can act only on the exposed surfaces of the food particles. Very fine particulation prevents excoriation of the lining of the tract, and the rate of digestion is dependent on the total surface area of food particle exposed.[8] General health teaching for children and adults should stress the reason behind thorough mastication of all food substances that are ingested.

Deglutition

Swallowing (deglutition) must be accomplished without compromising respiration. It consists of three phases, a voluntary phase in which the tongue forces the bolus of food into the pharynx, an involuntary pharyngeal phase in which the food moves into the upper esophagus, and an esophageal phase during which food moves from the pharynx down into the stomach. Food is prevented from passing into the trachea by the closing of the trachea and the opening of the esophagus.

Fig. 54-1. Location of digestive system organs. (From Anthony, C.P., and Thibodeau, G.A.: Textook of anatomy and physiology, ed. 11, St. Louis, 1982, The C.V. Mosby Co.)

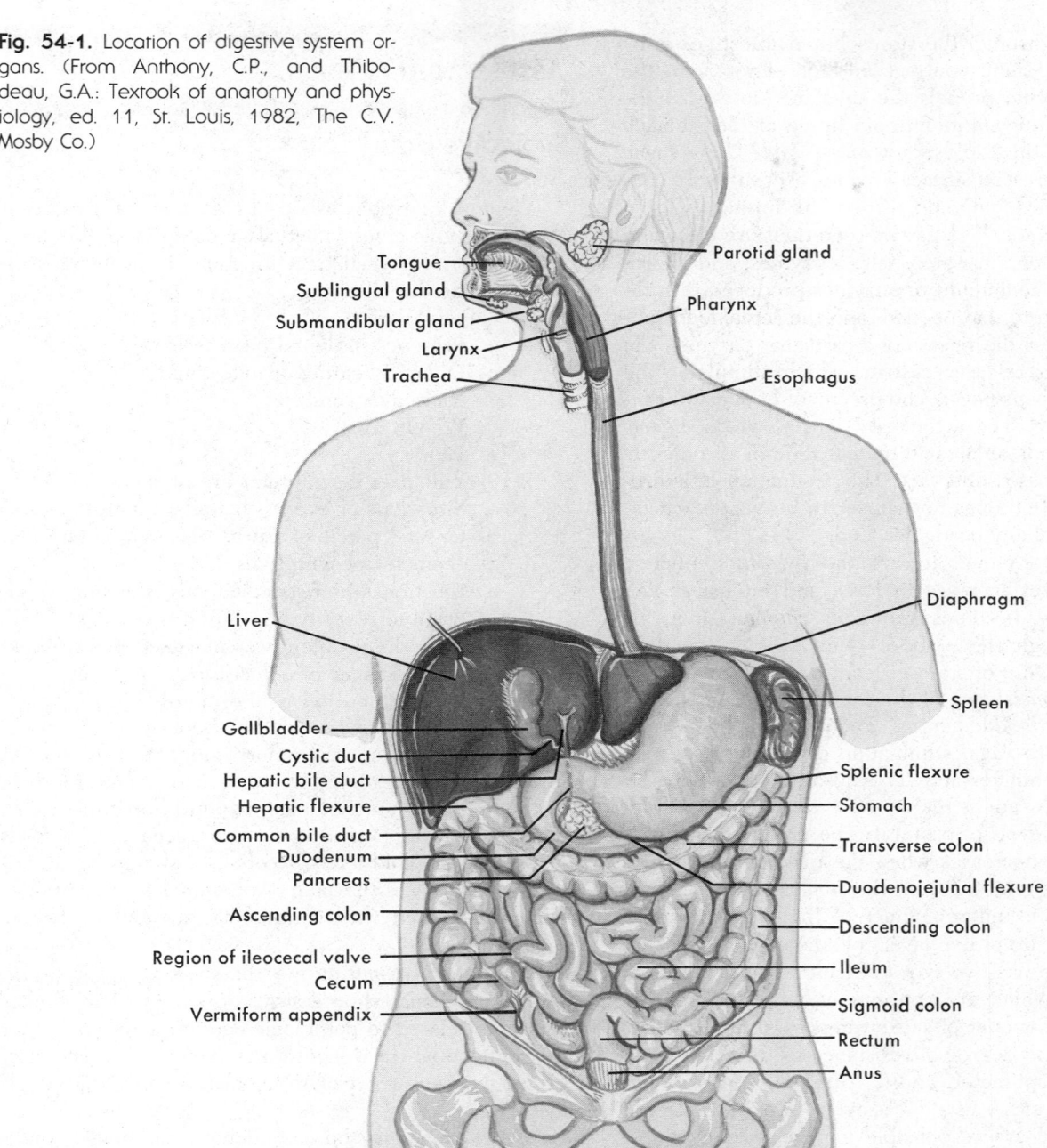

The esophagus is a hollow tube whose upper one third is composed of skeletal muscle and the remainder of smooth muscle. It is lined with mucous membrane, which secretes a mucoid substance for protection. The bolus of food arrives at the cardiac sphincter of the stomach within 5 to 10 seconds of ingestion.[8]

The cardiac sphincter prevents reflux of stomach contents back into the lower esophagus. This area is heavily layered with mucoid glands. The secretions adhere to the food particles and prevent actual contact with the wall mucosa. The coated particles adhere to each other, forming a bolus for digestion. These secretions act as a protective mechanism for the sphincter zone since they themselves are strongly resistant to digestion.

Stomach function

The food bolus enters the stomach, the largest dilated portion of the tract. There is relatively little muscular tone, allowing for increased distention. Movement of food through the stomach and intestines is by *peristalsis,* alternate contraction and relaxation of the muscle fibers that propels the substance in a wavelike motion. The mucous membrane lining of the stomach is arranged in thick folds known as *rugae.* These rugae provide an increased surface area for exposure and contain the gastric pit openings from the fundic, pyloric, and cardiac glands. The gastric secretions are clear and colorless and contain water, salts, enzymes, and hydrochloric acid. The amount of enzymes produced is in direct proportion to that needed, and the actual food substance stimulates the release of a particular enzyme. The gastric mucosa releases gastrin, which stimulates the production of *pepsinogen* (the precursor of pepsin), *rennin,* and *lipase.* The activity of pepsin, which digests protein, depends on an acid media. Rennin also digests protein, and lipase splits fats. The production of hydrochloric acid (HCl) does not appear to be dependent on the presence of any particular food.

As the food moves toward the pyloric sphincter, peristaltic waves increase in force and intensity. The fluid mass now becomes known as *chyme.* Chyme is pumped through the pyloric sphincter into the duodenum. Emptying of stomach contents is regulated by two factors: *consistency* of the fluid chyme and the *receptiveness of the duodenum.*[8] The pyloric sphincter activity stops with vagal stimulation of the *enterogastric* reflex. This sphincter activity is also slowed when the chyme requires an increased time for digestion (fatty foods or high levels of protein). The production of gastric secretions decreases when the pH falls and as enterogastrone is released from the small intestine.

The stomach and remainder of the gastrointestinal tract are made up of five layers of smooth muscle. This smooth muscle has two types of contractions: (1) *tonus* contractions, which are continuous and which determine both the amount of steady pressure exerted within the area and the degree of resistance to the movement of food at the sphincter, and (2) *rhythmic* contractions, which may be either as slow as every 2 to 3 minutes or very rapid and are responsible for the mixing of the food and peristaltic propulsion of it.

The entire tract is innervated through the intramural plexus, which begins in the wall of the esophagus and extends through the anus. The plexus is composed of two layers, *Auerbach's* plexus and *Meissner's* plexus. Stimulation to the plexus increases the tonic contractions and the intensity and rate of rhythmic contractions.[8] Innervation is accomplished through the vagus nerve and comprises both sympathetic and parasympathetic fibers.

Assessment

Subjective data

General questions asked of the client or significant other may give clues to actual or potential problems of upper gastrointestinal tract function. Data to be gathered include the following:
1. General data
   a. Presence of dental prosthesis
   b. Difficulty eating or digesting food
   c. Nausea or vomiting
   d. Weight loss
   e. Pain
2. Specific data if symptoms are present
   a. Situations or events that affect symptoms
   b. Onset, possible cause, location, duration, character of symptoms
   c. Relationship of specific foods, smoking, or alcohol to severity of symptoms
   d. How the problem was managed before seeking assistance of a health care provider

Pain may be reported in the mouth, throat, upper abdomen, or radiating from the abdomen to the back. Abdominal pain or discomfort may be reported as heartburn, indigestion, or stomachache and requires further clarification. The pain may interfere with chewing or swallowing food. Specific foods, such as spicy foods or very hot or cold foods, alcohol, or smoking may initiate or aggravate the pain. Abdominal pain may have been self-treated with commercial antacids or baking soda.

Nausea and *vomiting* may be caused by a gastrointestinal problem such as gastritis or by a number of other factors unrelated to pathologic conditions of the upper gastrointestinal tract. These may include side effects of drugs, fluid and electrolyte imbalances, or radiation effects.

Weight loss may be caused by a pathologic condition, nausea and vomiting, anorexia, or deliberate action on the part of the person to lose weight. Gradual weight loss and lack of appetite in the older person are not necessarily abnormal findings but bear investigation.

All persons should be asked about the presence of *dental prostheses.* It is important to ascertain if the person has any artificial dentures (bridges, partial or full plates), if the prosthesis is being worn, and if it fits and is comfortable. Chewing and digestion can be impaired if the person does not wear the prosthesis. If during the physical inspection of the mouth the teeth are noted to have caries, data are obtained concerning regularity of dental checkups for use in health teaching.

Objective data

Mouth and pharynx

Physical examination of the mouth (Fig. 54-2) will provide data indicating ability to salivate, masticate, and swallow as well as signs of local or systemic disease that can interfere with nutrition. A tongue blade and flashlight are needed for the examination of the oral cavity. The person should be seated comfortably on a level with the examiner and should remove any dental appliances and makeup.

Lips. The person is asked to purse his or her lips, which are observed for symmetry in form and function and for color, moisture, swelling, cracks, or lesions (Fig. 54-3). Asymmetry is often accompanied by drooling and may be the result of facial nerve paralysis from peripheral or central nervous system involvement.[17] If noted, the ability to masticate and swallow is assessed. A congenital malformation such as cleft lip may be observed, or there may be signs of residual dysfunction if this condition has been surgically corrected.

The lips are normally reddish in color and are good indicators of pallor or cyanosis (p. 1783). Dryness may indicate dehydration. Swelling is usually the result of edema of the inflammatory response such as with allergy. Cracks or fissures can occur with overdryness or exposure to cold or, if in the corners of the mouth (*an-gular stomatitis*), from lack of dentures, poorly fitting dentures, or a riboflavin deficiency.

Lesions may be benign or malignant. A frequently encountered benign lesion is *herpes simplex* (cold sore, fever blister), which is caused by a virus and which can create enough discomfort to limit mastication. Any lesion on the lip that does not heal should be referred to the physician for tests for possible malignancy.

Teeth. A full set of teeth consists of 20 teeth in children and 32 teeth in adults. The enamel surface should be white but will darken with surface stains (tea, coffee, tobacco). Commonly found abnormalities include caries, loose teeth, absence of some or all teeth, failure of a tooth to erupt, resulting in swelling and possible discomfort, and worn crown surfaces. These conditions may impair adequate mastication.

Gums. The gums, or *gingivae*, are normally pink in color, attach to the teeth, and fill the interdental surfaces. If the person is edentulous, the gingivae are examined for areas of redness caused by improperly fitting dentures. The person is then asked to insert the dentures to assess correct fit and comfort for adequate mastication. Recession of the gum line is not uncommon in the older individual. Bleeding of the gums may occur with improper teeth brushing, dental calculus, oral infections, or blood dyscrasias. Painful gums may interfere with mastication.

Mucosa. A tongue blade is inserted between the

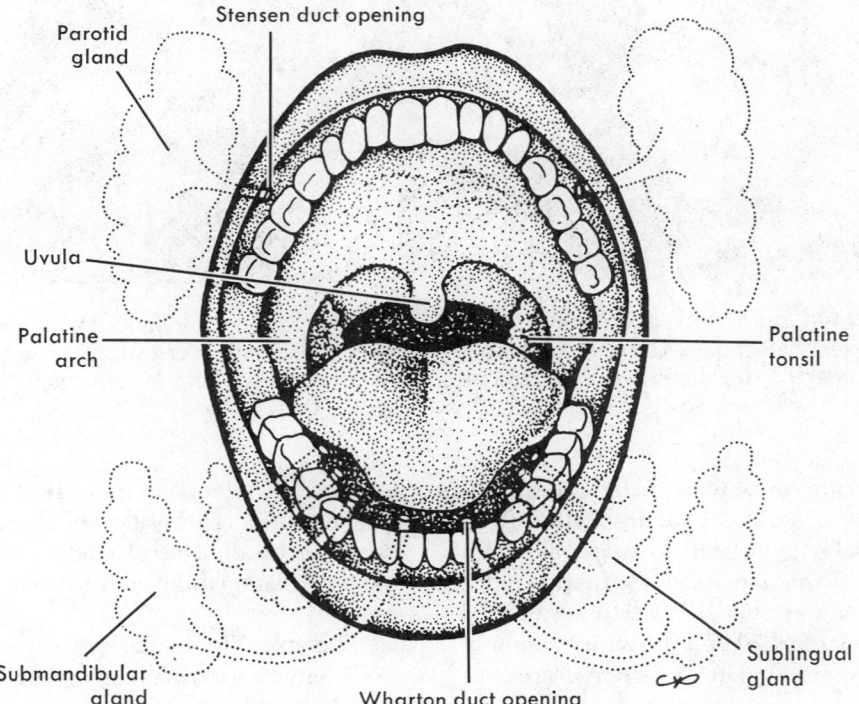

Fig. 54-2. Structures of mouth. (From Malasanos, L., et al.: Health assessment, ed. 2, St. Louis, 1981, The C.V. Mosby Co.)

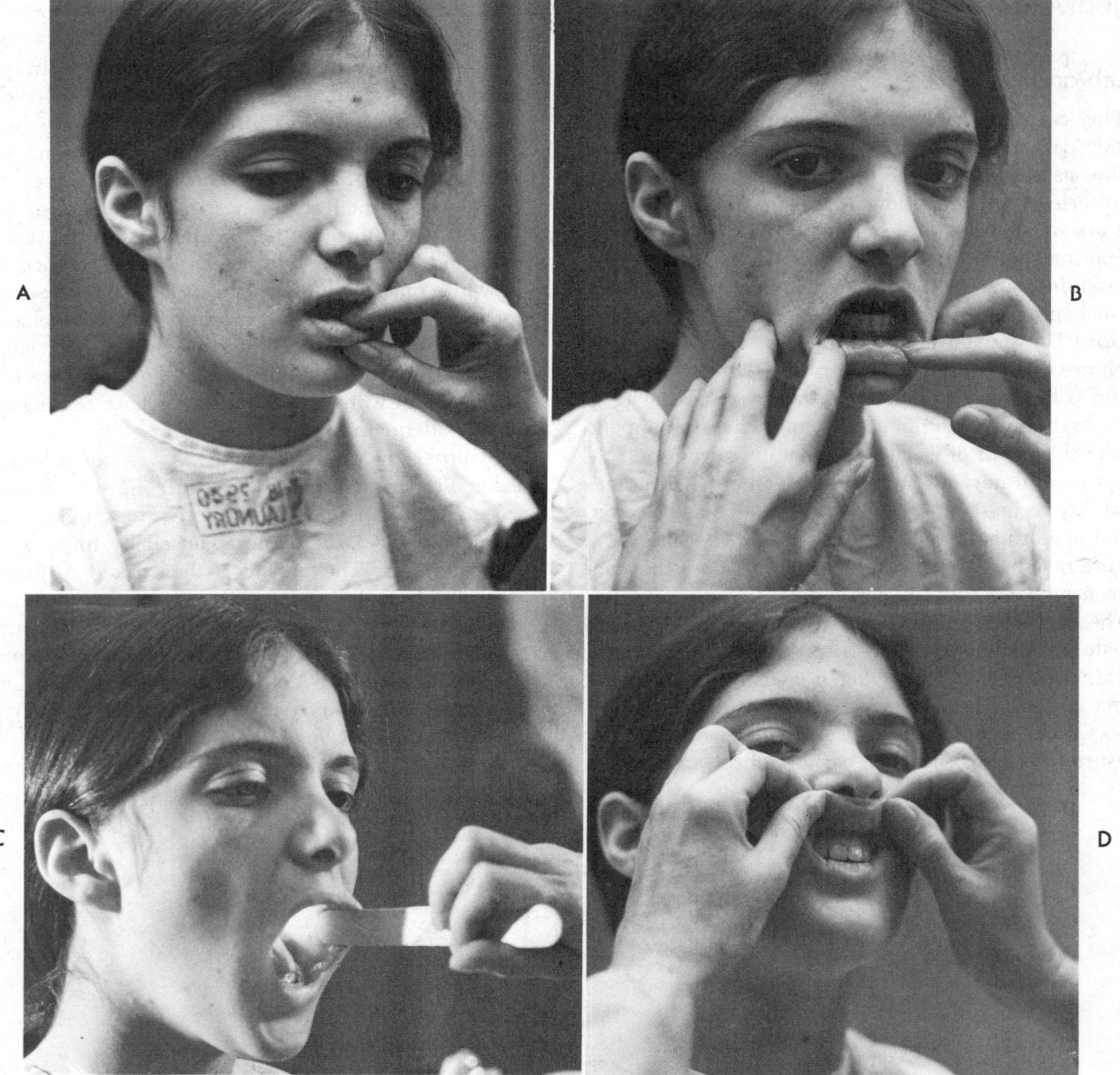

Fig. 54-3. Examination of lips and oral mucosa. **A,** Palpation of lips. **B,** Inspection of mucosa of lower anterior area. **C,** Inspection of mucosa of each cheek with identification of Stensen's duct opening. **D,** Inspection of mucosa of upper anterior area. (From Malasanos, L., et al.: Health assessment, ed. 2, St. Louis, 1981, The C.V. Mosby Co.)

cheek pockets and tooth surfaces, and the buccal mucosa is illuminated by a flashlight for inspection (Fig. 54-3, *C*). The mucosa is light pink in color, although patchy pigmentation is seen in blacks.[1] In the older person the mucosa may appear shiny as a result of a less vascular, thinner surface. The mucosa is examined for moisture, white spots or patches, debris, areas of bleeding, or ulcers. Dryness and debris may indicate dehydration. White curdy patches, which are removable with some effort, may be caused by *moniliasis* (thrush).[1] A round or oval white ulcer surrounded by

an area of redness is indicative of an *aphthous ulcer* (canker sore). The orifice of the parotid gland can be observed on the buccal mucosa near the upper second molar; inflammation of the parotid gland occurs with mumps.

Pharynx. The uvula, soft palate, tonsils, and posterior pharynx are usually observed at this time while the examiner still has the tongue blade. The middle of the tongue is pressed down firmly while the client says "Ah." This raises the soft palate, and symmetry should be noted (necessary for effective swallowing). The areas are examined for signs of inflammation (redness, edema, ulceration, thick yellowish secretions), and the size of the uvula is noted. A swollen uvula can cause pain and can limit swallowing. Changes in signs are reported to the physician.

Tongue. Tongue mobility and function are essential to mastication, taste, and swallowing. Inspection of the tongue is accomplished in two steps. First, the person is asked to protrude the tongue and rotate it in all four directions. Normally, there is no limitation in movement in any direction, but the tongue will deviate to the paralyzed side with paralysis of the twelfth cranial (hypoglossal) nerve. Second, the person is asked to protrude the tongue so that the dorsal surface can be observed and to elevate the tongue for inspection of the ventral surface and floor of the mouth. A thin white coating and the presence of large papillae on the dorsum are normal findings. A thick coating indicates poor oral hygiene, and a smooth red surface suggests a nutritional deficiency.[17] The ventral surface is examined for leukoplakia (a thickened white patch that is not removable), ulceration, or nodules, which may indicate malignancy.

Breath. Any distinctive odor of the breath is noted. A foul odor, *fetor oris*, may occur with poor oral hygiene or with dental or oral infections. Odors may occur after certain foods such as garlic or alcohol or with some systemic diseases (odor of acetone in diabetes, ammonia in liver disease).

Jaws

Examination for jaw articulation is generally performed last. The examiner places the fingertips of each hand at the angle of the temporomandibular joint (Fig. 54-4). The person is instructed to open and close the mouth slowly. Normally, the mandible may be felt to slide forward and down with ease. A normal sound of "cracking" may be heard when the person opens the mouth widely. Limitation of motion will affect mastication.

Stomach

Physical examination of the stomach is usually carried out in conjunction with assessment of the abdomen (p. 1435). Since most of the stomach lies beneath the ribs and liver, it is not usually palpable. Percussion is also of limited value. Pain elicited from palpation of the epigastric region may represent referred pain such as from acute appendicitis or hiatal hernia.

Diagnostic tests

Many of the examinations and tests performed for diagnosis of problems of the upper gastrointestinal system are both time consuming and vaguely unpleasant.

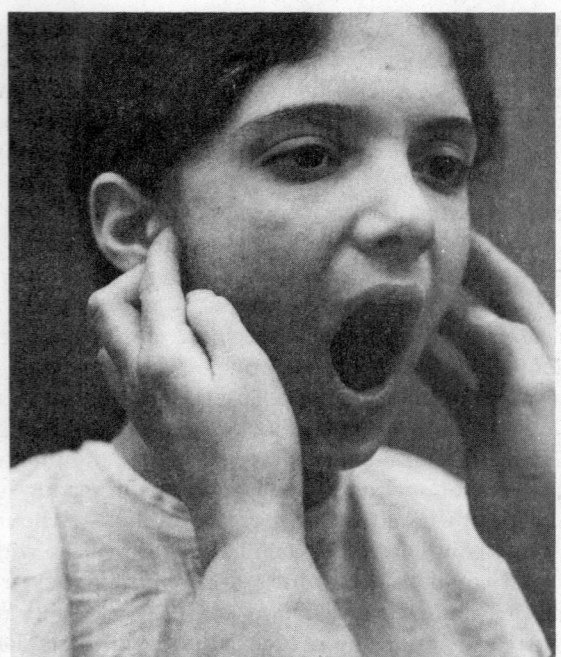

Fig. 54-4. Palpation of temporomandibular joint. (From Malasanos, L., et al.: Health assessment, ed. 2, St. Louis, 1981, The C.V. Mosby Co.)

Several of the tests are intrusive procedures and as such may present added stress for the individual and family.

The individual may already be physically debilitated because of poor nutritional intake and may be vomiting and experiencing acute or chronic pain. These data are utilized to plan for thorough and complete explanation of the tests and examinations to be done so that the patient or significant others may offer the optimal cooperation.

In many institutions the responsibility for explaining the procedures to the patient has been assumed by representatives from the radiology department or laboratory. Prepared literature that explains the procedures is also available for the patient and family. This approach, however, does not relieve the nurse from the responsibility of understanding the rationale and technique for each procedure, assessing the patient's understanding, and answering questions that the patient or family may have. The various tests and procedures are scheduled so that the time expended by the patient is best utilized; for example, a gastric analysis should be scheduled before a barium swallow, since the stomach must be empty for the gastric analysis.

The person's ability to tolerate discomfort before and during the examination is assessed. Narcotics and many sedatives will depress gastric emptying; therefore a notation to the radiologist or physician is made if these drugs are given before diagnostic tests of the stomach.

If the radiologist is aware that a narcotic has been given within 2 hours before the ingestion of barium, the decreased emptying time of the stomach would not necessarily be attributed to a definite pathologic problem. In this way inadvertent errors may be avoided as well as unnecessary repetition of time-consuming and expensive examinations.

Radiographic studies

Dental radiographs. Dental x-ray examinations are most frequently carried out as part of routine dental hygiene. The person needs no specific preparation for the examination. Radiographs are taken either of all the teeth (full-mouth) or of specific teeth.

The results of dental radiographs show the integrity of the enamel surface as well as the root shadow and alignment of the individual teeth in the bony structure. The most common abnormalities include caries within the internal tooth structure, pulp abnormalities from infection, abnormal alignment of the tooth and root structure, and the presence of nonerupted teeth. Dental radiographs may also be done for the hospitalized patient to determine the possible cause for dental pain and before dental extractions.

Facial bone radiographs. Facial bone x-ray examinations are most commonly used to determine alignment of the bone structure when trauma has occurred. The radiographs will be done soon after the initial trauma. The patient is usually experiencing pain; therefore gentleness in movement, proper administration of analgesics, and monitoring for adequacy of airway are guidelines to be implemented in the nursing care.

Gastrointestinal series. A gastrointestinal series consists of several radiographs of the stomach and intestinal tract and is used to detect tumors, ulcerations, or inflammation of the stomach and duodenum and to reveal any abnormal anatomy or malposition of these organs. As the person swallows barium (a radiopaque substance), the radiologist makes a fluoroscopic examination and then takes radiographs of the stomach and the duodenum. Since the barium tastes like chalk, it is often flavored to make it more palatable. After the person has drunk the barium, he or she is asked to assume various positions on the x-ray table, and the table may be tilted so that the barium will outline the stomach wall and flow by gravity into the intestinal loops as the radiologist, using the fluoroscope, watches the television monitor and takes the radiographs. Successive films are taken as the barium moves into the areas to be observed or into the large bowel, thus completing the visualization of the upper gastrointestinal tract, the ileum, or the small intestine. If the person has a spastic duodenal bulb or increased peristalsis in the duodenal area, atropine may be administered before the radiograph to slow down the action of the small intestine, permitting better visualization of the area. This procedure is called hypotonic duodenography.

Explanation of the procedure is given to the person before a gastrointestinal series. No food or fluids are permitted for 6 to 8 hours before the examination since the food in the stomach prevents the barium from outlining all of the stomach wall, and the radiographs will be inconclusive and misleading. If the person eats, the radiographic examination is usually postponed until the next day. The person can be assured that the test will not cause discomfort and that food may be eaten when the series is completed; however, breakfast will probably be omitted and lunch may be delayed. After a gastrointestinal series, a cathartic may be ordered to speed the elimination of barium from the intestines to prevent a fecal impaction.

Angiography. Arterial roentgenographs are especially useful in localizing bleeding sites in acute upper gastrointestinal bleeding. A contrast medium is injected through an arterial catheter for better visualization of bleeding areas and for differentiation between normal and tumor vessels. Following the procedure the femoral insertion site is observed for signs of bleeding, and vital signs are taken at frequent intervals.

Endoscopy

The esophageal and gastric mucosa may be visualized directly through an endoscope. By means of endoscopy a disease process may be located and inspected and a specimen of tissue may be obtained for microscopic study. Gastroscopy is especially useful for identifying upper gastrointestinal bleeding and for differentiating benign ulcers from gastric malignancies.

The *fiberscope*, a type of gastroscope, has a shaft made of rubber or plastic that allows for flexibility and permits visualization of the greater curvature of the stomach, the antrum, the pylorus, and the duodenal bulb. Glass fibers incorporated into the shaft of the instrument transmit light to the mucosa and the image back to the examiner. Cameras may be attached for the purpose of taking pictures of abnormalities of the gastric mucosa during the examination (Fig. 54-5).

Preprocedure intervention. Explanations are given to the person before the procedure. Food and fluids are withheld for 6 to 8 hours before the examination so that the patient does not regurgitate as the instrument is passed through the mouth into the esophagus and so that the lining of the stomach is visible. Occasionally, an esophagoscopy or a gastroscopy must be performed as an emergency measure to remove a foreign object such as a bone or a pin. In such an emergency the stomach cannot be emptied, but suction should be available for use to prevent aspiration of regurgitated food or fluid.

Eyeglasses and dentures are removed to prevent their being broken. The patient should void before the examination to prevent discomfort or embarrassment. Pajama bottoms may be worn to prevent inadvertent ex-

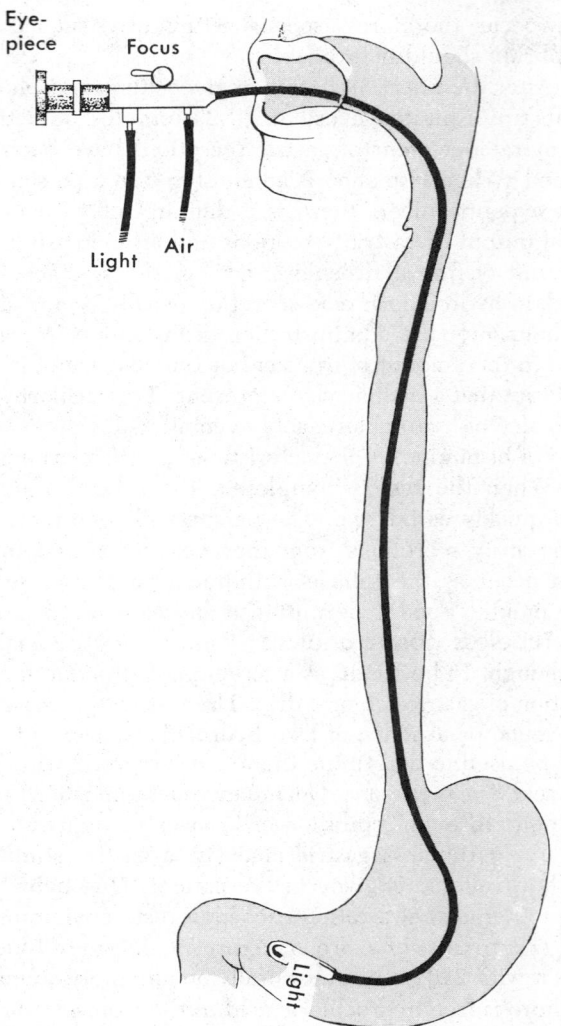

Eye-piece

Focus

Light   Air

Light

Fig. 54-5. Interior of stomach may be visualized by means of fiberscope.

posure during the procedure. The patient's written permission is obtained before this examination is performed.

Meperidine or diazepam (Valium) may be given by injection 30 minutes before the examination or at the time of the examination to lessen apprehension and to decrease awareness of the passage of the instrument. Although these procedures are not actually painful, a feeling of pressure and discomfort may be experienced in addition to exhaustion. To decrease secretions, atropine sulfate may be administered.

Procedure. Cooperation of the patient facilitates the procedure; therefore explanations are provided both before and during the examination. The patient is unable to speak and may be very frustrated by the inability to communicate. The gag reflex is inactivated by spraying the posterior pharynx with a local anesthetic

or by asking the patient to gargle with a solution containing the local anesthetic.

For passage of the fiberscope the patient sits or lies on the side of the bed or table facing the physician. The fiberscope is introduced through the mouth and advanced slowly through the esophagus to the stomach. Air is insufflated through the scope to permit better visualization of the mucosa. If tissue is removed for pathologic examinations, it is placed immediately into a specimen bottle and correctly labeled.

Postprocedure intervention. When the examination is finished, the patient is instructed not to eat or drink until the gag reflex returns, lest fluid be aspirated into the lungs. The gag reflex usually returns in 2 to 4 hours and can be tested for return by gently tickling the back of the throat with a tongue depressor.

Tests for malignancy

Exfoliative cytology. Exfoliative cytology is the study of the individual cells or clumps of cells to identify or to exclude the presence of malignancy. Because malignant cells tend to exfoliate (separate from the tumor), methods of accelerating exfoliation are used. This is accomplished by passing a Levin tube and lavaging the stomach vigorously with quantities of saline solution. *Chymotrypsin* may be administered to digest the overlying protective coat of mucus and thereby expose the mucosa to the irrigating solution. All the aspirated irrigating solution, cells, and bits of tissue obtained are sent to the laboratory for study.

Exfoliative cytology may also provide data concerning pernicious anemia, gastritis, and granulomatous diseases.[5] Barium may interfere with cell evaluation; therefore no barium studies using oral barium should be planned within 24 hours before exfoliative cytologic testing.

Biopsy. A biopsy of the oral cavity or tongue may be done on any lesion or ulcerated area that requires a differential diagnosis. This procedure is most generally carried out with the patient under local anesthesia. Following the biopsy the biopsy site is assessed for bleeding. Planned oral hygiene utilizing a neutral mouth wash solution is implemented at least every 4 hours until drainage from the site has ceased and at least three times a day thereafter. Biopsy of the stomach is performed during fiberoptic endoscopy.

Tests of gastric function

Gastric analysis (with histamine). Examination of the fasting contents of the stomach is helpful in establishing a diagnosis of gastric disease. For example, an unusual amount of gastric secretions containing food ingested the night before suggests pyloric obstruction. An absence of free hydrochloric acid in the stomach contents may indicate the presence of gastric malignancy or pernicious anemia, whereas an increased amount of free hydrochloric acid suggests a duodenal ulcer. In a gastric ulcer the amount of acid may be either decreased or normal in amount.

To obtain fasting stomach secretions, a nasogastric tube must be passed. The procedure must be explained to the patient, and food and fluids are withheld for 6 to 8 hours before the test is to be done. Anticholinergic drugs are omitted for 24 hours before the test. Smoking is prohibited the morning before the test, since smoking stimulates secretory action of gastric cells.

The procedure may be performed with the person seated comfortably in a secure chair and the head hyperextended for greater ease in inserting the tube. If the person is in bed, this position can be accomplished by raising the head of the bed to high Fowler's position and arranging pillows under the shoulders, allowing the head to rest on the mattress, The head is then slightly flexed to a more normal position as the person swallows the tube. The person's clothing or gown is protected, with a towel or plastic apron, and an emesis basin and paper tissues are provided.

A nasogastric tube (Levin no. 12, 14, or 16) is used. The tip of the tube is lubricated with a water-soluble lubricant and inserted through the nose (or mouth) into the posterior pharynx. The person is asked to swallow hard and repeatedly, and sips of water may be given as the tube is advanced quickly into the stomach. A syringe is then fitted onto the end of the tube, and all the stomach contents are aspirated and placed in a specimen bottle. The reactions of the aspirated secretions may be tested by using litmus paper. Blue litmus turns pink in the presence of acid. The tube is then secured to the nose and to the forehead with adhesive tape. Care should be taken that the tube does not pull or press against the nostril or cross in front of the eye. The end of the tube is closed with a clamp or with an elastic band to prevent leaking. Most patients are inclined to hold themselves very rigid while the tube is in the stomach, and they may be afraid to move. They are encouraged to assume any position that is most comfortable and instructed to expectorate saliva because it may act as a buffer and invalidate the examination.

After a fasting specimen has been collected, betazole hydrochloride (Histalog) or histamine phosphate is given subcutaneously. *Histamine is not given to persons with a history of allergy*. A skin test is carried out before the test is initiated if histamine is to be given. Betazole hydrochloride produces fewer side effects than histamine and is the preferred method. Pulse and blood pressure are taken immediately after drug administration; normally the pulse is increased and the blood pressure is slightly lowered.[9] Persons having a gastric analysis are told that they will look and feel flushed and warm and that they may develop headaches. These symptoms are caused by the vasodilating effects of histamine and will subside fairly rapidly. Vasogenic shock

may occur; therefore vasoconstricting drugs such as epinephrine should be available.

After the injection has been given, the stomach contents are aspirated every 10 to 20 minutes until three or more specimens of gastric secretions have been obtained. When histamine is administered to a person who has a peptic ulcer, there is a definite increase in the total output of gastric secretions and an increase in the amount of free hydrochloric acid in the stomach. The peak in hydrochloric acid secretion usually occurs about ½ hour after the administration of histamine. A reduction in the amount of free acid or the absence of it may indicate that a malignancy is present. True achlorhydria (absence of hydrochloric acid even after the administration of histamine) is characteristic of pernicious anemia.

When the test is completed, the tube is clamped and quickly withdrawn. The person will need tissues to wipe away secretions from the eyes, nose, and throat that occur as the tube is withdrawn, and to rinse out the mouth. Food is permitted if nausea is not present.

Tubeless gastric analysis. Tubeless gastric analysis is thought to be useful as a screening technique for detection of gastric achlorhydria. The test will indicate the presence or absence of free hydrochloric acid but cannot be used to determine the *amount* of free hydrochloric acid if it is present. Quantitative determinations must be done through aspiration of stomach contents.

For a tubeless gastric analysis, a gastric stimulant such as caffeine is given to the patient. One hour later 2 g (30 grains) of a cation exchange resin containing 90 mg (1½ grains) of azure A (Azuresin, Diagnex Blue) is given with 240 ml of water orally on an empty stomach. If there is free hydrochloric acid in the stomach, on the introduction of this resin a substance will be released in the stomach that will be absorbed from the small intestine and excreted by the kidneys within 2 hours. Absence of detectable amounts of dye in the urine indicates that free hydrochloric acid probably was not secreted.

Insulin tolerance test. An insulin tolerance test is another test used to evaluate the secreting action of the gastric mucosa. The test is carried out in the same way as a gastric analysis, except that instead of histamine a specified amount of regular insulin is administered intravenously. The drop in blood sugar produced by the insulin stimulates the vagus nerve, and the flow of gastric secretions may be increased. A normal stomach responds only slightly to stimulation of the vagus nerve, and there will be no significant increase in the gastric secretions. In the patient with a peptic ulcer, however, there will be a marked increase in the total gastric output and in the amount of free hydrochloric acid. The insulin tolerance test may be used to determine the success of a resection of the vagus nerve in decreasing the hyperactivity of the stomach. It is therefore often performed before and after vagotomy. In the event that symptoms of insulin reaction appear, orange or other fruit juice should be available as well as 50% glucose for intravenous injection.

REFERENCES AND SELECTED READINGS
Contemporary

1. *Bates, B.: A guide to physical examination, ed. 2, Philadelphia, 1979, J.B. Lippincott Co.
2. Bockus, H.L.: Gastroenterology, ed. 3, vol. 1, Philadelphia, 1974, W.B. Saunders Co.
3. Davidsohn, I., and Henry, J.B.: Todd-Sanford clinical diagnosis by laboratory methods, ed. 16, Philadelphia, 1979, W.B. Saunders Co.
4. DeGowin, E., and DeGowin, R.: Bedside diagnostic examination, ed. 3, London, 1976, Macmillan Publishing Co., Inc.

---

*References preceded by an asterisk are particularly well suited for student reading.

5. Fischbach, F.T.: A manual of laboratory diagnostic tests, Philadelphia, 1980, J.B. Lippincott Co.
6. French, R.: Guide to diagnostic procedures, ed. 5, New York, 1980, McGraw-Hill Book Co.
7. *Given, R., and Simmons, S.: Gastroenterology in clinical nursing, ed. 3, St. Louis, 1979, The C.V. Mosby Co.
8. Guyton, A.: Textbook of medical physiology, ed. 6, Philadelphia, 1981, W.B. Saunders Co.
9. Hahn, A.B., Barkin, R.L., and Oestreich, S.J.K.: Pharmacology in nursing, ed. 15, St. Louis, 1982, The C.V. Mosby Co.
10. Krupp, M., and Chatton, M.: Current medical diagnosis and treatment, Los Altos, Calif., 1980, Lange Medical Publications, Inc.
11. *Malasanos, L., et al.: Health assessment, ed. 2, St. Louis, 1981, The C.V. Mosby Co.
12. Sleisinger, M., and Fordtram, J.: Gastrointestinal disease: pathophysiology, diagnosis, management, ed. 2, Philadelphia, 1978, W.B. Saunders Co.
13. Sodeman, W., and Sodeman, W.: Pathologic physiology, ed. 6, Philadelphia, 1979, W.B. Saunders Co.
14. Spiro, H.M.: Clinical gastroenterology, New York, 1970, Macmillan Publishing Co., Inc.
15. Sweiger, J.L., Lang, J.W., and Sweiger, J.W.: Oral assessment: how to do it, Am. J. Nurs. **80:**654-657, 1980.
16. Thompson, J.M., and Bowers, A.C.: Clinical manual of health assessment, St. Louis, 1980, The C.V. Mosby Co.

Classic

17. Judge, R., and Zuidema, G.: Physical diagnosis: a physiological approach to the clinical examination, ed. 2, Boston, 1963, Little, Brown & Co.

CHAPTER 55

INTERVENTION FOR THE PERSON WITH DIGESTIVE DISORDERS

BARBARA C. LONG

Disorders of the upper gastrointestinal tract interfere in some manner and to some degree with the normal maintenance of gastrointestinal function and hence the nutritional status of the individual. Teeth that are in poor condition can interfere with chewing, the first step in the digestive process. Complaints of difficulty in swallowing (dysphagia), heartburn, and nausea and vomiting are common and numerous. People often turn to the nurse for assistance in coping with these discomforts. Changes in gastrointestinal tract functioning can affect absorption of medications as well as food.

Persons who have upper gastrointestinal disturbances often require nasogastric intubation for gastric decompression or tube feedings. A gastrostomy tube inserted directly into the stomach may also be used for tube feedings. Surgery may be performed for numerous reasons on the esophagus, stomach, and upper small intestine where digestion and absorption of nutrients occur. Interventions for persons with these conditions or undergoing these procedures are discussed in this chapter. Interventions for persons with specific pathophysiologic conditions of the upper gastrointestinal tract are discussed in Chapter 56.

Dental care

Teaching about care of the teeth is an important part of health education because of the relationship between nutrition and dental care. Poor dental hygiene influences the adequacy of nutritional intake; nutri-

tion, on the other hand, affects the growth and quality of teeth.

Dietary influences on teeth

Foods supply the calcium, protein, and vitamin D needed for tooth development. There is no evidence that calcium is removed from the mother's teeth during pregnancy and lactation regardless of how deficient in calcium her diet may be. There is, however, abundant evidence that a diet adequate in calcium, phosphorus, and other essential elements during pregnancy contributes to good tooth formation in the growing fetus and that a diet rich in these substances is essential during the years of life when the permanent teeth are being formed. Calcium is deposited in the buds of the permanent teeth almost immediately after birth. A high-calcium diet after teeth have erupted probably has no effect on their preservation.

A major influence on the development of dental caries is the consumption of refined carbohydrates, particularly sucrose. The frequency of ingestion of refined carbohydrate foods is more important than the amount consumed. Between-meal snacks of sucrose-containing foods, especially those that remain in the mouth for periods of time, such as sticky candies, sugar-containing chewing gum, and lollipops, are especially injurious to the teeth. The European custom of ending the meal with fresh fruit is an excellent one, since fresh fruit sugars and unrefined starches contain properties that inhibit bacterial enzyme action in the mouth. In fact, eating a raw apple before retiring is an excellent way to clean one's teeth.

Fluoridation

The use of fluoride has been shown conclusively to increase resistance of tooth enamel to bacterial action during the formative period of tooth growth in children. Fluoride may be added to drinking water, given by tablet, mixed in toothpaste, or applied topically to the teeth. Most urban communities in the United States fluoridate their water supplies. In areas where well water is used, fluoride should be taken in tablet form. The optimal dosage is 0.5 mg/day from birth to 3 years and 1 mg/day after 3 years of age. Use of fluoridated toothpaste is highly recommended by the American Dental Association. Local application is less effective and more expensive than fluoridation of water. Some dentists recommend the local application of fluoride to the teeth in addition to the systemic ingestion of fluoride as an extra protection against the development of caries.

Dental hygiene

Brushing the teeth or even rinsing the mouth with plain water immediately after ingestion of refined carbohydrate foods helps prevent decay. The times when most people brush their teeth are entirely wrong from the standpoint of prevention of dental caries. It is during the first half hour after eating refined carbohydrate that the most harm is done. Immediate rinsing of the mouth with plain water is more helpful than is thorough brushing of the teeth hours afterward when the bacterial damage has been done.

Brushing the teeth at least once a day is the most effective means of controlling the formation of plaque. *Bacterial plaque* is a soft, white mucoid material derived from the breakdown of saliva. Toxin-producing bacteria thrive in its matrix. Their enzymes and other products accumulate within the sulcus (crevice between the gingiva and the crown), causing inflammation and bleeding. Plaque that remains on the teeth for longer than 24 hours begins to mineralize or calcify, forming a hard, tenacious deposit known as calculus (tartar). Calculus has a consistency similar to sandpaper and causes abrasions and ulceration of the internal sulcus. It also has toxin-producing action.

Toothbrushes

Toothbrushes should be small enough to reach all tooth surfaces and should have soft bristles that conform to the tooth surface for effective cleansing. The electric-powered toothbrush is easy to use and safe to operate. Its use may encourage children to brush their teeth more often and may help incapacitated persons to clean their teeth more thoroughly. The individual, detachable brushes make it convenient for use in a family or hospital unit.

Dentifrices

Stannous fluoride has been officially recognized by the Council of Dental Therapeutics of the American Dental Association as an effective ingredient in dentifrices for the prevention of dental caries. Ammoniated dentifrices and those containing chlorophyll have been subject to much inquiry, but the results have been inconclusive or contradictory.

Mouth washes do not significantly inhibit bacterial growth in the mouth. They should not be used in an effort to treat an oral infection because they may be irritating to an infected mouth, and if used excessively they may be harmful to natural bacterial flora in the mouth. For the most part, however, they are harmless and are acceptable additions to oral hygiene if desired by the person. Most dentists suggest warm water and salt to rinse the mouth if occasional bleeding of the gums occurs.

Methods of cleansing teeth

Brushing the teeth should remove debris from between the teeth, stimulate the gums, and yet not traumatize the delicate gingival papillae between the teeth. Many people brush their teeth by passing the bristles quickly across the lateral surfaces of the teeth. This method damages the enamel, does not clean between the teeth, and may injure the gums. The brush should be placed along the gum line with the bristles toward the roots of the teeth. The bristles should then be brought down over the gum and teeth with a gentle sweep, using a downward and upward motion (Fig. 55-1). Although using a longer stroke is easier, it has a higher potential for traumatizing the gingiva or abrad-

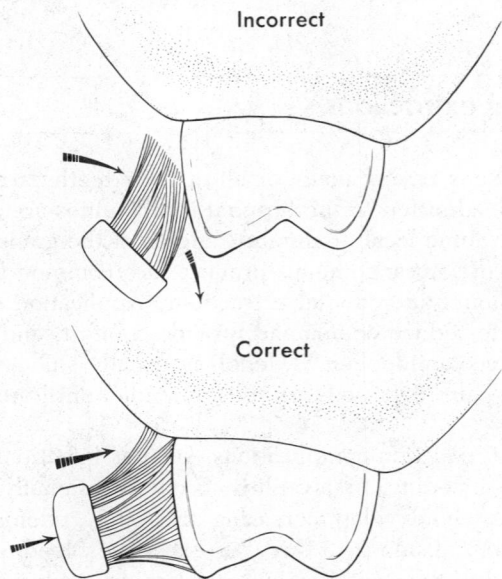

Fig. 55-1. Brushing teeth. Application of brush so that bristle ends slide gently under margin of gingiva.

ing tooth structure. Also, long strokes will generally pass over irregularly aligned teeth without cleansing adequately. Short strokes, on the other hand, may be more difficult for some patients to perform, since they require fine movements and coordination. They are more efficient in the cleansing process because the bristles bend or flex into malaligned or depressed areas. Crosswise motion should be reserved for the top grinding surfaces of the back teeth.

A toothbrush will cleanse most surfaces of the teeth adequately except the proximal surface (near the gum line). For cleaning this area dentists suggest the use of rubber tips, floss, and water irrigation. The *rubber tip* not only removes plaque from the proximal surface of the teeth but also massages as it cleans. It is used in every interdental space where there is room for it and inserted as far into the space as it will go without force. As the tip rests on the interdental tissue, the tip is activated in a gentle rotary motion so it rubs against the gingiva and proximal surfaces of the teeth.

Dental floss is highly recommended for cleaning plaque from interdental spaces. Unwaxed floss is preferable since it conforms well to crevice areas and does not leave wax on tooth surfaces. No matter how well instructed, when persons first use floss they tend to injure the gingiva as they pass the floss through tight contact areas. The tooth surface is cleansed by gently forcing the floss between the teeth with pressure exerted toward the side of the tooth and by moving the floss up and down the tooth surface for several seconds (Fig. 55-2). *Water irrigation* by means of the Water Pik is a useful and recommended aid. It acts by flushing away the plaque, food, and debris that has been loosened by the brush, rubber tip, or floss. Meticulous dental hygiene care should be maintained during orthodontic therapy.

Dental extractions

Persons having many or all of their teeth extracted may be admitted to the hospital if difficulties are anticipated. Some local discomfort, edema of the gums, and oozing of serosanguineous drainage are common for 24 to 48 hours after dental extractions. Application of ice will help reduce edema and provide comfort, and aspirin or acetaminophen (Tylenol) is usually sufficient to reduce pain. Soft foods are recommended until the gum heals.

Postextraction complications, such as infections, excessive bleeding, or alveolitis, occur occasionally, and patients who develop increasing discomfort, edema that does not subside in 3 days, or excessive bleeding are referred to the dentist. Alveolitis, or "dry socket," may occur particularly with removal of the third molar and is characterized by pain that is referred to the ear and

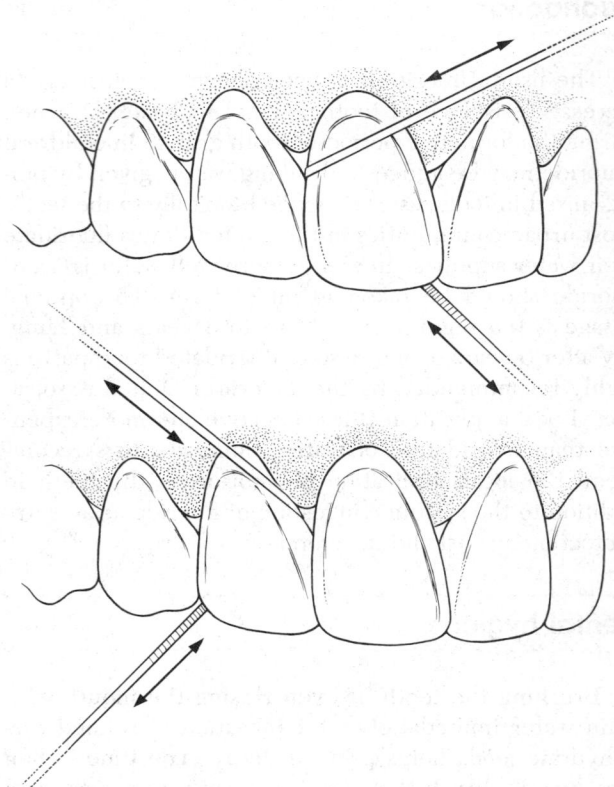

Fig. 55-2. Flossing. Proper placement of floss for effective interproximal cleaning.

that persists for several days. Treatment consists of packing the socket daily with gauze impregnated with a topical analgesic. If stitches are present, they are removed in 5 days.

Dental prostheses (dentures)

Partial dentures are important when several teeth are removed, since shifting of existing teeth leads to malocclusion. Complete dentures are necessary when all teeth are removed, not only for the esthetic effect, but also for ease in eating and speaking and for maintaining the maxillary-mandibular relationship.

Many people resist wearing complete dentures because of difficulties with adaptation. A young person may adapt to dentures within 10 days, but an older person may need 2 to 3 months to learn to adapt fully and comfortably. The tongue initially makes the dentures feel larger than they are, but this feeling subsides quickly. Adaptation to speech occurs more readily than to eating. The person can facilitate clearer speech by reading aloud and avoiding initially those words that are difficult to pronounce. Adapting to eating requires patience and persistence. The person begins with liquid or soft foods and then progresses to finely chopped foods before attempting more solid foods. Small frequent meals and small bites of food will facilitate learning to eat with

DENTURE CARE

1. Pad surface of sink or basin with washcloth (to prevent breakage if denture slips)
2. Brush denture with one of the following:
   a. Dentifrice
   b. Sodium bicarbonate in water
   c. Mild soap, such as Ivory
3. Rinse well under running warm water
4. Use one of the following immersion cleaners occasionally:
   a. Commercial preparation
   b. White vinegar, 1 tbsp in glass of water
   c. Bleach, 1 tbsp, and Calgon detergent, 2 tbsp, in glass of water

the new dentures. The person should chew slowly and deliberately and avoid foods that are sticky or fibrous or that have small seeds. An increase in salivation will be noted initially because of the presence of the teeth, perceived as "foreign objects," but salivation will return to normal with adaptation.

Insertion and removal of dentures. The tissue surfaces must be clean and moist for adherence of the denture. The upper (maxillary) dentures are inserted in an upward and backward movement and then pressed in place either by pressing with the thumb on the center of the palate or with both thumbs over the first molar. The lower (mandibular) dentures are pressed down and back by pressure of the index fingers over the first molars. The dentures are removed by sliding the tip of the index finger distally along the buccal surface with the mouth partially closed and then pulling the maxillary denture down and forward or the mandibular denture up in a rotating manner.

Preventive care. Dentures are cleaned after meals and after removal at night (see box above). Dentures require healthy supporting tissue for stability and retention and for comfort. The gums can be strengthened through stimulation by rubbing with the fingers, tongue, or soft toothbrush or by rinsing with alternating hot and cold liquids. Comfort can be facilitated by (1) rinsing the gums with warm isotonic solution, (2) removing the dentures daily (usually at night) to provide a rest period, and (3) correcting any broken or misfitting dentures. The gums gradually degenerate with aging as the tissue gets thinner and less keratinized. This leads to improper fitting, which requires new dentures, and to increased susceptibility to trauma and disease. The person needs to see the dentist for pain or difficulty with insertion or eating, presence of a persistent lesion, difficulty with denture retention, or broken dentures.

Outcome criteria for the person with a full-mouth extraction

The person or significant others can:
1. Demonstrate good mouth care.
2. Demonstrate proper technique for brushing artificial dentures.
3. Demonstrate proper techniques for cleansing the gums.
4. Describe the importance of removing food particles from the dentures at least twice a day.
5. Determine which dentifrice, soaking solution, or adhesive is most acceptable for personal needs.
6. State a specific plan for dental follow-up:
   a. State where dental services will be obtained.
   b. State situations under which the fit of the prosthesis may need to be adjusted (weight gain or loss, pain or tenderness in the gum area, slippage of the plate).

Dysphagia

Some persons have problems ingesting necessary nutrients because of difficulty in swallowing (*dysphagia*). If the person is unable to swallow, placement of liquids or solids in the posterior part of the throat may cause choking and aspiration of substances into the lungs. The underlying cause of the dysphagia influences the person's ability to swallow either solids or liquids or both.

Assessment

A person who gives a history of difficulty swallowing is questioned concerning the nature and circumstances of the dysphagia:

Is there greater dysphagia with liquids or with solids?
Is dysphagia intermittent or does it occur each time swallowing is attempted?
Are there other associated symptoms, such as pain with swallowing?
What approaches to eating has the client found most useful?

If dysphagia is suspected, a physical assessment is made of the person's ability to swallow. The mouth is observed for signs of drooling, as occurs with facial paralysis seen in the patient with a cerebrovascular accident or with Bell's palsy. The gag reflex is elicited by touching the posterior tongue or pharynx with a tongue blade. The person is asked to swallow and movement of the larynx is observed. A finger can be placed lightly over the larynx to facilitate detection of movement. If movement is limited and the gag reflex weak, a further assessment is made by placing 1 to 2 ml of water in the oropharynx and asking the patient to swallow.

Intervention for specific types of dysphagia

Dysphagia may result from interference with swallowing at the different phases of deglutition: the voluntary, pharyngeal, and esophageal phases.

Voluntary phase. In some situations, such as with upper motor neuron lesions (p. 762), the patient has the ability to swallow but has difficulty initiating and carrying out the function of swallowing. The patient may chew a mouthful for a period of time and then accept a second mouthful, unaware that swallowing has not occurred. Considerable amounts of food can collect between the cheek and gums. The patient may need direction to close the mouth when swallowing since it is difficult to swallow with an open mouth. Directions must be kept simple and extraneous conversation omitted so that the person can concentrate on swallowing.

Pharyngeal phase. Dysphagia resulting from interference with the pharyngeal phase of deglutition usually occurs with neuromuscular or neurologic disorders such as (1) diseases or trauma of cranial nerves V, IX, or X; (2) diseases that can affect the swallowing center in the brain, such as poliomyelitis and other CNS lesions; (3) diseases affecting neuromuscular transmission, such as myasthenia gravis and botulism; and (4) diseases affecting the striated muscle itself, such as myotonic dystrophy and polymyositis. Muscles may be severely weakened, resulting in difficulty moving the food from the oropharynx into the esophagus. Some function may be present so that swallowing can occur with difficulty.

Pharyngeal dysphagia is associated with immediate regurgitation.[3] *Fluids* are more difficult to swallow than soft foods, and there may be regurgitation of fluids through the nasal passages. Aspiration of feedings may occur from failure of the glottis to close. The patient must be closely supervised and suction equipment should be available for use with the severely dysphagic patient. A feeding syringe may be helpful when facial paralysis is present. The position of choice is the head-elevated position; if this is impossible, the patient is positioned on the *unaffected* side during feeding to ensure better control. If the ability to swallow is absent, tube feedings are usually instituted.

Esophageal phase. Dysphagia resulting from interference with the esophageal phase of deglutition may be either obstructive or motor in origin. *Obstruction* of the esophagus causes a decrease in the esphageal lumen and may be caused by (1) mechanical compression, such as that resulting from an enlarged thyroid or aneurysm, or (2) internal narrowing resulting from cancer of the esophagus, benign peptic stricture, narrowed lower esophageal ring, birth defects, or trauma causing esophageal strictures. Persons with obstructive lesions experience dysphagia primarily with *solids,* especially meat. If the dysphagia is mild, cutting solids into very small bites facilitates passage of the food. Some persons can take nutrients only in liquid form.

Esophageal dysphagia of *motor* origin results from involvement of the smooth muscles of the esophagus causing decreased esophageal peristaltic waves and an incompetent lower esophageal sphincter. This type of dysphagia is seen in persons with achalasia (p. 1412), esophageal spasm, and scleroderma. Difficulty in swallowing is experienced for both *solids* and *liquids*. Frequent small feedings are suggested. Some patients drink large amounts of fluid while swallowing solids to increase esophageal pressure, thus pushing the food into the stomach. Eating with the head elevated encourages movement of food through the esophagus by gravity. Regurgitation of food may occur several hours after eating, especially at night when the body is horizontal.

Psychologic dysphagia. Some persons may experience dysphagia without signs of organic lesions. This may occur with an anxiety or conversion reaction.[14] If the symptoms do not disappear after diagnostic workup, psychologic counseling may be indicated.

Common discomforts

Nausea and vomiting

Nausea and vomiting often are part of the body's response to insults to its integrity. They usually occur together, but occasionally, if the mechanism for vomiting is touched off by local pressure in the medulla, vomiting may be sudden and not preceded by nausea or any other warning sensation. Vomiting that occurs early in the morning may be related to pregnancy, metabolic states such as uremia, or chronic alcoholism.[3] Vomiting after meals is more likely associated with a gastric disturbance such as gastritis, food allergies, or food poisoning. Postoperative vomiting may occur at any time after surgery.

Pathophysiology

There are two centers in the medulla involved with vomiting: the chemoreceptor emetic trigger zone and the vomiting center. The *vomiting center* may be stimulated directly through the vagal or sympathetic nerves. Gastrointestinal irritants, distention or injury of any of the viscera, pain, and psychic trauma cause nausea and vomiting in this manner. Increased intracranial pressure may stimulate vomiting by direct local pressure. The vomiting center also may be stimulated indirectly through the *chemoreceptor emetic trigger zone*. Emetic agents such as morphine sulfate, meperidine hydrochloride (Demerol), ergot derivatives, digitalis preparations, and metabolic emetic substances resulting from uremia, infection, and radiation stimulate the chemoreceptor center to produce vomiting. Labyrinthine stimulation, the primary factor in the nausea and vomiting of motion sickness (seasickness, airsickness), is also believed to pass through the trigger center. It still is not clear by what route irritating gases such as those used in anesthesia affect the vomiting center or what specifically causes some women to vomit during the first trimester of pregnancy.

Nausea and vomiting are distressing to most people, but vomiting also can be a serious symptom. Prolonged and severe vomiting will interfere with nutrition and cause fluid and electrolyte imbalance, specifically dehydration and metabolic alkalosis with loss of potassium, chloride, and hydrogen ions (p. 356). The act of vomiting produces a strain on the abdominal muscles, and in some postoperative patients it may cause wound separation, wound dehiscence, or bleeding. Vomiting is especially dangerous for anesthetized patients, persons in coma, and infants because they are likely to aspirate the vomitus into the lungs. Aspiration may cause asphyxia, atelectasis, or pneumonitis, especially in the elderly person whose nasopharyngeal reflexes are less acute than those of a younger person.

Clinical picture

Persons who experience emesis on an empty stomach often vomit small amounts of gastric juices mixed with bitter-tasting, greenish yellow bile that has been forced back into the stomach. Retching, or "dry" emesis, may also occur. *Hematemesis* is the vomiting of blood. The color of the vomitus with hematemesis depends on the length of time that the blood has been in contact with gastric juices; thus bright red vomitus indicates overt bleeding of recent origin. It is important to ascertain whether the contents expelled from the mouth have been vomited from the stomach or coughed up from the lungs. Bloody sputum usually has a more frothy appearance than hematemesis. Blood that has been in the stomach for a period of time becomes partly digested by the gastric juices and has a dark brown "coffee-grounds" appearance. This blood may have originated in the stomach, or it may have been swallowed from the nose, mouth, or throat. Vomitus with a fecal odor indicates lower gastrointestinal obstruction.

Intervention

Treatment of nausea and vomiting depends on the cause. Medications or other substances known to cause nausea and vomiting are stopped, and fluid and electrolyte imbalances are treated. Most patients will have less vomiting if the emotional components of its cause are removed; therefore measures to reduce anxiety are instituted. Sedation may help to quiet the patient. Nausea and gagging sometimes are relieved by taking deep breaths through the mouth. Ginger ale and other effervescent drinks seem to have a remarkable effect in controlling postoperative nausea and vomiting and often can

be taken and retained long before other fluids are tolerated. Effervescent fluids also may be effective in controlling vomiting from other causes such as seasickness.

It must be recognized that certain odors or sights can cause the nurse to experience nausea while caring for a patient, especially one who is vomiting. The nurse's own sensations can be diminished by taking slow deep breaths through the mouth rather than the nose. Swallowing repeatedly helps to prevent gagging.

The patient's comfort is facilitated by keeping the emesis basin within easy reach, preferably out of sight, and emptying the basin immediately after vomiting has ceased. The person usually appreciates the opportunity to rinse the mouth after vomiting; a flavorful mouthwash is often preferred. The room is kept well ventilated since disagreeable odors can precipitate further emesis.

Antiemetic medications (Table 55-1) may be prescribed orally if the person is able to retain the tablets; in many instances, however, the medication must be given by rectal suppository or by *deep* intramuscular injection in order to be effective. Antihistamines such as dimenhydrinate (Dramamine), meclizine hydrochloride (Bonine), and trimethobenzamide hydrochloride (Tigan) are used widely in control of motion sickness such as is encountered in air and sea travel. These medications are effective prophylactically when taken about 30 minutes before the initial motion and then continued at regular intervals. They also are ordered with varying success in the nausea and vomiting associated with illness. Any of the antihistaminic drugs may cause drowsiness and dizziness, and the possibility of these reactions should be pointed out to persons who are taking them when traveling. They are especially dangerous to use when driving. Tigan and prochlorperazine (Compazine) are quite effective in controlling postoperative nausea and vomiting.

Very few antiemetics are significantly effective against nausea and vomiting induced by chemotherapeutic agents, although prochlorperazine (Compazine) does offer some relief. Recent interest has been shown in the use of delta-9-tetrahydrocannibol (THC), the active ingredient of marijuana. THC has more frequent central nervous system side effects than prochlorperazine, especially in the older population, but appears to be more effective in persons under 20 years of age.[24]

Heartburn

Heartburn is a common discomfort experienced either occasionally or frequently by some persons. It is caused by a reflux of acidic gastric contents back into the esophagus. If persistent, it can irritate the lower esophagus and lead to esophagitis.

TABLE 55-1. Antiemetic medications

Generic name	Trade name	Dosage	Usage for nausea and vomiting
Antihistamines			
Cyclizine hydrochloride	Marezine	50 mg	Motion sickness; postoperative nausea and vomiting
Dimenhydrinate	Dramamine	50 mg	Motion sickness
Hydroxyzine hydrochloride	Atarax, Vistaril	25-100 mg	Upper gastrointestinal disturbances; Meniere's syndrome; postoperative nausea and vomiting
Meclizine hydrochloride	Bonine, Antivert	25-50 mg	Motion sickness
Phenothiazines			
Chlorpromazine	Thorazine	10-25 mg	General use
Perphenazine	Trilafon	5 mg, IM	Severe nausea and vomiting
Prochlorperazine	Compazine	5-10 mg	General use
Promethazine hydrochloride	Phenergan, ZiPAN	12-25 mg	Motion sickness; postoperative nausea and vomiting
Triethylperazine	Torecan	10 mg	Postoperative
Triflupromazine hydrochloride	Vesprin	5-10 mg, IM	Severe nausea and vomiting
Miscellaneous			
Benzquinamide hydrochloride	Emete-Con	50 mg, IM	Postoperative nausea and vomiting
Buclizine hydrochloride	Bucladin-S	50-150 mg	Motion sickness; Meniere's syndrome
Doxylamine succinate and pyridoxine hydrochloride	Bendectin	2 tablets hs	Pregnancy
Diphenidol	Vontrol	20-50 mg	Labyrinthine disturbances
Trimethobenzamide hydrochloride	Tigan	200-250 mg	General use
Levulose, dextrose, and orthophosphoric acid	Emetrol	1-2 tbsp	Upper gastrointestinal disturbances; pregnancy; motion sickness

Pathophysiology

At the junction of the esophagus and stomach, the esophageal muscle encircling the esophagus is slightly hypertrophied and has a high resting wall tension as a result of its usual contracted state.[25] The muscle at this point is called the lower esophageal sphincter (LES). When food enters the pharynx and esophagus, the LES relaxes to permit the food to pass into the stomach. At all other times the LES is contracted to prevent reflux of gastric material back into the esophagus.

Some persons have an idiopathic incompetent LES; that is, the LES pressure is lower than it should be and reflux occurs. LES pressure is increased by gastrin release in the stomach and is decreased by secretin and cholecystokinin from the small intestine. Other substances that decrease LES pressure include anticholinergics, caffeine, theobromine, ethyl alcohol, and smoking. An incompetent LES may also occur with collagen vascular diseases associated with Raynaud's phenomenon.[3] Increased abdominal pressure may lead to reflux of gastric contents; thus heartburn may accompany pregnancy, ascites, or obesity. Reflux is more likely to occur when gravitational pull is decreased, such as when the person is lying down.

Clinical picture

Persons with heartburn experience a substernal "burning" sensation that may be referred to the neck or back if severe. It is frequently accompanied by a sour regurgitation of gastric contents into the mouth but is not accompanied by nausea.

An incompetent LES can be diagnosed by roentgenograms in Trendelenburg's position or by fluoroscopy. A water siphon test is a fluoroscopic examination in which barium is swallowed followed by plain water. If the LES is incompetent, the barium will be seen to reflux back into the esophagus. Overnight pH recordings measured from swallowed glass electrodes will demonstrate periods of increased gastric reflux.[3]

Intervention

Prevention is the best approach to the treatment of heartburn. The diet can be planned to include foods high in proteins, which stimulate gastrin release, and low in fats, which stimulate release of cholecystokinin. Foods containing caffeine (coffee, tea, colas), theobromine (chocolate), and alcohol should be avoided. Small frequent meals will prevent stomach distention and resulting gastric acid secretion.[34] Smoking should also be avoided.

To promote gravity drainage and thus prevent reflux, the person who is susceptible to heartburn should not lie down within 2 to 3 hours after eating and should avoid bending over. Raising the head of the bed on blocks about 15 cm (6 in.) is helpful. Avoidance of lifting and wearing tight belts or girdles following eating will help prevent increased abdominal pressure.

In the person with heartburn, acidity can be decreased by administration of 30 ml of a liquid antacid taken 1 hour after meals, at bedtime, and whenever heartburn occurs. Gaviscon, which is a mixture of antacids with alginic acid, was developed as a low-density x-ray contrast medium but has been found to be effective in alleviating heartburn. Two to four tablets, when *chewed* thoroughly and then swallowed, produce a viscous antacid foam that coats the esophagus and floats on the gastric contents. If antacids are not effective, medications that increase LES contraction may be prescribed; these include bethanechol chloride (Urecholine), 10 to 25 mg, or metoclopramide, 15 mg, to be taken 30 minutes before meals and at bedtime. Anticholinergic medications are avoided.

Effects of upper gastrointestinal changes on drug absorption

The presence or absence of food in the stomach can affect the absorption of medications taken by the oral route. Foods can interfere with drug absorption through changes in gastrointestinal motility and pH, through changes in ionization or solubility of the drug, or through interaction of a food component with the drug.

Drugs are absorbed more readily if the gastrointestinal tract is free of food. Drugs taken with water when the stomach is empty move rapidly into the small intestine, where much drug absorption takes place. Fatty foods delay gastric emptying for as much as 2 hours; therefore drugs that are absorbed in the small intestine have delayed absorption if taken with a meal high in fats. Whenever drug absorption is reduced by food, serum therapeutic levels of the drug may not be achieved, or there may be a sustained release, thus prolonging the drug effects. Food particularly delays the absorption of antimicrobial drugs, specifically the tetracyclines, the penicillins, and the sulfonamides. On the other hand, medications that have a gastric irritant effect may be enhanced if taken with food (see box above, at right).

Drugs that are normally slightly acidic, such as aspirin or barbiturates, usually ionize and are absorbed in the stomach. If the stomach pH is increased, such as by milk or antacids, the rate and extent of absorption of

---

MEDICATIONS TO BE TAKEN WITH FOOD

Aminophylline

Chlorothiazide (Diuril)

Ferrous sulfate

Indomethacin (Indocin)

Mitronidazole (Flagyl)

Nitrofurantoin (Macrodantin)

Phenylbutazone (Butazolidin)

Phenytoin (Dilantin)

Prednisolone

Reserpine (Serpasil)

Tramterene (Dyrenium)

---

these drugs will be decreased. Alteration in stomach acidity may also break down the protective coating of spansules or enteric-coated tablets, resulting in premature release of the contents.[5] Acid liquids, such as lemon, pineapple, or cranberry juices, or dry ginger ale may inactivate acid-unstable drugs such as ampicillin, penicillin G, cloxacillin, and erythromycin.

Food components can interact with oral medications by the chemical or physical binding of one substance on another (complexation), thus interfering with absorption of either the food component or the drug. Tetracycline becomes bound with calcium, aluminum, or magnesim ions when taken with milk or antacids, resulting in decreased absorption of tetracycline. Foods containing tyramine (cheeses, wines) may interact with monoamine oxidase (MAO) inhibitors, such as phenelzine (Nardil) or tranylcypromine (Parnate), which are depressants, causing hypertensive reactions.

Nasogastric intubation

Nasogastric tubes are inserted for (1) tests of gastric analysis (p. 1383), (2) tube feedings (p. 1373), (3) decompression of the stomach when gastric motility is severely decreased, and (4) removal of gastric contents following gastric hemorrhage or perforation.

One of the more common uses of nasogastric intubation is for decompression of the stomach following gastrointestinal surgery, since a marked decrease in gastrointestinal tract motility may occur fullowing manipulation of the viscera during abdominal surgery.

The nasogastric tube may be inserted before surgery

and removed after normal peristalsis returns (usually in 48 to 78 hours), or it may be inserted only if signs of distention occur after surgery. Tubes used in conjunction with gastric or esophageal surgery are carefully placed by the surgeon during surgery so that the tube does not intrude on the suture line. These tubes are not manipulated lest injury result. If there is some question about the tube's position or function, the surgeon should be consulted.

Nasogastric intubation is also used whenever there is cessation of peristalsis in the gastrointestinal tract (*ileus*), such as occurs with intestinal obstruction or peritonitis. The length of time that the tube remains in the stomach depends on the reason for its use and the physician's opinion of the physiologic effects of intubation on electrolyte balance and the psychologic effects on the patient.

Pathophysiology of ileus

When peristalsis ceases, the stomach or small intestine (depending on the site of obstruction) becomes distended by large quantities of fluids and gas. The se-

creted fluid has a high electrolyte content and is acid if in the stomach or alkaline if in the small intestine. Gas in the stomach results primarily from swallowed air. Gas in the small intestine may result from swallowed air or from gas that has diffused from blood vessels of the gastrointestinal tract. As the fluid and gas collect, the resulting distention causes edema of tissues of the gut wall with subsequent impairment of circulation and, if not removed, may cause rupture of the stomach or intestine. Shock occurs from excessive protein loss.

Nursing interventions

Prevention of injury. The purpose of continuous intubation is explained to both the patient and family to lessen apprehension and to prevent forceful removal of the tube with subsequent discomfort and possible injury to the mucosa. A Levin tube (Fig. 55-3) is most commonly used for continuous nasogastric intubation; however, because it is a single-lumen tube, damage to the mucosa may result even with intermittent suction. A less traumatic approach is the use of the double-lumen Salem sump tube (Fig. 55-4). The larger lumen

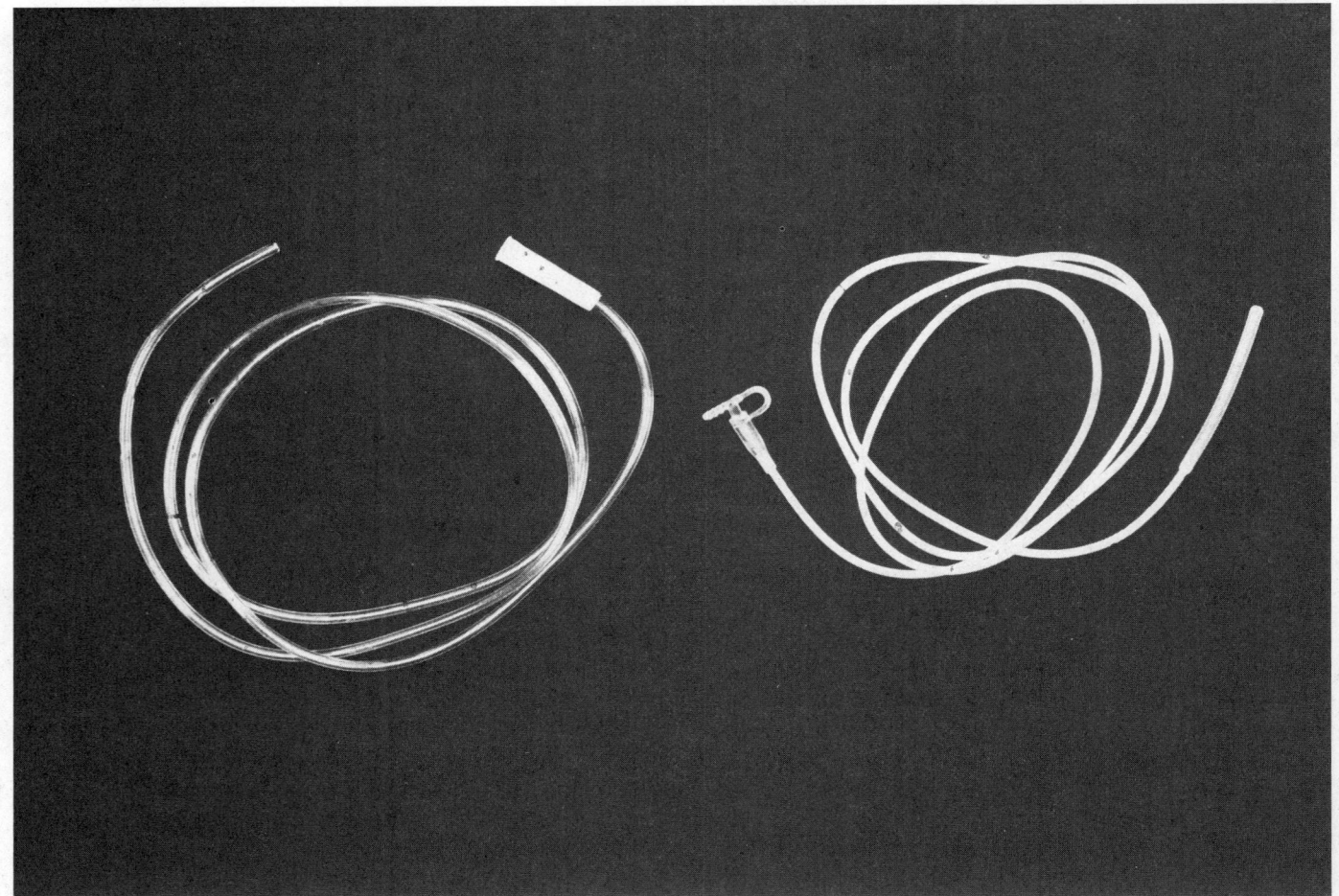

Fig. 55-3. A, Levin tube used for nasogastric intubation. **B,** Vivonex tube for nasogastric feeding.

drains the area while the smaller lumen provides a continuous flow of air at atmospheric pressure, thus maintaining the suction at a lower level and preventing tissue grab. The end of the smaller-lumen tube is positioned above the patient's midline to prevent gastric reflux.[26] (Passage of the nasogastric tube is described on p. 1384.) To prevent necrosis of the nares from constant pressure, the tube is taped securely so that it does not press against the nostril or obstruct vision. It is then pinned loosely to the clothing to support the weight of the tube and to permit free movement of the head.

Comfort measures. The presence of the tube in the nasopharynx causes local discomfort, and the patient may complain of a lump in the throat, difficulty in swallowing, sore throat, hoarseness, earache, or irritation of the nostril. Many patients report that discomfort from the tube far exceeds that from the incision. Excess secretions around the nares are removed, and a *water-soluble* lubricant, such as K-Y jelly, is applied to the tube and to the nostril to prevent crusting of secretions. Warm saline solution gargles may relieve dryness and soreness of the throat, and throat lozenges may be prescribed.

Phenylephrine (Neo-Synephrine), 0.25%, nose drops are sometimes helpful in relieving nasal stuffiness. Frequent changing of the patient's position helps to relieve pressure from the tube on any one area in the throat. Unless contraindicated, elevation of the bed to 30 degrees helps to prevent esophageal reflux and subsequent esophagitis.

When the tube is in the nostril, the patient tends to breathe through the mouth, and the lips, mouth, and tongue may become dry and cracked. *Good mouth care is essential* (for further information on mouth care, see p. 1405). Fluids are usually restricted, but the patient may chew gum or suck sour-ball candies to increase salivation. This helps maintain moisture of the mucous membrane and prevent infection of the parotid gland. Although ice chips are sometimes permitted, they should be used sparingly since large amounts may result in ingestion of a hypotonic solution that may increase electrolyte loss through gastric drainage.

Nasogastric tube suction. Nasogastric tubes for continuous intubation are attached to suction to ensure drainage, since the stomach contents must flow against

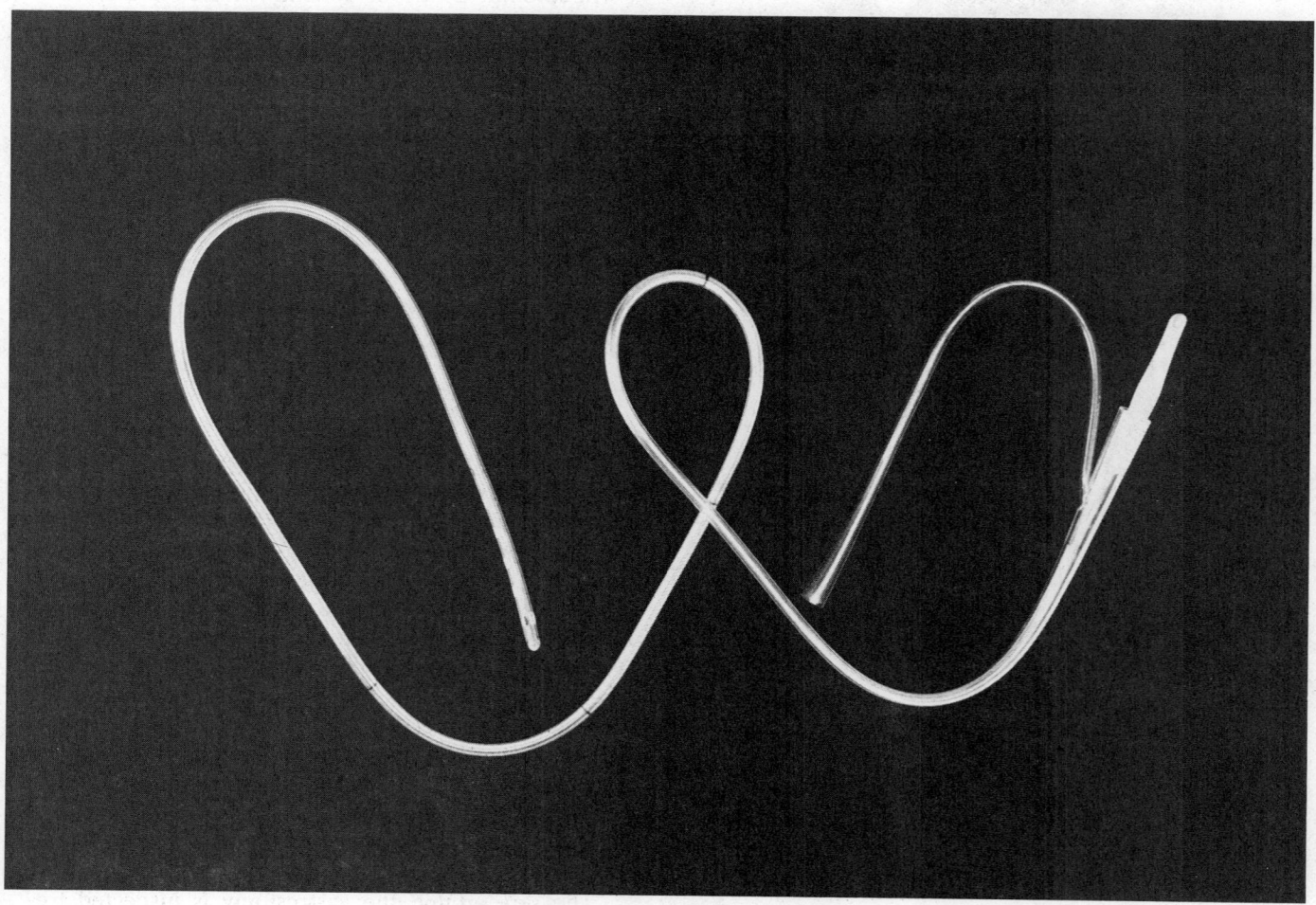

Fig. 55-4. Salem sump pump.

gravity. Intermittent suction at a low pressure setting is commonly ordered for Levin tubes, since constant suction could damage the mucosal wall if a section of the wall were to be pulled continually against the drainage holes of the gastric tube. Intermittent suction permits the wall to drop away from the tube during periods when suction is not occurring. The Salem sump pump may be used with intermittent suction set at high pressure or with continuous suction set at low pressure.[26]

The tubing from the suction apparatus (Fig. 55-5) is attached by a connecting tube to the nasogastric tube, permitting observation of the fluid being removed from the stomach. With intermittent suction, the fluid does not flow continuously. Mechanical failure of the suction apparatus or blockage of the drainage tubing or of the nasogastric tube itself may stop the suction, impeding drainage and causing distention, discomfort, and sometimes vomiting. The apparatus is checked frequently to minimize this possibility.

Irrigation of the nasogastric tube. The physician may wish the tube irrigated with small amounts (30 ml) of *normal saline solution* at specified intervals to keep the lumen of the tube open and free from mucus plugs or blood clots. Use of a hypotonic solution such as water would increase electrolyte loss through irrigation. After the fluid is inserted into the tube it should be aspirated if possible. Fluid that is instilled but not immediately withdrawn will be removed by suction. If the fluid does not flow easily into the tube or return by aspiration or suction, the sucking ports may be obstructed or the tube may be curled in the stomach. The tube can be rotated or pulled back 2 to 3 cm (1 to 1½ in.), or the patient may be asked to shift position to the opposite side. If the tubing remains blocked, the physician is consulted.

The Salem sump tube may be irrigated either through the smaller vent lumen without interrupting the suction or through the drainage lumen. When the irrigation by either lumen is completed, air is injected through the vent lumen during suction to ensure air patency.[26]

Recording. Gastric secretions collected in the drainage bottle are measured every 24 hours. The amount of fluid instilled by irrigation but not immediately withdrawn is subtracted from the 24-hour total in order to determine the actual amount of gastric secretion lost through drainage. The total amount of fluid and electrolytes lost through drainage must be replaced by parenteral routes.

Interventions for the person with a gastrostomy

Gastrostomy is an alternative approach to nasogastric tube feedings when the person is unable to swallow for a long period of time. The procedure is often performed under local anesthesia. A small incision is made in the left upper abdominal quadrant, and the stomach is exposed. A catheter is laid on and sutured to the exterior surface of the greater curvature of the stomach (Fig. 55-6). The tip of the anchored catheter is then inserted into the stomach and secured with purse-string sutures. The connecting end of the catheter is brought to the surface through either the incision or a separate stab wound. The main incision is closed and the catheter is sutured and taped to the skin.

Skin care

The skin around the gastrostomy is inspected frequently, because if leakage of gastric secretions around the tube occurs, the skin will become irritated and ex-

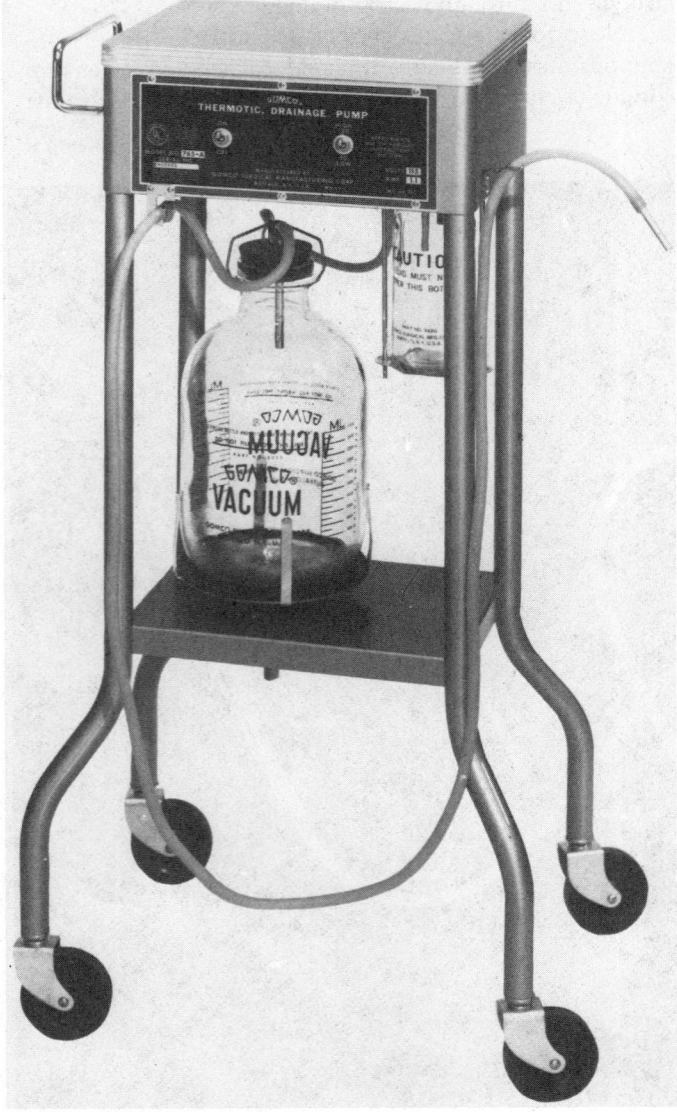

Fig. 55-5. Intermittent suction machine (Gomco). (Courtesy Chemetron Medical Products Co., St. Louis.)

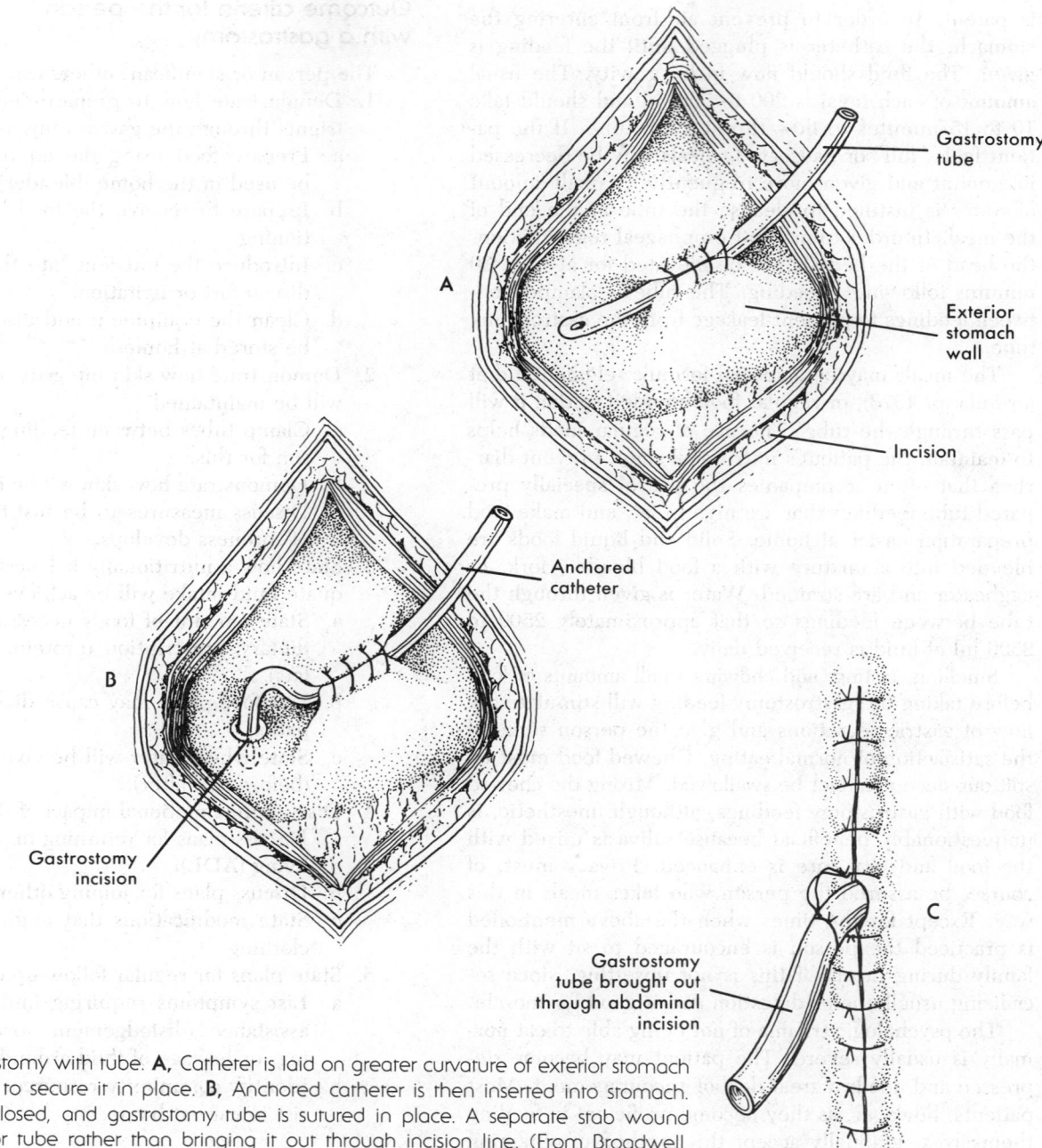

Fig. 55-6. Gastrostomy with tube. **A,** Catheter is laid on greater curvature of exterior stomach wall and sutured to secure it in place. **B,** Anchored catheter is then inserted into stomach. **C,** Abdomen is closed, and gastrostomy tube is sutured in place. A separate stab wound may be made for tube rather than bringing it out through incision line. (From Broadwell, D.C., and Jackson, B.L.: Principles of ostomy care, St. Louis, 1981, The C.V. Mosby Co.)

coriated from the action of the digestive enzymes. The skin is kept clean with frequent use of soap and water and is kept dry; a protective ointment such as zinc oxide or petrolatum gauze may be applied around the tube. After 10 to 14 days the tube may be removed and reinserted 10 to 15 cm (4 to 6 in.) only when food is given. The tube is kept clean by washing it with soap and water after each meal following removal.

Food and fluids

Following surgery the gastrostomy tube may be ordered attached to low intermittent suction for 24 hours, or fluids may be started the first day. The initial meal, consisting of a small amount of tap water or glucose in water, is given followed by fluids every 4 hours. If there is no leakage of fluid around the tube and if the patient appears to tolerate the clear fluids, foods blended into a mixture may be added until a full diet is eventually given through the tube. The meal is warmed to room or body temperature before it is given and is diluted if too thick.

A funnel is used to introduce the liquid into the catheter. Before the meal is given, a small amount of water is introduced through the tube to make sure it is patent. In order to prevent air from entering the stomach, the catheter is plugged until the feeding is given. The fluid should flow in by gravity. The usual amount of each meal is 200 to 500 ml and should take 10 to 15 minutes to flow through the tube. If the patient feels "full" or nauseated, meals may be decreased in amount and given more frequently. A small amount of water is instilled to cleanse the tube at the end of the meal. In order to prevent esophageal regurgitation, the head of the bed should be elevated for at least 30 minutes following a feeding. The tube is clamped between feedings to prevent leakage from the gastrostomy tube.

The meals may be a special formula, elemental diet formula (p. 1373), or regular food blended so that it will pass through the tube. The use of regular foods helps to maintain the patient's nutritional state, prevent diarrhea that often accompanies the use of specially prepared tube feedings that are high in fat, and make food preparation easier at home. Solid and liquid foods are blended into a mixture with a food blender, fork, or eggbeater and are strained. Water is given through the tube between feedings so that approximately 2500 to 3500 ml of fluid is received daily.

Smelling, tasting, and chewing small amounts of food before taking the gastrostomy feeding will stimulate the flow of gastric secretions and give the person some of the satisfaction of normal eating. Chewed food must be spit out since it cannot be swallowed. Mixing the chewed food with gastrostomy feedings, although unesthetic, is unquestionably beneficial because saliva is mixed with the food and oral care is enhanced. Privacy must, of course, be assured the person who takes meals in this way. Except for the times when the above mentioned is practiced the person is encouraged to sit with the family during meals, if this is not upsetting, since socializing usually helps digestion and is good for morale.

The psychologic trauma of not being able to eat normally is usually severe. The patient may become depressed and needs a great deal of encouragement. Most patients, however, as they become proficient in feeding themselves, gradually accept this method of obtaining nourishment as inevitable and adjust remarkably well.

Teaching

Both the patient and family should learn how to care for the skin and the tube and how to prepare the liquid meals as well as how to insert the tube and instill the nourishment through it. They should be told of the need for close medical supervision, and they should be encouraged to consult the physician, the nurse, or the dietitian when problems arise. It may be desirable for a community health nurse to visit the patient at home to supervise the initial preparation of food and giving of the feeding and to answer any other questions in regard to the patient's care.

Outcome criteria for the person with a gastrostomy

The person or significant others can:
1. Demonstrate how to prepare and introduce nutrients through the gastrostomy tube.
   a. Prepare food using the equipment that will be used in the home (blender).
   b. Prepare to receive the food by proper positioning.
   c. Introduce the nutrient into the tube without discomfort or irritation.
   d. Clean the equipment and discuss how it will be stored at home.
2. Demonstrate how skin integrity around the tube will be maintained.
   a. Clamp tubes between feedings and state reason for this.
   b. Demonstrate how skin wil be inspected daily.
   c. Discuss measures to be instituted if redness of soreness develops.
3. State how a nutritionally balanced diet and adequate fluid intake will be achieved.
   a. State amount of foods necessary to meet the dietary prescription (protein, carbohydrates, fats).
   b. List foods that may cause diarrhea or constipation.
   c. State when water will be given with feedings (before and after).
4. Discuss the emotional impact of the gastrostomy.
   a. Discuss plans for returning to activities of daily living (ADL).
   b. Discuss plans for joining others at mealtimes.
   c. State modifications that might be needed in clothing.
5. State plans for regular follow-up care.
   a. List symptoms requiring immediate medical assistance (dislodgement, occlusion, bleeding, or leakage of fluid around the opening).
   b. Identify community resources available to assist in care at home.

Interventions for the person with a cervical esophagostomy

An additional method for providing tube feedings in addition to nasogastric and gastrostomy approaches is a cervical esophagostomy, an artificial opening (stoma) directly into the esophagus at the neck. The benefits of cervical esophagostomy over gastrostomy are decreased skin excoriation, avoidance of intrusion of the peritoneum, and an easier feeding position.[10]

The surgery may be performed under general or local anesthesia. A nasogastric tube is inserted before surgery to serve as a landmark. An incision is made in the esophageal wall slightly above the left clavicle at the anterior border of the sternocleidomastoid muscle, the nasogastric tube is removed, and a Levin tube is inserted through the opening and advanced to the stomach. The Levin tube is sutured in position for 7 to 10 days. After healing of the tissue, the tube may be removed and reinserted through the stoma for each feeding.[10]

During the early postoperative period the patient is observed for signs of hoarseness or inability to cough, indicating possible tenth cranial nerve damage. The skin around the incision may become reddened for 2 to 3 days after surgery as a result of irritation from saliva that may drain around the tube. Tube feedings may be started as soon as the gastrointestinal tract is functioning. The same guidelines as for all tube feedings are followed (p. 1373).

Once the stoma is patent, the tube is inserted for the feeding and then removed. The person sits in an upright position. The tube is lubricated with a water-soluble lubricant and inserted in the stoma aimed in the direction of the opposite axilla.[10] The tube may be inserted for 15 to 20 cm (6 to 8 in.) if the feeding is to be placed in the lower esophagus to maintain lower esophageal sphincter (LES) pressure or for 25 to 35 cm (12 to 17 in.) if the feeding is to be placed into the stomach. The irrigating syringe is then attached to the tube and the feeding is given. When all fluid has been inserted, the tube is pinched closed, removed, and rinsed with tap water. The person should remain in an upright position for at least 1 hour to prevent regurgitation and aspiration.[10]

Patients and/or significant others are taught as soon as possible how to insert and remove the tube, give the feedings, and maintain the equipment.

Surgery of the esophagus and stomach

Surgery is one method of treatment used (1) to maintain patency of the upper gastrointestinal tract, (2) to provide a method for ingestion of food when esophageal patency is impaired, (3) to correct esophageal or gastric defects, or (4) to remove ulcerations or tumors. The term *-ostomy* means "an opening into"; thus a gastrostomy refers to an opening into the stomach. If only one prefix precedes the term -ostomy, then the surgical opening is made from the exterior, such as a gastrostomy. When two prefixes precede the term -ostomy, the surgery consists of an opening made (*anastomosis*) between two organs; for example, a gastroenterostomy is an anastomosis of a portion of the stomach (*gastro*) with a portion of the small intestine (*entero*). Other examples are listed in Table 55-2.

TABLE 55-2. Surgeries of the upper gastrointestinal tract

Name	Description	Comments
Esophagectomy	Removal of a section of esophagus	Usually combined with esophagoplasty
Esophagoplasty	Repair of esophagus	Usually involves insertion of a tissue or Dacron graft
Esophagogastrostomy	Anastomosis of esophagus and stomach	Usually involves removal of lower one third of esophagus; tissue graft may be used
Esophagojejunostomy	Removal of stomach (total gastrectomy) and anastomosis of esophagus to jejunum	Two portions of jejunum meeting esophagus are sometimes joined to form a reservoir for food
Gastrectomy	Removal of part (subtotal) or all (total) of stomach	Remaining portions are anastomosed to small intestine
Gastrostomy	Insertion of tube through abdominal wall into stomach	Permits esophageal bypass allowing for nutritional feedings into gastrointestinal tract
Gastroduodenostomy	Formation of new opening between stomach and duodenum	In Billroth I surgery (Fig. 56-7) part of stomach is removed and remaining portion is anastomosed to duodenum
Gastrojejunostomy	Anastomosis of stomach with jejunum	In Billroth II surgery (Fig. 56-7) duodenal stump is closed after excision of lower part of stomach
Antrectomy	Removal of entire antrum (lower portion) of stomach	Usually followed by gastroduodenostomy
Pyloroplasty	Repair of pyloric opening of stomach	To enlarge opening and facilitate emptying of stomach
Gastric partitioning	Stapling of stomach to reduce size	Staples applied in two rows partially across stomach for control of massive obesity

Preoperative care

Nutrition

If the nutritional status of the patient is poor, as may be seen in some persons with esophageal disorders or with malignancies of the upper gastrointestinal tract, an attempt is made preoperatively to improve nutrition. Hyperalimentation (p. 349) or a temporary gastrostomy (p. 1396) may be necessary. If the patient is to have surgery for an ulcer, any special dietary prescriptions are continued through the preoperative period.

Mouth care

Special mouth care is indicated for patients with esophageal disorders who have a foul breath. The patient may be spitting up a mixture of pus, blood, and decomposed food, and thus the emesis basin requires immediate emptying. Mouth washes are useful in making the mouth feel fresher and should be offered to the patient before eating. They should be varied from time to time unless the patient has a preference, because sometimes the flavor of the solution becomes identified with the unpleasant throat secretions and becomes almost as distasteful as the secretions.

Teaching

In addition to the general preoperative teaching, special preoperative teaching given before any thoracic surgery (p. 1251) is instituted if the planned surgery will involve a thoracic approach. Since the incision for gastric surgery is high in the abdomen, special emphasis is placed on teaching the patient breathing exercises preoperatively. Most patients having esophageal or gastric surgery have a nasogastric tube in place for several days postoperatively because of decreased peristalsis from manipulation of the gastrointestinal tract organs during surgery and to prevent trauma or pressure on suture lines. Patients need to learn preoperatively that a nasogastric tube may be inserted and that they will be receiving fluids and nourishment intravenously for several days until peristalsis is reestablished.

Postoperative care

The immediate postoperative care for the patient who has had esophageal or gastric surgery centers about the maintenance of an airway, prevention of respiratory difficulties, protection from injury, care of the chest drainage system (p. 1253) if used, and care of the nasogastric tube (p. 1393).

Respiratory care

Because of the neck, chest, or upper abdominal incision, patients with esophageal or gastric surgery are inclined to lie still and to breathe shallowly to limit incisional pain. The prescribed pain medications are given as indicated and special attention is given to encouraging the patient to turn, to breathe deeply, and to cough productively every 2 hours or more frequently as indicated during the first few days. A modified Fowler's position provides for comfort and increased chest expansion. Ambulation is encouraged when permitted.

Gastric drainage

Drainage from the nasogastric tube after surgery usually contains some blood for the first 6 to 12 hours, but bright red blood, large amounts of blood, or excessive bloody drainage is reported to the surgeon at once. If the nasogastric tube stops draining, the surgeon is also notified immediately since a buildup of gas or fluid can cause pressure on the suture line resulting in rupture or dislodgement of the sutures. It is the responsibility of the surgeon to adjust the placement of the nasogastric tube so that inadvertent dislodgement of the sutures is prevented. In esophageal surgery the tube is usually left in place until complete healing of the esophageal anastomosis has occurred because esophageal tissue is very friable and because the anastomosis may be under tension.

Food and fluids

While the nasogastric tube is used and until peristalsis resumes, fluids by mouth are restricted. Mouth care is therefore needed frequently to keep the mucous membranes of the throat and mouth moist and clean.

Until the tube is removed and until the patient is able to drink enough nutritious fluids, fluids are given parenterally. The average patient is given about 3500 ml of fluids intravenously each day (2500 ml for normal body needs plus enough to replace fluids lost through the gastric drainage and vomitus). It is important that gastric drainage and urinary output be accurately measured and recorded.

Vitamins are usually prescribed until the patient is eating a full, well-balanced diet. Fluids by mouth are restricted for about 12 to 24 hours after the nasogastric tube is removed. Small amounts of fluid are then given frequently and the patient is observed for signs of leakage, such as difficulty in breathing, pain, or rise in temperature. If water is well tolerated, small amounts of bland food may be added until the patient is able to eat six small meals a day and to drink 120 ml of fluid every hour between meals. The dietary regimen must be adapted to the individual since some persons tolerate increasing amounts of food and fluids better than others.

If an esophagogastrostomy has been performed, the patient may complain of a feeling of fullness in the chest or difficulty in breathing after eating. Smaller, more frequent meals often help to relieve these problems. When the cardia of the stomach has been removed, some patients complain of nausea and vomiting. This difficulty is usually caused by irritation of the esophageal mucosa by the gastric juices that reflux into the esophagus when the patient lies flat. The patient is advised to elevate the head when lying down.

Early satiety is a common problem after gastric surgery. Regurgitation after meals also occurs and may be caused by eating too fast, by eating too much, or by postoperative edema about the suture line that prevents the food from passing into the intestines. If regurgitation occurs, the patient is encouraged to eat more slowly and the size of the meals is decreased temporarily. If the gastric retention continues, it is probably caused by edema about the suture line, and food and fluids by mouth are discontinued for a time. A nasogastric tube may be passed and attached to a suction apparatus, and fluids will be administered parenterally until the edema subsides.

After a gastric resection the *dumping syndrome* sometimes occurs. It may also occur in patients who had a vagotomy, antrectomy, or gastroenterostomy. Mild symptoms occur in approximately 20% of patients and usually disappear in a few months to a year. They remain troublesome in approximately 7% of all patients who undergo gastric resection.[3] The onset may occur during the meal or from 5 to 30 minutes after the meal. The duration of the attack may last 20 to 60 minutes.[20] The patient complains of weakness, faintness, palpitations of the heart, and diaphoresis. A feeling of fullness, discomfort, and nausea often occurs, and diarrhea may also develop. These symptoms are thought to be caused by the entrance of food directly into the jejunum without undergoing usual changes and dilution in the stomach. The food mixture, more hyperosmolar than the jejunal secretions, causes fluid to be drawn from the bloodstream to the jejunum. The reaction appears to be greater after the ingestion of sugar, since sugar is the most osmotically active food. The symptoms just described are also attributed to the sudden rise in blood sugar (hyperglycemia), with the entrance of glucose into the bloodstream, and the subsequent fall in the blood sugar level. Blood glucose falls to subnormal levels, producing the symptoms of hypoglycemia. The rapid gastric emptying and the propulsion of chyme into the small intestine are felt to initiate an intensive gastrocolic reflex and cause diarrhea and a feeling of fullness and discomfort. Therapy for dumping syndrome consists of a low-carbohydrate, high-fat, high-protein diet with fluids restricted to between meals. Anticholinergic drugs and serotonin antagonists may be helpful.

Weight loss

Weight loss is common after gastric surgery as a result of the decreased caloric intake with early satiety, fear of postprandial symptoms, or mild interference of fat absorption with resultant steatorrhea. The person is advised to eat frequent, small, dry meals high in protein and complex carbohydrates, to avoid concentrated sugars that are rapidly dissolved, and to avoid drinking fluids with meals and for about 2 hours after eating.

Discharge planning

Before discharge, radiographic studies may be done to observe functioning of the remaining portions of the upper gastrointestinal tract. The patient may still be eating six small meals a day or may be tolerating three larger meals. The person is advised to eat slowly and to decrease the size of the meals and amount of fluids with meals if discomfort occurs after eating. The remaining stomach gradually is able to accept larger amounts of food and fluids.

Special needs after total gastrectomy

The nursing care of the patient who has had a total gastrectomy (esophagojejunostomy) differs in some ways from that of patients undergoing other types of gastric surgery. A thoracic approach is used, and the nursing care will be that for the patient who has had chest surgery (p. 1249). Drains are usually inserted from the site of the anastomosis, and there may be serosanguineous drainage. There is little or no drainage from the nasogastric tube because there is no longer any reservoir in which secretions may collect, and there is no stomach mucosa left to secrete.

Following a total gastrectomy the maintenance of good nutrition is difficult because the patient can no longer eat regular meals and because the food that is taken is poorly digested and therefore poorly absorbed from the intestines. Since the patient also becomes anemic, ferrous sulfate, folate, and vitamin B_{12} are often prescribed. Patients who have had a total gastrectomy rarely regain normal strength. Most of them are semiinvalids as long as they live.

Outcome criteria for the person who has had esophageal surgery

The person or significant others can:
1. Determine a specific plan for dietary modification that maintains an adequate intake of nutrients and fluids.
2. State specific position and activity requirements (see outcome criteria for esophageal disorders, p. 1415).
3. List name, dosage, frequency, action, and side effects of medications to be taken at home.
4. Demonstrate exercises to be done at home (exercises to be followed after thoracic surgery).
5. Discuss the emotional impact of the surgery and plan for the future.
6. State plans for follow-up care. State signs or symptoms requiring institution of specific therapy or contact with physician (respiratory infec-

tion, pain, hemoptysis, hematemesis, weight loss, increasing dysphagia).

Outcome criteria for the person who has had gastric surgery

The person or significant others can:
1. State a specific plan for dietary modifications following discharge.
   a. List specific types of fluids and foods to be avoided.
   b. Determine a specific plan for small frequent feedings that maintain optimal nutrition.
   c. Determine daily fluid requirements and state a plan for intake of fluids before, during, and after meals.
   d. Explain the need for planned rest periods following food ingestion.
2. Describe any medication or treatment program (antibiotics, iron and vitamins, antacids) to be followed at home.
3. State plans for follow-up care.
   a. Describe how the surgical procedure relates to the dietary and fluid modifications.
   b. List symptoms requiring medical follow-up (vomiting after meals, increasing feeling of abdominal fullness, increasing weakness, hematemesis, tarry stools, pain, increased temperature, persistent diarrhea).
4. Discuss the emotional impact of surgery.
   a. State a specific plan for returning to activities of daily living (ADL) and work (as appropriate).
   b. State situations within the environment that may produce increased stress and determine a plan to cope effectively with these.
5. Describe how to obtain professional and community resources necessary to structure a satisfactory life-style.

REFERENCES AND SELECTED READINGS

1. *Andrysiak, T., Carroll, R.M., and Ungerleider, J.T.: Marijuana for the oncology patient, Am. J. Nurs. **79**:1396-1398, 1979.
2. Bastiaan, R.J.: Dental sore mouth: etiological aspects and treatment, Oral Health **68**:12-16, 1978.
3. Beeson, P.B., McDermott, W., and Wyngaarden, J.B., editors: Textbook of medicine, ed. 15, Philadelphia, 1979, W.B. Saunders Co.
4. Bernier, J.L., and Muhler, J.C.: Improving dental practice through preventive measures, ed. 3, St. Louis, 1975, The C.V. Mosby Co.
5. *Black, C.D., Popovich, N.G., and Black, M.C.: Drug interactions in the GI tract, Am. J. Nurs. **77**:1426-1429, 1977.
6. *Block, P.L.: Dental health in hospitalized patients, Am. J. Nurs. **76**:1162-1164, 1976.

7. Bockus, H.L.: Gastroenterology, ed. 3, Philadelphia, 1974, W.B. Saunders Co.
8. Bond, J.H., and Levitt, M.D.: Gaseousness and intestinal gas, Med. Clin. North Am. **62**:155-163, 1978.
9. *Bruya, M., and Madeira, N.: Stomatitis after chemotherapy, Am. J. Nurs. **75**:1349-1452, 1975.
10. *Bush, J.: Cervical esophagostomy to provide nutrition, Am. J. Nurs. **79**:107-109, 1979.
11. Caldwell, R.C., and Stallard, R.E.: A textbook of preventive dentistry, Philadelphia, 1977, W.B. Saunders Co.
12. Chang, A.E., et al.: Delta-9-tetrahydrocannibol as an antiemetic in cancer patients receiving high-dose methotrexate, Ann. Intern. Med. **91**:819-824, 1979.
13. Cohen, S.: The diagnosis and management of gastroesophageal reflux, Adv. Intern. Med. **21**:47-75, 1976.
14. Conn, H.F.: Current therapy 1980, Philadelphia, 1980, W.B. Saunders Co.
15. Cooperman, A.M.: Highly selective vagotomy, Surg. Clin. North Am. **55**:1089-1101, 1975.
16. Cooperman, A.M., and Hoerr, S.O.: Pyloroplasty, Surg. Clin. North Am. **55**:1019-1024, 1975.
17. *Drucker, D.B.: Sweetening agents in food, drinks, and medicine: cariogenic potential and adverse effects, J. Hum. Nutr. **33**:114-124, 1979.
18. Dworken, H.J.: The alimentary tract, Philadelphia, 1974, W.B. Saunders Co.
19. *Dyer, E., Monson, M.A., and Cope, M.J.: Dental health in adults, Am. J. Nurs. **76**:1156-1159, 1976.
20. Egdahl, R.H., and Mannick, J.A.: Modern surgery, New York, 1970, Grune & Stratton, Inc.
21. Everhart, D.L.: Immunity and dental caries, N.Y. J. Dent. **48**(8):243-245, 1978.
22. Fisher, R.S., and Cohen, S.: Gastroesophageal reflux, Med. Clin. North Am. **62**(1):3-20, 1978.
23. *Franks, A.S.: The mouth in old age, Nurs. Times **69**:1292-1293, 1973.
24. Frytak, S., et al.: Delta-9-tetrahydrocannibol as an antiemetic for patients receiving cancer chemotherapy, Ann. Intern. Med. **91**:825-830, 1979.
25. Ganong, W.F.: Review of medical physiology, ed. 9, Los Altos, Calif., 1979, Lange Medical Publications.
26. Given, B., and Simmons, S.: Gastroenterology in clinical nursing, ed. 3, St. Louis, 1979, The C.V. Mosby Co.
27. Glickman, I.: Clinical periodontology, ed. 4, Philadelphia, 1972, W.B. Saunders Co.
28. *Griggs, B.A., and Hoppe, M.C.: Update: nasogastric tube feeding, Am. J. Nurs. **79**:481-485, 1979.
29. Hahn, A.B., Barkin, R.L., and Oestreich, S.J.K.: Pharmacology in nursing, ed. 15, St. Louis, 1982, The C.V. Mosby Co.
30. Hartwell, S.W., Jr.: Surgical treatment of cervical esophagostomy, Surg. Clin. North Am. **55**:1103-1105, 1975.
31. Jaffe, P.E.: Dental cleansing tape, N.Y. J. Dent. **43**:245-247, 1973.
32. *Johnson, N.: Teaching dental health to children, Pediat. Nurs. **4**(2):20-23, 1978.
33. *Kagawa-Busby, K.S., et al.: Effects of diet temperature on tolerance of enteral feedings, Nurs. Res. **29**:276-280, 1980.
34. Krause, M.V., and Mahan, L.K.: Food, nutrition and diet therapy, ed. 6, Philadelphia, 1979, W.B. Saunders Co.
35. *Lambert, M.L.: Drug and diet interactions, Am. J. Nurs. **75**:402-406, 1975.
36. *LeMaitre, G.D., and Finnegan, J.A.: The patient in surgery: a guide for nurses, ed. 4, Philadelphia, 1980, W.B. Saunders Co.
37. *Less, W.: Mechanics of teaching plaque control, Dent. Clin. North Am. **16**:647-659, 1972.
38. *McConnell, E.A.: Ensuring safer stomach suctioning with the Salem sump tube, Nurs. '77 **77**(9):54-57, 1977.

*References preceded by an asterisk are particularly well suited for student reading.

39. *McConnell, E.A.: Ten problems with nasogastric tubes and how to solve them, Nurs. '79 **79**(4):78-81, 1979.

40. Newbrun, E.: Dietary fluoride supplementation for the prevention of caries Pediatrics **62**:733-737, 1978.

41. Ostrom, C.A.: Effectiveness of a preventive dentistry delivery system, Oral Health **69**(2):39-43, 1979.

42. *Reitz, M., and Pope, W.: Mouth care, Am. J. Nurs. **73**:1728-1730, 1973.

43. Sabiston, D.C., editor: Davis-Christopher textbook of surgery, ed. 11, Philadelphia, 1977, W.B. Saunders Co.

44. Sallan, S.E., et al.: Antiemetics in patients receiving chemotherapy for cancer, N. Engl. J. Med. **302**(3):135-138, 1980.

45. *Schweiger, J.L., Lang, J.W., and Schweiger, J.W.: Oral assessment: how to do it, Am. J. Nurs. **80**:654-657, 1980.

46. *Scogna, D.M., and Smalley, R.: Chemotherapy-induced nausea and vomiting, Am. J. Nurs. **79**:1562-1565, 1979.

47. Siefkin, A.D., and Bolt, R.J.: Preoperative evaluation of the patient with gastrointestinal or liver disease, Med. Clin. North Am. **63**:1309-1320, 1979.

48. Welling, P.: How food and fluid affect drug absorption, Postgrad. Med. **62**:73-82, 1977.

49. Williams, S.R.: Nutrition and diet therapy, ed. 4, St. Louis, 1982, The C.V. Mosby Co.

CHAPTER 56

PROBLEMS OF THE UPPER GASTROINTESTINAL TRACT

BARBARA C. LONG

Disorders of the upper gastrointestinal tract may be acute or chronic and may lead to malnutrition through interference with ingestion or digestion. The disorders include infections, obstructions such as by tumors or strictures, alterations in motility, and alterations in the structure or integrity of the mucosa and underlying tissues.

Oral and dental conditions

The mouth has special emotional significance for every individual, perhaps because it is associated in infancy with food, sucking, warmth, love, and security. It continues to be associated throughout life with survival through the intake of food and with pleasurable sensations related to love and companionship, acceptance and belonging. Therefore severe emotional reactions frequently occur when treatment involving the mouth is necessary. The patient may refuse to visit the dentist, may go into complete panic when the jaws must be wired and normal eating is impossible, and may refuse to accept the fact that a lesion of the mouth is any threat to health. An understanding of what may be some of the patient's unspoken and often unrealized fears will enable the nurse to provide better care. Patience in explaining tests and treatments often helps. Sometimes merely taking time to explain to the patient the feeding method following oral surgery may make the difference between acceptance or rejection of the procedure. Sometimes the patient needs time to accept the need for referral to an oral surgeon and to accept the suggested treatment.

Infections of the mouth

Etiology

The mouth is an excellent barometer of general health, reflecting general disease and debility as well as good health. Specific diseases of the mouth most often occur when general nutrition and oral hygiene are poor, when people neglect their teeth, when smoking is excessive, and when broken teeth irritate the tissues.

Infections can occur in the buccal mucosa or the salivary glands. *Stomatitis* is an inflammation of the buccal mucosa occurring as a result of pathogenic organisms (bacteria, viruses, fungi), mechanical trauma, irritants (tobacco, alcohol, excessively spicy foods), nutritional disorders (vitamin deficiencies), disease (liver, kidney, blood dyscrasias), or following chemotherapy.

Aphthous stomatitis or canker sore is usually caused by biting the cheek or by a recurrent virus that can remain inactive in the mucosa for a period of years. The virus of *herpes simplex* can cause inflammation of the mouth with vesicle formation or may be limited to lips or nose (cold sore, fever blister). A combination of the *Bacillus fusiformis*, which resembles the spirochete of syphilis, and *Borrelia vincentii* causes *ulceromembranous stomatitis*, or Vincent's angina. During World War I this disease was so common that the name "trench mouth" was acquired. *Streptococcus* is the causative organism of Ludwig's angina, a rare deep and serious infection of the tissue of the floor of the mouth around the submaxillary gland. The fungus *Candida albicans* causes thrush which is sometimes seen following treatment with antibiotics over a period of time. It is thought that the antibiotic eliminates the bacteria permitting the existing fungus to flourish.

Parotitis is an inflammation of the parotid gland, a

salivary gland. Acute communicable parotitis (epidemic mumps) is caused by a virus that is transmitted by direct contact with the saliva. Noncommunicable parotitis occurs in debilitated persons whose oral hygiene is poor, whose mouths have been permitted to become dry, and who have not chewed solid foods regularly. Elderly persons are more susceptible than younger ones. Usually the *Staphylococcus* organism is present.

Prevention

Infections of the mouth can be prevented in many instances by adequate nutrition, maintenance of moist mucous membranes, and good oral hygiene. Excessive use of tobacco or hot spicy foods is discouraged for persons who have an increased risk of developing stomatitis. Prevention of nutritional deficiencies, especially vitamin deficiencies, will help prevent stomatitis, and emphasis on restoring nutritional balance of the debilitated patient will decrease the incidence of mouth infections.

In addition to maintaining the nutrition of the cells, the mucous membranes must be kept moist to prevent infection. Adequate hydration is therefore important. Mouth breathing and oxygen administration may lead to dry mucous membranes. Patients who are not permitted to drink fluids should have frequent mouth care to keep the mouth clean and the mucous membranes moist. Persons whose normal habits include poor mouth or dental care need health teaching.

The importance of good mouth care cannot be overemphasized. If self-care is inadequate the nurse must intervene. In situations where the mouth is in poor condition and a fetid odor is present, the task is disagreeable and thus unfortunately is often not carried out as frequently as is needed. Patients who are at high risk of developing infections need mouth care several times a day, and those whose mouths are in poor condition and who are on the verge of developing stomatitis may need attention to oral hygiene as often as every 1 to 2 hours while awake.

Clinical picture

In patients at high risk of developing infections the mouth is assessed daily for signs of developing or healing infection. Signs and symptoms may include mild erythema and edema of the mucous membranes, ulcerations, increased or decreased salivation, pain (especially when inflamed or ulcerated areas are touched by the teeth or foods), fetid odor to the breath, and a foul taste. Bleeding of the gums and a gray membrane over the gums may occur with Vincent's angina. Fever and edema, which may lead to obstruction of the throat, may occur with Ludwig's angina. Redness around the orifice of the parotid gland is seen with parotitis. Thrush is characterized by white patches (resembling milk curds) over the inflamed mucous membranes.

In addition to assessing the condition of the mouth, the nurse needs to assess the ability of the patient to carry out oral hygiene. Assessment includes the patient's level of consciousness, ability to open the mouth, presence of mouth breathing, and ability to feed self or drink fluids.[9]

Intervention

Maintenance of adequate nutrition and hydration is as important after mouth infections develop as it is in prevention. If the mouth is very sore and painful, eating may be difficult, and the patient may need considerable encouragement. Soft foods, including strained meats and fish, pureed vegetables and fruits, cooked cereals, soups, jello, and ice cream, are best tolerated. Hot spicy foods are to be avoided; cold drinks may be soothing. High-protein, high-caloric drinks such as eggnog serve both nutritional and fluid needs.

Thorough and frequent *mouth care* is a must. The frequency of mouth care and the effectiveness of agents in relation to therapeutic outcomes have not yet been thoroughly studied. It has been suggested that for mild stomatitis, mouth care at least every 4 hours around the clock is essential and at least every 2 hours for very severe cases.[9] If dentures are present and are increasing pain, they should be removed. Alkaline mouth-wash solutions such as sodium bicarbonate or sodium perborate can be used. Hydrogen peroxide diluted with normal saline 1:4 is effective in treating anaerobic infections, since it is an oxidizing agent. It should be mixed immediately before use because it decomposes rapidly. If the tissues are not too painful, a soft toothbrush may be used. If pain is severe, one layer of gauze may be wrapped around a finger to gently wipe the gums and teeth. The mouth is then rinsed with the solution, followed by rinsing with tap water.

With severe Vincent's angina or with Ludwig's angina, antibiotics are ordered and should be given on time to maintain blood levels. If the patient has difficulty swallowing tablets, they are crushed if possible or the antibiotic may be given intramuscularly.

Pain may be partially relieved by good oral hygiene. Smoking is contraindicated. Cold drinks or sucking on frozen popsicles may be soothing. Analgesic drugs may be necessary, and lidocaine hydrochloride (Xylocaine) may be applied to provide topical anesthesia.

Outcome criteria for the person with a mouth infection

The person or significant others can:
1. State the underlying cause of the infection.
2. Describe a specific plan to avoid future infections that includes:
   a. Maintenance of a balanced nutritional and fluid intake.
   b. Avoidance of causative factors.

c. Good oral hygiene.
d. Semiannual dental examinations.
3. State the action, dosage, and side effects of medications to be taken at home including the need to complete antibiotic therapy.
4. State signs or symptoms necessitating medical follow-up.

Diseases of the teeth and gums

Dental caries

Etiology and pathophysiology. Tooth decay is probably the most common yet most neglected chronic ailment of modern times. Dental caries is a progressive disease of the teeth related to the consumption of refined carbohydrates. There is a genetic influence in host susceptibility to caries formation. Within 30 minutes after eating, microorganisms in the mouth act on the sucrose to form long-chain polysaccharides, which stick to the tooth enamel. Lactic acid is formed that can dissolve the tooth enamel leading to caries formation. When the carious process breaks through the enamel to the dentin the process is accelerated because of the lowered mineral content of the dentin.

If the cavity is not treated by a dentist, the tooth may disintegrate with or without pain, and loss of the tooth follows. Malocclusion gradually develops as teeth are lost and may result in a poor bite with unequal pressure on teeth. Further tooth decay may result.

Prevention. Methods to control and prevent dental caries include good oral hygiene, dental examinations every 6 months, nutritional foods including avoidance of refined sugars, and the use of fluorides (p. 1387).

Periapical abscess

A periapical abscess develops around the root of a tooth. It usually is an extension of an infection arising in the pulp caused by dental caries. The abscess may perforate along the gum margin, or it may travel medially to form an abscess over the palate or spread directly to the soft tissues, causing cellulitis and a severely swollen face.

Periapical abscess can cause severe local pain and systemic reactions, including malaise, nausea, and elevation of temperature. The treatment consists of drilling an opening into the pulp chamber of the tooth to establish drainage and to relieve pain. Penicillin may be administered, and warm saline mouth washes usually are ordered several times a day. After the acute phase the tooth may be extracted, or root canal therapy may be started if a sound, permanent tooth is involved.

Periodontal disease

Periodontal disease results from inflammation or degeneration of the tissues that support the teeth; it affects the gingivae, bone, cementum, and periodontal membrane (Fig. 56-1). After the age of 40 years, more people lose their teeth from periodontal disease than from dental caries.

Etiology. Many factors contribute to the development of periodontal disease, among them malocclusion, accumulation of tartar, poor nutrition including eating

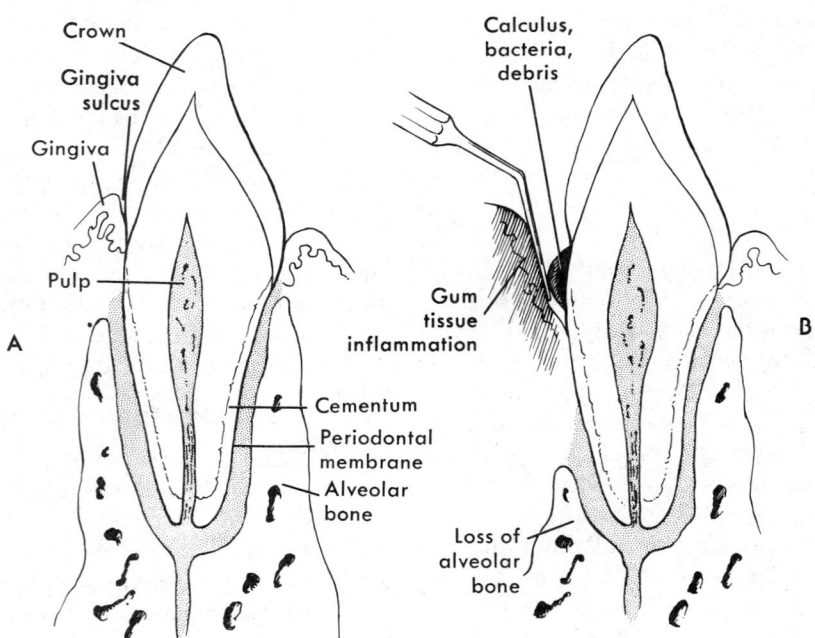

Fig. 56-1. A, Normal tooth with gum and root structure. **B,** Note presence of foreign materials along gum margin, which may lead to periodontal disease.

too much soft food instead of solid food that requires mastication, poor mouth hygiene, and improper brushing of the teeth. Certain systemic conditions may contribute to the development of periodontal disease. These include alcoholism, diabetes, thyroid imbalance, hormonal imbalance (menstruation and pregnancy), response to chemotherapy, blood dyscrasias, and debilitating diseases.

Pathophysiology. Nonmineralized plaque can form on the calculus surface and destroy the tiny tendrils holding the tooth in the socket. This situation eventually leads to unhealthy receding gums with lessened tooth support (Fig. 56-1). Poor nutrition, improper brushing of the teeth, and local infection may augment the destruction of gums and supportive gum structures to such a degree that they recede. The leverage of daily use then becomes too great on the teeth, and they loosen and finally have to be removed.

Clinical picture. Periodontal disease usually begins with *gingivitis,* a band of painless, reddened, inflamed tissue surrounding the roots. There may be bleeding on minimal injury, such as by vigorous brushing. The gingivitis progresses to *periodontitis* with pockets forming as the gums recede from the teeth and subsequent loosening of teeth. Debris collects in the periodontal pockets, and infection (pyorrhea) and pain may develop.

Intervention. Treatment of periodontal disease includes maintenance of oral hygiene and nutrition, control of local irritations and infections by regular visits to the dentist, removal of accumulations of tartar on the teeth, replacement of lost teeth, and correction of malocclusion. Even if treatment has been delayed until there is already a good deal of damage, care by an *orthodontist* (one who specializes in straightening teeth) may be surprisingly helpful. Sometimes bridgework and other forms of splinting can be used so that further erosion of bone and supportive tissue can be halted even if teeth cannot be straightened and the actual bite improved. Surgery may be required for large periodontal pockets.

Nutrition is so important for patients with periodontal disease that some periodontists have their patients keep weekly food-intake charts to determine what essentials of diet may be lacking. Intake should be evaluated carefully for inclusion of fresh citrus fruits and fresh vegetables, and protein consumption should be noted, since it is very important in gum healing and in gum health.

Tumors of the mouth

Epidemiology and etiology

The lips, the oral cavity, and the tongue are prone to develop malignant lesions. The largest number of these tumors are squamous cell epitheliomas that grow rap-

idly and metastasize to adjacent structures more quickly than do most malignant tumors of the skin. In the United States oral cancer accounts for 5% of the cancers in males and 3% in females.[1] Recent investigation has revealed a higher incidence of cancers of the mouth and throat among persons who are heavy drinkers and smokers. The combination of high alcohol consumption and smoking causes an apparent breakdown in the body's defense mechanism, as evidenced by an increase in the levels of immunoglobulin A (IgA) in saliva.[39]

The cure rate for cancer of the *lips* is high because the lesion is easily apparent to the patient and to others. Metastasis to regional lymph nodes has occurred in only 10% of persons when diagnosed. In some instances a lesion may spread rapidly and involve the mandible and the floor of the mouth by direct extension. Occasionally, the tumor may be a basal cell lesion that starts in the skin and spreads to the lip.

Cancer of the *anterior tongue* and *floor of the mouth* may seem to occur together because their spread to adjacent tissues is so rapid. Metastasis to the neck has already occurred in over 60% of the patients when the diagnosis is made because of the tongue's abundant vascular and lymphatic drainage. The mortality is high. Lesions about the base of the tongue may go unnoticed by the patient and may be far advanced when treatment is started.

Tumors of the *salivary glands* occur primarily in the parotid gland and are usually benign. Tumors of the submaxillary gland have a high incidence of malignancy. The malignant tumor grows more rapidly and may be accompanied by pain and impaired facial function.

Prevention

Avoidance of predisposing factors may decrease the potential for developing cancer of the mouth. This includes avoidance of excess exposure to sun and wind on the lips, elimination of smoking or chewing tobacco or betel leaf, and maintenance of good oral and dental care. There is a high correlation between the incidence of cancer of the mouth and cirrhosis of the liver associated with alcohol intake. Early detection of oral cancer can help increase the patient's chance of survival. Any person with a mouth lesion that does not heal within 2 to 3 weeks is urged to seek immediate medical care.

Clinical picture

Malignant lesions of the mouth are usually asymptomatic. *Leukoplakia,* white patches on the tongue and buccal mucosa that are not easily removed, are not cancerous but often become malignant. Early malignant lesions are difficult to detect since there may be an initial inflammatory response that frequently disappears, leaving only a small ulcer or growth. Cancer of the lips usually occurs on the lower lip as a fissure or a painless, indurated ulcer with raised edges. Cancer of the anterior tongue and floor of the mouth occurs as hard plaquelike or ulcerated areas that do not heal. Lesions are usually unilateral, and multiple lesions may occur.

Parotid tumors occur as painless lumps that can be palpated anterior to or directly below the ear. Biopsy of the parotid gland is not recommended because of the potential for tumor seeding; therefore the entire gland is usually removed for examination. If diagnosed as a malignancy, more extensive surgery may be indicated.

Intervention

Treatment consists of one or more approaches depending on the location, type, extent, and size of the tumor. Modalities include surgery, radiotherapy, cryotherapy, and chemotherapy.

Cancer of the lip may require excision and reconstructive surgery of jaw and mandible if extension to these areas has occurred. A radical neck dissection may be done if the lymph nodes are involved (p. 1284).

Cancer of the anterior tongue and floor of the mouth may require partial or total surgical excision of the tongue (*hemiglossectomy, glossectomy*) and a radical neck dissection if lymph nodes are involved. Intraarterial perfusion of antimetabolites into the site may be instituted before surgery (p. 506). Radiation treatment may be used instead of surgery or following surgery.

Surgery for cancer of the parotid gland may include removal of large amounts of surrounding tissue and nodes, but radical neck resection is not routine.[65] Radiation is only instituted for its palliative effect. Tumors of the submaxillary gland usually require complete excision of the gland and more radical surgery.

Preparation for therapy. Treatment for cancer of the mouth interferes with major oral functions such as eating and speaking and thus creates major changes in the person's life. The ability to speak will vary from some limitation to complete inability to speak depending on the amount of tissue resected or destroyed. Eating patterns will be changed in terms of the consistency of foods (soft or liquid) as well as methods of ingestion (assistance with moving foods to posterior pharynx or tube feedings). Patients may also have problems with choking and aspiration and with nasal returns and drooling. The person's facial appearance will also change depending on the extent of tissue removed or destroyed, and even with reconstructive surgery, noticeable changes will be present.

Thus one of the major problems that the person will have to cope with and adapt to is the change in body image. The person needs to know in advance the changes that will occur and the measures that will be taken to assist the person during the adjustment period. The impact of the loss may be slightly minimized when the grieving process begins early. The full emotional impact of the loss, however, occurs after therapy. (See Chapter 28 for further discussion on body image.)

Surgery

Preoperative care. Oral prophylactic treatment is given and antibiotics may be administered preoperatively to decrease the number of bacteria present in the mouth at the time of surgery. In addition to general preoperative teaching, the patient needs to know that suctioning will be necessary (except for surgery restricted to the lips) and that a nasogastric tube will be in place postoperatively.

Prostheses of the palate and jaw may be designed to replace portions of tissue that have been resected. If a prosthesis is to be made, impressions will be taken during the preoperative period; the prosthesis will be fitted when healing has occurred postoperatively. If a composite resection including a radical neck dissection (p. 1284) is to be performed, reconstructive surgery will be done, if possible, during the initial procedure; it may also be performed at a later date.

Postoperative care. The position of choice during the postanesthesia period is side-lying (or prone) to facilitate drainage from the mouth. When fully alert, the patient usually prefers Fowler's position. If a hemiglossectomy (excision of part of the tongue) has been performed, the patient will have difficulty in swallowing saliva or expectorating secretions, and the mouth may need to be suctioned frequently. Occasionally, a suction device such as is used by dentists is employed to carry away saliva as it accumulates. A gauze wick may be used to direct saliva into an emesis basin. A patient who cannot swallow requires constant attention. Bleeding and drainage from the suture line on the lip or tongue should be minimal, but because of the vascularity of the tongue, patients who have had a wide resection of the tongue are observed carefully for hemorrhage.

The seventh cranial (facial) nerve passes through the posterior portion of the parotid gland and may be affected by removal of this gland. Temporary facial paralysis frequently occurs, and permanent paralysis may occur after radical surgery. Facial weakness is assessed daily by asking the patient to pucker the lips, smile, show the teeth, and raise the eyebrows.[65] If the patient cannot close an eye, the cornea must be protected by lubricating eyedrops and patches while sleeping.

ORAL HYGIENE. Good mouth care is essential for comfort, prevention of infection, and promotion of healing. Teeth brushing is usually contraindicated because of discomfort and potential trauma. Uninvolved areas may be cleansed by using a cotton applicator moistened with hydrogen peroxide and saline. The mouth may be irrigated with sterile water, diluted hydrogen peroxide, normal saline, or a solution of sodium bicarbonate. Commercial mouth washes are too astringent. Sterile equipment is used to prevent introduction of exogenous organisms.

A catheter may be inserted along the side of the

mouth between the cheek and the teeth and solution injected with gentle pressure, or a spray may be used. Remaining fluid and mucus drains into an emesis basin or is removed with the suction apparatus. Dressings may be protected during this treatment by fitting a plastic sheet snugly over them. As soon as possible the patient is encouraged to assist with this part of care.

EATING. The method used to feed the patient will depend entirely on the extent and nature of the therapy. Most patients can suction and feed themselves a few days following mouth surgery and are happier doing so. An Asepto syringe with a catheter attached may be used, and from this apparatus the patient may progress to a feeding cup with a piece of rubber tubing attached. Through practice the patient will develop confidence in self-care and is often more adept than the nurse in placing the catheter or tube in a position where fluids can be received into the mouth and swallowed without difficulty. A mirror often helps. Privacy is essential during the initial period. The patient should not be hurried and is observed very carefully to determine how much assistance is needed. As the patient begins to take liquids and then soft, pureed foods, he or she is taught to follow all meals with clear water to cleanse the mouth and foster good oral hygiene.

The patient who has had a hemiglossectomy will be fed initially through a nasogastric tube (see p. 1373 for further information on tube feedings). When the tube is removed, the patient must learn to drink from a glass or cup since sucking is usually impossible because of the tissue loss. The patient is usually given prepared formula feedings initially; some persons must remain on a liquid diet for the remainder of their lives.

If the person is to be discharged on a liquid diet, the dietitian is consulted to assist the person in planning nutrient intake. Commercial preparations such as instant breakfast drinks are not suitable for long-term maintenance and often cause diarrhea or constipation. Gelatin preparations often create problems for patients with hemiglossectomies since the gelatin does not melt fast enough and creates unpleasant reactions with drooling or aspiration.[14] If used, gelatin preparations are best served in liquid form. Fruit-flavored yogurt preparations are less irritating to traumatized tissues than gelatin preparations and are more nutritious.[14] Solids prepared in a blender often require more than twice as much fluid as do other solids and result in excessive fluid volume being ingested.

The person who can progress to soft foods cannot chew properly without the tongue and has a problem in getting the food to the posterior pharynx. Sensation in the mouth is decreased and the person has difficulty locating the position of the food in the oral cavity. A spoon should be used rather than a fork, since the tines of the fork may traumatize the new tissue.[14] One method of eating is for the patient to use the forefinger to push

the food to the posterior pharynx. With sensory loss in the mouth, the person should avoid very hot or cold foods and can determine the temperature by touching the food before introducing it into the mouth. Very hot foods can injure new tissue, whereas very cold foods can cause severe facial or head pain or paralyze oral or throat functions.

SPEECH. The ability to speak is commonly lost for short or long periods of time after surgery, but if the vocal chords are intact, speech will eventually return. A Magic Slate may be used for communication; however, many patients have difficulty using this because of previous or present temporary visual impairments. Conversation can be carried out so that the patient's responses can be limited to affirmative or negative gestures. Loud noises are disturbing to the patient since the oral tissue loss may create a channel that amplifies sound; therefore the patient should be addressed in a soft clear voice.

As speech begins to return, the patient is encouraged to speak slowly and to use the throat rather than the lips to achieve clarity. The nurse needs to listen carefully and to validate what the patient is saying before initiating actions on requests. Speech retraining may be necessary, and a tape recorder may be useful for the patient to hear his or her own voice to work on improvements.

SOCIALIZATION. Because of difficulties with eating or talking or with disfigurement in the event of radical surgery, some patients may hesitate to move among strangers. A two-bed room provides contact with others while still maintaining some privacy. The patient is supported and encouraged to mingle with others as soon as clues indicating readiness are observed. Men are encouraged to shave using an electric razor as soon as this is permitted. Members of the family are encouraged to visit.

Radiation. Tumors of the mouth may be treated by radiation in various forms. Needles containing radium, radioactive cobalt, or other radioactive substances may be inserted and left in place for a prescribed time. Seeds containing emanations from radium or radioactive cobalt may be used and left in place indefinitely or else removed (see Fig. 25-8). External radiation treatment using x-rays or other radioactive substances may be prescribed.

Whatever the method of treatment chosen, it should be explained fully to the patient. If needles containing radioactive elements are used, the person must know that the needles are fastened to string that must not be pulled lest the dosage or direction of radiation be altered or the needle lost. Talking with the needles in place is difficult or impossible. Radioactive needles must be checked several times each day. Auxiliary personnel and all other persons in attendance should understand the need to watch all equipment carefully for needles that have been removed or dislodged (e.g., when emptying an emesis basin), lest radioactive materials be unwittingly discarded.

Radiation therapy produces secondary effects in the mouth that include mucositis, xerostomia (dryness), dental decay, and trismus (tightening of the jaw muscle).[68] Some of the changes may be permanent. The initial reaction is an inflammation of the mucous membrane (mucositis). Sloughing of the tissues may occur and cause a fetid odor. Dentures are not tolerated for some time thereafter because of the sensitivity of the tissues. When dentures are worn they should be checked frequently for fit and removed at night. Good oral hygiene is essential.

Because smoke is irritating to the mucous membranes, the patient should not smoke. Hot and cold foods or fluids should be avoided because the injured mucous membranes are extremely sensitive to changes in temperature. Solutions of local anesthetics or lozenges may be prescribed by the physician if discomfort in the mouth caused by the local irritation seriously interferes with eating.

Dryness of the mouth begins 1 to 2 weeks after radiation is started and may persist throughout life.[68] The dryness makes the mouth feel uncomfortable and gives an unpleasant taste. Frequent drinks of water, saline-peroxide mouth washes, and increased humidity in the room contribute to added moisture and comfort.

Decreased salivary secretion and altered pH of the saliva contribute to rapid dental decay, especially at the gingival margins. In the past all teeth were extracted before radiation of the mouth, but this is being done less commonly. An active control program is started before radiation therapy is initiated. Fluoride treatments to the teeth may be given and a conscientious teeth-brushing regimen using fluoride toothpaste, a soft toothbrush, and dental floss is instituted.

Persons who have had surgery in addition to radiation may be unable to open their mouths widely. This can interfere with talking, eating, or dental care.

Palliative care. Tissue necrosis and severe pain occur in advanced cancer of the mouth, either from failure of treatment or from death of tissue as a result of radiation. The patient is harassed by difficulty in swallowing, fear of choking, and the constant accumulation of foul-smelling secretions. The danger of severe, and even fatal, hemorrhage must always be considered. Nursing care of these patients includes the most careful and thoughtful attention to certain details; for example, secretions left in emesis basins or in suction bottles can be most upsetting to the patient. It is exceedingly difficult to induce patients with advanced carcinoma of the mouth to take sufficient nourishing fluids, and the nurse can often help by finding out specifically what fluids or foods the patient likes and believes are easiest to take.

Relatives may be permitted to prepare and bring special dishes to the hospital if the patient so desires. Sometimes gastrostomy is done to permit direct introduction of food into the stomach (p. 1396). Most physicians prescribe analgesic drugs freely for patients whose disease has progressed beyond medical control.

If the patient is to be cared for at home, the family is taught how to feed, suction, and otherwise care for the patient. Assistance and support can be provided by a community health nurse.

Outcome criteria for the person with a hemiglossectomy

The person or significant others can:
1. Describe preparation of a safe, nutritious fluid or soft diet.
2. Feed self through appropriate means.
3. State rationale and measures for promoting good oral hygiene.
4. Describe approaches to take for speech improvement.
5. Verbalize feelings about changes in life-style.
6. State plans for gradual resumption of activities involving other persons.
7. State plans for follow-up health care.
   a. Describe plans to stop smoking, if appropriate.
   b. State time of next medical appointment.
   c. State signs or symptoms indicating need for medical attention (pain, bleeding).
   d. Describe community resources that are available.

Trauma

Fracture of the jaw

Fracture of the jaw occurs quite frequently as a result of vehicular accidents and of combative physical encounters with others. Treatment consists of bringing the separated fragments together and immobilizing them. This is accomplished with wires that are attached to the upper and lower rows of teeth and twisted together or with arch bars fastened by rubber bands or tie wires (Fig. 56-2). Rubber bands are used most often since they can be removed readily and the degree of fixation can be adjusted easily. If an open operation is necessary, interosseous wiring or plating may be done. Because of the excellent blood supply to the jaw, fractures usually heal rapidly (5 to 8 weeks). Tetanus prophylaxis and antibiotic therapy are usually started on admission. Many times the patient with a fracture of the jaw can resume quite an active life during convalescence. Most patients are in the hospital a very short time or are treated on

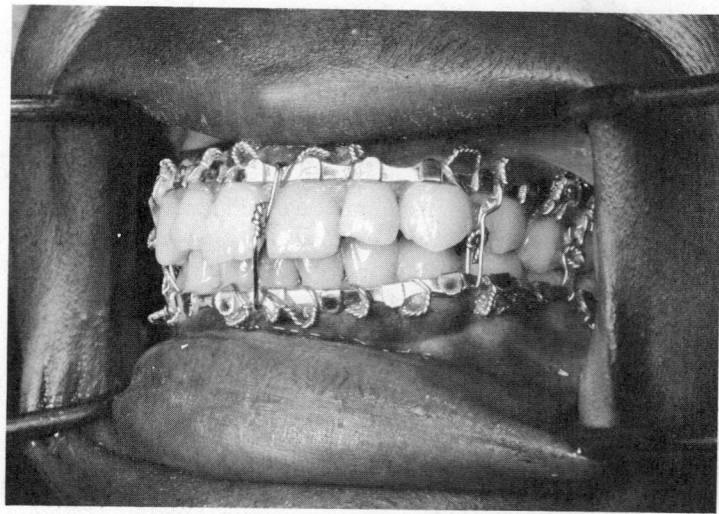

Fig. 56-2. One method of wiring jaw. (Courtesy Dr. Marsh Robinson.)

an ambulatory basis unless they have sustained other injuries.

Immediately following wiring of the teeth, the patient is watched for nausea and vomiting, which may be caused by emotional trauma, blood or other swallowed material, or anesthesia. Care must be taken to prevent aspiration of vomitus. Vomitus and secretions must be removed by suction, since the patient cannot expectorate them through the mouth. Usually a catheter can be inserted through the nasopharynx or into the mouth through a gap created by missing teeth or in the space behind the third molar. Scissors or a wire cutter should be at the bedside so that the wires can be cut or the elastic bands released if necessary. Specific orders should state the circumstances under which wires or rubber bands should be released.

Patients who have fixation by wiring need much the same care as is needed following surgery of the mouth. They must often subsist on liquids and must learn to take a high-caloric liquid diet through a catheter, an Asepto syringe, a feeding cup, or a straw. They need instructions about mouth hygiene, and they must be instructed to report any sudden swelling, pain, or other symptoms that may occur after dismissal from the hospital. Osteomyelitis is much less common now that antibiotics are available, but it can occur and is more likely to do so in the unusual cases of compound fracture in which bone fragments have penetrated either the outer skin or the inside of the mouth.

Outcome criteria for the person with immobilized jaws. The person or significant others can:
1. Describe situations that may require the establishment of an immediate clear airway (vomiting, increased secretions).

2. Describe methods of releasing the wires and re-establishing an airway if the airway becomes obstructed.
3. Describe the necessary dietary modifications (types of feedings, methods of preparation, foods to avoid that might cause vomiting or obstruction) and method of feeding.
4. Explain how to contact community or professional persons for assistance (counseling, vocational guidance).
5. State plans for follow-up care.

Injury to soft tissue

Injuries to soft tissues within the mouth usually are caused by pressure against teeth, direct trauma from a foreign object, or protrusion of bone through the buccal mucosa following fracture of the jaw. Breaks in the skin about the mouth often accompany these injuries. Treatment consists of thorough cleansing of the wounds. Usually an antibacterial solution is used and is followed by irrigation with sterile normal saline solution. Skin wounds are gently debrided and sutured with an extremely fine, nonabsorbable suture for best cosmetic results. Because of the vascularity of the scalp and face, infection is rare following traumatic injury to these areas.

Lacerations within the mouth are cleansed and sutured if their extent and location make these measures necessary. Hemorrhage must be watched for, especially if total injuries necessitate extensive dressing, which may hinder normal expectoration of blood and cause it to be swallowed. Edema may be pronounced following trauma to the mouth and may interfere with respirations. Usually the head of the bed is elevated in semi-Fowler's position to aid in venous drainage from the area and thereby lessen edema. Tight dressings about the face must be checked carefully, since they may contribute to development of edema and may cause headache.

Patients who have sustained penetrating wounds of the mouth are usually given antibiotics and tetanus serum prophylactically. The patient is questioned about a history of sensitivity to serum before treatment of prevention of tetanus is given. Mouth care and feeding of patients with these injuries present problems similar to those encountered following surgery or a fracture.

Outcome criteria for the person with sutures in the oral cavity. The person or significant others can:
1. Demonstrate techniques to keep the suture line clean (method, frequency, agents to avoid).
2. Describe any dietary modifications required during healing (soft, nonirritating foods).
3. State symptoms that require immediate medical supervision (increased temperature, swelling or redness of the suture line, drainage, loss of sutures).
4. State plans for follow-up care.

Esophageal disorders

Achalasia (cardiospasm, aperistalsis)

Achalasia is a condition in which there is an absence of peristalsis in the esophagus and the esophageal sphincter fails to relax following deglutition (swallowing), The cause is unknown, but the disorder is a direct result of disruption of the normal neuromuscular mechanism of the esophagus. The disease usually occurs between 20 and 50 years of age.

Pathophysiology

In the early phases of achalasia there is no gross lesion, but as the disease persists, the portion of the esophagus about the constriction dilates and the muscular walls become hypertrophied. The dilated area becomes atonic, and esophageal peristalsis may be absent so that little or no food can enter the stomach. While varying degrees of the condition exist, in extreme cases the esophagus above the constriction may hold a liter or more of fluid.

Clinical picture

Dysphagia for both liquids and solids is the major symptom. The onset is usually gradual over a period of months or years, and the person experiences increasing difficulty with swallowing, especially when anxious or tense. In time there is frank dysphagia with or without malnutrition. The person loses weight and may suffer from avitaminosis. Substernal chest pain may occur. As the condition progresses, there is regurgitation rather than vomiting of esophageal contents, which do not contain gastric acid, onto the pillow or into the larynx during sleep. The diagnosis is confirmed by radiographs taken as the person swallows barium and by esophagoscopy.

Intervention

Until treatment can be initiated, the person is encouraged to drink fluids with meals to increase lower esophageal sphincter (LES) pressure and help push the food beyond the LES. Treatment of achalasia consists of forceful dilation of the LES using pneumostatic or mechanical (Starck) dilators to impair sphincter contraction. Esophageal motility is not restored, but the open sphincter relieves the dysphagia in about 80% of patients. Repeated dilations may be necessary.

Surgical intervention consisting of a cardiomyotomy may be necessary if sphincter dilation is unsuccessful. The muscular layer is incised longitudinally down to but not through the mucosa. The incision is so done that two thirds of its length is in the esophagus and the remaining one third is in the stomach. This permits the mucosa to expand so that food can pass more easily into the stomach.

Postoperatively, the nursing care is the same as the routine care given any patient who has had chest surgery (p. 1252). A rare complication is accidental perforation of the esophageal mucosa so that leakage may contaminate the mediastinum. Regurgitation occasionally occurs after surgery but can usually be controlled by antacid medications. Since overflow may still occur at night, the patient is advised to refrain from food or fluid for several hours before retiring.

Esophageal diverticulum

Pathophysiology

An esophageal diverticulum is the bulging of the esophageal mucosa and submucosa through a weakened portion of the muscular layer of the esophagus. It is most often located at the pharyngoesophageal junction, in the lower end of the thoracic esophagus, or just above the diaphragm (epiphrenic diverticulum). As food is ingested, some of it may pass into the diverticulum. After a sufficient amount has accumulated in the pocket, it overflows into the esophagus and is regurgitated. There is always danger that some of the regurgitated material may be aspirated into the trachea and lungs during sleep or that the diverticulum may enlarge and cause esophageal obstruction.

Clinical picture

The patient may complain of pain on swallowing, of gurgling noises in the area, and of a cough caused by tracheal irritation. The breath usually has a foul odor caused by decomposition of food in the diverticulum. The odor can be alleviated somewhat by frequent brushing of the teeth and the use of aromatic mouthwashes.

Intervention

If the symptoms become severe, surgery is performed. The herniated sac is excised, and the resultant esophageal opening is closed. These procedures are well tolerated, and the administration of antibiotics makes postoperative infections rare. If a supraclavicular approach has been used, fluid are usually permitted as soon as nausea subsides. If a transthoracic approach is utilized, chest drainage may be used, and the patient usually is allowed nothing by mouth for several days.

Stricture of the esophagus

Etiology and pathophysiology

The deliberate or accidental swallowing of caustic materials such as lye may cause serious strictures in the esophagus as the mucosa heals. Unfortunately, many of the patients are small children, and they may suffer from the effects of such an accident for the remainder of their lives. Although the patient may be able to swallow fluids for a while after the accident, strictures develop as healing occurs, and sometimes no food can pass into the stomach.

Intervention

Careful attempts are made to dilate the stricture by passing bougies. Usually this is done under the fluoroscope so that danger of causing damage that would result in further stricture formation is lessened. If the destruction of the esophageal mucosa is extensive, a *gastrostomy* (permanent opening into the stomach) may be performed (p. 1396). Braided silk thread is then inserted through the mouth and esophagus into the stomach and brought out through the gastrostomy opening. The two ends of the thread are tied together to form a complete loop, and the thread is used for pulling bougies or beads tied to it through the esophagus to dilate it and to prevent complete closure of the lumen. Such treatment may be necessary for months or years after the ingesting of a caustic substance. If a satisfactory esophageal lumen cannot be maintained, surgery may be performed. The stricture may be resected or bypassed with a segment of jejunum or colon.

Outcome criteria for the person with esophageal disorders causing difficulty in swallowing

The person or significant others can:
1. Explain any dietary changes required after discharge.
   a. List specific foods to be avoided.
   b. State a plan for frequent small feedings that are soft and easily swallowed and will maintain nutrition.
   c. Determine daily fluid requirement and state a plan regarding intake of fluids before, during, and after food ingestion.
2. State plans for follow-up care.

Esophageal varices

The veins of the lower esophagus drain into the left gastric vein. When pressure in the portal system is increased, blood is shunted through the esophageal veins to the vena cava causing dilation of the esophageal veins. These varices may rupture and bleed profusely. Since this condition occurs primarily with liver disease, esophageal varices are discussed in detail in that section (p. 695).

Esophageal tumors

Epidemiology

Carcinoma is the most common condition causing obstruction of the esophagus and accounts for about 2% of all deaths from cancer in the United States. The incidence is increasing in nonwhite females, in persons with achalasia or hiatus hernia, and among alcoholics. The tumor may develop in any portion of the esophagus, but it is most common in the middle and lower thirds.

The only possible hope for successful treatment lies in very early diagnosis and surgical treatment. Any person who has difficulty in swallowing, no matter how trivial it may seem, should be urged to seek medical advice at once. This applies particularly to persons over 40 years of age, since cancer of the esophagus occurs more often in middle and later life than at younger ages. The incidence of cancer of the esophagus is more than twice as high in males as in females.

Clinical picture

Unfortunately, even if the person reports to a physician when the first symptoms appear, the disease is often already well established. The most common symptom is progressive dysphagia, first with solid food and eventually with liquids. As the esophagus becomes progressively obstructed, regurgitation may occur, and aspirated fluids may cause coughing and pneumonitis. The breath may have a foul odor, and the patient may complain of a foul taste.

The cancer may spread to adjoining areas by local invasion or by lymphatic spread. Neoplasms of the upper and middle esophagus may extend into the pulmonary system, and those of the lower esophagus may extend into the diaphragm, vertebrae, or heart.[6] Symptoms will depend on the area and extent of metastasis. Diagnosis is made by radiographs of the esophagus taken as the patient swallows barium (Fig. 56-3) or by examination of tumor cells obtained during esophagoscopy.

Intervention

Malignant lesions of the upper third of the esophagus are difficult to remove and are treated with high-voltage irradiation therapy. Lesions of the middle or lower third of the esophagus are removed surgically. For a middle esophageal neoplasm, an *esophagogastrostomy* (p. 1399) may be performed or a segment of colon may be anastomosed to the resected areas of the esophagus and stomach. Lower esophageal lesions are removed through a left thoracotomy or thoracic abdominal incision. The operation includes an *esophagogastrectomy*, splenectomy, and wide resection of lymph nodes. A major portion of the acid-secreting portion of the stomach is removed to reduce the occurrence of reflux esophagitis.

Since the malignant lesion is seldom completely removed, only a small percentage of persons live more than 5 years after the surgery, and many are chronic invalids during that time. Both the patient and significant others should be told of the need for close medical supervision. Persons with upper respiratory tract infections should be carefully avoided, and medical help should be sought at once if signs of even minor indisposition occur.

Some persons with cancer of the esophagus are not found to be suitable candidates for esophageal surgery. Their skin care, mouth care, and nutrition are similar to those described for the person being prepared for esophageal surgery.

Diaphragmatic hernia

Etiology and pathophysiology

Diaphragmatic hernia (hiatal hernia) refers to a protrusion of part of the stomach through the diaphragmatic hiatus into the thoracic cavity. The herniation may include the esophagogastric junction (*sliding hiatal hernia*) or a separate portion of the stomach excluding the esophagogastric junction (*paraesophageal hiatal hernia*) (Fig. 56-4). Sliding hiatal hernias occur in a large percentage of people and are often asymptomatic. Hiatal hernias may be congenital but usually develop in adult life. Contributing factors to the development of these hernias include obesity, trauma, and a general weakening of the supporting structures as a result of aging.

Clinical picture

Approximately 50% of persons with diaphragmatic hernias are asymptomatic. Heartburn resulting from reflux of gastric contents into the esophagus (p. 1391) is the predominant symptom. Dysphagia may also occur. An occasional complication includes incarceration of a portion of the stomach in the chest with constriction of the blood supply causing a sudden severe substernal pain and signs of upper gastrointestinal obstruction.

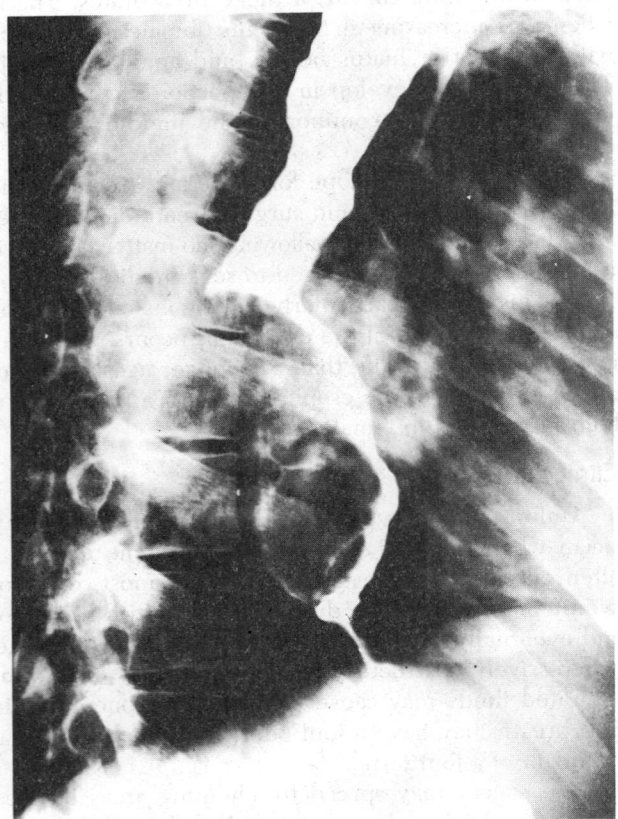

Fig. 56-3. Radiograph taken after patient had swallowed barium showing location of lesion in esophagus as it approaches stomach.

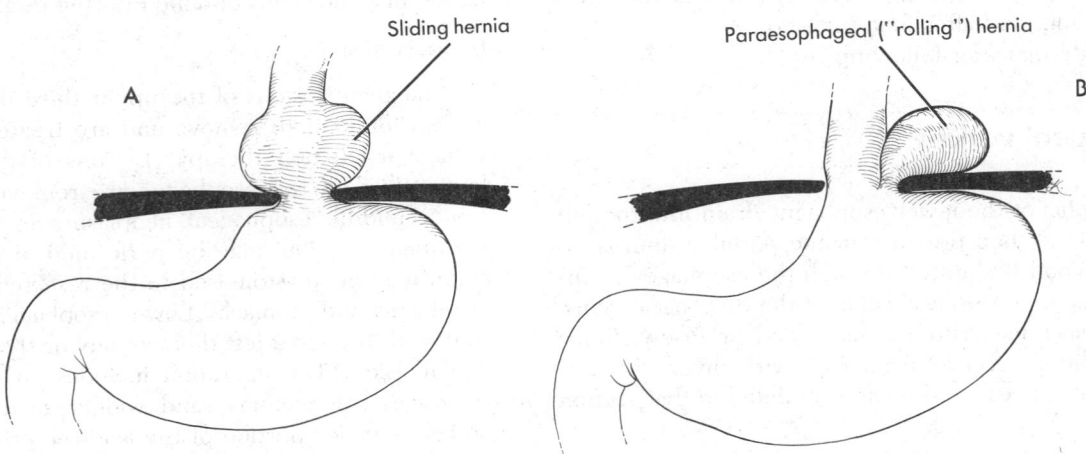

Fig. 56-4. Hiatal hernias. **A,** Sliding. **B,** Paraesophageal.

Intervention

Asymptomatic diaphragmatic hernias require no treatment. If heartburn is present, it is treated with a high-protein, low-fat diet, small frequent feedings, and antacids. Bending, lifting of heavy objects, or reclining after meals should be avoided (p. 1393). Incarcerated hernias or symptomatic paraesophageal hernias require surgery, which is performed either transthoracically or transabdominally.

Outcome criteria for the person with a diaphragmatic hernia

The person or significant others can:
1. Describe any dietary changes recommended.
   a. Plan a high-protein, low-fat diet.
   b. Keep weight at normal level and reduce weight if obese.
2. State body position and activity requirements.
   a. Avoid bending, lifting, or wearing tight, abdominal-constricting clothing.
   b. Avoid a supine position for 2 to 3 hours after eating.
   c. Elevate the head when sleeping.
3. State the action, dosage, frequency, and possible side effects of medication (antacids) to be taken at home.
4. State plans for follow-up care.

Gastric disorders

Gastritis

Etiology

Gastritis is an inflammation of the gastric mucosa and is the most common pathologic condition of the stomach. It may be acute or chronic, based on histologic criteria. Acute gastritis may be caused by exogenous or endogenous factors. The exogenous factors include (1) bacterial infections, especially staphylococcal endotoxins; (2) drugs such as alcohol, salicylates, indomethacin, sulfonamides, and steroids; (3) ingestion of corrosive substances (acid and alkali); (4) irritating foods; and (5) thermal or mechanical injuries. Endogenous factors include certain infectious diseases such as typhoid fever and viral hepatitis and allergic and systemic diseases that affect the cells of the gastric mucosa.

Pathophysiology

In acute gastritis the gastric mucosa appears red, inflamed, congested, and edematous. Acute episodes may become chronic, and various pathologic changes occur depending on the site involved. In *atrophic gastritis* there is atrophy of gastric glands and the appearance of patches of thin, gray or greenish gray mucosa and red or blue blood vessels of the submucosa on the fundus and body of the stomach. The loss of gastric mucosa will result in eventual diminution of gastric secretion and the development of pernicious anemia. Atrophic gastritis may be a precursor to gastric carcinoma.

Clinical picture

The symptoms depend on the cause of the gastritis and its severity. Some persons have only mild gastric discomfort or pain, while others have severe nausea and vomiting. In *acute hemorrhagic gastritis* the person complains of epigastric discomfort, nausea, hematemesis, and melena. There may be a severe drop in the hemoglobin and hematocrit levels. In *corrosive gastritis* caused by acid or lyes there will be bloody vomitus, bloody stools, and collapse. Death may occur secondary to blood loss or perforation of a viscus. Those who recover will have an obstruction later on. The diagnosis is made by histologic evidence obtained from gastric biopsy. The flexible, fiberoptic gastroscope makes repeated biopsies possible.

Intervention

The treatment will depend on the cause of the gastritis and the initial symptoms. Mild gastritis requires only a carminative antacid and rest. Belching and defecation often relieve the symptoms.

When nausea and vomiting are present, the person is given nothing by mouth until symptoms subside. With severe vomiting fluids and electrolytes will be replaced intravenously and a sedative such as sodium phenobarbital or an antinauseant such as prochlorperazine (Compazine) or trimethobenzamide (Tigan) will be given parenterally or by suppository. When vomiting subsides, tea, broth, and ginger ale are given orally every hour. Bland feedings of custard, gelatin, and cream soups are usually tolerated after 12 to 24 hours, and then other foods are added gradually. It may be 1 to 2 weeks before all symptoms subside and a normal diet can be resumed. Persons with epigastric discomfort will also receive antacids. When an infectious agent is the cause, appropriate antimicrobial therapy is prescribed. Persons with a positive Schilling test (p. 1195) will receive vitamin B_{12} for about 3 months.[13]

Persons with chronic superficial gastritis will usually respond to a diet that avoids highly seasoned or greasy foods and hot liquids.[13] Carbonated liquids are well tolerated.

Outcome criteria for the person with gastritis

The person or significant others can:
1. List substances that cause recurrence of the condition and should be avoided (alcohol, aspirin, spicy foods).

2. Discuss plans for a diet that meets nutritional requirements and is nonirritating.
3. Describe the medication program to be followed at home.
   a. State dosage, action, and side effects of prescribed medications such as antacids.
   b. List over-the-counter medications that are to be avoided such as apirin and aspirin-containing compounds such as Alka-Seltzer.
4. State plans for follow-up care.
   a. List community resources available to those with alcohol dependence if this is a problem.
   b. State signs and symptoms that indicate need for immediate medical assistance (recurrence of symptoms, especially nausea and vomiting, hematemesis, or bloody stools).

Peptic ulcer

A peptic ulcer is an ulceration involving the mucosa and deeper structure of the upper gastrointestinal tract and is due in part to action of the gastric juices containing acid and pepsin. The site of the peptic ulcer may be the distal esophagus, stomach, upper duodenum, or the jejunum (Fig. 56-5). Peptic ulcers are described as gastric or duodenal depending on their location. An ulcer (usually of the jejunum) occurring near the site of anastomosis is termed a *marginal* ulcer. Most *gastric ulcers* occur on the lesser curvature of the stomach. Such ulcers tend to be larger and deeper than duodenal ulcers, and they have a tendency to undergo malignant changes. *Duodenal ulcers* are not as well defined as gastric ulcers, but the pathologic condition is the same. Most of them occur on the first part of the duodenum, and they are more common than gastric ulcers.

Ulcers may be acute or chronic. Acute ulcers are usually superficial, involving only the mucosal layer. In most cases they heal within a relatively short time, but they may bleed, perforate, or become chronic. A chronic peptic ulcer is a deep crater with sharp edges and a "clean" base. It involves both the mucosa and the submucosa. If the ulcer penetrates the stomach wall and becomes adherent to an adjacent organ such as the pancreas, the organ may become the base of the ulcer.

Epidemiology

Peptic ulcer is a common disorder that occurs with varying frequencies in different geographic locations. In the United States peptic ulcer disease annually causes about 15,000 deaths and about 15 million days lost from work.[16] The incidence of peptic ulcers rose sharply from 1900 to 1914, remained relatively constant until 1955, and is now declining.[6,11] Men are affected more commonly than women, but the incidence of duodenal ulcers in women is increasing. Duodenal ulcers occur 7 to 10 times more frequently than gastric ulcers in younger adults but occur at essentially the same rate in older persons.

Etiology

Contributing to the development or delay in healing of peptic ulcers are a number of psychologic, environmental, and genetic factors.

Psychologic factors. Two common beliefs are that ulcers are more likely to occur in persons (1) experiencing stressful life events and (2) exhibiting certain traits such as tenseness or a striving for perfection or success. There is no conclusive evidence that directly relates these factors to the development of peptic ulcers although it is known that emotional tension can alter gastric function. One study in 1958 did demonstrate that persons with conflicts over dependency who also had high acid-pepsin secretory capacity had a higher tendency to develop duodenal ulcers.[6]

Environmental factors. Although the relationship between *smoking* and ulcer development is not clearly understood, cigarette smokers have a higher incidence of peptic ulcers and have delayed healing of gastric ulcers. *Diet* does not appear to be a predisposing factor although drinking coffee or cola may increase the risk whereas drinking milk may decrease the risk.

Ulcerogenic drugs such as corticosteroids, salicylates, indomethacin, and phenylbutazone (Butazolidin), when given in massive doses, may cause acute ulcers, but, with the exception of aspirin, there is no conclusive evidence that they cause chronic peptic diseases.[16] The mechanisms of these ulcerogenic drugs vary. With the antiinflammatory steroids, there is mucosal injury secondary to increased gastric secretion and reduced gastric mucus secretion. The latter is due to the steroid antiprotein synthetic action. With aspirin there is an increased exfoliation of mucous cells and a decrease in

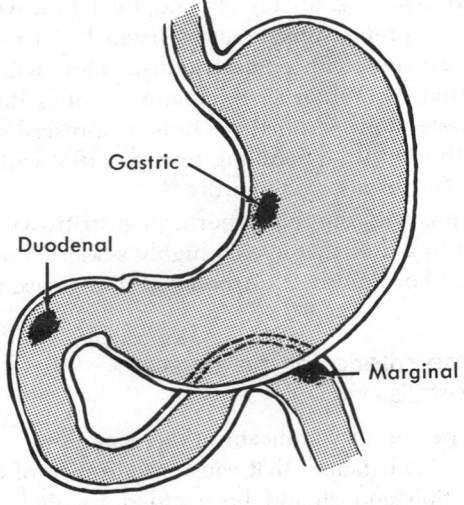

Fig. 56-5. Most common locations of peptic ulcers.

mucus production.[35] Ulcerogenic drugs may exacerbate an already existing chronic peptic ulcer.

Genetic factors. There appear to be certain intrinsic factors that are not related to environmental factors. The tendency for gastric or duodenal ulcers is inherited independently; that is, gastric ulcers occur three times more often when there is a family history of gastric ulcers, and duodenal ulcers occur three times more often with a family history of duodenal ulcers. Duodenal ulcers also occur more often in persons with type O blood and in those who are nonsecretory of blood group substances in their saliva.[11]

Pathophysiology

Gastric ulcers. Most persons with gastric ulcers have a normal gastric secretion and a normal emptying rate of the stomach. Ulceration appears to occur because of a decreased resistance of the gastric mucosa to acid-pepsin injury. Gastritis is usually present, resulting in shedding of the protective cells from the mucosal wall. A major causative factor in gastric ulcers appears to be increased *back diffusion* of gastric acid from the gastric lumen into the gastric mucosa. Free acid that has been secreted into the gastric lumen normally diffuses back into the tissues at a very slow rate. Rapid diffusion causes local histamine release with a subsequent inflammatory reaction, resulting in leakage of interstitial and plasma fluid into the gastric lumen, bleeding, and tissue damage. The natural barriers to back diffusion of gastric acid can be broken down by bile acids, alcohol, and salicylates. The greater reflux of bile-containing duodenal contents seen with gastric ulcers may be caused by deficient contractile response of the pylorus to cholecystokinin and secretin.[27] Cigarette smoking has been shown to increase bile reflux into the stomach.[11]

Duodenal ulcers. Persons with duodenal ulcers have an increase in gastric acid secretory rate. The capacity to secrete gastric acid is determined by the number of parietal cells in the gastric mucosa; these cells are increased in the person with a duodenal ulcer. A second reason for the increased gastric acid secretion is the change in gastrin levels. Gastrin, which is a peptide hormone released into the antrum by vagal stimulation, is a potent stimulator of gastric secretion. Gastrin levels are normal in persons with duodenal ulcers when the stomach is empty but increase postprandially. Thus both basal gastric acid secretion and postprandial gastric acid secretion are increased in the person with a duodenal ulcer.

In addition to increased gastric acid secretion with duodenal ulcer, there is a markedly increased rate of gastric emptying. Protein is a food substance that normally acts as a buffer for gastric acid. When the stomach empties more rapidly, this buffering mechanism is decreased and more gastric acid moves into the duodenum. The end result of the increased rate of gastric acid secretion and gastric emptying is an increased amount of acid content propelled into the duodenum causing irritation and breakdown of the duodenal mucosa.

Stress ulcers. Acute ulcers that are distinct from peptic ulcers may result when persons are experiencing life-threatening events such as severe trauma, burns, shock, sepsis, advanced carcinoma, or acute respiratory insufficiency. Possible causative factors have been identified as mucosal ischemia or mucus deficiency. *Cushing's ulcers,* which are associated with CNS lesions or injury such as brain injury, cerebrovascular accident, or brain tumors, more nearly resemble ordinary peptic ulcers in that increased levels of gastrin and gastric acid secretion are present. In all stress ulcers, hemorrhage and perforation usually occur without warning since pain is rare. Patients in intensive care units are monitored closely for signs of upper gastrointestinal bleeding, which usually occurs 7 to 10 days after the initial life-threatening insult to the body.

Zollinger-Ellison syndrome. Zollinger-Ellison syndrome, first described in 1955, refers to the peptic ulceration associated with a noninsulin-producing islet cell tumor of the pancreas. The syndrome is characterized by one or more peptic ulcerations occurring in the lower end of the esophagus, stomach, duodenum, and jejunum and by enormous gastric hypersecretion and acidity and the presence of nonbeta (non-β-) islet cell adenomas of the pancreas. Frequently, the syndrome is accompanied by diarrhea and steatorrhea. The latter is thought to be caused by lack of pancreatic lipase needed for fat digestion, whereas the diarrhea may result from large quantities of acid passing into the duodenum. Diarrhea of long duration can cause serious loss of electrolytes (potassium and sodium in particular) and may prove fatal.

These tumors of the pancreas have been found to produce enormous quantities of gastrin or a gastrinlike substance that is responsible for the excessive stimulation of gastric acid and the subsequent ulcerations. Because of the repeated reappearance of the peptic ulcers and the multiple and aberrant locations, it is usually impossible to resect all areas involved.

Clinical picture

The person who has a peptic ulcer usually complains of pain that is characteristic in its nature, intensity, radiation, location, and periodicity. Initial attacks of pain often occur in the spring and the fall, last for a few weeks, and then disappear. The pain is described as gnawing, aching, or burning. It is usually located in the upper abdomen, near the midline, and it is usually confined to a small area. However, it may radiate around the costal border or to the back. Pain usually starts 1 to 2 hours after eating, when the stomach begins to empty, and it may disappear spontaneously, after the ingestion of food, or after the ingestion of an antacid medication such as aluminum hydroxide gel. If the ulcer is severe it may cause pain at night. It is not unusual for the person to awaken with pain during the night, when gastric secretion is at its peak.

Although pain is felt at the site of the existing lesion, it is known that normal stomach mucosa does not have pain sensation. It is thought therefore that the inflamed mucosa around the ulcer must be sensitive to the gastric secretions because inflammation lowers the pain threshold. Some persons never experience pain, and the peptic ulcer may be discovered accidentally by x-ray or postmortem examination. Other less common symptoms include nausea, vomiting, or excessive salivation.

The diagnosis of peptic ulcer is made from the patient's history, a gastrointestinal series, a gastric analysis, and stool examinations for occult (hidden) blood. Direct visualization of the ulcer by endoscopy differentiates gastric ulcer from gastric carcinoma. Development of the flexible fiberoptic panendoscope (p. 1382) has greatly improved the diagnosis and evaluation of healing of gastric ulcers. Selective angiography is becoming useful in the diagnosis and evaluation of treatment of gastric hemorrhage when it is combined with endoscopy.

Intervention

Treatment is directed toward relief of symptoms, healing of the ulcer, prevention of complications, and prevention of recurrence. The majority of peptic ulcers heal under medical treatment. Surgery is used most often following a second or third recurrence and in the treatment of complications.

Treatment consists in the use of antacids and anticholinergic medications to relieve pain, avoidance of known causative or irritating drugs and foods, and an attempt to decrease stress by rest and counseling. New medications are showing some promise by increasing the rate of healing.

Antacids. Drugs that decrease ulcer pain by lowering the acidity of gastric secretions have been used for many years. Antacids reduce gastric acidity by physical absorption or by chemical neutralization. They do not hasten healing but do appear clinically to decrease pain. Antacids of choice are the nonsystemic antacids (Table 56-1), which are poorly absorbed from the stomach and therefore do not alter the pH of the blood or interfere with normal acid-base balance. Sodium bicarbonate is readily absorbed and therefore should be avoided as an antacid for relief of ulcer pain. Also the reaction of sodium bicarbonate and hydrochloric acid forms carbon dioxide, which may cause distention.

Antacids may be administered frequently, and if symptoms are severe it may be necessary to give them as often as every 30 to 60 minutes. When given in a fasting state, the buffering power is usually transitory. For maximal effectiveness antacids should be given *1 hour* after meals; this produces a buffering effect lasting approximately 3 to 4 hours. Liquids are more effective than tablets. If tablets are used they should be chewed slowly to permit complete pulverization. Aluminum hydroxide becomes less reactive over time and should not be given with anticholinergic drugs or with tetracycline since it interferes with absorption of these drugs.

Histamine antagonist. *Cimetidine* is a drug that decreases secretion of gastric acid by inhibiting the action of histamine at the histamine H_2 receptors of the parietal cells. Cimetidine is not an antihistamine drug. It has been demonstrated to produce an increased healing effect on ulcers in addition to a decrease of symptoms. No effect on the recurrence of ulcers has been noted, but both day and night pain are decreased, thus decreasing the use of antacids. For persons with Zollinger-Ellison syndrome, diarrhea and anorexia are decreased. Cimetidine therapy may extend for 8 weeks. Side effects include muscle pain, transient diarrhea, dizziness, and rash. Cimetidine is given in doses of 300 mg four times a day (with meals and at bedtime). The person should be encouraged to continue therapy for the prescribed period even when symptoms have abated.

Anticholinergic drugs. The usefulness of anticholinergic drugs in the treatment of peptic ulcer has not been shown conclusively. Anticholinergic drugs have theoretic value because they decrease gastric acid secretion and delay gastric emptying. In practice, however, they are less effective than antacids or cimetidine, although they appear to have an additive inhibiting effect when given with cimetidine.[6] Anticholinergic drugs may be useful in relief of nocturnal pain by delaying emptying of the evening snack. When given to relieve ulcer pain, anticholinergic drugs are usually prescribed in dosages that produce side effects such as dry mouth, blurring of vision, headache, constipation, or urinary retention. The more commonly used anticholinergic drugs include propantheline bromide (Pro-Banthine), glycopyrrolate (Robinul), and oxyphencyclimine hydrochloride (Daricon).

Other drugs. *Carbenoxolene,* an extract of licorice, has been reported to hasten gastric healing by increasing the production and viscosity of gastric mucus. The drug is structurally similar to aldosterone, and side effects include hypertension, fluid retention, and hypokalemia. A thiazide diuretic may be given to counteract the side effects.

Prostaglandins, which are under clinical study as a form of treatment for peptic ulcers, are naturally occurring unsaturated fatty acids found in various body tissues. They are divided into groups A, E, and F on the basis of their chemical structure. Prostaglandins of the E and A groups are potent inhibitors of gastric secretion and inhibit the formation of peptic ulcers in experimen-

TABLE 56-1. Commonly used antacids

Trade name	Drug composition	Comments
Maalox	Magnesium and aluminum hydroxide	Preferred antacid Good buffering effect Good taste Nonconstipating Low sodium content Can cause hypermagnesemia in persons with renal failure
Maalox Plus	Magnesium and aluminum hydroxide Simethicone	Same as above Antiflatus
Mylanta	Magnesium and aluminum hydroxide Simethicone	Same as Maalox Plus
Amphogel	Aluminum hydroxide gel	Constipating Can interfere with absorption of anticholinergic drugs Contains sodium Decreases absorption of phosphate Good antacid effect Give with water so that medication reaches stomach Can be given by continuous drip (1 part Amphogel to 2 or 3 parts water)
Gelusil	Magnesium trisilicate Magnesium and aluminum hydroxide	Slower buffering effect Gelatin effect in stomach to coat and protect the ulcer Nonconstipating
Riopan	Magaldrate (chemical combination of magnesium and aluminum hydroxide)	Rapid antacid action High acid-buffering effect No acid rebound Nonconstipating Low sodium content Can cause hypermagnesemia in persons with renal failure
Marblen	Magnesium and calcium carbonate Aluminum hydroxide Magnesium trisilicate	Neutralizes more acid than other antacids Nonconstipating Low sodium content
Alka-2	Calcium carbonate	Rapid neutralization of acid Constipating May cause hypercalcemia May cause acid rebound Not suitable for long-term therapy

tal animals.[27] Oral administration of a synthetic prostaglandin analogue has demonstrated beneficial effects in the healing of gastric ulcers during early clinical trials.[11] Side effects of high dosages include diarrhea and abdominal cramps.

Diet. Over the years many theories and diet prescriptions have been suggested for the treatment of peptic ulcers. Modified *Sippy* diets are based on the acid-buffering power of food proteins. Constant dilution and neutralization of stomach contents are achieved by giving whole milk, skim milk, and half milk–half cream punctually every hour. Bland foods are then added at specified intervals. *Bland* diets (diets that exclude "irritating" foods) have also been used. The interpretation of what constitutes a bland diet differs from hospital to hospital and from one part of the country to another.

There is no experimental evidence that modifying the diet accelerates healing of an uncomplicated peptic ulcer.[6] Spices such as pepper or roughage foods such as bran have not been shown to be ulcerogenic, although they may not be tolerated by some persons. Substances that have been demonstrated to increase acid secretions are caffeine-containing beverages such as coffee, tea, and cola drinks. Individuals may find that certain foods increase ulcer pain; if so, these foods should be avoided. Eating frequent small feedings provides an acid-neutralizing effect. Overdistention of the stomach should be avoided also since this predisposes to reflux.

If milk and antacids are given by continuous tube feeding for severe symptoms, the prescribed amount is spaced over the 24-hour period and must include sufficient water to supply the patient's daily needs. Only a small amount of milk is placed in the dispensing bag at one time to prevent the milk from becoming sour. A mechanical food pump may also be used.

Rest. If the person has severe pain or complications that do not respond to treatment at home, hospitalization will be necessary. Nursing care that provides a regular, smooth routine is the goal. Meals, medications, and treatments need to be given at correctly spaced intervals and on time. Noise, rush, confusion, and impatience on the part of members of the staff are avoided. Since rest means different things to different people, the person is assisted in identifying those activities that specifically achieve mental and physical rest for him or her.

Surgery. Emergency surgery is necessary when a peptic ulcer perforates and causes peritonitis or erodes a blood vessel causing severe hemorrhage. Elective surgery may be performed if the ulcer does not respond to the medical regimen and continues to produce symptoms, if it causes pyloric obstruction, or if a chronic recurring gastric ulcer is thought to be precancerous. The basic surgical procedures for treatment of peptic ulcers are (1) subtotal gastrectomy, which includes gastroduodenostomy or gastrojejunostomy, (2) vagotomy, (3) antrectomy, (4) pyloroplasty, and (5) total gastrectomy (esophagojejunostomy). Subtotal gastrectomy is now rarely performed alone but is usually combined with a form of vagotomy. Pyloroplasty is also combined with a vagotomy. The several common surgical combinations are listed in Table 56-2.

It is now generally accepted that surgical treatment of *duodenal* ulcers includes a vagotomy, which removes vagal stimulation to acid-pepsin stimulation and reduces the responsiveness of the parietal cells of the stomach. There are three types of vagotomy currently in use:

truncal, selective, and proximal. *Truncal vagotomy* consists of a resection of a small segment of each vagal nerve as it enters the abdomen on the distal esophagus (Fig. 56-6). *Selective vagotomy* severs the gastric branch of each vagus nerve just beyond the point where the nerve divides into the gastric and extragastric branches, thus preserving vagal stimulation of other organs.[16] With both truncal and selective vagotomies gastric emptying is inhibited; thus a pyloroplasty or antrectomy must be performed to prevent gastric stasis by enlarging the pyloric opening. *Proximal vagotomy* or *parietal cell vagotomy* is a procedure that has been used widely in Europe and increasingly in the United States.[6] Only those branches of the gastric portion of the vagal nerves that innervate the upper two thirds of the stomach are severed, thus maintaining effective gastric emptying. Since a pyloroplasty or antrectomy is unnecessary with a proximal vagotomy, there is no intrusion into the gastric lumen, and side effects, especially diarrhea, are reduced.

A *pyloroplasty* or drainage procedure widens the pyloric outlet. It is performed with a truncal or selective vagotomy to prevent gastric stasis. It may also be performed for pyloric stenosis (p. 1425). There are various types of pyloroplasties; in the United States the Heineke-Mikulicz pyloroplasty (Fig. 56-7) is most commonly selected.

Subtotal gastrectomy consists of removal of one half to two thirds of the lower part of the stomach with anastomosis of the remaining segment to the duodenum (Billroth I) or to the side of the proximal jejunum (Billroth II) (Fig. 56-8). The Billroth I procedure is the traditional procedure for a gastric ulcer whereas the Billroth II is usually preferred for a duodenal ulcer because of decreased duodenal ulcer recurrence. The duodenal stump is preserved to permit bile flow into the jejunum to mix with the food. Physiologically, subtotal gastrectomy removes the gastrin source in the antrum and some of the acid-pepsin secreting parietal cells. Side effects

TABLE 56-2. Comparison of different types of surgery for peptic ulcer

Type of surgery	Advantages	Disadvantages
Truncal vagotomy with pyloroplasty	Low operative mortality and morbidity	High recurrence rate
Selective vagotomy with pyloroplasty	Preservation of vagal innervation of viscus	More difficult to perform than truncal vagotomy
	Fewer side effects than truncal vagotomy	
Proximal vagotomy	Preserves gastric emptying; low recurrence rate; fewer side effects; no intrusion of gastrointestinal tract	Newer procedure; requires experienced surgeon
Vagotomy with antrectomy	Lower recurrence rate than for vagotomy with pyloroplasty	Higher operative mortality; Greater side effects

include loss of reservoir function with rapid emptying and dispersion of food through the small intestine, thus decreasing the effect of pancreatic enzymes.[6] Stasis with subsequent infection in the blind loop of the Billroth II may also occur. Both the rapid emptying and the blind loop stasis may produce malabsorption, leading to weight loss and vitamin B_{12} deficiency.

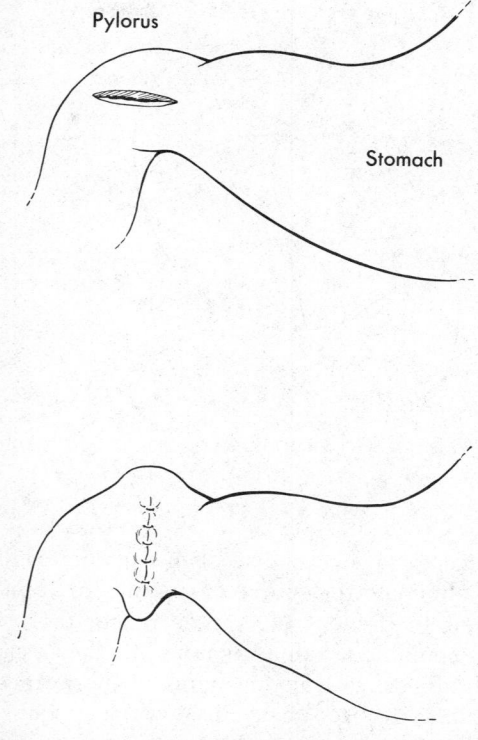

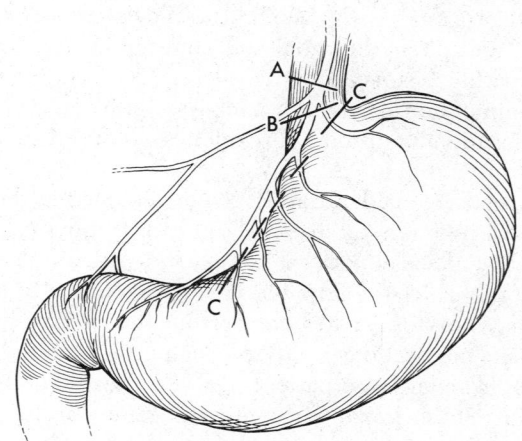

Fig. 56-6. Different types of vagotomies: truncal (*A*); selective (*B*); proximal or parietal cell (*C*).

Fig. 56-7. Heineke-Mikulicz pyloroplasty. A longitudinal incision across pylorus is pulled apart and closed in a transverse position to widen pyloric outlet.

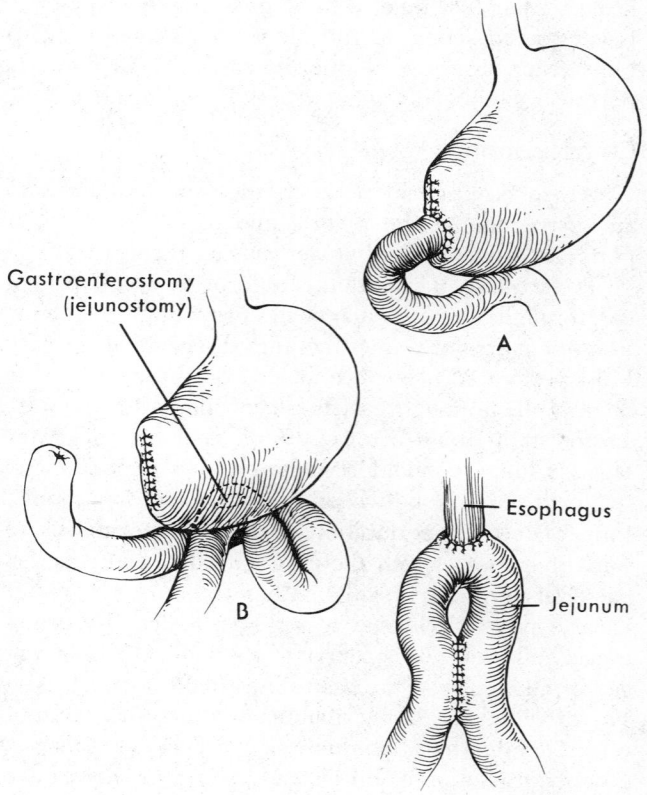

Fig. 56-8. Types of gastric resections and anastomoses. **A,** Gastric resection with anastomosis of remaining segment of stomach with duodenum (Billroth I). **B,** Gastric resection with closure of duodenum and anastomosis of remaining segment of stomach to jejunum (Billroth II). **C,** Total gastrectomy with anastomosis of esophagus to jejunum; duodenum has been closed.

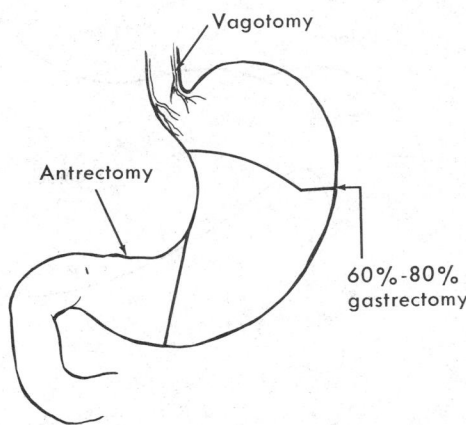

Fig. 56-9. Some surgical approaches used in treatment of peptic ulcer.

Antrectomy, or removal of the antrum of the stomach to eliminate the source of gastrin (Fig. 56-9), is not sufficient to prevent ulcer recurrence; therefore it is usually combined with a vagotomy. Either a gastroduodenostomy or gastrojejunostomy is performed. *Total gastrectomy* has too many disadvantages for the treatment of peptic ulcer (p. 1401).

For special considerations in the nursing care of persons undergoing gastric surgery, the reader is referred to p. 1399.

Preventive health teaching. The person with an ulcer needs to understand about factors that contribute to the development of ulcers and about excesses in lifestyle that may cause the ulcer to become reactivated. If removal from stressful environmental influences is impossible, the person must learn to cope with the stressful situations without reactivating the ulcer. Occasionally, the person is advised to obtain psychologic counseling to better understand his or her problems and thus be better able to cope with them.

The person should practice moderation in diet and activities of work and play. Dietary teaching should include avoidance of situations that cause emotional stress before and during meals. Meals should be eaten slowly in a quiet environment. The work situation sometimes makes the selection and eating of suitable meals difficult. If the selection of food is limited, the person can take milk in a vacuum bottle to supplement the limited selection. If situations at work or at home are emotionally upsetting, the person can eat frequent feedings and drink milk between meals. These measures may prevent a serious exacerbation of the ulcer. Alcohol should be avoided as much as possible since it tends to increase the secretion of acid and is irritating to the gastric mucosa, particularly if taken on an empty stomach. Some physicians allow their patients to take small amounts of alcohol with their meals.

Since there seems to be a relationship between smoking and irritation of a peptic ulcer, most physicians believe that the person who has a peptic ulcer should give up smoking permanently. To do so is often very difficult, since often the person's life and work situations as well as personality are such that a change of this sort is a major one. For some persons the stress of trying to give up smoking causes greater irritation of the ulcer than does the smoking. These persons are permitted to continue smoking, but moderation is strictly advised.

Ulcerogenic drugs such as salicylates, corticosteroids, and phenylbutazone are contraindicated for persons with a history of peptic ulcer. Medication such as acetaminophen (Tylenol) and Ascriptin (aspirin and magnesium aluminum hydroxide) can be used safely for relief of mild pain.

If every consideration is given to adjusting the prescribed regimen to fit the appropriate physical, economic, and social pattern, the person with an ulcer will be better able to follow the treatment. Some individuals may not appear to benefit from the dietary modifications, medications, and counseling, and they return to the hospital or outpatient health center several times a year. These persons require the same careful attention as that given to the newly diagnosed patient so that any underlying feelings of staff rejection are avoided.

The person who has had a symptomatic peptic ulcer must remain under medical supervision for about a year. Periodic x-ray examinations of the stomach may be advised to determine the extent to which the ulcer has healed. After that time, if healing is complete, the client is advised to report to the physician at once if symptoms reappear, since peptic ulcers can recur after the person has enjoyed several years of good health.

Complications

A peptic ulcer may perforate the stomach wall, cause an obstruction at the pyloric end of the stomach, or perforate a major blood vessel causing hemorrhage.

Perforation. Perforation is an erosion of a peptic ulcer through the muscular wall, providing an opening from the gastrointestinal tract into the peritoneal cavity. Most perforated ulcers are located on the anterior duodenal wall, although gastric ulcers may also perforate, and occur in about 5% to 10% of ulcer patients. Mortality is highest in older women and is dependent on the length of time between perforation and treatment.[16] Immediately on perforation a chemical peritonitis results from contact with the gastrointestinal contents, and bacterial peritonitis results within 12 hours.

The patient who has a perforated ulcer has symptoms similar to those occurring when any abdominal organ or other part of the gastrointestinal tract perforates. The extremely irritating qualities of the gastric contents released into the abdominal cavity, however, may be quite overwhelming and lead to prostration and severe shock in a short time. There is a sudden sharp pain that spreads quickly over the abdomen. Characteristically, the patient bends over with pain and draws up the knees to prevent pull on the abdominal wall. The person is reluctant to move, holds the body tense, and protests against having the abdomen touched. On palpation the abdomen is found to be boardlike and very tender. The patient usually perspires profusely, and the facial expression is one of agony and apprehension. Breathing is rapid and shallow to prevent pull on abdominal muscles. Body temperature is usually normal or subnormal, and the pulse is usually rapid and weak. A positive diagnosis is made by taking a radiograph of the abdomen with the patient standing. If the ulcer has perforated, air under the diaphragm is visible on the film. Patients taking corticosteroids may develop a peptic ulcer and perforation without exhibiting any of the usual symptoms.

Some perforations are minor and close within a short time or wall themselves off. However, most perforations require surgery and should be closed surgically as soon as possible. The longer the perforation exists, allowing the irritating (and infected) gastrointestinal secretions to pour into the abdominal cavity, the higher the mortality becomes.

Immediate therapy consists of passing a nasogastric tube, connecting it to continuous suction to drain gastric contents. Following the initial emptying of the stomach, the suction is generally returned to the intermittent level. Nothing is given orally. Parenteral fluids are given to combat fluid and electrolyte imbalance, and antibiotics are administered. The patient is kept in low Fowler's position so that the gastric contents that have escaped will collect in the pelvic cavity and will be more accessible surgically. The patient is very frightened and apprehensive, and the nurse should stay in the room to explain what is being done, and what will be done in surgery and to offer reassurance.

Surgery may consist of simple laparotomy with closure of the perforation and aspiration from the peritoneum of all escaped gastrointestinal fluid. A large majority of persons who have had a perforated ulcer, however, continue to have recurrences of ulcer symptoms; therefore most surgeons now perform definitive ulcer surgery, such as vagotomy with gastric resection or pyloroplasty, if the patient's condition permits.

Postoperatively, the patient is observed carefully for signs of continuing peritonitis and for abscess formation. Elevation of temperature, respiratory distress, continued abdominal pain, and signs of paralytic ileus such as distention, hyperactive or absent bowel sounds, and the inability to pass flatus or stool are reported to the physician. The physician may also perform periodic rectal examinations to determine the presence of pelvic masses caused by abscess formation. Such an abscess may need to be incised and drained. (A full discussion of the complications of peritonitis is given on p. 1482.)

Pyloric obstruction. Pyloric obstruction may be caused by edema of tissues around an ulcer or by scar tissue from a healed ulcer located near the pylorus. It may be only partial and cause dilation of the stomach, or it may be complete. Persons with this complication may have severe projectile vomiting that may or may not be preceded by nausea. A positive diagnosis is made by gastrointestinal tract x-ray examination and gastric analysis.

Obstruction caused by edema and spasm generally responds to medical management. The stomach is first decompressed by means of a large-bore tube to remove all food particles; this is then followed by 72 hours of gastric decompression with a standard nasogastric tube. During this period attention is given to correction of the metabolic alkalosis and dehydration that occur from loss of gastric contents.

At the end of the 72-hour period a *saline load test* is performed to assess the degree of gastric emptying; 700 ml of normal saline at room temperature is introduced through the nasogastric tube over a 3- to 5-minute period and the tube is then clamped. After 30 minutes the stomach is aspirated. A residual volume of more than 350 ml indicates continued pyloric obstruction, and surgery consisting of either a vagotomy with pyloroplasty or gastrectomy is considered. If the saline load test demonstrates improved gastric emptying, oral liquids and antacids are introduced with continued assessment of gastric emptying for several days. Solid foods are introduced gradually as tolerated.

Hemorrhage. Peptic ulcers cause bleeding in about 15% to 20% of all persons who have the disease.[6] If the ulcer has perforated a major blood vessel, the patient may have a severe hemorrhage, vomiting large amounts of blood and passing tarry stools. Vomiting of blood usually occurs with a gastric ulcer, whereas tarry stools are more common with a bleeding duodenal ulcer. It must be remembered, however, that the color of the stool may depend more on the length of time the blood has been within the intestine than on the actual source of the hemorrhage. About 25% of patients with hemorrhage have never had recognizable symptoms of ulcer previously.[6]

The patient may also complain of feeling faint, dizzy, and thirsty, and may become dyspneic, apprehensive, and restless as the blood volume is reduced, the blood pressure drops, the pulse rate increases, and signs of shock become apparent. The systemic signs of hemorrhage may appear before (or without) hematemesis and before passage of blood or tarry stools.

The patient with a bleeding ulcer is placed on bed rest and is given a sedative such as phenobarbital sodium to alleviate restlessness and apprehension. Morphine sulfate may be used, since it aids rest and also helps to slow down intestinal peristalsis. Anticholinergic drugs are not given because they obscure signs of bleeding (hyperactive bowel sounds). The blood pressure, pulse rate, and respirations are checked and recorded frequently (as often as every 15 minutes when acute bleeding is suspected). Blood transfusions are often given slowly to avoid increasing the blood pressure and thereby increasing the bleeding. Vital signs and urinary output are monitored frequently to determine the body's response to fluid replacement and possible continuation of the hemorrhage.

If the patient is not vomiting and only a small amount of blood is being passed rectally, milk is given every hour and antacids are prescribed. A full bland diet may be ordered because it maintains nutrition, neutralizes gastric acidity, reduces absorption of the formed clot, and slows peristalsis. If the patient is vomiting blood, however, nothing is given orally. All bloody vomitus is measured and described. The physician may wish it saved for inspection. A nasogastric tube may be passed and attached to suction to collect the blood so that it can be more accurately measured and replaced by transfusion. The fluid and electrolyte balance are maintained by infusions. Sometimes there is an order to irrigate the tube with iced physiologic saline solution or iced tap water or a combination of iced saline and water. If so, the irrigating fluid usually must be suctioned back, since the iced fluid causes blood to clot not only in the stomach but also within the tube. The patient who is vomiting blood will need special mouth care. A weak solution of hydrogen peroxide may be used to remove blood from the tongue, teeth, and gums more easily.

The number of tarry (or currant jelly–like) stools are also measured and recorded, and they may be saved for laboratory examination. Since the patient may be alarmed at the sight of blood, all evidence of bleeding is quickly removed from the bedside, and the linen is changed as needed without disturbing the patient any more than necessary. The patient should be told that blood transfusions are given to replace the lost blood and that rest and quiet will help stop the bleeding. The sedative or narcotic should be given regularly to allay anxiety and apprehension. If large doses of sedative and narcotic drugs are given, attention must be directed toward turning the patient hourly and encouraging deep breathing to prevent the possibility of respiratory congestion.

The mortality from upper gastrointestinal tract hemorrhage is about 10% and is more common in those over 50 years of age. Bleeding gastric ulcers are more likely to result in death than are bleeding duodenal ulcers because persons with gastric ulcers are usually older and the bleeding from gastric ulcers tends to be more severe. Of those who survive hemorrhage, 30% to 50% will hemorrhage again.

The question of which is the most effective surgery for the patient with a bleeding ulcer has been a source of controversy in the past. There is now convincing evidence that vagotomy with pyloroplasty, which has the advantage of simplicity and decreased mortality, is as effective in prevention of rebleeding as a gastrectomy.[16] If the bleeding is controlled by medical means but the patient has a second bleeding episode, elective surgery is considered.

The general principles of nursing a patient after gastric surgery are applicable (p. 1400). The drainage from the nasogastric tube is usually dark red for 6 to 12 hours after surgery but should turn greenish yellow within 24 hours. The patient may continue to pass tarry stools for several days postoperatively, but this is usually because the blood from the hemorrhage before surgery has not yet completely passed through the gastrointestinal tract. Stools may be guaiac positive for several days after bleeding stops.

Outcome criteria for the person with a peptic ulcer

The person or significant others can:
1. Describe plans for dietary management (not going for long times without eating, avoiding irritating foods).
2. Explain the need to be relaxed while eating (not eating on the run).
3. Explain the need for planned rest periods following food ingestion.
4. Describe medication program to be followed at home.
   a. Describe dosage, action, and possible side effects of medications (antacids, cimetidine).
   b. Discuss need to keep antacids at work or with them.
   c. State when the dosage and timing of the antacids may be safely and therapeutically increased (dietary indiscretion).
   d. List over-the-counter medications that are not used unless specifically ordered (aspirin products, scopolamine derivatives, bicarbonate of soda).
5. Discuss ways by which home and work environment can be structured so that stressors are kept at a reasonable level.
6. Describe how to obtain professional and community resources necessary to structure a satisfactory life-style.
7. List symptoms requiring medical follow-up (return of previous symptoms, onset of symptoms suggesting perforation or bleeding).
8. State plans for health maintenance and follow-up care.

Cancer of the stomach

Epidemiology and etiology

Almost all gastric tumors are malignant. The incidence of cancer of the stomach has decreased dramatically over the past 50 years; nevertheless, gastric cancer accounts for approximately 14,000 deaths each year in the United States and is the seventh most common cause of cancer-related mortality.[1] It affects men twice as often as women and occurs more frequently in blacks and Orientals than in whites. It rarely occurs under the age of 40 and is most frequent between the ages of 50 and 70.

The cause of gastric cancer remains unknown. Although no environmental or dietary factors have been directly implicated, epidemiologic studies have suggested influencing factors of low socioeconomic status, urban living, and dietary intakes high in salted fish or starches and low in vegetables or fruits.[6,16] Genetic factors have also been associated with a higher incidence. Persons with pernicious anemia have a 10% chance of developing gastric cancer.[6]

Pathophysiology

Cancer may develop in any part of the stomach but is found most often in the distal third. Most gastric cancers are adenocarcinomas and occur either in polypoid, ulcerative, or infiltrative forms. Growth of the tumors is either by expansion forming discrete tumor nodules or by individual cell infiltration. Gastric cancer may spread directly through the stomach wall into adjacent tissues, to the lymphatics, to the regional lymph nodes of the stomach, to the esophagus, spleen, pancreas, and liver, or through the bloodstream to the lungs or bones. Involvement of regional lymph nodes occurs early followed by involvement of the more distal nodes, such as supraclavicular (Virchow's) nodes. There is a tendency toward intraperitoneal seeding, particularly to the peritoneal cul-de-sac. Prognosis depends on the depth of invasion and extent of metastasis.

Clinical picture

Unfortunately, the person with cancer of the stomach usually has no symptoms until the growth spreads to adjacent organs. Symptoms may occur only after the disease has become incurable. Vague and persistent symptoms of gastric distress, flatulence, loss of appetite, nausea, gradual weight loss, and loss of strength may be the only complaints of the patient. These vague symptoms should never be ignored, and the person is encouraged to seek immediate medical advice. However, since such symptoms are not necessarily symptoms of cancer, the person should not be unduly frightened. Pain does not appear usually until late in the disease, and the absence of this symptom is often the reason for the delay in seeking medical help. If the disease progresses untreated, marked cachexia develops, and eventually a palpable mass can often be felt in the region of the stomach. Often no early gastric symptoms appear, and fatigue, persistent anemia, and weight loss may be the only signs.

A positive diagnosis of gastric carcinoma is usually made by means of a gastrointestinal tract x-ray series. The tumor may not be evident in its early stages, and the x-ray examinations may have to be repeated at intervals. Gastroscopy with biopsy is used to determine the type and site of the lesion. It also may identify small lesions not visible on x-ray film. An absence of free hydrochloric acid in stomach secretions obtained by gastric aspiration is suggestive of a gastric neoplasm. Gastric cytologic studies may demonstrate the presence of malignant cells in the stomach. Occult blood is frequently found in the stools.

Intervention

The cure rate for gastric carcinoma is very low, only about 10%, since metastasis is usually present when the diagnosis is made. The only curative treatment for gastric cancer is surgery; the type and extent of the surgery depend on the site and extent of the lesion. A subtotal gastrectomy is the most common procedure, usually a Billroth II (p. 1421). A proximal subtotal gastrectomy may be performed for tumors of the cardia or fundus of the stomach; total gastrectomy is now rarely performed. Palliative surgery is often indicated when metastasis is present. Surgery involves removal of adjacent infiltrated tissue, such as the omentum, and adjacent lymph nodes. Persons who have lost more than 10% of their body weight are usually given a course of total parenteral nutrition (TPN) before surgery. (For care of the person undergoing gastric surgery, see p. 1399.)

Combined drug chemotherapy has been found to prolong survival. Commonly used chemotherapeutic agents include 5-fluorouracil (5-FU) with mitomycin C, methyl-CCNU, BCNU, or cytosine arabinoside. Radiation therapy combined with chemotherapy may prolong survival in persons with inoperable gastric adenocarcinoma (see Chapter 25).

Pyloric stenosis

Etiology

Pyloric stenosis in the adult is usually the result of previous duodenal ulceration or carcinoma. It is one of the most common conditions requiring surgery in infancy. It occurs most often in infants of tense, apprehensive parents and is seen most often in firstborn children. In children the cause is hypertrophy of the sphincter muscle of the pylorus, which often may be felt as a tumor mass in the right upper quadrant of the infant's abdomen.

Clinical picture

Pyloric stenosis causes vomiting that usually is forceful and occurs soon after eating. The copious vomiting requires urgent attention because fluid and electrolyte loss follows rapidly. As the condition persists and loss of weight occurs, peristaltic waves can be seen passing across the abdomen from right to left and reversing immediately before vomiting. Symptoms in infants usually appear in the second or third week of life and seldom develop after 3 or 4 months of age.

Intervention

Pyloric stenosis is treated medically before surgery is considered. If it is treated early before hypertrophy is pronounced and malnutrition is severe, surgery may be avoided. Medical treatment consists of administering small amounts of sedative drugs such as phenobarbital or the alkaloids of belladonna such as atropine or methantheline bromide (Banthine) in regular doses several times a day, usually preceding meals, and modifying the diet. Smaller feedings may be given at more frequent intervals, and cereals may be substituted for some of the milk, since solid foods are less easily vomited. The infant needs a quiet, relaxed environment. Very gentle rocking before and immediately following meals sometimes helps. If the infant is at home, the community health nurse can often help the family to ensure a more relaxed environment for the infant. Sometimes, for example, it appears that a mother's fears about whether she is properly caring for her baby contribute to the infant's difficulties.

Surgical treatment for pyloric stenosis is used when the condition does not respond to medical treatment alone. It consists of incision into the sphincter muscle of the pylorus (pylorotomy, Ramstedt's operation), and the response to this treatment is almost uniformly good.

REFERENCES AND SELECTED READINGS

1. American Cancer Society, Inc.: 1980 Cancer facts and figures, New York, 1980, The Society.
2. American Medical Association drug evaluations, ed. 3, Acton, Mass., 1977, Publishing Sciences Group, Inc.
3. Arvanitakis, C.: Diet therapy in gastrointestinal disease: a commentary, J. Am. Diet. Assoc. 75:449-453, 1979.
4. Ayulo, J.A.: Hiatus hernia: a review, Am. J. Gastroenterol. 58:579-593, 1972.
5. Barreras, R.F.: Facts, anecdotes, and new horizons in the medical treatment of duodenal ulcers, Surg. Clin. North Am. 56:1243-1248, 1976.
6. Beeson, P.B., McDermott, W., and Wyngarden, J.B., editors: Textbook of medicine, ed 15, Philadelphia, 1979, W.B. Saunders Co.
7. Bockus, H.L.: Gastroenterology, ed. 3, Philadelphia, 1974, W.B. Saunders Co.
8. Brunner, L.S.: What to do (and what to teach your patient) about peptic ulcer, Nurs. '76 6(11):27-31, 1976.
9. *Bruya, M., and Madeira, N.: Stomatitis after chemotherapy, Am. J. Nurs. 75:1349-1452, 1975.
10. Bryant, L., et al.: Comparison of ice water and ice saline solution for gastric lavage in gastroduodenal hemorrhage, Am. J. Surg. 124:570-572, 1972.
11. Chapman, M.L.: Peptic ulcer: a medical perspective, Med. Clin. North Am. 62:39-49, 1978.
12. Christensen, E., et al.: Progress in gastroenterology: treatment of duodenal ulcer, Gastroenterology 73:1170-1182, 1977.
13. Conn, H.F.: Current therapy 1981, Philadelphia, 1981, W.B. Saunders Co.
14. *Daly, K.M.: Oral cancer: everyday concerns, Am. J. Nurs. 79:1415-1419, 1979.
15. Dodsworth, J.M., and Fisher, J.E.: Surgical therapy of chronic peptic ulcer, Surg. Clin. North Am. 54:529-543, 1974.
16. Dunphy, J.E., and Way, L.W., editors: Surgical diagnosis and treatment 1979, Los Altos, Calif., 1979, Lange Medical Publications.
17. Dworken, H.J.: The alimentary tract, Philadelphia, 1974, W.B. Saunders Co.
18. Dyck, W.P.: Cimetidine in the management of peptic ulcer disease, Surg. Clin. North Am. 59:863-867, 1979.
19. Ebeid, A.M., and Fischer, J.E.: Gastrin and ulcer disease: what is known, Surg. Clin. North Am. 56:1249-1265, 1976.
20. El-Domeiri, A.A., and Chaudhuri, P.: Management of oral and pharyngeal cancer: a multidisciplinary approach, Surg. Clin. North Am. 55:107-115, 1975.
21. Ellis, F.H., Jr.: Esophageal hiatal hernia, N. Engl. J. Med. 287:646-649, 1972.
22. Esselstyn, C.B.: Surgical management of actively bleeding duodenal ulcer, Surg. Clin. North Am. 56:1387-1392, 1976.
23. Fisher, R.S., and Cohen, S.: Gastroesophageal reflux, Med. Clin. North Am. 62:3-20, 1978.
24. Fleshler, B.: Medical management of bleeding duodenal ulcers, Surg. Clin. North Am. 56:1375-1386, 1976.
25. Fordtran, J.S.: Placebos, antacids and cimetidine for duodenal ulcer, N. Engl. J. Med. 288:923-928, 1978.
26. Fromm, D.: Stress ulcer, Hosp. Med. 14:58-61, 1978.
27. Ganong, W.F.: Review of medical physiology, ed. 9, Los Altos, Calif., 1979, Lange Medical Publications.
28. Given, B.A., and Simmons, S.J.: Gastroenterology in clinical nursing, ed. 3, St. Louis, 1979, The C.V. Mosby Co.
29. Glickman, I.: Clinical periodontology, ed. 5, Philadelphia, 1979, W.B. Saunders Co.
30. *Grossman, M.I., et al.: A new look at peptic ulcer, Ann. Intern. Med. 84:57-67, 1976.
31. Hahn, A.B., Barkin, R.L., and Oestreich, S.J.K.: Pharmacology in nursing, ed. 15, St. Louis, 1982, The C.V. Mosby Co.
32. Hallenbeck, G.A.: The natural history of duodenal ulcer disease, Surg. Clin. North Am. 56:1235-1242, 1976.
33. Heal, J.M., and Schein, P.S.: Management of gastrointestinal cancer, Med. Clin. North Am. 61:991-999, 1977.
34. *Herter, R.P.: Preparation of the bowel for surgery, Surg. Clin. North Am. 52:859-869, 1972.
35. Hunt, T.K.: Injury and repair in acute gastroduodenal ulceration, Am. J. Surg. 125:12-18, 1973.
36. Ippoliti, A.F., Maxwell, V., and Isenberg, J.I.: The effect of various forms of milk on gastric acid secretions, Ann. Intern. Med. 84:286-289, 1976.
37. Ippoliti, A., and Walsh, J.: Newer concepts in the pathogenesis of peptic ulcer disease, Surg. Clin. North Am. 56:1479-1483, 1976.
38. Ivey, K.J.: Anticholinergics: do they work in peptic ulcers, Gastroenterology 68:154-158, 1975.
39. Johnson, W.D., and Ballantyne, A.J.: Prognostic effect of tobacco and alcohol on tongue cancer, Am. J. Surg. 134:444-449, 1977.
40. Johnston, D., and Goligher, J.C.: Selective, highly selective, or truncal vagotomy, Surg. Clin. North Am. 56:1313-1321, 1976.
41. *Keogh, G., and Niebel, H.: Oral cancer detection, a nursing responsibility, Am. J. Nurs. 73:684-686, 1973.

*References preceded by an asterisk are particularly well suited for student reading.

42. *Kratzer, J.B., and Rauschenberger, D.S.: What to teach your patient about his duodenal ulcer, Nurs. '78 8(1):54-56, 1978.

43. Krause, M.V., and Mahan, L.K.: Food, nutrition and diet therapy, ed. 6, Philadelphia, 1979, W.B. Saunders Co.

44. Krupp, M., and Chatton, M.: Current medical diagnosis and treatment, Los Altos, Calif., 1978, Lange Medical Publications.

45. *Levine, P., et al.: Safeguarding your patients against periodontal disease, RN 36:38-41, 1973.

46. Lieberman, T.R., and Barnes, M.: Gastrointestinal fiberoptic endoscopy: diagnostic and therapeutic aspects, Surg. Clin. North Am. 59:787-795, 1979.

47. *Long, G.D.: G.I. bleeding: what to do and when, Nurs. '78 8:44-47, 1978.

48. McCredie, J.A.: Basic surgery, New York, 1977, Macmillan Publishing Co., Inc.

49. McDonald, R.E., and Avery, D.R.: Dentistry for the child and adolescent, ed. 3, St. Louis, 1978, The C.V. Mosby Co.

50. Moody, F.G., and Cheung, L.Y.: Stress ulcers: their pathogenesis, diagnosis, and treatment, Surg. Clin. North Am. 56:1469-1478, 1976.

51. Nankin, P., et al.: Hiatus hernia, Surg. Clin. North Am. 51:1347-1353, 1971.

52. Nelson, W.E.: Textbook of pediatrics, ed. 11, Philadelphia, 1979, W.B. Saunders Co.

53. Paparella, M.M., and Shumrick, D.A., editors: Otolaryngology, ed. 2, Philadelphia, 1980, W.B. Saunders Co.

54. Petersen, W.L., et al.: Healing of duodenal ulcer with an antacid regimen, N. Engl. J. Med. 297:341-346, 1977.

55. *Reitz, M., and Pope, W.: Mouth care, Am. J. Nurs. 73:1728-1730, 1973.

56. Rudick, J.: Peptic ulcer: surgical alternatives, Med. Clin. North Am. 62:53-57, 1978.

57. Sabiston, D.C., editor: Davis-Christopher textbook of surgery, ed. 11, Philadelphia, 1977, W.B. Saunders Co.

58. *Samborksy, V.: Drug therapy for peptic ulcer, Am. J. Nurs. 78:2064-2066, 1978.

59. Sandlow, L.J., and Spellberg, M.A.: Gastric hyperthermia for control of upper gastrointestinal bleeding, Am. J. Gastroenterol. 59:307-314, 1973.

60. Schwartz, S.I., et al.: Principles of surgery, ed. 3, New York, 1979, McGraw-Hill Book Co.

61. Schultz, R.C.: The nature of facial injury emergencies, Surg. Clin. North Am. 52:99-106, 1972.

62. Scopp, I.W.: Oral medicine, a clinical approach with basic science correlation, ed. 2, St. Louis, 1973, The C.V. Mosby Co.

63. Shklar, G., and Schwartz, S.M.: An approach to the diagnosis of disease of mouth and jaws, Dent. Clin. North Am. 18:55-75, 1974.

64. Sleisinger, M., and Fortran, J.S.: Gastrointestinal disease: pathology, diagnosis, management, ed. 2, Philadelphia, 1978, W.B. Saunders Co.

65. *Smith, M.: Parotidectomy, Am. J. Nurs. 76:422-425, 1976.

66. Spiro, H.M.: Clinical gastroenterology, ed. 2, New York, 1977, Macmillan Publishing Co., Inc.

67. Spouge, J.D.: Oral pathology, St. Louis, 1973, The C.V. Mosby Co.

68. *Trowbridge, J., and Carl, W.: Oral care of the patient having head and neck irradiation, Am. J. Nurs. 75:2146-2149, 1976.

69. Welsh, J.D.: Diet therapy of peptic ulcer disease, Gastroenterology 72:740-745, 1977.

70. Williams, S.R.: Nutrition and diet therapy, ed. 4, St. Louis, 1981, The C.V. Mosby Co.

71. Wintrobe, M.M., et al.: Harrison's principles of internal medicine, ed. 8, New York, 1977, McGraw-Hill Book Co.

72. Zollinger, R.M.: Surgical management of the ulcerogenic syndrome, Hosp. Pract. 9:72-79, 1974.

PROBLEMS OF ELIMINATION

Elimination of waste products is a basic physiologic need; a person cannot live long without the ability to get rid of waste products resulting from metabolic processes. There are several body systems involved with elimination, only two of which (urinary and bowel elimination) are discussed in this unit. The respiratory system eliminates carbon dioxide but is also involved with oxygen intake and is discussed in the unit on gas transportation. The skin is also an organ of elimination, but its primary function is that of protection from the environment, and it is therefore included in Unit XI.

The unit is divided into two parts, with *intestinal elimination* (Chapters 57 to 59) discussed first, followed by *urinary elimination* (Chapters 60 to 62). The same format is followed for each part. *Assessment* of lower gastrointestinal or urinary function is discussed first. This is followed by general *interventions* for persons with *impaired* intestinal or urinary functioning, including preventing dysfunction of the system, facilitating an open system for elimination of urine and feces, promoting adaptation to drainage through unnatural openings (stoma), promoting control of output (continence), and providing care for persons experiencing surgery of the intestinal or urinary tracts. Specific *problems* of the lower gastrointestinal tract and urinary tract (including the care of persons undergoing kidney dialysis and kidney transplantation) are discussed.

CHAPTER 57

ASSESSMENT OF LOWER GASTROINTESTINAL TRACT FUNCTION

BARBARA C. LONG
NANCY DURHAM

Anatomy and physiology of the lower gastrointestinal tract

Structure

The lower gastrointestinal tract consists of the small and large intestines. The small intestine is about 2.5 cm (1 in.) wide and 6 m (20 ft) long and fills most of the abdomen. It consists of three parts—the *duodenum,* which connects to the stomach; the *jejunum* or middle portion; and the *ileum,* which connects to the large intestine (see Fig. 54-1).

The large intestine is about 6 cm (2½ in.) wide and 1.5 m (5 ft) long. It consists of three parts—the *cecum,* which connects to the small intestine; the *colon*; and the *rectum.* The ileocecal valve prevents backward flow of fecal contents from the large intestine to the small intestine. The vermiform appendix, which has no function, is an appendage close to the ileocecal valve. The *colon* consists of four parts—the ascending, transverse, descending, and sigmoid colons. The points at which the colon changes direction are named for adjacent organs—the liver (hepatic flexure) and the spleen (splenic flexure). The *rectum* is 17 to 20 cm (7 to 8 in.) long, ending in the 2- to 3-cm anal canal. The opening (anus) is controlled by a smooth muscle internal sphincter and a striated muscle external sphincter.

The primary function of the small and large intestine is to receive the partially digested food components from the stomach and move these components forward to facilitate proper absorption of water, nutrients, electrolytes, and bile salts (Fig. 57-1). Secondary functions include secreting mucus, potassium, and bicarbonate and serving as a storage area before waste discharge.

Movement

Contents of the small intestine (*chyme*) are propelled analward by peristaltic movement, wavelike forward movements produced by alternating contraction and relaxation of the muscles of the intestinal wall. This movement also mixes the intestinal contents. Chyme moves slowly and normally takes 3 to 10 hours to move from the stomach to the ileocecal valve.

In the colon, the fecal contents are pushed forward by mass movements occurring only a few times each day. These mass movements are stimulated by gastrocolic reflexes initiated when food enters the duodenum from the stomach, especially after the first meal of the day. This is therefore the most frequent time of the day for defecation to occur.

The *defecation* reflex occurs when feces enter the rectum. Afferent impulses are transmitted to the sacral segments of the spinal cord from which reflex impulses are transmitted back to the colon, sigmoid, and rectum, initiating relaxation of the internal anal sphincter.

Secretion

Gastrointestinal tract secretions are specific to the type of food that is present and the amount that is needed. These secretions are stimulated in part by au-

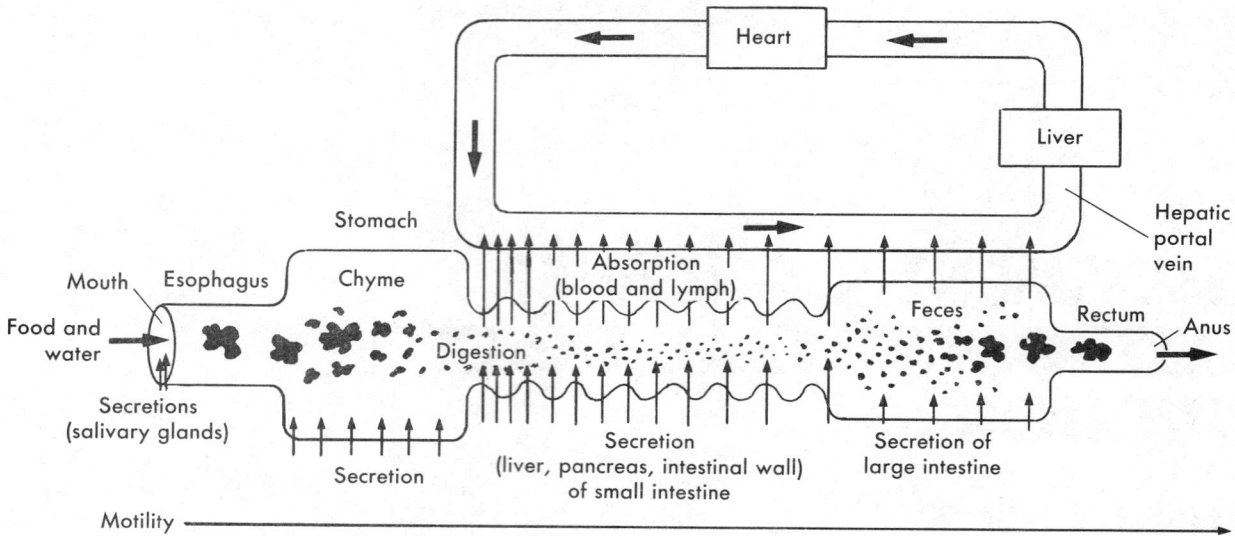

Fig. 57-1. Summary of gastrointestinal activity involving motility, secretion, digestion, and absorption. (From Human physiology, ed. 3, by Vander, A.J., et al. Copyright © 1980 by McGraw-Hill Book Co. Used with the permission of McGraw-Hill Book Co.)

tomatic *sympathetic* innervation, *hormonal* regulation, and local *mechanical pressure*.

Mucous secretion throughout the tract increases food adhesion, prevents contact of the food with the wall of the mucosa, enhances free passage of the food, neutralizes the small amounts of acid or alkali, and makes some particles more resistant to digestion.

Secretions of the small intestine provide for the final digestion of food. As chyme enters the small intestine, gastric secretion of hydrochloric acid is slowed and *secretin, pancreozymin,* and *cholecystokinin* are released.

Absorption

The intestinal wall has many folds, which are covered by fingerlike projections (villi). Epithelial cells cover the surface of each villus, and each cell has several microvilli projecting from its surface. The intestinal folds, villi, and microvilli thus greatly increase the absorptive area of the small intestine. In the center of each villi is a blind end lymph vessel (lacteal) for absorption into the lymphatic system. The lacteal is surrounded by capillaries, venules, and arterioles for absorption into the portal blood system (Fig. 57-2).

Ninety percent of absorption occurs within the small intestine either by active transport or diffusion. Many nutrients, such as amino acids, monosaccharides, sodium, and calcium, are transported by active transport, requiring metabolic energy expenditure. Other nutrients, such as fatty acids and water, diffuse passively across the cell membrane. Pancreatic lipase and conju-

gated bile salts must be present in the intestinal lumen for hydrolysis of fats into fatty acids to permit diffusion across the cell membranes of the villi.

Approximately 450 ml of chyme reaches the cecum per day. The transit time in the large bowel is slow, taking about 12 hours for material to reach the rectum. Reabsorption of water, electrolytes, and bile salts occurs predominantly in the ascending colon. The colon has the capacity to absorb six to eight times more fluid than is delivered to it daily. Approximately 100 ml of fluid contents remains to be mixed with the residue of feces. Normally, this residue (*feces*) is evacuated on a fairly regular schedule. This schedule differs for each individual and may vary from daily evacuation to evacuation every 3 to 4 days.

Physiologic changes with aging

Changes in the lower gastrointestinal tract may occur with aging but vary among individuals and may or may not cause altered functioning. Changes in the ability to digest and absorb foods are related to decreased secretion of most digestive enzymes and bile production. Absorption of fats and fat-soluble vitamins becomes impaired. The increased residue resulting from decreased digestion and absorption may lead to increased flatulence. Gas-forming foods may be less well tolerated than when the person was younger.

Decreased motility in the intestines may also occur as a result of decreased peristalsis, decreased muscular tone of the intestinal wall, and decreased abdominal muscle strength. Decreased anal sphincter tone may also

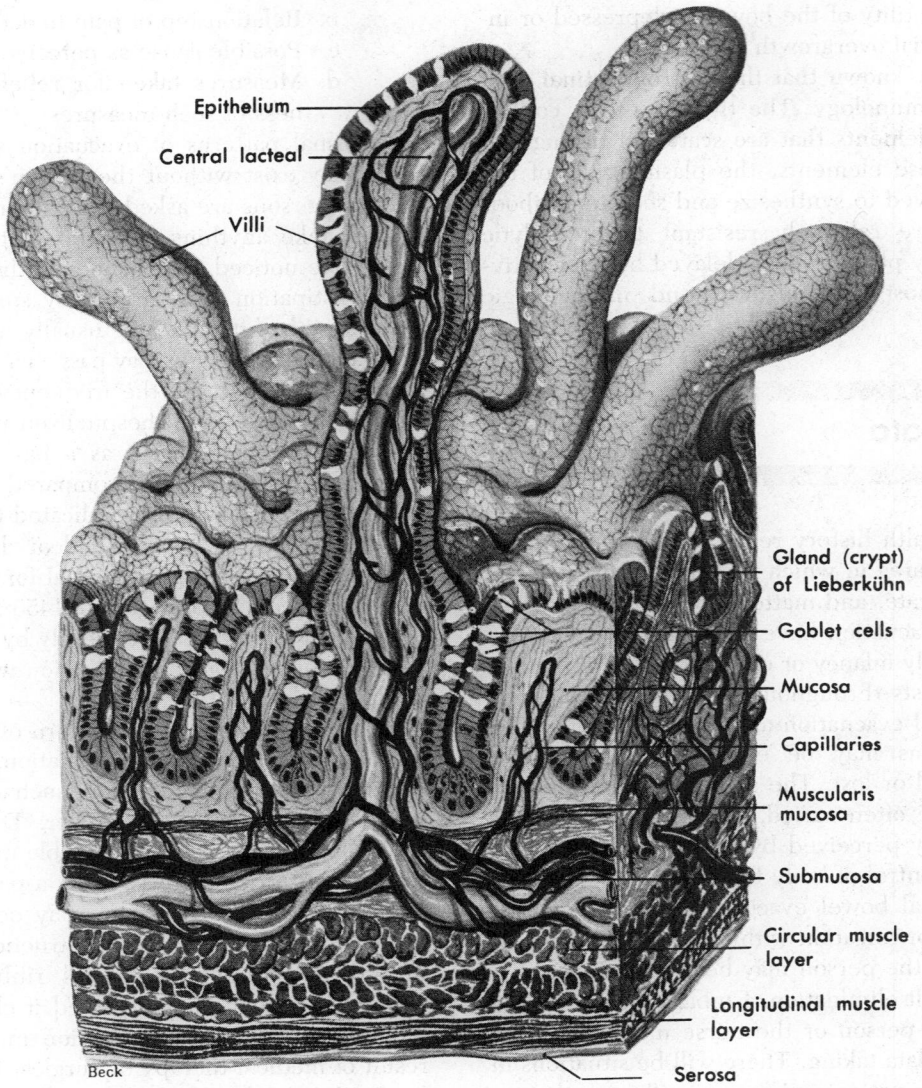

Epithelium

Central lacteal

Villi

Gland (crypt) of Lieberkühn

Goblet cells

Mucosa

Capillaries

Muscularis mucosa

Submucosa

Circular muscle layer

Longitudinal muscle layer

Beck

Serosa

Fig. 57-2. Section of intestinal mucosa. (From Anthony, C.P., and Kolthoff, N.J.: Textbook of anatomy and physiology, ed. 9, St. Louis, 1975, The C.V. Mosby Co.)

be present. These changes contribute to the increased occurrence of constipation in the older person.

Fluid and electrolyte balance

Pathologic alterations occur with the *loss* of particular segments of small or large bowel or when there is inability for proper reabsorption. The loss of small bowel contents precipitates metabolic acidosis and hypokalemia (p. 355). This problem may occur with drainage of small bowel contents through a suction tube or fistula or with persistent vomiting of the intestinal contents. Losses from the large intestine comprise mainly loss of water, sodium, and to a lesser extent chloride, resulting

in dehydration and hyponatremia. This occurs in conditions in which the rate of peristalsis is increased.

Bacteria

In addition to its role in nutrition, the alimentary tract supports bacterial growth that enhances digestive processes and has a role in antibody formation. Within 4 weeks after birth, the characteristic flora is established. The organisms are fewer in number in those portions of the bowel concerned with digestion and absorption. Certain disease conditions increase the breakdown of nonabsorbable carbohydrate, leading to the production of diarrhea. It is important to remember that whenever the motility of the bowel is depressed or interrupted, bacterial overgrowth will occur.

It is presently known that the gastrointestinal tract has a role in immunology. The thymus exerts control over lymphoid elements that are scattered throughout the tract. Of these elements, the plasma cells of the mucosa are believed to synthesize and secrete antibodies. The cells are relatively resistant to proteolytic digestion and may play a role in delayed hypersensitivity, graft and host relationships, and immunologic memory.

Subjective data

Eliciting a health history regarding bowel habits of the patient is an area in which the nurse must provide a tactful, considerate, and matter-of-fact approach. Patterns of bowel evacuation have in most instances been established in early infancy or childhood, and the effect of this training lasts throughout life. The infant learns to "control" bowel evacuation and is rewarded for this; therefore problems may be encountered when this function is altered or lost. The symptoms that the person may have are often varied, vague, and ill defined and are frequently perceived by the individual to represent a loss of control of body functions.

Because normal bowel evacuation is not usually a topic of general conversation within the family group or among strangers, the person may be hesitant about expressing data about elimination. Embarrassment on the part of either the person or the nurse may limit accurate or complete data taking. There will be situations in which the nurse must interview a significant other to obtain information regarding bowel functioning of the patient. Following is a listing of data obtained when eliciting a history of bowel function:

1. Normal pattern of bowel elimination
   a. Frequency and character of the stool
   b. Use of measures to encourage evacuation (e.g., specific food, laxatives, and enemas)
2. Recent changes in normal pattern
   a. Changes in character of stool (e.g., constipation, diarrhea, or alternating constipation or diarrhea)
   b. Changes in color of stool (if bleeding is present: stool mixed or streaked with blood, amount, rectal bleeding after evacuation, menstruation present)
   c. Drugs or medications being taken, if changes in elimination are present
   d. Measures taken to relieve symptoms
3. Pain in rectal area or abdomen
   a. Onset, frequency, location, and intensity
   b. Relationship of pain to activity or to foods
   c. Possible cause as perceived by person
   d. Measures taken for relief of pain; effectiveness of such measures

Normal patterns of evacuation vary greatly. Problems may exist without the person's awareness; therefore all persons are asked what their normal pattern is, if they take anything to maintain this pattern, and if they have noticed any changes in this pattern.

Constipation is identified by small hard dry stools passed with difficulty and usually at infrequent intervals, although a person may pass a constipated stool every day. Data concerning the frequency of bowel elimination is obtained on all hospitalized persons at the time of admission; this serves as a baseline against which subsequent elimination is compared. Continued assessment of frequency is also indicated on all persons who are inactive or who have fluid or diet restriction, because they have a high potential for developing constipation or fecal impaction (p. 1455). Information concerning measures used frequently by the person to help maintain normal bowel elimination will provide data for health teaching.

Changes in the normal pattern of bowel elimination may indicate a physiologic deviation, such as constipation, or a pathologic deviation, such as enteritis (inflammation of the bowel) or cancer. Diarrhea and stools containing mucus, pus, and possible undigested food may indicate enteritis or invasion by a parasite. Alternation of diarrhea and constipation may occur as a result of cancer of the colon. Partial obstruction of the descending colon may produce small ribbon-shaped stools, whereas no stool will be passed if obstruction is complete. Diarrhea and constipation may also occur as a result of medical therapy or surgical intervention.

Bright red blood in the stool indicates lower gastrointestinal bleeding. Blood from the upper gastrointestinal tract is changed by digestive secretions, and the stool appears black and sticky (tarry). Blood in the stool (*melena*) may be a recent or a chronic symptom and may result from erosion of the mucosa, leading to perforation of the muscle wall or rupture of a blood vessel.

Pain may be experienced as a general sensation throughout the abdomen, may be specifically directed to one particular quadrant, or may be referred to another somatic or skeletal part that shares the same innervation. The pain sensation is thought to arise from the distention or sudden contraction of a hollow viscus; therefore local stretching or traction on pain-sensitive structures will elicit the pain stimulus. The painful area may demonstrate local muscle guarding, which serves as a protective mechanism as the overlying muscles contract. Pain is frequently the reason given when seeking medical attention, despite the fact that pain by itself is not an early or common symptom of gastrointestinal disease.

Objective data

Examination of the abdomen may not follow a structured pattern, because signs are often found that require alteration in technique. The examination is supported by the attainment of a meaningful history describing the nature and site of pain and any alterations in bowel habits.

Examination will determine the presence or absence of (1) tenderness, (2) organ enlargement, (3) masses, (4) spasm or rigidity of the abdominal muscles, and (5) fluid or air in the abdominal cavity. During this part of the assessment, the examiner will be locating the hollow viscera (small intestine, colon, and urinary bladder). These are not normally palpable.

Examination of the abdomen requires knowledge of the terms used to designate the divisions of the abdomen (Fig. 57-3) and the anatomic structures located therein (see box at right).

ANATOMIC LOCATION OF VISCERA WITHIN EACH ABDOMINAL QUADRANT

Right upper quadrant (RUQ)	Left upper quadrant (LUQ)
Liver	Stomach
Gallbladder	Spleen
Duodenum	Left kidney
Right kidney	Pancreas
Hepatic flexure of colon	Splenic flexure of colon

Right lower quadrant (RLQ)	Left lower quadrant (LLQ)
Cecum	Sigmoid colon
Appendix	Left ovary and tube
Right ovary and tube	

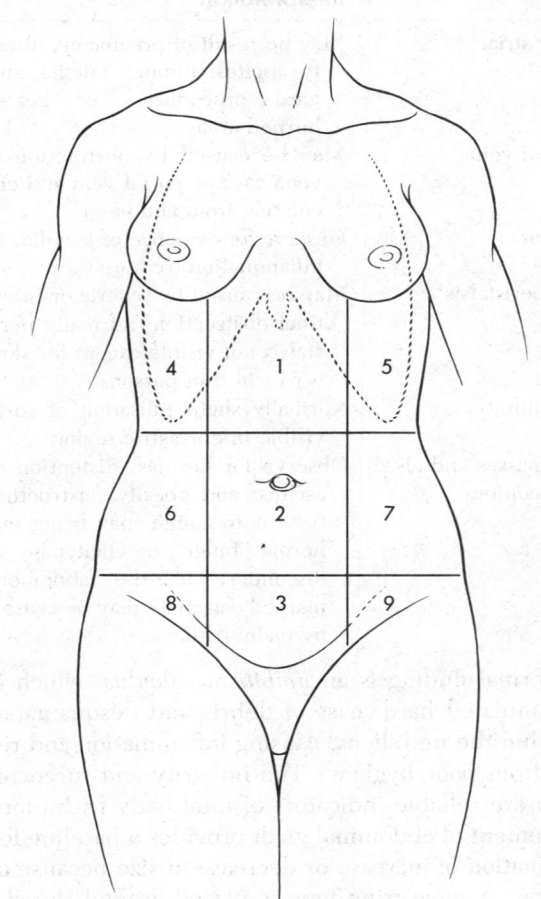

Fig. 57-3. Topographic division of abdomen commonly used to localize signs and symptoms, and anatomic location of viscera within abdomen. *1,* Epigastrium; *2,* umbilical; *3,* suprapubic (bladder and uterus); *4* and *5,* right and left hypocondrium; *6* and *7,* right and left lumbar or flank; *8* and *9,* right and left iliac or inguinal.

Normal findings are variable and will depend on general body build, the amount of abdominal fat, and the patient's ability to cooperate. Although the examination may be initiated in any quadrant, it is recommended that the lower quadrant be examined first, followed by upward movement toward the costal margins. The approach will need to be altered as necessaary, with painful areas being examined last. The examination is conducted in an unhurried manner. The methods for physical examination of the abdomen are performed in the following order: (1) inspection, (2) auscultation, (3) percussion, and (4) palpation.

Inspection

Arrange the illumination to shine across the abdomen and toward the examiner or have the light source lengthwise over the patient. Inspect the skin color and texture and observe for scars, engorged veins, visible peristalsis, masses, or abnormal contour.

Finding	Interpretation
Scars or striae	May be result of pregnancy, obesity, ascites, tumors, edema, surgical procedures, or healed burned areas
Engorged veins	May be caused by obstruction of vena cava or portal vein and circulation from abdomen
Skin color	Observe for evidence of jaundice of inflammation (redness)
Visible peristalsis	May be caused by pyloric or intestinal obstruction; normally peristalsis not visible except for slow waves in thin persons
Visible pulsations	Normally slight pulsation of aorta visible in epigastric region
Visible masses and altered contour	Observe for hernias, distention of ascites, and obesity; instructing patient to cough may bring out hernia "bulge" or elicit pain or discomfort in the abdomen; marked concavity may be caused by malnutrition

A normal finding is an *umbilical calculus,* which is an accumulated hard mass of debris and desquamated skin within the umbilicus, causing inflammation and resulting from poor hygiene. The integrity and turgor of the skin are reliable indicators of total body hydration. Measurement of abdominal girth provides a baseline for the evaluation of increase or decrease in size because of distention. A measuring tape is placed around the abdomen at the level of the umbilicus or 2.5 cm below, and the reading is taken. It is important that all subsequent measurements be taken at the same level for accurate evaluation.

Abdominal distention may be caused by air or fluid in the gastrointestinal tract or fluid in the peritoneal spaces (ascites). Air collects from the air that is swallowed, from gas formed by bacterial action, or from gas that has diffused from the blood.[8] Decreased peristalsis permits the air to collect in one portion of the gastrointestinal tract. Fluid accumulates in the tract as it becomes obstructed. Ascites usually results from increased portal hypertension secondary to liver or heart disease.

Auscultation

Auscultation is used primarily to determine the presence or absence of peristalsis and is done before percussion and palpation to avoid an increase or decrease of peristalsis secondary to disturbing the viscera and causing abnormal activity. Other sounds such as friction rubs or murmurs may be heard (Fig. 57-4). Using the diaphragm, the examiner places the stethoscope lightly over the abdominal wall. Most intestinal sounds occur at a rate of five or more per minute (although some may not be audible for up to 5 minutes) and are high pitched and gurgling in quality. A normal peristaltic wave produces audible sounds of air and fluid movement through the intestine. The stethoscope diaphragm is placed to the right and below the umbilicus where the sounds are the loudest.

Finding	Interpretation
Absence of sounds	Peritonitis, and paralytic ileus, pneumonia, and hypokalemia
Repeated, high-pitched sounds occurring at frequent intervals	Increased peristalsis heard in early pyloric obstruction, early intestinal obstruction, and diarrhea
Bruit	Presence of abnormal sounds (turbulence of blood flow through partially occluded or diseased aorta or renal artery)
Hum and friction rub	Heard over liver and splenic areas, indicating peritoneal inflammation

Percussion

Percussion of the abdomen (see Fig. 8-4) has relatively limited value. It is used primarily to confirm the size of various organs and to determine the presence of excessive amounts of fluid or air. Normally, per-

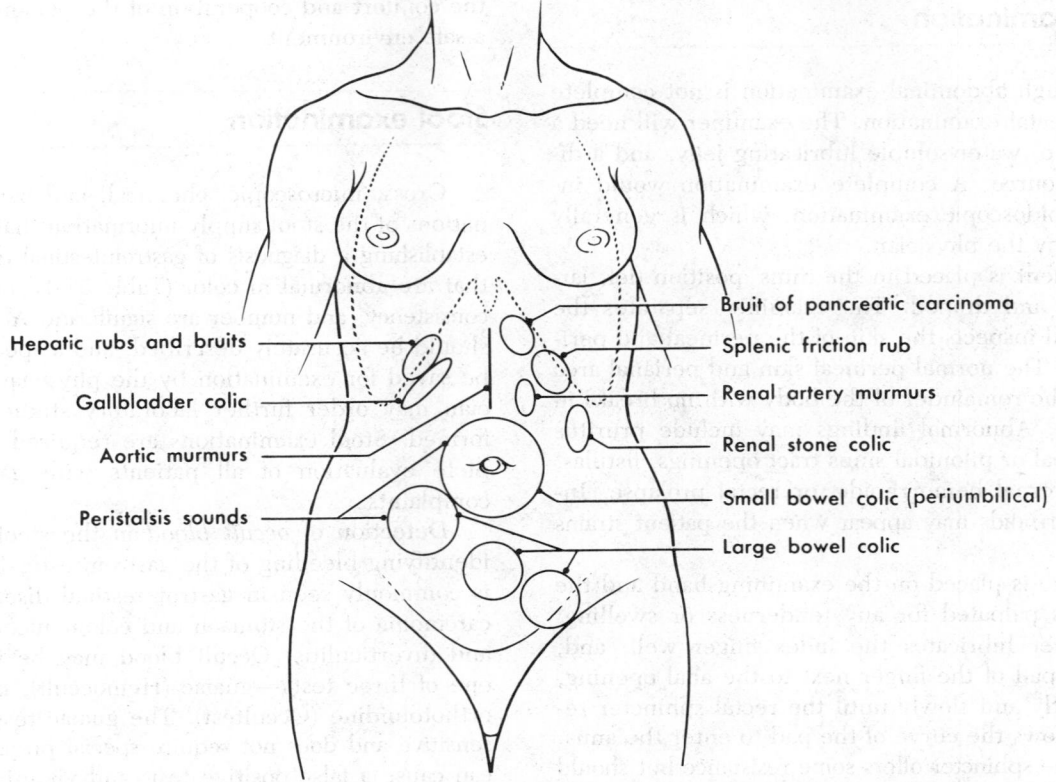

Fig. 57-4. Optimal areas for auscultation of various sounds in abdomen and localization of some types of pain. Note arrow from peristalsis sounds to small bowel and from large bowel colic to circle of ascending colon, which is the peristalsis sounds circle.

Labels (top to bottom, left side):
- Hepatic rubs and bruits
- Gallbladder colic
- Aortic murmurs
- Peristalsis sounds

Labels (top to bottom, right side):
- Bruit of pancreatic carcinoma
- Splenic friction rub
- Renal artery murmurs
- Renal stone colic
- Small bowel colic (periumbilical)
- Large bowel colic

cussion over the abdomen is tympanic because of the presence of a small amount of swallowed air within the gastrointestinal tract. A dull or flat percussion note will be found over a solid structure, such as a distended bladder or enlarged uterus, and over the lower border of the liver in the seventh interspace. Tympanic sounds should be heard beginning at the ninth interspace in the left upper quadrant of the abdomen (Traube's space). Dullness or flatness of tone in this area may be caused by some enlargement of the spleen or the left kidney.

The four quadrants are percussed beginning with the thorax area and moving downward systematically. The degree of soft to pronounced tympany determines gaseous bowel distention.

Palpation

Palpation is an important technique that aids in confirming the findings of inspection and history data. Palpation is of value in determining the outlines of the liver, spleen, kidneys, uterus, and bladder when these organs are enlarged and in determining the presence and char-

acteristics of abdominal masses and the degree of tenderness or muscle rigidity.

The examiner begins palpation at the pubis and works upward toward the costal margins. When moving from one quadrant to another, the entire hand is moved, avoiding a dragging motion across the skin surface, since this is generally an unpleasant or irritating feeling.[18] The entire palm and the extended fingers are placed lightly on the abdominal surface with the fingers approximated. With the palms and pads of the fingertips flat, pressure is applied gently to the depth of about 1 cm as each quadrant is palpated carefully. Normally no masses, swellings, or areas of tenderness will be encountered.

Abnormal findings may include (1) direct tenderness over an organ capsule, (2) rebound tenderness (Blumberg's sign), (3) muscular rigidity, or (4) masses that may be felt if they are sufficiently large enough or close enough to the surface. Distinction should be made between a distended abdomen that is firm to touch (indicating an active obstruction with fluid and gas accumulation) and an abdomen that is soft to touch (indicating a resolving obstruction or a normal occurrence).

Rectal examination

A thorough abdominal examination is not complete without a rectal examination. The examiner will need a rubber glove, water-soluble lubricating jelly, and a direct light source. A complete examination would include sigmoidoscopic examination, which is generally performed by the physician.

The patient is placed in the Sims' position (left lateral prone) and draped. The examiner separates the buttocks and inspects the skin of the perineal and perianal region. The normal perineal skin and perianal area resembles the remainder of the body with no breaks in its integrity. Abnormal findings may include pruritus ani, coccygeal or pilonidal sinus tract openings, fistulas, fissures, external hemorrhoids, or rectal prolapse. Internal hemorrhoids may appear when the patient strains down.

The glove is placed on the examining hand and the perineum is palpated for any tenderness or swelling. The examiner lubricates the index finger well, and, placing the pad of the finger next to the anal opening, presses gently and slowly until the rectal sphincter relaxes and allows the curve of the pad to enter the anus. Normally, the sphincter offers some resistance but should allow free passage of the examining finger. The walls should feel smooth with no areas of swelling or depressions. A normal occurrence is the presence of feces within the rectum. Possible pathologic conditions include stricture of the sphincter, a fixed or movable mass, and coccygeal tenderness.

At the completion of the rectal examination, the patient should have the perineal area cleansed and dried well.

Diagnostic tests

The examinations and procedures performed to rule out problems of the lower gastrointestinal tract are time consuming for the patient and may also be viewed as intrusive procedures. Frequently, the patient is elderly or debilitated, has some decrease in optimal motor function, or may have a chronic medical problem.

Preparations for the examinations (e.g., cathartics, suppositories, enemas, and restriction of food and fluid) frequently result in a decreased circulating volume, leading to weakness. Safety needs of the person assume priority. For example, the person who is having extensive testing may bathe more safely at the bedside than in the shower or may need to be transported by wheelchair. Consideration given to these needs will enhance the comfort and cooperation of the person and provide a safe environment.

Stool examination

Gross, microscopic, chemical, and bacterial examinations of the stool supply information that is helpful in establishing a diagnosis of gastrointestinal disease. Stools that are abnormal in color (Table 57-1), odor, amount, consistency, and number are significant. Abnormal stools should be accurately described, and a specimen should be saved for examination by the physician. The physician may order further laboratory studies to be performed. Stool examinations are required for the complete evaluation of all patients with gastrointestinal complaints.

Detection of *occult blood* in the stool is useful in identifying bleeding of the gastrointestinal tract, which is commonly seen in gastrointestinal diseases, such as carcinoma of the stomach and colon, ulcerative colitis, and diverticulitis. Occult blood may be identified by one of three tests—guaiac (Hemoccult), benzidine, or orthotoluidine (Occultest). The guaiac test is the least sensitive and does not require special preparation. Meat can cause a false-positive test, and vitamin C in quantities greater than 500 mg/day may cause a false-negative test; therefore these substances must be omitted from the diet for 4 days before testing with benzidine or orthotoluidine.[6]

The nurse is responsible for seeing that specimens are collected. A person who is ambulatory may be given a specimen box and spatula and instructed in obtaining a specimen. Otherwise, the specimen should be collected by the nursing personnel. The nurse should be familiar with and also inform auxiliary staff of any special techniques that are required to preserve stools for special examinations. For example, a specimen to be examined for amebae must be kept warm and taken immediately to the laboratory for examination. It can be kept warm by placing the specimen box in a pan of warm

TABLE 57-1. Interpretation of feces color

Color	Interpretation
White	Barium
Gray, tan (clay)	Lack of bile; biliary obstruction
Red	Lower gastrointestinal bleeding Beets
Black	
Tarry	Upper gastrointestinal bleeding
Dry	Iron

water or on a hot water bottle. If an enema must be given to collect a stool specimen, it is important that plain tap water or normal saline solution be used, since soaps or hypertonic solutions may change the consistency of the stool and alter any abnormal contents.

At any time during hospitalization that any abnormality in the color of the stool is noted, a specimen is collected and retained for physician inspection. This applies to all patients irrespective of their primary medical diagnosis.

Barium studies

A roentgenogram of the small intestine is most frequently performed in conjunction with the oral ingestion of contrast media to visualize the stomach (gastrointestinal series, p. 1382). The *barium enema* is performed after the gastrointestinal series, usually on the following day. A series of roentgenograms taken after a barium enema has been given is used to demonstrate the presence of polyps, tumors, and other lesions of the large intestine and to reveal any abnormal anatomy or malfunction of the bowel. As the barium is instilled through a rectal tube, the radiologist, using a fluoroscope and television monitoring screen, observes its passage into the large intestine. The barium must be retained for 15 to 30 minutes while roentgenograms of the intestines are taken. The person is then allowed to go to the bathroom to expel the barium, which may take as long as 30 minutes. After the barium is expelled another film is taken to see if any pockets of barium are retained. This procedure is commonly referred to as a lower GI (gastrointestinal) series.

The preparation for a barium enema includes an explanation of the x-ray procedure, of the importance of retaining the barium during the examination, and of the need for the preparatory regimen. For the barium to clearly outline the lumen of the bowel, the bowel must be empty. This is best accomplished by giving enemas, laxatives, or rectal suppositories as ordered. Food and fluids, including oral medications, are restricted after midnight. Persons may wish to take reading material with them so that they may read while expelling the barium.

Barium that is retained in the bowel becomes hard and difficult to expel. To ensure complete evacuation of the barium from the intestinal tract after this procedure, the physician may order an oil retention enema or a laxative such as magnesium citrate. The debilitated patient is usually exhausted after a barium enema and the subsequent cleansing regimen and should be permitted to rest. Petroleum jelly or, if ordered, a local analgesic ointment such as dibucaine (Nupercaine) may be applied to the anus to alleviate discomfort. If the patient is not too tired, a warm bath may also be soothing.

Endoscopy

Sigmoidoscopy and proctoscopy

The lowest portion of the gastrointestinal tract may be visualized by means of a proctoscope to examine the rectum or a sigmoidoscope to examine the sigmoid colon. Sigmoidoscopy is the most commonly used procedure and is indicated for screening of men over 40 years of age or persons with familial history of colonic cancer and for persons with symptoms of lower gastrointestinal bleeding or inflammatory disease of the colon. The sigmoidoscopic examination permits inspection of a segment of the bowel that is particularly difficult to examine satisfactorily with contrast media. Approximately 75% of all polyps and tumors of the large bowel are within the visualization of the sigmoidoscope.

Patient preparation. A light supper and a light breakfast are usually prescribed before the examination. Cathartics are seldom prescribed before the examination, because they may cause downward flow of fecal matter from the upper bowel when the test is performed. On the morning of the examination, enemas or cathartic rectal suppositories may be ordered to clear the bowel mucosa of fecal matter. An explanation of the preparation and of the procedure will facilitate patient comfort and cooperation during the examination.

Procedure. A new type of sigmoidoscope, the flexible fiberoptic sigmoidoscope, has been developed and is receiving greater use. The flexible sigmoidoscope (65 cm) is longer than the standard rigid sigmoidoscope (30 cm); therefore it permits greater visualization of the descending colon and is more tolerable for the patient.

The patient is placed in a knee-chest position, although a side-lying position (Sims') may be utilized for the elderly or very ill person who cannot assume or maintain the knee-chest position. The patient is draped and the rectum is examined first with a gloved finger. The lubricated instrument is then inserted and gently advanced. The patient feels the instrument as it is inserted and may experience an urge to defecate. Some discomfort consisting of a feeling of cramping may be experienced when the sigmoidoscope is advanced beyond the sigmoid flexure. Air is sometimes pumped into the bowel through the sigmoidoscope to distend the lumen of the bowel, thus permitting better visualization. The air may cause severe "gas" pains. If small amounts of fluid or stool are still present in the bowel, they are removed with cotton swabs and by suctioning.

As the instrument is removed, a careful observation of all of the mucosa is made. Normal variations include

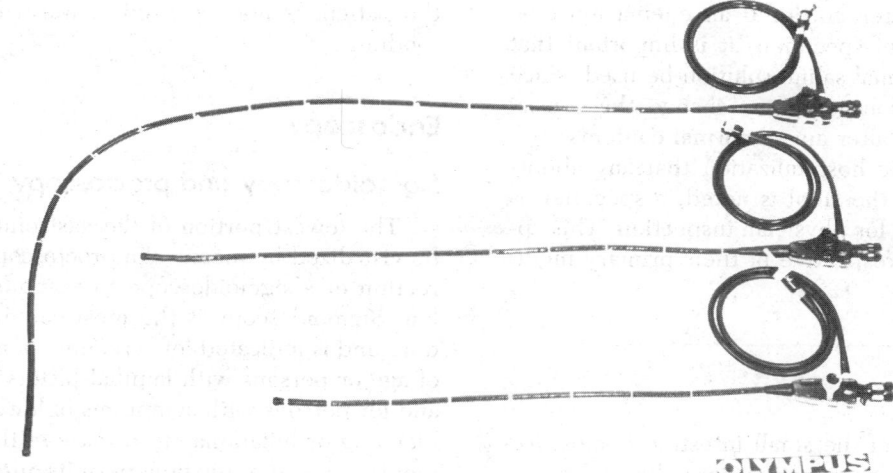

Fig. 57-5. Flexible colon fiberscopes. (From Given, B.A., and Simmons, S.J.: Gastroenterology in clinical nursing, ed. 3, St. Louis, 1979, The C.V. Mosby Co.)

(1) temporary hyperemia caused from the irritation of the enema solutions; (2) increased mucus production caused by inflammation, emotional disturbances, or sodium biphosphate found in commercial enema preparations; and (3) decreased mucus production resulting from habitual cathartic ingestion.

Common abnormalities noted include (1) local trauma caused by enema tips or instrumentation and enema solutions heated above 41° C (105° F); (2) diffuse hyperemia, edema, increased mucus, and a mucosa that bleeds easily (ulcerative colitis); (3) loss of valve edge sharpness, scars, strictures, and contractures (ulcerative colitis and pelvic irradiation); (4) discrete ulcers or polyps; and (5) evidence of an invasion by organisms or bacteria (tuberculosis, bacillary or amebic dysentery, and eggs of *Schistosomiasis* or *Balantidium* organisms).

Postexamination period. A proctoscopic procedure may be tiring, depending on the age and physical condition of the person. After the instrument is removed, excess lubricant is wiped from the anus. When indicated, the person is assisted back to bed and allowed to rest. The person who is examined in an outpatient setting may need to rest for an hour and have some food and fluid before leaving. This is especially important for the elderly or debilitated person.

Colonoscopy

In recent years, fiberoptic colonoscopy has been introduced for visualization of the entire colon up to the ileocecal valve. The colonoscope (Fig. 57-5) is 105 to 185 cm in length, and its use requires the skill of a specialist; but it has the advantage of permitting greater visualization than the sigmoidoscope. Fiberoptic colonoscopy is recommended for abnormalities of the colon that cannot be diagnosed by the usual means or for reexamination of an anastomosis of the colon following surgery for colonic cancer, but it is contraindicated when acute bleeding or inflammatory disease of the colon is present.

Patient preparation. A clear liquid diet is usually ordered for 3 days and nothing by mouth for 8 hours preceding the examination. Laxatives are prescribed for 1 to 3 days before the test, and enemas are given the night before.[6] Thorough bowel cleansing is important. A consent form must be signed by the patient. The patient is provided with explanations for the preparation and the procedure.

Procedure. The examination is performed under analgesia or light anesthesia. The patient needs to be alert enough to respond to the physician in order to describe any symptoms of possible complications. The patient is placed in Sims' position. Feelings of pressure but not pain may be experienced as the colonoscope is maneuvered around the various flexures of the colon. Intravenous anticholinergics may be given to relax bowel spasms. Air may be used to expand the walls of the colon, causing "gas" pains. Biopsy and snare cautery may be performed by looking through the colonoscope.

Postexamination period. Food and fluids may be given approximately 2 hours after completion of the test; however, a person who has had a polypectomy through the colonoscope is permitted only fluids the first day and a low-residue diet for 2 weeks.[3] Stools are observed for signs of bright red blood indicating colonic bleeding. The patient is monitored for signs of colon perforation as evidenced by a gradual onset of dull pain in the abdomen followed by a rise in body temperature. If the procedure is performed in an ambulatory care clinic,

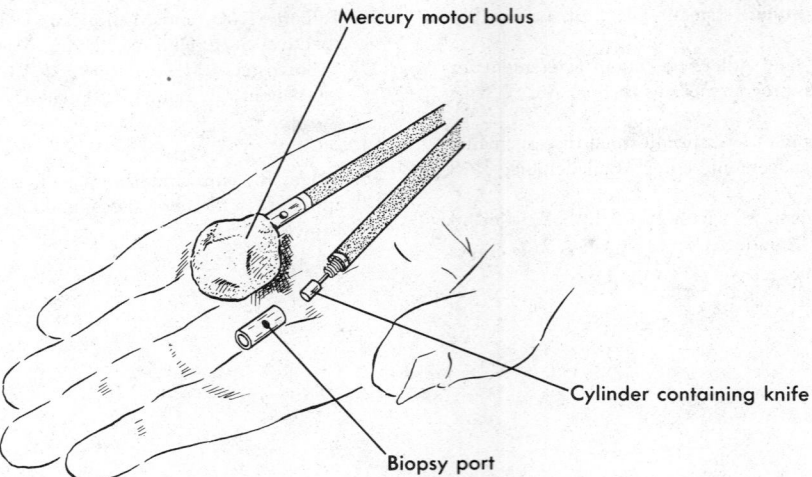

Mercury motor bolus

Cylinder containing knife

Biopsy port

Fig. 57-6. Multipurpose biopsy tube. Biopsy tube assembled and disassembled to show location of its parts. Note small size of tube in relation to human hand.

the patient is instructed about reporting signs of bleeding or perforation for 24 hours, if these signs should occur at home.

Biopsy

Biopsy of tissue includes rectal biopsy and peroral small bowel biopsy. In both instances tissue samples are removed and sent to the laboratory for definitive diagnosis.

Rectal biopsy

Biopsy of lesions, polyps, or tumors of the lower sigmoid colon, rectum, and anal canal is generally done at the time of the sigmoidoscopic examination. A knife blade or snare is used to obtain the tissue sample. The sample is placed on a slide or in a fixative solution and sent to the laboratory for analysis. The procedure is not generally painful, although a feeling of pressure may be experienced. Bleeding from the site of the biopsy is uncommon. The person is instructed to report immediately any signs of rectal bleeding and to curtail physical activity until examined by a physician.

Peroral small bowel biopsy

Biopsy of the mucosa and of lesions of the small intestines is possible through the passage of a biopsy capsule. The capsule consists of inner and outer shells that are attached to the distal end of a Miller-Abbott tube or to special tubes constructed for this purpose. The inner shell encloses a cylindric cavity that contains a blade. The biopsy opening is located in the distal end of the capsule (Fig. 57-6). The tube with the capsule is swallowed and, by peristaltic activity it reaches the bi-

opsy site as established by fluoroscopy. At this point, the biopsy port is opened, and the blade is operated by hydrostatic pressure and vacuum created by syringes attached to the double-lumen openings at the other end of the tube. The specimen is guillotined off and collected in the capsule. After the tube is removed, the tissue is sent to the laboratory for study.

REFERENCES AND SELECTED READINGS

1. *Bates, B.: A guide to physical examination, ed. 2, Philadelphia, 1979, J.B. Lippincott Co.
2. Bockus, H.L.: Gastroenterology, ed. 3, vol. 1, Philadelphia, 1974, W.B. Saunders Co.
3. *Curtis, C.: Colonoscopy: the nurse's role, Am. J. Nurs. **75**:430-432, 1975.
4. Davidsohn, I., and Henry, J.B.: Todd-Sanford clinical diagnosis by laboratory methods, ed. 16, Philadelphia, 1979, W.B. Saunders Co.
5. DeGowin, E., and DeGowin, R.: Bedside diagnostic examination, ed. 3, London, 1976, Macmillan Publishing Co., Inc.
6. Fischbach, R.: A manual of laboratory diagnostic tests, Philadelphia, 1980, J.B. Lippincott Co.
7. French, R.: Guide to diagnostic procedures, ed. 5, New York, 1980, McGraw-Hill Book Co.
8. Guyton, A.: Textbook of medical physiology, ed. 6, Philadelphia, 1981, W.B. Saunders Co.
9. *Holt, R.W., and Wherry, D.C.: Why flexible fiberoptic sigmoidoscopy is important in the geriatric patient, Geriatrics **34**:85-87, 1979.
10. Krupp, M., and Chatton, M.: Current medical diagnosis and treatment, Los Altos, Calif., 1980, Lange Medical Publications.
11. Lieberman, T.R., and Barnes, M.: Gastrointestinal fiberoptic endoscopy: diagnostic and therapeutic aspects, Surg. Clin. North Am. **59**:787-795, 1979.

*References preceded by an asterisk are particularly well suited for student reading.

12. *Malasanos, L., et al.: Health assessment, ed. 2, St. Louis, 1981, The C.V. Mosby Co.

13. *Mansell, E., Stokes, S., and Adler, J.: Patient assessment: examination of the abdomen: programmed instruction, Am. J. Nurs. 74:1679-1702, 1974.

14. Sleisinger, M., and Fortran, J.: Gastrointestinal disease: pathophysiology, diagnosis, management, ed. 2, Philadelphia, 1978, W.B. Saunders Co.

15. Sodeman, W., and Sodeman, W.: Pathologic physiology, ed. 6, Philadelphia, 1979, W.B. Saunders Co.

16. Talbott, T.M., and MacKeigan, J.M.: Colon endoscopy in perspective, Surg. Clin. North Am. 58:459-468, 1978.

17. *Thompson, J.M., and Bowers, A.C.: Clinical manual of health assessment, St. Louis, 1980, The C.V. Mosby Co.

Classic

18. Judge, R., and Zuidema, G.: Physical diagnosis: a physiological approach to the clinical examination, ed. 2, Boston, 1963, Little, Brown & Co.

CHAPTER 58

INTERVENTIONS FOR THE PERSON WITH IMPAIRED INTESTINAL ELIMINATION

BARBARA C. LONG
DEBRA C. BROADWELL

The normal pattern of bowel elimination may be altered for a number of reasons, which frequently results in an altered nutritional state or a fluid imbalance. Health teaching directed toward promotion of normal intestinal functioning can help prevent these physiologic alterations. Persons with intestinal dysfunctions may require intestinal tract decompression or bowel surgery. Some persons may require a diversion of the fecal stream through surgically created openings (ostomies) in the abdominal wall. Persons experiencing ostomy surgery may be assisted to lead healthy active lives despite this alteration in normal elimination. This chapter includes a discussion of factors promoting normal bowel elimination, common bowel dysfunctions, and the care of persons experiencing intestinal tract decompression, bowel surgery, or stomas for fecal diversion. Interventions for persons with specific pathophysiologic conditions of the lower gastrointestinal tract are discussed in Chapter 59.

Factors promoting normal elimination

The mechanisms involved in normal elimination are discussed in Chapter 57. There are a number of factors that promote the normal elimination of feces from the gastrointestinal tract.

Bowel habits

One of the primary interferences with normal elimination is poor bowel habits. The defecation reflex can be inhibited at will unless it is excessively strong, and persons learn to control evacuation in this way. The defecation reflex is stronger when natural impulses are followed, especially during the periods of mass movements (p. 1431). Persons who delay defecation as part of their natural patterns often become constipated; as the stool remains in the tract, additional water is reabsorbed, resulting in a hard stool.

Foods

Certain foods contain cellulose, which is indigestible and leaves a residue that is propelled through the gastrointestinal tract. The residue acts as an irritant to stimulate normal peristaltic movements and the defecation reflex. Examples of bulk or roughage foods are the skin and fibers of fruits and vegetables, and the coverings of grains in bran and whole wheat flours and cereals. Some foods such as prune juice promote peristalsis.

Fluids

An adequate fluid intake is necessary for maintenance of normal stool consistency. If the body lacks fluid (dehydration), the colon will reabsorb an increased amount of fluid from the chyme. The result will be a hardened stool.

Activity

Physical activity enhances normal peristaltic movements. Persons who are inactive have a higher incidence of constipation.

Emotional equilibrium

Stress affects gastrointestinal activity; therefore maintenance of normal bowel elimination includes taking measures to decrease stress. Stimulation of the sympathetic nervous system inhibits gastrointestinal activity, slowing peristalsis yet at the same time stimulating the internal anal sphincter. During a stressful situation, movement is temporarily halted, but incontinence can occur. Long-term stress effects are influenced by the parasympathetic system, which increases peristaltic activity, causing diarrhea; thus stress can cause incontinence, constipation, or diarrhea.

Common bowel dysfunctions

General dysfunction of bowel elimination includes slow passage of the fecal matter through the colon, resulting in a dry, hard stool usually passed infrequently (constipation) or rapid passage of chyme through the intestinal tract resulting in a watery stool (diarrhea). The causes of these dysfunctions are varied and may or may not be associated with pathologic conditions (Table 58-1). It can be noted in Table 58-1 that many causes of constipation are related to secondary factors that can be prevented, while most causes of diarrhea have a pathologic basis.

Constipation

Etiology and pathophysiology

Physiologically, constipation may result from decreased motility of the colon or from retention of feces in the lower colon or rectum. In either case, the longer

TABLE 58-1. Comparison of causes of diarrhea or constipation

Specific pathologic condition	Secondary factors	Medications
Diarrhea	Fecal impaction	Cathartics
Infections caused by pathogens and parasites	Food or fluids that promote hyperperistalsis	Cardiotonic drugs
Viral enteritis	Electrolyte imbalances	Antibiotics
Amebiasis		Antacids
Cathartic habituation		Other systemic medications
Gastrocolonic fistulas		
Malignant tumors		
Ulcerative colitis		
Malabsorption problems		
Pancreatic insufficiency		
Biliary tract disorders		
Diabetic neuropathy		
Tabes dorsalis		
Hyperthyroidism		
Extensive pelvic pathologic conditions		
Constipation	Inadequate fluid intake	Belladonna and derivatives
Colonic or rectal lesions	Low-residue or starvation diets	Narcotics (codeine)
Hypometabolism	Physical inactivity	Diuretics
Neuroses	Prolonged bed rest	Salts of bismuth, calcium, and iron
Intestinal obstruction	Fecal impaction	Aluminum hydroxide or aluminum phosphate gels
	Barium ingestion	

the time that the feces remain in the colon, the greater the reabsorption of water and the dryer the stool becomes. The stool is then more difficult to expel from the anus.

Defecation, which is initiated when the feces enter the rectum, can be voluntarily controlled by contraction of the external anal sphincter. If the defecation urge is not heeded, it soon disappears and the feces remain in the rectum. The defecation urge occurs most frequently following meals, particularly breakfast, as a result of stimulation of the gastrocolic reflex from food entering the stomach. Most people defecate on a regular pattern, but this pattern varies among persons from three times a day to once every 2 to 3 days.

Occasional constipation per se is not detrimental to health, although it can cause a feeling of general discomfort or abdominal fullness, anorexia, and anxiety in some persons. Intractable constipation is termed *obstipation*. Habitual constipation leads to decreased intestinal muscle tone, increased use of Valsalva's maneuver as the person bears down in the attempt to pass the hardened stool, and an increased incidence of hemorrhoids.

Intervention

Promotion of good bowel habits. Health teaching is one of the most important measures for prevention of constipation, since it is the individual who will need to carry out the suggested measures for the rest of his or her life. For the person who has been assessed as having poor bowel habits, an explanation is needed of the mechanisms underlying the need for a consistent time for defecation in order to maximize natural responses (after meals, especially breakfast). Travel, work schedules, or altered sleep patterns contribute to poor bowel habits. Daily schedules need to be planned so that time will be available for heeding the defecation urge when it occurs.

Diet. Fiber in the diet provides bulk, leaving a residue in the bowel after digestion that facilitates movement of the feces through the colon. High-fiber foods include vegetables and fruits (both raw and cooked), whole-grain cereal products, and nuts. Bran should be used in moderation, since it is a concentrated source of food fiber and may cause flatulence, loose stools, or intestinal blockage if taken in excess.[36] Prunes stimulate increased intestinal motility as a result of the presence of a laxative substance.

Fluids. One of the compensatory methods for conservation of body fluids is the reabsorption of water in the large intestine. Thus when fluid intake is decreased, more fluid wil be reabsorbed in the colon leading to formation of a dryer stool. A habitual intake of 8 to 10 glasses of fluid daily can help prevent the development of constipation.

Activity. Exercise promotes colonic motility and improves abdominal muscle tone necessary for defecation. Straight-leg-raising exercises also promote increased abdominal muscle strength.

Aids to defecation. The daily use of enemas and laxatives or cathartics is to be avoided, since these decrease the muscular tone and mucus production of the rectum and may result in water and electrolyte imbalances. They also become habit forming as the weakened muscle tone adds to the inability to expel the fecal contents, which then leads to the continued taking of enemas and laxatives. If persons experiencing bowel dysfunction are unsuccessful in initial attempts to regain normal function, they need encouragement to continue efforts, because considerable time may be needed to change a long-standing condition.

The hospitalized patient. For the person who is hospitalized and experiencing constipation, data analysis will identify potential causes. If the therapeutic diet is a contributing factor, consultation with the dietitian may be helpful. Measures to improve the intake of food (see Chapter 53) and fluids (see Chapter 21) are carried out as indicated. A constipating antacid may be exchanged with one that has a laxative effect. Ambulation is encouraged for all hospitalized patients as permitted. Privacy for bowel evacuation must be provided. Additional stimulation may be needed to increase peristalsis. For those persons who lack innervation of the rectum (paraplegics), digital stimulation of evacuation may be necessary. Various medications such as stool softeners or laxatives are frequently ordered, but efforts are made to promote normal bowel elimination.

Fecal impaction. If the stool is permitted to remain in the colon until it becomes exceedingly hard, a *fecal impaction* occurs. The impaction blocks the rectum and must be removed. If it cannot be softened and removed by oil and cleansing enemas, digital removal with a gloved finger may be necessary. This is an uncomfortable experience for the patient, and preventive measures must be instituted for all persons at high risk of developing impaction, including persons who are nutritionally depleted, dehydrated, receiving constipating medications, undergoing barium studies, or on prolonged bed rest. Preventive measures include identification and assessment of high-risk persons and carrying out measures to increase peristalsis.

Diarrhea

Etiology and pathophysiology

Diarrhea may result from disturbances in either the small or large intestine. The definition is based on the consistency of the stool and not the number expelled per day. Diarrhea may be caused by a change in the fecal contents (solutes exerting an osmotic effect or a

TABLE 58-2. Types of diarrhea

Type of diarrhea	Pathophysiology	Etiology
Secretory	Hypersecretion of water and salts in small or large intestine	Bacterial toxins (*Escherichia coli*, cholera); increased bile acids after ileal resection; caffeine
Exudative	Addition of plasma and mucus, which increases fluid content of feces	Crohn's disease; ulcerative colitis
Osmotic	Increased nonabsorbable solutes in bowel producing an osmotic effect	Saline laxatives; lactose intolerance; fat malabsorption; postgastrectomy syndrome
Rapid intestinal transit	Increased propulsive activity in colon leading to decreased water absorption	Irritable bowel syndrome; gastric and intestinal resection; surgical bypass; antibiotics; stress

fluid content increase) or may be caused by an increase in intestinal transit time so that less fluid is reabsorbed (Table 58-2). The end result is passage of feces high in water content.

Body water losses from diarrhea can be extensive, leading to dehydration, hyponatremia, hypokalemia, and metabolic alkalosis (see Chapter 20). Diarrhea can be distressing to the patient because it reflects loss of control of body function, interferes with other activities, and may lead to skin breakdown.

Diarrhea may be accompanied by abdominal cramping, abdominal distention, and borborygmi. It may also be painless, particularly as a result of stress. Defecation may be precipitated by the intake of food or may occur irrespective of time or situation.

Intervention

Since diarrhea is usually caused by a pathologic condition or is a side effect of medications, medical treatment consists primarily of correcting the underlying cause. Other measures include allowing the bowel to "rest," providing electrolyte replacement, and providing for patient comfort.

Medications. The most effective drugs for decreasing intestinal motility are opium derivatives, especially camphorated tincture of opium (paregoric). Diphenoxylate hydrochloride with atropine (Lomotil) is chemically related to meperidine and is commonly prescribed. Kaolin and pectate appear to be of limited value in the control of diarrhea. The fluidity of the stools may be decreased by providing bulk through the use of psyllium (Metamucil) or methylcellulose. If diarrhea occurs primarily after meals, antidiarrheal medications should be given 30 to 60 minutes before the meal to provide for maximal effectiveness.

Rest. Dietary restrictions decrease stimulation of the intestinal tract and prevent irritation of inflamed intestinal mucosa, thus permitting the bowel to rest. If diarrhea is severe, food may be withheld for 24 to 48 hours. When foods are permitted, a diet low in dietary fiber and high in protein and calories is recommended. Bed rest may provide symptomatic relief.[7] With extensive fluid and electrolyte loss, the person may become easily fatigued and require planned rest periods.

Fluid and electrolyte replacement. Since dehydration and electrolyte loss occur with diarrhea, fluids and electrolytes must be replaced. The person with moderate diarrhea may be given oral fluid replacement. Glucose is added to the fluid, since fluid and electrolytes will be absorbed more readily by osmosis with the glucose. An oral electrolyte preparation can be easily prepared at home by adding 1 teaspoon salt, 1 teaspoon bicarbonate of soda, and 4 teaspoons sugar to 1 L drinking water. If the diarrhea is severe, the person may require hospitalization for intravenous fluid replacement.

Comfort measures. Passage of frequent watery stools may be discomforting to the person, causing perineal irritation. Provision is made for personal hygiene after *each* loose stool, and the perineal area must be kept clean and dry to prevent skin breakdown. The environment must be conducive to privacy and free of odors.

Outcome criteria for the person with bowel dysfunction

The person or significant others can:
1. Explain the relationship of dietary and fluid intake to the formation of a normal stool.
2. Describe the relationship of activity to normal bowel evacuation.
3. Describe a plan incorporating good bowel habits.
4. Describe the effect of prescribed medications on bowel function.

5. State what to do when diarrhea or constipation occurs.

Flatulence

Etiology and pathophysiology

One of the most common gastrointestinal discomforts is abdominal distention or pain resulting from the presence of intestinal gas (flatus). This gas results from swallowed air, from gas formed by the action of intestinal bacteria, and from carbon dioxide formed by the action of bicarbonate with hydrochloric acid or fatty acids. Swallowed air that is not belched passes into the intestines and diffuses passively between the intestinal lumen and the blood stream depending on the partial pressure difference of the gas; thus different quantities of gas will be present in the intestinal lumen at different times.

Bacterial flora produces hydrogen through the action of the bacteria on ingested fermentable matter. Some vegetables (e.g., legumes), fruits (e.g., raw apples or melons), or whole grains contain some polysaccharides that cannot be digested; thus they serve as a substrate for bacterial action with the production of hydrogen.[8] Carbon dioxide can be produced during bacterial metabolism. Methane is also produced by bacteria in about one third of the adult population, and this appears to be a familial trait resulting from early environmental factors.[8] Persons who produce large amounts of methane have stools that float in water. Floating stools are also seen in persons with malabsorption syndromes because of the carbon dioxide and hydrogen produced from the unabsorbed food.

Persons experiencing abdominal distention or discomfort from gas may have problems with altered gastrointestinal motility or from malabsorption syndromes, and these conditions need to be ruled out if the person experiences marked discomfort. The distention or "bloating" may be functional and pain may be experienced by persons who have an increased pain response to intestinal distention.

Intervention

Some of the following interventions may help to decrease the intestinal gas volume when a pathologic condition is not present:

1. Avoid activities that increase repetitive swallowing of air.
2. Maintain an erect position after meals to facilitate gas rising to the fundus of the stomach and being expelled.
3. Eat a low-fat diet to decrease carbon dioxide production.
4. Take antacids containing hydroxide (e.g., Maalox) 1 hour after meals in order to neutralize hydrochloric acid.
5. Avoid gas-forming carbohydrates that the person identifies as producing more discomfort (e.g., selected vegetables or fruits and bran).
6. Ambulate to increase peristalsis to move the gas through the intestinal tract, if discomfort is present.

Fecal incontinence

Pathophysiology

The problem of fecal incontinence may be better understood if there is first an understanding of fecal continence. Normally, the contents of the bowel are moved by mass movements to the rectum. The rectum then stores this material until defecation occurs. Defecation may occur reflexly because of distention of the rectal musculature, or it may be inhibited voluntarily. Distention of the rectum initiates nerve signals that are transmitted to the spinal cord and then back to the descending colon, initiating peristaltic waves, which force more feces into the rectum. The internal anal sphincter relaxes and, if the external sphincter is also relaxed, defecation results. Voluntary control is under cortical control. Voluntary emptying of the rectum occurs when the external anal sphincter (under cortical control) is relaxed and the abdominal and pelvic muscles contract.

Defecation continues to occur even in the presence of most upper or lower motor neuron lesions because musculature of the bowel contains its own nerve centers that respond to distention through peristalsis. Peristalsis therefore persists or can be stimulated even when somatic paralysis is present. Defecation does not occur continually over 24 hours but occurs primarily during mass peristaltic movements following meals or whenever the rectum becomes distended.

Etiology

There are several causes of fecal incontinence. The external anal sphincter may be relaxed, the voluntary control of defecation may be interrupted in the central nervous system, or messages may not be transmitted to the brain because of a lesion within the cord or external pressure on the cord. The disorders causing breakdown of conscious control include cortical clouding or lesions, spinal cord lesions or trauma, and trauma to the anal sphincter (e.g., fistula, abscess, or surgery). Perineal relaxation and actual damage of the anal sphincter are often caused by injury during childbirth or during perineal operations. Relaxation usually increases with the general loss of muscle tone in aging. Perineal exercises similar to those used in urinary incontinence (p. 1544) may help some patients.

Assessment

Records are kept concerning the normal bowel habits, the frequency of defecations, the nature of the stool, the awareness of the need to defecate, the degree of sphincter control, and the ability to produce intraabdominal pressure to aid in expelling the feces. The person's general condition is also considered, as is willingness of the person and significant others to be involved in a bowel control program. In establishing a bowel control program, the nurse must bear in mind that feces may be expelled from the rectum by peristalsis as long as the stool is kept soft.

Intervention

Bowel training. If fecal incontinence is to be prevented, bowel training or a regular routine of stimulation of persitalsis and of going to the toilet should be carried out. In order to have an effective bowel program, it must be consistent; and it requires cooperation and diligence on the part of the staff as well as the individual and significant others. It is necessary to keep a daily record to determine whether the program is producing the desired results.

When establishing a bowel program, the person and a significant other are included in the planning. They can help determine whether a morning or evening program is best. The individual's previous habits and current and future activities are considered in the planning. The general welfare of the person benefits so much by automatic defecation that the time and energy expended to accomplish it are well spent. If "accidents" occur during the bowel training program, the person and significant other are reassured that these are temporary and do not indicate that the program is a failure.

Ordinarily, the bowel is trained to empty at regular intervals. Once a day or once every other day after breakfast is common. Food and fluids increase peristalsis, which may stimulate defecation. The taking of certain food or fluids may be associated with the accustomed time for defecation. For example, coffee or orange juice may provide the stimulus for some people. Most persons will be more relaxed and thus more likely to have a bowel movement if placed in as near the normal position as possible and if they have privacy.

Glycerin *suppositories* (usually two are needed) help stimulate evacuation of the bowel; they should be inserted about 2 hours before the usual time of defecation. They are lubricated with petrolatum and pushed well into the rectum against the mucosa with a gloved finger. If the person is unconscious or has disease of the spinal cord, it may be necessary to use the laxative suppository bisacodyl (Dulcolax). Suppositories are most effective if given following a meal, because the gastrocolic reflex will provide additional stimulus. Results from bisacodyl usually occur within a half hour. Care must be taken not to insert the suppository into a bolus of stool, since it is then ineffective.

Routine enemas and laxatives are to be avoided because they cause dependence, decrease the normal production of mucus, increase the possibility of trauma or perforation, and become less effective with prolonged use. At times, enemas may be necessary for the person with spinal cord injury; if so, no more than 500 ml of a nonirritating fluid is sufficient. Lying on the left side assists in retaining fluid. It may be necessary to pinch the buttocks together securely around the rectal tube to retain the fluid in the bowel. An indwelling catheter with a balloon may be used to prevent the fluid from being expelled until a sufficient amount has been instilled.

It is possible for persons with cord lesions to develop *automatic* defecation. Suppositories are given every day at the same time. If these persons are able to sit up, they should sit on the toilet. In addition to using suppositories, they may have to take stool softeners to keep the stool from becoming hard and causing an impaction. A diet that provides adequate bulk and a minimum of 3000 ml of fluids daily is a necessary part of the program. Massaging the abdomen toward the sigmoid area and digital rectal stimulation are additional measures that may be necessary to aid in evacuation. If results are obtained within an hour and impaction and incontinence do not occur, the schedule can be changed to every other day.

Diarrhea, which occurs in incontinent persons, may be a symptom of *fecal impaction*. Impaction is frequently a problem of the elderly. A rectal examination will identify the presence of an impaction in the rectum. The impaction is broken up through digital manipulation as necessary, and then an oil enema followed by a cleansing enema is given. If the leakage continues despite enemas and is liquid in consistency, a rectal tube (28 or 30 Fr) may be inserted into the rectum and anchored in the fold under the buttock with adhesive tape and attached to straight drainage. Fecal impaction may also cause urinary incontinence by creating pressure on the bladder. Such urinary incontinence will cease when the fecal impaction is removed. If the diarrhea is not caused by an impaction, other possible causes will need to be ascertained (p. 1445).

Uncontrolled fecal incontinence. If none of the above measures are appropriate or successful, measures are taken to maintain the person's integrity, both psychologic as well as physical. Loss of control over intestinal elimination may be associated with feelings of regression, inadequacy, guilt, and uncleanliness. The person needs to feel accepted as an adult and that the condition is accepted by others as a situational physical condition and not as personal inadequacy. Thus empathic communications by health care professionals are helpful. These persons are not treated as children but as adults, nor are they made to feel that they are the cause of the incontinence. Protective disposable pants are available and provide the person with a sense of security and dignity. Persons with incontinence are encouraged to participate in some or all of their own management to the extent that is possible, thus providing them with a sense of control.

Cleansing of the anal and perineal area as soon as possible after fecal incontinence helps to maintain skin integrity and removes a source of discomfort and odor. The patient's usual defecation pattern is monitored and plans can be made to place the patient on a commode, toilet, or bedpan at times that defecation is most likely to occur. The most common defecation time is after meals; thus the person may defecate in the usual manner, although control is not possible, and the skin is protected. Adequate intake of fiber foods and fluids assists in defecation of a normal stool at less frequent intervals. Uncontrolled fecal incontinence often occurs simultaneously with urinary incontinence (p. 1541).

Outcome criteria for the person with fecal incontinence

1. The person is free of perineal skin excoriation.
2. The person is free of fecal odor.
3. The person or significant other can:
   a. Describe the relationship of adequate hygiene to the maintenance of skin integrity.
   b. Describe the relationship of a diet containing adequate fiber foods and fluids to facilitate bowel training.
   c. Describe a bowel training program (if appropriate).

Decompression of the intestinal tract

Purpose

Decompression, or deflation, of the intestinal tract is accomplished by passing a tube through the nose or mouth into the intestine and attaching the tube to the suction apparatus. This procedure is used to drain fluids and gas that accumulate above a mechanical intestinal obstruction, to deflate the intestines during paralytic ileus, and to deflate the bowel before or after intestinal surgery.

Types of intestinal tubes

The tubes most often used for intestinal decompression are the Miller-Abbott tube and the Cantor tube. The length of these tubes permits their passage through the entire intestinal tract. There is a small balloon on the tip of each, which, when inflated with air or injected with water or mercury, acts like a bolus of food.

This balloon stimulates peristalsis, which advances it along the intestinal tract. If peristalsis is absent, the weight of the mercury in the balloon will usually carry it forward. When a Miller-Abbott tube is used, the mercury is inserted into the balloon of the tube after the tube is passed.

The choice of tube depends on the physician's preference. The Miller-Abbott tube is a double-lumen tube. One lumen leads to the balloon and the other has openings along its course, permitting drainage of intestinal contents and irrigation. The external end of the tube contains two openings—one for drainage of secretions and the other for inflating the balloon (Fig. 58-1). In irrigating this tube, the nurse must be careful that the correct opening is used—the one marked "suction." The other opening is for inflating or deflating the balloon. It should be clamped off and labeled "do not touch."

The Cantor tube, which is used less often, is a single tube with only one opening used for drainage. Before the tube is inserted, the balloon is injected with mercury with a needle and syringe. The needle opening is so small that the globules of mercury cannot escape through it. The mercury can be pushed about so that the balloon is elongated for easy insertion.

Insertion of tubes

Intestinal tubes are passed in the manner described under gastric analysis (p. 1383). The addition of the balloon on the tip of the tube makes its insertion through the nose doubly difficult for the patient. The tube can be mechanically inserted only into the stomach. Its passage along the remainder of the gastrointestinal tract is dependent on gravity and peristalsis. The weight of the mercury in the balloon helps propel the tube through the intestines. After the tube reaches the stomach, its passage through the pylorus and into the duodenum can be facilitated in many ways. Position and activity aid in its passage. After passage of the tube, the patient is usually encouraged to lie on the right side for 2 hours, on the back in Fowler's position for 2 hours, and then on the left side for 2 hours. Passage of the tube through the pylorus is usually ascertained by roentgenographic or fluoroscopic examination. After the tube has passed the pylorus, the patient may be encouraged to walk about to increase peristalsis and to speed the advancement of the tube through the intestines with the help of gravity. During this time, the physician or the nurse advances the tube 7 to 10 cm (3 to 4 in.) through the nose or mouth at specified intervals to provide slack for peristaltic action. The intestinal tube is not secured to the face until it has reached the desired point in the intestines, since taping the tube will prevent it from advancing with peristalsis. The pull of the mercury on the end of the tube may move the bowel along with the tube

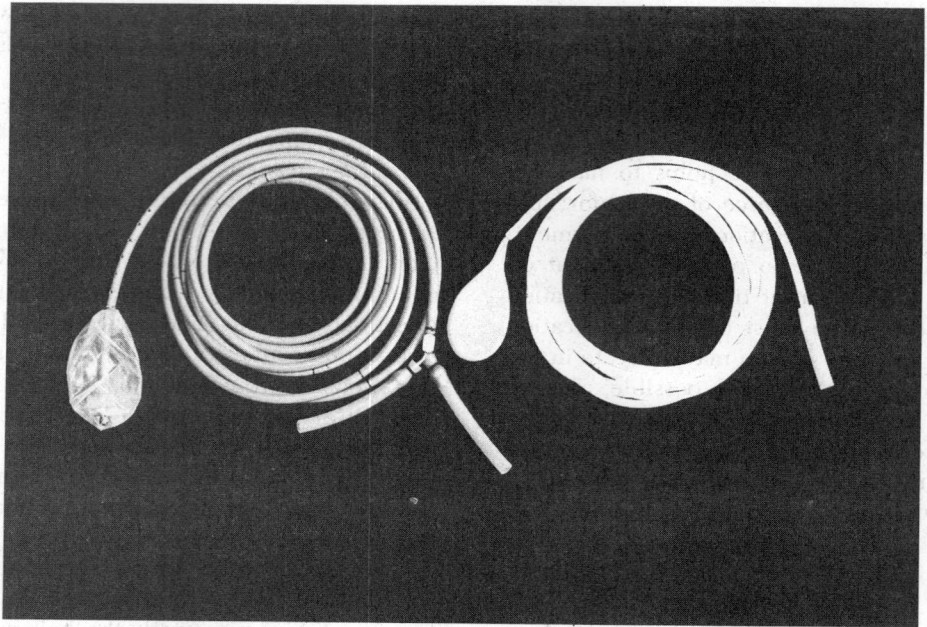

Fig. 58-1. Tubes for intestinal drainage. *Left,* Miller-Abbott tube. *Right,* Cantor tube.

and cause telescoping of the bowel. This results in *intussusception,* which is a serious complication. The tube should be monitored carefully by roentgenographic examination at least once daily to assure that coiling of the tube or telescoping of the bowel has not occurred. Extra tubing should be coiled on the bed or, if the patient is up, pinned to clothing.

Decompression is accomplished by attaching a suction apparatus to the tube either as the tube advances or after it has reached the obstructed portion of the bowel.

Care of the patient with an intestinal tube

Drainage is measured every 24 hours, and the fluid and electrolytes that are lost are replaced by the parenteral routes. If the tip of the tube is far down in the intestine and if the patient is not nauseated or vomiting, light foods such as clear or cream soups, custard, gelatins, milk, or fruit juice, all of which can be absorbed in the upper part of the small intestine, may be permitted.

The tube may require irrigation with normal saline to check its patency. Because the fluid has a longer distance to travel than in a nasogastric tube, it is difficult to aspirate the solution used. If no return flow can be obtained, only a small amount of fluid is used and the amount instilled is recorded.

Nasal and pharyngeal discomfort usually is pronounced, and the nursing measures described under gastric intubation are employed (p. 1395). Signs of the return of peristalsis (bowel sounds, passage of flatus rectally, or spontaneous bowel movement) are reported to the physician, since they usually indicate that the tube is no longer needed.

Removal of intestinal tubes

The intestinal tube is usually left in the intestine longer than the nasogastric tube remains in the stomach. It is always removed gradually several centimeters at a time. Some resistance may be felt as it is withdrawn because of the pull against peristalsis. The patient may feel a tugging sensation and become nauseated. When the tip of the tube reaches the posterior nasopharynx, it may be brought out through the mouth so that the balloon and mercury can be detached. The tube is then pulled through the nose. Since the tube usually has a fecal odor and may cause nausea, the tubing should be removed from sight at once and the patient is given oral care as soon as it is removed. For several days after removal of an intestinal tube, the patient's throat may be sore and hoarseness may result. Gargles and lozenges can be continued until these symptoms subside.

Occasionally, the balloon of an intestinal tube may extrude from the anus. If this occurs, the upper end of the tube is disconnected from suction and removed through the rectum. Removal is usually done slowly and with the help of peristaltic action.

Bowel surgery

Surgical intervention in the large or small intestine is usually performed in one of the following two ways: (1) the diseased portion of the bowel is removed (resected), and the remaining ends are joined together (anastomosis); or (2) the diseased portion of the bowel is removed, and the functioning end is brought out onto the abdominal surface forming a "stoma." The second method interrupts the normal continuity of the intestine but does allow maintenance of function. For example, an ileostomy is an opening into the ileum of the small intestine; a colostomy is an opening into the large intestine (colon).

Resection and anastomosis of the bowel

Preoperative care

Preoperative preparation of the person who is to have surgery of the bowel varies in some respects from preparation for other abdominal surgery.

Diet. During the preoperative period, a low-residue diet is given so that the bowel will contain little or no stool at the time of surgery. Bowel-cleansing methods, plus the inability of the bowel to absorb vitamins, require the administration of vitamins K and C. Parenteral fluids and electrolytes are given to replace losses from the bowel preparation, from the restricted food and oral fluid intake, and from the bowel absorptive failure. In the debilitated person, parenteral hyperalimentation may be used to administer fluid, electrolytes, and proteins and to prevent negative nitrogen balance in preparation for surgery (p. 402). Twenty-four hours before surgery a clear liquid diet may be given, if tolerated. The reasons for the diet restriction as well as for the intravenous fluids are explained to the individual and family.

Prevention of infection. Preparation of the bowel for surgery may be initiated several days before surgery, and a variety of mechanical (enemas) or chemical (drugs) approaches may be used. The purpose of the bowel preparation is to suppress bacterial growth in the colon and thus lessen the risk of postoperative peritoneal infection. Approximately 4 to 5 days preoperatively, a daily soapsuds enema may be given in addition to a daily laxative; 12 to 18 hours before surgery, oral antibiotic therapy is instituted. The antibiotic chosen is one that is not absorbed through the intestinal tract, has low toxicity, and has broad-spectrum activity against colonic bacteria.[39] Commonly used antibiotics include neomycin, erythromycin, succinylsulfathiazole (Sulfasuxidine), and phthalylsulfathiazole (Sulfathalidine). Systemic antibiotics are not recommended because they are ineffective against intraluminal colonic bacteria.[32] Mechanical and chemical measures are not instituted for patients with intestinal obstruction. Vigorous mechanical cleansing or purging may be poorly tolerated by some persons such as the acutely ill or elderly; therefore these approaches may be modified.

Intubation. A nasogastric or intestinal tube is inserted before the operation. Since the passage of a tube into the intestines may take as long as 24 hours, intestinal intubation is usually started the day before surgery. As the tube passes through the small intestine, the bowel becomes "threaded" on it, and thus is compactly held together and shortened while the operation is performed. Before and after surgery, the intestinal tube is usually attached to a suction apparatus for the aspiration of intestinal contents. This prevents the accumulation of gas and intestinal fluid around the suture line. If a nasogastric tube is used, it is inserted the morning the operation is scheduled.

An indwelling Foley catheter is usually inserted preoperatively to maintain bladder decompression during surgery so that bladder trauma does not occur. Urinary retention is a common postoperative complication following surgery of the distal colon and rectum, and thus the Foley catheter may be left in place for up to 1 week following surgery in these instances.

Postoperative care

Extensive handling of the gastrointestinal organs during surgery causes a marked inhibition of peristalsis—either cessation of movement (*paralytic ileus*) or weak ineffectual movements (*adynamic ileus*). Care during the early postoperative period is therefore directed at preventing the buildup of gas or fluid in the gastrointestinal tract, which can cause excessive fluid and electrolyte disturbances, pressure on the suture line, or inhibition of respiration by elevation of the diaphragm.

Fluid and electrolyte balance. Until peristalsis returns and the anastomosis is partially healed, the nasogastric or intestinal tube is used, and special attention is given to keeping the tube draining and to maintaining fluid and electrolyte balance. The surgeon carefully checks the amount of fluid needed and reviews the daily output from voiding and from gastric drainage. Recording of these fluids must be accurate. Electrolytes lost through the gastric drainage are replaced with the parenteral fluids.

Until the intestinal tube is removed, nothing is given by mouth. The patient needs frequent mouth care. If an intestinal tube is used, an antibiotic solution may be ordered for mouth care, since colon bacteria may travel up the tube by capillary action. After the tube is removed, foods are added gradually until a full diet is resumed. Occasionally, bland foods may be ordered for some time following surgery.

Oxygenation. Pain in the incision may be severe and may interfere with full respiratory excursion. Narcotics are administered as necessary for pain, and the patient is encouraged to cough, to breathe deeply, and to change position every hour to two. Encouragement and assistance are often necessary in doing so during the first day or two postoperatively. The incidence of pulmonary embolism is greater when pelvic surgery is performed than when surgery is performed higher in the abdomen. Pulmonary embolism and infarction are most apt to occur 7 to 10 days after surgery and are suspected if the person experiences an increased respiratory and pulse rate out of proportion to the degree of fever. Hemoptysis and pleuritic pain are experienced in less than 10% of persons with pulmonary emboli.[19]

Elimination. The length of time required for peristalsis to return depends on the extent of bowel manipulation. Presence of bowel sounds or passage of gas signals the return of function. A rectal tube can be inserted to facilitate the passage of flatus. Drugs to stimulate expulsion of flatus, such as dexpanthenol (Ilopan) or neostigmine (Prostigmin), may be administered. Since ambulation is of great assistance for encouraging peristalsis, the patient is assisted out of bed a day or two after surgery, even while the nasogastric or intestinal tube is still in use. The passage of gas or stool rectally should be reported to the surgeon at once, since it usually indicates the return of peristalsis and means that oral intake can be resumed and that the intestinal tube can be removed.

It is not unusual after a resection of the bowel for diarrhea to occur after peristalsis returns. Usually it is temporary and soon disappears. When the stool becomes normal, the patient is advised to avoid becoming constipated, because a hard stool and straining to expel it could possibly injure the anastomosis, depending on its location. Persons who have a tendency to develop constipation postoperatively are advised to try drinking fruit juice and water before breakfast or to take a glass of prune juice daily. They should not take laxatives without medical approval. Stool softeners or a mild bulk cathartic such as psyllium (Metamucil) is prescribed frequently.

Temporary cecostomy

A cecostomy, or opening into the cecum, may be performed as a temporary measure to decompress the colon when there is an obstructing lesion of the left colon and the situation (e.g., aged person or poor-risk patient with marked distention) does not permit more extensive surgery at the time.[19] With the use of local anesthetic to control pain, an opening is made into the

cecum through a small incision in the right lower quadrant of the abdomen, and a catheter is inserted into the bowel. The catheter is sutured to the skin and provides an outlet for feces, which is still fluid in the ascending colon. Tubing is attached to the catheter, which is attached to a container that is capped to control odors but that is provided with an air vent so that drainage can occur. The tubing should be long enough so that persons can move about freely. In order to keep the tube open, it is usually irrigated every 4 hours with a physiologic solution of sodium chloride. The fluid is allowed to run in by gravity and flows out by inverting the syringe or funnel or by aspiration.

The dressings around the tube are changed as frequently as necessary, and the skin is kept clean and dry. After the tube is removed, skin care and changes of dressing are continued until all drainage ceases. Occasionally, an ileostomy bag is used to keep drainage off the skin. A water-soluble chlorophyll derivative (Chloresium) may be applied for its soothing, antipruritic, and deodorizing effects.

Abdominoperineal resection of the bowel

Abdominal resection of the bowel may be performed for malignant growths in the rectum. The operation is performed through two incisions: a low midline incision of the abdomen and a wide elliptic incision about the anus. Through the abdominal incision, the sigmoid colon is divided and the lower portion is freed from its attachments and temporarily left beneath the peritoneum of the pelvic floor. The proximal end of the sigmoid is then brought out through a small stab wound on the abdominal wall and becomes the permanent colostomy. Through the perineal incision, the anus and rectum are freed from the perineal muscles; and the anus, the rectum containing the growth, and the distal portion of sigmoid are removed. The perineal wound may be closed around Penrose drains, or it may be left wide open and packed with gauze and a rubber dam to cause it to heal slowly from the inside outward (Fig. 58-2).

Preoperative care

Preoperative nursing care is similar to that for other intestinal surgery. Some surgeons pass ureteral catheters preoperatively so that the ureters are not inadvertently tied off during surgery. A Foley catheter is inserted into the bladder and attached to a straight drainage system to keep the bladder empty during surgery and thus prevent operative injury. In addition to the preoperative teaching about the stoma (p. 1459), the patient will need to know about the perineal incision. This will heal by secondary intention (p. 442) and therefore will take much longer to heal than a usual incision.

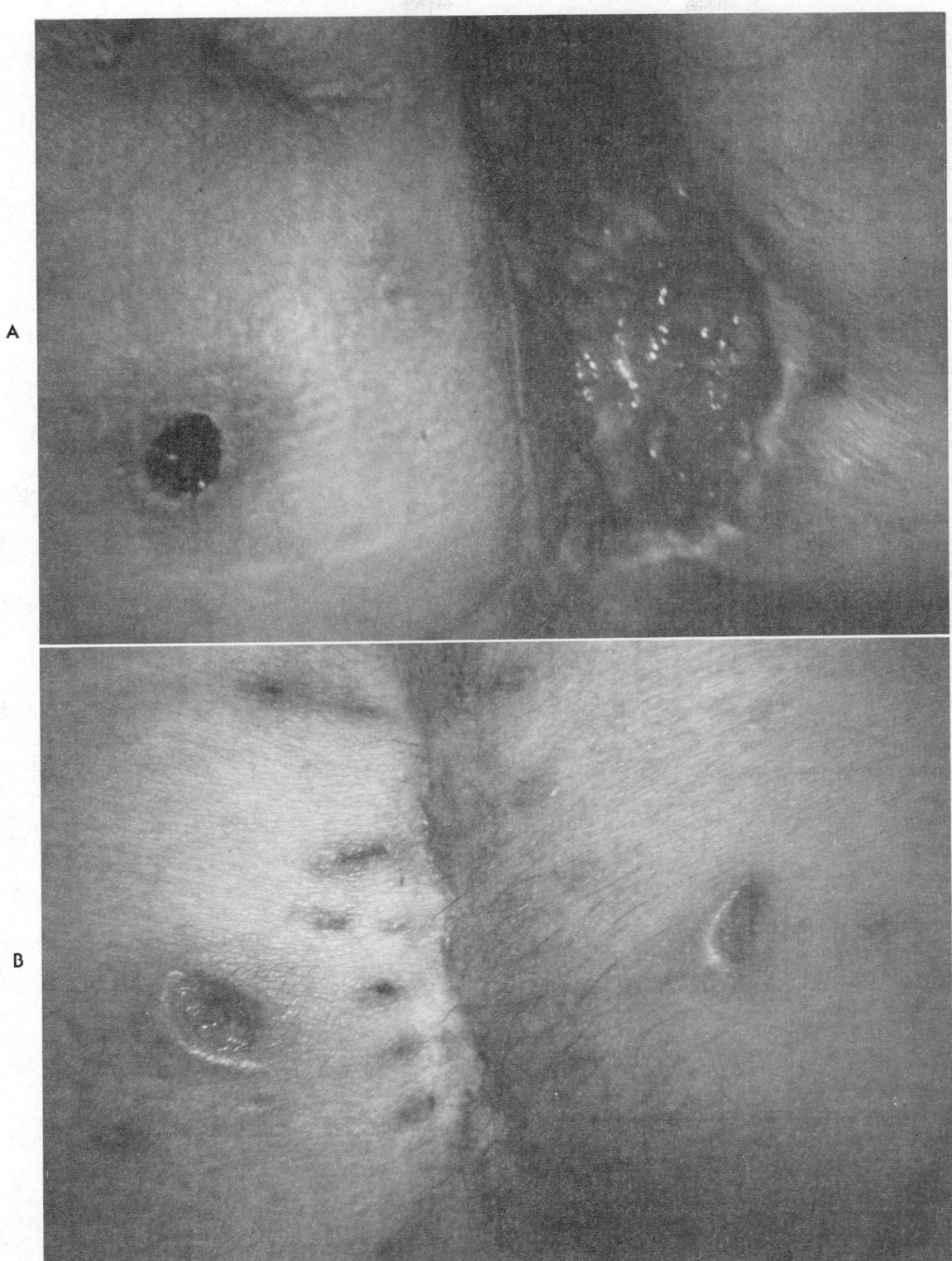

Fig. 58-2. Perineal wound following an anteroposterior resection for cancer in rectum. **A,** Postsurgical wound; note site of sump drain to left of wound. **B,** Following healing; perineum is completely closed; shape of buttocks looks normal.

Postoperative care

Shock. Postoperative shock is a frequent occurrence because of the large amount of tissue removed at the time of surgery. Measures to monitor and treat shock are therefore instituted (p. 310).

Wound care. In the immediate postoperative period, rectal dressings are observed carefully for signs of excessive bleeding. The usual drainage is serosanguineous and profuse, and the dressing may have to be reinforced during the first few hours postoperatively. Disposable pads are placed under the hips and are changed frequently. If sump catheters have been used, they are attached to low continuous suction.

After the surgeon has changed the first dressing (usually 24 hours postoperatively), the dressing is changed by the nurse as necessary. Since the dressing requires frequent changing, a T-binder is used to hold the dressing in place and to give support without causing skin irritation. Care of the colostomy is described on p. 1463. If the perineal wound has been packed, the packing is frequently changed. The wound is usually irrigated several times a day to remove secretions and tissue debris, to prevent abscesses from forming in the dead space that may be left, and to help ensure healing of the wound from the inside outward. If a catheter is to be inserted into the wound for the irrigation, the nurse should ascertain from the surgeon how deep it can be inserted and in what direction to insert it. Normal saline solution is frequently used as the irrigating solution. A hand-held shower massage or Water Pik with the jet on lowest pressure may also be used for irrigation.[25] The power spray washes away the debris and stimulates the circulation in the tissue to enhance healing. Precise directions as to how to do the irrigation should be recorded on the nursing care plan.

When the patient is permitted out of bed, sitz baths may be substituted for the irrigations, and as drainage from the wound decreases, a perineal pad may be substituted for the dressing. A rubber ring may be used during the sitz bath so that water can flow freely around the incision. The response in healing is often quite remarkable when this is done. Since the patient is usually ready to leave the hospital before the perineal wound has completely closed, arrangements must be made to continue with the sitz baths at home. If a bathtub is not available, a large basin may be used. Portable sitz baths are available and may be rented from hospital supply firms. They may be more comfortable to use than a regular tub.

Many patients complain of phantom rectal sensations and of feeling the necessity to defecate. An explanation of cortical perception and transmission of nerve impulses often helps the patient cope with these sensations.

Urinary elimination. The Foley catheter usually is left in the bladder postoperatively to prevent the blad-

der from becoming distended and from pressing against the repaired pelvic floor until it heals. Its use also eliminates the need for women to use the bedpan to void (a painful procedure after this operation) and prevents contamination of the wound and dressings with urine.

Urinary retention is a common occurrence following rectal excision, with approximately 50% of men experiencing some degree of adynamic bladder paralysis after the Foley catheter is removed.[2] Factors that influence urinary retention include loss of pelvic support, chronic urinary tract infection, enlarged prostate, or nerve injury. Symptoms of benign prostatic hypertrophy may have been masked following surgery; a subsequent prostatectomy may be required to relieve the symptoms. Loss of pelvic support increases problems with micturition when the patient is supine; thus micturition may improve with ambulation. If nerve injury is present, problems with urinary retention and urinary tract infections may persist for 6 to 8 months with partial resolution of retention but with urinary incontinence experienced at night.[2]

Special care should be taken that the catheter drains constantly so that residual urine does not remain in the bladder. When the catheter is removed, accurate intake and output records are necessary to monitor for possible residual urine that may lead to urinary tract infection.

Pain. A narcotic for pain is usually required at regular intervals for the first 2 to 3 days postoperatively.

Activity. Most patients prefer a side-lying position because of severe discomfort in the supine position. A soft foam pad may relieve pressure on the perineal area when the patient does lie supine. Frequent turning is encouraged, and considerable assistance may be necessary during the early postoperative period because of the incisional pain. Isometric exercises and quadriceps drills (p. 413) are encouraged. The potential for the development of postoperative thrombophlebitis is high.

Convalescence after an abdominal perineal resection is prolonged and may require many months. During this time the individual should remain under close supervision.

Surgical procedures for massive obesity

Obesity exists in two forms—*adult-onset* (hypertrophic) obesity and *lifelong* (hyperplastic-hypertrophic) obesity. Persons with adult-onset obesity (middle-aged spread) have a fixed number of fat cells, but each cell contains excessive fat. These persons respond well to weight reduction regimens. Persons with lifelong obesity not only have excessive fat in each cell but also have more fat cells and generally respond poorly to weight reduction regimens. Persons who become massively obese are usually of the lifelong type.[19]

Massively obese persons have an increased predisposition for numerous diseases (e.g., diabetes, hypertension, atherosclerotic heart disease, arthritis, pulmonary disease, and hernias). In addition, they have an increased mortality when these disorders occur, thus leading to a shortened life span.

Since medical treatment in the form of dietary restriction, medications for appetite control, as well as hypnosis and psychiatric therapy often is unsuccessful, surgical procedures have been tried in an attempt to alleviate the problem of massive obesity. Various surgical procedures have evolved in an effort to shunt or bypass a portion of the small intestine and limit the area available for absorption of fats and carbohydrates.

Intestinal bypass

In the jejunoileal bypass procedure, approximately 14 in. of the jejunum and 4 in. of the ileum are preserved for the bypass anastomosis. The 14 in. of the proximal jejunum are anastomosed to the side of the ileum 4 in. from the ileocecal valve (Fig. 58-3). The retention of the ileocecal area is an important factor in retarding the intestinal transit time and thus permitting longer contact of the chyme to the intestinal mucosa. The long length of bypassed jejunoileum is anastomosed with the ileal end to the transverse colon or sigmoid colon.

Persons selected for surgery are carefully evaluated physically and mentally. Studies are carried out with special attention being given to the cardiopulmonary and endocrine status as well as the gastrointestinal assessment of the stomach, small bowel, and colon function. Preoperative measurements of serum calcium, potassium, magnesium, and other electrolytes plus assessment of vitamins A, B_{12}, and C, and folic acid are made. *Psychologic evaluation* is considered essential in determining the individual's response to weight loss and change in body image and acceptance of the close surveillance of metabolic changes that may occur postoperatively. Despite the careful selection, many patients and their significant others experience long-range psychologic problems and difficulties in adjustments of lifestyle.

Diarrhea is usually a problem in the early postoperative period because of the increased transit time, but eventually most persons stabilize at about five semiformed stools per day.[19] Malabsorption of fat and fat-soluble vitamins usually occurs, and dietary supplements are usually necessary. Protein malnutrition may also occur and leads to hepatic dysfunction. Other complications include prolonged severe diarrhea, polyarthritis, intestinal inflammation, osteomalacia, and oxylate renal stones. Operative mortality rate is approximately 5%.

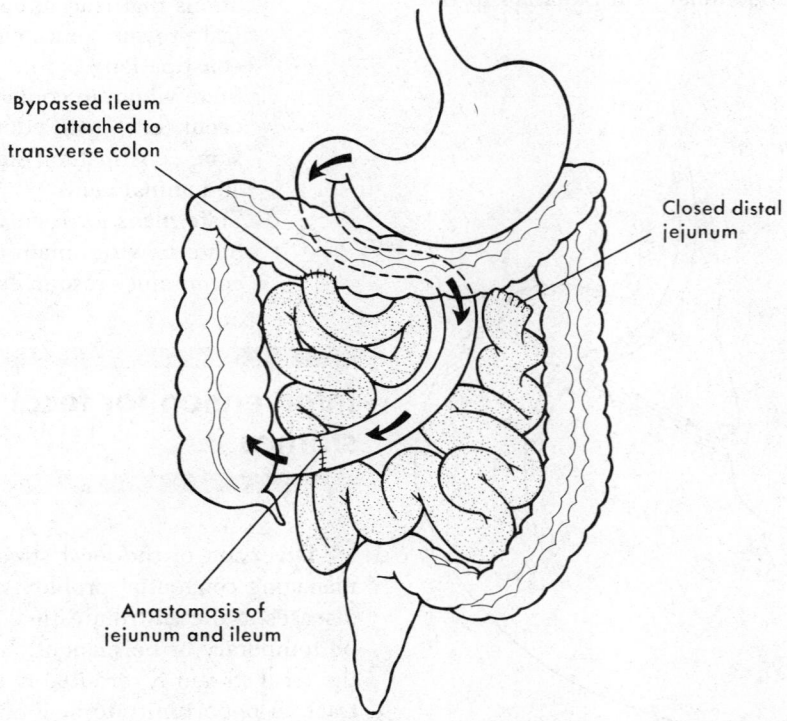

Bypassed ileum attached to transverse colon

Closed distal jejunum

Anastomosis of jejunum and ileum

Fig. 58-3. End-to-end jejunoileal anastomosis; 10 in. of jejunum is anastomosed to end of terminal ileum 20 in. from ileocecal valve. Proximal end of ileum is anastomosed to side of midtransverse colon. Distal end of jejunum is closed and sutured to mesentery. (From Given, B.A., and Simmons, S.J.: Gastroenterology in clinical nursing, ed. 3, St. Louis, 1979, The C.V. Mosby Co.)

Weekly follow-up is essential in the immediate postoperative period, and periodic clinical evaluation in the subsequent years must be impressed on the person. After discharge, rehabilitation and desired loss of weight is achieved by the physician's long-range metabolic and nutritional follow-up.

Gastric stapling

A newer surgical approach to the control of massive obesity is gastric stapling. In this procedure, a row of staples is placed across the upper end of the stomach with a small opening left for the slow passage of food into the remainder of the stomach (Fig. 58-4). A small pouch is thus formed that limits the amount of food the person can take without experiencing pain and vomiting. This type of surgery has fewer consequences than bypass surgery since the gastrointestinal tract is not opened and remains intact.

Drainage from a nasogastric tube inserted postoperatively is small (approximately 300 ml). If irrigation is necessary, only a small amount of fluid (300 ml) is used. Clear fluids are introduced about the third day and, if tolerated, the diet is advanced to pureed foods. A blenderized diet is followed for 8 weeks, at which time small amounts of soft bland foods are introduced gradually. The patient is monitored in the postoperative period for perforation of the stomach by the staples, which is evidenced by upper abdominal pain radiating to the left shoulder.

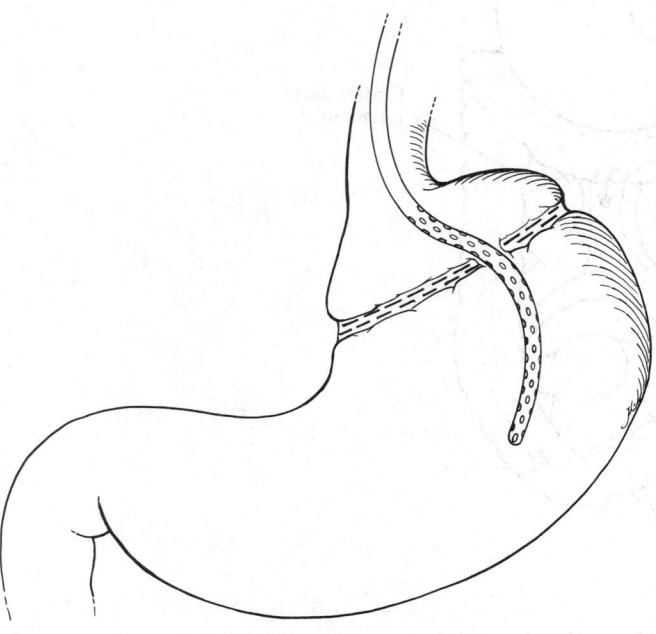

Fig. 58-4. Gastric stapling with a postoperative nasogastric tube for drainage. Stomach is partially closed by double row of staples.

Outcome criteria for the person who has had intestinal surgery

The person or significant others can:
1. Describe any medication or treatment program to be followed at home.
   a. State dosage, frequency, action, and side effects of medications (e.g., antibiotics and stool softeners).
   b. Demonstrate correct technique for cleansing of incisional area (if drainage or stoma is present) and the application of a dressing or appliance.
2. Describe a plan for any dietary modifications needed.
   a. State means of meeting fluid and nutrient requirements.
   b. List specific foods to be avoided if applicable (e.g., high roughage).
3. Describe the health maintenance or follow-up program.
   a. Explain the basic pathologic condition and overall treatment program in his or her own words.
   b. Explain the rationale for avoidance of situations that lead to an increase in intraabdominal pressure (e.g., chronic or acute cough and constipation.)
   c. State whom to contact if additional symptoms occur (e.g., red, edematous, or draining incision; constipation; signs of systemic infection; abdominal pain).
   d. State plans for regular follow-up care.
   e. State how to obtain any necessary or desired community resources.

Intervention for fecal diversion: stomas

Diversion of the fecal stream may be indicated for managing congenital problems, traumatic injuries, and diseases in the gastrointestinal tract. The diversion may be temporary or permanent. In a *temporary diversion,* the fecal stream is rerouted to allow the gastrointestinal tract an opportunity to heal or to provide an outlet for the stool when an obstruction is present. A *permanent diversion* implies that the intestine cannot or will not be reconnected; thus a return to a normal elimination mode will not occur.

Surgical procedures

There are three types of surgical procedures: an end stoma, a loop stoma, or a double-barrel ostomy.

When an *end stoma* is created surgically, the functioning proximal bowel is brought out through the abdominal wall to form a single stoma. The stoma is formed by bringing the intestine through an opening in the abdominal wall. The bowel is then folded on itself (forming a cuff) and sutured. The stomal surface is the mucosal lining layer of the intestinal wall. It is an absorbing surface and contains numerous small capillaries. The remaining (distal) bowel is surgically removed or the bowel is oversewn, forming a Hartmann's pouch. The most common fecal diversion is an end sigmoid colostomy for cancer of the rectum. An abdominal perineal resection is done, and the rectum and anus are removed (p. 1452).

The *loop stoma* is created by bringing the bowel through an abdominal incision, sliding a support under the bowel, and opening the upper wall of the bowel. The posterior wall remains intact. There is one stoma, but there are two openings—proximal and distal (Fig. 58-5). The loop ostomy is generally a temporary procedure. It is often done in an emergency situation (e.g., gunshot or stab wounds or for complications of diverticulitis or intestinal obstruction.

The *double-barrel ostomy* is created by bringing the proximal and distal bowel through the abdominal wall creating two stomas. This may be done as a planned temporary procedure for an inflamed or diseased bowel to permit the distal portion to "rest" or to heal (Fig. 58-6).

Patients who do not receive a bowel preparation before an emergency procedure in which a loop procedure is done or who are inadequately "prepped" for a double-barrel ostomy may have a bowel evacuation through the rectum. Patients should be told this may occur. Also after discharge, patients may experience the urge to defecate through the rectum. They should attempt to defecate, and generally mucus is passed. When a cleansing enema is given through the distal bowel for closure, the returns will be by way of the rectum.

Colostomy surgery

The surgical diversion of the large colon will result in a colostomy. The anatomic location of the ostomy in the large colon will determine the name, that is, *ascending* colostomy, *transverse* colostomy, or *sigmoid* colostomy. The nursing care and patient needs are different for each type of colostomy (Table 58-3).

Temporary colostomies are often done for complications of diverticulitis, volvulus, ischemia of bowel, perforations, and traumatic injuries from gunshot or stab wounds. The "temporary" colostomy is done to divert the stool from the injured or diseased bowel. The length

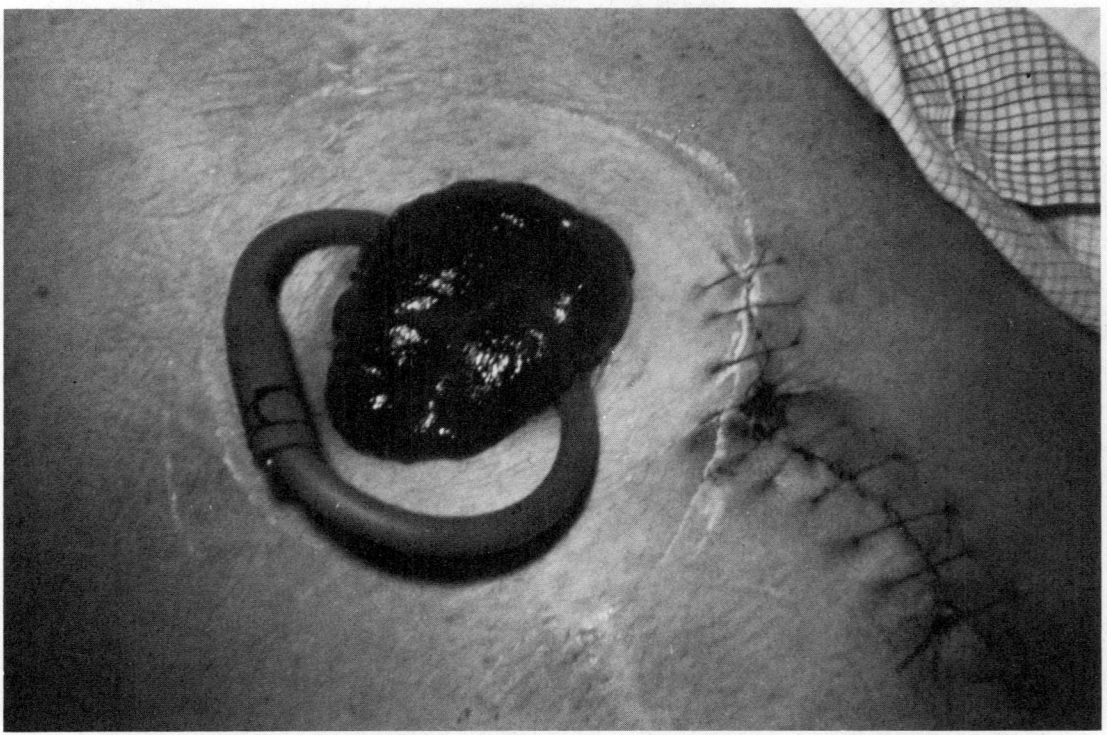

Fig. 58-5. Loop transverse colostomy.

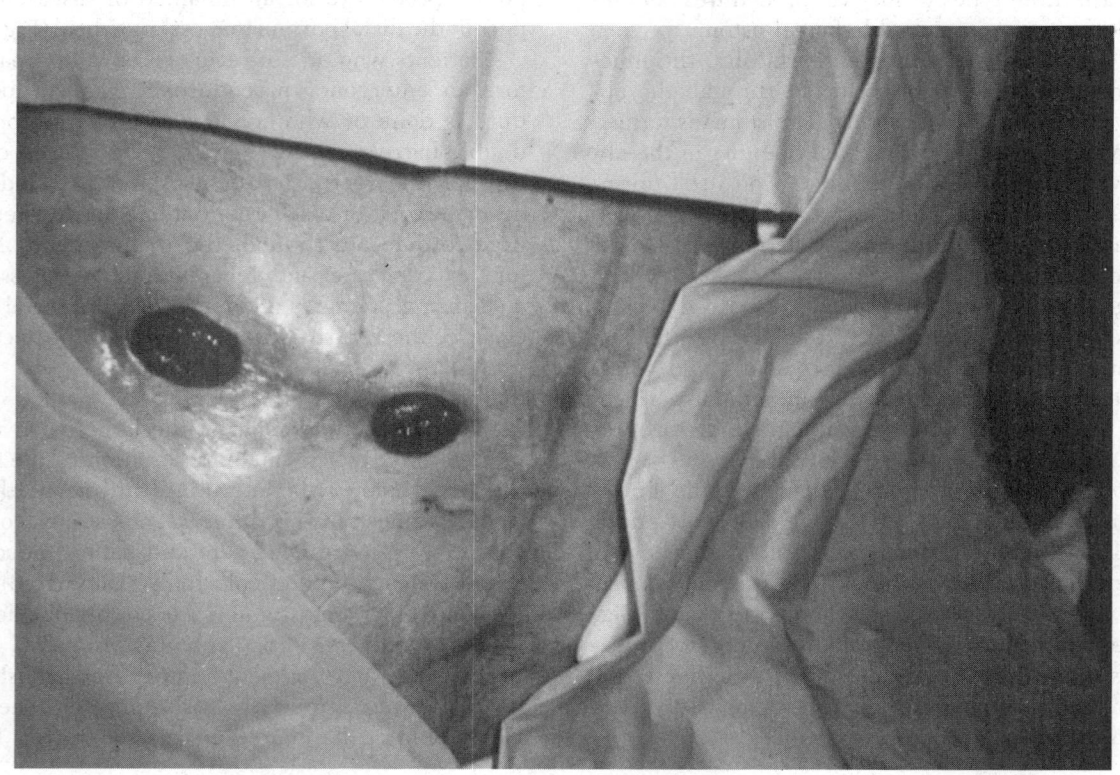

Fig. 58-6. Double-barrel colostomy.

TABLE 58-3. Comparison of ileostomy and colostomies

	Ileostomy	Ascending colostomy	Transverse colostomy	Sigmoid colostomy
Location	Ileum (terminal end of small intestine)	Ascending colon	Transverse colon	Sigmoid colon
Type of drainage	Initial: liquid; 3-6 mo: "toothpaste" consistency	Liquid to soft	Soft	Formed
Bowel regulation	No	No	No	Yes
Fluid and electrolyte imbalance	Occurs frequently with illness and diagnostic procedures	Same as for ileostomy	Less possibility than with ileostomy but may occur more readily than normal	No different from a person with intact colon
Skin irritation	Irritation occurs easily from digestive enzymes	Same as for ileostomy	Some skin irritation from constant moisture	Irritation may occur occasionally
Other complications	Stricture or inversion of stoma; diarrhea with antibiotic therapy; food blockage	Stricture or inversion of stoma	Stricture or inversion of stoma	Stricture or inversion of stoma

of time a person has a temporary ostomy will vary. A person is carefully reassessed before closure, and occasionally a temporary colostomy is never closed. Permanent colostomies are most often done for cancer of the colon, and the rectum is usually removed. In the person with an inoperable tumor, a loop colostomy is done as a permanent diversion.

Ileostomy surgery

When the small bowel (ileum) is the site of diversion, the ostomy is referred to as an ileostomy. The most frequent indications for an ileostomy in an adult are ulcerative colitis and Crohn's (granulomatous) colitis. In neonates, necrotizing enterocolitis commonly results in a temporary ileostomy.

There are several types of ileostomy procedures performed, including the end ileostomy (Brooke's procedure), loop ileostomy (Turnbull's procedure), and the continent ileostomy. Brooke's and Turnbull's procedures require the use of ostomy pouches postoperatively (Fig. 58-7). The continent ileostomy is a different surgical procedure in which an internal pouch is created, and the person must intubate the pouch to drain the effluent (p. 1485). The continent ileostomy can be done in patients with ulcerative colitis and familial polyposis.

Stoma site

The location of the stoma on the abdominal wall is selected preoperatively by an enterostomal therapist or a surgeon. It is imperative that the stoma site be marked after the abdomen is observed in lying, sitting, and standing positions (Fig. 58-8). It should be easily visible to the patient, and all bony prominences, folds, creases, scars, and the umbilicus should be avoided. The stoma is located within the rectus muscle. The selection of the stoma site is a serious decision and influences the postoperative rehabilitation. A person who is unable to manage the stoma or keep a pouch seal because of a poor location will have a difficult time returning to physical activities and social interactions.

Preoperative care

When the physician first tells the person of the probable need for an ostomy, the immediate reaction is likely to be shock and disbelief. Whether the ostomy is to be temporary or permanent, it is difficult for most people to accept. Knowledge that it is a lifesaving measure, confidence in the surgeon, and sometimes explanation and acceptance of the proposed operation by significant others may assist in the decision to have the operation. It is not unusual for the patient to be sad, withdrawn, and depressed after learning of the need for ostomy surgery.

The nurse should know what the patient has been told by the physician and should be prepared to supplement information and assess how much information to give the patient preoperatively on care of the ostomy. Some patients definitely benefit from discussing the care, reading materials, seeing equipment, and talking to persons who are living normal lives following ostomy surgery. Other patients find this approach upsetting.

The nurse should first assess the individual patient. Often asking patients what they would like to know is a place to begin. Patients may feel they do not know enough to ask questions. The following are some general guidelines for the nurse to use:

1. Provide a simple explanation of the anatomy of the gastrointestinal tract.
2. Use a simple drawing to demonstrate the anatomic sections.
3. Explain what portions of the colon will be removed and the effect on normal bowel function.
4. Explain that you will be available after surgery to help learn to care for the stoma.
5. Define terms such as ileostomy, colostomy, stool, feces, and pouch.
6. Offer services of an Ostomy Visitor.

While implementing the preoperative teaching, the nurse should constantly observe the patient. The nurse should not overwhelm the patient or go into deep explanations that are not required by the patient. It is best if preoperative counseling can take place over two or more consecutive days. Also, the patient should not be given reading material that the nurse has not read; sections that do not apply to the patient should be deleted.

During the preoperative period, effort should be made to augment patients' confidence in the members of the medical and nursing staff, since patients who have complete confidence in the persons who will treat and provide care are more likely to accept their situation postoperatively and be more willing to start to learn self-care. Patients watch every facial expression or gesture of the nurses and are extremely sensitive to evidence of distaste. If other persons accept the ostomy as not unusual, it helps patients feel that it is not a calamity that has happened to them alone.

The importance of significant others in the total planning with the patient cannot be forgotten. They must be encouraged and given the opportunity to discuss freely their own feelings and reactions to the surgery. They are given an opportunity to grieve for the patient's alteration and then are gently guided to recognize those areas in which they may provide support to the patient. The nurse gathers data at this time to anticipate how to include the significant others in the total care program, plan for specific transmission of information, plan the opportunity for ongoing discussion of feelings, and identify those areas in which the significant others may

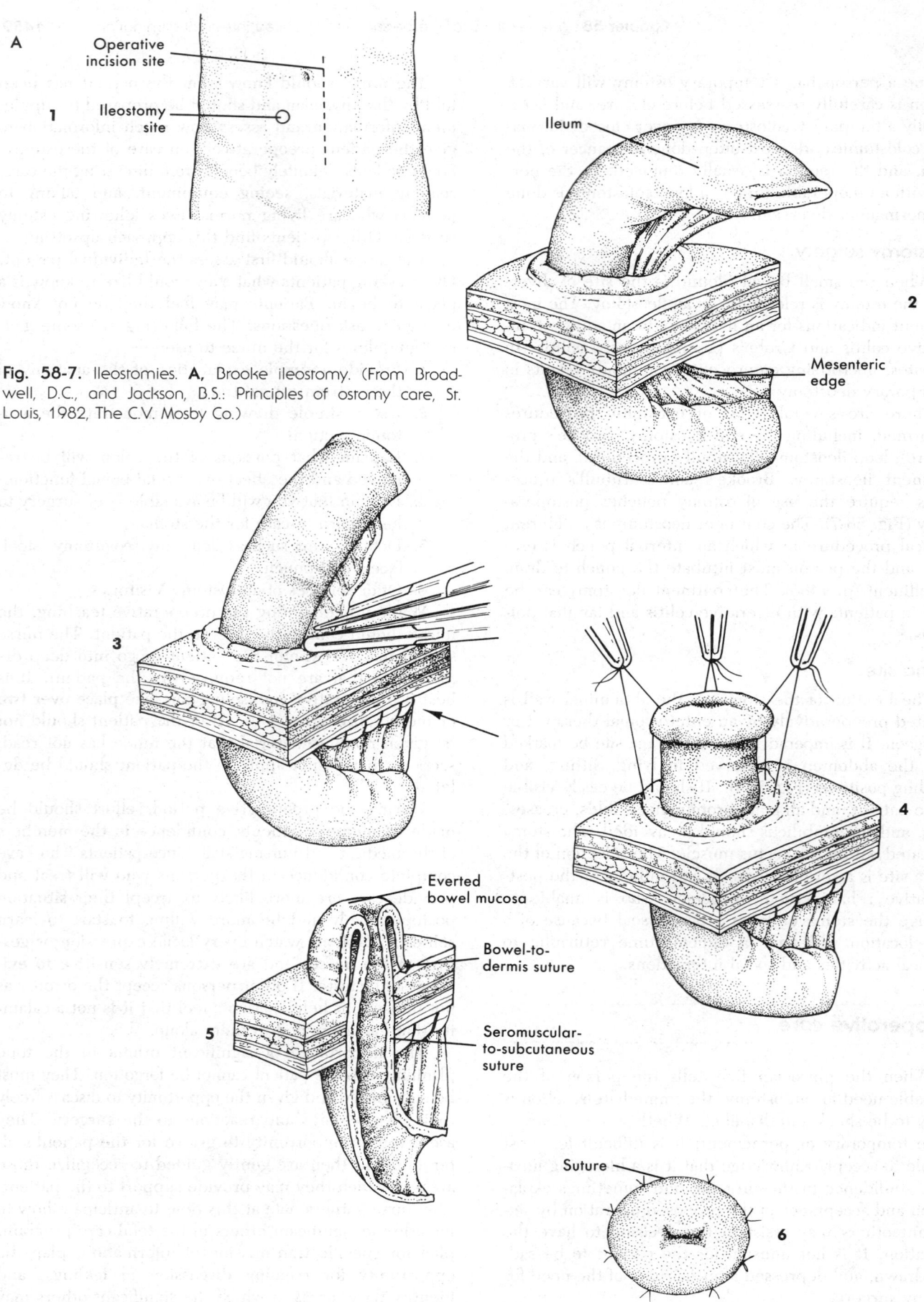

Fig. 58-7. Ileostomies. **A,** Brooke ileostomy. (From Broadwell, D.C., and Jackson, B.S.: Principles of ostomy care, St. Louis, 1982, The C.V. Mosby Co.)

Operative incision site

Ileostomy site

Ileum

Mesenteric edge

Everted bowel mucosa

Bowel-to-dermis suture

Seromuscular-to-subcutaneous suture

Suture

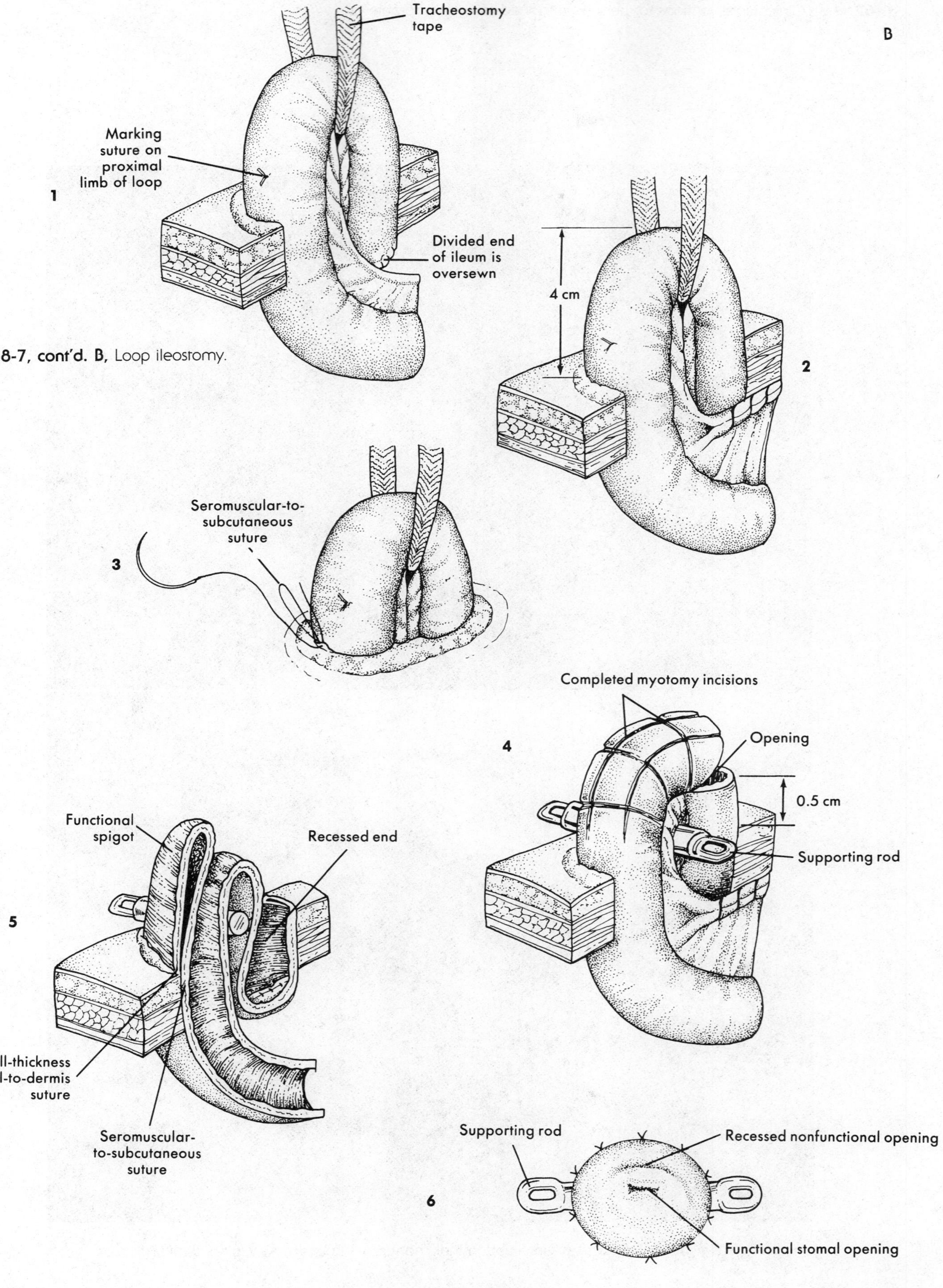

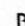

B

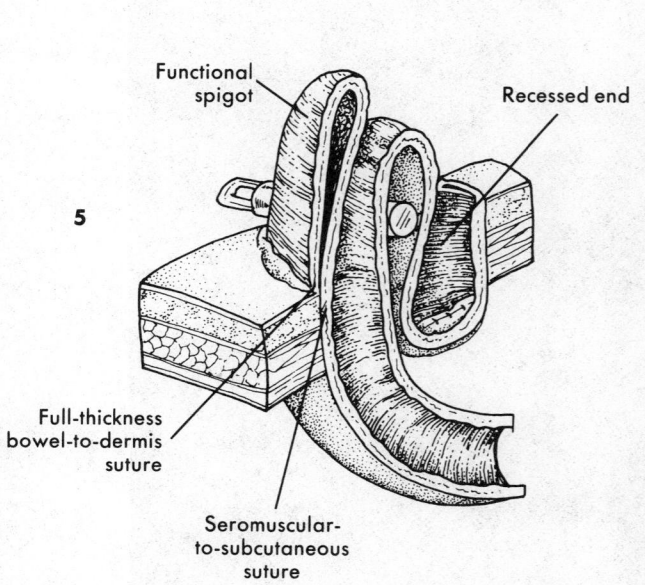

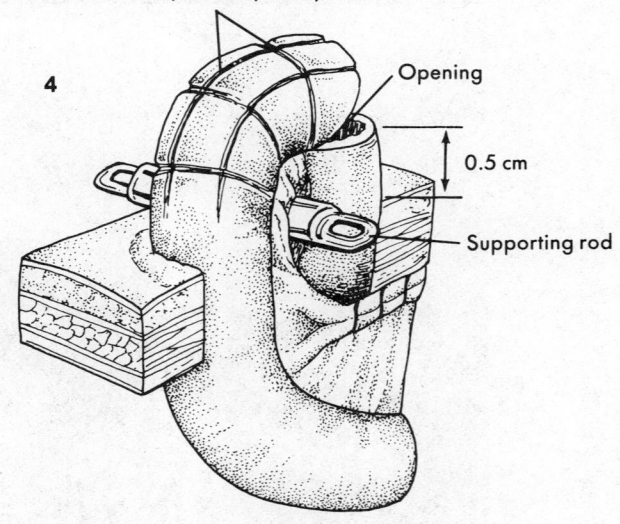

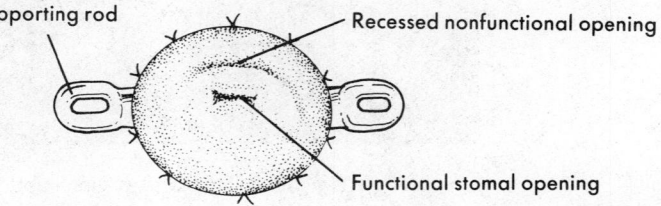

1 Marking suture on proximal limb of loop

Tracheostomy tape

Divided end of ileum is oversewn

2 4 cm

3 Seromuscular-to-subcutaneous suture

Fig. 58-7, cont'd. B, Loop ileostomy.

4 Completed myotomy incisions

Opening

0.5 cm

Supporting rod

5 Functional spigot

Recessed end

Full-thickness bowel-to-dermis suture

Seromuscular-to-subcutaneous suture

6 Supporting rod

Recessed nonfunctional opening

Functional stomal opening

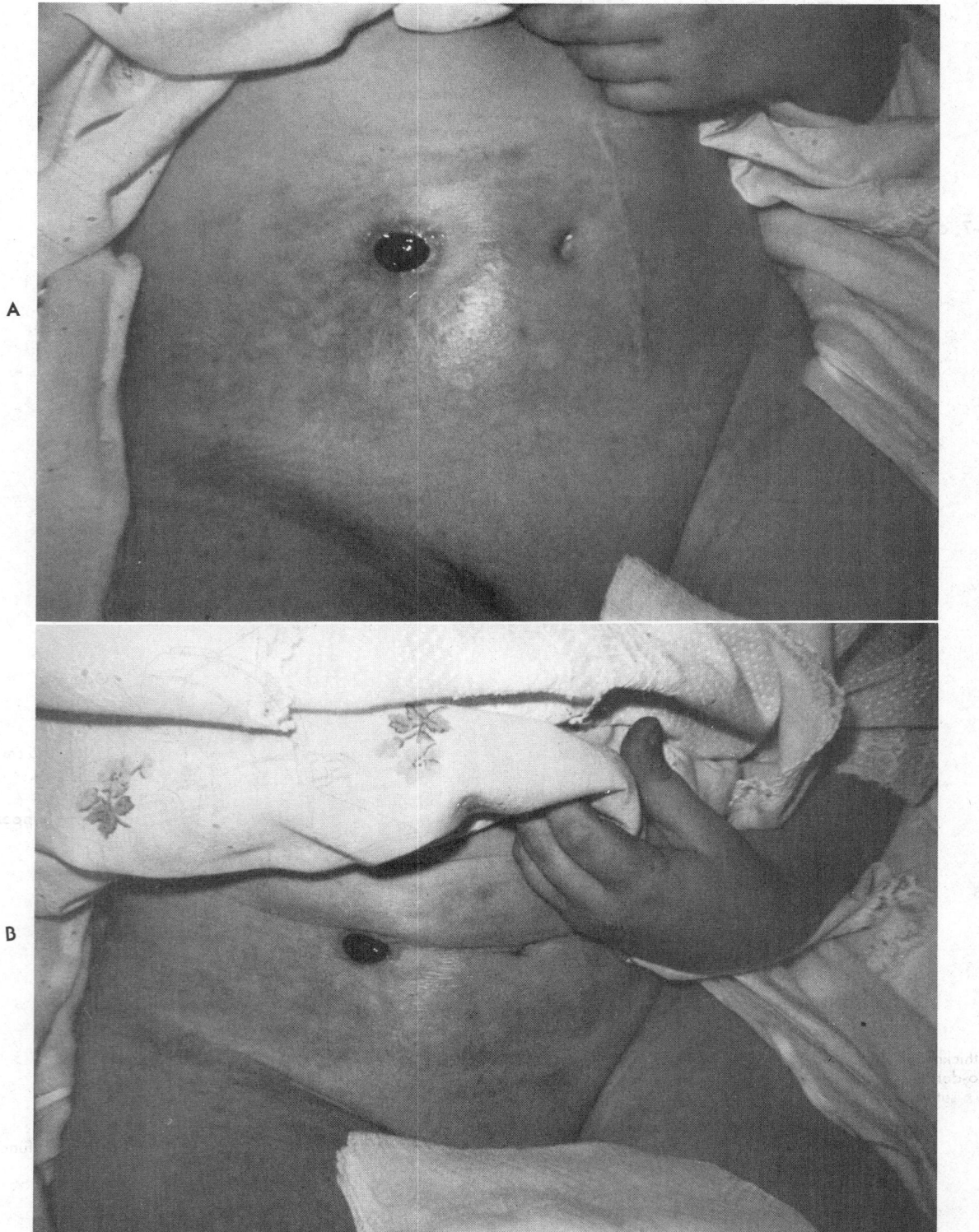

Fig. 58-8. Stoma sites. Note abdominal change with patient **A,** Supine. **B,** Sitting.

not be able to contribute. Significant others who provide support, acceptance, and reassurance will enhance the direct acceptance of the alteration by the patient.

Intraoperative care

At the beginning of the surgical procedure, most surgeons will scratch the stoma site that has been marked preoperatively. The patient is asleep and will not be aware of this. This step alleviates the problems that arise when the stoma site mark is scrubbed off the skin during the surgical preparation.

At the close of the operation, an appliance is applied over the stoma opening. In most cases, a clear disposable pouch is used. The stoma should be observed regularly for color (denoting viability) and to ensure the mucocutaneous suture line remains intact. The early use of a pouch allows for collection of the initial serosanguineous drainage and prevents possible contamination of the surgical incision.

Postoperative care

The immediate postoperative care for the colostomy or ileostomy patient follows the guidelines for bowel surgery (p. 1451). Hemorrhage through or around the stoma is rare, and if it occurs, it is reported immediately.

Stoma drainage

The stoma secretes mucus immediately following surgery and will also continue to produce mucus. During the first 24 to 48 hours, the stoma drainage is mucoid and serosanguineous. Then as the intestinal function returns, flatus is produced. An odor-proof pouch will contain the flatus, which is regularly emptied from the bottom of the pouch. Pinholes in a pouch will destroy the odor-proof quality of the material, and there will be a constant odor in the room. This can be upsetting for a person who is undergoing so many new experiences. Odor is common when a bowel movement occurs or a pouch is emptied. This should be explained so that, as the flatus is released from the pouch, the patient is aware that the odor is controlled at other times.

The fecal drainage from the stoma begins within 72 hours. With an ileostomy, the drainage is liquid and may be constant. The improved surgical techniques and alimentation procedures have changed the pattern of ileostomy output seen previously. Patients seldom experience high volumes of output with ileostomies. Commonly, patients will have approximately 1500 ml/24 hr, although it may go slightly higher. Within 10 to 15 days, the ileostomy effluent will be a soft, slightly formed stool. The terminal ileum adapts to the loss of the colon and begins to reabsorb water. Patients with ileostomies have "toothpaste" consistency stools within 3 to 6 months after the adaptation of the ileum, patients with ileostomies generally have drainage 2 to 4 hours after a meal, although there may be a small amount of effluent intermittently throughout the day.

Exceptions to the above pattern of ileostomy elimination are seen in patients who have had previous bowel resections or resections of the ileum for Crohn's (granulomatous) colitis. The more small intestine that is lost, the greater the chance of a high volume of very liquid output with resultant dehydration.

A person with a sigmoid colostomy has very little change in the function of the large colon, and there is adequate storage of waste and reabsorption of water. The stool is initially liquid and quickly changes to formed bowel movements as the diet progresses from clear liquids to solid foods.

The loop colostomy stoma may be opened in the operating room, or the surgeon may choose to open the loop of bowel in the patient's room within 72 hours postoperatively. A cautery is used to make an incision into the teniae coli on the external wall of the bowel. The bowel is then opened, and both proximal and distal bowel can be visualized. There are two pathways or openings in *one* stoma. The patient should be reassured that there will be no feeling of pain during the procedure, since there are no sensory (only motor) nerves in the stoma. There is, however, a very distinctive burning odor, and adequate ventilation during and following the procedure is required. A supporting rod of a loop stoma is removed 7 to 10 days postoperatively. At this time, adhesions have formed that prevent the loop from retracting through the incision.

The stool from a transverse colostomy is liquid initially and will eventually become soft. The stool drains several times a day from the stoma and thus requires the use of a drainable pouch.

Initial teaching

Teaching the patient regarding anticipated independent care of the stoma begins in the immediate postoperative phase. Each time the dressing and pouch are changed the patient is informed of the state of the skin and the incision healing as well as being given a description of the stoma. A concise explanation of each step in the procedure provides information to the patient. The nursing care plan includes detailed information regarding the approaches and techniques used so that consistency of approach is used by all nurses caring for the patient.

The nurse observes the patient's personal reaction to the information being shared and decides whether to continue with this approach or modify it until the patient indicates more readiness for learning. The word *stoma* is used consistently by the nurse when talking with the patient. This familiarizes the patient with the correct terminology and assists in the acceptance of the altered part of the body into the person's self-concept, thus decreasing distortion or fantasy.

Patient feelings

Not only will the nurse describe what is being observed during the pouch and dressing change, but also the nurse may reflect what the patient may be feeling (e.g., apathy, interest, disgust, or avoidance). This provides an opportunity for the patient to begin to verbalize and explore feelings early in the postoperative course.

Removal of any part of the body involves a sense of loss; therefore the patient may experience grief and mourning over the lost part, which includes shock, denial, anger, and depression. (See Chapter 17 for a discussion of these reactions.) In addition, because the surgery results in fecal contents being expelled through an unnatural opening in the abdomen, the patient will experience changes in body image and may have feelings of guilt, shame, disgust, and withdrawal. These are discussed in Chapter 28. Usually the formation of the stoma is viewed as mutilating surgery, but for some individuals the surgery may be a relief or release from coping with chronic pain, diarrhea, or debility. No matter what reaction is expressed, patients need time and support of others to work through their feelings.

Most persons do not wish to look at the stoma immediately, and if they are in the shock-denial phase of grieving, they will not hear what is being described about it. Patients are not pushed to look at the stoma but are gently encouraged to look at it as they evidence interest in doing so. Some patients will look at the stoma if they are left alone. The nurse can deliberately leave the room for a minute, leaving the stoma exposed and be ready on return to provide emotional support to the patient. It is helpful to set a mirror on the bedside table so the patient can watch the procedure without special emphasis placed on it. Patients often will begin to ask questions that indicate they have looked at the stoma. The nurse can then touch the stoma and describe what it feels like. The nurse does not require (or even request) the patient to touch the stoma, but if the nurse touches the stoma, the patient is shown (1) that there is no pain, although the stoma is red, (2) that touching the stoma will not damage or hurt the stoma, and (3) that the nurse is not disgusted by the stoma.

If it is acceptable to both the significant other and the patient, the significant other is included as an observer as the nurse implements care throughout the entire teaching program.

A patient who is unable (or refuses) to participate in self-care creates a management problem. The patient, significant other, nurse, and physician need to discuss the problem openly. Most patients are discharged within 10 to 14 days. Someone must be prepared to care for the stoma. If a patient cannot accept the surgery, and if he or she is unwilling to assume an active role, an early consultation with a psychiatric nurse specialist may be helpful.

Rehabilitation

Rehabilitation, an optimal return to presurgical lifestyle, does not occur immediately after discharge. It may take up to a full year for a person to reach an optimal level of functioning. Learning self-care, which generally occurs during hospitalization, is the first step in rehabilitation.

A planned systematic teaching protocol enhances the patient's ability to learn to manage the ostomy. Honesty is essential. A person with an ileostomy or an ascending or a transverse colostomy cannot regulate bowel movements; thus a drainable pouch and skin barrier are required. A person with a sigmoid colostomy may be able to regulate bowel evacuations.

The place of instruction, the methodology, and the content are important. A person who is taught to change a pouch while lying in bed will always do so; therefore patients should be sitting up as they learn. They should be taught to empty their pouches while sitting on the toilet in the usual manner (not backwards). Some people need to read instructions, others need to be shown the techniques, and some need both. Written instructions for discharge are imperative.

Teaching should include the following areas: maintenance of fluid and electrolyte balance, skin care, selection and application of pouches, colostomy irrigation, diet, activity, sexuality, community resources, and complications.

Maintenance of fluid and electrolyte balance

Attention to fluid and electrolyte balance is of extreme importance for the patient with an ileostomy. This individual no longer has a large bowel for absorption of water, and if the person becomes sick (e.g., flu or reaction to medications), an excessive loss of fluids through the stoma may occur. Diarrhea for a person with an ileostomy (who may normally have unformed stools) is defined as very hot liquid output in which the pouch must be emptied hourly or more frequently. Diarrhea accompanied by nausea and vomiting can rapidly progress to dehydration. Patients are taught to observe signs of dehydration and electrolyte imbalance. They should know how to replace fluids and electrolytes as well as when to seek medical attention.

Persons with ileostomies may become severely ill during routine diagnostic procedures. It is important to remember that this patient does not have a large colon and should *never* be given a laxative as a routine preparation. The ileostomy stoma should *never* be irrigated (as one would a colostomy stoma). Bowel preparation for the person with an ileostomy may be obtained by a clear liquid diet for 24 hours.

Medications, which are enteric-coated, time-released, or hard tablets, may not be absorbed with an ileostomy. Liquid or chewable forms of medications are preferred. The ileostomy does develop a bacterial flora, and diarrhea may develop with antibiotic therapy.

The person with a sigmoid colostomy is no more prone to fluid and electrolyte imbalance than a person with an intact colon. The ascending colostomy is similiar to the ileostomy, and the person with an ascending colostomy should be carefully instructed about fluid and electrolyte balance.

Skin care

The skin around the stoma should appear as normal and healthy as any other abdominal skin. Any change from the normal skin should be considered a problem and require proper identification of the cause and treatment. *Prevention* of skin breakdown is easier and less expensive than treatment and less painful for the patient. The condition of the peristomal skin plays an important role in the selection of pouching systems (Fig. 58-9).

Watt[56] has identified nine variables that influence peristomal skin integrity: (1) composition of effluent, (2) consistency of effluent, (3) quantity of effluent, (4) underlying disease and treatment, (5) medications, (6) surgical construction and location of stomas, (7) skill of those caring for the patient, (8) skill and interest of the patient in self-care, and (9) availability of proper supplies.

Ileostomy drainage contains residual digestive enzymes that will quickly break down the skin. The ascending colostomy effluent may also contain a small amount of residual enzymes and is also a very moist stool which, if it remains on the skin, will result in skin irritation. The stool from a transverse colostomy may cause skin irritation from constant moisture against the skin. The effluent from a sigmoid colostomy is least likely to irritate the skin.

In addition to the irritation from the effluent, the skin may be damaged from frequent removal of pouch adhesives from the skin. It is often the rough removal or changes of pouches rather than the emptying that first breaks down the skin's integrity.

There are several basic principles that protect the skin and limit peristomal skin irritation:

1. The skin should be gently cleansed and patted dry.
2. A skin barrier should be used to protect the ⅛ in. of skin exposed by pouch openings.
3. A skin sealant should be used under all tapes applied to the skin.
4. When a pouch seal leaks, the pouch should be immediately changed, not taped. Stool held against the skin can quickly result in severe irritation.

Skin barriers. Skin barriers include such products as karaya, Stomahesive (Squibb), Hollihesive (Hollister), Crixilene (Bard), and Colly-Seel (Mason). Skin barriers attached to the pouches are available as a one- or two-piece system and as single-use items that can be used with any pouch.

There are several basic forms in which one may obtain skin barriers: powder, paste, washer, or 4-in. × 4-in. squares. The use of powder as a basic skin protector was the first available product. Powder must be used correctly. A pouch will not adhere to powder, cream, or ointment; therefore if powder is applied to the skin, it must be sealed in before the pouch can be applied. Karaya powder releases acetic acid when applied to irritated skin and thus may result in a temporary stinging of the skin.

Paste (karaya, Stomahesive, or Hollihesive) is available for use around the stoma, to fill in creases or folds, and to supplement wafer skin barriers for a longer seal. The use of paste has made it easier to keep a pouch seal intact in poor locations.

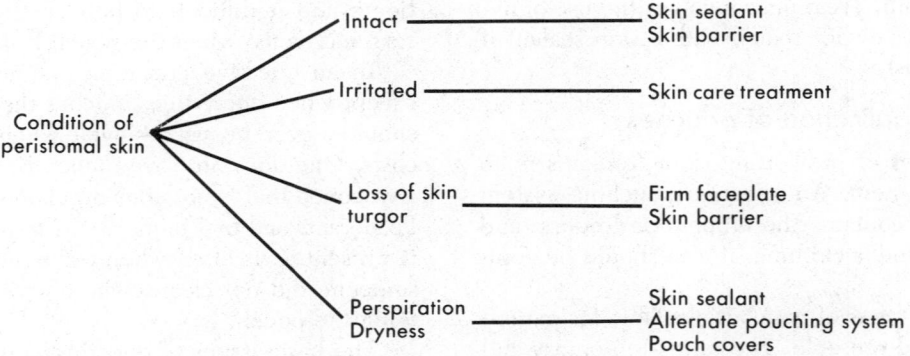

Fig. 58-9. Decision tree: selection of pouching system based on condition of peristomal skin. (From Broadwell, D.C., and Jackson, B.S.: Principles of ostomy care, St. Louis, 1982, The C.V. Mosby Co.)

Pectin-based wafers (e.g., Stomahesive and Hollihesive) have provided an innovative method of skin-care prevention. The wafers may be used with a variety of pouches and protect the skin from the effluent. The opening in the wafer is carefully prepared so that it fits at the base of the stoma without "riding up" onto the stoma. Warming the wafer (e.g., under the patient's back or between the hands) to the body temperature often will help the wafer adhere to the skin.

Skin sealants come in sprays, liquids, gels, and wipes. These products coat the skin with a clear film. They are useful under pouch adhesives, window-facing tape, and other areas where tape is used. When tape is removed from the skin, it removes the stratum corneum layer of the skin. When a skin sealant is used under the tape, the removal of tape removes the skin sealant leaving the skin intact.

Any patient may have a sensitivity to a product; therefore, it is appropriate to *patch test* patients to various products before surgery. A small amount of the product is applied to the upper back, covered with an occlusive dressing, and left in place for 48 hours. The dressing is removed, and after 30 minutes the test area is observed for skin reactions.

Intervention for skin breakdown. If the skin does become irritated, careful and systematic treatment should begin. The use of antacids on the skin should be avoided since they change the skin pH and may result in a bacterial secondary infection. Also, products containing large quantities of alcohol (e.g., benzoin) should be omitted.

The first step is to dry the skin. A heat lamp with a 60-watt bulb placed 30 cm (12 in.) away from the skin may be used to help dry the skin. A small piece of moist gauze should be used to cover the stoma. Table 58-4 presents steps in treating skin problems.

Peristomal skin infections may be bacterial or fungal. The most common is a yeast infection from *Candida albicans*. The skin is a bright erythema with papular lesions in an irregular area; secondary skin changes occur as the process continues and dry, scaling areas develop. The skin lesion may be diagnosed by a potassium hydroxide stain. Treatment involves the use of nystatin (Mycostatin) powder sealed with a skin sealant if the skin is not moist.

Selection and application of pouches

The best means of preventing skin problems is an effective pouch system. An effective pouching system protects the skin, contains the effluent and odors, and is inconspicuous under clothing; it also should be comfortable.[9]

There are two types of pouches available for patient use: disposable and reusable. The terms temporary and permanent have become obsolete. Disposable pouches are better made and are often used throughout hospitalization as well as after hospitalization. By definition,

TABLE 58-4. Management of skin breakdown*

Erythematous skin	Eroded skin
Remove appliance every 24-48 hr	Remove appliance every 24 hr
Cleanse skin with warm water, pat dry	Cleanse skin with warm water, pat dry
Expose irritated skin to air, light, and heat for 20-30 min; light and heat may be supplied by 60-watt bulb, 12-16 in. from stoma	Apply aluminum acetate (Burow's solution) compresses for 30 min
Cover all irritated skin with hypoallergenic skin barrier (Stomahesive or Hollihesive) to which patient is not sensitive; opening in skin barrier must be cut to exact size and shape of stoma; pouch opening is ⅛ in. larger than stoma	Expose irritated skin to light, air, and heat for 30 min
Select appliance, clamp, or belt of different materials if any were allergens	Apply Orabase to eroded areas
	Cover all irritated skin with hypoallergenic skin barrier (Stomahesive or Hollihesive) to which patient is not sensitive
	Select appliance, clamp, or belt to which patient is not sensitive
	Adhesive tapes or disks should not come in contact with eroded skin

*From Watt, R.: Pathophysiology of peristomal skin. In Broadwell, D.C., and Jackson, B.S.: Principles of ostomy care, St. Louis, 1981, The C.V. Mosby Co.

disposable pouches are worn once and discarded. They are available in one- and two-piece systems, with skin barriers attached, and in a variety of materials (Figs. 58-10 and 58-11). Reusable pouches are those that are worn, cleansed, and worn again. They are also available in one- and two-piece systems and are available in a variety of materials with a variety of faceplates.

The most important phase of nursing care is the careful selection and application of an effective pouching system. When the pouching system does not work, other processes of rehabilitation are often halted. Patients find it difficult to believe they can work, enjoy sex, and dance when the pouch leaks constantly.

In an effective pouching system, there is no odor except when emptying. Pouches that are not odor proof should never be used—even when attempting to cut costs. One does not save money by using a less expensive pouch that is not odor proof and then adding pouch deodorants and oral preparations to reduce odors. If odor is present, it is often when the pouch seal is leaking or someone did not cleanse the opening spout after emptying the pouch.

The basic issues of selecting equipment include the type of ostomy; the size and contour of the abdomen; the peristomal skin condition; and the patient's physical and mental status, physical activities, financial situa-

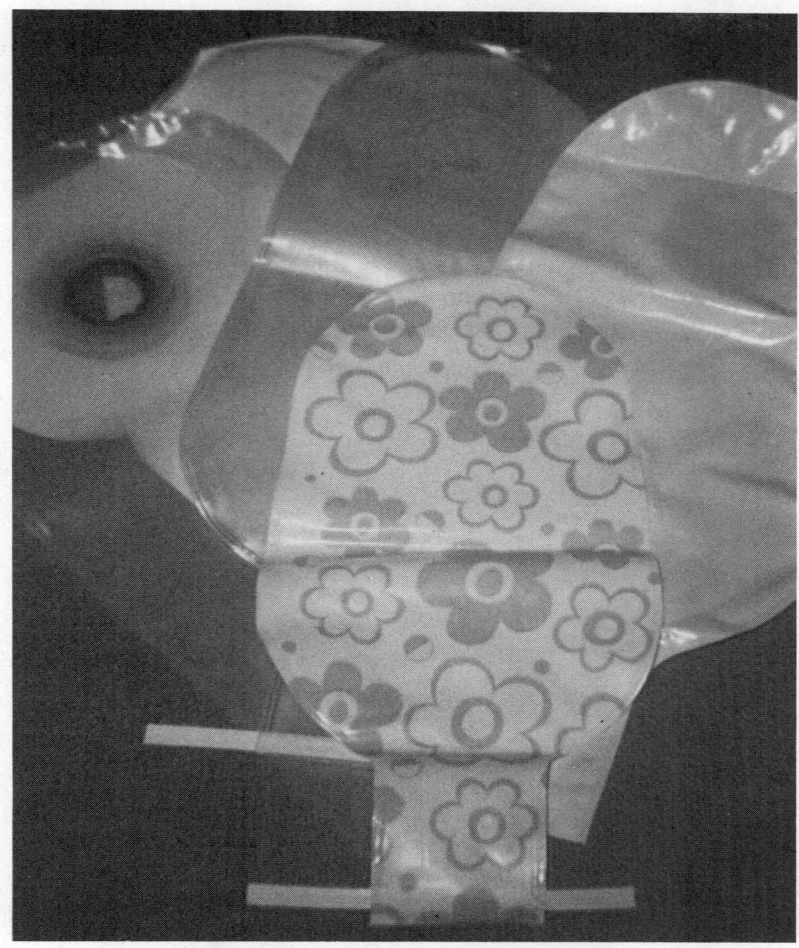

Fig. 58-10. Open and drainable pouches.

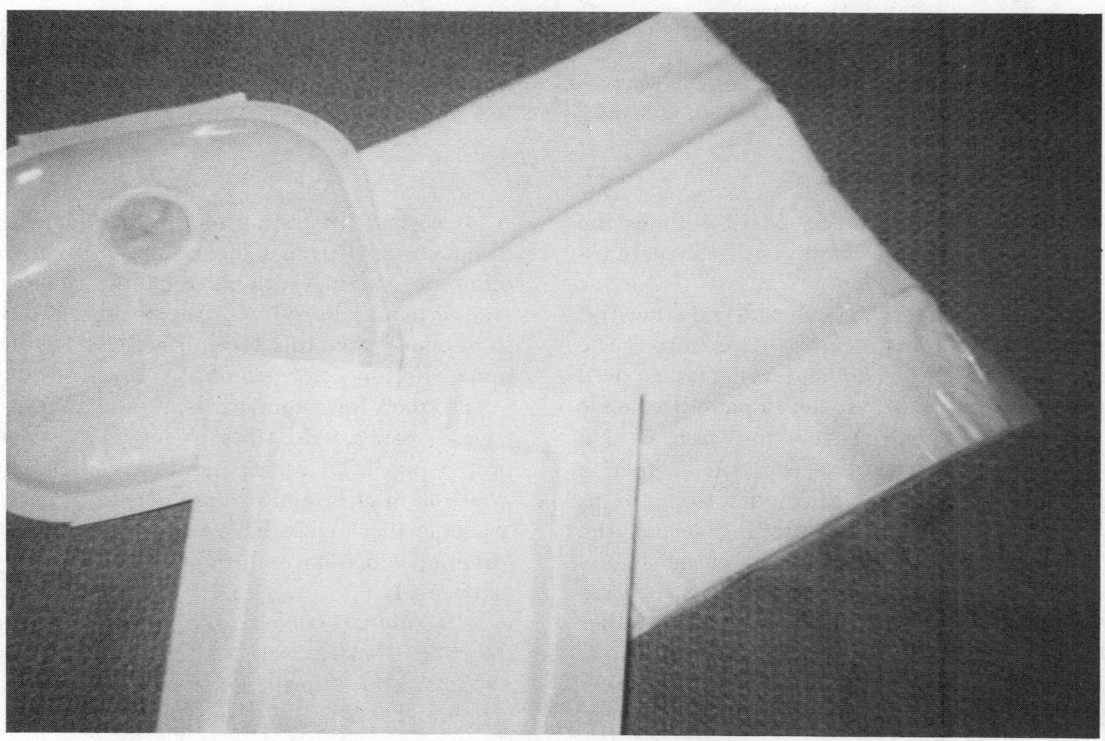

Fig. 58-11. Two piece pouch systems: pouch and skin barrier. (From Broadwell, D.C., and Jackson, B.S.: Principles of ostomy care, St. Louis, 1982, The C.V. Mosby Co.)

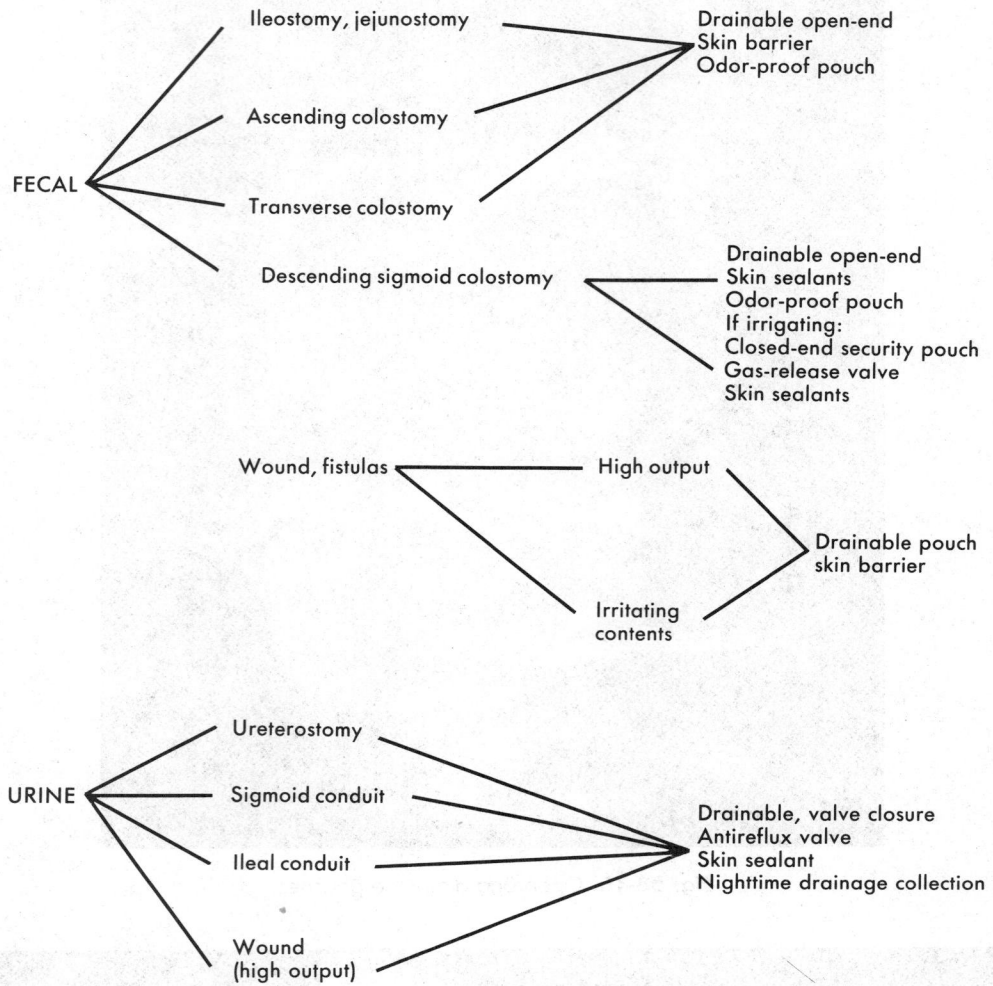

Fig. 58-12. Decision tree: selection of pouching system based on type of ostomy or wound. (From Broadwell, D.B., and Jackson, B.S.: Principles of ostomy care, St. Louis, 1982, The C.V. Mosby Co.)

tion, and personal preference. Fig. 58-12 outlines the selection of a pouching system based on the type of ostomy.

Once a pouching system (pouch and skin barrier) has been selected, the stoma is carefully measured. The skin barrier should "hug" the stoma, leaving no exposed skin. If the stoma is not exactly round, a pattern is made for repeated changes. It will prevent the waste of skin barriers inappropriately prepared. The pouch opening should be 3 mm (⅛ in.) larger than the stoma. This prevents lacerations of the stoma rubbing against the pouch faceplate with peristaltic movements of the stoma.

When pouching systems are not working, it is more effective to problem-solve what may be happening rather than just to try another pouch. Often pouches are misapplied and would work if more time were taken during the application process. The more careful one is to ensure that the surface area (skin) is clean and dry, the more likely it is that the pouch will adhere.

It is very frustrating for the patient when the type of pouch used is changed because the nurse prefers a different system. Patients relate stories of the pouch system being altered with the change of nursing shifts. It is hoped that this type of activity has decreased as nurses become more comfortable with ostomy care.

Products for ostomy care are available in a variety of styles, shapes, and sizes. Now, more than ever, the proper pouch for each patient is available. Pouches are available in clear and opaque plastics. Pouch covers are available that make the wearing of a pouch more comfortable. Pouch covers can also be made simply and inexpensively.

A written procedure for pouch change is given to the patient before discharge, since often the patient does not retain the information that had been taught in the hospital. The stresses of having surgery, the newness of the stoma, and anxieties and fears may result in minimal retention of even the best teaching plan. The box

POUCH APPLIANCE PROCEDURE*

Pattern

1. The pattern should be ⅛ in. larger than the stoma.
2. A paper towel may be used to trace a pattern.
3. Always label the pattern for "top" or "skin" side.

Stomahesive, Hollihesive, Reliaseal, or Colly-Seel (skin barrier)

1. You may use ¼, ½, or full wafer depending on the size of the stoma and the abdomen.
2. Round the corners to conform to the shape of the adhesive on the pouch.
3. Trace the pattern on the paper side.
4. Cut hole on pattern line; your line will not be visible when it is cut.
5. Smooth sides of the opening with your finger.

Pouch

1. Pouch opening should be slightly larger than the opening of the skin barrier (paper can cut the stoma).
2. Trace pattern on the paper side of the pouch (use the opening from the skin barrier that has already been cut).
3. Cut the hole larger than the line of the pattern (cut outside of the line).
4. The edges around the opening should be smooth.
5. Remove paper backing from the pouch, center the openings, and apply the shiny side of the skin barrier to the pouch.

Applying the system

1. Remove the pouch and skin barrier carefully.
2. Cleanse the skin with warm water.
3. Pat the skin dry.
4. Warm the skin barrier (the pouch is already attached).
5. Remove the backing; save this paper, because it can be used as your pattern in the future.
6. Center opening with the stoma; press and seal to the skin; hold your hand against the pouch to help seal the skin barrier to the skin.
7. Close the bottom.

*From Broadhurst, B.B., and Broadwell, D.C.: Ostomy care for children. Copyright © 1981 by Debra C. Broadwell.

above is a sample step-by-step procedure for one patient. The patient should also be given a written list of all the equipment needed and locations where the equipment can be obtained. A month's supply of equipment is usually given at the time of the patient's discharge.

If a person with an ostomy is readmitted, the nurse asks what assistance is needed with ostomy care and maintains any pattern of care that is effectively working. Reusable equipment is not discarded since it is expensive to replace. Also, the patient's skin is observed and the effectiveness of the system is assessed. The nurse may suggest new items that would be beneficial but should not force persons to change. If patients have worked for years to obtain a system they can trust, they may be unwilling to experiment.

Colostomy irrigation

Irrigation, or an enema, may be ordered after a sigmoid colostomy. There is controversy about the long-term effects of irrigations. The purpose of regular colostomy irrigations is to stimulate emptying of the colon at a convenient and regular time. A patient who is free of stool between irrigations will not need to wear a pouch but may wear a stoma covering (Fig. 58-13).

The decision to irrigate a colostomy should take into consideration the following factors: whether the colostomy is temporary or permanent, the length of bowel above the colostomy, stomal complications, personal preference of the patient, and physical and mental status of the patient. Persons who respond unfavorably to colostomy irrigation include those who respond to stress with diarrhea, have an abdominoperineal resection (p.

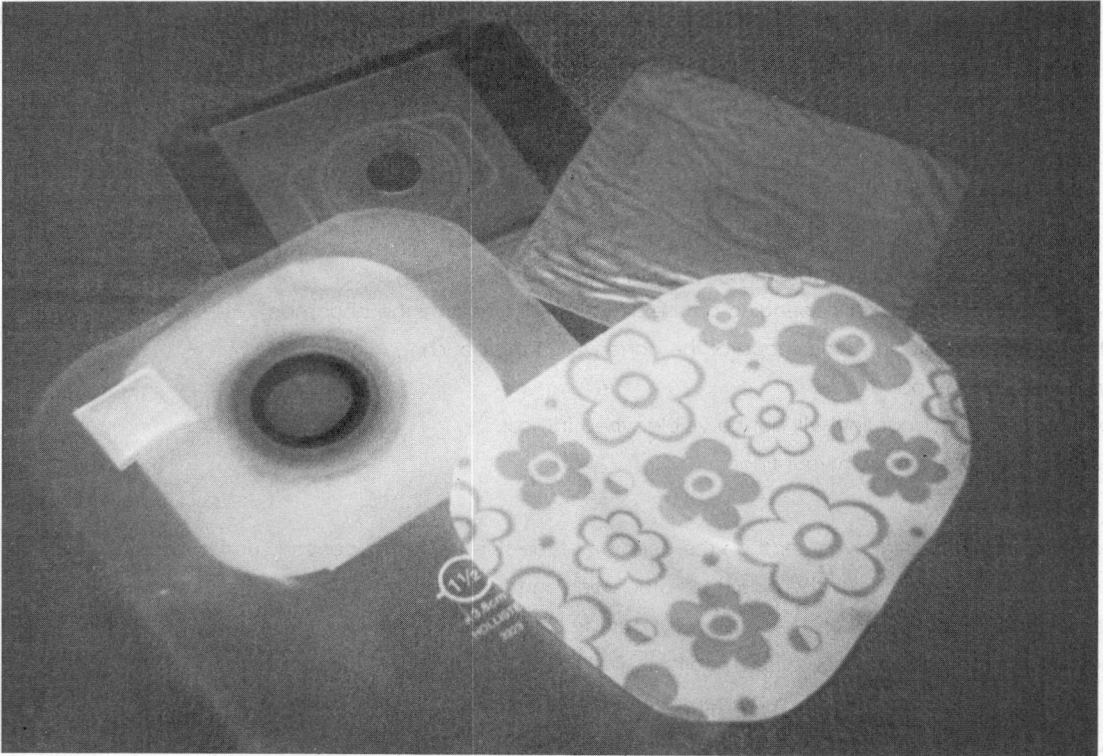

Fig. 58-13. Coverage for regulated stomas.

1452) followed by radiation therapy, have a poor prognosis, have a previous history of inflammatory bowel disease or radiation enteritis, have a stoma stenosis or parastomal hernia, or fear the procedure or resent having the procedure done.

Persons who have irrigated their colostomies successfully for years may develop irregular results with irrigation secondary to aging. As one ages, there is a decrease in mucus production and peristalsis. This is often frustrating for patients who may feel they have failed, because the elimination pattern is unpredictable.

Various types of commercial irrigation sets are available, and they all require similar supplies: an irrigation sleeve, which fits over the stoma and is long enough to drain into the toilet; a cone tip for the insertion of water into the stoma; an enema bag to contain the solution; and clips to close the top and bottom of the sleeve. A cone is used almost universally for insertion of the irrigation solution. Bowel perforations of the colon during colostomy irrigations are rarely seen because of the advancements of the cone. A catheter may be indicated for a stenosed stoma.

When ordered, irrigations are begun after the bowel has begun to function and the stool is beginning to become soft, usually between the fifth and seventh postoperative day. A digital examination of the stoma (insertion of a gloved, well-lubricated little finger) is done to assess the direction of the bowel. This is done only once, at the time of the first irrigation. The procedure for irrigation is described in Table 58-5.

The first irrigation is often performed in bed using 500 ml of warm tap water. This provides patients an opportunity to observe the procedure and experience the sensations. After this, patients are taken to the bathroom. They may wish to sit on a chair, with a pillow, facing the commode until the perineal wound heals. Subsequently, the patient sits on the commode (Fig. 58-14). The instillation and drainage of fluid take approximately 30 minutes. The end of the sleeve is then cleansed, dried and closed. Ambulation is encouraged to further stimulate peristalsis.

Cramping during an irrigation may be caused from inserting water too rapidly or from water that is too cold. If the water is too hot, the bowel mucosa can be injured.

If regularity occurs, small dressings are commercially available to wear over the stoma. There are also many closed-end security pouches with a deodorizing gas release valve, which may be worn by a person with a regulated colostomy. Since flatus cannot be eliminated or controlled, most people with colostomies prefer these small odor-proof pouches.

The loop colostomy, or double-barrel colostomy, is irrigated before closure. Irrigation sleeves and cones are

TABLE 58-5. General guidelines and tips for colostomy irrigation procedure*

Guidelines	Tips

Assemble all equipment
  Water container and water
  Irrigating sleeve and belt
  Items to clean skin and stoma
  Way to dispose of old pouch
  Clean, prepared pouch to reapply
  Skin-care items
	Try to keep all equipment together to facilitate daily routine

Remove old pouch and dispose of it	Plastic bag is odor proof and handy to put pouch in
Clean skin and stoma with water; let dry (NOTE: Observe condition and color of skin and stoma.)	May use washcloth, toilet paper, or tissue
Apply irrigating sleeve and belt securely (not too tight) (NOTE: If using karaya washer, dampen and apply this first.)	Sleeve should be long enough to reach toilet; excess may be cut off
Fill irrigating container with about 1 qt tepid water when ready to begin; (NOTE: Hot water traumatizes [burns] bowel and cold water causes cramping.)	
Suspend irrigating container so bottom of container is even with top of shoulder (NOTE: At lower height, water may not flow easily, and higher height will give too much force to water and cause cramping or incomplete results [Fig. 58-14].	Hang container to be on side of dominant hand; it will drape easily and be more manageable; can use hook or coat hanger to get proper height
Remove air from tubing (NOTE: This helps prevent air from increasing gas pains.)	Do not use large amount of irrigating water, or irrigation container will need to be refilled

Gently insert irrigating cone into stoma, holding it parallel to floor; start water slowly; NOTE: if water does not flow easily, try or check following:
  Slightly change position or angle of cone
  Check for kinks in tubing from irrigating container
  Check height of irrigating container
	Cone should fit snugly enough to block water in bowel; do *not* try to force it
	Cone opening maybe blocked by loop of bowel

Have patient take deep breaths	Deep breaths will relax abdominal muscles
Stool immediately under skin level may be slightly hard and blocking water flow; instill *small* amount of water to loosen it	Introduce water at slow rate, so it can penetrate behind stool and propel it out; fast rate of flow will spill out as it meets resistance of stool

Variations in water for irrigations
  People vary in amount of water they can hold at one time; some can take all at once, and others can tolerate small amount at one time
  Amount of water used can vary daily
	Use approximately 500 ml for first irrigation and increase by 250 ml until 1000 ml (1 qt) irrigation is reached

Cleanse as much of fecal matter out as possible without making patient uncomfortable	Ask patient to identify "full" feeling or need to expel stool
Do *not* force water into bowel if (1) cramping occurs, (2) flow of water stops, or (3) water is forcefully returning around irrigating cone or catheter; stop flow of water	
If patient complains of feeling bloated or constipated, irrigate with additional 500 ml water in same day or provide mild laxative	People who have always had problems with constipation will continue to have; diet (fruits), high fluid intake, stool softeners, or laxatives may be used
Majority of stool will return in about 15 min	Patient should remain seated on toilet
When most of stool has been expelled, rinse sleeve with water, dry bottom edge, roll out, close up end, and encourage activities for about 30-45 min to allow bowel adequate time to finish emptying	Activity will stimulate peristalsis and allow for thorough results
When irrigation is complete, assemble and apply clean pouch and skin barrier	
Rinse out irrigation sleeve, hang it up to dry, and put away other equipment	Rinse out with warm water to decrease odor; water may be run through sleeve by using irrigation container and tubing; sleeve could also be sprayed with cleansers (Peri-Wash or Uni-Wash) that help stool slide through sleeve, make cleaning easier, and decrease odor
Check supplies and reorder as necessary	Do not wait until supplies are depleted to reorder; it will take time for them to come
Try to irrigate within same 2- or 3-hr period each day so patient can become regulated; if possible, try to irrigate close to time bowels moved before surgery	

*From Broadwell, D.C., and Sorrells, S.L.: Summary of your colostomy care. Copyright © 1976 by Debra C. Broadwell.

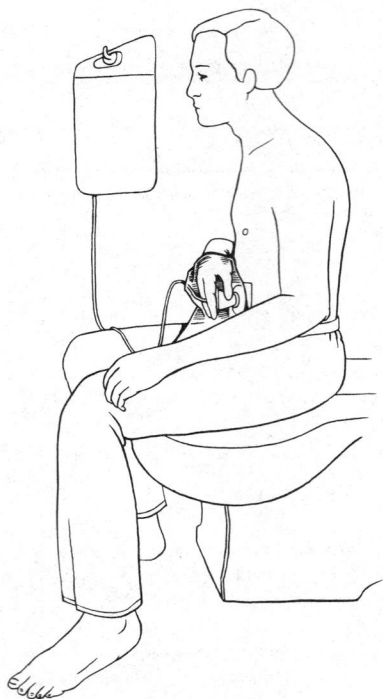

Fig. 58-14. Position for colostomy irrigation.

available as separate items from most companies. The irrigation sleeve and cone can be used with a hospital enema bucket for these irrigations. Several companies are now making inexpensive irrigation sets for this group of patients. The sets contain sleeves, cone, and solution container for in-hospital use.

Diet

The diet of a person with a colostomy should not be restricted. People know which foods cause them to have more gas, diarrhea, or constipation. Persons have the right to choose whether or not they will eat gas-forming foods and have gas. There are excellent odor-proof pouches and gas-release valves that make the previous problem of gas less of a problem. Odor and gas can be controlled.

Patients may be kept on low-residue diets for 6 weeks to decrease the amount of bulky and undigested foods as the intestinal tract recovers from the surgical intervention. Then the patient begins to add foods to the diet. It is strongly recommended that persons with ileostomies add only one high-fiber food at a time and chew their food well. Foods should not be eliminated from the diet unless the person is unable to tolerate them after two or three trials.

Following a colostomy or ileostomy, people tend to notice undigested foods that pass through the stoma. Seeds, kernels, peanuts, and other undigested residue usually do not alarm patients if they know this is normal.

Food blockage, or a large mass of undigested food, especially high-fiber foods, may occur with an ileostomy. The mass becomes lodged at a kink, or narrowing, in the bowel and blocks the lumen (Table 58-6), resulting in a mechanical bowel obstruction. Blockage most commonly occurs when a person eats several high-fiber foods in one meal or does not chew the foods properly. Coconut and corn cause the most problems. Following ileostomy surgery, some persons will discover they can only eat coconut, corn, celery, or Chinese foods in limited amounts. If the ileostomy becomes blocked, the person should get into a knee-chest position and gently massage the area below the stoma. Stomal edema will develop with a food blockage, and the pouch should be changed to accommodate the swelling. Diarrhea usually follows the removal of the obstruction, and the patient will need to replace fluids. Abdominal pain in the peristomal area is generally present for 3 to 5 days after obstruction.

If the obstruction is not passed following the use of the knee-chest position, the patient should notify the physician. It is often necessary for the person to be admitted for an ileostomy lavage, which is the gentle insertion of normal saline through the stoma, using a small catheter and a bulb syringe. Careful measurement of the fluid inserted and obtained is required. An irrigation sleeve is applied over the stoma to collect the fluid behind the obstruction, then a 14 or 16 Fr catheter is lubricated and inserted into the stoma until resistance is met. By using a bulb syringe, 30 to 50 ml of normal saline is inserted. This procedure is repeated until the obstruction is released. If the person has had the food blockage for a long time, nasogastric suctioning and intravenous fluids may be required.

Activity

For most persons whose condition warrants it, optimal recovery is achieved within 3 months, and they can return to their normal activities, including work. The person may participate in sports, although it is advisable to avoid direct-contact sports such as football. People find ways to return to those activities they enjoy. A young man who played professional football before surgery was able to return to professional football by playing a limited contact position—he is a place-kicker.

Swimming, playing tennis, and participating in planned exercise programs are all possible. The person is encouraged to socialize and continue those activities that resulted in satisfaction before the surgery. No one knows who has an ostomy unless they are informed. Proper pouching systems cannot be seen. People need to know that they can take baths and showers.

Traveling is also possible for the ostomate. Seat belts are worn above or below the stoma. Regular ostomy supplies should be carried by hand on airplanes or trains

TABLE 58-6. Signs and symptoms of food blockage in an ileostomy*

Symptoms of blockage	Causes of symptoms
Discharge changes from semisolid to thin liquid	Food is blocked, but water passes around it
Total volume of output increases and stoma functions almost constantly	Water is drawn from bloodstream in attempt to rid itself of blockage, and intestines become hyperactive
Objectional odor	Bacterial overgrowth occurs at blockage and causes fermentation of food stuff
Cramping, usually followed by increase in watery output	Increased bowel activity to rid itself of blockage
Distended abdomen	Blockage traps gas and liquids in bowel lumen
Vomiting	Further attempts of body to rid itself of blockage by traveling in direction of least resistance
No ileostomy output	Complete blockage

*From Broadwell, D.C. and Sorrells, S.L.: Summary of your ileostomy care. Copyright © 1976 by Debra C. Broadwell.

(rather than checked through with luggage) to facilitate maintenance of regimens if luggage should become delayed or misplaced. Plastic bags are useful for disposal of used supplies. Extra supplies should be taken for unanticipated events requiring extra days or increased use. Eating moderately and using restraint when eating different foods are suggested. The ostomate needs to be especially careful about water intake, particularly when traveling in areas where "traveler's" diarrhea is a high risk. The person with an ileostomy needs to maintain the required fluid intake; therefore bottled water should be used, and uncooked fruits and vegetables should be avoided. If the ostomate develops diarrhea that cannot be easily controlled, a physician needs to be consulted.

Sexuality

The opportunity for the patient and significant other to ask questions regarding the return to normal sexual functioning needs to be provided. It is most often the nurse who hears cues such as "I guess I'll never be able . . . " or "I wonder what my spouse. . . ." The nurse takes this opportunity to clarify this concern with the person. Arrangements can be made, if desired by the patient, for the significant other to be present when a frank discussion of sexual functioning is carried out by the nurse or physician. Many persons will not verbalize their concerns about sexuality so that a deliberate meeting must be planned to facilitate expression of these concerns. The patient and sexual partner can be assisted to consider sexual positions that may be more facilitating and less problematic if a bag is worn. An ileostomy bag is emptied before foreplay.

About 15% of male ostomates have decreased sexual activity that may be related either to nerve injury or to psychologic reasons.[51] The successful return to sexual activity depends on psychosexual functioning before surgery and adaptation and coping following surgery. Counseling may be helpful if nerve injury is not present

and sexual difficulties are being experienced. Female ostomates have a decreased incidence of nerve injury because of the larger pelvis.[51] Ostomy surgery does not interfere with contraception, pregnancy, or delivery; pregnancy seldom produces complications with stoma care. A pamphlet entilted *Sex and the Ostomate* is available from the United Ostomy Association.*

Community resources

During hospitalization, there are additional resources available to the patient and significant others to assist in adapting and coping with the ostomy. A representative from the local "Ostomy Group" who has been through the same experience may be helpful during both the preoperative and the postoperative period and will visit the patient if requested to do so. The enterostomal therapist, social worker, clinical nurse specialist, dietitian, and clergy may all be consulted as the needs are presented.

The patient and significant others should also be informed of the United Ostomy Association. The patient may become a member and through group sharing learn how others in the local community are effectively dealing with their alteration. The American Cancer Society will also provide assistance with information about home supplies, medications, and transportation.

Complications

Before hospital discharge teaching should include knowledge of common complications that should be reported directly to the health care provider. The more common complications include persistent diarrhea, constipation, or stricture of the stoma. Less common complications include bleeding from or around the stoma,

*United Ostomy Association, Inc., 1111 Wilshire Blvd., Los Angeles, CA 90017.

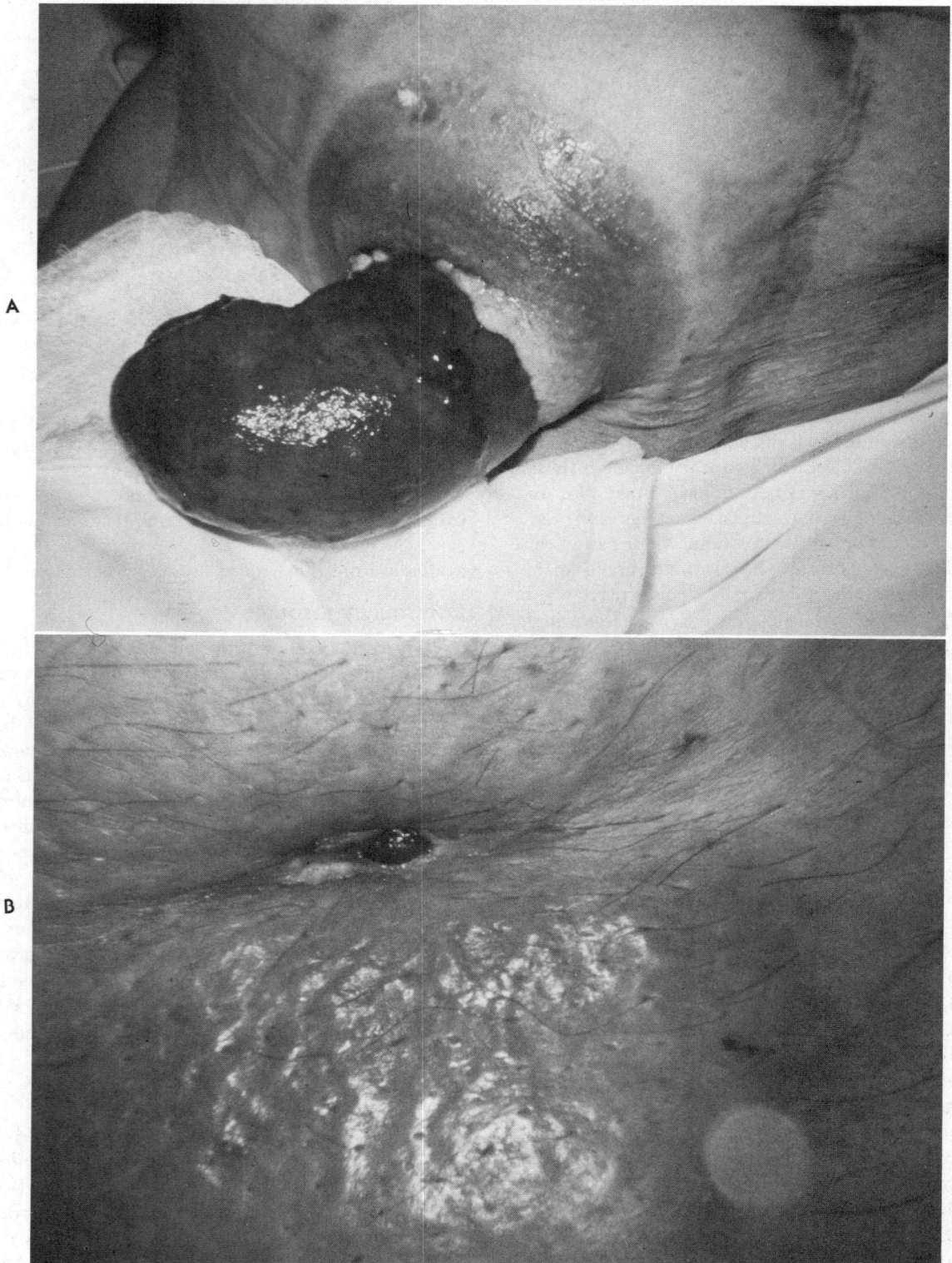

Fig. 58-15. Stomal complications. **A,** Stomal prolapse. **B,** Stomal stenosis.

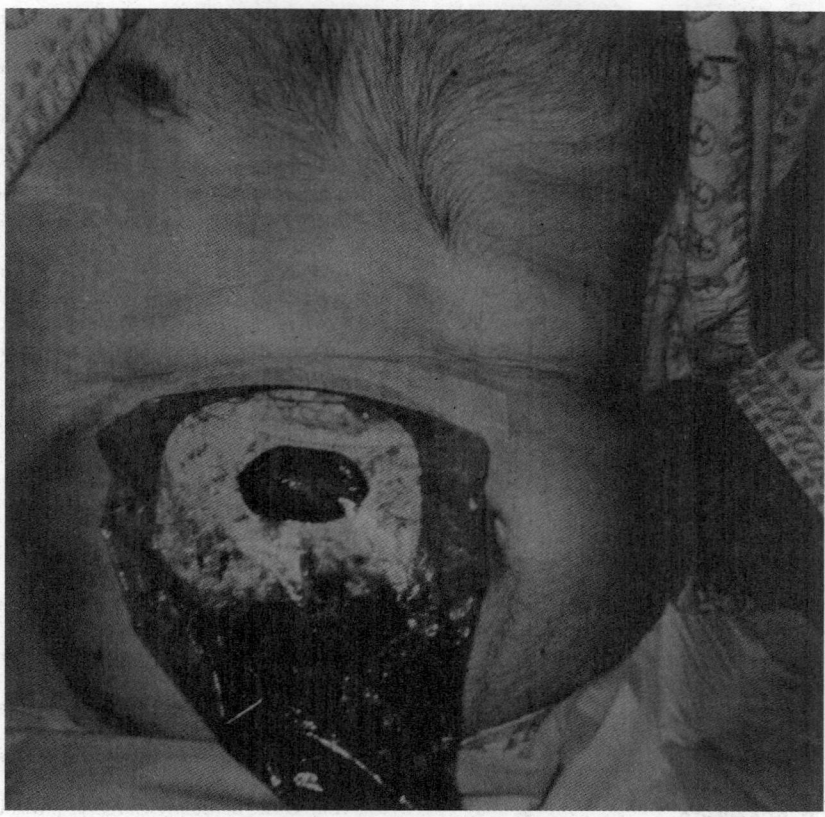

Fig. 58-16. Peristomal hernia. (From Broadwell, D.C., and Jackson, B.S.: Principles of ostomy care, St. Louis, 1982, The C.V. Mosby Co.)

prolapse or inversion of the stoma (Fig. 58-15), peristomal hernia (Fig. 58-16), or changes in the stomal color.

An enterostomal therapist should be consulted for pouching or skin problems. This nurse specialist has been prepared to manage the technical and the biopsychosocial aspects of persons undergoing ostomy surgery.

Closure of the colostomy

If the colostomy was performed to relieve obstruction or to divert the fecal stream to permit healing of a portion of the bowel, the person will be readmitted to the hospital at a later date for a further examination and for possible resection of the diseased portion of the bowel. The opening may subsequently be closed.

In preparation for a resection of the bowel and closure of the colostomy, the physician may order irrigations of both openings in the loop. Fluid, usually normal saline solution, is instilled into each opening through a catheter or cone. For this irrigation, the patient should sit on the bedpan or on the toilet; unless there is complete obstruction, the solution into the distal loop will be expelled through the rectum. Mucus and shreds of necrotic tissue may be passed. The returns should be inspected before discarded. A nonabsorbable sulfonamide derivative (e.g., phthalylsulfathiazole) dissolved in a small amount of water may be slowly instilled into the distal loop and rectum after the irrigation. The patient should retain this solution as long as possible, since the antibiotic lowers the bacterial count of the bowel contents and lessens the risk of postoperative infection. The patient will be unable to retain any solution inserted into the proximal bowel. Oral sulfonamides are also given before surgery.

Outcome criteria for the person with a surgical diversion of the fecal stream

The person or significant others can:
1. Describe the relationship of adequate dietary and fluid intake to the formation of a normal stool.
2. Describe the relationship of activity to normal bowel evacuation.
3. Demonstrate the correct use of stomal appliance: removal, cleansing of stoma, inspection of skin, application of appliance, and ordering of new equipment.
4. Demonstrate, if needed, the correct technique for colostomy irrigation.

5. Determine a specific time of day for anticipated normal evacuation, if colostomy is regulated.
6. State how to obtain available professional and community resources.
7. Utilize a resource person with whom they may share their thoughts and feelings regarding the alteration and its impact on the future.
8. State plans for regular follow-up care and symptoms that necessitate physician or nurse enterostomal therapist contact.
   a. Changes in configuration, color, consistency, or odor of stool.
   b. Bleeding through stoma or rectum.
   c. Persistent diarrhea; or lack of stool evacuation despite medications, treatment, fluids, diet, and exercise program.
   d. Persistent skin irritation despite treatment.
   e. Changes in contour of the stoma (e.g., prolapse or inversion) or signs of infection.
   f. Persistent leakage around the appliance.
   g. Signs of dehydration and electrolyte imbalance.
   h. Signs and symptoms of a food blockage with an ileostomy.

REFERENCES AND SELECTED READINGS

1. *Auld, L.S.: Pseudo-ostomy: an experiment, Am. J. Nurs. **78**:1525, 1978.
2. Bartizal, J., and Slosberg, P.: Combined abdominoperineal resection, Surg. Clin. North Am. **57**:1253-1261, 1977.
3. *Baum, M.E.: Enterostomal therapy in the hospital, Sup. Nurse **7**:11-14, 1976.
4. *Baum, M.E., and Fletcher, J.C.: Porcine dressing for ileostomy retraction, Am. J. Nurs. **76**:760-761, 1976.
5. *Beart, R.W., and Curlee, F.: Intestinal stomas: managing the "unmentionable," Geriatrics **33**(11):45-48, 1978.
6. *Beber, C.R.: Freedom for the incontinent, Am. J. Nurs. **80**:483-484, 1980.
7. Beeson, P.B., McDermott, W., and Wyngaarden, J.B.: Textbook of medicine, ed. 15, Philadelphia, 1979, W.B. Saunders Co.
8. Bond, J.H., and Levitt, M.D.: Gaseousness and intestinal gas, Med. Clin. North Am. **62**:155-163, 1978.
9. Broadwell, D.C., and Jackson, B.S.: Principles of ostomy care, St. Louis, 1982, The C.V. Mosby Co.
10. *Broadwell, D.C., and Sorrells, S.L.: Loop transverse colostomy, Am. J. Nurs. **78**:1029-1031, 1978.
11. Carpenter, C.C.: Mechanisms of bacterial diarrheas, Am. J. Med. **68**:313-315, 1980.
12. *Chandler, J.G.: Surgical treatment of massive obesity, Postgrad. Med. **56**:124-132, 1974.
13. Conn, H.F.: Current therapy 1981, Philadelphia, 1981, W.B. Saunders Co.
14. *Corman, M.L., Veidenheimer, M.C., and Coller, J.A.: Cathartics, Am. J. Nurs. **75**:273-279, 1975.
15. *Dericks, V.C., and Donovan, C.T.: The ostomy patient really needs you, Nurs. '76 **6**(9):30-32, 1976.
16. *Dericks, V.C.: The psychological hurdles of new ostomates: helping them up and over, Nurs. '74 **4**(9):52-55, 1974.
17. De Wind, L., and Payne, H.: Intestinal bypass surgery for morbid obesity, J.A.M.A. **236**:2298-2300, 1976.
18. Donovan, C., and Lenneberg, E.: Guidelines for the rehabilitation of ostomy patients, Glenville, Ill., 1975, International Association of Enterostomal Therapy, Inc.
19. Dunphy, J.E., and Way, L.W.: Current surgical diagnosis and treatment 1979, Los Altos, Calif., 1979, Lange Medical Publications.
20. Ferguson, J.A., editor: Symposium on colon and anorectal surgery, Surg. Clin. North Am. **58**:457-654, 1978.
21. *Fowler, E., Jeter, K.F., and Schwartz, A.A.: How to cope when your patient has an enterocutaneous fistula, Am. J. Nurs. **80**:426-429, 1980.
22. Gallagher, A.M.: Body image changes in the patient with a colostomy, Nurs. Clin. North Am. **7**:669-676, 1972.
23. *Geels, W., et al.: The enterocutaneous fistula: supplanting surgery with meticulous nursing care, Nurs. '78 **8**(4):52-55, 1978.
24. Gibbs, G.E., and White, M.: Stomal care, Am. J. Nurs. **72**:268-271, 1972.
25. *Given, B.A., and Simmons, S.J.: Gastroenterology in clinical nursing, ed. 3, St. Louis, 1979, The C.V. Mosby Co.
26. Grant, M., and Kubo, W.: Assessing a patient's hydration status, Am. J. Nurs. **75**:1306-1311, 1975.
27. Gutowski, F.: Ostomy procedure: nursing care before and after, Am. J. Nurs. **72**:262-267, 1972.
28. *Heindel, M.: How to protect your ostomy patients from post-op skin problems, RN **41**(1):43-45, 1978.
29. *Heydman, A.: Intestinal bypass for obesity, Am. J. Nurs. **74**:1102-1104, 1974.
30. Hill, G.L.: Ileostomy: surgery, physiology and management, New York, 1976, Grune & Stratton, Inc.
31. Hines, J., and Harris, G.: Colostomy and colostomy closure, Surg. Clin. North Am. **57**:1379-1392, 1977.
32. Hurley, D.L., Howard, P., Jr., and Hahn, H.H.: Perioperative prophylactic antibiotics in abdominal surgery, Surg. Clin. North Am. **59**:919-930, 1979.
33. *Hyman, E., et al.: The pouch ileostomy, Nurs. '77 **7**(9):44-47, 1977.
34. *Jensen, V.: Better techniques for bagging stomas. I. Urinary ostomies, Nurs. '74 **4**(7):60-64, 1974.
35. *Kodner, I.J.: Colostomy and ileostomy, Clin. Symp. **30**(5):1-36, 1978.
36. Krause, M.V., and Mahan, L.K.: Food, nutrition and diet therapy, Philadelphia, 1979, W.B. Saunders Co.
37. *Lamanske, J.: Helping the ileostomy patient to help himself, Nurs. '77 **7**(1):34-37, 1977.
38. Lasser, R.B., Bond, J.H., and Levitt, M.D.: The role of intestinal gas in functional abdominal pain, N. Engl. J. Med. **293**:524-528, 1975.
39. LeMaitre, G.D., and Finnegan, J.A.: The patient in surgery: a guide for nurses, ed. 4, Philadelphia, 1980, W.B. Saunders Co.
40. *Lyons, A.S., and Brockmeier, M.J.: Mechanical management of the ileostomy stoma, Surg. Clin. North Am. **52**:979-990, 1972.
41. MacLean, L.D., and Shibata, H.R.: The present status of bypass operations for obesity, Surg. Annu. **9**:213-230, 1977.
42. Mahoney, J.M.: Guide to ostomy care, Boston, 1976, Little, Brown & Co.
43. Matt, R., and Nundy, S.: Rectal carcinoma, abdominoperineal and anterior resection, Surg. Clin. North An. **54**:741-749, 1974.
44. Ostomate guide to government and private insurance services, St. Louis, 1977, Danal Laboratories Inc.
45. *Rush, A.: Cancer and the ostomy patient, Nurs. Clin. North Am. **11**:405-415, 1976.
46. Rusk, H.A.: Rehabilitation medicine: a textbook on physical medicine and rehabilitation, ed. 4, St. Louis, 1977, The C.V. Mosby Co.

*References preceded by an asterisk are particularly well suited for student reading.

47. Siefkin, A.D., and Bolt, R.J.: Preoperative evaluation of the patient with gastrointestinal and liver disease, Med. Clin. North Am. 63:1309-1320, 1979.

48. *United Ostomy Association, Inc.: Sex, courtship, and the single ostomate, Los Angeles, 1973, The Association.

49. *United Ostomy Association, Inc.: Sex and the male ostomate, Los Angeles, 1973, The Association.

50. *United Ostomy Association, Inc.: Sex, pregnancy, and the female ostomate, Los Angeles, 1972, The Association.

51. *Vukovich, V., and Grubb, R.D.: Care of the ostomy patient, St. Louis, ed. 2, 1977, The C.V. Mosby Co.

52. Walker, F.C.: Modern stoma care, New York, 1976, Churchill Livingstone, Inc.

53. *Watson, P.G., et al.: Comprehensive care of the ileostomy patient, Nurs. Clin. North Am. 11:427-444, 1976.

54. *Watt, R.: Irrigation—yes or no? Am. J. Nurs. 77:442-444, 1977.

55. *Watt, R.: Ostomies: why, how and where—an overview, Nurs. Clin. North Am. 11:393-404, 1976.

56. Watt, R.C.: Pathophysiology of peristomal skin. In Broadwell, D.C., and Jackson, B.S.: Principles of ostomy care, St. Louis, 1982, The C.V Mosby Co.

57. *Wentworth, A., and Cox, B.: Nursing management of the patient with a continent ileostomy, Am. J. Nurs. 77:1424-1428, 1976.

58. Yahle, M.: An ostomy information clinic, Nurs. Clin. North Am. 11:457-467, 1976.

AUDIOVISUAL RESOURCE

Trainex Corp.: Bowel and bladder retraining, Garden Grove, Calif., 1967, Trainex Corp. (Filmstrip, cassette, and script.)

CHAPTER 59

PROBLEMS OF THE LOWER GASTROINTESTINAL TRACT

BARBARA C. LONG

Problems that affect the lower gastrointestinal tract present a mosaic of symptoms in the individual. Some of these result in temporary dysfunction and as such may require no specific intervention from health personnel (e.g., diarrhea). The symptoms may be ignored by the person through choice or through lack of understanding of their possible significance. Other problems may present no particular symptoms until the disease has become one of extensive alteration in function. Whatever the alteration may be, it will in one way or another alter the normal absorptive function of the gastrointestinal tract and in this way alter nutrition, elimination, and fluid and electrolyte balance.

Prevention of problems of the lower gastrointestinal tract is not always possible since the cause of many of the particular diseases is unknown. Of increasing emphasis in prevention is the ongoing research related to cancer of the colon and rectum. Although the overall incidence rates have changed little over the last few years, there does appear to be an increase in the rate among nonwhite men.

Prevention of bowel problems is important not only in relation to mortality but also to work productivity. "Intestinal flu," diarrhea, and recuperation from bowel surgery account for an increasingly higher percentage of work time lost. Intensive health education beginning in childhood should assist in reducing the incidence of some of the more common problems of the lower gastrointestinal tract.

Malabsorption syndrome

Malabsorption syndrome is a group of signs and symptoms resulting from inadequate absorption of fat in the small intestine. Since fat-soluble vitamins (A, D, E, and K) require fat for absorption, decreasing absorption of these vitamins usually accompanies fat malabsorption. In addition, fat malabsorption often is accompanied by decreased absorption of protein, carbohydrate, and minerals. Different signs and symptoms specific to various nutrients result from malabsorption of nutrients other than fat.

Etiology and pathophysiology

Malabsorption results when there are (1) alterations of digestion so that nutrients are not broken down into a form that can be transported across the cell membranes of the villi, (2) alterations in the transportation of nutrients across the cell membranes of the villi so that nutrients cannot be absorbed, and (3) alterations in the transport of nutrients, particularly fat, from the villi through the lymphatic or circulatory systems (Table 59-1).

Gastrointestinal surgery can affect fat absorption in the following ways. (1) Following subtotal gastrectomy, gastric contents are emptied rapidly into the small intestine, thus decreasing the amount of secreted pancreatic enzyme necessary for fat absorption.[6] (2) Overgrowth of bacteria may occur in the duodenal blind loop formed during Billroth II surgery (p. 1421) interfering with fat and vitamin B absorption. (3) Although most of the fat absorption occurs in the proximal portion of the small intestine, ileal resection can also result in fat malabsorption. Most of the bile salts excreted into the intestines for fat absorption are absorbed primarily in the ileum and are returned to the liver for reexcretion. Thus if the ileum is removed, there will be increased bile loss in the feces and less bile available for fat absorption. Removal of short segments of the jejunum or ileum do not cause malabsorption; however, when more than

TABLE 59-1. Causes of intestinal malabsorption

Factors affecting absorption	Mechanism	Examples
Altered digestion (intraluminal phase)	Decreased gastric function	Subtotal gastrectomy
	Decreased pancreatic lipase	Pancreatic insufficiency: pancreatitis, cancer of pancreas, cystic fibrosis, Zollinger-Ellison syndrome
	Decreased conjugated bile salts	Liver disease, biliary tract obstruction, enteric fistulas
		Drugs that precipitate bile salts (neomycin, cholestyramine)
Altered mucosal cell transport (mucosal phase)	Genetic abnormalities	Lactase deficiency
	Small bowel disease	Crohn's disease, celiac disease, tropical sprue, Whipple's disease, infectious or allergic enteritis, parasitic infections, small bowel ischemia
	Inadequate surface	Intestinal resection or bypass
	Drugs	Para-aminosalicylic acid, colchicine, irritant laxatives, neomycin
	Radiation	Radiation enteritis
Altered lymph/blood transport (transit phase)	Lymphatic obstruction	Lymphoma
	Altered blood supply	Superior mesenteric thrombosis

50% of the small intestine is resected or bypassed, nutrient absorption is severely compromised.

Clinical picture

The characteristic sign of malabsorption syndrome is *steatorrhea,* or excessive loss of fat in the stool. The fat gives the stool a light, greasy, bulky, mushy appearance and a foul odor. The stools float because of their low specific gravity and because of gas produced by action of intestinal bacteria on the undigested fat. Stools may be limited to one bulky stool a day or may be frequent. Steatorrhea causes flatulence with borborygmi and abdominal distention. The decreased fat absorption leads to weight loss, weakness, fatigue, and anorexia.

Signs and symptoms of vitamin deficiencies include bleeding (ecchymoses, hematuria), bone pain, fractures, hypocalcemia, anemia, glossitis, ceilosis, muscle tenderness, peripheral neuritis, and dermatitis.[6] Protein deficiency results in edema, hypoalbuminemia, and loss of muscle mass. The person with malabsorption syndrome appears pale and emaciated and has dry scaly skin, which may be hyperpigmented.

Intervention

Medical treatment is based on the underlying cause of the malabsorption syndrome. Some specific malabsorption diseases are discussed below; other conditions leading to malabsorption can be found elsewhere in the text.

If acute generalized malabsorption is present, treatment consists of total parenteral nutrition; intravenous albumin, calcium, magnesium, and potassium; and packed red cells as necessary.[20] The patient is observed for signs of bleeding, tetany, and skin breakdown. Good mouth care, measures to prevent skin breakdown, and gentle handling to prevent pathologic fractures are important nursing measures.

Adult lactase deficiency

Epidemiology and etiology

Lactase deficiency is a common disorder found among most populations of the world with the exception of Northern European Caucasians and their descendants. In North America, blacks, Jews, Orientals, American Indians, Eskimos, and Mexicans are frequently affected. Lactase deficiency is usually a congenital disorder, although symptoms may not occur immediately. It also occurs occasionally after a subtotal gastrectomy.

Pathophysiology

Lactose, a disaccharide found in milk, is hydrolyzed by action of the enzyme *lactase* into glucose and galactose for absorption into the bloodstream. When insufficient lactase is present, the undigested lactose remains in the gut and acts (1) as an osmotic agent drawing water into the intestinal lumen and (2) as a substrate for bacterial fermentation generating lactic and other organic acids, carbon dioxide, and hydrogen gas. The increased fluid load leads to increased peristalsis resulting in malabsorption of other nutrients.

Clinical picture

The person with an intolerance to lactose has a history of gastrointestinal symptoms after the ingestion of milk. Symptoms include abdominal distention, discomfort or cramps, borborygmi, and a watery fermentive diarrhea. Diagnosis is made by a lactose tolerance test, a breath test, or jejunal biopsy specimen. In the lactose tolerance test, a rise in the blood glucose level of less than 20 mg/100 ml after the oral ingestion of 50 to 100 g of lactose following an overnight fast suggests lactose intolerance. The breath test measures an increase in exhaled hydrogen gas.

Intervention

Symptoms of lactase deficiency disappear when milk and other lactose-containing foods are removed from the diet. Foods that generally must be avoided are dairy products and any baked or processed foods that contain milk, butter, or added lactose. Labels of commercially prepared foods must be read carefully since some are processed with lactose, including some fruits and vegetables. Milk substitutes are available, and vegetable oils may be used in place of butter. Some margarines are prepared with lactose.

All lactose-containing foods are removed from the diet until symptoms disappear. Some persons can tolerate some cheeses and yogurt, and these foods can be introduced slowly to determine the tolerance. Adherence to the diet must be followed throughout life.

Outcome criteria for the person with adult lactase deficiency

The person or significant others can:
1. Explain basis of dietary requirements (relationship to symptoms).
2. Explain dietary changes required.
   a. List specific lactose-containing foods to be avoided.
   b. State plan to examine all food labels for the presence of lactose or milk.
3. Explain health maintenance and therapeutic follow-up programs.
   a. List signs and symptoms requiring reevaluation of diet (abdominal distention, abdominal discomfort, watery diarrhea).
   b. Explain plans for follow-up care until condition has stabilized.

Adult celiac disease

Etiology and pathophysiology

Adult celiac disease (also known as gluten enteropathy, celiac sprue, and nontropical sprue) results from an intolerance to the gliadin fraction of wheat or rye gluten, causing an atrophy of the intestinal villi and microvilli. The jejunum is more affected than the ileum. The disease is thought to be a hypersensitivity response and is familial with a high incidence of childhood celiac disease or evidence of disease in relatives.[6] Symptoms of childhood celiac disease usually disappear in later childhood.

Clinical picture

Symptoms usually appear between 30 and 60 years of age and may vary from mild diarrhea and anemia to severe signs typically seen in malabsorption syndrome. Hypotension and abdominal distention frequently oc-cur. Diagnosis is usually made by a symptom-abating response to a gluten-free diet.

Intervention

The anatomic and clinical changes of adult celiac disease can be reversed by a well-balanced, gluten-free diet. The diet eliminates all cereal grains (wheat, rye, oats, barley) except for rice. Corn, soybean, and gluten-free wheat flours must be used in baking and cooking, and all commercial baked goods are excluded. All food labels must be read carefully before the product is used; for example, pastas, commercial salad dressings, ice cream, and candies all contain gluten products. Beer and ale must be avoided but tea, carbonated beverages, and whiskies are permitted. Instant coffee labels must be examined since some contain wheat flour as filler.

During the initial treatment, secondary vitamin and mineral deficiencies are treated with replacement therapy. Symptoms will recur with dietary indiscretions; thus the person must plan for a permanent change in dietary habits.

Outcome criteria for the person with adult celiac disease

The person or significant others can:
1. Explain basis of dietary requirements (relationship to symptoms).
2. Explain dietary changes required.
   a. List specific gluten-containing foods to be avoided.
   b. State plan to examine all food labels for presence of substances containing gluten.
3. Explain health maintenance and therapeutic follow-up programs.
   a. List signs and symptoms requiring reevaluation of diet (steatorrhea, flatulence with abdominal distention, diarrhea).
   b. Explain plans for follow-up care until condition has stabilized.

Tropical sprue

Tropical sprue differs from celiac sprue. It is endemic to the Caribbean, Southeast Asia, and India. The cause is unknown but appears to have both a nutritional and an infectious basis. The initial symptoms are fatigue, diarrhea, and anorexia, followed by further signs of malabsorption syndrome after weeks to months. Symptoms are variable. Remission of symptoms occurs with treatment by broad-spectrum antibiotics, folic acid therapy, and a balanced diet high in protein and normal in fat. Folic acid is usually continued as maintenance therapy after symptoms have abated.[6]

Whipple's disease

Whipple's disease is a systemic disorder characterized by intestinal lipodystrophy that affects men 40 to 70 years of age. The cause is unknown. Although Whipple's disease responds to antibiotic therapy, no organism has been identified and the disease is thought to be caused by an immunologic deficit. Signs and symptoms of fever, arthritis, and lymphadenopathy occur in addition to those of malabsorption syndrome. Symptoms and pathologic manifestations disappear with oral antibiotic therapy. Long-term antibiotic therapy may be indicated.

Inflammation or infection of the intestinal tract

Pathophysiology

The mucous membrane of the intestinal tract responds to the process of inflammation in a manner similar to that of other tissues. The mucosa becomes reddened and edematous, has an increased temperature, is painful to touch, and loses some of its functional ability. As the surface of the mucosal membrane alters, the cells are exposed to an environment that includes lytic enzymes, pathogens, and trauma from food particles. This may cause further cellular damage. If pathogenic microorganisms or parasites are present, infection may occur.

At times pathogens or particles of feces will become lodged within small areas of the mucosa, multiply, and break down, resulting in fistulous tracts as seen in diverticulitis. These tracts or passageways may connect from one area of the gastrointestinal tract to another, to another organ, or to the outside of the body.

As the inflammation or infectious process resolves, the mucosal layer heals and muscular damage is replaced with scar tissue. This scarring will often draw the surrounding tissue closer together and shorten the length of the tract. Since scar tissue loses its secretory and absorptive properties, some function is lost, and the tissue is more easily traumatized, leading to local areas of bleeding. This scarring and bleeding is seen in *ulcerative colitis* and *Crohn's disease*.

Acute inflammations

Appendicitis

Epidemiology, etiology, and pathophysiology. Appendicitis is an inflammatory lesion of the vermiform appendix. It is more common among males, and it occurs most frequently between the ages of 10 and 30 years, although it may occur at any age. Although there is no certain cause of the disease, occlusion of the lumen of the appendix by hardened feces (fecaliths), by foreign objects, or by kinking of the appendix may impair the circulation and lower resistance to organisms within the body such as the colon bacilli or the streptococcus organisms. A small part of the appendix may be edematous or necrotic, or the entire appendix may be involved. An abscess may develop in the appendiceal wall or in the surrounding tissue. The serious danger is that the appendix will rupture and cause generalized peritonitis.

Prevention. In the United States there are still some deaths each year from appendicitis. If symptoms had not been neglected or if the individual had not been given a cathartic, some of these deaths might have been prevented. It is important therefore that the nurse continue to help teach the public that symptoms of right lower quadrant or periumbilical pain accompanied by loss of appetite, elevation of temperature, and possibly nausea, vomiting, and diarrhea should be reported to a physician. Persons with these symptoms should not be treated at home by local heat, enemas, or cathartics.

Clinical picture. The typical symptoms of acute appendicitis are pain about the umbilicus and throughout the abdomen (which may soon become localized at a point known as *McBurney's point* exactly halfway between the umbilicus and the crest of the right ilium) and nausea, anorexia, and vomiting. Light palpation of the abdomen will elicit pain in the right lower quadrant. Rebound tenderness is a common finding. The abdominal musculature overlying the area may feel tense as a result of voluntary rigidity. Rigidity noted over the entire abdomen is generally an indication of rupture of the appendix with resultant peritonitis. The person will often be noted to be lying on the side or back with knees flexed in an attempt to decrease muscular strain on the abdominal wall.

Acute appendicitis is remarkable for the suddenness of its onset. The person may have felt quite well an hour or two before the onset of severe pain. Approximately 90% of these persons will have a white cell count above 10,000/cu mm, and approximately three fourths will have a neutrophil count above 75%. The temperature usually ranges from 38° to 38.5° C and is accompanied by an increase in pulse. These symptoms are present in about 60% of persons with acute appendicitis.

There will be an area of hyperesthetic skin over the inflamed appendix before perforation. This response may be elicited by stroking the skin surface over the right lower quadrant with the point of a pin or by lightly grasping the skin over the right lower quadrant between the thumb and forefinger and gently pulling the fold upward. Both measures will elicit a verbal or facial pain response.

Other persons have less well-defined local symptoms because of the location of the appendix. It may be retrocecal, or it may lie adjacent to the ureter. If the symptoms are questionable, urinalysis and an intravenous pyelogram may be performed to rule out acute pyelitis or a ureteral stone. Many other diseases produce symptoms similar to appendicitis, and they sometimes need to be ruled out before a positive diagnosis can be made. Some of these are acute salpingitis, regional ileitis, mesenteric lymphadenitis, and biliary colic.

The older person with acute appendicitis may experience only dull pain. Children who develop appendicitis may have only slight abdominal pain, although usually they vomit. Because the abdominal omentum is not well developed in children, if the appendix perforates, peritonitis can develop easily because the infection cannot be walled off so quickly. It is recommended therefore that the ill child who refuses food and who vomits be taken to a physician for diagnosis and treatment. A cathartic should *never* be given for these complaints.

Intervention. When appendicitis is suspected, the person usually is hospitalized at once and placed on bed rest for observation and the necessary diagnostic procedures that must be performed. Since an operation may be performed shortly after admission nothing is given by mouth while reports of the blood count are awaited. Parenteral fluids may be given during this time. Narcotics are not given until the cause of the pain has been determined, since they would mask signs or symptoms. An ice bag to the abdomen may be ordered to help relieve pain.

An appendectomy is usually scheduled as an emergency operation. A general or regional anesthetic is used, and the appendix is removed through a small incision over McBurney's point or through a right paramedial incision. The incision usually heals with no drainage. Drains are used when an abscess is discovered, when the appendix has ruptured and peritonitis has developed, and sometimes when the appendix was edematous and ready to rupture and was surrounded by clear fluid.

Bowel function is usually normal soon after surgery. Nausea and vomiting disappear with surgical treatment, and the patient is permitted food as tolerated. Convalescence is usually short.

Peritonitis

Etiology. Peritonitis is an inflammatory involvement of the peritoneum caused by trauma or by rupture of an organ containing bacteria, which are then introduced into the abdominal cavity. Some of the organisms found are *Escherichia coli,* streptococci (both aerobic and anaerobic), staphylococci, pneumococci, and gonococci.

Peritonitis also can be caused by chemical response to irritating substances such as might occur following rupture of the fallopian tube in an ectopic pregnancy, perforation of a gastric ulcer, or traumatic rupture of the spleen or liver. Inflammation from chemical causes, however, is so closely followed by invasion of blood-borne bacteria that it is only a few hours before organisms may be isolated from most fluids that accumulate in peritonitis.

Pathophysiology. Natural barriers are used in the body's attempt to control the inflammation. Adhesions quickly form in an attempt to wall off the infection, and the omentum helps to enclose areas of inflammation. These processes may result in involvement of only part of the abdominal cavity and may finally narrow the infected area to a small, enclosed one (abscess). As healing occurs, fibrous adhesions may shrink and disappear entirely so that no trace of infection can be found on surgical exploration of the abdomen at a much later date, or they may persist as constrictions that may permanently bind the involved structures together. Sometimes they cause an intestinal obstruction by occluding the lumen of the bowel. If abscesses form, they are usually in the lower abdomen. They may, however, be walled off elsewhere. For example, abscess formation following a ruptured appendix may develop under the diaphragm and may even perforate that structure and cause empyema.

Clinical picture. Local reactions of the peritoneum include redness, inflammation, and the production of large amounts of fluid containing electrolytes and proteins. Hypovolemia, electrolyte imbalance, dehydration, and finally shock develop as a result of the loss of the fluid, electrolytes, and proteins into the peritoneal cavity. The fluid usually becomes purulent as the condition progresses and as bacteria become more numerous. Peristalsis is halted by the severe peritoneal infection, and all the symptoms of acute intestinal obstruction (p. 1492) may occur. Nausea, vomiting, pain in the abdomen on palpation, severe distention with absence of bowel sounds, rigidity of the abdomen, and failure to pass anything rectally occur. Peritonitis also causes serious systemic symptoms including high temperature, high white blood cell count, tachycardia, weakness, diaphoresis, pallor, and all other signs of severe systemic reaction and shock. Symptoms may be masked in elderly persons or in those receiving corticosteroids. Peritonitis was a very serious condition that had an extremely high mortality before antimicrobial and bacteriostatic drugs and other modern treatment became available.

Intervention. Intervention usually consists of immediate measures to reestablish fluid and electrolyte balance and to combat infection. Nasogastric intubation is usually instituted with restriction of oral intake. Fluids and electrolytes are given intravenously. Infection is controlled by large parenteral doses of antibiotics. Narcotics and sedatives are given for severe pain and apprehension as soon as the diagnosis is confirmed and there is no danger of masking symptoms.

Mouth care is given, and protection is needed to prevent drying and cracking of the lips, since dehydration is usually marked. Usually the person is placed in semi-Fowler's position so that gravity may help localize pus in the lower abdomen or the pelvis. Also in this position deeper breaths to prevent respiratory complications can be taken with less pain.

If the peritonitis is caused by a perforation that is releasing irritating or infected material into the abdominal cavity, surgery is performed as soon as the patient's condition permits. However, if the patient is in shock it may be several hours before shock can be relieved and before surgery can be safely performed. The operation usually consists of closure of the abnormal opening into the abdominal cavity and removal of the fluid that has accumulated.

Meckel's diverticulum

Meckel's diverticulum is a congenital sac or appendage that is occasionally found in the ileum 60 to 90 cm proximal to the ileocecal valve. Inflammation and perforation may occur with symptoms closely resembling those of appendicitis. Surgical excision is done at any time that Meckel's diverticulum is discovered during surgery for other reasons or when symptoms of inflammation occur.

Chronic inflammations

Crohn's disease: regional enterocolitis

Crohn's disease is a nonspecific inflammation that can affect any area of the small or large intestine. The most commonly involved areas are the terminal ileum, cecum, and ascending colon. The disease may occur in several segments separated by normal mucosa. Differences between Crohn's disease and ulcerative colitis are illustrated in Table 59-2.

Epidemiology. Crohn's disease occurs most frequently in the young adult between the ages of 20 and 30 years. The incidence peaks again between 40 and 50 years of age. There is a high rate of recurrence, and the mortality is 5% to 18%.[6] There is a high incidence among the English and a low incidence in the nonemergent societies. The incidence rate appears to be increasing in American blacks and in emergent societies, indicating the possible relationship of stress to the onset of symptoms.

Etiology. The cause of Crohn's disease is unclear. There is conflicting data relating to environmental or genetic factors as etiologic factors. No specific causative agents have been found. Some evidence suggests a

TABLE 59-2. Comparison of Crohn's disease and ulcerative colitis

	Crohn's disease	Ulcerative colitis
General appearance	Usually normal	May feel and look ill
Age	Bimodal: 20-30 yr and 40-50 yr	Mostly young adults
Area affected	Mainly terminal ileum, cecum, and ascending colon (right side)	Colon only, primarily the descending colon (left side)
Extent of involvement	Segmental areas of involvement	Continuous, diffuse areas of involvement
Inflammation	Mostly submucosal	Mostly mucosal
Mucosal appearance	Cobblestone effect; granulomas	Ulcerations
Cancer potential	Normal incidence	Increased incidence
Character of stools	No blood; may have some fat; three to four semisoft per day	Blood present; no fat; frequent liquid stools
Reasons for surgery	Fistulas; intestinal obstruction	Poor response to medical therapy; hemorrhage; perforation
Complications	Fistulas; perianal disease; strictures; vitamin and iron deficiencies; fistulas to other organs	Pseudopolyps; hemorrhage; toxic megacolon; cachexia; perforation less often, causes peritonitis

transmissible agent with a long latent period as a possible causative factor in susceptible persons.[6] Many persons with Crohn's disease manifest defects in their cellular immune system.[55]

Pathophysiology. Crohn's disease is characterized by cobblestone ulcerations along the mucosa, a thickening of the intestinal wall, and the formation of scar tissue. The ulcers are likely to perforate and form fistulas that connect with the abdominal wall or with any hollow viscus such as the bladder, colon, or vagina. Scar tissue may form as the ulcers heal, preventing the normal absorption of food, and strictures may form, causing intestinal obstruction. Mesenteric lymph nodes are enlarged and firm.

Clinical picture. The person with *acute* Crohn's disease usually has severe abdominal pain or cramps localized in the right lower quadrant, malaise, moderate fever, and mild diarrhea. The white blood cell count is elevated. Often the disease is diagnosed as acute appendicitis, but on exploratory surgery a normal appendix but an inflamed ileum is found.

Chronic Crohn's disease is characterized by a long

history of diarrhea, abdominal pain, loss of weight, anemia, fistula formation, and finally intestinal obstruction. Weight loss and anemia result from chronic persistent inflammation of the bowel, decreased food intake, and malabsorption. The diarrhea may consist of three or four semisolid stools daily containing mucus and pus but no blood. Steatorrhea may also be present if the ulceration extends high in the small intestine. The abdominal colicky pain is relieved with a bowel movement. A mass sometimes can be felt in the area of the appendix or cecum. Perineal suppuration and strictures at the anus and rectosigmoid junction may be noted on sigmoidoscopy.

Radiographs of the small and large intestine confirm the diagnosis. Ureteral calculi and hydronephrosis may occur as a result of obstruction at the ureterovesical junction from the inflammatory mass. Intravenous pyelography may be used to identify the presence of these complications.

Intervention. There is no specific therapy for Crohn's disease, and treatment is mainly supportive care. Activity may be somewhat restricted with rest periods suggested to conserve energy.

DIET. A well-balanced, high-calorie high-protein diet is encouraged. Fats or high-fiber foods may be poorly tolerated by some persons, and their diets will need appropriate modifications. Fad diets are to be avoided. If food intake is decreased, vitamin supplements are added. Replacement vitamin B_{12} is given when there is a marked loss of ileum. When anemia is present, iron-dextran (Imferon) is given by Z-track injection, since oral intake of iron is ineffective because of the intestinal ulceration. Total parenteral nutrition is helpful for the cachectic patient.

MEDICATIONS. Analgesic and anticholinergic drugs may be given on a temporary basis to decrease abdominal pain and intestinal motility. Intestinal antibiotics such as phthalysulfathiazole (Sulfathalidine) may be administered orally to treat local suppurative infections. Sulfasalazine (Azulfidine) appears useful for short-term therapy. Steroids have not demonstrated any long-term influence in the course of the disease, although they may be helpful in an acute episode. Azathioprine (Imuran), an immunosuppresive agent, has been shown to have a steroid-sparing effect, to be as beneficial as sulfasalazine, and in some cases to be beneficial in the healing of fistulas.[55]

SURGERY. If intestinal obstruction occurs or if there are fistulas, especially to the bladder, surgery is indicated. The involved portion of the intestines is removed, and the proximal portion is anastomosed to the remaining colon (ileoascending or ileotransverse colostomy). Unfortunately, the recurrence rate of the disease is high (50% at 5 years, 75% at 10 years).[6] Surgery may be helpful in young persons in the hope that they will be among the 25% in whom recurrence does not occur.

A diversionary temporary ileostomy procedure to permit rest of the inflamed portion of the intestinal tract is no longer being performed.

Ulcerative colitis

Epidemiology. Ulcerative colitis is a nonspecific inflammatory disease of the colon. It may occur at any age but is found most often at two peak periods, between 20 to 25 and 50 to 60 years of age. The disease appears to be more frequent in women than in men and has a higher incidence among Jews than non-Jews.

Etiology. The cause of ulcerative colitis is unknown, and numerous theories have been suggested. No specific organisms have been implicated. One theory emphasizes a psychosomatic relationship stressing an obsessive-compulsive immaturity of some patients, but this theory has been challenged.[6] More recent studies are pursuing the immunologic mechanisms as potential etiologic factors. The disease varies in severity, and the person may be symptom free between periods of acute distress. A severe attack may be brought on by an acute infection, stress, or unknown factors.

Pathophysiology. In the early stages of ulcerative colitis only the rectum or rectosigmoid colon is affected, with the rectal mucosa containing many superficial bleeding points. As the disease progresses, advancing up the colon, the bowel mucosa becomes edematous and thickened. The superficial bleeding points gradually enlarge and become ulcerated. The ulcers may bleed or perforate, causing abscess formation or peritonitis. The edematous mucosa may undergo changes and form pseudopolyps which may become cancerous. The continuous healing process, with formation of scar tissue between the frequent relapses, may cause the colon to lose its normal elasticity and its absorptive capability. Normal mucosa is replaced by scar tissue, and the colon becomes thickened, rigid, and pipelike.

Clinical picture. The diagnosis of ulcerative colitis is based on the history and symptoms, on results obtained from barium enemas, on proctoscopic and sigmoidoscopic examinations, and on failure to find any causative organisms in the stools.

The main symptom of an acute attack of the disease is diarrhea. There may be as many as 15 to 20 liquid stools a day containing blood, mucus, and pus. Abdominal cramps may or may not occur before the bowel movement. As the scarring within the bowel progresses, the feeling of the urge to defecate is lost leading to involuntary leakage of stool. There may be loss of appetite, low-grade fever, and occasionally nausea and vomiting. With the persistence of these symptoms as well as the marked depression of colonic absorption, weakness, dehydration, debility, and cachexia occur. Hypokalemia and hypoproteinemia are common. A distended abdomen is suggestive of *toxic megacolon*, a marked dilation of the colon that may result in rupture of the colon.

Intervention. The person with ulcerative colitis may be admitted to the hospital for immediate supportive treatment during an acute exacerbation of the disease or for preparation for surgery during a remission. Medical treatment for ulcerative colitis is directed toward restoring nutrition, combating infection, and reducing the motility of the inflamed bowel.

EMOTIONAL SUPPORT. If the disease is of long duration the patient is usually thin, nervous, and apprehensive and is inclined to be preoccupied with physical symptoms. Insecurity, dependency, and depressed or hostile behavior may be present, and empathic communication over time is usually needed to establish effective nurse-patient relationships (see Chapter 14). The patient needs to be included in the planning of care, which should incorporate those activities the patient has found helpful in the past.

COMFORT AND REST. Bed rest may be prescribed for the acutely ill patient, and care must be taken for thin persons that bony prominences are protected by an alternating-pressure mattress, foam pad, or sheepskin. Measures to ensure rest are explored with the patient. Sedatives or tranquilizers are often prescribed to alleviate nervous tension.

DIET. A high-protein, high-caloric, high-vitamin diet is usually urged to help the person regain nutritional losses and to foster healing. Because there is no conclusive evidence that the diet affects the condition, often any desired food is permitted.

ELIMINATION. It is crucial that a record be kept of the number, amount, and character of the stools and that specimens of stool be sent to the labroatory as requested. Antispasmodic drugs such as belladonna preparations may be given to slow peristalsis. Medications such as kaolin and bismuth (bismuth subcarbonate) may be used to help coat and protect the irritated intestinal mucosa and to give better consistency to the stools, and paregoric or diphenoxylate (Lomotil) may be used to lessen the frequency of stools.

Although each bowel movement may be very small, the commode or bedpan should be emptied as often as it is used. The patient wants the bedpan accessible at all times and may even insist on keeping it in bed. Room deodorizers are sometimes used to dispel unpleasant odors. Patients who brace themselves on the bedpan by leaning on their elbows, thereby causing pressure areas, will need these areas massaged frequently with a lubricant. If the patient spends much time on the bedpan, it can be padded with foam rubber, or a fracture pan can be used. If the commode is used it can also be padded. Linen is kept fresh, and the patient's perineum, buttocks, and anal region are washed thoroughly several times a day. Dibucaine (Nupercaine) or other prescribed ointment may be applied to the anus to relieve discomfort. Sitz baths are beneficial to the skin and circulation and are often permitted two or three times a day.

MEDICATIONS. Antibiotics may be ordered to prevent or to treat secondary infection. Sulfasalazine (Azulfidine) is now widely used in the treatment of ulcerative colitis, and many physicians consider it the drug of choice. The side effects of oliguria and crystalluria are particularly apt to be a problem in patients with ulcerative colitis unless they maintain a liberal fluid intake.

Adrenocorticotropic hormone (ACTH) and the adrenal steroids such as prednisone may be prescribed in the treatment of ulcerative colitis. They often produce dramatic results in severe cases of the disease by decreasing the toxemia and fever; diminishing diarrhea, bleeding, and rectal urgency; and promoting a sense of well-being. It should be understood, however, that while corticotropin and the corticosterioids suppress the inflammation associated with ulcerative colitis, they do not cure the disease.

In mild ulcerative colitis confined to the distal colon, rectal instillations may be prescribed. Commercially prepared enemas containing hydrocortisone or prednisolone phosphate are available and are given as retention enemas at bedtime.[6] Steroids are given orally to moderately ill patients and intravenously to acutely ill patients. (For care of persons receiving steroid therapy, see p. 958.)

Immunosuppressive drugs such as azathioprine (Imuran) or 6-mercaptopurine have been used for some patients with ulcerative colitis who cannot tolerate other therapies or who are unable to have surgery. They are given only as a short-term measure because of their high toxicity and are not recommended for routine use.

SURGERY. Ulcerative colitis can be cured by surgery. The trend is toward earlier surgical intervention for the acutely ill person and for persons experiencing frequent exacerbations. Surgery is clearly indicated when complications are present, including massive hemorrhage, perforation of the colon, strictures, and medically unresponsive toxic megacolon.

The most common surgical procedure is a total proctocolectomy through an abdominal perineal incision, leaving the patient with a permanent ileostomy. (For the care of the patient with an ileostomy, refer to Chapter 58.) If the rectum is only mildly diseased, an ileorectal anatomosis may be performed with preservation of rectal function.

A different type of surgical approach is the "continent ileostomy" or "Koch's pouch" (Fig. 59-1). An intraabdominal reservoir with a "nipple valve" is formed from the distal ileum to provide continence. The capacity of the pouch increases slowly over months until it can hold approximately 500 ml. Contents of the pouch are removed several times a day by catheterization. Difficulties have occurred with valve failure and in

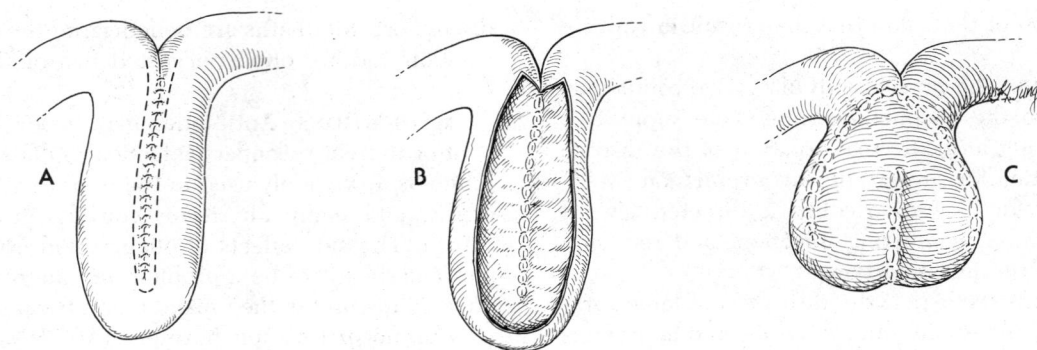

Fig. 59-1. Continent ileostomy. A reservoir is made by, **A,** suturing a loop of bowel together and then cutting around sutures; **B,** opening out incised area; and, **C,** folding open area end-to-end and suturing. Distal end of ileum is brought out through abdominal wall.

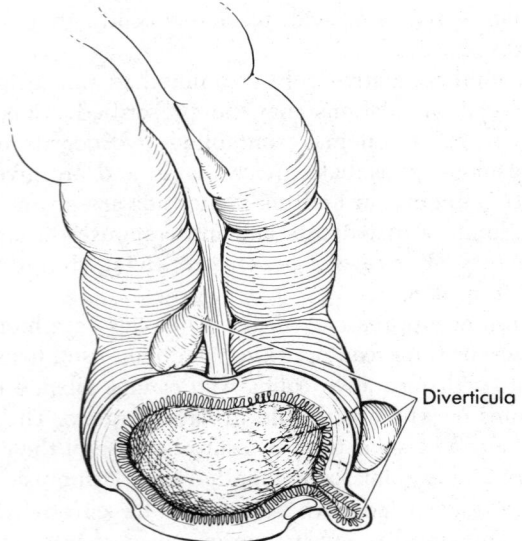

Fig. 59-2. Diverticuli of colon.

keeping the ileal contents from becoming too thick and plugging up the stoma. Only selected persons at this time are considered suitable candidates for this type of procedure. The procedure eliminates the need for wearing an external ileostomy bag.

Diverticular disease of the colon

Epidemiology and etiology. Diverticula are small mucosal outpouchings or sacs through defects in the muscular wall of the colon (Fig. 59-2). The presence of diverticuli is termed *diverticulosis*. They rarely occur before 35 years of age but increase progressively with age to about a 50% incidence in the elderly person. The number of persons who have diverticulosis of the colon is unknown since many persons with diverticulosis are asymptomatic. The term *diverticular disease* is used to describe symptomatic diverticula.

Diverticulosis has been described as a disease of Western civilization because of the high incidence in Western developed countries and the low incidence in nonindustrialized countries and Japan. The cause is thought to be the low intake of dietary fiber foods in developed countries. Symptoms appear when diverticula become inflamed (*diverticulitis*), when painful spasms associated with the diverticula occur, or when complications occur such as perforation, obstruction, or hemorrhage.

Clinical picture. Diverticulosis is usually asymptomatic. When diverticular disease is present, the patient complains of left lower quadrant abdominal pain of varying severity and quality. The pain, which is caused by muscular spasms of the sigmoid colon, is often aggravated by emotional tension or by eating. The patient may have constipation or constipation alternating with diarrhea. Excessive bleeding may result but usually resolves spontaneously. Fever and leukocytosis occur only with diverticulitis.

Intervention. The current treatment of asymptomatic diverticulosis is a diet high in vegetable fiber. Unprocessed wheat bran may be added to foods but should be started with a small amount and increased slowly over a 4- to 6-week period to 10 to 25 g/day.[1] Bran initially causes abdominal distention and excess flatus. The purpose of the high-fiber diet is to increase stool bulk, thus increasing the diameter of the colon leading to decreased intraluminal pressure. Hydrophilic colloids such as psyllium seed (Metamucil) or methylcellulose may also be prescribed to increase stool bulk.

High-fiber diets are also prescribed when diverticular disease occurs, except with diverticulitis. Measures to relieve pain include an analgesic such as pentazocine (Talwin), an antispasmodic such as dicyclomine hydrochloride (Bentyl) or propantheline (Pro-Banthine), or local application of heat. Antibiotics such as ampicillin or gentamicin may be prescribed for diverticulitis. When

TABLE 59-3. Common anal lesions

Lesion	Description	Symptoms	Treatment
Anal fissure	Slitlike ulceration in epithelium of anal canal	Pain with defecation; bleeding; constipation	Stool softeners; analgesic ointments; sitz baths; surgical removal of fissure if medical therapy ineffective
Anal abscess	Abscess in tissue around anus	Persistent throbbing anal pain with walking, sitting, defecation; systemic signs of infection	Incision and drainage of abscess
Anal fistula	Hollow track leading through anal tisuse from anorectal canal through skin near anus	Purulent discharge near anus	Fistulectomy or fistulotomy
Hemorrhoids	Varicosities of lower rectum and anus	Bleeding with defecation; pain if thrombosed	Analgesic ointments for mild discomfort; injection, ligation, or hemorrhoidectomy for severe discomfort

hemorrhage or severe diverticulitis occurs, the prescription is bed rest, sedation, and either intravenous fluids or a clear liquid diet to give the bowel a rest. Blood transfusions may be necessary if blood loss is extensive.

Since emotional tension often precipitates diverticular disease, the patient may need assistance in learning how to reduce emotional tension. Relaxation techniques, planned rest periods, and regular sleeping hours may prove helpful.

Surgery is often indicated for the person who has recurrent attacks of uncomplicated diverticulitis or when complications such as perforation or obstruction occur. The surgical procedure of choice is resection of the sigmoid with an end-to-end anastomosis.

Outcome criteria for the person with a chronic inflammatory disease of the lower gastrointestinal tract

The person or significant others can:
1. Describe the dietary modifications needed after discharge.
   a. Plan a diet that includes adequate protein, calories, and vitamins.
   b. List any specific foods to be encouraged or avoided (high roughage, fats).
2. Explain any medication program to be followed at home.
   a. State action, dosage, frequency, and side effects of medications (antibiotics, antidiarrheals, antispasmodics).
   b. Describe the use of medications to be taken as needed for discomfort.
3. Describe the health maintenance follow-up program.
   a Explain in own words the basic pathologic condition and overall treatment program.
   b. Describe the need to avoid infectious agents in the environment.

c. List signs requiring immediate contact with health care provider (abdominal pain or distention, increasing diarrhea, presence of blood or pus in the stool, signs and symptoms of systemic infection, constipation).
   d. State plans for regular follow-up care.
4. Describe measures for supportive care.
   a. Verbalize the relationship between compliance with therapy and optimal health.
   b. Identify a source for an ongoing supportive relationship.
   c. Verbalize awareness of potential surgery.

Anal fissure

An anal fissure is a slitlike ulcer resembling a crack in the lining of the anal canal at or below the anorectal line (Table 59-3). Usually it is the result of trauma caused by passage of hard-formed stool that overstretches the anal lining. The ulcer does not heal readily. Defecation initiates spasm of the anal sphincter causing severe pain that lasts for some time. Slight bleeding may occur, and constipation is usually caused by restraining of bowel movements to avoid pain.

Anal examination causes muscle spasm of the sphincter. Since spasm results in pain, the fissure must be examined with the patient under anesthesia. Treatment usually consists of digital dilation of the sphincter, or the anal ulcer may be surgically excised.

Local pain and spasm sometimes can be relieved by warm compresses, sitz baths, and use of analgesic ointments. Docusate sodium (Colace) is usually ordered to lubricate the canal and to soften the stool. Postoperatively, the care is similar to that given following a hemorrhoidectomy (p. 1495).

Anal abscess

An anal abscess is located in tissues around the anus. It is caused by infection from the anal canal and may follow an anal fissure. If the abscess involves the anal, paraanal, or perineal tissues, there is throbbing local pain caused by pressure on the somatic sensory nerves in the perineum and local signs of inflammation. The person finds it difficult to sit or lie on the area. In fact, any position is uncomfortable because reflected pain is common.

If the abscess is located deep in the ischiorectal tissues, however, the person is aware only of vague discomfort until the disease spreads into an area where there are nerve fibers. The person with an *ischiorectal abscess* is usually very ill. Fever, chills, and malaise are present, and the abscess must be incised and drained.

Postoperative care. Postoperatively, patients usually prefer to lie on their side or abdomen. Because some difficulty in voiding is common, nursing measures should be initiated to prevent bladder distention.

There is usually a large amount of seropurulent drainage from the wound. Until all drainage disappears, a dressing is worn, held in place with a T-binder. The wound should heal from the bottom outward. If the wound is located near the anus, the patient is advised to cleanse the area carefully after defecation and to take a sitz bath after each defecation. Sitz baths promote comfort and wound healing. A stool softener may be given to prevent or treat constipation. Antibiotics usually are administered.

The patient is often discharged from the hospital before the wound has completely healed. Sitz baths are continued at home. Any difficulties that are encountered should be reported to the physician.

Anal fistula

An anal fistula is an inflammatory sinus or tract with a primary opening in an anal crypt and with a secondary opening on the anal, paraanal, or perineal skin or in the rectal mucous membrane. It results from the rupture or drainage of an anal abscess. The individual has a periodic drainage that stains underclothing. An anal fistula is usually a chronic condition, and unfortunately many persons attempt to treat themselves with over-the-counter remedies before they seek competent medical care. The person is encouraged to have a gastrointestinal tract examination to rule out regional enteritis or other colon diseases.

The treatment for an anal fistula is a *fistulectomy* or a *fistulotomy*. A fistulectomy consists of an excision of the entire fistulous tract. The overhanging edges, if any, are trimmed away to leave an open, saucer-shaped wound. This procedure is usually performed when the fistula is quite straight and somewhat superficial. When a fistulotomy is performed, the entire tract is laid open and the overlying skin margins are excised to leave a wide, saucer-shaped wound. The membranous lining of the remaining half of the fistulous tract quickly acquires a covering of granulation tissue. This procedure is usually used when a deep fistulous tract exists.

Postoperative care. Postoperatively, a stool softener or mild laxative may be given orally daily until the first bowel movement occurs, and sitz baths are prescribed to keep the area clean and to relieve discomfort. The patient who has had an operation for a fistula is more comfortable sitting on a protected pillow or a piece of very thick foam rubber rather than on a rubber ring.

Parasitic infections

Amebiases

Etiology and pathophysiology. Amebiases is caused by the protozoan parasite *Entamoeba histolytica*, which primarily invades the large intestine and secondarily invades the liver. The active, motile form of the protozoa, the trophozoite, is not infectious and if ingested is easily destroyed by digestive enzymes. The inactive form, or cyst, however, is highly resistant to extremes in temperature, most chemicals, and the digestive juices. When the cyst is swallowed in fecally contaminated food or water, it easily passes into the intestines, where the active trophozoite is released and enters the intestinal wall. Here it feeds on the mucosal cells, causing ulceration of the intestinal mucosa.

Prevention. It is estimated that at least 10% of the population of the United States have amebiasis in the acute, chronic, or asymptomatic stages.[6] Although the disease exists chiefly in tropical countries, it also prevails wherever sanitation is poor. The cyst, which is the infectious agent, can survive for long periods outside the body, and it is transmitted by direct contact from person to person, by insects, and by contaminated water, milk, and other foods. For this reason persons traveling in tropical countries should drink only boiled water and eat only cooked foods. The most infectious agent is the "carrier," who, although having few or no symptoms of the disease, passes the cysts in stools. A food handler with poor hygienic habits can easily transmit the cysts in foods prepared for consumption by others.

Clinical picture. Most persons with amebiasis are asymptomatic and become carriers. Symptoms usually begin several months after infection and depend on the extent of tissue invasion. With mild involvement, the patient may experience abdominal cramps, intermittent diarrhea and constipation, and flatulence. With greater tissue involvement, there may be frequent semiliquid or liquid stools containing blood and mucus. This is followed by fever, colicky abdominal pains, and tenesmus. Hepatomegaly with tenderness over the liver often occurs. Complications include liver abscess and bowel perforation.

If either the trophozoite or the cyst can be found in the stool, a positive diagnosis of amebiasis can be made and definitive treatment started. It is easier to find the parasite in the stool during the acute stage of the disease than later. Immediately after defecation a warm stool should be sent to the laboratory for examination. Several stool specimens from successive bowel movements may be requested. If the laboratory is at a distance, the specimen container should be transported on a hot water bottle or in a pan of warm water. When special laboratory facilities are required, a fresh stool can be placed in a preservative and sent to the Centers for Disease Contol, Atlanta, for diagnosis.

Intervention. The person with a mild or asymptomatic form of amebiasis is treated on an outpatient basis; 90% of all persons usually respond to a course of amebicidal therapy. If the halogenated hydroquinolines such as di-iodohydroxyquinoline (Diodoquin) are given, the person may have some diarrhea. Neurotoxicity to this agent has been reported. The drug is administered in a dose of 650 mg three times a day for 20 days. Tetracycline may be prescribed alone or in combination with di-iodohydroxyquinoline. The maximum daily dose of tetracycline is 2 g/daily for 7 days.

Metronidazole (Flagyl) is the drug of choice for acute amebiasis, both for intestinal and hepatic involvement. The usual dosage is 750 mg orally three times daily for 5 to 10 days. Emetine hydrochloride may also be used for severe disease, especially when liver abscess is present. The patient receiving emetine hydrochloride is placed on strict bed rest, and pulse rate and blood pressure are watched carefully because the drug is very toxic. Some of the many signs of toxicity to this drug include nausea, vomiting, diarrhea, generalized weakness, cardiac irregularity, fall in blood pressure, neuritis, desquamation of the skin, loss of the sense of taste, and mental depression. Emetine hydrochloride usually is given for 7 to 10 days. Injections can cause tissue necrosis; therefore injection sites are carefully rotated.

Amebiasis is a disease with remissions and exacerbations, and it may persist for years. During acute exacerbations the person may become dehydrated, exhausted, or anemic and require hospitalization. Infusions and blood transfusions are often necessary. A bland low-residue, high-protein diet is commonly prescribed, and the person may be advised to avoid alcohol and tobacco.

A careful record of intake and output is kept, and generous amounts of oral fluids are encouraged. The number and character of the stools should be described. Excretion precautions are observed, and the bedpan is sterilized after each use. In handling the bedpan precautions are taken because some cysts are usually passed. Cleanliness should be stressed, and patients should know why it is so important to wash their hands after bowel movements. Particular emphasis is placed on careful washing of hands before meals to avoid reinfection.

Persons known to be exposed to amebiasis should have stool examinations weekly for 3 weeks. If infected, they are treated as described for the asymptomatic form of the disease.

Trichinosis

Etiology and pathophysiology. Trichinosis (trichinellosis, trichiniasis) is caused by the larvae of a species of roundworm, *Trichinella spiralis*, which become encysted in the striated muscles of humans, hogs, and other animals, particularly those (e.g., rodents) that consume infected pork in garbage. Trichinosis is found worldwide with the highest incidence occurring in Europe and the United States. Autopsy reports show that at least 5% of the population of the United States is affected with trichinosis. It occurs much more often in hogs that have been fed garbage than in those fed on grain. The larvae do not form cysts in pork. Therefore they are not visible to the naked eye and cannot be seen by food inspectors.

Trichinosis is transmitted through inadequately cooked food. Pork is the most common source of infection. When infected food is eaten, live encysted larvae develop within the intestine of the host; they mate and produce eggs that hatch in the uterus of the female worm. The larvae are discharged in huge numbers (approximately 1500 per worm) into the lymphatics and lacteals of the host's small intestine at the rate of about two an hour for about 6 weeks. They pass to the muscles of the host, where they become encysted by the reaction of the host's body and may remain for 10 years or longer (Fig. 59-3).

Prevention. No immunization for trichinosis is available, yet the disease could be eradicated with the knowledge that we now possess. Basic scientific facts necessary for the complete prevention of the disease in human beings have been known for years. Trichinae can be killed by cooking at a temperature of 60° C (140° F) for 30 minutes per pound of meat and by freezing at a temperature of -18° C (0° F) for 24 hours. They are not killed by smoking, pickling, or other methods of processing. Sausage and other infected pork products carelessly prepared are a common source of infection in humans. Other meats ground in the same machine without thorough cleaning or cut on the same meat block may also cause infection. There is a need for thorough cooking of all pork products consumed at home regardless of how sanitary the local meat market may appear to be.

Clinical picture. Signs and symptoms of trichinosis are varied. Although the reason is unknown, edema appears as puffiness about the eyes, particularly involving the upper lids. If a very large number of larvae have been ingested, nausea, vomiting, and diarrhea caused by intestinal irritation usually occur about 4 days after the infected food has been eaten. On about the seventh day, when the larvae migrate throughout the body to

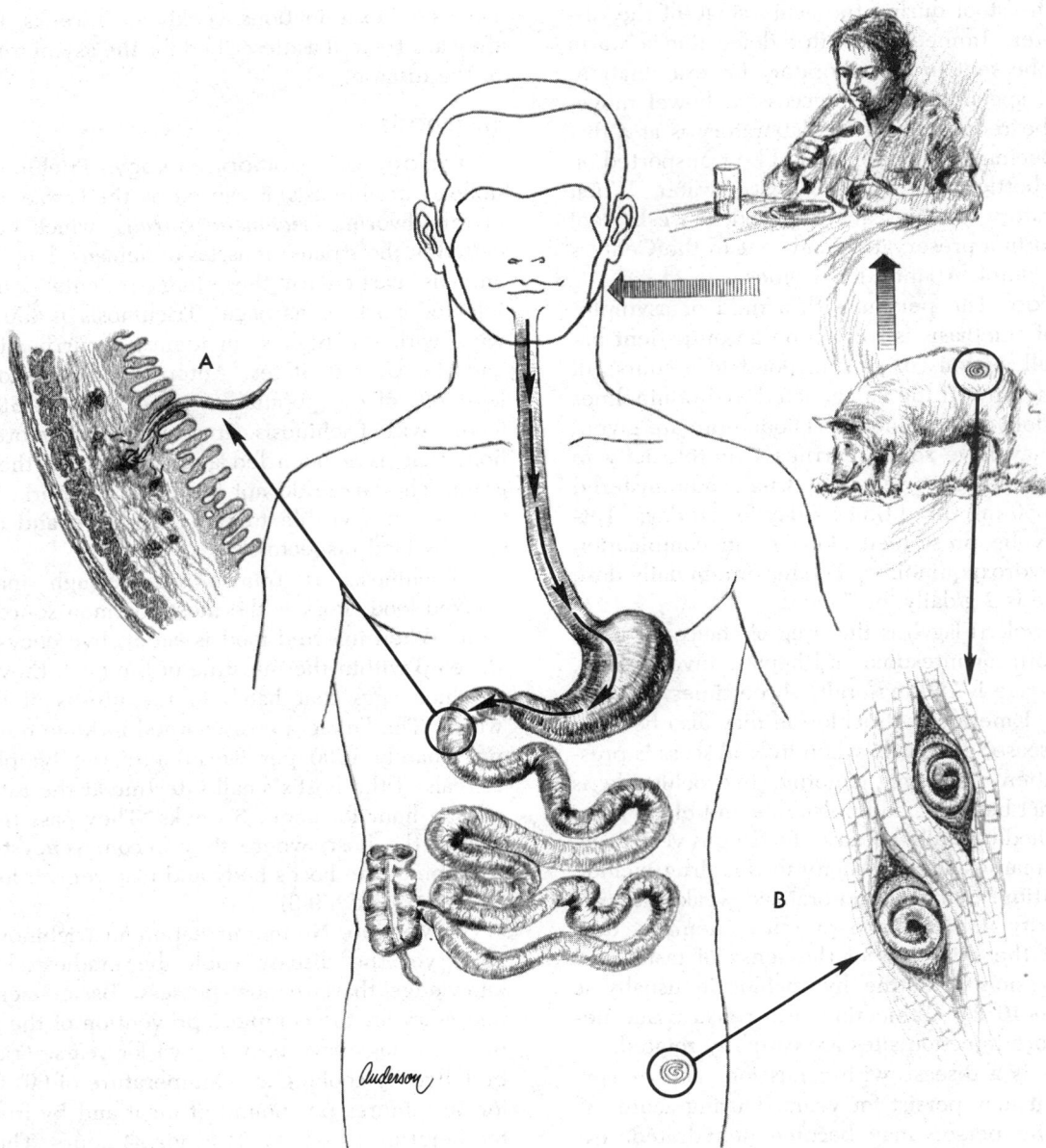

Fig. 59-3. Life cycle of *Trichinella spiralis*. Infective larvae, encysted in pork and other meat when ingested, become adult worms in small intestine. **A,** Female burrows into mucosa and deposits larvae into lacteals and blood vessels. **B,** Circulating larvae eventually penetrate skeletal muscle and become encysted. In humans these larvae are at a dead end, but in the pig and other animals they become a source of infection. (From Beck, J.W., and Davies, J.E.: Medical parasitology, ed. 2, St. Louis, 1976, The C.V. Mosby Co.)

the muscles, there are usually muscle stiffness, weakness, and remittent fever. The extent of these symptoms depends on the number of larvae present and the resistance of the host. There may be pain in the back, the muscles of the eyeballs, the muscles of chewing, and elsewhere in the body. Muscles of the diaphragm are often affected, causing pain on breathing. The di-

agnosis is confirmed by finding larvae in a biopsy specimen taken from the deltoid or gastrocnemius muscle in the fourth week of infection. An increase in the eosinophil count is a characteristic finding in trichinosis and persists for several weeks after the onset of acute symptoms. Persistent fever may also be present.

Intervention. Treatment is symptomatic. Usually the

person is confined to bed and placed on a high-caloric, high-protein diet. Analgesics are given for muscle pain, and antiinflammatory steroids such as prednisone or dexamethasone may relieve fever, edema, and muscle pain. Symptoms may also be relieved by thiabendazole, 25 mg/kg for 5 to 7 days.

In the acutely ill person circulatory collapse can occur if hypoproteinemia is present. Trichinosis can cause death, which usually occurs from pneumonia or cachexia from 4 to 6 weeks following the onset of symptoms. Death may also occur from paralysis of the respiratory muscles.

Outcome criteria for the person with a parasitic infection of the gastrointestinal tract

The person or significant others can:
1. Describe specific substances to be avoided (alcohol, tobacco).
2. Describe the health maintenance and follow-up program.
   a. Demonstrate correct hand-washing technique.
   b. State the basis for proper disposal of stool.
   c. Describe the basis for ongoing periodic stool examination and method of providing the specimen.
   d. State plans for follow-up care.
   e. Identify other family members who may require medical examination.

Irritable bowel syndrome

The irritable bowel syndrome (also known as spastic colon and mucous colitis) refers to symptoms of abdominal pain and altered bowel habits of diarrhea with constipation in the absence of detectable organic disease.[6]

Epidemiology

Irritable bowel syndrome accounts for almost 50% of all gastrointestinal illness in the United States.[6] It is seen most frequently in young adults between 20 and 50 years of age, although in some persons symptoms begin before 20 years of age. Women are more often affected than men.

Etiology and pathophysiology

The underlying mechanism appears to be a disorder of intestinal motility. Motility is increased in the proximal small bowel, and there is an increase in the frequency and amplitude of muscular contractions in the colon. The cause is unknown, although the symptoms in a susceptible person are usually precipitated by stress.

The personality makeup of many persons with irritable bowel syndrome demonstrates a behavior pattern of being sensitive and fastidious, demanding structured perfection in their life activities. They attempt to be in full control of situations and often become angry and frustrated, or depressed.

Clinical picture

Symptoms occur intermittently and vary among persons, although each person has a characteristic pattern. There appear to be two major symptom patterns: (1) spastic colon type, characterized by colicky abdominal pain relieved by passing gas or stool and by periodic constipation and diarrhea; and (2) painless diarrhea type, characterized by urgent diarrhea during or after meals. The stool of either type may contain excess mucus, but all other physical findings are negative.

Intervention

Persons with irritable bowel syndrome need empathic support from health care providers and assistance in coping with stress in their life experiences that may precipitate symptoms. Since the need for control is important to them, they need to be included in decision making regarding their care. The irritable bowel syndrome diagnosis is made by the physician after ruling out other pathologic conditions, and the person needs to know that the condition is benign and is related to bowel irritability induced by stress. A planned schedule of regular physical activity and relaxation periods may be helpful.

Spastic contractions of the colon may be reduced by increasing the intake of dietary fibers, particularly bran foods, and by hydrophilic colloids (Metamucil, methylcellulose) that add bulk to the stool. When abdominal pains occur, spasmolytic drugs such as dicyclomine hydrochloride (Bentyl) or propantheline bromide (Pro-Banthine) may be prescribed along with an analgesic such as pentazocine (Talwin) and local heat. Hydrophilic colloids are useful for painless diarrhea to solidify the stool.

Outcome criteria for the person with irritable bowel syndrome

The person or significant others can:
1. Explain the relationship of stress to occurrence of symptoms.
2. Describe a plan for regular physical activity and relaxation periods.
3. Describe health maintenance and follow-up program.
   a. Explain medication program (dose, when taken, side effects).
   b. Describe health care resources for assistance in coping with stress, if necessary.
   c. Describe symptoms (change in usual pattern) necessitating medical follow-up.

Intestinal obstruction

Etiology

Intestinal obstruction refers to blockage in movement of intestinal contents through the small or large intestines. Obstruction may occur from *mechanical* causes that physically impede passage of intestinal contents or from *paralytic* causes in which the passageway is open but peristalsis ceases. Many different conditions may cause intestinal obstruction (see box below), but the most common causes are adhesions, strangulated hernias, or neoplasms. Neoplasms may be within the intestines or extrinsic, entrapping loops of the bowel. *Volvulus*, a twisting of the bowel (Fig. 59-4), usually results from congenital anomalies or acquired adhesions.[25] *Intussusception* is a telescoping of a segment of the bowel within itself and is seen mostly in children. *Paralytic ileus* is seen frequently following abdominal surgery as a result of handling of the intestines. Peristalsis is inhibited from the effect of toxins or trauma on autonomic control of intestinal motility.

Pathophysiology

When intestinal obstruction occurs, there is an increase in peristaltic waves proximal to the area of obstruction in an effort to move the intestinal contents past the area of obstruction. Intraluminal pressure increases, the proximal intestine dilates, the smooth muscle becomes atonic, and peristalsis ceases. Large amounts of isotonic fluid move from the plasma and intestinal spaces into the distended gut and the normal reabsorp-

tion of intestinal fluid and gas is impeded by edema of the tissues and decreased mucosal blood flow from the increased intraluminal pressure. Large amounts of gas collect in the distended area from swallowed air or from gas produced by bacteria that multiply as a result of stasis of intestinal contents. The net result is loss of large amounts of fluids and electrolytes producing severe dehydration, hypovolemia, and electrolyte imbalances. Complications of a distended gut include perforation with peritonitis and strangulation or volvulus that further compromises blood flow to the intestine, resulting in gangrene of the tissue. A gangrenous intestine will bleed into both the intestinal lumen and the peritoneal cavity and eventually will perforate. Some of the toxic fluid may be absorbed into the bloodstream, causing septic shock.

Clinical picture

The symptoms of intestinal obstruction vary with the site and degree of obstruction. During partial or early phases of mechanical obstruction, auscultation of the abdomen will reveal loud, frequent, *high-pitched* sounds, but when smooth muscle atony occurs, bowel sounds will be absent. Obstruction of the proximal small bowel results in profuse nonfecal vomiting and upper abdominal pain, whereas obstruction of the distal bowel results in less frequent fecal-type vomitus and cramping, poorly localized abdominal pain, and distention. When obstruction is complete, the bowel distal to the obstruc-

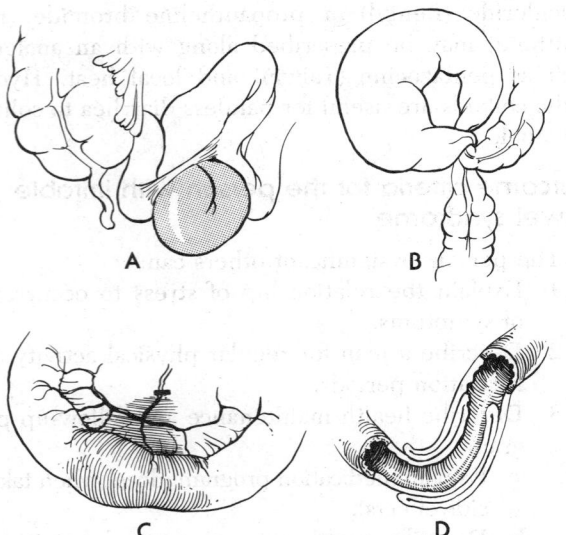

Fig. 59-4. Some causes of intestinal obstruction. **A,** Constriction by adhesions. **B,** Volvulus. **C,** Mesenteric thrombosis. **D,** Intussusception.

CAUSES OF INTESTINAL OBSTRUCTION

Mechanical

Adhesions
Hernias
Neoplasms
Inflammatory bowel disease
Foreign bodies, gallstones
Fecal impaction
Congenital strictures
Radiation strictures
Intussusception
Volvulus

Paralytic

Abdominal surgery
Abdominal trauma
Hypokalemia
Myocardial infarction
Pneumonia
Spinal injuries
Peritonitis
Vascular insufficiency

tion remains empty and obstipation (no passage of stool or gas) results. In paralytic ileus, vomiting occurs less frequently and bowel sounds are decreased or absent.

In early stages, vital signs and laboratory results are normal. As dehydration ensues, urinary output decreases, temperature increases, and there is hemoconcentration, leukocytosis, and electrolyte changes including hyponatremia, hypokalemia, and increases in plasma bicarbonate, pH, and BUN (blood urea nitrogen). Later signs include tachycardia, fever, and hypotension or shock. Air and fluid filled areas of obstruction are visualized by x-ray examination.

Intervention

The treatment for intestinal obstruction is nasogastric intubation, the administration of fluids and electrolytes by infusion, and the relief of mechanical and vascular obstruction by surgery. Intestinal intubation may be necessary. Paralytic ileus is not treated surgically unless gangrene of a portion of the bowel has occurred. The operative procedure varies with the cause and the location of the obstruction and the general condition of the patient. If constricting bands or adhesions are found, they are cut, and it may be necessary to resect the occluded bowel and to anastomose the remaining segments.

Nursing interventions include maintaining intestinal decompression and keeping an accurate record of all intake and output. Intravenous fluids are ordered to maintain fluid and electrolyte balance. Central venous pressure is monitored to avoid fluid overload. Total parenteral nutrition may be prescribed for the person who is nutritionally depleted. Any increase in temperature may indicate more obstruction or peritonitis and is reported. Good supportive care is necessary. Pain and vomiting often leave the patient physically and emotionally exhausted. Assistance in simple activities such as turning in bed may be necessary, and encouragement and assurance that the intubation and other treatments usually result in lessening of symptoms within a short time are helpful. Skin care and mouth care are essential. Any vomitus is immediately removed from the bedside, since its foul odor may increase nausea.

Pulmonary ventilation should receive the nurse's careful attention. Since intestinal distention may cause respiratory distress, Fowler's position is usually more comfortable for the patient, who is encouraged to breathe through the nose and not to swallow air because it increases the distention and discomfort.

The nurse assesses the return of peristalsis by listening for bowel sounds and evaluates the resolution of abdominal distention by measuring the abdominal girth. Passage of flatus or any abnormal substances such as blood or mucus is reported to the physician. Urinary retention caused by pressure on the bladder may occur, and the patient is monitored for the amount of urine at each voiding. An indwelling catheter may be inserted into the bladder to monitor urinary output, especially if shock is a possibility. A total 24-hour urinary output below 500 ml is reported to the physician.

Vascular occlusions

Mesenteric vascular occlusion

Etiology

Mesenteric vascular occlusion is common, occurring frequently in persons with heart disease resulting in emboli to the intestines. Often the patient is elderly. It also may occur in patients who are recovering from recent abdominal surgery. Thrombosis of the mesenteric vein may occur as a complication of cirrhosis of the liver, following splenectomy, or as a result of an extension of a thrombophlebitic process in the ileocolic veins. The superior mesenteric arteries usually are occluded. Causes other than atherosclerosis or intravascular thromboses of the mesenteric vessels include polycythemia, sickle cell disease, other blood dyscrasias, and connective tissue disorders.

Pathophysiology

The blood supply to the lower part of the jejunum and ileum is usually interrupted by a mesenteric vascular occlusion. The walls of the intestine become thickened and edematous, then reddened, and finally black and gangrenous. Infarction of the small bowel may develop over a period of several weeks or may appear suddenly.

Clinical picture

In partial blockage of the superior mesenteric artery by an atherosclerotic plaque, pain is crampy and colicky in nature and may last for several hours after a meal. The pain is associated with the demand for oxygen needed for the increased intestinal muscular activity. In the event of sudden occlusion, the patient complains of an acute onset of sharp abdominal pain between the xiphoid process and umbilicus and nausea and vomiting. There is disturbed bowel function. The white blood cell count is elevated. Occasionally, a tender mass may be palpable in the epigastrium. The abdomen may be distended, and there will be an absence of bowel sounds. If there has been hemorrhage into the peritoneal cavity, generalized abdominal rigidity will be noted. The patient may be in shock when first seen, even when the condition is reported at the onset of symptoms.

Intervention

Immediate hospitalization is required. Nothing is given orally, and a nasogastric tube is inserted and attached to suction. Parenteral fluids are started. Treatment depends on the suddenness and cause of the occlusion. If a clot can be found and removed after opening the superior mesenteric artery, the blood flow will be restored. If necessary, damaged bowel tissue is removed surgically. Chronic occlusion may be corrected by endarterectomy or a bypass procedure.

The patient who has surgery for vascular occlusion usually is given heparin and bishydroxycoumarin (Dicumarol) or sodium warfarin (Coumadin). Antispasmodic drugs such as papaverine hydrochloride may also be given. The patient may be very ill both preoperatively and postoperatively and may need constant nursing care. The mortality from mesenteric vascular occlusion is high, particularly among elderly persons.

Hemorrhoids

Etiology and pathophysiology

Hemorrhoids are one of the most common afflictions of humans, and they cause an enormous amount of pain and discomfort. Congestion occurs in the veins of the hemorrhoidal plexus and leads to varicosities within the lower rectum and the anus. The cause of this condition is not definitely known, but many factors seem to be involved. Heredity, occupations requiring long periods of standing or sitting, the erect posture assumed by human beings, structural absence of valves in the hemorrhoidal veins, increase of intraabdominal pressure caused by constipation, straining at defecation, and pregnancy are factors predisposing to development of hemorrhoids.

Clinical picture

Internal hemorrhoids appear above the internal sphincter and are not apparent to the individual unless they become so large that they protrude through the anus, where they may become constricted and painful. Internal hemorrhoids often bleed on defecation, and although the amount of blood lost may be small, continuous oozing over a long period of time may cause iron-deficiency anemia. *External hemorrhoids* appear outside the anal sphincter. They bleed relatively rarely and seldom cause pain unless a hemorrhoidal vein ruptures and a so-called thrombosis occurs. If this occurs the hemorrhoid becomes inflamed and extremely painful.

Many persons have both internal and external hemorrhoids. Constipation often predisposes to the development of hemorrhoids and usually becomes worse after the hemorrhoids occur because the person tries to restrain bowel movements that produce pain or bleeding. Other people resort to laxatives without competent medical supervision. Although hemorrhoids rarely undergo malignant degeneration, constipation and bleeding are symptoms of cancer of the rectum. For this rea-

son all persons with these symptoms should have a medical examination to rule out cancer. The nurse is often in a position to advise persons who have what they assume to be painless bleeding hemorrhoids of long duration to visit their physician.

Intervention

The treatment of hemorrhoids consists of local treatment, sclerosing by injection, ligation, or surgery.

Local treatment. The local application of ice, warm compresses, or analgesic ointments such as dibucaine (Nupercaine) gives temporary relief from pain and reduces the edema around external hemorrhoids or prolapsed internal ones. Sitz baths are also extremely helpful in relieving pain. The physician may prescribe agents to soften the stool. Thrombosed external hemorrhoids usually respond to this treatment with lessening of pain and absorption of the confined blood. Finally, only a painless skin tag remains, and it is not removed surgically unless it causes strictures or its presence interferes with cleanliness enough to cause serious aggravation. If a thrombosed external hemorrhoid does not respond to medical treatment, it may be incised to release the encased blood. This procedure usually is performed in a physician's office and results in immediate relief of pain.

Injection. Injection is used in the treatment of moderate-sized internal hemorrhoids that cause bleeding or are protruding. A sclerosing solution such as 5% phenol in oil is injected carefully into the submucous areolar tissue in which the hemorrhoidal veins lie to produce an inflammatory reaction. Fibrous induration, which surrounds and constricts the veins, occurs at the site of the injection in 2 or 3 weeks. Bleeding from the hemorrhoids usually stops within 24 to 48 hours. There is some local pain at the time of the injection but there usually is no limitation of activity following this treatment.

Ligation. Internal hemorrhoids may be treated by ligating them with rubber bands. The hemorrhoid is grasped with a forceps and pulled down into a special instrument which, when the trigger handle is pressed, slips an elastic band over it. The rubber band constricts the circulation and causes necrosis. The destroyed tissue usually sloughs off within a week. An enema is given before the treatment to prevent a bowel movement for 24 hours so that there is no straining that would cause the rubber band to break or slip off. No anesthesia is required, and the procedure usually is performed in the physician's office. Local discomfort is minimal and usually is relieved by aspirin or acetaminophen (Tylenol).

Surgery. Surgical excision with ligation (*hemorrhoidectomy*) is the treatment used for external or internal hemorrhoids that do not respond well to sclerosing or ligation. There are several methods by which a hemorrhoidectomy may be performed. However, the classic procedure involves excising each hemorrhoid and tying the pedicle with a ligature. The raw areas in the anus then heal by secondary intention.

Preoperatively, the patient may be given a laxative and is encouraged to eat a full, normal diet until a few hours before the anesthetic is given. Stool softeners are often given to soften the stool and facilitate its passage through the rectum postoperatively, and a bulk laxative such as psyllium (Metamucil) may be given to increase the bulk of the stool.

Postoperatively, the patient's vital signs are monitored to rule out internal bleeding. During the first 24 hours after surgery a ligature on one of the pedicles may slip off, causing a hemorrhage that may go undetected because blood will gather in the anal canal and not be expelled immediately. This can also occur during the seventh to tenth day after surgery when the suture may slough off and separate from the pedicle. If bleeding is severe, the physician is notified. In certain situations the ligature may have to be reapplied.

Comfort. Because the operation is usually considered minor and dressings may not be used, there may be a tendency to minimize this operative procedure. In reality it can cause more discomfort than some more serious operations, and the patient assumes a position of least discomfort. When lying supine a support such as a flotation pad under the buttocks will help to distribute the pressure and relieve discomfort. Ice packs, warm wet compresses, analgesic ointments, and narcotics may be given. Sitz baths usually are ordered to be taken at least twice a day for relief of pain and discomfort. The patient is monitored frequently during the initial sitz baths since hypotension may occur secondary to dilation of the pelvic blood vessels in the early postoperative period.

Elimination. The patient often has difficulty voiding after a hemorrhoidectomy. This difficulty can usually be overcome by getting the patient out of bed to urinate. Sitz baths also stimulate voiding.

Stool softeners are continued as preoperatively, and the patient is encouraged to have a bowel movement as soon as the inclination occurs. Passing a stool of normal consistency as soon as possible after surgery prevents the formation of strictures and preserves the normal lumen of the anus. The incidence of wound infection is slight after rectal surgery because of local tissue resistance to the bacteria normally present in the rectum. It is most likely to occur if bowel action has been delayed and healing tissues have become adherent. If the patient complains of much pain about the area and is fearful of having a bowel movement, an analgesic may be taken a short time before a bowel movement is attempted. The patient needs careful nursing attention when attempting the first bowel movement, since it may cause dizziness and even fainting.

If a spontaneous bowel movement does not occur within 2 or 3 days postoperatively, laxatives are in-

creased and an oil-retention enema followed by a cleansing enema may be given through a small rectal tube. The patient is advised to take a sitz bath after each bowel movement to keep the operative area clean and to relieve local irritation. This practice should be continued until a return visit to the physician (usually within 1 or 2 weeks).

Following a hemorrhoidectomy the patient is advised to avoid constipation by eating a diet containing adequate fiber, exercising moderately, drinking plenty of fluids, and establishing a regular time for daily bowel movements. Stool softeners or a mild laxative may be prescribed to be taken daily or every other day for some time.

Outcome criteria for the person who has had rectal surgery

The person or significant others can:
1. Describe a plan to enhance evacuation of a soft stool including sufficient fluids, bulk-producing foods, and regular exercise.
2. Explain the rationale for thorough cleansing of the rectal area after each stool evacuation until healing has occurred.
3. State symptoms requiring medical follow-up (rectal bleeding, continued pain on defecation, constipation, suppurative drainage on dressings).
4. State plans for regular follow-up care.

Cancer of the bowel

Epidemiology

Malignant tumors of the colon and rectum are among the most commonly occurring malignancies in the United States, second only to cancer of the lung in men and cancer of the breast in women. Each year over 110,000 Americans develop cancer of the colon and rectum and over 50,000 will die.[4] There have been only small changes in the incidence or death rates in recent years. The incidence of bowel cancer is significantly higher in developed countries whose inhabitants are of Northern European descent, and it is lower in Japan, India, Africa, and some Latin American countries.[6]

The incidence of bowel cancer increases with age and reaches a peak in the late 70s. Sixty percent of the malignancies occur in the lower portion of the colon and rectum (Table 59-4). Overall, cancer of the colon occurs twice as often as cancer of the rectum. Cancer of the colon occurs more frequently in women, whereas rectal cancer is seen more frequently in men.

Etiology

Although the cause of cancer of the bowel remains unknown, environmental and genetic factors and preex-

TABLE 59-4. Comparison of cancer of colon by site

	Ascending colon	Descending colon	Sigmoid colon and rectum
Type of lesion	Polypoid	Annular	Annular
Incidence	20%	5%	25% in sigmoid colon; 35% in rectum
Symptoms	Occult blood in feces; anemia; nausea and vomiting; right upper quandrant pain; palpable mass	Gross blood in feces; progressive constipation; pencil-shaped stools	Gross blood in feces; altered bowel pattern (constipation, diarrhea); sensation of incomplete bowel evacuation
Surgery	Right colectomy with anastomosis	Left colectomy with anastomosis	Sigmoid: left colectomy with anastomosis Upper rectum: resection with sutured or stapled anastomosis Lower rectum: abdominal-perineal resection with colostomy

isting disease appear to be influential. The high incidence of colorectal cancer in industrial countries relates to a diet high in animal fat, protein, and refined carbohydrates, which are low in dietary fiber. Diets low in fiber appear to increase the number of anaerobic colon bacteria that transform bile acids into potential carcinogens. Low-roughage diets also decrease colonic transit time, potentially increasing contact of endogenous or exogenous carcinogens with the bowel mucosa. Popular literature often suggests certain foods as carcinogenic; however, research has not yet identified specific foods as carcinogenic for bowel cancer. Genetically, some "cancer families" have been identified in which cancers of certain body areas, including the bowel, are transmitted as dominant traits. Persons with familial polyposis have a high incidence of bowel cancer. Polypoid adenomas and ulcerative colitis also predispose persons to cancer of the bowel.

Pathophysiology

Cancer of the colon may develop in one of two ways. In the cecum and ascending colon the lesions tend to develop initially as polyps that grow as cauliflower-like masses protruding into the lumen of the colon. These lesions may ulcerate, but obstruction of the colon is un-

common. Eventually, the lesions penetrate the colon wall and extend into surrounding tissue.

In the descending colon, especially the rectosigmoid portion, an annular lesion is more common. The early lesion is a small polypoid mass that becomes plaquelike. The plaque grows circumferentially, encircling the colon wall, and then contracts, causing narrowing of the lumen. Obstruction may result from formed stool on the left side unable to pass through the narrowed lumen. These lesions also eventually penetrate the colon wall, extending into adjacent tissue.

Cancer of the colon may spread by direct extension or through the lymphatic or circulatory systems, seeding at distant points in the peritoneum or at distant points in the colon. The liver is the major organ of metastasis. Most of the colorectal cancers are adenocarcinomas.

Prevention

Since dietary factors have a significant role in the incidence of bowel cancer, a diet that is high in dietary fibers and low in animal protein, fats, and refined carbohydrates may offer some protection against bowel cancer.[59] Although colorectal cancer cannot be prevented, early diagnosis and treatment offer a fairly good chance for cure. Anyone who develops a change in bowel patterns such as constipation, diarrhea, or alternating constipation and diarrhea, a change in the shape of the stool, or the passing of blood should consult a physician.

The American Cancer Society recommends a proctoscopic examination as routine in regular checkups for persons over 40 years of age. Since adenomas grow slowly over a 5- to 10-year period and since patient acceptance of the rigid proctoscopic examination is low, it has been suggested that the proctoscopic examination be performed in persons over 40 years old every 3 to 5 years.[16,59] The more acceptable screening technique by the client is occult blood testing of the stool, which could be done annually (p. 1438).

Clinical picture

Symptoms of cancer of the colon vary with the location of the growth. Carcinoma of the colon on the right side (*ascending colon*) causes severe anemia, nausea, vomiting, and alternating constipation and diarrhea. A mass is usually palpable on the right side of the abdomen. There are no symptoms of obstruction as a rule because the fecal contents in this portion of the colon are still liquid and able to flow past the growth.

Carcinoma of the colon on the left side (*descending colon*) often produces symptoms of partial obstruction. Because the stool in the bowel on the left side is formed, it has difficulty passing by the tumor and through the stenosed area. Progressive constipation occurs, and the stool may be small or flattened, "pencil shaped," or "ribbon-shaped." Blood, mucus, and pus may be passed

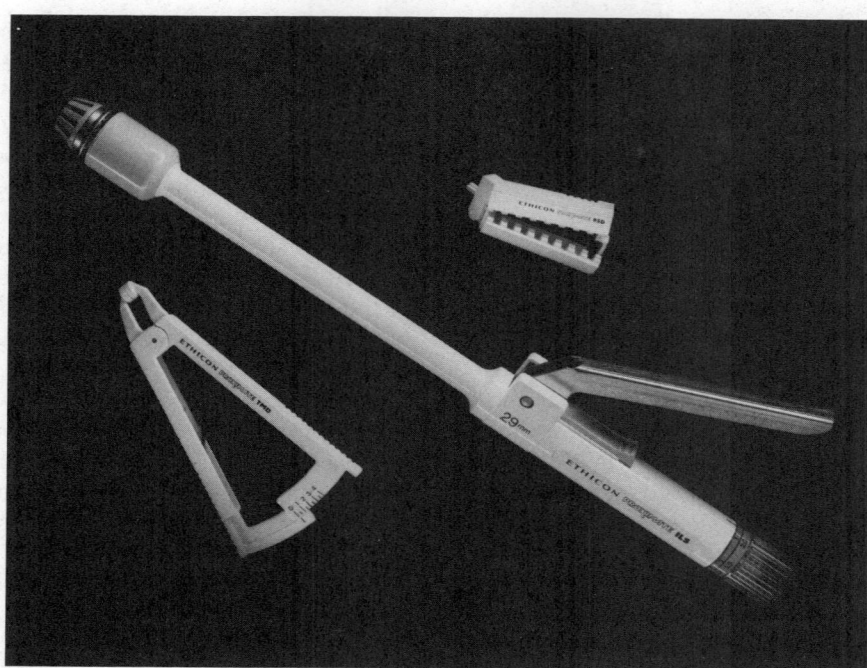

Fig. 59-5. Proximate intraluminal stapling system for colorectal anastomoses. (Courtesy Ethicon, Inc. Somerville, N.J.)

with the bowel movement. The abdomen may become distended, and rumbling of flatus and fluid may be heard.

Carcinoma of the *rectum* usually produces symptoms of alteration in bowel habits, rectal bleeding, a sensation of incomplete evacuation, and a palpable tumor that can be visualized in the proctoscopic examination.

The most common symptoms of cancer of the sigmoid colon and rectum are the passage of small amounts of bright red blood in the stool and an alteration in bowel habits. Either constipation or diarrhea may occur, or these two conditions may alternate. Pain does not occur until the disease is far advanced.

Carcinoma of the colon may cause a complete obstruction, and the acute symptoms of obstruction may be the first indication that anything is wrong. Occasionally, the tumor perforates into the peritoneal cavity and peritonitis occurs before any other signs of illness have been noticed by the individual (p. 1482).

Diagnosis of cancer of the colon is made by physical examination, sigmoidoscopy, colonoscopy, and barium enema examination. Cancer of the rectum can be accurately diagnosed by pathologic examination of a biopsy specimen of the lesion taken during a proctoscopic examination.

Intervention

The treatment of cancer of the colon is always surgical, and the tumor, surrounding colon, and lymph nodes are resected. If possible, the remaining portions of the bowel are anastomosed. If cancer of the ascending colon is found, the colon on the right side is entirely removed (*right colectomy*), and the ileum is anastomosed to the transverse colon (*ileotransverse colostomy*). Growths of the descending colon or upper sigmoid are removed by a *left colectomy*, and the remaining sigmoid is anastomosed to the transverse colon. Usually, growths in the middle and lower third of the rectum require removal of the entire rectum (abdominoperineal resection, p. 1452), leaving the patient with a permanent colostomy. For growths in the upper third of the rectum it may be possible to resect that portion containing the tumor and then anastomose the remaining segments so that the anal sphincter is maintained and normal bowel evacuation is possible.

A newer approach in the surgical treatment of colorectal cancer is the *anterior colonic* resection with a stapled anastomosis. Anastomosis by stapling has been performed for more than a decade; however, it has only come into general use since 1978. The procedure is performed with the use of an end-to-end anastomosis stapler gun (Fig. 59-5) that is inserted through the rectum after resection of the diseased portion of the colon through an abdominal incision. The two cut ends of the colon and rectum are stapled together by a double row of stainless steel staples and the end-to-end anastomosis stapler is then withdrawn. In very low resections or when blood supply is poor, a proximal temporary colostomy may be performed to prevent leakage during healing. The colostomy is subsequently closed in about 6 weeks.

Use of the stapled anastomosis permits resections lower in the rectum, thus providing an alternative approach to anteroposterior resections with permanent colostomies in a number of situations.

Preoperative preparation consists of a thorough cleaning of the colon and rectum. Both antibiotic preparation and mechanical preparation with purgatives and enemas are necessary. The major complication in the early postoperative period is leakage of intestinal contents into the pelvic cavity with development of a pelvic abscess. Signs of shock, increased temperature, or patient reports of increased abdominal pain are reported immediately to the physician. There is a greater incidence of intestinal leakage with low anastomoses, those that are between 2.5 and 5 cm above the anal margin. Late complications include stenosis and incontinence, primarily of flatus, but these effects usually resolve without further surgery.

If the cancerous growth is such that it is not resectable, or if the growth has caused an obstruction with accompanying inflammation, an opening may be made into the cecum (*cecostomy*) or into the transverse colon (*transverse colostomy*, p. 1457) as a palliative measure to permit the escape of fecal contents. When the edema and the inflammation around the tumor subside, the growth is resected, the bowel sections are anastomosed, and the cecostomy or colostomy usually is closed.

Although the overall 5-year survival rate has remained fairly constant at 50%, there is a small trend upward as a result of more extensive preoperative staging of the growth, more precise preoperative preparation, improvement in surgical techniques, and use of additional therapies (radiation, chemotherapy, and immunotherapy).[39] Preoperative radiation retards cell growth so that cells that may be accidentally dislodged during surgery do not seed themselves at other locations. Hyperthermia may be given concurrently with radiation to decrease the radiation dosage. Additional chemotherapy has been restricted to the use of 5-fluorouracil alone in the past, but new combinations, especially with methyl-CCNU, are being evaluated. Immunostimulation with bacille Calmette Guérin (BCG) is aimed at increasing the patient's immune response and combating the immunosuppresive effect of surgery.[39] It is hoped that the adjunct therapies will increase the 5-year survival rate.

Benign tumors of the bowel

The most common benign growths in the colon and rectum are *adenomatous polyps*, small masses of tissue that project into the lumen of the bowel. They may be single or, more commonly, multiple, and they may be pedunculated (stemlike base) or sessile (broad base). Adenomatous polyps may cause bleeding but are rarely painful. About one third of the polyps are thought to become malignant. Pedunculated or small sessile polyps are usually removed by electrocautery and fulguration. Large sessile polyps are excised surgically. *Familial polyposis* is a rare genetic disorder characterized by numerous adenomatous polyps in the lower bowel that usually become malignant. For these persons removal of the colon leaving the rectum intact is recommended before malignancy occurs. The rectum is then examined on a regular basis and suspicious lesions are excised.

Other benign tumors of the bowel, such as lymphomas, lymphosarcomas, and leiomyomas, are uncommon and occur mostly in the rectum. They are often asymptomatic but are removed if they cause pain or obstruction.

Hernia

Pathophysiology

A hernia is a protrusion of an organ or structure from its normal cavity through a congenital or acquired defect. Depending on its location, the hernia may contain peritoneal fat, a loop of bowel, a section of bladder, or a portion of the stomach. If the protruding structure of the organ can be returned by manipulation to its own cavity, it is called a *reducible* hernia. If it cannot, it is called an *irreducible* or an *incarcerated* hernia. The size of the defect through which the structure or organ passes (the neck of the hernia) determines largely whether the hernia can be reduced. When the blood supply to the structure within the hernia becomes occluded, the hernia is said to be *strangulated*.

Types of hernias

An *indirect inguinal hernia* is one in which a loop of intestine passes through the abdominal ring and follows the course of the spermatic cord into the inguinal canal (Fig. 59-6). The descent of the hernia may end in the inguinal canal, or it may proceed into the scrotum (and occasionally into the labia). It is caused by the intestines being forced by increased intraabdominal pressure into a congenital defect resulting from failure of the processus vaginalis to close after the descent of the testes in the male and after fixation of the ovaries in the female. Indirect hernias are much more common in men than in women. This higher incidence in men may be explained by the size of the testes, which must pass through the inguinal ring during fetal life.

A *direct inguinal hernia* is one that passes through the posterior inguinal wall. It is caused by increased intraabdominal pressure against a weak posterior inguinal wall. These hernias are more common in men.

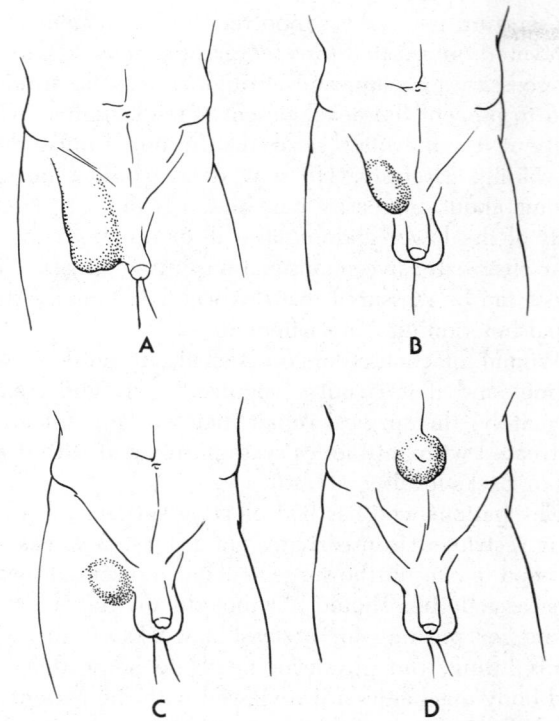

Fig. 59-6. Types of hernias. **A,** Large, indirect inguinal hernia. **B,** Direct inguinal hernia. **C,** Femoral hernia. **D,** Umbilical hernia.

They are the most difficult to repair and are likely to recur after surgery.

A *femoral hernia* is one in which a loop of intestine passes through the femoral ring and down the femoral canal. It appears as a round bulge below the inguinal ligament and is thought to be caused by a congenital weakness in the femoral ring. Increased intraabdominal pressure as a result of pregnancy or obesity probably causes the herniation through weakened muscle. Femoral hernias are more common in women than in men, and the incidence of strangulated hernia is high. This is thought to be because of the inclination of the female pelvis.

An *umbilical hernia* is one in which a loop of intestine passes through the umbilical ring. It is caused either by the failure of the umbilicus to close at birth or by a defect in the umbilical scar, which opens in adult life when there is increased intraabdominal pressure such as occurs in pregnancy, intestinal obstruction, chronic cough, or chronic obstructive pulmonary disease (COPD). Infantile umbilical hernias occur frequently in nonwhite babies. Umbilical hernias that occur in adults are seen most often in elderly, obese women.

An *incisional hernia* is one that occurs through an old surgical incision. It is caused by the failure of the resected and approximated muscles and fascial tissues to heal properly because of wound infections, drains, or

poor physical condition. As a result of increased intraabdominal pressure a portion of the intestine or other organs and tissues may protrude through the weakened scar.

Clinical picture

The person with a hernia complains of a lump in the groin, around the umbilicus, or protruding from an old surgical incision. The swelling may have always been present, or it may have appeared suddenly after coughing, straining, lifting, or other vigorous exertion.

Palpation of the herniated area will reveal the contents of the sac as soft and nodular (omentum) or smooth and fluctuant (bowel). Fingertip palpation is utilized to feel the edges of the ring and its contents by inserting the examining fingertip into the ring and feeling for the impulse as the person coughs. At no time should the examiner attempt to replace (reduce) the sac in the ring, since the result may be the rupture of the strangulated contents or a reduction in the mass without relief of strangulation.

A femoral hernia may be palpated by placing the index finger over the femoral artery. The middle finger will then overlie the femoral vein and the ring finger overlies the femoral canal. As the person coughs, the examiner's fingertips will feel the sensation if the herniated sac is in the canal area.

A hernia may cause no symptoms except swelling that disappears when the person lies down and reappears on standing or coughing. If pain is present it may be caused by local irritation of the parietal peritoneum or by traction on the omentum. An incarcerated hernia may become strangulated, causing severe pain and symptoms of intestinal obstruction such as nausea, vomiting, and distention. These complications require emergency surgery, and a portion of bowel may have to be resected if it has become gangrenous from impairment of its circulation.

Intervention

The person can very often reduce the hernia (return it to its normal position) by lying down with the feet elevated or by lying in a tub of warm water and pushing the mass gently back toward the abdominal cavity. If the person's physical condition does not permit surgery, the physician sometimes advocates the use of a *truss* to keep the hernia reduced. However, this device is not a cure, and its use is somewhat rare today. A truss is a pad made of firm material that is placed over the opening through which the hernia protrudes and is held in place with a belt. The truss should be applied before getting out of bed and after the hernia has been reduced. If the hernia cannot be reduced, the truss should not be applied, and the physician should be consulted.

The only cure for a hernia is surgical treatment. The

herniating tissues are returned to the abdominal cavity, and the defect in the fascia or muscle is closed with sutures (*herniorrhaphy*). To prevent recurrence of the hernia and to facilitate closure of the defect, a *hernioplasty* may be performed using fascia, filigree wire, tantalum mesh, stainless steel mesh, or a variety of plastic materials to strengthen the muscle wall.

Preoperative care. The preoperative preparation for a hernia repair includes examination to detect any diseases of the respiratory system that might cause increased intraabdominal pressure postoperatively. A chronic cough from excessive smoking or other causes or excessive sneezing from an allergy might cause weakening of the repair before the incision has completely healed. The operation is postponed until the respiratory disorder is under control. The nurse should report to the surgeon any signs of incipient upper respiratory tract infection, since such an infection may occur after the patient has been examined.

Postoperative care. In addition to good general postoperative care, the nurse who in caring for the patient who has had an operation for a hernia should prevent tension on the newly repaired tissues. If a cough occurs, medications are usually prescribed to depress the cough reflex. They are given as ordered to prevent paroxysms of coughing and subsequent strain on the repair. The patient is instructed to hold one hand firmly over the operative area when coughing or sneezing.

Since urinary retention may occur after a herniorrhaphy, appropriate nursing measures are taken to prevent the bladder from becoming overdistended. Catheterization is sometimes necessary. The patient is usually permitted to get out of bed to void on the operative day, and full ambulatory privileges are granted after the first operative day.

The person who has elective surgery for a hernia usually is permitted a full diet as soon as it is tolerated. If a spinal anesthetic is used and the abdominal cavity is not entered, there is usually no loss of peristalsis, and the patient is able to eat normally at once. When an *umbilical* or a *large incisional hernia* has been repaired, a nasogastric tube attached to suction may be used to prevent postoperative vomiting and distention with subsequent strain on the suture line. Fluids are given parenterally, and food and fluids by mouth are restricted. Abdominal distention following a hernia repair is reported at once. A nasogastric tube may be passed or a rectal tube inserted. Mild cathartics may be prescribed, since straining during defecation increases intraabdominal pressure and should be avoided.

Because of postoperative inflammation, edema, and hemorrhage, *swelling of the scrotum* often occurs after repair of an indirect inguinal hernia. This complication is extremely painful, and any movement of the patient causes discomfort. It is difficult to turn, to get into or out of bed, and to walk. Ice bags help to relieve pain.

The scrotum is usually supported with a suspensory or is elevated on a rolled towel. Narcotics may sometimes be necessary for pain, and antibiotics may be administered to prevent the development of epididymitis. When a patient has a swollen scrotum, the nurse must check his voiding carefully. He may delay voiding because moving about increases pain and discomfort. Ecchymosis of the lower abdominal wall or upper thigh may occur after extensive manipulation during surgery. The patient can be reassured that this will fade in a few days. Sexual functioning is not affected.

Wound infection occurs occasionally. It interferes with healing, and if it is not recognized early and treated adequately, the surgical repair may weaken. Infections are treated with antibiotics systemically and with dressings or packs locally.

The patient who has had elective surgery for a hernia is restricted from driving for at least 2 weeks and will need to consult the surgeon about returning to work. Physical activities should not include any heavy lifting, pulling, or pushing for at least 6 weeks. If the work entails lifting, the physician needs to know this, and good body mechanics are reviewed with the patient before discharge.

Outcome criteria for the person who has had a herniorrhaphy

The person or significant others can:
1. State plans for gradual resumption of physical activities.
2. State signs and symptoms of wound infection and need to report these to the physician for treatment.
3. State plans for follow-up care.

REFERENCES AND SELECTED READINGS

1. Almy, T.P., and Howell, D.A.: Diverticular disease of the colon, N. Engl. J. Med. **302:**324-330, 1980.
2. Alpers, D., and Avioli, L.: Inflammatory bowel disease (ulcerative colitis), Arch. Intern. Med. **138:**284-291, 1978.
3. American Academy of Pediatrics: Report of the Committee on Infectious Diseases, ed. 17, Evanston, Ill., 1974, The Academy.
4. American Cancer Society, Inc.: 1980 Cancer facts and figures, New York, 1980, The Society.
5. Arvanitakis, C.: Diet therapy in gastrointestinal disease: a commentary, J. Am. Diet. Assoc. **75:**449-453, 1979.
6. Beeson, P.B., McDermott, W., and Wyngaarden, J.B.: Textbook of medicine, ed. 15, Philadelphia, 1979, W.B. Saunders Co.
7. Berk, J.G., and Goldberg, S.M.: Modern management of hemorrhoids, Surg. Clin. North Am. **58:**469-478, 1978.
8. Binder, S.C., and Katz, B.: Regional enteritis: a review of the literature, Ohio State Med. J. **73:**661-666, 1977.
9. Block, G.E.: Surgical management of Crohn's colitis, N. Engl. J. Med. **302:**1068-1070, 1980.
10. Block, G.E., and Guliano, A.: Operations for inflammatory bowel disease, Surg. Clin. North Am. **57:**1235-1250, 1977.
11. Bockus, H.L.: Gastroenterology, ed. 3, vol. 1, Philadelphia, 1974, W.B. Saunders Co.

12. Bowman, H.E.: Colon-rectal cancer: health organizations and government regulations, Surg. Clin. North Am. **58**:633-636, 1978.

13. Burkitt, D.P., Walker, A.R.P., and Painter, N.S.: Dietary fiber and diseases, J.A.M.A. **229**:1068-1073, 1974.

14. *Burns, N.: Cancer chemotherapy: a systemic approach, Nurs. '78 **8**(2):56-58, 1978.

15. Byrne, J.J., and Hennessy, V.L.: Diverticulitis of the colon, Surg. Clin. North Am. **52**:991-999, 1972.

16. *Cancer of the colon and rectum, CA **30**:208-215, 1980.

17. Castro, A.F., and Tuxen, P.: Inflammatory bowel disease, Surg. Clin. North Am. **58**:573-582, 1978.

18. Cole, J.W.: Carcinogens and carcinogenesis in the colon, Hosp. Pract. **8**:123-130, 1973.

19. *Cole, W.H.: Cancer of the colon and rectum, Surg. Clin. North Am. **52**:871-881, 1972.

20. Conn, H.F.: Current therapy 1980, Philadelphia, 1980, W.B. Saunders Co.

21. Connell, A.M.: Pathogenesis of diverticular disease of the colon, Adv. Intern. Med. **22**:377-395, 1977.

22. *Cullen, P.P.: Patients with colorectal cancer: how to assess and meet their needs, Nurs. '76 **6**(9):42-45, 1976.

23. *deLuca, J.: The ulcerative colitis personality, Nurs. Clin. North Am. **5**:22-23, 1970.

24. Driscoll, R., Jr., and Rosenberg, R.: Total parenteral nutrition in inflammatory bowel disease, Med. Clin. North Am. **62**:185-201, 1978.

25. Dunphy, J.E., and Way, L.W.: Current surgical diagnosis and treatment 1979, Los Altos, Calif., 1979, Lange Medical Publications.

26. Dworken, H.J.: The alimentary tract, Philadelphia, 1974, W.B. Saunders Co.

27. Enker, W.: Carcinoma of the colon and rectum, Surg. Clin. North Am. **56**:175-187, 1976.

28. Ferguson, J.A., editor: Symposium on colon and anorectal surgery, Surg. Clin. North Am. **58**:459-636, 1978.

29. Ferguson, J.H.: Acute intestinal obstruction, Practitioner **209**:164-169, 1972.

30. Gianella, R.A., Broitman, S.A., and Zamcheck, N.: Salmonella enteritis. I. Role of reduced gastric secretion in pathogenesis, Am. J. Dig. Dis. **16**:1000-1013, 1971.

31. Gianella, R.A., Broitman, S.A., and Zamcheck, N.: Salmonella enteritis. II. Fulminant diarrhea in and effects on the small intestine, Am. J. Dig. Dis. **16**:1000-1013, 1971.

32. *Given, B., and Simmons, S.: Gastroenterology in clinical nursing, ed. 3, St. Louis, 1979, The C.V. Mosby Co.

33. Green, J.B., and Trowbridge, A.A.: The use of carcinoembryonic antigen in the clinical management of colorectal cancer, Surg. Clin. North Am. **59**:831-839, 1979.

34. Heal, J.M., and Schein, P.S.: Management of gastrointestinal cancer, Med. Clin. North Am. **61**:991-999, 1977.

35. Herrera, A.F.: Medical therapy of colonic diverticular disease, Postgrad. Med. **60**:107-112, 1977.

36. High fiber diets and colonic disease, Am. J. Nurs. **77**:255, 1977.

37. *Hongladarom, G.C., and Russell, M.: An ethnic difference—lactose intolerance, Nurs. Outlook **24**:764-765, 1976.

38. Irwin, M., et al.: The reservoir ileostomy, Ann. Surg. **185**:179-184, 1977.

39. Jackson, B.: Contemporary management of rectal cancer, Cancer **40**:2365-2372, 1977.

40. Kirsner, J.B.: Observation on the medical treatment of inflammatory bowel disease, J.A.M.A. **243**:557-563, 1980.

41. Krause, M.V., and Mahan, L.K.: Food, nutrition and diet therapy, Philadelphia, 1979, W.B. Saunders Co.

42. Krupp, M., and Chatton, M.: Current medical diagnosis and treatment, Los Altos, Calif., 1978, Lange Medical Publications.

43. *Literte, J.W.: Nursing care of patients with intestinal obstruction, Am. J. Nurs. **77**:1003-1006, 1977.

44. McKechnie, J.D.: Outdated and updated diets for G.I. disease, Consultant **18**(9):82-86, 1978.

45. Mendeloff, A.I.: Dietary fiber and gastrointestinal diseases, Med. Clin. North Am. **62**:165-171, 1978.

46. Nankin, P., Jacobson, M., and Evans, R.: Hiatus hernia, Surg. Clin. North Am. **51**:1347-1353, 1971.

47. Painter, N.: Diverticular disease of the colon: a bane of the elderly, Geriatrics **31**:89-94, 1976.

48. Payne, J.H., et al.: Surgical treatment of morbid obesity: sixteen years of experience, Arch. Surg. **106**:432-437, 1973.

49. *Plumley, P.F., and Francis, B.: Dietary management of diverticular disease, J. Am. Diet. Assoc. **63**:527-530, 1973.

50. Rhoads, J.E.: The control of large bowel cancer, Cancer **36**:2314-2318, 1975.

51. Roberts, J.W.: Continent ileostomy, Surg. Clin. North Am. **59**:853-862, 1979.

52. Robinson, C.: Normal and therapeutic nutrition, ed. 15, New York, 1977, Macmillan Publishing Co., Inc.

53. *Rosenberg, F.H.: Lactose intolerance, Am. J. Nurs. **77**:823-824, 1977.

54. Sabiston, D.C., editor: Christopher's textbook of surgery, ed. 11, Philadelphia, 1977, W.B. Saunders Co.

55. Sachar, D.B., and Present, D.H.: Immunotherapy in inflammatory bowel disease, Med. Clin. North Am. **62**:173-181, 1978.

56. Schwartz, A.I., et al.: Principles of surgery, ed. 3, New York, 1979, McGraw-Hill Book Co.

57. Scott, H.W., Jr., et al.: Considerations in use of jejunoileal bypass in patients with morbid obesity, Ann. Surg. **177**:723-735, 1973.

58. Sheridan, J.L.: Obstructions of the intestinal tract, Nurs. Clin. North Am. **10**:147-155, 1975.

59. Sherlock, P., Lipkin, M., and Winawer, S.J.: The prevention of colon cancer, Am. J. Med. **68**:917-931, 1980.

60. Sleisinger, M.H.: How should we treat Crohn's disease? N. Engl. J. Med. **302**:1024-1025, 1980.

61. Sleisenger, M.H., and Fordtran, J.S.: Gastrointestinal diseases: pathology-diagnosis-management, ed. 2, Philadelphia, 1978, W.B. Saunders Co.

62. Smith, A., editor: Diverticular disease, Clin. Gastroenterol. **4**:3-219, Jan. 1975.

63. Spiro, H.M.: Clinical gastroenterology, ed. 2, New York, 1977, Macmillan Publishing Co., Inc.

64. *Stahlgren, L.H., and Morris, N.W.: Intestinal obstruction, Am. J. Nurs. **77**:999-1002, 1977.

65. Stearns, M.W.: Benign and malignant neoplasms of colon and rectum, Surg. Clin. North Am. **58**:605-618, 1978.

66. *Valdivieso, M., et al.: Chemoimmunotherapy of metastatic large bowel cancer, Cancer **40**:2731-2742, 1977.

67. Vendenheimer, M.C., Nugent, F.W., and Haggitt, R.C.: Ulcerative colitis or Crohn's disease: is differentiation needed? Surg. Clin. North Am. **56**:721-726, 1976.

68. Williams, S.R.: Nutrition and diet therapy, ed. 4, St. Louis, 1981, The C.V. Mosby Co.

69. Winship, D.H., editor: Symposium on inflammatory bowel disease, Med. Clin. North Am. **64**:1021-1231, 1980.

70. Wintrobe, M.M., et al., editors: Harrison's principles of internal medicine, ed. 8, New York, 1977, McGraw-Hill Book Co.

71. Zimmerman, W.J., and Zinter, D.E.: The prevalence of trichiniasis in swine in the United States, 1966-1970, HSMHA Health Rep. **86**:937-945, 1971.

*References preceded by an asterisk are particularly well suited for student reading.

CHAPTER 60

ASSESSMENT OF URINARY FUNCTION

PAULA LAMBRECHT MILLER

In maintaining an internal environment compatible with life, the body must be able to regulate fluid volume, electrolyte composition, and acid-base balance and to maintain a means for excreting metabolic wastes. Primary effectors of these regulatory functions are the organs and structures of the urinary system (Fig. 60-1) The kidneys control the composition of body fluids, waste, and electrolytes and maintain these substances in the body within a narrow and critical range. The kidneys also are the primary organs responsible for maintaining the acid-base balance in the body. Additionally, the kidneys are important in the production of red blood cells, control of blood pressure, and calcium metabolism. These functions are accomplished through various hormones that are produced or modified by kidney tissue and that affect various other tissues throughout the body. The box below summarizes the major regulatory functions of the kidneys.

MAJOR REGULATORY FUNCTIONS OF THE KIDNEY

1. Regulation of volume and composition of body fluid
   a. Fluid volume control
   b. Electrolyte regulation
   c. Excretion of metabolic waste, toxins, and drugs
2. Regulation of acid-base balance
3. Regulation of body processes
   a. Blood pressure regulation
   b. Erythropoietin production
   c. Calcium phosphate metabolism

The reserve capacity of the kidneys to maintain the internal environment is quite remarkable; during progressive chronic illness where nephrons are destroyed gradually, the sheer number of nephrons and their capacity to hypertrophy allow the individual to maintain a fairly normal internal environment until 80% of all functional kidney tissue has been destroyed.

The ureters, bladder, and urethra serve as the mechanism whereby waste that is filtered and secreted by the kidneys is eliminated. In assessment of elimination from the urinary tract, both the upper urinary tract that produces the urine and the lower urinary tract that removes the urine need to be considered.

Structure and function of the urinary system

Kidneys

Structure

The kidneys are two bean-shaped organs that lie behind the parietal peritoneum at the costovertebral angle. The organs are composed of nephrons, a vascular system, an interstitium, and the kidney pelvis. The *nephron* is the functional unit of the kidney, and each kidney contains approximately one million of these units. The structures of the nephron involved in the process of urine formation include the glomerulus and Bowman's capsule, the proximal convoluted tubule, the loop of Henle, the distal convoluted tubule, and the collecting tubule (Fig. 60-2). Bowman's capsule and both convoluted tubules lie in the cortex of the kidney, whereas the loop of Henle and collecting tubules are in the medulla. Urine from many collecting tubules drains into larger tubules that form the pyramids seen in the me-

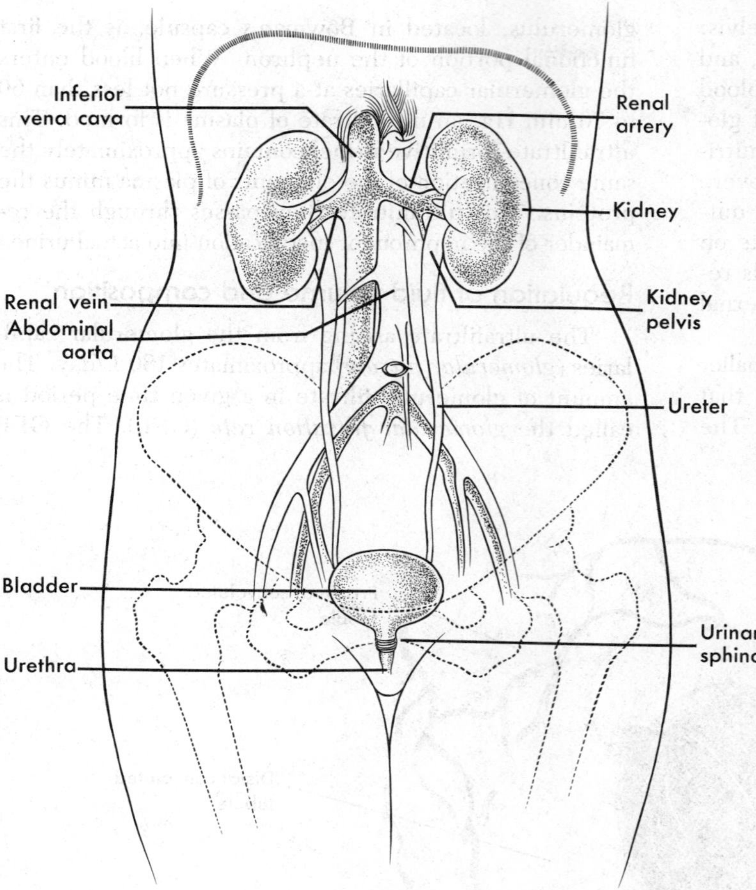

Inferior
vena cava

Renal
artery

Kidney

Renal vein

Kidney
pelvis

Abdominal
aorta

Ureter

Fig. 60-1. Organs and structures of urinary system.

Bladder

Urethra

Urinary
sphincter

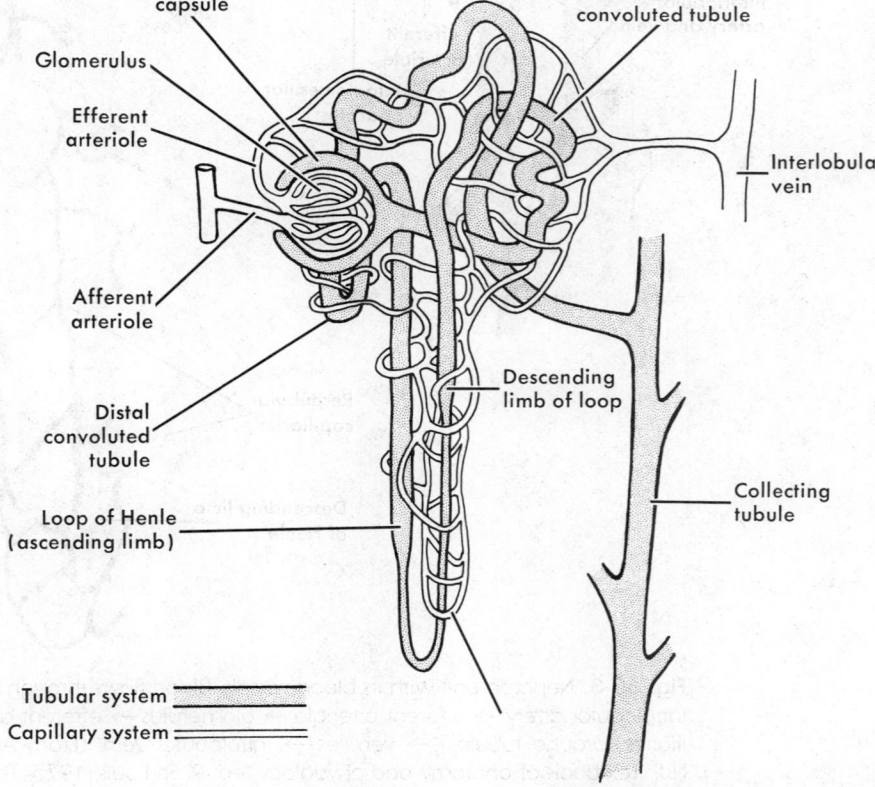

Bowman
capsule

Proximal
convoluted tubule

Glomerulus

Efferent
arteriole

Interlobular
vein

Afferent
arteriole

Fig. 60-2. Nephron. (From Groër, M.E., and
Shekleton, M.E.: Basic pathophysiology: a
conceptual approach, ed. 2, St. Louis,
1983, The C.V. Mosby Co.)

Descending
limb of loop

Distal
convoluted
tubule

Loop of Henle
(ascending limb)

Collecting
tubule

Tubular system

Capillary system

Pelvis of kidney

dulla (Fig. 60-3) and then drains into the kidney pelvis.

The kidneys receive 25% of the cardiac output, and renal blood flow approximates 600 ml/min. This blood supply to the kidneys is basic to the formation of glomerular filtrate, or beginning urine, and to the nutrition and respiration requirement of kidney cells. Severe and prolonged problems with maintaining cardiac output and renal perfusion will have profound effects on the formation of urine and the viability of the cells responsible for maintaining consistency in the internal environment.

After passing through a series of progressively smaller arteries, the blood enters the afferent arteriole that branches into the glomerular capillaries (Fig. 60-4). The glomerulus, located in Bowman's capsule, is the first functional portion of the nephron. When blood enters the glomerular capillaries at a pressure not less than 60 to 70 mm Hg, an ultrafiltrate of plasma is formed. This ultrafiltrate (primitive urine) contains approximately the same concentration of the elements of plasma minus the proteins. This ultrafiltrate then passes through the remainder of the nephron for modification into actual urine.

Regulation of fluid volume and composition

The ultrafiltrate arising from the glomerular capillaries (*glomerular filtrate*) approximates 180 L/day. The amount of glomerular filtrate in a given time period is called the *glomerular filtration rate* (GFR). The GFR

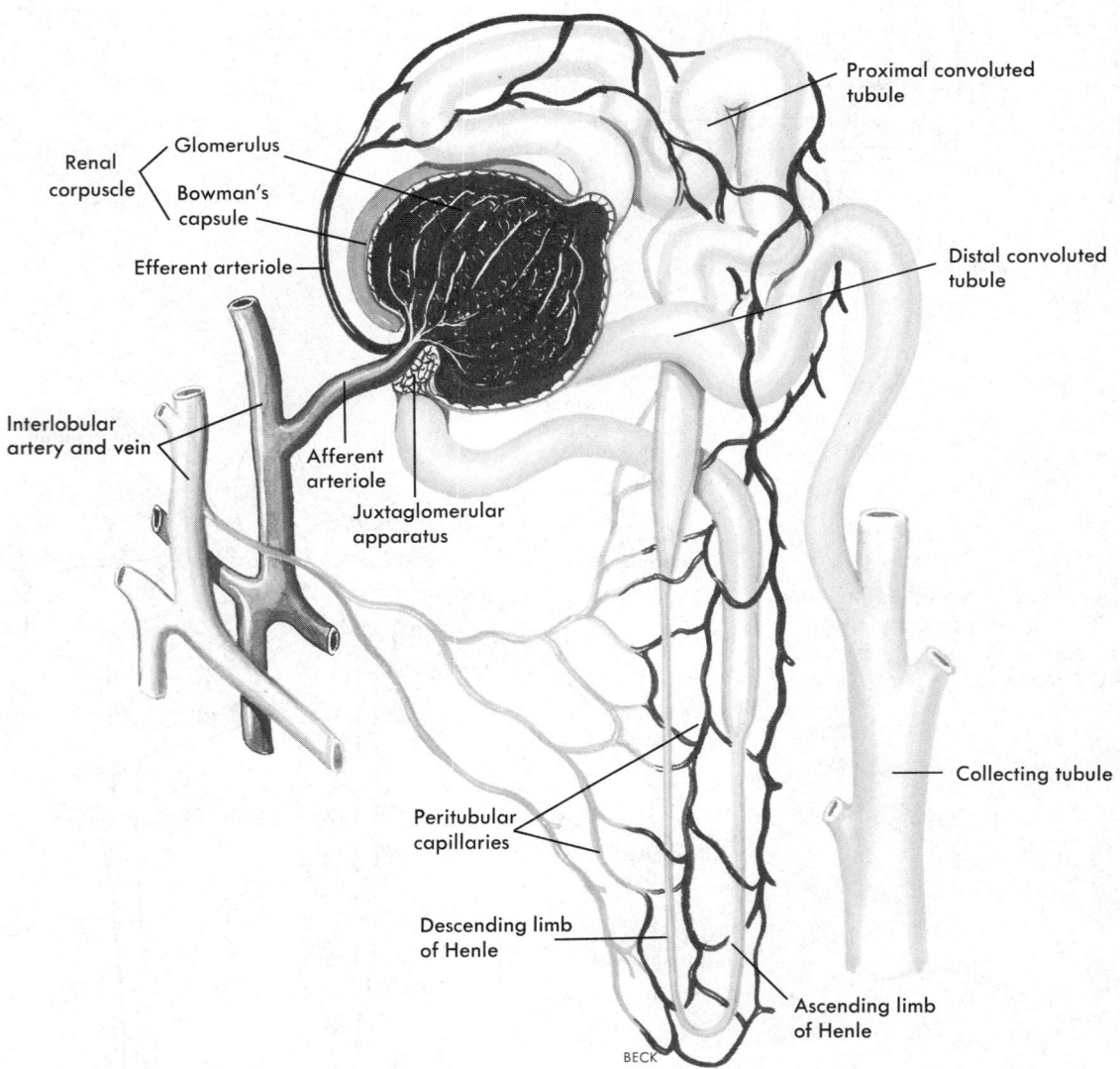

Fig. 60-3. Nephron unit with its blood vessels. Blood flows through nephron vessels as follows: intralobular artery → afferent arteriole → glomerulus → efferent arteriole → peritubular capillaries (around tubules) → venules → intralobular vein. (From Anthony, C.P., and Kolthoff, N.J.: Textbook of anatomy and physiology, ed. 9, St. Louis, 1975, The C.V. Mosby Co.)

in an average-sized man is approximately 125 ml/min (7.5 L/hr) or the equal in 1 day of about 60 times the plasma volume. The average GFR in a woman is about 10% less. The same forces that affect fluid transport between vascular and interstitial spaces in other parts of

the body (p. 301) also affect filtration in the glomerular capsule. GFR is affected by changes in hydrostatic pressure (e.g., with decreased renal blood flow in shock or with arteriolar constriction from sympathetic stimulation or medications) or by changes in osmotic pressure (e.g., with hypoproteinemia).

Were it not for some conserving mechanism in the kidneys, a person would be depleted of fluid and salts within 3 to 4 minutes. The proximal convoluted tubule reabsorbs up to 85% to 90% of water in the ultrafiltrate, up to 80% of filtered sodium, and the majority of filtered potassium, bicarbonate, chloride, phosphate, glucose, and protein.

Dehydration would still occur if the body did not have an additional mechanism within the kidneys to conserved filtered water. This mechanism allows urine to be concentrated to less than 1% of the daily filtered volume. The kidneys can vary the amount of fluid excreted so precisely that intake over that required for normal fluid balance is excreted and intake under that required for normal fluid balance leads to further concentration of the urine. The mechanisms responsible for this increased urine concentrating ability and precision in excreting appropriate urine volume exist in the loop of Henle and the distal convoluted and collecting tubules (Fig. 60-5). The loop of Henle reaches into the medullary portion of the kidney, which is very hypertonic in comparison to the filtrate. In the descending portion of the loop, sodium diffuses into the filtrate as the tubule passes deeper into the medullary area, and

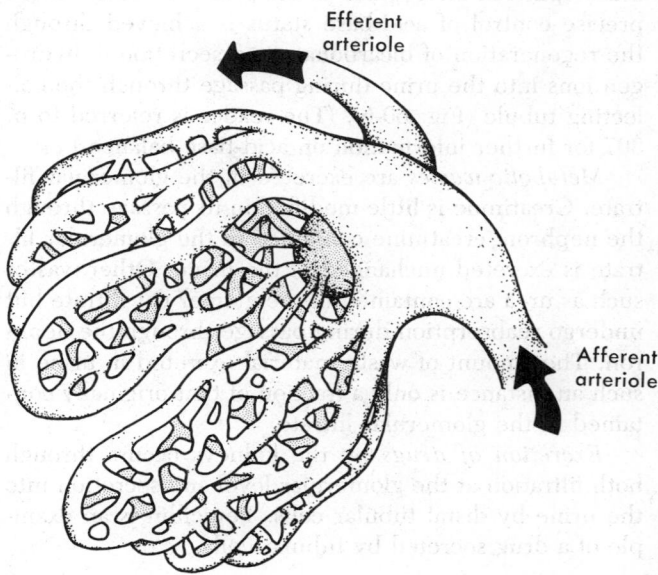

Fig. 60-4. Glomerulus, illustrating arrangement of glomerular capillaries between afferent and efferent arterioles (arrows indicate direction of blood flow). (From Elias, H., et al.: J. Urol. **83**:790-798, 1960. Copyright 1960 The Williams & Wilkins Co., Baltimore.)

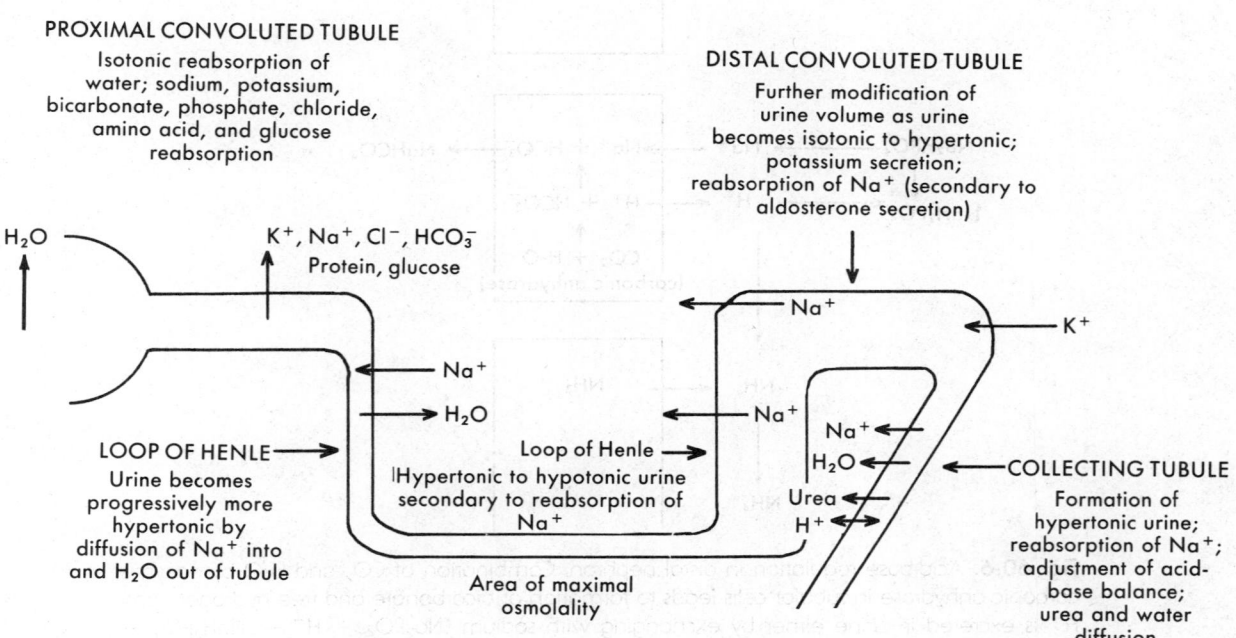

Fig. 60-5. Sites in nephron at which various changes occur in transforming primitive glomerular filtrate into definitive urine. (Adapted from Hamburger, J.: Structure and function of the kidney, Philadelphia, 1971, W.B. Saunders Co.)

water moves out of the primitive urine in response to the high sodium concentration. The result is a reduction in volume of the glomerular filtrate and a dramatic increase in its osmolality. In the ascending limb of the loop of Henle, sodium is reabsorbed into the interstitium (Fig. 60-5), but the loop is impermeable to the movement of water either into or out of the tubule. The primitive urine now presented to the distal convoluted and collecting tubules is greatly reduced in volume, but hypotonic from the reabsorption of sodium. The influence of antidiuretic hormone (ADH) upon these last two segments of the tubule allows water to be reabsorbed into the interstitium in an amount compatible with maintenance of proper fluid balance. The reabsorption of water from the forming urine increases osmolality and results in the excretion of a hypertonic urine.

Electrolyte balance is achieved mainly in the distal convoluted and collecting tubule portions of the nephron. As with fluid, the major conservation site for electrolytes is the proximal convoluted tubule where the vast majority of all filtered electrolytes are reabsorbed, thus preventing rapid depletion of these substances. The precise regulation of body electrolyte composition occurs in the distal tubular segments. Depending upon the concentrations of electrolytes presented to the tubular cells in the primitive urine and the concentrations of these substances in the interstitium, tubular cells secrete or further reabsorb electrolytes into the urine.

Acid-base balance is maintained partially through the reabsorption of bicarbonate in the proximal tubule. More precise control of acid-base status is achieved through the regeneration of bicarbonate and secretion of hydrogen ions into the urine during passage through the collecting tubule (Fig. 60-6). (The reader is referred to p. 307 for further information on acid-base balance.)

Metabolic wastes are excreted in the glomerular filtrate. Creatinine is little modified in its passage through the nephron; creatinine contained in the glomerular filtrate is excreted unchanged in the urine. Other wastes such as urea are contained in the glomerular filtrate but undergo reabsorption during passage through the nephron. The amount of waste material excreted in urine in such an instance is only a fraction of that originally contained in the glomerular filtrate.

Excretion of drugs by the kidneys occurs through both filtration at the glomerular level and secretion into the urine by distal tubular cells. Penicillin is an example of a drug secreted by tubular cells.

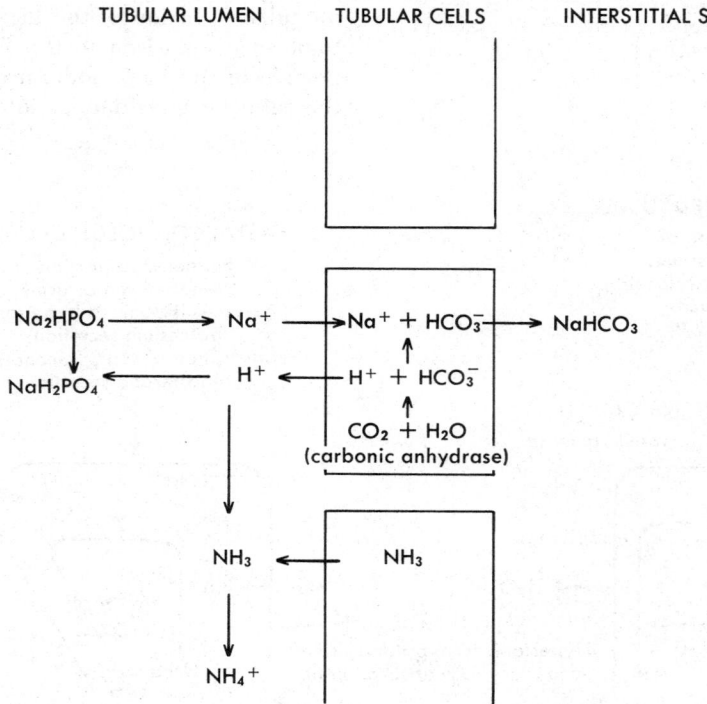

Fig. 60-6. Acid-base regulation in distal nephron. Combination of CO_2 and H_2O by enzyme carbonic anhydrase in tubular cells leads to formation of bicarbonate and free hydrogen ions. H^+ is excreted in urine either by exchanging with sodium ($Na_2PO_4 + H^+ \rightarrow NaH_2PO_4 + Na^+$) or by combining with NH_3 to form NH_4. Bicarbonate combines with reabsorbed sodium and diffuses back into interstitial spaces. (Adapted from Hamburger, J.: Structure and function of the kidney, Philadelphia, 1971, W.B. Saunders Co.)

Additional kidney functions

Major endocrine functions of the kidney include stimulation of red cell production, regulation of blood pressure, and metabolism of calcium. Red cell *production* is influenced through secretion of erythropoietin. This hormone directly stimulates stem cells to produce erythropoetic cells. For persons with chronic end-stage renal failure, serum hematocrit values of 20 to 30 are typical (normal values are 42 to 47). The lowering of the hematocrit in this patient population largely results from decreased secretion of erythropoietin from severely damaged kidneys compounded by bone marrow toxicity, decreased red blood cell survival time, and increased loss from bleeding, all of which are associated with the altered metabolic state present in chronic renal failure.

Renal regulation of blood pressure is controlled by the *renin-angiotensin-aldosterone system*. This system is involved in maintaining systemic blood pressure when states of sodium depletion or acute hypovolemia occur (see Chapter 20). The systemic hypertension associated with renal artery occlusion, chronic renal failure, and acute transplant rejection occurs because of inappropriate activation of this system. In these conditions the circulating blood volume is adequate but renal perfusion is diminished and the renin-angiotension-aldosterone system is stimulated. *Renin* is a hormone released in the juxtaglomerular apparatus in response to sodium depletion, reduction in renal arterial perfusion, and stimulation of renal nerves through the sympathetic pathway. *Angiotensinogen* is activated in the presence of renin to *angiotensin I*, which is converted to *angiotensin II* in the lungs. Angiotensin II is a powerful vasoconstrictor and stimulates aldosterone secretion. Although renin synthesis is enhanced by many renal prostaglandins, a direct role for renal prostaglandins as a systemic vasopressor is doubtful. Additionally, renal prostaglandins that possess vasodilating properties do not appear to have a systemic effect on blood pressure regulation. Rather, renal prostaglandins seem to be locally active vasodilators and constrictors that serve to maintain renal blood flow and GFR in response to a variety of perfusion and endocrine changes.[4]

Renocortical tissue is the site for conversion of the vitamin D prohormone to its most active form. Absorption of calcium from the gut, its deposition in bone matrix, and renal handling of calcium and phosphorus are major metabolic processes under the control of this hormone. The hydroxylation of vitamin D that occurs in the kidney is so important to the activity of vitamin D that in children vitamin D must be supplemented to produce growth. Deficiency of the active vitamin D form also leads to the secondary hyperparathyroidism and the altered calcium-phosphate ion balance seen in persons with end-stage renal disease.

Ureters, bladder, and urethra

The ureters arise as extensions of the kidney pelvices and empty into the bladder in an area called the trigone. These small tubes are composed of smooth muscle; their function is to propel the urine from the kidneys into the bladder. Spasm and severe colic-type pain result from obstruction of the ureters. The bladder, situated behind the symphysis pubis, can retain urine until an appropriate time for urination arises. This voluntary control is based on the learned inhibition of reflex pathway messages arising from the bladder walls. The urethral sphincter operating under voluntary control allows the urine to pass into the urethra for discharge from the body.

Data collection

General assessment of urinary functioning

Subjective data

Obtaining baseline data concerning the person's usual voiding patterns, such as the frequency and general amount of urine voided, is helpful when changes are anticipated. Persons who are admitted to a hospital or other nursing care facility are questioned about their ability to carry out toileting independently. All persons are asked initially if any changes have been noted in voiding patterns. If changes have occurred, further data are obtained pertaining to onset, duration, and measures taken.

When asking questions about urination, it is important to recognize that some persons may be somewhat reluctant to answer, either because of embarrassment or misunderstanding. A calm, matter-of-fact approach by the interviewer will assist in putting the person at ease. Many persons are not familiar with terms such as "voiding" or "urination" and more colloquial words may need to be used in certain situations.

Specific questions are directed at eliciting the presence of abnormal findings (see box, p. 1508). *Dysuria* (painful urination) is usually described as "burning with urination" and is usually associated with frequency and urgency when urinary tract infection is present. *Frequency* of urination is voiding at frequent intervals, either in small or large amounts; therefore the approximate amount must be ascertained when this symptom is present. Small amounts may be caused by infection. Large amounts may be the result of an increased fluid intake or the effect of a diuretic. If frequency is associated with suprapubic discomfort and sense of fullness but not with dysuria, the cause may be retention of urine

POSSIBLE CAUSES OF URINARY SYMPTOMS

Dysuria	Urinary tract infection
Frequency of urination	Urinary tract infection, retention with overflow, excess fluid intake
Urgency	Bladder irritation as a result of inflammation, trauma, tumor
Nocturia	Increased fluid intake, diuretics, enlarged prostate, early renal disease
Hesitancy	Partial urethral obstruction
Decreased force and flow of urinary stream	Partial urethral obstruction, weakened perineal muscles
Urinary incontinence	Stress, spinal cord damage, CNS disease, urinary tract infection, urethral obstruction, injury during childbirth or prostatectomy

in the bladder with frequent overflow of the excess amounts. *Urgency* refers to the need to void immediately. It commonly accompanies frequency in persons with urinary tract infections. A person with *nocturia* awakens at night with the need to urinate. Additional data include the number of times this occurs per night, the amount of fluid intake over 24 hours, and whether this is a change in the usual pattern.

Hesitancy refers to difficulty in initiating voiding. This is often accompanied by a decrease in the force and flow of the urinary stream. Persons with difficulties in this area are asked if they have to strain to start or maintain the urinary flow. In men the most common partial obstruction is an enlarged prostate (p. 1559) whereas in women there may be weakened perineal muscles or meatal stenosis.

Urinary incontinence is assessed by determining the specific nature of the problem: whether it occurs continually or only with stress, the presence of a sensation of fullness before voiding, health conditions associated with the incontinence, and the person's awareness of an feelings regarding the incontinence. Methods used by the person or family for controlling the incontinence are identified.

Pain resulting from urinary disorders is located in different areas depending on the organ involved. Pain from the kidney is usually experienced over the kidney site in the back between the twelfth rib and the iliac crest (costovertebral angle). Pain from the ureters may begin over the kidney area but then radiate to the front along the course of the ureter and down into the groin. Pain from the bladder is usually suprapubic. Any dis-

comfort from prostatic disease is usually felt in the perineum.

Objective data

Urinary output. Most persons have a urinary output approximately equal to their fluid intake (see Chapter 21). *Polyuria* (urinary output greater than 2500 ml/day) may occur with an intake greater than 2500 ml/day, uncontrolled diabetes mellitus, or renal disease. *Oliguria* (urinary output less than 400 ml/day) may be the result of *suppression* of urine formation by the kidney (prerenal or renal factors) or to *retention* of urine in the bladder (postrenal factors). When urinary retention is present, the person experiences suprapubic discomfort and the enlarged bladder may be palpated above the symphysis pubis. Small amounts of urine being voided frequently is often a sign of retention with overflow. *Anuria* (urinary output less than 100 ml/day) is associated with renal failure.

Obtaining an accurate assessment of urinary output is often difficult in a hospital setting because urine is sometimes discarded inadvertently or the patient voids into the toilet. When an accurate assessment is urgent, such as with shock or acute renal failure, an indwelling urinary catheter is usually inserted.

Urine characteristics. The urine is inspected for gross changes. Normal urine color varies from pale to deep yellow depending on the specific gravity. A very dark shade suggests that the urine may be concentrated (high specific gravity) or that there may be an increased excretion of bilirubin. Certain medications and foods may change the color of urine.

Hematuria, blood in the urine, may be detected overtly or may be present microscopically without visual signs. If blood is observed in the urine of a woman having her menstrual period, the vaginal orifice can be blocked with cotton balls and an additional specimen obtained to ascertain the source of the blood. Hematuria without pain is usually caused by disease of the kidney, bladder, or prostate. Hematuria with pain may be the result of calculi, a clot from renal bleeding, or bladder infection.

Cloudy urine may result from precipitation of phosphate salts in an alkaline urine or from bacterial growth. A urinary or vaginal discharge may also give the urine a cloudy appearance. (The method used to collect urine specimens is described under the section on diagnostic tests.)

Renal disease

Health problems that arise for persons with renal disease are varied in number and extent and depend on both the type and severity of the underlying disease. Some persons may appear well and have little or no physiologic dysfunction while others with advanced renal disease will reflect changes in every organ system and in all aspects of their daily living.

The following data are useful in making a nursing assessment of a person with renal disease:

1. Person's perception of illness
   a. Factors leading person to the seeking of health care
   b. Knowledge of health status and care needs
   c. Expectations regarding current health care
   d. Knowledge of significant others about person's health status
2. Previous or concurrent illness
   a. Other chronic health problems
   b. Medications currently taken
3. Social needs
   a. Resources for assistance as needed
   b. Current occupation; capacity to continue present work
4. Fluid balance
   a. Subjective
      (1) Shortness of breath (relate to position of comfort; activity tolerance)
      (2) Visual changes
      (3) Headaches
   b. Objective
      (1) Apprehension
      (2) Blood pressure (related to normal levels for the person; postural blood pressure)
      (3) Central venous pressure
      (4) Respirations (rate; depth)
      (5) Breath sounds
      (6) Pulse irregularities
      (7) Pericardial friction rub
      (8) Peripheral edema (location and extent)
      (9) Weight (direction of change; rate and extent of change)
      (10) Output (amount per hour; amount per day; related to intake)
      (11) Urine specific gravity
5. Electrolyte balance
   a. Subjective
      (1) Lethargy
      (2) Memory function
      (3) Parasthesias
      (4) Vague muscle weakness
   b. Objective
      (1) Behavior (observe for changes)
      (2) Level of alertness and orientation
      (3) Kussmaul's respirations
      (4) Blood pH
      (5) Serum electrolytes
      (6) ECG pattern
6. Nutrition
   a. Subjective

   (1) Anorexia, nausea, or vomiting
   (2) Aids to food tolerance
   (3) History of special diets
   (4) Knowledge of diet restrictions
   (5) Normal meal pattern
   b. Objective
      (1) Diet order (Na$^+$; K$^+$; protein)
7. Elimination
   a. Subjective
      (1) Bowel pattern
      (2) Laxative use
      (3) Nocturia
      (4) Symptoms of urinary tract infection
   b. Objective
      (1) Urinalysis
      (2) Urine culture
      (3) Serum creatinine
      (4) Serum urea nitrogen
      (5) Stool guaiac
8. Skin and hygiene habits
   a. Subjective
      (1) Bathing pattern
      (2) History of dental care
   b. Objective
      (1) Lesions (skin, mucous membranes)
      (2) Moisture (skin, mucous membranes)
      (3) Parotitis
      (4) Condition of teeth
9. Comfort; rest; sleep
   a. Subjective
      (1) Puritus (extent, relief measures)
      (2) Sleep pattern (adequacy of rest)
      (3) Pain (nature, extent, etc)
      (4) Breath odor (control measures)
   b. Objective
      (1) Scratching
      (2) Sleeping during day
      (3) Nonverbal signs of pain
      (4) Fever
10. Mobility; functional ability
    a. Subjective
       (1) Fatigue (extent; recovery with rest)
       (2) Weakness of an extremity
       (3) Numbness; tingling
    b. Objective
       (1) Balance
       (2) Gait
       (3) Muscle tone
       (4) Decreased sensation
11. Sexuality
    a. Subjective
       (1) Menses (pattern)
       (2) Concerns regarding sexual function and reproduction
    b. Objective
       (1) Behavior when with significant others

Palpation of the kidney

Palpation of the kidney is performed while assessing the organs of the abdomen. Normally the left kidney is not palpable; occasionally, the lower pole of the right kidney can be felt. To examine the kidney the individual lies in a supine position with the examiner on the right side of the examining table or bed. Each kidney is examined in the following manner: (1) the flank is elevated anteriorly with one hand; (2) the kidney is palpated lightly with the palmar surface of the hand; and (3) the individual is asked to inspire during palpation. Sometimes the lower pole of the right kidney can be felt as a rounded smooth mass that descends with inspiration.

An enlarged spleen can be mistaken for an enlarged left kidney. To differentiate between the two, percussion is necessary (see Fig. 8-4). An enlarged spleen has a dull percussive note, while resonance is heard over the kidney.

Diagnostic studies

Special examinations of the urinary system are performed to identify the location and nature of existing disease. The accuracy of findings in many of the following tests is dependent on the assistance of the person in restricting or augmenting intake of fluids or in collecting specimens at designated time intervals. The person is given clear, precise directions, and written instructions are a valuable supplement to verbal directions. Some examinations are performed under sedation. If the person is to return home after such a procedure, prior discussion includes making arrangements for someone to accompany the person home following the procedure.

Examination of the urine

Urinalysis

In identifying disease of the urinary tract, one of the first tests performed is the urinalysis. This test yields information about probable locations and causes of urinary disease and some information as to the extent of the illness. Urinalysis is a test that assists in establishing tentative diagnoses and predicting additional tests and observations required to make precise diagnoses. Urinalysis also indicates abnormalities of nonrenal and nonurologic origin (e.g., diabetes mellitus). Table 60-1 indicates possible normal and abnormal findings.

Clean-catch specimens. Ideally, the urine specimen is collected from the first voiding of the day. This

TABLE 60-1. Urine constituents identified on a urinalysis test: normal and abnormal findings

Test	Normal	Abnormal
Color	Amber-yellow	Red indicates hematuria (possible urinary obstruction, renal calculi, tumor, renal failure)
Clarity	Clear	Cloudy: debris, bacterial sediment (urinary infection)
pH	4.6-8.0 (average 6.0)	Alkaline on standing or with urinary tract infection (UTI) Increased acidity with renal tubular acidosis
Specific gravity	1.003-1.035	Usually reflects fluid intake; the less the fluid intake, the higher the specific gravity If specific gravity remains low (1.010-1.014), renal disease is suspected
Protein	0-8 mg/100 ml	Proteinuria may occur with high-protein diet and exercise (particularly prolonged) Seen in renal disease
Sugar	0	Glycosuria occurs after a high intake of sugar or with diabetes mellitus
Ketones	0	Ketonuria occurs with starvation and diabetic ketoacidosis
Red blood cells	0-4	Injury to kidney tissue (see hematuria)
White blood cells	0-5	UTI
Casts	0	UTI, renal disease

sample is preferable because it is concentrated and abnormal constituents are more likely to be present. The person is given a clean container in which to catch urine. Cleansing the meatus before collecting the specimen decreases likelihood of external contamination; mild soap followed by water or a special cleansing solution may be used. At least 50 to 100 ml of urine is collected for the test to ensure a sufficient amount to determine specific gravity in addition to microscopic analysis. If analysis of the urine cannot be performed immediately, the specimen must be refrigerated to retard bacterial growth.

Multiple-glass test. The multiple-glass test is performed on a man when infection of the lower urinary tract is to be evaluated. A full bladder is required for this test since a number of samples will be taken during a single voiding. The man cleanses the area about the meatus with an antiseptic solution before specimen collection, with care being taken throughout the procedure to avoid introducing new bacteria into the specimens. The man is asked to void about 100 ml into a container; this sample contains organisms and sediment "washed" from the urethra. Without interrupting the urinary stream, another 100 ml of urine is voided into a second container. This urine contains organisms and sediment representative of that in the bladder and kidney. The man is then instructed to stop voiding and the physician gently massages the prostate; a third specimen, which contains secretions from the prostate gland is then collected.

Composite specimens. A specimen of all the urine excreted over a specific period of time is often required for the urologic diagnosis. The duration of urine collections may vary from 2 to 24 hours. Specimens are examined for sugar, protein, sediment (blood cells and casts), 17-ketosteroids, electrolytes, catecholamines, and breakdown products of protein metabolism. These tests provide information regarding (1) the ability of the kidneys to excrete and conserve various solutes; (2) the production in the body of excessive hormones that are excreted in the urine; (3) changes in the body's regulation of glucose metabolism; (4) identification of organisms difficult to recognize through routine urine cultures; and (5) presence of abnormal cells and debris in the urine.

The accuracy of findings in this type of test is in most instances entirely dependent on cooperation of the patient. Whether the specimen is to be obtained in the hospital or in the home, the person needs to be told exactly how to collect it. Instructions must include the following:

1. The bladder is emptied and the urine *discarded* at the appointed time to start the test.
2. Urine from *all* subsequent voidings is saved.
3. Specific directions for storing the urine should be given. Some specimens need to be kept cold during the collection period; some need preservatives added; some need no special care.
4. The person should void into a separate receptacle before defecation to prevent contamination of the specimen.
5. The bladder is emptied and the urine *added* to the collection at the appointed time to end the test.
6. The designated amount (properly labeled) is sent to the laboratory.
7. If an aliquot (5 to 10 ml sample of the total specimen) is the designated amount, the total amount collected is (1) measured and recorded on the specimen requisition and (2) mixed well before the aliquot is selected.

Composite urine tests may also involve collecting urine from multiple sources from the body. For instance, the person may pass urine from the urethra and also have a nephrostomy tube from which urine drains. Ureteral catheters may also be in place, with urine being collected from each kidney separately. Depending on the function of the test, whether the purpose is to measure the identified element in the urine as a whole or to measure separately the excretion of this element from each kidney, the urine collected from each source might

be combined into one specimen container or collected into separate appropriately labeled containers.

Urine culture

Urine cultures are obtained to confirm suspected infections, identify causative organisms, and determine appropriate antimicrobial therapy. Cultures are also obtained for periodic screening of urine when the threat of urinary tract infection persists.

Urine in a properly collected and stored sample is considered to be normal if it contains 10,000 or fewer organisms per milliliter. Organisms of this magnitude are the result of normal urethral flora and do not signify urinary tract infection. A urinary tract infection is diagnosed when bacterial counts in a properly collected and stored sample reach 100,000 or more organisms per milliliter and the organisms are of one or very largely one bacterial type.[23] Contamination of the urine specimen during collection is most likely when bacterial counts include predominant colonies of *Staphylococcus, Streptococcus,* and diphtheroids, when two or more organisms contribute significantly to the total bacterial count, or when repeated cultures yield differing results. All of these results are indications of a need to repeat the culture, paying particular attention to the collection of the specimen and to its handling.

Specimens for urine culture may be obtained either by catheterization or midstream voiding. It should be made clear, however, that *urethral catheterization should never be used routinely in collecting urine for culture because of the risk of introducing additional bacteria into the bladder*. Catheterization may be necessary to obtain a sterile urine specimen when the person is unable to void even after being adequately hydrated or if the person is incontinent of urine. When a catheter is passed, meticulous attention is given to nontraumatic aseptic technique. After urine flow from the catheter is established, 5 to 10 ml of urine should be collected directly into a sterile specimen container. Care must be taken to ensure that the rim and the inside of the container are not touched by the catheter or by the hands. If a culture tube with a cotton plug is used as specimen container, care must be taken to keep the tube upright to prevent moistening the cotton and thereby contaminating the specimen. Cultures may also be ordered on the urine taken from the renal pelvis during ureteral catheterization or when ureterostomy or nephrostomy tubes are in place.

In collecting a voided specimen for culture, the nurse must decide if the patient is capable of independently obtaining the specimen or if nursing or medical personnel will need to collect a midstream specimen. Most persons who are ambulatory and are given precise and unhurried direction will be able to collect their own midstream urine specimen (see box, p. 1512).

The first voided specimen of the day should be used

DIRECTIONS FOR COLLECTING A MIDSTREAM URINE SPECIMEN

Equipment needed

Sterile container for the urine

Three sponges (cotton or gauze) saturated with cleansing solution

General directions

Only outside of collecting container is touched

Urine is collected in container well after urinary stream is started

Special directions

Female

Labia are kept separated throughout procedure

Meatus is cleansed with one front-to-back motion with each of the three cleansing sponges

Male

Foreskin is retracted if man is uncircumcised

Glans is cleansed with each of the three cleansing sponges

---

whenever possible because bacteria will be more numerous. If the specimen is not cultured immediately, refrigeration is mandatory to prevent growth of organisms in the specimen.

Evaluation of bladder function

Measurement of residual urine

Normally the bladder contains little or no urine after voiding; however, certain disease states inhibit the bladder from emptying completely. Some common conditions in which incomplete emptying of the bladder occurs are benign prostatic hypertrophy, urethral strictures, and interruptions in bladder innervation. Urine left in the bladder after voiding is called *residual urine*.

One way to determine the amount of residual urine is to *catheterize* the person immediately after voiding. This may be ordered by the physician on a one-time or on a serial basis. Before catheterizing the person, the physician is consulted regarding the plan for establishing urinary drainage. If a large residual urine is suspected, the physician may wish the catheter to be left in place in the bladder. *Residual urine volumes of 50 ml or less indicate near-normal or returning bladder function.*

To avoid passing a catheter to measure residual urine volumes, roentgenographic examination of retained urine may be performed. In this procedure a radiopaque sub-

stance excreted by the kidneys is injected intravenously. As the dye is excreted in the urine, it passes into the bladder. A sufficient amount of urine containing the radiopaque material is allowed to accumulate in the bladder before the person is instructed to void. Immediately after voiding a roentgenogram is taken. Any urine retained in the bladder will be visualized on the radiograph. This means of determining residual urine is used in conjunction with other studies requiring visualization of the urinary tract.

Cystometrogram

Cystometric examination is performed to evaluate bladder tone. In general, the examination is indicated when incontinence is present or when there is evidence of suspicion of neurologic dysfunction of the bladder. The *cystometrogram* provides data on (1) the presence of a spastic of flaccid muscular tone, (2) the presence of fullness and urgency sensations, (3) the effect of drug therapy in establishing or changing bladder tone, (4) the rate of change in bladder tone with a progressive illness, such as multiple sclerosis, (5) the person's ability to generate sufficient pressure to expel urine using Credé's or Valsalva's maneuver, (6) the intactness and innervation of the urinary sphincter, and (7) the residual urine volume. This data assists in diagnosis and in planning effective management of the dysfunction.

A Foley catheter is inserted before the examination. After the person assumes a supine position, a liter bottle of normal saline or sterile distilled water and a cystometer are connected to the catheter. Fluid is instilled at a constant and specified rate; measurements of the pressure exerted on the fluid by the bladder musculature are taken and recorded after the instillation of every 50 ml of fluid. The person is asked to report feelings of fullness, the need to void, and any urgency or discomfort. Fluid is instilled until urgency occurs, or is discontinued after determining that sensation is absent. During cystometric examination, bethanechol chloride (Urecholine) may be administered to determine its effect on enhancing the tone of a flaccid bladder, or an anticholingergic medication may be given to assess relaxation in a hyperactive bladder. There is no specific care required by person after cystometric examination.

Electromyography (p. 938) may be used to evaluate sphincter tone and intactness of nerve pathways.

Evaluation of renal functioning

Tests of renal function are carried out when findings in the general physical evaluation of the person or in the urinalysis suggest renal disease. The best overview of the person's clinical condition is obtained when the results of a number of tests are compared.

Clearance tests

When renal disease is suspected, the physician will want to determine the amount of damage, if any, that has already occurred. The most practical and efficient way to identify losses in renal function is by means of clearance tests. These tests measure the amount of blood that an individual's kidneys can "clear" of a substance in a given amount of time. When the person's values are compared to normal values, changes in renal function become apparent. Clearance tests are also used to monitor the direction of change and the rate of change in renal function over time.

The *creatinine clearance* test is the most practical and widely used of all clearance tests. Creatinine is a substance that results from the breakdown of muscle tissue. It is produced at a relatively fixed and uniform rate throughout the day, it can be measured readily in the blood, and it is not influenced by dietary intake. Creatinine is excreted through the kidneys; it is filtered in the glomerulus and passes practically unchanged through the renal tubules. It is an ideal naturally occurring substance that, when blood and urine values are compared, allows one to estimate changes in glomerular filtration rates and overall kidney function. The creatinine clearance value for an individual is expressed in terms of milliliters per minute and is determined according to the following equation:

$$\text{Creatinine clearance (ml/min)} =$$
$$\text{Urine volume (ml/min)} \times$$
$$\frac{\text{Urine creatinine concentration (mg/ml)}}{\text{Plasma creatinine concentration (mg/ml)}}$$

For this test, a morning-to-morning 24-hour urine collection is obtained. (Refer to collection of composite urine specimens on p. 1511.) Immediately after the final urine specimen is collected, a blood specimen is drawn to determine the serum creatinine level. Both blood and urine specimens are sent together for anlaysis. Analysis of the total urine volume for the test period is essential for accurate determination of renal function. If one voiding is accidentally discarded, the test must be repeated. A shorter period of time may be used in instances when collection of accurate urine collections over a 24-hour period are next to impossible.

Normal *clearance* values for creatinine are approximately 95 to 140 ml/min for men and 85 to 125 ml/min for women. In individuals with depressed renal function these values will be decreased.

The *urea clearance* test is seldom used anymore, since it is influenced by the rate of urine formation, state of liver function, and protein intake and breakdown and is less accurate than the creatinine clearance test.

The *sodium excretion* test measures tubular function. Specifically, this test provides information as to the kidneys' ability to appropriately excrete or conserve this electrolyte; in chronic renal failure either inappropriate retention or excretion of sodium can occur. Knowledge of urinary excretion of this electrolyte is helpful in calculating sodium intake requirements of the patient. In order to determine change in direction and degree of tubular functions, comparison of current and past sodium excretion studies should be made. The test is performed by analyzing the sodium content of a 24-hour urine collection.

The *phenolsulfonphthalein (PSP) excretion* test measures tubular secretion. The normal kidney will excrete 30% to 50% of the PSP dye within 15 minutes of injection. If the renal tubules are damaged by disease or if blood flow to the kidneys is markedly reduced, as in shock, less dye will be excreted during the first 15-minute period. A damaged kidney may excrete the same amount of dye as the normal kidney in a 60-minute period, but the percentage in the first 15 minutes will be much less. If blood flow is decreased, the kidney will secrete the remainder of the dye over a longer period of time.

The person is asked to drink 8 to 10 glasses of water and is then given 1 ml of PSP dye intravenously. Specimens are collected at 15-, 30-, and 60-minute intervals. The exact time of voiding is recorded, and the entire volume voided each time is sent to the laboratory.

Blood chemistry tests

A major function of the kidney is excretion of by-products of metabolism. The two most commonly ordered tests of renal function, *serum creatinine* and *blood urea nitrogen* (BUN) tests, are measures of the kidneys' ability to excrete metabolic wastes. Specifically, these tests measure serum concentrations of nitrogenous products derived from protein breakdown. In health, serum creatinine concentration approximates 0.9 to 1.5 mg/100 ml, and blood urea nitrogen ranges from 10 to 20 mg/100 ml. In the later stages of renal insufficiency, nitrogen products are retained and serum values are markedly elevated. No special preparation is required for these tests. In interpreting test results, however, it should be remembered that high-protein diets, strenuous, prolonged muscular activity, and rapid cellular destruction from trauma, infection, and fever increase urea nitrogen waste levels. In addition, diminished cardiac function may decrease renal blood flow and cause a decrease in excretion of urea nitrogen and an increase in BUN even through no actual renal dysfunction is present. Longstanding diminished cardiac function will cause irreversible renal damage, and then both the serum creatinine and BUN will be elevated. Abnormally high laboratory values of urea nitrogen occur in these states and may not reflect the person's true level of renal function.

Since the kidneys are also responsible for regulating

the *concentration of electrolytes* in the extracellular fluid compartment, analysis of the levels of these electrolytes yields information about kidney function. The electrolytes most frequently evaluated include potassium (3.5 to 5.0 mEq/L of blood), sodium (138 to 148 mEq/L), calcium (9.0 to 11.0 mg/100 ml), chloride (100 to 106 mEq/L), and phosphorus (3.0 to 4.5 mg/100 ml). Levels of serum electrolytes in persons with renal disease are dependent on the location and severity of pathologic conditions of the kidneys and hence can be quite varied from person to person.

Urinary chemistry tests

In kidney disease involving the glomeruli, loss of *plasma proteins* may occur. It has been demonstrated that various types of glomerular lesions exist and that these lesions allow passage of different amounts and types of plasma proteins into the glomerular filtrate. Serum determinations of plasma protein fractions and total protein content can assist in evaluating the nature and extent of the renal disease. Urinary electrolytes, particularly sodium, are also diagnostic of renal disorders. Urinary electrolyte values are correlated with the patient's serum electrolyte values.

Urine concentration tests

The ability of the kidneys to concentrate urine permits simultaneous excretion of waste materials and conservation of needed body fluid. This concentrating ability is lost early in renal disease when damage occurs in the medullary portion of the kidneys and impairs tubular functions.

Specific gravity. The specific gravity of urine is one indicator of concentrating ability, especially after periods of limited fluid intake such as occurs with the first voiding of the morning. In a healthy person the specific gravity of the first morning voiding is toward the middle to high end of the normal range (1.010 to 1.026). As nephrons are destroyed, the specific gravity of the urine falls. In severe renal disease, where a small remaining population of nephrons attempts to excrete proportionally larger volumes of fluid and waste materials, specific gravity falls to the 1.010 to 1.012 range and remains "fixed" at this level.

Fishberg concentration test. The Fishberg concentration test involves a controlled effort to determine the ability of the kidneys to conserve fluid. Clinically the test is useful in making a differential diagnosis between diabetes insipidus (p. 621) and psychogenic polydipsia. The test involves a period of dehydration for the person (usually 8 to 12 hours overnight). During the test no fluid is taken. Morning specimens ensure maximal concentrations of substances in the urine. Three hourly urine specimens are collected to determine volume, specific gravity, and osmolality. Normal findings include a urine volume of up to 300 ml, specific gravity of 1.024 or

higher, and osmolality of greater than 850 milliosmoles. The person is carefully observed for signs of vascular collapse, indicating severe dehydration.

Visualization tests of the urinary tract

Patient preparation

Visualization tests measure both structure and function of organs and tissues in the urinary system. They are used *both* in initially *diagnosing* and in *evaluating response to treatment* over a period of time.

Several of these tests are dependent on radiographs for visualization of the urinary tract. Since the kidneys lie retroperitoneally, any accumulation of flatus or feces in the intestines could obstruct the view of the kidneys on a radiograph. To assure visualization, emptying of the bowel is carried out before the examination. The person's age and state of health are considered in determining the extensiveness of the bowel preparation.

Infants, young children, elderly people, and physically debilitated individuals should not be subjected to vigorous bowel preparation as dehydration and serious electrolyte disturbances may ensue. Some instances of preexisting conditions in which bowel cleansing is especially hazardous are severe nutritional deficiencies, colitis, presence of an ileostomy, fluid and electrolyte disturbances, and renal insufficiency or failure. Bowel preparation for individuals with any of these conditions should be discussed with the patient's physician or the radiologist.

Preparation usually includes a cathartic such as 60 ml of castor oil or bisacodyl (Dulcolax) tablets the night before the test and nothing by mouth after midnight. A bisacodyl suppository or enema may be given in the morning. Ineffectiveness of these efforts is communicated to the physician and the radiology department well before the time scheduled for examination.

Physical safety of the person must be ensured when vigorous cathartics are employed. Urgency, fatigue, and weakness are common following bowel cleansing; falls and accidents easily occur in these states. Sedation, which slows reaction time and makes walking even more unsteady, should be withheld. Before sleep the person should become familiar with the surroundings and with the location of the call light. Close observation is provided throughout the night, with assistance provided as indicated.

Radiographs of the urinary tract may be ordered in conjunction with other abdominal studies. Problems may arise in visualizing the urinary system if barium studies have been recently carried out. This problem is prevented by scheduling tests so that examination of the urinary tract precedes barium swallows, gastrointestinal series, and barium enemas.

Direct visualization: cystoscopy

Cystoscopy is the examination of the inside of the bladder through an instrument called a cystoscope (Fig. 60-7). The instrument is connected to an illuminating source, thus enabling direct visualization of the bladder wall. This procedure is indicated for patients who have or have had hematuria. Although blood in the urine can result from numerous causes, it is one of the earliest signs of malignancy of the urinary tract. Cystoscopic examination may be performed as part of a series of diagnostic tests or as an emergency measure in locating the source of and controlling heavy bleeding.

Most hospitals require a signed permit before cystoscopy after the person is given an explanation of what is to occur. Fluids are usually forced for several hours before the procedure. This ensures a continuous flow of urine in the event specimens need to be collected and aids in preventing multiplication of bacteria that may be introduced during the procedure. If general anesthesia is to be used, fluids may be administered intravenously. If radiographs are to be taken during the procedure, bowel preparation may be ordered.

The cystoscopic examination may be performed with or without anesthetics. General anesthetics are required for cytoscopy when the person is quite apprehensive or when much manipulation is anticipated. In these instances, anesthesia reduces the possibility of trauma to the urethra or perforation of the bladder caused by sudden vigorous movement by the patient during the examination. Children are usually given a general anesthetic for this procedure.

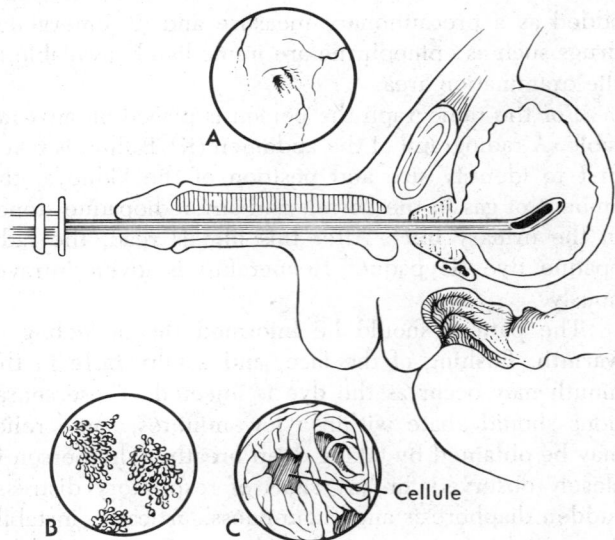

Fig. 60-7. Cystoscope inserted for examination of bladder. **A,** Appearance of normal ureteral orifice as seen through cystoscope. **B,** Appearance of papillomas of bladder as seen through cystoscope. **C,** Appearance of trabeculated bladder as seen through cystoscope. Note formation of cellules.

Much of the discomfort felt during this procedure is the result of contraction or spasm of the bladder sphincters; this can be decreased through deep-breathing exercises and general relaxation on the part of the patient. A sedative such as diazepam (Valium) and a narcotic such as morphine or meperidine hydrochloride (Demerol) are usually given an hour before the examination.

If the patient is relatively comfortable, the cystoscope should be passed with little pain, provided there is no obstruction in the urethra. A local anesthetic such as procaine (usually 4%) may be instilled into the urethra before insertion of the cystoscope.

When the patient is awake, passing the instrument will be followed immediately by a strong desire to void. This occurs as a result of the pressure the instrument exerts against the internal sphincter. During the examination the bladder is distended with distilled water to make visualization more effective. As the bladder becomes increasingly distended, the urge to void increases.

During cystoscopy a number of tests may be performed on the urinary system. Cystography involves the injection of a radiopaque dye such as methiodal (Skiodan) or air as a contrast medium to visualize the bladder and determine its size, shape, and any irregularities. Bladder capacity may be measured through instillation of distilled water. A *voiding cystourethrogram* can reveal reflux of urine into the ureters on voiding, a bladder malfunction that can lead to pyelonephritis.

Ureteral catheterization (with a nylon, radiopaque, size 4 to 6 Fr catheter) can be performed through the cystoscope. The catheter is inserted into the ureteral opening in the bladder, into the ureter, and into the renal pelvis (Fig. 60-8). This procedure may involve one or both ureters. It is performed (1) when culture and analysis of urine from individual kidneys is required, (2) when tests of renal function are to be performed on the kidneys separately, and (3) when visualization of the urinary tract is desired and intravenous pyelogram visualization (p. 1516) has been inadequate, obstruction is present, or sensitivity to intravenous radiopaque material is noted.

Care should be taken that the person does not stand or walk alone immediately after cystoscopy. Blood that has drained from the legs while in the lithotomy position will flow back into the vessels of the feet and legs as standing is assumed. Accidents caused by dizziness and fainting can occur from the sudden change in distribution of blood.

Three complications of cystoscopy that need to be monitored are bleeding, perforation of the bladder, and spread of infection throughout the urinary tract or into the bloodstream (sepsis). Observation for frank bleeding (pink-tinged urine is normal) is necessary. Urinary output and voiding pattern are monitored to detect obstruction, and fluid intake is increased to prevent stasis.

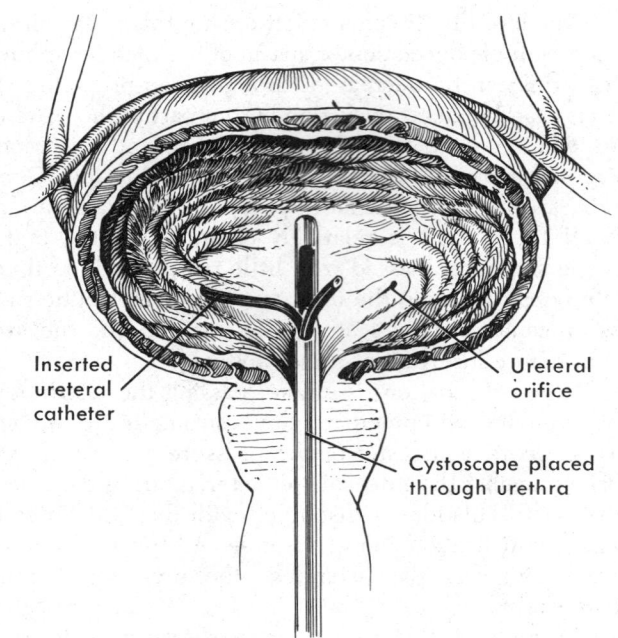

Fig. 60-8. Ureteral catheterization through cystoscope. Note ureteral catheter inserted into right orifice. Left ureteral catheter is ready to be inserted.

Inserted ureteral catheter

Ureteral orifice

Cystoscope placed through urethra

Mild analgesics are given for discomfort, and warmth is provided if the patient complains of being chilly. Vital signs are monitored as necessary.

Radiologic tests

Retrograde pyelography. Visualization of the urinary tract through ureteral catheterization is termed *retrograde pyelography*. This involves injecting 4 to 8 ml of radiopaque material (Hypaque, Renografin) gently into the ureteral catheter. While the solution is being injected, the patient who is awake may feel slight discomfort in the kidney region. Pain should not be experienced unless too much of the solution is injected, and the renal pelvis becomes overdistended. Radiographs are taken and demonstrate filling of the renal collecting structures. As the catheter is withdrawn, more of the contrast medium is injected, filling the ureter. Immediately another radiograph is made to outline the ureteral structure.

Urethrography involves instilling 20 ml of radiopaque water-soluble lubricant into the urethra in order to visualize urethral irregularities of size and shape.

Radiologic examination of the abdomen (KUB). A flat plate film of the abdomen to visualize kidneys, ureters, and bladder (KUB) can reveal gross structural changes in the kidneys and urinary system. The size, shape, and placement of the kidneys can be determined, and calcifications or stones located in a kidney, pelvis, or ureter can be visualized. Bowel preparation

may or may not be ordered for this examination.

Intravenous pyelography (excretory urogram). In the intravenous pyelogram (IVP) a radiograph can demonstrate the size and location of the kidneys, cysts or tumors within the kidneys, filling of the renal pelves, and the outline of the ureters and bladder. This is accomplished through the excretion by the kidneys of a radiopaque dye that has been injected intravenously. The IVP determines kidney excretory function and the patency of the urinary tract. This test may be performed in a clinic or hospital setting.

Preparation for the examination includes bowel cleansing and withholding of fluids for up to 8 hours before testing to produce slight dehydration and a greater concentration of dye in the kidneys and urinary system. However, patients with multiple myeloma should never be dehydrated before this test. The hypercalcemia and increased urinary proteins found in patients with multiple myeloma may precipitate acute renal failure in the dehydrated patient.[1] The renal failure is thought to be the result of intrarenal obstruction caused by deposition of calcium crystals in collecting ducts and in the renal papillae or inspissation of the proteinaceous materials in the lumen of tubules.

Before examination an attempt is made to learn whether the person is sensitive to iodine, as the radiopaque material injected intravenously contains this substance. The test should not be performed on individuals with known sensitivity to iodine because anaphylaxis can result. At times it is difficult to determine sensitivity before use. Two precautions are taken to prevent serious reactions to the dye during IVP examination: (1) most dye preparations have an antihistamine added as a precautionary measure and (2) emergency drugs such as epinephrine are immediately available in the examination area.

For the radiograph the person is placed on an x-ray table. A radiograph of the abdomen (KUB film) is taken first to identify size and position of the kidneys, the amount of gas in the bowel, and any radiopaque stones in the urinary tract. After this film is read, the radiopaque dye (Hypaque, Renografin) is given intravenously.

The patient should be informed that a feeling of warmth, flushing of the face, and a salty taste in the mouth may occur as the dye is injected. These sensations should abate within a few minutes; some relief may be obtained by taking deep breaths. The person is closely observed for any signs of respiratory distress, sudden diaphoresis and clamminess, urticaria, instability in vital signs, or any unusual sensation; any of these may indicate a reaction to the contrast medium. Tripelennamine (Pyribenzamine), diphenhydramine hydrochloride (Benadryl), epinephrine (Adrenalin), oxygen, and cardiopulmonary resuscitation equipment should be available for immediate use.

Sometimes a large plastic ball is strapped firmly on the abdomen to prevent dye from passing freely down the ureters until after radiographs of the kidneys have been taken. Films are usually taken at 3, 5, 10, and 20 minutes after the dye has been injected. If obstruction or poor renal function is present, additional films may be taken 1 and 2 hours later.

Computed tomography. Whole-body computed tomography (CT) scanners can be used to take pictures that clearly outline the kidneys and renal blood vessels and distinguish them from surrounding tissues. The study can be done without a contrast dye, or contrast can be provided by intravenous injection of a radiopaque dye (Hypaque, Renografin). When dye is used, care during the procedure is similar to that given a patient having a renogram. CT scanning is used to detect renal tumors, cysts, trauma, and hydronephrosis.

Renography. Renography tests involve scintillation scanning or photography techniques in visualizing the urinary tract. Diagnostically these tests can measure renal blood flow and renal tubular or excretory function. Therefore they are useful tests in (1) detecting obstructions in the upper urinary tract, (2) detecting renal vascular disease in hypertensive patients, (3) detecting acute renal failure within 48 hours of onset of oliguria, (4) monitoring the function of transplanted kidneys and detecting early signs of rejection, and (5) general follow-up of patients with renal disease and evaluation of the effectiveness of their treatment.

In radiorenography a preparation containing a radioactive isotope such as iodohippurate sodium (Hippuran) tagged with ^{131}I or ^{125}I is injected intravenously. No precautions need to be taken against radioactivity, as only tracer doses of the isotope are used. When iodine isotopes are used, Lugol's solution need not be given before the examination to prevent thyroid damage because the isotopes used are bound to large molecules that prevent their uptake by the thyroid gland. There are no dietary or activity restrictions before testing. The test lasts only minutes and can be repeated a number of times.

In performing the test the patient is placed on an x-ray table and scintillating probes are placed over the kidney or kidneys being examined. The radioisotope is injected and scanning or photographic recording is begun. The patient should feel no pain or discomfort as the test is being carried out.

Renal angiography. The renal angiogram provides an outline of the vascularization of the kidneys. The examination is particularly useful in attempting to evaluate the possibility of renal artery stenosis as a causative factor in hypertension and in demonstrating renal neoplasms and abnormal renal vessels.

Preparation of the individual is similar to that for the IVP. In addition, sedation of the patient is often carried out using secobarbital or similar medication.

When sedation is used, attention must be given to safety of the person.

In this test a contrast material similar to that used in intravenous pyelography is injected. Precautions should be taken against iodine sensitivity reactions. As the dye is injected and passes into the renal vasculature, radiographs are taken in rapid succession. The dye may be injected intravenously, in which case circulation time is calculated to ensure proper timing in taking the roentgenograms, or it may be injected intraarterially. The latter technique is more widely performed and is termed aortography. In *translumbar aortography* the radiopaque dye is injected into the aorta by way of a long needle inserted through the soft tissue in the lumbar region. If a *femoral percutaneous aortogram* is performed, a catheter is threaded from a puncture of the femoral artery upward to the level of the renal arteries; dye is then injected through this catheter. After the roentgenograms have been taken and the catheter or needle removed, a pressure dressing is applied to the puncture site.

Care after the procedure includes observing the site for bleeding, especially within the first 4 hours after the procedure. The dressing is observed for fresh bleeding, the puncture area is checked for swelling and increasing tenderness, vital signs are monitored frequently, and distal pulses are taken if femoral percutaneous aortography has been performed. Bed rest is indicated for at least 8 hours after the test, and the pressure dressing is left in place until the following morning.

Venocavography. Venocavography determines patency in the venous system and can detect masses in the renal veins. A contrast medium is injected into the inferior vena cava via the femoral vein, and radiographs are taken. Preparation of the patient and precautions observed during and after the test are similar to those for angiography.

Retroperitoneal pneumography. The retroperitoneal pneumogram is an x-ray examination performed to diagnose adrenal or retroperitoneal tumors not visible on a flat plate examination. In this test the patient is placed in a side-lying position, and 400 to 800 ml of gas is injected in the retroperitoneal space as a contrast medium. Carbon dioxide is the gas most commonly used as it is rapidly absorbed into the bloodstream.

Preparation for this examination is similar to that carried out for the IVP. The patient is sedated, as discomfort, abdominal cramping, and nausea and vomiting may occur as the gas is injected. Following this test the patient should be kept in bed for a few hours and comfort maintained. Bleeding should not be precipitated by this procedure.

Ultrasound

Ultrasound is a noninvasive procedure that involves passing sound waves into internal body structures and recreating images of these structures. This is accomplished through a computer that interprets tissue density based upon sound waves and displays this information in picture form. The procedure is painless and requires no preparation other than explanation.

Ultrasound is particularly useful in distinguishing between abnormal fluid collections and solid masses. It is frequently performed as a follow-up to abnormal findings first noted during IVP in asymptomatic persons. Commonly, ultrasound differentiates obstructions in the kidney pelvis, or ureter and renal cysts from tumors. Ultrasound is also useful in detecting abscesses in persons with fevers of undetermined origin and in detecting abcesses, ureteral leaks, and ureteral obstructions in renal transplant recipients. It cannot be used when the structures to be examined lie behind bony tissue, since this tissue prevents passage of the sound waves to deeper structures.

Renal biopsy

Renal biopsy is potentially the most accurate diagnostic test for determining both the type and the stage of progression of renal pathologic conditions. Specifically, this test aids in differentiating diagnoses, in following the progression of disease, in choosing therapy most beneficial to the patient, and in determining prognosis of the illness. The biopsy can be performed either through a skin puncture (closed biopsy) or through an incision (open biopsy).

Inherent in taking a biopsy specimen of this vascular tissue is a potential threat of hemorrhage. Throughout the procedure, care is given to prevent and to detect early loss of blood. Before biopsy is performed, a thorough medical evaluation with particular attention to detection of any abnormality in bleeding or coagulation time is carried out. The patient's blood is usually typed and cross-matched with 2 units of blood; the blood is held for the patient until any threat of bleeding has passed.

An open biopsy carries less risk of hemorrhage and provides better visualization of the kidney; however, the risk of infection is increased, and a longer period of recovery is required.

Preparation before biopsy also includes discussing the procedure with the patient. Topics covered include the necessity for the examination, the procedure itself, the care to be anticipated, and any questions of concern to the patient. The preparation of the patient is shared by the physician and the nurse. In most institutions it is necessary to have the patient sign a special permit before having the biopsy performed. The biopsy may be carried out in the patient's room, in the radiology department, or in the operating room.

The procedure for *percutaneous (closed) biopsy* is as follows: Before the biopsy, the patient is taken to the radiology department for localization of the kidney. This is accomplished with a plain film, a dye contrast film, or fluoroscopic location. The position of the kidney in relation to body landmarks is marked on the skin in ink. The lower pole of the kidney is located, this being the site for biopsy, since it contains the fewest number of large vessels. The patient is then transported to the area where the biopsy will be performed. Sedation is usually not required except for children or adults who are restless and unable to relax sufficiently to follow necessary instructions during the test. The patient is placed prone over a sandbag or firm pillow and an additional soft pillow. The body should be bent at the level of the diaphragm, with the shoulders on the bed and the spine in straight alignment. Blood pressure and pulse rate are determined at this point and are recorded. Cleansing of the skin is carried out to remove as many surface contaminants as possible. The physician identifies the location for biopsy, and a local anesthetic agent is injected. As the biopsy is being taken, the patient is instructed to hold his or her breath. Pain may be felt in the kidney region as the tissue sample is taken. The needle is withdrawn immediately, and direct pressure is applied to the site for 20 minutes. A pressure bandage is then applied, and the patient is turned supine and is kept flat (one small pillow may be used under the head) and motionless for the next 4 hours. Coughing and any activity that increases abdominal venous pressure is to be avoided during this time. Blood pressure and pulse should be taken every 15 minutes for 1 hour, every 30 minutes during the next hour, and every hour for an additional 2 to 3 hours. The patient should remain in bed for at least 24 hours. All urine is observed for hematuria, and bed rest is maintained until the urine is clear. Initially, the patient's urine is likely to demonstrate blood, but this rarely continues after a 24-hour period. Once out of bed, the patient should be cautioned against any heavy lifting for a period of 10 days.

REFERENCES AND SELECTED READINGS

1. Beeson, P., and McDermott, W., editors: Cecil-Loeb textbook of medicine, ed. 15, Philadelphia, 1980, W.B. Saunders Co.
2. Black, D.A.K.: The measure of renal function, Am. Heart J. 85:147–152, 1973.
3. Brenner, B.M., and Rector, F.C., Jr., editors: The kidney, ed. 2, vols. 1 and 2, Philadelphia, 1981, W.B. Saunders Co.
4. Dunn, M.: Renal prostaglandins' influences on excretion of sodium and water, the renin-angiotensin system, renal blood flow, and hypertension. In Brenner, B., and Stein, J., editors: Hormonal function and the kidney, Edinburgh, 1979, Churchill Livingstone.
5. *Dutcher, I.E., and Hardenbure, H.C.: Water and electrolyte

---

*References preceded by an asterisk are particularly well suited for student reading.

imbalances. In Meltzer, L.E., et al., editors: Concepts and practices of intensive care for nurse specialists, ed. 2, Bowie, Md., 1976, The Charles Press.

6. *Fennell, S.: Percutaneous renal biopsy, Am. J. Nurs. **75:**1292-1294, 1975.

7. French, R.: Guide to diagnostic procedures, ed. 5, New York, 1980, McGraw-Hill Book Co.

8. Garb, S.: Laboratory tests in common use, ed. 6, New York, 1976, Springer Publishing Co., Inc.

9. *Goldberger, E.: A primer of water, electrolyte, and acid-base syndromes, ed. 6, Philadelphia, 1980, W.B. Saunders Co.

10. *Juliani, L.: Assessing renal function, Nurs. '78 **8**(1):34-35, 1978.

11. Kellerman, E.: Ultrasonic echography in renal disease, Hosp. Pract. **11:**109-116, 1976.

12. Korobkin, M., and Palubinskas, A.J.: CT of the urinary tract, Appl. Radiol. **7:**47-49, 1978.

13. *Kunin, C.M.: Detection, prevention and management of urinary tract infections, ed. 3, Philadelphia, 1979, Lea & Febiger.

14. Lingard, D.A., and Lawson, T.L.: Accuracy of ultrasound in predicting the nature of renal masses, J. Urol. **122:**724-727, 1979.

15. Marshall, S.: Flank pain, hematuria, and allergy to intravenous pyelogram dye. Real or contrived? J.A.M.A. **245:**1557, 1981.

16. Munzig, N.C.: Why physical assessment? Nephrol. Nurse **2:**56, 1980.

17. Papper, S.: The effects of age in reducing renal function, Geriatrics **28:**83-87, 1973.

18. *Pillay, V.: Clinical testing of renal function, Med. Clin. North Am. **55:**231-241, 1971.

19. Pitts, R.F.: Physiology of the kidney and body fluids, ed. 3, Chicago, 1974, Year Book Medical Publishers, Inc.

20. *Roberts, S.L.: Renal assessment: a nursing point of view, Heart Lung **8:**105-113, 1979.

21. *Steele, B.W.: Interpretation of renal function tests, Geriatrics **29:**63-66, 69-71, 1974.

22. *Stroot, V.R., et al.: Fluids and electrolytes: a practical approach, ed. 2, Philadelphia, 1977, F.A. Davis Co.

23. U.S. Department of Health, Education, and Welfare, Center for Disease Control: Outline for surveillance and control of nosocomial infections, Atlanta, 1974.

24. Vander, A.: Renal physiology, New York, 1975, McGraw-Hill Book Co.

AUDIOVISUAL RESOURCES

National Medical Audiovisual Center: Infections of the kidney and the urinary tract, Atlanta, 1974, National Medical Audiovisual Center. (Cassette tape, filmstrip, guide, workbook.)

Medcom: Ultrasound evaluation of the kidney, New York, 1981, Medcom. (Cassette tape, slides, guide.)

CHAPTER 61

INTERVENTION FOR THE PERSON WITH IMPAIRED URINARY ELIMINATION

PAULA LAMBRECHT MILLER
REBECCA ROBERTS
DEBRA C. BROADWELL
PATRICIA BUERGIN

An alteration in urinary elimination is manifested by symptoms such as a marked change in urinary output, hematuria, flank pain, dysuria, urgency, or incontinence of urine. In this chapter factors promoting normal urination will be reviewed, along with the factors causing an alteration in urination and the interventions necessary to achieve desired outcomes.

Factors promoting normal urinary function

Normal urinary output varies depending on a number of factors, such as the amount of fluid intake, the amount of fluid loss from sources other than the kidney (p. 303), the amount of solutes excreted in the urine, or the action of the antidiuretic hormone. An adequate amount of urine must be produced daily in order for the kidney to carry out its functions. A urinary output of 100 to 400 ml/day is termed *oliguria;* less than 100 ml/day is termed *anuria*.

Under normal conditions the person eating an adequate diet has a urinary output essentially equal to fluid input. Inadequate urinary output may occur because of two major reasons, either the kidney is not producing urine *(urinary suppression)* or the flow of urine is blocked between the kidneys and the urethral opening *(urinary retention)*. Disease conditions influencing production of urine are discussed in Chapter 62. Measures that can

be taken when inadequate fluid intake (dehydration) is present can be found in Chapter 21.

Urinary retention

Causes

Causes of urinary retention may be categorized as either mechanical or functional. Mechanical obstruction refers to an anatomic blockage of urine flow at any level in the urinary tract. Such mechanical obstructions may be congenital (urethral stricture) or acquired (calculus, inflammation, injury, tumor or hyperplasia, pregnancy). Functional obstruction refers to the impairment of urine flow in the absence of mechanical obstruction, such as neurogenic bladder dysfunction, ureterovesical reflux, or decreased peristaltic activity of the ureter. For assessment of inability to void, see p. 1507.

Intervention

Interventions for urinary retention are aimed at reestablishment of urine flow. Some mechanical obstructions must be corrected by surgical intervention; others, such as that caused by an enlarged prostate, may require temporary urethral catheter drainage. If the person is having difficulty eliminating urine from the bladder in the absence of mechanical obstruction, measures that encourage voiding are attempted before catheterization is instituted. These measures may include assuring a position that facilitates voiding (positional stimuli), running water or blowing bubbles in water (auditory stimuli), or pouring water over the perineum or placing the hands in water (tactile stimuli). Sitting in lukewarm water may help relax the urinary sphincters. Bethanechol chloride (Urecholine) may be given to initiate voiding by stimulation of the detrusor muscle of the bladder. Persons having long-term problems may be taught to carry out intermittent catheterization rather than maintaining an indwelling catheter.

Assisted urinary drainage

Assisted urinary drainage is utilized in a variety of clinical situations in both acute and chronic care. Following are major reasons for catheter drainage of some part of the urinary system:

1. Relieve temporary anatomic or physiologic obstruction
2. Permit healing of various parts of the urinary system postoperatively
3. Permit accurate measurement of urinary output in severely ill patients
4. Relieve inability to void
5. Achieve continence
6. Prevent retention of urine in certain persons with neurogenic bladder dysfunction
7. Permit irrigation to prevent obstruction of urine flow

Reestablishment of the flow of urine is an immediate treatment goal. The type of catheter used to provide drainage in the presence of obstruction will depend on the location of the blockage.

Catheters are used in urinary tract surgery to facilitate healing of some portion of the urinary tract by diverting urine from above the operative site or by "splinting" a narrow portion of the tract to prevent stricture until healing occurs. In critical care settings where hourly fluid balance assessments are necessary, urethral catheter drainage may be employed until the patient's condition has stabilized.

Temporary inability to void accompanies spinal cord injury, and postoperative patients may also experience temporary urinary retention and may require one or two urethral catheterizations until their usual voiding pattern is resumed. Persons who have urogenital surgery and some women following childbirth may have urinary retention secondary to edema of surrounding tissues.

In certain circumstances urethral catheterization may be used to control urinary incontinence. Incontinence itself is not adequate reason for continuous catheter drainage unless urine retention is present or the integrity of the skin is threatened despite all possible nursing measures to manage the incontinence. Generally, the dangers of catheterization (infection) outweigh the advantages. Intermittent catheterization, however, is utilized as a means of continence for certain persons with neurogenic bladder dysfunction associated with birth defects, chronic illness, and spinal cord trauma. Not only can it offer continence to these persons, but it also can decrease urinary tract infections in persons who otherwise retain large amounts of residual urine in the bladder.

Urethral catheterization may be performed to provide irrigation of the bladder or to prevent excessive clot formation in the presence of bleeding. Irrigation may be ordered intermittently. If irrigation is required continuously or more often than every 3 hours, a special closed three-way irrigation system should be used.

Types of catheters

Catheters are hollow tubes made of rubber, nylon, silk, plastic, metal, or glass. The circumference measurement is used to designate the size of the catheters and is specified in French units. One French (Fr) unit is equal to 1 mm in circumference. The size of the catheter to be used depends on the purpose for which it is used as well as the size and age of the patient. Appropriate urethral catheter sizes for adult men are 16 to 22 Fr, and for women, 14 to 20 Fr. Adult *ureters* are generally intubated with sizes 4 to 6 Fr.

Straight catheters include the following: (1) the *Robinson* catheter, which is made of rubber or plastic, has a hollow tip with two or more openings, and is the catheter most frequently used for intermittent catheterizations (Fig. 61-1, *B*); (2) the *coudé* catheter, which has a curved tip and is used for older men or when hypertrophy of the prostate is suspected in order to avoid trauma to the gland (Fig. 61-1, *D*); (3) the *whistle-tip* catheter, which has a whistle-shaped opening at the tip that is ideal for use when hematuria and blood clots are present (Fig. 61-1, *A*); and (4) the *filiform* catheter, which is a stiff catheter used when a urethral stricture is present.

Self-retaining, or indwelling, catheters are employed when continuous drainage is required and are made of latex rubber, silicone-coated latex, or silicone. For short-term use any of the three types is satisfactory. For long-term use silicone-coated or silicone catheters are preferred if encrustation is a problem. Self-retaining catheters include the following:

1. The *Foley* catheter, the most frequently used, has a double lumen with an inflatable balloon near its tip. The balloon is inflated with either normal saline or sterile water after it has been placed well within the bladder (Fig. 61-1, *C*). These catheters are constructed with either a 5-ml balloon (for routine use) or a 30-ml balloon (for use when hemostasis is required) and may have one

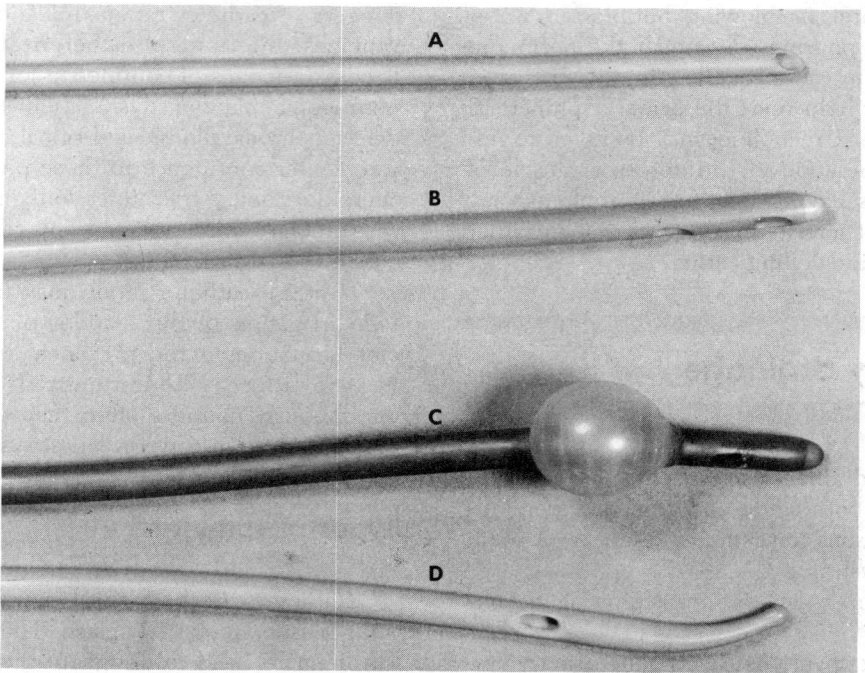

Fig. 61-1. Urethral catheters. **A**, Whistle-tip catheter. **B**, Many-eyed Robinson catheter. **C**, Foley catheter, **D**, Coudé catheter.

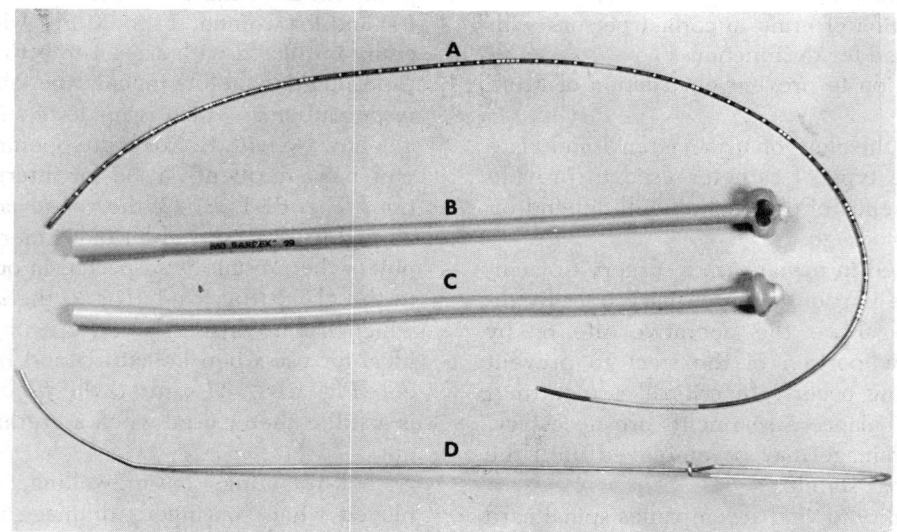

Fig. 61-2. A to **C**, Catheters used to drain renal pelvis. **A**, Ureteral catheters. **B**, Malecot (batwing) catheter. **C**, Pezzer (mushroom) catheter. **D**, Stylet used to insert urethral catheter into male patient.

or two openings. They may be straight or have a curved tip (coudé shaped) and may have a short or long tip. A three-way Foley catheter has a third lumen that is used for the inflow of irrigating fluids. A disadvantage of the Foley catheter is the small lumen of its outlet channel compared to its external diameter.

2. The *Malecot* catheter (Fig. 61-2, *B*), made of rubber or plastic, has a large single channel, and its tip is in the shape of two or four rings that collapse into the shape of a tube when traction is applied as during its removal.

3. The *Pezzer,* or *mushroom,* catheter is similar to

the Malecot except that its tip forms a noncollapsible mushroom shape (Fig. 61-2, *C*).

Ureteral catheters are much smaller and longer than urethral catheters (Fig. 61-2, *A*) and are made of nylon, polyethylene, Teflon, Dacron, silicone, woven silk, or rubber.

Drainage systems

Catheters that have been placed in the urinary system are usually allowed to drain by gravity. The procedure of connecting a catheter to a collecting device and allowing drainage to flow by gravitational force is called *straight drainage*. *Closed drainage* refers to the design of the collection set-up and indicates that the drainage tube is sealed to the collection container; this lessens the chance for contamination of the set-up and decreases the risk of urinary tract infection. Most closed urinary drainage systems employ disposable plastic drainage bags and tubing.

Proper maintenance of the drainage system is a nursing function. Attention to the following points will help to maintain drainage and decrease the entry of organisms into the system: (1) Once the catheter has been connected to the drainage system it should not be disconnected except to perform ordered irrigations. Samples of urine should be obtained by inserting a small-bore needle into a drainage port that has been cleansed with alcohol or povidone-iodine (Fig. 61-3). (2) The drainage bag must not be elevated above the level of the patient's bladder or the cavity being drained because reflux of urine will occur. Drainage bags are also available with antireflux valves to decrease accidental reflux. Bags should be suspended from the bed frame when the patient is recumbent, suspended from the frame of the cart when a patient is being transported, and from below the knee level when the patient is ambulatory. (3) Drainage bags and tubing should not be allowed to rest on the floor. (4) Kinks or loops of tubing below the level of the drainage container should be avoided; to prevent interference with flow of urine, excess tubing may be clipped to and coiled on the bed. The patency of all tubes should be checked each time a patient is repositioned. (5) The drainage container should not be held upside down when being emptied since this causes reflux of urine into the drainage tubing and bladder. (6) The drainage bag should be emptied into a measuring container that is only used for that patient. The container should be cleaned or replaced regularly to decrease contamination of specimens. (7) Cultures of the urine should be taken at frequent intervals when a patient has an indwelling drainage tube. (8) The collecting system should be checked daily for signs of sediment and leaks. The presence of either indicates the need for a new collection system.

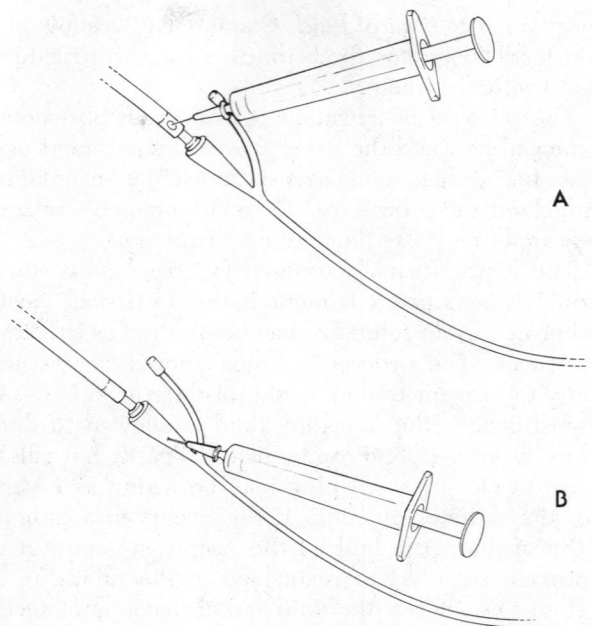

Fig. 61-3. Aspiration of sterile specimen from Foley catheter connected to closed drainage system. **A,** Aspiration from drainage port. **B,** Aspiration from Foley catheter.

Since the purpose of the catheter is to promote drainage of urine, *patency* of the system must be ensured. The flow of urine from a catheter is checked hourly when urine is bloody and at least every 2 hours when there is no evidence of bleeding or disturbance in drainage. Common causes of obstruction of urine flow may be internal or external. Hemorrhage leads to formation of clots that may plug a catheter, and infection increases sediment in the urine that may clog the drainage system. Any evidence of bleeding or change in the amount of bleeding is reported to the physician. To detect the buildup of sediment in the drainage system, the catheter may be rolled between the fingers to detect gritty accumulation, and the drainage tubing is visually inspected. External causes of obstruction in urine flow include kinking and dependent loops in the tubing. If correction of these problems fails to restore the flow of urine, irrigation, if ordered, may be done. In the event that none of these measures restores the flow of urine, the physician is notified.

Catheter irrigation

Catheters should be irrigated only with a physician's order. The physician should specify the quantity, frequency, and type of irrigating solution. When a catheter is to be irrigated, the size of the cavity into which the fluid is being instilled should be considered. *The renal pelvis of an adult should never be irrigated with more than 4 to 6 ml of fluid*. Commonly, 30 to 60 ml of fluid instilled two or three times is used to irrigate an adult urethral catheter.

The purpose of irrigation is to prevent obstruction of the catheter and the urine flow. All equipment used must be sterile, and asepsis must be maintained throughout the procedure. Therefore opened irrigation sets cannot be reused for the next irrigation.

The solution usually ordered for irrigation is sterile normal saline since it is nonirritating to tissues. Acetic acid or neomycin solutions may be ordered as irrigating substances. The ordered solution should be instilled gently to prevent trauma to the bladder or kidney. After instillation, the irrigating fluid is allowed to drain out by gravity. If fluid can be instilled easily but fails to return, a clot or small plug may be acting as a valve over the catheter opening. If this occurs in a catheter to the bladder, the bulb of the Asepto syringe can be depressed slightly and reattached to the tubing in an attempt to withdraw the fluid and obstructing material. If fluid is not returned, the nurse can instill a small amount of fluid in an attempt to dislodge the clot. If the fluid again does not drain, the nurse should discontinue the irrigation and reconnect the tubing. If after a 10- to 15-minute period the catheter is not draining properly, the physician is notified.

When frequent irrigation of a urethral catheter appears necessary, intermittent bladder irrigation should be considered. This involves alternately instilling fluid from a reservoir (usually suspended above patient level) into the bladder through the catheter and allowing the solution to return freely to the collecting bag. Intermittent irrigation is not recommended for irrigation of the kidney because control of inflow in 4- to 6-ml amounts is difficult and instillation of larger amounts into the renal pelvis may lead to tissue damage.

Another variation in bladder irrigation involves the use of a three-way Foley catheter. Constant irrigation involves continuous and simultaneous inflow and outflow of irrigating solution for the bladder. The system is used more frequently after surgery of the bladder or prostate when bleeding is expected and clot formation with obstruction of the bladder outlet is a threat.

In calculating the patient's output when either intermittent or continuous irrigation of the bladder is employed, the amount of irrigating fluid is subtracted from the total volume of urinary drainage obtained in the same time period. The difference between these two values is the patient's actual urinary output.

Drainage of the kidney, pelvis, and ureters

If a ureter becomes obstructed, a catheter must be placed directly into the renal pelvis. This prevents renal

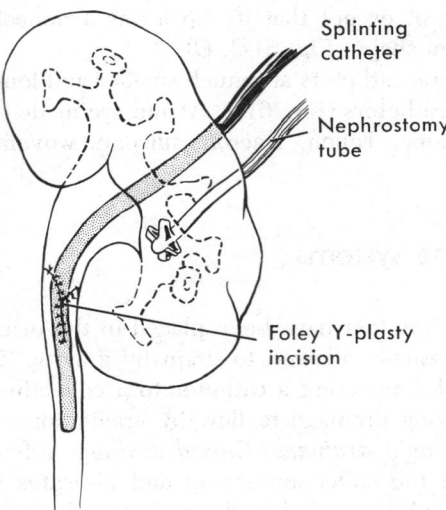

Fig. 61-4. Placement of splinting catheter after repair of ureteropelvic stricture. Note use of nephrostomy tube from drainage of urine during healing of anastomosis.

damage that otherwise would occur as pressure in the kidney increases because of continued urine formation. When there is complete obstruction of a ureter, a *nephrostomy* or *pyelostomy* tube may be inserted surgically into the renal pelvis. The surgical incision is located laterally and posteriorly in the kidney region. Catheters used as nephrostomy or pyelostomy tubes are usually of the Pezzar (mushroom) or Malecot (batwing) types (Fig. 61-2). An alternate form of drainage for a ureteral obstruction is the surgical placement of a ureterostomy tube (a whistle-tip or many-eyed Robinson catheter, size 6 or 8 Fr) that is passed through an incision in the upper outer quadrant of the abdomen into the ureter above the obstruction. The catheter is then passed through the ureter to the renal pelvis.

If the ureter is unobstructed or partially obstructed, the renal pelvis may be drained by a ureteral catheter, which is passed up the ureter to the renal pelvis by means of a cystoscope (see Fig. 60-8). Ureteral catheterization is performed before gynecologic and lower abdominal surgery when there is danger of not recognizing and accidentally injuring the ureter during the operation. Ureteral catheterization is also used after surgery involving the ureters in order to prevent stricture as the ureter heals. When used for this purpose, the catheter is referred to as a *splinting catheter* (Fig. 61-4). Whether it is expected to drain urine will depend on its relation to other catheters used.

Adequate anchorage of *nephrostomy* and *ureteral* catheters must be provided to prevent accidental dislodgment and trauma to the tissues in which they lie (Fig. 61-5). The openings made for these tubes are essentially fistulas that rapidly decrease in size on removal of the catheter. Even 30 minutes after removal

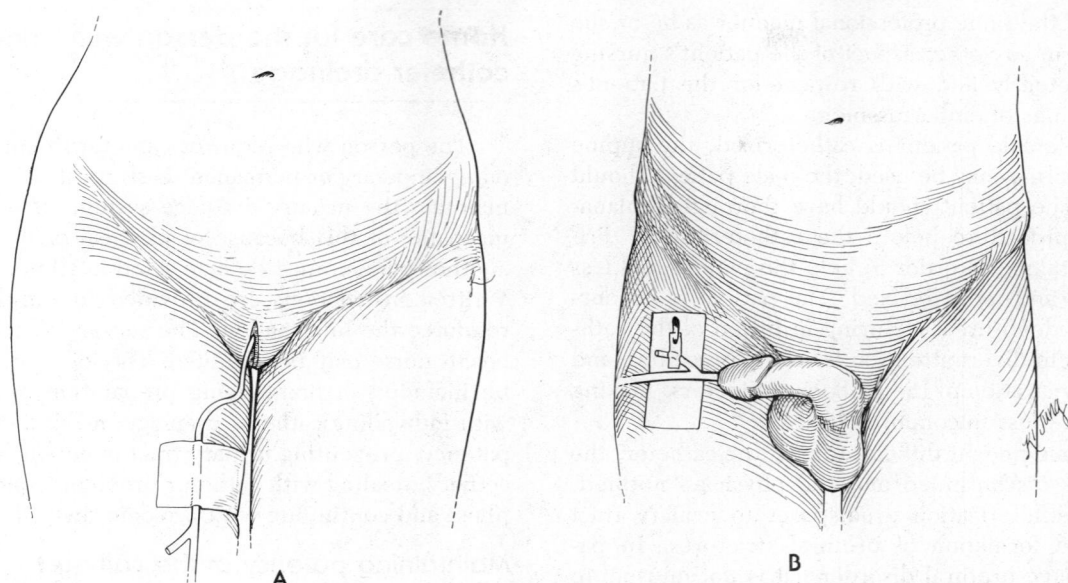

Fig. 61-5. Anchoring of Foley catheter. **A,** In female patient. **B,** In male patient. Proper anchoring prevents accidental traction that could result in injury to bladder or urethra and yet keeps catheter from moving in and out of urethra.

of this type of catheter it is often impossible to reinsert a similar-sized tube. When a catheter is inserted during surgery, it is usually sutured in place. In this case, additional anchorage consists of affixing the tube to the skin with adhesive tape after the skin has been cleansed. When the tube is not sutured in place, it should be anchored to the skin at *two points* using adhesive—with some slack in the tubing between the anchor points.

Free drainage of catheters leading to the renal pelvis is of the utmost importance. Since the normal renal pelvis has only a 5- to 8-ml capacity, great pressure can be exerted on renal structures even when these catheters are obstructed for only a few minutes. Care must be taken to prevent kinking of the tubes while the patient is in the side-lying position in bed.

In some cases nephrostomy tubes may be left in place for several months, with the patient returning to the hospital later for their removal. Occasionally, the nephrostomy tube serves a form of urinary diversion for long-term use. The person at home with a catheter draining the kidney pelvis must know how to obtain medical assistance quickly should the catheter obstruct or become dislodged.

Drainage of the bladder

When obstruction occurs below the bladder, constant drainage must be provided to prevent renal damage, which may occur because of inadequate emptying of the lower urinary system. One means of providing drainage is by the use of a *cystostomy* tube (usually a Foley, Malecot, or Pezzer catheter), which is placed directly into the bladder through a suprapubic incision. This method is usually used when the urethra is completely obstructed or when the prolonged use of a urethral catheter is to be avoided in a male patient. During some operative procedures both a cystostomy tube and a small urethral catheter will be inserted to drain the bladder. Both catheters must be monitored for patency. If patency is assured, it is not necessary to record the output from each catheter separately, since both tubes drain the bladder. The catheters will not necessarily drain equal amounts of urine. As is true with nephrostomy and ureteral catheters, secure anchorage of these catheters is also necessary.

Urethral catheterization is the most common means of draining the bladder, and insertion of this type of catheter is a nursing responsibility in many settings. The Foley catheter is most frequently used for this purpose.

Catheterization is a major cause of urinary tract infections, and strict asepsis should be practiced by anyone carrying out this procedure or assembling the drainage equipment. The need for urethral catheterization must be carefully evaluated; use of urethral catheter drainage only for nursing convenience is not appropriate. Institutional policies differ in regard to whether female nursing personnel may catheterize male patients; however, catheterization of a patient of either sex may be performed by a health care professional of either sex in the same professional manner as he or she would perform any other aspect of the patient's nursing care—competently and with respect for the patient's possible feelings of embarrassment.

When a female patient is catheterized, the supine or lateral position may be used; the male patient should be supine. The patient should have thorough explanation of the procedure before the catheterization. Privacy is maintained in order to help the patient feel less embarrassed and more relaxed. The patient is encouraged to take deep breaths during insertion of the catheter in order to divert attention from the procedure and to increase relaxation of the bladder sphincters, making the procedure less uncomfortable.

If the nurse finds it difficult to pass the catheter, the procedure is discontinued and the physician notified. Traumatic catheterization predisposes to urinary tract infection and formation of urethral strictures. In patients who have urethral disorders, it is not unusual to be unable to pass a standard catheter; special equipment such as catheter directors, filiform catheters, or sounds may be needed. The introduction of such equipment into the urinary tract is not a nursing procedure; neither is catheterization of a patient in the immediate postoperative period following surgery of the urethra or bladder. (For specific information on the catheterization procedure refer to a fundamentals of nursing or urologic nursing text.)

In addition to the previously discussed basic principles of catheter drainage maintenance, the meatal-catheter junction is gently cleansed twice a day with soap and water to prevent urinary tract infections. Vigorous cleaning is avoided, since this predisposes to infection by causing irritation and by removing protective microorganisms. Irrigation of the catheter may be necessary when urine flow is sluggish but is not recommended on a routine basis.

The urethral catheter is anchored securely, not only for patient comfort, but also to prevent complications. For the female the catheter is taped to the inner thigh, allowing sufficient slack to prevent tension at the bladder neck. For the male the catheter should be taped on either side between the groin and iliac crest or on the lower abdomen, so that the penile-scrotal angle is straightened. This avoids pressure and friction that can lead to necrosis of tissue and the formation of urethral ulceration and fistulas. In all patients the catheter should be securely anchored so that it does not move in and out of the urethra and track bacteria into the urethra (p. 372).

The urethral catheter is changed when it is in danger of becoming obstructed by encrustations within its lumen. The person who will have an indwelling urethral catheter at home will either have to be able to learn to change the catheter or have someone to do this when needed.

Home care for the person with urinary catheter drainage

The person who requires catheter drainage at home on a temporary or permanent basis must be able to safely maintain the urinary drainage system. If the person is incapable of this because of physical or mental status, another person must be instructed in all necessary care. Written instructions are provided to supplement and reinforce the information. The services of a community health nurse may be indicated. The following areas must be included in home-going preparation of any person with indwelling catheter drainage: maintaining catheter patency, preventing urinary tract infection, maintaining activity, dealing with catheter problems, obtaining supplies, and continuing with urologic surveillance.

Maintaining patency of the catheter

The person (or care provider) must know how to check for kinks in the tubing and should be aware of the most appropriate way to secure the catheter to prevent kinking. An adequate fluid intake of 2 to 3 L of fluid per day should be encouraged unless contraindicated by the person's condition. Persons who will be irrigating their own catheters at home should practice this under supervision several times before discharge.

Preventing urinary tract infection

The person (or care provider) must be helped to understand the importance of cleanliness as a means of preventing complications. Instruction includes the necessity of good hand washing before and after working with the catheter. Instruction also includes cleansing the meatal-catheter junction with soap and water twice daily. The person should be reassured that cleansing the meatal-catheter junction will not dislodge or pull out the catheter. Ideally, frequent disconnection of the catheter and drainage tubing should be avoided. However, the person at home must disconnect the tubing at night to change from a leg bag to the overnight drainage bag and again in the morning to resume leg-bag drainage. To lessen the risk of contamination, the person is taught to wash the hands and then wipe the catheter and tubing with 70% alcohol before disconnection and reconnection. The disconnected ends of the drainage bags are protected with sterile gauze secured in place with a rubber band or a connector cap.

When equipment must be sterilized at home, instruction is given in how to do this properly. Before use the equipment, which has been washed with soap and water, is boiled for a full 10 minutes in a pan of water. Other parts of the system such as collection bags and tubing should be kept as clean as possible by daily washing with soap and water followed by 15 minutes of soaking in a solution of equal parts of vinegar and water (half-strength vinegar). Teaching also includes the need to keep the drainage collection receptacle at a level lower than the cavity being drained.

Promoting activity

The person needs to be well informed about the adaptations that can be made with the urinary drainage system to allow return to an optimal level of activity. A shower or tub bath with a catheter in place is generally permitted unless there is an unhealed surgical incision. The adhesive tape holding the catheter in place will need to be replaced after bathing. Leg bags are available in a variety of sizes and are concealed by clothing. There is no need for men or women to remove an indwelling catheter before intercourse—a question persons may be hesitant to ask. The male can fold the indwelling catheter over the penis to facilitate insertion during intercourse.[49] Questions pertaining to resumption of usual life-style activities should be encouraged so that the person can be as well prepared as possible for self-care at home.

Dealing with catheter problems

The patient (or care provider) should be informed about how to handle problems such as obstruction of the catheter or displacement of the catheter. The person needs to know whether to contact the physician or to seek help through a clinic or emergency room. The amount of time that can safely elapse before obtaining help will depend on the type of catheter and its location.

Obtaining supplies

At discharge the patient should be provided with adequate supplies for at least a few days. A list of names, addresses, and phone numbers of where additional supplies may be obtained and what resources are available to assist with payment if necessary should be given to the person before discharge. A written list of the specific supplies needed should be provided to aid the person, who is likely to be confused by the many products available.

Providing ongoing care

The person with a urinary catheter of any type will need continued urologic surveillance. Instruction includes the need to contact the physician if back pain, fever, or other urinary tract symptoms are present and to plan for regular examination by the physician as well.

Intervention for the patient after removal of a catheter

It is normal to note some dribbling of urine for a few hours after a urethral catheter has been removed because of dilation of the sphincter muscles by the catheter. Dribbling of urine that persists longer than a few hours should be reported to the physician; this symptom may indicate damage to the sphincters. In determining the type of intervention necessary to reestablish bladder control, information about the nature of the incontinency is gathered. Incontinence is described as complete (constant dribbling) or occurring only on urgency or stress. It should also be observed whether incontinence is present in all positions (lying, sitting, standing). If muscular weakness of the sphincters is the major problem, incontinence is least likely to occur when the person is in a prone position and most likely to be a problem when standing or walking. Perineal exercises (p. 1544) may help to regain control of voiding.

Another problem that may arise after removal of a catheter is inability to void. The patient should be encouraged to drink fluids and then attempt to void. The nurse carefully assesses the patient's bladder for distention. Efforts are made to provide comfortable positioning and privacy to facilitate voiding. No patient with an adequate intake should go longer than 8 hours without voiding. It is not uncommon for a patient with edema of the bladder neck to require temporary reinsertion of a catheter to facilitate urinary output. It is the nurse's responsibility to accurately determine and record all spontaneous voidings of the patient until adequacy of output has been well established.

Color and consistency of the urine are noted. *Cystitis* (inflammation of the bladder) may develop after catheter removal because of incomplete emptying of the bladder as muscle tone is being reestablished. Any abnormalities in color, odor, or sediment in the urine are reported.

Education of the patient about signs and symptoms of urinary retention, changes in the color and consistency of the urine, and incontinence and dysuria is undertaken when bladder drainage is discontinued. Often the first indicators of dysfunction are subjective judgments offered by the patient. This information greatly increases the ability to detect early recurrence of urinary drainage problems and should be sought and clearly recorded.

Outcome criteria for the person with an indwelling catheter

The person:
1. Maintains free flow of urine through the catheter.
2. Does not acquire a urinary tract infection.

The person or significant others can:
1. Explain the purpose and expected duration of the catheter.
2. Demonstrate aseptic technique in care of the catheter.

3. State how to arrange for reestablishment of urine flow should failure of adequate flow occur.
4. State where to obtain needed supplies.
5. Describe signs and symptoms of urinary tract infection requiring medical attention.
6. State plans for follow-up care.

Intermittent catheter drainage

Intermittent catheterization of the urinary bladder is being used with increasing frequency in the treatment of neurogenic bladder dysfunction secondary to spinal cord trauma, birth defects, urinary retention, and some chronic diseases. Originally it was carried out only as a sterile procedure used in hospital settings. A clean, unsterile technique that facilitates home use of this method has been adapted by some urologists.[46]

Because periodic complete emptying of the bladder eliminates residual urine (an excellent culture medium for multiplication of bacteria) and maintains a good blood supply to the bladder wall by avoiding high intrabladder pressures, infections are often decreased, even when only a clean technique is used.

Individuals are evaluated for their appropriateness for this form of management by the urologist. Potential for success with this form of therapy should be further evaluated, utilizing input from the nurse, psychologist, social worker, and other involved health care professionals. Teaching, however, is generally a nursing responsibility in either an inpatient or outpatient setting. Before a teaching plan can be made, the nurse must know whether a clean or sterile technique is to be taught and the frequency with which it is to be used. Knowledge of the person's physical, mental, and emotional status as well as usual life-style must also be utilized in planning a program suitable for each person.

The hospitalized patient previously on an established intermittent catheterization program at home may require catheterization by nursing personnel during an acute illness but may be encouraged to continue self-care as able.

The goals of intermittent catheterization may vary from patient to patient but are generally to prevent urinary retention and its sequelae (urinary tract infection and renal damage) and to achieve continence. The patient should know exactly what is expected of the treatment plan in order to elicit full cooperation.

Intervention

The hospitalized patient with intermittent catheter drainage of the bladder may be one for whom the treatment is temporary (as in the early phases of spinal cord trauma), one who is learning the technique for home use, or one who has been using intermittent catheterization before admission. Even though the clean technique is suitable for home use, sterile technique is necessary during hospitalization to decrease the possibility of hospital-acquired infection when the catheterization is performed by hospital personnel. When hospitalized, the patient who customarily performs self-catheterization may continue to use clean technique if this method is used at home, but preferably a sterile catheter will be used each time or special precautions are taken to store the reusable catheter in a closed container. Specimens for culture must be obtained by the usual sterile catheterization technique to avoid contamination of the specimen. The patient is informed about the reasons why sterile precautions are necessary in the hospital setting.

A size 14 Fr Robinson catheter is generally used for an adult. The volume of urine obtained with each catheterization is recorded to assure that schedule adjustments can be made if necessary. The adult bladder should not be permitted to hold more than 300 ml at any time, since greater amounts lead to overdistention of the bladder with greater susceptibility to infection. The frequency of catheterization is determined by the amount of residual urine. The person first attempts to void and then performs self-catheterization. A large amount of residual urine (more than 200 ml) means that more frequent catheterization is necessary. Usually such individuals will need catheterization every 4 to 6 hours. A small amount of residual urine (less than 200 ml) after voiding means that the person will only need to do self-catheterization every 8 to 12 hours. Some persons eventually will be able to manage with once-a-day catheterization.[35] Some individuals may also have to catheterize themselves at night if they have a large output of urine at night. It is important to realize that the person who normally does not perform self-catheterization at night at home may need to do so during periods where the fluid intake is greater than usual, as with intravenous fluid administration.

In some instances the physician will prescribe the frequency of catheterizations; in other instances, adjustment of the schedule may be a nursing judgment. If the nurse notes that excess volumes of urine are being obtained with a prescribed schedule, the physician is consulted about the need to alter the schedule.

Color, clarity, and odor of the urine are noted and any symptoms of urinary tract infection reported. Periodic urine specimens are obtained and sent for culture and sensitivity. Some individuals are given long-term antibiotic therapy prophylactically.

The person is helped to understand the rationale for intermittent catheter drainage, and the regularity of bladder emptying must be stressed. Basic anatomy of the genitalia and urinary tract is pointed out to aid the person to understand where the catheter is inserted and to alleviate fears of causing damage by misplacement of the catheter.

In most cases, clean (not sterile) catheterization technique is prescribed for home use. Hand washing is advised before each catheterization, and the meatal area is cleansed with soap and water. After inserting the catheter and draining the bladder, the catheter is removed and washed with soap and water before being stored in a clean, closed container for the next use. The catheter is reused until it becomes either too soft or too hard to be directed properly.

Most individuals require much support during the actual teaching but very quickly become comfortable with the procedure. Initially, a mirror is used to teach women where to place the catheter. The woman should learn to catheterize while sitting on the commode, using palpation to locate the urethral meatus. Men may sit or stand to catheterize themselves. It is important that they use generous amounts of lubricant to avoid urethral irritation; women generally do not require lubrication of the catheter.

If the person, because of age or physical limitations, is unable to perform self-catheterization, a care provider may be instructed in the technique. The individual or care provider must know where additional catheters may be obtained.

If sterile catheterization technique is needed for home use, more time and practice will be required in order to learn good sterile technique. Careful explanation of sterilization of equipment must be provided, and planning for adapting sterile intermittent self-catheterization to the individual's usual life-style must be worked out with the person.

If teaching of self-catheterization is performed on an outpatient basis or if hospitalization is short, follow-up for adjustment of schedule and other concerns of adaptation to home routine should be provided. This may be done by the primary nurse, by the physician, or by referral to a visiting nurse. Ongoing urologic care with periodic urine cultures is essential.

Outcome criteria for the person who is using the intermittent catheter drainage technique

The person or significant others can:
1. Explain the reason for the intermittent catheter drainage.
2. State the need for regular, periodic, complete emptying of the bladder.
3. Demonstrate self-catheterization using clean technique unless sterile technique is prescribed.
4. Describe how to adapt the catheterization routine to the individual life-style.
5. State how to obtain needed supplies.
6. Describe symptoms of urinary tract infection requiring medical care.
7. State plans for ongoing urologic care.

Intervention for fluid imbalance in persons with urinary problems

Management of fluid balance is a fundamental and common problem for persons requiring urologic procedures and nephrology care. Maintaining normal fluid balance helps to (1) preserve renal function in individuals having ongoing kidney insufficiency or failure, (2) prevent the development of acute renal failure caused by fluid depletion, (3) prevent inadequate tissue perfusion and shock from depletion of blood volume, (4) provide continuous urine formation to help alleviate stasis of urine and bacterial growth, and (5) prevent fluid overload, which would increase the work of the heart and lead to peripheral and cerebral edema. The potential for altered states of fluid balance in urologic and renal patients commonly involves both abnormal losses and gains of fluid.

Accurate assessment of a patient's hydration state depends on a thorough physical examination and carefully kept records of fluid losses and gains. Most often fluid balance records and patient observations are obtained by nursing personnel. The following information should provide some direction to nurses regarding crucial observations to be made and data to be recorded, and specific instances in urologic and nephrology nursing where problems of fluid balance are likely to arise. For general information on fluid and electrolyte balance the reader is referred to Chapter 21; for common electrolyte problems accompanying renal disease the reader is referred to Chapter 62.

Prevention

In order to prevent the occurrence of fluid imbalance, three considerations are important to nursing practice. First, persons prone to developing fluid imbalances and the specific nature of their potential fluid problems require identification. Individuals predisposed to developing *fluid overload* include (1) those with acute renal failure where kidney shutdown and oliguria are the rule; (2) those with bilateral obstructive disease attributed to strictures, tumors, or calculi, who present with anuria or severely decreased urinary output; and (3) those with chronic renal failure characterized by limited and fixed ability to excrete fluid through the kidneys. The common defect in the above situations is an inability to excrete more than a low and fixed volume of urine per day, regardless of fluid intake.

Individuals susceptible to *fluid depletion* or *dehydration* include (1) those recovering from acute renal failure and in a phase of the illness where the kidneys do not appropriately conserve body fluid; (2) those with chronic renal failure whose urinary output per day is fixed at a high volume (2000 ml/day or greater) and who are unable to obtain or retain fluids sufficient to replace those lost through the kidneys; and (3) persons on diuretic therapy whose oral intake does not keep up with renal and other body fluid losses. The kidneys of these persons are unable to conserve fluid when intake is low or when extrarenal losses are high. Such situations occur, for example, when there is vomiting or diarrhea over prolonged periods, when fluids are restricted for several diagnostic tests in succession, when there is sudden sodium restriction or loss, which decrease thirst, or when individuals become weak and unable to replace fluid losses on their own.

In addition, certain urologic situations make it very difficult to measure fluid output accurately. These include copious wound drainage or continuous bladder irrigation following urologic surgery, ill-fitting urinary appliances, and incontinence.

A second consideration in preventing fluid imbalances involves collecting appropriate baseline data and continuing to monitor the patient who is at risk of developing fluid problems. Such data will assist both in diagnosing imbalances and in the ongoing management of these problems. For example, when the diagnosis is chronic renal failure, the nurse would wish to obtain information regarding the ability to excrete fluid. Fluid intake and output measurements along with daily weights will help to identify the ability of the person to regulate body fluid balance.

Prevention of fluid imbalances is also achieved through efforts to educate individuals about potential problems they may have in handling fluids. Persons with chronic renal failure and those on diuretic therapy in particular will need to be given guidelines about current goals for fluid management, potential problems with fluid balance, signs and symptoms indicating a problem, and mechanisms for correcting fluid problems or in receiving assistance when they cannot manage the problems on their own.

Outcome criteria for the person having fluid imbalance associated with urinary problems

The person will:
1. Exhibit no signs of abnormal fluid loss or gain.
   a. No peripheral edema.
   b. No orthostatic hypotension.
   c. Blood pressure stable and within normal range.

The person or significant others can:
1. Explain any dietary (sodium) and fluid intake restrictions.
2. Explain how these restrictions will be met.

Urologic surgery

General intervention

Before discussing in detail particular types of surgery of the urinary tract, general principles of care of the patient requiring urologic surgery will be described.

Preoperative care

The focus of preoperative care is to prepare the patient for the impending surgery through instructions and to carry out the medical regimen including medications, shaving of the operative site, and preparation of the skin. Much of the patient's concern depends on the type of surgery and diagnosis. Since the surgery will temporarily or permanently alter urinary elimination, the person will be concerned about the degree of change that will be present.

Preoperative instructions include a discussion of the type and length of surgery, type of anesthesia, and the need for an intravenous line, catheter, or other drains. Instructions in coughing and deep breathing are crucial since ventilation is a frequent problem postoperatively. The patient is informed of the pain medication routine—whether or not it will be offered or if it must be requested. A description of methods of decreasing pain, such as by splinting the incision, should be offered. The patient is assessed for understanding and acceptance of the surgery at the beginning and conclusion of instruction.

The evening before surgery the person receives a shave, skin preparation, and/or a medicated shower, depending on the type of surgery. The woman patient may also receive a medicated douche to cleanse the perineal area. The person is given nothing by mouth after midnight. Persons having a urinary diversion will also require bowel preparation (p. 1534).

Postoperative care

The basic needs of the patient requiring urologic surgery are the same as those of any other surgical patient. Special emphasis must be placed on promotion of ventilation and adequate urinary output, prevention of distention and hemorrhage, and attention to drainage tubes and dressings.

Ventilation. Surgery of the kidney or upper ureters usually involves a flank incision that can influence respiratory status. Because the incision is directly below the diaphragm, deep breathing is painful and the patient is reluctant to take deep breaths or to move about. Splinting of the chest is common, and therefore atelectasis or other respiratory complications must be guarded against. In addition, because of the placement of the incision there is a greater incisional pull every time the person moves, as compared with an abdominal incision. The patient is often reluctant to turn in bed or to get up to ambulate. Most patients will be more comfortable turning themselves if they are given time, side rails to hold onto, and encouragement. Incisional pain usually requires a narcotic every 3 to 4 hours for 24 to 48 hours after surgery, and turning, ambulation, and deep breathing exercises can be planned so that these activities occur at the time the analgesic has the greatest effect. Patients may lie on the affected side unless a nephrostomy tube is in place. Even then they can be tilted to the affected side with pillows placed at the back for support. It must be ascertained that the tube is not kinked and that there is no traction on it.

Urinary output. The urinary output is monitored carefully for several days postoperatively to ascertain adequate renal functioning and drainage. The output should be at least 50 ml/hr, preferably greater in order to prevent urinary stasis and subsequent infection. A urinary output of 20 to 30 ml/hr in a patient with satisfactory fluid intake (at least 1200 ml/day) and in the absence of signs of urinary retention is reported immediately to the physician. Urinary output includes drainage from nephrostomy or cystostomy tubes, urethral or ureteral catheters, and an estimate from urine-soaked dressings. Daily weights are compared with the preoperative weight and with each other to identify fluid retention.

Distention. Following kidney surgery most patients have some abdominal distention that may result in part from pressure on the stomach and intestinal tract during surgery. Patients who have had renal colic before surgery frequently develop paralytic ileus postoperatively. This condition may be related to the reflex gastrointestinal tract symptoms caused by postoperative pain. Because of the problem of abdominal distention following renal surgery, food and fluids by mouth are often restricted for 24 to 48 hours postoperatively. By the fourth postoperative day most patients tolerate a regular diet. Fluids are usually forced to 3000 ml/day.

Hemorrhage. Hemorrhage may follow such operative procedures as prostatectomy, nephrolithotomy, or nephrectomy. It occurs most often when the highly vascular parenchyma of the kidney has been incised. The bleeding may occur on the day of surgery, or it may occur 8 to 12 days postoperatively, during the period when tissue sloughing normally occurs with healing. The presence of bright red blood on the dressing or in the urine is reported immediately to the physician. The patient is observed for signs of shock. Since many patients with urologic disease have hypertension, the blood pressure may be relatively high but still represent a marked drop for the individual. Comparisons should therefore be made with baseline data.

If hemorrhage occurs, a pressure dressing is applied over the incision while awaiting the physician's arrival. Measures to prevent shock are instituted (p. 321). Several liters of sterile physiologic saline solution for irrigation should be available.

Dressings. There may be large amounts of urinary drainage following urologic surgery except after nephrectomy. The drainage may be pink or dark red but should not be bright red. If the surgery involves a flank incision, drainage is usually the heaviest on the posterior edge of the dressing because of gravity flow. It is important therefore to turn the patient on the side opposite the surgery to examine the posterior edge of the dressing. When a suprapubic incision is present, drainage is heaviest on the side and in the inguinal region.

The dressings are usually held in place by Montgomery straps and must be changed frequently. Urinary drainage irritates the skin, has an unpleasant odor, and leads to discomfort. If a drain is present, the end of the drain should be placed over dressings, then covered with additional dressings to absorb the drainage. If a drainage tube is present, presence of large amounts of drainage on the dressing with little drainage coming from the tube indicates blockage of the tube. If a large amount of drainage is present, a disposable drainage bag used for urinary stomas (p. 1538) may be applied over the drainage site.

Drainage tubes. A catheter is usually inserted during surgery to drain urine from the operative area and permit healing to occur. Different types of drainage tubes may be inserted, and each tube is connected to a separate drainage system. It is important to know the purpose of the catheter and the area to be drained.

Outcome criteria for the person having urologic surgery

The person will:
1. Maintain adequate urinary drainage.
2. Maintain clear breath sounds and normal respiratory rate and depth.
3. Maintain good skin integrity surrounding the surgical incision.

The person or significant others can:
1. Describe maintenance of drainage and sterility of any indwelling drainage tube on discharge from the hospital.
2. State plans for follow-up care.

Specific types of urologic surgery

Surgery of the kidney

Removal of a kidney (*nephrectomy*) may be indicated for some congenital anomalies or for irreparable damage to kidney tissue from trauma or diseases such as renal hypertension, tumor, multiple cysts, or kidney stones. Adequate waste removal can be maintained by the remaining kidney or by even less than half of one healthy kidney. In some instances only a portion of a diseased kidney is removed (*partial nephrectomy*). If an entire kidney is removed, a drain may be placed to remove serous fluid from the space previously occupied by the kidney. In this situation there will be no urinary drainage. Urinary drainage will occur with a partial nephrectomy.

The kidney may also be incised for removal of calculi, either through the pelvis of the kidney (*pyelolithotomy*) (p. 1557) or through the parenchyma (*nephrolithotomy*). There is usually a large amount of urinary drainage following these surgeries.

A kidney may become loosened and "float" or become displaced (*nephroptosis*). If symptoms of obstruction occur, the kidney may be sutured to its anatomic site (*nephropexy*). Postoperatively, the patient is positioned with the hips elevated to prevent tension on the sutures.

Surgery of the ureters and bladder

Removal of stones (*calculi*) blocking a ureter is termed *ureterolithotomy* (p. 1557). The root word "lith" refers to stones. Obstruction at the ureteropelvic junction is corrected by means of a *pyeloplasty* (plastic repair of the renal pelvis).

The bladder may be incised (*cystotomy*) for removal of calculi or as part of one method of prostate removal (suprapubic prostatectomy) (p. 1561). A *cystostomy* (note the "s" in the middle of the word) is an opening made in the bladder for drainage, usually by means of a tube.

Partial removal of the bladder (*segmental resection*) is usually performed for tumors of the bladder (p. 1558). Bladder capacity will be small initially with a capacity of no more than 60 ml immediately postoperatively, but the elastic tissue of the bladder will regenerate so that the patient is able to retain from 200 to 400 ml of urine within several months.

The decreased size of the bladder, however, is of major importance in the postoperative period. The patient will return from surgery with catheters draining the bladder both from a cystostomy opening and from the urethra. This is to obviate the possibility of obstruction of drainage, since it would take only a very short time for the bladder to become distended and there would be danger of disrupting the suture line on the bladder. Because the bladder capacity is limited, the catheters usually cause severe bladder spasm. The urethral catheter is usually removed 3 weeks after surgery, but it may be left in place longer if the cystotomy wound is not well healed.

As soon as the urethral catheter is removed, the patient becomes acutely aware of the small capacity of the bladder. Most patients will need to void at least every 20 minutes, and they need to be reassured that the bladder capacity will gradually increase. Meanwhile they should be urged to force fluids to 3000 ml but should be advised to space the fluids so that time spent in the bathroom is not an inconvenience. They also should not take large quantities of fluids at one time, should limit fluids for several hours before planning to go out, and should take no fluids after 6 PM.

If the entire bladder is removed (*cystectomy*), diversion of the urinary tract is necessary. Immediately after the cystectomy the patient is usually acutely ill, since not only the bladder but also large amounts of surrounding tissue will be removed if the diagnosis is a malignant tumor. These patients may have a circulatory disturbance and should be monitored for signs and symptoms of shock, thrombosis, or cardiac decompensation. There is a long vertical or transverse abdominal incision, and there may be a perineal incision. The patient is given nothing by mouth for several days, and a nasogastric tube is inserted. The nursing care is the same as that given any patient after major abdominal surgery plus the routine care for a perineal wound and the care of the diverted urinary drainage.

Urinary diversion procedures

Purpose and types

Urinary diversion procedures are required to treat malignancies of the urinary tract, birth defects, neurogenic bladder dysfunction, chronic progressive pyelonephritis, and irreparable trauma to the urinary tract. Several years ago urinary diversions were done for neurogenic bladder dysfunction, acquired and congenital. However, the development of intermittent clean catheterization has resulted in this method becoming the treatment of choice in this patient population. The most frequent urinary diversion procedures are ureterostomy, ileal conduit, and colonic or sigmoid conduit, all of which result in external stomas and the need for ostomy pouches. New surgical advances being studied include the continent ileal conduit, the continent vesicostomy, and the carbon conduit.

Cutaneous ureterostomy is employed when the physical condition prohibits more extensive surgical procedures. One or both ureters are excised from the bladder and brought out through the skin either on the flank or the anterior abdominal wall to create a small stoma. When both ureters are involved, each may be brought out to the skin surface separately, resulting in two stomas, or they may be joined at some point and brought out through the abdominal wall to form only one stoma. Initially following surgery ureterostomy stomas are pink, but they will turn very pale in several weeks. Unless the ureters are dilated from chronic reflux, the ureterostomy stoma will be very small (Fig. 61-6) and will tend to become stenosed and to develop strictures. The complications associated with ureterostomy stoma stenosis are inadequate drainage of the kidney resulting in hydronephrosis, infection, and progres-

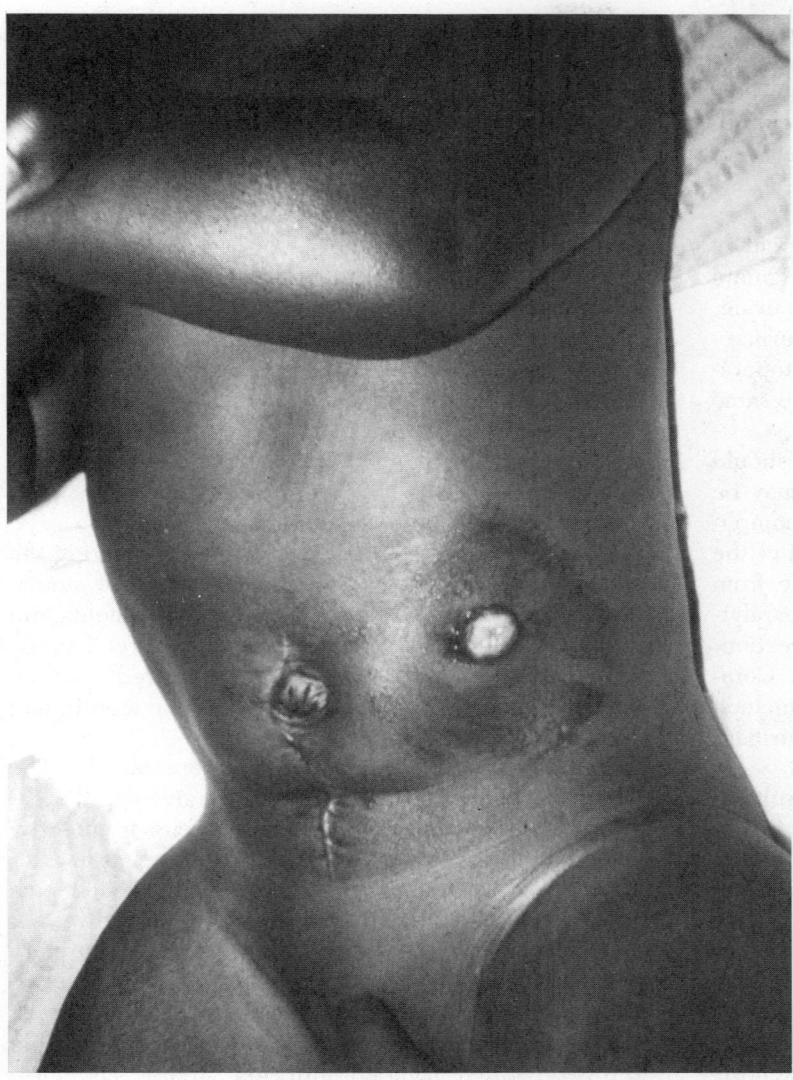

Fig. 61-6. Normal functioning ureterostomy in child with a myelomenigocele.

sive renal damage. Urinary tract infection in persons with ureterostomy is common because of the ease of reflux of the urine from the stoma to the kidney.

The *ureteroileocutaneous anastomosis* (also called an *ileal conduit, ileal loop,* or Bricker procedure) is the most common form of permanent urinary diversion. During the surgical procedure, the ureters are excised from the bladder and transplanted into one end of a 15- to 20-cm (6- or 8-in.) segment of ileum that has been resected from the intestinal tract with its mesentery, which contains the blood supply. The remaining intestinal segments are anastomosed, and gastrointestinal function is expected to return to its normal preoperative state after healing. The end of the resected ileum into which the ureters are connected is sutured closed and the other end is brought through the abdominal wall to the skin surface to create a stoma (Fig. 61-7). The urinary bladder may be resected or left intact, depending upon the reason for the diversion.

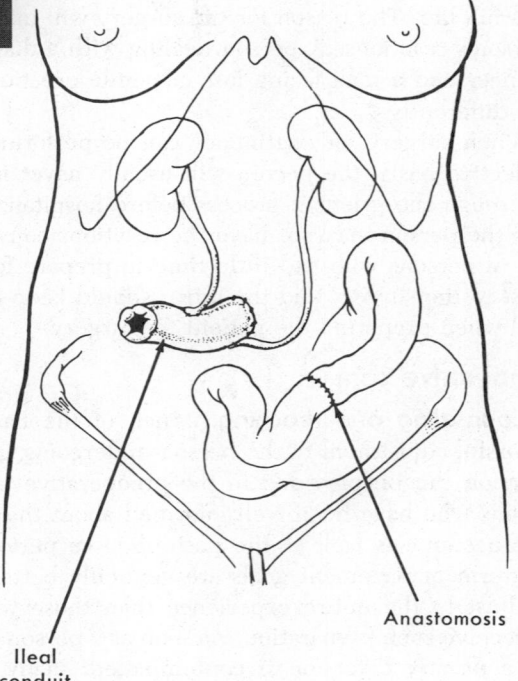

Ileal conduit

Anastomosis

Fig. 61-7. Ileal conduit or ileal loop.

The ileal segment is intended to serve as a passageway for urinary flow rather than as a reservoir; therefore in an ileal conduit urine flow is continuous. Electrolyte imbalance caused by reabsorption of waste products from the urine in the ileal segment is generally not a problem in a well-functioning ileal conduit.

The colonic conduit (colonic loop) is basically performed like an ileal conduit except that a segment of colon (ascending, descending, transverse, or sigmoid colon) instead of ileum acts as the conduit for the urine. The colonic loop has reduced the incidence of urinary reflux for some persons.[33] Preoperative and postoperative nursing care and ongoing managment are the same as those for ileal conduit surgery.

The ileal conduit and colonic conduit stomas should be a bright red color. Peristalsis of the stoma may be visualized when the pouch is removed. Early complications following the surgery include breakdown of the anastomosis in the gastrointestinal tract, leakage from the ureteroileal or ureterosigmoid anastomosis, paralytic ileus, obstruction of the ureters, wound infection, mucocutaneous separation, and stomal necrosis. Complications that may occur after hospitalization include stomal problems (retraction, prolapse, hernia), urinary infections, crystal formation, and stones.

Any procedure for diversion of urine that results in an external stoma leads to a significant change in the person's body image. Reactions may vary depending upon the reason for the procedure, but virtually every person will require time and much nursing support while adapting to the altered means of urine elimination.

A person may never like having an ostomy, but one does not have to like a situation to adapt to it and to live a full life. The reason for the surgery will influence a person's reactions. A person dealing with a diagnosis of cancer and a man facing loss of penile erection will react differently.

When surgery for continency can be performed on an elective basis, the person will usually have time to go through the grieving process before hospitalization. Thus the person may not have the reactions commonly seen in persons who had little time to prepare for and adjust to the surgery and the nurse should keep this in mind when preparing the patient for surgery.

Preoperative care

Counseling and teaching. Much of the basis for successful adjustment of the person undergoing urinary diversion can be provided in the preoperative period. Persons who have been well informed about the surgical procedure as well as the postoperative period and long-term management goals are generally better able to adjust to the entire experience than those who do not receive such preparation. As soon as a person learns that a urinary diversion is contemplated, many questions arise, and it is important that accurate answers be given at this time. The well-informed nurse in any setting recognizes that concerns are present and encourages verbalization of them. The nurse in the outpatient urology clinic, for example, can begin preoperative preparation even before hospital admission.

The important aspect of preoperative counseling is that the patient's questions are answered truthfully. The nurse's goals for preoperative teaching must reflect the individual patient's needs. Not every one wants to see a stoma model or a pouch. However, certain basic information needs to be included. An assessment of the patient will determine how much of the basic information is provided preoperatively. The patient should be able to describe the surgical procedure in terms of what will be done and should know that a pouch will have to be worn postoperatively. The patient should also understand that work, hobbies, physical activities, diet, and clothing will not change following surgery.

Preoperative instruction also involves preparing the person for the surgery and the appearance of the stoma. An anatomy chart or simple drawing supplements and clarifies explanations of the surgical procedure. The patient should be told that the stoma will be red, that the tissue is similar to the mucosal lining in the mouth, and that it will not be painful.

Terminology is also important preoperatively. The definitions of various terms should be given to the patient. Urine is not something people discuss frequently. Some patients will not know what urinary output is or what to call the surgery. The nurse should define such terms as urine, stoma, and pouch for the patient.

Booklets designed for the person having a urinary diversion may be given to the patient preoperatively.* Some persons need this additional information to assist them in accepting the surgery. Others may be unable to review written materials until after surgery. The nurse needs to be very sensitive to the wishes of the patient in this regard. When the patient indicates a desire to have written materials, the nurse should be present to carefully review the content with the patient.

If the person is willing, a urostomy appliance should be shown (Fig. 61-8). Usually viewing the appliance and learning how it adheres to the body will dispel any misconceptions about the pouch. Assurance is given that the nurse will provide stoma care immediately after surgery and that the patient will be assisted to master self-care before discharge.

Physical preparation. Physical preparation for surgery for ureterostomy is similar to that for any abdominal surgery. Before an ileal or colonic conduit diversion there is usually a complete cleansing of the bowel to reduce the possibility of fecal contamination when the bowel is resected. The cleansing routine

---

Living with your ureterostomy, New York, 1979, American Cancer Society; *Managing a urostomy . . . so it doesn't manage you*, Chicago, 1974, Hollister, Inc.; *Urinary ostomies: a guidebook for patients*, ed. 2, Los Angeles, 1978, United Ostomy Association.

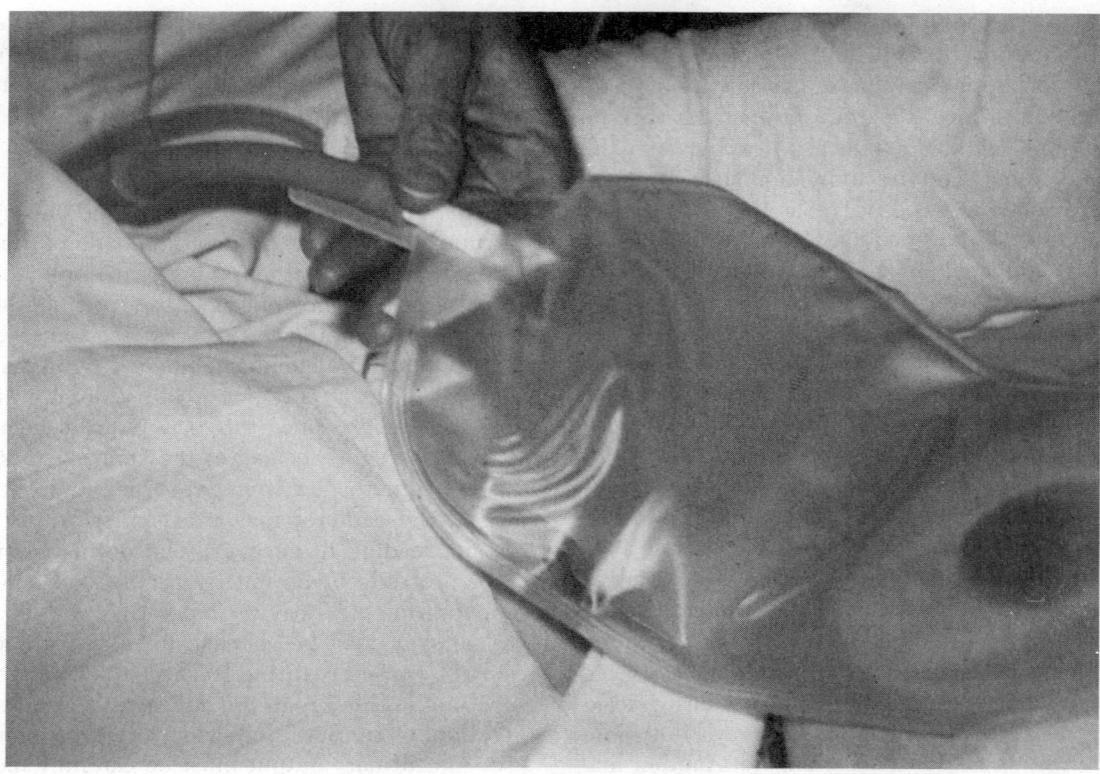

Fig. 61-8. Urinary appliances should be connected to bedside drainage at night. Tongue blade may be used to splint connection and prevent twisting of tubing.

generally consists of a clear liquid diet for about 3 days, followed by nothing by mouth for at least 8 hours before surgery. Cleansing enemas are usually ordered until returns are clear, and an intestinal antibiotic such as neomycin is administered by mouth or by enema. If surgery is delayed for any reason, the surgeon needs to be consulted before continuing with the regimen, since vitamin B and K deficiencies may result and fungus infection may occur secondary to changes in intestinal flora.

The stoma for the ileal conduit is usually constructed on the right side of the abdomen below the waist. The stoma for the colonic conduit is located according to the portion of large intestine selected and may be on the right or left side of the abdomen. Determination of the exact placement for the stoma site is ideally made before surgery and should include evaluation of the person's body when in the lying, sitting, and standing positions. Since a smooth, even skin surface surrounding the stoma is important for optimal adherence of an appliance, it is important that the site selected by free from scars, skin folds, and bony prominences.

Postoperative care

Following a *cutaneous ureterostomy*, the person generally returns from surgery with catheters inserted through the ureters to drain the renal pelves. These are usually left in place for 7 to 14 days. Patency of the catheters must be maintained because hydronephrosis can rapidly ensue if obstruction occurs.

Following an *ileal or colonic conduit* procedure there may or may not be splinting catheters in place in the stoma for the first few days postoperatively. A nasogastric tube with gastric suction will be used for 3 to 5 days to allow for the return of effective intestinal peristalsis and the healing of the intestinal anastomosis site. Adequate drainage through the nasogastric tube is maintained to prevent pressure on the intestinal anastomosis. Nothing by mouth is permitted until peristalsis has resumed; then a normal diet is gradually resumed, beginning with small amounts of water. Intravenous fluids are continued until an adequate diet is possible. A regular diet is resumed in simple ureterostomies, since the procedure does not involve the intestinal tract.

Skin care. In any type of urinary diversion, care must be taken to prevent urine leakage onto the surrounding skin. If all the urine is draining from the catheters in the stoma, skin care should present little problem for the first few days, especially when the catheter is connected to constant drainage.

If there is urine drainage around the catheters, if no catheters were used, or when catheters have been removed, a temporary postoperative drainage bag is applied over the stoma to collect the continuous urine drainage. An appropriate appliance has an opening hole cut so that the appliance fits around the stoma with no more than 3 mm (⅛ in.) of skin exposed between the appliance and stoma. The urostomy appliance designed for urinary diversions has a valve at the bottom that permits emptying of the pouch at frequent intervals. It also allows the appliance to be attached to drainage tubing and a collection bag.

For better adherence of the appliance and for skin protection, a skin sealant product, such as United's "Skin-Prep" or Hollister's "Skin-Gel," may be used. Some of the skin sealant products contain alcohol and will cause burning and discomfort if applied to excoriated skin. Tincture of benzoin should be used with caution because it can cause allergic skin reactions in some individuals. A skin barrier product, such as "Stomahesive" or "Hollihesive," may be used during the postoperative period to prevent skin excoriation or to protect excoriated skin.

Appliances with karaya rings are generally *not* used since urine gradually erodes the karaya, causing leakage. Appliances with rings similar to karaya but more resistant to urine breakdown are available. Another feature available in some urostomy appliances is an antireflux chamber to reduce the backflow of urine.

The appliance should be changed to visualize the stoma and assess the mucocutaneous suture line. During the hospitalization, the pouch is changed whenever it leaks or when a teaching session is planned. In the active phases of teaching, the pouch is removed more frequently than is recommended following discharge. The procedure for changing the pouch is a clean, not sterile, procedure.

1. Assemble all supplies.
2. Empty the pouch and gently remove the appliance from the skin.
3. Cleanse the skin surrounding the stoma with mild soap and water. Rinse and pat dry. Mucous secretions should be washed off the stoma gently.
4. Place a rolled piece of gauze or cotton balls over the stomal opening to absorb draining urine while the skin is being cared for.
5. Measure the diameter of the stoma and cut a corresponding opening in the skin barrier (if used) and the appliance or select the corresponding size of precut appliance.
6. Apply skin sealant around the stoma if desired. Allow the area to dry completely.
7. Attach the appliance to the skin barrier. The pouch and skin barrier may be applied to the skin separately or together. In the early postoperative period it is easier to attach the pouch to the skin barrier and then to apply the system in one piece to the skin.
8. Apply the appliance and skin barrier around the stoma, keeping the adhesive area free of wrinkles or creases. Press gently but firmly into place for 30 secomds. The valve at the bottom of the pouch must be closed or attached to drainage tubing and a collection bag.

In the early postoperative period the appliance is positioned so that it drains to the side of the bed, facilitating drainage and emptying of the appliance. During each change of the appliance, the condition of the stoma and the surrounding skin is assessed for bleeding and excoriation. The stoma should be bright pink or red—any evidence of gray or black discoloration is reported to the surgeon, since this may indicate necrosis of the stoma. Careful checking of the stoma that is in contact with a catheter is imperative, since improper positioning of the catheter may exert pressure on the stomal tissue, leading to necrosis. The normal stoma may either protrude or be flush with the skin, and edema is common in the early postoperative period. The peristomal skin must be checked for signs of irritation that may be caused by urine leakage, too large an appliance opening, or allergy to the adhesive backing or tape.

Urinary output. Following any type of urinary diversion, urinary output must be carefully monitored in the postoperative phase. Edema of the stoma or of the ureteral anastomosis site may cause failure of adequate urine drainage that may lead to hydronephrosis or to a break in the anastomosis. Other complications that may first be detected by a decreased urinary output include dehydration, obstruction of the ureters, ileal loop ileus, or compromised renal function.

Decreased urinary output associated with symptoms of peritonitis (fever, abdominal distention, and pain) should alert the nurse to the possibility of intraperitoneal leakage caused by a leak at either the intestinal or ureterointestinal anastomosis. If this occurs, emergency surgery is required to repair the leak.

The color and nature of the urinary output are also noted. Blood in the urine is expected in the early postoperative period with gradual clearing. Mucus, a normal discharge from the intestinal segment, is normally secreted from an ileal or colonic conduit. However, mucous threads in the urine from an ureterostomy are abnormal and may indicate the presence of an infection.

The abdominal incision is observed *at least daily* for healing of the suture line. Care of this incision is sometimes complicated by the possibility of urine leakage onto it. An appropriate postoperative drainage bag will minimize this problem.

Body image. A person having a urinary diversion will need time and assistance in adjusting to the change in his or her body, to the loss of the "normal" pattern of elimination, and to the presence of an external pouch. An opportunity for the patient to explore feelings and to begin to cope with all the changes should be provided. Competent physical nursing care is also important, since the person who experiences constant urine leakage and skin breakdown will most likely feel discouraged and depressed. If a person's life is "saved" and the appliance is leaking all the time, it is difficult for the person to believe it possible to resume all presurgical activities. The patient gains a sense of control and independence when the management of the ostomy and its drainage is mastered.

A man undergoing a radical cystectomy for cancer of the bladder will most likely be impotent. There will be a loss of erection, ejaculation, and orgasm. The patient and his sexual partner need help in coping with this information. A referral to a counselor for alternate means of sexual expression may be very helpful.

Self-care. As soon as a person feels able to do so, he or she is encouraged to begin to participate in stomal care with adequate supervision and support. During the appliance changing procedures and related nursing care, the nurse can explain important aspects of ongoing management. This all cannot be accomplished in a day or two before discharge! If possible, one nurse should coordinate the care and teaching. Having one well-informed person responsible for nursing care assists in the development of a trusting relationship that allows the person to feel free to discuss any concerns.

Appliances. Measurement for a permanent appliance occurs about 7 days after surgery when the major edema has subsided. Continued shrinkage of the stoma will probably occur in the following 6 to 8 weeks, so that a check for appropriate fit is required at that time. Several manufacturers provide measuring cards with various-sized holes than can be placed around the stoma to determine the size that will allow 1.5 to 3 mm of skin to show around the stoma. An alternative method is to measure the diameter of the stoma and add 3 to 6 mm to the measurement to obtain the proper size for ordering. The person should be taught how to measure the stoma before discharge. Too large an opening size is a frequent cause of skin excoriation for persons with an ileal loop. Too small an opening in the appliance may restrict circulation or cause trauma to the stoma.

Several types of appliances are available (Figs. 61-9 and 61-10). All have two things in common—a pouch to collect the urine and an outlet at the bottom for easy emptying every 3 or 4 hours. *The basic types of bags are (1) permanent appliances that can be washed and reused, (2) semidisposable bags that fit onto a permanent disk, and (3) one-piece disposable appliances that are discarded after use.* All adhere to the body with some form of adhesive to form a watertight seal. The type of appliance used depends on the individual's preference, body build, and special needs, such as physical or visual impairment. The person is informed of the choices available, but much direction and guidance in selecting the most appropriate appliance may be required. Cost comparisons for the various types of appliances can be made by comparing the expected life of the bag with the current price.

The individual (or care provider) must learn how to manage the assembly, application, emptying, cleaning, and changing of whatever appliance is chosen. The permanent appliance is obtained before discharge so that the person can demonstrate the ability to assemble and apply the appliance. A family member or friend is included in the teaching to provide support at home, but the individual, unless limited physically, is encouraged to be responsible for self-care.

The permanent appliance should be one that will remain in place and free of leakage for at least 24 hours. Most persons can wear an appliance 3 to 5 days between changes; an interval longer than 7 days should be discouraged because of potential odor and crystallization problems. An appropriate schedule that eliminates leakage and odor problems will need to be determined. For example, if the appliance tends to leak on the fifth day, it will need to be changed every 4 days, before leakage occurs. The appliance must be cleaned once or twice a day whether or not it is being replaced.

Proper cleaning of reusable equipment is essential for odor control, general hygiene, and prevention of stomal complications. Manufacturers include cleaning instructions with their equipment. Following are the principles for proper cleaning of reusable urinary appliances:

1. Clean equipment promptly.
2. Use adhesive remover as necessary to remove residue.
3. Avoid soaking equipment for prolonged periods of time (20 to 30 minutes in soap and water is sufficient). Longer soaking speeds deterioration of many appliances.
4. For odor problems soak appliance in half-strength vinegar water for an additional 20 to 30 minutes.

Problems. Odor is generally not a problem in persons with urinary diversions. Deodorants are not recommended for routine use because they cover up odors. If an odor is present, it usually signifies a urinary tract infection, alkaline urine, or inadequate cleansing of the equipment. All of these need correction as soon as possible.

Full- or half-strength vinegar (10 ml) should be inserted into the pouch twice a day. The vinegar is allowed to flow up into the pouch. Vinegar decreases urinary odor and will assist in disinfecting the pouch.[70] A pouch with an antireflux valve is recommended to prevent infections from bacteria found in the pouch.

Stomal problems include bleeding, lacerations, crystal formations, stenosis, hernia, and prolapse. A small amount of bleeding is not uncommon when the stoma is cleansed. This generally clears up immediately.

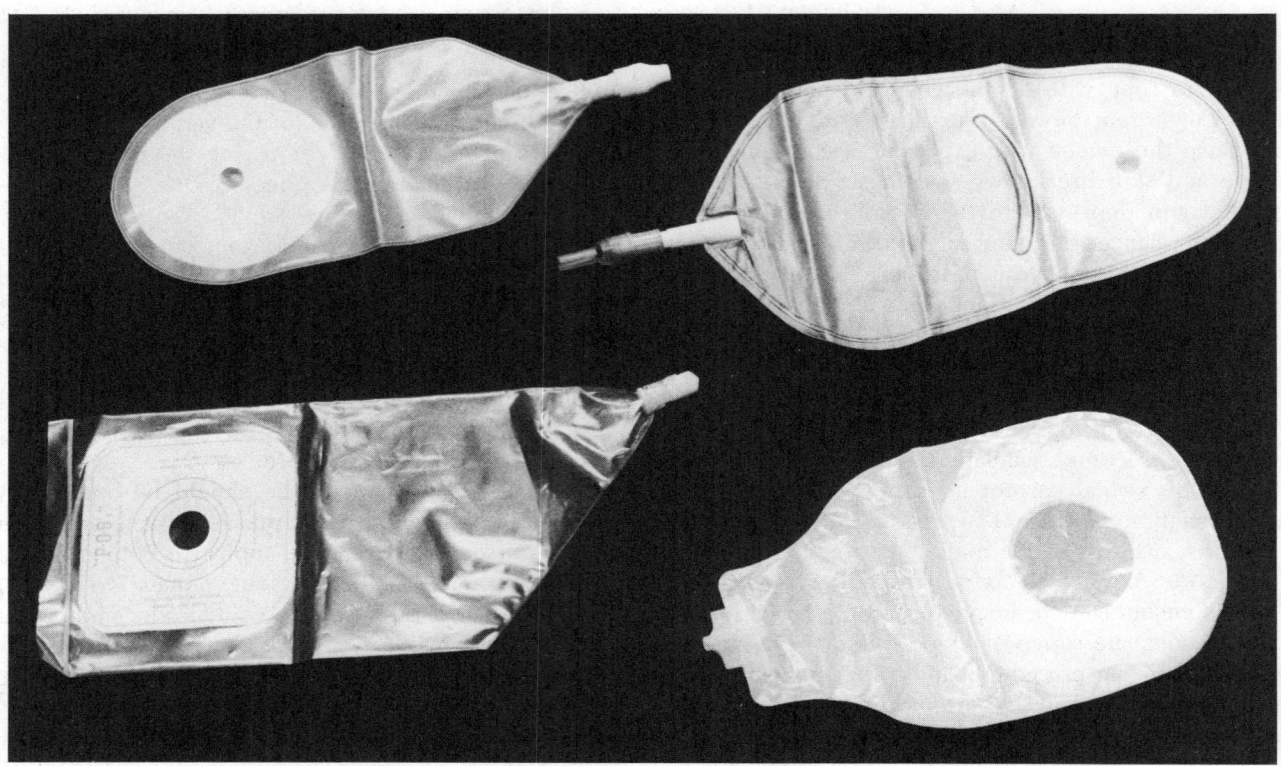

Fig. 61-9. Examples of postoperative drainage bags for urinary stoma.

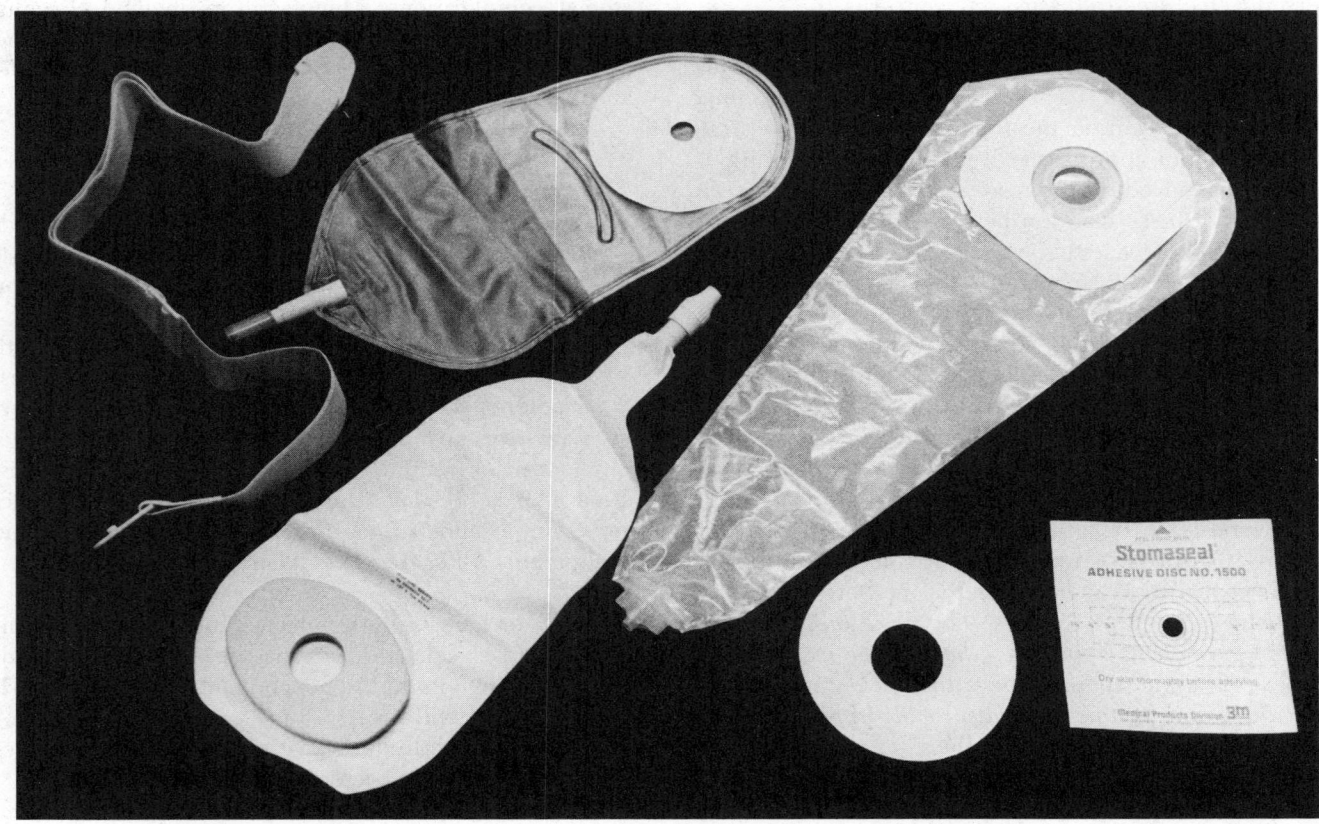

Fig. 61-10. Some examples of urinary appliances used by persons for long-term management of urinary tract diversion. Adhesive tape disks and belt are also shown.

However, a stoma may be traumatized from a sharp blow to the abdomen, such as from the steering wheel in an auto accident. If bleeding occurs, a cold washcloth may be held against the stoma or, with the pouch in place, an ice bag may be used. If bleeding persists or is unusually severe, the physician is notified. The blood can be originating from the urinary tract and may be related to complications such as infection or calculi. Patients also need to be forewarned before taking medications that will discolor the urine. For example, doxorubicin (Adriamycin) will produce red urine.

A stoma may be lacerated by a pouch opening that is too small, a pouch that is misapplied and lies on the stoma, or the misuse of belts. If the source of the irritation is removed, the laceration will heal. If the laceration is through the entire thickness of the stoma and into the lumen, creating a fistula, surgical intervention is required.

Crystal formation on the stoma or peristomal skin is usually related to alkaline urine. However, acidic crystals occur in a small number of patients. Crystals may also result in stomal bleeding. The urine pH should be checked before any treatment is initiated. A sample of the crystals may be sent to the laboratory to determine the chemical composition. Alkaline crystals may be treated with vinegar soaks, acidification of the urine, and disposable pouches. Vinegar (full or half strength) may be applied as a wet soak to the stoma with pouch changes or through the bottom of a pouch with no antireflux valve. If the crystals are formed in acid urine, a solution of bicarbonate may be used. Rubber pouches are more often associated with crystal formation than vinyl or plastic pouches. The crystals collect in the pores of the rubber, and the pouch will feel gritty. The pouch can be cleaned with vinegar or with United's "Urikleen."

Alkaline urine is associated with crystals, recurrent urinary infections, stomal and loop stenosis, and hyperkeratosis of the skin. Alkaline urine has been associated with urea-splitting organisms. The stenosis, according to Hardy et al.,[34] is thought to be the result of an inflamed ileal segment secondary to the presence of alkaline urine. If the surgeon orders stomal dilation, the patient should be instructed to insert a sterile, gloved, lubricated finger gently into the stoma. The hyperkeratosis consists of raised, often painful lesions around the stoma. The skin problem is usually related to an improperly fitted faceplate and alkaline urine. The exposed skin is covered by recalibrating the stomal opening and treating the skin (see box below).

Peristomal hernias and stomal prolapses may occur after hospitalization. These require surgical intervention as the primary treatment. Some patients may elect not to have a hernia or prolapse repaired.

Electrolyte imbalance may develop if the urine is retained in the conduit because of stomal or loop ste-

---

TREATMENT OF SKIN PROBLEMS*

Rash

Location: Rash can be located under tape, under faceplate, and on any part of skin where pouch comes in contact with skin. Generalized reddish appearance that covers an entire area, similiar to diaper rash, will be seen.

Cause:
1. Leaking appliance.
2. Perspiration.
3. Allergies to tape.
4. Hair follicle irritation.

Remedy:
1. Use heat lamp† and/or hair dryer to dry skin.
2. Use Colly-Seel, Stomahesive, Holliseal, or Reliaseal between skin and faceplate until skin clears. Try to leave on 24 to 48 hr.
3. Powder skin on which pouch lies (not under faceplate).
4. Make or buy pouch cover.
5. Wearing pouch belt that is too tight may break seal.

6. If rash does not clear up in 5 to 7 days, consult an enterostomal therapist.

Cement or solvent burns

Location: Burns can be located anywhere under faceplate but usually are found at outside edges.

Cause: Agents in cement or solvent were not allowed to evaporate off skin surface before applying pouch, and/or cement was too thick and was unable to dry completely. Directions on these products should be carefully followed. Patients should be patch tested with the products before application.

Remedy:
1. Use heat lamp and/or hair dryer for weeping skin.
2. Cover burn with Colly-Seel, Holliseal, Stomahesive, or Reliaseal and apply pouch in usual way. Try to leave pouch on 24 to 48 hr.
3. If burn does not clear up in 5 to 7 days, consult an enterostomal therapist.

---

*From Broadwell, D.C., and Sorrells, S.L.: Summary of your urinary diversion care. Copyright © 1976 by Debra C. Broadwell.
†NOTE: Heat lamp refers to a lamp with a 60-watt bulb, 1 ft away from the stoma for 10 to 15 min. Never use a sunlamp. Never use a heat lamp on radiated skin. A hair dryer should be set on a cool setting. *Continued.*

TREATMENT OF SKIN PROBLEMS—cont'd

Ulcerated area on stoma

Location: Anywhere on stoma.

Cause: Opening of pouch was too small or activities were causing faceplate to rub or cut into stoma.

Remedy: 1. Enlarge size of pouch opening. (Opening should be at least ⅛ in. larger than stoma.)
2. Evaluate patient's activities; a different size or shaped faceplate may be necessary.
3. Loosen belt; if too tight, belt may cause faceplate to ride into stoma.
4. If the ulcerated area does not clear up in 5 to 7 days, consult an enterostomal therapist.

Infected or irritated hair follicles

Location: Under faceplate, raised reddened areas (similar to acne) at shaft of hair follicle.

Cause: Not keeping area under faceplate shaved.

Remedy: 1. Must let the irritation improve before removing any more hair by shaving or cutting.
2. Use hair dryer and/or heat lamp to dry area if it is oozing.
3. Use Colly-Seel, Hollihesive, Stomahesive, or Reliaseal between the skin and faceplate until irritation improves. Try to leave on 24 to 48 hr.
4. If irritation does not clear up in 5 to 7 days, consult an enterostomal therapist.

Water-logged skin

Location: Between opening of faceplate and stoma.

Cause: Too much skin exposed between stoma and faceplate opening, and thus urine pools on skin.

Remedy: 1. Use hair dryer and/or heat lamp to dry.
2. Use Colly-Seel, Stomahesive, or ReliaSeal under faceplate, firmly hugging stoma.
3. Decrease size of faceplate opening.
4. If this condition does not clear up in 5 to 7 days, consult an enterostomal therapist.

Monilial infection

Location: On exposed skin between stoma and faceplate and possibly spreading under faceplate.

Cause: Yeast infection is often seen when patient is on antibiotics, which alter normal bacterial flora.

Remedy: 1. Use heat lamp and/or hair dryer for the area.
2. Apply nystatin (Mycostatin) powder to area, if prescribed, blow off excess powder, and seal this in with a thin coat of a skin sealant. Apply pouch in usual manner. (You will need a prescription for nystatin.)
3. Drink lots of fluids.
4. If infection does not clear up in 5 to 7 days, consult an enterostomal therapist.

Alkaline crystals

Location: One stoma and/or around stoma base.

Cause: Alkaline urine and predisposition to stone formation.

Remedy: 1. Vinegar compresses on the stoma when changing the pouch.
2. Insert vinegar into pouch while wearing it. For a minor formation, insert twice a day; for an excessive formation, insert four times a day.
   a. Empty pouch.
   b. Instill 1 to 2 oz. of vinegar solution into pouch.
   c. Lie down so solution will bathe inside of pouch and stoma for approximately 20 min.
   d. Empty pouch and rinse with cool water. NOTE: The vinegar solution may discolor stoma, making it appear "blanched" or "white." It will return to its normal red color in a few minutes.
3. Use vinyl or plastic pouches until condition clears, or use new rubber pouches. Rubber pouches tend to precipitate crystals inside pouch, which may cause bleeding and irritation to stoma.

---

nosis. The mucosa of the conduit reabsorbs chlorides from the urine, and the patient may develop a metabolic hyperchloremic acidosis. A person with good renal function has no difficulty excreting the reabsorbed chlorides. When the renal function is compromised, the patient is more likely to develop electrolyte problems.[64]

Discharge planning. Before discharge from the hospital the nurse must be certain that the individual can manage the urinary drainage and can detect any deviations from normal. At least one return visit or an opportunity for telephone consultation with the primary nurse involved in the teaching is extremely helpful so that questions that arise after returning home can be discussed. Visiting nurse assistance may be required for a period of time. Ongoing urologic care will be required, including urine cultures, which are correctly obtained by catheter from the ileal or sigmoid loop stoma. A specimen taken from the pouch is likely to be contaminated. Catheterization of a ureterostomy stoma is generally performed by the physician unless nurses have been instructed in the procedure.

Outcome criteria for the person with a urinary stoma

The person or significant others can:

1. Explain rationale for urinary diversion and de-

scribe anatomic variation created by diversion.

2. Describe any necessary activity restrictions and duration of limits (avoidance of heavy lifting).

3. Recognize normal stomal and peristomal skin conditions, and state changes requiring medical assistance:
   a. Keep stoma pink, moist, patent, clean, and free of infection.
   b. Keep peristomal skin intact and free of infection.

4. Describe potential for return to preoperative sexual performance and fertility.

5. Demonstrate care of appliance:
   a. Change and empty appliance.
   b. State how often to empty and change appliance.
   c. Describe principles of care of appliance including cleaning and maintenance.
   d. Describe types of appliances available and where to seek help in selecting appropriate appliances.
   e. Review written list of where and how to order appropriate appliances and supplies.
   f. Demonstrate how to measure stoma for optimal appliance fit.

6. Describe signs and symptoms of a urinary tract infection and the necessity of notifying the physician.

7. State plans for follow-up care and continued urologic surveillance.

Intervention for the incontinent person

Urinary incontinence, the involuntary expulsion of urine, may be encountered in a number of temporary and permanent conditions. Inability to control urination is a problem that frequently leads to emotional distress and can seriously impair an individual's socialization patterns if not managed in a suitable manner. Incontinence must be managed either by the person or by others in a way that makes the person feel physically and emotionally comfortable and socially acceptable.

Persons with incontinence often present baffling management problems. Solutions require that the nurse understand the physiologic basis of incontinence.

Factors promoting urinary continence

Bladder sphincter control is necessary to have urinary continence. Such control requires normal voluntary and involuntary muscle action coordinated by a normal urethrobladder reflex. Understanding this coordinated sequence of nerve stimuli and muscle action will help the nurse understand how continence is maintained.

As bladder filling occurs, the pressure within the bladder gradually increases. The detrusor muscle (the three-layered bladder wall) responds by relaxing to accommodate the greater volume. When a certain point of filling is reached, usually 150 to 200 ml of urine, the parasympathetic stretch receptors located in the bladder wall are stimulated. The stimuli are transmitted through the afferent fibers of the reflex arc to the reflex center for micturition. This reflex center is located in the S2 to S4 segments of the spinal cord (Fig. 61-11). Impulses are then carried through the efferent fibers of the reflex arc to the bladder, causing reflex contraction of the detrusor muscle. The internal sphincter, which is normally closed, reciprocally opens and the urine enters the posterior urethra. Relaxation of the external sphincter and perineal muscles follows, and the bladder content is released. Completion of this reflex act can be interrupted and voiding postponed through release of inhibitory impulses from the cortical center, which results in voluntary contraction of the external sphincter. If any part of this complex function is upset, there is apt to be incontinence of urine.

Urinary incontinence

Etiology and pathopysiology

The five major causes of urinary incontinence and the nature of the incontinence they cause are outlined in Table 61-1.

Cerebral clouding is most common in the aged. In many instances the very elderly person is incontinent because of a lack of awareness of the need to empty the bladder. This type of incontinence is often not associated with any definite pathologic problem at the cerebral level. Cerebral clouding also occurs in acutely ill persons, who may be so ill that cerebration is dulled. They may not be able to think or may not have the energy to exercise voluntary control. Likewise a person who is comatose is incontinent because of loss of the ability to control voluntarily the opening of the external sphincter. As soon as urine is released into the posterior urethra, the bladder contracts and empties. This is the reason why voiding sometimes occurs under anesthesia.

Infection anywhere in the urinary tract may lead to incontinence, since bacteria in the urine cause irritation of the mucosa of the bladder and *stimulate* the *urethrobladder reflex abnormally*.

Disturbance of the central nervous system pathways may occur in diseases such as *cerebral embolus, cerebral hemorrhage, brain tumor, meningitis,* or *traumatic*

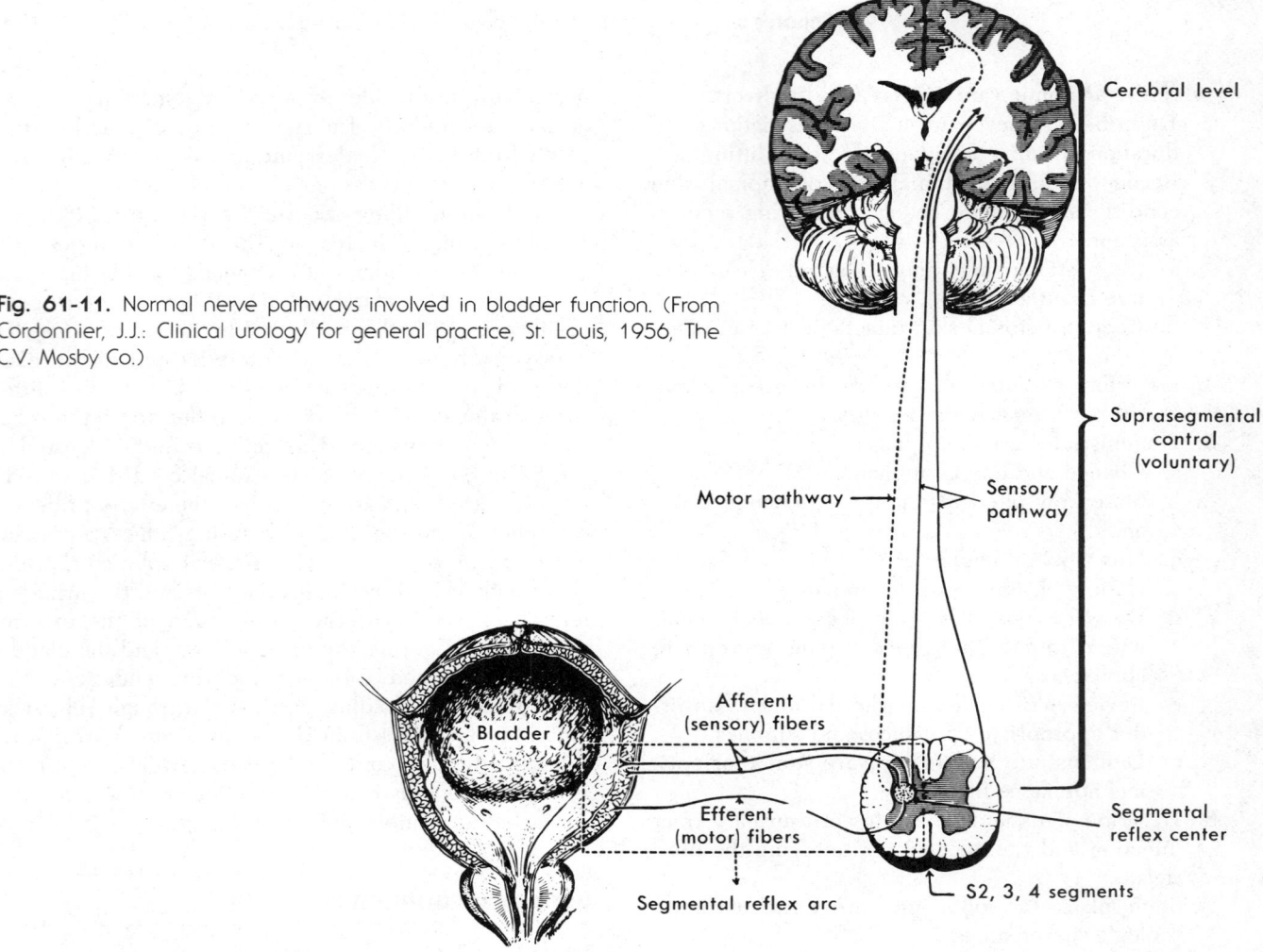

Fig. 61-11. Normal nerve pathways involved in bladder function. (From Cordonnier, J.J.: Clinical urology for general practice, St. Louis, 1956, The C.V. Mosby Co.)

TABLE 61-1. Major causes of urinary incontinence

| Cause of urinary incontinence | Factors involved | | | | |
	Awareness of need to void	Cortical ability to inhibit voiding	Reflex arc	Bladder response to filling	Result
Cerebral clouding	Impaired	Impaired	Intact	Normal	Uncontrolled voiding because of reflex response
Infection	Intact	Intact, but overcome by strong reflex response	Abnormally stimulated	Heightened	Voiding because of strong reflex response (urgency)
Disturbance of CNS pathways (cortical lesions)	Diminished	Impaired	Intact	Heightened	Voiding because of reflex response
Disturbance of urethrobladder reflex					
Upper motor neuron lesion	Destroyed	Destroyed	Intact but deranged	Heightened	Voiding because of reflex response
Lower motor neuron lesion	Destroyed	Destroyed	Destroyed or impaired	Diminished to absent	Distention or incomplete emptying
Tissue damage	Intact	Intact, but not functional because of poor muscle response	Intact	Normal	Loss of control of voiding because of muscular impairment

injury of the brain. Adequate voluntary (cortical or cerebral) control of bladder function is prevented in these situations. Urgency incontinence may be present as a result of the inability to inhibit completion of the urethrobladder reflex by the higher centers.

Disturbance of the urethrobladder reflex may result from *lesions of the spinal cord or damage to peripheral nerves of the bladder*. This form of incontinence may be seen in persons with spinal cord malformations, injuries, or tumors, and those with compression of the cord caused by fractures of the vertebrae, herniated disk, metastatic tumor, or postoperative edema of the spinal cord. This type of difficulty can result in two types of responses known as *neurogenic bladder*. The person with a neurogenic bladder has no way of knowing when voiding is occurring.

Lesions above the S2 level of the spinal cord or impairment of the cerebrocortical centers do not destroy the reflex arc for voiding, although they may derange it. Such lesions destroy the potential for cortical control to inhibit the reflex. The result is an "upper motor neuron" or "automatic" bladder. The bladder is hypertonic and has a small capacity (less than 150 ml). The increased detrusor tone and increased sensitivity to small amounts of urine present in the bladder result in precipitous voiding and the potential for vesicoureteral reflux.

Damage to nerves in the cauda equina or sacral segments of the spinal cord may cause destruction of the reflex arc by interruption of its afferent, efferent, or central components. The result is a "lower motor neuron" or "flaccid" bladder. The bladder is hypotonic with capacities of 500 ml or more. Overflow incontinence, retention of residual urine, and the potential for vesicoureteral reflux are problems imposed by a hypotonic bladder.

Overflow incontinence is considered to be caused by pressure exerted on the distended bladder by the abdominal muscles. Residual urine, urine remaining in the bladder after incomplete emptying, provides a medium for the growth of bacteria, and urinary tract infections are common.

Tissue damage to the sphincters of the bladder from instrumentation, surgery, or accidents, scarring following urethral infections, lesions involving the sphincter, or relaxation of the perineal structures may cause urinary incontinence. The latter cause of incontinence is seen occasionally following childbirth. The problem is local in nature and does not involve the nervous system.

Assessment

Until the cause of a patient's urinary incontinence is understood, the question of whether rehabilitation of the bladder is possible cannot be answered. The nurse's role in the assessment includes accurate recording of intake and output, amount and frequency of voiding, symptoms of urgency, indications of the state of awareness of the need to void, and the appearance of the urine. In the assessment the nurse must also include general data concerning the person's condition, ability to follow directions, and any other factors that may predispose to or directly cause urinary incontinence.

After all available data concerning incontinence have been collected and a reasonable cause for the incontinence determined, a program of appropriate management may be instituted. If the incontinence has been a long-standing problem well managed by the person or the family, continuation of usual methods of management is facilitated. In these instances, particularly in a hospital or other institutional setting, the nurse should ascertain the method used by the person and provide whatever equipment or assistance is needed during the stay. Although the person may be managing well, additional suggestions may be offered by the nurse concerning newer equipment available, less costly equipment, and so on as appropriate. The patient may wish to try alternative methods even after discharge from the setting.

Control of urinary incontinence

No program of bladder retraining or management of uncontrolled incontinence is likely to be successful without the cooperation of the individual involved. The probable outcomes of the management program should be included in planning for implementation of the program.

Control of urinary incontinence is largely dependent on its cause. Measures include treatment of associated conditions, programs of bladder retraining, surgical procedures, or the use of internal or external drainage devices. Both the person and nurse need to know that rehabilitation may take weeks or months to accomplish. The person often becomes discouraged by recurring accidental voiding and needs a great deal of encouragement. It is often helpful to teach the physiology of voiding so that there is better understanding of the problem. Consistency in carrying out any plan for bladder control is often the key to success.

Intervention related to cause

Sphincter dysfunction. Repair of a sphincter that has been cut is almost impossible. When the *external sphincter* has been damaged, the person will be incontinent on urgency. A voiding schedule can be planned so that voiding occurs before the bladder is full enough to exert sufficient pressure to open the internal sphincter involuntarily. When the *internal sphincter* is damaged, there may be no acute feeling of the need to void. Here the problem is not one of incontinence but of retention. To assure regular emptying of the bladder, a regular voiding schedule is necessary. *If both sphinc-*

ters are damaged, there will be total incontinence.

Stress incontinence. Urinary *incontinence* that occurs during *coughing, straining,* or *heavy lifting* is termed *stress incontinence*. It is seen primarily in women who have relaxed pelvic musculature, but it may also occur in men following prostatectomy. When bladder pressure is suddenly increased, urine enters the proximal third of the urethra then returns to the bladder when the pressure is decreased after exertion. Some of the urine escapes through the urethra. The person is continent at night because bladder pressure is decreased in the recumbent position. A woman who has a cystocele (p. 1691) may not be aware of the problem until after the cystocele is repaired.[44]

Perineal exercises are helpful in controlling mild stress incontinence. The exercises consist in tightening and relaxing perineal and gluteal muscles and can be performed in a number of ways. Much of the problem of incontinence caused by a relaxed perineum in women can be prevented if perineal exercises are taught before and following childbirth. These exercises also may be included as part of the health teaching of any woman. Following are different methods for performing perineal exercises:

1. Tighten the perineal muscles as if to prevent voiding. Hold for 3 seconds, then relax.
2. Inhale through pursed lips while tightening perineal muscles.
3. Bear down as if to have a bowel movement. Relax then tighten perineal muscles.
4. Hold a pencil in the fold between the buttock and thigh.
5. Sit on the toilet with knees held wide apart. Start and stop the urinary stream.

Surgery may be indicated for severe stress incontinence. A *vesicourethropexy* (Marshal-Marchetti operation) consists of fixation of the urethra to the fascia of the rectus muscle of the abdomen with support given to the neck of the bladder. A suprapubic incison is usually made, but a transvaginal repair may be carried out if there is scar tissue around the urethra from vaginal surgery. A urethral catheter is inserted postoperatively and maintained for 5 to 6 days. The urine may be pink, but the urethral catheter is not irrigated as a rule. It is not uncommon for difficulty in voiding to be experienced immediately after the indwelling catheter is removed. The woman is observed for signs of vaginal bleeding. Straining and use of Valsalva's maneuver should be avoided until healing has occurred, and mild laxatives may be given to prevent straining from constipation. Surgeons differ in the amount of activity permitted in the early postoperative period.

Urgency. Incontinence caused by urinary tract infection is generally temporary, responding to treatment of the infection by systemic antibiotics. Specific causes of infection such as obstruction must be identified and corrected where possible. Provision must be made for adequate fluid intake of 3000 ml or more per day unless contraindicated by the person's medical condition. Because of heightened bladder sensitivity to even small amounts of urine, urgency to void demands rapid response by the nurse to the request for help to void.

The person who has a brain tumor, meningitis, or traumatic injury to the brain that prevents adequate voluntary control of bladder function and causes urgency incontinence by inhibiting cortical control over the urethrobladder reflex may also respond to a bladder retraining program. If the person's condition or response prohibits such a program, an internal or external drainage divice should be used.

Neurogenic bladder dysfunction. Persons with injuries of the spinal cord experience a transitory period of "spinal shock" in which urinary retention occurs (p. 821). This is treated with continuous or intermittent catheter drainage that aims to prevent urinary tract infection and overdistention of the bladder. Following this acute stage, further management depends upon the exact nature of any residual neurogenic bladder dysfunction. Persons with a lesion above the sacral segments and who have an intact urethrobladder reflex may initiate voiding by pinching or stroking trigger areas of the thighs or suprapubic area. In persons with a lower motor neuron lesion the use of the *Credé method*, which consists of exerting manual pressure over the bladder, may be ordered to provide for more complete bladder emptying. The appropriateness of this technique must be determined by the physician based upon the person's complete urologic status. An increasing number of persons with neurogenic bladder dysfunction are being taught intermittent self-catheterization using clean technique to prevent infection and manage incontinence (p. 1528). Maintenance of a regular schedule is stressed, and the frequency of catheterization is determined on an individual basis.

Certain medications are sometimes utilized alone or in conjunction with an intermittent catheterization program in the management of incontinence related to neurogenic bladder dysfunction. Alpha adrenergic drugs such as ephedrine sulfate are used to increase urethral resistance. Anticholinergic drugs such as propantheline (Pro-Banthine) are prescribed to control the reflex bladder activity.

General intervention

Bladder retraining. When incontinence is caused by dulled cerebration in the elderly, by confusion, or by acute illness, control can usually be established if a persistent retraining schedule is carried out. A voiding schedule is developed and strictly adhered to until the person gradually relearns to recognize and react appropriately to the feeling of having to void. A successful program of this type, leading to complete rehabilitation, or continence, requires mental competence of the individual. Otherwise someone else must always remind the person to follow the schedule.

People ordinarily void on awakening, before retiring, and before or after meals. If a diuretic such as coffee has been taken it is usually necessary to void about 30 minutes later. Using this knowledge, the nurse can begin to set up a schedule for placing the person on a bedpan or taking the person to the toilet. Then, if a record is kept for a few days of the times the person voids involuntarily, it is usually possible to determine the normal voiding pattern. If the schedule based on the pattern of incontinence is not successful, toileting every 1 to 2 hours should be carried out on a 24-hour basis.

During the retraining program, *mobilization* of the individual, attention to the *position* assumed for voiding, and adequate *fluid intake* contribute to reduction of the possibility of infection. Complete emptying of the bladder eliminates the possibility of residual urine acting as a medium for bacterial growth, while a high fluid intake provides for internal bladder irrigation.

Elderly persons isolated from their families and familiar surroundings, confused by institutionalization, or suffering feelings of loss of self-esteen frequently respond well to mobilization in bladder retraining programs. Their circulation is enhanced by the imposed mobility, their awareness is increased, and they respond to the attention given them. In instances where nurses believe that it is easier to change bed linen than it is to establish an appropriate bladder retraining program, a disservice is done to the individual and more work is actually created for the nurse. The person becomes subject to urinary tract infection and skin breakdown, and feelings of worthlessness are increased. For those who can be continent, incontinence is an indignity.

When it is possible, toileting should be carried out in surroundings that will remind the person of the voiding function; that is, the person should be taken to the bathroom where the toilet can be used. If this is not possible, a bedside commode can be an adequate substitute. Many men can void into a urinal more easily if allowed to stand at the bedside. The use of a bedpan is unfamiliar and distasteful to most persons, but in instances where women must remain in bed, voiding into a bedpan can be facilitated if the head of the bed is rolled up as high as allowed. This kind of positioning is more consistent with the position normally assumed for voiding and facilitates complete emptying of the bladder. Few persons can void adequately in the supine position.

Providing adequate amounts of fluids, a minimum of 3000 ml per day, is necessary to ensure that there will be adequate amounts of urine produced and present in the bladder to stimulate the voiding reflex at the proper times. Fluids may be given at scheduled times, the largest portion being given during the day before 4:00 PM to decrease the frequency of voiding through the night. Persons on fluid restriction because of medical problems should, of course, receive no more fluids than the amount prescribed.

External urinary drainage. Occasionally there are justifications for the use of an indwelling catheter for the incontinent patient. Such reasons include the need to protect a surgical incision or to permit healing of a decubitus ulcer in the area. Indwelling catheterization, however, presents many potential dangers such as urinary tract infection, urethritis, epididymitis, and urethral fistulas. All other means to manage the incontinence should be tried before resorting to catheterization. (Refer to p. 1521 for details of catheter management.)

For the man external drainage can be easily accomplished by applying a watertight apparatus to the penis. The following is one method. Select a condom of the correct size. Puncture a hole in the closed end of the condom with an applicator stick. Attach the punctured end of the condom to a firm rubber or plastic drainage tube with either a 3-mm (1/8-in.) piece of rubber tubing or a strip of adhesive tape (Fig. 61-12). Before applying the condom, clean and dry the penis thoroughly and check it for edema, skin breaks, or discoloration. Invert the condom and roll it onto the penis. There should be no roll at the top that could cause constriction. At least 2.5 cm (1 in.) of the condom should remain between the meatus and drainage tube to allow for penile erection. There should not be so much slack as to cause

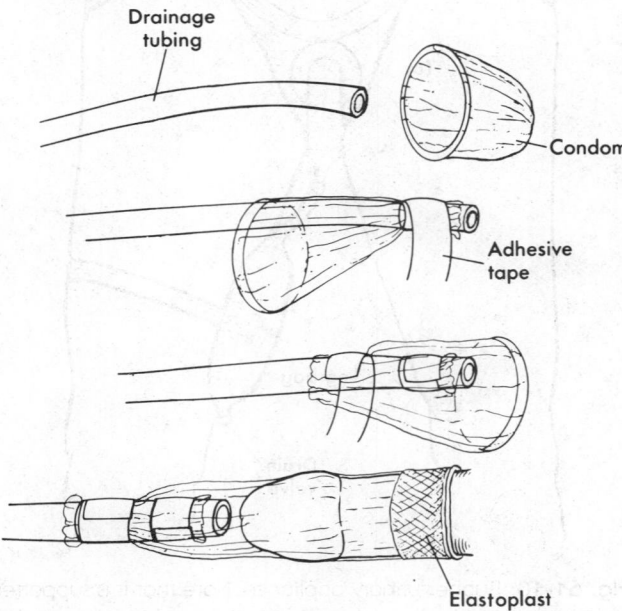

Fig. 61-12. One method of making an external drainage apparatus.

twisting and subsequent interference with drainage. Elastoplast is then applied over the condom and around the penis (never touching the skin). *Under no circumstances should adhesive tape be used.* The Elastoplast must not be constricting.

The external catheter should be removed daily and the skin washed and checked. Frequent checking is necessary to determine whether edema or irritation is present and to ensure proper drainage. This is especially important in men with loss of sensation. The external device is attached to straight drainage or to a leg bag.

For persons who need external catheter drainage indefinitely, a rubber urinary appliance (sometimes called an incontinence urinal) may be used (Fig. 61-13). There are several models available, and the one best suited to the person's needs is selected. Two appliances are recommended to allow for cleaning and drying. They should be washed in mild soap, turned inside out, and thoroughly dried before application.

Most persons prefer to manage their own incontinence if they are at all able to do so. The nurse supports and encourages this, offering assistance as necessary and instruction in basic principles of skin care, equipment selection, and maintenance. The choice of management method should take into account the person's ability to manage as independently as is possible.

Artificial sphincter. A relatively new surgical procedure, implantation of an artificial urinary sphincter, can be utilized to achieve continence when other methods have failed. In this procedure a hydraulically activated sphincter mechanism is placed around the urethra or bladder neck. The sphincter is made to open and close at will be squeezing one of two bulbs implanted under the skin of the labia or scrotum (Fig. 61-14). Postoperative nursing care of the person with such an implant includes observation for and reporting of fever or pain on inflation of the device, swelling of the genitalia, and recurrence of incontinence. Complications of the procedure include erosion of the urethra, abscess, cellulitis, and mechanical malfunctions in the system. Men have had more success with the artificial sphincter than have women.

Uncontrolled urinary incontinence

In some instances none of the above measures are appropriate or successful. Therefore, nursing goals of assisting the person to remain clean, free of odor, and free of ducubiti may require external urinary protection; the type varies with the sex, functional status, and physical status of the person.

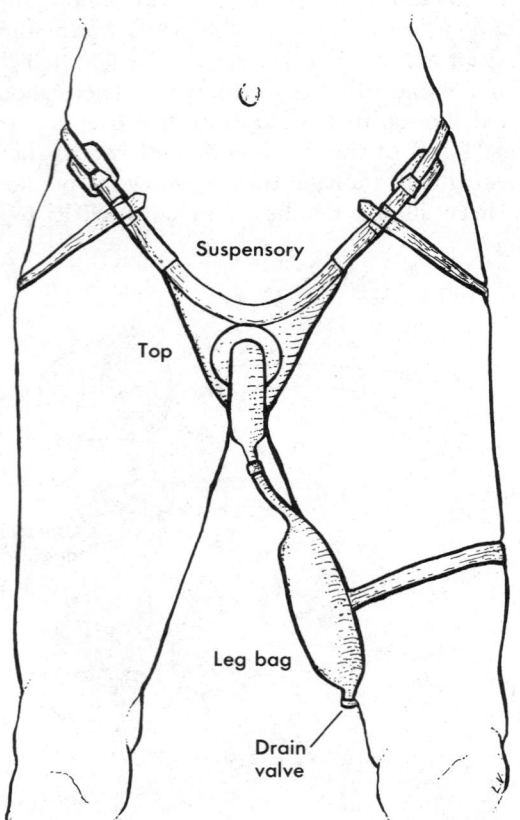

Fig. 61-13. Rubber urinary appliance. Note that it is supported by strap around waist and under buttock and is connected to drainage bag strapped to leg. Drain valve at bottom of bag is removed for emptying.

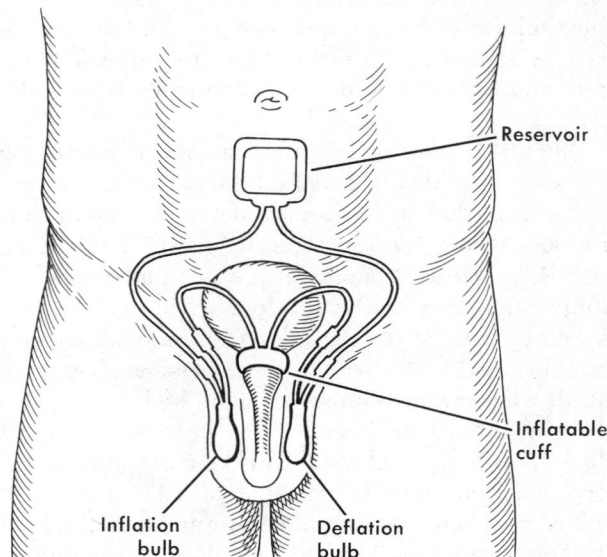

Fig. 61-14. Artificial bladder sphincter. Compression and release of inflation pump bulb inflates cuff surrounding urethra stopping urine flow. Compression and release of delflation pump bulb deflates inflatable cuff, returning fluid to storage reservoir. This releases urethral constriction, permitting urine to flow.

Those who are incapacitated by critical illness or unconsciousness are dependent upon the nursing staff to manage their incontinence by protective pants or external catheter drainage. Others may be capable of some or all of their own management. Men and woman may wear protective waterproof pants that are lined by disposable or washable absorbent pads. A resourceful person may be able to improvise equipment that is as comfortable and is less costly than commercially available pants. Zippers, Velcro, elastic, and a variety of waterproof materials may be used. Bedding and furniture can be protected with waterproof materials such as the squares of absorbent cellucotton backed with light plastic that are commercially available.

Whatever the type of padding, liners, or pants used, frequent changing is required for skin protection and comfort. The perineal and genital areas are thoroughly washed with soap and water and dried well at each changing. If possible, the person should be bathed in a tub of warm water at least once a day. Periodic exposure of the perineal area to the air is beneficial. Zinc oxide powder can be applied to lessen irritation. Excess amounts of powder are avoided, as this will cake on the skin, causing irritation. Deodorant sprays for use on dressings and liners are valuable, but they may cause skin irritation in persons who develop hypersensitivity to them. Deodorant room fresheners may be helpful if the odor is strong.

Special bed arrangements are helpful for persons who are confined to bed for long periods of time. A *Bradford frame* with an opening under which a pan or urinal can be placed is helpful for a person who is incontinent. A similar arrangement can be improvised by building the bed up with padding so that there is a depressed area in which a receptacle for drainage can be placed. This arrangement should be made so that the receptacle does not come in contact with the patient's skin. Sometimes, if the problem is expected to go on for years, a circular hole can be cut in the mattress, the edges padded, and a funnel and collection bottle placed beneath the opening. A *Stryker frame, Foster bed,* or *CircOlectric bed* also can be modified to accommodate the incontinent person.

If the person can be up, his or her favorite chair can be equipped with a commode seat. Special commode wheelchairs are also available, making it possible for the person to be more comfortable and to mingle socially with others.

Outcome criteria for the person who is incontinent

1. The person is free of perineal skin excoriation.
2. The person is free of urinary odor.
3. The person or significant others can:

   a. Describe the relationship of adequate hygiene to the mainteneance of skin integrity.
   b. Describe the relationship of adequate fluid intake to facilitate bladder training.
   c. Describe the bladder training plan.
   d. Describe how to care for minor skin problems if they occur.
   e. State how to obtain professional and community resources.
     (1) Agencies that are available when necessary.
     (2) How to obtain and maintain any needed supplies and equipment (drainage systems, commodes, protective padding, special beds).
     (3) Where and when to seek assistance if problems are encountered.
   f. State plans for follow-up care.

REFERENCES AND SELECTED READINGS
Contemporary

1. American Cancer Society, Inc.: Living with your urostomy (urinary diversion), New York, 1979, The Society.
2. American Cancer Society, Inc.: Colostomy, ileostomy and ureterostomy care: a guide of practical information for nurses, New York, 1977, The Society.
3. Anderson, R.U.: Response of bladder and urethral mucosa to catheterization, J.A.M.A. **242:**451-453, 1979.
4. *Baum, M.E.: I want to be dry, Nurs. '78 **8:**75-78, Feb. 1978.
5. *Beaumont, E.: Urinary drainage system, Nurs. '74 **4:**52-60, Jan. 1974.
6. Beber, C.R.: Freedom for the incontinent, Am. J. Nurs. **80:**482-484, 1980.
7. *Bellfly, L.: You can improve your catheterized patient's care, RN **40:**33-35, 1977.
8. Bielski, M.: Symposium on infection control: preventing infection in the catheterized patient, Nurs. Clin. North Am. **15:**703-713, 1980.
9. Birum, L., and Zimmerman, D.: Catheter plugs as a source of infection, Am. J. Nurs. **71:**2150-2152, 1971.
10. Broadwell, D.C., and Jackson, B.S.: Principles of ostomy care, St. Louis, 1982, The C.V. Mosby Co.
11. Broadwell, D.C., and Sorrells, S.L.: Summary of your urinary diversion care, unpublished material, 1976.
12. Brundage, D.J.: Nursing management of renal problems, ed. 2, St. Louis, 1980, The C.V. Mosby Co.
13. *Champion, V.: Clean technique for intermittent self-catheterization, Nurs. Res. **25:**13-18, 1976.
14. *Chezem, J.: Urinary diversion: select aspects of nursing management, Nurs. Clin. North Am. **11:**445-456, 1976.
15. *Cleland, V., et al.: Prevention of bateriuria in female patients with indwelling catheters, Nurs. Res. **20:**309-318, 1971.
16. *DeGroot, J.: Catheter-induced urinary tract infections: how can we prevent them? Nurs. '76 **6:**34-37, Aug. 1976.
17. DeGroot, J., and Kunin, C.: Indwelling catheters, Am. J. Nurs. **75:**448-449, 1975.
18. Dericks, V.: The psychological hurdles of new ostomates: helping them up and over, Nurs. '74 **4:**52-55, Oct. 1974.

*References preceded by an asterisk are particularly well suited for student reading.

19. Dericks, V., and Donovan, C.: The ostomy patient really needs you, Nurs. '76 **6**:30-33, Sept. 1976.

20. Diokno, A., and Taub, M.: Experience with the artificial urinary sphincter at Michigan, J. Urol. **116**:496-500, 1976.

21. *Dobbins, J., and Aliet, C.: Experience with the lateral position for catheterization, Nurs. Clin. North Am. **6**:373-379, 1971.

22. Donovan, C., and Lenneberg, E.: Guidelines for the rehabilitation of ostomy patients, Glenville, Ill., 1975, International Association of Enterostomal Therapy, Inc.

23. Dowd, J.B.: Urinary diversion: alternatives and techniques, Surg. Clin. North Am. **60**:687-702, 1980.

24. *Garner, J.: Urinary catheter care, Nurs. '74 **4**:54-56, Feb. 1974.

25. Gault, P.: Six patients with bladder cancer and how they fared after surgery, Nurs. '77 **7**:48-55, Nov. 1977.

26. Glenn, J.F., editor: Urologic surgery, ed. 2, Hagerstown, Md., 1975, Harper & Row, Publishers.

27. Gonzalez, R., and DeWolf, W.: The artificial bladder sphincter AS-721 for the treatment of incontinence in patients with neurogenic bladder, J. Urol. **121**:71-72, 1979.

28. Graham, S.D.: Present urological treatments of spinal cord injury patients, J. Urol. **126**:1-3, 1981.

29. Grant, M., and Kubo, W.: Assessing a patient's hydration status, Am. J. Nurs. **75**:1306-1311, 1975.

30. Gross, P.A., et al.: The fallacy of cultures of the tips of Foley catheters, Surg. Gynecol. Obstet. **139**:597-598, 1974.

31. *Gurevich, I.: The new urine meters, Nurs. '80 **10**:47-52, Dec. 1980.

32. Gurevich, I.: Selection criteria for closed urinary drainage systems, Superv. Nurse **10**:39-46, 1979.

33. Hagen-Cook, K., and Althausen, A.: Early observations on 31 adults with non-refluxing colon conduits, J. Urol. **121**:13-16, 1979.

34. Hardy, B.E., et al.: Strictures of the ileal loop, J. Urol. **117**:358-361, 1977.

35. Hartman, M.: Intermittent self catheterization, Nurs. '78 **8**:72-75, Nov. 1978.

36. Hinkle, M.T., and Bowditch, R.R.: The great stent mystery: can you solve it? Nurs. '81 **11**:94-95, April 1981.

37. Hollister, Incorporated: Managing a urostomy . . . so it doesn't manage you, Spokane, Wash., 1974, Hollister.

38. Hurd, J.K., Jr.: Urinary stress incontinence, Surg. Clin. North Am. **60**:425-433, 1980.

39. *Jensen, V.: Better techniques for bagging stomas. I. Urinary ostomies, Nurs. '74 **4**:60-64, July 1974.

40. Johnson, J.H.: Rehabilitative aspects of neurologic bladder dysfunction, Nurs. Clin. North Am. **15**:293-307, 1980.

41. King, A.W.: Nursing management of stomas of the genitourinary system. In Broadwell, D.C., and Jackson, B.S., editors: Principles of ostomy care, St. Louis, 1982, The C.V. Mosby Co.

42. *Kunin, C.: Detection, prevention and management of urinary tract infections, ed. 3, Philadelphia, 1979, Lea & Febiger.

43. *Langford, T.: Nursing problem: bacteriuria and indwelling catheter, Am. J. Nurs. **72**:113-115, 1972.

44. Lapides, J.: Fundamentals of urology, Philadelphia, 1976, W.B. Saunders Co.

45. Lapides, J., et al.: Further observations on self-catheterization, J. Urol. **116**:169-171, 1976.

46. Lapides, J., et al.: Clean, intermittent self-catheterization in the treatment of urinary tract disease, Trans. Am. Assoc. Genitourin. Surg. **63**:92-95, 1971.

47. Mahoney, J.M.: Guide to ostomy care, Boston, 1976, Little, Brown & Co.

47a. Mahoney, J.M.: What you should know about ostomies, Nurs. '78 **8**:74-84, May 1978.

48. Mooney, T.O., Cole, T., and Chilgren, R.: Sexual options for paraplegics and quadriplegics, Boston, 1975, Little, Brown & Co.

49. *Murray, B.S., Elmore, J., and Sawyer, J.R.: The patient has an ileal conduit, Am. J. Nurs. **71**:1560-1565, 1971.

50. Patterson, D., and Schuster, P.A.: Artificial urinary sphincter, Can. Nurse **71**(11):27-31, 1975.

51. Paulson, D.: Carcinoma of the bladder and urethra, Hosp. Med. **11**:63-68, 1975.

52. Pickering, L., and Robbins, D.: Fluid, electrolyte, and acid-base balance in the renal patient, Nurs. Clin. North Am. **15**:577-592, 1980.

53. Pitts, W.R., and Muscke, E.C.: A 20-year experience with ileal conduits: the fate of the kidneys, J. Urol. **122**:154-157, 1979.

54. *Rush, A.: Cancer and the ostomy patient, Nurs. Clin. North Am. **11**:405-415, 1976.

55. Rusk, H.A.: Rehabilitation medicine: a textbook on physical medicine and rehabilitation, ed. 4, St. Louis, 1977, The C.V. Mosby Co.

56. Scott, R.B., Bradley, W.E., and Timm, G.W.: Treatment of urinary incontinence by an implanted urinary sphincter, J. Urol. **112**:75-82, 1974.

57. *Shapbell, N.J., and Sweigart, J.E.: A urinary device for patients with problem stomas, Nurs. Clin. North Am. **9**:383-386, 1974.

58. Spraggon, E.: Urinary diversion stomas: a guide for patients and nurses, ed. 2, Edinburgh, 1975, Churchill Livingstone.

59. Stamm, W.: Guidelines for prevention of catheter-associated urinary tract infections, Ann. Intern. Med. **82**:386-390, 1975.

60. Tebeau, J.L.: Fluid, electrolyte, and acid-base balance: special considerations in gastrointestinal and urinary diversions. In Broadwell, D.C., and Jackson, B.S., editors: Principles of ostomy care, St. Louis, 1982, The C.V. Mosby Co.

61. *Tobieson, S.: Benign prostatic hypertrophy, Am. J. Nurs. **79**:286-290, 1979.

62. Underwood, M.A.: Urinary tract infections, Crit. Care Q. **3**:63-70, 1980.

63. *United Ostomy Association, Inc.: Urinary ostomies: a guidebook for patients, Los Angeles, 1978, The Association.

64. *United Ostomy Association, Inc.: Sex and the male ostomate, Los Angeles, 1973, The Association.

65. *United Ostomy Association, Inc.: Sex, courtship, and the single ostomate, Los Angeles, 1973, The Association.

66. *United Ostomy Association, Inc.: Sex, pregnancy, and the female ostomate, Los Angeles, 1972, The Association.

67. Voegl, C.: Keeping patients alive in spite of postobstructive diuresis, Nurs. '79 **9**:50-56, March 1979.

68. *Vukovich, V., and Grubb, R.D.: Care of the ostomy patient, ed. 2, St. Louis, 1977, The C.V. Mosby Co.

69. *Watt, R.: Urinary diversion, Am. J. Nurs. **74**:1806-1811, 1974.

70. Watt, R.C., and Thomas, E.: Relating urinary diversion and appliance bacteriology, E.T.J. **5**:5-12, 1978.

71. Whyte, J., and Thistle, N.: Male incontinence: the inside story on external collection, Nurs. '76 **6**:66-67, Sept. 1976.

72. Wilpizesk, M.C.: Helping the ostomate return to normal life, Nurs. '81 **11**:62-66, March 1981.

73. Winter, C.C., and Morel, A.: Nursing care of patients with urologic diseases, ed. 4, St. Louis, 1977, The C.V. Mosby Co.

74. Wyker, A., and Gillenwater, J.: Methods of urology, Baltimore, 1975, The Williams & Wilkins Co.

75. Yahle, M.: An ostomy information clinic, Nurs. Clin. North Am. **11**:457-467, 1976.

Classic

76. Licht, S., editor: Rehabilitation and medicine, New Haven, Conn., 1968, Elizabeth Licht Publishing Co.

AUDIOVISUAL RESOURCE

Trainex Corp.: Bowel and bladder retraining, Garden Grove, Calif., 1967, Trainex Corp. (Filmstrip, cassette, script.)

CHAPTER 62

PROBLEMS OF THE URINARY SYSTEM

PAULA LAMBRECHT MILLER

Disease of the urinary system is a major cause of morbidity and a significant cause of mortality in the United States. Mortality from disease of the urinary system is generally associated with destruction of renal tissue. When disease involves the kidneys, renal function is directly threatened. When disease occurs in the lower urinary tract, it not only affects tissue locally but can threaten renal function through spread of infection and obstruction of urine flow. The primary objective for treatment of disease in any part of the urinary tract should be early detection and adequate therapy directed toward preserving or improving renal function, for without renal function life can continue for only a few days.

During the last two decades some of the most striking developments in treatment of individuals with disease of the urinary system have been in the area of prolonging life after renal function has ceased. Dialysis and transplantation have given hundreds of people each year a continued, though somewhat uncertain, life expectancy. Technical, physical, and psychosocial components of the new life-style of these individuals demand the nurse's attention.

Nurses can assist in significantly reducing the morbidity of the urinary system. This can be achieved through increasing public awareness of preventive measures, assisting in early detection of signs and symptoms of disease, and providing long-term care to the growing population of chronically ill individuals with urinary tract disease. This chapter defines common problems of the person with disease of the urinary system and identifies rquirements for nursing care before and during the acute and chronic phases of illness.

Infection of urinary tract

Urinary tract infections (UTI) are a significant source of morbidity in the United States. These infections contribute to illness during the acute infection and also are significant in the development of chronic renal failure. Infection occurs in both acute and chronic stages in all portions of the urinary tract.

Etiology and epidemiology

Table 62-1 summarizes factors contributing to infection of the urinary tract. Although the great majority of noncomplicated urinary infections are asymptomatic and clear spontaneously, there remains a portion significant enough to warrant consideration as a health problem. There is no controversy among those practicing preventive health care regarding the question of the need for screening of asymptomatic infections; however, there exists difficulty in identifying the specific risk groups in which the detection and treatment of these infections yield significant improvement in the person's health. As the health care of our population becomes more oriented toward prevention of health problems, specific target populations will be better defined and the number of screening programs for asymptomatic urinary tract infection will increase.

Females seem more predisposed to urinary tract infections than males. Factors postulated in their higher infection rates include a shorter urethra with a close proximity to the rectum and the lack of prostatic fluid protection present in the male. Infection rates for females approximate 1% of school-aged girls and 4% of women

TABLE 62-1. Risk factors associated with development of urinary tract infection

Risk factor	Common examples
Female population	
Structural abnormality	Strictures
	Incompetent ureterovesical junction anomalies
Obstruction	Tumors
	Prostatic hypertrophy
	Calculi
	Iatrogenic causes
Impaired bladder innervation	Congenital spinal cord malformation
	Spinal cord injury
	Multiple sclerosis
Chronic disease	Gout
	Diabetes mellitus
	Hypertension
	Sickle cell disease
	Chronic renal disease
Instrumentation	Catheterization
	Diagnostic procedures

through the childbearing years.[46] Incidence of infection in females increases directly with sexual activity and aging. Pregnancy does not seem to increase infection rates, although spontaneous clearing of infections is decreased during pregnancy and there is a higher incidence of acute kidney infections progressing from the lower urinary tract.

Structural and functional abnormalities of the urinary tract, obstruction to the flow of urine, and impaired bladder innervation promote infection of the urinary tract. Mechanisms involved include stasis of urine, which provides a culture medium for bacteria; reflux of infected urine higher into the urinary tract; and increasing hydrostatic pressure.

Certain chronic health problems predispose to urinary tract infection by changing the metabolism of tissues, creating extrarenal obstructions, and altering the function and structure of kidney tissue. Common among these health problems are diabetes mellitus, gout, hypertension, polycystic kidney disease, multiple myeloma, and glomerulonephritis.

Instrumentation of the urinary tract is associated with high rates of infection. Catheterization, even when performed without break in asepsis, results in significant infection of the bladder. Nosocomial infections account for a sizable percentage of all urinary tract infections. Drug-resistant strains of *Staphylococcus* and *Pseudomonas*, along with various other organisms commonly found in hospitals, are frequently those involved in nosocomial urinary tract infections. Prevention and control

of all urinary tract infections can be most significantly influenced through a lowering of this nosocomial infection rate (p. 368).

Infections of the lower urinary tract involve the urinary bladder *(cystitis)* and the urethra *(urethritis)*. In the upper urinary tract, infection involves the kidney (pyelonephritis). The etiologic factors and general preventive and mangement principles are the same for infection anywhere in the urinary tract. Pyelonephritis is discussed in greater detail on p. 1567.

Pathophysiology

Most infections of the urinary tract result from gram-negative organisms, such as *Escherichia coli, Klebsiella, Proteus, Enterobacter,* or *Pseudomonas,* that originate in the person's own intestinal tract and ascend through the urethra to the bladder. During micturition, urine may flow back up the ureters *(vesicoureteral reflux)* and carry bacteria present in the bladder up through the ureters to the kidney pelvis. Whenever stasis of urine occurs, such as with incomplete emptying of the bladder, renal calculi, or genitourinary obstructions, the bacteria have a greater opportunity to grow and a more alkaline media, which favors their growth and multiplication.

Urinary tract infections occur primarily when host resistance is impaired. The major factors in preventing urinary tract infections are tissue integrity and blood supply.[51] A break in the surface of the mucous membrane lining permits the bacteria to invade the tissue and cause infection. Breaks in tissue integrity result from erosions caused by tips of indwelling catheters or rough-edged renal stones, from neoplasms, or from invasion of the tissue by parasites such as *Schistosoma*.[51] In the bladder, blood supply to the tissues can be compromised when the pressure within the bladder is markedly increased, as may occur with overdistention of the bladder, contracture of the bladder neck, or obstruction of the urethra by an enlarged prostate, metastatic growth, or urethral stricture.

Prevention

Three considerations are important in preventing infection of the lower urinary tract: (1) preventing or minimizing morbidity that can accompany these infections, (2) preventing recurrence of the infection, and (3) preventing renal damage from untreated or inadequately treated ascending infection. Since individuals with lower urinary tract infections seek medical attention as a result of symptoms or are identified through routine urinalysis or screening of populations at high risk, both education of the public and community health case finding assist in decreasing urinary tract infection and its complications. *Public education should center on (1) the need for prompt medical attention for symptoms, (2) the need to continue with drug therapy*

even though symptoms abate, (3) the importance of fol-
low-up care and repeated urine cultures, and (4) main-
tenance of fluid intake of 3 to 4 L/day if the person's
health permits.

Clinical picture

The symptoms that bring the person to medical attention typically include urgency, burning on urination (dysuria), and slight to gross hematuria. Most persons, however, are asymptomatic or minimally symptomatic, the infection being identified only on routine examination of the urine. Bacteriuria and positive urine cultures serve as the basis for diagnosing lower urinary tract infections. Growth of a single pathogen in excess of 1×10^5 organisms/ml of urine in a properly obtained and stored midstream specimen (p. 1510) indicates infection.

Intervention

Treatment goals for lower urinary tract infections include sterilizing the urine and identifying any illness or urinary tract abnormality that may be contributing to the infection. After culture and sensitivity studies a 10- to 14-day course of antibiotic therapy is instituted. It is crucial that urine culture be obtained before initiating drug therapy to ensure appropriateness of antimicrobial medication and to decrease the development of resistant strains of organisms. The urine should be recultured every few months during the following year to reconfirm urine sterility.

A more extensive urologic workup including intravenous pyelogram (IVP) and voiding cystogram may be performed for men and young children after a repeated, or even first, urinary tract infection or when infection does not abate. This workup is performed on women when infection occurs repeatedly or cannot be cleared up with treatment. The rationale for this extensive workup is that urinary tract infections are not common in men and children and that a significant portion of infection in these populations, and in women with persistent infection, involves abnormality of the urinary tract.

Medications commonly used in the treatment of urinary tract infection include urinary antiseptics such as sulfisoxazole (Gantrisin) or nitrofurantoin (Furadantin) and systemic antibiotics. Sulfonamides are widely used; they are usually effective against the organisms causing a large percentage of urinary tract infections, are safe, and are less likely than most systemic antibiotics to contribute to growth of resistant organisms. Urinary antiseptics that contain analgesic properties (trimethoprim and sulfamethoxazole [Bactrim]) may be prescribed for the patient when burning is a problem.

Additional treatment includes increasing fluid intake to 3 to 4 L/day unless contraindicated. Increased fluids help to dilute the urine, which lessens irritations and burning, and provide a continual flow of urine to discourage stasis and multiplication of bacteria in the urinary tract. Sitz baths may provide comfort for individuals with urethritis. Patient education concerning the problem, the requirements for drug therapy, and follow-up care should facilitate early identification of recurrence and completion of drug regimens for eradication of bacteria. Success in both of these areas is directly dependent on patient follow-through and comprises the means by which the patient is able to assist in overcoming this health problem.

For individuals with chronic bacteriuria, urine-acidifying agents may be prescribed. The effect of these medications is to provide a less suitable environment for bacterial growth and to enhance the effectiveness of antibiotic and urinary antiseptics. When bacteriuria becomes constant, prophylaxis may be undertaken with antimicrobial drugs.

Outcome criteria for the person with urinary tract infection

The person will:
1. Have relief of symptoms.
2. Show no further damage in kidney function; current damage is arrested.
3. Have sterile urine or bacterial urine count of less than 1×10^4 to 1×10^5.
4. Have identified or corrected any disease or abnormality that would contribute to reinfection or relapse.

The patient or significant other can:
1. State signs and symptoms of lower urinary tract infection.
2. Explain when and how to take prescribed medication.
3. State plan for follow-up urine cultures.
4. State rationale and means of increasing fluid intake to 3 to 4 L/day.

Congenital malformations of urinary tract

Variation from the normal anatomic structure of the urinary tract occurs in about 10% to 15% of the population.[51] These deviations range from minor, easily correctable anomalies to those incompatible with life.

The following congenital malformations are included in this text because of their potential influence on urinary tract function in adult life. The reader is referred to other specialty texts for information about additional defects that can be repaired in early life without expected residual urologic sequelae or those that result in death before adulthood.[70,72]

Partial or complete duplication of the ureters is a relatively common anomaly of the urinary tract. Unilateral duplication occurs in about one of 200 births, while bilateral duplication occurs in about one in 1200 births.[51] This defect includes duplication of the renal pelvis as well as the ureters. A *complete duplication* refers to the occurrence of two separate ureters from one kidney. More common is a *partial duplication* in which the duplicate ureters unite at some point between the kidney and bladder. The clinical significance of duplication of the ureter is dependent on the presence of obstruction or reflux. Obstruction at the point where the two ureters join or reflux from one ureter into the other in a partial duplication may lead to dilation of the ureter, hydronephrosis, and persistent or recurrent urinary tract infections. In the case of complete duplication the ureter draining the upper pole of the kidney may open either into the bladder or into the vulva, urethra, or seminal vesicle. If the ureter drains ectopically (outside the bladder), incontinence and obstruction are generally present. Surgical intervention when necessitated by obstruction or reflux may include reimplantation of an ectopic ureter into the bladder, resection of the duplicated ureter, resection of the hydronephrotic portion of the kidney, or nephrectomy if severe renal damage has occurred. *Triplication of the ureters* occurs infrequently, and management is the same as for duplication.

Horseshoe kidney refers to fusion of the kidneys, usually at their lower poles. The incidence varies between 1 in 600 and 1 in 1800 births.[51] Potential problems that may arise because of anterior angulation of the ureters include stasis, hydronephrosis, and possible calculus formation. Surgical treatment when indicated because of obstruction consists of division of the fused part. Cases uncomplicated by obstruction or calculi are generally not treated surgically.

Hydroureter, dilation of the ureter, may result from obstruction in the lower urinary tract, from vesicoureteral reflux, or from an atonic lower ureteral segment, all of which may be congenital. In some cases of severe ureteral dilation, peristalsis in the lower ureter is decreased secondary to atony. Urinary diversion for a time may allow the ureter to become amenable to future repair and reimplantation into the bladder. If such attempts fail, urinary diversion is permanent. Congenital deficiency of abdominal musculature, or prune belly syndrome, is rare and includes extreme hydronephrosis and dilated ureters. Treatment usually necessitates permanent urinary diversion.

Exstrophy of the bladder and *epispadias* are developmental anomalies that often occur together. They result from failure of the midline to close adequately during fetal development and may vary a great deal in their severity.

Epispadias is a failure of closure on the dorsal surface

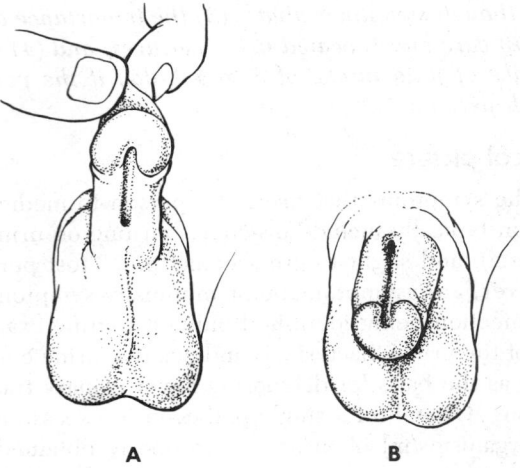

Fig. 62-1. A, Hypospadias. **B,** Epispadias.

of the penis and may extend from the glans to the perineum (Fig. 62-1, *B*). The defect often extends to the urinary sphincter, causing incontinence. If surgical correction involving the urinary sphincter is not successful, urinary diversion may be performed.

Exstrophy of the bladder, which occurs in approximately 1 in 40,000 births, may consist only of a small fistula leading to the surface of the abdominal wall that drains urine, or it may be so extensive that most of the interior of the bladder is everted on the outer abdominal wall. Usually the sphincter muscles of the urethra are faulty and epispadias is present. The muscles below the umbilicus are separated, and the pubic rami are not joined. Operations for exstrophy of the bladder may include attempts to reconstruct sphincter muscles of the urethra and to close the bladder and abdominal walls. If satisfactory repair cannot be made, as is frequently the case in complete exstrophy, permanent urinary diversion may be necessary. If untreated, the bladder wall undergoes squamous metaplastic changes that predispose the patient to adenocarcinoma in later life.

Hypospadias is a common anomaly in which the urethra opens in the male at any ventral point on the penis between the glans and perineum (Fig. 62-1, *A*). It is almost always accompanied by *chordee*, fibrous bands causing curvature of the penis. In the female the urethra opens into the vagina. Very slight anomalies require no intervention; when treatment is indicated, surgical reconstruction of the urethra (and release of chordee in the male) is done. Postoperative strictures may occur, which require further treatment.

Congenital malformations of the spinal cord such as myelomeningocele and sacral agenesis frequently cause bladder dysfunction as a result of disturbances of innervation (neurogenic bladder). Complications arising from neurogenic bladder dysfunction include infection, hydronephrosis, and calculus formation. Treatment is aimed

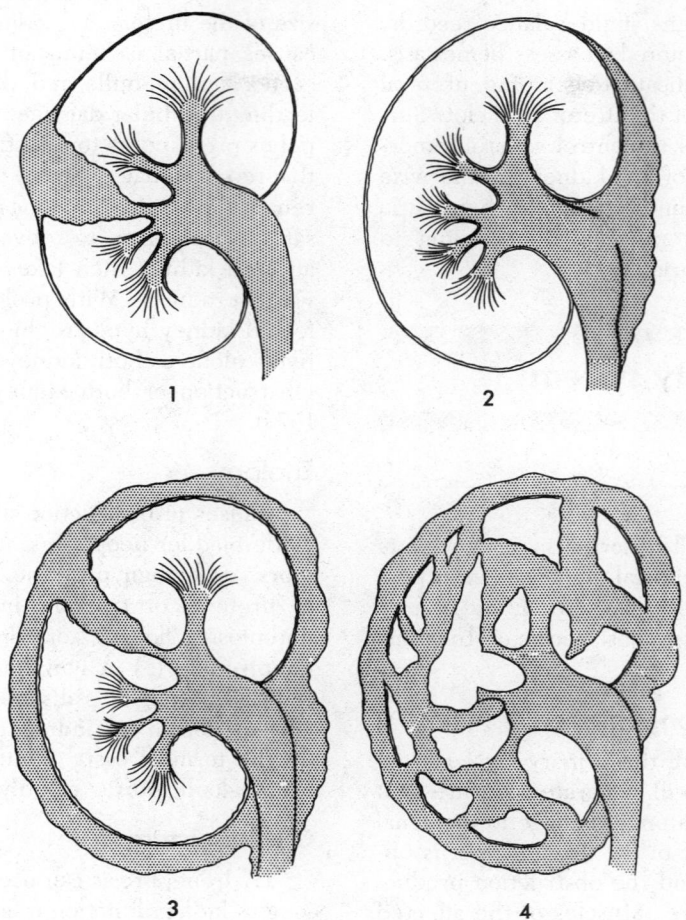

Fig. 62-2. Four degrees of renal trauma. *1,* Urine is extravasating from split in renal parenchyma but confined under renal capsule. *2,* Urine is extravasating through tear in renal pelvis. *3,* Urine is extravasating through rent in kidney and capsule and surrounds kidney and renal pelvis. *4,* Kidney is shattered and urine is extravasating in all areas. (From Winter, C.C., and Morel, A.: Nursing care of patients with urologic diseases, ed. 4, St. Louis, 1977, The C.V. Mosby Co.)

at controlling incontinence and preserving renal function and may include such methods as Credé maneuver of the bladder, intermittent catheterization, systemic medications, or urinary diversion or other forms of surgical treatment.

For details in the care of the person having surgical treatment[84] of the urinary tract, see Chapter 61.

Trauma to urinary tract

Assessing intactness of urinary tract structures must be part of the evaluation of any person with traumatic injury to the lower trunk. Injuries particularly related to urinary tract damage include fractures of the pelvis and sharp blows to the body.

Trauma of the lower urinary tract. Pelvic fractures may result in *bladder perforation* and *ureteral* and *urethral tearing.* Following these injuries urinary output may be scant or absent, the urine may be bloody, and symptoms of peritonitis may appear. Treatment is directed toward stabilizing the patient and surgically repairing the perforation or laceration. Before stabilizing the patient, a cystotomy may be performed to provide urinary drainage when injury involves the bladder or urethra.

Kidney trauma. A sharp blow to the body, particularly to the lower back, may result in *contusion, tearing,* or *rupture of a kidney* (Fig. 62-2). Signs and symptoms include *hematuria and pain* and *tenderness of the upper abdominal quadrant and flank* on the involved side. Signs of shock may be present or absent depending on the extent of hemorrhage. Treatment includes control of bleeding, prevention of shock, and promoting drainage of the urinary tract. Vital signs, fluid balance records, and hematocrit level are monitored to assess hemostasis. Complaints of pain may indicate developing ureteral colic, signifying obstruction of the ureter by a clot. Surgical intervention is required to control severe hemorrhage. Spontaneous healing of the kidney is otherwise permitted. Bed rest is maintained until gross hematuria clears; thereafter activity is progressed according to continued absence of hematuria.

Obstruction of urinary system

General obstruction

The following section will describe major concepts related to pathophysiology, clinical picture seen in persons with obstruction of the urinary system, and care of such patients. In subsequent sections specific obstructions will be discussed in detail.

Pathophysiology of hydronephrosis

Obstruction of any part of the urinary system from the kidney to the urethra will generate pressure that may cause functional and anatomic damage to the renal parenchyma. When any part of the urinary tract is obstructed, urine collects behind the obstruction producing a dilation of the structure. Muscles of the affected area contract in an effort to push the urine around the obstruction. Partial obstruction may produce slow dilatation of structures above the obstruction without functional impairment. As the obstruction increases, however, pressure builds up in the tubular system behind the obstruction causing a backflow of urine and dilation of ureter (*hydroureter*). The urine backup eventually reaches the kidney causing dilation of the kidney pelvis (*hydronephrosis*). Pressure buildup in the renal pelvis leads to destruction of kidney tissue and eventual renal failure.

With obstruction urine flow is decreased even to the point of stagnation. This stagnant urine provides a good culture medium for bacterial growth, and rarely is obstruction seen without some infection. The specific effects that occur with obstruction will depend on the location of the obstruction, the extent of obstruction (partial or complete), and the duration. Obstruction in the *lower* urinary tract causes bladder distention. If this is prolonged, muscle fibers become hypertrophied and *diverticuli* (herniated sacs of bladder mucosa) develop between the hypertrophied muscle bands. Since the diverticulum holds stagnant urine, infection often occurs, and bladder stones may form.

Obstruction of the *upper* urinary tract leads even more quickly to hydronephrosis because of the small size of the ureters and kidney pelvis. Increased pressure causes partial ischemia of arteries between the renal cortex and medulla and dilation of the renal tubules leading to tubular damage. Stasis of urine in the dilated pelvis predisposes to infection and calculi, which add to the renal damage. Some urine can flow back up the renal tubule into the veins and lymphatics as a compensatory mechanism to prevent kidney damage. The unaffected kidney then takes on increased elimination of waste products. With prolonged obstruction the unaffected kidney hypertrophies and may function as effectively alone as both kidneys did before the obstruction. Obstruction of both kidneys leads to renal failure (p. 1570).

Etiology

Causes of obstruction of the lower urinary tract include bladder neoplasms, urethral stricture, calculi, tumors, or benign prostatic hypertrophy (BPH). Causes of ureteral obstruction include calculi, trauma, nephroptosis ("floating" or "dropped" kidney), an enlarged lymph node (as in lymphosarcoma, reticulum cell sarcoma, or Hodgkin's disease), or a congenital anomaly. Obstruction in the kidney can occur at the tubule level (in the form of casts or inflammation) or in the pelvis from calculi, ptosis, or polycystic disease.

Clinical picture

Hydronephrosis can occur without any symptoms as long as kidney function is adequate and urine can drain. An acute upper urinary tract obstruction will cause pain, nausea, vomiting, local tenderness, spasm of the abdominal muscles, and a mass in the kidney region. The pain is caused by the stretching of the tissues and by hyperperistalsis. Since the amount of pain is proportionate to the rate of stretching, a slowly developing hydronephrosis may cause only a dull flank pain, whereas a sudden blockage of the ureter such as may occur from a stone causes a severe stabbing (colicky) pain in the flank or abdomen. The pain may radiate to the genitalia and thigh and is caused by the increased peristaltic action of the smooth muscle of the ureter in an effort to dislodge the obstruction and force urine past it.

The nausea and vomiting frequently associated with acute ureteral obstruction are caused by a reflex reaction to the pain and will usually be relieved as soon as pain is relieved. A markedly dilated kidney, however, may press on the stomach causing continued gastrointestinal symptoms. If the renal function has been seriously impaired, nausea and vomiting may be symptoms of impending uremia. (See p. 1572 for discussion of uremia and renal failure.)

When the bladder is distended from lower urinary tract obstruction, the person will experience lower abdominal discomfort and a feeling of the need to void although voiding may not be possible. The bladder may be palpated above the symphysis pubis. With partial obstruction such as by benign prostatic hypertrophy the man first complains of increasing urinary frequency because the bladder fails to empty completely at each voiding and therefore refills more quickly to the amount that causes the urge to void (usually 250 to 500 ml). Nocturia may also be present.

Diagnostic examinations may include cystoscopy and retrograde pyelography (p. 1516) to identify the source of the obstruction. Selection of other diagnostic tests will depend on the probable cause (see Chapter 60).

Intervention

When obstruction occurs the treatment consists of reestablishing adequate drainage from the urinary system. This may be temporarily accomplished by placing a catheter above the point of obstruction. Sometimes surgery must be performed to insert a catheter (nephrostomy, ureterostomy, suprapubic cystostomy). Later, definitive treatment is dependent on the cause. The infection is treated with antibiotics, fluids, and rest. Urinary antiseptics may also be given.

The person with a sudden obstruction is frequently acutely ill and may have severe colic but will not be able to remain in bed until the pain has been relieved. It is not unusual to see a person with acute renal colic walking the floor "doubled up" and vomiting. Narcotics such as morphine and meperidine and antispasmodic drugs such as propantheline bromide (Pro-Banthine) and belladonna preparations are usually necessary to relieve severe colicky pain. After narcotics have been given, the patient will be dizzy and must be protected from injury. As the pain eases the patient can usually be made relatively comfortable in bed. As soon as the nausea subsides large amounts of fluids are urged.

Outcome criteria for the person with obstruction of the urinary system

The person is free of infection or is maintaining therapy to eradicate infection.

The person or significant others:
1. Understand the need to maintain fluid intake of 3000 ml/day.
2. Maintain adequate urinary drainage.
3. Can state plans for follow-up care.

Renal calculi

Urinary stones (*urolithiasis*) may develop at any level in the urinary system but are most commonly found within the kidney (*nephrolithiasis*). Renal stones are crystallizations of minerals around a mucoprotein (organic) matrix that may be pus, blood, devitalized tissue, crystals, or tumors. The mineral compositions of renal calculi vary. About three fourths of the stones are calcium oxalates; other stones are calcium phosphate, magnesium ammonium phosphate, uric acid, or cystine.

Etiology and pathophysiology

No demonstrable cause (idiopathic) can be found for over half of the renal stones that occur. A major predisposing factor is the presence of a urinary tract infection (p. 1549). Infection increases the presence of organic matter around which the minerals can precipitate and increases the alkalinity of the urine (by the production of ammonia), resulting in precipitation of calcium phosphate and magnesium ammonium phosphate. Stasis of urine also permits precipitation of organic matter and minerals.

Since most stones are calcium oxalates, anything that leads to hypercalciuria is a predisposing factor to renal stones. In those persons for whom no underlying cause can be identified, the hypercalciuria may result from an increased absorption of calcium from the intestine with subsequent increased elimination in the urine or from decreased reabsorption of calcium by the kidney tubules. These persons do not have hypercalcemia. Hypercalcemia leading to hypercalciuria may be present with an increased calcium intake (milk, alkali); prolonged immobilization (loss of bone calcium), hypervitaminosis D (increased calcium absorption from the intestines); hyperparathyroidism, multiple myeloma, Paget's disease, or cancer (loss of bone calcium); Cushing's syndrome or prolonged intake of corticosteroids (loss of bone calcium); and renal tubular acidosis (increased calcium secondary to defective ammonia formation). Increased uric acid in the urine leading to uric acid stones may be seen with gout, with some leukemias, or in patients treated with cancer chemotherapeutic agents. Cystine stones usually result from a genetic defect. Both uric acid and cystine precipitate in acid urine.

Prevention

Measures can be taken to decrease the potential for renal stones in persons at high risk. Adequate hydration (intake of 2500 ml/day or more unless contraindicated) will help to prevent urinary stasis that can lead not only to stone formation but also to urinary tract infection. Persons restricted to bed should be encouraged to turn and move frequently, exercising their arms if the legs are immobilized. Changing the body position of a bedfast patient by means of a CircOlectric bed or tilt table or by sitting up in a wheelchair (if permitted) can help to prevent urinary stasis. Even with exercises and the use of a wheelchair, however, paraplegics and quadriplegics often develop renal calculi. *Persons with indwelling catheters need scrupulous aseptic technique in catheter care to prevent infection and require adequate hydration and good catheter drainage to wash away minerals that can be deposited at the tip of the catheter.*

TABLE 62-2. Acid and alkaline ash food groups*

Acid ash	Alkaline ash	Neutral
Meat	Milk	Sugars
Whole grains	Vegetables	Fats
Egg	Fruit (except cranberries,	Beverages (coffee, tea)
Cheese	prunes, plums)	fee, tea)
Cranberries		
Prunes		
Plums		

*From Williams, S.R.: Nutrition and diet therapy, ed. 4, St. Louis, 1982, The C.V. Mosby Co.

Persons at risk for developing calcium oxalate or phosphate or magnesium ammonium phosphate stones may be placed on an acid ash diet (Table 62-2) to promote excretion of an acid urine. Catheter irrigations using acetic acid solution or Renacidin help provide an acid environment and thus decrease precipitation of calcium and phosphates.

Clinical picture

Pain *(renal colic)* is the primary symptom in an acute episode of renal calculi. The location of the pain depends on the location of the stone. If the stone is in the pelvis of the kidney, the pain is due to hydronephrosis and is more dull and constant in character, occurring primarily in the costovertebral angle. As the stone moves along the ureter the pain can be excruciating and is intermittent in character. It is caused by spasm of the ureter and anoxia of the wall of the ureter from the pressure of the stone. The pain follows the anterior course of the ureter down to the suprapubic area and radiates to the external genitalia. Nausea and vomiting often accompany renal colic.

Gross hematuria may occur if the stone has rough edges, and microhematuria usually is present. Signs of urinary tract infection (p. 1551) may also be present. Often a stone is "silent," causing no symptoms for years. This is especially true of very large renal stones. Extremely small smooth stones may be passed without awareness of the person.

Diagnostic tests are performed to determine the presence of one or more stones. Calcium stones are radiopaque, but uric acid stones usually cannot be visualized in radiographic studies. Intravenous pyelography may demonstrate dilation of the ureter above an obstructing stone. Very small stones may be washed away during the radiographic studies. Urinalysis will show the presence of red blood cells and sometimes the minerals involved in stone formation.

Because recurrence of renal calculi is common, additional studies are carried out after the acute episode has subsided. Successive determinations of serum calcium, phosphorus, protein, electrolytes, and uric acid are performed to determine presence of underlying disease that can influence stone formation. The urinary pH should be measured with pH paper each time the person voids to ascertain the acidity or alkalinity. A *nitroprusside urine test* may be performed to check the presence of cystine. An accurate *24-hour urine collection* is made to measure calcium, oxalate, phosphorus, and uric acid levels. The 24-hour urine collection may be made with the patient eating a normal diet or following a 3-day low-calcium, low-phosphorus diet.

Intervention

Acute care. About 90% of urinary calculi are passed spontaneously. Therefore *the urine of all patients with relatively small stones should be strained*. Urine can be strained easily by placing two opened 4-in. × 8-in. gauze sponges over a funnel. The urine from each voiding is strained, and one needs to watch closely for the stone because it may be no bigger than the head of a pin and the patient may not realize that it has been passed.

Stones smaller than 5 mm have a good chance of being passed. If there is no infection or obstruction, the stone may be left in the ureter for several months. The person is observed closely but permitted to carry out usual activities. A person who is up and about is more likely to pass a stone than one who is in bed. Fluids should be taken freely (2500 ml/day or more) to promote passage of the stone and prevent infection.

Patients frequently have two or three attacks of acute renal colic before the stone passes. This is probably because the stone gets lodged at a narrow point in the ureter causing temporary obstruction. The ureters are normally narrower at the ureteropelvic and ureterovesical junctions and at the point where they pass over the iliac crest into the pelvis. If the stone is to pass along the ureter by peristaltic action, the patient will have some pain. The patient is involved in determining when medication is needed. Drugs used include morphine sulfate and meperidine hydrochloride (Demerol) for direct pain and atropine, methantheline bromide (Banthine), and propantheline bromide (Pro-Banthine) to depress the smooth muscles of the ureter and lessen pain from spasm.

If the stone fails to pass, one or two ureteral catheters may be passed through a cystoscope up the ureter and left in place for 24 hours. The catheters dilate the ureter, and when they are removed the stone may pass into the bladder.

If there are *signs of infection*, an attempt is made to pass a ureteral catheter past the stone into the renal pelvis. If such an attempt is successful, the catheter is left as a drain, since pyelonephritis will quickly follow if adequate urinary drainage is not reestablished. When there is a catheter in each ureter, each catheter is labeled and should drain into a separate drainage bag. The catheters must be checked frequently to see that

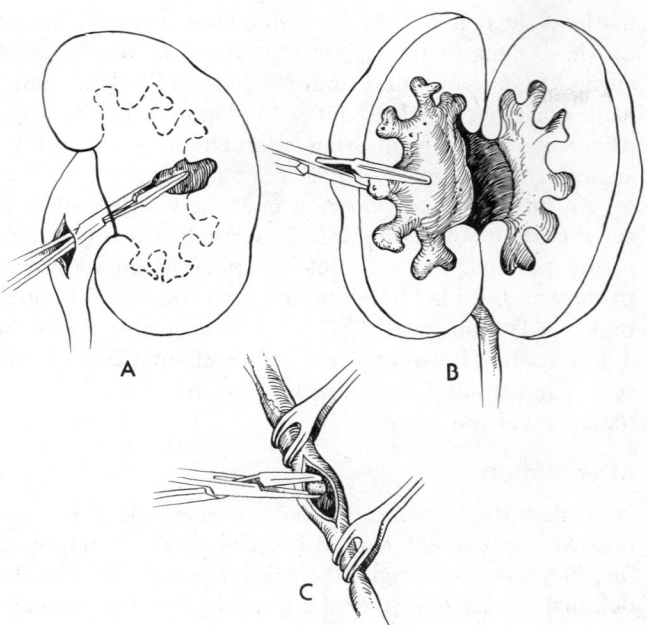

Fig. 62-3. Location and methods of removing renal calculi from upper urinary tract. **A,** Pyelolithotomy, removal of stone through renal pelvis. **B,** Nephrolithotomy, removal of stag-horn calculus from renal parenchyma (kidney split). **C,** Ureterolithotomy, removal of stone from ureter.

they are draining. Patients with ureteral catheters are usually confined to bed to prevent possible dislodgement of the catheters.

If the stone has passed to the lower third of the ureter, it can sometimes be removed by *manipulation*. Special catheters with corkscrew tips, expanding baskets, and loops are passed through the cystoscope, and an attempt is made to "snare" the stone. This procedure is performed with the patient under anesthesia. The aftercare of a patient on whom manipulation has been carried out is the same as that following cystoscopy. Any signs suggestive of peritonitis or a decreased urinary output are carefully watched for, since the ureter occasionally is perforated during manipulation.

Surgery. Surgical intervention is indicated when a large stone (greater than 1 cm) is producing pain, obstruction, or infection. The operation for removal of a stone from the ureter is a *ureterolithotomy* (Fig. 62-3, *C*). A radiograph is taken immediately preceding surgery, since the stone may have moved, and it is desirable to make the incision into the ureter directly over the stone. If the stone is in the lower third of the ureter, a rectus incision is made. If it is in the upper two thirds, a flank approach is used. If the patient has a ureteral stricture that causes stones to form, a plastic surgery procedure to relieve the stricture may be carried out as part of the operation.

Removal of a stone through or from the renal pelvis is known as a *pyelolithotomy* (Fig. 62-3, *A*). Removal of

a stone through the parenchyma is a *nephrolithotomy* (Fig. 62-3, *B*). Occasionally, the kidney may have to be split from end to end (a kidney split) to remove the stone. Patients in whom such a split is done may have severe hemorrhage following surgery.

Bladder stones may be removed through a suprapubic incision, or they may be crushed with a lithotrite (stone crusher) that is passed transurethrally. This procedure is known as a *litholapaxy*. Following bladder stone removal, the bladder may be irrigated (intermittently or constantly) with an acid solution such as magnesium and sodium citrate (G solution) or Renacidin to counteract the alkalinity caused by the infection and to help wash out the remaining particles of stone. If there has been a suprapubic incision, the care of the incision is similar to that following a suprapubic prostatectomy. (See p. 1561 for care of the patient requiring urologic surgery.)

Long-term care. Persons who have recurrent renal calculi benefit from ongoing prophylactic therapy, which is determined by the type of stone being produced. *All persons with recurrent renal stones should drink fluids in sufficient quantity to produce very dilute urine and nocturia.* This may amount to a daily intake of up to 4 to 5 L of fluid.[66] The purpose of the increased fluid intake is to rinse away any precipitates that can serve as a nidus for stone formation.

Any underlying identifiable cause of calciuria is treated to prevent recurrence of calcium stones. Hydrochlorothiazide (HCTZ) in doses of 50 mg twice a day may be prescribed for persons with hypercalciuria to decrease urinary excretion of calcium. Persons receiving HCTZ therapy must be monitored carefully for signs of electrolyte imbalances especially hypokalemia.

As previously stated, more than 50% of calcium stones are idiopathic. Foods high in calcium are sometimes restricted, but a very low–calcium diet is usually unsatisfactory because it is unpalatable. The solubility of oxalate salts is not pH dependent; therefore manipulation of pH is not useful. Sodium or potassium phosphate, 1.5 to 2.0 g/day, may be prescribed to decrease urinary calcium.

Phosphatic calculi develop in alkaline urine; therefore their prevention depends on keeping the urine acid and preventing urinary tract infection. Medications such as ascorbic acid or ammonium chloride may be given for a time to increase urine acidity.

The Shorr regimen has given beneficial results in the prevention of phosphatic calculi. A diet containing only 1300 mg of phosphorus daily is prescribed, and 40 ml of aluminum hydroxide gel is taken after meals and at bedtime. The aluminum combines with the excess phosphorus, causing it to be excreted through the bowel instead of through the kidney, thus decreasing the possibility of stone formation. Constipation frequently results from this regimen.

Prophylaxis for *uric acid* stones consists in alkalinizing

the urine by the administration of sodium bicarbonate and acetazolamide (Diamox) sufficient to maintain a urine pH of 6.0 to 6.5. Allopurinol (Zyloprim) usually is prescribed to inhibit synthesis of uric acid.

Outcome criteria for the person with recurrent renal calculi

The person or significant others can:
1. Describe a plan to achieve a daily fluid intake of 4 to 5 L, sufficient to maintain a dilute urine.
2. Describe the need to be as active as possible and prevent long periods of immobilization.
3. Plan menus to include any dietary restrictions.
4. State name, dosage, desired action, and side effects of medications prescribed to acidify or alkalinize the urine.
5. State plans for follow-up care.
   a. Describe signs of recurrence of calculi (pain in costovertebral angle or radiating anteriorly to external genitalia).
   b. Describe assessment and prevention of urinary tract infection.

Tumors of the kidney

Epidemiology

Malignant renal tumors, primarily adenocarcinomas, account for 3% of all cancers. Small benign renal tumors (adenomas) may occur without causing significant damage or symptoms. Renal cell carcinomas rarely occur before the age of 30 years, are more commonly seen in the 50- to 70-year age range, and occur twice as often in men as in women.

Pathophysiology

Renal carcinomas usually develop unilaterally but may be bilateral. In stage I the tumor margins are well defined (encapsulated) and compress the kidney parenchyma during growth rather than infiltrating it. The upper pole of the kidney is usually involved, and the tumor is usually large at the time of diagnosis. In stage II the tumor invades the fat surrounding the kidney. Stage III consists of local metastasis either through direct extension or through the renal vein or lymphatics (lymph node involvement). Distant metastases during stage IV are found primarily in the lungs or bone, but other areas, such as the liver, spleen, or brain, may also be involved.

Clinical picture

Hematuria is the most frequent symptom of renal cell carcinoma. Unfortunately, the hematuria is often intermittent, lessening the person's concern and causing procrastination in seeking medical care. Any person with hematuria should have a complete urologic examination, since it is only by immediate investigation of the first signs of hematuria that there is any hope of cure. Other symptoms may include dull flank pain, flank mass, weight loss, fever, and polycythemia. Hypertension may result from stimulation of the renin-angiotensin system.

An intravenous pyelogram may show a distortion of renal outline suggesting a kidney tumor. Small tumors in the parenchyma may not be apparent on a routine pyelogram but may be identified by a computed tomography (CT) scan (p. 1517). A CT scan is also useful in differentiating between renal cell carcinoma and a renal cyst. Angiography may also be performed to differentiate a cyst from a tumor.

Intervention

Unless the person is a poor surgical risk or has extensive metastases, the diseased kidney is removed (*nephrectomy*) through a transabdominal, thoracoabdominal, or retroperitoneal approach. The first two approaches are preferred in order to secure the renal artery and vein and prevent any spread of malignant cells. (See p. 1530 for care of the person requiring urologic surgery.)

Following surgery for a malignant tumor that is radiosensitive, the patient is usually given a course of x-ray therapy. Hospitalization is not always necessary during this time. Radiation may also be used over the metastatic sites as palliative treatment for the person with an inoperable tumor. Chemotherapy has not yet proved of value in the treatment of renal cell carcinomas. The survival rate after therapy depends on the extent of metastasis. The 10-year survival rate is very low, especially since many persons do not seek initial treatment until the disease is far advanced.

Wilms' tumor

Children under the age of 7 years may develop an embryonal type of highly malignant renal growth called Wilms tumor. It metastasizes early. A mass in the abdomen may be the first sign, and later hematuria and anemia may occur. Excellent therapeutic results have been obtained by a combination of nephrectomy, radiation, and chemotherapy.

Tumors of the bladder

Epidemiology

The most common site of cancer in the urinary tract is the bladder. Cancer of the bladder occurs three times more often in males than in females and multiple tumors are common, with about 25% of patients having more than one lesion at the time of diagnosis. This figure increases to about 50% in patients with papilloma, grade I carcinoma, over a 5-year period. Approximately 40%

of the tumors involve the trigone, and an additional 45% involve the posterior and lateral bladder walls.

Etiology

Known factors predisposing to bladder cancer are exposure to the chemicals beta-naphthylamine and xenylamine, infestation with *Schistoma haematobium,* and cigarette smoking.

Pathophysiology

Tumors of the bladder range from small benign papillomas to large invasive carcinomas. Most of the neoplasms are of the transitional cell type since the urinary tract is covered with transitional epithelium. These neoplasms begin as papillomas; therefore all papillomas of the bladder are considered premalignant and are removed when identified. Squamous cell carcinoma occurs less frequently and has a poorer prognosis. Other neoplasias include adenocarcinoma (which is often inoperable) and rhabdomyosarcoma (seen in infants).

Grades I (well differentiated) and II (medially differentiated) bladder tumors are usually superficial, while grades III (poorly differentiated and IV (anaplastic) tumors are usually invasive. Bladder cancers are *staged* according to the depth of invasiveness:

Stage 0: mucosa
Stage A: submucosa
Stage B: muscle
Stage C: perivesical fat
Stage D: lymph nodes

Clinical picture

Painless hematuria is the first symptom in the majority of bladder tumors. It is usually intermittent, and the individual may fail to seek treatment. Painless hematuria occurs also in nonmalignant urinary tract disease and in cancer of the kidney; therefore any hematuria should be investigated. Cystitis (p. 1550) may be the first symptom of a bladder tumor, since the tumor may act as a foreign body in the bladder. Renal failure from obstruction of the ureters sometimes is the reason given for seeking medical care. Vesicovaginal fistulas may occur before other symptoms develop. The last two conditions indicate a poor prognosis because usually the tumor has infiltrated widely.

Cytologic examination of the urine may identify malignant cells before the lesion can be visualized by cystoscopy. The diagnosis is established by cystoscopic visualization of the bladder with biopsy. Clinical determination of the invasiveness of the tumor is important in establishing a therapeutic regimen and in predicting the prognosis. Any person who has had a papilloma removed should have a cystoscopic examination every 3 months for 2 years and then at less frequent intervals if there is no evidence of a new lesion. Repeated cystoscopies may seem unacceptable to patients who dread them. The necessity for frequent examination should be fully explained by the urologist and the explanation reinforced by the nurse. Emphasis should be placed on the necessity for repeated cystoscopies, since papillomas tend to recur without symptoms until they are far-advanced tumors.

Intervention

The treatment for bladder tumors depends on the size of the lesion and the depth of the tissue involvement.

Surgery. Small tumors with minimal tissue layer involvement may be adequately treated with *transurethral fulguration* or *excision*. A Foley catheter may or may not be inserted after surgery. The urine may be pink tinged, but gross bleeding is unusual. Burning on urination may be relieved by forcing fluids and applying heat over the bladder region by means of a heating pad or a sitz bath. The patient is discharged within a few days after surgery.

If the tumor involves the dome of the bladder, a *segmental resection* of the bladder (p. 1532) may be carried out. Over half of the bladder may be resected. A *cystectomy,* or complete removal of the bladder (p. 1532), usually is performed only when the disease appears curable. Complete removal of the bladder requires permanent urinary diversion.

Radiation. *External cobalt radiation of large invasive tumors* is often given before surgery to retard tumor growth. Supervoltage irradiation can be given when the patient physically cannot tolerate surgery. Radiation is not curative and has little value in patient management if the tumor is deemed inoperable. Internal radiation (radioisotopes or radon seeds) is rarely used since the introduction of better methods of external radiation.

Chemotherapy. Chemotherapy is primarily palliative. 5-Fluorouracil (5-FU) and doxorubicin (Adriamycin) are the most commonly used agents. Thio-TEPA may be instilled into the bladder as a topical treatment. The patient is dehydrated 8 to 12 hours before thio-TEPA treatment, and the drug remains in the bladder for 2 hours.

Benign prostatic hypertrophy

Epidemiology

Benign prostatic hypertrophy or hyperplasia (BPH) is an adenomatous enlargement of the prostate gland. The prostate is an encapsulated gland weighing about 20 g that encircles the male urethra below the bladder neck. When the middle lobe of the gland enlarges, it causes narrowing of the urethra. More than half of all men over 50 years of age and 75% of men over 70 have some symptoms of prostatic enlargement. The cause is not known but appears to be related to the presence of male hormones.

Clinical picture

One of the early symptoms of benign prostatic hypertrophy is *nocturia* (awakening at night to void) and urinary frequency in general. The man notices that the urinary stream is smaller and more difficult to start (*hesitancy*). The bladder muscle must contract more forcibly to push the urine past the partial obstruction, and the overworked muscles hypertrophy. Stagnant urine is held in trabeculae, or cellules, formed by sagging of the atonic mucous membranes between hypertrophied muscle bands. The bladder will not empty completely at each voiding (*residual urine*); this urine becomes alkaline from stasis and is a fertile medium for bacterial growth. The man will then complain of symptoms of cystitis (frequency, urgency), and bladder stones may occur. Some men develop hematuria from rupture of blood vessels that have become overstretched. Destruction of renal function can eventually occur from back pressure up the ureter to the kidney. Acute urinary retention is not uncommon.

Enlargement of the lateral lobes of the prostate gland may be palpated by digital rectal examination. Enlargement of the middle lobe is diagnosed by signs of partial obstruction of the urethra and visualization of the obstruction and bladder trabeculae by cystoscopy.

Intervention

Surgery is the primary treatment for benign prostatic hypertrophy. During surgery the capsule of the prostate gland is left intact, and the adenomatous soft tissue is removed by one of four surgical routes: transurethral, suprapubic, retropubic, or perineal. See Table 62-3 for a comparison of the different approaches.

Transurethral prostatectomy. Transurethral prostatic resection (TURP) is performed when the major enlargement exists in the medial lobe that directly surrounds the urethra. There must be a relatively small amount of tissue requiring resection so that excessive bleeding will not occur and the time required to complete the surgery will not be prolonged. A resectoscope (an instrument similar to a cystoscope but equipped with a cutting and cauterization loop attached to electric current) is passed through the urethra. The bladder is irrigated continuously during the procedure. The patient is grounded against electric shocks by a lubricated metal plate placed under his hips. Tiny pieces of tissue are cut away, and the bleeding points are sealed by cauterization (Fig. 62-4). A transurethral prostatectomy may be performed with the patient under general or spinal anesthesia.

Following a TURP, a large (24 Fr) three-way Foley catheter with a 30-ml baloon is usually inserted into the urethra. After the retention balloon of the catheter is inflated, the catheter is pulled down so that the bag

TABLE 62-3. Comparison of types of prostatic surgery

	Transurethral resection	Suprapubic resection	Retropubic resection	Perineal resection	Radical perineal resection
Reason for surgery	Enlargement of medial lobe surrounding urethra	Extremely large mass of obstructing tissue	Large mass located high in pelvic area	Large mass located low in pelvic area	Cancer of prostate gland
Location of incision	No incision; removal by way of urethra	Low midline abdominal incision through bladder to prostate gland	Low midline abdominal incision into prostate gland (bladder not incised)	Incision between scrotum and rectum	Large perineal incision between scrotum and rectum
Drainage tubes	Three-way Foley catheter with 30-ml bag in urethra, constant irrigation for 24 hr	Cystotomy tube or drain through incision; Foley catheter with 30-ml bag in urethra	Foley catheter with 30-ml bag in urethra, constant irrigation for 24 hr	Foley catheter with 30-ml bag in urethra	Foley catheter with 30-ml bag in urethra; drain in incision
Bladder spasms	Yes	Yes	Few	Few	Few
Dressing	No dressing	Abdominal dressing easily soaked with urinary drainage	Abdominal dressing; no urinary drainage	Perineal dressing; no urinary drainage	Perineal dressing; urinary drainage
Complications	Hemorrhage; water intoxication; incontinence	Hemorrhage; wound infection	Hemorrhage; wound infection	Hemorrhage; wound infection	Urinary incontinence; wound infection; impotence; sterility

rests in the prostatic fossa and provides hemostasis. Traction may be applied to the Foley catheter to increase pressure on the operative area to control bleeding. The large size catheter (24 Fr) is used to facilitate removal of clots from the bladder. Since the catheter retention balloon exerts pressure on the internal sphincter of the bladder, the patient continually feels the urge to void. If the catheter is draining properly, the strongest of these sensations usually passes momentarily. Attempting to void around the catheter causes the bladder muscles to contract and results in a painful "bladder spasm."

The nurse should discuss the physiology of the "need to void" with the patient preoperatively so that spasms will be seen as an expected event and not an abnormal complication. The patient is taught that the catheter produces the sensation of fullness and that not straining to pass urine around the catheter and drinking large amounts of fluids will reduce irritation and spasm. Narcotics are given to lessen the pain sensation; belladonna and opium suppositories are prescribed to relieve bladder spasms. As the nerve endings become fatigued, the frequency and severity of spasms decrease. This usually occurs by the end of 24 to 48 hours.

The bladder is constantly irrigated by a three-way drip apparatus with normal saline or another solution prescribed by the surgeon. The purpose of constant irrigation is to keep the bladder free of clots that would block the drainage of urine.

A full bladder increases pressure on the outside of the prostatic fossa "milking" the bleeding vessels. Straining to have a bowel movement may also cause prostatic hemorrhage as can enemas, rectal tubes, and rectal thermometers, all of which are avoided for about a week postoperatively.

Persistent bladder discomfort, bladder spasms, or

failure of a catheter to drain properly usually signifies one of the following serious complications, which require immediate medical attention: (1) hemorrhage and clot retention, (2) displacement of the catheter, or (3) unsuspected perforation of the bladder during surgery.

Sometimes patients develop *water intoxication*, formerly known as transurethral resection (TUR) syndrome, as a result of excessive irrigating solution being absorbed into the venous sinusoids during surgery. Cerebral edema may result. Confusion and agitation on the part of the patient may be the first signs of this condition.

Constant bladder irrigation is usually discontinued after 24 hours if no clots are draining from the bladder. The catheter may then be manually irrigated every 4 hours until removed, usually 3 to 5 days after surgery.

Following removal of the catheter, the patient should measure and record the time and amount of each voiding. The patient may not be able to void after removal of the catheter because of urethral edema. When this occurs, the catheter may need to be reinserted. Continence should also be assessed since the internal and external sphincters lie above and below the prostate, close to the operative area, and may have been disturbed during surgery.

About 2 weeks after TURP when desiccated tissue is sloughed out, there may be a secondary hemorrhage. The patient, who probably is home at this time, must contact the physician immediately should there be any bleeding.

Suprapubic prostatectomy. The alternate methods of prostatectomy are open operations. In the *suprapubic resection* the prostate gland is removed from the urethra by way of the bladder; this type of resection is performed when a large mass of tissue must be resected. The usual method of draining urine following surgery is illustrated in Fig. 62-5, *A*. There will be some type of hemostatic agent placed in the prostatic fossa and urine will be drained by Foley catheter or cystotomy tube or both.

Hemorrhage is a possible complication, and the precautions are the same as those taken following TURP. Since there is some oozing of blood from the prostatic fossa, continuous bladder irrigations are usually ordered for the first 24 hours.

Cystotomy tubes are usually removed 3 to 4 days postoperatively; urethral catheters generally remain until the suprapubic wound is well healed. After the urethral catheter has been removed, the nursing care of the patient is similar to that for the patient undergoing transurethral resection. If the suprapubic wound should reopen and drain, a urethral catheter is usually reinserted.

Retropubic prostatectomy. In a retropubic prostatectomy a low abdominal incision similar to that used

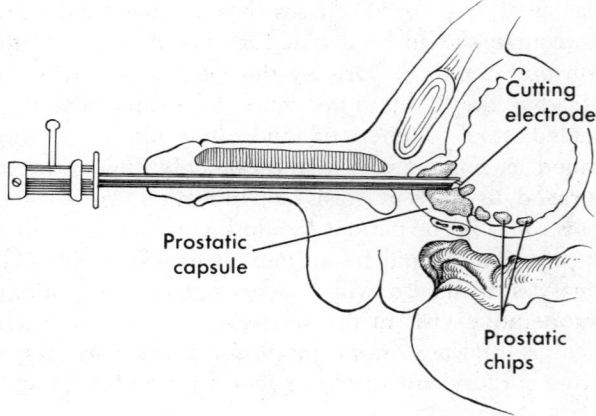

Fig. 62-4. Transurethral resection of prostate gland by means of resectoscope. Note cutting and cauterizing loop of instrument, enlarged prostate gland surrounding urethra, and tiny pieces of prostatic tissue that have been cut away.

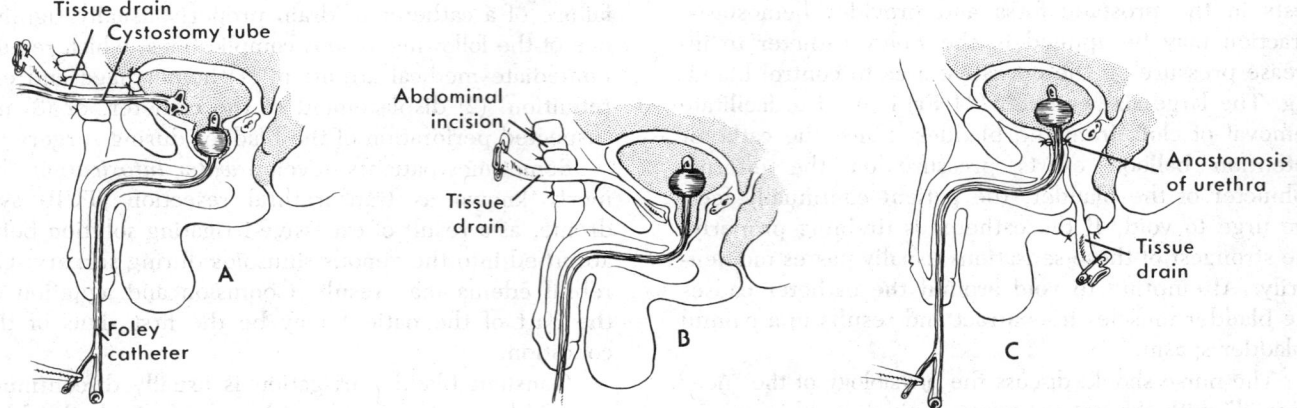

Fig. 62-5. Three methods of surgical removal of prostate gland. **A,** Suprapubic prostatectomy. Note placement of tissue drain, cystostomy tube, and inflated Foley catheter in prostatic fossa. **B,** Retropubic prostatectomy. Note intact bladder, placement of tissue drain, and retention catheter. **C,** Radical perineal prostatectomy. Note placement of tissue drain in incision between scrotum and rectum and anastomosis of urethra made necessary by excision of prostate gland and its capsule.

for suprapubic prostatectomy is made, but the bladder is not opened. Rather, it is retracted and the adenomatous prostatic tissue is removed through an incision in the anterior prostatic capsule (Fig. 62-5, *B*).

Sphincter muscles are seldom damaged by retropubic prostatectomy, and there is no urine fistula. A large Foley catheter is inserted postoperatively, but bladder spasms are not usually a problem. When the Foley catheter is removed, the patient seldom has difficulty voiding. Hemorrhage from the prostatic fossa and wound infection may complicate the surgery; therefore precautions to prevent bleeding as discussed under TURP are taken. There should be no urinary drainage on the abdominal dressing. If urine, purulent drainage, fever, or increased pain with ambulation occurs, the physician should be notified since these symptoms may indicate deep wound infection or pelvic abscess. Hospitalization generally is required for about 1 week after a retropubic prostatectomy.

Perineal prostatectomy. The perineal approach is used primarily for confirmed or suspected cancer of the prostate (Fig. 62-5, *C*). The incision is made between the scrotum and rectum. In addition to removal of the adenomatous prostate tissue, adjacent tissue may be excised when cancer is confirmed. Preoperative and postoperative care is similar to that given a patient having radical perineal surgery (p. 1704).

Patient concerns. Common to all patient undergoing prostatectomy are concerns regarding *sexual functioning* and the *ability to be continent of urine*. The nurse may need to provide opportunity during interactions with the patient to promote expressions of these concerns by the patient. Impotence occurs physiologically when the

perineal nerves are cut during a radical perineal prostatectomy and not with the other types of prostatectomies. If the man believes that the surgery will or may produce impotence, however, this may occur because of psychologic influences. Urinary incontinence frequently follows radical perineal prostatectomy but only occasionally follows transurethral or suprapubic prostatectomy. Most men have some difficulty with continence after any type of prostatectomy. The patient should understand that this is normal for a period after surgery, and he should be taught perineal exercises (p. 1544) to hasten recovery of control over voiding.

Discharge planning. The following points should be included in preparing the patient for discharge from the hospital: (1) Vigorous exercises, heavy lifting, and sexual intercourse should be avoided for about 3 weeks after returning home. (2) Driving during this period is also not advised. (3) Straining with defecation should be avoided; stool softeners or mild cathartics may be prescribed as home-going medication. (4) Fluids are encouraged to prevent stasis and infection and to keep stools soft. (5) The patient should be instructed to notify his physician should his urinary stream diminish. The urinary stream also will be checked on the patient's postoperative visit to the physician. This is important since urethral mucosa in the prostatic area is destroyed during surgery and strictures may form with healing.

Outcome criteria for the man following prostatectomy

The patient or significant others can:
1. Explain care of the catheter if discharged with an indwelling catheter.

2. Describe perineal exercises if mild incontinence is present.
3. State measures to prevent constipation.
4. Describe signs of wound infection, urinary retention, or excessive bleeding requiring medical intervention.
5. State plans for medical follow-up.
6. State activities to be avoided because of possible bleeding (sexual intercourse, heavy lifting, straining at stool) until medical permission to perform them is given (about 3 weeks).

Renal disease

Although kidney disease is often equated with a severe life-threatening illness without reversibility, this picture is seen in only a very small percentage of individuals in whom kidney disease has been diagnosed. Renal problems are extremely varied (1) in cause and potential for a cure as compared with control of the illness; (2) in the signs and symptoms the patient shows that reflect differences in the kidney structures involved and the functions impaired; (3) in the event or progression of the illness and the "sickness" of the patient; and (4) in the onset of the problem, which can be sudden, occur gradually, or be entirely unknown to the person.

The overall goal for managing renal problems is to preserve renal function. This must be achieved through prompt recognition of the illness, cure of those problems that can be eradicated, and control of those problems that cannot be reversed.

The National Kidney Foundation,* through state and local offices, provides assistance to those concerned with kidney disease. Services of this organization include direct service to patients, public education, and funding for research.

Classification of renal disease

Renal disease usually alters the functional ability of one of the major structural parts of the kidney: the glomeruli, the tubules, the vascular bed, or the interstitial tissue (Table 62-4). When disease is persistent or severe in nature, all of the kidney structures may become affected and the kidney becomes nonfunctional. In the following section on common diseases of the kidney an illness involving each of the major renal structures is discussed.

*Two Park Ave., New York, NY 10016.

TABLE 62-4. Effect of kidney disease on structure and function

Site of disease	Renal process affected	Effect on function
Glomeruli	Alters filtration process in capillary tufts	Loss of large amounts of protein and red blood cells
Tubules	Destroys ability to modify fluid	Interferes with conservation of electrolytes and elimination of waste materials
Vascular bed	Decreased blood supply to glomeruli and tubules	Decreased function depending on structure affected
Interstitial tissue	Destroys kidney tissue by pressure as cysts fill and scar tissue forms	Decreased function depending on structure affected

Illness can occur that influences renal function without directly involving kidney tissue. Problems of this nature are seen when urinary output decreases and the clearance of materials normally excreted by the kidneys falls. *Problems commonly involve either a reduction in blood supply to the kidneys (prerenal disease) or an obstruction in the flow of urine within the urinary tract (postrenal disease).* The signs and symptoms of renal failure that these conditions precipitate may disappear as the underlying extrarenal problems are resolved. The classification of renal disease is given in Table 62-5.

Within the broad area of kidney disease, certain illnesses are more amenable than others to prevention, as follows:

Glomerular disease
Acute poststreptococcal glomerulonephritis
Infective endocarditis
Toxemia of pregnancy

Vascular disease
Nephrosclerosis
Hypersensitivity angiitis

Tubular disease
Acute tubular insufficiency
Hypokalemic nephropathy
Hypercalcemic nephropathy
Obstructive nephropathy

Interstitial disease
Pyelonephritis
Drug and heavy-metal poisoning
Urate nephropathy[60]

TABLE 62-5. Classification of renal disease

Prerenal (poor kidney perfusion)	Renal (primary kidney pathologic condition)	Postrenal (obstructive disorders)
Hypovolemia	Glomerular	Calculi
Blood or plasma loss	Nephritis: acute and	Tumor
Sodium or	chronic	Benign prostatic
water loss	Diabetic sclerosis	hypertrophy
Cardiac failure	Lupus erythematosus	Cancer
Myocardial infarct	Nephrotic syndrome	Strictures or ste-
Congestive failure	Vascular	nosis
Arrhythmias	Nephrosclerosis	
Septic shock	Vasculitis	
	Tubular	
	Toxins or poisons	
	Ischemic injury	
	Congenital dysfunction	
	Interstitial	
	Pyelonephritis	
	Tuberculosis	
	Analgesic or heavy-	
	metal toxicity	
	Tumors or cysts	
	Polycystic disease	
	Benign or malignant	
	tumors	

Acute glomerulonephritis

Etiology

Glomerulonephritis is a disease that affects the glomeruli of both kidneys. Etiologic factors are many and varied; they include immunologic reactions (lupus erythematosus, streptococcal infection), vascular injury (hypertension), metabolic disease (diabetes mellitus), and disseminated intravascular coagulation (DIC). Glomerulonephritis exists in acute, latent, and chronic forms. The most common form of *acute glomerulonephritis* occurs after a streptococcal infection. Common sites of infection include the throat (tonsillitis, strep throat) and the skin (impetigo).

Epidemiology

Children of preschool and grade-school age are most likely to develop the illness. Of all individuals developing acute poststreptococcal glomerulonephritis, approximately 1% to 2% will develop end-stage renal failure in which dialysis or transplantation is required to maintain life. Approximately 90% of children and 50% of adults with acute glomerulonephritis attain full recovery from illness, although recovery may require up to 2 years.[60] Little inference regarding prognosis can be made on the severity of the acute episode. Persons with mild illness may develop chronic disease, and those with severe ill-

ness may completely recover and have no recurrence of the illness.

Pathophysiology

Acute poststreptococcal glomerulonephritis is a result of an antigen-antibody reaction with glomerular tissue that produces swelling and death of capillary cells. The antigen-antibody reaction activates the complement pathway (p. 278) resulting in chemotaxis of polymorphonuclear (PMN) leukocytes with release of lysosomal enzymes that attack the glomerular basement membrane (GBM). The response in the membrane is an increase in the three types of glomerular cells (endothelial, mesangial, and epithelial) causing an increase in membrane porosity with resultant proteinemia and hematuria. Renal function is depressed by scarring in the glomerulus causing oliguria and retention of water, sodium, and nitrogenous waste products, leading to edema and azotemia.

Prevention

Prevention of acute poststreptococcal glomerulonephritis involves prompt medical treatment of sore throats and upper respiratory tract infections. Cultures should be obtained, and when indicated appropriate antibiotics are prescribed.

Clinical picture

Common complaints are shortness of breath, mild headache, weakness, and anorexia. Usual signs include proteinuria, hematuria, increased urine specific gravity, dependent edema, and an elevated antistreptolysin O titer. Additionally, signs of elevation in blood pressure, decreased urinary output, and elevation in serum urea nitrogen and creatine levels may be present. Signs and symptoms reflect damage to the glomeruli with leaking of protein and red cells into the urine, varying degrees of decreased glomerular filtration with retention of wastes, and fluid overloading of varying severity.

Intervention

Control of infection. Persistent infection is treated promptly to help further decrease antigen-antibody complex formation. Persons with poststreptococcal glomerulonephritis are given a prophylactic antibiotic; the drug of choice is penicillin. Rationale for this therapy is based on preventing further infections that could reactivate the nephritis. Prophylactic therapy may be continued for months after the acute phase of illness. Exposure to any infection must be avoided, since even mild infections may reactivate nephritis.

Activity. Bed rest is instituted until clinical signs disappear; this may involve a period of several months. Ambulation is allowed when blood sedimentation rates and blood pressure are normal and edema abates. If ambulation causes an increase in proteinuria or hematuria, bed rest is reinstituted. Since the period of bed rest may be long and the person usually does not feel ill, the nurse may need to continue reinforcing the importance of bed rest and assist in planning diversionary activities and the constructive use of time. For small children this can present no small problem. When bed rest is reinstituted after periods of ambulation, the person may become depressed. Helping the person to express concerns and feelings can serve as a basis for helping make realistic plans about the illness and its sequelae.

Maintenance of fluid balance. Edema and fluid overloading are anticipated and treated initially with dietary sodium restrictions. The amount of restriction depends on the severity of fluid retention, and it is maintained until dependent edema and circulatory overload are no longer a problem. Diuretics are generally reserved for managing severe fluid overload and pulmonary edema. The nurse is constantly alert for signs of fluid overload (p. 333). Blood pressure elevation is treated with antihypertensive drugs only after fluid control has proved unsuccessful in contolling hypertension. Dietary protein is reduced only when blood urea nitrogen and creatinine levels are elevated. The diet should contain sufficient carbohydrate to prevent protein being used for energy. This helps maintain nitrogen balance.

Long-term care. Up to 2 years may be required for resolution of the illness. During this time proteinuria, hematuria, and cellular debris may exist microscopically. The person generally shows little to no change from normal in renal function. At this point normal activities may be continued, although fatigue, trauma, and infection need to be avoided as they exacerbate illness. Good general health measures are stressed. Since these persons usually feel well, they often must be convinced of the need to continue prescribed treatment and to return for routine follow-up health care. They should understand which signs and symptoms are significant and indicate a need for medical attention. They need to be encouraged to pursue care even though they were thoroughly examined only a short time previously.

Chronic glomerulonephritis

Etiology

Although chronic glomerulonephritis (CGN) may follow the acute disease, the majority of persons give no history of the disease. In most instances no evidence of predisposing infection can be found. The course of chronic glomerulonephritis is extremely varied. Some persons with minimal impairment in renal function continue to feel well and show little progression of disease. With other individuals the progression of renal deterioration may be slow but steady and end in renal failure.

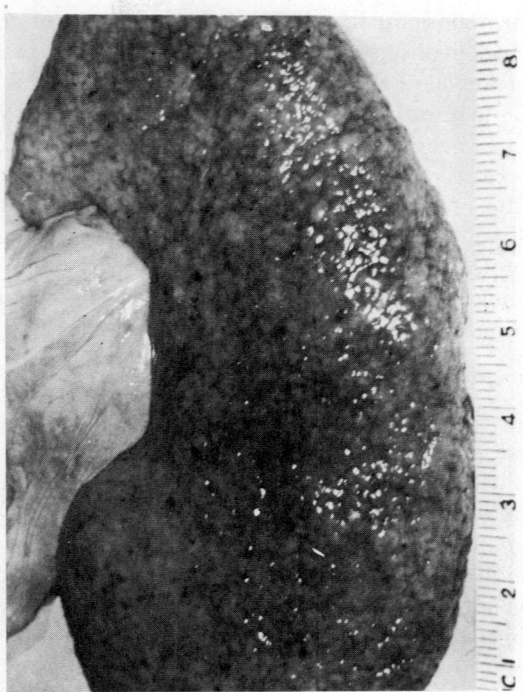

Fig. 62-6. End-stage chronic glomerulonephritis. Note pebbly surface corresponding to surviving hypertrophied nephrons amid atrophy. (From Anderson, W.A.D., and Kissane, J.M.: Pathology, ed. 7, St. Louis, 1977, The C.V. Mosby Co.)

In still other individuals the progression of disease is rapid.

Pathophysiology

Chronic glomerulonephritis is characterized by slow progressive destruction (sclerosis) of glomeruli and gradual loss of renal function. The glomeruli have varying degrees of hypercellularity and become sclerosed (hardened). The kidney decreases in size and eventually there is tubular atrophy, chronic interstitial inflammation, and arteriosclerosis[51] (Fig. 62-6).

Clinical picture

Various symptoms of failing renal function, none of which may seem severe, may lead the person to seek health care. There may be a slow onset of recurrent dependent edema, or there may be mild headache, especially in the morning. Dyspnea on exertion or difficulty sleeping in a flat position may be noted. Blurring of vision may lead the person to an ophthalmologist, who may be the first to suspect chronic renal disease based on ocular vascular changes. Nocturia is a common complaint. Occasionally, chronic nephritis is discovered during routine physical examination or may be discovered by a school nurse who observes marked visual changes and lassitude in a student. Weakness, fatigue, and weight loss are common but nonspecific symptoms of chronic glomerulonephritis. Early in the disease urinalysis shows the presence of albumin, casts, and blood. At this point renal function tests may be normal. The ability of the kidneys to regulate the internal environment will begin to decrease as more and more glomeruli become scarred and the amount of functional renal tissue is reduced. Finally, when few intact nephrons remain, hematuria and proteinuria decrease, the specific gravity of the urine becomes fixed, and the nonprotein nitrogen level in the blood increases.

Intervention

No specific therapy exists to arrest or reverse the disease process. With some forms of chronic glomerulonephritis steroid therapy may be attempted, although results of this therapy in arresting disease are not well documented. Care involves teaching the person to live healthfully: to avoid infections, to eat a balanced diet within modifications of sodium intake if prescribed, to appropriately administer medications, and to maintain follow-up health care visits and report to the physician any exacerbations in signs and symptoms. Treatment of renal failure (p. 1570) begins when the illness destroys so much kidney tissue that the individual's kidneys are no longer able to independently control his or her internal environment.

With any exacerbation of hematuria, hypertension, and edema, the person is put to bed, and treatment similar to that for acute glomerulonephritis is instituted. Signs of pulmonary edema and congestive failure are monitored for when caring for these persons. Treatment is symptomatic and supportive.

Women with chronic glomerulonephritis who become pregnant appear to be susceptible to toxemia and to spontaneous abortion. The woman who has had nephritis of any nature should be urged to see a physician if she plans on pregnancy. When pregnancy does occur, she should remain under close health supervision.

Outcome criteria for the person with glomerulonephritis

The person or significant others can:
1. Explain the rationale for therapy (prolongation of bed rest, maintenance of fluid balance).
2. Explain dietary changes (decreased sodium intake, adequate caloric intake, controlled protein intake if prescribed).
3. Explain medication program to be followed at home (prophylactic penicillin therapy).
4. Explain health maintenance program.
   a. Measures to prevent further infection.
   b. Signs that require immediate medical attention (hematuria, hypertension, edema, headaches).
   c. Plans for continued follow-up health care.

Nephrotic syndrome (nephrosis)

Etiology and epidemiology

Nephrotic syndrome is a condition involving damage to the glomeruli where quantities of protein are lost in the urine. This condition has been associated with allergic reactions (insect bites, pollen, acute glomerulonephritis), infections (herpes zoster), systemic disease (diabetes mellitus, sickle cell disease), circulatory problems (severe congestive heart failure, chronic constrictive pericarditis), and pregnancy. Known glomerular disease is the most common precipitating event in adults; in children the syndrome appears frequently with no evidence of a causative factor. In approximately 25% of children and 50% to 75% of adults who develop nephrosis the disease progresses to renal failure within 5 years.[9] In other individuals (particularly children) there may be remissions, or nephrosis may exist in a chronic form. Other than treating underlying illness, little can be done to prevent the occurrence or recurrence of nephrosis.

Pathophysiology

The initial change in nephrotic syndrome is a derangement of cells in the glomerular basement membrane resulting in increased membrane porosity with loss of large amounts of protein into the urine (proteinuria). As protein continues to be excreted, serum albumin is decreased (hypoalbuminemia) decreasing the serum osmotic pressure. The capillary hydrostatic fluid (push) pressure in all body tissues becomes greater than the capillary osmotic (pull) pressure, and generalized edema results (Fig. 62-7). As fluid is lost into the tissues, the plasma volume decreases, stimulating secretion of aldosterone to retain more sodium and water and decreasing the glomerular filtration rate to retain water. This additional fluid also passes out of the capillaries into the tissue, leading to even greater edema.

Clinical picture

Characteristic manifestations of the nephrotic syndrome include *severe generalized edema* that is particularly noticeable in dependent areas, pronounced *proteinuria* that contains *albumin* and *globulin* protein fractions, and *hypoalbuminemia*. Serum lipids are often elevated; hypertension and hematuria occur when glomerulonephritis is the underlying disease. Urine volumes and renal function may be either normal or markedly altered. Altered renal function and development of renal failure occur as a result of progressing glomerulonephritis.

Loss of appetite and fatigue are common. Women usually have amenorrhea or other disturbances in their reproductive cycle.

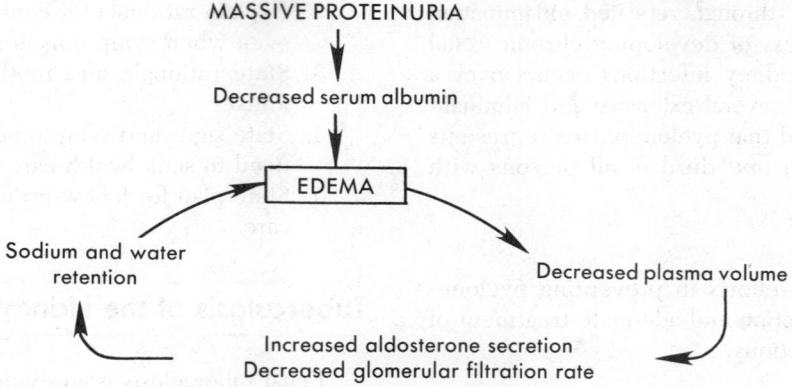

Fig. 62-7. Pathophysiologic changes in nephrotic syndrome.

Intervention

Treatment of nephrotic syndrome is directed toward reducing albuminuria, controlling edema, and promoting general health. Corticosteroids may be useful in controlling the illness, but the response to them will vary from remission of nephrosis to no response. Prednisone is the steroid preparation most frequently prescribed. The diet should contain normal to increased amounts of protein (1 g/kg body weight per day) and be high in calories. Periodic determination of proteinuria and measures of renal function enable the physician to monitor response to treatment and level of kidney function.

To control edema, sodium intake is reduced and diuretics are employed to increase excretion of fluid. When diuretics are administered over prolonged periods, hypokalemia usually results (p. 337). Potassium may be supplemented through dietary intake; medication supplements should be initiated only after attempts to increase serum potassium through dietary means have failed. Bed rest is usually ordered when edema is severe; however, immobility is contraindicated for prolonged periods.

Persons with nephrosis need to direct particular attention toward preventing infection, since body defenses are impaired by urinary protein losses and edematous tissues are particularly susceptible to injury. When infection is suspected, it is important to give immediate attention to the problem. Culture and sensitivity studies are done and appropriate antibiotics are prescribed. The person is informed of the importance of prescribed medication and diet therapy and of the need for follow-up health care.

Outcome criteria for the person with nephrotic syndrome

1. Independence in activities of daily living is maintained.
2. The person remains free of infection.
3. Edema and blood pressure are controlled; pul-

monary edema and congestive heart failure do not occur.

The person or significant others can:
1. Describe measures to prevent infection.
2. State name, dosage, frequency, and side effects of prescribed medications (steroids, diuretics).
3. State dietary prescription (increased calories, adequate protein, decreased sodium) and plan appropriate meals.
4. State plans requiring immediate attention (increase in edema, fatigue, headache, presence of infection).
5. State plans for follow-up health care.

Pyelonephritis

Etiology

Pyelonephritis refers to bacterial infection of kidney tissue. This infection usually begins in the lower urinary tract and ascends into the kidneys. Lower urinary tract infection may be asymptomatic, and kidney involvement may be the first indication of lower (urinary) tract disease. Often the diagnostic workup of a person with pyelonephritis reveals previously unknown urinary tract obstruction or the presence of other chronic kidney disease. *Escherichia coli* is the most common organism identified in pyelonephritis, and resistance to antibiotic therapy rarely results. Pyelonephritis is most commonly associated with (1) pregnancy; (2) obstruction, instrumentation or trauma of the urinary tract; and (3) chronic health problems including diabetes, analgesic abuse, polycystic kidney disease, and hypertensive kidney disease.

Pathophysiology

Infection of the kidney occurs in both acute and chronic forms. Although acute pyelonephritis may temporarily affect renal function, rarely does this progress to a level of renal failure. Chronic pyelonephritis destroys renal tissue permanently through repeated inflammation and scarring. The process of developing chronic renal failure from repeated kidney infections occurs over a number of years or after several extensive and fulminant infections. It is estimated that pyelonephritis represents the original diagnosis in one third of all persons with chronic renal disease.[80]

Prevention

The most significant efforts in preventing pyelonephritis are through detection and adequate treatment of lower urinary tract infections.

Clinical picture

Signs and symptoms of pyelonephritis usually include those associated with lower urinary tract infection (p. 1551), along with fever, chills, malaise, costovertebral tenderness, and leukocytosis. The urine shows white blood cells, white blood cell casts, and bacteria. Signs and symptoms of renal failure may be present when nephron damage is extensive (p. 1571).

Intervention

Optimal treatment includes early detection of the illness, antibacterial therapy based on urine cultures, and correction and treatment of any underlying systemic disease or urinary tract abnormality. Anyone with symptoms of dysuria, cloudy urine, or frequent small voidings should be examined for urinary tract infection and appropriately treated. Persons complaining of fever and costovertebral tenderness should be encouraged to seek medical attention.

The course of antibiotic therapy may extend over weeks, and the person may need to be reminded of the necessity to continue taking the medication even when symptoms disappear and he or she begins to feel better. Continuing drug therapy to eradicate all infection and prevent development of resistant strains of organisms is stressed. The urine is recultured 2 weeks after drug therapy has been discontinued and every month thereafter for the next several months. Increasing fluid intake to 3 L/day in persons capable of excreting this amount of fluid is desirable to prevent stasis of urine and further bacterial growth. Should infection become chronic, drug therapy may continue indefinitely; the goal is to reduce and control the bacterial population of the urinary tract so that renal damage is prevented. Urine cultures should be repeated periodically and the person should be instructed in the signs and symptoms indicating reactivation of infection and the need for medical attention.

Outcome criteria for the person with pyelonephritis

The person or significant others can:
1. State name, dosage, frequency, and side effects of antibiotic therapy.
2. Explain rationale for continued antibiotic therapy even when symptoms are no longer present.
3. State rationale and method for increasing fluid intake.
4. State signs and symptoms of kidney infection and need to seek health care when symptoms recur.
5. State plan for follow-up urine cultures and health care.

Tuberculosis of the kidney

Renal tuberculosis is an example of a kidney infection that is secondary to an infection in a different site (pulmonary tuberculosis). It is acquired by hematogenous spread from the lung and is most common in men between 20 and 40 years of age. Treatment is primarily medical and consists of antituberculosis medication therapy coupled with rest and good nutrition. Respiratory isolation is not necessary.

Hypertensive renal disease (nephrosclerosis)

Etiology and epidemiology

Hypertension is a major precipitating factor of renal damage. It is estimated that approximately 10% of individuals with essential hypertension develop severe renal damage, and approximately 1% will develop end-stage renal failure and die unless supportive care is provided.[59]

Pathophysiology

Regardless of origin (essential or renal), hypertension that is untreated over a period of time leads to the sclerosing of renal arterioles. The blood supply to glomeruli, tubules, and interstitium gradually decreases. Scarring and death of kidney tissue occur, and signs of renal insufficiency develop when damage to the kidneys has become extensive. *Nephrosclerosis* is the term given to this destructive process.

Prevention

Preventive care includes greater screening efforts to detect persons with elevated blood pressure, adequate treatment and follow-up for those with hypertension, and education regarding the nature of the illness, the diet and medications, and the importance of periodic follow-up health care. Yearly blood pressure monitoring of persons with elevated blood pressure is a minimal preventive care measure.

Clinical picture

By the time signs and symptoms indicating kidney involvement develop, the disease has progressed to an extreme point. Deterioration in renal function progresses gradually unless an acute or malignant phase of hypertension (p. 1177) occurs to accelerate the process. Signs and symptoms are those of chronic renal failure (p. 1577).

Intervention

Treatment of nephrosclerosis is directed toward early detection and treatment of hypertension. Causative factors are sought, and treatment to lower blood pressure is begun (p. 1179). When significant renal damage exists, stabilizing the person's current level of function or slowing deterioration of kidney tissue is the goal. Control of hypertension is continued, and management of end-stage disease and uremic symptoms provides for comfort and increased independence in daily living, although renal function may not improve.

Polycystic kidney disease

Etiology and epidemiology

Polycystic kidney disease is an inherited defect that involves the kidneys bilaterally. Cysts develop that compress and destroy functional renal tissue. Polycystic disease occurs primarily in two distinct age groups, infancy and middle age. Infants developing this illness typically die within a few months. Adults in the 40- to 50-year range generally become symptomatic and develop end-stage disease 10 to 15 years after symptoms arise. Males and females seem equally affected (Fig. 62-8).

There is no preventive care for the illness. Early detection and medical care that prevents and controls infection retard the development of renal failure.

Pathophysiology

Polycystic disease of the newborn (Fig. 62-8, *A*) is characterized by fully developed cysts that are essentially closed sacs into which the glomerular filtrate flows. In the adult, cysts develop slowly in the nephron over a period of years and are open cysts through which the filtrate flows. Gradually, the increasing size of the cysts creates pressure on the surrounding parenchyma causing ischemic atrophy (Fig. 62-8, *B*).

Clinical picture

Signs and symptoms of polycystic disease include discomfort and pain in the flank; the awareness of a "mass," which is the enlarged cystic kidney; fever, chills, and malaise when infection occurs; and hematuria with rupturing of cysts. Colicky pain may be experienced when clots are passed down the ureter. Signs and symptoms of uremia occur when renal function deteriorates to the point of the end-stage renal disease. When the diagnosis of polycystic kidney disease is made, tests of renal function are obtained. These serve to evaluate current renal status and provide a baseline for detecting future changes in kidney function.

Intervention

Intervention for the person with polycystic disease centers largely on preventing infection or bleeding and on dealing with the emotional impact of having a genetically determined illness. Infection is difficult to eradicate in polycystic kidneys, and when uncontrolled it leads to further destruction of kidney tissue. Frequent culture of the urine is performed, and instru-

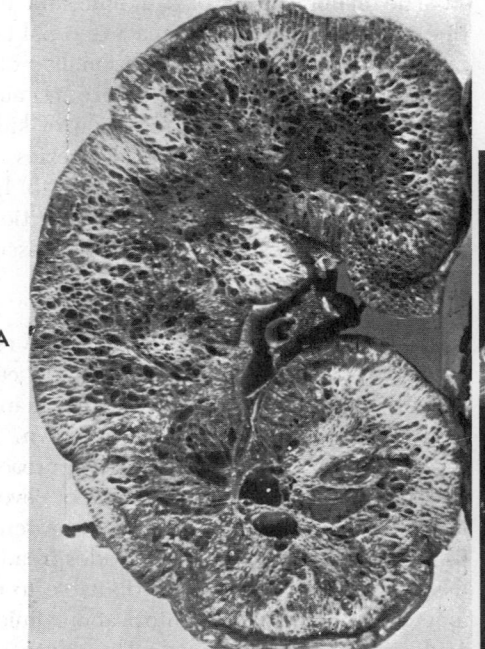
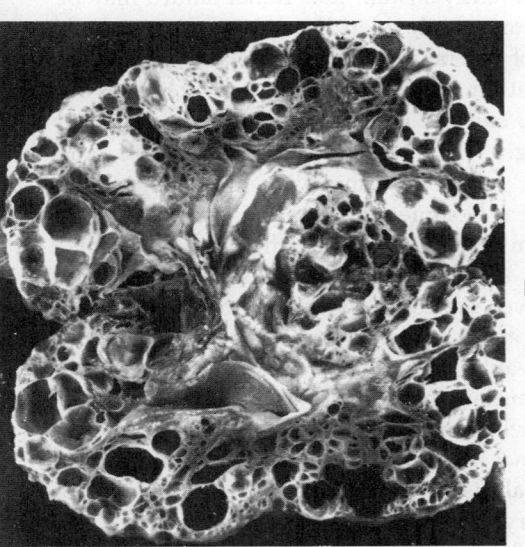

Fig. 62-8. Polycystic disease of kidney. **A,** Newborn infant. **B,** Adult. (From Anderson, W.A.D., and Kissane, J.M.: Pathology, ed. 7, St. Louis, 1977, The C.V. Mosby Co.)

mentation of the urinary tract is avoided whenever possible. Bleeding occurs with rupture of cysts and varies from microscopic to gross hematuria. Bed rest is instituted when bleeding is sufficient to turn the urine from pink to red. Nephrectomy may be required to control continuing, severe bleeding. Treatment for renal failure is instituted when signs and symptoms of uremia appear.

The emotional overtones of this illness can be severe for both the individual and the family. Challenge exists in helping a person deal with an illness on an individual basis when relatives have died of the same disease and children have not yet developed symptoms. Counseling regarding family health care and the person's role in passing on a potentially fatal disease to children will at some time be required.

Outcome criteria for the person with polycystic kidney disease

The person or significant others can:
1. State signs and symptoms of infection and blood loss requiring medical attention.
2. State plans for follow-up health care.
3. Describe appropriate health screening and follow-up care for children.

Renal failure

Renal failure indicates a state of total or nearly total loss of the kidney's ability to excrete waste products and to maintain fluid and electrolyte balance. Laboratory tests reflect the changes in the internal environment, and the person appears clinically ill. The person in renal failure cannot independently sustain life. Renal failure may be acute in onset or may develop slowly and progressively over a course of several years. When renal failure occurs suddenly, as within a few days, biochemical changes are often dramatic, and the person has little time to adjust to these changes. The person becomes very ill, and hospitalization, frequently involving placement in a critical care area, becomes necessary.

When renal failure occurs as the end result of a chronic kidney illness where kidney tissue is destroyed progressively over the course of several months or years, control of symptoms and preservation of functional abilities are achievable goals. Dietary adjustment, medications, and attention to preventing additional illnesses compensate for loss of kidney function in early stages of progressing renal failure. As renal function continues to deteriorate, dialysis or transplantation additionally becomes necessary to support life.

Renal insufficiency designates significant loss of renal function but with enough function remaining to maintain an internal environment consistent with life, providing no additional stressors to health occur. The individual may appear and feel well although laboratory data reflect a deterioration in renal function. Renal insufficiency occurs as a phase in gradually and chronically progressive renal disease.

Acute renal failure

Pathophysiology

Acute renal failure occurs as a sudden and frequently reversible decrease or cessation of kidney function. It generally follows an identifiable trauma of either toxic or ischemic nature. The health of the individual before the insult is usually good to adequate. Renal *ischemia* occurs when blood flow to the kidneys is reduced. The response of the normal kidney is vasoconstriction, which compounds the problem of reduced renal blood flow and increases renal ischemia. Perfusion problems affect both kidneys. When ischemia is prolonged, renal tubular tissue dies and frank renal failure develops.

A variety of substances are *toxic* to the cells of the renal tubules. The kidney with its large blood flow, ability to concentrate solute inside the tubules, and ability to concentrate fluid in the medullary portion of the kidney (where the tubules are located) creates conditions where exposure of tubular cells to toxins is maximized. The kidneys are affected bilaterally.

Etiology

The major causes of ischemic and toxic injuries to the kidney that may lead to acute renal failure are listed in the box on p. 1571. Additionally, other conditions can precipitate acute renal failure: (1) acute glomerular disease, (2) acute severe infection of kidney tissue, (3) bilateral occlusion of the renal arteries, (4) mechanical obstructions in the urinary tract, and (5) hemoglobinemia and myoglobinemia. All of these conditions lead to massive and rapid destruction of kidney tissue.

Prognosis

Recovery from an episode of acute renal failure depends on the underlying illness, the condition of the patient, and the careful, supportive management given during the period of kidney shutdown. Mortality associated with acute tubular necrosis approaches 40%; these statistics largely reflect the deaths of severely ill persons in whom renal failure is a sequela to extensive underlying illness. Owing to the more widespread availability of dialysis, mortality directly attributable to decreased renal function from potassium intoxication, fluid overload, and acidosis has been reduced. The potential for recovery of renal function for those who survive the acute episode of tubular insufficiency is good. Although recovery sta-

CONDITIONS AND SUBSTANCES THAT PRODUCE ISCHEMIC OR NEPHROTOXIC INJURY TO THE KIDNEY

Ischemic*

Hypovolemia

Blood loss (surgery, trauma)

Plasma loss (burns, surgery, acute pancreatitis)

Sodium and water loss (prolonged diarrhea or vomiting, gastrointestinal tract drainage, sustained high fever)

Cardiac failure

Myocardial infarction

Cardiac arrhythmias

Congestive heart failure

Septic shock

Toxic†

Solvents (carbon tetrachloride, methanol, ethylene glycol)

Heavy metals (lead, arsenic, mercury)

Antibiotics (kanamycin, gentamicin, polymyxin B, amphotericin B, colistin, neomycin, phenazopyridine)

Pesticides

Mushrooms

*Inadequate perfusion of the kidney.
†Injury to kidney cells.

tistics indicate that kidney tissue may regenerate more completely after toxic injury in comparison with ischemic injury, follow-up studies of persons years after episodes of acute tubular insufficiency show normal to near normal renal function.[59]

For those in whom acute renal failure has been caused by glomerular disease or severe infection of kidney tissue, the prognosis may not be as favorable. Return of renal function is determined by the extent of scarring and obliteration of functional renal tissue that has occurred during the acute episode of kidney failure. A significant number of adults who develop acute glomerulonephritis show some decrease in renal function, which may remain at a level not producing biochemical abnormalities or may progress to a chronic form of renal failure.

Prevention

The incidence of acute renal failure can be reduced through identification and observation of populations at risk and identification and control of environmental risk factors. *The greatest incidence of acute renal failure occurs in persons who have undergone major trauma, extensive burns, aortic surgery, massive blood loss, or severe myocardial infarction with or without associated arrhythmia*. Acute renal failure also frequently occurs in patients with *sepsis* and in those having abnormal intravascular coagulation, such as *DIC*, since these acutely ill persons are prime candidates for inadequate kidney perfusion. Frequent monitoring of urinary output and detection of excessive losses of body fluid will help to identify instances of inadequate renal perfusion before development of renal failure.

Significant factors in preventive care for the general population include control of nephrotoxic drugs, increased medical supervision of persons with sore throats and upper respiratory tract infections, and increased case finding and treatment of individuals with bacteriuria and obstructive disease of the urinary system. Attempts to control the distribution and identification of nephrotoxic drugs and chemicals is largely accomplished through the Food and Drug Administration (FDA). Identification of nephrotoxic drugs and chemicals, enforced labeling of these substances, and drug dispensing by prescription only are examples of this agency's attempts to promote the public health. Proper labeling and storage of potentially toxic drugs and chemicals in the home can reduce further the number of accidental ingestions of nephrotoxic substances.

Clinical picture

Signs and symptoms indicating the onset of acute renal failure appear rapidly and are a direct result of retention of fluids, electrolytes, and waste materials (Table 62-6). Typically, the person is acutely ill; in addition to the renal failure frequently being superimposed on an already severely compromised individual, biochemical changes occur rapidly and give the person little time to adjust to the altered internal environment. Either *oliguria* (urinary output below 400 ml/day) or *anuria* (urinary output below 100 ml/day) may be present, although oliguria is more common. Classically, the patient in acute renal failure shows a fall in urinary output within 1 to 2 days to between 50 and 400 ml/day. The specific gravity of the urine is low (1.010), and the osmolality of the urine approaches that of the person's serum (280 to 320 milliosmoles). Specific gravity and urine osmolality remain within this fixed range and reflect tubular damage with loss of concentrating ability. Additionally, the urine may show a higher concentration of sodium than would be expected in the case of dehydration or low circulating blood volume. This finding reflects the damaged kidneys' inability to conserve sodium ions and is an important consideration in diagnosing the existence of acute renal failure.

Fluid intake in excess of the diminished urinary output and insensible losses is retained in the body, resulting in edema. When fluid overload is excessive, signs of congestive failure and pulmonary edema are present. Hypertension accompanies acute renal failure when the

TABLE 62-6. Symptoms caused by physiologic changes in acute renal failure

Physiologic effects	Findings	Symptoms
Oliguric phase		
Inability to excrete metabolic wastes	Increased serum urea nitrogen and creatinine	Nausea; vomiting; drowsiness; confusion; coma; gastrointestinal bleeding; asterixis; pericarditis
Inability to regulate electrolytes	Hyperkalemia; hyponatremia; acidosis	Nausea; vomiting; cardiac arrhythmias; Kussmaul's breathing; drowsiness; confusion; coma
Inability to excrete fluid loads	Fluid overload: hypervolemia	Edema; congestive heart failure; pulmonary edema; hypertension
Diuretic phase		
Increased production of urine	Hypovolemia; loss of sodium and potassium in urine	Urinary output of up to 4-5 L/day; postural hypotension; tachycardia
Slowly increasing excretion of metabolic wastes	Initially, high BUN (fluid loss greater than solute loss); gradual return of BUN to normal	Increasing mental alertness and activity

person is hypervolemic, although this is usually not a finding when fluid balance is controlled.

Retention of electrolytes and waste materials from cellular metabolism produces typical signs and symptoms often referred to as *uremia*. Serum potassium, urea nitrogen, and creatinine values rise sharply. In the person who has already sustained illness and trauma, urea nitrogen values may increase at a rate of 30 mg/100 ml/day. As urinary excretion of the acid end products of metabolism decreases, acidosis occurs, carbon dioxide values decline to 15 mEq/L or less, and Kussmaul's breathing occurs (p. 356). Symptoms attributable to retained wastes and altered electrolyte balance include nausea, vomiting, drowsiness, fatigue, and shortness of breath with fluid overloading. Signs produced by these internal changes include confusion, convulsions, coma, gastrointestinal tract bleeding, and asterixis (p. 699).

Additional problems that may beset the person with acute renal failure are pericarditis and infection. Pericarditis is thought to develop as a result of pericardial irritation from accumulated metabolic wastes. It is diagnosed by the presence of a cardiac friction rub and pleuritic-like pain over the precordium. Fever often accompanies pericarditis. When fluid accumulates in the pericardial sac, the rub becomes less intense or absent and *pulsus paradoxus* (pulse weaker during inspiration)

is likely to be present. Pericardial effusion can be confirmed by echocardiography. Infection frequently develops in response to lowered host resistance, multiple trauma, and immobility during the course of the illness.

When oliguria or rising creatinine and urea nitrogen values are noted, the physician must determine whether the decreased output and decreased renal function are the results of inadequate renal perfusion or of frank renal failure. This distinction directs treatment. In instances of poor kidney perfusion, restoring circulating volume by adding fluids and otherwise increasing cardiac output prevents death of kidney tissue and subsequent renal failure. In contrast, the treatment of true renal failure is supportive and is based on careful balance of input and output of fluid, electrolytes, and wastes. In addition to the urine sodium concentration as a diagnostic sign, the physician may wish to challenge the patient's ability to excrete fluid. In this instance usually 100 to 500 ml of fluid is given as rapidly as possible intravenously. A poorly perfused but intact kidney should respond with increased urinary output. During this treatment the patient must be closely monitored for signs and symptoms of cardiac failure and pulmonary edema (p. 1127). The kidney in acute failure will be unable to produce a greater urine flow in response to this fluid challenge. The physician may give furosemide, 40 to 80 mg intravenously, in an attempt to produce a greater flow of urine. The test may be repeated if there is no response to the initial trial, although subsequent attempts to produce urine in this manner are contraindicated.

When the cause of a sudden acute decline in renal function cannot be identified, particularly when anuria is present, cystoscopy and retrograde pyelography may be used to detect the presence of any obstructive urinary tract disease.

The course of acute renal failure is usually characterized by *an initial oliguric phase followed in a number of days to a few weeks by a diuretic period. Major patient care problems during the oliguric phase* of illness include (1) inability to excrete metabolic wastes, (2) inability to regulate electrolytes, (3) inability to excrete fluid loads, (4) difficulty maintaining adequate nutrition, (5) increased potential for injury, and (6) discomfort. *Major patient care problems arising during the diuretic portion of the illness* include (1) inability to appropriately conserve fluid and (2) inability to appropriately conserve electrolytes.

Intervention: oliguric phase

During the oliguric phase of acute renal failure, development of hyperkalemia, severe acidosis, severe fluid overload and pulmonary edema, infection, convulsions, or pericarditis connotes some urgency for control or resolution. Included among these problems are the major causes of death resulting from acute kidney failure. These conditions and their management are outlined in the box at right and discussed below.

Control and excretion of metabolic waste buildup. Because the patient's ability to excrete metabolic wastes (nonprotein nitrogen products and acids) cannot keep pace with production of these substances, alternative routes of excretion and control over production of these materials must be found. Means available to accomplish this include providing carbohydrate to spare protein stores, preventing additional tissue trauma, and increasing excretion of wastes through the lungs and through renal dialysis. Of these, dialysis is by far the most efficient and is the only true means available for controlling the internal environment of the severely ill hypercatabolic person. Daily laboratory tests will determine blood nonprotein nitrogens and bicarbonate levels, which serve as a guide for determining the frequency of dialysis (p. 1584).

Decreasing the production of metabolic wastes can be influenced through dietary means. Calories in the form of carbohydrates and fats provide energy and spare body protein stores, thus decreasing nonprotein nitrogen production. The body recycles urea to synthesize amino acids for protein building so that some regeneration of tissues can occur even though protein intake is curtailed.

Preventing infections and tissue breakdown decreases production of metabolic wastes. Aseptic technique should be rigorously pursued in all treatments performed on the patient. Indwelling lines and catheters are a common source of infection and are to be avoided when possible. *The patient should be isolated from anyone with an infection, including other patients, health care personnel, and visitors.* Detecting existent infections early so that treatment can be instituted promptly decreases tissue breakdown. When the patient is extremely weak and immobile, frequent turning and repositioning to prevent decubiti must be performed. Skin care for patients with edematous tissues should include observation and prevention of pressure and trauma; these tissues are particularly prone to breakdown.

Acidosis develops when hydrogen ion secretion and bicarbonate ion production diminish in the tubular cells. The pH of the blood decreases, the carbon dioxide content decreases, and central nervous system symptoms of drowsiness progressing to stupor and coma may appear. Although the lungs are unable to compensate totally for the increasing acid load, they help determine the rate at which acidosis develops and the frequency or need for dialysis. In compensating for increased metabolic acid loads, the lungs attempt to excrete more carbon dioxide (p. 356). To maximize this pathway for acid excretion, pulmonary hygiene should be carried out. Preventing atelectasis and maintaining maximal lung expansion are goals of nursing care.

INTERVENTIONS FOR PERSON IN OLIGURIC PHASE OF ACUTE RENAL FAILURE

Control and excretion of metabolic waste buildup	Dialysis; protein-sparing diet; prevent infection and tissue breakdown; provide pulmonary hygiene
Regulation of electrolytes	Monitor for changes: *Hyperkalemia:* decrease intake (low-potassium diet); increase excretion (exchange resin) *Hyponatremia:* dialysis to remove fluids and drugs
Control of fluids	Monitor for overload; control fluid intake; conserve energy
Maintenance of adequate nutrition	Diet high in carbohydrates and fat, low in potassium
Prevention of injury	Control environment to prevent falls; maintain good surgical and medical asepsis; prevent drug toxicity
Promotion of comfort	Control nausea, pain, thirst
Provision of emotional support	Maintain orientation; support significant others during changes in patient behavior

Regulation of electrolytes. Some common electrolyte disturbances occurring in acute renal failure are *hyperkalemia, hyponatremia (usually indicative of overhydration),* and increased body sodium content. The rate of accumulation of electrolytes varies greatly in acute renal failure; each patient must be managed individually. Daily or more frequent assessment of laboratory data and clinical signs and symptoms is needed to determine current electrolyte abnormalities and need for treatment.

HYPERKALEMIA. Patients in renal failure with extensive tissue trauma, infection, or bleeding are at a high risk of developing hyperkalemia. In the normal individual the potassium ion is exchanged in the distal convoluted tubule of the nephron for either sodium or hydrogen ions; *for the healthy person there is no mechanism in the body to conserve the potassium ion. However, in the individual with acute renal failure in whom a large number of tubular cells are no longer functional, there exists no mechanism to remove potassium from the body.* Hyperkalemia is said to exist when the serum concentration of this ion reaches a level of 5.5 mEq/L or higher. Serum concentrations of 7 to 10 mEq/L can be quickly reached in acute renal failure and are incompatible with normal cardiac function and life.

In monitoring for signs of potassium toxicity, electrocardiography and laboratory determinations of serum potassium are the most reliable indicators. *Rarely does the patient become symptomatic, and pulse changes must not be relied on to indicate the degree of rise of potassium in the patient's system.*

Interventions to control the rise of serum potassium and prevent cardiac arrest include those that (1) decrease the intake of potassium, (2) decrease the liberation of potassium from body tissues, (3) protect the cardiovascular system, and (4) assist in removal of potassium from the body by nonrenal means.

Decreasing the intake of potassium is achieved by administering intravenous feedings or a diet in which potassium content is very low or absent. All fluids and drugs that the patient receives intravenously should be checked for potassium content. Some medications (e.g., most penicillin preparations) contain large amounts of this ion.

Controlling the breakdown of body tissues is extremely important in preventing a rapid rise in serum potassium.

Preventing infection, trauma, bleeding, and *pressure sores* should be major goals for nursing care.

Protecting the cardiovascular system from high levels of extracellular potassium is essential. When high K^+ levels occur and the patient is exhibiting cardiovascular effects, renal dialysis is required. Because it takes several hours to get the dialysis treatment underway and for the K^+ to be reduced to safe levels other therapy is instituted. Hypertonic glucose (25%) may be given with 1 unit of regular insulin per 2 g of glucose. Over a 30-minute period, 200 to 300 ml of fluid is given to promote the movement of K^+ back into the cells. This lowers the serum K^+ level and reduces cardiac instability resulting from the high serum K^+ levels. The K^+ levels will begin to fall in 1 hour and will remain lowered for 4 to 6 hours.[38] In addition to hypertonic glucose, calcium gluconate may be given intravenously to reduce the irritability of cardiac cells caused by the hyperkalemia.

To *promote the excretion of potassium* from the body when the kidneys are nonfunctional, an exchange resin such as polystyrene sodium sulfonate (Kayexalate) may be ordered for the patient as a temporary measure before a dialysis treatment when (1) the serum K^+ level is high and rising rapidly; (2) the serum K^+ level is rising, although at a controlled rate, and other metabolic disturbances do not necessitate dialysis; or (3) control of a rising serum K^+ is required before a patient's transfer to an acute care area where dialysis can be provided. This drug reduces serum potassium by exchanging sodium for potassium ions in the intestinal tract. It can be administered orally, through a nasogastric tube, or by enema. The medication is given orally when the patient's condition permits; oral daily doses range from 15

to 60 g/day. When sodium sulfonate is administered in enema form, the usual dose is 50 g of exchange resin for each enema; it may be repeated daily or as necessary to lower serum potassium. The medication is a powder that when mixed becomes a thick paste within a few seconds; therefore preparation should take place at the bedside just before administration. Often mannitol is used to mix the powdered sodium sulfonate, since it induces an osmotic shift of fluid into the bowel producing diarrhea, which helps to expel the medication, additional K^+ from the gastrointestinal tract, and additional fluid from the hypervolemic patient. If spontaneous bowel movements do not occur, a cathartic or cleansing enema can be given to ensure the elimination of potassium from the bowel.

HYPONATREMIA. Hyponatremia in acute renal failure most commonly develops with overhydration of the patient. The oliguric patient cannot excrete large volumes of urine; when the administration of sodium-free or low-sodium intravenous or oral fluids continues in such an individual, the serum is diluted and the serum concentration of sodium falls.

In this situation hyponatremia is accompanied or caused by *hypervolemia.* In the very acutely ill, the situation commonly occurs when the patient receives numerous drugs and fluids in an attempt to treat coexisting life-threatening problems. When the volume of drugs and fluids cannot be reduced to a safe level, dialysis is required to remove the excess fluid and restore sodium balance.

Signs and symptoms of hyponatremia include warm, moist, flushed skin, muscle weakness, muscle twitching, and behavioral changes involving confusion, delirium, coma, and convulsions. Serum sodium concentrations will be below 130 mEq/L. The hematocrit and hemoglobin values suddenly fall without evidence of bleeding; this is caused by hemodilution.

INCREASED BODY SODIUM CONTENT. Increases in total body content of sodium also occur in acute renal failure. Commonly, this occurs when the patient is receiving medications high in sodium content and excess sodium in the diet. *Edema and increasing blood pressure indicate retention of sodium and fluids even though the serum sodium concentration is normal or below normal.*

Control of fluids. The oliguric or anuric patient is unable to excrete more than minimal amounts of fluid. Nursing care is directed toward three broad objectives: (1) monitoring for signs of fluid overload, (2) maintaining the patient's energy expenditure at a level compatible with the individual's state of health, and (3) controlling or helping the patient to control fluid intake.

All observations regarding the patient's state of hydration need to be recorded so that hour-to-hour and day-to-day comparisons can be made. Any finding indicating retention of fluids is reported to the physician.

Edema can first be noted in dependent areas such as the feet and legs, in the presacral area, and around the eyes. The patient is observed carefully for signs of pulmonary edema (p. 1135) and congestive heart failure (p. 1127). Central venous or arterial monitoring lines will help to provide data for short-term comparisons in managing the fluid balance of the critically ill person. Accurate recording of intake and output is extremely important as are daily weight records.

The patient in renal failure is unable to excrete fluid loads, and much energy is expended just to maintain current functional status. Positioning and activity are determined daily based on assessment of the energy level and ability to ventilate adequately.

Controlling fluid intake is essential when the ability to excrete fluid is limited. All fluid (parenteral and oral) must total only slightly more than daily output if severe overhydration is to be avoided. When the patient is neither to gain nor lose additional body fluid, the physician will calculate the patient's fluid replacement using the following as a guide: intake will approximate 500 ml/day plus urinary output and adjustments for additional fluid lost through fever, diarrhea, and wound drainage. Thirst is a problem that can defy control of fluid intake. Fortunately, when sodium intake is controlled, extreme thirst does not develop.

Devices that allow 50 to 150 ml of fluid to be isolated from the main intravenous solution container and drip chambers that allow precise control of fluids through administration of smaller drops of fluid are added safety measures when giving fluids parenterally to anuric or oliguric individuals. Accuracy in fluid balance records is essential. For the patient who is unable to take medications with small amounts of fluid, medications may be given in soft foods such as applesauce.

Maintenance of adequate nutrition. Most persons in acute renal failure are too ill to tolerate oral feedings either initially or for sustained periods of time. Some patients who are able to tolerate fluids orally find that eating food compounds the nausea they experience as a result of an altered biochemical environment and accompanying gastrointestinal tract irritation. Intravenous hypertonic glucose in amounts of 100 g/day or more provides a temporary source of energy that slows the burning of the body's own protein stores. For patients who are severely ill or nauseated, maintaining positive nitrogen balance is not feasible. It is suggested that glucose solutions not be administered in concentrations greater than 10% and that these be administerd into large veins to prevent sclerosing of veins.[59] The amount of fluid that can be given within a 24-hour period will influence the total caloric intake provided to the patient. The patient receiving 100 g of intravenous glucose a day will burn approximately 225 g (8 oz) of body tissue per day.[80]

If the patient is able to tolerate oral feedings, dietary protein and potassium are avoided unless dialysis has been initiated. In this case modest amounts of protein and potassium are allowed, thus increasing protein available for tissue building and increasing the palatability of the diet. Foods high in carbohydrate and fat content are encouraged. A total intake of 2000 calories per day is desired although often not achieved because of anorexia and nausea.

Prevention of injury. Monitoring safety is a major nursing responsibility. Specific care for the person with acute renal failure should include preventing falls and physical trauma, preventing infection, and assisting with prevention of drug toxicity by monitoring medication therapy.

The person in acute renal failure is weak, may be confused, and may have visual changes. The amount of supervision required during daily care must be assessed continually. Falls from a bed, from a chair, and during transfer can be prevented by judicious assessment of the person's behavior and capabilities. Convulsions may be precipitated by dialysis, occur as the result of metabolic and electrolyte imbalances, or be the result of co-existing central nervous system disease.

Infection is a leading cause of mortality in persons with acute renal failure. Nosocomial infections (p. 368) are readily contracted by patients whose ability to resist invading organisms is low. Protective isolation is used in some medical centers, while in others this is not thought necessary. Strict attention to aseptic technique must be maintained.

Monitoring prescribed medications is a shared nursing and medical responsibility. The route of excretion and signs of toxicity should be known for all medications that the patient receives. *The potential for drug toxicity exists when medications normally excreted by the kidneys are retained in the body as a result of renal damage.* Commonly used drugs that fall into this category include antibiotics, cardiac glycosides, and analgesics.[6] Drugs should also be monitored for potassium and sodium content; large increases in daily intake of these ions can result from medications.

Promotion of comfort. Major *discomforts* that the alert patient commonly experiences *include nausea, pain, and thirst.* Nausea is generally a result of the renal failure through disturbances in the body's internal environment. The only truly effective treatment is control of uremia with dialysis and good supportive care, which involves correction of electrolyte abnormalities, nonprotein nitrogen levels, and acid-base imbalance. Antiemetic medications at best seem to provide only partial and short-lived relief of nausea and may be contraindicated for patients with liver disease in addition to renal failure.

Pain is a common experience for most acutely ill patients with renal failure. The origins of pain are not related to the renal failure itself but to the trauma, surgery, and insertion of multiple tubes and lines that most of these acutely ill patients undergo. Pain can be controlled safely through the use of narcotic and synthetic narcotic medications. When giving these medications, a judgment needs to be made regarding existing level of central nervous system depression, a common finding in acute acidotic uremia. Medication within "normal" drug dosages can bring about severe respiratory depression, unconsciousness, and death because of the synergistic effects of the person's metabolic state and the actions of the analgesic. It is always safer to determine the patient's tolerance to medication by starting with smaller doses of the medication, which can then be augmented. The respiratory rate and level of awareness provide data as to the patient's tolerance of the analgesic.

Thirst becomes a problem for the alert patient when oral intake is dramatically reduced and the majority of fluid intake is parenteral. Thirst does not become as great a problem when sodium intake is controlled, although for the person who is mouth breathing it is still a discomfort. Fluid that is allowed may be given as ice chips and spaced throughout the day. Meticulous oral care should provide additional relief.

Integrating the emotional aspects of the acute illness. During the acute phase of the illness, biochemical aberrations will generally cause alterations in both the level of awareness and personality of the patient. The family members and occasionally the patient will be aware of these changes such as faltering memory or an inability to think clearly. The biochemical changes may be extensive enough to cause coma. When the patient is sufficiently alert to begin relating to the environment, it should be anticipated that the confusion contributed by the altered internal environment will increase the patient's difficulty in processing information about his or her condition and surroundings. Simple conversations that attempt to structure the environment and the situation are useful in assisting the person to maintain orientation. These conversations with the patient may require frequent repetition. The patient who perceives a decreased memory or ability to think clearly is assisted to express these concerns and is given reassurance that mental capacities will return with recovery of physical health.

Belligerent, vocal, angry behavior may be seen in previously docile patients. Often this is a source of embarrassment to the family; the patient is generally quite ill and probably unaware of the behavior. Reassurance may be provided to the family, indicating that personalities return to previous states when biochemical alterations are corrected.

Outcome criteria for the person in renal failure during the oliguric phase. The person demonstrates control of internal environment through:

1. Absence of pulmonary edema.

2. Absence or control of peripheral edema.
3. Control of blood pressure (range between 170/100 and 100/60 mm Hg).
4. Restored or maintained mental alertness.
5. Control of electrolyte balance.
   a. Sodium range of 125 to 145 mEq/L.
   b. Potassium range of 3.0 to 6.0 mEq/L.
   c. Bicarbonate above 14 mEq/L.
6. Control of protein catabolism.
   a. Urea nitrogen below 100 mg/100 ml.
   b. Creatinine below 12 mg/100 ml.
   c. Absence of skin breakdown.
7. Absence of bleeding.
8. Resolution or control of intercurrent illness (congestive heart failure, shock).

The person is free of:
1. Infection.
2. Injury resulting from decreased level of awareness and strength.
3. Toxicity from inadequately excreted medication.

Intervention: diuretic phase

After a period of oliguria or anuria, which may last a few days to 2 weeks, patients recovering renal function pass into another distinct phase of illness characterized by increased urinary output. Increased output indicates that the damaged nephrons are healing and are able to begin excreting urine. At first daily urine volume increases slowly, although within 1 to 2 days diuresis up to or exceeding 4 to 5 L/day may occur. Although fluid can be excreted, the kidneys are not yet healed. Often there is inability to excrete proportional amounts of waste materials, and serum concentrations of urea nitrogen may rise or remain elevated as urine volume increases. At times excessive excretion of sodium and potassium occurs during diuresis. *Complete recovery of renal function is slow and requires anywhere from days to a few weeks. Return of the renal function to normal or near normal levels is evidenced when the kidney can both conserve and dilute urine and when serum electrolytes and nonprotein nitrogen levels become normal.*

Nursing care during the diuretic phase is directed toward detecting fluid losses and electrolyte imbalances. Much of the fluid excreted during diuresis in excess of an amount proportional to the patient's intake may be fluid that has accumulated in the body during the oliguric phase of illness. However, serious fluid and electrolyte depletion can occur. In addition to detecting fluid and electrolyte imbalances, several nursing care objectives established during the oliguric phase should be continued. These include maintaining nutritional intake, maintaining safety of the patient, and preventing infection.

Nursing observations and recording needed in judging the adequacy of hydration and serum sodium of the pa-

tient include (1) changes in mental awareness and activity; (2) degree of thirst; (3) moistness of mucous membranes; (4) development of skin turgor; (5) development of tachycardia and postural hypotension; and (6) accurate daily weight, fluid balance, and vital signs.

Outcome criteria for the person with renal failure during the diuretic phase. The person or significant others can:

1. State extent of recovery of kidney function.
2. Identify any preventable environmental or health factor involved in generating the illness.
3. Plan a diet to maintain positive nitrogen balance and sufficient caloric intake.
4. Identify signs and symptoms of dehydration and sodium and potassium loss.
5. Describe plans for prevention of infection.
6. State plans for follow-up health care.

Chronic renal failure

Etiology and epidemiology

Chronic renal failure exists when the kidneys are no longer capable of maintaining an internal environment consistent with life and when return of function is not anticipated. For the majority of individuals the transition from health to a state of chronic or permanent disease is a slow one extending over a number of years. Recurrent infections and exacerbations of nephritis, obstruction of the urinary tract, and destruction of vessels from diabetes and long-standing hypertension lead to scarring of kidney tissue and progressive loss of renal function. Some individuals, however, develop total irreversible loss of renal function acutely; such loss of renal function usually develops in a matter of a few hours or days and follows a direct traumatic insult to the kidneys.

Chronic renal failure exists as a major health problem in the United States. Approximately 8 million individuals now have chronic kidney disease; approximately 60,000 persons die each year as the result of renal failure.[80]

Pathophysiology

During chronic renal failure some of the nephrons (including the glomerulus and tubules) are thought to remain intact while others are destroyed (intact nephron hypothesis). The intact nephrons hypertrophy and produce an increased volume of filtrate with increased tubular reabsorption in spite of a decreased glomerular filtration rate. This adaptive method permits the kidney to function until about three fourths of the nephrons become destroyed. The solute load then becomes greater than can be reabsorbed, producing an osmotic diuresis with polyuria and thirst. Eventually, as more nephrons are damaged, oliguria occurs with retention of waste products.

Prognosis

The individual with chronic renal failure can to some extent control and manage the symptoms of the disease. Although renal function that has been lost as a result of destruction of kidney tissue cannot be recovered, the life of the person can be maintained by limiting the intake of substances that require excretion and by providing alternative routes of excretion from the body for waste and electrolytes. By adhering to a prescribed management routine, albeit quite strict and demanding, life may be sustained. For some individuals medication and diet therapy alone may control uremic symptoms; other individuals may require in addition dialysis or transplantation to control the symptoms of their disease.

Prevention

Obstruction and infection of the urinary tract and hypertensive disease are common and often asymptomatic causes of renal damage and renal failure. A significant reduction in the incidence of renal failure can be effected through increasing attention to general health promotion. Yearly physical examinations in which blood pressure is determined, urinalysis is performed, and the person is questioned about dysuria or pain in the urinary tract assist in early detection of disease that may lead to renal failure.

General health maintenance can reduce the number of individuals progressing from renal insufficiency into frank renal failure. Care is aimed toward adequately treating medical problems and closely supervising the person's health status in times of stress (infection, pregnancy).

Clinical picture

Although the clinical course of chronic renal disease varies from individual to individual, there are common features of the illness. Signs and symptoms result from disordered fluid and electrolyte balance, alterations in regulatory functions of the body, and retention of solutes. *Azotemia* (excess nitrogenous products in the blood), *anemia*, and *acidosis* are always present. Potassium and hydrogen ion excretion is impaired. Fluid and sodium balance is abnormal and may involve either abnormal retention or secretion of sodium and water; thus urinary volume can be decreased, normal, or increased. With end-stage renal disease, hyperuricemia is a common finding, although the varied serum levels of uric acid seem to have no definite relationship to the exact level of kidney function.[60] Increased levels of serum phosphate are characteristic, and calcium levels may be low or normal. These findings result from decreased renal excretions of phosphate and simultaneous reduction in ionized serum calcium. Through increased production of parathormone the body may reestablish a normal serum calcium level, although this is accomplished at the expense of the individual's bone matrix.

Hypertension may or may not be present. Often with the development of end-stage renal disease blood pressure is elevated and seems to be the result of increased total body water, a renally released vasopressor, or an inadequately secreted vasodepressor.[9] Glucose intolerance may be seen although usually not of sufficient severity to warrant treatment. The rising blood sugar level appears to be the result of an altered biochemical environment produced by the failing kidneys and does not signify the development of diabetes mellitus. As renal failure progresses the patient develops increased pigmentation of the skin; the skin becomes sallow or brownish in tone. With more advanced and insufficiently treated renal failure the patient may develop muscular twitching, numbness in the feet and legs, pericarditis, and pleuritis. These signs will disappear with restabilization of the patient with diet and medication or with the additional assistance of dialysis.

The symptoms of uremia usually develop so slowly that the patient and family often do not recall the time of onset of the illness. Symptoms generally noticed as uremia develops include lethargy, headaches, physical and mental fatigue, weight loss, irritability, and depression. Anorexia, persistent nausea and vomiting, shortness of breath on either mild or no exertion, and pitting edema are symptomatic of severe loss of renal function. Pruritus may be absent, mild, or severe.

The point at which the patient becomes obviously symptomatic and displays signs typical of renal failure occurs when approximately 80% to 90% of renal function has been lost (Fig. 62-9). At this level of renal function creatinine clearance values will fall to 15 ml/min or less.

Alterations in fertility. As end-stage renal failure develops, most women note changes in their menstrual cycle. Bleeding may occur at more widely spaced intervals, may be heavier or lighter in flow than normal, or may cease all together. This obvious change in reproductive cycle is usually accompanied by changes in fertility. Ovulation may occur normally or may occur only a few times a year. *Pregnancy in uremic women is of much lower incidence than in the normal population. In men impotence may occur as chronic renal failure progresses toward end-stage disease.* Dialysis or more vigorous treatment of uremia is indicated to return or maximize reproductive function. It should be stressed that sexual activity of some persons with chronic renal failure may remain quite normal even though changes in reproductive ability are present.

Intervention

Major problems for the patient in chronic renal failure include (1) inability to appropriately control fluid balance; (2) inability to regulate electrolyte balance; (3) inability to excrete metabolic wastes; (4) inability to transport oxygen to cells; (5) inability to maintain normal rest and

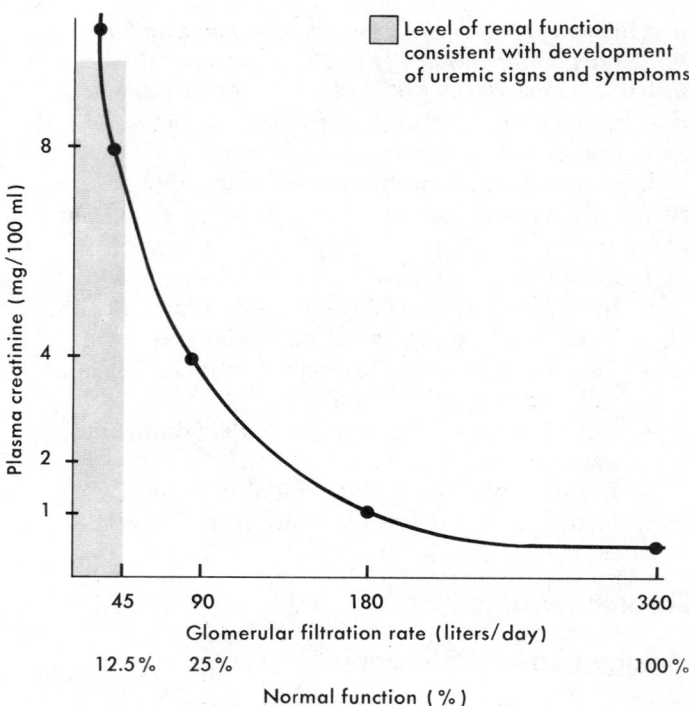

Fig. 62-9. Glomerular filtration and plasma creatinine level.

sleep patterns; (6) difficulty in maintaining adequate nutrition; (7) increased potential for physical injury; (8) discomfort; (9) alterations in fertility; and (10) changes in life-style, group membership, and feelings regarding the self. Interventions and treatment goals for the person with chronic renal failure are listed in the boxes on p. 1579.

Control of fluid balance. The ability to excrete sodium and water in the urine varies considerably in chronic renal failure. Although volume problems for most patients with chronic end-stage renal failure involve *hypervolemia* resulting from a marked inability to excrete sodium and water, some patients are unable to conserve these substances and are subject to *hypovolemic* states. With either marked inability to excrete or conserve body fluid, the patient can develop severe fluid imbalances in a relatively short period of time. Care is directed toward identifying fluid imbalances and in providing an intake of sodium and water equivalent to the amounts of these substances excreted. The desired effect of this care is to maintain the patient in a normotensive, normovolemic state. (For further information on assessment and intervention of hypervolemia and hypovolemia, see Chapter 21.)

Controlling sodium intake can be an extremely challenging problem for both the nurse and the patient. Any sudden increase in weight indicates accumulating fluid, and the source of this fluid must be sought with the patient. Often when the person is not acutely ill

INTERVENTIONS FOR PERSONS WITH CHRONIC RENAL FAILURE

Control of fluid balance	Monitor changes; control sodium and water intake
Regulation of electrolyte balance	Monitor for potassium and phosphorus excess:
	Hyperkalemia: exchange resins; decreased potassium intake; prevent tissue breakdown
	Hyperphosphatemia: aluminum hydroxide to bind phosphorus
	Hypocalcemia: calcium supplement; activated vitamin D
Prevention of metabolic waste buildup	*Decrease metabolic waste products:* dietary protein restriction; prevent infection
	Maintain pulmonary function; monitor for acidosis
Maintenance of oxygen transport to cells	Conserve energy; prevent blood loss
Promotion of comfort, rest, and sleep	*Pruritus:* control environment; emollient baths; antipruritics
	Muscle cramping: therapy for control of uremia and electrolyte balance; heat; massage
	Ocular irritation: control phosphate excess; artificial tears
	Insomnia: measures to promote sleep and control pruritus
Maintenance of adequate nutrition	Oral hygiene before meals; antacids for gastrointestinal irritation; measures to encourage eating balanced diet within the protein, sodium, and water limitations prescribed
Promotion of safety	Maintain good medical/surgical asepsis; avoid exposure to known infectious agents; avoid fatigue
	Facilitate awareness of environment to prevent injury
	Teach about medication therapy
Coping with changes in life-style and feelings about self	Promote hope; assist with identification of problems and resources

TREATMENT GOALS FOR THE PERSON WITH CHRONIC RENAL FAILURE

1. *Stabilization of the internal environment* as demonstrated by:
   a. Mental alertness, attention span, and appropriate interaction with the environment.
   b. Absence or control of peripheral edema, absence of pulmonary edema.
   c. Control of electrolyte balance:

Sodium	125 to 145 mEq/L
Potassium	3 to 6 mEq/L
Bicarbonate	> 15 mEq/L
Calcium	9 to 11 mg/100 ml
Phosphate	3 to 5 mg/100 ml

   d. Serum albumin > 2 g/100 ml
   e. Control of protein catabolism and protein breakdown products:

Urea nitrogen	<100 mg/100 ml
Creatinine	<15 mg/100 ml
Uric acid	<12 mg/100 ml

   f. Absence of joint inflammation and pain.
2. *Infection and abnormal bleeding are not present.*
3. *Blood pressure is controlled at less than 160/100 mm Hg sitting and less than 30 mm Hg postural change on standing.*
4. *Anorexia, nausea, and pruritus are absent or controlled.*
5. *Intercurrent illness is resolved or controlled* (heart failure, infection, dehydration).
6. *There is no toxicity from inadequately excreted medication.*
7. *Nutrient intake is sufficient to maintain positive nitrogen balance.*

purchasing commercially prepared foods. The words "sodium" and "salt" should be sought on food labels when the person is on a severely sodium-restricted diet, and these foods should be avoided. At times the person is unable to offer an explanation for increasing thirst and sodium ingestion. At this point the question of home self-medication (e.g., sodium bicarbonate for indigestion) should be raised. After failure to uncover increased intake of either sodium or fluid to explain hypervolemia, the person is asked to list for a period of 3 consecutive days all foods and fluids ingested. This list can then be reviewed with the individual and used not only to uncover instances of dietary indiscretion but also as a teaching tool.

Regulation of electrolyte balance. Potassium and phosphorus retention occur in chronic renal failure.

and is responsible for control of intake, the problem can be traced to excess sodium ingestion, which produces thirst. In helping to avoid this cycle of thirst leading to increased fluid ingestion and overhydration, the patient is carefully taught the allowances of sodium and fluid in the diet and what restrictions are to be observed in

Nursing care is aimed at identifying signs and symptoms of *hyperkalemia* and *hyperphosphatemia* and reducing intake and providing alternative routes of excretion for these substances from the body.

Signs of potassium intoxication and the role of cation exchange resins in utilizing the intestinal tract as an alternative route of excretion are discussed on p. 1574. Serum potassium can be at least partially controlled in chronic renal failure by decreasing dietary and drug intake. Thorough diet teaching of the patient and all persons responsible for food preparation is essential. This teaching should help the patient identify the foods that are high in potassium and the methods of cooking that can reduce the potassium content of the diet. *Salt substitutes should be avoided by all patients with chronic renal disease since they contain large amounts of potassium.* Medications that are prescribed for the patient should be reviewed for potassium content.

Significant rises in serum potassium can be averted by preventing tissue breakdown. Potassium is largely an intracellular cation, and extensive tissue damage can liberate a lethal amount of this ion into the system of the patient with chronic renal failure. Patients should be advised to seek medical attention when symptoms of infection, gastrointestinal bleeding, or other problems first appear.

When the kidneys fail, the ability to excrete phosphorus decreases. This leads to a vicious cycle whereby Ca^{++} decreases, parathormone is stimulated, and bone demineralization occurs. Because the excess phosphorus is not excreted, calcium and phosphorus precipitate out in soft tissue. The serum phosphorus level again rises, the calcium level falls, and the cycle continues. Severe bone demineralization may develop, and if the problem continues unabated hyperparathyroidism can occur. Serum levels show elevated phosphorus with low to normal levels of Ca^{++}. Treatment is aimed at decreasing serum phosphorus levels. Aluminum hydroxide preparations that bind phosphorus in the intestinal tract and allow it to be eliminated are given in doses ranging from 1 to 5 g daily.

Aluminum hydroxide is best taken at mealtimes. It should not be taken with other medications because it can bind drugs in the intestinal tract. Aluminum hydroxide is constipating, and stool softeners or laxatives may have to be given to patients receiving large doses of it. Depressed serum levels of Ca^{++} may result not only from elevated levels of phosphorus but also from the inability of the diseased kidney to activate vitamin D. In the absence of vitamin D there is poor absorption of Ca^{++} from the intestinal tract. In some instances activated vitamin D or calcium supplements or both are prescribed.

Prevention of metabolic waste buildup. *Azotemia* and *acidosis* occur in all patients with chronic renal failure, although the severity of the problems and the degree to which the person has developed tolerance to the altered internal environment vary considerably. *Nursing care should be directed toward (1) decreasing the production of metabolic wastes, (2) promoting excretion of volatile acids by the lungs, and (3) detecting increasing acidosis and its clinical effect on the patient.*

Metabolic waste production can be significantly reduced by controlling dietary protein intake and by preventing catabolism of existing protein stores. The amount of protein allowed in the diet for the person with chronic renal failure can vary from 20 to 80 g/day. The specific level of protein intake prescribed depends on the presence of some means for clearing the products of protein breakdown from the patient's system. Dietary protein intake is more liberal for persons who have some ability to excrete wastes in their urine and for those being treated with dialysis. When restricting dietary protein, the quality of that allowed must be high. The persons must be taught to select foods that contain all of the essential amino acids. When calories are provided in the form of carbohydrate and fat for immediate energy needs, smaller amounts of protein can suffice for cellular growth and repair. Catabolism of existing protein stores liberates nitrogenous wastes. For this reason sources of potential infection such as indwelling catheters are avoided, and when infection is noted, it is immediately treated.

In chronic renal failure the kidneys are unable to excrete hydrogen ions and to manufacture bicarbonate. *Metabolic acidosis* results. On the basis of laboratory data acidosis may appear to be severe; however, persons with chronic renal failure adjust to lowered serum bicarbonate levels and often do not become acutely symptomatic even when bicarbonate levels reach values of 15 to 16 mEq/L. Because of this adjustment, treatment with bicarbonate is not routine. The lungs assume a prominent role in regulating acid-base balance, and helping the individual to maintain pulmonary function becomes an important objective for nursing care.

Determining patient tolerance of a state of acidosis that can fluctuate from moderate to critical levels (as additional stressors such as infection and blood loss occur) is important in the nursing care given the patient. Severe acidosis results in central nervous system depression (p. 356).

Maintenance of oxygen transport to cells. Anemia universally accompanies chronic renal disease. Hematocrit values of 16% to 22% are not abnormal for these individuals. Anemia results from both a decreased production of red blood cells and a decrease in longevity of the cells in circulation. Although oral iron supplements may be tried, iron is not well absorbed by the gastrointestinal tract in chronic renal failure, and in some individuals it may cause nausea and vomiting. Since dietary sources of folate (folic acid) may be restricted in chronic renal failure, and food preparation may further decrease the amount of folate ingested, this vitamin may be given as a medication. A sufficient dose is 1 mg/day. Transfusions are not generally given unless the hematocrit level becomes extremely low and the patient is grossly symptomatic. The reason for this is that when transfusions are given frequently, the patient's own stimulus to red cell production is decreased.

The severely anemic person complains of extreme fatigue and shortness of breath. Because of a lack of red cells there is an inability to transport sufficient oxygen to cells for energy production. Milder complaints of the anemic person include an inability to work or play without extended rest periods. Nursing activities can be directed toward helping identify activities essential to daily living and helping the person to modify these activities according to existing energy level. Preventing the accumulation of excess fluid in a person with a very low hematocrit level allows energy to be used for activities of daily living rather than for carrying extra fluid.

Other important nursing activities include helping the person to control blood losses. A soft toothbrush is recommended for oral care. Antacids taken at regular and frequent intervals can reduce gastrointestinal tract bleeding. The person is instructed to observe for melena and to report this finding to the physician without delay. Anabolic steroids may be used, but their side effects of fluid retention, masculinization, and hirsutism may limit their usefulness.

Some degree of peripheral neuropathy occurs in almost all persons with chronic renal failure. Numbness, tingling, and burning of the extremities are common complaints. Treatment that is effective in controlling these symptoms consists of more intensive management of the uremic state.

Promotion of comfort, rest, and sleep. Rarely does the person with chronic renal failure have acute sharp pain; however, these individuals are subject to a wide variety of chronic discomforts. *Most commonly these discomforts include pruritus, muscle cramping, numbness and tingling in the hands and feet, thirst, headaches, and irritation of the eyes*. Most persons with end-stage renal disease develop pruritus. Patients relate that itching is of a deep sensation. Factors that seem to exacerbate the itching include increasing levels of serum phosphorus, dry skin, warm moist heat, and emotional stress. Itching is largely symptomatic, and measures that are effective in controlling it vary from individual to individual. Reducing levels of serum phosphorus with aluminum hydroxide preparations decreases itching for most patients. Keeping the skin moist and supple through use of lotions and bath oils, controlling the room temperature during sleep to prevent excessive warmth, emollient baths, and bathing with a vinegar solution are measures alone or in combination that may provide some relief from itching. Medications such as trimeprazine tartrate (Temaril) are

also prescribed as necessary and for some individuals provide much relief from itching. Since emotional stress seems to increase the itching, helping the person verbalize feelings may provide for some resolution of conflict and help decrease these manifestations of psychologic stress. The urge to scratch the skin is acute in some persons. Because scratching is often vigorous, injury to the skin with subsequent infection can result. Fingernails are trimmed closely. In preference to fingernails, a soft cloth should be used to scratch the skin.

Muscle cramping in the lower extremities and the *hands* is common in renal failure. Often cramping can be correlated with sodium depletion. Primary treatment for muscle cramping involves controlling the state of uremia and fluid and electrolyte balance. Temporary measures of heat and massage are effective for some persons.

Headaches in chronic renal failure result from a variety of causes. These include increasing blood pressure, progressing uremia, and rapid changes in osmotic gradients between cellular, interstitial, and intravascular compartments. Treatment of these problems has been discussed previously.

Ocular irritation in chronic renal failure is caused by calcium deposits in the conjunctiva that cause burning and watering of the eyes. Treatment involves controlling the plasma phosphate level through administration of oral aluminum hydroxide preparations. "Artificial tears" (methylcellulose) placed in the conjunctival sac every few hours also help to reduce irritation.

Insomnia and *chronic daytime fatigue* are common complaints of persons with chronic renal failure. This reversal of normal sleep patterns has been attributed to a variety of causes. These include (1) recurring preoccupation with thoughts concerning the disease state and changes in life-style required by the illness, (2) pruritus, and (3) the state of uremia itself. Reduction of high serum levels of urea nitrogen and creatinine through decreasing dietary intake of protein or dialysis may bring sleep patterns more toward normal. When control of uremia fails to cure insomnia, mild central nervous system depressants may be ordered.

General comfort at bedtime is needed to induce sleep at any time and is especially important whenever sleeping problems arise. Comfort measures can include warm baths, pursuing quiet activities an hour or two before bedtime, controlling itching, or anything the patient finds calming and soothing.

The individual who is awake a significant portion of the night may need to plan for rest periods during the day. These rest periods should be taken far enough ahead of bedtime to prevent compounding sleeplessness.

Maintenance of adequate nutrition. Maintaining a good nutritional intake can be difficult for persons with chronic renal failure. Anorexia, nausea, and vomiting frequently occur, and diets can be so severely restricted that they bear little resemblance to normal dietary patterns. In uremia, disturbances in fluid, electrolyte, and waste composition of body fluids occur and produce changes in osmotic gradients in all cells. When these changes occur in the cells of the gastrointestinal tract and the central nervous system, anorexia, nausea, and vomiting result. Persons with uremia are prone to bleeding of the gastrointestinal tract and the oral cavity. Urea is broken down to ammonia by the action of intestinal bacteria. Since ammonia is a mucosal irritant, ulceration and bleeding can occur. In addition to the gastrointestinal tract problems that lead to nausea and vomiting, there is a decreased salivary flow in persons with chronic renal disease. An ammonia smell and taste can accumulate in the mouth quickly and can further compound anorexia. Treatment includes administering antacids every 2 to 4 hours to decrease gastrointestinal irritation. Dietary control of uremia, perhaps augmented by dialysis, should help to control disturbances in fluid, electrolyte, and waste composition of body fluids and thus help to control nausea and vomiting. Oral hygiene, especially before meals, is important to combat anorexia.

Modifying the diet as possible to the preferences of the individual can also help to maintain intake of food. Dietary teaching and meal planning can be approached according to an exchange system similar to that used for individuals with diabetes. With this approach there is greater ability to modify the diet according to personal preferences. The pattern of meals during the day is also a matter of personal preference. Some individuals prefer two or three meals a day. When eating patterns are known and used in dietary instruction and meal planning, intake of food is likely to increase.

Actual eating of prepared food can be promoted through attempting to decrease emotional tension at the dinner table. Periods other than mealtime should be used to discuss family and individual problems. Food that is attractively arranged and well flavored is likely to be more acceptable to the patient. Spices and other flavorings can add variety to foods that are prepared without sodium. It is interesting that most persons relate that their taste for salt disappears once they have adhered to a low-sodium diet for several weeks. When the gastrointestinal tract is ulcerated, bland foods may be tried in an attempt to increase ingestion of food.

Promotion of safety. Common injuries to the person in chronic renal failure include infection, accidents caused by decreased mental and visual awareness of the environment, and improper usage of medications. In chronic renal failure resistance to infection is decreased. Control of infection is essentially similar to that described in the section on care of the patient in acute renal failure. In addition, the person is counseled to avoid exposure to individuals with known infections and to avoid extreme fatigue, which lowers body resistance.

The buildup of osmotically active particles and fluid in the body that occurs in uremia produces changes in the cells of the brain that may lead to confusion and impairment in decision-making ability. In some instances convulsions and coma may result from the changed internal environment. Fluid accumulation and hypertension can produce visual changes. Nursing care should include assessing and helping the family to assess decisions made by the patient. The patient's awareness of the environment also needs assessment.

At times the person may need to be helped in limiting activities to a level commensurate with mental processes and level of awareness. For instance, *blurred* vision and *delayed reaction time* contraindicate driving an automobile. *Convulsions* and *coma* may result from severe fluid, electrolyte, and waste imbalances. In most instances when the person is subject to developing these complications hospitalization is necessary. Individuals caring for the patient need to be aware of the possibility of seizure activity and take appropriate precautions. Correcting abnormal body chemistry is the most important measure for preventing coma or convulsions.

Education about medications is carried out with the person in the areas of both prescribed medications and over-the-counter or folk medicines. The use of common popular medications that are sold without prescription must be discouraged. All medications should be prescribed by the physician. Aspirin is dangerous because it is normally excreted by the kidneys and may rapidly build to toxic levels and prolong bleeding time. Ingestion of sodium bicarbonate (baking soda) to treat indigestion can result in extremely large intakes of sodium. Many cold preparations also contain large amounts of sodium. Remembering to take prescribed medications can be a problem for the person who may have to take over two dozen pills each day. Correlating pill-taking times with major activities of the day is often helpful. Medications that are frequently given to those with chronic renal failure are listed in the box on p. 1583.

Coping with changes in life-style group membership, and feelings regarding self. Numerous alterations in life-style, group membership, and feelings regarding the self occur for the person with chronic renal failure. The numerous physical changes that occur often make it difficult to carry on activities that were once normally pursued. *Chronic fatigue* may make it impossible for the person to continue to be employed. Because the patient is often tired and not feeling well, it may be difficult to plan in advance for social events. The former roles of the sick member of the family must often be taken on by another. When roles cannot easily be changed or additionally assumed by other members of the family, serious threats to the organization of the family group occur. Physical appearance also changes and is of much concern to most persons. As uremia progresses, the individual often becomes thin and weaker

COMMONLY PRESCRIBED MEDICATIONS FOR PERSONS WITH CHRONIC RENAL FAILURE

1. Drugs that increase intake of essential substances
   a. Vitamins
   b. Folic acid
   c. Calcium
   d. Bicarbonate
   e. Iron
2. Drugs that promote excretion of nonessential or excessive substances
   a. Diuretics (sodium and water)
   b. Phosphate binders
   c. Exchange resins (potassium)
   d. Allopurinol (uric acid)
3. Drugs that regulate body processes
   a. Antihypertensives (↓ blood pressure)
   b. Cardiac glycosides (↑ rate; ↓ arrhythmias)
   c. Steroids (↓ inflammatory response)
   d. Laxatives or stool softeners (↓ constipation)
   e. Androgens (↑ red blood cell production)
4. Drugs that promote comfort and rest
   a. Mild analgesics (without aspirin)
   b. Trimeprazine (Temaril)
   c. Diazepam (Valium)
   d. Mild hypnotics

and appears sallow. Thoughts concerning death and the quality of this changed life are common.

Denial often becomes a chief defense mechanism for the patient. With it the individual can periodically forget the constant threat of life. The use of this mental mechanism for the person with chronic renal failure can be quite appropriate as long as it is not manifested by maladaptive or harmful behavior. Inappropriate uses of denial involve continuous dietary indiscretion and failure to take prescribed medications.

The patient with chronic renal failure needs the hope and encouragement that with treatment discomfort will be lessened and continued existence to pursue what seems most productive and important will be provided. Hope should not be focused on cure but on learning to manage a new style of life. In managing the changes that occur as a result of chronic renal failure, the patient should be encouraged to be as independent and as active as possible. The patient should be taught to manage the treatment and should be given the responsibility of doing so. Nursing care should be provided as part of the team approach that assists the patient in identifying problems and resources and helps the patient and family adjust to the changing style of life.

Outcome criteria for the person with chronic renal failure

The person or significant others can:
1. Explain the dietary program.
   a. State means of identifying content of foods.
   b. Explain use of small frequent feedings to maintain nutrient intake when anorexic or nauseated.
   c. State fluid prescription and identify sources of fluid in diet.
2. Demonstrate measurement of fluid intake and output and accurate recording of intake and output.
3. State name, dosage, frequency, purpose, and side effects of medications.
4. Describe measures useful in controlling common discomforts (pruritus, insomnia).
5. Describe preventive health care measures (good oral hygiene, prevention of infection, avoidance of bleeding).
6. Relate a plan for gradual increase in physical activity including need for rest periods and measures to conserve energy.
7. Describe plan for health care follow-up.
   a. State signs and symptoms of progressing disease that require immediate medical attention.
   b. Explain the goals of health care.
   c. Explain plans for continued management of other chronic health problems and relate changes in management required as a result of kidney failure.

Intervention for the person dying of renal failure

At times nursing care must be provided for the patient who is dying from renal failure. Major objectives should be maintaining the comfort and the safety of the patient and providing opportunity for the patient and family to vent feelings and arrive at some degree of emotional comfort. In providing physical comfort to the patient, diets may be liberalized. Frequent turning and repositioning are necessary to prevent skin excoriation and breakdown. Oral care is extremely important, since sores in the mouth, once developed, are almost impossible to cure. Mineral oil is an acceptable protective lubricant for the alert patient. A water-soluble lubricant with a vegetable base (e.g., K-Y jelly) is preferable for the stuporous patient. Hydrogen peroxide is helpful in removing blood from the mouth and the nose.

As death approaches, the patient often becomes severely confused or comatose. As the patient's level of awareness and ability to control the environment decrease, it becomes the responsibility of the nursing staff to provide safety for the patient. The specific care required for the unconscious patient is described in Chapter 27.

Providing an opportunity for the patient and family to ventilate feelings is one of the more important aspects of nursing care for a patient with either acute or chronic onset of uremia. Thoughts concerning death and alarm over treatments produce considerable anxiety. The wishes of the patient and family regarding spiritual counseling should be determined. Through demonstrating interest in the patient's needs and providing comfort measures the nurse can do a great deal to help the patient and family accept the patient's ultimate death.

Dialysis and renal transplantation

Development and usage

During the 1960s, the technology and understanding required to make dialysis and transplantation practical solutions for extending life developed rapidly. Presently, most research and development focus on adapting this technology to a more comfortable and convenient lifestyle for those with end-stage renal disease. Advances have been made in (1) the development of more efficient dialysis treatments to shorten dialysis time; (2) the development of alternatives to hospital-based dialysis; and (3) the development of a better understanding of the body's immune mechanism and response to drug therapy, which has increased success in transplantation. Congress has made the federal government a full partner with the health care community in supporting the end-stage renal program. Title 18 of the Social Security Act granted financial support to those requiring dialysis or transplantation; in 1979, congressional action extended further financial support to those persons treated in home dialysis programs.

The following statistics reflect somewhat the nature and scope of the current end-stage renal disease program in the United States. Approximately 14 of every 100,000 people are affected with chronic kidney disease severe enough to require dialysis or transplantation. Of individuals on long-term dialysis, approximately 85% are dialyzed in hospitals or community-based centers and 15% elect home dialysis. In 1970, the total dialysis population approached 2000 individuals. By 1978, the number of individuals receiving dialysis increased to more than 35,000. The average age of these individuals approaches 50 years. There have been between 3000 and 4000 transplants performed or about 16 per million population during the past few years.[83] The major disease entities responsible for progression to end-stage renal failure are glomerulonephritis (41%), cardiovascular and hypertensive disease (13%), diabetes mellitus (7%), and pyelonephritis (6%).[12]

Dialysis

Dialysis involves the movement of fluid and particles across a semipermeable membrane. It is a treatment that can help restore normal fluid and electrolyte balance, control acid-base balance, and remove waste and toxic material from the body. It is a treatment that can sustain life successfully in both acute and chronic situations where substitution for or augmentation of normal renal function is needed. Specifically, dialysis is used to remove excessive amounts of drugs and toxins in poisonings of both an intentional and accidental nature, to correct serious electrolyte and acid-base imbalances, to maintain kidney function when renal shutdown occurs as a result of transfusion reactions, to temporarily replace renal function in persons with acute renal failure of various origins, and to permanently substitute for loss of renal function in persons with chronic end-stage kidney disease.

Physiologic principles of dialysis. Dialysis is based on three principles: diffusion, osmosis, and ultrafiltration (Fig. 62-10). *Diffusion* involves the movement of particles from an area of greater to an area of lesser concentration. In the body this usually occurs across a semipermeable membrane. Diffusion is involved in the clearance of solute from the patient's body in both hemodialysis and peritoneal dialysis. Diffusion results in the movement of urea, creatinine, and uric acid from the patient's blood into the dialysate solution. This solution contains fewer particles to be removed from the bloodstream and higher concentrations of particles to be added to the blood (Fig. 62-11). Since the dialysate contains no protein waste products, the concentration of these substances in the blood will decrease because of random movement of the particles across the semipermeable membrane into the dialysate. The same principle applies to the movement of potassium ions. Although the concentration of red blood cells and protein is high in blood, these molecules are quite large and do not diffuse through the membrane pores; hence they are not lost from the blood.

Osmosis involves the movement of fluid across a semipermeable membrane from an area of lesser to an area of greater concentration of particles. Osmosis is responsible for movement of extra fluid from the patient, particularly in peritoneal dialysis. Fig. 62-11 shows that glucose has been added to the dialysate to make its particle concentration greater than that of the patient's blood. Fluid will then move through the pores of the membrane from the patient's blood to the dialysate.

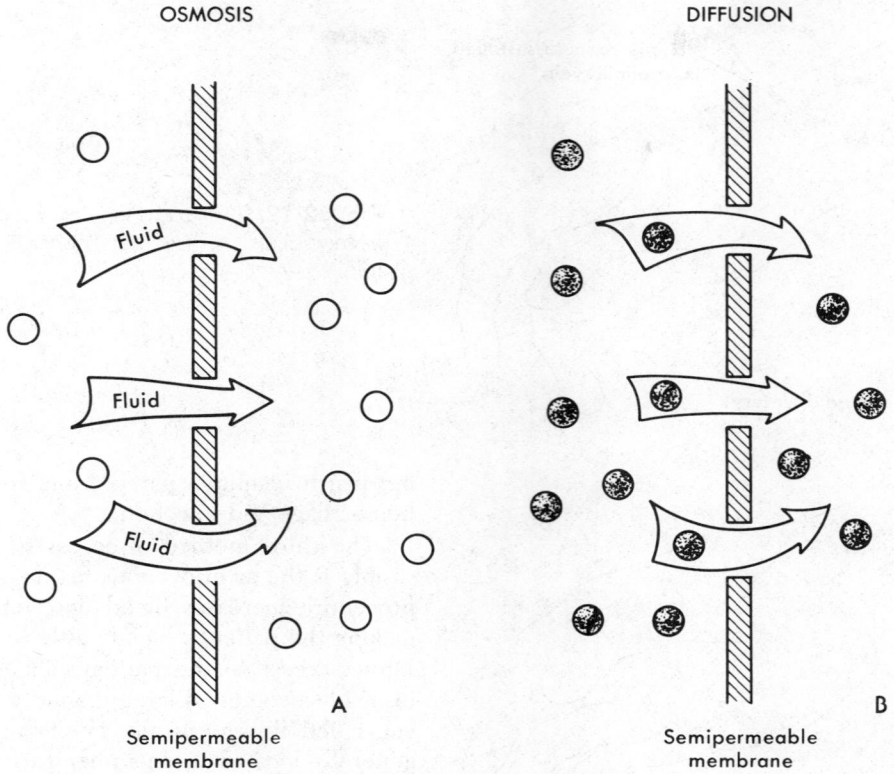

Fig. 62-10. A, Process of osmosis. **B,** Process of diffusion.

Ultrafiltration involves the movement of fluid across a semipermeable membrane as a result of an artificially created pressure gradient. Ultrafiltration is more efficient than osmosis for removal of fluid and is used in hemodialysis for this purpose. During dialysis osmosis and diffusion or ultrafiltration and diffusion occur simultaneously.

Hemodialysis

PROCEDURE. Hemodialysis involves shunting the patient's blood from the body through a dialyzer in which diffusion and ultrafiltration occur and back into the patient's circulation. In order to perform hemodialysis there must be an access to the patient's blood, a mechanism to transport the blood to and from the dialyzer, and a dialyzer (area in which the exchange of fluid electrolytes and waste products occurs).

Presently, the major means for gaining access to the patient's bloodstream include an arteriovenous fistula, an external shunt, and femoral vein catheterization. Use of an external shunt is largely restricted to situations requiring immediate access to the patient (in terms of hours) and is an alternative to femoral vein catheterization. The external shunt (Fig. 62-12, A) is constructed by placing two cannulas through a skin incision into a large vein and a large artery that lie close to each other. Generally, the shunt is placed in an upper extremity.

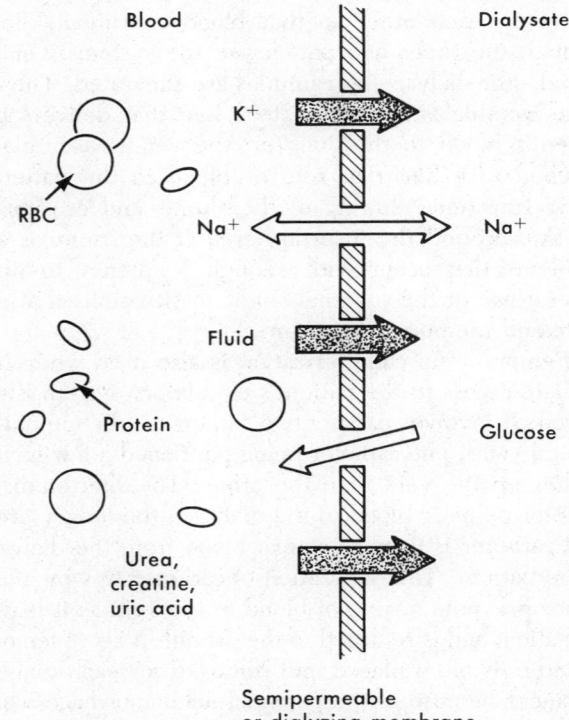

Fig. 62-11. Osmosis and diffusion in dialysis. Net movement of major particles and fluid is illustrated.

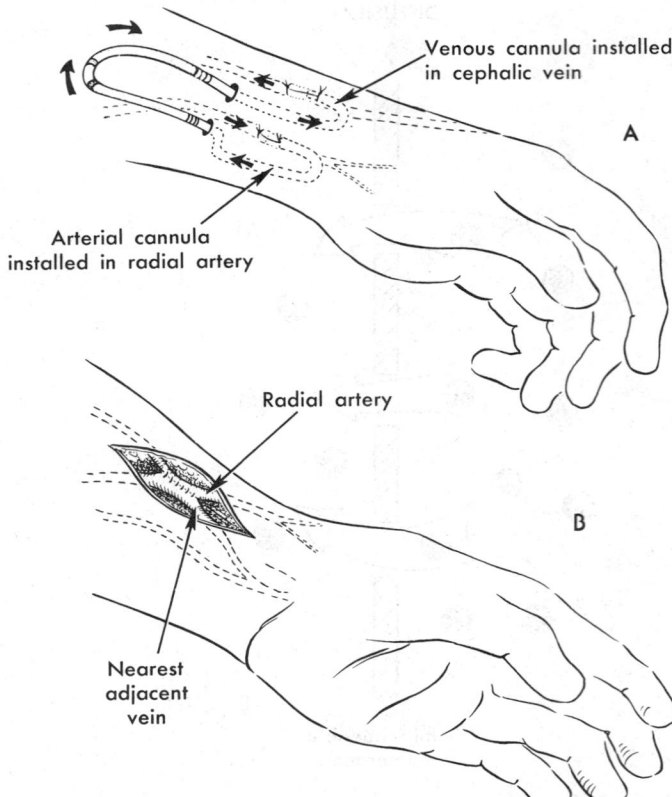

Venous cannula installed
in cephalic vein

A

Arterial cannula
installed in radial artery

Radial artery

B

Nearest
adjacent
vein

Fig. 62-12. Two common forms of venous access for hemodialysis. **A,** External shunt. **B,** Arteriovenous fistula.

When dialysis is not occurring, the cannulas are connected to each other so that blood continually flows through the tubes and patency of the system is maintained. For dialysis the cannulas are separated. The arterial cannula is connected to a line that delivers the patient's blood to the dialyzer; the venous cannula is attached to a line that returns blood to the patient's body. Infection, clotting of the shunt, and erosion of the skin around the insertion area of the cannulas are problems that occur with enough frequency to limit general use of the external shunt to situations that are acute and temporary in nature.

Femoral vein catheterization is also used when immediate access to the patient's circulatory system is required. It involves passing two catheters into one of the femoral veins, one catheter being positioned a few inches further up the vein than the other. The shorter distal catheter delivers blood to the dialyzer; the longer proximal catheter is used to return blood from the dialyzer to the patient. This separation of catheter tips by a few inches prevents mixing of blood in the vein as it leaves the patient and is returned to the patient. A set of femoral catheters is often placed and removed for each dialysis treatment because of the potential for hemorrhage when left in place for subsequent treatments. Occasionally, when placement has been difficult, well-secured catheters are left in place. These catheters require injection of

heparin to maintain patency and frequent checking for hemorrhage and infection.

The third method of access to the patient's blood supply is the arteriovenous fistula (Fig. 62-12, *B*). This procedure increases blood flow into superficial veins, making the patient's blood easily accessible for dialysis. Direct access to the patient's blood is established by inserting needles of large diameter into the superficial veins "fed" by the fistula. The fistula, like the shunt, is generally located in an upper extremity, although the legs may also be used.

Precautions must be taken to maintain the patency of a shunt or fistula. During the patient's hospitalization it is the nurse who is the most consistent observer of the shunt or fistula and the individual most able to see that precautionary measures are followed by all individuals dealing with the patient. To ensure proper maintenance of the shunt or fistula in the home, the same care that the nurse provides in the hospital must be taught to the patient or family.

Decreasing the flow of blood through the shunt or fistula for even short periods can result in clotting. Decreased blood flow results from (1) systemic hypotension, (2) infection of the shunt or fistula, (3) compression of the shunt or fistula, (4) tight bandages or restrictive clothing, (5) phlebitis from punctures of the involved veins, and (6) prolonged inflation of the blood pressure cuff when taking the blood pressure. All of these must be avoided.

Because the external shunt involves a break in the surface of the skin, special attention is given to preventing infection. A dry, sterile dressing that is changed daily should cover the shunt. The cannula insertion sites should be observed for any signs of infection. Any redness, tenderness, swelling, or excessive warmth of the skin in these areas is reported to the physician.

Clotting of the shunt or fistula can be detected by an absence of the palpable or audible *bruit* along the venous portion of the shunt or fistula. Since blood can be observed as it flows through a shunt, clotting may also be detected by the presence of dark or separated

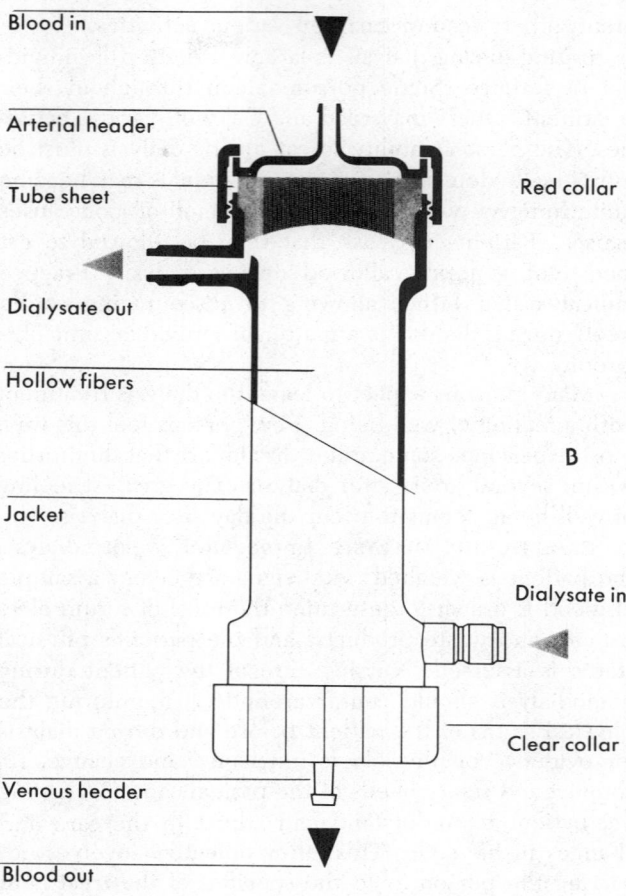

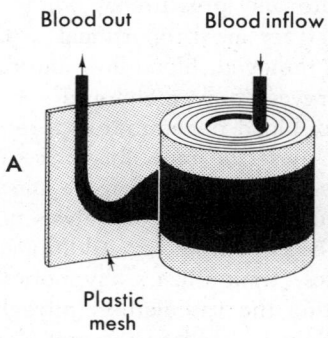

Fig. 62-13. Examples of dialyzers. **A,** Coil dialyzers. **B,** Hollow-fiber artificial kidney. (From Gutch, C.F., and Stoner, M.H.: Review of hemodialysis for nurses and dialysis personnel, ed. 3, St. Louis, 1979, The C.V. Mosby Co.)

blood in the tubing. When it is suspected that a shunt has clotted, the physician should be notified immediately since it may be possible to clear the shunt.

Several types of hemodialyzers are currently in use (Fig. 62-13). Although quite different in appearance, all artificial kidneys function similarly.

PRETREATMENT CARE. Before the procedure, patients should have an opportunity to become familiar with the dialysis unit. They should be given an explanation of what will happen and what will be expected of them during the treatment. Patients often want to know (1) what types of pain will be experienced during the treatment, (2) how long and how often the dialysis will be, (3) what they should feel like during and after the treatment, (4) what they will be allowed to do during dialysis, and (5) if family members may be present during the therapy.

When the patient has an external shunt, no pain should be experienced during initiation of dialysis. However, pain of a moderate degree may be present when venipuncture is performed in an arteriovenous fistula. A local anesthetic is used in most dialysis centers before insertion of the needles.

Patients should be told that they may experience some headache and nausea during the treatment and for a few hours afterward. Headache and nausea result from changes in fluid, acid-base, and waste balance during dialysis. The symptoms should never be extreme, and relief should be attained from rest and sleep, mild analgesics, or antiemetics. Postural hypotension may also occur following dialysis; it is transitory in nature and caused by a relative depletion of intravascular volume secondary to fluid removal. The hypotension may produce dizziness and faintness. Relief should be obtained within a few hours with rest. The patient is assured that all of these symptoms will abate and that frequent monitoring during the procedure will help to control the degree of change that occurs during dialysis and the development of these symptoms.

A dialysis treatment lasts from 3 to 5 hours, depending on the type of dialyzer used and the time necessary to correct the fluid, electrolyte, acid-base, and waste problems that are present. Dialysis for an acute problem may be carried out daily or as often as the condition of the patient warrants. Hemodialysis for chronic renal failure is usually performed two or three times a week. Activity during dialysis is largely a matter of individual preference. Some persons sleep throughout their treatment; others read or carry on various activities.

Eating during dialysis is largely a matter of individual preference. Some persons sleep throughout their treatment; others may read and carry on various activities. The person's ability to eat during dialysis must be individually determined. Some individuals may become quite hungry, while for others the smell of food causes nausea. Patients may ask that they be allowed to eat foods not generally allowed during dialysis. Practice indicates that either allowing or discouraging eating freely during dialysis is a matter of individual unit philosophy.

Many persons expect to leave the dialysis treatment with a feeling of well-being. Few persons feel this way; most experience some minor discomfort that diminishes within several hours after dialysis. The greatest feeling of well-being seems to occur the day after dialysis.

CARE DURING DIALYSIS. Immediately before dialysis the patient is weighed, vital signs are taken, a sample of blood is drawn to determine the level of serum electrolytes and waste products, and the patient's physical status is assessed. Nursing care of the patient during hemodialysis should center around (1) monitoring the physical status of the patient before and during dialysis for evidence of physiologic imbalance and change, (2) comfort and safety needs of the patient, and (3) helping the patient to understand and adjust to the care and changes in life-style. This latter objective involves educating the person as to the specifics of the treatment program (diet and medications in particular) and how these relate to altered kidney function. The person is encouraged to express concerns and feelings, and attempts must be made to help the individual work through these feelings (Fig. 62-14). If dialysis is performed at home, the patient and back-up person must be able to institute all the care described.

Physiologic imbalances. Most physical problems that occur during dialysis are related to hypotension from removal of fluid and disequilibrium from a rapid reduction in extracellular electrolytes and wastes. *Hypovolemia* and *shock* can occur during dialysis as a result of rapid removal of fluid from the intravascular compartment. Since this can occur faster than reequilibration of intracellular and intravascular volume relationships, the person may appear edematous and yet exhibit signs of shock. Signs and symptoms that indicate that the intravascular volume is being rapidly depleted are anxiety, restlessness, dizziness, nausea and vomiting, diaphoresis, tachycardia, and hypotension.

To avoid depleting the intravascular space and producing shock, the blood pressure and pulse rate are checked every 30 to 60 minutes, more frequently when the patient shows any of the previously mentioned signs and symptoms. Blood pressure readings should show only a slight gradual drop during the course of dialysis. Because the rate and pressure at which blood flows through the dialyzer are proportional to the rate and amount of fluid removed, blood flow and dialyzer pressure settings are carefully monitored. (A flow rate of 200 to 250 ml of blood per minute is a reasonable rate for an adult.) Unless the individual is severely hypertensive, rapid-acting antihypertensive medications are usually withheld the morning of dialysis until after the treatment has been completed. Additionally, sedative drugs (analgesics, tranquilizers, hypnotics) and those primarily affecting the vasculature (nitroglycerin) predispose the patient to hypotensive episodes. Self-medication with these agents before and during dialysis must be carefully reviewed with each patient.

In treating a patient who shows signs of hypovolemia, initial nursing measures include determining the blood pressure and pulse, placing the head of the bed in a flat

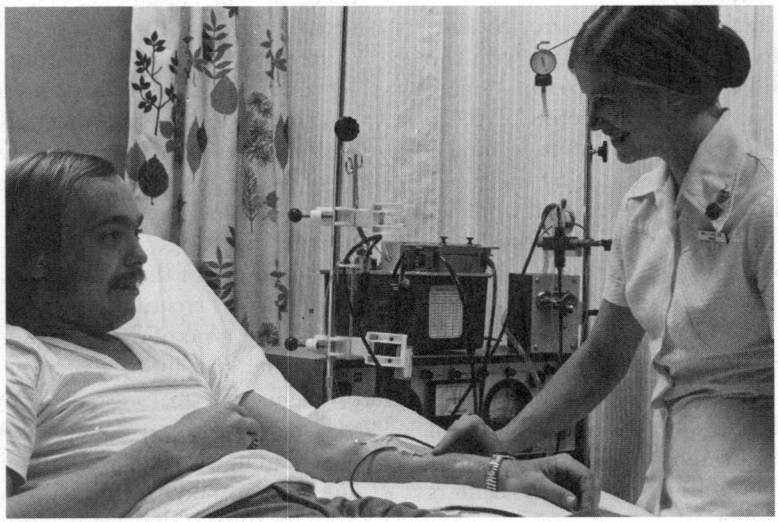

Fig. 62-14. Professional nurse must provide physical and emotional support to patient receiving hemodialysis.

position, and raising the patient's feet. Administration of normal saline solution may be necessary to restore blood pressure. Throughout a hypotensive episode vital signs, level of consciousness, and any complaints offered are closely monitored. It is important for the nurse to know that vomiting frequently accompanies hypotension. Because an upper extremity must be maintained fairly immobile during the dialysis, it may be awkward for the patient to clear the mouth if vomiting should occur. The patient is helped to a safe position so that aspiration is avoided.

The patient is weighed before and after dialysis to determine the amount of fluid loss during treatment. When the weight losses of several dialysis treatments are correlated with the patient's blood pressure, pulse, and other indications of hypovolemia, an individual pattern of the patient's tolerance to fluid removal can be determined. This trend or pattern can be used to help adjust the rate and overall effect of the dialysis in keeping with the patient's physiologic tolerance.

A *disequilibrium phenomenon* occurs for many dialysis patients. This syndrome occurs toward the end of or after dialysis. Disequilibrium results when excess solutes are cleared from the blood more rapidly than they can diffuse from the body's cells, particularly those of the central nervous system, into the vascular compartment. Hence, disequilibrium exists in the concentration of solute inside and outside the cells. Since particle content is greater inside the cells, water is taken in and edema results. Intracellular pH changes are also present. To some degree this process occurs with all patients with each dialysis procedure and helps to explain why patients do not feel their best immediately after treatment. *Severe disequilibrium* or *disequilibrium phenomenon* is most likely to be seen in the person whose blood chemistry values are exceptionally high before dialysis. Signs and symptoms of disequilibrium include *headache, restlessness, mental confusion,* and *nausea* and *vomiting.* Severe disequilibrium may result in convulsions, especially in children when blood urea nitrogen levels exceed the concentration of 100 mg/ml.

Treatment includes anticipation that severe disequilibrium may occur. Often when a patient is beginning dialysis treatments, the procedures are kept short and may be spaced more frequently than normal during the first week. This allows solute to be cleared from the body without producing the extremely wide swings in body chemistry that would result in severe disequilibrium. Keeping the patient quiet, reducing environmental discomfort such as temperature extremes and bright lights, and closely supervising the patient to ensure physical safety are nursing care requirements. Mild analgesics may help to relieve headache. If disequilibrium becomes severe and the patient is still on dialysis, the therapy may be discontinued.

Care of the patient on dialysis should also include preventing *blood loss.* To prevent the patient's blood from clotting as it flows through the dialyzer, heparin is administered. Protamine sulfate is not generally given to the patient to counteract the effect of heparin. The patient is watched for signs of bleeding anywhere in the body. At the end of the treatment when dialysis needles are removed from the fistula, pressure dressings are applied to the puncture sites. They are observed at frequent intervals to detect hemorrhage. During and shortly after dialysis, treatments that cause tissue trauma should not be performed. These commonly include venipuncture and intramuscular injections. The patient who has had recent surgery, dental extractions, or recent trauma to soft tissues will have clotting times frequently monitored during dialysis to prevent hemorrhage. These patients need to be closely observed for signs of bleeding.

Comfort. Nursing care should also include measures to increase the patient's physical comfort. Lying relatively immobile for even a few hours can produce pressure over bony prominences and general restlessness. Changing the patient's position increases tolerance to limited movement. Mouth care is required if the patient is nauseated and vomiting. Because an upper extremity is generally kept immobile during dialysis, the patient may need help with activities requiring the use of both hands.

Changes in the life-style. Much has been written in the literature concerning the changing style of life of the person receiving dialysis treatment and adaptation patterns that commonly arise for coping with required adjustments. The literature also contains much regarding nursing measures most helpful in assisting persons to incorporate their treatment into their style of living. The reader is referred to references 11, 53, and 70.

Peritoneal dialysis. In peritoneal dialysis the dialyzing fluid is instilled into the peritoneal cavity and the peritoneum becomes the dialyzing membrane (Fig. 62-15). In comparison with hemodialysis treatments, which last 3 to 6 hours, peritoneal dialysis is maintained continuously for up to 36 hours. The procedure, once instituted, becomes largely a nursing responsibility. Peritoneal dialysis is used in treating acute and chronic renal failure. It can be performed in the hospital or at home.

PROCEDURE. Access to the peritoneum is gained through introduction of a catheter into the peritoneal space. For acutely ill patients and those who are chronically ill and require sporadic dialysis, a sterile catheter is inserted for each procedure. For the chronically ill person treated on a routine basis, a special catheter can be placed into the peritoneal space; the catheter remains until it malfunctions or another form of treatment is selected for the patient. These catheters present a continued potential entrance for organisms into the peritoneum. Each patient must be thoroughly instructed in the care of the catheter and the signs and symptoms indicative of local or peritoneal infection. These must be reported to the physician.

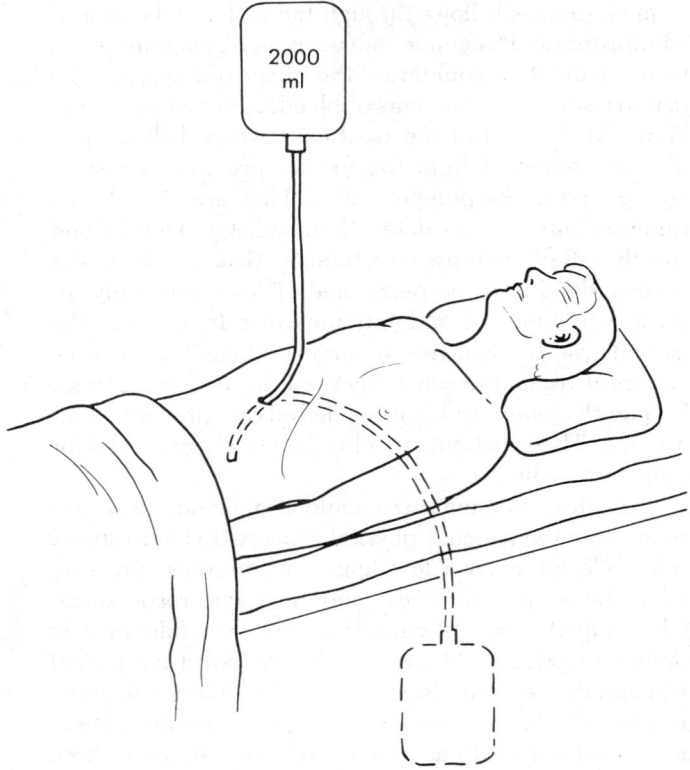

Fig. 62-15. Peritoneal dialysis.

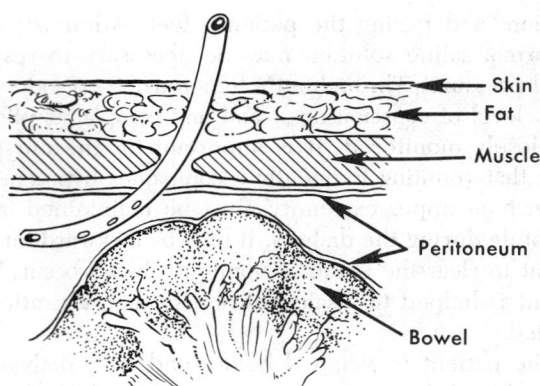

Fig. 62-16. Catheter in place in peritoneal cavity.

For all patients, weight, blood pressure, and pulse are recorded before initiating the procedure. These values serve as baseline information to assess changes in the patient's condition. For persons undergoing insertion of a peritoneal catheter before dialysis, assessment should be made of their knowledge of the procedure and their anxiety level. A mild sedative may help the severely anxious person to better tolerate the insertion of the catheter. It is important that these patients void just before catheter insertion; this decompresses the bladder and prevents accidental puncture during catheter placement.

To insert a peritoneal catheter, the physician cleanses the abdomen and anesthetizes a small area in the midline of the abdomen about 5 cm (2 in.) below the umbilicus. A small incision is made, and the many-eyed nylon catheter is inserted into the peritoneal cavity (Fig. 62-16). A dressing is placed around the protruding catheter. Dialysis is initiated for the person with a permanent catheter by carefully cleansing the catheter and surrounding skin with a bactericidal agent before the catheter is connected to the dialysate line. Approximately 2 L of sterile dialysate warmed to body temperature is attached by tubing to the catheter and allowed to run into the peritoneal cavity as rapidly as possible. This usually takes about 10 minutes. The tubing is then clamped, and 10 to 30 minutes are allowed for osmosis of fluid and diffusion of particles into the dialyzing solution. At the end of the dwell time the tubing is unclamped and the fluid is allowed to flow by gravity from the abdomen. Fluid should drain in a steady stream. Drainage time should average about 10 to 15 minutes. The first drainage may be pink tinged as a result of the trauma of catheter insertion; however, this should clear with the second or third drainage. At no time should fluid draining from the abdomen appear grossly bloody. After fluid has drained from the abdomen, another cycle is started immediately. After the dialysis has been completed, the permanent catheter is again cleansed and a sterile cap is applied to the tip; the temporary catheter is removed, and the incision is covered with a dry sterile dressing. The small abdominal wound from the catheter should heal completely in 1 to 2 days.

CARE DURING PERITONEAL DIALYSIS. Complications most commonly associated with peritoneal dialysis include hypotension and hypovolemia, inadequate drainage of fluid from the peritoneal space, pain, atelectasis, respiratory distress, and peritonitis. As with hemodialysis, *hypotension* is most likely to result from rapid removal of fluid from the intravascular space. In addition to checking vital signs and observing the patient's behavior, records of fluid balance are crucial in determining the amount of fluid that has been removed. The net gain or loss of fluid from the abdomen should be determined at the completion of each cycle. To decrease the amount of fluid that is being removed from the vascular space, the physician may decrease the hypertonicity of the dialysate and may increase the rate at which fluid is administered through an intravenous line.

Drainage of fluid from the abdomen can be slow or impossible to start. Generally, this problem results when the tip of the catheter has become lodged against abdominal tissues. It may also result from plugging of the catheter with blood or fibrin that has accumulated as a result of tissue trauma. A small amount of heparin may be added to the dialysate to decrease the chance of a clot forming in the catheter. When the dialysate does not drain freely from the abdomen, the patient should be turned from side to side in an attempt to reposition the catheter in the peritoneal cavity. In addition, firm pressure may be applied to the abdomen with both hands and the head of the bed may be raised. If the flow of the dialysate does not increase, the physician is called to irrigate the catheter or reposition it.

Severe pain should not be experienced during peritoneal dialysis. Moderate levels of pain are often experienced as fluid is instilled and withdrawn from the peritoneal cavity. Procaine hydrochloride may be instilled with the dialysate in an attempt to control the patient's discomfort. Mild analgesics may be ordered for administration at 3- to 4-hour intervals during the procedure.

When the patient is markedly overhydrated and shows evidence of congestive failure and pulmonary edema, *respiratory difficulty* may be encountered as the dialyzing fluid infuses. The quality and rate of respiration should be closely observed. The head of the bed can be raised to decrease the pressure of the dialysate on the diaphragm. The amount of dialyzing fluid used for each cycle may be decreased when respiratory distress becomes prolonged and severe. The patient, although encouraged to eat while being dialyzed, may find that this increases respiratory difficulty. To help overcome additional pressure created by a full stomach, frequent small meals may be provided.

Peritonitis is an ever present threat during peritoneal dialysis. Aseptic technique must be rigidly maintained during insertion of the catheter and throughout the procedure. Care should be taken to avoid contaminating the solution or the tubing when dialysate solution is hung. Cultures of the dialysate fluid are performed routinely to ensure continued attention to asepsis and to identify organisms if peritonitis should develop subsequently. The patient should be observed for signs of peritonitis. These include an elevated temperature and tenderness or pain of the abdomen.

Although the patient is generally confined to a recumbent position for the length of the dialysis, comfort and diversion can be provided. The patient may turn from side to side and move about in bed as desired as long as the catheter remains undisturbed. The patient may be provided assistance with oral care and bathing as needed. Visiting and other diversional activity should be encouraged when the patient's physical condition permits. If peritoneal dialysis is carried out at home, the patient and a backup person need to be able to do all steps described above.

In the future it is probable that conventional peritoneal dialysis will be used increasingly in both home and in-center dialysis settings. Advances in the man-

agement of patients with chronic end-stage renal disease will likely reflect greater emphasis on home and self-dialysis. Continuous ambulatory peritoneal dialysis (CAPD)[63,65] is one new development that should make self-dialysis increasingly acceptable to patients, safe, useful, and practical. Basically, CAPD involves *continuous contact* of dialysate and peritoneal membrane. Two liters of dialysate are maintained intraperitoneally and exchanged by the patient through a permanent peritoneal catheter four to five times each day. *Major advantages* of this treatment form include (1) steady state of blood chemistry values, (2) reduction in cost of dialysis, (3) patient can dialyze alone in any location without need for machinery and continuous technical supervision, (4) shorter patient training period, and (5) fewer restrictions on life-style.

Although peritonitis is the major problem associated with CAPD, refinement in techniques during exchange of dialysate should reduce the incidence of this problem and make CAPD a practical home procedure.

Outcome criteria for the person experiencing dialysis. The person or significant others can:

1. Explain the process of dialysis and relate work of dialysis to own body needs.
2. State observations required of the shunt or fistula for hemodialysis regarding infection and clotting and state means of obtaining care when these occur.
3. State observation indicating infection of the peritoneal cavity or catheter and state means of obtaining care when these occur.
4. Demonstrate appropriate care of venous access or permanent peritoneal catheter.
5. Relate common side effects of treatment, means for controlling mild symptoms, and means of obtaining medical attention for severe or persistent complications.
6. Explain changes in medication schedule required before and after dialysis.
7. Plan a work and activity schedule as physical capabilities permit with minimal interference from scheduled dialysis time.

Kidney transplantation

Kidney transplants are being performed with increasing frequency in an effort to prolong the lives of persons with chronic renal failure. At present the ability to completely overcome the body's tendency to reject the grafted kidney has not been achieved. Persons undergoing kidney transplantation in essence exchange a program of chronic hemodialysis and its limitations for a new problem. Unless the kidney has been donated by an identical twin, the body senses the graft as a foreign tissue and attempts to destroy it.

Donor selection. Kidney allografts may be obtained from cadavers, matched family members, or an identical twin. Although more than half of the transplanted kidneys are from cadavers, better results are obtained from related donors. Currently, success rates 1 year after transplantation are 50% when a cadaveric kidney is used, 65% to 70% when a matched sibling or parent donates the kidney, and 90% when an identical twin is the organ donor. Many cadaver donors are persons who have irreversible brain damage requiring life support. This has created new definitions of "death" with many legal ramifications.

The major requirement for the donated kidney is histocompatibility. Rejection occurs from a cell-mediated (type IV hypersensitivity) response (p. 289) or from a humoral (type II cytotoxic hypersensitivity) response (p. 288). The important antigens are the human leukocyte antigen (HLA) and the ABO blood groups. For the ABO groups the same rules apply as for blood transfusions (p. 1868). Survival of the kidney depends on suppression of the body's biologic defense mechanisms. Immunosuppressive medications include azathioprine (Imuran) and prednisone. Antilymphocyte serum (ALS) (p. 511) is being used in some medical centers.

A new procedure currently being tested that researchers hope will significantly increase graft survival from living related donors is that of *donor-specific transfusion*. Shortly before transplantation the recipient receives three transfusions of the donor's blood, each 2 weeks apart. After these transfusions, if the recipient and donor blood cross match is still compatible, transplantation is peformed. The purposes of donor-specific transfusion are (1) to identify those recipients who would respond *unfavorably* to the donated organ and (2) to desensitize the recipient to the donor's tissue. Preliminary results of this procedure are encouraging.[69]

Related donors must be in good health, be highly motivated to be a donor, have good mental health, and not be receiving drugs such as barbiturates, which depress reflexes and electrical brain activity.[51] The donor is given a complete medical evaluation and in some cases may be referred to a psychiatrist for further evaluation. Cadavers should be free of renal disease, neoplasms (excluding those of the central nervous system and skin), and sepsis.[51] Permission for cadaver donation is given by next of kin or by persons who plan in advance to donate their organs.

Viability of the donor kidney must be maintained until the time of transplantation surgery. Preservation times of 24 to 72 hours have been reported with proper technique. Methods include washing out the formed blood elements and perfusing a heparinized electrolyte solution at 2° to 4° C. Use of a pulsatile flow pump and oxygenator helps to preserve the kidney beyond 6 to 12 hours.

Preoperative care. Nursing care of the patient in the preoperative phase includes physical and emotional preparation for the surgery. The patient and family should understand the outcomes expected from the surgery and the follow-up care that will be required. They should be prepared for the possibility of the kidney not functioning after transplantation.

The nature of the surgery and location of the kidney, the possible need for postoperative dialysis, the use of immunosuppressive drugs, and the need for infection prevention after surgery must be explained to the patient and family. As with any surgical patient, the individual should know of any drainage tubes that will be inserted during surgery, that medication will be given for relief of pain, and that after only a few hours moving about, coughing, and deep breathing will be necessary.

Throughout the period from the patient's acceptance as a transplant candidate to the time of surgery, the concerns and anxieties of the patient and family regarding transplantation need to be identified. As appropriate, the nurse and other members of the health team are called to help in dealing with these concerns and anxieties.

The patient must be in optimal physical condition for transplantation. Dialysis may be required before transplantation to ensure optimal fluid and electrolyte balance, acid-base balance, and removal of wastes. The integrity of the fistula must be maintained. Before surgery the extremity containing the fistula may be wrapped to draw attention to it and identify it as containing the patient's access for dialysis. This identification will help all individuals caring for the person to avoid using the affected extremity for blood pressure determinations, drawing of blood, or intravenous infusions.

Surgery. During surgery the transplanted kidney is placed in the fossa (Fig. 62-17). Generally, the peritoneal cavity is not entered. The patient's own kidneys are not disturbed unless they are infected or are the cause of significant hypertension. In this case, the recipient undergoes bilateral nephrectomy before transplant surgery. The donor ureter is used to the extent that is possible. If long enough, it is connected to the bladder in such a way as to prevent reflux of urine (Fig. 62-18). If the ureter is short, a ureteroureterostomy may be performed. A catheter is placed in the wound to promote drainage of accumulating fluid.

Postoperative care. Immediate postoperative care includes maintaining drainage of the urinary bladder, assessing the adequacy of fluid and electrolyte balance, protecting the patient from infection, observing for signs and symptoms of rejection and other complications, and identifying the effects of medications that have been administered throughout the entire care cycle. A free flow of communication must be maintained with the patient and significant others regarding the individual's progress.

In the operating room a Foley catheter is inserted into the bladder to promote drainage of urine and to prevent bladder distention and pressure on the newly

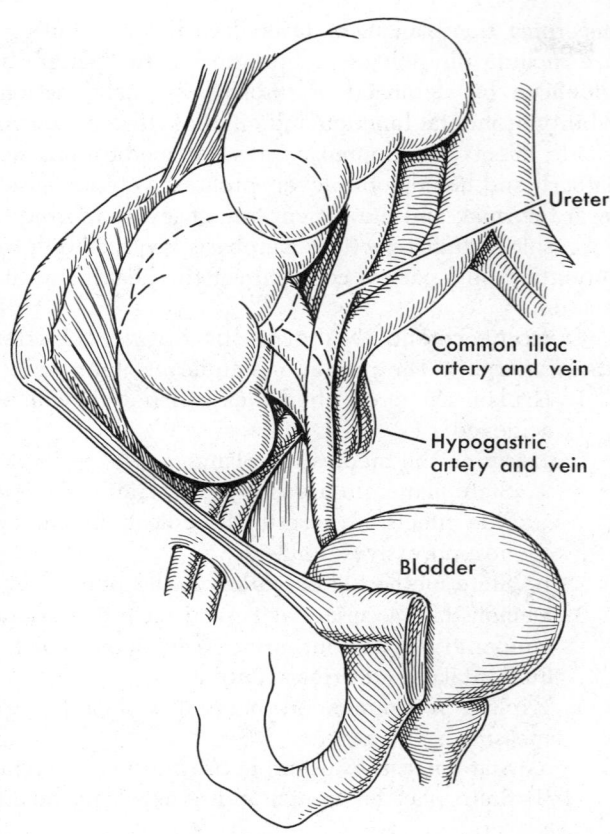

Fig. 62-17. Various positions for placement of homografted kidney. (Redrawn from Starzl, T.E., et al.: Techniques of renal homotransplantation, Arch. Surg. **89**:87, 1964. Copyright 1964, American Medical Association.)

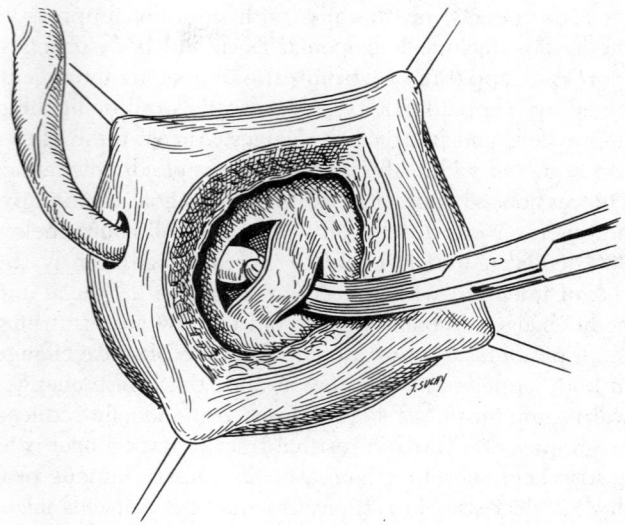

Fig. 62-18. Extraction of intravesical ureter through performed submucosal tunnel. (Redrawn from Starzl, T.E., et al.: Techniques of renal homotransplantation, Arch. Surg. **89**:87, 1964. Copyright 1964, American Medical Association.)

anastomosed ureter. If gross hematuria or clots are noted in the drainage system, the physician should be notified immediately.

As with any surgical patient, the possibility of hemorrhage and hypovolemia exists. Blood pressure and pulse are determined frequently. Because the patient may have little or no urinary output for a number of hours to weeks after transplantation, fluid and electrolyte balance must be monitored carefully. Parameters indicating disturbed fluid and electrolyte balance are listed in the discussion of care of the patient with chronic renal failure (p. 1577). Any drainage from dressing or tubes should be carefully calculated into the patient's fluid balance record.

Rejection, the leading cause of graft failure, may occur as a *hyperacute event* (difficulty as the new kidney is anastomosed into the renal function), as an *acute event,* or as a slow and *progressive decline* in renal function. In a hyperacute event, the graft is completely destroyed and it must be removed immediately. Acute rejection usually occurs within the first 2 weeks following transplantation but may occur at any time. Rejection is caused by a cell-mediated immune response. The delay in the

occurrence of the first attack is related to the time it takes for T-lymphocytes to become sensitized.

Signs and symptoms indicating acute rejection include rising serum creatine level; decreasing renal clearance of creatinine; decreasing urinary output; fever, pain, or tenderness over the kidney; and malaise. Treatment of acute rejection involves increasing steroid doses. Acute rejection episodes are treated with Solu-Medrol (methylprednisolone) intravenously. Most rejection episodes are suppressed successfully, although two or three events in succession indicate a poor prognosis for the new kidney. The person should be helped to feel that although rejection is always a serious medical event, it should not be equated with unequivocal loss of the graft.

Chronic rejection is a slow progressive process. It occurs secondary to both *cell-mediated* and *humoral immune responses*. The signs and symptoms are similar to those that occur in acute rejection, but they develop more slowly. Treatment may include increasing doses of steroids, but in most instances the patient will eventually lose all renal function.

Since the person is *immunosuppressed*, it is imperative to provide protection from infection. Reverse isolation is not commonly practiced in most institutions. A system of closed drainage is meticulously maintained for the catheter draining the bladder. Cleansing of the perineum is performed once every 8 hours to help prevent bacteria from entering the meatus and bladder. Special attention is also given to any line or tube inserted into the patient since these are potential sources of infection. Good pulmonary hygiene to prevent pulmonary infection is also required.

Side effects of therapy with immunosuppressive medication include leukopenia, facial and body changes, increased appetite, gastrointestinal tract irritation and bleeding, hepatotoxicity, decreased wound healing, depression, and personality changes. Any of these effects can be noted within the first few weeks of administration. Depression of white cell count is the goal of therapy; however, severe depression with white cell counts below 3000 cells/cu mm is likely to increase significantly the risk of infection with the potential of death. Facial and body changes secondary to steroid therapy are disturbing to all patients. Support during the time of acute change in body appearance and reassurance that these changes will be minimized as steroid doses are gradually reduced are important. Gastrointestinal tract irritation occurs as gastric acid secretion increases and gastric mucus production decreases in response to steroids. Antacids taken between meals can reduce this irritation. *Hepatotoxicity* with symptoms of hepatitis can result from azathioprine (Imuran) administration. This side effect requires a change in immunosuppressive medication. Because of the side effects of azathioprine and the steroids, research is on-going for immunosuppressive drug therapy with fewer side effects.

Anxiety and fear of losing control may occur as the person perceives changes in mood and behavior. It is helpful for the patient to know that steroids are capable of producing these changes. Psychiatric intervention may be required when behavior becomes maladaptive.

Steroid dosage is gradually reduced to the lowest level compatible with preservation of renal function. Alternate-day prednisone therapy is used in most transplant centers to minimize the effects of chronic steroid administration. The adult dose is 20 mg every other day. To ensure that the steroid level is effective in suppressing rejection, the patient's serum creatinine and creatinine clearance are carefully monitored during reduction of the steroids and at specific intervals thereafter.

Early in the postoperative course the patient should begin to become involved in learning to manage self-care. By the time of discharge from the hospital, the patient should understand the following aspects of care: (1) dietary limitations; (2) medications, their dosage, and effects; (3) how to care for the incision; (4) any precautions necessary in regard to activity and preventing trauma to the graft site; (5) how to measure own intake and output and record daily weights; (6) how to take his or her temperature; (7) how to collect a 24-hour urine specimen; (8) signs and symptoms of rejection; and (9) means of contacting health care personnel.

The importance of regular follow-up visits and close medical supervision cannot be overemphasized. Subsequent health visits should include physiologic evaluation of the person and opportunity to raise questions regarding present life-style and new health concerns. These visits should also include continuation of patient education

concerning transplantation. Overall goals for ambulatory care include physiologic stabilization of the patient as evidenced by stabilized or improving renal function, stability in mental function and emotional state, control of side effects of immunosuppressive medication, hematocrit and hemoglobin levels progressively increased toward normal, and the patient free of severe morbidity as a result of graft rejection. Emphasis is placed on promoting maximal patient control over the health and life situation.

Outcome criteria for the person having a kidney transplantation. The person or significant others can:
1. Explain the prescribed diet and how it will be achieved.
2. Describe the medication plan.
    a. State name, dosage, frequency, rationale, and side effects of prescribed medications (immunosuppressives, antacids).
    b. State method of obtaining medications.
3. Demonstrate accurate taking and recording of oral temperature, 24-hour urine specimens, weight, fluid intake, and urinary output.
4. Explain recommended preventive health care measures.
    a. State measures useful in preventing infection.
    b. State plan for dental and gynecologic health care.
    c. State need to avoid immunization with live-virus vaccines.
5. Relate a program for continued health supervision.
    a. Explain concept of immunosuppression and relate this to health care needs.
    b. Describe signs and symptoms requiring immediate medical attention.
    c. Relate appropriate information regarding sexual functioning and family planning.
    d. State need to preserve dialysis access.
    e. State resources available for assistance with illness and rehabilitative concerns and means of contact with resources.
    f. Explain specific plans for follow-up health care.

REFERENCES AND SELECTED READINGS

1. *Analgesic abuse and the kidney, Kidney Int. **17:**250-260, 1980.
2. Anderson, C.F., et al.: Nutritional therapy for adults with renal disease, J.A.M.A. **223:**68-72, 1973.
3. Asscher, A.: The detection and natural history of urinary infection. In Blandy, J.F., editor: Lecture notes on urology, Oxford, England, 1976, Blackwell Scientific Publications, Ltd.
4. Bailey, G.L., editor: Hemodialysis: principles and practice, New York, 1972, Academic Press, Inc.

*References preceded by an asterisk are particularly well suited for student reading.

5. Beard, M.P.: The impact of hemodialysis and transplantation on the family, Crit. Care Q. **1**:87-91, 1978.

6. Bennett, W.M., editor: Symposium on clinical pharmacology and the kidney patient, Dialysis and Transplantation **8**:7-72, 1979.

7. Bergstein, J.M.: Acute renal failure in children, Crit. Care Q. **1**:41-51, 1978.

8. *Bernbeck, L.: Conservative care of patients with renal failure. In Schlotter, L., editor: Nursing and the nephrology patient, Flushing, N.Y., 1973, Medical Examination Publishing Co., Inc.

9. Black, D.A.K., editor: Renal disease, ed. 4, Oxford, England, 1979, Blackwell Scientific Publications, Ltd.

10. *Blount, M., and Kinney, A.: Chronic steroid therapy, Am. J. Nurs. **74**:1626-1631, 1974.

11. Brundage, D.: Nursing management of renal problems, ed. 2, St. Louis, 1980, The C.V. Mosby Co.

12. Bryan, F.A.: Final report of National Dialysis Registry. Artificial Kidney–Chronic Uremia Program, NIH report no. AK-8-7-1387-F, PB2591741 AS, Aug. 1976.

13. *Burton, B.: Current concepts of nutrition and diet in diseases of the kidney, J. Am. Diet. Assoc. **65**:623-633, 1974.

14. *Campbell, J.D., and Campbell, A.R.: The social and economic cost of end-stage renal disease: a patient's perspective, N. Engl. J. Med. **229**:386-392, 1978.

15. Campbell, M., and Harrison, J., editors: Urology, ed. 4, vols. 1 to 3, Philadelphia, 1978-79, W.B. Saunders Co.

16. Castelnuovo-Tedesco, P., editor: Psychiatric aspects of organ transplantation, New York, 1971, Grune & Stratton, Inc.

17. Center for Disease Control, Hospital Infections Section: Outline for surveillance and control of nosocomial infections, Atlanta, 1974, Center for Disease Control, Bureau of Edpidemiology.

18. Chapman, W.H., et al., editors: The urinary system, Philadelphia, 1973, W.B. Saunders Co.

19. Chatteryee, V., et al.: Perspectives in organ transplantation, Surg. Clin. North Am. **58**:221-451, 1978.

20. Cimino, J.: Diagnosis and management of urinary tract infection, Hosp. Med. **10**:59-62, 1974.

21. *Cohen, S.: Metabolic acid-base disorders. II. Physiologic abnormalities and nursing actions. Programmed instruction, Am. J. Nurs. **78**(suppl.):1-20, 1978.

22. *Cohen, S.: Metabolic acid-base disorders. I. Chemistry and physiology. Programmed instruction, Am. J. Nurs. **77**(suppl.):1-32, 1977.

23. Cooper, H., and Robinson, E.: Treatment of genitourinary tuberculosis: report after 24 years, J. Urol. **108**:136-142, 1972.

23a. *Davis, V., and La Vandero, R.: Caring for the catheter carefully . . . before, during, and after peritoneal dialysis. II, Nurs. '80 **10**:67-71, Dec. 1980.

24. *deGreco, F., and Krumlovsky, F.: Chronic renal failure: clinical and therapeutic considerations, Postgrad. Med. **52**:176-183, 1972.

25. Denniston, D.J., and Burns, K.T.: Home peritoneal dialysis, Am. J. Nurs. **80**:2022-2026, 1980.

26. Dolan, P., and Greene, H.: Renal failure and peritoneal dialysis, Nurs.'75 **5**:41-49, July 1975.

27. *Fellows, B., and Blagg, C.: Acute renal failure and renal dialysis. In Meltzer, L., Abdellah, F., and Kitchell, J., editors: Concepts and practices of intensive care for nurse specialists, ed. 2, Bowie, Md., 1976, The Charles Press.

28. Flamenbaum, W.: Pathophysiology of acture renal failure, Arch. Intern. Med. **131**:911-928, 1973.

29. Foster, J.K.: Dialysis: a treatment modality in renal failure, Crit. Care Q. **1**:25-39, 1978.

30. Fox, R., and Swazey, J.: The courage to fail: a social view of organ transplants and dialysis, Chicago, 1974, The University of Chicago Press.

31. Freedman, P.: Acute renal failure, Heart Lung **4**:873-878, 1975.

32. Froom, J.: The spectrum of urinary tract infections in family practice, J. Fam. Pract. **11**:385-391, 1980.

33. Galloway, A.L., Jr.: Emotional aspects of dialysis and transplantation, Crit. Care Q. **1**:75-85, 1978.

34. *Gault, P.: How to break the kidney stone cycle, Nurs. '78 **8**:24-31, Dec. 1978.

35. *Gault, P.: The prostate: coping with dangerous and distressing complications, Nur. '77 **7**:34-38, April 1977.

36. Gleckman, R., et al.: Therapy of recurrent invasive urinary tract infections of men, N. Engl. J. Med. **301**:878-880, 1979.

37. Gleckman, R.D.: Recurrent urinary tract infections: therapeutic considerations, Postgrad. Med. **65**:156-159, 1979.

38. Goldberger, E.: A primer of water, electrolyte and acid-base syndromes, ed. 6, Philadelphia, 1980, Lea & Febiger.

39. Goodman, L., and Gilman, A., editors: The pharmacological basis of therapeutics, ed. 6, New York, 1980, Macmillan Publishing Co., Inc.

40. Gutch, C., and Stoner, M.: Review of hemodialysis for nurses and dialysis personnel, ed. 3, St. Louis, 1979, The C.V. Mosby Co.

41. Hansen, G.L.: Caring for patients with chronic renal disease, Philadelphia, 1974, J.B. Lippincott Co.

42. Hunsicker, L., et al.: Transfusion and renal allograft and survival, Arch. Surg. **115**:737-741, 1980.

43. Johnson, K., et al.: Nursing care of the patient with acute renal failure, Nurs. Clin. North Am. **10**:421-430, 1975.

44. *Juliani, L.: Kidney transplant: your role in aftercare, Nurs. '77 **7**:46-53, Oct. 1977.

45. Kark, R.: Symposium on diseases of the kidney, Med. Clin. North Am. **55**:1-241, 1971.

46. Kass, E.H., and Brunfitt, W., editors: Infections of the urinary tract, Chicago, 1978, The University of Chicago Press.

47. *Kemp, G., and Kemp, D.: Diuretics, Am. J. Nurs. **78**:1006-1010, 1978.

48. *Kobrzychi, P.: Renal transplant: complications, Am. J. Nurs. **77**:641-643, 1977.

49. Kunin, C.: Detection, prevention and management of urinary tract infections, ed. 3, Philadelphia, 1979, Lea & Febiger.

50. Lang, G., and Levin, S.: Diagnosis and treatment of urinary tract infections, Med. Clin. North Am. **55**:1439-1456, 1971.

51. Lapides, J., editor: Fundamentals of urology, Philadelphia, 1976, W.B. Saunders Co.

52. *La Vandero, R., and Davis, V.: Caring for the catheter carefully . . . before, during, and after peritoneal dialysis. I, Nurs. '80 **10**:73-79, Nov. 1980.

53. Levy, N.: Living or dying: adaptation to hemodialysis, Springfield, Ill., 1974, Charles C Thomas, Publisher.

54. Licina, M.G., Adler, S., and Bruns, F.J.: Acute renal failure in a patient with polycystic kidney disease, J.A.M.A. **245**:1664-1665, 1981.

55. Luke, B.: Nutrition in renal disease: the adult on dialysis, Am. J. Nurs. **79**:2155-2157, 1979.

56. Oestreich, S.J.: Rational nursing care in chronic renal disease, Am. J. Nurs. **79**:1096-1099, 1979.

57. *O'Neil, M., editor: Symposium on care of the patient with renal disease, Nurs. Clin. North Am. **10**:411-516, 1975.

58. Oreopoulos, D.G., et al.: Continuous ambulatory peritoneal dialysis: a new era in the treatment of chronic renal failure, Clin. Nephrol. **11**:125-128, 1979.

59. Papper, S.: Clinical nephrology, ed. 2, Boston, 1978, Little, Brown & Co.

60. *Papper, S.: Renal failure, Med. Clin. North Am. **55**:335-357, 1971.

61. Penn, I., et al.: Parenthood in renal homograft recipients, J.A.M.A. **216**:1755-1761, 1971.

62. Pollak, V., and Mendoza, N.: Rapidly progressive glomerulonephritis, Med. Clin. North Am. **55**:1397-1416, 1971.

63. *Popovitch, R.P., et al.: Continuous ambulatory peritoneal dialysis, Ann. Intern. Med. **88:**449-456, 1978.

64. *Pullman, T., and Coe, F.: Chronic renal failure, Clin. Symp. **25:**1-32, 1973.

65. *Robson, M.D., and Oreopoulos, D.G.: Continuous ambulatory peritoneal dialysis: a revolution in the treatment of chronic renal failure, Dialysis and Transplantation **7:**999-1003, 1978.

66. Rous, S.N.: Urology in primary care, St. Louis, 1976, The C.V. Mosby Co.

67. Sabath, L.D., and Charles, D.: Urinary tract infections in the female, Obstet Gynecol. **55:**1625-1705, 1980.

68. *Sachs, B.: Renal transplantation: a nursing perspective, Flushing, N.Y., 1977, Medical Examination Publishing Co., Inc.

69. *Salvatierra, O., et al.: Deliberate donor-specific blood transfusions prior to living related renal transplantation, Ann. Surg. **192:**543-522, 1980.

70. *Schlotter, L., editor: Nursing and the nephrology patient: a symposium on current trends and issues, Flushing, N.Y., 1973, Medical Examination Publishing Co., Inc.

71. *Schumann, D.: The renal donor, Am. J. Nurs. **74:**105-110, 1974.

72. Scott, R., et al.: Urology illustrated, Edinburgh, 1975, Churchill Livingstone.

73. Smith, J.W., et al.: Recurrent urinary tract infections in men: characteristics and response to therapy, Ann. Intern. Med. **91:**544-548, 1979.

74. Smith, S.: Concepts in renal transplantation, Crit. Care Q. **1:**53-73, 1978.

75. Sorrels, A.J.: Continuous ambulatory peritoneal dialysis, Am. J. Nurs. **79:**1400-1401, 1979.

76. Stamm, W.E., et al.: Is antimicrobial prophylaxis of urinary tract infections cost effective? Ann. Intern. Med. **94:**251-255, 1981.

77. Strauss, M.B., and Gottschalk, C.W., editors: Diseases of the kidney, ed. 3, vols. 1 and 2, Boston, 1979, Little, Brown & Co.

78. Szwed, J.J.: Pathophysiology of acute renal failure: rationale for signs and symptoms, Crit. Care Q. **1:**1-9, 1978.

79. Turk, M.: Renal disease at a glance: analgesic nephropathy. A case study including symptoms, diagnoses, and prognosis, Nephrol. Nurse **2:**37, 1980.

80. U.S. Department of Health, Education and Welfare: Outline for surveillance and control of nosocomial infections, Atlanta, 1974, Center for Disease Control, Bureau of Epidemiology.

81. Williams, H.: Nephrolithiasis, N. Engl. J. Med. **290:**33-38, 1974.

82. Williams, S.R.: Nutrition and diet therapy, ed. 4, St. Louis, 1981, The C.V. Mosby Co.

83. *Wineman, R.J.: End-stage renal disease, Dialysis and Transplantation **7:**1034-1037, 1064, 1978.

84. *Winter, C.C., and Morel, A.: Nursing care of patients with urologic diseases, ed. 4, St. Louis, 1977, The C.V. Mosby Co.

85. *Wolf, Z.R.: What patients awaiting kidney transplant want to know, Am. J. Nurs. **76:**92-94, 1976.

86. Woodrow, M., Wilsey, G., and Wiley, N.: Suprapubic catheters. I. A direct line to better drainage, Nurs. '76 **6:**40-45, Oct. 1976.

87. Woodrow, M., Wilsey, G., and Wiley, N.: Suprapubic catheters. II. A direct line to better drainage, Nurs. '76 **6:**40-42, Nov. 1976.

AUDIOVISUAL RESOURCES

Acute renal failure, Ann Arbor, Mich., 1978, University of Michigan Medical Center. (Cassette tape, slides.)

Chronic renal failure, Ann Arbor, Mich., 1978, University of Michigan Medical Center. (Cassette tape, slides, guide.)

Chronic renal failure: predialytic or conservative management, Baltimore, 1980, Norwich-Eaton Pharmaceutical Film Library. (Cassette tape, slides.)

Infections of the kidney and the urinary tract, Atlanta, 1974, National Medical Audiovisual Center. (Cassette tape, slides, script.)

Nursing care of the patient undergoing peritoneal dialysis, Buffalo, N.Y., 1977, District I, New York State Nurses Association. (Cassette tape, sound recording, guide.)

Polycystic kidney disease and other cystic disorders, New York, 1978, Medcom. (Cassette tape, slides, guide.)

Preventable forms of kidney disease, Ann Arbor, Mich., 1978, University of Michigan Medical Center. (Cassette tape, slides, guide.)

Principles of hemodialysis, Garden Grove, Calif., 1971, Trainex Corp. (Cassette tape, filmstrip, guide, workbook.)

Psychosocial aspects of hemodialysis and kidney transplantation, Fort Sam Houston, Tex., 1975, Academy of Health Sciences. (Videorecording, cassette.)

Vidt, D.: Peritoneal dialysis: a bedside procedure, 1971, Abbott Laboratories. (Film.)

PROBLEMS RELATED TO SEXUALITY AND REPRODUCTION

Sexuality and reproductive concerns are being presented to nurses with increasing frequency. Persons are becoming more aware of their sexual and reproductive health and are more comfortable about discussing sexual and reproductive issues. It is becoming increasingly necessary for nurses to provide counseling and education to persons with concerns related to family planning, sexuality, venereal diseases, malignancies of the reproductive system, and the changes in sexual and reproductive experiences throughout the life cycle.

Assessment of the reproductive and sexual systems is described first in this unit. Common approaches to *management of the person with a reproductive or sexual problem* follow. A discussion of *reproductive problems, problems of the breast, and problems of sexuality* concludes the unit.

CHAPTER 63

ASSESSMENT OF THE REPRODUCTIVE AND SEXUAL SYSTEMS

GREER GLAZER
NANCY FUGATE WOODS
ELLA CINKOTA

Conditions affecting healthful functioning of the reproductive systems of men and women take a high toll in terms of loss of life and acute and chronic physical and emotional stress. The nurse has a responsibility to assist in general health education, to refer patients to good medical care, and to understand the treatment available and the nursing care needed when disease develops. A sound knowledge of the structure and functions of the reproductive system is essential to the assessment process.

Anatomy and physiology

Pelvis

The bones of the pelvis are shown in Fig. 63-1. The pelvis is the weight-bearing structure of the upper body and trunk. The pelvic bones consist of the innominate bones, the sacrum, and the coccyx. The two innominate bones are made up of the pubic bone, ilium, and ischium. Anteriorly, the pubic bones join at the symphysis pubis. The inferior borders of the pubic bones and symphysis form an inverted V, called the pubic arch. The sacrum and coccyx come together at the sacrococcygeal joint, which is movable. The sacral hiatus is the site of administration of caudal anesthetics.

The pelvis is divided into two parts (the true and the false pelvis) by a bony ridge called the pelvic brim. The false pelvis is the broad, expanded portion above the pelvic brim. The narrow part below the pelvic brim is the true pelvis. The true pelvis is further described as having an inlet and an outlet. The inlet is located at the pelvic brim, and the outlet is at the base of the pelvis. The iliac spines mark the midpoint between the inlet and the outlet. The distances between the bones of the true pelvis have special significance during childbirth, since it is through this bony canal that the baby must pass to be born.

Like other bones of the skeletal system, the pelvic bones undergo changes during periods of growth and development until maturity is reached. The major differences between the pelves of men and women are in the contour of the pelvis and thickness of the bones. While variations are seen in both sexes, the female pelvis is more delicate because the bones are thinner and lighter in weight. The female pelvis is wider and more shallow because of the flaring of the iliac bones; the male pelvis tends to be narrow and deep. In women, the sacrum is shorter, wider, and less curved, and the coccyx is more movable. The pubic arch is wider and more rounded in women, and the ischial spines are less prominent. Pelvic dimensions vary with age and race in addition to sex. The typical architecture of the female pelvis is especially suited for childbirth.

Female genital system

External structures

Fig. 63-2 shows the external genitalia of a female. Collectively, the external genitalia are often referred to as the vulva, and consist of the mons pubis (mons veneris), labia majora, labia minora, clitoris, prepuce,

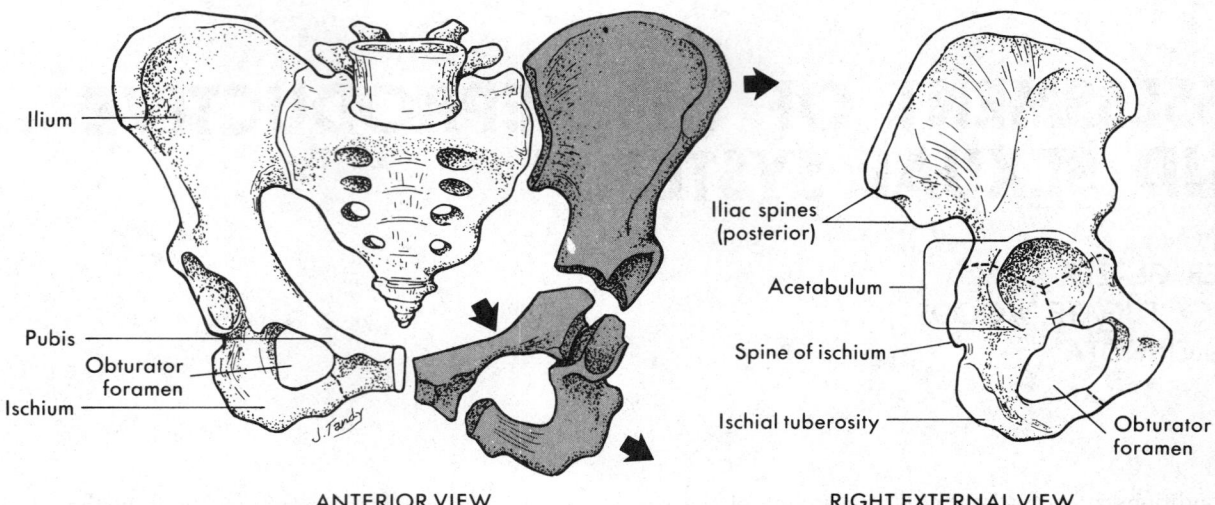

Ilium

Pubis

Obturator
foramen

Ischium

J. Tandy

ANTERIOR VIEW

Iliac spines
(posterior)

Acetabulum

Spine of ischium

Ischial tuberosity

Obturator
foramen

RIGHT EXTERNAL VIEW

Fig. 63-1. Adult female pelvis, showing origin of parts from separate embryonic bones. (From Jensen, M.D., Benson, R.C., and Bobak, I.M.: Maternity care: the nurse and the family, ed. 2, St. Louis, 1981, The C.V. Mosby Co.)

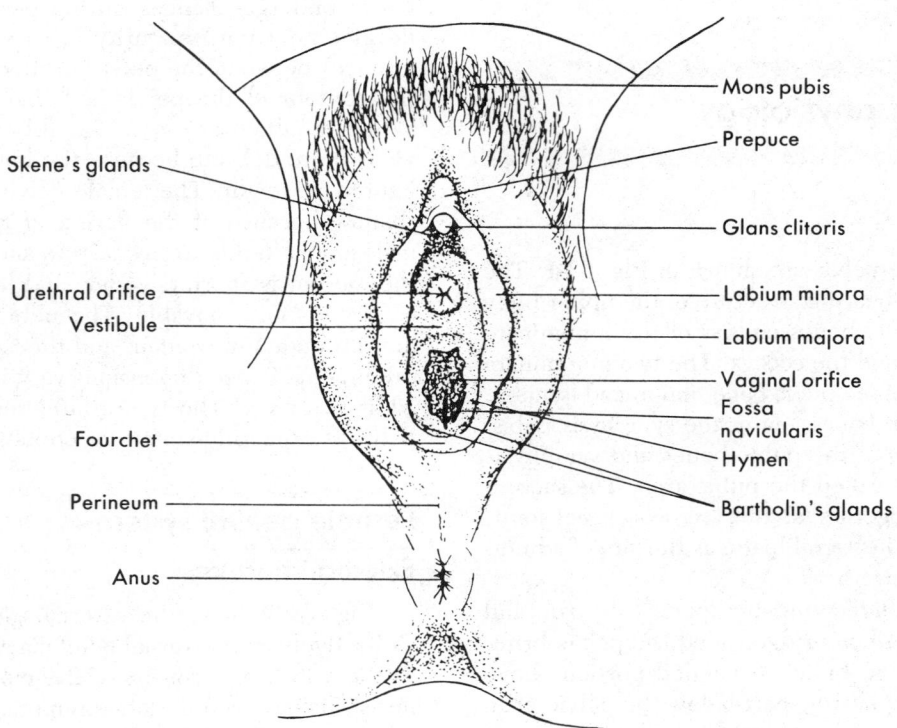

Skene's glands

Urethral orifice

Vestibule

Fourchet

Perineum

Anus

Mons pubis

Prepuce

Glans clitoris

Labium minora

Labium majora

Vaginal orifice

Fossa
navicularis

Hymen

Bartholin's glands

Fig. 63-2. External female genitalia.

frenulum, vestibule, urethral meatus, Skene's (paraurethral) glands, vaginal orifice, hymen, fossa navicularis, Bartholin's (vulvovaginal) glands, fourchet, perineum, and escutcheon. The escutcheon is the triangular pubic hair pattern from the upper portion of the pubic bone to the lateral areas of the labia majora. The *mons pubis* is the rounded area in front of the symphysis pubis. It consists of a collection of fatty tissue beneath the skin and is covered with hair after puberty.

The *labia majora* are two prominent, longitudinal folds of tissue extending back from the mons pubis. These labia are thicker in front, gradually become thinner as they extend back, and appear to flatten out as they merge with the adjacent tissues in the area of the perineum. The labia majora have two surfaces. The outer surface is covered by a thin layer of skin containing hair follicles and sebaceous and sweat glands. The inner surfaces are smooth, lack hair, and are supplied with a large number of sebaceous follicles. The labia are homologous to the male scrotum.

The *labia minora* are two smaller folds of tissue that are parallel to the labia majora and are sometimes concealed between the folds of the labia majora. In sexually active women and in women who have borne children, the labia minora may project beyond the labia majora. The labia minora join near the prepuce, which covers the clitoris, extend backward to enclose the urethral and vaginal openings, and merge with the labia majora in the perineum. The labia minora are made up of connective and elastic tissue and contain little fatty tissue. Sweat glands and hair follicles are absent from the labia minora, but sebaceous glands are present. Abnormal sexual differentiation is possible with maldevelopment or fusion of the labia. Vulvovaginitis affects the labia minora.

The *clitoris* is situated near the anterior folds of the labia minora. The glans of the clitoris is a small, rounded area consisting of erectile tissue enclosed in a layer of fibrous membrane. Although it is often compared with or said to be homologous to the penis in males because it consists of the glans, corpus, and crura, the clitoris is unique in that its sole physiologic functions are initiation and elevation of sexual tension levels. The clitoris serves as both receptor and transformer of sexual stimuli. Sexual stimulation initiates a process whereby the clitoris becomes enlarged, erect, and very sensitive to sexual stimuli. Female orgasm can occur from stimulation of the clitoris but also results from stimulation of other sites; in fact, female orgasm has been documented in instances where the clitoris had been surgically removed. Inflammation of the lower genital tract or cancer may develop on the clitoris.

The *vestibule* is a boat-shaped fossa formed between the labia minora, clitoris, and fourchet. The *fossa navicularis* is a small depression between the fourchet and hymen. On opening the labia minora, the vaginal and urethral orifice can be visualized. These surfaces are thin, easily irritated, and especially subject to laceration during childbirth.

The *hymen* is an irregular membranous fold of connective tissue of varying thickness that partially covers the vaginal orifice. The hymen may be avulsed (broken) by coitus, digital examination, vigorous exercise, or surgery. Absence of the hymen does not denote lack of virginity. Remnants of the hymen usually persist after avulsion and form an irregular border around the vaginal opening.

The location of *Skene's* (paraurethral) glands and *Bartholin's* (vulvovaginal) glands should be noted, because they are common sites of infection. Skene's glands are located on each side of the urethral meatus. Bartholin's glands are situated at each side of the vaginal opening near the bases of the labia. Since both Skene's glands and Bartholin's glands are very small, their openings are just visible. They may not be palpable unless the woman is very thin or unless the glands are enlarged because of infection.

The *perineum* is the area between the vagina and anus. It is composed of muscles and subdermal and dermal tissue.

The appearance of the vulvar structures varies with age. Before puberty, the external genitalia are characterized by absence of pubic hair, and the labia minora are more prominent than the labia majora. With deposit of body fat and hormone effects during puberty, the labia majora increase in thickness and pubic hair appears. With the onset of the menopause and gradual withdrawal of hormones, the external genitalia again become less prominent and the pubic hair begins to thin. In elderly women, the vulva may appear wrinkled, shrunken, and almost flat. During the life span, congenital defects, childbirth, infection or other diseases, and surgery may alter the structure and appearance of the external genitalia.

Internal organs

The female internal reproductive organs are shown in Fig. 63-3. In relation to the skeletal system, the internal reproductive organs are located in the true pelvis. Unless their size is increased by a disease process or by pregnancy, the internal organs of reproduction remain within the cavity of the true pelvis. An exception is noted during sexual response when the uterus elevates into the false pelvis.

Vagina. The vaginal orifice serves as the boundary between the external structures and the internal organs. The vagina is a musculofascial tube that connects the vulva with the cervix and uterus. The functions of the vagina are to receive the penis during intercourse, allow for childbirth, and permit discharge of the menstrual flow. The vagina is located between the rectum and urethra and is a soft, tubular structure that extends upward and back from the vaginal opening.

The length of the vaginal canal varies, and the pos-

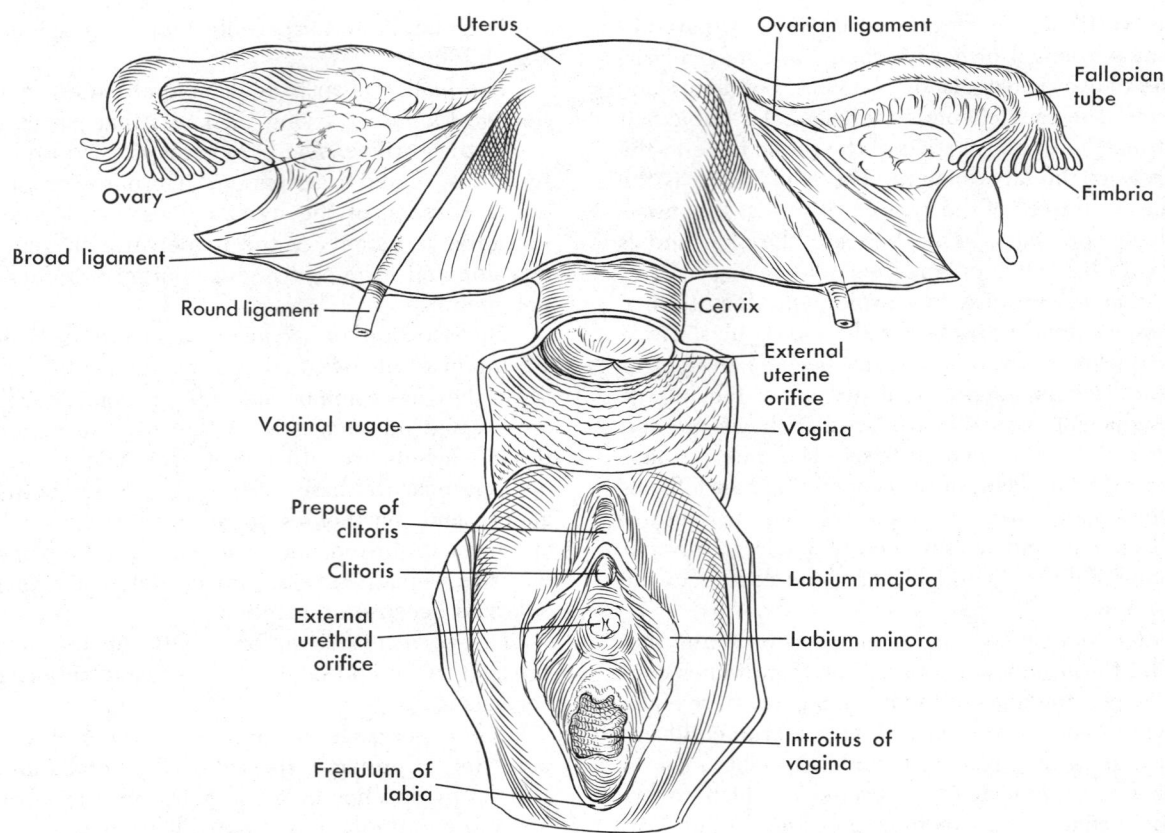

Fig. 63-3. Female internal organs of reproduction. Major ligaments are shown.

terior wall is longer than the anterior wall. The anterior wall averages 6 to 8 cm in length, while the posterior wall averages 8 to 9 cm.

The vagina is lined with pink mucous membrane arranged in folds called *rugae*. Physiologic events (e.g., pregnancy) and pathologic conditions (e.g., infections) often alter the color of the vaginal mucosa because of congestion with blood. The rugae make it possible for the vagina to distend and to stretch during coitus and childbirth. The rugated appearance of the vaginal canal is prominent during adolescence and tends to disappear with multiparity.

The vaginal walls end in a blind pouch *around* the cervix. Note that the vaginal epithelium is continuous with the epithelium of the cervix and that the cervix projects into the upper vagina. The groove formed by the termination of the vagina around the cervix is called the *vaginal vault*.

A cup-shaped *fornix* is formed by the protrusion of the cervix into the superior portion of the vagina. The fornix is divided into anterior, posterior, and lateral fornices.

The vagina is lubricated by secretions from its own cells and by secretions from the cervix and Bartholin's glands. The combined vaginal secretions are normally

acid during the years of ovarian function. The presence of Döderlein bacilli and estrogen influences the acidity of the vagina. When adequate estrogen stimulation is present, the cells of the vagina and cervix contain glycogen. Lactic acid is produced by breakdown of glycogen, and the degree of glycogen breakdown is related to acidity of the vagina. Before puberty, the vaginal pH tends to be neutral. With the onset of puberty, the vaginal pH varies between 4.0 and 5.0, depending on the phase of the menstrual cycle and the level of estrogen. The pH is lowest at the time of ovulation and just before menstruation. During pregnancy, a pH of 4.0 or less is common. Neutral or alkaline values are normally found in postmenopausal women. The importance of vaginal acidity is demonstrated by the fact that most pathogenic bacteria produce signs of vaginal infection when the pH falls below 4.0 or rises above 5.0.

Until puberty, the vaginal epithelium is thin. The epithelium thickens at the time of puberty, and this state persists through the reproductive years until the menopause, when the epithelium again becomes thin. The thickness of the vaginal epithelium is closely related to estrogen levels.

The natural barriers to infection (thickness of the vaginal epithelium and acidity of the vagina) are minimal before puberty and after menopause, predisposing females in these age groups to vaginal infections and trauma of the vaginal mucosa.

Uterus. The uterus is a hollow, muscular organ located between the urinary bladder and rectum. It consists of two portions—the corpus (body) and the cervix. The body is composed of the fundus, which is the thick muscular region above insertion of the fallopian tubes; the body, which is the main portion of the uterus; and the isthmus, which is the lower region. The cervix is located between the isthmus and the vagina. The size of the uterus decreases from the fundus to the cervix, giving the contour of the uterus a triangular, pear-shaped appearance. The size of the uterus varies among women, ranging from 5.5 to 9 cm long, 3.5 to 6 cm wide, and 2 to 4 cm thick in nonparous women. All dimensions may be 2 to 3 cm larger in multiparas.

The position, shape, and size of the uterus vary at different periods of life and under different circumstances. Minor developmental abnormalities, probably the result of embryonic error, are relatively common. During infancy, the uterus is an abdominal organ, and the cervix is larger than the corpus. By puberty, the uterus has increased in size and has descended into the pelvic cavity. In women, the position of the uterus is subject to considerable variation (see Fig. 65-2). The uterus is usually anteverted and slightly anteflexed, although it may be retroverted, retroflexed, or in midposition. During pregnancy, the uterus changes remarkably in size, shape, structure, and position and returns to its prepregnancy state within 6 to 8 weeks following delivery. During menopause, the uterus begins to hypertrophy and decreases in size.

The body of the uterus is normally bent forward over the bladder so that the fundus is behind the symphysis pubis. The uterus is in direct contact with the bladder and may also touch the rectum, sigmoid colon, and small intestines.

The cervix curves forward. The relationship between the corpus and the cervix produces an angle of about 90 degrees. The angle is decreased as the urinary bladder fills and elevates the corpus.

The outer surfaces of the uterus are covered by peritoneum, which is reflected from the abdominal wall. The anterior and posterior reflections of the peritoneum join at the sides to enclose the fallopian tubes and ovaries. Reflection of the peritoneum over the top of the pelvic organs creates spaces between the uterus and bladder anteriorly and the uterus and rectum posteriorly. the posterior space is known as the cul-de-sac of Douglas and is clinically important in that the peritoneal cavity can be entered through the posterior vaginal wall with little risk of damaging adjacent organs or structures. The cul-de-sac of Douglas is a common entry site for culdoscopy, culpotomy, and surgical drainage of the peritoneal cavity.

The uterus has three functional layers—the parametrium, which is the peritoneal and fascial outer layer; the myometrium, which is the middle muscular layer; and the endometrium, which is the mucous membrane–type tissue. The endometrial lining is thickest before the beginning of menstruation and thinnest after menstruation. The cavity of the uterus is continuous with the cervical canal and has an average capacity of 3 to 8 ml. Near the fundus, the uterus opens into the lumen of the fallopian tubes. Thus there is a direct route from the vagina through the cervix, uterus, and fallopian tubes to the peritoneum. This is important in prevention of infection and its spread by continuity of tissue.

The cervix is firm, smooth, and round. It is primarily made up of elastic and fibrous connective tissue and smooth muscle. Its color is usually lighter pink than that of the vagina. The lower portion of the cervix protrudes into the vagina, and in the center of the vaginal portion of the cervix is the external os. Extending upward from the external os is the cervical canal, which averages 2 to 3 cm in length. The cervical canal terminates as it joins the corpus, and the junction of the cervical canal and the corpus is termed the internal cervical os. The functions of the cervix are to secrete mucus to facilitate transport of sperm, to dilate during labor, and to provide a channel for discharge of the menstrual flow. During the birth experience, cervical lacerations are almost inevitable.

Changes in the physical properties and in the pH of the cervical mucus are significant in the treatment of infertility and in fertility control (p. 1658). At the time of ovulation, the cervical mucus becomes thinner and more elastic. These changes enhance penetration of the cervical mucus by sperm. The viscosity of the cervical mucus can be determined by studies of mucous flow and elasticity. The term *spinnbarkeit* is applied to describe the characteristic ability of the cervical mucus to stretch and recoil.

Fallopian tubes. The fallopian tubes are two narrow, muscular canals ranging from 8 to 14 cm in length. They extend outward from the corpus near the fundus at the cornua and are enclosed in the folds of the broad ligaments. The tubes are divided into three portions: the isthmus is the proximal portion of the tube nearest the cornu; the ampulla is the longer, middle portion where fertilization usually occurs; and the farthest, distal portion of the tube is fimbriated.

The walls of the fallopian tubes contain smooth muscles possessing peristaltic properties. Mucous membrane containing cilia lines the fallopian tubes. At the time of ovulation, peristaltic action and ciliary action increase, and it is likely that these combined actions provide the mechanism for ovum transport.

The functions of the fallopian tubes are to serve as a site for union of the sperm and ovum and to transport the ovum to the uterus. Fertilization of the ovum occurs in the distal third of the fallopian tube. If a stricture of the fallopian tube exists in the proximal portion, the fertilized ovum may not be able to pass the point of obstruction and an ectopic (tubal) pregnancy may result.

Ovaries. The ovaries are endocrine glands as well as reproductive organs. There are normally two almond-shaped ovaries, ranging from 3 to 4 cm long, 2 cm wide, and 1 to 2 cm thick, each lying near the fimbriae of the fallopian tubes. They are partly enclosed by the broad ligaments. Each ovary contains an outer portion (cortex) and an inner portion (medulla). The term *adnexa* refers to the ovaries, fallopian tubes, and supporting tissues. The functions of the ovaries are to store primordial follicles; to produce mature ova; and to produce and secrete estrogen, progesterone, and androgens. Ovarian functions are readily disturbed by acute and chronic diseases. The functions can also be altered or interrupted by surgery, radiation, and the ingestion of drugs such as oral contraceptives.

The ovaries undergo histologic changes resulting from endocrine stimulation as well as physical changes in position, size, and shape during the life span. At birth, the ovaries are very small, round, smooth, and light pink and are located in the false pelvis. Between infancy and puberty the ovaries increase in size, become more flattened, assume a grayish color, and descend into the true pelvis. During the childbearing years, the ovaries appear long and flat, have a nodular surface caused by the presence of follicles, and lie close to the pelvic walls. During pregnancy, the ovaries are lifted out of the pelvis by the enlarging uterus, but they descend into the pelvis after childbirth. After menopause, the ovaries undergo rapid regressive changes. They decrease in size, their surfaces become wrinkled, and the color fades from gray to white. In most postmenopausal women, the ovaries are so small that they cannot be palpated during vaginal examination.

After puberty, the surfaces of the ovaries are covered by connective tissue fibers that form a layer called the *tunica albuginea*. Immediately below the connective tissue is the ovarian cortex containing a large number of minute vesicles, the primordial follicles. Each primordial follicle contains an undeveloped ovum having the capacity to respond to stimulation by pituitary hormones. It is estimated that each ovary contains 500,000 primordial follicles at the time of birth. Many of the primordial follicles disintegrate before puberty, and the process of disintegration continues throughout the childbearing years. Consequently, few if any primordial follicles are found in the ovaries after menopause.

Unlike sperm, which are produced constantly by males, only one ovum matures at a time, and the process of ovum maturation requires an average of 28 days. When the ovum reaches maturity, it leaves the ovary by the process of ovulation.

Male genital system

The male reproductive organs and associated structures are shown in Fig. 63-4. The male reproductive organs produce sperm, suspend the sperm in a liquid, and deliver the sperm into the vagina to fertilize an ovum. Another important function is secretion of male hormones, the androgens. The male genitalia include the testes, vas deferens, seminal vesicles, ejaculatory ducts, and penis, along with the prostate and bulbourethral glands, which are accessory structures.

Testes. The testes produce the sperm. During fetal life the testes are located in the abdominal cavity behind the peritoneum. Before birth, the testes descend through the inguinal canals and inguinal rings into the scrotum and are suspended in position by the spermatic cords. The testes are oval. The spermatic cords are attached to the posterior borders of the testes. At the lateral edge of each spermatic cord is the epididymis, which appears as a narrow, flattened structure.

The testes are composed of glandular tissue covered by fibrous tissue. The glandular tissue is composed of many lobules differing in size according to their location. The lobules consist of 600 to 1200 small convoluted structures, the seminiferous tubules. The seminiferous tubules produce the sperm, and spermatozoa in different stages of development can be seen along the cells of the tubules.

After puberty, the lining of the seminiferous tubules continually forms millions of sperm. Approximately 74 days are required for conversion of immature sperm to mature sperm. Each mature sperm has a whiplike tail making it possible for the sperm to move freely in the proper environment. Because of the environment of the testes, the sperm are passive. Some of the sperm are moved by peristaltic action in the epididymis and vas deferens to the prostate gland. The seminal vesicles and prostate gland produce most of the fluid in which the sperm can be suspended and made motile.

In addition to producing sperm, the testes function as an endocrine gland. The male hormone testosterone is produced by the interstitial cells of the testes and is responsible for development of the genitalia during puberty and for maintaining the genitalia in a functional state during life. Androgenic hormones are also responsible for the development of secondary sex characteristics including growth of body hair and thickening of the vocal cords.

Spermatic cords. The spermatic cords extend from the deep inguinal rings and consist of arteries, veins, lymphatics, nerves, and the excretory duct of the testes held together by the spermatic fascia. At the deep inguinal rings, the structures of the spermatic cords converge with the structures of the testes. The spermatic cords then pass through the inguinal canals, emerge through the superficial inguinal rings, and pass downward into the scrotum.

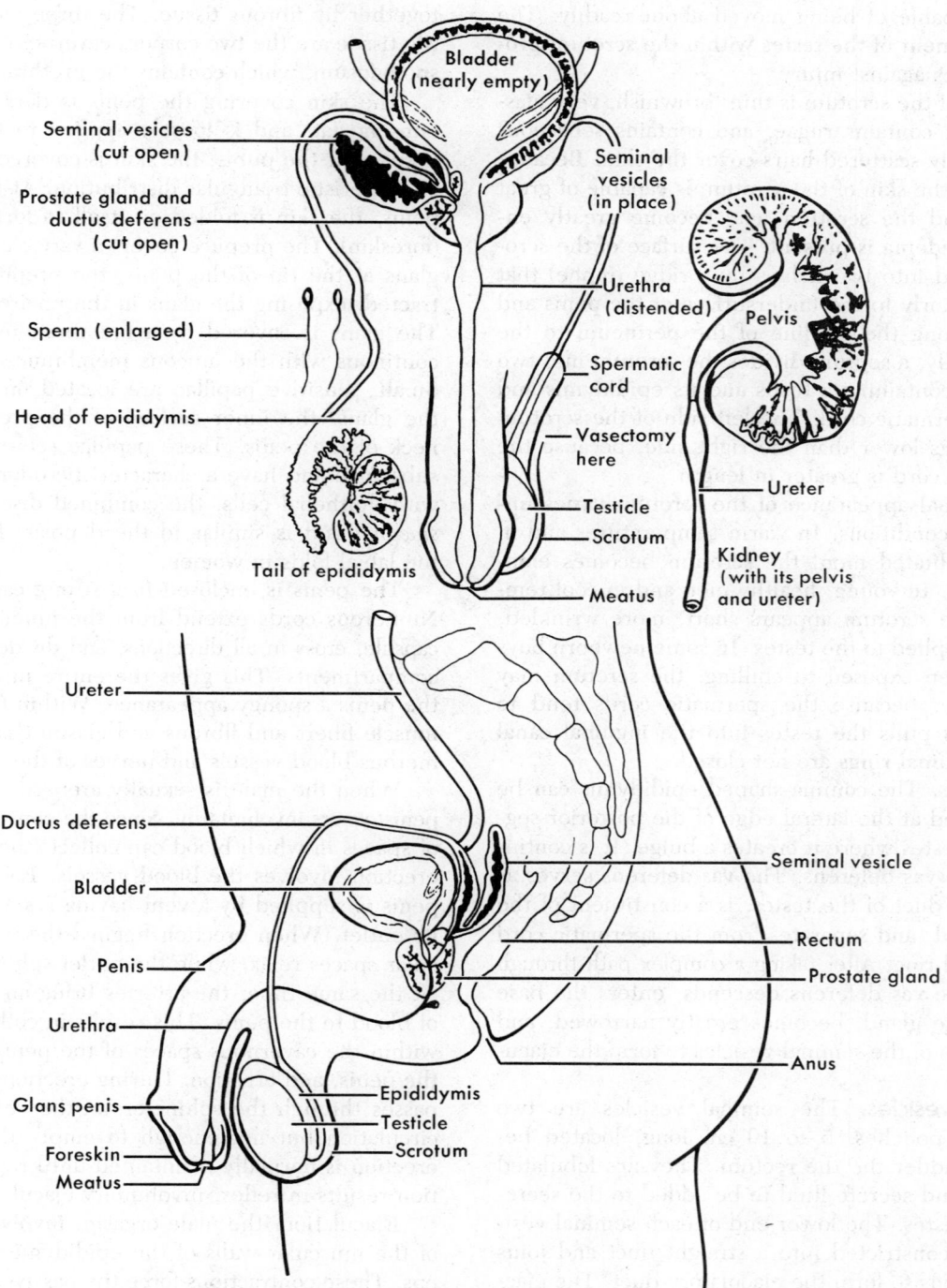

Fig. 63-4. Male organs of reproduction. Note relatively large size of seminal vesicle as compared with testicle.

Bladder (nearly empty)

Seminal vesicles (cut open)

Prostate gland and ductus deferens (cut open)

Sperm (enlarged)

Head of epididymis

Tail of epididymis

Seminal vesicles (in place)

Urethra (distended)

Pelvis

Spermatic cord

Vasectomy here

Testicle

Scrotum

Ureter

Meatus

Kidney (with its pelvis and ureter)

Ureter

Ductus deferens

Bladder

Penis

Urethra

Glans penis

Foreskin

Meatus

Seminal vesicle

Rectum

Prostate gland

Anus

Epididymis

Testicle

Scrotum

Scrotum. The scrotum is a cutaneous pouch that covers and protects the testes and spermatic cords. Because the testes are surrounded by serous membrane and are suspended in the cavity of the scrotum, the testes are capable of being moved about readily. The ease of movement of the testes within the scrotum protects the testes against injury.

The skin of the scrotum is thin, brownish, very elastic because it contains rugae, and contains sebaceous follicles. Thinly scattered hairs cover the skin. Because of the rugae, the skin of the scrotum is capable of great distention, and the scrotum may become greatly enlarged when edema is present. The surface of the scrotum is divided into two halves by a ridge (raphe) that extends anteriorly to the undersurface of the penis and posteriorly along the midline of the perineum to the anus. Internally, a septum divides the scrotum into two halves, each containing a testis and its epididymis and portion of spermatic cord. The left side of the scrotum normally hangs lower than the right side, because the left spermatic cord is greater in length.

The external appearance of the scrotum varies under different conditions. In warm temperatures and in older or debilitated men, the scrotum becomes elongated and flat. In young, healthy men and in cool temperatures, the scrotum appears short, more wrinkled, and closely applied to the testes. In some newborn boys who have been exposed to chilling, the scrotum may appear empty, because the spermatic cords tend to contract. This pulls the testes into the inguinal canal when the inguinal rings are not closed.

Epididymis. The comma-shaped epididymis can be visually located at the lateral edge of the posterior segment of the testes where it creates a bulge. It is continuous with the vas deferens. The vas deferens serves as the excretory duct of the testes, is a constituent of the spermatic cord, and separates from the spermatic cord at the inguinal ring. After taking a complex path through the pelvis, the vas deferens descends, enters the base of the prostate gland, becomes greatly narrowed, and joins the ducts of the seminal vesicles to form the ejaculatory duct.

Seminal vesicles. The seminal vesicles are two membranous pouches, 5 to 10 cm long, located between the bladder the the rectum. They are lobulated in structure and secrete fluid to be added to the secretions of the testes. The lower end of each seminal vesicle becomes constricted into a straight duct and joins the vas deferens to form the ejaculatory duct. The ejaculatory duct begins at the base of the prostate gland, runs posteriorly and downward, and enters the prostate gland in the midline. In the prostate gland, the ejaculatory duct opens into the prostatic portion of the urethra.

Penis. The penis is a conduit for elimination of ejaculate and urine through the urethral opening. It is attached to the front and sides of the pubic arch. When flaccid, the penis is cylindric in shape; when erect, it assumes a triangular shape with rounded angles. The penis consists of three masses of cavernous tissue held together by fibrous tissue. The three columns of erectile tissue are the two corpora cavernosa and the corpus spongiosum, which contains the urethra.

The skin covering the penis is dark in color, contains no fat, and is loosely applied to the underlying tissues. At the pubis, the skin is covered with hair in a characteristic triangular distribution. At the neck of the penis, the skin is folded on itself to form the prepuce (foreskin). The prepuce covers a variable amount of the glans at the tip of the penis; the prepuce may be retracted, exposing the glans in the uncircumcized male. The glans is covered by a membranous tissue that is continous with the mucous membrane of the urethra. Small, sensitive papillae are located on the surface of the glans, the inner surface of the prepuce, and the neck of the penis. These papillae secrete a sebaceous substance and have a characteristic odor. When mixed with epithelial cells, the combined discharge is called *smegma* and is similar to the deposits found between the labial folds in women.

The penis is enclosed in a strong capsule of fascia. Numerous cords extend from the inner surface of the capsule, cross in all directions, and divide the penis into compartments. This gives the entire inner structure of the penis a spongy appearance. Within the structure of muscle fibers and fibrous and elastic tissue are the numerous blood vessels and nerves of the penis.

When the male is sexually aroused, erection of the penis occurs involuntarily. Since the penis consists largely of spaces in which blood can collect, the mechanism of erection involves the blood vessels. Each space in the penis is supplied by a vein having a small sphincter at its outlet. When erection begins, the walls of the vascular spaces relax, while the outlet sphincters contract. At the same time, the arteries bring an increased flow of blood to the penis. This results in collection of blood within the cavernous spaces of the penis, hardening of the penis, and erection. During erection, enough blood passes through the sphincters of the veins to maintain circulation but not enough to empty the spaces. The erection is normally maintained until repeated stimulation results in reflex, involuntary ejaculation.

Ejaculation, the male orgasm, involves contractions of the muscular walls of the epididymis and vas deferens. These contractions force the passive sperm upward to the prostate gland. The seminal vesicles, which also have muscular walls, contract and force their contents into the urethra with the sperm. The fluid secreted by the seminal vesicles makes up most of the volume of the ejaculate. In the seminal fluid, the sperm become motile and begin to move about actively. As the seminal fluid moves into the prostatic portion of the urethra, the urethral walls begin peristaltic movement. The semen is thus forced down the urethra and through the urinary meatus in short series of spurts, called ejaculation. Shortly following ejaculation, erection of the penis begins to subside. The vascular spaces relax, causing the blood to flow freely from the spaces within the penis. The walls of the vascular spaces contract as they empty of blood, and the body of the penis returns to its flaccid state.

Prostate gland. The prostate gland is located below the internal urethral orifice, behind the symphysis pubis, and close to the rectal wall. It is so situated that it extends around the beginning of the urethra. The prostate gland averages 4 cm in width at its base, 3 cm from top to bottom, 2 cm from front to back, and 20 g in weight.

The prostate gland, which grows to the size and shape of a walnut during puberty, is enveloped in a firm, adherent capsule. Internally, the prostate gland is partly muscular and partly glandular. The glandular substance of the prostate gland consists of numerous follicular pouches that open into long canals. These canals join to form 12 to 20 small excretory ducts. The prostatic ducts open into the prostatic portion of the urethra, thus adding the prostatic secretion to the seminal fluid.

Clinically, the prostate gland is important because of its affinity for congestive, inflammatory, hyperplastic, and malignant diseases. Since the prostate gland is close to the rectal wall, it is easily palpable by rectal examination, and this makes diagnosis of problems at an early stage possible. Because of the anatomic relationship of the prostate gland to the urethra, most prostatic diseases present urinary tract symptoms.

Cowper's glands. Cowper's (bulbourethral) glands are two small, round bodies located at the sides and to the back of the membranous portion of the urethra. They are enclosed by the transverse fibers of the sphincter muscles of the urethra. Each gland has an excretory duct that opens into the urethra. The main excretory duct of a Cowper gland represents the joining of many ducts from the internal glandular tissue substance. Cowper's glands secrete an alkaline substance into the semen to counteract vaginal and urethral acidity.

Pelvic ligaments and muscles

The internal and external reproductive structures are maintained in their positions by groups of ligaments and muscles (Fig. 63-3). In the female, the broad ligaments (consisting of peritoneum) extend from the surfaces of the uterus to the sides of the pelvis and support the uterus in a horizontal position. The free margins of the broad ligament enclose and support the fallopian tubes and ovaries. The ovaries are suspended from the broad ligament by the ovarian ligaments.

The round ligaments extend laterally from the an-

terior surface of the uterine fundus. They pass through the abdominal wall, inguinal canals, and inguinal rings and terminate by dissemination of their fibers in the labia majora and surrounding tissues, holding the corpus forward over the urinary bladder. These ligaments are capable of stretching to allow for increase in size and alteration of position of the uterus during pregnancy. They appear to keep the uterus in an anteverted position.

The uterosacral ligaments originate from the posterior surface of the uterus at the level of the internal os. They arch posteriorly and are inserted into the sacrum at the level of the second and third sacral vertebrae. Because the uterosacral ligaments exert backward tension on the cervix, they maintain the cervix and vagina at right angles to each other. The uterosacral ligaments thus prevent prolapse of the uterus by preventing the corpus from taking a position in line with the vagina. It is likely that uterosacral ligaments contain sensory nerve fibers, which may contribute to dysmenorrhea.

The cardinal ligaments arise from the base of the broad ligaments. They integrate with the uterosacral ligaments and with the pelvic fascia and fan outward around the base of the uterus. The cardinal ligaments provide the chief support for the cervix and upper vagina, preventing descent of these structures.

The pubocervical ligaments extend from the posterior surface of the pubis to the anterolateral portion of the cervix. They provide some support to the bladder and cervix.

The muscles that actively and passively support the pelvic floor are shown in Fig. 63-5. The pelvic diaphragm consists of the levator ani and coccygeus muscles together with the pelvic fascia and stretches across the bottom of the pelvic cavity. The anal cavity, the urethra, and in females the vagina, pierce the pelvic diaphragm. The levator ani muscles contain striated muscle fibers that enable the vaginal and anal openings to be closed voluntarily. The pubococcygeus muscle (part of the levator ani muscle) is especially important to women in sexual functioning, in relaxation of the perineum, in expulsion of the fetus in birthing, and for bladder control.

The muscles of the perineum, commonly called the perineal body or perineal center, reinforce the support provided by the levator ani and coccygeus muscles. The perineal body consists of a mass of several muscles extending across the center of the pelvic outlet. It is located between the anus and bulb in males and between the anus and vagina in females. Together the pelvic diaphragm and perineum support the pelvic organs and external genitalia from below.

In females, the perineum is wider and thicker than it is in males. The muscles of the perineal body are the means of approach to the bladder and prostate gland in

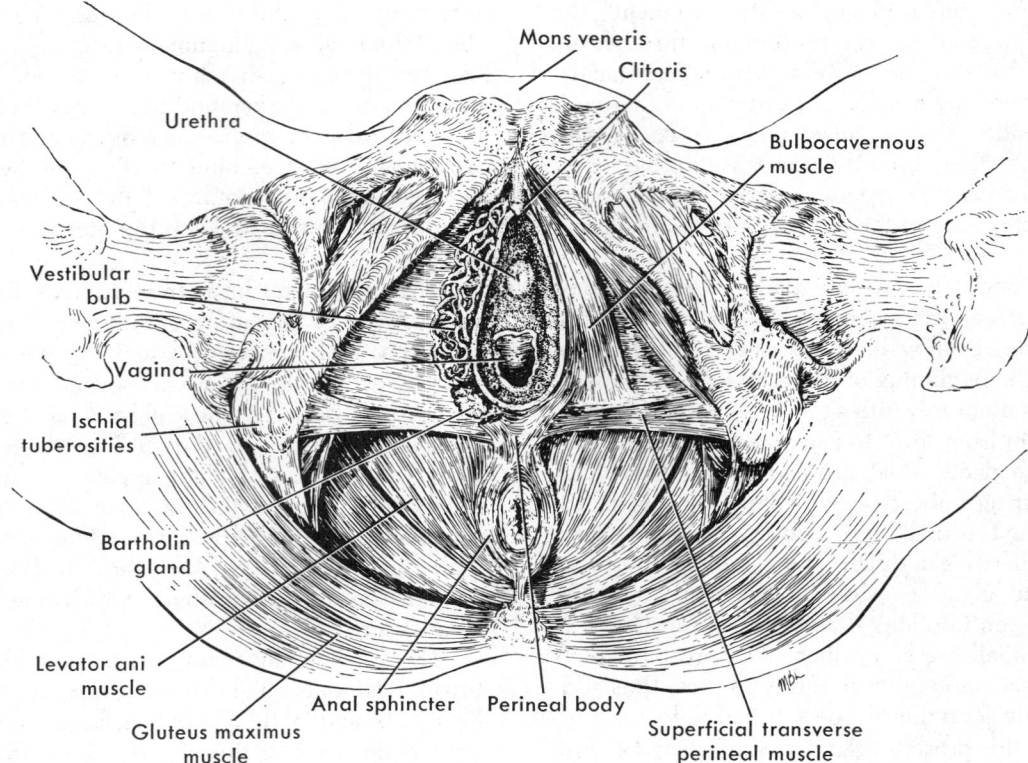

Fig. 63-5. Female pelvic floor in dissection from below. Coccygeus muscle is obscured by gluteus maximus muscle. (From Ingalls, A.J., and Salerno, C.: Maternal and child health nursing, ed. 4, St. Louis, 1979, The C.V. Mosby Co.)

males, and they are the site of perineal incisions and lacerations during childbirth.

Blood, lymph, and nerve supply

In males and females the organs of reproduction are supplied with blood from the aorta as it branches downward and divides into the internal iliac (hypogastric) artery.

The ovarian and uterine arteries anastomose to furnish the ovaries with blood. The venous drainage is similar to the arterial supply to the reproductive organs, with the blood vessels emptying into the vena cava.

In males, blood is similarly supplied to and drained from the reproductive organs. The pudendal branches of the aorta divide into the testicular arteries, and arteries supplying the seminal vesicles are derived from the inferior vesical and middle rectal arteries. Most of the blood to the penis is furnished through the internal pudendal artery. Venous return is similar to the arterial supply. Blood from the penis, testes, and prostate gland is returned to the internal iliac vein and then to the vena cava.

In both males and females, lymphatic drainage of the external and internal organs of reproduction is extensive. Both superficial and deep lymphatics empty into the external iliac, internal iliac, and preaortic lymph nodes. Nerve supply is derived from sympathetic and parasympathetic fibers of the autonomic nervous system and by spinal nerve pathways.

Endocrine functions

The major hormones produced by the ovaries are estrogen and progesterone. Estrogen is the hormone responsible for the development of secondary sex characteristics at the time of puberty. After puberty, the primary function of estrogen is to cause development of the endometrium in preparation for implantation of a fertilized ovum. Progesterone enhances the preceding action of estrogen on the endometrium.

Like production of a mature ovum, secretion of ovarian hormones occurs in a cyclic fashion, with each cycle requiring an average of 28 days. Unless stimulated by pituitary hormones, however, the ovaries do not fulfill their hormone-secreting and ovum-producing functions.

The menstrual cycle is divided into phases accord-

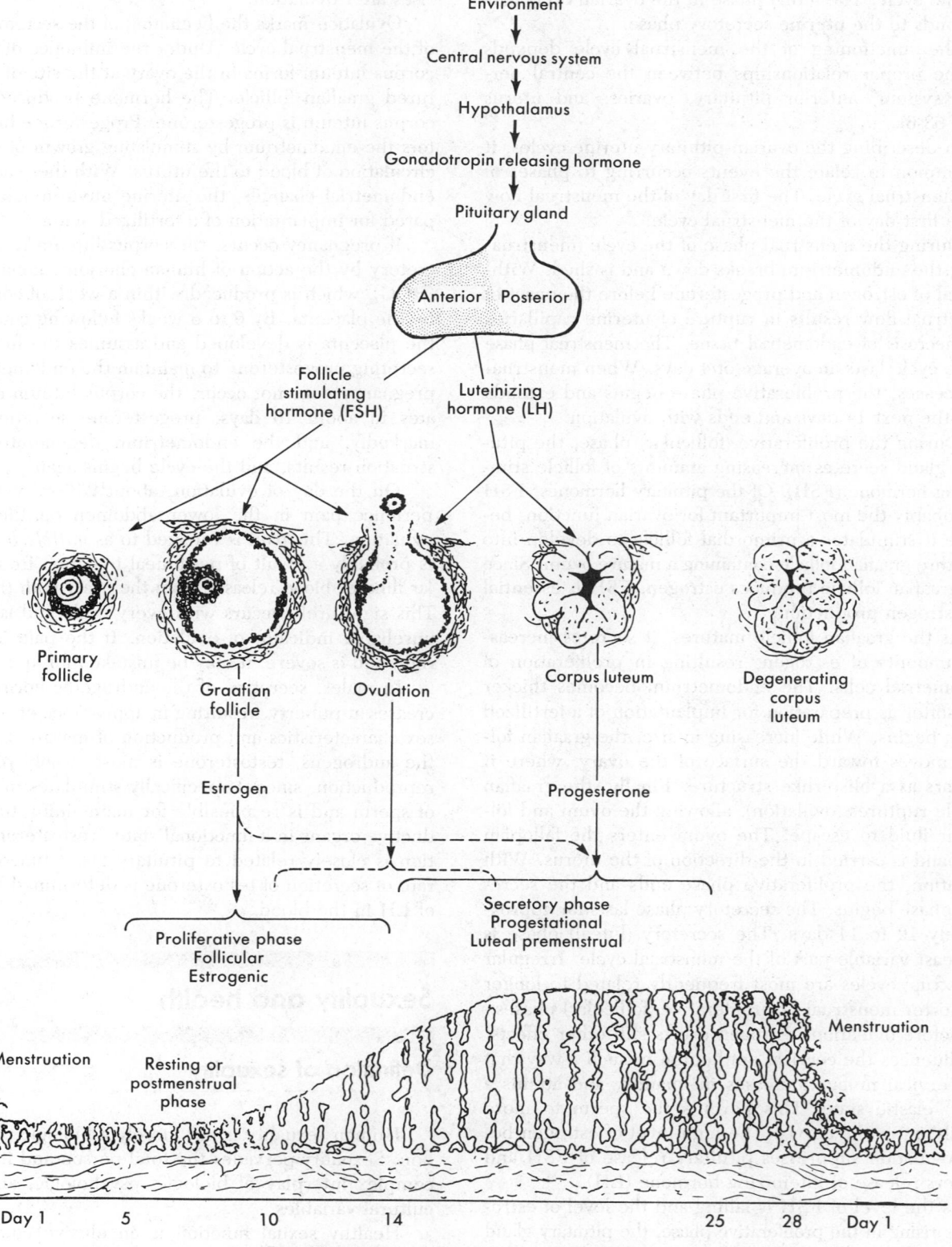

Fig. 63-6. Hormone control of menstrual cycle.

ing to uterine or ovarian changes. The uterine cycle consists of the menstrual, proliferative, and secretory phases. The follicular phase in the ovarian cycle corresponds to the menstrual and proliferative phases of the uterine cycle. The luteal phase in the ovarian cycle corresponds to the uterine secretory phase.

The functioning of the menstrual cycle depends on the proper relationships between the central nervous system, anterior pituitary, ovaries, and uterus (Fig. 63-6).

In describing the ovarian-pituitary-uterine cycles, it is common to relate the events occurring to phases of the menstrual cycle. The first day of the menstrual flow is the first day of the menstrual cycle.

During the menstrual phase of the cycle (menstruation), the endometrium breaks down and is shed. Withdrawal of estrogen and progesterone before the onset of menstrual flow results in rupture of uterine capillaries and necrosis of endometrial tissue. The menstrual phase of the cycle lasts an average of 4 days. When menstruation ceases, the proliferative phase begins and extends over the next 14 days and ends with ovulation.

During the proliferative (follicular) phase, the pituitary gland secretes increasing amounts of follicle stimulating hormone (FSH). Of the pituitary hormones, FSH is probably the most important for ovarian function, because it stimulates a primordial follicle to develop into a mature graafian follicle containing a mature ovum. Since the graafian follicle produces estrogen, FSH is essential for estrogen production.

As the graafian follicle matures, it secretes increasing amounts of estrogen, resulting in proliferation of endometrial cells. The endometrium becomes thicker and softer as preparation for implantation of a fertilized ovum begins. While increasing in size, the graafian follicle moves toward the surface of the ovary, where it appears as a blisterlike structure. Finally, the graafian follicle ruptures (ovulation), allowing the ovum and follicular fluid to escape. The ovum enters the fallopian tube and is carried in the direction of the uterus. With ovulation, the proliferative phase ends and the secretory phase begins. The secretory phase lasts for approximately 10 to 14 days. The secretory (luteal) phase is the least variable part of the menstrual cycle. Irregular menstrual cycles are most frequently related to longer or shorter menstrual or proliferative (follicular) phases.

Before ovulation, estrogen exerts still other effects. It influences the cervical epithelium in such a way that the cervical mucus increases in quantity and attains a clear, elastic state. This permits the sperm to more readily enter the cervix. The high level of estrogen before ovulation suppresses pituitary release of FSH and triggers release of luteinizing hormone (LH).

As the level of FSH is falling and the level of estrogen is rising in the proliferative phase, the pituitary gland secretes increasing amounts of LH. There is a sharp rise in LH levels 12 to 24 hours before ovulation, followed by a peak level about 8 hours after ovulation. This change in hormone levels is reflected in the basal body temperature, which drops just before ovulation and rises after ovulation.

Ovulation marks the beginning of the secretory phase of the menstrual cycle. Under the influence of LH, the corpus luteum forms in the ovary at the site of the ruptured graafian follicle. The hormone produced by the corpus luteum is progesterone. Progesterone further alters the endometrium by stimulating growth of cells and circulation of blood to the uterus. With these additional endometrial changes, the uterine environment is prepared for implantation of a fertilized ovum.

If pregnancy occurs, the corpus luteum remains secretory by the action of human chorionic gonadotropin (HCG), which is produced within a week of conception by the placenta. By 6 to 8 weeks following conception, the placenta is developed and assumes the function of secreting progesterone to maintain the endometrium. If pregnancy does not occur, the corpus luteum degenerates in about 10 days, progesterone secretion drops markedly, and the endometrium degenerates; menstruation results, and the cycle begins again.

On the day of ovulation, about 25% of women experience pain in the lower abdomen on the side of ovulation. This pain is referred to as *mittelschmerz* and is probably a result of peritoneal irritation from follicular fluid or blood released from the ovary with the ovum. This sign rarely occurs with every cycle and is thus an unreliable indicator of ovulation. If the pain is on the right and is severe, it may be mistaken for appendicitis.

In males, secretion of the androgenic hormones increases at puberty, resulting in appearance of secondary sex characteristics and production of mature sperm. Of the androgens, testosterone is most closely related to reproduction, since it specifically stimulates maturation of sperm and is responsible for maintaining the reproductive organs in a functional state. Testosterone secretion is closely related to pituitary gland function. The rate of secretion of testosterone is determined by levels of LH in the blood.

Sexuality and health

Definition of sexuality

Human sexuality is not merely a biologic phenomenon. Sexuality pervades the total person and involves a complex interplay of biologic, psychologic, and sociocultural variables.

Healthy sexual function is an elusive concept, its definition involving a person's unique combination of feelings, attitudes, and values that shape what is "healthy" at a given moment and in specific social situations. The World Health Organization's "Report on Education and Treatment in Human Sexuality" asserts that: "Sexual health is the integration of the somatic, emotional, intellectual, and social aspects of sexual being, in ways that are positively enriching and that enhance personality, communication, and love."[20]

As with many definitions of health, sexual health is not restricted to a discrete state, but it encompasses a range of behaviors, functions, and experiences. One way of thinking about sexual health involves a consideration of the possible mechanisms by which altered health states can influence sexuality, including *sexual function, sexual self-concept, and sexual relationships*. Sexual function implies the person's capacity to engage in and to experience pleasure from sexual activity. Although emphasis is frequently placed on ability to experience orgasm or to pleasure a partner, sexual function includes a wide variety of behaviors that make up the unique repertoire of that individual. Sexual self-concept pertains to the image we have of ourselves as men or women. It is evident in our feelings of adequacy, our masculinity, and our femininity. It is influenced by our body image, which is the mental image we have of our physical selves. Sexual relationships are those interpersonal relationships with others in which sexual activity is shared. This may include, but is not restricted to, marriage or long-term relationships.

Sexual origins

We are sexual beings from the moment we are conceived. This event establishes chromosomal sex and is the first of a series of developmental influences on our sexuality. The paternal sperm contributes either an X or a Y chromosome, which combines with the maternal X chromosome; this results in the XX (female) or XY (male) combination. (There are, however, disorders in which some other combinations occur).[50] Indeed, the X or Y chromosome from the paternal sperm sets in motion a process analogous to a relay race; that is, each component has control of the process for a time, eventually yielding control to another.[50]

After fertilization, there are two other critical points in the evolution of gender identity. The first is the induction of development of internal and external genitalia, and the second is the process by which the hypothalamus takes on a male or female pattern. At about 5 to 6 weeks of fetal life, the XX or XY chromosomal combination determines whether the undifferentiated fetal gonads will develop as ovaries or testes. Further differentiation occurs in response to the secretion of fetal androgen in the male fetus. If androgens are not present at critical periods and in appropriate amounts,

male structures will not develop from the wolffian ducts; thus it is possible for a fetus with XY chromosomes to develop female genitalia. It is also believed that a müllerian-inhibiting substance is necessary in males to prevent development of the female (müllerian) duct system. Lack of müllerian-inhibiting substance is thought to be responsible for some males being born with both male and female internal genitalia (e.g., ovaries, tubes, and uterus). In the absence of fetal gonadal hormones, female reproductive structures will begin to develop from the müllerian ducts, regardless of the chromosomal sex of the fetus. By the twelfth week of fetal life, biologic sex is well established. Although there does not appear to be a hormone necessary for induction of the ovarian function in female fetuses, estrogen is necessary for full development of female genitalia.[50]

Another critical stage probably occurs just before or soon after birth, at which time another set of sexual controls is introduced. Testosterone is thought to influence the hypothalamus in such a way that the male hypothalamus develops a male acyclic pattern for the release of pituitary gonadotropins. In the female, a cyclic pattern of gonadotropin release is established. Although the infant is born with an established biologic sex (gender), gender identity and gender role are yet to be established. Gender identity is the feeling that one is male, female, or ambivalent. Typically, the child is deemed male or female by the parents or other caretakers shortly after birth, and their subsequent behavior confirms and reinforces the child's sense of maleness or femaleness. Gender identity is probably solidified in children by the time they are 3 years of age.[50] Gender role is the outward expression of one's gender and is learned early in life. The distinctions between appropriate masculine and feminine behavior vary with the culture. In Western cultures, these distinctions are becoming less clear. Recently, Western societies have begun to appreciate the optimal characteristics of both sexes. Indeed, being androgynous (possessing characteristics once associated with both women and men) is now nearly synonymous with mentally healthy sex-role behavior.[9] If the processes described above proceed without interference, the person's biologic sex (female or male) will be congruent with gender identity (person sees herself or himself as a woman or a man) and gender role (outward manifestations of masculinity or femininity). (Consequences of lack of congruence between sex, gender identity, and gender role are explored briefly in Chapter 67.)

This complex set of biologic and psychosocial variables set in motion by the event of conception has a pervasive influence on the remainder of our lives. The biologic component of sexuality, sexual function or expression, constantly interacts with the psychological components of gender identity, cognition, and affect as well as with social factors such as sanctioned roles and mores and folkways regulating sexual expression. Such complexity mandates a holistic approach to conceptualizing clients' sexual problems and concerns.

Human sexual response

Throughout life, various components of biologic sexual function develop and change. Many of the basic sexual functions are evident in infants and children (e.g., the ability to have erections and orgasms) and persist well into the last decades of life. Human sexual response represents an opportunity for the integration of biologic sexuality with our thoughts, feelings, and interpersonal relationships.

Masters and Johnson,[71] pioneers in the scientific study of the physiologic aspects of sexual behavior, demonstrated that sexual response is a cyclic phenomenon consisting of four phases. The *excitement phase*, the initial component of the cycle, develops from sexually arousing stimuli such as touch; an increase in sexual tension is observed during this phase. Next, a consolidation period, the *plateau phase*, occurs, during which sexual tension becomes intensified. The involuntary climax of sexual tension, *orgasm*, follows and involves only a small portion of the sexual response cycle. During this period, changes attributable to muscular tension and congestion of blood vessels reach a peak and begin to dissipate. During the *resolution phase*, an involutionary period, the changes involving the blood vessels, sexual organs, and muscular tension are reversed. Women may at this time begin another sexual response cycle immediately; men must observe an obligatory period during which they cannot be restimulated to higher levels of sexual tension.

The physiologic changes seen during human sexual response depend on two main principles: myotonia and vasocongestion. The congestion of pelvic blood vessels and involuntary muscular contractions in the pelvic organs and other parts of the body are responsible for orgasmic experience. It should also be noted that sexual response is a total body response. The phase-specific descriptions of the sexual response cycle that follow illustrate the widespread involvement in this phenomenon.

Excitement

The hallmark of sexual arousal in the woman is vaginal lubrication. Believed to result from transudation of a mucoidlike substance across the vaginal mucosa, lubrication appears within seconds of sexual stimulation. The vaginal barrel becomes longer and wider as the uterus begins to elevate in the pelvis. Vasocongestive changes are also seen in the external genitalia: the clitoris becomes longer and wider, and the labia minora flatten and separate from the vaginal opening. As the labia minora become vasocongested, they actually extend outward, lengthening the vaginal barrel. The man's penis rapidly becomes erect, tensing of the scrotal sac is noted, and the testes begin to rise toward the perineum.

Extragenital changes are also seen with sexual excitement: the woman's nipples become erect, the areolae become engorged, venous patterns in the breast become more evident, and breast size actually increases. The sex flush, which looks like a red, maculopapular rash, appears over the chest in some persons. The man's nipples may also become erect. An increase in both the heart rate and blood pressure is evident, paralleling the level of sexual excitement.[71]

Plateau

During the plateau phase, the clitoris retracts upward beneath the clitoral hood. Clitoral stimulation may still occur indirectly as the penis exerts traction on the labia while moving in and out of the vagina. The orgasmic platform, the extremely vascular tissue at the outer portion of the vagina and the labia minora, becomes increasingly congested. The uterus continues to elevate in the pelvis, which creates a tenting effect in the innermost portion of the vagina. Externally, the labia majora become more congested, and the labia minora deepen in color as a result of vasocongestion. A few drops of mucoidlike material are secreted from Bartholin's glands, probably to assist with the lubrication of the outermost portion of the vagina. The diameter of the penis continues to increase, especially at the coronal ridge, and the testes increase in size to 50% over their unstimulated state as they elevate closer to the perineum. A few drops of mucoid material are secreted from Cowper's glands.

The woman's areolae are now so engorged that it is difficult to see the erect nipple. The sex flush continues to spread, sometimes involving the neck, face, and arms. Hyperventilation occurs in both sexes, along with heart rates of 100 to 175 beats/min. There is elevation of systolic blood pressure (20 to 60 mm Hg for women, 20 to 80 mm Hg for men) and diastolic blood pressure (10 to 20 mm Hg for women, 10 to 40 mm Hg for men).

Orgasm

Orgasm involves the climactic release of sexual tension and is evident in contractions throughout the body. The woman's orgasmic platform contracts rapidly, and expulsive contractions along the entire male urethra propel semen from the vas out through the penis. During orgasm, the internal bladder sphincter in men contracts, thus preventing semen from being propelled backward into the bladder. Uterine contractions are also noted in women with orgasm, much like those characteristic of labor. The rectal sphincter also contracts rapidly in both men and women during orgasm.

Resolution

During this phase, vasocongestion is gradually lost from the clitoris and breasts but rapidly lost from the orgasmic platform. The clitoris quickly returns to its usual position from under the clitoral hood. Vasocongestion of the labia dissipates, nipple erection recedes, and the uterus descends to its usual position in the pelvis. Cardiovascular and respiratory rates quickly return to normal. In the man, there is initially a rapid loss of erection to 1 to 1.5 times the size of the penis in its unstimulated state. Later there is a slower resolution of vasocongestion until the penis returns to prestimulation size. The scrotum and testes lose their vasocongestive changes, and the testes rapidly descend into the scrotum. Occasionally, a thin film of perspiration may appear over the entire body.

Triphasic concept of human sexual response

Recently, Kaplan[33] has suggested a triphasic concept of human sexual response. She delineates three phases—desire, excitement, and orgasm—that are related components of sexual response but are governed by separate neurophysiologic systems. This notion has utility for understanding not only the physiology of sexual response, but also the consequences of pathophysiologic conditions, the etiology of sexual dysfunction, and appropriate therapies.

The *desire phase* refers to the experiences of sexual appetite or drive produced by the activation of a neural system in the brain. Sexual desire is experienced as sensations that move the person to seek sexual experiences. Although the precise neural circuitry involved in sexual desire is unknown, it is believed to involve the limbic system and the preoptic nuclei of the hypothalamus. It is likely that the sexual centers of the brain have either neural or chemical connections with the pleasure and pain centers of the brain. The pleasure centers are stimulated when we have sex, which accounts for the pleasurable quality of sexual behavior. On the other hand, the pain centers can inhibit the sexual system. Some persons suggest that the pleasure center is stimulated by release of endorphins in sexual behavior. If a sexual object or situation produces pain, then it will cease to evoke desire.

Testosterone is important in mediating sexual desire in both men and women. Luteinizing hormone also may be important in mediating sexual desire. Two neurotransmitters, serotonin (5HT) and dopamine, are also believed to be important in mediating sexual desire. Serotonin acts as an inhibitor, and dopamine acts as a stimulant to the sexual centers of the brain. Bonding to another person and love are powerful stimuli to sexual desire. There seem to be many stimuli capable of evoking sexual desire, such as sight, smell, and other sensory cues, and some of these are conditioned by the culture. Fear and pain, however, are potent inhibitors.

The connections between the sex center and other parts of the brain also make it possible for people to "turn off" sexual desire when other stimuli are more important or when it is not to the individual's advantage to pursue sexual activity. Hypoactive desire and inhibited sexual desire are common problems of the sexual desire phase.

The *excitement phase* of sexual response is similar to the excitement and plateau phases described by Masters and Johnson and is produced by reflex vasodilation of the genital blood vessels. Two centers in the spinal cord—S2 to S4 and T11 to L2—cause the arterioles to dilate. This vasodilation causes the genitalia to swell and changes their shape to adapt to their reproductive function. The vasocongestion is primarily a parasympathetically mediated response, and the intense sympathetic response such as that produced by fear and anxiety can instantly lead to loss of erection. It is believed that erection is governed by two spinal reflex centers. The thoracolumbar center (psychogenic) appears to respond more to psychic stimuli, whereas the sacral center is stimulated from tactile input to the genitalia. It is believed that the spinal reflex centers and the higher neural connections are analogous in men and women. *Disorders of the excitement phase* include difficulty in attaining or maintaining erection in men and difficulty with swelling and lubrication in women.

The *orgasm phase* of sexual response, which corresponds to orgasm as described by Masters and Johnson, is also a genital reflex governed by spinal neural centers, but it consists of reflex contractions of certain genital muscles. Sensory influences, which trigger orgasm, enter the cord in the pudendal nerve at the sacral level and the efferents are T11 to L2. *Disorders of the orgasm phase* include inadequate ejaculatory control (premature ejaculation) and retarded ejaculation in men and orgasmic dysfunction in women. Other disorders include painful intercourse and sexual phobias.

Subjective experience of sexual response

The persons in the sample studied by Masters and Johnson[71] were polled with regard to the subjective experience associated with orgasm. Three distinct stages of women's orgasmic experiences were found. The first stage of orgasm begins as a sensation of "stoppage" or "suspension." This instantaneous sensation is followed by an intense sensual awareness oriented to the clitoris. A loss of sensory acuity has been described during this period. Some women described a sense of bearing down occurring simultaneously with the clitoral-pelvic sensation. A feeling of receptive opening has also been expressed by parous women. This sensation has also been compared to sensations felt during the second stage of labor.

The second stage of the female orgasmic response is described as a feeling of warmth that pervades the pelvis and then spreads throughout the body. The third stage of subjective experience is a feeling of involuntary contraction of the vagina followed by a sensation of pelvic throbbing; however, the female experience is highly individual and varied.

The Singers[59] have recently described three types of orgasmic experience for women—the vulval, uterine, and blended organsms. The vulval orgasm involves involuntary contractions of the orgasmic platform, as described by Masters and Johnson. The uterine orgasm depends on deep stimulation of the cervix that displaces the uterus, thus stimulating the peritoneum; it is characterized by a gasping type of breathing, eventually culminating in an explosive type of exhalation. The blended orgasm combines features of both the vulval and uterine variety.

Men in Masters and Johnson's study reported two stages of the subjective orgasmic experience. The first stage is a feeling of ejaculatory inevitability that develops as seminal fluid collects in the prostatic urethra. Distention of the urethral bulb may also contribute to this sensation. The second stage of subjective experience involves two phases—the sensation of contractions of the urethral sphincter and the perception of the volume of seminal fluid as it is expelled through the penile urethra.

Variations in sexual expression

People experience sexual pleasure in a variety of ways. Usually one's culture influences both the forms of sexual expression deemed acceptable and one's value system about sexual behavior. Indeed, what is normal varies widely among cultures. Comfort[14] suggests that the health professional should not use his or her own concept of normal but rather should consider the meaning that a behavior has for any individual, whether it impoverishes or enriches the lives of that person and any others with whom the sexual relations are shared, and finally, whether the behavior is tolerable to the society.

Sexual pleasuring

Each culture provides for a variety of erotic behaviors, but nearly all are concerned with sexual modesty. Incest taboos are common to most societies, but the definition of incest varies among cultures. Each society has some form of legal system to regulate sexual behavior.

Ford and Beach[69] found that the approaches to sexual pleasuring were highly variable among and within cultures. Positions used for intercourse include the woman astride (on top), man astride, side-to-side, or squatting. Women are expected to initiate sexual activity in some cultures, but in other cultures only men are

expected to do so. The duration of sexual acts is also regulated by the culture. In some cultures, men are encouraged to ejaculate rapidly; whereas in others the man's ability to prolong intromission is valued. Forms of sexual stimulation are also highly variable. Although kissing is nearly ubiquitous, some cultures deem it unsanitary. Stimulation of the female breasts either manually or orally is common. Manipulation of the female genitalia by the male is a common prelude to intromission. Oral stimulation of the woman's genitalia (cunnilingus) is common to many cultures, and somewhat less common is oral stimulation of the male's genitalia (fellatio). Painful stimulation is sometimes used to enhance arousal. Although the circumstances surrounding coitus vary among cultures, usually privacy is important. Sexual frequency is also often governed by cultural norms; for example, intercourse may be prohibited during menses, lactation, pregnancy, and in some cultures before hunts or wars.

Although heterosexuality is the most prevalent form of sexual expression in the cultures that have been studied, it is rarely the only type of sexual behavior in which people engage.

Sexual behavior

There are many variations in sexual behavior. Heterosexuals choose partners of the opposite sex, while homosexuals seek partners of the same sex. Bisexuals enjoy both same- and opposite-sexed partners at various points in time. The pedophile experiences sexual arousal with a child, whereas those who practice "swinging sex" have sexual relations as a couple with another person or persons. Incest implies having sexual relations with a close relative. In zoophilia, the sexual object is an animal; in fetishism, it is an inanimate object; and in necrophilia, it is a dead body. Transvestites experience sexual pleasure by dressing in clothes of the opposite sex. Some persons experience sexual pleasure from watching others (voyeurism), exposing their genitalia (exhibitionism), inflicting pain (sadism), or receiving pain (masochism).

Homosexuality

The Institute for Sex Research recently conducted a study of 979 homosexual men and women and a comparison group of 477 heterosexuals from the San Francisco area. Through an extensive interview, these investigators determined that homosexuality involved more than just sexual practices. Homosexuals varied in the degree to which they were involved in homosexual and heterosexual experiences, ranging along a continuum from those with exclusively homosexual feelings and behaviors to those with more heterosexual than homosexual feelings and behaviors. They were predominantly covert about their homosexuality, although frequently their families were aware of their sexual preferences. Many common assumptions about homosexuality were not supported by this study. Homosexuals could not be typified as sexually hyperactive or hypoactive. The investigation made clear the uniqueness of homosexual life-styles and the differences in life-style for men and women. For example, cruising (purposefully searching for a partner) was common among men but less common among women. Men tended to have more partners than women, but both men and women preferred a relatively steady relationship with a lover.

The men and women in this study used a variety of sexual techniques. Men most frequently used fellatio, hand-genital contact, and anal intercourse; and women most frequently participated in masturbation and cunnilingus with their partners. Sexual problems were more commonly reported by men than by women and included difficulty meeting a partner and meeting the partner's sexual requests. Venereal disease was a common health problem for men, but this was not the case for women.

Bell and Weinberg[8] found that the homosexuals they interviewed were involved in a variety of relationships ranging from a quasimarriage to having multiple short-term contacts. Some were not involved in a relationship, had little sexual interest, and regretted their homosexuality.

When psychologic adjustment of the homosexual group was compared with that of the heterosexual group, it was apparent that the homosexuals who were in dysfunctional sexual relationships or situations and who were asexual were less well adjusted than heterosexuals. However, when the comparison was restricted to those who were functional (had little regret about homosexuality) or were in a coupled relationship, the homosexuals were no more distressed than the heterosexuals.

Masters and Johnson[44] recently compared the physiology of sexual response in homosexuals and heterosexuals in the laboratory setting. They found no significant difference in the homosexual and heterosexual subjects' facility for orgasm in response to masturbation, partner manipulation, fellatio, or cunnilingus nor were there demonstrable physiologic differences in the sexual response cycles of homosexuals and heterosexuals.

Aging and sexuality

It is commonly assumed that sexuality is not a concern for older people, and some consider that an aged person's interest in sex is perverse. Research on sexuality and aging disconfirms the sterotypes of the elderly as either disinterested in sex or abnormally obsessed with it. Instead, it appears that for many aging persons, sexuality is an important dimension of being alive. There is no single point in the life cycle at which sexual activity must cease, although there is a decline in reports on sexual interest and activity with increasing age. Even

so, investigators have demonstrated that both sexual interest and activity persist well into the seventh, eighth, and ninth decades of life.[53,70,73] One study estimated that 40% to 65% of those persons 60 to 71 years of age engaged in intercourse fairly frequently, while 10% to 20% of those over 78 years of age were sexually active. Indeed, 13% to 15% of the older persons in one study actually showed *increased* patterns of sexual activity interest with age.[73]

If one were to compare sexual response in young men and women with their middle-aged and older counterparts, there would be more similarities than differences. The processes essential for sexual response occur more slowly with age, and the phase-specific changes may appear somewhat less intense. Nevertheless, the capacity for sexual pleasure exists in many aging persons.

As women age, there is a gradual change in their genitalia and breasts paralleling the change in estrogen levels associated with menopause. There is often a delay in the production of vaginal lubrication, although this appears to be much less a problem for women who have been consistently sexually active throughout their lives. As women age, the vagina becomes smaller in both length and diameter.

As women age, there is less marked elevation and tenting of the uterus during sexual excitement and less evidence of vasocongestive changes in the labia and breasts. Vasocongestion of the orgasmic platform is less apparent; and during orgasm, the frequency of contraction of the orgasmic platform is less than that for younger women. Indeed, some women report uncomfortable uterine contractions during orgasm. The resolution of sexual tension proceeds more slowly than in younger women.[71]

Age-related changes in sexual response in men parallel those changes in women. The time period necessary to experience an erection increases, and the erection is likely to be less full than earlier in life. There is usually less profound evidence of vasocongestion in the scrotum and testes. Because the plateau phase of the sexual response cycle becomes prolonged, the aging man attains better control of ejaculation. Orgasm encompasses a shorter time span. The intensity of the ejaculation decreases, and the man may feel satisfied ejaculating every second or third intercourse.[71]

A gap between interest and sexual activity has been found for middle-aged persons. Usually the gap is much wider for men than women, with men exhibiting more interest in sexual activity than actual activity. An explanation for this gap was that men had impaired sexual function as a result of poor health. The absence of such a gap for women was attributed to their adaptively inhibiting sexual interest because of lack of opportunity—usually the result of the loss of a partner or the partner's sexual dysfunction.[53]

Assessment

Subjective data

Men and women who present themselves for a checkup or with a complaint related to the genital tract should have a complete history taken. Some persons who at first appear to have no symptoms indicating involvement of the reproductive organs may be found to have a problem of the genital system. Careful eliciting of information will help define the problem or problems so that immediate attention can be directed to relieving the cause of the complaint or preventing problems from occurring.

Many of the problems that individuals bring to the attention of nurses and physicians concern subjects or body areas that they are hesitant to discuss. Careful, tactful questioning can assist them to feel more at ease, and often they are relieved that the topic has been raised by someone else. Establishment of a trusting relationship between the nurse and the patient is imperative and should lead to open communication. Sympathy and understanding, along with respect for personal feelings, are essential in obtaining information that individuals might omit because of fear, tension, or embarrassment. Listening with attention and interest is reassuring to the individuals and helps them to be more open and free in expression.

Personal data

Sociocultural information will be helpful in determining the patient's frame of reference. The data includes the person's age, socioeconomic status, educational background, occupation, religion, ethnic group, living arrangements, family network, and support systems. Many superstitions related to the reproductive system are culture specific.

Past medical history

The person's history of previous illnesses is carefully recorded and includes any previous treatment for conditions that might influence functioning of the reproductive organs. Past history or surgery is recorded and includes the type and date of surgery, the preoperative and postoperative diagnoses and any complications that occurred.

Men are questioned about their past history concerning pain or swelling of the scrotum, testes, sores on the penis, discharges from the urethra, urinary tract problems, ability to achieve and maintain an erection, and previous surgery or treatments for problems of the genitourinary tract. Both men and women should be questioned about a history of discharge, syphilis, gonorrhea, or other venereal diseases.

Family history

The incidence of such diseases as diabetes, hypertension, coronary occlusion, and cancer should be obtained and recorded. Some chronic diseases that tend to recur in families influence functioning of the reproductive organs. A history of the mother's past pregnancies is important especially if it involved use of diethylstilbestrol (DES), which leads to vaginal adenosis.

Gynecologic-obstetric history

In securing information for the gynecologic history, as with other aspects of the history, it is important to assess the person's level of understanding and to use words that are readily understood. Many persons are hesitant to give information because they lack knowledge of medical terms and are embarrassed because of this. Questions should be clearly stated so that accurate answers will be given. For example, few women can answer questions about *menarche*, but most could answer the question, "How old were you when your periods began?"

When the nurse takes the history, it is usual to begin with previous illnesses or surgery related to the reproductive organs. The gynecologic-obstetric history is outlined in the box below.

Because countless women are using some form of contraception, and since some of the contraceptives in use may affect the state of reproductive health, a complete contraceptive history should be taken if the woman has been determined to be heterosexually active and of reproductive age. Information includes types of contraceptives used in the past and at present, how long each type was used, why a specific method was discontinued

---

GYNECOLOGIC-OBSTETRIC HISTORY

Previous illness or surgery involving the reproductive organs

Menstrual history
  Age at menarche
  Interval and duration of menstrual periods
  Pain with menstruation, including days of cycle on which it occurs, duration, and factors that intensify or alleviate it
  Amount of flow (number of tampons or pads)
  Presence of clots, their size, and dates on which they appear
  Dates of onset of last two menstrual periods and duration of flow

Obstetric history
  Pregnancies (dates, length of gestation, type of delivery, birth weight, complications during or after pregnancy)
  Abortions, miscarriages (length of pregnancy, method of abortion, physical or psychologic complications)

and another substituted, and any problems that occurred during the use of contraception.

Urinary and gastrointestinal symptoms

Urinary and gastrointestinal symptoms are frequently reported by women and may be associated with various gynecologic disorders. Urinary symptoms that should be explored further are pain on urination, increased frequency of urination, hematuria, nocturia, and incontinence. Gastrointestinal symptoms that may relate to gynecologic disease are nausea and vomiting, constipation, bloating, discomfort after eating, and heartburn.

Patient's complaint

The patient's complaint should be recorded in the patient's own language in order to direct the questioning and to assess the urgency of any problem. The data should include location of the symptoms, duration, severity, treatment by a physician, and attempts the patient has made to relieve the problem.

Once a general statement or description of the patient's chief complaint is obtained, more specific questioning can follow. If pain is a complaint, the patient is asked to describe it in clear terms (e.g., sharp, dull, cramping, steady, or intermittent). The site of the pain can usually be determined by asking the patient to show where it is. Identification of events or activities that increase or decrease the pain is important. Such facts as the use of heat or cold, self-medication, alterations in position, coughing, or having intercourse and their influence on the pain should be obtained.

When the patient complains of bleeding, as much specific information should be obtained as possible. If a woman complains of bleeding, vague statements such as "irregular periods" or "intermittent bleeding" are inadequate. Data about the last two menstrual periods should be obtained. If the menstrual periods are irregular, the range of the cycles and duration of flow are recorded. Bleeding between menstrual periods is described in terms of number of days before or after a menstrual period and duration of bleeding at these times. In addition, characteristics of the blood lost are obtained and recorded.

In men, complaints of bleeding are often related to the presence of blood in the urine, and other symptoms such as pain on voiding may be present. Frank bleeding may be present in the form of bright or dark blood on the underwear, and the patient is questioned about this. Associated symptoms of other types of discharge, burning or itching of the genitalia, and ability to initiate urination are determined.

In a similar way, specific descriptions of complaints of a tumor, mass, swelling, sore on the genitalia, discharges other than bleeding, and symptoms related to the bladder and rectum are obtained by questioning the patient.

Since the reproductive tract is sensitive to endocrine functioning and the use of medications, all patients are questioned about these. In women, it is especially important to determine whether hormones or contraceptive pills are being taken.

Sexual history

Many health care providers may not be experienced in eliciting a sexual history and may initially be uneasy when doing so. No doubt this uneasiness is conditioned by social prohibitions about discussing intimate matters such as sexual experiences or behavior. However, health professionals are expected to be informed, willing to discuss sexual matters openly with clients, and prepared to educate and counsel clients appropriately. Nurses who are hesitant to deal with sexual matters with clients will be helped by working through their own feelings about sex and sexual matters. Seeking counsel from other nurses or health professionals who are comfortable with the topic is often helpful. Recently, special courses and workshops on sexuality for nurses have become available, and some nurses may find it helpful to attend one of these. During the past decade, the public has been exposed to explicit portrayals of sex and sexuality. Although sometimes criticized, this candor has had salutory effects: more people are willing and able to discuss their sexual concerns. As a result, health professionals are increasingly expected to be informed, willing to discuss these concerns, and able to educate and counsel clients.

Although there is no single approach to taking a sexual history, application of certain principles will facilitate both the client's and the practitioner's comfort. Absolute requirements for history taking include provision of privacy, such as in a closed room; an atmosphere of trust between client and practitioner, such as assurance of confidentiality for the client; and comfort on the part of the practitioner with her or his own sexuality.

Some principles for promoting client-practitioner comfort follow. First, obtaining the sexual history early in the therapeutic relationship conveys to the client that sexuality is a legitimate component of health and that it is normal and usual for it to be examined in the context of a physical examination or health history. Next, the sexual history itself may be therapeutic. Within the context of obtaining the data, the practitioner can provide permission for the client to discuss her or his concerns, provide limited information or suggestions, or validate the normalcy and acceptability of the client's concerns and practices. Avoiding overreaction, such as shock and horror, to the information related by the client, as well as underreaction, such as boredom, facilitates truthful history giving on the part of the client. Use of language that the client understands and with which the practitioner is comfortable will also facilitate obtaining an adequate picture of the client's concerns. It may be necessary for both the client and the practitioner to define their terms; "street" language may be unfamiliar to the nurse, and highly technical language may be confusing to the client. The nurse may need to become familiar with some commonly used street language in order to be sure what the client is reporting.[42,67] The technique of moving from less sensitive to more sensitive areas paves the way for both the client and practitioner. For example, the nurse may explore a woman's sexual role before discussing her ability to have orgasm, her menstrual history before her experience with sexual variations, and her personal experiences with sex education before her actual sexual experiences.

"Unloading the question" is another technique useful in obtaining a sexual history. This consists of prefacing the question with a statement referring to the known variation in or prevalence of a specific behavior. For example, the question related to frequency of intercourse may be asked in the following fashion: "Some women have intercourse many times a week, some a few times a week, and still others not at all. On the average, how often do you have intercourse?" This approach conveys to the client that no matter what her practices, they fit into the framework of known behavioral patterns.

Referring to the ubiquity of sexual practices is another useful strategy. This consists of asking clients "how" or "when" they began certain sexual practices as opposed to the more threatening "did you ever?" approach. Prefacing an inquiry by a statement such as "Many people experience. . . ." conveys to the client that his or her practices or experiences are not too unusual to relate.

Following the life cycle chronology is another useful technique inasmuch as it provides for a logical unfolding of events. Finally, terminating the sexual history by inquiring whether the client has additional questions or issues to discuss conveys a willingness on the part of the practitioner to further explore sexual matters.

Brief sexual assessment. A brief assessment can be incorporated in the nursing history by means of three questions. The first of these deals with the person's *role,* the second with the *affective-cognitional elements* of sexuality, and the third with *biologic aspects* of sexual function. These questions may be modified to deal with illness, hospitalization, life events, or any other relevant entity that may influence or interfere with sexual health.

Has your (illness, pregnancy, hospitalization) interfered with your being a (husband, wife, father, mother)? Has your (abortion, heart attack) changed the way you see yourself as a (woman, man)? Has your (colostomy, hysterectomy) changed your ability to function sexually (or your sex life)? These questions may also be adapted to elicit the client's expectations of changes resulting

from procedures or hospitalization that he or she is about to experience. Similar questions may be found in the format for the nursing history described by McPhetridge.[72] These brief items invite the client to explore sexual concerns. Often it is unnecessary for the practitioner to ask the second and third questions, because many clients proceed to state their concerns about masculinity, femininity, and sexual functioning without further prompting.

Sexual problem history. The sexual problem history may be used in conjunction with the brief history described above or alone in the context of sexual counseling or therapy. Although the parameters explored in a sexual problem history will vary with the theoretical framework guiding the nurses' practice, there are commonalities to be explored regardless of the approach to therapy. The approach described below has been suggested by Annon.[4]

The first component of the sexual problem history is a *description,* in the client's terms, of the current problem or concern.

Next, the *onset and course* of the problem are explored. The practitioner may wish to inquire about the age of the client when the problem began, whether it had an insidious onset or occurred suddenly, whether the client can identify any precipitating events, and whether there are other life events associated with the sexual problem. The course of the sexual problem can be described in terms of its fluctuations over time, such as with the changing intensity of a disease process, and whether the problem has any functional relationships to phenomena such as medication or alcohol use.

Of great importance is the *client's conception of the cause and persistence of the problem.* This data will enable the nurse to respond directly to the client's concerns rather than dealing with them indirectly.

Past attempts at treatment and their results may be explored, including evaluations by other health practitioners (e.g., physicians), the use of other professional help (e.g., counselors), and finally the attempts that the client has made to cope with the problem.

The last component of the sexual problem history includes an examination of the *client's current expectations and the goals* identified for treatment. A woman complaining of inability to have orgasm may have the expectations of having orgasm with intercourse rather than by self-stimulation. If her expectations are not stated precisely, the practitioner may inappropriately treat her with the latter goal in mind or refer her to a practitioner whose approach to therapy would not be congruent with her goals.

Alternative approaches. Although the two approaches to obtaining sexual history data described above are probably most appropriate for nurses, several alternatives exist. For further information about these alternatives the reader is referred to references 4, 32, 39, 46, and 56.

Diagnosing sexual problems is frequently difficult. Often sexual problems are entangled in problems with relationships or with intrapersonal problems. As a consequence, the sexual problem may be a symptom of another problem such as a power struggle in a relationship or depression. Careful description of the problem is therefore essential.

Objective data

Physical examination

When patients present themselves for a checkup or because of a problem of the genital tract, a complete physical examination should be done. Men should have a rectal examination, and woman should have a pelvic examination and thorough examination of the breasts. General items that should be assessed are the patient's weight, height, body build, thyroid gland, heart, lungs, hair distribution, blood pressure, pulse, and urine for protein, glucose, and bacteria.

Both men and women may delay medical examinations of the reproductive tract, since this type of examination may cause intense emotional reactions. Fear, embarrassment, and cultural mores play an important part in this emotional distress. In our culture, people frequently fear that their anxieties concerning carcinoma, venereal disease, sterility, or the climacteric will be verified. Many patients are embarrassed by the required exposure of the external genitalia during examination. Many patients also may be fearful that some condition will be discovered that will require surgery resulting in sterility or impotence. The nurse who is sensitive to the many thoughts and fears that may trouble patients will be better prepared to help them accept the necessary examination.

Men should be encouraged to have a yearly rectal examination to detect early prostatic disease. The positive aspects of such an examination should be pointed out. It is customary in some areas for male practitioners to request a female "chaperone" to be present during the female patient's pelvic examination. However, it is customary for men to be examined without the presence of a chaperone.

Whether the physical examination is to be performed by a nurse or a physician, it is a function of the nurse to prepare the patient for the examination. Preparation includes informing the patient of what is to be done, by whom and why, what the patient needs to do in preparation for the examination and why, what the patient can do to feel more relaxed and comfortable during the examination, and when the patient will be informed of findings of the examination.

Abdominal examination

Information related to the reproductive organs is obtained by inspection, palpation, percussion, and auscultation of the lower abdomen. *Inspection* is done first because pressure on the bowel by palpation and percussion alter bowel motility and heighten sounds. The abdomen is inspected for the presence of scars and for size and contour. If scars are noted, the patient is questioned about these, even though information may have been obtained during the history taking. Any localized areas of prominence are noted, since these may indicate enlargement of the reproductive organs or adjacent structures. The skin of the abdomen and pubic area is inspected for amount, distribution, and character of hair; abnormal pigmentation; and lesions. Abdominal muscle tone is assessed by having the patient cough or raise the head. Such actions reveal muscle weakness by producing bulging around the umbilicus, inguinal region, or in the midline between the rectus muscles. Women who have been pregnant are more likely to have diastasis recti. In men, hernias most often are evident in the inguinal areas.

Abdominal *palpation* follows inspection. Since the reproductive organs are normally situated in the pelvic cavity, they are usually not palpable through the abdominal wall. Therefore abdominal palpation is done for the purpose of ruling out or discovering abnormalities. If an abdominal mass is felt, it is described in relation to its position and relationship to any pelvic or abdominal organ, size, shape, consistency, contour, tenderness, and movability. Palpation should be light at first, then followed by deep palpation (p. 1437). An estimate of the amount of pressure needed to palpate can be obtained by gently picking up the skin in either lower quadrant to estimate the thickness of the abdominal wall.

If the patient has complained of pain, the site of pain should never be palpated first. Instead, palpation is started in the farthest removed quadrants, and the area of pain is gradually and gently approached. Observation of the patient for responses indicating pain or tenderness on palpation is necessary. For patients who are nonreactive, it is advisable to seek verbal confirmation of the absence of pain or tenderness. The site and degree of any pain or tenderness should be recorded.

Enlargement of the uterus is detected by palpating in the midline of the lower abdomen. Palpation is started just below the umbilicus and continued in the direction of the symphysis pubis. In contrast to a full bladder, which feels soft, an enlarged uterus feels firm and may be round or asymmetric. During pregnancy, the uterus is not palpable as an abdominal organ until about the end of the third month. A firm, isolated area of enlargement may be caused by the presence of a tumor of the uterus. In men, a distended bladder after voiding requires further evaluation, as does bulging in either or both inguinal areas.

Enlargement of the fallopian tubes and ovaries may be detected by palpation of the right and left lower quadrants. Even when enlarged, these organs are not always palpable through the abdominal wall. However, enlargement is often associated with pain or tenderness on palpation of the lower quadrants. The round ligaments are often palpable in the lower quadrants, stretching from the iliac crests to the pubic bones, and they should not be confused with the fallopian tubes.

Percussion of the lower abdomen is directed chiefly to the organs or masses that are palpable. A tumor, such as an ovarian cyst, or fibroid tumor of the uterus produces a flat note (dullness), over the area; while a uterus enlarged because of pregnancy usually produces a hollow note. The increased risk of benign liver tumors in women who use oral contraceptives necessitates palpation and percussion of the liver.

Auscultation is used to determine the presence and quality of peristaltic movement. During pregnancy, it is possible to hear the fetal heartbeat through the abdominal wall by the twentieth week if an ordinary stethoscope is used. If devices with Doppler signals and amplification are used, the fetal heartbeat may be heard at least 8 weeks earlier.

Pelvic examination

While some nurses perform pelvic examinations as part of their practices, in some instances the nurse's involvement includes acting as a chaperone during the examination when it is performed by a man, encouraging the woman to relax and providing assistance as necessary. The nurse assisting with a pelvic examination has an ideal opportunity to create an educational atmosphere, encouraging the woman to learn more about her body and her sexuality and to explore concerns about her body and its functions. Following the examination, nurses can reinforce findings, discuss treatment plans, or provide necessary health education.

Preparation. For female patients, visual aids are useful when a pelvic examination is to be done. Models of the pelvic organs, pamphlets, and films such as *The Gynecologic Examination** assist with the presentation of information about the purposes of the examination, what is done, and what to expect.

In order to make the pelvic examination a positive experience, there must be open communication between the examiner and the patient. The examiner explains the procedure and answers questions before the patient is undressed and on the examination table. Some patients may need to see and touch the speculum before it is inserted. The patient should have the option to use or not use drapes to cover her perineum. Some women feel that drapes prevent embarrassment and protect their modesty, while others feel that draping indicates something mysterious or shameful about the pelvic examination. During the examination, the ex-

*Your Health, Educational Division, 5841 S. Maryland Ave., Chicago, IL 60637.

aminer tells the patient what will be done next and informs her of the findings. The patient is told to relax *specific* tense body parts rather than generally to relax throughout the examination. The patient's face is monitored for responses. After the pelvic examination, the examiner reviews findings and answers any patient questions. The pelvic examination is a unique opportunity to teach anatomy and physiology as well as to discuss health practices.

Women who are scheduled ahead of time for pelvic examination should be advised to avoid douching and applying any vaginal preparations (medicinal or deodorant) for at least 24 hours before examination. Patients should void immediately before examination, since an empty bladder makes palpation of the pelvic organs easier, decreases patient discomfort, eliminates possible distortion of the position of pelvic organs caused by a full bladder, and obviates the danger of incontinence during examination. The patient should be in the supine position with a small pillow under her head for comfort and under her knees to maintain slight leg flexion. The arms are at the sides.

The following equipment may be necessary for the pelvic examination:

1. Bivalve vaginal specula (various sizes)
2. Uterine tenaculum forceps
3. Sponge forceps
4. Biopsy forceps (sterile)
5. Cautery unit with tips
6. Uterine sounds and probes (sterile)
7. Gloves (disposable rubber or plastic)
8. Lubricant (water soluble, vegetable base)
9. Aspirator or wooden blade for Pap smear
10. Cotton applicators
11. Cotton balls
12. Gauze sponges
13. Topical antiseptic solution
14. Specimen bottles with fixative solution
15. Glass microscope slides
16. Test tubes and culture tubes

Good lighting is important for a pelvic examination. Probably the best lighting is obtained with a head mirror.

A lighted speculum can be used for the pelvic examination. A mirror used by the examiner enables the woman to visualize her genitalia, often correcting myths about the vagina and other structures. This educational approach to the pelvic examination may provide many women with their first opportunity to view and identify their genitalia.

Positions for pelvic examinations. Several positions may be used for the pelvic examination. Arthritis and other conditions that limit the woman's mobility may preclude some of these positions. Furthermore, some positions, such as the knee-chest position, are both uncomfortable and embarrassing for women of almost any

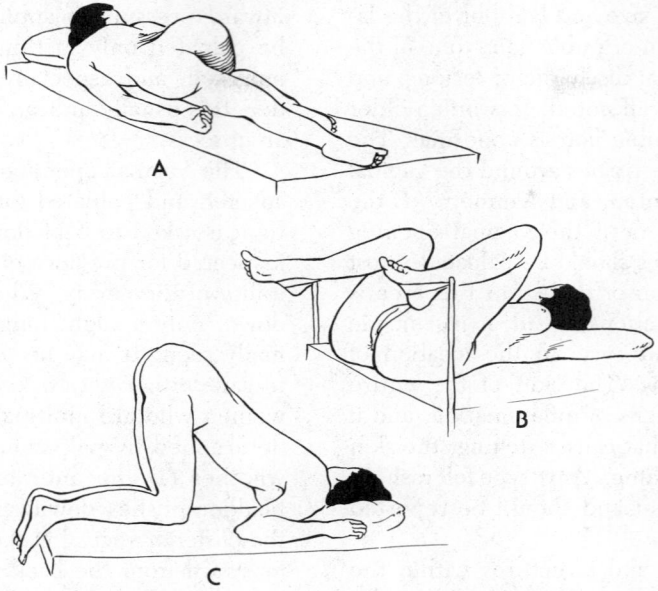

Fig. 63-7. Various positions that can be assumed for examination of rectum and vagina. **A,** Sims's (lateral) position. Note position of left arm and right leg. **B,** Lithotomy position. Note position of buttocks on edge of examining table and support of feet. **C,** Knee-chest (genupectoral) position. Note placement of shoulders and head.

age or physical condition. Nurses can interpret the necessity for such positions.

In *Sims' position (used for rectal examination)* (Fig. 63-7, *A*) the woman is placed on her left side with her left arm and hand behind her. The left thigh is only slightly flexed, and the right knee is flexed sharply on the abdomen.

For the *dorsal recumbent position (lithotomy position)* (Fig. 63-7, *B*) the lower leaf of the examining table should be dropped before the woman gets onto the table, since dropping it may be frightening to her after her feet have been placed in the stirrups. There should be a footstool handy so that she can be guided to step on the stool, sit down on the edge of the table, and then lie back. Most women are able to place their own legs in the stirrups; they should be told to raise both legs and put them in the stirrups simultaneously. When a woman needs help, two persons may assist, with one on each side of the patient so that both can hold one leg and simultaneously place them in position without abruptly lifting the lower extremities. Gentleness and gradual positioning are essential to prevent strain or twisting of the hip joint. Metal stirrups are the most satisfactory; however, if they are used, the patient should wear her shoes because the heels help to hold the feet in the stirrups.

Care must be taken to see that there is no pressure on the legs when sling stirrups are used, since nerve damage and impairment of circulation can occur. The buttocks need to be moved down so that they are even

with the end of the table. The pillow under the head is pulled down at the same time to assure comfort for the patient.

The pelvic examination can be done with the woman in bed if it is inadvisable for her to be moved to an examining table. The woman can be helped to assume a position across the bed, and her feet can be supported on the seats of two straight chairs. Some practitioners find this a useful adaptation when the pelvic examination is done at home.

For the *knee-chest position* (Fig. 63-7, *C*), first the lower end of the examination table is dropped; then the woman is helped to get on her hands and knees on the table. Her buttocks will be uppermost, and her thighs will be sharply flexed on her trunk. The woman's head is turned to one side and rests on the table. Her arms are flexed and resting well forward (often above her head), and her knees are apart. Her feet extend over the lower edge of the table to prevent pressure on her toes. This examination can also be done by positioning the woman crosswise on the bed.

Inspection and palpation of female external genitalia. This portion of the pelvic examination is done before internal examination. Protective gloves are usually worn throughout the examination. Inspection and palpation of the external genitalia include examination of the mons pubis, labia minora, labia majora, clitoris, urethral meatus, Skene's and Bartholin's glands, vaginal orifice, hymen, escutcheon, and perineum.

The external genitalia are first inspected for gross

deviations from normal. The size and contour of the labia, presence and distribution of pubic hair, tone of the perineum, presence of vaginal discharge or lesions, and presence of hemorrhoids are all noted. In women older than 16 years, absence of pubic hair is abnormal. The opening of the vagina and the tissues around the vaginal opening are inspected for contour and symmetry. If the structures appear distorted, or if the vaginal opening appears asymmetric, the tissues should be palpated. Most often irregularity or distortion of tissues in this area is the result of scars from lacerations, an ulcer just inside the vagina, or infections and cysts in the location of Skene's or Bartholin's glands. The skin of the entire vulvar area is observed for signs of inflammation, and if there is a vaginal discharge that causes itching, the skin may be broken from scratching. Any type of rash or lesion of the skin is significant and should be reported to the physician.

Inspection of the tissues and structures within the labial folds is important. To expose the area adequately, the labia minora are separated using two fingers as when a catheterization is being performed. This maneuver makes the clitoris, urinary meatus, vaginal opening, and tissues around these structures more readily visible. Clitoral enlargement or atrophy is abnormal. The clitoris is frequently a site for malignant lesions in older women and syphilitic chancres in younger women. Abnormalities of the urethral meatus include erythema, exudates, and masses. The labia must be inspected for the following abnormalities: asymmetry, enlargement, atrophy before menopause, exudates, parasites, altered pigmentation, ulcerations, varicosities, and leukoplakia (white adherent patches).

Especially important is the presence of a spontaneous purulent discharge from the meatus. If there is reason to suspect a urethral infection without evidence of urethral discharge, the urethra may be "stripped." This is done by placing the forefinger into the vagina for about half the finger's length. The finger is then bent so that its tip touches the anterior wall of the vagina in the midline behind the urethra. While exerting gentle pressure, the finger is then slowly withdrawn. This maneuver forces any accumulation of discharge out through the meatus and should not be painful. A culture should be taken whenever a purulent discharge from the urethra is present.

Skene's and Bartholin's glands are closely inspected and palpated. These are common sites of infection, especially from the gonococcus organisms. If there is a purulent discharge from either of these glands, a smear or culture should be taken. Bartholin's glands are palpated by placing one finger inside the base of the vagina and a thumb on the outside of the labia majora near the perineum. Pressure is made by bringing the finger and thumb together. To palpate Skene's glands, a finger is placed over the site of the glands, and gentle,

inward pressure is applied. Usually, these glands can be palpated only in thin women; therefore if they are enlarged, and especially if they are enlarged and tender, this usually indicates cystic formation, infection, or an abscess.

The vaginal opening and perineum are further inspected and palpated for loss of muscle tone. The patient is asked to bear down, and the vaginal opening is inspected for prolapse of tissue into the vagina and visibility of the cervix. When the patient is asked to bear down, only a slight bulging of the entire vulva is normally seen. It may be observed that the vagina seems to gape either with or without straining, particularly in women who are multiparous. If this is so, it should be determined by palpation with one finger in the vagina whether (1) the anterior vaginal wall appears as the bladder pushes downward in the front (cystocele), (2) the posterior vaginal wall appears as the rectum is pushed forward from the back (rectocele), or (3) both the anterior and posterior vaginal walls protrude into the vagina (uterine prolapse).

Perineal muscle tone is further tested by inserting two fingers into the vagina and asking the patient to tighten her muscles. The muscles can be felt to contract around the fingers if there is normal muscle tone but not if the muscles are weakened. An additional estimate of muscle tone can be made by placing two fingers inside the vagina. The fingers are slightly spread, and traction is applied against the tissues by pressing toward the examiner. Urinary stress incontinence will be observed if present. If the muscle tone is normal, the tissues cannot be displaced more than a finger's breadth. If the muscles of the perineum are weak, the tissues can be readily depressed. The perineum of a woman who has had an episiotomy will feel thinner and more rigid than that of a woman who has not had an episiotomy.

Inspection and palpation of internal organs. It is now considered good practice first to perform a speculum examination of the vagina and cervix before introducing lubricated fingers to palpate. It has been shown that some lubricants in common use prevent securing of adequate specimens from the cervix and might alter laboratory findings.[28] Lubricants are bacteriostatic and alter cells on Papanicolaou (Pap) smears. Methods for obtaining cervical and vaginal specimens are discussed later in this chapter.

SPECULUM EXAMINATION. In order to provide for inspection of the vagina and cervix, it is necessary to select the size and type of speculum the provides the best exposure without producing undue discomfort for the woman. The examiner determines the correct type and size of speculum after inspection of the external genitalia and through the subjective assessment. The two types of specula are Grave's speculum and the Pederson speculum. Grave's speculum is most often used with multiparous and sexually active adult women. It varies in length from 9 to 12 cm and in width from 2 to 4 cm. The Pederson speculum, which is flatter and more narrow, is frequently used with nulliparous and nonsexually active women, children, and postmenopausal women with contracted vaginal orifices.

The speculum is lubricated with warm water. The woman is told she will feel pressure in her vagina but that it should not be painful. The examiner asks her to bear down to additionally open the vaginal orifice and relax the perineal muscles. The labia minora are separated and held in this position with the index and middle fingers of one hand, while the speculum is introduced with the other hand. The speculum is held so that the blades are firmly closed to avoid pinching of tissues and so that the blades are vertical with the handles of the speculum to one side. This position of the speculum allows the instrument to fit better the contour of the vagina. (Some examiners contend that inserting and subsequently turning the speculum create discomfort. They recommend inserting the speculum with the blades parallel to the examination table.)

The speculum is advanced into the vagina close to the rectal wall, while slight downward pressure is exerted on the posterior vaginal wall to avoid the more sensitive urethra and anterior vaginal wall. When the speculum blades are about three fourths their length inside the vagina, the speculum is turned so that the handle is downward within the palm of the hand. The lever is pressed to open the blades, and an attempt is made to visualize the cervix. The cervix is almost immediately visible, and the external os can readily be seen. If the cervix is not visualized, the speculum is withdrawn slightly until the cervix comes into view (Fig. 63-8). The screw on the speculum is tightened to hold the blades in the open position.

The Pap smear and gonorrhea culture are collected at this point. Currently, there is controversy about how often Pap smears are needed. Women who are at high risk for developing cervical neoplasms (those with abnormal Pap smears or history of intercourse at an early age or with multiple partners) should have Pap tests every year. The American Cancer Society now recommends Pap tests every 3 years for women at low risk for developing cervical neoplasia and who have had two normal Pap tests 1 year apart. If a woman has been exposed to gonorrhea or has symptoms of gonorrhea, a gonorrhea culture should be obtained before insertion of an intrauterine device (IUD) and at the first prenatal appointment. The optimal time to obtain the Pap smear is 5 to 6 days after the end of menstruation, although it can be taken at any time. The menstrual flow may obscure atypical cells and make the interpretation more difficult.

The cervix is inspected for color, contour, position, size, symmetry, surface characteristics, discharge, projection into vaginal vault, consistency, shape, and patency of the external os. In nulliparous women the external os appears as a round depressed area (Fig. 63-9). In multiparous women the cervical os usually appears as a transverse slit in the center of the cervix. The color of the cervix varies but is usually pink. It becomes pale after menopause and cyanotic either during pregnancy or with any condition causing venous congestion or hypoxia.

The surface of the cervix is inspected to determine whether it is smooth, irregular, or raw and whether there is any purulent or other type of discharge from the os. It is not uncommon to see a red, somewhat raw appearing area (an erosion) on the surface of the cervix. There may be scars appearing as white or reddened slits radiating from the cervical os. These are lacerations of the cervix and are often present in women who have borne children (Fig. 63-9). Occasionally, a stalked polyp may be seen extending through the cervical os as a bright or dark red mass. These polyps frequently cause bleeding and require further study.

After inspection of the cervix, the screw on the speculum is loosened and the speculum is slowly withdrawn. Pressure on the lever is maintained to make inspection of the vagina possible. As the speculum is withdrawn, the cervix is checked to see whether contact with the cervix has caused bleeding. Slight spotting from collection of cervical specimens may be present. However, frank bleeding that ceases only with application of pressure is significant. The walls of the vagina are inspected as the speculum is withdrawn. The vaginal mucosa is observed for color, consistency, inflammation, ulcers, masses, presence of rugae, discharge, and odor. The vaginal wall is normally pink in color but is usually pallid after menopause.

PALPATION. Palpation of the internal reproductive organs follows speculum examination. Lubricant should be used on the first and middle fingers of the examining hand. The hand is held so that the first and middle fingers are straight and close together. The thumb is stretched straight up, and the ring and small fingers are curled into the palm of the hand. Throughout the examination, the examiner's wrist is held in a rigid, straight line.

The labia minora are separated, and the first and middle fingers are slowly but firmly introduced into the vaginal canal. As the fingers are advanced, the elbow is raised slightly so that the fingers can follow the normal curve of the posterior vaginal wall. The fingers are advanced until the cervix is felt. Usually, the cervix is located with ease. In nonpregnant women, the cervix normally has a consistency similar to the tip of the nose. It feels smooth and round, is about 2.54 cm in diameter, and under normal circumstances moves easily in all directions. Normally, the cervix is situated in the midline.

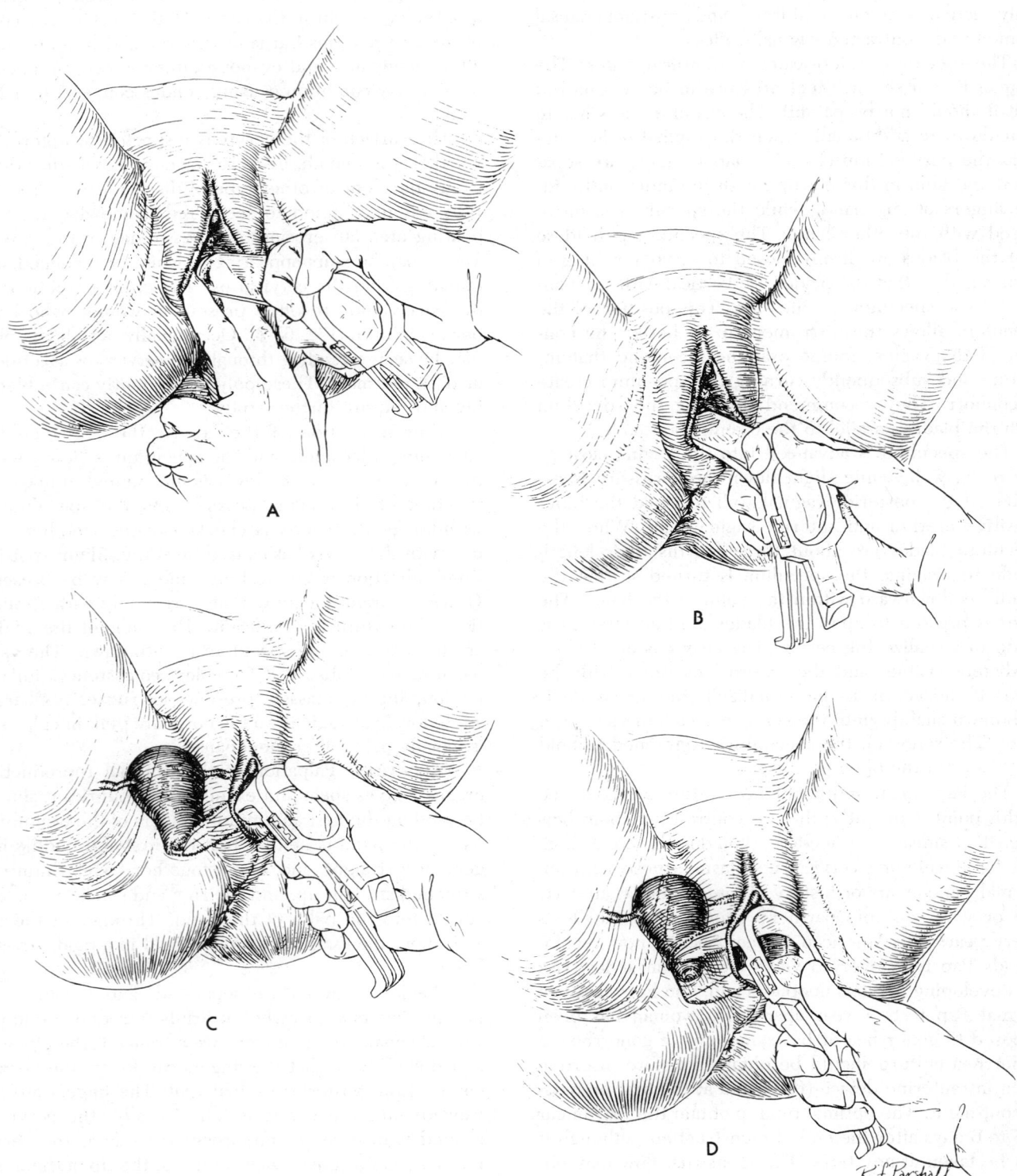

Fig. 63-8. Procedure for speculum examination. **A,** Opening of introitus. **B,** Oblique insertion of speculum. **C,** Final insertion of speculum. **D,** Opening of speculum blades. (From Malasanos, L., et al.: Health assessment, ed. 2, St. Louis, 1981, The C.V. Mosby Co.)

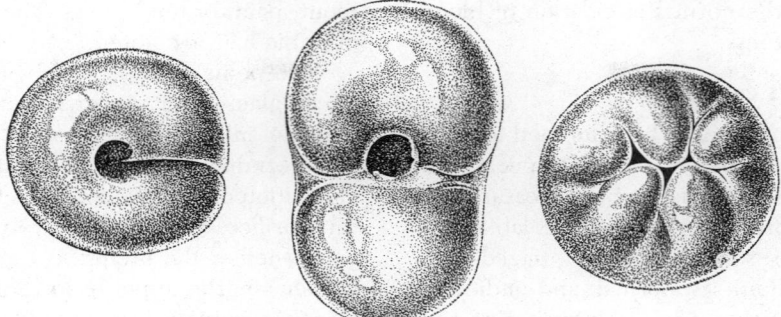

Fig. 63-9. Nulliparous cervix and laceration of cervix. (From Malasanos, L., et al.: Health assessment, ed. 2, St. Louis, 1981, The C.V. Mosby Co.)

The cervix is palpated for consistency and contour. It is noted whether the cervix feels softer or harder than normal and whether the surface and shape feel regular or irregular. The cervix feels softer with pregnancy and harder with tumors. Areas of irregularity and abnormal tension should be carefully noted in terms of site. For example, abnormalities can be described as being in position 12 o'clock, 6 o'clock, 9 o'clock.

An attempt is made to insert a finger into the cervical os to detect masses, but excessive force should not be used. In nulliparous women, the cervix is usually closed. In multiparous women, the cervix may admit one or two fingers. Movability of the cervix in all directions is checked, and any restrictions of movement are noted. The vaginal vault is palpated for areas of tenderness and presence of masses. Feces in the rectum may be palpated, and this can later be verified by rectal examination.

Bimanual palpation follows palpation of the cervix. The purpose of the bimanual examination is palpation of the internal reproductive organs and assessment of pelvic supports. The gloved fingers are placed behind the cervix, and the ungloved hand is placed palm down on the abdomen with the fingertips just below the umbilicus. The wrist is bent, and the fingers are pressed into the abdominal wall. The hand is then pulled toward the examiner so that the uterus is forced against the fingers inside the vagina. The palmar surfaces of the fingers are used to palpate rather than the tips or dorsal surfaces, which are less sensitive. The position of the uterus is determined first. It may be anteverted, midpositioned, retroverted, anteflexed, or retroflexed. Usually, the fundus can be felt anterior to the cervix between the two hands. If not, the uterus may lie posteriorly and be palpated through the posterior vaginal vault. The size, shape, and regularity of the uterine surface are palpated. Normally, the uterus feels firm and the fundus is round. The uterus is softer during pregnancy and firmer during menopause. Localized areas of enlargement are noted, and the approximate size and

shape of masses are determined. Because the uterus is normally movable and easy to displace, loss of movability is readily detected. This, too, is noted and recorded.

The areas around the fallopian tubes and ovaries require deep palpation. Normally, the fallopian tubes are not palpable, and therefore any enlargement is significant. An enlarged fallopian tube resembles an enlarged ovary to a great extent, and it may not be possible to distinguish between the two.

On bimanual examination, the ovaries are normally slightly tender to palpation and are not always palpable, especially in obese women. When palpable, the ovaries feel smooth and oval in shape if no pathologic condition exists. Any readily palpable mass in the area of the fallopian tubes and ovaries that feels irregular, round, or very firm indicates a possible deviation from normal. Because the ovaries atrophy during the menopause, any mass felt in the areas of the ovaries in postmenopausal women is usually a sign of a problem.

The rectovaginal examination is done to confirm uterine position, to reassess the adnexal areas, to follow up on complaints of pain or bleeding, and to determine rectal sphincter tone. The woman is told that it may be uncomfortable and she may feel as though she has to have a bowel movement. Hemorrhoids, fistulas, and fissures can be observed.

Rectal examination is usually done in order to palpate masses in the rectum (p. 1438). If it is necessary for any reason to repeat any part of the examination requiring insertion of fingers into the vagina, the glove is changed following rectal examination to avoid contamination.

Terminating pelvic examination. Following the pelvic examination, a woman may need assistance with removing lubricating jelly or discharge that may be on her genitalia, removing her legs from the stirrups, and getting down from the table. Some women may also require assistance with dressing. Elderly women merit careful assistance following the pelvic examination, since unnatural positions such as the knee-chest and lithotomy positions may alter the normal circulation of blood sufficiently to cause faintness.

Examination of infants and girls

At birth, female infants should be examined for evidence of any abnormalities detectable by inspection of the external genitalia. The clitoris, urinary meatus, and labia minora normally protrude beyond the labia majora. A mucous discharge, sometimes lightly tinged with blood (pseudomenstruation), is normal and indicates withdrawal of hormones present in the intrauterine milieu. Hospital and community health nurses should be certain that mothers know what is normal. Girls born to mothers who have taken diethylstilbestrol (DES) during pregnancy should be observed with particular care, since large doses of this hormone have been associated with vaginal and cervical cancer in the offspring. (A national registry for vaginal adenocarcinoma was established in 1973.) Without alarming the mother, the nurse can advise her to bring any abnormality observed in the child to the physician's attention, particularly abnormal perimenarchial bleeding.

Unless there are definite indications making examination necessary, detailed examination of the internal reproductive organs is usually delayed until after puberty. When examination is necessary, it may be done with the child under anesthesia. A urethroscope may be used to visualize the cervix when a speculum cannot be used.

Examination of males

As with women, men should have an examination of the genital system during physical examination. Examination of the male genitourinary system includes inspection and palpation of the lower abdomen, inspection and palpation of the external genitalia, and palpation of the prostate gland by rectal examination.

Sometimes male patients are requested not to void until they are seen by the physician. This allows the physician to evaluate ability to start and maintain a stream and to assess characteristics of the urinary stream by observing the patient during voiding.

The abdomen is palpated above the symphysis pubis to determine whether the bladder is distended; if so, as evidenced by a soft, palpable mass, the patient is questioned regarding the time of last voiding.

The inguinal area is inspected for areas of bulging caused by hernias. The man is requested to hold his breath and to bear down in order to make presence of herniation more evident. Straining is preferable to coughing because it produces more steady sustained pressure. The load test is used if a hernia is not palpated despite complaints of hernia symptoms. The man lifts something heavy, while the inguinal area is inspected.

The inguinal lymph nodes are palpated for enlargement, pain, or tenderness. The amount and distribution of pubic hair are noted.

The penis is inspected for abnormalities of the prepuce, glans, and urethral meatus and for visible evidence of infection and masses. The prepuce is retracted to determine the presence and degree of phimosis, an elongation of the foreskin such that it constricts the urethral orifice and cannot be retracted. It is important to note whether the urethra is centrally located or whether it opens on the upper or lower surface of the glans. The urinary meatus is inspected for lesions, periurethral abscess, and purulent or bloody discharge. If a discharge is present, a specimen is obtained by milking the penis from the base to the urethra. The skin along the shaft of the penis is checked for lesions of any type and for general color.

The scrotum is observed for general appearance, color of the skin, tension of the skin surfaces, size, symmetry, and the presence of lesions on the skin surfaces.

The left testis is lower than the right testis, which causes the scrotum to appear asymmetric under normal conditions. Scrotal size is determined by the tone of the dartos muscle. The scrotum may look pendulous in older age as the dartos muscle becomes atonic and in warm temperatures with relaxation of the dartos muscle. Cold temperatures cause the dartos muscle to contract and the scrotum shrinks. The testes are inspected for shape, size, consistency, and response to pressure by simultaneous palpation between the thumb and first two fingers. The spermatic cords are palpated between the thumb and forefinger. Unilateral or bilateral enlargement usually indicates presence of a mass or edema.

Palpation of the scrotum is necessary to distinguish between enlargement caused by a mass and swelling caused by collection of fluid. The size, shape, location, tenderness, and consistency of any mass are carefully noted. Transillumination of the scrotum, by placing a flashlight behind the scrotal area in a dark room, is attempted to differentiate the cause of the scrotal mass. Serous fluid will transilluminate or produce a red glow; tissue and blood will not transilluminate.

The prostate gland is palpated by means of a rectal examination with the patient standing (Fig. 63-10). Rectal examination on a regular basis is the most important step in the diagnosis of prostatic disease, especially carcinoma. Cancer of the prostate gland may start as a localized, hard nodule, palpable by rectal examination, before proceeding to an advanced, inoperable, or incurable stage. For this reason, it is recommended that all men, especially those over the age of 50 years, have a rectal examination at least once a year.[51]

All newborn male infants should be examined shortly after birth for visible evidence of problems related to the urogenital system. The prepuce of most infants extends beyond the glans, and the excess is frequently removed by circumcision. Mothers are instructed in care

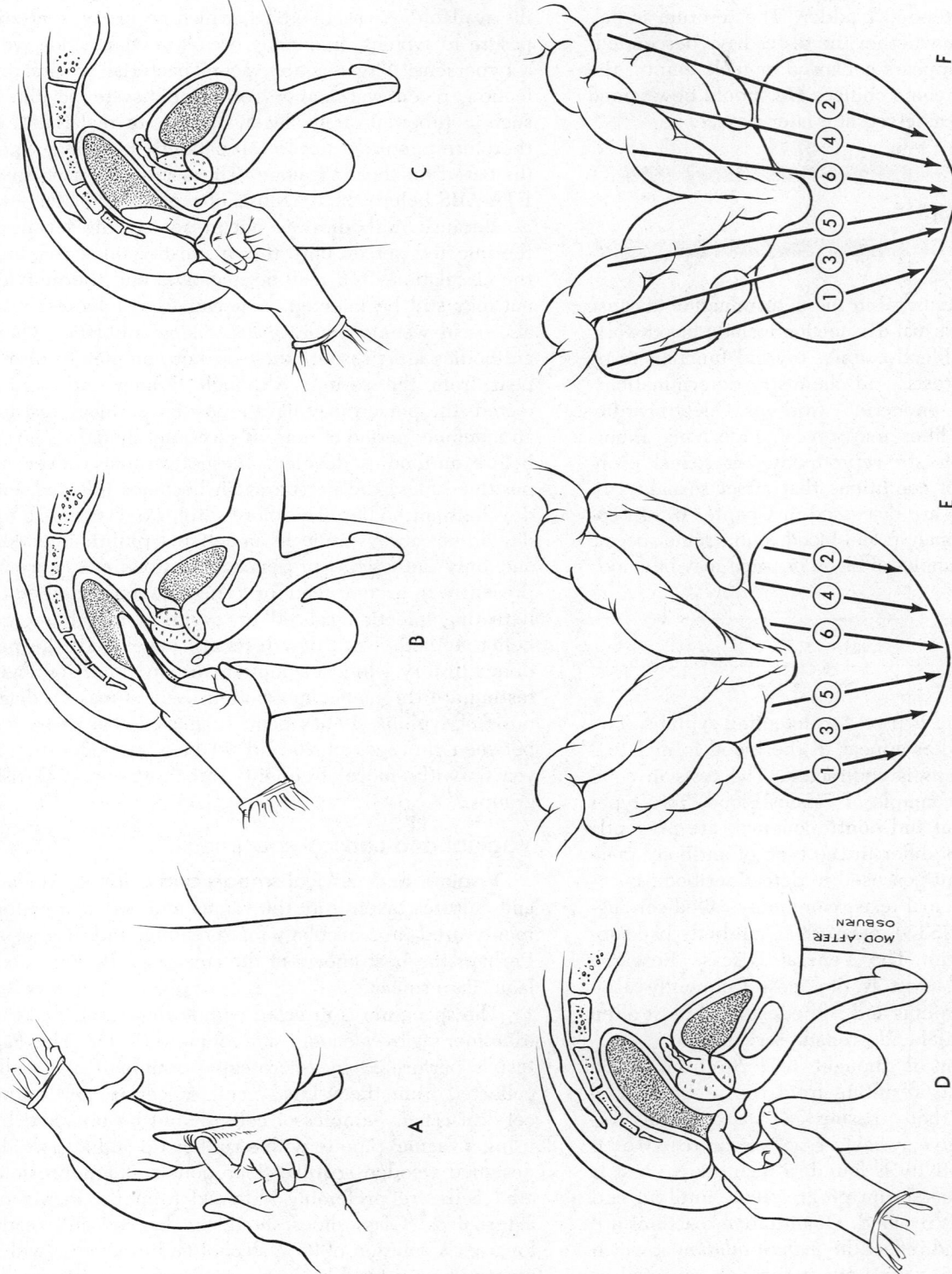

Fig. 63-10. Rectal examination. **A,** Introduction of protected, well-lubricated finger. **B,** Palpation of prostate gland and seminal vesicles, lateral view. **C,** Palpation of anterior surface of sacrum and coccyx. **D,** Palpation of Cowper's glands. **E,** Massage of prostate gland for specimen collection or treatment; order of strokes is indicated by gradually working toward center (verumontanum). **F,** Massage of seminal vesicles and prostate gland. (From Campbell, M.F., and Harrison, J.H.: Urology, vol. 1, ed. 3, Philadelphia, 1970, W.B. Saunders Co.)

MOD. AFTER OSBURN

of the circumcised area to prevent infection. The infant is closely observed for voiding. If the urethral opening is on the upper or lower surface of the glans and if the prepuce is long, the infant may be unable to void and will develop a distended bladder. The scrotum is palpated to determine whether the testes have descended. If the scrotal sac appears collapsed or feels empty, the infant may have become chilled. He should be warmed and the scrotum reassessed at a later time.

Diagnostic tests

Laboratory data useful in the determination of cause of reproductive or sexual dysfunction include blood work, such as complete blood counts, thyroid function tests, glucose tolerance tests, and chemistry determinations. Vaginal cytology, endocrine workups, electrocardiograms, and chest films may reveal underlying abnormalities responsible for reproductive or sexual problems. A number of conditions that affect sexuality directly or indirectly are discussed in Chapter 67. In addition to routine urinalysis and blood count, some specific studies requiring samples of blood or urine may be done.

Routine tests

Tests for syphilis

Serologic testing is used for detecting syphilis. Two identifiable antibodies appear in the blood from 1 to 4 months after syphilis is contracted. The tests in common use require a sample of venous blood. Two types of tests, treponemal and nontreponemal, are presently available. The tests differ in the type of antibody measured and in the antigen used to detect antibodies.

The nontreponemal tests, commonly called serologic tests for syphilis (STS), measure an antibody-like substance called reagin. The Veneral Disease Research Laboratory (VDRL) test is the most frequently used serologic test for syphilis and is the test used most often for routine premarital and prenatal screening.

Syphilitic reagin is thought to form from tissue breakdown products resulting from the interaction of the organism and body tissues. STS are usually reported as nonreactive, weakly reactive, or reactive. If any degree of reactivity is found, a quantitative test is done by diluting the serum progressively until an end point of reactivity is reached. Quantitative reactions are reported in ratios and reflect the *highest dilution* at which the serum reacts. For example, a reaction reported as 1:16 means that the person's serum was diluted 16 times and still produced reaction, but no reaction occurred when the serum was diluted more than 16 times.

A reactive STS is confirmed by alternate serologic tests. For this purpose, the fluorescent treponemal antibody–absorption test (FTA-ABS) is most often used, since it is the most sensitive and specific test for syphilis available. A reactive STS, which occurs with no exposure to syphilis, frequently occurs in conjunction with a hypersensitivity reaction, acute bacterial or viral infection, recent vaccination, or chronic systemic illness such as tuberculosis, collagen disease, or malaria. It is therefore important not to tell patients they have syphilis based on the STS alone. There must be a positive FTA-ABS before the diagnosis of syphilis is made.

Because antibodies are not present in the serum of the infected person until the organism gains entry into the circulation, STS may be negative, and the individual may still be infected. A negative syphilis test may also occur when an individual is taking antibiotics. Once antibodies are present, they do not completely disappear from the serum. Although treated and noninfected, the person may have a positive serology test for an indefinite period of time. If successful therapy is given before antibodies develop, these tests may never be positive unless the person again becomes infected and develops antibodies. Therefore serologic tests in use today do not always indicate an active syphilitic infection and only detect the presence of antibodies. There is presently an urgent need for a specific, rapid method of detecting infection caused by syphilis, and these are being studied. Until new tests are developed, the patient's history, clinical symptoms (if any), and serologic testing are the means most often used to make a diagnosis of syphilis. It has been suggested that everyone between the ages of 20 and 50 be screened every 6 years, with more frequent screening of high-risk groups.[44]

Vaginal and cervical specimens

Vaginal and cervical smears and cultures. Smears and cultures taken from the vagina and cervix are commonly used in gynecology for screening and diagnosis. Perhaps the best known of the smears is the Papanicolaou (Pap) smear.

The speculum is inserted without lubricant, and the examiner's gloves should not contain powder. The Pap test is performed by microscopic examination of cells collected from the vaginal pool, exocervix, and endocervical canal. Samples of cells should be obtained by using a vaginal pipette with a rubber tip and a specially designed wooden spatula. Secretions containing exfoliated cells are preferably obtained from the cervix or external os. Glass slides should be labeled and ready for use. A solution of 95% alcohol and ether in a wide-mouthed jar is used because rapid fixation of the smear is essential. The secretions are collected, smeared on the glass slide, and immediately placed in the fixative solution to prevent drying out and cell distortion. Only a small amount of material is needed, but there should be enough to make a distinct blur on the slide. Most experts believe samples from both cervical aspiration and cervical scraping must be taken to increase the chances of detecting abnormal cells.[57]

It should be noted that the Pap test makes it possible to detect abnormal cells, not all of which are cancerous. However, the Pap test has made it possible through routine use to detect precancerous conditions and cancer of the cervix early enough to make treatment of these conditions almost 100% successful.[58] For detection of atypical cells, the Pap test is 95% accurate. False-negative reports, which should not exceed 10%, are most frequently the result of an inadequate sample or improperly fixed slide.[22]

When the Pap test is positive, additional tissue studies are indicated. The woman should understand that the Pap test is not necessarily conclusive and that biopsy or even surgery may be necessary to verify the diagnosis of premalignancy or malignancy. The false-positive rate is 5%.[43]

Many women are familiar with the Pap test because of the vast amount of publicity it has received. Securing the specimen does not cause pain. Since the procedure can be used to obtain cell samples for study in cases of infertility or when women are taking estrogen preparations, the woman may be required to learn how to take the smear herself. It is imperative that the woman be taught how to insert the aspirator or spatula deeply enough to reach the cervix, how to prepare the slide, and how to place the slide in the fixative.

Do-it-yourself Pap tests are available. These can be used by women who are reluctant or unable to visit a physician for examination. The same instruction is required for an adequate specimen to be obtained. The Pap test alone is not a substitute for the more complete history and examination necessary for preventive care, and women should be encouraged to have a yearly pelvic examination.

To ensure that an adequate and reliable specimen is taken, certain precautions must be observed. These precautions apply to all Pap smears, whether they are taken by a physician, a nurse, or the patient. The ideal time to obtain a Pap smear is 5 to 6 days following menstrual termination. Although the smear can be taken any time, it is preferable to collect the specimen when a woman is not menstruating. Menses makes interpretation difficult and may camouflage atypical cells. A tub bath or douche of any type should not be taken for at least 48 hours before the Pap test. Cauterization of the cervix produces distortion of the cells of the cervix, and this may persist for 6 weeks. Radiation produces distortion of cells for a much longer period. The Pap test should be delayed for at least 1 month after use of topical antibiotics because they produce rapid, heavy shedding of cells. Systemic antibiotics do not produce this effect. The two specimens must be carefully labeled for site and placed in the solution so that the unsmeared sides are back to back.

Many women experience some vaginal bleeding in the form of spotting after a Pap smear has been taken. They should be advised that this is expected and normal, but that any bleeding in excess of spotting is abnormal and should be reported to the health care provider.

Smears or cultures are also taken from various sites when symptoms of infection are present. Most infectious diseases of the reproductive tract produce a purulent discharge. In men, the most common site of purulent discharge is the urinary meatus. The cervix, urethra, Skene's glands, and Bartholin's glands are the most common sites of infection in women. Smears or cultures of the discharge are usually successful in identification of the organism responsible for the infection. The sexually transmitted diseases require a number of different diagnostic studies, and these are discussed in Chapter 65.

Schiller's test. Schiller's test is a simple test that helps the physician to decide whether other diagnostic procedures should be performed when cervical disease is suspected. For example, Schiller's test assists with identifying the area from which a cervical biopsy specimen should be taken.

Schiller's test reveals the presence of atypical cervical cells. A solution of 3.5% iodine or Lugol's solution is applied to the cervix. Atypical cells, both malignant and benign, do not contain glycogen and will fail to stain. Early cancerous lesions and also benign lesions such as cervicitis may appear as glistening areas of a lighter color than surrounding tissue. The tissue having lighter color indicates, for example, the site from which a biopsy specimen should be taken.

Cervical biopsy. In the event that the physician wishes to send a piece of cervical tissue to the laboratory for pathologic examination, a cervical biopsy is done. This procedure usually can be performed safely on an outpatient basis. The biopsy should be scheduled for a week after the end of a menstrual period, since the cervix is more vascular before and after menstruation. The woman should know what is to be done and why. She should be told that there may be momentary discomfort, but that an anesthetic will not be required.

A cervical biopsy specimen can be secured by using a scalpel, but most often a special punch-biopsy forceps is used. A speculum is used to expose the cervix, and a small piece of the cervix is excised. Bleeding is minimal following a punch biopsy but is usually checked by use of electric cautery, silver nitrate, or vaginal packing.

Following the procedure, the nurse ascertains that the woman understands the physician's instructions. Sometimes the main points are written out. Instructions will vary, but they usually include the following:

1. Rest more than usual for the next 24 hours; avoid lifting and marked exertion.
2. Leave the tampon or packing in place as long as the physician advises (usually 8 to 24 hours).
3. Report to the hospital or physician's office if bleeding is excessive; usually more than occurs during normal menses is considered excessive.
4. Do not use an internal douche or have sexual relations until the next visit to the physician, unless specific instructions have been given as to when intercourse can be safely resumed.

Conization of cervix. If the suspected cervical lesion is widespread or the location of abnormal cells found on the Pap smear cannot be located, conization of the cervix may be performed. This method of obtaining tissue from the cervix is also preferred when cancer of the cervix is suspected. Conization of the cervix is sometimes performed as a therapeutic measure in cases of chronic cervical infections in which the inflammatory process has involved the deep tissues of the cervix.

Women may be hospitalized for a conization procedure or may have the procedure done as outpatients. A local or general anesthetic is administered. A cone-shaped portion of the cervix containing the suspected malignant or infected tissue is removed. Bleeding from the site of conization is greater than that occurring from punch biopsy. If the bleeding is excessive or if hemorrhage seems likely, the cervix is sutured to control loss of blood. Oozing is controlled by packing to be kept in place for 24 to 48 hours. The nursing care is basically the same as that required after a dilation and curettage (D and C) (p. 1633).

Following the procedure, the woman needs to know that her next two or three menstrual periods may be heavy and prolonged. If conization was done for carcinoma in situ, the woman will be observed by her physician more frequently, probably every 4 to 8 months. She will need support from the nurse to cope with the diagnosis, prognosis, and future implications of carcinoma.

Special tests

Pregnancy tests

Testing for pregnancy is commonly employed so that management can be started as soon as possible. This is true whether a woman intends to deliver her baby, whether she elects to have an abortion, or whether the physician suspects an ectopic pregnancy. Most of the commonly used pregnancy tests are based on two facts. First, human chorionic gonadotropin (HCG) is present in the serum of pregnant women within 10 to 14 days after the first missed menstrual period. Second, HCG produces antisera. Currently available methods of pregnancy testing fall into four groups: biologic, immuno-

logic, radioimmunoassay, and radioreceptor assay tests.

Biologic tests for pregnancy were first available in the mid-1920s. Among the better-known biologic tests are the *Ascheim-Zondek* test, the *Friedman* test, and the *Hogben* test. These tests require that an early morning voided urine specimen from the woman be injected into a laboratory animal. If HCG is present in the urine, the test is positive as indicated by rapid maturational changes in the ovaries of the laboratory animal. Biologic tests for pregnancy are 95% accurate after 2 weeks following the first missed menstrual period. Because of their relative lack of sensitivity and difficulty doing them, biologic pregnancy tests are no longer used.

Since the early 1960s, a number of commercial *immunologic tests* for pregnancy have become available (*Ortho, Hyland,* and *Roche*). Depending on the specific test, blood or urine specimens are required from the woman. Results are obtained within 2 minutes to 2 hours depending on the test used. The short period for obtaining results is an advantage of immunologic tests. However, these tests are not as sensitive in detecting pregnancy as are other tests. When used in women in whom menstruation is delayed for up to 2 weeks, they show positive results 53.3% of the time.[36] Immunologic pregnancy tests are valuable in screening women who are possibly pregnant. It is generally believed that women with negative immunologic tests should have further examination for pregnancy.

In 1972, the *radioimmunoassay* test for pregnancy became available. This test requires a sample of blood from the woman and detects HCG as early as 7 to 9 days following ovulation. However, the test requires 72 hours for reliable results, which is a greater period of time than is needed for any other test. For this reason, the radioimmunoassay test has not gained popularity.

The *radioreceptor assay* test for pregnancy was developed in 1974 and is reported to be a rapid and reliable test for pregnancy.[55] The test can be performed in 1 hour and is 99% accurate by 6 to 8 days following ovulation.[48] A sample of blood from the finger is used in performing the test. This test has proved to be very reliable clinically.

"Do-it-yourself" pregnancy tests are available to women through department and drug stores. Although a self-performed early pregnancy test is of utility in detecting one's pregnancy shortly after a missed period, tests of this type need to be improved to provide a greater degree of accuracy and reliability.

Two conditions, *hydatidiform mole* and *choriocarcinoma,* produce false-positive pregnancy tests. In both of these conditions, trophoblastic tissue secretes chorionic gonadotropin in abundance.

Infertility studies

Semen analysis. Analysis of the semen is indicated in evaluation of male and female infertility. It is also used to follow up male sterilization by vasectomy.

Multiple semen examinations are done to determine the presence, number, maturity, shape, and motility of sperm. The man may be instructed to secure a specimen of semen at home by masturbation or by coitus interruptus, but because of rapid deterioration of sperm, most physicians prefer a fresh sample collected in the physician's office or in the laboratory. If collected at home, the specimen of semen should be taken to the office or laboratory within 2 to 3 hours.

The semen is usually collected following a period of abstinence corresponding to the man's usual frequency of intercourse. The specimen is ejaculated into a clean, widemouthed jar supplied by the laboratory or physician. The dates of the last emission and of the current specimen are recorded.

A gross examination of the semen for its physical properties is first carried out. Semen is normally a highly viscous, opaque, grayish white fluid that spontaneously liquefies by prostatic enzymes within 10 to 45 minutes after ejaculation. After this time, the semen appears translucent, turbid, and viscous. Semen is normally slightly alkaline, with a pH of about 7.7, which protects sperm from the acid environment in the vagina. The normal volume in an ejaculation of semen is 3 to 5 ml.

After the semen liquefies, a sperm count is taken. A count repeatedly greater than 20 million/ml is considered to be associated with normal fertility if other parameters are normal. The sperm are also examined for motility and presence and number of abnormal forms. It is generally accepted that normal semen contains more than 70% motile sperm and fewer than 30% abnormal forms. A sperm count of less than 20 million/ml of semen, sperm motility under 40%, and abnormal sperm forms over 25% are known to lower the chance of fertilization of an ovum. Also, men who are infertile may have an increased, rather than a decreased, volume of semen, and the increased volume of semen is often associated with a significantly decreased sperm count.

Postcoital test. The postcoital test involves examination of the cervical mucus of women following intercourse to measure both the ability of sperm to penetrate the mucus and remain active and the quality of the cervical mucus. This test is valuable in evaluation of infertility. Similar tests are done in cases of rape, where secretions from the vagina and cervix are examined for the presence of sperm.

For the postcoital test, mucus is aspirated from the cervical canal and examined for the presence and number of sperm. Characteristics of the cervical mucus (spinnbarkeit) are also studied. At the time of ovulation under normal circumstances, the amount of cervical mucus is maximal, but the viscosity is decreased. This facilitates penetration of the cervical mucus by the sperm. If the cervical mucus lacks the characteristics normally associated with ovulation and large numbers of sperm are found in the cervix, it indicates that the sperm are unable to enter the cervix in the number required for an ovum to be fertilized.

The woman who is to have a postcoital test is advised to abstain from intercourse 48 hours before the test and to see the physician 12 hours after intercourse. The woman should be informed of how the specimen is to be collected for examination. After the examination, the woman should be instructed in additional studies to be done or measures to be taken at home.

Rubin test. The Rubin test (uterotubal insufflation) is done to determine whether the fallopian tubes are patent, and this test may be part of the study done in cases of infertility. The procedure is considered highly safe and is most often done on an outpatient basis.

Various devices and instruments for the test are available. The majority of these require a constant source of carbon dioxide, a flow meter and pressure gauge, and an apparatus to record the degree of tubal peristaltic action and resistance. The woman is prepared as for a pelvic examination; and under sterile technique, carbon dioxide is forced into the uterus. The woman usually feels pain under the scapula if the fallopian tubes are open.

With normal tubal patency, the pressure of gas flow rises to a height of 60 to 120 mm Hg and then falls to a constant level. If tubal obstruction is present, there is a steady rise of gas pressure to 200 mm Hg.

It is important that the Rubin test be scheduled to avoid ovulation so that fertilization of an ovum is not prevented by the test. The optimal time for performing the test is 3 to 4 days following the last day of a menstrual period. Since the test is usually done on an outpatient basis, instruction of the woman in preparation for the test is important. She is usually advised to take a laxative the night before the test. On the morning of the test, the woman is given an enema or bisacodyl (Dulcolax) suppository. Before the test, the procedure should be explained, and the woman should be told what she can expect to feel. When the cervix is dilated, the woman may experience pain; and if gas passes through the fallopian tubes, pain in the shoulder usually occurs.

Hysterosalpingogram. The uterus and fallopian tubes can be visualized when a contrast medium is used with roentgenography. A sterile, opaque, aqueous contrast medium is injected through the cervix into the uterus for a hysterogram. For a hysterosalpingogram, the dye is also injected into the fallopian tubes. Radiographs are then taken to observe the structure of the uterus and fallopian tubes. As with the Rubin test, these studies are preferably done 3 or 4 days after the end of a menstrual period to avoid interfering with ovum transport. Preparation for these studies is similar to preparation for a Rubin test.

Screening for prostatic and testicular problems

Prostatic smears and biopsy specimens. When the prostate gland is enlarged or when a suspect prostatic lesion is palpated by rectal examination, a biopsy of the prostate gland or a smear of the prostatic secretions may be done.

For a *prostatic smear,* the physician first massages the prostate gland (Fig. 63-10). The next voided urine specimen is collected, and a smear is prepared in the laboratory. It is possible to detect some cases of cancer and tuberculosis of the prostate gland by this method.

Most often, biopsy specimens of the prostate gland are used for diagnosis. Various methods are used to obtain tissue specimens from the prostate gland.

For a *perineal needle biopsy,* the patient is placed in the lithotomy position (Fig. 63-7, *B*), and a finger is inserted into the rectum to identify the area from which the biopsy specimen is to be taken. The biopsy needle is inserted through the perineum into the prostate gland, and a core of tissue is removed. This technique is considered a minor procedure and can be done on an outpatient basis. The specimen of tissue obtained by perineal needle biopsy is very small and is about 95% accurate for obtaining cells adequate for study.[21]

A *transrectal needle biopsy* is performed in a manner similar to a perineal needle biopsy. The major difference is that the biopsy needle is inserted through the rectal wall into the prostate gland. Because the needle can be inserted more directly into the prostate gland, this method is slightly more accurate in obtaining tissue specimens than is the perineal needle biopsy method.

When a *transurethral biopsy* is done, the biopsy needle is inserted through the urethra toward the prostate gland. This method is used least and is usually confined to cases where the prostatic lesion is producing bladder obstruction. Of all the methods, transurethral biopsy is the least adequate for obtaining specimens.

To obtain a specimen of tissue by *open perineal biopsy,* a small incision is made in the perineum between the anus and the scrotum. This technique gives the greatest accuracy, since the suspect lesion can be clearly identified and multiple specimens can be taken from the prostate gland.

The needle techniques may or may not be done as inpatient procedures. A local or general anesthetic is most often given. Dressings are not required when needle biopsy specimens are taken. Patients should be cautioned to watch for bright red bleeding and to report the occurrence to the physician.

A dressing is required following open perineal biopsy and can be held in place for about 24 hours with a two-tailed binder. The patient is instructed not to contaminate the incision while cleansing himself following defecation by wiping from front to back. Cleansing by perineal irrigation is sometimes advised for both cleanliness and comfort. Unless the physician prescribes a solution, warm water poured from front to back over the incision can be used. A heat lamp with a 60-watt bulb placed 30 cm from the perineum is often used two or three times a day to encourage healing and for comfort. The man must be in a position in which the scrotum is elevated so that the heat strikes the incision. One method is to allow the scrotum to rest on a wide piece of adhesive tape extending from thigh to thigh. Alternately, exaggerated Sims' position (Fig. 63-7, *A*) gives satisfactory wound exposure. After sutures are removed, sitz baths may be used instead of the heat lamp, and they add a great deal to the general comfort of the patient. The man usually remains hospitalized after an open perineal biopsy until the laboratory findings are reported. If he is not hospitalized, he requires instruction in self-care, including signs to report, prevention of infection of the incision, use of heat lamp, and sitz baths.

Testicular smears and biopsy specimens. Smears or biopsy specimens from the testes can be obtained by the needle method or by an incision made through the scrotum. Most often an incision is used. After a local or general anesthetic has been administered, a small incision about 2.5 cm long is made, and a small piece of the testis is removed. A dressing is applied, and postoperative management is similar to that after open perineal prostatic biopsy. Testicular biopsy specimens are sometimes used in evaluation of fertility. If sperm are present in the biopsy tissue but are absent from the semen, absence of the sperm is most often the result of stricture of tubal systems beyond the testes.

Enzyme values. Enzyme values play a role in diagnosis of cancer of the prostate gland. The enzyme tests of most value are phosphatase levels. The phosphatases are secreted in the serum of the tumor mass in the prostate gland and are reflected in changes in the blood chemistry. The phosphatases are labeled as acid or alkaline, depending on the optimal pH. Acid phosphatase usually has a pH of 4.0 to 6.0, while alkaline phosphatase usually ranges between a pH of 8.5 to 9.5.[51] A rise in phosphatase value is indicative of cancer of the prostate gland but is not conclusively diagnostic. Usually the phosphatase values are repeated for reliability, since such events as rectal examination, prostate massage, or recent episodes of fever may cause either an elevation or drop in phosphatase level. Additional studies such as prostatic biopsy are done to confirm the diagnosis.

Screening for endometrial cancer

With the decline of mortality from cervical cancer, greater attention has been directed toward developing mass screening techniques to detect early cancer of the endometrium (uterus). An ideal method for mass screening has not yet been developed, but continued refinement of available methods and development of new methods will probably make it possible for screening for uterine cancer to become part of every woman's health care program. Since women over the age of 50 years are more likely to develop cancer of the uterus, screening of postmenopausal women assumes greater significance.

A variety of methods for screening and diagnosis of uterine cancer are now in use. It is generally agreed that the Pap test is not ideal for detecting uterine cancer. The best results are obtained when cervical aspiration is conscientiously done as part of the Pap test. Variation in the reported rates of accuracy is probably caused by a combination of factors, including the site from which samples are taken, clinical grade of the uterine malignancy, and care exercised in obtaining specimens. Less than one half of women with uterine cancer have an abnormal Pap test at the time of routine screening. Probably the main reason the Pap test is inadequate is that cells rarely exfoliate from the endometrium in the early stages of uterine cancer.

Endometrial cells obtained by *aspiration smear* show malignant changes between 75% and 92% of the time when uterine cancer exists.[12] The aspiration method is popular because of its simplicity. In this method, a small cannula is inserted through the cervix into the uterine cavity and suction is applied by means of a syringe attached to the cannula. The specimen obtained is prepared as for a Pap smear.

The *endometrial biopsy* is similar to a cervical biopsy in that small samples of tissue are obtained with a biopsy forceps. The specimens are taken from several sites of the uterine cavity to increase the chances of obtaining malignant cells. For diagnosis of endometrial cancer, the biopsy method is reported to be 90.6% accurate.[15]

Obtaining endometrial cells by *jet washings* of the uterine cavity is another method for screening and diagnosing cancer of the uterus. The irrigating device is inserted into the uterus, and the uterine cavity is irrigated with about 30 ml of normal saline solution. The normal saline solution containing cells from the uterine cavity is returned by suction into a collecting chamber. The cells are then centrifuged out, stained, and examined microscopically. Studies indicate that washing of the uterine cavity results in obtaining malignant cells in 91.5% of the cases.[15]

Vacuum curettage of the endometrium is still another method used in screening and diagnosis. The procedure and apparatus used are similar to those used in suction curettage for performing an abortion. The cervix is dilated, and the suction tip is inserted through the cervix into the uterus. Suction is applied, and the entire uterine cavity is suctioned to secure specimens. The literature reports small numbers of patients studied using this method, and further study is needed before conclusions can be reached regarding its accuracy as a diagnostic method for cancer.

Dilation and curettage. The most prevalent and preferred method of obtaining endometrial cells for study is dilation and curettage (D and C). Since the entire uterine cavity is "scraped," a large tissue sample is obtained. This makes the likelihood of missing malignant cells minimal. In addition to suspected malignancy, endometrial tissue may be studied for influence of ovarian hormones on the endometrial cells and evaluation of other causes of infertility. D and C is sometimes used for the treatment of excessive or prolonged uterine bleeding. This procedure is often carried out to induce abortion and is frequently used following a spontaneous abortion to reduce the chances of hemorrhage. Occasionally, dilation alone is done to treat dysmenorrhea or to correct a stricture or stenosis of the cervical canal. Most of the procedures used for screening and diagnosis of endometrial cancer require some dilation of the cervix in order to introduce instruments into the uterus.

For a D and C, metal dilators of graduated sizes are inserted into the cervical canal. Once the cervix is dilated, curettes having a sharp surface are used to remove endometrial tissue. The major complications of a D and C are hemorrhage and perforation of the uterus. Perforation is a greater risk during pregnancy because the uterus is much softer than in the nonpregnant state. Preoperative care includes informing the woman what will be done and why and preparing her for anesthesia. She may or may not have a perineal shave done in preparation for the procedure. Most physicians now believe that shaving is not necessary and that the discomfort from regrowth of pubic hair can be avoided.

After a D and C, the woman is observed for excessive bleeding. A perineal pad is placed over the perineum. To ensure that all blood loss will be absorbed by the pad and to add to the woman's comfort, the pad is anchored with a sanitary belt. The amount of bleeding is checked at least every 15 minutes for 2 hours. Thereafter, blood loss is assessed as indicated by the woman's condition, and such observations may need to be made every hour for about 8 hours if active bleeding continues. The blood loss should always be recorded in estimated milliliters. A blood loss of at least 60 ml is required to saturate a perineal pad. It is important to record each pad change as well as blood loss. Any excessive bleeding should be reported to the physician. Vital signs are taken every 15 minutes until the patient is stable.

The woman having a D and C may experience mild cramping postoperatively. Mild analgesics such as codeine sulfate and acetylsalicylic acid are usually ordered to relieve pain. Abdominal pain that is continuous, sharp, and not relieved by analgesics should be reported at once, since this type of pain may indicate perforation of the uterus.

After a D and C, women are observed for voiding; usually, no problems are experienced. Most women are permitted to ambulate as soon as they recover from anesthesia and vital signs are stable; most are discharged on the day following surgery, and some are discharged on the day of surgery. These women can resume most of their normal daily activities, increasing to normal activity in about a week. The degree of activity permitted is partly dependent on the reason for the D and C. Vigorous exercising is discouraged, and the woman is usually told to abstain from intercourse until her return visit to the physician, at which time she is advised as to when intercourse can safely be resumed. The menstrual cycle usually is not upset by a D and C. All vaginal bleeding should disappear in a week to 10 days. Women should be advised to report recurrence of bright red blood or the development of a vaginal discharge with an unpleasant odor.

Ultrasonography

Ultrasonography (ultrasound) has become a useful diagnostic tool for gynecologic problems. It can be used to locate pelvic masses, IUDs, and ectopic pregnancies. The *CT* (computed tomography) *scan* is not widely used but may be helpful in identification of very small lesions.

Endoscopy

The pelvic organs and surrounding tissues can be visualized directly by endoscopy. The procedures by which this can be accomplished are colposcopy, culdoscopy, peritoneoscopy (laparoscopy), and hysteroscopy. Depending on the organs and structures inspected, these methods are valuable for determining the cause of abnormal bleeding, in evaluating the stage of malignancies, and for inspecting organs for size, shape, and position.

Colposcopy is the technique in which a low-power microscope with a light source offers magnifications of 6 to 40 times the visible part of the cervix. The procedure is useful to evaluate women with abnormal Pap tests; to study neoplastic changes in the vulva, vagina, and cervix; and to follow up patients after radiation therapy.

Culdoscopy is an examination in which a culdoscope is inserted through the posterior vaginal vault into the cul-de-sac of Douglas (Fig. 63-11). The fallopian tubes and ovaries can be seen as well as the presence of pus, blood, or other abnormal fluids in the cul-de-sac. If such fluids are observed, the physician may perform a *culdocentesis* by inserting a needle into the site and aspirating a specimen for laboratory study.

Laparoscopy, which has replaced culdoscopy, is a procedure by which the pelvic organs are studied by insertion of a laparoscope through the abdominal wall, which is insufflated with carbon dioxide (Fig. 63-12). A local anesthetic is injected before insertion of the instrument. Laparoscopy is useful in inspecting the outer surfaces of the uterus, the fallopian tubes, and the ovaries for appearance. For example, a tubal pregnancy can be seen. In addition to inspection of the pelvic structures, the laparoscope is used for sterilization by tubal ligation.

Hysteroscopy is the procedure used to inspect the inside of the uterus and sometimes to treat adhesions. The hysteroscope is inserted through the cervix rather than the abdomen. This procedure is contraindicated whenever a pregnancy is suspected.

Most of the procedures used for visualizing the pelvic organs can be performed as outpatient procedures. Since direct inspection by hysteroscopy and laparosco-

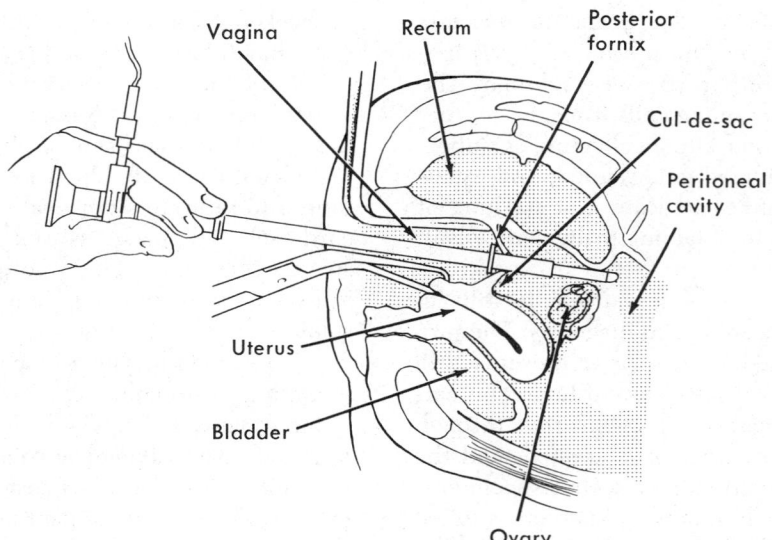

Fig. 63-11. With patient in knee-chest position, culdoscope is inserted through posterior fornix of vagina into cul-de-sac of Douglas. Note that ovaries can be seen.

py are relatively new procedures in gynecology, many patients are hospitalized for the procedure. Maintaining asepsis throughout any of these procedures is important in preventing infection. During the procedures, air may enter the abdominal cavity and cause discomfort. Placing the woman in a prone position with a pillow under the abdomen may decrease discomfort. Douching and intercourse should be avoided for about 1 week following a culdoscopy. Complications such as hemorrhage and infection are rare following these procedures, but women should be cautioned to report fever or pain in the lower abdomen.

Methods most often used for visualization of the male reproductive organs and related structures include cystoscopy and visualization of the seminal vesicles. *Cystoscopic examination* allows the physician to inspect the condition of the urethral and bladder mucosa and to detect prostatic encroachment on the urethra (p. 1515).

Radiographs are used to diagnose obstruction of the seminal vesicles. Two techniques are in use. One method utilizes a specially designed panendoscope through which catheters are passed into the ejaculatory ducts. The second method requires surgical exposure of the vas through an incision in the scrotum and introduction of small plastic catheters into the vas. For both methods, radiographs are taken to inspect the positions of the catheters.

Endocrine studies

Because the endocrine system is so closely related to reproductive function, almost any study for endocrine function may be ordered, for example, thyroid function tests. In women having menstrual problems and in cases of infertility, ovarian function is often studied.

Endocrine studies may include determination of estrogen secretion and estrogen levels in women. Secretion of estrogen in the secretory phase of the menstrual cycle can be estimated by study of the elasticity of the cervical mucus. Quantitative determinations of estriol levels is accomplished by measuring the amount of estriol in a 24-hour collection of urine. The same studies are done during pregnancy to measure indirectly the placental secretion of hormones. All of the urine voided in a 24-hour period is collected in one container and kept cold until it is sent to the laboratory. If the woman is to collect the urine at home, she is provided with a container, told to save all her urine for 24 hours, instructed to keep the urine cold by refrigeration or by

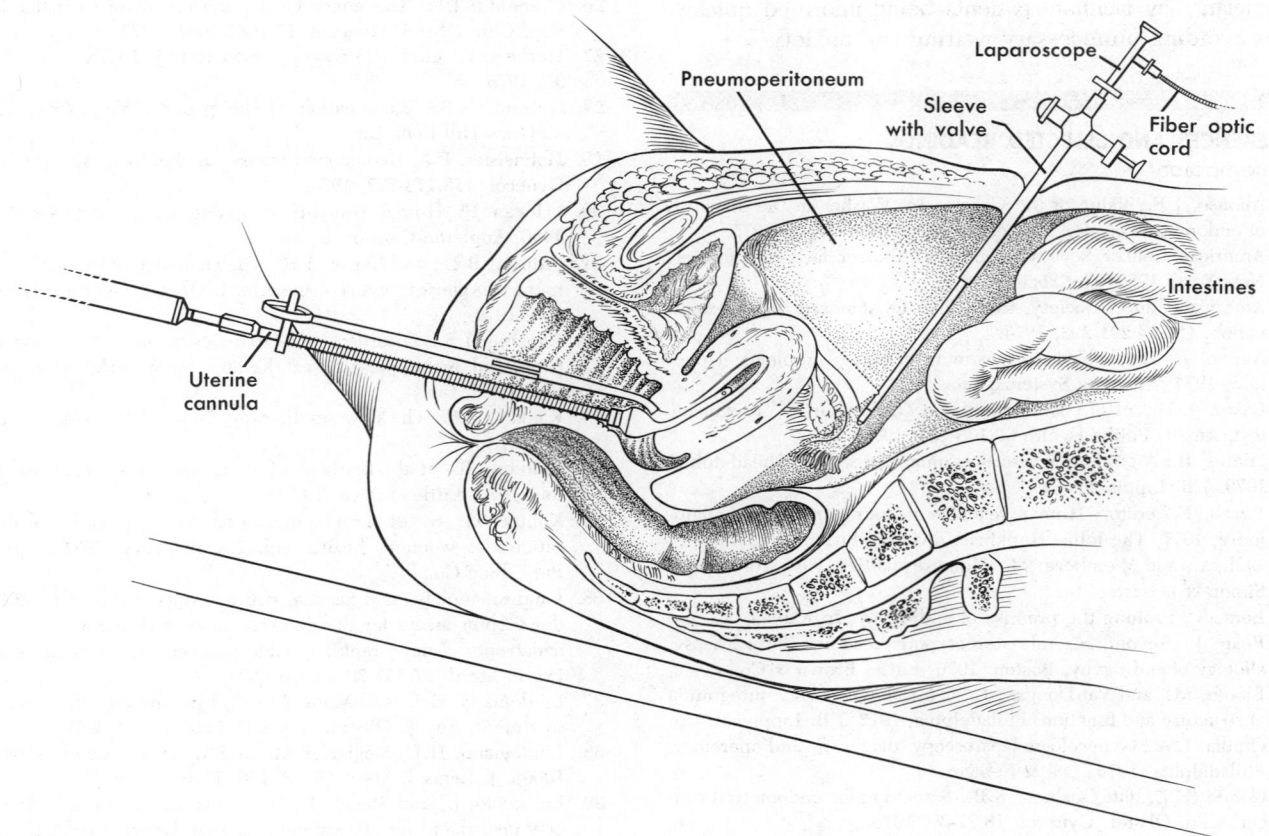

Fig. 63-12. Schema of gynecologic laparoscopy. (From Cohen, M.R.: Laparoscopy, culdoscopy and gynecography: techniques and atlas, vol. 1, Philadelphia, 1970, W.B. Saunders Co.)

surrounding the urine container with ice in a basin, and to bring the urine specimen to the laboratory when the 24 hours elapse.

In addition to infertility, estrogen level determination may be valuable in discovering whether amenorrhea is from pituitary, ovarian, or uterine failure of function. With pituitary or ovarian problems, the estrogen level is low; with uterine problems, the estrogen level is normal. A combination of urinary estriol levels with endometrial tissue studies helps to pinpoint failure of the uterus to respond to estrogen stimulation.

Determination of male hormone levels is sometimes helpful in treating fertility problems. The levels of 17-ketosteroids, pituitary gonadotropins, and corticosteroids may be determined. A 24-hour sample of urine is required, and the procedure for collection is the same as for urinary estriols.

Frequently, men and women show signs of anxiety and depression following diagnostic studies and procedures that necessitate waiting for pathologic reports. Fear about the findings and the possible ways in which sexuality and fertility might be affected is common. Many times, patients are poorly informed and worry needlessly. Nurses can reduce the distress associated with many of these procedures by providing factual information and avoiding hedging. Collaboration with the physician may facilitate patients being informed quickly, thus avoiding unnecessary waiting and anxiety.

REFERENCES AND SELECTED READINGS
Contemporary

1. Alfonso, J.F.: Value of the Gravlee Jet Washer in the diagnosis of endometrial cancer, Obstet. Gynecol. 46:141-146, 1975.
2. American Cancer Society, Inc.: 1981 Cancer facts and figures, New York, 1981, The Society.
3. American Cancer Society, Inc.: Close-up standard breast examination, CA 24:291-293, 1974.
4. Annon, J.: The behavioral treatment of sexual problems, Honolulu, 1974, Enabling Systems, Inc.
5. Baker, L.D., et al.: Evaluation of a "do-it-yourself" pregnancy test, Am. J. Public Health 66:166-167, 1976.
6. *Bates, B.: A guide to physical examination, ed. 2, Philadelphia, 1979, J.B. Lippincott Co.
7. Beach, F., editor: Human sexuality in four perspectives, Baltimore, 1977, The Johns Hopkins University Press.
8. Bell, A., and Weinberg, M.: Homosexualities, New York, 1978, Simon & Schuster, Inc.
9. Bem, S.: Probing the promise of androgyny. In Kaplan, A., and Bean, J.: Beyond sex role stereotyping: readings toward a psychology of androgyny, Boston, 1976, Little, Brown & Co.
10. Bloom, M., and VanDongan, L.: Clinical gynecology: integration of structure and function, Philadelphia, 1972, J.B. Lippincott Co.
11. Cibilia, L.A.: Gynecologic laparoscopy: diagnostic and operatory, Philadelphia, 1976, Lea & Febiger.
12. Cohen, C.J., and Gusberg, S.B.: Screening for endometrial cancer, Clin. Obstet. Gynecol. 18:27-39, 1975.
13. Cohen, M.R.: Laparoscopy, culdoscopy, and gynecography: techniques and atlas, vol. 1, Philadelphia, 1970, W.B. Saunders Co.
14. Comfort, A.: The normal in sexual behavior: an ethological view, J. Sex. Educ. Ther. 2:1-7, 1975.
15. Creasman, W.T., and Weed, J.C.: Screening techniques in endometrial cancer, CA 38(suppl.):436-440, 1976.
16. Curnow, R.N.: The use of additional information in estimating disease risks from family histories, Biometrics 30:655-665, 1974.
17. Dan, A., Graham, E., and Beecher, C.: The menstrual cycle: a synthesis of interdisciplinary research, vol. 1, New York, 1981, Springer Publishing Co.
18. Denis, R., Jr., Barnett, J.M., and Forbes, S.E.: Diagnostic suction curettage, Obstet. Gynecol. 42:301-303, 1973.
19. DePetrillo, A.D., et al.: Gravlee Jet Washer effectiveness as performed by obstetric-gynecologic paramedical personnel, Am. J. Obstet. Gynecol. 117:371-374, 1974.
20. Education and treatment in human sexuality: the training of health professionals: report of a WHO meeting, Geneva, 1975, World Health Organization.
21. Flocks, R.H., and Culp, D.A.: Surgical urology, ed. 4, Chicago, 1975, Year Book Medical Publishers, Inc.
22. Fogel, C.I., and Woods, N.F.: Health care of women: a nursing perspective, St. Louis, 1981, The C.V. Mosby Co.
23. Galask, R.P., Larsen, B., and Ohm, M.J.: Vaginal flora and its role in disease entities, Clin. Obstet. Gynecol. 19:61-81, 1976.
24. *Gillies, D.A., and Alyn, I.B.: Patient assessment and management by the nurse practitioner, Philadelphia, 1976, W.B. Saunders Co.
25. Green, R.: Taking a sexual history. In Green, R., editor: Human sexuality: a health practitioner's test, Baltimore, 1975, The Williams & Wilkins Co.
26. Greenhill, J.P.: The nonsurgical management of vaginal relaxation, Clin. Obstet. Gynecol. 15:1083-1097, 1972.
27. Herbert, P., et al.: Colposcopy: what is it? J.O.G.N. Nurs. 5:29-32, 1976.
28. Hobson, L.B.: Examination of the patient, New York, 1975, McGraw-Hill Book Co.
29. Hofmeister, F.J.: Endometrial biopsy: another look, Am. J. Obstet. Gynecol. 118:773-777, 1974.
30. *Hogan, R.: Human sexuality: a nursing perspective, New York, 1980, Appleton-Century-Crofts.
31. *Kaiser, B.L., and Kaiser, I.H.: The challenge of women's movement to American gynecology, Am. J. Obstet. Gynecol. 120:652-665, 1974.
32. Kaplan, H.S.: Disorders of sexual desire and other new concepts and techniques in sex therapy, New York, 1979, Brunner/Mazel, Inc.
33. Kaplan, H.S.: The new sex therapy, New York, 1974, Brunner/Mazel, Inc.
34. Kolodny, R., et al.: Textbook of human sexuality for nurses, Boston, 1979, Little, Brown & Co.
35. Komnenich, R., et al.: The menstrual cycle: research and implications for women's health, vol. 2, New York, 1981, Springer Publishing Co.
36. Landesmann, R., and Saxena, B.B.: Results of the first 1,000 radioreceptor assays for the determination of human chorionic gonadatropin: a new, rapid, reliable and sensitive pregnancy test, Fertil. Steril. 27:357-368, 1976.
37. Lindemann, H.J., and Mohr, J.: CO_2 hysteroscopy: diagnosis and treatment, Am. J. Obstet. Gynecol. 124:129-133, 1976.
38. Lindemann, H.J., Siegler, A.M., and Mohr, J.: The hysteroflator 1000S, J. Reprod. Med. 16:145-146, 1976.
39. LoPiccolo, J., and Steger, J.: The sexual interaction inventory: a new instrument for assessment of sexual dysfunction, Arch. Sex. Behav. 3:585-593, 1974.
40. *Lytle, N.: Nursing of women in the age of liberation, Dubuque, Ia., 1977, William C. Brown Co., Publishers.

*References preceded by an asterisk are particularly well suited for student reading.

41. *Malasanos, L., et al.: Health assessment, ed. 2, St. Louis, 1981, The C.V. Mosby Co.

42. Mandetta, A., and Gustaveson, P.: Abortion to zoophilia, Chapel Hill, N.C., 1976, Carolina Population Center.

43. Martin, L.: Health care of women, Philadelphia, 1978, J.B. Lippincott Co.

44. Masters, W., and Johnson, V.: Ten sexual myths explored. In Barbour, J.R., editor: Focus: human sexuality 77/78, Guilford, Conn., 1978, Dushkin Publishing Group, Inc.

45. Masters, W., and Johnson, V.: Principles of the new sex therapy, Am. J. Psychol. **133:**548-584, 1976.

46. Masters, W., and Johnson, V.: Human sexual inadequacy, Boston, 1970, Little, Brown & Co.

47. McGowan, L.: Cytologic methods for the detection of endometrial carcinoma, Gynecol. Oncol. **2:**272-278, 1974.

48. McNally, L.K., and Galeener, J.T.: Current practice in obstetric and gynecologic nursing, vol. 1, St. Louis, 1976, The C.V. Mosby Co.

49. *Mims, F., and Swenson, M.: Sexuality: a nursing perspective, New York, 1980, McGraw-Hill Book Co.

50. Money, J., and Erhardt, A.: Man, woman, boy, girl, Baltimore, 1972, The Johns Hopkins University Press.

51. Murphy, G.P.: The diagnosis of prostatic cancer, Cancer **37**(suppl.):589-596, 1976.

52. Novak, E.R., Jones, G.S., and Jones, H.W., Jr.: Novak's textbook of gynecology, ed. 9, Baltimore, 1975, The Williams & Wilkins Co.

53. Pfeiffer, E., Verwoerdt, A., and Davis, G.C.: Sexual behavior in middle life, Am. J. Psychiatry **128:**1262-1267, 1972.

54. Phillips, J.M.: The impact of laparoscopy, hysteroscopy, fetoscopy and culdoscopy of gynecologic practice, J. Reprod. Med. **16:**187-190, 1976.

55. Radioreceptor assay: a new pregnancy test, Am. J. Nurs. **76:**1281, 1976.

56. Schiller, P.: Creative approach to sex education and counseling, New York, 1974, Association Press.

57. Schulman, J.J., et al.: The Pap smear: take two, Am. J. Obstet. Gynecol. **121:**1024-1028, 1975.

58. Silverberg, E., and Holleb, A.I.: Major trends in cancer: 25 year survey, CA **25:**2-7, 1975.

59. Singer, J., and Singer, J.: Types of female orgasm, J. Sex Res. **8:**255-267, 1972.

60. Skydel, B., and Crowder, A.S.: Diagnostic procedures: a reference for health practitioners and a guide for patient counseling, Boston, 1975, Little, Brown & Co.

61. Strand, M.M., and Elmer, L.A.: Clinical laboratory tests: a manual for nurses, St. Louis, 1976, The C.V. Mosby Co.

62. Tovell, H.M.: Cone biopsy of the cervix, Clin. Obstet. Gynecol. **19:**2-15, 1976.

63. Villee, D.B.: Human endocrinology: a developmental approach, Philadelphia, 1975, W.B. Saunders Co.

64. *Watts, R.: Dimensions of sexual health, Am. J. Nurs. **79:**1568-1572, 1979.

65. Webb, M.J., and Gaffey, T.A.: Outpatient diagnostic aspiration curettage, Obstet. Gynecol. **47:**239-242, 1976.

66. *Whitley, M., and Willingham, D.: Adding a sexual assessment to the health interview, J. Psychiatr. Nurs. Mental Health Serv. **5**(4):17-22, 1978.

67. Wilson R.: Introduction to sexual counseling, Chapel Hill, N.C., 1974, Carolina Population Center.

68. *Woods, N.F.: Human sexuality in health and illness, ed. 2, St. Louis, 1979, The C.V. Mosby Co.

Classic

69. Ford, C., and Beach, F.: Patterns of sexual behavior, New York, 1951, Harper & Row, Publishers.

70. Kinsey, A.C., et al.: Sexual behavior in the human male, Philadelphia, 1948, W.B. Saunders Co.

71. Masters, W., and Johnson, V.: Human sexual response, Boston, 1966, Little, Brown & Co.

72. McPhetridge, L.M.: Nursing history: one means to personalize care, Am. J. Nurs. **68:**68-75, 1968.

73. Pfeiffer, E., Verwoerdt, A., and Wang, H.S.: The natural history of sexual behavior in a biologically advantaged group of aged individuals, J. Gerontol. **23:**193-198, 1969.

AUDIOVISUAL RESOURCES

Controversies in laparoscopy, Audio-Digest Foundation, 1250 S. Glendale Ave., Glendale, CA 91205. (Audiotape and slides, module no. 5.)

Laparoscopy—what's new, Audio-Digest Foundation, 1250 S. Glendale Ave., Glendale, CA 91205. (Audiotape and slides, module no. 15.)

The nurse and homosexuality, Concept Media Series on Human Sexuality and Nursing Practice, Concept Media, Inc., 1500 Adams Ave., Costa Mesa, CA 92626. (Filmstrip.)

Operative laparoscopy in gynecology, Materials Utilization Branch, National Medical Audiovisual Center (Annex), Station K, Atlanta, GA 33024. (Film.)

Ovulation, Audio-Digest Foundation, 1250 S. Glendale Ave., Glendale, CA 91205. (Audiotape and slides, module no. 4.)

Physical assessment of the well adult: abdomen, Wiley Biomedical, John Wiley & Sons, Inc., 605 Third Ave., New York, NY 10016. (Audiotape and slides, module V.)

Physical assessment of the well adult: rectum and genitalia, Wiley Biomedical, John Wiley & Sons, Inc., 605 Third Ave., New York, NY 10016. (Audiotape and slides, module VI.)

Physiological responses of the sexually stimulated female in the laboratory; Physiological responses of the sexually stimulated male in the laboratory; Sexual intercourse, Focus International, Inc., 505 West End Ave., New York, NY 10024. (Film.)

Sex in today's world, The American Journal of Nursing Co., Educational Services Division, 10 Columbus Circle, New York, NY 10019. (Film.)

CHAPTER 64

INTERVENTION FOR THE PERSON WITH A REPRODUCTIVE OR SEXUAL PROBLEM

GREER GLAZER

NANCY FUGATE WOODS

ELLA CINKOTA

Although people now discuss reproductive and sexual matters more openly than in the past, many people still find it difficult to ask questions about the reproductive organs and sex. People thus often act on the basis of incomplete information or misinformation received from uninformed sources. This means that many reproductive or sexual problems may be disregarded or treatment may be delayed.

Nurses are in a strategic position to give information based on sound knowledge and can give cues to people indicating willingness to discuss sexual and reproductive matters with them. By listening to people express their thoughts, ideas, beliefs, and attitudes, nurses can assess the extent of their knowledge, can recognize deviations from normal, and can determine needs for help. By treating the topics of sexuality and reproduction in a serious, objective way, nurses can put people at ease and can encourage a climate in which questioning is encouraged.

In some instances people are more comfortable discussing matters related to reproduction and sexuality with someone of their own sex. The woman's movement in particular has emphasized the need for women to better understand their own bodies and has raised questions about the insensitivity of some male physicians to female problems.[7] For this reason female nurses and physicians may be preferred sources of information and other help for some women. Obtaining factual information at an early age may prevent physical, emotional, reproductive, and sexual problems in later years.

Preparation for puberty

Sex education

Sex education begins when a child is born. From that moment on infants begin to experience the self as a sexual being, responding to and absorbing the attitudes of those in the environment. From the way they are touched and handled, infants sense the importance of all parts of the body. They touch themselves and feel and learn from their own exploration and from the responses of others to the exploration. Infants learn from the way they are bathed. Therefore the genitalia should be bathed as carefully and tenderly as the rest of the body, for bathing is perhaps the most important introduction to sex education that the infant receives.

Sex education involves more than teaching the facts of life, for sexuality is the sum total of the self and the experiences of the self. Thus sex education teaches one how to be a responsible human being. As children grow, they experience attitudes and relationships and begin to interact with those around them and with the environment. During these early years the child quite naturally incorporates the attitudes of surrounding persons and starts to behave like them. Since parents are usually the most influential persons to the very young child, it is necessary that they have healthy attitudes to accompany the facts that are needed for teaching children how to live.

Parents often ask nurses questions about sex, and frequently they want to know how and what to teach their children. Nurses not only can help parents understand the anatomy and physiology of the reproductive system but also can help them see the importance of their own attitudes and the importance of how they behave toward each other and how they relate to their children. For example, parents need to understand that young children do not want lengthy explanations but do need direct and truthful answers to questions.

Although many schools have added sex education to their curricula, the subject has aroused much controversy among parents and educators. It is hoped that careful planning with parents about course content will avoid misunderstandings, and it may help parents to learn facts that they need to know before they can teach their children themselves. Thus in addition to teaching parents individually, nurses can work with various community groups. The school nurse and the public health nurse are most likely to have this opportunity, but in small communities any nurse may be asked to help with sex education. Nurses may participate in parent-teacher programs and by using drawings, filmstrips, and films can explain anatomy and the reproductive processes. Nurses may also help others to confront their own feelings, beliefs, and attitudes about sexuality. Church groups as well as organizations such as the Girl Scouts that include courses in sex education and personal hygiene as a part of their programs provide nurses with opportunities to participate in community programs. The school nurse may be asked to help physical education teachers cover course content and sometimes teach or help teach classes in hygiene for children.

Nurses can evaluate articles in daily papers and popular magazines in order to advise parents on the use of this information. Often books for parents can be recommended to help them answer children's questions about sex. Books specifically for children can also be recommended. There are many pamphlets and books on sex education, but only a few can be mentioned here. Most state departments of health supply material. *When Children Ask About Sex,* * *Your Child and Sex: A Guide for Parents,†* and *Sexuality in Childhood and Adolescence‡* are useful references for parents in answering questions about sex and reproduction commonly asked by children. For people contemplating marriage and for adults, *Fundamentals of Human Sexuality§* and *Human Sexuality‖* offer accurate information.

---

*Child Study Association of America, New York, 1974, Child Study Association.
†Pomeroy, W.B.: New York, 1974, Delacorte Press.
‡DeLora, J., Warren, C., and Ellison, C.: Boston, 1980, Houghton Mifflin Co.
§Katchadourian, H., and Lunde, D.: New York, 1980, Holt, Rinehart, & Winston Inc.
‖McCary, J.: New York, 1978, Van Nostrand Reinhold Co.

Sexual activity

In most social organizations the family is the basic unit of society. The family continues to serve the same basic human needs although its structure may vary across cultures and between generations.

Like the family, the institution of marriage is timeless and complex. Traditional monogamous marriages remain the norm, although different forms of marriage and family life-styles are practiced by some people. The communal living group in which people pool their resources and share the responsibilities of family life is one example. Single couples living together as husband and wife is another. Still a different notion is that of renewable marriages in which marriage is on a limited-term contract with an option to renew the contract by mutual consent at the end of a specified time.

Single young people are experiencing a new sense of sexual freedom, and this has led to frequent sexual intercourse for its own sake rather than in association with love and marriage. Studies indicate that sexual behavior patterns are changing. In 1978, 79% of young men and 68% of young women in the United States had sexual intercourse before they reached 19 years of age.* An increasing number of unmarried couples no longer consider marriage as a prerequisite for sexual relationships. There is, among many of these couples, however, a mutual commitment to a love relationship before sexual intercourse. Among many of them there is also contemplation of marriage.

It is advisable for couples planning sexual relationships, marriage, and childbearing to have complete physical examinations, including a serologic test for syphilis (now compulsory in most states). Women should have a pelvic examination. At this time a tight hymenal ring, which could make intercourse difficult, can be dilated or incised, provided this procedure is psychologically and culturally acceptable to both the woman and her partner.

Before marriage the couple can talk freely with their physician, their religious adviser, and particularly with each other concerning the physical, psychologic, and religious implications of sex. It is important that cultural differences be considered and that questions or differences about intercourse and size and spacing of the prospective family be discussed at this time.

Women often ask female nurses about intercourse. Tremendous variation exists in the sexual activity of married couples. With adequate knowledge, patience, and understanding, a couple can find a frequency satisfactory to both. Frequency of intercourse may vary from one or more times a day to once a month or less.

---

*From *The Plain Dealer,* Oct. 4, 1981. From study by Alan Guttmacher Institute of New York.

The frequency normally drops considerably after the first year or two of marriage.

From 25% to 50% of married couples have some difficulty in intercourse, often as a result of worry or guilt feelings related to sex, inability to meet cultural standards for satisfactory intercourse, or fear of an unplanned or unwanted pregnancy. This may result in sexual dysfunction (see Chapter 67). The couple can discuss these problems frankly with a health professional or spiritual adviser, since reassurance and additional sex education may relieve the situation. A few persons may need psychiatric help.

Absence of menstruation (amenorrhea) in the sexually active female who is not practicing effective conception prevention and who has a history of normal menstrual cycles usually indicates pregnancy. It is important to note that conception occurs approximately 14 to 16 days *before* a woman misses her first period. By this time the fertilized ovum has become implanted in the uterus. From the standpoint of healthful embryonic development and the changing health needs of the pregnant woman, it is essential that women become knowledgeable about the importance of health care as soon as pregnancy is suspected. Regardless of the cause of amenorrhea, assistance from a health professional should be sought at once.

Some women may have a slight vaginal discharge following intercourse. If it is irritating, a douche with plain water or with 15 ml of white vinegar to 1 L of water may be used from 1 to 3 hours after intercourse. For marked discharge not alleviated by this means, further advice should be sought. Normally, douches are not needed for cleanliness, and it is inadvisable to douche routinely because excessive douching alters the pH of the vagina and predisposes to acute and chronic infections.

Menstruation

Puberty and menarche

The onset of menstruation in young girls is called *menarche*. Menarche is the external phenomenon used to identify the point of true puberty, the time when reproduction is first possible. The average age of the menarche, which has decreased over the past 100 years, is 12.5 to 12.8 years, with the normal range between 9.5 and 15.5 years. The onset of menstruation occurs at an earlier age in the southern hemisphere. Other factors affecting the onset of menstruation are heredity, health, nutritional status, and weight.[56]

It is not possible to predict the exact time at which the first menstrual period will occur. Menarche is caused by cyclic changes in estrogen levels. In general, most girls experience the following progression of somatic changes several months before the menarche: apocrine and other glandular development, increased diameter of the internal pelvis, growth of the ovaries and uterus, breast enlargement, appearance of pubic hair, and growth of the labia and vagina. Some irregularity in duration of menstrual cycles and in the amount of flow is normal for the first few years. The irregularity is probably caused by the lack of progesterone since progesterone is not produced until ovulation begins. By the age of 18 to 20 years the menstrual cycle usually assumes a rhythmic pattern with minor variations. Theoretically, conception is possible with the menarche, but anovulatory cycles are common during the early years of menstruation.

Normal menstruation

There is normal variation among women in the intervals between menstrual periods. Menstruation occurs on an average of every 28 days, but most cycles occur within a normal range of 26 to 34 days. Sixty percent of women have cycles that normally vary in length by up to 5 days.[59] The menstrual flow usually lasts for 3 to 7 days, with an average of 4 days. The menstrual flow can be divided into 3 phases: premenstrual discharge, major discharge, and postmenstrual discharge. Some women do not experience a premenstrual or postmenstrual flow. The premenstrual flow is initially light, lasting up to 1 or 1½ days and is pink mucoid to dark brown. The major discharge is the heaviest flow, lasts 3 to 5 days, and is bright red. The postmenstrual discharge gradually subsides in up to 2 days and may be pink mucoid, yellow-brown, red, or brown.

Some women have heavier flows than others. Normally, there is a loss of from 30 to 180 ml of menstrual fluid during the period, with an average blood loss of 44 ml (1½ oz). One half to three fourths of the fluid is blood, and the remainder is mucus, fragments of endometrial cells, and desquamated vaginal epithelium. The average woman needs approximately one dozen pads or one dozen tampons for the entire period; however, this is highly variable in relation to both the amount of flow and esthetic concern. Normally, menstrual fluid does not clot unless it is retained in the uterus or vagina for a prolonged time. It is believed that the endometrium produces an anticoagulant that prevents clotting of blood in the uterus. An occasional very small "clot" may occur during the first 24 hours, and this is probably a particle of endometrial tissue. Large clots or pus is never normal in the menstrual flow.

During pregnancy menstruation ceases and then returns within 6 to 8 weeks following delivery, although lactation suppresses the menses for varying periods of time. Unless disease occurs, the menstrual periods recur during adult life until the woman reaches menopause. The pattern of the menstrual cycle may be upset by such things as changes in climate, changes in working hours, emotional trauma, fatigue, exercise, and acute or chronic illness. Any of these factors may alter the lifestyle temporarily and produce change in the menstrual cycle by way of the nerve centers of the hypothalamus that influence the rate and timing of pituitary stimulation of the ovaries. A period that is missed, earlier or later than expected, or shorter or longer than usual is not significant if it occurs for only 1 month. If any of these irregularities continue, a health professional should be consulted.

Before and during menstruation a variety of discomforts may be present, and these are considered normal. Fluid retention, with up to a 5-lb weight gain, is very common. The excess fluid is lost through increased urine production during the first few days after menstruation begins. Slight aching in the lower back, legs, and pelvis, especially on the day of onset of the flow, occurs frequently. A slight tendency toward fatigue during the menses is common, and many women experience a spurt of energy a few days before the period begins. Fatigue, dizziness, and nausea may result from hypoglycemia. Breast changes are also often noticed. These changes are usually noticed before the menses begin and last for 1 to 2 days after the flow starts. They include sensations of tingling, fullness, tenderness, and increase in size of the breasts. Breast changes associated with menstruation reflect the influence of estrogen during the ovarian cycle. Other physical symptoms that some women experience are sweating, weakness, constipation, and diarrhea. Some women note mood changes premenstrually. The exact role of cultural expectations in the cause of premenstrual tension is being explored.

Lower abdominal cramps caused by decreased uterine blood flow and increased contractility of the uterus are often associated with menstruation. Painful menstruation, called dysmenorrhea, is discussed later in this chapter.

Promoting positive attitudes

Menstruation is a manifestation of normal body function and should be treated as such. The "period" and "monthly period" are sensible and accurate terms to use if the individual does not wish to say, "I am menstruating." Because of the negative connotations engendered by such terms as "being sick," "on the rag," or "having the curse," girls and women can be encouraged to avoid using them and to use appropriate terms instead. Some women consider the menstrual periods a time of great inconvenience, perhaps because of inadequate knowledge of the physiology of menstruation, inadequate information about how it is possible to main-

tain usual physical, mental, and social activities, sociocultural conditioning, or in some instances, because of symptoms. Menstruating women have been viewed as dangerous, vulnerable, sick, and contaminated throughout history.

Health teaching

Before engaging in any discussion of menstruation, the nurse first assesses the individual's knowledge and level of understanding. Once this is done, a teaching plan can be designed to meet the specific learning needs of the person. All information can be given in an open, factual manner, but latitude must be allowed for individuals to express their feelings, thoughts, beliefs, and concerns.

Girls and women often want and need information about menstruation. Their understanding may be limited or inaccurate because of word-of-mouth information passed along by peers, parents, and others who are poorly informed. On the other hand, nurses may find women who know about the entire menstrual cycle but have difficulty in accepting it as a normal process. Women need to know the physiology of menstruation. They also need to know what discomforts are normally associated with the menstrual period and what measures can be taken to relieve them. They need to know what signs indicate deviations from normal and what actions to take regarding possible problems.

Nurses are often questioned about methods of sanitary protection during menstruation. Either pads or tampons can be used, depending on which is most comfortable and acceptable. Tampon use has been associated with an increased risk of developing toxic shock syndrome (see Chapter 65). Women should be encouraged to wear pads on their first menstrual day, to use regular tampons instead of super tampons, and to change tampons frequently during their menstrual period. If tampons are of the correct size and are properly inserted, there should be no discomfort when they are worn. If the tampons are not easily inserted or if they produce pain when in place, a health professional should be consulted.

In order to increase knowledge and to reduce fear and anxiety, women can be informed of the events that may temporarily alter the menstrual cycle. However, they also need to be informed of symptoms indicating potential problems so that medical attention can be sought. In order to become knowledgeable about the patterns of their menstrual cycles, women can be encouraged to keep a written record. Establishing this habit makes it possible to predict the onset of the next menstrual period and to determine the range of cycles and duration of flow. Should it be necessary to seek the attention of a health professional for any reason, the date of onset of the last menstrual period (LMP) would be known.

Some women have marked discomfort during menstruation and take a variety of medications to relieve the symptoms. Women can be advised to treat minor discomforts with rest, warmth, and small amounts of acetylsalicylic acid. Use of patent medications and other nonprescribed remedies is discouraged, and women should be urged to seek medical evaluation if discomfort is incapacitating.

Daily bathing and frequent changing of sanitary devices add greatly to comfort and hygiene during menstruation. An unpleasant odor develops when the menstrual flow comes into contact with the air. The sanitary devices can serve as breeding areas for bacteria, and pads or tampons should be changed often to prevent distasteful odors, infection, and toxic shock syndrome. A warm tub bath often relieves slight pelvic discomfort, although many women prefer to take showers during the menstrual period. Cold baths and showers may increase discomfort, but many women use tampons and go swimming during their periods with no ill effects.

Daily activities may be continued for both physical and mental health. If fatigue is associated with menstruation, exercise may need to be modified to provide for additional rest. Fatigue should be avoided, and exercises or activities that are more vigorous than usually practiced can be postponed until after menstruation.

The diets of women of childbearing age are often inadequate, and after reviewing their diets with them, suggestions can be made about ways to make their diets more adequate. Most women experience some fluid retention preceding menstruation, and many notice weight gain that may be controlled to some extent by restricting the intake of salt and other foods high in sodium. Edema from other causes can be ruled out by having the woman observe her weight on a daily basis. If edema is present at times other than the premenstrual and menstrual periods, the woman should be advised to consult a physician. The preceding statements about health counseling in relation to menstruation apply not only to women but to young girls as well, since many of them can benefit from accurate and useful information.

Outcome criteria

As a result of instruction, women can:
1. Gather information about their menstrual cycles.
2. Judge whether their menstrual cycles are normal.
3. Distinguish between occasional irregularity in the menstrual cycle and symptoms indicating problems.
4. If a problem exists:
   a. Seek health care.
   b. Give well-informed answers to questions about their problems.
5. Exercise judgment regarding self-medication and practices of folk medicine.

Investigation of major complaints

Problems related to the menstrual cycle are common. They include a variety of symptoms directly or indirectly related to the pelvic organs and may result from any one or a combination of causes.

Women who seek care because of absence of menstruation (*amenorrhea*), irregular periods, excessive flow, or *dysmenorrhea* should have a complete history taken and a physical examination done. Close questioning about the menstrual periods and sexual activity is important (p. 1616). The history should include use of medication including tranquilizers and hormones, since these often disrupt the menstrual cycle.

A pelvic examination to assess the state of the reproductive organs is essential. If a sexually active woman complains of amenorrhea, a pregnancy test is usually done. Urinalysis, complete blood count, study of cervical and endometrial tissue, hormone assays, or visualization of the pelvic organs may be indicated to determine the cause of the problem.

Dilation and curettage (D and C) is often the method selected for obtaining endometrial tissue for study. In many cases, a D and C is temporarily therapeutic because it removes hypertrophied endometrium. Unless the direct cause of the menstrual problem is found, however, and unless treatment for the cause is instituted, symptoms tend to recur. Women having a D and C should understand the purpose of the procedure and should be urged to remain under medical care even though the D and C has helped the problem (p. 1633).

Dysmenorrhea

Pathophysiology. Uterine pain with menstruation, commonly called "menstrual cramps," is properly termed *dysmenorrhea*. Primary dysmenorrhea usually develops when ovulatory function is established and occurs in the absence of organic disease. It often disappears after pregnancy or by age 25. Secondary dysmenorrhea is painful menstruation caused by organic disease, usually pelvic inflammatory disease, endometriosis, or cervical stenosis, or rarely by a malpositioned uterus. The pain is produced by a high concentration of uterine prostaglandin. Although estimates vary, it is generally believed that greater than 50% of menstruating women have some degree of dysmenorrhea. Studies in industry and schools have shown dysmenorrhea to be the greatest single cause of absenteeism among women.[95] Dysmenorrhea is one of the most common health problems for which women seek treatment.

Dysmenorrhea is commonly described as colicky, cyclic, cramping pain in the lower abdomen. The pain may also be perceived as nagging, dull, and aching, and backache is also commonly present. The pain may occur before the menstrual flow begins or during the first 2 days of the period. Most often the pain begins to subside with the onset of the flow. Many women also experience systemic symptoms of breast tenderness, abdominal distention, nausea and vomiting, headache, dizziness, palpitation, perspiration, and flushing. The systemic symptoms are thought to result from systemic prostaglandin absorption into the bloodstream.[24,47,95]

Dysmenorrhea has most often been attributed to contractions of the uterus, although other factors may be involved. Hormone dysfunctions, infections, displacements of the uterus, endometriosis, stricture of the cervical canal, uterine hypoplasia, psychogenic factors, and constipation have been previously associated with dysmenorrhea. Poor posture and conditions that cause general debilitation, such as poor eating habits, minimal exercise, anemia, excessive fatigue, and chronic illness, are often related to dysmenorrhea. Recent studies strongly suggest the link between prostaglandins and dysmenorrhea. Prostaglandin $F_{2\alpha}$ stimulates the frequency and strength of uterine contractions. Prostaglandin $F_{2\alpha}$ has been found to be up to four times higher in the endometrium during menstruation in dysmenorrheic women. Menstrual fluid of dysmenorrheic women also had prostaglandin levels that were about 70% higher than values for nondysmenorrheic women.[18]

Prevention. Knowledge of predisposing factors resulting in dysmenorrhea is limited. Pathologic conditions resulting in dysmenorrhea cannot always be prevented. Advising women at an early age to maintain good posture, to exercise, and to practice good nutrition has not been found to reduce the incidence of dysmenorrhea. Prevention of pressure on the uterus from a full bladder or constipation can be corrected by teaching.

Positive attitudes can be encouraged, since a woman who regards menstruation as normal is less likely to experience it as an illness. Women who are consistently unable to engage in usual activities because of pain associated with menstruation should be urged to seek health care.

Assessment. Since the degree of pain perceived by individual women is subjective, dysmenorrhea is open to wide interpretation by patients, nurses, and physicians. Some women have minor cramping that they barely notice. Others require use of comfort measures such as decreased activity, local applications of heat, and mild analgesia. Still others are incapacitated and are unable to carry out their usual activities.

Nurses are often asked for practical suggestions to relieve dysmenorrhea. In helping with the immediate problem, an assessment is made to determine whether menstrual periods are in any way abnormal, to discover the degree of pain, and to help the client identify factors that exacerbate or alleviate dysmenorrhea. Once patterns can be identified, counseling the woman about nutrition, exercise, and rest may be appropriate.

Intervention. Treatment of secondary dysmenorrhea is aimed at the organic cause. If no organic cause of dysmenorrhea can be found, the woman is advised to try such measures as rest, moderate exercise, good nutrition, and avoidance of constipation. Local application of heat and mild analgesics are usually prescribed. Aspirin is a prostaglandin antagonist and heat causes vasodilation of blood vessels, thereby increasing the blood flow and relieving ischemia, increasing elimination of the menstrual flow, and decreasing hypertonus of the muscles. Prostaglandin inhibitors such as ibuprofen (Motrin), mefenamic acid (Ponstel), flufenamic acid, and indomethacin (Indocin) have been used successfully to alleviate dysmenorrhea in many women. The woman's individual response to side effects of the medications may affect compliance rates. Oral contraceptives have also been used to suppress ovulation by inhibiting prostaglandin levels.

Nurses can also counsel clients to explore the utility of nonpharmacologic measures such as systematic relaxation, exercise, muscle toning, massage, effleurage, breathing techniques, manual pressure on the abdomen, and orgasm. There are currently several investigations in progress to explore the utility of biofeedback and autogenic training in the treatment of dysmenorrhea.[2,26]

If the uterus is found to be in an abnormal position and can be manually returned to a normal position, a pessary may be inserted for a trial period to learn whether malposition is the cause of dysmenorrhea. Dilation of the cervical canal is done when a cervical stricture is found and thought to be the cause of dysmenorrhea.

Nurses must educate women to facilitate positive attitudes toward menstruation and to provide them with alternative interventions for dysmenorrhea. Women can then choose among the alternatives to select the ones most appealing and helpful.

Outcome criteria for the woman with dysmenorrhea. The woman can:

1. Examine her daily activities and evaluate them for necessary modifications.
2. Identify activities that relieve or aggravate dysmenorrhea.
3. Select from alternative interventions those most useful to her.
4. Explain the rationale for therapy, its expected and side effects, and actions to deal with side effects.
5. Evaluate the effectiveness of therapy.
6. Explain the effects on the reproductive functions of any necessary surgery and carry out prescribed self-care both preoperatively and postoperatively.

Amenorrhea

Amenorrhea (absent menstruation) is classified as primary or secondary. Primary amenorrhea is most often defined as lack of menstruation in a female 18 years or older who has never menstruated. Secondary amenorrhea is usually defined as cessation of menstruation for greater than 3 months in a woman who has had normal menstruation. Temporary amenorrhea, in which one period is missed, may be normal in the event of emotional stress, sudden changes of climate, strenuous exercise, or acute episodes of illness. Prolonged amenorrhea is common among athletes in training. This is thought to be a consequence of hypothalamic suppression. Consequences of prolonged amenorrhea are unknown. Some causes of primary and secondary amenorrhea are summarized in Table 64-1.

Aside from menopause, the most common cause of amenorrhea is pregnancy. In breast-feeding mothers amenorrhea may persist through lactation, leading to the common misconception that breast-feeding is a safe method of contraception.

Women who take oral contraceptives may have amenorrhea for up to 6 months after discontinuing the pill. Amenorrhea is also a consequence of removal of the uterus or removal of both ovaries. Frequently, amenorrhea is a symptom of a problem in the reproductive system such as a congenital defect, dysfunction of the ovaries, or another endocrine disorder. Nutritional anemia, wasting chronic illness such as tuberculosis, and psychogenic factors such as fear of pregnancy or desire for pregnancy may be associated with amenorrhea.

Instruction of girls and women of all ages can do much to encourage them to seek prompt health care in the event of amenorrhea. Knowledge of the conditions under which amenorrhea is normal and abnormal assists women to make better informed judgments about the need for health care. Amenorrhea may be very disturbing to some women and cause concern, fear, and a threat to their self-concept.

Assessment. Early diagnosis and prompt management are necessary if reproductive and genital problems of a more serious nature are to be prevented. Sexually active women need to be urged to see a physician as soon as a menstrual period is missed, since maintaining health during pregnancy is vital for both the mother and the fetus. For those women who do not wish to remain pregnant early diagnosis is important if the least traumatic methods are to be used in terminating pregnancy. Women who suspect their amenorrhea is caused by menopause can be examined to confirm their suspicions. A Papanicolaou (Pap) smear and endometrial tissue studies are necessary if premalignant and malignant conditions are to be diagnosed early.

Intervention. When a woman complains of amenorrhea, the usual complete history is taken and a physical examination is done. It is important to know whether menstruation has ever occurred, especially in young girls. The number of periods missed and whether amenorrhea was present previously are important. Recent use of medications and drugs needs to be determined. Women who have recently discontinued oral contraceptives and drug users[16,20,80] often have menstrual abnormalities, of which amenorrhea is common. Girls over 18 years of age who have not started to menstruate usually have a detailed history and pelvic examination to rule out congenital deformity such as absence of reproductive organs or imperforate hymen. Primary amenorrhea is also less frequently diagnosed by buccal smears to detect chromosomal alterations and by progesterone and estrogen-progesterone withdrawal tests.

Treatment of amenorrhea is dependent on the cause. If a pregnancy is not present, hormone therapy may be required except in women who have recently used oral contraceptives. Cystic disease of the ovaries is usually treated medically. Ovarian cysts and ovarian tumors are usually treated surgically, and some congenital defects can be surgically managed.

Most causes of primary amenorrhea are not amenable to therapy and lead to infertility. Only 20% of the women with primary amenorrhea are capable of men-

TABLE 64-1. Examples of causes of amenorrhea

Etiology	Primary amenorrhea	Secondary amenorrhea
Structural defect	Congenital absence of uterus or vagina	Hysterectomy
	Congenital obstruction (imperforate hymen, cervical stenosis)	
	Testicular feminization	
Ovarian dysfunction	Ovarian malformation	Oophorectomy
	Ovarian tumor	Ovarian cyst or tumor
Anterior pituitary dysfunction	Pituitary tumors	Pituitary tumors
	Panhypopituitarism	Postpartum pituitary necrosis
Systemic disorders		Nutritional disorders (anorexia nervosa, obesity)
		Adrenocortical disease
		Thyroid disease
		Tuberculosis
Other		Stress
		Pregnancy; prolonged lactation
		Medications: oral contraceptives, tranquilizers

struating.[20] These women need extensive counseling to deal with feelings about their infertility, lack of menstruation, and the significance it has to their present and future plans.

Outcome criteria for the woman with amenorrhea. The woman can:

1. State the health team's plan for determining its cause.
2. State what preparations for laboratory tests and clinical studies are necessary and carry out these preparations.
3. Make a decision about treatment when presented with its alternatives, consequences, and risks.
4. Participate in evaluating the effectiveness of treatment.

Abnormal vaginal bleeding

There are different types of abnormal vaginal bleeding. *Menorrhagia* (hypermenorrhea) is prolonged profuse menstrual flow during the regular period. A woman may soak a tampon or pad every few hours for up to 9 days. *Metrorrhagia* is bleeding between periods. *Polymenorrhea* is increased frequency of menstruation, and *dysfunctional uterine bleeding* is abnormal bleeding without any known organic cause.

Abnormal bleeding may be caused by a variety of factors (see box at right). The likely causes of abnormal bleeding differ in women during the childbearing years and in postmenopausal women. Thirty to forty percent of postmenopausal women with abnormal gynecologic bleeding have carcinoma.

Menorrhagia in an adolescent girl may be caused by a blood dyscrasia or an endocrine disturbance. This is called *functional bleeding*. Menorrhagia in adult women may be a symptom of an ovarian tumor, a uterine myoma, or pelvic inflammatory disease.

Abnormal bleeding from the vagina requires immediate medical attention. Any bleeding, even slight spotting, between periods is significant. Metrorrhagia may be a symptom of many disorders, including benign or malignant uterine tumors; pelvic inflammatory disease; abnormal conditions of pregnancy such as a threatened abortion, ectopic pregnancy, or hydatid mole; blood dyscrasias; and bleeding at ovulation caused by the withdrawal of estrogen. The wide use of combined ovarian hormones such as norethindrone to suppress ovulation sometimes causes bleeding at irregular times. When metrorrhagia is present, however, prompt medical examination is indicated even though the cause may not be serious. The cause, not the symptom, must be treated, and nurses have a responsibility to help disseminate this information to all women. Early diagnosis and treatment increase the possibility of cure even when the cause is a malignancy.

CAUSES OF ABNORMAL GYNECOLOGIC BLEEDING DURING THE CHILDBEARING AND POSTMENOPAUSAL YEARS*

Childbearing Years

Pregnancy complications

Anovulation

Oral contraceptives

Intrauterine contraceptive devices

Cervical erosion

Vaginal infections

Vaginal or cervical lacerations

Uterine fibroids (after age 25)

Cervical polyps (after age 25)

Medications: phenoziathines, hypothalamic depressants, anticoagulants, anticholinergics, thiazide diuretics

Systemic disease: hypothyroidism, blood dyscrasias

Psychogenic factors

Endometrial hyperplasia (after age 35)

Endometriosis and adenomyosis (after age 25)

Menopausal years

Carcinoma

Estrogen therapy

Endometrial hyperplasia

Polyps

Fibroids

Coital injuries caused by atrophy

Atrophic vaginitis

---

*From Fogel, C.I., and Woods, N.F.: Health care of women: a nursing perspective, St. Louis, 1981, The C.V. Mosby Co.

Reproductive system and aging process

New scientific knowledge concerning the reproductive system and the aging process is evolving; this knowledge is unbiased by sexism and ageism, unlike most past research. The *climacteric* is the transitional phase between reproductive and nonreproductive ability. Menopause is said to have occurred when there has been no menstrual flow for 1 year (although some women have periods even after 1 year of amenorrhea). During the climacteric, which usually lasts for 1 year to 18 months, there is a gradual decline in ovarian function. The ovaries gradually cease to produce ova and estrogen, and as a result the menses become scanty, irregular, and spaced farther apart. Finally, the menstrual periods stop altogether, and the menopause occurs. Men also have a climacteric, but it is usually less noticeable and occurs at a much older age; some men may never experience the climacteric.

Natural menopause may occur between 35 and 60 years of age with the average age being 51. Factors that have been associated with early menopause are excessive exposure to radiation, hard manual labor, poor general health, breast-feeding, inadequate spacing between pregnancies, frequent spontaneous or therapeutic abortions, and hypothyroidism with severe obesity.[7]

Physiology of menopause

With the climacteric and menopause there is a gradual reduction in fertility. However, the menopause does not mark the end of active sexual life. In fact, an active sex life appears to maintain pliability of the vaginal tissue. Since sexual function is not dependent on the release of ova or hormones, women can enjoy sexual activity during the climacteric and after the menopause. Men, too, often continue a fairly active sex life after many signs of normal aging such as hypertrophy of the prostate gland have occurred. Among women, changes are most striking in the vagina, in which the loss of estrogen results in a thinned, easily traumatized epithelium. The vagina loses its elasticity and becomes shorter and narrower because of the increased submucosal connective tissue. Vulvar changes also occur as evidenced by flattening of the labia, thinning of pubic hair, and shrinkage of the introitus.[45] These changes may lead to dyspareunia (painful coitus).

The menopause may be artificially induced by such procedures as irradiation of the ovaries, surgical removal of both ovaries, or hysterectomy. Each of these has one common consequence, namely, cessation of menstruation. Beyond this, however, differences occur. Since the menopause is induced by cessation of ovarian function, surgical removal of both ovaries results in menopause with all its physiologic changes. When the uterus is removed but the ovaries are left in place, menstruation ceases, but the ovaries continue to function provided the age of climacteric has not been reached.

Clinical picture

During the climacteric many women experience hot flashes (flushes), which are felt as waves of warmth accompanied by flushing of the skin, especially the face, neck, and arms and perspiration. The hot flash is the perception of the spread of heat from an anatomic point of origin on the body to other areas of the body. Hot flashes may be so mild that they are hardly noticed or

so severe that they produce distress. Situations of increased heat production such as exercise, excitement, eating, drinking alcoholic beverages, impairment of heat loss in hot weather, or excessive clothing may provoke hot flashes. Hot flashes last seconds to minutes, ranging from 0.5 to 60 minutes. Many women go through the climacteric with little awareness of its occurrence.

Intervention

Guidance and support. Most women have heard of the "change of life." The negative image of menopause is reinforced by the media, books, health professionals, and the general public. Depending on the climate in which they were reared and on their own changes in attitude toward normal functions of the reproductive organs, women may feel more or less free to discuss the menopause and their feelings and concerns during this period of life. Since many problems related to the reproductive organs occur in this age group, and since it is important for mental health that women be helped to make the menopause as comfortable as possible, it is important for nurses to identify women who can profit from interventions.

Education regarding the menopause should precede its onset. Understanding human behavior and the emotional impact cessation of reproductive ability may have and skill in using direct and indirect approaches assist in establishing a climate that permits open, honest discussion. Many women appreciate openings made by nurses to discuss the menopause. Women approaching the menopause, regardless of whether it is an event of normal aging or is artificially induced, need to know what the menopause is, why it occurs, the effects menopause has on reproductive and sexual ability, what can be done to make the menopause more comfortable, and what symptoms require medical attention. Anatomic teaching aids are usually useful. Publications that the patient can read may be very helpful and include *Our Bodies Ourselves,* The Menopause: A Positive Approach,†* and *Menstruation and Menopause.‡*

Some women feel they are less attractive after than before menopause. Moderate exercise to maintain muscle tone is beneficial to both health and physical appearance. Advice regarding diet to control weight is appreciated by many women. Feelings of depression and uselessness are common among women, particularly those who have been highly invested in the maternal role. Men sometimes have feelings of depression and uselessness if they perceive a decline in sexual and other abilities. They require the same explanation as women regarding what is happening to them and what

---

*Boston Women's Health Book Collective: New York, 1980, Simon & Schuster, Inc.
†Reitz, R.: Philadelphia, 1979, Chilton Book Co.
‡Weideger, P.: New York, 1976, Alfred A. Knopf, Inc.

they can do to maintain a healthful attitude and productive life. Peer support groups during menopause may be helpful.

Many men and women have heard of "change of life babies" and fear they may become pregnant during the menopause. When counseling menopausal women about contraception, it is important to remember that the menstrual cycles and ovulation are irregular and that if pregnancy is to be prevented a highly reliable contraceptive method is necessary. Contraception should be used for 1 year following a woman's last menstrual period. The rhythm method is unreliable during the menopause, because the menstrual cycles are irregular. There are some advantages to oral contraceptives during the menopause. They give excellent protection against pregnancy at an age when pregnancy is usually not desired, when pregnancy is more dangerous to the woman from an obstetric viewpoint, and when some types of fetal anomalies are more likely to occur. On the other hand, greater mortality as a result of thromboembolus and a higher incidence of cancer have been linked to the use of oral contraceptives at older ages. Therefore, when counseling about a contraceptive method, it is necessary to assess the chances of pregnancy occuring, the risks pregnancy might carry, alternatives should pregnancy occur, and the chances of a woman being able to successfully use an alternate method.

Because the incidence of cancer of the uterus and cancer of the prostate gland is higher in menopausal men and women, they should be urged to have physical examinations including screening for cancer at least once a year. All women should be advised that bleeding after the menopause, menstrual periods that become increasingly heavy, and contact bleeding noted after douching or intercourse require the attention of a health professional.

Relief of symptoms. Approximately 10% of women have pronounced symptoms during the menopause. Vasomotor reactions producing hot flashes and excessive perspiration may occur and are associated with lack of estrogen, increased luteinizing hormone (LH), increased prostaglandins, and high levels of follicle stimulating hormone (FSH).[9,15,49,64] Although other symptoms may occur, only the thinning of the vaginal mucosa and vasomotor spasms can be linked directly to hormonal changes. There is very little doubt that osteoporosis is related to estrogen deprivation. Other symptoms thought to be related to estrogen decrease are urinary frequency, painful urination, joint and muscle pain, and cardiovascular disorders.

VASOMOTOR REACTIONS. Most often estrogen is prescribed for the relief of hot flashes. Other natural methods reported to almost equal the effectiveness of estrogens in relieving hot flashes are vitamin E and ginseng.[72] The B-complex vitamins have also been used successfully to alleviate hot flashes. Vitamins E and B complexes can be added to the diet or taken by supplementation. Dietary sources of vitamin E are vegetable oils, soybeans, spinach, peanuts, and wheat germ. Good dietary sources of vitamin B complexes are whole grains, brewer's yeast, wheat germ, yogurt, liver, and milk.[87]

VAGINAL DISCOMFORT AND INFECTION. Women may have pain during intercourse (dyspareunia) because of thinning of the vaginal mucosa. This condition is most often treated by local application of a vaginal cream. Vaginal estrogens are absorbed in much greater amounts than when given systemically; thus they must be used with caution. Vitamin E has been effective over time in alleviating dryness of vaginal tissue.

Vaginal infections are common among women experiencing the menopause because of the lack of estrogen, which causes the vaginal secretions to become more alkaline. Women need to know the signs of vaginal infections and when to consult a physician. Such vaginal infections are treated according to the causative organism but frequently respond to vinegar douching. The best results from douching are achieved while lying in a bathtub rather than sitting on a toilet seat. The douche tip is inserted upward and backward and moved about to prevent fluid from being forced into the cervix and to ensure flushing of the posterior vaginal vault. For a vinegar douche, 30 ml (approximately 2 tbsp) of white vinegar is diluted in 2 L of warm water (40° C [105° F] unless otherwise ordered). If a medicated or hot douche is to be used, the labia are held together for a few minutes to allow the vagina to fill and thus benefit all areas.

Skeletal system changes. Estrogen decrease causes a negative nitrogen balance and muscle is replaced by fibrous tissue. About 25% of postmenopausal women develop osteoporosis. An imbalance in the calcium-phosphorus ratio may be the most significant factor in the development of osteoporosis. The phosphorus excess may be related to eating foods high in phosphorus, such as soft drinks, bread, and cereal, and to the reduced ability of older adults to absorb calcium from the intestines. Diets high in protein can cause bone loss and should be avoided. Increased calcium is removed from the bones to buffer the high nitrogen levels resulting from protein metabolism. Some rarely eaten foods that contain considerable calcium but no phosphorus are sesame seeds and seaweed. Turnip greens are a good source of calcium. As with other menopausal problems, changes in the skeletal system are usually treated with estrogen.

Estrogen therapy. Estrogen therapy during the menopause has long been in use, and over the years there has been much debate over the advantages and disadvantages of this therapy. Studies suggest that administration of estrogens to postmenopausal women is associated with an increased risk of endometrial cancer.[3,42,74,96] Since estrone, which has been linked to endometrial cancer, is made in adipose tissue of menopausal women, some persons feel that other types of synthetic estrogens such as estriol or estradiol preparations should be used in estrogen replacement therapy.[57]

In considering the benefits and risks of estrogen therapy, certain information is valuable. A study investigating the extent of estrogen use during the menopause suggests that estrogens are sometimes prescribed for trivial reasons and that estrogens are likely to be used by women for an extended time.[12] Only 26% of the women studied reported problems with hot flashes before therapy, yet 51% had taken estrogen for more than 3 months; the median period of estrogen use was 10 years.

The latent effects of estrogen therapy have caused some concern about the association of estrogen and uterine cancer.[68] Use of estrogens for treatment of the menopause became popular in the early 1960s. The latency period for human carcinogens is generally accepted to be about a decade. It is therefore possible that the results of years of estrogen treatment of the menopause are just beginning to emerge.

Whether estrogen should be used for prevention and management of osteoporosis in postmenopausal women is also being debated. It is believed by some people that estrogens may retard bone resorption temporarily[15,51] but that later reverses in bone formation may negate or reverse gains made by estrogen therapy.[5,15] Many people, however, feel that there is a permanent beneficial effect.

It has been suggested that when estrogen is used for relief of menopausal symptoms it should be administered in a cyclic manner, with the woman taking estrogen for 3 weeks and then abstaining from medication for 1 week.[68] Some health professionals are encouraging the use of a progestin during the last week to initiate shedding of the endometrial lining because of the association of endometrial hyperplasia with atypical adenomatous hyperplasia.[20] In general, it is desirable to use the lowest dose possible to relieve symptoms, with the eventual goal of gradual and complete withdrawal of medication. Absolute contraindications to estrogen replacement therapy are gallbladder, liver, cerebrovascular, and pancreatic disease; sickle cell anemia; and a history of myocardial infarction, deep vein thrombosis, pulmonary embolism, and estrogen-dependent tumors of the uterus and breasts.[38]

During estrogen therapy women should be seen at least every 6 months for examination and for review of menopausal symptoms. The examination should include the breasts and reproductive organs, Pap smear, and blood pressure.

Outcome criteria for the person experiencing menopause. As a consequence of health management during menopause, men and women can:

1. Make informed decisions about birth control.
2. Consider the possible consequences and alternatives if pregnancy occurs.
3. State the signs of menopause and self-care actions to safely maximize their comfort.
4. In the event that a health practitioner is consulted regarding problems of menopause, state the treatment regimen, its purpose, and anticipated results.

Family planning and contraception

Overpopulation and world hunger have become problems of such magnitude that they affect every living being. Ecologic insights force us to look at life and our environment in a different way than in previous decades. We now know that we have few choices left if we are to survive on this planet. Beyond the question of survival are questions of quality of life. Thus birth control and family planning not only become matters of personal concern but also take into consideration the rights of others.

For the first time in the history of humankind it is now possible to regulate conception with a high degree of reliability. During the past 20 to 30 years there has been a sharp decline in the birth rate in the United States and similarly developed nations. This drop is attributed to widespread use of highly effective fertility and birth control methods and new techniques for performing abortions and sterilizations.

Contraception remains a controversial issue. The incentives and imperatives for separating sexual and reproductive functions have been widely discussed from the standpoint of medical care, sociology, psychology, demography, economics, theology, and the law. Prevention of the birth of unwanted children and prevention of illness are two of the themes addressed pro and con in the literature.

Regardless of the personal and global issues involved, individuals and couples are required more than ever before to examine the consequences of their actions and to select from among the various alternatives the one most consistent with their beliefs, needs, and sense of responsibility. Bound into these issues and pressures for individual responsibility are controversies surrounding the use of particular methods of conception prevention, advantages and disadvantages of methods available for birth control, and the problems incurred by the use of individual methods of preventing pregnancy.

Mortality associated with the use of various methods of birth control has received much attention through the years. Reports continue to be made indicating that very low rates of mortality are associated with all *reversible* methods of fertility control as compared with mortality associated with pregnancy and childbirth.[83] The view that any type of contraception is better than pregnancy needs to be qualified because maternal mortality is influenced by a woman's health and socioeconomic status before becoming pregnant. Mortality reported for tubal ligation and hysterectomy for sterilization of women is higher than for any other form of birth control. However, these rates are still lower than mortality during pregnancy and childbirth. The mortality from hysterectomy is considerably higher than that for tubal sterilization. Hysterectomy is often an acceptable method to women who would not undergo tubal ligation for religious reasons but wish to terminate their ability to conceive. No mortality from vasectomy is reported in the literature.

Counseling of individuals and couples

People choose a method of preventing pregnancy for reasons other than risk to health or life. These reasons include effectiveness, convenience, reversibility, ethical considerations, cost, life-style, and noninterference with enjoyment of sexual intercourse. Much of the literature is devoted to the concerns of risk to health and life and very little to other factors, including risks attended by reproduction.

In order for people to make a fully meaningful and responsible choice, they need to be informed of all advantages and disadvantages of all methods or combinations of methods available for preventing pregnancy. With the flood of publicity in the media, especially regarding congressional hearings and actions, considerable anxiety and confusion on the part of the public has resulted. Usually the publicity is directed toward one aspect of health risks associated with one method of conception control, and the risks are not presented in comparison with risks associated with pregnancy and childbirth. In addition, certain biases are inherent in the lay and professional literature regarding which forms of contraception are most desirable. Many family planners have biased their responses about contraceptive effectiveness largely in favor of oral contraceptives and the intrauterine device (IUD). This biased approach dissuades people from using diaphragms, foam, condoms, and fertility awareness methods of conception control.[84] However, there seems to be a growing trend toward the lower risk methods. Thus health professionals are given the task of fitting pieces of information together to form a whole picture with meaning and perspective and of presenting the total block of information to persons seeking information, advice, and help.

Individuals who use a reversible method of birth control and then decide to change have two alternatives: they can choose an alternate method or not use any method of birth control. When the second alternative is chosen, pregnancy is very likely. Pregnancy then may lead to either an abortion or continuation of the pregnancy resulting in the birth of an unplanned child. It is therefore important that information be fully given, including risks to health and life and risks of pregnancy. Only in this way can people make an intelligent judgment of the risks they are willing to take and assume responsibility for their actions.

One of the greatest responsibilities of nurses is to assist sexually active people in making decisions regarding contraception, childbearing, and pregnancy spacing in a well-informed manner. Experience has shown that, on an individual basis, the best method of contraception is one that is acceptable and comfortable to both sexual partners, readily available, convenient and easy to use, effective and safe, and inexpensive, that does not interfere with the enjoyment of the sex act, and that will be used consistently and correctly. These factors should be explored with persons seeking assistance with birth control.

People are usually more concerned with effectiveness than any other factor when deciding among contraceptive methods. Before discussing effectiveness rates, the nurse must recognize the two types: theoretical effectiveness and actual use effectiveness. *Theoretical effectiveness* is the effectiveness of a method when used correctly, without error, and according to instructions. *Actual use effectiveness* takes into consideration those who use the method correctly and those who use it incorrectly. The theoretical and actual use effectiveness rates of reversible contraceptive methods are given in Table 64-2. Both types of effectiveness rates must be presented to people when providing contraceptive counseling.

Changes in the technology of contraceptives will change theoretical effectiveness rates in the future. Actual use effectiveness rate of a given contraceptive method may be lowered by the following factors: fear of the method, difficulty in remembering to use the method, past unsuccessful attempts with the method, inability to use the method as counseled, unanswered questions or concerns, cost, side effects, complications, embarrassment, or inconsistency with personal beliefs.

In many clinics nurses take an active role in managing birth control programs. The nurse's role includes history taking, physical examination, counseling, and evaluating the effectiveness of various methods of birth control during follow-up visits. In some settings nurses in extended roles prescribe the method of birth control. Outside of these settings nurses have many opportunities to seek out individuals and couples in need of birth control information.

Counseling individuals or couples regarding birth control goes beyond teaching them how to use a method correctly. If couples are to accept responsibility for conception control, the nurse needs to assess the extent to

TABLE 64-2. Reversible method effectiveness of contraceptives: theoretical and actual use rates*†

Method	Theoretical effectiveness	Actual use effectiveness
Abstinence	0	?
Oral contraceptive (combined)	0.34	4-10
IM long-acting progestin	0.25	5-10
Condom and spermicidal agent	<1	5
Low-dose oral progestin	1-1.5	5-10
IUD	1-3	5
Condom	3	10
Diaphragm (with spermicide)	3	17
Spermicidal foam	3	22
Spermicidal suppository	3	20-25
Coitus interruptus	9	20-25
Calendar	13	21
Basal body temperature	7	20
Basal body temperature with no intercourse before ovulation	1	—
Cervical mucus	2	25
Douche	?	40

*Adapted from Hatcher, R.A., et al.: Contraceptive technology, 1980-1981, ed. 10, New York, 1980, Irvington Publishers, Inc.
†This table provides the percentage of women who would become pregnant within 1 yr following initiation of use of the various contraceptive methods.

which misunderstanding, superstition, and fear exist and to take action by presenting facts about reproduction as well as facts about contraceptive methods. For example, lay people sometimes confuse contraception, which is temporary and reversible, with sterilization, and the differences need to be pointed to them.

People may have many questions about contraception, and the nurse can anticipate some that are frequently asked:
1. What methods are most effective in preventing pregnancy?
2. How safe are the available methods? Will they harm the couple, the individual, or a future child?
3. Will contraception interfere with sexual intercourse in any way?
4. Do the methods hamper or prevent later desired pregnancies?
5. How convenient are the different methods?
6. What is the cost of different methods?

Often nurses must initiate the discussion of conception control, although this is now a commonly expressed concern of clients. In many instances women who are hesitant to pose questions about birth control are relieved when nurses indicate that this is an acceptable concern.

Direct or indirect questions may be used to initiate discussions. Questions may be more direct; that is,

"Would you like help in planning your family?" "Do you want help in preventing pregnancy before you are ready for another child?" "Do you want information about birth control?" Also questions can be posed more indirectly and individualized for the patients' circumstances.

Pamphlets can be placed where patients have access to them, and this often gives the nurse a cue to the patient's interest. To verify this the nurse might say, "I noticed you looking at this pamphlet. What information or help can I give you?"

The various methods of contraception, their actions, effects, and contraindications are summarized in Table 64-3. Showing persons the actual birth control methods (Fig. 64-1) is valuable. Audiovisual materials such as *Family Planning Series** are very useful in giving individuals and couples information about methods of birth control.

The records of hospitalized patients are a source of information regarding the patient's history, physical condition, and reason for current hospitalization. The medical and nursing records should be reviewed before the nurse offers assistance with birth control and family planning.

During the interview and physical examination, the patient's reliability should be assessed. Ability to recall facts or to give information readily may give clues as to the most reliable method for the patient. For example, a woman who states she is taking vitamins but often forgets them, or a woman who when questioned about self-medication states she hates taking pills or does not believe in medicines, may not be the best candidate for oral contraceptives. Although judgment about reliability needs to be reserved until follow-up visits reveal a repeated pattern of missed pills, the initial interview will alert the nurse to question the woman carefully during future visits.

Physical examination is directed toward discovering conditions that indicate which methods of contraception should not be used and why. During the examination, opportunities for health teaching arise, and the nurse can take advantage of these. All women seeking assistance for conception prevention should have a Pap test and breast examination and should be encouraged to have an annual physical examination. In addition, serology and cervical smears and cultures are usually taken to detect infections, and individuals can be instructed at this time about how to prevent infection, how to recognize infection, and the need for medical care when infection occurs.

Finally, it is especially important that the woman's value system is respected even though it may not be congruent with that of the health provider. The decisions

*Milner Fenwick, Inc., 3800 Liberty Heights Ave., Baltimore, MD 21215.

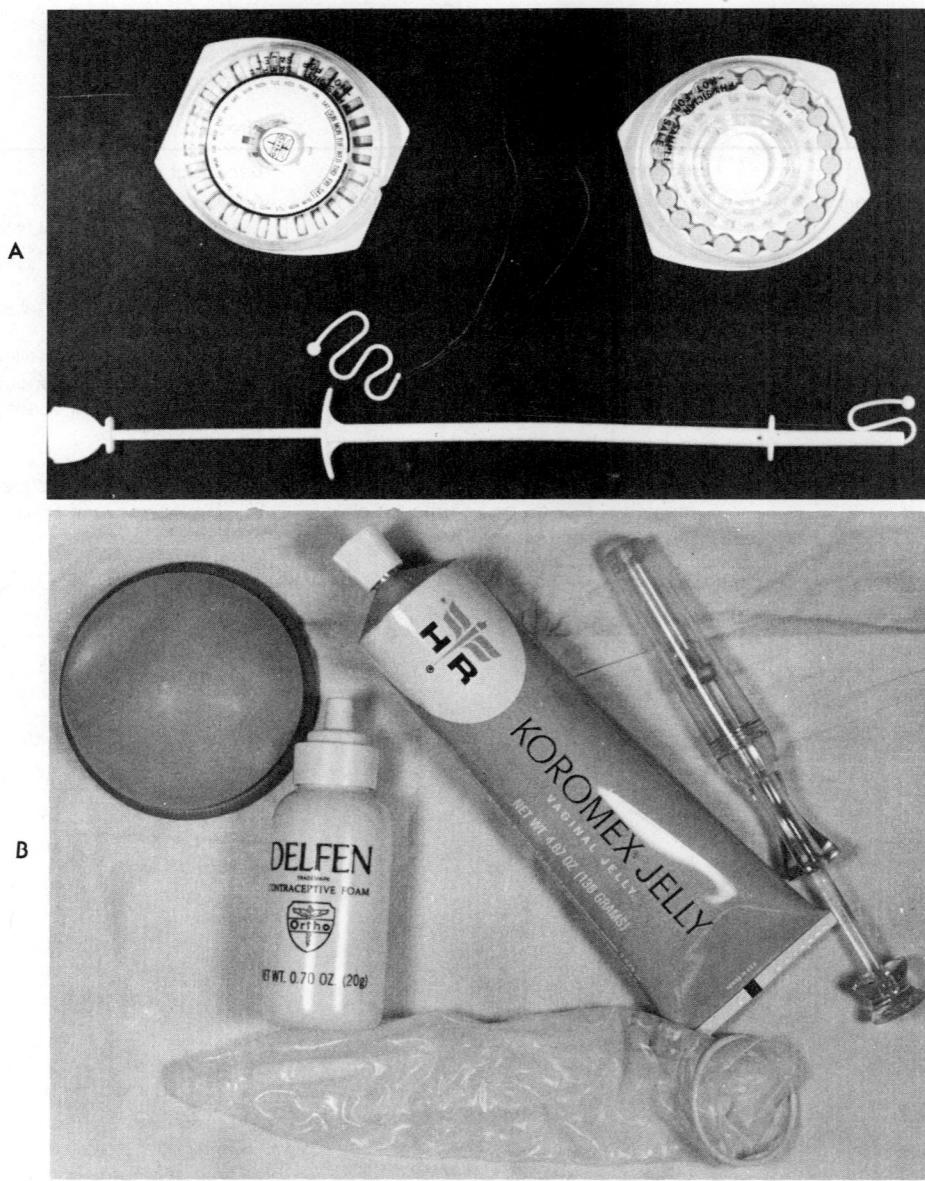

Fig. 64-1. A, Two types of oral contraceptives and Lippes loop with applicator. **B** *(left to right),* Diaphragm, contraceptive foam for vaginal application, contraceptive jelly and vaginal applicator, and condom.

regarding family size need to be made by the woman, not by the health professional.

Methods of contraception

When assisting people to select a method of birth control, personal beliefs and biases must be avoided. The nurse's personal opinions about preferred methods may be dangerous to the patient's health and may force the patient to follow a practice not really desired, and this in turn may result in the pregnancy the patient wishes to avoid. Information should be given about each method, how the method works, the degree

of protection against pregnancy provided by the method, self-care requirements, side effects of the method, contraindications to use, and the need for follow-up care (Tables 64-2 and 64-3). Information is repeated in the same way for each method. Once the person has selected a method, information about that method is reviewed again. The person should then demonstrate a complete understanding of the chosen contraceptive method.

Hormonal contraceptives. It has been estimated that 25 to 50 million women worldwide are using oral contraceptives ("the pill"), including 5 to 8 million women

TABLE 64-3. Summary of major reversible methods of conception control

Method	Action	Effects

Hormonal contraceptives
 	
Combination pill (estrogen and progestin)
IM long-acting progestin
Low-dose oral progestin
(minipill)
	Estrogenic effects
	Inhibit ovulation by suppression of pituitary FSH and LH
	Inhibit implantation by antiprogestational effect on uterus with high doses
	May accelerate ovum transport
	Prevent normal implantation and placental attachment by causing degeneration of corpus luteum and decreasing serum progesterone levels
	
	Progestin effects
	Produce hostile cervical mucus, hampering transport of sperm and decreasing ability of sperm to penetrate cervical mucus
	May inhibit implantation by altering FSH and LH peaks
	May inhibit ovulation via subtle disturbance in hypothalamic-pituitary ovarian functioning
		Beneficial effects
		Combination pill
		  Relief of premenstrual tension
		  Regulation of menstrual cycles
		  Relief of acne (80-90%)
		  Increased sex drive
		  Improved feeling of well-being
		  ↓ Incidence of functional ovarian cysts
		  ↓ Fibrocystic breast disease and breast fibroadenomas
		Pill and IM progestin
		  ↓ Incidence of iron deficiency anemia
		Pill, IM progestin, and minipill
		  Relief of dysmenorrhea (60-90%)
		  ↓ Amount of blood and number of days of bleeding
		
		Fairly minor side effects
		Pill
		  Nausea
		  ↑ Incidence of yeast infection
		  Chloasma
		Pill and IM progestin
		  Weight gain
		  Mild headache
		  Mood changes
		  Depression
		IM progestin
		  Decreased libido
		Pill, IM progestin, and minipill
		  Spotting
		  Missed periods
		
		Serious side effects
		Pill
		  Hypertension
		  Gallbladder disease
		  Thromboembolic disorders

IUDs
 	
Lippes loop
Saf-T-Coil
Copper-7
Copper-T
Progestasert-T
	Unknown
	Suggested mechanisms
	  ↑ Mobility of ovum in fallopian tube
	  Local foreign body inflammatory response preventing implantation and/or causing lysis of blastocyst
	  Immobilization of sperm
	  Inhibition of implantation by ↑ local prostaglandin production
	  Mechanical dislodging of implanted blastocyst
	  Copper may interfere with estrogen uptake and its intracellular effects on endometrium
		Spotting
		↑ Amount of blood and length of bleeding: hemorrhage, irregular menstrual flow
		Anemia
		Cramping pain
		May expel IUD
		Uterine perforation or embedding
		Cervical perforation
		Pelvic inflammatory disease: endometritis, salpingitis, oophoritis, peritonitis, tubo-ovarian abscess, sepsis

Condom Thin, comfortable plastic sheath worn over penis	Mechanical barrier to prevent transmission of semen into vagina	Reduced glans sensitivity Protection against transmission of venereal disease Possible prevention of cancer of cervix

Absolute contraindications	Strong relative contraindications	Other relative contraindications
All hormonal contraceptives	**Combination pill**	**Combination pill**
History of CVA, coronary artery disease, hepatic adenoma, malignancy of breast or reproductive tract, thromboembolic disorder	Diabetes mellitus or strong family history of diabetes	History of cardiac or renal disease
	Elective surgery within 4 wk	Unreliability to follow instructions (e.g., mental retardation)
Impaired liver function	Fibrocystic breast disease or breast fibroadenomas	History of taking pills incorrectly
Pregnancy	Gallbladder disease, cholecystotomy	Irregular menstrual cycle, infertility
Undiagnosed abnormal vaginal bleeding	Hypertension with resting diastolic pressure > 110	Lactation
	Long leg casts	Use with caution if history of depression, hypertension with resting diastolic pressure 90-100, asthma, epilepsy, acne, uterine fibromyomata, varicose veins, hair loss related to pregnancy
	Mononucleosis, with acute phase over age 35	
	Previous cholestasis during pregnancy	
	Severe vascular or migraine headaches	
	Sickle cell disease	
	Term pregnancy terminated within past 12-14 days	
Acute pelvic infection	Pelvic infection (recent or recurrent)	Cervical stenosis
Pregnancy	Acute cervicitis or vaginitis	Small or bicornuate uterus
Gonorrhea (known or suspected)	History of ectopic pregnancy	Endometriosis
	Valvular heart disease	Fibromyomata
	Abnormal Pap test	Endometrial polyps
	Cervical or uterine malignancy or premalignancy	Severe dysmenorrhea or menorrhagia (Progestasert-T may be helpful)
	Diabetes mellitus	Anemia
	Steroid therapy	Abnormal uterine bleeding
	Anticoagulant therapy	Psychologic or intellectual inability to check for danger signals
		Multiple sex partners
Allergy of either partner to rubber	None	Psychologic inability to enjoy intercourse
Inability of man to obtain an erection		

Continued.

TABLE 64-3. Summary of major reversible methods of conception control—cont'd

Method	Action	Effects
Diaphragm (with spermicide) Rubber dome attached to flexible metal ring; inserted into vagina to cover cervix	Mechanical barrier to ↓ contact between semen and cervix Spermicide kills sperm	Bladder pressure, pelvic discomfort, urethral irritation, urinary retention, uterine cramps May protect against sexually transmitted diseases May have some protective effect against development of cervical dysplasia Provides barrier to menstrual flow during intercourse
Chemical contraceptives: spermicides Foam, jelly, cream, suppository applied inside vagina by means of plunger-type applicator	Chemical immobilizes and kills sperm Contains medium to hold spermicide in vagina against cervix—mechanically blocks cervix and prevents entry of sperm	May irritate genitalia Unpleasant taste Foam decreases transmission of gonorrhea and trichomoniasis Provides vaginal lubrication
Fertility awareness Calendar method Basal body temperature Cervical mucus	Sexual abstinence around time of ovulation	↑ Understanding/appreciation of own body Frustration May have lack of sexual gratification during abstinence if other lovemaking techniques not used

in the United States. Twenty to forty percent of women of childbearing age in developed countries have used oral contraceptives to prevent conception.[60] Twenty-five to fifty-five percent of the women who begin taking birth control pills discontinue use of the pills within 1 year.[25] Because of the high rate of discontinuation, every woman receiving the pill should be encouraged to think about an alternative method and receive instructions in the proper use of that method.

Birth control pills today most commonly contain 30 to 50 μg of an estrogen and 1 mg or less of a progestin, compared to 100 to 150 μg of estrogen and 1 to 10 mg of a progestin used in the 1960s. Minipills do not contain estrogen and have less than 1 mg of a progestin. The two major synthetic estrogen steroids used in oral contraceptives are mestranol or ethinyl estradiol. Six types of progestins, all 19-nortestosterone derivatives, are used. Major progestins are either norgestrel or norethindrone. The mechanism of action between the naturally occurring and the synthetic hormones differs with respect to metabolism, binding properties, excretion, intracellular transport, and behavior in body fluids.[77]

Many individuals and couples are apprehensive about the safety of the pill because of reports linking the use of oral contraceptives to cancer and thromboembolic disease.[3,19,32,37,82] Although apprehensive, many women using the pill are incorrectly or poorly informed about the correct use and side effects of the drug. According to a study of women using oral contraceptives, most of them read the labeling and package insert and found the information useful, but after reading this information some women were still inadequately informed about correct usage and side effects. When questioned, these women preferred information about oral contraceptives from health professionals. This information indicates that merely handing printed information to clients and telling them to read it is inadequate. Such a procedure should be accompanied by verbal information and questioning to determine the accuracy and degree of knowledge about oral contraceptives. The printed information can then be utilized by the patient for future reference.

Women taking oral contraceptives require close supervision. Some laboratory tests, especially liver function and endocrine function tests, are altered by the use of birth control pills (Table 64-4). Phenytoin (Dilantin), phenobarbital, rifampin, ampicillin, and a variety of tranquilizers, antihistamines, and sedatives have been implicated in reducing the effectiveness of birth control pills. To ensure that women will return for periodic examination, they are given a prescription or supply of pills for only 1 to 3 months. The advantages of returning for checkups should be emphasized. When an oral contraceptive is prescribed, the woman should be told when to take it and what to do if she misses one or more days.

The pills should be started on the seventh day after menstruation begins. One pill is swallowed each day until the pack is finished. (Incidents have been reported

Absolute contraindications	Strong relative contraindications	Other relative contraindications
Allergy to rubber or spermicide Recurrent urinary tract infections Inability to obtain proper fitting as a result of uterine prolapse, cystocele, rectocele, extreme fixed uterine retroversion, vaginal fistula or septae	None	Inability of either partner to learn proper insertion technique Lack of motivation to use method correctly Aversion to touching genitalia
Allergy to spermicide	None	Lack of motivation to use at time of intercourse
None	Irregular menstrual cycles History of anovulatory cycle Irregular temperature charts	Unwillingness to abstain from intercourse during fertile period Inability or unwillingness to keep proper records

of women inserting the pills in their vagina or giving them to their partner.) Women using the 21-day pack should stop taking pills for 1 week and start the new pack the first day of the next week. Women using the 28-day pack, with a placebo for the last 7 days, should begin the new pack when the old one is completed.

Pills work best if taken at the same time every day since this keeps estrogen and progestin at a constant level. Many women find it easier to remember taking pills if they associate taking the pills with a daily activity such as before bedtime or at mealtime. A second birth control method should be used during the first month of taking the pill because the hormone levels may not be sufficient to suppress ovulation.

Most women will forget at some time to take one or more pills. Unfortunately "making up" pills can increase the risk of pregnancy. Low levels of estrogen and progestin resulting from missed pills may stimulate the pituitary gland to release FSH and LH, resulting in the development of a graafian follicle. If the woman takes two or three pills at one time, this causes a sharp rise in estrogen level and may trigger ovulation.

If one pill is missed, the woman should take the forgotten pill as soon as she remembers and then take the pill for the day at her regular time. If two pills are missed consecutively, two pills should be taken as soon as the woman remembers and two pills taken on the next day. Another method of contraception is necessary for the remainder of the cycle. If three or more pills

TABLE 64-4. Laboratory tests affected by birth control pills

Type of study	Increased (false-positive) results	Decreased (false-negative) results
Blood chemistry	Alkaline phosphate Bilirubin, icteric index Bromsulphalein (BSP) retention Cholesterol Glucose (fasting) Glucose tolerance curve ^{131}I thyroid uptake (estrogen) Iron, iron-binding capacity Lipids, total Lipoproteins Protein-bound iodine (PBI) Serum glutamic-oxaloacetic transaminase (SGOT), serum glutamic-pyruvic transaminase (SGPT) Sodium Thyroxine-binding globulin Thyroxine (T_4) uptake	 ^{131}I thyroid uptake (progesterone) Protein, total Triiodothyronine (T_3) uptake
Hematology	Leukocyte count Platelet count and aggregation Sedimentation rate (ESR)	Prothrombin time
Urine	Porphyrins	17-Ketosteroids

TABLE 64-5. Symptoms that may be associated with use of oral contraceptives*

Due to hormone excess		Due to hormone deficiency	
Estrogen	Progestogen	Estrogen	Progestogen
Nausea, vomiting	Increased appetite, weight gain	Breakthrough bleeding early in cycle	Breakthrough bleeding late in cycle
Headache	Fatigue	Absence of withdrawal bleeding	Menorrhagia with clotting
Edema, weight gain	Decrease in libido	Hot flashes, nervousness	Delay of withdrawal bleeding
Vertigo	Depression	Candidal vaginitis	Weight loss
Uterine cramps	Absence of withdrawal bleeding	Dyspareunia	
Breast changes, mastalgia	Headache†		
Cervical erosion	Breast fullness†		
Cervical mucorrhea	Cholestatic jaundice		
Vein complications (eg., thrombosis, phlebitis)	Increased tendency to thromboembolism		
Chloasma, acne, rashes	Hirsutism		
Increase in size of myoma (if present)	Loss of scalp hair		
Depression	Acneform rash		

*From Effler, S.B.: Postgrad. Med. **59:**164-170, 1976.
†During medication-free period.

TABLE 64-6. Symptoms that may indicate serious trouble when taking oral contraceptives*

Symptom	Possible problem
Severe abdominal pain	Gallbladder disease, hepatic adenoma, blood clot, pancreatitis
Severe chest pain or shortness of breath	Blood clot in lungs or myocardial infarction
Severe headaches	Stroke, hypertension, or migraine headache
Eye problems: blurred vision, flashing lights, or blindness	Stroke, hypertension, or temporary vascular problems of many possible sites
Severe leg pain (calf or thigh)	Blood clot in legs

*From Hatcher, R.A., et al.: Contraceptive technology, 1980-1981, ed. 10, New York, 1980, Irvington Publishers, Inc.

are missed, ovulation will probably occur. The old pack of pills should be thrown away. A new pack of pills is started after three or more pills have been missed, and another method of birth control should be used until the new package of pills is used for two weeks. In this case the woman should seriously consider whether oral contraception is a good method of birth control for her. Women who have had several days of severe diarrhea, which may retard absorption of the contraceptives, should also use another method of birth control for the remainder of that cycle.

Women should also be advised about storing pills used for contraception. Not only are they dangerous if ingested by children, but they are affected by extremes in temperature. High humidity may soften the pills and cause them to disintegrate, while extreme heat may decrease their potency.

During interim care the woman should be closely observed for side effects and emerging problems. Table 64-5 shows symptoms associated with oral contraceptives. The most serious side effects and many of the fairly minor but annoying side effects likely to result in discontinuation of oral contraceptives are estrogen related. This information can be used for instructing women about problems to report and as a guide for screening for problems during follow-up visits. Women are instructed to call their health care provider if they develop one of the five symptoms listed in Table 64-6, which may signify serious trouble. All women taking oral contraceptives should receive a copy of the symptoms and should discuss them with the nurse.

The incidence of vaginal infections is higher among women using oral contraceptives because the pill alters the natural environment of the vagina. If infections occur and persist, a different oral contraceptive or an entirely different method of birth control may be necessary.

Women who desire a pregnancy should discontinue use of the pill and use another contraceptive until they have three spontaneous normal menstrual periods.

Long-acting progestin injections ("the shot") are used by approximately 1 million women in 70 countries and have been close to receiving Food and Drug Administration (FDA) approval in the United States.[25] Medroxyprogesterone acetate (Depo-Provera), one of the most commonly used injectable progestins, was not approved in 1978 by the FDA because of possible teratogenicity of the drug, linkage to breast tumors in beagles, and the possible necessity to add estrogen supplementation to limit irregular bleeding. Despite lack of FDA approval, medroxyprogesterone acetate has been used widely in the United States. Women using this method receive an injection every 3 months. There is considerable controversy concerning the serious side effects of medroxyprogesterone acetate and the paternalism often involved in its prescription; as advocates, nurses cannot ignore these issues.

Intrauterine devices. Intrauterine devices (IUDs) are used by approximately 50 to 60 million women worldwide.[65] At the present time the IUDs that seem to be most widely used are the Lippes loop, Saf-T-Coil, Copper-T, Cooper-7, and Progestasert-T. Theoretical effectiveness rates for the different types of IUDs range from 95% to 99%. The differences in rates of effectiveness are caused by IUD characteristics, such as form, size, amount of copper or progesterone, and to IUD user characteristics, such as age, parity, uterine shape and size, and frequency of intercourse.

It is well known that women using IUDs have menstrual periods that are heavier and that they more often have intermenstrual spotting than do women using other methods of contraception. The bleeding experienced by women using IUDs may be due to spontaneous abortion. A recent report indicates that 12% to 19% of women using a copper-type IUD demonstrated human chorionic gonadotropin in their blood.[36] This adds to the evidence that the IUD probably interferes with pregnancy by producing degeneration of a fertilized ovum, that fertilization of the ovum can and does occur, and that tubal pregnancy occurs more often in women using the IUD.

Women who decide to use an IUD for contraception are given a thorough explanation of the insertion procedure as well as of the side effects and potential complications. There is a high incidence of pelvic inflammatory disease (PID) and tubal disease leading to infertility among IUD users. Some women experience cramping pain and/or nausea during and after insertion of the IUD. The discomforts can be relieved by bed rest, heat, and analgesics. Women using an IUD are required to feel for the string on the device before they leave the clinic or office to be sure it is still in place. The string is checked frequently (about once a week) in the first months and then after each period or if the woman is experiencing abdominal cramping. Two recent studies have suggested that IUDs should not have a string reaching into the vagina. It was found that the endometrial surfaces of IUD users may contain bacteria if the IUD has a string, thus the string facilitates ascending infections.[22,76]

Many women fear the device will get lost inside them, and occasionally this occurs. Showing them a model of the pelvis and how the device is situated when in place helps them overcome this fear. Informing the woman that the string becomes soft with body heat and that her sexual partner probably will not be aware of it

during intercourse is usually reassuring. Many women also welcome hearing that tampons can be used during the menstrual period when an IUD is in place.

Women should call their health care provider if they experience any of the following symptoms: severe abdominal pain, severe cramping, pelvic pain or tenderness, fever, chills, foul discharge, spotting, clots, or unusual vaginal bleeding. These symptoms may be signs of impending pelvic inflammatory diseases.

A Copper-T or Copper-7 device must be replaced every 3 to 5 years because the copper loses its effectiveness. The Progestasert-T must be replaced every year because the progesterone also loses its effectiveness. The Dalkon Shield was taken off the market; any woman still wearing one should have it removed immediately. The other IUDs (Lippes Loop and Saf-T-Coil) can remain in place indefinitely.

Diaphragm. Women choosing a diaphragm should receive written and verbal instructions, opportunity to practice insertion and removal, and assistance until placement is correct. Diaphragms must be used with contraceptive jelly or cream to provide maximal effectiveness. The diaphragm must be inspected for holes or defects each time before use. Approximately 1 tbsp of jelly or cream is placed into the dome and on the rim of the diaphragm up to 6 hours before intercourse. Placement of the diaphragm is checked to ascertain that the back rim of the diaphragm is below and behind the cervix and that the front edge is behind the pubic bone. Additional spermicide via an applicator is necessary after each act of intercourse. The diaphragm is not removed for 6 to 8 hours after intercourse. After removal, the diaphragm is washed in soapy water and dried before storage.

Women should see their health care providers if they experience one of the following signs indicating that the size of the diaphragm should possibly be changed: weight loss or gain greater than 5 kg (11 lb), birth, abortion, pelvic surgery, pain or discomfort caused by the diaphragm, or sensations of the diaphragm being too large or small.

The *cervical cap* is a miniature diaphragm with a dome that fits over the cervix and is held in place by suction. Cervical caps have been used in other countries for many years but have not been granted FDA approval in the United States. The cervical cap can be left in place for as long as 4 weeks. It has great potential for use with women who want to use a diaphragm but are unable to be fitted because of lax vaginal tone or marked cystocele or rectocele.

Condom. Condoms have been used for centuries to prevent pregnancy; nevertheless, the health care provider should never assume that the person does not need instructions to use condoms correctly. The condom is placed on the penis before insertion in the vagina, and the rim of the condom is rolled to the base of the penis.

One-half inch of empty space should be left at the tip unless the condom has a nipple tip to hold the semen. The condom is held as the penis is withdrawn. The penis should be withdrawn soon after ejaculation because loss of erection may cause the condom to slip off. If this occurs, contraceptive jelly or foam should be inserted immediately into the vagina.

Condoms may be stored away from heat for 2 years; those kept in wallets may deteriorate as a result of body heat. Petroleum jelly used as a lubricant will also cause the rubber to deteriorate. A new condom should be used each time a couple has intercourse.

Spermicidal foam and suppository. There is a significant difference between actual use effectiveness and theoretical effectiveness rates for both spermicidal foam and spermicidal suppositories (Table 64-2). It is therefore important that women be taught how to use these methods correctly and consistently.

FOAM. If the applicator is not preloaded, it is filled to the designated mark. By shaking the can 20 times before using, the spermicide will be mixed with the foam and there will be enough bubbles to form a barrier. The applicator is inserted 3 to 4 in. into the vagina until it cannot go any farther and then withdrawn about ½ in. The plunger is pushed to deposit the foam, and the applicator is then withdrawn. The foam is inserted no more than 30 minutes before intercourse, and additional foam must be added before each act of intercourse. The applicator is washed with soap and water.

SUPPOSITORY. The spermicidal suppository is inserted high in the vagina at least 10 minutes but no longer than 1 hour before intercourse. An additional suppository must be used with each subsequent act of intercourse. The woman may feel warmth in the vagina as the suppository disintegrates. The major problem with this method of contraception is its actual use effectiveness rate of 20% to 25%[25] (Table 64-2).

Fertility awareness. Cyclic fertility can be evidenced by covert and overt signs that occur in fertile women. Many women can become aware of the following signs that relate to their own fertility: basal body temperature patterns, cervical mucus changes, a recorded history of menstrual dates, mittelschmerz (pain during ovulation), breast changes, placement and consistency of the cervix, mood, and sexual desire.

CALENDAR METHOD. To be reliable, the calendar method (rhythm) requires that the woman be certain of the length of the menstrual cycles and the shortest and longest ranges of her cycles (Table 64-7). A woman records the length of her menstrual cycles over the preceding 8 months. The first day of bleeding is day one in each cycle. The earliest day that she is likely to be fertile is determined by subtracting 18 days from her shortest cycle. The last day she is likely to be fertile is computed by subtracting 11 days from the length of her longest cycle. The two numbers represent the beginning

TABLE 64-7. Ovulation and the menstrual cycle

Shortest cycle (in days)	First unsafe day	Longest cycle (in days)	Last unsafe day
20	2nd	20	9th
21	3rd	21	10th
22	4th	22	11th
23	5th	23	12th
24	6th	24	13th
25	7th	25	14th
26	8th	26	15th
27	9th	27	16th
28*	10th*	28	17th
29	11th	29	18th
30	12th	30*	19th*
31	13th	31	20th
32	14th	32	21st
33	15th	33	22nd
34	16th	34	23rd
35	17th	35	24th
36	18th	36	25th

*Example: A woman whose cycles range from 28 to 30 days has her first "unsafe" day on the tenth day after the start of any period and her last "unsafe" day on the nineteenth day after the start of any period.

and end of the woman's fertile period. During the fertile period a woman may either avoid intercourse or use another method of birth control. Calculation of the fertile period is based on the following assumptions: ovulation occurs 14 days before the beginning of menstruation; sperm can survive for 2 to 3 days; and the ovum remains viable for 24 hours.

BASAL BODY TEMPERATURE. The basal body temperature (BBT) is the lowest body temperature of a healthy person during waking hours. A woman can determine when she ovulates by taking her temperature daily immediately after waking and before any activity, and recording it on a chart for 3 to 4 months (Fig. 64-2). A special BBT thermometer should be used. This method is based on two temperature variations. Immediately preceding ovulation, some women's BBT drops slightly or remains the same. A noticeable rise in temperature occurs 24 to 72 hours after ovulation and remains elevated until menstruation.

A woman should avoid intercourse or use another contraceptive method until her temperature has remained elevated (a rise of 0.4° to 0.8° F above her normal BBT) for 3 consecutive days. Temperature elevations may not signify ovulation in cases of infections, irregular sleeping hours, or use of an electric blanket.

CERVICAL MUCUS. Cervical mucus changes in amount, color, viscosity, spinnbarkeit (ability to stretch), and ferning pattern throughout the menstrual cycle (Table 64-8). A woman can observe these physical changes to determine when she is fertile. During ovulation the

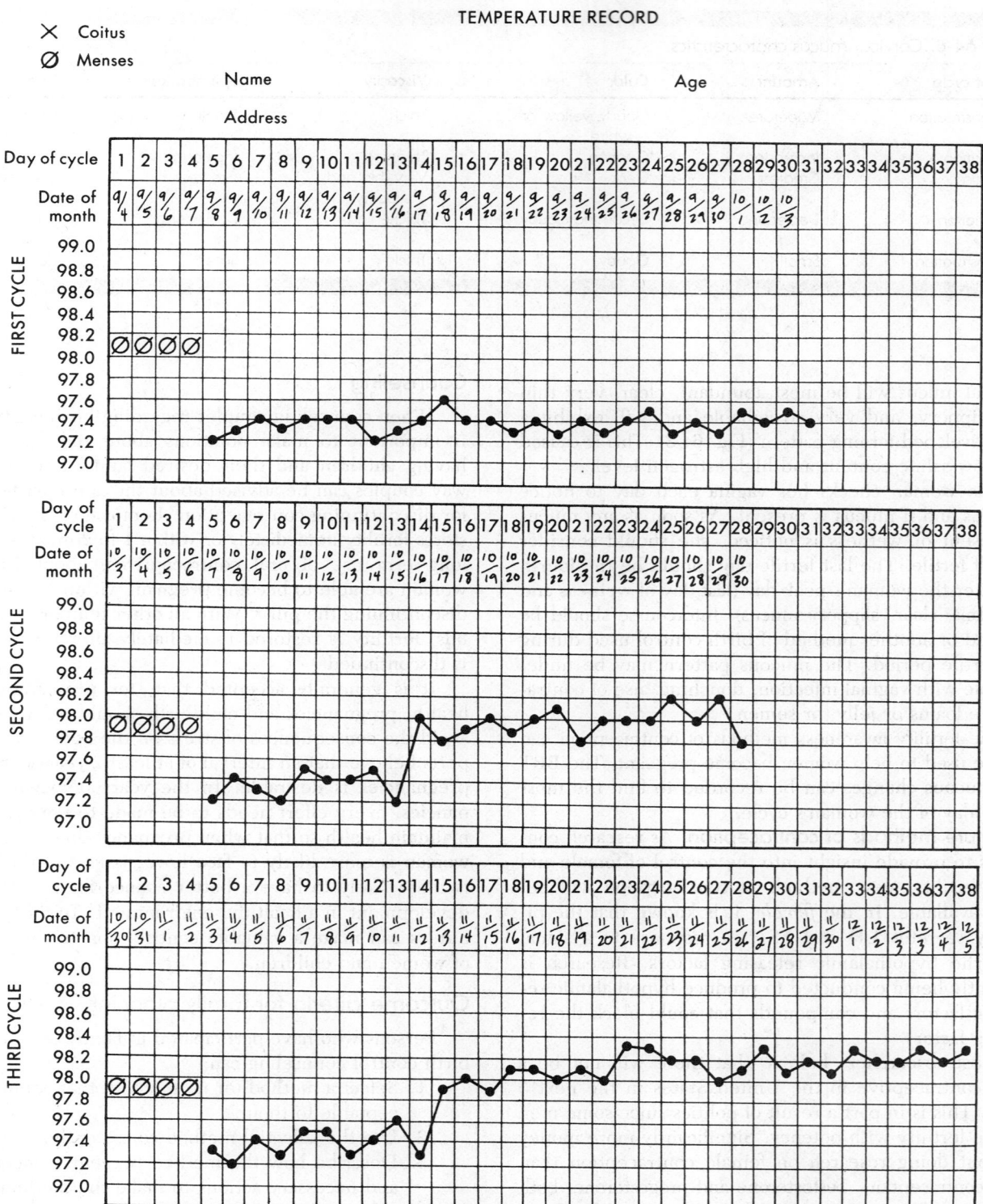

Fig. 64-2. Basal body temperature (BBT) chart illustrating determination of ovulation. First cycle shows no midcycle rise in BBT. Second cycle shows a drop followed by a rise in BBT. Third cycle shows a BBT pattern consistent with pregnancy. (From Fogel, C.I., and Woods, N.F.: Health care of women: a nursing perspective, St. Louis, 1981, The C.V. Mosby Co.)

TABLE 64-8. Cervical mucus characteristics

Time of cycle	Amount	Color	Viscosity	Spinnbarkeit	Ferning
Postmenstruation	Moderate	Cloudy, yellow or white	Thick	Small	None
Preovulation	Increasing	Clearing	Thinning	Increasing	Increasing
Ovulation	Greatest	Clear	Very thin and slippery	Greatest	Greatest
Postovulation	Decreasing	Becoming cloudy	Thickening	Decreasing	Decreasing or none
Premenstruation	Small	Cloudy	Thick	Small	None

cervical mucus will be most abundant, clear, very thin and slippery, and very stretchable and will exhibit a well-developed ferning pattern (Fig. 64-3). This is caused by a low saline content and high estrogen level.

The woman checks her vagina each day to notice wetness and if mucus is present. As soon as any mucus is present or wetness is noticed, she should consider herself fertile. The last fertile day should be the fourth day after the woman's peak day (last day of wetness and abundant, clear, slippery mucus). Intercourse should be avoided or another method of birth control used during the fertile period. The mucous pattern may be undetectable with vaginal infection, douching, use of contraceptive foams or jelly, or semen.

The fertility awareness methods of contraception can also be used to help women become pregnant. The BBT and mucous changes can be recorded to find the most fertile day of the woman's cycle.

Future methods of contraception. As research continues to provide insight into the control of female and male fertility, new methods of contraception will become available. In the *female*, it is known that the pituitary secretes LH and FSH in response to a signal from the hypothalamic releasing factors. Research is currently being conducted to produce hypothalamic releasing factors and compounds that could block the releasing factors.

Most researchers believe that there will not be a *male* contraceptive in the United States in the next 5 years. This is in part a result of politics since some men equate fertility with potency. Significantly more money is spent doing research on female contraception than male contraception. Testosterone and progesterone, both inhibitors of spermatogenesis, have been used but have the following complications: slow acting, diminished return of fertility, and difficulty in the administration method. Gossypol, a phenolic compound derived from the seed stem or roots of cotton plants, has been used successfully since 1972 in China as an oral antifertility agent for men. Potential side effects are hypokalemia, weakness, and rarely a decreased libido.

Counseling

When counseling couples regarding birth control, it is important to make notations about their plans for having children and their desired family size. In this way couples can be advised about the appropriate time for discontinuing contraception. Removal of an IUD restores fertility immediately or within 1 to 2 months. After long-term use of oral contraceptives, about 75% of women are able to become pregnant within 1 year after discontinuing the pill.[12] With all other temporary methods, fertility is restored immediately after the method is discontinued.

It is generally accepted that, for preservation of health, pregnancies and childbirth should be spaced to avoid the consequences of stress on the body. Most experts believe that an interval of at least 2 years between pregnancies is desirable. In the years between pregnancies, every effort needs to be made to improve and maintain health so that when pregnancy does occur the woman is more likely to face fewer risks and the fetus is more likely to have a better chance for growth and development in a healthful environment. To these ends nurses can make a valuable contribution to the health of women and children.

Outcome criteria for family planning

Persons who have participated in family planning or birth control counseling can:

1. Select a method (or no method) that is most acceptable to them.
2. Use the selected method consistently.
3. Describe how the method prevents conception and necessary actions to make the method reliable.
4. Compare the risks associated with the method with the risks of pregnancy.
5. State the side effects of the method.
6. State the complications of the method that require the attention of a health professional.
7. Describe self-care actions to relieve minor, common discomforts associated with the method.

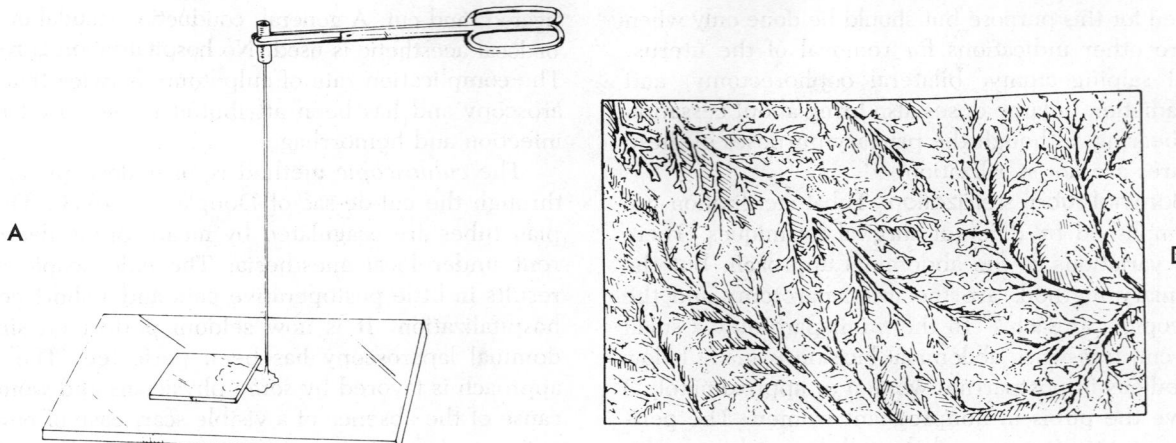

Fig. 64-3. A, Spinnbarkeit. At midcycle the mucus resembles raw egg white, being clear, stretchy, and slippery. It will stretch without breaking or spin a thread (spinnbarkeit). **B,** Ferning. When allowed to dry on a slide, the midcycle mucus gives a fern or palm-leaf pattern. (From Fogel, C.I., and Woods, N.F.: Health care of women, St. Louis, 1981, The C.V. Mosby Co.)

8. State the optimal time for a pregnancy.
9. If a pregnancy is desired, discontinue the birth control method.
10. If an alternative method is necessary, explain why this is desirable.
11. Describe the effects of temporary or permanent methods of fertility control on reproductive ability.

Sterilization

In addition to the conception control methods mentioned above, voluntary sterilization has become increasingly acceptable to both men and women as a method of preventing pregnancy. It is the most commonly used method of fertility control for married couples over 30 years of age.[11,93] It has been estimated that greater than 11.5 million adults have been sterilized in the United States, and every year approximately 100,000 American women elect surgical sterilization. In addition, each year between 500,000 and 1,000,000 American men have vasectomies.[78]

A profile of men and women seeking sterilization indicates they come from all strata of society, are between 25 and 50 years of age, are married, have large families, and are likely to be white and of the Protestant faith. The primary reason given by both men and women for wishing sterilization is a desire to limit family size.[1] Other reasons include financial inability to support a large family, concern over population growth, problems with other methods of contraception, and age, with some couples preferring personal freedom over risk of childbearing with advancing age.[1] More frequently than women, men give as an important reason for sterilization their wish for an effective contraceptive that does not interfere with sexual pleasure.[1] Also, men express concern over the health of their sex partners. Almost 83% of men whose sexual partners (including wives) used or were currently using oral contraceptives felt that the pill was actually or potentially harmful to the woman.[1]

Medical indications for sterilization broadly include any condition or situation in which pregnancy would be attended by risks to health or life of the woman or her infant. Included in this category are severe heart disease and diabetes and probable genetic defects in the infant.

The laws governing sterilization vary from state to state and have undergone many changes. In general, if the surgery does not violate specific state provisions and if written, informed consent is given by a man or woman legally capable of giving permission, the surgery can be performed by a physician. Since sterilization is a permanent method of contraception, it is absolutely necessary to obtain voluntary, informed consent. Patients using federal funds for sterilization must be at least 21 years old and mentally competent. There may be a prescribed waiting period for patients using medicaid funds before the sterilization procedure can take place.

Methods

Most methods of sterilization involve mechanical removal of a part of the male or female reproductive system so that the sperm and ovum cannot unite. The most common surgical procedure for elective sterilization of women is tubal sterilization. Hysterectomy is being performed for this purpose but should be done only when there are other indications for removal of the uterus. Bilateral salpingectomy, bilateral oophorectomy, and pelvic radiation in large doses also bring about cessation of childbearing, although the primary purposes of these procedures are not sterilization.

Abdominal tubal sterilization. Tubal sterilization can be accomplished by different surgical techniques. There are 100 variations of the abdominal approach, but the two primary methods are the minilaparotomy and the laparoscopic approach.[85] In the minilaparotomy a small (2- to 3-cm) transverse abdominal incision is made below the umbilicus in postpartum women or approximately 3 cm above the pubis in nonpregnant women. The peritoneal cavity is entered, and the fallopian tubes are located. A loop of the midportion of the tube is elevated and the loop is ligated at the base. Most often a bilateral partial salpingectomy is done to produce greater effectiveness. If this is the case, a small piece of each fallopian tube is excised. Cauterization can be performed, or the end of the tube may be tied off. This may be done as ambulatory surgery, or hospitalization for 2 to 4 days may be required. A local or general anesthetic is given. Complications following minilaparotomy are wound infection, hematoma, medication reaction, and bladder injury. The major advantages are the relatively nondestructive nature of the procedure and relatively good chance for future reanastomosis if sterilization reversal is requested.

Laparoscopic tubal sterilization requires only a very small subumbilical incision for the purpose of introducing the laparoscope through the abdominal wall. A segment of each tube is grasped with forceps, and an electric current is passed through the forceps to bring about coagulation of the tissues, or clips or rings are applied to the tube. A local or general anesthetic may be used, and postoperative pain is minimal. Advantages of laparoscopy are its safety, minimal discomfort, small amount of time required to perform the procedure and for recovery, and inexpensiveness as compared to those procedures requiring hospitalization.

Tubal sterilization using one of the abdominal approaches is often performed in the early postpartum period or at the time of cesarean section, since the fallopian tubes have not descended into the pelvis and are more readily accessible at this time. The abdominal approaches are favored by some physicians because most physicians are familiar with the female pelvic anatomy as viewed from the abdomen, and the oviducts are free and suspended in this position, which makes them easy to see, manipulate, and ligate or cauterize.

Vaginal tubal sterilization. Culpotomy and culdoscopy are the two types of vaginal approaches in tubal ligation. *Culpotomy* is performed by way of a small incision in the cul-de-sac of Douglas with the woman in the lithotomy position. Each oviduct is brought into view,

ligated, and cut. A general, conduction (caudal or spinal), or local anesthetic is used. No hospitalization is required. The complication rate of culpotomy is twice that of laparoscopy and has been attributed to increased rates of infection and hemorrhage.

The *culdoscopic* method is an endoscopic approach through the cul-de-sac of Douglas (p. 1634). The fallopian tubes are coagulated by means of an electric current under local anesthesia. The culdoscopic method results in little postoperative pain and a short period of hospitalization. It is now seldom performed since abdominal laparoscopy has been perfected. The vaginal approach is favored by some physicians and women because of the absence of a visible scar, ease of peritoneal entry, and rapid postoperative recovery; however, because of its higher complication rate, it is becoming less utilized.

Successful sterilization (conception prevented) is dependent on the technique used, the health professional's experience in performing the procedure, other surgical factors, and the length of tube removed.

The main causes of failure are recanalization of the fallopian tube, erroneous ligation, and pregnancy resulting from tuboperitoneal fistula. The failure rates reported vary from 1 in 57 to 1 in 340 women having tubal sterilization.[73]

Vasectomy. Bilateral vasectomy (Fig. 64-4) is the surgical procedure for accomplishing sterilization of men. At least 11 techniques are described to accomplish what is generally considered to be a safe, simple procedure. Two reasons probably account for the variety of techniques developed. The first is the tendency of the vas deferens to spontaneously rejoin, a distressing long-term complication. The second reason centers around developing techniques having potential reversibility.

Bilateral partial vasectomy is the surgical method most often used. Because of its safety and simplicity, the procedure is most often performed on an outpatient basis in a clinic or a physician's office using a local anesthetic. A small incision is made in the scrotum to expose the sheath of the vas. The sheath is opened, the vas deferens is exposed, and a segment measuring 0.63 to 1.27 cm is removed. The segmented ends of the vas are then ligated. Some physicians prefer to coagulate the severed ends of the vas to ensure sterility. The incision is then closed by suturing.

Complications following vasectomy are rare and of a minor nature when they do occur. Bruising, mild edema, and mild discomfort are common and usually subside without treatment. Infection of the wound occurs in about 3% of patients.[21,23] Hematoma, epididymitis, and granuloma formation may occur. The incidence of failure as a result of recanalization is reported to be between 0% and 6%.[22,78] The cause of spontaneous recanalization (reanastomosis) is unknown, but duplication of the vas has occasionally been noted. The literature does not re-

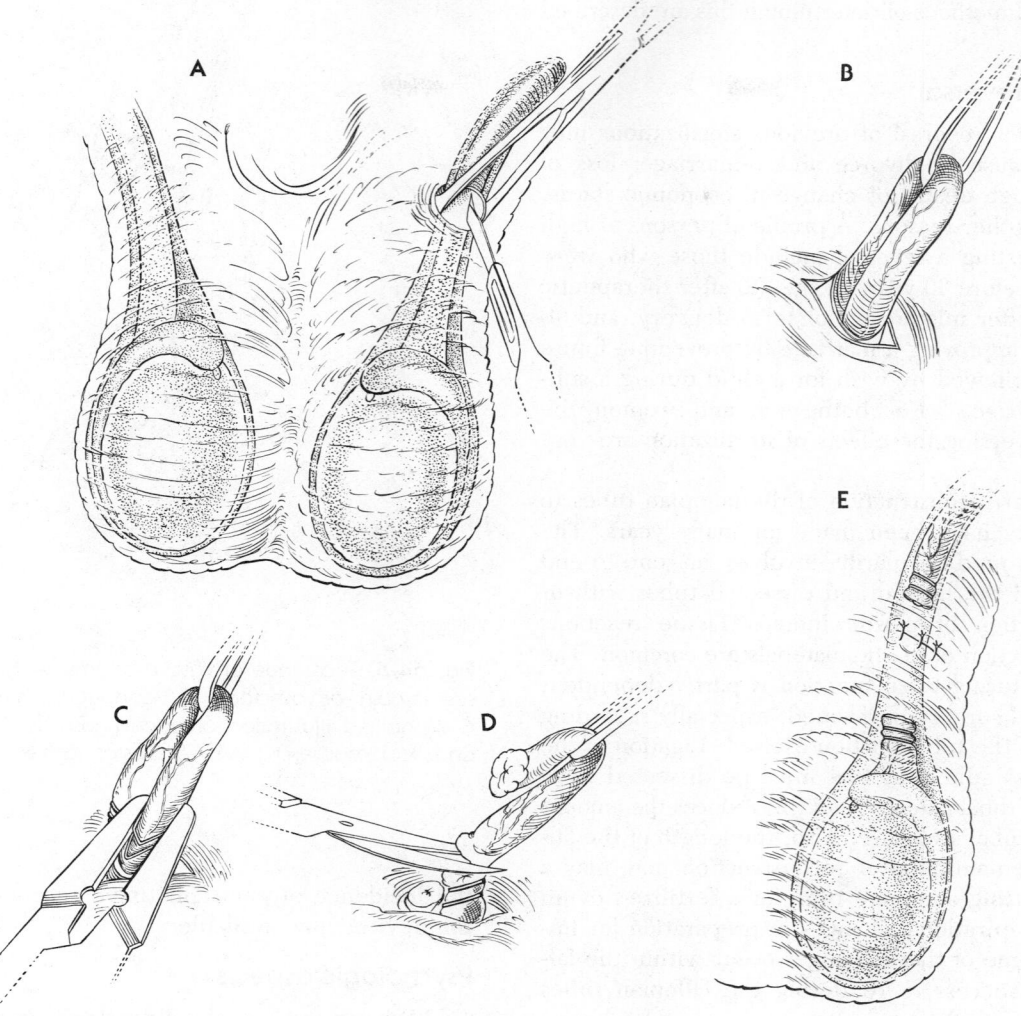

Fig. 64-4. Vasectomy procedure. **A,** Bilateral incision used to expose sheath. **B** and **C,** Vas exposed and occluded. **D,** Segment is excised. **E,** Vas is replaced in sheath and skin sutured. (Modified from Davis, J.E.: Am. J. Nurs. **72:**510, 1972.)

port any occurrences of mortality from vasectomy.

After vasectomy, antibodies to sperm develop in about 50% of men.[86] There has not been any relationship found in humans between the presence of sperm antibodies and any systemic pathologic condition. In some studies with samples of 5 to 10 monkeys, atherosclerosis has developed more extensively in vasectomized monkeys. It is hypothesized that antisperm antibodies formed after vasectomy may result in circulating immune complexes that exacerbate atherosclerosis.[10] Studies are currently underway to determine if men who have had vasectomies have a higher incidence of coronary heart disease.

Physiologic effects

While tubal sterilization usually terminates a woman's ability to bear children, ovarian hormones and menstrual functioning are not altered and an artificial menopause is not induced. Ability to derive satisfaction from sexual intercourse should not be impaired, and some women may experience greater enjoyment from intercourse with the removal of fear of pregnancy.

Since vasectomy interrupts the continuity of the vas deferens, sperm are prevented from being ejaculated with other components of the semen. However, sperm are still produced, and the ejaculate is not noticeably diminished in amount. Residual fertility lasting for a variable period is present because of sperm in the semen beyond the point of occlusion of the vas. Sperm *gradually* disappear from the ejaculate; thus conception is possible in the immediate postoperative period. Following a vasectomy it is important for the man to report for semen analysis as advised. Disappearance of the sperm from the semen and methods of determining this are described on p. 1630.

Sterilization reversal

Requests for reversal of previous sterilizations may be made because of divorce and remarriage, loss of children through death, or change in economic status, as well as for other reasons. A profile of persons at high risk for requesting a reversal include those who were sterilized (1) before 30 years of age, (2) after therapeutic abortion, (3) after miscarriage or term delivery, and (4) for reasons of improving a marriage by preventing future pregnancies followed by wish for a child during a subsequent marriage.[40] For both men and women the chances of reversing the effects of sterilization are very small.

Attempts at reconstruction of the fallopian tubes to restore fertility have been made for many years. The surgery performed primarily involves an end-to-end anastomosis of the ligated and dissected tubes with or without insertion of plastic lumen. Tissue reactions caused by rejection of plastic materials are common. The success of restoring tubal function is partly dependent on the original surgery performed, especially regarding the amount of the tubal portion excised. Ligation of the tubes produces adhesions that must be dissected away to the point of tubal patency, and this reduces the amount of remaining tubal structure. Also, the length of the fallopian tube remaining after reconstruction may play a role in permitting adequate time for a fertilized ovum to undergo maturational changes in preparation for implantation. Some of these changes occur within the fallopian tube. Success in rendering the fallopian tubes functional after sterilization is usually measured in terms of pregnancy rate following reconstruction. Reports of success range from 50% to 69%.[89]

A surgical attempt to restore male fertility following vasectomy is called a *vasovasostomy* (Fig. 64-5). An attempt is made to rejoin the severed ends of the vas deferens. Success is measured by the presence of sperm in semen specimens following reconstruction. Reports of success in restoring fertility range from 37% to 90%. A notable point is that although sperm reappear in the semen, the pregnancy rate following vasovasostomy is low, and the reason for this is unknown. Only 20% to 25% of vasovasostomies result in pregnancy.[13]

Considerable research is now in progress for the development of a reversible vasectomy device. One such device is shown in Fig. 64-6. Other devices include the vas plug, intravas device, and vas clips. Ideally, reversible vasectomy devices would effectively block the vas deferens, would permit simple and safe insertion and removal of the device, could be turned on and off to provide for timing of conception, would not cause discomfort when in place, and would not cause complications. The ideal vasectomy device has not been developed, and

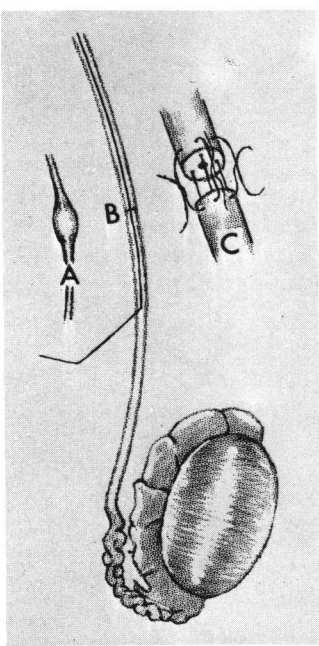

Fig. 64-5. Technique of vasovasostomy. *A,* Nodule of scar tissue at point of vasectomy. *B,* Reanastomosis over nylon splint. *C,* Magnified illustration of anastomosis. (From Hackett, R.E., and Waterhouse, K.: Am. J. Obstet. Gynecol. **116:**438-455, 1973.)

the incidence of pain and tissue reaction is high with the devices now available.

Psychologic aspects

Men and women who elect sterilization seem to have little or no regret after the surgery if they understand what to expect during and after the procedure and are able to express their feelings and have questions answered before the procedure.[67] One study reports that over 90% of women having tubal sterilization expressed no regret but that some women were disturbed emotionally by having been sterilized.[43] The method of elective sterilization seems to make little difference to women regarding their emotional responses. Depression, loss of self-esteem, physical complaints, feelings of guilt, and difficulty in sexual adjustment after surgery are reported to be some of the psychologic responses of women to sterilization even when the surgery is elective.[73] Psychologic studies have suggested that women who regretted having been sterilized had preexisting emotional problems.[73]

Women who were dissatisfied after sterilization describe themselves as having feelings of inferiority, weakness, emptiness, being torn up inside, being a damaged and changed person, and having less desire for and gratification from sexual intercourse. These emotional reactions are less likely to occur if a woman

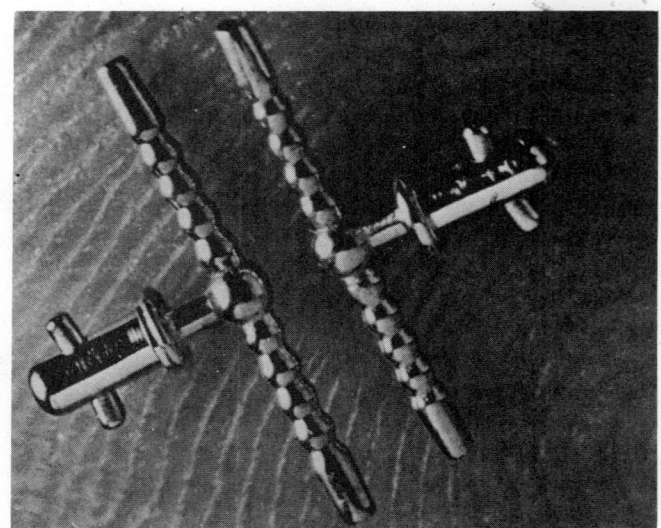

Fig. 64-6. Vas valve (Bionyx Control). (From Hackett, R.E., and Waterhouse, K.: Am. J. Obstet. Gynecol. **116:**438-455, 1973.)

requests sterilization and it is done for reasons of family size rather than for organic disease.[81]

Studies indicate that 95% to 99% of men are satisfied with the results of vasectomy and that, like women, some men have increased emotional difficulties after sterilization.[13] In a follow-up study of men who had vasectomies it was found that 70% were happier than before the surgery and that frequency of intercourse had increased.[97]

There is a need to recognize that tubal sterilization affects men as well as women and that vasectomies affect women as well as men when there is mutual caring and concern between them. This concern may be best illustrated by a woman who described her feelings when she and her husband selected vasectomy as their method of contraception:

> The worst part of the experience was that I had not anticipated the range of my reactions. Now it seems that these transitions may have been natural. Perhaps if I had known the experiences of others, I would have passed more easily through these feelings. We try to prepare husbands for childbirth; we should recognize the need to prepare wives for vasectomy.[30]

Intervention

Preoperative counseling and care. The findings of studies regarding the psychologic aspects of sterilization indicate a need to identify men and women before surgery who may later have strong regrets and emotional problems. One aim of counseling before surgery is to confirm that the decision for sterilization is made as objectively as possible. Asking hypothetical questions about the possibility of divorce, loss of the spouse, or loss of a child can assist in estimating whether the decision to be sterilized has been treated as a serious step.

INFORMED CONSENT GUIDELINES (FEDERAL) RELATING TO STERILIZATION

1. Choice is made by patient. No pressures are placed on choice (e.g., loss of welfare benefits, wrath of health care provider).

2. Benefits and risks of sterilization are described:

    a. Benefits: permanent, no further costs or decision making

    b. Risks: usual surgical risks, possibility of future pregnancy (i.e., not 100% effective)

3. Alternative contraceptive methods are described.

4. Patient is encouraged to ask questions.

5. Explanations are given about the entire sterilization procedure, costs, and possible side effects (effects of hormones, weight changes, menstrual changes, sexual response).

6. Written instructions and risk factors are given to patient.

7. A written consent to the procedure is signed by patient and witnessed.

Previous experience with other methods of contraception can be explored and reasons for dissatisfaction with the methods determined. It may be that an individual or couple lacks knowledge about contraceptive methods and with adequate information might choose something other than sterilization. Care must be taken, however, that persons who are knowledgeable and have made a firm, objective decision are not made to feel that their decision is a poor one or is unacceptable.

The discussion of sterilization methods should be based on the federal government's informed consent guidelines (see box above). The nature and consequences of the surgery must be explained to the patient. It is important to emphasize that the sterilization procedure does nothing to increase or decrease sexual performance or enjoyment but simply removes the chance of pregnancy. It is common for lay people to equate sterilization with castration and loss of femininity or masculinity. Even those patients who know the difference need reassurance.

Visual aids and models can be of great value in giving explanations about the surgery to patients. Films such as *Freedom from Pregnancy,** *Sterilization by Laparoscopy,†* and *Tubal Ligation†* and pamphlets such as *Voluntary Sterilization for Men and Women‡* are useful in increasing patients' understanding.

---

*Allend'or Productions, Inc., 3449 Cahuenga West, Hollywood, CA 90068.
†Milner Fenwick, Inc., 3800 Liberty Heights Ave., Baltimore, MD 21215.
‡Planned Parenthood World Population, 810 Seventh Ave., New York, NY 10019.

The facts of reversibility, including current success rates, are discussed. In the case of vasectomy the chance of recanalization with return of fertility should be pointed out. The man or couple also must be informed of progressive rather than immediate sterility following vasectomy, and alternate methods of protection until sterility results should be discussed.

For men having vasectomies, a preoperative specimen of semen is examined to serve as a baseline for interpreting sperm disappearance following surgery. The patient is instructed to shave the scrotal hair and to take a shower the night before surgery. He is advised to bring briefs-type underpants with him on the day of surgery to hold the postoperative dressing in place.

Postoperative care. Most women having tubal sterilization can be discharged when effects of the general anesthetic have disappeared and when vital signs are stable. Exceptions are women who have recently delivered a baby and those having tubal sterilization by other than the laparoscopic abdominal method. All women need to be advised of the signs of infection and the need to report persistent pain in the lower abdomen or pelvis. Women having culdoscopic sterilization probably should be advised to abstain from intercourse for about a week to reduce the chances of infection and trauma. Those having abdominal tubal sterilization may resume intercourse when healing has taken place and when pain does not prevent it. Women should rest for 24 to 48 hours after the procedure and abstain from lifting heavy objects for 1 week. All patients need to be advised when to report to the physician for follow-up examination or to call if they have a fever over 38° C (100° F), faint, or have persistent abdominal pain or bleeding from the incision after 12 hours.

Following vasectomy men are advised to expect slight swelling of the scrotum, minor pain, and a small amount of bleeding. Ice to the scrotal area, sitz baths, time, and rest will ameliorate these discomforts. They should be advised to report bleeding, increased swelling, hematoma, or persistent pain immediately. A 48-hour rest period with no showers or baths will decrease the incidence of complications. The man is instructed to wear a scrotal support day and night for 48 hours. Strenuous exercise should be avoided for 1 week. Intercourse can be resumed in 2 to 3 days, but an alternate method of contraception is needed until the physician reports that the semen no longer contains sperm.

Disappearance of sperm from the ejaculate following vasectomy and the methods for determining when sterility actually occurs have been studied extensively. The standard procedure has been to take a sperm count 4 weeks following vasectomy. Some experts believe that at least two consecutive sperm-free specimens must be found before the man can be considered sterile.[23] Others utilize the number of ejaculations required to render the semen free of sperm in establishing guidelines for sterility following vasectomy. It has been noted that after 12 ejaculations 65.5% of men become aspermatic, after 24 ejaculations 97.5% of men become aspermatic, and after 36 ejaculations all men (except those with spontaneous reanastomosis of the vas) become aspermatic.[43] Reanastomosis is suspected if sperm fail to disappear from the ejaculate despite an adequate number of ejaculations, if there is an increase in sperm in the semen after two successive sperm counts, if motile sperm are found in the semen beyond 3 months following vasectomy, and if, of course, pregnancy occurs.

In the postoperative period both men and women need opportunities to express their feelings about having been sterilized. Information previously given regarding sexual performance may need to be repeated. If the patient expresses feelings of regret or guilt, a review of the reasons for the sterilization may be of assistance in recognizing that the decision was made as objectively as possible.

Outcome criteria for the person who elects sterilization

The person can:
1. Describe the physiologic effects of sterilization and the small chances of reversing sterility.
2. Carry out self-care activities consistent with the surgery performed.
3. Describe how activities of daily living (ADL) need to be modified during the postoperative period.
4. State the signs of complications of surgery.
5. If complications of surgery occur, seek help from a clinician.

Infertility

It has been estimated that 10% to 15% of all couples in the United States are unwillingly childless. This represents about 10 million Americans.[51,77] Approximately 50% of the couples who undergo assessment and treatment for infertility in major infertility settings are likely to conceive. Although infertility is most often attributed to women, about 40% of infertile marriages result from infertility of men. Some of the major factors that account for infertility are failure of ovulation (10% to 15%), tubal pathologic conditions (10% to 30%), and cervical factors (5%). There is no known cause in 10% to 20% of infertility problems.[77]

Couples wishing to have children and who find themselves unable to do so experience immeasurable emotional distress. Feelings of inadequacy are common, as are anger and guilt. The infertile couple must confront feelings about lack of control, self-image, self-esteem, and sexuality. Couples who are informed that they will never be able to have children experience a life crisis with all of its ramifications and have a strong need to grieve. For those who are told they are a normal, fertile couple and for whom pregnancy does not result despite months or years of tests, studies, examinations, and advice, feelings of frustration alternating with hope are high. All of these couples require emotional support, including encouragement to grieve, to express their anger and other feelings in order to regain objectivity, and to avoid premature decisions and actions about alternatives. The urgent need for such support is reflected in the emergence of support groups organized by infertile individuals and couples.*

It is important that couples who wish to have children and are unsuccessful after about a year of trying to achieve pregnancy seek medical advice. Infertility evaluation often requires a long time. Sometimes infertility cannot be treated successfully, and alternatives such as adoption, artificial insemination, or child-free living are considered.

Definitions

Infertility is the inability to achieve a pregnancy within a stipulated period of time, usually within 1 year of regular unprotected sexual intercourse. Some authorities include the inability to carry pregnancies to a live birth. Infertility is classified as either primary or secondary. *Primary infertility* describes couples who have never conceived, whereas *secondary infertility* refers to couples who have previously conceived. *Sterility* is irreversible and refers to an individual who has an absolute factor preventing procreation.

Prevention

The fertility of a couple is affected by four factors: duration of pregnancy exposure, coital frequency, female's age, and male's age. In general, the likelihood of becoming pregnant is greater as the duration of exposure to pregnancy increases. Approximately 25% of women will become pregnant during the first month of non-contraceptive intercourse. Sixty-five percent become pregnant within 6 months, 75% within 9 months, 80% to 90% within 1 year, and 93% to 95% within 1½ years.[6]

Increased coital frequency enhances fertility to a point. In couples having intercourse four or five times a week, 83% become pregnant within 6 months, as compared to 16% of the couples having intercourse less than once a week.[58] Frequent ejaculation improves sperm motility unless ejaculation is excessive, resulting in depletion of available sperm.

Fertility in women is low during the early teenage

years, peaks at 24 years of age, and declines after age 30. An infertility rate of 31.8% has been reported for married women 35 to 40 years old and 70% for women over age 40.[98] Fertility reaches its peak at 25 years of age in men and subsequently declines, although some 80- to 90-year-old men are fertile.

There are many causes of infertility in men and women. Some of these are preventable, while others are not. Some causes of infertility can be corrected, while other causes do not respond to any form of treatment.

Infertility in women may be caused by diseases of the cervix and uterus that inhibit passage of active sperm, obstructions of the fallopian tubes that interfere with transport of ova, ovarian and other endocrine gland disturbances that inhibit release of ova, and hormonal problems that leave the endometrium unprepared for implantation.

One of the most common, preventable causes of infertility in women is infection of the pelvic organs, especially as a result of gonorrhea, which causes obstruction of fallopian tubes. An estimated 17% of women have symptoms of salpingitis as the first sign of gonorrheal infection, and during the course of treatment about 4.5% are surgically sterilized.[90] Such serious consequences are preventable through prophylactic use of penicillin for women exposed to gonorrhea and through early diagnosis and treatment of all vaginal and cervical infections. Gonococcal cultures should be obtained every 6 months for women with multiple partners. If infection is present and the women has an IUD, it should be removed.

Many of the ovarian and hormonal problems that cause infertility produce symptoms such as menstrual irregularities and ill health before a problem with conception is ever recognized. Many of these problems can be managed with hormone therapy, provided women seek help for such problems at an early age or as soon as deviations are noticed. Birth control pills should be avoided by women who have not established normal menses, have irregular menstrual cycles, or have used birth control pills for over 2 years. Some authorities suggest a break from prolonged usage of birth control pills to reactivate the hypothalamic controls.

In men infertility may be caused by obstruction of the vas deferens, destruction of the testicular tissue by disease, undescended testes, and hormonal deficiencies. Bilateral undescended testes (cryptorchism) should be corrected surgically before puberty. In later life cryptorchism may produce sterility because of failure of the testes to develop their sperm-producing function, even if the condition is surgically corrected. Destruction of testicular tissue by infectious processes can be prevented through prompt treatment when symptoms first appear. Prepubescent boys should be immunized for mumps to prevent orchitis.

---

*RESOLVE, Inc., P.O. Box 474, Belmont, MA 02178; and for child-free living, National Organization for Non-Parents, 806 Reistertown Rd., Baltimore, MD 21208.

Assessment and intervention

The purposes of an infertility evaluation are to establish the etiology of infertility and determine the diagnosis, to give a prognosis for future fertility, to provide a basis for medical or surgical treatment, and to plan for assisting the couple to accept their diagnosis, treatment, and future options. The assessment and intervention can be physically painful as well as emotionally and economically stressful.

Attempts to correct infertility are based on data obtained through a detailed history and physical examination as well as data obtained from laboratory tests and clinical studies. During the physical examination close attention is given to the individual's general health; development of secondary sex characteristics; size, position, and condition of the reproductive organs; and signs of metabolic diseases or infection. A sexual history is taken, and sexual practices are reviewed. Suggestions about sexual intercourse are given if this seems to be the problem. The couple should attempt to be at the first interview together since they share responsibility for infertility, information is needed by both partners, and this may be their first opportunity to confront their feelings about being infertile.

Examination of the man. Many physicians prefer to carry out examination of the man first, since it is more easily accomplished and less time consuming. The first special test done is multiple semen examinations (p. 1630) to determine the presence, number, maturity, and motility of sperm. Normal findings indicate fertility.

Absence of sperm in the semen may indicate a stricture along the vas deferens. A biopsy of the testes is done, and if sperm are being produced, there is a stricture. The stricture can sometimes be successfully repaired by plastic surgery (vasovasostomy). Varicoceles (dilated veins of the spermatic cord) are also associated with decreased sperm counts. A varicocelectomy may restore fertility in some men.

If the sperm count and motility rate of sperm are low, thyroid extract and vitamins may be prescribed, along with a well-balanced diet, rest, and moderate exercise. A lack of vitamins A and E in the diet may cause some atrophy of the sperm-producing structures. The couple are advised to have intercourse every other day during the fertile period (usually 12 to 16 days before the beginning of the next menstrual period). When the man is completely aspermatic, conception is impossible, and the couple should be counseled regarding the alternatives open to them.

Examination of the woman. If the man is found to be fertile, examination of the woman is carried out. A complete history and physical examination are done. If there is an infection of the reproductive tract, it is treated. A systematic check is then made of each organ that might affect the woman's reproductive ability.

If menstruation occurs regularly, this usually indicates that the ovaries are producing estrogen and progesterone but does not indicate that amounts are sufficient for ovulation. To determine whether ovulation is occurring, the woman is instructed to keep a basal body temperature chart to help determine the presence and time of ovulation. In the interim, cervical secretions are examined for pH and spinnbarkeit. A postcoital test is usually done. If sperm are being destroyed by vaginal and cervical secretions, smears from these sites are studied. If the secretions are too acid or too alkaline, medicated douches may be prescribed. A douche using sodium bicarbonate (15 ml to 1 L of water) taken just before intercourse has been found to increase the motility of sperm in many cases.

If a question remains regarding ovulation, endometrial biopsies and occasionally serum progesterone and estradiol levels may be done. Laparoscopic inspection of the ovaries may be carried out to determine if ovulation has, in fact, occurred. Laparoscopy is the only definitive way to know if ovulation occurs. Laparoscopy is planned for 1 or 2 days after ovulation. If an obstruction of the fallopian tubes is suspected, tubal patency studies by hysterosalpingography or laparoscopy are indicated.

Tubal strictures or obstructions are sometimes repaired by plastic surgery, but the rates of success in restoring tubal function are very low. If ovulation is occurring, the couple may require advice concerning timing of intercourse and ovulation. Metabolic disease processes can be detected by thyroid function tests, glucose tolerance tests, 17-ketosteroid assays or measures of circulating androgens, and prolactin assays to detect hyperprolactinemia, although most often extensive laboratory evaluation is not necessary.

Coping with infertility. Couples who are found to be infertile are confronted with the need to make choices from among available alternatives. Remaining childless or adopting a child are the usual alternatives from which they must select. First the couple must deal with their feelings and accept their infertility.

The couple needs objective guidance when making a decision, and they need help in making a sound decision to prevent regret stemming from premature and hastily made decisions. The couple needs time to cope with the crisis of being told they are infertile, and they need to be permitted to handle their grief (see Chapter 17). They may grieve for their loss of fertility, loss of future children, or loss of the pregnancy experience.[43,44] Once the initial crisis is dealt with, the couple is better prepared to discuss alternatives. Couples who elect to remain childless need to be informed that with advancing age there is increased difficulty in adopting children, should they change their minds at a later time, but this must be done in such a way that they will not feel guilty about not wanting to adopt a child.

Those couples deciding on adoption need to be presented with the facts concerning their chances of success in locating the child of their choice and the need to undergo still another long process before obtaining a child. These couples need information about reliable adoption agencies and may need help in dealing with frustration during adoption procedures. Organizations to support people seeking adoption are available.* Some couples will not be successful in their attempts to adopt a child and will need help in coping with still another crisis.

Artificial insemination. Artificial insemination is an alternative in some cases of infertility. This is a highly controversial topic, surrounded by deep personal feelings, and must be approached with tact. However, infertile couples should know about this alternative and should have an opportunity to make their own decision.

The major indication for artificial insemination is male infertility. Loss of children because of Rh or ABO incompatibility or severe hereditary defects transmitted by the man are other indications. Therefore artificial insemination is not reserved only for infertile couples.

Medically, the procedure of artificial insemination is simple, safe, inexpensive, and highly successful. Accepted routes for insemination are intrauterine (which is painful and rarely necessary to use), cervical-vaginal, and intra-cervical. A few drops of semen are injected as close to the time of ovulation as possible. Having intercourse around the time of insemination or mixing the partner's semen with the donor's may be emotionally satisfying for the couple.

Artificial insemination is *homologous* (AIH) when the partner's semen is used and *heterologous* (AID) when donor semen is used. Homologous insemination may be employed when there is a small volume of semen with normal density, oligospermia with normal sperm motility and morphology, impotence or refractory premature ejaculation, or congenital or acquired anomalies preventing adequate cervical insemination (procidentia, hypospadias, retrograde ejaculation, vaginismus, incompatible cervical mucus). Heterologous insemination is indicated in irreversible male infertility, a partner with a proven gene error, or an Rh incompatibility with a homozygous Rh-positive partner.

Donor selection in heterologous insemination is a very important part of the procedure. Criteria for donor selection is based on semen analysis as well as on a complete history and physical examination. AID couples are also concerned with intelligence. Attempts may be made to select donors who have similar physical characteristics to the partner. Donor candidates with venereal disease, diabetes, hepatitis, blood diseases,

prostatic infection, and a family history of hereditary disorders are excluded. Fertility of donors must be proved by semen analysis. The semen should show a sperm count of over 100 million/ml, have a predominance of normal sperm forms, and have a greater than 70% sperm motility.[55] Karyotyping has been advocated by some authorities.

Artificial insemination has not been widely practiced or publicized. Many people are poorly informed about it, and some people find the topic highly distressing or distasteful and refuse to discuss it. Others may not have considered artificial insemination, wish to have additional information, and welcome opportunities to discuss the subject.

Other infertility approaches. Two recent approaches to infertility management involve in vitro fertilization and surrogate mothers. *In vitro fertilization* (extracorporeal fertilization or fertilization outside the mother's body) has been performed successfully in England, Australia, the United States, and India. This method is still relatively new and has a poor success rate.

Surrogate mothers are women who contract to conceive by artificial insemination and give the baby to the semen donor after delivery. There are many social, moral, psychologic, and legal implications surrounding this approach. The U.S. courts are currently trying cases of legitimacy and parents' rights to the child.

Intervention for sexual problems

Health practitioners have demonstrated an increased awareness of their responsibilities for providing sex education and counseling to individuals as evidenced by the recent increase of nursing literature dealing with sexual issues. Even though the literature is beginning to reflect nursing's acknowledgement of the validity of these roles, many professional education programs have not yet emphasized sexual health to the same extent as other components of health. Consequently, many professionals feel unprepared for assuming the role of sex educator or counselor.

Scope of services for sexual health care

The report of a recent World Health Organization meeting dealing with education and treatment in human sexuality acknowledges that a variety of sexual health services is needed, ranging from dissemination of information to the community to intensive therapy for complex sexual dysfunctions. Participants in the conference recommended that sexual health education of the community and of other health practitioners receive first

---

*OURS (Oganization for a United Response), 3418 Humboldt Ave, South Minneapolis, MN 55408.

priority, since it would reach the largest number of people. Further, it was indicated that sex education was not only a part of preventive medicine but also an important component in assisting persons with sexual problems. The group also recommended that health professionals including nurses and other practitioners be able to provide counseling for individuals and couples with sexual problems. Finally, provision for sex therapy by professionals with special preparation was seen as an essential health service for those persons with complex problems.

Prerequisites for intervention

With the scope of sexual health services in mind, it is easy to see that each level of intervention requires a slightly different professional preparation. However, three prerequisites are common to each level of intervention. First, a knowledge base is required, including an understanding of sexual response, knowledge of the variety of sexual behaviors that exist in our society and their prevalence, an understanding of the types of sexual dysfunctions, and an awareness of the relationship between age, life events, pathologic conditions, behavioral problems, pharmaceutical agents, and sexual function. Without such a knowledge base the practitioner has no basis for discriminating between healthy and unhealthy responses or the interpretation of client's concerns, and thus no basis for education or counseling.

Although a knowledge base is essential to effective intervention, an awareness of the professional's own value system, including the biases and beliefs about appropriate and inappropriate sexual behavior, is also important. Unless the professional can accept her or his own sexuality and is comfortable with her or his own behavior, it will be difficult to convey comfort to others. Self-acceptance is seen as a prerequisite to the development of a nonjudgmental and tolerant approach. Just as individuals have belief systems related to sexual phenomena, so do professionals. This does not imply that the sex educator or counselor must condone every variety of sexual activity. Rather, it is essential that they be aware of their own feelings and values and attempt to keep them in perspective by acknowledging them. This will assist them to maintain a supportive climate that encourages sharing of feeling by clients and simultaneously permits professionals to acknowledge the validity of their own beliefs.[94]

Furthermore, there are some issues about which the professional has such strong beliefs that his or her own value system would interfere with effective intervention. An example encountered in practice is the health professional whose basic conviction is that homosexuality is an illness or deviation, rather than a variation in sexual expression or orientation. No matter how ex-

tensive the professional's training, knowledge base, and therapy skills, such a strong basic belief is likely to interfere greatly with the ability to relate objectively to a homosexual's sexual problems. Often professionals need to acknowledge their inability to deal with sexual problems because of their own value systems. Topics likely to elicit bias among health professionals include abortion, alternative life-styles, and sexual variations.

Finally, the professional needs to be able to communicate genuinely and therapeutically with clients. Often this involves using the client's own language, which may be quite different from that of the health professional. Without the ability to interact accurately and empathically with individuals, the most sophisticated knowledge base and objective attitudes are of little benefit. A framework for developing skills supportive of sex education and counseling includes the progression from active listening techniques to sophisticated psychotherapeutic skills.

Prevention of sexual problems

Nurses may prevent sexual problems among client populations through three strategies: education of client groups likely to have sexual concerns, provision of anticipatory guidance throughout the life cycle, and promotion of a milieu conducive to sexual health.

Education of client populations implies more than mere dissemination of information. As in the case of educating nurses to provide sex education, clients may also need assistance in exploring the attitudes and values that shape their sexual behavior and in developing the ability to communicate comfortably about sexual phenomena. Thus providing accurate knowledge about sex and sexuality is not synonymous with education for a healthy sexuality.

Nurses are often in strategic positions to provide *anticipatory guidance* at sensitive points in the life cycle. Adolescence and middle age are two life periods during which anxiety about sexuality is likely to surface. By informing individuals about the usual changes experienced at these points (e.g., nocturnal emissions or concerns about masturbation in adolescents and worry about effects of menopause on the ability to function sexually among middle-aged persons), nurses can assist individuals to cope realistically with major changes in their bodies. Adults with young children can also benefit from anticipatory guidance regarding their childrens' sexuality.

Finally, nurses can assist individuals to *provide a milieu conducive to sexual health*. Some approaches useful in developing such a milieu include minimizing guilt experienced in conjunction with sexual thoughts, feelings, and behavior. This may be accomplished by assisting persons to examine objectively the consequences of their activities within a reality-oriented framework. Reduction of performance anxiety, that is, concern about how well one is able to function, can be facilitated by helping individuals to understand the relationship between being attentive to their own performance at the expense of losing touch with their sexual feelings. "Spectatoring" refers to the habit of watching oneself or a partner perform. Just as in athletics, one cannot be both spectator and performer without minimizing the effectiveness of the performance.

Often individuals need to be advised to modify their environments to reduce competing stimuli. Use of anxiety-provoking settings or those prone to interruption can help to establish dysfunctional patterns. (The relationship between anxiety and orgasmic dysfunction and premature ejaculation has been well established.)

Finally, maintenance of good general health facilitates optimal sexual functioning. Fatigue, pain, and malaise are stimuli that compete with sexual pleasure.

Promotion of sexual health

Principles for promoting sexual health

Mims[52] cites some basic principles involved in the promotion of sexual health. The first of these acknowledges that there is no single set of appropriate sexual values in our society; rather, the professional needs to accept that major conflicts of values exist. A second principle basic to promotion of sexual health is that provision of accurate and adequate information is more helpful than indoctrination. Although it is often tempting to impose one's own solutions to sexual concerns or a values conflict on others, growth of the individual is more likely to be fostered by guidance rather than by indoctrination. Finally, it is suggested that individuals be assisted to make their own informed choices rather than conform to guidelines established by a professional or an agency. It is the individuals, and not the health professional, who will have to cope with the consequences of their choices.

Levels of intervention

Annon[2] presents an extremely useful distinction between the various levels of intervention possible for persons with sexual concerns or problems. He terms these levels *permission, limited information, specific suggestions,* and *intensive therapy.* These are listed in order of increasing sophistication, with permission giving requiring the most basic preparation and intensive

therapy requiring specific educational preparation in sex therapy theory and techniques. Annon's contention is that sexual problems may be resolved on a variety of levels and do not always require counseling or intensive therapy.

Permission

Often individuals merely want to know that they are normal, acceptable, and not "perverted," and they seek out the health professional for validation of their sexual normalcy. Permission is not merely a therapeutic measure but also a preventive one. It can be applied in a variety of community settings as well as in the hospital. Permission may be applied to thoughts, fantasies, dreams, and feelings as well as to overt sexual behaviors. At times nurses will be asked to provide individuals with permission *not* to engage in certain sexual behaviors if this is their choice. This may relieve individuals from feeling pressured to conform to someone else's standards for sexual behavior that are not necessarily their own.

Persons with disabling diseases that interefere with their usual forms of sexual expression may seek permission to discuss alternative approaches to sexual pleasure. For example, cord-injured persons may welcome the permission from staff members to discuss alternatives to penis-vagina intercourse. Women who do not experience orgasm with every act of intercourse may be seeking permission *not* to do so, even though some of their peers insist that "normal women do." The adolescent who is comparing his sexual prowess with that of peers may seek permission *not* to be sexually active. A common concern among young married couples is the normalcy of oral-genital sex. Often these couples merely seek reassurance that this variation is not perverted, or on the contrary that it is not necessary to engage in this practice unless both partners are comfortable with it.

In summary, permission giving can help individuals break associations between behaviors, thoughts, fantasies, dreams, and labels. Usually, these labels bear negative connotations such as "dirty," "perverted," or "abnormal."[2] Even though most sexual acts could be considered normal in some sense (e.g., statistically or phylogenetically), individuals do need to be aware of the consequences of their behavior. These consequences may include legal prosecution or social ostracism, and such concerns need to be explored with the individual before the counselor gives blanket permission to engage in such practices.

Limited information

The next level of intervention can also be therapeutic as well as preventive. It involves providing information to individuals that is directly relevant to their particular problems or concerns. Rather than condoning the individual's behavior, this approach may result in a change of behavior on the basis of an informed decision. Some common areas of sexual concern that may require only limited information include worry over breast and genital shape, configuration, and size; masturbation; sexual intercourse during menstruation; oral-genital sex. The nurse familiar with famous myths associated with each of these topics can appreciate that providing individuals with basic factual information regarding any of these concerns may be responsible for the resolution of their sexual worries.

A common concern among adolescent and young adult men is penis size. Giving the information that the smaller flaccid penis becomes about as large when erect as larger flaccid penises may be sufficient to relieve anxieties. A woman who is about to have a hysterectomy is often concerned that she will no longer be able to have intercourse or that she will have no more sexual desire. Informing the woman in advance of the surgery that this is not true may remove unnecessary barriers from the resumption of sexual activity. Similar information would be helpful to a man about to undergo a transurethral prostatectomy. Even though the man having a transurethral resection is likely to experience retrograde ejaculation, he may still have an erection and enjoy intercourse. Having this bit of information before surgery may avert dysfunctional sex later.

In sum, providing limited information can free the individual from anxieties connected with sexual performance or assumptions about negative effects of health-related conditions on sexual activity. Combating popular mythology with this approach is often a sufficient preventive or therapeutic measure.

Specific suggestions

Before giving individuals specific suggestions regarding direct attempts to help them change their behavior in order to reach a designated goal, it is essential to obtain a sexual problem history. This approach presupposes a brief approach to counseling individuals, with the understanding that if results are not achieved within a limited period, referral to someone prepared to provide intensive sexual therapy will be made. Again specific suggestions may be preventive as well as therapeutic. Some specific suggestions may relate to the conditions conducive to optimal sexual functioning, specific approaches to use given certain illnesses or surgeries, and directives for coping with some sexual dysfunctions.

One specific suggestion often incorporated in sexual counseling is that a couple having difficulties with intercourse abstain from it for a specified period. This admonition is designed to reduce the "pressure to perform" perceived by a member of the dysfunctional couple.

The counseling approach applied to persons who have

EXAMPLES OF SPECIFIC SUGGESTIONS FOR PERSONS RECOVERING FROM MYOCARDIAL INFARCTION

To minimize cardiac workload:

Avoid having intercourse in either very hot or very cold rooms.

Wait about 3 hours after eating a meal or drinking alcoholic beverages.

Allow plenty of time to rest afterwards.

Use positions that are comfortable.

Consult your health care provider if:

You have chest pain during or after intercourse.

You feel extremely tired after having intercourse.

You feel your heart beating very loudly for more than a few minutes after intercourse.

---

just had a myocardial infarction is outlined in the box above. These suggestions are designed to minimize the effects of cardiovascular problems during intercourse.* Similar specific suggestions can be given to cord-injured persons, including positions most likely to be comfortable, care of the catheter before and during intercourse, and techniques available to stimulate the noninjured partner. Use of imagery (fantasy) can also be incorporated as a specific suggestion.† Ostomy patients often have concerns about accidents involving their appliances during intercourse. Specific suggestions might include emptying the appliance before initiating sexual activity, employing cosmetic covers for the stoma bag, or avoiding excess pressure over the stoma site until the ostomy incision is well healed.‡

Finally, nurses can offer some rather simple directives for coping with specific sexual dysfunctions. The man with premature ejaculation can be taught to use the "squeeze technique" (p. 1766), or the partner may learn

---

*Clients can refer to Scheingold, L., and Wagner, N.: Sound sex and the aging heart, New York, 1974, Human Services Press.
†Clients can refer to Bregman, S.: Sexuality and the spinal cord injured woman, 1975, Sister Kenny Institute, Office of Continuing Education, Dept. 188, 1800 Chicago Ave., Minneapolis, MN 55404.
Mooney, T., Cole, T., and Chilgrin, R.: Sexual options for paraplegics and quadriplegics, Boston, 1975, Little, Brown & Co.
Toward intimacy: family planning and sexuality concerns of physically disabled women, Planned Parenthood of Snohomish County, 2730 Hoyt, Everett, WA 98201.
‡Clients can refer to the following: Binder, D.: Sex, courtship, and the single ostomate, Los Angeles, 1973, United Ostomy Association.
Gambrell, E.: Sex and the male ostomate, Los Angeles, 1973, United Ostomy Association.
Norris, C., and Gambrell, E.: Sex, pregnancy, and the female ostomate, Los Angeles, 1972, United Ostomy Association.

to apply it. Women who have inadequate lubrication and experience painful intercourse as a consequence of steroid changes during the postpartum period or menopause may benefit from the use of a water-soluble lubricant such as K-Y jelly.

Intensive sexual therapy

The intensive sexual therapy approach combines techniques and concepts of psychotherapy with special approaches to intervention for individuals or couples having sexual problems. Usually the problems involved are one or more of the sexual dysfunctions discussed in Chapter 67. Since a discussion of the many approaches to intensive therapy is beyond the scope of this text, interested readers are referred to the references.* These forms of therapy usually require intensive preparation beyond that provided in most schools of nursing. However, an awareness of the sexual dysfunctions discussed in Chapter 67 will enable nurses to refer clients with complex problems to trained therapists.

Contexts for intervention

One context in which nurses may intervene is the one-to-one relationship. Individuals may initiate questions about their sexual concerns or problems that do not require intervention with both partners. Others may not have a current partner, or a partner may be unwilling to be involved in counseling.

Often sexual issues may arise in the course of dealing with family problems. Some sexual issues may be appropriately addressed in the context of family therapy.[100] Sexual issues also may be addressed in group therapy settings where peer consultation and support are available to the individual. Finally, sexual issues are thought to be most profitably addressed in the context of the dyad. The assumption here is that there is never an uninvolved partner in a relationship where sexual problems exist.[45]

Mims and Swenson[53] point out that if nurses attempt to provide sexual health care based on their life experiences, their behaviors may be both destructive and intuitively helpful. Because nurses are exposed to the same confusing messages and misinformation about sexuality as others, they may perpetuate incorrect or destructive ideas about sexuality. Mims and Swenson describe three levels in the provision of sexual health care that are based on an increasingly sophisticated preparation. The first level is characterized by increasing awareness on the part of the nurse. Awareness is a product of the interactions between perceptions, attitudes, and cognitions, in other words, a consciousness-raising process. The next level incorporates communi-

cation, counseling, and teaching skills to give permission and to give information. The most advanced level includes suggestion giving, therapy, educational programs, and research projects. A basic course in human sexuality would permit many nurses to provide capably specific suggestions, whereas postbaccalaureate education is seen as necessary preparation for providing sex therapy, planning and conducting educational programs, and conducting sex research.

REFERENCES AND SELECTED READINGS
Contemporary

1. *Ager, J.W., et al.: Vasectomy: who gets one and why, Am. J. Public Health 64:680-686, 1974.
2. Annon, J.: The behavioral treatment of sexual problems, Honolulu, 1974, Enabling Systems, Inc.
3. Antunes, C., et al.: Endometrial cancer and estrogen use, N. Engl. J. Med. 300:9-13, 1979.
4. Banner, E.A.: The menopause and thereafter, Postgrad. Med. 59:174-178, 1976.
5. Bartuske, D.G.: Physiology of aging: metabolic changes during the climacteric and menopausal problems, Clin. Obstet. Gynecol. 20:105-112, 1977.
6. Behrman, S.J., and Kistner, R.W., editors: Progress in infertility, ed. 2, Boston, 1975, Little, Brown & Co.
8. Budoff, P.: Use of mefenamic acid in the treatment of primary dysmenorrhea, J.A.M.A. 241:2713-2716, 1979.
9. Casper, R.F., Yen, S.S., and Wilkes, M.M.: Menopausal flushes: a neuroendocrine link with pulsatile luteinizing hormone secretion, Science 205:823-825, 1979.
10. Clarkson, T.I., and Alexander, N.: Long-term vasectomy: effects on the occurrence and extent of atherosclerosis in rhesus monkeys, J. Clin. Invest. 65:15-25, 1980.
11. Contraceptive utilization among currently married women 15-44 years of age: United States, 1973, National Survey of Family Growth Data from the National Center for Health Statistics, Monthly Vital Statistics Report 25(suppl.), 1976.
12. *Cowart, M., and Newton, D.W.: Oral contraceptives: how best to explain their effects to patients, Nurs. '76 6(6):44-48, 1976.
13. *Davis, J.E.: Vasectomy, Am. J. Nurs. 72:509-513, 1972.
14. Delaney, J., Lupton, M.J., and Toth, E.: The curse: a cultural history of menstruation, New York, 1976, New American Library.
15. Detre, T., et al.: Management of the menopause, Ann. Intern. Med. 88:373-378, 1978.
16. *Effer, S.: Gynecologic aspects of the "routine" checkup, Postgrad. Med. 59:164-170, 1976.
17. Evans, M.I., Mukherjee, A.B., and Schulman, J.D.: Human in vitro fertilization, Obstet. Gynecol. Surv. 35:71-81, 1980.
18. Expanding the clinical potential of prostaglandins, Contemp. Obstet. Gynecol. 16(3):133-140, 1980.
19. Fleischauer, M.L.: A modified Lamaze approach in the treatment of primary dysmenorrhea, J. Am. Coll. Health Assoc. 25:273-275, 1977.
20. *Fogel, C.I., and Woods, N.F.: Health care of women: a nursing perspective, St. Louis, 1981, The C.V. Mosby Co.
21. Goldacre, M., et al.: Follow-up of vasectomy using medical record linkage, Am. J. Epidemiol. 108:176-180, 1978.
22. Guilleband, J.: Pelvic inflammatory disease and IUCD's, Br. J. Fam. Plann. 4:25-31, 1978.

---

*References 2, 34, 35, 39, 45.

*References preceded by an asterisk are particularly well suited for student reading.

23. Hackett, R.E., and Waterhouse, K.: Vasectomy reviewed, Am. J. Obstet. Gynecol. **116**:438-455, 1973.

24. Halbert, D.R., Demers, L.M., and Darnell Jones, D.E.: Dysmenorrhea and prostaglandins, Obstet. Gynecol. Surv. **31**(1):77-81, 1976.

25. Hatcher, R.A., et al.: Contraceptive technology, 1980-1981, ed. 10, New York, 1980, John Wiley & Sons, Inc.

26. Heczey, M.D.: Effects of biofeedback and autogenic training on dysmenorrhea, paper presented at The Menstrual Cycle: An Interdisciplinary Conference, Chicago, June 27-28, 1977, University of Illinois.

27. Henderson, S.: Reversal of female sterilization: comparison of microsurgical and gross surgical techniques for tubal anastomosis, Am. J. Obstet. Gynecol. **139**:73-79, 1981.

28. *Hogan, R.: Human sexuality: a nursing perspective, New York, 1980, Appleton-Century-Crofts.

29. Hoover, R., et al.: Menopausal estrogens and breast cancer, N. Engl. J. Med. **295**:401-405, 1976.

30. *Houghton, B.: Vasectomies affect women, too, Am. J. Nurs. **73**:821-825, 1981.

31. *Huxall, L.: Today's pill and the individual woman, M.C.N. **2**:359-363, 1977.

32. *Jelovsek, F.R., et al.: Risk of exogenous estrogen therapy and endometrial cancer, Am. J. Obstet. Gynecol. **137**:85-91, 1980.

33. Jowsey, J.: Why is mineral nutrition important in osteoporosis? Geriatrics **33**(8):39-52, 1978.

34. Kaplan, H.S.: Disorders of sexual desire and other new concepts and techniques in sex therapy, New York, 1979, Simon & Schuster, Inc.

35. Kaplan, H.S.: The new sex therapy, New York, 1974, Brunner/Mazel, Inc.

36. Landesman, R., and Saxena, B.B.: Results of the first 1,000 radioreceptor assays for the determination of human chorionic gonadotropin: a new, rapid, reliable and sensitive pregnancy test, Fertil. Steril. **27**:357-368, 1976.

37. *Langer, A., et al.: Choice of an oral contraceptive, Am. J. Obstet. Gynecol. **126**:153-157, 1976.

38. Lauritzen, C.: Management of the patient at risk with estrogen therapy, Front. Horm. Res. **5**:230-247, 1978.

39. Lo Piccolo, J., and Lo Piccolo, L., editors: Handbook of sex therapy, New York, 1978, Plenum Press.

40. Loffer, F.: Anticipating complications of laparoscopic sterilization, Contemp. Obstet. Gynecol. **17**(3):41-51, 1981.

41. Lovesky, J.: Menstruation: alternatives to pharmacologic therapy for menstrual distress, J. Nurse Midwife. **23**:34-44, 1978.

42. Mack, T.M., et al.: Estrogens and endometrial cancer in a retirement community, N. Engl. J. Med. **294**:1262-1267, 1976.

43. Marshall, S., and Lyon, R.P.: Variability of sperm disappearance from the ejaculate following vasectomy, J. Urol. **107**:815-817, 1972.

44. Martin, L.: Health care of women, Philadelphia, 1978, J.B. Lippincott Co.

45. Masters, W., and Johnson, V.: Human sexual inadequacy, Boston, 1970, Little, Brown & Co.

46. McCarthy, B., Ryan, B.M., and Johnson, F.: Sexual awareness: a practical approach, San Francisco, 1975, Boyd & Fraser Publishing Co.

47. Meckler, J., and Jordan, J.: The relationship of life change events, social supports, and symptoms of dysmenorrhea, master's report, Chapel Hill, 1980, University of North Carolina.

48. Meema, H.E., and Meema, S.: Involutional (physiologic) bone loss in women and the feasibility of preventing structural failure, J. Am. Geriatr. Soc. **22**:443-452, 1974.

49. Meldrum, D.R., et al.: Gonadotropins, estrogens, and andrenal steroids during the menopausal hot flash, J. Clin. Endocrinol. Metab. **50**:685-689, 1980.

50. *Menning, B.E.: Counseling infertile couples, Contemp. Obstet. Gynecol. **13**:101-108, 1979.

51. Menning, B.E.: Infertility: a guide for the childless couple, Englewood Cliffs, N.J., 1977, Prentice-Hall, Inc.

52. *Mims, F.: Sexual health education and counseling, Nurs. Clin. North Am. **10**:519-528, 1975.

53. *Mims, F., and Swenson, M.: Sexuality: a nursing perspective, New York, 1980, Appleton-Century-Crofts.

54. Moghissi, K., et al.: Homologous artificial insemination, Am. J. Obstet. Gynecol. **129**:909-913, 1977.

55. Murray, R., and Zentner, J.: Nursing assessment and health promotion through the life span, Englewood Cliffs, N.J., 1975, Prentice-Hall, Inc.

56. Notelovitz, M.: Gynecologic problems of menopausal women, I. Changes in genital tissue, Geriatrics **33**(8):24-32, 1978.

57. Notelovitz, M.: Gynecologic problems of menopausal women. II. Treating estrogen deficiency, Geriatrics **33**(9):35-38, 1978.

58. Novak, E.R., Jones, G.S., and Jones, H.W., Jr.: Novak's textbook of gynecology, ed. 10, Baltimore, 1981, The Williams & Wilkins Co.

59. Oral contraceptives, Federal Register, part II, Jan. 31, 1978.

60. Oral contraceptives, Population Reports (A), no. 1, Jan. 1974.

61. Ory, H., et al.: Contraceptive choice and prevalence of cervical dysplasia and carcinoma in situ, Am. J. Obstet. Gynecol. **124**:573-577, 1976.

62. *Patient information: what you should know about infertility, Contemp. Obstet. Gynecol **15**:101-105, 1980.

63. Pfeffer, R.: Estrogen use in postmenopausal women, Am. J. Epidemiol. **105**:21-29, 1977.

64. Phillips, W.S., and Lightman, S.L.: Is cutaneous flushing prostaglandin mediated? Lancet **1**:754-756, 1981.

65. Pietrow, P., Rinehart, W., and Schmidt, J.: Intrauterine devices, Population Reports (B) no. 3, May 1979.

66. Proudfit, C.M.: Estrogens and menopause, J.A.M.A. **236**:939-940, 1976.

67. Recommendations for minimizing adverse psychological results, paper presented at the Second International Conference on Sterilization, Geneva, 1973.

68. Reeder, S.R., Mastroianni, L., and Martin, L.: Maternity nursing, ed. 14, Philadelphia, 1980, J.B. Lippincott Co.

69. Riggs, B.L., et al.: Short- and long-term effects of estrogen and synthetic anabolic hormones in postmenopausal osteoporosis, J. Clin. Invest. **51**:1659-1663, 1972.

70. Sandelowski, M.: Women, health and choice, Englewood Cliffs, N.J., 1981, Prentice-Hall, Inc.

71. Sawatzky, M.: Tasks of infertile couples, J.O.G.N. Nurs. **10**:132-133, 1981.

72. Seaman, B., and Seaman, G.: Women and the crisis in sex hormones, New York, 1977, Rawson Associates.

73. *Siegler, A.M.: Tubal sterilization, Am. J. Nurs. **72**:1624-1629, 1972.

74. Smith, D.C., et al.: Association of estrogen and endometrial carcinoma, N. Engl. J. Med. **293**:1164-1167, 1975.

75. Smith, R.P., and Powell, J.R.: The objective evaluation of dysmenorrhea therapy, Am. J. Obstet. Gynecol. **137**:314-319, 1980.

76. Sparks, R., et al.: The bacteriology of the cervical canal in relation to the use of an intrauterine device. Proceedings of the workshop The Uterine Cervix in Human Reproduction, Stuttgart, W. Germany, 1977, Georg Thieme Verlag KG.

77. Speroff, L, Glass, R.H., and Kase, N.: Clinical gynecologic endocrinology and infertility, ed. 2, Baltimore, 1978, The Williams & Wilkins Co.

78. Squires, J.W., Barb, M.W., and Pinch, L.W.: The morbidity of vasectomy, Surg. Gynecol. Obstet. **143**:237-240, 1976.

79. Stadel, B.V., and Weiss, N.: Characteristics of menopausal women: a survey of King and Pierce counties in Washington, 1973-1974, Am. J. Epidemiol. **102**:209-210, 1975.

80. Taylor, R.N., et al.: Changes in menstrual cycle length and regularity after using oral contraceptives, J. Gynecol. Obstet. **15**:55-59, 1977.

81. Thompson, B., and Baird, D.: Follow-up of 186 sterilized women, Lancet **1**:1023-1027, 1968.

82. Tietze, C.: The pill and mortality from cardiovascular disease: another look, Fam. Plann. Perspect. **11**(12):80-89, 1979.

83. Tietze, C., Bongaarts, J., and Schearer, B.: Mortality associated with the control of fertility, Fam. Plann. Perspect. **8**(1):6-14, 1976.

84. Trussell, T.J., Faden, R., and Hatcher, R.A.: Efficacy information in contraceptive counseling: those little white lies, Am. J. Public Health **66**:761-767, 1976.

85. Tubal sterilization: review of methods, Population Reports (C), no. 7, May 1976.

86. Tung, K.: Human sperm antigens and antisperm antibodies. I. Study on vasectomized patients, Clin. Exp. Immunol. **20**:93-104, 1975.

87. *Tyson, M.C.: Let's talk about menopause, Nurs. '78 **8**(8):34-36, 1978.

88. Ulfelder, H.: The stilbestrol-adenosis-carcinoma syndrome, CA **38**(suppl.):426-431, 1976.

89. Umezaki, C., Katayama, K.P., and Jones, H.W., Jr.: Pregnancy rates after reconstructive surgery on the fallopian tubes, Obstet. Gynecol. **43**:418-424, 1974.

90. U.S. Department of Health, Education and Welfare, Public Health Service: VD fact sheet, ed. 32, DHEW pub. no. (CDC) 76-8195, Atlanta, 1976, Center for Disease Control.

91. Walker, A., et al.: Hospitalization rates in vasectomized men, J.A.M.A. **245**:2315-2318, 1981.

92. Weinstein, L.: Sterilization via the mini-laparotomy technique, Clin. Obstet. Gynecol. **23**:273-280, 1980.

93. Westoff, C.: The modernization of U.S. contraceptive practice, Fam. Plann. Perspect. **4**(3):9-12, 1977.

94. *Woods, J.S.: Drug effects on human sexual behavior. In Woods, N.F.: Human sexuality in health and illness, ed. 3, St. Louis, 1983, The C.V. Mosby Co.

95. Ylikorkala, O., and Dawood, M.Y.: New concepts in dysmenorrhea, Am. J. Obstet. Gynecol. **130**:833-847, 1978.

96. Ziel, H., and Finkle, W.: Increased risk of endometrial carcinoma among users of conjugated estrogens, N. Engl. J. Med. **293**:1167-1170, 1975.

Classic

97. Feber, A.S., Tietze, C., and Lewit, C.: Men with vasectomies: a study of medical, sexual, and psychosocial changes, Psychosom. Med. **29**:354-366, 1967.

98. Guttmacher, A.: Fertility of man, Fertil. Steril. **3**:281, 1952.

99. Lu, T., and Chin, D.: A long-term follow-up of 1,055 cases of postpartum tubal ligation, J. Obstet. Gynecol. Br. Commonw. **74**:875-880, 1967.

100. Satir, V.: Conjoint family therapy, rev. ed., Palo Alto, Calif., 1967, Science and Behavior Books, Inc.

AUDIOVISUAL RESOURCES

Communicating family planning: speak, they are listening, Media Resources Branch, National Medical Ausiovisual Center (Annex), Station K, Atlanta, GA 30324. (Motion picture.)

Infertility and sterility, The American Journal of Nursing Co., Educational Services Division, 10 Columbus Circle, New York, NY 10019. (Motion picture on audiotape and slides.)

The nurse's role in family planning, The American Journal of Nursing Co., Educational Services Division, 10 Columbus Circle, New York, NY 10019. (Film.)

CHAPTER 65

PROBLEMS OF THE REPRODUCTIVE SYSTEM

MARGARET LAMB
DEBORAH POWER
NANCY FUGATE WOODS
ELLA CINKOTA

Since both professionals and lay people have become more enlightened about prevention of problems of the reproductive system, there is heightened awareness of the importance of illness prevention and health promotion throughout the life span. This increased awareness has led many persons to initiate requests for information about or treatment of reproductive system problems.

Although men and women are better informed today about matters relating to reproductive health than they were previously, many neglect preventive measures and ignore signs or symptoms of illness because of embarassment and the special significance that they attach to the reproductive organs.

In spite of advanced in medicine, science, and technology, diseases and disorders of the genital system continue to threaten the lives and the physical and emotional health of men and women, sometimes needlessly. Many of these problems are preventable; many of them can be treated and cured. Nurses occupy a unique position because their daily contacts with men and women provide opportunities to actively seek out persons in need of information and other forms of assistance, help people find necessary information, seek solutions to their problems, increase their awareness of health-promoting measures, and promote their comfort in discussing problems related to reproduction and their prevention and treatment.

PROBLEMS AFFECTING WOMEN

Infectious processes

Infections of the vulva and vagina

Epidemiology, etiology, and pathophysiology

Although the vulva and vagina are considered to be relatively resistant to infection, infections are quite common. Many organisms play a causative role, including streptococci, staphylococci, Pseudomonas, *Escherichia coli, Candida albicans, Trichomonas vaginalis, Treponema pallidum, Neisseria gonorrhoeae*, chlamydiae, *Trachomatis, Gardnerella vaginalis*, and the virus of herpes simplex. (Parasites such as pinworms, mechanical irritants, and contact allergens can also cause vaginal discharge.) It is possible, however, for women to harbor many of these organisms without developing infection. Thus one must consider the factors associated with increased risk of infection in some women.

Normally, the vagina is protected from infection by its pH and the presence of *Döderlein's bacilli*. If the vaginal pH is altered, if the invading organisms are numerous, or if the woman's resistance is decreased by aging, malnutrition, stress, disease, or the use of drugs, the woman's risk of infection is increased. Yeast organisms grow best in an acid pH less than 4.7, whereas *Trichomonas* and organisms causing nonspecific vaginitis thrive in a pH greater than 5.

Organisms causing infection of the vulva and vagina are most often introduced from outside sources such as clothing, hands, douche nozzles, or other contaminated articles or during intercourse. In sexually active women, reinfection may occur following treatment unless their sexual partners are also successfully treated. Because vaginitis produced by *Candida albicans*, trichomonas, and *Gardnerella vaginalis* is considered a sexually transmitted disease, it will be discussed in greater detail later in this chapter (p. 1722).

Nonspecific vaginitis is a superficial vaginal infection that may be caused by *Gardnerella vaginalis* or unidentified organisms (p. 1735).

Vaginitis in mature women. Women of menopausal and postmenopausal ages often develop vaginitis (some refer to this as atrophic or senile vaginitis; we prefer a less negative diagnostic label). Pyogenic bacterial invasion of the thin vaginal mucosa produces symptoms of burning, pruritus, and leukorrhea. Vaginitis is usually treated with warm douches of a weak acid solution such as vinegar and water (15 ml [1 tbsp] vinegar to 1 L [1 qt] water). An estrogenic preparation, given orally or applied intravaginally as an ointment, may help to restore the vaginal epithelium to a normal state. Because of the link between estrogen use in menopausal women and endometrial cancer, this therapy should be used with caution.

Bartholinitis. Invasion of Bartholin's glands by streptococci, staphylococci, gonococci, *E. coli*, or anaerobes may result in infection. The infection is usually unilateral but may be bilateral. With infection, the duct from the gland becomes partially or completely obstructed, resulting in severe redness, enlargement of the gland, and edema of the surrounding tissues. The area becomes tender, and walking may become difficult because of the pain. Sometimes the abscess that forms ruptures and affords almost immediate relief of pain. Most often, however, this is followed by recurrence of symptoms. The usual course of the infectious process results in an abscess that does not rupture and requires surgical incision and drainage. A smear or culture is usually taken to identify the causative organism, and an appropriate antibiotic is prescribed. The cervix should be cultured for gonococci.

Occasionally, acute bartholinitis subsides, leaving fibrotic or scar tissue. When this occurs, Bartholin's cyst develops. The cyst may vary in size from a few centimeters in diameter to the size of a hen's egg, is mobile, and is not tender. If the cyst grows to be of sufficient size to interfere with walking or intercourse, or if it shows signs of inflammation, it may be excised surgically.

Skene's glands are less often infected than are Bartholin's glands. When infection does occur, the local symptoms include redness, enlargement of the gland, tenderness, and accumulation of pus. These also may spontaneously rupture or require incision and drainage. Identification of the causative organism by smear or culture is important in determining the need for antibiotic therapy. Infections proven to be or strongly suspected of being sexually transmitted are discussed in the section on sexually transmitted diseases.

Prevention

Recognition of predisposing factors is important in the prevention of vulvar and vaginal infections. Risk factors associated with vulvar and vaginal infections include pregnancy, premenarchal age, menopausal and postmenopausal status, allergies, diabetes, oral contraceptives, inadequate hygiene, excessive douching or use of vaginal inserts, treatment with broad-spectrum antibiotics, and intercourse with an infected partner. Those women in whom the natural barriers to infection (low estrogen levels, thinness of the vaginal epithelium, or reduced acidity of the vagina) are at a minimum are at greatest risk.

Some women may require instruction in daily health and hygiene practices. In particular, it is important that women wipe from front to back after bowel movements to avoid fecal contamination of the vulva. Maintaining cleanliness of the vulva and vagina without altering vaginal pH is essential. Frequent douching may alter vaginal pH, and using a high-pressure douche may irritate vaginal tissues and facilitate the spread of infection into the pelvis. In general, women should not douche unless advised to do so for treatment. Women can also be advised to void shortly after having intercourse, thus removing organisms from the urethra and vulva. Women also may need to know the characteristics of normal vaginal discharges and how to distinguish between these and abnormal discharges. They need to be informed of the other signs of vulvar and vaginal infections and the particular significance of lesions on the vulva. Sexually active women may require information about how to recognize signs of infection in their partners and the importance of seeking medical attention when they suspect the partner is infected. Pregnant and diabetic women need to know about their predisposition to infections and how to prevent infection from occurring, and they need to be urged to seek professional help as soon as signs of infection develop.

Clinical picture

The patient is asked to give a detailed account of her symptoms including duration and what she has done to relieve them. The history should include sexual practices (including the last sexual exposure so that the incubation period can be calculated) and information about signs of infection in the sex partner. The history and physical examination may reveal predisposing factors, patterns of repeated infections, or evidence of concurrent problems. In such cases, further examination, laboratory tests, or clinical studies may be indicated.

The vulva and vagina are inspected and palpated (see Chapter 63). A smear or culture is taken from the vagina, and a Papanicolaou (Pap) smear may also be taken. Palpation of the internal organs of reproduction will help to determine whether upward extension of infection has occurred.

The common signs of infection of the vulva and vagina are inflammation of the tissues; abnormal discharge from the vagina, urethra, or Bartholin's glands; and itching (pruritus). The discharge may be purulent, white, and curdlike or grayish white. *Leukorrhea*, a white vaginal discharge, is a symptom of vaginal infections, but it is also associated with erosions of the cervix. This discharge differs from the normal vaginal discharge occurring just before menstruation in that it is more abundant and thicker and is associated with inflammation and pruritus.

Each of the organisms producing vaginitis is usually associated with a specific type of vaginal discharge (Table 65-1). In addition, each organism may produce slightly different symptoms. Itching is common to most, but *Trichomonas* is usually associated with intense itching of the vulva. Severe itching may be present because of menopausal changes in the epithelium, vitamin A deficiency, irritation from chronic discharge, high urinary sugar content as in diabetes mellitus, pediculosis pubis, scabies, allergies, pinworms, and cancer of the vulva. With severe pruritus there are usually excoriations of the skin caused by scratching, and secondary infection may result. Dysuria may occur as a consequence of local irritation of the urinary meatus. Abdominal cramps and abdominal or pelvic fullness may also be associated with vaginal infections.

Lesions of various types may be seen on the vulva, between the labial folds, or inside the vagina. These may appear as macules, papules, boils, abscesses, vesicles, ulcers, or eroded areas. Skene's or Bartholin's glands may be enlarged because of accumulation of pus.

Intervention

Since most women having vulvar and vaginal infections are treated on an outpatient basis, it is imperative that they be actively involved in decisions and plans related to therapy.

A variety of methods are available for management

TABLE 65-1. Common causes of vaginal discharge, symptoms, diagnostic measures, and treatment*

Cause	Symptoms	Diagnostic measures	Treatment
Infections			
Candida albicans (<50% of all vaginitis)	White, curdlike, cheesy discharge; characteristic patches on vaginal walls and cervix; itching; inflamed vagina and cervix	KOH slide shows hyphae and/or spores; Nickerson culture	Miconazole (Monistat) cream used daily for 14 days Nystatin suppositories daily or bid for 14 days
Trichomonas vaginalis	Yellowish to greenish, frothy, copious discharge; "strawberry spots" on cervix; foul odor; severe burning, itching and dyspareunia	Saline wet smears show *Trichomonas*	Metronidazole (Flagyl), 250 mg tid for 7 days *or* 2 g stat for both partners Symptomatic therapy
Gardnerella vaginalis	Grayish white, homogeneous discharge; scant amount; fishy or foul odor	Saline wet smear demonstrates typical "clue" cells	Oral antibiotics for both partners: ampicillin, 500 mg qid for 5 days; metronidazole (Flagyl), 250 mg tid for 7 days
Foreign body	Blood tinged, serosanguineous, or purulent discharge; usually foul odor; discharge may be thick or thin	Visualization of object	Removal of object; antibiotics specific to secondary infection
Allergens or irritants	Increase in usual type and amount of secretions; itching, burning, rash	By exclusion of other possible causes; identification of possible allergen or irritant	Removal of possible allergen or irritant; topical steroid ointment as needed
Cervicitis	Yellow, mucopurulent discharge; erosion seen on cervix; cervix appears inflamed and irritated with varying amounts of ulceration; nabothian cysts; mucosa around os everted	Pap smear; visualization of cervical lesions; gonorrhea or other culture to identify infecting organism	Cauterization; antibiotics; conization of cervix For *Chlamydia* infection: tetracycline, 250 mg qid for 14 days for both partners

*From Fogel, C.I., and Woods, N.F.: Health care of women: a nursing perspective, St. Louis, 1981, The C.V. Mosby Co.

and treatment of vulvar and vaginal infections. The major goals are to cure the infection, prevent reinfection, prevent complications associated with infections of the reproductive tract, and prevent infection of the sexual partner or partners. In fact, with *Trichomonas* or persistent nonspecific vaginitis, the partner is often treated as a contact although he has no signs or symptoms. Usual methods for treating vaginal infections are given in Table 65-1. Some alternative therapies developed by women themselves are included in Table 65-2.

Abscesses require incision and drainage, and this is usually done at the time the woman first seeks medical attention. Antibiotics may be given if cervicitis or systemic effects of another infection are present. The woman needs to be advised to expect a small amount of purulent drainage that may be slightly tinged with blood and to promptly report any active, bright red bleeding. Relief from pain occurs almost immediately following incision and drainage. The woman may experience soreness or mild pain for about a day. Perineal irrigations serve the purposes of cleansing and giving comfort. Nurses can suggest that women use warm water to cleanse the involved area after each voiding or bowel movement.

Douching (p. 1640) is frequently prescribed for treatment of vaginal infections; for example, povidone-iodine (Betadine) douches are recommended for *Trichomonas* when metronidazole is contraindicated. Local applications in the form of vaginal suppositories, ointments, or creams are commonly employed when vaginal infection occurs. A model of the pelvis is of value in showing women how to use these preparations. The woman is advised of the importance of hand washing before and after each application. Because the substances used to treat vaginitis melt with body heat, the patient is advised to lie down after insertion to facilitate distri-

bution of the medication in the vaginal canal and to prevent loss of medication from the vagina. Women are advised not to douche but to wear a minipad.

When douche equipment is necessary, it is essential that women understand how to clean and disinfect their equipment. Douche equipment should be washed and soaked in diluted bleach for approximately 30 minutes.

Most of the suppositories, creams, and ointments used contain an antibiotic or a drug specific to the causative organism. Estrogenic preparations are sometimes prescribed. The patient is cautioned to report aggravation of any symptoms or appearance of symptoms not previously noted.

Heat increases circulation, promotes healing, and provides comfort. Applications of heat may be prescribed in the form of hot soaks, douches, perineal irrigations, or sitz baths. The patient may require instruction in any of these procedures. If both heat and local applications of medications are prescribed, the patient is instructed to use the medication after application of heat.

Most women who have vaginal infections are advised to abstain from intercourse during the period of treatment. The extent to which abstinence is possible should be explored, and if this is not feasible for the woman, use of a condom by the male partner until symptoms of infection disappear can be suggested.

Women taking oral contraceptives should be carefully screened and examined during interim visits to the physician for signs of vaginal infection. If repeated episodes of infection occur, it may be necessary for the patient to try an alternate brand of pill used as a contraceptive. If infections continue, it usually becomes necessary for the woman to use an entirely different method of birth control (see Chapter 64).

When pruritus is present, the patient needs to know

TABLE 65-2. Alternative therapies for vaginitis*

Infection	Intervention	Dosage	Administration
Monilia	Gentian violet	Few drops/qt water 0.25% to 2% (over-the-counter drug)	Douche or local application
	Vinegar (white)	1 tbsp/1 pt water	Douche every day for 5-7 days; twice daily for 2 days
	Acidophilus culture	2 tbsp/1 pt water	Douche twice daily
	Acidophilus yogurt	1 application hourly and as needed to labia	
	Plain yogurt	for symptom relief	
Trichomonas	1 handful chapparel chamomile	Steep in 1 qt water for 20 min	Douche 2-3 times/wk for 2 wk
Nonspecific vaginitis	Vinegar douche	5 tbsp/2 qt water	Every other day for 1 wk
	Salt (sea)	1 tbsp/1 qt water	Every other day for 1 wk
	1 tsp goldenseal and		
	1 clove minced garlic	Steep in 1 qt boiling water	Douche every day for 1 wk
	1 tsp goldenseal	Steep in 1 pt water; strain with cloth	Douche every day for 1 wk
	Povidone-iodine (Betadine) gel		Twice daily for 1 wk

*From Fogel, C.I., and Woods, N.F.: Health care of women: a nursing perspective, St. Louis, 1981, The C.V. Mosby Co.

that any irritation such as scratching can aggravate the itching and predispose to secondary infection. Frequent bathing, sitz baths, and careful cleansing are essential for comfort as well as prevention of complications. Soothing lotions are sometimes prescribed to relieve itching. If the pruritus is severe enough to interfere with sleep, the physician may prescribe a mild sedative.

All patients need to know when to return for follow-up care and what steps to take in preparation for examination at the time of the return visit.

Women need to know what observations to make regarding success of treatment and what signs to report indicating problems.

Outcome criteria for the woman with a vulvar or vaginal infection

The woman can:
1. Demonstrate an increase in knowledge about her body and promoting her health.
2. Practice habits that improve or promote her health.
3. Describe how infections occur and are spread.
4. Identify ways to prevent reinfection.
5. State how changes in daily practices influence control of infection.

When the woman must employ therapies at home, she should be able to:
1. State the limitations imposed by the infection and self-care activities.
2. Describe a realistic schedule of therapy and necessary modifications of daily living.
3. Cite alternative ways in which the needs of family members can be met.

When the woman who has a vulvar or vaginal infection is presented with alternatives of therapy, she will be able to:
1. State reasons for her choice of therapy.
2. Describe the rationale and expected results of the treatment.
3. Describe use and methods of cleaning and storing special equipment, if cleaning and storage are required.

Cervicitis

Epidemiology, etiology, and pathophysiology

Cervicitis, infection of the cervix, is the most common gynecologic disorder, affecting over half of all women. The gonococcus, streptococcus, staphylococcus, a variety of other aerobic and anaerobic organisms, herpes virus, and chlamydia may be responsible for the infection. There are two forms of cervicitis—acute and chronic. Chronic cervicitis is the most frequent of all the pathologic conditions of the cervix. Cervicitis usually progresses from the acute to the chronic form if not treated, and it

may go undetected for a long period of time. In fact, the cervix may heal and appear quite healthy after the disease has spread upward. This condition presents few symptoms, and those symptoms that occur do not ordinarily lead women to seek medical attention. Leukorrhea may be the only sign, and if it is a small amount of discharge, the woman may not become concerned. Pain does not usually occur unless the infection extends upward and involves the uterus or adjacent pelvic structures. A long history of leukorrhea may lead the nurse or physician to suspect cervicitis.

Cervicitis may follow childbirth or abortion, or it may be caused by infection of a cervical laceration or erosion. In untreated cervicitis, the tissues are constantly irritated, and there is some evidence that this irritation predisposes to cancer.

Prevention

If the practice of a careful 6-week postpartum examination were adhered to and if women presented themselves for yearly examinations, much acute and chronic cervicitis could be prevented. During childbirth, the cervix is frequently lacerated as it stretches and thins to allow the baby to pass through the birth canal. These torn surfaces do not always heal properly and thus serve as foci for infection. At the 6-week postpartum examination, improperly healed lacerations of the cervix and cervical erosions can be easily detected and treated.

Prompt detection and treatment of infections of the vulva and vagina can prevent upward spread of infection resulting in cervicitis. The preventive aspects discussed under infection of the vulva and vagina are applicable to prevention of cervical infections. Opportunities similarly arise for teaching women about desirable health habits and prescribed therapy.

Clinical picture

Acute cervicitis may be present without subjective symptoms. When inspected, however, the cervix is grossly erythematous and edematous, and the mucosa around the external os shows hypertrophic ectopy and looks everted. There is usually a mucoid, purulent discharge from the cervix, but the amount may be so small that it is not noticed by the patient. A smear or culture of the discharge is taken to determine the causative organism, as well as the number of white blood cells.

Chronic cervicitis is a common cause of leukorrhea. On examination, a laceration or eversion of the cervix may be seen. Purulent discharge from the cervix is common, and erythema and hypertrophy of the cervix are usually present. Inclusion cysts, appearing as gray or white vesicles, may be seen on the surface of the cervix. A reddened, irritated area (an erosion) may or may not be present. Hyperemia of the infected cervix may produce intermenstrual or postcoital spotting. Some women may merely complain of infertility as a result of the thick, viscid cervical mucus interrupting sperm transport, pruritus, or vulvar burning; others may experience lower abdominal pain or dyspareunia as a result of pelvic congestion.

A Pap smear or cervical biopsy specimen is frequently taken when patients have cervicitis. This is usually done as a precautionary measure to rule out malignancy.

Intervention

In acute cervicitis, the associated vaginitis is usually treated first, and then the condition of the cervix is evaluated. Acute gonococcal cervicitis is usually treated with procaine penicillin G, 4.8 million units, given intramuscularly. Women who are allergic to penicillin can be treated with tetracycline, 1.5 g followed by 0.5 g four times daily for 3 days. Usually the cervix is recultured in a week and serologic tests for syphilis performed 6 to 9 weeks later. Women with trichomoniasis are given metronidazole (Flagyl), 250 mg orally three times daily for 10 days. Their partners are simultaneously treated with metronidazole, 250 mg two times daily for 10 days. For candidal infections, nystatin vaginal suppositories (100 mg) are used twice daily for 10 days, or miconazole (Monistat) cream may be used. Sultrin cream is usually prescribed for *Gardnerella* infections. Some physicians advocate treatment of acute cervicitis with tetracycline, 2 g daily for 7 days. In chronic cervicitis, the infection has extended deeper into the tissues, and the patient may need to have conization of the cervix performed (p. 1700).

When cervical lacerations or erosions are present, the area is usually cauterized. Silver nitrate sticks may be used to remove very small lesions. For larger areas requiring cauterization, an electric cautery unit is used. The woman is informed that a small, lubricated sheet of lead will be placed against the skin under the lumbar areas as a safety device for grounding electrical charges and that there will be slight bleeding, which will be controlled by a tampon or packing that will be inserted by the physician. The odor of burning tissue when cautery is used is distressing to some patients. They should be told to expect an odor but that the odor is insignificant and that the procedure is over quickly.

Following cauterization, the nurse can ascertain that the patient understands instructions for follow-up care. Directions will vary, but they usually include the following:

1. Leave the tampon or packing in place as long as the physician advises (usually 8 to 24 hours).
2. Report to the hospital or physician's office if bleeding is excessive (more than occurs during a normal menses is considered excessive).
3. Do not use a douche or have sexual relations until the next visit to the physician unless specific instructions have been given as to when intercourse can be safely resumed.
4. An unpleasant discharge caused by sloughing of destroyed cells may appear 4 to 5 days following cauterization; a warm bath several times a day will help this condition, which should not last more than a few days.

Additional opportunities for teaching and counseling may arise during the course of treatment of cervicitis.

Pelvic inflammatory disease

Epidemiology and etiology

Pelvic inflammatory disease (PID) is an infectious process involving the fallopian tubes, ovaries, pelvic peritoneum, pelvic veins, or pelvic connective tissue. The infection may be confined to one structure, or it may be widespread and involve all of the pelvic structures. Inflammation of the fallopian tube is known as *salpingitis*, and inflammation of the ovary is known as *oophoritis*. (The routes of pelvic infection are shown in Fig. 65-1.)

In addition to the gonococcus, chlamydia, coliforms,

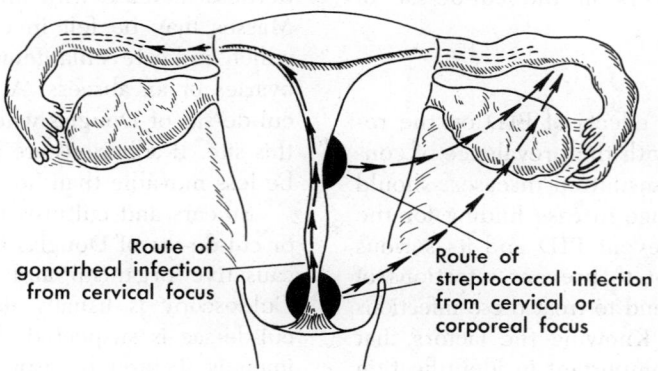

Fig. 65-1. Two chief routes of pelvic infection. (From Novak, E.R., Jones, G.J., and Jones, H.W., Jr.: Novak's textbook of gynecology, ed. 9, © 1975 The Williams & Wilkins Co., Baltimore.)

Haemophilus, streptococcus, mycoplasma, and anaerobes have been implicated in severe or recurrent salpingitis. These pathogens may invade the pelvic organs during sexual intercourse, childbirth, or the postpartum period or when an abortion is done. The rupture of any adjacent structure may spill organisms into the pelvic cavity, thus producing secondary infection. For example, when the appendix perforates, pelvic peritonitis may follow. PID is reported to occur five times more often among women using intrauterine devices as a method for birth control than among women using other methods. These women need to be urged to have regular checkups for signs of infection. Instruction in prevention of infection and signs of infection is important.

Pathophysiology

Pathogenic organisms are usually introduced from outside the body and pass up the cervical canal into the uterus. They seem to cause little trouble in the uterus but pass into the pelvis by way of the fallopian tubes through thrombosed uterine veins or through the lymphatics of the uterus. The invaded structures become involved in an acute or chronic inflammatory process. Many of the pathogens causing PID lodge in the fallopian tubes. Purulent material collects in the tubes, adhesions form, strictures may occur, and sterility is a frequent result. Infertility is one of the most serious consequences of PID. Although tubal surgery is available for correcting tubal adhesions, fertility after tubal surgery is not assured. Obstruction of the fallopian tubes because of the results of inflammation may be complete or partial. Complete obstruction of the tubes makes conception impossible. Partial tubal obstruction predisposes the woman to ectopic pregnancy, since the fertilized ovum cannot reach the uterus, although the sperm has been able to pass the stricture and produce conception. Adhesions resulting from inflammation may cause such distress that complete removal of the uterus, fallopian tubes, and ovaries may be necessary. Although generalized peritonitis can occur, the infection usually remains confined to the lower abdomen and pelvis. An abscess in the cul-de-sac of Douglas is common.

Prevention

The potential destructive effects of PID on the reproductive organs, coupled with the prevalence of gonorrhea and other sexually transmitted diseases, should mobilize every nurse to engage in case finding for the purpose of education. To prevent PID and its serious consequences, it is important to prevent infections of the vulva, vagina, and cervix and to treat these infections promptly when they occur. Knowing the factors that predipose women to PID is important in identification of the population at risk.

Hospitalized women usually have decreased resistance and need protection against infection. Gynecologic disorders of long duration are especially debilitating. Surgery of the reproductive tract, childbearing, and abortion lower resistance and provide portals of entry for organisms. Cleanliness and asepsis are important in giving care to these women, and every attempt should be made to prevent introduction of organisms into the reproductive tract.

Every sexually active women having a physical examination should have a routine cervical smear or culture taken to screen for gonorrhea. Women need to be informed of methods of preventing infection, how to recognize infection in their sexual partners, and what to do when they suspect infection has occurred.

Clinical picture

Signs and symptoms of *acute* PID include severe abdominal pain (or pressure and fullness), lower abdominal cramps, intermenstrual spotting, dyspareunia, fever and chills, malaise, nausea, and vomiting. There may be a foul-smelling purulent vaginal discharge. These symptoms last for a variable period of time. If they are mild and the woman ignores them, the symptoms may temporarily subside. Some cases of acute PID are never reported to a nurse or physician.

Chronic PID is generally considered to be a result of undiagnosed, inadequately treated, or neglected acute PID. This type of pelvic inflammation is characterized by chronic, dull, aching pain in the lower abdomen; backache; constipation; malaise; low-grade fever; and disturbances of menstruation. During periods of exacerbation, acute symptoms return. Occasionally, a patient may be labeled neurotic because of the repeated, nonspecific nature of her complaints. The diagnosis of PID may be made when the patient seeks medical care for another problem, such as menstrual irregularity or infertility.

Abdominal palpation usually reveals the presence of pain and tenderness in the lower abdomen and lower quadrants. Most often, both lower quadrants are painful on palpation. On vaginal examination, the pain and tenderness increase with movement of the pelvic organs. Masses may be felt in either one or both quadrants, which indicate enlargement of the fallopian tubes or ovaries or an abscess. A mass may be palpated in the cul-de-sac of Douglas when abscess formation occurs in this site. If adhesions are present, the pelvic organs may be less movable than normal.

Smears and cultures taken from the vagina, cervix, or cul-de-sac of Douglas may aid in identification of the causative organism and its sensitivity to antibiotics. Culdoscopy is usually done when an abscess in the cul-de-sac is suspected. If an abscess is seen, a specimen is secured by aspiration. Laparoscopy has gained popularity in the diagnosis of PID, since it permits visualization of the reproductive organs and adjacent tissues.

Intervention

Treatment for outpatients is tetracycline, 500 mg four times daily for 10 days. Some patients with PID are hospitalized. They are usually placed on bed rest in mid-Fowler's position to provide dependent drainage so that abscesses will not form high in the abdomen where they might rupture and cause generalized peritonitis. Intravenous fluids may be indicated. It is recommended that sexual partners of women with PID be treated the same as contacts.

Heat (a hot-water bottle or electric heating pad) applied to the abdomen may promote circulation and comfort. Analgesics may be necessary to alleviate pain. The woman is instructed to observe the amount, color, consistency, and odor of any vaginal discharge and changes in pain level. Her temperature is usually monitored every 4 hours until fever subsides. In some instances, women may need to be hospitalized for therapy.

Salpingectomy may be necessary in the event of tubal abscess, and all of the reproductive organs may require removal in severe cases of chronic inflammation. Surgery of the reproductive organs is discussed on p. 1700.

Outcome criteria for the woman with early pelvic inflammatory disease

The woman can:
1. Describe the potentially undesirable effects of such infections on her general health and functioning of the reproductive organs.
2. Participate in the program of care by carrying out prescribed self-care measures.
3. Describe how organisms gain entry to the reproductive organs and how infection can spread by continuity of tissue.
4. State the signs that indicate improvement or lack of response to therapy.
5. Seek health care when problems of care and therapy arise.
6. If treated on an outpatient basis, the woman should be able to:
   a. Order her activities based on priorities.
   b. Present plans for modification in daily activities to provide for self-care requirements.

Puerperal infection

Epidemiology and etiology

Puerperal (postpartum) infection refers to infections of the reproductive organs and pelvic tissues that occur following childbirth or a spontaneous or induced abortion. Most often, the uterus (as in endometritis) is the organ involved. Infection is most often caused by streptococci, anaerobes, or coliforms. The usual route for infections is through the vagina and cervix. Patients who have been delivered by cesarean section also develop puerperal infection.

With improved obstetrics and availability of antibiotics, deaths from puerperal infection have declined markedly during this century. However, despite these advances, the incidence of puerperal infection has not decreased during the past 20 years. Because of the varying criteria used to diagnose puerperal infection, the reported incidence ranges between 1% and 8% of all deliveries. Postpartum infections continue to rank among the three leading causes of mortality in obstetrics.

Endometritis following full-term delivery or abortion is usually attributable to pyogenic organisms. In acute puerperal sepsis, the endometrium as well as other pelvic structures is involved. The severity of the local infection depends on the virulence of the organisms. In mild forms, the endometrium is swollen, hyperemic, and edematous with polymorphonuclear leukocytic infiltration. In severe forms, the bacterial toxins may bring about necrosis of the endometrium and ulceration. The inflammation also may involve the myometrium and parametrium. In severe forms, thrombophlebitis of the uterine and pelvic vessels may occur. With antibiotic therapy, postpartum endometritis usually does not result in septic emboli, but clostridium infections may lead to septicemia and death.

Prevention

Prevention of infection has become a major goal in the management of pregnant and postpartum women. Women at risk for postpartum infection include those who have poor nutrition, develop obstetric complications during the childbearing cycle, have prolonged labor, have premature rupture of the membranes, are delivered by cesarean section, have chronic diseases, have preexisting infection of the reproductive tract, or who are delivered without the benefit of aseptic technique. In addition to good nutrition, adequate rest and exercise, and treatment of preexisting infection, antibiotics may be given to prevent infection in women who are at risk.

Clinical picture

Fever, cramping or dull pain in the lower abdomen, pain and tenderness on palpation of the abdomen over the uterus, foul-smelling vaginal discharge (lochia), and malaise are characteristic signs of puerperal infection.

Intervention

When signs of infection appear, the woman is placed on bed rest, fluids are urged, infusions may be given, and antibiotic therapy is instituted. In some hospitals, infected mothers may be separated from other patients and from the newborn infant to prevent spread of infection. This is not necessary, however, unless group A streptococci are involved. In the case of herpes, the virus is destroyed by soap and water, and careful hand washing is advised. The psychologic aspect of mother-infant bonding and the effects of separating mothers and newborn infants need to be carefully considered when making the decision to isolate the mother from her child.

Because of short hospitalization following delivery and abortion, signs of infection may not appear until after the patient is discharged. Therefore patients need to be informed of the signs indicating puerperal infection, and they should be encouraged to insist on being examined, since even episiotomy infections may lead to death if neglected. If signs do not clear promptly, women should insist on being seen by the physician. To prevent infection following discharge, women should be instructed in self-care, including perineal irrigation, expected changes in lochia, rest, nutrition, exercise, and the importance of having an examination during the postpartum period.

Toxic shock syndrome

Epidemiology, etiology, and pathophysiology

Toxic shock syndrome (TSS) is a severe acute disease associated with strains of staphylococci of phage group I, which produce a unique epidermal toxin. The incidence of TSS is markedly greater among women during menstruation and among women using tampons (particularly superabsorbent tampons). TSS recurs in some women during subsequent menstrual periods, although treatment of TSS with beta (β-) lactamase–resistant antibiotics (e.g., cephalosporins and penicillinase-resistant pencillins) may decrease the likelihood of recurrence.[46,168] TSS may also occur in men. It is suggested that the organism gains entry to the circulation through lesions in the vagina produced by tampons. Superabsorbent tampons maintain a milieu favorable to bacterial growth, since they can contain a large amount of menstrual blood and may be left in place several hours. Sepsis ensues and produces the clinical picture described below.

Prevention

The primary means for preventing TSS in women is through prevention of the introduction of organisms. Following hygienic principles for cleaning the perineum, caring for douche equipment, and handling tampons aseptically may help prevent vaginal colonization with *Staphylococcus aureus*. In addition, women can modify their use of tampons by avoiding superabsorbent brands, or they can use sanitary napkins instead of tampons. Tampon manufacturers now recommend that women use only the absorbency necessary, change tampons at least every 4 to 6 hours, and use sanitary napkins at night. More frequent changing of tampons may produce ulcerations, thus actually increasing the risk of infection. Recurrent TSS can be limited by use of the β-lactamase–resistant antibiotics. Women who carry *S. aureus* should be advised of this so they can make informed choices regarding menstrual hygiene.

Clinical picture

The woman experiencing TSS exhibits a fever above 38.9° C (102° F), palmar or diffuse erythroderma followed by desquamation of the skin of the hands and feet, hypotension or orthostatic dizziness, hyperemia of the conjunctivae or mucous membranes, and multisystem dysfunction including symptoms such as vomiting or diarrhea, alterations in consciousness, and impaired renal, hepatic, or cardiopulmonary function. TSS has caused death in some women. The diagnosis of TSS is usually confirmed by cultures for *Staphylococcus aureus*.[46,168]

Intervention

Women who are menstruating and develop a sudden high fever accompanied by vomiting or diarrhea should be counseled to seek immediate treatment. If the woman is wearing a tampon, she should remove it immediately. Treatment of TSS involves use of β-lactamase–resistant antiobitics. Women who are acutely ill with TSS require careful monitoring and supportive therapy similar to that given patients with septic shock (p. 310).

Pregnancy-related problems

Abortion

The obstetric and legal definition of abortion is termination of a pregnancy before the twenty-sixth week of gestation (viability). There is consensus that *viability* means a state of development that theoretically is compatible with survival outside of the uterus. Arguments continue, however, as to when viability actually occurs. The definition used in reporting perinatal statistics is that fetal weight of 500 g or less constitutes an abortion.

There are several types of abortion, which are usually classified as follows:
1. Spontaneous abortion
   a. Threatened abortion
   b. Inevitable abortion
   c. Incomplete abortion
   d. Complete abortion
   e. Missed abortion
   f. Habitual abortion
2. Induced abortion

Spontaneous abortion

Epidemiology, etiology, and pathophysiology. Spontaneous abortions result from "natural" causes, that is, without the aid of mechanical or medicinal intervention. Estimates of the incidence of spontaneous abortions range from 10% to 20% of all pregnancies. The wide range of estimate is partially a result of the belief that many women may experience an abortion without ever being aware conception had occurred. These women probably have very minor symptoms that they do not recognize as signs of an abortion and that do not require hospitalization.

It is known that a large number of embryos spontaneously aborted in the first 12 weeks of gestation are abnormal. In addition to defective embryos, an intrauterine environment that is not adequate for sustaining embryonic and fetal development may result from inadequate nutrition, injuries and anomalies of the reproductive tract, endocrine disorders, and acute and chronic illnesses. For the past 30 years, the incompetent cervix has been considered a cause of abortions occurring during the second trimester of pregnancy, usually between 14 and 16 weeks. The etiology of diminished resistance of the internal cervical os to the increasing weight of the embryo is unknown. Both congenital and traumatic causes have been implicated. There is increasing evidence that women having repeated induced abortions are predisposed to incompetent cervix with future pregnancies.[21,188]

Spontaneous abortions are classified according to a sequence of progression of severity of symptoms. Medical or surgical intervention at any point in the sequence may alter the progression.

In *threatened abortion*, the process has presumably started, as evidenced by vaginal bleeding or spotting, minor cramping from uterine contractions, and mild backache. The cervix has not started to dilate, and the process may or may not respond to treatment. Management consists of bed rest and evaluation of the effects of blood loss. Mild sedatives and progesterone may be prescribed in an attempt to conserve the pregnancy.

In an *inevitable abortion*, the process has progressed so far that it is impossible to salvage the pregnancy. The symptoms include copious vaginal bleeding, rupture of the amniotic sac, severe abdominal cramping, and dilation of the cervix. Supportive treatment consists of bed rest, monitoring for effects of blood loss, blood transfusion as indicated, and medications for relief of pain. Medical intervention may take a variety of forms, depending on the patient's general condition. The process may be permitted to terminate spontaneously and be followed by a dilation and curettage. Oxytocin may be administered to hasten the process and to decrease blood loss, and this may be followed by a dilation and curettage, or a dilation and curettage may be performed first with oxytocin administered concomitantly.

An *incomplete abortion* is one in which part of the products of conception (usually the embryo) is expelled and part is retained. There is abdominal pain from uterine contractions. Vaginal bleeding is usually moderate to heavy and continues until all the retained products are passed spontaneously or are removed by dilation and curettage. Oxytocic drugs are administered to control blood loss, and transfusion may be required.

When all of the products of conception are expelled spontaneously, a *complete abortion* has occurred. Bleeding is usually minimal, but oxytocic drugs may be given and a dilation and curettage performed.

A *missed abortion* is one in which the products of conception are not spontaneously expelled after embryonic death occurs. The term is usually applied when at least 2 months elapse between embryonic death and expulsion. The uterus fails to increase in size, and the changes anticipated with advancing pregnancy do not appear. There is some difference of opinion regarding management of the patient when the diagnosis is made. Some physicians feel that it is better to wait for spontaneous abortion to follow. Infection and hemorrhage are rare, but the idea of "carrying a dead baby" is distressing to many women. Occasionally, hypofibrinogenemia may occur as a consequence of entry into the maternal circulation of thromboplastin from the uterus and placenta. For this reason, as well as for the resulting emotional stress, many physicians believe the uterus should be evacuated as soon as possible. This may be accomplished by different methods, depending on the period of gestation reached when embryonic death occurs. If it is less than 12 weeks, a dilation and curettage may be performed, or the abortion process may be induced with oxytocin. Induction with oxytocin may be carried out after the twelfth week.

Habitual abortion refers to a condition in which spontaneous abortion occurs in three or more consecutive pregnancies. The causes are similar to those stated for spontaneous abortion. Treatment is dependent on the point in the abortive process reached and on determining the causative factors.

Prevention. Application of knowledge of the factors predisposing women to spontaneous abortion and educating women at an early age regarding desirable health habits can assist in preventing spontaneous abortions. Establishing a healthful intrauterine environment and maintaining such an environment must begin in the years before childbearing is undertaken. Good nutrition, prevention of illness and disease, prompt prenatal care, and supervision of a physician during pregnancy all increase the chance of successful childbearing.

Assisting couples to select a method of contraception other than abortion after two or more abortions have been done may decrease the chances of development of incompetent cervix.

During the prenatal period, it is important for women to seek prompt prenatal care, remain under care of a nurse or physician, and to follow advice about self-care. Women need to be advised of the signs of abortion and the need to contact the physician immediately. Hospitalization is sometimes necessary if attempts are to be made to conserve the pregnancy.

Clinical picture. In order to determine treatment required, it is necessary to determine the extent to which the abortive process has progressed. A menstrual history is taken to estimate the duration of pregnancy. The time of onset of symptoms, the amount and type of vaginal discharge, and the degree, duration, and site of pain are assessed. If clots are passed, they should be saved for examination to determine whether they contain embryonic or placental tissue. The vital signs are taken to estimate effects of blood loss. A vaginal examination may or may not be done to determine the extent of cervical dilation. In general, the greater the blood loss, pain, and cervical dilation, the less chance there is of salvaging the pregnancy.

The patient's psychologic response must also be assessed in order that emotional support can be given. Many women, especially those experiencing repeated disappointments because of spontaneous abortion and those highly motivated to have a baby, experience feelings of guilt and tend to associate the abortion with some forbidden event or act. They require factual information about the causes of abortion. During the abortion process, women are more concerned with the present rather than the future and their ability to bear children. Therefore emphasis should be placed on what is happening and what the woman can do to help herself at the present time.

Intervention. Women having three or more consecutive spontaneous abortions should be carefully screened beforehand and followed during subsequent pregnancies to establish a diagnosis. At the present time, most experts agree that a positive diagnosis of incompetent cervix is best made by the finding of progressive, painless cervical dilation with bulging of the membranes through the cervix after the twelfth week of pregnancy in a woman with a history of repeated abortions. In some cases, the diagnosis is confirmed at a time when cervical dilation has progressed to the extent that it is not possible to prevent abortion. Once the diagnosis is made, however, surgical intervention is highly successful in preventing future spontaneous abortions. Repeated spontaneous abortions may be a consequence of infections or chromosomal or structural anomalies as well as incompetent cervix. Therefore cultures for chlamydia, cytomegalovirus, and other organisms, chromosomal analysis, and a hysterosalpingogram are performed early in the workup.

The surgery for incompetent cervix consists of closing the internal os of the cervix by suturing in a purse-string (drawstring) fashion. Timing of the surgery is debated, and there are proponents of the interim repair (repair of the cervix between pregnancies) and proponents of the more usual repair during pregnancy.

There is a need for standardization in selecting patients for surgery and for evaluating the results of surgery performed at different times. A scoring system using five criteria for cervical cerclage has been suggested.[21] To apply the scoring system, a value of 1 is given for each criterion met by the patient. The patient receives a total score between 1 and 5. It is reported that as the total score increases, the average number of weeks between surgery and delivery increases; that is, the higher the score, the better are the chances of successful surgery. The scoring system also has prognostic value in predicting the outcome of future pregnancies.

The treatments for specific types of spontaneous abortion have been discussed previously. In general, the earlier in the process the woman is treated, the better are the chances of conserving the pregnancy. Assisting women to cope with the crisis of loss of a pregnancy is important for their emotional health. Opportunities for counseling individuals and couples about family planning and desirable health practices often arise. Usually, women are counseled not to become pregnant for at least 6 months after a spontaneous abortion has occurred.

Outcome criteria for the woman having a spontaneous abortion

1. The woman treated on an outpatient basis can:
   a. Identify how her usual activities will need to be modified in order to follow advice and instructions.
   b. Determine alternatives for meeting the needs of other family members when necessary.
2. The woman treated at home can state and recognize the signs of progression or regression of the abortion process and give information related to the signs.
3. The woman hospitalized for spontaneous abortion can:
   a. Explain the medical and nursing plans of care.
   b. Take measures to restrict activity and reduce stress.
   c. State the chances for successful treatment and alternatives necessary if treatment is not successful.
4. The woman who has completed the abortion process will recognize her loss and her need to grieve. She will:
   a. Identify supportive persons in her environment.
   b. Seek help from appropriate people.

c. Be able to discuss how the abortion came about.

d. Begin to resolve any feelings of guilt.

e. Decide when she wishes to undertake another pregnancy.

f. Select a method of preventing pregnancy until the desired time for conception.

5. On discharge from the hospital, the woman can:

a. State what modifications in activities and health practices are required, the signs of complications, and the need to report them.

b. State when she is expected to return for a follow-up visit and the purposes of such visits.

Induced abortion

Epidemiology, etiology, and pathophysiology. The topic of abortion has received great attention for hundreds of years. Volumes have been written about the types of abortion, ranging from medical aspects to legal, sociologic, psychologic, moral, and economic aspects.

Estimates of the number of abortions that are self-induced or performed by nonmedical persons range from 500,000 to 1,500,000 per year. The availability of elective abortion services seems to have reduced the use of self-induced abortion. This is partly reflected by the decreased numbers of women being admitted to hospitals with symptoms of sepsis resulting from self-induced abortions.[99]

Attempts to bring about a self-induced abortion are generally made by ingestion of quinine, douching with soap and water, or inserting lye or potassium permanganate crystals into the vagina. These rarely act as abortifacients. Instead, they can cause serious toxicity or local trauma and may even result in death. Insertion of foreign bodies such as catheters, knitting needles, and metal coat hangers into the uterus is another common method by which abortions are attempted. While these are more effective, they are attended by highly serious consequences, including perforation of the uterus, hemorrhage, infection, permanent infertility resulting from infection, and death from blood loss or infection.

Legal aspects. Whether induced abortions should or could be prevented remains a question open to personal opinion and considerable debate. In the United States, the legality of abortions and the circumstances under which they might be justifiably performed by physicians became a major area of controversy by 1968, and by 1972 the legality and morality of abortions had assumed extremely unclear aspects. On January 22, 1973, the U.S. Supreme Court, in an unprecedented action, reached a decision regarding legalization of abortions. It ruled that a state could not intervene in the abortion decision between a woman and her physician during the first 12 weeks of pregnancy.[161] Although the Supreme Court did not take the position that a woman has an absolute right to abortion regardless of period of gestation or individual circumstances, its decision regarding the first trimester renders all previous original and reform laws unconstitutional.

The major ground for the Supreme Court decision is based on personal liberty provided by the Fourteenth Amendment to the U.S. Constitution. In essence, this means the woman has a right to privacy, which includes the right to decide whether to terminate her pregnancy.

Not all the issues, however, were settled by the Supreme Court's action. After the end of the first trimester, the states reserve rights to enact legislation and other regulations to protect maternal health. The states are now required to adopt statues specifying the circumstances under which abortions can be legally performed.

Despite the Supreme Court ruling, arguments continue. Many states have not revised laws to provide for second- and third-trimester abortions, and the laws vary greatly. Various attitudes, beliefs, and values are evident in the variety of terms used today. "Therapeutic" abortion no longer simply means an abortion performed by a physician when the mother's life is threatened by serious physiopathologic conditions. The term has gradually been broadened to include threats to health, both physical and emotional. However, some state laws have not clearly defined what constitutes a threat to health. "Abortion on demand," "legalized abortion," "abortion on request," "elective abortion," and "social abortion" are some of the terms in common use.

Indications for abortions. Therapeutic abortions for purely medical reasons (the presence of serious physiopathologic conditions) have become more rare as the science of obstetrics has developed. Severe heart disease, pulmonary hypertension, and malignancy may be reasons for terminating pregnancy by abortion. With increased effectiveness of conception control and availability of sterilization, fewer women who are at risk of developing life-threatening conditions during pregnancy are becoming pregnant. Because of improved medical management of high-risk pregnancies, many women with diabetes, heart disease, and other health problems are able to carry pregnancies to term without jeopardizing their own health.

Today, many induced abortions are performed for "social" reasons. Social and economic pressures for small families are strong. There is an increased tendency among people to see abortion as an alternative method of birth control. Despite advances in the effectiveness of methods available for conception control, the continued demand for elective abortion indicates that many women see abortion as a means of birth control and possibly that deficiencies in knowledge, motivation, or availability of contraceptive services continues to be a problem.[153]

"Medically sound" reasons for performing abortions

have been expanded to include such aspects as the fate of the unwanted child after birth, psychologic stress, history of genetic abnormalities, the effects of teratogens (agents causing embryonic defects), maternal and fetal blood incompatibility, rape, and incest.

Effects of abortions. The continued liberalization and acceptance of induced abortion as a means of birth control have raised concern over the effects of repeated induced abortions on women electing this method. There is growing concern over the late sequelae of repeat induced abortion including cervical incompetence, ectopic pregnancy, secondary sterility, Rh immunization, infections, and uterine rupture.[140,141,149,188] Women utilizing abortion as a means of birth control need to be informed of these possible consequences in order to make informed choices.

Almost universally, when abortion is liberalized and legalized and made available, the maternal mortality drops and the incidence of septic and incomplete abortions decreases.[99] To point out the low risk to maternal life associated with induced abortions, comparisons have been made with other causes of mortality (Table 65-3).

Both the physical and psychologic long-term effects of induced abortions require continued study. Psychologic studies indicate that adverse reactions to an abortion experience are influenced by legal, moral, and social antiabortion climates in that such a climate is punitive to the woman. Cultural attitudes have a pervasive effect and are likely to influence the way a woman reacts to an abortion. Attitudes of health care professionals influence the woman's feeling about herself and the abortion experience. The nurse's feelings and values about abortions, and identification with the roles of women, can influence the patient's response to abortion and perceptions of herself as a woman.[30]

Counseling. Counseling women regarding abortion is an appropriate function for nurses to assume, provided the nurse has the knowledge, skills, and abilities to assist individual women to cope with a situation that may have both immediate and long-term effects.

Preabortion counseling includes assisting the woman to make a decision regarding her state of pregnancy. This requires that the patient be helped with identifying the alternatives available to her and the consequences of the various alternatives and selecting the alternative that is best for her in her circumstances. If this process is employed, the woman is more likely to arrive at a decision she feels is the best one she could make and less likely to experience excessive emotional distress. Therefore it is important in the counseling process to avoid telling the woman what to do or expressing opinions about what is best for her. For those women who seem unable to reach a decision, the nurse may arrange for referral to a counselor or social worker for further assistance.

For patients who decide to have an abortion, it is necessary that the nurse be able to explain the methods that will most likely be used, where an abortion may be obtained, and what will be required in terms of finances and time. It may be important that other health team members become involved in assisting the woman with planning. Preabortion counseling may also involve beginning explorations about conception control and family planning. Depending on her readiness to pursue these topics, the woman may be given information about the availability of services and methods. Otherwise, she can be reassured the topic can be discussed at a later time.

In counseling, the nurse will usually find that an objective approach, utilizing facts and terms the woman can understand, and conveying an attitude of willingness and readiness to assist her will encourage the woman to remain as objective as possible. Continuity in care seems to be particularly important to people in stressful situations, and it may be helpful to inform the woman about the personnel she is likely to encounter. Nursing care plans should be available to other nurses who will be participating in the patient's care whenever this is possible.

When hospitalized for an abortion, patients feel some degree of anxiety, and their behaviors must be interpreted with care. If a patient begins to ask questions or verbalize feelings, it does not necessarily mean she has "changed her mind." It might mean that, under anxiety, she cannot recall what she was told would be done and needs to have this information repeated. Nurses cannot assume that the patient was not informed of the procedure and its consequences or that the patient has made a poor decision. Those patients who seem to be expressing "second thoughts" or seem to be doubtful about whether their decision should be carried out usually find it helpful to review how they initially reached the decision.

In the postabortion period, a variety of emotional responses may be seen. Relief that the problem has been solved might be mingled with some minor feelings of guilt. Those women who express regret and guilt can be helped by again reviewing with them their decision-making process. They may need to be aware that such

TABLE 65-3. Comparison of mortality for childbirth, abortion, and contraceptive use

Causes of mortality	Mortality
Maternal mortality from childbirth	20/100,000 pregnancies
Self-induced abortion	100/100,000 abortions
Legal abortion	3/100,000 abortions
Thromboembolic disorders from use of oral contraceptives	3/100,000 users

feelings may recur from time to time and that remembering how and why they reached the decision to have an abortion may help. Postabortion patients are candidates for conception control information. Many of these patients wish to learn more about reproduction and prevention of pregnancy. The approaches and methods described previously will be of assistance to the nurse engaged in counseling about conception control.

The date of the last menstrual period is important to ascertain, since the method selected for inducing abortion is partly determined by the period of gestation reached. The woman's physical and emotional states are also important. Although the methods for inducing abortion are generally considered very safe, some methods require greater physical and emotional energy.

A pregnancy test (p. 1630) is usually done to confirm pregnancy and to rule out other causes of amenorrhea. A vaginal or cervical smear should be done to detect infection, and a pelvic examination is usually done to confirm the length of gestation and to rule out diseases of the reproductive tract. A routine urinalysis and complete blood count are done.

The extent to which patients are able to handle the crisis of having a pregnancy terminated by induced abortion is partially dependent on the timing and quality of medical and nursing interventions. Women seeking abortion will engage in problem solving and select from the various alternatives available to them that alternative which is most advantageous to them in terms of physical, emotional, social, and economic resources. The decision made will be based on factual information, and patients will be better able to make an objective choice. Women having an induced abortion will understand the procedure to be used, length of hospitalization required, cost, and potential effects on physical and emotional health. They will realize that deep feelings are involved, regardless of the degree of objectivity involved in the decision to have an abortion. Knowing this, women will be better prepared to handle such feelings when they do arise. They will identify supportive persons with whom they can discuss their feelings following discharge from the hospital or clinic.

Intervention. Several methods are available for inducing abortion. The particular method selected for a patient is highly dependent on the length of gestation at the time a woman seeks an abortion. As the pregnancy progresses, the methods required to be effective increase in complexity, are attended by greater risks to the woman, are more time consuming in terms of length of hospitalization, are more expensive, and are perhaps more emotionally traumatic.

In the first trimester, abortion is performed in special clinics as an outpatient procedure or in acute-care settings. Many special abortion clinics have opened as a result of the demand for abortion in the early weeks of pregnancy. Some clinics provide counseling and referral services; others have facilities in which abortions can be performed. If admitted to an acute-care setting, the woman may be admitted and discharged on the same day or remain only one night.

VACUUM ASPIRATION. Vacuum aspiration (suction curettage) has increased in popularity because of its ease and safety in bringing about termination of pregnancy in the first few weeks. It has become the method of choice for inducing abortions in clinics and hospitals providing abortions for large numbers of patients.

Vacuum aspiration can be performed as soon as pregnancy is documented. The equipment used is similar to that used for suction curettage. The cervix is dilated, and the uterus is evacuated by means of a vacuum suction machine. When vacuum aspiration is employed immediately after the first menses is missed, a soft catheter of 5 to 6 mm in diameter is used, and very little cervical dilation is required. *Menstrual extraction* and *minisuction* are terms also used when vacuum aspirations is done following the first missed menstrual period.

The procedure can be performed under either local or general anesthesia. The patient is observed for excess bleeding and pain immediately following the procedure and can be discharged as soon as the vital signs are stable and effects of anesthesia have subsided. There is a low incidence of complications of vacuum aspiration. An incidence of 1.4% major complications, including uterine perforation, fever lasting 3 days or more, and retained tissue, is reported.[91]

DILATION AND CURETTAGE. Dilation and curettage is an alternative method for accomplishing abortion in the first 12 to 14 weeks. The products of conception and superficial layer of the endometrium are scraped from the walls of the uterus. A paracervical block or general anesthesia is used. Oxytocin is usually administered intramuscularly or in an intravenous infusion after the procedure is completed. Blood loss is usually minimal, and physical care is similar to that for any patient having a dilation and curettage.

INTRAAMNIOTIC INJECTION. Intraamniotic injection (saline injection or "salting out") is the method most often used after the sixteenth week of gestation. Occasionally, it may be attempted as early as the fourteenth week, but the chances of failure are greater, since the amniotic sac is not well distended.

Since the woman must be responsive to detect adverse effects, general anesthesia is not used. Sedatives, analgesics, and tranquilizing agents are usually administered before the procedure, and a local anesthetic is used. The procedure is performed under aseptic conditions. The local anesthetic is injected into the skin and abdominal wall in the midline below the umbilicus. A 17- or 18-gauge spinal length needle is introduced through the abdominal and uterine walls into the amniotic sac. The stylet is removed, and the physician observes for the flow of amniotic fluid from the needle. When the amniotic fluid appears, a syringe is attached to the needle and the amniotic fluid is aspirated. An alternative method of using a size 14 trocar and cannula to which a short length of rubber or plastic tubing is attached may be preferred by the physician. The total amount of amniotic fluid aspirated averages 200 ml for this period of gestation but may vary by about 50 ml. The amniotic fluid is replaced by 20% sodium chloride solution, and the amount injected is at least equivalent to the amount of amniotic fluid aspirated. Some physicians prefer to inject an additional 50 ml over the amount of amniotic fluid withdrawn, since there is some evidence that the additional fluid injected has a distending effect on the uterus. Most physicians elect to alternately withdraw and inject 15 to 20 ml of fluid and sodium chloride solution to prevent collapse of the amniotic sac that might result from withdrawal of all of the amniotic fluid.

During introduction of the needle, the injection is made slowly, and care is taken to avoid insertion into the placenta or a blood vessel. The patient is closely observed during the procedure and for at least 1 hour afterward for untoward effects. These include shocklike symptoms or vascular collapse and abdominal pain resulting from injection into a blood vessel or the placenta.

The action of hypertonic solutions inducing labor is not completely clear. The hypertonic solution disrupts the placenta, and this result alone produces an intrauterine environment incompatible with life. Disruption of the placenta may also release the progesterone block, causing uterine contractions to result. The volume of fluid in the uterus may be significant in that the body attempts to balance the effects of the hypertonic solution. In doing so, the volume of intraamniotic fluid is increased. This expands the uterus beyond its normal size for gestation and probably triggers stretch receptors and pacemakers within the uterus.

The abortive process (labor) begins 12 to 36 hours after the injection of sodium chloride solution. The patient is hospitalized throughout this time and observed for late untoward effects as well as the onset of abortion. The products of conception are most often expelled as in a spontaneous, complete abortion. Once the symptoms of abortion appear (abdominal pain, vaginal bleeding, rupture of the amniotic sac), oxytocin may be administered by infusion to hasten the process and minimize blood loss. Because the woman having a second trimester abortion experiences feelings similar to increased labor, she needs emotional support and needs to work on how to cope with discomfort from contractions. A dilation and curettage may be performed after the abortion is completed as a precaution against excessive blood loss. If labor does not ensue within 36 to 48 hours following

the injection, oxytocin by infusion is usually administered to initiate contractions of the uterus.

The thirteenth to sixteenth weeks of pregnancy pose difficulties for patients seeking an abortion. Most physicians consider this time to be too late for safe curettage and too early for intraamniotic injection.

HYSTEROTOMY. An abortion may also be performed by hysterotomy. This method is usually selected for terminating pregnancies that have advanced to 16 weeks or more, or when a tubal sterilization is to be carried out at the same time. Hysterotomy involves incision through the abdominal wall and uterus to remove the products of conception. A general or spinal anesthesia is administered, and the patient has a longer period of hospitalization because of the surgical procedure. The postoperative complications that might occur are similar to those occurring after any abdominal surgery.

EXPERIMENTAL DRUG. While an abortion pill, systemic abortion injection, or uterine insert to produce an abortion has not been developed as yet, it is quite likely that much simpler methods of inducing abortion will evolve if the current trend of increasing demand for elective abortion continues.

One group of drugs, the prostaglandins, is currently undergoing study. Intraamniotic injection of prostaglandins has been associated with a high incidence of complications, including fall in hematocrit, failure to abort within 48 hours after injection, infection requiring antibiotic therapy, cervical lacerations, and uterine rupture.[54] There is additional concern that with intraamniotic injection of saline, cervical incompetence may develop in future pregnancies because of atypical cervical dilatation.

Intravaginal administration of prostaglandins is also being studied and is reported to have a high success rate of inducing abortion within 12 hours and a low complication rate. Complications are less serious with intravaginal administration of prostaglandins but are distressing to the patient and include fever, nausea and vomiting, and diarrhea during administration. In some instances, fetuses with signs of viability are expelled, thus creating serious ethical conflicts for health professionals.

Outcome criteria for the woman experiencing an induced abortion. The woman can:
1. Describe methods of limiting family size other than abortion.
2. Have literature about these methods available for her use at home.
3. State her needs for health care follow-up.
    a. List signs of complications that need to be reported.
    b. State method of obtaining nursing or medical assistance.
    c. State the appropriate time to report for her follow-up examination and counseling.

4. Describe available community resources for family planning.

Ectopic pregnancy

Epidemiology and etiology

An ectopic pregnancy is one in which the fertilized ovum becomes embedded outside the body of the uterus. Since it is almost always located in the fallopian tube, the term *tubal pregnancy* is often used.

Ectopic pregnancy is an increasing problem in gynecology. The incidence of tubal pregnancy has risen since 1970. Factors contributing to ectopic pregnancy include presence of an intrauterine device, pelvic infection, oral contraceptives containing only progesterone, induced abortion, and tubal surgery including sterilization.

Pathophysiology

Ectopic pregnancy occurs frequently in women who have a narrowed fallopian tube caused either by inflammation or by a congenital stricture. The sperm may be small enough to pass through the stricture, but the larger fertilized ovum may be unable to do so. The ovum may then attach itself to the tubal wall and develop into an embryo. As the embryo grows, the fallopian tube stretches and finally may rupture. Frequently, however, early diagnosis and surgery prevent rupture of the tube. This rupture usually occurs within the first 6 weeks of pregnancy.

Clinical picture

The woman experiences a sudden severe pain on one side of the abdomen in conjunction with a history of amenorrhea and often of suspected pregnancy. She may go into shock quickly after the onset of pain because of massive hemorrhage into the peritoneal cavity.

Because of its frequency, ruptured tubal pregnancy is one of the most common surgical emergencies in women. Laparoscopy may be performed to make the diagnosis. The radioreceptor assay test for pregnancy may have some value in diagnosing pregnancy. It has been noted that women are usually operated on within 2 hours following admission to the hospital.[162] Because the radioreceptor assay can be performed in 1 hour, pregnancy can be quickly confirmed. The test, however, does not reveal the site of pregnancy, and the patient's history and complaints on admission are important.

Intervention

Emergency treatment for shock and hemorrhage is given. Early treatment of a ruptured ectopic pregnancy is imperative to prevent death from hemorrhage. Immediately on diagnosis, the woman is prepared for a salpingectomy. The primary purpose of surgery for tubal pregnancy is saving of the woman's life. In some cases, however, tuboplasty can be attempted to salvage the fallopian tube. The surgery also affects the woman's future fertility and her risk of future ectopic pregnancy. Estimates of impaired fertility following tubal surgery for ectopic pregnancy range from 33% to 60%.[163]

If there has been prolonged bleeding preoperatively, the postoperative course may be complicated by peritonitis, since the blood in the abdomen becomes infected with organisms.

The nursing care combines the aspects of emergency treatment of a patient who has sustained a severe hemorrhage, general care of a patient who has had major abdominal surgery and who may have peritonitis, and care of a woman whose pregnancy has been terminted prematurely.

Structural problems

Uterine displacement

Pathophysiology and etiology

Displacement of the uterus, bladder, and rectum can be congenital or acquired because of stretching of the ligaments supporting the uterus and stretching of the muscles of the perineal floor. Acquired displacement of these structures usually results from unrepaired lacerations during childbirth and ill-advised bearing down during labor. Repeated, close pregnancies especially predispose to loss of muscle tone and displacement of the uterus and other pelvic structures.

With better obstetric care, use of episiotomies to prevent tearing of the pelvic muscles, immediate repair of all tears, and the trend toward fewer pregnancies and births per woman, fewer women should require vaginal wall repairs late in life. Perineal exercises practiced following delivery help to prevent relaxation. Apparently relaxation may also be caused by a congenital weakness of the muscles of the pelvis because it occurs occasionally in women who have had no children.

As the uterus begins to drop, the vaginal walls become relaxed, and a fold of vaginal mucosa may protrude outside the vaginal orifice. This is known as a *colpocele*. With the relaxation of the vaginal walls, the bladder may herniate into the vagina (*a cystocele*), or the rectal wall may herniate into the vagina (*a rectocele*) (Fig. 65-2). Both conditions may occur simultaneously.

Older women may have suffered from these conditions for years and yet may not have sought medical attention. They may remember that their mothers had a similar condition and think that it is to be expected in women who have borne children. Since they are not

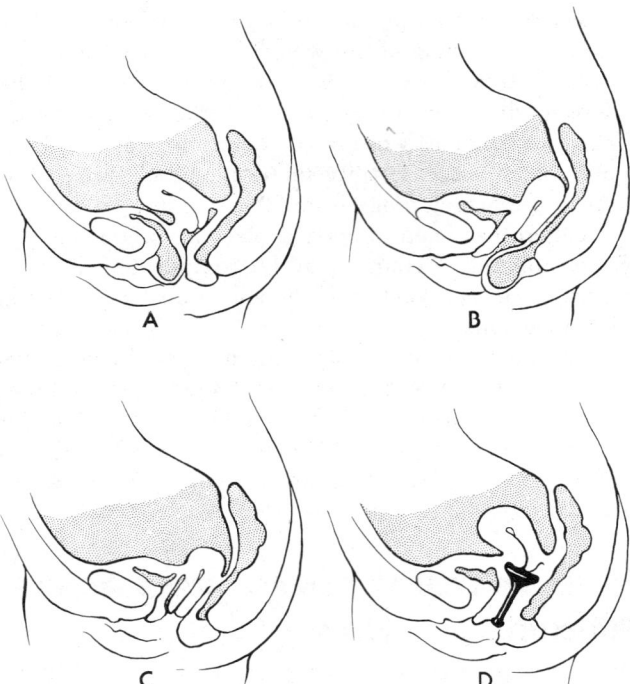

Fig. 65-2. Abnormalities of vagina. **A,** Cystocele: downward displacement of bladder toward vaginal orifice. **B,** Rectocele: pouching of rectum into posterior wall of vagina. **C,** Prolapse of uterus into vaginal canal. **D,** Stem pessary in place to maintain normal anatomic position of uterus.

incapacitated, some may decide not to have reparative surgery that they know is available. Some delay seeking treatment because they dread surgery or because of the expense. However, untreated displacements of the uterus may cause complications such as cervical ulceration and infection, cystitis, and hemorrhoids.

Clinical picture

A sign of relaxation of the pelvic musculature is a dragging pain in the back and in the pelvis. It is made worse by standing or walking. The woman who has a cystocele may complain of urinary incontinence accompanying activity that increases intraabdominal pressure such as coughing, laughing, walking, or lifting (stress incontinence). The cystocele may become so pronounced that in order for the patient to void, the bladder must be pushed back into place by holding the finger against the anterior vaginal wall. If the patient has a rectocele, she may complain of constipation and resultant hemorrhoids.

Intervention

Cystoceles and rectoceles are treated by plastic operations designed to tighten the vaginal wall. The operation is done through the vagina. The repair for a cys-

tocele is called an *anterior colporrhaphy;* the repair for rectocele is called a *posterior colporrhaphy.* Old tears of the pelvic floor, usually caused by childbearing, may also be repaired. Such repair is called a *perineorrhaphy.*

General surgical care. As part of the preoperative preparation, a cleansing douche is frequently ordered the morning of surgery. When surgery involving the vagina is performed, postoperative nursing care includes prevention of pressure on the vaginal suture line and prevention of wound infection. Perineal dressings are seldom used.

Perineal care is given at least twice a day and after each voiding or defecation. Sterile cotton balls moistened with benzalkonium chloride, bichloride of mercury, or normal saline solution may be used, or the patient may be placed on a douche pan and the solution poured over the perineum. Cleansing is always done away from the vagina toward the rectum so that contamination is avoided. An indwelling catheter may be inserted and attached to continuous drainage for 24 to 48 hours. After removal, the usual methods to encourage voiding can be employed.

A heat lamp may be used for 15 to 20 minutes two or three times a day to encourage healing of the perineum. The heat lamp should be used after perineal care to help dry the area and thereby prevent sloughing of tissue. If the patient complains of perineal discomfort, an ice pack applied locally helps to reduce swelling and give relief. A plastic bag or disposable glove filled with ice, firmly tied and covered, makes an adaptable pack. When sutures have been removed, sitz baths are usually ordered.

About 1 week after surgery, daily vaginal douches with normal saline solution may be prescribed. Occasionally, douches are ordered during the immediate postoperative period. Sterile equipment and sterile solution should then be used. The douche nozzle should be very gently inserted and very carefully rotated.

After discharge, the woman who has had a vaginal repair should continue to take a daily douche and a daily tub bath. A laxative may be prescribed to be taken each night to prevent constipation and excessive stress on the surgical site. When she returns to the clinic or to the physician's office, the woman is told when to discontinue the douches and laxative and when it is safe for her to resume sexual intercourse. Women who have had vaginal repair procedures, like other patients having gynecologic surgery, need to avoid jarring activities and heavy lifting for at least 6 weeks postoperatively.

Posterior colporrhaphy. Women who are having a posterior colporrhaphy are given a cathartic approximately 24 hours before surgery, and several enemas usually are given preoperatively to help ensure an empty bowel at the time of surgery and immediately thereafter. Up to 24 hours preoperatively, she may be permitted only clear liquids orally to further reduce bowel contents. Postoperatively, the patient may be kept flat in bed or in low Fowler's position to prevent increased intraabdominal pressure or strain on the wound. Special attention must be given to exercise for the patient's legs, to having her turn frequently, and to having her cough deeply. For 5 days, only liquids are permitted orally, and camphorated tincture of opium (paregoric) is also given to inhibit bowel function. At the end of this time, mineral oil is given each night, and an oil-retention enema is given the morning after the first laxative is given. Only a soft rectal tube and small amount of oil (200 ml) should be used. Straining to produce a bowel movement is discouraged. Enemas for relieving flatus and for cleansing the bowel usually are not given until at least a week postoperatively.

Anterior colporrhaphy. After an anterior colporrhaphy, an indwelling catheter is usually left in the bladder for about 4 days. The catheter should keep the bladder completely empty. If a catheter is not used and if the patient is taking sufficient fluid, voiding should be checked at least every 4 hours. No more than 100 ml of urine should be allowed to accumulate in the bladder. It is usually very difficult to catheterize a patient following a vaginal repair, since the urethral orifice may be distorted and edematous. Having the patient take deep breaths may help in locating the orifice because it dilates slightly with each breath. A soft rubber catheter should be used. Ambulation is begun immediately after surgery. A regular diet is given, and mineral oil is taken each night to lessen the need to strain on defecation.

Urethral suspension. Sometimes a vaginal plastic procedure does not relieve the *stress incontinence* caused by a cystocele and by general relaxation of the pelvic floor. When this happens, the ligaments about the bladder neck may be shortened in such a way that the bladder drops less easily into the vagina. The degree of incontinence may be tested by filling the bladder to various levels with sterile normal saline solution and then having the patient cough or strain while standing. If the incontinence is marked, the patient may be placed in a lithotomy position, while the physician fills the bladder with normal saline solution and supports the bladder neck with a finger or with a clamp in the vagina to test the effectiveness of the bladder with this support. If the patient can cough and strain down without being incontinent, she is considered a good candidate for the operation. The surgery consists of a retropubic urethral suspension and is usually combined with further vaginal repair. A urethral catheter is inserted, and the nursing care is similar to that following a vaginal repair. If the catheter does not drain freely or if the patient without a catheter does not void within 4 to 6 hours, the physician should be notified. Pressure from a full bladder may disrupt the repair.

Prolapse of the uterus

Pathophysiology

Prolapse of the uterus, or procidentia uteri, is a marked downward displacement of the uterus. The severity of the displacement is designated as first, second, or third degree. In a first-degree prolapse, the cervix is still within the vagina. In a second-degree prolapse, the cervix protrudes from the vaginal orifice. In a third-degree prolapse, the entire uterus, which is suspended by its stretched ligaments, hangs below the vaginal orifice. In both second-degree and third-degree prolapses, the cervix becomes irritated from clothing, the circulation becomes impaired, and ulceration often follows.

Clinical picture

Displacement of the uterus may cause dysmenorrhea, although many women with known displacements have no pain. Some women with displacement complain of chronic backache, pelvic pressure, easy fatigue, and leukorrhea in addition to painful menstruation.

Common kinds of displacement are *anteflexion, retroflexion,* and *retroversion* of the uterus caused by congenitally weak uterine ligaments, adhesions following infections or surgery in the pelvic region, or the strain of pregnancy on the ligaments. A space-filling lesion in this region or even a full bladder or rectum may also displace the uterus enough to cause symptoms. Normally, the body of the uterus flexes forward at a 45-degree angle at the cervix. In retroflexion, this angle is increased; in anteflexion, it is decreased; in retroversion, the whole uterus is tipped backward (Fig. 65-3).

Intervention

If the displacement is not caused by some coexistent pelvic disease, various pelvic exercises may be recommended in an attempt to return the uterus to a normal position. These exercises, employing the principles of gravity, stretch or strengthen the uterine ligaments. Some exercises used are knee-chest exercises, the "monkey trot," lying on the abdomen 2 hours a day, and premenstrual exercises. Corrective exercises for poor posture may also be prescribed.

In doing knee-chest exercises, the woman is instructed to assume a knee-chest position (Fig. 63-7) and to separate the labia to allow air to enter the vagina, since this helps to produce normal positioning of the uterus. This position should be maintained for 5 minutes two or three times a day.

In doing the monkey trot, the woman is instructed to walk about on her hands and feet, keeping the knees straight. This should be done for 5 minutes two or three times a day.

The usual treatment for a uterine prolapse is hysterectomy. This procedure may sometimes be done by the vaginal route. If any operation is contraindicated because of the age or general condition of the patient, a pessary may be inserted to hold the uterus up in the pelvis (Fig. 65-4). A string should be attached to the pessary, and after its insertion the woman pins the string to her underclothing. This type of pessary occasionally becomes displaced and might cause the patient embarrassment.

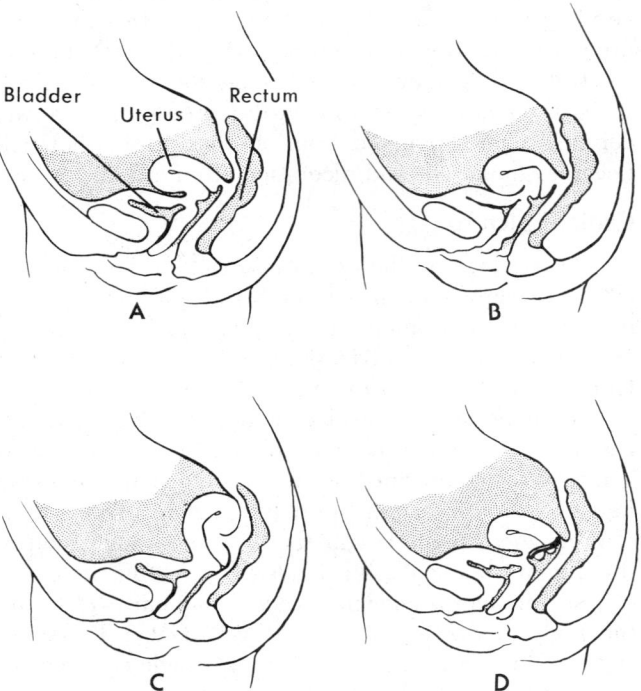

Fig. 65-3. Normal and abnormal positions of uterus. **A,** Normal anatomic position of uterus in relation to adjacent structures. **B,** Anterior displacement of uterus. **C,** Retroversion or backward displacement of uterus. **D,** Normal anatomic position of uterus maintained by use of rubber S-shaped pessary.

Fistulas

Fistulas can occur in several locations (Fig. 65-5). They may occur when a malignant lesion has spread or when radiation treatment has been used for a malignancy, or they may be caused by trauma at surgery or delivery.

Women with vesicovaginal or rectovaginal fistulas may become withdrawn because of embarrassment about odors and soiling of their clothing. Sometimes women become immune to the odors associated with a fistula. Chlorine solution (e.g., 5 ml [1 tsp] chlorine household bleach to 1 L [1 qt] water) makes a satisfactory deodorizing douche, and this solution is also excellent for external perineal irrigation. Sitz baths and thorough cleansing of the surrounding skin with mild soap and water are helpful. Deodorizing powders such as sodium borate can be used. Care is time consuming and must be repeated at regular intervals to ensure cleanliness. Protective pants can be worn.

The patient needs encouragement from the medical and nursing staff, and she needs assurance that they understand her problem. When fistulas persist, couples have special problems that require patience and understanding. Husband and wife should be encouraged to communicate with one another regarding interference with their sexual relationship.

Ureterovaginal fistulas

Ureterovaginal fistulas complicate gynecologic treatment frequently. In treating cancer of the uterus, either by radiation or surgery or occasionally when a hysterectomy is done, the blood supply to the ureter may be impaired, or other damage may occur. The ureteral wall sloughs, and a fistula opens from the ureter to the vagina. This causes a constant drip of urine through the vagina. A ureterovaginal fistula usually heals spontaneously after

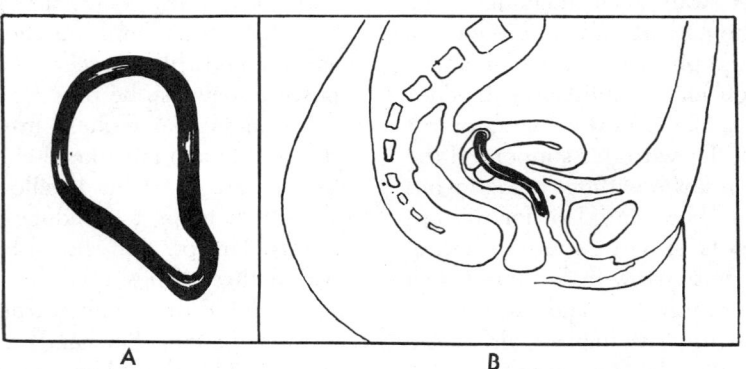

Fig. 65-4. A, Albert Smith pessary. **B,** Pessary in place to hold posterior vaginal fornix, and with it attached cervix, well backward and upward in pelvis. (From Beacham, D.W., and Beacham, W.D.: Synopsis of gynecology, ed. 10, St. Louis, 1982, The C.V. Mosby Co.)

a period of time. If it does not, repair procedures may be attempted, and occasionally an ileobladder must be made (p. 1533).

Vesicovaginal fistulas

Vesicovaginal fistulas, or fistulas between the bladder and the vagina, and urethrovaginal fistulas, between the urethra and the vagina, may follow radiation of the cervix, gynecologic surgery, or trauma during delivery. It is impossible to perform surgery to repair the fistula until the inflammation and induration have subsided. This may take 3 to 4 months. A suprapubic incision is made into the bladder, the fistula tract is dissected out, and the defect is closed by primary closure or by using a graft from the bladder or adjacent mucosal wall.

Postoperatively, usually both a suprapubic tube and a urethral catheter are inserted to drain the bladder. These tubes are sometimes attached to a "bubble" suction drainage apparatus in order to ensure that the bladder is kept empty. Bladder drainage is maintained for about 1 week or until the wound is completely healed. The catheters should not be irrigated unless it is absolutely necessary, and only very gentle pressure should be used when irrigating them. Signs of urinary drainage from the vagina should be noted. There is normally a small amount of serosanguineous drainage from the vagina for a few days postoperatively. Vaginal douches may be ordered and should be given gently and with little pressure from the fluid. Women may need to stay in bed for several days or may need to remain in their rooms if bubble suction is being used. Such confinement is tiring, and visitors, television, radio, reading materials, and a

variety of occupational therapy activities may help to pass the time satisfactorily.

The results of repair operations for fistulas are not always successful. The patient must sometimes have several operations, and each successive hospitalization increases her anxiety about the outcome of surgery and lessens her ability to accept the discomforts and inconveniences entailed. All possible nursing measures should be taken to prevent infection and to be certain that free drainage of urine is ensured. Obstruction of drainage tubes may place pressure against the newly repaired vesicovaginal wall and cause healing tissue to break down, resulting in return of the fistula.

Rectovaginal fistulas

Rectovaginal fistulas are less common than vesicovaginal fistulas. The constant escape of flatus and fecal material through the vagina is particularly distressing to the patient, especially so because rectovaginal fistulas are quite resistant to satisfactory surgical treatment. They may be the result of the same causes as vesicovaginal fistulas. Surgical repair is usually done through the rectum. It may not be satisfactory, and operations may have to be repeated. The nursing care is similar to that needed by patients following surgery for other types of rectal fistulas (p. 1488). In addition, the patient will need sympathetic understanding and encouragement, since the emotional reactions are often severe.

If there is dribbling of fecal material into the vagina, it may be temporarily lessened by giving a high enema, and the woman at home is encouraged to do this before going out. After surgery, of course, enemas are never permitted until healing is complete. They may be given during the preoperative period. A soft rubber catheter should be used and should be directed carefully on the side of the rectum opposite the fistula. The catheter must go beyond the fistulous opening, or the fluid will return through the vagina and no benefit will be derived from the treatment. While a constipating diet will temporarily prevent fecal material from going into the vagina, it eventually will cause pressure and may aggravate the condition and increase the size of the fistula. The woman therefore is advised against restricting diet and fluids in an effort to control bowel action.

Outcome criteria for the woman with a structural problem of the reproductive system

The woman or her significant others can:
1. State the sexual and reproductive consequences of the condition.
2. Perform the self-care measures needed to manage the condition.
3. State signs and symptoms indicating a need to seek professional care.
4. Seek help from a professional when necessary, within an appropriate time period.

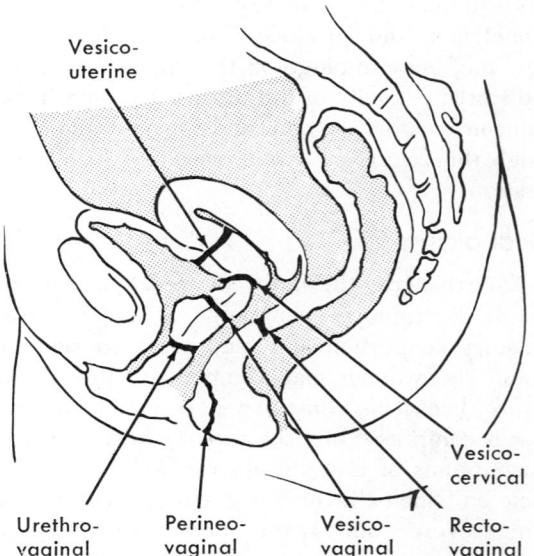

Vesico-uterine

Vesico-cervical

Urethro-vaginal Perineo-vaginal Vesico-vaginal Recto-vaginal

Fig. 65-5. Types of fistulas that may develop in vagina and uterus.

Benign tumors of the female genital tract

Ovarian tumors and cysts

Epidemiology and pathophysiology

There are many types of benign neoplasms affecting the female reproductive tract. Neoplasms of the ovary alone account for several varieties. Almost a third of women have no symptoms of ovarian tumors at the time of diagnosis. Nearly 80% of these are discovered during routine pelvic examination.[76] Women between the ages of 45 and 60 years are at greatest risk for developing ovarian tumors.

Benign neoplasms of the ovary include serous cystadenomas, mucinous adenomas, endometroid benign cysts, and benign mesonephric tumors. In addition, nonneoplastic cysts originating in the graafian follicle, cysts derived from the ruptured follicle (corpus luteum cyst), and simple cysts may occur. The follicle cysts are thin walled and translucent, arising during the evolution or involution of the graafian follicle and do not grow autonomously. Corpus luteum cysts result from an abnormal persistence or exaggeration of the process of formation and resorption of the corpus luteum. After resorption, the cavity is normally distended with hemorrhagic or clear fluid. When exaggerated, the process results in the corpus luteum taking on a cystic structure. Simple cysts, thin-walled structures containing serous fluid, occur frequently during menopause. Polycystic ovarian (Stein-Leventhal) disease is characterized by enlargement of the ovaries, with numerous cystic follicles encased in a fibrotic capsule. Effects of these tumors are often not noted unless there is compression of a neighboring organ or blood supply, a menstrual disorder, or infertility.

Clinical picture

Symptoms are usually nonspecific. With rapidly growing cysts or tumors of the ovary, the first symptom may be an increase in abdominal size. Complaints of fatigue and sensations of weight, fullness, or pressure in the pelvis are common. Pain is an unusual symptom in the absence of acute complications such as twisting of an ovarian cyst on its pedicle. An increase in the size of the tumor may cause pressure symptoms such as urinary frequency and constipation, and backache may be present. Ovarian tumors and cysts are a frequent cause of menstrual irregularities.

Palpation of reproductive organs during pelvic examination usually reveals a mass or enlargement of the ovary. One or both ovaries normally atrophy and become nonpalpable after the menopause; any mass palpated in the area of the ovaries requires further evaluation. Laparoscopy or exploratory laparotomy is usually done to confirm the diagnosis.

Intervention

Ovarian tumors and cysts are treated surgically, and most often an oophorectomy is performed.

Fibroid tumors

Epidemiology and etiology

It has been estimated that 20% to 25% of women over 30 years of age develop uterine fibroid tumors (myomas).[136] Uterine myomas are more common in black women and in women who have never been pregnant. They rarely become malignant. Because their growth is stimulated by ovarian hormones, fibroid tumors of the uterus tend to disappear spontaneously with the advent of the menopause.

Pathophysiology

The cause of uterine myomas is unknown. They do not appear to be transmitted genetically. Because uterine myomas regress after menopause, it has been suggested that they are stimulated by estrogen. The sizes of myomas are variable. Most are found in the body of the uterus (corporeal), but some occur in the cervix or may involve the broad ligament. Subserous growths may extend outward into the folds of the broad ligament, cresting as intraligamentary tumors that burrow outward to form retroperitoneal masses. Intramural growths may cause no change in the contour of the uterus if they are small. When the growths are larger, they may produce an actual uterine enlargement. Submucous tumors may impinge on the blood vessels of the endometrium and produce bleeding. As they grow larger, they may impinge on the opposite uterine wall and distort the cavity of the uterus. In some instances, submucous tumors develop pedicles and may protrude through the vagina or cervix, resulting in infection or ulcerations.

Clinical picture

Menorrhagia is the most common symptom of myomas. If the tumor is very large, it may cause pelvic circulatory congestion and may press on surrounding viscera. The woman may complain of low abdominal pressure, backache, constipation, or dysmenorrhea. If a ureter is compressed by the tumor, there may be signs and symptoms of ureteral obstruction. Sometimes the pedicle on which a myoma is growing becomes twisted, causing severe pain. Large tumors growing into the opening of the fallopian tubes may cause sterility, those in the body of the uterus may cause spontaneous abortions, and those near the cervical opening may make the delivery of a baby difficult and may contribute to hemorrhage postpartally.

Intervention

The treatment of fibroid tumors depends on the symptoms and the age of the patient, on whether more children are desired, and on how near she is to the menopause. If the symptoms are not severe, the woman may simply need close health supervision. If the tumor is near the outer wall of the uterus, a *myomectomy* (surgical removal of the tumor) may be performed. This operation leaves the muscle walls of the uterus relatively intact. If there is severe bleeding or obstruction, a hysterectomy is usually necessary. Occasionally, if surgery is contraindicated or if the woman is approaching the menopause, x-ray therapy or radiation is used to reduce the size of the tumor and to stop vaginal bleeding.

Endometriosis

Pathophysiology

Endometriosis is a condition in which endometrial cells that normally line the uterus are seeded throughout the pelvis and occasionally extend to as distant a location as the umbilicus (Fig. 65-6). The disease appears to be increasing, although the increased incidence may be a result of better diagnosis and recognition of the condition.

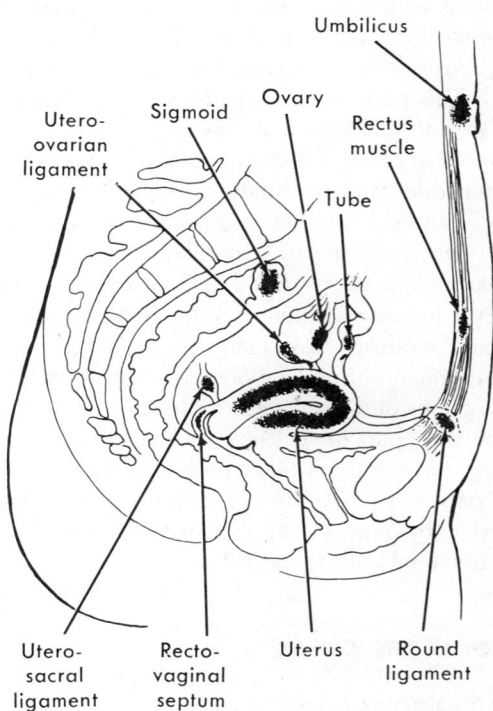

Fig. 65-6. Sites of endometrial implants.

It is not known how endometriosis first develops. Theories include congenital presence of endometrial cells out of their normal location, their transfer by means of blood vessels or the lymphatic system, and reflux of menstrual fluid containing endometrial cells up the fallopian tubes and into the pelvic cavity. None of these theories has been proved. With each menstrual period, the endometrial cells are stimulated by the ovarian hormones and bleed into the surrounding areas, causing an inflammation. Subsequent adhesions may be so severe that pelvic organs may become fused together, occasionally causing a stricture of the bowel or interference with bladder function. Encased blood may lead to palpable tumor masses, which often occur on the ovary and are known as *chocolate cysts*. Occasionally, these cysts rupture and spread endometrial cells still farther throughout the pelvis.

Clinical picture

Usually endometriosis progresses gradually and does not produce symptoms until the age of 30 to 40. Occasionally, however, symptoms appear when the woman is in her teens. The characteristic symptom of endometriosis is pain and general discomfort accompanying menstruation that becomes progressively worse and that was not present at the onset of the menses. This one characteristic feature should alert the nurse to urge that the woman see a gynecologist at once. Many women with severe pain related to menstruation have been judged to be neurotic, when in reality, they were suffering from endometriosis. Other symptoms of endometriosis are a feeling of fullness in the lower abdomen, dyspareunia, menorrhagia, irregular menstrual cycles, prostration, and general poor health. Sometimes the disease is far advanced and yet has caused no symptoms at all. Approximately 40% to 50% of women are infertile, and endometriosis is sometimes first detected when a woman presents herself with the complaint of inability to conceive. On pelvic examination (done preferably during the first 24 hours of menses), tender, nodular, uterosacral ligaments and sometimes fixed uterine retroversion are found. With endometriosis, the uterus is enlarged, nodular, and tender, but the cul-de-sac of Douglas is usually normal.

Intervention

Although a great deal of study of endometriosis is under way at present, its response to treatment is still variable and poorly understood. For this reason, treatment is highly individualized. If the woman is young and wants to have children, the treatment for endometriosis is usually as conservative as possible. Pregnancy is beneficial, because menstruation ceases during this time. If a young women has endometriosis, she and her husband usually are advised to have their family early, because the fertility rate is low, sterility caused by adhesions may occur, and a hysterectomy may have to be done within a reasonable period of time. Nursing the infant is also recommended, because it delays the onset of menstruation following delivery.

Because they imitate the state of pregnancy by inducing the ovaries to become anovulatory, antiovulatory drugs are frequently prescribed. Oral contraceptives with potent progestins and minimal amounts of estrogen are used for prolonged periods of time to produce endometrial atrophy and to lessen endometrial flow into the peritoneal cavity. The disadvantages of this treatment are that irregular bleeding may occur and that the symptoms of early pregnancy, including nausea, vomiting, depression, and fatigue, may be troublesome.

Drugs having reversible antigonadotropic action by suppressing ovarian activity (danazol) have recently become available.[56] These drugs are given in a dose of 200 mg twice a day for 3 to 6 months. Treatment can be extended up to 9 months if necessary, or it can be reinstituted if symptoms recur. Danazol is used to arrest proliferation of the endometrium, to prevent ovulation, and to thus produce atrophy of the ectopic endometrium. This therapy is expensive (often $100/month), and may create hot flashes, dry vagina, and depression and foster weight gain. Antigonadotropic drugs are contraindicated if the woman has undiagnosed abnormal vaginal bleeding; has impaired hepatic, renal, or cardiac function; is pregnant; or is breast-feeding an infant. Some women find their endometriosis disappears spontaneously, and some who become pregnant remain asymptomatic thereafter. For minimal symptoms, treatment with mild analgesics may be adequate. Regular pelvic examinations (every 6 months) are recommended to monitor the progress of endometriosis.

When the involvement is severe and does not respond to hormonal treatment, surgery may be necessary. A total hysterectomy, oophorectomy, and salpingectomy may be done. Removal of the ovaries prevents further bleeding of endometrial implants that cannot be removed. If the woman is premenopausal and the ovaries must be removed, she may be given very small amounts of estrogen. Menopause stops the progress of this condition.

Cervical polyps

Cervical polyps form when an area of the cervical mucosa proliferates. These growths are usually visible at the cervical os as bright red, vascular, fragile areas. They are most often pedunculated and appear to protrude from the cervical canal. Polyps may occur singly or in clusters.

Because of the vascularity of the polyp, bleeding is a common symptom. Generally, no other symptom is present. The characteristics of the bleeding associated with polyps closely resemble the signs of early cancer of the cervix. The bleeding is small in amount and occurs between menstrual periods. Especially characteristic is the contact bleeding produced by coitus, by douching, or by vaginal examination.

The pedicle by which the polyp is attached is usually quite small so that the polyp can easily be removed by twisting the pedicle at its base or by use of a biopsy forceps or sharp curette.[6] Tissue examination of removed polyps is essential, since epidermoid cancer arises from cervical polyps in a small percentage of cases.

Cancer of the female genital tract

There are only three avenues by which the toll of gynecologic cancer morbidity and mortality can be controlled and reduced—prevention, early detection, and improvements in treatment.[125] Fortunately, many of the gynecologic malignancies have an associated high "cure" rate. This has been at least in part a result of the development of diagnostic techniques that can identify precancerous conditions, the ability to apply highly effective treatments that are more restricted elsewhere in the body, better understanding of disease spread patterns, and more sophisticated and effective treatment in cancers that previously had poor prognoses.[51] Thus the patient with a gynecologic malignancy may look forward to earlier diagnosis, more effective treatment, and subsequently longer survival than was previously experienced. This optimism should be realistically transferred to the patient and significant others.

The nurse caring for the gynecologic oncology patient is responsible for coordination of patient care, which includes physical, psychosocial, and discharge planning needs. The nurse must understand that women with gynecologic cancers are faced with anxieties precipitated by threats to survival, body image, personal and cultural roles, and modesty. For many patients, genital cancer may symbolize cultural taboos or retribution for sexual transgressions and may cause embarrassment and reluctance on their part to verbalize these concerns. Therefore the nurse must address these problems, placing emphasis on the patient's perception of femininity, the stigma associated with gynecologic cancer, and fears regarding future personal and sexual roles.[9]

Cancer of the cervix

Epidemiology and etiology

Twenty-five percent of all malignant diseases in women arise in the genital tract, and half of these malignancies arise in the cervix.[50] The annual mortality for cancer of the cervix has fallen steadily over the past 40 years. This decline has been attributed to early detection through annual examinations (including a Pap smear) and improved surgical and radiotherapeutic techniques. Nevertheless, despite these improved diagnostic and therapeutic techniques, the estimated mortality from cervical cancer in 1981 was 7200 with an estimated incidence of 16,000 new cases.[1]

The age of patients with carcinoma "in situ" is, on the average, 10 years less than the average patient with invasive cancer of the cervix. The average age of patients with invasive cancer of the cervix is 45 years. There are, however, many exceptions; and in the past 20 years, there has been an increasing number of young women (late teens and early 20s) diagnosed with invasive cancer of the cervix. The risk factors associated with cancer of the cervix include the following: first coitus at an early age, multiple sexual partners, low socioeconomic group, and exposure to herpesvirus type 2. There is no correlation with frequency of sexual intercourse.[51]

Pathophysiology

Cervical carcinomas may arise in one of two cell types—squamous carcinomas (epidermal layer of the cervix) make up 95% of all cervical cancers; adenocarcinomas (cervical mucus–producing gland cells) primarily make up the remaining 5%.

The precursor lesions of cervical squamous cell carcinoma have been identified as dysplasia. Cervical intraepithelial neoplasia (CIN) is the term commonly used to define the precursor state. CIN has been subdivided into the following three stages:

CIN I   Mild to moderate dysplasia
CIN II   Moderate to severe dysplasia
CIN III Severe dysplasia to carcinoma in situ[11]

It is generally agreed that patients with the earlier stages of CIN (the dysplasias) may have one of three courses—regression, persistence, or progression to carcinoma in situ or invasive carcinoma.[3]

Adenocarcinoma arises from the mucus-producing gland cells of the cervix. Unlike squamous cell carcinoma of the cervix, adenocarcinoma is not preceded by a well-recognized, prolonged precursor state, and because of its origin within the cervix, it may be present for a considerable time before it can be clinically detected.[51]

Prevention and early detection

Dramatic decreases in deaths from cancer are associated with early detection and treatment. The decline in deaths from cervical cancer is primarily because of increased use of the Pap smear for mass screening combined with more frequent and more thorough gynecologic examinations.

To salvage more lives through diagnosis and treat-

ment, it is important first to determine the population at risk and then to provide them with the means by which frequent, inexpensive screening can be accomplished. The risk factors associated with cervical cancer have been cited. Application of this knowledge in practice assists with identification of specific individuals at high risk for cancer.

Cervical cancer deaths could be greatly reduced if every adult woman had an annual physical examination, including a Pap smear. Many older women, especially those in rural areas, have not had a physical examination since their childbearing years. The American Cancer Society, in its report on *The Cancer-Related Health Checkup*, recommended the following:

. . . that all asymptomatic women age 20 and over, and those under 20 who are sexually active, have a Pap test annually for two negative examinations and then at least every three years until the age of 65. A pelvic examination should be done as part of a general physical examination every three years from age 20 to 40 and annually thereafter; women who are at a high risk of developing cervical cancer because of early age at first intercourse, multiple sexual partners, or other risk factors may need to be tested more frequently. Women who are relatively inactive sexually may prefer a less frequent interval.[2]

This report by the American Cancer Society has caused considerable concern about its possible adverse effect on the current successful cancer control in this country. In response to this report, the American College of Obstetricians and Gynecologists recommended the continuation of annual cytologic screening for cervical neoplasia. A summation of this report states the following*:

The dramatic fall in cervical cancer incidence and death rates has been brought about largely as a result of annual cytologic screening. There is no existing clinical experience which can provide assurance that such reductions could be maintained with a program of less frequent screening. Any change in this pattern should take into account the following facts: the Papanicolaou smear is an inexpensive procedure, has no discernible morbidity, is easily obtained, and has the potential for a high degree of sensitivity.

The choice of a screening interval is arbitrary and is based on a subjective assessment of cost-effectiveness. Lengthening the screening interval inevitably detects the cancers or precancerous states at a later stage and inevitably trades lives for dollars.

The Pap smear has an inherent false-negative rate of 15% to 40%. This problem has its greatest impact on the high-risk patient. Any screening interval that fails to recognize this fact, introduces some increased risk to the individual woman's health and life.

The earlier that cervical neoplasia is detected, the more amenable it is to local, office-based treatment. Later stages,

---

*From American College of Obstetricians and Gynecologists, Washington, D.C., 1980, The College.

even of the cancer precursors, may require surgery (conization or hysterectomy) for diagnosis or therapy.

It has been recommended that high-risk women (those who have had early sexual intercourse, have had several sexual partners, or multiple marital events) should be screened annually.

Since a substantial proportion of women in the United States are at high risk for developing cervical neoplasia, they should be made aware of those factors that result in high-risk status.

Although the annual screening interval has been arrived at arbitrarily, it has served as a convenient benchmark. Abandoning this traditional interval may result in an increase in untreated cervical neoplasia. The annual interval may be too short for some populations and too long for others. Further attempts to codify this decision are potentially dangerous and may lead to an increase in cancer deaths.[4]

Clinical picture

The 5-year survival rate for CIN is 100%; the 5-year survival rate for cervical cancer stage IV is 8%. In the early stages, cervical cancer is asymptomatic. With progression of disease, a slight watery vaginal discharge may appear, occasional bloody spotting following intercourse or between periods may occur, and as the disease progresses, a foul discharge or pain may develop.

Intervention

Cervical cancer is treated according to the stage of the disease (Table 65-4), the woman's age and general health, and the presence of complications.

Treatment of carcinoma in situ may consist of an excisional conization of the cervix (or cryosurgery in some institutions) if the woman is young, wishes to have more children, and invasive cancer has been ruled out. In other women, simple hysterectomy is preferred to radiotherapy, particularly for those in whom preservation of ovarian function is desirable.

Invasive cancer of the cervix can be treated by means of surgery or radiotherapy (Table 65-5). Usually the tumors above stages I and II are treated with radiotherapy. Surgery for stage I and early stage II disease may be reserved in some institutions for those women

desiring preservation of ovarian function. Comparable cure rates are obtained with either surgery or radiotherapy; however, the morbidity associated with both approaches is considered in light of the individual and her problem.

Surgery. The surgery recommended for stage I and early stage II is a radical hysterectomy with pelvic lymph node dissection (Fig. 65-7). The structures that are removed in this procedure are the uterus, the nearby supporting tissues, the uppermost part of the vagina, and the pelvic lymph nodes. This surgery is more extensive than a simple hysterectomy, and the nursing care is more involved. (Fig. 65-8 shows comparison with other types of hysterectomies.)

If a radical hysterectomy is to be performed, the preoperative physical preparation is the same as that for any other abdominal surgery. A vaginal douche may be given. Postoperatively, the patient has an abdominal dressing and wears a perineal pad. The dressings should be observed for any sign of bleeding every 15 minutes for 2 hours and then at least every hour for 8 hours. There is normally a moderate amount of serosanguineous drainage. Two catheters connected to hemovacs (p. 437) are placed below the incision to drain excess fluid from the surgical site. These drains are left in place until there is only a minimal amount of drainage from them (3 to 5 days).

TABLE 65-4. Stages of cancer of the cervix

Stage	Involvement
0	Confined within epithelium of cervix
I	Completely confined to cervix
II	Extends outside cervix but does not involve pelvic wall or lower third of vagina
III	Involves pelvic wall and lower third of vagina
IV	Extends beyond stage III; involves bladder, rectum, or metastatic spread

TABLE 65-5. Summary of treatment options for cervical cancer

Clinical stage	Treatment options	5-year survival (%)
Dysplasia CIN	Cryosurgery/conization Simple hysterectomy*	100
Ia Microinvasive (3mm below basement membrane)	Simple hysterectomy or radiation (cesium implant)	95-100
Microinvasive 3-5 mm depth	Radical hysterectomy with nodes or radiotherapy (external and implant)	95-98
Ib and IIa	Radical hysterectomy with nodes or radiotherapy	75-90
IIb	Radiation	50-60
IIIa and IIIb	Radiation	30-40
IV	Radiation or chemotherapy	5-14
Recurrent	Pelvic exenteration, if operable	Varies according to site and extent of recurrence

Following a hysterectomy, especially one in which there has been extensive nodal and parametrial resection, the *bladder* may be temporarily *atonic* as a result of nerve trauma, and a Foley catheter is used to maintain constant drainage of the bladder. If no catheter is used and if the woman is unable to void within 8 hours, she is usually catheterized. The catheter is usually left in place for 2 to 3 weeks. After catheter removal, the woman is catheterized after voiding to check residual urine. If the residual urine is more than 100 ml, the catheter is left in place for an additional 1 to 2 weeks and is then rechecked.

Abdominal distention may complicate a hysterectomy. It is caused by nerve damage or by handling of the viscera during operation. Some physicians insert a nasogastric tube prophylactically following surgery, and most physicians restrict food and fluids orally for 24 to 48 hours. Fleet's enema may be given on the second or third postoperative day. When peristalsis returns, fluids and food are started gradually.

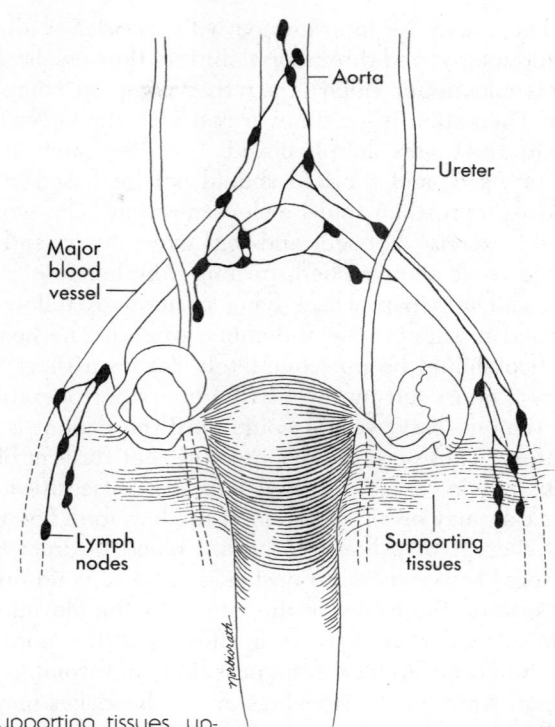

Fig. 65-7. Radical hysterectomy includes removal of uterus, nearby supporting tissues, uppermost part of vagina, and pelvic lymph nodes.

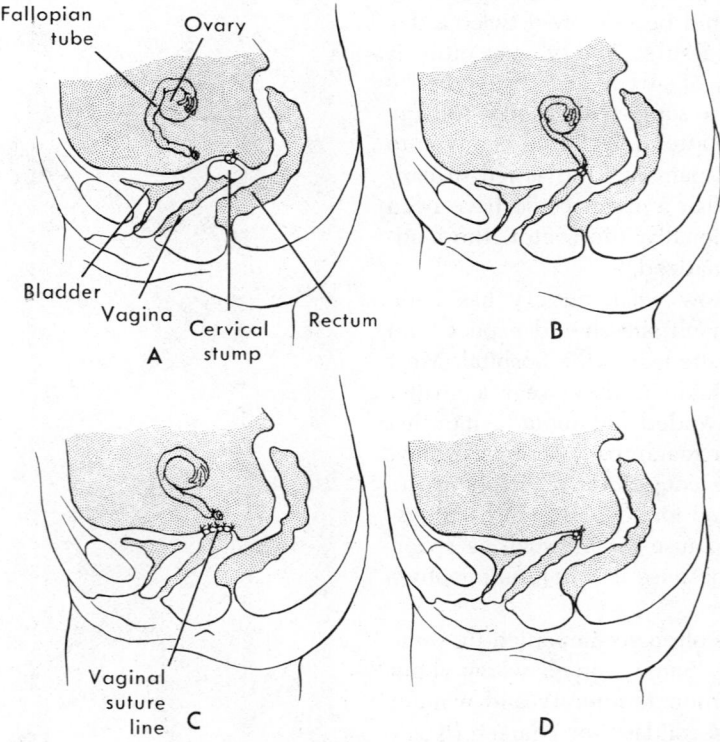

Fig. 65-8. A, Cross-section of subtotal hysterectomy. Note that cervical stump, fallopian tubes, and ovaries remain. **B,** Cross-section of total hysterectomy. Note that fallopian tubes and ovaries remain. **C,** Cross-section of vaginal hysterectomy. Note that fallopian tubes and ovaries remain. **D,** Total hysterectomy, salpingectomy, and oophorectomy. Note that uterus, fallopian tubes, and ovaries are completely removed.

There may be interference with *circulation* during hysterectomy, and thrombophlebitis of the vessels of the pelvis and upper thigh is a rather common complication. The patient should never rest with the knees bent or with the thighs sharply flexed. The knee gatch should not be used, and the bed should not be raised at the head to more than mid-Fowler's position. The woman should exercise her feet and legs every hour, and she should move about in bed, turning from her side to her back and to a partial face-lying position. A pillow can be used to support the abdominal wound. The head of the bed should be put completely flat for a short time every 2 hours during the first 24 hours postoperatively and then at least every 4 hours until the patient is ambulatory. These precautions help prevent stasis of blood in the pelvic vessels. If the woman has varicosities, the physician may order elevation of the legs for a few minutes every 2 or 3 hours to permit blood to drain from the legs. Nurses need to ensure that there is no undue pressure on the calves of the legs, that the elevation is uniform, and that there is no flexing at the popliteal region in order to lessen the possibility of thrombus formation. Antiembolic stockings or Ace bandages may be applied from the toes to just below the knee, excluding the popliteal region. Recent research on thrombophlebitis has indicated that improperly applied Ace bandages are a major cause of postoperative thrombus formation. The bandages should be reapplied twice a day to ensure a snug, even pressure. The woman often is permitted out of bed the day of surgery.

Other nursing care is the same as that following any abdominal surgery. Special attention should be given to any complaint of low back pain or to lessened urinary output, since it is possible that a ureter could have been accidentally ligated. Occasionally, the ureter, the bladder, or the rectum is traumatized.

The woman should know what surgery has been done, what changes in herself she should expect, and what care she needs when she leaves the hospital. Most patients are more comfortable if they wear a girdle. Heavy lifting should be avoided for about 2 months. Activities such as riding over rough roads, walking swiftly, and dancing tend to cause congestion of blood in the pelvis and should be avoided for several months. Physical activity that does not cause strain, such as swimming, may be engaged in because it is helpful for physical and mental well-being.

Radical hysterectomy is often accompanied by some degree of emotional upset. Some women worry about the effect it will have on their femininity and wonder about possible changes in secondary sex characteristics. Young women may feel bitterly disappointed because they can no longer have children; others may be relieved from the fear of becoming pregnant. Some women worry about gaining weight, although weight gain is most often caused by overeating rather than by hormonal changes.

It is true that the childbearing function will be terminated, but usually the vagina is intact so that 4 to 6 weeks following surgery women can resume normal sexual intercourse.

Older women may be less upset by the prospects of surgery of this kind than are those who have not reached the menopause. Postoperatively, however, almost all patients feel depressed for several days. The patient often is unable to explain why she is depressed and crying. Grieflike responses to loss of a body part may appear as they do following surgery in other cases. Feelings of guilt, shame, and remorse are not uncommon. Encouraging the woman to continue activities associated with being feminine, such as using makeup, arranging her hair, and wearing her own clothing, often helps the woman to regain her feminine perspective. During this period, she needs understanding and sympathetic care. Families need to be helped to accept these responses

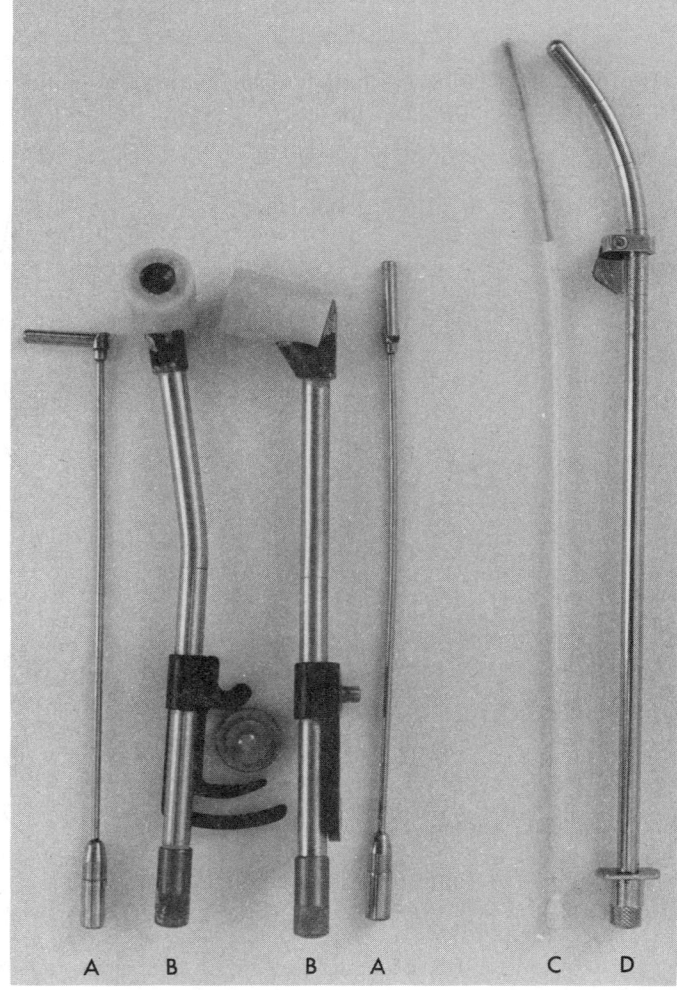

Fig. 65-9. Intracavitary implant. *A,* Inserts for colpostats to insert radium or cesium. *B,* Colpostats. *C,* Teflon tubing to insert radium or cesium into tandem. *D,* Tandem.

calmly, and a husband may need help in understanding her need for reassurance of his continued love and affection.

Radiotherapy. The radiotherapy employed in the treatment of cervical cancer usually consists of whole pelvis irradiation as well as two intracavitary implants (Figs. 65-9 to 65-11). The amount of radioactive substance used and the number of hours it is left in place are determined by the amount of radiation needed to kill the less resistant cancer cells without damaging nor-

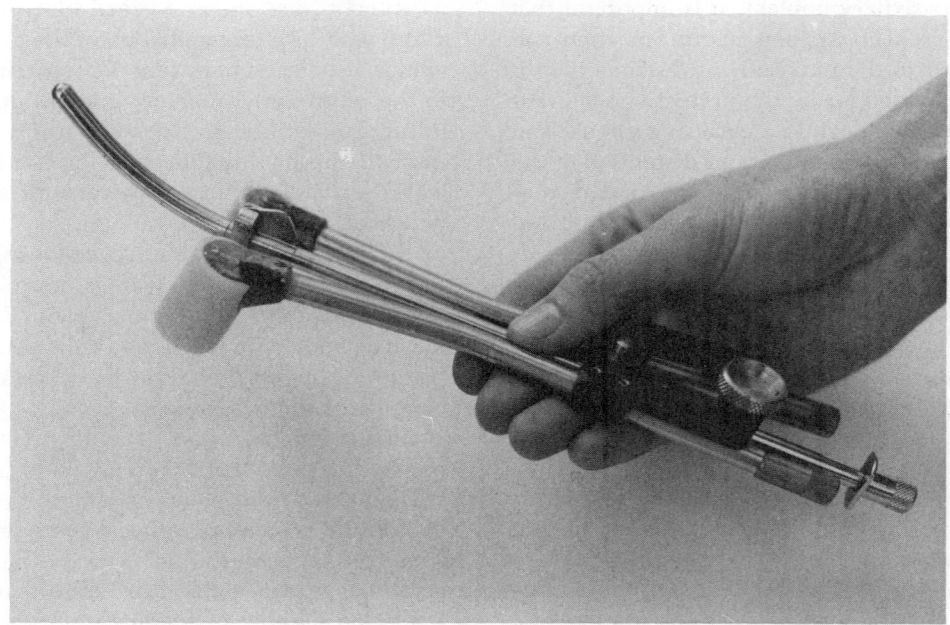

Fig. 65-10. Assembled configuration of tandem and colpostat before placement.

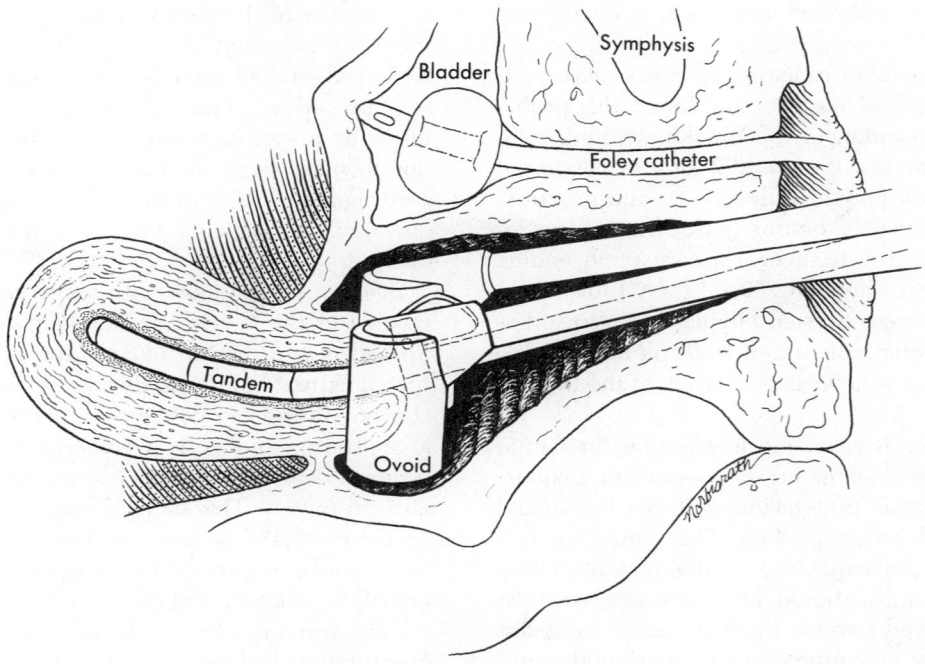

Fig. 65-11. Placement of tandem and colpostats before vaginal packing.

mal cells. (For a discussion of radiation treatment and the general nursing care and precautions involved, see p. 490.)

Premenopausal women who receive pelvic irradiation will lose their ovarian function. Counseling regarding use of hormones, vaginal lubricants, and other methods to prevent or alleviate menopausal symptoms is indicated.

During an intracavitary implant, it is important that all normal tissues remain in their natural position and do not come nearer to the radioactive substance than is anticipated and provided for by the protective materials used. Before treatment begins, a cleansing enema and a low-residue diet are given to prevent distention of the bowel. A catheter may be inserted to prevent distention of the bladder. Gauze packing is usually inserted into the vagina to push both the rectum and the bladder away from the area being irradiated. Cleansing enemas are not given during the treatment. To prevent any displacement of the radioactive substance, the patient is kept flat in bed and is allowed to turn only from side to side. A roentgenogram is taken before the radioactive substance is inserted to determine its exact location.

Since the presence of anything in the cervix stimulates uterine contractions, the woman who has a tandem or intrauterine applicator in place may have severe uterine contractions as a result of dilation of the cervix. She should know that they will occur. Often a narcotic is given at regular intervals while the applicator is in place. There will be foul-smelling vaginal discharge from the destruction of cells. Good perineal care is essential, and it must be remembered that since the patient must lie on her back, she will need assistance. A deodorizer is helpful.

Patients may develop radiation sickness, with nausea, vomiting, diarrhea, malaise, and fever; this probably is a systemic reaction to the breakdown and reabsorption of cell proteins. (See p. 492 for a discussion of care.) Local reaction may include cystitis and proctitis. Camphorated tincture of opium (paregoric) helps relieve the diarrhea. If it is severe, a cornstarch enema (15 ml [1 tbsp] cornstarch to 250 ml [1 C] lukewarm water) may be ordered. Steroid enemas are also sometimes given. The woman is urged to drink at least 3 L of fluid a day to help relieve any irritation of the urinary system.

The woman who is receiving intracavitary radiation treatments often feels alienated, depressed, or anxious. Nurses can spend some time talking with her but should remain at a safe distance (p. 497). The reason for this precaution should be explained to the patient. Close members of the family should be encouraged to visit when it is considered safe for them to do so. Pregnant nurses, visitors, or any other personnel should avoid contact with the patient while the implant is in place.

Following removal of the radioactive agent, the catheter is removed, a cleansing enema is given, and the woman is allowed out of bed. Vaginal discharge will continue for some time, and the patient may need to take douches for as long as the odor and vaginal discharge persist. Usually douches are ordered twice a day. The woman who is returning home needs detailed instructions in how to give herself douches and what solutions to use. Some vaginal bleeding may occur for 1 to 3 months after irradiation of the cervix. The woman who is at home should report persistent rectal irritation to the physician. Emollient enemas may be prescribed to be taken at home. The woman is usually discharged from the hospital within a day or two after the applicators are removed but may return for another course of radiation.

Complications to watch for following radiation of the uterus are vesicovaginal fistulas, ureterovaginal fistulas, cystitis, phlebitis, and hemorrhage. Each is caused by the radiation or by extension of the disease process. The patient is urged to report even minor symptoms or complaints to her physician.

Pelvic exenteration. The natural history of many pelvic cancers is that they may be locally advanced but still limited to the pelvis; therefore they may be cured by radical resection. Pelvic exenterative surgery was subjected to severe initial criticism but is currently accepted as a respectable procedure that can offer life to a selected number of patients where no other possibility of cure exists.[51]

Although pelvic exenteration has been implemented for various pelvic malignancies, its greatest and most important role is in the treatment of advanced or recurrent cancer of the cervix. Total exenteration entails removal of the pelvic viscera, including the bladder, rectosigmoid, and all reproductive organs. In selected cases, the procedure may be limited to either an anterior or posterior exenteration. An anterior exenteration involves removal of all the pelvic viscera except the rectosigmoid. A posterior exenteration involves removal of all the pelvic viscera with preservation of the bladder.

Only a few patients with recurrent or advanced carcinoma of the cervix are candidates for the operation. Spread of the disease outside the pelvis, which is detected either before or during surgery, is an absolute contraindication to pelvic exenteration. The decision to abort the procedure is a grave prognostic sign. The 5-year survival rate after pelvic exenteration varies from 20% to 62%.[51] The survival rates are most influenced by the criteria of patient selection. For instance, survival rates can be improved by excluding the elderly obese, heavily irradiated, and other high-risk patients.

The nursing care of the patient undergoing pelvic exenteration includes the care given the patient having a hysterectomy (p. 1701), the care given the patient having an abdominal perineal resection of the bowel (p. 1452), and the care given the patient having an ileobladder with transplantation of the ureters (p. 1533). An essential aspect in the nursing care of the exenteration patient is teaching. It is essential that each patient be cognizant of the indications, goal, and scope of the surgical procedure. Explanations regarding female anatomy, alteration in body function, and impact on sexual function should be included in the preoperative teaching sessions. Also helpful are introductions to other members of the health care team who will be involved in postoperative care (e.g., enterostomal therapist, social worker, and dietitian). Excellent teaching plans for patients undergoing pelvic exenteration are available.[37,189] The psychosocial aspects of undergoing a pelvic exenteration are understandably immense. The psychosexual adjustment to this radical surgery encompasses psychologic, social, and sexual factors. Adaptation includes changes in body image, social life-style, and sexual relations. Nurses have the professional responsibility of nurturing these women so they redevelop and adjust their life to what they consider an acceptable and worthwhile level.

Chemotherapy. The control or cure of metastatic cancer of the cervix has not significantly improved with the progress of modern chemotherapy. This may be caused, in part, by the the fact that most cervical cancers (95%) are of the squamous cell variety, which are generally the least responsive to most chemotherapeutic agents. In addition to cell type, often recurrent cancers appear within a previously irradiated area that is fibrotic and avascular. The perfusion of this area is marginal, and therefore it is difficult to obtain a high tissue concentration of the drug in the recurrent neoplasm. The drugs most commonly employed are mitomycin C, vincristine, bleomycin, doxorubicin (Adriamycin), cisplatin, 5-fluorouracil, cyclophosphamide, and methotrexate. These can be given alone or in various combinations at regular intervals. (For the nursing care of patients receiving these drugs, see p. 497.)

Cancer of the endometrium

Epidemiology and etiology

Cancer of the endometrium (uterine corpus) afflicts mostly mature women; this diagnosis is most common in women between the ages of 50 and 64 years. The yearly estimated incidence of new cases in the United States is 38,000; the estimated mortality is 3100.[1] Seventy-five percent of all endometrial cancers occur in postmenopausal women.

Multiple risk factors for endometrial cancer have been identified. The most common risk factors are obesity, nulliparity, late menopause (after 52 years of age), diabetes mellitus, and hypertension. Use of exogenous estrogens has also been implicated as a risk factor.

Pathophysiology

Uterine hyperplasia is somewhat analogous to dysplasia of the cervix. Some of these lesions revert to normal, some persist as hyperplasia, and a few progress to endometrial adenocarcinoma. Unfortunately, unlike cervical dysplasia, there is no reliable commonly used screening method for endometrial hyperplasia. Most women with this condition are diagnosed because they present for medical care with symptoms of abnormal uterine bleeding. The diagnosis of endometrial hyperplasia can be made only on pathologic examination of uterine tissue.

Prevention and early detection

Cancer of the endometrium is a slow-growing form of cancer and is very amenable to treatment if detected early. Women who are in the high-risk category (e.g., obesity, late menopause, diabetes mellitus, and hypertension) for developing endometrial cancer often have endometrial tissue samples taken. This can be done either as an outpatient in an ambulatory clinic, in a physician's office, or as an inpatient. The tissue samples can be obtained in a variety of ways (Table 65-6) with varying effectiveness.

Clinical picture

The most common symptom associated with endometrial cancer is abnormal spotting and bleeding. Any postmenopausal woman with uterine bleeding should be evaluated for endometrial cancer. In the premenopausal woman, or one who is currently going through menopause, these symptoms may be interpreted as normal menopausal symptoms. During this time in a woman's life, the menstrual periods should become lighter and farther apart. Any other bleeding pattern should be evaluated.[51]

Other more vague symptoms include abdominal pain or pressure, nausea, and vomiting. These are late symptoms, however, and patients who present with these symptoms and have the subsequent diagnosis of uterine cancer usually have a history of abnormal bleeding.

TABLE 65-6. Methods for detection of endometrial cancer

Method	Effectiveness (%)
Endometrial aspirations	70-80
Endometrial washings	80-90
D and C (fractional curettage)	85-90
Pap smear	45-50
Combination of above	90

Intervention

Endometrial cancer is treated according to the stage of the disease (Table 65-7).

The treatment for cancer of the corpus is most commonly total abdominal hysterectomy and bilateral salpingo-oophorectomy (TAH/BSO). The nursing care for women who undergo a TAH/BSO is similar to that of any other patient receiving major abdominal surgery (see Chapter 24). If, on analysis of the tissue, the tumor has deeply invaded the uterus or spread to the pelvic lymph nodes, postoperative radiation will be given. In advanced stages, preoperative radiation is used (intrauterine radiation and external whole pelvic irradiation). This treatment can also be done preoperatively to shrink the tumor and decrease the amount of local infection so that the operation will be safer and easier to perform. Since endometrial cancer often occurs in later life, some women who are poor operative risks will be given radiation therapy as opposed to being exposed to the risk of surgery. The nursing care of patients receiving radiation therapy for endometrial cancer is similar to the care given any patient receiving external radiation with a subsequent radium implant (p. 493).

Treatment of patients with stage III or stage IV disease usually includes hormonal treatment and chemotherapy in addition to surgery and radiation. Progestins have been used for more than 20 years with good response, especially in patients with well-differentiated tumors. Progestin therapy may be administered in several different ways. Medroxyprogesterone acetate (Depo-Provera), 400 mg intramuscularly at weekly intervals; oral medroxyprogesterone in the range of 150 mg/day; or megestrolacetate (Megace), 160 mg/day. The side effects from these medications are rare. Most women tolerate this form of hormonal manipulation extremely well.

For patients who do not respond to progestins, doxorubicin, cyclophosphamide, and 5-fluorouracil have been employed, either singularly or in combination. The effectiveness of these agents varies. (For the nursing care of patients receiving these drugs, see p. 497.)

Cancer of the ovary

Epidemiology and etiology

Ovarian cancer causes more deaths than any other female genital cancer. There are about 18,000 new cases diagnosed each year in the United States with about 11,400 deaths annually. Cancer of the ovary is the fourth most frequent fatal cancer in women in the United States.[51] Malignant neoplasms of the ovaries occur at all ages, including infancy and childhood. The major histologic types occur in distinctive age ranges. Malignant germ cells are most common in women under the age of 20, whereas epithelial cancers of the ovary are primarily seen in women over 50 years. The greatest number of cases is found in the age group of 50 to 59 years.

There are no known specific risk factors for ovarian cancer. The nonspecific risk factors most commonly seen are familial history and environmental factors. The highest rates of ovarian cancer are seen in highly industrialized countries, which suggests exposure to physical or chemical products of industry. The etiology of ovarian neoplasms is poorly understood. The mechanisms of development are virtually a mystery. Many retrospective studies are currently underway to determine preexisting gynecologic abnormalities.

Pathophysiology

The pathophysiology of ovarian cancer is complex. Ovarian cancer is a broad term that can be divided into many categories depending on the cell type of origin. The four main types of ovarian neoplasms are shown in Table 65-8.

Clinical picture

The early diagnosis of an ovarian neoplasm is usually by chance rather than a result of frequent screening. There is no known method for detecting ovarian cancer at an early stage. The signs and symptoms of advancing disease include abdominal girth enlargement, abdominal pain and pressure, nausea and vomiting, constipation, and urinary frequency. Any ovarian enlargement should be suspected of being an ovarian malignancy. Palpable ovaries in premenarchal or postmenopausal women are an abnormal physical finding.

Intervention

Ovarian cancer is diagnosed and staged at the time of exploratory laparotomy. A total abdominal hysterectomy with bilateral salpingo-oophorectomy is most commonly done in addition to the removal of as much of the tumor as possible. Any ascites encountered during the surgery is submitted for cytology and, if there is no ascitic fluid, "washings" will be taken by lavaging the peritoneal cavity with normal saline and submitting this fluid for analysis. Often the omentum is removed as well as samples of the paraaortic and pelvic lymph nodes. All of the remaining tissue in the pelvis and abdomen is carefully scrutinized and a biopsy is done of any suspicious areas.

TABLE 65-7. Stages of cancer of the endometrium

Stage	Involvement
I	Confined to corpus
II	Involves corpus and cervix
III	Extends outside corpus but not outside pelvis (vaginal wall but not bladder or rectum)
IV	Involves bladder, rectum, or outside pelvis

TABLE 65-8. Classification of ovarian neoplasms

Source of neoplasm	Examples
Epithelium	Serous, mucinous, endometrioid
Germ cell	Teratoma (mature and immature), dysgerminoma
Gonadal stroma	Granulosa-theca, Sertoli-Leydig
Mesenchyme	Fibroma, lymphoma, sarcoma

TABLE 65-9. Stages of cancer of the ovary

Stage	Involvement
I	Limited to ovaries
II	Involving one or both ovaries with pelvic extension
III	Involving one or both ovaries with intraperitoneal metastasis outside pelvis or positive lymph nodes
IV	Involving one or both ovaries with distant metastasis (e.g., liver, lungs)

Ovarian cancer is surgically staged (unlike cervical and endometrial cancer, which are clinically staged). The staging of ovarian cancer is included in Table 65-9.

In addition to surgery, some form of adjuvant therapy is often recommended. The adjuvant therapy employed is usually based on the stage of the disease. The long-term survival is dependent on the stage of the disease, the grade of differentiation of the tumor, the amount of tumor left after surgery, and the additional treatment used after surgery.

Additional or adjuvant therapy usually suggested for stage I disease is chemotherapy with an alkylating agent, such as melphalan, or intraperitoneal instillation of radioactive phosphorus (32-P). For the nursing care of patients who have had 32-P instilled, see p. 506.

Patients with stage II disease may be offered a variety of adjuvant therapies. The most common options include instillation of 32-P, external abdominal and pelvic irradiation, or systemic combined chemotherapy. Often, after completion of systemic chemotherapy, a "second-look" operation is done to determine if there is any remaining disease. This surgery is done only if the patient is clinically free of disease. If no disease is found during this procedure, no further therapy is given.

Patients with stage III or stage IV ovarian cancer have as much of the tumor removed as possible. It has been found that the survival rates of patients with stage III and stage IV disease is directly related to the amount of residual disease. Patients with minimal residual disease appear to have a better prognosis with adjuvant therapy.

The adjuvant therapy used in stage III and stage IV ovarian cancer is most commonly combined chemotherapy. Occasionally, in stage III disease, whole abdominal irradiation is implemented. For patients who cannot tolerate aggressive chemotherapy or radiation, a single alkylating agent such as melphalan is employed.

The nursing care for any patient with ovarian cancer includes management similar to those patients undergoing major abdominal surgery (see Chapter 24). The nursing care for patients receiving external radiation therapy can be found on p. 493; the care of patients receiving chemotherapy is found on p. 497. Patients who receive the recommended number of courses of chemotherapy and who are clinically free of disease usually undergo a "second-look" operation to determine if the disease has been completely eradicated.

Cancer of the vulva

Epidemiology and etiology

Cancer of the vulva is the fourth most common malignant tumor of the female genital tract; cervical, uterine, and ovarian cancers are more frequent. Cancer of the vulva accounts for 3% to 4% of all primary malignancies of the female genital tract.[50] It is most often a disease of elderly women; approximately 85% of the cases occur after the menopause, particularly after 65 years of age.

Little is known of the etiology of vulvar cancer. Parity, marital status, and racial differences have no etiologic relationship to this cancer.[11]

Pathophysiology

The majority of all cancers of the vulva are squamous in origin. Approximately 86% of reported vulvar cancers are of the squamous cell type.[51] The vulva is covered with a layer of skin; therefore any malignancy that appears elsewhere on the skin can occur in this area. The initial lesion often arises from an area of intraepithelial neoplasia, which can eventually form a firm nodule that can ulcerate. The diagnosis of vulvar cancer can only be made by biopsy and histologic examination of the tissue.

Prevention and early detection

Since the etiology of vulvar cancer is vague, its prevention is difficult. Cancer of the vulva is usually (60% of the time) diagnosed in the localized stage.[11] Any mass, pigmented lesion, ulcer, or hypertrophic process of the vulva should be suspected of being vulvar cancer, and therefore a biopsy should be done. The 5-year survival rate for vulvar cancer diagnosed and treated in an early stage approaches 90%. This emphasizes the importance of early diagnosis and treatment. Many women delay seeking medical attention for vulvar problems. There are many reasons for these delays—economic concerns, modesty, denial, and neglect. Occasionally, some patients are treated with topical creams or ointments without being initially examined.

Clinical picture

The lesion can develop anywhere on the vulva. Seventy percent of vulvar cancers arise on the labia. The disease is usually localized and well demarcated. The most common complaints are vulvar itching (pruritus) and burning. On inspection, an ulcer may be noted; abnormal pigmentation or lack thereof (leukoplakia) and asymmetry may also be detected.

Intervention

Surgery is the most common form of treatment employed in vulvar cancer. Over 80% of patients are treated primarily by surgery.[11] A radical vulvectomy is often the treatment of choice for invasive disease. This involves dissection of bilateral inguinal lymph nodes, excision of the mons pubis and terminal portion of the urethra and vagina, and excision of portions of the round ligments and saphenous veins. In some instances, much less radical surgery is performed. Patients with cancer of the vulva are often poor surgical risks because of concurrent physical disease.

The woman requiring a vulvectomy has some special nursing needs in addition to routine preoperative and postoperative care. Preoperatively, she is given enemas; and postoperatively, she is given a low-residue diet. Measures are taken to obviate the need for straining to defecate and help prevent contamination of the vulvar wound. A Foley catheter usually is employed to provide urinary drainage. When the catheter is removed, the patient may be unable to void because of difficulty in relaxing the perineum; sitz baths may help. If the inguinal nodes have been dissected, a heat lamp may be directed to the groin. After all the sutures are removed, sitz baths may be substituted for the heat lamp. Large amounts of tissues are removed from the vulva and the groin during the operation, and the sutures are usually taut, leading to severe discomfort. The patient will usually need analgesic medication at frequent intervals during the 2 or 3 weeks before sutures can be removed. Following an inguinal node dissection, pillows need to be arranged to prevent undue pulling on the taut inguinal sutures when the patient moves. If the patient is lying on her side, she will be more comfortable if her upper leg is supported by a pillow. If she is lying on her back, low Fowler's position puts less tension on the sutures. Wound breakdown is often a complication.

The vulvar wound is frequently left exposed, but if a dressing is used, it is held in place with a T binder. The wound is cleansed twice a day with solutions such as hydrogen peroxide, normal saline solution, benzalkonium chloride, or other antiseptic solutions. Follow-

ing this, a heat lamp is used to dry the area. The heat also improves local circulation, thus stimulating healing.

The wounds following a vulvectomy or an inguinal node dissection also heal slowly, and the woman may become quite discouraged. Diversional activities and socializing with other patients may help her to pass the time. Privacy should be ensured, and women should be encouraged to express their feelings concerning this disfiguring surgery. Some women feel that their femininity has been irreparably damaged or that the disfigurement may end their sexual life. Actually, by the time of hospital discharge the wounds are usually healed, and the convalescence will be similar to that following any surgical procedure. Sexual intercourse can usually be resumed after complete wound healing has been achieved (approximately 4 weeks).[167]

Gestational trophoblastic neoplasia

Epidemiology and etiology

Gestational trophoblastic neoplasia (GTN) is the term now commonly applied to hydatidiform mole, molar pregnancy, invasive mole, and choriocarcinoma.[51] GTN is recognized as one of the most curable gynecologic malignancies. This is mainly because this neoplasm is extremely sensitive to various chemotherapeutic agents. The reported incidence of GTN varies significantly in different regions of the world—in the Far East, it is about 1 in 120 pregnancies; in the United States, it is about 1 in 1200 pregnancies.

The etiology of GTN is not thoroughly understood. Nutrition and socioeconomic factors have been correlated; however, no conclusive evidence has been found to directly relate these factors to the incidence of the disease.

Pathophysiology

GTN is an abnormal pregnancy characterized by a degeneration, or an abnormal growth, of the trophoblastic tissue of the placenta. This anomaly of the placental tissue usually is associated with the absence of an intact fetus. One of the most important characteristics of GTN is the serum marker this tumor produces—human chorionic gonadotropin (HCG). The amount of this hormone present in the serum is directly related to the number of viable tumor cells.[51] Therefore even in the absence of clinical disease, levels of serum HCG can determine the presence of recurrence of disease in minute amounts.

Clinical picture

There is no known prevention for GTN, except to avoid conception. Early stages of GTN may be similar to normal pregnancy. As the disease progresses, most women will have uterine bleeding. Uterine growth more rapid than gestational age, anemia, nausea, and vomiting are also common symptoms of this disease process. The diagnosis of GTN is usually by pathologic examination of the products of conception. Before evaluation, amniography or ultrasonography can determine the presence of a molar pregnancy. Serum HCG titers are also routinely done before evacuation of the uterus.

Intervention

Suction curettage is the most common method employed for evacuation of a molar pregnancy. After a moderate amount of tissue has been removed, intravenous oxytocin (Pitocin) is begun. If the patient does not desire future pregnancies, a primary hysterectomy may be done as opposed to a suction dilation and curettage (D & C). After the removal of the molar tissue, weekly serum HCG titers are drawn. This test is continued weekly until 2 consecutive weeks of normal values are reached. This indicates a spontaneous remission and should occur in 80% of the patients.[51] The HCG titer should then be continued monthly for 6 months, then every month up to a year. After a full year without an elevated HCG titer, the woman may become pregnant. Pregnancy is not advised before this time, since HCG is also secreted during normal pregnancy. If a patient becomes pregnant before 1 year has elapsed, it would be difficult to determine whether this hormone was being secreted by a normal pregnancy or by remaining molar tissue. Therefore it is essential to have patients use a reliable method of birth control.

If the HCG titer plateaus, or rises, during the observation period, this indicates persistent or recurrent GTN, and the patient will be evaluated and started on chemotherapy. The pretreatment evaluation includes a physical examination and a chest x-ray film. Persistent disease can metastasize, and GTN usually disseminates widely by way of the bloodstream. The most common sites of metastasis are the lung, vagina, pelvis, brain, and liver.

Chemotherapy is employed in the treatment of recurrent or persistent GTN. Methotrexate intravenously or intramuscularly for 5 days every 14 days, or actinomycin D intravenously for 5 days every 14 days are the regimens most often used (p. 501). Patients receive their courses of chemotherapy until the HCG titer returns to normal. Most institutions give one or two additional courses after a normal HCG titer is reached. Women who do not respond to single agent chemotherapy may be given a multiple-drug regimen, surgery (e.g., hysterectomy or lobectomy), or radiation.

There is a great need to address the social and emotional impact of the disease process on both the patient and her family. CTN is a unique neoplastic process since it is an aberration of pregnancy. Therefore it can not only raise concerns about malignancy and death but also influence feelings about self-worth, self-image, future sexual relationships, and plans for future pregnancies. Patient and family teaching should include an understanding of the disease process compatible with the level of education and desire for knowledge, future pregnancies, change in body image, effect of chemotherapy (if given) on future children, chance of GTN developing with future pregnancy, and need for effective birth control.

PROBLEMS AFFECTING MEN

The female nurse must be particularly sensitive to the reactions and feelings of male patients who have diseases of the reproductive system. The patient may feel more comfortable discussing his problems with a male nurse or male physician. However, it is incumbent on all nurses to provide a comfortable environment in which these patients can verbalize their concerns and feelings. The nurse, male or female, must be alert to comments with subtle sexual connotations that reveal concerns the patient has regarding his sexuality and often must give permission to the patient to discuss them. The patient may "try out" his sexuality on a female nurse. Rejection from her may be perceived by the patient as less threatening than rejection by a loved one. The nurse should give the patient permission to verbalize his concerns. The nurse must also be aware of the implications of various diagnoses, diagnostic procedures, and therapeutic modalities on a man's sexuality in order to be able to discuss the impact of the disease on his life-style (Table 65-10).

TABLE 65-10. Problems affecting the male reproductive organs

Organ	Infections	Structural problems	Neoplasms
Penis	Phimosis Paraphimosis		Penile
Urethra	Nonspecific urethritis		
Scrotum		Hydrocele Varicocele Spermatocele	
Testes	Orchitis	Torsion of testicle	Seminomatous Nonseminomatous
Epididymis	Epididymitis		
Prostate	Prostatitis		Prostatic

Infectious processes

Etiology

Nonspecific pyogenic organisms as well as specific organisms such as the gonococci and tubercle bacilli may cause stubborn infections of the male reproductive system. Urethritis, prostatitis, seminal vesiculitis, and epididymitis are the most common infections. Infecting organisms may reach the genital organs by direct spread through the urethra, or they may be borne by blood or lymph.

Diagnostic tests

The site of the infection will influence treatment. The physician may obtain segmented bacteriologic localization cultures to make the determination. Four sterile culture tubes are used for collection. The patient must be well hydrated, have a full bladder, and be able to cooperate. The first 5 to 10 ml of a voiding is collected and labeled VB1 (voided bladder 1). After approximately 200 ml, a 5- to 10-ml midstream specimen (VB2) is collected. The patient is asked to stop voiding, then the prostate is massaged rectally until the secretions (EPS [expressed prostatic secretions]) are collected. The next 5 to 10 ml of urine (VB3) is collected and the bladder emptied. The specimens must be refrigerated and taken to the laboratory for culture within 4 hours. If VB2 is profusely infected, the other specimens probably will be also. Antibiotics are given to sterilize the urine (eradicate cystitis, if present), and the segmented bacteriologic localization cultures are repeated.

Prevention

Because urethral infection spreads so readily to the genital organs, men should not be catheterized unless it is absolutely necessary. Every means should be used to help them void normally. They are often allowed to stand to void even when they are to be on bed rest otherwise. Because of the length and curvature of the male urethra, some trauma to the urethral mucosa is likely to accompany catheterization or the passage of instruments such as a cystoscope. The distal part of the urethra is not sterile, and trauma makes the urethra susceptible to attack from the bacteria present. Fluids should be given liberally following passage of instruments through the urethra.

Nonspecific urethritis

Nonspecific (nongonococcal) urethritis is an inflammation of the urethra caused by such organisms as *Chlamydia trachomatis*, *Ureaplasma urealyticum*, *Trichomonas vaginalis*, *Candida albicans*, the herpes virus, or coliforms. The patient complains of urgency, frequency, and burning on urination, and there may be a purulent urethral discharge. Treatment of nonspecific urethritis is discussed in the section of this chapter dealing with sexually transmitted diseases (p. 1722).

Prostatitis

Clinical picture

The patient with prostatitis usually has acute symptoms of urinary obstruction. He suddenly has difficulty in voiding, perineal tenderness and pain, and elevation of temperature. There may be hematuria.

Rotating specimens (also called *serial urine specimens* or *racking*) are collected to determine the change in the character of the urine (Fig. 65-12). Three or more test tubes are used. Urine is voided into a container and mixed thoroughly; then a portion is poured into one of the test tubes and placed in a rack (hence its name). At the next voiding, the procedure is repeated; the first tube is moved toward the center of the rack, and the second specimen is placed at the end. The procedure is repeated a third time or until all test tubes and the rack are full. The first specimen is discarded at the subsequent voiding to make room for fresher specimens. Subtle changes in the degree of hematuria, cloudiness, sediment, and so on may be detected more easily without constant laboratory analysis, whereas if the specimens were discarded at the time of voiding, important signs might not be noticed.

Intervention

Treatment is usually conservative, consisting of antibiotics for 30 days to prevent chronic infection, chemotherapy, forcing fluids, physical rest, stool softeners to decrease rectal irritation of the prostate, and local application of heat by sitz baths or lower rectal irrigations. Before having a rectal irrigation, the patient should have a cleansing enema. Then, by means of a Y connector on the rectal tube, tap water is allowed to flow alternately in and out of the rectum. The use of 2 L of 115° F (46° C) water and the insertion of the tube only 7.5 to 10 cm (3 to 4 in.) into the rectum will concentrate heat in the area of the prostate gland.

Prompt treatment of prostatitis may prevent edema of the prostate with resultant obstruction of the urethra. If severe urinary retention occurs, suprapubic needle aspiration is safer than urethral straight or indwelling catheterization which would increase the risk of epidid-

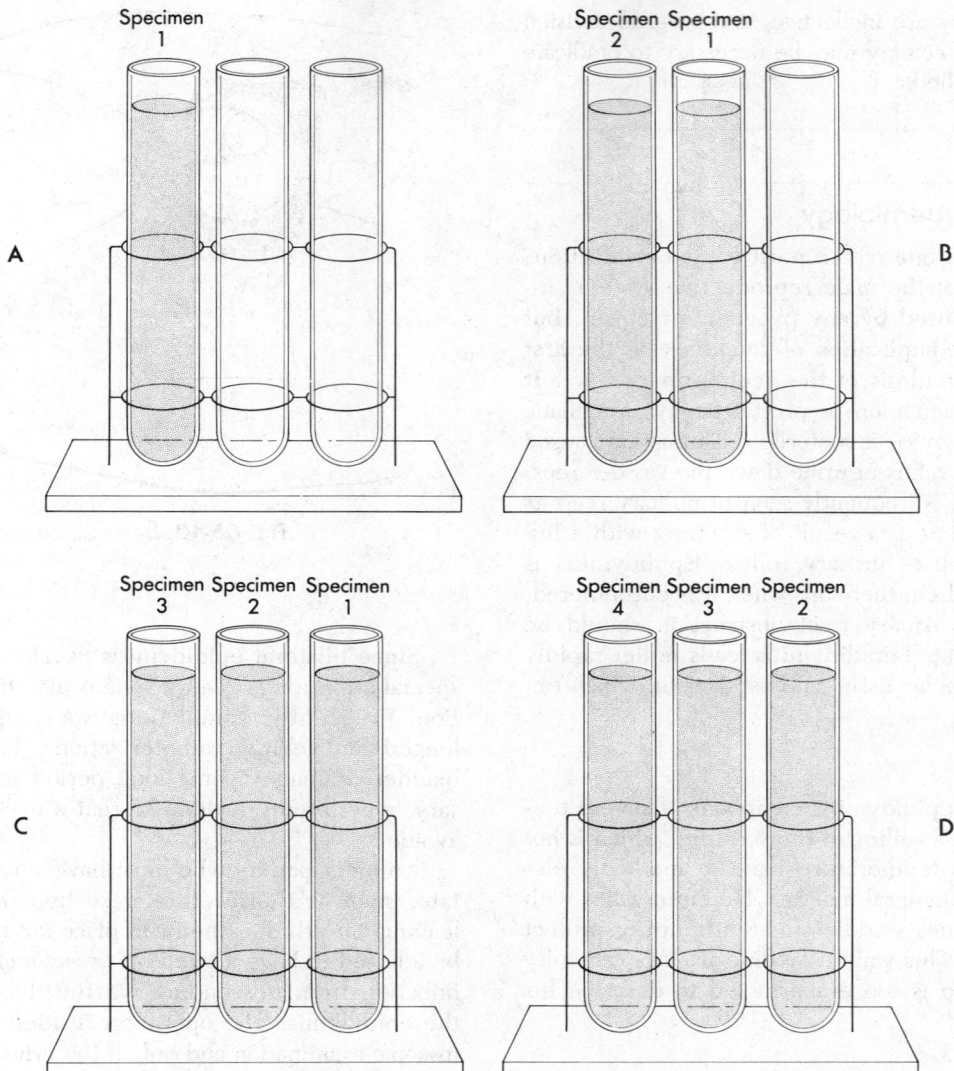

Specimen
1

A

Specimen Specimen
2   1

B

Specimen Specimen Specimen
3   2   1

C

Specimen Specimen Specimen
4   3   2

D

Fig. 65-12. Rotating specimens. **A,** Specimen is obtained and placed in rack. **B,** Specimen 1 is moved to right when specimen 2 is obtained. **C,** Specimens 1 and 2 are moved to right when specimen 3 is obtained. **D,** Specimens 2 and 3 are moved to right and specimen 1 is discarded when specimen 4 is obtained.

ymitis. Prostatic massage to eliminate residual pus pockets is contraindicated during the acute phase since it may cause bacteremia, although it may be used after the acute attack subsides. Because congestion of glandular secretions may also cause prostatitis, sexual intercourse is helpful in reducing the congestion.

Recurrent episodes of acute prostatitis may cause fibrotic tissue to form. The fibrosis causes a hardening of the prostate, which may initially be confused with carcinoma. In the granulomatous form of prostatitis, the enlargement may take 3 to 6 months to resolve.

Inadequate treatment of acute infection may result in chronic prostatitis. A subacute infection may also de-

velop into a chronic prostatitis that remains asymptomatic. Therefore prostatic secretions should be examined routinely to detect infection and to prevent complications such as acute or chronic cystitis, pyelonephritis, or epididymitis. It is believed that inflammation permits entry of antibiotics that normally do not diffuse into the prostatic fluid. Although they may be used during an acute infection, they are ineffective in a chronic condition. Trimethoprim is the only antibiotic that diffuses into the prostatic fluid and is therefore the drug of choice in chronic prostatitis. Occasionally, *prostatic abscesses* complicate the clinical course and may have to be drained surgically. If prostatic calculi are present, they may be infected. Antibiotics are ineffective, and surgical excision is required. Prostatectomy may be necessary to eradicate the infection (p. 1560).

Epididymitis

Etiology and epidemiology

Epididymitis is one of the most common infections or inflammations of the male reproductive system. Infection may be caused by any pyogenic organism, but it is frequently a complication of gonorrhea or the first indication of tuberculosis of the genitourinary tract. It may follow instrumentation or prostatectomy. Traumatic or chemical epididymitis is a sterile inflammation caused by direct injury or reflux of urine down the vas deferens. The chemical form is frequently seen in military recruits during basic training as a result of straining with a full bladder, which causes urinary reflux. Epididymitis is uncommon in children; therefore when it is encountered, the possibility of urinary tract obstruction should be considered. Untreated epididymitis leads rather rapidly to necrosis of testicular tissue and septicemia, which can be fatal.

Clinical picture

The man with epididymitis complains of severe tenderness, pain, and swelling of the scrotum, which is hot to the touch. His temperature may be markedly elevated, and he has general malaise. He often walks with a characteristic "duck waddle" in an attempt to protect the affected part. This walk may first disclose difficulty in the patient who is too embarrassed to describe his trouble.

Intervention

The patient with epididymitis is usually put to bed and the scrotum elevated either on towel rolls or with adhesive strapping known as a Bellevue bridge (Fig. 65-13). Ice is used to help reduce the swelling and to relieve the pain and discomfort. Heat is usually contraindicated because the normal temperature of the scrotal contents is below normal body temperature, and excessive exposure to heat may cause destruction of sperm cells. If an ice cap is used, it should be placed under the scrotum and should be removed for short intervals every hour to prevent ice burns. A plastic glove may also be filled with ice. With the palm of the glove placed under the scrotum, the fingers provide cold to the sides. Antibiotic therapy is given. Narcotic analgesics, antiinflammatory agents, and local anesthetics may also be used. Surgical excision (epididymectomy) may be required for severe or recurrent infection. If the testis is involved, an orchiectomy may be performed. The patient should drink at least 3 L of fluid daily. When the patient is pain free, he is allowed out of bed, at which time he should wear a scrotal support.

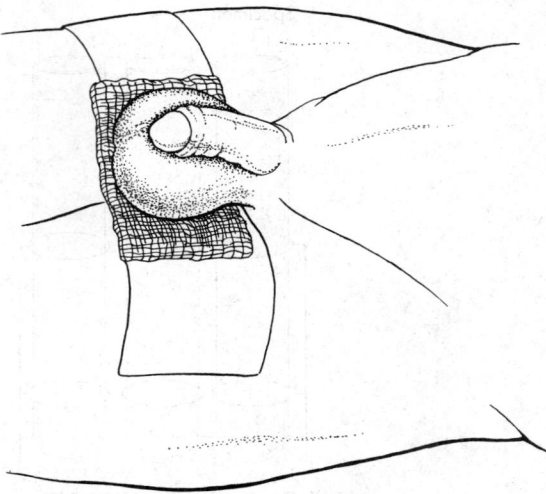

Fig. 65-13. Bellevue bridge.

Since bilateral epididymitis usually causes sterility, special attention is given to the prevention of this infection. Frequently, epididymitis is a complication of prolonged indwelling catheterization. Therefore, when bladder drainage over a long period of time is necessary, a cystotomy is done so that a urethral catheter is avoided.

An older patient who must have surgery of the prostate, such as transurethral resection that will require leaving a urethral catheter in place for a long time, may be advised to have a *bilateral vasectomy* to prevent any infection from descending via the ductus deferens to the epididymis. The operation is done before any cystoscopic examination and only if the urine is sterile. Since bilateral vasectomy causes sterility, permission to perform the surgery must be granted by the patient. The vasectomies are done through two very small incisions in the scrotum or in the groins. Local anesthesia is used. Postoperatively, the patient should still be watched for symptoms of epididymitis, since the organisms may have invaded the epididymis before the vasectomy.

Vasovasostomies are being done in an attempt to restore fertility in men who have had vasectomies. This currently results in a 90% to 96% sperm count and a 45% to 56% pregnancy rate. The operation takes 2½ hours, so although it could be done in a physician's office, it is usually performed in the hospital.[127]

Phimosis

Phimosis is condition in which the opening of the prepuce or foreskin is unable to be retracted behind the glans (Fig. 65-14, A). It may be congenital or acquired as a result of inflammation or infection. Constriction may interfere with adequate hygiene. There may be a buildup

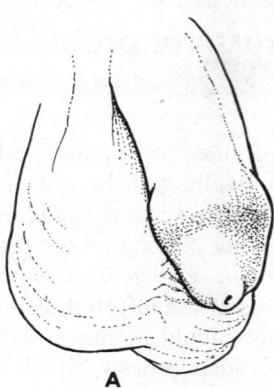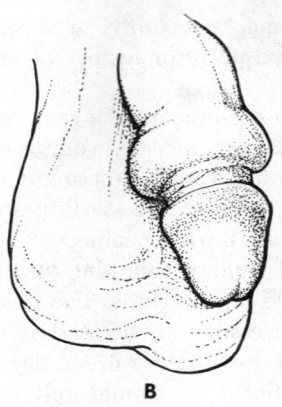

Fig. 65-14. A, Phimosis. Note pinpoint opening of foreskin. **B,** Paraphimosis. Note foreskin is retracted but has become constricting band around penis.

of smegma, urine may be trapped in the preputial sac, and calculi may form, irritating the glans and predisposing to infection. Chronic irritation may be a cause of penile carcinoma. Healing is by fibrosis, which causes the acquired phimosis. If the constriction is severe enough, it causes a urinary obstruction with straining and painful urination. This condition may be fatal in infants. Treatment for mild irritation and infection is hot soaks and antibiotics. If severe, a dorsal slit or two lateral slits of the prepuce may be necessary. Circumcision, the surgical excision of the prepuce, should be performed when the tissue has returned to normal.

Treatment of congenital phimosis is stretching of the prepuce and repeated retraction behind the glans. If this does not permit adequate retraction, circumcision is the preferred treatment.

Paraphimosis

Paraphimosis is a condition in which the prepuce is retracted over the glans and forms a constriction that is sometimes impossible to reduce as edema develops in the glans (Fig. 65-14, *B*). Cool compresses are applied to the penis, and it is elevated for a short time before a gentle attempt is made to reduce the prepuce. If this measure fails, emergency surgery must be done. A dorsal slit is made in the prepuce to prevent necrosis of the glans caused by impairment of its blood supply.

Circumcision is usually done later to prevent recurrences. If the operation is performed a few days after birth, no general anesthetic is needed. Older patients, even if they need anesthesia, are not hospitalized for more than a few hours for this operation. The wound is covered with gauze generously impregnated with petrolatum. Bleeding usually is controlled by applying a pressure dressing that may be bulky and that sometimes must be removed before the patient can void. It should be removed cautiously and replaced after void-

ing with a petrolatum dressing. If the patient goes home on the same day as the surgery (or after the surgery), he, or his mother if the patient is a child, is taught to change the dressing at each voiding for a few days and to try to avoid fecal contamination of the area. An antibiotic ointment may be prescribed for the older child or adult. Instruction is also given to be alert for signs of bleeding. If severe bleeding occurs, a firm dressing should be applied to the penis and the patient should be taken at once to the physician's office or the hospital emergency room. Very occasionally, if bleeding persists, it is necessary to resuture the wound. An estrogen preparation may be prescribed for adult patients for several days after surgery to prevent painful penile erections.

Orchitis

An inflammation or infection of the testicle is known as orchitis. It may be caused by pyogenic bacteria, gonnococci, or tubercle bacilli, or it may follow any septicemia. It rarely involves only the testis; usually the epididymis is also involved (epididymoorchitis). In children, torsion may be misdiagnosed as orchitis. When mumps are contracted after puberty, approximately 18% of the cases are complicated by orchitis with symptom development 4 to 6 days after parotitis. If the case is mild, there may be no symptoms before the onset of orchitis. The testis atrophies to some degree 30% to 50% of the time, but it does not appear to be related to the severity of the orchitis. If the orchitis is bilateral, it usually causes sterility. Any postpubertal boy or man who is exposed to mumps usually is given gamma globulin immediately unless he has already had the disease. If there is any doubt, globulin usually is given. Although it may not prevent mumps, the disease is likely to be less severe with less likelihood of complications. Impotence and sterility are now rare sequelae. Traumatic orchitis may follow trauma, vasectomy, or surgical manipulation. There may be no prior history of inflammation or disease.

The signs and symptoms of orchitis are the same as those of epididymitis; there is also nausea, vomiting, and pain radiating to the inguinal canal. Treatment is the same for both conditions. Atrophy and sterility are caused by the fibrosis that occurs during healing.

Hydrocele (a collection of fluid within the tunica vaginalis) is frequently associated with orchitis. The fluid may be aspirated to reduce pressure on the testis. If the hydrocele is surgically tapped within the first 2 days, it may decrease the atrophy, but a tap should only be done in cases where edema is persistent. Although effectiveness is questionable, stilbestrol (which inhibits normal testicular function), cortisone, and antibiotics may be given to reduce the severity of the disease. Abscesses of the testis require orchiectomy. A testicular prosthesis composed of Silastic gel is available for cosmetic purposes.[73] Possible complications of the prosthesis include infection and rejection. Unilateral orchiectomy may result in impotence and subfertility. Sexual counseling might be indicated.

Lesions of the external genitalia

Any lesion of the external genitalia requires medical attention, and no ulcer of the genitalia should be treated by the patient before seeing a physician lest the diagnosis be obscured. Although lesions are present in a wide variety of conditions, they should always be considered infectious until proved otherwise, since each of the sexually transmitted diseases, with the exception of gonorrhea, produces a genital lesion or ulceration. These lesions will be discussed in the section that deals with the sexually transmitted diseases.

Outcome criteria for the person with infection or inflammation of the male reproductive organs

The person or significant others can:
1. Explain the source and factors contributing to the infection.
2. State the name, dose, reasons for drug therapy, and possible side effects.
3. Explain the need for compliance and continuation of drug therapy.
4. State implications for sexual activity during acute and chronic conditions.
5. State significance and effect of condition on reproductive function.
6. State signs and symptoms for seeking immediate health care.

Structural problems

Immediate medical attention should be sought for any swelling of the scrotum or the testes within it. Any acute swelling of sudden onset must be considered twisting (torsion) of the testicles until proved otherwise. Torsion, as discussed below, leads to ischemia and necrosis of the affected testicle. Therefore scrotal enlargement should be diagnosed, not treated symptomatically with suspensories, which give relief and encourage procrastination about seeking appropriate medical care.

Hydrocele

Hydrocele, a common condition, is a benign, painless collection of clear, amber fluid within the tunica vaginalis that leads to swelling of the scrotum. It occurs fairly often in infant boys as well as in adult men. The cause of hydrocele is usually unknown, but it may be associated with trauma, acute nonspecific or tuberculous epididymitis, or orchitis. Hydrocele transilluminates when examined in a darkened room using a fiberoptic light.

If uncomplicated by other scrotal abnormalities, hydrocele is treated by aspirating the fluid and injecting a sclerosing drug such as urea hydrochloride into the scrotal sac. There is no pain, and only a Bandaid is required. Thirty percent of hydroceles recur and thus require repeated injections. Excision of the tunica vaginalis (hydrocelectomy) produces a permanent resolution. Postoperatively, a pressure dressing is applied on the scrotum, which is elevated. The patient should be observed carefully for any symptoms of hemorrhage. Bleeding may not be external. The patient needs a scrotal support when he is out of bed and may still require one after he is discharged from the hospital. He should have two scrotal suspensories, since they should be washed each day. Immediately after surgery or following an infection, most patients require an extra large suspensory or perhaps an athletic support (jockstrap).

Spermatocele

A spermatocele is a nontender cystic mass attached to the epididymis and containing a milky fluid and sperm. Since it also transilluminates, it should be distinguished from a hydrocele by the color of the fluid on aspiration. Because the lesion is benign and there are usually few symptoms, excision is rarely necessary. Occasionally, the patient is uncomfortable because of the size or heaviness of the cyst. Since excision of the cyst may affect fertility, if the patient desires children, he is usually advised to wear a scrotal support to prevent undue discomfort until after he has a family. Large masses may then be excised.

Varicocele

Varicocele is a dilation of the spermatic vein and is commonly seen on the left side only, probably because the left spermatic vein is much longer than the right. The venous valves are incompetent resulting in pooling of blood. A varicocele on the right side only is suggestive of an abdominal tumor. One third of men with subfertility or infertility have varicoceles. The decreased blood flow is thought to cause a rise in intrascrotal temperature, which interferes with spermatogenesis. The ipsilateral testes may be atrophied. Ligation of the spermatic vein has been shown to improve semen quality with a pregnancy rate of 17% to 62%. Otherwise, unless severe, a scrotal support is usually all that is necessary to relieve any dragging sensation.

Torsion of the testes

Etiology and pathophysiology

Torsion of the testes or kinking of the spermatic artery causes a sudden onset of severe pain, tenderness, and swelling of the testes. The affected testis will be elevated. It often follows activity that puts a sudden pull on the cremasteric muscle such as may occur from jumping into cold water, blunt trauma during sporting events, or riding a bicycle. In severe trauma, rupture of the testis is the expected finding and torsion of the testis is often not considered, leading to misdiagnosis and inappropriate treatment. It may also occur spontaneously. In 40% of the cases, the individual is awakened at night by pain. Although torsion may occur at any age including infancy, the incidence is highest between 12 and 18 years of age. As the testis becomes larger and heavier, the steadying action and support of the cremasteric muscle decrease and thus predispose the individual to torsion.

Clinical picture

Torsion interrupts the blood supply leading to ischemia and severe pain that is not relieved and may be aggravated by elevation. Absence of pain indicates infarction and necrosis. Gangrene may be a serious sequela. The patient experiences nausea and vomiting but is afebrile even if the testis is gangrenous. The scrotum may be red and swollen and look infected, but there are no urinary symptoms, that is, the urinalysis is normal as are blood tests. An orchiogram, or testicular scan, which is performed in the nuclear medicine department, qual-

itatively measures the blood flow to the testis and differentiates between torsion and acute epididymitis.[183] If an orchiogram cannot be performed, surgical exploration is necessary.

Intervention

Detorsion may be attempted manually. If detorsion is unsuccessful, surgical intervention is imperative within 6 to 12 hours to maintain viability of the testis. Even so, the testis may atrophy. Unless the testis is gangrenous, it is not excised since it may still produce hormones, even if spermatogenesis is destroyed. The testis is fixed surgically to the scrotal wall (orchiopexy). The contralateral testis is usually fixed prophylactically at the same time. A small Penrose drain may be placed in the scrotum. Ice bags to reduce swelling and elevation of the scrotum may be ordered. Observation for signs of testicular necrosis and fever is continued. Body image disturbances may include fears of castration, loss of masculinity, sterility, and impotence. The possibility of these fears being justified depends on the degree of insult to the testis and the functioning of the remaining testicle.

Following scrotal surgery, the patient should be instructed to limit stair climbing to two flights and not to lift or carry heavy objects for 4 weeks. He is to refrain from sexual activity for 6 weeks unless otherwise instructed by his physician. The use of a scrotal support for at least 3 weeks is recommended to control edema. Sitz baths may help relieve any discomfort.

Outcome criteria for the man with a structural problem of the reproductive system

The person or significant others can:
1. State the sexual and reproductive implications of the condition.
2. State management of the condition when appropriate.
3. State signs and symptoms for seeking health care.
4. Seek health care within an appropriate time frame.

Neoplasms of the male reproductive tract

Cancer of the testes

Epidemiology

Cancer of the testes is the second most common malignancy in men between the ages of 25 and 34 and is the second most common cause of death from cancer in this age group. On the whole, testicular neoplasms are relatively rare, affecting only two to three men per 100,000, but the frequency is increasing. Testicular cancer will most often be found in infancy, between 20 and 40 years of age, and over the age of 60. If testicular cancer is untreated, death occurs in 2 to 3 years. If it is detected and treated early, there is a 90% to 100% chance of cure.

Etiology and pathophysiology

The causes of testicular cancer are still unknown. Acquired causes being investigated are chemical carcinogens, trauma, and orchitis. Environmental factors are also being considered since there is a greater incidence of testicular cancer in rural than in urban areas. Congenital causes implicated are familial predisposition, gonadal dysgenesis (developmental abnormality), and cryptorchidism.

Cryptorchidism is the failure of the testis to descend at birth. Most testes will descend within the first year. The incidence of true cryptorchidism (the undescended testes after 1 year of age) is 0.4%. However, the probability of developing testicular cancer is 30 to 50 times greater than in the normally descended testis. It may not be the failure to descend but a developmental abnormality in the testis that is the predisposing factor. Orchiopexy (a surgical procedure to bring the testis into the scrotum) is being recommended between the ages of 1 and 2 years. Hormonal therapy may also be used to cause the testes to descend. In some cases descent is spontaneous. The effect of early treatment on the probability of cancer is not known at this time. Although the likelihood of cancer in the testis that descends after the age of 5 or 6 years is comparable to the likelihood of cancer in the testis that has always been outside the scrotum, regular examination of the descended testis does increase the chance of early cancer detection: the site of the testis makes no difference in the risk of developing cancer. Patients with current cryptorchidism or a history of cryptorchidism should be observed yearly, and then after a 20-year latency period when testicular cancer is prone to develop, they should be examined every 6 months. Orchiectomy instead of orchiopexy is recommended in adults with cryptorchidism as a prophylaxis against cancer.

Prevention

Regular *testicular self-examination* (TSE) is recommended to detect cancer in its early stages when it is most likely to be localized and most curable. The best time to perform TSE is after a bath or shower when the scrotum is warm and most relaxed. Each testis is examined by holding and feeling it between the thumb and fingers of both hands (Fig. 65-15). The testis should feel smooth, egg shaped, and firm to the touch, without any lumps. The epididymis is found behind the testis

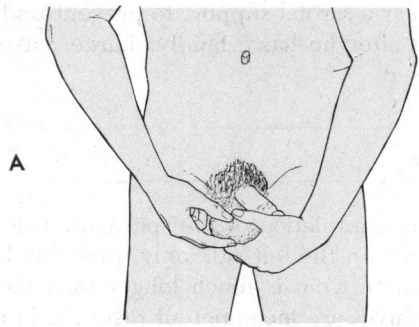

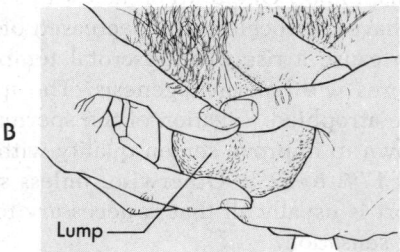

Fig. 65-15. Testicular self-examination. **A,** Grasp testis with both hands; palpate gently between thumb and fingers. **B,** Abnormal lumps or irregularities are reported to physician. (Adapted from Fred Hutchinson Cancer Research Center, Cancer Control Program: Self breast and testicular exam [grant no. 2 R18-CA 16404], Seattle 1980, Cancer Control Program.)

and feels like a soft tube. By performing TSE routinely, each man can get to know what is normal for him and more readily identify any lumps or abnormalities. Anything that is not normal for that individual should be examined by a physician. Nine out of ten testicular cancers are detected by the patient or his sexual partner. Nurses should include knowledge about testicular cancer in assessment of all adolescent and adult male patients and include TSE in patient teaching.

Clinical picture

Frequently, a lump or swelling of the testis will be noted after bathing or following trauma, although trauma is not usually the cause. Other symptoms include a heaviness or dragging sensation in the scrotum, a dull ache in the lower abdomen or inguinal area, and occasionally pain. A small or atrophied testis may grow to normal size. Pride (or embarrassment) may prevent the individual from seeking medical advice.

Testicular neoplasms are divided into two classifications: germinal and nongerminal. Germinal cancers make up 90% to 95% of all testicular neoplasms and are further divided into two groups: seminomatous (40%) and nonseminomatous (60%) tumors. This division is crucial for diagnosis and treatment. Diagnostic workup includes chest x-ray films, computed tomograms, an intravenous pyelogram, skeletal surveys in the presence

STAGING OF TESTICULAR NEOPLASIA

Stage I   No metastasis

Stage II   Metastasis to retroperitoneal lymph nodes or other subdiaphragmatic areas

Stage III Metastasis to mediastinal and supraclavicular nodes or other areas above diaphragm

of an elevated alkaline phosphatase, and lymphangiography. Lymphangiography decreases pulmonary function by 10% because of oil embolism; therefore general anesthesia is contraindicated for 48 hours after the procedure. *Biopsy of the testis is contraindicated* because of the highly metastatic character of testicular carcinoma. Laboratory tests include evaluation of alphafetoprotein (AFP), human chorionic gonadotropin (HCG), carcinoembryonic antigen (CEA), luteinizing hormone (LH), and serum and urine estrogen levels. AFP, HCG, CEA, and LH are considered *markers* that indicate the presence of nonseminomatous disease. The level of one or more may be elevated in any combination. There is no one combination of elevated and normal markers to specifically indicate testicular neoplasm. These are monitored throughout the course of therapy to determine appropriate therapeutic regimens.

Intervention

In any suspected testicular cancer, the testis is always removed immediately. *Orchiectomy* consists of en bloc excision of the spermatic cord, the contents of the inguinal canal, and the testis with the tunicae attached. The adjacent area is explored for metastases. The specimens are then examined to determine the type of cancer. Staging of the disease (see box above), as well as pathologic findings, determines the course of treatment.

Seminoma is highly responsive to radiation therapy. For stage I seminoma, irradiation is started to the retroperitoneal nodes. In stage II, irradiation of the mediastinal and supraclavicular nodes is indicated. Chemotherapy is added for stage III. If markers are elevated after irradiation, nonseminomatous involvement must be suspected. Seminoma can metastasize in a different type of cancer. It is possible to develop a second primary lesion in the remaining testis. The prognosis in that case is the same as if it were the first lesion.

Nonseminomatous neoplasms are radioresistant. Therefore retroperitoneal lymphadenectomy or radical node dissection is performed immediately. If the nodes are free of metastases, careful follow-up every 2 months is mandatory. Chemotherapy is given for clinical, radio-

logic, or tumor marker evidence of metastasis. If the lymph nodes dissection is positive, the patient has stage II disease. Cyclic combination chemotherapy is started for 2 years with adjuvant surgery. If in either stage I or II there is a history of scrotal surgery (i.e., orchiopexy), ipsilateral pelvic lymphadenectomy and hemiscrotectomy are indicated. In stage III, intensive cyclic combination chemotherapy is instituted for 10 to 12 months, followed by surgical excision of all metastatic sites. Mithramycin, a cytotoxic agent, may greatly improve the survival rate for persons with advanced nonseminomatous tumors.

Following a *radical node dissection,* there is danger of hemorrhage. Active movement may be contraindicated, since nodes may have been resected from around many large abdominal vessels, but gentle passive turning and leg and arm movement are essential to prevent postoperative pneumonia and thrombosis. Deep breathing should be encouraged at hourly intervals. A turning sheet and a chest support are usually helpful. The patient is extremely uncomfortable and needs frequent and large doses of narcotics and sedative drugs.

Nongerminal testicular tumors are rare. Treatment consists of various combinations of the four modes of treatment (orchiectomy, radiation, lymphadenectomy, and chemotherapy) used in germinal neoplasms depending on the specific type.

Prognosis

Seminoma has the best prognosis of any of the germinal neoplasms. Five-year survival rates are as follows: for stage I, 95% to 100%; for stage II, 70% to 90%; for stage III, 50% to 60%. For nonseminomatous neoplasms, 5-year survival rates are as follows: for stage I 90%; for stage II, 60% to 85%; and for stage III, 30% to 40%.[86]

Complications of treatment

Radiation sickness and adverse reactions to chemotherapeutic agents have been addressed elsewhere (see Chapter 25). Although the normal testis is shielded during external radiation, it does receive radiation scattered from the abdomen and thighs. A period of 70 days is required to determine if spermatogenesis has been affected. Spermatogenesis may be decreased for 7 months to 5 years or more. Although genetic defects are possible following irradiation, there is currently no evidence to cause serious concern. Genetic counseling may be helpful for those couples desiring children. Orchiectomy alone does not result in impotence if the contralateral testis is normal. The remaining testis undergoes hyperplasia, producing sufficient testosterone to maintain sexual function, drive, and characteristics. Retroperitoneal lymphadenectomy results in decreased ejaculation in 90% of the patients as a result of disruption of the sympathetic nervous system pathways. Ejaculation is independent of other sexual functions; orgasm is still possible. The patient's perception of sexuality must be considered as well as his physiologic capabilities.

Cancer of the prostate gland

Epidemiology, etiology, and pathophysiology

The prostate gland is the second most common site of cancer among men, with 17% of all cancers in men occurring here; it is responsible for 10% of all deaths from cancer in men.[1] Prostatic cancer rarely occurs before the age of 50, incidence increases with age, and there is an increased familial risk. Its incidence has increased by more than 20% since 1940.[171] The increased incidence may reflect greater attention to the need for early diagnosis, improved diagnostic methods, and the fact that men are better informed about cancer than in the past. There is a geographic distribution of prostatic cancer, so environmental factors may be causative. It may be caused by an oncogenic virus. Industrial exposure to cadmium has been implicated.

No classification system for the stages of prostatic cancer has been accepted. However, the information in the box below represents a sampling of classification systems most often used.[47]

Cancer of the prostate may start as a discrete, localized, hard nodule, often in areas of senile atrophy. Although it can start anywhere and may be multifocal in origin, it usually arises in the peripheral lobes causing a palpable nodule before progressing to an advanced, inoperable, and incurable stage. For this reason, there is agreement that all men near and over the age of 50 should have an annual rectal examination.

The younger the patient with prostatic cancer, the more lethal the disease. Sixty-nine percent of men under 50 years of age die within 3 years. With radiation therapy,

30% under the age of 60 survive 10 years compared with 84% of those over 60 years of age.[86] Overall, 5-year survival rates are 70% for stages I and II, 61% for stage III, and 20% for stage IV.[1]

Clinical picture

Cancer of the prostate gland is most often diagnosed when the man seeks medical advice because of symptoms of urethral obstruction or because of sciatica (low back, hip, and leg pain). The pain is caused by metastasis of the cancer to the bones via the blood system. The pelvis, lumbar spine, and femur are the most common sites. This form of cancer frequently occurs concurrently with benign prostatic hypertrophy (p. 1559). The relationship between the two is controversial. Benign prostatic hypertrophy causes urethral obstruction. However, the cancer itself may be so far advanced as to cause obstruction.

Most cancers of the prostate gland are adjacent to the rectal wall and can be detected by rectal examination before symptoms appear. Diagnosis is confirmed by biopsy. If the transrectal route is used, no bowel preparation is required. Prophylactic antibiotics are used only for high-risk patients. Vital signs should be monitored for possible hemorrhage because of the high vascularity of the gland. Bleeding may be from the urethra or the bladder and may be internal. Rotating urine specimens (p. 1710) should be utilized to monitor the amount of hematuria. Bacteremia is usually transient following transrectal biopsy[55]; however, the patient should be observed for fever and septicemia. Other complications include acute urinary retention, rectal bleeding, and epididymoorchitis. If the biopsy is done on an outpatient basis, the patient should be informed of possible complications and instructed to notify his physician if any symptoms are persistent or severe. During biopsy, especially needle biopsy, or during suprapubic or retropubic prostatectomy, if seminal vesicle tissue is obtained, its histologic similarity to prostatic adenocarcinoma may result in misdiagnosis.[177]

Intervention

In patients in whom a diagnosis is made before local extension of the cancer or distant metastasis, a radical resection of the prostate gland usually is curative. The entire prostate gland, including the capsule and the adjacent tissue, is removed. The remaining urethra is then anastomosed to the bladder neck.

Since the internal and external sphincters of the bladder lie in close approximation to the prostate gland, it is not unusual for the patient to have urinary incontinence following this type of surgery. The perineal approach is most used, but the procedure may be accomplished by the retropubic route (Fig. 62-5, *B* and *C*).

Preoperative care. If the patient is to have a perineal approach in surgery, he is given a bowel preparation,

---

STAGING OF PROSTATIC NEOPLASIA

Stage I	Microscopic lesions found in the prostate removed because of benign hypertrophy
Stage II	Nodules confined to the prostate gland; no capsular adherence or urethral involvement; normal serum acid phosphatase level
Stage III	Carcinoma involving prostatic capsule, seminal vesicles, urethra, bladder, and pelvic lymph nodes, or a malignant tumor of a lesser extent with an elevated serum acid phosphatase level
Stage IV	Findings as in stage III plus evidence of extrapelvic lesions or osseous involvement

which includes enemas, cathartics, and phthalylsulfathiazole (Sulfathalidine) or neomycin preoperatively and only clear fluids the day before surgery to prevent fecal contamination of the operative site. Postoperatively, when food is permitted, a low-residue diet may be given until wound healing is well advanced. Camphorated tincture of opium may be prescribed to inhibit bowel action. If the retropubic approach is used, the preoperative care is similar to that of any patient having major surgery.

Postoperative care. Regardless of the surgical approach, the patient returns from surgery with a urethral catheter inserted. A large amount of urinary drainage on the dressing for a number of hours is not unusual. This can be managed by use of an ostomy bag around the dressing. Urinary drainage should decrease rapidly, however. There should not be the amount of bleeding that follows other prostatic surgery. Since the catheter is not being used for hemostasis, the patient usually has little bladder spasm. The catheter is used both for urinary drainage and as a splint for the urethral anastomosis; therefore care should be taken that it does not become dislodged or blocked. Clinically, the risk of blockage from clots is greatest during the first hour. The catheter may be irrigated intermittently or continuously as ordered by the physician. The catheter is usually left in the bladder for 2 or 3 weeks.

The care of the perineal wound is the same as that following a perineal biopsy except that healing is usually slower. If there has been a retropubic surgical approach, the wound and possible wound complications are the same as for a simple retropubic prostatectomy (p. 1561).

Since perineal surgery causes relaxation of the perineal musculature, the patient may suddenly have fecal incontinence. It is disturbing to the patient and sometimes can be avoided by starting perineal exercises (p. 1544) within a day or two after surgery. Control of the rectal sphincter usually returns readily. Perineal exercises should be continued even after rectal sphincter control returns, since they also strengthen the bladder sphincters and, unless the bladder sphincters have been permanently damaged, the patient will retain urinary control more readily on removal of the catheter.

The patient with cancer of the prostate gland is often very depressed after radical prostatectomy because he suddenly realizes the implications of being impotent and perhaps permanently incontinent. He usually has been told by the physician before the operation that these consequences are possible, but he may not have fully comprehended their meaning. A penile prosthesis may be considered to treat the impotence (erectile dysfunction) (p. 1765). He needs to be encouraged, and provisions should be made to keep him dry so that he will feel able to be up and to socialize with others without fear of having obvious incontinence (see p. 1541 for

ways to manage incontinence). Until the physician has ascertained that return of urinary sphincter control is unlikely, a method that gives only partial protection, such as the use of a bathing cap, is preferable since the patient is more likely to attempt to regain voluntary control.

Prostatic prosthesis. If voluntary urinary control has not been regained within 6 months to a year, a prostatic prosthesis is available to control urinary incontinence.[33,102] This puts pressure on the urethra, and if the pressure is too great, urethral erosion can occur. This will interfere with other forms of incontinence control, such as, artificial sphincters. Therefore intraurethral pressure is measured during surgery. The prosthesis consists of a silicone gel–filled sac placed at the base of the penis. Four tapes of polypropylene mesh are stapled to the pelvic rami or sutured to the periosteum to secure the prosthesis in place (Fig. 65-16). If the pressure decreases within the prosthesis, injections may be used to increase it. There is a 60% success rate. Although it is better for the prosthesis to be applied loosely rather than too tight, if it is too loose it will fail. It may be repositioned surgically.

Patients who have undergone radiation therapy have a greater risk of osteomyelitis as well as wound complications; therefore they are not candidates for prostatic prosthesis. The prerequisite for surgery is a sterile urine culture. Preoperative antibiotics are given prophylactically and continued for 7 days postoperatively. An indwelling catheter is inserted during surgery and left for 48 hours. If difficulty with voiding persists, the patient may be discharged with the indwelling catheter or taught

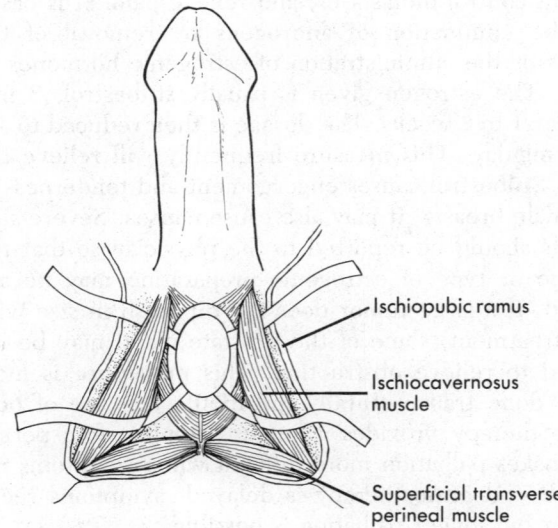

Fig. 65-16. Placement of silicone gel prostatic prosthesis. Tapes are stapled to pubic rami or sutured to periosteum. (Adapted from Kauffman, J.J.: Urol. Clin. North Am. **5**:395, 1978.)

intermittent self-catheterization (p. 1528). Residual urine of 50 to 100 ml may persist for a few weeks. A urinary antiseptic is given after the initial course of antibiotics and continued until the patient is voiding well.

Radiation therapy. Irradiation is an alternate therapy for prostatic cancer. It may be delivered by external beam or by implant. The testes are shielded during external radiation. [125]Iodine retropubic prostatic implantation may be used initially or after failure of external radiation therapy. The mortality and morbidity of internal irradiation when coupled with lymphadenectomy are less than for radical prostatectomy. Complications of [125]iodine implantation include blood loss from multiple needle punctures during implantation, deep vein thrombosis, pulmonary emboli, hematomas, and abscesses. Potency is retained. There is a greater risk of complications if radioactive implants are used after external beam radiation.[38] Risk of incontinence and serious rectal complications such as rectourethral fistulas increases with the size of the gland and the intensity of the implant seed.

Hormone therapy. When cancer of the prostate gland is inoperable, or when signs of metastasis occur following surgery, medical treatment is given. Relief from conservative treatment is quite dramatic in many patients and may last for 10 years or more in some instances. Usually, the response is quite good for about 1 year and then the patient's condition begins to deteriorate. Cytotoxic drugs are not indicated in prostatic cancer because they are most effective against rapidly proliferating cells whereas prostatic cancer has a slow growth rate. Also, the elderly tolerate the side effects of these drugs poorly.

Huggins' treatment may be used for inoperable cancer of the prostate gland to cause atrophy of the local lesion, control metastases, and relieve pain. It is based on the elimination of androgens by removal of the testes or the administration of estrogenic hormones or both. The estrogen given is usually stilbestrol, 3 mg/day for 1 to 2 weeks. The dosage is then reduced to 1.5 to 3 mg/day. This measure frequently will relieve the pain. Stilbestrol causes engorgement and tenderness of the male breasts. It may also cause nausea. Severe side effects should be reported to the physician so that the dosage or type of estrogenic preparation may be adjusted. If a large tumor does not diminish in size with this treatment, some of the prostate gland may be resected to relieve obstruction. This procedure is most often done transurethrally (p. 1560). The use of hormone therapy provides a longer symptom-free period but makes palliation more difficult when symptoms recur. If endocrine therapy is delayed, symptoms recur earlier but longer palliation is possible.

When symptoms begin to recur, or if the patient is very uncomfortable and needs immediate relief when the diagnosis of cancer is first made, a bilateral orchiectomy (castration) may be done. This operative procedure is technically minor and is often done under local anesthesia, but it may cause the patient considerable psychologic distress. The man's permission for sterilization must be obtained. If he is married, he is usually urged to discuss the operation with his wife. This surgery eliminates the testicular source of male hormones and seems to cause regression or at least slow the cancer growth. Very occasionally, a hypophysectomy may be done to further reduce hormonal stimulation.

Sexual dysfunction

As stated briefly above, sexual dysfunction is an adverse effect of prostatic surgery. Following transurethral resection of the prostate (TURP), erectile incompetence is largely the result of psychologic factors. Retrograde ejaculation is common after TURP. If the patient equates ejaculation with sexual competence, the decreased or absent fluid emission may be interpreted as impotence with concomitant dysfunction.

Total prostatectomy, which includes bilateral pelvic lymphadenectomy, results in physiologic sexual dysfunction as a result of disruption of genital innervation. Ninety percent of patients lose emission, ejaculation, and erectile potency. Ten percent do have satisfactory erections, possibly because some nerves escaped damage during surgery.

External radiation therapy causes erectile dysfunction more than lymphadenectomy. Erectile impotence is not an automatic consequence of castration since adult levels of testosterone are not required to maintain an erection. Erectile dysfunction during cytotoxic chemotherapy is felt to be caused more by the general ill health of the individual than by specific effects on sexual physiology. A test for nocturnal penile tumescence may be performed to help distinguish between psychologically and organically based erectile dysfunction. A penile implant (p. 1765) may be a viable option.

Any time a procedure may result in loss of sexual function, the wife should be consulted. Recent court decisions have awarded compensation to wives who have lost conjugal relationships with their husbands as a result of medical therapy. Therefore the wife should sign a consent form for procedures that may result in sterility or impotence.[177,183]

Cancer of the penis

Epidemiology and etiology

In America, penile cancer accounts for 0.5% to 1.5% of all male malignancies. It is most common between the ages of 50 and 70, but it can occur in younger men and has been reported in children. There is a higher incidence in blacks than whites, possibly because of a lower incidence of circumcision. Penile cancer accounts for 10% to 20% of all male malignancies among African and Asian peoples.

The incidence of penile cancer is highly dependent on hygienic standards as well as cultural and religious practices. It almost never occurs in a male who was circumcised at birth. Circumcision after puberty does not decrease the risk of cancer when compared with the incidence among uncircumcised males. Circumcision removes the prepuce, or foreskin, which provides a haven for bacteria. The bacteria act on desquamated cells producing smegma, which is irritating to the tissue of the glans penis and the prepuce. This chronic irritation is considered to be carcinogenic. Therefore adequate hygiene is theoretically sufficient prophylaxis against penile cancer, making circumcision unnecessary. In clinical practice this has not been substantiated and requires further study. Trauma and sexually transmitted diseases are felt to be coincidental to penile cancer rather than causative.

The box below shows the stages of penile cancer.

Pathophysiology

Penile cancer starts as a small lesion usually on the glans and extends until the entire glans and shaft are involved. It becomes autoamputative. If penile cancer is left untreated, death occurs in 2 to 3 years. The lesion may be papillary and exophytic (flowery). It may be a small bump or resemble a pimple or wart. It may also occur as a nonhealing ulcer with the edges rolled inward. The latter is associated with earlier metastases and a poorer 5-year survival. Phimosis (p. 1712), which occurs in 25% to 75% of penile cancer cases, may obscure the lesion. The lesion may then cause erosion through the prepuce with a foul odor and discharge. Bleeding may or may not be present. Urethral and bladder involvement is rare.

Clinical picture

Presenting complaints include weakness, fatigue, malaise, and weight loss. A delay of 1 year before seeking treatment is common in 15% to 50% of the cases. Biopsy is performed to establish the diagnosis; however, benign penile lesions are uncommon. Results of laboratory tests will indicate prolonged illness and chronic infection. Metastasis usually occurs at the regional femoral and iliac nodes and is associated with a significantly worse prognosis. Five-year survival with inguinal node involvement is 20% to 25%. If radiation therapy is instituted, the survival rate may approach 50%.

Intervention

Treatment is usually surgical. Irradiation as the initial mode of treatment is indicated only in younger patients in whom sexual function is important and who have small superficial lesions.

If the lesion is confined to the prepuce, circumcision may be adequate. If the lesion is on the glans, partial penectomy or amputation of the penis is required. If the shaft of the penis is involved, total amputation may be necessary. The decision is based on the amount of penis remaining after excision with an adequate tumor-free margin. The remaining penis must be long enough for the patient to void standing, direct the stream, and not void on himself. If this is possible, the sexual function will probably be retained. If total amputation is required, a perineal urethrostomy is performed in which the urethra is redirected to an opening between the scrotum and the anus. With spread of the cancer to the scrotal contents, radical removal is required, either hemipelvectomy or hemicorporectomy.

Radiation therapy is used as adjuvant therapy at all stages. Aside from common adverse reactions to irradiation, specific genitourinary reactions include penile necrosis (10%) and urethral strictures (30%).

Lymphadenectomy is indicated for lymph node involvement. Accurate detection of metastases is difficult since enlarged lymph nodes may be free of cancerous tissue whereas normal-sized lymph nodes may contain metastatic lesions. Either may contain undetectable lesions. Lymphedema of the lower extremities may be a debilitating complication of lymphadenectomy.

Bleomycin, a chemotherapeutic agent, has been used with some success. Dose-related pulmonary toxicity resulting in interstitial fibrosis and possible fatal pulmonary insufficiency limits its use. Methotrexate given intravenously has been somewhat successful. Other chemotherapeutic agents have not been effective. If the disease is confined to the penis, 5-year survival is 80% to 85% with amputation. With metastasis to the lymph nodes, it is only 20%.

Sexual counseling is indicated for the patient with a total penectomy. Some patients with a urethrostomy have experienced orgasm and ejaculation following stimulation of the perineal, scrotal, and testicular regions.

STAGES OF PENILE CANCER

Stage A   Lesions confined to glans or foreskin

Stage B   Shaft or corpora cavernosa invaded by tumors

Stage C   Shaft involvement; lymph nodes involved but operable

Stage D   Shaft involvement; lymph nodes inoperable; metastases to distant sites

---

Outcome criteria for the man with a neoplasm of the reproductive organs

---

The person or significant others can:

1. Demonstrate or describe testicular self-examination (TSE).

2. Perform regular TSE.
3. Seek health care for conditions unusual for him.
4. State expected effects of treatment and ways to manage distressing effects.
5. State reasons for continued monitoring of condition.
6. State plans for appropriate follow-up health care.
7. Verbalize understanding that cancer is not sexually transmissible.
8. Seek sexual counseling if needed.

SEXUALLY TRANSMITTED DISEASES

Epidemiology and etiology

Sexually transmitted diseases (STDs) are diseases that are *usually* or *can* be transmitted from one person to another with heterosexual or homosexual intercourse or intimate contact with the genitalia, mouth, or rectum. In addition to the five classic venereal diseases (syphilis, gonorrhea, chancroid, lymphogranuloma venereum, and granuloma inguinale), the STD category includes genital herpes infection, nonspecific urethritis, trichomoniasis, candidiasis, pediculosis pubic (crabs), scabies, genital or venereal warts, hepatitis b infections, molluscum contagiosum, and *Gardnerella vaginalis* (previously referred to as *Cornybacterium vaginalis* or *Haemophilus vaginalis*) vaginitis.

These latter STDs might be considered the "new generation" of STDs, although they have probably existed since antiquity. Because of improved laboratory and epidemiologic methods, their prevalence, modes of transmission, and clinical consequences are better understood than in earlier decades. In addition, many of the newly recognized STDs have become epidemic or hyperendemic as a consequence of changing sexual behavior patterns. Not only has the incidence of many STDs increased, but for agents with multiple modes of transmission (e.g., hepatitis B virus, enteric pathogens), the proportion of infections that are transmitted sexually has also increased. In addition to the immediate consequences of STDs, there are newly recognized effects on maternal and infant morbidity as well as on human reproduction and fertility.

All states require that each case of syphilis and gonorrhea be reported to the state or local health officer. Chancroid, granuloma inguinale, and lymphogranuloma venereum are reportable in most states. Herpes genitalis, trichomoniasis, and candidiasis are not reportable in any state. The true incidence of STDs is not known because of variable reporting requirements and also because many cases are not reported by the clinicians who treat them.

In explaining the trends of reported cases of STDs in the United States, three changes occurring in recent years are often referred to in the literature. The first of these concerns use of antibiotics and changes in the antibiotic susceptibility of pathogenic organisms. The widespread, perhaps indiscriminate, use of penicillin and other antibiotics between the late 1940s and early 1950s parallels the decline in both syphilis and gonorrhea. It is said that the organisms developed a greater resistance to antibiotics over time and that antibiotics have therefore become less effective than previously. There is no firm evidence to indicate a decrease in effectiveness of penicillin against syphilis. However, the gonococcus tends to develop resistance to antibiotics.[42]

A second explanation for the rise in incidence of STDs is that they are more likely to occur if a social system is permissive. During times of war and other catastrophes it is easier for agencies to control interpersonal behavior, while in times of peace and absence of national crisis, civil liberties tend to flourish. The incidence curve of syphilis and gonorrhea (Fig. 65-17) after the years of World War II seems to support this thesis.

The third explanation centers around sexual behavior patterns and includes permissiveness. Concern has been particularly expressed about the prevalence of gonorrhea among adolescents who are considered to be promiscuous. In fact, rates for gonorrhea show young adults of 20 to 24 years of age to be at greatest risk for acquiring gonorrhea, with the second highest risk group being teenagers 15 to 19.[22] The incidence of syphilis according to age indicates that young adults are at the greatest risk but that teenagers are the fourth highest risk group by age.[181]

The above discussion makes an assumption of sexual promiscuity, and in doing so, requires acknowledgement of advances in contraceptive technology, especially "the pill." These social changes are often termed the three Ps (permissiveness, promiscuity, and the pill).[43] The underlying idea is that, with the advent of antibiotics and the pill, people began to lose fear of untreated venereal disease and pregnancy and that sexual promiscuity increased significantly, leading to increased exposure to infection.

If the definition of promiscuity is that sexual relations are not restricted to one partner, studies show that patients diagnosed in clinics as having STD are not promiscuous. In one study 66.4% of patients having an STD named only one sexual contact.[43] It must be realized, however, that persons may hesitate to admit to having more than one sex partner for any number of reasons.

In the past, prostitution has been considered a major force in the transmission of STDs. Before World War II it was estimated that approximately 75% of all STDs could be traced to prostitutes and that at least 10% of all prostitutes had contracted an STD at least once. Today

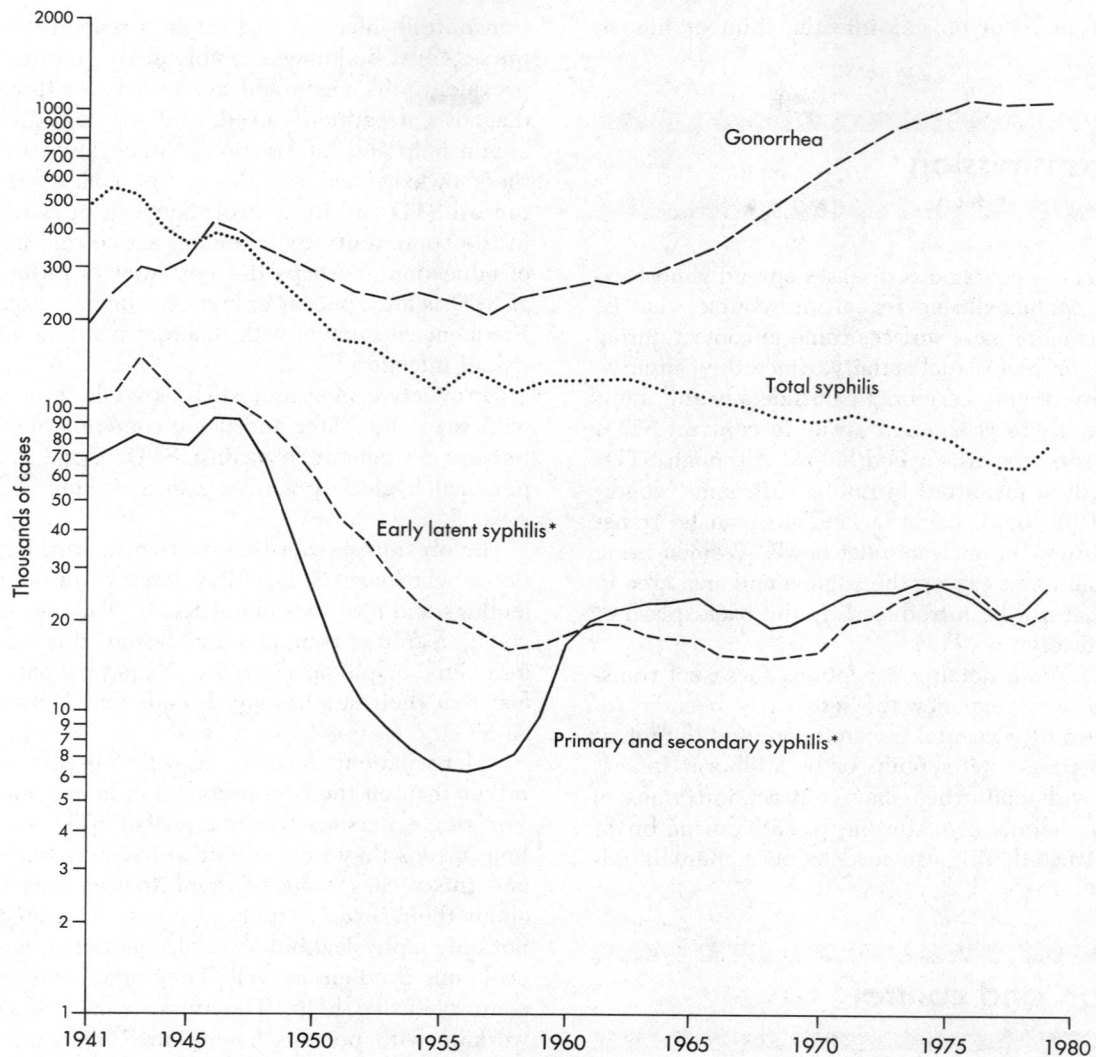

Fig. 65-17. Reported cases (by diagnosis) of syphilis and gonorrhea in the United States, 1941 to 1979. Asterisks indicate that incidence for 1941 to 1946 is for the fiscal year (12-month period ending June 30). Figures for 1947 to 1979 are for the calendar year.

less than 5% of patients with syphilis can be classed as prostitutes. Also, most persons with gonorrhea are single and under 25 years of age, and most clients of prostitutes are usually older, married men.[22] *Chlamydia trachomatis* and herpes are two STDs that are very common in middle-class America.

Before 1960, homosexuals were rarely mentioned in the literature as carriers of STDs. By 1972, however, it was noted that about 14.4% of all syphilitic infections are spread by persons who name only sexual partners of the same sex.[16] In 1975, two instances of outbreaks of gonorrhea were reported.[16] One of these occurred in a large county jail, where 10 cases of gonorrhea were traced to an infected homosexual inmate. Homosexual men carry pathogens in the rectum and colon, including

gonococcus, *Giardia*, ameba, *Shigella*, and *Campylobacter*.

The condom was the main method of contraception used before the advent of antibiotics and oral contraceptives. The use of the condom may have discouraged spread of the STDs by providing a mechanical barrier to the organisms. The pill has almost revolutionized contraception practices, and it has been noted that neutralization of the vaginal and cervical environment by estrogenic substances predisposes to infection. It would appear that individual characteristics of persons engaging in sexual activity need to be more closely studied before any conclusions about permissiveness, promiscuity, and use of the pill can be made.

Currently, it is not unusual for the same person to

have two or more organisms infecting him or her simultaneously.

Sexual transmission

The STDs are contagious diseases spread almost exclusively by contact during sexual intercourse, that is, when mucous membrane surfaces come in contact during genital, oral, or anal sexual activity. Since the causative organisms survive only very briefly outside a warm, moist environment, there is almost no way to contract STDs from toilet seats, towels, or bed linens. Although STDs are not usually transmitted in public restrooms, conditions caused by fungi, bacteria, and lice can be transmitted from water in unclean toilet bowls. Women using a conventional toilet expose the vaginal and anal area to pathogens that can be introduced by the back splash of contaminated toilet water.

There are some notable exceptions to sexual transmission. During pregnancy the fetus may become infected in utero by placental transmission, and the infant may acquire congenital syphilis or be stillborn. Infants of mothers with gonorrhea may contract infections of the eyes (ophthalmia neonatorum, p. 888) during birth, and unless treated, this can lead to permanent blindness.

Prevention and control

Prevention and control measures for STDs include three levels of prevention. Primary prevention is directed at preventing the disease. This includes educating uninfected persons so that they can avoid contact with an infected person, identification and treatment of exposed persons who are asymptomatic, interviewing patients with infection for identification of contacts, examination and preventive treatment of contacts, educational programs for the public, and active involvement of professionals in programs of control. The goal of these efforts includes eradication of the reservoir of disease in the population. Secondary prevention is directed toward prevention of complications, and tertiary prevention focuses on decreasing the effects of complications.

Education

The nurse's first responsibility in STD control is to educate patients who may develop or have a sexually transmitted infection. To act in a responsible manner, nurses must be knowledgeable about the diseases most prevalent, the signs and symptoms, methods used in diagnosis, treatments used, and where individuals can obtain help and information. Nurses also can influence the knowledge and attitudes of their colleagues and peers toward STD and its control. Nurses can exert influence in the community by taking an active role in programs of education. Perhaps the best way to reduce the risk of STD is for a person to know his or her sexual partner. Frequent encounters with different partners increase the risk of infection.

Preventive measures such as washing or showering with soap and water and using condoms may also help but are no guarantee against STD. Good laundry and personal hygiene practices also may help reduce STD risk.

Before nurses can be effective in working with patients who have STDs, they must confront their own feelings and attitudes about STDs. The patient is often young, fearful of pain, and unaccustomed to surroundings in a clinic or physician's office. Young patients especially fear that their families and friends may learn they have an STD.

Many patients focus on how the diseases are spread rather than on the consequences of having an infection. For single persons, contracting an STD and securing help means they must admit to having sexual relations, and this means some of them at least may feel guilty about their sexual activity. Patients with an STD have not only a physical but a social, emotional, and perhaps economic problem as well. They need constructive and comprehensive help. The nurse who is successful in working with persons having an STD is one who can create an atmosphere of trust in which the person feels free to discuss all aspects of the problem.

Persons who seek help recognize they have a problem; they want to get better and stay well. Because of this they are highly motivated to do what is necessary, are receptive to information and advice, and are attentive when advice is given. Nurses can take advantage of the patient's readiness to learn and motivation to improve and maintain health.

A careful history and physical examination are important. Previous episodes of genital infection, chronic health problems, and factors predisposing to venereal diseases may be revealed. Careful documentation of the person's present problem aids in the diagnosis, treatment, and follow-up. Pelvic examination is necessary for determining the extent of the infection. The person should be informed of the purposes and importance of the history, examination, and laboratory tests so that greater cooperation, especially in giving information, can be obtained.

Once the diagnosis, tentative or conclusive, is made, focus should first be placed on obtaining a cure and preventing complications and reinfection. Many lay people know the treatment for syphilis and gonorrhea is penicillin but they may not be fully informed about this and other aspects of treatment. Because some of the diseases respond to penicillin or other antibiotics, many people believe that all genital infections can be cured simply, and this is not so. Some people believe that antibiotics not only cure an infection but that they produce immunity against reinfection as well. Persons receiving an antibiotic or other medications for STDs must be informed of the action of the drug, its duration of effectiveness, side effects, chances of cure, and the need for follow-up. They need to be advised that treatment failures do occur and that reinfection rates are high. Return visits should be encouraged whenever possible, since adequacy of treatment of all of the STDs is evaluated best by laboratory analysis for the specific organism.

Persons treated for sexually transmitted infections need information about self-care. To understand their therapy and to responsibly engage in self-care, they must be informed about the venereal nature of the infection, how it is transmitted, and the possibility of reinfection and infection of their sexual partner or partners. The patient needs to know that it is important for sexual partners to be checked for signs of infection, to be advised of what the signs are, and have a culture done for asymptomatic infection. Patients should be advised to abstain from intercourse until cured. If sexual intercourse cannot be avoided, a condom should be used by the man to prevent the possibility of infection or reinfection.

Education of patients regarding hygiene and personal health practices is beneficial for reducing the chances of secondary infection, recurrence, and infections of various types in the future. Frequent bathing and hand washing are indicated. It is known that many of the organisms causing STDs are destroyed by soap and water. For women, douching is contraindicated unless it is prescribed for the purpose of applying heat or applying medication. All women should be informed that, for personal cleanliness, frequent douching at any time is not advisable, since this may disturb the vaginal and cervical environments and predispose the woman to infection. If douching is prescribed by the physician, the patient should be instructed in the procedure (p. 1640).

If lesions are present on body surfaces, the patient should be instructed in their care. Unless contraindicated, a hot bath is taken two to three times a day, and lesions are kept as dry as possible between bathings. Both men and women should be advised to wear cotton underwear, and women should be advised to avoid using pantyhose, since they tend to trap moisture and prevent circulation of air. Unless they are specifically prescribed as local medications, the patient should not apply any lotion, cream, or ointment to any of the lesions associated with STDs.

Opportunities to engage in instruction regarding diet, exercise, nutrition, contraception, and reproduction often arise when persons are being treated for an STD. Nurses can pursue any of these opportunities.

Opportunities for promoting health attitudes about sexual activity and STDs also frequently arise. These topics are approached tactfully and with consideration of the patient's feelings. Adolescents especially require an approach that indicates understanding balanced with ability to help them set limits. Developmental tasks of adolescence requie that young people find means of sexual gratification within the context of meaningful sexual relationships. In their search, adolescents need to be reassured that mutually rewarding relationships involving sexual gratification can be fulfilling. However, within this context, adolescents need to recognize that consequences of their behavior may include unwanted pregnancy and STD. Nurses may not always feel comfortable in exploring the meaning of sexual experiences with adolescents who they know are, or suspect of being, sexually active. Despite this, nurses do have an obligation to provide patients with information about STD prevention.

Many films are available from local and state health departments including *VD: Old Bugs, New Problems,* and *VD: A Newer Focus.*

Contact investigation

In the prevention and control of STDs, especially gonorrhea, emphasis was once placed on interviewing for information regarding sexual contacts. The named contacts were sought out for examination and treatment. Lay people knowledgeable about the required reporting to the local health department of some of the diseases were very hesitant to name their sexual contacts. Young people often feared that their parents and the parents of the sexual partner would find out about their infection. Minors need to know that they can probably obtain treatment without parental consent. Presently most states permit physicians to treat minors for STD without obtaining parental consent, and several states are proposing changes in existing legislation restricting treatment of minors.[6] Lay people also may perceive reporting of STDs as a threat from an official agency and may hesitate to name their contacts out of a sense of protection if they do not know that no punishment is involved.

Interviewing the patient for contacts is done at the time of the initial visit in the event that the patient does not return for follow-up. This interview is probably best done after the patient is examined, the type of infection is determined, and treatment is prescribed. If assessment is accompanied by information giving, the patient should be better informed about STDs and how they are treated after the examination is over. It is hoped that the patient will be less concerned about self and more willing and able to give information about sexual contacts.

Interviewing for contacts involves two aspects. The patient is first asked to name sexual contacts. Second, the patient is interviewed for "cluster suspects," who are friends or acquaintances who may have been exposed to the same contacts, or who have symptoms of an STD. Since one focus of STD control is on increasing self-referrals, the patient is asked to advise known contacts and cluster suspects to present themselves for examination and preventive treatment. Confidentiality is stressed. There is reason to believe that patients do not name all their contacts at the time of the first interview and that a reinterview, after the patient has reflected, will usually result in additional names of contacts. Because of the understandable reluctance of many people to name their sexual contacts, in many areas the patient is given the responsibility of informing the contacts and advising them of their need for treatment. (The contacts are not named, but instead cards that permit both examination and treatment without identification are given to the contact by the patient.) The local health departments cooperate in locating, culturing, and treating these contacts as necessary.

Whenever possible, the contacts of the infected person are located and advised to have an examination and tests as soon as possible. If the sexual contacts do not have symptoms of infection at the time of the first examination, treatment is instituted to abort infection. Giving preventive treatment to named contacts who have no clinical evidence of infection has gained popularity and acceptance in the United States, and indications are present that this same approach is being used more often in management of patients having the "minor" STDs.

Current and future needs

The epidemic nature of some STDs makes it evident that measures for control of spread need to be even more vigorously applied and that new measures may be necessary to check the spread of infection. Efforts to implement mass education and screening programs need to be continued. Program efforts are directed toward creating public awareness of the problem of STDs and their control methods and informing the public of the possible serious consequences of these diseases. There also is a need to expand screening, contact treatment, and diagnostic and treatment programs.

Little is known about some of the STDs. Surveil-lance over some of them is inadequate, so that even the true incidence of several sexually transmitted infections is not known. Treatment of several of these diseases is poorly understood because knowledge of the natural history of the causative organisms is inadequate. Such knowledge is necessary to understand the epidemiology of the spread of these diseases so that treatment and prevention can be better directed than is now possible. Diagnostic methods need to be improved so that they are more reliable and can be carried out inexpensively for large numbers of people. Alternative therapies for prophylaxis require development of agents to be used specifically and with discretion for treatment of exposed individuals, for treatment of persons sensitive to specific drugs, and for the management of pregnant women.

In order to better understand the modes of transmission and circumstances surrounding spread of the STDs, knowledge of human behavior is required. Considerable research has been done in recent years regarding sexual behavior patterns, contraceptive practices, and permissiveness. While this has been helpful, there is little consensus about whether these variables influence the incidence and spread of STDs. Further study will add to the pool of knowledge, which can be applied in programs of detection, treatment, and prevention.

Development of prophylactic vaccines, especially for gonorrhea and syphilis, needs to be given high priority. To accomplish this, techniques for growing the organisms need to be developed, and this in turn requires knowledge of the natural history and evolution of specific organisms, including viruses.

History has revealed that treatment alone has never conquered any of the major communicable diseases, but that programs through which the public becomes better informed and demands services, as well as the development of protective vaccines, have almost always been universally successful in preventing disease.

Gonorrhea

Epidemiology, etiology, and pathophysiology

Over 1 million cases of gonorrhea were reported in the United States in 1979 and 1980 (Fig. 65-17), making it the most commonly reported communicable disease in the country.[181] In view of the fact that only 25% to 50% of the patients with gonorrhea treated by private physicians are reported, and that women have little or no evidence of infection so that underdiagnosis may occur, the true incidence is probably more than 2 million cases. Young adults 20 to 24 years of age are at highest risk of acquiring gonorrhea, with the next highest rates found among teenagers 15 to 19 years of age. In fact, 1 of every 30 teenagers in this age group will acquire gonorrhea each year.[179]

It is estimated that the total cost of gonorrhea to the United States in 1979 was $1 billion. Women and their offspring suffer the major physical, emotional, and economic burden. Pelvic inflammatory diseases occur in 10% to 20% of women with gonorrhea, and even when treated, these women are likely to suffer from recurrent salpingitis, ectopic pregnancy, infertility, and menstrual abnormalities and may face surgical removal of the pelvic organs as well as fetal loss.[179]

Asymptomatic persons or those with few symptoms are an important reservoir for gonorrhea since they usually remain untreated As many as 10% to 40% of gonorrheal infections in men are asymptomatic, and in women as many as 80% of infections are a symptomatic. Homosexual men can harbor reservoirs of anorectal and pharyngeal infections.[179]

Gonorrhea, often referred to as "GC" or "the clap" by lay people, is caused by *Neisseria gonorrhoeae*. Gonorrhea is of great concern because of its epidemic rise, high reinfection rate, and seriousness of residual effects. The incubation period is 3 to 30 days in men and 3 days to an indefinite period in women.

Clinical picture

In *men*, the gonococcus is introduced into the anterior urethra during sexual activity. In about 90% of infected men, urethritis is the first symptom to appear and often is indicated by severe dysuria, particularly intense in the first morning voiding. Other symptoms quickly follow and include purulent discharge from the urethra, dysuria, and rarely, swelling of the penis and balanitis. Because of the distress produced by the symptoms, men usually present themselves for examination early in the disease. As a result, diagnosis is made and treatment instituted early, and complications and residual effects of gonorrhea are uncommon among men. Sterility from orchitis or epididymitis can occur as a residual effect, but this is rare.

The incidence of asymptomatic gonorrhea in men is believed to be low; however, there is an increasing awareness of the importance of men with asymptomatic infection in the transmission of gonorrhea. Some men have been found to have no symptoms of infection despite positive tests for gonorrhea 2 weeks after exposure.[6]

In contrast to men, *women* rarely have early, distressing symptoms of gonorrhea. The early signs include a slight purulent discharge, a vague feeling of fullness in the pelvis, and discomfort or aching in the abdomen. Since these signs are not perceived as severe, women may disregard them. If the bladder is involved, there is burning, frequency, and urgency of urination, and women are more likely to seek medical assistance because of discomfort. Bartholin's glands may become infected, resulting in distention and swelling that make walking or sitting painful. These symptoms may also lead the woman to see a physician.

Gonorrhea in women most often begins as asymptomatic cervicitis, and the infection can be present for extended periods without causing noticeable signs. Hence there are a high number of infected, asymptomatic women. These women do not receive treatment unless gonorrhea is diagnosed through screening or unless the woman is identified by the sexual partner and presents herself for treatment. Frequently, complications are the first indicators of gonorrhea in women. Salpingitis is the most common complication with 10% to 20% of women presenting themselves with symptoms of salpingitis as the first sign of infection.[179] During the course of treatment for salpingitis, many women are surgically sterilized. In cases of untreated gonorrhea, the residual effects of chronic pelvic inflammatory disease, infertility, and ectopic pregnancy are well known.

Other complications of untreated gonorrhea in both men and women include dermatitis, carditis, meningitis, and arthritis. The incidence of these complications is higher among women because of the prolonged period of infection without symptoms.

Gonorrheal infection may be suspected on the basis of history, symptoms, and clinical evidence obtained by physical examination. However, identification of the organism is necessary to confirm the diagnosis and to rule out other problems. In men the diagnosis is confirmed by gram-stained smear of the discharge from the penis. Culture of the discharge from the penis is usually reserved for those whose smears are negative in the presence of strong clinical evidence.

Gram-stained cervical smears are inadequate for diagnosing gonorrhea in women. These smears are negative in about 50% of women having gonorrhea and are falsely positive in some cases. Therefore cultures from the cervix, urethra, throat, and anus are usually taken. Because of the great length of time required to obtain reports of cultures for gonorrhea, treatment is usually instituted on a presumptive basis.

Prevention

Prevention of gonorrhea and its complications can be achieved in three stages. The first and most crucial stage is prevention of the disease. The second stage involves prevention of complications of the disease, such as pelvic inflammatory disease. The third stage is reversal of the damage caused by the disease, such as by tubal reconstruction.

Early treatment of infected persons is currently the most effective measure to prevent new infection of sexual partners. Mechanical methods, such as condoms, appear effective when used. Education to acquaint people with the symptoms of gonorrhea, the efficacy of condoms, and the availability of diagnostic and treatment resources is also important. Early detection through contact tracing and screening can reduce the serious complications of gonorrhea. Experiments are currently in progress to develop and test an effective vaccine for gonorrhea.

Intervention

Therapy for gonorrhea presents a greater problem than for syphilis because the gonococcus tends to develop resistance to antibiotics. It also is believed that inadequate therapy is common in the United States. Several drug regimens are in use with emphasis on single-dose treatment to avoid problems in follow-up and patient cooperation. Uncomplicated gonococcal infections in men and women are usually treated with 4.8 million units of aqueous procaine penicillin G injected intramuscularly in two sites, with 1.0 g of probenecid by mouth just before injection. This regimen is preferred in men with anorectal or pharyngeal infections, and the single-dose treatment is recommended for those who are unlikely to complete a multiple-dose schedule. Alternatively, tetracycline hydrochloride, 0.5 g by mouth four times a day for 5 days, for a total dose of 10 g, may be given. The tetracycline regimen is effective against nongonococcal organisms such as chlamydiae, as well as gonococcus, but should not be given to pregnant women or children under 8 years of age.

Those who are allergic to penicillins or probenecid or who cannot tolerate tetracycline may be given spectinomycin, 2 g in one injection, ampicillin, 3.5 g, or amoxicillin, 3 g, all with 1 g of probenecid by mouth. Spectinomycin is the drug of choice for penicillinase-producing *Neisseria gonorrhoeae*. The most common and clinically significant reactions to penicillin are allergic reactions, of which urticaria is the most common. Before initiating treatment it is important to screen for a history of previous reaction to penicillin. Symptoms of life-threatening reactions such as anaphylaxis most often occur within 30 minutes after injection, and although such reactions are rare, it may be advisable to detain patients for this period of time after parenteral administration of penicillin.[159]

In addition, some individuals may experience a procaine reaction, indicated by disorientation, agitation, a "high" feeling, hallucinations, or combativeness. This reaction usually begins 5 minutes after the injection and resolves within 20 to 30 minutes. Monitoring the blood pressure and attempting to calm the individual are important.

Syphilis

Epidemiology, etiology, and pathophysiology

Although the total number of cases of syphilis has decreased steadily since about 1963 (Fig. 65-17), the number of reported cases of primary and secondary syphilis has increased since 1975. The highest incidence of syphilis is found among 20- to 24-year-olds. The number of early latent cases of syphilis reported seems to have leveled off since about 1973. The current statistics for late syphilis indicate a decrease of 74% between 1943 and 1979. This decrease partly reflects control programs in effect between 1955 and 1965 and therefore a decrease in the late consequences of syphilis. An increase in the incidence of reported syphilis may be seen shortly because of an influx of refugees with positive VDRL (Venereal Disease Research Laboratories) tests, which may be due not only to syphilis but also to pinta or yaws. Because it is impossible to determine the cause of the positive VDRL test, most of these cases are diagnosed and treated as syphilis.

Intensive screening of pregnant women and increased prenatal care have resulted in dramatic decreases in the incidence of congenital syphilis. A decrease of 21.5% in the incidence of congenital syphilis in infants occurred between 1978 and 1979. It is felt that of all the methods by which syphilis can be acquired, congenital syphilis is the most preventable, yet 130 cases were reported in infants in 1979.[179]

The greatest percentage of cases of syphilis is believed to be unreported. It has been estimated that close to 100,000 new cases of syphilis actually occurred in 1980 and that a reservoir of more than 350,000 untreated patients exists.[179]

Syphilis is caused by a spirochete, *Treponema pallidum*, that gains entry into the body through either the mucous membrane or skin during intercourse. The organism is readily destroyed by physical and chemical agents including heat, drying, and mild disinfectants such as soap and water.

The incubation period for syphilis is usually 3 weeks. However, symptoms can appear as early as 9 days or as long as 3 months after exposure; this is the case for rectal infections in homosexual men. If untreated, the disease progresses through four identifiable stages (Table 65-11).

Prevention

As with gonorrhea, three levels of prevention are important. The first is prevention of the initial infection by finding and treating those with the disease. Secondary prevention is directed at early treatment of cases to prevent late syphilis or congenital syphilis. Finally, efforts can be made to treat the complications of syphilis when they occur.

Clinical picture

Syphilis is most often diagnosed by standard serologic tests. Massive screening programs in the past made serologic diagnosis of syphilis very common. Mass screening

TABLE 65-11. Stage of syphilis

	Primary	Secondary	Latent	Late
Duration	2-8 wk	Appears 2-4 wk after chancre appears; extends over 2-4 yr	5-20 yr	Terminal if not treated
Clinical signs	Hard sore or pimple on vulva or penis that breaks and forms painless, draining chancre; may be a single chancre or groups of more than one; may be present also on lips, tongue, hands, rectum, or nipples; chancre heals leaving almost invisible scar	Depends on site; low-grade fever, headache, anorexia, weight loss, anemia, sore throat, hoarseness, reddened and sore eyes, jaundice with or without hepatitis, aching of joints, muscles, long bones; sores on body or generalized fine rash; condylomata lata (venereal warts) on rectum or genitalia	No clinical signs	Tumorlike masses, gumma, on any area of body; damage to heart valves and blood vessels; meningitis, paralysis, lack of coordination, paresis, insomnia, confusion, delusions, impaired judgment, slurred speech
Communicability	Exudates from lesions and chancre highly contagious	Exudates from lesions highly contagious; blood contains organisms	Contagious for about 2 yr; not contagious to others after that; blood contains organisms; may be transmitted placentally	Noncontagious; spinal fluid may contain organisms

TABLE 65-12. Serologic tests for syphilis (STSs)

Type	Description	Examples	Comments
Flocculation	Antibody-antigen reaction produces a precipitation (fluocculation)	VDRL RPR	Used primarily for screening; performed in standard laboratories
Complement fixation	Complement (p. 278) is used up in antigen-antibody reaction (fixed); hemolysis occurs	Reiter (Wasserman outdated)	Nonspecific; used less frequently; performed in standard laboratories
Fluorescent antibody	Antigen of killed *Treponema pallidum* is labeled with a fluorescent dye	FTA FTA-ABS	More specific than flocculation or complement-fixation tests; differentiates false-positive from true syphilis positive results; performed in special laboratoryies
Treponema pallidum immobilization	Serum is mixed with live *Treponema pallidum*; presence of antibody decreases organism mobility	TPI	Most sensitive test; performed at CDC laboratory in Atlanta

using the VDRL test is no longer practiced except on high-risk populations, pregnant women, sexually active women, and couples who are applying for a marriage license. Dark-field microscopic examination of tissue scrapings from lesions or material obtained by aspiration of regional lymph nodes also reveals the presence of the spirochete, especially during the primary and secondary stages. A presumptive diagnosis is made on the basis of suspicious lesions, positive serologic tests, known exposure to infection, and involvement of regional lymph nodes. False-positive VDRL reactions are common among persons previously treated for syphilis, but fluorescent treponemal antibody (FTA) and absorption (ABS) tests are more specific (Table 65-12). Also, once a VDRL test is positive, it remains so and is not useful for identifying reinfection. Infectious mononucleosis, hepatitis, pregnancy, viral pneumonia, malaria, chickenpox, measles and smallpox vaccination, narcotic addiction, and terminal malignancy have also been associated with false-positive VDRL results.

Intervention

Syphilis can be successfully treated at any stage of the disease, although treatment may have to be more prolonged in latent and late syphilis. While syphilis can be cured in late stages, the damage to the body is much less easily managed.

Because penicillin continues to be effective in the treatment of syphilis, it remains the drug of choice. All types of penicillin are effective, but penicillin G benzathine is preferred because it is long acting and can be given in a limited number of injections.

Patients with primary, secondary, and latent syphilis (and their contacts) are usually given 2.4 million units of penicillin intramuscularly. Patients with late syphilis are generally given 2.4 million units intramuscularly at 7-day intervals until a total of 7.2 to 9.6 million units has been given. When the use of penicillin is contraindicated because of drug sensitivity, tetracycline in a total dose of 30 g over a period of 15 days is effective (and over 30 days for late syphilis).

Pregnant women with penicillin sensitivity pose problems for treatment. In the large dosage required to treat syphilis, tetracycline produces mottling and staining of fetal dentition, and possible abnormal bone formation may occur. If given the usual adult dose, inadequate placental transfer of tetracycline is likely and congenital syphilis would probably develop. Erythromycin in a dose of 30 g over a period of 15 days seems to be the best alternative treatment for pregnant women with syphilis. Neurosyphilis is treated with intravenous penicillin. Contacts are treated with 2.4 million units of penicillin G benzathine.

Herpes genitalis

Epidemiology, etiology, and pathophysiology

Herpes genitalis (genital herpes, HVH-2) is caused by infection with *Herpesvirus hominis* type 2 (HVH-2). Herpes genitalis is the most important STD of the past decade. Its chronicity, frequent recurrences, and difficult treatment and prevention distinguish it from other STDs. It is estimated that about 300,000 to 500,000 new cases occur annually.[181] Conservative estimates are that 15% to 20% of Americans now suffer from genital herpes, and it is believed that because of poor control measures the number of cases is increasing dramatically.[179] Its peak incidence parallels the young age groups affected by other STDs. Herpes genitalis is a lifelong disease once acquired and carries with it not only intense and recurrent discomfort, but also anxieties about future childbearing, malignancy, and sexual and marital function. In early pregnancy women infected with herpes have an increased chance of miscarriage. Because genital herpetic lesions endanger the fetus during delivery, caesarean delivery is often necessitated. Genital herpes has also been associated with cervical cancer. It is now generally accepted that HVH-2 is spread by sexual contact.

The incubation period is 3 to 14 days. The primary lesion appears as a vesicle on the external genitalia in men, often on the rectum in homosexual men, and on the vagina, cervix, or external genitalia in women. These lesions often ulcerate, especially when located on moist surfaces. Following primary herpes, the virus persists in a latent or unrecognized form in most patients. It believed that latent infections are localized in the ganglia of sensory nerves to the genitalia. When the host factors favor it, the latent infection becomes clinically apparent as recurrent herpes.

Prevention

Primary prevention of herpes depends on limiting sexual contact between infected individuals and uninfected partners. There is preliminary evidence that the herpes virus may survive on towels for up to 20 minutes, therefore it is important to use separate linens. Refraining from sexual intercourse while lesions are present is essential. Youths should be taught to look at themselves and prospective partners for such lesions. In some communities there are groups of individuals with herpes who have chosen to restrict themselves to sexual contact only with others who already have been exposed to herpes. Condoms may be helpful. Transmission to the fetus may be prevented by caesarean section. Infected neonates may develop subsequent mental retardation or die. If drug therapy for HVH-2 is effective, it will help limit new infections by eradicating at least some of the reservoir of infected individuals by preventing reactivation of HVH-2.

Secondary prevention is aimed at reducing or eliminating complications such as cervical cancer. Another important complication of the disease is its ability to create great psychologic pain and anxiety, to disrupt normal social and sexual relationships, and to stigmatize its victims. In the event that secondary prevention is not possible, efforts are essential to detect and treat cervical cancer in its early stages. Attenuation of the psychologic complications induced by herpes is also crucial.

Clinical picture

Primary infections are associated with local inflammation, pain, enlargement of the inguinal lymph nodes, and generalized signs of infection, such as photophobia, headaches, and flulike symptoms. Although primary herpetic lesions begin as single or multiple reddish papules that then develop into clear, fluid-filled vesicles, once they rupture they form ulcerations that may fuse with other lesions to form large ulcerated areas. The disease tends to be more extensive in women than in men. In some women cervical infection accompanies the external lesions, and in certain cases it may be the only infected site. Cervical involvement may be mild or severe with extensive ulceration and pus. Genital lesions often worsen during the first 10 to 15 days but usually heal within 3 to 4 weeks. These symptoms usually lead the individual to seek medical attention.

Vaginal discharge is common among women, and discharge from the urethra is usual in men having primary infections. Urinary tract involvement may occur and is reflected in symptoms of dysuria or urinary retention. The lesions can cause severe pain, requiring hospitalization for parenteral analgesia. Subclinical infections in which patients are unaware of any problem occur in only about 10% of the cases of genital herpes. Unfortunately, about 75% of all patients have at least one recurrence. Fortunately, recurrent infections are usually milder and of shorter duration than primary infections and usually produce local rather than systemic reaction. The patient experiencing a recurrent infection often has prodromal signs of paresthesia and burning at the site where the lesion will erupt. Factors known to predispose to recurrent infection include fever, emotional upsets, premenstrual states, and overexposure to heat and sunshine. While the mode of recurrent infection is not clear, it has been theorized that during primary infection the virus ascends sensory nerve sheaths, localizing in corresponding nerve ganglia, and that when the environment becomes favorable, the virus is reactivated. Recurrent herpes usually begins with abnormal sensation or itching of a localized genital area. Lesions of recurrent infections usually occur in the site of primary infection. Herpes encephalitis may also occur.

Diagnosis of herpes genitalis is made by isolation of the virus from specimens obtained from lesions. Pap smears or fluid from the vesicles collected in transport medium demonstrates cellular characteristics of viruses.

Intervention

Treatment for genital herpes has most often been symptomatic, since there is presently no known cure for the disease. Currently, trials are being conducted with acyclovir, a drug that appears capable of suppressing herpetic infections. The drug appears capable of inhibiting the replication of herpetic viruses in vitro, and in clinical trials with patients who had antibodies against herpes simplex viruses acyclovir prevented active herpes infections.[160] A topical form of acyclovir may be marketed in 1982.

Symptomatic treatment consists of using Burow's solution or hydrogen peroxide and soap and water to cleanse the lesions. The involved areas are blown dry

with a hair dryer, and the skin is then dusted with cornstarch. Use of cream or ointment is avoided since it may spread the virus. Women are advised to use a mirror to examine the vulva, vagina, and cervix for hidden lesions.

Chlamydial infection

Epidemiology, etiology, and pathophysiology

Chlamydia trachomatis is a bacteria-like organism. Its incubation period averages 10 days. It is estimated that each year more than 3 million Americans suffer from epidemic chlamydial infections. *Chlamydia trachomatis* is the major cause of nongonococcal urethritis in men* and probably causes more than 50% of the 500,000 annual cases of epididymitis (p. 1712), a potentially painful and sterilizing condition. In women, chlamydiae produce not only urethritis and cervicitis (p. 1680) but also pelvic inflammatory diseases (p. 1681) with consequent infertility. Chlamydial infections are responsible for about 20% of diagnosed pelvic inflammatory disease cases, and it is estimated that about 11,000 women each year become involuntarily sterilized and 3600 suffer ectopic pregnancies as a result of this organism.[179] Chlamydial infections can be transmitted to infants during delivery, causing conjunctivitis and pneumonia in many.

Prevention

Primary prevention of chlamydial infections consists of limiting sexual contact with infected partners. Secondary prevention requires early diagnosis and treatment.

Clinical picture

Chlamydial infections are usually diagnosed on the basis of history and pelvic examination. Women notice painful or difficult urination, abnormal vaginal discharge or bleeding, and possibly dyspareunia or other pelvic pain. Other women, however, are asymptomatic. Men usually have nonspecific urethritis or may seek treatment for epididymitis. Chlamydia can be diagnosed by culture, but the test currently is expensive and inaccessible to many facilities.

Intervention

Urethritis is usually treated with tetracycline, 500 mg four times daily for 7 days. It is strongly recommended that partners of infected persons also be treated.

---

*Nongonococcal urethritis may also be caused by *Ureaplasma urealyticum*, *Trichonomonas vaginalis*, *Candida albicans*, HVS-2, chlamydiae or coliforms, with chlamydiae and *Ureaplasma urealyticum* each accounting for about 40% of cases.

Lymphogranuloma venereum

Epidemiology, etiology, and pathophysiology

Lymphogranuloma venereum (LGV) is a systemic, sexually transmitted disease caused by *Chlamydia* organisms. Other species of *chlamydia* are the causative organisms of trachoma and psittacosis. The disease is contracted by vaginal, anal, or oral intercourse, and primary inoculation with the organism may occur at any site involved in close contact. The incubation period is 7 to 12 days. Lymphadenitis of regional lymph nodes draining the site of primary infection occurs, and the disease spreads by way of the lymphatic system.

LGV occurs with relative infrequency in the United States, but it is prevalent in Southeast Asia. It is thought to be endemic among blacks in the United States,[150] but epidemiologic studies are needed to determine its true incidence. Reports of the incidence of LGV indicate less than 1000 cases annually. The symptoms of LGV resemble those of other sexually transmitted diseases, and its reported incidence may be influenced by this.

Clinical picture

There are three clinical phases of infection in LGV: (1) inoculation and appearance of the primary lesions, (2) lymphatic spread and generalized symptoms, and (3) late complications. In individual cases any one of the phases may be absent or go unnoticed.

The primary lesion, which is transient, appears as a papule, small erosion, or vesicle. The most common sites of the primary lesion are the prepuce and glans in men and the vagina and cervix in women. Since it is painless, the primary lesion may go unnoticed, especially in women. Localized edema may be present. If the rectum is infected, there is a bloody discharge followed by a mucopurulent discharge, diarrhea, and cramping.

Involvement of the lymphatics follows appearance of the primary lesion in 1 to 4 weeks. If the primary lesion is on the penis, anal margin, clitoris, or upper vulva, the superficial inguinal lymph nodes are involved. Infection of the vagina or cervix as the primary site produces involvement of the deep iliac and anorectal lymph nodes. The buboes that appear are firm and lobular. The skin over the superficial nodes is bluish red and adheres to the nodes. The first indication of infection in most patients is a feeling of stiffness and aching in the groin followed by swelling in the inguinal area. Symptoms of nongonococcal urethritis may be present. Constitutional symptoms of infection may or may not appear at this time. The involved lymph nodes may suppurate, causing extensive scarring. Obstruction of the lymphatics may result, leading to chronic edema and ulceration. Lymphatic spread of the infection is accompanied by generalized symptoms that vary. Mild to severe fever, malaise, nausea, and vomiting may occur. Abdominal pain, symptoms of cystitis, and urinary retention are common when pelvic lymph nodes are involved. Acute proctocolitis is common in homosexual men.

Among the most severe complications of LGV are development of perianal abscesses, rectovaginal or rectovesical fistulas, and rectal strictures. In the last clinical phase, generalized infection is indicated by blood values showing anemia, leukocytosis, and elevated sedimentation rate.

LGV is isolated from aspirate from an affected lymph node. The LGV complement-fixation test (LGV-CFT) requires that the organism be isolated in tissue culture and has gained increased use because it is 90% to 95% sensitive.[75] It is a nonspecific test, but it can be titrated, and a rising titer over several weeks is of diagnostic value. Specific tests for LGV, including immunofluorescence and neutralization tests, have been developed, but they are not widely available and have had only limited evaluation for accuracy in diagnosis. A positive LGV-CFT test along with a careful history and physical examination affords the best chances for diagnosing LGV.

Intervention

Early antibiotic therapy is essential for controlling and reducing morbidity from LGV, and it is generally agreed that treatment should not be delayed until diagnostic test results are obtained. Tetracycline in a dosage of 500 mg four times a day for at least 3 weeks is the treatment of choice. If drug sensitivity or pregnancy precludes use of tetracycline, erythromycin, 500 mg four times daily for 2 to 6 weeks, is used. Flocculent lymph nodes may be aspirated to prevent scarring and destruction of lymphatic channels. This is usually done in conjunction with antibiotic therapy. Surgical removal of the lymph nodes is not advised, since this may increase lymphedema and elephantiasis.[150]

If rectal stricture supervenes, rectal dilation at 2-week intervals may be attempted. Development of fistulas is especially distressing and requires that surgical repair be accomplished. LGV is a disease characterized by remissions and exacerbations, and thorough surveillance is important. Antibiotic therapy should be reinstituted as soon as symptoms of reactivation occur. Biopsy of lesions and lymph nodes is advised in chronic cases of LGV, since cancer may develop in the ulcerative lesions and may be overlooked as a result of similarity in appearance.

Chancroid

Epidemiology, etiology, and pathophysiology

Chancroid is a sexually transmitted disease caused by a gram-negative bacillus, *Haemophilus ducreyi*. Although chancroid rarely occurs in the United States, with only about 1000 cases reported annually, there is a need for surveillance to determine an increase in incidence. Although it is found worldwide, chancroid is most prevalent in tropical and semitropical areas in Asia, Africa, and Latin America. The disease occurs more often in men than in women and more often among nonwhite than white people. Repeated references to the relationship between chancroid and the poor, socially deprived, and unhygienic can be misleading. In American troops in Korea the incidence of chancroid was as great as that of syphilis, and in troops in Vietnam chancroid ranked second in incidence to gonorrhea.[180] It is possible that returning military personnel may have introduced the disease into areas where it did not previously exist.

The incubation period varies from 1 to 14 days and averages 4 to 5 days. The primary lesion appears as an inflamed macule that rapidly progresses to vesicle and pustule stages. By the time the patient seeks medical care the lesions have usually become ulcerated. Multiple lesions in various stages of progression may be seen and are caused by rupture of vesicles and pustules and autoinoculation. There may be single or multiple ulcers that are nonindurated and painful. Inguinal lymphadenopathy may or may not be present.

Clinical picture

In women, the lesions of chancroid are most often found on the labia, anus, clitoris, vagina, and cervix. A few women do not have any lesions but may have signs of mild vaginitis. In men the lesions appear on the prepuce, glans, or shaft of the penis.

The ulcers found in chancroid are typically ragged and irregular. They appear excavated, have a granulating, purulent surface, and are painful. Often, edema of the surrounding tissues is present. Involvement of the inguinal lymph nodes occurs in about 50% of all cases of chancroid within 2 weeks after appearance of the primary lesion.[150] The enlarged lymph nodes, called buboes, are most often unilateral, painful, and spheric in shape. The skin over the buboes is inflamed. The buboes tend to become softer as abscesses form. These abscesses in turn may suppurate and rupture, further spreading the infection. Generalized symptoms of infection usually appear when inguinal abscesses form.

Diagnosis of chancroid depends on demonstration of the organism. A specimen is collected by aspiration of

a vesicle, pustule, or lymph node, or from the margin of an ulcer. A gram-stained smear is prepared and visualized by microscopy.

Intervention

Treatment consists of oral sulfonamides given in doses of 1 g every 6 hours for 10 to 14 days. For persons with allergies to sulfonamides, tetracycline, 500 mg four times daily for 7 days, is recommended.

Local therapy for chancroid is beneficial for comfort and prevention of complications. Cleansing the lesions with a debriding solution three times a day aids in removing necrotic tissue and provides comfort as well. In men with ulcers of the glans or prepuce, the prepuce should be retracted during treatment unless there is edema of the prepuce. This site of ulceration may lead to phimosis (p. 1712), requiring circumcision once the lesions are healed. Cleanliness is essential for prevention of secondary infection.

Donovanosis

Epidemiology and etiology

Donovanosis, commonly called granuloma inguinale or granuloma venereum, is believed to be most often transmitted by sexual contact. The infection is caused by a gram-negative bacillus, *Calymmatobacterium (Donovania) granulomatis*, widely referred to as Donovan bacillus. The incubation period is unknown but is estimated to be 8 to 12 weeks.[150]

Donovanosis is common in tropical and subtropical areas and rarely occurs in the United States. It is very common in New Guinea, India, and the Caribbean. The disease, however, is mildly contagious and probably requires repeated exposures for spread of infection. Predisposing factors are poorly understood. The disease is more common in men than women and is especially common among homosexual men.[150]

Clinical picture

In donovanosis lesions appear on the genitalia and in the perianal area. The most common sites of lesions are the prepuce and glans in men and the vagina and labia in women. The infection first appears with development of subcutaneous nodules. These elevated areas eventually ulcerate, producing sharply defined, painless lesions. The ulcers enlarge slowly and bleed on contact. With ulceration, the infection tends to spread along the pubic region. Involvement of the lymph nodes is uncommon but can occur and produce occlusion of the lymphatics, resulting in elephantiasis.

Smears of exudates taken from the lesions do not always demonstrate the causative organism, even when donovanosis is present. Therefore a sample of tissue is taken from the lesion, is crushed between two slides, and is stained. The specimen is examined for the presence of Donovan bodies, which represent the intracellular stage of the causative organism. Examination of a tissue sample also makes it possible to differentiate between donovanosis and cancer.

Intervention

Penicillin is of limited value in the treatment of donovanosis.[150] Tetracyclines are sometimes effective when given in doses of 500 mg orally four times a day for 2 weeks. Resistance to these drugs, however, may develop. If the infection does not respond to tetracyclines, gentamicin, 40 mg daily for 2 weeks, or chloramphenicol, 500 mg three times a day for 2 weeks, is usually effective. If an antibiotic is effective, clinical response is usually evident in a week.

Trichomoniasis

Epidemiology, etiology, and pathophysiology

A protozoan Trichomonas vaginalis, is the causative organism of trichomoniasis. Evidence suggests that the incubation period ranges between 4 and 28 days.[150] Trichomoniasis may well be the most frequently acquired sexually transmitted disease in the United States, with an estimated incidence of 3 million cases occurring annually.[179] The Trichomonas vaginalis organisms are found in 3% to 15% of women under the care of private physicians, 13% to 23% of women attending gynecologic clinics,[150] and 50% of women who have gonorrhea. There is no documentation of the rate at which asymptomatic carriers become symptomatic. Older women who experience changes in vaginal pH often exhibit the disease in the absence of new sexual contact.

Trichomoniasis is frequently viewed as an innocuous infection, yet there are serious implications for health. During the postpartum period in women who have trichomoniasis, the rate of persistent fever, prolonged vaginal discharge, and endometritis is twice as high as in women who do not habor the organism. About 90% of patients with trichomoniasis have cervical erosions and leukorrhea, and it has been suggested that chronic irritation may predispose to cervical cancer. Interpretation of cervical cytology, as in the Pap test, is unreliable in the presence of trichomoniasis, since the infection produces atypical cervical cells. Unless repeated cervical smears are taken, cancer of the cervix may be missed. Trichomoniasis results in urethritis; it also causes prostatitis in men 40% of the time; and, finally, reversible sterility can occur as a result of inhibition of sperm motility by toxins produced by the organism.

Clinical picture

Only 25% of women harboring the organism are asymptomatic. Pruritus of the vulva and vagina is the predominant symptom among women. The itching may be so severe as to awaken the patient, and excoriation from scratching is common. Secondary infection of the broken skin may result.

Classically, the symptoms of trichomoniasis in women are a copious, frothy, green or greenish-yellow vaginal discharge, inflammation of the labia minora and lower vagina, and a red-speckled appearance of the vaginal canal and cervix. A small number of patients present this classic picture, usually presented in texts. Most patients have a vaginal discharge, but it is small in amount and yellow, and there is some inflammation of the labia and vagina. Itching is almost universally present, however, and dyspareunia, dysuria, and urinary frequency may also occur.

In men, urethritis and its symptoms of purulent discharge, itching, burning, and inflammation are the signs of trichomoniasis most often seen. Prostatitis, epididymitis, and urethral stricture may occur as complications among men. However, these consequences of trichomoniasis have not been extensively studied and are not well documented.

Diagnosis of trichomoniasis is most often made by preparing a hanging drop slide containing a specimen of the discharge and observing the motile organism under the microscope. Serologic and skin tests are currently being investigated but lack reliability so far. Because of the high incidence of coexisting gonorrhea, smears or cultures for gonococci should also be taken.

Intervention

The treatment of choice for trichomoniasis is metronidazole (Flagyl), 2 g orally immediately, and if the organisms are resistant, 500 mg twice daily for 5 days is used. In stable relationships, both partners should be treated simultaneously to prevent reinfection by the untreated partner at a later date. Vaginal inserts of metronidazole are less effective. The drug is known to cross the placental barrier, but the effects of metronidazole on the fetus have not been established. Therefore the treatment of choice for pregnant women is a povidone-iodine (Betadine) douche (1 tbsp of Betadine per quart of water). Claims that iodine from the douche causes goiter in the fetus are unsubstantiated.

Candidiasis

Epidemiology, etiology, and pathophysiology

Candidiasis, commonly called monilial infection or monilial vaginitis, is an infection caused by a yeast form,

Candida albicans. The overall incidence of candidiasis in the United States is unknown. There is disagreement about whether yeast infections such as candidiasis should be classed as venereal. The organism is commonly found on mucous membrane surfaces in women who have no symptoms of infection. The greatest incidence of candidiasis occurs during the ages of maximal sexual activity. The causative organism is frequently cultured from the urethra of regular male sexual partners, and urethritis and balanitis (inflammation of the glans penis) occur in up to 10% of men who engage in sexual activity with infected women.[150] Women who respond to therapy and become reinfected are usually married women having one sex partner.

Candida albicans is found in the mouth, gastrointestinal tract, and vagina of 25% to 50% of women. Differentiation between colonization and true infection may be difficult in some cases. Colonization rate and the chance of true infection increase in diabetic persons, during pregnancy, and with diseases or therapies that impair body defenses (use of broad-spectrum antibiotics, corticosteroids, and oral contraceptives).

Clinical picture

Women having symptoms of candidiasis most often complain of pruritus of the vulva. A vaginal discharge that is thick, white, and curdlike is characteristic. The vulva appears inflamed and edematous, and excoriations from scratching are often present. White patches that appear to adhere to the mucosal surfaces are often seen in the vagina. Similar white, curdlike patches appear on the mucous membrane surfaces and tongue in newborn infants infected by the organism, causing a condition known as thrush.

Little is known about candidiasis ocurring among men. Symptoms of balanitis may be present, especially in uncircumcised men. Asymptomatic urethritis occurs in up to 10% of infected men.

Diagnosis may be suspected from the patient's history of predisposing factors and symptoms, but it is usually made by microscopic examination of a smear of the discharge.

Intervention

Therapy consists of nystatin (Mycostatin) vaginal suppositories inserted twice a day for 10 to 14 days. When nystatin fails, one vaginal applicator of clotrimazole, 1% nightly for 7 days is recommended. Men with balanitis should be treated with clotrimazole ointment applied to the glans several times a day. A solution of 1% gentian violet applied to the vagina or gentian violet suppositories have been popular for several years because of the effectiveness of gentian violet. However, because it stains clothing, gentian violet lacks patient acceptance and may not be effective if the patient does not use it as directed.

Gardnerella vaginalis

Etiology

Gardnerella vaginalis (previously known as *Cornyebacterium vaginalis* or *Haemophilus vaginalis*) can be cultured from 23% to 96% of women with vaginitis and is recovered from up to 50% of asymptomatic women.

Clinical picture

Gardnerella vaginalis infection is characterized by a small amount of homogeneous gray or grayish white discharge. The discharge usually has a disagreeable odor, and since it is less irritating than discharges caused by other organisms, pruritus is mild or absent. On inspection, the vaginal walls are slightly reddened and the discharge appears to adhere to the mucosal lining. Some women are asymptomatic despite positive cultures. Diagnosis is confirmed by microscopic examination of a smear or culture of the vaginal discharge.

Intervention

Treatment of *Gardnerella vaginalis* consists of oral ampicillin given four times a day for 5 days; cephalosporin, 500 mg four times a day for 7 to 10 days; tetracycline, 500 mg four times a day for 14 days; or oral metronidazole, 250 mg three times a day for 7 days. Many physicians recommend treating the patient's sexual partner at the same time.

Other sexually transmitted diseases

In addition to those diseases already enumerated, genital warts, hepatitis B infection, pediculosis pubis, and scabies are also considered to be sexually transmitted diseases.

Genital warts (condylomata acuminata) caused by a papilloma virus are the fourth most common sexually transmitted disease in men and the third most common in women. There are approximately 500,000 cases per year in the United States.[179] Genital warts occur in or around the vulva, vagina, cervix, perineum, anal canal, urethra, and glans penis. Their diagnosis is made by clinical appearance or histologic examination. Recommended treatment is podophyllum, 10% to 25% in tincture of benzoin applied weekly, or electrocautery. Recurrences are common. Genital warts enlarge during pregnancy and may cause hemorrhage or obstruction during delivery. They also sometimes undergo malignant change.

Viral hepatitis (see Chapter 33), including A, B, and non-A, non-B, is more prevalent among homosexuals and prostitutes than the rest of the population, and is believed to transmitted by sexual contact.[179]

Pediculosis pubis, also known as "crabs," is caused by pubic lice (p. 1830). Although lice can be transmitted by bedding or clothing they are often transmitted during sexual contact. They produce erythematous, itchy papules. The lice adhere to hair around the pubic area, anus, abdomen, and thighs. Diagnosis is made by observation of lice or microscopic observation of nits at the base of hair. Recommended treatment is 1% Kwell lotion or shampoo. One treatment per episode is necessary, but itching may persist.

Scabies, caused by mites known as *Sarcoptes scabiei,* is transmitted by close body contact, bedding, and clothing (p. 1831). Diagnosis is made from linear burrows, often characterized by a reddened papule containing the mite. Common sites are finger webs, wrists, elbows, ankles, and the penis. Nocturnal itching is common. A one-time use of 1% Kwell shampoo is recommended. Family, household, and sexual contacts should also be treated.

Outcome criteria for the person with a sexually transmitted disease

The person and/or partner can:
1. Explain the etiology and factors contributing to the sexually transmitted disease (STD).
2. State the name, dosage, and schedule of administration of drug therapy as well as its possible side effects.
3. Explain the need for compliance with the entire treatment regimen.
4. State the implications for sexual activity during the infectious stages of the STD.
5. State effects of the STD on the reproductive system of oneself and one's partner.
6. State indications for seeking immediate health care.
7. Explain necessity for treatment of sexual partner or partners.

REFERENCES AND SELECTED READINGS
1. American Cancer Society: 1981 cancer facts and figures, New York, 1981, The Society.
2. American Cancer Society: Report on the cancer-related health check-up, New York, 1980, The Society.
3. American Cancer Society: Clinical oncology for medical students and physicians: a multidisciplinary approach, New York, 1978, The Society.
4. American College of Obstetricians and Gynecologists: Periodic cancer screening for women: statement of policy, Washington, D. C., 1980, The College.
5. American Nurses Association: A report on the hearings on the unmet health needs of children and youth (no.G-140), Kansas City, Mo., 1979, The Association.
6. American Social Health Association: Today's VD control program, New York, 1975, The Association.
7. Ananth, J.: Hysterectomy and depression, Obstet. Gynecol. **52**:524-730, 1978.
8. Baden, M.F., and Baden, E.E.: Cervical incompetence: repair during pregnancy, Am. J. Obstet. Gynecol. **74**:241-245, 1975.
9. Ballon, S.: Gynecologic oncology: controversies in cancer treatment, Boston, 1981, G.K. Hall & Co.
10. Baluk, U., et al.: Health professionals' perceptions of the psychological consequences of abortion, Am. J. Community Psychol. **8**(2):67-75, 1980.
11. Barber, H.: Manual of gynecologic oncology, Philadelphia, 1980, J.B. Lippincott Co.
12. Barrett, F.: Changes in attitudes toward abortion in a large population of Canadian university students between 1968 and 1978, Can. J. Public Health **71**:195-200, 1980.
13. Batata, M.A., et al.: Cryptorchidism and testicular cancer, J. Urol. **124**:382-387, 1980.
14. Benditt, J.: Second-trimester abortion in the United States, Fam. Plann. Perspect. **11**:358-361, 1979.
15. Benedet, J., et al.: Squamous carcinoma of the vulva: results of treatment, 1938-1976, Am. J. Obstet. Gynecol. **134**:201-207, 1979.
16. Berger, M., and Goldstein, D.: Impaired reproductive performance in DES-exposed women, Obstet. Gynecol. **55**:25-27, 1980.
17. Berkowitz, R., et al.: Psychological and social impact of gestational trophoblastic neoplasia, J. Reprod. Med. **25**:14-16, 1980.
18. Berkus, M., and Daly, J.: Cone biopsy: an outpatient procedure, Am. J. Obstet. Gynecol. **137**:953-958, 1980.
19. Betts, J., and Buttram, V.: A plan for managing endometriosis, Contemp. Obstet. Gynecol. **15**:121-129, 1980.
20. Blaustein, A.: Pathology of the female genital tract, New York, 1976, Springer-Verlag New York, Inc.
21. Block, M.F., and Rahhal, D.K.: Cervical incompetence: a diagnostic and prognostic scoring system, Obstet. Gynecol. **47**:279-281, 1976.
22. *Blount, J.H., Darrow, W.W., and Johnson, R.E.: Venereal disease in adolescents, Pediatr. Clin. North Am. **20**:1021-1033, 1973.
23. *Bouchard, R., and Owens, N.F.: Nursing care of the cancer patient, ed. 4, St. Louis, 1980, The C.V. Mosby Co.
24. *Brown, L.: Toxic shock syndrome, M.C.N. **6**:57-59, 1981.
25. Brown, Z., and Stenchever, M.: Genital herpes and the FTA-ABS, Obstet. Gynecol. **51**:186-187, 1978.
26. Bygdeman, M.: Comparison of prostaglandin and hypertonic saline for termination of pregnancy, Obstet. Gynecol. **52**:424-429, 1978.
27. Callahan, D.: Abortion and government policy, Fam. Plann. Perspect. **11**:275-279, 1979.
28. *Campbell, C., and Herten, R.: VD to STD: redefining venereal disease, Am. J. Nurs. **81**:1629-1634, 1981.
29. Carr, M., Hanna, L., and Jawetz, E.: Chlamydiae, cervicitis and abnormal Papanicolaou smears, Obstet. Gynecol. **53**:27-30, 1979.
30. *Char, W.J.: Abortion and acute identity crisis in nurses, Am. J. Psychiatry **128**:66-71, 1975.
31. Chlamydial infection in neonates, Briefs **43**:157-158, 1979.
32. Cohen, C.J., and Gusberg, S.B.: Screening for endometrial cancer, Clin. Obstet. Gynecol. **18**:27-39, 1975.

*References preceded by an asterisk are particularly well suited for student reading.

33. *Confer, D.J., and Beall, M.E.: Evolved improvements in placement of the silicone gel prosthesis for post-prostatectomy incontinence, J. Urol. **126**:605-608, 1981.

34. *Cosper, B., Fuller, S., and Robinson, G.: Characteristics of posthospitalization recovery following hysterectomy, J.O.G.N. Nurs. **7**:7-11, 1978.

35. Creasman, W.T., and Weed, J.C.: Screening techniques in endometrial cancer, Can **38**(suppl.):436-440, 1976.

36. *Cronewett, L.R., and Choyce, J.M.: Saline abortion, Am. J. Nurs. **71**:1754-1757, 1971.

37. *Crosson, K.: A patient teaching aid for the pelvic exenteration patient, Oncol. Nurs. Forum **8**:53-56, 1981.

38. Cumes, D.M., et al.: Complications of ^{125}iodine implantation and pelvic lymphadenectomy for prostatic cancer with special reference to patients who had failed external beam therapy as their initial mode of therapy, J. Urol. **126**:620-622, 1981.

39. Cunanan, R., Courey, N., and Lippes, J.: Complications of laparoscopic tubal sterilization, Obstet. Gynecol. **55**:501-516, 1980.

40. Curran, J.: Economic consequences of pelvic inflammatory disease in the United States, Am. J. Obstet. Gynecol. **138**:848-851, 1980.

41. Cutler, S.J., and Young, J.: Third national cancer survey: incidence data. National Cancer Institute monograph no. 41. DHEW pub. no. (NIH) 75-787, Washington, D.C., 1975, U.S. Government Printing Office.

42. *Darrow, W.W.: Approaches to the problem of venereal disease prevention, Prev. Med. **5**:165-175, 1976.

43. *Darrow, W.W.: Changes in sexual behavior and venereal diseases, Clin. Obstet. Gynecol. **18**:255-267, 1975.

44. David, H., et al.: Postpartum and postabortion psychotic reactions, Fam. Plann. Perspect. **13**:88-89, 1981.

45. *Davis, A.: Competing ethical claims in abortion, Am. J. Nurs. **80**:1359, 1980.

46. Davis, J., et al.: Toxic shock syndrome: epidemiologic features, recurrence, risk factors, and prevention, N. Engl. J. Med. **303**:1429-1435, 1980.

47. Del Regato, J.A.: Cancer of the prostate, J.A.M.A. **235**:1727-1730, 1976.

48. *Dewhurst, J.E., and Weeks, A.R.: Occult manifestations of septic abortion, Nurs. Mirror **142**:62-63, 1975.

49. Dimowski, W.P., and Cohen, M.R.: Treatment of endometriosis with an antigonadotropin, danazol: a laparoscopic and histologic evaulation, Obstet. Gynecol. **46**:147-154, 1975.

50. DiSaia, P.J., et al.: Synopsis of gynecologic oncology, New York, 1975, John Wiley & Sons, Inc.

51. DiSaia, P.J., and Creasman, W.T.: Clinical gynecologic oncology, St. Louis, 1981, The C.V. Mosby Co.

52. Dosoretz, D.E., et al.: Megavoltage irradiation for pure testicular seminoma: results and patterns of failure, Cancer **48**:2184-2190, 1981.

53. Droegemueller, W., Weinstein, L., and Milzer, G.: Low-dose prostaglandins for second-trimester abortion, Contemp. Obstet. Gynecol. **15**:19-23, 1980.

54. Duenholter, J.H., and Gant, N.F.: Complications following prostaglandin $F_{2\alpha}$-induced midtrimester abortion, Obstet. Gynecol. **46**:247-250, 1975.

55. Eaton, A.C.: The safety of transrectal biopsy of the prostate as an outpatient investigation, Br. J. Urol. **53**:144-146, 1981.

56. Effer, S.: Gynecologic aspects of the "routine" checkup, Postgrad. Med. **59**:164-170, 1976.

57. Ekman, E.P., and Edsmyr, F.: Chemotherapy in nonseminomatous testicular tumors, stage I, Br. J. Urol. **53**:184-187, 1981.

58. Emans, S., and Goldstein, D.: Pediatric and adolescent gynecology, Boston, 1977, Little, Brown & Co.

59. Eschenbach, D.: Recognizing chlamydial infections, Contemp. Obstet. Gynecol. **16**:15-30, 1980.

60. *Faulkner, W.L., and Ory, H.W.: Intrauterine devices and acute pelvic inflammatory disease, J.A.M.A. **235**:1851-1853, 1976.

61. Felman, J., and Nikitas, J.: Nongonococcal urethritis: a clinical review, J.A.M.A. **245**:381-386, 1981.

62. *Finch, J.: Law and the nurse. V. From all points of view: the legal position of the nurse in relation to abortion practice, Nurs. Mirror **153**(1):29-30, 1981.

63. Fisher, R., and Goodpasture, H.: Toxic shock syndrome in menstruating women, Ann. Intern. Med. **94**:156-163, 1981.

64. Flesh, G., et al.: The intrauterine contraceptive device and acute salpingitis, Am. J. Obstet. Gynecol. **78**:402-408, 1979.

65. *Fogel, C.I., and Woods, N.F.: Health care of women: a nursing perspective, St. Louis, 1981, The C.V. Mosby Co.

66. Forrest, D., et al.: Abortion in the United States, 1977-1978, Fam. Plann. Perspect. **11**:329-335, 1979.

67. Fred Hutchinson Cancer Research Center, Cancer Control Program: Self breast and testicular exam (grant no. 2 R18 CA 16404), Seattle, 1980, Cancer Control Program.

68. Freeman, E., et al.: Emotional distress patterns among women having first or repeat abortions, Obstet. Gynecol. **55**:630-636, 1980.

69. Friedman, C.M., Greenspan, R., and Mittleman, F.: The decision-making process and the outcome of therapeutic abortion, Am. J. Psychiatry **131**:1332-1337, 1974.

70. Galask, R.P., Larsen, F., and Ohm, M.J.: Vaginal flora and its role in disease entities, Clin. Obstet. Gynecol. **19**:61-81, 1976.

71. *Gardner, H.: Herpes genitalis: our most important venereal disease, Am. J. Obstet. Gynecol. **135**:553-554, 1979.

72. Gibbs, R.S., and Weinstein, A.J.: Puerperal infection in the antibiotic era, Am. J. Obstet. Gynecol. **124**:769-787, 1976.

73. *Goldman: L.: Anorchia. In Kauffman, J.J.: Current urologic therapy, Philadelphia, 1980, W.B. Saunders Co.

74. Graduate education, gonorrhea: CDC recommended treatment schedules, 1979, Obstet. Gynecol. **55**:255-258, 1980.

75. Greenhill, J.P.: The nonsurgical management of vaginal relaxation, Clin. Obstet. Gynecol. **15**:1083-1097, 1972.

76. Greenwald, E.F.: Ovarian tumors, Clin. Obstet. Gynecol. **18**:61-86, 1975.

77. Grimes, D., and Cates, W.: The brief for hypertonic saline, Contemp. Obstet. Gynecol. **15**:29-38, 1980.

78. Grimes, D., and Cates, W.: Complications from legally-induced abortion: a review, Obstet. Gynecol. Surv. **34**:177-191, 1979.

79. Grimes, D., Cates, W., and Tyler, C.: Comparative risk of death from legally induced abortion in hospitals and nonhospital facilities, Obstet. Gynecol. **51**:323-326, 1978.

80. Gromko, L.: Intrauterine devices, Nurse Pract. **5**(5):17-20, 1980.

81. Grossman, R., et al.: Management of genital herpes simplex infection during pregnancy, Obstet. Gynecol. **58**:1-4, 1981.

82. Hacker, S., et al.: Factors influencing the success of a community VD program held in a university facility, Public Health Rep. **95**:247-252, 1980.

83. Hale, R.W., et al.: Office termination of pregnancy by "menstrual aspiration," Am. J. Obstet. Gynecol. **134**:213-218, 1979.

84. *Hall, R.E.: The Supreme Court decision on abortion, Am. J. Obstet. Gynecol. **116**:1-8, 1973.

85. Harrison, J.H., et al.: Campbell's urology, ed. 4, vol. 1, Philadelphia, 1978, W.B. Saunders Co.

86. Harrison, J.H., et al.: Campbell's urology, ed. 4, vol. 2, Philadelphia, 1979, W.B. Saunders Co.

87. Hauerwas, S.: Abortion: why the arguments fail, Hosp. Prog. **61**:38-49, 1980.

88. *Heath, M.: The abortion debate: nurses for LIFE, Nurs. Times **75**:2145-2146, 1979.

89. Heller, M.: The gay bowel syndrome: a common problem of homosexual patients in the emergency department, Ann. Emerg. Med. **9**:487-493, 1980.

90. Herpes on delivery, Emerg. Med. **12**:105-108, 1980.
91. Hodgson, J.E., and Portmann, K.C.: Complications of 10,453 consective first-trimester abortions: a perspective study, Am. J. Obstet. Gynecol. **120**:802-807, 1974.
92. Hoke, A.: Sexually transmitted diseases, chancroid, LGV, and GI, part of the VD differential (pictorial), Consultant **19**:128-129, 1979.
93. Holmes, K., et al.: Chlamydial genital infections: a growing problem (pictorial), Hosp. Pract. **14**:(12)105-110, 1979.
94. Howe, B., et al.: Repeat abortions: blaming the victims, Am. J. Public Health **69**:1242-1246, 1979.
95. IUD users may have higher risk of contracting PID, Fam. Plann. Perspect. **12**:206-208, 1980.
96. *Iveson-Iveson, J.: Prevention: how to stay healthy. X. Risks of promiscuous sexual activity, Nurs. Mirror **149**(20):24-25, 1979.
97. Jelovsek, F., et al.: Risk of exogenous estrogen therapy and endometrial cancer, Am. J. Obstet. Gynecol. **137**:85-91, 1980.
98. Johannisson, G., Lowhagen, G., and Lycke, E.: Genital *Chlamydia trachomatis* infection in women, Obstet. Gynecol. **56**:671-675, 1980.
99. Kahan, R.S., Baker, L.D., and Freeman, M.G.: The effect of legalized abortion on morbidity resulting from criminal abortion, Am. J. Obstet. Gynecol. **121**:114-116, 1975.
100. *Kane, F.J., Jr., et al.: Motivational factors in abortion patients, Am. J. Psychiatry **130**:290-293, 1973.
101. Kauffman, J.J., editor: Current urologic therapy, Philadelphia, 1980, W.B. Saunders Co.
102. Kauffman, J.J.: The silicone-gel prosthesis for the treatment of male urinary incontinence, Urol. Clin. North Am. **5**:393-404, 1978.
103. Kaufman, D., et al.: Intrauterine contraceptive device use and pelvic inflammatory disease, Am. J. Obstet. Gynecol. **136**:159-162, 1980.
104. Kaufman, R.H., et al.: Upper genital tract changes and pregnancy outcome in offspring exposed in utero to diethylstilbestrol, Am. J. Obstet. Gynecol. **137**:299-308, 1980.
105. Kessler, I.I.: Perspectives on the epidemiology of cervical cancer with special reference to the herpesvirus hypothesis, Clin. Orthop. **99**:1091-1110, 1974.
106. Kessler, I.I., and Aurelian, L.: Uterine cervix cancer. In Schottenfeld, D.: Cancer epidemiology and prevention: current concepts, Springfield, Ill., 1975, Charles C Thomas, Publisher.
107. Kramer, M., et al.: Self-reported behavior patterns of patients attending a sexually transmitted disease clinic, Am. J. Public Health **70**:997-1000, 1980.
108. Kraus, S.J.: Complications of gonococcal infection, Med. Clin. North Am. **56**:1115-1125, 1972.
109. *Kuczynski, H.: Pros and cons of douching: the nurse's role in counseling, J.O.G.N. Nurs. **9**:90-93, 1980.
110. Kursh, E.D.: Traumatic torsion of testicle, Urology 1981 **17**:441-442, 1981.
111. Larsen, B., and Galask, R.: Vaginal microbial flora: practical and theoretic relevance, Obstet. Gynecol. **55**(suppl.):100-113, 1980.
112. Lindheim, B.: Services, policies and costs in U.S. abortion facilities, Fam. Plann. Perspect. **11**:283-289, 1979.
113. Loffer, F., and Pent, D.: Pregnancy after laparoscopic sterilization, Obstet. Gynecol. **55**:643-648, 1980.
114. Lupfer, M., et al.: How patients view mandatory waiting periods for abortion, Fam. Plann. Perspect. **13**:75-79, 1981.
115. Mack, T.M., et al.: Estrogens and endometrial cancer in a retirement community, N. Engl. J. Med. **294**:1262-1267, 1976.
116. MacMahon, B.: Risk factors for endometrial cancer, Gynecol. Oncol. **2**:122-129, 1974.
117. Maine, D.: Special report: NAF sets sights on quality care, Fam. Plann. Perspect. **11**:303-304, 1979.
118. Malkosian, G., Annegers, J., and Fountain, K.: Carcinoma of the endometrium: stage 1, Am. J. Obstet. Gynecol. **136**:872-888, 1980.
119. Maunes, P., et al.: Early diagnosis of neonatal syphilis: evaluation of a gamma M-fluorescent treponemal antibody test, Am. J. Dis. Child. **120**:17-21, 1970.
120. Mardh, P.: An overview of infectious agents of salpingitis, their biology, and recent advances in methods of detection, Am. J. Obstet. Gynecol. **138**:933-951, 1980.
121. Marrs, R., et al.: Disappearance of human chorionic gonadotropin and resumption of ovulation following abortion, Am. J. Obstet. Gynecol. **135**:731-736, 1979.
122. Martin, D.C.: Testis (editorial), J. Urol. **124**:388, 1980.
123. Martin, L.: Health care of women, Philadelphia, 1978, J.B. Lippincott Co.
124. McDaniel, S., et al.: Estimates of the rate of illegal abortion and the effects of eliminating therapeutic abortion, Alberta 1973-74 Can. J. Public Health **70**:393-398, 1979.
125. McGowan, L.: Gynecologic oncology, New York, 1978, Appleton-Century-Crofts.
126. McGowan, L.: Cytologic methods for the detection of endometrial carcinoma, Gynecol. Oncol. **2**:272-278, 1974.
127. *McLoughlin, M.G.: Obstructive sterility. In Kauffman, J.J.: Current urologic therapy, Philadelphia, 1980, W.B. Saunders Co.
128. Meheus, A.: Surveillance, prevention, and control of sexually transmitted disease, Am. J. Obstet. Gynecol. **138**:1064-1070, 1980.
129. Meisels, A.: Is condyloma virus a potential human oncogen? Contemp. Obstet. Gynecol. **16**(3):99-106, 1980.
130. Miles, P.: Sexually transmissible diseases: fourteen sexually transmissible diseases currently recognized by the Center for Disease Control, Atlanta, Georgia, J.E.N. **6**(3):6-12, 1980.
131. Nahimas, A., et al.: Perinatal risk associated with maternal genital herpes simplex virus infection, Am. J. Obstet. Gynecol. **110**:825-837, 1971.
132. Nahmias, A., et al.: Infection of the newborn with herpes-virus hominis, Adv. Pediatr. **17**:185-226, 1970.
133. Nahmias, A.M.L., Naib, Z.M., and Josey, W.E.: Epidemiological studies relating genital herpetic infection to cervical carcinoma, Clin. Orthop. **99**:1111-1117, 1974.
134. Nathanson, C., et al.: Obstetricians' attitudes and hospital abortion services, Fam. Plann. Perspect. **12**:26-32, 1980.
135. Novak, E.R., Jones, G.S., and Jones, H.W., Jr.: Novak's textbook of gynecology, ed. 10, Baltimore, 1980, The Williams & Wilkins Co.
136. Novak, E.R., and Woodruff, J.D.: Novak's gynecologic and obstetric pathology with clinical and endocrine relations, ed. 7, Philadelphia, 1974, W.B. Saunders Co.
137. Oill, P.: Herpesvirus type 2 infection of the genital tract, J.E.N. **6**(3):13-16, 1980.
138. Olson, M.: Helping staff nurses care for women seeking saline abortions, J.O.G.N. Nurs. **9**:170-174, 1980.
139. Ory, H., et al.: Contraceptive choice and prevalence of cervical dysplasia and carcinoma in situ, Am. J. Obstet. Gynecol. **124**:573-577, 1976.
140. Panayotou, P.P.: Induced abortion and ectopic pregnancy, Am. J. Obstet. Gynecol. **114**:507-510, 1972.
141. Pantelakis, S.N., Stefanos, C.G., and Doxiadis, S.A.: Influence of induced and spotaneous abortions on the outcome of subsequent pregnancies, Am. J. Obstet. Gynecol. **116**:799-805, 1973.
142. Pasquale, S., et al.: A dose-response study with Monistat cream, Obstet. Gynecol. **53**:250-253, 1979.
143. Payton, T., and Beilman, A.A.: Caring for the urologic surgery patient. In West, R.S., Waring, K.S., and Lawson, P.K.: Implementing urologic procedures, Horsham, Pa., 1981, Nursing '81 Books, Intermed Communications, Inc.

144. *Pettyjohn, R.: Health care of the gay individual, Nurs. Forum 18:366-393, 1979.

145. *Raisler, J.: Abortion 1980: battleground for reproductive rights, J. Nurse Midwife. 25(2):23-27, 1980.

146. Rawls, W.E., Gardner, E., and Herman, L.: Herpes genitalis: venereal aspects, Clin. Obstet. Gynecol. 15:913-917, 1972.

147. Rawls, W.E., Gardner, H.L., and Kaufman, R.L.: Antibodies to genital herpes virus in patients with carcinoma of the cervix, Am. J. Obstet. Gynecol. 107:710-716, 1970.

148. Rees, E.: The treatment of pelvic inflammatory disease, Am. J. Obstet. Gynecol. 138:1042-1047, 1980.

149. Reid, E.P.: Rh sensitization following abortion, Can. Med. Assoc. J. 111:1182, 1974.

150. Rein, M.F., and Chapel, T.A.: Trichomoniasis, candidiasis, and the other minor venereal diseases, Clin. Obstet. Gynecol. 18:73-88, 1975.

151. Renaer, M., et al.: Psychological aspects of chronic pelvic pain in women, Am. J. Obstet. Gynecol. 134:75-80, 1979.

152. Ridenour, N.: Chlamydia, Nurse Pract. 5(5):45-48, 1980.

153. Robins, J., and Surrago, E.: Alternatives in midtrimester abortion induction, Obstet. Gynecol. 56:716-722, 1980.

154. *Rodriguez, D.B.: The problem for the nurse. In Von Eschenbach, A.C., and Rodriguez, D.B.: Sexual rehabilitation of the urologic cancer patient, Boston, 1981, G.K. Hall & Co.

155. Rosenfeld, D., and Bronson, R.: Reproductive problems in the DES-exposed female, Obstet. Gynecol. 55:453-456, 1980.

156. Rosoff, J.: Judge Dooling's decision: ". . . allied to her right to be," Fam. Plann. Perspect. 12:4-8, 1980.

157. *Ross, T.: The abortion debate: facing up to reality, Nurs. Mirror 150(4):40-41, 1980.

158. Rothman, C.M., Newmark, H., and Karson, R.A.: The recurrent varicocele: a poorly recognized problem, Fertil. Steril. 35:552-556, 1981.

159. Rudolph, A.H., and Price, E.V.: Penicillin reactions among patients in venereal disease clinics: a national survey, J.A.M.A. 223:499-501, 1973.

160. Saral, R., et al.: Acyclovir prophylaxis of herpes-simplex virus infections: a randomized, double-blind, controlled trial in bone marrow transplant recipients, N. Engl. J. Med. 305:63-67, 1981.

161. Sarvis, B., and Rodman, H.: The abortion controversy, New York, 1973, Columbia University Press.

162. Saxena, B.B., and Landesman, R.: The use of radioreceptor assay of human chorionic gonadotropin for the diagnosis and management of ectopic pregnancy, Fertil, Steril. 26:397-404, 1975.

163. Schenker, J.G., Eyal, F., and Polishuk, E.J.: Fertility after tubal pregnancy, Surg. Gynecol. Obstet. 135:74-76, 1972.

164. *Scouller, A., et al.: The abortion debate: nurses for a woman's right to choose, Nurs. Times 75:2144-2145, 1979.

165. Seibel, M., Freeman, M., and Graves, W.: Carcinoma of the cervix and sexual function, Obstet. Gynecol. 55:484-487, 1980.

166. Seims, S.: Abortion availability in the United States, Fam. Plann. Perspect. 12:88-91, 1980.

167. *Servantius, D., et al.: Easing the shock of radical vulvectomy, Nurs. '75 5:26-31, 1975.

168. Shands, K., et al.: Toxic shock syndrome in menstruating women: association with tampon use and *Staphylococcus aureus* and clinical features in 52 cases, N. Engl. J. Med. 303:1436-1442, 1980.

169. Sherman, A., and Brown, S.: The precursors of endometrial carcinoma, Am. J. Obstet. Gynecol. 135:947-956, 1979.

170. Shives, V.: Coping with a miscarriage, Parents 55:56-59, Nov. 1980.

171. Silverberg, E., and Holleb, A.: Cancer statistics, 1975, Cancer 25:8-21, 1975.

172. Smith, D.R.: General urology, ed. 9, Los Altos, Calif., 1978, Lange Medical Publishers.

173. Termination of pregnancy by medical induction: new DHSS guidelines, Midwives Chron. 93:112-113, 1980.

174. Thompson, S., et al.: The microbiology and therapy of acute pelvic inflammatory disease in hospitalized patients, Am. J. Obstet. Gynecol. 136:179-186, 1980.

175. Toffe, R., and Williams, D.: Toxic shock syndrome: clinical and laboratory features in 15 patients, Ann. Intern. Med. 94:149-155, 1981.

176. Trandel-Korenchuk, D., et al.: Minor consent in birth control and abortion. I, Nurse Pract. 5(2):47-49, 1980.

177. Tsuang, M.T., Weiss, M.A., and Evans, A.T.: Transurethral resection of the prostate with partial resection of the seminal vesicle, J. Urol. 126:615-617, 1981.

178. Ulfelder, H.: The stilbestrol-adenosis-carcinoma syndrome, Cancer 38(suppl.):426-431, 1976.

179. U.S. Department of Health, Education and Welfare, Public Health Service: Summary and recommendations of the National Institute of Allergy and Infectious Diseases study group on sexually transmitted diseases, Bethesda, Md. 1980, National Institute of Allergy and Infectious Diseases.

180. U.S. Department of Health, Education and Welfare, Public Health Service: Chancroid, donovanosis, lymphogranuloma venereum, DHEW pub. no. (CDC) 75-8302, Atlanta, 1975, Center for Disease Control.

181. U.S. Department of Health and Human Services, Public Health Service: STD fact sheet edition 35, HHS pub. no. (CDC) 81-8195, Atlanta, 1981, Center for Disease Control.

182. Von Eschenbach, A.C., and Rodriguez, D.B.: Sexual rehabilitation of the urologic cancer patient, Boston, 1981, G.K. Hall & Co.

183. Vordermark, J.S., et al.: The testicular scan use in diagnosis and management of acute epididymitis, J.A.M.A. 245:2512-2514, 1981.

184. Walker, A., and Jick, H.: Declining rates of endometrial cancer, Obstet. Gynecol. 56:733-736, 1980.

185. Whitehead, S.L.: Nursing care of the adult urology patient, New York, 1970, Appleton-Century-Crofts.

186. Widdicombe, J., et al.: Abortion: legal, medical and social perspectives, Fam. Commun. Health 2:17-28, Nov. 1979.

187. Winter, C.C., and Morel, A.: Nursing care of patients with urologic diseases, ed. 4, St. Louis, 1977, The C.V. Mosby Co.

188. Wright, C.S., Campbell, S., and Beazley, J.: Second-trimester abortion after vaginal termination of pregnancy, Lancet 1:1278-1279, 1972.

189. *Yarborough, B.: Teaching plan for the patient undergoing total pelvic exenteration, Oncol. Nurs. Forum 8:36-40, 1981.

190. Zarins, O.: Thoughts on abortion, Midwives Chron. 92:425, 1979.

191. Ziel, H.K., and Finkle, W.D.: Increased risk of endometrial carcinoma among users of conjugated estrogens, N. Engl. J. Med. 293:1167-1170, 1975.

CHAPTER 66

PROBLEMS OF THE BREAST

BARBARA C. LONG
DORIS M. MOLBO

The breasts are associated functionally with the reproductive system as an organ for milk production in the postpartum woman. The female sex hormones influence the development of the breasts and the production of milk (and the specific hormone prolactin). The breasts are also associated with feelings of sexuality and are an integral component of sexual behavior. The development of the breasts in the female adolescent indicates to her the approach of womanhood and emphasizes her femininity. The breasts, especially the nipples, which are erectile tissue, are erogenous areas in sexual activity. The advertising media emphasizes the desirability of the female breast; femininity is typified by a fashion model's curved breasts, whereas masculinity is typified by the flat, expansive chest of the lifeguard. Diseases of the breast therefore evoke varied feelings and cause fears and concerns that influence the practice of breast self-examination or the seeking of diagnostic and therapeutic care without delay.

The most common diseases of the breast are dysplasia (fibrocystic disease), fibroadenoma, cancer, and infections. Although these diseases occur primarily in women, *they can also occur in men*. Cancer requires the most extensive nursing care and is discussed in greater detail than the other diseases.

Malignancies of the breast

Nurses play a vital role in regard to cancer of the breast. Their responsibilities include (1) educating women so that breast cancer may be discovered and treated early; (2) caring for the patient who has had primary therapy for the cancer; (3) assisting the patient with physical and emotional rehabilitation; and (4) caring for and assisting the patient when metastasis has occurred and adjuvant therapy, chemotherapy, hormonal therapy, or irradiation is needed.

Currently, major changes are being made in the modes of treatment and rehabilitation for the person with breast cancer. Nurses therefore have two additional and important responsibilities: (1) nurses must feel a real commitment to read and to keep current with the imminent controversies and actual changes taking place in the whole field of breast cancer so that the implications for women are understood; (2) nurses are expected to be able to explain to the woman the many options she has heard about, differing detection methods, primary therapies, options for reconstructive surgery, and other rehabilitative resources. This often also means assisting the woman to most effectively discuss these issues with her physician and to be able to ask those necessary questions so that wise choices for her future are made. Women today read current and accurate information about breast cancer in magazines and other publications. Nurses cannot be less informed. Since breast cancer is not one disease, the nurse can also assist a woman to accept the physician's professional advice that considering *her* disease all options may not be appropriate or adequate for her.

Epidemiology

The cancers of the breast, carcinoma and sarcoma, are the most common malignancies in women and the leading cause of *cancer* mortality in women, as well as the leading cause of death in women aged 40 to 50 years. It is estimated that 1 out of 11 women in the United

States will develop cancer of the breast, and the probability increases with age. The chance of a 70-year-old woman developing breast cancer is six times greater than that of a 40-year-old woman. The American Cancer Society estimates that 112,000 new cases will be discovered in the United States yearly and that 37,300 women will die from the disease. The incidence of breast cancer has been increasing by 1% per year for at least the last 10 years; there has been a steeper rise for women under 40 years of age.[7] In black women breast cancer has surpassed cervical cancer as the most frequent cancerous site.

The mortality for cancer of the breast in the United States has remained about the same for the past 40 years, with the rate fixed at 26 to 27 per 100,000. The present 5-year survival rate for all patients with cancer of the breast, whether treated or untreated, is approximately 68%. This low survival rate is caused in part by the frequent failure to detect the early lesion and the delay in seeking medical treatment as soon as a lesion is discovered. Studies show that approximately 88% of all women treated when the lesion appears localized have a 5-year life expectancy compared with 52% for those with obvious regional involvement at the time of treatment.[7] As with any malignancy, however, survival at the end of 5 years cannot be considered synonymous with cure. Lower survival rates for black women have been attributed to the later stage of disease at diagnosis. The average size of a breast tumor at diagnosis in black women is 5.5 cm. Tumors that are 1 cm or smaller are present at diagnosis in 21% of white women; only 8.3% of black women present with such minimal-sized lesions.[33,51]

Breast cancer occurs in both premenopausal and postmenopausal women; peak incidence occurs between ages 45 and 49 and at age 65. It must be stressed, however, that when the comparison is made between the number of diagnosed breast cancer patients of a certain age and the total number of women in the population of that age, the resulting ratio will show a steady rise in incidence as age increases (e.g., 1 of every 420 women aged 45 years has breast cancer; 1 of every 110 women aged 70 years has breast cancer[44]) (Fig. 66-1). In addition, breast cancer is not one disease but many, depending on the tissue of the breast involved, its estrogen dependency, and the age at onset. Premonopausal breast malignancy is different from postmenopausal malignancy. Treatment response and prognosis differ with all malignancies.

Causes of breast cancer are not known but appear to include a number of factors rather than just one. High-risk factors are those factors that increase the possibility that breast cancer will occur. Whites have a slightly higher incidence of breast cancer than blacks, especially postmenopausal disease. The obese, hypertensive, diabetic person also appears to have a higher risk. When

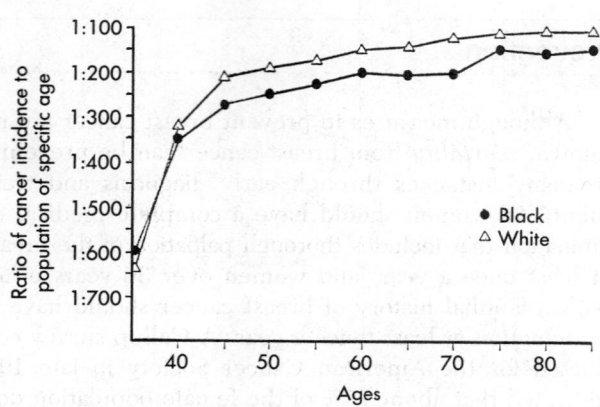

Fig. 66-1. Ratio of breast cancer incidence to age-specific populations by 5-year cohorts. (Based on National Cancer Institute data, 1975. From Carnevali, D., and Patrick, M.: Nursing management for the elderly, Philadelphia, 1979, J.B. Lippincott Co.)

breast cancer occurs in the male, it is usually after 55 years of age.

Breast-feeding or breast injury does *not* influence the incidence of breast cancer. Often a neoplasm is discovered after a minor injury was already present, but the woman had not previously examined herself. A palpable hematoma could result from trauma, however. Preparations of estrogen for menopausal symptoms do not increase the potential for the development of breast cancer but can accelerate preexisting cancer. Whether or not estrogen preparations are used with at-risk women will be a decision reached between the patient and her physician.

Prognosis

Favorable prognosis in cancer of the breast depends on early diagnosis, the type of cancer present, host factors, and complete therapeutic destruction or removal of all tissues containing malignant cells before metastasis occurs. It is estimated that approximately one third of all patients who seek medical attention for cancer of the breast are incurable at the time of the initial examination. This is particularly true of black women; stage II disease is present at the time of diagnosis in 32% and stage III is present in 29% of these women.[33] Breast malignancy in men also is often found and diagnosed at a later stage. Since the disease develops in a relatively accessible part of the body, it is unfortunate that early diagnosis is not made more often so that more lives might be saved. At the present time, the American Cancer Society acknowledges the several primary therapies: surgery of a varying extent and radiation therapy, as well as chemotherapy or hormonal manipulation used in combination.

Prevention

Although measures to prevent breast cancer are not known, *mortality* from breast cancer can be prevented in many instances through early diagnosis and treatment. All women should have a complete medical examination that includes thorough palpation of the breasts at least once a year, and women over 30 years of age with a familial history of breast cancer should have an examination at least twice a year. A Gallup survey conducted for the American Cancer Society in late 1977 indicated that about 75% of the female population does have an annual breast examination by a physician. However it was reported at the International Conference on Cancer in Black Populations that only 10% of black women have regular breast examinations by physician.[51] The lack of examination is more prevalent among older women, poorly educated women, low-income women, and black women. For those in low-income levels, health-seeking services are on a crisis priority. The elderly also refrain from annual checkups in the absence of symptoms. Further, the message to black women and to white and black elderly women has been inadequately delivered. Neither blacks nor the elderly population are aware of the rising incidence of breast cancer in their populations and the need for vigilance by each woman personally and by her health provider. The most accessible tool to detect early breast lesions is breast self-examination.

Women should be taught that the prognosis for cancer of the breast is much better *if the cancer is discovered early and treatment instituted immediately*. Although 90% of all breast cancers are discovered by self-examination, many are not reported for several months. Fear of mutilation or of death are the two main reasons why some women delay seeking medical advice and treatment and hesitate to risk confirmation of their fears when a tumor is discovered. Publicized national statistics on death from cancer of the breast or a relative or a friend who died from the disease causes the fear to be even more acute. Unfortunately, the average woman may tell only her closest friends when a breast cancer has been successfully treated. As a result, deaths from the disease are much better known than cures with no recurrence. A National Cancer Institute study has found that black women fear breast cancer more than any other disease and that both black and Hispanic women are more concerned about the changes in their lives that breast cancer would cause than were the white women studied.[51] Some women wish to avoid the expense or embarrassment of an examination, or they rationalize that their trouble would appear trivial to the busy physician. Sometimes instead they seek the advice of nurses. It then becomes the responsibility of the nurse to stress the urgency of getting medical advice at once. The pub-

licized mastectomies of prominent women in recent years and their continued activity in life has encouraged other women to obtain breast examinations.

In an attempt to improve and assess the relative effectiveness of early detection of breast cancer, the National Cancer Institute and the American Cancer Society in 1973 jointly funded 27 screening centers around the country to provide free diagnostic services to a population of presumed asymptomatic women. The objective of the program was to evaluate the ability of mammography, thermography, and palpation to find *early* breast cancers. A decision was made in 1977 to continue the nationwide screening project despite the controversy over the use of roentgenography examinations used in the screening process (p. 1745). The screening centers during the first 3 years of the project detected 1800 breast cancers in 280,000 women examined. The program did demonstrate that screening for early breast cancer is feasible and valuable.

Breast self-examination

All women, beginning with high school age, should know how to carry out breast self-examination and should practice this monthly as a health habit. The 1973 Gallup survey reported that only 18% of the 1000 women sampled carried out monthly breast examinations. This was attributed to lack of knowledge of the importance of and the method for doing breast self-examination and fears concerning possible findings.[23] More recent studies in compliance have revealed that despite being taught breast self-examination, women state they do not know what they are feeling.[64]

In response to the finding that women are confused by the lumpiness of their breasts, or that they cannot know whether they have a pathologic lump each month or not, a new teaching approach to breast self-examination was begun in 1976. Called the Breast Health Program, and initiated in Seattle and Washington state, it emphasizes a positive health approach and individually teaches each woman to distinguish her own healthy breast tissues from month to month. If she feels something that she knows is not her normal tissue, she confidently contacts her physician. A high rate of monthly breast self-examination compliance (81%) has been achieved with this program.[5] (Specific details may be obtained from address given in the references.)

Nurses working in the hospital or community settings have the responsibility of teaching women how to examine their breasts and of explaining why it is necessary. When working with groups of women, arrangements can be made with the American Cancer Society or the local health department for showing movies developed for the general public describing the traditional method of self-examination. Specialized volunteers from the American Cancer Society, nurses, and other health care providers have been trained and certified in the

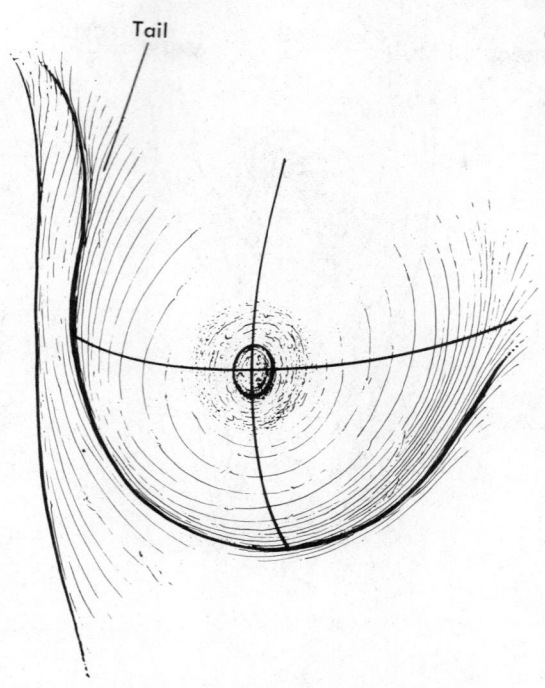

Tail

Fig. 66-2. Breast mass includes "tail" that extends from upper, outer quadrant toward axilla. (From Malasanos, L., et al.: Health assessment, ed. 2, St. Louis, 1981, The C.V. Mosby Co.)

traditional teaching of breast self-examination to the public. The nurse follows through by teaching the women the actual breast self-examination and by answering questions. The woman then practices palpation of lumps on models of the breast.

Self-examination of the breasts should be done regularly *each month*. The best time is at the conclusion of or a few days following the menstrual period. Some women have engorgement of the breast premenstrually, and the breasts normally may have a lumpy consistency at the time. This condition usually disappears a few days after the onset of menstruation. Because of this possible change, it is important that the breasts be examined at the same time each month in relation to the menstrual cycle. Women who have passed the menopause should examine their breasts at a set time each month.

There are several approaches that can be followed when carrying out breast self-examination. All approaches follow these general guidelines: (1) the approached used is systematic; (2) the entire breast tissue is examined, including the tail (Fig. 66-2) and the nipple; (3) examination is carried out in both the horizontal and vertical body positions; and (4) the flat parts of the fingers are used for palpation.

There are essentially three different approaches that are most commonly employed for breast self-examination: (1) dividing the breast into quadrants and examining the area in each quadrant from the outer perim-

eter toward the nipple, (2) palpating the inner half and then the outer half of the breast, or (3) palpating in concentric circles beginning at the outer rim of breast tissue and moving toward the nipple (Fig. 66-3). The method of approach suggested by the American Cancer Society is described in Fig. 66-3.

Some women need help in learning self-examination; they may, for example, feel a rib when examining the medial half of the breast and become alarmed. However, most women learn the technique of palpation quite readily. If a lump of any kind is discovered, it should not be rubbed or touched excessively. It should be left alone, and the advice of a physician should be sought at once. It is therefore important for women to be taught to discriminate the normal texture of glandular and fat tissues from that which feels different.

It will be interesting to see if women will be less reluctant to perform self-examination of their breasts and seek medical advice concerning lumps in the breasts now that cancer of the breast has received such widespread publicity in the United States and now that the women's movement stresses self-health and awareness of one's body. Rosenstock[57] states that a person will take a medication or will practice a health procedure if (1) it is important to her to do it, (2) she can learn it, and (3) she is confident in her ability to do it. Many women report that they do breast self-examination not at all or infrequently because they are not confident that they

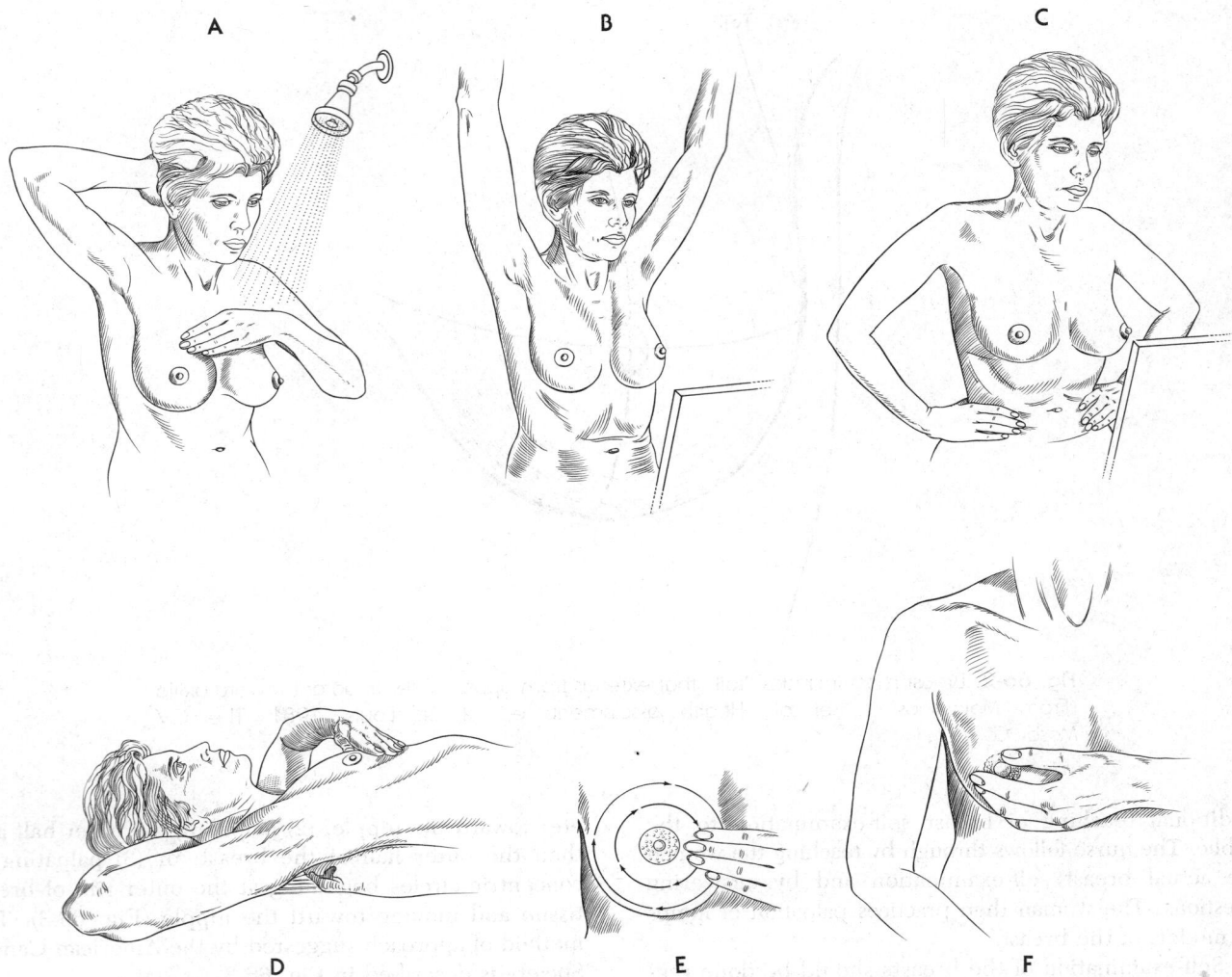

Fig. 66-3. Breast self-examination. **A,** Examine breasts during bath or shower since flat fingers glide easily over wet skin. Use right hand to examine left breast and vice versa. **B,** Sit or stand before a mirror. Inspect breasts with hands at sides then raised overhead. Look for changes in contour or dimpling of skin. **C,** Place hands on hips and press down firmly to flex chest muscles. **D,** Lie down with one hand under head and pillow or folded towel under that scapula. **E,** Palpate that breast with other hand using concentric circle method. It usually takes three circles to cover all breast tissue. Include the tail of the breast and the axilla. Repeat with other breast. **F,** End in a sitting position. Palpate the areola areas of both breasts, and inspect and squeeze nipples to check for discharge.

are competent enough to carry out this monthly responsibility.[5,64]

Assessment

Subjective data

If the woman is at high risk for breast cancer (see box on p. 1745), it is important to ascertain her knowledge of risk factors, breast self-examination practices, and feelings concerning breast cancer. This data pro-

vides a base for health teaching and exploring of feelings. *All* women should be questioned concerning their knowledge and practices related to monthly breast self-examination.

If the client has been suspected of or diagnosed as having a breast tumor that is or may be malignant, the following additional data is obtained as a baseline for planning:

1. Identification of family relationships and the existence and availability of support persons
2. Usual coping mechanisms

HIGH-RISK FACTORS ASSOCIATED WITH BREAST CANCER

Sex	Female (99% in women)
Age	Over age 50 (80% over age 35)
Familial history	Mother/sister, especially with premenopausal or bilateral breast cancer
Parity	First live birth after age 30, or nullipara
Personal history	Primary breast cancer (7 times risk for a second primary cancer in breast)
	Uterine cancer
	Benign breast disease
	Menarche before age 11
	Menopause after age 50

---

3. Feelings and thoughts about her own sexuality and the relationship of the breast to these feelings
4. Thoughts about feelings of sex partner (if appropriate) concerning forthcoming diagnostic procedures or potential therapy options
5. Future goals, life expectancies, zest for living, actual or perceived responsibilities to others

If possible, data is obtained from the sex partner (if appropriate) regarding his feelings about the forthcoming surgery. This identifies possible conflicts in perceptions, the degree of support that can be anticipated from the sex partner, and the potential effects of the partner's feelings on the client's adaptation and relationships.

Objective data

The woman's breasts are inspected to determine size and symmetry, contour, and appearance of the skin. Although there is often some difference in breast size, that is, the left breast may be smaller than the right, they usually are relatively symmetric. Variations in breast contour may include the presence of masses, dimpling, or flattening. The color of the skin, presence of thickened areas, or abnormalities of the venous pattern may be indicative of a pathologic condition. The nipple may be inverted; this is usually not pathologic unless it has not been previously present; the direction in which the nipples are pointing may provide clues to masses. Discharge from the nipple may be indicative of an abnormal condition; a clear fluid resembling colostrum may be present in certain women with monthly hormonal fluctuation. Nipple discharges unrelated to lactation should be evaluated by the physician without delay. Ul-

cerated areas and other lesions of the nipple require further exploration.

The only early sign of cancer of the breast is a small palpable mass. It is the primary sign of 90% of women with breast cancer. Dimpling of the skin, puckering of the skin, changes in the color of the skin over the lesion, alteration in the contour of the breast, distortion of the nipple, serous or bloody discharge from the nipple, and unusual scaling or inversion of the nipple are signs that the lesion is well established and has invaded surrounding tissues. (An infrequent but very aggressive breast malignancy, inflammatory carcinoma, invades the mammary lymphatics early and presents as a totally edematous, red, hot breast. In the absence of mastitis associated with lactation, the woman should be *quickly* referred to her physician. Currently, radiation therapy is the primary therapy and is begun immediately.) In the advanced phases of neglected cases there may be ulceration of the skin and underlying tissue with subsequent infection of necrotic tissue. Spread to the axillary lymph nodes occurs early. Because of the distribution of lymph vessels, malignant cells may spread rapidly with metastasis to bone, lung, or brain. Discovery of enlarged lymph nodes or pain in the ribs or vertebrae may be the first indication to the patient that anything is wrong, particularly when the lesion is deep in the breast tissue or routine monthly breast self-examination or medical palpation of the breast has not been carried out. It is now believed that the finding of a subsequent malignancy in the contralateral or ipsilateral breast is a primary tumor rather than a metastatic one and that the subsequent malignancy was probably present at the time of the first malignancy but was undetectable because of size or location.

Diagnostic tests

Mammography is an x-ray examination of the breast used to detect early lesions before they are palpable (Fig. 66-4). Early cancers are often easily seen on the developed films as small densities with stippled calcifications within. Mammography is about 80% to 97% accurate in detecting early breast cancer. Mammography does have limitations, particularly in the penetration of dense breasts as in adolescents, young nulliparous women, or women with large breasts.

Controversy still exists concerning the use of mammography as a screening device for women under 35 years of age. The routine screening of women under age 50 by mammography is questioned by some authorities including the National Cancer Institute because of the increased hazard of radiation carcinogenesis.[44] The American Cancer Society, however, has asserted that improved mammography techniques have decreased radiation dosage to low levels and that the positive potential for diagnosing breast cancer is considerably greater than the inherent risk. Mammography is recommended

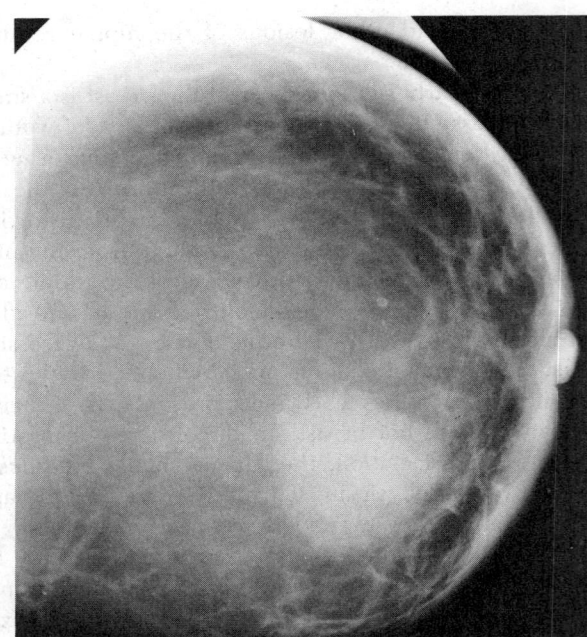

Fig. 66-4. Mammogram of patient with area of density indicating carcinoma. (From Cramer, L.M., and Lapayowker, M.S.: Applied anatomy of the female breast: surgical, radiographic, and thermographic. In Masters, F.W., and Lewis, J.R., Jr., editors: Symposium on aesthetic surgery of the face, eyelid, and breast, vol. 4, St. Louis, 1972, The C.V. Mosby Co.)

by the American Cancer Society for women in whom breast cancer is suspected and for high-risk women regardless of age. Further, annual mammography is recommended for all women over age 50. *Guidelines for the Cancer-Related Checkup: Recommendations and Rationale* should be in the possession of all nurses. It can be obtained free from the American Cancer Society.

Xeroradiography (Fig. 66-5) is a variation of mammography. In xeroradiography an aluminum plate with an electrically charged selenium layer is used in the place of the familiar black and white mammogram x-ray film. It is exposed in the usual manner using special mammoradiographic equipment. The resulting film is blue and white.

Thermography is a less valuable screening device. In this procedure an infrared scanner is used to measure the heat emissions coming from the breast. Abnormal variations in an area because of increased vascularization may indicate the presence of benign or malignant neoplasm. It is infrequently used in the United States because of the high numbers of false-positive results.

Ultrasonography (ultrasound) is currently being evaluated for its possible value in detecting lesions in the dense breasts of young women. Although ultrasonography can differentiate the presence of a cystic mass, it does not indicate calcium deposits or tissue configu-

rations, factors that are considered important in diagnosis and that are readable in mammograms. The future value of ultrasonography is yet undetermined.

The only way to determine conclusively whether a tumor is benign or malignant is by microscopic examination of a section of the tumor obtained by *biopsy* (p. 488). Rarely, a palpable axillary node may be excised for microscopic study. Most surgeons believe that if there is the slightest possibility of cancer, it is safer to remove the entire tumor mass. Pieces of a tumor are seldom removed surgically because of the release of malignant cells into the blood and lymphatic systems at the time of the operation.

The success of mammography (and xeroradiography) to detect early nonpalpable lesions or to detect areas of calcification results in more and earlier biopsies. Sometimes the small size makes location of the lesion difficult or uncertain when biopsy is attempted. Therefore to locate areas for surgical biopsy a small methylene blue dye marker is made within the area of the breast using a syringe and needle during mammographic monitoring. This is done in the diagnostic radiography department a few hours before the surgical biopsy, and the marker is made with the patient under local anesthesia. No color disfiguration is apparent on the breast surface as a result of this procedure, but it ensures that the biopsy tissue corresponds to the site identified by mammogram. This procedure requires preinstruction to the patient and support in the radiology department. To the woman it is not routine, but a "tagging of the enemy within," during which she is consciously involved. Denial here is very difficult; the woman feels very helpless and vulnerable.

Until recently the most common approach has been to remove the tumor and examine a frozen section of the tissue under the microscope. If the tumor was found to be malignant, the surgical setup was completely changed, and the more extensive operation was performed. In this approach to surgery, when the patient went for a biopsy, she did not know in advance whether it was necessary for the breast to be removed or the extent of surgery that would be performed.

An increasing number of surgeons are now scheduling the patient for a biopsy alone. The patient then goes home and awaits the biopsy results. She thus has time to make decisions and prepare herself psychologically for the more extensive surgery if a malignancy is found. The disadvantage of this approach is the stress of waiting for the diagnostic results and then facing the prospect of a repeat hospital admission and a second surgical procedure. In the Gallup survey of 1973, 47% of the women indicated they would prefer to sign the consent for surgery along with the consent for biopsy (the first approach described above), while 48% would prefer the second approach in order to get other opinions (20%) or to discuss the situation after diagnosis

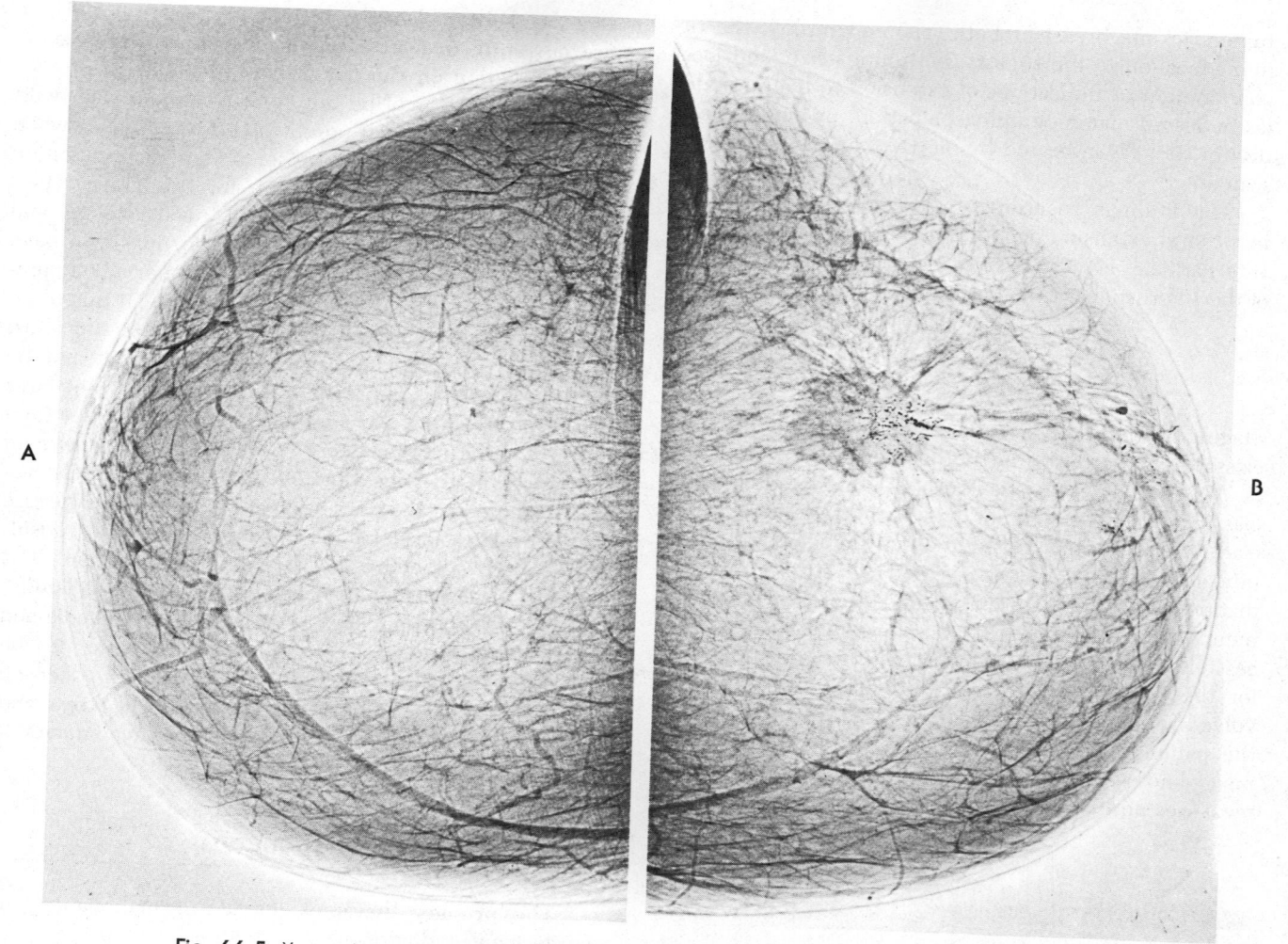

Fig. 66-5. Xeroradiographs. **A,** Normal left breast. **B,** Right breast shows mass with spiculated margins characteristic of neoplasm. (Courtesy University Hospitals of Cleveland.)

(28%).[23] Since today there are not only several surgery options to be considered but also a therapy option that is nonsurgical, these figures may not reflect current thought. A National Cancer Institute study in 1980 reported 41% of white women would consent to a mastectomy at the time of biopsy, but 55% would want the two-stage biopsy and treatment decision making (the latter figure 52% for Hispanic women and 48% for black women).[44] It is believed that there is an understandable difference between a young woman's choice and an older woman's choice in this matter as well.

In either of the above approaches, after excision of the tumor masses the pathologist will send tissue to a special laboratory for determination of estrogen receptors (estrogen receptor assay test [ERA]). Such studies are helpful in future management of the patient. The hormone assay test (ERA) identifies those breast cancers that are hormone dependent; that is, their growth is stimulated by estrogen. Postmenopausal women have a higher incidence of hormone-dependent breast cancers. Later treatment such as removal of the ovaries (oophorectomy) or endocrine chemotherapy (hormonal therapy) or adrenalectomy (see Chapter 25) removes the source of estrogen and thereby can retard growth and spread of the tumor. A negative ERA indicates that the breast cancer is not hormone dependent and therefore reduction of estrogen production is of no consequence to the later course of the malignancy.

Therapy planning

The therapy to be proposed to the patient is planned and based on a number of factors: the tissue involved and indications of its aggressiveness (histopathology of the biopsy specimen); the hormonal milieu, that is, premenopausal, postmenopausal, estrogen dependent (history and ERA); the identification of multifocal primary tumors in one breast or both (mammography); the tumor's location in the breast; the tumor's size; and local containment or indications of extension to lymph nodes (as indicated mammography, palpation, or biopsy) or to distant sites (as indicated by biopsy, bone scan, or liver scan).

The findings regarding tumor size, node involvement, and extension or metastasis are expressed by the International TNM Classification (a result of the work of the International Union against Cancer [UICC] where

$$T = \text{Tumor size}$$
$$N = \text{Node involvement}$$
$$M = \text{Metastasis}$$

Staging of the breast malignancy incorporates the TNM classification as shown in the box below.[27]

When the diagnostic work is completed and the classification of the tumor has been made, the physician, often with the consultation advantages of the hospital tumor board members (medical, surgical and radiation oncologists), discusses and proposes the treatment protocol by which the tumor would be most successfully destroyed and which offers the best prognosis for the patient. The patient and family are often involved at some point in this treatment decision plan. If the patient is not involved, she should request to be made knowledgeable of the findings of the diagnostic measures and of the determinations considered in set-

ting the therapy plan now being described to her. There are currently many treatments for breast malignancy. Yet depending on the factors known about her tumor (p. 1747), there may be only one treatment plan with no alternative plans and no options. (For example, when inflammatory carcinoma is present, immediate radiation therapy is *the specific treatment* for this grave type.) However, if the malignancy is small, nonaggressive, and present in a young woman, she may, for instance, have several options for therapy, which offer her a comparable prognosis with the knowledge available at this time. Every woman should realize, however, that the latest therapy written up in magazines may or may not be *best* for her. If it is not best for her or does not have the same advantages as another therapy offers, it is then not an option for her decision making. Nurses have an advantage in assisting a patient to understand these factors involved in the decision making from the expertise of the medical professional but still taking into consideration the subjective hesitations of the woman. The roles of teacher and advocate to both patient, family, and physician are important today when both media and medical professionals voice controversial issues in the treatment of breast malignancy. Although decision making is always difficult during periods of stress and crisis, for the woman today with a breast malignancy it has never been harder.

Primary therapy interventions

The primary therapies for breast malignancy are surgery and radiation.

Surgery

Surgery in the past has been the treatment of choice unless extensive metastasis has occurred or the tumor is very large, ulcerated, and inoperable.

Types of surgery. Different types of surgeries can be performed:

1. *Lumpectomy:* simple removal of the tumor mass
2. *Partial mastectomy:* removal of the tumor mass and 2.5 to 7.5 cm (1 to 3 in.) of surrounding tissue
3. *Subcutaneous mastectomy (adenomammectomy):* removal of all underlying breast tissue, leaving skin, areola, and nipple intact
4. *Simple mastectomy:* removal of entire breast but not axillary lymph nodes
5. *Modified radical mastectomy:* complete removal of breast and pectoralis minor and removal of some axillary lymph nodes
6. *Radical mastectomy:* complete removal of breast, axillary lymph nodes, pectoralis muscles (minor and major), and adjacent fat and fascia
7. *Extended radical mastectomy (supraradical):* same

STAGING AND TNM CLASSIFICATION

Stage 1 T_1 (tumor 2 cm or less)
         N_0 (no palpable axillary nodes)
         M_0 (no evident metastasis)

Stage 2 T_0 (no palpable tumor)
         T_1 (tumor 2 cm or less)
         T_2 (tumor less than 5 cm)
         N_1 (palpable axillary nodes with histologic evidence of breast malignancy)
         M_0

Stage 3 T_3 (tumor more than 5 cm; may be fixed to muscle or fascia)
         N_1 or N_2 (fixed nodes)
         M_0

Stage 4 T_4 (tumor any size with fixation to chest wall or skin; presence of edema, including peau d'orange; ulceration; skin nodules; inflammatory carcinoma)
         N_3 (supraclavicular or intraclavicular nodes or arm edema)
         M_1 (distant metastasis present or suspected)

as radical mastectomy plus removal of parasternal lymph nodes[70]

Recently, there has been considerable professional controversy in lay periodicals and in medical journals about the surgical treatment of cancer of the breast. It is suggested by some that a lumpectomy is sufficient to treat small cancers of the breast and that a mastectomy is not necessary. At this time there is insufficient data to compare survival rates or the instance of metastatic disease for lumpectomy vs. simple or modified radical mastectomy.

A *modified* radical mastectomy is often performed for early, well-localized, small lesions of the breast. It offers comparable therapy prognosis to the classic radical mastectomy. In the *radical* mastectomy the judgment of the surgeon regarding the amount of overlying skin that can safely be left to cover the defect determines whether a skin graft will be necessary. Preoperatively, the surgeon may order the skin of the anterior surface of one thigh shaved and prepared surgically in case the need for a graft should arise. If the lesion is located in the medial quadrant of the breast, particularly the upper medial quadrant, an *extended* radical mastectomy may be performed, since lesions of the medial quadrant tend to metastasize to the internal mammary chain of lymph nodes. A *simple* mastectomy sometimes is performed if cancer is believed to be limited to the breast or as a palliative measure to remove an ulcerated cancer of the breast in disease that is known to be advanced.

Radiation therapy

Radiation therapy is the specific primary therapy of choice for inflammatory carcinoma and is also chosen as therapy for those whose physical condition could not tolerate anesthesia and surgery.

For the past 8 years, Bonnadonna and others in Europe have been doing a two-stage radiation therapy procedure for women with stage I or stage II disease. The therapy is done after biopsy of the lesion (and sometimes the axillary nodes) is performed. As an outpatient, the woman is given external beam therapy to the breast daily (Monday through Friday) for 5 weeks. This is followed by a hospitalization period of 3 or 4 days when iridium needles are implanted in the breast under anesthesia. They are removed in 2 or 3 days, and the therapy is concluded. The data collected and reported by these European oncologists seem to show similar therapy results for the modified radical surgery *when* comparable-sized lesions and aggressiveness of tissue are compared.[2,35] It must be remembered, however, that treatment data are not yet available to tell us the comparative survival rate over 10 years or the incidence of metastasis or additional primary cancers after this radiation therapy protocol. This treatment protocol is now being given in various parts of the United States,

most often in connection with one of the cancer research centers. It seems to be gaining the attention and enthusiasm of many U.S. oncologists and their patients.[2,20]

Adjuvant therapy

Today there are many combination therapies given to women with breast malignancies. Since many of the therapy protocols are under study by regional cancer research groups, the specific timing of the therapies in use, or the specific cytotoxic agent or agents and dosage in chemotherapy or hormonal therapy, may vary in different parts of the country. It is important therefore to know what protocols are being used in your region. It is also necessary to keep *current* in this knowledge. The burgeoning field of oncology and especially the growing amount of information within the area of breast malignancy require professionals to assume responsibility for reliable and current reading sources. Thus in general today, chemotherapy may be given after surgery, chemotherapy may be given after radiation therapy, there may be a combination of all three modes of therapy, or hormonal therapy may also be used. This complex therapeutic planning is rationally based on those factors cited on p. 1747 as well as clinical indicators as the patient passes through the prescribed therapy or therapies.

Patient care for primary therapies

Surgery

PREOPERATIVE CARE. Since much emphasis is placed on the breast as a symbol of attractiveness, the thought of losing a breast becomes almost intolerable to many women. This is particularly true of those who depend largely on physical attractiveness for their work, for example, models, to hold the esteem of others and to secure gratification of their emotional needs. Psychologists have pointed out that there is a symbolic connection between the breasts and motherhood that is severely threatened when a breast must be removed. It is understandable that women may be seriously threatened emotionally by the loss of a part of the body that is so closely associated with sexual attractiveness and motherliness. Cancer of the breast often occurs at the menopause or soon after when some women feel that they have lost much of their sexual attractiveness. Surgical removal of the breast may save a woman's life, but it also may cause her to feel less feminine.

Although she may try to conceal fear, any woman who is hospitalized for removal of a breast tumor is always anxious, and some may be in a state of near panic. Most of the fears are related to sexual acceptance, social isolation, disfigurement, recurrence, and death. Many of these women have been unable to discuss their worries and feelings with their significant others, including their spouse. The nurse can help the patient to express feelings and can help her to understand what breast surgery means to her as a person. The woman who is having breast surgery has a special need to feel understood and accepted by all persons who are giving preoperative care.

Simple explanations with repetition may decrease the patient's fear of the unknown. If it seems that the patient does not fully comprehend the surgeon's explanation, as the surgeon discusses the diagnosis and treatment with the patient and significant others the nurse can repeat the explanation and report this to the surgeon, who in turn can talk with the patient again and clarify any misconceptions, alleviating needless anxiety. Since attention span, memory, and perception are limited when anxiety levels are high, it is helpful if the nurse can be present when information is given to the patient. The nurse can then repeat, reinforce, or clarify given information.

The American Cancer Society sponsors a volunteer program, Reach to Recovery, in which the patient has an opportunity to visit with a woman who has had a mastectomy. This encourages the patient, and she will receive practical help from someone who has made a satisfactory adjustment to the same operation. Although most of the patient visits by the volunteer from Reach to Recovery occur during the postoperative period, preoperative visits may be very helpful to some women and can be requested.

Additional testing may be done. If a diagnosis of a malignancy is almost a certainty, x-ray examinations such as bone, lung, or liver scans or liver function studies may be ordered to rule out the possibility of metastases to these areas of the body or as baseline data for the future. Preparing the patient for procedures that will take place before and after surgery is of utmost importance in allaying her fears as well as in setting the stage for successful rehabilitation.

Preoperative teaching should include the following information if a mastectomy is planned: a dressing may be applied to the incision, and a catheter attached to suction may be used. The arm will be elevated. The woman should practice sitting up and turning to the side opposite the proposed surgery by *pushing* up on the unaffected elbow. Postoperative exercises will be started early.

POSTOPERATIVE ACTIVITY AND EXERCISE. If the breast is removed, there will be a tendency for the shoulder to droop on that side because of the inequality of weight; this can be prevented by close attention to posture and a properly weighted and fitted prosthesis. Exercises will be taught postoperatively to help maintain posture and to strengthen muscles. Telling the patient about the exercises helps to give her the feeling that there is something in the situation that she can control and contribute to, and thus she will begin to have a positive attitude toward rehabilitation. There will always be some vigilance required of her in protecting the arm on the

side of the surgery. This will begin postoperatively as she too monitors that no blood pressure or blood drawing or injections are done on that arm. It is easier to prevent lymphedema than to treat it.

Arm measurements are taken by the nurse *preoperatively* as baseline data; these measurements are also taken *postoperatively*, and the patient will continue to take them monthly. Measurements are made with a tape measure at the olecranon, at 6 in. above and at 6 in. below the olecranon. These measurements should be taken in both arms and the findings recorded in a permanent portion of the patient's record.

It is often possible for the nurse to prepare the patient for the visits of resident or attending physicians, the anesthesiologist, the laboratory technicians, the hospital chaplain, and various nursing staff on the night before surgery or the morning before surgery. The patient then can also plan some time for her family or those significant to her.

POSTOPERATIVE CARE

Wound care. Following the completion of the mastectomy and closure, a stab wound may be made and a catheter inserted and attached to a low constant suction, such as that provided by a Hemovac (see Fig. 24-12) or other low-suction system. The purpose of the catheter is to remove blood and serum that may collect under the skin flaps and that would prevent healing and predispose the woman to infection. The Hemovac must be checked frequently and emptied when half full to maintain constant suction through the catheter and prevent buildup of fluid under the skin flaps. There is usually no drainage from around the incision when a catheter is draining properly. The catheter may be clamped for short periods of ambulation and is usually removed within 3 to 5 days or when the amount of drainage is less than 5 to 10 ml in 24 hours.

At one time pressure dressings rather than a catheter were used to prevent the accumulation of fluid under the skin. Many surgeons now believe that the use of a catheter and a smaller dressing is preferable to the use of a large pressure dressing. This corresponds to the change from the radical procedure to the modified radical procedure.

The dressing is checked often for the first few hours to detect hemorrhage or excessive serous oozing. The bed clothes under the patient must be examined for blood that may flow down from the operated region. Any evidence of bleeding is reported to the surgeon. If the wound is not covered with a dressing, a cradle may be used to protect it from the bed covers. The arm is usually elevated on a pillow. Signs of circulatory obstruction, such as swelling and numbness of the lower arm or inability to move the fingers, must be reported at once. Any dressings should not be loosened without specific instruction from the surgeon.

Dressings may be removed in 24 hours, or they may

not be changed for several days after the operation. The skin sutures are often removed on the sixth to the eighth postoperative day. Usually this is after the patient's discharge from the hospital.

If a graft has been taken from the thigh, this area may be covered with a firm pressure dressing or fine mesh gauze and the wound exposed to the air. The patient may complain of severe discomfort in this donor site as soon as she recovers from anesthesia.

Comfort. Pain in the operated area also may be referred to the affected arm or shoulder. Sensations of numbness and tingling over the chest that is painful may cause her to take short, shallow breaths. She should be kept comfortable with analgesics and a cough–deep breathe routine started. Each chest excursion may painfully discourage compliance. The empathic nurse works *with* the patient.

When the patient recovers from the effects of anesthesia, she is usually only comfortable lying on her back with the head end of the bed elevated. If the operated arm is not incorporated in the dressing, the arm is elevated to enhance circulation and prevent edema. The pillows are arranged so that the hand is higher than the arm and the arm is above the level of the right atrium. *No blood pressure readings, injections, or blood testing* should be done on the *affected* arm because of potential circulatory impairment or infection (to prevent lymphedema). A sign or tape should be placed on this side of the bed with this message. The patient and family should be taught to be firm and aggressive in refusing procedures to the arm. The patient will be more comfortable sitting up straight during back care, since turning toward the affected side will be exceedingly painful and place pressure on the area. To turn to the opposite side and to sit up, she should be taught to *push up on the elbow of the unaffected side* rather than pull up. *She should lie down by using that arm in the same way.*

Nutrition. During the initial postoperative period of metabolic (adrenergic and mineralocorticoid) readjustment to the anesthesia and surgery the patient probably will have little interest in food (1 to 1½ days). Relief that the surgery is over will collide with the impact of the nature of the surgery and its meaning to her. For some women the assurance of removal of the malignancy will counterbalance the change in breast size and contour or total absence of the breast or breasts. For others, grieving focuses on these results of the surgery. Such depression becomes superimposed on the same period postoperatively (mineralocorticoid period) when, normally, the patient feels down, tearful, introspective, and socially disinterested. Thirst would be assuaged; hunger, somewhat thought about, if even present; appetite absent.

During this period the goals of nutrition for wound healing and esthetics for the feminine patient can be combined in *small* trays containing a *very nourishing* beverage, soup, or dessert, not all given at once but offered at short, *unexpected* intervals. The tray cover, a colorful napkin, a flower, or a note from the family not only restores to this patient protein nourishment but also reattaches her to the love of her family and friends *and* the realization that she still responds to gifts of beauty and surprise in a very feminine way.

In the wisdom of the body's conservation, wound healing has priority for all utilization of nutrients and energy. When the next postoperative metabolic (glucocorticoid) phase is reached (only in the absence of infection), the nurse can emphasize through teaching the importance of balanced nutrition and she can assess and discuss with the patient her menu choices while she is hospitalized. Nutrition is *very* important to the cancer patient in treatment and after treatment (no matter what modality), and it has been found that nutrition beneficially influences the success of the therapeutic outcome when optimal nutrition was present before therapy and maintained during therapy. For the woman who has the primary therapy of surgery to be followed by chemotherapy, nutrition is especially important. For the woman who has surgical biopsies, to be followed by radiation therapy, wound healing and therefore good nutrition are imperative. Excellent cookbooks for cancer patients are available free from the National Cancer Institute. *Something's Got to Taste Good*[62] is in most public libraries, and a cookbook by Aker and Lesson[1] is available at nominal cost from the Hutchinson Cancer Center, Seattle. Nutrition introduced, learned, and reinforced during the initial therapy experience should be a patient care goal. Patients should be introduced at that time also to the literature available.[45]

Energy. In the first few days after any surgery, energy reserve is accepted by patient, family, and staff to be limited and transitory. When the patient is also greatly grieving, lack of energy reserve is even more apparent. This must be acknowledged by staff and explained to family. One mastectomy patient cannot be compared to another.

During these 1 or 2 days of quick fatigue, more ambulation is required and increasing exercise expected. It is during this time that the nurse teaches the patient to plan for and to anticipate those time spans when energy will be needed. The nurse teaches the patient to conserve her energy for what is required, to recognize the early signs of tiredness that are uniquely hers, and the importance of stopping activity *before fatigue*. When the patient becomes fatigued, she is energy bankrupt and, closely following, emotionally distraught. Fatigue is unnecessary and detrimental. To be tired is to appreciate the support of a chair or the rest offered by a bed after the woman has achieved her *realistic* activity or exercise or social visiting goals for that time period. After rest she is motivated to continue again.

A more difficult time to tolerate decreased energy

reserves begins about the third postoperative day and extends for about a 5- to 6- week period. During this glucocorticoid phase, the patient begins making and receiving more phone calls. She bathes and dresses and prepares her hair and face and hands as she is accustomed to. This *costs energy*. She walks further, talks and visits with others, has visitors come to see her, and plays hostess: cost of energy. She still grieves: cost of energy. She eats and has the dressing changed and the catheter removed: cost of energy. She views the surgical site: cost of energy. She exercises, hears about prostheses, and considers going home: cost of energy. This time in the hospital and extending to 6 weeks postoperatively can be discouraging *if* the woman is not prepared during this time to know that her energy now is more available. She feels better and better, but *it is normal* that her energy is capricious. Realistic plans, short tasks, and single interests and endeavors are necessary, all interspersed with planned rest periods. It is a pitfall of the period for her to feel she is not up to expectations, that something is wrong and that she should not wilt so suddenly in the midst of activity. This is very important patient teaching to patient and family members alike. The priority of the body resources is for healing. She can initiate and partake in more and more energy-using activities, but this energy is limited until healing is fully completed.

Sleep at night should be facilitated in the hospital, with rest or sleep periods during the day. It is, however, important that she establish a distinct day-night activity and sleep routine and that she gives this priority when she goes home as well. Sleeplessness or 3 AM awakening with insomnia is often symptomatic of grieving and can be a rewarding time for the night nurse to practice crisis intervention.

Activity and exercise. Exercises are essential to prevent shortening of muscles, stiffness, and contracture of the shoulder girdle and to preserve muscle tone so that the affected arm can be used without limitations. To prevent additional deformities, exercises should be bilateral ones with the patient using both arms simultaneously. When specific postoperative exercises should be started will depend on the extent of the operation and whether skin grafting has been necessary. This can be a commonly shared knowledge between doctor and nurse, and the *skilled* nurse can anticipate when exercises can begin.

Slings are to be avoided. Gentle exercises started early in the postoperative course help decrease muscle tension as well as regain muscle function more quickly. Usually the patient is encouraged to flex and extend her fingers immediately on return to her room. She should also be encouraged to pronate and supinate her forearm; simply turning the palm up and down will do this. Squeezing a rubber ball is often started on the first postoperative day. Brushing the teeth and hair are en-

couraged later but as soon as they can be tolerated. The patient is encouraged under close supervision to exercise each day more and more to the limits of incisional pulling and pain. A specific exercise schedule planned by nurse and patient together is imperative. It is an important aspect of nursing care to this patient.

Continuing exercises are shown in the box below. With exercise, full range of motion will return; that is, both arms can be extended equally high above the head. This will not be achieved before the patient leaves the hospital; therefore the patient must learn and be motivated in the hospital so she will continue exercises at

---

POSTMASTECTOMY ARM EXERCISES*

Exercise: Climbing the wall

1. Stand facing wall with toes close to wall.
2. Bend elbows and place palms of hands against wall at shoulder level.
3. Move both hands parallel to each other up the wall as far as possible until incisional pull or pain occur.
4. Move both hands down to starting position.
5. Goal is complete extension with elbow straight.
6. Activities that utilize the same action: reaching top shelves, hanging out clothes, washing windows, hanging curtains, setting hair.

Exercise: Arm swinging

1. Bend forward from waist, permitting both arms to relax and hang naturally.
2. Swing arms together left to right (motion comes from shoulder).
3. Swing arms in circles parallel to floor, clockwise and counterclockwise.
4. Stand up slowly.

Exercise: Rope pull

1. Attach a rope over a shower rod or hook.
2. Grasp each end of rope, alternately pulling on each end, raising affected arm to a point of incisional pull or pain.
3. Shorten rope over time until affected arm is raised almost directly overhead.

Exercise: Elbow spread

1. Clasp hands behind neck.
2. Raise elbows to chin level, holding head erect. Move slowly and rest when incisional pull or pain occur.
3. Gradually spread elbows apart. Rest when pull or pain occur.

*From American Cancer Society: Reach to recovery, New York, The Society.

home on a regular basis. Following radical mastectomy, full muscle power for horizontal adduction may be less.

Participation in classes with others who have undergone the same operation may stimulate the patient to learn the prescribed exercises. However, for most women this is best done individually while other teaching and grief work can be coordinated. As soon as possible, normal activities supplement the exercises, and the patient is taught how particular exercises can be accomplished by specific tasks. The patient must know what motion is intended in each exercise. For example, the patient may brush her hair with the arm on the affected side, but she may lower her head and hunch her shoulders in such a way that she does not get normal use of the shoulder girdle. The whole intent of the exercise may therefore be lost. A small handbook entitled *Reach to Recovery*[53] is given to the patient by the American Cancer Society Reach to Recovery volunteers and will be used by the nurse in teaching and reinforcing the exercising. In addition to the book of exercises, the Reach to Recovery volunteer, as a woman who has had surgical therapy for breast malignancy, will give a colorful gift bag to the patient containing a rubber ball, a rope for exercising, and in most states, a temporary soft padded bra of her size for going home (to be used until it is time to be fitted for a weighted prosthesis in the store). The Reach to Recovery volunteer holds the potential of motivating the patient, extending hope, providing visible evidence that femininity, personality, and activity can be retained, and proves to be a good resource person as the patient moves from hospital to community. All nurses should be familiar with the volunteers and should sponsor the program. Often whether or not the patient has the opportunity to use this resource depends on a nurse's initiating the contact.

Later, after the patient returns to the community, swimming is excellent exercise. Bathing suits used with prostheses are available in retail stores. (Reach to Recovery volunteers also supply a current regional guide to such stores.[53]) Some areas have swimming rehabilitation programs for women with mastectomies. The ENCORE program is sponsored by the YMCA or YWCA.

Emotional support. Loss of a breast involves two major concepts: change in body image and mourning over loss. This reflects a physical loss and a sexuality loss, as well as changes in goals, plans, and life span. The patient is trying to cope with the fear of cancer and its potential spread and death. Removal of a breast for cancer is therefore an extremely stressful situation. The initial response is usually shock. Denial may take the form of the woman speaking about "the cancer" and the "mastectomy" but never dealing with her loss or her fears on a feeling level. Denial here is a conservation of energy. If she is to express herself on a feeling level, she must have someone who is capable and responsible to support her according to *her* need. If she does not

receive this professional assistance, the impact of her loss occurs at a later date when support systems may not be available.

Phantom symptoms of the missing breast occur in women with painful breasts or nipples before surgery.

Avoidance of looking at the dressing or incision can be expected initially. The incision is large, and the feeling experienced by most women is that of mutilation. Postponing looking at the incision delays the impact that the breast is indeed gone. Preparing the woman in advance concerning the size of the incision is helpful, but she still needs considerable support when viewing the incision and her new image. She is usually physically capable when she feels stronger and begins to socially respond to others (third day: glucocorticoid phase). She is encouraged to look at the incision several times before discharge from the hospital, while health professionals are available for support.

Feelings of anger and resentment may occur and if present frequently are projected on female staff or friends. Families may also express anger or anxiety and may complain without cause about the care the patient is receiving. Feelings of decreased self-worth and self-esteem on the part of the patient plus increased dependency needs often produce depression. (For a more detailed discussion on mourning and body image, see Chapters 17 and 28.) The feeling of being isolated and alone during this experience can be helped by interaction with others who have had the same experience, such as a visitor from the Reach to Recovery program.

After the patient is discharged, she may experience periods of depression if she perceives her recovery is slow or if she tries to reenter her previous activities and responsibilities sooner than her energy reserves return. Fatigue will always give rise to depression. She may have difficulty sleeping or concentrating if she is still acutely grieving with little recognition or little support. Although she will be aware of this, she usually will be inexpressive of her needs; significant others can be told of her continuing need for support and patience and can help to extend the kind of support needed. Sometimes it is possible for the nurse to assess how the newly discharged patient is coping when she makes a home discharge telephone call. Often simple misunderstandings or forgotten discharge information can discourage, frighten, or depress a patient during the first days at home. Some patients remain at home, avoid their friends, and hesitate to engage in social activities. The reasons for withdrawal from social participation may include fatigue and fear of rejection by others because of loss of body intactness. Healing of the incision and the underlying area so that she is able to wear a fitted brassiere and prosthesis usually reassures the woman and encourages her to participate in home and social activities. It must unfortunately also be recognized that the woman's fear of rejection may be real. *Cancer patients do lose friends, female and male. They also lose their jobs sometimes or their place on the ladder.* In general, cancer patients need professionals to advocate for them in these arenas.[75]

Sexual adaptation. Woods[71] has identified a number of factors that can influence sexual adaptation following mastectomy (Fig. 66-6). Women with very small or very large breasts may have long unresolved feelings about breast size and may also experience more difficulty in obtaining a satisfactory breast prosthesis. The woman who perceives the surgery as mutilating may withdraw from the sexual relationship, fearing rejection from her partner. Women who felt sexually inadequate before surgery may find these feelings enhanced postoperatively and use the surgery as a reason for withdrawing from sexual relationships. Sexual and marital counseling is helpful for couples who are unable to communicate their feelings openly with each other. The patient with a new mastectomy (or radiation therapy) has a changed tactile perception over the operated site as well as part of the upper arm for sometimes 3 to 6 months. *She needs to be touched.* This should be discussed and begun by her spouse in the hospital. It is too much to leave for the initial period at home.

Breast prostheses and clothing. Information about breast prostheses is given to the patient whenever she asks about them or appears interested; this may occur preoperatively but usually occurs postoperatively. The volunteer from Reach to Recovery provides current information and suggestions concerning prostheses and clothing, where it can be purchased, and current prices.[53] The volunteer is often of great assistance in accompanying the patient as she shops for her first prosthesis. It is often very difficult for her to request a prosthesis at a busy counter filled with two-breasted women. The volunteer supports her; she does not recommend kinds of prostheses. They are a very individual choice and require fitting. Breast prostheses are not fitted until at least 6 weeks postoperatively or until the incision is healed and is no longer tender.

Until the incision is well healed, the woman is advised to wear one of her own brassieres, which can be lightly padded with a soft, fluffy filling (Fig. 66-7), or a temporary soft prosthesis, which will not shift and embarrass her and which is available from the Reach to Recovery volunteer. Knowing her brassiere size, a friend could also purchase one of these for her home trip if she desires that. Plain cotton can be covered with gauze and lightly tacked to the inside of the brassiere. Opaque, loose-hanging gowns are usually most acceptable to the patient. Both gown and robe should have wide armholes to prevent constriction of the underarm. When

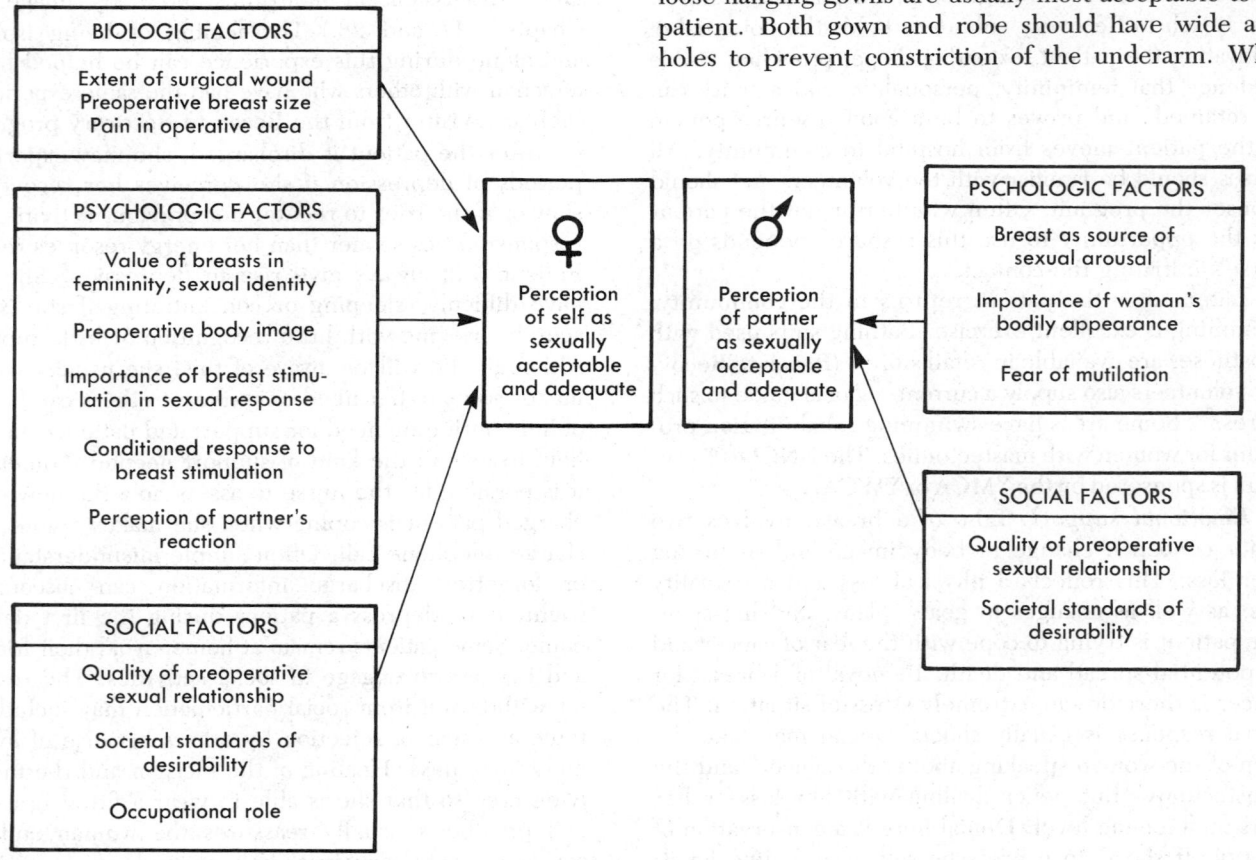

Fig. 66-6. Factors influencing a couple's sexual adaptation to mastectomy. (From Woods, N.F.: J. Obstet. Gynecol. Neonatal Nurs. **4:**34, 1975.)

the woman goes home, loose-fitting clothes with wide armholes are suggested.

Breast prostheses vary in price, type, and weight (Fig. 66-8). All women will want the prosthesis to make them look bilaterally symmetric and *feel* bilaterally weighted. Even the small-breasted woman will change posture if weighting is not balanced. All women need the assurance that the prosthesis will not shift and, unbeknownst to her, create some odd position beneath her clothing. Firm, molded prostheses have a disadvan-

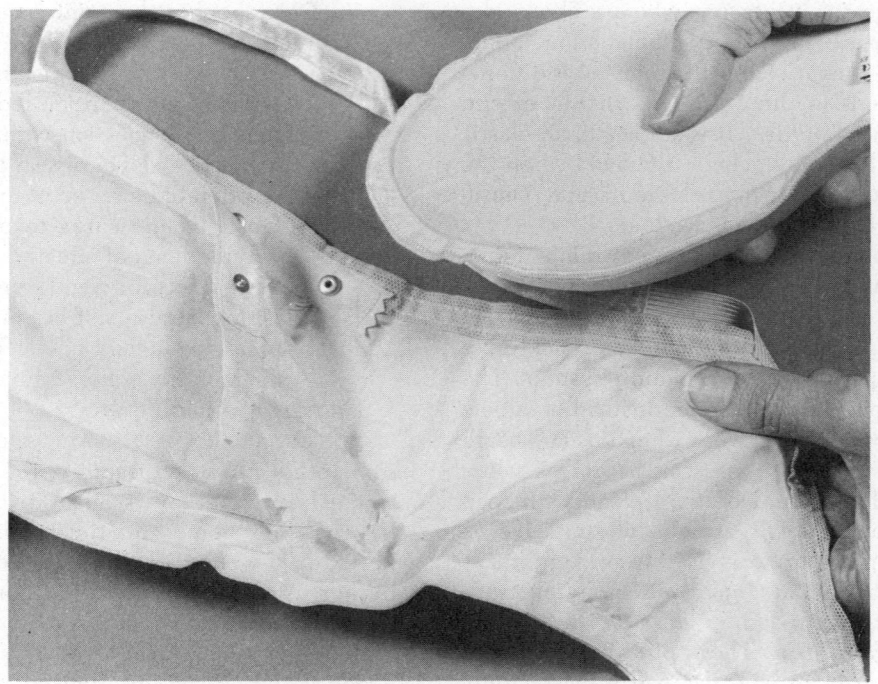

Fig. 66-7. Inner pocket that will hold padding or prosthesis securely can be made in patient's own brassiere. Note snaps that simplify removal of padding.

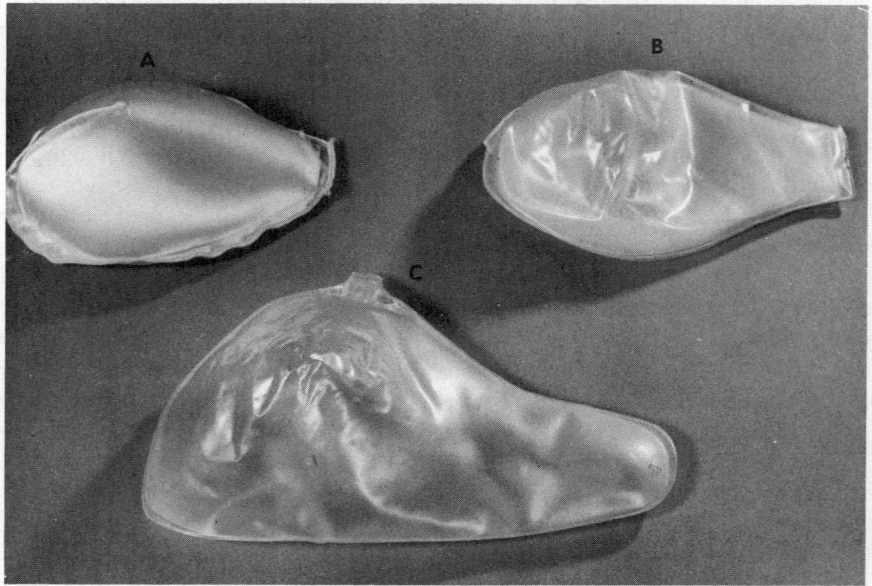

Fig. 66-8. Several types of breast prostheses are available. **A,** Foam rubber prosthesis. **B,** Prosthesis containing fluid. **C,** Prosthesis containing air.

tage of remaining elevated when the woman is lying supine, whereas fluid types have a more natural look.

Lymphedema. Many patients develop a slight edema of the upper arm that disappears within a week. A few patients, however, develop a severe edema that persists, that may become permanent, and that is caused by surgical interruption of lymph channels and nodes. The incidence is greater in persons who are obese, develop infections, or are subjected to irradiation. Some surgeons order an elastic sleeve that gives additional support to the vessels in the arm. This should extend from the wrist to the shoulder. It is similar to an elastic support stocking and usually may be removed when the patient is in bed. A diuretic such as chlorothiazide (Diuril) may be ordered to help relieve the edema.

Special care must be taken to prevent minor infections of the hands and arms in patients with lymphedema, and if they do occur, medical treatment should be sought at once, since the infection spreads quickly because of the improper functioning lymph system. The patient is advised to use cuticle cream instead of cuticle scissors, to wear rubber gloves when using harsh household products, and to wear canvas gloves when gardening. The axillae should be kept clean with soap and water, deodorants used sparingly, and an electric razor used for shaving. Care is advised to prevent burns of the affected arm and hand. *Injections, blood pressure measurements, and constricting clothing are to be avoided on the affected arm.* These precautions should be taught to every woman who has had a mastectomy (and radiation therapy) since they are also important to *prevent* lymphedema for the rest of her life.

LONG-TERM ADAPTATION. During the recovery period at home, many women experience varied symptoms that may last for several years. In a study of 49 women in North Carolina interviewed 4 years following a mastectomy, 53% reported one or more of the following symptoms still existing: swelling, weakness, stiffness, trouble moving and numbness of the arm, poor healing, and pain.[73] About three fourths of the sample experienced symptoms immediately following surgery, especially weakness and stiffness of the arm. The study also reported that women with a high number of physical symptoms were more likely to have a high number of symptoms of depression. Measures that can be taken to prevent the symptoms from developing may assist the woman in her adaptation to the loss of the breast. She also needs to be prepared for potential occurrence of these symptoms.

OUTCOME CRITERIA FOR THE WOMAN WHO HAS HAD A MASTECTOMY. The patient or significant others can:

1. Identify feelings related to loss of the breast; state feelings about having a malignancy.
2. Describe and demonstrate exercises to be continued until full range of motion to the affected shoulder returns.
3. State types of breast prostheses available and where these may be obtained.
4. Describe types of clothing to be avoided (constricting of arm).
5. Describe plans for return to social activities as carried out before surgery.
6. Describe plans for avoidance of fatigue.
7. Describe health maintenance or follow-up program.
   a. State symptoms indicating need for immediate medical attention (edema of affected arm, redness or infection within or surrounding the scar, breakdown of scar tissue, mass in axillae or operated area or in unaffected breast.)
   b. Describe measures to prevent infection and lymphedema of affected arm.
   c. State plans for regular medical follow-up.
   d. Demonstrate self-examination of remaining breast tissue and operated side and state plans for monthly self-examination.

Primary radiation therapy

EXTERNAL BEAM THERAPY. Unless complicated by some other physical disability, the patient receiving external beam therapy is an outpatient, travelling daily between her home and the hospital for therapy for a period of 5 weeks. Thus while she may be surrounded by her usual support group at home, she may also try to carry full responsibilities at home. Often the outpatient is not recognized to be sick or to have as many needs as the person hospitalized. The woman receiving external beam therapy will have an extended period of waning energy and transient depression. After all, daily destruction of malignant and some normal tissue is taking place in her breast area; this controlled catabolic phase necessarily affects her. In addition to reduced energy, she may experience some nausea, sometimes some reflux discomfort (heartburn) associated with a transient esophagitis, or a cough toward the end of the therapy span. This dry cough is frightening to her, for she usually has heard and read enough media coverage on breast cancer to conclude that her cough is indicative of the extension of the cancer. She should be quickly reassured that the pneumonitis cough is a transient result of minor exposure (unavoidable) of a small part of the lower lung to the beam. To allay fears of such symptoms since they may begin over a weekend, it is best to prepare the patient before therapy by relating some of the ways some other patients have experienced the treatment. The nurse's role in teaching and supporting these patients is very important.[52] The patient requires explanation and assistance with handling nausea, good nutrition intake, fluctuating energies, possibly cough and sleeping position change, as well as the ever present awareness that "I have cancer" and the attendant anxiety and grieving for her future.

This patient may also require assistance in the transportation aspect of her therapy. Nurses should be aware of the American Cancer Society's Transportation Program and offer this resource *before* the patient becomes exhausted and considers dropping therapy. One of the greatest lessons of illness and convalescence is to be able to recognize that no one is independent or dependent; if we are mature individuals, we are interdependent. The nurse must help patients to be aware of the helping resources available for them and help them to accept resources without feeling immature, inefficient, or losing face in their own eyes and others. The Washington Division of the American Cancer Society has started a Share-a-Ride Program through the offices of radiation oncologists. The Washington division also provides free housing at their Seattle headquarters for those who cannot make a daily trip involving 50 or more miles even with volunteer drivers. Details of these programs for patients may be obtained from the division office in Seattle.

The patient receiving external beam therapy for breast malignancy should receive the same considerations, emotional support, and teaching as she would have with surgery as primary therapy. A maliganancy is present in her breast; it threatens her. Her breast may or may not ever look the same; it will not feel the same; she will mourn.

All the teaching, arm measurements, and precautions for lymphedema pertain to the patient receiving external beam therapy. Since it is infrequent that many nurses work in the outpatient radiation therapy department, this teaching is being missed. The importance of exercise is also lacking. All should be started for the patient's future benefit.

The patient may receive only external beam therapy, or she may in addition receive interstitial therapy.

INTERSTITIAL THERAPY. Interstitial therapy is the second part of the radiation therapy protocol for primary therapy of small lesions.

The patient may begin this phase immediately after completing the 5 weeks of external beam therapy. She will be hospitalized in a room alone, and under anesthesia in the operating room, iridium needles will be placed within the breast tissue (iridium IR 192). Her postanesthesia period is easy, and she will be up and about in her room with little discomfort. The needles will be removed (by a physician) in her room after 3 days and she is discharged. Far from being a patient with few needs, this woman requires support, teaching, sometimes crisis intervention, and always assistance with the isolating aspect that radiation safety policies impose on her, her visitors, and the staff. (See discussion of radiation safety precautions on p. 490.)

Breast reconstruction. Mastectomy is the surgery women (especially black and Hispanic women) fear most; reconstructive surgery is the surgery women never thought possible.[62]

Reconstruction mammoplasty is a possibility for some women following a mastectomy. Both physical assessment and psychologic assessment are indicated before the procedure is considered. The patient must be realistic in what she thinks will be accomplished. The "you can be whole again" evangelism is detrimental. Preexisting psychosocial problems will not be solved by the surgery. Nor do all women feel it is important or necessary to have a reconstruction. For some women, it is not essential to their positive self-image and esteem, femininity, or sexual experience. Many do not want the added surgery and attendant anesthesia, the costliness of time or money, or the pain. They are comfortable and active and successful without the added surgery. However, every woman should know about the options of reconstruction, whether it is appropriate for her stage of disease, as well as those facts that tell her what it can and cannot do. She should have the opportunity to talk and read about breast reconstruction so she can determine its meaning for her. An excellent pamphlet, *Breast Reconstruction following Mastectomy for Cancer*, is available free of charge from the American Cancer Society.[6] Attractive in format, it answers questions about insurance coverage, cost, how many operations are necessary, can a nipple be banked for later use, can a nipple be reconstructed too, and so on. The pamphlet is designed for patient use but has been assessed for its readability at grade 13.[54] Since the woman contemplating breast surgery for a malignancy, whether educated or not, will have difficulty in concentrating on anything but the shortest words and sentences, this excellent pamphlet can be used to best advantage by nurses and patients speaking together, reading and interpreting the questions and answers in the brochure together. It is recommended that all hospital units have a supply of this pamphlet and that professionals be familiar with it before discussion with patients.

In a study reported by Shain,[61] no difference was found in the degree of self-esteem, activity, or satisfaction with sex and "zest for living" between women who had reconstructive surgery and those who did not. The difference between these two groups of women lay in how the individual woman felt about her body nude. Reasons given by women who had reconstructive surgery were as follows: desire for a nipple, desire for greater freedom than an external prosthesis afforded in order to energetically play tennis, swim, and so on; desire for a feeling of normal contour when nude; desire to wear clothing that revealed breast cleavage; and desire to wear a wide range of clothes with no restrictions. Breast reconstruction is contraindicated when there is an aggressive tumor, a probability that metastasis has occurred, a concern about adequate healing being impaired, or unrealistic psychosocial expectations.

Reconstruction can be performed at the time of the mastectomy, or, as is preferred by many plastic reconstruction surgeons, the reconstruction can take place some months later after some psychologic readjustment and physical strength and energy reserves have been achieved.

An early consultation with a plastic reconstruction surgeon is preferred; ideally, the consultation should be one where the plastic surgeon and the oncologic surgeon work together. For the woman who makes her decision before her mastectomy, the plastic surgeon is often present at the time of the mastectomy, when he can recommend incisional approaches, tissue salvage, or tissue banking, as is sometimes done for a later use of the woman's nipple *if* the nipple is free of disease. The surgery consists of a Silastic implant filled with silicone or saline placed under the subcutaneous tissue. A nipple can be reconstructed if necessary from labial tissue, or in the absence of malignant cells, the patient's own nipple is sometimes banked on her inner thigh and salvaged at the appropriate time for reimplanting.

A brassiere is worn postoperatively in order to maintain implant position and alignment. Presurgery and postsurgery activity and exercise are individually prescribed by the plastic surgeon.

There are certain possible complications: more anesthesia time for a person who recently had extensive surgery; infection; necrosis of the flaps, fibrotic contractures, or hardening of tissue around implant; and asymmetry in relation to the existing breast.

Shain[61] reports that women who have reconstruction surgery immediately after the mastectomy are less satisfied with reconstruction than those who have surgery after an interval of 6 months. It is possible that this is a result of not enough time to grieve for loss and to see loss. Grief cannot be hurried. A significant loss warrants significant grieving and a time interval before a replacement is made.

The patient should have frequent medical checks by her physician and should know how to do a very thorough monthly breast self-examination. She and her physician are somewhat handicapped since tissue in back of the implants cannot be palpated nor visualized by mammography. However, there seems to be no current data that would identify this as a risk to early detection of recurrent disease.

The American Cancer Society is adding a program on breast reconstruction to their rehabilitation visitation program, Reach to Recovery. It will entail volunteers who have themselves had reconstruction because of cancer, who have been carefully screened as volunteers for the program, and who are carefully trained, supervised, and periodically evaluated. This will be an additional resource for patients and professionals. As the program emerges within the fall and winter of 1982-83, it is hoped that hospital and community professionals will learn about it, initiate contact, and use it as a beneficial resource for women before or after therapy for breast cancer. (Reach to Recovery is also adding volunteers who have had chemotherapy after their surgery and those who have had primary radiation therapy. This is important so that they will fully recognize the anxieties and questions of the patient.)

Metastatic disease

The progress of breast malignancy is from the primary mass foci (often more than one) through intramammary lymphatics to regional nodes and then to systemic dissemination or from primary mass to extension of local structures (skin, rib) and then to systemic disseminated disease.

The most usual metastasis of breast malignancy is to bone, lung, or brain. One of the hard concepts to live with when you have any kind of cancer is the knowlege that it may metastasize. "Cancer cure" of 5, 10, or more years means cancer control for 5, 10, or more years. Thus all patients should be made knowledgeable about early symptoms they might find that signal disseminated disease and their responsibility to not delay further treatment (and often a different therapy protocol than before). This is difficult for a cancer patient and family because a cough along with coryza alerts spoken or unspoken anxiety: "Is it more than a cold?" Aching in a different area than the common arthritic pain may alert an older patient to wonder, "Is it more arthritis, or is it more than that?" Health providers must create initial relationships with patients that make it comfortable and easy for them to recontact the professional for such anxious, nebulous, but often first perceived symptoms of disseminated disease. Guilt at treatment delay with initial disease need not be repeated again if relationships with the oncology team have been open and therapeutic.

Therapy for disseminated breast cancer is specific to the area involved. If the metastasis is found in the lung, surgical ablation, chemotherapy, and/or radiation may be used. The tumor board again becomes activated for the benefit of the patient's clinical management. Single and in-combination therapies will be used. If the tumor was estrogen dependent, hormonal therapy, adrenalectomy, ablation of the ovaries (by surgery or radiation), or hypophysectomy may be performed. The sequelae of all these therapy interventions require further physiologic and psychologic adaptations. This is why strong coping mechanisms and good supporting individuals and groups are necessary for the cancer patient and family. They live with cancer. Most patients today also believe they do live, not only exist in a perpetual sick role.

New battles must be fought by the patient's family with the occurrence of new therapies and their sequelae. For the first time the woman may have chemotherapy[14] and a new adversary to her femininity met: alopecia. The time to address this problem is when the chemotherapy protocol is planned; if alopecia is an expected or "could be" possibility, she needs a wig prepared according to her hair and style. She should begin wearing it *before* she needs it, and she should wear it when she needs it. She may have new problems with eating because of stomatitis. Patients need in their hands the cookbooks especially written for cancer patients. Bone metastasis will mean changes or cautions in ambulation and often means pain. Adequate, round-the-clock, systematic administration of medication by patient or family is necessary for this deep, suffering pain. Radiation to the bone involved is also used to reduce pain.

The cancer patient is vulnerable to many infections, especially when metastatic disease has occurred. She must protect herself from others about her with infections and seek help from her physician at the early symptoms of infection in herself.

This is a heavy burden. Patient and family may become overwhelmed with the disappointing hopes of successful therapy, a hiatus period of promise and then recurrent symptoms. Hopelessness and giving up occur when coping is inappropriate or unsupported. The little engine in the children's story struggled all alone to get up the mountain with toys for the children; but the patients cannot go it alone in their struggle up their mountain. They need help. Giving up and suicide ideation reflect perceived (and often real) inadequacy of help offered or given, often help by professionals themselves. Support groups offer one kind of assistance to the patient and family. These may be held in the hospital setting or in the community by professional nurses or social workers. Helpful interventions by American Cancer Society volunteers, many of whom are physicians, nurses, and social workers, are also possible when the need is recognized and the helper alerted. Many communities have crisis clinics or crisis telephone hot lines. Use of the direct-dial Cancer Information Service through the American Cancer Society and the National Cancer Institute furnishes patients and families with immediate answers to their questions and their need of resources. Reading material can also be sent to them; community resources for care, supplies, transportation, housing during treatment, assistance with insurance forms, and seeking financial assistance are services to patients by the American Cancer Society in every state in the United States. There are also two other programs needed by and available to the patient and family: (1) learning how to live with cancer, given in an 8-week group program called *I Can Cope*; and (2) a support group of trained patients with cancer in a program called *Can Survive*. Information is available at all local American Cancer Society offices.

There are many things that we do not yet know about metastatic cancer. Some of these involve the influences of the interacting psychologies and spiritual and social aspects of the patient herself on the metastatic process, as well as the influence of the interfacing aspects of family, friends, and the helping-healing professionals on the patient and the metastatic process.

Cancer often kills. Yet there seem to be times when getting cancer can become the beginning of living. The search for one's own being, the discovery of the life one needs to live, can be one of the strongest weapons. . . . Several years ago walking along a city street, I saw a familiar face in the crowd moving towards me. It was a woman patient I had not seen or heard from for over a year. She had had a terminal malignancy. . . . She was (now) walking so quickly with such a light but determined stride that she almost passed me by before she noticed me. She smiled happily, hugged me briefly, and then with a wave of her hand as she went her way, said she was in a hurry and shouted back to me, "I've been too busy *living* to get in touch with you." I watched her as she disappeared again. Going somewhere important; on her way. Alive. Living.*

Nonmalignant disease of the breast

Dysplasia

Dysplasia (fibrocystic disease) is characterized by thickened nodular areas in the breast that usually become painful during or before menstruation. The process is almost always bilateral. It occurs mostly in women between 30 years of age and menopause. The condition is thought to be caused by hormonal imbalance during the monthly cyclic changes with failure of normal involution following the reaction of the breasts to the monthly cyclic activity of the female sex hormones, estrogen and progesterone. The nodules or cysts may be singular or multiple and may increase in size or stay the same. They are usually fairly soft and tender on palpation and are movable, sliding under the examining fingers.

The woman who discovers such mass (or masses) in her breast should seek the advice of a physician, who will decide whether the lesion should be measured and checked at frequent intervals or whether aspiration or biopsy should be considered. There is little evidence that dysplasia predisposes to the development of malignancy, but these women are considered more at risk than those who do not have fibrocystic disease. The presence of nodular tissue in the breast makes the early detection of malignant lesions more difficult. For this reason some physicians suggest periodic mammography or xeroradiography of the breast to detect any changes. Such women should be taught to recognize the tactile

---

*From You Can Fight for Your Life by Lawrence LeShan. Copyright © 1977 by Lawrence LeShan. Reprinted by permission of the publisher, M. Evans & Co., Inc., New York.

discrimination of their normal breast tissue and the location and size of the areas of dysplasia; they should be capable of mapping,[5] and *they should be encouraged to do a monthly* breast self-examination. It is *extremely* important for them.

Fibroadenomas

Fibroadenomas are tumors of fibroblastic and epithelial origin that are thought to be caused by hyperestrinism. These tumors are usually firm, round, freely movable, nontender, and encapsulated; they occur most often in women under 25 years of age.

The woman who discovers such a mass should not delay in seeking medical consultation. Usually the tumor will be removed with the woman under local anesthesia and will be examined microscopically to be sure it is not malignant. Although the hospital stay for excision of an adenoma is short and the patient returns to the surgeon's office or clinic for the sutures to be removed, she needs thoughtful nursing care, since she naturally is extremely fearful of cancer until the histology report reassures her otherwise.

Gynecomastia

Gynecomastia is a hyperplasia (overdevelopment) of the stroma and ducts in the mammary glands in the *male*. It occurs most commonly during puberty and after 40 years of age. The cause is thought to be an abnormally large estrogen secretion. A gonadotropin (CG-beta) determination should be obtained, as well as chest and mediastinum x-ray films and a careful testes examination, since germ cell testicular malignancy or lung cancer may show signs of gynecomastia and elevated CG-beta. It is also frequently seen following estrogen therapy for cancer of the prostate. Gynecomastia is a nonmalignant lesion, but physicians may suggest a biopsy specimen of the breast, since older men occasionally develop cancer of the breast.

The male is fraught with anxiety about the condition, which is little reduced by the information that it is a benign condition. This is the ultimate assault to the *male* self-image—enlarged breasts. The greater freedom of the male to be "topless" in the sun, at home, in construction work, and in recreation activities makes the developing and existent condition visible and joke provoking. In a like manner, the infrequent male (900 persons estimated in the United States in 1982) who develops breast cancer (unrelated to the dysplasia) and who has primary surgical therapy has a publicly visible mastectomy, and the asymmetry is very apparent. Heretofore the problems and unmet needs of this patient have not been recognized.

Common problems of the breast in women

Periodic tender, painful, or enlarged breasts

Although it is upsetting and uncomfortable to women, tender, painful, or enlarged breasts are normal functional changes in the breasts that respond to the monthly cyclic changes in estrogen and progesterone. Women who experience this "normal problem" require reassurance, but above all they need health teaching about the normal changes that regularly occur in all women with functional ovaries or who have hormonal replacement (p. 611). A reduction of dietary salt during the premenstrual period of time may be beneficial for some women.

Breast pain

There is a small population of women who experience almost constant pain in one or both breasts. Careful assessment should be made to assure such a woman that there is an absence of infection or fibrocystic disease, or rarely, a tumor mass. This woman needs patient listening, understanding, and support from her physician and nurse health providers. Breast pain is a problem unrelieved and unexplained to the woman who has it and is an idiopathic problem to the health professional who currently can offer only symptomatic relief.

Clogged ducts during lactation

Sometimes tender, small, red, "lumps" are palpable on the surface of the breasts. These are milk ducts, temporarily occluded by pressure (position, brassiere, or nursing child). If the baby does not nurse long enough, the breasts should be manually pumped.

Infection

Infection of the skin

Women who wear no brassiere or who have large or pendulous breasts often have problems with yeast (*Candida albicans*) or *Staphylococcus aureus* infections, particularly during hot weather. This most commonly occurs under the breasts, where skin breakdown and maceration can occur quickly in the presence of heat, perspiration, and touching skin surfaces. It is attended by pruritus and bright, sharp pain and has often been present for a period of weeks before medical assistance is sought. Prevention could be taught to all women in addition to teaching breast self-examination. This would include encouraging frequent bathing of the breasts during hot weather, use of cornstarch to keep the areas under the breasts dry, and use of a supporting brassiere to reduce skin surfaces touching.

Infection of the areolar area

Some hair normally grows around the areola. If the hairs are plucked or if a depilatory is used, follicular infection by *Staphyloccoccus aureus* or group A streptococcus may occur. Women should be cautioned not to pluck hairs on their breast (rather to cut them close if unwanted) nor to squeeze any other pimple or skin lesion temporarily present on the breast. The local infection could progress to a breast cellulitis (mastitis).

Infection of the nipple

Infection usually results from cracks in the nipple during lactation. This condition is less common than previously, because women are taught to "toughen" the nipple during pregnancy so that cracking during breast-feeding is less likely to occur. Since this infection often occurs when the new mother is at home, discharge teaching should involve care of the nipples, vigilance for problems that might develop, and encouragement for early treatment from her health provider. The most common organisms involved are *Staphylococcus aureus,* group A streptococcus, and *Candida albicans* (rarely *Escherichia coli*); thus the *untreated* nursing mother can transmit the organisms to the feeding infant.

Infection of the breast

An infection can occur in the breast by direct spread from cracked or infected nipples, thus creating a cellulitis through the extensive breast lymphatic system. The pathogens may be transmitted to the mother's breast from the nasopharynx of the newborn infant who has been exposed to infected infants and hospital personnel or from the hands of the patient or hospital personnel. Staphylococcal and group A streptococcal infections are most common.

Infections of the breast cause pain, redness, swelling, and elevation of temperature. The woman's breasts will feel "heavy" and "feverish," and the condition will not be relieved by the baby's feeding; thus the symptoms are different from the engorged breast or "clogged ducts." The treatment is usually conservative. Antibiotics are usually given systemically. If the condition does not subside with conservative treatment and becomes localized to form an abscess, surgical drainage is necessary. To help prevent infections of the breast, there is a continued need for strict aseptic techniques in nurseries for newborn infants, thus preventing infected persons (carriers) from coming in contact with mothers and babies; and breast health teaching for all women is important. Nurses must be vigilant to early signs and symptoms and committed to *early* documentation and

verbal reporting so that early treatment can begin. This is particularly imperative during long holiday weekends when access to a woman's own physician may not be possible.

Mastitis is a physical complication for the nursing mother. It is a psychologic complication to her as well, making her anxious about her baby's health and her own and thereby stealing energies meant for postpartum adaptations and mothering pleasures. The nursing mother with mastitis requires high-protein nutrition, longer rest periods, and greater considerations of caring from her husband, family, friends, and professionals. Because infections of this magnitude reverse a person into a mineralocorticoid phase, she will be tearful. Explain to her that it is normal and empathize with the occurrence.

REFERENCES AND SELECTED READINGS*

1. Aker, S., and Lesson, P.: A guide to good nutrition: during and after chemotherapy and radiation, Seattle, 1980, Fred Hutchison Cancer Research Center.
2. Amelric, R., et al.: Radiation therapy with or without primary limited surgery for operable breast cancer, Ca **49:**1, 1982.
3. The American Cancer Society: what it is, what it does, how it began, where it's going, New York, 1978, American Cancer Society.
4. Black Americans' attitudes toward cancer and cancer tests: highlights of a study, Ca **31:**4, 1981.
5. Breast Health Program, Seattle, Univ. Washington. (Doris Molbo, SM-28 School of Nursing.)
6. Breast reconstruction following mastectomy for cancer: questions and answers, New York, 1979, American Cancer Society and the American Society of Plastic and Reconstructive Surgeons.
7. Cancer facts and figures, 1982, New York, 1982, American Cancer Society.
8. Cancer screening and diagnosis: an annotated bibliography of public and patient education materials (NIH pub. no. 81-2153), Bethesda, Md., 1981.
9. Cancer Surmount Program, New York, 1979, American Cancer Society.
10. Cancer treatment: an annotated bibliography of patient education materials (NIH pub. no. 81-2152), Bethesda, Md., 1981, National Institutes of Health, Office of Cancer Communications.
11. Cancer treatment, medicine for the layman, 1980, National Cancer Institute Publication.
12. Cancer Word Book, New York, American Cancer Society.
13. Cantor, R.C.: And a time to live: toward emotional well-being during the crisis of cancer, New York, 1978, Harper & Row.
14. Chemotherapy and you: a Guide to self-help during treatment (NIH pub. no. 81-1136), Bethesda, Md., 1981.
15. Choices: realistic alternatives in cancer treatment, New York, 1980, Avon Books.

*NOTE: 1. Unless otherwise indicated American Cancer Society materials can be obtained from your local or state office at no expense. 2. All National Institutes of Health (NIH) and National Cancer Institute (NCI) materials can be obtained by writing to: Office of Cancer Communications, NCI, Building 31, Room 10A18, Bethesda, MD 20205. 3. A way to keep updated is with *Ca: A Cancer Journal for Clinicians,* published by American Cancer Society, 6 issues per year. Free to nurses through American Cancer Society division (state) offices.

16. The clergy and the cancer patient, New York, 1976, American Cancer Society.

17. Copeland, E., Van Eys, J., and Shils, M.: Nutrition and cancer, New York, 1979, American Cancer Society.

18. Coping with cancer: an annotated bibliography of public, patient and professional information and education materials. (NIH pub. no. 80-2080), Bethesda, Md., 1980, National Institutes of Health.

19. Coping with cancer: a resource for the professional, Bethesda, Md., 1980, National Cancer Institute Publication.

20. Deffebach, R.R., et al.: Lampectomy and irradiation in the treatment of early carcinoma of the breast, West. J. Med. **4:**136, 1982.

21. Developing patient education programs: an annotated bibliography of methods and resources for Cancer education (NIH pub. no. 81-2234). Bethesda, Md. 1980, National Institutes of Health, Office of Cancer Communications.

22. Dietz, J.H.: Rehabilitation oncology, New York, 1981, John Wiley & Sons, Inc.

22a. Eating hints, recipes, and tips for better nutrition during cancer treatment (NIH pub. no. 82-2079), Bethesda, Md., 1982.

22b. Fishman, J., and Anrod, B.: Something's got to taste good: the cancer patient's cookbook, Farway, Kan., 1981, Andrews & McMeel, Inc. Also published by Signet Books (New York) in 1981.

23. Gallup polls women on attitudes on breast cancer, Am. J. Nurs. **74:**124, 1974.

24. Gant, T.D., and Vasconez, L.O.: Post-mastectomy reconstruction, Baltimore, 1981, The Williams & Wilkins Co.

25. Goin, M.K., et al.: Midlife reactions to mastectomy and subsequent breast reconstruction, Arch. Gen. Psychiatry **38:**2, 1981.

26. Guidelines for the cancer-related check-up: recommendations and rationale, New York, 1980, American Cancer Society.

27. Hellman, S., et al.: Cancer of the breast. In DeVita, V., et al.: Cancer: principles and practice of oncology, Philadelphia, 1982, J.B. Lippincott Co.

28. Hofland, S.: Post mastectomy lymphedema: incidence and etiological factors, unpublished thesis, Seattle, 1979, University of Washington.

29. Holland, J.: Understanding the cancer patient, New York, 1980, American Cancer Society Professional Education Publication.

30. Holland, J., and Frei, E.: Cancer, Philadelphia, 1982, W.B. Saunders Co.

31. Kaufman, R.J.: Advanced breast cancer: additive hormonal therapy, New York, 1981, American Cancer Society Professional Education Publication.

32. LeShan, L.: You Can Fight for Your Life: emotional factors in the treatment of cancer, New York, 1980, M. Evans & Co. Inc.

33. Leffall, L.D.: Breast cancer in black women, Ca **31:**4, 1981.

34. Lesnick, G.J.: Detection of breast cancer in young women, J.A.M.A. **237:**967-969, 1977.

35. Levene, M.B., Harris, J.R., and Hellman, S.: Treatment of carcinoma of the breast by radiation therapy, CA **29**(suppl.):2840-2845, 1977.

36. Levene, M.B.: A new role for radiation therapy, Am. J. Nurs. **77:**1443-1444, 1977.

37. Lubin, J.H., et al.: Risk factors for breast cancer in women in Alberta, Canada, J. N. C. I. **68:**2, 1982.

38. McCorkle, M.R.: Coping with physical symptoms in metastatic breast cancer, Am. J. Nurs. **73:**1034-1038, 1973.

39. Molbo, D.M.: Cancer. In Carnivalli, D., and Patrick, M., editors: Nursing management for the elderly, Philadelphia, 1979, J.B. Lippincott Co.

40. Morris, T.: Psychological adjustment to mastectomy, Cancer Treatment Reviews, **6:**41, 1979.

41. Mouridsen, H.T., and Palshof, T.: Breast cancer: experimental and clinical aspects, Oxford, England, 1980, Pergamon Press, Inc. (Three selected papers on hormone and adjuvant chemotherapy available free from Stuart Pharmaceuticals, Div. of ICI Americas, P.O. Box 751, Wilmington, DE 19897)

42. Myers, W.P.: Hypercalcemia and cancer, Ca **27:**5, 1977.

43. National conference on breast cancer—proceedings of American Cancer Society: 1979 and 1981. (compilation of current management.)

44. National survey on breast cancer: a measure of progress in public understanding, (NIH pub. no. 81-2306), Bethesda, Md., 1980, National Cancer Institute.

45. Nutrition and the cancer patient: an annotated bibliography of patient and professional information and educational materials (NIH pub. no. 81-1511), ed. 2, Bethesda, Md., 1981, National Institutes of Health.

46. Patient rights: an annotated bibliography of cancer education materials for the public, patient and professional (NIH pub. no. 81-2134), Bethesda, Md., 1981, National Institutes of Health, Office of Cancer Communications.

47. Peterson, B.H., et al.: Aging and cancer management, New York, 1979, American Cancer Society.

48. Planning public education programs: an annotated bibliography of methods and resources for cancer education, Bethesda, Md., 1981, National Cancer Institute.

49. Poliby, J.: Psychological effects of radical mastectomy, Public Health Rev. **4:**279-295, 1975.

50. Preece, P.E., et al.: Tamofixen as initial sole treatment of localized breast cancer in elderly women, Br. Med. J. **284:**6319, 1982.

51. Proceedings of the American Cancer Society National Conference: meeting the challenge of cancer among black Americans, Washington D.C., 1979, American Cancer Society.

52. Radiation therapy and you: a guide to self-help during treatment (NIH pub. no. 80-2227), Washington, D.C., 1980, National Institutes of Health.

53. Reach to recovery. 1. Exercises. 2. Current prices and retail stores for prostheses in regional communities, American Cancer Society.

54. Readability testing in cancer communications (NIH pub. no. 81-1689), Washington, D.C., 1981, National Institutes of Health.

55. Reich, D.: Estrogen receptors and advanced breast cancer, Ca. Nurs. **4**(3):247-248, 1981.

56. Rosenbaum, E.: A comprehensive guide for cancer patients and their families, Palo Alto, Calif., 1981, Bull Publishing Co.

57. Rosenstock, I.: The health belief model and personal health behavior, Thorofare, N.J., 1974, Charles Slack, Inc.

58. Rubin, P., editor: Metastases and disseminated cancer, New York, 1979, American Cancer Society.

59. Sanger, C., and Pezmikoff, M.: A comparison of the psychological effects of breast-saving procedures with the modified radical mastectomy, Ca **48:**2341, 1981.

60. Schmale, A.: Psychological reactions to recurrences, metastases or disseminated cancer. In Rubin, P., editor: Metastases and disseminated cancer, New York, 1979, American Cancer Society.

61. Shain, W.: Facts every woman should know about breast reconstruction, New York, 1979, American Cancer Society.

62. Shain, W.: Reconstruction issues. In Proceedings of the Western States Conference on Cancer Rehabilitation, San Francisco, 1982.

63. Speaker's guide on breast cancer: for PACE, Priority Activities in Cancer Education, New York, 1981, American Cancer Society.

64. Stillman, M.J.: Women's health beliefs about breast cancer and breast self-examination, Nurs. Res. **26:**121-127, 1977.

65. Taking time: support for people with cancer and the people who care about them, (NIH pub. no. 80-2059), Bethesda, Md., 1980, National Cancer Institute.

65a. Third National Cancer Survey: Incidence data: monograph 41 (DHEW pub. no. 75-787 NIH), Bethesda, Md., 1975.

66. Thomas, S.G., and Yates, M.M.: Breast reconstruction after mastectomy, Am. J. Nurs. **77:**1438-1442, 1977.

67. Thomas, S.G.: Breast cancer: the psychosocial issues, Ca. Nurs. **1:**53, 1978.

67a. TNM classification of malignant tumours, Geneva, 1974, UICC.

68. Vredevoe, D.L., et al.: Concepts of oncology nursing, Englewood Cliffs, N.J., 1981, Prentice-Hall, Inc.

69. Winkler, W.A.: Choosing the prosthesis and clothing, Am. J. Nurs. 77:1433-1436, 1977.

70. Women's health and medical guide, Des Moines, Iowa, 1981, Better Homes and Gardens. (Excellent diagrams of various breast surgery procedures and appearance implications; a book for all women, health oriented.)

71. Woods, N.F.: Influences on sexual adaptation to mastectomy, J. Obstet. Gynecol. Neonatal Nurs. 4:33-37, 1975.

72. Woods, N.F.: Psychologic aspects of breast cancer: review of literature, J. Gynecol. Nurs. 4:1522, 1975.

73. Woods, N.F., and Earp, J.A.: Women with cured breast cancer: a description of women's experiences four years after mastectomy, Unpublished manuscript.

74. Woods, N.F., and Earp, J.A.: Women with cured breast cancer: a study of mastectomy patients in North Carolina, Nurs. Res. 27:5, 1978.

75. Work and cancer health histories: a study of recovered patients' experiences, 1980, American Cancer Society, California division.

76. Your xeroradiographic mammogram (brochure), American Cancer Society, local office or Xerox Corporation, 125 N. Vinedo St., Pasadena, CA 91107.

AUDIOVISUAL RESOURCE

Breast self-examination: a life time habit (you have a lot to live for), New York, The City of New York, Maternity, Infant Care Family Planning Project. Brochures and 16-mm film. (The most accurate and health oriented breast self-examination film.)

CHAPTER 67

PROBLEMS OF SEXUALITY

NANCY FUGATE WOODS

This chapter will examine the common etiologies of sexual problems, describe common sexual problems and the approaches to their treatment, and explore the influence of altered health states on sexual health. It will also present outcome criteria for interventions with clients experiencing sexual problems.

Etiologies of sexual problems

Just as most diseases, which were once viewed from a monoetiologic framework, are now recognized to be determined by a multiplicity of factors, so it is also recognized that sexual problems have multiple etiologies. Three classes of etiologic variables to be explored here are the biologic, psychologic, and socioenvironmental.

Biologic etiologies

Biologic determinants of sexual problems may relate to illness, use of pharmacologic agents, and the aging process. Although these variables may negatively influence an individual's sexual function, it should be kept in mind that even given optimal health, sexual response remains vulnerable to interference from behavioral and socioenvironmental factors. Kaplan[48] estimates that the number of sexually dysfunctional patients whose dysfunction is purely organic ranges from only 3% to 20%.

Interferences with the processes of vasocongestion and myotonia may be a direct result of diseases affecting the nervous system or circulatory system, as well as of pharmacologic agents that act in a similar fashion. Additionally, pathologic or pharmacologically induced processes that reduce the individual's androgen level interfere with libido in both sexes and impair male erection. Any entity that causes painful sensations with either stimulation or intercourse can interfere with sexual function. Although aging often leads to concerns about sexual response, experts agree that there need not be a decrease in interest in sex or in sexual activity.[48]

Psychologic etiologies

There are a number of theories to explain the psychologic origins of sexual dysfunction. While there is no agreement regarding the nature of the behavioral factors involved, there is general agreement that the majority of sexual difficulties are attributable to experiential factors. Psychoanalysts believe that unconscious conflicts resulting from childhood experiences are the roots of sexual problems, whereas systems theorists attribute sexual dysfunction to unhealthy transactions between sexual partners. The learning theorists and behavioral school accord the blame for such problems to conditioning.

Recently, Kaplan[47] has suggested that on one level all sexual dysfunctions are caused by a single factor: anxiety. Indeed, she suggests that sexual anxiety may well be the final common pathway through which many psychopathogens produce sexual dysfunctions. While this anxiety is evoked by sex, it is not specific in its content or intensity, and it may be the product of unconscious conflict as well as simple fears of performance. The person may be conscious of the anxiety or totally unaware of the cause of his or her sexual dysfunction. The *time* at which anxiety is evoked, its quality or intensity, and specific defenses against sexually related anxiety together determine the type of sexual dysfunction.

Socioenvironmental etiologies

Several schools of sex therapy focus primarily on interpersonal components of sexual problems, treating both partners or the relationship as the client. Their approach is based on the assumption that neither partner is uninvolved in the etiology and treatment of the dysfunction. This dyadic approach to therapy recognizes the power of social stimuli to create and maintain a sexually dysfunctional relationship.[60]

Environmental stimuli may lead to sexual problems or inability to express oneself sexually; these may include the presence of stimuli that compete with sexual sensation, the absence of a partner, or obstacles to interacting sexually with a partner. An example of the former is competing environmental noises, and an example of the latter is institutionalization.[102]

Thus while sexual concerns and problems may result from any one of these variables, it is likely that a combination of these contribute to the problems of an individual.

Definitions and types of sexual concerns and problems

People experience a variety of sexual problems ranging from concerns about sexual phenomena to sexual dysfunctions. Each type of problem is the consequence of different antecedents, and each requires somewhat different therapeutic approaches. *Sexual concerns* constitute a source of worry, dissatisfaction, or discomfort for clients but do not produce difficulty in sexual function, profound problems in the sexual relationship, or a greatly altered sexual self-concept. Sexual concerns often arise because of misinformation or lack of information, conflicting values, difficulty communicating about sexual issues, and anxiety or guilt about sexual phenomena. These concerns are usually amenable to sex education strategies such as permission giving, provision of limited information, values clarification exercises, rehearsal of communication, validation of normalcy, and provision of anticipatory guidance.

Sexual difficulties create discomfort in the sexual relationship, may occasionally interfere with sexual function, and sometimes may challenge the person's sexual self-image. Sexual difficulties include the inability to relax, disinterest in sexual activity, sexual dissatisfaction, inability to please or be pleased by a partner, and problems in the timing of sexual activities. These difficulties are amenable to counseling approaches, including relaxation training, exploration of alternatives in the sexual repertoire, provision of specific suggestions, and training in communication skills.

Sexual dysfunctions usually result not only in disruption of sexual function but also in severe strains on the sexual relationship and a threatened sexual self-image. There are three categories of sexual dysfunctions:

Disorders of sexual desire
Disorders of arousal
Disorders of orgasm[47]

There are also two other categories of sexual dysfunction. The first includes disorders from involuntary painful spasms of genital and reproductive organ muscles resulting in vaginismus in women and ejaculatory pain in men. Sexual phobias constitute the second category.

Disorders of the desire phase include hypoactive sexual desire and inhibited sexual desire. The person with hypoactive sexual desire loses interest in sexual matters, does not pursue sexual gratification, and is not likely to avail himself or herself of sexual opportunities. Individuals with inhibited sexual desire may be able to experience lubrication or erection but do not experience much pleasure.

Disorders of arousal (the excitement phase) include inability to have an erection in men and difficulty with lubrication and swelling in women (general sexual dysfunction). Erectile dysfunction probably affects most men at least once in their lifetimes, and transient episodes are estimated to occur in 50% of all men. These fleeting episodes are considered within the range of normal. Impotence occurs in varying degrees: some men experience total inability to attain an erection of sufficient hardness. This frustrating, humiliating condition may lead to decreased self-esteem and consequent depression. Impotence is described as primary if the man has never been able to achieve or maintain an erection that would permit intercourse. Secondary impotence, a more common phenomenon, occurs situationally and is likely to be seen in conjunction with pathophysiologically and pharmacologically induced states.

The penile prosthetic implant has recently been devised as a method of treatment for organic impotence in men. There are two types of penile prostheses (Fig. 67-1). The older type consists of the implantation of two sponge-filled silicone rods in the corpora cavernosa. This maintains the penis in a constant semierect position. The newer and more acceptable method for many men is the inflatable penile prosthesis. Both types of prostheses are implanted surgically and do not interfere with normal urinary elimination. The silicone implants are inserted through perineal or penile incisions and the inflatable prostheses through perineal and abdominal incisions. Penile edema is minimal, but scrotal edema may occur with the inflatable type. Pain may be severe during the first week, and mild pain may continue for several weeks after surgery.[101] As with any prosthetic

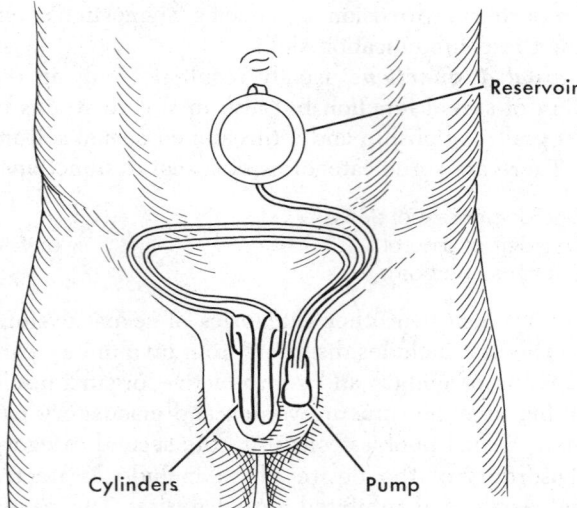

Fig. 67-1. Inflatable penile prosthetic implant. Reservoir is implanted under abdominal muscles, inflatable cylinders in each corpus cavernosum, and pump inside scrotum. Man can compress pump to fill cylinders from reservoir, producing penile erection. Small release valve in lower portion of pump bulb releases fluid to return the penis to flaccid state.

device, there is a need to integrate it into one's self-image *and* the relationship.

Disorders of the orgasmic phase include inadequate ejaculatory control or premature ejaculation, retarded ejaculation, and orgasmic dysfunction in women. Premature ejaculation occurs when the man cannot inhibit his ejaculation for a long enough period of time to permit his partner to experience orgasm in at least half of their attempts at intercourse. This is thought likely to be a conditioned response to hurried circumstances and is treated quite successfully by means of the "squeeze technique." This technique requires the man or his partner to place the thumb and second and third fingers at the coronal ridge of the glans, exerting enough pressure over this area for 3 or 4 seconds to relieve the feeling of ejaculatory inevitability. Retarded ejaculation, also known as ejaculatory incompetence, implies that despite the amount and quality of stimulation of the penis, intravaginal ejaculation either does not occur or is so delayed that the couple experiences pelvic irritation and fatigue as a result.

Primary orgasmic dysfunction occurs in the woman who has not experienced orgasm with sexual activity, including intercourse or masturbation. Secondary orgasmic dysfunction is characterized by inability to experience orgasm under certain conditions. The woman with secondary orgasmic dysfunction has experienced orgasmic sensations with one form of stimulation at some point in her life. This problem does not preclude the woman from experiencing sexual arousal and its physiologic accompaniments. Rather, only the orgasmic portion of the sexual response cycle seems impaired. Vag-

inismus is a relatively rare sexual problem characterized by an involuntary, conditioned spasm of the vaginal outlet, thus causing it to shut tightly. This problem precludes sexual intercourse, but vaginismic women may be orgasmic with alternative methods of sexual stimulation. Dyspareunia, or painful intercourse, may be attributable to a number of factors ranging from a full lower bowel to feelings of aversion toward sexual intercourse. It is sometimes experienced by women with steroid alterations, for example, the postpartum mother and the postmenopausal woman.

Masters and Johnson[61] have also conducted clinical studies with homosexual men and woman who had a sexual dysfunction or were sexually dissatisfied. There appeared to be more similarity than difference in the kinds of sexual dysfunctions homosexuals and heterosexuals experienced. For a highly motivated segment of the homosexual population that desires conversion or reversion to heterosexuality, a therapy approach was described that may be effective.

Nursing practice framework for identifying persons at risk of sexual concerns or problems

Although many persons, themselves, will identify their sexual concerns and problems, in some instances nurses need to initiate discussion of issues of potential concern to the individual. In the context of clinical nursing practice, many persons are "at risk" of experiencing sexual concerns or problems. A framework for understanding the effects of altered health states on human sexuality will be described and illustrative examples given.

Influences of altered health states on sexual health

Altered health states and their treatment can influence sexuality in several ways, some of which are direct and some of which are mediated by other variables. Some may have the ability to enhance sexuality, whereas others may interfere with sexual health. Some may affect the person's ability to engage in sexual activity, some may change the image the person has of himself or herself as a sexual being, and others may induce changes in the sexual relationship. Some effects may pertain only to the client whereas others affect the partner.

Enhancing influences. Although it may seem ironic, some illnesses and their therapies may improve sexual health. Confrontation with a critical illness or one that has a bad prognosis may lead couples to reassess the importance of their relationship and may be the prelude to a renewed closeness. Some therapies may lead to an enhanced feeling of general well-being and may even reverse sexual dysfunctions such as problems getting an erection. This can occur when a debilitating disease is arrested or when the therapy itself improves well-being, as is sometimes the case with the use of steroids. In both examples the mechanisms are probably indirect, but one or more of the components of sexual health are enhanced.

Interfering influences. Several mechanisms do exist whereby altered health states can interfere with the sexual health of the client and the partner. Potential threats to sexual health include structural changes in anatomy, physiologic interferences, body image distortion, environmentally induced problems, and behavioral problems. Superimposed on these may be variations in life events and changes throughout the life cycle.

Anatomic structural changes are probably best exemplified by the spinal cord–injured person who has sustained irreversible damage to neural pathways and consequently has interference with usual methods of sexual function. *Physiologic interferences,* such as those associated with diabetes and circulatory insufficiency, probably alter the individual's ability to respond to sexual stimuli by interfering with the processes of vasocongestion and sensorimotor conduction essential to sexual response. *Pharmacologic agents* are capable of inducing sexual problems by interfering with hormonal, neurologic, and circulatory mechanisms. *Body image distortion* may accompany surgery or traumatic injury. Having an altered image of oneself may interfere with sexual expression and alter the person's current sexual relationship. *Environmental restrictions* may minimize sexual opportunity or accessibility of a partner. *Life events,* such as pregnancy or menopause, although not pathologic entities in themselves, require adaptation to changes in biology as well as emotional response. Certain parts of the *life cycle* bring sexual issues to the forefront, for example, adolescence and middlescence. Finally, *behavioral problems* such as inability to form a relationship with another person may result in inappropriate sexual expression or thwart the client's attempts at sexual expression. Those problems most likely to be encountered in medical-surgical nursing practice will be explored in more detail.

Structural changes interfering with sexual health

The person with a spinal cord injury best exemplifies the sexual consequences of structural alterations. Other conditions resulting in sexual problems or concerns as a result of structural changes are listed in Table 67-1.

The literature on sexual function following cord injury* confirms that men and women alike are anxious to know about the future of their sexuality. Shortly after cord injury, it may be difficult to determine the extent to which sexual activity will return. However, after spinal shock subsides, many men regain their ability to have an erection.

One major difference between sexual response in spinal cord–injured persons and those who are not disabled in this manner is that genital sexual functioning and cerebral or cognitional eroticism become separated. In those persons who have complete transections of the cord, an erection or swelling may not be perceived unless the person can visualize it.

Often questions are raised about the likelihood of any form of sexual function among cord-injured persons. In general, the higher the lesion, the more likely men will be able to experience an erection. Men with cervical lesions are able to achieve erections in a greater percentage of cases that those with lumbar or sacral lesions. In fact, if there is injury to the sacral cord, the nerves supplying the pelvis and involved in the reflex arc permitting erection are likely to be damaged, and thus reflexogenic erections often are not possible. When the lower motor neuron is damaged, there is sometimes the potential for psychogenically induced erections. In this case, thoughts or feelings perceived at higher levels of the cortex may trigger erections.

The major complication of cord injury is the decreased likelihood of experiencing ejaculation. Generally, ejaculation is infrequent and is much less frequent in men with complete transections than in those with partial lesions.

Thus a person's sexual function after cord injury depends on two biologic variables: the number of fibers that were severed (complete vs. incomplete lesions) and the level of the injury (cervical, thoracic, lumbar, or sacral). Erection can occur in response to local stimulation, which produces it reflexly, or in response to psychogenic stimuli. In the latter case, impulses from the brain can sometimes bypass the injured portion of the cord via the autonomic nervous system. Indeed, some men with complete denervation of the genitalia report experiencing erection and orgasm. Usually psychogenic erections are much less common than reflexogenic erections. Ejaculation usually cannot occur.[107]

Because of the sensory losses associated with cord injury, the experience of orgasm as it occurred before injury is usually impossible. However, there are many cord-injured persons who report what is an orgasmlike experience in other parts of their bodies. This sensation is commonly referred to the breasts in women. Additionally, recent work with imagery or fantasy seems promising. In this technique the person's thoughts and

TABLE 67-1. Anatomic changes and their hypothesized interferences with sexual health*

System	Hypothesized mechanism of interference
Central and peripheral nervous systems	
Spinal cord injury	Disrupts integrity of peripheral nerves and spinal cord reflexes involved in sexual response (e.g., erection)
Spinal cord tumors	
Herniated disk	
Multiple sclerosis	
Spina bifida	
Amyotrophic lateral sclerosis	
Tumors of frontal or temporal lobes	May interfere with function of centers controlling sexual drive
Cerebrovascular accident	
Trauma to frontal or temporal lobes	
Cardiovascular system	
Thrombus formation in vessels of penis	May interfere with blood supply to penis, thus interfering with erection
Leriche's syndrome	
Sickle cell disorders	
Leukemia	
Trauma to vasculature supplying sexual organs	
Reproductive/sexual system	
Prostatectomy, radical perineal	May destroy nerve supply, interfering with sensory and motor aspects of sexual response
Abdominal perineal resection	
Lumbar sympathectomy	May result in disturbed ejaculation
Rhizotomy	May result in impotence as well as disturbed ejaculation
Absence of penis or penile injury	Precludes or discourages intromission
Penectomy	
Imperforate hymen	
Congenital absence of vagina	
Pelvic exenteration	
Vaginectomy	
Obstetric trauma or poor episiotomy	Leaves gaping vaginal opening or painful scarring, thus discouraging intercourse
Damage to pubococcygeus muscle	

*See references 1, 5, 9-11, 15-21, 24, 27, 33, 35, 38, 39, 43, 44, 53, 57, 64, 80, 81, 87, 98, 107.

feelings are channeled to produce a psychic experience similar to orgasm.[16]

Sexual options available to the cord-injured person depend on numerous factors, including their sexual value systems, muscle strength in the upper extremities, presence of hip flexors and extensors, the presence of appliances, and access to a partner. The first of these, the individual's sexual value system, in conjunction with a partner's, determines what range of behaviors is acceptable. For example, oral genital stimulation is a viable means for a cord-injured man to stimulate his partner, but this may be prohibited within the couple's sexual value system. The muscle strength of the arms will determine to what extent the person can support the body weight, thus determining the variety of positions that can be used. The ability to flex and extend the hips may enable the man or woman to take a more active role in intercourse by thrusting the pelvis. Weakness in these muscles can be compensated by use of a water bed, which amplifies movement (and also decreases skin problems). The presence of a urinary appliance may not be a problem. Condom catheters and leg bags can be removed before intercourse, Foley catheters can be taped in place and left in the bladder, or the urinary collection system can be positioned in such a way that it is not likely to become clamped off or ruptured by the partner's weight. If the patient has an indwelling catheter, the woman with adequate vaginal lubrication usually does not have trouble accommodating the catheter in her vagina.[64]

With orgasmic release, some cord-injured persons experience violent muscle spasms. These can sometimes be managed with medication, but there is a trade-off involved—some antispasmodics precipitate sexual dysfunction.

For those cord-injured men who cannot obtain a full erection, the "stuffing" technique may be a useful approach. The penis is literally stuffed in the partner's vagina. By then contracting her pubococcygeus muscle, the woman can experience sexual sensations similar to those previously associated with penile thrusting.[63]

Although not much has been written about adaptation of homosexuals to cord injury, probably similar concerns and options are appropriate. For those not currently involved in a relationship, opportunity is likely to be a problem just as it is for heterosexuals.

Perhaps one of the greatest assets the cord-injured person can have is the presence of a caring partner. Those who are not involved in a caring relationship at the time of their injuries are faced with the problems of developing new relationships as well as experimenting with new sexual options.

Fertility is usually unimpaired in cord-injured women, but because of a number of factors, sperm may not be viable in cord-injured men. Use of artificial insemination (either with the man's own or a donor's semen) is a possibility for those who want children. Normal pregnancy is possible for women with cord injuries. Careful health monitoring is essential since the incidence of urinary tract infections may be greater in cord-injured women during pregnancy, they may fail to perceive the beginnings of labor because of loss of sensation, and in a few instances cesarean section may be necessitated.

Although in the past much emphasis has been placed on the cord-injured person's ability to help the partner achieve sexual gratification, new techniques, such as imagery, actively seek to help the disabled person adapt to the sexual changes experienced. Nurses as health professionals may be involved in long-term relationships with these persons and have an excellent opportunity to assess their sexual concerns and intervene by teaching or counseling.

Other structural changes that influence sexual health are those directly affecting the reproductive/sexual system. Penectomy and vaginectomy are obvious examples, but structural changes in the pelvis from obstetric trauma or abdominal-perineal resection for bowel malignancies also may impair sexual function.

Physiologic interference with sexual health

Many illnesses alter physiologic processes essential to the sexual response, including nervous transmission, vasocongestion, hormonal metabolism, myotonia, and perception of pleasurable sensation. Pharmacologic agents that interfere with these basic physiologic activities have the potential to affect sexual drive as well as performance. Table 67-2 illustrates some illnesses and Table 67-3 some drugs that have the potential to interfere with sexual response and the hypothesized mechanism by which they limit sexual response.

In general, it appears that the extent of a physiologic disorder and its chronicity determine relative frequency of sexual problems. For example, frequency of sexual dysfunction among women with diabetes in-

creases with the duration of the disease, although no correlation exists between sexual dysfunction and actual complications of the disease.[50] This relationship between chronicity and dysfunction is also observed in men with diabetes.[121] A high incidence of impotence is found among diabetic men during the first year after diagnosis. It is believed that in this instance the lack of diabetic control (physiologic derangement) is responsible for the sexual dysfunction.[120]

Often a change in health is accompanied by malaise or fatigue. As a consequence, the person experiences a decrease in sexual desire or difficulty becoming aroused. This effect may not be a direct function of the disease itself, but the consequence of "feeling bad" being incompatible with the stimulating thoughts and feelings an individual finds necessary for sexual response.

Other altered health states involve endocrine or metabolic changes. For example, both men and women experience a decrease in sexual desire when testosterone is absent. Erection and vaginal lubrication are diminished when the appropriate hormonal milieu is not present and sometimes orgasm and ejaculation may be impaired as well.

Painful conditions may make it difficult for the client to be physically close to a partner or may require special attention to the use of positioning; for example, in arthritic individuals the person's mobility may be limited, and he or she may require assistance with positioning or other preparations for lovemaking. Depression is an appropriate response to illness for some, and depression is often accompanied by decreased interest in sexual function and in some instances inability to function sexually.

The relationship between extent of physiologic derangement and degree of sexual dysfunction is also demonstrated by pharmacologically induced changes. For example, alcohol induces transiently positive changes; in small doses it initially promotes relaxation and release of inhibitions as do other psychoactive drugs. However, in larger doses alcohol has negative effects on sexual function, leading to central nervous system depression and interference with motor activity.[121]

Several categories of drugs have demonstrable negative effects on sexual function. These include antihypertensives, antidepressants, antihistamines, antispasmodics, sedatives and tranquilizers, ethyl alcohol, some sex hormone preparations, and some narcotics and psychoactive drugs. Examples of these drugs are listed in Table 67-3.

Although some medical-surgical conditions do not interfere directly with sexual function, their perceived seriousness or the presence of symptoms discourages persons from engaging in their usual sexual practices. One very common example is associated with cardiac disease, more specifically myocardial infarction. Although marital coitus probably does not demand a great

TABLE 67-2. Physiologic interferences with sexual health*

Physiologic interferences	Hypothesized mechanism of action	Physiologic interferences	Hypothesized mechanism of action
Systemic diseases			
Pulmonary disease	Debility, pain, and depression probably interfere with sexual libido as well as expression	Trauma to penis	
Renal disease		Vaginal infections	
Malignancies		Senile vaginitis	
Infections		Vulvitis	
Degenerative diseases		Leukoplakia	
Some cardiovascular diseases		Bartholin's cyst	
		Allergic response to vaginal sprays and deodorants	
Metabolic disruptions		Vaginitis following radiation therapy	
Cirrhosis	Hepatic problems in men result in estrogen buildup from inability of liver to conjugate estrogens; similar processes occur in women along with general debility	Pelvic inflammatory disease	
Mononucleosis		Fibroadenomas	
Hepatitis		Endometriosis	
		Uterine prolapse	
		Anal fissures, hemorrhoids	
Hypothyroidism	By depression of CNS function, general debilitation, and depression, libido may be decreased, and impaired erectile abilities in men may result	Pelvis masses	
Addison's disease		Ovarian cysts	
Hypogonadism		Prostatitis	Local irritability, damage to genitalia, and consequent interference with reflex mechanisms involved in erection and ejaculation
Hypopituitarism		Urethritis	
Acromegaly			
Feminizing tumors			
Cushing's disease			
Diabetes mellitus			
		Medical or surgical castration	
Diseases of the genitalia		Orchiectomy	Lowered androgen levels depress libido and lead to impotence, retarded ejaculation, or impaired sexual responsiveness
Priapism	Each of these problems involves damage to genital organs, which may result in painful intercourse	Radiation therapy	
Peyronie's disease		Oophorectomy, adrenalectomy	
Balantitis			
Phimosis			
Genital herpes			

*See references 2-4, 7, 8, 22, 25, 28-30, 42, 45, 46, 49, 50, 52, 54-59, 66, 67, 70, 73, 75, 77, 81, 83, 85, 88-91, 94, 106, 114-116, 118, 121, 124.

energy expenditure, many persons are fearful of attempting intercourse after having a heart attack. One study of married men who had had myocardial infarctions demonstrated that heart rates with orgasm were much lower in this group (about 117 beats/min on the average) than among the younger group studied by Masters and Johnson.[42] An active physical conditioning program did produce significant improvments in the frequency and quality of sexual activity for men who had had a myocardial infarction. The energy expenditure associated with sex seemed to be better tolerated by those who exercised regularly.

In general, the literature indicates that the post–myocardial infarction patient may return to regular sexual activity provided there are no symptoms of congestive heart failure. However, certain conditions that increase energy expenditure during coitus are to be avoided. These include having intercourse shortly after a meal or soon after alcohol consumption, since both increase the heart rate and metabolic demands, and avoiding extremes in temperatures and anxiety-provoking or secretive situations. (Sample instructions for cardiac patients appear in the boxed material on p. 1672.)

Body image changes

The extent to which distortion of body image influences sexuality often depends on the perceptions of at least two persons: oneself and a significant other. Multiple variables may influence the body image of a woman who has had a mastectomy. Among these are factors such as extent of the surgical procedure, the value she assigns to her breasts, her preoperative body image, and social factors such as the quality of her preoperative sexual relationship. A sexual partner's reaction may be similarly affected.[102]

The *visibility* of a defect plays an important role in sexual adaptation. Goffman refers to individuals with "spoiled identities" whose interactions with others are

TABLE 67-3. Pharmacologic interferences by drug or drug category*

Drug	Mechanism of action	Drug	Mechanism of action
Antihypertensives Alpha-methyldopa (Aldomet) Guanethidine (Ismelin) Hydralazine hydrochloride (Apresoline) Reserpine (Serpasil) Mecamylamine (Inversine) Clonidine hydrochloride (Catapres) Trimethaphan (Arfonad) Spironolactone (Aldactone)	Peripheral blockade of nervous innervation of sex glands	Marijuana LSD Methadone (Amidone, Dolophine)	Release of inhibitions; increased suggestibility; relaxation; improvement of well-being Can impair fertility by reducing size and secretory activity of secondary sex organs, resulting in extremely low ejaculate volume and low sperm motility
Antidepressants Imipramine (Tofranil) Desipramine (Norpramin, Pertofrane) Amitriptyline (Elavil) Nortriptyline (Aventyl) Protriptyline (Vivactil) Phenelzine sulfate (Nardil) Tranylcypromine sulfate (Parnate) Pargyline (Eutonyl)	Central depression; peripheral blockade of nervous innervation of sex glands	**Barbiturates** Amobarbital (Amytal) Pentobarbital (Nembutal) Secobarbital (Seconal) Thiopental sodium (Penothal)	General depressant effects on all nervous tissues
Antihistamines Diphenhydramine (Benadryl) Promethazine (Phenergan) Chlorpheniramine (Chlor-trimeton)	Blockade of parasympathetic nervous innervation of sex glands	**Amphetamines** Amphetamine sulfate (Benzedrine) Dextroamphetamine sulfate (Dexedrine) Methamphetamine hydrochloride (Methedrine)	Central stimulation with heightened mood followed by nervousness and insomnia with prolonged use; peripheral sympathomimetic effects
Antispasmodics Methantheline (Banthine) Glycopyrrolate (Robinul) Hexocyclium (Tral) Poldine (Nacton)	Ganglionic blockage of nervous innervation of sex glands	**Antiparkinsonism drugs** Trihexyphenidyl (Artane, Tremin) Biperiden (Akineton) Benztropine (Cogentin) L-Dopa	Peripheral blockade of parasympathetic nervous innervation of sex glands Central stimulation with improvements of wellbeing

Sedatives and tranquilizers
Chlorpromazine (Thorazine, Megaphen)
Prochlorperazine (Compazine)
Meprobamate (Miltown, Equanil)
Thioridazine (Mellaril)
Mesoridazine (Serentil)
Chlordiazepoxide (Librium)
Diazepam (Valium)
Benperidol
Phenoxybenzamine (Dibenzyline)
Chlorprothixene (Taractan)
Methaqualone (Quaalude)
	Central sedation; blockade of autonomic innervation of sex glands; suppression of hypothalmic and pituitary function; tranquilization and relaxation	**Diuretic agents**
		Thiazide diuretics
		  Bendroflumethiazide (Naturetin)
		  Chlorothiazide (Diuril)
		  Cyclothiazide (Anhydron)
		Nonthiazide diuretics
		  Ethacrynic acid (Edecrin)
		  Furosemide (Lasix)
			Possible impotency from hyperglycemia or potassium depletion (hyperkalemia)

Ethyl alcohol	Central depression; suppression of motor activity; diuresis; release of inhibitions; relaxation	**Anticonvulsants** Phenytoin sodium (Dilantin) Ethotoin (Peganone)	Central depression
Sex hormone preparations Cyproterone acetate Methandrostenolone (Dianabol) Nandrolone phenpropionate (Durabolin) Norethandrolone (Nilevar)	Antiandrogenic effects on sexual function; loss of libido; decreased potency	**Miscellaneous drugs** Amyl nitrite Disulfiram (Antabuse) Lithium carbonate Sodium nitrite	Peripheral vasodilation Impotence; nausea when taken with ethanol Impotence associated with endocrine changes Peripheral vasodilation
Narcotics and psychoactive drugs Morphine Heroin Cocaine	Central depression; decreased libido and impaired potency		

*Adapted from Woods, J.S.: Drug effects of human sexual behavior. In Woods, N.F.: Human sexuality in health and illness, ed. 2, St. Louis, 1979, The C. V. Mosby Co.

TABLE 67-4. Some health problems resulting in body image changes that may raise sexual concerns*

Surgically induced	Traumatically induced	Others
Mastectomy	Burns	Dermatologic disorders
Ostomy	Lacerations, scarring	Obesity
Hysterectomy		Congenital anomalies of sexual organs (e.g., absence of penis, hypospadias)
Amputation of limb or limbs	Amputations	Unusual breast size, including immaturity or hypertrophy

*See references 6, 10, 11, 13, 26, 31, 32, 34, 51, 68, 74, 76, 85, 95, 99, 102, 103, 108-112, 122, 123.

marked by disgrace and rejection and who may elicit withdrawal on the part of others.[113] Visibility of a disability seems to be just as disruptive of marital and family relations as it is of other social relationships.[104]

The *meaning* and *significance* one attaches to a changed body part may interfere with sexual behavior. The male amputee who views his loss as castration, the woman who sees her hysterectomy as a neutering surgery, and the person who equates an ostomy with loss of adult control are likely to experience problems with self-image and, in turn, sexual adjustment. Some common health problems resulting in body image change are listed in Table 67-4.

Environmental restrictions

Environmental factors such as privacy, competing stimuli, and segregation interfere with sexual expression. Institutionalization rarely affords sufficient privacy for sexual expression. As indicated by Masters and Johnson's work, the presence of incongruous stimuli is capable of interfering with the progression of sexual arousal.[117] Finally, many institutions segregate persons on the basis of sex. For whatever reason this may be done, the act of segregation may elicit a range of adaptation including masturbation, homosexual activity, or withdrawal from human warmth. Often these adaptive behaviors are punished, and those who resort to them are stigmatized. In some institutions staff members may assume an in loco parentis stance, treating even aging persons as if they required protection from their sexual inclinations.

Other effects of illness

Some individuals may not be able to integrate their sexuality with the role changes that accompany being ill. Other individuals may see their illnesses as punishment and therefore not feel they "deserve" sexual expression.

The partner of the person with an altered health can also experience changes in sexuality. For some, there may be no acceptable opportunity for sexual expression. When the client is ill, the partner may be forced to inhibit his or her sexual interest. This is often frequently the case for aging women. In some instances the partner may feel guilty about initiating sexual acitivity, particularly if he or she perceives the client as vulnerable to injury. Sometimes the partner may express guilt for being interested in sex when the client is not. In other instances the partner may experience role confusion when he or she is expected to be caretaker as well as lover. For example, the partner may not be able to integrate helping with a bowel program with being sexually involved with the client.

Aging process

Changes in sexual function become accentuated during middle age, although their onset is gradual and they probably begin long before they are perceived. Men need more time to attain an erection, and once attained, it is likely to be less full than in earlier years. The testes elevate more slowly with sexual excitement, and vasocongestive changes in the scrotum and testes are less noticeable. With prolongation of the plateau phase of the sexual response cycle, the middle-aged man actually achieves much better control over ejaculation than he had as a young adult.[117]

Orgasm is perceived as happening more quickly, and feelings of ejaculatory inevitability may disappear entirely. Resolution of sexual tension becomes more rapid with age, and the obligatory refractory period (a period during which men cannot be restimulated to orgasm) becomes longer. With aging, men actually gain better control of ejaculation, and because of reduced ejaculatory demand, they may be satisfied not to ejaculate with each intercourse.[117]

Menopausal changes ensue in women: the vaginal epithelium thins, and there is a delay in production of vaginal lubrication and diminished expansion of the vaginal barrel. Loss of fatty tissue in external genitalia as well as the breasts is apparent. The woman's orgasmic experience becomes shorter, and resolution occurs more rapidly.[40,117]

Studies of healthy aging individuals indicate that a decline in overall interest and activity is seen with age.[91] However, men from each age range tend to report greater interest and activity than women in each respective age range. For men, past sexual experience, age, objective and subjective health factors, and social class influence sexual interest and activity. For women, the most important factors were marital status, age, and the enjoyment they derived from sex during younger years. Level of sexual activity in youth appears to be related to that in older years.[73,119]

As men age, an interest-activity gap appears. That is, they desire more sexual activity than they are able to experience. This gap grows as men age; however, it remains small for women. It is suggested that women without a socially acceptable partner adaptively inhibit their sexual interest.[119] Another explanation is that men have been socialized to express a strong sexual desire and they continue to do so despite their experiences of dysfunction. Other social factors, such as the role loss associated with children leaving the parents' home and retirement, are likely to influence the aging person's sexual interests.

Gender disorders

Although many gender disorders exist, they are encountered less often in medical-surgical practice than the problems discussed earlier. Recently, the media have called attention to one gender identity problem, transsexualism, which may be encountered in many medical-surgical services.

Transsexualism refers to the condition of people who are convinced that they are "trapped in the body of the wrong sex." These persons believe that they belong to the opposite sex and desire the body, appearance, and social status of the opposite sex. Many actually live in the role of the opposite sex before treatment. Male-to-female transsexuals are usually treated initially with hormonal therapy, and later surgical revision of their genitalia is performed. The surgery involves removal of the male genitalia and revision of the scrotal and neighboring tissue to resemble the female genitalia. Usually, the surgery is cosmetically successful, and an artificial but functional vagina can be created. These women are, of course, sterile, since they have neither ovaries nor uteri.[62]

The female-to-male transsexual has a less cosmetically effective and functional surgical transformation. In a series of procedures, the breasts and the vulva are revised and a phallus is created. Hormonal therapy is also used to effect the transformation. Often the creation of the penis requires extensive grafting and surgical revision, and the female-to-male transformation is consequently more difficult and usually less satisfactory. After the transformation these men are also sterile.

Both men and women electing transsexual surgery require considerable emotional support. Usually, they have careful psychologic assessments before and following surgery. Because of their cultural conditioning, nurses sometimes find it difficult to relate appropriately to the transsexual. Often it is necessary to analyze one's attitudes and values carefully in order to be accepting of these patients.

Transsexualism should not be confused with transvestism, the act of dressing in the clothing of the opposite sex. Additionally, transsexuals are not to be assumed to be homosexuals.

Hermaphroditism is a congenital condition in which the reproductive structures appear ambiguous. Early life experiences seem to have profound impact on our gender identities. Therefore it is important that sexual assignment be correctly established very early in life to prevent gender confusion later on.[62]

Rape and sexual molestation are problems frequently presented to nurses, especially those employed in emergency care facilities (see Chapter 73 for a further discussion of these problems).

Coping with special client-staff problems

Nurses must sometimes confront (1) clients whose actions are overtly and inappropriately sexual, (2) gender differences between nurse and client that can lead to embarrassing situations, and (3) their own sexual feelings as nurses for particular clients.

Clients may expose their genitalia or make sexual overtures to nurses. Often these behaviors are manifestations of the client's need for some validation of his or her sexuality, a need for feeling some control over a situation in which they feel dependent and out of control, or to attract attention. Some patients may simply be expressing sexual deprivation. Nurses can respond to clients in a way that addresses these concerns, validating their client's sexuality while simultaneously respecting their own integrity. It is important for nurses to assert their rights to have their own body boundaries respected as well as to empathize with the client. It is also important that nurses do not automatically assume they were responsible for eliciting the client's sexual behavior.

Because of the intimate contact sanctioned by the nurse-patient relationship, many potentially embarrassing situations can occur, such as those in which nurses provide direct care to patients of the opposite gender. Maintaining privacy and preventing shaming experiences where possible can help protect the patient from unnecessary anxiety. It is often useful to acknowledge uncomfortable feelings and discuss them instead of denying their existence.

It is not unusual for nurses to have sexual feelings for clients, and these feelings are often anxiety provoking. Professional ethics discourage sexual involvement with patients since they are in a vulnerable position. When sexual feelings interfere with one's practice, it is helpful to acknowledge this and request help for the patient from another professional. Nurses may feel sexually aroused, have physical manifestations of sexual arousal, or have a desire for and fantasies about the patient. It is important that nurses recognize the difference between having these feelings and acting on them. Discussing these feelings with a peer often helps put them into perspective.

Outcome criteria for the person experiencing sexual concerns or problems

The person can:
1. Express sexuality in a manner comfortable and rewarding to both partners.
2. Identify erotically pleasing stimuli that facilitate sexual arousal.
3. Maintain, with cooperation of the partner, a relationship conducive to sexual functioning.
4. Express sexual feelings in a manner consistent with personal values and beliefs.
5. Relate knowledge of STD prevention and family planning to personal sexual relationships.
6. Accurately describe how medical or surgical problems or treatment is likely or not likely to interfere with sexual functioning.
7. Explore with the partner any adaptations in sexual behavior necessitated by illness, hospitalization, or medication.

The first four criteria are applicable to persons of all ages and health statuses. The last three are particularly relevant to those persons hospitalized for medical-surgical problems.

REFERENCES AND SELECTED READINGS
Contemporary

1. Abitol, M.N., and Davenport, J.H.: Sexual dysfunction after therapy for cervical carcinoma, Am. J. Obstet. Gynecol. **119:**181-189, 1974.
2. Abram, H.S., et al.: Sexual functioning in patients with chronic renal failure, J. Nerv. Ment. Dis. **160:**220-226, 1975.
3. Abramov, L.A.: Sexual life and sexual frigidity among women developing acute myocardial infarction, Psychosom. Med. **38:**418-425, 1976.
4. Barlow, D.: Sexually transmitted diseases: the facts, New York, 1979, Oxford University Press.
5. Berkman, A.H., et al.: Sexual adjustment of the spinal cord injured veterans living in the community, Arch. Phys. Med. Rehabil. **59:**29-33, 1978.
6. Binder, D.: Sex, courtship and the single ostomate, Los Angeles, 1973, United Ostomy Association, Inc.
7. Block, A., Maider, J.P., and Haissly, J.E.: Sexual problems after myocardial infarctions, Am. Heart J. **90:**536-537, 1975.
8. Bommer, J., et al.: Sexual behavior of hemodialyzed patients, Clin. Nephrol. **6:**315-318, 1976.
9. Bregman, S.: Sexuality and the spinal cord injured woman, 1975, Sister Kenny Institute, Office of Continuing Education, Dept. 188, 1800 Chicago Ave., Minneapolis, MN 55404.
10. Brouillette, J.N., Pryor, E., and Fox, T.: Evaluation of sexual dysfunction in the female following rectal resection and intestinal stoma, Dis. Colon Rectum **24:**96-102, 1981.
11. Brown, R.S., et al.: Social and psychological adjustment following pelvic exenteration, Am. J. Obstet. Gynecol. **114:**162-171, 1972.
12. Burgess, A., and Holmstrom, L.: Rape: sexual disruption and recovery, Am. J. Orthopsychiatry **49:**648-657, 1979.
13. Burnham, W.R., Lennard-Jones, J.E., and Brooke, B.N.: Sexual problems among married ileostomists, GUT **18:**673-677, 1977.
14. Cassem, H.H., and Hackett, T.P.: Psychiatric consultation in a coronary care unit, Ann. Intern. Med. **75:**9-14, 1971.
15. Cole, T.M.: Sexuality and physical disabilities, Arch. Sex. Behav. **4:**389-403, 1975.
16. Cole, T.M., Chilgren, R.A., and Rosenberg, P.: A new programme of sex education and counseling for spinal cord injured adults and health care professionals, Paraplegia **11:**111-124, Aug. 1973.
17. Comarr, A.E.: Sexual concepts in traumatic cord and equina lesions, J. Urol. **106:**375-378, 1971.
18. Comarr, A.E.: Sexual function among patients with spinal cord injury, Urol. Int. **25:**134-168, 1970.
19. Comarr, A.E., and Vigue, M.: Sexual counseling among male and female patients with spinal cord and/or cauda equina injury, Am. J. Phys. Med. **57:**107-122, 1978.
20. Comarr, A.E., and Vigue, M.: Sexual counseling among male and female patients with spinal cord and/or cauda equina injury. II. Results of interview and neurological examinations of females, Am. J. Phys. Med. **57:**215-227, 1978.
21. Comfort, A., editor: Sexual consequences and disability, Philadelphia, 1978, George F. Stickley Co.
22. Confortini, P., et al.: Full term pregnancy and successful delivery in a patient on chronic hemodialysis, Proc. Eur. Dialysis Transplant Assoc. **8:**74-78, 1971.
23. Craft, M., and Craft, A.: Sex and the mentally handicapped, London, 1978, Routledge and Kegan Paul, Ltd.
24. deBaker, E., et al.: Sexual behavior after prostatectomy, Eur. Urol. **3:**295-298, 1977.
25. DeNour, A.K.: Hemodialysis: sexual functioning, Psychosomatics **19**(4):229-235, 1978.
26. Dlin, B.A., and Perlman, A.: Emotional response to ileostomy and colostomy in patients over the age of 50, Geriatrics **26:**112-118, 1971.
27. Eisenberg, M.G., and Rustad, L.C.: Sex and the spinal cord injured: some questions and answers, Cleveland Veterans Administration Hospital, 1975.
28. Ellenberg, M.: Sex and diabetes: a comparison between men and women, diabetes care **2**(1):4-8, 1979.
29. Ellenberg, M.: Sexual aspects of the female diabetic, M. Sinai J. Med. **44:**495-500, 1977.
30. Ellenberg, M.: Impotence in diabetes: the neurologic factor, Ann. Intern. Med. **75:**213-219, 1971.
31. Fazio, V., Fletcher, J., and Montague, D.: Prospective study of the effect of resection of the rectum on male sexual function, World J. Surg. **4:**149-152, 1980.
32. Fisher, S.: Psychosexual adjustment following total pelvic exenteration, Cancer Nurs., pp. 219-225, June 1979.
33. Fitting, M.D., et al.: Self concept and the sexuality of spinal cord injured women, Arch. Sex. Behav. **7:**43-156, 1978.
34. Gambrell, E.: Sex and the male ostomate, Los Angeles, 1973, United Ostomy Association, Inc.
35. Glass, D.D., et al.: Sexual adjustment in the handicapped, J. Rehabil. **44:**43-47, 1978.

36. Green, R.: Sexual identity conflict in children and adults, New York, 1974, Basic Books, Inc., Publishers.

37. Griffith, C.: Sexuality and the cardiac patient, Heart Lung **2**:70-73, 1973.

38. Griffith, E.R., and Trieschmann, R.B.: Sexual functioning in women with spinal cord injury, Arch. Phys. Med. Rehabil. **56**:18-21, 1975.

39. Griffith, E.R., et al.: Sexual dysfunction associated with physical disabilities, Arch. Phys. Med. Rehabil. **56**:8-13, 1975.

40. Hallstrom, T.: Sexuality of women in middle age: the Goteborg study, J. Biosoc. Sci. **6**(suppl.):165-175, 1979.

41. Hanson, R., and Franklin, M.: Sexual loss in relation to other functional losses for spinal cord injured males, Arch. Phys. Med. Rehabil. **57**:291-293, 1976.

42. Hellerstein, H., and Friedman, E.G.: Sexual activity and the postcoronary patient, Arch. Intern. Med. **125**:987-999, 1970.

43. Heslinga, K., Schellen, A., and Verkuyl, A.: Not made of stone: the problems of handicapped people, Springfield, Ill., 1974, Charles C Thomas, Publisher.

44. Hohmann, G.W.: Reactions of the individual with a disability complicated by a sexual problem, Arch. Phys. Med. Reabil. **56**:9-10, 1975.

45. Holdsworth, S., Atkins, R.C., and DeKretser, D.M.: The pituitary testicular axis in men with chronic renal failure, N. Engl. J. Med. **296**:1245-1249, 1977.

46. Howard, E.J.: Sexual expenditure in patients with hypertensive disease, Med. Aspects Hum. Sex. **7**:82-92, 1973.

47. Kaplan, H.S.: Disorders of sexual desire and other new concepts and techniques in sex therapy, New York, 1979, Simon & Schuster, Inc.

48. Kaplan, H.S.: The new sex therapy, New York, 1974, Brunner/Mazel, Inc.

49. Kavanagh, T., and Shepard, R.J.: Sexual activity after myocardial infarction, Can. Med. Assoc. J. **116**:1250-1253, 1977.

50. Kolodny, R.C.: Sexual dysfunction in diabetic females, Diabetes **20**:557-559, 1971.

51. Krueger, J.C., et al.: Relationship between nurse counseling and sexual adjustment after hysterectomy, Nurs. Res. **28**:145-150, 1979.

52. Kushnir, B., et al.: Primary ventricular fibrillation and resumption of work, sexual activity, and driving after first acute myocardial infarction, Br. Med. J. **4**:609-611, 1975.

53. Lamont, J.K., et al.: Psychosexual rehabilitation after exenterative surgery, Gynecol. Oncol. **6**:236, 1978.

54. Larson, J.: Heart rate and blood pressure: responses of coronary artery disease patients during sexual activity and a two-flight stair climbing test, master's thesis, Seattle, 1978, University of Washington.

55. Levy, N.B.: Coping with maintenance hemodialysis: psychological considerations in the care of patients. In Massry, S.G., and Sellers, A.L.: Clinical aspects of uremia and dialysis, Springfield, Ill., 1976, Charles C Thomas, Publisher.

56. Levy, N.B.: Sexual adjustment to maintenance hemodialysis and renal transplantation: national survey by questionnaire: preliminary report, Trans. Am. Soc. Artif. Intern. Organs **19**:138-143, 1973.

57. Lilius, H.G., and Wikstrom, J.: Sexual problems of patients suffering from multiple sclerosis, Scand. J. Soc. Med. **4**:41-44, 1976.

58. Lim, V.S., and Fang, V.S.: Restoration of plasma testosterone levels in uremic men with clomiphene citrate, J. Clin. Endocrinol. Metab. **43**:1370-1377, 1976.

59. Malik, M.: Sudden coronary deaths associated with sexual activity, J. Forensic Sci. **24**:216-220, 1979.

60. Masters, W., and Johnson, V.: Human sexual inadequacy, 1970, Boston, Little, Brown & Co.

61. Masters, W., and Johnson, V.: Homosexuality in perspective, Boston, 1979, Little, Brown & Co.

62. Money J., and Ehrhardt, A.: Man and woman, boy and girl, Baltimore, 1972, The Johns Hopkins University Press.

63. Mooney, T., Cole, T., and Chilgren, R.: Sexual options for paraplegics and quadriplegics, Boston, 1975, Little, Brown & Co.

64. Morgan, S. Sexuality after hysterectomy and castration, Women and Health **3**(1):5-10, 1978.

65. Nagel, T.C., et al.: Gynecomastia, prolactin, and other peptide hormones in patients undergoing chronic hemodialysis, J. Clin. Endocrinol. Metab. **36**:428-432, 1973.

66. National Institute of Allergy and Infectious Diseases study group report: Sexually transmitted diseases: summary and recommendation, U.S. Department of Health, Education and Welfare, 1980.

67. Naughton, J.: Stress involved in masturbation vs. coitus, Med. Aspects Hum. Sex. **10**:94, 1974.

68. Norris, C., and Gambrell, E.: Sex, pregnancy and the female ostomate, Los Angeles; 1972, United Ostomy Association, Inc.

69. Oaks, W., Melchiode, G., and Ficher, I.: Sex and the life cycle, New York, 1976, Grune & Stratton, Inc.

70. O'Brien, K.M., et al.: Sexual dysfunction in uremia, Proc. Clin. Dial. Transplant Form **5**:98-101, 1975.

71. Orifer, A.P.: Loss of sexual function in the male. In Schoenberg, B., et al., editors: Loss and grief: psychological management in medical practice, New York, 1970, Columbia University Press.

72. Papadopoulos, C., et al.: Sexual concerns and needs of the postcoronary patient's wife, Arch. Intern. Med. **140**:38-41, 1980.

73. Pfeiffer, E., and Davis, G.C.: Determinants of sexual behavior in middle and old age, J. Am. Geriatr. Soc. **20**:151-158, 1972.

74. Pluchinotta, A., and Fabris, G.: Sexual function after abdominoperineal resection of the rectum, Am. J. Proctol. Gastroenterol. Colon Rect. Surg. **31**(6):18-21, 1980.

75. Procci, W.R., et. al.: Sexual functioning of renal transplant recipients, J. Nerv. Ment. Dis. **166**:402-407, 1978.

76. Reach to recovery: for women who have had breast surgery, ed. 2, New York, American Cancer Society, New York City Division, and Memorial Sloan-Kettering Cancer Center.

77. Rhodes, E.N.: Blood pressure and heart rate responses during sexual activity, master's thesis, Seattle, 1974, University of Washington.

78. Roberts, N.: Advising patients on sex after surgery, A.O.R.N. J. **32**:55-61, 1980.

79. Robinault, I.: Sex, society and the disabled: a developmental inquiry into roles, reactions and responsibilities, New York, 1978, Harper & Row, Publishers.

80. Romano, M.D.: Sexuality and the disabled female, Accent on Living, pp. 26-34, Winter 1973.

81. Romm, M.E.: Loss of sexual function in the female. In Schoenberg, B., et al., editors: Loss and grief: psychological management in medical practice, New York, 1970, Columbia University Press.

82. Sadoughi, W., Leshner, M., and Fine, H.: Sexual adjustment in a chronically ill and physically disabled population: a pilot study, Arch. Phys. Med. Rehabil. **52**:311-317, 1971.

83. Scalzi, C., et al.: Sexual counseling of coronary patients, Heart Lung **7**:840-845, 1978.

84. Schiavi, R., and Hogan, B.: Sexual problems in diabetes mellitus: psychological aspects, Diabetes Care **2**(1):9-17, 1979.

85. Seibel, M.: Hysterectomy for carcinoma in situ and sexual function, Gynecol. Oncol. **11**:195-199, 1981.

86. Senior, D.: Adjustment, sexual behavior, and concerns of spinal cord injured women: a pilot study, master's thesis, Seattle, 1977, University of Washington.

87. Sex and Disability Project: Who cares? A handbook on sex education and counseling services for disabled people, Washington, D.C., 1979, George Washington University.

88. Sherman, F.P.: Impotence in patients with chronic renal failure on dialysis: its frequency and etiology, Fertil. Steril. **26:**221-223, 1975.

89. Shulka, G., Srivastava, O., and Katiyar, B.: Sexual disturbances in temporal lobe epilepsy: a controlled study, Br. J. Psychiatry **134:**288-292, 1979.

90. Soloff, L.A.: Sexual activity in the heart patient, Psychosomatics **18:**(4)23-38, 1977.

91. Vermeulen, A.: Decline in sexual activity in aging men: correlation with sex hormone levels and testicular changes, J. Biosoc. Sci. **6**(suppl.):5-18, 1979.

92. Wagner, N.N.: Some sexual aspects of the rehabilitation of cardiac patients. In Stocksmeir, R., editor: Psychological approach to the rehabilitation of coronary patients, New York, 1976, Springer-Verlag New York, Inc.

93. Wasow, M.: Human sexuality and terminal illness, Health and Social Work **2**(2):105-121, 1977.

94. Watts, R.J.: Sexuality and the middle-aged cardiac patient, Nurs. Clin. North Am. **2:**349-359, 1976.

95. Williams, J., and Slack, W.: A prospective study of sexual function after major colorectal surgery, Br. J. Surg. **67:**722-724, 1980.

96. Williams, M.A.: Cultural patterning of the feminine role: a factor in response to hysterectomy, Nurs. Forum **12:**378-387, 1973.

97. Wise, T.: Sexual difficulties with concurrent physical problems, Psychosomatics **18**(4):56-64, 1977.

98. Within reach: providing family planning services to physically disabled women, Planned Parenthood of Snohomish County, 2730 Hoyt, Everett, WA 98201.

99. Witkin, M.H.: Sex therapy and mastectomy, J. Sex Martial Ther. **1:**290-304, 1975.

100. Wood, R.Y., and Rose, K.: Penile implants for impotency, Am. J. Nurs. **78:**234-238, 1978.

101. Woods, N.F.: Human sexuality in health and illness, ed. 2, St. Louis, 1979, The C.V. Mosby Co.

102. Woods, N.F.: Influences on sexual adaptation to mastectomy, J.O.G.N. Nurs. **4:**33-37, 1975.

103. Woods, N.F., and Earp, J.A.L.: Women with cured breast cancer: a study of mastectomy patients in North Carolina, Nurs. Res. **27:**279-285, 1978.

104. Zahn, M.A.: Incapacity, impotence, and invisible impairment: their effects upon interpersonal relations, J. Health Soc. Behav. **14:**115-123, 1973.

Classic

105. Babbott, D., Rubin, A., and Ginsburg, S.J.: Reproductive characteristics of diabetic men, Diabetes **7:**469-472, 1958.

106. Bard, M., and Sutherland, A.: Psychological impact of cancer and its treatment, Cancer **8:**656-672, 1955.

107. Bors, E., and Comarr, A.E.: Neurological disturbances of sexual function with special reference to 529 patients with spinal cord injury, Urol. Surv. **10:**191-222, 1960.

108. Dlin, B.A., Perlman, A., and Ringold, E.: Psychosexual responses to ileostomy and colostomy, A.O.R.N. J. **34:**77-84, 1969.

109. Drellich, M., and Bieber, J.: The psychologic importance of a uterus and its functions: some psychoanalytic implications of hysterectomy, J. Nerv. Ment. Dis. **126:**322-336, 1958.

110. Druss, R.G., et al.: Psychologic response to colectomy, Arch. Gen. Psychiatry **18:**53-59, 1968.

111. Druss, R.G., O'Connor, J.F., and Stern, L.O.: Psychological response to colectomy. II. Adjustment to a permanent colostomy, Arch. Gen. Psychiatry **20:**419-427, 1969.

112. Dyk, R.B., and Sutherland, A.: Adaptation of the spouse and other family members to the colostomy patient, Cancer **9:**123-138, 1956.

113. Goffman, E.: Stigma: notes on the management of spoiled identity, Englewood Cliffs, N.J., 1963, Prentice-Hall, Inc.

114. Goodwin, N.J., et al.: Effects of uremia and chronic hemodialysis on the reproductive cycle, Am. J. Obstet. Gynecol. **100:**528-535, 1968.

115. Greene, L.F., Panayotis, P.K., and Weeks, R.E.: Retrograde ejaculation of semen due to diabetic neuropathy, Fertil. Steril. **14:**617-625, 1963.

116. Kalliomaki, J.L., Markkanne, T.K., and Mustonen, V.A.: Sexual behavior after CVA: a study on patients below the age of 60 years, Fertil. Steril. **12:**156-158, 1961.

117. Masters, W., and Johnson, V.: Human sexual response, Boston, 1966, Little, Brown & Co.

118. Oken, D.E.: Chronic renal diseases and pregnancy: a review, Am. J. Obstet. Gynecol. **94:**1023-1043, 1966.

119. Pfeiffer, E., Verwoerdt, A., and Wang, H.S.: The natural history of sexual behavior in a biologically advantaged group of aged individuals, J. Gerontol. **24:**193-198, 1969.

120. Rubin, A., and Babbott, D.: Impotence and diabetes mellitus, J.A.M.A. **168:**498-500, 1958.

121. Schöffling, K., et al.: Disorders of sexual function in male diabetics, Diabetes **12:**519-527, 1963.

122. Stahlgren, L.H., and Fergusson, L.K.: Influence on sexual function of abdominoperineal resection of ulcerative colitis, N. Engl. J. Med. **259:**873-875, 1958.

123. Sutherland, A., et al. The psychological impact of cancer and cancer surgery, Cancer **5:**857-872, 1952.

124. Tuttle, W.B., Cook, W.L., and Fitch, E.: Sexual behavior in postmyocardial infarction patients, Am. J. Cardiol. **13:**140, 1964.

125. Ueno, M.: The so-called coition death, Jpn. J. Legal Med. **17:**330, 1963.

AUDIOVISUAL RESOURCE

Sexuality and nursing concerns, Concept Media, 1500 Adams Ave., Costa Mesa, CA 92626. ([1] Sexual behavior: nursing reactions—discusses certain sexual behavior with which the nurse might be confronted in hospital setting. [2] Medical conditions: impact on sexuality—discusses how heart attack and diabetes can affect sexual functioning. [3] Disabling and deforming conditions: impact on sexuality—discusses rheumatoid arthritis and spinal cord injury with emphasis on adaptation to chronic disease.)

PROBLEMS RELATED TO IMPAIRED PROTECTIVE MECHANISMS

Protection from the environment involves an intact integument and an ability to defend oneself from foreign matter that has the potential to harm the outer skin barrier. The skin is a visible organ and can be assessed without the use of involved or invasive equipment. Assessment of the skin provides the nurse and other health personnel with additional data concerning other functions of the body such as nutrition (including fluid hydration) and elimination.

Persons with problems of the integument or immune system are at risk with the environment. Many of the skin conditions have been known for many years because of the obvious evidence presented to the naked eye. Because of the overtness of skin lesions, including burns, persons afflicted with these problems may experience psychologic problems. Nurses need to be cognizant of the problems to assist the person with coping and adaptation. The underlying bases of problems of the immune system are relatively new and more complex, although the symptoms of conditions such as allergies have been known for many years. Lives are now being saved through a better understanding of the bases of immunodeficiency diseases.

This unit begins with *assessment* of the integument and immune status. The next two chapters discuss the *general nursing care* requirements of the person with a *dermatologic* problem or with *burns*. The last two chapters deal with specific *problems of the integument and immune response*.

CHAPTER 68

ASSESSMENT OF THE INTEGUMENT AND IMMUNE STATUS

BARBARA C. LONG

The integument, or skin, is the largest organ of the body. It is exposed to the external environment and provides the first line of defense of the body; yet at the same time it is affected by changes in the internal environment. (See Chapter 19 for a review of biologic defense mechanisms.) Assessment of the integument and immune response provides data about how the person is affected by and is coping with both external and internal environments. Data obtained in the assessment provide the bases for identification of nursing problems related to the skin, potential for infection, fluid and electrolyte imbalances, nutritional imbalances, or inadequate oxygenation of tissues. Baseline observations are useful for identifying changes that may occur.

Anatomy and physiology of the skin

Structure of the skin

The skin is composed of two main layers, the epidermis and the dermis (Fig. 68-1). The *epidermis* is composed of two parts, a thin layer of closely packed dead squamous cells covering a second layer of cells containing melanin, which gives skin its color. The dead cells are constantly being shed and replaced by deeper cells. Blood vessels do not reach into the epidermis.

The second main layer, the *dermis* or corium, is connected to the epidermis by a convoluted layer of cells that produce new cells for the epidermis. The dermis is composed of bundles of collagen fibers that act to support the epidermis. It is well supplied with nerves and blood vessels and contains the sweat glands, sebaceous glands, and hair follicles.

Thickness of the skin varies over different areas of the body. Exposed areas such as the hands and face are usually thicker. The skin on the inner aspect of the arms is thinner and therefore more sensitive to heat.

Sweat glands excrete directly to the surface of the skin and are under control of the sympathetic nervous system. There are two types of sweat glands, *eccrine* and *apocrine*. The eccrine glands are distributed throughout the body and are more abundant in the forehead, palms, and soles of the feet. Eccrine glands assist in the heat-regulating mechanisms of the body. The apocrine glands are found mainly in the axillary and genital regions. Some of the protoplasm of these secretory cells is secreted with the fluid, and it is bacterial decomposition of the sweat from these glands that is responsible for body odor.[3] Sweat glands of the axilla, palms, and soles are mostly under psychic control.

Sebaceous glands secrete an oily, odorless fluid (*sebum*) into the hair follicles. Ear wax is sebum from glands in the external ear canal. Sebum protects the hair follicle from infection and lubricates the skin.

Beneath the skin is the subcutaneous tissue composed of loose connective tissue filled with fat cells. Fat conducts heat only one fourth as rapidly as do other tissues and thus serves as the heat insulator of the body.

Functions of the skin

Protection. The outermost layer of the epidermis, the stratum corneum, is a relatively impermeable layer of tightly packed flat cells that provide protection of the underlying tissue from the outer environment. There

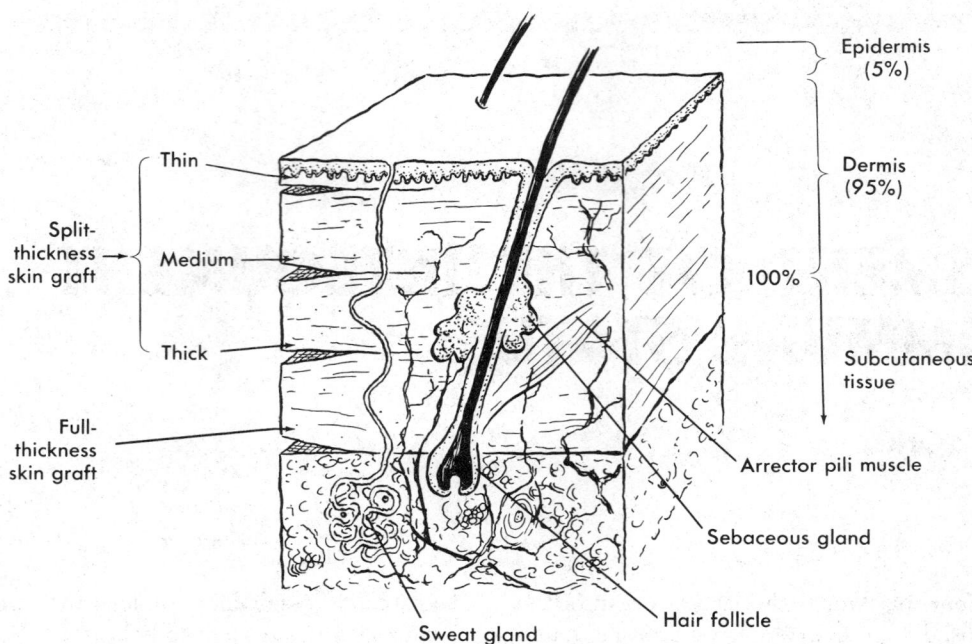

Fig. 68-1. Layers of skin involved in various types of skin grafts. Thickness of epidermis and dermis pictured here is typical of that found on lateral thigh of adult. (Redrawn from Graab, W.S., and Smith, J.W.: Plastic surgery, Boston, 1968, Little, Brown & Co.)

are numerous nonpathogenic bacteria on the outer surface of the skin, but the dryness of the surface keeps the number small since microorganisms require moisture for growth. Bacteria that penetrate hair follicles are usually removed by the sebum. Fat-soluble substances can penetrate the skin by passing through the hair follicles and sebaceous glands. Atrophic or senile skin contains fewer hair follicles; thus permeability of fat-soluble substances through the skin is decreased in the elderly.

An intact skin is the first line of defense against bacterial and foreign substance invasion, slight physical trauma, heat, or rays. The epidermis can be weakened by scraping or stripping the surface, such as by dry razors or by removal of tape. Once the barrier has weakened, permeability to bacteria, drugs, and so forth is increased. Large amounts of drugs can be absorbed by extensive denuded skin areas. Epidermis that becomes overdry may crack and lead to breaks in the surface. If it remains wet for long periods of time, it becomes macerated and the moisture provides a medium for bacterial growth.

The stratum corneum is not found in mucous membranes since these areas are somewhat protected from the external environment. Fluids and other substances such as certain drugs can be absorbed through the mucous membranes.

Heat regulation. Body temperature is controlled by *radiation* of heat from the surface of the skin, *conduction* of heat from skin to other objects or air, removal of heat by air currents on the skin (*convection*), or *evaporation* of water from skin surfaces. Insensible water evaporation from the skin and lungs occurs at a rate of 600 to 1000 ml/day. On a hot day the only way the body can lose heat is by evaporation, and anything that restricts evaporation under these conditions will increase body temperature. Blood vessels of the skin assist in control of body temperature by constriction in cold environments to promote conservation of heat, and dilation in warm environments to promote loss of heat by radiation. These mechanisms help maintain a constant internal body temperature.

Sensory perception. Receptors for pain, touch, heat, and cold are present in the skin.

Excretion. Water lost through the skin is a factor in maintaining water balance in the body. Salt is lost through excessive sweating in addition to water. A person can become acclimatized to a continually hot environment, however, and the amount of salt lost decreases over time.

Vitamin D production. Synthesis of vitamin D takes place in the skin by the effect of sunlight (ultraviolet rays). Vitamin D is necessary in the metabolism of calcium and phosphorus (p. 340).

Expression. Since the skin is the part of the body that is visible to others, it serves as a means of communicating feelings. Also, because of its visibility, skin is largely involved in a person's feelings of *body image*. Individuals become concerned when there is fear of or presence of disfigurement. (The reader is referred to Chapter 28 for a discussion of body image.)

Subjective data

Data to be obtained from a person on an initial health history are of two types: (1) information to identify a potential dermatologic or immune problem and (2) information specific to a skin condition or allergy that is already present.

General information

1. *History of dermatologic disease:* identification of any skin conditions that may be familial or that may recur (allergy)
2. *History of recurrent infections:* identification of a possible decreased immune response
3. *Nutritional status:* a history of weight loss and underweight may indicate a possible protein-calorie malnutrition, which can affect the immune response (p. 1857)
4. *Occupation:* contact with potential skin irritants such as arsenic, lead, chromium, strong acids or bases (contact dermatitis); abnormal heat or unhygienic environment (infections, insect infestations); hands constantly in water (dermatitis)
5. *Seasonal factors:* exposure to excessive sun (burn, skin cancer) or cold (frostbite); pollens (allergies, hay fever)
6. *Recreational activities:* for example, painting, camping, yard work, exposure to paint compounds, poison ivy, poison oak, or poison sumac (dermatitis venenata)
7. *Travel to foreign countries:* exposure to contagious disease
8. *Drugs:* steroids (glucocorticoids) are antiinflammatory and may produce a false-negative response to skin testing; antimetabolites may depress bone marrow, resulting in thrombocytopenia (potential for hemorrhage) or leukopenia (potential for infection)
9. *Radiation therapy:* radiation decreases the immune response (p. 1858)

Specific information

1. *Onset of the problem:* initial sites; when were changes first noticed; skin appearance at onset; any other symptoms noted at time of onset such

as pain, itching, sneezing, rhinitis; any specific known cause such as contact with poison ivy, exposure to a known allergen, stress
2. *Changes since onset:* changes in location of lesions; changes in appearance; new symptoms such as pain or itching
3. *If cause is unknown:* recent exposure to sensitizing substances such as metals, toxic inhalants, animal dander, foods, poisonous plants, pollens (depending on symptoms); new drug prescriptions such as penicillin
4. *Alleviating factors:* physician-prescribed or self-prescribed treatment
5. *If cause is an allergen:* previous history including pattern and sequence of symptoms and signs, preventive or desensitization measures, medical follow-up (continual or symptomatic)
6. *Psychologic reaction to problem:* withdrawal from social activities; cosmetics for cover up; feelings concerning self in view of the problem (body image)

Objective data

Methods of assessment

The skin is an organ that can be examined by *direct inspection* and *observation* with no tools but a good light. *Palpation* is also used in gathering data related to certain types of lesions.

Considerable data can be obtained from physical assessment of the skin, not only concerning dermatologic problems, but also concerning the health status of the individual. A systematic head-to-toe skin assessment is usually carried out while gathering other significant data in the initial interview and physical assessment of the person. Specific areas of the skin are reassessed as potential or existing problems are identified.

Guidelines for skin assessment

1. Be prepared; have a good light available. If the lighting is inadequate, lesions may be missed or described inaccurately.
2. Be systematic: if only some parts of the skin are inspected, an important parameter may be omitted or a lesion missed.
3. Be thorough: look at all areas carefully. If the person is lying down, be sure to examine the back, especially the sacral area. Lift folds of tissue, such as under the breasts or gluteal folds. Embarrassment by the examiner or anticipated embarrass-

TABLE 68-1. Skin color changes

Color	Physiology	Conditions
Redness	Vasodilation: more rapid blood flow, more oxygenated blood giving a reddish hue (erythema)	Blushing, heat, inflammation, fever, alcohol ingestion, extreme cold (below 15 C),[10] hot flushes
Whiteness (pallor)	Vasoconstriction: slower blood flow, less blood in capillaries	Cold, fear, shock
	Partially obstructed blood flow: less blood in capillaries	Vasospasm, thrombus, narrowed vessels
	Fluid between blood vessels and skin surface	Edema
	Decreased oxygenation of blood from decreased hemoglobin	Anemia
	Loss of melanin	Vitiligo
Bluish	Deoxygenated hemoglobin (cyanosis) seen in earlobes, lips, mucous membranes of mouth, nail beds	Heart or lung disease, inadequate respiration, peripheral blood vessel obstruction
Yellow	Increased bile pigment in blood eventually distributed to skin and mucous membranes and to sclera of eye	Liver disease, obstruction of bile ducts, chronic uremia, rapid hemolysis
Brown	Increased melanin deposits: normal in brown-black races	Aging, sunburn
Dullness	Vasoconstriction in dark skin	Cold, fear, shock

ment of the examinee may result in inadequate data.

4. Be specific: when lesions are identified, describe the lesions using the metric system and established parameters (e.g., color, size, shape).

5. Compare right side with left side: when observing changes in skin color or tissue shape, always compare one side of the body with the other to differentiate structural from pathologic changes.

6. Record the data: unrecorded data is lost data. Baseline observations indicating normality or abnormality are needed for comparison with subsequent findings. Changes need to be recorded to determine progress toward achieving desired outcomes.

Parameters of general skin assessment

The objective data to be collected when examining the skin for general health status include skin color, temperature, moisture, elasticity, turgor, texture, and odor.

Color. Changes in skin color are best observed in the lips, mucous membranes of the mouth, earlobes, fingernails and toenails, and the extremities. The lips show rapid color changes.

Color of the skin varies with the amount of *melanin* in the cells and with the *blood supply* (Table 68-1). Melanin formation requires the amino acid tyrosine, the enzyme tyrosinase, and molecular oxygen. Variations of general pigmentation are seen within one individual; an increase in pigmentation is usually seen on exposed surfaces and in the areola of the nipples. Conversely, decreased pigmentation is seen on unexposed surfaces and on the palms and soles of dark-skinned persons.

Hyperpigmentation occurs normally in some persons as a genetic factor (dark skin). Light-skinned persons may have increased pigmentation from the effects of sunlight (tanning). Melanin is formed in the basal cells of the stratum basale and then gradually moves to the surface, where it is cast off and the tan fades. Elderly light-skinned persons may normally develop irregular brown patches (Fig. 68-2). Hyperpigmentation may be seen with x-ray therapy as a result of activation of tyrosinase. This type of hyperpigmentation fades slowly but may be long lasting. Hydroquinone with salicylic acid or with retinoic acid (Artra) inhibits the tyrosinase reaction. Hyperpigmentation also occurs with inflammations, acne vulgaris, drug eruptions, neurodermatitis, and pityriasis rosea.

Hypopigmentation occurs normally in some persons as a genetic factor (light skin). Albinos have a congenital inability to produce melanin. Severe trauma can destroy cells producing melanin and result in hypopigmentation (scar tissue). Some healthy persons develop a condition called *vitiligo* in which there is a failure of melanin formation in certain areas, primarily around orifices and hairy areas, producing sharply demarcated white patches. Vitiligo can also occur with hyperthyroidism, pernicious anemia, and adrenocortical insufficiency. One treatment for small patches of vitiligo is methoxypsoralen orally plus exposure to sunlight or longwave ultraviolet light.

The degree of blood supplied to the skin produces color changes. The rate of blood flow through the skin is highly variable because of its function in heat control. The blood vessels are innervated by the sympathetic nervous system; thus vasoconstriction occurs with the stress response. With vasoconstriction, smaller amounts of blood pass through the vessels, producing decreased redness; a dark skin becomes duller and a light skin whiter (pallor). Vasodilation increases the amount of oxygenated blood flow, and the skin acquires a reddish color (erythema). Vascular flush areas of the body are the "butterfly" band from cheek to cheek across the nose

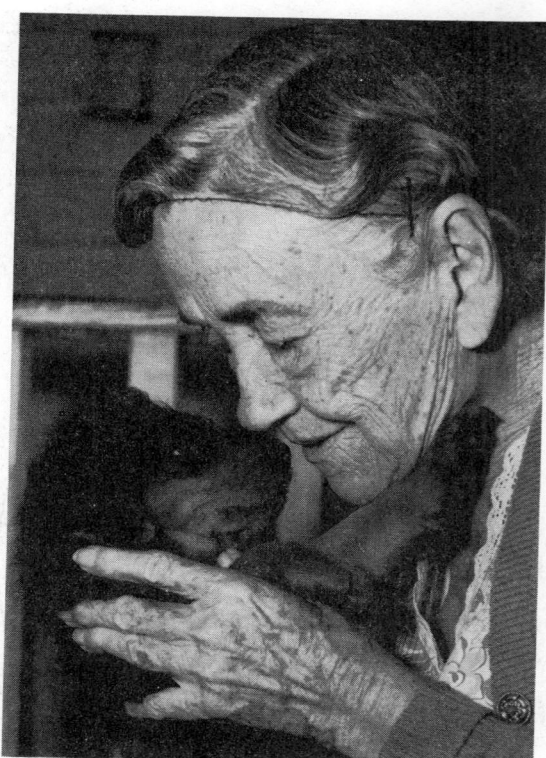

Fig. 68-2. Elderly patients have skin changes. Note discolored spots on skin and tiny raised area on this woman's eyelid. (VanDerMeid from Monkmeyer Press Photo Service.)

the neck, upper chest, flexor surfaces of the extremities, and genital areas.[27]

Changes in blood composition can also alter skin color. Excess deoxygenated hemoglobin gives a bluish tint (*cyanosis*) to the skin and mucous membranes. An excess of bile pigment results in a yellowish tint to the skin and sclera of the eyes.

Temperature. The temperature of the skin is regulated by vasoconstriction or vasodilation. If an excess amount of heat is being produced within the body such as with fever or exercise, or if heat from the external environment increases, the sympathetic centers in the hypothalamus are inhibited and vasodilation occurs. An increase in the amount of blood flow creates a sensation of warmth on the skin. A local inflammation of the skin or underlying tissue also produces vasodilation; this is part of the inflammatory response (p. 280). Cold skin is caused by vasoconstriction as a result of sympathetic stimulation. To assess the temperature of the skin, the backs of the fingers, which are more sensitive than the finger tips, should be used.

Moisture. Skin is assessed as being dry, moist, or oily. *Dry skin* is frequently seen in the elderly person because of decreased activity of the sebaceous glands. Dry skin and mucous membranes are also seen in persons who are dehydrated as water moves from the cells

into the intravascular compartments. Persons with hypothyroidism have thick, dry, leathery skin.

Moist skin is caused by the presence of water or sweat on the surface. Overheating produces sweating. Persons with hyperthyroidism have moist, smooth skin. Some persons have more effective sweat mechanisms than others. Stress, shock, or any situation that stimulates the sympathetic nervous system will cause increased fluid loss through the sweat glands. Since vasoconstriction is also occurring with stimulation of the sympathetic nervous system, the skin is cold and wet (clammy).

Oily skin is frequently seen in the adolescent. An excess amount of sebum formation by the sebaceous glands may lead to blocking of the follicular orifices, resulting in blackheads (*comedo*), acne, or sebaceous cysts.

Elasticity, mobility, and turgor. The skin is very elastic and moves freely over most areas. It loses its mobility when it becomes stretched; this occurs with edema when the interstitial spaces become filled with fluid and swelling occurs. Skin becomes rigid in the person with scleroderma, a collagen disease, as a result of collagenous fibrosis of the tissue. *Turgor* is the speed of skin return to normal position of fullness after it has been stretched. Decreased turgor indicates dehydration of the tissue. To assess elasticity and turgor, a portion of skin over the sternum is picked up (elasticity) and the speed of return to normal is assessed (turgor). Skin that has decreased turgor will remain for a few seconds in a fold before returning slowly to normal (Fig. 68-3).

Texture. Roughness may occur normally on exposed areas, especially elbows and the soles of the feet. The skin of an infant is usually soft and smooth, while that of an elderly person may be rough and lack underlying tissue substance (atrophy). Roughness may occur with hypothyroidism.

Odor. Normal clean skin is usually free of odor except for areas containing apocrine sweat glands. Odor occurs because of bacterial decomposition of protein matter. Some draining skin lesions may produce an odor.

Accessory structures

Hair. If the person is wearing a wig or other hairpiece, this should be removed temporarily for inspection of the hair and scalp. It is easy to miss lesions on the scalp, and the person can assist by indicating areas of itching, pain, or roughness.

Hair growth, pattern, and distribution are indicators of the general state of health of an individual.[10] Excessive hair growth (*hirsutism*) is usually related to hormonal changes. Hair loss (*alopecia*) occurs normally with age, especially in some men. Abnormal hair loss may

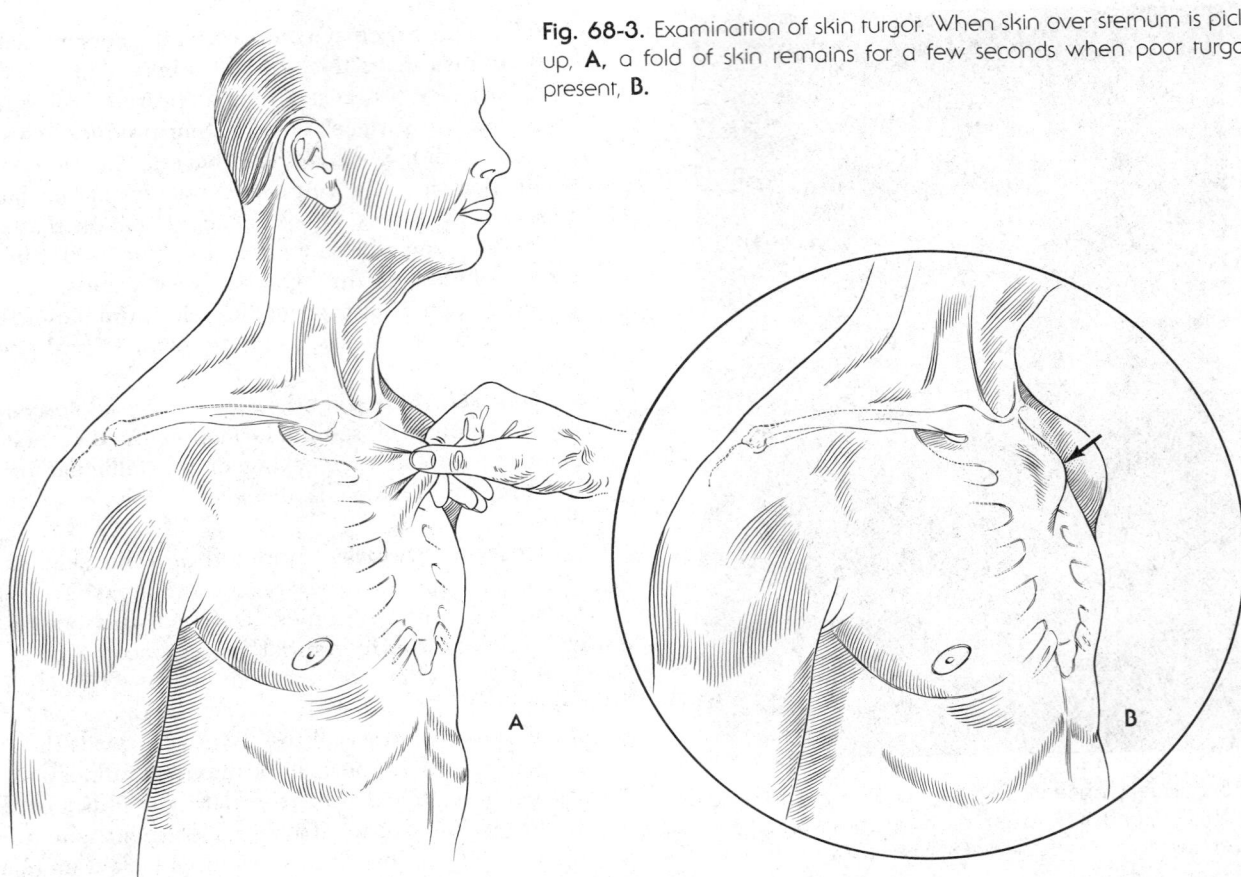

Fig. 68-3. Examination of skin turgor. When skin over sternum is picked up, **A,** a fold of skin remains for a few seconds when poor turgor is present, **B.**

be caused by hormonal imbalance, general ill health, infections of the scalp, typhoid fever, chronic liver disease, stress, or drugs (antimetabolites, heparin). Changes in hair distribution on the body may be caused by hormonal changes. Hair loss on the dorsum of the toes may be indicative of decreased arterial circulation. Contrary to popular belief, shaving does not promote the growth of dark coarse hairs, singing hair does not alter growth, brushing and massaging does not increase hair growth, nor does hair "turn gray overnight."[16] The hair shaft is an inert structure, and changes occur over time as a result of hormonal activity and the availability of nutrients to the bulb at the base of the hair root.

Hair should also be free of lice or nits. Nits are the eggs of the lice and are usually found embedded on hair strands behind the ears. They are observed as small, glistening, grayish specks along the hair shaft near the scalp.

Nails. The appearance of the nails changes with age and with ill health. Changes in hardness, brittleness, roughness, or shape may be indicative of some metabolic diseases, nutritional imbalances including vitamin deficiencies, or digestive disturbances. Pale nail beds and poor capillary return (slow return to normal color after the nail is pinched) may indicate hypoxia or anemia. Clubbing of the nails refers to the elimination of the small concave portion at the base of the nail by soft

tissue growth; this occurs with certain pulmonary diseases (Fig. 68-4).

The epithelial lining of the nail bed is usually inert. The nail is affixed to the nail bed, and both move outward as the nail grows. The epithelial lining of the nail bed loses its inert quality in the presence of inflammatory lesions of the nail bed, such as occur with psoriasis or ringworm, and the nail bed begins to keratinize. Horny masses collect under the nail, resulting in a thickening deformity of the nail and possible separation from the nail bed.[16]

Infections of the tissue around the nail may occur (*paronychia*) characterized by red, shiny skin and painful swelling around the edge of the nail. The infection may result from trauma or from certain diseases such as psoriasis or dermatitis. If the nail is lost, it will usually grow back unless the nail bed has been injured.

Lesions

When lesions are observed, the following parameters are used for description: type, color, size, shape and configuration, texture, effect of pressure, distribution, arrangement, and variety.

Type. Use of medical terminology facilitates communication (Table 68-2). For example, use of the term

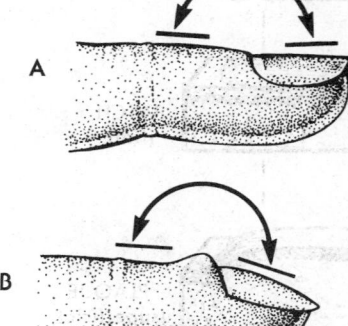

Fig. 68-4. Diagram showing clubbing of finger. **A,** Normal angle of nail. **B,** Abnormal angle of nail seen in late clubbing. (From Malasanos, L., et al.: Health assessment, ed. 2, St. Louis, 1981, The C.V. Mosby Co.)

TABLE 68-2. Types of skin lesions

Observed skin changes	Differentiation	Term	Example
Change in color or texture			
Spot	Circumscribed; flat; color change	Macule	Freckle
Discoloration (reddish purple)	Bleeding beneath the surface; injury to tissue	Contusion	Bruise
Soft whitening	Caused by repeated wetting of skin	Maceration	Between toes after soaking
Flake	Dry cells of surface	Scale	Dandruff; psoriasis
Roughness from dried fluid	Dry exudate over lesions	Crust	Eczema; impetigo
Roughness from cells	Leathery thickening of outer skin layer	Lichenification	Callus on foot
Change in shape			
Fluid-filled lesions	Less than 1 cm; clear fluid	Vesicle	Blister; chickenpox
	Greater than 1 cm; clear fluid	Bulla	Large blister; pemphigus
	Small, thick yellowish fluid (pus)	Pustule	Acne
Solid mass, *cellular* growth	Less than 5 mm	Papule	Small mole; raised rash
	5 mm to 2 cm	Nodule	Enlarged lymph node
	Greater than 2 cm	Tumor	Benign or malignant tumor
	Excess connective tissue over scar	Keloid	Overgrown scar
Swelling of tissue	Generalized swelling; fluid between cells	Edema	Inflammation; swelling of feet
	Circumscribed surface edema; transient; some itching	Wheal	Allergic reaction
Breaks in skin surfaces			
Oozing, scraped surface	Loss of superficial surface of skin	Abrasion	"Floor burn"; scrape
Scooped-out depression	Loss of deeper layers of skin	Ulcer	Decubitus or stasis ulcer
Superficial linear skin breaks	Scratch marks, frequently by finger nails	Excoriations	Scratching
Linear crack or cleft	Slit or splitting of skin layers	Fissure	Athlete's foot
Jagged cut	Tearing of skin surface	Laceration	Accidental cut by blunt object
Linear cut, edges approximated	Cutting by sharp instrument	Incision	Knife cut
Vascular lesions			
Small, flat, round, purplish red spot	Intradermal or submucous hemorrhage	Petechia	Bleeding tendency; vitamin C deficiency
Spiderlike, red, small	Dilation of capillaries, arterioles, or venules	Telangiectasis	Liver disease; vitamin B deficiency
Discoloration, reddish purple	Escape of blood into tissue	Ecchymosis	Trauma to blood vessels

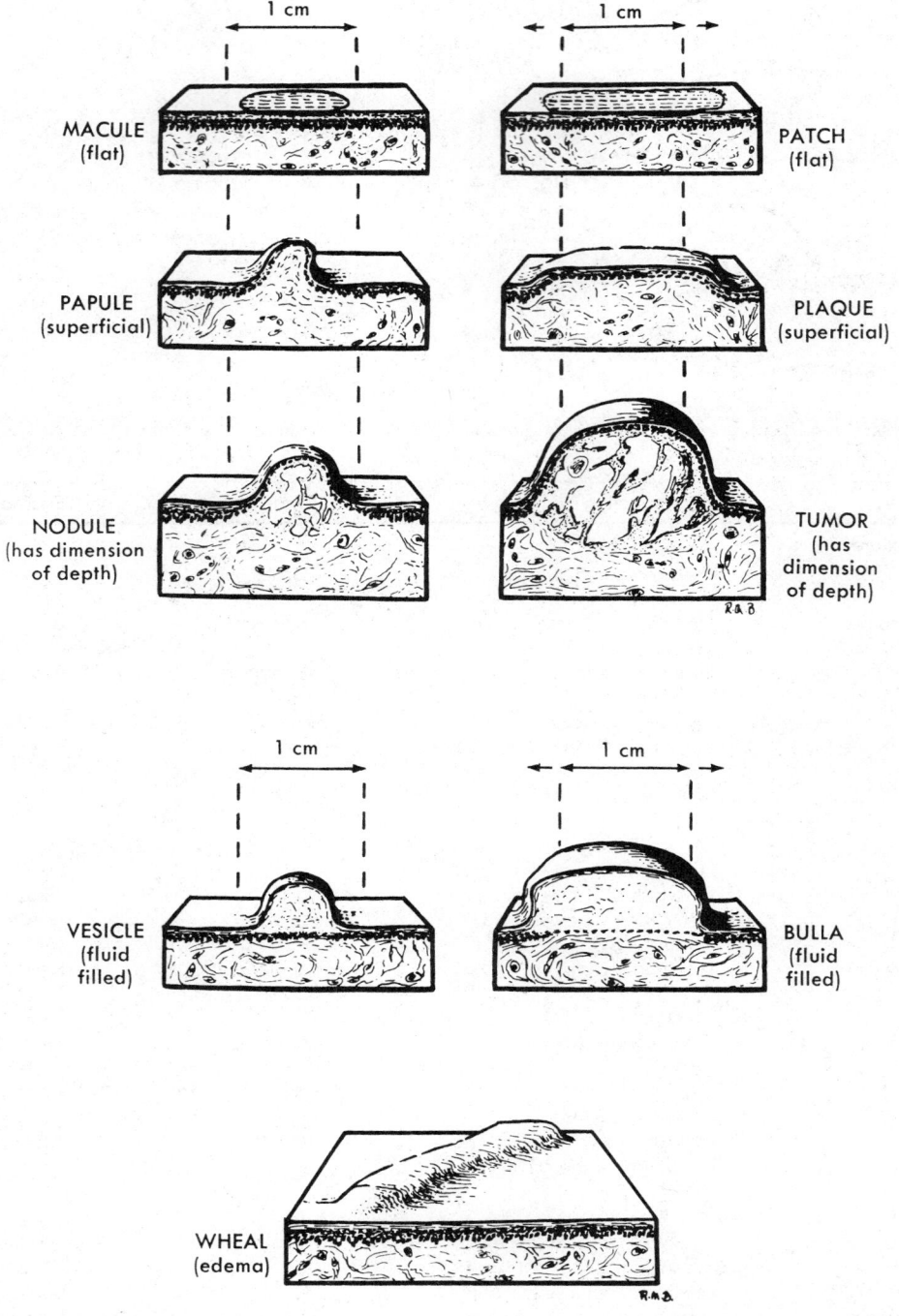

Fig. 68-5. Skin lesions (From Stewart, W.D., Danto, J.L., and Madden, S.: Dermatology: diagnosis and treatment of cutaneous disorders, ed. 4, St. Louis, 1978. The C.V. Mosby Co.)

vesicle will immediately establish the lesion as a clear, fluid-filled lesion smaller than 1 cm (Fig. 68-5).

Size. The metric system is used for descriptions. A helpful hint is to measure a portion of one's own fingers, such as the distance from the tip of the right thumb to the first joint, or the width of the nail on the right little finger. This can then be used as a gauge for estimating the size of a lesion.

Shape and configuration. Shape can be described as round, oval, and so on. Configuration refers to the sharpness of demarcation of the lesion; that is, is it discrete or diffuse.

Texture. The lesion is described as rough or smooth, dry or moist, and on the surface or deeply penetrating into the tissue.

Effect of pressure. Some vascular lesions blanch when pressure is applied and then return to their original color. Other lesions remain the same with pressure.

Arrangement. Some lesions occur in patches while others occur diffusely over the body. This is an important parameter when describing rashes.

Distribution. Some lesions occur in certain parts of the body, such as on exposed areas as with contact dermatitis, or on main body areas as in chickenpox. The lesions may follow the area of distribution of one of the spinal nerves as in herpes zoster.

Variety. In some diseases, such as smallpox, the lesions may all occur at the same time, whereas in chickenpox the lesions occur in crops so that there may be lesions at different stages of development occurring at the same time.

Assessment of dark skin

Assessment of dark-skinned persons is more difficult than that of light-skinned persons because color changes are less obvious. Often other signs and symptoms must be used to reach a conclusion. For example, when a skin area is inflamed, the erythema may not be noticeable and the involved area must be palpated for warmth and edema. Rashes may not be visible and must be determined by palpation if the rash is papular or by patient reports of pruritus.

Melanin, which gives skin its general color, is produced by melanocytes. The skin of darkly pigmented persons does not contain more melanocytes, but the melanocytes are larger and produce more melanin.[16] Pigmented skin offers more protection from ultraviolet radiation; hence dark skin reacts less to sunlight and skin cancers occur less frequently.

Baseline skin assessments of dark-skinned persons are important in order to gather data for future comparison. Skin color changes will be seen best in areas of lesser pigmentation, which include the lips, areas around the mouth, mucous membranes, conjunctiva, earlobes, nail beds, palms, and soles. The sclera of many dark-skinned persons contains fatty deposits with carotene, giving the sclera a yellowish tinge.[18] In these persons, jaundice will have to be concluded by other signs, such as bile in the urine or feces.

Pallor is seen as a grayish or dull tone of the skin caused by the loss of redness provided by the blood. This sign may be difficult to observe by the untrained eye. Pallor can be visualized best in the lips, mucous membranes, conjunctivae, and nail beds. *Cyanosis* also

gives the skin a grayish or dull tone because of loss of redness. All of the areas of lesser pigmentation, including the earlobes, palms, and soles, are assessed for signs of cyanosis.

Integumentary changes with aging

As people grow older changes occur in the skin and accessory structures (Table 68-3) that make assessment more difficult in differentiating normal from abnormal. The changes result primarily from loss of subcutaneous tissue, degeneration of collagen and elastic fibers, loss of melanocytes, increased capillary fragility, decreased secretion of sweat glands, hormonal changes, and overexposure to environmental elements. The elderly person is also more likely to have one or more chronic diseases and be taking medications that can cause skin changes. Dry skin may cause itching and may lead to skin breakdown if the person scratches. Toenails become thickened and difficult to trim; fingernails become more brittle and develop longitudinal ridges. Body hair changes in consistency and distribution.

Since part of the skin is highly visible to others, senile skin changes may be disturbing to some persons, especially to those who have placed great emphasis on their appearance when younger. Because the changes occur slowly over time, however, most people are able to cope with their changed body image.

TABLE 68-3. Normal skin and hair changes seen in elderly persons

Assessment parameters	Changes caused by aging
Skin	
Color	Hyperpigmentation in exposed areas
	Hypopigmented areas
Moisture	Dry skin (sometimes scaly)
	Decreased perspiration
Elasticity, turgor	Decreased elasticity
	Loose folds
	Decreased turgor
Texture	Some rough areas
	Thinner, more transparent skin
Lesions	Skin tags on face and neck
	Seborrheic keratoses
	Senile angiomas
	Stasis dermatitis
	Bruises (capillary fragility)
Hair	
Consistency	Thinner on head and body
	More bristly on face, in nose
Distribution	Loss of hair on head and body
	Increased hair on face

Diagnostic tests

Diagnostic tests for dermatologic problems

Diascopy

Pigmented lesions resulting from increased blood in dilated vessels (e.g., erythema, spider angiomas, telangiectasis) can be differentiated from other lesions resulting from blood that has escaped into the tissue (e.g., petechiae, ecchymoses) or resulting from melanin changes. Diascopy consists of pressing a transparent object such as a glass slide over a pigmented lesion. The lesion resulting from dilated blood vessels will whiten with pressure as the blood is pushed to other areas, whereas the other lesions will not change in color.

Skin biopsy

Biopsy specimens of skin lesions may be obtained either by incision and suturing or by punch biopsy, which does not require suturing. A biopsy punch has a sharp edge that cuts through previously anesthetized skin and removes a core from the lesion for analysis. Bleeding may be stopped by direct pressure or by electrodesiccation (p. 1798).

Culture

If a lesion is draining and there are symptoms of infection, a culture may be taken to identify the causative organism. If the causative factor is believed to be a fungus, a potassium hydroxide (KOH) examination may be carried out. The lesion is scraped with a knife blade, and the scraping is placed on a slide and put into a KOH solution for microscopic analysis.

Wood's light

In order to assist in the diagnoses of certain conditions, such as tinea of the scalp, a fungal infection, the hair is illuminated by a special filter (Wood's light) attached to an ultraviolet lamp. The infected hairs fluoresce or appear luminous under the light.

Diagnostic tests for immune problems

There are many different diagnostic tests used in evaluation of host defense defects but many of these tests are available only at major medical centers or in specialized laboratories.[4] Some of the tests that are more commonly used are listed below.

Bone marrow production tests

A white blood cell (WBC) count and differential count will identify the presence of leukopenia and lympho-penia. Leukopenia is a reduction in leukocyte serum levels below 4000/cu mm. The normal range of serum lymphocytes is 1500 to 3000/cu mm. A transient lymphopenia below 1500/cu mm occurs with stress, but a chronic lymphopenia is observed in persons with defective cellular immunity. Bone marrow aspiration and biopsy (p. 1188) may be performed to obtain further data on marrow production.

T cell (cellular) deficiency

T cell function (p. 287) can be screened by delayed hypersensitivity skin testing to common antigens. Specific antigens, including purified protein derivative (PPD), *Candida*, mumps antigen, streptokinase, and streptodornase, are injected intradermally. Reactions are read at 24 and 48 hours to determine hypersensitivity. The test is to determine the hypersensitivity, not the presence of disease. A person who does not react to any of these antigens is said to be *anergic*. Sensitization with dinitrochlorobenzene (DNCB) is an additional test for suspected anergic patients. DCNB is a chemical to which natural sensitivity does not occur. Following application of DCNB to the skin, contact sensitivity can be elicited after 1 to 2 weeks if T cell function is present.

B cell (humoral) deficiency

Electrophoresis. The movement of colloid (protein) particles in an electrical field is called electrophoresis. In an applied electrical field, different proteins migrate at different rates because of their different sizes and shapes, and this property can be utilized to analyze plasma protein content. The plasma proteins consist of albumin and globulin, which can be further divided into alpha (α-) globulins, beta (β-) globulins, and gamma (γ-) globulins (immunoglobulins). The serum proteins are subjected to electrophoresis in a medium that stabilizes the migration so that the proteins can be stained and examined. A densitometer records the color densities on graph paper. Fig. 68-6 illustrates typical patterns seen in persons with normal protein levels, with decreased γ-globulin level, and with increased γ-globulin levels. In immune disorders, the immunoglobulins may be either increased or decreased.

Quantitative immunoglobulin test. Three of the immunoglobulins, IgG, IgA, and IgM, can be measured quantitatively whereas IgD and IgE are present in amounts too small to measure. (See Chapter 19 for a discussion of immunoglobulins.) The levels of the immunoglobulins are assessed by immunodiffusion on agar plates prepared with specific antisera to each of the immunoglobulins. The normal values of the three major immunoglobulins vary with age. The adult normal levels are as follows: IgG, 600 to 1600 mg/100 ml; IgA, 20 to 500 mg/100 ml; and IgM, 60 to 200 mg/100 ml.

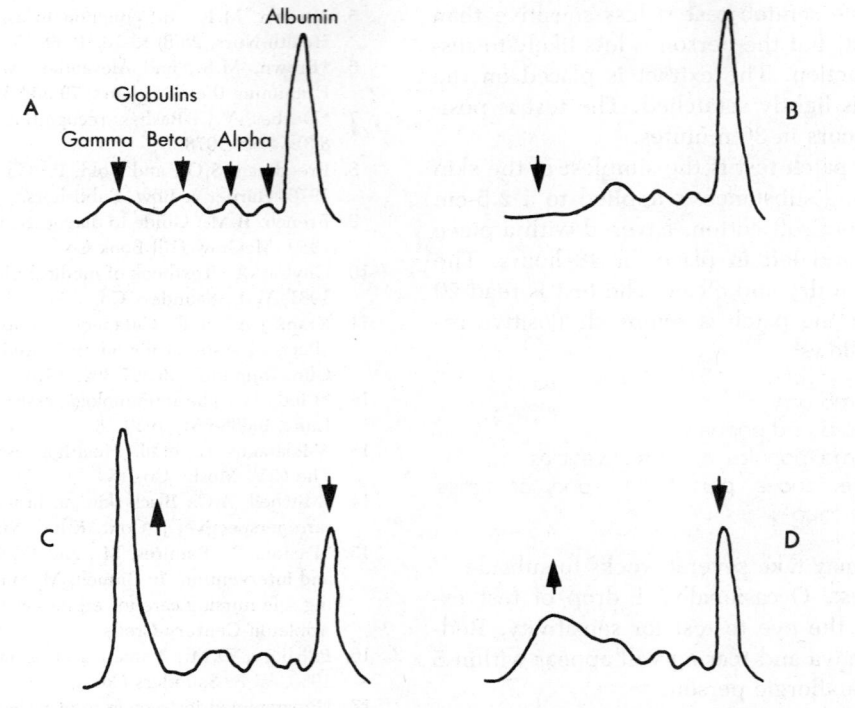

Fig. 68-6. Electrophoretic patterns **A,** Normal. **B,** Hypogammaglobinemia. **C,** Monoclonal gammopathy. **D,** Polyclonal gammopathy.

Specific antigen-antibody tests

There are numerous in vitro tests to measure specific antigen-antibody responses including radioimmunoassay tests, immunofluorescent techniques, agglutination tests, and complement-fixation tests.

Radioimmunoassay test. The radioimmunoassay (RIA) test consists of adding the unknown antigen to the antibody, followed by incubation. A radioactive-labeled antigen is then added, and the preparation is incubated again. If the unknown antigen is similar to the labeled antigen, both antigens will compete for the same antibody. The antibody-antigens are then separated, and the amount of radioactivity of the preparation is determined to identify the amount of free radioactive-labeled antigen remaining. Minute quantities of antigen can be detected by this method.

Immunofluorescence test. The immunofluorescence test consists of attaching fluorescein dye to antibodies and then mixing this with the antigen to be tested. The excess antibody is removed and the substance examined under a microscope with the aid of ultraviolet light to make the dye fluoresce.

Agglutination test. The agglutination test is used to determine the presence of antigens located on the surfaces of red blood cells or on microorganisms. Dilutions of antiserum are mixed with a solution containing the suspected antigen. The antigen and antibody react by agglutination or clumping of the cells.

Complement-fixation test. A standard amount of complement is added to a mixture of an antigen and its corresponding antibody. Since complement is essential to the antibody-antigen reaction, a subsequent antibody-antigen test will not yield a reaction.

Allergy tests

Hypersensitivity to specific antigens can be tested in vivo by skin tests or by the use test. In skin testing, the antigens are administered to the skin either through intradermal, scratch, or patch tests, or an allergen may be instilled in the eye.

Intradermal test. Small amounts of extracts of various allergenic substances to which sensitivity is suspected are injected intradermally at spaced intervals, usually on the forearm or in the scapular region. Control tests with the diluent alone are carried out concurrently. The test is positive if a wheal with surrounding erythema appears in 15 to 30 minutes but not in the control test. The test is begun with highly diluted solutions and then repeated with stronger extracts if the results are negative, in order to avoid a systemic reaction. The person should be observed for signs of anaphylactic shock.

Scratch test. The scratch test is less sensitive than the intradermal test, but the person is less likely to sustain a systemic reaction. The extract is placed on the skin and the skin is lightly scratched. The test is positive if erythema occurs in 30 minutes.

Patch test. The patch test is the simplest of the skin tests. The sensitizing substance is applied to a 2.5-cm (1-in.) square piece of soft cotton, covered with a piece of occlusive tape, and left in place for 48 hours. The patches must remain dry and clean. The test is read 20 to 30 minutes after the patch is removed. Positive results are read as follows:

+	Erythema only
+ +	Erythema and papules
+ + +	Erythema, papules, and small vesicles
+ + + +	All the above plus bullae and at times ulceration[1]

Positive reactions may take several weeks to subside.

Conjunctival test. Occasionally, 1 drop of test extract is instilled in the eye to test for sensitivity. Redness of the conjunctiva and tearing will appear within 5 to 15 minutes in an allergic person.

Use test. Substances such as foods, cosmetics, or fabrics to which a person is suspected of being allergic are eliminated from use and then added individually according to a set schedule. Reaction to the use test may be immediate or over a period of time. Some persons become discouraged during the testing and may need encouragement to adhere to the testing schedule.

REFERENCES AND SELECTED READINGS
Contemporary

1. Arndt, K.: Manual of dermatologic therapeutics, Boston, 1974, Little, Brown & Co.
2. Barber, H.R.: Immunobiology for the clinician, New York, 1977, John Wiley & Sons, Inc.
3. *Bates, B.: A guide to physical examination, ed. 2, Philadelphia, 1979, J.B. Lippincott Co.
4. Beeson, P., and McDermott, W., editors: Cecil-Loeb textbook of medicine, ed. 15, Philadelphia, 1979, W.B. Saunders Co.
5. *Brown, M.E.: Introduction to assessment of the skin, Occup. Health Nurs. 28(8):13-16, 1980.
6. *Brown, M.S., and Alexander, M.: Physical examination. III. Examining the skin, Nurs.'73 3(9):39-43, 1973.
7. *Derbes, V.J.: Rashes: recognition and management, Nurs. '78 8(3):54-59, 1978.
8. Freedman, S.O., and Gold, P.: Clinical immunology, New York, 1976, Harper & Row, Publishers.
9. French, R.M.: Guide to diagnostic procedures, ed. 5, New York, 1980, McGraw-Hill Book Co.
10. Guyton, A.: Textbook of medical physiology, ed. 6, Philadelphia, 1981, W.B. Saunders Co.
11. Kram, J.A., et al.: Cutaneous immediate hypersensitivity in man: effects of systemically administered adrenergic drugs, J. Allergy Clin. Immunol. 56:387-392, 1975.
12. *Lind, M.: The immunologic assessment: a nursing focus, Heart Lung, 9:658-661, 1980.
13. *Malasanos, L., et al.: Health assessment, ed. 2, St. Louis, 1981, The C.V. Mosby Co.
14. *Mitchell, A.C.: Black skin: an historical, psychological and health care perspective, J. Cont. Educ. Nurs. 10(6):28-33, 1979.
15. *Paxton, P., Ramires, M., and Wolloch, E.: Nursing assessment and intervention. In Branch, M., and Paxton, P., editors: Providing safe nursing care for ethnic people of color, New York, 1976, Appleton-Century-Crofts.
16. Pillsbury, D.M.: A manual of dermatology, ed. 2, Philadelphia, 1980, W.B. Saunders Co.
17. *Programmed instruction: skin rashes in infants and children, Am. J. Nurs. 78(6):1-32, 1978.
18. *Roach, L.B.: Color changes in dark skin, Nurs. '77 7(1):48-51, 1977.
19. *Roach, L.B.: Assessing skin changes—the subtle and the obvious, Nurs. '74 4(3):64-67, 1974.
20. *Roberts, S.: Skin assessment for color and temperature, Am. J. Nurs. 75:610-613, 1975.
21. *Rubin, B.A.: Black skin, J. Sch. Health 47:365-367, 1977.
22. *Sana, J., and Judge, R.: Physical appraisal methods in nursing practice, Boston, 1975, Little, Brown & Co.
23. Sherman, J., and Fields, S.: Guide to patient evaluation, Flushing, N.Y., 1974, Medical Examination Publishing Co., Inc.
24. *Thompson, J.M., and Bowers, A.C.: Clinical manual of health assessment, St. Louis, 1980, The C.V. Mosby Co.
25. *Uhler, D.M.: Common skin changes in the elderly, Am. J. Nurs. 78:1342-1344, 1978.
26. Waisman, M.: A clinical look at the aging skin, Postgrad Med. 66:87-96, 1979.

Classic

27. Judge, R., and Zuidema, G.: Physical diagnosis: a physiological approach to the clinical examination, ed. 2, Boston, 1963, Little, Brown & Co.

*References preceded by an asterisk are particularly well suited for student reading.

CHAPTER 69

INTERVENTION FOR THE PERSON WITH A DERMATOLOGIC PROBLEM

BARBARA C. LONG

The specific management of persons with dermatologic problems varies with each disease entity. There are general principles, however, that the nurse should follow in the care of these individuals.

Prevention of dermatologic conditions not only relieves the patient of discomfort but is cost effective since many skin conditions are chronic. This chapter discusses methods of prevention, measures to alleviate common patient discomforts, care of skin lesions, and care of persons experiencing dermatologic or plastic surgery. Interventions for persons with specific dermatologic problems are discussed in Chapter 71.

Prevention of dermatologic disorders

Avoidance of causative agents

The first step in prevention of dermatologic conditions may be directed toward avoidance of the causative agent. This may be a specific antigen, contact irritant, microorganism, trauma, or insect. Instructing the person to avoid a known causative agent is preventive medicine; however, it may not be that simple. Many dermatologic diseases have no known cause or are hereditary, or once the mechanism of the disease is known, it is not always possible to remove the trigger factors. Finally, symptoms may persist long after the agent is removed. Therefore the nurse's responsibility is one of educating the patient about good skin care, the importance of rest and avoidance of emotional stress, good nutrition, and, lastly, close observation to determine changes in skin conditions.

Cleansing

The outer layer of skin cells and the perspiration are acid in reaction, and their presence inhibits the life and growth of bacteria. Strong soaps that are alkaline in reaction may neutralize this protective acid condition of the skin. They may also remove the oily secretion of the sebaceous glands, which lubricate the outer skin layers and contribute to their health. It is sometimes necessary to remove excess oil and scale or debris to facilitate the absorption of medication, promote healing, and enhance the appearance of the skin. In psoriasis, for example, removal of scale by mechanical means and slowing of skin metabolism are prime objectives.

Normal skin should be washed often enough to remove excess oils and excretions and to prevent odor. Care must be taken not to cause drying or irritation. Maintaining a proper degree of hydration in the skin will prevent dryness and itching, which may lead to scratching, excoriation, and further trauma. Hydrating the stratum corneum, or outer layer of skin, may be accomplished by soaking in a tub of water for 20 to 30 minutes and then immediately applying a lubricating lotion or cream. This application of a cream prevents the rapid loss of water from the skin surface.

Nutrition

Good diet and nutrition play an important role in preventing the occurrence of skin lesions. Some skin lesions may be directly associated with dietary intake. Excessive dryness of the skin and thickening of the stratum corneum at the hair follicle openings may be caused by nutritional deficiencies. Elevated blood lipids secondary to hyperlipoproteinemia may take the form of xanthomas on the skin surface. Restriction of sodium in patients who are on steroids may lessen or prevent edema as a side effect.

Hypersensitive individuals may be placed on restrictive diets to exclude intake of known causative agents or as a diagnostic tool to identify causative agents. Whatever the product or food additive the hypersensitive person is to avoid, food labels should be read carefully. It also may be necessary to request information from the manufacturer if questions about food additives arise. The patient should know the type of diet to be followed. This includes knowledge of any restrictions, methods of preparing these foods, if necessary, and the duration of the prescribed diet.

Rest

Rest and relief from emotional stress may prevent exacerbations of existing diseases. *Alopecia areata,* which is a circumscribed patch of hair loss, has frequently been seen to follow several weeks after a real or threatened loss of a loved one. The direct relationship of emotional stress has not been explained.

Persons should be made aware that lack of rest or emotional tension can be a trigger factor in the development of skin conditions. For example, a woman may be able to cite the fact that she was tense from the recent preparation for her daughter's wedding and that this may have precipitated a flare-up of her psoriasis.

Observations of changes

Care of normal skin includes regular observation of pigmented skin areas, moles, or other apparently minor skin lesions. Any change in size, color, or general appearance should be reported to a physician at once since a change in moles or new skin growths is one of the danger signals of cancer. Ultraviolet irradiation seems to be the most common, least disputed exogenous factor in the etiology of skin cancer. Basal cell carcinoma has been found to occur more frequently in sunny climates, in fair-skinned persons, in older people, and in those who work outdoors.

Patients should be instructed to avoid the sun if they have been diagnosed as having a skin condition that is aggravated by ultraviolet light. This is accomplished by the use of sunscreen lotions when outside, covering exposed skin surfaces by use of long sleeves and a hat, and most important, by regular medical follow-up.

Dangers of self-treatment

People should be urged to seek competent medical help when skin conditions develop. Although skin dis-

eases rarely cause death, they may be reflections of serious systemic illness and can account for much human discomfort and for serious interruption of work and other activities. Many persons are inclined to rely on the advice of friends or the local druggist or on medications they may have on hand. Each individual's skin reacts differently to treatment, and the skin that is already irritated or diseased may respond violently to inexpert treatment. Because of changes in the skin, medications prescribed even for a similar skin ailment in the same patient some time previously may not produce a favorable response. Medications may deteriorate, and for this reason old medications are not safe. The person may be spared much discomfort and expense by consulting a specialist when symptoms first develop and before a mild skin condition becomes a real problem.

Psychologic effects of dermatologic problems

There is a certain degree of "beauty orientation" in Western culture. Beauty pageants are popular, advertisements in the media use beautiful models to attract the reader, and in public groups, heads turn as a good-looking person walks by. Cosmetics to enhance good looks are extensively used by men as well as women. It is no wonder, therefore, that skin diseases or physical defects that detract from "good looks" produce psychologic reactions.

A person's emotional reaction to a deformity or defect must not be underestimated. One's pride in oneself, the ability to think well of oneself, and to regard oneself favorably in comparison with others are essential to the development and maintenance of a well-integrated personality. Every person who has a defect or a handicap, particularly if it is conspicuous to others, suffers from some threat to emotional security. The extent of the emotional reaction and the amount of maladjustment that follows depend on the individual's makeup and ability to cope with emotional insults. Disfigurements almost invariably lead to disturbing experiences. The child who has webbed fingers may be ridiculed at school; the adolescent girl who has acne scars may be self-conscious and avoid social situations; and the young man with a posttraumatic scar on his face may be refused a salesman's job. Under any of these circumstances it is not unusual for the individual to withdraw from a society that is unkind. The defect may be used to justify failure to assume responsibility or to justify striking out against an unkind society by such reactions as becoming a "problem child" or, in some extreme cases, a criminal.

Skin diseases that produce marked disfigurement of

visible body surfaces can therefore effect alterations in body image, as described in Chapter 28. Feelings of decreased worth by persons with large draining lesions or with severe disfigurement are reinforced during interactions with others. Some people are repelled when viewing persons with severe skin diseases, or they may experience a threat to their own body integrity and physically withdraw to avoid interaction. Persons may also frequently experience nonverbal messages of disgust when others view them for the first time. This is markedly poignant when those nonverbal messages are sent by significant others or by health professionals.

The person with severe facial disfigurement may also experience job discrimination. One woman was moved sequentially from a large office to a smaller office to a single office and finally to the evening hours in a lonely room so that co-workers could avoid looking at her. She lived alone and was increasingly deprived of social contacts with others. It was only after her eyesight failed and she was encouraged to attend groups for the blind that she was able to develop meaningful relationships again.

In working with the person with severe skin disease, the nurse first examines his or her own feelings that could be expressed nonverbally in a negative manner. Measures to assist the patient and family to deal with and cope with their feelings are described in Chapters 16 and 28.

General intervention

Relief of pruritus

Pruritus or itching is a cutaneous symptom that provokes the desire to scratch. It is caused by repetitive low-frequency stimulation of C fibers that are similar to but different from C fibers that transmit pain stimuli. Itching can be produced by mechanical stimulation of the skin or by chemical mediators, primarily the kinins.[6] Itching occurs only in the skin, certain mucous membranes, and the eyes. The areas most sensitive to itching are the nostrils, mucocutaneous junctions, external ear canals, and perineum.[31]

Pruritus can be caused by any irritating substance that interrupts the stratum corneum layer of the skin, or it can be a result of certain systemic diseases (see box in next column). Not all infectious diseases producing rashes cause itching. One of the most common causes is dry skin, sometimes occurring as a result of excessive bathing, particularly with "bubble bath," which has a drying effect. Factors that can intensify itching include vasodilation, tissue anoxia, and stasis of circulation. Whatever the cause, pruritus ranges from an annoyance

---

COMMON CAUSES OF ITCHING

Dry skin

Skin irritants: plastic or glass fibers, wool, plant products, insects

Drug reactions

Psychogenic reactions

Infectious diseases

Infestation: hookworm

Systemic diseases: obstructive biliary disease, uremia, diabetes mellitus

Neoplasia: Hodgkin's disease, leukemia, lymphoma

---

to a severe, distressing, or exhausting symptom.

Pruritus leads to the motor response of scratching. Persons with very intense itching may excoriate the skin severely by digging deeply into the skin with their fingernails when trying to alleviate the itch. Persons with generalized itching may be observed to be in almost constant motion—twisting, rubbing, and scratching.

A major step in treating pruritus is to attempt to remove the itch stimuli and break the itch-scratch cycle. Cold causes vasoconstriction and will provide some relief. Hydration in a tepid bath followed by the application of an emollient lotion is helpful. Cornstarch or oatmeal preparations (p. 1794) may be added to the bath. Topical corticosteroids decrease inflammation leading to vasoconstriction. In some persons antihistamines are of some value as are tranquilizers.

The awareness of pruritus may be more acute during the night because of a decrease in diverting stimuli. Cool, light, nonrestrictive bed clothing may help allay itching. Excessive drying of the skin caused by high room temperature, and low humidity can also increase pruritus. It occurs readily in the elderly person who already has a dry skin. Usually a room temperature of 20° C (68° to 70° F) and humidity of 30% to 40% are best for the person with pruritus.

Temperature control

The individual who has a generalized flush, or erythema, and the one who has an extensive exfoliative dermatitis may be losing body heat at an abnormally increased rate and may need a room temperature of 32.2° C (90° F) or more to maintain normal body temperature. Care must be taken to avoid chilling, particularly after baths, when compresses are used, or when parts of the body are exposed.

Hygienic measures: baths and soaks

The patient admitted to the hospital with skin disease should not bathe until examination by a physician has been completed. Clothing, dressings, and the lesions themselves with crusts or exudates should be left undisturbed unless a definite order has been given for their care. Exudate may be removed on order of a physician, and a specific method of removal should be prescribed. Hard crust or thickened exudates often are soaked with physiologic solution of sodium chloride, peroxide, pHisoHex in water, or a mild solution of tincture of green soap in warm water. Clean techniques should be used unless sterile technique is indicated. Care should be taken to avoid reinfection from soiled outer dressings or other sources.

Tub baths are a frequent means of cleansing the body and are part of the treatment in many dermatologic conditions. Depending on the skin condition being treated, the additives to bath water will vary. Many times persons with psoriasis who are using crude coal tar are permitted to wash with pHisoHex or Dial soap while in the tub. This will help prevent folliculitis because of the antibacterial properties within the soap. Special attention should be paid to intertriginous areas (areas between skin surfaces such as between fingers or toes) where creams and topical medications may collect. Tub baths or soaks to a specific body part are soothing and antipruritic. Baths are an effective means of rehydrating the skin. The tub soak should last 20 to 30 minutes with a water temperature between 32° to 38° C (90° to 100° F). If creams or ointments are to be applied after a bath, it should be done immediately, since this lessens itching, retains moisture, and prevents "drying out" of the outer layer of skin. Patients should be assisted in and out of the tub when additives are added to the water. A rubber mat should be used and special attention given to the potential for slipping when oils are used.

Many persons with arthropathic psoriasis find it difficult to use a tub because of their limited mobility. If a lift is not available to lower the patient into the tub or if the lift is too difficult to maneuver in the bathroom, sitting on a chair under a gentle shower is the next best alternative. After a bath the skin should be patted dry; vigorous rubbing is avoided.

Substances may be added to the bath for specific therapeutic effects (Table 69-1). *Oatmeal, soybean* powder, and soluble *cornstarch* may be added to lessen pruritus or when soap is contraindicated (see box below).

Potassium permanganate ($KMnO_4$) is used in a bath or soak to deodorize and dry lesions for such conditions as pyoderma gangrenosum or slow-healing ulcers and to help prevent infection in pemphigus lesions. The dilution is ordered by the physician, usually at a 1:32,000 or 1:16,000 dilution. If tablets of $KMnO_4$ are used in preparing the solution, the *pulverized* tablets should be strained through gauze to filter out any undissolved particles that may cause irritation.

DIRECTIONS FOR PREPARATION OF A COLLOIDAL BATH

1. Add 0.45 kg (2 C) of cereal (oatmeal, soybean, or bran) to 480 ml (2 C) of boiling water.

2. Stir cereal while boiling for 5 minutes.

3. Fill tub one-half to three fourths full with *tepid* water (35° C [95° F]).

4. Pour the cooked cereal into a mesh or gauze bag and stir the bag through the bath for a few minutes until the water becomes opalescent.

5. The bag may also be used as a mop to gently pat the skin to remove crusts and debris.

TABLE 69-1. Preparations commonly used for baths or soaks

Substance	Effect	Suggested actions
Colloids: oatmeal, cornstarch, soybean powder	Antipruritic, drying	Tub surfaces become very slippery; support person to prevent falls
Potassium permanganate	Antifungal, drying, deodorizing	Strain pulverized tablet through cheesecloth to prevent irritation; stains surfaces and linens
Burow's solution (aluminum acetate)	Antibacterial, drying	Commonly used for soaks
Sulfur bath suspension	Antibacterial	Rinse body with tepid water after bath to remove residual sulfur particles
Tar preparations	Antipruritic, moisturizing	Do not use soap with tar baths
Bath oils: Alpha-Keri, Jeri-Bath, Domol	Antipruritic, moisturizing	Tub surfaces may become slippery

Sulfur acts as an antibacterial agent for such conditions as acne or hidradenitis suppurativa. If a sulfur bath suspension is used, it is important to rinse the body with tepid water to remove any residual particles of sulfur.

Tar baths are used frequently before ultraviolet light therapy in persons with psoriasis. Balnetar Bath Oil, Zetar, Alma-Tar, and Polytar Bath are popular brand names used for this purpose. Tar residual is thought to enhance the effect the ultraviolet light has on the skin.

The tub used for a medicated bath should be disinfected after each use by pouring 240 ml (1 C) of bleach into the used tub water, letting it stand for 5 minutes, then wiping the sides and bottom of the tub. The tub is then drained and cleaned in the usual fashion. If the bath is to be taken at home, the person should know how to prepare any treatment tub bath prescribed by the physician. This would include gathering supplies, mixing solutions if necessary, and special precautions to be followed with the specific treatment.

Topical medications

Application of medications to the skin surface may take many forms. Wet dressings, creams, pastes, ointments, or lotion can be used. The nurse should know the purpose for which a local application is ordered, the drug (or drugs) contained in the preparation, and any toxic signs that may occur from its use.

Types of topical medications. There are many different topical medications used for persons with dermatologic problems. *Steroids* are among the most commonly used for their antiinflammatory, vasoconstrictive, and antipruritic effects. Occlusive dressings are sometimes prescribed over local steroid applications to enhance the steroid absorption. There are a large variety of steroid preparations. Cortisone is ineffective when applied topically but hydrocortisone is effective. Fluorinated corticosteroids are powerful agents but have greater side effects than do nonfluorinated corticosteroids.[31] Adverse reactions include (1) burning, itching, and irritation; (2) folliculitis; (3) secondary infection; and (4) telangiectasia, striae, and hypopigmentation. Contact sensitivity may occur, especially in persons with a history of hypersensitivity. Topical steroids should not be used in the presence of viral infections. *Antibacterial* or *antifungal* topical medications (Table 69-2) are used rather than steroids for bacterial or fungal infections.

Open wet dressings

Wet dressings are used frequently over various skin lesions for cooling, drying, antipruritic, vasoconstricting, or debriding effects. Plain tap water or physiologic

TABLE 69-2. Some common topical antibiotic and antifungal medications

Generic name	Trade name	Vehicle	Comments
Antibacterial			
Bacitracin	Bacitracin	Ointment	Effective against gram-positive organisms (nonprescription)
Neomycin, bacitracin, and polymyxin B	Neosporin	Powder, cream, ointment	Broad-spectrum antibiotic effect
Bacitracin and polymyxin B	Polysporin	Ointment	Same as Neosporin
Gentamicin	Garamycin	Cream, ointment	Broad-spectrum antibiotic
Chloramphenicol	Chloromycetin	Cream	Broad-spectrum antibiotic
Clioquinol	Vioform	Powder, cream, ointment	Has both antibacterial and antifungal effects, useful for eczema and tinea
Nitrofurazone	Furacin	Powder, solution, cream	Broad-spectrum antibiotic
Povidone-iodine	Betadine	Solution	Kills gram-negative and gram-positive organisms, fungi, viruses, protozoa, yeasts
Mafenide	Sulfamylon	Cream	Effective against both gram-positive and gram-negative bacteria; used for burns
Silver sulfadiazine	Silvadene	Cream	Effective against bacteria and yeast; used for burns
Antifungal			
Tolnaftate	Tinactin	Powder, cream, ointment	Useful for tinea
Nystatin	Mycostatin Nilstat	Powder, cream, ointment	Useful against wide variety of yeasts, especially *Candida*
Amphotericin B	Fungizone	Lotion, cream, ointment	Effective against *Candida*
Clotrimazole	Lotrimin	Cream, solution	Broad-spectrum antifungal
Haloprogin	Halotex	Cream, solution	Synthetic agent useful for superficial fungal infections
Miconazole nitrate	Micatin	Cream	Synthetic agent useful for tinea

saline may be used, or medications may be added. An astringent effect may be obtained through the use of *Burow's* solution (Domeboro, Buro-Sol, Bluboro), 1:20 or 1:40 dilution. *Potassium permanganate* ($KMnO_4$), one 300 mg tablet in 1500 ml (1:5000) or one 300 mg tablet in 3000 ml (1:10,000), has an antimicrobial and drying effect. All tablet crystals must be thoroughly dissolved to prevent chemical burning of the skin. Potassium permanganate should not be used on the face. *Silver nitrate* ($AgNO_3$), 0.5%, is also an antimicrobial and is often used in the treatment of burns. Both $KMnO_4$ and $AgNO_3$ stain skin and cloth.

The type of dressing material used for a wet dressing should be one without cotton filling, since cotton leaves particles and a residue on the skin, which may cause irritation. Several layers of fine mesh gauze are ideal, and roller gauze or Kerlix may be used for extremities. A mask for the face may be designed by cutting out openings for the eyes, nose, and mouth from several thicknesses of gauze. At home the person can use muslin-type cotton material such as old clean sheets, handkerchiefs, cloth diapers, or muslin dish towels that are lint free. These materials need not be sterilized but should be washed or discarded every 24 hours.[43]

The best effects of wet dressings are obtained by several treatment periods spaced across the person's waking hours.[43] The solution is applied at room temperature (see box below) to prevent the marked vasoconstriction with subsequent vasodilation that occurs with cold solutions. Although the dressings can be kept wet by adding solution with the dressings in place, this practice usually leads to excessive dripping. Dressings *must* be removed, soaked, and reapplied when $KMnO_4$ or $AgNO_3$ is used since evaporation can increase the solute on the dressings, increasing the dosage and causing

a chemical burn or irritation. Occlusive plastic wraps should be avoided unless specifically ordered by the physician.

Closed wet dressings

Wet dressings can be covered with a nonpermeable material such as plastic wrap specifically to retain heat if an early abscess is present, to soften excessive keratinized tissue, or to enhance penetration of a topical medication. This method is not used frequently since interference with evaporation contributes to skin maceration.

Wet-to-dry dressings

Wet-to-dry dressings are used to *debride* wounds or ulcerations. A fine mesh gauze is moistened with the prescribed solution, placed over the lesion, and allowed to dry. The crust and debris are removed as the dressing is pulled off dry. This process is usually repeated every 4 to 8 hours. Half-strength Dakin's solution is frequently used for this purpose.

Vehicles for topical medication

Topical medications can be prepared in a variety of bases (Table 69-3). *Powders* are effective in reducing friction and moisture in intertriginous areas. *Lotions* must be shaken well, since the insoluble powder may settle out. The addition of alcohol increases the cooling effect of a lotion. *Ointments* do not usually leave an oily residue on the skin unless they have a petrolatum base. A nonporous covering such as plastic should not be used over an ointment unless so prescribed, because the heat retention may increase percutaneous absorption of the medication.

Application of topical medications

Powders should first be sprinkled into the hand, then applied to the skin to avoid getting excess powder into

---

APPLICATION OF OPEN WET DRESSINGS

1. Prepare solution to be applied at room temperature. Sterility is not required.
2. Soak dressing thoroughly in solution.
3. Protect bed or clothing with towels, bath blanket, flannel squares, etc.
4. Wring out dressings—they should be wet but not dripping.
5. Apply dressings in smooth layers (two to four layers) to involved areas. Wrap fingers and toes separately, and wrap joints so that they can bend.
6. Remove, soak, and reapply dressings *before* they dry (i.e., every 3 to 5 min).
7. Continue treatment for 20 to 30 min.
8. Pat skin dry.

TABLE 69-3. Comparison of vehicles for topical medications

Type	Base	Effect
Powder	Dry	Drying by absorbing moisture; cooling by evaporating moisture
Lotion	Powder suspended in water or oil	Protective, cleansing, cooling, antipruritic effect depending on drug and base used
Creams and ointments	Emulsions of oil and water	Occlusive covering over skin to prolong contact of medication with skin—good skin penetration; warming effect
Paste	50% or more powder in ointment base	Holds medication for longer period of time with slower skin penetration

the air and thus causing irritation to the mucous membrane. Powders should be used sparingly to prevent caking. Powders should not be used on wet surfaces since this leads to caking. Cornstarch is *not* suggested since it encourages growth of yeast, bacteria, and fungi.[43]

Lotions with a water or alcohol base are applied by patting gently. A gauze pledget should be used for extremely thin lotions. Lotions with an oily base are applied thinly and evenly with the palm of the hand. A small area of skin is often tested to determine if the person will tolerate the cream or lotion over the entire body. The topical medication is applied to a small area (silver-dollar size) on the person's forearm. The time and the exact location of the trial are recorded, and the skin response to the trial medication is read 24 hours later. Crude coal tar is frequently tested in this manner.

Ointments may be applied with gloved hands or with the bare palm, depending on the type of ointment used. If a dressing is to be applied, the ointment may be spread on the dressing with a tongue blade before application to the skin. Anthralin may be caustic to normal skin, so gloves should be worn. Crude coal tar is always applied in firm, long, downward strokes to prevent folliculitis, since tar is an irritant. Creams, as opposed to ointments, may be rubbed in.

Some topical medications such as crude coal tar are often removed before other treatment. Crude coal tar must be removed in the morning before ultraviolet light therapy (following the Goeckerman regimen). This is done by applying corn oil in long downward strokes over the skin surface and then wiping with gauze pledgets, leaving only a thin film of tar. A general rule to remember is to remove only the excess ointment or ointments having a consistency of cold cream before a bath or wet dressing. Cottonseed oil may be used to remove caked, oily-based lotions, using a gauze pledget.

Teaching of self-help skills

Many persons with skin disease are not hospitalized. In the home and in the clinic the nurse must be specific in instructions to the person or to the family member who will be responsible for the person's care. It is best to write out instructions specifically. A common mistake that some persons make when at home is to believe that if some is good, much is better. While a skin ailment may respond to an ointment rubbed on very gently and lightly, trauma from vigorous rubbing may counteract all benefit and may even make the condition worse. The individual, eager to cure the condition, may not realize how vigorous his or her own administrations are. The nurse can help the patient to improvise needed equipment.

The nurse should always assume initial responsibility for the application of topical medications and various treatments. At some point in the patient's hospitalization these responsibilities should be transferred to the patient. There may be a need for a visiting nurse to assist the person at home, and this should be determined before discharge.

Many times the person may use old linen such as napkins, pillowcases, and socks for dressings. A plastic shower cap may be used on the scalp as an occlusive covering at night. The person may have a plastic occlusion suit to wear at bedtime. These are usually worn over a steroid cream. Instructions for the care of this suit should include daily washing to prevent the caking of creams and collection of scales and exudate.

Outcome criteria for the person with a dermatologic condition

The person or significant others can:
1. Explain the rationale for the prescribed treatments.
2. Demonstrate prescribed baths, soaks, or medicated dressings.
3. Describe any special precautions to be observed during treatments, including:
   a. Avoidance of nonporous coverings over dressings unless so ordered.
   b. Complete dissolving of tablets or crystals in baths or soaks.
   c. Avoidance of excessive rubbing of medications over lesions.
   d. Application of thin layers of lotions or powders.
4. Describe the prescribed medication routine: route of administration, vehicle to be used, dosage, frequency, duration of topical application, side effects, and where supplies can be obtained.
5. Describe plans for socialization with others.

Dermatologic surgery

Treatment of skin lesions by dermatologists sometimes includes removal of skin lesions or hair by means of curettage, surgical diathermy (electric current), or cryosurgery (freezing).

Curettage

Skin lesions may be removed by incision followed by suturing or by curettage followed by electrodesiccation

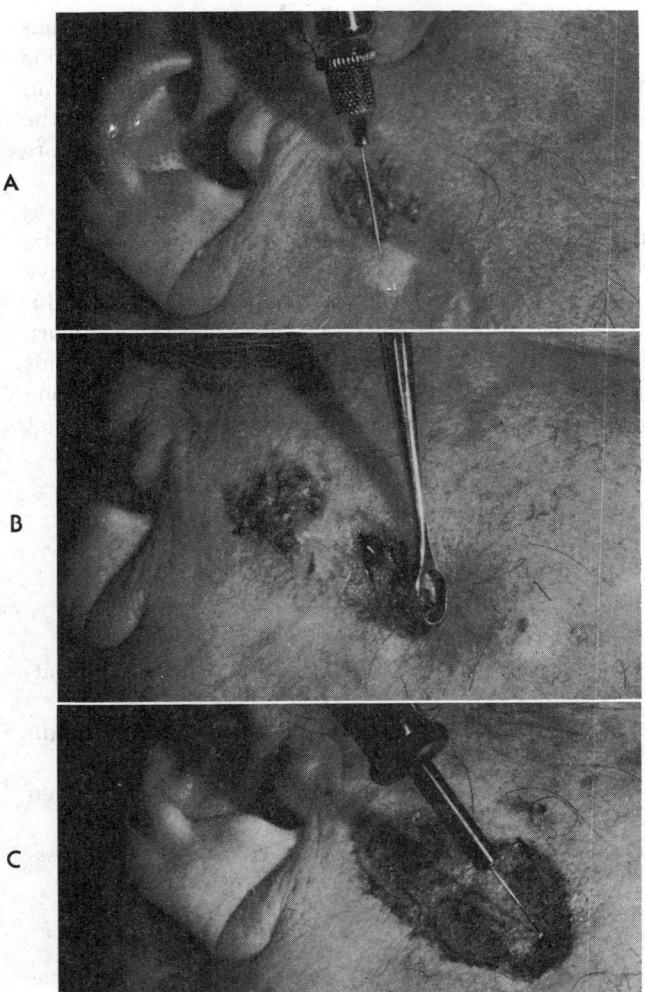

Fig. 69-1. A, Infiltration with local anesthetic. **B,** Curettage. **C,** Electrodesiccation for hemostasis. (From Stewart, W.D., Danto, J.L., and Maddin, S.: Dermatology: diagnosis and treatment of cutaneous disorders, ed. 4, St. Louis, 1978, The C.V. Mosby Co.)

(Fig. 69-1). The curet, which is a spoon-shaped instrument with sharp edges, is applied in a downward scraping motion across the lesion. A local anesthetic is usually injected around the lesion before curettage. Lesions that may be removed by curettage and desiccation include seborrheic keratoses, actinic keratoses, basal cell epitheliomas, leukoplakia, warts, and nevi.

Surgical diathermy

Electrosurgery

Electric current may be used in dermatologic surgery to remove tissue and to control bleeding. *Electrodesiccation* is the drying of tissue by means of a monopolar current through a needle electrode. *Electrofulguration* is a form of electrodesiccation in which the needle electrode is held close to the tissue rather than inserted into the tissue, thus spraying the area with sparks. Bipolar current is used for *electrocoagulation*, which coagulates the tissue, curtailing capillary bleeding, and for *electrosection*, which cuts the tissue. Electrodesiccation or electrocoagulation is often used in conjunction with electrosection. Delayed bleeding may occur especially from electrocoagulation and may alarm the unprepared patient. The bleeding can be easily controlled by direct pressure.

Electrosurgery is usually performed under local anesthesia. Sedation is rarely necessary. Following most uses of electrosurgery the wound is left exposed for air drying. Dressings may be used if the area is subject to frequent trauma or rubbing or if oozing is present. The wound may be wiped with 70% alcohol to hasten drying. A hemostatic nonocclusive dressing may be made by covering the wound with Gelfoam powder and Micropore tape.[30]

Epilation

Hair removal can be effected by means of electrolysis. Different methods may be used. High-frequency alternating electrical current, which is safer, less painful, and less likely to produce scarring than other methods, requires more skill and is the procedure of choice by dermatologists. Lay persons use a direct current method. Self-epilation may be carried out by a hand-held galvanic epilator (Perma-Tweez). The skin should be clean before epilation is attempted. Approximately 20% to 30% of hairs may regrow after diathermy epilation and require removal.[30]

Cryosurgery

Tissue can be destroyed by rapid freezing with substances such as liquid oxygen, carbon dioxide snow or gas, liquid nitrogen, dichlorodifluoromethane (Freon), or nitrous oxide. Carbon dioxide snow and liquid nitrogen are used most frequently. The rapid freezing causes formation of intracellular ice, which destroys the cell membranes and produces cell dehydration. Cryosurgery is frequently used for removal of skin tumors (benign and malignant), warts, and keloids.

Although the procedure is not usually painful, a tingling pain occurs when the freezing substance is applied and may be uncomfortable to some persons, particularly if multiple lesions are treated. Local anesthesia may be necessary. Analgesics may be helpful during thawing.

Tissue necrosis may not be evident until 24 hours after cryosurgery. A clear or hemorrhagic bulla forms during the first day, but inflammatory reactions and bleeding are usually absent. A serous exudate occurs during the first week, followed by eschar or crust formation. The crust drops off in 3 to 4 weeks as the underlying tissue heals. Scarring usually results. Hypopigmentation may occur because melanocytes are highly vulnerable to freezing.

Plastic surgery

Plastic surgery is surgery that is performed to improve the appearance or function of the visual parts of the body. Plastic surgery has been attempted for centuries. Surgery of this kind was performed before the era of the Roman Empire. Hindu records describe some good results from efforts to alter deformities caused by disease or other misfortune. In the sixteenth century, Italian surgeons did remarkable work in plastic surgery, and there was interest in the emotional aspects of facial deformities. The discovery of anesthetics and of the cause of infection enabled surgeons to make strides in this field. Disfigurements resulting from World Wars I and II challenged the imagination of surgeons so that new techniques were developed.

Purposes of plastic surgery

The main purposes of plastic surgery are to restore function, prevent further loss of function, and cosmetically improve the defects caused by deformities present at birth, from disease, or from trauma. Plastic surgery such as skin grafting may be performed as an emergency measure in severe burns. It is also performed for esthetic improvement.

Although medical science has made progress in learning the causes of some developmental anomalies (e.g., German measles contracted during the first trimester of pregnancy may cause anomalies in the infant), it is not possible at the present time to prevent the occurrence of many defects at birth. Many birth defects such as cleft lip and cleft palate require plastic surgery. The cause of cancer is still unknown, and extensive surgery will continue to be used until a better method of treatment is discovered. Following surgical treatment for this disease, plastic surgery often is necessary. Trauma such as that sustained in automobile accidents often necessitates plastic surgery, and it seems likely that the number of people requiring such treatment will increase. Plastic surgery is often needed following loss of skin and scarring from burns. *Keloid tissue*, the thick, weltlike masses of overgrowth of scar tissue, which most commonly occur in dark-skinned persons, will often require plastic surgery. Posttraumatic scars in which subcutaneous tissues are separated

from, or are adherent to, underlying structures such as bone may be corrected by plastic surgery.

The two aspects of plastic surgery, *reconstruction* and *correction,* are evident in most plastic surgery treatment. Often several medical specialists care for patients needing reconstructive and corrective surgery. The dental surgeon, the ear, nose, and throat specialist, and the plastic surgeon may all work together, for example, in treatment of the child who has a cleft lip and a cleft palate.

Directing the person in seeking appropriate care

Many people do not know that it is possible to correct a congenital defect. Some parents may delay seeking medical care for a child with a defect caused by a congenital anomaly because of their own guilt feelings. They may hope that somehow, miraculously, the child will "outgrow" the condition. Often they do not realize that the normal development of the child depends on the early treatment of some conditions. A defect may interfere with the use of a part of the body so that normal growth does not take place. This result follows the principle that form follows function; for instance, a child's deformed and therefore unused hand does not grow at the same rate as the hand that is used normally. Contractures of joints and atrophy of muscles occur with disuse, thus increasing the defect and handicap; for example, facial asymmetry can result from contractures in the neck that prevent uniform action of the muscles of both sides of the face even though the muscles themselves are not affected.

Parents need to know that healthy emotional development in the child is dependent on normal physical appearance. When a defect is allowed to persist, there may be emotional maladjustment that will affect the child's entire life. For example, conspicuous patches of brightly discolored skin present at birth and known as birthmarks or port-wine stains are quite common. These stains, particularly if they are on the face or neck, cause the child great emotional distress and sometimes lead to serious personality maladjustment.

Plastic surgery may require repeated and long hospitalizations that may place serious financial strain on the patient and family if they must assume responsibility for the major part of the expense. Clinic nurses, community health nurses, social workers, and welfare agency personnel can help in preparing the patient for this problem and in helping him or her to meet it. If the patient is an adult, leaves from employment, financial support while undergoing treatment, and plans for convalescent care and rehabilitation are examples of problems that must be faced in many instances. The person should be encouraged to discuss problems freely, since their solution does affect medical treatment.

Many parents do not know that financial resources are available to cover costs of plastic surgery for children. Every state in the country has a plan for medical care of crippled children. This program is partially supported by matching funds from the federal government, administered by the Office of Child Development (formerly the Children's Bureau) of the Department of Health and Human Services, which was created soon after the first White House Conference on Child Care, held in Washington, DC, in 1909. Children and adolescents up to 21 years of age with defects requiring plastic surgery are eligible for care under this plan. If the nurse encounters a child who might benefit from medical treatment, the family can be encouraged to discuss this with their physician. If the family has no personal physician, the local hospital may conduct a clinic or may recommend a physician designated to care for eligible children in the area or the state. Small community hospitals may not have clinics of their own but may refer patients to larger hospitals or special clinics in nearby cities. In larger communities the school nurse is usually well informed about available resources.

General intervention for the person experiencing plastic surgery

Emotional factors related to surgery

It is believed that any plastic surgery for an obvious defect is justified if it helps people feel they have a better chance for recognition among other persons. The plastic surgeon may reshape a nose or repair a deformed hand so that an emotionally stable person will have more assurance among others. It is foolish to assume, however, that reconstructive surgery alone will correct a basic personality problem. Some people blame an apparently trivial physical defect for a long series of failures in their lives when the major defect lies within their personalities. Because of this possibility, the person is usually studied before surgery is planned. It is necessary to know what the person expects the surgery to accomplish before the physician can decide whether such expectations are realistic and if surgery should be performed.

It is also necessary to learn about the social standards and cultural mores of the community and the person's adjustment to them. Assessment should be made of the person's characteristic pattern in interpersonal relationships and whether previous medical treatment of the particular problem has been sought. The nurse and the social worker are often called on to assist the surgeon in efforts to learn as much as possible about the patient. Sometimes the help of specialists in psychology and psychiatry is sought.

Before surgery the surgeon will tell the patient what probably can be done and what changes are possible. It is important that the nurse know what the patient has been told so that misunderstandings and misinterpretations can be avoided. It is frequently necessary to reinforce repeatedly the fact that immediate results may not meet the patient's expectations. Preparation is necessary for the normal appearance of skin grafts and reconstructed tissue immediately after surgery. Postoperative tissue reaction may distort normal contours, suture lines may be reddened, and the color of the newly transplanted skin may differ somewhat from that of surrounding skin. The appearance of the surgical area changes as the edema decreases and the suture line becomes less reddened and indurated. Six months after surgery the scar will be less noticeable than at 6 days or 6 weeks postoperatively.

The patient who is admitted to the hospital for plastic surgery may have extensive scarring and deformity and may be exceedingly sensitive to scrutiny. On the other hand, the patient may have little apparent deformity, and it may be difficult to understand why the patient wishes to have surgery. The nurse cannot know what the disfigurement means to the individual person and should avoid judgment concerning the necessity of surgery.

Diet

A diet high in protein and vitamins before elective surgery is thought to help in the "take" or healing of a graft. Hemoglobin and clotting times are usually determined, and the blood protein level is assayed because a normal blood protein level has been found to be necessary for satisfactory growth of grafted tissue.

Postoperative care

Many plastic surgeons prefer that the patient not see the operative site until the initial edema and inflammation subside since the initial view is distorted compared to the end result. For this reason the patient is discouraged from looking into a mirror until healing begins to occur, and the surgeon may leave the incision covered for longer periods than necessary to prevent patient discouragement. The patient frequently needs support when seeing the operative site for the first time. The nurse is present when dressings are removed and assesses the reaction of the patient so that immediate and future nursing intervention can be planned and implemented. Members of the family should also know what to expect so that they will not be unduly worried and so that they can give support to the patient if apprehension occurs.

Corrective surgery

Implants

In plastic surgery the surgeon may use, in addition to the patient's own tissues, inert materials and tissues from other human beings. Inert substances must meet several criteria. They must not be irritating or contribute to the development of cancer, they should be an appropriate consistency for their intended use, and they should not deteriorate or change their shape and form with time. A large variety of substances have been used in the past, including wax, metal, ivory, and bone that has been rendered inert by boiling. In recent years materials such as Teflon and silicone have been used extensively, since they appear to be nonirritating and they retain their form indefinitely.

For many years reconstructive procedures have been attempted in which the tissues of other human beings are used. Whenever these tissues are used, however, there is the potential of rejection of the tissue because of the body's immune response (p. 1872). The least difficulty is encountered with tissues such as the cornea of the eye that have a very limited blood supply.

Grafts

The most common procedure used in plastic surgery is grafting, or the transplantation of skin and other tissue from one part of the body to another part or from a donor.

Graft sources. An *autograft* is skin, bone, cartilage, fat, fascia, muscle, or nerves that are moved from one part of the body to another.

Tissue transplanted from another person is called a *homograft (allograft)*. It can be obtained from living persons, or it can be taken from persons shortly after death. Tissue taken under the latter circumstances can be used only if cancer or an infectious disease was not present. The use of homografts may be necessary when the patient's condition is poor and autografting is impossible. For example, the patient may be in shock but require the covering of large burned areas by grafted skin. The survival time of homografts varies from a few days to a number of weeks. Depending on the tissue used and the recipient site, the transplanted tissue will then die and slough or be absorbed and replaced by the host's own developing tissues. They are used only as temporary grafts.

Heterografts (xenografts) consist of tissue from another species. They are rejected by the recipient and are used only in special cases. For example, if tissue in banks is not readily available, it may be more feasible to use heterografts to cover the open wounds of patients with massive burns. The transplant acts as an antigen, and the body forms antibodies against it that prevent growth and function of the graft. When bone, cartilage, or blood vessels are obtained from sources other than the patient, they do not become part of the patient's body but act as a framework around which the body usually lays down cells of its own. The graft is then gradually absorbed over a period of time.

Grafting procedures. Plastic surgery may be performed by means of free grafting—cutting tissue from one part of the body and moving it directly to another part. It may also be done by leaving one end of the graft attached to the body to provide a blood supply for the graft until blood vessels form at the new place of attachment. The surgeon selects skin for grafting that is similar in texture and thickness to that which has been lost and studies the normal lines of the skin and its elasticity to avoid noticeable scars. Scar tissue contracts with time, and in normal circumstances this process is good because it produces a complete closure of the line of injury. However, in some cases scar tissue may contract in such a way that surrounding tissues are pulled out of normal contour, and distortion may result.

FREE GRAFTS. Free grafts are those that are lifted completely from one site and placed at another site. There are several types of free grafts, each with its advantages and limitations (Table 69-4). Split-thickness grafts consist of the epidermis and varying thicknesses of the dermis. Full-thickness grafts include the entire dermis and epidermis (see Fig. 68-1).

Thin split-thickness grafts (Ollier-Thiersch grafts), which have only a very thin layer of the dermis, are of limited use because they contract easily, often become shiny and discolored, and have poor wearing qualities. They may be used to replace mucous membrane in reconstructive surgery of such areas as the mouth and vagina. Appropriate means to prevent excessive contraction of the graft as it heals must be taken. Thin split-thickness homografts may be used to cover large burned areas to reduce the loss of body fluids. Within a few weeks the grafts can be removed and replaced with intermediate or thick split-thickness autografts.

Intermediate and *thick split-thickness grafts* are widely used. These grafts have a thicker layer of dermis attached to the epidermis and do not wrinkle, contract, or become discolored as easily as the thin split-thickness graft. The donor site is able to reepithelialize completely, since the deeper layers of the dermis have been left intact. These split-thickness grafts can be used to cover almost any part of the body. They can be cut into large pieces with a dermatome set to ensure a uniform thickness of the graft, and these can then be cut into smaller pieces to correspond to the size of the area to be grafted.

Meshed grafts are either thin or intermediate split-thickness grafts that have been placed through a perforating machine that creates a mesh. Meshed grafts are elastic and can be used to cover larger areas than the original size. They also conform more easily to irregular surfaces and can be placed over less clean bases than regular split-thickness grafts. Cosmetic appearance is poor. Meshed grafts are used frequently to cover large burned skin areas.

Full-thickness grafts (Wolfe's grafts) are used primarily to cover small areas where matching skin color and texture is important, such as on the face. One disadvantage of the full-thickness graft is that only a moderate-sized

TABLE 69-4. Various types of skin grafts

Type of graft	Description	Use	Comments
Free grafts			
Split-thickness: thin	Epidermis and thin layer of dermis (0.25-0.30 mm)	Burns	Becomes vascularized quickly Survives transplantation readily Donor sites heal quickly Poor cosmetic results Considerable postgraft contraction Does not withstand trauma
Split-thickness: intermediate or thick	Epidermis and thicker layer of dermis (0.40-0.45 or 0.55-0.60 mm)	Widely used over large wounds	Less contraction Better cosmetic results Epithelialization of donor site occurs completely but more slowly
Full-thickness	Epidermis and all of dermis	For small areas where matching skin color and texture is important	Best cosmetic results No contraction Donor site must be sutured (no epithelialization) Limited donor sites Lowest transplantation survival
Flap grafts	Skin and subcutaneous tissue; one end remains attached to donor site for vascularization	Large areas of defect; over avascular areas	More complex, requires greater skill Are bulky May introduce hair into nonhairy areas

piece of full-thickness skin can survive as a free graft under the best circumstances because the blood supply cannot become established quickly enough to provide essential nutrition. For nourishment these grafts depend entirely on existing lymph until their own blood supply can be established. It takes at least 2 weeks for blood supply to become established, although it is usually possible to tell within a week whether the graft is going to survive. If the graft dies, the skin is irretrievably lost to the body, since regeneration of skin at the donor site is not possible. If possible, the surrounding skin at the donor site is usually undermined so that the skin edges can be brought together, and grafting of the donor site is not necessary. This means that full advantage may have been taken of the elastic quality of the skin, and another graft probably cannot be taken from the same place for some time.

FLAP GRAFTS. Flap grafts are not moved entirely to another area as are free grafts but always have one end left attached to the primary site to provide vascularization. Flap grafts are used to cover larger defects than can be covered by free grafts.

There are several different types of flap grafts. *Transposed flaps* are rectangular sections of tissue moved from a site adjacent to the defect. The flap is cut along two long sides and one short side and then slid sideways to cover the defect. If the skin is loose enough, the donor site can be sutured; if it is not loose, a split-thickness free graft is used to cover the donor site. A *rotation* flap is similar to the transposed flap except that

a semicircle of tissue is cut and then rotated over the defect.

Island flaps are narrow strips of neurovascular tissue from which the skin has been removed. The flap is transferred to a distant site through a tunnel made *under* the skin. The only scars that remain are at the donor and recipient sites. *Tube pedicle grafts* are formed by suturing the long sides of the graft together to form a tube and then suturing the end to another area of the body. For example, the end can be sutured to the forearm, which then serves as a "carrier" (Fig. 69-2). After the graft has taken, the original site is freed and the graft is sutured to the recipient site. When this second-stage graft has taken, the graft is freed from the forearm. Pedicle grafts are used less frequently since the advent of microsurgery.

Preoperative skin care. The wound that is to receive a graft must be free from infections that would delay healing, lead to more scar tissue formation, or cause death of the graft. Infection is treated by the administration of local and systemic antibiotics and by the use of warm soaks and compresses. A sterile physiologic solution of sodium chloride is the solution most often used. Before skin grafting is attempted, any dead tissue that is adherent to the wound is removed by debridement; otherwise, this tissue will interfere with the graft's healing.

The *donor site* (the area from which skin is to be taken) is washed with a germicidal soap the evening before surgery, and this cleansing may be repeated the

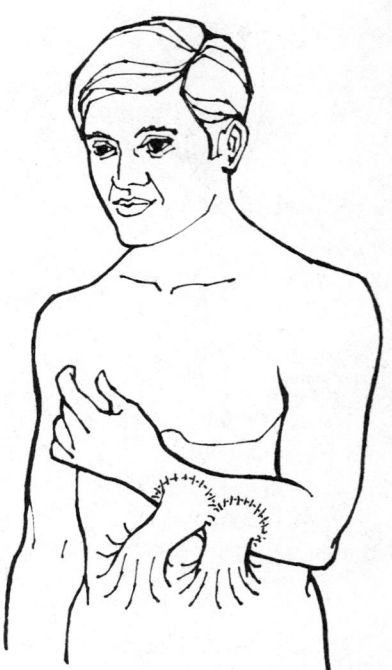

Fig. 69-2. Bilateral tubed pedicle flaps from abdomen to forearm. At later operation they will be detached from forearm and spread to cover burned areas on trunk.

morning of operation. Frequently, the site is shaved in the operating room after the patient is anesthetized so that the damage of cutting the skin is minimized. Strong antiseptics are avoided because they may irritate the skin. If the *recipient site* (the area that is to receive the graft) is not an open wound, it is cleansed in the same way.

Postoperative care of the recipient site. There are four conditions that are necessary for a graft to survive: adequate vascularization of the recipient site, constant contact with the underlying tissue, immobilization, and freedom from infection.[4] Tissue that has had advanced radiation damage or that is infected is a poor base for the graft and must be cleaned or scraped to remove debris or avascular tissue before a graft can be attempted.

Anything that comes between the undersurface of the graft and the recipient area such as a discharge caused by infection, excess serous fluid, or blood will float the graft away from close contact and may cause it to die. To prevent floating, some surgeons insert the drains at strategic spots along the edges of the graft, or a small catheter is inserted on the edge of the graft under the recipient skin and attached to suction to remove the fluid.

If the recipient site is a clean wound with no infection, the graft usually is sutured with many fine sutures to hold it in place and in contact with the normal skin adjacent to it. The area is inspected frequently to see if the skin is adhering to the underlying tissue. If fluid

collects under the skin graft, it is removed by aspiration with a sterile needle and syringe or the fluid is rolled to the wound edge with a sterile applicator.

A wide variety of materials are used as dressings. The choice depends on the kind of graft and the surgeon's preference. Petrolatum, Adaptic gauze, or Telfa dressings are often selected. Often the graft is covered with a piece of coarse mesh gauze that is anchored to the adjacent skin edges with an elastic bandage to give firm, gentle pressure and to immobilize the area. The first dressing may be covered with a compress of sterile normal saline solution. Because the compress is moist, it fits the contour of the wound better. Continuous pressure is necessary to keep the graft adherent to the recipient bed, but pressure should not be so firm as to cause death of the graft. Occasionally, the sutures anchoring the graft at the skin edges are left uncut and brought over a pressure dressing to hold it firmly against the graft (Fig. 69-3). This type of dressing, called a *stent* dressing, is especially useful for areas where movement cannot be controlled.

The graft site is elevated when possible and protected from pressure and motion. The nurse should be certain that dressings do not become loosened so that pressure is reduced and that the patient *does not lie on these dressings* or in any other way increase the pressure on them. When flap grafts are used, slings and casts may ensure immobilization and help to keep parts of the body in the correct relationship for healing (Fig. 69-4).

Some surgeons believe that grafts are stimulated in their effort to establish blood supply by the use of *warm, moist compresses,* and sterile normal saline solution is usually ordered for this purpose. The greatest care must be taken that infection is not introduced when compresses are being changed and moistened. Hands must be washed before dressings are handled or compresses changed. Meticulous technique is followed so that infection does not occur. Care is taken so that the newly grafted skin is not traumatized. The temperature of the compress solution should not be over 40.5° C (105° F), and compresses should be applied with sterile forceps. Compresses may sometimes be covered with a sterile petroleum jelly dressing and moistened by gently directing fluid from a sterile Asepto syringe under the edge of the dressings. Sterile tubes with tiny openings (Dakin's tubes) may also be placed through the outer compresses to provide a means of moistening the inner dressings without disturbing them and without introducing infection.

Inner dressings on the recipient site are usually changed by the surgeon 1 to 2 days after surgery, and it is usually possible to know then whether the result of the operation is satisfactory. Sutures may be removed at this time.

Postoperative care of the donor site. Following surgery a layer of fine mesh Xeroform gauze is placed

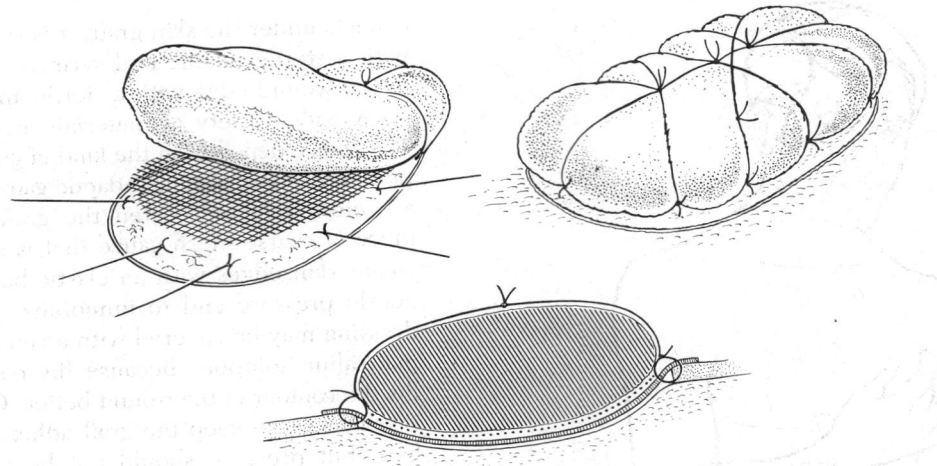

Fig. 69-3. Tie-over (stent) dressing used as pressure dressing on skin graft. (Modified from McGregor, I.A.: Fundamental techniques of plastic surgery and their surgical applications, ed. 4, Baltimore, 1969, The Williams & Wilkins Co.)

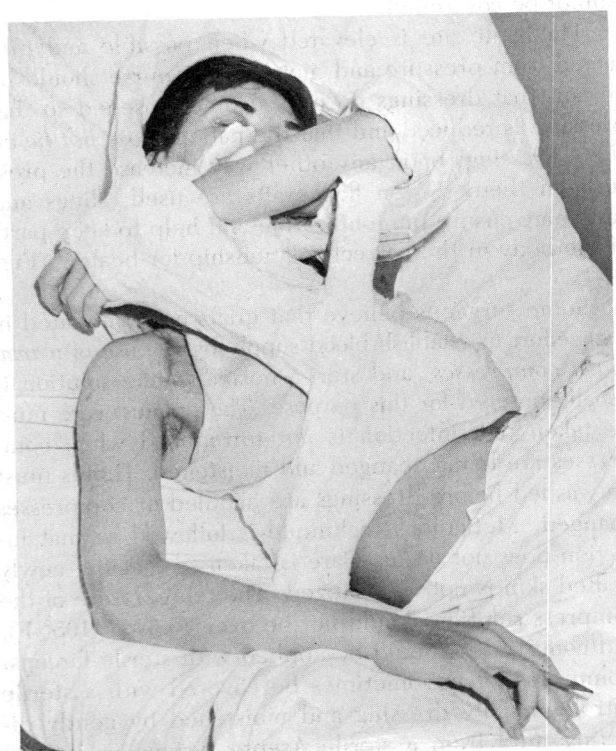

Fig. 69-4. Plastic operations sometimes require patient to be in extremely awkward positions. Eating, mouth hygiene, and communicating with others are problems in caring for this patient. Note pencil used for communicating.

on the donor site and is covered by fluffy sterile dressings to absorb the serum that oozes from the site. The donor site is left uncovered after 24 hours following removal of a thin section of tissue and 48 hours after a thick graft. The dressing over the donor site for a thick graft is changed after the first 24 hours. A heat lamp may be used with caution to hasten drying of the donor site. A bed cradle may be used to protect the donor site and allow more air circulation for drying. As the donor site heals, the edges of the fine mesh gauze are trimmed as they loosen until the gauze drops off.

When split-thickness grafts have been used, the donor site (often the anterior surface of the thigh) may be a greater source of discomfort to the patient than the recipient site. Analgesics may be necessary during the first few postoperative days.

Cast care. The general care of the patient with a cast is similar to that of patients with casts following other types of surgery (p. 964). The cast is applied in this case to support a graft. Immediately after application and frequently thereafter the cast must be examined for cracks or breaks that will interfere with support for the graft, and it must be carefully checked to make certain that no excessive pressure is being exerted. Pillows can be used to give support and to lessen strain on body parts.

One major difference in cast care following plastic surgery is that the patient is sometimes placed in very awkward positions, especially after pedicle flap surgery (see Fig. 69-4). Arrangements should be made for the patient to see what goes on in the surrounding environment. Sometimes this is made possible by changing the patient's position in bed or the position of the bed in the room. In some instances putting the patient "head to foot" in the bed is helpful. A mirror may be attached to the bed and arranged at such an angle that the patient can see at least a part of the room if the head, neck, and shoulder movements are restricted by a cast.

Procedures for contractures

Plastic surgeons make excellent use of the natural elastic quality of normal skin. Operations known as Z-*plasty* and Y-*plasty* are often performed. Scar tissue can

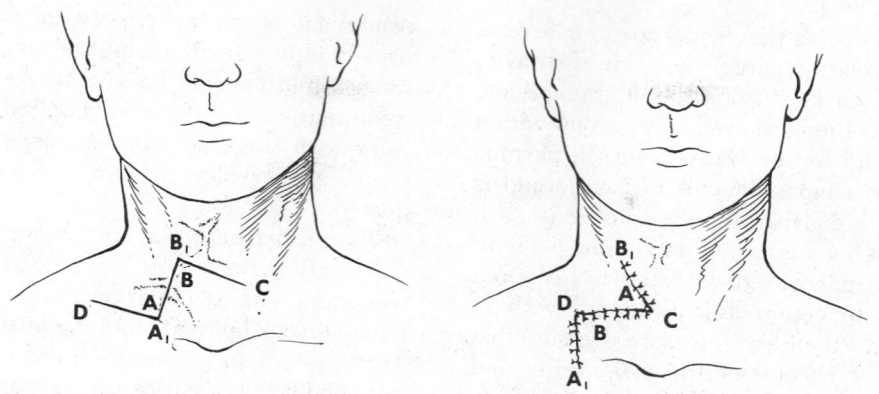

Fig. 69-5. By means of Z-plasty operations, scar tissue can be removed and defects can be covered without need to transplant skin.

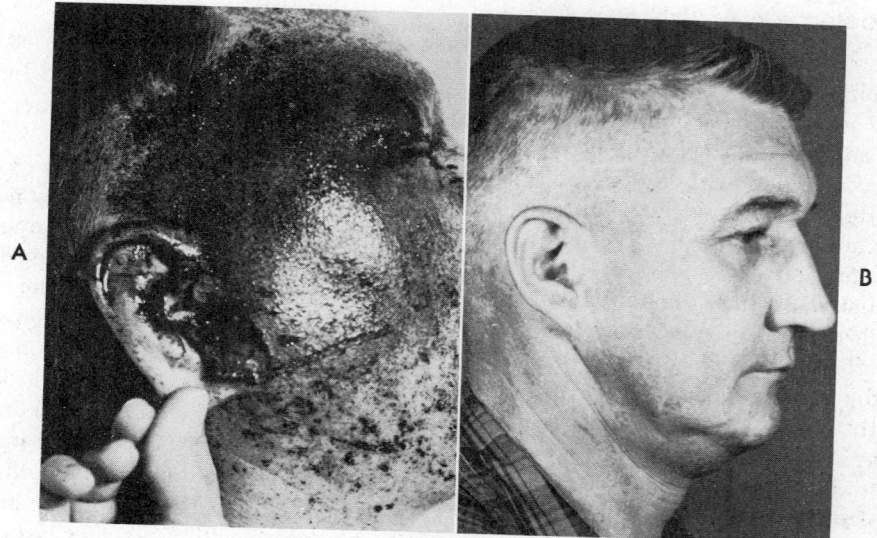

Fig. 69-6. A, Meticulous cleansing and dermabrasion were required to remove impregnated bits of galvanized metal. **B,** Postoperative view of patient 17 years after dermabrasion. (From Saunders, W.H., et al.: Nursing care in eye, ear, nose, and throat disorders, ed. 4, St. Louis, 1979, The C.V. Mosby Co.)

often be removed, and the Z- or Y-shaped incision enables the surgeon to undermine adjacent skin, draw the edges together, and cover the defect without using skin from another part of the body (Fig. 69-5). These procedures are naturally limited by the size of the scar and its location, since elasticity of skin varies in different parts of the body. Z-plasty and Y-plasty procedures are suitable for such locations as the axilla, the inner aspects of the elbow, and the neck and throat. They are not so useful in treating defects on the back or on the palmar surfaces of the hand because the skin in these areas cannot be undermined and stretched.

Dermabrasion

Pockmarks, scars from acne, and certain other disfiguring marks may be removed from the skin by abrasive action. The variable results depend on the type and extent of the condition and the age of the patient (Fig. 69-6). Preoperatively, the patient is prepared by the surgeon for the degree of improvement to be expected so that expectations are realistic. The patient is also informed about postoperative swelling, discomfort, crusting, and erythema, which may persist for several weeks. The procedure is performed under local or general anesthesia depending on the size of the area to be treated, the individual patient, and the preference of the surgeon. It may be done in the clinic, the surgeon's office, or the hospital, again depending on the extent of the procedure, type of anesthetic, and the preference of the physician. Contraindications to dermabrasion include deep skin defects and a history of keloid formation.

The skin is washed with germicidal soap for several days before surgery. During surgery the skin is sprayed with a refrigerant such as dichlorotetrafluoromethane (Freon II), and this is then followed by abrasion with a wire brush or diamond fraise. The wire brush permits deeper abrasion but is more difficult to handle and is more likely to cut and dig than the diamond fraise.[30] If the procedure has not been extensive and oozing is slight, the area may be left uncovered. Usually it is covered with an ointment or by compresses moistened with an antiseptic solution and then by a pressure dressing that covers the entire face except for the eyes, nose, and mouth. Prepared dressings that adhere less readily to the skin surface, such as Telfa dressings, are also used. Dermabrasion may be done in stages. At least 2 weeks and often longer may intervene between treatments.

Medical dermatattooing

Tattooing has been found useful in plastic surgery for changing the color of grafted skin so that it more closely resembles the surrounding skin. This treatment is usually given on an ambulatory basis. Pigment is carefully selected and blended with the normal skin coloring by a skilled technician who then impregnates the grafted skin, using a tattooing needle. The procedure is painful, since no anesthetic is used. Sometimes the patient is given a sedative such as phenobarbital or is instructed to take such medication approximately 1 hour before coming to the clinic or the physician's office. Before the tattooing, the skin is cleansed with a gauze sponge moistened with alcohol or normal saline solution. There may be a slight serous oozing from the skin after the treatment, and it should be left to dry and crust. Sometimes a piece of sterile gauze can be placed over the tattooed area, and an ice bag may be applied if severe discomfort follows the treatment.

Tattooing is usually done in several stages. The amount done at one time depends on individual circumstances such as the location of the part treated and the emotional reactions of the patient. For example, treatment of the skin close to the eye is often quite painful and is extremely trying for the patient. Therefore usually only a small amount of tattooing is done at one time. Children may be given a general anesthetic for treatment around the eyes. Grafted skin may change in color with time, so tattooing done for the purpose of changing the color of grafted skin may have to be repeated.

Port-wine stains that are too large to treat by excision and grafting have also responded to this method of treatment with excellent results. Treatments are carried out at 4-week intervals until the final results are achieved. This is a tedious procedure if the stain is large and dark but, finally, in some cases the stain is barely apparent to the casual observer.

Reconstructive surgery

Reconstructive surgery is carried out to correct birth defects, repair tissues destroyed by trauma or disease, or replace tissue removed by other surgeries.

Birth defects

Birth defects can occur in any part of the body. Providing they are treated at the proper time in the child's life, most of them can be improved a great deal by reconstructive procedures and some can be corrected entirely. Among the more common defects are cleft lip and cleft palate, urogenital anomalies (p. 1551), and musculoskeletal defects. (Musculoskeletal anomalies are discussed fully in orthopedic nursing texts.)

Cleft lip (Figs. 69-7 and 69-8) may involve the nostril floor and lip on either one or both sides. Repair of the cleft lip is best performed in the infant some time after the tenth to twelfth week after birth, providing the infant weighs more than 5 kg and has a hemoglobin level of 10 g/100 ml or more.[4] The older the child when the cleft lip is repaired, the greater the possibility of needed secondary revisions. The *cleft palate* is not repaired until some time between the first and second year of life, since more tissue is available then for a successful repair.

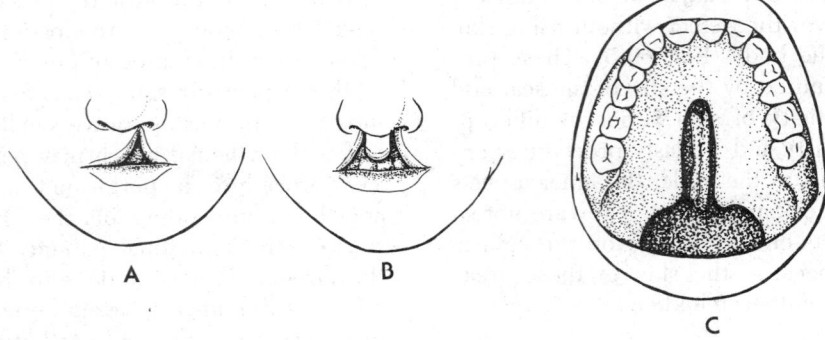

Fig. 69-7. Cleft lip and palate. **A,** Single cleft of lip. **B,** Double cleft of lip. **C,** Cleft of posterior palate.

Repair of the cleft palate should be done before the child begins regular speech. Satisfactory speech after repair occurs in 70% to 90% of cases.[4] Feeding of the infant with a cleft palate can be a problem, and the mother may require considerable help and guidance by the nurse. Measures to facilitate feedings are covered in detail in most pediatric nursing texts.

Maxillofacial surgery

Maxillofacial surgery received impetus as a result of injuries sustained in World War II and the increase in radical surgery for malignancies of the head and neck (p. 1284). The surgeon works closely with the dental surgeon and with the specialist in problems of the nose and throat. When damage has been so great that reconstruction with living tissue is impossible, it is sometimes possible to construct prosthetic parts of the face that are so true to natural color and contour that they are not easily detectable. For example, a side of the nose may be replaced by a prosthetic part that is colored to match the patient's skin and disguised with marking to resemble skin.

Rhinoplasty. Reconstructive surgery of the nose can be done either to correct an anatomic problem (p. 1270) or for cosmetic reasons. Bone and cartilage may be removed from the nose if it is irregular, or they may be inserted if a defect such as a saddle nose is being corrected (Fig. 69-9). A local anesthetic is usually used for these procedures. The incision is usually made at the end of the nose inside the nostril so that it is not conspicuous. A nasal splint made of plaster, tongue blades, or crinoline may be used for protection. There will be ecchymosis and swelling around the eyes and nose for 10 to 14 days after surgery. Ice compresses and an ice bag may be used to hasten fluid reabsorption. The patient must anticipate waiting several weeks before evaluating the final result of the surgery.

Otoplasty. Another common operation, usually for purely cosmetic reasons, is the removal of some of the cartilage from the ears in order to flatten them against the head. This procedure is relatively simple and requires only a short hospitalization.

Rhytidoplasty. "Face-lifting" is also performed primarily for cosmetic reasons. An incision is made at the hairline, and excess skin is separated from its underlying tissue and removed. The remaining skin is pulled up and sutured at the hairline, thus removing wrinkles and giving firmness and smoothness to the face. A gentle pressure dressing is then applied and left in place for 24 to 48 hours. The patient is often discharged at this time, and sutures are removed later in the surgeon's office. The patient frequently needs medication for pain in the postoperative period because of the extent to which the tissue has been undermined. The surgery may be repeated at a later date.

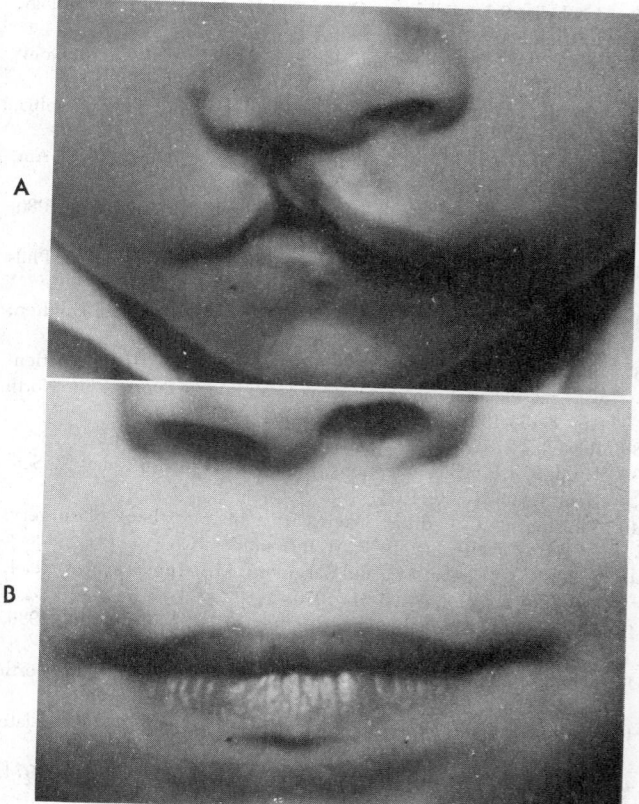

Fig. 69-8. A, Patient with almost complete cleft lip. **B,** Three years after surgery. (From Brauer, R.O.: Repair of the unilateral cleft lip. In Georgiade, N.G., editor: Symposium on management of cleft lip and palate and associated deformities, vol. 8, St. Louis, 1974, The C.V. Mosby Co.)

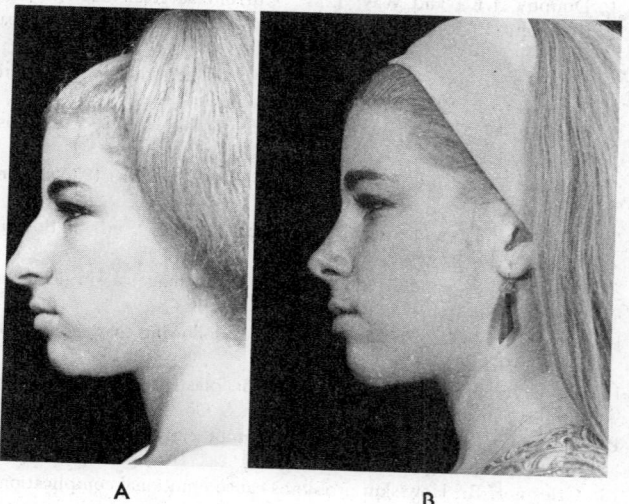

Fig. 69-9. A, Preoperative appearance of 16-year-old girl. **B,** Postoperative appearance 1 year after rhinoplasty. (From Peck, G.C.: Surgery of the nasal tip. In Masters, F.W., and Lewis, J.R., Jr., editors: Symposium on aesthetic surgery of the nose, ears, and chin, vol. 6, St. Louis, 1973, The C.V. Mosby Co.)

Mammoplasty

Mammoplasty, or reconstructive breast surgery, may be done to replace breast tissue removed by surgery (p. 1757) or to improve the appearance of a woman's breasts. Some women develop conspicuously large and pendulous breasts that they wish to have reduced in size. Large breasts are embarrassing to some women and make it difficult for them to participate in sports, maintain good posture, and buy clothes that fit. Such women often respond to reconstructive surgery remarkably well. Cosmetic surgery of the breast may also be done to make unusually small breasts larger. A variety of plastic materials may be used for this procedure.

Outcome criteria for the person having plastic surgery

The person or significant others can:
1. Explain the time interval necessary before results are achieved.
2. Describe care of wound sites and the necessity for prevention of infection.
3. Describe the need for follow-up care until healing has occurred.

REFERENCES AND SELECTED READINGS

1. Converse, J.M., editor: Reconstruction plastic surgery: principles and procedures in correction, reconstruction and transplantation, ed. 2, Philadelphia, 1977, W.B. Saunders Co.
2. Cronin, T.D., and Brauer, R.O.: Augmentation mammoplasty, Surg. Clin. North Am. 51:441-452, 1971.
3. Dison, N.: Clinical nursing techniques, ed. 4, St. Louis, 1979, The C.V. Mosby Co.
4. Dunphy, J.E., and Way, L.W.: Current surgical diagnosis and treatment 1979, Los Altos, Calif., 1979, Lange Medical Publications.
5. Fitzpatrick, T.B., et al.: Dermatology in general medicine, ed. 2, New York, 1979, McGraw-Hill Book Co.
6. Ganong, W.F.: Review of medical physiology, ed. 9, Los Altos, Calif., 1979, Lange Medical Publications.
7. Grabb, W.C., and Myers, M.B.: Skin flaps, Boston, 1975, Little, Brown & Co.
8. Grabb, W.C., and Smith, J.W.: Plastic surgery, ed. 3, Boston, 1979, Little, Brown & Co.
9. Grazer, F.M., and Klingbeil, J.R.: Body image: a surgical perspective, St. Louis, 1980, The C.V. Mosby Co.
10. Georgiade, N.G.: Breast reconstruction following mastectomy, St. Louis, 1979, The C.V. Mosby Co.
11. Goldwyn, R.M.: Long-term results in plastic and reconstructive surgery, Boston, 1980, Little, Brown & Co.
12. Griesmer, R.: How emotional trauma causes skin problems, Medical Insights, Dec. 1971.
13. Griesmer, R.: How skin problems cause emotional complications, Medical Insights, Nov. 1971.
14. Grossman, A.R.: Augmentation mammoplasty, Springfield, Ill., 1976, Charles C Thomas, Publisher.
15. Hahn, A.B., Barkin, R.L., and Oestrich, S.J.: Pharmacology in nursing, ed. 15, St. Louis, 1982, The C.V. Mosby Co.
16. Hardy, J.D., editor: Textbook of surgery: principles and practice, ed. 5, Philadelphia, 1977, J.B. Lippincott Co.
17. *Hawkins, K.: Wet dressings: putting the damper on dermatitis, Nurs. '78 8(2):64-67, 1978.
18. Hurwitz, A.: About faces, Am. J. Nurs. 71:2168-2171, 1971.
19. Jones, F.A.: The skin—a mirror of the gut, Geriatrics 28:75-81, 1973.
20. *Kinmont, P.D.: Pruritus as a dermatological problem, Practitioner 208:622-632, 1972.
21. Korting, G.W.: Diseases of the skin in children and adolescents, ed. 3, Philadelphia, 1979, W.B. Saunders Co.
22. Leider, M.: Some principles of dermatologic nursing, RN 35:48-53, 1972.
23. *Macgregor, F.C.: Selection of cosmetic surgery patients, Surg. Clin. North Am. 51:289-298, 1971.
24. *Management of common skin problems, Postgrad. Med. 52:63-194, 1972.
25. Marlow, D.R.: Textbook of pediatric nursing, ed. 5, Philadelphia, 1977, W.B. Saunders Co.
26. Mathes, S.J., and Nahai, F.: Clinical atlas of muscle and musculocutaneous flaps, St. Louis, 1979, The C.V. Mosby Co.
27. Mathews, K.P.: A current view of urticaria, Med. Clin. North Am. 58:185-205, 1974.
28. McGregor, I.A.: Fundamental techniques of plastic surgery, ed. 7, Baltimore, 1980, The Williams & Wilkins Co.
29. *Miller, S.H.: Breast reconstruction following mastectomy, A.O.R.N. J. 25:945-952, 1977.
30. Moschella, S.L., Pillsbury, D.M., and Hurley, H.J.: Dermatology, Philadelphia, 1975, W.B. Saunders Co.
31. Parrish, J.: Dermatology and skin care, New York, 1975, McGraw-Hill Book Co.
32. Pillsbury, D.M.: A manual of dermatology, ed. 2, Philadelphia, 1980, W.B. Saunders Co.
33. Rees, T.D., editor: Cosmetic surgery, Surg. Clin. North Am. 51:265-531, 1971.
34. Rees, T.D., et al.: Aesthetic plastic surgery, Philadelphia, 1980, W.B. Saunders Co.
35. Rhoads, J.E., et al.: Surgery: principles and practice, ed. 5, Philadelphia, 1977, J.B. Lippincott Co.
36. Robin, M.: How emotions affect skin problems in school children, J. Sch. Health 43:370-373, 1973.
37. *Rosillo, R.H., Welty, M.J., and Graham, W.P., III: The patient with maxillofacial cancer: psychological aspects, Nurs. Clin. North Am. 8:153-158, 1973.
38. Rowell, N.: Urticaria, Practitioner 208:614-621, 1972.
39. *Ruppe, J.P.: Skin infections: their role in health today, J. Sch. Health 43:373-380, 1973.
40. Sabiston, D.C., editor: Davis-Christopher textbook of surgery, ed. 11, Philadelphia, 1977, W.B. Saunders Co.
41. Saitoh, M., Uzuka, M., and Sakamoto, M.: Human hair cycle, J. Invest. Dermatol. 54:65-61, 1970.
42. Sauer, G.C.: Manual of skin diseases, ed. 4, Philadelphia, 1980, J.B. Lippincott Co.
43. Schmidt, L.M.: Topical dermatologic therapy, Pediatr. Clin. North Am. 25:191-209, 1978.
44. *Shapiro, C.S., et al.: Nursing care of the cleft-lip/cleft-palate child, RN 36:46-60, 1973.
45. Shelley, W.B.: Consultations in dermatology, Philadelphia, 1974, W.B. Saunders Co.

*References preceded by an asterisk are particularly well suited for student reading.

46. Stuart, M.S.: Skin flaps and grafts after head and neck surgery, Am. J. Nurs. **78:**1368-1373, 1978.
47. *Tierney, E.A.: Accepting disfigurement when death is the alternative, Am. J. Nurs. **75:**2149-2150, 1975.
48. *Topical therapy: choosing and using the proper vehicle, Nurs. '77 **7**(11):9-10, 1977.
49. *Welty, M.J., Graham, W.P., III, and Rosillo, R.H.: The patient with maxillofacial cancer: surgical treatment and nursing care, Nurs. Clin. North Am. **8:**137-151, 1973.
50. Williams, S.R.: Nutrition and diet therapy, ed. 4, St. Louis, 1981, The C.V. Mosby Co.
51. Woods, J.E., and Payne, W.S.: Contour restoration following simple or modified radical mastectomy, J.A.M.A. **235:**1588-1589, 1976.

CHAPTER 70

INTERVENTION FOR THE PERSON WITH BURNS

PENNY O'MALLEY

Epidemiology and etiology

Burns are wounds caused by dry or moist heat, chemicals, electricity, radiation, and other rays such as x-rays. The most common cause of burns is fire, which kills 13,200 and scars and injures 300,000 Americans each year, including 50,000 persons who must be hospitalized for periods of 6 weeks to 2 years. Many of these deaths could have been prevented. Knowledge, patience, and understanding are needed in the nursing care of severely burned persons during the acute and the long-term recovery phases. Principles of burn care remain the same regardless of etiology.

Classification

Burns are classified as first, second, and third degree, depending on their depth. First- and second-degree burns are classified as *partial-thickness* burns, whereas third-degree burns are *full-thickness* burns (Fig. 70-1). A *first-degree* burn is one in which the outer layer of skin is injured and reddened without blister formation; mild sunburn is a good example. A *second-degree* burn injures all of the epidermis and much of the corium. Blister formation is characteristic, and there is usually considerable subcutaneous edema. The deeper layers of the corium are not destroyed and regeneration can occur. First-degree and second-degree burns are likely to be painful, because nerve endings have been injured and exposed. During the healing phase, the person experiences dryness and itching caused by increased vascularization of sebaceous glands, reduction of secretions, and decreased perspiration.

A *third-degree* burn is one in which all layers of skin are destroyed, thus making regeneration impossible. Nerves, muscles, bone, and blood supply also may be injured or destroyed in third-degree burns. Nerves are destroyed, resulting in a painless wound. The destroyed tissue will be unable to epithelialize; therefore these areas must be covered either by skin growing from normal skin around the edges of the burned area, by scar tissue, or by skin grafts. Skin grafting is preferred for its esthetic advantages.

Pathophysiology of severe burns

As a result of burns, normal skin function is diminished, resulting in physiologic alterations. These include (1) loss of protective barriers against infection, (2) escape of body fluids, (3) lack of temperature control, (4) destroyed sweat and sebaceous glands, and (5) a diminished number of sensory receptors. The severity of these alterations will depend on the extent of the burn and the depth to which damage has occurred.

Increased knowledge of the physiologic changes that occur during severe burns has led to the saving of many lives. There are three stages that occur following *severe* burns: the immediate hypovolemic stage, the diuretic stage, and the long-term rehabilitative stage. Fig. 70-2 presents an overview of the pathophysiologic changes seen in a severe burn.

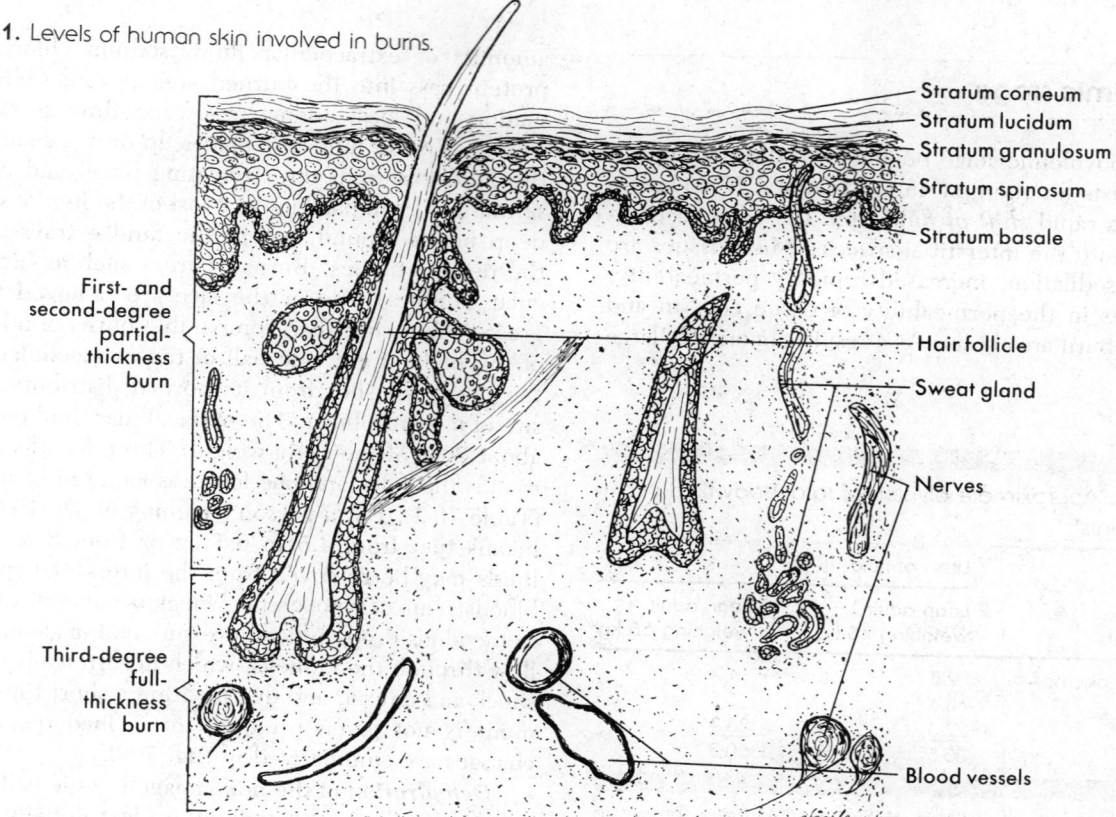

Fig. 70-1. Levels of human skin involved in burns.

Stratum corneum
Stratum lucidum
Stratum granulosum
Stratum spinosum
Stratum basale

First- and second-degree partial-thickness burn

Hair follicle

Sweat gland

Nerves

Third-degree full-thickness burn

Blood vessels

Fig. 70-2. Overview of pathophysiology of a major burn.

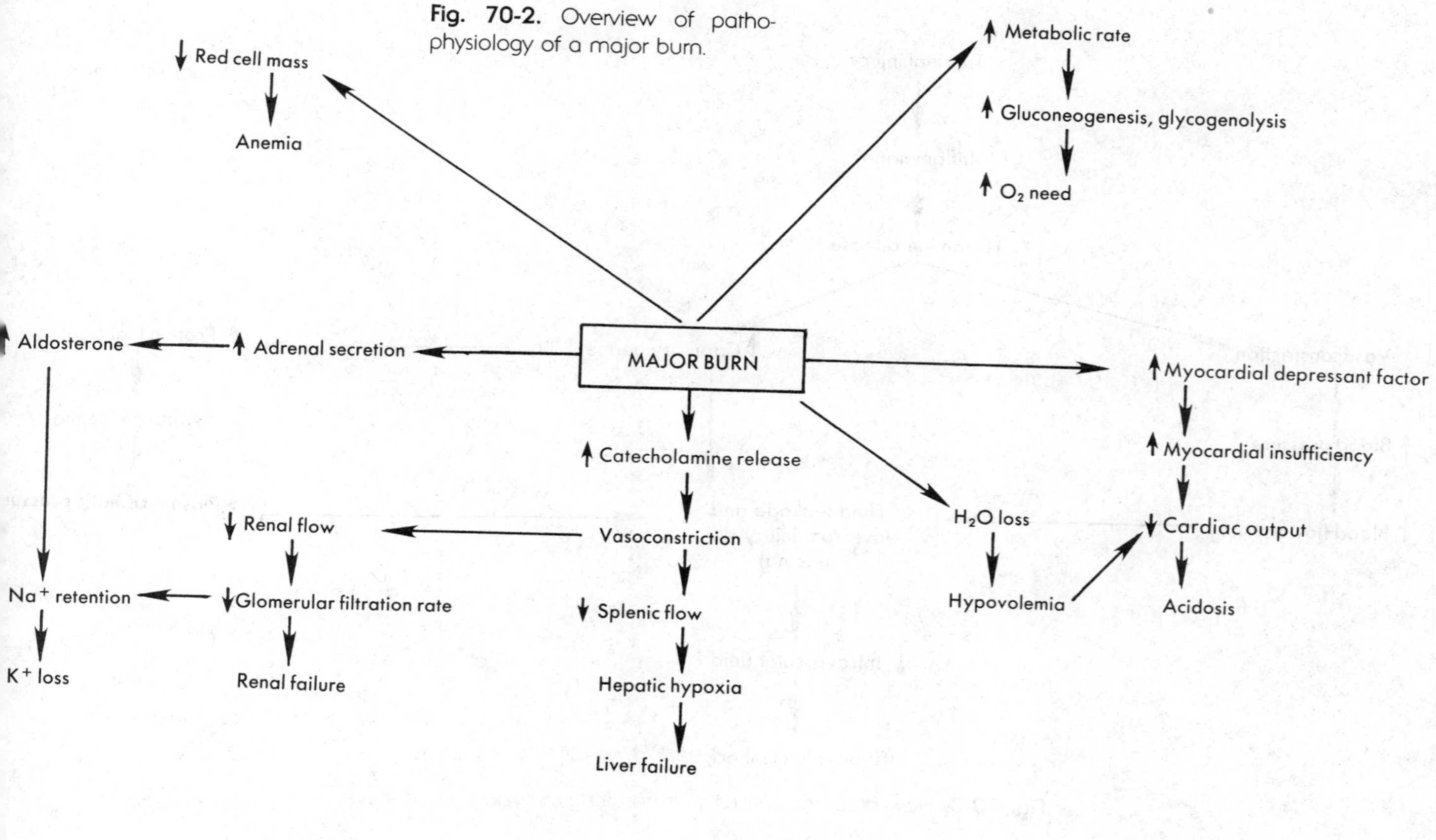

↓ Red cell mass

Anemia

↑ Metabolic rate

↑ Gluconeogenesis, glycogenolysis

↑ O_2 need

↑ Aldosterone ← ↑ Adrenal secretion ← **MAJOR BURN** → ↑ Myocardial depressant factor

↑ Myocardial insufficiency

↑ Catecholamine release

↓ Renal flow ← Vasoconstriction

H_2O loss

↓ Cardiac output

Na$^+$ retention ← ↓ Glomerular filtration rate

↓ Splenic flow

Hypovolemia

Acidosis

K$^+$ loss

Renal failure

Hepatic hypoxia

Liver failure

Hypovolemic stage

The hypovolemic stage begins from the time of the burn and lasts for the first 48 to 72 hours. It is characterized by a rapid *shift of fluid* from the vascular compartments into the interstitial spaces. When tissues are burned, vasodilation, increased capillary permeability, and changes in the permeability of tissue cells in and around the burn area occur. As a result, abnormally large

TABLE 70-1. Approximate division of total body fluid into compartments*

Body fluid compartments	Liters of fluid	
	Lean adult weighing 45 kg	Lean adult weighing 68 kg
Intravascular (plasma)	2.8	4.2
Interstitial	8.4	12.5
Intracellular	22.3	33.3
TOTAL	33.5	50.0

*Note that the smaller the individual, the less fluid he or she has in each compartment and that plasma is reduced most markedly with decrease in size. The normal size and body type of the individual are considered when fluid replacement is ordered.

amounts of extracellular fluid, sodium chloride, and protein pass into the burned area to cause blister formation and local edema or escape through the open wound. Visible fluid loss makes up only a small part of the fluid lost from the circulating blood and other essential fluid compartments. Most of the fluid loss occurs deep in the wound, where the fluid extravasates into the deeper tissues. Burns of areas such as highly vascular muscle tissue or the face are believed to cause greater fluid shift than comparable burns of other parts of the body. Fully one half of the extracellular fluid of the body can shift from its normal distribution to the site of a severe burn. The extracellular fluid constitutes about 20% of the body weight. Three fourths of it surrounds the cells, and one fourth is found in blood plasma (Table 70-1). For a person weighing 68 kg (150 lb), this means that from 4.5 to 6.5 kg or from 5 to 7.5 L of fluids may be removed from the interstitial spaces and bloodstream. Hypovolemic shock occurs, resulting in a tremendous drop in blood pressure and inadequate blood flow through the kidneys, which in turn leads to further shock and anuria, and death within a short time if treatment is not given promptly or is inadequate. These changes are summarized in Fig. 70-3.

Dehydration of the nondamaged tissue cells may result. More fluids and sodium are lost initially from the capillaries than is protein. This increases the capillary osmotic pressure, leading to dehydration with pro-

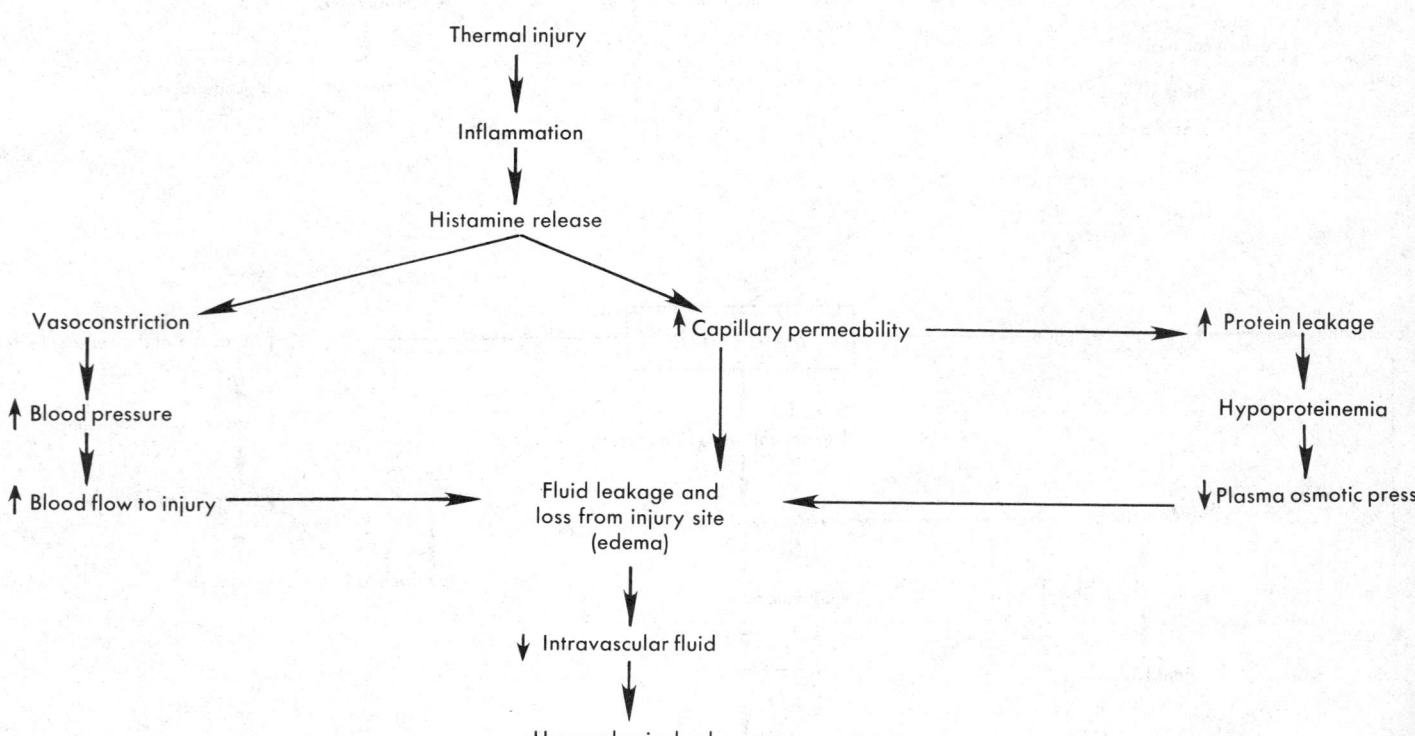

Fig. 70-3. Flow diagram of fluid shifts resulting in hypovolemic shock.

nounced edema in the burned area. As protein continues to be lost into the burned area because of the increased capillary permeability, *hypoproteinemia* results. The increased amount of protein in the tissue spaces is a further contributing factor to edema formation. Proteins may be lost through the open wound; and nitrogen is lost through the kidney from catabolism, leading to a significant negative nitrogen balance. The blood urea nitrogen (BUN) is elevated when oliguria is present.

With loss of fluid from the vascular system, *hemoconcentration* occurs and the hematocrit rises. Blood flow becomes sluggish in the burned area and cellular nutrition decreases. Large numbers of red blood cells become trapped in the burned area and are hemolyzed. Renal damage and hematuria may occur as a result of reduced blood volume and passage of the end products of the hemolyzed cells through the glomeruli. The decreased renal blood flow leads to *oliguria*.

Electrolyte imbalances also occur. *Hyperkalemia* (excessive serum potassium) results from injury to the tissue cells and red blood cells, and from the diminished urinary output, and may lead to heart block and ventricular failure. Potassium may be encouraged to move back into the cells by the administration of insulin, since potassium is transported back into the cells along with glucose. Sodium is retained by the body as a result of the endocrine response to stress. Aldosterone is increased, leading to sodium reabsorption by the kidney. This sodium, however, quickly passes into the interstitial spaces of the burn area with the fluid shift; therefore despite the increased amount of sodium in the body, most of the sodium is trapped in the edema fluid, and a *sodium deficit* occurs. Inadequate tissue perfusion results in anaerobic metabolism, and the acid end products are retained because of the decreased kidney function. *Metabolic acidosis* may then occur.

Respiratory distress may result from burns of the airway or from the effects of hypovolemic shock. Most airway burns are of the upper airway, since this is where incoming air is normally cooled and humidified.[12]

Diuretic stage

The diuretic stage begins about 48 to 72 hours after the person was burned, and the changes may occur rapidly. A *fluid shift* occurs in the opposite direction from the initial stage, and the edema fluid returns to the vascular system. Blood volume increases, leading to increased renal blood flow and diuresis unless renal damage has occurred. Serum electrolyte and hematocrit levels will be decreased because of the *hemodilution*. *This phase requires extreme caution in administration of intravenous fluids*. Fluid overload may occur as fluids shift from the interstitial spaces. The patient's vital signs, breath

sounds, and urinary output are utilized to determine the amount of intravenous fluid replacement. *Dehydration* may occur if rapid urinary fluid losses deplete the intravascular reserve. Sodium is lost with diuresis, and a *sodium deficit* may occur. *Hypokalemia* results from potassium moving back into the cells or being excreted in the urine. Protein continues to be lost from the wounds. *Metabolic acidosis* remains a possibility because of the loss of sodium bicarbonate in the urine and the increased fat metabolism secondary to a decreased carbohydrate intake.

Following the period of fluid shifts, the patient remains acutely ill. This period is characterized by anemia and malnutrition. *Anemia* develops from the loss of red blood cells. *Negative nitrogen balance* begins at the onset of the burn and is the result of tissue destruction, protein loss, and the stress response. It continues throughout the acute period and is secondary to continued loss of protein from the wound, from tissue catabolism resulting from immobility, and from decreased protein intake. *Hypovitaminosis* may also occur from the decreased intake of vitamins. Special attention to the nutritional needs of the patient is an integral part of the comprehensive care during this time. Increased metabolism from loss of water and heat from the wound, loss of fluid during diuresis, and catabolism during tissue breakdown lead to *weight loss*.

Rehabilitative stage

The rehabilitative stage begins when the burned area is reduced to less than 20% of the body surface. The person is now in an *anabolic phase*.

Prevention

Nurses can help prevent accidental burns by participating in health education programs that stress fire prevention and the consequences of fires such as burns, deformities, and death, and by promoting legislation that would control hazardous practices and make working and living environments safer. Community health nurses are in an unusually advantageous position to recognize unsafe practices in the home and to help families develop safe habits of living.

Approximately 80% of accidental burns occur in the home and primarily are caused by ignorance, carelessness, and curiosity of children. Infants and children are the most common victims of fires in and about the home. Young children should be supervised in their play and should never be left at home alone. Children should be taught at an early age about the hazards of fire such as

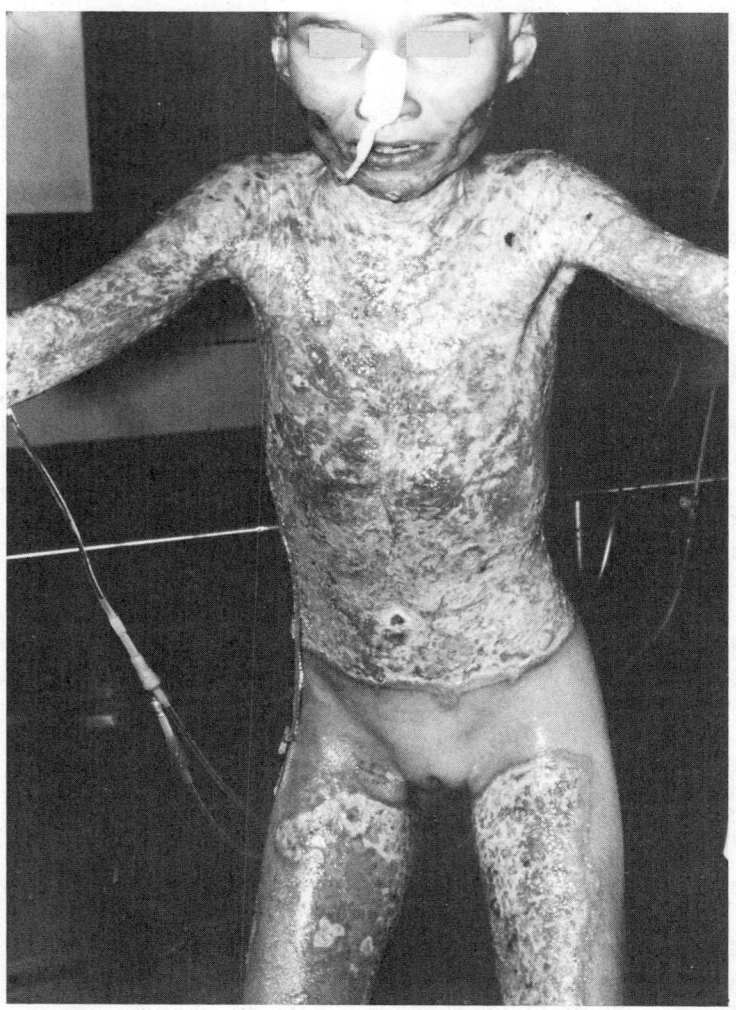

Fig. 70-4. Child with a 90% burn. She had been playing with matches while hiding in a closet. (Courtesy Burn Center, Cleveland Metropolitan General Hospital.)

playing with matches (Fig. 70-4). Parents must carefully check play areas for all fire hazards such as live extension wires, matches, and unprotected floor heaters and should remove them. Many pamphlets are available to parents that provide information on child proofing their home for safety. Serious burns to children often result from pot handles that project beyond the stove top or appliance cords within the reach of toddlers. A large number of children have been burned to death or permanently disabled or disfigured by fireworks. Legislation in many states now prohibits the sale of fireworks, but violations of the law and accidents still occur. Approximately 1000 serious burns occur every year from fireworks.

A high incidence of burn injuries affecting adults are related to accidents while cooking or smoking or otherwise using matches. Burns commonly occur when the person is distracted while cooking or falls asleep while smoking. Activities that persons were engaged in when they caught on fire in their homes are shown in Table 70-2.

Each year brings increased demand for careful inspection and regulation of places in which the ill and infirmed are housed. Aged persons frequently are housed in old and poorly equipped structures, and many of them have been burned to death. Nurses can bring necessary pressures to bear to ensure adequate protection and planned evacuation if a fire occurs. The American Burn Association suggests all health facilities conduct one mock evacuation drill each year. Attention is being focused on places where large numbers of people congregate. Laws require that doors in public buildings be hinged to swing outward, that draperies and decorations be fireproof, and that stairways with special fire doors be used in new apartment buildings and hotels. Smoke detectors and sprinkler systems are also required in new buildings and residential health care facilities. Nurses working in institutions need to encour-

TABLE 70-2. Activities of persons burned by fire*

Activity	Number	Percent
Playing with matches/lighter	175	11.3†
Smoking	152	10.0
Using matches/lighter	116	7.5
Fell asleep while smoking	100	6.4
Reaching across stove	86	5.5
Sleeping	77	5.0
Standing too close to stove	64	4.1
Leaning against stove	47	3.0

*From Flammable fabric investigations, Washington, D.C., 1973, Department of Health, Education, and Welfare, Food and Drug Administration, Bureau of Product Safety, FY66-FY72.
†Percent based on 1554 cases in which activity is known.

age and participate in fire prevention programs.

Rigid enforcement of laws requiring that industrial products be labeled when known to be flammable and that new products be tested carefully for their flammable qualities before being placed on the market is further evidence of government efforts to protect the public from accident by fire. Industry can be made safer by constant vigilance by management in cooperation with fire safety officers and health care professionals to identify hazards and implement a safety program. All chemicals should be labeled, and antidotes should be identified and available. A core of every work force should be versed in emergency treatment of all types of burns for the protection of every employee.

Recent statistics indicate a rise in the number of chemical injuries as a result of "homemade" solutions for cleaning and home remodeling.

Sunburn should be cautioned against, since even a relatively mild first-degree burn of a large part of the body can cause change of fluid distribution and kidney damage. Camp nurses should keep this in mind in their educational programs for children and camp counselors. There are many newer sunscreen products available that are very effective and should be used in times of exposure.

Intervention

Prehospitalization emergency care

The initial care for major burns is outlined in the box above at right.

If flame is involved and clothing is on fire, the victim's first reactions is to run, which only fans the flame. Rolling the burning person in a blanket on the ground to exclude oxygen, thereby putting out the fire, is one

---

INITIAL CARE FOR MAJOR BURNS

1. Extinguish flame.
2. Remove nonadherent *smoldering* clothing.
3. Establish patency of airway. Assess for inhalation burns (singed nasal hair, mouth burns, sooty cough, dyspnea). Give oxygen if available.
4. Assess and initiate treatment for injuries requiring immediate attention.
5. Remove tight-fitting jewelry or clothing.
6. Cover burn with moist sterile or clean cover.
7. Cover unburned areas with warm dry cover to prevent heat loss.
8. Transport victim to nearest medical facility.

of the best procedures. Any water source can be used to extinguish flames. The person whose clothing is aflame should never stand, since this increases the danger of inhalation burns in which heat and smoke are drawn into the lungs.

Once all flame is extinguished, it is important that the burning agent be removed and the wound cooled. Clothing and gross debris are carefully removed, avoiding the removal of any clothing that adheres to the burned area. Tepid water (or saline if available) is used in copious amounts until the wound is cool to the touch. Once the wound is cooled, the victim may be wrapped for transport to a medical facility.

Chemicals should be identified, and copious flushing with water is initiated. As much as 20 to 30 minutes of continuous flushing may be necessary to ensure complete removal of the destructive agent. Burns occurring about the eyes should also be lavaged with copious amounts of cool, clean water, and if the burn was caused by acids, the procedure should be repeated in 10 to 15 minutes.

Persons who are burned on the face and neck or those who have inhaled flame, steam, or smoke should be observed closely for signs of laryngeal edema and airway obstruction. Data indicating potential or existing airway burns include (1) singed nasal hair, (2) burns of the mouth or throat, (3) brassy-sounding or sooty cough, and (4) respiratory distress. Immediate arrangements should be made to transport these patients to a hospital or burn center if one is available. Often burns are more severe than they first appear to be. Thus all persons with burns, even if the burns appear to be superficial, should be seen by a physician. The hospital or burn center should be notified, so that preparations can be made for the arrival of the patient, since a well-prepared and well-equipped team of personnel needs to be assembled to care for the severely burned person.

According to the 1981 American Burn Association Directory, 185 hospitals in the United States reported the presence of a specialized burn care service. Of these 185 hospitals, only 148 reported that they had a special burn unit. These burn units are located throughout the United States and many of them are located in major medical centers in urban areas. The Association estimates that there are 70,000 annual acute inpatient burn admissions in the United States. Only about 21,500 (or 30%) of these patients are cared for in specialized units. The American Burn Association publishes a list of specialized burn care services every year.*

While awaiting transportation to a medical facility, the burned person be kept quiet and lying down. Exposed burned surfaces should be covered with sterile dressings or with the cleanest material available, such as clean sheets. These coverings may be soaked in cool water to ease the pain, reduce the edema, and prevent evaporation of body water. Ice should be avoided, because sudden vasoconstriction causes severe shifting of fluid. *Oils, salves, and ointments should not be used on burns,* since these materials hamper treatment. Pain in extensive burns is best controlled by gentle and minimal handling and by the application of dressings to exclude air from the burned skin surfaces. Deep, third-degree burns are usually painless, since nerve endings have been destroyed, and for the first few minutes the person may appear not too badly affected. A burn should never be underestimated. In most cases, however, first- and second-degree burns will accompany third-degree burns, causing discomfort to the person.

For obviously small burns, fluids may be given by mouth with caution. Large burns are accompanied by decreased peristalsis; therefore nothing should be given by mouth. Patients with large burns or smoke inhalation may vomit, and particular attention is given to preventing them from aspirating vomitus.

Comprehensive team approach

Comprehensive care of the burn patient can best be provided by a multidisciplinary team approach. This is a desirable method designed to meet the complex and varied needs of the patient. The nurse's role in the team is to coordinate the interactions of the various disciplines and to incorporate the team's suggestions and approaches into an effective plan of care. Because this type of care is most likely to be available in specialized burn units and centers, patients are frequently moved to these units when it is safe to transport them. Generally accepted criteria for admission to these specialized care

facilities include burns of the head, neck, and face; burns of the perineum or joints; burns that involve more than 25% of the body; and burns of children under age 2 years and adults over age 60 years. When such specialized care is not available, the nurse may be able to serve as a catalyst and suggest that as many disciplines as are available be actively involved in the care of the patient.

Inpatient assessment

On arrival at the hospital, the remaining clothes of the patient are removed and the patient's condition is assessed. Respiratory status is evaluated first and immediate treatment initiated as indicated. Vital signs are taken for baseline data and for identification of hypovolemic shock. *The patient should be weighed.* This measurement will be used to determine fluid therapy and to evaluate progress. Venous and arterial blood samples are taken to determine protein, electrolyte, red blood cell, pH, and blood gas levels.

The following five factors are used to determine the severity of the burn: (1) size of the burn; (2) depth of the burn injury; (3) age of the patient; (4) history of cardiac, pulmonary, renal, or hepatic disease, or trauma such as fracture or internal injuries sustained at the time of the burn; and (5) the part of the body involved.

For adults, the "rule of nines" is used (Fig. 70-5) in determining the size of the burn. Calculations are mod-

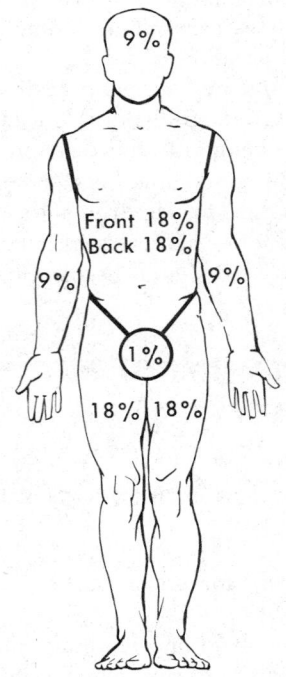

Fig. 70-5. "Rule of nines" is used to estimate amount of skin surface burned.

*American Burn Association: Joseph A. Moylan, M.D., Duke University Medical Center, Box 30, Durham, NC 27710.

ified for infants and children under 10 years of age because of their relatively larger head and smaller bodies. (See pediatric textbooks for these figures.)

The depth of the burn injury is summarized in Table 70-3.

Infants under 2 years of age and adults over 60 years of age have a higher mortality than persons in other age groups with a similar size injury.[45]

Immediate inpatient intervention

Rapid and efficient care can be provided by anticipation of patient needs and having an organized admission area to treat burns (see box below at left). If any respiratory distress is present, an airway should be es-

tablished. Prophylactic intubation should be initiated if any heat or smoke has been inhaled, or if the head, neck, or face is involved (Fig. 70-6). Inhalation injuries are best managed with controlled ventilation, because swelling of the upper airway can progress to obstruction. Endotracheal intubation is preferred over a tracheostomy, because edema of the respiratory passages frequently subsides within a few days and avoidance of surgical trauma is desired. Depending on the severity of symptoms, emergency treatment may include oxygen, suctioning, and postural drainage.

A nasogastric tube should be inserted to prevent gastric distention. A Foley catheter is also inserted so that there can be accurate monitoring of urinary output. A central venous line will be required to permit fluid replacement and monitoring of fluid volume. Morphine

TABLE 70-3. Factors used in determining depth of burn injury.

Degree	Depth	Sensation	Blisters	Color	Texture
First (minor)	Epidermis only	Painful	None	Increased redness	Normal
Second (partial thickness)	Involvement of epidermis and dermis	Very painful	Large, thick walled; usually will increase in size	If vesicles are ruptured, skin may be mottled in color but demonstrates capillary refill on pressure	Normal or somewhat firm
Third (full thickness)	Destruction of all layers of skin into subcutaneous tissue including fascia, muscle, and bone	Little or no pain	None or if present, thin walled; do not increase in size	Skin may be charred, white, brown, or red; does not demonstrate capillary refill	Firm and leathery

INITIAL TREATMENT OF MAJOR BURNS IN EMERGENCY ROOM

1. Establish an airway.

2. Initiate fluid therapy by intravenous catheters.

3. Insert indwelling catheter for hourly urine measurement.

4. Insert nasogastric tube to remove stomach contents, prevent aspiration, and provide fluids.

5. Insert central venous pressure (CVP) and pulmonary wedge pressure (PWP) catheters.

6. Manage pain by intravenous narcotics in small, frequent doses.

7. Weigh patient for baseline measurement.

8. Initially treat burn wounds.

9. Initiate tetanus prophylaxis.

10. Initiate protective isolation measures.

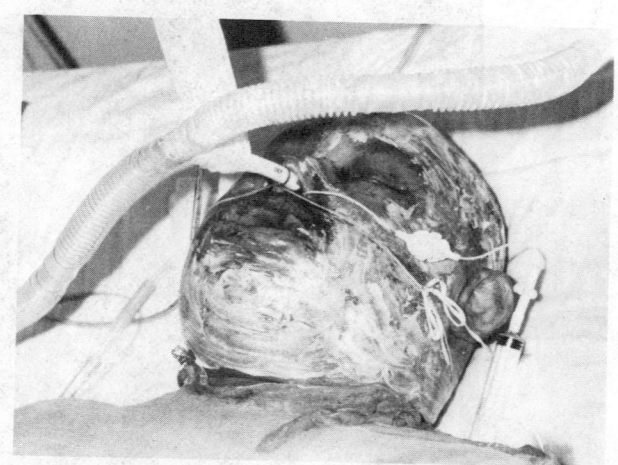

Fig. 70-6. Patient with severe edema 5 hours after burn occurred. Airway was managed with endotracheal intubation. Edema subsided, and patient was extubated 4 days after admission. (Courtesy Burn Center, Cleveland Metropolitan General Hospital.)

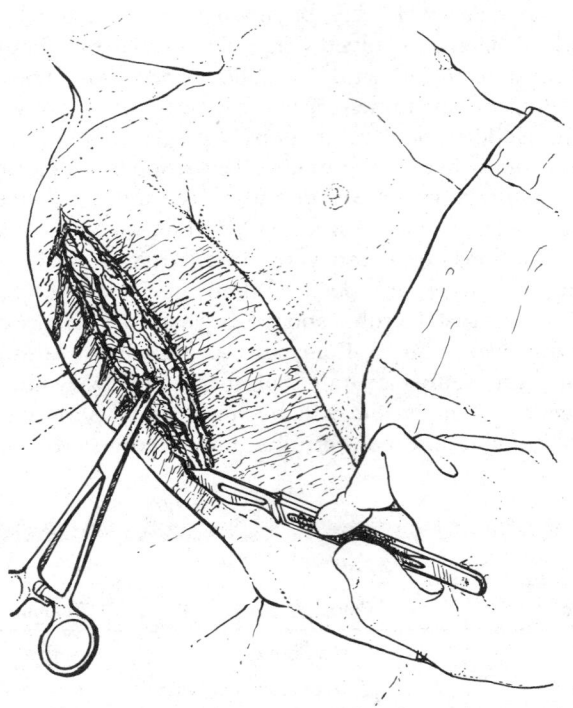

Fig. 70-7. Escharotomy surgically performed for circumferential burn of upper arm.

sulfate or meperidine hydrochloride is often given intravenously to the patient with an extensive burn. The intravenous route is used because of inadequate absorption at peripheral sites. Large doses of sedatives and analgesics are avoided because of the danger of respiratory depression and because they may mask other symptoms.

All debris and loose skin are removed from the burn wound, and the area is cleansed with a solution of 2 L normal saline, 16 oz hydrogen peroxide, and 1 tbsp Dreft detergent. Dressings with the selected topical preparation are applied. Tetanus prophylaxis is initiated. Tetanus toxoid is given to persons who have been immunized within 4 to 5 years; other persons are given a dose of tetanus immune globulin (human) (TIGH) and then an active tetanus immunization program is begun. Frequent observations of chest excursion in addition to respiratory rate are necessary to determine respiratory restriction. Pulses must be checked every 15 minutes to ensure uninterrupted vascular flow to all extremities. Particular caution is necessary with the presence of a circumferential burn. An *escharotomy* (linear incision of constricting eschar) may be necessary when constriction of circulation or respiration is evident (Figs. 70-7 and 70-8). *Eschar* (a crust formed on the burn wound) from a third-degree burns rapidly contracts, causing restriction to soft tissues, vessels, and underlying organs.

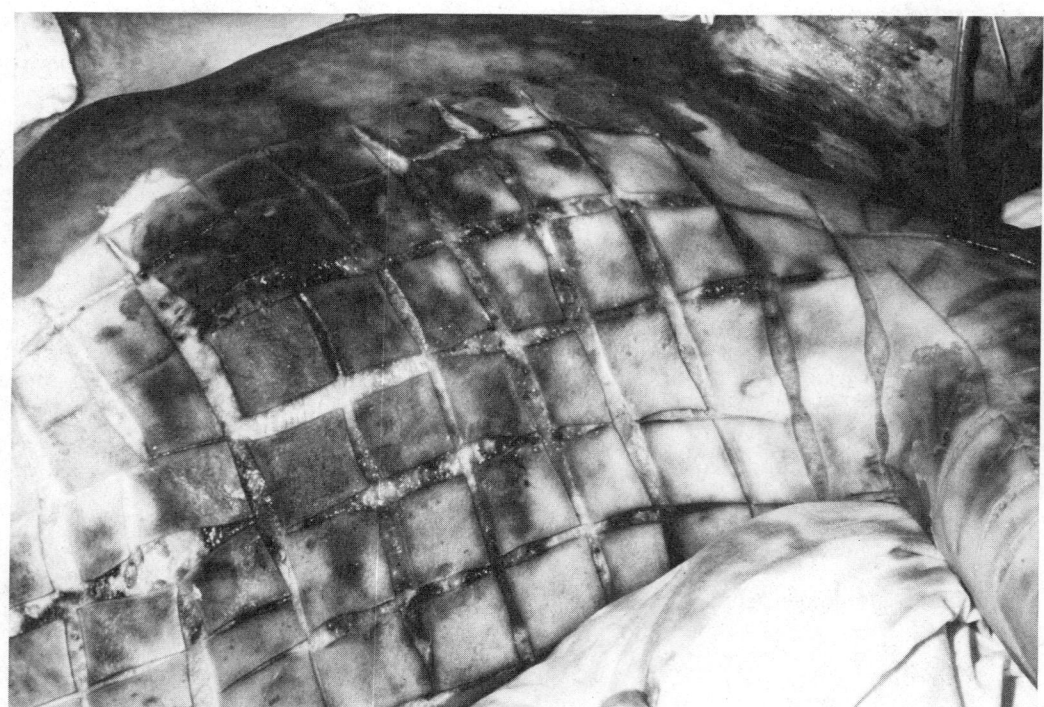

Fig. 70-8. Grid escharotomy used to alleviate circulatory and pulmonary constriction. (Courtesy Burn Center, Cleveland Metropolitan General Hospital.)

Replacement of body fluids

Replacement of fluids and electrolytes is an essential part of the treatment and is instituted as soon as the extent of the burn and the patient's condition have been determined. Ideally, fluid therapy is started within an hour following a severe burn. Insertion of a large-bore central venous line permits the rapid administration of fluids and electrolytes.

Three types of fluid are considered in calculating the needs of the patient: (1) colloids, including plasma and plasma expanders such as dextran; (2) electrolytes, such as physiologic solution of sodium chloride, Ringer's solution, Hartmann's solution, and Tyrode's solution; and (3) nonelectrolyte fluids, such as distilled water with 5% glucose. Medical authorities do not agree as to the proportion of colloid and electrolyte fluids needed. Several formulas are described in the medical literature to guide physicians in determining the type and amount of fluids to be administered, based on the patient's weight and age and the percentage of the body burned.[12, 16] The present trend is to administer balanced salt solutions (e.g., Ringer's), water, and plasma, and to use whole blood only if a large number of red cells are destroyed or if anemia develops.

Fluids administered during the first 48 hours are given to maintain circulating blood volume. Additional fluids and electrolytes are added to replace losses from vomiting or from nasogastric drainage. The amount of fluid replacement required during the first 48 hours is determined by assessment of several factors; these include urinary output, serum electrolyte levels, blood gas findings, central venous pressure, body weight, desire to maintain the hematocrit at slightly above normal levels, level of consciousness, and vital signs. Fluid needs for the first 24 hours are calculated from the time of the burn. Usually the patient receives *one half of the total amount in the first 8 hours,* one fourth in the second 8 hours, and one fourth in the third 8 hours. One half of the total amount given on the first day is given in the second 24 hours.

Patients complain of moderate to severe thirst. Aggressive oral hygiene may alleviate patient discomfort. If oral fluids are permitted, accurate recording of ingested fluids is important. Unlimited oral intake and failure to measure it may result in too much fluid in the circulating blood, resulting in water intoxication. A Swan-Ganz catheter may be inserted to monitor pulmonary arterial and capillary wedge pressure (p. 1056) in the severely burned patient for identification of hypovolemia or hypervolemia and to assist in evaluating fluid therapy.

The rate of urinary output is a reliable measure of determining the adequacy of fluid therapy during the first 48 hours. Hourly checking and measuring of urinary output are responsibility of the nurse. Usually, a retention catheter is inserted and drained into a calibrated container. The amount of urine is measured and recorded every hour. The care of the patient with an indwelling catheter is discussed on p. 1521. The urine should be observed for color and analyzed for a positive hematocrit level. The physician is notified if hematuria or a positive Hemastix reaction is present. A urine flow of 30 to 50 ml/hr is adequate for an adult. The urine flow should be at least 15 ml/hr for infants and 25 ml/hr for older children. *If the urinary output rises above or falls below these figures, the physician is notified immediately.* Fluid therapy will need to be adjusted accordingly. Lack of urinary output may indicate insufficient fluids or acute tubular necrosis. All efforts must be taken to provide sufficient fluid to protect vital organs.

After the first 48 to 72 hours, the urinary output is no longer a reliable guide to fluid needs, since water deprivation may occur even when the urinary output for adults is 1000 ml/day or more. Severely burned patients require a large fluid intake to compensate for the loss of fluid into the tissues and from the wound. Fluid needs then are determined by measuring serum electrolyte levels. Fluid replacement during the diuretic stage is based on individual assessment. Parenteral fluids may be discontinued if serum electrolyte levels return to normal. If dehydration occurs from the diuresis, fluid replacement therapy may be continued until blood volume is stabilized. The patient is observed closely for signs of water intoxication (p. 329) or pulmonary edema (p. 1135).

The hyperkalemia of the first stage can change to hypokalemia within a very few hours during diuresis or as the potassium moves back into cells. The serum levels of potassium are monitored closely, and potassium is replaced parenterally when hypokalemia results. Compromised renal function significantly complicates potassium management, since potassium is excreted by the kidney.

Prevention of infection

A major principle in the care of the burned person is the prevention of infection. Local and systemic infections (septicemia) are the most common complications of burns and are a major cause of death, particularly in burns covering more than 25% of the body. Autogenous sources are the primary sources of infection initially, although the wound is highly susceptible to infection from exogenous sources. The person's own bacteria become trapped under the eschar, and aggressive wound management is necessary. Daily tubbings and mechanical debridement must be done to remove wound exudate and debris from the wound. Washing and friction removes build-up of debris and supports healthy tissue regeneration. Topical agents are more effective in preventing local infection because impairment of the vasculature in the burn area prevents systemic antibiotics from reaching the wound. Antibiotics may be given prophylactically, or they may be withheld until an infection does occur.

The organisms that usually infect burn wounds are *Staphylococcus aureus, Pseudomonas aeruginosa,* and the coliform bacilli. In the past few years there has been a high incidence of fungal infections resulting from the use of broad-spectrum antibiotics. *Candida albicans,* which normally is found in the gastrointestinal tract, accounts for the majority of the fungal infections. Cultures of the patient's nose, throat, wound, and unburned skin, and a punch biopsy specimen may be taken on admission and at biweekly intervals to determine the bacteria present and their sensitivity to antibiotics.

All persons who approach the patient should wear gowns and masks to prevent the introduction of their organisms into the wound. Persons with upper respiratory tract infections should not be permitted near the patient. Surgical aseptic technique and sterile gloves are used when applying dressings. Hydrotherapy tanks used for aggressive cleansing of burn wounds need particular attention to prevent infection of burn wounds when the tanks are used by different patients.

The extent of local cleansing depends on the severity of the burn and the judgment of the physician. Detergents or antiseptic preparations, such as povidone-iodine (Betadine), are effective cleansing agents. A rather extensive debridement may be carried out at the initial cleansing. The wounds are then treated by the open or closed methods as determined by the physician. Hair on skin areas adjacent to burn tissue is shaved as necessary.

Care of severely burned persons in special burn units can contribute to decreased infection because the environment is specifically geared to infection control. If the patient is cared for on a general hospital unit, a private room is essential, and all equipment needed by the patient should remain in the room. Reverse isolation precautions are implemented (p. 374).

Methods of treatment of burned areas

There are several methods of treating the burned area, depending on the location of the burn, its size and depth, the facilities available, and the patient's response to the therapy. One method may be started and then replaced with another during the course of treatment. Only those commonly used today are described.

Open, or exposure, method. The exposure method of treatment was accidentally discovered to be effective in 1888 when, during a serious steamboat fire on the Mississippi River, those in attendance ran out of bandages and later observed that the neglected persons fared

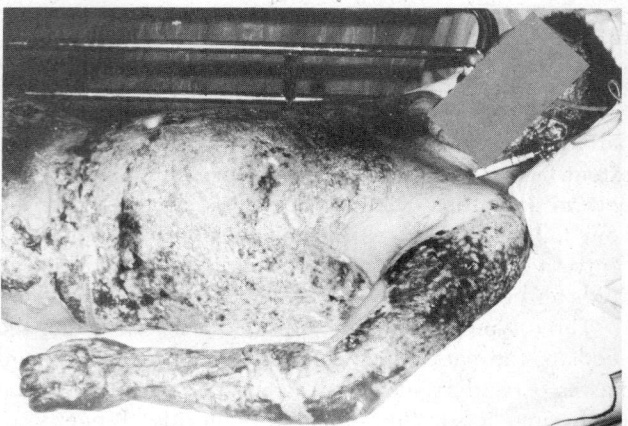

Fig. 70-9. Severely burned man being treated by open method. (Courtesy Burn Center, Cleveland Metropolitan General Hospital.)

better than those who received more intensive local treatment.[47] Today, the exposure method is used most often in the treatment of burns involving the face, neck, perineum, and broad areas of the trunk. The burned area is cleansed and exposed to the air (Fig. 70-9). The exudate of a partial-thickness burn dries in 48 to 72 hours and forms a hard crust that protects the wound. Epithelialization occurs beneath this crust and may be complete in 14 to 21 days. The crust then falls off spontaneously, leaving a healed, unscarred surface. The dead skin of a full-thickness burn is dehydrated and converted to an eschar (black, leathery dead tissue covering) in 48 to 72 hours. Loose eschar may be gradually removed through the use of whirlpool baths or debridement (Fig. 70-10). Uninfected eschar acts as a protective covering. The danger of infection exists as bacteria proliferate beneath the eschar. Spontaneous separation, produced by bacterial action, occurs unless surgical debridement is performed first.

Isolation technique is essential when the exposure method is used. The nurse caring for the patient should wear a sterile gown and mask, and sterile linen may be used on the patient's bed. Infants may need to have their hands restrained to prevent them from picking off crusts. Until the wounds are healed, children's toys need to be sterilized to prevent them from causing infection.

A cradle may be used on the bed since no clothing or bedclothes are allowed directly over burned areas. If the burn is extensive, a CircOlectric bed draped with a sheet is an ideal way to care for the patient (Fig. 70-11). The burned person can be kept from embarrassing exposure by wearing a halter and loin cloth. Lights or heat lamps may be used with caution to provide warmth, and with these the patient has maximal freedom to move about and perform exercises for the prevention of contracture and the improvement of circulation.

Patients having exposure treatment complain of pain

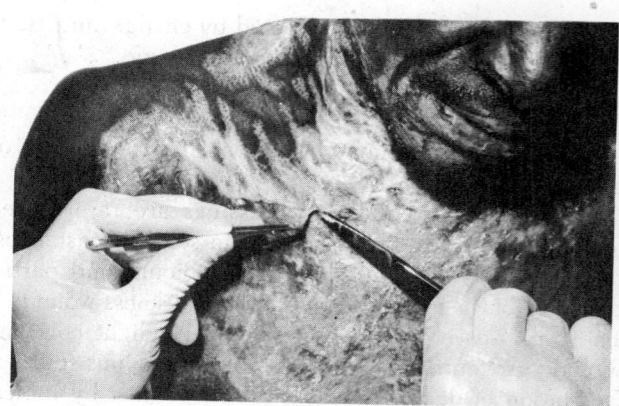

Fig. 70-10. Nurse's role in burn centers may include debridement of patient's eschar. (Courtesy Burn Unit, Cook County Hospital, Chicago.)

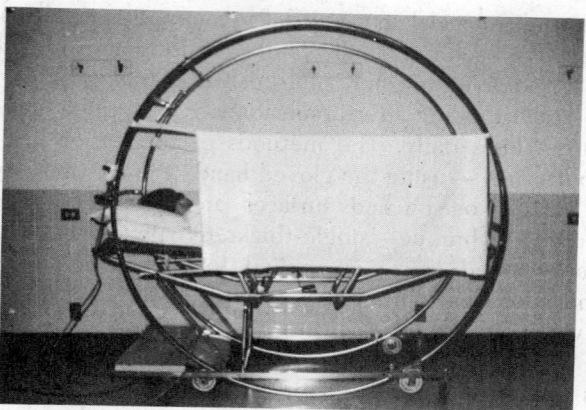

Fig. 70-11. Another exposure method of treating burns. A sheet is draped over CircOlectric bed so that burned areas are not touched. (Courtesy Burn Unit, Cook County Hospital, Chicago.)

and chilling. Pain may be controlled by administering morphine sulfate, meperidine hydrochloride (Demerol), or salicylates as ordered. Discomfort can be decreased if drafts are avoided and the temperature of the room is kept at 24.4° C (85° F). Patients lose more heat from burned surfaces than from the normal skin surfaces, since the vascular bed that normally contracts and retains heat in the body is lost. The humidity of the room also should be controlled. A humidity of 40% to 50% usually is considered satisfactory. Portable electric humidifiers and dehumidifers can be used to achieve and maintain this level.

Closed method. In the closed method of burn treatment, the wounds are washed; and dressings are changed at least once each day, or in some instances, once each shift. Commonly, the dressing consists of gauze impregnated with topical ointments and a gauze wrap. When a dressing is in place, nursing observation should include checking for signs of impaired circulation, such as numbness, pain, and tingling, and being alert for signs of infection (odor on dressings and elevated temperature and pulse rate).

Hydrotherapy. Hydrotherapy is a valuable adjunct to therapy and should be used when available in the care of the burned person. It is a more painless method for removal of dressings, aids in the cleansing of the wound by removal of loose eschar and other debris, and facilitates range-of-motion exercises with minimal energy expenditure and discomfort. Tubbing is usually performed once or twice daily for 20 to 30 minutes and is started after the patient's vital signs and fluid balance have stabilized. Tubbings are limited to no more than 30 minutes to prevent unneccessary exposure and chilling. The patient must receive careful personal care before being placed in the tub so that fecal contamination is minimal. Those in attendance should wear gowns and gloves until the patient's wounds are healed. The pa-

tient is never left unattended during the procedure because fainting and injury may occur.

Topical applications. The application of topical agents to the burned area has helped to decrease infection and hasten healing. There are a number of agents currently being used, and each has certain advantages and disadvantages. The ideal agent has not yet been developed.

MAFENIDE. Mafenide (Sulfamylon) is a white cream containing sulfonamide. It diffuses through devascularized areas and is an effective bacteriostatic agent against many gram-negative as well as gram-positive microorganisms. The cream is applied with a sterile gloved hand in a thin layer just enough to cover the burn completely. The wound is usually left open to the air. Washing of the wound and reapplication of the cream are necessary when the wound is no longer covered with ointment. Metabolic acidosis may result when impaired renal function is present because mafenide inhibits carbonic anhydrase. Side effects include pain and allergic manifestations. Treatment is usually continued until healing occurs or the wound is ready for grafting.

SILVER SULFADIAZINE. Silver sulfadiazine (Silvadene) is a white cream with bactericidal action against many gram-negative and gram-positive bacteria, as well as against *Candida albicans*. It does not result in metabolic acidosis, but some persons develop sensitivity reactions. The patient is observed for side effects common with sulfonamide drugs. The wound may develop a slimy, grayish appearance simulating an infection, despite negative cultures.[20] The ointment is applied in a thin layer with a sterile gloved hand to cover the burn after wound cleansings. The wound may be covered with a dressing or left exposed.

POVIDONE-IODINE. Povidone-iodine (Betadine) ointment is a reddish brown germicidal preparation of 10% povidone-iodine (1% available iodine) with broad-spectrum microbicidal action. It kills gram-positive and gram-negative bacteria, fungi, yeasts, viruses, and protozoa. It is nonirritating and nonsensitizing and permits air to reach the site after application. It is applied at least three times daily. The methods of application are (1) "buttering"—using the gloved hand, a ¼-in. thick layer is spread on burned surfaces and (2) the modified closed technique—single-thickness povidone-iodine–impregnated gauze is applied to the affected areas, and additional ointment is spread on top of the gauze layer.

SILVER NITRATE TREATMENT. Although silver nitrate is being used less often than in the past, some physicians still prescribe it. In this treatment, thick gauze dressings are saturated with a 0.5% solution of silver nitrate, and the dressings are kept wet so that the solution remains in constant contact with burned surfaces. The purpose of these dressings is to retain moisture and heat and to reduce evaporation. The proponents of this method of treatment believe that it reduces mortality, lessens pain, eliminates odors, and has a bacteriostatic effect.[16] The dressings are removed every 12 to 24 hours, and the patient may be placed in a bath of salt solution with the temperature carefully maintained at the same level as that of the body. When skin grafts are applied, silver nitrate dressings are placed over the graft and donor sites on the first postoperative day. Because the silver nitrate solution is hypotonic, electrolytes are lost into the wound. Therefore throughout treatment, frequent determinations of blood sodium levels are necessary, and sodium that is lost may need to be replaced.

Isolation technique is not required when the burn is treated with silver nitrate dressings, but clean dressings and sterile gloves and instruments are used. Because everything that comes in contact with the silver nitrate solution is stained black, the nurse wears a gown and gloves when applying the solution to protect skin, nails, and clothing. Although linen can be specially treated to remove stains, great care must be taken to prevent splashing the solution on the furniture, walls, and floors.

OTHER TOPICAL APPLICATIONS. *Neomycin* is a bactericidal agent that causes miscoding in the messenger RNA of bacterial cells. It is effective against most organisms but has serious toxic effects and can cause irreversible hearing loss or kidney failure when used over a long period of time.

In addition to ointments, two other solutions are used frequently in burn care; these are sodium chloride solution and a mixture of equal parts of acetic acid, peroxide, and normal saline solution, commonly referred to as "thirds." *Normal* or balanced *saline* solutions are applied to clean granulation tissue or to new grafts to maintain moisture or are used with fine mesh gauze to provide for slight debridement. The *"thirds" solution* has limited antimicrobial action and is most effective

against organisms that are affected by changes in pH. It is also used to clean dirty granulation tissue.

Wound coverings

The burn wound may be covered with dressings or grafts.

Dressings. Large, bulky dressings are rarely used today for large-scale burns except in selected instances, because infection control is more difficult, and partial thickness burns may develop into full-thickness wounds.[12] The purposes of applying some type of light covering include prevention of infection from exogenous sources, facilitation of debridement, maximal contact by topical agents, and prevention of fluid evaporation with loss of body heat. The type of dressing that is usually applied consists of a single layer of fine mesh gauze held in place by a wrapping of a coarse gauze such as Kerlix.

The dressing change may be a painful procedure, and if analgesics are required, they should be given 30 minutes before the procedure for maximal effectiveness. Most dressing changes are performed after tubbing, because this facilitates dressing removal and is less painful. Additional debridement of eschar and dead tissue may be performed before the new dressing is applied.

Wet dressings may be used such as with silver nitrate or normal saline applications. A single layer of fine mesh gauze is usually placed over the wound, covered with thick gauze pads to maintain moisture, and held in place with a gauze wrapping. The dressings must be kept wet. Plastic wrap should *not* be used to cover the dressings, since this prevents any fluid evaporation, causes increased heat at the wound site and results in patient discomfort and increased tissue destruction and infection.

Skin grafts. Skin grafts are applied to cover the burn wound and speed healing, to prevent contractures, and to shorten convalescence. Successful grafting reduces the patient's vulnerability to infection and prevents the loss of body heat and water vapor from the open wound or eschar. Most skin grafts are applied between the fifth and twenty-first day after the initial injury, depending on the depth and extent of the burn and the condition of the base. Small areas of third-degree burns such as those that occur on the dorsum of the hand may be excised and skin grafted during the first 24 to 48 hours to hasten healing and to help restore function more quickly. The wound is prepared for the graft as described on p. 1802.

Split-thickness grafts usually are used (Fig. 70-12). These grafts include the upper layer of the skin and part of the under layer but are not taken so deep as to prevent regeneration of the skin at the site from which they are taken (donor site). They grow as normal skin on the burned areas (recipient sites). These grafts are removed with a dermatome from almost any unburned

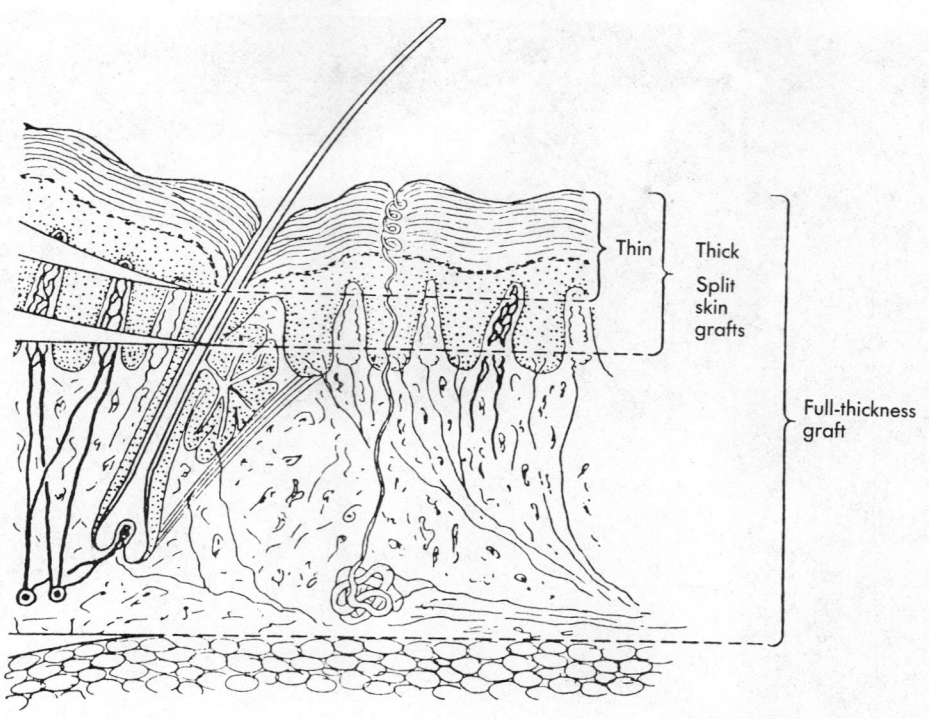

Fig. 70-12. Levels of the skin involved in thin and thick split skin grafts, and full-thickness grafts.

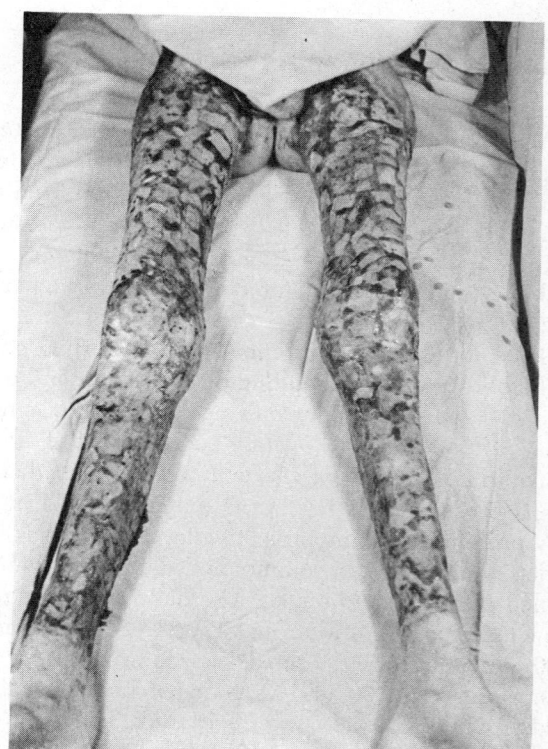

Fig. 70-13. Postage stamp grafts have been cut from split-thickness graft and have been used to partially cover large burned areas on lower limbs. (From Artz, C.P., and Reiss, E.: The treatment of burns, Philadelphia, 1957, W.B. Saunders Co.)

part of the body. They may be removed in strips or small squares (postage stamps) (Fig. 70-13). Another type of split-thickness graft is the *mesh graft*, which is used when few donor sites are available and there are large areas of burned body surface to be covered. The graft is removed with a dermatome and then meshed with a special instrument. The meshing of the graft makes it more distensible, and thus it can be used to cover wider areas of the body surface (Fig. 70-14). Grafts may be laid on the burn wounds and held in place with dressings or sutured into place and left exposed. Pressure dressings may be applied to secure the graft, provide even compression, and act as a splint. If the loss of skin

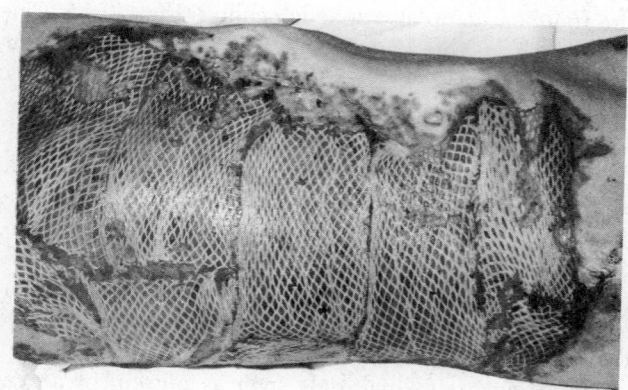

Fig. 70-14. Mesh graft covering full-thickness burn. (Courtesy Burn Unit, Cook County Hospital, Chicago.)

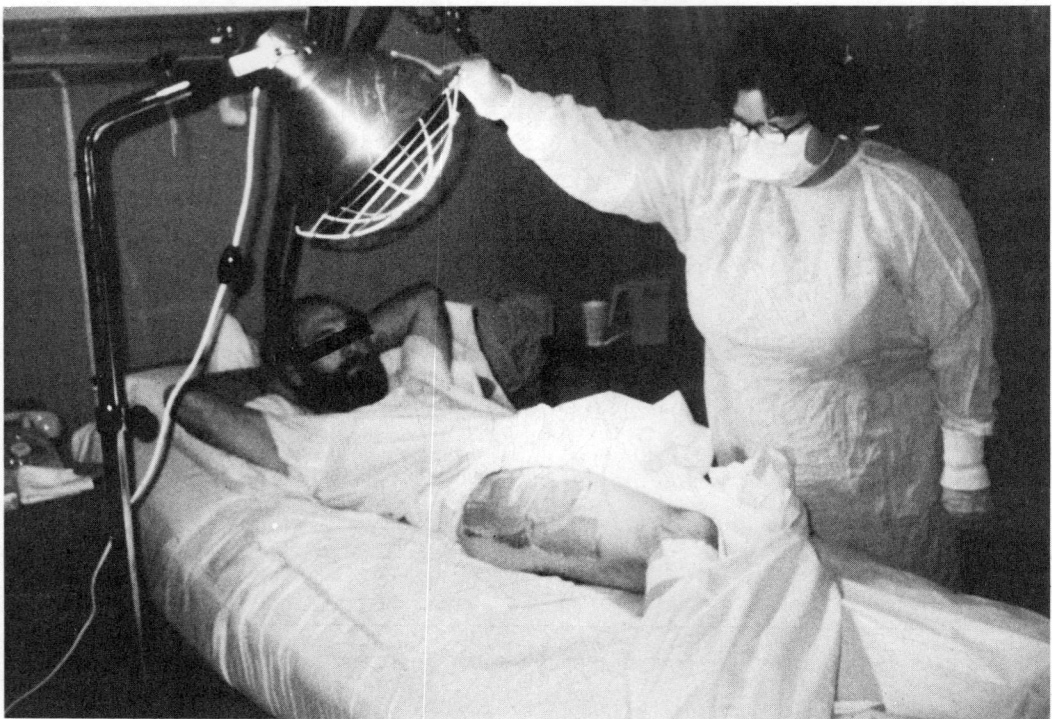

Fig. 70-15. Heat lamp used to dry donor site to promote epithelialization from deep layers and prevent infection. (Courtesy Burn Center, Cleveland Metropolitan General Hospital.)

is so great that life is threatened, the skin of other persons (that of recently deceased persons or stored postmortem skin) is taken to cover burned surfaces (*homografts*). The use of homografts helps to limit infection and loss of water, electrolytes, and protein and helps to reduce pain in the burn wound. Homografts may survive 4 to 5 weeks before being rejected, but they usually are needed only about 10 days if applied to cover a large granulating wound.[45]

The donor site, which presents an oozing, painful surface, may be covered with sterile gauze and a pressure dressing or it may be covered with a fine mesh gauze and left exposed to the air. Exposing the donor site to a heat lamp also speeds healing (Fig. 70-15). The drainage from the wound dries and serves as a protective covering. The wound usually heals within 2 weeks. Many patients complain of severe pain in the donor site, and the nurse should not hesitate to give medications that are ordered for pain. The pain should subside within a day or two. Sometimes an odor develops from the dead tissue at either the donor site or the recipient site, which is distressing to the patient and should be reported to the physician. If infection has developed, antibiotics may be administered and the wound treated with wet dressings.

Heterografts of materials such as pigskin or a synthetic substitute are being used commonly to provide temporary protection to wounds, reduce pain, promote granulation, and reduce surface bacterial count.

Provision of nutritional requirements

Metabolism is increased following moderate to severe burns as a result of stress, fluid loss, fever, infection, hypercatabolism, and immobility. Uninjured cells have increased metabolic activity initially as a result of decreased oxygenation because of hypovolemia. The catabolic phase may last for 30 to 40 days in persons with extensive injury.[12]

The protein and caloric needs of the burned person are highly variable, depending on the extent and depth of injury and on the person's age and preburn nutritional state. The daily *protein* requirement is greater than normal because of the negative nitrogen balance that is present following burns (p. 1813). The normal daily protein requirement is 0.8 g/kg of body weight for adults, whereas the recommended daily intake for the burned person is 2 to 4 g/kg. The daily *caloric* requirement increases from a normal 1700 to 3000 calories to 3500 to 5000 calories. The caloric requirement for children varies from 90 to 100 cal/kg of body weight for children under 3 years of age to 70 cal/kg of body weight for children between 4 and 12 years of age.

Supplemental vitamins are needed. Vitamin C promotes healing (p. 443), and the daily requirement in the burn patient increases from a normal of 45 mg to 1 to 2 g. The B-complex vitamins are necessary for the metabolism of the increased protein and carbohydrate intake. Sodium chloride, potassium, and calcium preparations also may be administed intravenously or orally, depending on the extent of the burned area and serum electrolyte levels. Iron preparations are required for persons who become anemic.

Weight loss and gain are monitored for evaluation of nutritional status of the severely burned person. Weight gain occurs initially because of the fluid retention. Following diuresis, there is a marked loss of weight caused by loss of fluid and negative nitrogen balance. The weight curve will level out at a point below the preburn weight, and weight gain does not begin until the wounds are nearly all grafted.[12]

The person with large-scale burns may develop paralytic ileus because of the neuroendocrine response to stress, or may have nausea and vomiting to such an extent that nutrition must be provided entirely by the parenteral route. Intravenous fluids are given during the hypovolemic stage (p. 1812). When fluid balance is achieved, efforts are directed to meet the increased nutritional requirements. If the person is unable to eat the quantities of necessary nutrients, total parenteral nutrition (TPN) (p. 349) or tube feedings may be necessary. If nausea is present, a chilled solution containing 3 to 4 g (1½ tsp) of table salt and 1.5 to 2 g (½ tsp) of sodium bicarbonate in 1 L (1 qt) of water flavored with lemon juice (Haldane's solution) can often be retained while supplying needed electrolytes. Carbonated beverages are also an acceptable means of supplying some necessary electrolytes as well as sugar. Salty solutions such as meat broths often are given to help replace sodium chloride that is lost into the tissues and in wound exudate, but broths or fruit juices that contain potassium are withheld for 48 hours or until the serum potassium levels go down.

If the patient is able to eat without assistance, appetite may improve. It is important that painful and disagreeable changes of dressings and other treatments be timed so that they do not immediately precede meals.

High-protein powdered milk preparations are valuable in increasing the amount of protein taken and often seem to leave the patient with less of a feeling of oversatiation than may result from large servings of meats that are often high in fat.

The diet is advanced as quickly as possible to a regular one, but because of the patient's poor appetite, the utmost imagination and ingenuity on the part of the dietitian and the nurse are needed to motivate the patient to eat the food necessary to meet nutritional requirements. Sometimes relatives are helpful in suggesting favorite foods. Milkshakes supply large amounts of nourishment. They are also valuable because very ill patients can take fluids more easily than they can chew and swallow solid foods.

Bulk foods and fruit juices must be stressed in the diet of the severely burned patient because they aid in elimination. Fecal impaction is a common problem for burn patients. Bulk-forming laxatives such as preparations of the psyllium seed (Metamucil) may be given, or a fecal softener such as dioctyl sodium sulfosuccinate (Colace) may be ordered.

Prevention of limitations of mobility

Contractures are among the most serious long-term complications of burns. Two major types of contractures occur—those caused by muscle and joint stiffening and those occurring after skin grafting. Many patients must undergo painful reconstructive surgery that would not have been necessary if those in attendance had been alert to the prevention of contractures. A large responsibility for the prevention of contractures rests with the nurse, who is with the patient more than anyone else. Nursing care should be planned so that the patient's position is changed regularly during the day and night. Early skin grafting prevents many contractures by mobilizing the patient sometimes months earlier than would otherwise be possible.

Burned patients often have severe pain as healing progresses. They are anemic, debilitated, and very often in a state of depression. The patient must be helped to maintain range of joint motion and thus prevent scars from healing in positions that will result in deformity. It is important that patients understand why ambulation or motion is necessary even though it may be painful. Constant encouragement can be provided by setting short-term achievable goals. Since normal skin and normal tissues grow while scar tissue shrinks, children are more likely to develop deformities than adults, and what begins as a minor deformity in childhood may become a major one with increased growth.

For a definite interval of time each day, patients with burns should lie prone and also flat on their backs with no pillow or elevation of the head of the bed. This can be accomplished more easily if the patient is placed on a Stryker frame, a Foster bed, or a CircOlectric bed. These beds facilitate the use of the bedpan and urinal, permit change of position with a minimum of handling and permit larger skin surfaces to remain free from body pressure than is possible when the patient lies in bed. These special beds are particularly useful when both the back and front of the trunk, thighs, and legs have been burned. The beds allow turning of the patient with a minimum of handling and thus help decrease pain.

Prolonged rest in semi-Fowler's position or with the pillow pushing the head foward must be avoided. Many patients like this position because it enables them to see about the room better. The bed can often be turned so that the patient can look about without having to assume positions that may lead to the formation of contractures. It is often advisable to change the bedside table from one side of the bed to the other at intervals. Mirrors help these patients keep in better touch with their environment, provided that they are able to cope with their appearance.

If burns have been sustained about the neck, chin, and face, the patient should always lie in a position of hyperextension of the neck for most of each day. A pillow may be placed under the shoulders and the bed lowered to a level position. Facial exercises are encouraged to prevent scars from tightening as they form. Chewing gum and blowing up balloons provide exercise that helps to prevent facial contractures.

Burns of the hand can easily result in contractures. Differences of opinion exist about methods of positioning that best preserve function and prevent contractures, therefore consultation with the physiatrist (rehabilitation specialist) and physician is recommended. Burns on the dorsal surfaces of the hand are frequently positioned in a flexed position of function, whereas the hand with burns of the palmar surface may be positioned in hyperextension. Total hand burns are splinted as for dorsal burns.[12] Various types of splints (p. 954) may be used. Some physicians prefer to use the open method of treatment, providing for frequent exercise to prevent contractures.

Exercises for prevention and correction of contractures are begun as soon as the patient's vital signs are stable. Supervision by a physical therapist is desirable. When burns are completely covered (by healing or by graft), exercises may be performed more easily in an occupational therapy or physical therapy department where the patient also may benefit from a change in environment. In the department of physical medicine, exercises often are performed in water. A Hubbard tank may be used for this purpose. The occupational therapist may help the patient to improve range of motion in a satisfying and efficient fashion by teaching functional activities of daily living and crafts suitable for particular needs such as typing, weaving, or a host of other activities. The nurse must know what the patient is being taught by the physical therapist and the occupational therapist so that progress can be continued on the nursing unit.

The patient who is not hospitalized and the one who returns home early because of skin grafting needs instruction in how to prevent contractures from developing. Contracture clinics are available for burn patients and are associated with some burn centers. If community health nursing services are available, a physical therapist or occupational therapist may be called on to assist the patient at home. If this service is not available, the nurse in the hospital or the community health agency may have to take responsibility for teaching the patient how to prevent contractures from developing.

Emotional responses to severe burns

The emotional impact of severe burns is enormous and reality based. During the first few days, the patient is too ill to fully comprehend what has happened. Patients fear that they may not survive, and the fear of death is a major concern. Other fears include pain and suffering, disfigurement, prolonged hospitalization, and disruption of life-style. Patients who are severely burned usually are exhausted and often demoralized by the pain, treatment, and frequent dressing changes. Many defense mechanisms may be evident as the patient attempts to control pain. Care givers need to be supportive, although they may find the patient's behavior unacceptable. Support and understanding will allow the patient to develop more acceptable means of coping with the stressful situation. Diazepam (Valium) may be helpful in decreasing anxiety and providing muscle relaxation. The pain can be minimized by clear explanations that gain the patient's cooperation, planned use of analgesics, careful sterile technique, gentle handling, and permitting the patient to participate in the treatment whenever possible. Depending on the age of the patient and the extent of the pain, distracting activities may be helpful.

After the initial period, the long healing period begins, accompanied by the realization of endless implications for the future. Patients' reactions are determined by their personality makeup, by their degree of total adjustment to life, and by the extent and location of the burns. Burns on the face make adjustment particularly difficult. All kinds of fears arise to harrass the patient. "Will my spouse still care for me? Can I ever let my children see me?" To the adolescent, the thought of being different or conspicuous may be unbearable. Fears about not being taken back on the job often haunt the wage earner who is badly burned. If possible, the patient should see facial burns only after being prepared for the experience. Support and understanding will be needed in order for the patient to cope with what will be seen in the mirror. The patient will exhibit readiness by asking to look in the mirror. Interaction with other burned patients who are further along in their healing process may help the patient feel that recovery is possible. In some instances, the recovery is incredible, and although differences in skin pigmentation remain, the redness that accompanies burns and newly healed skin often fades considerably within a few months. Pigmentation problems are more acute for persons with brown or black skin. Their skin may be a different shade, freckled, or whitish in color.

Clinical observation indicates that the burned individual experiences concern about changes in appearance and its effect on others. Since the skin, peripheral blood vessels, and lymph vessels are damaged, the

DISCHARGE INSTRUCTIONS FOR BURN PATIENT*

We on the burn team are happy to see that you are able to go home. To ensure you the speediest possible recovery, it is important that you are able to care for yourself and recognize problems that may interfere with your complete recovery.

If any of the following occur, please call the hospital and ask for the burn clinic. The nurse will be able to assist you.

1. Healed area breaking open. Cover with clean dressing.
2. Formation of blisters.
3. Signs of infection:
   a. Fever, temperature over 37.2° C (99° F).
   b. Redness, pain, swelling, hardness, or warmth in or around wound or any other part of body.
   c. Increased or foul-smelling drainage from wound.
4. Problems with your Ace bandages or Jobst garment such as improper fit, formation of blisters, or opening of healed area underneath.

Your first clinic appointment will be on _____. If a family member can come with you they can register for you and you may go to the burn clinic waiting room.

Skin care for healed burn

These are your guidelines for your daily skin care of a healed burn. When you do your skin care, this is the time to look at the involved areas and note if there are any changes that need to be reported.

1. Wash healed area every day with solution of 2 tbsp Dreft (or Ivory Snow) and water.
2. Wash gently with washcloth to remove dead skin.
3. Rinse skin well after washing.
4. Dry thoroughly.
5. Apply Nivea lightly twice a day and more frequently if the skin is dry and flaked.
6. Do not put Nivea on open areas.
7. You can purchase Nivea at your local drugstore.

Care for burn wound

These are your guidelines for the care of your burn wound. When you do your care, this is the time to look at the involved areas and note if there are any changes that need to be reported.

Procedure for burn wound care

1. Wash hands.
2. Remove dressing and dispose of in paper bag or wrap in newspaper.
3. Wash hands.
4. Wash open area with gauze using solution of Dreft (or Ivory Snow) and water. Add 1 tbsp Dreft to a basin of water; 2 tbsp Dreft, if you use the bathtub. Use a clean towel and washcloth with each dressing change.
5. Rinse skin well.
6. Wash hands.

7. Apply dressing as described below.
8. Wear gloves. Wash basin or bathtub with a disinfectant such as Lysol.
9. Wash hands.

Care of clothing

When you are discharged, you may find that healed burn areas are sensitive to harsh detergents, fabric softeners, and clothing dyes. If you are sensitive, we suggest the following:

1. Launder new clothing before use by machine or hand with Dreft or Ivory Snow.
2. Rinse clothes twice.
3. Do not use fabric softeners.
4. If you have open burns or a healed area that opens, wash all clothes separately from other family members.
5. Scarlet red ointment will permanently stain clothing.
6. If dyes used in clothing cause irritation, wear white articles.

Ace bandages

You have been taught to put on your own Ace bandages while in the hospital; but if you do have a problem with this, please notify the burn clinic. It is also important that you know how to care for them and understand problems that occur.

1. If they are too loose, they will be ineffective and must be rewrapped.
2. If they are too tight, they will cause discomfort, numbness, tingling, and puffiness and must be rewrapped.
3. They must be worn for a long period of time, probably 6-12 mo to be effective, so please do not stop wearing them until your doctor tells you.
4. To care for your Ace bandages:
   a. Hand wash with Dreft or Ivory Snow in cold water.
   b. Towel dry.
   c. Lay flat or place over rod or clothesline.
   d. Do not use clothespins.

Jobst garment

You have been taught how to put on your Jobst garment while in the hospital; but if you have a problem with this, please notify the burn clinic. It also is important that you know how to care for it and understand problems that can occur.

1. If it is too loose, it will be ineffective and you will require a new garment.
2. If it is too tight, it will cause discomfort, numbness, and tingling. Do not wear it if this occurs, but notify the burn clinic as soon as possible.
3. To care for your Jobst garment:
   a. Hand wash with Dreft or Ivory Snow in cold water.
   b. Towel dry.
   c. Lay flat or place over rod or clothesline.
   d. Do not use clothespins.

*Courtesy Cleveland Metropolitan General Hospital Department of Nursing Service.

burned patient's sense of body boundary probably is altered. Patients undergoing debridement following loosening of burn eschar describe sensations of having their skin torn away from them. It has been asserted that persons who perceive their body boundaries as being well defined tend to be more confident and have a higher goal and task completion drives. (See Chapter 28.) It is therefore possible that those who lose a part of that sense of definiteness will tend to take a more languid approach to life with less successful interactions with others.[51]

The patient should have an opportunity to talk about any problems and fears. Some patients may discuss these with the nurse when they cannot express them to relatives, and the nurse must be prepared to listen and help the individual accept necessary changes in life style. (See reference 51 for further discussion.) Almost every burned patient and the family need the help of the social worker. The nurse should recognize this need and initiate the referral. Visiting hours can be used to talk with relatives who may be able to give information that will clarify the patient's needs and resources. This time also provides opportunity for the nurse to help relatives and friends accept their loved one's change in appearance and to help them plan for the return of the loved one to the community.

Special teaching needs

Patients have a great need for education so that they may take increasing responsibility for their own care. They need to learn (1) care of the healed burn wound, (2) nutritional needs, (3) prevention of injury, (4) recognition of signs and symptoms of complications, and (5) methods of coping with resocialization. Complete and comprehensive instructions followed by return demonstrations contribute to learning the necessary skills to be independent and prudent in self-care activities after discharge (see box, p. 1827). Patients should not be discharged from the hospital until they can care for themselves physically and are prepared to meet the stresses involved in returning to their former living patterns. Accentuation of strengths of the individual and focus on effective coping mechanisms will overshadow the limitations the person may be experiencing.

Rehabilitation

Complete recovery and rehabilitation of the severely burned patient constitute a long and costly process. Many industries have compensation insurance to cover part of the cost, and the patient should be encouraged to discuss financial problems with the physician and with the social worker if one is available. Patients under 21 years of age are eligible for care financed in part by the Office of Child Development (formerly the Children's Bureau) through its aid to states for their programs for crippled children. This care will cover surgical procedures and care, special rehabilitative services, and social service.

Patients who have been burned should have medical checkups at regular intervals indefinitely, and they should be advised to report any unusual change in the burn scar at once. There is a fairly high frequency of malignant degeneration of scar tissue following burns. This is particularly true when the burn is caused by electricity or by x-rays.

Outcome criteria for the person with burns

1. Following the acute phase, the person will:
   a. Be in a state of homeostasis (normal blood volume, normal serum electrolytes, vital signs at preburn levels).
   b. Be in a state of positive nitrogen balance.
   c. Be free of infection.
   d. Have intact integumentation.
   e. Be free of contractures.
   f. Be mobile and independent in self-care.
2. At discharge, the person or significant others can:
   a. Demonstrate care of the burn wound.
   b. State name, dosage, frequency, desired effect, and side effects of topical or systemic antibiotics.
   c. Demonstrate range-of-motion exercises to prevent contractures.
   d. Plan a diet high in protein, calories, vitamins, and minerals.
   e. Describe injuries that can occur to the healing wound or graft and methods of prevention of injury.
   f. Describe plans for return to former activities (work, social activities).
   g. Describe plans for follow-up health care.
      (1) State signs and symptoms requiring intervention (wound infection, loss of weight, contractures, changes in scar tissue).
      (2) State plans for continued medical care until wounds are fully healed.

REFERENCES AND SELECTED READINGS
Contemporary

1. *Andereasen, N.J., et al.: Management of emotional reactions in seriously burned adults, N. Engl. J. Med. **286**:65-69, 1972.
2. Artz, C.P., and Yarbourgh, D.R., III: Major body burn, J.A.M.A. **223**:1355-1357, 1973.
3. Bell, J.G.: Bitsy was so little. . .and her problems so big, Nurs. '77 **7**(6):35-37, 1977.
4. Bowden, M.L., and Feller, I.: Family reaction to a severe burn, Am. J. Nurs. **73**:316-319, 1973.
5. Busby, H.C.: Nursing management of the acute burn patient and nursing management of optimal burn recovery, J. Contin. Educ. Nurs. **10**:16-30, 1979.
6. Campbell, L.: Special behavioral problems of the burned child, Am. J. Nurs. **76**:220-224, 1976.
7. Castillo, J.: Treatment of thermal injuries, Surg. Clin. North Am. **53**:627-637, 1973.
8. *deTornay, R., and Doswell, W.M.: Nursing decisions: experiences in clinical problem solving, series 2, no. 7: Kare A., a patient with burns, RN **40**(5):59-68, 1977.
9. Dyer, C.: Burn care in the emergent period, J. Emerg. Nurs. **6**:9-16, 1980.
10. *Emig, E., and Lloyd, J.R.: How to get burned children home sooner, RN **40**(7):37-39, 1977.
11. Feist, C.: Reprieve, Nurs. '79 **9**(10):144, 1979.
12. *Feller, I., and Archanbeault, C.: Nursing the burned patient, Ann Arbor, Mich., 1973, Institute for Burn Medicine Press.
13. Finlayson, J.: Emergent care of the burn patient, Crit. Care Update **7**:18-19, 22-23, 1980.
14. Gaston, S.F., and Schumann, L.L.: Burn wound management, Crit. Care Update **7**:5-17, 1980.
15. *Hadley, R.D.: Knowledge, understanding: keys to burn patient care, Am. Nurse **9**:9-10, 1977.
16. Hardy, J.D., editor: Textbook of surgery: principles and practice, ed. 5, Philadelphia, 1977, J.B. Lippincott Co.
17. Hartford, C.E.: The early treatment of burns, Nurs. Clin. North Am. **8**:447-455, 1973.
18. Iveson-Iveson, J.: Burn—a continuing battle, Nurs. Mirror **151**:31-32, 1980.
19. Jacoby, F.G.: Individualized burn wound dressings, Nurs. '77 **7**(6):62-63, 1977.
20. *Jacoby, F.G.: Nursing care of the patient with burns, ed. 2, St. Louis, 1976, The C.V. Mosby Co.
21. Jones, C.A., and Feller, I.: Burns: the home stretch . . . rehabilitation, Nurs. '77 **7**(12):54-57, 1977.
22. *Jones, C.S., and Feller, I.: Burns: what to do during the first crucial hours, Nurs. '77 **7**(3):22-31, 1977.
23. Kavanagh, C.: The severely burned child: a portrait of need and giving, Matern. Child Nurs. **2**:223, 1977.
24. Kenner, C., and Manning, S.: Emergency care of the burn patient, Crit. Care Update **7**:24-27, 30-33, 1980.
25. Kessler, R.L.: Nursing care study: care of a scalded child, Nurs. Times **75**:619-624, 1979.
26. Kinzie, Y., and Lau, C.: What to do for the severely burned, RN **43**(4):46-51, 104-110, 1980.

27. *Moncrief, J.A.: Burns, N. Engl. J. Med. **288**:444-454, 1973.
28. Nelson, W.E., et al.: Textbook of pediatrics, ed. 11, Philadelphia, 1980, W.B. Saunders Co.
29. Nursing grand rounds: realistic goals don't mean failure, Nurs. '79 **9**(5):54-59, 1979.
30. Polk, H., and Stone, H.H., editors: Contemporary burn management, Boston, 1971, Little, Brown & Co.
31. *Quinly, S., et al.: Identity problems and the adaptation of nurses to severely burned children, Am. J. Psychiatry **128**:58-63, 1971.
32. Reyes, M., et al.: Burns. In Meltzer, L.E., Abdellah, F.G., and Kutchell, J.R., editors: Concepts and practices of intensive care for nurse specialists, ed. 2, Bowie, Md., 1976, The Charles Press.
33. *Rogenes, P.R., and Moylan, J.: Restoring fluid balance in the patient with severe burns, Am. J. Nurs. **76**:1952-1957, 1976.
34. Sabiston, D.C., editor: Davis-Christopher textbook of surgery, ed. 11, Philadelphia, 1977, W.B. Saunders Co.
35. *Savedra, M.: Coping with pain: strategies of severely burned children, Matern. Child Nurs. J. **5**:197-203, 1976.
36. Schumann, L., and Gaston, S.: Common sense guide to topical burn therapy, Nurs. '79 **9**(3):34-39, 1979.
37. *Septic shock in a burn patient, nursing grand rounds, Nurs. '76 **6**:39-43, Jan. 1976.
38. Severely burned patients: anticipating their emotional needs, nursing grand rounds, Nurs. '80 **10**(9):47-50, 1980.
39. Silver, H.K., et al.: Handbook of pediatrics, ed. 12, Los Altos, Calif., 1977, Lange Medical Publications.
40. Singletary, Y.: More than skin deep, J. Psychiatr. Nurs. **15**:7-13, 1977.
41. *Tichy, A.M.: Stress of hospitalization: perspectives of burn care, Commun. Nurs. Res. **9**:23-39, 1977.
42. *Wagner, M.: Emergency care of the burned patient, Am. J. Nurs. **77**:1788-1791, 1977.
43. *Williams, B.P.: The burned patient's need for teaching, Nurs. Clin. North Am. **6**:615-639, 1971.
44. Williams, S.R.: Nutrition and diet therapy, ed. 4, St. Louis, 1981, The C.V. Mosby Co.

Classic

45. Artz, C.P., and Moncrief, J.A.: The treatment of burns, ed. 2, Philadelphia, 1969, W.B. Saunders.
46. Boswick, J.A., and Stone, N.H.: Methods and materials in managing the severely burned patient, Surg. Clin. North Am. **48**:177-190, 1968.
47. Cockshott, W.P.: The history of the treatment of burns, Surg. Gynecol. Obstet. **102**:116-124, 1956.
48. Fox, C.L., Rappole, B.W., and Stanford, W.: Control of pseudomonas infection in burns by silver sulfadiazine, Surg. Gynecol. Obstet. **128**:1021-1026, 1969.
49. Korloff, B.: Social and economic consequences of deep burns. In Wallace, A.B., and Wilkinson, A.W., editors: Second international congress on research in burns, Edinburgh, 1966, E. & S. Livingstone, Ltd.
50. Smith, C.A., editor: Profiles of burn management, Miami, 1969, Industrial Medicine Publishing Co., Inc. (Reprinted from Industrial Medicine and Surgery, Aug.-Dec., 1968.)
51. Williams, B.P.: The problems and life-style of a severely burned man. In Bergersen, B., et al., editors: Current concepts in clinical nursing, vol. 2, St. Louis, 1969, The C.V. Mosby Co.

*References preceded by an asterisk are particularly well suited for student reading.

CHAPTER 71

PROBLEMS OF THE INTEGUMENT

BARBARA C. LONG

Skin problems may result from various causes, such as parasitic infestations, fungal, bacterial, or viral infections, reactions to substances encountered externally or taken internally, or new growths. Many of the skin manifestations have no known cause, while others are hereditary. This chapter provides an overview of the more common dermatologic disorders.

Parasitic infestations

Pediculosis

Etiology

Pediculi (lice) are most often found among individuals who have poor personal hygiene habits. Lice are not restricted to low-income urban populations, however, and many children get head lice from their classmates or from people on crowded buses. Control and treatment of pediculosis (lice infestation) in middle- or upper-income populations can be hampered by refusal of parents to admit that their children have pediculosis. The incidence of pediculosis is 36 times higher in whites than in blacks and occurs mostly among children.[24]

Lice obtain their nutrition by sucking blood from the skin. They leave their eggs on the skin surface attached to hair shafts, and this results in the transference from person to person.

There are three types of lice that infest humans: the head louse, the body louse, and the pubic louse. The head louse (Pediculosis capitis) attaches itself to the hair shaft, laying about eight eggs a day. The eggs, or nits, are firmly attached to the hair or threads of clothing. They may be viewed with a hand lens and appear as grayish, glistening oval bodies. The head louse is usually confined to the scalp and beard.

The body louse (Pediculosis corporis) resides chiefly in the seams of clothing around the neck, waist, and thighs. The bite causes minute hemorrhagic points and severe itching. Transmission is by direct contact or by way of clothing, bedding, and towels.

The pubic louse (Phthirus pubis) differs slightly from the head and body louse. It resembles a tiny crab, having clawlike pincers that attach firmly to the pubic hair. Nits are visible in the pubic hair. Phthirus pubis is transmitted by sexual contact, bed clothing, towels, and occasionally toilet seats.

Clinical picture

Diagnosis is made by finding nits or lice on a person who also has pinpoint erythema, raised macules, and a complaint of pruritus. Intense itching is caused from the bite of the insect with contamination from saliva, head parts, and feces of the lice. Scratching may lead to further trauma with the possibility of secondary infection and enlarged cervical lymph nodes.

Intervention

Treatment is topical, and the effective agents are gamma (γ-) benzene hexachloride (Kwell) or benzyl benzoate. Kwell comes in shampoo, lotion, or cream. There may be a need to repeat treatment in severe cases. Treatment of head lice consists of shampooing vigorously with the medication. A fine-toothed comb may be used to remove remaining nits. The hair may be shampooed with regular shampoo in 24 hours. Treatment of body lice consists of an initial cleansing bath followed by application of a thin layer of lotion or cream. After 24 hours the person bathes and redresses in clean clothes. If eyelashes are infested, nits are removed and petroleum jelly is applied to smother the lice. A local application of 0.25% physostigmine (Eserine) may also be used.

Clothing, linen, and towels should be washed in very hot water or dry cleaned. Garments that have been stored for 1 month will not be infested.

Scabies

Epidemiology

Scabies is highly prevalent during periods of overcrowding, such as that seen in Europe during World War II or in other war-torn areas. During the 1950s and 1960s, the incidence of scabies decreased, but during the 1970s there was a rise in the incidence of scabies worldwide. The reason for the current pandemic is unknown and is thought to be multifactorial, including poverty, sexual promiscuity, increased worldwide travel, and ecologic changes.[47]

Etiology

Scabies is caused by the female itch mite *(Sarcoptes scabiei)*, which penetrates the stratum corneum and burrows into the skin. Within several hours after skin penetration, the itch mite lays enormous eggs and deposits fecal material. The larvae mature in 10 days and move to the skin surface where the female is impregnated; then the cycle repeats itself. The incubation period varies, but there is often a long period of time before symptoms are noted. Delayed hypersensitivity is thought to be a major factor.[47] Scabies is usually transmitted with prolonged contact, so that it is frequently observed among several members of a family. Young adults may transmit it by sleeping together as opposed to a brief sexual contact. Scabies occurs among all age groups and socioeconomic levels.

Clinical picture

The *classic* symptoms of scabies include lesions that resemble wavy, brownish, threadlike lines occurring most frequently on the hands (especially the interdigital webs), flexor surface of the wrists, posterior inner surface of the elbows, anterior axillary folds, nipples in the female, belt line, gluteal creases, and male genitalia. The head and neck are rarely involved. Pruritus may be severe, especially at night. Secondary infections with excoriations and pustules may result from scratching.

In the recent pandemic, the classic symptoms have been less frequently seen and the lesions may imitate different dermatoses. Distribution of lesions has also been atypical.[47] Scabies can be suspected if several family members have similar symptoms.

Diagnosis is made by identifying the itch mite. Skin scrapings are made by placing mineral oil on a recently developed lesion, scraping the lesion vigorously with a blade, and transferring the oil and scraped material onto a glass slide for microscopic examination.

PATIENT DIRECTIONS FOR SCABICIDE TREATMENT

1. Take a prolonged tub bath, scrubbing affected areas well with soap.
2. Apply a *thin* layer of scabicide lotion over the *entire body below the head*, paying special attention to fingers and toes. Lotion is left on the skin for 24 hours.
3. Shower or bathe thoroughly after 24 hours to remove the medication.
4. Machine wash clothing and bed linens, and then iron them or dry them in an automatic dryer. No special precautions are needed for other objects since the mites do not live for long away from the host.

Intervention

Scabies that is left untreated may result in severe disabling skin lesions with infections. Treatment with a scabicide is effective if the patient follow directions carefully (see box above). The most commonly used scabicide is lindane (γ-benzene hexachloride) as found in Kwell. One application is usually sufficient. Eurax (Crotamiton) is more irritating, especially over severely inflamed skin. Two 24-hour applications of eurax are necessary, with bathing at the end of the first and second 24-hour periods. Sulfur ointment is the treatment that has been used for centuries, but it is messier to use since it stains and has an odor. Three 24-hour applications are necessary when sulfur is used.

Symptoms do not disappear immediately after treatment, and the patient may need reassurance that further scabicide treatment is not usually necessary and that contagion does not occur after treatment. A soothing lotion such as a hydrocortisone preparation may provide symptomatic relief after therapy. Oral antipruritic agents, antihistamines, or salicylates may help to decrease the pruritus.

Bedbugs

The bite of *Cimex lectularius* produces purpuric spots often occurring in clusters of four or more. Itching and burning are experienced over the ankle and lower leg, the most frequent site of the bite. Bedbugs often can be detected if the bed covers are thrown back at night in a lighted room; they can be seen most frequently at the foot of the bed. They may also be found along the seams of mattresses and in cracks in the bed frame. Spraying with benzene hexachloride over the mattress, floor, and walls is usually sufficient for control of bedbugs.

Outcome criteria for the person with a parasitic infestation

The person or significant others can:
1. Describe preventive hygiene measures.
2. Explain method of transmission of the parasite.
3. Describe care of clothing and linens (washing in hot water or dry cleaning).
4. Explain medication and treatment program: desired effect of drug, areas of application, number of applications.

Fungal infections

Fungi are larger and more complex than bacteria. They may be unicellular, such as yeasts, or multicellular, such as molds. Many types are pathogenic to humans, causing common skin disorders or serious systemic diseases such as blastomycosis. Certain types of fungi cause few symptoms, while others produce inflammatory or hypersensitivity reactions.

Candidiasis

Etiology

Candida albicans, a yeastlike fungus, normally inhabits the gastrointestinal tract, mouth, and vagina but not usually the skin. Candidiasis (moniliasis), the inflammation associated with the organism's overgrowth on the skin, is caused by the toxins that are released. Some predisposing factors causing an overgrowth of *Candida albicans* are pregnancy, use of birth control pills, poor nutrition, antibiotic therapy, diabetes mellitus, other endocrine diseases, and immunosuppressed conditions. Yeast thrives in a warm, moist environment such as the perineum and intertriginous areas.

Clinical picture

Thrush is candidiasis of the mucous membrane. The lesions are white spots like milk curd on the buccal mucosa and may extend down the esophagus. Vaginal thrush causes intense itching with a cheesy vaginal discharge. Skin lesions appear as pruritic, eroded, moist, inflamed areas with vesicles and pustules. Diagnosis of candidiasis at any site is made by clinical appearance and microscopic examination.

Intervention

Treatment is aimed at the precipitating factors. Other measures include keeping the skin dry to avoid maceration, wearing loose, absorbent clothing, and using topical medications such as powders that help to keep the skin dry. Nystatin (Mycostatin), an antibiotic available in tablets, powder, or vaginal suppositories, and amphotericin are very effective against yeast infections.

Dermatophytoses

There are several different types of dermatophytoses (tinea), or superficial fungal infections of the skin and its appendages. The most common types are tinea capitis, tinea corporis, tinea cruris, and tinea pedis.

Tinea capitis

Tinea capitis, inappropriately called ringworm of the scalp, has a worldwide distribution, primarily among prepubertal children. It can be caused either by the species of *Microsporum* or by *Trichophyton fungi*. The most common type in the United States is *Microsporum audouini*. The infection is transmitted readily, especially in crowded conditions where poor hygiene exists, although many children show a high resistance. Minor scalp trauma facilitates implantation of the spores; hence the infection can be spread by contaminated barber's instruments, combs, or sharp brushes.

The characteristic lesion is round, with erythema, a slight scaling, and some pustules appearing at the edge of the lesion (Fig. 71-1, *A*). Hair loss occurs, with the hair shaft broken off at skin level. The hair loss is only temporary, since the lesions usually heal without scarring. Although tinea capitis is usually noninflammatory, a painful inflammatory condition called a *kerion* may develop. Infected hairs placed under Wood's light will fluoresce blue-green.

Intervention. Griseofulvin is an effective antifungal agent in the treatment of all the dermatophytoses. The adult dose for tinea capitis is 500 mg orally, and absorption is enhanced when the medication is administered after a high-fat meal. Four to six weeks are usually necessary before the infection is resolved.

The scalp should be shampooed at least twice a week. Cutting the hair short facilitates shampooing but may pose psychologic trauma for some children and is then best left at an acceptable length. A mild antifungal agent, such as tolnaftate (1%) or haloprogin, may be applied topically twice daily. If inflammation occurs, the scalp is shampooed daily.

Tinea corporis and tinea cruris

Tinea corporis is a dermatophytic infection of nonhairy parts of the body, commonly seen in children living in hot humid climates. Typical lesions appear flat with an erythematous scaling border and clearing center (Fig. 71-1, *B*). Tinea cruris, commonly referred to as "jock itch," occurs in warm moist intertriginous areas of the groin. It occurs frequently in men, especially those

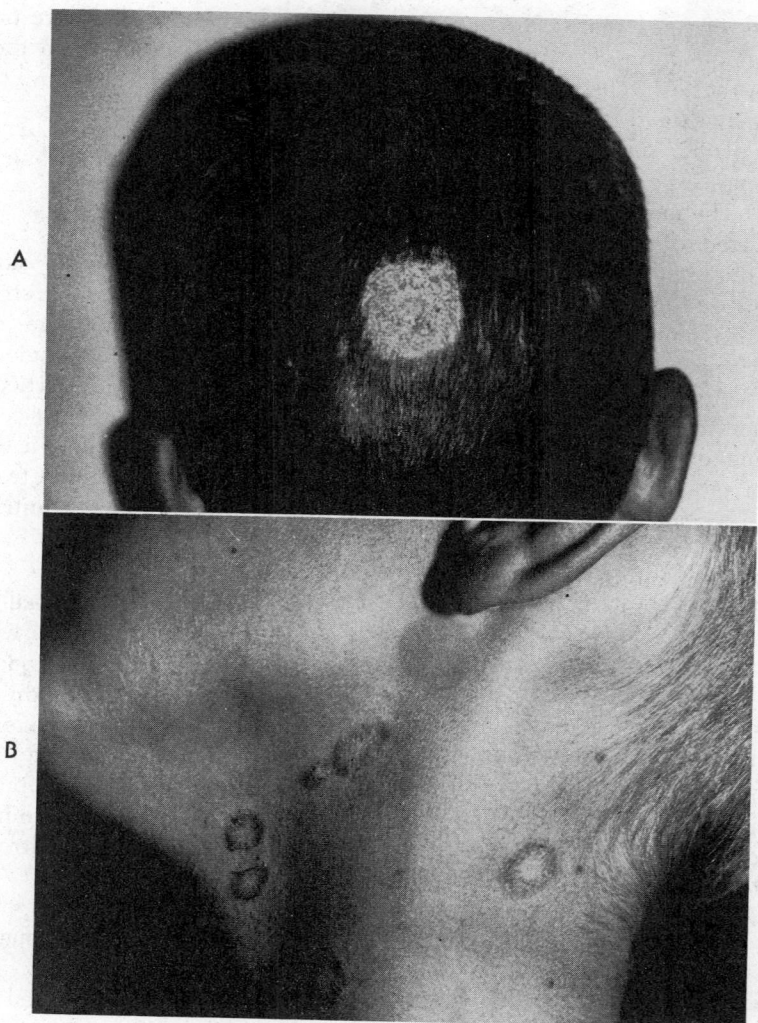

Fig. 71-1. A, Tinea capitis. **B,** Tinea corporis. (From Stewart, W.D., Danto, J.L., and Maddin, S.: Dermatology: diagnosis and treatment of cutaneous disorders, ed. 4, St. Louis, 1978, The C.V. Mosby Co.)

who have tinea pedis and those who frequently wear athletic supporters or tight shorts, but it is being seen more frequently in women who wear tight pantyhose or slacks. The lesions are bilateral and extend outward from the groin along the inner thigh. The color ranges from brown to red, scaling is absent, and pruritus is usually present.

Intervention. Griseofulvin, 500 mg given over a 2- to 4-week period, is usually effective. Topical application of haloprogin or tolnaftate may hasten healing. Loose pants should be worn by susceptible persons.

Tinea pedis

The most common dermatophytosis is tinea pedis, or athlete's foot. There are many misconceptions about prevention and treatment of athlete's foot. It is rarely seen in children or women but is widespread among young men, especially those wearing shoes in hot climates. It is often confused with other foot eruptions such as simple intertrigo (chronic bacterial infection of the intertriginous areas of the toes), contact dermatitis, or psoriasis. Walking barefoot in gymnasiums or around swimming pools will not necessarily lead to a tinea infection, but susceptible persons will acquire it regardless of their activities. Preventive actions commonly taken, such as prophylactic foot baths in public places, are ineffective. Wearing white socks does not affect the course of the infection.[41] Factors that may lessen infection include wearing sandal-type shoes or going barefoot (to decrease tissue moisture), and using good foot hygiene that includes washing the feet frequently and drying well between the toes.

There are several forms of tinea pedis, the most common being the intertriginous form. The fungus involvement usually begins in the toe webs, especially in the fourth interspace, and may extend to the undersurface of the toes or onto the plantar surface. The person may be asymptomatic or may experience itching and burning in the affected area. The nails may become discolored, thickened, or distorted (onychomycosis).

Intervention. The daily dose of griseofulvin for tinea pedis is usually 1.0 g given over 4 to 8 weeks, but treatment may extend to almost 4 months if the nails are involved. The person with tinea pedis needs to carry out meticulous foot hygiene. After drying the toes thoroughly, a light dusting of antifungal powder is applied to promote dryness. Caking of the powder is to be avoided. Socks should be of an absorbent material such as cotton and may have to be changed more than once daily to promote dryness. If marked inflammation is present, excessive foot activity should be restricted and foot soaks with Burow's solution may be helpful.

Outcome criteria for the person with a fungal infection

The person or significant others can:
1. Describe drug name, dosage, route, desired effect, frequency, and duration of treatment.
2. Describe proper foot care, avoidance of moisture and heat, use of own toilet articles, and wearing of loose clothing.
3. Describe plans for medical follow-up for severe infections.

Bacterial infections

Skin infections may result from loss of skin integrity or from altered host resistance. Most bacteria that normally inhabit the skin are nonpathogenic. Pathogenic bacteria that penetrate the outer skin layer may cause a superficial skin infection such as impetigo or superficial folliculitis, or they may penetrate deeper causing a deep folliculitis or a furuncle.

General principles of treatment for bacterial skin infections include cleansing the skin well and applying a topical antibiotic. The skin is cleansed with soap and water or with hexachlorophene. Water or saline compresses may be used to dry the horny layer of the skin or apply heat. Topical antibiotics commonly used include the hydroxyquinilones such as Vioform; neomycin, bacitracin, or polymyxin (Polysporin) either alone or in combination; and gentamicin or erythromycin. Systemic antibiotics are used only when systemic signs

such as fever and malaise are present, when the infection is widespread, or when there is an epidemic, especially among children.[41]

Impetigo

Etiology

Impetigo is a common skin infection caused by staphylococci or β-hemolytic streptococci. Although impetigo may occur at any age, children are most often affected. It is highly contagious among newborns or young infants but is not particularly contagious among older children or adults.[41] It occurs more commonly in the summer or early fall. Factors that promote development of impetigo include tropical climates, uncleanliness, poor hygiene, poor nutrition, and poor health.

Clinical picture

Impetigo begins as a small thin-walled vesicle that ruptures easily and leaves a weeping denuded spot. It becomes pustular and dries to form a honey-colored crust that appears stuck on the skin (Fig. 71-2). The process, which is superficial, may extend below the crust. Impetigo is usually confined to the face but may occur elsewhere. If untreated, impetigo may last for several weeks with new lesions forming. Glomerulonephritis is a serious complication of untreated impetigo.

Intervention

Treatment consists of maintaining cleanliness and applying topical antibiotics. The crusts must be removed and the lesions washed gently two to three times daily to prevent further crust formation. Warm soaks or saline compresses may be necessary to soften crusts that adhere firmly. Topical antibiotics are rubbed in thoroughly at least three times daily. Systemic antibiotics are given only if specifically indicated.

Family or health care providers should wash their hands thoroughly with a bacteriostatic soap after contact.

Folliculitis

Bacterial infections of the hair follicle may be superficial in the epidermis around the hair follicle or deep in the tissue surrounding both the lower and upper portions of the hair follicle. *Superficial folliculitis* is usually caused by a staphylococcus organism, but occasionally it is caused by other bacteria, both gram negative and gram positive. The infection may occur secondary to drainage from other infected lesions. Predisposing factors include uncleanliness, maceration, exposure to oils and solvent, traction of hair by tar therapy, or occlusion therapy. Treatment of superficial folliculitis

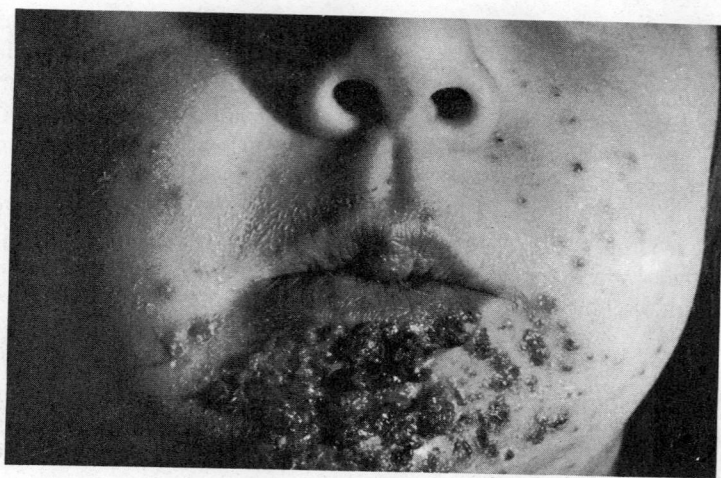

Fig. 71-2. Impetigo contagiosa. (From Stewart, W.D., Danto, J.L., and Maddin, S.: Dermatology: diagnosis and treatment of cutaneous disorders, ed. 4, St. Louis, 1978, The C.V. Mosby Co.)

includes cleansing with soap and water and application of topical antibiotics.

Deep folliculitis produces a more severe inflammatory response. *Sycosis barbae* (barber's itch) is a deep folliculitis of the beard. The hairs do not fall out or break, such as occurs with tinea barbae. *Hordeolum* (stye) is a deep folliculitis of the cilia of the eyelids. There is usually swelling of the surrounding eyelid with crusting along the edge of the eyelid. Warm compresses are applied to encourage resolution. Topical antibiotics such as Neosporin hasten healing.

Furuncles and carbuncles

Furuncles (boils) are a deep folliculitis that originate either from a superficial folliculitis or as a deep nodule around the hair follicle. *Furunculosis* is the appearance of several furuncles. An infection that involves several surrounding hair follicles is termed a *carbuncle*.

Furuncles are likely to occur on the face, neck, forearms, groin, and legs, whereas carbuncles are usually limited to the nape of the neck and the back. Both occur most often in obese, poorly nourished, fatigued, or otherwise susceptible persons whose hygiene may be poor, in debilitated elderly people, and in persons who have inadequately treated diabetes mellitus.

Clinical picture

Local swelling and redness occur, and there is severe local pain, which is decreased by moving the involved part as little as possible. Within 3 to 5 days the lesion becomes elevated or "points up," the surrounding skin becomes shiny, and the center or "core" turns yellow (p. 281). A carbuncle has several cores. The boil will usually rupture spontaneously, but it may be surgically incised and drained. As drainage occurs, the pain is immediately relieved. The drainage soon changes from a yellow purulent material to a serosanguineous discharge. All drainage usually subsides within a few hours to a few days; the redness and swelling subside gradually.

Intervention

Hot, wet dressings are used to help bring the boil to a head, but these dressings are discontinued as soon as drainage occurs in order to prevent skin maceration and spread of infection. As the boil drains, care must be taken to keep the infected drainage off the surrounding skin, since organisms may be harbored in hair follicles and furunculosis may recur. Persons are cautioned to keep their hands away from the drainage to prevent spread of infection.

If the person is hospitalized, wound isolation procedures are followed until the drainage subsides lest the organism be carried to others. Health personnel should wash their hands thoroughly after caring for the patient and should avoid getting the drainage on their own skin.

The person who is at home must be taught to be scrupulously careful in hygiene practices to prevent accidentally passing the organisms to others in the family or to persons at work. It is not uncommon for entire families to have some type of staphylococcal infection after one member has had a boil. Both the patient and the family should bathe and shampoo daily with bacteriostatic soap for as long as infection is present. Razor blades should be discarded after each use. Each family member needs separate bath linens that are changed daily to prevent the spread of infection.

Furuncles and carbuncles tend to recur in susceptible individuals, and the staphylococci causing them often are resistant to local treatment and to antibiotics.

Erysipelas

Erysipelas is an acute febrile disease caused by the hemolytic streptococcus and characterized by localized inflammation and swelling of the skin and subcutaneous tissues, usually of the face. A bright, sharp line separates the diseased skin from the normal skin. Elderly people with poor resistance are most often affected. Erysipelas was a serious disease before the advent of antibiotics; penicillin is the drug of choice.

Outcome criteria for the person with a bacterial skin infection

The person or significant others can:
1. Describe measures to avoid bacterial spread by:
   a. Avoidance of contamination from drainage.
   b. Cleansing practices.
   c. Disposal of contaminated articles.
2. Describe the medical treatment program.
   a. Demonstrate use of hot compresses, if appropriate.
   b. State name of drug, dosage, purpose, route, frequency, and side effects.
   c. State plans for health care follow-up.

Viral diseases

Warts

Warts are benign skin growths that develop from hypertrophy of epidermal cells as a result of a viral infection. The infection is not highly contagious but does spread along the dermis through autoinfection. It is seen most commonly in older children and young adults.

Warts grow in a variety of shapes. The common wart is a small, circumscribed, painless, hyperkeratotic papule commonly seen on the extremities, especially the hands. *Filiform warts* are slender fingerlike projections occurring mostly on the face and neck. *Plantar warts* grow inward from the pressure on the soles of the foot and are frequently painful. They are differentiated from calluses by lack of skin lines over the surface. Warts that develop in the anogenital region have a lighter-colored surface and a cauliflower-like appearance, and they may cause itching. Anogenital warts may be spread either by sexual activity or by other means.

Intervention

There are numerous treatments for warts but no one major effective method. Warts sometimes disappear spontaneously or under psychologic suggestion, thus creating a basis for numerous folktales concerning how to get rid of warts. If only a few painless warts are present, no treatment is necessary and the warts will probably disappear in time.

The most commonly used therapeutic measures for common warts are electrodesiccation and cryosurgery. In electrodesiccation the top of the wart is seared gently for softening of the keratinized surface, and then the wart is curetted off and the bleeding points cauterized. This method is not used for plantar warts. Cryosurgery consists of freezing the lesion with a substance such as liquid nitrogen. Cauterant chemicals such as formalin, phenol, nitric acid, salicylic acid, or podophyllum may also be used. X-ray therapy has been used in the past, but serious sequelae that may occur have discouraged its use. Surgical excision is seldom used since painful scarring may result.

Herpes simplex

One of the most common viruses found in humans is the herpes simplex virus (HSV). It occurs as two similar yet serologically different strains, type 1 and type 2. The type 1 virus is found primarily in lesions of the face and mouth (fever blister, cold sore), eye (keratitis), and brain (encephalitis). Type 2 is associated with a lesion of the genitalia that can be transmitted by sexual contact. HSV has a DNA-containing core surrounded by a phospholipid covering. Factors that may precipitate recurrence of herpes simplex lesions include fever, upper respiratory tract infection, exhaustion, and nervous tension. Lesions also are more common during the menses or following direct exposure to the sun's rays.

Clinical picture

Most persons experience the initial contact with HSV as a young child. The HSV remains in the cells of the sensory nerves that supply the affected areas and cause recurrent lesions when the person is subjected to stresses. The appearance of vesicles is preceded by several hours by a sensation of burning or itching. A cluster of vesicles on an erythematous base appears at the mucocutaneous junctions of the lips or nose or as an inflammation of the cornea of one eye with photophobia and tearing. The type 2 virus lesions occur in the vagina or cervix of the woman or on the penile skin of the man. The lesions are painful and frequently crack open. A crust gradually forms, and the lesions heal in about 10 days.

Intervention

There is no safe, effective, systemic approach at this time to treatment of recurrent herpes simplex of the face or genitalia. Local treatment is the most effective if given *early* to prevent the virus from multiplying and thus hasten healing for general comfort. The vesicles on the face can be opened and 70% alcohol applied every 1 to 2 hours to break down the fat-soluble covering of the virus, thus inactivating it. Ether has also been used as a solvent. The drug 5-iodo-2-deoxyuridine (idoxuridine) that inhibits viral DNA is effective in the treatment of HSV-induced keratitis. Disagreement exists as to the effectiveness of idoxuridine for skin manifestations, but some positive results have been achieved with early hourly applications.[62]

Another controversial method of treatment is photoinactivation. A heterocyclic dye (neutral red, proflavine, methylene blue) is applied to vesicles that have been opened, and the area is then subjected to exposure to an ordinary fluorescent light for 15 minutes. The light exposure is repeated for 30 minutes at 8 hours and again at 36 hours after dye application.[62] The dye binds to the viral nucleic acid in the presence of light, thus destroying it. Controversy over use of photoinactivation centers on the potential oncogenicity of the dyes.

After the initial phase of vesicle eruption, the goal of therapy is promotion of comfort. Pain may be relieved by analgesics such as aspirin or by application of warm, moist compresses. Spirits of camphor applied as a liquid or in small tubes of camphorated lip ice may be helpful.

Herpes zoster

Herpes zoster, or shingles, is caused by the same virus (V-Z) that causes varicella (chickenpox). Varicella is believed to be the primary infection in a nonimmune host, while herpes zoster is thought to be the response in a partially immune host. Although herpes zoster is far less communicable than chickenpox, persons who have not had chickenpox may develop it after exposure to the vesicular lesions of persons with herpes zoster. For this reason, susceptible persons should not care for patients with herpes zoster.

Herpes zoster can be a serious condition in any adult and may even lead to death from exhaustion in elderly debilitated individuals. It is one of the most drawn out and exasperating conditions found in elderly patients and leads to discouragement and demoralization. Contrary to popular thought, one episode of herpes zoster does *not* provide immunity, and the disease may recur.[4] Herpes zoster often occurs in persons with Hodgkin's disease and in those with lymphoid and some bone cancers because of reduced cell-mediated immunity.

Clinical picture

In herpes zoster, clusters of small vesicles usually form in a line. They follow the course of the peripheral sensory nerves and often are unilateral (Fig. 71-3). Since they follow nerve pathways, the lesions never cross the midline of the body, however, nerves on both sides of the body can be involved. Two thirds of persons with herpes zoster develop lesions over thoracic dermatomes, and the remainder show involvement of the trigeminal nerve with lesions on the face, eye, and scalp. The rash develops first as macules but progresses rapidly to vesicles. The fluid becomes turbid, and crusts develop and drop off in about 10 days.

Malaise, fever, itching, and pain over the involved area may precede the eruption of the lesions. If vesicles develop within 1 or 2 days after the initial pain symptoms, the lesions usually clear in 2 to 3 weeks, but if the vesicles develop over the period of a week, a prolonged course can be expected.[41]

Discomfort from pain and itching is the major prob-

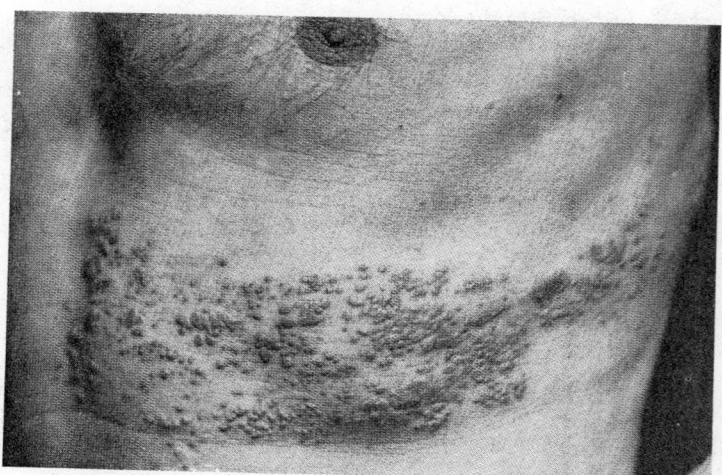

Fig. 71-3. Herpes zoster. Note abrupt cessation at midline. (From Stewart, W.D., Danto, J.L., and Maddin, S.: Dermatology: diagnosis and treatment of cutaneous disorders, ed. 4, St. Louis, 1978, The C.V. Mosby Co.)

lem with herpes zoster. The pain may vary from a light burning sensation to a deep visceral-type pain, and it may be intermittent or constant. It usually persists for up to 4 weeks. In approximately 30% of persons over age 40, the pain may last for months or years, especially in the elderly.[4] Enlargement of the lymph nodes may also occur with the rash.

Intervention

There is no specific therapy for the treatment of herpes zoster, and the care is primarily symptomatic. If discomfort is severe, the person may benefit from a short period of rest, especially if malaise and fever have occurred. Loose clothing is suggested to minimize contact with the affected area. Pruritus may be relieved by the application of calamine lotion or collodion over the vesicular area. Analgesics are usually necessary. Corticosteroids such as methylprednisolone (Medrol) may be given to shorten the period of acute pain, but they have no effect on healing of the skin lesions.

Postherpetic neuralgia presents difficulties in obtaining relief of pain because of limited results from the usual analgesics. Narcotics should be avoided because of the persistency of the pain and potential for addiction. Medications that have proved useful for some persons include carbamazepine (Tegretol), phenothiazines such as chlorpromazine (Thorazine), or sedatives. The cooling effect of ethyl chloride spray may provide some temporary relief. Rhizotomy and cordotomy are usually ineffective.

Outcome criteria for the person with a herpes infection

The person or significant others can:
1. Describe the nature of the condition and the probability of recurrence.
2. Describe measures that can be taken to decrease discomfort (alcohol, camphor, or moist compresses over lesions of herpes simplex; calamine lotion or collodion over lesions of herpes zoster; analgesics).

Acne

Acne vulgaris

Etiology

Acne vulgaris is a very common skin disease seen in 80% of adolescents. The cause of acne is still unknown but is thought to be multifactorial. Some of the common causes that have been postulated are free fatty ac-

ids, endocrine effects, stress, diet, heredity, and infection. Diet has been essentially ruled out as a causative factor, but none of the other factors have been demonstrated conclusively. Acne occurs at puberty when the sebaceous glands are stimulated by androgens, and it is often found occurring within families. Acne is more quiescent in summer months.

Prevention

The lesions in acne develop when the pilosebaceous follicles become plugged; therefore activities that contribute to occlusion of the follicles are to be avoided (see box below). Hair and hands should be kept away from the face. Loose clothing prevents pressure over the follicles, and tight collars should not be worn. The skin should be kept clean. Greasy, oil-based cosmetics may be occlusive and plug up the follicles. Any food that appears to cause acne flare-ups in a given individual is best avoided.

In the past there have been numerous practices attributed to causing acne, such as staying up late or masturbating. Often the practice in question is one of concern to parents; and acne has been used as a means to discourage the undesired practice, although there is no relationship between acne and these practices.

Pathophysiology

At puberty sebaceous glands undergo enlargement from androgen stimulation. When sebum is released it passes through the follicular canal, where it is combined with sebaceous gland cell fragments, epidermal cells (keratin), and bacteria. At this time the triglycerides in the sebum are hydrolyzed to glycerol and free fatty acids. The sebum and debris may become plugged in the hair follicle (Fig. 71-4) to form an open comedo (blackhead) if it is at the surface or a closed comedo

---

GUIDELINES FOR PERSONS WITH ACNE VULGARIS

1. Avoid touching or squeezing lesions.
2. Keep hair and hands away from face.
3. Avoid constricting clothing over lesions.
4. Shampoo hair and scalp regularly (at least twice a week).
5. Wash skin frequently (at least twice a day) using a drying medicated soap; avoid use of creams or moisturizers.
6. Use water-based rather than cream-based makeup preparations.
7. Expose skin to sunlight, as possible (in moderation).

(whitehead) if it is below the surface. The dark color of the blackhead is melanin, not dirt, and results from passage of melanin from the adjoining epidermal cells.

Inflammatory lesions develop apparently from escape of sebum into the dermis, which then serves as an irritant causing an inflammatory reaction. Free fatty acids may also be an irritant in the follicle itself.

Clinical picture

Acne occurs mostly on the face and neck, upper chest, and back, although the upper arms, buttocks, and thighs may also be involved. Comedones are the first visible signs, and the skin is characteristically oily. The inflammatory lesions include papules, pustules, nodules, and cysts. Superficial lesions may resolve in 5 to 10 days without scarring, but large lesions last for several weeks and often result in scarring. The typical scar resembles an old volcano (ice-pick scar); however, many other sizes and shapes may result, depending on the depth and extent of the inflammatory lesions.

There is great variability among adolescents in the extent of the lesions. Some persons have only a few small lesions. Many adolescents have several lesions that peak at ages 16 to 18 and then slowly resolve. A few persons develop severe nodular acne that may not resolve for 10 to 15 years.[53]

Intervention

Treatment of acne requires full compliance by the patient for effectiveness. It is therefore important that the patient (1) understand the physiologic basis of acne to correct misconceptions and enhance compliance with therapy, (2) understand the therapy to be used and the need to avoid adding other self-remedies at the same time, (3) be aware of the length of time needed (usually at least 4 to 6 weeks) for any one therapy to begin to demonstrate marked improvement, and (4) know expected side effects so that therapy is not interrupted before positive results can be achieved.[53] Treatment usually consists of a combination of several agents or approaches.

Skin cleansing. The skin should be washed frequently with regular or medicated soap to remove the excess oil on the skin surface and to effect drying of the skin with erythema and peeling. Alcohol may also be used as an astringent.

Topical therapy. Most topical agents are keratolytic, causing erythema and peeling or desquamation. If no scaling occurs, the agent is ineffective; if discomfort is present, the agent is too strong.[49] Medications are applied gradually in increasing doses until tolerance is reached. Commonly used keratolytic agents are available in the form of powders, lotions, creams, or cakes

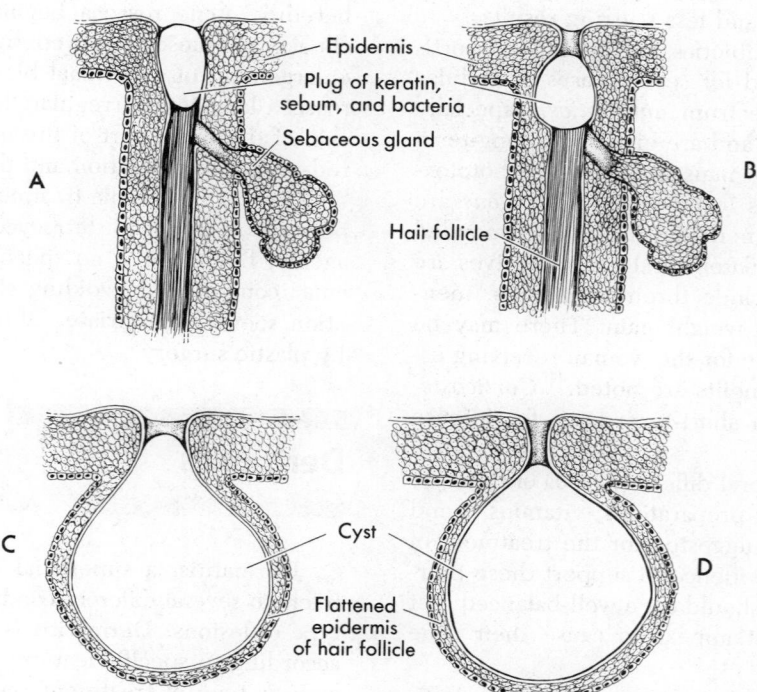

Fig. 71-4. Formation of lesions in acne vulgaris. **A,** Open comedo (blackhead), early stage. **B,** Closed comedo (whitehead), early stage. **C,** Cyst formation in open comedo, advanced stage. **D,** Cyst formation in closed comedo, advanced stage. (From Dermatology and skin care by J.H. Parrish. Copyright © 1975 by McGraw-Hill Book Co. Used with the permission of McGraw-Hill Book Co.)

and include resorcinol, benzoyl peroxide, salicylic acid, and sulfur. A topical vitamin A acid (retinoic acid) loosens comedones and prevents new ones from forming. Small doses of retinoic acid causing some irritation are as effective as the keratolytic agents. Large doses initially cause an increased inflammatory response followed by striking improvement.[49]

Ultraviolet light therapy. Acne improves in the summer from the effect of ultraviolet rays from the sun, which produce erythema and peeling of the skin. Use of artificial sources of ultraviolet light is controversial regarding its effect. Precautions to take when using ultraviolet light include (1) protecting the eyes from the light to prevent conjunctival inflammation, (2) using a timer to prevent overexposure, and (3) maintaining the specified distance from the light to prevent burning.

Mechanical drainage. Open comedones (blackheads) can be removed by the use of the bulb from the end of a plastic eyedropper. The bulb is removed and the smaller end applied with gentle pressure over the comedo.[53] The skin is cleansed well before removal of the comedo. The person is instructed never to use the fingers to push out the open comedo since this leads to tissue irritation and inflammation.

Intralesional therapy. Severe nodular or cystic acne can be treated by injecting the lesions with a corticosteroid using a syringe and small-bore needle or an injector without a needle.[41] Lesions respond rapidly to intralesional corticosteroid, and less scarring results.

Systemic therapy. Antibiotics, estrogens, and corticosteroids have been used for severe cases of nodular or cystic acne. Broad-spectrum *antibiotics,* especially tetracycline, are effective and are given on a long-term basis. Side effects include nausea, diarrhea, phototoxicity, and yeast infections (candidiasis). *Estrogens* are used only in selected women who have not responded to other therapies. Anovulatory oral contraceptives are used, but side effects include thrombophlebitis, menstrual abnormalities, and weight gain. There may be initial flare-ups of the acne for the woman receiving estrogen therapy before benefits are noted.[41] *Corticosteroids* are used only on a short-term basis for intense inflammatory reactions.

Other therapies. Several different types of therapy, such as diuretics, thyroid preparations, vitamins A and E, and zinc, have been suggested for the treatment of acne, but there is little evidence to support these therapies. Persons with acne should eat a well-balanced diet and avoid any foods that appear to cause their acne flare-ups.

After the acne is under control, dermabrasion (p. 1805) may be used to lessen the pitting and scarring; the effectiveness is approximately 50%. Some complications of dermabrasion are hyperpigmentation, infection, and persistent erythema. A technique of injecting fibrin into areas of pitting may help minimize the defect.

Outcome criteria for the person with acne vulgaris

The person or significant others can:
1. Explain the basis of skin lesion development.
2. Describe preventive measures (keeping hands and hair away from face, wearing loose clothing, washing skin frequently, avoiding greasy cosmetics).
3. Describe the medical treatment.
   a. State the type, frequency, and effect (peeling, erythema) of the topical application to be used.
   b. Describe the necessity to continue treatment for several weeks or longer as prescribed.
   c. State plan to avoid self-medication in conjunction with prescribed treatment.
   d. State drug name, dose, frequency, duration of treatment, and side effects.
4. Describe plan for medical follow-up for severe inflammatory acne.

Acne rosacea

Acne rosacea is a skin condition that usually affects people over 25 years of age. The actual cause is unknown. Over the years many causative factors have been suggested, including bacteria, vitamin deficiency, hormonal imbalance, alcohol, caffeine, psychic factors, and heredity. Acne rosacea begins with redness over the cheeks and nose, followed by papules, pustules, and enlargement of superficial blood vessels. Years of acne rosacea lead to an irregular, bulbous thickening of the skin of the distal part of the nose (rhinophyma), with a red-purple discoloration and dilated follicles.

There is no specific treatment for acne rosacea. Some persons respond to tetracycline and topical peeling agents, but there is no specific treatment for the vascular component. Avoiding stimuli that cause vasodilation seems appropriate. Rhinophyma may be treated by plastic surgery.

Dermatitis

Dermatitis, a superficial inflammation of the skin, refers to several different conditions resulting in the same type of lesions. Dermatitis is often classified arbitrarily according to specific features such as etiology, pattern, age, or type of treatment required. Some of the common types of dermatitis are listed in Table 71-1 and are discussed in more detail in succeeding paragraphs. The term *eczema* is often used synonymously with dermatitis but frequently refers to the chronic type.

Regardless of the etiology, the lesions in any der-

TABLE 71-1. Types of dermatitis

Type	Cause	Characteristics
Contact	External agents	Site and pattern of lesions depend on exposure pattern (linear, angular, etc.) Itching a major symptom
Atopic	Hypersensitivity reaction, hereditary	Itching a major symptom Lesions caused by scratching
Lichen simplex chronicus	Stasis, irritants, psychic factors	Itching a major symptom Lesions caused by scratching
Seborrheic	Unknown	Erythematous, scaly (e.g., dandruff)
Nummular	Unknown	Coin-shaped lesions Severe itching
Stasis	Decreased circulation	Erythema, edema Lesions may develop from trauma Itching may be severe

TABLE 71-2. Common causes of contact dermatitis of different areas*

Area	Cause
Face	Cosmetics, hair sprays, hair dyes, airborne contactants
Earlobes	Nickel
Ears	
Pinnae	Photosensitizers
Canals	Medications
Eyelids	Cosmetics, airborne sensitizers, transfer by hands
Nose (bridge)	Metal or plastic spectacle supports
Lips and perioral area	Toothpaste, lipstick
Neck	Perfumes, clothing (especially wool)
Axillae	Deodorants, clothing, perfumes
Scapular area	Nickel in clasps on straps
Breasts	Elastic and other brassiere material
Waist	Elastic
Perianal area	Dibucaine (Nupercaine) and other medications, excessive use of cleansers
Arms and legs	Poison ivy and other plants
Wrists	Nickel, etc. in watchbands
Hands	Detergents and other cleansers, gloves
Feet	Medication for "athlete's foot," shoes

*From Moschella, S.L., Pillsbury, D.M., and Hurley, H.J.: Dermatology, Philadelphia, 1975, W.B. Saunders Co.

matitis follow a characteristic pattern. Initially, there is erythema and local edema, which is followed by vesicle formation with oozing and then crusting and scaling. If the dermatitis persists, there will be evidence of excoriation from scratching and thickening of the skin, and the color becomes more brownish. Secondary infection may result.

Contact dermatitis

Etiology

Contact dermatitis is caused by external agents and may affect various parts of the body (Table 71-2). There are two types of contact dermatitis, irritant and allergic. *Irritant contact dermatitis* can occur in any person on contact with a sufficient concentration of an irritant. Mechanical irritation may result from wool or glass fibers. Chemical irritants include acids, alkalies, solvents, detergents, or oils commonly found in cleaning compounds, insecticides, or industrial compounds. Biologic irritants include urine, fecal drainage, and toxins from insects or aquatic plants. People who are exposed to constant wetting of the hands or feet often develop irritant contact dermatitis.

Allergic contact dermatitis is a cell-mediated hypersensitivity immune reaction from contact with a specific antigen (p. 1872). There are many compounds that are capable of causing sensitization under specified conditions. Typical antigens include poison ivy, synthetics, industrial chemicals, drugs (e.g., sulfanilamide or penicillin), and metals (especially nickel and chromate). Once the skin has been sensitized, further contact with the sensitizing substance will produce an eczematous reaction. The sensitizing allergen may reach the site by direct contact; by indirect contact such as transmission by animals, from one part of the body to the other by the hands, or on clothing; or by the air such as in smoke.

Prevention

Contact dermatitis may be prevented by avoiding the irritating or sensitizing substance whenever possible. People should know how to recognize the leaves of poisonous plants such as poison ivy, poison oak, or poison sumac that grow where they live (Fig. 71-5). Persons walking in areas where poison ivy grows need to protect the skin by clothing. If contact with poison ivy is suspected, symptoms may possibly be averted by immediately lathering the skin several times with an alkaline soap and rinsing well each time with running water to remove the resin before skin penetration occurs.

The person who develops a sensitivity to material encountered in the living or working environment may need to consider a permanent change of environment if other measures are unsuccessful. Gloves may be used if the person is handling irritant or allergenic substances. Persons sensitive to detergents may need to wash their clothes and to bathe with a mild soap such as Ivory.

Clinical picture

The characteristic dermatitis lesions appear sooner in irritant contact dermatitis than in the allergic type;

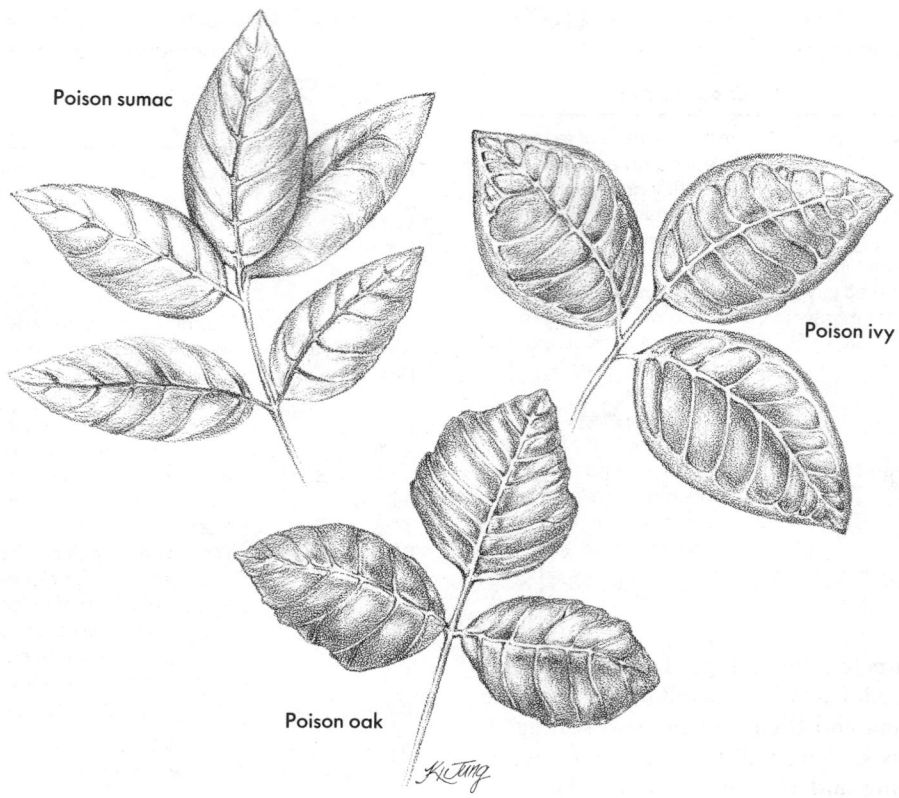

Fig. 71-5. Typical leaves of poison sumac, poison ivy, and poison oak.

however, the onset and appearance vary depending on the type and concentration of the irritant. The lesions develop on the exposed areas, particularly the more sensitive areas such as the dorsal rather than the palmar surface of the hands. If the irritant can be spread by the hands, such as in poison ivy, lesions may involve other nonexposed areas.

When contact dermatitis is suspected but the agent is unknown, patch testing (p. 1790) may be carried out or the environment may be manipulated to exclude suspected agents.

Intervention

Weeping uninfected lesions respond rapidly to wet dressings with Burow's solution (1:40 dilution of aluminum acetate) for 20 minutes four times daily. Crusts and scales are not removed but are allowed to drop off naturally as the skin heals. Topical corticosteroids are applied to dry lesions. Systemic corticosteroids may be given in acute extensive exacerbations but are not used to treat a mild contact dermatitis. Systemic antibiotics are prescribed when infection is present. Severe pruritus may be eased by sedatives, tranquilizers, or colloidal baths.

Atopic dermatitis

Etiology

Atopy refers to a type I hypersensitivity that is hereditary (p. 1865) and includes asthma, hay fever, and eczema (atopic dermatitis). About 50% of persons with atopic dermatitis develop asthma or hay fever. The person who has inherited the tendency to eczema may not necessarily demonstrate symptoms. Exacerbating factors include sudden changes in temperature or humidity; exercise; psychologic stress; fibers such as wool, fur, or nylon; detergents; and perfumes.[41]

Pathophysiology

Persons with atopic dermatitis have a dry, highly sensitive skin with a lowered threshold to pruritus so that minor stimuli cause intense itching. There is a marked tendency toward vasoconstriction of superficial blood vessels and the skin blanches readily.[52] Cold and low humidity are poorly tolerated. Heat and high humidity are also poorly tolerated because vasodilation increases the inflammatory reaction, thus aggravating the dermatitis and causing increased itching and discomfort.

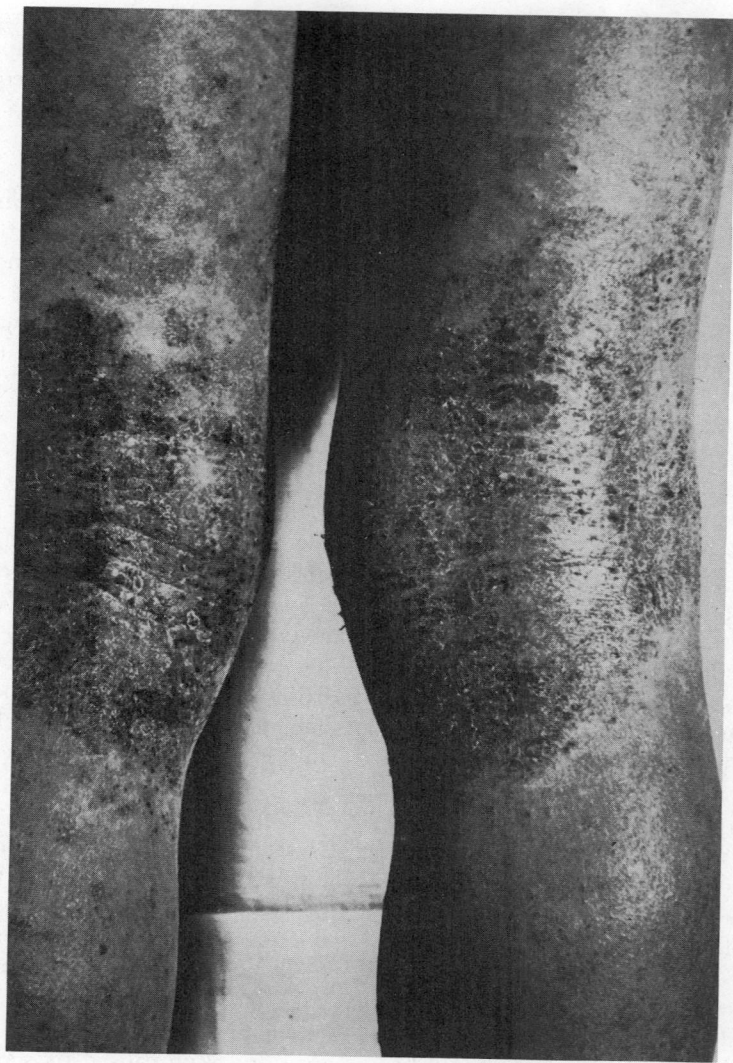

Fig. 71-6. Atopic dermatitis with characteristic flexural involvement and crusting. (From Stewart, W.D., Danto, J.L., and Maddin, S.: Dermatology: diagnosis and treatment of cutaneous disorders, ed. 4, St. Louis, 1978, The C.V. Mosby Co.)

Clinical picture

The major symptom of atopic dermatitis is pruritus. Chronic scratching leads to eczematous lesions and subsequent lichenification. Healing usually occurs without scarring but hypopigmentation or hyperpigmentation may result.

Atopic dermatitis is usually first noted in the infant about the third month. The lesions are moderately erythematous and may be dry or weeping. They usually involve the face, especially the cheeks, but they may also occur on other parts of the body except the palms and soles. Atopic dermatitis usually disappears or becomes less severe about the age of 2 to 3 years, but it recurs in late childhood or adolescence in a large num-

ber of persons. The lesions become localized to the flexor surfaces of the neck, to the eyelids, behind the ears, in the antecubital and popliteal areas (Fig. 71-6), and at the wrists. The erythema is now dusky in color, and excoriations may become secondarily infected. By the late 20s or early 30s the lesions usually disappear, but they may recur at a later date as chronic hand or foot eczema.[41]

Persons with atopic dermatitis are highly susceptible to viral infections, especially herpes, and to bacterial infections such as those caused by staphylococcus or β-hemolytic streptococcus. There is also an increased incidence of fungal infections such as tinea. Lymph nodes draining affected areas may be enlarged.

Intervention

There is no cure for atopic dermatitis, but symptoms can be controlled. The focus of therapy is relief of pruritus in order to break the itch-scratch cycle that leads to lesions. The major form of *topical* therapy consists of corticosteroid cream or ointment. Fluorinated corticosteroids may be used for localized lesions in adults but are used less often in children and *never on the face*. An occlusion wrap over the steroid in adults may enhance the steroid effect but may lead to folliculitis. Topical antibiotics are rarely used. Cool compresses with Burow's solution are helpful for acute phases when weeping lesions are present.

Systemic therapy includes sedation or antihistamines at night when itching is more intense. Antibiotics such as penicillin or erythromycin may be given systemically for bacterial infections. Systemic corticosteroids are rarely used because once started they are difficult to stop and the side effects preclude long-term therapy for this chronic condition.[41]

Persons with atopic dermatitis have dry skin; therefore baths and showers are best kept at a minimum and the water should be at skin temperature because of the person's intolerance to extremes of temperature. Detergents, which are drying to the skin, should be avoided and soap used minimally. Soaking in the bath water (to which oil may be added) for about 25 minutes and then applying a steroid cream will promote skin hydration. The person will experience some pruritus when leaving the bath.

Wool, nylon, or fur clothing should be avoided, since these irritate the sensitive skin and lead to pruritus. Strenuous exercise, especially outdoors, also leads to itching and should be limited. Whenever possible, extremely cold winters or hot humid summers should be avoided. Sunlight, however, improves the condition.

Other types of dermatitis

Lichen simplex chronicus

Lichen simplex chronicus (LSC), or circumscribed neurodermatitis, is a chronic skin condition that results from repeated scratching. Although it is more common in females and Orientals, it may occur in both sexes and all races. Itching initiates the condition in normal skin and may occur as a result of stasis or an irritant, or it may occur without any known cause. Psychic factors are thought to be involved. LSC is more commonly found in the occipital region of the scalp, hands, perineum, and legs.

Once itching starts, the itch-scratch cycle is initiated and scratching becomes a habit. The skin becomes excoriated, and lichenified plaques result. Lesions disappear if scratching ceases, but it is difficult for the person to stop scratching. Itching is often worse at night. Top-

ical corticosteroids are the treatment of choice. In nonhairy areas corticosteroid tape (Cordran tape) is effective if the medicated tape covers the area so that further excoriation is reduced.

Seborrheic dermatitis

Dermatitis may occur primarily in areas of increased sebaceous gland activity on the face, ears, scalp, chest, and back. The cause is unknown. Mild seborrheic dermatitis is often seen in the scalp in the form of erythema and dandruff and can be controlled easily by shampooing with selenium sulfide (Selsun Blue) shampoo. More extensive seborrheic dermatitis leads to red scaly plaques and is treated with topical hydrocortisone.

Nummular dermatitis

The lesions of nummular dermatitis are coin shaped and are found on the dorsum of the hand, the extensor surfaces of the extremities, and the buttocks. It occurs most frequently in middle-aged or older men. The cause is uncertain, and the condition is chronic. Itching is often severe. The skin is usually dry; therefore frequent bathing is inadvisable. Exposure to sunlight may be helpful. Treatment consists of topical corticosteroids and antibiotic therapy if bacteria are isolated by culture.

Stasis dermatitis

Stasis dermatitis is a common skin condition of the lower extremities in older persons. It is usually preceded by varicosities and poor circulation. With the reduction in venous return from the legs, substances normally carried away by the circulation remain in the tissues and irritate them. The skin is often reddened and edematous. Pruritus may be quite severe. Breaks in the skin are often caused by scratching, and infection then is introduced by the hands, clothing, and other sources.

The most important treatment for stasis dermatitis is prevention by careful attention to the treatment of peripheral vascular conditions and preventing the constriction of the circulation to the extremities. When acute weeping lesions are present, wet compresses and elevation of the leg are advised.

Outcome criteria for the person with dermatitis

The person or significant others can:
1. State causative agents (if known), source of the agent, and method of contact.
2. Describe measures to prevent further contacts.
3. Describe problems of self-treatment and the need for medical follow-up.
4. Describe medical treatment program.
   a. State name of medication, purpose, dosage, route and frequency, and side effects.

b. Demonstrate treatment measures to be carried out at home.

Skin reactions from systemic factors

Dermatitis medicamentosa

Many skin eruptions result from the large number of drugs now being used in the treatment of disease. There are a wide variety of skin responses simulating skin diseases. The reaction to drugs may occur through toxic, metabolic, or allergic mechanisms.[12] Many of the drug reactions are hypersensitivity reactions, either type I (anaphylactic), type II (cytotoxic), or type III (immune complex). The most common forms are the type III reactions; signs include fever, urticaria, rashes, erythema, and vasculitis.[12] The rash is often bright red, semiconfluent, macular and papular, generalized, and bilateral. It can appear at any time, but the onset is usually sudden.[49] Hypersensitivity occurs early when previous sensitization has taken place.

Photosensitivity may occur in some persons taking phenothiazines, thiazides, tetracycline, griseofulvin, or sulfonamides. The skin develops the appearance of a sunburn. People taking these drugs should not be exposed to direct sunlight for any period of time.

Exfoliative dermatitis

Exfoliative dermatitis is a rare generalized dermatitis characterized by erythema and marked scaling. In most cases, the cause is unknown, but the disease may be associated with other types of dermatitis or with a lymphoma, or it may be the result of a drug reaction.

The onset may be rapid or insidious and consists of an elevated temperature and a generalized erythema followed by extensive scaling (exfoliation). Pruritus may be present, and the lesions often become infected. Loss of large amounts of water and protein from the skin leads to hypoproteinemia, weight loss, and difficulty with temperature control. Heart failure may occur in elderly patients. Death may result from overwhelming infection or circulatory collapse.

Therapy consists of maintaining fluid balance and preventing infection. Methods used to prevent infection in patients with burns are applicable (see Chapter 70). All drugs are discontinued as potential etiologic factors, although antibiotics may be started after culture and sensitivity tests of infected lesions. Oral corticosteroids are only given for severe cases. Daily baths followed by application of petrolatum to the skin promote comfort.

Erythema multiforme

Erythema multiforme is a skin condition believed to occur secondary to an underlying systemic disease such as an infection. The skin eruption is characterized by red to purple macules, papules, and vesicles. Most often the lesions occur on the wrists, back of the hands, ankles, tops of the feet, knees, elbows, face, palms, and sole of the feet; the entire body may be involved. The skin eruption may be preceded by fever, chest pain, and arthralgia. The treatment is to seek out the underlying cause and eliminate it if possible. Other treatment is supportive, and corticosteroids are often used. Local treatment includes baths, soaks, and dressings. If lesions appear in the mouth, special mouth care is indicated, including irrigations with warm salt solution.

Infectious diseases

Communicable diseases such as measles, chickenpox, smallpox, scarlet fever, and typhoid fever produce skin reactions (Table 71-3). Nodes and hemorrhagic spots in the skin also accompany severe acute rheumatic fever.

Lupus erythematosus

One of the more common tissue diseases that may result in skin conditions is lupus erythematosus (LE), which occurs in two forms, systemic (SLE) (see p. 1845) and discoid (DLE). *Discoid lupus erythematosus* is a chronic, relatively benign skin condition that has worldwide distribution among all races and that occurs most often in the fourth decade of life. It is rarely seen in children or the elderly. Precipitating factors include physical trauma and stress. Less than 1% of persons with DLE develop SLE, but almost 10% of persons with SLE develop DLE.[49]

The lesions of DLE are well demarcated and erythematous, have a characteristic scaly border with an atrophied center, and vary in size. The most common sites are the cheeks (butterfly pattern), nose, ears, scalp, and chest, although other parts of the body, including mucous membranes, may also be involved. In addition to the skin lesions, the person may have leukopenia, an increased sedimentation rate, a positive rheumatoid factor test, a positive serologic test for syphilis (STS), and a low titer of antinuclear factors.

Preventive measures include avoiding physical trauma, such as by using protective lotions to prevent sunburn, and wearing warm clothing to protect against cold and wind. If stress is a precipitating factor, measures to reduce stress (see Chapter 13) can be instituted. There is no cure for DLE. Palliative measures

TABLE 71-3. Skin reactions of some communicable diseases

Disease	Cause	Incubation period (days)	Place of rash origin	Skin lesions
Measles (rubeola)	Rubeola virus	11 (8-14)	Face	Pink macular-papular rash; lesions coalesce
German measles; 3-day measles (rubella)	Rubella virus	14-21	Face	Pink macular-papular rash; lesions usually discrete, may coalesce
Scarlet fever (scarlatina)	Hemolytic strepto-coccus	1-3	Neck, chest	Bright red (scarlet) mac-ules (pinpoint)
Chickenpox (varicella)	V-Z virus	14-21	Back, chest	Macule, papule, vesicle, crust, lesions at differ-ent stages
Smallpox (variola)	Variola virus	12 (7-21)	Face	Macule, papule, vesicle, crust, lesions all at same stage
Typhoid fever	*Salmonella typhosa*	14 (7-21)	Abdomen	Macular rash

include topical steroid therapy under occlusive wraps, intralesional steroid therapy, or antimalarial therapy with chloroquine (Aralen), hydroxychloroquine sulfate (Plaquenil), or quinacrine hydrochloride (Atabrine).

Papulosquamous diseases

Psoriasis

Psoriasis is a genetically determined, chronic, epidermal proliferative disease. It is not infectious or contagious and is not a nervous disorder. Approximately 1% to 2% of the population of the United States have psoriasis; 5% of this group have associated inflammatory arthritis. There is a higher incidence of psoriasis among whites and a lower incidence among the Japanese, American Indians, and blacks of West African origin. Men and women are equally affected. Psoriasis occurs in all ages but is less common among children and the elderly. There are no specific precipitating factors for the majority of persons; however, some people may develop exacerbations following climatic changes, stress, trauma, or infections. Pregnant women often see a remission of symptoms.

Clinical picture

The turnover time for normal skin is 28 days. After the basal cell divides, it normally takes 14 days to reach the stratum corneum and an additional 14 days for this cell to be sloughed off. In psoriasis the time is accelerated to 4 to 7 days.

The lesions of psoriasis are elevated, erythematous, sharply circumscribed, scaling plaques. The primary lesion is a papule; these papules then join to form plaques. In the black person the plaques may appear to be purple. Lesions may occur over the entire body but are found more commonly on the scalp, elbows, shins, and trunk. Beefy red lesions may be observed in an acute flare-up. The nails of persons with psoriasis have characteristic involvement; there may be pitting of the nails, yellowish discoloration, and onycholysis (separation of the nail from the nail bed).

Psoriasis takes many forms. *Arthropathic psoriasis* is one of the cruelest forms and may produce crippling. The nails are always involved and show denting and pitting. *Pustular psoriasis* (von Zumbusch) may present with fever, tenderness of the skin, and sterile pustules.

Intervention

Because of the overproduction of skin in psoriasis, treatment is based on slowing mitotic activity. Initially, the lesions may be treated with topical steroids with occlusive wraps and wet dressings to decrease inflammation. Topical medications such as crude coal tar, anthralin, and related compounds are frequently used because they appear to have a keratolytic effect. The combination of tar and ultraviolet light known as the Goeckerman regimen (see box, p. 1847) is one of the oldest forms of therapy for psoriasis; it is quite effective and is still widely used today in modified forms. Anthralin, a distillate of crude coal tar, is used over stubborn plaques of psoriasis. Gloves should be worn during application because of anthralin's irritating effect. Folliculitis may result from coal tar therapy.

Methotrexate, an antimetabolite, is reserved for those cases of psoriasis that are resistant to topical treatment. When used appropriately, it has shown a good to excel-

---

GOECKERMAN REGIMEN FOR PSORIASIS

1. Apply crude coal tar two to three times a day over all affected areas.

2. Remove tar with corn oil before ultraviolet therapy, leaving a thin film on skin.

3. Give ultraviolet light therapy.

4. Give tub bath with soap and oil. Shampoo scalp.

5. Reapply tar to skin and lotion to scalp.

6. Have person wear pajamas for 3 days to act as a dressing.

---

lent clearing of lesions in 80% of the patients. The person receiving methotrexate should be monitored closely. An initial liver biopsy and a creatinine clearance level are done and repeated at intervals to determine liver and renal function. Hematologic toxicity is a side effect that can be monitored by periodic blood counts.

A more recent treatment in psoriasis is the combination of orally administered methoxsalen (Psoralen) and long-wave ultraviolet light (UVA), hence the name PUVA therapy. Methoxsalen is a photosensitizing agent and does not produce systemic toxicity as may occur with methotrexate. The results of PUVA therapy in one study showed complete clearing of lesions in 90% of the patients.[71] Some side effects of PUVA therapy include pruritus, erythema, localized blistering, a moderate flare-up of psoriasis (Koebner's phenomenon), and transient nausea. The dosage schedules vary and are calculated according to body weight. The person is exposed to long-wave ultraviolet light (320 to 400 nm) 2 hours after ingestion of the methoxsalen. Photochemotherapy in psoriasis causes inhibition of increased DNA synthesis within the psoriatic lesion. Since the skin remains photosensitive until methoxsalen is excreted, persons receiving this treatment are warned to avoid exposure to the sun for at least 8 hours after ingestion of the medication.[71]

Since the lesions are commonly found in visible skin areas, persons with psoriasis are faced with a socially disabling disease. They may need help in identifying and coping with their feelings and with changes that may occur in their life-style (see Chapter 28).

Lesions may fade with treatment, only to recur eventually in the same area or elsewhere. The disease is not curable and may wax and wane continuously. Persons who are not aware of this may lose confidence in the physician and may seek a quick cure. Because psoriasis is so common and so stubborn in response to treatment, manufacturers of patent remedies find a lu-

crative field for their products among persons who have the disease.

Outcome criteria for the person with psoriasis

The person or significant others can:

1. Describe the nature of the condition (noncurable, recurrence of symptoms).

2. Describe the prescribed treatment program.

3. State the problems of self-medication.

4. Describe plans for medical follow-up.

5. Describe plans for socialization with others.

Pityriasis rosea

Pityriasis rosea is a common skin condition with worldwide distribution affecting all races. It occurs more commonly in women and in adolescents and young adults. The cause is thought to be viral, but the disease is not contagious.

The initial symptom is usually a single oval lesion with a thin scaly border and yellowish center appearing most often on the trunk, upper arm, or thigh. This lesion is followed within a few hours, days, or weeks by similar smaller erythematous lesions with the long axis of the oval lesion along lines of skin cleavage and by scaling of the peripheral borders. The skin usually clears in 6 to 8 weeks, and the condition does not recur.

Treatment is essentially symptomatic and includes topical steroids and antihistamines or colloid baths if itching is present. Systemic corticosteroids are effective for more severe cases.

Lichen planus

Lichen planus is a relatively common papulosquamous eruption of unknown origin. Lesions occur initially as shiny flat-topped papules on the flexor surfaces of the wrist, ankles, trunk, mucous membranes, and genitalia. The mouth is frequently involved. Bullous or hypertrophic lesions may also occur. Itching is severe, and new lesions may occur at the scratched sites. Nails may become distorted. Oral or hypertrophic lesions may become chronic. A number of drugs (streptomycin, para-aminosalicylic acid, methyldopa, thiazides, antimalarials) may also cause lichen planus–like eruptions.

Treatment of lichen planus is essentially symptomatic. Corticosteroids may be given as topical therapy under occlusive wraps or as intralesional or systemic therapy. Persons with oral lesions should avoid smoking or ingesting hot or irritating foods or liquids. Acute lichen planus usually resolves in 6 to 18 months, but the chronic types frequently last for more than 10 to 15 years.[41]

Bullous diseases

Pemphigus

Pemphigus is a skin condition characterized by enormous bullae that appear all over the body and on the mucous membranes. The lesions break and are followed by crusts that heal and leave scars. The disease is characterized histologically by acantholysis (cells slip past one another and fluid accumulates between the cells). By placing the thumb firmly on the skin and exerting lateral sliding pressure, the upper epidermis can be dislodged, resulting in erosion or blister (Nikolsky's sign).

The cause of pemphigus is unknown, but it is thought by some to be a type of autoimmune disease. It usually manifests itself in middle age. In more than one-half the patients the first lesion appears in the mouth, and pain from oral lesions may prevent adequate food intake. The treatment of choice for severe pemphigus is systemic corticosteroid therapy. Corticosteroids are initiated early in large doses until the disease is controlled, and then the dose is reduced to an effective maintenance level. Immunosuppressants, such as methotrexate, azathioprine, and cyclophosphamide, may be added to reduce the corticosteroid dose or may be given alone for early localized lesions or for maintenance therapy.

Nursing care of a person with severe pemphigus is very difficult. Foster or Stryker frames may be used in an effort to move the patient as painlessly as possible and prevent weight bearing on raw surfaces. Dakin's solution compresses may be applied to oozing lesions to help control odors and infection. Reverse isolation may be indicated. Special mouth care is usually necessary, and bland diets are more easily tolerated.

Emotional support and encouragement of both the patient and family are extremely important. Patients may fear rejection by others because of their appearance, and they need evidence of continued interest and attention by family and staff. The potential for social isolation is high in this situation. Family and friends can be prepared in advance concerning the patient's appearance, and they are encouraged to visit often and to maintain usual relationships.

Dermatitis herpetiformis

Dermatitis herpetiformis is a chronic skin condition usually seen in men. The lesion is a vesicular, papular, pruritic eruption of unknown cause. There is a characteristic distribution of lesions, usually symmetric, bilateral, and appearing over the surfaces of the limbs, on the buttocks, and on the scalp. Scarring and hyperpigmentation may occur after the lesions heal. Some persons have associated atrophy of the villi of the small intestine that may or may not be accompanied by signs of malabsorption. Treatment is with systemic sulfones, and the response is often diagnostic because of the improvement. Antipruritic medications may or may not relieve the intense pruritus.

Tumors of the skin

Growths of skin cells may develop from the epidermis, from sebaceous or sweat glands, from the melanocyte system, or from mesodermal tissue (e.g., connective or vascular tissue). Most skin tumors are benign, and even those that are malignant, with the exception of some tumors such as malignant melanoma, are often of less serious consequence than tumors elsewhere in the body.

Keratoses

The term *keratosis* refers to any cornification or growth of the horny layer of the skin. There are several different types of keratoses, including corns and calluses, warts (p. 1836), seborrheic and actinic (senile) keratoses.

Corns and calluses

Corns are thickened skin lesions with a center core that thickens inwardly and causes acute pain on pressure. They are often caused by the pressure of ill-fitting shoes and occur on the toes. A corn is best treated by correction of shoes and by placing a small felt pad with a hole in the center over it to relieve pressure. Popular corn remedies seldom produce a cure, since their active ingredient is usually salicylic acid, which only dissolves the outer layer of skin. As soon as the medicated pad is removed, a new layer of skin forms unless pressure is relieved.

Calluses, or thickening of circumscribed areas of the horny layer of the skin, often appear on the plantar surface of the foot when the metatarsal arch has fallen and there is constant pressure against the sole of the shoe. They are often successfully treated by relief of the pressure and by regular massage with softening lotions and creams.

Seborrheic keratoses

The most common benign keratotic tumors seen in older persons are the seborrheic keratoses. The lesions, which resemble large, darkened, greasy warts, are usu-

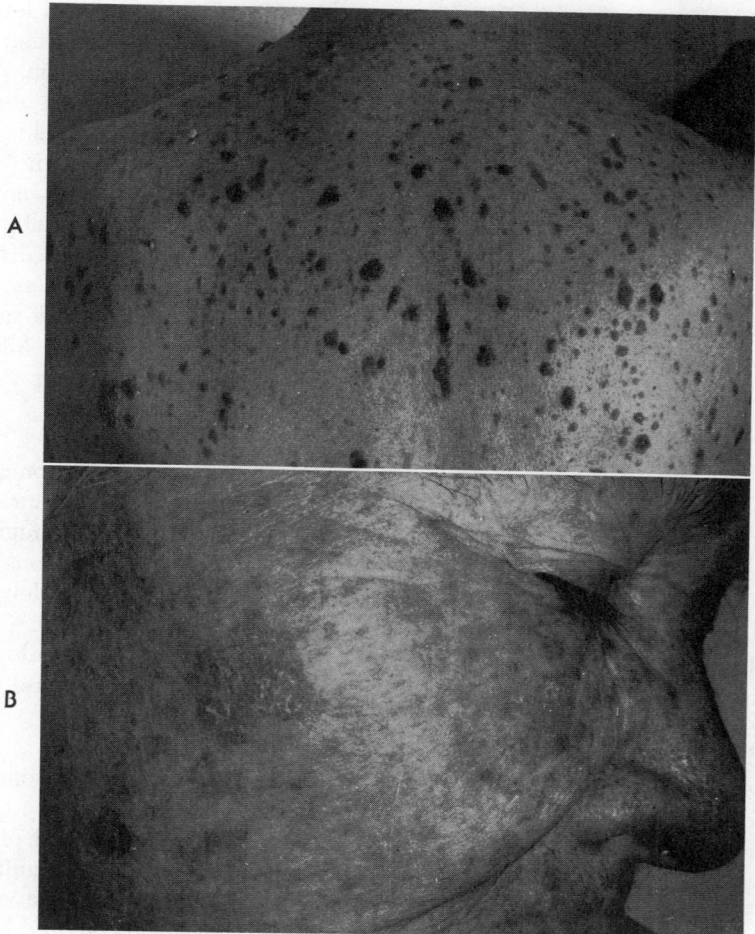

Fig. 71-7. A, Seborrheic keratosis. **B,** Actinic (senile) keratoses. (From Stewart, W.D., Danto, J.L., and Maddin, S.: Dermatology: diagnosis and treatment of cutaneous disorders, ed. 4, St. Louis, 1978, The C.V. Mosby Co.)

ally seen on the trunk but may also occur on the face, scalp, and proximal extremities (Fig. 71-7, *A*). Development of malignancy from seborrheic keratoses is rare, but a sudden increase in the number and size of the lesions may indicate an internal gastrointestinal malignancy. Blacks at an earlier age develop a type of seborrheic keratosis called *dermatosis papulosa nigra* with lesions that are small, pedunculated, and heavily pigmented.[41]

Most seborrheic keratoses do not require treatment except for cosmetic reasons or at areas of frequent irritation. They may be removed with a curette followed by light electrodesiccation or by application of liquid nitrogen.

Actinic keratoses

Actinic (senile, solar) keratoses result from exposure of the skin to irradiation, primarily solar. They are noted most often on exposed skin areas of persons who work outdoors and on older persons. Light-skinned persons are more vulnerable to skin changes from irradiation. The number of lesions can be restricted by the use of clothing and sunscreen lotions over skin areas frequently exposed to the sun. The skin lesions are round or irregular, are red-brown to gray in color, and have a dry, scaly appearance. The surrounding skin is usually dry and wrinkled from overexposure to the sun (Fig. 71-7, *B*).

About 25% of the lesions become malignant (squamous cell carcinoma), evidenced by inflammation and a rapid increase in size of the lesion. The lesions of actinic keratoses are removed by curettage and light electrodesiccation or by cryotherapy with solid carbon dioxide or liquid nitrogen. Large lesions or lesions suspected of possible malignancy are removed by excision. Multiple lesions may be treated with a topical application of a 1% to 5% 5-fluorouracil cream.

Hemangiomas

Hemangiomas are common benign tumors of vascular origin that are present at birth or develop shortly thereafter. There are various types of hemangiomas. Capillary hemangiomas include the nevus flammeus and the strawberry hemangioma. The *nevus flammeus,* or port-wine stain, is a flat lesion commonly found over the forehead and eyelids or at the nape of the neck. Color varies from faint pink to deep purple and is intensified by crying or on exposure to heat or cold. As the child grows, the lesions grow proportionately and may become papular. Treatment for cosmetic purposes is unsatisfactory. Tattooing with flesh-colored pigment may be attempted. Best cosmetic results are usually obtained by covering up the lesion with an opaque make-up.

Strawberry hemangiomas are the most common type and occur primarily on the head, neck, and trunk. Most persons have only one lesion. The tumors grow rapidly during the first 3 to 6 months after birth, becoming bright red lobular masses, and then gradually disappear. Unless ulceration occurs, the lesions heal without scarring. Treatment is instituted only if the growth because of its size produces a gross deformity, develops severe ulcerations, or occludes body orifices. Treatment, which is not entirely satisfactory, may include cryotherapy with carbon dioxide snow, selected irradiation, or systemic corticosteroids.

Senile, or cherry, hemangiomas occur mostly on the trunk of older persons and are small, smooth, bright red to purple, dome-shaped lesions. They usually do not require treatment but can be removed for cosmetic reasons by excision with cautery and electrodesiccation.

Cavernous hemangiomas are composed of large dilated blood vessels and connective and fatty tissue. The color ranges from bright red to blue depending on the depth of the lesion. The lesions do not regress spontaneously. Treatment is unsatisfactory. Plastic surgery may be attempted for grossly disfiguring lesions on the face.

Premalignant lesions

Skin lesions that may lead to malignancy include actinic keratoses (p. 1849), leukoplakia, Bowen's disease, and pigmented moles. The term *premalignant* does *not* infer that *all* of the lesions become malignant but that the tendency to become malignant exists.

Leukoplakia

The mucous membranes of the mouth or vagina may develop a thickened white patch of keratinized cells, which may eventually develop into invasive squamous cell carcinoma. External irritants that appear to have an etiologic relationship to oral leukoplakia include poorly fitting dentures, cheek biting, and pipe or cigarette smoking. Chronic maceration, friction, and senile atrophy may lead to leukoplakia of the vagina.[41]

Preventive measures include removal of potentially causative factors. Persons who continue to smoke need to inspect their mouths for signs of changes. Dentures should fit firmly and comfortably, and dental care should be sought for any rough-edged teeth. Persons with small lesions should seek medical attention for continued observation. Large lesions are usually surgically excised and a biopsy is performed. Benign lesions may be removed by electrodesiccation.

Bowen's disease

Bowen's disease is a chronic skin disease that can be considered as carcinoma *in situ.* It occurs mostly in older light-skinned men and is thought to be related to chemical carcinogens.[49] The lesions are sharply demarcated brown plaques that are widely distributed, although a single lesion may be present. Persons with Bowen's disease are at high risk for developing other malignant disease. Treatment is by surgical excision.

Pigmented nevi

Almost all persons have some pigmented nevi (moles), which usually develop during childhood, becoming more raised and prominent, and often contain hair. Moles, per se, are not generally significant except for cosmetic reasons or for those that develop into malignant melanomas. Small evenly colored brown moles with hair are benign. A blue or greenish-black color does not usually indicate malignancy if the color is even. Changes in moles that should be reported immediately to the physician for further diagnosis include (1) development of a ring of new pigment around the base, (2) development of uneven pigmentation, (3) sudden growth in size, (4) loss of hair in a mole, or (5) bleeding in a mole.[52]

Malignant lesions

Squamous cell carcinoma

Squamous cell carcinoma is a malignant tumor of the surface epidermis that may appear on the exposed skin surface of older persons or at areas of chronic irritation or skin damaged from irradiation or burns. If the growth developed from actinic keratosis, Bowen's disease, or leukoplakia, the lesion will be indurated and surrounded by an inflammatory base. If it is a new lesion, it appears as a firm keratotic nodule with an indurated base (Fig. 71-8). Lesions that develop on hair-bearing skin rarely metastasize, but lesions of the lip or ear frequently metastasize to regional lymph nodes.

Protection of the skin from excessive solar radiation and early detection of lesions are important preventive

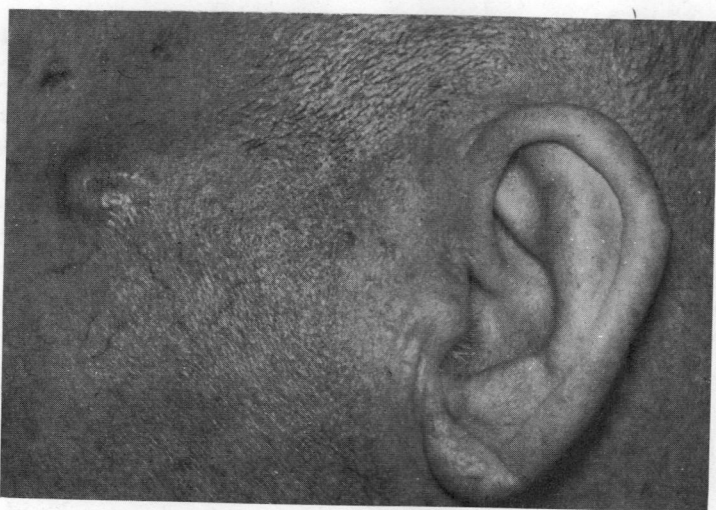

Fig. 71-8. Squamous cell carcinoma in infratemporal area, one of the commonest sites for this tumor. (From Stewart, W.D., Danto, J.L., and Maddin, S.: Dermatology: diagnosis and treatment of cutaneous disorders, ed. 4, St. Louis, 1978, The C.V. Mosby Co.)

measures. Lesions may be removed by surgical excision, curettage with electrodesiccation, irradiation, or chemosurgery. *Chemosurgery* involves application of a dressing with a fixative paste such as zinc chloride and then removal of the dressing with some tissue fixed to it. Reapplication is often necessary until all malignant tissue has been removed. Chemosurgery is used only for tumors without well-defined borders.[41]

Keratoacanthoma

Keratoacanthoma is a skin tumor that has microscopic characteristics similar to squamous cell carcinoma but that is relatively noninvasive and does not metastasize. The lesions occur mostly on normal skin areas exposed to sun, tar, and oils. The tumor grows rapidly to a 1- to 2-cm size, remains quiescent for 2 to 8 weeks, and then begins to regress spontaneously.[41] The dome-shaped, shiny, pink lesion is filled with a keratinous plug that is expelled as the nodule shrinks. The lesion is usually excised and a biopsy is done because of its similarity to squamous cell carcinoma.

Basal cell epithelioma

Basal cell epithelioma or carcinoma is the most common malignant tumor affecting light-skinned people over 40 years of age. It is uncommon among blacks or Orientals. It occurs primarily over hairy areas, those containing pilosebaceous follicles. The growths initially have a characteristic translucent appearance ranging from flesh color to a pale pink with a few telangiectatic vessels across the surface. Since the lesion grows slowly, the center becomes indurated. Basal cell epitheliomas rarely metastasize, but untreated tumors can become locally invasive with severe tissue destruction, infection, and hemorrhage.

Treatment of basal cell epitheliomas depends on the site and extent of the tumor. The four treatment modalities include curettage with electrodesiccation, surgical excision, irradiation, and chemosurgery.

Malignant melanoma

Malignant melanoma is one of the most serious of malignant tumors but is relatively uncommon, occurring in 3% of all skin cancers. It is seen more often in whites than blacks, especially in those who have had frequent exposure to the sun. It may develop from a pigmented nevus or arise from healthy skin and occurs mostly on the head, neck, and lower extremities. The lesions vary considerably in appearance, some with deep pigmentation, irregular borders, and surrounding erythema, and others with irregular pigmentation (yellow, blue, black) and irregular surfaces. The rate of growth is variable. Late changes include bleeding and ulceration. The incidence of metastasis from malignant melanoma is high and depends on the depth of invasion. Metastasis occurs first to the regional lymph nodes and then by hematogenous spread to the lungs and liver and to other areas.

Early diagnosis leads to a more favorable prognosis. Treatment consists of total wide excision, and skin grafts may be needed to cover the defect. Chemotherapy by regional perfusion or systemic therapy, or immunotherapy may be given when metastasis has occurred.

Mycosis fungoides

Mycosis fungoides is an uncommon chronic lymphoma of the skin. The cause is unknown. It occurs in all races, primarily from 40 to 60 years of age. Skin lesions initially resemble those of psoriasis or eczema, but they eventually become indurated and are followed by plaque formation, nodules, and tumors. Pruritus may be present. Lymph nodes finally become involved, and metastasis results. The course of the disease varies among individuals and is often unpredictable.

Early stages of mycosis fungoides can be treated with topical steroids under occlusive wrap or topical nitrogen mustard, intralesional steroids, superficial radiation therapy, electron beam therapy, or ultraviolet light used with or without photoactive medications. More advanced nodular or tumor stages are treated with deeper radiation therapy and systemic chemotherapy.

Skin disorders in blacks

The reported incidence of dermatologic disorders varies among different races, and some disorders are reported to be higher among blacks. Socioeconomic conditions must be considered when intrepreting the data, and the reported incidence may actually reflect poor hygiene, poor diet, or poor health care rather than a racial difference.[49] Disorders that are commonly seen among blacks include lichen planus, follicular syphilis, acne, follicular eczema, and psoriasis. Since the pigment of black skin screens out the sun's rays, those disorders that are affected by solar irradiation, such as squamous cell carcinoma, keratoacanthoma, and basal cell epithelioma, rarely occur.

Pigmentary changes more commonly result from dermatologic disorders in blacks than whites because of the greater amount of melanin present. *Hyperpigmentation* is commonly seen after acne vulgaris, drug eruptions, lichen simplex chronicus, and pityriasis rosea. *Hypopigmentation* may result from atopic dermatitis, tinea, and pityriasis alba. Some dermatologic disorders that are unique to blacks include traumatic alopecia, pseudofolliculitis barbae, keloids, dermatosis papulosa nigra, and perifolliculitis abscedens.

Traumatic alopecia

Black hair shafts are highly susceptible to breakage, and hair loss may result from hair care practices sometimes used by blacks, such as tight hair curlers, cornrow braiding, hot combing, or the use of picks. Wetting or "softening" the hair before the use of a pick may help prevent trauma to the hair. The hair usually grows back when the specific hair practice is discontinued.

Pseudofolliculitis barbae

Hair follicles in blacks are curved rather than straight; therefore the hair curls back as it grows. After shaving, the sharpened point of the hair shaft (especially if a straight razor has been used) acts like a hook and reenters the skin, causing an inflammatory response. The most commonly affected areas include the chin and upper anterior neck. The legs and axilla may also develop pseudofolliculitis from shaving.

The lesions consist of papules and pustules, with some postinflammatory hyperpigmentation. Treatment consists of growing a beard or shaving with a safety razor set at a coarse setting. As the beard is growing, a brush or rough washcloth may be used to dislodge ingrowing hairs. A mild depilatory may be used in place of shaving.

Keloids

Although keloids are seen in all races, they are much more prevalent in blacks than whites. Keloids are hard, raised, shiny growths of collagen tissue that usually originate from a scar and then grow beyond the wound, often with clawlike projections. Keloids occur most often in young adults but may require many years to reach full growth. Highly susceptible areas for keloid growth include the sternum, mandible, ear, and neck. Keloids may recur after simple excision; therefore surgery is often followed by intralesional steroid therapy, radiation therapy, or electron beam therapy.

Dermatosis papulosa nigra

Almost 35% of blacks develop a seborrheic keratosis consisting of small (5-mm) brown or black papules appearing in varying numbers primarily on the face but also on the neck, chest, and upper back. Pruritus may occur but is usually absent. Treatment consists of light electrodesiccation or cryotherapy.

Perifolliculitis abscedens

Perifolliculitis abscedens is a rare, chronic skin disorder seen in black males. It occurs on the scalp, and the lesions consist of numerous firm or fluctuant small nodules connected by purulent sinus tracts. Alopecia and scarring occur in the affected areas. Treatment is difficult. Antibiotics are ineffective, and intralesional steroid therapy provides only temporary relief. X-ray therapy is more effective, but in severe cases scalp excision with split-thickness grafting may be necessary.[41]

REFERENCES AND SELECTED READINGS

1. Arndt, K.A.: Manual of dermatologic therapeutics, ed. 2, Boston, 1978, Little, Brown & Co.
2. Arnold, V., and Rose, S.: Photochemotherapy for psoriasis, Am. J. Nurs. **79:**466-468, 1979.
3. Barnowe, K., et al.: Round table discussion: skin diseases in a rural practice, Nurse Pract. **1:**11-14, 1976.
4. Beeson, P.B., and McDermott, W., editors: Textbook of medicine, ed. 15, Philadelphia, 1979, W.B. Saunders Co.
5. Bergstresser, P.R., Schreiber, S.H., and Weinstein, G.D.: Systemic chemotherapy for psoriasis, Arch. Dermatol. **112:**977-981, 1976.
6. *Billstein, S.: Diagnosis and treatment of lice, J. Sch. Health **47:**356-357, 1977.
7. Black skin problems, Am. J. Nurs. **79:**1092-1094, 1979.
8. Bluefarb, S.M.: Dermatology, Kalamazoo, Mich., 1978, The Upjohn Co.
9. Callen, J.P.: Manual of dermatology: introduction to diagnosis and therapy, Chicago, 1980, Year Book Medical Publishers, Inc.
10. Criep, L.H.: Dermatologic allergy: immunology, diagnosis, management, Philadelphia, 1970, W.B. Saunders Co.
11. *Dobson, R.L.: Diagnosis and treatment of eczema, J.A.M.A. **235:**2228-2229, 1976.
12. Dunagin, W.G., and Millikan, L.E.: Drug eruptions, Med. Clin. North Am. **64:**983-1002, 1980.
13. Felber, T.D., et al.: Photodynamic inactivation of herpes simplex, J.A.M.A. **223:**289-292, 1973.
14. Fischer, R.G.: Acne vulgaris: a common disease, Pediatr. Nurs. **4:**9-14, 1978.
15. Fisher, A.A.: Contact dermatitis, ed. 2, Philadelphia, 1973, Lea & Febiger.
16. Fitzpatrick, T.B., et al.: Dermatology in general medicine ed. 2, New York, 1979, McGraw-Hill Book Co.
17. Goodwin, P., Hamilton, S., and Fry, L.: The cell cycle in psoriasis, Br. J. Dermatol. **90:**517-521, 1974.
18. Hahn, A.B., Barkin, R.L., and Oestrich, S.J.: Pharmacology in nursing, ed. 15, St. Louis, 1982, The C.V. Mosby Co.
19. Hanifin, J.M., and Lobitz, W.C.: Newer concepts of atopic dermatitis, Arch. Dermatol. **113:**663-669, 1977.
20. Hodge, L., et al.: Photochemotherapy in mycosis fungoides, Br. Med. J. **2:**1258-1259, 1977.
21. *Jacobs, P.: Fungal infections in childhood, Pediatr. Clin. North Am. **25:**357-370, 1978.
22. *Jarratt, M.: Viral infections of the skin, Pediatr. Clin. North Am. **25:**339-355, 1978.
23. Johnson, H.A., editor: Symposium on plastic surgery for general surgeons, Surg. Clin. North Am. **57:**847-1131, 1977.
24. *Juranek, D.D.: Epidemiology of lice, J. Sch. Health **47:**352-355, 1977.
25. Kenny, J.A.: Dermatoses common in blacks, Postgrad. Med. **61**(6):122-127, 1977.
26. Kligman, A.M., Mills, O.H., Jr., and Leyden, J.J.: Acne vulgaris: a treatable disease, Postgrad. Med. **55:**99-105, 1974.
27. *Koblenzer, P.: Common bacterial infections of the skin in children, Pediatr. Clin. North Am. **25:**321-337, 1978.
28. Korting, G.W.: Diseases of the skin in children and adolescents, ed. 3, Philadelphia 1979, W.B. Saunders Co.
29. Lever, W.F.: Immunosuppressants and prednisone in pemphigus vulgaris, Arch. Dermatol. **113:**1236-1241, 1977.
30. Levine, G.M., and Calvan, C.D.: Color atlas of dermatology, Chicago, 1973, Year Book Medical Publishers, Inc.
31. *Maher, A.: Mycosis fungoides: nursing care study, Nurs. Times **74:**830-832, 1978.
32. Management of common skin problems, Postgrad. Med. **52:**63-194, 1972.
33. Marisco, A.R.: Ultraviolet light and tar in the Goeckerman treatment of psoriasis, Arch. Dermatol. **112:**1249-1250, 1976.
34. Marlow, D.R.: Textbook of pediatric nursing, ed. 5, Philadelphia, 1977, W.B. Saunders Co.
35. Mathews, K.P.: A current view of urticaria, Med. Clin. North Am. **58:**185-205, 1974.
36. *McNab, W.L.: The "other" venereal diseases: herpes simplex, trichimoniasis, and candidiasis, J. Sch. Health **49:**79-83, 1979.
37. Michaélsson, G., Pettersson, L., and Juhlin, L.: Purpura caused by food and drug additives, Arch. Dermatol. **109:**49-52, 1974.
38. Mihm, M.C., Jr.: Early detection of primary cutaneous malignant melanoma: a color atlas, N. Engl. J. Med. **289:**989-996, 1973.
39. Millikan, L.E.: Superficial and cutaneous fungal infections: diagnosis and treatment, Postgrad. Med. **60:**52-58, 1976.
40. Mohs, F.E.: Chemosurgery for melanoma, Arch. Dermatol. **113:**285-291, 1977.
41. Moschella, S.L., Pillsbury, D.M., and Hurley, H.J.: Dermatology, Philadelphia, 1975, W.B. Saunders Co.
42. *Moss, E.M.: Atopic dermatitis, Pediatr. Clin. North Am. **25:**229-237, 1978.
43. Myers, M.C., Photodynamic inactivation in recurrent infections with herpes simplex virus, J. Infect. Dis. **133**(suppl.):A145-A150, 1976.
44. Nahmias, A.J., and Roizman, B.: Infection with herpes-simplex viruses 1 and 2 N. Engl. J. Med. **289:**667-674, 719-725, 781-789, 1973.
45. Nelson, W.E., editor: Textbook of pediatrics, ed. 11, Philadelphia, 1979, W.B. Saunders Co.
46. North, C., and Weinstein, G.: Treatment of psoriasis, Am. J. Nurs. **76:**410-412, 1976.
47. *Orkin, M., and Maibach, H.I.: Scabies, a current pandemic, Postgrad. Med. **66:**53-62, 1979.
48. *Orkin, M., and Maibach, H.I.: Scabies in children, Pediatr. Clin. North Am. **25:**371-385, 1978.
49. *Parrish, J.H.: Dermatology and skin care, New York, 1975, McGraw-Hill Book Co.
50. Parrish, J.H., et al.: Photochemotherapy of psoriasis with oral methoxsalen and longwave ultraviolet light, N. Engl. J. Med. **291:**1207-1213, 1974.
51. *Pearson, L.B.: Acne: a common clinical entity for the nurse practitioner, Nurse Pract. **2:**28-29, 1977.
52. *Pillsbury, D.M.: A manual of dermatology, ed. 2, Philadelphia, 1980, W.B. Saunders Co.
53. *Rasmussen, J.E.: A new look at old acne, Pediatr. Clin. North Am. **25:**285-301, 1978.
54. Reisner, R.M.: Acne vulgaris, Pediatr. Clin. North Am. **21:**851-864, 1973.
55. Robin, M.: How emotions affect skin problems in school children, J. Sch. Health **43:**370-373, 1973.
56. Rowel, N.: Urticaria, Practitioner **208:**614-621, 1972.
57. *Ruppe, J.P.: Skin infections: their role in health today, J. Sch. Health **43:**373-380, 1973.
58. Sauer, G.C.: Manual of skin diseases, ed. 4 Philadelphia, 1980, J.B. Lippincott Co.
59. *Schmidt, L.M.: Topical dermatologic therapy, Pediatr. Clin. North Am. **25:**191-209, 1978.
60. Shelley, W.B.: Consultations in dermatology II, Philadelphia, 1974, W.B. Saunders Co.
61. *Slonka, G.G.: Life cycle and biology of lice, J. Sch. Health **47:**349-351, 1977.
62. Smith, E.B.: Management of herpes simplex infections of the skin, J.A.M.A. **235:**1731-1733, 1976.

---

*References preceded by an asterisk are particularly well suited for student reading.

63. Smith, J.G.: Letter: treatment of psoriasis with PUVA, J.A.M.A. **239**:525-526, 1978.

64. Soter, N.A., Wilkinson, D.S., and Fitzpatrick, T.B.: Clinical dermatology, N. Engl. J. Med. **289**:189-195, 242-249, 296-302, 1973.

65. Spangler, A.S.: Treatment of depressed scars with fibrin foam—seventeen year study, J. Dermatol. Surg. **4**:65-69, 1975.

66. *Sullivan, B.P.: Patient responses to BCG therapy for malignant melanoma, Am. J. Nurs. **79**:320-324, 1979.

67. Systemic antibiotics for treatment of acne vulgaris, Arch. Dermatol. **111**:1630-1636, 1975.

68. Weinstein, G.D.: Managing psoriasis, Postgrad. Med. **52**:190-194, 1972.

69. *Welch, L.B.: Pediculosis at summer camp, Am. J. Nurs. **79**:1073, 1979.

70. *Willis, I.: Sunlight, aging, and skin cancer, Geriatrics **33**:33-36, 1978.

71. Wolf, K., et al.: Photochemotherapy for psoriasis with orally administered methoxsalen, Arch. Dermatol. **112**:943-950, 1976.

CHAPTER 72

PROBLEMS ASSOCIATED WITH IMPAIRED IMMUNE RESPONSE

BARBARA C. LONG
E. RONALD WRIGHT
WILMA J. PHIPPS

Immunologic alterations occur in a wide variety of diseases, and although knowledge concerning the immunologic bases of these diseases is expanding rapidly, much remains obscured. In some disorders, the immunologic basis is clear cut, such as in allergic disorders, thyroiditis, and immunodeficiency diseases. In some instances, as in systemic lupus erythematosus or pemphigus, immunologic response is known to have a role, but the relative significance of the immunologic factors as compared to other factors is not clear. In still other disorders such as neoplasias the role of the immunologic response as the causative agent of the accompanying pathology is even less well documented.

The biologic basis of the immune system is discussed in Chapter 19. Because immunologic factors are operative in such a wide variety of disorders, much of the information about the disorders is found elsewhere in the text. This chapter will describe the various categories of immune disorders and will discuss in more detail those disorders not described elsewhere.

Classification of immunologic disorders

In the interrelated complex system providing immunologic defense, there are innumerable points at which the system may malfunction. The immunologic disorders that have been characterized reflect nonresponsiveness, blocked responsiveness, misdirected responsiveness, and overresponsiveness. The underlying causes of the disorders may be attributed to genetic or developmental defect, infection, malignancy, trauma, altered metabolic states, or pharmacologic intervention. The severity of the disorders ranges from creation of a minor nuisance (e.g., mild hay fever) to an immediate life-threatening situation (e.g., anaphylactic shock) to a chronic debilitating condition (e.g., rheumatoid arthritis). The disorders may be classified into the following general categories:

1. Immunodeficiencies—deficiencies in the proper expression of the immune response system, parts of the system, or individual cell types within the system
2. Gammopathies—abnormal production of immunoglobulins
3. Hypersensitivities—exaggerated or inappropriate response to specific antigens
4. Autoimmunities—the immunologic attack on self-antigens

Immunodeficiencies

Pathophysiology

Protection of the host depends on an intact immune system. Interference with *development* of cells and tissues of the immune response leads to immunodeficient disorders. Since the cells and tissues of the immune response system develop in sequential fashion, if a defect in that development appears, the se-

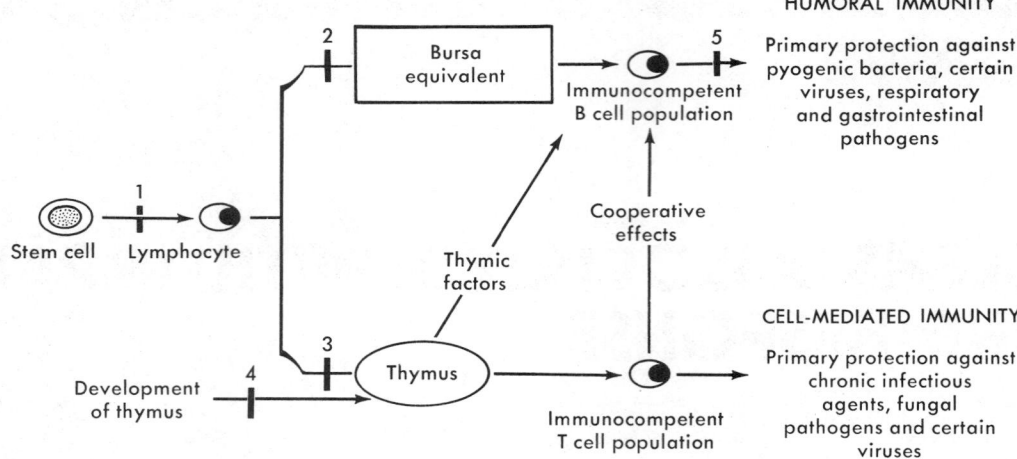

Fig. 72-1. Causes of immunodeficiencies. Abnormalities at *1* result in combined humoral and cell-mediated immunodeficiency. Blockage at *2* produces agammaglobulinemia. Blockage at *3* or *4* results in drastic reduction in T cell—mediated function and, because of cooperative effects on B cell system, some reduction in humoral response. Abnormalities in synthesis of specific immunoglobulin classes are reflected by blockage at *5*. While some blockages result in complete deficiency, others show up as reduction in response.

verity of the resulting deficiency reflects the stage of development at which the abnormality arose (Fig. 72-1). Deficiencies exist in immunoglobulin synthesis, cellular immune functions, a combination of deficiencies, or phagocytosis. The deficiencies resulting from the improper development of the immunoresponsive cells and tissues are termed *primary immunodeficiencies*. The nonspecific depression of immune responsiveness as a secondary result of some interference with the immune system produces a *secondary immunodeficiency*.

Primary immunodeficiencies

The basis of the primary immunodeficiencies and the possible approach to therapy are summarized in Table 72-1. The primary immunodeficiencies are mainly genetic disorders seen in children.

T cell deficiency

DiGeorge's syndrome (thymic hypoplasia) is a classic example of T cell deficiency. The basis of the disease is the absence of the thymus in the neonate. Stem cells cannot differentiate to become T-lymphocytes; therefore the T cell areas of the lymph nodes are underdeveloped. Circulating antibodies are present but at a somewhat reduced level.

Infants with DiGeorge's syndrome usually have hypocalcemia, anomalies of the great blood vessels, notched low-set ears, down-slanting eyes, and a small mouth. Most infants die young. Sometimes the defect is revers-

ible by the transplant of a fetal thymus into the immunodeficient neonate.

B cell deficiency

Bruton-type agammaglobulinemia. In the severe B cell deficiency known as *infantile sex-linked agammaglobulinemia* (Bruton type), the production of all immunoglobulin is grossly depressed and the follicular areas of the lymph nodes lack plasma cells. This disease is found only in boys and is manifested in childhood by multiple infections with pyogenic bacteria. Respiratory tract infections, sinusitis, pneumonia, otitis media, dermatitis, osteomyelitis, and meningitis are common and recurrent in these children. Because the cell-mediated response is intact, these children respond well to antibiotics. Gamma (γ-) globulin is administered prophylactically.

Common variable immunodeficiencies. Some immunoglobulin deficiencies may not become evident until the person is an adult, and these are termed common variable immunodeficiencies (CVI). The deficiencies differ among persons having CVI; these deficiencies are primarily IgA or IgM, although most persons have sufficient IgA. Persons with CVI develop recurrent virulent infections and display a high incidence of malignancies, hematologic disorders, and autoimmune diseases. γ-Globulin may be given during acute episodes, but recurrent pulmonary infections often lead to death from pulmonary insufficiency.[4] Early recognition of infection and immediate antimicrobial therapy for bacterial or fungal infections are important. Pulmonary disease may be prevented by prophylactic regimens

TABLE 72-1. Classification, characterization, and potential reconstitution of primary immunodeficiencies

Deficiency	Basis of deficiency	Potential reconstitution
T cell deficiency		
Nezelof's syndrome	Congenital failure of embryonic thymic development	Bone marrow or thymus grafts
DiGeorge's syndrome	Nongenetic failure of thymic development	Bone marrow or thymus grafts
B cell deficiency		
Bruton-type agamma-globulinemia	Sex-linked depression of all immuno-globulin classes	Human γ-globulin
Common variable im-munodeficiency	Variable degree of ability to synthe-size primarily IgA or IgM in adults	Human γ-globulin
Combined B and T cell deficiency		
Swiss-type immunodefi-ciency	Non-sex-linked defi-ciency of circular-ing antibodies or cell-mediated re-sponse	Transfer factor plus human γ-globu-lin or bone marrow and thymus graft
Wiskoff-Aldrich syn-drome	Sex-linked IgM and T cell deficiency in males	
Ataxia-telangiectasia	Autosomally inher-ited deficity in IgA and IgE	
Phagocytotic cell deficiency		
Chronic granulomatous disease	Sex-linked recessive genetic disease in males producing lack of destruction of phagocytized organisms and particles	None; antibiotic therapy

similar to the pulmonary toilet for cystic fibrosis (e.g., postural drainage, breathing exercises, and inhalation therapy).

Severe combined immunodeficiency disease

The most severe type of immunodeficiency is a combined type in which there is a lack of responsive-ness from both immune systems. *Lymphopenic agam-maglobulinemia*, also known as *Swiss-type immunodefi-ciency syndrome*, characterizes this type of defect. Nei-ther T cells nor B cells develop, and the infant is im-munologically incompetent. On any exposure to the environment, even nonpathogenic organisms can initi-ate a fatal infection. The basis of this deficiency is a stem cell defect that creates an inability to develop

lymphocytes. Until recently, treatment has been pri-marily symptomatic and most children died within 1 to 2 years of life. Success has been obtained in some in-stances by bone marrow transplants with complete res-toration of both T cell and B cell immunity systems.[9]

Phagocytic defects

Chronic granulomatous disease (CGD) in children is an example of a defect in phagocytosis. The disease is characterized by the development of abscesses and granulomas containing plasma cells and macrophages. In persons exhibiting this defect, the polymorphonu-clear leukocytes will ingest organisms and particles, but because they lack a specific digestive enzyme, killing and digestion do not occur. The defect is a sex-linked recessive genetic characteristic appearing only in males; however, the female carriers of the trait have somewhat reduced leukocytic activity. In recent years, some per-sons with CGD have survived to young adult life through treatment of infections with high-dose, long-term anti-biotic therapy and surgical drainage and excision of the abscesses and granulomas.

Secondary immunodeficiencies

Any factor that can interfere with the normal growth or expression of the immune response system can lead to a secondary immunodeficiency. In the nursing care of the adult, these types of immunodeficiencies, al-though not as dramatic, are of greater significance than the primary deficiencies. Secondary immunodeficien-cies are present to one degree or another in most of the major disease conditions experienced by persons in ad-dition to the normal response to aging. Thus when car-ing for a person beyond the age of 60 years or with any acute disease condition, the concepts of immunodefi-ciency must be considered. Situations in which immu-nodeficiency plays a major role include protein-calorie malnutrition, alcoholism, infections (especially viral), autoimmune diseases, lymphomas (including Hodgkin's disease), neoplasia, allergies, trauma, and transplanta-tions. Major stress of any type may affect the immune response as a result of increased corticosteroid produc-tion and alterations in protein metabolism. *Immuno-suppression* may result from medical therapies includ-ing irradiation and drug therapy.

Nutrition and immunity

Malnutrition leads to an increased susceptibility to infection, and conversely, infection leads to increased nutritional requirements. *Protein-calorie malnutrition* is associated with thymic atrophy and reduction in lym-phoid tissue. Primary immune responses and delayed hypersensitivity responses are affected. Persons expe-riencing large-scale burns or other trauma develop protein deficiency, which affects their immune response. Attention to the nutritional requirements of all acutely ill persons can help to prevent acquired immunologic abnormalities.[4] Vitamin deficiencies can also affect the immune response. Vitamin B_6 (pyridoxine) and pantothenic acid deficiencies depress antibody formation and cause delayed hypersensitivity reactions. Vitamin C influences infection primarily by its effect in the healing process.

Induced immunosuppression

There are several ways in which unwanted immune responses can be suppressed by artificial manipulation. Some of these approaches include (1) administration of antigen, (2) administration of specific antibodies, (3) antilymphocyte serum, (4) irradiation, (5) steroid and cytotoxic drugs, and (6) surgical excision of lymphoid tissue.

Antigen administration. Specific antigens can be administered to a hypersensitive person in small amounts over a period of time. The antigenic stimulation forms circulating antibodies of the IgG class that combine with the antigen to block contact with the immunocompetent cells or IgE coated mast cells, thus suppressing the immune response. An adaptation of this method is used by allergists to desensitize persons allergic to specific antigens such as pollens.

Antibody administration. A slightly different method is to administer the specific antibody which then combines with the antigen to block contact with the immunocompetent cell. This method has been used successfully in obstetrics to prevent the sensitive Rh-negative mother from responding to the Rh-positive fetus during pregnancy.

Antilymphocyte serum. The antilymphocyte serum (ALS) is prepared by immunizing a nonhuman species (e.g., a horse) with human lymphocytic tissues (lymph, thymus, or spleen). The ALS is then prepared from the horse serum. The mode of action of ALS seems to be associated with the preferential elimination of lymphocytes from the blood and lymph nodes. This produces a lymphocytopenia; thus fewer cells are available to initiate an immune response. Although this method is effective, its use clinically has been restricted because of the serious side effects of serum sickness, anaphylactic shock, and nephritis.

Irradiation. Both primary and secondary immune responses (p. 288) may be suppressed by irradiation, but suppression of primary sensitization is more effective than suppression of immunologic memory (secondary immune response, p. 290). Irradiation destroys lymphocytes, either directly or through depletion of the precursor stem cells (p. 286). It may be directed at local areas or at the total body. *Local irradiation* of renal allografts has been effective in only selected instances. Local irradiation results in a local destruction of the cel-

lular elements (primarily T cell response) immediately involved in allograft rejection. The best results are obtained by pretreatment of the donor organ.

The effect of *total body irradiation* depends on the size of the radiation dose. The hematopoietic, gastrointestinal, and central nervous systems are affected in that order as the dosage is increased.[34] Unfortunately, the hematopoeitic system is affected at the same dosage level as the lymphoid tissues; hence a sufficient dosage to decrease lymphoid activity will create problems in the hematopoietic system. To achieve sufficient immunosuppression by irradiation, such as before an organ transplantation, bone marrow atrophy leading to pancytopenia usually results.[34]

Drug immunosuppression. A number of drugs affect the immune system (Table 72-2). *Corticosteroids* produce a decreased immune response. The immunosuppressive action is related to several potentially effective mechanisms associated with both natural steroids and synthetic steroid compounds (prednisone and prednisolone). Steroids can cause lysis of lymphocytes, especially in T cell populations. The compounds also serve to inhibit DNA, RNA, and protein synthesis in lymphocytes as well as in macrophages and neutrophils. As a result, the corticosteroids are the most widely used immunosuppressive agents.

Corticosteroids are given for therapy in a large number of diseases. If infections are present, the severity of the infection may increase despite the minimizing of symptoms, as a result of the antiinflammatory effects of the steroids. Persons receiving corticosteroid therapy are highly susceptible to superimposed infections.

Cytotoxic drugs have the potential for *destroying* any cell that is replicating; therefore immunosuppression occurs with the destruction of the rapidly dividing immunologically stimulated cells. Cytotoxic drugs (e.g., antimetabolites, alkylating agents, and selected antibiotics) act by interfering with the basic metabolic processes. B cell reduction is greater than T cell reduction.

Antimetabolites are frequently given in combination with steroids for immunosuppression therapy in order to decrease the dosage of both antimetabolites and steroids, thereby decreasing serious side effects. Azathioprine is the antimetabolite of choice for persons receiving kidney transplantation.

Surgical excision of lymphoid tissue. Removal of the thymus in the neonate alters the immune response; because permanent immunosuppression results, this procedure is rarely done. Removal of the spleen or lymph nodes as a means of immunosuppression is controversial. Splenectomy has been performed for immunosuppression with clinical transplantation, but there is actually little clinical evidence that this alters the immune response.[4,29]

TABLE 72-2. Effect of selected drugs on the immune system

Drug	Immune system impairment	Indications for immunosuppressive therapy
Corticosteroids	Impairment of T cell function Catabolism of immunoglobulins (decreased IgG) Lymphocytopenia Type I hypersensitivity: vasoconstriction, eosinopenia Type III hypersensitivity: decreased vascular permeability Type IV hypersensitivity: decreased macrophage function	Diseases where immune disorder is unknown Tissue and organ transplantation Autoimmune diseases
Antimetabolites (azathioprine)	Interference with RNA, DNA, and protein synthesis Depression of bone marrow and antibody reproduction Decreased primary immune response	Autoimmune diseases Tissue transplantation Dermatologic disease (pemphigus, psoriasis) Neoplasia
Alkylating agents (cyclophosphamide)	Interference with DNA, RNA, and protein synthesis Lymphocytolytic effect Suppression of primary immune response	Autoimmune disease Tissue transplantation Inflammatory disease of unknown cause
Antilymphocytic serum (ALS, ALG)	Inhibition of lymphocyte stimulation by specific antigens Inhibition of lymphocyte mobility Agglutination and lysis of lymphocytes in the presence of complement	Renal transplantation Bone marrow transplantation Autoimmune diseases
Antibiotics (actinomycin D, chloramphenicol, tetracycline)	Interference with DNA-directed RNA synthesis Suppression of primary immune response Inhibition of protein synthesis	None

Assessment

Persons with recurrent infections or who are suspected of having an immunodeficiency should receive a thorough medical evaluation. The type of recurrent infection may give a clue as to the type of deficiency. Recurrent *viral* or *fungal* infections are suggestive of *T cell*–mediated deficiencies. Lymphopenia is often present. Delayed-type hypersensitivity skin tests such as (purified protein derivative) (PPD) or *Candida* antigen or node biopsy may help to establish the diagnosis of a T cell deficiency. Persons with recurrent *bacterial* infections may have an underlying *B cell* (humoral) deficiency. Tests for the presence of B cell deficiency include measurement of serum immunoglobulin levels, skin tests with inactivated vaccines (diphtheria, pertussis, tetanus [DPT] and Schick), and bone marrow studies. Persons concerned about the skin tests can be told that the tests indicate the ability of the body to react to the foreign proteins and that the specific diseases are not thought to be present.

Intervention

Replacement therapy

Treatment of secondary immunodeficiencies consists primarily in treatment of the underlying condition that has affected the immune response. Specific replacement therapy may be given for primary immunodeficiencies. When B cell deficiency is present, γ-globulin or fresh-frozen plasma free of HB$_s$Ag (hepatitis antigen) may be given at monthly intervals. γ-*Globulin* is a purified concentrated solution of antibodies found in normal plasma. It can be given as a prophylactic measure against viral diseases such as measles, German measles, poliomyelitis, mumps, and hepatitis. A dose of 0.01 ml/lb body weight is injected *intramuscularly*. Some localized reaction (tenderness, erythema) may be experienced. For the treatment of immunodeficiency, much larger doses must be given (0.25 to 0.45 ml/lb body weight), and these large volumes are more painful and less well tolerated. When giving γ-globulin intramuscularly, a large-bore (18 to 20) needle is recommended, and the solution should be injected slowly. Large amounts need to be divided and given at separate sites. *Plasma therapy* is better tolerated by the individual than large doses of γ-globulin, and all five immunoglobulins are included in the plasma. Homologous serum hepatitis and transfusion reactions, however, are potential risks with plasma therapy.

Replacement therapy for T cell–mediated immune deficiencies is more complex. *Transfer factor* extracted from the lymphocytes of humans who have demonstrated delayed hypersensitivity reactions has benefitted some persons. Repeated injections are required. *Thymosin*, a thymic hormone, has been effective in some instances in which the T cell precursors are already present. Bone marrow transplants have also been used. Immunotherapy for neoplasia is discussed on p. 509.

Protection from infection

The most important factor in the care of the immunodeficient or immunosuppressed person is protection from infection. If the degree of immunosuppression is *minimal*, careful *medical asepsis* techniques may be the only requirements. This involves good hygiene practices, careful hand washing before touching body areas, and avoidance by the person of other individuals with infections. The person should learn to avoid bumping or breaking the skin, and even minor skin breaks should receive meticulous cleaning and protection. Medical attention should be sought for small skin lesions that do not heal quickly or for larger skin lesions. Skin areas must be examined daily for signs of symptom-free lesions. Injections should be avoided as much as possible, since this involves penetration of the protective skin barrier. Nutrition must be maintained at an optimal level with special emphasis on adequate protein, vitamin, and mineral intake. Fluid intake should also be adequate to prevent tissue dehydration or low urinary output that can lead to skin or urinary tract infections.·

Hospitalized patients with *moderate* immunosuppression who demonstrate leukopenia or lymphopenia are sometimes placed in *reverse* (protective) isolation, although there is question about the effectiveness of this system. The person is placed in a single room with the door closed, and all who enter wear mask and gown and carry out isolation technique. If the person is acutely ill, good mouth care, perineal care, and pulmonary hygiene are important for prevention of infection.

Persons with *severe* immunodeficiency require the highest degree of protection from infection. *Life islands* consist of plastic tents that completely surround the patient's bed. Sterile objects are passed through portholes irradiated by ultraviolet light. Patient care is given by special arm gloves built into the plastic wall. Life islands are more confining for the patient and are used less frequently since the advent of the *laminar air flow units* (see Fig. 25-13). Air flow across the unit is laminar (in layers) to decrease microorganisms moving toward the patient, and the air is filtered continuously through microfilters. Persons who remain downstream from the patient need not wear protection, but anyone approaching or giving care to the patient wears cap, mask, and gown. All equipment is sterilized before entry to the room. It is imperative that measures be carried out to prevent social isolation of the patient. Infants born with severe immunodeficiency disease have been maintained in laminar air flow units for long periods until therapy is successful so that they may survive in the normal environment.

Gammopathies

Pathophysiology

Gammopathies, better termed *hypergammaglobulinemias*, are elevated levels of γ-globulin in serum resulting from the overproduction of whole γ-globulin or nonassociated heavy chains (H chains) or nonassociated light chains (L chains) (p. 284). The normal synthesis of an immunoglobulin is the result of the proliferation and plasma cell differentiation of a single clone of B cells in response to an antigenic signal. In gammopathies, a single clone or multiple clones of plasma cells begin to overproduce immunoglobulin product. If the gammopathy involves a single B cell clone, it is termed a *monoclonal gammopathy,* and the electrophoretic pattern will be characterized by a single sharp peak in the γ-globulin region (Fig. 72-2). *Polyclonal gammopathies* involve the overproduction of virtually all classes of immunoglobulins in response to inappropriate antigenic stimulation. The electrophoretic pattern of polyclonal gammopathies is characterized by a diffuse increase in the γ-globulin curve.

Monoclonal gammopathies

Monoclonal gammopathies (M-type) are commonly referred to as plasma cell dyscrasias. Some plasma cell dyscrasias, such as multiple myeloma and macroglobulinemia, have distinctive clinical patterns. In some instances, electrophoretic changes resembling the clinical forms can be identified but no symptoms are present, and these can be classified as plasma cell dyscrasias of unknown significance (PCDUS).

Multiple myeloma

Multiple myeloma is a monoclonal plasma cell malignancy seen in both men and women and peaking about the mid 50s. It is characterized by widespread bone destruction, anemia, hypercalcemia, and hyperuricemia. These symptoms are traced to the proliferation of plasma cell tumors from the bone marrow into the hard bone tissue causing an erosion of the bone. Frequent recurrent infections (especially of the respiratory tract) and spontaneous pathologic fractures occur because of the production of ineffective immunoglobulins that in turn depress the production of normal antibodies. Renal failure may result from precipitation of urate and calcium crystals.

Supportive care. Ambulation and adequate hydration are vitally important to prevent renal complications from the increased amounts of urates and calcium being excreted in the urine. Fluid intake should be sufficient

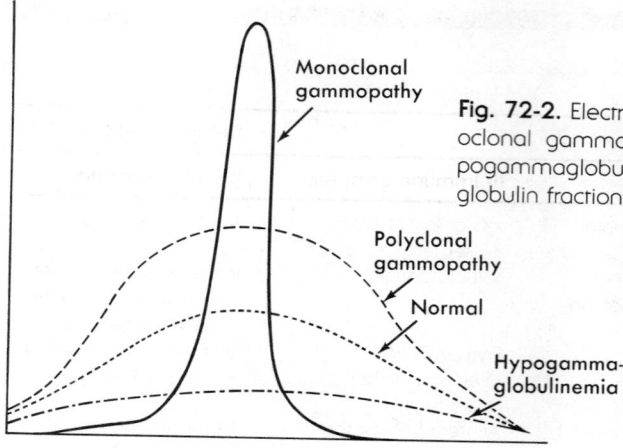

Fig. 72-2. Electrophoretic peaks of γ-globulin fractions in monoclonal gammopathies, polyclonal gammopathies, and hypogammaglobulinemia. Obtained by electrophoresis of γ-globulin fraction of serum.

to ensure a urinary output of a *minimum* of 1500 ml/24 hr. Ambulation may be difficult because of the skeletal pain and the possibility of fractures. A light-weight spinal brace, analgesics, and local radiotherapy may facilitate ambulation.

Measures to prevent infection should be instituted and include avoidance of persons with upper respiratory tract infections. Medical attention should be sought for any signs of infection, and antibiotics are often given since infections are usually caused by gram-positive organisms. Rest periods are planned if fatigue from anemia is present.

Medical intervention. Chemotherapy is the major treatment for multiple myeloma. The alkylating agents melphalan and cyclophosphamide (Cytoxan) are the two drugs most commonly used and may be given alone or sequentially. Several weeks may elapse between the initiation of therapy and signs of improvement. Periods of remission of 6 years or more have been obtained with chemotherapy.

Macroglobulinemia

Macroglobulinemia is a plasma cell dyscrasia involving the overproduction of IgM globulins. Symptoms usually begin in the fifth or sixth decade of life and include fatigue and weakness from anemia, weight loss, and bleeding (mucosal, epistaxis). Blood viscosity is increased because of the increased globulins. Disease progression is similar to a lymphoma (p. 1206). Medical therapy includes plasmapheresis to decrease blood viscosity and chemotherapy with chlorambucil (Leukeran).

Polyclonal gammopathies

Polyclonal gammopathies refer to a diffuse increase in antibody synthesis as a result of inappropriate antigen stimulation. The major causes of the hypergammaglobinemia are infectious diseases (especially chronic bacterial infections such as lung abscess and osteomyelitis), connective tissue diseases (such as SLE and rheumatoid arthritis), and chronic active liver disease. IgG and IgM are the most commonly involved immunoglobulins, and the degree of immunoglobulin levels reflects the severity of the diseases.

The development of high levels of dysfunctional γ-globulins depresses the synthesis of normal immunoglobulins. This renders the person with hypergammaglobulinemia susceptible to infection; therefore carrying out measures and teaching the patient how to prevent infection are major nursing responsibilities.

Hypersensitivity reactions

Pathophysiology

The immune response system that has been immunologically primed or sensitized is designed to provide an immediate, effective, protective reaction to subsequent encounter with the sensitizing antigen. This of course is a positive factor in the provision of immunity; however, under a given set of conditions or because of an idiotypic reactivity to a particular antigen, the response of the immune system may produce detrimental effects. This inappropriate response is usually manifested as a tissue-damaging overreaction to the antigen; thus it is termed *hypersensitivity*, or allergy. The antigenic stimulants invoking the reactions are referred to as *allergens*. Hypersensitivities, then, are classic expressions of the immune system, but they take place in inappropriate sites, in excessive amounts, or with inappropriate involvement of nonspecific tissues. Whether an allergic response occurs and to what degree is dependent on a combination of interrelated factors:

1. *Responsiveness of the host to the allergen*. If the host's sensitivity is extremely high, there is a far greater chance that a tissue-damaging reaction will occur.

2. *Amount of the allergen*. Generally, the greater

TABLE 72-3. Summary of hypersensitivity reactions

Property	Hypersensitivity type			
	Immediate (humoral)			Delayed (cellular)
	I Anaphylactic	II Cytotoxic	III Immune complex	IV Cell mediated
Immune system mediators	IgE (IgG) bound to mast cells	IgG or IgM (+ complement)	IgG or IgM + complement	T cells, macrophages
Allergens	Exogenous antigens	Foreign cells or alteration of cell surface antigens	Soluble antigens	Infectious agent, contact allergens, foreign tissues, cancer cells
Response to intradermal skin test	Wheal and flare within 30 min, edema	Not done	Erythema and edema within 3-8 hr	Erythema and induration within 24-48 hr
Pathophysiologic effects	Release of histamines, kinins, SRS-A from mast cells, which affect smooth muscle shock organs	Direct cytotoxic destruction of cells	Acute inflammatory reaction; primarily polymorphonuclear neutrophil leukocytes	Tissue destruction, primarily lymphocytes and macrophages
Examples	Systemic anaphylaxis, atopic allergies, hayfever, insect sting reactions	Hemolytic disease of the newborn (Rh), transfusion reactions	Serum sickness, Arthus reaction, glomerulonephritis	Tuberculin reaction, skin graft rejection, poison ivy

the amount of allergen contacted, the more severe the reaction.

3. *Nature of the allergen.* Most are complex, high–molecular weight, multivalent proteins, but some may be low–molecular weight nonprotein materials, which exert a haptenic effect when coupled with a normal tissue protein carrier.

4. *Route of entrance of the allergen.* The greatest proportion of allergens enter through the respiratory tract; however, others may enter by epidermal or mucosal contact, injection, or through the digestive tract.

5. *Timing of exposure to the allergen.* If the host's contacts with the allergen are widely separated (e.g., years apart), the immunologic mediators (antibodies or sensitized cells) may be so dilute that there will be less response.

6. *Site of the allergen–immune mediator reaction.* If certain antigen-antibody reactions occur in the tissues, there is no untoward effect; whereas the same reaction occurring within the bloodstream can lead to intravascular inflammation.

Hypersensitivities can be broadly divided into two categories based on the components of the immune system involved in mediating the hypersensitivity reaction: humoral response (B cell mediated) or cellular response (T cell mediated) (Table 72-3). This basic division corresponds with the older clinical symptom division of *immediate* and *delayed,* which was developed before the elucidation of the mechanisms. The terms immediate or delayed were assigned to describe the timing of the appearance of clinical symptoms and the

speed of skin test reactions when a host was challenged with various allergens. This terminology is still used today, but it has taken on new significance in relation to the understanding of the basic mechanisms at work.

It is possible to subcategorize the different manifestations of the humorally mediated hypersensitivities. The most widely used scheme of classification is presented in Table 72-3. As can be seen from this table, the type I, II, and III reactions are mediated by the humoral system, while type IV reactions are those of the cell-mediated system. Since type I, II, and III hypersensitivities are the result of interactions involving circulating antibodies, these reactions can be transferred from a sensitized host to a nonsensitized host by serum transfer. Type IV sensitivities can be transferred by lymphocyte exchange only.

Type I hypersensitivities

Pathophysiology

The most serious life-threatening (anaphylactic and IgE-dependent) hypersensitivity diseases are associated with the reactions mediated by the IgE class of immunoglobulins. These antibodies, also called *reaginic antibodies,* have a predilection for attachment to the surface of mast cells and basophils. The mast cells are found in virtually all tissues of the body and often in close proximity to blood vessels, while the basophils found circulating as one of the leukocytes within the blood. Mast cells are particularly abundant in the skin, nasal region, and lungs. Both mast cells and basophils harbor

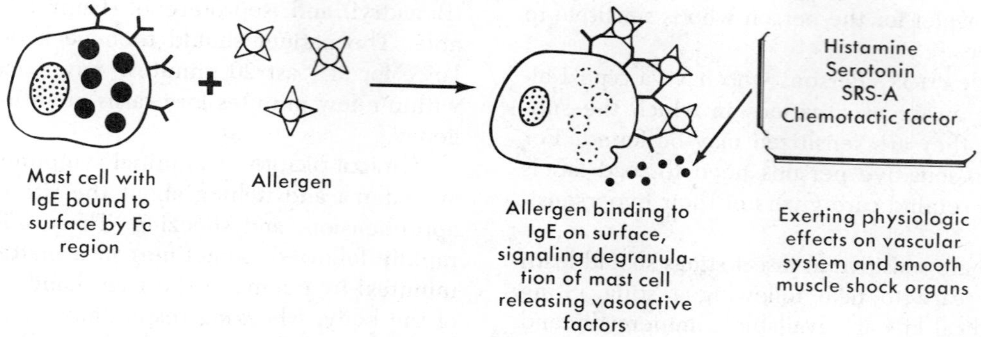

Fig. 72-3. Mediators of type I hypersensitivity.

within their cells numerous, membrane-bound vacuoles containing potent, pharmacologically active substances (histamine, bradykinin, serotonin, and other vasoactive amines). When IgE immunoglobulins bind to the surface of these cells by the Fc portion of the immunoglobulin molecule, the antigen-binding site of the molecule is left exposed to bind the allergen at the surface of the cell (Fig. 72-3). When the allergen is bound to the IgE, the cell is induced to undergo *degranulation*, which releases the internal agents into the environment of the mast cell or basophil. These mediators then cause increased vascular permeability and smooth-muscle contraction.

Of the agents released, histamine seems to be the most important. The direct injection of histamine can mimic many of the symptoms of the type I hypersensitivity, and in the hypersensitive individual a reaction may be assuaged by antihistamines. Other physiologically similar substances are released as well. Thus in type I reactions, the detrimental symptoms are not at the site of the antigen-antibody reaction but at the site of the *shock organs* where the pharmacologically active *anaphylactic mediators* exert their action. If those mediators remain confined to a local area, the tissue reactions remain localized and are referred to as *local anaphylaxis*. The local hypersensitivity that most people demonstrate to a mosquito bite is the classic example of this type of reaction; the intradermal injection of the mosquito anticoagulants produces a wheal-flare type of reaction within a matter of minutes. If, on the other hand, the mediators become released systemically, the response is known as *systemic anaphylaxis*, which can produce *anaphylactic shock*. As is illustrated by the mosquito bite, the mediators are quickly broken down in the body and their effects are reversible.

For type I reactions to occur, the hypersensitive individual must initially come into contact with the allergen that triggers the synthesis of the specific antiallergenic IgE antibodies. This primary contact is known as a *sensitizing dose*. With the synthesis of the IgE antibodies and their attachment to mast cells and basophils,

the individual is rendered hypersensitive. On subsequent contact with the allergen (termed the *shocking* or *challenging dose*), the individual exhibits the symptoms of type I sensitivity. The severity of those symptoms depends on a number of factors: the amount and route of entrance of the sensitizing dose, the amount and distribution of the IgE antibodies, and the amount and route of entrance of the shocking dose.

Anaphylaxis

Etiology. The most severe form of type I hypersensivity in humans is systemic anaphylaxis. Antigens that commonly induce anaphylaxis are drugs such as penicillin or heterologous antiserum, insect stings, pollen, and iodinated contrast media used in selected roentgenographic studies. Persons also have been known to develop anaphylactic reactions to acetylsalicylic acid (aspirin) as it is absorbed into the bloodstream.

Prevention. Severe anaphylactic reactions can be prevented through (1) identification of high-risk persons, (2) patient education concerning avoidance of antigens and actions to take if sensitization occurs, (3) desensitization, and (4) precautionary actions.

IDENTIFICATION OF HIGH-RISK PERSONS. Since persons with a history of allergies are more likely to develop anaphylactic reactions to drugs than those without such a history, all patients should be questioned about allergies and sensitivities to drugs before drug therapy is initiated. If there is any positive history, the physician is consulted before a new drug is given, and if it is given, the patient is watched closely for allergic responses. High-risk persons should wear an identity bracelet or tag at all times that indicates the known allergy. These tags may be obtained commercially.* Hospitalized persons who are sensitive to certain substances should be identified, and the information should be posted conspicuously outside of the room or on the medical order sheets of the patient's record or in both places. In addition, many hospitals use a special color

---

*Medic-Alert Foundation, 1000 N. Palm St., Turlock, CA 95380.

identification bracelet for the person who is sensitive to certain substances.

PATIENT EDUCATION. Persons who have a type I allergy should be aware of situations in which the substance to which they are sensitized may be found. For example, aspirin-sensitive persons need to read labels carefully and to remind care givers of their hypersensitivity.

Persons who are sensitive to insect stings should learn the emergency care to take following a sting. Sting emergency medical kits are available commercially and should be readily available. If a sting occurs, the person should immediately swallow the uncoated antihistamine tablet and place the isoproterenol tablet under the tongue. A family member or friend should know how to inject the 1:1000 epinephrine hydrochloride available in the ampule. Immediate medical help should be sought.

DESENSITIZATION. Persons known to have hypersensitivity of insect stings are recommended to obtain immunizing injections with Hymenoptera extract. The approach is similar to desensitization for atopic allergies (p. 1867).

PRECAUTIONARY ACTIONS. Persons who are known to be allergic or who have received a specific type of animal serum and who must receive antiserum should be given another type, if it is available, in order to lessen the possibility of an allergic response. When it is necessary to use animal serum, the individual should first be tested for sensitivity to the substance. An intradermal skin test preceded by a scratch or eye test is recommended.

If animal sera, allergenic extracts, or contrast media containing iodide are given, a syringe containing 1:1000 epinephrine hydrochloride should be readily available; in addition, an antihistamine such as diphenhydramine (Benadryl) and isoproterenol (Isuprel) should be available. The patient should then be kept under surveillance for at least 20 minutes. Any reaction that occurs within a few minutes forewarns of an impending emergency.

Clinical picture. The initial symptoms of anaphylaxis are edema and itching about the site of the injection, apprehension, and sneezing. These mild reactions are rapidly followed (sometimes in a matter of seconds or minutes) by edema of the face, hands, and other parts of the body; wheezing respirations; dyspnea, and signs of vascular collapse with shock (rapid and weak pulse, falling blood pressure, cyanosis). Death may ensue unless rapid action is taken.

Intervention. At the first sign of anaphylaxis, epinephrine hydrochloride (1:1000), 0.3 to 0.5 ml (less for children), is given subcutaneously. A tourniquet may be applied proximal to the injection site, and epinephrine may be injected into the site. Diphenhydramine hydrochloride (Benadryl), 50 to 100 mg, is injected intramuscularly. Aminophylline may be given to relax bronchial spasm, and tracheal intubation may be necessary to maintain an airway if tracheal edema results. Because shock ensues with severe anaphylaxis, measures to control shock are taken (p. 317).

Urticaria

Urticaria (hives) may occur as an IgE-mediated local anaphylactic response. The pruritic lesions are characterized by a pale pink elevated edge (wheal) on an erythematous background (Fig. 72-4). The lesions are transient and may reappear in different body areas. The allergic form of urticaria is usually caused by foods, especially eggs, fish, and nuts, or by drugs such as penicillins.

Urticaria may also occur in a chronic form from causes

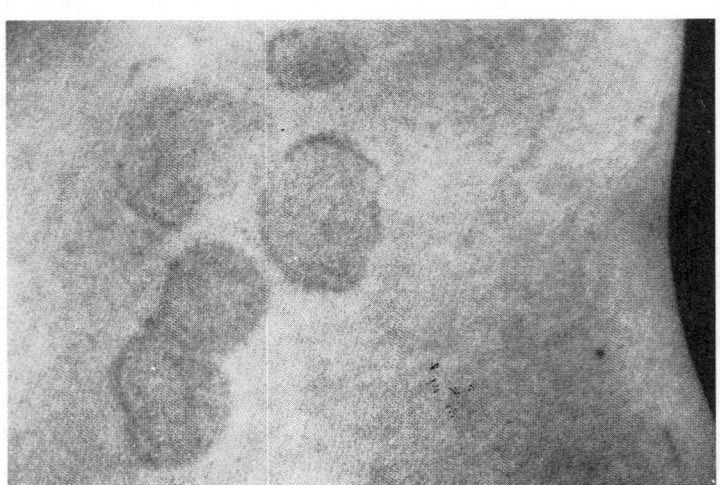

Fig. 72-4. Urticaria. (From Stewart, W.D., Danto, J.L., and Maddin, S.: Dermatology: diagnosis and treatment of cutaneous disorders, ed. 4, St. Louis, 1978, The C.V. Mosby Co.)

other than IgE-mediated hypersensitivity. Etiologic factors in the chronic form include exposure to cold, heat, or various light waves. Another form, cholinergic urticaria, occurs as a response to stress or physical exertion.

Since urticaria is usually self-limiting, treatment is often not required. Known offending agents are removed if possible. Epinephrine and antihistamines may be given to hasten resolution and to prevent further histamine reaction.

Atopic allergy

A less severe form of type I hypersensitivity than anaphylaxis is exhibited in atopic allergies, which have hereditary influences.

Epidemiology and etiology. About 10% to 20% of the population react to antigens that are not antigens for the remainder of the population. These individuals are referred to as being "atopic." This tendency to become hypersensitive is inherited as a dominant trait. If both parents are atopic, there is a high probability that the children will be atopic. What these individuals become hypersensitive to, however, will be determined by the allergens to which they are exposed. Three factors are helpful in understanding atopy: (1) atopic individuals will not form antibodies unless they are exposed to a substance that is antigenic for them; (2) an atopic child is like a blank sheet; that is, the child does not inherit a specific allergy such as hay fever or asthma, but the allergy will manifest itself in response to the allergen or allergens to which the child is exposed; and (3) atopic allergies are the most common form of allergy. The most common allergens for the atopic person are:

1. Foods, which are primarily a problem from birth to 2 years of age and manifested primarily as infantile eczema. Between 80% to 85% of these allergies disappear by age 2 years.
2. Environmental inhalants such as house dust and animal dander, which are primarily a problem from age 2 to 6 years.
3. Seasonal inhalants such as tree and grass pollens and fungus spores, which mainly affect those over age 6 years.

Children who develop eczema from food allergy are highly allergic individuals, and the majority of them (80% to 85%) will develop hay fever or asthma before the age of 6 years.

Environmental and seasonal inhalants are about equally important allergens, but environmental inhalants are easier to control by providing a controlled environment in the home (discussed later in this section).

In order to determine if seasonal inhalants are the cause of an allergic response, one needs to know when trees, grasses, and molds are pollenating in that geographic area. One also needs to know which trees and grasses are insect pollenated and therefore seldom cause an allergic response.

There are several facts about allergens that are helpful for the nurse to understand:

1. Persons who believe they have "rose fever" are really allergic to pollenating grasses; persons who believe they are allergic to goldenrod are really allergic to ragweed; both roses and goldenrod are insect pollenated.
2. Persons may be allergic to the pollen of one tree and not another; therefore there is need to know which tree is pollenating at the time symptoms appear.
3. Persons who are allergic to pollenating grasses will have the same symptoms no matter which grass is pollenating. If they move from one geographic area to another, they will become sensitized to whatever grasses are present in that area. For example, *ragweed* is a grass that causes an allergic response in many persons. It is not present in all parts of the United States, but atopic individuals moving into the ragweed belt of the Great Lakes Basin will become sensitized to it. If these persons later move to an area of the country such as the Pacific Northwest where there is no ragweed, they will become sensitized to another type of pollenating grass.
4. Persons may be allergic to spores of molds and not realize it. A careful history detailing where molds are most likely to be found may be helpful, including (1) inside the house: basements that are warm and damp or, when there is no basement, in crawl spaces under the house; (2) outside the house: leaves of certain trees, wheat, and corn. For both pollens and spores, the highest counts (amounts in the air) occur between 12 midnight and 8 AM.

Clinical picture. Histamine that is released by the mast cells has three main effects: (1) it constricts smooth muscle such as in the bronchi, resulting in bronchospasm and constriction of conducting airways; (2) it increases vascular permeability, resulting in such conditions as hives or mucosal edema in asthma; and (3) it increases mucous gland secretions, resulting in increased mucus production as occurs in hay fever and asthma. Factors influencing an allergic response are summarized in the box on p. 1866. The symptoms seen in the person with a type I hypersensitivity reaction will be determined by the organ affected. The person with hay fever will have sneezing, tearing of the eyes, and watery discharge from the nose; the individual who has asthma will wheeze when the bronchial muscles are constricted; and the person with a skin manifestation will have hives, urticaria, and skin rash. Nausea, vomiting, and diarrhea may also be allergic manifestations (Fig. 72-5).

Assessment

HISTORY. It usually is possible to determine the specific allergens to which a person is hypersensitive by taking a detailed history (see Chapter 68) and then testing for sensitivity.

SKIN TESTING. *Skin tests* are often used to determine whether a person has a sensitivity to certain substances in the external environment. Several methods of testing are used. Small amounts of extracts of various allergenic substances to which the person is suspected to have a sensitivity may be injected intradermally at spaced intervals, usually on the outer surface of the upper arm, on the forearm, or in the scapular region. The extract also may be placed on the skin and the skin scratched lightly *(scratch test)*. These two methods are

used most often to test for sensitivity to pollen, feathers, dander, and dust. They also may be used to test for sensitivity to foods, but the results are often inaccurate. When clothing or other material is the suspected allergen, a small piece of it may be put against the skin under an airtight patch for 48 to 72 hours *(patch test)*. Sensitivity to soaps and other cleaning agents such as detergents is often tested in this way. An infant may be tested indirectly by injecting his or her blood serum at spaced intervals under the skin of a nonallergic person. Twenty-four hours later the extract of the suspected allergenic substance is injected at these sites. Tests for allergenic substances usually are done in series; for example, pollens from trees are tested first and then pollens from grasses. Positive reactions to allergens are indicated by the appearance of a *wheal* or redness at the test site. Occasionally, 1 drop of a test extract is instilled into the eye to test for sensitivity *(conjunctival test)*. Redness of the conjunctiva and tearing will appear within 5 to 15 minutes in an allergic person.

SERUM TESTING. With the recognition of the central role of IgE in atopic hypersensitivities and the development of laboratory tests to quantitate IgE in the serum, clinical laboratory testing procedures may soon replace skin testing. Procedures for identification of total serum IgE or IgE specific for selected antigens may prove to be more quantitative and safer than other techniques.

FOOD DIARY. A person with a food allergy is asked to keep a food diary for at least a week. On the basis of this diary, suspect foods such as milk, wheat products, and eggs may be removed from the diet (elimination

---

FACTORS THAT INFLUENCE AN ATOPIC ALLERGIC RESPONSE (AMOUNT OF REACTION)

Allergen: amount and type

Antibodies: number

Histamine: amount liberated

Tissue: adequacy in preventing histamine from reaching sites

Response: tissue to histamine and other substances released

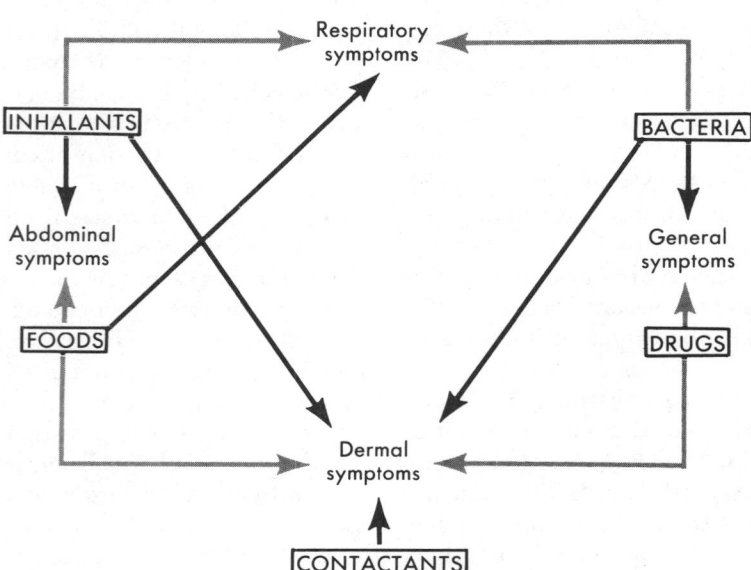

Fig. 72-5. Causes of allergic responses and symptoms produced.

diet) until symptoms subside and then added one at a time in an attempt to identify the offending foods. Babies on this diet often must be given a special nonmilk formula made of products such as soybeans or barley. The mothers need instructions in preparing the formula. A similar elimination process may be used to test for allergy to other substances such as cosmetics or fabrics.

SPECIAL HOSPITAL ROOMS. Some hospitals now have environmentally controlled rooms that may be used to remove a highly allergic person from the usual environment and thus facilitate the search for the substances to which the individual is sensitive. The room is kept free from substances most likely to be allergenic and is air conditioned to prevent inflow of pollens through open windows. The rooms may also be used for treatment. When the symptoms have subsided, various articles used at home may be introduced one at a time to see if they cause symptoms. Only a limited number of staff members are allowed to enter the room, and they may be requested to avoid the use of cosmetics and to wear special gowns.

The nurse may be helpful by providing encouragement to the person who may have to undergo tests that may continue for weeks or months. By suggesting common allergenic substances, the nurse may help the person give a more complete history. Nurses are often called on to help the person plan for elimination testing.

Intervention. The best treatment for an allergy is to prevent the person from coming in contact with the allergen or allergens to which he or she is sensitive. If the allergen is a *food,* it should be eliminated from the diet. Often infants who have food allergies outgrow them by 2 years of age. Infants who could not tolerate cow's milk can often drink it as they grow older. Persons who are sensitive to environmental or seasonal inhalants should be taught how to control exposure to these allergens. This is most often accomplished by having a controlled room (usually the bedroom) in which the person can spend much of his or her time when at home.

PREPARATION OF AN ENVIRONMENTALLY CONTROLLED ROOM. A properly prepared room is especially important for atopic children, since they are apt to be hypersensitive to a variety of allergens.

Persons whose allergies are caused by *environmental* inhalants will need a room free of house dust, animal dander, fungus spores, and other allergens. Because 90% of the airborne particles in the house (e.g., house dust) are 5 μm or less in size, an electrostatic filter will be necessary. An electrostatic filter attracts particles by means of highly charged metal plates, which can be removed for cleaning. These filters come in portable models for room use or can be attached to the central heating system.

The room should also have wooden floors or be covered with linoleum or plastic tile. No rugs other than

cotton throw rugs that can be washed frequently should be used, since carpets trap materials that produce house dust. Closet doors should be rendered airtight by applying weather stripping around the door. It is also recommended that clothes be placed in plastic bags. The closet should be cleaned frequently to prevent accumulation of house dust. Atopic children and adults are often allergic to animal dander, and most allergists will not allow them to have any fur-bearing pets. Goldfish may be a suitable substitute pet. Persons who are allergic to animal dander must also avoid feather pillows and other inanimate articles that may contain animal dander. Only cotton curtains that are made of smooth material and can be easily washed should be used. The bed should have a mattress made from an allergen-free material, such as foam rubber, or be completely encased in an allergen-proof cover. Pillows should be made of a nonallergenic substance such as foam rubber, Dacron, or Acrilan. A room air conditioner may add to the comfort of the individual and is often prescribed by the physician. *Daily damp dusting* of the room should be done to lessen the amount of dust in the air.

The person who is sensitive to *seasonal* inhalants (tree and grass pollens and fungus spores) will benefit from eliminating all outside air from the bedroom. This can be achieved by sealing the windows and installing an air conditioner or an electrostatic window filter. The cost of electrostatic filters and air conditioners prescribed by a physician is an income tax–deductible medical expense.

AVOIDANCE OF ALLERGENS. In addition, some persons with allergies such as those caused by ragweed may be advised to vacation outside of the ragweed area during the peak of the pollenating season. This is possible for many persons and prevents them from having seasonal attacks of hay fever or asthma.

Usually the individual with hay fever will find relief from symptoms after about 30 minutes in an environmentally controlled room; however, the symptoms of the individual with asthma will not be relieved until all antigenic inhalants are removed from the environment. This may take days or weeks to accomplish. Experience has shown that individuals who understand what they are hypersensitive to can remain symptom free for years if they avoid these allergens. Since the antibodies to the allergens are always present in the body, the individual will have symptoms if he or she comes in contact with the offending allergen. This is especially true of animal dander, and parents should understand that atopic children can probably never have a fur-bearing pet.

DESENSITIZATION. Sometimes an attempt is made to slowly desensitize a patient by injecting small but increasingly larger doses of the allergen at regular intervals (usually 1 to 4 weeks) over a long period. This treatment may take years, or it may have to be continued indefinitely. It is about 80% effective against hay fever but less effective against asthma and dermatitis. It is essential that the individual (or the parents, if the patient is a child) understand that desensitization is of little value until the environment is controlled; otherwise the constant exposure to allergens will only increase antibody response.

When a person has been desensitized to a particular food, the food may be resumed, but only small amounts should be taken at first. If any symptoms develop, the food is stopped and the physician is notified.

Specific care of the patient with asthma is discussed on p. 1327; care for the patient with allergic dermatitis is discussed on p. 1842.

MEDICATIONS. Persons who are allergic may take maintenance medications to prevent an allergic attack or will require medication during an attack. Medications used to prevent an attack include preparations such as ephedrine, aerosolizide bronchodilating agents, and cromolyn sodium (Aarane). All of these drugs may be prescribed for persons with asthma. Cromolyn sodium has been found to be effective in the treatment of patients with chronic asthma. It works by partially or completely preventing the release of histamine and slow-reacting substance of anaphylaxis (SRS-A) from mast cells coated with IgE, which is sensitive to the offending allergen. *Cromolyn sodium should not be used to treat an asthmatic attack*, since the histamine and SRS-A have already been released.

Antihistamines are commonly used to prevent and treat hay fever. They have a tendency to produce drowsiness and should be taken at times when alertness is not essential. Persons taking antihistamines should not drive motor vehicles or operate machinery.

During an acute allergic reaction, epinephrine (Adrenalin) is commonly administered. The corticosteroids also may be given. These compounds tend to (1) inhibit degranulation of and histamine release from mast cells, (2) decrease edema, (3) relax smooth muscles, and (4) relieve constriction of bronchial mucosae. When corticosteroids are prescribed, the person should be tuberculin tested first; if results are positive, the person should be given isoniazid therapy (see p. 1303 for discussion of this precaution).

Outcome criteria for the person with atopic allergy. The person or significant others can:

1. Explain what substances are allergens and must be avoided.
2. Describe in detail how to prepare an environmentally controlled room.
3. Describe measures to be taken during periods of high pollen counts (restrict periods out of doors, remain in air-conditioned environment).
4. Describe dietary restriction, if any; relate how daily nutritional needs will be met.
5. Explain each medication prescribed in terms of expected action, route and frequency of administration, expected side effects, and precautions to be observed when taking medications.
6. List signs and symptoms that require immediate medical intervention (asthma attack not relieved by usual means).
7. Describe plans for ongoing health care.

Type II hypersensitivities

Pathophysiology

The underlying mechanism of type II, (cytotoxic) hypersensitivities involves the direct binding of IgG or IgM immunoglobulins to an antigen on the surface of a cell. This antibody labeling then triggers the destruction of the cell by phagocytic attack, nonspecific lymphocytic attack, or lysis of the cell through the operation of the full complement cascade (p. 278).

Blood transfusion reactions

The type II hypersensitivity is classically illustrated by the reactions that occur in mismatched blood transfusion reactions. Blood replacement therapy is used when there has been excessive blood loss (whole blood or blood components) or in treatment of diseases of the hematopoietic system. Replacement therapy may be whole blood or one or more of the blood components (Table 72-4). Blood transfusions are not without dangers to the recipient; therefore the transfusion of 1 unit (500 ml) of blood for minor therapy is not usually recommended.

Pathophysiology. There are many antigens on the surface of red blood cells, but there are two major systems that are significant clinically in terms of potential immunologic reactions—the ABO system and the Rh system.

ABO SYSTEM. There are four major blood groups that exist in humans: *A*, when antigen A is present; *B*, when

TABLE 72-4. Types of blood replacement

Component	Indications
Whole blood	Loss of blood volume (trauma, surgery)
Packed red cells	Anemias
	Liver and kidney disease
Washed red cells	Febrile reaction after receiving leukocyte-poor red cells
Leukocyte-poor red cells	Febrile transfusion reactions
Frozen red cells (leukocyte free)	Prospective transplant recipients
Platelet concentrate	Thrombocytopenia
Cryoprecipitate (antihemophilic factor)	Hemophilia
γ-Globulin	Prophylaxis for certain virus diseases
	Immunodeficiency disease
Plasma	Shock
Fresh-frozen plasma	Immunodeficiency disease

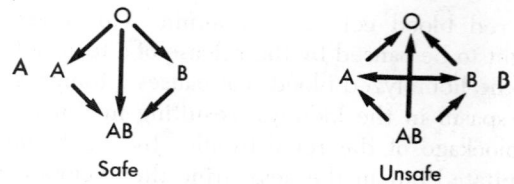

Fig. 72-6. Blood groups and the groups each can receive blood from and give blood to. **A,** Safe. **B,** Unsafe.

antigen B is present; *AB*, when both of the antigens A and B are present; and *O*, when neither antigens A nor B are present. Since type AB blood contains both antigens, persons with type AB may receive blood from any type (Fig. 72-6). Persons with type *O* may donate blood to other types, but since both antigens are absent in type *O*, they may not receive another type without experiencing a reaction.

Within the serum, individuals possess naturally occurring antibodies to the red blood cell surface antigens of the ABO blood groups that are not present on their own erythrocytes. Thus a person with type A blood will possess anti-B antibodies within the serum. These antibodies, called *isohemagglutinins*, are usually of the IgM class. They are thought to arise through a natural immunization to the glycopeptide antigens on the red blood cell surface through contact with similar glycopeptide found on the surface of the cell walls of bacteria that make up the natural flora of the gut. Antibodies formed in this way are capable of cross-reacting with the A or B antigens on the surface of the "foreign" ABO types. Since these antibodies are naturally present in the serum, on transfusion mismatched blood will be immediately coated by the isohemagglutinins, causing agglutination of the introduced cells and the rapid lysis of the cells by complement. The products released by the lysed cells are then dumped into the bloodstream.

RH SYSTEM. The Rh system is more complex because there are at least 27 different antigens in this system. The D antigen is the most significant clinically since it is more immunogenic than any other Rh antigen, and it is usually the antigen involved in hemolytic disease of the newborn. When the term *Rh positive* is used, the presence of antigen Rh-D is implied; *Rh negative* indicates the absence of antigen D. Approximately 85% of the population have Rh-positive blood.

When an Rh-negative person is first exposed to Rh-positive blood, Rh antibodies are formed. On subsequent exposures to Rh-positive blood, the Rh antibody binds to its corresponding antigen on the surface of the red blood cells containing the Rh antigen. The Rh antibodies do not usually fix complement; therefore there is no immediate hemolysis as occurs in the ABO system. Instead, the Rh-antigen red blood cells are rapidly broken down by macrophages in the spleen, with conversion of hemoglobin to bilirubin resulting in jaundice.

HLA SYSTEM. Another system that has clinical signif-

icance in blood transfusions is the human leukocyte antigen (HLA) system (p. 1873). HLAs are found on many types of tissue cells and on blood leukocytes and platelets. The system is more complex than the red blood cell antigen systems, and there are literally thousands of combinations of the antigens that may occur.[50] Sensitization may occur through pregnancy or through exposure to platelets and white blood cells during transfusions. Repeated transfusions of blood cells may lead to transfusion reactions.

Prevention of reactions. The frequency of blood transfusion reactions is unknown but is estimated to be 2% to 3%. Approximately 8 million units of blood are administered in the United States annually; therefore over 160,000 transfusion reactions can be expected yearly.[9] Measures to prevent reactions thus assume major importance, since acute hemolytic reactions can be fatal.

DONOR PRESCREENING. Prescreening of potential blood donors is essential. Blood received from volunteer donors through the American Red Cross Blood Service or hospital blood banks is preferable to that of paid donors, because paid donors may be less likely to report present or previous diseases that may affect the recipient. Requirements have been delineated that include guidelines for persons with heart, lung, liver, or kidney disease. Persons who are not accepted as donors include those with a history of (1) infectious diseases such as hepatitis, tuberculosis, syphilis, or malaria; (2) malignant disease; (3) allergies or asthma; and (4) polycythemia vera or abnormal bleeding tendencies. Temporary deferments include pregnancy, recent major surgery, hypotension, and anemia. The donor's hemoglobin level is tested before giving blood, and the hemoglobin acceptance level should be above 13.5 g/100 ml for men and 12.5 g/100 ml for women.[26] Temperature, pulse, and blood pressure should be within normal ranges. Children and elderly persons are also excluded in order to protect the donor from adverse effects of blood loss. Donors should allow at least 8 weeks between blood donations and should not give blood more than five times a year.

After the blood has been collected, the blood group and subgroups including Rh typing are identified, and the blood is tested for syphilis and hepatitis. The blood *must* be cross-matched with blood from the recipient in order to determine compatibility to prevent an acute hemolytic reaction. Crossmatching consists of mixing samples of the donor's blood and the recipient's blood and examining for cell clumping or hemolysis. A major crossmatch is between recipient serum and donor cells; a minor crossmatch is between recipient cells and donor serum. The minor crossmatch is rarely performed, because donor antibodies are greatly diluted by the recipient's plasma; therefore the major crossmatch usually suffices.

ADMINISTRATION SAFEGUARDS. Most of the serious reactions that now occur during transfusions are the result of human error. Crossmatching and testing in the laboratory must be accurate. Blood must be kept cold until ready to use. If blood has remained at room temperature for more than 30 minutes, it should not be returned to refrigeration and then reissued; this contributes to growth of gram-negative organisms that can produce serious septicemia.[38] Blood being administered to the patient should be given within a 4-hour period. The unit of blood must be labeled with the name of the person for whom it is intended, and this label must be checked against the patient's wristband before the blood is administered. The patient must be monitored throughout the administration of the blood. All blood products should be administered through filters.

Complications of blood transfusions

IMMUNOLOGIC TRANSFUSION REACTIONS. Several immunologic reactions can occur with the administration of blood; these reactions are listed in Table 72-5. The most serious reaction is the acute hemolytic reaction, which occurs during administration of the first 50 ml of blood transfusion. If symptoms appear, the blood flow is stopped immediately, but an intravenous line is kept open with normal saline solution in the event that shock occurs. Several hours after a hemolytic transfusion reaction, the urine becomes red (port-wine urine), and the urinary output is diminished. The urine contains red blood cells and albumin. This reactions is thought to be caused by the release of a toxic substance from the hemolyzed blood that causes a temporary vascular spasm in the kidneys, resulting in renal damage and blockage of the renal tubules by the hemoglobin precipitated out in the acid urine (hemoglobinuria). If the patient receives more than 100 ml of incompatible blood, irreversible shock with complete renal failure may occur, and death may follow.

As blood cells disintegrate (lyse), large amounts of potassium are released into the bloodstream; and if the renal function is impaired, hyperkalemia will develop. If this condition occurs, the patient may be treated with renal dialysis (p. 1584). Shock, disseminated intravascular coagulation (DIC) (p. 1201), and renal shutdown are treated as they occur. Since fever is a sign of both acute hemolytic reaction and the less serious pyrogenic reaction, the transfusion is stopped until the diagnosis is made. If an allergic reaction is present, the transfusion is usually continued with concomitant therapy (antihistamines, epinephrine).

Symptoms of transfusion reactions are nonspecific; therefore errors may be made in diagnosis. Persons receiving blood transfusions are usually seriously ill, and many of the symptoms may be caused by the underlying medical condition. Persons are monitored carefully for any changes in existing symptoms, and these are reported immediately to the physician.

TABLE 72-5. Immunologic reactions to blood transfusions

Reaction	Cause	Mechanism	Symptoms	Occurrence	Action
Acute hemolytic	Recipient has antibody with which transfused red cells are incompatible	Red cells agglutinate, rapid hemolysis Capillary plugging (type II hypersensitivity)	Headache Lumbar pain Constriction of chest Nausea, vomiting Chills, fever Hemoglobinuria Signs of shock, DIC, renal shutdown	Shortly after initiation of transfusion	Transfusion stopped Saline continued IV Blood unit and blood sample from patient sent to laboratory for immediate testing Treat for shock, DIC, renal shutdown as they occur.
Delayed hemolytic	Anamnestic immune response	Slow hemolysis	Jaundice Anemia	Days to weeks after transfusion	Monitor adequacy of urinary output and degree of anemia
Allergic	Transfer of an antigen or a reaginic antibody from donor to recipient	Immune sensitivity to foreign serum protein (type I hypersensitivity)	Urticaria Wheezing Dyspnea Bronchospasm	Within 30 min after initiation of transfusion	Mild: give antihistamine, continue transfusion Severe: give aqueous epinephrine (0.5 ml of 1:1,000 IM)
Pyrogenic	Reaction of antigen other than on RBC (WBC, platelets) Bacterial contamination	Leukocyte agglutination Bacterial pyrogens	Fever, chills Flushing Palpitations Tachycardia	Within 30-90 min after initiation of transfusion	Stop transfusion Treat symptomatically (antipyretics) after ascertaining that acute hemolytic reaction is not occurring Transfuse with leukocyte-poor blood or washed RBC

NONIMMUNOLOGIC REACTIONS. Complications other than those of immunologic origin may also occur. *Fluid volume overload* (p. 333) is one of the more frequent reactions, especially in children, elderly persons, persons with congestive heart failure, or persons who are severely anemic (less than 4 to 5 g/100 ml).[9] Fluid overload may be prevented by the use of packed cells in place of whole blood. If symptoms of hypervolemia occur, the rate of the infusion is slowed or stopped depending on the severity of symptoms.

Air embolism may result when blood is administered under air pressure following severe blood loss. If an embolus should occur, the transfusion is stopped immediately, and the patient is positioned in left side-lying Trendelenburg's position to divert the air away from the pulmonary artery. *Disease transmission* of hepatitis, malaria, syphilis, and cytomegalovirus disease may also result from blood transfusions.

COMPLICATIONS OF MASSIVE BLOOD REPLACEMENT. When blood is administered in large amounts over a short period of time (exchange of one blood volume within 24 hours),[38] additional problems may occur. Platelets deteriorate rapidly in stored blood, and *thrombocytopenia* with abnormal bleeding may result. Infusions of cold blood may stimulate *cardiac arrhythmias;* therefore large amounts of blood given rapidly should be warmed during administration. Blood-warming equipment consisting of coils that warm the blood can be used, or the blood may be warmed by placing part of the transfusion tubing in a water bath warmed to body temperature (37° C [98.6° F]).

Electrolyte imbalances may also result from transfusion of large amounts of stored blood preserved by the addition of acid citrate dextrose (ACD). Increased potassium that results from the breakdown of red blood cells can be a severe problem in the person with renal insufficiency. *Hypocalcemia* may result from the binding of the sodium citrate with serum calcium ions. This can be aggravated by preexisting liver disease or by hypothermia.[38]

Pheresis therapy. A newer therapy (pheresis) involves the separation and removal of selected blood components from an individuals's blood.[60] Persons may experience overproduction or malfunctions of one or more blood components. Blood may be removed, centrifuged to remove selected components, and then returned to the person. This can be done manually, removing not more than 500 ml at one time, or by means of a continuous-flow centrifuge machine (blood-cell separator). The continuous-flow centrifuge machine pumps blood from the patient's arm, through the centrifuge machine, and then back into the other arm.[60] The patient is monitored for signs of hemorrhage, pyrogenic reaction, hypovolemia or hypervolemia, and electrolyte imbalance.

Type III hypersensitivities

Pathophysiology

The pathogenesis of the type III (immune complex) hypersensitivities lies in the union of soluble antigen and immunoglobulins of the IgM and IgG classes. The complexes formed in these interactions are not properly cleared by the reticuloendothelial system because of the small size of the complexes, which tend to defy phagocytosis. They are deposited in the body tissues. The complexes can then bind complement with all the attendant reactions of an internal, often intravascular, inflammatory response. The chemotactic factors released with the involvement of complement lead to an influx of phagocytes, which tend to intensify the inflammation. The clinical symptoms observed are the result of the amounts and relative proportions of the antigens and antibodies and the distribution of the complexes within the body.

Arthus reaction

The repeated subcutaneous injection of a highly antigenic soluble antigen can lead to the formation of such *immune complexes*, which trigger a localized inflammatory response known as *Arthus reaction*. The region exhibiting Arthus reaction shows the following sequential tissue changes: reduction of blood flow, development of microthrombi in the venules, increased permeability of the venule to the point that red blood cells escape into the surrounding tissues, development of edema, massive infiltration of the site by polymorphonuclear neutrophil leukocytes, and tissue destruction. Arthus' reactions are not of great clinical importance, since strongly antigenic substances are not usually administered in repeated subcutaneous injections. However, a disseminated type of intravascular inflammation, known as allergic vasculitis, sometimes occurs in patients undergoing therapy with certain drugs (e.g., sulfonamides, iodides, thioureas, and penicillin).

Serum sickness

Etiology. A type III hypersensitivity of clinical significance is serum sickness, which can develop from 1 to 3 weeks after the administration of a large amount of foreign serum (e.g., horse serum). This classic type of serum sickness occurs less frequently than in the past with the decreasing use of foreign serum administration; however, serum sickness reactions may also occur with the administration of certain drugs, particularly antimicrobials such as penicillin.

Pathophysiology. The critical factor in this hypersensitivity reaction is a large amount of a persisting soluble antigen, the foreign serum proteins. The antigen initiates an immune response, and the resultant antibodies begin to appear in the blood about 1 week later where they interact with the antigen still present in the bloodstream. The complexes are deposited within the blood vessel walls. Complement is bound, and an intravascular inflammation occurs.

Clinical picture. Itching and discomfort at the injection site are usually the first symptoms noted. These are followed by lymphadenopathy, fever, urticaria or erythematous rash, angioedema of the face, and joint pain. Splenomegaly, abdominal pain, headache, nausea, and vomiting may also occur. Objective signs of arthritis may be present.

Intervention. Serum sickness is a self-limiting disease. Mild symptoms respond well to antihistamines and salicylates. More severe symptoms are treated with a steroid such as prednisone, with relief of symptoms often obtained within hours. Epinephrine is given if an anaphylactic reaction occurs.

Type IV hypersensitivities

Pathophysiology

Type IV hypersensitivities are cell mediated (delayed type), involving T cells. Antigens identified as "foreign" to the body can cause a reaction in two ways—by direct or by indirect action. The T-lymphocyte can destroy the antigen directly by attaching itself to the antigen cell wall, breaking down the cell membrane and causing lysis and death of the cell. This direct action approach appears to be a major factor in allograft rejections.[4] The indirect approach consists of activating nonspecific phagocytic cells (macrophages and polymorphonuclear leukocytes) through release of lymphokines by the sensitized T-lymphocytes (p. 289).

The cell-mediated immune mechanisms function in host defense against chronic bacterial and fungal infections, in rejection of foreign tissue cells, and in surveillance for cancer cells; however, they can also produce adverse effects in the form of delayed-type hypersensitivity. Three major areas of clinical concern are (1) hypersensitivity reactions in response to infections by certain bacteria, fungi, or viruses; (2) contact dermatitis reactions; and (3) tissue transplant rejections.

Hypersensitivity reactions in certain infections

The body's reaction to the tubercle bacillus (*Mycobacterium tuberculosis*) is a classic example of a type IV hypersensitivity. The organism itself is not directly toxic to human cells or tissues. As a result, the tubercle bacillus may invade the tissues of a nonsensitized host and establish residence in the host tissues, causing virtually no damage. However, in the course of time, as the organism sheds antigenic material, the cell-mediated immune response system is triggered. The sensitized lymphocytes and the activated macrophages attack not only the organism but also the tissues sur-

rounding the organism. This process is aimed at destroying the foreign organism; but in the course of the attack, tissue destruction may result. The lesions associated with tuberculosis (such as caseation necrosis cavitation) and general toxemia are results of the hypersensitivity.

Following the initial sensitization with the infectious organism, subsequent contact with the tuberculosis organism or even an extract of a purified protein from the organism will elicit a hypersensitivity reaction. This is the basis of the Mantoux tuberculin skin test (p. 1303). The skin rashes of smallpox and measles and the lesions of herpes simplex virus and tuberculoid leprosy have all been attributed to an infectious type IV hypersensitivity.

Allergic contact dermatitis

Allergic contact dermatitis is one of the most commonly encountered types of human allergic disease. Usually, both the route of sensitization and the display of symptoms are produced by direct dermal contact with the allergen. Many simple chemicals can serve as contact allergens. Among those most often implicated are industrial chemicals, topical ointments, soaps, dinitrochlorobenzene (DNCB), nickel, mercury, topical antibiotics, cosmetics, and the catechols of poison ivy, poison oak, and poison sumac.

Many of the contact allergens are of a size (less than 10,000 molecular weight) and structure that do not allow them to serve as a complete antigen (p. 283). It is most probable that the compound attaches to proteins of the skin and functions as a hapten to stimulate the proliferation of a T cell population sensitized to the compound. Following sensitization, subsequent contact with the contact allergen leads to the formation of an erythematous, vesiculated (blistered) lesion. The inflamed area itches, burns, or stings. Scratching the lesion may further spread the allergen or infect the site. There is often a serous exudate. (For care of the person with contact dermatitis, see p. 1841.)

Tissue transplantation rejection

The rejection of foreign cells and tissues by the body is a beneficial function of the immune system primarily mediated by a type IV hypersensitivity. If it were not for this mechanism, the human body would be a haven for the inappropriate establishment of growth of any animal cell that penetrated the external defense mechanisms; however, this process is regarded as a disservice when it operates to prevent the positive aspects of the exchange of tissues between hosts.

The transfer of healthy tissues and organs from one individual to replace damaged or diseased tissues of another has been surgically possible for many years. The early attempts at tissue graft failed because of the rejection process. With the growing knowledge of the immune response, the mechanisms of this rejection process became more apparent, and it is now possible to make judgments and predictions concerning the likelihood of success of such an endeavor. Recently, with this newly acquired knowledge it has become possible to control the course of the graft transfer process to favor the acceptance of the transplanted tissues. Today certain tissues can be transferred with a high expectation for success if the "rules" for prevention of rejection are followed.

The following terminology has been derived to describe transplants between individuals and species. It is based on the genetically derived discrepancies and similarities between the donor and the recipient.

autograft Transfer of tissue from one site on an individual to another site; since this simply means the rearrangement of self, immunologically there is little concern.

isograft Transfer of tissue between syngeneic (identical genetic makeup) individuals, such as identical twins; since there is no genetic discrepancy in antigens, the immunologic factors favor success.

allograft Transfer of tissues between allogeneic (same species but exhibiting different genetic makeup) individuals; since the tissues of the donor are foreign to the recipient, they are antigenic and subject to rejection.

xenograft Transfer of tissues between xenogeneic (different species) individuals; since the genetic differences are enormous, there is virtually no chance of avoiding immunorejection.

The allograft tissue transfer offers the most promise for organ and tissue replacement and is the one currently receiving the most experimental attention. Blood transfusion is the most common allografting procedure used today, and notwithstanding the problems associated with transfusion (p. 1868), it is carried out daily with success. Solid-tissue grafts such as skin and organs, however, introduce considerably greater problems.

Pathophysiology. The antigenic determinants of the tissues that lead to graft rejection are primarily found on the surface of the cells within the transplanted tissues. These antigens are known as *histocompatibility antigens* and are controlled by independently segregating genes within the chromosomal structure of the animal. They are also called HLAs (human leukocyte antigens). Some of the histocompatability antigens are more antigenic than are others; thus some antigens are referred to as major and others as minor. The major transplantation antigens are those of the ABO and Rh blood groups and the HLAs.

Tissue typing. In preparation for an allograft the closest match of donor-recipient transplantation antigens is sought. This is done by *tissue typing* for the major antigenic determinants (ABO, Rh, and HLA). If there are no significant discrepancies in these antigens, the recipient's serum is mixed with the lymphocytes from the donor, or the lymphocytes from the donor and recipient are cultured together to detect minor (but significant) cross-reactions. This is known as a *mixed lymphocyte reaction* (MLR).

Clinical picture. The process of graft rejection is as complicated and exquisite as the immune response system that brings it about. It has been best characterized in the case of skin allograft rejections. In this case, when the nonmatched skin is transferred to the new host, it settles down and becomes vascularized within 2 to 3 days; however, within 6 to 10 days, sensitized lymphocytes appear in the regional lymph nodes, and the lymph nodes begin to enlarge. The initial signs of rejection appear in about 10 to 14 days with the appearance first of sensitized lymphocytes and then macrophages at the site. Within 12 to 14 days, the vascular bed begins to deteriorate and the graft becomes necrotic and is sloughed off. This is known as *first-set rejection*. If another skin graft is taken from the *same* donor and is transplanted to a different site on the same recipient, the graft rejection is more rapid. This accelerated reaction, known as *second-set rejection*, is so rapid that the graft may never be vascularized before it is sloughed. In second-set rejection, circulating antibodies as well as the sensitized lymphocytes play a role. The antibodies create a direct cytotoxic attack on the graft. This is analogous to a type II immediate hypersensitivity reaction.

Some allografts circumvent immunorejection because of their site in the body. Corneal grafts survive without the need for immunosuppression because the site is avascular. Cartilage grafts enjoy the same privilege. Grafts into these types of sites are referred to as *privileged-site grafts*. By some (as yet unknown) mechanism, the fetus developing within the uterus enjoys this privileged-site status.

Intervention

IMMUNOSUPPRESSION. Graft rejection can be minimized by the use of chemical or physical agents that nonspecifically or specifically interfere with the development of an immune response reaction against the allograft. Clinically, three types of immunosuppressive agents are effective in providing the transitional protection needed to promote the graft establishment.

Antimetabolites and *alkylating agents*, such as *azathioprine* (Imuran) and *cyclophosphamide* (Cytoxan), act nonspecifically against rapidly dividing cells within the body; for this reason, they are also used for cancer chemotherapy. They interfere with DNA synthesis. Azathioprine, which is the most commonly used and least toxic, has both immunosuppressive and antiinflammatory actions. The major toxic effect is bone marrow depression. Both agents nonspecifically interfere with both the B cell and T cell systems.

Glucocorticosteroids, especially *prednisone*, are significantly antiinflammatory and impair lymphocyte (B cell and T cell) activation and function. Prednisone exerts a wide spectrum of activity against all immune response and inflammatory response mechanisms. Although it suppresses the cell-mediated system to a greater degree than the humoral system, the continued high dosage needed to maintain cell-mediated suppression creates significant risks in reducing the responsiveness of the humoral system. Other side effects (fluid retention, hypertension, behavior alterations, peptic ulcers, and osteoporosis) also obviate its use for prolonged periods at high dosage. Often lower dosages of prednisone and azathioprine are used together because they seem to act synergistically.

A more specific immunosuppression of the T cell system is achieved with the use of *antilymphocytic serum* (ALS) or more specifically, the antilymphocyte globulin (ALG). The antiserum is prepared by immunizing horses with human fetal thymocytes obtained from aborted fetuses. The antibody-containing globulin fraction is extracted and used to block the action of the sensitized cells in circulation, while leaving the lymph node B cell system only slightly suppressed. This leaves the host with protection against the humorally protected infectious agents, while providing protection against the most active rejection system. ALG is often given prophylactically against rejection for 1 to 2 weeks postoperatively. Since ALS contains foreign proteins itself and since it must be administered in fairly high repeated dosages, an Arthus reaction (p. 1871) frequently occurs. Other adverse effects include thrombocytopenia and allergic reactions.

PREVENTION OF INFECTION. Because persons experiencing organ transplantation are given immunosuppressive therapy to prevent tissue rejection, prevention of infection is as important as with any immunodeficiency (p. 1860). Invasive procedures such as venipunctures, catheterizations, or gastrointestinal intubation are performed as seldom as possible, and invasive catheters are removed as soon as feasible. Meticulous care is given to insertion sites, such as cleansing venipuncture sites with povidone-iodine preparations, using aseptic dressing changes around central venous catheter insertion sites, and giving good perineal care to patients with indwelling catheters. Irrigation of indwelling nasogastric tubes or urinary catheters is performed carefully to avoid traumatizing mucous membranes. Antibiotic solutions may be prescribed for urinary catheter irrigations.

Maintenance of skin integrity is important to prevent a breakdown of the first line of defense, since the immune defense is deficient. Frequent assessment of skin and mucous membranes is carried out, and vigorous preventive measures are immediately instituted for any early signs of skin breakdown. Classic signs and symptoms of infection may not occur because of the immunosuppression. Preventive isolation may be instituted if leukopenia occurs.

Autoimmune diseases

Individuals sometimes respond immunologically to some of their own antigens. When the mechanisms for recognition of self vs. nonself are subverted or altered, immune attack of self may result. The chance that the control mechanisms will be lost increases with the age of the individual. The symptoms of such a self-attack are referred to as *autoimmune disease* or *autohypersensitivity*. For the most part, these self-reactions are not immunologically initiated; the etiologic (causative) agent lies outside the immune system, but the immune response serves as the pathogenic mechanism.

The meaning of the demonstration of *autoantibodies* and *autosensitive T cell clones* is not always clear. These self-reactive immunoglobulins are often associated with certain pathologic states in the body but many times can also be isolated from the serum of "normal" individuals as well, especially in older persons. Autoantibodies have been demonstrated against nuclear material in systemic lupus erythematosus, against γ-globulins in rheumatoid arthritis, against gastric parietal cells in pernicious anemia, and against platelets in autoimmune thrombocytopenia. Sensitized lymphocytes have been demonstrated in the Guillain-Barré syndrome and autoimmune thyroiditis.

Some of the theoretical mechanisms by which the immunologic tolerance to self-antigens might be broken include:

1. *Release of sequestered antigens*. If an antigen does not come into contact with the immune system during fetal development when the tolerance to self normally develops (either because of anatomic site or later development), it is not registered as a self-antigen, and clones of immunoresponsive cells to that antigen remain reactive. As a result of trauma or infection, these antigens may be exposed to the immune system. If this occurs, they will elicit an immune response. Examples include thyroiditis, aspermia (male infertility) and uveitis.

2. *Activation of suppressed clones*. If one of the functions of the suppressor T cell is to suppress the activation of certain clones of potentially self-reactive T cells or B cells, it is possible through some loss of suppressor function that these "forbidden" clones are allowed to proliferate. There is no currently identified experimental disease model to support this hypothesis, but it is theoretically feasible.

3. *Synthesis of cross-reactive antibodies*. Antibodies synthesized in response to certain foreign anti-

TABLE 72-6. Some diseases with autoimmune aspects

Disease	Autoantigen	Comments
Pernicious anemia	Intrinsic factors of parietal cells	Specific autoantibodies detectable
Autoimmune hemolytic anemia	Antigens on the surface of RBC	RBC surface antigens may be altered by drugs
Systemic lupus erythematosus	Nucleoproteins, DNA, many other antigens	Multiple autoimmune responses
Guillain-Barré syndrome	Myelin	
Glomerulonephritis	Cross-reactive streptococcal antigens	May also result from direct attack of glomerular basement membrane
Rheumatic fever	Cross-reactive streptococcal antigens	
	Immunoglobulin G	
Rheumatoid arthritis		Rheumatoid factor is IgM that reacts with IgG
Ulcerative colitis	Colon cells	
Myasthenia gravis	Skeletal and heart muscle	Thymectomy improves
Male infertility	Sperm cell	Agglutinins formed against sperm cells
Multiple sclerosis	Brain cells	Not proved to be autoimmune
Sympathetic uveitis	Uveal tissues	Release of sequestered uveal antigen
Autoimmune thyroiditis	Thyroid hormones and tissues	Autoantibodies and sensitized lymphocytes

gens may have cross-reactivity with some similar antigenic components within human tissues. Contact with antigens called *heterophile antigens* may trigger the production of autoantibodies. This seems to be a mechanism of rheumatic heart disease, in which the antibodies produced against certain streptococcal antigens during scarlet fever, streptococcal sore throat, or other streptococcal infections cross-react with myocardial tissue, producing a myocardial inflammation.

4. *Alteration of self-antigens.* Normal body proteins may be altered by chemicals, infectious organisms, or therapeutic drugs to present new antigenically active groups to the immune system. The autoimmune hemolytic anemia associated with alpha-methyldopa (Aldomet) treatment of hypertension probably results from the alteration of the Rh antigens of the red blood cell rendering it antigenic. Certain antibiotics such as the penicillins and cephalosporins can have the same effect.

Many diseases for which no etiologic agent could be identified have been classified as autoimmune, only to be removed from that category when some cryptic, latent, or slow-growing agent was identified within the cells or tissue under attack. Some of the diseases listed as autoimmune-associated diseases in Table 72-6 will probably be removed from that list as the initiating factor or microorganism is identified. (The care of persons experiencing these diseases is discussed elsewhere in the text.)

REFERENCES AND SELECTED READINGS

1. Abdou, N.I., et al.: The thymus in myasthenia gravis: evidence for altered cell populations, N. Engl. J. Med. **291**:1271, 1975.

2. Acherson, G.F.: Immunodeficiency disorders, Practitioner **214**:494, 1975.

3. Aisner, J.: Platelet transfusion therapy, Med. Clin. North Am. **61**:1133-1145, 1977.

4. Alexander, J.W., and Good, R.A.: Fundamentals of clinical immunology, Philadelphia, 1977, W.B. Saunders Co.

5. Amos, H.E.: Allergic drug reactions, London, 1976, Edward Arnold, Ltd.

6. Asher, I.M., editor: Inadvertent modification of the immune response. Proceedings of the Fourth FDA Science Symposium, HHS Publication no. (FDA) 80-1074, Washington, D.C., 1980, U.S. Government Printing Office.

7. Barber, H.R.: Immunology for the clinician, New York, 1977, John Wiley & Sons, Inc.

8. *Barr, S.E.: Allergy to hymenoptera stings, J.A.M.A. **228**:718, 1974.

9. Beeson, P.B., editor: Textbook of medicine, ed. 15, Philadelphia, 1979, W.B. Saunders Co.

10. Benacerraf, B.: Immunogenetics and immunodeficiency, Baltimore, 1975, University Park Press.

11. Blood transfusions today: what you should know and do, Nurs. '78 **8**(2):68-72, 1978.

12. Booth, B., et al.: Modern concepts in clinical allergy, New York, 1973, Medcom Books, Inc.

13. Bridgewater, S.C., Voignier, R.R., and Smith, C.S.: Allergies in children: recognition, Am. J. Nurs. **78**:614-616, 1978.

14. Brown, S.M., et al.: Immunologic dysfunction in heroin addicts, Arch. Intern. Med. **134**:1001, 1974.

15. Buckley, R.H.: Plasma therapy in immunodeficiency disease, Birth Defects **11**:347-349, 1975.

16. *Buickus, B.A.: Blood therapy: administering blood components, Am. J. Nurs. **79**:937-941, 1979.

17. Burnet, F.M.: Auto-immunity and autoimmune disease, Philadelphia, 1972, F.A. Davis Co.

18. Chapman, R.G.: Leukocytes help clear confusion about transfusions, Lab World **30**:14-19, 1979.

19. *Child, J., Collins, D., and Collins, J.: Blood transfusions, Am. J. Nurs. **72**:1602, 1972.

20. Cochrane, C.G., and Koffler, D.: Immune complex disease in

*References preceded by an asterisk are particularly well suited for student reading.

experimental animals and man, Adv. Immunol. **16**:186, 1973.

21. *Craven, R.F.: Anaphylactic shock, Am. J. Nurs. **72**:718, 1972.
22. Criep, L.H.: Allergy and clinical immunology, New York, 1976, Grune & Stratton, Inc.
23. *Cullins, L.C.: Blood therapy: preventing and treating transfusion reactions, Am. J. Nurs. **79**:935-936, 1979.
24. *Cunningham, B.A.: The structure and function of histocompatibility antigens, Sci. Am. **237**:96, 1977.
25. Danilevicius, Z.: HL-A system and rheumatic disease, J.A.M.A. **231**:283, 1975.
26. Davidsohn, I., and Henry, J.B.: Todd-Sanford clinical diagnosis by laboratory methods, ed. 16, Philadelphia 1979, W.B. Saunders Co.
27. Dharan, M.: Immunoglobulin abnormalities, Am. J. Nurs. **76**:1626-1628, 1976.
28. *Donley, D.L.: Nursing the patient who is immunosuppressed, Am. J. Nurs. **76**:1619-1625, 1976.
29. Dunphy, J.E., and Way, L.W.: Surgical diagnosis and treatment, Los Altos, Calif. 1979, Lange Medical Publications.
30. Elpern, E.H.: Asthma update: pathophysiology and treatment, Heart Lung **9**:665-670, 1980.
31. Ern, M.: Immunology: bone marrow transplantation, Ca. Nurs. **3**:387-400, 1980.
32. Faktor, M.A., et al.: Hypersensitivity to tetanus toxoid, J. Allergy Clin. Immunol. **52**:1, 1973.
33. *Faulk, W.P., Demaeyer, E.M., and Davies, A.J.: Some effects of malnutrition on immune response in man, Am. J. Clin. Nutr. **27**:638, 1974.
34. Freedman, S.O., and Gold, P.: Clinical immunology, ed. 2, Hagerstown, Md., 1976, Harper & Row, Publishers, Inc.
35. Fruth, R.: Anaphylaxis and drug reactions: guidelines for detection and care, Heart Lung **9**:662-664, 1980.
36. Fudenberg, H.H., editor: Basic and clinical immunology, ed. 3, Los Altos, Calif., 1980, Lange Medical Publications.
37. Glaser, R.S.: The body is the hero, New York, 1976, Random House.
38. Grindon, A.J.: Untoward reactions to blood transfusion. In Conn, H.F.: Current therapy, Philadelphia, 1980, W.B. Saunders Co.
39. *Groenwald, S.L.: Physiology of the immune system, Heart Lung **9**:645-650, 1980.
40. Harris, J., editor: Symposium on clinical immunology, Med. Clin. North Am. **56**:1-575, 1972.
41. Hitzig, W.H., and Muntener, V.: Conventional immunoglobin therapy, Birth Defects **11**:339-342, 1975.
42. Hood, L.E., Weissman, I.L., and Wood, W.B.: Immunology, Menlo Park, Calif., 1978, Benjamin/Cummings Co.
43. Jones, J.V.: Plasmapheresis: current research and success, Heart Lung **9**:671-674, 1980.
44. Jones, W.R.: Immunological infertility: fact or fiction? Fertil. Steril. **33**:577-582, 1980.
45. *Kazak, A.: Blood therapy: processing blood for transfusion reactions, Am. J. Nurs. **79**:935-936, 1979.
46. *Kelly, J.F., and Patterson, R.: Anaphylaxis, course, mechanisms, and treatment, J.A.M.A. **227**:1431, 1974.
47. Kirkpatrick, C.H.: Therapeutic potential of transfer factor, N. Engl. J. Med. **303**:390-394, 1980.
48. Lind, M.: The immunologic assessment: a nursing focus, Heart Lung **9**:658-661, 1980.
49. *McAllen, M.K.: Hayfever, Nurs. Mirror **138**:63, 1974.
50. McLeod, B.C.: Immunologic factors in reactions to blood transfusions, Heart Lung **9**:675-681, 1980.
51. McPhaul, J.J., Jr.: IgA-associated glomerulonephritis, Ann. Rev. Med. **28**:37-42, 1977.

52. *Moody, L.: Asthma: physiology and patient care, Am. J. Nurs. **73**:1212, 1973.
53. Old, L.S.: Cancer immunology, Sci. Am. **236**:62-79, 1977.
54. Park, A.K., et al.: Immunosuppressive effect of surgery, Lancet **1**:53, 1971.
55. *Parker, A.L.: Blood therapy: massive transfusions, Am. J. Nurs. **79**:944-948, 1979.
56. Parker, C.W., editor: Clinical immunology, Philadelphia, 1980, W.B. Saunders Co.
57. Rana, A.N., and Luskin, A.: Immunosuppression, autoimmunity, and hypersensitivity, Heart Lung **9**:651-657, 1980.
58. Remington, J.S.: The compromised host, Hosp. Pract. **7**:59, 1972.
59. Roberts-Thomson, I.C., et al.: Aging, immune response and mortality, Lancet ·**2**:368, 1974.
60. *Rossman, M., Slavin, R., and Taft, E.G.: Pheresis therapy: patient care, Am. J. Nurs. **77**:1135-1141, 1977.
61. *Rutman, R., et al.: Blood therapy: screening donors and the phlebotomy procedure, Am. J. Nurs. **79**:926-930, 1979.
62. Samter, M.: Immunological diseases, ed. 3, Boston, 1978, Little, Brown & Co.
63. Samter, M., editor: Syposium on immunotherapy in malignant disease, Med. Clin. North Am. **60**:1-648, 1976.
64. Sell, S.: Immunology, immunopathology and immunity, ed. 3, Hagerstown, Md., 1980, Harper & Row, Publishers, Inc.
65. Solomon, G.F., and Amkraut, A.A.: Emotions, stress and immunity, Front. Rad. Ther. Onc. **7**:84, 1974.
66. Sophie, L.R.: Meeting the immunologic challenge of transplant nursing, Heart Lung **9**:690-694, 1980.
67. Stiller, C.R., Russell, A.S., and Dosseter, J.B.: Autoimmunity: present concepts, Ann. Intern. Med. **82**:405-410, 1975.
68. Tarnawski, A., and Balko, B.: Antibiotics and immune processes. Lancet **1**:674-675, 1973.
69. *Tenczynski, J.: Leukapheresis: the process, Am. J. Nurs. **77**:1133-1134, 1977.
70. Terry, W.D., editor: Symposium on immunotherapy in malignant disease, Med. Clin. North Am. **60**:1-648, 1976.
71. Terry, W.D.: Immunotherapy of malignant melanoma, N. Engl. J. Med. **303**:1174-1178, 1980.
72. Thaler, M.S., Klausner, R.D., and Cohen, H.S.: Medical immunology, Philadelphia, 1977, J.B. Lippincott Co.
73. *Thomas, S.: Blood therapy: transfusing granulocytes, Am. J. Nurs. **79**:942-943, 1979.
74. *Voignier, R.R., and Bridgewater, S.C.: Allergies in children: testing and treating, Am. J. Nurs. **78**:617-619, 1978.
75. Waldman, R.H.: Clinical concepts of immunology, Baltimore, 1979, The Williams & Wilkins Co.
76. Weiss, H.J.: Aspirin: a dangerous drug? J.A.M.A. **229**:1221, 1974.
77. Yunis, E.J., Fernandes, G., and Greenberg, L.J.: Tumor immunology, autoimmunity and aging, J. Am. Geriatr. **24**:253, 1976.

AUDIOVISUAL RESOURCES

Autoimmune diseases, New York, 1973, Medcom Products. (Color slides and audiocassette.)

Autoimmunity and disease, West Point, Pa., 1968, Merck, Sharp and Dohme. (Film, 16 mm color, 33 min.)

Immune complexes and disease, Washington, D.C., 1974, National Medical Audiovisual Center. (Color slides and audiocassette.)

Transplantation immunology, Baltimore, 1972, University Park Press. (Color slides and audiocassette.)

SPECIAL ENVIRONMENTS OF CARE

The nurse working or living in a community may be called on to provide *emergency care* for trauma or medical conditions at normal times or during *disasters*. The overwhelming effects of disasters need also to be considered and are discussed in Chapter 73.

The final three chapters explore the nature of care in *critical* care units. Critical illness occurs when problems that individually may not be intense enough to culminate in crises interact to cause major disturbances in a person's physiologic equilibrium. The complex interrelationship among these problems leads to disturbances or failure of several systems, and in turn this multisystem failure aggravates the complexity of the problems. Critical illness usually is a life-threatening event that endangers or involves the respiratory, cardiovascular, renal, and central nervous systems as well as each person's self-concept.

A critically ill person is in crisis or at a turning point with potentially negative outcomes. Multiple physiologic, psychologic, and social stressors impinge on critically ill patients and their significant others. Whether a critical illness experience will culminate in a crisis for the patient and the significant others depends on their perceptions of the event, the support systems available to them, and their previous coping skills.

The stressors imposed by critical illness threaten the equilibrium of both the patient and the significant others because of sudden actual or potential losses that disrupt the individual's current life-style. Patients may face loss of life, loss of biologic function and body integrity, and loss of independence and control over their bodily functions as well as their immediate destinies. They also face potential loss of identity and feelings of self-worth as life-threatening physiologic problems assume the priority and attention of the health care team. In addition, they may lose financial security and the potential to retain or to regain their premorbid life-style. Significant others lose the ability to change or alter the events that present hazards to the well-being of loved ones and are faced with the very real threat of permanent loss through death. Within a systems perspective these stressors become input that influence the patient's and significant others' behavior and their ability to cope with the losses threatened by critical illness.

The nurse caring for a person who is critically ill is in a position to reestablish a state of equilibrium through the use of crisis and systems theories integrated with refined decision-making skills. The essence of critical care nursing lies in the decision-making process and the willingness of the nurse to act on the decisions. The decision-making process is founded on highly developed and integrated assessment and management skills that (1) reduce the impact of losses and subsequent stressors experienced by a critically ill patient and significant others, (2) promote realistic perceptions of the illness experience for the individual and the significant others, (3) identify support systems, (4) provide support to previously learned coping behaviors, and (5) foster the learning of new coping skills.

Chapters 74 to 76 discuss the assessment and management of critically ill patients as physiologic, psychologic, and social beings. The first chapter presents a framework for data collection and recording and guidelines for *assessment*. The second chapter discusses *managing patients who are critically ill* in terms of preventive, supportive, and restorative interventions directed toward alleviation of physiologic, psychologic, and social stressors. In the third and final chapter assessment and management principles are applied to an actual *case study of a patient who suffers multisystem failure*.

CHAPTER 73

EMERGENCIES AND DISASTERS

BARBARA C. LONG

Nurses are frequently called on to provide emergency care in the community or in settings where medical help is not immediately available; therefore all nurses need to know the basics of emergency care. Nurses whose primary focus is the delivery of emergency care in specialized settings, such as the hospital emergency care department, require additional knowledge and skills that are beyond the scope of this chapter, and there are a number of texts available that deal with this topic alone (see references). The purpose of this chapter is to identify major points in the delivery of emergency care in the community, in assessment and intervention for common emergencies, and in principles of management in disasters.

Epidemiology

Accidents in the United States claim more than 100,000 lives each year. Of these deaths, 50% are due to motor vehicle accidents; 13% to falls; 5% each to fires, drowning, poisoning, and industrial accidents; and 16% to other types of accidents.[97] Motor vehicle deaths dropped sharply in 1974 at the time that the 55-mph speed limit was imposed. Since 1975, however, deaths from motor vehicles have shown an increase (Fig. 73-1). Accidents are the leading cause of death in the 1- to 44-year-old age group and the third leading cause of death in the 45- to 64-year-old age group.

In terms of morbidity, approximately *60 million* persons are injured in the United States every year, or about 30 of every 100 persons. Approximately 13% are injured at work, 37% at home, and 50% in motor vehicle accidents.[97] Billions of dollars are spent annually on medical expenses, property damage, and administra-

tive costs related to accidents. Money lost from potential earnings or disability adds to this figure.

Accidents that result in injury or death involve human suffering that cannot be measured in dollars and includes pain, long-term rehabilitation, disabilities (temporary or permanent), loss and grief, and family disruption. Accidents are for the most part preventable and require attention of health care professionals not only as to their causes and the environment in which they occur but also to the victim's physical, social, and psychologic state and readiness to avoid accidents.

Delivery of emergency care

Health crises that demand immediate interventions can occur anywhere—in the home, in other parts of the community, or in the hospital itself. The nurse may be the sole giver of care until medical care is available, or the nurse may be working with other paramedical personnel.

Community

In recent years there has been an increased awareness by communities of inadequacies in the delivery of emergency care. In the past, persons who usually responded to emergency calls were either police or drivers from funeral homes who also doubled as private ambulance drivers. The preparation for care of the injured varied from nothing to elementary first aid training. Victims who might have survived if more advanced care had been available have died on the way to a hospital.

Many communities are now preparing and utilizing

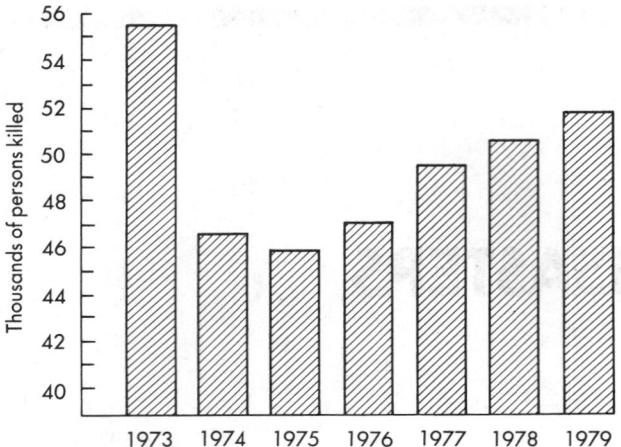

Fig. 73-1. Yearly motor vehicle deaths in the United States.

emergency medical technicians (EMTs) or paramedics to respond to emergency calls. EMTs have had preparation beyond basic first aid training but do not carry out invasive procedures. Paramedics have had more training than EMTs and can carry out such skills as starting intravenous fluids, giving medications, defibrillation, and intubation. The preparedness of personnel responding to emergency calls and the responsibilities that are legally permissible vary among states and communities within each state.

The National Safety Act of 1966 requires each county to appoint an emergency medical care committee. The effectiveness of these committees varies greatly, influenced to a large extent by citizen interest and political activity.[107] Every community needs an organized emergency care system with support and input from community health organizations and community political elements. Once an organization is established there should be continued evaluation of the effectiveness of the emergency care provided. Nurses should become actively involved in all phases of activities that can influence the level of emergency care in their own communities.

The American Heart Association has been instrumental in developing a program to educate large numbers of persons who are certified to administer cardiopulmonary resuscitation (CPR). This increases the possibility of a trained person being available to initiate resuscitation early in a larger number of emergency situations.

Hospitals

Hospitals that receive financial support from government sources are required to provide emergency departments open to the public. In many emergency departments more than half of the persons seeking medical attention are not actually in need of emergency care. These are persons who do not have a private physician or are unable to obtain the services of their physician at the hour or day when they feel they need medical attention. Persons requiring immediate care are treated first. If there are a large number of patients, those with nonacute symptoms often have to wait a considerable time. Newer approaches to delivery of both emergency and nonacute health care are being explored.

Many emergency departments have direct radio communication with rescue personnel in the community. Treatment can be initiated at the site of injury under medical direction and hospital personnel can be better prepared to receive the injured. This helps to eliminate some of the delays in initiation of care.

The role of the nurse in the emergency department has changed considerably in recent years as a result of the increased utilization of emergency departments by persons seeking medical attention and the increased sophistication of therapeutic management. Emergency department (ED) nurses are developing skills in assessment and *triage* (sorting patients to determine priority of need for medical attention); in management of persons with high levels of anxiety; and in carrying out specialized technical skills such as initiating parenteral fluids, defibrillation, resuscitation, intubation, or operating monitoring devices, and interpreting selected laboratory findings and electrocardiograms and acting on these findings.

Legal aspects of emergency care

Nurses who intervene to assist victims in an emergency situation should be aware of the legal ramifications that can ensue as a result of their actions. Many states have enacted "Good Samaritan" laws in an effort to protect health personnel who aid accident victims. These laws vary in coverage among states as to the classes of people who are protected from liability, types of situations, geographic limits, and extent of immunity.[32] The classification of persons covered varies in specificity from any person who stops at the scene of an accident to only those registered nurses licensed in that state. Thus in the latter situation giving nursing care in an emergency situation could be construed in that state to practicing nursing without a license. One state (Vermont) allows criminal penalties for failure to stop and give assistance, although the victim cannot sue if the nurse fails to stop.

Good Samaritan laws serve to identify in statutory

language those persons or situations that provide some degree of immunity from liability, many of which already exist by common law. Persons are judged as not liable unless they act willfully with gross negligence.[32] Negligence is the key word. Negligence, according to common law, involves four concepts: duty, breach of duty, damage, and proximal cause.[32] In an emergency a nurse is not duty bound to stop and render aid (except in Vermont) unless the nurse was the cause of the accident. The moral issue of whether to stop and render aid is the nurse's decision. If the nurse does render aid, then duty is implied and failure to continue rendering aid until the victim is released to another competent person can result in breach of duty (abandonment). Some Good Samaritan laws permit releasing the care of the victim to a qualified ambulance attendant (EMT). Damage must occur if negligence is to be proved, and the actions of the nurse must be the proximal cause of the damage.

"Reasonable care" provided by the nurse at the scene of an accident is usually judged as that care given by another similar nurse *under the prevailing situation*. Thus the care provided on a back road on a dark rainy night would not be judged the same as that given in an emergency room. In an emergency situation a nurse can perform medical acts to save life. It may be necessary later, however, to prove that a true emergency did exist. Good Samaritan laws will not protect the nurse in this situation.[32] Malpractice and liability claims can be filed even if Good Samaritan laws exist.

Nurses who work in hospital emergency departments need to be aware of legal implications of care provided in that setting, such as the care given to minors when parents are not present to give consent, and actions that may be taken in helping police officers gather evidence.[20]

Prevention of accidents

Accident prevention is a major public health goal, and both the Public Health Service and the American Public Health Association (APHA) are active in promoting accident prevention. Community groups can be helpful in investigating accident statistics in their local area and in disseminating information to encourage accident prevention. Nurses have an important role in accident prevention, both through their roles as professionals and as residents of a community. The influence of nurses can be extended in many areas because nurses are represented in schools, industry, community nursing programs, and hospitals.

There are a number of resources for information concerning accident prevention. The *Statistical Ab-*

HOME SAFETY FEATURES FOR ELDERLY PERSONS

Floors	Large rugs and carpets anchored
	Small rugs with nonskid backing
	Avoidance of floor wax (unless nonskid)
Stairs	Uniform height
	Nonskid treads
	Risers marked with contrasting color
	Strong handrails
	Adequate lighting
Bathroom	Handrail at tub or shower
	Skid-proof bath mats
	Treads in tub or on shower floor
	Seat in shower

stracts published by the U.S. Bureau of the Census is a helpful reference. Local health departments can provide local data, health education materials, and other resource materials. Engineers can be a valuable resource for consultation on safety hazards in the home, hospital, or community.

Home

Accidents in and about the home cause almost one third of all accidental deaths each year. Falls account for about half the number, and fires and poisonings account for most of the remainder. Many aged persons who fall do so when walking from room to room. Some fall because of heavily waxed floors, loose rugs, poor lighting, scattered toys, and other conditions that could have been corrected (see box above). People fall from roofs, windows, high ladders, and steps and are fatally burned or otherwise injured while using solvents and cleansing agents without proper knowledge of their hazards.

The number of electric appliances used in the home has increased the danger of electric shock and fire from overloaded circuits. Many persons die in fires caused by burning cigarette ashes dropped on furniture or rugs or discarded in waste containers and by cigarettes that are dropped as the smoker falls asleep. Attention needs to be given to teaching homeowners with older heating systems to have the equipment checked periodically for gas leaks and other unsafe features. All persons in a household should be aware of what to do in the event of fire, and fire evacuation drills are encouraged. Homes should be equipped with smoke alarms in strategic places, such as the kitchen, bedrooms, hallways, and basement.

Homes with young children should be made as accident proof as possible. Prevention of poisoning is discussed on p. 1890. Safety rules should be taught to children at an early age. Children sustain injuries during their play and exploring activities. The possibility of child abuse must be considered, however, when children, especially those under the age of 3 years, are seen with injuries such as bruises, fractures, or burns. When child abuse is suspected, health care professionals have a responsibility to protect the child from further injury by reporting their suspicions. At the same time it is important that help be sought for the parent or parents involved. In several communities, groups have been organized for parents who are child abusers. Since it has been found that most parents who abuse their children were abused as children themselves, this form of group therapy is often helpful in assisting parents to ventilate deep-seated feelings. Information about local groups can be obtained from child welfare agencies. One group working in this area is CALM (Child Abuse and Listening Mediation, Inc.), located in California.* Another group, Parents Anonymous, has local chapters in many cities (p. 209).

The community health nurse has an opportunity to assess safety hazards during home visits and to teach not only the client but also members of the family about general accident prevention as well as specific measures for the safety of the ill person.

Community

Community action can best be effected by group action, but it often takes persistent individuals to interest and stimulate group action. Parent-teacher associations, recreational associations, and religious and social groups are usually interested in accident control. Support by governmental groups is important. Efforts should be made to use existing agencies and groups and to work with them in order that the sincere efforts of small groups of enthusiastic citizens will not be dissipated. Phases of accident prevention that should be of community interest include (1) teaching of accident prevention in the public schools, (2) better control and inspection of homes for the aged and prisons, (3) rigid enforcement of driving regulations, (4) improvement of street lighting and traffic signals at busy intersections, (5) periodic inspection of all automobiles, and (6) promotion of laws pertaining to fire-proofing of buildings and laws protecting the public from flammable clothing, potentially harmful toys, and similar items.

*PO Box 718, Santa Barbara, CA 93102.

Hospital

Assessing the need for safety in the general environment and for the safety of specific patients, and taking measures to prevent injury are important functions of the nurse. The nurse can participate in policy making and safety monitoring through membership on hospital safety committees.

Falls

The major cause of hospital-incurred injury is falling. Hospitalized persons are in unfamiliar surroundings with strange furniture and equipment, may be weak for many reasons, or may become confused, all of which may contribute to falls. Elderly persons are at high risk for falls. All patients should be assessed for the potential of falling, and preventive measures should be instituted.

The following safety measures help to prevent falls. Handrails in hospital corridors and in bathrooms give weak persons something to hold onto for support. Chairs with arms are safer than armless chairs. Stools in showers and adjacent to tubs provide safety for patients who become tired or who develop hypotension from vasodilation. There should be call systems in the bathrooms and lounges as well as the patient's bedside. Hi-Lo beds should be used whenever possible, and the bed should be in low position when the patient is ambulatory.

Elderly persons often become confused at night, a time when sensory input is decreased. Sedation may increase the confusion. A night light in the room can be useful for sensory input. The bed should be in low position; in the event that the patient attempts to climb out of bed, the bed will be at the same height as his or her bed at home. The use of the side rails is a nursing decision. Side rails should be kept raised for all infants and unconscious patients. A confused patient may attempt to climb over the side rail and thus have farther to fall; a jacket restraint may be more useful.

Patients who are weak may need frequent reminders to seek assistance before ambulating. Some patients do not want to "bother the nurse" and attempt to walk to the bathroom unaided, especially at night. All patients should use supportive slippers; paper slippers can be a hazard.

Fire

All hospitals and nursing homes must have established fire prevention routines and all personnel must be familiar with these routines. Participation in fire drills should be taken seriously, and evaluation should follow each drill.

Fires usually occur from smoking or faulty electrical equipment. Since smoking is also hazardous to one's health, many hospitals are restricting smoking in patient's rooms and in many public areas. If smoking is permitted in the patient's room, ashtrays should be available and the patient and visitors instructed about not emptying them. Patients who are careless smokers or who may drop a cigarette or ash are to be monitored while smoking. Faulty electrical equipment is not used. Any questions about smoke should be investigated and reported immediately.

If a fire should occur, the nurse in charge who is most familiar with the patients' conditions should be in charge of any evacuation. Until evacuation is necessary, the doors and windows of all patient rooms are closed. If evacuation is deemed advisable, patients closest to the fire are evacuated to the opposite end of the floor (horizontal evacuation), then downward by the stairway (vertical evacuation) if necessary. Death usually occurs from inhaling the smoke. Doors that are excessively hot should not be opened. The rescuer should keep as low as possible and, if necessary, use wet cloths around the nose and mouth if the air is hot.

Assessment

When an emergency occurs or on arriving at the emergency scene, it is important to assess the situation, the patient, and the environment before initiating action. Some conclusions can be drawn from the immediate environment. If there is multiple victim trauma, all victims should be assessed before any but lifesaving interventions are initiated. Overt clues such as an automobile accident, report of falling, or ingestion of poison can give direction to probable types of injuries. A complete head-to-toe assessment is carried out, if possible, before moving the victim so that additional injuries or conditions requiring intervention can be identified.

Data collection

A person who is not breathing, who has no palpable pulse, or who is hemorrhaging needs immediate assistance. Obtaining data to identify these circumstances is the first priority in assessment (see box above). This is sometimes referred to as the ABCs of emergency assessment (*a*irway, *b*reathing, *c*irculation). Assessing the general level of consciousness can be done as the approach is made to the victim. The carotid pulse can be checked at the same time as breathing is checked. If pulse and breathing are absent, CPR is initiated (p. 1080).

Hemorrhage is treated with direct pressure to the wound, and if shock is present the legs are assessed and then elevated if there are no signs of fracture. The victim is protected from chilling. Before the victim is moved

---

PRIORITY ASSESSMENT

Airway
Presence of respirations
Presence of foreign body, vomitus, loose dentures in mouth

Breathing
Respiration rate, depth, character
Use of accessory muscles for breathing
Tracheal deviation

Circulation
Presence of carotid pulse
Pulse rate, strength, rhythm
Presence of hemorrhage
Skin color, temperature, moisture

Level of consciousness
Response to voice and touch (or painful stimulus)
Pupillary response
If unconscious, presence of Medic-Alert tag

---

or turned, it is important to assess for possible fracture of the neck and spine (see box, p. 1884).

Before starting the head-to-toe assessment, observe the victim's general position, any obvious deformities or asymmetry, or any purposeful movements. Ask the person to indicate any pain or discomfort and assess these areas first. During the overall assessment continue to monitor for changes in level of consciousness and respiratory status. Ask the victim or any relatives or friends present to describe the preceding events; the presence of any medical conditions such as heart or lung disease, epilepsy, or diabetes; or any special medications taken by the victim that may have a bearing on the present situation.

If there is more than one person on the scene, the nurse or paramedic should remain with the victim while others are given directions to assess the environment for additional signs of danger and to call for any needed transportation.

Data analysis

Patient data

Level of consciousness. Determine whether the person responds immediately to voice and touch, responds only to painful stimuli, or does not respond.

HEAD-TO-TOE ASSESSMENT

Head and neck

Assess airway

Assess pupils

Examine ears, nose, mouth for bleeding, other drainage, foreign body

Palpate* cervical spine for pain (do not move head)

Examine head for bleeding, lacerations, contusions, depression of skull

Palpate jaw for fracture (pain, deformity)

Ask about stiffness of neck (if no history of trauma, assess movement)

Examine neck for distended neck veins, presence of tracheal stoma, tracheal deviation

Chest and spine

Observe chest movements for symmetry of expansion and character of respirations

Palpate clavicles for fracture (pain, deformity)

Examine chest for external injury

Palpate ribs for fracture (pain)

Palpate spine for point tenderness (do not move victim)

Abdomen and pelvis

Palpate pelvis for pain in groin when pressure applied over pelvis

Ask about abdominal pain

Examine abdomen for external injury, rigidity, distention, penetrating objects

Extremities

Examine for signs of external injury

Ask about pain in extremities

If no obvious injury, ask victim to move each limb

Test for sensation in each limb

Assess presence and strength of peripheral pulses

*All palpations should be carried out gently.

POSSIBLE CAUSES OF UNCONSCIOUSNESS

1. Hypoxia (decreased oxygen to brain)
   a. Respiratory insufficiency
      (1) Airway obstruction from foreign body, secretions
      (2) Pneumothorax
      (3) Spinal cord injury
   b. Shock
      (1) Cardiogenic: cardiac arrest
      (2) Hypovolemic: hemorrhage
2. Metabolic (chemical brain depressants)
   a. Extrinsic
      (1) Drugs: alcohol, narcotics, barbiturates, antihistamines, tranquilizers
      (2) Poisons: carbon monoxide, carbon tetrachloride, hydrocarbons, methane gas
   b. Intrinsic
      (1) Ketones: diabetic ketoacidosis, starvation
      (2) Glucose: hypoglycemia, hyperglycemia
      (3) Ammonia: liver failure
      (4) Urea: kidney failure
      (5) Hormonal hypofunction: hypothyroidism, Addison's disease
      (6) Electrolyte imbalance: sodium, potassium, calcium, hydrogen ions
3. Brain pathologic conditions
   a. Trauma: concussion, brain stem contusion, intracranial hematoma
   b. Seizures: epilepsy, tumors, idiopathology
   c. Cerebrovascular accident: cerebral hemorrhage, thrombosis
   d. Tumors: benign, malignant
   e. Infections: meningitis, encephalitis

Unconsciousness may be due to many causes (see box above at right).

When shock or respiratory insufficiency occurs, there is decreased oxygenation of the brain, either because there is an insufficient amount of blood to carry the oxygen or because there is decreased oxygen taken in. This can lead to loss of consciousness, and the pupils will be equal and may be dilated.

When unconsciousness occurs because of the effect of drugs or chemicals, the pupils are equal and may be constricted or dilated depending on the effect of the specific drug. Information from relatives may elicit data concerning history of diabetes, liver or kidney disease, and medication taken by the victim. Environmental data such as an empty pill container can be useful in the identification of unconsciousness from drug overdose.

If there has been trauma to the brain, it is important to ascertain level of consciousness at different times. Temporary loss of consciousness followed by alertness and equal pupils usually indicates a concussion. If there is no skull fracture present, the patient is simply observed for 24 hours. Alertness after injury followed by increasing loss of consciousness usually indicates an intracranial hematoma. The pupils are usually *unequal*. Medical attention is urgent if an intracranial hematoma is suspected. The pupils may also be unequal if the patient has had a cerebrovascular accident (stroke).

An unconscious person should be placed in a position that facilitates patency of the airway (side-lying position is preferred unless contraindicated), and the respiratory status should be constantly monitored (see Chapter 27).

Respirations. The rate, depth, and character of respiration provide clues to the presence of ventilatory, central nervous system, or metabolic problems. Most trauma victims breathe a little faster than normal (18 to 24/min).[41] If the person shows signs of respiratory effort (nasal flaring; suprasternal, intercostal, or substernal retractions), the airway may be partially obstructed. The type of noise accompanying respirations may indicate the degree and location of a partial obstruction. The following findings are suggestive of specific emergency care problems:

1. Rate
   a. Slow (below 10/min): ventilatory or central nervous system problems
   b. Rapid (above 26/min): hypoxia, acidosis, shock
2. Depth
   a. Shallow: shock, chest pain
   b. Deep: hypoxia, hypoglycemia, metabolic acidosis
3. Sounds
   a. Inspiratory stridor: upper airway obstruction (above tracheal bifurcation)
   b. Expiratory wheezes/stridor: lower airway obstruction
4. Frothy, blood-tinged sputum: lung injury, pulmonary edema, pulmonary embolus

Shock. Victims who sustain major trauma or a major stressor to the system such as a myocardial infarction usually develop shock (p. 310). Signs of shock include restlessness, pale, cold, moist skin, rapid thready pulse, and rapid shallow respirations. Nausea and vomiting may occur. With anaphylactic shock the victim may complain of itching or burning of the skin, a tightness in the chest, and difficulty in breathing. Wheals may develop on the skin, and the face and tongue may develop edema (p. 1863).

Sensation. Trauma may result in *pain* if there is soft-tissue injury, fracture, or visceral damage. Pain may also occur with tissue anoxia, such as with obstruction of blood vessels or frostbite. Data are obtained from the patient concerning location (region), severity, quality, onset and duration, and provoking factors. One suggested approach for evaluating these parameters is the use of the mnemonic *PQRST*[20]:

P—provoking factors: what makes the pain worse or relieves it
Q—quality: dull, sharp, crushing, etc.
R—region or radiation: site and radiation to other areas
S—severity (on a scale of 1 to 10, where 1 is no pain and 10 is the worst imaginable pain)
T—time: onset, duration, constancy

For a further discussion of pain, see Chapter 23.

Loss of sensation may result from injury to peripheral nerves or injury to nerves in the central nervous system. Peripheral nerve injuries may occur with fractures, lacerations, penetrating wounds, or dislocations. Loss of sensation concurrent with loss of movement and absence of local tissue or bone injury indicates central nervous system injury, such as spinal cord injury or cerebral hemorrhage.

Other data

Analysis of the data should include the type of injury or medical emergency that has probably occurred, the urgency of the need for medical attention, the availability of resources for carrying out necessary interventions, the availability of transportation, and the time factor before medical attention can be obtained. For example, the type of interventions that will be carried out for someone with a fractured tibia when splints are available and an ambulance is standing by for transportation to a nearby hospital may be quite different than if the same injury occurs during a wilderness hiking expedition.

General intervention

Some general principles of management when accidental injuries or sudden illnesses occur serve as guidelines when giving first aid:

1. Remain calm and think before acting.
2. Identify oneself as a nurse to victim and bystanders.
3. Do a rapid assessment for *priority* data (cessation of breathing or heartbeat, interference with breathing, hemorrhage, poisoning).
4. Carry out lifesaving measures as indicated by the priority assessment.
5. Do a head-to-toe assessment before initiating *general* first aid measures.
6. Keep the victim lying down or in the position in which he or she is found (unless orthopnea is present), protected from dampness or cold.
7. If victim is conscious, explain what is occurring. Assure him or her that help will be given.
8. Avoid unnecessary handling or moving of the victim; move the victim only if danger is present.
9. Do not give fluids if there is a possibility of abdominal injury or if anesthesia will be necessary within a short time.

10. Do not transport the victim until all first aid measures have been carried out and appropriate transportation is available.

Lifesaving measures (described on succeeding pages) are carried out first when the initial assessment indicates the presence of breathing or circulatory difficulties. After breathing has been reestablished and excessive bleeding controlled, other interventions are carried out when the head-to-toe assessment is completed.

The victim is kept in a supine or sitting position, depending on symptoms, until all necessary interventions are carried out. Wounds are covered and fractures splinted before the victim is transported. Since shock is a possibility when major injuries occur, the victim should be protected from chilling. On a cold day, protection may be needed underneath the victim with sufficient covering to prevent loss of body heat but not cause vasodilation. Oral fluids are given only to a conscious person showing signs of shock if there will be a considerable delay before medical care can be obtained and if abdominal injury is not present.

Psychologic needs of victims and significant others

Trauma is anxiety producing. It may be perceived by the victim as life threatening and a source of pain and disability. The person may be unsure of what is happening, leading to a fear of the unknown. There may be concern about economic problems such as the cost of medical care and loss of time from work. In addition, many persons have been found to have already been experiencing some other temporary anxiety and were under stress immediately before the time of the accident.

The very nature of the experiences following the emergency contribute additional anxieties. The victim is transported, perhaps by strangers, in an ambulance to a hospital emergency department. Significant others are relegated to long periods in a waiting room with little information provided. Victims see or hear other persons who are upset. They may be alone. They may wait for long periods for medical attention, while other higher priority victims are receiving care, and for results of tests or treatment. Small incidents become blown out of proportion, and a casual remark may be misinterpreted. Five minutes can seem like an hour.

Health personnel who work with accident victims from the primary point of input into the health care system until the emergency is over are prepared to meet the physical life-threatening needs. Because these needs assume priority, it is easy to overlook the psychologic needs of the victim and significant others. A calm, interested approach that conveys concern to the victim as a person is helpful. Giving information frequently dur-

ing all phases of emergency care to both victim and significant others will help them understand what is occurring and that help is being provided, thus decreasing some of the anxiety.

Varying levels of tolerance to stress are found in different individuals. The highly anxious person may need someone to stay with him or her. At the scene of an accident a calm bystander can be helpful. Some hospitals provide selected volunteers for that purpose. All health personnel need to evaluate frequently their own effectiveness in assessing anxiety and in conveying understanding and emotional support to the victim and significant others during an emergency.

Cardiopulmonary problems

For life to be maintained, oxygen must be taken in by the lungs and pumped to the tissues; carbon dioxide must be returned from the tissues to the lung and exhaled. Thus any obstruction that interferes with the diffusion of these gases, failure of the heart as a pump, or inadequate blood to carry the oxygen to the tissues is a threat to life and demands immediate emergency intervention. Airway patency, breathing facilitation, and circulation maintenance are the ABCs of emergency care and take first priority in assessment and intervention.

Airway obstruction and breathing difficulties

Asphyxia occurs if the airway is obstructed suddenly by foreign bodies or the tongue, by edema of the tissues (as with smoke inhalation or inflammation of airway passages), or by laryngospasm occurring with croup. Interference with respiration can also occur if an open chest wound, tension pneumothorax, or flail chest (p. 1235) is present. In an open wound air rushes into the pleural cavity between the lung and chest wall, creating positive pressure rather than the normal negative pressure, and the lung cannot expand to take in air. In tension pneumothorax (p. 1898), air enters the pleural space with each breath but cannot escape. The resultant increase in intrapleural pressure compromises both respirations and thoracic blood flow. A flail chest is a closed chest injury in which ribs are broken creating an unstable chest wall. Paradoxical movement of the chest wall will occur and leads to hypoxia.

Presence of fluid in the alveoli can interfere with diffusion of gases to and from the circulation in the lung. This can occur with near-drowning, secretions from infection (pneumonia), or pulmonary edema (p. 1135). Hypoxia can also occur if there is depression of the respiratory center in the brain such as with drug overdose.

Assessment

Pupils that constrict when exposed to light indicate adequate oxygenation of the brain. This will not occur with some drugs or in some elderly persons.

Signs of hypoxia are related to the efforts made by the victim to take in air. As the anoxic condition persists, signs of decreased oxygenation to tissue occur. The person with asphyxia will be dyspneic. Neck muscles will be prominent, but little or no air may be moving in or out of the nose and mouth. Intercostal rib retractions will occur as the intercostal muscles pull against resistance. Infants may show sternal retraction. If the passageway is not totally blocked, respirations will be noisy, and wheezing or stridor may be heard as the air moves through the narrowed passageway. As less oxygen is taken in, skin color will become first pale and then eventually cyanotic (grayish blue). This can be observed first in mucous membranes, lips, and nail beds.

If an open chest wound is present, a sucking noise may be heard with inspiration. The chest should be inspected for signs of bleeding or a wound. Paradoxical chest movement is denoted by the fact that the chest cage at the site of fractures moves in the direction opposite from normal during inspiration and expiration (p. 1235). Noisy respirations, rales, or rhonchi may be heard with auscultation if fluid is present in the alveoli. Excess fluid may be coughed up; secretions will be mucoid with infection, watery and frothy or blood tinged with pulmonary edema. Dyspnea will be present.

Depression of the respiratory center will be evidenced by bradycardia and slow shallow respirations. In respiratory arrest, breathing ceases completely.

Intervention

Open airway. A conscious victim may need assistance to facilitate removal of a foreign body obstructing the airway. Four forceful blows to the back between the shoulder blades may dislodge the object. If this is not effective, the Heimlich abdominal thrust maneuver may be attempted (Fig. 73-2). The rescuer stands behind the victim encircling one arm around the victim's waist. The rescuer then places a fist between the umbilicus and the xiphoid process with the thumb against the abdomen. The fist is grasped with the other hand and pressed into the abdomen with quick upward thrusts. Unless it is known positively that there is a foreign body obstructing the trachea, time should not be wasted examining for one.

The first step in assisting a person who is not breathing or is having extreme difficulty breathing is to position him or her to ensure a maximal airway. If the person is unconscious, the neck may be observed to be in a position of flexion with the back of the tongue obstructing the airway (see Fig. 24-8). If there is no trauma suggesting a neck fracture, the neck is extended by placing one hand on the forehead and the other hand

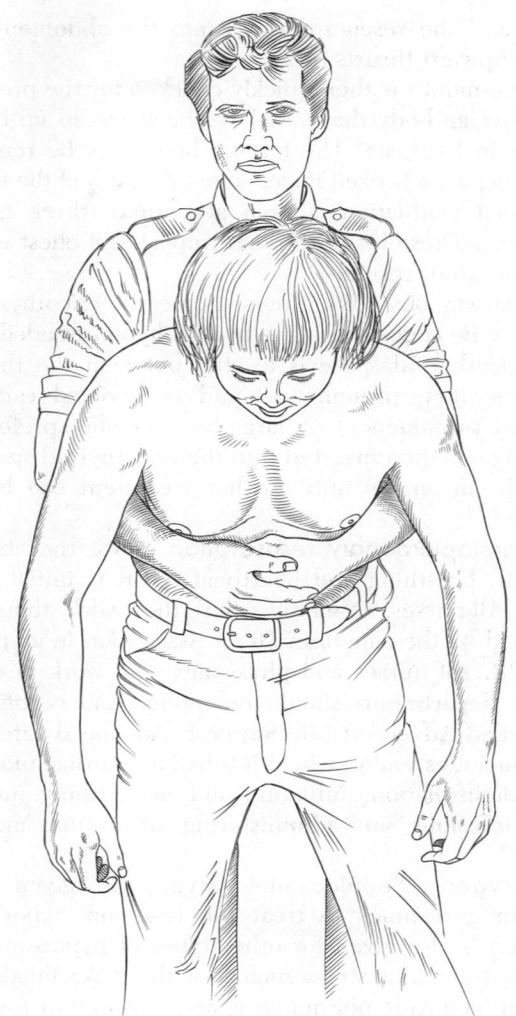

Fig. 73-2. Heimlich abdominal thrust maneuver. Rescuer places fist between umbilicus and xiphoid process with thumb pressed against abdomen.

under the neck and tilting the head back (see Fig. 44-20). If a neck fracture is suspected, the jaw can be pulled forward while the neck remains in a stable position. Either of these maneuvers will pull the back of the tongue away from the pharynx. Sometimes this maneuver alone may be enough to open the airway.

If extension of the head and neck does not initiate breathing, artificial ventilation must be initiated immediately (p. 1081). Failure of the chest to rise with ventilation indicates that the airway is obstructed by a foreign body. The victim is rolled onto one side and given four sharp blows between the shoulder blades. If this fails to dislodge the object, the victim is turned on the back and given a series of eight abdominal thrusts. The rescuer kneels at the victim's hips and places the heel of one hand between the xiphoid process and the umbilicus. The second hand is placed on top of the first hand and the rescuer presses into the abdomen with quick upward thrusts.

The mouth is then quickly checked for the presence of a foreign body that may have been forced up by the abdominal thrusts. The foreign body may be removed by sweeping a hooked finger across the back of the throat. Artificial ventilation is then attempted (three to five breaths). These maneuvers are repeated if chest expansion does not resume.

If airway obstruction persists, needle cricothyreotomy may be considered. The neck is hyperextended, and the cricothyroid space is located between the thyroid cartilage (first prominence) and the cricoid cartilage (second prominence). A large-bore needle (preferably 10 gauge) is then inserted into the cricothyroid space to provide an airway until further treatment can be instituted.[14]

Cardiopulmonary resuscitation. With the absence of both breathing and heartbeat, CPR is initiated (p. 1080). All nurses, no matter where they work, should be certified by the American Heart Association in all phases of CPR. All nurses and physicians who work in emergency departments should be trained and certified in Basic and Advanced Life Support. Advanced Life Support includes endotracheal intubation, cardiac monitoring, defibrillation, initiating and maintaining intravenous infusions, and administering intravenous medications.

Oxygen. Supplemental oxygen is given after breathing resumes to treat the resultant hypoxemia. Oxygen is also given for other types of hypoxemia following trauma or stress such as with smoke inhalation, carbon monoxide poisoning, near-drowning, or myocardial infarction. Oxygen is given following all major trauma, especially chest injuries.

Special cardiopulmonary problems

Myocardial infarction

The person suspected of experiencing a myocardial infarction needs immediate attention. The greatest risk of mortality occurs within the first 2 hours after onset.[96] Some communities have established mobile coronary units that respond immediately in these situations with advanced life-support systems. In the absence of such a unit the victim needs immediate safe transport to a medical center. If the heart ceases to beat, CPR is instituted immediately. If the patient is breathing, he or she may be more comfortable in a well-supported sitting position. Oxygen should be given if available. A calm atmosphere is of utmost importance, and the patient should never be left alone. Fear will add an additional stress to the already overburdened heart (see Chapter 45).

Near-drowning

Approximately 5800 people die from drowning in the United States each year,[97] over half in home swimming pools. *Near-drowning* is the term that refers to asphyxiation or partial asphyxiation from a fluid medium, with the person either recovering spontaneously or resuscitated at least temporarily.[14] There are three types of drowning: wet, dry, and secondary.[20] *Wet* drowning is the most common type and refers to asphyxiation from the aspiration of fluid into the lungs, inhaled as the person panics and gasps for breath. *Dry* drowning refers to asphyxiation from laryngospasm that prevents both air and water from entering the lungs. *Secondary* drowning is the recurrence of respiratory distress following recovery from the initial incident.[20] This may occur from a few minutes to several days later.

The effect of water aspirated into the lungs depends on the amount and type of water. Saltwater produces more severe changes than fresh water. Fresh water is rapidly absorbed into the circulation causing a temporary hypervolemia and hemodilution. Saltwater, because of its hypertonicity, pulls fluids into the alveoli, causing persistent hypovolemia with hemoconcentration, and pulmonary edema. Asphyxiation results in arterial hypoxemia and metabolic acidosis.

If the victim of near-drowning has ceased breathing, artificial ventilation is initiated as soon as possible, even before the victim has been completely removed from the water (see Chapter 44). If the carotid pulse is absent, cardiac resuscitation is started as soon as possible. Time should not be wasted trying to remove water from the lungs. The person removed from saltwater should be placed in a head-lowered position if possible. If distention of the abdomen from swallowed water is present and is interfering with adequate ventilation, the victim can be rolled onto the stomach and lifted with pressure over the stomach to force the water out.[96]

Persons who have experienced near-drowning need close observation for at least 24 hours, even if they indicate that they feel all right. Pulmonary edema can develop several hours later.

Electrical injuries

Electricity can cause injury in a number of ways. Depression of the respiratory center results in temporary or prolonged paralysis of respiration. Ventricular fibrillation occurs when the electric current passes through the heart at the end of the refractory period. This can occur with a low current. Powerful muscle contraction from the effect of the electric current can cause bone fractures or muscle injury that may persist for many months. Since the body acts as a conductor, electricity has an entrance point, travels through the body, and exits at a distant point. Burns with resultant necrosis of tissue occur at both entrance and exit points and possibly along the path of the current.

The extent of injury from electricity depends on the point in the heartbeat cycle that is stimulated by the electricity, the intensity of the current, and skin resistance. Moisture decreases skin resistance; therefore greater damage occurs when skin is moist with water or perspiration.

The victim must be removed from the source of electricity with the rescuer being careful to avoid contact with the electric charge. The rescuer must never have direct contact with the body of the victim because the charge may be transmitted. The rescuer should use a long, dry stick and stand on a dry board to roll the victim away from the electric charge. Asbestos or heavy dry gloves are needed if the victim must be moved away from an electric wire. CPR is started immediately (if breathing and pulse are absent) and continued even when there is no evidence of response. Defibrillation is indicated for ventricular fibrillation.

Hemorrhage

As stated earlier, maintenance of an adequate blood flow to carry oxygen to the tissues is vital to support life. External bleeding is readily visible, and if bleeding is profuse, it needs immediate attention. It can occur with lacerations, crushing injuries, amputations, fractures, and nosebleeds. Internal bleeding is more difficult to identify and can occur with chest or abdominal trauma such as a ruptured spleen, trauma to large muscle masses of the extremity (thigh), or certain medical conditions such as esophageal varices or bleeding ulcers.

When a blood vessel is severed, there is an immediate contraction of the vessel wall reducing the size of the opening and decreasing blood loss. Platelets begin to adhere to the roughened edges until a platelet plug is formed. A clot begins to form within 1 to 2 minutes. By 3 to 6 minutes that clot has filled the end of the blood vessel, blocking blood flow.[51] Direct pressure over a bleeding vessel for 5 to 6 minutes will help stop the blood flow to permit clot formation. If a major artery is severed, ligation (tying off) of the artery may be necessary for continued cessation of bleeding. Pressure (digital pressure or tourniquet) applied to an artery proximal to the wound may also slow or stop the blood flow. This also slows or stops blood perfusion to the tissue between the pressure point and the wound producing tissue damage. Direct pressure over the bleeding vessel is therefore the action of choice unless bleeding cannot be controlled in this manner. Large arteries have musculature that can produce considerable vasospasms.

Amputation of a leg, for example, may produce minimal bleeding. Veins and capillaries have thinner walls, and bleeding of these vessels can usually be controlled by direct pressure.

Assessment

External bleeding, if excessive, will saturate the clothing and be readily visible. If the person is wearing bulky outer garments, bleeding may be concealed. The examiner should run the hands quickly over the entire body under the outer clothing, being sure to check underneath the victim. Saturated clothing may need to be cut away to examine the area of bleeding. Three types of bleeding can be observed: spurting of bright red blood indicates arterial bleeding, continuous flow of darker blood indicates venous bleeding, and oozing indicates capillary bleeding. The scalp is very vascular, and what appears to be considerable bleeding may occur from a small scalp laceration.

Internal bleeding may be difficult to identify. Bleeding into the thorax (hemothorax) may inhibit respirations, and chest pain may be present. Abdominal bleeding may be evidenced by rigidity of abdominal muscles and abdominal pain. Hemoptysis or hematemesis indicates internal bleeding.

Shock occurs with severe internal or external bleeding. The victim is assessed for weak rapid pulse, slow shallow respiration, cold clammy skin, anxiety, restlessness, and thirst. The pupils are equal, may be dilated, and respond slowly to light.

Intervention

Direct pressure is applied to the site of external bleeding. If a sterile dressing is not available, a clean handkerchief, sanitary pad, or clean cloth may be used. The dressing is held in place by a tight bandage for continued pressure. The bare hand can be used to apply direct pressure until an adequate dressing is available. If severe arterial bleeding cannot be controlled by direct pressure, or if direct pressure cannot be applied, pressure-point control over a bony prominence proximal to the point of hemorrhage can be attempted (Fig. 73-3).

Tourniquets are rarely necessary since they may cause further damage and can result in loss of an arm or leg. If a tourniquet must be used, it should be applied with the following precautions. A triangular bandage should be folded at least 3 to 4 in. wide, six to eight layers thick, and wrapped twice around the extremity.[3] A stick or similar object is tied on by the ends of the bandage and twisted to tighten the tourniquet just enough to stop the bleeding but no tighter. A blood pressure cuff makes a useful tourniquet. Once the tourniquet is applied, it should be released only by a physician. The tourniquet is never covered, and a notation

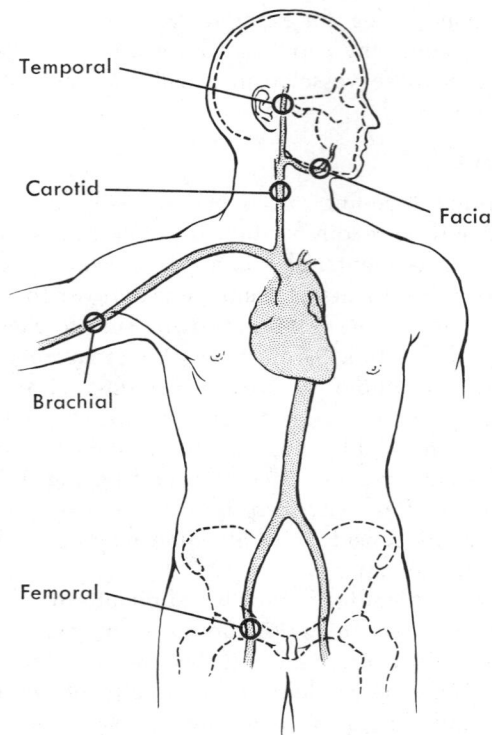

Fig. 73-3. Pressure points—locations at which large blood vessels may be compressed against bones to help control hemorrhage.

is made and attached to the patient giving the location and time of application.

Poisoning

Poisoning, either unintentional or deliberate, remains a major cause of deaths from accidents. On the average there are 5000 deaths from poisoning in the United States each year.[97]

Poisoning among children usually results from accidental ingestion. Children are naturally curious, and as they begin to crawl and walk they explore their widening horizons. Bottles or containers containing brightly colored pills or liquids are examined, and if the container can be opened the substance is put into the mouth and swallowed. Older children mimic the pill taking of adults either in their play activities or as a relief of symptoms for which they have received medication in the past. They may also take pills as an attention-getting device.

Poisoning in adults commonly occurs from not checking medication labels (overdose or wrong medi-

cation), from lack of knowledge (e.g., taking alcohol and sedatives together), by taking an excess amount in an attempt to obtain a desired effect, or as a suicide attempt.

Prevention

There has been a decrease in the number of fatalities from poisoning in children under the age of 5 years. This has been the result of safety packaging of medications and to better education of the public about preventive measures. The Food and Drug Administration established regulations in 1970 that require that hazardous medicines be enclosed in containers with child-proof safety closure caps. The cap must be squeezed in or pushed down before it can be released.

Education of the public is directed toward increasing their awareness of safety hazards in the home. Medicine cabinets, kitchen cupboards, and laundry closets are the places from which children most often take poisons. Sleeping pills and tranquilizer tablets left on bedside tables and in handbags also are a potential source of poisoning. Cleaning compounds should be kept away from food storage areas and out of reach of children. Nonpotable liquids should be kept in their original containers, tightly capped, and *never* placed in a soft-drink bottle, drinking glass, or cup.

Aspirin remains the substance most often ingested in quantity by children. There has been a decrease in the ingestion of insecticides and bleaches but an increase in the ingestion of soaps, detergents, plants, perfumes, vitamins, and cold medicines by children.[79] Lead poisoning remains a problem in preschool children in low economic areas who live in pre–World War II housing, a time when lead-based paints were commonly used.[26]

In recent years education about drug abuse has been aimed at school-aged children. A comparison of four studies of an existing drug education program indicated that drug education at the secondary school level may fail to decrease the illegal use of drugs. Drug abuse education should be aimed at younger children, who appear more easily influenced by drug education than older students. During the 1960s there was a rapid increase in the number of persons using hallucinogenic drugs, but this leveled off by the mid 1970s. A considerable number of young persons become addicted and may experience overdoses (see Chapter 15).

Assessment

A *rapid* assessment is made to determine whether poisoning or overdose has occurred so that immediate action can be taken to prevent or diminish the effects of the poison or drug. It is important to identify (1) cues that poisoning is a possibility and (2) the type and quantity of the poisonous agent.

Poisoning is suspected when there is a sudden onset of symptoms, especially in a very young child. These symptoms may include nausea and vomiting, abdominal pain, convulsions, change of consciousness, and decreased respirations or pulse rate. If poisoning is suspected, the lips and mouth are examined for signs of burns, excessive salivation, or difficulty in swallowing. The breath is noted for an odor such as from petroleum products or cleaning compounds.

If the victim is conscious he or she should be questioned for information concerning what and how much was taken. The victim may not be conscious, since coma occurs with many drug overdoses. Not much time should be spent looking for needle marks since drugs may be injected by addicts in unusual places such as the penis or feet.[44] Identification of the poison or drug can be facilitated by asking others to look for clues while you are examining the victim. Empty containers, spilled fluids, open medication bottles, or syringes may provide needed information. *All* potential agents should be gathered in their original containers and taken to the hospital with the victim. The physician may need to know the ingredients of the agent for those situations when an antidote is indicated. Assessment data should also include the expected time before medical help can be obtained.

Common accidental poisoning

Immediate action is necessary if poisoning is suspected; in some instances delay of a few minutes may make a difference between life and death. An *unconscious* victim must be transported *without delay* to the nearest medical facility.

If the victim is *conscious*, ascertain age and identify the type, method, and estimated amount of poison or drug taken. Have someone call a physician immediately if possible. If a private physician is not available, a *poison control center* can give rapid and accurate information. Most large cities have poison control centers, which maintain an extensive file on the most common substances and drugs. The telephone number is usually easily obtained from a list of emergency numbers in the front of the telephone directory.

Management consists of stopping absorption of the poisonous substance or drug. Poisonous substances can be inhaled, absorbed from the skin or mucous membranes, ingested, or injected. The type of intervention depends on the method by which the poison entered the system.

Inhaled poison

Persons who have inhaled a toxic gas first need to be removed from the site to fresh air and given oxygen if available. As in any emergency, cardiopulmonary status should be assessed and resuscitation started if indicated. The victim is transported immediately to a medical center.

Carbon monoxide is one of the more common of the toxic gases. It is odorless and occurs as a result of incomplete combustion such as during fires or from automobile exhaust. It cannot be filtered by the use of a cloth face mask. Toxicity occurs because of the higher affinity of hemoglobin for carbon monoxide than for oxygen. The victim becomes profoundly hypoxic and loses consciousness. Carboxyhemoglobin has a deep red color and is seen in the mucous membranes of all victims and by a red coloring of white or light-colored skin.

Contact poison

Poisonous substances absorbed through the skin or mucous membranes should be rinsed off immediately with copious amounts of water without taking time to remove garments. Following this the garments containing the substance are removed and the skin is rinsed again.

Ingested poison

The most common form of poisoning is by ingestion of a poisonous substance or an excessive amount of a drug. Absorption of the agent can be prevented by inducing vomiting or by lavage to eliminate the agent and by giving a substance that will make the poisonous agent inert.

Elimination of the poison. The first treatment objective is removal of the ingested poison (except with ingestion of caustics or low volatile hydrocarbons). *Vomiting* is the best method since gastric lavage does not remove substances in stomach pouches that are inaccessible to lavage.[15] Lavage with a cuffed endotracheal tube to prevent aspiration is indicated for unconscious persons.

The recommended method of inducing vomiting is by the oral administration of *syrup of ipecac,* 15 ml for a child and 30 ml for adolescents and adults. The dose may be repeated once in 15 to 20 minutes if necessary. The victim is encouraged to drink a small glass of fluid 3 to 5 minutes after administration of the syrup of ipecac to promote complete emptying of the stomach. Mechanically induced vomiting, such as tickling the back of the throat, is usually ineffective since only a small amount is vomited.[70] The use of mustard or salt mixed with water is ineffective for inducing vomiting, and the ingested salt may produce a hypernatremia.[39]

Caustic substances such as lye erode the esophagus as they are ingested and frequently result in esophageal perforation and subsequent esophageal stenosis. Drinking acidic substances such as vinegar or citrus juices to counteract the basic property of lye is now *not* recommended since this may result in an exothermic reaction causing additional pain and burning.[39] Emergency care consists in giving a small amount of milk or water and seeking immediate medical attention.

Hydrocarbons, which are found in all petroleum products, produce a severe pneumonia from direct aspiration into the lungs during ingestion.[15] The question of whether vomiting should be induced is controversial. It is now thought that highly volatile hydrocarbons such as charcoal lighter fluid, which may cause a central nervous system depression, should be eliminated by vomiting but that low volatile hydrocarbons should not be immediately eliminated, and medical attention should be obtained.[15]

Inactivation of the poison. In recent years there has been renewed interest in the use of activated charcoal, which is usually given after the victim has vomited. Activated charcoal will adsorb a drug and prevent it from being absorbed into the body by way of the gastrointestinal tract. It varies in its adsorptive action but has a high affinity for analgesics (especially aspirin), barbiturates and other hypnotics, and amphetamines. Activated charcoal should be administered within 30 minutes of poisoning to achieve maximal effect but can be given later with good results.

Activated charcoal, which is not the same as a blackened piece of toast, can be purchased at a drugstore. (Nuchar A, Norit A, Activated Charcoal by Merck). It is given as a powder, not a tablet, and the major drawback is the color of the solution. Children will drink it, however, if it is presented with a positive approach. The child's dose is 0.5 to 1 g/kg, and the adult dose is 30 to 50 g, both are given in 60 to 90 ml of water. Saline cathartics are then given to remove the adsorbed poison.

Cathartics are now seldom used except with activated charcoal since ipecac itself will usually cause catharsis and the ingested poison will also often cause diarrhea.[15]

Antidotes. If it is known exactly what poisonous substance or drug has been ingested, a specific antidote may be given in some cases by the physician. (Common poisons and antidotes are discussed in pharmacology and toxicology texts.) The use of a "universal antidote" has not proved to be effective.

Injected poison

Toxic substances can be injected through the skin, such as by insect bites or by needle injection. Drugs most commonly injected are heroin, barbiturates, and amphetamines. Stimulants such as the amphetamines produce hyperactivity and "uncooperative" behavior. Overdose may produce tachycardia, chills, and col-

lapse. Depressants such as heroin or barbiturates produce respiratory depression resulting in coma and death. Overdose often occurs because the victim is unaware of the potency of the drug purchased illegally.

Insect bites. The most common insect bites that can produce severe reactions are those of wasps and bees. Death can occur either because of the multiplicity of bites (especially in young children) or from anaphylactic shock if the victim is allergic to the protein in the venom. The reaction may be slow in developing or sudden and acute. Sensitized persons should avoid areas where bees and wasps are found, should carry tablets of isoproterenol for sublingual use and uncoated antihistamine tablets for immediate oral use, and should have epinephrine (Adrenalin) available for immediate use parenterally if anaphylaxis occurs. The wearing of a Medic-Alert tag facilitates emergency care if the victim is unconscious.

When a person is stung by a bee, the stinger with the venom bag is left in the skin. The stinger should be removed immediately because venom continues to be pumped into the skin from the bag. Removal of the stinger by grasping and pulling is to be avoided, since this pushes more venom into the skin. The stinger is removed by a scraping motion.[107] Ice can be applied to prevent absorption of the venom (heat should be avoided). A paste of sodium bicarbonate and water or a weak solution of ammonia may help by counteracting the formic acid present in the venom.

Tick bites can cause tick fever by transmission of a toxin, a virus as in Colorado tick fever, or rickettsiae as in Rocky Mountain spotted fever. Sudden removal of a tick will result in its mouthpiece remaining. Applying gasoline or turpentine to the head of a tick or applying the hot end of a previously lighted match to the body will cause the tick to drop off within 10 minutes. Ice can be applied to reduce absorption of toxin.

Supportive care

Good nursing care of the acutely poisoned patient may make the difference between a favorable and a fatal outcome. The patient is kept warm enough to prevent chilling and observed extremely closely for changes in physical signs such as rapid thready pulse, respiratory distress, cyanosis, diaphoresis and other signs of collapse, vasogenic shock, or impending death. Changes are reported to the physician immediately. Vital signs are usually monitored at least every 15 minutes for several hours. Nausea, vomiting, and abdominal pain are recorded, and all vomitus is observed for signs of blood and saved for study. Stools and urine are checked for abnormal constituents such as blood. Intravenous fluids are usually prescribed.

If the patient has marked depression of respiration, oxygen may be given, and sometimes a mechanical ventilator is necessary. A suction machine should be on hand at all times since suctioning of the bronchial tree may be necessary. Unconscious patients are turned frequently to provide drainage from each bronchus.

If the poisoning was a suicide attempt, adequate safety precautions are instituted. A psychiatric consultation is often recommended. Persons addicted to heroin or morphine derivatives who have overdosed should be observed for signs of withdrawal. Symptoms usually appear within 12 to 18 hours and include yawning, sweating, shaking, vomiting, diarrhea, lacrimation, runny nose, abdominal pain, backache, and other flu-type symptoms.

Food poisoning

A number of toxicants occur in plants and animals ingested as food. Some toxicants are introduced by mistake as pesticides during plant growth, as food additives, or as part of food packaging. Commercially packaged foods are monitored closely, and products are withdrawn from the market if contamination is suspected.

Plant poisoning

Poisoning from plants is usually not a problem, because people have learned to identify poisonous foods. Mushroom poisoning still occurs, however, when people eat uncultivated mushrooms thinking that they are of a safe variety. Two types of mushroom poisoning can occur. One type contains the alkaloid muscarine, which has a parasympathetic effect. Symptoms develop immediately after eating and are characterized by sweating, lacrimation, salivation, dyspnea, vomiting, and muscle tremors. Respiratory and circulatory depression may occur. The second type of mushroom poisoning has an atropine-like effect. Symptoms occur 6 to 24 hours after ingestion and are characterized by nausea and vomiting, bloody diarrhea, dehydration, and muscle weakness. Circulatory system collapse and central nervous system involvement may occur.

First aid treatment for mushroom poisoning is the same as for drug poisoning: induce vomiting with syrup of ipecac, give fluids, and then give activated charcoal. After the ipecac, 30 mg of magnesium sulfate (Epsom salts) is given in water by mouth to hasten evacuation. Medical care should be obtained.

Bacterial food poisoning

Food poisoning occurs more frequently than is reported because the majority of persons recover quickly without treatment.[50] The incidence of food poisoning from commercially prepared foods has become relatively uncommon in the United States, but food poisoning from home-cooked foods or improper handling of foods still occurs.

Bacteria such as *Staphylococcus aureus* or *Clostridium botulinum* can produce a toxin that acts as a poison causing acute gastrointestinal tract upset. The toxin of *Staphylococcus aureus* does not spread through the body, and the symptoms are therefore limited. The toxin of *Clostridium botulinum* does spread and can be fatal (Table 73-1). *Salmonella* organisms introduced in food multiply in the intestines causing acute gastrointestinal tract upset and infection. Food poisoning is not caused by food that has spoiled or decomposed unless the food

TABLE 73-1. Bacterial food poisoning

Symptoms	Causative agent	Source	Comments
Nausea and vomiting, abdominal pain, lowered temperature, diarrhea is variable	*Staphylococcus aureus:* enterotoxin	Fish and meats (especially ham), dehydrated milk, unrefrigerated mayonnaise and cream-filled foods; skin and respiratory tract of food handlers	Mortality low Toxin heat stable Incubation of 1-6 hr Symptoms last 8-24 hr Treatment: bed rest, fluids
Nausea and vomiting, diarrhea, abdominal pain, chills and fever, weakness	*Salmonella:* multiply in gut and produce toxin	Inadequately cooked eggs, poultry, meat (especially pork)	Mortality low Organism killed by heat Incubation of 10-48 hr Symptoms last 2-5 days Treatment: bed rest, fluids (no antibiotics; they produce resistant strains)
Nausea and vomiting; double vision; flaccid paralysis of face, eyes, mouth, throat; dryness of skin, mouth, throat	*Clostridium botulinum:* exotoxin; spores germinate under anaerobic conditions and produce toxin	Improperly canned vegetables, meat (low-acid foods); spiced, smoked, vacuum-packed, or canned alkaline foods eaten without cooking	Mortality high Toxin heat labile Incubation of 12-36 hr Death from respiratory failure

happens to contain disease-causing bacteria. The majority of food poisonings are caused by *Staphylococcus aureus*.

Prevention

Acute food poisoning can be prevented. Rigid controls of slaughterhouse practices have decreased the incidence of food poisoning. Pasteurization of milk destroys salmonellae. Rigorous enforcement of sanitary practices by food handlers can decrease food poisoning by *Staphylococcus* and *Salmonella* organisms. Food handlers should not be allowed to work if they have even minor infections on their hands or do not adhere to the requirements for hand washing after using the toilet. Toilets should not be adjacent to kitchens.

Health teaching should include the proper handling and cooling of foods. Home canning has become increasingly popular, but many people are unaware of the need to process low-acid foods (foods other than tomatoes or fruits) under pressure to prevent botulism. The U.S. Department of Agriculture, state agricultural departments, the home economics departments of schools, or newspapers may have booklets available on home canning methods. Any can that is bulging should be discarded.

Additional measures to prevent food poisoning include avoiding slow cooling of meat dishes; avoiding cooking of extremely large chunks of meat (especially pork) unless a meat thermometer is used that measures the heat of the core of the meat; or allowing meats, fish, mayonnaise, or cream-filled foods to remain unrefrigerated for periods of time. Foods that are rewarmed should be boiled, since merely warming will rapidly increase bacterial growth.

Intervention

If abdominal pain and diarrhea accompany the nausea and vomiting, with or without fever, the causative organisms are either *Staphylococcus* or *Salmonella*. If the symptoms are very mild, no interventions are indicated. If fluid loss is severe, fluid balance should be restored and bed rest may be indicated. Fluids such as tea or broth may be well tolerated. If severe dehydration occurs, intravenous fluids may be necessary.

There is no emergency first aid treatment suitable for *Clostridium botulinum* poisoning. The victim should be taken to a hospital for medical care. Data should be obtained concerning the source of the poisoning, and any other persons who might have eaten the contaminated food should be contacted immediately. Medical treatment consists of supportive therapy and the administration of botulinum antitoxin. Antitoxin cannot undo damage that has already occurred but can prevent further damage. Approximately 65% of these patients die within 3 to 16 days after onset of symptoms. Fortunately, this type of poisoning is now quite rare.

Environmental injuries: heat, cold, radiation

Exposure to extremes of temperature affects both the general reaction of the body to the stress and the local reaction of the skin. General reactions occur more readily when the individual has not been conditioned to the extremes in temperature. Incidences of overexposure to heat, for example, occur more often in the early part of a hot spell before the individual is acclimated.

General reactions to heat and cold

Three general reactions can occur with heat: heat cramps, heat exhaustion, and heatstroke (sunstroke). Cold produces a general cooling of the body (hypothermia).

Heat cramps

Heat cramps are sudden muscle pains caused by loss of sodium chloride in perspiration during strenuous exercise in hot weather. The best treatment is prevention by taking extra salt and water or drinking a balanced salt-containing fluid such as Gatorade when severe exertion is anticipated. The immediate treatment consists of salty fluids and foods by mouth, extra water, and rest for a few hours.

Heat exhaustion

Heat exhaustion is vasomotor collapse caused by the inability of the body to supply the peripheral vessels adequately with sufficient fluids to produce the perspiration needed for cooling and yet meet vital tissue requirements. The condition usually follows an extended period of vigorous exercise in hot weather, particularly when an individual has not had a period of acclimatization. The symptoms are faintness, weakness, headache, and sometimes nausea and vomiting. The skin is pale and moist. Body temperature is slightly above normal. Heat exhaustion can often be prevented by taking extra salt and extra fluid during hot weather and by tempering physical activity during very hot weather. Emergency care consists of treating for shock and transporting the victim to a medical center. Fluids should be given, preferably containing salt, although the condition is not primarily caused by lack of salt.[3]

Heatstroke

Heatstroke (sunstroke) is a serious condition in which excessive body heat is retained, and it requires immediate emergency treatment. It is caused by a failure of the perspiration-regulating mechanism in the hypothalamus. Persons at high risk are those who are elderly or obese, have not become acclimatized, or have had a recent infectious disease.[15] Heatstroke is typically seen during a heat wave but also occurs in healthy young persons who exercise vigorously in hot weather. The person undergoing vigorous exercise in intense heat may perspire profusely for some time and then become dehydrated and fail to produce sufficient perspiration to maintain normal body temperature. The skin is dry, hot, and flushed in contrast to the pale, moist skin of the person suffering from heat exhaustion. The victim becomes confused, dizzy, and faint and may quickly lose consciousness. Body temperature is above 40° C (104° F).

Without treatment most heatstroke victims will die, but with prompt and vigorous treatment almost all will recover. Treatment consists of actions to reduce the body temperature immediately while transporting the victim to a medical center. The victim should be placed in a cool place, such as an air-conditioned room, while awaiting transportation. Cold, moist applications to the body and a fan to increase evaporation are helpful. These measures are continued during transportation.

If the elevated temperature is allowed to persist, serious permanent damage is done to the brain and the entire nervous system. Treatment should be continued until the temperature has been lowered to at least 39° C (102° F), and the temperature must then be checked carefully for several hours for sudden rise. The patient should respond when the temperature lowers. Failure to do so may indicate that brain damage has occurred. Persons do not recover from heatstroke as quickly as from heat exhaustion. Often there is faulty heat regulation for days and a lowered tolerance to heat for years and sometimes for the rest of the individual's life. The person who has had a heatstroke should be advised to plan his or her living so that repeated long exposures to heat are avoided.

Accidental hypothermia

The extent of the cooling effect that occurs with exposure to extreme cold depends on the temperature and exposure time, the thermal conductivity of the environment, and the amount of air current present. Moisture is a good conductor; air is not. Wet clothing therefore contributes to increased cooling of the body. Several light layers of clothing to provide air insulation will keep a person warmer than one heavy layer. Air movement contributes to heat loss; thus lower environmental temperatures can be tolerated better in the absence of wind (windchill factor).

When the body is exposed to cold, shivering occurs to produce heat by increased metabolism. As the cold increases, shivering ceases and heat loss exceeds heat production. The individual becomes listless, apathetic, and sleepy and may become indifferent to the sur-roundings and not seek adequate protection. Pulse and respirations become slower as metabolism decreases. Freezing of the extremities, unconsciousness, and finally death will result if help is not received.

The victim needs to be kept warm while being transferred to a medical facility. Wet clothing is removed immediately and warmed blankets applied. If a tub bath is given, the temperature should be approximately 40° to 42° C (104° to 108° F). Warmer temperatures can cause skin damage from the decreased circulation to the skin.[51] Rubbing of the skin is to be avoided since this can also cause skin damage. Warm liquids may be given if the victim is conscious.

The person suffering hypothermia should be monitored closely during rewarming. Hypovolemic shock can occur from vasodilation. If intravenous fluids are given, overloading of the circulation is a potential complication. Vital signs are monitored for sudden changes. Cardiac monitoring may also be indicated during the rewarming period for signs of ventricular fibrillation and cardiac arrest.

Local reactions to heat and cold

Burns

Burns may be caused by direct heat, chemicals, electricity, or radiation (sun or nuclear rays). Heat burns are treated by immersion in cool water or application of clean, cool wet packs. Clothing should not be removed nor ointments applied. Shock may occur with severe burns as a result of fluid shifts. (For more detailed information on burns, see Chapter 70.)

Frostbite

Cellular injury occurs with exposure to extreme cold. Cell water freezes, and the resulting ice crystals damage the cell. The degree of injury depends on the depth of freezing. Frostbite occurs most frequently in exposed areas such as the nose, cheeks, ears, and fingers and can be prevented by adequate covering with loose-fitting dry clothing. Toes are also susceptible because of dampness and tight pressure from shoes or boots. Persons with circulatory problems are more prone to develop frostbite.

Frostbite can be classified as incipient, superficial, or deep.[3] *Incipient frostbite* often goes unnoticed and is evidence by paleness or loss of color of the skin. Removing the victim to a warm room, cupping the injured part with the hands, or placing fingers in the armpit for warmth may be all that is needed. Tingling occurs with warming.

Superficial frostbite may develop if incipient frostbite is not noticed. Freezing extends into the superficial tissue below the skin. The frozen part is soft, and white skin does not redden with pressure. Dark skin has a dull ashen shade. The frozen part may be warmed by covering. Heat is not applied since this may damage the injured tissue, but the frozen part may be immersed gently in warm water (43° C [110° F]). Contrary to popular belief, the frozen part should never be rubbed with snow because this increases the trauma to the injured tissue.

Deep frostbite is evidenced by hardness of the frozen tissue because deep subcutaneous tissue is injured. After thawing, the skin becomes hyperemic and edematous with blister formation. The edema subsides in 24 to 48 hours, and tissue breakdown with necrosis results. The frozen part should be covered to warm it, and the victim should be taken to a medical center as soon as possible. The care is then similar to that for vascular disease of the extremities (p. 1146). Efforts are made to decrease the oxygen needs of the tissues while healing takes place, to improve blood supply by the use of drugs, and to prevent infection of open lesions. Necrotic tissue may have to be debrided for healing to occur.

Radiation exposure and injury

Accidental injury through radiation is an ever present potential as a result of nuclear energy and the use of nuclear materials in industry. Considerable precautions are employed in areas where nuclear materials are used. The likelihood of accidental injury is greater while these materials are being transported from one area to another.[3]

Radiation injury is caused by exposure to gamma (γ-) rays and neutrons from radioactive material. Persons can become contaminated by the rays as a result of a nuclear explosion or directly through the air from unshielded radioactive material or inhaled or swallowed on particles of contaminated dust or smoke. The amount of radiation that a person receives depends on the strength of the radiation source, the distance of the victim from the source, the duration of the exposure, the area of the body exposed to the radiation source, and the amount and type of shielding that are present.

Prevention

Special precautionary measures should be used whenever radioactive materials are being utilized. All persons having contact with these materials should become knowledgeable concerning preventive measures. Exposure to radiation is carefully monitored; for example, personnel who work with radioactive materials or x-rays (γ- rays) wear special monitoring badges.

Rescue workers who must remove a victim from an area of radioactivity need to protect themselves from radiation exposure. Since radioactive particles can be carried on dust, all skin areas must be covered and a filtering mask worn by rescue workers following an explosion involving nuclear materials. The greater the time of exposure, the greater the potential for injury; therefore the victim must be removed immediately to a less hazardous environment. Some of the basic principles of emergency care may have to be violated when there is danger of other explosions or when fires occur. The rescue worker should remove all contaminated clothing at the edge of the contaminated area, and any exposed skin areas are washed throughly. A shower should be taken as soon as possible as an additional preventive measure.[3]

Intervention

Radiation rays can cause a local inflammatory reaction of the skin similar to a burn. The involved area may be washed gently with soap and water and a dry sterile dressing applied. No antiseptic or disinfectant solutions should be used, and no debridement should be attempted.[37]

Radiation sickness will not become apparent until several days after exposure. There may be nausea and vomiting shortly after exposure, but this ceases spontaneously. Because radiation affects the body's immune response, later symptoms may include severe inflammation and sometimes sloughing and hemorrhage of the mucous membranes of the mouth and throat, bloody diarrhea, purpura (hemorrhagic spots under the skin), and alopecia (loss of hair). A severe leukopenia quickly follows exposure to large amounts of radiation.

There is no specific treatment for radiation sickness. The patient needs the same care as one who receives radiation treatment (p. 493). This care includes rest, protection from superimposed infection, good mouth care, fluid and electrolyte replacement, and a high-calorie diet.

Musculoskeletal injuries

Soft-tissue injuries

Injury to soft tissue may result in either open or closed wounds. Types of open wounds include abrasions, avulsions, incisions or lacerations, and puncture wounds. In a closed wound the skin is not broken, but there is injury to underlying tissue. A contusion (bruise) is a closed wound.

Open wounds usually become infected. This develops 1 to 2 days after injury, but in grossly contaminated wounds signs of infection can be observed in 8 to 12 hours. Signs of infection include erythema, edema, and pain, and a purulent exudate is present. The patient may develop fever and lymphadenopathy.

General management of open wounds consists of

control of bleeding, thorough cleansing with soap and water to prevent infection, irrigation of deep wounds to remove foreign material, and suturing, if possible, to approximate skin edges and hasten healing.

Types of wounds

Abrasions. An abrasion is a scraping of the skin surface commonly referred to as a "floor burn" or "brush burn." It involves only a partial thickness of the skin. Abrasions are commonly experienced by active children and athletes and in motorcycle accidents. When a large area of skin has been denuded, an abrasion can be painful. Good cleaning of the wound with soap and water is important to remove all pieces of embedded foreign matter, which can delay healing and cause scarring. A topical antibiotic ointment can be applied. If the wound can be kept clean, no covering is necessary. Covering with a sterile dressing may be indicated for children.

Avulsions. A flap of skin and subcutaneous tissue that has been torn loose is called an avulsion. Large flaps can be torn loose from any part of the body, especially the head and extremities. Avulsions must be cleaned thoroughly and irrigated well to remove any foreign material before they are sutured.

Lacerations. A jagged cut through skin and other tissue is termed a laceration. A sharp knife will produce a straight cut, or *incision*. Lacerations or incisions vary in depth and may involve muscles and tendons.

The laceration or incision is cleaned well and sutured through each layer. Any gap left through nonapproximation of the wound may delay healing. Incisions usually heal more quickly with less scar formation than lacerations because the edges can be better approximated. Suturing should be carried out within the first few hours after injury to obtain maximal healing with fewer complications or scarring. If the wound is grossly contaminated, the decision may be made to delay suturing for a few days to permit thorough cleansing. Healing then occurs by tertiary intention (p. 442). Suturing may not be necessary for superficial lacerations. The edges of the wound can be approximated by the use of one or more butterfly adhesive strips (Fig. 73-4).

Puncture wounds. A puncture wound is caused by a sharp, pointed, narrow object such as a nail, pin, bullet, splinter of wood, or animal bite. As the tissues are penetrated by the object, pathogenic organisms may be introduced. Since the skin quickly seals over, the wound rarely bleeds enough to wash out organisms. Bacteria such as *Clostridium tetani*, which thrive without air, may infect these wounds. Because anaerobic bacterial infections are extremely serious, a physician should be consulted if the puncture was made by a dirty object.

Puncture wounds received from objects such as contaminated needles used for any parenteral treatment also should be reported to the physician since viral hepatitis may be contracted from this type in injury. Immune

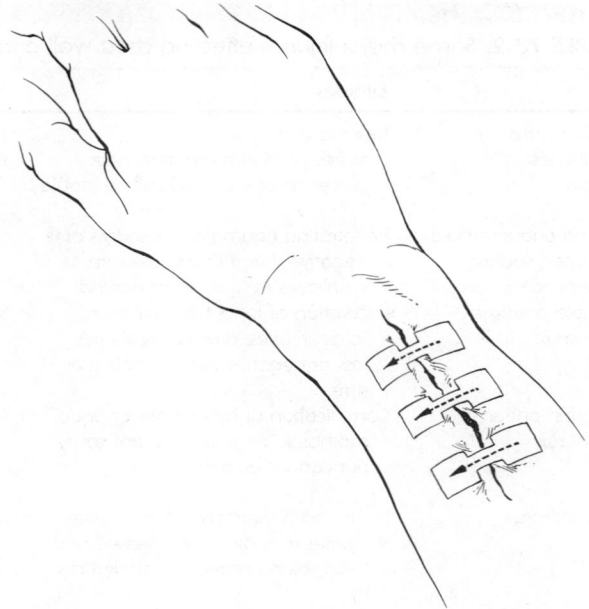

Fig. 73-4. Use of butterfly adhesive strips to approximate skin edges in laceration of forearm. Note irregular wound edges and placement of adhesive. Arrows indicate direction of pull used to partially close wound.

serum globulin may be given as prophylaxis.

Puncture wounds are treated by soaks. A small amount of bleeding is encouraged in small puncture wounds to assist in washing out microorganisms. The wound should be observed for signs of infection. Prophylaxis against tetanus is instituted (p. 1902).

Stab wounds are a form of puncture wound. An object such as a knife, stick, or piece of glass can become impaled in the body. The impaled object should *not* be removed except by a physician in a medical facility, usually in the operating room. If there is severe bleeding, pressure points may be used to control loss of blood. The object should be stabilized before transportation to prevent accidental dislodgement and further trauma.

Contusions. Blunt objects may injure underlying tissue without breaking the skin. Edema may develop from trauma to the injured cells; this is usually "brawny" edema because it does not "pit." Blood vessels usually rupture, and the blood seeps into the tissue creating a hematoma. The skin acquires a black-and-blue appearance from the extravasated blood. Pain is usually present. Rest of the injured part is advised, and analgesics may be helpful if pain is severe. Application of ice during the first 24 to 48 hours encourages vasoconstriction, decreasing blood seepage and edema.

Special wounds

Chest injuries. Injuries to the chest may result in open chest wounds, fractured ribs, or injuries to the

TABLE 73-2. Some major injuries affecting chest wall and pleural cavity

Injury	Etiology	Signs and symptoms	Initial emergency care
Rib fracture	Blow to chest	Pain on inspiration; local tenderness	Transport
Flail chest	Ribs fractured in more than one place; chest wall becomes unstable	Paradoxical respirations; respiratory distress; chest pain	Apply external pressure: sandbags, pillow, your hand; give oxygen; transport with flail side down
Open pneumothorax (open sucking wound)	Penetrating trauma to chest; loss of negative intrathoracic pressure as air moves in and out of wound	Sucking sound on chest wall during inspiration; tracheal deviation	Cover wound with occlusive dressing during exhalation; give oxygen
Simple pneumo-thorax	Laceration of lung, hyperinflation (blast injuries, driving accidents), loss of negative intrathoracic pressure	Sudden onset of chest pain; decreased breath sounds of affected area; dyspnea, tachypnea	Semi-Fowler's or Fowler's position; give oxygen
Tension pneumo-thorax	Complication of other types of pneumothorax; air enters pleural cavity but cannot escape	Respiratory distress; paradoxical chest movements; neck vein distention; tracheal deviation to unaffected side	Maintain airway and breathing; give oxygen (needle thoracotomy by trained person)
Hemothorax	Blunt and penetrating chest injuries; injuries to major blood vessels and heart; blood collects in pleural cavity	Decreased breath sounds; dyspnea (cyanosis and signs of shock if severe)	Treat for shock; give oxygen

respiratory tract or to the heart. Some of the major injuries include flail chest, open sucking wounds, tension pneumothorax, hemothorax, and cardiac tamponade (Table 73-2). These conditions are described in more detail elsewhere in the text.

Open wounds of the chest create a problem if there is intrusion into the pleural cavity. Air is drawn into the pleural space because of the existing negative pressure. The resultant positive pressure causes *pneumothorax* (collapse of the lung) (p. 1237). A sucking noise is heard as the air is drawn in. Respirations are impaired. Immediate action is indicated to cover the opening. A nonporous material must be used since air can pass through a standard dressing or material. Plastic wrap, which is not only nonporous but tends to cling to the skin, is excellent. Aluminum foil or the cellophane covering of a cigarette pack can also be used. If a dressing is used, it must be covered with petrolatum to create an air barrier. After the chest wound has been sealed, a pressure dressing is applied. Continual monitoring of respirations is indicated.

Flail chest results when multiple adjacent ribs are fractured in two places. The chest wall becomes unstable and responds paradoxically during inspiration; that is, the affected side falls with inspiration while the unaffected side rises. The opposite effect occurs with expiration.

With *tension pneumothorax* air enters the pleural cavity with inspiration but the wound edges serve as a one-way flap valve, not permitting escape of the air during expiration. Air pressure builds up in the pleural space and effects a shift in mediastinal structures away from the affected side. This results in compression of the unaffected lung and decreased venous return to the heart (Fig. 73-5).

Cardiac tamponade is a compression of the heart resulting from leakage of blood into the pericardial sac. The accumulating blood cannot escape and exerts pressure against the heart, interfering with cardiac pumping. Symptoms include neck vein distention from increased venous pressure, a paradoxical pulse (weaker during inspiration), dyspnea, and Kussmaul breathing. The victim is placed in high Fowler's position and transported to the hospital. Treatment is pericardiocentesis.

Persons with chest trauma are considered to have sustained serious injury until proved otherwise.[20] Primary consideration in emergency management is maintenance of an open airway, breathing, and circulation. *Oxygen* is administered at high flow. Rapid transport after initial emergency measures is essential.

Abdominal wounds. Blows to the abdomen can rupture underlying organs. The spleen is often lacerated, and the intestines, liver, kidney, and bladder may also sustain injury. Symptoms may include abdominal pain and rigidity, nausea and vomiting, shock, and contusions on the abdominal wall. The victim may assume a position with knees drawn up toward the abdomen. If severe shock is present, the use of antishock trousers (if available) is indicated before transport. The trousers extend from the ankle to below the lowest rib. After application the trousers are inflated to apply pressure on the lower half of the body, decreasing the size of the vascular system and redirecting blood flow to vital areas (Fig. 73-6).

If there is an open wound, evisceration may occur.

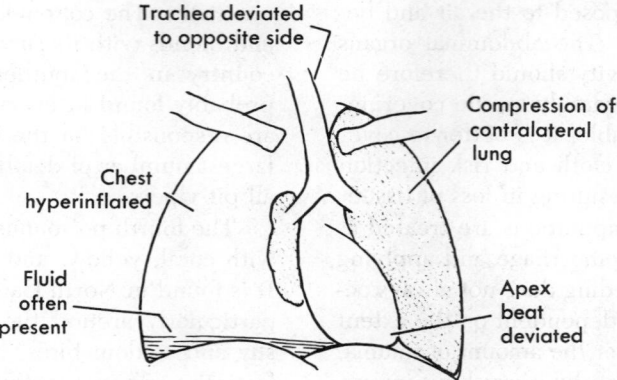

Fig. 73-5. Physiology of tension pneumothorax. (From Effler, D.B., editor: Blades' surgical diseases of the chest, ed. 4, St. Louis, 1978, The C.V. Mosby Co.)

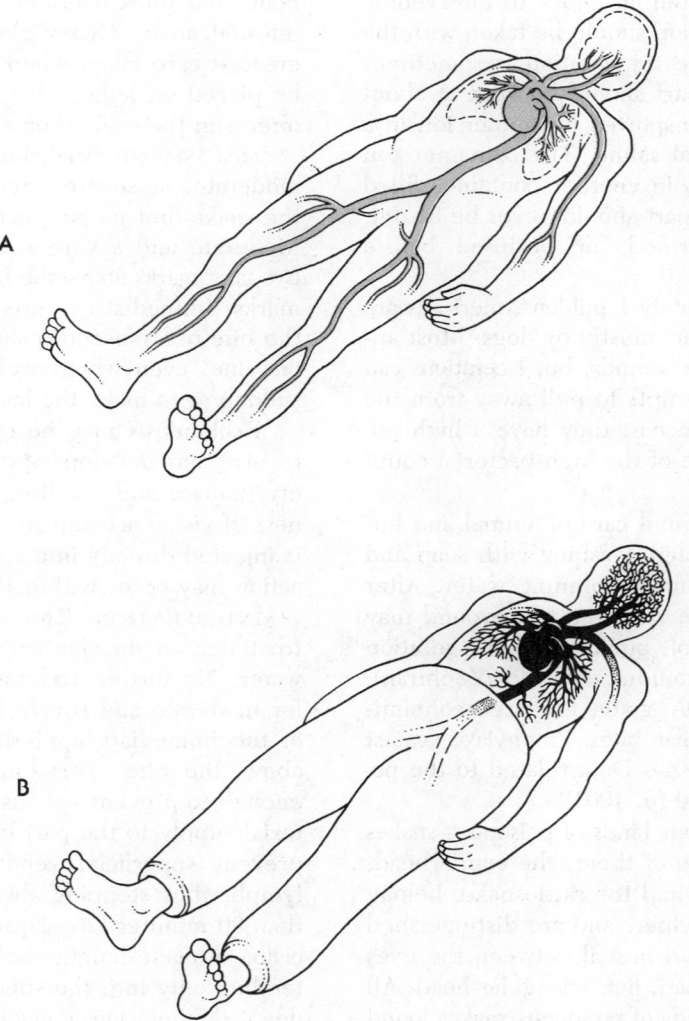

Fig. 73-6. In shock states, perfusion of vital organs is greatly enhanced by antishock trousers. **A,** Before application. **B,** After application. (From Budassi, S., and Barber, J: Emergency nursing: principles and practice, St. Louis, 1981, The C.V. Mosby Co.)

If the abdominal organs are exposed to the air and become dry, necrosis can result. The abdominal organs lying outside the abdominal cavity should therefore be covered by a warm, moist, preferably sterile covering. If a sterile dressing is not available, it is better to cover the organs with a clean moist cloth and risk infection than not to cover the organs, resulting in loss of tissue.

Amputations. Traumatic amputations are treated as other wounds by controlling hemorrhage and applying pressure dressings. Severe bleeding does not always occur. The amount of bleeding is dependent on the extent of trauma that occurs. The greater the amount of trauma, such as the amputation of a limb by a crushing injury, the greater will be the amount of muscle spasm in the arterial walls (vascular spasm).[51] This causes the artery to contract, and bleeding is decreased. A limb or appendage that is severed cleanly by a sharp object such as a knife will bleed more profusely. If a tourniquet is necessary, it should be applied close to the site of the amputation to decrease potential injury to intervening tissue. The amputated portion should be taken with the victim to the hospital since replantation is sometimes possible. The amputated part should be kept at about 5° C (40° F). It can be transported by immersion in a container filled with normal saline. The container can be kept cold by placing it in another container filled with ice.[20] The amputated part should never be frozen, cleaned, disinfected, debrided, or perfused before transportation.[63]

Animal bites. Approximately 1 million Americans are bitten by animals every year, mostly by dogs. Most animal bites produce puncture wounds, but lacerations can occur as the individual attempts to pull away from the animal. Human bites also occur; they have a high potential for infection because of the high bacterial count in the human mouth.

The immediate local wound care of animal and human bites consists in thorough washing with soap and water and copious rinsing under running water. After all traces of soap have been removed, the wound may be flushed with 70% alcohol, povidone-iodine solution (Betadine), or 1% benzalkonium chloride (Zephiran). Antibiotic therapy is usually given for large contaminated animal bites or for human bites. Prophylaxis against tetanus is also given (p. 1902). Data related to the potential for rabies is collected (p. 1901).

Snakebites. There are four kinds of poisonous snakes in the United States. Three of them, the copperhead, the cottonmouth moccasin, and the rattlesnake, belong to the group known as pit vipers and are distinguished by a pit resembling a second nostril between the eyes and the nostril and by a broad, flat, triangular head. All persons should know the kinds of poisonous snakes found in the part of the country in which they live and how to recognize them. The copperhead, named for its color, is about 3 ft long and is found in the eastern and southern states. The cottonmouth moccasin is grayish in color and blends with its surroundings. It is found in marshy country in the southeastern states. Rattlesnakes are probably found in every state in the United States and are responsible for the largest number of bites and the largest number of deaths. One antivenin is effective for all pit vipers.

The fourth poisonous snake, the coral snake, is small with coral, yellow, and black rings encircling its body. It is found in North Carolina and other southern states, particularly around the Gulf of Mexico. The snake is shy and seldom bites, but its venom is deadly and affects the nervous system. No specific antivenin is prepared for the bite of the coral snake, but cobra antivenin, kept in most zoos, is effective.

PREVENTION. Poisonous snakes in North America will almost always move away when disturbed and will not bite unless suddenly molested without warning. Snakebites can often be prevented by wearing high leather boots and thick trousers when walking through snake-infested areas. Heavy gloves should be worn and the greatest care taken when climbing because hands may be placed on ledges that cannot be seen, and reptiles often sun themselves on rocky ledges.

ASSESSMENT. Snakebites can be classified as mild, moderate, or severe.[5] Scratches made by the teeth of the snake (but no fang marks) are visible in mild cases. Moderate and severe snakebites are distinguished by two fang marks above the horseshoe-shaped array of tooth marks. Immediate severe *pain* and *swelling* distinguish the bite of a poisonous snake from that of a nonpoisonous one, even when swelling and discoloration are so sudden as to make the fang marks impossible to see.

Ecchymosis may be extensive, and bullae and petechiae may develop. Systemic symptoms such as anxiety, nausea and vomiting, vertigo, dyspnea, and dimness of vision accompany the severe bite. If the venom is injected directly into a major blood vessel, a fatal reaction may occur within 15 minutes.

INTERVENTION. The mild bite (no fang marks) is treated as an abrasion with good cleaning with soap and water. No further treatment is necessary.[5] Treatment for moderate and severe poisonous snakebites consists of the immediate application of a flat tourniquet just above the bite. This tourniquet should not be tight enough to prevent venous return in deep vessels or arterial supply to the part but should be tight enough to prevent superficial venous circulation of blood and lymph, thus stopping absorption of the poison. If less than 30 minutes has elapsed since the bite, a ½-in. incision is made lengthwise through the fang marks, extending only into the subcutaneous tissue about ¼ in. deep. (No incision is made if the bite marks are near a major blood vessel.) If emergency snakebite equipment is not available, suction must be applied by mouth. This procedure is safe unless there are open lesions in the rescuer's mouth, since the venom is not poisonous if swallowed. Constant suctioning is continued for 20 to 30 minutes.

Antivenin, if available, is given only for severe snakebites, since severe reactions to the antivenin can occur. Antivenin is given intravenously, not injected into the tissue around the bite, since is will not neutralize the venom.

The victim of the moderate or severe snakebite should lie very quietly to lessen circulatory flow and absorption of the poison. He or she should be observed for signs of shock. If no nausea or vomiting is present, warm but not hot fluids can be given. Alcohol is contraindicated, since it increases circulation and thus speeds up the absorption of the poison. The injured limb should be placed in a dependent position. Cold but not ice may be applied; cold will diminish circulation, but ice may freeze the injured tissue.

The victim should be transported quickly to the hospital. Antivenin treatment will be given if indicated. Tetanus prophylaxis is instituted, and antibiotics are given to combat infection. Analgesics are given for pain; however, the initial severe pain may diminish to a numbness after a few hours. Fluid balance is monitored and therapy for shock instituted as indicated. Oxygen should be available for use as needed. Massive sloughing of the tissues may occur following snakebite. The skin under the large bullae that form may resemble a severe burn.[107] Frequent dressing changes may be indicated. Snakebite wounds heal slowly, and in severe cases amputation may be necessary.

Rabies

Rabies is an acute infectious viral disease that affects the nervous system, primarily the brain. The disease has been known for centuries. In the twentieth century BC the Eshnunna code of ancient Mesopotamia set forth strict regulations about the obligations of dog owners who let mad dogs bite persons, thereby causing death. Rabies is usually fatal, although there have been a few documented survivals.

The rabies virus is transmitted to humans through bites of carnivorous animals. The most frequent source in the United States since the advent of required inoculation of dogs is wild animals, primarily skunks, foxes, bats, and raccoons. Bats can frequently be found in urban as well as rural areas. Rabies does not usually occur following bites by members of the rodent family (rats, squirrels, chipmunks, or rabbits). There has been an increase in the incidence of rabies found in cattle. The virus can also be transmitted from the saliva of the rabid animal to a person through an existing break in the victim's skin.

Not all rabies-infected animals are mad. There are two types of rabies. In one type the animal may be restless, barking, and biting. In the other, so-called dumb rabies, the animal may be quiet and stay close to its master. In the latter type, paralysis, which begins in the throat and lower jaw, may lead the animal's owner to suspect that something harmful has been swallowed. If the owner tries to investigate the trouble, some of the highly infectious saliva may enter an abrasion on the hand.

Prevention. The control of rabies is a public health responsibility. The police and health departments must be notified at once if it is thought that a rabid animal is at large. In England and the Scandinavian countries the disease has been almost entirely eliminated by rigid enforcement of laws that prohibit allowing dogs to run about unleashed. Rabies could be controlled by compulsory vaccination of all dogs and cats kept as household pets, capture and confinement of stray animals, and destruction of wild animal reservoirs of infection under the supervision of wildlife experts. How long the immunity lasts following vaccination is not known for certain. Immunization in humans is thought to last about 12 months and in animals up to 39 months.

Rabies can be prevented in humans by immunization whenever the possibility of developing rabies is present. The decision for postexposure prophylaxis is made by the physician after comparing the potential for developing rabies with the potential for serious reaction to prophylaxis. Prophylaxis is initiated if the bite was from a wild animal, from an unprovoked attack by a domestic animal that cannot be observed for 10 days, or from an animal observed to develop signs of rabies. Every attempt is made to capture the animal by competent authorities, and wild animals are killed for analysis. The presence of *Negri bodies* in the brain of an animal is conclusive evidence of rabies. The effectiveness of postexposure prophylaxis decreases over time; therefore a prompt decision to start treatment for prevention of rabies is important.[25]

The United States Public Health Service Advisory Committee on Immunization Practices has developed standards for prophylactic treatment. There are two types of prophylactic treatment for rabies: antirabies serum and rabies vaccine. In most situations both the serum and the vaccine are given to the victim. The vaccine may be given alone for nonbite exposures to escaped cats and dogs.[24]

Hyperimmune rabies *serum* is a form of passive immunity for rabies. Until recently the antirabies serum (ARS), a horse serum, has been the recommended serum. Since horse serum causes allergic reactions in at least 20% of those receiving it, hypersensitivity testing must be done before it is administered. Serum sickness occurs in 15% of children and 40% of adults who receive ARS.[24] At least half of the ARS given is used to infiltrate around the wound, and the remainder is given intramuscularly. There is a new hyperimmune rabies immune globulin (HRIG), but it is not yet readily available.[24] The benefit of the new serum is that it is not a horse serum so the danger of anaphylaxis is not present.

Rabies *vaccine* produces active immunity. Two vaccines are in common use at this time, and one new vaccine is being tested. Nerve tissue vaccine (NTV) is used worldwide but seldom in the United States, since it is associated with central nervous system reactions. The vaccine approved for use in the United States at this time is duck embryo vaccine (DEV). Injections are given subcutaneously in rotating sites in the abdomen or lateral aspects of the thighs for 21 doses over 14 to 21 days, followed by two booster doses on the tenth and twentieth days after the initial series is completed. Anaphylaxis occurs in 0.9% of persons and systemic reaction (fever, malaise, myalgia) in 33%.[82] All patients experience local reactions (pain, erythema). Major complications are uncommon, but central nervous system reactions can occur.

The new human diploid cell vaccine (HDCV) shows promise as a possible replacement for DEV. Since the origin is from human cells, anaphylaxis is prevented. Systemic reactions occur in a smaller number of persons. The vaccine has been found to produce effective antibody titers after a four-dose schedule.[82] HDCV vaccine is given intramuscularly, and local soreness does develop as with DEV.

Corticosteroids should not be given to the person receiving any type of rabies vaccine unless the situation is life threatening.[24] Corticosteroids are antiinflammatory and interfere with the development of active immunity.

Clinical picture. The incubation period of the disease in humans is from 10 days to more than a year.[15] The involvement, as in animals, is in the central nervous system. The disease is ushered in with a few days of melancholia, depression, pain at the site of the animal bite, and a feeling of impending danger. Acute symptoms (difficulty in swallowing, excessive salivation, muscle spasm, often maniacal fear, difficulty in breathing, and convulsions) then appear. A terrific, painful spasm of the muscle of deglutition occurs when there is an attempt to swallow water, hence the name hydrophobia. Even the mention of water is often enough to bring on an attack. Aerophobia is also present, and convulsions can be produced by a draft of air on the skin. Death from rabies has been reduced in the United States to several cases per year.

Intervention. There is no specific therapy for rabies. Treatment is symptomatic, and most nursing care of the patient with acute rabies is difficult but of short duration. Most patients die from heart failure or respiratory difficulty within 3 or 4 days of the acute onset of symptoms. The patient is restless, irritable, and fearful, with episodes of uncontrolled fear and mania alternating with periods of calm. Every effort is made to keep the patient quiet. The room is darkened, and the noises in the halls outside the room should be eliminated. Side

rails are placed on the bed and sometimes padded to help prevent injury during episodes of uncontrolled thrashing about. Sedatives, including chloral hydrate, morphine, and the barbiturates, are given. Anesthetics may be given intravenously. Fluids often are given intravenously, and it is important to bandage the arm securely on a board to prevent injury in the event of a convulsion or an attack of mania while a needle is in the vein. The head of the bed is sometimes lowered in an attempt to facilitate drainage of saliva, and often suctioning must be used. All persons caring for the patient should be aware of contamination from saliva, and a gown and rubber gloves should be worn.[4] Relatives of the patient must be prepared for the fact that the patient cannot talk. Sometimes the visits of relatives bring on severe painful muscle spasm in the throat of the patient, who is usually conscious up to the time of death even though unable to speak.

Tetanus

Tetanus, or lockjaw, is an infectious disease caused by the gram-positive anaerobic spore-producing bacteria *Clostridium tetani*, which are normal inhabitants of the intestinal tracts of humans and other animals and which can survive for years in soil and dirt. They enter the bloodstream of human beings through wounds and travel to the central nervous system. They produce a powerful toxin that acts at the myoneural junction causing prolonged muscular contractions. Tetanus is a highly fatal disease; almost one fourth of persons who develop tetanus die, even with rigorous treatment.

Prevention. The only sure method of prevention of tetanus is through immunization. Tetanus prophylaxis is part of the planned immunization program for children. Booster doses are given after a person sustains a contaminated or deep puncture wound (Table 73-3). If more than 10 years have passed of if the person has never been immunized, instructions are given to the

TABLE 73-3. Tetanus prophylaxis following injury*

Booster date	Wound size	Prophylaxis
Within past 10 yr	Small, moderate	0.5 ml toxoid†
	Severe, or more than 24 hr old	0.5 ml toxoid 250 units of TIGH‡
More than 10 yr or none	Small	0.5 ml toxoid (start series)
	Moderate	0.5 ml toxoid (start series)
		250 units of TIGH
	Severe	0.5 ml toxoid (start series)
		500 units of TIGH

*Recommended by the American College of Surgeons.
†Absorbed tetanus toxoid.
‡Tetanus immune globulin (human).

patient to complete the immunization series. In addition, tetanus immune globulin (human) (TIGH) is given for severe wounds as a means of passive immunization.

Clinical picture. The symptoms of tetanus appear from 2 days to several weeks after introduction of the clostridia into the wound. Symptoms of mild tetanus include mild muscle rigidity and some tonic spasms of the jaw muscles (trismus). When moderate tetanus is present, the trismus is more pronounced so that the person can hardly open the mouth, and this produces the characteristic sardonic smile (risus sardonicus). The person has difficulty swallowing because of pharyngeal spasms. The abdominal and lumbar muscles also become rigid, and opisthotonos (arching of the back) occurs. In severe tetanus the muscle spasms are so severe that fractures may result and respirations are compromised. Painful muscle spasms may occur on the slightest stimulation.

Intervention. Treatment is directed at neutralization of toxin that has not yet affected central nervous system cells. Large doses (3000 to 6000 units) of TIGH are administered intramuscularly. A program of active immunization with absorbed tetanus toxoid is initiated. Penicillin or tetracycline is given for its antibacterial effect on any remaining clostridia and to prevent secondary infections. A wound that is identified as the source of the infection is debrided.

Care is provided in a single room of an intensive care unit. Ventilatory measures are used to provide adequate ventilation as indicated. Sedatives, tranquilizers, and muscle relaxants may be given to prevent muscle spasms. Maintenance of fluid balance and adequate nutrition is essential but may be difficult because of the muscle spasms. Some persons may be able to ingest fluids and soft foods orally, but if trismus is severe, tube feedings or parenteral feedings are instituted.

Frequent position changes help to prevent pulmonary complications, and side-lying positions are recommended to promote pulmonary drainage. Urinary retention may result from bladder spasms, and an indwelling catheter may be necessary if the patient cannot void.

Fractures

Injury to the musculoskeletal system may result in fractures or dislocations of the bones, strained muscles, or torn ligaments (see Chapter 42 for a complete discussion of these injuries). Emergency care consists in assessment of injury and interventions to prevent further trauma until medical help is available.

Assessment

Pain localized over a bone or joint should be considered a fracture until a definitive diagnosis is made. Obvious deformity can be either a dislocation (if at a joint) or a fracture. In a compound fracture the bone may be protruding through the skin. Ecchymosis (bluish discoloration) of the skin may occur with any musculoskeletal injury as a result of rupture of blood vessels at the time of injury. The ability to move an extremity or digit does not negate a fracture, although the victim usually refrains from movement because of pain. Shock may occur with severe fractures, either from the stress of the trauma or from blood loss such as the extravasation of blood in the thigh following injury.

The victim should not be moved when being examined for fracture of the spine (neck or back). The examiner slides his or her hand under the victim and checks for point tenderness along the length of the spine. Bruises on the head may indicate that a force has been exerted that could cause a neck fracture. Bruises on the shoulder, back, or abdomen are frequently seen with back fractures, but a spinal fracture can be present in the absence of any bruises. If the spinal cord has been damaged, there may be loss of movement or sensation of the extremities.

Skull fractures may vary from a small linear fracture with few symptoms to severe depression of bone fragments into the brain. Basilar skull fractures may be accompanied by bleeding or draining serous fluid from the nose or ears or both. Fractures of facial bones may interfere with respiration if the air passages become blocked.

Pain or deformity at the hip can be caused by either a fracture or dislocation. The leg will be shortened in both instances but turned outward if there is a fracture and inward with a dislocation. Fractures of the extremities may be accompanied by loss of circulation or sensation if blood vessels or nerves are pinched by the bone fragment. Circulation distal to the fracture is assessed by observing skin color and presence of pulses. A neurologic check for sensation and circulatory system checks should be repeated after splinting and during transportation.

Intervention

General management of fractures. Dressings are applied to an open wound at the site of a fracture before splinting is carried out in order to prevent infection and minimize bleeding. The fractured bone should be well supported and moved as little as possible during application of dressing and splint. Unless there is imminent danger of further accidental injury, such as by fire or explosion, the victim is not moved until the fracture is splinted.

Fractures are splinted as they are found with the exception of severely angulated fractures of the *shafts* of bones of the extremities. The severe angulation is straightened by placing one hand just below the fracture and the other farther down the extremity and applying gentle traction.[3] The purpose of straightening a severe angulation is not to reduce the fracture but to decrease the spasm of the muscles and prevent damage to blood vessels and nerves. The sooner the traction is applied, the less the discomfort to the victim, since some numbness occurs immediately following the injury.[3] Traction is maintained until the extremity is splinted. Deformities of a joint (shoulder, elbow, wrist, knee) are *never* straightened because of the presence of major blood vessels and nerves at a joint.

Splints are applied to include the joint above and below the fracture. Rigid splints such as boards or cardboard are padded for comfort and to prevent pressure areas. Soft splints such as pillows can be reinforced by a rigid material such as boards or magazines for added firmness. Air splints, if available, are inflated only by the mouth, not a pump, to a point where the thumb makes a slight dent. Toes and fingers should remain free for assessment of circulation. Gentleness and support of the fractured part are imperative during handling, since careless handling can add to the severity of the original injury and increase the potential for shock.

Fracture of the spine. Any questionable injury to the head, neck, or back is treated as a fracture of the spine. Two problems can occur from a fractured spine: damage to the spinal cord and neurogenic shock. If the cervical spine is fractured, there may be interference with respiration so that respirations must be continually monitored. The victim may use diaphragmatic breathing for a short period of time but be unable to sustain this. Artificial ventilation is more difficult because the neck cannot be hyperextended because this can cause further injury to the spinal cord. The head can be extended by gentle traction and the jaw pulled forward to open the airway. Traction must be maintained until the neck can be supported in this position. The neck should never be flexed, twisted, or hyperextended. If the victim is not having difficulty with respiration, the neck can be splinted in the position in which it was found.

Transportation of a person with a potential spine fracture must be on a firm base, preferably a back board. Forward or backward flexion of the spine is to be avoided to prevent further trauma to the spinal cord. The victim should be slid, not rolled, in straight alignment onto the back board. It takes several persons working together to move the victim safely. The victim remains on the back board during the initial diagnostic tests in the emergency room.

Rape

Rape is one of the violent crimes for which an increasing number of people, primarily women, are seeking help. Despite the increasing number of rapes being reported, it is estimated that unreported rape ranges from 200% to 300% more than reported rape.[92] There are many reasons why women do not report rape. In the past, women who were raped were often thought to have encouraged it or to have been secretly desiring rape. This belief still persists among some people.

In past years if the victim pursued the matter of rape in the courts, she was often embarrassed and humiliated; the rapist would then often be acquitted. The rise of the feminist movement has provided an impetus to make changes. These changes are occurring, more rapidly in some places than in others, but there is still much to be accomplished.[86] Legal definitions are being changed. The court procedure is still one of great trauma psychologically for the victim, and she needs to know what is actually involved before she makes the decision to press charges.

Rape crisis centers have been formed in many large cities. These centers differ in their functions but usually have one or all of three main functions: (1) victim service, (2) service to professional agencies (health, law), and (3) community education. The victim service is the primary role for which the centers have been formed. Since this service is not adequate to change the system for the victim, services for education of professionals serving rape victims and education of the community to increase public awareness of the problems of rape victims are being pursued. The victim service consists of volunteers, many of whom have been raped themselves, who serve as victim advocate through the medical examination and police interview. Some form of follow-up service such as counseling may be available. Some rape crisis centers have volunteer attorneys who can offer the victim legal advice or representation.

It is difficult to obtain statistics concerning the sociologic variables relating to rape because of the large number of unreported cases. There are many misconceptions concerning rape. The facts are that rape is common to all classes (there is a higher incidence of reported rape among the lower class), that rape occurs mostly *intra*racially rather than interracially, and that a majority of rapes are committed by someone the victim knows.[8] This latter reason is one major factor why many rapes go unreported. Often the victim fears for her own safety, is made to feel that she is the cause of the incident, or fears the stigma involved. The majority of rape victims are females, but males, especially young boys, may also be rape victims. The attacker is usually another male. Rape of males is a major problem in prisons in the United States. Some prison reform groups are actively addressing this problem with the major emphasis being on protecting the young and the vulnerable from attack.

Trauma of rape

Rape is a traumatic event for the victim physically, psychologically, and socially. Physical force is often employed; a weapon may be used either as a threat or to injure the victim, or the hands or fists may be used to beat the victim or threaten choking. Injury can also occur as the victim is attempting to defend herself or is struggling on the ground or floor. The vagina and perineum may be injured by force used during the sexual attack, and the rectum may also be lacerated if anal sex has been attempted. The latter is more common in rape of males.

Psychologic trauma is usually severe; the rape victim is in a state of crisis. Fear is a dominant theme as the victim perceives the event as life threatening.[61] Other feelings expressed by victims are depersonalization, shame, degradation, defilement, violation, guilt, humiliation, and anger.[22,92] The victim has not only been under threat of harm but has also been subjected in many instances to multiple sexual assaults, some natural, some perverted, by one or more persons. Fellatio (oral sex) is frequently demanded by the rapist. Some rapists will urinate on the victim before leaving her.

The rape victim also experiences a sociologic crisis. If the woman is married, marital relationships may be affected. If she is single she is often in fear of repeated occurrences and may feel the need to move, especially if the attack occurred in her home or apartment. Decisions have to be made concerning whom to tell about the incident, since loss of needed support by significant others may occur. Job security or relationships with coworkers may be threatened. If a child is the victim, social relationships within the family may be altered. Problems of a sociologic nature take considerable time to be resolved, but concerns related to these potential problems may occur in the initial emergency period.

Types of rape victimization

Burgess and Holmstrom[22] have identified three types of rape victimization from their research: (1) rape or sex without consent, (2) accessory to sex or inability to give consent, and (3) sex stress situation or sex with initial consent. The first type is easily identified as rape; the victim is attacked suddenly (blitz rape) or the rapist gains the victim's confidence but then takes advantage of her. Some persons are unable to give consent because of their cognitive or personality development. They are lured by the rapist by offers of material goods such as candy or by offers of pleasure or human contact. In the third group are persons who agree to a sexual relationship, but either perversion occurs or the victim or family becomes worried later concerning possible consequences. All of these situations produce victims in need of help.

Prevention

All women need to know the measures they can take to help prevent rape from occurring (see box). It would

---

RAPE PREVENTIVE MEASURES

Prevention of attack

Set house lights to go on and off by timer

Keep light on at all entrances

Place safety locks on windows and doors

Have key ready before reaching door of house or car

Look in car before entering

Insist on identification before letting a stranger in house; check identification with agency if suspicious

Do not list first name on mailbox or in telephone directory

Make arrangements with neighbor for needed assistance

Be alert when walking in street; walk in lighted areas

Walk down center of street if possible

Avoid lonely or enclosed areas

If attacked

Run toward a lighted house; yell, "Fire"

Spit in rapist's face; act bizarre; vomit

Rip off rapist's glasses

Step hard on his foot (instep)

Aim at eyes—try to gouge eyes, scrape face

Hit throat at Adam's apple (larynx)

Use fighting and screaming with caution; this may scare some rapists, encourage others

Try talking to avoid rape

If powerless, make close observations about rapist, car, location

---

also be helpful for every woman to learn methods of self-defense. Some communities are beginning to introduce both the issue of rape and self-defense into secondary school curricula. Many YWCAs teach classes in self-defense. Rape crisis centers can provide information on availability of classes in the community. Women learning physical defense skills need to learn to value themselves so they can justify the need for self-defense and have confidence in their ability to defend themselves.

Health care

Persons who are raped may seek medical help directly or call the police, who will then take the victim for medical examination. Some victims fear reprisal by the rapist or are unwilling for others to know about the rape and therefore do not seek medical attention. Victims need to be encouraged to report the incident. They need considerable support during both the acute emergency and the long-term consequences, and knowledgeable nurses are able to provide appropriate support.

Many hospitals have developed protocols for care of the rape victim in the emergency department. If such a protocol does not exist, it behooves the nurses in the emergency department to work toward development of a protocol. Rape crisis centers can be helpful in this regard. The protocol includes high priority in triage, provisions for privacy without leaving the victim alone, provision of a victim advocate such as a woman from a rape crisis center if desired, continual emotional support by nonjudgmental health personnel, and routines to ensure the protection and comfort of the victim. These routines delineate which personnel have priority for contacts with the victim. If no injury is present that threatens life, the nurse may be designated to have primary contact with the victim and make the decision as to when the victim is ready for medical examination or police interview. Large city police departments often have women police officers assigned to interview rape victims, since many girls and women become very upset when asked to talk with a male police officer.

Assessment

Subjective data

The person who has been raped goes through the same phases as any person facing a crisis situation (p. 182). The initial phase is one of shock and disbelief that rape has occurred and of emotional disequilibrium manifested in many different ways. After the initial acute phase there is a period of pseudoequilibrium when the victim rationalizes the event or attempts to suppress thoughts concerning the rape. During the long-term phase there are periods of depression, phobic reactions, nightmares, and changes in life style.[22,37]

The victim will be asked many questions by the physician to identify the type of assault and potential for injury. If the victim has been threatened, she may have succumbed through fear, and this needs to be elicited. Victims often talk freely to the nurse about their feelings; their fears concerning injury, mutilation, or death at the time of assault; or present fears concerning pregnancy or venereal disease. Other feelings of degradation, feeling "dirty," shame, guilt, and so forth, may be expressed. Anger may be directed at the assailant or projected toward medical care or personnel. Pain may be local at the site of assault or generalized and diffuse. The victim may complain of a sore throat if choking was used as a threat or following oral sex. Nausea may also be reported.

Objective data

One of the myths concerning rape is that all women are hysterical after rape. Burgess and Holmstrom[22] in their research identified two different types of responses with about half of the victims falling in each category. The first type they labeled "expressed style." These women were emotionally labile as evidenced by crying, shaking, restlessness, tenseness, and smiling or laughing inappropriately. The other group, labeled "controlled style," appeared calm, composed, or subdued. The full impact of the experience often hit them at a later time.

A head-to-toe assessment for signs of physical trauma is usually carried out by the physician. The clothing will be inspected and described and is often requested by the police for evidence. Clothing should not be washed or discarded. Other data needed by the police usually include samples of the assailant's hair from combing of pubic hair and fingernail deposits for samples of the assailant's tissue.

Tests

Papanicolaou smears of the vagina, mouth, or rectum and saline suspensions are done to test for the presence of sperm. An acid phosphatase test will demonstrate recency of intercourse. Tests will be inconclusive if the victim has bathed or douched since the rape. Tests for venereal disease are done at the initial visit to obtain baseline information for comparison at 3 to 6 weeks.

Intervention

All personnel who have contact with the rape victim need to refine their skills in providing support to the victim using a nonjudgmental approach. Knowledge of the problems and experiences of other victims as well as rapists is helpful in understanding what is being experienced by the victim (see references listed at the end of the chapter). Interdisciplinary conferences involving health care providers, volunteers from rape crisis centers, and the police help clarify issues and problems.

Emotional support

Initially, the victim needs time to marshal her coping responses. Most victims have a need to talk and a need to know that someone cares what is happening to them. The nurse utilizes crisis intervention theory as the basis for deciding how best to help the victim (see Chapter 14). Many hospitals have contacts with a rape crisis center. The victim is given the choice of having a victim advocate from the center be with her during the entire procedure, and medical examination or interviews by the police are not begun until the volunteer arrives.

Preparation for the physical examination is carried out in advance. Having a pelvic examination after a sexual assault can be a traumatic experience for the victim, and some girls or women have never had a pelvic examination previously.

Comfort

After the victim has been examined, she will probably have a need to wash herself. Mouthwash is appreciated, especially if there has been oral sex. A change of clothing may be needed if the police want her clothing for evidence, which is not uncommon.

Sexuality

The victim has many concerns related to her sexuality. Time is needed to work through these concerns, and long-term counseling is helpful to many victims.

Concern about possible pregnancy depends on the circumstances: whether she is in the childbearing years, whether birth control is in effect at the time of sexual attack, and at what point in the menstrual period the rape occurs. If pregnancy is a possibility, diethylstilbestrol (DES) may be given. Side effects may include nausea, vomiting, and cramplike chest pains. Menstrual aspiration for a delayed, expected menstrual period may be done in place of giving DES.

Concern about venereal disease is common. An antibiotic is given following the initial examination as a preventive measure. The victim needs to know that medical follow-up is important and that she should be retested for venereal disease in about 3 weeks unless symptoms occur earlier. In addition, the victim may experience vaginal discharge, itching, and a burning sensation caused by an acute vaginal infection (vaginitis). This infection may become chronic.[22]

Discharge

The victim should not go home to an empty house or apartment. The volunteer from the rape crisis center, the social worker, or police can all facilitate arrangements for transportation to her home or to the home of family or friends. Frequently, the victim goes to the police station after medical care is completed to follow up with the police report. The victim needs to know about the availability of follow-up medical services and counseling services. In some medical centers there are psychiatrists who are especially interested in assisting rape victims with counseling as desired.

Outcome criteria for the woman who has been raped

The victim:
1. Has means for transportation and someone to accompany her to a self-designated destination.

2. Can state why, when, and where to obtain medical follow-up for venereal disease.
3. Knows resources for obtaining temporary and long-term support or counseling.

Disasters

Disasters are sudden catastrophic events that disrupt patterns of life and in which there is possible loss of life and property in addition to multiple injuries. Disasters can be either natural phenomena or caused by people (see box).

There are essentially three types of disasters: multiple patient, multiple casualty, and mass casualty.[20] *Multiple patient* disasters involve up to 10 people and occur with events such as multiple vehicle crashes, bus crashes, bomb explosions, or fires. Rescue squads apportion victims to different hospitals, if possible, to prevent overload on any one hospital emergency department. In *multiple casualty* disasters as many as 100 people may be injured in events such as air crashes, riots, tornadoes, hurricanes, minor earthquakes, and dam breaks.[20] Heavy demands are placed on available hospital emergency departments. *Mass casualty* disasters are large-scale disasters resulting in large numbers (over 100) of injured persons and disruption of community services and resources. Mass casualty disasters, such as unusually severe hurricanes, large-scale earthquakes, or war bombings, fortunately rarely occur, but the possibilities exist and community preparedness is essential.

CAUSES OF DISASTERS

Natural	Man-made
Air	*Transportation*
Tornado	Air
Hurricane	Land
Blizzard	Water
Land	*Fire*
Earthquake	Housing
Volcanic eruption	Forest
Avalanches	Explosions
Cave-ins	*Disease*
Water	Epidemics
Floods: slow rising and flash floods	*Civil disorders*
	Riots
Tidal waves	Wars (nuclear attack)

Effect of disasters

The effects of disasters are multiple. People are killed or injured and separated from their families. Many become homeless. In a large-scale disaster confusion and chaos occur during the early stages. Panic rarely occurs, but when it does it is because the involved persons believe that escape routes are limited and may be closing off. Effective leadership and communication can usually prevent panic from occurring.

Transportation difficulties are created as streets and roads become clogged by persons trying to get away from the impact area or others trying to get in. Persons within the area are trying to flee or to find friends, family, or medical assistance. Persons outside of the disaster area are either trying to move in to help, to find relatives, or just because of curiosity. Sightseers can present a serious problem to maintenance of open roads in and out of the area and should be deterred from entering the disaster area.

Food and water supplies can become contaminated or nonexistent. Medical supplies can be inadequate to meet the sudden increased need. Utilities can become disrupted. Law enforcement is necessary to prevent looting and other civil disorders. Establishment of a communication system takes first priority to prevent chaos.

Roles of nurses in disasters

The actual role assumed by a given nurse at a disaster will depend on (1) the abilities of the nurse and (2) the specific situation. The nurse may not be able to reach a specific location where his or her services may be most useful, so the needs of victims may then be better served by the nurse functioning in a different capacity.

Nurses can participate in a disaster in many ways. Nurses with leadership ability and experience may be needed to serve in this capacity. Any nurse may be in a position of being the only health care provider in a given area and be responsible for giving initial first aid treatment or supervising the activities of others. It therefore behooves nurses to continually update their first aid skills. Because of their education and experience in assessment and intervention for psychosocial problems, professional nurses can be especially helpful in aiding victims to cope with their emotional reactions to the disaster. Nurses may be asked to serve at emergency morgues for support of families experiencing loss of loved ones.

As shelters are established, nurses are needed to staff the shelters to help meet the health needs of victims separated from their homes and families. The American Red Cross, which assumes an active role during disasters along with governmental agencies, operates shelters for victims. They provide supplies and food as well as service personnel (shelter manager, nurses, physicians, food helpers). Nurses interested in serving during diasters at home or in other parts of the country may contact the local American Red Cross office. Other services provided by the American Red Cross include emergency services on an individual family basis and aid for recovery.

When the disaster occurs in the nurse's own geographic area, the ability of the nurse to function is influenced by the impact of the disaster on self and on family. The nurse may be unable to contact or reach his or her own family and may be in a position of having to provide health care while actively concerned about the family's safety and welfare. The nurse may also be experiencing the emotional impact of the crisis situation, and this may limit the effectiveness of the care provided.

Prevention

Preparedness for disasters includes community planning to identify and, it is hoped, to prevent disasters that can occur and education of the public to minimize the number of casualties.

Community planning

Most states have disaster service agencies, which are outgrowths of civil defense organizations. These agencies act as coordinating agencies for the local agencies. Every community should have a disaster planning group as part of the emergency medical care committee. There should be representation by all groups who will be active participants if a disaster occurs. This would include governmental groups (political, law enforcement, fire), health groups (hospitals, physicians, nurses, pharmacists, social workers), official groups (American Red Cross), and nonofficial groups (telephone company, parent-teacher organization, religious organizations). The disaster planning committee identifies the types of disasters that may occur in the local community, organizes a plan to be followed for different situations and arranges for simulated drills to test the effectiveness of the plans, and determines need for education or updating of necessary skills of participants. Nurses need to be active participants in the planning, implementation, and evaluation phases.

During a disaster the local hospitals become actively involved and need their own disaster plan to cope with the sudden influx of persons needing emergency care. Any time a large number of injured persons are in need of emergency care, hospital disaster plans are put into effect. Testing of hospital disaster plans at specified intervals by simulated drills is necessary for determining if the plans are effective and what changes, if any, are needed.

Public education

Public awareness of potential community disasters is needed for effective community preparedness for disasters. Disaster planning committees need support and participation by community members. Individual persons need to know what they should do in the event of a disaster. Most radio and television stations regularly notify communities of potential disasters and give directions for preventive actions to be taken and for methods of obtaining further information should the disaster occur. Since electricity may be cut off, battery-operated radios should be available in all homes for continued communication.

All homes should have an emergency food cabinet with sufficient nonperishable foods to meet nutritional needs for several days. Supplies are rotated with current supplies to prevent these supplies from spoiling or becoming outdated.

Assessment

Triage

There are essentially two different approaches to triage of victims during a disaster. The *military* triage system, which may be initiated during a mass casualty disaster, is based on the philosophy of doing the "best for the most with the least by the fewest." Victims with injuries of such magnitude that there is question of survival are given low priority for transportation. In this system the numbers of critically injured must greatly outnumber the health and transportation personnel available. Victims are reclassified as the emergency situation changes. Priority is then given to those victims with the greatest chance of survival.

The more commonly used *civilian* triage system is used during multiple patient or multiple casualty disasters. There are several victim-sorting methods that can be used for triage, but essentially all methods give most priority to life-threatening injuries and least priority to minimal injuries (see box).

Disaster syndrome

The behavior of victims following the impact of disaster can be characterized as progressing through phases of shock, awareness, euphoria, and anger. The victims are experiencing loss; therefore the phases are similar to those experienced by others during any kind of loss (grieving).

The shock phase may last only a few minutes or up to several hours after impact. The victim is dazed, un-

---

FOUR-COLOR CODED TRIAGE SYSTEM*

0—Black: Dead

1—Red: Critical or life-threatening

These victims have a reasonable chance of survival only if they receive immediate treatment. Emergency treatment is initiated immediately and continued during transportation. This category includes victims with respiratory insufficiency, cardiac arrest, hemorrhage, and severe abdominal injury.

2—Yellow: Serious

These victims can wait for transportation after they receive initial emergency treatment. They include victims with immobilized closed fractures, soft-tissue injuries without hemorrhage, and burns on less than 40% of the body.

3—Green: Minimal

Victims in this category are ambulatory, have minor tissue injuries, and may be dazed. They can be treated by nonprofessionals and held for observation if necessary.

---

*Adapted version of Four-Color Triage System reprinted from *Topics in Emergency Medicine* 1:1/May 1979 by Baker, F.J., by permission of Aspen Systems Corporation ©.

---

able to comprehend what is occurring, and cannot follow even simple directions. Persons prepared to function in emergencies are less apt to spend much time in the shock phase.

The awareness phase may last up to several days. The victim becomes aware of survival and tries to help others, minimizing his or her own injuries or losses. During this stage guilt feelings may arise because others died while he or she survived. The victim is highly suggestible, can follow simple directions, but cannot carry out problem solving effectively. For example, following one major earthquake a young woman who had run outdoors on a chilly night clad only in a thin nightgown was told to put on something warm. Her solution was to wrap a warm scarf around her neck.

The euphoria phase may last for several weeks. The victim feels a sense of brotherhood with the community and participates willingly in helping others with plans for recovery.

Before resolution occurs, the victim may go through the "Why me?" or anger phase that occurs because of the experienced loss. The anger is often projected against helping persons from the outside who were not personally affected by the disaster. It is especially important for nurses who may be assisting victims during the recovery phase to understand that the anger is part of the loss experience. As the victim copes with the losses incurred by the disaster and life returns to more normal patterns, the anger will disappear.

Intervention

Emergency aid stations

The number, size, and staffing of emergency aid stations depend on the type and extent of the disaster. There must be one person who is designated as the leader and who is responsible for making decisions for maximal effectiveness of the unit. Medical supplies and food for personnel must be available. One person is designated for triage. In the absence of a physician, a nurse assumes leadership of emergency care that is rendered. Transportation teams will bring some victims to the station and transport victims to a medical center for follow-up care. Unfortunately, many victims will go directly to a medical center, bypassing a first aid unit and thus creating a logistics problem at the medical center and decreasing the effectiveness of the care that can be given.

The types of injuries that occur will depend on the type of disaster. Soft-tissue and bone injuries are common in most natural disasters. Respiratory insufficiency may occur with airway injuries. Fear resulting from the disaster can precipitate cardiac arrests. Childbirth may also be precipitated. If the weather is inclement, additional injuries and disease may occur after the immediate crisis is over. If tear gas has been used, the victim should not be placed in a closed environment near other victims. Health personnel will be unable to function if they are affected by the tear gas.

Victims are not transported until first aid care has been given, as in any emergency. If hemorrhage has not been controlled or fractures splinted, the victim may arrive at the medical center in shock that could have been prevented or minimized, and surgical intervention will not take place until measures to treat shock are instituted and the patient's condition is stable. If first aid measures are instituted before transportation, the victim can be taken to surgery at the earliest opportunity. Records indicating all treatment given at an emergency aid center *must* accompany a victim who is referred or transported to a medical center or any other health care facility. The information, which is attached to the victim who is not responsible, should include name, age, address, name of nearest relative, assessment made, and treatment.

Shelters

Most shelters are set up in schools, which can house a large number of people. Toilet facilities, running water, and cooking facilities must be available. The role of the nurse in a shelter is to assess and provide for health needs of the shelter population. Persons with infectious diseases need to be isolated from other persons.

Elderly persons may become confused by the rapidly changing events and strange surroundings. Many elderly have chronic illnesses, and very often their medications have been left at home. They may not be able to see well if their glasses have been lost or eat well if dentures are missing. Because elderly persons may have decreased resistance, they are more susceptible to disease following a disaster.

Any victims who have chronic illnesses must be identified. If they are receiving replacement therapy such as insulin, this must be obtained. Arrangements must be made for the care of pregnant women and infants. Formulas must be obtained and special dietary needs arranged. Immunization of shelter occupants may also be necessary. Occupants should be monitored for signs of developing health problems.

Assessment of safety factors in the environment is also a nursing responsibility. The nurse is part of the shelter team and advises the shelter manager of any potential health hazards. The care of victims in a disaster is a team effort, and the nurse is an important member of this team.

Adaptation to loss after disasters

Adaptation to loss following large-scale community disasters may differ from adaptation to losses under normal life situations because of the lack of *individual* support systems as a result of (1) death of usual support persons or (2) inability of usual support persons to provide support because of their own personal losses. There may also be a loss of *community* support systems.

Immediately following a disaster there is usually an immediate outpouring of material assistance and personnel services from people outside the community. This diminishes with the passing of time, and the victims are often faced with having to work through their grief with less support than usual and sometimes with visual environmental reminders of the loss. It is important that long-term counseling sevices be made available in these situations to persons of all ages, including children. Group therapy can be a useful method of providing support by helping the victim realize that he or she is not alone and that others understand what the victim is experiencing and by aiding in problem solving through group efforts.

REFERENCES AND SELECTED READINGS

1. Accident facts, Chicago, 1980, National Safety Council.
2. Affeldt, J.E.: Newly revised emergency services standards, Hospitals **52:**14-18, 1978.
3. American Academy of Orthopedic Surgeons, Committee on Injuries: Emergency care and transportation of the sick and injured, Chicago, 1971, The Academy.
4. American Academy of Pediatrics, Committee on Accident and Poisoning Prevention: Handbook on accident prevention and injury control for children and youth, Hagerstown, Md., 1980, Harper & Row, Publishers, Inc.
5. American College of Surgeons, Committee on Trauma: Early

care of the injured patient, ed. 2, Philadelphia, 1976, W.B. Saunders Co.

6. American Council of Life Insurance: Life insurance fact book, New York, 1981, The Council.

7. American Hospital Association: Principles of disaster preparedness for hospitals, rev. ed., Chicago, 1971, The Association.

8. Amir, M.: Forcible rape. In Schultz, L.: Rape victimology, Springfield, Ill., 1975, Charles C Thomas, Publisher.

9. Arena, J.M.: The treatment of poisoning, Clin. Symp. 30(2):3-46, 1978.

10. Baer, E.: Civil disorder: mass emergency of the 70's, Am. J. Nurs. 72:1072-1076, 1972.

11. Bailey, J.A.: Development of a regional trauma center, Nurs. Clin. North Am. 13:255-265, 1978.

12. Baker, F.J.: The management of mass casualty disasters, Topics Emerg. Med. 1:149-157, 1979.

13. Barber, J.M., and Budassi, S.A.: Mosby's manual of emergency care: practices and procedures, St. Louis, 1979, The C.V. Mosby Co.

14. Barry, J.: Emergency nursing, New York, 1978, McGraw-Hill Book Co.

15. Beeson, P.B., and McDermott, W., editors: Textbook of medicine, ed. 15, Philadelphia, 1979, W.B. Saunders Co.

16. Bhatt, D.: Human rabies, Am. J. Dis. Child 127:862-869, 1974.

17. *Bishop, G., and Hynek, R.: Rape. In The Boston Women's Health Book Collective, editors: our bodies, ourselves: a book by and for women, ed. 2, New York, 1976, Simon & Schuster, Inc.

18. *Brandenburg, J.: Inhalation injury: carbon monoxide poisoning. Am. J. Nurs. 80:98-100, 1980.

19. Brody, D.M.: Running injuries, Clin. Symp. 32(4):2-36, 1980.

20. *Budassi, S.A., and Barber, J.M.: Emergency nursing: principles and practice, St. Louis, 1981, The C.V. Mosby Co.

21. Burgess, A., and Holmstrom, L.: Crisis and counseling requests of rape victims, Nurs. Res. 23:196-202, 1974.

22. Burgess, A., and Holmstrom, L.: Rape: victims of crisis, Bowie, Md., 1974, Robert J. Brady Co.

23. Burgess, A., and Holmstrom, L.: The rape victim in the emergency ward, Am. J. Nurs. 73:1741-1745, 1973.

24. Corey, L., and Hattwick, M.: Treatment of persons exposed to rabies, J.A.M.A. 232:272-276, 1975.

25. Cosgriff, J.H., Jr., and Anderson, D.: The practice of emergency nursing, Philadelphia, 1975, J.B. Lippincott Co.

26. Croft, H., and Frenkel, S.: Children and lead poisoning, Am. J. Nurs. 75:102-104, 1975.

27. *Crooks, L., Corn, M., and DeAtley, C.: Disaster planning: a team effort, A.O.R.N. J. 28:395-410, 1978.

28. *DeLapp, T.D.: Taking the bite out of frostbite and other cold weather injuries, Am. J. Nurs. 80:56-60, 1980.

29. Di Vasto, P., et al.: Caring for rape victims: its impact on providers, J. Community Health 5:204-208, 1980.

30. Dreisbach, R.H.: Handbook of of poisoning, diagnosis and treatment, ed. 9, Los Altos, Calif., 1977, Lange Medical Publications.

31. Eckert, C.: Emergency room care, ed. 3, Boston, 1976, Little, Brown & Co.

32. Ede, L., and Nelson, R.: The "Good Samaritan" law and the nurse's immunity for emergency care, Occup. Health Nurs. 20:10-15, 1972.

33. Erdman, K.: Keeping the consumer informed, FDA, Ohio's Health, vol. 19-22, July-Aug. 1973.

34. Erilson, K.T.: Disaster at Buffalo Creek: loss of communality at Buffalo Creek, Am. J. Psychiatry 133:320-305, 1976.

35. Farrell, J.: Illustrated guide to orthopedic nursing, Philadelphia, 1977, J.B. Lippincott Co.

36. Feins, N.R.: Multiple trauma, Pediatr. Clin. North Am. 26:759-771, 1979.

37. Flint, T. and Cain, H.D.: Emergency treatment and management, ed. 6, Philadelphia, 1980, W.B. Saunders Co.

38. Ford, A.H.: Use of automobile restraining devices for infants, Nurs. Res. 29:281-284, 1980.

39. Ford, P.S.: Management of pediatric poisoning: update on first aid management, Pediatr. Nurs. 6(5):35-36, 1980.

40. Fox, S., and Scherl, D.: Crisis intervention with victims of rape. In Schultz, L.: Rape victimology, Springfield, Ill., 1975, Charles C Thomas, Publisher.

41. Furgurson, J.E., and Meislin, H.W.: Airway problems in the trauma victim, Topics Emerg. Med. 1:9-28, 1979.

42. *Furste, WL., and Aguirre, A.: Preventing tetanus, AM. J. Nurs. 78:834-837, 1978.

43. *Gaston, S.F., and Schumann, L.L.: Inhalation injury: smoke inhalation, Am. J. Nurs. 80:94-97, 1980.

44. Gay, G.: Immediate care in the drug scene. In Stephenson, H.E., Jr.: Immediate care of the acutely ill and injured, ed. 2, St. Louis, 1978, The C.V. Mosby Co.

45. Genigeorgis, C., and Riemann, H.: Food safety and food poisoning, World Rev. Nutr. Diet. 16:363-397, 1973.

46. *George, O.G.: Anatomy and physiology of CPR, A.O.R.N. J. 27:992-996, 1978.

47. *Gilroy, A., and Caldwell, E.: Initial assessment of the multiple injured patient, Nurs. Clin. North Am. 13:177-190, 1978.

48. Goodwin, R.H.: Child-resistant locks in poison control, Pediatrics 61:79-86, 1978.

49. *Gosselin, T., et al.: Clinical toxicology of commercial products, ed. 4, Baltimore, 1976, The Williams & Wilkins Co.

50. *Gunn, A.: Food poisoning, Nurs. Times 72:842-844, 1976.

51. Guyton, A.: Textbook of medical physiology, ed. 5, Philadelphia, 1979, W.B. Saunders Co.

52. Hahn, A.B., Barkin, R.L., and Oestrich, S.J.K.: Pharmacology in nursing, ed. 15, St. Louis, 1982, The C.V. Mosby Co.

53. *Hargreaves, A.G.: Coping with disaster, Am. J. Nurs. 80:683, 1980.

54. *Hargreaves, A.G., et al.: Blizzard '78: dealing with disaster, Am. J. Nurs. 79:268-271, 1979.

55. Heimlich, H.J.: Death from food-choking prevented by a new life-saving maneuver, Heart Lung 5:755-758, 1976.

56. Heimlich, H.J.: Pop goes the café coronary, Emergency Med. 6:154-155, 1974.

57. Heimlich, H.J., and Uhley, M.H.: The Heimlich maneuver, Clin. Symp. 31(3):3-31, 1979.

58. *Hendrix, M.J., LaGodna, G.E., and Bohen, C.A.: The battered wife, Am. J. Nurs. 78:650-653, 1978.

59. Hill, G.J., II, editor: Out-patient surgery, ed. 2, Philadelphia, 1980, W.B. Saunders Co.

60. Holmstrom, L.L., and Burgess, A.W.: The victim of rape: institutional reactions, New York, 1978, John Wiley & Sons, Inc.

61. *Holmstrom, L.L., and Burgess, A.W.: Assessing trauma in the rape victim, Am. J. Nurs. 75:1288-1291, 1975.

62. Ipema, D.K.: Rape: the process of recovery, Nurs. Res. 28:272-275, 1979.

63. Jaffe, S., et al.: Replantation of amputated extremities: report of five cases, Ohio State Med. J. 71:381-386, 1975.

64. Kerr, A.: Orthopedic nursing procedures, ed. 3, New York, 1980, Springer Publishing Co., Inc.

65. Kohn, M.S.: Management of chest injuries, Topics Emerg. Med. 1:79-94, 1979.

66. Lanros, N.: Assessment and intervention in emergency nursing, section I, Bowie, Md., 1978, Robert J. Brady Co.

67. *Lee, J.M.: Emotional reactions to trauma, Nurs. Clin. North Am. 5:577-587, 1970.

*References preceded by an asterisk are particularly well suited for student reading.

68. Lifton, R.J., and Olson, E.: The human meaning of total disaster: the Buffalo Creek experience, Psychiatry **39**(2):1-18, 1976.

69. Lovejoy, F.H., and Berenberg, W.: Poisoning in children under age 5: identification and treatment, Postgrad. Med. **63**:79-86, 1978.

70. Lovejoy, F.H., and Easom, J.M.: Efficacy and safety of gastrointestinal decontamination in the treatment of oral poisoning, Pediatr. Clin. North Am. **26**:827-836, 1979.

71. MacDonald, J.: Rape: offenders and their victims, Springfield, Ill., 1971, Charles C Thomas, Publisher.

72. Mancine, M.: Liability in the emergency room, Am. J. Nurs. **78**:1083-1084, 1978.

73. Marcum, L.N., Box, C.L., and Waeckerle, J.F.: Priorities in multiple system injuries, Topics Emerg. Med. **1**:1-8, 1979.

74. *McKeel, N.L.: Child abuse can be prevented, Am. J. Nurs. **78**:1478-1482, 1978.

75. *Meyd, C.J.: Acute brain trauma, Am. J. Nurs. **78**:40-44, 1978.

76. *Miller, M.E.: Cycle trauma: nursing's three key roles, Nurs. '80 **8**(7):26-31, 1980.

77. Miller, R.H.: Textbook of basic emergency medicine, ed. 2, St. Louis, 1980, The C.V. Mosby Co.

78. Mofenson, H., and Greensher, J.: Keeping up with the trends in childhood poisoning, Clin. Pediatr. **14**:621, 1975.

79. Mofenson, H., and Greensher, J.: The unknown poison, Pediatrics **54**:336-342, 1974.

80. Moore, M.: Medical emergency manual: differential diagnosis and treatment, Baltimore, 1972, The Williams & Wilkins Co.

81. *Palmer, E.L.: Student reactions to disaster, Am. J. Nurs. **80**:680-682, 1980.

82. Plotkin, S., et al.: Immunization schedules for the new human diploid cell vaccine against rabies, Am. J. Epidemiol. **103**:75-80, 1976.

83. Rauckhorst, L.M., Stokes, S.A., and Mezey, M.D.: Community and health assessment, J. Gerontol. Nurs. **6**:319-327, 1980.

84. Reece, R.M.: Manual of emergency pediatrics, ed. 2, Philadelphia, 1978, W.B. Saunders Co.

85. Replantation of digits, Point of View (Sommerville, N.J., Ethicon, Inc.) **13**:11, 1976.

86. Report of District of Columbia Task Force on Rape. In Schultz, L.: Rape victimology, Springfield, Ill., 1975, Charles C Thomas, Publisher.

87. Roberts, J.R.: Pathophysiology, diagnoses, and treatment of head trauma, Topics Emerg. Med. **1**:41-62, 1979.

88. Roberts, J.R.: Trauma of the cervical spine, Topics Emerg. Med. **1**:63-78, 1979.

89. Romano, T.: Trauma nurse specialist, Am. J. Nurs. **73**:1008-1011, 1973.

90. Romano, T., and Boyd, D.: Illinois trauma program, Am. J. Nurs. **73**;1004-1007, 1973.

91. Rothstein, R.J.: Hemorrhagic shock in multiple trauma, Topics Emerg. Med. **1**:29-40, 1979.

92. Schultz, L.: Rape victimology, Springfield, Ill., 1975, Charles C Thomas, Publisher.

93. Shires, G.R., editor: Care of the trauma patient, ed. 2, New York, 1979, McGraw-Hill Book Co.

94. Slater, R.R.: Triage nurse in the emergency department, Hospitals **44**:50-52, 1970.

95. Sovie, M., and Fruehan, C.: Protecting the patient from electrical hazards, Nurs. Clin. North Am. **7**:469-480, 1972.

96. Standards for cardiopulmonary resuscitation and emergency cardiac care, J.A.M.A. **244**:453-508, 1980.

97. Statistical abstract of the United States, 1980, ed. 80, Washington, D.C., 1980, U.S. Bureau of the Census.

98. Stephenson, H.E., Jr., editor: Immediate care of the acutely ill and injured, ed. 2, St. Louis, 1978, The C.V. Mosby Co.

99. Sternbach, G.: Fractures and dislocations, Topics Emerg. Med. **1**:119-132, 1979.

100. *Symposium on Trauma, Nurs. Clin. North Am. **13**:175-265, 1978.

101. Symposium on Trauma, Surg. Clin. North Am. **57**:1-226, 1977.

102. Talento, B.N., and Fernandez, J.C.: Nursing care for rape victims, A.O.R.N. J. **27**:1408-1418, 1978.

103. Tennant, F.S., Jr., Weaver, S.C., and Lewis, C.E.: Outcomes of drug education: four case studies, Pediatrics **52**:246-251, 1973.

104. Tomlanovich, M.C., et al.: Abdominal trauma, Topics Emerg. Med. **1**:95-118, 1979.

105. *Wagner, M., guest editor: Emergency nursing, Nurs. Clin. North Am. **1**:377-466, 1973.

106. Walker, L.: Why do patients use the emergency room? Hosp. Topics **53**:19-21, 1975.

107. Warner, C., editor: Emergency care: assessment and intervention, ed. 3, St. Louis, 1982, The C.V. Mosby Co.

108. Watson, G.S., Zador, P.L., and Wilks, A.: The repeal of helmet use laws and increased motorcyclist mortality in the United States, 1975-1978, Am. J. Public Health **70**:579-585, 1980.

109. White, K.M.: Evaluating the trauma of gunshot wounds, Am. J. Nurs. **77**:1589-1593, 1977.

110. Wintrobe, M.M., et al.: editors: Harrison's principles of internal medicine, ed. 8, New York, 1977, McGraw-Hill Book Co.

AUDIOVISUAL RESOURCES

Acute poisoning and drug overdose, New York, 1980, MEDCOM. (64 slides, 1 audiotape.)

Basic and advanced life support, New York, 1980, MEDCOM. (62 slides, 1 audiotape.)

The Heimlich maneuver, Cincinnati, 1976, Edumed Corp. (33 slides, 1 audiotape.)

Major wounds and multiple injuries, Garden Grove, Calif., 1974, Trainex Corp. (Filmstrip.)

Triage, New York, 1980, MEDCOM. (42 slides, 1 audiotape.)

CHAPTER 74

ASSESSMENT OF THE CRITICALLY ILL PATIENT

MARY K. KIRKPATRICK

The assessment process for the critically ill patients differs from the assessment of other patients in terms of the number of supportive devices available to assist in data collection, the constantly changing data from laboratory parameters, the constant and sometimes rapidly changing physiologic status of the patient, the complexity and the magnitude of interrelated problems, and the time constraint within which the nurse collects data and makes decisions. One of the distinguishing features of the assessment of the critically ill patient stems from the predicament of the patient who may be in a potential life-death situation.

Even when a life-death situation is not present, other limitations may be imposed on nursing assessment. For example, the patient's diminished mental status or the presence of an endotracheal or tracheostomy tube may preclude verbal communication. The assessment of critically ill patients is often limited by their close proximity to other patients, the shorter amount of time available to the nurse to elicit information, and the presence of machines and other devices that may hamper the assessment process. The numerous pieces of equipment and the use of invasive monitoring techniques such as pressure devices also contribute to the crisis environment that surrounds the critically ill patient. Another significant aspect of these patients is the constant change in priorities that results from changes in their biologic status. Often the physiologic assessment takes precedence over the psychologic assessment because of the critical state of the patient.

Although eliciting the patient's collaboration in the assessment process is imperative in all settings, the nature of the critically ill patient's physiologic and psychologic status often prohibits subjective input. Because of the patient's condition, nurses may first elicit input from the significant others. Nevertheless, this in no way negates the advantages of eliciting subjective data from the patient when feasible.

Baseline assessment

After receiving a detailed report of the patient's current physical and emotional status and any interventions that were instituted and their effects, the nurse proceeds to the patient's bedside to make a firsthand assessment of the patient. Using the flow sheet to record the routine measurements and observations (chart on pp. 1914-1915) and the narrative notes to summarize the patient's status at the beginning and at the end of each shift, the nurse documents (1) the patient's vital signs; (2) a head-to-toe assessment (see Chapter 8); (3) physiologic measurements such as central venous pressure (CVP) and intraarterial blood pressure; (4) color, amount, and consistency of drainage and secretions; and (5) observations about mental status. Physiologic measurements such as vital signs are obtained periodically throughout a 24-hour period, whereas other observations are recorded only if they represent a change from the initial baseline assessment. For example, hourly CVP readings may be recorded, although the patient's behavior will not be recorded unless there is a marked change.

Nursing notes will depict pertinent changes in the patient's status, significant interventions, and observations about the reactions of significant others. Changes in a patient's condition are often reflected in several parameters over a period of time. An isolated observa-

SURGICAL INTENSIVE CARE UNIT FLOW SHEET

Surgical procedure: _____ 7 AM weight: _____ kg

Date Time	T	P	R	BP	CVP	MAP	PAP	MPAP	Wedge	CO	Set FIO$_2$ / Meas. FIO$_2$	pH	PCO$_2$	PO$_2$	HCO$_3$	Base Sat.
8-hr total: 3 PM																
8-hr total: 11 PM																
8-hr total: 7 AM																
24-hr total																

Vital signs

Blood gases

Pulmonary function								Ventilator parameters		
Time	TV	V̇	VC	Qs/Qt	Vd/Vt	FRC	NIF	TV	V̇	Infla. pres.

Intake							Output						Chest tube			
CVP line		Periph. IV						Sp. Gr.								
Type	Amt.	Type	Amt.	Oral	Amt.	Urine		SPOT					In	Out	Bal.	Patient notes

Total intake: Total output:

tion has limited usefulness for accurately predicting or validating a problem. For example, a sudden and moderate fall in a patient's blood pressure can result from the effects of a narcotic, a change of position, or circulating blood volume. The change in blood pressure along with an increasing pulse rate, falling CVP, diminishing urinary output, and deterioration of the patient's mental status is a more accurate predictor of a low circulating blood volume than any one measure alone.

At the conclusion of the nurse's workday, a summary is written about the patient's status as depicted in the data collected over a period of time. Interpretative statements as well as evaluative remarks regarding the effectiveness of interventions during the shift are made; for example, "Mr. Jones shows progressive signs of congestive heart failure: increased peripheral edema, decreased urinary output, jugular vein distention." Documentation is a continuous process when caring for the critically ill patient.

Approach to bedside

The nurse caring for a critically ill patient is in a unique position to correlate the bedside assessment of the patient's signs and symptoms with data from the monitors. *It is imperative to note the danger of complete dependency on a monitor. This may cause adequate and reliable data obtained directly from the patient to be missed.*

The nurse approaching the bedside is able to inspect the critically ill patient and the surroundings in order to elicit significant data. Critical illness always endangers and involves the ventilatory, circulatory, renal, and neurologic subsystems as well as the self-esteem of the person; therefore the nurse needs to be alert to changes in these subsystems. For example, cardiac or respiratory distress can be assessed by the position a patient assumes in bed or the number of pillows required for the patient to gain maximal function of the ventilatory system. The patient who is short of breath will sit up, or if already sitting up will lean forward in order to facilitate breathing. Facial expressions are also helpful in assessing the patient. The patient who is in pain may grimace or grit the teeth. The patient's expression may reveal fright, sadness, or other feelings.

In addition, specific input from supportive or monitoring devices contributes significant data to the assessment process. An example of specific input from the ventilator elicited while the nurse is en route to the bedside is the flashing yellow light on the MA-1 respirator, indicating the patient's capability to assist the ventilator, or the flashing red light accompanied by a constant noise that is indicative of obstruction in the airway.

Cardiac monitors, intracranial pressure monitors, and intraarterial blood pressure devices are commonly used for continuous surveillance of the patient's status. Although monitors are not to be completely relied on for accuracy, the electrocardiogram, intracranial pressure monitors, arterial pressure monitors, and other devices afford the nurse a moment-to-moment assessment of vital signs or subsystem parameter readings. Listening to the sounds of the monitor as well as viewing the oscilloscope provides constant data to the nurse.

Another clue is the presence of an odor. The nurse may smell the acetone breath of the unconscious patient in ketosis or the aroma of alcohol from an accident victim. The odor from a tracheostomy tube or an incision may sometimes be the first clue to an infection.

Assessment of vital functions

Assessment priorities for the critically ill involve the vital functions of ventilatory, circulatory, neurologic, and renal subsystems. Although standard techniques may be used to obtain data, the data collection is focused on early signs and symptoms of multisystem complications. These are likely to be evident in data obtained from vital signs, records of fluid intake and output, blood gas analyses, and other physiologic indices.

Because nursing and medical interventions occur so frequently, observations of their impact on vital functions are made at frequent intervals. The effects of interventions may be monitored by responses in the physiologic parameters discussed below.

Ventilatory subsystems

Constant observation of ventilatory function as well as the effectiveness of ventilatory supports is essential. Data used to measure ventilatory function include changing mental status, pulmonary rate and rhythm, quality of breath sounds, skin color, and changing circulatory status.

Changes in the person's mental status may provide early clues to hypoxia; cyanosis is one of the last changes to occur with hypoxia. Hypoxia resulting from ventilatory impairment may be further aggravated by a decreased hemoglobin level. Tachycardia and other cardiac arrhythmias are often prominent symptoms of hypoxia. The importance of respiratory rate and rhythm is addressed elsewhere (p. 1216). The quality of breath sounds may indicate the presence of atelectasis as well as the effectiveness of pulmonary toilet. Adventitious sounds may indicate the need for devices such as blowbottles or three-ball inspirometry. Laboratory data such as arterial blood gas values, chest radiographs, or tidal volume measurements are used to validate observations.

The patient often requires ventilatory support such as a respirator attached to an endotracheal or tracheostomy tube. These supports mandate observations of the equipment itself as well as the impact of the support on the patient's status. The effectiveness of ventilatory equipment is usually monitored by periodic blood gas analyses. For example, the use of PEEP (positive end-expiratory pressure) should increase the oxygen content of the patient's blood. When chest tubes are present, their patency, the color and amount of drainage, absence or presence of bubbling of the fluid in the collection bottle, and presence of crepitus around the tube site must be ascertained (see p. 1253 for discussion of care of patients with chest tubes). When a mechanical ventilator is used, nurses must be alert to potential complications such as pneumothorax, infection, atelectasis, decreased cardiac output, and gastrointestinal tract bleeding from a stress ulcer. Therefore changes in vital signs and in breath and bowel sounds must be constantly monitored. The presence of occult blood in the stool or nasogastric drainage may indicate gastrointestinal tract bleeding. Thus ventilatory assessment implies more than observation of pulmonary status alone.

Cardiovascular subsystems

A format for cardiovascular assessment similar to that described in Chapters 8 and 43 may be used in the critical care unit. However, observations are made at frequent intervals, and particular attention is devoted to the assessment of arrhythmias. In addition, cardiovascular pressures are frequently monitored.

The cardioscope can be used to validate data obtained by palpation or auscultation. For example, the skipped beat in a patient's apical pulse may be depicted as a premature ventricular contraction on the monitor. Data obtained from the cardioscope should include the basic rhythm, the type of cardiac arrhythmia, and its frequency and duration. The cardioscope can also be used to evaluate the person's electrolyte status (potassium level) as well as the effects of medications such as sympathomimetic agents like isoproterenol (Isuprel). The cardioscope may also provide data about the effectiveness of an internal pacemaker.

Data other than that obtained with the cardioscope are crucial in the evaluation of an arrhythmia. The blood pressure, level of consciousness, renal output, electrolyte levels, and blood levels of drugs may provide clues to the cause as well as the effects of the arrhythmia.

In addition to observing the cardioscope, the nurse measures various pressures to evaluate the circulatory status. Although the CVP reflects the functioning of the right atrium and vascular volume, the pulmonary capillary wedge pressure obtained through the use of a Swan-Ganz catheter more readily indicates left ventricular function (see Figs. 43-18 to 43-20). Measurement of the intraarterial blood pressure enables the nurse to assess vascular volume, a *pulsus alternans* reflecting ventricular failure, or a *pulsus paradoxus* reflecting cardiac tamponade. The measurement of cardiac output also provides important data about the pumping function of the heart.

What is "normal" for one patient may not be normal for another; therefore serial readings of these values must be obtained to evaluate a patient's status. In addition to the level of these pressures, nurses consider the position of the patient when the measurements were made, the previous pressure readings as well as the normal range, the amount and type of intravenous infusions, the underlying cardiovascular dysfunction, the type of medications the patient is receiving, and the functioning of the vascular lines.[34]

Other parameters to assess in evaluating the cardiovascular subsystem are urinary output; blood loss from chest tubes; the difference between the arterial and venous oxygen saturation; hemoglobin and hemotocrit levels; enzyme levels, especially CPK (creatine phosphokinase), LDH (lactic dehydrogenase), and SGOT (serum glutamic-oxalacetic transaminase); and electrolyte levels including calcium, sodium, and potassium.

Renal subsystems

The guidelines for assessing the renal subsystem are noted in Chapters 8 and 60. Laboratory findings as well as other patient data are used to monitor renal function. The monitoring of hourly urinary output is often accompanied by determination of specific gravity of the urine. Serum and urinary osmolality, blood urea nitrogen, creatinine levels, and sodium and potassium levels are commonly used as indices of renal function. Changes in renal status often precipitate changes in the patient's weight and mental status. Signs and symptoms of renal dysfunction may also include cardiovascular changes such as edema, distention of neck veins, adventitious breath sounds, gallop rhythm, and changes in pulse and blood pressure.[15]

The nurse also assesses the inputs likely to influence renal parameters. These include the type and amount of additives in intravenous fluids as well as irrigating solutions. The urinary output is obviously influenced by fluid input as well as by many medicatons such as digitalis and diuretics.

Other subsystem dysfunctions such as dehydration, hypervolemia or hypovolemia, ADH (antidiuretic hormone) changes, or osmotic diuresis induced by total parenteral nutrition (hyperalimentation) may alter renal output, since they influence the renal function of the critically ill person.

A final mediating factor is the presence of an indwelling urinary catheter. Although it facilitates obtaining an accurate record of urinary output, inattention to its patency or a urinary tract infection may interfere with the accurate assessment of renal outputs.

Neurologic subsystems

While the nurse assesses other subsystems, clues are elicited to provide information regarding the critically ill patient's orientation to time, place, and person and the appropriateness of responses to either verbal or tactile stimuli. Determining the intactness of the cranial nerves as well as the functional status of the musculoskeletal system, which is dependent on innervation, is essentially the same as for other patients (see Chapters 8 and 40).

Although determining the presence or absence of a neurologic sign remains significant, it is the returning or the diminishing of a sign that is often more relevant in critical care settings. Subtle and slight changes, such as the return of reflexes following anesthesia or trauma or even a slight decrease in the level of consciousness, may be extremely significant.

In addition to recognizing and interpreting neurologic changes, the evaluation of parameters that alter the patient's neurologic status becomes imperative. Although assessing the appropriate or inappropriate behavioral response to stimuli continues to be important, assessing the types of posturing or ventilatory pattern provides valuable information with respect to the physiologic basis of the neurologic dysfunction. For example, metabolic changes resulting from vital subsystem dysfunction, as in the case of ventilatory insufficiency, may alter the patient's level of consciousness; therefore the integration of data from the assessment of other subsystems is paramount.

For the critically ill patient, the assessment of the neurologic subsystem is complicated by the environment as well as by the use of medications. Because of the lack of sensory input, such as absence of a clock or an overload of sensory input such as constant noise and bright lights, a patient's disorientation may not necessarily reflect a neurologic deficit. Drugs can alter a patient's thought processes as well as perceptions, gait, and responsiveness. In no other part of the assessment can concomitant clues provide such essential information. Often it is necessary to continuously arouse the patient to the highest level of consciousness, and a painful stimulus may be the only way to elicit a response.

The *late* signs and symptoms of increased intracranial pressure are apt to be more readily encountered among critically ill patients. In addition to the vital signs and the neurologic assessment, data regarding intracranial pressure can be obtained by means of the subarachnoid screw, which directly measures changes in the intracranial pressure.

It is not enough merely to assess the neurologic status in relation to the other subsystems, but recording the observations so that they are available for ongoing comparison is imperative. Establishing a data base, following the sequence of events frequently, and recognizing subtle and concomitant clues are of great significance in the care of the critically ill patient.

Assessment of other physiologic parameters

Integumentary and musculoskeletal status

The importance of assessing the integument, which protects the body from the external environment, is intensified in the care of the critically ill patient because there is often inadequate circulation, oxygenation, and nutrition along with long periods of immobility. Factors that enhance physiologic inadequacies and immobility must be considered, including pain and the presence of monitoring devices or equipment that necessitates that a patient lie in a supine position or that interferes with position change. Also prevalent in the critical care setting are factors that intensify the hazards of immobility such as the use of vasoconstrictor drugs, which predispose a patient to skin breakdown. The length of time that the critically ill person is confined to bed, the state of debilitation, inadequate hydration, effects of medications, and changes in ingestion and digestion patterns further predispose the individual to contractures and skin breakdown.

Assessing the range of motion and muscle tone of all extremities for any bedridden patient is imperative. However, in the critically ill patient, complications of procedures themselves often affect the musculoskeletal and integumentary systems. For example, the insertion of a transvenous pacemaker can result in a "frozen" or stiff shoulder if appropriate range of motion is not maintained. In addition, the restraints on or contraindications to moving a patient, such as the placement of tubes or catheters in the femoral area, impose barriers to movement. Restrictions often increase with the amount of equipment and are unrelated to the patient's mental status. When immobility is not required, the usual assessment of activity tolerance as reflected in the patient's pulse, fatigue, shortness of breath, and other symptoms guides the nurse.

Fluid and electrolyte balance

Disturbances of fluid and electrolyte balance are common to the critically ill patient and are secondary to a dysfunctional subsystem, therapeutic regimens such as a nasogastric tube and suction, the presence of pain, and prolonged periods of stress. While assessment of the functional capacity of the renal subsystem provides a major part of the data regarding fluid and electrolyte balance, it is imperative to recognize the interrelatedness of electrolyte balance with other subsystems. For example, renal dysfunction changes the level of circulating potassium, and in turn this electrolyte potentiates cardiovascular dysfunction. Electrolyte balance is even more crucial because of an already weakened subsystem. Because therapeutic regimens may entail a number of devices, such as a nasogastric tube and the use of medications that deplete the body of fluids and electrolytes, fluid and electrolyte disturbances may be compounded. For example, the loss of potassium through the nasogastric tube, as well as its excretion in response to certain diuretics, may potentiate electrolyte disturbances, thus necessitating frequent and constant monitoring. Although critically ill patients usually receive intravenous fluids that contain electrolyte supplements such as potassium, elevated or lowered electrolyte levels must be carefully monitored. This is especially so since electrolytes such as potassium are known to be depleted during surgery and other periods of stress. The signs and symptoms of the *hypo* and *hyper* electrolyte states, urine and serum levels of electrolytes, and electrocardiographic changes caused by electrolyte disturbance provide diagnostic indications (see Chapter 21). Because of the complexity of the critically ill patient's problems, physical signs and symptoms may be masked or difficult to determine; therefore validation of electrolyte imbalance by the use of laboratory values is necessary. Electrolytes most commonly assessed because of their importance and their continually changing levels are potassium, sodium, and chloride.

Often critically ill patients receive multiple intravenous infusions simultaneously. In addition to the usual assessment of type and amount of fluid and the additives being infused, the signs and symptoms of overhydration and dehydration as reflected by integumentary signs, weight changes, and subsystem changes are noted. Hourly measurements of intake and output are mandated by the critical state of the patient. Although weighing patients daily provides the most accurate data about fluid balance, it is essential that weight changes be examined in light of any variation in the weighing procedure required by the presence of life-support equipment.

Nutritional and elimination status

During the time that the nutritional demands for repair of the debilitated state are greatly increased, the critically ill patient commonly is unable to take nutritional supplements orally. With increasing complications, the caloric, nitrogen, and fluid requirements are increased, and nutritional supplementation by an intravenous or central line is required. The patient's catabolic state mandates that special attention be given to protein and caloric intake.

To assess the nutritional status of the critically ill person, it is necessary to determine (1) present condition, (2) the length of time nutritional status has been impaired or is expected to be impaired, (3) daily vitamin and caloric needs, (4) nitrogen balance, (5) changes in body weight, and (6) the means by which the nutritional status is maintained (gastrostomy or intravenous routes). Complications of these nutritional supplements as well as changes in subsystems that may cause a supplement to become a potential hazard necessitate constant surveillance.

With increased excretion of solute or in the presence of a potential osmotic diuretic state, assessment of the patient's tolerance of amino acids, presence of hyperglycemia manifested by glycosuria, or potential hypoglycemic reaction is essential. Often these nursing assessments may indicate the need for immediate cessation of the prescribed therapy. In addition, careful observation of the hydration status is essential for patients receiving nutritional supplements parentally.

Inspection of the condition of mucous membranes of the mouth and the tongue is of particular significance. The presence of nasogastric and endotracheal tubes hampers oral hygiene. The use of medications such as anticoagulants and some chemotherapeutic agents predisposes patients to oral problems such as bleeding gums. Other factors to assess with respect to the nutritional status of the critically ill patient include abdominal distention, bowel sounds, pain that inhibits the patient's desire for food, tolerance and preference for food, and the patient's elimination status.

A gastrointestinal tract complication well known to the nurse in the critical care area is bleeding secondary to a stress ulcer resulting from intense and prolonged stress. Although the observation of the patient's pale color and fatigued appearance increases the nurse's level of suspicion, the objective assessment of occult blood in stools or gastrointestinal tract drainage, the drop in hematocrit and hemoglobin levels, and the presence of abdominal pain validate this suspicion. Predisposition of patients to stress ulcers can be assessed from past history as well as current use of anticoagulant agents including aspirin, warfarin sodium (Coumadin), or heparin and the prolonged use of mechanical ventilators. An antacid regimen is commonly prescribed to prevent or treat this complication.

Although bowel elimination often receives less attention than other vital functions, it may precipitate major complications. Not only is the patient's elimination pattern disrupted as a result of a medical or surgical procedure or prohibited intake of food, but the common use of medications such as meperidine (Demerol) or codeine, which predispose the patient to constipation, and the long periods of immobility, the effect of continued stress, and fluid and electrolyte disturbances exacerbate elimination problems.

Use of the bedpan or bedside commode, with only a curtain serving as a means of separation from the patient in the next bed, decreases the amount of privacy available to the patient and may interfere with elimination. In addition to assessing the effects of the previously mentioned factors on a patient's elimination status, it is important to determine the most effective position for elimination, the optimal time for elimination, and the utility of a regimen to facilitate a normal bowel movement. When appliances are used for elimination (e.g., with a colostomy), it is imperative that the nurse monitor complications from such appliances (e.g., skin breakdown under the colostomy bag). The patient's tolerance or energy expenditure while using a bedpan or a bedside commode can also be assessed. Helping the patient learn positions that facilitate elimination, as well as breathing techniques that minimize Valsalva's maneuver, are especially significant in the care of patients who are vulnerable to the negative effects of straining when attempting to have a bowel movement.

Assessing the impact of the critical care environment

Environment

The environment of most critical care units is considerably different from the environment in general care units. The critically ill patient is not only forced into a state of dependency but is also maintained in an environment conducive to both sensory deprivation and sensory overload (see Chapter 26). The openness of some critical care areas and the close proximity of patients reduce privacy, while the number of procedures and almost constant presence of artificial light in addition to the noise in critical care areas demand constant assessment of the type and amount of sensory input. Eliciting input regarding a patient's usual routine and how the routine can be altered to maintain individual preferences and foster normal body rhythms is very significant. For example, critically ill persons may have time lapses of days or weeks during which they are not aware of the date, the time, or the place. It is imperative that the patient's orientation and the situations that enhance meaningful stimulation be assessed daily. Varying the time or amount of visiting hours for significant others may increase patterned input.

The amount of sensory overload and sensory deprivation increases relative to the severity of illness and the needs of the patient. Consequently, constant observations for signs and symptoms of delirium or postoperative psychosis is essential. It is not enough to identify the signs and symptoms of these disorders. Steps should be taken to determine the factors causing the disorders; these include therapeutic and idiosyncratic causes as well as environmental factors. The effects of medications, constant interventions by personnel, the individual's own emotional state and age, as well as the status of the critical subsystems, may all contribute to altered behavioral states.

A factor common to the critical care environment is the noise level. The nurse assesses the noise with respect to the equipment, staff, and patients' input as well as to extraneous sources such as a radio. Critical analysis of the source, the amount, and the level of stimuli is essential; what may be advantageous for one patient is often disadvantageous for another. Means by which to individualize such input require constant attention.

Complications of therapy

Infection is an ever present problem. The critically ill patient's debilitated state increases vulnerability to infection. In addition, invasive procedures, exposure to many personnel, and the administration of steroids all increase the risk of infection. At the same time, steroids and prophylactic antibiotics may mask the presence of an infection. For these reasons, personnel in critical care units must be particularly vigilant in maintaining sterile and nontraumatic techniques, especially when suctioning tubes or inserting or irrigating catheters. (See Chapter 22 for further information on infection control.)

Careful assessment is made of the skin surrounding each tube or catheter entrance for increased tenderness and warmth. An increase in the white blood cell count or the growth of organisms from cultures of secretions validates the presence of an infection. When an infection occurs, nurses investigate the potential causes of the infection such as inadequate aseptic technique or cross-contamination through shared equipment, and appropriate steps are taken to prevent such hazards from occurring in the future.

Comfort

Because of the many lifesaving measures that must be instituted when patients are in an intensive care unit, comfort of the patient may not be a major priority. Yet patients in these areas may be extremely uncomfortable because of their dependent states and the many factors that can predispose them to prolonged discomfort.

Hygiene

Because the patient cannot meet personal hygiene needs, this responsibility is assumed by the nurse. Meticulous and frequent mouth care is important, especially for patients who have nasogastric tubes. The presence of an indwelling catheter requires careful perineal care. One study suggests that the care of the perineum should not be too vigorous, since such a practice may increase rather than decrease urinary tract infections.[19] The position of urinary catheters and means for maintaining the position are ascertained in order to provide comfort and to prevent complications. (See Chapter 22 for further information.)

Body alignment

A critically ill person requires more frequent turning to prevent complications such as skin breakdown and atelectasis. It is the nurse's responsibility to assess the patient's capability to turn, to determine the frequency of position change, contraindications to turning (e.g., possible malfunctioning of a monitor when a patient turns), effects of a position on the patient's physical state, and need for passive and active range of motion. Care to prevent complications such as skin breakdown must begin in the critical care setting.

Pain

The critically ill patient may have multiple painful sites. When the patient is unable to talk, the cause of pain must be determined without benefit of the patient's description. Pharmacologic agents to relieve the pain may be administered more frequently to critically ill patients than to those persons less ill. Pain medications are commonly given intravenously; this necessitates astute observation of the effects of the medications, since they act rapidly and can lead to dangerous side effects. To avoid potentiating the effects of anesthesia or previously administered medications, the time that anesthesia or other medications were given is noted before an analgesic is administered. Identifying factors that influence pain, such as treatments, body positions, fatigue, or annoying sounds from machinery, is as essential as noting the effectiveness of pain medications. Immediate feedback about the presence of pain may be elicited from the monitors, which indicate an elevated blood pressure or pulse rate in the presence of pain.

Safety

Many factors in the critical care setting make this environment potentially hazardous. Frequently, the patient is confused, or the patient's sensorium is depressed from medications and anesthesia. The patient who is confused may resist therapy and may attempt to remove catheters and other tubes. This often necessitates confining the patient with soft restraints. The effects of restraints on the circulation, nerve functioning, and the patient's behavior are assessed to ensure that protective devices are not creating further problems.

Most critical care units are air conditioned, and the cool room temperature may impede an already poor circulation and cause the patient to receive diminished effects of medications or to slow down their excretion. The critically ill patient may have few bed covers because of an already elevated body temperature and should be observed for chilling, which would result in undesirable demands on an already taxed metabolism.

Another major hazard is the presence of much electrical equipment. Considerable information is available about electrical hazards and safety, and it is a nursing responsibility to ensure that hazards are recognized, that equipment is in good working order, that safety practices are observed, and that all equipment is properly grounded to reduce the possibility of electrical shock.

Assessment of psychologic status

The admission of a patient who is critically ill produces anxiety or fear in the patient and significant others. The patient may be threatened with a number of losses: life itself; impairment, if not severance, of the functional capacity of a subsystem; insult to body integrity caused by the state of disability or helplessness; and loss of comfort as the result of pain. The predicament becomes that of forced dependency, immobilization, and lack of control in an unfamiliar, if not frightening, environment that may depersonalize and assault the person while affording few, if any, means for the person to respond to this crisis. No longer can significant others afford support by their physical presence. The patient is usually isolated and removed from familiar faces except for brief periods each day. Even in the short visits with significant others, the patient may be deprived of usual means of communication because he or she is intubated.

The patient's response to critical illness will be determined by factors that influence behavior. These include basic personality, perceptions of the illness and what is happening, usual mode of coping, cultural background, the reaction of significant others, and the openness or closedness of the critical care unit.

Perceptions

It is imperative to assess the patient's perception of the situation and its meaning. The critical care setting is an intense one with respect to the pace of activity as well as the person's physical condition and the potentially fatal outcome of the person's illness. Consequently, the patient's emotional responses may be more intense than those observed in less ill patients. The patient may react with greater anger or hostility or may experience prolonged periods of depression, shock, and disbelief.

Culture can influence perceptions of the critical care environment. The dramatization of emergency or life-threatening situations in the mass media may cause the patient to perceive his or her situation as more serious than it really is. Previous illnesses and hospitalizations also influence the patient's perceptions. For individuals who have no experience with illness or hospitalization the anxiety may be even greater, since they have no idea of what to expect from the environment or the personnel caring for them.

The assessment of the patients' perception is made by observing, listening, and eliciting from them or others their views or feelings about what is occurring. When a patient is unable to communicate verbally, assessment is restricted to nonverbal clues such as facial expressions, hand gestures, body movements, and muscle tone. If physical status does not permit the patient to communicate the input of significant others is imperative. Because the environmental stimuli are so numerous, it is often difficult to differentiate between a patient's perception of physical status and the perception of the environment or therapeutic regimen.

Coping behaviors

In addition to assessing the general regulators of behavior, it is necessary to assess three main characteristics of response of the critically ill person: the *emotional*, the *behavioral*, and the *physiologic*. These apply to both the patient and the significant others.

An *emotional response* to either a psychologic or social loss may be similar to the adaptation to illness. The nurse's assessment of a patient's emotional response should include possible explanations for the feelings of anxiety or depression. Anxiety caused by a fear of dying may be intensified by pain or dyspnea or by nursing and medical measures. A critically ill person and the significant others may also experience helplessness, hopelessness, and powerlessness intensified by their isolation.[29]

Behavioral responses that indicate anxiety and a fear of dying may include unwillingness to participate in personal care when able to do so, withdrawal from interactions with others, and facial or postural expressions of no longer caring, or giving up. The nurse can validate inferences about these responses by urging the patient or family to ventilate their feelings.

The behavioral modes of dissipating excess energy or discharging stress are greatly limited by the patient's health status as well as by the environment.[26] Consequently, excess energy may be evidenced by hyperactive, anxious, angry, or talkative states, while energy deficits are manifested by fatigue, depression, or withdrawal.

Determining whether a response is physiologic or behavioral is often difficult because of the confounding variables of the environment, the patient's physical state, and the effects of medication. For example, a patient may be lethargic and unresponsive to a procedure because of a hypoxic or medicated state or hyperactive and overresponsive to the same procedure because of a sensory overload from the environment.

It is imperative in judging whether behavior is adaptive or maladaptive to consider both the appropriateness of the behavior relative to the situation and the previous behavior patterns of the individual. For example, a patient may experience confusion or loss of sense of time when the natural body rhythms are disrupted. This is a common experience of patients in intensive care units who are kept awake day and night by constant noise, bright lights, and frequent procedures. An analogy is the "jet lag" experienced by travelers.

Altered *physiologic responses,* including those of the autonomic nervous system, such as increased or abnormal heart rate, dilated pupils, increased respirations, and dizziness, may also denote the adaptation to crisis (see Chapter 14). Other physiologic responses may include weight loss, constipation, and insomnia.

Communication problems

Nurses need to assess the patient's and significant others' desire to talk and to express feelings. Input from significant others will assist the nurse in interpreting what the critical illness means to them and to the patient and their usual means of coping with crises.

If the patient's usual modes of communication are altered, it is necessary to assess the utility of alternative ways to communicate such as writing, using sign language or alphabet charts, and lipreading. It is also necessary for the nurse to assess the effect of alternate means of communication on the patient who becomes upset over the amount of time required for the interpretation of sign language.

Knowledge assessment

In addition to identifying the patient's and significant others' reaction to the illness, it is necessary to assess the effect that the environment has on each of them. Determining what each of them knows about monitors, machines, tubes, and procedures as well as their readiness to learn about the equipment, the rationales for the regimens, and information about objectives of care guides the amount of teaching that is given. It is necessary to assess the patient's mental status to determine how often information needs to be repeated. Repetition is often necessary because pain, physical status, and the psychologic adjustment of the patient may interfere with learning. Recognizing that the patient may not retain data, the nurse continually observes the effect that information has on him or her and whether it relieves or increases anxiety. The need for information sharing with the critically ill patient has been documented.[5]

The observance of the patient's rights is just as important in a critical care setting as in other hospital areas. These rights are the right to be informed, right to have interpretations, right to have someone listen, right to question, right to see family, and right to deny. The guiding principle is prefacing each nursing action with an explanation to facilitate the patient's rights.[32]

The perceptions of a patient and significant others depend on the information that they have or are given about the patient's physical status, the procedures and routines of the critical care environment, the objectives of care, and the prognosis. Often the frequency of nursing tasks and the pace of the unit limit the amount of communication with the patient and significant others. The nurse needs to determine that the perceptions of the patient and significant others are accurate, since often they misinterpret the patient's condition and the purpose of equipment. In addition, the nurse needs to constantly assess the readiness of the patient and significant others for additional information and should plan an appropriate time to meet with them.

Assessment of sociologic stressors

Although the assessment of the social systems is the same for the critically ill patient as for any other patient, certain aspects may not take precedence until after physiologic stability is achieved. Often in a life-threatening situation, the patient or significant others may request the presence and support of the hospital chaplain or another clergyperson; their presence can give support to the patient and significant others and is especially important, since the efforts of physicians and nurses are directed toward maintaining the patient's life.

Another aspect of the social system to be assessed is the interaction and continuity of the relationship beginning between the patient and significant others. Those characteristics that make the assessment different are the imposed restrictions (sometimes unnecessarily placed) on the visiting privileges of significant others, the specialized areas (often behind closed doors) that serve to separate the critically ill from other patients as well as from significant others, and the lack of involvement of significant others in the care of the patient. It is necessary to assess the frequency and the quality of interactions between the client and significant others, the strengths and limitations of the significant others, the availability of significant others, and the state of stress or crisis in which the significant others find themselves. The impact of the crisis and the continued stress on the significant others can be assessed by observing their facial expressions, their attentiveness or lack of it, and their coping behaviors. It is necessary for the nurse to identify factors that increase or decrease the stress of the significant others. For example, lack of information regarding a patient's status, inability to visit frequently, and the general emotional climate in the waiting room may increase the significant others' discomfort. Family members commonly spend the night in the waiting rooms or sleep in the hospital lobby, since they desire to be present if anything adverse happens to the patient. Consequently, they may be exhausted at a time when continuously high levels of energy are demanded.

It is also important to assess the problem-solving ability of the significant others in the midst of stress. The identification of the coping mechanisms on which significant others rely as well as their ability to begin to act and to make decisions regarding changed roles, lifestyles, and responsibilities is imperative. The prescribed role of the patient, such as head of the family, often must be assumed by another family member. The nurse can be instrumental in assessing the willingness of the significant others to identify and utilize other resources and support systems. For example, the critical illness of a small child may require unlimited time of one or both parents, requiring that a grandparent or another adult assume the parental role in the home.

The nurse obtains much of the data about the strengths and limitations of the family through observation of their emotional and behavioral responses to the situation as well as by talking to other family members. The assessment of the family with respect to mental status, communication patterns, emotional stability, physical status, affection and cohesion among family members, and socialization with each other is similar to an assessment of a family in another situation. However, the duration of stress associated with having a critically ill family member, the abrupt change in family roles, and isolation from the loved one creates additional stressors for the family. The reality of a change in life-style for the patient and its effect on the life-style of the significant others must be assessed from the beginning to prepare them for the anticipated outcomes.

In summary, the principles that govern the assessment of any patient are applicable to the assessment of the critically ill person. The collaboration with the patient and family, the explanation of each nursing activity, and the recognition of increased psychophysiologic vulnerability because of the severity of the illness may provide the opportunity for growth for all concerned. The interaction that takes place during this period of crisis may strengthen relationships between the patient and significant others and may also determine their ability to cope with future crises.

REFERENCES AND SELECTED READINGS
Contemporary

1. Aguilera, D.C., and Messick, J.M.: Crisis intervention: theory and methodology, ed. 4, St. Louis, 1982, The C.V. Mosby Co.
2. Auger, J.R.: Behavioral systems and nursing behavioral assessment and nursing, Englewood Cliffs, 1976, Prentice-Hall Inc.
3. *Bolin, R.H.: Sensory deprivation: an overview, Nurs. Forum 13:241-258, 1974.
4. Byrne, M.L., and Thompson, L.F.: Key concepts for the study and practice of nursing, ed. 2, St. Louis, 1978, The C.V. Mosby Co.
5. *Cassem, N.H., Hackett, T., and Bascon, C.: Reactions of coronary patients to the C.C.U. nurse, Am. J. Nurs. 70:312-319, 1970.
6. *Codd, J., and Grohar, M.E.: Postoperative pulmonary complications, Nurs. Clin. North Am. 10:5-15, 1975.
7. *Corbell, M.: Nursing process for a patient with a body image disturbance, Nurs. Clin. North Am. 6:155-163, 1971.
8. Davis, M.Z.: Socioemotional components of coronary care, Am. J. Nurs. 72:705-709, 1972.
9. *Dodd, M.J.: Assessing mental status, Am. J. Nurs. 78:1500-1503, 1978.
10. Downs, F.S.: Bedrest and sensory disturbances, Am. J. Nurs. 74:434-438, 1974.
11. Fitzgerald, L.M.: Mechanical ventilation, Heart Lung 5:945-949, 1976.
12. *Garrett, J.J.: Oliguria in postoperative patients, Nurs. Clin. North Am. 10:59-67, 1975.
13. *Gordon, M.: Assessing activity tolerance, Am. J. Nurs. 76:72-75, 1975.
14. Hamilton, W.P.: Common cardiovascular problems in the postoperative period, Nurs. Clin. North Am. 10:27-41, 1975.
15. *Heath, J.K.: A conceptual basis for assessing body water status, Nurs. Clin. North Am. 6:189-198, 1971.

16. Hudak, C.M., Gallo, B.M., and Lohr, T.: Critical care nursing, Philadelphia, 1973, J.B. Lippincott Co.
17. Kiely, W.F., and Procci, W.R.: Psychiatric aspects of critical care. In Zschoche, D.A.: Mosby's comprehensive review of critical care, ed. 2, St. Louis, 1981, The C.V. Mosby Co.
18. Kuenzi, S.H., and Fenton, M.V.: Crisis intervention in acute care areas, Am. J. Nurs. 75:830-834, 1975.
19. Kumin, C.M.: Detection, prevention and management of urinary tract infections, ed. 2, Philadelphia, 1974, Lea & Febiger.
20. Lawson, B.N.: Clinical assessment of cardiac patients in acute care facilities, Nurs. Clin. North Am. 7:431-434, 1972.
21. Laycock, J.: Nursing the patient on the ventilator, Nurs. Clin. North Am. 10:17-25, 1975.
22. Lewis, L.: Systematic assessment: what it can do for the hospitalized patient, Med. Arts Sci. 27:39-50, 1973.
23. *Maykoski, K., and Fabre, D.: Nursing assessment of the surgical intensive care patient, Nurs. Clin. North Am. 10:83-106, 1975.
24. McVan, B.: Odors: what the nose knows, Nurs. '77 7:46-49, 1977.
25. Methery, N.A.: Water and electrolyte balance in the postoperative patient, Nurs. Clin. North Am. 10:49-57, 1975.
26. Murray, R.L.E.: Assessment of psychological status in the surgical I.C.U. patients, Nurs. Clin. North Am. 10:69-81, 1975.
27. Obier, K., and Haywood, L.J.: Enhancing therapeutic communication with acutely ill patients, Heart Lung 2:49-53, 1973.
28. *Reynolds, M.T., and Walters, W.J.: Physical assessment of the critically ill. In Daly, B.J., editor: Intensive care nursing, Garden City, N.Y., 1980, Medical Examination Publishing Co., Inc.
29. Roberts, S.L.: Behavioral concepts and the critically ill patients, Englewood Cliffs, N.J., 1976, Prentice-Hall, Inc.
30. Roberts, S.L.: Systems approach in assessing behavioral problems of critical care patients, Heart Lung 4:593-598, 1975.
31. *Smith, R.N.: Invasive pressure monitoring, Am. J. Nurs. 78:1514-1521, 1978.
32. Storlie, F.: Patient teaching in critical care, New York, 1975, Appleton-Century-Crofts.
33. Woods, N.F., and Falk, S.A.: Noise stimuli in the acute care area, Nurs. Res. 23:144-150, 1974.
34. Woods, S.L.: Monitoring PA pressures, Am. J. Nurs. 76:1765-1771, 1976.
35. Zetterland, J.E.: An evaluation of visiting policies for intensive and coronary care units. In Duffey, M., et al.: Current concepts in clinical nursing, vol. 3, St. Louis, 1971, The C.V. Mosby Co.

Classic

36. Klein, R., Kliner, W., and Lipos, D.: Transfer from a coronary care unit: some adverse responses, Arch. Intern. Med. 122:104-108, 1968.
37. Strauss, A.: The intensive care unit: its characteristics and social relationships, Nurs. Clin. North Am. 3:7-15, 1968.

*References preceded by an asterisk are particularly well suited for student reading.

CHAPTER 75

INTERVENTIONS FOR THE CRITICALLY ILL PATIENT

SALLY SCHAFER TODD

The nursing process is the same in critical care situations as it is in any other patient care setting. Management of critically ill patients requires establishing a data base, identifying problems and potential problems, delineating priorities, defining outcome criteria, determining goals for intervention, carrying out the planned interventions, evaluating the effects of interventions, and modifying goals and plans as necessary. Management of critically ill patients differs from management of other patients because of an ever changing data base; a larger number of complex, interrelated problems; frequent reordering of priorities; and time limitations imposed by the rapidity with which the data base changes.

Nurses in critical care settings are called on to make decisions rapidly and to act on those decisions based on discriminating observations, understanding of the interrelationship among phenomena observed, and a current and comprehensive assessment of the situation. It is essential to keep pace with the constant input of new data in order to identify new problems as they arise, make predictions about potential problems that might occur, and intervene according to appropriate priorities and goals.

The ultimate goal of nursing intervention for any patient, regardless of the nature of the illness, is to promote, sustain, and restore optimal level of physiologic, psychologic, and social functioning. However, in a critical care setting the immediate goal of ensuring a patient's survival initially determines the priorities for intervention. Once the question of a patient's survival has been determined, priorities are reordered and other problems can be addressed.

The life-threatening and potentially life-threatening events that are a part of critical illness require constant vigilance by members of the critical care team in order to maintain a patient in a homeokinetic state, to prevent complications, and to restore optimal function. Since nurses are in 24-hour attendance, they are the first to recognize changes in a patient's condition. In most critical care units there is one nurse for every one to three patients, depending on each patient's physiologic stability, numbers of personnel available, and care requirements.

When assuming responsibility for the care of a critically ill patient, the nurse receives a detailed report of significant changes that have occurred, interventions that were instituted and their effects, and a summary of the patient's current physical and emotional status. A well-organized comprehensive report will highlight problems and priorities and will help the nurse establish initial goals for intervention.

Having received this report, the nurse proceeds to the patient's bedside, where introductions are made either by the nurse or by the nurse who has been with the patient during the previous shift. The patient is engaged in discussion as to concerns and perceptions of his or her condition. This approach to the patient can accomplish several purposes. It reinforces the fact that the patient is seen first as a worthwhile person and second as a patient who is critically ill.

There are advantages in having the nurse who has been with the patient and the nurse who is new to the situation go through the initial interaction with the patient together. First, the patient is not only aware that an exchange of information has taken place but participates in the exchange. The patient can see that the new nurse is familiar with and understands the patient's problems and concerns, which in turn allays anxieties and helps develop trust in the new nurse. Second, the new nurse can validate initial observations with the nurse who is more familiar with the patient's condition. And finally, the nurse leaving the setting can orient the new nurse to procedures and equipment at the bedside that may be new or unfamiliar.

Several factors inherent in critical care situations may require altering the approach described. The nurse who has been caring for the patient may be unavailable; the patient may be intubated or have a tracheostomy, either of which would make communication more difficult; the patient may be disoriented or his or her level of consciousness may hamper or preclude effective interaction or there may be a change in the patient's condition requiring immediate action. Nevertheless, whenever possible the nurse entering the critical care setting considers an approach to the patient that will convey respect for the patient as a worthwhile human being, recognize the patient's need for input and some control over care, foster feelings of security and trust in the nurse, and give the nurse an opportunity to make meaningful observations about the patient.

Following the initial interaction the nurse continues to collect data for a baseline assessment of the patient's physical condition, psychologic status, and immediate environment and comparing these findings with those already reported. The nurse reviews medical and nursing orders and the most recent progress notes, observes the frequency of routines and treatments, and notes pertinent laboratory data and test results. From this assessment appropriate priorities for patient care are established. The frequency of routines, observations, and treatments as ordered by physicians and other nurses provides input but does not determine priorities. The critically ill patient's condition changes rapidly, and the therapeutic regimen must be altered to meet those changing needs. Taking vital signs every hour may not be sufficient if a patient has a labile blood pressure but may be too often if the patient's condition is stable and he or she needs rest. In many instances nursing judgment will determine the appropriate frequency of routines and treatments, such as the patient's readiness for ambulation, change in diet, or the need for tranquilizers, sedatives, or analgesics.

Problems that initially require the most attention are usually physiologic in nature. However, when a patient's survival is not in immediate jeopardy, that is, when the patient's condition is stable either from a return in function of the patient's own homeokinetic mechanisms or from support of medical and nursing therapies, problems of a psychosocial nature may assume equal if not primary emphasis.

With problems identified and priorities established, the nurse reviews the data pertinent to each problem and determines the desired outcomes of interventions. Despite varying pathologic conditions the commonalities among critically ill patients help to identify desired behaviors for patients and their significant others. These behaviors become the criteria by which the effectiveness of patient care is evaluated. In order to reach the desired outcomes, specific interventions are determined for each problem. The following outcome criteria and goals for intervention are relevant for all critically ill patients; however, the emphasis and priority each receives will be determined by the nature and number of physiologic, psychologic, and social stressors in each patient situation.

Alleviation and prevention of physiologic and physical stressors

Patient outcomes

The patient should:
1. Show improvement of signs and symptoms from the primary insult.
2. Show no signs or symptoms indicative of severe physiologic reaction to stress or to the therapeutic regimen such as hyperglycemia, stress ulcer, colitis, paralytic ileus, hypertension, myocardial infarction, cerebrovascular accident, infection, injuries, altered neurologic function, renal failure, extreme fatigue.
3. Be free of complications from prolonged immobility or restricted activity.
4. Experience maintenance and improvement in all vital functions such as respiratory, circulatory, neurologic, and renal.
5. Maintain an adequate nutritional status.
6. Be free of extreme physical discomfort.

Goals of intervention

Restore and support vital functions

Of primary concern is the patient's cardiovascular, respiratory, renal, and neurologic function. Among interventions receiving major emphasis are those directed toward preventing hypoxia by maintaining a patent airway and supporting respiratory function, preventing circulatory collapse and supporting cardiac output and peripheral perfusion, maintaining adequate glomerular filtration, and preventing renal failure.

One of the most important nursing responsibilities is monitoring of vital functions by means of direct observation and by direct and indirect measurement of physiologic parameters. Ongoing physical assessment, measurement of vital signs, determination of cardiac and respiratory function, precise recording of intake and output, and collection of specimens of urine, blood, secretions, and drainage for analysis are routine nursing functions in critical care areas. In most instances critical care is primarily preventive care accomplished through intensive physical and mechanical monitoring, astute observations, and early intervention by nurses.

Promote physical comfort and protect from personal injury

Critical illness leaves many patients dependent and unable to take care of their basic physical needs. They are also vulnerable to actual and potential dangers in the environment. The patient's comfort is primarily the responsibility of the nurse, and care will include attention to personal hygiene and grooming, frequent repositioning, maintaining proper body alignment, appropriate use of analgesics, sedatives, and tranquilizers, and emphasis on all measures to promote rest. Critically ill patients are bombarded with routine monitoring procedures, tests, treatments, and interactions with many different members of the health care team, all of which may be important to the patient's well-being but allow little time for rest. When setting priorities, the nurse plans direct care activities and coordinates activities and services of other health care workers to provide the patient with uninterrupted periods of rest. The nurse's attention to comfort measures not only adds to a patient's feelings of well-being but also conveys the nurse's concern and respect for the patient as a human being, thereby engendering a sense of trust.

Ensuring a patient's safety requires adequate numbers of personnel to meet a patient's needs for observation, monitoring, and prompt intervention. Safety measures also include ensuring that electrical equipment is safe and functioning properly. It is not unusual for critically ill patients to be disoriented or confused as a result of physiologic or psychologic disturbances or from effects of analgesics, sedatives, and tranquilizers. Side rails need to be in place when a patient is unattended, and measures need to be taken to ensure a patient's safety when out of bed.

Critically ill patients frequently receive vasopressor, cardiotonic, and antiarrhythmic medications to support their faltering homeokinetic mechanisms. The dosages of these medications have a small margin of safety and even when administered within that safety range can cause severe side effects. Accurate administration, validation of dosages with colleagues, and close observation for untoward effects of medications are necessary. The fluid balance of the patient whose conditions is critical is often tenuous and requires constant attention. The amount of fluid administered must be balanced with output in order to prevent fluid overload or dehydration.

Infection is a potential problem in the critically ill. In addition to being debilitated, many patients receive a variety of antibiotics that potentially may allow resistant organisms to multiply. In addition, some patients receive steroids that make them more vulnerable to infection and also mask signs and symptoms of infection, which then may go untreated. Invasive procedures and disruption of skin integrity as with the insertion of intravenous catheters increase the risk of infection. Because of the openness of many critical care units and the close proximity of patients, it is especially important that there be adequate air exchange in the unit. In order to prevent infection, stringent hand-washing policies and strict sterile technique in all procedures including suctioning of tubes and irrigation of catheters are required. Also, the patient is observed carefully for signs or symptoms of infection such as an elevated white blood cell count, elevated temperature, or change in amount, consistency, or odor of body secretions or drainage. (See Chapter 22 for information on infection control.)

Preserve and maintain musculoskeletal function

Most critically ill patients are confined to bed for varying lengths of time and are hampered further in movements by pain, presence of tubing, and connection to equipment such as a respirator. Preserving function of weight-bearing muscles, maintaining joint mobility, and preventing skin breakdown are real challenges to nurses caring for these patients. All of the preventive and supportive nursing care techniques used for any bedridden patient are appropriate in this situation (see Chapter 29). A primary nursing responsibility is to help determine a patient's readiness for increased activity. This decision is based on an assessment of the patient's ability to tolerate activity without undue stress on the cardiovascular and respiratory systems rather than being based on the nature or number of tubes and pieces of equipment surrounding the patient. If vital signs and blood pressure are stable, the patient is conscious, and if it is not contrary to medical therapy, the patient will benefit both physiologically and psychologically from being out of bed. Physical support from several staff members may be required at first, but every effort needs to be made to help the patient bear some, if not all, of his or her weight, since *lifting* the patient from a bed to a chair will *not* exercise weight-bearing muscles or prevent decalcification of bones.

Promote and maintain fluid and electrolyte balance

Critically ill patients are very vulnerable to fluid and electrolyte alterations. Pain and apprehension aggravate the body's physiologic response to stress, resulting in sodium and chloride retention, potassium excretion, and decreased urinary output. Many patients have temporary or permanent alterations in ingestion, elimination, and metabolism caused by renal failure or insufficiency, ostomies, injuries to the digestive tract, paralytic ileus, nausea, vomiting, diarrhea, or increased insensible water loss, all of which compound existing fluid and electrolyte disturbances. Disturbances in fluid and electrolyte balance secondary to medical and nursing interventions and therapies such as surgery, nasogastric suction, irrigations, and diuretics are also common occurrences.

To prevent potential disturbances and to promote fluid and electrolyte balance the nurse monitors several parameters. Meticulous intake and output records are kept, including fluids received by all routes (oral, intravenous, arterial line, irrigations, nasogastric) and drainage from all sources (bladder, bowel, ostomy, surgical drains) (see flow sheet, p. 1914). The patient is weighed daily, and the specific gravity of urine is measured at least every 4 hours. Vital signs and central venous pressure (CVP) are monitored, and the patient is observed for specific signs and symptoms of dehydration or fluid overload. All laboratory data reporting fluid and electrolyte status are reviewed as soon as they are available.

In addition to collecting these data, the nurse administers fluids and supplemental electrolytes as ordered. When the patient has several sources of intake, it is a nursing responsibility to maintain ordered fluid intake. Fluid orders are often written in relationship to output, and the nurse must adjust intravenous intake in accord with urinary output.

Maintain adequate nutritional status and normal bowel function

Critically ill patients are subject to nutritional deficits caused by alterations in amount and type of nutrients ingested; disturbances in ingestion, digestion, absorption, and elimination; and the increased demand for energy than many aspects of critical illness impose. Patients are often not allowed anything by mouth or are anorexic. Their caloric and nutritional requirements may be partially or totally supplied depending on the type of intravenous fluids prescribed. Concurrently, immobility-induced catabolism causes negative nitrogen balance at a time when many patients need extra protein to rebuild cells broken down by surgery, injuries, or disease. The energy required to cope physically with multisystem failure makes extraordinary demands on the body. Severely burned patients experience high energy demands with decreased mobility, enormous tissue damage and cellular breakdown, loss of protein, and alterations in ingestion imposed by the injury or by medical therapy. Critically ill patients with respiratory insufficiency and secondary respiratory infection who require frequent and vigorous pulmonary care to mobilize secretions also experience extreme weakness and fatigue and need high-protein, high-caloric nutrition.

To maintain positive nitrogen balance nursing interventions may include supplying patients who are able to eat with high-protein, high-calorie foods in frequent small amounts. In order to combat anorexia, these meals need to reflect the patient's food preferences. Vitamin supplements are ordered routinely in intravenous solutions. The nurse may be responsible for administering total parenteral nutrition (hyperalimentation) intravenously or prepared formulas given through nasogastric or gastrostomy tubes for patients unable to take food by mouth. Observing and monitoring for the side effects and complications of total parenteral nutrition become part of the nurse's routine patient assessment. (See Chapter 21 for more information on fluids and electrolytes.)

Bowel dysfunction may be caused by disruption in integrity of the gastrointestinal tract from disease, surgery, injury, immobility, altered dietary patterns, and lack of privacy or the opportunity to use regular bathroom facilities. Except for patients with loss of integrity in the gastrointestinal tract, normal bowel function can be promoted by ensuring adequate fluid intake and giving stool softeners or laxatives. These medications combat constipation and impaction resulting from loss of muscle tone and the defecation reflex. Providing as much privacy as possible and helping the patient to assume the most normal position for defecation are simple but important nursing actions. If the patient is able to be out of bed, the bedside commode can be used while the patient is up.

Alleviation and prevention of physiologic and environmental stressors by disease, trauma, and the therapeutic regimen initially may be the major although not exclusive emphasis in the care of the critically ill. When vital functions are stable, the outcome of a critical illness is determined largely by preventive and restorative nursing interventions that have as their goal the preservation and maintenance of optimal functional status. Since physiologic and psychosocial stressors conjointly influence the attainment of the optimal level of functioning by the critically ill patient and significant others, it is essential that nursing intervention be directed toward all these stressors concurrently.

Alleviation and prevention of psychologic stressors for the patient and significant others

Patient outcomes

The patient should:
1. Show no signs of symptoms indicative of severe psychologic reactions to stress (i.e., inappropriate affect, distortion of reality).
2. Experience no disturbances in sensation or perception related to the environment.
3. Be able to state plans for medical and nursing care.

4. Be able to state plans for transfer from the critical care unit.

Goals of intervention

Determine patient's or significant other's perceptions of the illness and therapeutic regimen

Psychologic response to illness or injury experienced by a patient and significant others will be determined by their perception of the situation and its meaning to them. Their perception depends on their premorbid personalities, current psychologic status, and adequacy of coping mechanisms.

Misperception or misinterpretation of elements in the environment such as the presence of a cardiac monitor often results in adding unnecessary stressors. Because it is the *perception* of the event or element that in part determines the degree of stress caused, not merely the event or element itself, nurses need to frequently determine the perceptions of the patient and significant others about what is happening.

Another major determinant of when and if a crisis will ensue is the ability of the patient and significant others to cope with the perceived stressor. The patient's perceptions and ability to cope with stressors are assessed with psychologic and physiologic monitoring.

Psychologic monitoring entails eliciting information from the patient and significant others about how the patient is perceiving the environment, his or her physical condition, and the procedures and routines being performed. Techniques used to elicit this information might include asking open-ended questions such as, "How are things going for you today?" or, to the significant others, "How does he (she) seem to you today?"; recognizing and following up on nonverbal cues: "You look worried (uncomfortable, nervous)"; and interpreting the patient's or significant others' behavior such as anger, withdrawal, uncooperativeness, or passiveness as clues to their psychologic states. Awareness of popular public and cultural misconceptions about hospitals, specific diseases, and treatments aids in understanding the patient's misperceptions and misconceptions.

Acknowledge, accept, and encourage patient and significant others to air their feelings

The psychologic impact of critical illness is a major influence on a patient's immediate and eventual survival and a crucial factor in defining his or her optimal level of wellness. The critically ill person is partially or totally isolated from the usual support system, is alienated from familiar surroundings and daily living patterns, and is dependent on others to meet basic needs, not the least of which is survival itself. A critically ill person has limited alternatives with which to cope with these stressors, and depending on past experiences may have few appropriate coping behaviors in his or her repertoire. Feelings of helplessness, powerlessness, loneliness, and depersonalization and disturbances in body image are common. Modes of dissipating the frustration, anger, hostility, depression, and anxiety generated by these feelings are circumscribed by physical limitations and the therapeutic regimen.

Health care providers can provide many of these patients with means of coping with multiple stressors by maintaining an atmosphere of openness and acceptance that encourages them to talk about their feelings. A basic need of these patients is to share difficult experiences with others and to identify problems.[28] Talking with patients openly and honestly decreases feelings of depersonalization and anxiety and prevents isolation and alienation. Expressing emotionally laden materal in an atmosphere of acceptance discharges stress while maintaining the patient's self-esteem. Recognizing that anger and hostility are often indicative of fear and anxiety and that depression and withdrawal may be signs of hopelessness, loneliness, powerlessness, or loss assist the nurse in accepting these feelings as normal and expected in this situation. The nurse who encourages the patient to talk about feelings provides an avenue for relieving tension and promotes psychologic well-being. Encouraging the patient to express feelings helps him or her to identify the reasons behind feeling and behaving in a manner that may be unusual and anxiety provoking; at the same time it gives the person permission to feel and act that way. Using cognitive feedback such as, "It's normal in this situation for you to be angry," invites an expression of feelings. Health team members who are helping a patient to talk about feelings need to be ready to accept whatever emotionally laden material may be expressed.[22] Often a hospital chaplain or member of the clergy from the community can help health care providers develop the ability to handle this aspect of patient care comfortably.

Patients who are intubated are unable to express their feelings even though they are alert and oriented, and therefore they are particularly vulnerable to psychologic stressors. To help prevent feelings of isolation and alienation in the person who is unable to communicate verbally, paper and pencil or a magic slate are placed within easy reach. However, writing about concerns, anxieties, and feelings is time consuming and cumbersome. Not all patients are willing to write out their feelings, either because it requires more energy than they have or they are unsure about how to express their feelings in writing. Nurses need to be particularly sensitive to stressors in the environment, to recognize behavior as clues to a patient's psychologic state, and to verbalize feelings for the patient that are common to most patients in similar situations and thus validate with the patient that he or she too is experiencing some of these feelings. Being empathetic with the patient conveys acceptance and understanding and counteracts feelings of depersonalization, isolation, loneliness, and powerlessness.

Provide information and clarify misconceptions about physical status and plans and goals of treatment

As already mentioned, the patient's *perception* of stress and not the stress itself determines his or her reaction to illness and the intensive care environment. Failure to give simple explanations and adequate information results in the patient's perceiving the condition and the rationale for procedures and treatments as far more threatening than actually may be the case. Care given without explanations and communication may falsely impress the patient and significant others with the severity of illness and the patient's total dependence on lifesaving equipment. The cardiac monitor may be believed to keep the heart beating rather than monitoring the heartbeat. Administering blood as a precautionary measure may be perceived as a lifesaving intervention for what is thought to be a deteriorating condition.

Much of what a patient learns about his or her health problems and their relation to self-image depends on what is taught directly and indirectly by the health care team.[28] Patient teaching in critical care requires short-term goals. Pain, discomfort, weakness, anxiety, noise, and confusion are some of the obstacles to learning experienced by these patients. Despite such obstacles, patients and significant others need explanations of procedures and purposes of treatments. A patient may not believe what he or she is told the first time or may be coping with the situation by denying the problems. In either case there needs to be reinterpretation and reiteration of previous explanations regarding diagnosis, prognosis, and current physical status. Keeping the patient and significant others apprised of the condition and treatment plans helps them perceive the situation accurately, enhances their ability to cope realistically and effectively, and promotes their cooperation by making them members of the health care team.

Encourage and support involvement of patient and significant others in decision making and care

The essence of crisis intervention is to help people cope with a major life crisis such as a critical illness. The patient is assisted to formulate individual goals and is helped to reach them. When the patient and significant others are knowledgeable about goals and the rationale for treatments and understand the patient's current physical status and prognosis, they can be involved in many aspects of care and can make decisions and set goals consistent with the treatment regimen. Involving the significant others in care and decision making serves at least two purposes. First, involvement decreases feelings of helplessness, powerlessness, and anxiety. Second, when significant others understand treatment goals and support them and are involved in the patient's care, they are able to continue this behavior after the patient is transfered from the intensive care unit. Significant others can make valuable contributions in the care of the patient in a variety of ways. Even when a patient is unconscious, visits by significant others who talk to and touch the patient may be supportive to the patient and help decrease the helpless feelings of the significant others.

An alert patient can be involved in making a schedule for activities and treatments throughout the day. If the patient is taking food by mouth, he or she and significant others can help make choices in planning the menu. Significant others can assist a patient at mealtime if help is needed. They can encourage a postoperative patient to deep breathe and help support the incision during coughing, and they can remind the patient of fluid limits or offer fluids frequently depending on the goals of therapy. Significant others can be very helpful as they reiterate and reinforce explanations about physical status, prognosis, and treatments.

Promote and maintain a sensory-regulated environment

The environment of critical care units is a major stressor with which the patient must cope. The many sources of external stress and the methods to assess such stressors have been reviewed in Chapter 74. Although some environmental factors cannot be altered, there are some measures the nurse can implement to address this problem.

Providing a sensory-regulated environment requires attention to the lack of meaningful stimulation to the patient as well as to overstimulation by disruptive activities and noise. Environmental stressors contribute to a patient's experiencing sensory deprivation or emotional touch deprivation. The spatially confined environment and limited mobility of the patient are among factors common to all critically ill patients. Limited mobility reduces the quantity and quality of sensory input. The alert patient has decreased interactions with the environment, and this causes disturbances in time, pattern, form, and temperature perception and discrimination. The technical environment and language further reduce the meaningfulness of stimulation. In some instances there is reduction in the intensity of stimulation, as with patients with hearing loss, patients without glasses who have poor sight, patients who cannot eat or who are on bland, monotonous diets that do not stimulate the sense of taste, or patients who are not stimulated by their own voices because they are intubated and cannot speak.

Reducing the amount of disturbing sensory bombardment and providing meaningful sensory input for patients are crucial to promoting rest and preventing disturbances in patients' reality orientations. Not all disruptive input can be eliminated, but actions can be taken to limit the amount of input, thus reducing the intensity of environmental stressors. Bedside conversations that exclude patient participation should be limited to essential interactions. Spacing patients as far apart as possible and placing alert, stable patients in the most quiet area of an open unit helps reduce noise generated by the care of other patients. Limiting the frequency of taking vital signs and disruptive observations, particularly at night, and planning care to provide for the least disturbance of the patient encourage rest. One study suggests (1) reducing the noise level by using tactile stimuli in arousing patients rather than calling their names; (2) turning the surface of a bedside monitor with the amplifier away from the patient and turning the sound off if the oscilloscope is easily visible to staff; (3) positioning an MA-1 respirator with bellows away from the patient's ear; (4) refraining from using bedpan washers and hoppers at night; (5) using carpet and draperies to absorb sound in utility areas and nursing stations; and (6) placing staff lounges away from patient care areas.[43] If someone is always present in the nursing station, a telephone with a flashing light instead of a bell can be used to limit noise.

To provide meaningful sensory input that will help maintain orientation, wall clocks and calendars that are large enough to be seen easily by patients are essential. If surroundings permit, keeping familiar objects at the bedside, listening to a radio over earphones, displaying cards from friends, or being in a bed near a window also help to maintain a patient's reality orientation.

Frequent orientation of a patient to person, place, time, and physical status has been shown to diminish the sensory distortion that leads to delirium in postoperative cardiac patients.[9] Patients with tracheostomies need to be encouraged to talk whenever the cuff of the tracheostomy tube is deflated so they can hear their own voices. Patients need to be engaged in self-care when possible in order to keep them involved purposefully with themselves and their environment. Visits from significant others who bring news about family, friends, and current events keep the patient in touch with social realities and need to be emphasized as important contributions to the patient's total care.

Promote and maintain the patient's reality orientation

Despite attempts to control stress-producing environmental factors and to provide a sensory-regulated environment, some patients will exhibit disturbed thought processes, indicated by confusion, impaired judgment, delusions and phobias, and perceptual disturbances such as illusions, hallucinations, and pares-

thesia. Factors other than environmental that contribute to these problems are certain medications, premorbid psychologic status and physical condition, metabolic state as indicated by blood chemistry and blood gas levels, and age. Patients receiving narcotics and barbiturates, highly anxious patients, patients with multiple, interrelated, debilitating physical problems, patients with disturbed metabolic and respiratory function, patients deprived of sleep, and older patients are most prone to disturbed thought processes and perceptual distortions.

Some patients are aware of intermittent breaks from reality and disturbances in thought processes but are reluctant to share these with the health care team. Being aware of possible attempts by patients to conceal thought and perceptual distortions, nurses need to assess patients' behavior for clues that these are occurring. Patients who seem indifferent to people and events, who are unusually preoccupied, who sleep poorly, whose conversation is disjointed, whose attention span is brief, and whose affect seems inappropriate may be experiencing reality disturbances.

Patients affected by reality disturbances and their significant others need to be reassured that these disturbances are transient and are not unusual in such circumstances. Significant others can be involved in providing meaningful sensory input by orienting and reorienting the patient to person, time, place, physical status, events occurring in the vicinity, and physical characteristics of the environment. Changing medications, correcting disturbed metabolic phenomena, and permitting uninterrupted sleep when possible are other actions to be taken to help resolve the problem and minimize deleterious effects.

Prepare patient or significant others for transfer from critical care unit

For many patients and their significant others transfer from the critical care area is a time of considerable psychologic stress. The critical care area with its sophisticated electronic equipment and attentive, knowledgeable, and highly skilled personnel connotes security and protection. Discharge from this area to an area with less nursing personnel per patient, with less frequent interaction with staff, and where the patient is expected to be more independent often seems premature to the patient and significant others, particularly if they have misconceptions regarding the patient's physical status and care requirements. The anxiety precipitated by the transfer can be prevented or reduced if the patient or significant others are taught to interpret the meaning of particular signs and symptoms and helped to understand the purpose of equipment and routines. Signs that indicate progress need to be pointed out continuously. Informing the patient and significant others of plans for transfer as soon as such plans begin to be discussed (not waiting until the day of transfer) helps them adjust to the idea gradually and gives them time to plan for it. They need to know the projected date of transfer, what to expect on the new unit, and what will be expected of them. Ideally, a nurse from the receiving unit is introduced to the patient and significant others before transfer. After transfer, visits from members of the critical care unit staff are helpful in conveying continued concern for the patient's welfare and in promoting trust in the nursing staff in the new setting. This is accomplished by validating with the patient that attention and care are appropriate to his or her improved status.

Alleviation and prevention of social stressors for the patient and significant others

Patient outcomes

The patient and significant others should:
1. Maintain continuity in their relationship.
2. Make knowledgeable decisions for instituting changes in therapy, life-style established family roles, and relationships.

Goals of intervention

Promote continuity in relationship between the patient and significant others

As mentioned previously, in the critical care setting a patient's physiologic needs often assume priority over psychologic needs, and the patient's social being is marginally recognized and less seldom addressed. Limited visiting hours and the strange technical environment and language of the critical care unit isolate patients from their significant others and prevent them from assuming their usual social roles. For the most part, a person who is critically ill is approached exclusively in the context of his or her role as patient. Efforts need to be made to retain a link between the patient and significant others while the patient is physically removed from them.

Some of the same techniques described above that involve significant others with the patient's care serve to promote continuity in their relationship. The patient is able to maintain identity with roles other than that of patient when significant others are involved in supporting the therapeutic regimen, explaining and reinterpreting information about the patient's physical status and progress, and keeping the patient informed about people and events in the premorbid social environment. Including significant others when teaching the patient promotes consistency of the information given and prevents misunderstandings and misinterpretations between the patient, significant others, and staff. Relaying messages between patients and significant others by telephone helps maintain contact.

One of the most effective and important ways to prevent disruption in relationships is to prepare significant others for their first visit with the patient in the critical care unit. Before the significant others enter the area, the patient's physical appearance and the environment should be described to them. They need to know the patient's level of consciousness, ability to communicate, and ability to understand their communication. They need to realize the importance of their presence to the patient and the patient's need for their support. When the significant others approach the bedside, a staff member should stay with them and facilitate the initial interaction between them and the patient. At each subsequent visit the nurse responsible for the patient's care should meet with the significant others to answer questions and apprise them of the patient's status and progress.

Support changes in roles and relationships between the patient and significant others

While efforts need to be made to help a patient maintain identity with his or her premorbid social roles, the patient cannot fulfill the obligations and responsibilities of those roles during illness. Roles of parent, spouse, breadwinner, sexual partner, decision maker, employer or employee, and leader may be altered, reversed, or eliminated. The responsibilities of the patient need to be assumed by family and friends. Depending on the length of the illness and period of recovery, it may be some time, if ever, before a patient can function fully in those roles. Dwindling or absent financial resources may result in changes in social status, social mobility, and life-style.

During the critical phase of illness the significant others will be attempting to cope with precipitous role changes and may need help working through problems that arise as family members and friends assume or fail to assume additional responsibilities. When disintegration among significant others occurs and no one assumes the role formerly held by the patient, members of the health care team may need to be directive in helping the family to reorganize themselves and their resources. The most stable family member may be designated as the decision maker or the one to be called first in case of emergency. The family may need help in planning visiting schedules that will be least disruptive to their daily lives and still meet their needs and those of the patient. They may also need assistance in identifying supportive figures within and without the immediate family who can be called on for assistance.

Documentation of patient care

An integral part of all nursing intervention is reporting and recording of pertinent data about the patient's physical, physiologic, and emotional status, response to medical and nursing therapies, and plans for changing or continuing with nursing interventions. Written and verbal communication promotes continuity and consistency in patient care in any setting; however, in critical care settings where the variety and intensity of physiologic and psychosocial stressors interact to produce multiple problems and frequently changing priorities, reporting of new data and documentation of the effect of interventions on a patient's condition are crucial. Because of the large amount of data collected and the time available for recording, most critical care areas use a flow sheet as an efficient and organized means of reporting information (p. 1914).

At the conclusion of each shift a summary is written that highlights the patient's primary problems as reflected by the pattern of data collected throughout the shift. Included in the summary are a range of the patient's vital signs and other physiologic measurements, intake and output totals, the patient's response to treatments and procedures, plans for further observations and interventions, and comments about the patient's reaction to and interactions during visits from significant others.

Although the evaluation *process* is the same in the critical care unit as it is in other patient care areas, multisystem embarrassment, constant fluctuation in the data base, rapidly changing priorities, and shorter periods between interventions impose constraints that influence the nature of evaluation.

A general systems perspective negates a cause-effect relationship because of the number of intervening variables introduced by suprasystems and subsystems. When a patient suffers multisystem failure, interventions directed at one system have direct as well as indirect effects on other systems. As a result an outcome is obtained that may be different from one that the same interventions might have produced in isolation. Decisions about modifying a plan of action based on generalizations about the impact of a single intervention are usually inappropriate and unwise.

Goals for intervention in critical care areas are short term and fluctuate according to the patient's changing condition. Evaluation of those goals likewise is short term and often narrowed to specific interventions. For example, the outcome of an intermittent positive pressure breathing (IPPB) treatment is evaluated in terms of its immediate effect on breath sounds, ability to mobilize secretions, and general ventilatory status. Because of the instability of a patient's condition, an intervention that is effective at one time may not bring about the desired outcome at another time. For example, if a patient's ventilatory status deteriorates, an IPPB treatment may not be effective, and more aggressive therapy may be needed to maintain ventilatory function. In order to keep pace with the continuous reassessment and reordering of priorities, the frequency of evaluation in critical care areas is increased, resulting in less time between evaluation and modification of interventions. Many times the opportunity to repeat the intervention and to observe for the same or different outcomes is limited. Because of sophisticated monitoring devices, decisions can be based on a data base that is larger and collected in a shorter time.

In most critical care areas nurses have more flexibility and autonomy in decision making and intervention than do nurses on general care divisions. This increased latitude in role functions coexists with the responsibility and accountability for making sound decisions based on accurate interpretation of the data base and the changes in a patient's physiologic and emotional behavior.

REFERENCES AND SELECTED READINGS

1. *Adams, M., et al.: Psychological response in critical care units, Am. J. Nurs. **78:**1504-1512, 1978.
2. Adams, N.R., editor: Hemodynamic monitoring, Crit. Care Q. **2:**1-55, 1979.
3. Aguilera, D.C., and Messick, J.M.: Crisis intervention: theory and methodology, ed. 4, St. Louis, 1982, The C.V. Mosby Co.
4. Black, S.K.: Social isolation and the nursing process, Nurs. Clin. North Am. **8:**575-586, 1973.
5. *Bolin, R.H.: Sensory deprivation: an overview, Nurs. Forum **13:**240-258, 1974.
6. Borg, N., et al.: Care curriculum for critical care nursing, Philadelphia, 1981, W.B. Saunders Co.
7. *Brantigan, C.O.: Hemodynamic monitoring: interpreting values, Am. J. Nurs. **82:**86-89, 1982.
8. *Breu, C., and Dracup, K.: Helping the spouses of critically ill patients, Am. J. Nurs. **78:**50-53, 1978.
9. *Budd, S., and Brown, W.: Effect of reorientation technique on postcardiotomy delirium, Nurs. Res. **23:**341-348, 1974.
10. *Codd, J., and Grohar, M.E.: Postoperative pulmonary complications, Nurs. Clin. North Am. **10:**5-15, 1975.
11. *Daly, B.J., editor: Intensive care nursing, Garden City, N.Y., 1980, Medical Examination Publishing Co., Inc.
12. *Davis, M.Z.: Socioemotional components of coronary care, Am. J. Nurs. **72:**705-709, 1972.
13. *Ellis, R.: Unusual sensory and thought disturbances after cardiac surgery, Am. J. Nurs. **72:**2021-2025, 1972.
14. Gentry, W.D., Musante, G., and Haney, T.: Anxiety and urinary sodium/potassium as stress indicators on admission to coronary-care unit, Heart Lung **2:**875-877, 1973.
15. *Hamilton, W.P.: Common cardiovascular problems in the postoperative period, Nurs. Clin. North Am. **10:**27-41, 1975.
16. *Haughey, B.: CVP lines: monitoring and maintaining, Am. J. Nurs. **78:**635-638, 1978.

*References preceded by an asterisk are particularly well suited for student reading.

17. Holloway, N.M.: Nursing the critically ill adult, Menlo Park, Calif., 1979, Addison-Wesley Publishing Co., Inc.

18. Hudak, C.M., Gallo, B.M., and Lohr, T.: Critical care nursing, ed. 2, Philadelphia, 1977, J.B. Lippincott Co.

19. *Humbrecht, B., and Van Parys, E.: From assessment to intervention: how to use heart and breath sounds as part of your nursing care plan, Nurs. '82 **12**(4):34-42, 1982.

20. *ICU psychosis (nursing grand rounds), Nurs. '82 **12**(1):58-63, 1982.

21. Kiely, W.F., and Procci, W.R.: Psychiatric aspects of critical care. In Zschoche, D.A., editor: Mosby's comprehensive review of critical care, ed. 2, St. Louis, 1980, The C.V. Mosby Co.

22. *Kuenzi, S.H., and Fenton, M.V.: Crisis intervention in acute care areas, Am. J. Nurs. **75**:830-834, 1975.

23. Meltzer, L.E., Abdellah, F.G., and Kitchen, J.R.: Concepts and practices of intensive care for nurse specialists, ed. 2, Bowie, Md., 1976, The Charles Press.

24. *Metheny, N.A.: Water and electrolyte balance in the postoperative patient, Nurse. Clin. North Am. **10**:49-75, 1975.

25. *Murray, R.: Assessment of psychological status in the surgical ICU patient, Nurs. Clin. North Am. **10**:69-81, 1975.

26. *Nielsen, L.: Mechanical ventilation: patient assessment and nursing care, Am. J. Nurs. **80**:2191-2196, 1980.

27. Nursing critically ill patients confidently, Horsham, Pa., 1979, InterMed Communications, Inc.

28. *Obier, K., and Haywood, L.J.: Enhancing therapeutic communication with acutely ill patients, Heart Lung **2**:49-53, 1973.

29. Olson, E.V.: The impact of serious illness on the family system, Postgrad. Med. **47**:169-174, 1970.

30. *Pulmonary function tests in patient care, programmed instruction, Am. J. Nurs. **80**:1135-1161, 1980.

31. Rau, J.L.: Continuous mechanical ventilation. I, Crit. Care Update 8(1):10-29, 1981.

32. Rau, J.L.: Continuous mechanical ventilation. II, Crit. Care Update 8(2):5-20, 1981.

33. *Risser, N.L.: Preoperative and postoperative care to prevent pulmonary complications, Heart Lung **9**:57-67, 1980.

34. Roberts, S.L.: Behavioral concepts and the critically ill patient, Englewood Cliffs, N.J., 1976, Prentice-Hall, Inc.

35. Shoemaker, W.C., and Thompson, W.L.: Critical care: state of the art, vol 1, Fullerton, Calif., 1980, Society of Critical Care Medicine.

36. *Spicer, M.R.: What about the patient? Patient-centered management in an intensive care area, Nurs. Clin. North Am. **7**:313-322, 1972.

37. *Stanford, J.L., Flener, J.M., and Arensberg, D.: Antiarrhythmic drug therapy, Am. J. Nurs. **80**:1288-1295, 1980.

38. *Stephenson, C.A.: Stress in the critically ill patient, Am. J. Nurs. **77**:1806-1809, 1977.

39. Storlie, F.: Patient teaching in critical care, New York, 1975, Appleton-Century-Crofts.

40. *Visalli, F., and Evans, P.: The Swan-Ganz catheter, Nurs. '81 **11**(1):42-47, 1981.

41. *Visich, M.A.: Knowing what you hear: a guide to assessing heart and breath sounds, Nurs. '81 **11**(11):64-79, 1981.

42. Waisbren, B.A.: Critical care manual: a systems approach method, Garden City, N.Y., 1972, Medical Examination Publishing Co., Inc.

43. Walker, B.J.: Nursing care to assess and prevent common cardiovascular problems, Nurs. Clin. North Am. **10**:43-48, 1975.

44. Woods, N.F., and Falk, S.A.: Noise stimuli in the acute care area, Nurs. Res. **23**:144-150, 1974.

CHAPTER 76

CASE STUDY OF A CRITICALLY ILL PATIENT

SALLY SCHAFER TODD
MARY K. KIRKPATRICK

This chapter presents a case study of a young girl with multisystem trauma after an automobile accident. The format follows the systems approach. Changing priorities and emphases in care as the patient progresses along the recovery continuum are presented. Nursing diagnosis of patient stressors is identified at two phases: on admission and before transfer from the critical care unit. Appropriate patient outcomes and nursing orders are given for each nursing diagnosis.

Admission note

Sandy J. is an 18-year-old, single student who was admitted after an automobile accident. She was transferred from a rural hospital to a medical center about 100 miles away after she developed respiratory insufficiency. This is her first hospitalization. Her father and older brother accompanied her to the medical center.

Sandy sustained multisystem trauma including circulatory instability with possible ruptured spleen, pulmonary contusions with bilateral and partial pneumothorax, head trauma with facial lacerations and contusions, and fractures of the right ilium and left femur, tibia, and fibula. Immediate medical intervention included a tracheostomy, closed reduction of all fractures with application of a left long leg cast and traction, and suturing of facial lacerations.

On admission to the critical care unit, Sandy is in respiratory distress (rate 32, Po_2 43, Pco_2 46, HCO_3 30, pH 7.32). She is hypotensive (BP 80-90/50) and has tachycardia (pulse 120, regular). She also is oliguric (10 ml of urine last hour), febrile (38.2° C), and alternately agitated and somnolent. She has a cuffed tracheostomy tube, a urinary retention catheter, nasogastric tube, central venous pressure (CVP) catheter, intravenous infusions including a dopamine drip, and a long leg cast with balanced traction on her left leg.

Assessment data

Physiologic data

Further nursing assessment reveals that Sandy's pupils are equal and reactive to light. She moves all extremities spontaneously, follows simple commands and responds appropriately to verbal and painful stimuli when fully aroused, and becomes less agitated when verbal reassurance is offered and contact is maintained through touching her, as when holding her hand. Her general color is pale including her lips and nail beds. Her facial lacerations are dry and well approximated. Without ventilatory assistance her respirations are slightly labored at rest with the head of the bed elevated 30 degrees. Her respiratory rate increases and substernal and intercostal retractions are apparent when she is agitated. Her chest movement is symmetric, and breath sounds are equal but diminished in the lower lobes with diffuse rales throughout all lobes. A moderate amount of thick white secretions is suctioned through the tracheostomy. Sandy tolerates suctioning without arrhythmias or significant change in color. She is receiving ventilatory assistance from a volume ventilator (patient triggered, 50% oxygen with 12-cm positive end-expiratory pressure [PEEP], 20 cm of water pressure, 800 ml volume). Her apical pulse is regular without extra heart sounds, and the cardiac monitor shows a sinus tachycardia. Occasionally, bowel sounds are auscultated, and her abdomen is firm and moderately distended with diffuse tenderness on palpation. Her abdominal girth is 81.2 cm. Her peripheral pulses are equally palpable bilaterally but weak, and her extremities are cool to touch, pale in color, with good movement and sensation. Skin surrounding the cast and intravenous infusion sites is dry without evidence of inflammation. The nasogastric tube is draining a moderate amount of green-brown fluid (200 ml since leaving the previous hospital) and irrigates freely. Urinary drainage is clear yellow with a specific gravity of 1.022; the catheter irrigates freely. CVP reads 5 cm of water. A solution of 5% dextrose in water is infusing through the CVP line at 60 drops/min. An IV solution of 500 D5W with 400 mg dopamine at 23 ml/hr is currently maintaining a systolic pressure of greater than 100 mm Hg (5 µg/kg/min for 60-kg weight).

Laboratory values on admission were K^+ 3.7, Na^+ 142, Cl^- 99, BUN 24, hemoglobin 10.1, Hct 34, CO_2 33 mEq/liter, and glucose 150.

Behavioral data

Sandy makes no attempt to communicate verbally. Her facial expression is strained and sad, and her wide eyes stare at each movement of the health team members. She is confused regarding the date and time but nonverbally confirms the admission to the medical center by nodding her head when explanations are given. She is restless and agitated when aroused, but this subsides with explanations and reassurance. Family interaction appears warm and reassuring and elicits her increased cooperation.

Sociocultural background

Sandy is 18 years old. Her mother died in childbirth, and she has been reared primarily by her father with assistance from an aunt. She lives with her father and brother on a farm in a small rural town in the South. She has been reared in the Protestant faith. Her father has adequate insurance coverage.

On Sandy's admission her father and brother stood in the doorway of the waiting room adjacent to the critical care unit quietly watching the activities of the health care team members who were caring for Sandy.

The immediate admitting patient care orders are shown in the box at right.

The nursing diagnoses, patient outcomes, nursing goals, and orders shown in Table 76-1 were developed from the admission nursing assessment.

Text continued on p. 1941.

ADMITTING ORDERS

NPO
NG to intermittent low Gomco suction
Measure abdominal girth q 1 hr
Vital signs q 15 min, temperature q 4 hr
CVP q 30 min
Hourly I & O with specific gravity (24-hr totals)
Foley catheter to straight drainage
Circulation checks q 15 min until stable, then q ½ hr
Neurologic checks q 15 min
Volume ventilator with 50% O_2 with 12-cm PEEP
Suction q 1 hr prn with tracheostomy care
Passive range of motion (ROM) q 4 hr
Cardiac monitor: mount ECG strip
Bed rails up at all times
Left leg to balanced suspension traction with Thomas splint

Laboratory

Arterial blood gases q 1 hr
Hct q 2 hr, monitor WBC, creatinine clearance
Coagulation studies (PTT, APTT) stat, then every morning
Electrolytes stat, chem. 6 q 4 hr × 2, then every morning
Type and cross-match two units of blood
CBC
X-ray (portable) of chest, skull, KUB stat
ECG stat

Intravenous fluids

D5W, 500 ml with 400 mg dopamine to keep systolic BP above 100 mm Hg and free of signs and symptoms of extreme peripheral vasoconstriction
Replace NG drainage ml/ml with D5 ½ NS (each bottle with 20 mEq KCL)
CVP line with 1000 D5W to keep open (TKO)
5% Dextrose in Ringer's lactate, 1000 ml q 8 hr alternating with 1000 ml D5 ½ NS (each bottle with 20 mEq KCL)
Dextran 70, 500 ml/day

Medications

Lasix, 40 mg IV stat and q 6 hr unless K^+ falls below 3.5 mEq/L
Ancef, 1 g q 8 hr
Tylenol, 650 mg per rectum now and q 4 hr for temp of 38.5° C
Solu-Medrol, 80 mg IV q 6 hr
Valium, 5 mg IM q 2-3 hr prn for agitation
Riopan, 60 ml q 2 hr via NG tube and clamp for 15 min
Morphine sulfate, 1-3 mg IV push q 2-3 hr prn
Garamycin, 60 mg IV tid

TABLE 76-1. Nursing plan on admission

Input	Throughput	
Nursing diagnosis of stressors	**Predicted patient outcomes**	**Nursing orders**

1. Effects of primary insult

a. Altered level of consciousness and agitation related to head trauma, ventilatory insufficiency, or anxiety

1. Improvement in signs and symptoms of the primary insult (head trauma)
   a. Alert and oriented
      Moves all uninjured extremities
      Quiet when undisturbed; easily aroused

Goal: *Restore and support vital functions*

a. Neurologic checks q 15 min, arouse to highest level of consciousness
   Orient to surroundings and events
   Monitor pulse pressure
   Monitor vital signs
   Maintain unobstructed airway
   Provide reassurance; explain procedures; use touch to enhance verbal communication

b. Shock related to possible internal hemorrhage

b. Vital signs stable: pulse, 80/120; BP, 100 systolic; RR, 12-20
   CVP > 5 cm H_2O pressure
   Hct and hemoglobin within normal limits
   Color pink
   Skin warm, dry
   Peripheral pulses present
   Urinary output, 30 ml/hr
   No increase in abdominal girth

b. Monitor vital signs q 15 min
   Monitor CVP q 1 hr
   Measure and monitor abdominal girth q 30 min
   Measure urinary output with specific gravity q 1 hr
   Titrate dopamine infusion to keep systolic BP 100 mm Hg
   Monitor Hct and hemoglobin

c. Ventilatory insufficiency related to lung contusions, pneumothorax, and head trauma

c. Maintains open airway
   Maintains arterial blood gases within normal range
   Maintains pulmonary function parameters within normal range (shunt, dead space, inspiratory force, tidal and minute volumes)

c. Suction tracheostomy q 1 hr and prn
   Auscultate breath sounds before and after suctioning and cuff deflation
   Monitor central and peripheral color continuously
   Note characteristics and changes in respiratory pattern, increases in tracheal secretions
   Monitor ABG
   Measure pulmonary function q shift: tidal volume (TV) and minute volume (MV)

d. Oliguria related to trauma or decreased circulatory volume

d. Maintains urinary output > 30 ml/hr

d. Measure urinary output q 1 hr, note color and characteristics
   Test specific gravity q 1 hr
   Maintain IV infusion rates as ordered
   Titrate dopamine infusion to keep systolic BP > 100 mm Hg

2. Effects of critical illness

Potential physiologic reactions (hyperglycemia, gastrointestinal ulcer) related to stress secondary to multisystem failure

2. No signs or symptoms of severe physiologic reactions to stress
   Free of signs and symptoms of diabetes mellitus
   Free of signs and symptoms of gastrointestinal ulcer

Goal: *Restore and support vital functions*

Monitor urine for sugar and acetone
Monitor amount of urinary output (O > I may indicate hyperglycemic osmotic diuresis)
Monitor NG drainage and stools for frank and occult blood
Monitor Hct
Check for abdominal distention
Administer antacid (Riopan) as ordered

Goal: *Protect from injury*

3. Untoward effects of treatment

a. Potential untoward effects related to medications

3. No signs or symptoms of toxic or untoward physiologic reactions to therapy
   a. Tolerates medications and is free of signs and symptoms of side effects from:
      Dextran 70
      Morphine sulfate
      Solu-Medrol
      Garamycin

a. Maintain dextran infusion at consistent rate to prevent interstitial-to-plasma fluid shift
   Morphine sulfate: monitor respirations
   Solu-Medrol: give Riopan as ordered; continue psychologic assessment
   Garamycin: monitor BUN, creatinine clearance; note and record allergic response

Continued.

TABLE 76-1. Nursing plan on admission—cont'd

Input	Throughput	
Nursing diagnosis of stressors	**Predicted patient outcomes**	**Nursing orders**
b. Potential circulatory impairment and skin irritation related to long leg cast	b. Maintains adequate circulation to immobilized extremity Free of skin excoriation, disruption, and inflammation surrounding cast	b. Circulation checks q 2 hr Adhesive tape to rough cast edges Protection of cast and surrounding skin from moisture and drainage
c. Potential infection related to invasive procedures	c. Maintains normal body temperature Maintains WBC within normal range Free of purulent drainage	c. Check temperature q 4 hr; if 38.5° C (R) check q 2 hr; if 39° C (R), check q 1 hr Check WBC daily Note consistency, color, odor, and amounts of all drainage Anchor catheter securely to prevent movement Change IV tubing q 24 hr Change IV dressing q 24 hr
d. Potential stress ulcer related to ventilatory assistance	d. See Outcome 2	d. See Order 2
e. Potential tracheal erosion related to cuff pressure of tracheostomy tube	e. Maintains closed airway system with consistent cuff volume	e. Use minimal inflating volume necessary to maintain seal Check cuff volume and pressure every shift Record cuff volume and pressure every shift Use swivel adapter on endotracheal tube to prevent traction or pull on tubes
4. Problems related to fractures	4. Free of complications of immobility-restricted activity	**Goal:** *Preserve and maintain musculoskel-*
a. Potential emboli related to thrombus formation or fracture	a. Free of sudden, sharp chest pain Maintains adequate ventilation Free of signs and symptoms of local inflammation of extremities Absence of pink frothy secretions	a. Check for signs and symptoms of phlebitis Check for pink frothy secretions Assess ventilatory status including signs and symptoms of hypoxia Do passive range of motion q 4 hr Give dextran as ordered
b. Potential skin breakdown related to immobility	b. Skin integrity maintained without signs of circulatory impairment (redness, tenderness) over bony prominences	b. Keep skin dry Use alternating-air-pressure mattress Tilt, prop with pillows q 2 hr Massage bony prominences and apply lubricating lotions liberally each shift
5. Nutritional deficits Catabolism and negative nitrogen balance related to trauma, immobility, increased metabolic rate	5. Maintains nutritional status Stable weight	**Goal:** *Maintain adequate nutritional status* Decrease negative effects of immobility: Exercises: active-passive ROM and resistive exercises q 4 hr to decrease loss of calcium from bone Scrupulous hygienic care and prevention of skin disruption to decrease tissue breakdown Control increase in metabolic rate: Controlled environmental temperature and appropriate use of covers to prevent increased body temperature Use of antipyretics prn Careful hand washing and strict aseptic technique to decrease infection risk Vitamin supplements per IV or NG Weight daily

TABLE 76-1. Nursing plan on admission—cont'd

Input	Throughput	
Nursing diagnosis of stressors	**Predicted patient outcomes**	**Nursing orders**
6. Fluid and electrolyte imbalance Potential fluid and electrolyte imbalance related to NG drainage, stress reaction, increased insensible H_2O loss per ventilatory system	6. Maintains fluid and electrolyte balance Intake equals output Na^+, K^+, Cl^- within normal limits Weight stable Skin turgor normal Moist mucous membranes Respiratory rate within normal limits Absence of ECG changes related to electrolyte imbalance Absence of muscular cramps	**Goal:** *Promote and maintain fluid and electrolyte balance* Replace NG drainage ml/ml with 5% dextrose in 0.45 NS (each bottle with 20 mEq KCL) Monitor electrolyte laboratory values Weigh daily Assess skin turgor and mucous membranes Monitor respiratory rate Check specific gravity q 4 hr Checks signs and symptoms of fluid overload and dehydration Monitor ECG
7. Pain Pain at sites of injuries	7. Free of extreme physical discomfort a. With use of analgesics and progressive relaxation techniques, is able to tolerate position changes and procedures involved in therapeutic regimen b. Rests quietly when undisturbed	**Goal:** *Promote physical comfort and protect from personal injury* Move slowly when positioning Maintain body alignment Assess need and effectiveness of analgesic Assist patient in using progressive relaxation techniques to control pain Check traction for alignment and free movement Assess environment for potential dangers to safety and discomfort Give medication for pain before procedures such as bed change, bath
8. Impairment of vital functions a. Potential CNS disturbances related to head trauma b. Potential systemic infection related to debilitation, iatrogenic factors	8. Maintenance and improvement of vital functions a. Remains alert and oriented to person, place, time Maintains stable vital signs b. Maintains normal body temperature Maintains WBC within normal range Cultures remain negative	**Goal:** *Restore and support vital functions* a. Neurologic checks q 1 hr including signs and symptoms of increased intracranial pressure Vital signs q 1 hr b. Check temp q 4 hr if 38.5° C (R); if 39° C (R) check q 1 hr Check WBC daily Prevent skin disruptions Use sterile tracheostomy suctioning technique Avoid cross-contamination from other patients Inspect IV sites, apply Betadine, and maintain sterile dressings every day Do Foley care every shift Give Garamycin
9. Psychologic response to illness and therapy a. Potential disorientation related to medication effects and trauma b. Anxiety related to unfamiliar environment and procedures	9. Shows no signs or symptoms of severe psychologic reactions to stress a. Oriented to person, time, place, surroundings, activities b. Rests quietly when undisturbed Is able to cooperate and follow directions	**Goal:** *Promote and maintain reality orientation, minimize anxiety* a. Use open-ended questions Recognize nonverbal cues Observe behavior b. Recognize nonverbal cues and behavior as indicative of perception Use cognitive feedback Provide reassurance Explain all procedures Identify self and other care givers Enlist Sandy's cooperation in care (e.g., turning, taking deep breaths, coughing, lying quietly for procedures) Remain with Sandy when physical care or monitoring is not required Use touch at times other than for purposes of physical care (e.g., when talking with patient)

Continued.

TABLE 76-1. Nursing plan on admission—cont'd

Input	Throughput	
Nursing diagnosis of stressors	**Predicted patient outcomes**	**Nursing orders**
c. Inability to communicate verbally because of tracheostomy	c. Shows no signs or symptoms of severe psychologic reaction to stress Communicates effectively (i.e., gets basic needs met through means other than speech)	c. Anticipate needs Provide pad and pencil, magic slate, alphabet chart, pictures Ask questions to be answered yes or no Speak slowly Reassure that her inability to talk is temporary (i.e., there is nothing wrong with her voice)
d. Potential delusions/hallucinations related to inappropriate environmental stimulation and extreme fatigue	d. Experiences no disturbances in sensation or perception related to the environment Oriented to reality Communicates coherently Cooperates with care Follows directions	d. Reduce sensory overload Provide meaningful sensory input Orient to person, place, time, surroundings, activities When possible, try not to awaken if she's sleeping (after frequent neurologic checks are no longer needed)
10. Family's response to crisis		**Goal:** *Determine father's and brother's perceptions of the situation*
a. Father's and brother's lack of knowledge related to unfamiliar environment and confusion about Sandy's condition	a. Significant others able to state plans for medical and nursing care State all of Sandy's current major problems (e.g., respiratory, neurologic, orthopedic injuries, shock) Describe nursing and medical care emphasis State rationale for potential surgery	Recognize nonverbal and verbal cues as indications of their perceptions Determine their previous experience with similar situations **Goal:** *Provide information and clarify misconceptions* Discuss Sandy's condition with significant others in terms of nursing priorities and interventions (i.e., major nursing care emphases at this time are to monitor her condition, facilitate optimal ventilation, regulate medication to keep her blood pressure stable, promote optimal comfort, and decrease her fear and anxiety) Facilitate a meeting with the physician to clarify medical problems and treatment Sandy's major medical problem is difficulty breathing as a result of lung damage from the accident and low blood pressure from possible bleeding in her abdomen Major medical interventions will be to assist her breathing until she can breathe on her own and to support her vital functions Drowsiness and confusion are not unusual for patients in Sandy's situation and will be temporary Explain purposes of equipment in the environment
b. Anxiety of father and brother related to unfamiliar environment and confusion about Sandy's condition	b. Significant others able to discuss feelings and fears with members of health care team Demonstrate behaviors indicative of lowered anxiety (e.g., sit quietly between visits with Sandy, demonstrate more relaxed facial expression and body posture) Demonstrate constructive means for dealing with anxiety, (e.g., take walks between visits, talk with chaplain, eat meals regularly, communicate with relatives about Sandy's condition)	**Goal:** *Acknowledge, accept, and encourage ventilation of feelings by father and brother* Anticipate feelings of helplessness, powerlessness, frustration Identify behaviors indicative of grieving process (shock, disbelief, anger) Use therapeutic means of communication to facilitate verbalization of feelings Identify need for chaplain referral Allow flexibility in length and frequency of visiting periods

TABLE 76-1. Nursing plan on admission—cont'd

Input	Throughput	
Nursing diagnosis of stressors	Predicted patient outcomes	Nursing orders
c. Separation from significant others	c. Maintains continuity in relationship with significant others Acknowledges significant others' presence during visiting periods Attempts to communicate by touching significant others	**Goal:** *Promote continuity in relationship between Sandy and significant others* Inform Sandy that father and brother are in waiting room Provide flexibility in length and frequency of visiting periods Continually reassure that family are nearby Facilitate interactions between Sandy and family during visiting periods
d. Family stress related to indecision about immediate changes in daily living patterns	d. Make knowledgeable decisions for instituting changes in therapy, life-style, established family roles and relationships Make realistic decisions consistent with Sandy's condition (e.g., stay in nearby motel at least for first 24 hours; father makes arrangements for assistance on the farm for several days)	**Goal:** *Support decisions for temporary life-style changes* Explore viable options regarding the assumption of responsibility for the care of the farm, making sleeping and eating arrangements, acquisition of personal belongings **Goal:** *Provide information and clarify misconceptions* See Diagnosis 10a

Progress note (actual outcome)

Four weeks following admission Sandy's vital functions are self-sustaining and her recovery has progressed to where she will be transferred from the critical care unit within the next several days.

Sandy is alert and oriented. Her vital signs are stable and within normal limits except for a low-grade fever (37.5° C). Her respirations are easy without ventilatory support or oxygen therapy (arterial blood gases: pH 7.41, Pco_2 38, Po_2 90, HCO_3 24, saturation 96%, Hct 40, and hemoglobin 14). She receives continuous humidification to her tracheostomy, intermittent positive pressure breathing (IPPB) treatments every 4 hours, and clapping and modified postural drainage every 4 hours by the physical therapist. Her secretions are thick, yellow, and moderate in amount. Cultures reveal a *Pseudomonas* infection. She is able to clear most secretions from her tracheostomy with vigorous coughing, requiring suctioning more frequently after IPPB treatments and on awakening in the morning. Her breath sounds are equal bilaterally, audible with scattered rales and rhonchi in all lobes, which clear with coughing or suctioning. Her apical pulse is regular; peripheral pulses are equal and strong bilaterally. Bowel sounds are audible, and her abdomen is soft. She had a splenectomy the day after admission. Her abdominal incision is dry and well approximated without sutures. She has not had a bowel movement for several days. The nasogastric tube has been discontinued, and she is eating a regular diet, although because of anorexia she eats very little solid food. She has lost 6.8 kg (15 lb) since admission. All intravenous infusions and the arterial line have been discontinued. The condition of her skin is good without areas of disruption. Healed facial lacerations are without sutures, but suture lines are visible with ecchymotic areas remaining. She is voiding in sufficient quantities; her urine is clear yellow, and specific gravities are within the normal range.

Sandy's behavior indicates a labile psychologic status with intermittent periods of withdrawal, crying, and anger. She communicates by writing and mouthing words but at times becomes very frustrated with these procedures and withdraws. Some days she is interested and involved in her care and is able to assume increasing responsibility for self-care. She has been told that the current medical treatment emphasis is to clear up her pneumonia, and it is important that accumulated secretions not be retained in her lungs. She consistently requests to be suctioned if she is unable to clear her respiratory tract by coughing. She has also been told that she can further assist in her recovery process by improving her strength through increasing her daily activity and eating high-calorie, high-protein foods. She is hesitant to get out of bed because of discomfort with movement, and she requests to return to bed because of fatigue after sitting in a chair for a brief period. Sandy will agree to transfer to a chair after receiving medication for pain and has remained out of bed for increasing lengths of time each day. Her oral intake remains very poor, consisting primarily of clear liquids.

Having asked for a mirror several days ago and inspected her face, Sandy has become more withdrawn,

---

PATIENT CARE ORDERS

Vital signs q 4 hr except when asleep (temperature q 4 hr 37°-38.5° C; q 2 hr 38.5° C; q 1 hr > 39° C)

Discontinue IV

Regular diet (high protein, high caloric) with supplemental feedings

Advance activity as tolerated

IPPB q 4 hr

Physical therapist for percussion q 4 hr

Digital occlusion intermittently of tracheostomy for communication

Colace, 100 mg daily

Tylenol, 650 mg q 4 hr for temperature of 38.5° C

Keflex, 250 mg PO q 6 hr

Multivitamin with iron every day

Chest x-ray examination every AM

WBC daily

Sputum culture daily

---

irritable, passive, and less cooperative in her care. She denies that viewing her face bothers her and refuses to discuss the expected changes.

Information gained during periods when Sandy communicates more freely indicates that she has been a typical teenager with average academic and social pursuits. A recent high-school graduate, Sandy planned to attend a nearby community college in the fall and has a full-time summer job to help absorb the burden of that expense. Recently, Sandy has realized that classes begin in 1 month and that she will be unable physically and financially to attend.

Sandy's father, brother, and aunt visit every other weekend now that her condition is stable. She is most communicative and interested in her care immediately before, during, and after their visits.

At the time of this progress note, the patient care orders are shown in the box above.

The nursing diagnoses, patient outcomes, nursing goals and orders at the time of transfer from the critical care unit are shown in Table 76-2.

Evaluation

Comparing the *actual* outcomes of Sandy's medical and nursing interventions since admission with those *predicted* on admission reveals that Sandy experienced both improvement of signs and symptoms from the primary insult (automobile accident) and restoration and maintenance of vital functions. She developed no signs or symptoms indicative of severe physiologic stress (gastrointestinal tract bleeding, diabetes). Laboratory values and physical assessment indicate fluid and electrolyte balance. She is generally free of physical discomfort, complaining of pain only when transferring between bed and chair. She has had neither prolonged nor severe psychologic reactions to stress nor displayed any thought disturbances, hallucinations, or delusions that would indicate disturbances in sensation or perception. A respiratory tract infection (low-grade fever and positive sputum cultures) is not surprising in light of her general debility and the presence of a tracheostomy tube.

Increased catabolism from restricted activity and increased metabolic demands from a low-grade fever along with anorexia led to weight loss and concern about her nutritional status. Bed rest and an essentially liquid diet contributed to mild constipation. Restricted activity and prolonged immobility resulted in some loss of muscle tone and muscle weakness despite active and passive exercises.

Frustration from cumbersome alternatives to verbal communication and withdrawal secondary to depression made it impossible for Sandy to verbalize her feelings and her fears about her physical appearance, prolonged recovery, and changes in her life-style.

Before her depression and increasing withdrawal, Sandy seemed to understand the medical and nursing treatment goals and rationale for her care, as was evidenced by her cooperation in her pulmonary care and other daily activities.

As she became less withdrawn, her spirits improved around the time of her family's visits. Unfortunately, they are able to visit only every other weekend, and during their absence she experiences loneliness from separation, which compounds her depression.

Summary

For the patient and significant others, critical illness is a time of crisis, usually involving severe physiologic, psychologic, and social stressors. The foregoing patient study illustrates that the initial focus of the critical care team is on patient survival and support of significant others in their attempt to cope with the situation. The case study also illustrates the changes in priorities as the patient progresses toward recovery. The emphasis of the health care team then changes to assist the patient and significant others in adjusting to temporary

Table 76-2. Nursing plan at time of transfer from critical care unit

Input	Throughput	
Nursing diagnosis of stressors	Predicted patient outcomes	Nursing orders
1. Respiratory tract infection related to invasive procedures, restricted activity, and debilitation	1. Without signs and symptoms of physiologic reaction to therapy Sputum culture free of pathogenic organisms Clear breath sounds Temperature normal	**Goal:** *Promote physical comfort; protect from personal injury* Administer tracheostomy care q 4 hr Adhere to sterile tracheostomy suctioning Determine food technique Monitor amount, consistency, and odor of secretions Collect secretions for culture and sensitivity before and after every AM Avoid cross-contamination from other patients (do not exchange IPPB machine with other patients) Avoid assigning personnel with URI to care for Sandy Ensure as much uninterrupted rest as possible **Goal:** *Restore and maintain vital functions* Deep-breathing exercises with percussion q 4 hr Change position q 2 hr OOB to chair four times a day **Goal:** *Promote adequate nutritional status* Determine food preferences of high-calorie, high-protein content
2. Muscle weakness related to restricted activity	2. Free of complications of immobility-restricted activity Assumes responsibility for increasing number of self-care activities Tolerates sitting in a chair for increasing periods of time	**Goal:** *Preserve and maintain musculoskeletal function* Continue active ROM q 4 hr Assess activity tolerance Promote independence in self-care activities
3. Inadeqate nutritional intake related to anorexia, increased metabolic demands (infection, trauma), immobility	3. Maintains nutritional status Maintains or gains weight Increases caloric and protein intake	**Goal:** *Maintain adequate nutritional status* Determine food preferences Monitor calories daily **Goal:** *Promote physical comfort* Give oral hygiene before and after meals Provide esthetic environment Control environmental temperature and administer Tylenol as ordered to decrease metabolic demands **Goal:** *Preserve and maintain musculoskeletal functions* Assist back to bed, OOB four times a day Continue active ROM exercises q 4 hr
4. Constipation related to low-roughage diet, decreased activity, difficulty using bedpan	4. Maintains normal bowel function Has stool of normal frequency, color, and consistency every other day. Soft, nontender abdomen	**Goal:** *Promote normal elimination* Offer warm beverage, offer bedpan in 20 minutes Push fluids to 3000 ml/day Determine food preferences of high-roughage content **Goal:** *Preserve and maintain musculoskeletal function* Continue exercise regimen **Goal:** *Promote physical comfort* Ensure privacy when using bedpan Use room deodorizer after use of bedpan Hygienic measures after bowel movement Position patient to facilitate elimination

Continued.

Table 76-2. Nursing plan at time of transfer from critical care unit—cont'd

Input	Throughput	
Nursing diagnosis of stressors	**Predicted patient outcomes**	**Nursing orders**
5. Pain in fracture sites related to movement and therapeutic regimen	5. Free from extreme physical discomfort Tolerates increasing activity without change in vital signs Tolerates increasing activity with decreasing amounts of analgesics Tolerates activity with assistance of progressive relaxation techniques	**Goal:** *Promote physical comfort and protect from personal injury* Give analgesic before movement and procedures Clarify reasons for pain and acknowledge as normal Reassess effectiveness of analgesic Differentiate types of pain Assist Sandy in learning progressive relaxation techniques to control pain
6. Altered body image related to injuries and tracheostomy	6. Sandy will show no indication of negative reaction to change in appearance Discusses feelings with supportive person	**Goal:** *Acknowledge, accept, and encourage ventilation of feelings by Sandy* Determine perception and explore with Sandy extent of physical limitations now and in the future Provide information and clarify misconceptions
7. Potential anxiety and intensified feelings of loss related to transfer from critical care unit (CCU)	7. Sandy able to state plans for transfer from CCU States day of anticipated transfer States name of receiving unit Describes differences in routines between CCU and receiving unit Recognizes staff members from receiving unit Discusses fears with supportive person Free from signs and symptoms of severe physiologic or psychologic reaction to stress	**Goal:** *Prepare Sandy and significant others for her transfer* Support Sandy's involvement in decision making regarding transfer, private or semiprivate room, means of transportation for transfer (e.g., wheelchair, stretcher) Introduce Sandy to at least one staff member from receiving unit before transfer Inform Sandy on initial consideration for transfer Promote independence in self-care **Goal:** *Acknowledge, accept, and encourage ventilation of feelings* Point out improvement in condition and impending transfer as signs of recovery Emphasize positive aspects of transfer (e.g., increased privacy, less disruption of rest and sleep, more flexible visiting hours, indication of improvement in physical condition) See Order 6
8. Depression related to loneliness (loss of significant other's support), lack of diversion (boredom), hopelessness (discouraged about slow recovery)	8a. Sandy able to discuss feelings and fears with members of health care team Demonstrates behaviors reflective of decreased withdrawal, increased involvement in self-care b. Sandy and significant others maintain continuity in relationships Communicates with family weekly by telephone or letter with assistance from nurse	**Goal:** *Acknowledge, accept, and encourage ventilation of feelings by Sandy and significant others* Suggest sending of cards by family and friends Explore types of diversional activities of interest to Sandy Promote continuity in relationship between patient and significant others (father, brother, aunt, cousins) Flexible family visiting hours. Facilitate continuity in relationships with peer group (e.g., ask family to bring news of friends, explore possibility of including friends in family visit)

and permanent life-style changes and in making knowledgeable decisions and plans in order to progress to maximal recovery. Progression toward recovery means that the patient and significant others must cope with other aspects of illness such as rehabilitation and the adjustment to temporary and permanent changes in lifestyle. The emphasis of health professionals also changes as they assist the patient and significant others to make knowledgeable decisions and plans for the future.

REFERENCES AND SELECTED READINGS

1. *Aspinall, M.J.: Nursing diagnosis: the weak link, Nurs. Outlook 24:433-437, 1976.
2. Daly, B.J., editor: Intensive care nursing, Garden City, N.Y., 1980, Medical Examination Publishing Co., Inc.
3. *Gebbie, K., and Lavin, M.A.: Classifying nursing diagnosis, Am. J. Nurs. 74:250-253, 1974.
4. *Gordon, M.: Nursing diagnosis and the diagnostic process, Am. J. Nurs. 76:1298-1300, 1976.
5. *Mundinger, M.O., and Jauron, G.D.: Developing a nursing diagnosis, Nurs. Outlook 75:94-98, 1975.

*References preceded by an asterisk are particularly well suited for student reading.

INDEX

A

A bands, 916
AA; *see* Alcoholics Anonymous
Aarane; *see* Cromolyn sodium
Ab; *see* Antibodies
ABCs of emergency assessment, 1883
Abdomen
  bleeding in, 1889
  blood disorders and, 1188
  cramps in, 1641, 1642-1643
  distention of, 1436, 1437; *see also* Ascites
    after aneurysmectomy, 1139
    casts and, 967
    diarrhea and, 1446
    hernia repair and, 1500
    hysterectomy and, 1701
    postoperative, 455
    spinal cord trauma and, 822
    sympathectomy and, 1165
    ulcerative colitis and, 1484
    urologic surgery and, 1531
  engorged veins in, 1436
  examination of, 1435-1436, 1619
    auscultation in, 1436, 1437, 1620
    bruit in, 1436
    friction rub in, 1436
    palpation in, 1437, 1619-1620, 1626
    percussion in, 1436-1437, 1620
    radiologic, 1516
    reproductive disorders and, 1619-1620
    skin color in, 1436
    striae in, 1436
    visible disturbances in, 1436
  pain in, 1434; *see also* Pain
    abdominoperineal resection and, 1454
    cholecystitis and, 701
    cirrhosis and, 689
    history of, 1378
    pancreatic malignancies and, 711
    pancreatitis and, 708, 709
  scars of, 1436
  support for, 1238
  tenderness of, 1553
  topographic division of, 1435
  tubal sterilization and, 1662, 1664-1666
  wounds of, 1898, 1900
Abdominal breathing
  augmented, 1242, 1243
  chronic obstructive pulmonary disease and, 1326
  after thoracic surgery, 1253
Abdominal thrust maneuver, 1887
Abdominal wall fistulas, 1483

Abdominoperineal resection of bowel, 1452-1454, 1497
Abducens nerve, 731
ABO system, 1868-1869
Abortion, 1684-1691
  dilation and curettage and, 1633
  values and, 149
Abortion clinics, 1689
Above-the-knee amputations, 1167
Abramson drain, 438
Abrasion, 1785, 1897
  prevention of, 941-943
Abscesses, 282
  anal, 1487-1488
    lymphogranuloma venereum and, 1732
  appendiceal, 282
  bacteria and, 281
  bartholinitis and, 1677
  brain, 753, 809-810
  breast, 1761
  chronic granulomatous disease and, 1857
  endocarditis and, 1104
  ischiorectal, 1488
  liver, 676-677, 1488
  of lung, 1307-1308
    lobectomy and, 1250, 1251
  pelvic
    colorectal surgery and, 1498
    inflammatory disease and, 1682
    prostatectomy and, 1562
  periapical, 1406
  peritonitis and, 1482
  prostatic, 1711
  renal ultrasound and, 1518
  in synovium, 1002
  of testis, 1714
  vulvar, 1679
Absenteeism, school, 38
Absorption disorders; *see* Malabsorption syndrome
Abstractions, 216, 755
Abuse
  child, 209, 1882
  of drugs, 198-201
    adolescents and, 226
    education about, 1890
ABVD; *see* Doxorubicin with bleomycin, vinblastine, and dacarbazine
Acantholysis, 1848
Acceptance
  aged and, 244
  critical illness and, 1929
  dying and, 253
  maladaptive behavior and, 186, 189, 193

Accessory muscles of respiration, 1215, 1216
Accessory structures, 1783-1784
Accidents, 1881-1883; *see also* Safety
  of adolescents, 225
  aging and, 237
  automobile, 1234-1235
    adolescence and, 225
    children and, 213
    critical care and, 1935
  body image and, 545, 546, 547
  head injury and, 811
  incidence of, 1879
  middle-aged adults and, 233
  poisoning and, 1890-1894; *see also* Poisons
  vision impairment and, 864-865
Acclimatization, 1227
Accommodation, 839, 841
Accountability, 131
ACD; *see* Acid citrate dextrose
Ace bandages; *see* Elastic bandages or stockings
Acetabulum, 1021
Acetaminophen, 387-388
  back pain and, 397
  brain surgery and, 777
  interferon and, 512
  migraine and, 749
  peptic ulcer and, 1422
  rheumatic diseases and, 958
  sinusitis and, 1265
  teeth extraction and, 1388
  tonsillectomy and, 1277
Acetanilid, 388
Acetazolamide, 865
  glaucoma and, 897, 898
  hepatic coma and, 699
  Ménière's disease and, 910
  metabolic alkalosis and, 357
  ototoxicity of, 873
  renal calculi and, 1558
Acetest, 599
Acetic acid
  burns and, 1822
  catheter irrigations and, 1556
  denture care and, 1389
  for douches, 1647, 1677, 1679
  itching and, 1581
  otitis and, 903
  stomal crystals and, 1539
  of sweat, 274
  synovial fluid and, 936
  urinary appliance and, 1537
Acetohexamide, 658
Acetone, 599, 658